Fifth Edition

MEDICAL TERMINOLOGY

A LIVING LANGUAGE

Bonnie F. Fremgen, PhD

Suzanne S. Frucht, PhD
Associate Professor Emeritus
Northwest Missouri State University
Maryville, MO

PEARSON

Boston Columbus Indianapolis New York San Francisco Upper Saddle River
Amsterdam Cape Town Dubai London Madrid Milan Munich Paris Montreal Toronto
Delhi Mexico City Sao Paulo Sydney Hong Kong Seoul Singapore Taipei Tokyo

Publisher: Julie Levin Alexander
Publisher's Assistant: Regina Bruno
Editor-in-Chief: Mark Cohen
Development Editor: Danielle Doller
Associate Editor: Melissa Kerian
Director of Marketing: David Gesell
Executive Marketing Manager: Katrin Beacom
Marketing Coordinator: Michael Sirinides
Senior Managing Editor: Patrick Walsh
Project Manager: Christina Zingone-Luethje
Senior Operations Supervisor: Ilene Sanford
Operations Specialist: Lisa McDowell
Illustrator: Body Scientific International, LLC.
Art Director: Christopher Weigand
Cover and Interior Designer: Rachael Cronin
Media Editor: Amy Peltier
Lead Media Project Manager: Lorena Cerisano
Full-Service Project Management: Amy L. Saucier
Composition: Laserwords
Printer/Binder: Courier/Kendallville
Cover Printer: Lehigh-Phoenix/Hagerstown
Cover Image: Sebastian Kaulitzki/Shutterstock
Text Font: Meridien

Dedication

To my husband for his love and encouragement.

Bonnie Fremgen

To my husband, Rick, and my daughter,
Kristin, for their love, support, and friendship.

Suzanne Frucht

Notice: Care has been taken to confirm the accuracy of the information presented in this book. The authors, editors, and the publisher, however, cannot accept any responsibility for errors or omissions or for the consequences of the application of the information in this book and make no warranty, express or implied, with respect to its contents.

The authors and the publisher have exerted every effort to ensure that drug elections and dosages set forth in this text are in accord with current recommendations and practice at time of publication. However, in view of ongoing research, changes in government regulations, and the constant flow of information relating to drug therapy and drug reactions, the reader is urged to check the package inserts of all drugs for any change in indications of dosage and for added warnings and precautions. This is particularly important when the recommended agent is a new and/or infrequently employed drug.

The authors and publisher disclaim all responsibility for any liability, loss, injury, or damage incurred as a consequence, directly or indirectly, of the use and application of any of the contents of this volume.

Library of Congress Cataloging-in-Publication Data

Fremgen, Bonnie F.
  Medical terminology : a living language / Bonnie F. Fremgen,
Suzanne S. Frucht.—5th ed.
     p. ; cm.
  Includes bibliographical references and index.
  ISBN-13: 978-0-13-284347-8
  ISBN-10: 0-13-284347-1
I. Frucht, Suzanne S. II. Title.
  [DNLM: 1. Medicine—Terminology—English. W 15]
  610.1'4—dc23
                       2011048322

10 9 8 7 6 5 4 3 2 1

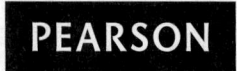

ISBN-13: 978-0-13-284347-8
ISBN-10: 0-13-284347-1

Welcome!

Welcome to the fascinating study of medical language—a vital part of your preparation for a career as a health professional. We are glad that you have joined us. Throughout your career, in a variety of settings, you will use medical terminology to communicate with co-workers and patients. Employing a carefully constructed learning system, *Medical Terminology: A Living Language* has helped thousands of readers gain a successful grasp of medical language within a real-world context.

In developing this book we had seven goals in mind:

1. To provide a clear introduction to the basic rules of using word parts to form medical terms.
2. To use phonetic pronunciations that will help you easily pronounce terms by spelling out the word part according to the way it sounds.
3. To help you understand medical terminology within the context of the human body systems. Realizing that this book is designed for a terminology course and not an anatomy & physiology course, we have aimed to stick to only the basics.
4. To help you develop a full range of Latin and Greek word parts used to build medical terms so that you will be able to interpret unfamiliar terms you encounter in the future.
5. To help you visualize medical language with an abundance of real-life photographs and accurate illustrations.
6. To provide you with a wealth of practice applications at the end of each chapter to help you review and master the content as you go along.
7. To create rich multimedia practice opportunities for you by way of Medical Terminology Interactive.

Please turn the page to get a visual glimpse of what makes this book an ideal guide to your exploration of medical terminology.

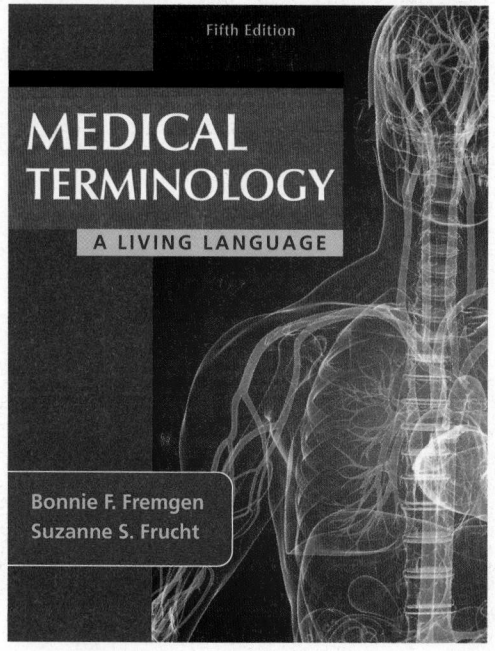

A Guide to What Makes This Book Special

Streamlined Content

14 chapters and only the most essential anatomy & physiology coverage makes this book a perfect mid-sized fit for a one-term course.

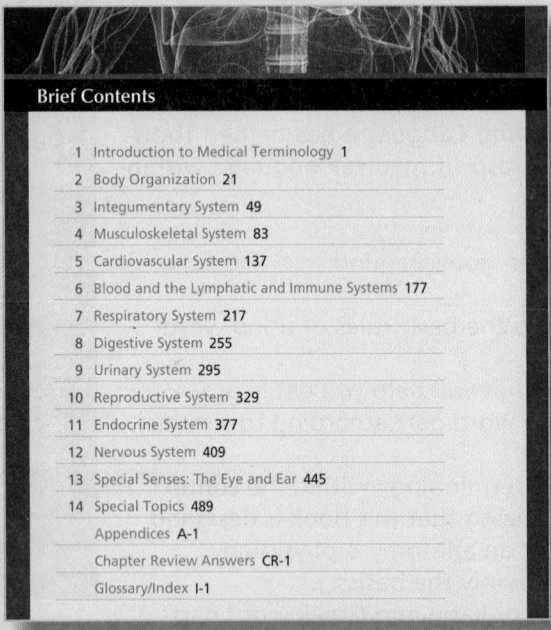

Brief Contents

1 Introduction to Medical Terminology 1
2 Body Organization 21
3 Integumentary System 49
4 Musculoskeletal System 83
5 Cardiovascular System 137
6 Blood and the Lymphatic and Immune Systems 177
7 Respiratory System 217
8 Digestive System 255
9 Urinary System 295
10 Reproductive System 329
11 Endocrine System 377
12 Nervous System 409
13 Special Senses: The Eye and Ear 445
14 Special Topics 489
   Appendices A-1
   Chapter Review Answers CR-1
   Glossary/Index I-1

Chapter-Opening Page Spreads

"At a Glance" and "Illustrated" pages begin each chapter, providing a quick, visual snapshot of what's covered.

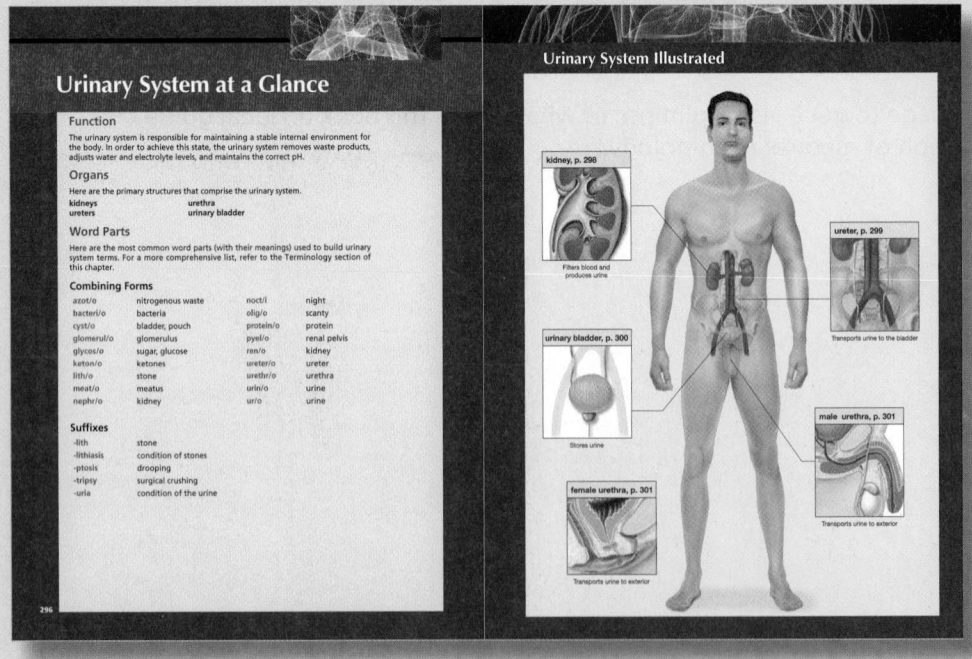

Key Terms and Pronunciations

Every subsection starts with a list of key terms and pronunciations for those words that will be covered in that section. This sets the stage for comprehension and mastery.

Med Term Tips

This popular feature offers tidbits of noteworthy information about medical terms that engage learners.

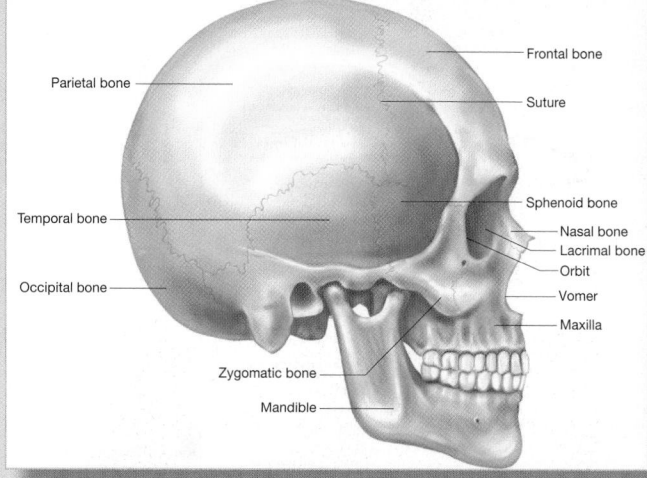

Medically-Accurate Illustrations

Concepts come to life with vibrant, clear, consistent, and scientifically precise images.

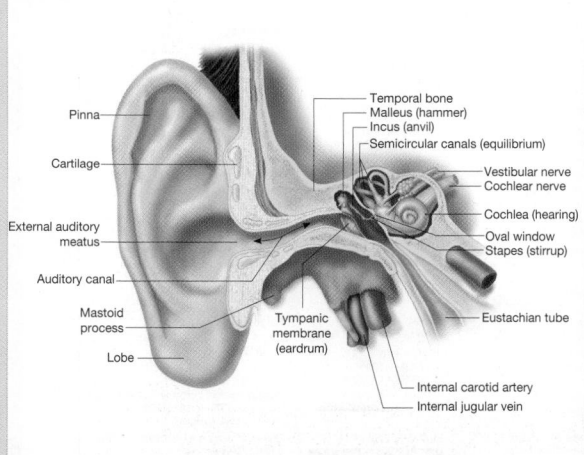

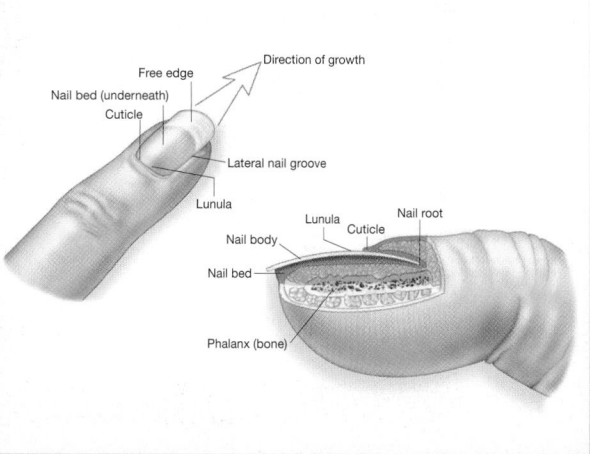

Word Tables

Study lists are categorized and presented in a clear, logical, color-coded format that eases the learning process.

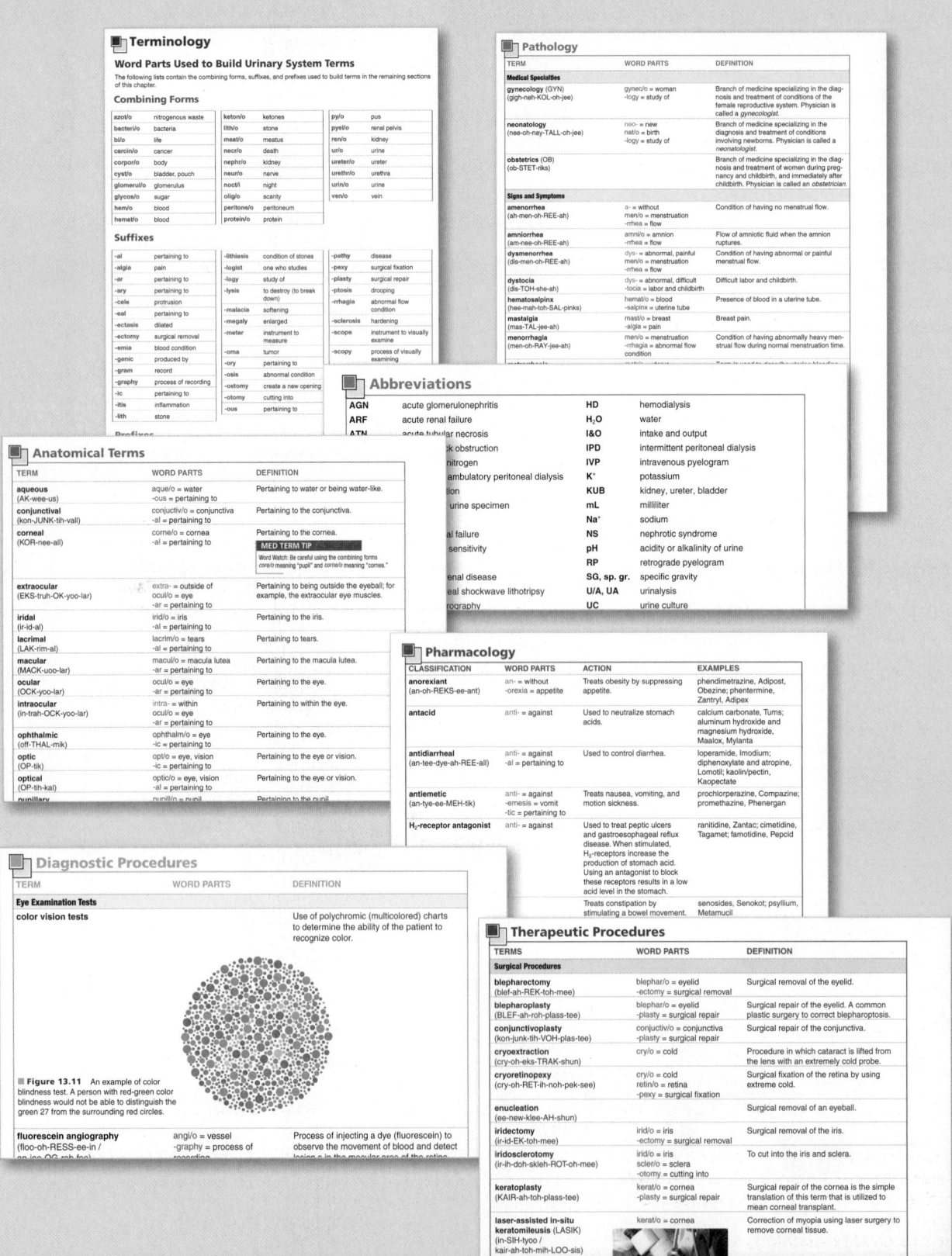

Workbook Sections

A wide array of exercises at the end of each chapter serve as a fun and challenging study review.
Here are some examples:

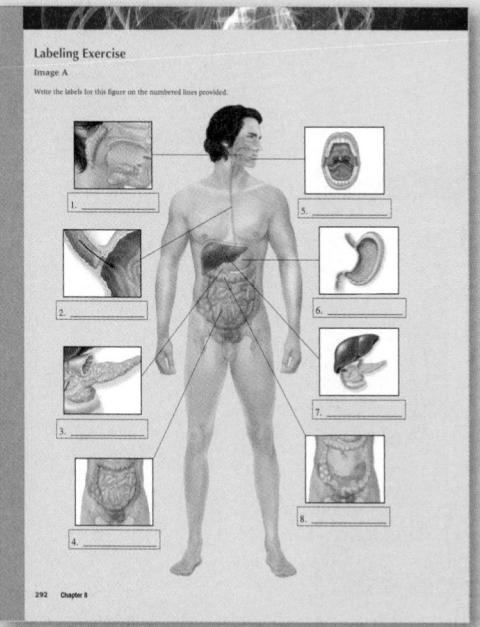

Labeling Exercises—A visual challenge to
reinforce students' grasp of anatomy &
physiology concepts.

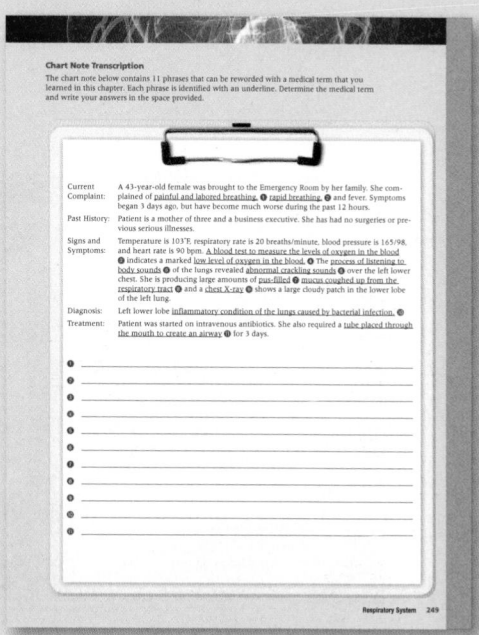

Chart Note Transcription—Slice-of-real-life
exercise that asks students to replace lay
terms in a medical chart with the proper
medical term.

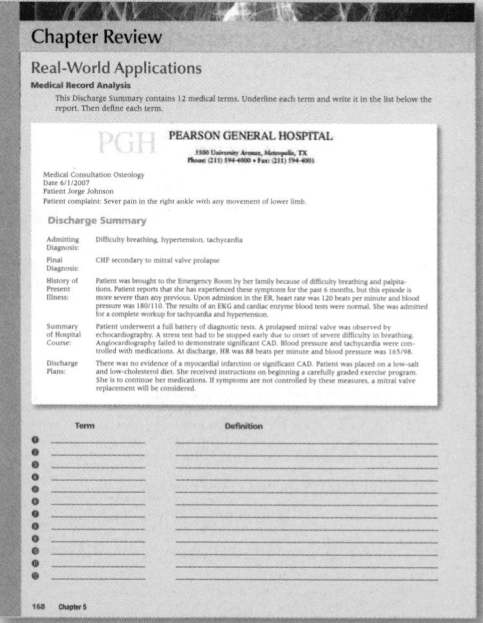

Medical Record Analysis—Exercises that
challenge students to read examples of
real medical records and then to apply
their medical terminology knowledge in
answering related questions.

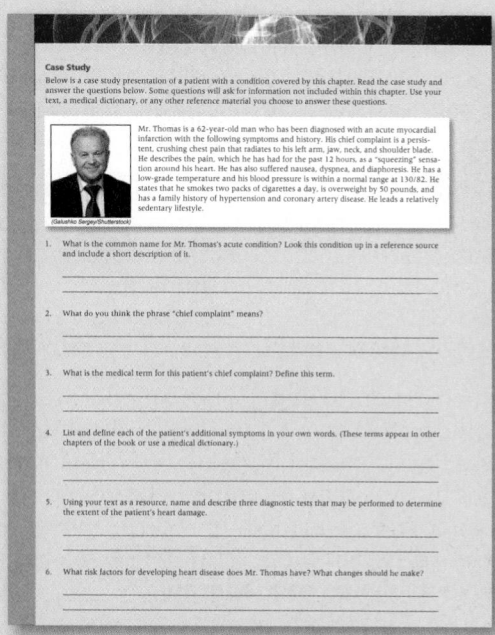

Case Study—Scenarios that use critical
thinking questions to help students
develop a firmer understanding of the
terminology in context.

The Total Teaching and Learning Package

We are committed to providing students and instructors with exactly the tools they need to be successful in the classroom and beyond. To this end, *Medical Terminology: A Living Language* is supported by the most complete and dynamic set of resources available today.

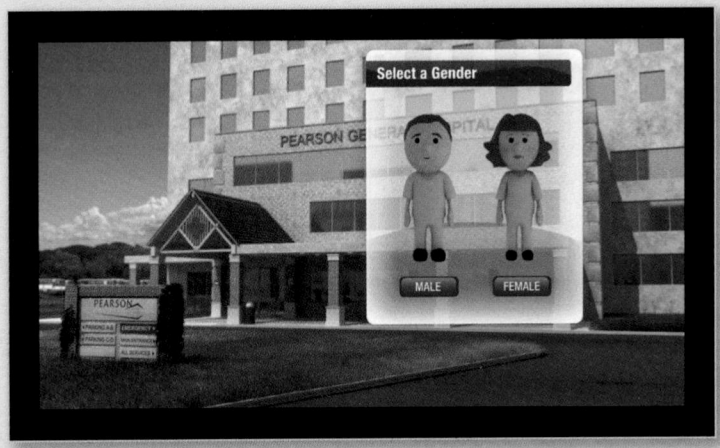

Medical Terminology Interactive

The ultimate personalized learning tool is available at **www.pearsonhighered.com/mti**. This online course correlates with the textbook and is available for purchase separately or for a discount when packaged with the book. Medical Terminology Interactive is an immersive study experience that takes place within Pearson General Hospital—a virtual world of fun quizzes, word games, videos, flashcards, learning modules, and other self-study challenges. The system allows learners to track their own progress through the course to achieve success.

Medical Terminology Interactive saves instructors time by gathering all student results in a class grade book. This can be exported to any learning management system, and instructor resources all in one place. It offers instructors the flexibility to make technology an integral part of their course, or a supplementary resource for students.

Comprehensive Instructional Package

Perhaps the most gratifying part of an educator's work is the "aha" learning moment when the light bulb goes off and a student truly understands a concept—when a connection is made. Along these lines, Pearson is pleased to help instructors foster more of these educational connections by providing a complete battery of resources to support teaching and learning. Qualified adopters are eligible to receive a wealth of materials designed to help instructors prepare, present, and assess. For more information, please contact your Pearson sales representative or visit **www.pearsonhighered.com/educator**.

Since the first edition of *Medical Terminology: A Living Language* was published it has been noted for its "clean" and logical format that promotes learning. In this revised edition, we have built upon this strength by enhancing many features to make this text an ideal choice for semester-or quarter-length courses.

Features of this Edition

This new fifth edition contains features that facilitate student mastery, while maintaining the best aspects of previous editions. Each chapter is arranged in a similar format and the content is organized with an emphasis on maintaining consistency and accuracy. All terms have been evaluated to ensure they remain in current use and reflect the newest technologies and procedures.

We have revised *Medical Terminology: A Living Language* so that it provides for an even more valuable teaching and learning experience. Here are the enhancements we have made:

- The Terminology section includes a comprehensive list of all combining forms, suffixes, and prefixes used to build terms in the remaining sections of the chapter.

- The Signs and Symptoms subsection within the Pathology table contains disease-related terms grouped by organ. This allows terms to be categorized into smaller groups, therefore making learning easier.

- Improved three-column format in the word building sections allows for the term (with pronunciation and/or abbreviation), word parts (if appropriate), and definitions to be displayed. The Pharmacology table also includes word parts in a new fourth column.

- The Anatomical Terms section includes anatomical terms as well as adjective forms of organs.

- Color-coded word parts—red combining forms, blue suffixes, and green prefixes allow for quick recognition throughout the book.

- The Real World Applications section now contains three critical thinking activities (Medical Record Analysis, Chart Note Transcription, and a new Case Study) to allow readers to apply their knowledge to real world situations.

Organization of the Book

Introductory Chapter

Chapter 1 contains information necessary for an understanding of how medical terms are formed. This includes learning about word roots, combining forms, prefixes, and suffixes, and general rules for building medical terms. Readers will also learn about terminology for medical records and the different health care settings. Chapter 2 presents terminology relating to the body organization, including organs and body systems. Here readers will first encounter word building tables, a feature found in each remaining chapter that lists medical terms and their respective word parts.

Anatomy and Physiology Chapters

Chapters 3 through 13 are organized by body system. Each chapter begins with a System At A Glance which lists combining forms, prefixes, and/or suffixes with their meanings and is followed by System Illustrated overview of the organs in the system. The anatomy and physiology section is divided into the various components of the system, and each subsection begins with a list of key medical terms accompanied by a pronunciation guide. Key terms are boldfaced the first time they appear in the narrative. The Terminology section of each chapter begins with a list of all word parts used within the chapter. For ease of learning, the medical terms are divided into five separate sections: anatomical terms, pathology, diagnostic procedures, therapeutic procedures, and pharmacology. The word parts used to build terms are highlighted within each table. An abbreviations section then follows to complete the chapter.

Special Topics Chapter

Chapter 14 contains timely information and appropriate medical terms relevant to the following medical specialties: pharmacology, mental health, diagnostic imaging, rehabilitation services, surgery, and oncology. Knowledge of these topics is necessary for the well-rounded health care worker.

Appendices

The appendices contain helpful reference lists of word parts and definitions. This information is intended for quick access. There are three appendices: Word Parts Arranged Alphabetically and Defined, Word Parts Arranged Alphabetically by Definition and Abbreviations. Finally, all of the key terms appear again in the glossary/index at the end of the text.

About the Authors

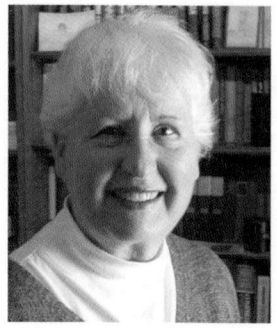

Bonnie F. Fremgen

Bonnie F. Fremgen is a former associate dean of the Allied Health Program at Robert Morris College. She has taught medical law and ethics courses as well as clinical and administrative topics. In addition, she has served as an advisor for students' career planning. She has broad interests and experiences in the health care field, including hospitals, nursing homes, and physicians' offices.

Dr. Fremgen holds a nursing degree as well as a master's in health care administration. She received her PhD from the College of Education at the University of Illinois. She has performed postdoctoral studies in Medical Law at Loyola University Law School in Chicago. She has authored five textbooks with Pearson.

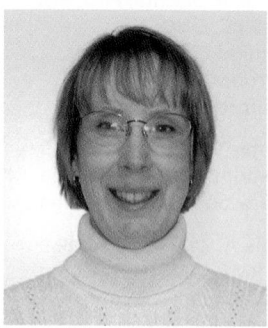

Suzanne S. Frucht

Suzanne S. Frucht is an Associate Professor Emeritus of Anatomy and Physiology at Northwest Missouri State University (NWMSU). She holds baccalaureate degrees in biological sciences and physical therapy from Indiana University, an MS in biological sciences at NWMSU, and a PhD in molecular biology and biochemistry from the University of Missouri-Kansas City.

For 14 years she worked full-time as a physical therapist in various health care settings, including acute care hospitals, extended care facilities, and home health. Based on her educational and clinical experience she was invited to teach medical terminology part-time in 1988 and became a full-time faculty member three years later as she discovered her love for the challenge of teaching. She taught a variety of courses including medical terminology, human anatomy, human physiology, and animal anatomy and physiology. She received the Governor's Award for Excellence in Teaching in 2003. After retiring from teaching in 2008, she continues to be active in student learning through writing medical terminology texts and anatomy and physiology laboratory manuals.

About the Illustrators

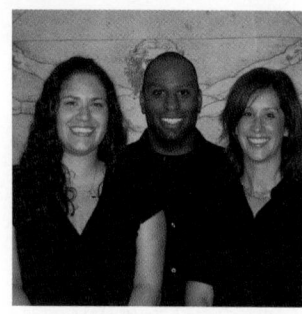

Marcelo Oliver is president and founder of Body Scientific International LLC. He holds an MFA degree in Medical and Biological Illustration from University of Michigan. For the past 15 years, his passion has been to condense complex anatomical information into visual education tools for students, patients, and medical professionals. For seven years he worked as a medical illustrator and creative director developing anatomical charts used for student and patient education. In the years that followed, he created educational and marketing tools for medical device companies prior to founding Body Scientific International, LLC.

Body Scientific's lead artists in this publication were medical illustrators Liana Bauman and Katie Burgess. Both hold an Master of Science degrees in Biomedical Visualization degree from the University of Illinois at Chicago. Their contribution in the publication was key in the creation and editing of artwork throughout.

Our Development Team

We would like to express deep gratitude to our 105 colleagues from schools across the country that have provided us with hundreds of hours of their time over the years to help us tailor this book to suit the dynamic needs of instructors and students. These individuals have reviewed manuscript chapters and illustrations for content, accuracy, level, and utility. We sincerely thank you and feel that *Medical Terminology: A Living Language* has benefited immeasurably from your efforts, insights, encouragement, and selfless willingness to share your expertise as educators.

Reviewers of the 5th Edition

Dr. Pam Besser Ph.D
Jefferson Community and
Technical College
Louisville, Kentucky

Jeannie Bower, BS, NRCAMA
Central Penn College
Summerdale, Pennsylvania

Karen R. Hardney, M.S. Ed
Chicago State University
Chicago, Illinois

Holly Jodon, MPAS, PA-C
Gannon University
Erie, Pensylvania

Francesca L. Langlow, BS
Delgado Community College
New Orleans, Louisiana

**Bridgit R. Moore, EdD,
MT(ASCP), CPC**
McLennan Community College
Waco, Texas

Christine J. Moore, M Ed
Armstrong Atlantic
State University
Savannah, Georgia

Lisa J. Pierce, MSA, RRT
Augusta Technical College
Augusta, Georgia

**Georgette Rosenfeld, Ph.D,
RRT, RN**
Indian River State College
Fort Pierce, Florida

**Donna J. Slovensky, PhD,
RHIA, FAHIMA**
University of Alabama at
Birmingham
Birmingham, Alabama

Jodi Taylor, A.A.S, LPN, RMA
Terra State Community College
Fremont, Ohio

Scott Throneberry, BS, NREMTP
Calhoun Community College
Decatur, Alabama

**Patricia A. Slachta, PhD, RN,
ACNS-BC, CWOCN**
Technical College of the
Lowcountry
Beaufort, South Carolina

Lenette Thompson, CST, AS
Piedmont Technical College
Greenwood, South Carolina

**Carole A. Zeglin, MSEd, BS,
MT, RMA (AMT)**
Westmoreland County
Community College
Youngwood, Pennsylvania

Reviewers of Earlier Editions

Yvonne Alles, MBA, RMT
Davenport University
Grand Rapids, Michigan

**Rachael C. Alstatter, Program
Director**
Southern Ohio College
Fairfield, Ohio

Steve Arinder, BS, MPH
Meridian Community College
Meridian, Mississippi

**K. William Avery, BSMT,
JD, PhD**
City College
Gainesville, Florida

Beverly A. Baker, DA, CST
Western Iowa Technical
Community College
Sioux City, Iowa

Michael Battaglia, MS
Greenville Technical College
Taylors, South Carolina

**Nancy Ridinger Bean, Health
Assistant Instructor**
Wythe County Vocational
School
Wytheville, Virginia

Deborah J. Bedford, CMA, AAS
North Seattle Community
College
Seattle, Washington

Barbara J Behrens, PTA, MS
Mercer County Community
College
Trenton, New Jersey

Pam Besser, Ph.D.
Jefferson Community College
Louisville, Kentucky

Norma J Bird, M.Ed., BS, CMA
Idaho State University College
of Technology
Pocatello, Idaho

Trina Blaschko, RHIT
Chippewa Valley Technical
College
Eau Claire, Wisconsin

Richard T. Boan, PhD
Midlands Technical College
Columbia, South Carolina

Susan W. Boggs, RN, BSN, CNOR
Piedmont Technical College
Greenwood, South Carolina

Bradley S. Bowden, PhD
Alfred University
Alfred, New York

Joan Walker Brittingham
Sussex Tech Adult Division
Georgetown, Delaware

**Phyills J. Broughton,
Curriculum Coordinator**
Pitt Community College
Greenville, North Carolina

Barbara Bussard, Instructor
Southwestern Michigan College
Dowagiac, Michigan

Toni Cade, MBA, RHIA, CCS
University of Louisiana at
Lafayette
Lafayette, Louisiana

Gloria H. Coats, RN, MSN
Modesto Junior College
Modesto, California

Lyndal M. Curry, M.A., R.P.
University of South Alabama
Mobile, Alabama

Nancy Dancs, P.T.
Waukesha County Technical
College
Pewaukee, Wisconsin

Antoinette Deshaies, RN, BSPA
Glendale Community College
Glendale, Arizona

Theresa H. deBeche, RN, MN, CNS
Louisiana State University at Eunice
Eunice, Louisiana

Bonnie Deister, MS, BSN, CMA-C
Broome Community College
Binghamton, New York

Carol Eckert, RN, MSN
Southwestern Illinois College
Belleville, Illinois

Jamie Erskine, Ph.D., R.D.
University of Northern Colorado
Greeley, Colorado

Mildred K. Fuller, Ph.D., MT(ASCP), CLS(NCA)
Norfolk State University
Norfolk, Virginia

Deborah Galanski-Maciak
Davenport University
Grand Rapids, Michigan

Debra Getting, Practical Nursing Instructor
Norwest Iowa Community College
Sheldon, Iowa

Ann Queen Giles, MHS, CMA
Western Piedmont Community College
Morganton, North Carolina

Brenda L. Gleason, MSN
Iowa Central Community College
Fort Dodge, Iowa

Steven B. Goldschmidt, DC, CCFC
North Hennepin Community College
Brooklyn Park, Minnesota

Linda S. Gott, RN, MS
Pensacola High School
Pensacola, Florida

Martha Grove, Staff Educator
Mercy Regional Health System
Cincinnati, Ohio

Kathryn Gruber
Globe College
Oakdale, Minnesota

Karen R. Hardney, M.S., Ed.
Chicago State University
Chicago, Illinois

Mary Hartman, MS, OTR/L
Genesee Community College
Batavia, New York

Joyce B. Harvey, Ph.D, RHIA
Norfolk State University
Norfolk, Virginia

Beulah A. Hofmann, RN, BSN, MSN, CMA
Ivy Tech Community College of Indiana
Greencastle, Indiana

Kimberley Hontz , RN
Antonelli Medical and Professional Institute
Pottstown, Pennsylvania

Pamela S. Huber, M.S., MT(ASCP)
Erie Community College
Williamsville, New York

Eva I. Irwin
Ivy Tech State College
Indianapolis, Indiana

Susan Jackson, EdS
Valdosta Technical College
Valdosta, Georgia

Mark Jaffe, DPM, MHSA
Nova Southeastern University
Ft. Lauderdale, Florida

Carol Lee Jarrell, MLT,AHI
Brown Mackie College
Merrillville, Indiana

Virginia J. Johnson, CMA
Lakeland Academy
Minneapolis, Minnesota

Marcie C. Jones, BS, CMA
Gwinnett Technical Institute
Lawrenceville, Georgia

Robin Jones, RHIA
Meridian Community College
Meridian, Mississippi

Gertrude A. Kenny, BSN, RN, CMA
Baker College of Muskegon
Muskegon, Michigan

Dianne K. Kuiti, RN
Duluth Business University
Duluth, Minnesota

Andrew La Marca, EMT-P
Mobile Life Support Services
Middletown, New York

Julie A. Leu, CPC
Creighton University
Omaha, Nebraska

Norma Longoria, BS, COI
South Texas Community College
McAllen, Texas

Jeanne W. Lovelock, RN, MSN
Piedmont Virginia Community College
Charlottesville, Virginia

Jan Martin, R.T.(R)
Ogeechee Tech College
Statesboro, Georgia

Leslie M. Mazzola, MA
Cuyahoga Community College
Parma, Ohio

Michelle C. McCranie, CPhT
Ogeechee Technical College
Statesboro, Georgia

Lola McGourty, MSN, RN
Bossier Parish Community College
Bossier City, Louisiana

Connie Morgan
Ivy Tech State College
Kokomo., Indiana

Katrina B. Myricks
Holmes Community College
Ridgeland, Mississippi

Patricia Moody, RN
Athens Technical College
Athens, Georgia

Catherine Moran, Ph.D.
Breyer State University
Birmingham, Alabama

Pam Ncu, CMA
International Business College
Fort Wayne, Indiana

Judy Ortiz MHS, MS, PA-C
Pacific University
Hillsboro, Oregon

Tina M. Peer, BSN, RN
College of Southern Idaho
Twin Falls, ID
Sylvania, Ohio

Dave Peruski, RN, MSA, MSN
Delta College
University Center, Michigan

Sister Marguerite Polcyn, OSF, PhD
Lourdes College
Sylvania, Ohio

Vicki Prater, CMA, RMA, RAHA
Concorde Career Institute
San Bernardino, California

Carolyn Ragsdale CST, BS
Parkland College
Champaign, Illinois

LuAnn Reicks, RNC, BS, MSN
Iowa Central Community College
Fort Dodge, Iowa

Linda Reigel
Glenville State College
Glenville, West Virginia

Ellen Rosen, RN, MN
Glendale Community College
Glendale, California

Georgette Rosenfeld, Ph.D., RN, RRT
Indian River Community College
Fort Pierce, Florida

Brian L. Rutledge, MHSA
Hinds Community College
Jackson, Mississippi

Sue Shibley, M.Ed., CMT, CCS-P, CPC
North Idaho College
Coeur d'Alene, Idaho

Misty Shuler, RHIA
Asheville Buncombe Technical Community College
Asheville, North Carolina

Connie Smith, RPh
University of Louisiana at Monroe School of Pharmacy
Monroe, Louisiana

Karen Snipe, CPhT, ASBA, MAEd
Trident Technical College
Charleston, South Carolina

Donna Stern
University of California San Diego Extension
La Jolla, California

Janet Stehling, RHIA
McLennan College
Lorena, Texas

Annmary Thomas, MEd, NREMT-P
Community College of Philadelphia
Philadelphia, Pennsylvania

Marilyn Turner, RN, CMA
Ogeechee Technical College
Statesboro, Georgia

Joan Ann Verderame, RN, MA
Bergen Community College
Paramus, New Jersey

Kathy Wallington
Phillips Junior College
Campbell, California

Twila Wallace, MEd
Central Community College
Columbus, Nebraska

Linda Walter, RN, MSN
Northwestern Michigan College
Traverse City, Michigan

Jean Watson, PhD
Clark College
Vancouver, Washington

Twila Weiszbrod, MPA
College of the Sequoias
Visalia, California

Sara J. Wellman, RHIT
Indiana University Northwest
Gary, Indiana

Leesa Whicker, BA, CMA
Central Piedmont Community College
Charlotte, NC

Lynn C. Wimett, RN, ANP, EdD
Regis University
Denver, Colorado

Kathy Zaiken, Pharm.D.
Massachusetts College of Pharmacy and Health Sciences
Boston, Massachusetts

A Commitment to Accuracy

As a student embarking on a career in health care you probably already know how critically important it is to be precise in your work. Patients and co-workers will be counting on you to avoid errors on a daily basis. Likewise, we owe it to you—the reader—to ensure accuracy in this book. We have gone to great lengths to verify that the information provided in *Medical Terminology: A Living Language* is complete and correct. To this end, here are the steps we have taken:

1. **Editorial Review**—We have assembled a large team of developmental consultants (listed on the preceding pages) to critique every word and every image in this book. No fewer than 10 content experts have read each chapter for accuracy.

2. **Medical Illustrations**—A team of medically-trained illustrators was hired to prepare each piece of art that graces the pages of this book. These illustrators have a higher level of scientific education than the artists for most textbooks, and they worked directly with the authors and members of our development team to make sure that their work was clear, correct, and consistent with what is described in the text.

3. **Accurate Ancillaries**—Realizing that the teaching and learning ancillaries are often as vital to instruction as the book itself, we took extra steps to ensure accuracy and consistency within these components. We assigned some members of our development team to specifically focus on critiquing every bit of content that comprises the instructional ancillary resources to confirm accuracy.

While our intent and actions have been directed at creating an error-free text, we have established a process for correcting any mistakes that may have slipped past our editors. Pearson takes this issue seriously and therefore welcomes any and all feedback that you can provide along the lines of helping us enhance the accuracy of this text. If you identify any errors that need to be corrected in a subsequent printing, please send them to:

Pearson Health Editorial
Medical Terminology Corrections
One Lake Street
Upper Saddle River, NJ 07458

Thank you for helping Pearson to reach its goal of providing the most accurate medical terminology textbooks available.

Contents

Welcome iii

A Guide to What Makes This Book Special iv

The Total Teaching and Learning Package viii

Preface ix

About the Authors xi

About the Illustrators xi

Our Development Team xii

A Commitment to Accuracy xiv

1 Introduction to Medical Terminology 1

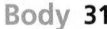

Learning Objectives 1

Medical Terminology at a Glance 2

Building Medical Terms from Word Parts 3

Word Roots 3

Combining Vowel/Form 3

Prefixes 4

Suffixes 6

Word Building 9

Interpreting Medical Terms 9

Singular and Plural Endings 10

Abbreviations 11

The Medical Record 11

Healthcare Settings 13

Confidentiality 14

Chapter Review 15

Practice Exercises 15

2 Body Organization 21

Learning Objectives 21

Body Organization at a Glance 22

Body Organization Illustrated 23

Levels of Body Organization 24

Cells 24

Tissues 25

Organs and Systems 27

Body 31

Body Planes 32

Body Regions 33

Body Cavities 34

Directional and Positional Terms 35

Terminology 38

Anatomical Terms 39

Abbreviations 41

Chapter Review 42

Practice Exercises 42

Labeling Exercise 47

3 Integumentary System 49

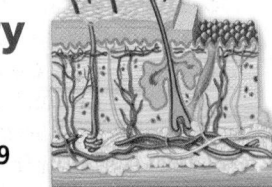

Learning Objectives 49

Integumentary System at a Glance 50

Integumentary System Illustrated 51

Anatomy and Physiology of the Integumentary System 52

The Skin 52

Accessory Organs 54

Terminology 56

Word Parts Used to Build Integumentary System Terms 56

Anatomical Terms 57

Pathology 58

Diagnostic Procedures 70

Therapeutic Procedures 70

Pharmacology 72

Abbreviations 72

Chapter Review 73

Real-World Applications 73

Practice Exercises 76

Labeling Exercise 81

4 Musculoskeletal System 83

Learning Objectives 83

SECTION I: SKELETAL SYSTEM AT A GLANCE 84

Skeletal System Illustrated 85
Anatomy and Physiology of the Skeletal System 86
  Bones 86
  Skeleton 89
  Joints 95
Terminology 97
  Word Parts Used to Build Skeletal System Terms 97
Anatomical Terms 98
Pathology 99
Diagnostic Procedures 106
Therapeutic Procedures 107
Pharmacology 109
Abbreviations 110

SECTION II: MUSCULAR SYSTEM AT A GLANCE 111

Muscular System Illustrated 112
Anatomy and Physiology of the Muscular System 113
  Types of Muscles 113
  Skeletal Muscle 114
  Naming Skeletal Muscles 115
  Skeletal Muscle Actions 115
Terminology 119
  Word Parts Used to Build Muscular System Terms 119
Anatomical Terms 119
Pathology 120
Diagnostic Procedures 122
Therapeutic Procedures 122
Pharmacology 123
Abbreviations 123
Chapter Review 124
  Real-World Applications 124
  Practice Exercises 127
  Labeling Exercise 134

5 Cardiovascular System 137

Learning Objectives 137
Cardiovascular System at a Glance 138
Cardiovascular System Illustrated 139
Anatomy and Physiology of the Cardiovascular System 140
  Heart 141
  Blood Vessels 146
Terminology 151
  Word Parts Used to Build Cardiovascular System Terms 151
Anatomical Terms 152
Pathology 152
Diagnostic Procedures 159
Therapeutic Procedures 161
Pharmacology 163
Abbreviations 164
Chapter Review 166
  Real-World Applications 166
  Practice Exercises 169
  Labeling Exercise 175

6 Blood and the Lymphatic and Immune Systems 177

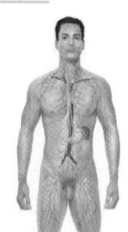

Learning Objectives 177

SECTION I: BLOOD AT A GLANCE 178

Blood Illustrated 179
Anatomy and Physiology of Blood 180
  Plasma 180
  Erythrocytes 180
  Leukocytes 181
  Platelets 182
  Blood Typing 182
Terminology 183
  Word Parts Used to Build Blood Terms 183
Anatomical Terms 184
Pathology 184

Diagnostic Procedures **187**
Therapeutic Procedures **189**
Pharmacology **189**
Abbreviations **190**

**SECTION II: THE LYMPHATIC AND IMMUNE
SYSTEMS AT A GLANCE 191**

The Lymphatic and Immune Systems
Illustrated **192**
Anatomy and Physiology of the
Lymphatic and Immune Systems **193**
Lymphatic Vessels **193**
Lymph Nodes **194**
Tonsils **196**
Spleen **196**
Thymus Gland **196**
Immunity **196**
Terminology **199**
Word Parts Used to Build Lymphatic
and Immune System Terms **199**
Anatomical Terms **199**
Pathology **200**
Diagnostic Procedures **203**
Therapeutic Procedures **204**
Pharmacology **205**
Abbreviations **205**
Chapter Review **206**
Real-World Applications **206**
Practice Exercises **209**
Labeling Exercise **215**

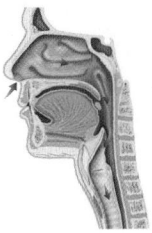

7 Respiratory System 217

Learning Objectives **217**
Respiratory System at a Glance **218**
Respiratory System Illustrated **219**
Anatomy and Physiology of the
Respiratory System **220**
Nasal Cavity **220**
Pharynx **222**
Larynx **222**
Trachea **223**
Bronchial Tubes **223**
Lungs **224**
Lung Volumes and Capacities **225**

Respiratory Muscles **226**
Respiratory Rate **227**
Terminology **227**
Word Parts Used to Build Respiratory
System Terms **227**
Anatomical Terms **228**
Pathology **229**
Diagnostic Procedures **238**
Therapeutic Procedures **240**
Pharmacology **242**
Abbreviations **243**
Chapter Review **244**
Real-World Applications **244**
Practice Exercises **247**
Labeling Exercise **253**

8 Digestive System 255

Learning Objectives **255**
Digestive System at a Glance **256**
Digestive System Illustrated **257**
Anatomy and Physiology of the Digestive
System **258**
Oral Cavity **258**
Pharynx **261**
Esophagus **261**
Stomach **262**
Small Intestine **262**
Colon **263**
Accessory Organs of the Digestive
System **264**
Terminology **266**
Word Parts Used to Build Digestive
System Terms **266**
Anatomical Terms **267**
Pathology **268**
Diagnostic Procedures **276**
Therapeutic Procedures **279**
Pharmacology **281**
Abbreviations **282**
Chapter Review **283**
Real-World Applications **283**
Practice Exercises **286**
Labeling Exercise **292**

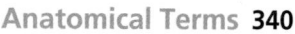

9 Urinary System 295

Learning Objectives 295
Urinary System at a Glance 296
Urinary System Illustrated 297
Anatomy and Physiology of the Urinary
  System 298
  Kidneys 298
  Ureters 299
  Urinary Bladder 300
  Urethra 301
  Role of Kidneys in Homeostasis 301
  Stages of Urine Production 302
  Urine 303
Terminology 304
  Word Parts Used to Build Urinary System
    Terms 304
Anatomical Terms 305
Pathology 306
Diagnostic Procedures 310
Therapeutic Procedures 312
Pharmacology 315
Abbreviations 316
Chapter Review 317
  Real-World Applications 317
  Practice Exercises 320
  Labeling Exercise 326

10 Reproductive System 329

Learning Objectives 329

SECTION I: FEMALE REPRODUCTIVE SYSTEM AT A GLANCE 330

Female Reproductive System
  Illustrated 331
Anatomy and Physiology of the Female
  Reproductive System 332
  Internal Genitalia 332
  Vulva 335
  Breast 336
  Pregnancy 336
Terminology 339
  Word Parts Used to Build Female
    Reproductive System Terms 339

Anatomical Terms 340
Pregnancy Terms 341
Pathology 342
Diagnostic Procedures 347
Therapeutic Procedures 349
Pharmacology 351
Abbreviations 351

SECTION II: MALE REPRODUCTIVE SYSTEM AT A GLANCE 352

Male Reproductive System Illustrated 353
Anatomy and Physiology of the Male
  Reproductive System 354
  External Organs of Reproduction 354
  Internal Organs of Reproduction 356
Terminology 356
  Word Parts Used to Build Male Reproductive
    System Terms 356
Anatomical Terms 357
Pathology 358
Diagnostic Procedures 360
Therapeutic Procedures 361
Pharmacology 362
Abbreviations 363
Chapter Review 364
  Real-World Applications 364
  Practice Exercises 367
  Labeling Exercise 374

11 Endocrine System 377

Learning Objectives 377
Endocrine System at a Glance 378
Endocrine System Illustrated 379
Anatomy and Physiology of the Endocrine
  System 380
  Adrenal Glands 382
  Ovaries 382
  Pancreas 383
  Parathyroid Glands 384
  Pineal Gland 384
  Pituitary Gland 384
  Testes 386
  Thymus Gland 387
  Thyroid Gland 387
Terminology 388
  Word Parts Used to Build Endocrine System
    Terms 388

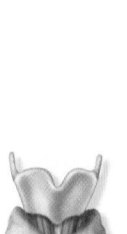

Anatomical Terms 389
Pathology 390
Diagnostic Procedures 395
Therapeutic Procedures 396
Pharmacology 397
Abbreviations 398
Chapter Review 399
 Real-World Applications 399
 Practice Exercises 402
 Labeling Exercise 407

12 Nervous System 409

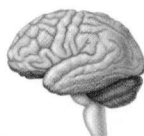

Learning Objectives 409
Nervous System at a Glance 410
Nervous System Illustrated 411
Anatomy and Physiology of the Nervous
 System 412
 Nervous Tissue 412
 Central Nervous System 413
 Peripheral Nervous System 418
Terminology 420
 Word Parts Used to Build Nervous System
 Terms 420
Anatomical Terms 421
Pathology 422
Diagnostic Procedures 430
Therapeutic Procedures 432
Pharmacology 432
Abbreviations 433
Chapter Review 434
 Real-World Applications 434
 Practice Exercises 437
 Labeling Exercise 443

13 Special Senses: The Eye and Ear 445

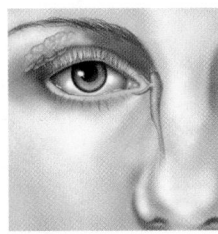

Learning Objectives 445

SECTION I: THE EYE AT A GLANCE 446

The Eye Illustrated 447
Anatomy and Physiology of the Eye 448
 The Eyeball 448
 Muscles of the Eye 450
 The Eyelids 451
 Conjunctiva 451
 Lacrimal Apparatus 451
 How We See 452
Terminology 453
 Word Parts Used to Build Eye Terms 453
Anatomical Terms 454
Pathology 455
Diagnostic Procedures 460
Therapeutic Procedures 462
Pharmacology 463
Abbreviations 464

SECTION II: THE EAR AT A GLANCE 465

The Ear Illustrated 466
Anatomy and Physiology of the Ear 467
 External Ear 467
 Middle Ear 468
 Inner Ear 468
 How We Hear 469
Terminology 470
 Word Parts Used to Build Ear Terms 470
Anatomical Terms 470
Pathology 471
Diagnostic Procedures 473
Therapeutic Procedures 475
Pharmacology 476
Abbreviations 477
Chapter Review 478
 Real-World Applications 478
 Practice Exercises 481
 Labeling Exercise 488

14 Special Topics 489

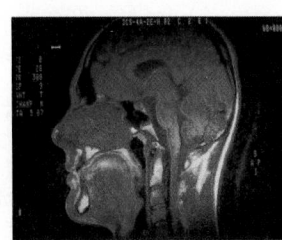

Learning
 Objectives 489
Introduction 490

SECTION I: PHARMACOLOGY AT A GLANCE 490

Pharmacology 491
 Drug Names 491
 Legal Classification of Drugs 492
 How to Read a Prescription 493
 Routes and Methods of Drug
 Administration 494

Pharmacology Terms **496**
Abbreviations **498**

**SECTION II: MENTAL HEALTH
             AT A GLANCE 499**

Mental Health Disciplines **500**
  Psychology 500
  Psychiatry 500
Pathology **500**
Therapeutic Procedures **504**
Abbreviations **505**

**SECTION III: DIAGNOSTIC IMAGING
              AT A GLANCE 506**

Diagnostic Imaging **507**
Diagnostic Imaging Terms **507**
Diagnostic Imaging Procedures **508**
Abbreviations **511**

**SECTION IV: REHABILITATION SERVICES
             AT A GLANCE 513**

Rehabilitation Services **514**
  Physical Therapy 514
  Occupational Therapy 514
Rehabilitation Services Terms **514**
Therapeutic Procedures **516**
Abbreviations **518**

SECTION V: SURGERY AT A GLANCE 519

Surgery **520**
  Anesthesia 520

Surgical Instruments 520
Surgical Positions 522
Surgery Terms **523**
Abbreviations **524**

SECTION VI: ONCOLOGY AT A GLANCE 525

Oncology **526**
  Staging Tumors 526
Oncology Terms **527**
Diagnostic Procedures **529**
Therapeutic Procedures **529**
Abbreviations **530**
Chapter Review **531**
  Real-World Applications 531
  Practice Exercises 533

Appendicies A-1

Appendix I: Word Parts Arranged
  Alphabetically and Defined **A-1**
Appendix II: Word Parts Arranged
  Alphabetically by Definition **A-8**
Appendix III: Abbreviations **A-15**
Chapter Review Answers **CR-1**
Glossary/Index **I-1**

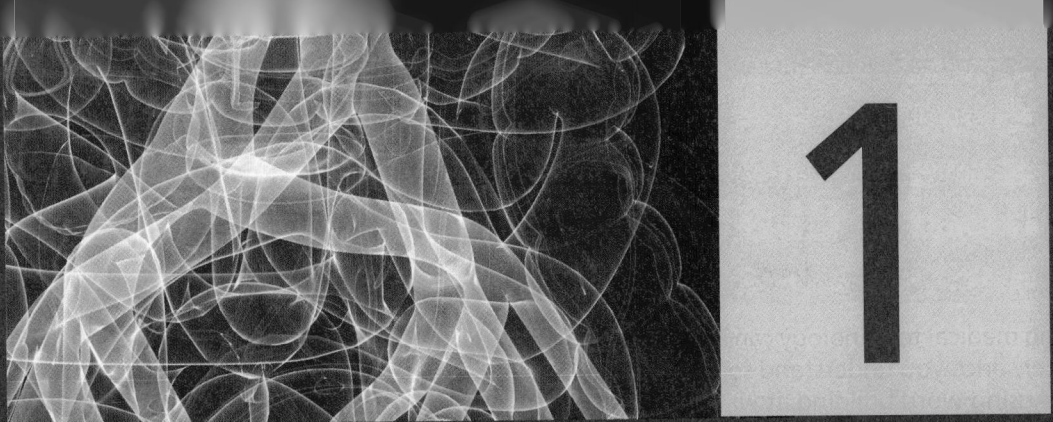

Learning Objectives

Upon completion of this chapter, you will be able to

- Discuss the four parts of medical terms.
- Recognize word roots and combining forms.
- Identify the most common prefixes and suffixes.
- Define word building and describe a strategy for translating medical terms.
- State the importance of correct spelling of medical terms.
- State the rules for determining singular and plural endings.
- Discuss the importance of using caution with abbreviations.
- Recognize the documents found in a medical record.
- Recognize the different healthcare settings.
- Understand the importance of confidentiality.

INTRODUCTION TO MEDICAL TERMINOLOGY

1

Medical Terminology at a Glance

Learning medical terminology can initially seem like studying a strange new language. However, once you understand some of the basic rules about how medical terms are formed using word building, it will become much like piecing together a puzzle. The general guidelines for forming words; an understanding of word roots, combining forms, prefixes, and suffixes; pronunciation; and spelling are discussed in this chapter. Chapter 2 introduces you to terms used to describe the body as a whole. Chapters 3–13 each focus on a specific body system and present new combining forms, prefixes, and suffixes, as well as exercises to help you gain experience building new medical terms. Finally, Chapter 14 includes the terminology for several important areas of patient care. In addition, "Med Term Tips" are sprinkled throughout all chapters to assist in clarifying some of the material. New medical terms discussed in each section are listed separately at the beginning of the section, and each chapter contains numerous pathological, diagnostic, treatment, and surgical terms. You can use these lists as an additional study tool for previewing and reviewing terms.

Understanding medical terms requires you being able to put words together or build words from their parts. It is impossible to memorize thousands of medical terms; however, once you understand the basics, you can distinguish the meaning of medical terms by analyzing their prefixes, suffixes, and word roots. Remember that there will always be some exceptions to every rule, and medical terminology is no different. We attempt to point out these exceptions where they exist. Most medical terms, however, do follow the general rule that there is a **word root** or fundamental meaning for the word, a **prefix** and a **suffix** that modify the meaning of the word root, and sometimes a **combining vowel** to connect other word parts. You will be amazed at the seemingly difficult words you will be able to build and understand when you follow the simple steps in word building (see Figure 1.1 ■).

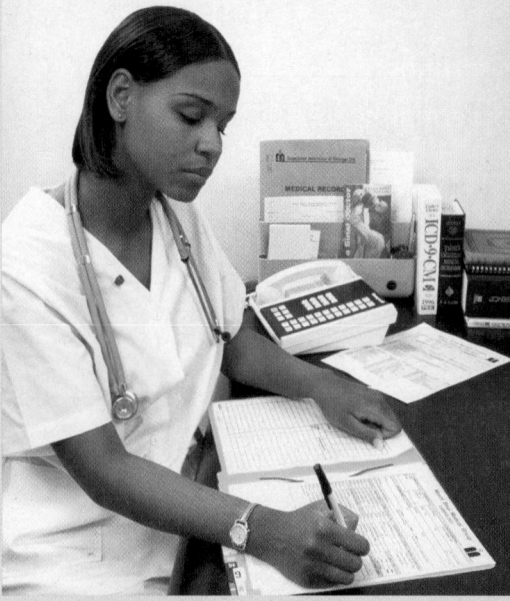

■ **Figure 1.1** Nurse completing a patient report. Healthcare workers use medical terminology in order to accurately and efficiently communicate patient information to each other.

Building Medical Terms from Word Parts

Four different word parts or elements can be used to construct medical terms:

1. The **word root** is the foundation of the word.
2. A **prefix** is at the beginning of the word.
3. A **suffix** is at the end of the word.
4. The **combining vowel** is a vowel (usually *o*) that links the word root to another word root or a suffix.

cardiogram = record of the heart

pericardium = around the heart
card**itis** = inflammation of the heart
cardi**o**my**o**pathy = disease of the heart muscle

The following sections on word roots, combining vowels and forms, prefixes, and suffixes will consider each of these word parts in more detail and present examples of some of those most commonly used.

Word Roots

The word root is the foundation of a medical term and provides the general meaning of the word. The word root often indicates the body system or part of the body being discussed, such as *cardi* for heart. At other times the word root may be an action. For example, the word root *cis* means to cut (as in incision).

A term may have more than one word root. For example, **osteoarthritis** (oss-tee-oh-ar-THRY-tis) combines the word root *oste* meaning bone and *arthr* meaning the joints. When the suffix *-itis*, meaning inflammation, is added, we have the entire word, meaning an inflammation involving bone at the joints.

Combining Vowel/Form

To make it possible to pronounce long medical terms with ease and to combine several word parts, a combining vowel is used. This is most often the vowel *o*. Combining vowels are utilized in two places: between a word root and a suffix or between two word roots.

To decide whether or not to use a combining vowel between a word root and a suffix, first look at the suffix. If it begins with a vowel, do not use the combining vowel. If, however, the suffix begins with a consonant, then use a combining vowel. For example: To combine *arthr* with *-scope* will require a combining vowel: **arthroscope** (AR-throh-scope). But to combine *arthr* with *-itis* does not require a combining vowel: **arthritis** (ar-THRY-tis).

The combining vowel is typically kept between two word roots, even if the second word root begins with a vowel. For example, in forming the term **gastroenteritis** (gas-troh-en-ter-EYE-tis) the combining vowel is kept between the two word roots *gastr* and *enter* (gastrenteritis is incorrect). As you can tell from pronouncing these two terms, the combining vowel makes the pronunciation easier.

When writing a word root by itself, its **combining form** is typically used. This consists of the word root and its combining vowel written in a word root/vowel form, for example, *cardi/o*. Since it is often simpler to pronounce word roots when they appear in their combining form, this format is used throughout this book.

Common Combining Forms

Some commonly used word roots in their combining form, their meaning, and examples of their use follow. Review the examples to observe when a combining vowel was kept and when it was dropped according to the rules presented on the preceding page.

COMBINING FORM	MEANING	EXAMPLE (DEFINITION)
aden/o	gland	adenopathy (gland disease)
carcin/o	cancer	carcinoma (cancerous tumor)
cardi/o	heart	cardiac (pertaining to the heart)
chem/o	chemical	chemotherapy (treatment with chemicals)
cis/o	to cut	incision (process of cutting into)
dermat/o	skin	dermatology (study of the skin)
enter/o	small intestine	enteric (pertaining to the small intestine)
gastr/o	stomach	gastric (pertaining to the stomach)
gynec/o	female	gynecology (study of females)
hemat/o	blood	hematic (pertaining to the blood)
hydr/o	water	hydrocele (protrusion of water [in the scrotum])
immun/o	immunity	immunology (study of immunity)
laryng/o	voice box	laryngeal (pertaining to the voice box)
nephr/o	kidney	nephromegaly (enlarged kidney)
neur/o	nerve	neural (pertaining to a nerve)
ophthalm/o	eye	ophthalmic (pertaining to the eye)
ot/o	ear	otic (pertaining to the ear)
path/o	disease	pathology (study of disease)
pulmon/o	lung	pulmonary (pertaining to the lungs)
rhin/o	nose	rhinoplasty (surgical repair of the nose)

Prefixes

A new medical term is formed when a prefix is added to the front of the term. Prefixes frequently give information about the location of an organ, the number of parts, or the time (frequency). For example, the prefix *bi-* stands for two of something, such as **bilateral** (bye-LAH-ter-al), meaning to have two sides. However, not every term will have a prefix.

Common Prefixes

Some of the more common prefixes, their meanings, and examples of their use follow. When written by themselves, prefixes are followed by a hyphen.

PREFIX	MEANING	EXAMPLE (DEFINITION)
a-	without, away from	aphasia (without speech)
an-	without	anoxia (without oxygen)
ante-	before, in front of	antepartum (before birth)
anti-	against	antibiotic (against life)
auto-	self	autograft (a graft from one's own body)
brady-	slow	bradycardia (slow heartbeat)
contra-	against	contraception (against conception)
de-	without	depigmentation (without pigment)
dys-	painful, difficult, abnormal	dyspnea (difficulty breathing)
endo-	within, inner	endoscope (instrument to view within)
epi-	upon, over	epigastric (upon or over the stomach)
eso-	inward	esotropia (inward turning)
eu-	normal, good	eupnea (normal breathing)
ex-	external, outward	exostosis (condition of external bone)
exo-	outward	exotropia (outward turning)
extra-	outside of	extracorporeal (outside of the body)
hetero-	different	heterograft (graft [like a skin graft] from another species)
homo-	same	homograft (graft [like a skin graft] from the same species)
hydro-	water	hydrotherapy (water therapy)
hyper-	over, above	hypertrophy (overdevelopment)
hypo-	under, below	hypodermic (under the skin)
in-	not; inward	infertility (not fertile); inhalation (to breathe in)
inter-	among, between	intervertebral (between the vertebrae)
intra-	within, inside	intravenous (inside, within a vein)
macro-	large	macrotia (having large ears)
micro-	small	microtia (having small ears)
myo-	to shut	myopia (to shut eyes/squint)
neo-	new	neonatology (study of the newborn)
pan-	all	pansinusitis (inflammation of all the sinuses)
para-	beside, near; abnormal; two like parts of a pair	paranasal (beside the nose); paresthesia (abnormal sensation); paraplegia (paralysis of two like parts of a pair/the legs)
per-	through	percutaneous (through the skin)
peri-	around	pericardial (around the heart)
post-	after	postpartum (after birth)
pre-	before, in front of	preoperative (before a surgical operation)
pro-	before	prolactin (before milk)
pseudo-	false	pseudocyesis (false pregnancy)

> **MED TERM TIP**
>
> Be very careful with prefixes; many have similar spellings but very different meanings. For example:
>
> *anti-* means "against"; *ante-* means "before"
>
> *inter-* means "between"; *intra-* means "inside"
>
> *per-* means "through"; *peri-* means "around"

PREFIX	MEANING	EXAMPLE (DEFINITION)
retro-	backward, behind	retroperitoneal (behind the peritoneum)
sub-	below, under	subcutaneous (under, below the skin)
supra-	above	suprapubic (above the pubic bone)
tachy-	rapid, fast	tachycardia (fast heartbeat)
trans-	through, across	transurethral (across the urethra)
ultra-	beyond, excess	ultrasound (high-frequency sound waves)
un-	not	unconscious (not conscious)

Number Prefixes

Some common prefixes pertaining to the number of items or measurement, their meanings, and examples of their use follow.

PREFIX	MEANING	EXAMPLE (DEFINITION)
bi-	two	bilateral (two sides)
hemi-	half	hemiplegia (paralysis of one side/half of the body)
mono-	one	monoplegia (paralysis of one extremity)
multi-	many	multigravida (woman pregnant more than once)
nulli-	none	nulligravida (woman with no pregnancies)
poly-	many	polyuria (large amounts of urine)
primi-	first	primigravida (first pregnancy)
quadri-	four	quadriplegia (paralysis of all four limbs)
semi-	partial, half	semiconscious (partially conscious)
tetra-	four	tetraplegia (paralysis of all four limbs)
tri-	three	triceps (muscle with three heads)

Suffixes

A suffix is attached to the end of a word to add meaning, such as a condition, disease, or procedure. For example, the suffix *-itis,* meaning inflammation, when added to *cardi-* forms the new word **carditis** (car-DYE-tis), meaning inflammation of the heart. Every medical term *must* have a suffix. Most often the suffix is added to a word root, as in carditis above; however, terms can also be built from a suffix added directly to a prefix, without a word root. For example, the term **dystrophy** (DIS-troh-fee), meaning abnormal development, is built from the prefix *dys-* (meaning abnormal) and the suffix *-trophy* (meaning development).

Common Suffixes

Some common suffixes, their meanings, and examples of their use follow. When written by themselves, suffixes are preceded by a hyphen.

SUFFIX	MEANING	EXAMPLE (DEFINITION)
-algia	pain	gastralgia (stomach pain)
-cele	hernia, protrusion	cystocele (protrusion of the bladder)

MED TERM TIP

Remember, if a suffix begins with a vowel, the combining vowel is dropped; for example, *mastitis* rather than *mast**o**itis.*

SUFFIX	MEANING	EXAMPLE (DEFINITION)
-cyte	cell	erythrocyte (red cell)
-dynia	pain	cardiodynia (heart pain)
-ectasis	dilation	bronchiectasis (dilated bronchi)
-gen	that which produces	pathogen (that which produces disease)
-genesis	produces, generates	spermatogenesis (produces sperm)
-genic	producing, produced by	carcinogenic (producing cancer)
-ia	state, condition	bradycardia (condition of slow heart)
-iasis	abnormal condition	lithiasis (abnormal condition of stones)
-iatry	medical treatment	podiatry (medical treatment for the foot)
-ism	state of	hypothyroidism (state of low thyroid)
-itis	inflammation	dermatitis (inflammation of skin)
-logist	one who studies	cardiologist (one who studies the heart)
-logy	study of	cardiology (study of the heart)
-lysis	destruction	hemolysis (blood destruction)
-lytic	destruction	thrombolytic (clot destruction)
-malacia	abnormal softening	chondromalacia (abnormal cartilage softening)
-megaly	enlargement, large	cardiomegaly (enlarged heart)
-oid	resembling	fibroid (resembling fibers)
-oma	tumor, mass, swelling	carcinoma (cancerous tumor)
-osis	abnormal condition	cyanosis (abnormal condition of being blue)
-pathy	disease	myopathy (muscle disease)
-phobia	fear	photophobia (fear of light)
-plasia	development, growth	hyperplasia (excessive development)
-plasm	formation, development	neoplasm (new formation)
-ptosis	drooping	blepharoptosis (drooping eyelid)
-rrhage	excessive, abnormal flow	hemorrhage (excessive bleeding)
-rrhagia	abnormal flow condition	cystorrhagia (abnormal flow from the bladder)
-rrhea	discharge, flow	rhinorrhea (discharge from the nose)
-rrhexis	rupture	hysterorrhexis (ruptured uterus)
-sclerosis	hardening	arteriosclerosis (hardening of an artery)
-stenosis	narrowing	angiostenosis (narrowing of a vessel)
-therapy	treatment	chemotherapy (treatment with chemicals)
-trophy	nourishment, development	hypertrophy (excessive development)
-ule	small	venule (small vein)

Adjective Suffixes

The following suffixes are used to convert a word root into an adjective. These suffixes usually are translated as *pertaining to*.

SUFFIX	MEANING	EXAMPLE (DEFINITION)
-ac	pertaining to	cardiac (pertaining to the heart)
-al	pertaining to	duodenal (pertaining to the duodenum)
-an	pertaining to	ovarian (pertaining to the ovary)
-ar	pertaining to	ventricular (pertaining to a ventricle)
-ary	pertaining to	pulmonary (pertaining to the lungs)
-atic	pertaining to	lymphatic (pertaining to lymph)
-eal	pertaining to	esophageal (pertaining to the esophagus)
-iac	pertaining to	chondriac (pertaining to cartilage)
-ic	pertaining to	gastric (pertaining to the stomach)
-ile	pertaining to	penile (pertaining to the penis)
-ine	pertaining to	uterine (pertaining to the uterus)
-ior	pertaining to	superior (pertaining to above)
-nic	pertaining to	embryonic (pertaining to an embryo)
-ory	pertaining to	auditory (pertaining to hearing)
-ose	pertaining to	adipose (pertaining to fat)
-ous	pertaining to	intravenous (pertaining to within a vein)
-tic	pertaining to	acoustic (pertaining to hearing)

Surgical Suffixes

The following suffixes indicate surgical procedures.

MED TERM TIP

Surgical suffixes have very specific meanings:

-*otomy* means "to cut into"
-*ostomy* means "to create a new opening"
-*ectomy* means "to cut out" or "remove"

SUFFIX	MEANING	EXAMPLE (DEFINITION)
-centesis	puncture to withdraw fluid	arthrocentesis (puncture to withdraw fluid from a joint)
-ectomy	surgical removal	gastrectomy (surgically remove the stomach)
-ostomy	surgically create an opening	colostomy (surgically create an opening for the colon [through the abdominal wall])
-otomy	cutting into	thoracotomy (cutting into the chest)
-pexy	surgical fixation	nephropexy (surgical fixation of a kidney)
-plasty	surgical repair	dermatoplasty (surgical repair of the skin)
-rrhaphy	suture	myorrhaphy (suture together muscle)

Procedural Suffixes

The following suffixes indicate procedural processes or instruments.

SUFFIX	MEANING	EXAMPLE (DEFINITION)
-gram	record or picture	electrocardiogram (record of heart's electricity)
-graph	instrument for recording	electrocardiograph (instrument for recording the heart's electrical activity)

SUFFIX	MEANING	EXAMPLE (DEFINITION)
-graphy	process of recording	electrocardiography (process of recording the heart's electrical activity)
-meter	instrument for measuring	audiometer (instrument to measure hearing)
-metry	process of measuring	audiometry (process of measuring hearing)
-scope	instrument for viewing	gastroscope (instrument to view stomach)
-scopy	process of visually examining	gastroscopy (process of visually examining the stomach)

Word Building

Word building consists of putting together two or more word elements to form a variety of terms. Prefixes and suffixes may be added to a combining form to create a new descriptive term. For example, adding the prefix *hypo-* (meaning below) and the suffix *-ic* (meaning pertaining to) to the combining form *derm/o* (meaning skin) forms **hypodermic** (high-poh-DER-mik), pertaining to below the skin.

Interpreting Medical Terms

The following strategy is a reliable method for puzzling out the meaning of an unfamiliar medical term.

STEP	EXAMPLE
1. Divide the term into its word parts.	gastr/o/enter/o/logy
2. Define each word part.	**gastr** = stomach
	o = combining vowel, no meaning
	enter = small intestine
	o = combining vowel, no meaning
	-logy = study
3. Combine the meaning of the word parts.	stomach, small intestine, study of

> **MED TERM TIP**
>
> To gain a quick understanding of a term, it may be helpful to you to read from the end of the word (or the suffix) back to the beginning (the prefix), and then pick up the word root. For example, *pericarditis* reads inflammation (*-itis*) surrounding (*peri-*) the heart (*cardi/o*).

Pronunciation

You will hear different pronunciations for the same terms depending on where people were born or educated. As long as it is clear which term people are discussing, differing pronunciations are acceptable. Some people are difficult to understand over the telephone or on a transcription tape. If you have any doubt about a term being discussed, ask for the term to be spelled. For example, it is often difficult to hear the difference between the terms **abduction** and **adduction.** However, since the terms refer to opposite directions of movement, it is very important to double-check if there is any question about which term was used.

Each new term in this book is introduced in boldface type, with the phonetic or "sounds like" pronunciation in parentheses immediately following. The part of the word that should receive the greatest emphasis during pronunciation appears in capital letters: for example, **pericarditis** (per-ih-car-DYE-tis). Each

term presented in this book is also pronounced on the CD-ROM packaged with the book. Listen to each word, then pronounce it silently to yourself or out loud.

Spelling

Although you will hear differing pronunciations of the same term, there will be only one correct spelling. If you have any doubt about the spelling of a term or of its meaning, always look it up in a medical dictionary. If only one letter of the word is changed, it could make a critical difference for the patient. For example, imagine the problem that could arise if you note for insurance purposes that a portion of a patient's **ileum,** or small intestine, was removed when in reality he had surgery for removal of a piece of his **ilium,** or hip bone.

Some words have the same beginning sounds but are spelled differently. Examples include:

Sounds like *si*

psy	**psychiatry** (sigh-KIGH-ah-tree)
cy	**cytology** (sigh-TALL-oh-gee)

Sounds like *dis*

dys	**dyspepsia** (dis-PEP-see-ah)
dis	**dislocation** (dis-low-KAY-shun)

 # Singular and Plural Endings

Many medical terms originate from Greek and Latin words. The rules for forming the singular and plural forms of some words follow the rules of these languages rather than English. For example, the heart has a left atrium and a right atrium for a total of two *atria*, not two *atriums*. Other words, such as *virus* and *viruses,* are changed from singular to plural by following English rules. Each medical term needs to be considered individually when changing from the singular to the plural form. The following examples illustrate how to form plurals.

Words ending in	Singular	Plural
-a	vertebra	vertebrae
-ax	thorax	thoraces
-ex or -ix	appendix	appendices
-is	metastasis	metastases
-ma	sarcoma	sarcomata
-nx	phalanx	phalanges
-on	ganglion	ganglia
-us	nucleus	nuclei
-um	ovum	ova
-y	biopsy	biopsies

Abbreviations

Abbreviations are commonly used in the medical profession as a way of saving time. However, some abbreviations can be confusing, such as *SM* for simple mastectomy and *sm* for small. Use of the incorrect abbreviation can result in problems for a patient, as well as with insurance records and processing. If you have any concern that you will confuse someone by using an abbreviation, spell out the word instead. It is never acceptable to use made-up abbreviations. All types of healthcare facilities will have a list of approved abbreviations, and it is extremely important that you become familiar with this list and follow it closely. Throughout the book abbreviations are included, when possible, immediately following terms. In addition, a list of common abbreviations for each body system is given in each chapter. Finally, Appendix I provides a complete alphabetical listing of all the abbreviations used in this text.

The Medical Record

The **medical record** or chart documents the details of a patient's hospital stay. Each healthcare professional who has contact with the patient in any capacity completes the appropriate report of that contact and adds it to the medical chart. This results in a permanent physical record of the patient's day-to-day condition, when and what services he or she received, and the response to treatment. Each institution adopts a specific format for each document and its location within the chart. This is necessary because each healthcare professional must be able to locate quickly and efficiently the information he or she needs in order to provide proper care for the patient. The medical record is also a legal document. Therefore, it is essential that all chart components be completely filled out and signed. Each page must contain the proper patient identification information: the patient's name, age, gender, physician, admission date, and identification number.

While the patient is still in the hospital, a unit clerk is usually responsible for placing documents in the proper place. After discharge, the medical records department ensures that all documents are present, complete, signed, and in the correct order. If a person is readmitted, especially for the same diagnosis, parts of this previous chart can be pulled and added to the current chart for reference (see Figure 1.2 ■). Physicians' offices and other outpatient care providers such as clinics and therapists also maintain a medical record detailing each patient's visit to their facility.

The digital revolution has also impacted healthcare with the increasing use of the **Electronic Medical Record** (EMR). A software program is used to enter patient information into a computer which then organizes and stores the information. Information may be entered either at a centralized workstation or by using mobile devices at the point of care. Once digitally stored, the information may be analyzed and monitored to detect and prevent potential errors. Since the records are digitally stored, they can be easily accessed and shared between healthcare providers which will reduce repeating tests unnecessarily and inadvertent medication errors. The following list includes the most common elements of a paper chart with a brief description.

History and Physical—Written or dictated by admitting physician; details patient's history, results of physician's examination, initial diagnoses, and physician's plan of treatment

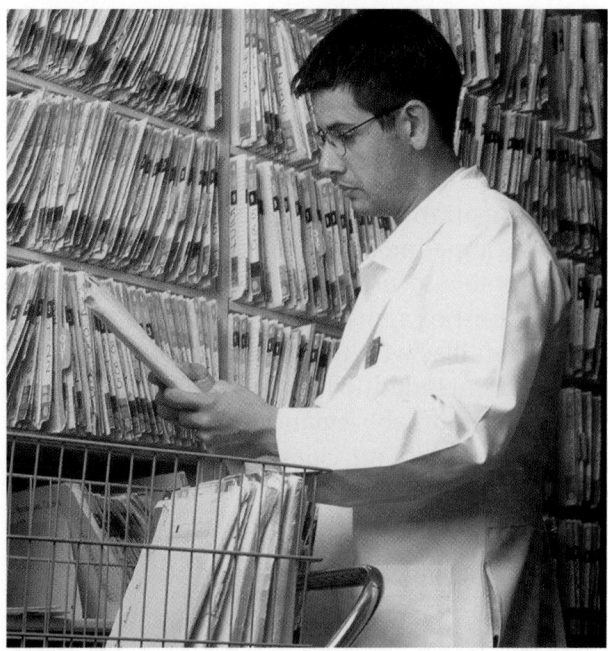

Figure 1.2 Health information professionals maintain accurate, orderly, and permanent patient records. Medical records are securely stored and available for future reference.

Physician's Orders—Complete list of care, medications, tests, and treatments physician orders for patient

Nurse's Notes—Record of patient's care throughout the day; includes vital signs, treatment specifics, patient's response to treatment, and patient's condition

Physician's Progress Notes—Physician's daily record of patient's condition, results of physician's examinations, summary of test results, updated assessment and diagnoses, and further plans for patient's care

Consultation Reports—Reports given by specialists whom physician has asked to evaluate patient

Ancillary Reports—Reports from various treatments and therapies patient has received, such as rehabilitation, social services, or respiratory therapy

Diagnostic Reports—Results of diagnostic tests performed on patient, principally from clinical lab (e.g., blood tests) and medical imaging (e.g., X-rays and ultrasound)

Informed Consent—Document voluntarily signed by patient or a responsible party that clearly describes purpose, methods, procedures, benefits, and risks of a diagnostic or treatment procedure

Operative Report—Report from surgeon detailing an operation; includes pre- and postoperative diagnosis, specific details of surgical procedure itself, and how patient tolerated procedure

Anesthesiologist's Report—Relates details regarding substances (such as medications and fluids) given to patient, patient's response to anesthesia, and vital signs during surgery

Pathologist's Report—Report given by pathologist who studies tissue removed from patient (e.g., bone marrow, blood, or tissue biopsy)

Discharge Summary—Comprehensive outline of patient's entire hospital stay; includes condition at time of admission, admitting diagnosis, test results, treatments and patient's response, final diagnosis, and follow-up plans

■ Healthcare Settings

The use of medical terminology is widespread. It provides healthcare professionals with a precise and efficient method of communicating very specific patient information to one another, regardless of whether they are in the same type of facility (see Figure 1.3 ■). Descriptions follow of the different types of settings where medical terminology is used.

Acute Care or General Hospitals—Provide services to diagnose (laboratory, diagnostic imaging) and treat (surgery, medications, therapy) diseases for a short period of time; in addition, they usually provide emergency and obstetrical care

Specialty Care Hospitals—Provide care for very specific types of diseases; for example, a psychiatric hospital

Nursing Homes or Long-Term Care Facilities—Provide long-term care for patients needing extra time to recover from illness or injury before returning home, or for persons who can no longer care for themselves

Ambulatory Care Centers, Surgical Centers, or Outpatient Clinics—Provide services not requiring overnight hospitalization; services range from simple surgeries to diagnostic testing or therapy

Physicians' Offices—Provide diagnostic and treatment services in a private office setting

Health Maintenance Organization (HMO)—Provides wide range of services by a group of primary-care physicians, specialists, and other healthcare professionals in a prepaid system

Home Health Care—Provides nursing, therapy, personal care, or housekeeping services in patient's own home

Rehabilitation Centers—Provide intensive physical and occupational therapy; includes inpatient and outpatient treatment

Hospices—Provide supportive treatment to terminally ill patients and their families

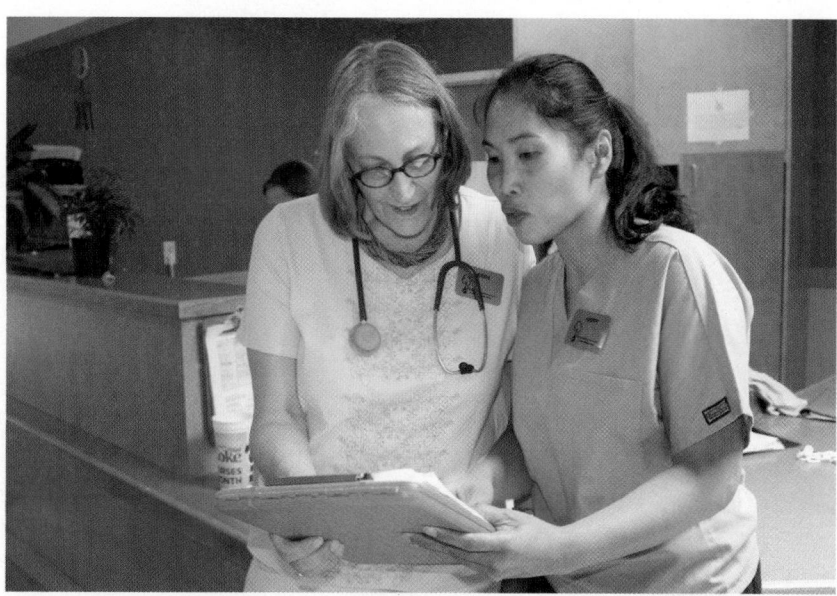

■ **Figure 1.3** A nurse and medical assistant review a patient's chart and plan his or her daily care.

Confidentiality

Anyone working with medical terminology and involved in the medical profession must have a firm understanding of confidentiality. Any information or record relating to a patient must be considered privileged. This means that you have a moral and legal responsibility to keep all information about the patient confidential. If you are asked to supply documentation relating to a patient, the proper authorization form must be signed by the patient. Give only the specific information that the patient has authorized. The Health Insurance Portability and Accountability Act of 1996 (HIPAA) set federal standards providing patients with more protection of their medical records and health information, better access to their own records, and greater control over how their health information is used and to whom it is disclosed.

Chapter Review

Practice Exercises

A. Complete the Statement

1. The combination of a word root and the combining vowel is called a(n) _____.

2. The vowel that connects two word roots or a suffix with a word root is usually a(n) _____.

3. A word part used at the end of a word root to change the meaning of the word is called a(n) _____.

4. A(n) _____ is used at the beginning of a word to indicate number, location, or time.

5. Although the pronunciation of medical terms may differ slightly from one person to another, the

   _____ must never change.

6. The four components of a medical term are _____, _____,

   _____, and _____.

B. Terminology Matching

Match each definition to its term.

1. _____ Provides services for a short period of time
2. _____ Complete outline of a patient's entire hospital stay
3. _____ Describes purpose, methods, benefits, and risks of procedure
4. _____ Contains updated assessment, diagnoses, and further plans for care
5. _____ Provides supportive care to terminally ill patients and families
6. _____ Written by the admitting physician
7. _____ Reports results from study of tissue removed from the patient
8. _____ Written by the surgeon
9. _____ Provides services not requiring overnight hospital stay
10. _____ Report given by a specialist
11. _____ Record of a patient's care through the day
12. _____ Clinical lab and medical imaging reports
13. _____ Provides intensive physical and occupational therapy
14. _____ Report of treatment/therapy the patient received
15. _____ Provides care for patients who need more time to recover

a. rehabilitation center
b. nurse's notes
c. ancillary report
d. hospice
e. discharge summary
f. physician's progress notes
g. ambulatory care center
h. diagnostic report
i. long-term care facility
j. informed consent
k. history and physical
l. acute care hospital
m. pathologist's report
n. consultation report
o. operative report

C. Define the Suffix

1. -plasty _____

2. -stenosis _____

3. -itis _____

4. -al _____

5. -algia _____

6. -otomy _____

7. -megaly _____

8. -ectomy _____

9. -rrhage _____

10. -centesis _____

11. -gram _____

12. -ac _____

13. -malacia _____

14. -ism _____

15. -rrhaphy _____

16. -ostomy _____

17. -pexy _____

18. -rrhea _____

19. -scopy _____

20. -oma _____

D. Combining Form and Suffix Practice

Join a combining form and a suffix to form words with the following meanings.

1. study of lungs _____

2. pain relating to a nerve _____

3. nose discharge or flow _____

4. abnormal softening of a kidney _____

5. enlarged heart _____

6. cutting into the stomach _____

7. inflammation of the skin _____

8. surgical removal of the voice box _____

9. surgical repair of a joint _____

10. gland disease _____

E. Name That Prefix

1. within, inside _____

2. large _____

3. before, in front of _____

4. around _____

5. new _____

6. without _____

7. half _____

8. painful, difficult _____

9. above _____

10. over, above _____

11. many _____

12. slow _____

13. self _____

14. across _____

15. two _____

F. Prefix Practice

Circle the prefixes in the following terms and define in the space provided.

1. tachycardia _____

2. pseudocyesis _____

3. hypoglycemia _____

4. intercostal _____

5. eupnea _____

6. postoperative _____

7. monoplegia _____

8. subcutaneous _____

G. Make It Plural

Change the following singular terms to plural terms.

1. metastasis _____

2. ovum _____

3. diverticulum _____

4. atrium _____

5. diagnosis _____

6. vertebra _____

H. Name That Term

Use the suffix -ology to write a term for each medical specialty.

1. heart _____

2. stomach _____

3. skin _____

4. eye _____

5. immunity _____

6. kidney _____

7. blood _____

8. female _____

9. nerve _____

10. disease _____

MEDICAL TERMINOLOGY INTERACTIVE

Medical Terminology Interactive is a premium online homework management system that includes a host of features to help you study. Registered users will find:

- Fun games and activities built within a virtual hospital
- Powerful tools that track and analyze your results—allowing you to create a personalized learning experience
- Videos, flashcards, and audio pronunciations to help enrich your progress
- Streaming lesson presentations and self-paced learning modules

www.pearsonhighered.com/mti

I. Building Medical Terms

Build a medical term by combining the word parts requested in each question.

For example, use the combining form for *spleen* with the suffix meaning *enlargement* to form a word meaning *enlargement of the spleen* (answer: *splenomegaly*).

1. combining form for *heart* _____

   suffix meaning *abnormal softening* _____ ⎤
   ⎦ term meaning *softening of the heart*

2. word root form for *stomach* _____

   suffix meaning *to surgically create an opening* _____ ⎤
   ⎦ term meaning *creating an opening into the stomach*

3. combining form for *nose* _____

   suffix meaning *surgical repair* _____ ⎤
   ⎦ term meaning *surgical repair of the nose*

4. prefix meaning *over, above* _____

   suffix meaning *nourishment, development* _____ ⎤
   ⎦ term meaning *overdevelopment*

5. combining form meaning *disease* _____

   suffix meaning *the study of* _____ ⎤
   ⎦ term meaning *the study of disease*

6. word root meaning *gland* _____

   suffix for *tumor/mass* _____ ⎤
   ⎦ term meaning *gland tumor or mass*

7. combining form meaning *stomach* _____

   combining form meaning *small intestine* _____

   suffix meaning *study of* _____ ⎤
   ⎦ term meaning *study of stomach and small intestine*

8. word root meaning *ear* _____

   suffix meaning *inflammation* _____ ⎤
   ⎦ term meaning *ear inflammation*

9. prefix meaning *water* _____

   suffix meaning *treatment* _____ ⎤
   ⎦ term meaning *water treatment*

10. combining form meaning *cancer* _____

   suffix meaning *that which produces* _____ ⎤
   ⎦ term meaning *that which produces cancer*

J. Define the Combining Form

1. aden/o _____

2. carcin/o _____

3. cardi/o _____

4. chem/o _____

5. cis/o _____

6. dermat/o _____

7. enter/o _____

8. gastr/o _____

9. gynec/o _____

10. hemat/o _____

11. hydr/o _____

12. immun/o _____

13. laryng/o _____

14. path/o _____

15. nephr/o _____

16. neur/o _____

17. ophthalm/o _____

18. ot/o _____

19. pulmon/o _____

20. rhin/o _____

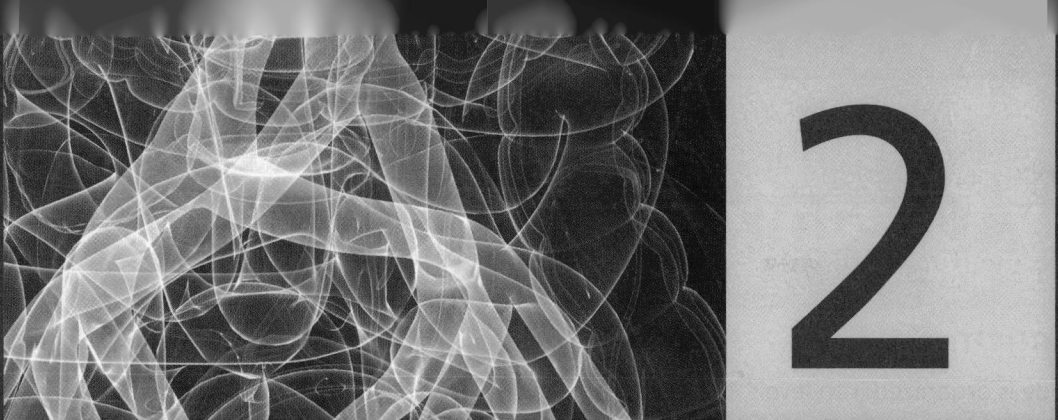

2

BODY ORGANIZATION

Learning Objectives

Upon completion of this chapter, you will be able to

- Recognize the combining forms introduced in this chapter.
- Correctly spell and pronounce medical terms and anatomical structures relating to body structure.
- Discuss the organization of the body in terms of cells, tissues, organs, and systems.
- Describe the common features of cells.
- Define the four types of tissues.
- List the major organs found in the 12 organ systems.
- Describe the anatomical position.
- Define the body planes.
- Identify regions of the body.
- Define directional and positional terms.
- List the body cavities and their contents.
- Locate and describe the nine anatomical and four clinical divisions of the abdomen.
- Build body organization medical terms from word parts.
- Interpret abbreviations associated with body organization.

Body Organization at a Glance

Arrangement

The body is organized into levels; each is built from the one below it. In other words, the body as a whole is composed of systems, a system is composed of organs, an organ is composed of tissues, and tissues are composed of cells.

Levels

cells   tissues   organs   systems   body

Word Parts

Presented here are some of the more common combining forms used to build body organizational terms. For a list of the prefixes and suffixes used, refer to the Terminology section of this chapter.

Combining Forms

abdomin/o	abdomen	later/o	side
adip/o	fat	lumb/o	loin
anter/o	front	lymph/o	lymph
brachi/o	arm	medi/o	middle
cardi/o	heart	muscul/o	muscles
caud/o	tail	nephr/o	kidney
cephal/o	head	neur/o	nerve
cervic/o	neck	ophthalm/o	eye
chondr/o	cartilage	ot/o	ear
crani/o	skull	pelv/o	pelvis
crin/o	to secrete	peritone/o	peritoneum
crur/o	leg	pleur/o	pleura
cyt/o	cell	poster/o	back
dermat/o	skin	proct/o	rectum and anus
dist/o	away from	proxim/o	near to
dors/o	back of body	pub/o	genital region
enter/o	small intestine	pulmon/o	lung
epitheli/o	epithelium	rhin/o	nose
gastr/o	stomach	spin/o	spine
glute/o	buttock	super/o	above
gynec/o	woman	thorac/o	chest
hemat/o	blood	ur/o	urine
hist/o	tissue	vascul/o	blood vessel
immun/o	protection	ventr/o	belly
infer/o	below	vertebr/o	vertebra
laryng/o	larynx	viscer/o	internal organ

Body Organization Illustrated

cell, p. 24

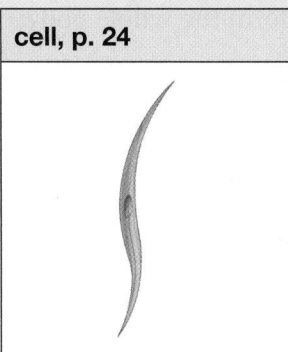

Basic unit of life

tissues, p. 25

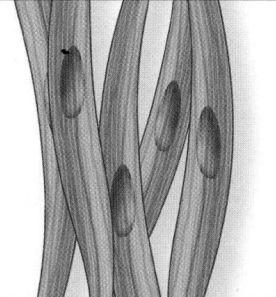

Group of identical cells
working together

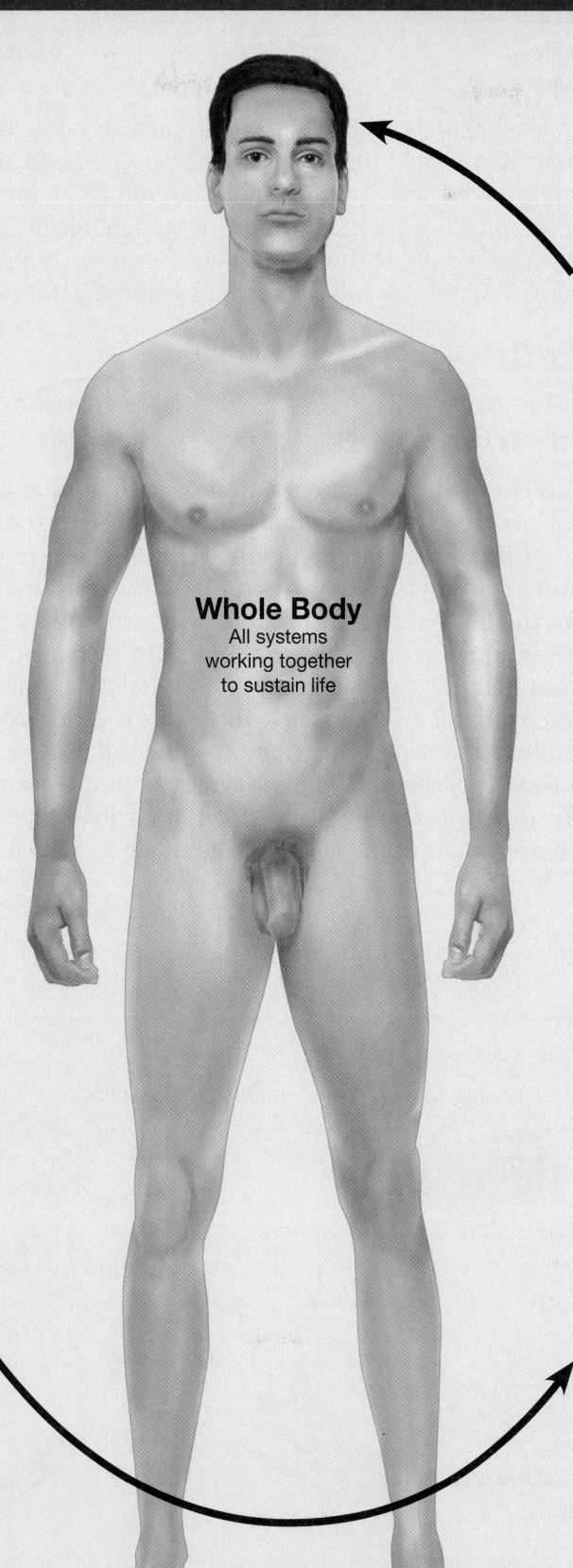

Whole Body
All systems
working together
to sustain life

systems, p. 27

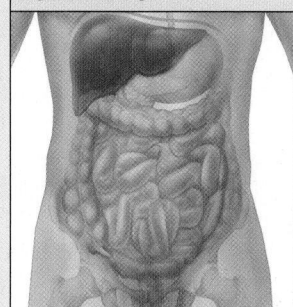

Collection of organs
working together

organs, p. 27

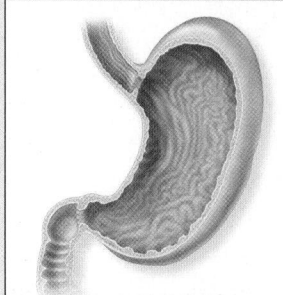

Composed of two or
more types of tissue

Levels of Body Organization

body   **organs**   **tissues**
cells   **systems**

Before taking a look at the whole human body, we need to examine its component parts. The human **body** is composed of **cells, tissues, organs,** and **systems.** These components are arranged in a hierarchical manner. That is, parts from a lower level come together to form the next higher level. In that way, cells come together to form tissues, tissues come together to form organs, organs come together to form systems, and all the systems come together to form the whole body.

Cells

cell membrane   **cytoplasm** (SIGH-toh-plazm)
cytology (sigh-TALL-oh-jee)   **nucleus**

The cell is the fundamental unit of all living things. That is to say, it is the smallest structure of a body that has all the properties of being alive: responding to stimuli, engaging in metabolic activities, and reproducing itself. All the tissues and organs in the body are composed of cells. Individual cells perform functions for the body such as reproduction, hormone secretion, energy production, and excretion. Special cells are also able to carry out very specific functions, such as contraction by muscle cells and electrical impulse transmission by nerve cells. The study of cells and their functions is called **cytology.** No matter the difference in their shape and function, at some point during their life cycle all cells have a **nucleus, cytoplasm,** and a **cell membrane** (see Figure 2.1 ■). The cell membrane is the outermost boundary of a cell. It encloses the cytoplasm, the watery internal environment of the cell, and the nucleus, which contains the cell's DNA.

MED TERM TIP

Cells were first seen by Robert Hooke over 300 years ago. To him, the rectangular shapes looked like prison cells, so he named them cells. It was a common practice for early anatomists to name an organ solely on its appearance.

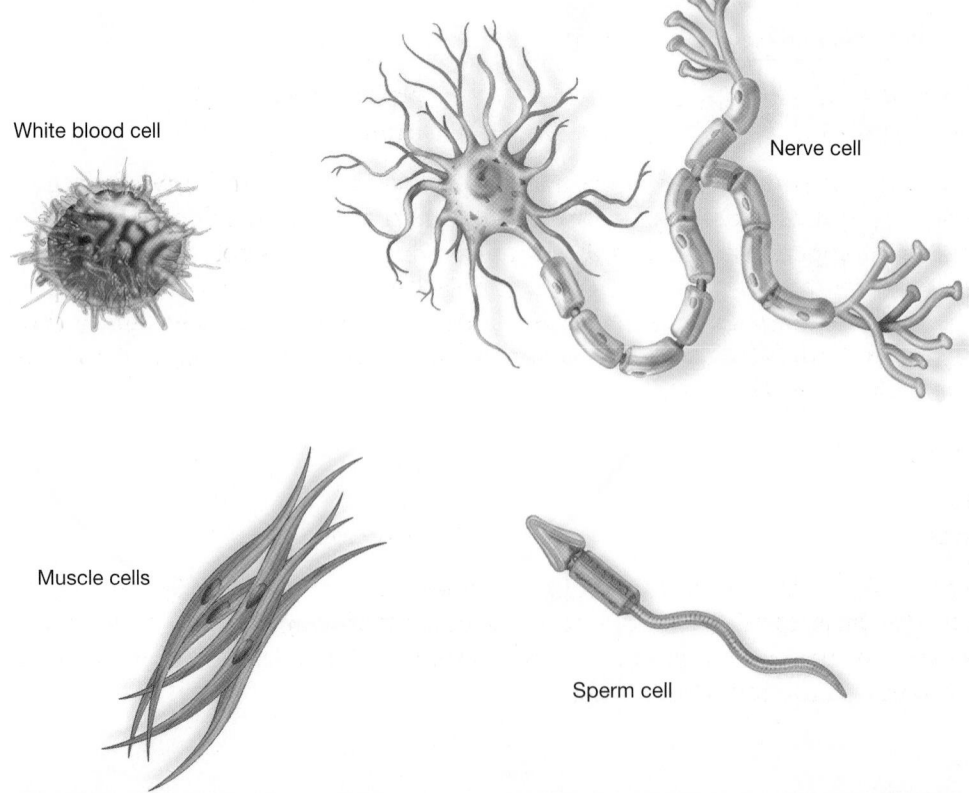

White blood cell

Nerve cell

Muscle cells

Sperm cell

■ **Figure 2.1** Examples of four different types of cells from the body. Although each cell has a cell membrane, nucleus, and cytoplasm, each has a unique shape depending on its location and function.

Tissues

connective tissue

epithelial tissue (ep-ih-THEE-lee-al)

histology (hiss-TALL-oh-jee)

muscle tissue

nervous tissue

Histology is the study of tissue. A tissue is formed when like cells are grouped together and function together to perform a specific activity. The body has four types of tissue: **muscle tissue, epithelial tissue, connective tissue,** and **nervous tissue** (see Figure 2.2 ■).

Muscle Tissue

cardiac muscle

smooth muscle

muscle fibers

skeletal muscle

Muscle tissue produces movement in the body through contraction, or shortening in length, and is composed of individual muscle cells called **muscle fibers.** Muscle tissue forms one of three basic types of muscles: **skeletal muscle, smooth muscle,** or **cardiac muscle.** Skeletal muscle is attached to bone. Smooth muscle is found in internal organs such as the intestine, uterus, and blood vessels. Cardiac muscle is found only in the heart.

Epithelial Tissue

epithelium (ep-ih-THEE-lee-um)

Epithelial tissue, or **epithelium,** is found throughout the body and is composed of close-packed cells that form the covering for and lining of body structures. For example, both the top layer of skin and the lining of the stomach are epithelial tissue (see Figure 2.2). In addition to forming a protective barrier, epithelial tissue may be specialized to absorb substances (such as nutrients from the intestine), secrete substances (such as sweat glands), or excrete wastes (such as the kidney tubules).

> **MED TERM TIP**
>
> The term *epithelium* comes from the prefix *epi-* meaning "on top of" and the combining form *theli/o* meaning "nipple" (referring to any projection from the surface).

Connective Tissue

adipose (ADD-ih-pohs)

bone

cartilage (CAR-tih-lij)

tendons

Connective tissue is the supporting and protecting tissue in body structures. Because connective tissue performs many different functions depending on its location, it appears in many different forms so that each is able to perform the task required at that location. For example, **bone** provides structural support for the whole body. **Cartilage** is the shock absorber in joints. **Tendons** tightly connect skeletal muscles to bones. **Adipose** provides protective padding around body structures (see Figure 2.2).

Nervous Tissue

brain

nerves

neurons

spinal cord

Nervous tissue is composed of cells called **neurons** (see Figure 2.2). This tissue forms the **brain, spinal cord,** and a network of **nerves** throughout the entire body, allowing for the conduction of electrical impulses to send information between the brain and the rest of the body.

Figure 2.2 The appearance of different types of tissues—muscle, epithelial, nervous, connective—and their location within the body.

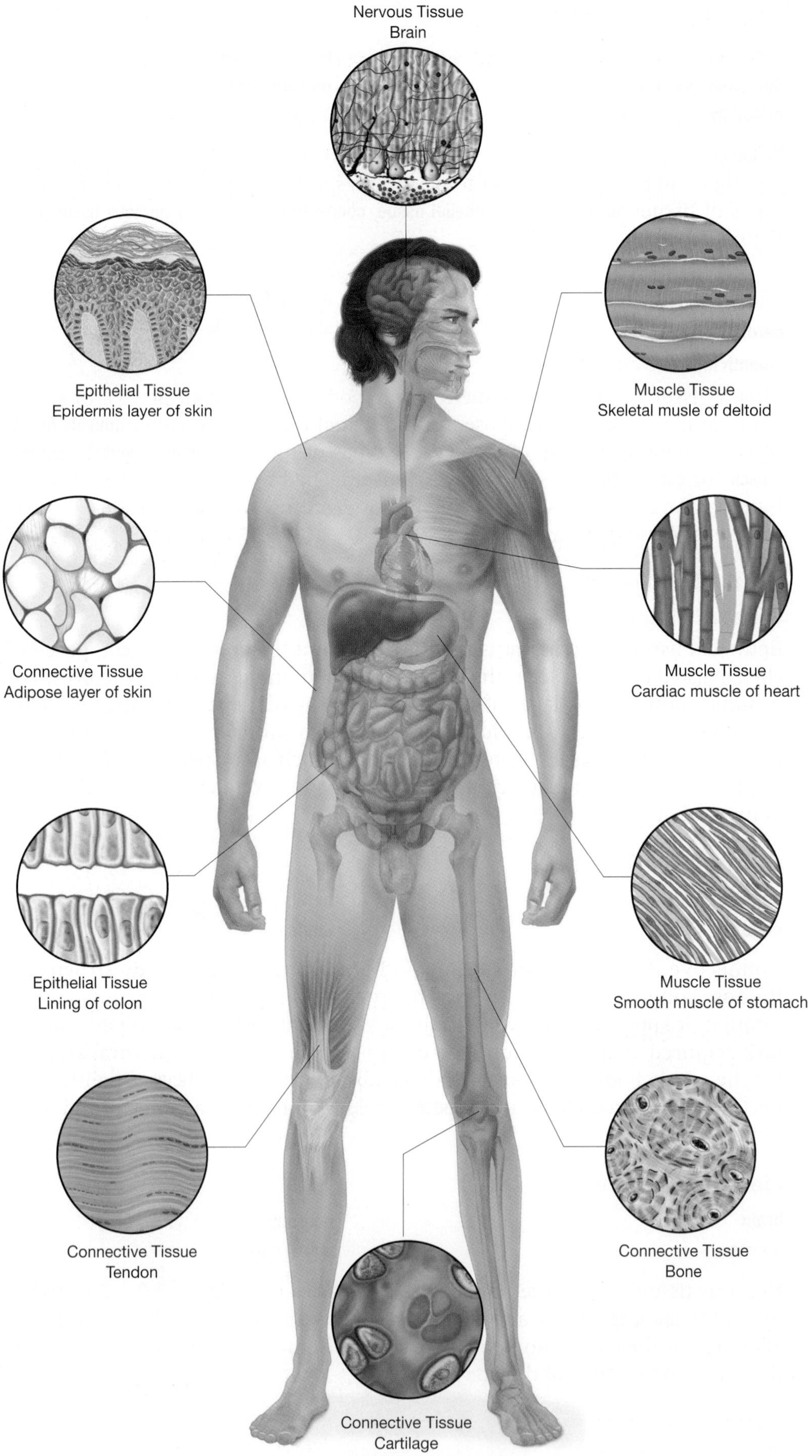

Nervous Tissue
Brain

Epithelial Tissue
Epidermis layer of skin

Muscle Tissue
Skeletal musle of deltoid

Connective Tissue
Adipose layer of skin

Muscle Tissue
Cardiac muscle of heart

Epithelial Tissue
Lining of colon

Muscle Tissue
Smooth muscle of stomach

Connective Tissue
Tendon

Connective Tissue
Bone

Connective Tissue
Cartilage

Organs and Systems

Organs are composed of several different types of tissue that work as a unit to perform special functions. For example, the stomach contains smooth muscle tissue, nervous tissue, and epithelial tissue that allow it to contract to mix food with digestive juices.

A system is composed of several organs working in a coordinated manner to perform a complex function or functions. To continue our example, the stomach plus the other digestive system organs—the oral cavity, esophagus, liver, pancreas, small intestine, and colon—work together to ingest, digest, and absorb our food.

Table 2.1 ■ presents the organ systems that are discussed in this book along with the major organs found in each system, the system functions, and the medical specialties that treat conditions of that system.

Table 2.1	Organ Systems of the Human Body		
SYSTEM/MEDICAL SPECIALTY	**STRUCTURES**		**FUNCTIONS**
Integumentary System (in-teg-you-MEN-tah-ree) **dermatology** (der-mah-TALL-oh-jee)	• skin • hair • nails • sweat glands • sebaceous glands		Forms protective two-way barrier and aids in temperature regulation.
Musculoskeletal System (MS) (mus-qu-low-SKEL-et-all) **orthopedics** (or-thoh-PEE-diks) **orthopedic surgery** (or-the-PEE-dik)	• bones • joints • muscles		Skeleton supports and protects the body, forms blood cells, and stores minerals. Muscles produce movement.

(Continued)

Table 2.1   Organ Systems of the Human Body (continued)

SYSTEM/MEDICAL SPECIALTY	STRUCTURES	FUNCTIONS
Cardiovascular System (CV) (car-dee-oh-VAS-kew-lar) **cardiology** (car-dee-ALL-oh-jee)	• heart • arteries • veins	Pumps blood throughout the entire body to transport nutrients, oxygen, and wastes.
Blood (Hematic System) (he-MAT-tik) **hematology** (hee-mah-TALL-oh-jee)	• plasma • erythrocytes • leukocytes • platelets	Transports oxygen, protects against pathogens, and controls bleeding.
Lymphatic System (lim-FAT-ik) **immunology** (im-yoo-NALL-oh-jee)	• lymph nodes • lymphatic vessels • spleen • thymus gland • tonsils	Protects the body from disease and invasion from pathogens.

Table 2.1   Organ Systems of the Human Body (continued)

SYSTEM/MEDICAL SPECIALTY	STRUCTURES	FUNCTIONS
Respiratory System **otorhinolaryngology** (ENT) (oh-toh-rye-noh- lair-ing-GALL-oh-jee) **pulmonology** (pull-mon-ALL-oh-jee) **thoracic surgery** (tho-RASS-ik)	• nasal cavity • pharynx • larynx • trachea • bronchial tubes • lungs 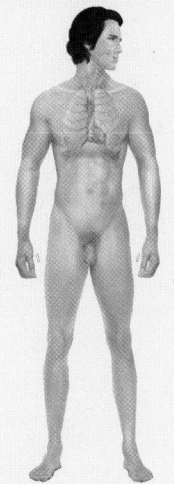	Obtains oxygen and removes carbon dioxide from the body.
Digestive or **Gastrointestinal System** (GI) **gastroenterology** (gas-troh-en-ter-ALL-oh-jee) **proctology** (prok-TOL-oh-jee)	• oral cavity • pharynx • esophagus • stomach • small intestine • colon • liver • gallbladder • pancreas • salivary glands 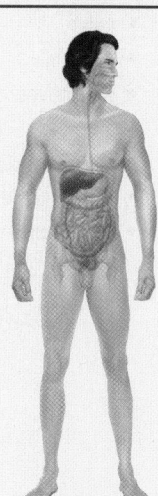	Ingests, digests, and absorbs nutrients for the body.
Urinary System (YOO-rih-nair-ee) **nephrology** (neh-FROL-oh-jee) **urology** (yoo-RALL-oh-jee)	• kidneys • ureters • urinary bladder • urethra 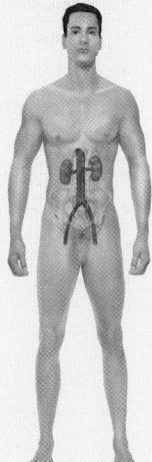	Filters waste products out of the blood and removes them from the body.

(Continued)

Table 2.1   Organ Systems of the Human Body (continued)

SYSTEM/MEDICAL SPECIALTY	STRUCTURES	FUNCTIONS
Female Reproductive System **gynecology** (GYN) (gigh-neh-KOL- oh-jee) **obstetrics** (OB) (ob-STET-riks)	• ovary • fallopian tubes • uterus • vagina • vulva • breasts	Produces eggs for reproduction and provides place for growing baby.
Male Reproductive System **urology** (yoo-RALL-oh-jee)	• testes • epididymis • vas deferens • penis • seminal vesicles • prostate gland • bulbourethral gland	Produces sperm for reproduction.
Endocrine System (EN-doh-krin) **endocrinology** (en-doh-krin-ALL-oh-jee)	• pituitary gland • pineal gland • thyroid gland • parathyroid glands • thymus gland • adrenal glands • pancreas • ovaries • testes	Regulates metabolic activities of the body.

Table 2.1	Organ Systems of the Human Body (continued)	
SYSTEM/MEDICAL SPECIALTY	STRUCTURES	FUNCTIONS
Nervous System **neurology** (noo-RAL-oh-jee) **neurosurgery** (noo-roh-SIR-jer-ee)	• brain • spinal cord • nerves	Receives sensory information and coordinates the body's response.
Special Senses **ophthalmology** (off-thal-MALL-oh-jee)	• eye	Vision
otorhinolaryngology (ENT) (oh-toh-rye-noh-lair- ing-GALL-oh-jee)	• ear	Hearing and balance

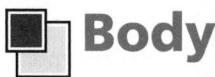

Body

anatomical position

As seen from the previous sections, the body is the sum of all the systems, organs, tissues, and cells found in it. It is important to learn the anatomical terminology that applies to the body as a whole in order to correctly identify specific locations and directions when dealing with patients. The **anatomical position** is used when describing the positions and relationships of structures in the human body. A body in the anatomical position is standing erect with the arms at the sides of the body, the palms of the hands facing forward, and the eyes looking straight ahead. In addition, the legs are parallel with the feet, and the toes are pointing forward (see Figure 2.3 ■). For descriptive purposes the assumption is always that the person is in the anatomical position even if the body or parts of the body are in any other position.

Body Planes

coronal plane (kor-RONE-al)	**longitudinal section**
coronal section	**median plane**
cross-section	**sagittal plane** (SAJ-ih-tal)
frontal plane	**sagittal section**
frontal section	**transverse plane**
horizontal plane	**transverse section**

The terminology for body planes is used to assist medical personnel in describing the body and its parts. To understand body planes, imagine cuts slicing through the body at various angles. This imaginary slicing allows us to use more specific language when describing parts of the body. These body planes, illustrated in Figure 2.4 ■, include the following:

1. **Sagittal plane:** This vertical plane runs lengthwise from front to back and divides the body or any of its parts into right and left portions. The right and left sides do not have to be equal. If the sagittal plane passes through the middle of the body, thus dividing it into equal right and left halves, it is called a **midsagittal** or **median plane.** A cut along the sagittal plane yields a **sagittal section** view of the inside of the body.

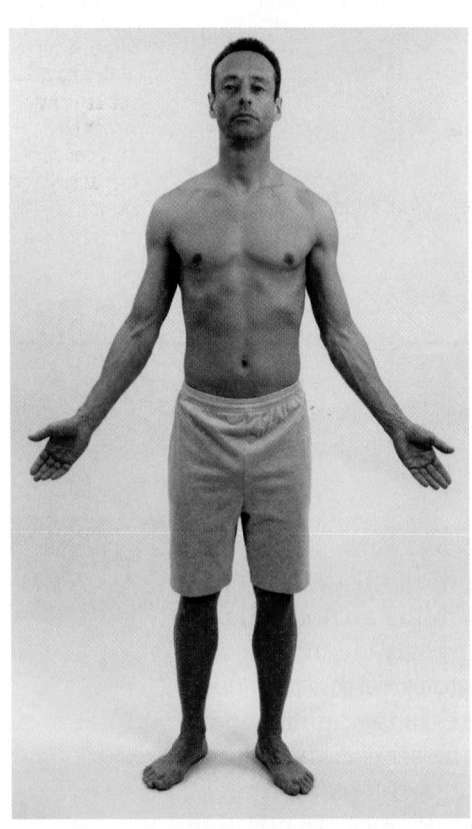

■ **Figure 2.3** The anatomical position: standing erect, gazing straight ahead, arms down at sides, palms facing forward, fingers extended, legs together, and toes pointing forward.

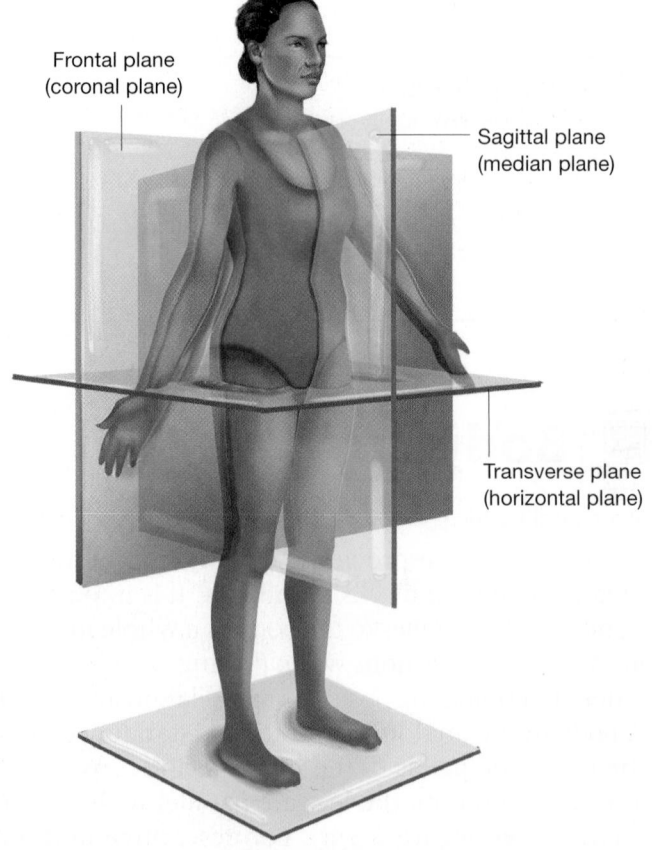

Frontal plane
(coronal plane)

Sagittal plane
(median plane)

Transverse plane
(horizontal plane)

■ **Figure 2.4** The planes of the body. The sagittal plane is vertical from front to back, the frontal plane is vertical from left to right, and the transverse plane is horizontal.

2. **Frontal plane:** The frontal, or **coronal plane,** divides the body into front and back portions; a vertical lengthwise plane is running from side to side. A cut along the frontal plane yields a **frontal** or **coronal section** view of the inside of the body.

3. **Transverse plane:** The transverse, or **horizontal plane,** is a crosswise plane that runs parallel to the ground. This imaginary cut would divide the body or its parts into upper and lower portions. A cut along the transverse plane yields a **transverse section** view of the inside of the body.

The terms **cross-section** and **longitudinal section** are frequently used to describe internal views of structures. A longitudinal section is produced by a lengthwise slice along the long axis of a structure. A cross-section view is produced by a slice perpendicular to the long axis of the structure.

Body Regions

abdominal region (ab-DOM-ih-nal)

brachial region (BRAY-kee-all)

cephalic region (she-FAL-ik)

cervical region (SER-vih-kal)

crural region (KREW-ral)

dorsum (DOOR-sum)

gluteal region (GLOO-tee-all)

lower extremities

pelvic region (PELL-vik)

pubic region (PEW-bik)

thoracic region (tho-RASS-ik)

trunk

upper extremities

vertebral region (VER-tee-bral)

The body is divided into large regions that can easily be identified externally. The **cephalic region** is the entire head. The neck is the **cervical region** and connects the head to the **trunk** (the torso). The trunk is further subdivided into different anterior and posterior regions. The anterior side consists of the **thoracic** (the chest), **abdominal, pelvic,** and **pubic** (genital) **regions.** The posterior side consists of the **dorsum** (the back), **vertebral region,** and **gluteal** (buttock) **region.** The **upper extremities** (UE) and **lower extremities** (LE) are attached to the trunk. The upper extremities or **brachial regions** are the arms. The lower extremities or **crural regions** are the legs. See Figure 2.5 ■ to locate each region on the body.

> **MED TERM TIP**
>
> As you learn medical terminology, it is important that you remember not to use common phrases and terms any longer. Many people commonly use the term *stomach* (an organ) when they actually mean *abdomen* (a body region).

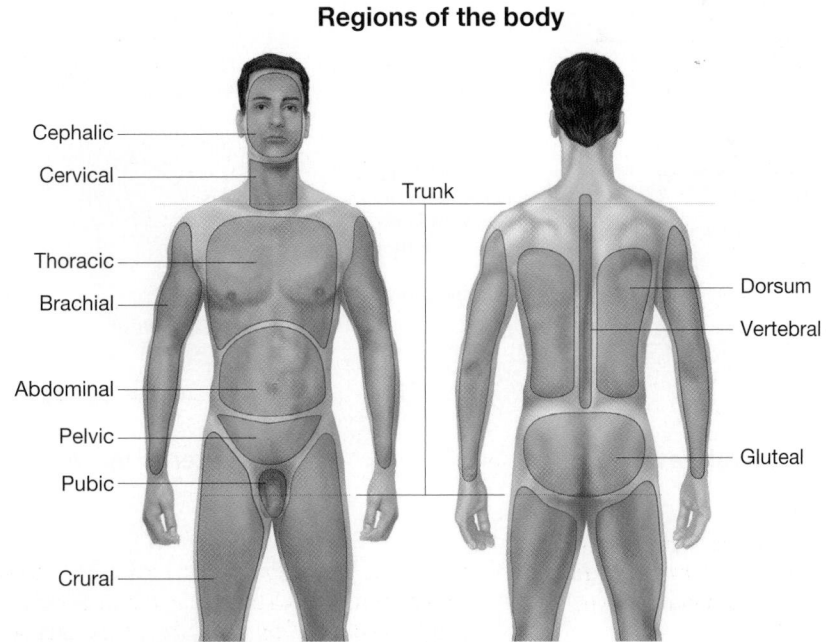

Regions of the body

Cephalic — Cervical — Trunk — Thoracic — Brachial — Abdominal — Pelvic — Pubic — Crural — Dorsum — Vertebral — Gluteal

■ **Figure 2.5** Anterior and posterior views of the body illustrating the location of various body regions.

Body Cavities

abdominal cavity

abdominopelvic cavity
(ab-dom-ih-noh-PELL-vik)

cranial cavity (KRAY-nee-al)

diaphragm (DYE-ah-fram)

mediastinum (mee-dee-ass-TYE-num)

parietal layer (pah-RYE-eh-tal)

parietal peritoneum

parietal pleura

pelvic cavity

pericardial cavity (pair-ih-CAR-dee-al)

peritoneum (pair-ih-toh-NEE-um)

pleura (PLOO-rah)

pleural cavity (PLOO-ral)

spinal cavity

thoracic cavity

viscera (VISS-er-ah)

visceral layer (VISS-er-al)

visceral peritoneum

visceral pleura

The body is not a solid structure; it has many open spaces or cavities. The cavities are part of the normal body structure and are illustrated in Figure 2.6 ■. We can divide the body into four major cavities—two dorsal cavities and two ventral cavities.

The dorsal cavities include the **cranial cavity,** containing the brain, and the **spinal cavity,** containing the spinal cord.

The ventral cavities include the **thoracic cavity** and the **abdominopelvic cavity.** The thoracic cavity contains the two lungs and a central region between them called the **mediastinum.** The heart, aorta, esophagus, trachea, and thymus gland are some of the structures located in the mediastinum. There is an actual physical wall between the thoracic cavity and the abdominopelvic cavity called the **diaphragm.** The diaphragm is a muscle used for breathing. The abdominopelvic cavity is generally subdivided into a superior **abdominal cavity** and an inferior **pelvic cavity.** The organs of the digestive, excretory, and reproductive systems are located in

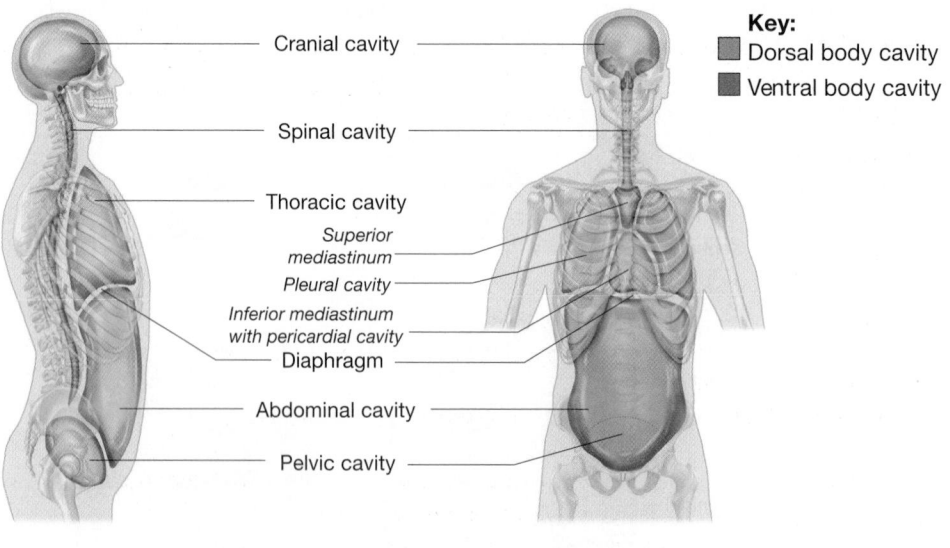

Key:
■ Dorsal body cavity
■ Ventral body cavity

Cranial cavity

Spinal cavity

Thoracic cavity

Superior mediastinum

Pleural cavity

Inferior mediastinum with pericardial cavity

Diaphragm

Abdominal cavity

Pelvic cavity

Lateral view

Anterior view

■ **Figure 2.6** The dorsal (red) and ventral (blue) body cavities.

these cavities. The organs within the ventral cavities are referred to as a group as the internal organs or **viscera.** Table 2.2 ■ describes the body cavities and their major organs.

All of the cavities are lined by, and the viscera are encased in, a two-layer membrane called the **pleura** in the thoracic cavity and the **peritoneum** in the abdominopelvic cavity. The outer layer that lines the cavities is called the **parietal layer** (i.e., **parietal pleura** and **parietal peritoneum**), and the inner layer that encases the viscera is called the **visceral layer** (i.e., **visceral pleura** and **visceral peritoneum**).

Within the thoracic cavity, the pleura is subdivided, forming the **pleural cavity,** containing the lungs, and the **pericardial cavity,** containing the heart. The larger abdominopelvic cavity is usually subdivided into regions so different areas can be precisely referred to. Two different methods of subdividing this cavity are used: the anatomical divisions and the clinical divisions. Choose a method partly on personal preference and partly on which system best describes the patient's condition. See Table 2.3 ■ for a description of these methods for dividing the abdominopelvic cavity.

Directional and Positional Terms

Directional terms assist medical personnel in discussing the position or location of a patient's complaint. Directional or positional terms also help to describe one process, organ, or system as it relates to another. Table 2.4 ■ presents commonly used terms for describing the position of the body or its parts. They are listed in pairs that have opposite meanings; for example, superior versus inferior, anterior versus posterior, medial versus lateral, proximal versus distal, superficial versus deep, and supine versus prone. Directional terms are illustrated in Figure 2.7 ■.

> **MED TERM TIP**
>
> The kidneys are the only major abdominopelvic organ located outside the sac formed by the peritoneum. Because they are found behind this sac, their position is referred to as *retroperitoneal* (retro- = behind; peritone/o = peritoneum; -al = pertaining to).

> **MED TERM TIP**
>
> Remember when using location or direction terms, it is assumed that the patient is in the anatomical position unless otherwise noted.

Table 2.2	Body Cavities and Their Major Organs
CAVITY	**MAJOR ORGANS**
Dorsal cavities	
Cranial cavity	Brain
Spinal cavity	Spinal cord
Ventral cavities	
Thoracic cavity	Pleural cavity: lungs
	Pericardial cavity: heart
	Mediastinum: heart, esophagus, trachea, thymus gland, aorta
Abdominopelvic cavity	
Abdominal cavity	Stomach, spleen, liver, gallbladder, pancreas, and portions of the small intestines and colon
Pelvic cavity	Urinary bladder, ureters, urethra, and portions of the small intestines and colon
	Female: uterus, ovaries, fallopian tubes, vagina
	Male: prostate gland, seminal vesicles, portion of the vas deferens

Table 2.3   Methods of Subdividing the Abdominopelvic Cavity

Anatomical Divisions of the Abdomen

- **Right hypochondriac** (high-poh-KON-dree-ak): Right lateral region of upper row beneath the lower ribs
- **Epigastric** (ep-ih-GAS-trik): Middle area of upper row above the stomach
- **Left hypochondriac:** Left lateral region of the upper row beneath the lower ribs
- **Right lumbar:** Right lateral region of the middle row at the waist
- **Umbilical** (um-BILL-ih-kal): Central area over the navel
- **Left lumbar:** Left lateral region of the middle row at the waist
- **Right iliac** (ILL-ee-ak): Right lateral region of the lower row at the groin
- **Hypogastric** (high-poh-GAS-trik): Middle region of the lower row beneath the navel
- **Left iliac:** Left lateral region of the lower row at the groin

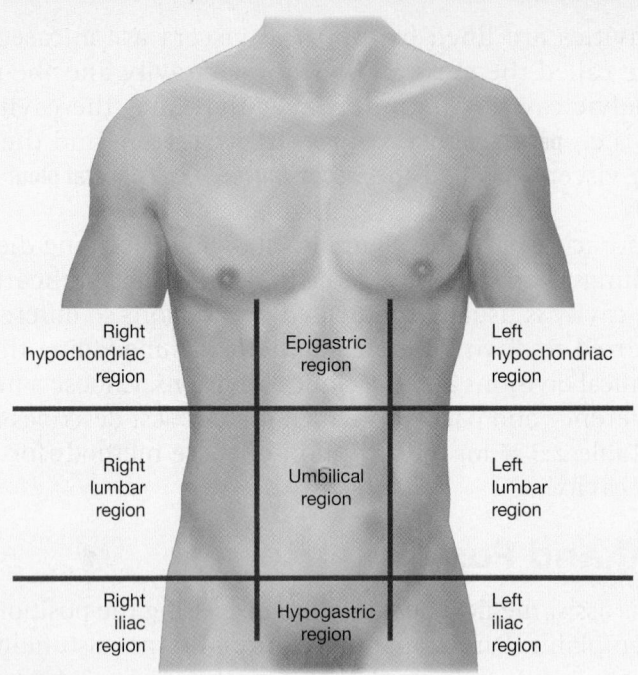

Right hypochondriac region | Epigastric region | Left hypochondriac region

Right lumbar region | Umbilical region | Left lumbar region

Right iliac region | Hypogastric region | Left iliac region

MED TERM TIP

To visualize the nine anatomical divisions, imagine a tic-tac-toe diagram over this region.

MED TERM TIP

The term *hypochondriac,* literally meaning "under the cartilage" (of the ribs), has come to refer to a person who believes he or she is sick when there is no obvious cause for illness. These patients commonly complain of aches and pains in the hypochondriac region.

Clinical Divisions of the Abdomen

- **Right upper quadrant (RUQ):** Contains majority of liver, gallbladder, small portion of pancreas, right kidney, small intestines, and colon
- **Right lower quadrant (RLQ):** Contains small intestines and colon, right ovary and fallopian tube, appendix, and right ureter
- **Left upper quadrant (LUQ):** Contains small portion of liver, spleen, stomach, majority of pancreas, left kidney, small intestines, and colon
- **Left lower quadrant (LLQ):** Contains small intestines and colon, left ovary and fallopian tube, and left ureter
- Midline organs: uterus, bladder, prostate gland

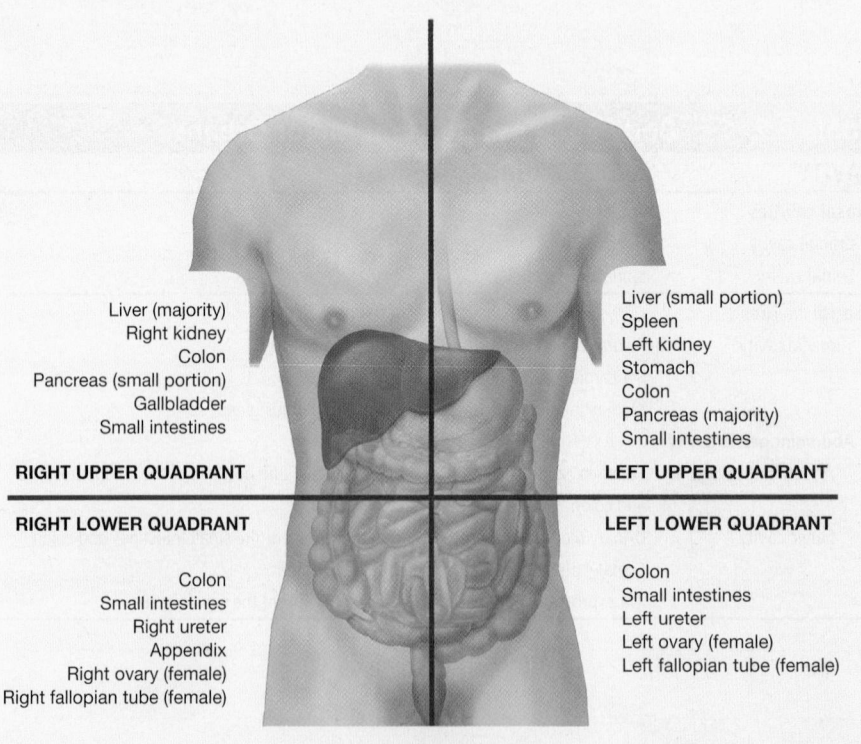

Liver (majority)
Right kidney
Colon
Pancreas (small portion)
Gallbladder
Small intestines
RIGHT UPPER QUADRANT

Liver (small portion)
Spleen
Left kidney
Stomach
Colon
Pancreas (majority)
Small intestines
LEFT UPPER QUADRANT

RIGHT LOWER QUADRANT

LEFT LOWER QUADRANT

Colon
Small intestines
Right ureter
Appendix
Right ovary (female)
Right fallopian tube (female)

Colon
Small intestines
Left ureter
Left ovary (female)
Left fallopian tube (female)

MIDLINE AREA
Bladder - Uterus (female) - Prostate (male)

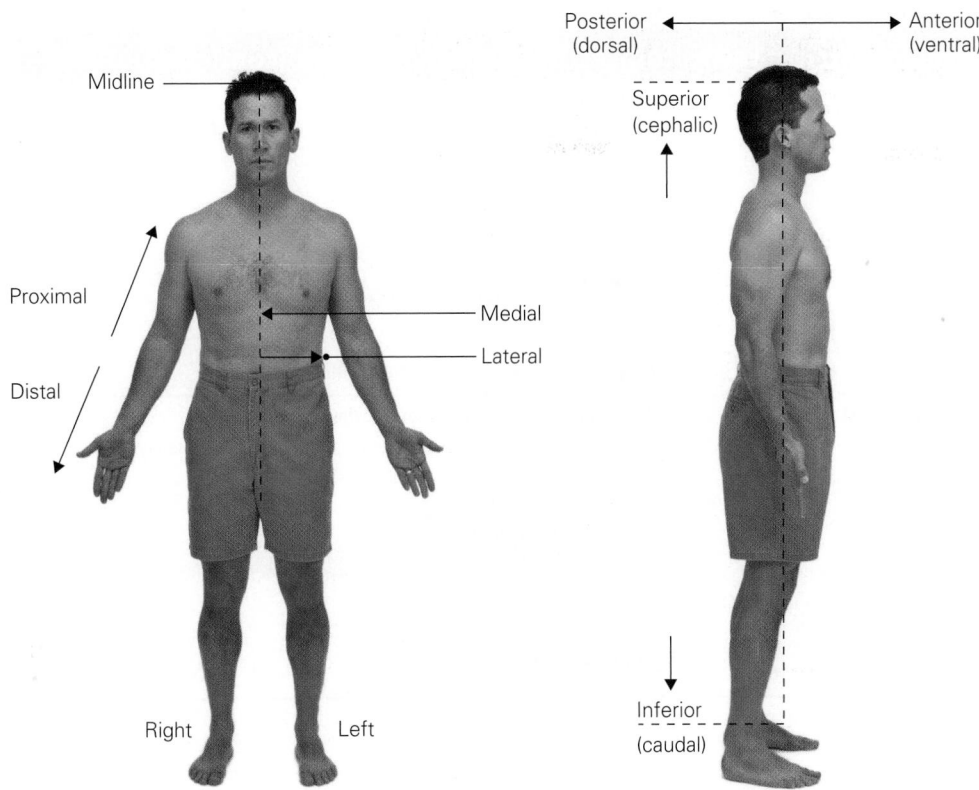

Table 2.4	Terms for Describing Body Position
superior (soo-PEE-ree-or) or **cephalic** (seh-FAL-ik)	More toward the head, or above another structure. *Example:* The adrenal glands are superior to the kidneys.
inferior (in-FEE-ree-or) or **caudal** (KAWD-al)	More toward the feet or tail, or below another structure. *Example:* The intestine is inferior to the heart.
anterior (an-TEE-ree-or) or **ventral** (VEN-tral)	More toward the front or belly-side of the body. *Example:* The navel is located on the anterior surface of the body.
posterior (poss-TEE-ree-or) or **dorsal** (DOR-sal)	More toward the back or spinal cord side of the body. *Example:* The posterior wall of the right kidney was excised.
medial (MEE-dee-al)	Refers to the middle or near the middle of the body or the structure. *Example:* The heart is medially located in the chest cavity.
lateral (lat) (LAT-er-al)	Refers to the side. *Example:* The ovaries are located lateral to the uterus.
proximal (PROK-sim-al)	Located nearer to the point of attachment to the body. *Example:* In the anatomical position, the elbow is proximal to the hand.
distal (DISS-tal)	Located farther away from the point of attachment to the body. *Example:* The hand is distal to the elbow.
apex (AY-peks)	Tip or summit of an organ. *Example:* We hear the heart beat by listening over the apex of the heart.
base	Bottom or lower part of an organ. *Example:* On the X-ray, a fracture was noted at the base of the skull.
superficial	More toward the surface of the body. *Example:* The cut was superficial.
deep	Further away from the surface of the body. *Example:* An incision into an abdominal organ is a deep incision.

(Continued)

Table 2.4	Terms for Describing Body Position (continued)
supine (soo-PINE)	The body lying horizontally and facing upward. *Example:* The patient is in the supine position for abdominal surgery. 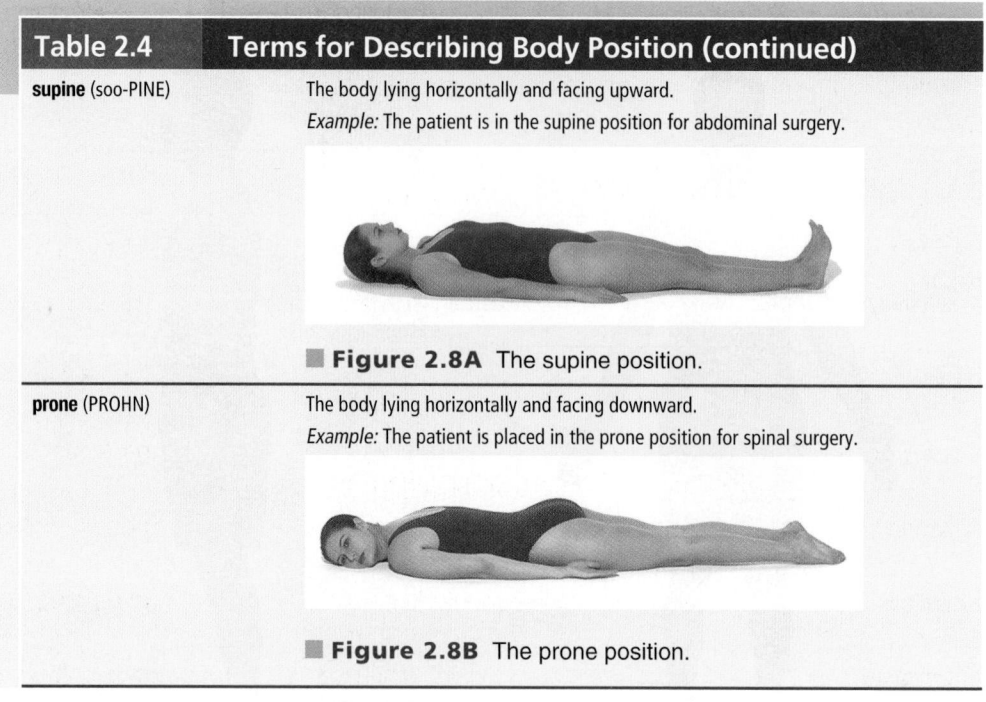 ■ **Figure 2.8A** The supine position.
prone (PROHN)	The body lying horizontally and facing downward. *Example:* The patient is placed in the prone position for spinal surgery. ■ **Figure 2.8B** The prone position.

MED TERM TIP

The prefixes and suffixes introduced in Chapter 1 will be used over and over again in your medical terminology course, making it easier to recognize new terms more quickly.

Terminology

The following lists contain the suffixes and prefixes used to build terms in the remaining section of this chapter. The combining forms were introduced on page 22 of this of this chapter.

Suffixes

-ac	pertaining to	-atic	pertaining to	-logy	study of
-al	pertaining to	-iac	pertaining to	-ose	resembling
-ar	pertaining to	-ic	pertaining to		
-ary	pertaining to	-ior	pertaining to		

Prefixes

endo-	within	**hypo-**	under	**retro-**	behind
epi-	above	**peri-**	around		

The terms below, introduced in this chapter, are built directly from word parts following the rules given in Chapter 1. Review these terms in order to begin to familiarize yourself with how medical terms are built.

Anatomical Terms

TERM	WORD PARTS	DEFINITION
abdominal	abdomin/o = abdomen -al = pertaining to	pertaining to the abdomen
adipose	adip/o = fat -ose = resembling	resembling fat
anterior	anter/o = front -ior = pertaining to	pertaining to the front
brachial	brachi/o = arm -al = pertaining to	pertaining to the arm
cardiac	cardi/o = heart -ac = pertaining to	pertaining to the heart
cardiology	cardi/o = heart -logy = study of	study of the heart
cardiovascular	cardi/o = heart vascul/o = blood vessel -ar = pertaining to	pertaining to the heart and blood vessel
caudal	caud/o = tail -al = pertaining to	pertaining to the tail
cephalic	cephal/o = head -ic = pertaining to	pertaining to the head
cervical	cervic/o = neck -al = pertaining to	pertaining to the neck
cranial	crani/o = skull -al = pertaining to	pertaining to the skull
crural	crur/o = leg -al = pertaining to	pertaining to the leg
cytology	cyt/o = cell -logy = study of	study of the cell
dermatology	dermat/o = skin -logy = study of	study of the skin
distal	dist/o = away from -al = pertaining to	pertaining to away from
dorsal	dors/o = back of body -al = pertaining to	pertaining to the back of body
endocrinology	endo- = within crin/o = to secrete -logy = study of	study of secreting within [endocrine system]
epigastric	epi- = above gastr/o = stomach -ic = pertaining to	pertaining to above the stomach
epithelial	epitheli/o = epithelium -al = pertaining to	pertaining to the epithelium

◼ Anatomical Terms *(continued)*

TERM	WORD PARTS	DEFINITION
gastroenterology	gastr/o = stomach enter/o = small intestine -logy = study of	study of the stomach and small intestine
gluteal	glute/o = buttock -al = pertaining to	pertaining to the buttocks
gynecology	gynec/o = woman -logy = study of	study of women
hematic	hemat/o = blood -ic = pertaining to	pertaining to the blood
hematology	hemat/o = blood -logy = study of	study of the blood
histology	hist/o = tissue -logy = study of	study of tissue
hypochondriac	hypo- = under chondr/o = cartilage -iac = pertaining to	pertaining to under the cartilage
hypogastric	hypo- = under gastr/o = stomach -ic = pertaining to	pertaining to under the stomach
immunology	immun/o = protection -logy = study of	study of protection [immune system]
inferior	infer/o = below -ior = pertaining to	pertaining to below
lateral	later/o = side -al = pertaining to	pertaining to the side
lumbar	lumb/o = loin -ar = pertaining to	pertaining to the loin [side and back between ribs and pelvic bones]
lymphatic	lymph/o = lymph -atic = pertaining to	pertaining to lymph
medial	medi/o = middle -al = pertaining to	pertaining to the middle
muscular	muscul/o = muscles -ar = pertaining to	pertaining to muscles
nephrology	nephr/o = kidney -logy = study of	study of the kidney
neurology	neur/o = nerve -logy = study of	study of nerves
ophthalmology	ophthalm/o = eye -logy = study of	study of the eye
otorhinolaryngology	ot/o = ear rhin/o = nose laryng/o = larynx -logy = study of	study of ear, nose, and larynx
pelvic	pelv/o = pelvis -ic = pertaining to	pertaining to the pelvis
peritoneal	peritone/o = peritoneum -al = pertaining to	pertaining to the peritoneum

Anatomical Terms *(continued)*

TERM	WORD PARTS	DEFINITION
pleural	pleur/o = pleura -al = pertaining to	pertaining to the pleura
posterior	poster/o = back -ior = pertaining to	pertaining to the back
proctology	proct/o = rectum and anus -logy = study of	study of the rectum and anus
proximal	proxim/o = near to -al = pertaining to	pertaining to near to
pubic	pub/o = genital region -ic = pertaining to	pertaining to the genital region
pulmonology	pulmon/o = lung -logy = study of	study of the lungs
spinal	spin/o = spine -al = pertaining to	pertaining to the spine
superior	super/o = above -ior = pertaining to	pertaining to above
thoracic	thorac/o = chest -ic = pertaining to	pertaining to the chest
urology	ur/o = urine -logy = study of	study of urine
ventral	ventr/o = belly -al = pertaining to	pertaining to the belly [side]
vertebral	vertebr/o = vertebra -al = pertaining to	pertaining to the vertebrae
visceral	viscer/o = internal organ -al = pertaining to	pertaining to internal organs

 ## Abbreviations

AP	anteroposterior	**LUQ**	left upper quadrant
CV	cardiovascular	**MS**	musculoskeletal
ENT	ear, nose, and throat	**OB**	obstetrics
GI	gastrointestinal	**PA**	posteroanterior
GYN	gynecology	**RLQ**	right lower quadrant
lat	lateral	**RUQ**	right upper quadrant
LE	lower extremity	**UE**	upper extremity
LLQ	left lower quadrant		

D. Terminology Matching

Match each term to its definition.

1. _____ distal

2. _____ prone

3. _____ lateral

4. _____ inferior

5. _____ deep

6. _____ apex

7. _____ base

8. _____ posterior

9. _____ superficial

10. _____ supine

11. _____ anterior

12. _____ medial

13. _____ proximal

14. _____ superior

a. away from the surface

b. toward the surface

c. located closer to point of attachment to the body

d. caudal

e. tip or summit of an organ

f. lying face down

g. cephalic

h. ventral

i. dorsal

j. lying face up

k. to the side

l. middle

m. bottom or lower part of an organ

n. located further away from point of attachment to the body

E. What's the Abbreviation?

1. musculoskeletal _____

2. lateral _____

3. right upper quadrant _____

4. cardiovascular _____

5. gastrointestinal _____

6. anteroposterior _____

7. obstetrics _____

8. left lower quadrant _____

H. Organ System and Function Challenge

For each organ listed below, identify the name of the system it belongs to and then match it to its function.

Organ   **System**

1. _____ skin   _____   a. supports the body

2. _____ heart   _____   b. provides place for growing baby

3. _____ stomach   _____   c. filters waste products from blood

4. _____ uterus   _____   d. provides two-way barrier

5. _____ bones   _____   e. produces movement

6. _____ lungs   _____   f. produces sperm

7. _____ kidney   _____   g. ingest, digest, absorb nutrients

8. _____ testes   _____   h. coordinates body's response

9. _____ brain   _____   i. pumps blood through blood vessels

10. _____ muscles   _____   j. obtains oxygen

I. Body Region Practice

For each term below, write the corresponding body region.

1. head _____

2. genitals _____

3. leg _____

4. buttocks _____

5. neck _____

6. arm _____

7. back _____

8. chest _____

J. Terminology Matching

Match each organ to its body cavity.

1. _____ gallbladder
2. _____ appendix
3. _____ urinary bladder
4. _____ small intestines
5. _____ right kidney
6. _____ left ovary
7. _____ stomach
8. _____ colon
9. _____ right ureter
10. _____ pancreas (majority)

a. right upper quadrant

b. left upper quadrant

c. right lower quadrant

d. left lower quadrant

e. all quadrants

f. midline structure

K. Fill in the Blank

cardiology	otorhinolaryngology	urology	gynecology
ophthalmology	gastroenterology	dermatology	orthopedics

1. John is a musician who plays an electric bass guitar and is experiencing difficulty in hearing soft voices. He would consult a physician in _____.

2. Ruth is a stock trader with the Chicago Board of Trade. She has had a pounding and racing heartbeat. She would consult a physician specializing in _____.

3. Mary Ann is experiencing excessive bleeding from the uterus. She would consult a _____ doctor.

4. José has fractured his wrist in a fall. He would be seen for an examination by a physician in _____.

5. A physician who performs eye exams specializes in the field of _____.

6. When her daughter had repeated bladder infections, Mrs. Cortez sought the opinion of a specialist in _____.

7. Martha could not get rid of a persistent skin rash with over-the-counter creams. She decided to make an appointment with a specialist in _____.

8. After reviewing his X-ray, the specialist in _____ informed Mr. Sparks that he had a stomach ulcer.

Labeling Exercise

Image A

1. Write the labels for this figure on the numbered lines provided.

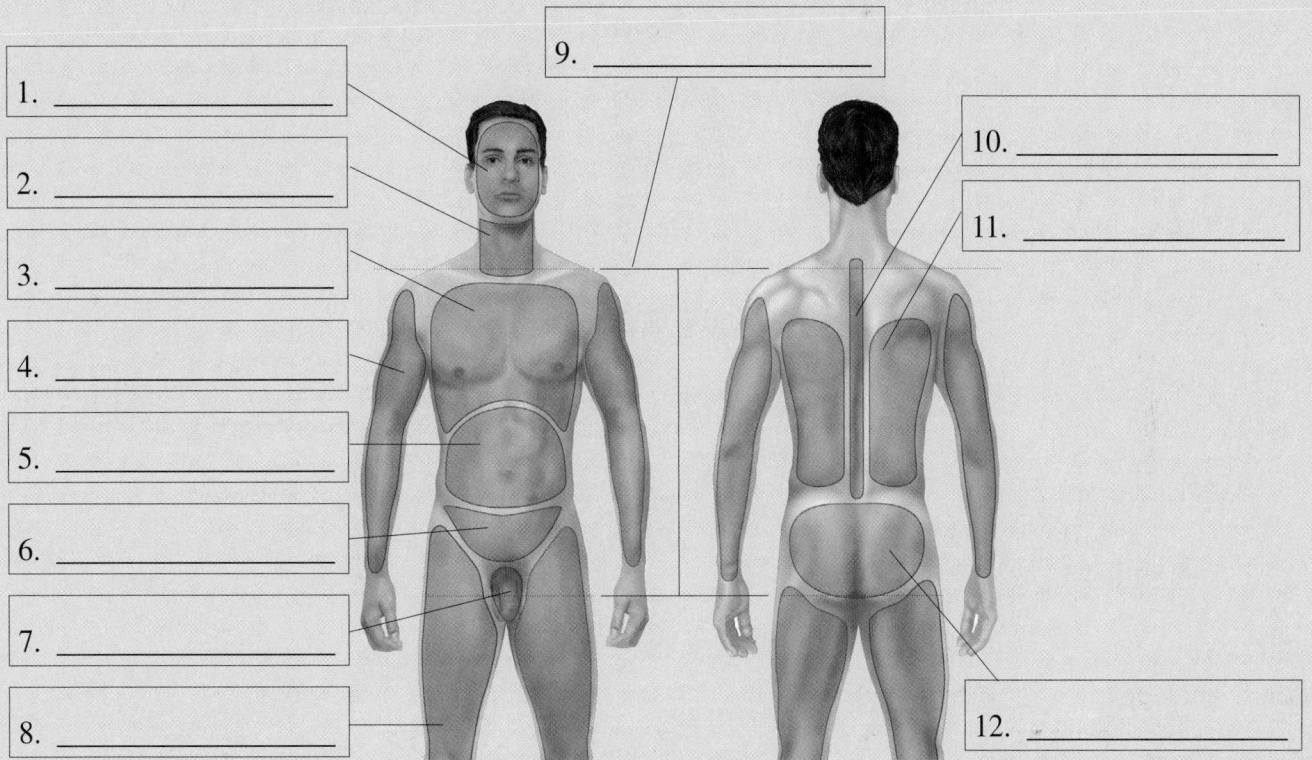

1. _____

2. _____

3. _____

4. _____

5. _____

6. _____

7. _____

8. _____

9. _____

10. _____

11. _____

12. _____

Image B

2. Write the labels for this figure on the numbered lines provided.

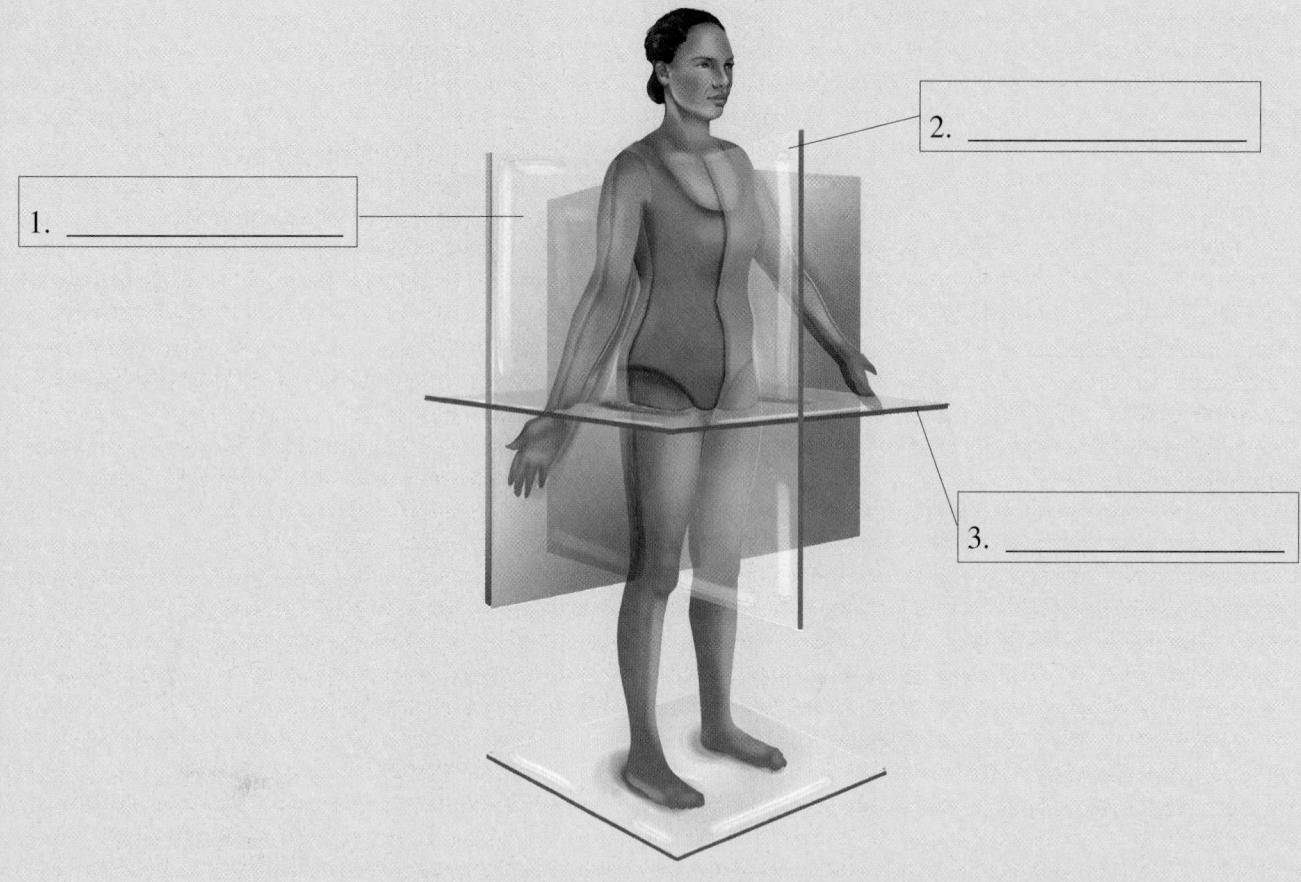

1. _____

2. _____

3. _____

MEDICAL TERMINOLOGY INTERACTIVE

Medical Terminology Interactive is a premium online homework management system that includes a host of features to help you study. Registered users will find:

- Fun games and activities built within a virtual hospital
- Powerful tools that track and analyze your results—allowing you to create a personalized learning experience
- Videos, flashcards, and audio pronunciations to help enrich your progress
- Streaming video lesson presentations and self-paced learning modules

www.pearsonhighered.com/mti

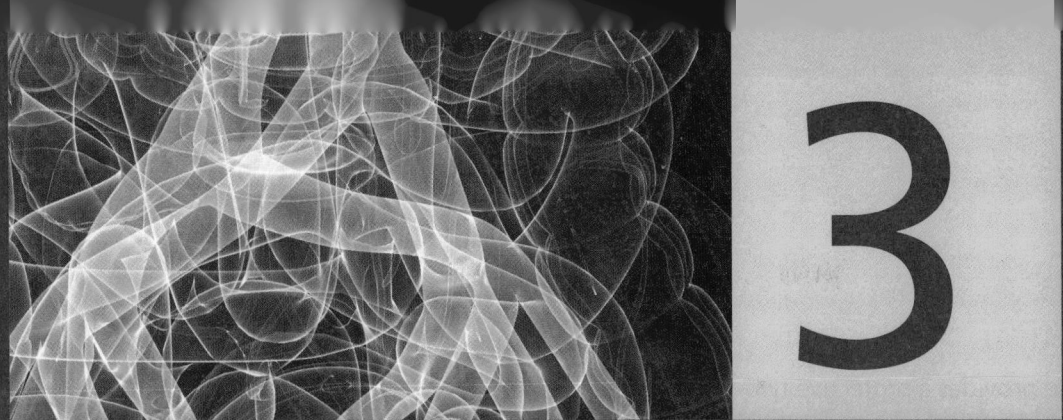

3

INTEGUMENTARY SYSTEM

Learning Objectives

Upon completion of this chapter, you will be able to

- Identify and define the combining forms, prefixes, and suffixes introduced in this chapter.
- Correctly spell and pronounce medical terms and major anatomical structures relating to the integumentary system.
- List and describe the three layers of skin and their functions.
- List and describe the four purposes of the skin.
- List and describe the accessory organs of the skin.
- Identify and define integumentary system anatomical terms.
- Identify and define selected integumentary system pathology terms.
- Identify and define selected integumentary system diagnostic procedures.
- Identify and define selected integumentary system therapeutic procedures.
- Identify and define selected medications relating to the integumentary system.
- Define selected abbreviations associated with the integumentary system.

Integumentary System at a Glance

Function

The skin provides a protective two-way barrier between our internal environment and the outside world. It also plays an important role in temperature regulation, houses sensory receptors to detect the environment around us, and secretes important fluids.

Organs

Here are the primary structures that comprise the integumentary system.

skin　　**hair**　　**nails**　　**sebaceous glands**　　**sweat glands**

Word Parts

Here are the most common word parts (with their meanings) used to build integumentary system terms. For a more comprehensive list, refer to the Terminology section of this chapter.

Combining Forms

albin/o	white	melan/o	black
bi/o	life	myc/o	fungus
cry/o	cold	necr/o	death
cutane/o	skin	onych/o	nail
cyan/o	blue	pedicul/o	lice
derm/o	skin	phot/o	light
dermat/o	skin	py/o	pus
diaphor/o	profuse sweating	rhytid/o	wrinkle
electr/o	electricity	scler/o	hard
erythr/o	red	seb/o	oil
hidr/o	sweat	trich/o	hair
ichthy/o	scaly, dry	ungu/o	nail
kerat/o	hard, horny	vesic/o	bladder
leuk/o	white	xer/o	dry
lip/o	fat		

Suffixes

-derma	skin condition
-opsy	view of
-tome	instrument used to cut

Prefixes

allo-	other, different from usual
xeno-	strange, foreign

Integumentary System Illustrated

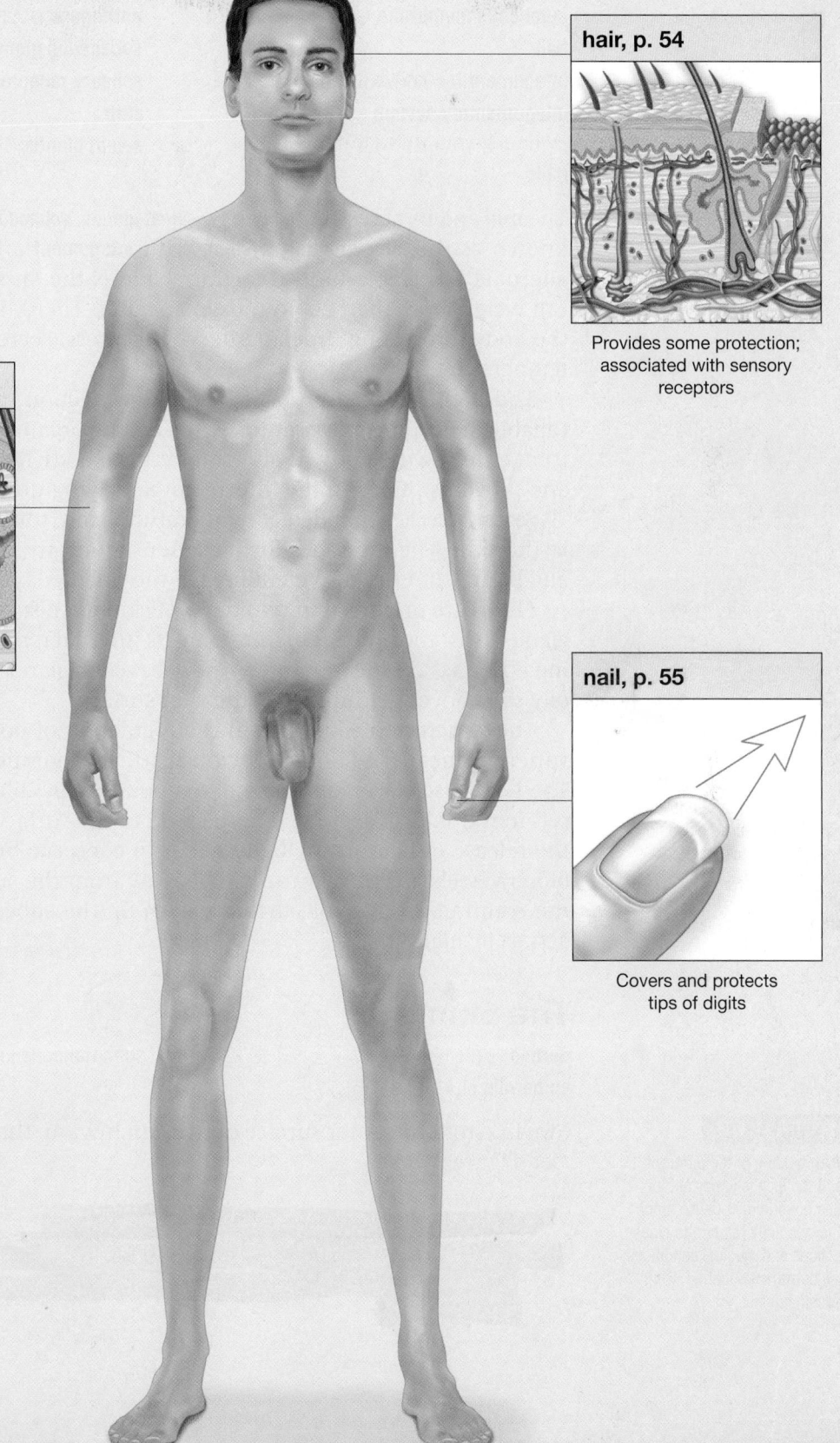

hair, p. 54

Provides some protection; associated with sensory receptors

skin, p. 52

Protective barrier, houses sensory receptors, secretes sweat and sebum, temperature regulation

nail, p. 55

Covers and protects tips of digits

■ Anatomy and Physiology of the Integumentary System

cutaneous membrane (kew-TAY-nee-us)	**pathogens** (PATH-oh-jenz)
hair	**sebaceous glands** (see-BAY-shus)
integument (in-TEG-you-mint)	**sensory receptors**
integumentary system	**skin**
(in-teg-you-MEN-tah-ree)	**sweat glands**
nails	

The **skin** and its accessory organs—**sweat glands, sebaceous glands, hair,** and **nails**—are known as the **integumentary system,** with **integument** and **cutaneous membrane** being alternate terms for skin. In fact, the skin is the largest organ of the body and can weigh more than 20 pounds in an adult. The skin serves many purposes for the body: protecting, housing nerve receptors, secreting fluids, and regulating temperature.

The primary function of the skin is protection. It forms a two-way barrier capable of keeping **pathogens** (disease-causing organisms) and harmful chemicals from entering the body. It also stops critical body fluids from escaping the body and prevents injury to the internal organs lying underneath the skin.

Sensory receptors that detect temperature, pain, touch, and pressure are located in the skin. The messages for these sensations are conveyed to the spinal cord and brain from the nerve endings in the middle layer of the skin.

Fluids are produced in two types of skin glands: sweat and sebaceous. Sweat glands assist the body in maintaining its internal temperature by creating a cooling effect as sweat evaporates. The sebaceous glands, or oil glands, produce an oily substance that lubricates the skin surface.

The structure of skin aids in the regulation of body temperature through a variety of means. As noted previously, the evaporation of sweat cools the body. The body also lowers its internal temperature by dilating superficial blood vessels in the skin. This brings more blood to the surface of the skin, which allows the release of heat. If the body needs to conserve heat, it constricts superficial blood vessels, keeping warm blood away from the surface of the body. Finally, the continuous layer of fat that makes up the subcutaneous layer of the skin acts as insulation.

> **MED TERM TIP**
>
> Flushing of the skin, a normal response to an increase in environmental temperature or to a fever, is caused by an increased blood flow to the skin of the face and neck. However, in some people, it is also a response to embarrassment called blushing and is not easily controlled.

The Skin

dermis (DER-mis)	**subcutaneous layer**
epidermis (ep-ih-DER-mis)	(sub-kyoo-TAY-nee-us)

Moving from the outer surface of the skin inward, the three layers are as follows (see Figure 3.1 ■):

1. **Epidermis** is the thin, outer membrane layer.
2. **Dermis** is the middle, fibrous connective tissue layer.
3. The **subcutaneous layer** (Subcu, Subq) is the innermost layer, containing fatty tissue.

> **MED TERM TIP**
>
> An understanding of the different layers of the skin is important for healthcare workers because much of the terminology relating to types of injections and medical conditions, such as burns, is described using these designations.

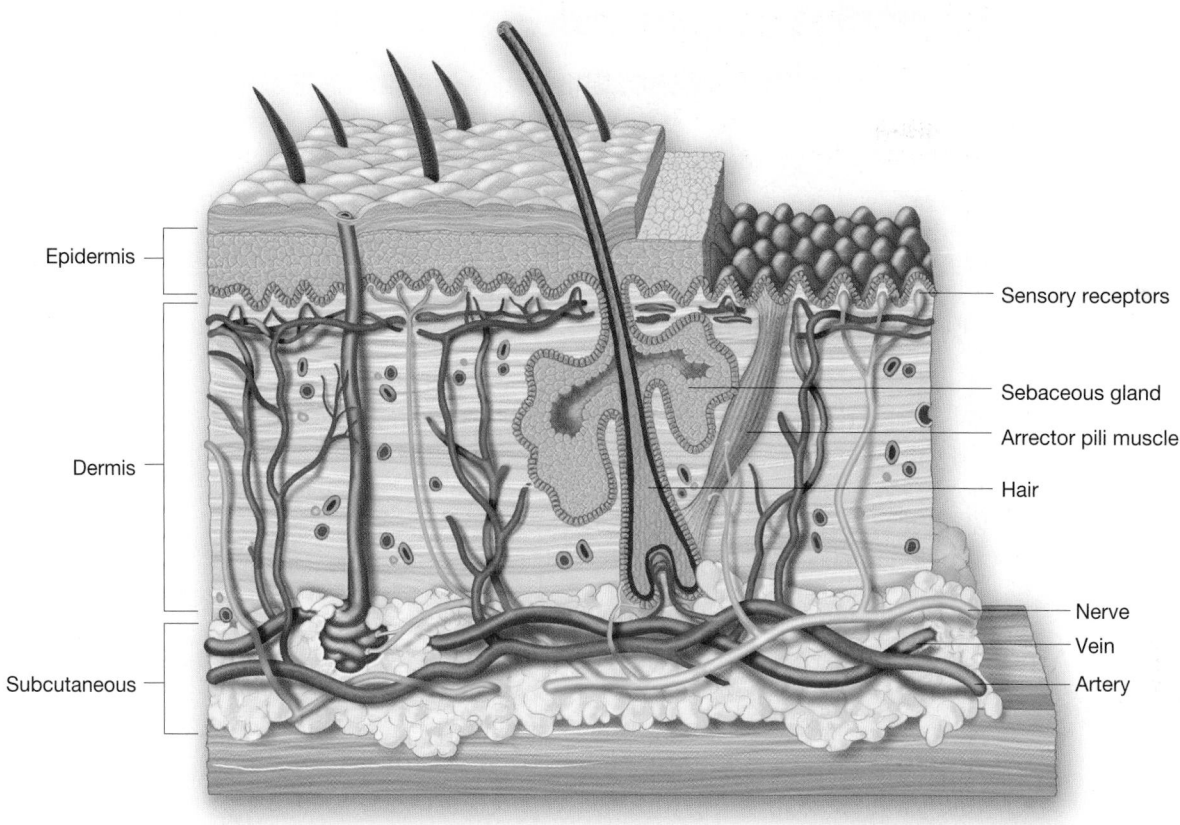

■ **Figure 3.1** Skin structure, including the three layers of the skin and the accessory organs: sweat gland, sebaceous gland, and hair.

Epidermis

basal layer (BAY-sal)
keratin (KAIR-ah-tin)
melanin (MEL-ah-nin)

melanocytes (mel-AN-oh-sights)
stratified squamous epithelium (STRAT-ih-fyde
  / SKWAY-mus / ep-ih-THEE-lee-um)

The epidermis is composed of **stratified squamous epithelium** (see Figure 3.2 ■). This type of epithelial tissue consists of flat scale-like cells arranged in overlapping layers or strata. The epidermis does not have a blood supply or any connective tissue, so it is dependent for nourishment on the deeper layers of skin.

The deepest layer within the epidermis is called the **basal layer.** Cells in this layer continually grow and multiply. New cells that are forming push the old cells toward the outer layer of the epidermis. During this process the cells shrink, die, and become filled with a hard protein called **keratin.** These dead, overlapping, keratinized cells allow the skin to act as an effective barrier to infection and also make it waterproof.

The basal layer also contains special cells called **melanocytes,** which produce the black pigment **melanin.** Not only is this pigment responsible for the color of the skin, but it also protects against damage from the ultraviolet rays of the sun. This damage may be in the form of leatherlike skin and wrinkles, which are not hazardous, or it may be one of several forms of skin cancer. Dark-skinned people have more melanin and are generally less likely to get wrinkles or skin cancer.

MED TERM TIP

We lose 30,000-50,000 old, dead skin cells per minute and replace them with new, younger cells. In fact, because of this process, the epidermis is completely replaced every 25 days.

MED TERM TIP

A suntan can be thought of as a protective response to the rays of the sun. However, when the melanin in the skin is not able to absorb all the rays of the sun, the skin burns and DNA may be permanently and dangerously damaged.

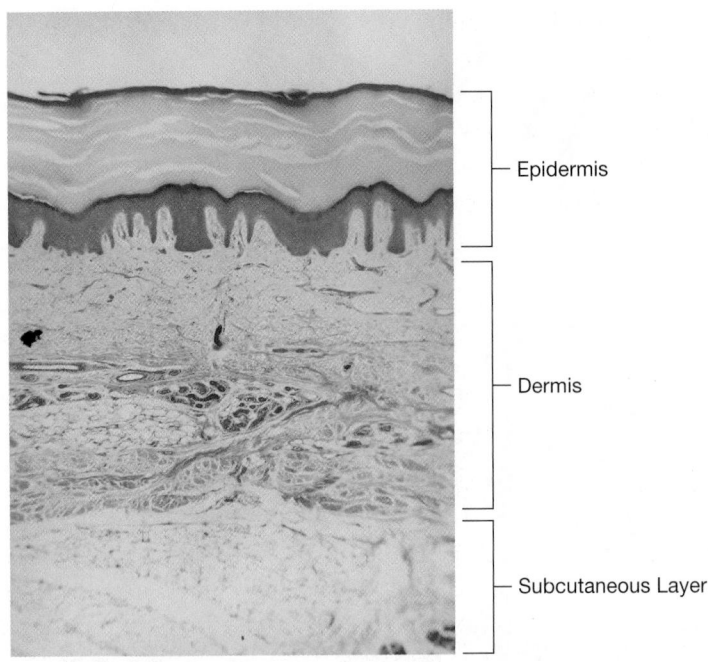

- Epidermis
- Dermis
- Subcutaneous Layer

Dermis

collagen fibers (KOL-ah-jen)   **corium** (KOH-ree-um)

The dermis, also referred to as the **corium,** is the middle layer of skin, located between the epidermis and the subcutaneous layer (see Figure 3.2). Its name means "true skin." Unlike the thinner epidermis, the dermis is living tissue with a very good blood supply. The dermis itself is composed of connective tissue and **collagen fibers.** Collagen fibers are made from a strong, fibrous protein present in connective tissue, forming a flexible "glue" that gives connective tissue its strength. The dermis houses hair follicles, sweat glands, sebaceous glands, blood vessels, lymph vessels, sensory receptors, nerve fibers, and muscle fibers.

Subcutaneous Layer

hypodermis (high-poh-DER-mis)   **lipocytes** (LIP-oh-sights)

The third and deepest layer of the skin is the subcutaneous layer, also called the **hypodermis.** This layer of tissue, composed of fat cells called **lipocytes,** protects the deeper tissues of the body and acts as insulation for heat and cold. (see Figure 3.2)

Accessory Organs

The accessory organs of the skin are the anatomical structures located within the dermis, including the hair, nails, sebaceous glands, and sweat glands.

Hair

arrector pili (ah-REK-tor / pee-lie)   **hair root**
hair follicle (FALL-ikl)   **hair shaft**

The fibers that make up hair are composed of the protein keratin, the same hard protein material that fills the cells of the epidermis. The process of hair formation

is much like the process of growth in the epidermal layer of the skin. The deeper cells in the **hair root** force older keratinized cells to move upward, forming the **hair shaft.** The hair shaft grows toward the skin surface within the **hair follicle.** Melanin gives hair its color. Sebaceous glands release oil directly into the hair follicle. Each hair has a small slip of smooth muscle attached to it called the **arrector pili muscle** (see Figure 3.3 ■). When this muscle contracts the hair shaft stands up and results in "goose bumps."

Nails

cuticle (KEW-tikl)	**nail bed**
free edge	**nail body**
lunula (LOO-nyoo-lah)	**nail root**

Nails are a flat plate of keratin called the **nail body** that covers the ends of fingers and toes. The nail body is connected to the tissue underneath by the **nail bed.** Nails grow longer from the **nail root,** which is found at the base of the nail and is covered and protected by the soft tissue **cuticle.** The **free edge** is the exposed edge that is trimmed when nails become too long. The light-colored half-moon area at the base of the nail is the **lunula** (see Figure 3.4 ■).

Sebaceous Glands

sebum

Sebaceous glands, found in the dermis, secrete the oil **sebum,** which lubricates the hair and skin, thereby helping to prevent drying and cracking. These glands secrete sebum directly into hair follicles, rather than a duct (see Figure 3.1). Secretion from the sebaceous glands increases during adolescence, playing a role in the development of acne. Sebum secretion begins to diminish as age increases. A loss of sebum in old age, along with sun exposure, can account for wrinkles and dry skin.

> **MED TERM TIP**
>
> Because of its rich blood supply and light color, the nail bed is an excellent place to check patients for low oxygen levels in their blood. Deoxygenated blood is a very dark purple-red and gives skin a bluish tinge called *cyanosis.*

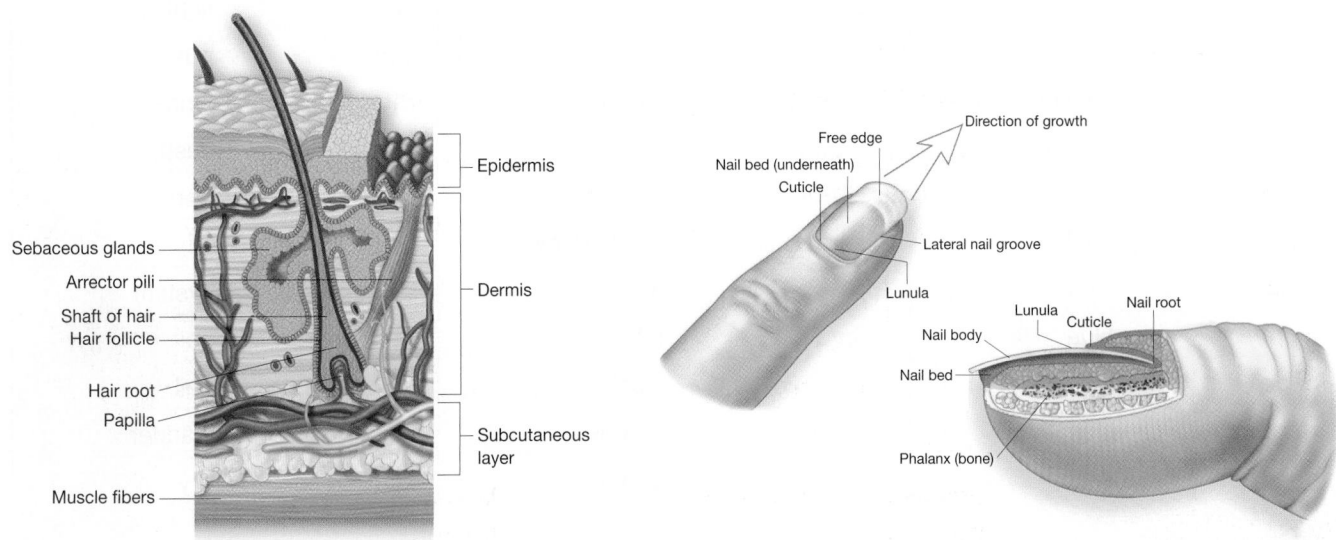

■ **Figure 3.3** Structure of a hair and its associated sebaceous gland.

■ **Figure 3.4** External and internal structures of nails.

Sweat Glands

apocrine glands (APP-oh-krin)	**sweat duct**
perspiration	**sweat pore**
sudoriferous glands (sue-doh-RIF-er-us)	

About 2 million sweat glands, also called **sudoriferous glands,** are found throughout the body. These highly coiled glands are located in the dermis. Sweat travels to the surface of the skin in a **sweat duct.** The surface opening of a sweat duct is called a **sweat pore** (see Figure 3.1).

Sweat glands function to cool the body as sweat evaporates. Sweat or **perspiration** contains a small amount of waste product but is normally colorless and odorless. However, there are sweat glands called **apocrine glands** in the pubic and underarm areas that secrete a thicker sweat, which can produce an odor when it comes into contact with bacteria on the skin. This is what we recognize as body odor.

> **MED TERM TIP**
>
> Word Watch: Be careful when using *hydro-* meaning "water" and *hidr/o* meaning "sweat."

Terminology

Word Parts Used to Build Integumentary System Terms

The following lists contain the combining forms, suffixes, and prefixes used to build terms in the remaining sections of this chapter.

Combining Forms

albin/o	white	**diaphor/o**	profuse sweating	**onych/o**	nail
angi/o	vessel	**electr/o**	electricity	**pedicul/o**	lice
bas/o	the base	**erythr/o**	red	**phot/o**	light
bi/o	life	**esthesi/o**	feeling	**py/o**	pus
carcin/o	cancer	**hem/o**	blood	**rhytid/o**	wrinkle
chem/o	chemical	**hidr/o**	sweat	**sarc/o**	flesh
cis/o	to cut	**ichthy/o**	scaly, dry	**scler/o**	hard
cry/o	cold	**kerat/o**	hard, horny	**seb/o**	oil
cutane/o	skin	**leuk/o**	white	**system/o**	system
cyan/o	blue	**lip/o**	fat	**trich/o**	hair
cyt/o	cell	**melan/o**	black	**ungu/o**	nail
derm/o	skin	**myc/o**	fungus	**vesic/o**	bladder
dermat/o	skin	**necr/o**	death	**xer/o**	dry

Suffixes

-al	pertaining to	-itis	inflammation	-ous	pertaining to
-derma	skin condition	-logy	study of	-phagia	eating
-ectomy	surgical removal	-malacia	softening	-plasty	surgical repair
-emia	blood condition	-oma	mass	-rrhea	discharge
-ia	state, condition	-opsy	to view	-tic	pertaining to
-ic	pertaining to	-osis	abnormal condition	-tome	instrument to cut
-ism	state of			-ule	small

Prefixes

allo-	other	de-	without	intra-	within
an-	without	epi-	upon	para-	beside
anti-	against	hyper-	excessive	sub-	under
auto-	self	hypo-	under	xeno-	strange, foreign

Anatomical Terms

TERM	WORD PARTS	DEFINITION
cutaneous (kyoo-TAY-nee-us)	cutane/o = skin -ous = pertaining to	pertaining to the skin
dermal (DER-mal)	derm/o = skin -al = pertaining to	pertaining to the skin
epidermal (ep-ih-DER-mal)	epi- = upon derm/o = skin -al = pertaining to	pertaining to upon the skin
hypodermic (high-poh-DER-mik)	hypo- = under derm/o = skin -ic = pertaining to	pertaining to under the skin
intradermal (in-trah-DER-mal)	intra- = within derm/o = skin -al = pertaining to	pertaining to within the skin
subcutaneous (sub-kyoo-TAY-nee-us)	sub- = under cutane/o = skin -ous = pertaining to	pertaining to under the skin
ungual (UNG-gwal)	ungu/o = nail -al = pertaining to	pertaining to the nails

Pathology

TERM	WORD PARTS	DEFINITION
Medical Specialties		
dermatology (Derm, derm) (der-mah-TALL-oh-jee)	dermat/o = skin -logy = study of	Branch of medicine involving diagnosis and treatment of conditions and diseases of the integumentary system. Physician is a *dermatologist.*
plastic surgery		Surgical specialty involved in repair, reconstruction, or improvement of body structures such as the skin that are damaged, missing, or misshapen. Physician is a *plastic surgeon.*
Signs and Symptoms		
abrasion (ah-BRAY-zhun)		A scraping away of the skin surface by friction.
anhidrosis (an-hi-DROH-sis)	an- = without hidr/o = sweat -osis = abnormal condition	Abnormal condition of no sweat.
comedo (KOM-ee-do)		Collection of hardened sebum in hair follicle. Also called a *blackhead.*
contusion		Injury caused by a blow to the body; causes swelling, pain, and bruising. The skin is not broken.
cyanosis (sigh-ah-NOH-sis)	cyan/o = blue -osis = abnormal condition	Bluish tint to the skin caused by deoxygenated blood.

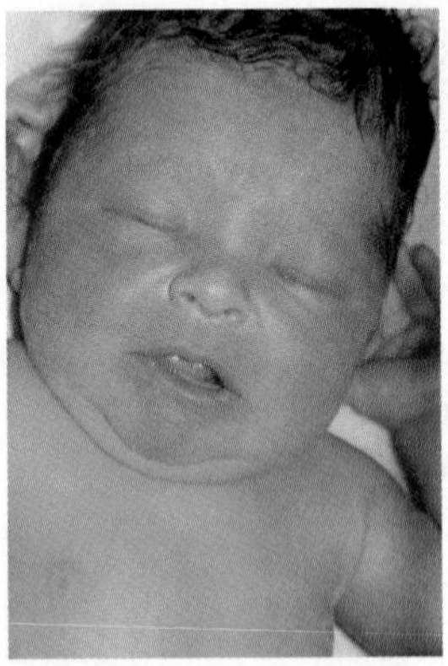

■ **Figure 3.5** A cyanotic infant. Note the bluish tinge to the skin around the lips, chin, and nose. *(St. Bartholomew's Hospital, London/Photo Researchers, Inc.)*

cyst (SIST)		Fluid-filled sac under the skin.

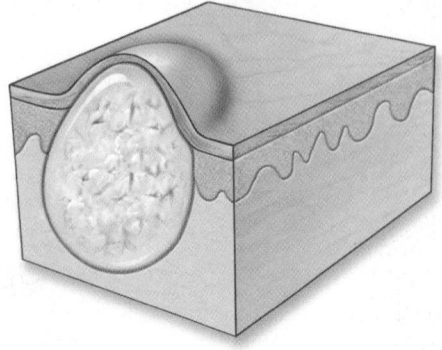

■ **Figure 3.6** Cyst.

■ Pathology *(continued)*

TERM	WORD PARTS	DEFINITION
depigmentation (dee-pig-men-TAY-shun)	de- = without	Loss of normal skin color or pigment.
diaphoresis (dye-ah-for-REE-sis)	diaphor/o = profuse sweating	Profuse sweating.
ecchymosis (ek-ih-MOH-sis)	-osis = abnormal condition	Skin discoloration caused by blood collecting under the skin following blunt trauma to the skin. A bruise.

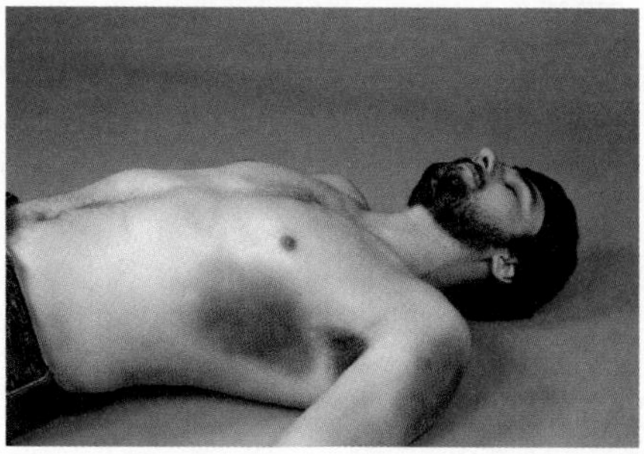

■ **Figure 3.7** Male lying supine with large ecchymosis on lateral rib cage and shoulder.

TERM	WORD PARTS	DEFINITION
erythema (er-ih-THEE-mah)	erythr/o = red hem/o = blood	Redness or flushing of the skin.
erythroderma (eh-rith-roh-DER-mah)	erythr/o = red -derma = skin condition	The condition of having reddened or flushed skin.
eschar (ESH-shar)		A thick layer of dead tissue and tissue fluid that develops over a deep burn area.
fissure (FISH-er)		Crack-like lesion or groove on the skin.

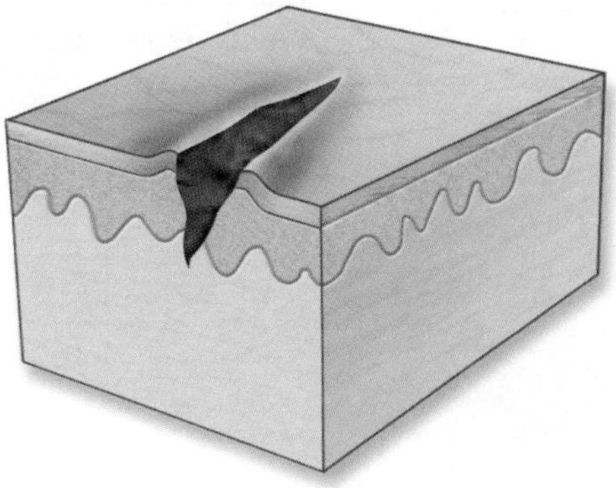

■ **Figure 3.8** Fissure.

TERM	WORD PARTS	DEFINITION
hirsutism (HER-soot-izm)		Excessive hair growth over the body.
hyperemia (high-per-EE-mee-ah)	hyper- = excessive -emia = blood condition	Redness of the skin due to increased blood flow.
hyperhidrosis (high-per-hi-DROH-sis)	hyper- = excessive hidr/o = sweat -osis = abnormal condition	Abnormal condition of excessive sweat.
hyperpigmentation (high-per-pig-men-TAY-shun)	hyper- = excessive	Abnormal amount of pigmentation in the skin.
ichthyoderma (ick-thee-oh-DER-mah)	ichthy/o = scaly, dry -derma = skin condition	The condition of having scaly and dry skin.

Pathology *(continued)*

TERM	WORD PARTS	DEFINITION
lesion (LEE-shun)		A general term for a wound, injury, or abnormality.
leukoderma (loo-koh-DER-mah)	leuk/o = white -derma = skin condition	Having skin that appears white because the normal skin pigment is absent. May be all the skin or just in some areas.
lipoma (lip-OH-mah)	lip/o = fat -oma = mass	Fatty mass.
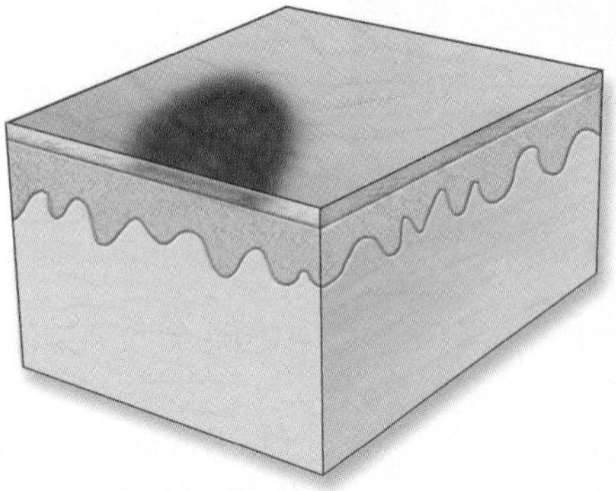 **macule** (MACK-yool)	-ule = small	Flat, discolored area that is flush with the skin surface. An example would be a freckle or a birthmark.

■ **Figure 3.9** Macule.

TERM	WORD PARTS	DEFINITION
necrosis (neh-KROH-sis)	necr/o = death -osis = abnormal condition	Abnormal condition of death.
nevus (NEV-us)		Pigmented skin blemish, birthmark, or mole. Usually benign but may become cancerous.
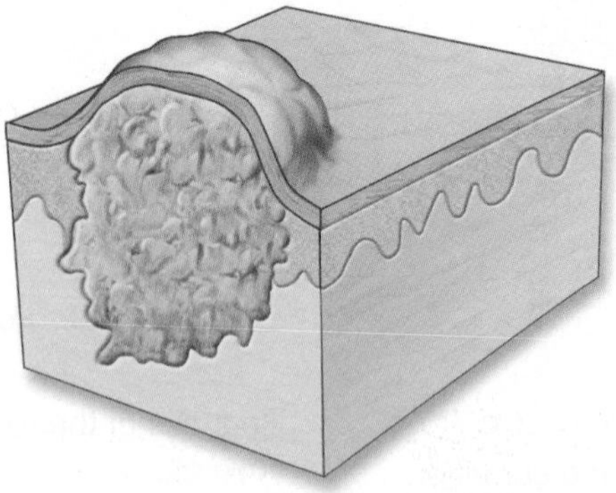 **nodule** (NOD-yool)	-ule = small	Firm, solid mass of cells in the skin larger than 0.5 cm in diameter.

■ **Figure 3.10** Nodule.

TERM	WORD PARTS	DEFINITION
onychomalacia (on-ih-koh-mah-LAY-she-ah)	onych/o = nail -malacia = softening	Softening of the nails.
pallor (PAL-or)		Abnormal paleness of the skin.

Pathology *(continued)*

TERM	WORD PARTS	DEFINITION
papule (PAP-yool)	-ule = small	Small, solid, circular raised spot on the surface of the skin less than 0.5 cm in diameter.

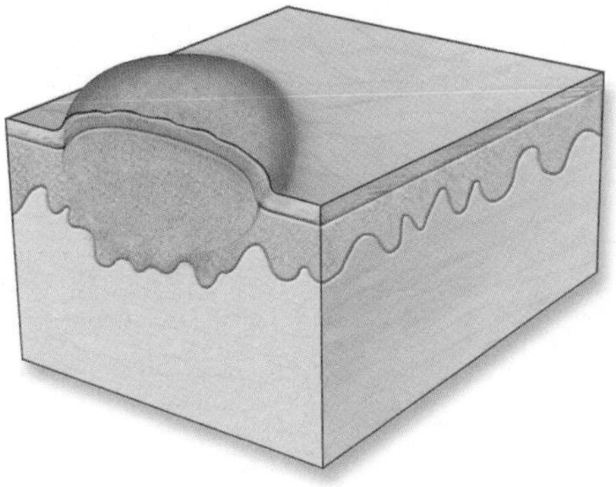

Figure 3.11 Papule.

| **petechiae**
(peh-TEE-kee-eye) | | Pinpoint purple or red spots from minute hemorrhages under the skin. |

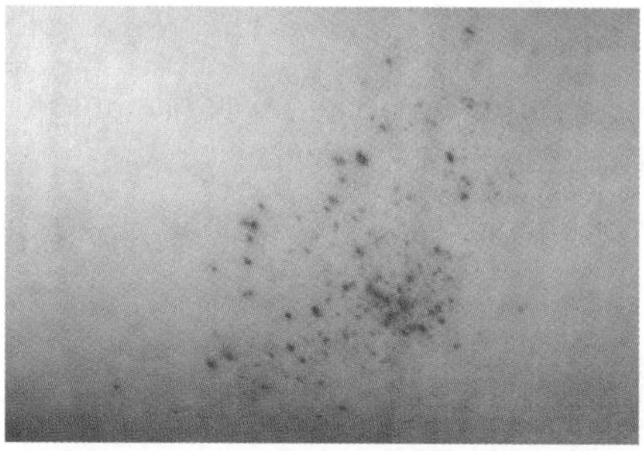

Figure 3.12 Petechiae, pinpoint skin hemorrhages. *(Custom Medical Stock)*

photosensitivity (foh-toh-sen-sih-TIH-vih-tee)	phot/o = light	Condition in which the skin reacts abnormally when exposed to light, such as the ultraviolet (UV) rays of the sun.
pruritus (proo-RIGH-tus)		Severe itching.
purpura (PER-pew-rah)		Hemorrhages into the skin due to fragile blood vessels. Commonly seen in older adults.

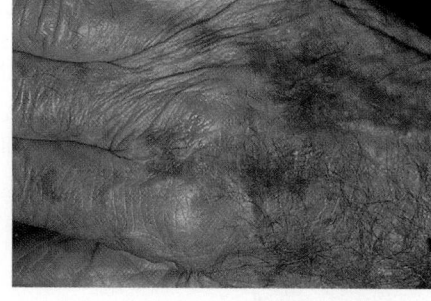

Figure 3.13 Purpura, hemorrhaging into the skin due to fragile blood vessels. *(Caroll H. Weiss/Camera M.D. Studios)*

MED TERM TIP

Purpura comes from the Latin word for "purple," which refers to the color of these pinpoint hemorrhages.

| **purulent**
(PYUR-yoo-lent) | | Containing pus or an infection that is producing pus. Pus consists of dead bacteria, white blood cells, and tissue debris. |

◼ **Pathology** *(continued)*

TERM	WORD PARTS	DEFINITION
pustule (PUS-tyool)	-ule = small	Raised spot on the skin containing pus.

◼ **Figure 3.14** Pustule.

TERM	WORD PARTS	DEFINITION
pyoderma (pye-oh-DER-mah)	py/o = pus -derma = skin condition	The presence of pus on or in the layers of skin. A sign of a bacterial infection.
scleroderma (sklair-ah-DER-mah)	scler/o = hard -derma = skin condition	A condition in which the skin has lost its elasticity and become hardened.
seborrhea (seb-or-EE-ah)	seb/o = oil -rrhea = discharge	Oily discharge.
suppurative (SUP-pure-a-tiv)		Containing or producing pus.
ulcer (ULL-ser)		Open sore or lesion in skin or mucous membrane.

◼ **Figure 3.15** Ulcer.

TERM	WORD PARTS	DEFINITION
urticaria (er-tih-KAY-ree-ah)		Also called *hives;* a skin eruption of pale reddish wheals with severe itching. Usually associated with food allergy, stress, or drug reactions.
vesicle (VESS-ikl)	vesic/o = bladder	A blister; small, fluid-filled raised spot on the skin.

◼ **Figure 3.16** Vesicle.

Pathology *(continued)*

TERM	WORD PARTS	DEFINITION
wheal (WEEL)		Small, round, swollen area on the skin; typically seen in allergic skin reactions such as *hives* and usually accompanied by urticaria.

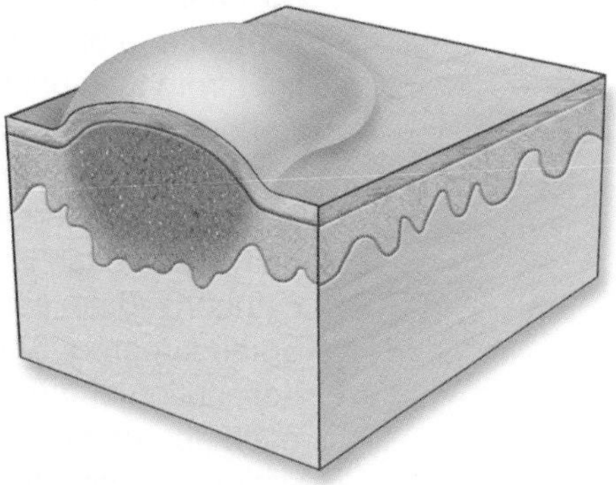

Figure 3.17 Wheal.

TERM	WORD PARTS	DEFINITION
xeroderma (zee-roh-DER-mah)	xer/o = dry -derma = skin condition	Condition in which the skin is abnormally dry.

Skin

TERM	WORD PARTS	DEFINITION
abscess (AB-sess)		A collection of pus in the skin.
acne (ACK-nee)		Inflammatory disease of the sebaceous glands and hair follicles resulting in papules and pustules.
acne rosacea (ACK-nee roh-ZAY-she-ah)		Chronic form of acne seen in adults involving redness, tiny pimples, and broken blood vessels, primarily on the nose and cheeks.
acne vulgaris (ACK-nee vul-GAY-ris)		Common form of acne seen in teenagers. Characterized by comedo, papules, and pustules.
albinism (al-BIH-nizm)	albin/o = white -ism = state of	A genetic condition in which the body is unable to make melanin. Characterized by white hair and skin and red pupils due to the lack of pigment. The person with albinism is called an *albino*.
basal cell carcinoma (BCC) (BAY-sal / sell / kar-sin-NOH-ma)	bas/o = the base -al = pertaining to carcin/o = cancer -oma = tumor	Cancerous tumor of the basal cell layer of the epidermis. A frequent type of skin cancer that rarely metastasizes or spreads. These cancers can arise on sun-exposed skin.

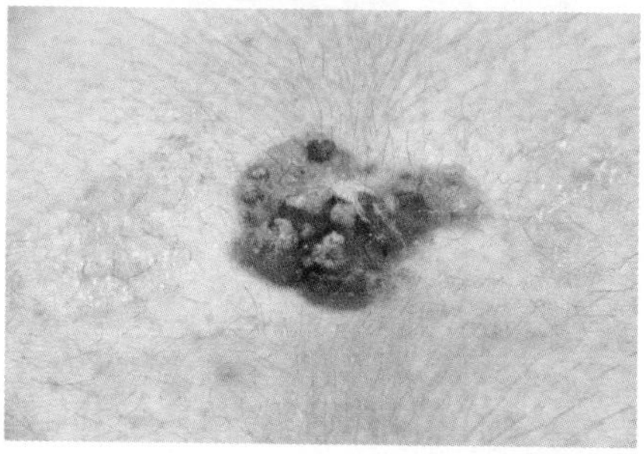

Figure 3.18 Basal cell carcinoma, a frequent type of skin cancer that rarely metastasizes. *(Bob Craig/CDC)*

▪ Pathology *(continued)*

TERM	WORD PARTS	DEFINITION
burn		Damage to the skin that can result from exposure to open fire, electricity, ultraviolet light from the sun, or caustic chemicals. Seriousness depends on the amount of body surface involved and the depth of the burn as determined by the amount of damage to each layer. Skin and burns are categorized as first degree, second degree, or third degree. See Figure 3.19 ▪ for a description of the damage associated with each degree of burn. Extent of a burn is estimated using the Rule of Nines (see Figure 3.20 ▪).

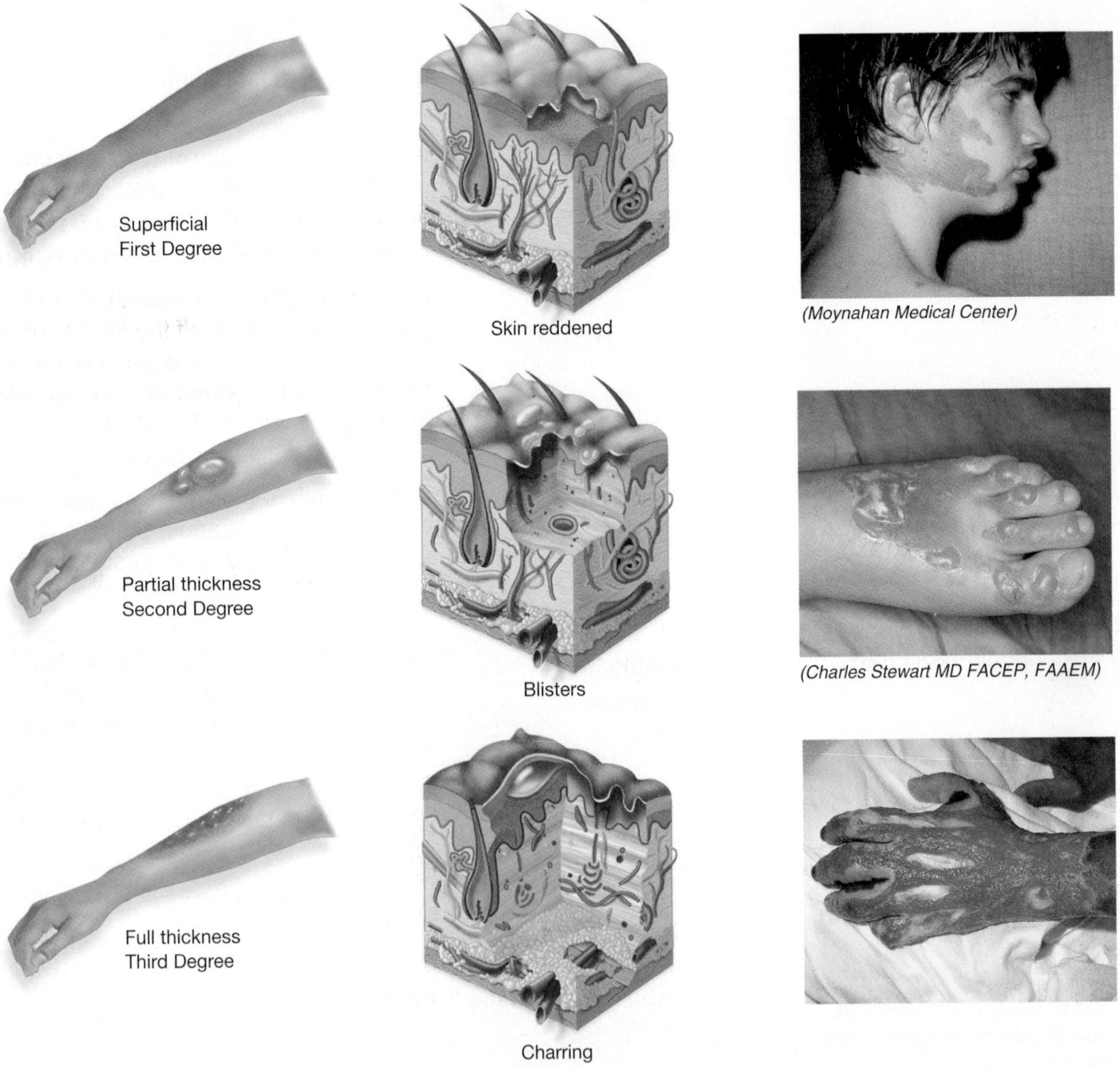

Superficial
First Degree

Skin reddened

(Moynahan Medical Center)

Partial thickness
Second Degree

Blisters

(Charles Stewart MD FACEP, FAAEM)

Full thickness
Third Degree

Charring

▪ **Figure 3.19** Comparison of the level of skin damage as a result of the three different degrees of burns.

▣ **Pathology** *(continued)*

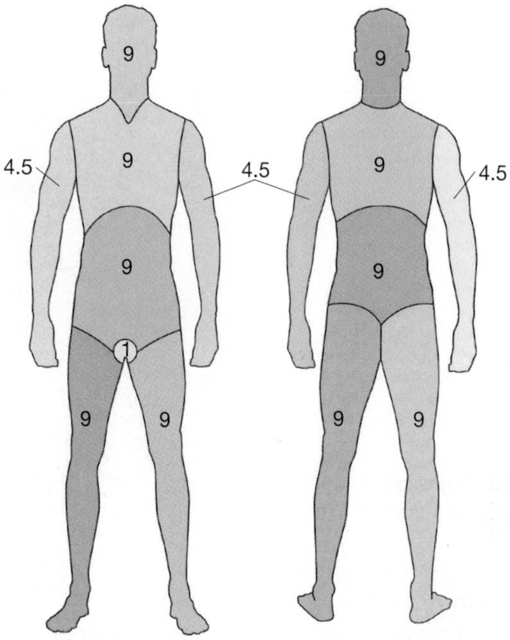

TERM	WORD PARTS	DEFINITION

■ **Figure 3.20** Rule of Nines. A method for determining percentage of body burned. Each different-colored section represents a percentage of the body surface. All sections added together will equal 100%.

TERM	WORD PARTS	DEFINITION
cellulitis (sell-you-LYE-tis)	-itis = inflammation	A diffuse, acute infection and inflammation of the connective tissue found in the skin.
decubitus ulcer (decub) (dee-KYOO-bih-tus)	**MED TERM TIP** *Decubitus* comes from the Latin word *decumbo,* meaning "lying down," which leads to the use of the term for a bedsore or pressure sore.	Open sore caused by pressure over bony prominences cutting off the blood flow to the overlying skin. These can appear in bedridden patients who lie in one position too long and can be difficult to heal. Also called *bedsore* or *pressure sore*.
dermatitis (der-mah-TYE-tis)	dermat/o = skin -itis = inflammation	Inflammation of the skin.
dermatosis (der-mah-TOH-sis)	dermat/o = skin -osis = abnormal condition	A general term indicating the presence of an abnormal skin condition.
dry gangrene (GANG-green)		Late stages of gangrene characterized by the affected area becoming dried, blackened, and shriveled; referred to as *mummified*.
eczema (EK-zeh-mah)		Superficial dermatitis of unknown cause accompanied by redness, vesicles, itching, and crusting.
gangrene (GANG-green)		Tissue necrosis usually due to deficient blood supply.
ichthyosis (ick-thee-OH-sis)	ichthy/o = scaly, dry -osis = abnormal condition	Condition in which the skin becomes dry, scaly, and keratinized.

Pathology *(continued)*

TERM	WORD PARTS	DEFINITION
impetigo (im-peh-TYE-goh)		A highly infectious bacterial infection of the skin with pustules that rupture and become crusted over.

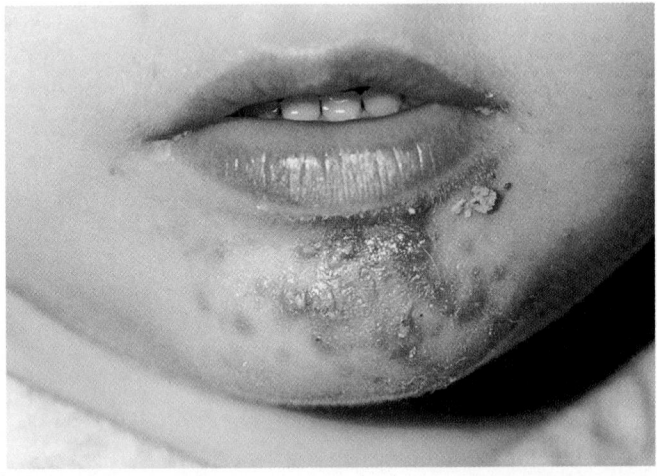

■ **Figure 3.21** Impetigo, a highly contagious bacterial infection. *(Dr. Jason L. Smith)*

TERM	WORD PARTS	DEFINITION
Kaposi's sarcoma (KAP-oh-seez / sar-KOH-mah)	sarc/o = flesh -oma = tumor	Form of skin cancer frequently seen in acquired immunodeficiency syndrome (AIDS) patients. Consists of brownish-purple papules that spread from the skin and metastasize to internal organs.
keloid (KEE-loyd)		Formation of a raised and thickened hypertrophic scar after an injury or surgery.

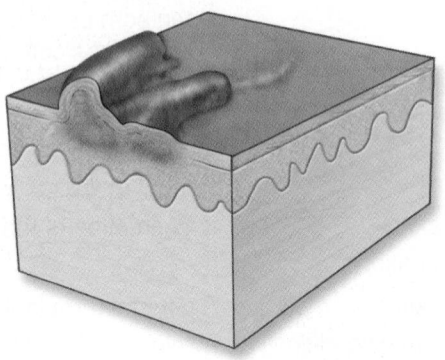

■ **Figure 3.22** Keloid.

TERM	WORD PARTS	DEFINITION
keratosis (kair-ah-TOH-sis)	kerat/o = hard, horny -osis = abnormal condition	Term for any skin condition involving an over-growth and thickening of the epidermis layer.
laceration		A torn or jagged wound; incorrectly used to describe a cut.
malignant melanoma (MM) (mah-LIG-nant / mel-a-NOH-ma)	melan/o = black -oma = tumor	Dangerous form of skin cancer caused by an uncontrolled growth of melanocytes. May quickly metastasize or spread to internal organs.

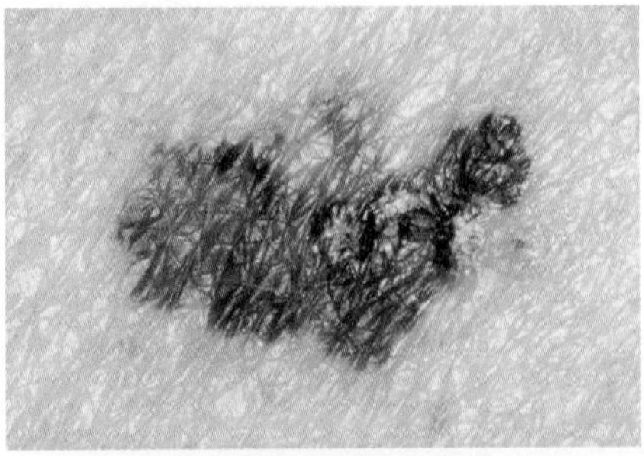

■ **Figure 3.23** Malignant melanoma. This photograph demonstrates the highly characteristic color of this tumor. *(Skin Cancer Foundation/National Cancer Institute)*

■ Pathology *(continued)*

TERM	WORD PARTS	DEFINITION
pediculosis (peh-dik-you-LOH-sis)	pedicul/o = lice -osis = abnormal condition	Infestation with lice. The eggs laid by the lice are called nits and cling tightly to hair.
psoriasis (soh-RYE-ah-sis)		Chronic inflammatory condition consisting of papules forming "silvery scale" patches with circular borders.

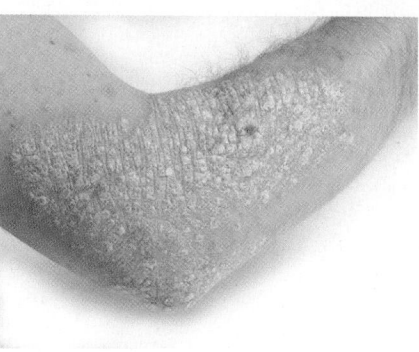

■ Figure 3.24 Psoriasis. This photograph demonstrates the characteristic white skin patches of this condition. *(kenxro/Shutterstock)*

TERM	WORD PARTS	DEFINITION
rubella (roo-BELL-ah)		Contagious viral skin infection. Commonly called *German measles.*
scabies (SKAY-bees)		Contagious skin disease caused by an egg-laying mite that burrows through the skin and causes redness and intense itching; often seen in children.
sebaceous cyst (see-BAY-shus / SIST)	seb/o = oil	Sac under the skin filled with sebum or oil from a sebaceous gland. This can grow to a large size and may need to be excised.
cicatrix (SICK-ah-trix)		A scar.
squamous cell carcinoma (SCC) (SKWAY-mus / sell / kar-sih-NOH-mah)	carcin/o = cancer -oma = tumor	Cancer of the epidermis layer of skin that may invade deeper tissue and metastasize. Often begins as a sore that does not heal.

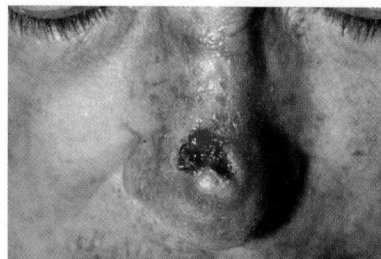

■ Figure 3.25 Squamous cell carcinoma. *(National Cancer Institute)*

Pathology *(continued)*

TERM	WORD PARTS	DEFINITION
strawberry hemangioma (hee-man-jee-OH-ma)	hem/o = blood angi/o = vessel -oma = tumor	Congenital collection of dilated blood vessels causing a red birthmark that fades a few months after birth.

■ **Figure 3.26** Strawberry hemangioma, a birthmark caused by a collection of blood vessels in the skin. *(H.C. Robinson/Science Photo Library/ Photo Researchers)*

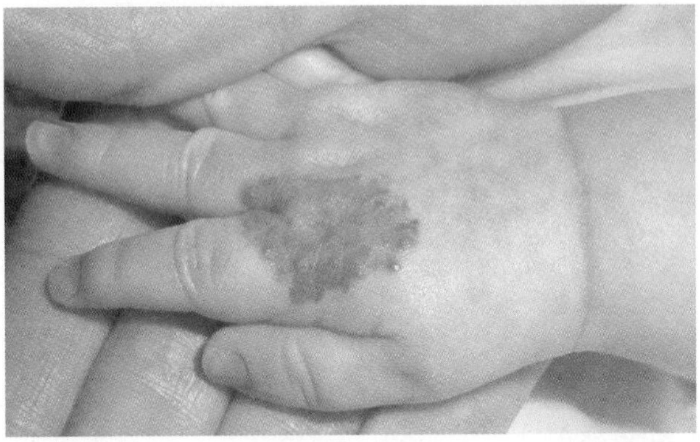

TERM	WORD PARTS	DEFINITION
systemic lupus erythematosus (SLE) (sis-TEM-ik / LOO-pus / air-ih-them-ah-TOH-sis)	system/o = system -ic = pertaining to erythr/o = red	Chronic disease of the connective tissue that injures the skin, joints, kidneys, nervous system, and mucous membranes. This is an autoimmune condition meaning that the body's own immune system attacks normal tissue of the body. May produce a characteristic red, scaly butterfly rash across the cheeks and nose.
tinea (TIN-ee-ah)		Fungal skin disease resulting in itching, scaling lesions.
tinea capitis (TIN-ee-ah / CAP-it-is)	*capitis* is the Latin term for the head	Fungal infection of the scalp. Commonly called *ringworm.*
tinea pedis (TIN-ee-ah / PED-is)	*pedis* is the Latin term for the foot	Fungal infection of the foot. Commonly called *athlete's foot.*
varicella (VAIR-ih-chell-a)	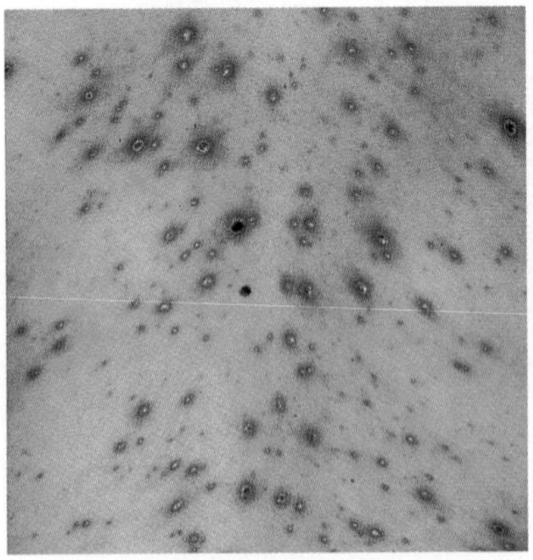	Contagious viral skin infection. Commonly called *chickenpox.*

■ **Figure 3.27** Varicella or chickenpox, a viral skin infection. In this photograph, the rash is beginning to form scabs.

TERM	WORD PARTS	DEFINITION
verruca (ver-ROO-kah)		Commonly called *warts;* a benign growth caused by a virus. Has a rough surface that is removed by chemicals and/or laser therapy.

■ Pathology *(continued)*

TERM	WORD PARTS	DEFINITION
vitiligo (vit-ill-EYE-go)		Disappearance of pigment from the skin in patches, causing a milk-white appearance. Also called *leukoderma*.
wet gangrene (GANG-green)		An area of gangrene that becomes secondarily infected by pus-producing bacteria.
Hair		
alopecia (al-oh-PEE-she-ah)		Absence or loss of hair, especially of the head. Commonly called *baldness*.
carbuncle (CAR-bung-kl)		Furuncle involving several hair follicles.
furuncle (FOO-rung-kl)		Bacterial infection of a hair follicle. Characterized by redness, pain, and swelling. Also called a *boil*.
trichomycosis (trik-oh-my-KOH-sis)	trich/o = hair myc/o = fungus -osis = abnormal condition	Abnormal condition of hair fungus.
Nails		
onychia (oh-NICK-ee-ah)	onych/o = nail -ia = state, condition	Infected nail bed.
onychomycosis (on-ih-koh-my-KOH-sis)	onych/o = nail myc/o = fungus -osis = abnormal condition	Abnormal condition of nail fungus.
onychophagia (on-ih-koh-FAY-jee-ah)	onych/o = nail -phagia = eating	Nail eating (nail biting).
paronychia (pair-oh-NICK-ee-ah)	para- = beside onych/o = nail -ia = state, condition	Infection of the skin fold around a nail.

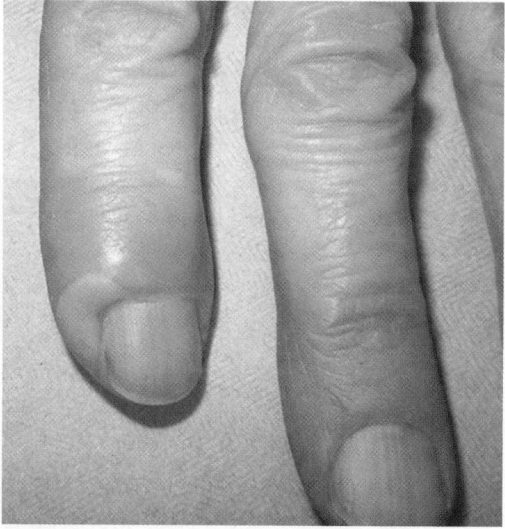

■ **Figure 3.28** Paronychia.
(Local Images Inc.)

Diagnostic Procedures

TERM	WORD PARTS	DEFINITION
Clinical Laboratory Tests		
culture and sensitivity (C&S)		Laboratory test that grows a colony of bacteria removed from an infected area in order to identify the specific infecting bacteria and then determine its sensitivity to a variety of antibiotics.
Biopsy Procedures		
biopsy (BX, bx) (BYE-op-see) **MED TERM TIP** Word Watch: Be careful when using *bi-* meaning "two" and *bi/o* meaning "life."	bi/o = life -opsy = to view	Piece of tissue removed by syringe and needle, knife, punch, or brush to examine under a microscope. Used to aid in diagnosis.
exfoliative cytology (ex-FOH-lee-ah-tiv / sigh-TALL-oh-jee)	cyt/o = cell -logy = study of	Scraping cells from tissue and then examining them under a microscope.
frozen section (FS)		Thin piece of tissue cut from a frozen specimen for rapid examination under a microscope.
fungal scrapings	-al = pertaining to	Scrapings, taken with a curette or scraper, of tissue from lesions are placed on a growth medium and examined under a microscope to identify fungal growth.

Therapeutic Procedures

TERM	WORD PARTS	DEFINITION
Skin Grafting		
allograft (AL-oh-graft)	allo- = other	Skin graft from one person to another; donor is usually a cadaver. Also called *homograft* (homo = same).
autograft (AW-toh-graft)	auto- = self	Skin graft from a person's own body.
dermatome (DER-mah-tohm)	derm/o = skin -tome = instrument to cut	Instrument for cutting the skin or thin transplants of skin.

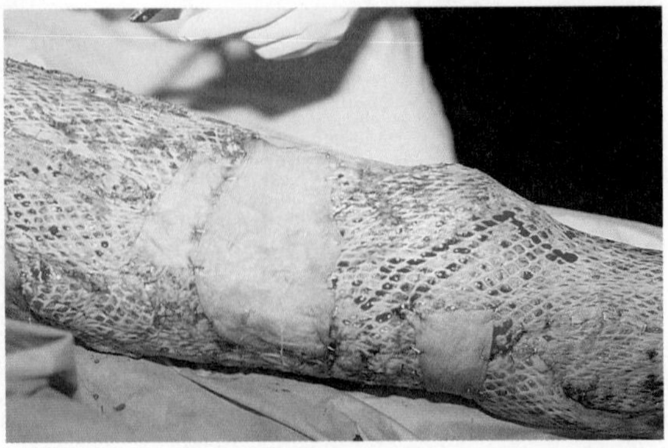

■ **Figure 3.29** A freshly applied autograft. Note that the donor skin has been perforated so that it can be stretched to cover a larger burned area. *(Courtesy of Dr. William Dominic, Community Regional Medical Center)*

Therapeutic Procedures *(continued)*

TERM	WORD PARTS	DEFINITION
dermatoplasty (DER-mah-toh-plas-tee)	dermat/o = skin -plasty = surgical repair	Skin grafting; transplantation of skin.
skin graft (SG)		Transfer of skin from a normal area to cover another site. Used to treat burn victims and after some surgical procedures. Also called *dermatoplasty*.
xenograft (ZEN-oh-graft)	xeno- = strange, foreign	Skin graft from an animal of another species (usually a pig) to a human. Also called *heterograft* (hetero- = other).
Surgical Procedures		
cauterization (kaw-ter-ih-ZAY-shun)		Destruction of tissue by using caustic chemicals, electric currents, heat, or by freezing.
cryosurgery (cry-oh-SER-jer-ee)	cry/o = cold	Use of extreme cold to freeze and destroy tissue.
curettage (koo-REH-tahz)		Removal of superficial skin lesions with a curette (surgical instrument shaped like a spoon) or scraper.
debridement (de-BREED-mint)		Removal of foreign material and dead or damaged tissue from a wound.
electrocautery (ee-leck-troh-KAW-teh-ree)	electr/o = electricity	To destroy tissue with an electric current.
incision and drainage (I&D)	cis/o = to cut	Making an incision to create an opening for the drainage of material such as pus.
onychectomy (on-ee-KECK-toh-mee)	onych/o = nail -ectomy = surgical removal	Removal of a nail.
Plastic Surgery Procedures		
chemabrasion (kee-moh-BRAY-zhun)	chem/o = chemical	Abrasion using chemicals. Also called a *chemical peel*.
dermabrasion (DERM-ah-bray-shun)	derm/o = skin	Abrasion or rubbing using wire brushes or sandpaper. Performed to remove acne scars, tattoos, and scar tissue.
laser therapy		Removal of skin lesions and birthmarks using a laser beam that emits intense heat and power at a close range. The laser converts frequencies of light into one small, powerful beam.
liposuction (LIP-oh-suck-shun)	lip/o = fat	Removal of fat beneath the skin by means of suction.
rhytidectomy (rit-ih-DECK-toh-mee)	rhytid/o = wrinkle -ectomy = surgical removal	Surgical removal of excess skin to eliminate wrinkles. Commonly referred to as a *face lift*.

Pharmacology

CLASSIFICATION	WORD PARTS	ACTION	EXAMPLES
anesthetic (an-es-THET-tic)	an- = without esthesi/o = feeling -ic = pertaining to	Applied to the skin to deaden pain.	lidocaine, Xylocaine; procaine, Novocain
antibiotic (an-tye-bye-AW-tic)	anti- = against bi/o = life -tic = pertaining to	Kill bacteria causing skin infections.	bacitracin/neomycin/polymix-inB, Neosporin ointment
antifungal (an-tye-FUNG-all)	anti- = against -al = pertaining to	Kill fungi infecting the skin.	miconazole, Monistat; clotrim-azole, Lotrimin
antiparasitic (an-tye-pair-ah-SIT-tic)	anti- = against -ic = pertaining to	Kill mites or lice.	lindane, Kwell; permethrin, Nix
antipruritic (an-tye-proo-RIGH-tik)	anti- = against -ic = pertaining to	Reduce severe itching.	diphenhydramine, Benadryl; camphor/pramoxine/zinc, Caladryl
antiseptic (an-tye-SEP-tic)	anti- = against -tic = pertaining to	Used to kill bacteria in skin cuts and wounds or at a surgical site.	isopropyl alcohol; hydrogen peroxide
antivirals	anti- = against	Treats herpes simplex infection.	valacyclovir, Valtrex; fam-cyclovir, Famvir; acyclovir, Zovirax
corticosteroid cream		Specific type of powerful anti-inflammatory cream.	hydrocortisone, Cortaid; tri-amcinolone, Kenalog

Abbreviations

BCC	basal cell carcinoma	**MM**	malignant melanoma
BX, bx	biopsy	**SCC**	squamous cell carcinoma
C&S	culture and sensitivity	**SG**	skin graft
decub	decubitus ulcer	**SLE**	systemic lupus erythematosus
Derm, derm	dermatology	**STSG**	split-thickness skin graft
FS	frozen section	**subcu, SC,**	subcutaneous
HSV	herpes simplex virus	**sc, subq**	
I&D	incision and drainage	**UV**	ultraviolet
ID	intradermal		

> **MED TERM TIP**
>
> Word Watch: Be careful when using the abbreviation *ID* meaning "intradermal" and *I&D* meaning "incision and drainage."

Chapter Review

Real-World Applications

Medical Record Analysis

This Dermatology Consultation Report contains 11 medical terms. Underline each term and write it in the list below the report. Then define each term.

Dermatology Consultation Report

Reason for Consultation: Possible recurrence of basal cell carcinoma, left cheek.

History of Present Illness: Patient is a 74-year-old male first seen by his regular physician 5 years ago for persistent facial lesions. Biopsies revealed basal cell carcinoma in two lesions, one on the nasal tip and the other on the left cheek. These were successfully excised. The patient noted that the left cheek lesion returned approximately one year ago. Patient reports pruritus and states the lesion is growing larger.

Results of Physical Exam: Examination revealed a 10 × 14 mm lesion on left cheek 20 mm anterior to the ear. The lesion displays marked erythema and poorly defined borders. The area immediately around the lesion shows depigmentation with vesicles.

Assessment: Recurrence of basal cell carcinoma.

Recommendations: Due to the lesion's size, shape, and reoccurrence, deep excision of the carcinoma through the epidermis and dermis layers followed by dermatoplasty is recommended.

	Term	Definition
1	_____	_____
2	_____	_____
3	_____	_____
4	_____	_____
5	_____	_____
6	_____	_____
7	_____	_____
8	_____	_____
9	_____	_____
10	_____	_____
11	_____	_____

Chart Note Transcription

The chart note below contains 10 phrases that can be reworded with a medical term that you learned in this chapter. Each phrase is identified with an underline. Determine the medical term and write your answers in the spaces provided.

Current Complaint: A 64-year-old female with an <u>open sore</u> ❶ on her right leg is seen by the <u>specialist in treating diseases of the skin.</u> ❷

Past History: Patient states she first noticed an area of pain, <u>severe itching,</u> ❸ and <u>redness of the skin</u> ❹ just below her right knee about 6 weeks ago. One week later <u>raised spots containing pus</u> ❺ appeared. Patient states the raised spots containing pus ruptured and the open sore appeared.

Signs and Symptoms: Patient has a deep open sore 5 × 3 cm: It is 4 cm distal to the knee on the lateral aspect of the right leg. It appears to extend into the <u>middle skin layer,</u> ❻ and the edges show signs of <u>tissue death.</u> ❼ The open sore has a small amount of drainage but there is no odor. A <u>sample of the drainage that was grown in the lab to identify the microorganism and determine the best antibiotic</u> ❽ of the drainage revealed *Staphylococcus* bacteria in the open sore.

Diagnosis: <u>Inflammation of connective tissue in the skin.</u> ❾

Treatment: <u>Removal of damaged tissue</u> ❿ of the open sore followed by application of an antibiotic cream. Patient was instructed to return to the skin disease specialist's office in 2 weeks, or sooner if the open sore does not heal, or if it begins draining pus.

❶ _____

❷ _____

❸ _____

❹ _____

❺ _____

❻ _____

❼ _____

❽ _____

❾ _____

❿ _____

Case Study

Below is a case study presentation of a patient with a condition discussed in this chapter. Read the case study and answer the questions below. Some questions will ask for information not included within this chapter. Use your text, a medical dictionary, or any other reference material you choose to answer these questions.

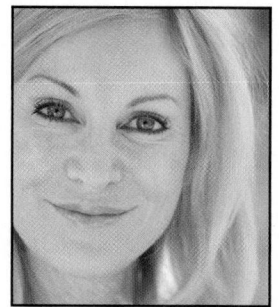

A 40-year-old female is seen in the dermatologist's office, upon the recommendation of her internist, for a workup for suspected SLE. Her presenting symptoms include erythema rash across her cheeks and nose, photosensitivity resulting in raised rash in sun-exposed areas, patches of alopecia, and pain and stiffness in her joints. The dermatologist examines the patient and orders exfoliative cytology and fungal scrapings to rule out other sources of the rash. Her internist had already placed the patient on oral anti-inflammatory medication for joint pain. The dermatologist orders corticosteroid cream for the rash. The patient is advised to use a sunscreen and make a follow-up appointment for results of the biopsy.

(Monkey Business Images/Shutterstock)

1. What pathological condition does the internist think this patient might have? Look this condition up in a reference source, and include a short description of it. SLE is an autoimmune disease. Use a reference source to look up the name of another autoimmune disease.

_____

_____

2. List and define each of the patient's presenting symptoms in your own words.

_____

_____

3. What diagnostic tests did the dermatologist perform? Describe it in your own words. Why were they important in helping the dermatologist make a diagnosis?

_____

_____

4. Each physician initiated a treatment. Describe them in your own words.

_____

_____

5. What do you think the term "workup" means?

_____

_____

Practice Exercises

A. Complete the Statement

1. The three layers of skin in order starting with the most superficial layer are _____, _____, and _____.

2. The _____ layer is the only living layer of the epidermis.

3. The subcutaneous layer of skin is composed primarily of _____.

4. Sensory receptors are located in the _____ layer of skin.

5. Nails and hair are composed of a hard protein called _____.

6. _____ is the pigment that gives skin its color.

7. Another name for the dermis is _____.

8. The nail body is connected to underlying tissue by the _____.

9. _____ glands release their product directly into hair follicles while _____ glands release their product into a duct.

10. _____ glands are sweat glands found in the underarm and pubic areas.

B. Define the Combining Form

	Definition	Example from Chapter
1. cry/o		
2. cutane/o		
3. diaphor/o		
4. py/o		
5. cyan/o		
6. ungu/o		
7. lip/o		
8. hidr/o		
9. rhytid/o		
10. seb/o		
11. trich/o		
12. necr/o		

C. Describe the Type of Burn

1. first degree _____

2. second degree _____

3. third degree _____

D. Terminology Matching

Match each term to its definition.

1. _____ eczema   a. decubitus ulcer

2. _____ nevus   b. lack of skin pigment

3. _____ lipoma   c. acne commonly seen in adults

4. _____ urticaria   d. hardened skin

5. _____ bedsore   e. redness, vesicles, itching, crusts

6. _____ acne rosacea   f. birthmark

7. _____ acne vulgaris   g. excessive hair growth

8. _____ hirsutism   h. caused by deficient blood supply

9. _____ alopecia   i. fatty tumor

10. _____ gangrene   j. hives

11. _____ scleroderma   k. baldness

12. _____ albinism   l. acne of adolescence

E. Define the Term

1. macule _____

2. papule _____

3. cyst _____

4. fissure _____

5. pustule _____

6. wheal _____

7. vesicle _____

8. ulcer _____

9. nodule _____

10. laceration _____

F. Combining Form Practice

The combining form **dermat/o** refers to the skin. Use it to write a term that means:

1. inflammation of the skin _____

2. any abnormal skin condition _____

3. an instrument for cutting the skin _____

4. specialist in skin _____

5. surgical repair of the skin _____

6. study of the skin _____

The combining form **melan/o** means black. Use it to write a term that means a:

7. black tumor _____

8. black cell _____

The suffix **-derma** means skin. Use it to write a term that means:

9. scaly skin _____

10. white skin _____

11. red skin _____

The combining form **onych/o** refers to the nail. Use it to write a term that means:

12. softening of the nails _____

13. infection around the nail _____

14. nail eating (biting) _____

15. removal of the nail _____

G. Procedure Matching

Match each procedure to its definition.

1. _____ debridement   a. surgical removal of wrinkled skin

2. _____ cauterization   b. instrument to cut thin slices of skin

3. _____ chemabrasion   c. removal of fat with suction

4. _____ dermatoplasty   d. use of extreme cold to destroy tissue

5. _____ liposuction   e. skin grafting

6. _____ rhytidectomy   f. removal of lesions with scraper

7. _____ curettage   g. removal of skin with brushes

8. _____ dermabrasion   h. removal of damaged skin

9. _____ dermatome   i. destruction of tissue with electric current

10. _____ cryosurgery   j. chemical peel

H. What's the Abbreviation?

1. frozen section _____

2. incision and drainage _____

3. intradermal _____

4. subcutaneous _____

5. ultraviolet _____

6. biopsy _____

I. What Does it Stand For?

1. C&S _____

2. BCC _____

3. derm _____

4. SG _____

5. decub _____

6. MM _____

J. Fill in the Blank

impetigo	tinea	keloid	exfoliative cytology	xeroderma
petechiae	frozen section	paronychia	scabies	Kaposi's sarcoma

1. The winter climates can cause dry skin. The medical term for this is _____.

2. Kim has experienced small pinpoint purplish spots caused by bleeding under the skin. This is called _____.

3. Janet has a fungal skin disease. This is called _____.

4. A contagious skin disease caused by a mite is _____.

5. An infection around the entire nail is called _____.

6. A form of skin cancer affecting AIDS patients is called _____.

7. Latrivia has a bacterial skin infection that results in pustules crusting and rupturing. It is called _____.

8. James's burn scar became a hypertrophic _____.

9. For a(n) _____ test, cells scraped off the skin are examined under a microscope.

10. During surgery a _____ was ordered for a rapid exam of tissue cut from a tumor.

K. Pharmacology Challenge

Fill in the classification for each drug description, then match the brand name.

Drug Description	Classification	Brand Name
1. _____ kills fungi	_____	a. Kwell
2. _____ reduces severe itching	_____	b. Cortaid
3. _____ kills mites and lice	_____	c. Valtrex
4. _____ treats herpes simplex infection	_____	d. Benadryl
5. _____ powerful anti-inflammatory	_____	e. Neosporin
6. _____ deadens pain	_____	f. Monistat
7. _____ kills bacteria	_____	g. Xylocaine

Labeling Exercise

Image A

Write the labels for this figure on the numbered lines provided.

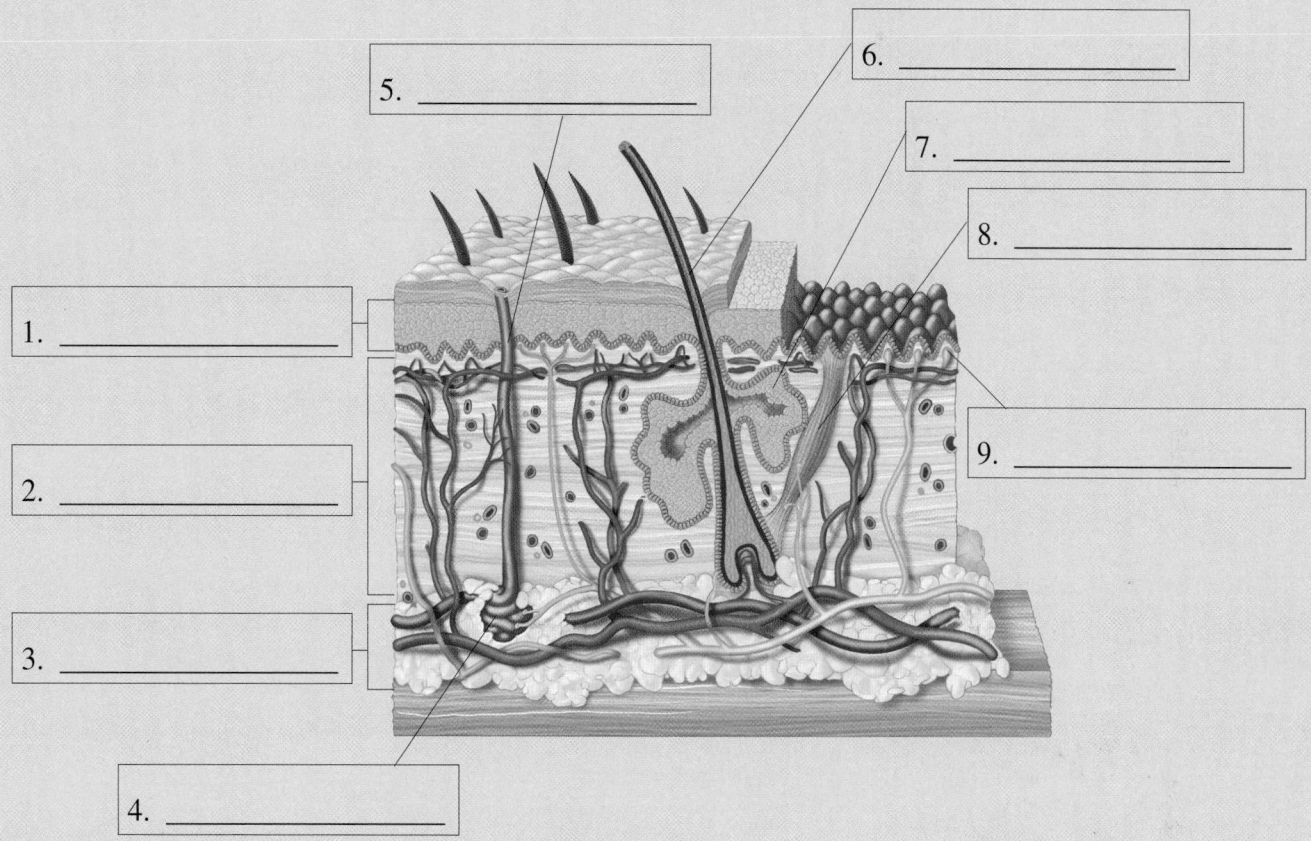

5. _____

6. _____

7. _____

8. _____

1. _____

2. _____

3. _____

9. _____

4. _____

Image B

Write the labels for this figure on the numbered lines provided.

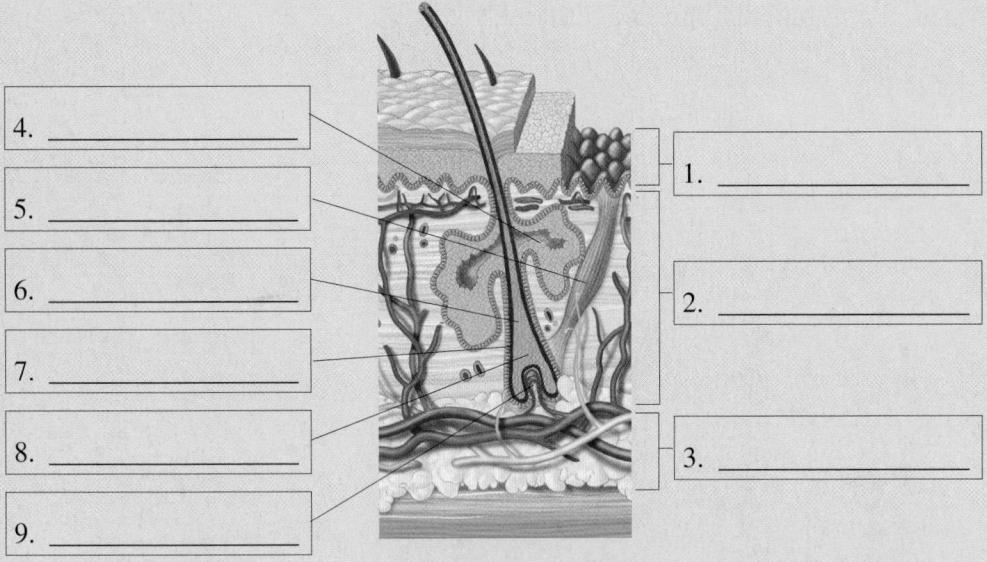

4. _____

5. _____

6. _____

7. _____

8. _____

9. _____

1. _____

2. _____

3. _____

Image C

Write the labels for this figure on the numbered lines provided.

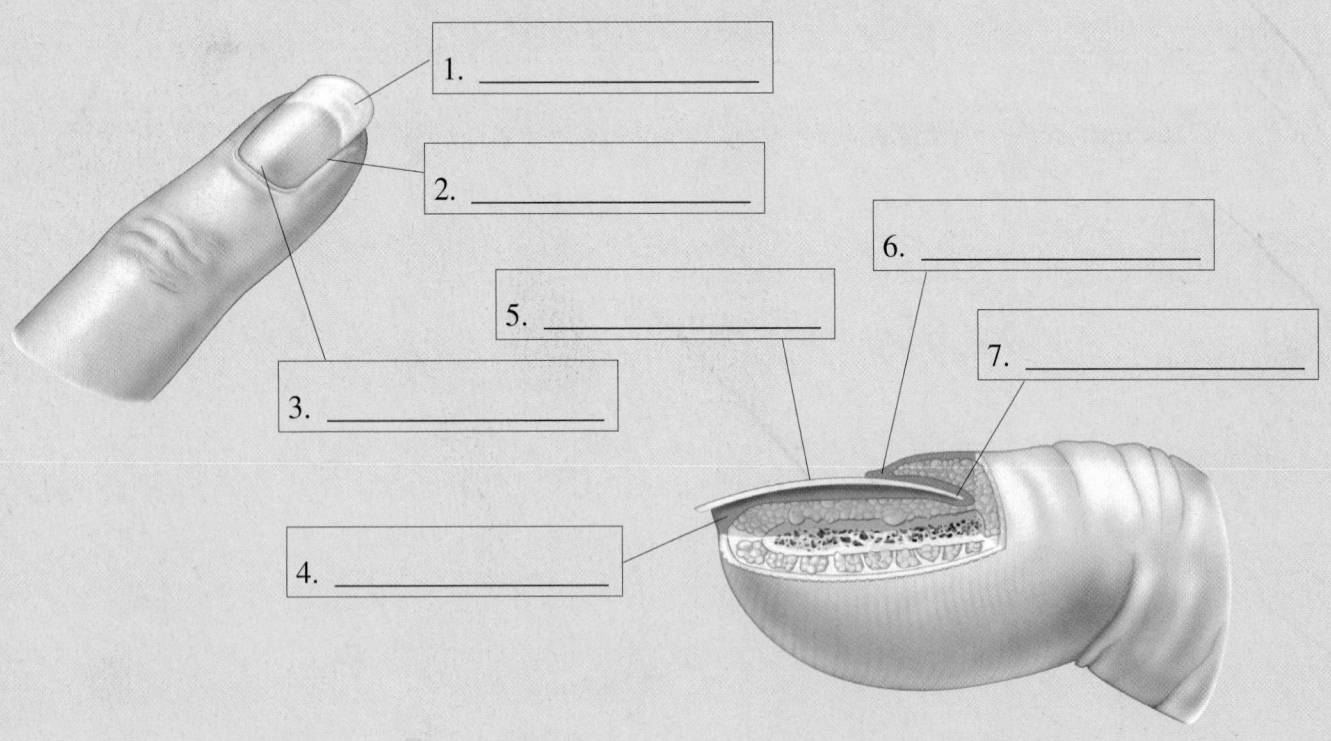

1. _____

2. _____

3. _____

4. _____

5. _____

6. _____

7. _____

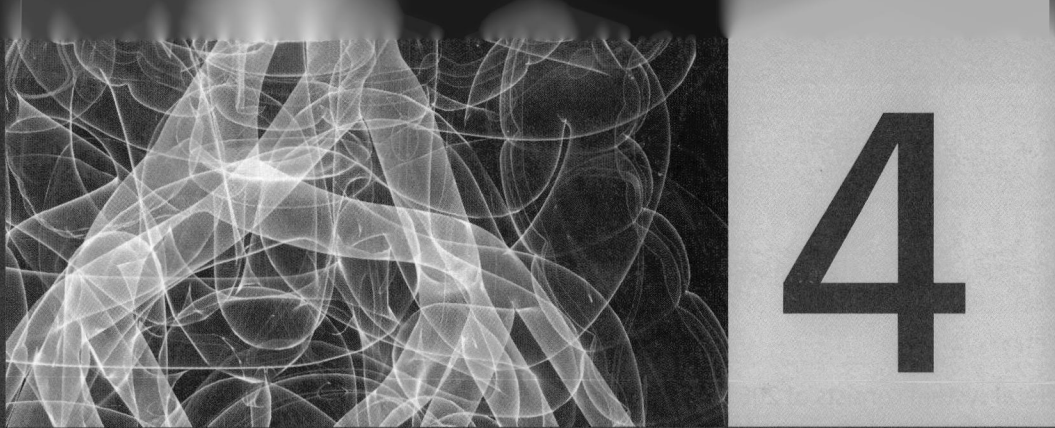

4

MUSCULOSKELETAL SYSTEM

Learning Objectives

Upon completion of this chapter, you will be able to

- Identify and define the combining forms, prefixes, and suffixes introduced in this chapter.
- Correctly spell and pronounce medical terms and major anatomical structures relating to the musculoskeletal system.
- Locate and describe the major organs of the musculoskeletal system and their functions.
- Correctly place bones in either the axial or the appendicular skeleton.
- List and describe the components of a long bone.
- Identify bony projections and depressions.
- Identify the parts of a synovial joint.
- Describe the characteristics of the three types of muscle tissue.
- Use movement terminology correctly.
- Identify and define musculoskeletal system anatomical terms.
- Identify and define selected musculoskeletal system pathology terms.
- Identify and define selected musculoskeletal system diagnostic procedures.
- Identify and define selected musculoskeletal system therapeutic procedures.
- Identify and define selected medications relating to the musculoskeletal system.
- Define selected abbreviations associated with the musculoskeletal system.

Section I: Skeletal System at a Glance

Function

The skeletal system consists of 206 bones that make up the internal framework of the body, called the skeleton. The skeleton supports the body, protects internal organs, serves as a point of attachment for skeletal muscles for body movement, produces blood cells, and stores minerals.

Organs

Here are the primary structures that comprise the skeletal system.

bones   **joints**

Word Parts

Here are the most common word parts (with their meanings) used to build skeletal system terms. For a more comprehensive list, refer to the Terminology section of this chapter.

Combining Forms

ankyl/o	stiff joint	myel/o	bone marrow, spinal cord
arthr/o	joint	orth/o	straight
articul/o	joint	oste/o	bone
burs/o	sac	patell/o	patella
carp/o	wrist	ped/o	child, foot
cervic/o	neck	pelv/o	pelvis
chondr/o	cartilage	phalang/o	phalanges
clavicul/o	clavicle	pod/o	foot
coccyg/o	coccyx	prosthet/o	addition
cortic/o	outer portion	pub/o	pubis
cost/o	rib	radi/o	radius, ray (X-ray)
crani/o	skull	sacr/o	sacrum
femor/o	femur	sarc/o	flesh (muscular substance)
fibul/o	fibula	scapul/o	scapula
humer/o	humerus	scoli/o	crooked, bent
ili/o	ilium	spin/o	spine
ischi/o	ischium	spondyl/o	vertebrae
kyph/o	hump	stern/o	sternum
lamin/o	lamina, part of vertebra	synovi/o	synovial membrane
lord/o	bent backwards	synov/o	synovial membrane
lumb/o	low back, loin	tars/o	ankle
mandibul/o	mandible	thorac/o	chest
maxill/o	maxilla	tibi/o	tibia
medull/o	inner portion	uln/o	ulna
metacarp/o	metacarpals	vertebr/o	vertebra
metatars/o	metatarsals		

Suffixes

-blast	immature, embryonic	-listhesis	slipping
-clasia	to surgically break	-porosis	porous
-desis	stabilize, fuse		

Skeletal System Illustrated

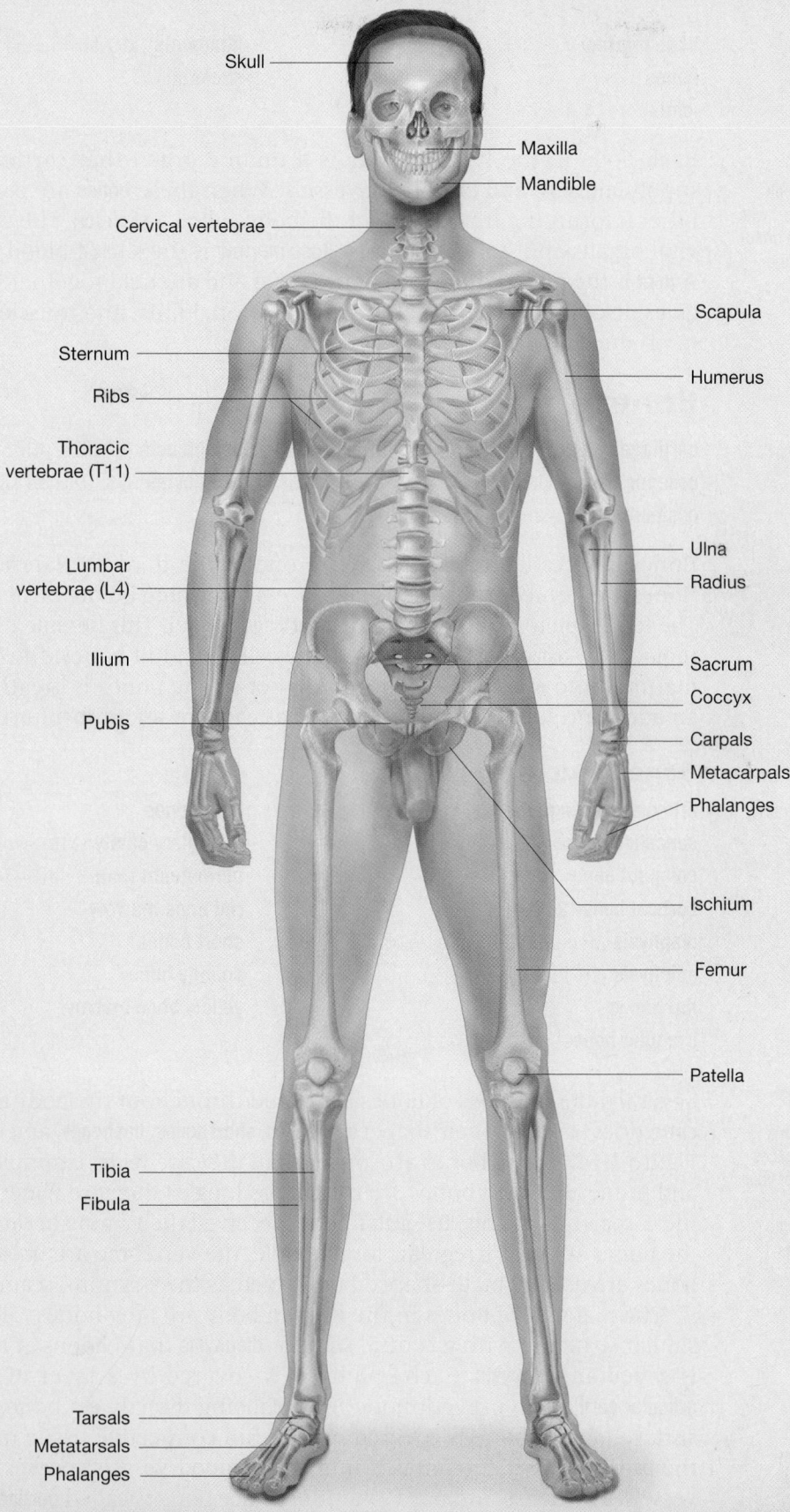

Skull

Maxilla

Mandible

Cervical vertebrae

Scapula

Sternum

Humerus

Ribs

Thoracic
vertebrae (T11)

Lumbar
vertebrae (L4)

Ulna

Radius

Ilium

Sacrum

Coccyx

Pubis

Carpals

Metacarpals

Phalanges

Ischium

Femur

Patella

Tibia

Fibula

Tarsals

Metatarsals

Phalanges

Anatomy and Physiology of the Skeletal System

bone marrow	**ligaments** (LIG-ah-ments)
bones	**skeleton**
joints	

Each bone in the human body is a unique organ that carries its own blood supply, nerves, and lymphatic vessels. When these **bones** are connected to each other it forms the framework of the body called a **skeleton.** The skeleton protects vital organs and stores minerals. **Bone marrow** is the site of blood cell production. A **joint** is the place where two bones meet and are held together by **ligaments.** This gives flexibility to the skeleton. The skeleton, joints, and muscles work together to produce movement.

Bones

cartilage (CAR-tih-lij)	**osteoblasts** (OSS-tee-oh-blasts)
osseous tissue (OSS-ee-us)	**osteocytes** (OSS-tee-oh-sights)
ossification (oss-sih-fih-KAY-shun)	

Bones, also called **osseous tissue,** are one of the hardest materials in the body. Bones are formed from a gradual process beginning before birth called **ossification.** The fetal skeleton is formed from a **cartilage** model. This flexible tissue is gradually replaced by **osteoblasts,** immature bone cells. In adult bones, the osteoblasts have matured into **osteocytes.** The formation of strong bones is greatly dependent on an adequate supply of minerals such as calcium and phosphorus.

Bone Structure

articular cartilage (ar-TIK-yoo-lar)	**long bones**
cancellous bone (CAN-sell-us)	**medullary cavity** (MED-you-lair-ee)
compact bone	**periosteum** (pair-ee-AH-stee-um)
cortical bone (KOR-ti-kal)	**red bone marrow**
diaphysis (dye-AFF-ih-sis)	**short bones**
epiphysis (eh-PIFF-ih-sis)	**spongy bone**
flat bones	**yellow bone marrow**
irregular bones	

Several different types of bones are found throughout the body and fall into four categories based on their shape: **long bones, short bones, flat bones,** and **irregular bones** (see Figure 4.1 ▇). Long bones are longer than they are wide; examples are the femur and humerus. Short bones are roughly as long as they are wide; examples being the carpals and tarsals. Irregular bones received their name because the shapes of the bones are very irregular; for example, the vertebrae are irregular bones. Flat bones are usually plate-shaped bones such as the sternum, scapulae, and pelvis.

The majority of bones in the human body are long bones. These bones have similar structure with a central shaft or **diaphysis** that widens at each end, which is called an **epiphysis.** Each epiphysis is covered by a layer of cartilage called **articular cartilage** to prevent bone from rubbing directly on bone. The remaining surface of each bone is covered with a thin connective tissue membrane called the **periosteum,** which contains numerous blood vessels, nerves, and lymphatic vessels. The dense and hard exterior surface bone is called **cortical** or **compact bone. Cancellous** or **spongy bone** is found inside the bone. As its name indicates, spongy

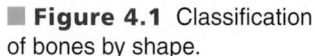 **Figure 4.1** Classification of bones by shape.

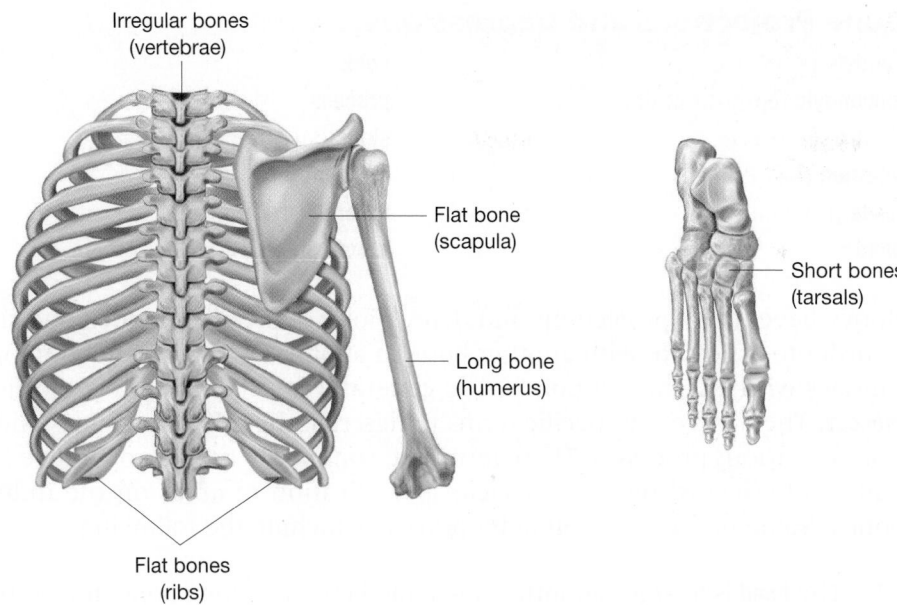

Irregular bones
(vertebrae)

Flat bone
(scapula)

Short bones
(tarsals)

Long bone
(humerus)

Flat bones
(ribs)

bone has spaces in it, giving it a spongelike appearance. These spaces contain **red bone marrow,** which manufactures most of the blood cells and is found in some parts of all bones.

The center of the diaphysis contains an open canal called the **medullary cavity.** Early in life this cavity also contains red bone marrow, but as we age the red bone marrow of the medullary cavity gradually converts to **yellow bone marrow,** which consists primarily of fat cells. Figure 4.2 ■ contains an illustration of the structure of long bones.

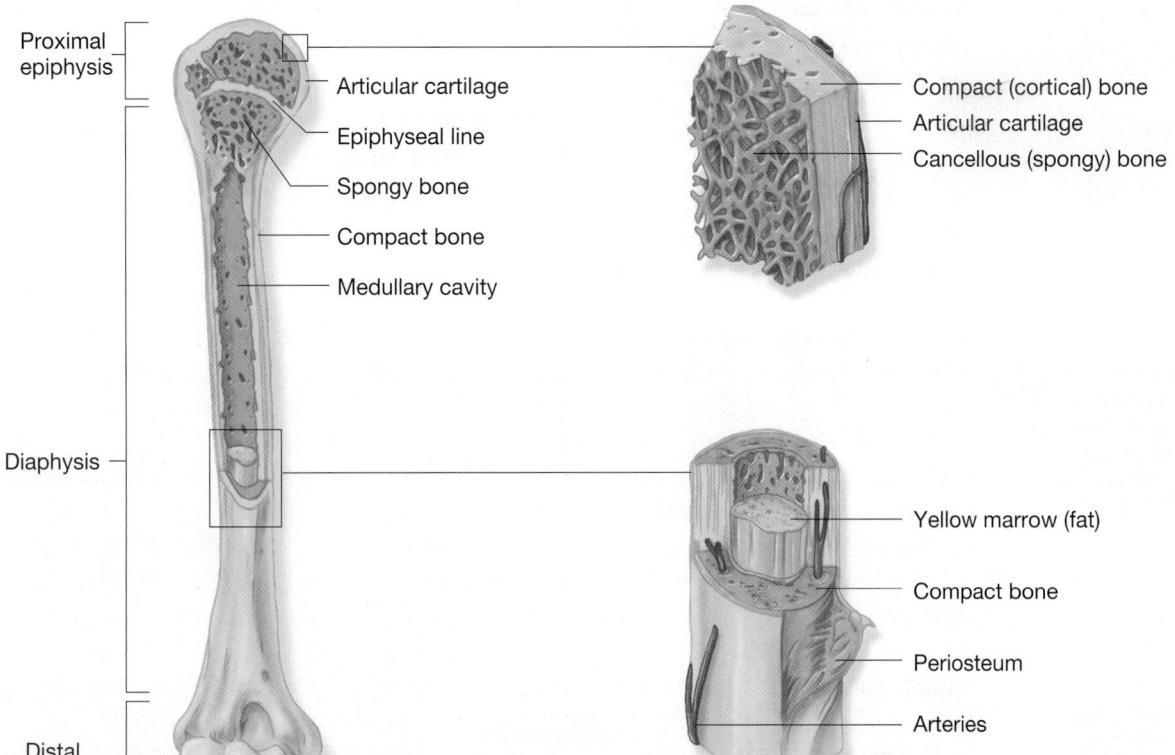

Proximal epiphysis

Articular cartilage

Epiphyseal line

Spongy bone

Compact bone

Medullary cavity

Compact (cortical) bone

Articular cartilage

Cancellous (spongy) bone

Diaphysis

Yellow marrow (fat)

Compact bone

Periosteum

Distal

Arteries

■ **Figure 4.2** Components of a long bone. The entire long bone is on the left side accompanied by a blowup of the proximal epiphysis and a section of the diaphysis.

Bone Projections and Depressions

condyle (KON-dile)	**neck**
epicondyle (ep-ih-KON-dile)	**process**
fissure (FISH-er)	**sinus** (SIGH-nus)
foramen (for-AY-men)	**trochanter** (tro-KAN-ter)
fossa (FOSS-ah)	**tubercle** (TOO-ber-kl)
head	**tuberosity** (too-ber-OSS-ih-tee)

MED TERM TIP

The elbow, commonly referred to as the *funny bone*, is actually a projection of the ulna called the olecranon process.

Bones have many projections and depressions; some are rounded and smooth in order to articulate with another bone in a joint. Others are rough to provide muscles with attachment points. The general term for any bony projection is a **process.** Then there are specific terms to describe the different shapes and locations of various processes. These terms are commonly used on operative reports and in physicians' records for clear identification of areas on the individual bones. Some of the common bony processes include the following:

1. The **head** is a large, smooth, ball-shaped end on a long bone. It may be separated from the body or shaft of the bone by a narrow area called the **neck.**
2. A **condyle** refers to a smooth, rounded portion at the end of a bone.
3. The **epicondyle** is a projection located above or on a condyle.
4. The **trochanter** refers to a large rough process for the attachment of a muscle.
5. A **tubercle** is a small, rough process that provides the attachment for tendons and muscles.
6. The **tuberosity** is a large, rough process that provides the attachment of tendons and muscles.

See Figure 4.3 ■ for an illustration of the processes found on the femur.

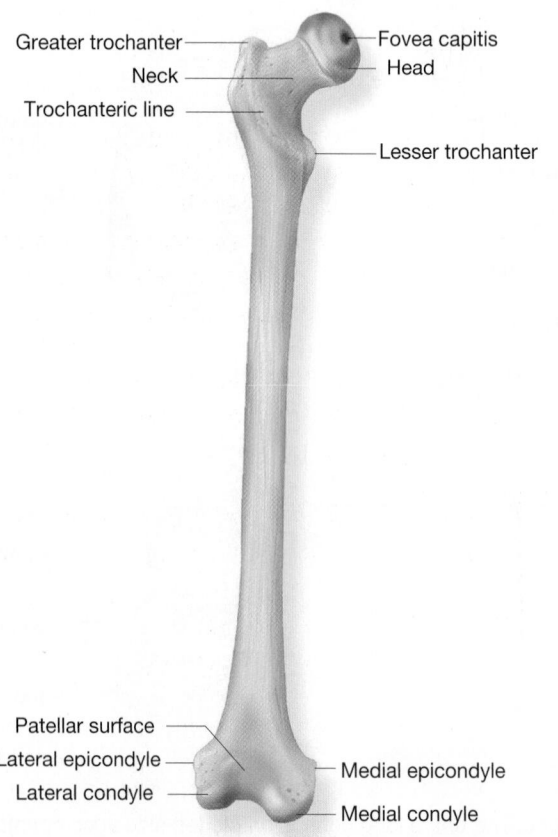

Greater trochanter — Fovea capitis
Neck — Head
Trochanteric line —
Lesser trochanter

Patellar surface —
Lateral epicondyle — Medial epicondyle
Lateral condyle — Medial condyle

■ **Figure 4.3** Bony processes found on the femur.

Additionally, bones have hollow regions or depressions. The most common depressions are the:

1. **Sinus** is a hollow cavity within a bone.
2. **Foramen** is a smooth, round opening for nerves and blood vessels.
3. **Fossa** consists of a shallow cavity or depression on the surface of a bone.
4. **Fissure** is a slit-type opening.

Skeleton

appendicular skeleton (app-en-DIK-yoo-lar)   **axial skeleton** (AK-see-al)

The human skeleton has two divisions: the **axial skeleton** and the **appendicular skeleton**. Figures 4.4 and 4.8 illustrate the axial and appendicular skeletons.

MED TERM TIP

Newborn infants have about 300 bones at birth that will fuse into 206 bones as an adult.

Axial Skeleton

cervical vertebrae	**occipital bone** (ock-SIP-eh-tal)
coccyx (COCK-six)	**palatine bone** (PAL-ah-tine)
cranium (KRAY-nee-um)	**parietal bone** (pah-RYE-eh-tal)
ethmoid bone (ETH-moyd)	**rib cage**
facial bones	**sacrum** (SAY-crum)
frontal bone	**sphenoid bone** (SFEE-noyd)
hyoid bone (HIGH-oyd)	**sternum** (STER-num)
intervertebral disc (in-ter-VER-teh-bral)	**temporal bone** (TEM-por-al)
lacrimal bone (LACK-rim-al)	**thoracic vertebrae**
lumbar vertebrae	**vertebral column** (VER-teh-bral)
mandible (MAN-dih-bl)	**vomer bone** (VOH-mer)
maxilla (mack-SIH-lah)	**zygomatic bone** (zeye-go-MAT-ik)
nasal bone	

The axial skeleton includes the bones of the head, neck, spine, chest, and trunk of the body (see Figure 4.4 ■). These bones form the central axis for the whole body and protect many of the internal organs such as the brain, lungs, and heart.

The head or skull is divided into two parts consisting of the **cranium** and **facial bones.** These bones surround and protect the brain, eyes, ears, nasal cavity, and oral cavity from injury. The muscles for chewing and moving the head are attached to the cranial bones. The cranium encases the brain and consists of the **frontal, parietal, temporal, ethmoid, sphenoid,** and **occipital bones.** The facial bones surround the mouth, nose, and eyes and include the **mandible, maxilla, zygomatic, vomer, palatine, nasal,** and **lacrimal bones.** The cranial and facial bones are illustrated in Figure 4.5 ■ and described in Table 4.1 ■.

The **hyoid bone** is a single U-shaped bone suspended in the neck between the mandible and larynx. It is a point of attachment for swallowing and speech muscles.

■ **Figure 4.4** Bones of the axial skeleton.

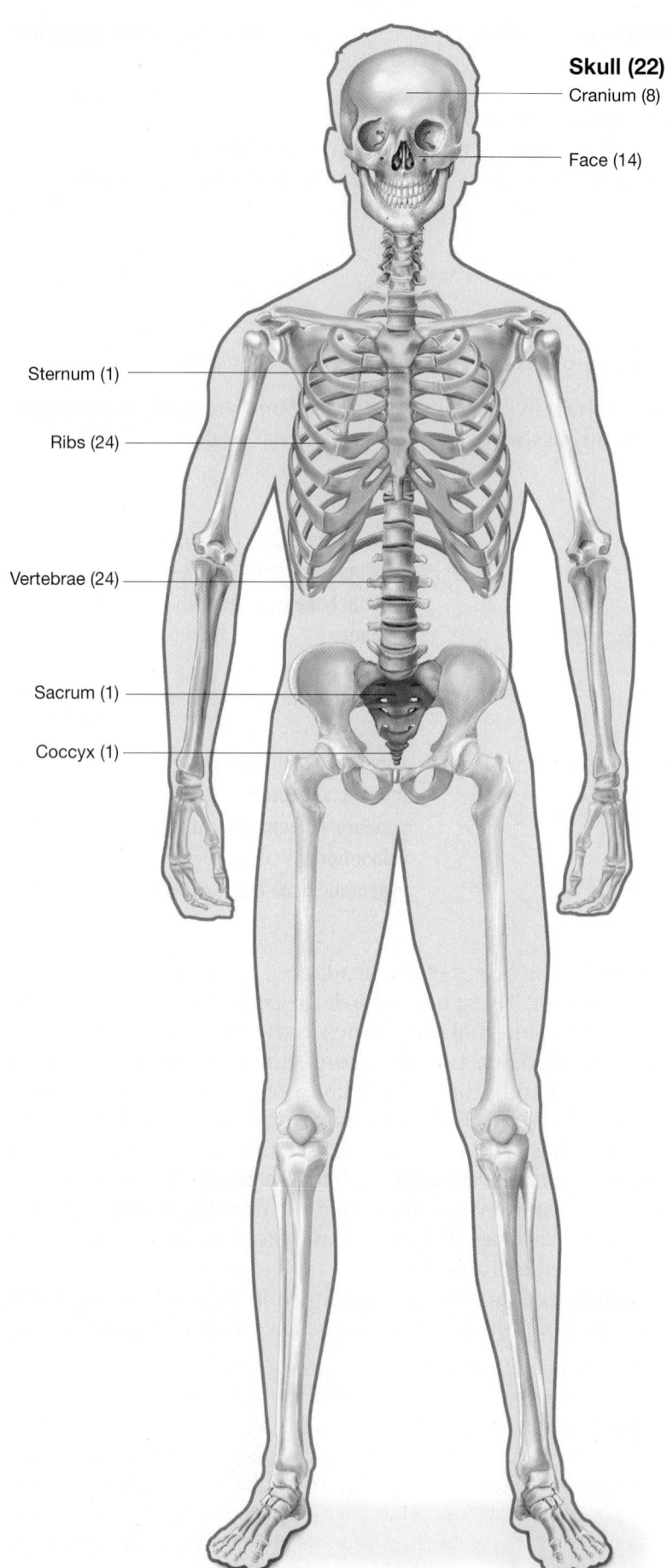

Skull (22)
Cranium (8)

Face (14)

Sternum (1)

Ribs (24)

Vertebrae (24)

Sacrum (1)

Coccyx (1)

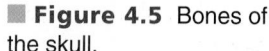

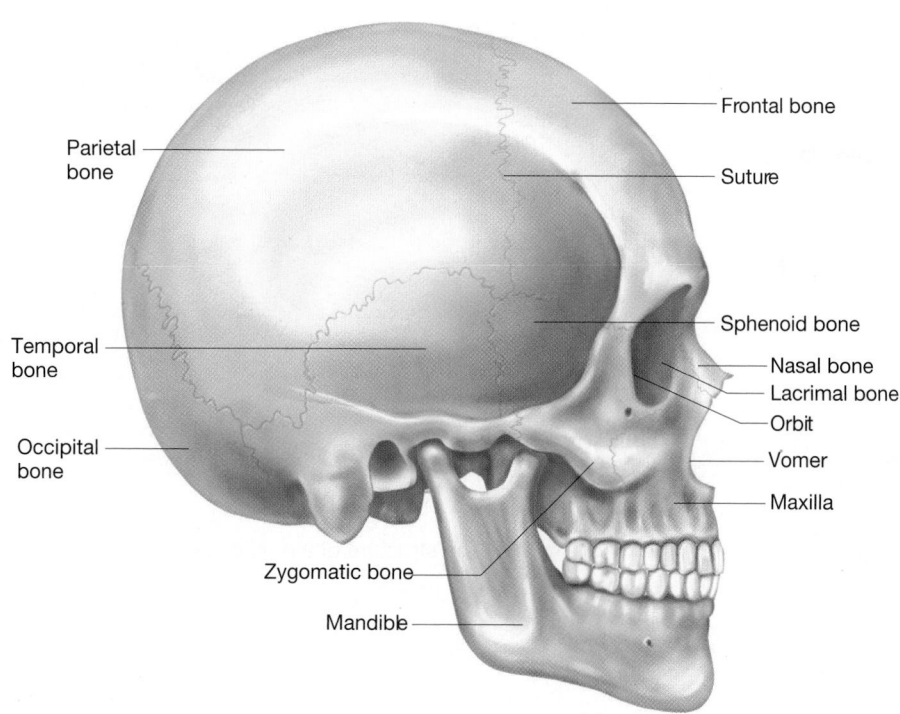

Table 4.1		Bones of the Skull
NAME	**NUMBER**	**DESCRIPTION**
Cranial Bones		
Frontal bone	1	Forehead
Parietal bone	2	Upper sides of cranium and roof of skull
Occipital bone	1	Back and base of skull
Temporal bone	2	Sides and base of cranium
Sphenoid bone	1	Bat-shaped bone that forms part of the base of the skull, floor, and sides of eye orbit
Ethmoid bone	1	Forms part of eye orbit, nose, and floor of cranium
Facial Bones		
Lacrimal bone	2	Inner corner of each eye
Nasal bone	2	Form part of nasal septum and support bridge of nose
Maxilla	1	Upper jaw
Mandible	1	Lower jawbone; only movable bone of the skull
Zygomatic bone	2	Cheekbones
Vomer bone	1	Base of nasal septum
Palatine bone	1	Hard palate (PAH lat) roof of oral cavity and floor of nasal cavity

The trunk of the body consists of the **vertebral column, sternum,** and **rib cage.** The vertebral or spinal column is divided into five sections: **cervical vertebrae, thoracic vertebrae, lumbar vertebrae, sacrum,** and **coccyx** (see Figure 4.6 ■ and Table 4.2 ■). Located between each pair of vertebrae, from the cervical through the lumbar regions, is an **intervertebral disc.** Each disc is composed of fibrocartilage to provide a cushion between the vertebrae. The rib cage has twelve pairs of ribs attached at the back to the vertebral column. Ten of the pairs are also attached to the sternum in the front (see Figure 4.7 ■). The lowest two pairs are called *floating ribs* and are attached only to the vertebral column. The rib cage serves to provide support for organs, such as the heart and lungs.

MED TERM TIP

The term *coccyx* comes from the Greek word for the cuckoo because the shape of these small bones extending off the sacrum resembles this bird's bill.

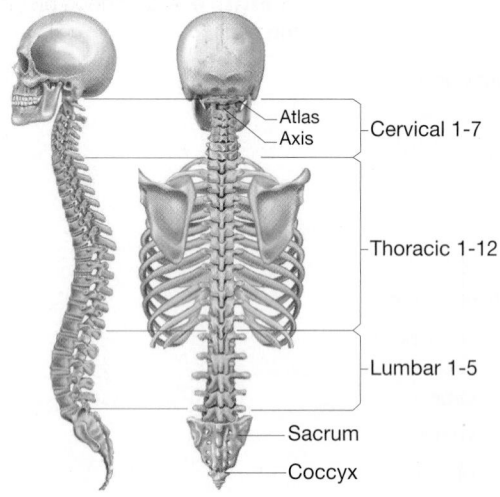

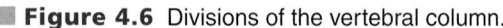

Figure 4.6 Divisions of the vertebral column.

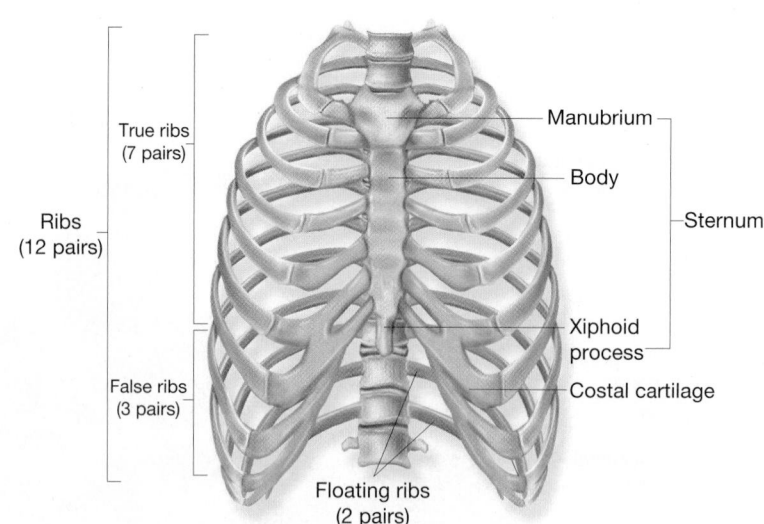

Figure 4.7 The structure of the rib cage.

Table 4.2		Bones of the Vertebral/Spinal Column
NAME	**NUMBER**	**DESCRIPTION**
Cervical vertebra	7	Vertebrae in the neck region
Thoracic vertebra	12	Vertebrae in the chest region with ribs attached
Lumbar vertebra	5	Vertebrae in the small of the back, about waist level
Sacrum	1	Five vertebrae that become fused into one triangular-shaped flat bone at the base of the vertebral column
Coccyx	1	Three to five very small vertebrae attached to the sacrum, often become fused

Appendicular Skeleton

carpals (CAR-pals)
clavicle (CLAV-ih-kl)
femur (FEE-mer)
fibula (FIB-yoo-lah)
humerus (HYOO-mer-us)
ilium (ILL-ee-um)
innominate bone (ih-NOM-ih-nayt)
ischium (ISS-kee-um)
lower extremities
metacarpals (met-ah-CAR-pals)
metatarsals (met-ah-TAHR-sals)
os coxae (OSS / KOK-sigh)

patella (pah-TELL-ah)
pectoral girdle
pelvic girdle
phalanges (fah-LAN-jeez)
pubis (PYOO-bis)
radius (RAY-dee-us)
scapula (SKAP-yoo-lah)
tarsals (TAHR-sals)
tibia (TIB-ee-ah)
ulna (UHL-nah)
upper extremities

MED TERM TIP

The term *girdle,* meaning something that encircles or confines, refers to the entire bony structure of the shoulder and the pelvis. If just one bone from these areas is being discussed, like the ilium of the pelvis, it would be named as such. If, however, the entire pelvis is being discussed, it would be called the pelvic girdle.

The appendicular skeleton consists of the **pectoral girdle, upper extremities, pelvic girdle,** and **lower extremities** (see Figure 4.8 ■). These are the bones for our appendages or limbs and along with the muscles attached to them, they are responsible for body movement.

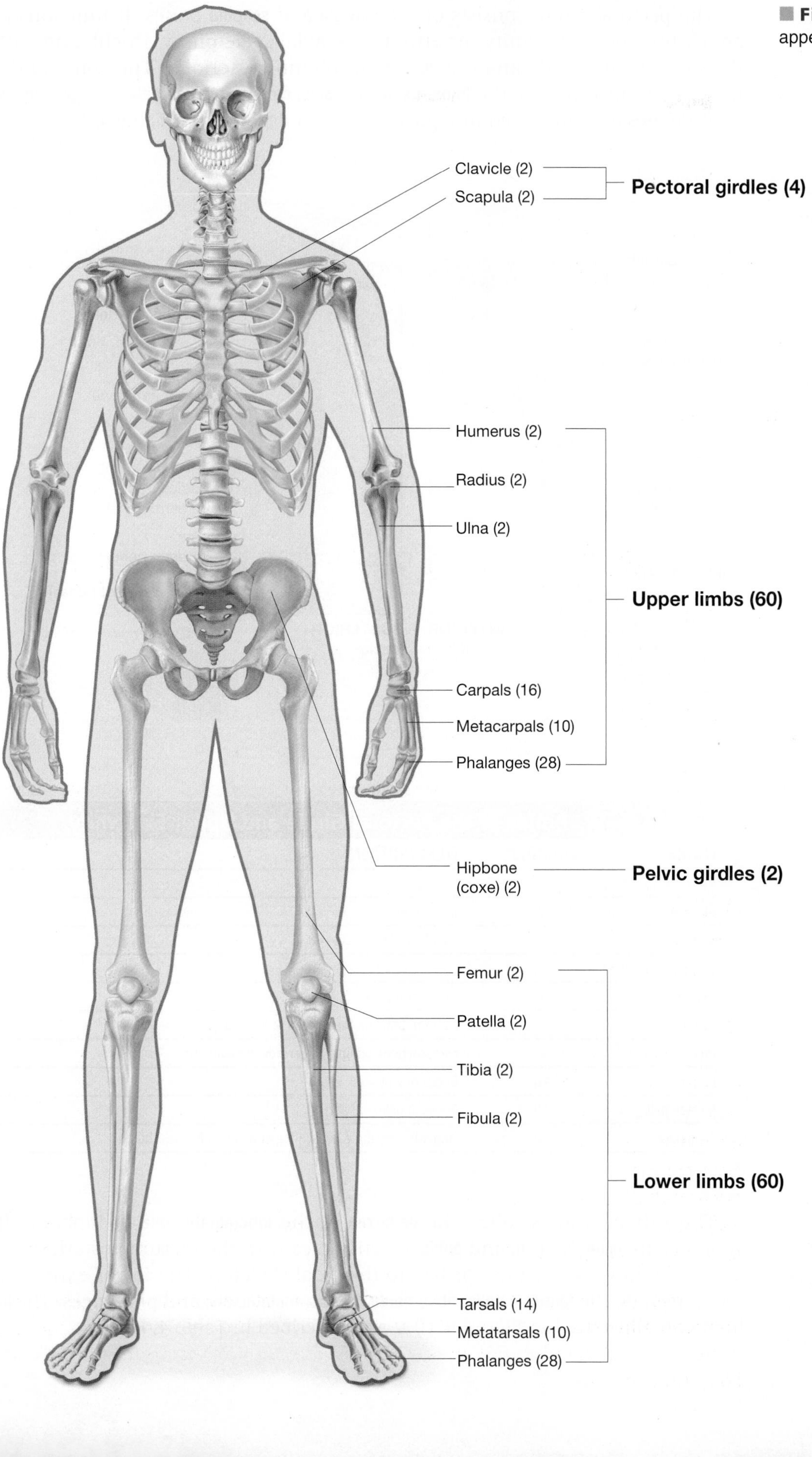

Figure 4.8 Bones of the appendicular skeleton.

Clavicle (2)

Scapula (2)

Pectoral girdles (4)

Humerus (2)

Radius (2)

Ulna (2)

Upper limbs (60)

Carpals (16)

Metacarpals (10)

Phalanges (28)

Hipbone (coxe) (2)

Pelvic girdles (2)

Femur (2)

Patella (2)

Tibia (2)

Fibula (2)

Lower limbs (60)

Tarsals (14)

Metatarsals (10)

Phalanges (28)

The pectoral girdle consists of the **clavicle** and **scapula** bones. It functions to attach the upper extremity, or arm, to the axial skeleton by articulating with the sternum anteriorly and the vertebral column posteriorly. The bones of the upper extremity include the **humerus, ulna, radius, carpals, metacarpals,** and **phalanges.** These bones are illustrated in Figure 4.9 ■ and described in Table 4.3 ■.

■ **Figure 4.9** Anatomical and common names for the pectoral girdle and upper extremity.

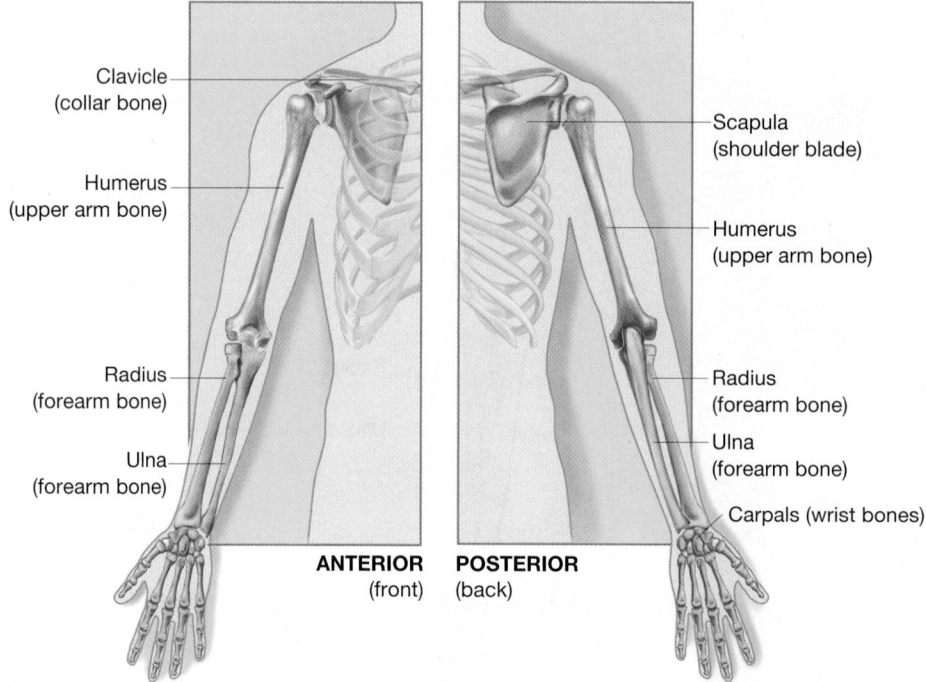

Table 4.3	Bones of the Pectoral Girdle and Upper Extremity	
NAME	**NUMBER**	**DESCRIPTION**
Pectoral Girdle		
Clavicle	2	Collar bone
Scapula	2	Shoulder blade
Upper Extremity		
Humerus	2	Upper arm bone
Radius	2	Forearm bone on thumb side of lower arm
Ulna	2	Forearm bone on little finger side of lower arm
Carpal	16	Bones of wrist
Metacarpals	10	Bones in palm of hand
Phalanges	28	Finger bones; three in each finger and two in each thumb

The pelvic girdle is called the **os coxae** or the **innominate bone** or hipbone. It contains the **ilium, ischium,** and **pubis.** It articulates with the sacrum posteriorly to attach the lower extremity, or leg, to the axial skeleton. The lower extremity bones include the **femur, patella, tibia, fibula, tarsals, metatarsals,** and phalanges. These bones are illustrated in Figure 4.10 ■ and described in Table 4.4 ■.

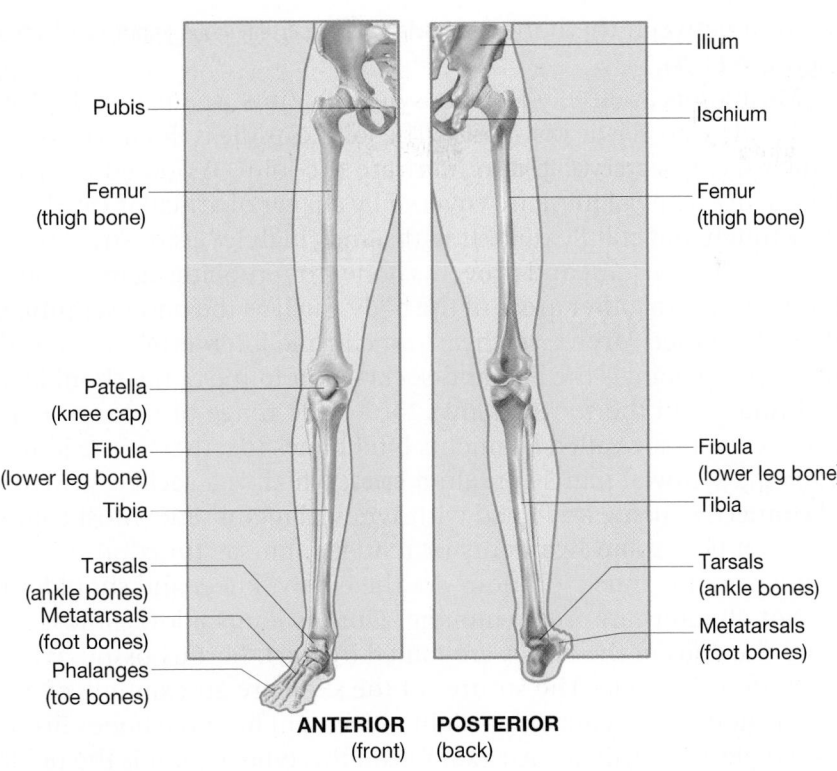

Pubis

Femur
(thigh bone)

Patella
(knee cap)

Fibula
(lower leg bone)

Tibia

Tarsals
(ankle bones)

Metatarsals
(foot bones)

Phalanges
(toe bones)

ANTERIOR
(front)

Ilium

Ischium

Femur
(thigh bone)

Fibula
(lower leg bone)

Tibia

Tarsals
(ankle bones)

Metatarsals
(foot bones)

POSTERIOR
(back)

Figure 4.10 Anatomical and common names for the pelvic girdle and lower extremity.

Table 4.4	Bones of the Pelvic Girdle and Lower Extremity	
NAME	**NUMBER**	**DESCRIPTION**
Pelvic Girdle/Os Coxae		
Ilium	2	Part of the hipbone
Ischium	2	Part of the hipbone
Pubis	2	Part of the hipbone
Lower Extremity		
Femur	2	Upper leg bone; thigh bone
Patella	2	Knee cap
Tibia	2	Shin bone; thicker lower leg bone
Fibula	2	Thinner, long bone in lateral side of lower leg
Tarsals	14	Ankle and heel bones
Metatarsals	10	Forefoot bones
Phalanges	28	Toe bones; three in each toe and two in each great toe

Joints

articulation (ar-tik-yoo-LAY-shun)
bursa (BER-sah)
cartilaginous joints (car-tih-LAJ-ih-nus)
fibrous joints (FYE-bruss)

joint capsule
synovial fluid
synovial joint (sin-OH-vee-al)
synovial membrane

Joints are formed when two or more bones meet. This is also referred to as an **articulation.** There are three types of joints based on the amount of movement

allowed between the bones: **synovial joints, cartilaginous joints,** and **fibrous joints** (see Figure 4.11 ■).

Most joints are freely moving synovial joints (see Figure 4.12 ■), which are enclosed by an elastic **joint capsule.** The joint capsule is lined with **synovial membrane,** which secretes **synovial fluid** to lubricate the joint. As noted earlier, the ends of bones in a synovial joint are covered by a layer of articular cartilage. Cartilage is very tough, but still flexible. It withstands high levels of stress to act as a shock absorber for the joint and prevents bone from rubbing against bone. Cartilage is found in several other areas of the body, such as the nasal septum, external ear, eustachian tube, larynx, trachea, bronchi, and intervertebral disks. One example of a synovial joint is the ball-and-socket joint found at the shoulder and hip. The ball rotating in the socket allows for a wide range of motion. Bands of strong connective tissue called ligaments bind bones together at the joint.

Some synovial joints contain a **bursa,** which is a saclike structure composed of connective tissue and lined with synovial membrane. Most commonly found between bones and ligaments or tendons, bursas function to reduce friction. Some common bursa locations are the elbow, knee, and shoulder joints.

Not all joints are freely moving. Fibrous joints allow almost no movement since the ends of the bones are joined by thick fibrous tissue, which may even fuse into solid bone. The sutures of the skull are an example of a fibrous joint. Cartilaginous joints allow for slight movement but hold bones firmly in place by a solid piece of cartilage. An example of this type of joint is the pubic symphysis, the point at which the left and right pubic bones meet in the front of the lower abdomen.

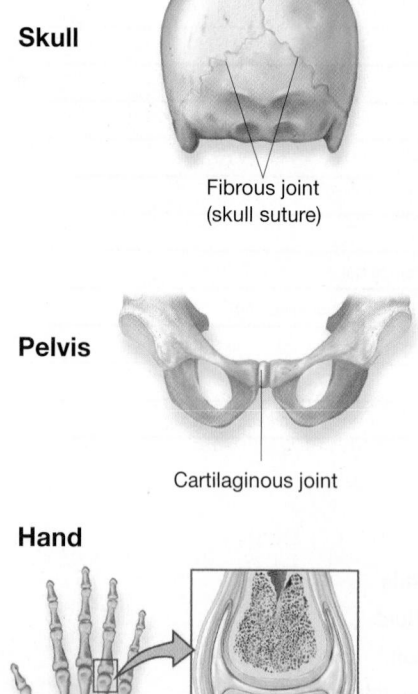

Skull

Fibrous joint
(skull suture)

Pelvis

Cartilaginous joint

Hand

Synovial joint

■ **Figure 4.11** Examples of three types of joints found in the body.

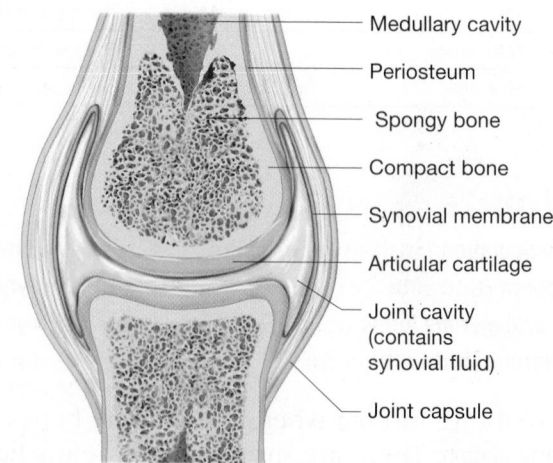

Medullary cavity

Periosteum

Spongy bone

Compact bone

Synovial membrane

Articular cartilage

Joint cavity
(contains
synovial fluid)

Joint capsule

■ **Figure 4.12** Structure of a generalized synovial joint.

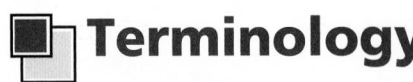
Terminology

Word Parts Used to Build Skeletal System Terms

The following lists contain the combining forms, suffixes, and prefixes used to build terms in the remaining sections of this chapter.

Combining Forms

ankyl/o	stiff joint	**kyph/o**	hump	**prosthet/o**	addition
arthr/o	joint	**lamin/o**	lamina, part of vertebra	**pub/o**	pubis
articul/o	joint	**lord/o**	bent backwards	**radi/o**	radius, ray (X-ray)
burs/o	bursa	**lumb/o**	low back	**sacr/o**	sacrum
carp/o	carpus	**mandibul/o**	mandible	**sarc/o**	flesh
cervic/o	neck	**maxill/o**	maxilla	**scapul/o**	scapula
chondr/o	cartilage	**medull/o**	inner portion	**scoli/o**	crooked, bent
clavicul/o	clavicle	**metacarp/o**	metacarpus	**spin/o**	spine
coccyg/o	coccyx	**metatars/o**	metatarsus	**spondyl/o**	vertebra
cortic/o	outer portion	**myel/o**	bone marrow	**stern/o**	sternum
cost/o	rib	**orth/o**	straight	**synovi/o**	synovial membrane
crani/o	skull	**oste/o**	bone	**synov/o**	synovial membrane
cutane/o	skin	**patell/o**	patella	**system/o**	system
erythr/o	red	**path/o**	disease	**tars/o**	tarsus
femor/o	femur	**ped/o**	child, foot	**thorac/o**	thorax
fibul/o	fibula	**pelv/o**	pelvis	**tibi/o**	tibia
humer/o	humerus	**phalang/o**	phalanges	**uln/o**	ulna
ili/o	ilium	**pod/o**	foot	**vertebr/o**	vertebra
ischi/o	ischium				

Suffixes

-ac	pertaining to	-gram	record	-otomy	cutting into
-al	pertaining to	-graphy	process of recording	-ous	pertaining to
-algia	pain	-iatry	medical treatment	-pathy	disease
-ar	pertaining to	-ic	pertaining to	-plasty	surgical repair
-ary	pertaining to	-itis	inflammation	-porosis	porous
-centesis	puncture to withdraw fluid	-listhesis	slipping	-scope	instrument for viewing
-clasia	surgically break	-logy	study	-scopy	process of visually examining
-desis	fuse	-malacia	softening		
-eal	pertaining to	-metry	process of measuring	-stenosis	narrowing
-ectomy	surgical removal	-oma	tumor	-tic	pertaining to
-genic	producing	-ory	pertaining to	-tome	instrument used to cut
		-osis	abnormal condition		

Prefixes

anti-	against	inter-	between	per-	through
bi-	two	intra-	inside	sub-	below, under
ex-	external, outward				

Anatomical Terms

TERM	WORD PARTS	DEFINITION
articular (ar-TIK-yoo-lar)	articul/o = joint -ar = pertaining to	pertaining to a joint
carpal (CAR-pal)	carp/o = carpus -al = pertaining to	pertaining to the carpus
cervical (CER-vih-kal)	cervic/o = neck -al = pertaining to	pertaining to the neck
clavicular (cla-VIK-yoo-lar)	clavicul/o = clavicle -ar = pertaining to	pertaining to the clavicle
coccygeal (cock-eh-JEE-all)	coccyg/o = coccyx -eal = pertaining to	pertaining to the coccyx
cortical (KOR-ti-kal)	cortic/o = outer portion -al = petaining to	pertaining to the outer portion
costal (COAST-all)	cost/o = rib -al = pertaining to	pertaining to the rib
cranial (KRAY-nee-all)	crani/o = skull -al = pertaining to	pertaining to the skull
femoral (FEM-or-all)	femor/o = femur -al = pertaining to	pertaining to the femur
fibular (FIB-yoo-lar)	fibul/o = fibula -ar = pertaining to	pertaining to the fibula
humeral (HYOO-mer-all)	humer/o = humerus -al = pertaining to	pertaining to the humerus
iliac (ILL-ee-ack)	ili/o = ilium -ac = pertaining to	pertaining to the ilium
intervertebral (in-ter-VER-teh-bral)	inter- = between vertebr/o = vertebra -al = pertaining to	pertaining to between vertebrae
intracranial (in-trah-KRAY-nee-al)	intra- = inside crani/o = skull -al = pertaining to	pertaining to inside the skull
ischial (ISH-ee-all)	ischi/o = ischium -al = pertaining to	pertaining to the ischium
lumbar (LUM-bar)	lumb/o = low back -ar = pertaining to	pertaining to the low back
mandibular (man-DIB-yoo-lar)	mandibul/o = mandible -ar = pertaining to	pertaining to the mandible
maxillary (mack-sih-LAIR-ree)	maxill/o = maxilla -ary = pertaining to	pertaining to the maxilla

Anatomical Terms *(continued)*

TERM	WORD PARTS	DEFINITION
medullary (MED-you-lair-ee)	medull/o = inner portion -ary = pertaining to	pertaining to the inner portion
metacarpal (met-ah-CAR-pal)	metacarp/o = metacarpus -al = pertaining to	pertaining to the metacarpus
metatarsal (met-ah-TAHR-sal)	metatars/o = metatarsus -al = pertaining to	pertaining to the metatarsus
patellar (pa-TELL-ar)	patell/o = patella -ar = pertaining to	pertaining to the patella
pelvic (PEL-vik)	pelv/o = pelvis -ic = pertaining to	pertaining to the pelvis
phalangeal (fay-lan-JEE-all)	phalang/o = phalanges -eal = pertaining to	pertaining to the phalanges
pubic (PYOO-bik)	pub/o = pubis -ic = pertaining to	pertaining to the pubis
radial (RAY-dee-all)	radi/o = radius -al = pertaining to	pertaining to the radius
sacral (SAY-kral)	sacr/o = sacrum -al = pertaining to	pertaining to the sacrum
scapular (SKAP-yoo-lar)	scapul/o = scapula -ar = pertaining to	pertaining to the scapula
sternal (STER-nal)	stern/o = sternum -al = pertaining to	pertaining to the sternum
synovial (sin-OH-vee-al)	synovi/o = synovial membrane -al = pertaining to	pertaining to the synovial membrane
tarsal (TAHR-sal)	tars/o = tarsus -al = pertaining to	pertaining to the tarsus
thoracic (tho-RASS-ik)	thorac/o = thorax -ic = pertaining to	pertaining to the thorax
tibial (TIB-ee-all)	tibi/o = tibia -al = pertaining to	pertaining to the tibia
ulnar (UHL-nar)	uln/o = ulna -ar = pertaining to	pertaining to the ulna

Pathology

TERM	WORD PARTS	DEFINITION
Medical Specialties		
chiropractic (ki-roh-PRAK-tik)	-tic = pertaining to	Healthcare profession concerned with diagnosis and treatment of malalignment conditions of the spine and musculoskeletal system with the intention of affecting the nervous system and improving health. Healthcare professional is a *chiropractor*.

Pathology *(continued)*

TERM	WORD PARTS	DEFINITION
orthopedics (or-thoh-PEE-diks)	orth/o = straight ped/o = child, foot -ic = pertaining to	Branch of medicine specializing in the diagnosis and treatment of conditions of the musculoskeletal system; also called *orthopedic surgery*. Physician is an *orthopedist* or *orthopedic surgeon*. Name derived from straightening (*orth/o*) deformities in children (*ped/o*).
orthotics (or-THOT-iks)	orth/o = straight -tic = pertaining to	Healthcare profession specializing in making orthopedic appliances such as braces and splints. Person skilled in making and adjusting these appliances is an *orthotist*.
podiatry (po-DYE-ah-tree)	pod/o = foot -iatry = medical treatment	Healthcare profession specializing in diagnosis and treatment of disorders of the feet and lower legs. Healthcare professional is a *podiatrist*.
prosthetics (pross-THET-iks)	prosthet/o = addition -ic = pertaining to	Healthcare profession specializing in making artificial body parts. Person skilled in making and adjusting prostheses is a *prosthetist*.

Signs and Symptoms

TERM	WORD PARTS	DEFINITION
arthralgia (ar-THRAL-jee-ah)	arthr/o = joint -algia = pain	joint pain
bursitis (ber-SIGH-tis)	burs/o = bursa -itis = inflammation	inflammation of a bursa
callus (KAL-us)		The mass of bone tissue that forms at a fracture site during its healing.
chondromalacia (kon-droh-mah-LAY-she-ah)	chondr/o = cartilage -malacia = softening	softening of the cartilage
crepitation (krep-ih-TAY-shun)		The noise produced by bones or cartilage rubbing together in conditions such as arthritis. Also called *crepitus*.
ostealgia (oss-tee-AL-jee-ah)	oste/o = bone -algia = pain	bone pain
osteomyelitis (oss-tee-oh-mi-ell-EYE-tis)	oste/o = bone myel/o = bone marrow -itis = inflammation	inflammation of bone and bone marrow
synovitis (sih-no-VI-tis)	synov/o = synovial membrane -itis = inflammation	inflammation of synovial membrane

Fractures

TERM	WORD PARTS	DEFINITION
closed fracture		Fracture in which there is no open skin wound. Also called a *simple fracture*.

Pathology *(continued)*

TERM	WORD PARTS	DEFINITION

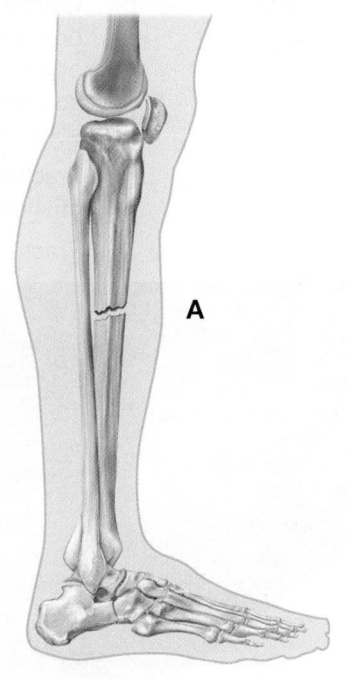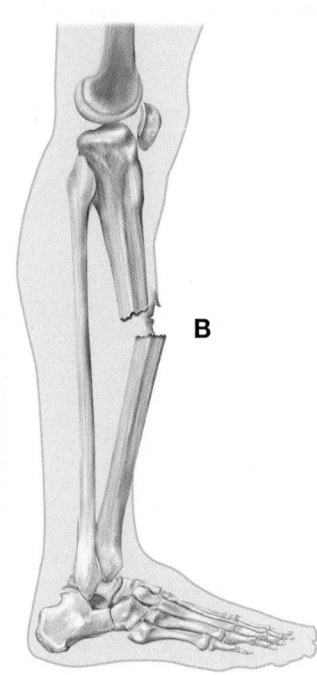

■ **Figure 4.13** (A) Closed (or simple) fracture and (B) open (or compound) fracture.

Colles'
(COL-eez) **fracture**

A common type of wrist fracture.

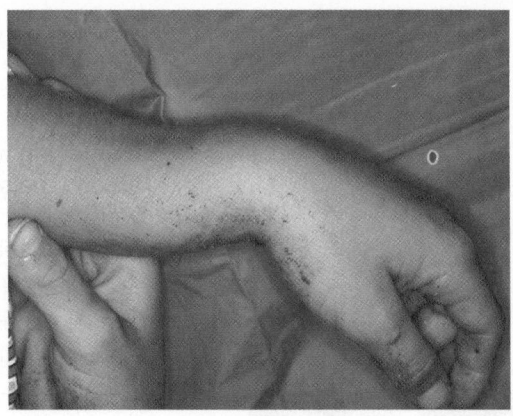

■ **Figure 4.14** Colles' fracture.
(Charles Stewart MD FACEP, FAAEM)

---

comminuted fracture
(kom-ih-NYOOT-ed)

Fracture in which the bone is shattered, splintered, or crushed into many small pieces or fragments.

---

compound fracture

Fracture in which the skin has been broken through to the fracture. Also called an *open fracture* (see Figure 4.13B ■).

---

compression fracture

Fracture involving loss of height of a vertebral body. It may be the result of trauma, but in older people, especially women, it may be caused by conditions like osteoporosis.

---

fracture
(FX, Fx)

A broken bone.

Pathology *(continued)*

TERM	WORD PARTS	DEFINITION
greenstick fracture		Fracture in which there is an incomplete break; one side of bone is broken and the other side is bent. This type of fracture is commonly found in children due to their softer and more pliable bone structure.
impacted fracture		Fracture in which bone fragments are pushed into each other.
oblique (oh-BLEEK) fracture		Fracture at an angle to the bone.

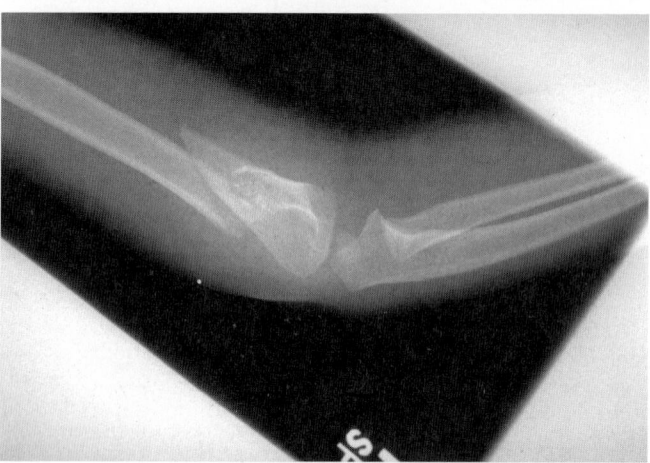

Figure 4.15 X-ray showing oblique fracture of the humerus. *(Charles Stewart MD)*

TERM	WORD PARTS	DEFINITION
pathologic (path-a-LOJ-ik) fracture	path/o = disease -logy = study -ic = pertaining to	Fracture caused by diseased or weakened bone.
spiral fracture		Fracture in which the fracture line spirals around the shaft of the bone. Can be caused by a twisting injury and is often slower to heal than other types of fractures.
stress fracture		A slight fracture caused by repetitive low-impact forces, like running, rather than a single forceful impact.
transverse fracture		Complete fracture that is straight across the bone at right angles to the long axis of the bone.

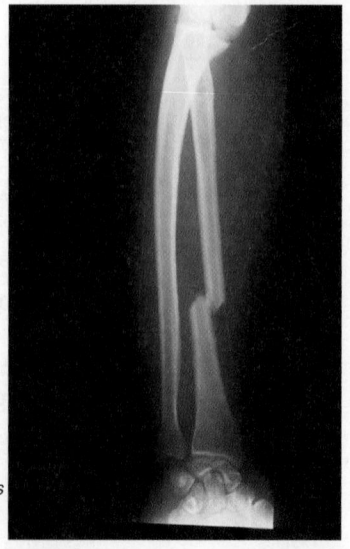

Figure 4.16 X-ray showing transverse fracture of radius. *(James Stevenson/Science Photo Library/Photo Researchers, Inc.)*

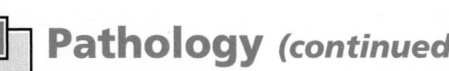

Pathology *(continued)*

TERM	WORD PARTS	DEFINITION
Bones		
chondroma (kon-DROH-mah)	chondr/o = cartilage -oma = tumor	A tumor, usually benign, that forms in cartilage.
Ewing's sarcoma (YOO-wings / sar-KOH-mah)	sarc/o = flesh -oma = tumor	Malignant growth found in the shaft of long bones that spreads through the periosteum. Removal is the treatment of choice because this tumor will metastasize or spread to other organs.
exostosis (eck-sos-TOH-sis)	ex- = external, outward oste/o = bone -osis = abnormal condition	A bone spur.
myeloma (my-ah-LOH-mah)	myel/o = bone marrow -oma = tumor	A tumor that forms in bone marrow tissue.
osteochondroma (oss-tee-oh-kon-DROH-mah)	oste/o = bone chondr/o = cartilage -oma = tumor	A tumor, usually benign, that consists of both bone and cartilage tissue.
osteogenic sarcoma (oss-tee-oh-GIN-ik / sark-OH-mah)	oste/o = bone -genic = producing sarc/o = flesh -oma = tumor	The most common type of bone cancer. Usually begins in osteocytes found at the ends of long bones.
osteomalacia (oss-tee-oh-mah-LAY-she-ah)	oste/o = bone -malacia = softening	Softening of the bones caused by a deficiency of calcium. It is thought to be caused by insufficient sunlight and vitamin D in children.
osteopathy (oss-tee-OPP-ah-thee)	oste/o = bone -pathy = disease	A general term for bone disease.
osteoporosis (oss-tee-oh-por-ROH-sis)	oste/o = bone -porosis = porous	Decrease in bone mass producing a thinning and weakening of the bone with resulting fractures. The bone becomes more porous, especially in the spine and pelvis.
Paget's disease (PAH-jets)		A fairly common metabolic disease of the bone from unknown causes. It usually attacks middle-aged and older adults and is characterized by bone destruction and deformity. Named for Sir James Paget, a British surgeon.
rickets (RIK-ets)		Deficiency in calcium and vitamin D found in early childhood that results in bone deformities, especially bowed legs.
Spinal Column		
ankylosing spondylitis (ang-kih-LOH-sing / spon-dih-LYE-tis)	ankyl/o = stiff joint spondyl/o = vertebra -itis = inflammation	Inflammatory spinal condition resembling rheumatoid arthritis and results in gradual stiffening and fusion of the vertebrae. More common in men than women.

Pathology *(continued)*

TERM	WORD PARTS	DEFINITION
herniated nucleus pulposus (HNP) (HER-nee-ated / NOO-klee-us / pull-POH-sus)		Herniation or protrusion of an intervertebral disk; also called *herniated disk* or *ruptured disk*. May require surgery.

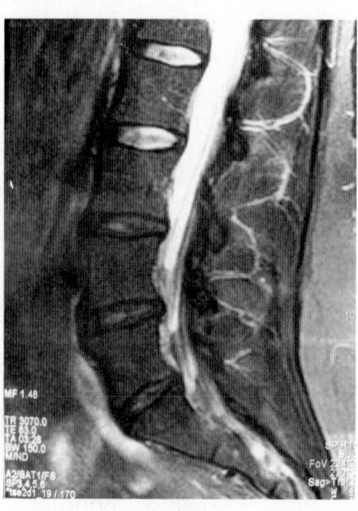

■ **Figure 4.17** Magnetic resonance imaging (MRI) image demonstrating a back herniated disk. *(Michelle Milano/ Shutterstock)*

| **kyphosis** (ki-FOH-sis) | kyph/o = hump -osis = abnormal condition | Abnormal increase in the outward curvature of the thoracic spine. Also known as *hunchback* or *humpback*. See Figure 4.18 ■ for an illustration of abnormal spine curvatures. |

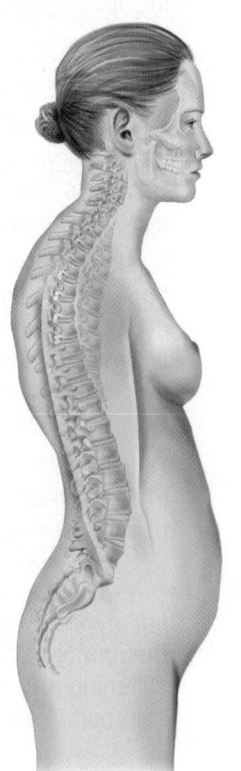
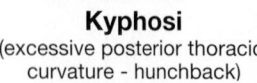
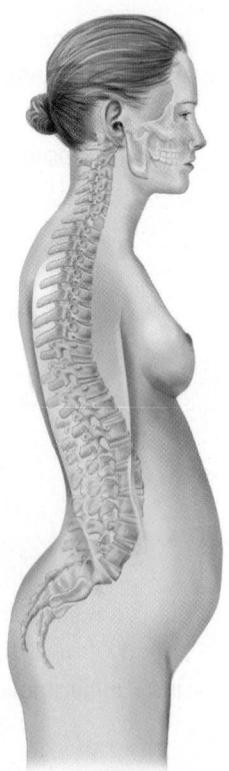
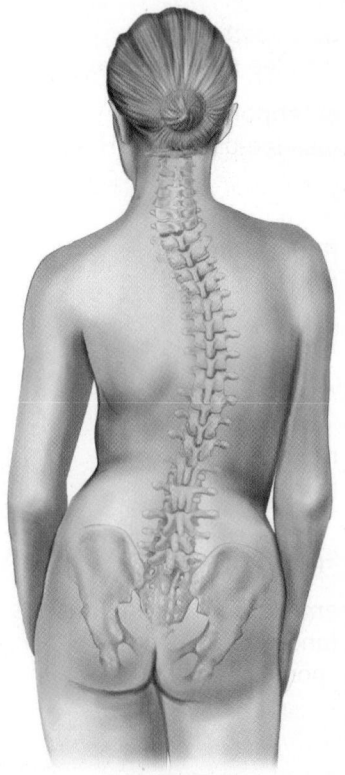

■ **Figure 4.18** Abnormal spinal curvatures: kyphosis, lordosis, and scoliosis.

Kyphosi
(excessive posterior thoracic curvature - hunchback)

Lordosis
(excessive anterior lumbar curvature - swayback)

Scoliosis
(lateral curvature)

◼ Pathology *(continued)*

TERM	WORD PARTS	DEFINITION
lordosis (lor-DOH-sis)	lord/o = bent backwards -osis = abnormal condition	Abnormal increase in the forward curvature of the lumbar spine. Also known as *swayback*. See again Figure 4.18 for an illustration of abnormal spine curvatures.
scoliosis (skoh-lee-OH-sis)	scoli/o = crooked, bent -osis = abnormal condition	Abnormal lateral curvature of the spine. See again Figure 4.18 for an illustration of abnormal spine curvatures.
spina bifida (SPY-nah / BIF-ih-dah)	spin/o = spine bi- = two	Congenital anomaly occurring when a vertebra fails to fully form around the spinal cord.
spinal stenosis (ste-NOH-sis)	spin/o = spine -al = pertaining to	Narrowing of the spinal canal causing pressure on the cord and nerves.
spondylolisthesis (spon-dih-loh-liss-THEE-sis)	spondyl/o = vertebra -listhesis = slipping	The forward sliding of a lumbar vertebra over the vertebra below it.
spondylosis (spon-dih-LOH-sis)	spondyl/o = vertebra -osis = abnormal condition	Specifically refers to ankylosing of the spine, but commonly used in reference to any degenerative condition of the vertebral column.
whiplash		Cervical muscle and ligament sprain or strain as a result of a sudden movement forward and backward of the head and neck. Can occur as a result of a rear-end auto collision.
Joints		
bunion (BUN-yun)		Inflammation of the bursa of the first metatarsophalangeal joint (base of the big toe).
dislocation		Occurs when the bones in a joint are displaced from their normal alignment and the ends of the bones are no longer in contact.
osteoarthritis (OA) (oss-tee-oh-ar-THRY-tis)	oste/o = bone arthr/o = joint -itis = inflammation	Arthritis resulting in degeneration of the bones and joints, especially those bearing weight. Results in bone rubbing against bone.
rheumatoid arthritis (RA) (ROO-mah-toyd / ar-THRY-tis)	arthr/o = joint -itis = inflammation	Chronic form of arthritis with inflammation of the joints, swelling, stiffness, pain, and changes in the cartilage that can result in crippling deformities; considered to be an autoimmune disease.

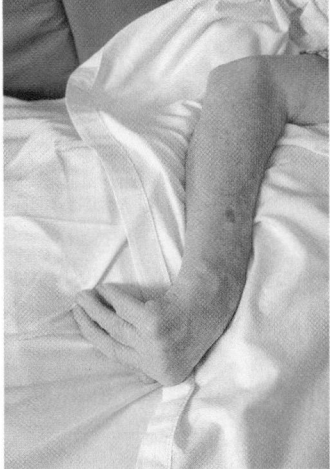

◼ **Figure 4.19** Patient with typical rheumatoid arthritis contractures.

Pathology *(continued)*

TERM	WORD PARTS	DEFINITION
sprain		Damage to the ligaments surrounding a joint due to overstretching, but no dislocation of the joint or fracture of the bone.
subluxation (sub-LUCKS-a-shun)	sub- = below, under	An incomplete dislocation, the joint alignment is disrupted, but the ends of the bones remain in contact.
systemic lupus erythematosus (SLE) (sis-TEM-ik / LOOP-us / air-ih-them-ah-TOH-sis)	system/o = system -ic = pertaining to erythr/o = red	Chronic inflammatory autoimmune disease of connective tissue affecting many systems that may include joint pain and arthritis. May be mistaken for rheumatoid arthritis.
talipes (TAL-ih-peez)		Congenital deformity causing misalignment of the ankle joint and foot. Also referred to as a *clubfoot*.

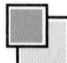

Diagnostic Procedures

TERM	WORD PART	DEFINITION
Diagnostic Imaging		
arthrogram (AR-throh-gram)	arthr/o = joint -gram = record	X-ray record of a joint; usually taken after the joint has been injected by a contrast medium.
arthrography (ar-THROG-rah-fee)	arthr/o = joint -graphy = process of recording	Process of X-raying a joint; usually after injection of a contrast medium into the joint space.
bone scan		Nuclear medicine procedure in which the patient is given a radioactive dye and then scanning equipment is used to visualize bones. It is especially useful in identifying stress fractures, observing progress of treatment for osteomyelitis, and locating cancer metastases to the bone.
dual-energy absorptiometry (DXA) (ab-sorp-she-AHM-eh-tree)	-metry = process of measuring	Measurement of bone density using low-dose X-ray for the purpose of detecting osteoporosis.
myelography (my-eh-LOG-rah-fee)	myel/o = bone marrow -graphy = process of recording	Study of the spinal column after injecting opaque contrast material; particularly useful in identifying herniated nucleus pulposus pinching a spinal nerve.
radiography	radi/o = ray (X-ray) -graphy = process of recording	Diagnostic imaging procedure using X-rays to study the internal structure of the body; especially useful for visualizing bones and joints.
Endoscopic Procedures		
arthroscope (AR-throw-skop)	arthr/o = joint -scope = instrument for viewing	Instrument used to view inside a joint.

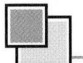 ## Diagnostic Procedures *(continued)*

TERM	WORD PART	DEFINITION
arthroscopy (ar-THROS-koh-pee)	arthr/o = joint -scopy = process of visually examining	Examination of the interior of a joint by entering the joint with an *arthroscope.* The arthroscope contains a small television camera that allows the physician to view the interior of the joint on a monitor during the procedure. Some joint conditions can be repaired during arthroscopy.

 # Therapeutic Procedures

TERM	WORD PART	DEFINITION
Medical Treatments		
arthrocentesis (ar-thro-sen-TEE-sis)	arthr/o = joint -centesis = puncture to withdraw fluid	Involves the insertion of a needle into the joint cavity in order to remove or aspirate fluid. May be done to remove excess fluid from a joint or to obtain fluid for examination.
orthotic (or-THOT-ik)	orth/o = straight -tic = pertaining to	Orthopedic appliance, such as a brace or splint, used to prevent or correct deformities.
prosthesis (pross-THEE-sis)	prosthet/o = addition	Artificial device used as a substitute for a body part that is either congenitally missing or absent as a result of accident or disease. An example would be an artificial leg.
Surgical Procedures		
amputation (am-pew-TAY-shun)		Partial or complete removal of a limb for a variety of reasons, including tumors, gangrene, intractable pain, crushing injury, or uncontrollable infection.
arthroclasia (ar-throh-KLAY-see-ah)	arthr/o = joint -clasia = surgically break	To forcibly break loose a fused joint while the patient is under anesthetic. Fusion is usually caused by the buildup of scar tissue or adhesions.
arthrodesis (ar-throh-DEE-sis)	arthr/o = joint -desis = fuse	Procedure to stabilize a joint by fusing the bones together.
arthroscopic surgery (ar-throh-SKOP-ic)	arthr/o = joint -scopy = process of visually examining -ic = pertaining to	Performing a surgical procedure while using an arthroscope to view the internal structure, such as a joint.
arthrotomy (ar-THROT-oh-mee)	arthr/o = joint -otomy = cutting into	Surgical procedure that cuts into a joint capsule.
bone graft		Piece of bone taken from the patient used to take the place of a removed bone or a bony defect at another site.
bunionectomy (bun-yun-ECK-toh-mee)	-ectomy = surgical removal	Removal of the bursa at the joint of the great toe.

◼◻ Therapeutic Procedures *(continued)*

TERM	WORD PART	DEFINITION
bursectomy (ber-SEK-toh-mee)	burs/o = bursa -ectomy = surgical removal	Surgical removal of a bursa.
chondrectomy (kon-DREK-toh-mee)	chondr/o = cartilage -ectomy = surgical removal	Surgical removal of cartilage.
chondroplasty (KON-droh-plas-tee)	chondr/o = cartilage -plasty = surgical repair	Surgical repair of cartilage.
craniotomy (kray-nee-OTT-oh-mee)	chondr/o = cartilage -otomy = cutting into	Surgical procedure that cuts into the skull.
laminectomy (lam-ih-NEK-toh-mee)	lamin/o = lamina, part of vertebra -ectomy = surgical removal	Removal of the vertebral posterior arch to correct severe back problems and pain caused by compression of a spinal nerve.
osteoclasia (oss-tee-oh-KLAY-see-ah)	oste/o = bone -clasia = surgically break	Surgical procedure involving the intentional breaking of a bone to correct a deformity.
osteotome (OSS-tee-oh-tohm)	oste/o = bone -tome = instrument used to cut	Instrument used to cut bone.
osteotomy (oss-tee-OTT-ah-me)	oste/o = bone -otomy = cutting into	Surgical procedure that cuts into a bone.
percutaneous diskectomy (per-kyou-TAY-nee-us / disk-EK-toh-mee)	per- = through cutane/o = skin -ous = pertaining to -ectomy = surgical removal	A thin catheter tube is inserted into the intervertebral disk through the skin and the herniated or ruptured disk material is sucked out or a laser is used to vaporize it.
spinal fusion	spin/o = spine -al = pertaining to	Surgical immobilization of adjacent vertebrae. This may be done for several reasons, including correction for a herniated disk.
synovectomy (sih-no-VEK-toh-mee)	synov/o = synovial membrane -ectomy = surgical removal	Surgical removal of the synovial membrane.
total hip arthroplasty (THA) (ar-thro-PLAS-tee)	arthr/o = joint -plasty = surgical repair	Surgical reconstruction of a hip by implanting a prosthetic or artificial hip joint. Also called *total hip replacement (THR)*.

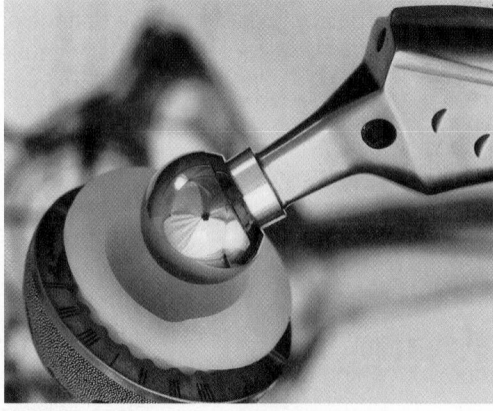

◼ **Figure 4.20** Prosthetic hip joint. *(Lawrence Livermore National Library/Science Photo Library/Photo Researchers, Inc.)*

total knee arthroplasty (TKA) (ar-thro-PLAS-tee)	arthr/o = joint -plasty = surgical repair	Surgical reconstruction of a knee joint by implanting a prosthetic knee joint. Also called *total knee replacement (TKR)*.

■ Therapeutic Procedures *(continued)*

TERM	WORD PART	DEFINITION
Fracture Care		
cast		Application of a solid material to immobilize an extremity or portion of the body as a result of a fracture, dislocation, or severe injury. It may be made of plaster of Paris or fiberglass.
fixation		Procedure to stabilize a fractured bone while it heals. *External fixation* includes casts, splints, and pins inserted through the skin. *Internal fixation* includes pins, plates, rods, screws, and wires that are applied during an *open reduction*.
reduction		Correcting a fracture by realigning the bone fragments. *Closed reduction* is doing this manipulation without entering the body. *Open reduction* is the process of making a surgical incision at the site of the fracture to do the reduction. This is necessary when bony fragments need to be removed or *internal fixation* such as plates or pins are required.
traction		Applying a pulling force on a fractured or dislocated limb or the vertebral column in order to restore normal alignment.

■ Pharmacology

CLASSIFICATION	WORD PARTS	ACTION	EXAMPLES
bone reabsorption inhibitors		Conditions that result in weak and fragile bones, such as osteoporosis and Paget's disease, are improved by medications that reduce the reabsorption of bones.	alendronate, Fosamax; ibandronate, Boniva
calcium supplements and vitamin D therapy		Maintaining high blood levels of calcium in association with vitamin D helps maintain bone density; used to treat osteomalacia, osteoporosis, and rickets.	calcium carbonate, Oystercal, Tums; calcium citrate, Cal-Citrate, Citracal
corticosteroids	cortic/o = outer portion	A hormone produced by the adrenal cortex that has very strong anti-inflammatory properties. It is particularly useful in treating rheumatoid arthritis.	prednisone; methylprednisolone, Medrol; dexamethasone, Decadron
nonsteroidal anti-inflammatory drugs (NSAIDs)	-al = pertaining to anti- = against -ory = pertaining to	A large group of drugs that provide mild pain relief and anti-inflammatory benefits for conditions such as arthritis.	ibuprofen, Advil, Motrin; naproxen, Aleve, Naprosyn; salicylates, Aspirin

Abbreviations

AE	above elbow	**LLE**	left lower extremity
AK	above knee	**LUE**	left upper extremity
BDT	bone density testing	**NSAID**	nonsteroidal anti-inflammatory drug
BE	below elbow	**OA**	osteoarthritis
BK	below knee	**ORIF**	open reduction–internal fixation
BMD	bone mineral density	**Orth, ortho**	orthopedics
C1, C2, etc.	first cervical vertebra, second cervical vertebra, etc.	**RA**	rheumatoid arthritis
		RLE	right lower extremity
Ca	calcium	**RUE**	right upper extremity
DJD	degenerative joint disease	**SLE**	systemic lupus erythematosus
DXA	dual-energy absorptiometry	**T1, T2, etc.**	first thoracic vertebra, second thoracic vertebra, etc.
FX, Fx	fracture		
HNP	herniated nucleus pulposus	**THA**	total hip arthroplasty
JRA	juvenile rheumatoid arthritis	**THR**	total hip replacement
L1, L2, etc.	first lumbar vertebra, second lumbar vertebra, etc.	**TKA**	total knee arthroplasty
		TKR	total knee replacement
LE	lower extremity	**UE**	upper extremity

Section II: Muscular System at a Glance

Function

Muscles are bundles, sheets, or rings of tissue that produce movement by contracting and pulling on the structures to which they are attached.

Organs

Here is the primary structure that comprises the muscular system.
muscles

Word Parts

Here are the most common word parts (with their meanings) used to build muscular system terms. For a more comprehensive list, refer to the Terminology section of this chapter.

Combining Forms

duct/o	to bring	myocardi/o	heart muscle
extens/o	to stretch out	myos/o	muscle
fasci/o	fibrous band	plant/o	sole of foot
fibr/o	fibers	rotat/o	to revolve
flex/o	to bend	ten/o	tendon
kinesi/o	movement	tend/o	tendon
muscul/o	muscle	tendin/o	tendon
my/o	muscle	vers/o	to turn

Suffixes

-asthenia	weakness
-ion	action, condition
-kinesia	movement
-tonia	tone

Prefixes

ab-	away from
ad-	toward
circum-	around
e-	outward, without
in-	inward, without

Muscular System Illustrated

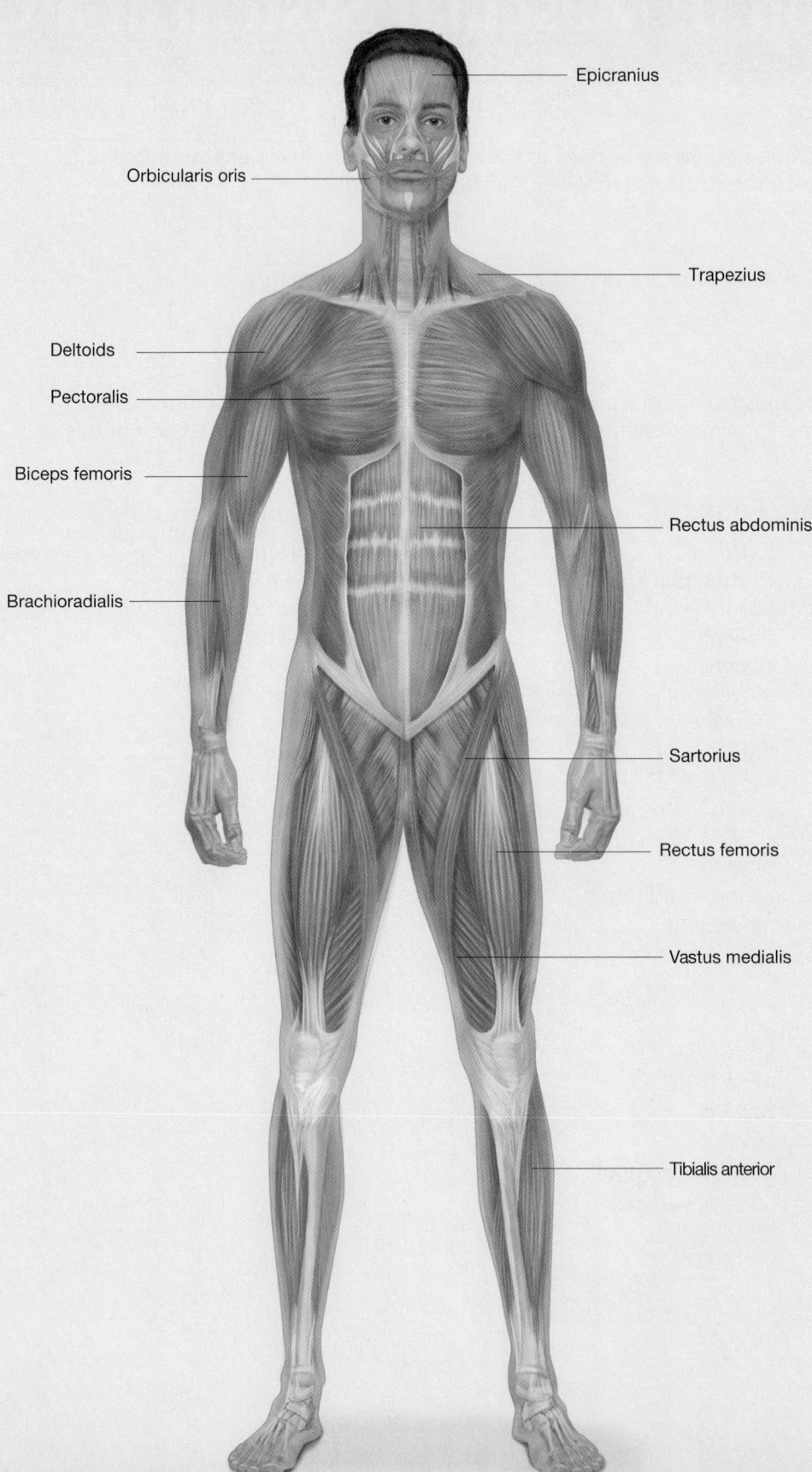

- Epicranius
- Orbicularis oris
- Trapezius
- Deltoids
- Pectoralis
- Biceps femoris
- Rectus abdominis
- Brachioradialis
- Sartorius
- Rectus femoris
- Vastus medialis
- Tibialis anterior

Anatomy and Physiology of the Muscular System

muscle tissue fibers   **muscles**

Muscles are bundles of parallel **muscle tissue fibers.** As these fibers contract (shorten in length) they produce movement of or within the body. The movement may take the form of bringing two bones closer together, pushing food through the digestive system, or pumping blood through blood vessels. In addition to producing movement, muscles also hold the body erect and generate heat.

Types of Muscles

cardiac muscle   **smooth muscle**
involuntary muscles   **voluntary muscles**
skeletal muscle

The three types of muscle tissue are **skeletal muscle, smooth muscle,** and **cardiac muscle** (see Figure 4.21 ■). Muscle tissue may be either voluntary or involuntary. **Voluntary muscles** are those muscles for which a person consciously chooses to contract and for how long and how hard to contract them. The skeletal muscles of the arm and leg are examples of this type of muscle. **Involuntary muscles** are the muscles under the control of the subconscious regions of the brain. The smooth muscles found in internal organs and cardiac muscles are examples of involuntary muscle tissue.

> **MED TERM TIP**
>
> The term *muscle* is the diminutive form of the Latin word *mus* or "little mouse." This is thought to describe how the skin ripples when a muscle contracts, like a little mouse running.

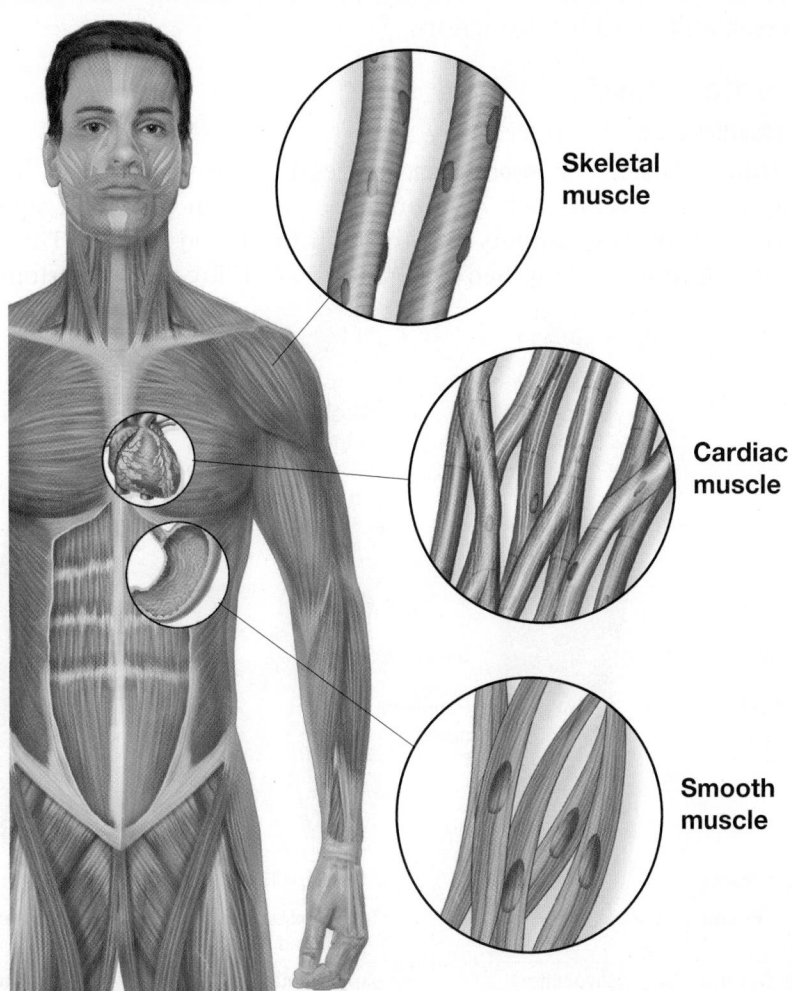

Skeletal muscle

Cardiac muscle

Smooth muscle

■ **Figure 4.21** The three types of muscles: skeletal, smooth, and cardiac.

Skeletal Muscle

fascia (FASH-ee-ah)   **striated muscles** (stry-a-ted)
motor neurons   **tendon** (TEN-dun)
myoneural junction (MY-oh-NOO-rall)

A skeletal muscle is directly or indirectly attached to a bone and produces voluntary movement of the skeleton. It is also referred to as a **striated muscle** because of its striped appearance under the microscope (see Figure 4.22 ■). Each muscle is wrapped in layers of fibrous connective tissue called **fascia.** The fascia tapers at each end of a skeletal muscle to form a very strong **tendon.** The tendon then inserts into the periosteum covering a bone to anchor the muscle to the bone. Skeletal muscles are stimulated by **motor neurons** of the nervous system. The point at which the motor nerve contacts a muscle fiber is called the **myoneural junction.**

Smooth Muscle

visceral muscle (vis-she-ral)

Smooth muscle tissue is found in association with internal organs. For this reason, it is also referred to as **visceral muscle.** The name smooth muscle refers to the muscle's microscopic appearance; it lacks the striations of skeletal muscle (see again Figure 4.22). Smooth muscle is found in the walls of the hollow organs, such as the stomach, tube-shaped organs, such as the respiratory airways, and blood vessels. It is responsible for the involuntary muscle action associated with movement of the internal organs, such as churning food, constricting a blood vessel, and uterine contractions.

Cardiac Muscle

myocardium (my-oh-CAR-dee-um)

Cardiac muscle, or **myocardium,** makes up the wall of the heart (see again Figure 4.22). With each involuntary contraction the heart squeezes to pump blood out of its chambers and through the blood vessels. This muscle will be more thoroughly described in Chapter 5, Cardiovascular System.

■ **Figure 4.22**
Characteristics of the three types of muscles.

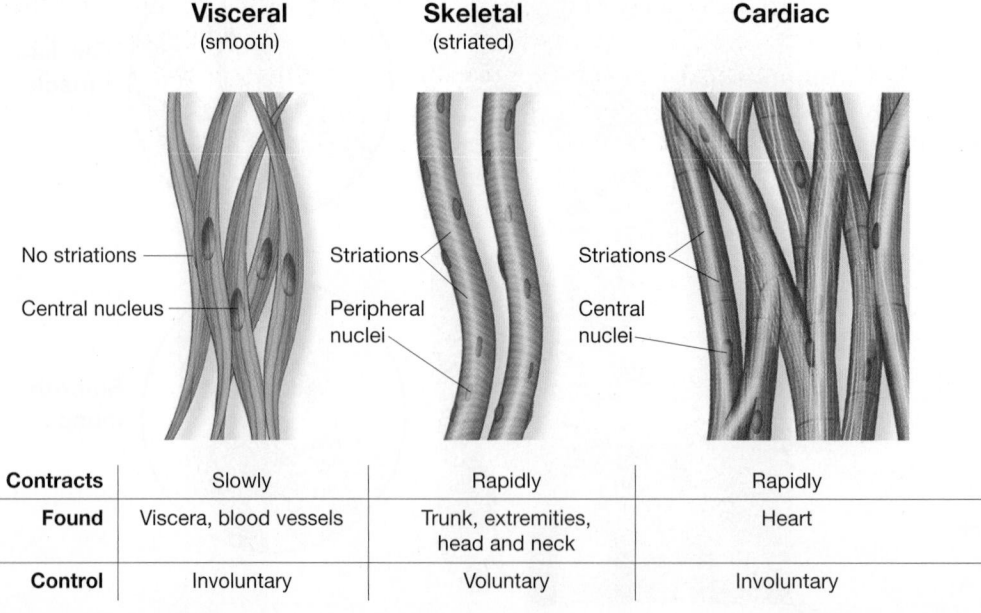

	Visceral (smooth)	Skeletal (striated)	Cardiac
Contracts	Slowly	Rapidly	Rapidly
Found	Viscera, blood vessels	Trunk, extremities, head and neck	Heart
Control	Involuntary	Voluntary	Involuntary

Naming Skeletal Muscles

biceps (BYE-seps)

extensor carpi

external oblique

flexor carpi

gluteus maximus (GLOO-tee-us / MACKS-ih-mus)

rectus abdominis (REK-tus / ab-DOM-ih-nis)

sternocleidomastoid (STER-noh-KLY-doh-MASS-toid)

The name of a muscle often reflects its location, origin and insertion, size, action, fiber direction, or number of attachment points, as illustrated by the following examples:

- **Location:** the term **rectus abdominis** means straight (rectus) abdominal muscle.
- **Origin and insertion:** the **sternocleidomastoid** is named for its two origins (stern/o for sternum and cleid/o for clavicle) and single insertion (mastoid process).
- **Size:** when gluteus, meaning rump area, is combined with maximus, meaning large, we have the term **gluteus maximus.**
- **Action:** the **flexor carpi** and **extensor carpi** muscles are named as such because they produce flexion and extension at the wrist.
- **Fiber direction:** the **external oblique** muscle is an abdominal muscle whose fibers run at an oblique angle.
- **Number of attachment points:** the term *bi,* meaning two, can form the medical term **biceps,** which refers to the muscle in the upper arm that has two heads or connecting points.

Skeletal Muscle Actions

action

antagonistic pairs

insertion

origin

Skeletal muscles are attached to two different bones and overlap a joint. When a muscle contracts, the two bones move, but not usually equally. The less movable of the two bones is considered to be the starting point of the muscle and is called the **origin.** The more movable bone is considered to be where the muscle ends and is called the **insertion.** The type of movement a muscle produces is called its **action.** Muscles are often arranged around joints in **antagonistic pairs,** meaning that they produce opposite actions. For example, one muscle will bend a joint while its antagonist is responsible for straightening the joint. Some common terminology for muscle actions are described in Table 4.5 ■.

Table 4.5   Muscle Actions Grouped by Antagonistic Pairs

ACTION	WORD PARTS	DESCRIPTION
abduction (ab-DUCK-shun)	ab- = away from duct/o = to bring -ion = action, condition	Movement away from midline of the body (see Figure 4.23 ▮)
adduction (ah-DUCK-shun)	ad- = toward duct/o = to bring -ion = action, condition	Movement toward midline of the body (see again Figure 4.23)
flexion (FLEK-shun)	flex/o = to bend -ion = action, condition	Act of bending or being bent (see Figure 4.24 ▮)
extension (eks-TEN-shun)	extens/o = to stretch out -ion = action, condition	Movement that brings limb into or toward a straight condition (see again Figure 4.24)
dorsiflexion (dor-see-FLEK-shun)	dors/o = back of body flex/o = to bend -ion = action, condition	Backward bending, as of hand or foot (see Figure 4.25A ▮)
plantar flexion (PLAN-tar / FLEK-shun)	plant/o = sole of foot -ar = pertaining to flex/o = to bend -ion = action, condition	Bending sole of foot; pointing toes downward (see Figure 4.25B ▮)

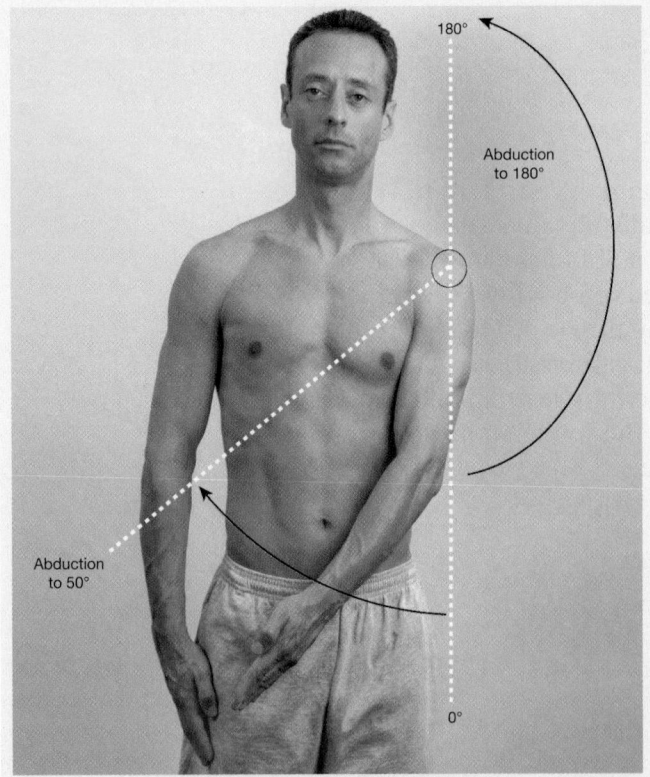

■ **Figure 4.23** Abduction and adduction of the shoulder joint.

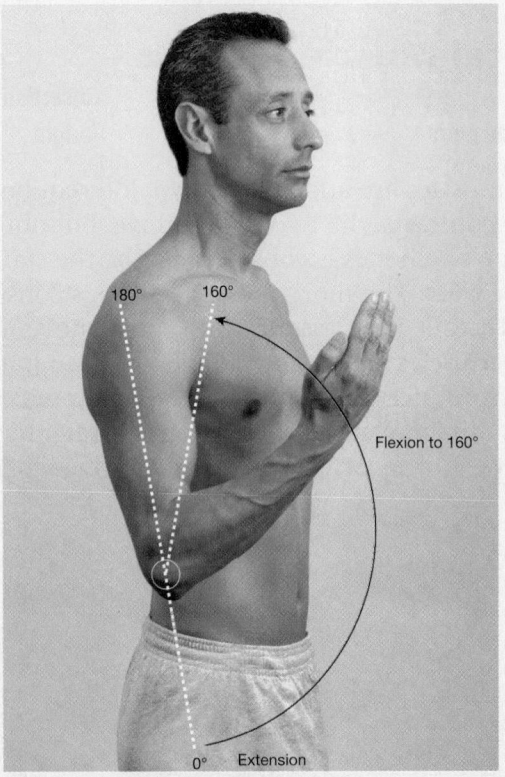

■ **Figure 4.24** Flexion and extension of the elbow joint.

Table 4.5	Muscle Actions Grouped by Antagonistic Pairs (continued)	
ACTION	**WORD PARTS**	**DESCRIPTION**
eversion (ee-VER-zhun)	e- = outward, without vers/o = to turn -ion = action, condition	Turning outward (see Figure 4.26 ▪)
inversion (in-VER-zhun)	in- = inward, without vers/o = to turn -ion = action, condition	Turning inward (see again Figure 4.26)

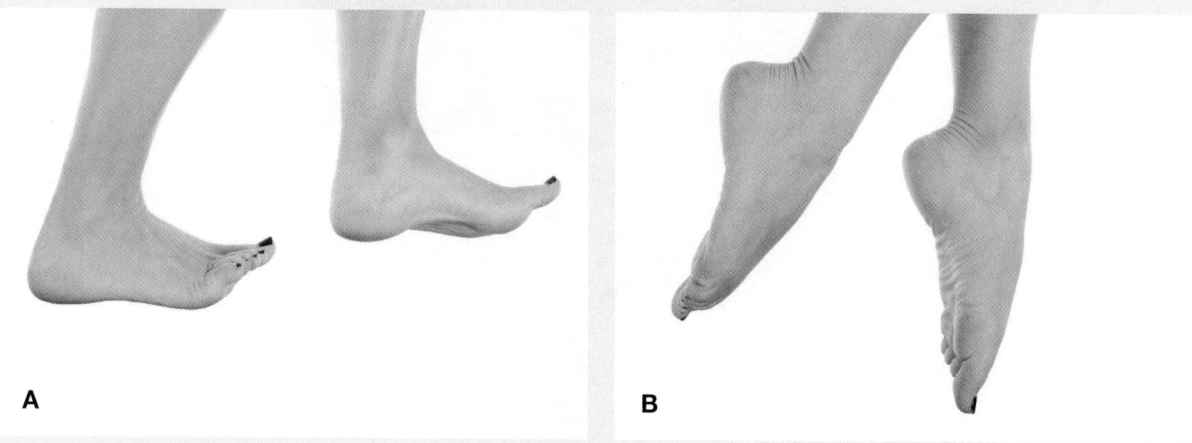

A   **B**

■ **Figure 4.25** Dorsiflexion (A) and plantar flexion (B) of the ankle joint. *(Poulsons Photography/Shutterstock)*

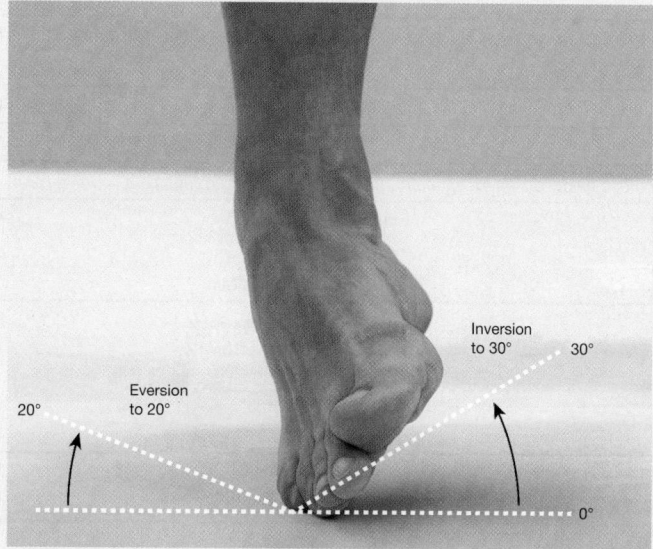

20°   Eversion to 20°   Inversion to 30°   30°

0°

■ **Figure 4.26** Eversion and inversion of the foot.

(Continued)

Table 4.5   Muscle Actions Grouped by Antagonistic Pairs (continued)

ACTION	WORD PARTS	DESCRIPTION
pronation (proh-NAY-shun)		To turn downward or backward as with the hand or foot (see Figure 4.27 ■)

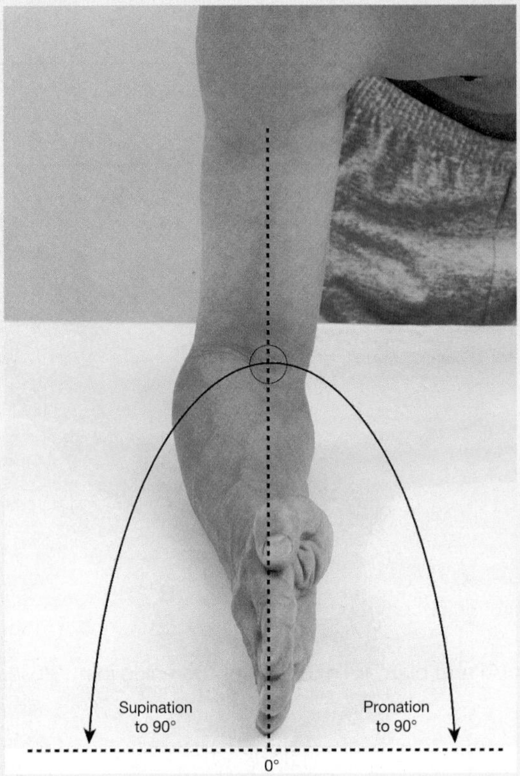

■ Figure 4.27 Pronation and supination of the forearm.

ACTION	WORD PARTS	DESCRIPTION
supination (soo-pin-NAY-shun)		Turning the palm or foot upward (see again Figure 4.27)
elevation		To raise a body part, as in shrugging the shoulders
depression		A downward movement, as in dropping the shoulders
The circular actions described below are an exception to the antagonistic pair arrangement.		
circumduction (sir-kum-DUCK-shun)	circum- = around duct/o = to bring -ion = action, condition	Movement in a circular direction from a central point as if drawing a large, imaginary circle in the air
opposition		Moving thumb away from palm; the ability to move the thumb into contact with the other fingers
rotation	rotat/o = to revolve -ion = action, condition	Moving around a central axis

MED TERM TIP

Primates are the only animals with opposable thumbs.

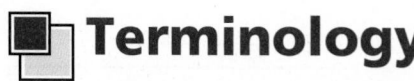

Terminology

Word Parts Used to Build Muscular System Terms

The following lists contain the combining forms, suffixes, and prefixes used to build terms in the remaining sections of this chapter.

Combining Forms

bi/o = life	**kinesi/o** = movement	**myos/o** = muscle
carp/o = wrist	**later/o** = side	**ten/o** = tendon
electr/o = electricity	**muscul/o**–muscle	**tend/o** = tendon
fasci/o = fibrous band	**my/o** = muscle	**tendin/o** = tendon
fibr/o = fibers	**myocardi/o** = heart muscle	

Suffixes

-al = pertaining to	**-graphy** = process of recording	**-pathy** = disease
-algia = pain	**-itis** = inflammation	**-plasty** = surgical repair
-ar = pertaining to	**-kinesia** = movement	**-rrhaphy** = suture
-asthenia = weakness	**-logy** = study of	**-rrhexis** = rupture
-desis = fuse	**-opsy** = view of	**-tonia** = tone
-dynia = pain	**-otomy** = cutting into	**-trophy** = development
-gram = record	**-ous** = pertaining to	

Prefixes

a- = without	**epi-** = over	**poly-** = many
brady- = slow	**hyper-** = excessive	**pseudo-** = false
dys- = abnormal, difficult, painful	**hypo-** = insufficient	

 ## Anatomical Terms

TERM	WORD PARTS	DEFINITION
fascial (FAS-ee-all)	fasci/o = fibrous band -al = pertaining to	pertaining to fascia
muscular (MUSS-kew-lar)	muscul/o = muscle -ar = pertaining to	pertaining to muscles
myocardial (my-oh-CAR-dee-al)	myocardi/o = heart muscle -al = pertaining to	pertaining to heart muscle
skeletal (SKEL-eh-tal)	-al = pertaining to	pertaining to the skeleton
tendinous (TEN-din-us)	tendin/o = tendon -ous = pertaining to	pertaining to tendons

Pathology

TERM	WORD PARTS	DEFINITION
Medical Specialties		
kinesiology (kih-NEE-see-oh-loh-jee)	kinesi/o = movement -logy = study of	The science that studies movement, how it is produced, and the muscles involved.
Signs and Symptoms		
adhesion		Scar tissue forming in the fascia surrounding a muscle, making it difficult to stretch the muscle.
atonia	a- = without -tonia = tone	The lack of muscle tone.
atrophy (AT-rah-fee)	a- = without -trophy = development	Poor muscle development as a result of muscle disease, nervous system disease, or lack of use; commonly referred to as *muscle wasting.*
bradykinesia (brad-ee-kih-NEE-see-ah)	brady- = slow -kinesia = movement	Having slow movements.
contracture (kon-TRACK-chur)		Abnormal shortening of muscle fibers, tendons, or fascia, making it difficult to stretch the muscle.
dyskinesia (dis-kih-NEE-see-ah)	dys- = difficult, painful -kinesia = movement	Having difficult or painful movement.
dystonia	dys- = abnormal -tonia = tone	Having abnormal muscle tone.
hyperkinesia (high-per-kih-NEE-see-ah)	hyper- = excessive -kinesia = movement	Having an excessive amount of movement.
hypertonia	hyper- = excessive -tonia = tone	Having excessive muscle tone.
hypertrophy (high-PER-troh-fee)	hyper- = excessive -trophy = development	Increase in muscle bulk as a result of use, as with lifting weights.
hypokinesia (HI-poh-kih-NEE-see-ah)	hypo- = insufficient -kinesia = movement	Having an insufficient amount of movement.
hypotonia	hypo- = insufficient -tonia = tone	Having insufficient muscle tone.
intermittent claudication (klaw-dih-KAY-shun)		Attacks of severe pain and lameness caused by ischemia of the muscles, typically the calf muscles; brought on by walking even very short distances.
myalgia (my-AL-jee-ah)	my/o = muscle -algia = pain	Muscle pain.
myasthenia (my-ass-THEE-nee-ah)	my/o = muscle -asthenia = weakness	Muscle weakness.
myotonia	my/o = muscle -tonia = tone	Muscle tone.
spasm		Sudden, involuntary, strong muscle contraction.

Pathology *(continued)*

TERM	WORD PARTS	DEFINITION
tenodynia (ten-oh-DIN-ee-ah)	ten/o = tendon -dynia = pain	Tendon pain.
Muscles		
fasciitis (fas-ee-EYE-tis)	fasci/o = fibrous band -itis = inflammation	Inflammation of fascia.
fibromyalgia (figh-broh-my-AL-jee-ah)	fibr/o = fibers my/o = muscle -algia = pain	Condition with widespread aching and pain in the muscles and soft tissue.
lateral epicondylitis (ep-ih-kon-dih-LYE-tis)	later/o = side -al = pertaining to epi- = over -itis = inflammation	Inflammation of the muscle attachment to the lateral epicondyle of the elbow. Often caused by strongly gripping. Commonly called *tennis elbow.*
muscular dystrophy (MD) (MUSS-kew-ler / DIS-troh-fee)	muscul/o = muscle -ar = pertaining to dys- = abnormal -trophy = development	Inherited disease causing a progressive muscle degeneration, weakness, and atrophy.
myopathy (my-OPP-ah-thee)	my/o = muscle -pathy = disease	A general term for muscle disease.
myorrhexis (my-oh-REK-sis)	my/o = muscle -rrhexis = rupture	Tearing a muscle.
polymyositis (pol-ee-my-oh-SIGH-tis)	poly- = many myos/o = muscle -itis = inflammation	The simultaneous inflammation of two or more muscles.
pseudohypertrophic muscular dystrophy (soo-doh-HIGH-per-troh-fic)	pseudo- = false hyper- = excessive -trophy = development muscul/o = muscle -ar = pertaining to dys- = abnormal -trophy = development	A type of inherited muscular dystrophy in which the muscle tissue is gradually replaced by fatty tissue, making the muscle look strong. Also called *Duchenne's muscular dystrophy.*
torticollis (tore-tih-KOLL-iss)		Severe neck spasms pulling the head to one side. Commonly called *wryneck* or a *crick in the neck.*
Tendons, Muscles, and/or Ligaments		
carpal tunnel syndrome (CTS)	carp/o = wrist -al = pertaining to	Repetitive motion disorder with pain caused by compression of the finger flexor tendons and median nerve as they pass through the carpal tunnel of the wrist.
ganglion cyst (GANG-lee-on)		Cyst that forms on tendon sheath, usually on hand, wrist, or ankle.
repetitive motion disorder		Group of chronic disorders involving the tendon, muscle, joint, and nerve damage, resulting from the tissue being subjected to pressure, vibration, or repetitive movements for prolonged periods.

Pathology *(continued)*

TERM	WORD PARTS	DEFINITION
rotator cuff injury		The rotator cuff consists of the joint capsule of the shoulder joint reinforced by the tendons from several shoulder muscles. The high degree of flexibility at the shoulder joint puts the rotator cuff at risk for strain and tearing.
strain		Damage to the muscle, tendons, or ligaments due to overuse or overstretching.
tendinitis (ten-dih-NIGH-tis)	tendin/o = tendon -itis = inflammation	Inflammation of a tendon.

Diagnostic Procedures

TERM	WORD PARTS	DEFINITION
Clinical Laboratory Test		
creatine phosphokinase (CPK) (KREE-ah-teen / foss-foe-KYE-nase)		Muscle enzyme found in skeletal muscle and cardiac muscle. Blood levels become elevated in disorders such as heart attack, muscular dystrophy, and other skeletal muscle pathologies.
Additional Diagnostic Procedures		
deep tendon reflexes (DTR)		Muscle contraction in response to a stretch caused by striking the muscle tendon with a reflex hammer. Test used to determine if muscles are responding properly.
electromyogram (EMG) (ee-lek-troh-MY-oh-gram)	electr/o = electricity my/o = muscle -gram = record	The hardcopy record produced by electromyography.
electromyography (EMG) (ee-lek-troh-my-OG-rah-fee)	electr/o = electricity my/o = muscle -graphy = process of recording	Study and record of the strength and quality of muscle contractions as a result of electrical stimulation.
muscle biopsy (BYE-op-see)	bi/o = life -opsy = view of	Removal of muscle tissue for pathological examination.

Therapeutic Procedures

TERM	WORD PARTS	DEFINITION
Surgical Procedures		
carpal tunnel release	carp/o = wrist -al = pertaining to	Surgical cutting of the ligament in the wrist to relieve nerve pressure caused by carpal tunnel syndrome, which can result from repetitive motion such as typing.
fasciotomy (fas-ee-OT-oh-mee)	fasci/o = fibrous band -otomy = cutting into	A surgical procedure that cuts into fascia.

Therapeutic Procedures *(continued)*

TERM	WORD PARTS	DEFINITION
myoplasty (MY-oh-plas-tee)	my/o = muscle -plasty = surgical repair	A surgical procedure to repair a muscle.
myorrhaphy (MY-or-ah-fee)	my/o = muscle -rrhaphy = suture	To suture a muscle.
tendoplasty (TEN-doh-plas-tee)	tend/o = tendon -plasty = surgical repair	A surgical procedure to repair a tendon.
tendotomy (tend-OT-oh-mee)	tend/o = tendon -otomy = cutting into	A surgical procedure that cuts into a tendon.
tenodesis (ten-oh-DEE-sis)	ten/o = tendon -desis = fuse	Surgical procedure to stabilize a joint by anchoring down the tendons of the muscles that move the joint.
tenoplasty (TEN-oh-plas-tee)	ten/o = tendon -plasty = surgical repair	A surgical procedure to repair a tendon.
tenorrhaphy (tah-NOR-ah-fee)	ten/o = tendon -rrhaphy = suture	To suture a tendon.

Pharmacology

CLASSIFICATION	WORD PARTS	ACTION	EXAMPLES
skeletal muscle relaxants	-al = pertaining to	Medication to relax skeletal muscles in order to reduce muscle spasms. Also called *antispasmodics.*	cyclobenzaprine, Flexeril; carisoprodol, Soma

Abbreviations

CTS	carpal tunnel syndrome	**EMG**	electromyogram
CPK	creatine phosphokinase	**IM**	intramuscular
DTR	deep tendon reflex	**MD**	muscular dystrophy

Chapter Review

Real-World Applications

Medical Record Analysis

This Discharge Summary contains 10 medical terms. Underline each term and write it in the list below the report. Then define each term. You will find Chapter 14 of your textbook helpful with the rehabilitation terms.

Discharge Summary

Admitting Diagnosis:	Osteoarthritis bilateral knees.
Final Diagnosis:	Osteoarthritis bilateral knees with right TKA
History of Present Illness:	Patient is a 68-year-old male. He reports he has experienced occasional knee pain and swelling since he injured his knees playing football in high school. These symptoms became worse while he was in his 50s and working on a concrete surface. The right knee has always been more painful than the left. He saw his orthopedic surgeon six months ago because of constant knee pain and swelling severe enough to interfere with sleep and all activities. He required a cane to walk. CT scan indicated severe bilateral osteoarthritis. He is admitted to the hospital at this time for TKR right knee.
Summary of Hospital Course:	Patient tolerated the surgical procedure well. He began intensive physical therapy for lower extremity ROM and strengthening exercises and gait training with a walker. He received occupational therapy instruction in ADLs, especially dressing and personal care. He was able to transfer himself out of bed by the third post-op day and was able to ambulate 150 ft with a walker and dress himself on the fifth post-op day.
Discharge Plans:	Patient was discharged home with his wife one week post-op. He will continue rehabilitation as an outpatient. Return to office for post-op checkup in one week.

Term	Definition
1 _____	_____
2 _____	_____
3 _____	_____
4 _____	_____
5 _____	_____
6 _____	_____
7 _____	_____
8 _____	_____
9 _____	_____
10 _____	_____

Chart Note Transcription

The chart note below contains 11 phrases that can be reworded with a medical term that you learned in this chapter. Each phrase is identified with an underline. Determine the medical term and write your answers in the space provided.

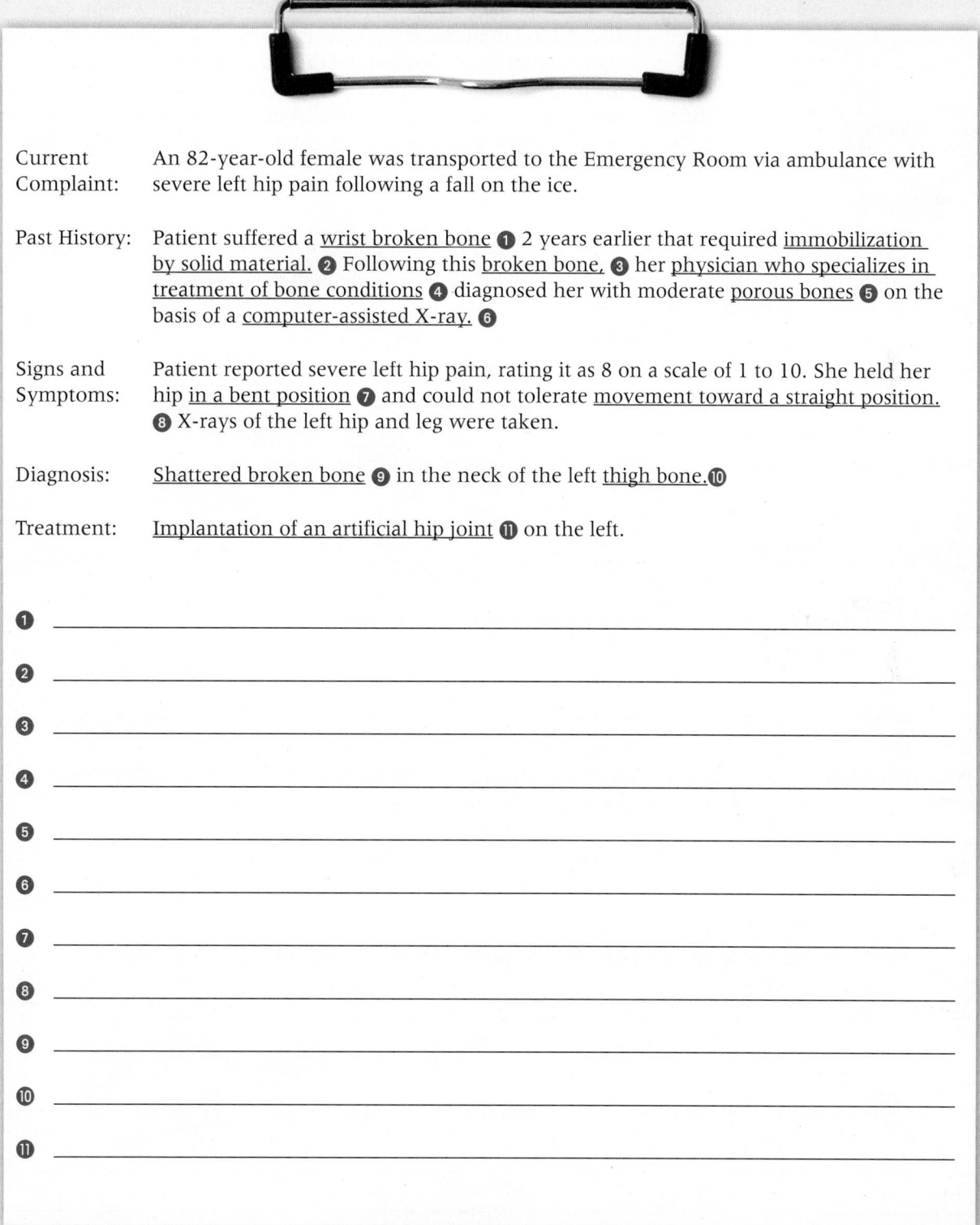

Current Complaint: An 82-year-old female was transported to the Emergency Room via ambulance with severe left hip pain following a fall on the ice.

Past History: Patient suffered a <u>wrist broken bone</u> **1** 2 years earlier that required <u>immobilization by solid material.</u> **2** Following this <u>broken bone,</u> **3** her <u>physician who specializes in treatment of bone conditions</u> **4** diagnosed her with moderate <u>porous bones</u> **5** on the basis of a <u>computer-assisted X-ray.</u> **6**

Signs and Symptoms: Patient reported severe left hip pain, rating it as 8 on a scale of 1 to 10. She held her hip <u>in a bent position</u> **7** and could not tolerate <u>movement toward a straight position.</u> **8** X-rays of the left hip and leg were taken.

Diagnosis: <u>Shattered broken bone</u> **9** in the neck of the left <u>thigh bone.</u>**10**

Treatment: <u>Implantation of an artificial hip joint</u> **11** on the left.

1 _____

2 _____

3 _____

4 _____

5 _____

6 _____

7 _____

8 _____

9 _____

10 _____

11 _____

Case Study

Below is a case study presentation of a patient with a condition covered by this chapter. Read the case study and answer the questions below. Some questions will ask for information not included within this chapter. Use your text, a medical dictionary, or any other reference material you choose to answer these questions.

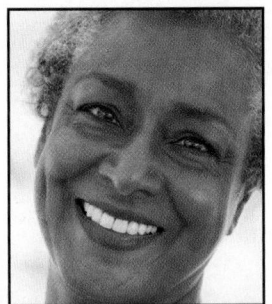

Mary Pearl, age 60, has come into the physician's office complaining of swelling, stiffness, and arthralgia, especially in her elbows, wrists, and hands. A bone scan revealed acute inflammation in multiple joints with damaged articular cartilage and an erythrocyte sedimentation rate blood test indicated a significant level of acute inflammation in the body. A diagnosis of acute episode of rheumatoid arthritis was made. The physician ordered nonsteroidal anti-inflammatory medication and physical therapy. The therapist initiated a treatment program of hydrotherapy and AROM exercises.

(Monkey Business Images/Shutterstock)

1. What pathological condition does this patient have? Look this condition up in a reference source and include a short description of it.

   _____

   _____

2. What type of long-term damage may occur in a patient with rheumatoid arthritis?

   _____

   _____

3. Describe the other major type of arthritis mentioned in your textbook.

   _____

   _____

4. What two diagnostic procedures did the physician order? Describe them in your own words. What were the results? (One of these procedures is described in Chapter 6 of your text.)

   _____

   _____

5. What treatments were ordered? Explain what the physical therapy procedures involve (refer to Chapter 14).

   _____

   _____

6. This patient is experiencing an acute episode. Explain what this phrase means and contrast it with chronic.

   _____

   _____

Practice Exercises

A. Complete the Statement

1. The two divisions of the human skeleton are the _____ and _____.

2. Another name for visceral muscle is _____ muscle.

3. The five functions of the skeletal system are to _____, _____, _____, _____, and _____.

4. Nerves contact skeletal muscle fibers at the _____ junction.

5. _____ bones are roughly as long as they are wide.

6. The membrane covering bones is called the _____.

7. A Colles' fracture occurs in the _____.

8. Another name for spongy bone is _____ bone.

9. _____ joints are the most common joints in the body.

10. The three types of muscle are _____, _____, and _____.

11. A _____ is a smooth, round opening in bones.

12. The _____ is the shaft of a long bone.

B. Adjective Form Practice

Give the adjective form for the following bones.

1. femur _____

2. sternum _____

3. clavicle _____

4. coccyx _____

5. maxilla _____

6. tibia _____

7. patella _____

8. phalanges _____

9. humerus _____

10. pubis _____

C. Combining Form Practice

The combining form **oste/o** refers to bone. Use it to write a term that means:

1. bone cell _____

2. embryonic bone cell _____

3. porous bone _____

4. disease of the bone _____

5. cutting into a bone _____

6. instrument to cut bone _____

7. inflammation of the bone and bone marrow _____

8. softening of the bones _____

9. tumor composed of both bone and cartilage _____

The combining form **my/o** refers to muscle. Use it to write a term that means:

10. muscle disease _____

11. surgical repair of muscle _____

12. suture of muscle _____

13. record of muscle electricity _____

14. muscle weakness _____

The combining form **ten/o** refers to tendons. Use it to write a term that means:

15. tendon pain _____

16. tendon suture _____

The combining form **arthr/o** refers to the joints. Use it to write a term that means:

17. surgical fusion of a joint _____

18. surgical repair of a joint _____

19. cutting into a joint _____

20. inflammation of a joint _____

21. puncture to withdraw fluid from a joint _____

22. pain in the joints _____

The combining form **chondr/o** refers to cartilage. Use it to write a term that means:

23. cartilage removal _____

24. cartilage tumor _____

25. cartilage softening _____

D. Name That Suffix

	Suffix	Example from Chapter
1. fuse	_____	_____
2. weakness	_____	_____
3. slipping	_____	_____
4. to surgically break	_____	_____
5. movement	_____	_____
6. porous	_____	_____

E. Spinal Column Practice

Name the five regions of the spinal column and indicate the number of bones in each area.

Name	Number of Bones
1. _____	_____
2. _____	_____
3. _____	_____
4. _____	_____
5. _____	_____

F. Prefix and Suffix Practice

Circle the prefix and/or suffix. Place a *P* for prefix or an *S* for suffix over these word parts then, define the term.

1. arthroscopy _____

2. intervertebral _____

3. chondromalacia _____

4. diskectomy _____

5. intracranial _____

6. subscapular _____

G. Define the Combining Form

	Definition	Example from Chapter
1. lamin/o	_____	_____
2. ankyl/o	_____	_____
3. chondr/o	_____	_____
4. spondyl/o	_____	_____
5. my/o	_____	_____
6. orth/o	_____	_____
7. kyph/o	_____	_____
8. tend/o	_____	_____
9. myel/o	_____	_____
10. articul/o	_____	_____

H. What's the Abbreviation?

1. intramuscular _____

2. total knee replacement _____

3. herniated nucleus pulposus _____

4. deep tendon reflex _____

5. upper extremity _____

6. fifth lumbar vertebra _____

7. bone density testing _____

8. above the knee _____

9. fracture _____

10. nonsteroidal anti-inflammatory drug _____

I. Define the Term

1. orthopedics _____

2. chiropractic _____

3. podiatry _____

4. orthotics _____

5. prosthetics _____

J. Terminology Matching

Match each term to its definition.

1. _____ abduction
2. _____ rotation
3. _____ plantar flexion
4. _____ extension
5. _____ dorsiflexion
6. _____ flexion
7. _____ adduction
8. _____ opposition

a. backward bending of the foot
b. bending the foot to point toes toward the ground
c. straightening motion
d. motion around a central axis
e. motion away from the body
f. moving the thumb away from the palm
g. motion toward the body
h. bending motion

K. Fill in the Blank

carpal tunnel syndrome	rickets	lateral epicondylitis	systemic lupus erythematosus
scoliosis	osteogenic sarcoma	pseudohypertrophic muscular dystrophy	
herniated nucleus pulposus	osteoporosis		
	spondylolisthesis		

1. Mrs. Lewis, age 84, broke her hip. Her physician will be running tests for what potential ailment? _____

2. Jamie, age 6 months, is being given orange juice and vitamin supplements to avoid what condition? _____

3. George has severe elbow pain after playing tennis four days in a row. He may have _____ .

4. Marshall's doctor told him that he had a ruptured disk. The medical term for this is _____ .

5. Mr. Jefferson's physician has discovered a tumor at the end of his femur. He has been admitted to the hospital for a biopsy to rule out what type of bone cancer? _____

6. The school nurse has asked Janelle to bend over so that she may examine her back to see if she is developing a lateral curve. What is the nurse looking for? _____

7. Gerald has experienced a gradual loss of muscle strength over the past 5 years even though his muscles look large and healthy. The doctors believe he has an inherited muscle disease. What is that disease? _____

8. Roberta has suddenly developed arthritis in her hands and knees. Rheumatoid arthritis had been ruled out, but what other auto-immune disease might Roberta have? _____

9. Mark's X-ray demonstrated forward sliding of a lumbar vertebra; the radiologist diagnosed _____ .

10. The orthopedist determined that Marcia's repetitive wrist movements at work caused her to develop _____ .

L. Fracture Type Matching

Match each fracture type to its definition.

1. _____ comminuted
2. _____ greenstick
3. _____ compound
4. _____ simple
5. _____ impacted
6. _____ transverse
7. _____ oblique
8. _____ spiral

a. fracture line is at an angle

b. fracture line curves around the bone

c. bone is splintered or crushed

d. bone is pressed into itself

e. fracture line is straight across bone

f. skin has been broken

g. no open wound

h. bone only partially broken

M. Name That Anatomical Name

1. knee cap _____

2. ankle bones _____

3. collar bone _____

4. thigh bone _____

5. toe bones _____

6. wrist bones _____

7. shin bone _____

8. shoulder blade _____

9. finger bones _____

N. What Does it Stand For?

1. DJD _____

2. EMG _____

3. C1 _____

4. T6 _____

5. IM _____

6. DTR _____

7. JRA _____

8. LLE _____

9. ortho _____

10. CTS _____

O. Define the Term

1. chondroplasty _____

2. bradykinesia _____

3. osteoporosis _____

4. lordosis _____

5. atrophy _____

6. myeloma _____

7. prosthesis _____

8. craniotomy _____

9. arthrocentesis _____

10. bursitis _____

P. Pharmacology Challenge

Fill in the classification for each drug description, then match the brand name.

Drug Description	Classification	Brand Name
1. _____ Treats mild pain and anti-inflammatory	_____	a. Flexeril
2. _____ Hormone with anti-inflammatory properties	_____	b. Aleve
3. _____ Reduces muscle spasms	_____	c. Fosamax
4. _____ Treats conditions of weakened bones	_____	d. Oystercal
5. _____ Maintains blood calcium levels	_____	e. Medrol

MEDICAL TERMINOLOGY INTERACTIVE

Medical Terminology Interactive is a premium online homework management system that includes a host of features to help you study. Registered users will find:

- Fun games and activities built within a virtual hospital
- Powerful tools that track and analyze your results—allowing you to create a personalized learning experience
- Videos, flashcards, and audio pronunciations to help enrich your progress
- Streaming video lesson presentations and self-paced learning modules

www.pearsonhighered.com/mti

Labeling Exercise

Image A

Write the labels for this figure on the numbered lines provided.

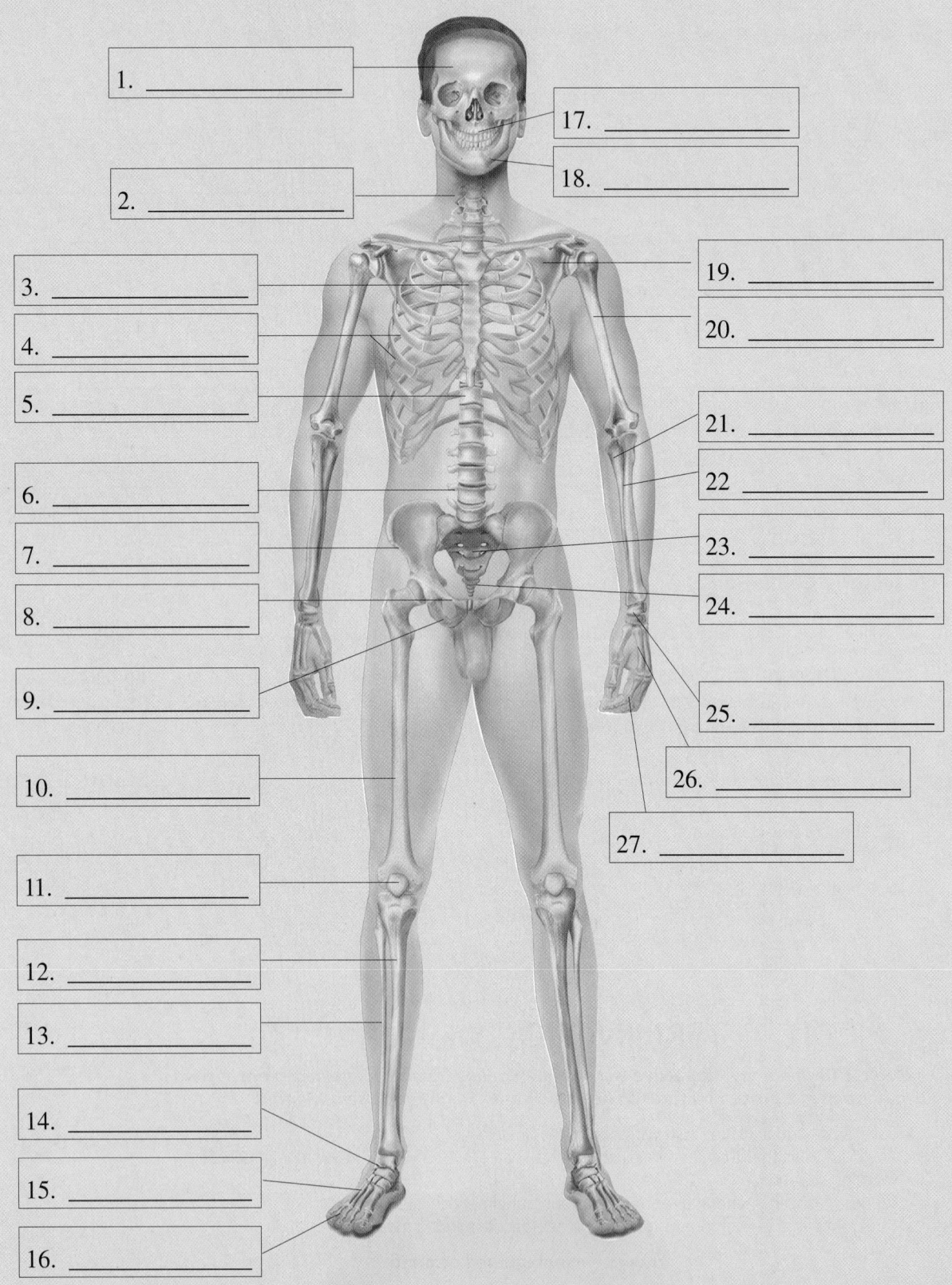

1. _____

2. _____

3. _____

4. _____

5. _____

6. _____

7. _____

8. _____

9. _____

10. _____

11. _____

12. _____

13. _____

14. _____

15. _____

16. _____

17. _____

18. _____

19. _____

20. _____

21. _____

22. _____

23. _____

24. _____

25. _____

26. _____

27. _____

Image B

Write the labels for this figure on the numbered lines provided.

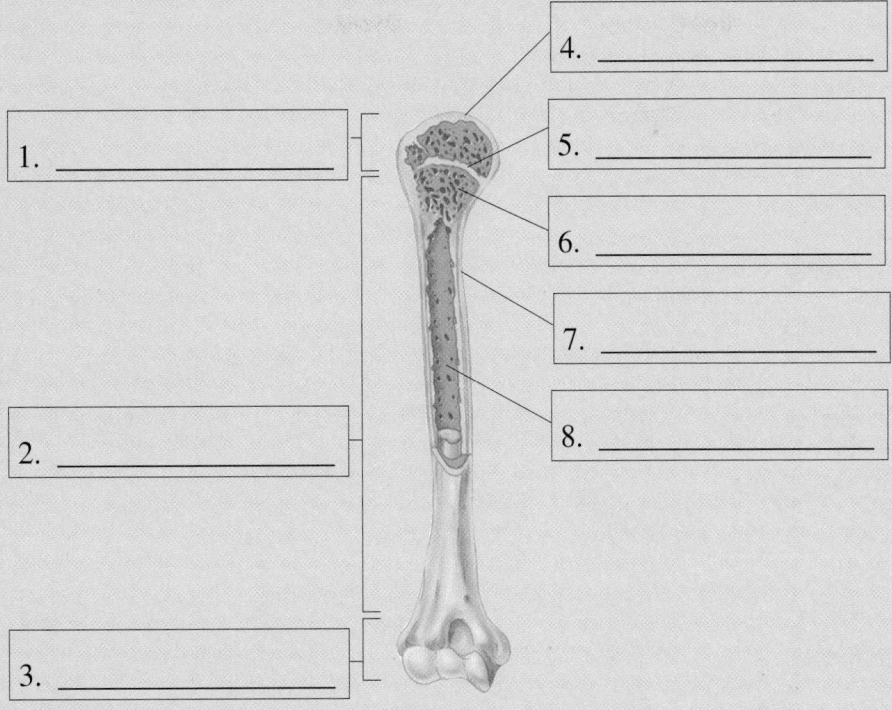

1. _____

2. _____

3. _____

4. _____

5. _____

6. _____

7. _____

8. _____

Image C

Write the labels for this figure on the numbered lines provided.

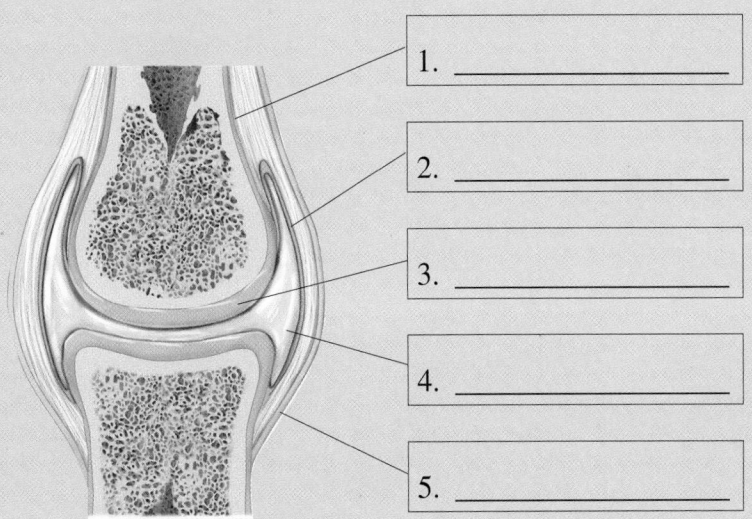

1. _____

2. _____

3. _____

4. _____

5. _____

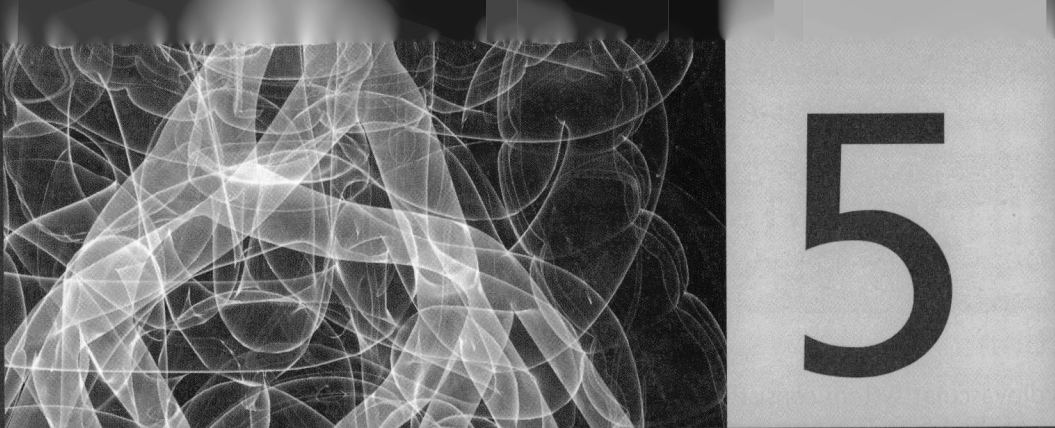

5

CARDIOVASCULAR SYSTEM

Learning Objectives

Upon completion of this chapter, you will be able to

- Identify and define the combining forms and suffixes introduced in this chapter.
- Correctly spell and pronounce medical terms and major anatomical structures relating to the cardiovascular system.
- Describe the major organs of the cardiovascular system and their functions.
- Describe the anatomy of the heart.
- Describe the flow of blood through the heart.
- Explain how the electrical conduction system controls the heartbeat.
- List and describe the characteristics of the three types of blood vessels.
- Define pulse and blood pressure.
- Identify and define cardiovascular system anatomical terms.
- Identify and define selected cardiovascular system pathology terms.
- Identify and define selected cardiovascular system diagnostic procedures.
- Identify and define selected cardiovascular system therapeutic procedures.
- Identify and define selected medications relating to the cardiovascular system.
- Define selected abbreviations associated with the cardiovascular system.

Cardiovascular System at a Glance

Function

The cardiovascular system consists of the pump and vessels that distribute blood to all areas of the body. This system allows for the delivery of needed substances to the cells of the body as well as for the removal of wastes.

Organs

Here are the primary structures that comprise the cardiovascular system.

blood vessels   **heart**
- arteries
- capillaries
- veins

Word Parts

Here are the most common word parts (with their meanings) used to build cardiovascular system terms. For a more comprehensive list, refer to the Terminology section of this chapter.

Combining Forms

angi/o	vessel	phleb/o	vein
aort/o	aorta	sphygm/o	pulse
arteri/o	artery	steth/o	chest
ather/o	fatty substance	thromb/o	clot
atri/o	atrium	valv/o	valve
cardi/o	heart	valvul/o	valve
coron/o	heart	varic/o	dilated vein
corpor/o	body	vascul/o	blood vessel
embol/o	plug	vas/o	vessel, duct
isch/o	to hold back	ven/o	vein
myocardi/o	heart muscle	ventricul/o	ventricle
pect/o	chest		

Suffixes

-manometer	instrument to measure pressure
-ole	small
-tension	pressure
-tonic	pertaining to tone
-ule	small

Cardiovascular System Illustrated

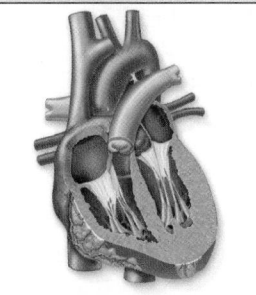

heart, p. 141

Pumps blood through
blood vessels

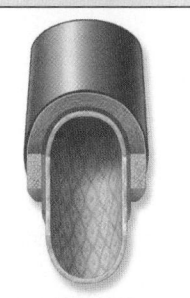

artery, p. 147

Carries blood away
from the heart

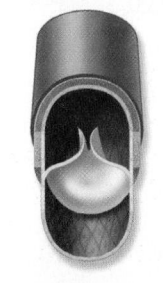

vein, p. 149

Carries blood
towards the heart

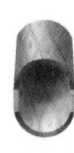

capillary, p. 149

Exchange site between
blood and tissues

Anatomy and Physiology of the Cardiovascular System

arteries

blood vessels

capillaries

carbon dioxide

circulatory system

deoxygenated (dee-OK-sih-jen-ay-ted)

heart

oxygen

oxygenated (OK-sih-jen-ay-ted)

pulmonary circulation
(PULL-mon-air-ee / ser-kew-LAY-shun)

systemic circulation
(sis-TEM-ik / ser-kew-LAY-shun)

veins

The cardiovascular (CV) system, also called the **circulatory system,** maintains the distribution of blood throughout the body and is composed of the **heart** and the **blood vessels—arteries, capillaries,** and **veins.**

The circulatory system is composed of two parts: the **pulmonary circulation** and the **systemic circulation.** The pulmonary circulation, between the heart and lungs, transports **deoxygenated** blood to the lungs to get oxygen, and then back to the heart. The systemic circulation carries **oxygenated** blood away from the heart to the tissues and cells, and then back to the heart (see Figure 5.1 ■). In this way all the body's cells receive blood and oxygen.

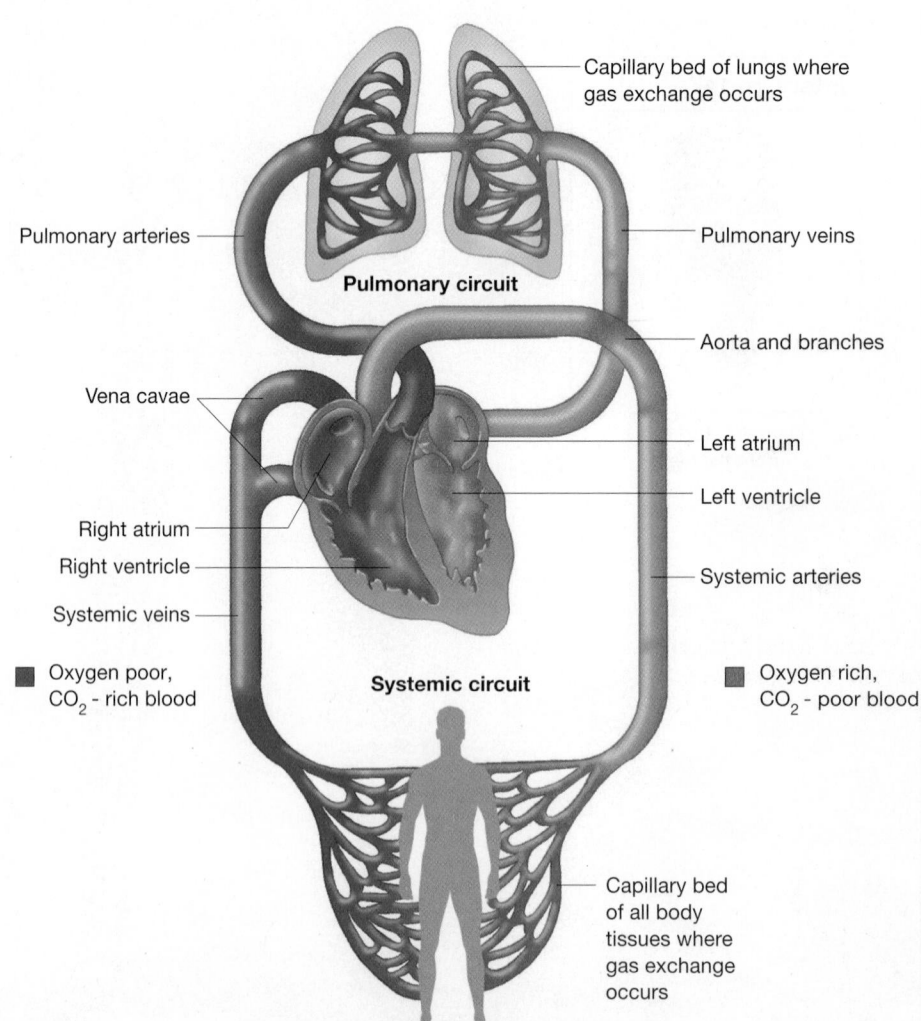

■ Figure 5.1 A schematic of the circulatory system illustrating the pulmonary circulation picking up oxygen from the lungs and the systemic circulation delivering oxygen to the body.

In addition to distributing **oxygen** and other nutrients, such as glucose and amino acids, the cardiovascular system also collects the waste products from the body's cells. **Carbon dioxide** and other waste products produced by metabolic reaction are transported by the cardiovascular system to the lungs, liver, and kidneys where they are eliminated from the body.

Heart

apex (AY-peks)   **cardiac muscle** (CAR-dee-ak)

The heart is a muscular pump made up of **cardiac muscle** fibers that could be considered a muscle rather than an organ. It has four chambers, or cavities, and beats an average of 60–100 beats per minute (bpm) or about 100,000 times in one day. Each time the cardiac muscle contracts, blood is ejected from the heart and pushed throughout the body within the blood vessels.

The heart is located in the mediastinum in the center of the chest cavity; however, it is not exactly centered; more of the heart is on the left side of the mediastinum than the right (see Figure 5.2 ■). At about the size of a fist and shaped like an upside-down pear, the heart lies directly behind the sternum. The tip of the heart at the lower edge is called the **apex**.

> **MED TERM TIP**
>
> Your heart is approximately the size of your clenched fist and pumps 4,000 gallons of blood each day. It will beat at least three billion times during your lifetime.

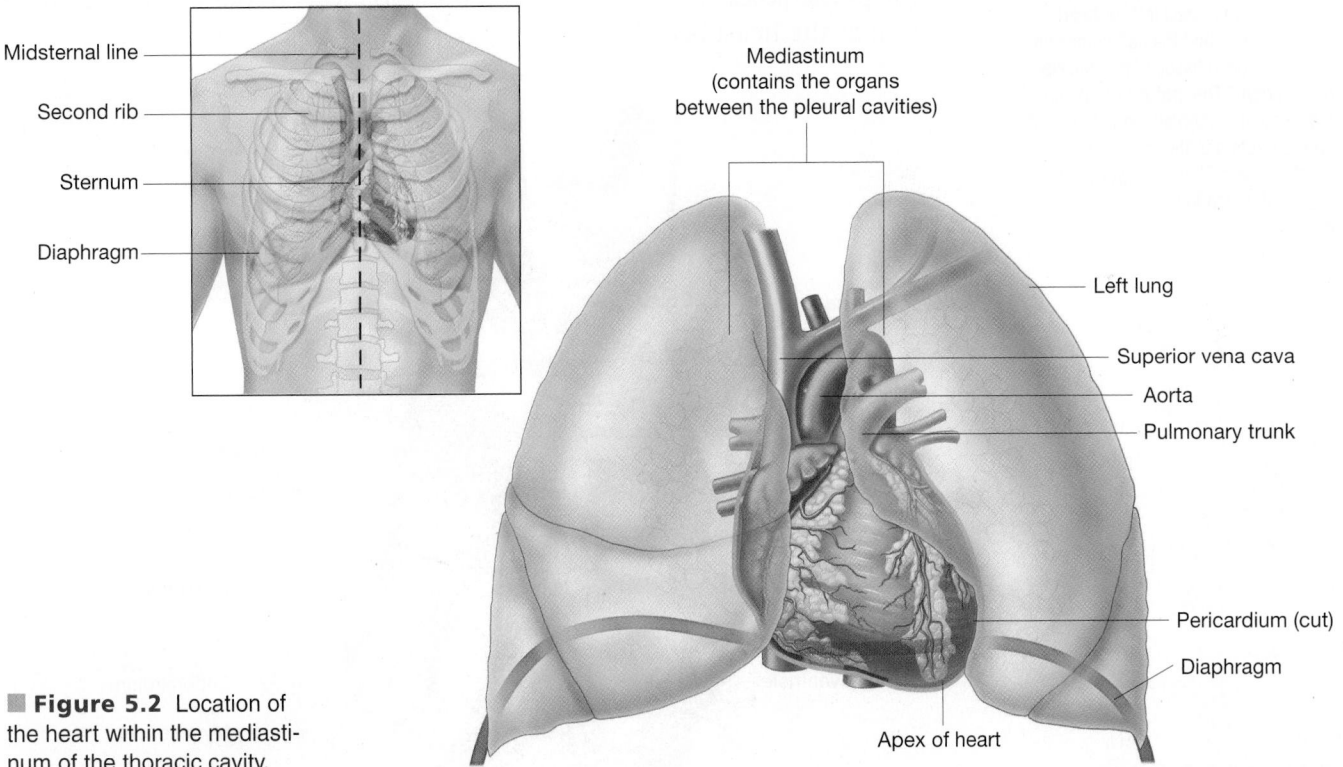

■ **Figure 5.2** Location of the heart within the mediastinum of the thoracic cavity.

Heart Layers

endocardium (en-doh-CAR-dee-um)
epicardium (ep-ih-CAR-dee-um)
myocardium (my-oh-CAR-dee-um)
parietal pericardium
   (pah-RYE-eh-tal / pair-ih-CAR-dee-um)

pericardium (pair-ih-CAR-dee-um)
visceral pericardium
   (VISS-er-al / pair-ih-CAR-dee-um)

The wall of the heart is quite thick and composed of three layers (see Figure 5.3 ■):

MED TERM TIP

These layers become important when studying the disease conditions affecting the heart. For instance, when the prefix *endo-* is added to *carditis*, forming *endocarditis*, we know that the inflammation is within the "inner layer of the heart." In discussing the muscular action of the heart, the prefix *myo-*, meaning "muscle," is added to *cardium* to form the word *myocardium*. The diagnosis *myocardial infarction* (MI), or heart attack, means that the patient has an infarct or "dead tissue in the muscle of the heart." The prefix *peri-*, meaning "around," when added to the word *cardium* refers to the sac "surrounding the heart." Therefore, *pericarditis* is an "inflammation of the outer sac of the heart."

1. The **endocardium** is the inner layer of the heart lining the heart chambers. It is a very smooth, thin layer that serves to reduce friction as the blood passes through the heart chambers.
2. The **myocardium** is the thick, muscular middle layer of the heart. Contraction of this muscle layer develops the pressure required to pump blood through the blood vessels.
3. The **epicardium** is the outer layer of the heart. The heart is enclosed within a double-layered pleural sac, called the **pericardium.** The epicardium is the **visceral pericardium,** or inner layer of the sac. The outer layer of the sac is the **parietal pericardium.** Fluid between the two layers of the sac reduces friction as the heart beats.

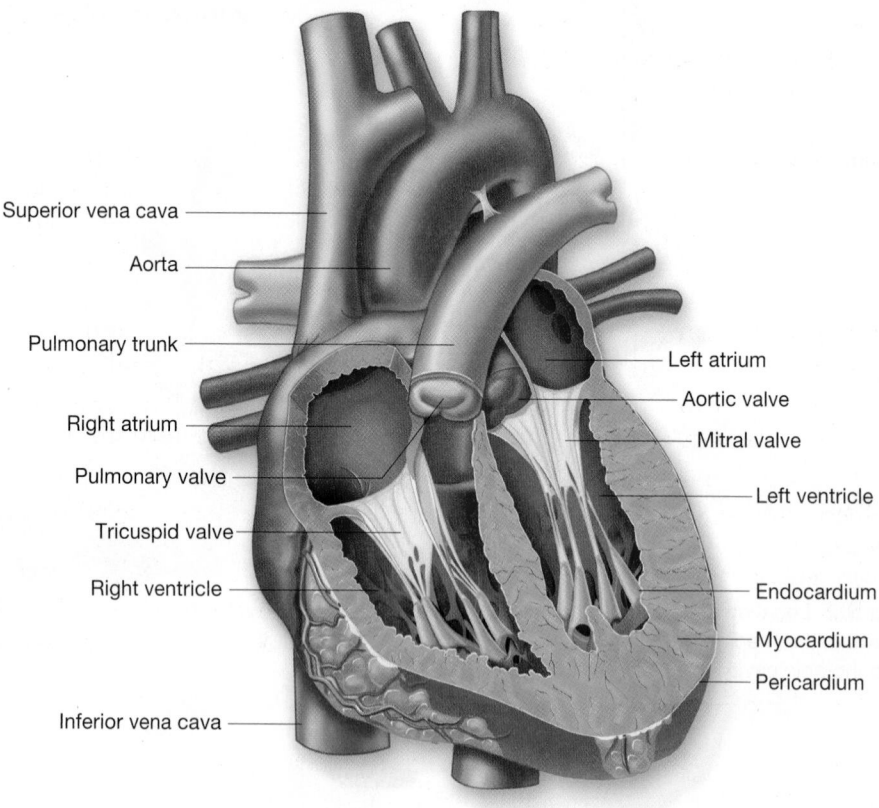

■ **Figure 5.3** Internal view of the heart illustrating the heart chambers, heart layers, and major blood vessels associated with the heart.

Heart Chambers

atria (AY-tree-ah)

interatrial septum
  (in-ter-AY-tree-al / SEP-tum)

interventricular septum
  (in-ter-ven-TRIK-yoo-lar / SEP-tum)

ventricles (VEN-trik-lz)

The heart is divided into four chambers or cavities (see Figures 5.3 and 5.4). There are two **atria,** or upper chambers, and two **ventricles,** or lower chambers. These chambers are divided into right and left sides by walls called the **interatrial septum** and the **interventricular septum.** The atria are the receiving chambers of the heart. Blood returning to the heart via veins first collects in the atria. The ventricles are the pumping chambers. They have a much thicker myocardium and their contraction ejects blood out of the heart and into the great arteries.

> **MED TERM TIP**
>
> The term *ventricle* comes from the Latin term *venter,* which means "little belly." Although it originally referred to the abdomen and then the stomach, it came to stand for any hollow region inside an organ.

Heart Valves

aortic valve (ay-OR-tik)

atrioventricular valve
  (ay-tree-oh-ven-TRIK-yoo-lar)

bicuspid valve (bye-CUSS-pid)

cusps

mitral valve (MY-tral)

pulmonary valve (PULL-mon-air-ee)

semilunar valve (sem-ih-LOO-nar)

tricuspid valve (try-CUSS-pid)

Four valves act as restraining gates to control the direction of blood flow. They are situated at the entrances and exits to the ventricles (see Figure 5.4 ■). Properly functioning valves allow blood to flow only in the forward direction by blocking it from returning to the previous chamber.

The four valves are as follows:

1. **Tricuspid valve:** an **atrioventricular valve** (AV), meaning that it controls the opening between the right atrium and the right ventricle. Once the blood enters the right ventricle, it cannot go back up into the atrium again. The prefix *tri-,* meaning three, indicates that this valve has three leaflets or **cusps.**
2. **Pulmonary valve:** a **semilunar valve.** The prefix *semi-,* meaning half, and the term **lunar,** meaning moon, indicate that this valve looks like a half moon. Located between the right ventricle and the pulmonary artery, this valve prevents blood that has been ejected into the pulmonary artery from returning to the right ventricle as it relaxes.
3. **Mitral valve:** also called the **bicuspid valve,** indicating that it has two cusps. Blood flows through this atrioventricular valve to the left ventricle and cannot go back up into the left atrium.
4. **Aortic valve:** a semilunar valve located between the left ventricle and the aorta. Blood leaves the left ventricle through this valve and cannot return to the left ventricle.

> **MED TERM TIP**
>
> The heart makes two distinct sounds referred to as "lub-dupp." These sounds are produced by the forceful snapping shut of the heart valves. *Lub* is the closing of the atrioventricular valves. *Dupp* is the closing of the semilunar valves.

Figure 5.4 Superior view of heart valves illustrating position, size, and shape of each valve.

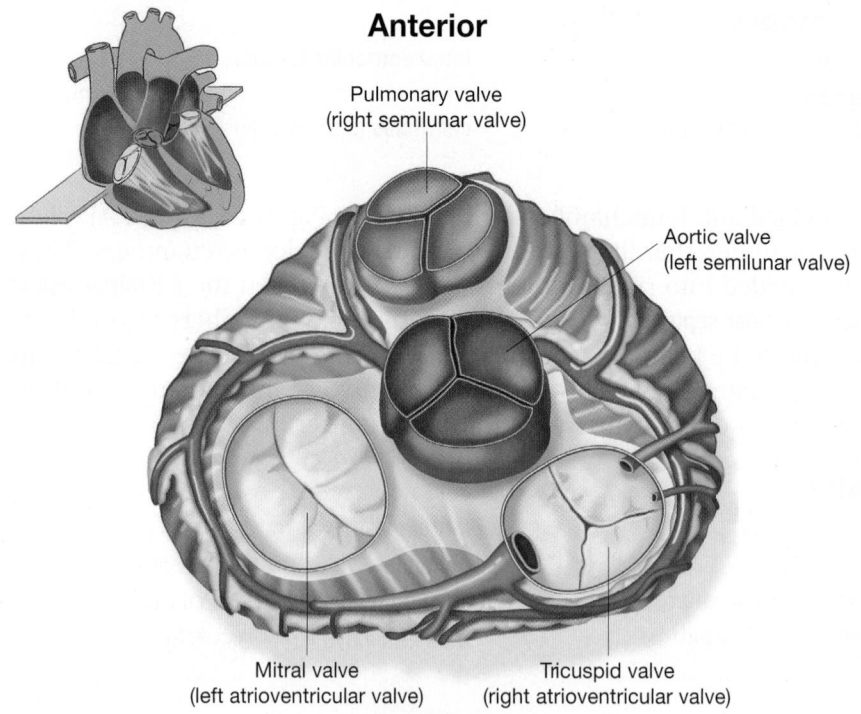

Anterior

Pulmonary valve
(right semilunar valve)

Aortic valve
(left semilunar valve)

Mitral valve
(left atrioventricular valve)

Tricuspid valve
(right atrioventricular valve)

Posterior

Blood Flow Through the Heart

aorta (ay-OR-tah)
diastole (dye-ASS-toe-lee)
inferior vena cava (VEE-nah / KAY-vah)
pulmonary artery (PULL-mon-air-ee)

pulmonary veins
superior vena cava
systole (SIS-toe-lee)

The flow of blood through the heart is very orderly (see Figure 5.5 ■). It progresses through the heart to the lungs, where it receives oxygen; then goes back to the heart; and then out to the body tissues and parts. The normal process of blood flow is:

1. Deoxygenated blood from all the tissues in the body enters a relaxed right atrium via two large veins called the **superior vena cava** and **inferior vena cava.**
2. The right atrium contracts and blood flows through the tricuspid valve into the relaxed right ventricle.
3. The right ventricle then contracts and blood is pumped through the pulmonary valve into the **pulmonary artery,** which carries it to the lungs for oxygenation.
4. The left atrium receives blood returning to the heart after being oxygenated by the lungs. This blood enters the relaxed left atrium from the four **pulmonary veins.**
5. The left atrium contracts and blood flows through the mitral valve into the relaxed left ventricle.
6. When the left ventricle contracts, the blood is pumped through the aortic valve and into the **aorta,** the largest artery in the body. The aorta carries blood to all parts of the body.

It can be seen that the heart chambers alternate between relaxing in order to fill and contracting to push blood forward. The period of time a chamber is relaxed is **diastole.** The contraction phase is **systole.**

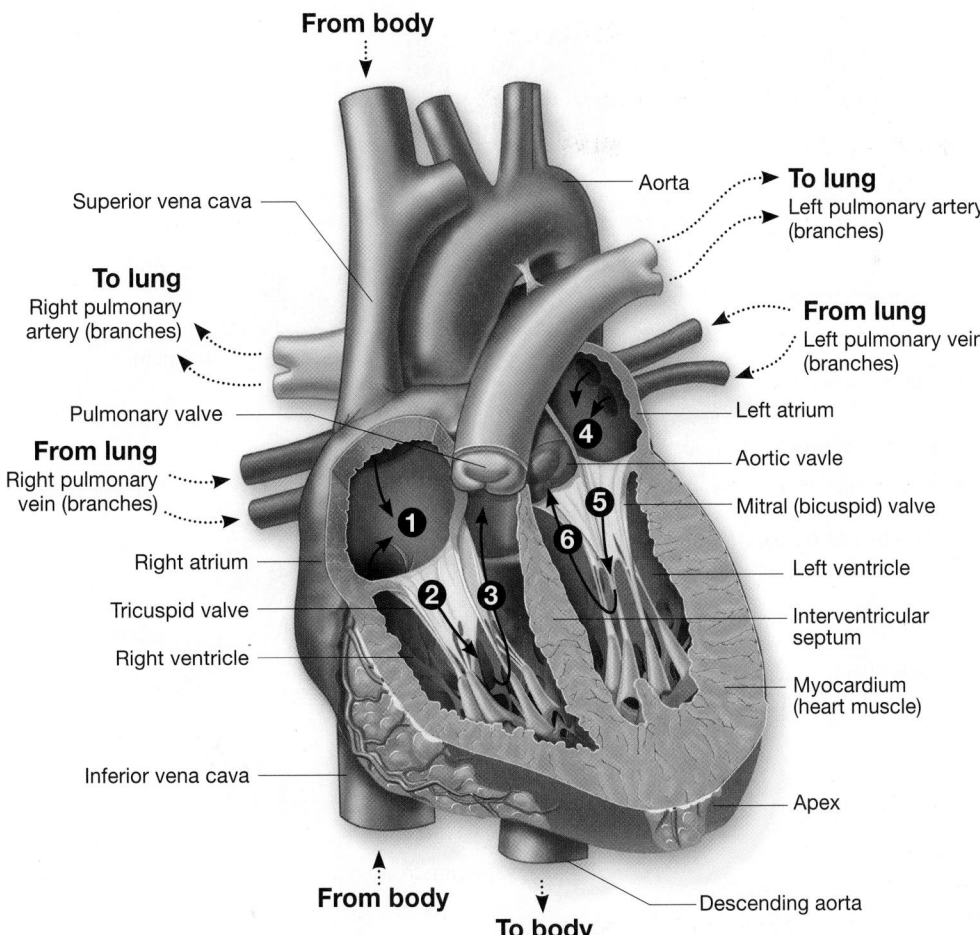

From body

Superior vena cava

Aorta

To lung
Left pulmonary artery
(branches)

To lung
Right pulmonary
artery (branches)

From lung
Left pulmonary vein
(branches)

Pulmonary valve

Left atrium

Aortic vavle

From lung
Right pulmonary
vein (branches)

Mitral (bicuspid) valve

Right atrium

Left ventricle

Tricuspid valve

Interventricular
septum

Right ventricle

Myocardium
(heart muscle)

Inferior vena cava

Apex

From body

Descending aorta

To body

■ **Figure 5.5** The path of blood flow through the chambers of the left and right side of the heart, including the veins delivering blood to the heart and arteries receiving blood ejected from the heart.

Conduction System of the Heart

atrioventricular bundle

atrioventricular node

autonomic nervous system
(aw-toh-NOM-ik / NER-vus / SIS-tem)

bundle branches

bundle of His

pacemaker

Purkinje fibers (per-KIN-gee)

sinoatrial node (sigh-noh-AY-tree-al)

The heart rate is regulated by the **autonomic nervous system;** therefore, we have no voluntary control over the beating of our heart. Special tissue within the heart is responsible for conducting an electrical impulse stimulating the different chambers to contract in the correct order.

The path that the impulses travel is as follows (see Figure 5.6 ■):

1. The **sinoatrial (SA) node,** or **pacemaker,** is where the electrical impulses begin. From the sinoatrial node a wave of electricity travels through the atria, causing them to contract, or go into systole.
2. The **atrioventricular node** is stimulated.
3. This node transfers the stimulation wave to the **atrioventricular bundle** (formerly called **bundle of His**).
4. The electrical signal next travels down the **bundle branches** within the interventricular septum.
5. The **Purkinje fibers** out in the ventricular myocardium are stimulated, resulting in ventricular systole.

■ **Figure 5.6** The conduction system of the heart; traces the path of the electrical impulse that stimulates the heart chambers to contract in the correct sequence.

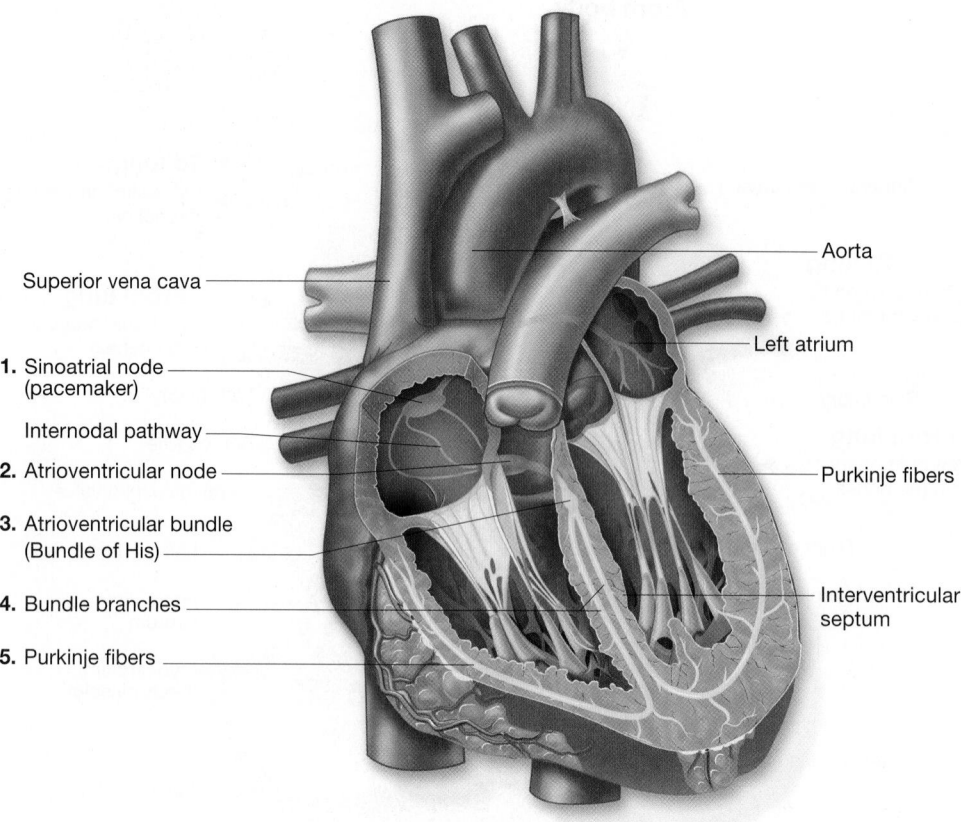

Superior vena cava

Aorta

Left atrium

1. Sinoatrial node (pacemaker)

Internodal pathway

2. Atrioventricular node

3. Atrioventricular bundle (Bundle of His)

4. Bundle branches

5. Purkinje fibers

Purkinje fibers

Interventricular septum

■ **Figure 5.7** An electrocardiogram (EKG) wave, a record of the electrical signal as it moves through the conduction system of the heart. This signal stimulates the chambers of the heart to contract and relax in the proper sequence.

MED TERM TIP

The electrocardiogram, referred to as an EKG or ECG, is a measurement of the electrical activity of the heart (see Figure 5.7 ■). This can give the physician information about the health of the heart, especially the myocardium.

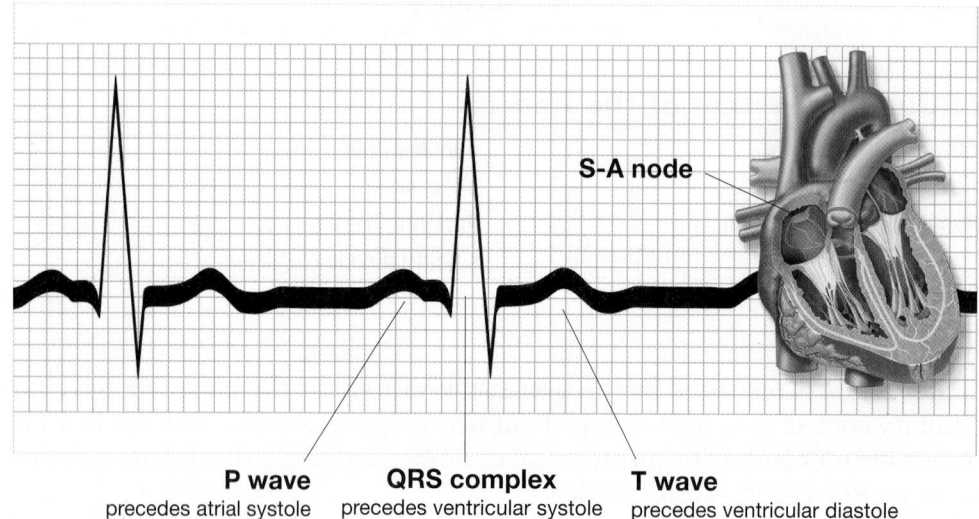

S-A node

P wave
precedes atrial systole

QRS complex
precedes ventricular systole

T wave
precedes ventricular diastole

Blood Vessels

lumen (LOO-men)

There are three types of blood vessels: arteries, capillaries, and veins (see Figure 5.8 ■). These are the pipes that circulate blood throughout the body. The **lumen** is the channel within these vessels through which blood flows.

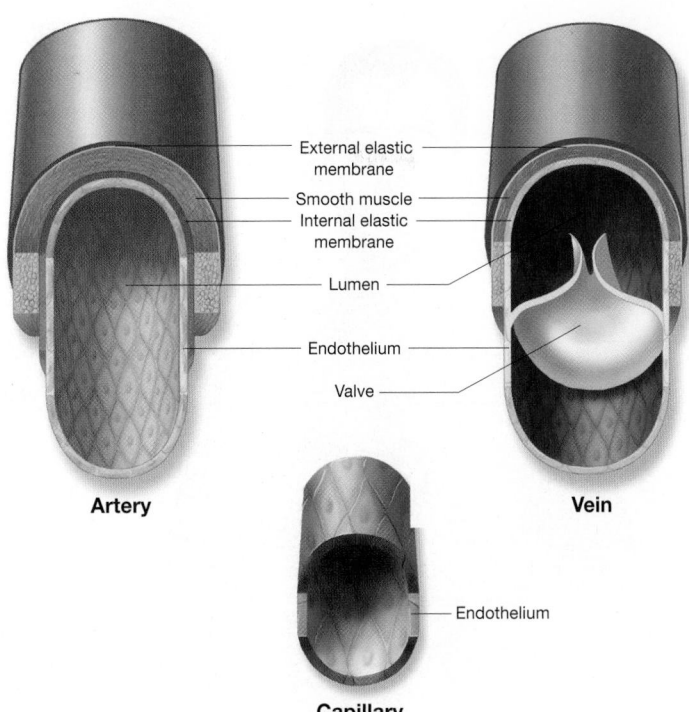

■ **Figure 5.8** Comparative structure of arteries, capillaries, and veins.

- External elastic membrane
- Smooth muscle
- Internal elastic membrane
- Lumen
- Endothelium
- Valve

Artery   **Vein**

- Endothelium

Capillary

Arteries

arterioles (ar-TEE-ree-ohlz)   **coronary arteries**
(KOR-ah-nair-ee / AR-te-reez)

The arteries are the large, thick-walled vessels that carry the blood away from the heart. The walls of arteries contain a thick layer of smooth muscle that can contract or relax to change the size of the arterial lumen. The pulmonary artery carries deoxygenated blood from the right ventricle to the lungs. The largest artery, the aorta, begins from the left ventricle of the heart and carries oxygenated blood to all the body systems. The **coronary arteries** then branch from the aorta and provide blood to the myocardium (see Figure 5.9 ■). As they travel through the body, the arteries branch into progressively smaller sized arteries. The smallest of the arteries, called **arterioles,** deliver blood to the capillaries. Figure 5.10 ■ illustrates the major systemic arteries.

> **MED TERM TIP**
>
> The term *coronary*, from the Latin word for crown, describes how the great vessels encircle the heart as they emerge from the top of the heart.

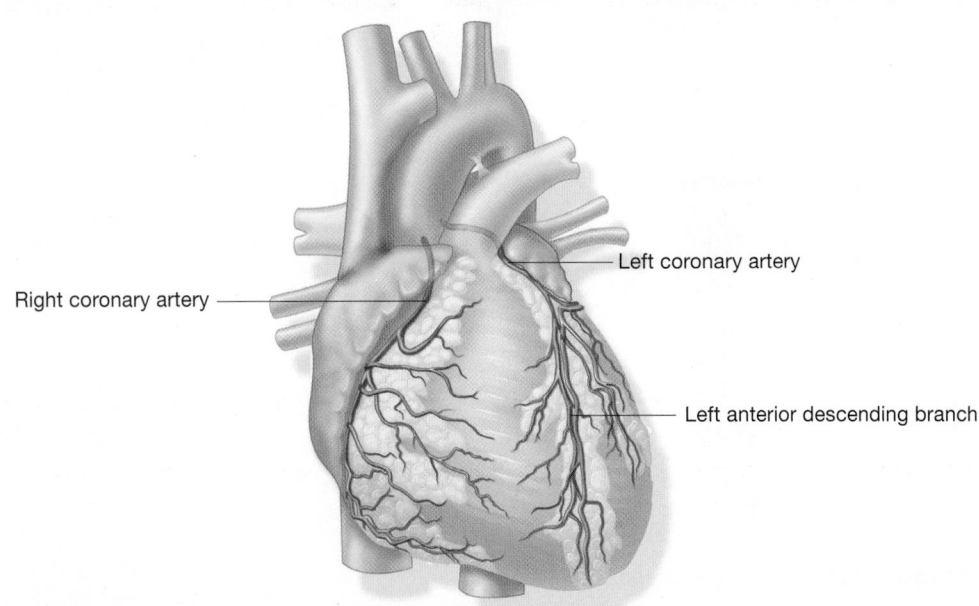

- Right coronary artery
- Left coronary artery
- Left anterior descending branch

■ **Figure 5.9** The coronary arteries.

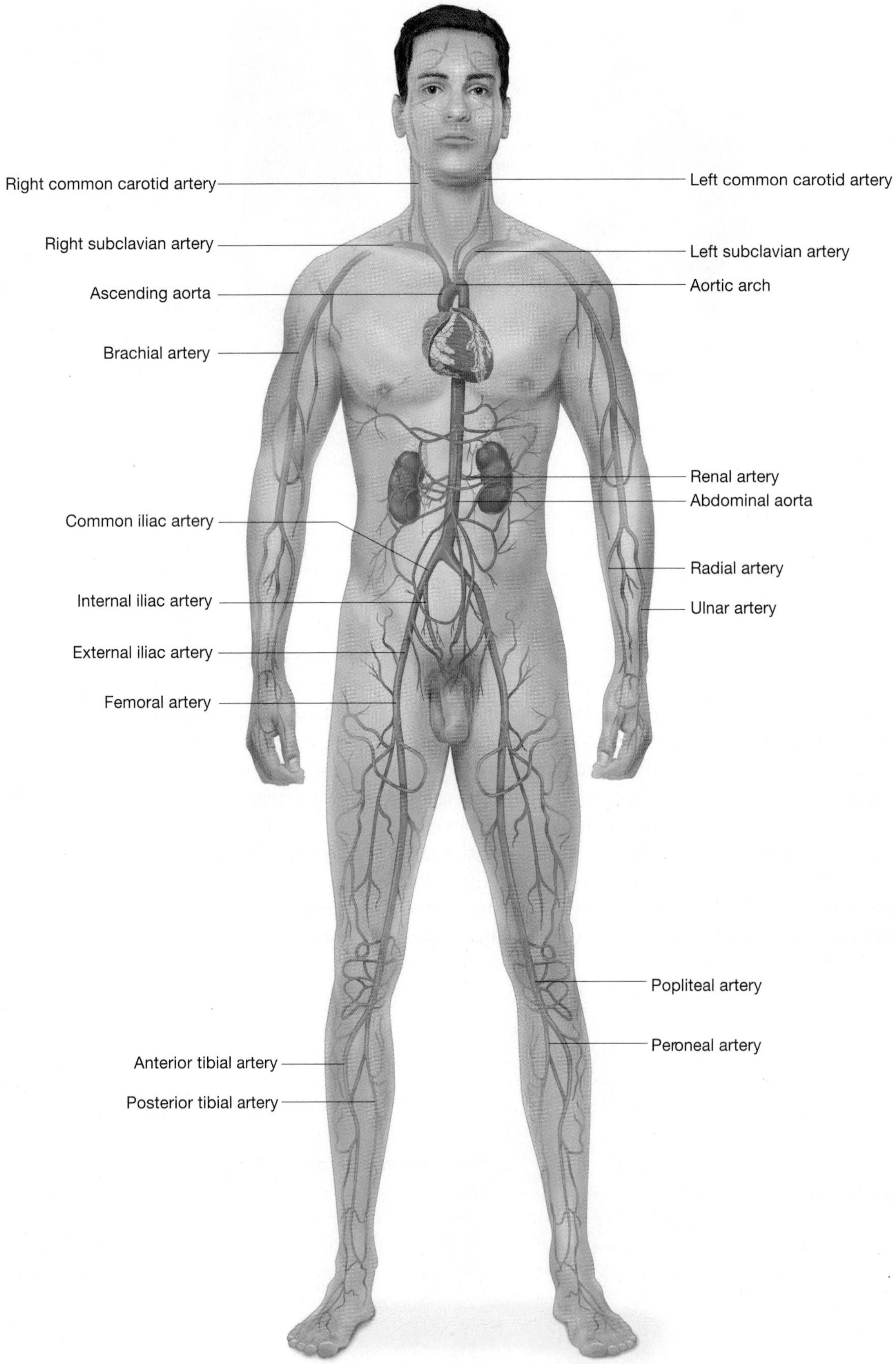

Right common carotid artery

Right subclavian artery

Ascending aorta

Brachial artery

Common iliac artery

Internal iliac artery

External iliac artery

Femoral artery

Anterior tibial artery

Posterior tibial artery

Left common carotid artery

Left subclavian artery

Aortic arch

Renal artery

Abdominal aorta

Radial artery

Ulnar artery

Popliteal artery

Peroneal artery

■ Figure 5.10 The major arteries of the body.

Capillaries
capillary bed

Capillaries are a network of tiny blood vessels referred to as a **capillary bed.** Arterial blood flows into a capillary bed, and venous blood flows back out. Capillaries are very thin walled, allowing for the diffusion of the oxygen and nutrients from the blood into the body tissues (see Figure 5.8). Likewise, carbon dioxide and waste products are able to diffuse out of the body tissues and into the bloodstream to be carried away. Since the capillaries are so small in diameter, the blood will not flow as quickly through them as it does through the arteries and veins. This means that the blood has time for an exchange of nutrients, oxygen, and waste material to take place. As blood exits a capillary bed, it returns to the heart through a vein.

Veins
venules (VEN-yools)

The veins carry blood back to the heart (see Figure 5.8). Blood leaving capillaries first enters small **venules,** which then merge into larger veins. Veins have much thinner walls than arteries, causing them to collapse easily. The veins also have valves that allow the blood to move only toward the heart. These valves prevent blood from backflowing, ensuring that blood always flows toward the heart. The two large veins that enter the heart are the superior vena cava, which carries blood from the upper body, and the inferior vena cava, which carries blood from the lower body. Blood pressure in the veins is much lower than in the arteries. Muscular action against the veins and skeletal muscle contractions help in the movement of blood. Figure 5.11 ■ illustrates the major systemic veins.

Pulse and Blood Pressure

blood pressure (BP)	**pulse**
diastolic pressure (dye-ah-STOL-ik)	**systolic pressure** (sis-TOL-ik)

Blood pressure (BP) is a measurement of the force exerted by blood against the wall of a blood vessel. During ventricular systole, blood is under a lot of pressure from the ventricular contraction, giving the highest blood pressure reading—the **systolic pressure.** The **pulse** felt at the wrist or throat is the surge of blood caused by the heart contraction. This is why pulse rate is normally equal to heart rate. During ventricular diastole, blood is not being pushed by the heart at all and the blood pressure reading drops to its lowest point—the **diastolic pressure.** Therefore, to see the full range of what is occurring with blood pressure, both numbers are required. Blood pressure is also affected by several other characteristics of the blood and the blood vessels. These include the elasticity of the arteries, the diameter of the blood vessels, the viscosity of the blood, the volume of blood flowing through the vessels, and the amount of resistance to blood flow.

MED TERM TIP

The instrument used to measure blood pressure is called a *sphygmomomanometer.* The combining form *sphygm/o* means "pulse" and the suffix *-manometer* means "instrument to measure pressure." A blood pressure reading is reported as two numbers, for example, 120/80. The 120 is the systolic pressure and the 80 is the diastolic pressure. There is no one "normal" blood pressure number. The normal blood pressure for an adult is a systolic pressure less than 120 and diastolic pressure less than 80.

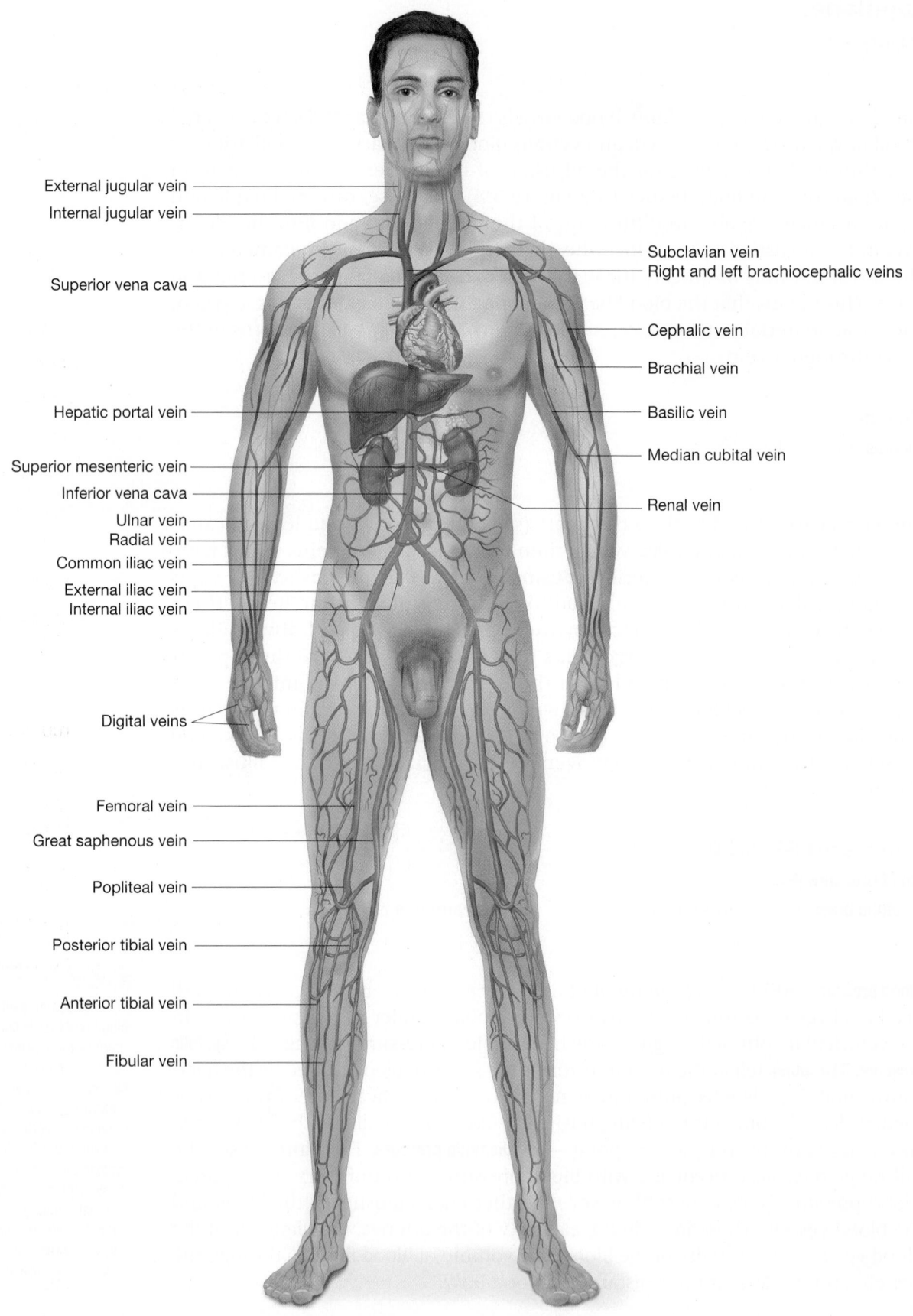

External jugular vein
Internal jugular vein
Superior vena cava
Hepatic portal vein
Superior mesenteric vein
Inferior vena cava
Ulnar vein
Radial vein
Common iliac vein
External iliac vein
Internal iliac vein
Digital veins
Femoral vein
Great saphenous vein
Popliteal vein
Posterior tibial vein
Anterior tibial vein
Fibular vein

Subclavian vein
Right and left brachiocephalic veins
Cephalic vein
Brachial vein
Basilic vein
Median cubital vein
Renal vein

■ **Figure 5.11** The major veins of the body.

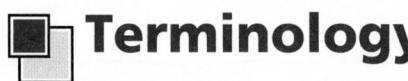
Terminology

Word Parts Used to Build Cardiovascular System Terms

The following lists contain the combining forms, suffixes, and prefixes used to build terms in the remaining sections of this chapter.

Combining Forms

aort/o	aorta	embol/o	plug	son/o	sound
angi/o	vessel	hem/o	blood	sphygm/o	pulse
arteri/o	artery	isch/o	to hold back	steth/o	chest
ather/o	fatty substance	lip/o	fat	thromb/o	clot
atri/o	atrium	my/o	muscle	valv/o	valve
cardi/o	heart	myocardi/o	heart muscle	valvul/o	valve
coron/o	heart	orth/o	straight	varic/o	dilated vein
corpor/o	body	pect/o	chest	vas/o	vessel
cutane/o	skin	phleb/o	vein	vascul/o	blood vessel
duct/o	to bring	pulmon/o	lung	ven/o	vein
electr/o	electricity	sept/o	a wall	ventricul/o	ventricle

Suffixes

-ac	pertaining to	-logy	study of	-rrhexis	rupture
-al	pertaining to	-lytic	destruction	-sclerosis	hardening
-ar	pertaining to	-manometer	instrument to measure pressure	-scope	instrument for viewing
-ary	pertaining to	-megaly	enlarged	-spasm	involuntary muscle contraction
-eal	pertaining to	-ole	small		
-ectomy	surgical removal	-oma	growth	-stenosis	narrowing
-gram	record	-ose	pertaining to	-tension	pressure
-graphy	process of recording	-ous	pertaining to	-tic	pertaining to
-ia	condition	-pathy	disease	-tonic	pertaining to tone
-ic	pertaining to	-plasty	surgical repair	-ule	small
-itis	inflammation				

Prefixes

a-	without	hyper-	excessive	poly-	many
anti-	against	hypo-	insufficient	tachy-	fast
brady-	slow	inter-	between	tetra-	four
de-	without	intra-	within	trans-	across
endo-	inner	per-	through	ultra-	beyond
extra-	outside of	peri-	around		

Anatomical Terms

TERM	WORD PARTS	DEFINITION
aortic (ay-OR-tik)	aort/o = aorta -ic = pertaining to	Pertaining to the aorta
arterial (ar-TEE-ree-al)	arteri/o = artery -al = pertaining to	Pertaining to an artery
arteriole (ar-TEE-ree-ohl)	arteri/o = artery -ole = small	A small (narrow in diameter) artery
atrial (AY-tree-al)	atri/o = atrium -al = pertaining to	Pertaining to the atrium
cardiac (CAR-dee-ak)	cardi/o = heart -ac = pertaining to	Pertaining to the heart
coronary (KOR-ah-nair-ee)	coron/o = heart -ary = pertaining to	Pertaining to the heart
interatrial (in-ter-AY-tree-al)	inter- = between atri/o = atrium -al = pertaining to	Pertaining to between the atria
interventricular (in-ter-ven-TRIK-yoo-lar)	inter- = between ventricul/o = ventricle -ar = pertaining to	Pertaining to between the ventricles
myocardial (my-oh-CAR-dee-al)	myocardi/o = heart muscle -al = pertaining to	Pertaining to heart muscle
valvular (VAL-view-lar)	valvul/o = valve -ar = pertaining to	Pertaining to a valve
vascular (VAS-kwee-lar)	vascul/o = blood vessel -ar = pertaining to	Pertaining to a blood vessel
venous (VEE-nus)	ven/o = vein -ous = pertaining to	Pertaining to a vein
ventricular (ven-TRIK-yoo-lar)	ventricul/o = ventricle -ar = pertaining to	Pertaining to a ventricle
venule (VEN-yool)	ven/o = vein -ule = small	A small (narrow in diameter) vein

Pathology

TERM	WORD PARTS	DEFINITION
Medical Specialties		
cardiology (car-dee-ALL-oh-jee)	cardi/o = heart -logy = study of	The branch of medicine involving diagnosis and treatment of conditions and diseases of the cardiovascular system. Physician is a *cardiologist*.
cardiovascular technician	cardi/o = heart vascul/o = blood vessel -ar = pertaining to	Healthcare professional trained to perform a variety of diagnostic and therapeutic procedures including electrocardiography, echocardiography, and exercise stress tests.

Pathology *(continued)*

TERM	WORD PARTS	DEFINITION
Signs and Symptoms		
angiitis (an-jee-EYE-tis)	angi/o = vessel -itis = inflammation	Inflammation of a vessel.
angiospasm (AN-jee-oh-spazm)	angi/o = vessel -spasm = involuntary muscle contraction	An involuntary muscle contraction of the smooth muscle in the wall of a vessel; narrows the vessel.
angiostenosis (an-jee-oh-sten-OH-sis)	angi/o = vessel -stenosis = narrowing	The narrowing of a vessel.
bradycardia (brad-ee-CAR-dee-ah)	brady- = slow cardi/o = heart -ia = condition	The condition of having a slow heart rate; typically less than 60 beats/minute; highly trained aerobic persons may normally have a slow heart rate.
embolus (EM-boh-lus)	embol/o = plug	The obstruction of a blood vessel by a blood clot that has broken off from a thrombus somewhere else in the body and traveled to the point of obstruction. If it occurs in a coronary artery, it may result in a myocardial infarction.

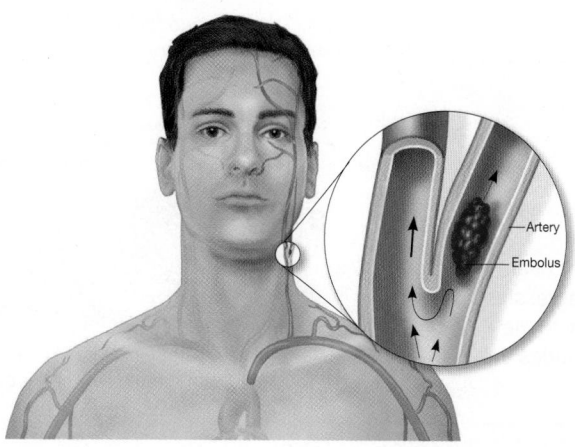

■ **Figure 5.12** Illustration of an embolus floating in an artery. The embolus will become lodged in a blood vessel that is smaller than it is, resulting in occlusion of that artery.

infarct (IN-farkt)		An area of tissue within an organ or part that undergoes necrosis (death) following the loss of its blood supply.
ischemia (is-KEYH-mee-ah)	isch/o = to hold back hem/o = blood -ia = condition	The localized and temporary deficiency of blood supply due to an obstruction to the circulation.
murmur (MUR-mur)		A sound, in addition to the normal heart sounds, arising from blood flowing through the heart. This extra sound may or may not indicate a heart abnormality.
orthostatic hypotension (or-thoh-STAT-ik)	orth/o = straight hypo- = insufficient -tension = pressure	The sudden drop in blood pressure a person experiences when standing straight up suddenly.
palpitations (pal-pih-TAY-shunz)		Pounding, racing heartbeats.

■ Pathology *(continued)*

TERM	WORD PARTS	DEFINITION
plaque (plak)		A yellow, fatty deposit of lipids in an artery that is the hallmark of atherosclerosis. Also called an *atheroma*.
regurgitation (re-ger-gih-TAY-shun)		To flow backwards. In the cardiovascular system this refers to the backflow of blood through a valve.
tachycardia (tak-ee-CAR-dee-ah)	tachy- = fast cardi/o = heart -ia = condition	The condition of having a fast heart rate; typically more than 100 beats/minute while at rest.
thrombus (THROM-bus)	thromb/o = clot	A blood clot forming within a blood vessel. May partially or completely occlude the blood vessel.

A

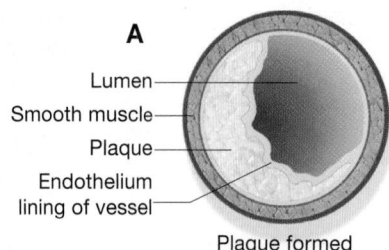 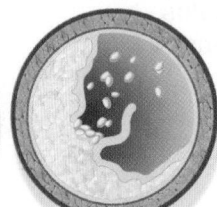

Lumen
Smooth muscle
Plaque
Endothelium lining of vessel

Plaque formed in artery wall   Damage to epithelium   Platelets and fibrin deposit on plaque forming a clot

B

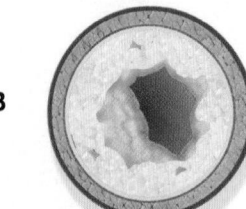 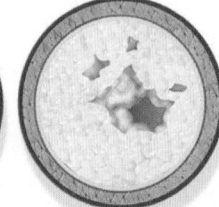 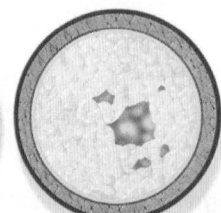

Moderate narrowing of lumen   Thrombus partially occluding lumen   Thrombus completely occluding lumen

■ **Figure 5.13** Development of an atherosclerotic plaque that progressively narrows the lumen of an artery to the point that a thrombus fully occludes the lumen.

Heart

TERM	WORD PARTS	DEFINITION
angina pectoris (an-JYE-nah / PECK-tor-is)	pect/o = chest	Condition in which there is severe pain with a sensation of constriction around the heart. Caused by a deficiency of oxygen to the heart muscle.
arrhythmia (ah-RITH-mee-ah)	a- = without -ia = condition	Irregularity in the heartbeat or action. Comes in many different forms; some are not serious, while others are life-threatening.
bundle branch block (BBB)		Occurs when the electrical impulse is blocked from traveling down the bundle of His or bundle branches. Results in the ventricles beating at a different rate than the atria. Also called a *heart block*.
cardiac arrest	cardi/o = heart -ac = pertaining to	Complete stopping of heart activity.
cardiomegaly (car-dee-oh-MEG-ah-lee)	cardi/o = heart -megaly = enlarged	An enlarged heart.

Pathology *(continued)*

TERM	WORD PARTS	DEFINITION
cardiomyopathy (car-dee-oh-my-OP-ah-thee)	cardi/o = heart my/o = muscle -pathy = disease	General term for a disease of the myocardium. Can be caused by alcohol abuse, parasites, viral infection, and congestive heart failure. One of the most common reasons a patient may require a heart transplant.
congenital septal defect (CSD)	sept/o = a wall -al = pertaining to	A hole, present at birth, in the septum between two heart chambers; results in a mixture of oxygenated and deoxygenated blood. There can be an *atrial septal defect* (ASD) and a *ventricular septal defect* (VSD).
congestive heart failure (CHF) (kon-JESS-tiv)		Pathological condition of the heart in which there is a reduced outflow of blood from the left side of the heart because the left ventricle myocardium has become too weak to efficiently pump blood. Results in weakness, breathlessness, and edema.
coronary artery disease (CAD) (KOR-ah-nair-ee)	coron/o = heart -ary = pertaining to	Insufficient blood supply to the heart muscle due to an obstruction of one or more coronary arteries. May be caused by atherosclerosis and may cause angina pectoris and myocardial infarction.

MED TERM TIP

All types of cardiovascular disease have been the number one killer of Americans since the 19th century. This disease kills more people annually than the next six causes of death combined.

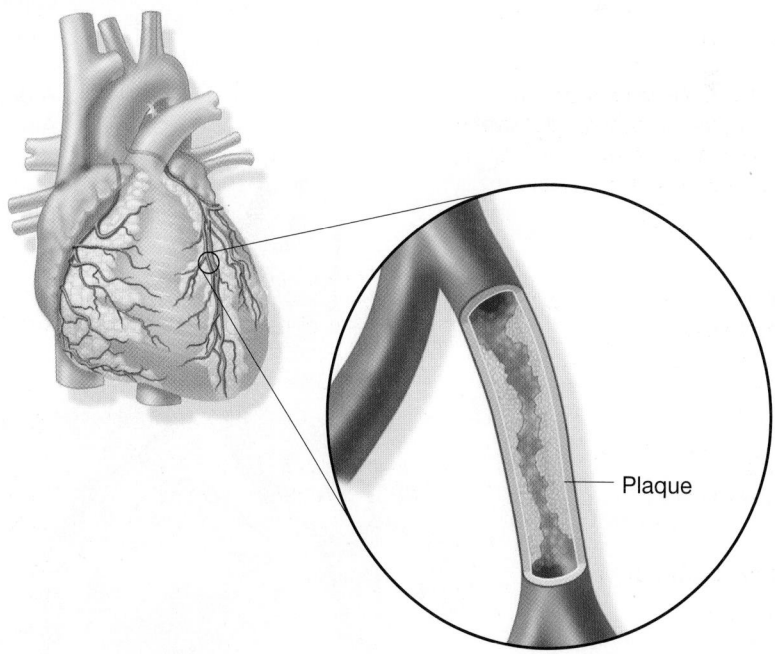

■ **Figure 5.14** Formation of an atherosclerotic plaque within a coronary artery; may lead to coronary artery disease, angina pectoris, and myocardial infarction.

TERM	WORD PARTS	DEFINITION
endocarditis (en-doh-car-DYE-tis)	endo- = inner cardi/o = heart -itis = inflammation	Inflammation of the lining membranes of the heart. May be due to bacteria or to an abnormal immunological response. In bacterial endocarditis, the mass of bacteria that forms is referred to as *vegetation*.

■ Pathology *(continued)*

TERM	WORD PARTS	DEFINITION
fibrillation (fih-brill-AY-shun)		An extremely serious arrhythmia characterized by an abnormal quivering or contraction of heart fibers. When this occurs in the ventricles, cardiac arrest and death can occur. Emergency equipment to defibrillate, or convert the heart to a normal beat, is necessary.
flutter		An arrhythmia in which the atria beat too rapidly, but in a regular pattern.
heart valve prolapse (PROH-laps)		Condition in which the cusps or flaps of the heart valve are too loose and fail to shut tightly, allowing blood to flow backward through the valve when the heart chamber contracts. Most commonly occurs in the mitral valve, but may affect any of the heart valves.
heart valve stenosis (steh-NOH-sis)	-stenosis = narrowing	The cusps or flaps of the heart valve are too stiff. Therefore, they are unable to open fully, making it difficult for blood to flow through, or shut tightly, allowing blood to flow backward. This condition may affect any of the heart valves.
myocardial infarction (MI) (my-oh-CAR-dee-al / in-FARC-shun)	myocardi/o = heart muscle -al = pertaining to	Condition caused by the partial or complete occlusion or closing of one or more of the coronary arteries. Symptoms include a squeezing pain or heavy pressure in the middle of the chest (angina pectoris). A delay in treatment could result in death. Also referred to as a *heart attack*.

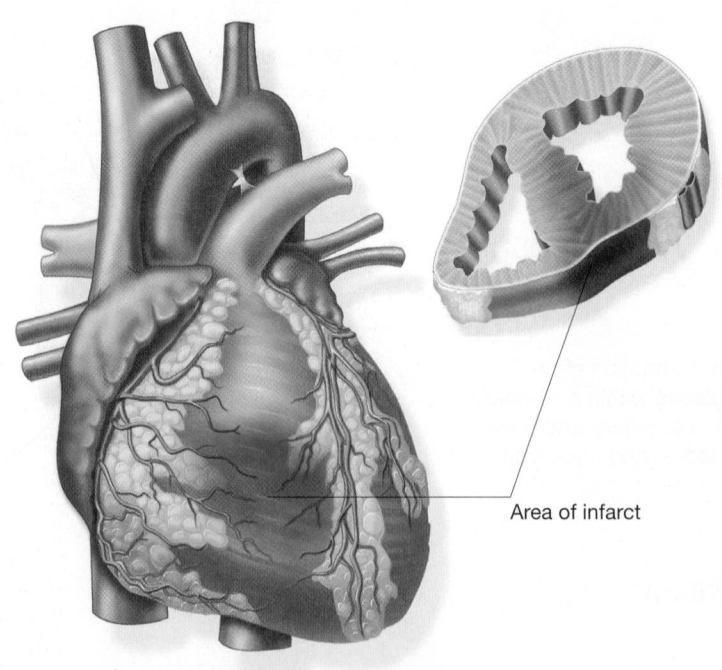

Area of infarct

■ **Figure 5.15** External and cross-sectional view of an infarct caused by a myocardial infarction.

Pathology *(continued)*

TERM	WORD PARTS	DEFINITION
myocarditis (my-oh-car-DYE-tis)	myocardi/o = heart muscle -itis = inflammation	Inflammation of the muscle layer of the heart wall.
pericarditis (pair-ih-car-DYE-tis)	peri- = around cardi/o = heart -itis = inflammation	Inflammation of the pericardial sac around the heart.
tetralogy of Fallot (teh-TRALL-oh-jee / fal-LOH)	tetra- = four -logy = study of	Combination of four congenital anomalies: pulmonary stenosis, an interventricular septal defect, improper placement of the aorta, and hypertrophy of the right ventricle. Needs immediate surgery to correct.
valvulitis (val-view-LYE-tis)	valvul/o = valve -itis = inflammation	The inflammation of a heart valve.

Blood Vessels

aneurysm (AN-yoo-rizm)		Weakness in the wall of an artery resulting in localized widening of the artery. Although an aneurysm may develop in any artery, common sites include the aorta in the abdomen and the cerebral arteries in the brain.

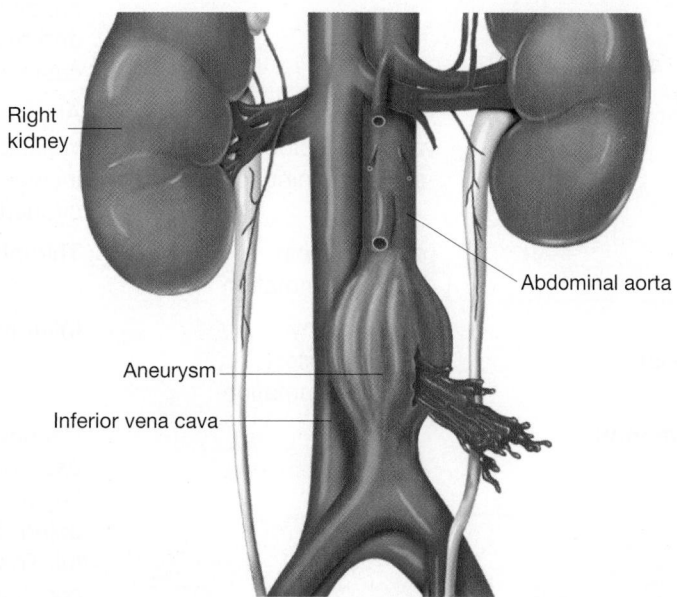

Right kidney

Abdominal aorta

Aneurysm

Inferior vena cava

■ **Figure 5.16** Illustration of a large aneurysm in the abdominal aorta that has ruptured.

arteriorrhexis (ar-tee-ree-oh-REK-sis)	arteri/o = artery -rrhexis = rupture	A ruptured artery; may occur if an aneurysm ruptures an arterial wall.
arteriosclerosis (ar-tee-ree-oh-skleh-ROH-sis)	arteri/o = artery -sclerosis = hardening	Thickening, hardening, and loss of elasticity of the walls of the arteries. Most often due to atherosclerosis.
atheroma (ath-er-OH-mah)	ather/o = fatty substance -oma = growth	A deposit of fatty substance in the wall of an artery that bulges into and narrows the lumen of the artery; a characteristic of atherosclerosis. Also called a *plaque*.

Pathology *(continued)*

TERM	WORD PARTS	DEFINITION
atherosclerosis (ath-er-oh-skleh-ROH-sis)	ather/o = fatty substance -sclerosis = hardening	The most common form of arteriosclerosis. Caused by the formation of yellowish plaques of cholesterol on the inner walls of arteries (see again Figures 5.13 & 5.14).
coarctation of the aorta (CoA) (koh-ark-TAY-shun)		Severe congenital narrowing of the aorta.
hemorrhoid (HIM-oh-royd)	hem/o = blood	Varicose veins in the anal region.
hypertension (HTN) (high-per-TEN-shun)	hyper- = excessive -tension = pressure	Blood pressure above the normal range. *Essential* or *primary hypertension* occurs directly from cardiovascular disease. *Secondary hypertension* refers to high blood pressure resulting from another disease such as kidney disease.
hypotension (high-poh-TEN-shun)	hypo- = insufficient -tension = pressure	Decrease in blood pressure. Can occur in shock, infection, cancer, anemia, or as death approaches.
patent ductus arteriosus (PDA) (PAY-tent / DUCK-tus / ar-tee-ree-OH-sis)	duct/o = to bring arteri/o = artery	Congenital heart anomaly in which the fetal connection between the pulmonary artery and the aorta fails to close at birth. This condition may be treated with medication and resolve with time. However, in some cases surgery is required.
peripheral vascular disease (PVD)	-al = pertaining to vascul/o = blood vessel -ar = pertaining to	Any abnormal condition affecting blood vessels outside the heart. Symptoms may include pain, pallor, numbness, and loss of circulation and pulses.
phlebitis (fleh-BYE-tis)	phleb/o = vein -itis = inflammation	The inflammation of a vein.
polyarteritis (pol-ee-ar-ter-EYE-tis)	poly- = many arteri/o = artery -itis = inflammation	Inflammation of several arteries.
Raynaud's phenomenon (ray-NOZ)		Periodic ischemic attacks affecting the extremities of the body, especially the fingers, toes, ears, and nose. The affected extremities become cyanotic and very painful. These attacks are brought on by arterial constriction due to extreme cold or emotional stress.
thrombophlebitis (throm-boh-fleh-BYE-tis)	thromb/o = clot phleb/o = vein -itis = inflammation	Inflammation of a vein resulting in the formation of blood clots within the vein.
varicose veins (VAIR-ih-kohs)	varic/o = dilated vein -ose = pertaining to	Swollen and distended veins, usually in the legs.

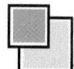

Diagnostic Procedures

TERM	WORD PARTS	DEFINITION
Medical Procedures		
auscultation (oss-kul-TAY-shun)		Process of listening to the sounds within the body by using a stethoscope.
sphygmomanometer (sfig-moh-mah-NOM-eh-ter)	sphygm/o = pulse -manometer = instrument to measure pressure	Instrument for measuring blood pressure. Also referred to as a *blood pressure cuff.*

Figure 5.17 Using a sphygmomanometer to measure blood pressure.

TERM	WORD PARTS	DEFINITION
stethoscope (STETH-oh-scope)	steth/o = chest -scope = instrument for viewing	Instrument for listening to body sounds (auscultation), such as the chest, heart, or intestines.
Clinical Laboratory Tests		
cardiac enzymes (CAR-dee-ak / EN-zyms)	cardi/o = heart -ac = pertaining to	Blood test to determine the level of enzymes specific to heart muscles in the blood. An increase in the enzymes may indicate heart muscle damage such as a myocardial infarction. These enzymes include creatine phosphokinase (CPK), lactate dehydrogenase (LDH), and glutamic oxaloacetic transaminase (GOT).
serum lipoprotein level (SEE-rum / lip-oh-PROH-teen)	lip/o = fat	Blood test to measure the amount of cholesterol and triglycerides in the blood. An indicator of atherosclerosis risk.
Diagnostic Imaging		
angiogram (AN-jee-oh-gram)	angi/o = vessel -gram = record	X-ray record of a vessel taken during angiography.
angiography (an-jee-OG-rah-fee)	angi/o = vessel -graphy = process of recording	X-rays taken after the injection of an opaque material into a blood vessel. Can be performed on the aorta as an aortic angiography, on the heart as angiocardiography, and on the brain as a cerebral angiography.
cardiac scan	cardi/o = heart -ac = pertaining to	Patient is given radioactive thallium intravenously and then scanning equipment is used to visualize the hear. It is especially useful in determining myocardial damage.

Diagnostic Procedures (continued)

TERM	WORD PARTS	DEFINITION
Doppler ultrasonography (DOP-ler / ul-trah-son-OG-rah-fee)	ultra- = beyond son/o = sound -graphy = process of recording	Measurement of sound-wave echoes as they bounce off tissues and organs to produce an image. In this system, used to measure velocity of blood moving through blood vessels to look for blood clots or deep vein thromboses.
echocardiography (ek-oh-car-dee-OG-rah-fee)	cardi/o = artery -graphy = process of recording	Noninvasive diagnostic method using ultrasound to visualize internal cardiac structures. Cardiac valve activity can be evaluated using this method.
Cardiac Function Tests		
catheter (KATH-eh-ter)		Flexible tube inserted into the body for the purpose of moving fluids into or out of the body. In the cardiovascular system a catheter is used to place dye into blood vessels so they may be visualized on x-rays.
cardiac catheterization (CAR-dee-ak / cath-eh-ter-ih-ZAY-shun)	cardi/o = heart -ac = pertaining to	Passage of a thin tube catheter through a blood vessel leading to the heart. Done to detect abnormalities, to collect cardiac blood samples, and to determine the blood pressure within the heart.
electrocardiogram (ee-lek-tro-CAR-dee-oh-gram)	electr/o = electricity cardi/o = heart -gram = record	Hard copy record produced by electrocardiography.
electrocardiography (ECG, EKG) (ee-lek-troh-car-dee-OG-rah-fee)	electr/o = electricity cardi/o = heart -graphy = process of recording	Process of recording the electrical activity of the heart. Useful in the diagnosis of abnormal cardiac rhythm and heart muscle (myocardium) damage.
Holter monitor		Portable ECG monitor worn by a patient for a period of a few hours to a few days to assess the heart and pulse activity as the person goes through the activities of daily living. Used to assess a patient who experiences chest pain and unusual heart activity during exercise and normal activities.
stress testing		Method for evaluating cardiovascular fitness. The patient is placed on a treadmill or a bicycle and then subjected to steadily increasing levels of work. An EKG and oxygen levels are taken while the patient exercises. The test is stopped if abnormalities occur on the EKG. Also called an *exercise test* or a *treadmill test*.

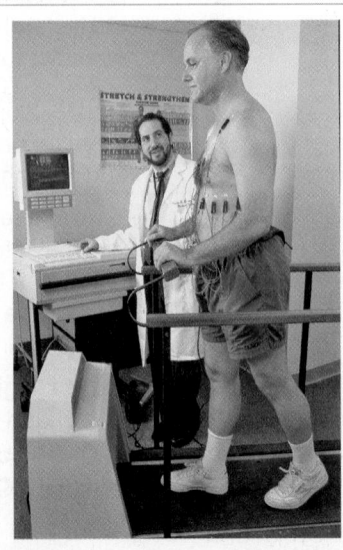

■ **Figure 5.18** Man undergoing a stress test on a treadmill while physician monitors his condition. *(Jonathan Nourok/PhotoEdit Inc.)*

Therapeutic Procedures

TERM	WORD PARTS	DEFINITION
Medical Procedures		
cardiopulmonary resuscitation (CPR) (car-dee-oh-PULL-mon-air-ee / ree-suss-ih-TAY-shun)	cardi/o = heart pulmon/o = lung -ary = pertaining to	Procedure to restore cardiac output and oxygenated air to the lungs for a person in cardiac arrest. A combination of chest compressions (to push blood out of the heart) and artificial respiration (to blow air into the lungs) performed by one or two CPR-trained rescuers.
defibrillation (dee-fib-rih-LAY-shun)	de- = without	Procedure that converts serious irregular heartbeats, such as fibrillation, by giving electric shocks to the heart using an instrument called a defibrillator. Also called *cardioversion*. Automated external defibrillators (AED) are portable devices that automatically detect life-threatening arrhythmias and deliver the appropriate electrical shock. They are designed to be used by nonmedical personnel and are found in public places such as shopping malls and schools.

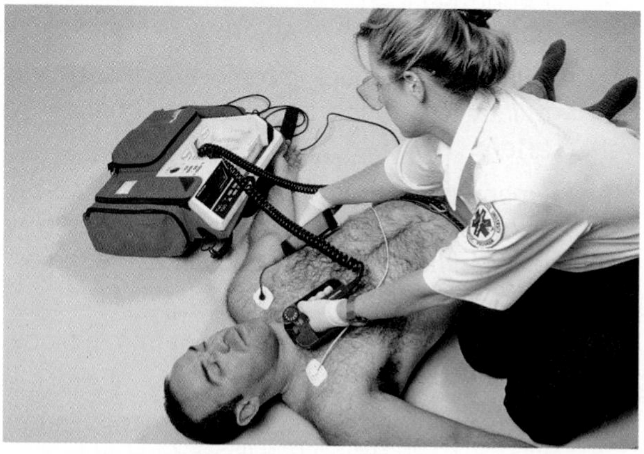

■ **Figure 5.19** An emergency medical technician positions defibrillator paddles on the chest of a supine male patient.

TERM	WORD PARTS	DEFINITION
extracorporeal circulation (ECC) (EX-tra-core-poor-EE-al)	extra- = outside of corpor/o = body -eal = pertaining to	During open-heart surgery, the routing of blood to a heart-lung machine so it can be oxygenated and pumped to the rest of the body.
implantable cardioverter-defibrillator (ICD) (CAR-dee-oh-ver-ter / de-FIB-rih-lay-tor)	cardi/o = heart de- = without	Device implanted in the heart that delivers an electrical shock to restore a normal heart rhythm. Particularly useful for persons who experience ventricular fibrillation.
pacemaker implantation		Electrical device that substitutes for the natural pacemaker of the heart. It controls the beating of the heart by a series of rhythmic electrical impulses. An external pacemaker has the electrodes on the outside of the body. An internal pacemaker has the electrodes surgically implanted within the chest wall.

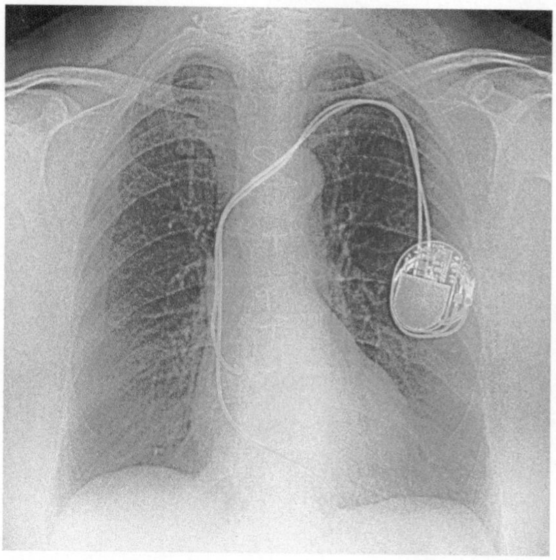

■ **Figure 5.20** Color enhanced X-ray showing a pacemaker implanted in the left side of the chest and the electrode wires running to the heart muscle. (*UHB Trust/Getty Images*)

Therapeutic Procedures *(continued)*

TERM	WORD PARTS	DEFINITION
thrombolytic therapy (throm-boh-LIT-ik / THAIR-ah-pee)	thromb/o = clot -lytic = destruction	Process in which drugs, such as streptoki-nase (SK) or tissue-type plasminogen acti-vator (tPA), are injected into a blood vessel to dissolve clots and restore blood flow.

Surgical Procedures

TERM	WORD PARTS	DEFINITION
aneurysmectomy (an-yoo-riz-MEK-toh-mee)	-ectomy = surgical removal	Surgical removal of the sac of an aneurysm.
arterial anastomosis (ar-TEE-ree-all / ah-nas-toe-MOE-sis)	arteri/o = artery -al = pertaining to	Surgical joining together of two arteries. Performed if an artery is severed or if a damaged section of an artery is removed.
atherectomy (ath-er-EK-toh-mee)	ather/o = fatty substance -ectomy = surgical removal	Surgical procedure to remove a deposit of fatty substance, an atheroma, from an artery.
coronary artery bypass graft (CABG) (KOR-ah-nair-ee)	coron/o = heart -ary = pertaining to	Open-heart surgery in which a blood vessel from another location in the body (often a leg vein) is grafted to route blood around a blocked coronary artery.
embolectomy (em-boh-LEK-toh-mee)	embol/o = plug -ectomy = surgical removal	Removal of an embolus or clot from a blood vessel.
endarterectomy (end-ar-teh-REK-toh-mee)	endo- = inner arteri/o = artery -ectomy = surgical removal	Removal of the diseased or damaged inner lining of an artery. Usually performed to remove atherosclerotic plaques.
heart transplantation		Replacement of a diseased or malfunction-ing heart with a donor's heart.
intracoronary artery stent (in-trah-KOR-ah-nair-ee / AR-ter-ee)	intra- = within coron/o = heart -ary = pertaining to	Placement of a stent within a coronary artery to treat coronary ischemia due to atherosclerosis.

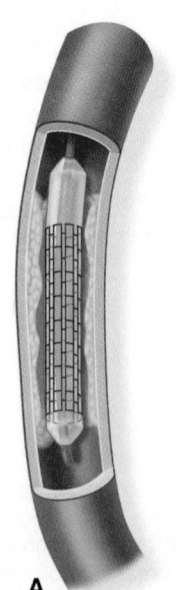 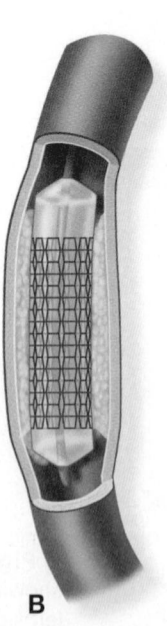 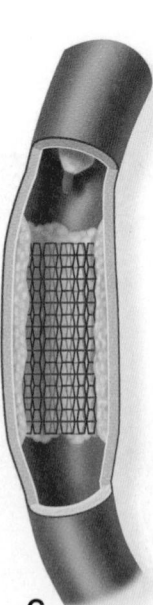

A   B   C

■ **Figure 5.21** The process of placing a stent in a blood vessel. (A) A catheter is used to place a collapsed stent next to an atherosclerotic plaque; (B) stent is expanded; (C) catheter is removed, leaving the expanded stent behind.

Therapeutic Procedures *(continued)*

TERM	WORD PARTS	DEFINITION
ligation and stripping (lye-GAY-shun)		Surgical treatment for varicose veins. The damaged vein is tied off (ligation) and removed (stripping).
percutaneous transluminal coronary angioplasty (PTCA) (per-kyoo-TAY-nee-us / trans-LOO-mih-nal / KOR-ah-nair-ee / AN-jee-oh-plas-tee)	per- = through cutane/o = skin -ous = pertaining to trans- = across -al = pertaining to angi/o = vessel -plasty = surgical repair	Method for treating localized coronary artery narrowing. A balloon catheter is inserted through the skin into the coronary artery and inflated to dilate the narrow blood vessel.

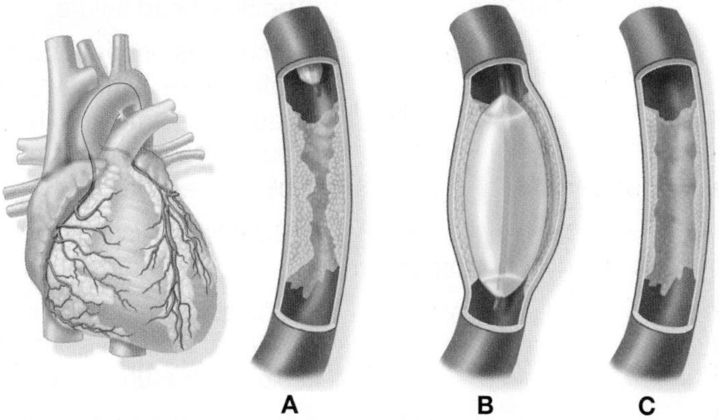

■ **Figure 5.22** Balloon angioplasty: (A) deflated balloon catheter is approaching an atherosclerotic plaque; (B) plaque is compressed by inflated balloon; (C) plaque remains compressed after balloon catheter is removed.

A   B   C

TERM	WORD PARTS	DEFINITION
stent		Stainless steel tube placed within a blood vessel or a duct to widen the lumen (see again Figure 5.21).
valve replacement		Removal of a diseased heart valve and replacement with an artificial valve.
valvoplasty (VAL-voh-plas-tee)	valv/o = valve -plasty = surgical repair	Surgical procedure to repair a heart valve.

 ## Pharmacology

CLASSIFICATION	WORD PARTS	ACTION	EXAMPLES
ACE inhibitor drugs		Produce vasodilation and decrease blood pressure.	benazepril, Lotensin; catopril, Capoten
antiarrhythmic (an-tye-a-RHYTH-mik)	anti- = against a- = without -ic = pertaining to	Reduces or prevents cardiac arrhythmias.	flecainide, Tambocor; ibutilide, Corvert
anticoagulant (an-tye-koh-AG-you-lant)	anti- = against	Prevents blood clot formation.	warfarin sodium, Coumadin, Warfarin
antilipidemic (an-tye-lip-ih-DEM-ik)	anti- = against lip/o = fat -ic = pertaining to	Reduces amount of cholesterol and lipids in the bloodstream; treats hyperlipidemia.	atorvastatin, Lipitor; simvastatin, Zocor
antiplatelet agents	anti- = against	Inhibits the ability of platelets to clump together as part of a blood clot.	clopidogrel, Plavix; aspirin; ticlopidine, Ticlid

■ Pharmacology *(continued)*

CLASSIFICATION	WORD PARTS	ACTION	EXAMPLES
beta-blocker drugs		Treats hypertension and angina pectoris by lowering the heart rate.	metoprolol, Lopressor; propranolol, Inderal
calcium channel blocker drugs		Treats hypertension, angina pectoris, and congestive heart failure by causing the heart to beat less forcefully and less often.	diltiazem, Cardizem; nifedipine, Procardia
cardiotonic (card-ee-oh-TAHN-ik)	cardi/o = heart -tonic = pertaining to tone	Increases the force of cardiac muscle contraction; treats congestive heart failure.	digoxin, Lanoxin
diuretic (dye-you-RET-ik)	-tic = pertaining to	Increases urine production by the kidneys, which works to reduce plasma and therefore blood volume, resulting in lower blood pressure.	furosemide, Lasix
thrombolytic (throm-boh-LIT-ik)	thromb/o = clot -lytic = destruction	Dissolves existing blood clots.	tissue plasminogen activator (tPA); alteplase, Activase
vasoconstrictor (vaz-oh-kon-STRICK-tor)	vas/o = vessel	Contracts smooth muscle in walls of blood vessels; raises blood pressure.	metaraminol, Aramine
vasodilator (vaz-oh-DYE-late-or)	vas/o = vessel	Relaxes the smooth muscle in the walls of arteries, thereby increasing diameter of the blood vessel. Used for two main purposes: increasing circulation to an ischemic area; reducing blood pressure.	nitroglycerine, Nitro-Dur; isoxsuprine, Vasodilan

■ Abbreviations

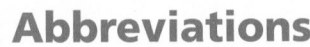

AED	automated external defibrillator	**CHF**	congestive heart failure
AF	atrial fibrillation	**CoA**	coarctation of the aorta
AMI	acute myocardial infarction	**CP**	chest pain
AS	arteriosclerosis	**CPR**	cardiopulmonary resuscitation
ASD	atrial septal defect	**CSD**	congenital septal defect
ASHD	arteriosclerotic heart disease	**CV**	cardiovascular
AV, A-V	atrioventricular	**DVT**	deep vein thrombosis
BBB	bundle branch block (L for left; R for right)	**ECC**	extracorporeal circulation
BP	blood pressure	**ECG, EKG**	electrocardiogram
bpm	beats per minute	**ECHO**	echocardiogram
CABG	coronary artery bypass graft	**GOT**	glutamic oxaloacetic transaminase
CAD	coronary artery disease	**HTN**	hypertension
cath	catheterization	**ICD**	implantable cardioverter-defibrillator
CC	cardiac catheterization, chief complaint	**ICU**	intensive care unit
CCU	coronary care unit	**IV**	intravenous

Abbreviations *(continued)*

LVAD	left ventricular assist device	**PDA**	patent ductus arteriosus
LVH	left ventricular hypertrophy	**PTCA**	percutaneous transluminal coronary angioplasty
MI	myocardial infarction, mitral insufficiency		
mm Hg	millimeters of mercury	**PVC**	premature ventricular contraction
MR	mitral regurgitation	**S1**	first heart sound
MS	mitral stenosis	**S2**	second heart sound
		SA, S-A	sinoatrial
		SK	streptokinase
		tPA	tissue-type plasminogen activator
		V fib	ventricular fibrillation
MVP	mitral valve prolapse	**VSD**	ventricular septal defect
P	pulse	**VT**	ventricular tachycardia
PAC	premature atrial contraction		

MED TERM TIP

Word Watch: Be careful using the abbreviation *MS*, which can mean either "mitral stenosis" or "multiple sclerosis."

Chapter Review

Real-World Applications

Medical Record Analysis

This Discharge Summary contains 12 medical terms. Underline each term and write it in the list below the report. Then define each term.

PGH PEARSON GENERAL HOSPITAL

5500 University Avenue, Metropolis, TX
Phone: (211) 594-4000 • Fax: (211) 594-4001

Medical Consultation Osteology
Date 6/1/2013
Patient Jorge Johnson
Patient complaint: Sever pain in the right ankle with any movement of lower limb.

Discharge Summary

Admitting Diagnosis:	Difficulty breathing, hypertension, tachycardia
Final Diagnosis:	CHF secondary to mitral valve prolapse
History of Present Illness:	Patient was brought to the Emergency Room by her family because of difficulty breathing and palpitations. Patient reports that she has experienced these symptoms for the past 6 months, but this episode is more severe than any previous. Upon admission in the ER, heart rate was 120 beats per minute and blood pressure was 180/110. The results of an EKG and cardiac enzyme blood tests were normal. She was admitted for a complete workup for tachycardia and hypertension.
Summary of Hospital Course:	Patient underwent a full battery of diagnostic tests. A prolapsed mitral valve was observed by echocardiography. A stress test had to be stopped early due to onset of severe difficulty in breathing. Angiocardiography failed to demonstrate significant CAD. Blood pressure and tachycardia were controlled with medications. At discharge, HR was 88 beats per minute and blood pressure was 165/98.
Discharge Plans:	There was no evidence of a myocardial infarction or significant CAD. Patient was placed on a low-salt and low-cholesterol diet. She received instructions on beginning a carefully graded exercise program. She is to continue her medications. If symptoms are not controlled by these measures, a mitral valve replacement will be considered.

Term	Definition
1 _____	_____
2 _____	_____
3 _____	_____
4 _____	_____
5 _____	_____
6 _____	_____
7 _____	_____
8 _____	_____
9 _____	_____
10 _____	_____
11 _____	_____
12 _____	_____

Chart Note Transcription

The chart note below contains 11 phrases that can be reworded with a medical term that you learned in this chapter. Each phrase is identified with an underline. Determine the medical term and write your answers in the space provided.

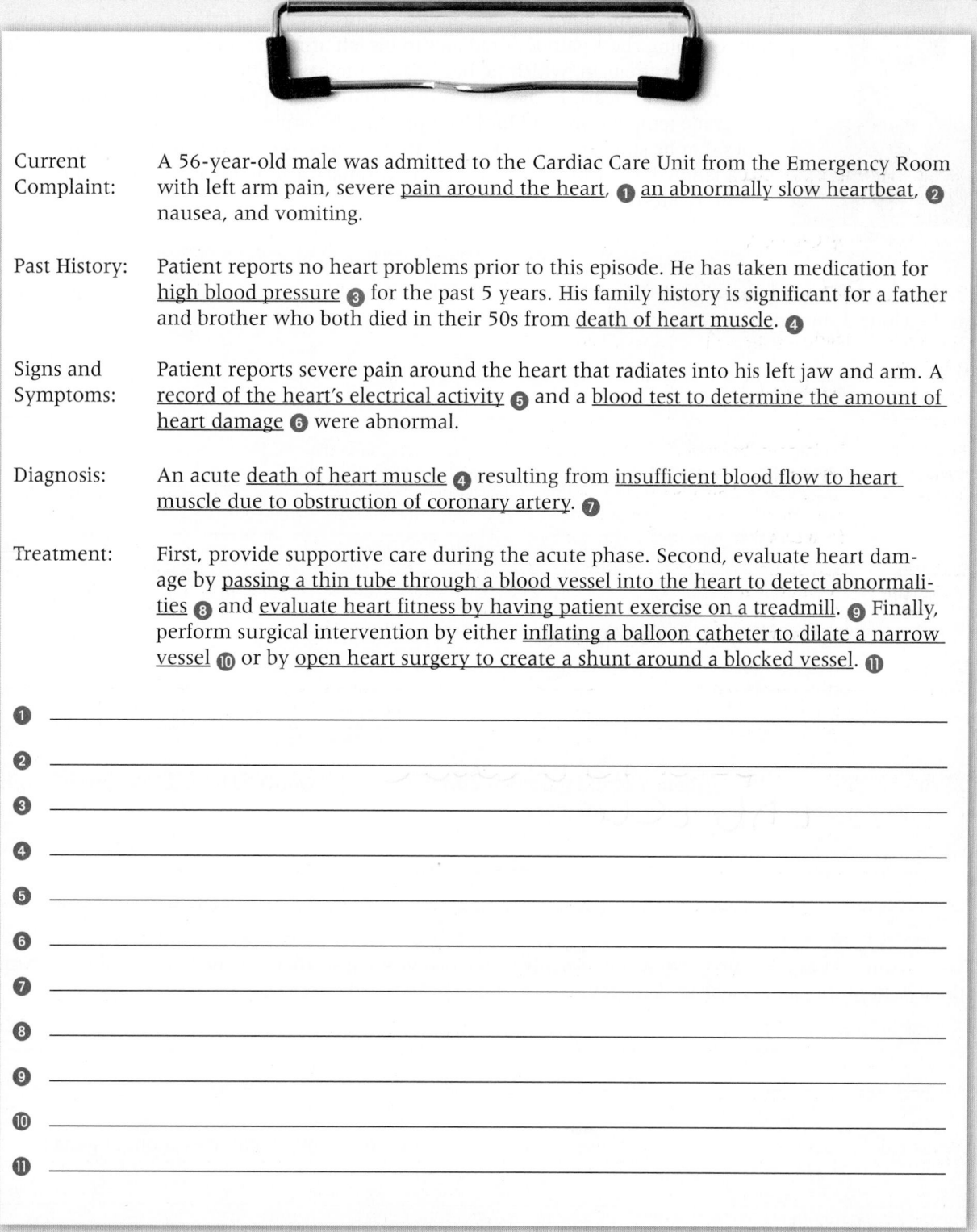

Current Complaint:
A 56-year-old male was admitted to the Cardiac Care Unit from the Emergency Room with left arm pain, severe <u>pain around the heart</u>, ❶ <u>an abnormally slow heartbeat</u>, ❷ nausea, and vomiting.

Past History:
Patient reports no heart problems prior to this episode. He has taken medication for <u>high blood pressure</u> ❸ for the past 5 years. His family history is significant for a father and brother who both died in their 50s from <u>death of heart muscle</u>. ❹

Signs and Symptoms:
Patient reports severe pain around the heart that radiates into his left jaw and arm. A <u>record of the heart's electrical activity</u> ❺ and a <u>blood test to determine the amount of heart damage</u> ❻ were abnormal.

Diagnosis:
An acute <u>death of heart muscle</u> ❹ resulting from <u>insufficient blood flow to heart muscle due to obstruction of coronary artery</u>. ❼

Treatment:
First, provide supportive care during the acute phase. Second, evaluate heart damage by <u>passing a thin tube through a blood vessel into the heart to detect abnormalities</u> ❽ and <u>evaluate heart fitness by having patient exercise on a treadmill</u>. ❾ Finally, perform surgical intervention by either <u>inflating a balloon catheter to dilate a narrow vessel</u> ❿ or by <u>open heart surgery to create a shunt around a blocked vessel</u>. ⓫

❶ _____

❷ _____

❸ _____

❹ _____

❺ _____

❻ _____

❼ _____

❽ _____

❾ _____

❿ _____

⓫ _____

Case Study

Below is a case study presentation of a patient with a condition covered by this chapter. Read the case study and answer the questions below. Some questions will ask for information not included within this chapter. Use your text, a medical dictionary, or any other reference material you choose to answer these questions.

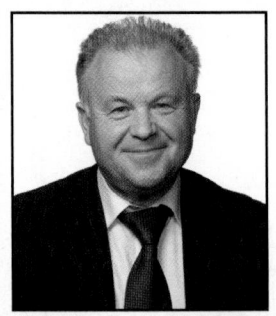

Mr. Thomas is a 62-year-old man who has been diagnosed with an acute myocardial infarction with the following symptoms and history. His chief complaint is a persistent, crushing chest pain that radiates to his left arm, jaw, neck, and shoulder blade. He describes the pain, which he has had for the past 12 hours, as a "squeezing" sensation around his heart. He has also suffered nausea, dyspnea, and diaphoresis. He has a low-grade temperature and his blood pressure is within a normal range at 130/82. He states that he smokes two packs of cigarettes a day, is overweight by 50 pounds, and has a family history of hypertension and coronary artery disease. He leads a relatively sedentary lifestyle.

(Galushko Sergey/Shutterstock)

1. What is the common name for Mr. Thomas's acute condition? Look this condition up in a reference source and include a short description of it.

    _____

    _____

2. What do you think the phrase "chief complaint" means?

    _____

    _____

3. What is the medical term for this patient's chief complaint? Define this term.

    _____

    _____

4. List and define each of the patient's additional symptoms in your own words. (These terms appear in other chapters of the book or use a medical dictionary.)

    _____

    _____

5. Using your text as a resource, name and describe three diagnostic tests that may be performed to determine the extent of the patient's heart damage.

    _____

    _____

6. What risk factors for developing heart disease does Mr. Thomas have? What changes should he make?

    _____

    _____

Practice Exercises

A. Complete the Statement

1. The study of the heart is called _____.

2. The three layers of the heart are _____, _____, and _____.

3. The impulse for the heartbeat (the pacemaker) originates in the _____.

4. Arteries carry blood _____ the heart.

5. The four heart valves are _____, _____, _____, and _____.

6. The _____ are the receiving chambers of the heart and the _____ are the pumping chambers.

7. The _____ circulation carries blood to and from the lungs.

8. The pointed tip of the heart is called the _____.

9. The _____ divides the heart into left and right halves.

10. _____ is the contraction phase of the heartbeat and _____ is the relaxation phase.

B. Combining Form Practice

The combining form **cardi/o** refers to the heart. Use it to write a term that means:

1. pertaining to the heart _____

2. disease of the heart muscle _____

3. enlargement of the heart _____

4. abnormally fast heart rate _____

5. abnormally slow heart rate _____

6. record of heart electricity _____

The combining form **angi/o** refers to the vessel. Use it to write a term that means:

7. vessel narrowing _____

8. vessel inflammation _____

9. involuntary muscle contraction of a vessel _____

The combining form **arteri/o** refers to the artery. Use it to write a term that means:

10. pertaining to an artery _____

11. hardening of an artery _____

12. small artery _____

C. Prefix Practice

Add the appropriate prefix to **-carditis** to form the term that matches each definition.

1. inflammation of the inner lining of the heart _____

2. inflammation of the outer layer of the heart _____

3. inflammation of the muscle of the heart _____

D. Define the Combining Form

	Definition	Example from Chapter
1. cardi/o	heart	
2. valvul/o	valve	
3. steth/o	stethoscope chest	
4. arteri/o	artery	
5. phleb/o	vein	
6. angi/o	vessel	
7. ventricul/o	ventricle	
8. thromb/o	clot	
9. atri/o	atrium	
10. ather/o	fatty substance	

E. Name That Term

1. pertaining to a vein Superior vena cavae _____

2. study of the heart EKG, ECG _____

3. record of a vein _____

4. process of recording electrical activity of the heart _____

5. high blood pressure _____

6. low blood pressure _____

7. surgical repair of valve _____

8. pertaining to between ventricles _____

9. removal of fatty substance _____

10. narrowing of the arteries _____

F. Name That Suffix

	Suffix	Example from Chapter
1. pressure	_____	_____
2. abnormal narrowing	_____	_____
3. instrument to measure pressure	_____	_____
4. small	_____	_____
5. hardening	_____	_____

G. Terminology Matching

Match each term to its definition.

1. _____ arrhythmia
2. _____ thrombus
3. _____ bradycardia
4. _g_ murmur
5. _____ phlebitis
6. _____ hypotension
7. _____ varicose vein
8. _____ tetralogy of Fallot
9. _e_ catheterization
10. _j_ sphygmomanometer

a. swollen, distended veins
b. inflammation of vein
c. serious congenital anomaly
d. slow heart rate
e. insertion of thin tubing
f. irregular heartbeat
g. an abnormal heart sound
h. clot in blood vessel
i. low blood pressure
j. blood pressure cuff

H. What Does it Stand For?

1. BP _Blood Pressure_
2. CHF _____
3. MI _____
4. CCU _____
5. PVC _____
6. CPR _____
7. CAD _____
8. CP _____
9. EKG _____
10. S1 _____

I. What's the Abbreviation?

1. mitral valve prolapse _____

2. ventricular septal defect _____

3. percutaneous transluminal coronary angioplasty _____

4. ventricular fibrillation _____

5. deep vein thrombosis _____

6. lactate dehydrogenase _____

7. coarctation of the aorta _____

8. tissue-type plasminogen activator _____

9. cardiovascular _____

10. extracorporeal circulation _____

J. Procedure Matching

Match each procedure to its definition.

1. _____ cardiac enzymes

2. _____ Doppler ultrasound

3. _____ Holter monitor

4. _____ cardiac scan

5. _____ stress testing

6. _____ echocardiography

7. _____ extracorporeal circulation

8. _____ ligation and stripping

9. _____ thrombolytic therapy

10. _____ PTAC

a. visualizes heart after patient is given radioactive thallium

b. uses ultrasound to visualize heart beating

c. blood test that indicates heart muscle damage

d. uses treadmill to evaluate cardiac fitness

e. removes varicose veins

f. clot-dissolving drugs

g. measures velocity of blood moving through blood vessels

h. balloon angioplasty

i. use of a heart-lung machine

j. portable EKG monitor

K. Define the Term

1. catheter _____

2. infarct _____

3. thrombus _____

4. palpitation _____

5. regurgitation _____

6. aneurysm _____

7. cardiac arrest _____

8. fibrillation _____

9. myocardial infarction _____

10. hemorrhoid _____

L. Fill in the Blank

angiography	murmur	varicose veins	echocardiogram
pacemaker	CHF	defibrillation	angina pectoris
Holter monitor	hypertension	MI	CCU

1. Tiffany was born with a congenital condition resulting in an abnormal heart sound called a(n) _____.

2. Joseph suffered an arrhythmia resulting in cardiac arrest. The emergency team used an instrument to give electric shocks to the heart to create a normal heart rhythm. This procedure is called _____.

3. Marguerite has been placed on a low-sodium diet and medication to bring her blood pressure down to a normal range. She suffers from _____.

4. Tony has had an artificial device called a(n) _____ inserted to control the beating of his heart by producing rhythmic electrical impulses.

5. Derrick's physician determined that he had _____ after examining his legs and finding swollen, tortuous veins.

6. Laura has persistent chest pains that require medication. The term for the pain is _____.

7. La Tonya will be admitted to what hospital unit after surgery to correct her heart condition? _____

8. Stephen is going to have a coronary artery bypass graft to correct the blockage in his coronary arteries. He recently suffered a heart attack as a result of this occlusion. His attack is called a(n) _____.

9. Stephen's physician scheduled a(n) _____, an X-ray to determine the extent of his blood vessel damage.

10. A patient scheduled to have a diagnostic procedure that uses ultrasound to produce an image of the heart valves is going to have a(n) _____.

11. Eric must wear a device for 24 hours that will keep track of his heart activity as he performs his normal daily routine. This device is called a(n) _____.

12. Lydia is 82 years old and is suffering from a heart condition that causes weakness, edema, and breathlessness. Her heart failure is the cause of her lung congestion. This condition is called _____.

M. Pharmacology Challenge

Fill in the classification for each drug description, then match the brand name.

Drug Description	Classification	Brand Name
1. _____ prevents arrhthymia	_____	a. tPA
2. _____ reduces cholesterol	_____	b. Coumadin
3. _____ increases force of heart contraction	_____	c. Cardizem
4. _____ increases urine production	_____	d. Nitro-Dur
5. _____ prevents blood clots	_____	e. Tambocor
6. _____ dissolves blood clots	_____	f. Lanoxin
7. _____ relaxes smooth muscle in artery wall	_____	g. Lipitor
8. _____ cause heart to beat less forcefully	_____	h. Lasix

MEDICAL TERMINOLOGY INTERACTIVE

Medical Terminology Interactive is a premium online homework management system that includes a host of features to help you study. Registered users will find:

- Fun games and activities built within a virtual hospital
- Powerful tools that track and analyze your results—allowing you to create a personalized learning experience
- Videos, flashcards, and audio pronunciations to help enrich your progress
- Streaming video lesson presentations and self-paced learning modules

www.pearsonhighered.com/mti

Labeling Exercise

Image A

Write the labels for this figure on the numbered lines provided.

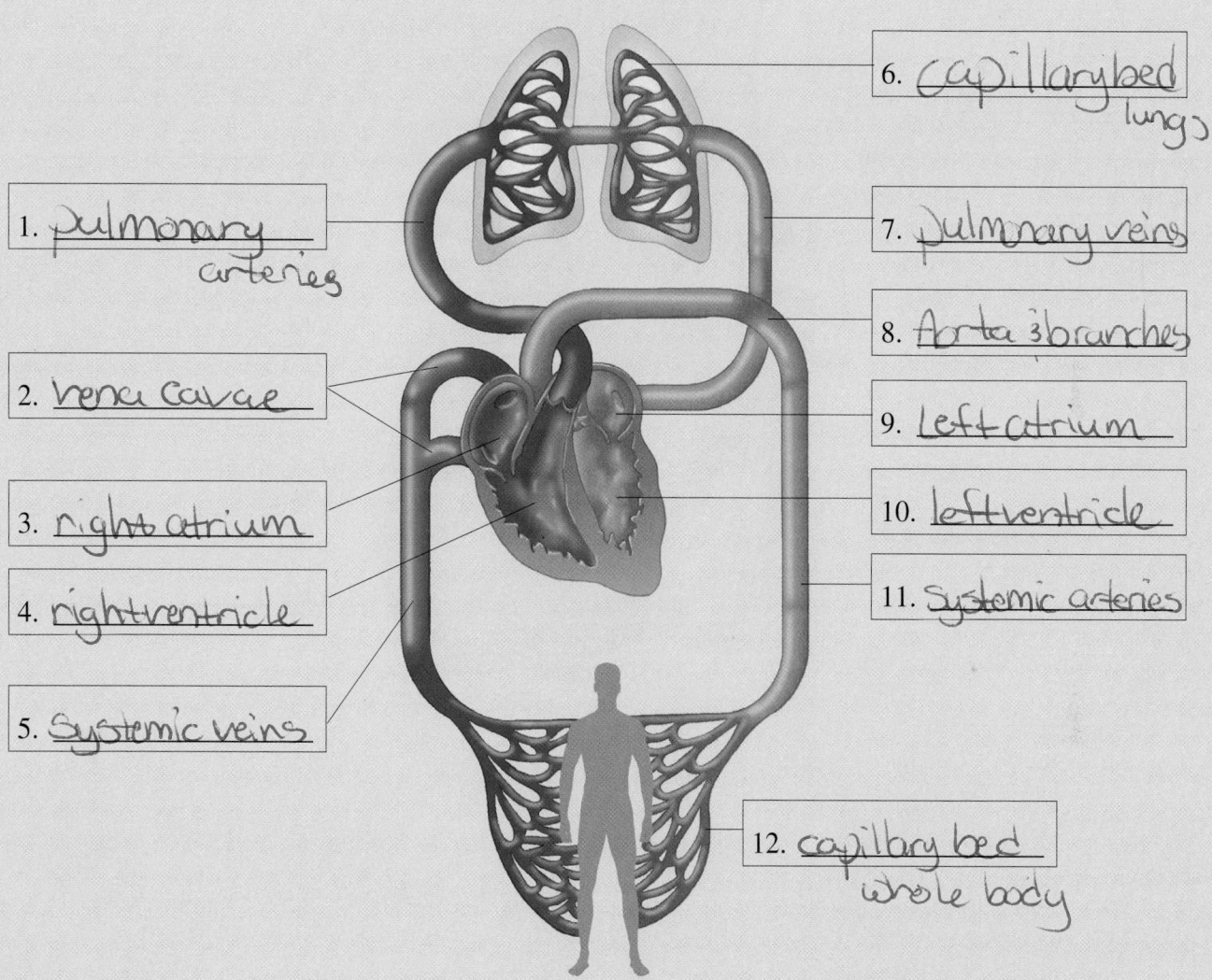

1. pulmonary arteries

2. vena cavae

3. right atrium

4. right ventricle

5. Systemic veins

6. capillary bed lungs

7. pulmonary veins

8. Aorta 3 branches

9. Left atrium

10. left ventricle

11. Systemic arteries

12. capillary bed whole body

Image B

Write the labels for this figure on the numbered lines provided.

1. _____

2. _____

3. _____

4. _____

5. _____

6. _____

7. _____

8. _____

9. _____

10. _____

11. _____

12. _____

13. _____

14. _____

15. _____

16. _____

17. _____

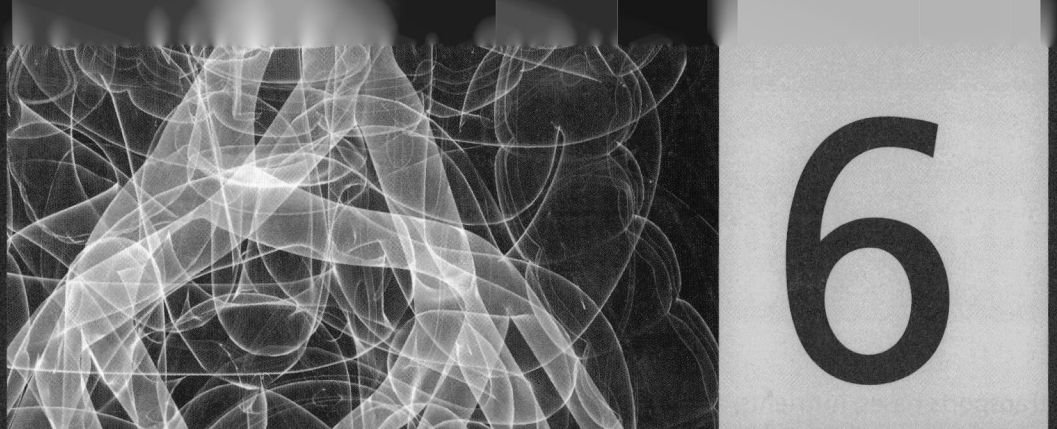

6

BLOOD AND THE LYMPHATIC AND IMMUNE SYSTEMS

Learning Objectives

Upon completion of this chapter, you will be able to

- Recognize the combining forms and suffixes introduced in this chapter.

- Gain the ability to pronounce medical terms and major anatomical structures.

- List the major components, structures, and organs of the blood and lymphatic and immune systems and their functions.

- Describe the blood typing systems.

- Discuss immunity, the immune response, and standard precautions.

- Identify and define blood and lymphatic and immune system anatomical terms.

- Identify and define selected blood and lymphatic and immune system pathology terms.

- Identify and define selected blood and lymphatic and immune system diagnostic procedures.

- Identify and define selected blood and lymphatic and immune system therapeutic procedures.

- Identify and define selected medications associated with blood and the lymphatic and immune systems.

- Define selected abbreviations associated with blood and the lymphatic and immune systems.

Section I: Blood at a Glance

Function

Blood transports gases, nutrients, and wastes to all areas of the body either attached to red blood cells or dissolved in the plasma. White blood cells fight infection and disease, and platelets initiate the blood clotting process.

Organs

Here are the primary components that comprise blood.

formed elements   **plasma**
- erythrocytes
- leukocytes
- platelets

Word Parts

Here are the most common word parts (with their meanings) used to build blood terms. For a more comprehensive list, refer to the Terminology section of this chapter.

Combining Forms

agglutin/o	clumping	hem/o	blood
bas/o	base	hemat/o	blood
chrom/o	color	leuk/o	white
coagul/o	clotting	lymph/o	lymph
cyt/o	cell	morph/o	shape
eosin/o	rosy red	neutr/o	neutral
erythr/o	red	phag/o	eat, swallow
fibrin/o	fibers, fibrous	sanguin/o	blood
fus/o	pouring	septic/o	infection
granul/o	granules	thromb/o	clot

Suffixes

-apheresis	removal, carry away
-crit	separation of
-cytosis	more than the normal number of cells
-emia	blood condition
-globin	protein
-penia	abnormal decrease, too few
-phil	attracted to
-poiesis	formation
-stasis	standing still

Blood Illustrated

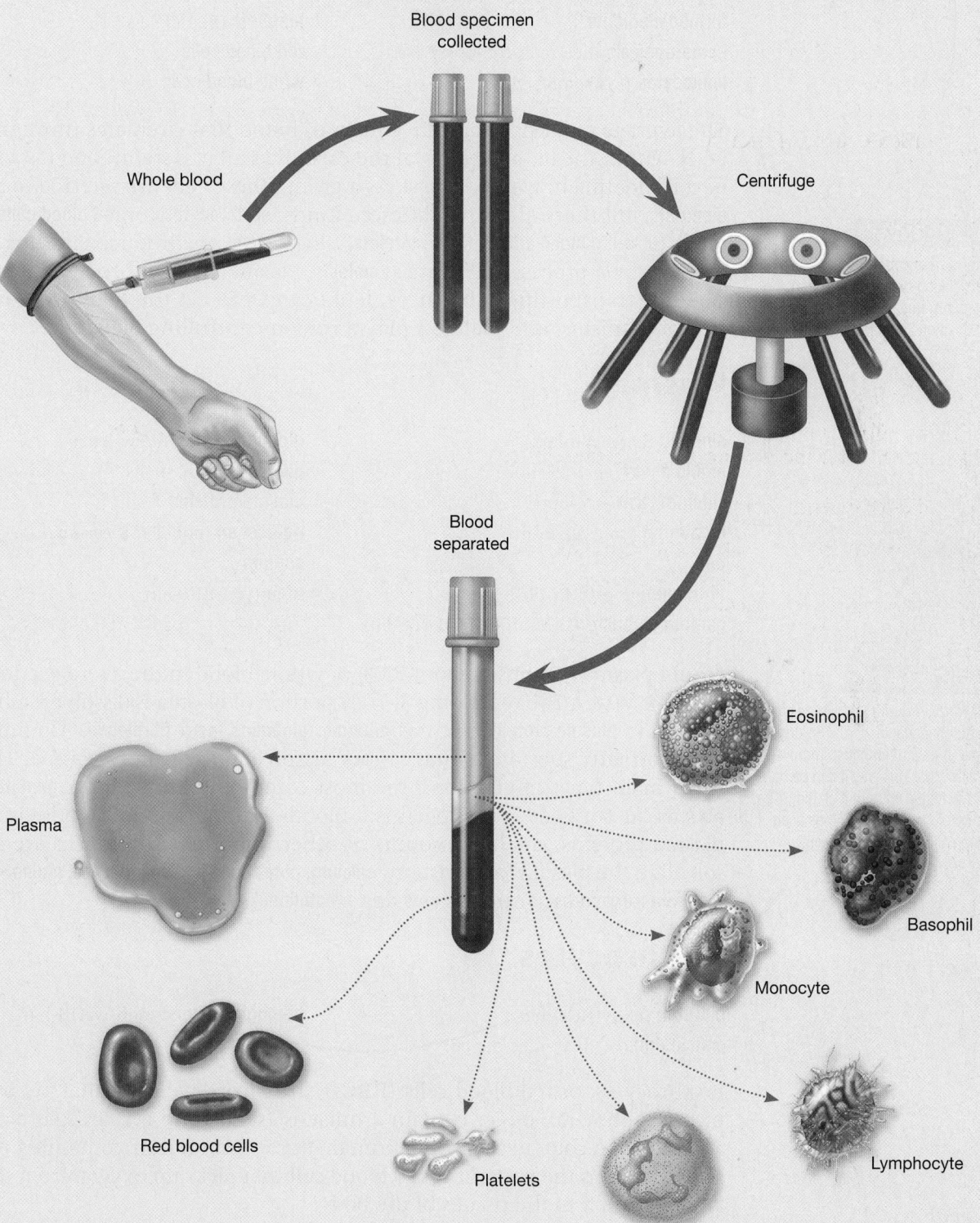

Whole blood

Blood specimen collected

Centrifuge

Blood separated

Plasma

Eosinophil

Basophil

Monocyte

Lymphocyte

Red blood cells

Platelets

Neutrophil

⬛ Anatomy and Physiology of Blood

erythrocytes (eh-RITH-roh-sights)   **plasma** (PLAZ-mah)

formed elements   **platelets** (PLAYT-lets)

hematopoiesis (hee-mah-toh-poy-EE-sis) **red blood cells**

leukocytes (LOO-koh-sights)   **white blood cells**

MED TERM TIP

The term *hematopoiesis* literally means "blood formation" by combining hemat/o (meaning blood) with -poiesis (meaning formation).

The average adult has about five liters of blood that circulates throughout the body within the blood vessels of the cardiovascular system. Blood is a mixture of cells floating in watery **plasma.** As a group, these cells are referred to as **formed elements,** but there are three different kinds: **erythrocytes** (or **red blood cells**), **leukocytes** (or **white blood cells**), and **platelets.** Blood cells are produced in the red bone marrow by a process called **hematopoiesis.** Plasma and erythrocytes are responsible for transporting substances, leukocytes protect the body from invading microorganisms, and platelets play a role in controlling bleeding.

Plasma

albumin (al-BEW-min)   **globulins** (GLOB-yew-lenz)

amino acids (ah-MEE-noh)   **glucose** (GLOO-kohs)

calcium (KAL-see-um)   **plasma proteins**

creatinine (kree-AT-in-in)   **potassium** (poh-TASS-ee-um)

fats   **sodium**

fibrinogen (fye-BRIN-oh-jen)   **urea** (yoo-REE-ah)

gamma globulin (GAM-ah / GLOB-yoo-lin)

MED TERM TIP

Word Watch: *Plasma* and *serum* are not interchangeable words. Serum is plasma, but with fibrinogen removed or inactivated. This way it can be handled and tested without it clotting. The term *serum* is also sometimes used to mean antiserum or antitoxin.

Liquid plasma composes about 55% of whole blood in the average adult and is 90–92% water. The remaining 8–10% portion of plasma is dissolved substances, especially **plasma proteins** such as **albumin, globulins,** and **fibrinogen.** Albumin helps transport fatty substances that cannot dissolve in the watery plasma. There are three main types of globulins; the most commonly known one, **gamma globulin,** acts as an antibody. Fibrinogen is a blood-clotting protein. In addition to the plasma proteins, smaller amounts of other important substances are also dissolved in the plasma for transport: **calcium, potassium, sodium, glucose, amino acids, fats,** and waste products such as **urea** and **creatinine.**

Erythrocytes

bilirubin (bil-ly-ROO-bin)   **hemoglobin** (hee-moh-GLOH-bin)

enucleated (ee-NEW-klee-ate-ed)

Erythrocytes, or red blood cells (RBCs), are biconcave disks that are **enucleated,** meaning they no longer contain a nucleus (see Figure 6.1 ⬛). Red blood cells appear red in color because they contain **hemoglobin,** an iron-containing pigment. Hemoglobin is the part of the red blood cell that picks up oxygen from the lungs and delivers it to the tissues of the body.

There are about 5 million erythrocytes per cubic millimeter of blood. The total number in an average-sized adult is 35 trillion, with males having more red blood cells than females. Erythrocytes have an average lifespan of 120 days,

Erythrocytes

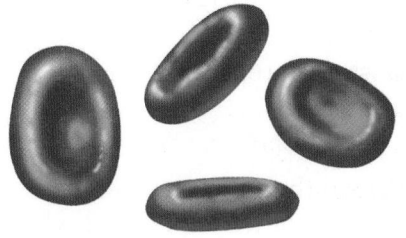

Red blood cells

■ **Figure 6.1** The biconcave disk shape of eryth-rocytes (red blood cells).

Leukocyctes

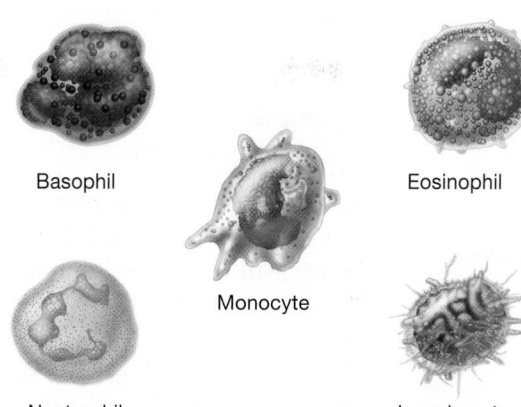

■ **Figure 6.2** The five different types of leukocytes (white blood cells).

and then the spleen removes the worn-out and damaged ones from circulation. Much of the red blood cell, such as the iron, can be reused, but one portion, **bilirubin,** is a waste product disposed of by the liver.

Leukocytes

agranulocytes (ah-GRAN-yew-loh-sights)   **pathogens** (PATH-oh-ginz)
granulocytes (GRAN-yew-loh-sights)

Leukocytes, also referred to as white blood cells (WBCs), provide protection against the invasion of **pathogens** such as bacteria, viruses, and other foreign material. In general, white blood cells have a spherical shape with a large nucleus, and there are about 8,000 per cubic millimeter of blood (see Figure 6.2 ■). There are five different types of white blood cells, each with its own strategy for protecting the body. The five can be subdivided into two categories: **granulocytes** (with granules in the cytoplasm) and **agranulocytes** (without granules in the cytoplasm). The name and function of each type is presented in Table 6.1 ■.

MED TERM TIP

Your body makes about 2 million erythrocytes every second. Of course, it must then destroy 2 million every second to maintain a relatively constant 30 trillion red blood cells.

MED TERM TIP

A *phagocyte* is a cell that has the ability to ingest (phag/o = eat; -cyte = cell) and digest bacteria and other foreign particles. This process, *phagocytosis*, is critical for the control of bacteria within the body.

Table 6.1	Leukocyte Classification
LEUKOCYTE	**FUNCTION**
Granulocytes	
Basophils (basos) (BAY-soh-fillz)	Release histamine and heparin to damaged tissues
Eosinophils (eosins) (ee-oh-SIN-oh-fillz)	Destroy parasites and increase during allergic reactions
Neutrophils (NOO-troh-fillz)	Engulfs foreign and damaged cells (phagocytosis); most numerous of the leukocytes
Agranulocytes	
Monocytes (monos) (MON-oh-sights)	Engulfs foreign and damaged cells (phagocytosis)
Lymphocytes (lymphs) (LIM-foh-sights)	Plays several different roles in immune response

Platelets

agglutinate	**prothrombin** (proh-THROM-bin)
(ah-GLOO-tih-nayt)	**thrombin** (THROM-bin)
fibrin (FYE-brin)	**thrombocyte** (THROM-boh-sight)
hemostasis	**thromboplastin**
(hee-moh-STAY-sis)	(throm-boh-PLAS-tin)

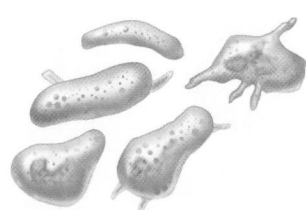

■ **Figure 6.3** Platelet structure.

Platelet, the modern term for **thrombocyte,** refers to the smallest of all the formed blood elements. Platelets are not whole cells, but rather are formed when the cytoplasm of a large precursor cell shatters into small plate-like fragments (see Figure 6.3 ■). There are between 200,000 and 300,000 per cubic millimeter in the body.

Platelets play a critical part in the blood-clotting process or **hemostasis.** They **agglutinate** or clump together into small clusters when a blood vessel is cut or damaged. Platelets also release a substance called **thromboplastin,** which, in the presence of calcium, reacts with **prothrombin** (a clotting protein in the blood) to form **thrombin.** Then thrombin, in turn, works to convert fibrinogen to **fibrin,** which eventually becomes the meshlike blood clot.

Blood Typing

ABO system	**Rh factor**
blood typing	

Each person's blood is different due to the presence of antigens or markers on the surface of erythrocytes. Before a person receives a blood transfusion, it is important to do **blood typing.** This laboratory test determines if the donated blood is compatible with the recipient's blood. There are many different subgroups of blood markers, but the two most important ones are the **ABO system** and **Rh factor.**

ABO System

type A	**type O**
type AB	**universal donor**
type B	**universal recipient**

In the ABO blood system there are two possible red blood cell markers, A and B. A marker is one method by which cells identify themselves. A person with an A marker is said to have **type A** blood. Type A blood produces anti-B antibodies that will attack type B blood. The presence of a B marker gives **type B** blood and anti-A antibodies (that will attack type A blood). If both markers are present, the blood is **type AB** and does not contain any antibodies. Therefore, type AB blood will not attack any other blood type. The absence of either an A or a B marker results in **type O** blood, which contains both anti-A and anti-B antibodies. Type O blood will attack all other blood types (A, B, and AB). For further information on antibodies, refer to the lymphatic section later in this chapter.

Because type O blood does not have either marker A or B, it will not react with anti-A or anti-B antibodies. For this reason, a person with type O blood is referred to as a **universal donor.** In extreme cases, type O blood may be given to a person with any of the other blood types. Similarly, type AB blood is the **universal recipient.** A person with type AB blood has no antibodies against the other blood types and, therefore, in extreme cases, can receive any type of blood.

Rh Factor

Rh-negative   **Rh-positive**

Rh factor is not as difficult to understand as the ABO system. A person with the Rh factor on his or her red blood cells is said to be **Rh-positive** (Rh+). Since this person has the factor, he or she will not make anti-Rh antibodies. A person without the Rh factor is **Rh-negative** (Rh−) and will produce anti-Rh antibodies. Therefore, an Rh+ person may receive both an Rh+ and an Rh− transfusion, but an Rh− person can receive only Rh− blood.

 # Terminology

Word Parts Used to Build Blood Terms

The following lists contain the combining forms, suffixes, and prefixes used to build terms in the remaining sections of this chapter.

Combining Forms

bas/o	base	**fibrin/o**	fibers	**lymph/o**	lymph
chrom/o	color	**fus/o**	pouring	**morph/o**	shape
coagul/o	clotting	**granul/o**	granules	**neutr/o**	neutral
cyt/o	cell	**hem/o**	blood	**phleb/o**	vein
eosin/o	rosy red	**hemat/o**	blood	**sanguin/o**	blood
erythr/o	red	**leuk/o**	white	**septic/o**	infection
		lip/o	fat	**thromb/o**	clot

Suffixes

-apheresis	removal, carry away	**-ia**	condition	**-ous**	pertaining to
-crit	separation of	**-ic**	pertaining to	**-penia**	too few
-cyte	cell	**-ion**	action	**-phil**	attracted to
-cytosis	more than the normal number of cells	**-logy**	study of	**-plastic**	pertaining to development
		-lytic	destruction		
-emia	blood condition	**-oma**	growth	**-rrhage**	abnormal flow
-globin	protein	**-otomy**	cutting into	**-rrhagic**	pertaining to abnormal flow

Prefixes

a-	without	**dys-**	abnormal	**mono-**	one
an-	without	**homo-**	same	**pan-**	all
anti-	against	**hyper-**	excessive	**poly-**	many
auto-	self	**hypo-**	insufficient	**trans-**	across

Anatomical Terms

TERM	WORD PARTS	DEFINITION
agranulocyte (ah-GRAN-yew-loh-sight)	a- = without granul/o = granules -cyte = cell	A leukocyte without granules in its cytoplasm; monocytes and lymphocytes.
basophil (BAY-soh-fill)	bas/o = base -phil = attracted to	A granulocytic leukocyte that attracts a basic pH stain.
eosinophil (ee-oh-SIN-oh-fill)	eosin/o = rosy red -phil = attracted to	A granulocytic leukocyte that attracts a rosy red stain.
erythrocyte (eh-RITH-roh-sight)	erythr/o = red -cyte = cell	A red blood cell.
fibrinous (fye-brin-us)	fibrin/o = fibers -ous = pertaining to	Pertaining to fibers.
granulocyte (GRAN-yew-loh-sight)	granul/o = granules -cyte = cell	A leukocyte with granules in its cytoplasm; basophils, eosinophils, neutrophils.
hematic (hee-MAT-ik)	hemat/o = blood -ic = pertaining to	Pertaining to blood.
leukocyte (LOO-koh-sight)	leuk/o = white -cyte = cell	A white blood cell.
lymphocyte (LIM-foh-sight)	lymph/o = lymph -cyte = cell	An agranulocytic leukocyte formed in lymphatic tissue.
monocyte (MON-oh-sight)	mono- = one -cyte = cell	An agranulocytic leukocyte with a single, large nucleus.
neutrophil (NOO-troh-fill)	neutr/o = neutral -phil = attracted to	A granulocytic leukocyte that attracts a neutral pH stain.
sanguinous (SANG-gwih-nus)	sanguin/o = blood -ous = pertaining to	Pertaining to blood.
thrombocyte (THROM-boh-sight)	thromb/o = clot -cyte = cell	A clotting cell; a platelet.

Pathology

TERM	WORD PARTS	DEFINITION
Medical Specialties		
hematology (hee-mah-TALL-oh-jee)	hemat/o = blood -logy = study of	The branch of medicine specializing in treatment of diseases and conditions of the blood. Physician is a *hematologist*.
Signs and Symptoms		
blood clot		The hard collection of fibrin, blood cells, and tissue debris that is the end result of hemostasis or the blood-clotting process (see Figure 6.4 ■).

■ Pathology *(continued)*

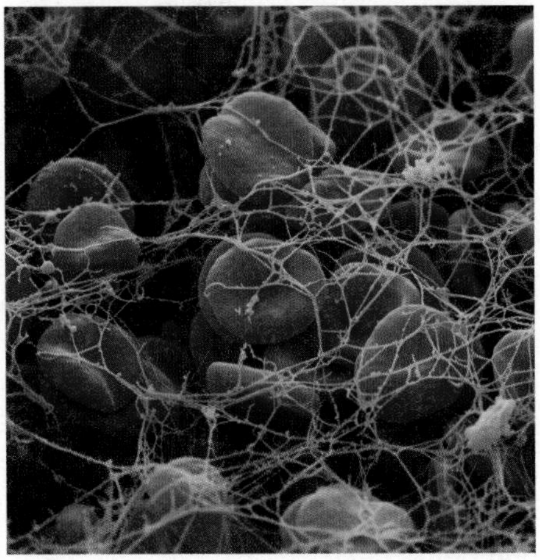

TERM	WORD PARTS	DEFINITION

■ **Figure 6.4** Electronmicrograph showing a blood clot composed of fibrin, red blood cells, and tissue debris. *(Eye of Science/Photo Researchers, Inc.)*

TERM	WORD PARTS	DEFINITION
coagulate (koh-ag-YOO-late)	coagul/o = clotting	To convert from a liquid to a gel or solid, as in blood coagulation.
dyscrasia (dis-CRAZ-ee-ah)	dys- = abnormal -ia = condition	A general term indicating the presence of a disease affecting blood.
hematoma (hee-mah-TOH-mah)	hemat/o = blood -oma = growth	The collection of blood under the skin as the result of blood escaping into the tissue from damaged blood vessels. Commonly referred to as a *bruise*.

> **MED TERM TIP**
>
> Word Watch: The term *hematoma* is confusing. Its simple translation is "blood tumor." However, it is used to refer to blood that has leaked out of a blood vessel and has pooled in the tissues.

TERM	WORD PARTS	DEFINITION
hemorrhage (HEM-er-rij)	hem/o = blood -rrhage = abnormal flow	Rapid flow of blood.

Blood

TERM	WORD PARTS	DEFINITION
hemophilia (hee-moh-FILL-ee-ah)	hem/o = blood -phil = attracted to -ia = condition	Hereditary blood disease in which blood-clotting time is prolonged due to a lack of one vital clotting factor. It is transmitted by a sex-linked trait from females to males, appearing almost exclusively in males.
hyperlipidemia (HYE-per-lip-id-ee-mee-ah)	hyper- = excessive lip/o = fat -emia = blood condition	Condition of having too high a level of lipids such as cholesterol in the bloodstream. A risk factor for developing atherosclerosis and coronary artery disease.
pancytopenia (pan-sigh-toe-PEN-ee-ah)	pan- = all cyt/o = cell -penia = too few	Having too few of all cells.
septicemia (sep-tih-SEE-mee-ah)	septic/o = infection -emia = blood condition	Having bacteria or their toxins in the bloodstream. *Sepsis* is a term that means putrefaction or infection. Commonly referred to as *blood poisoning*.

Pathology *(continued)*

TERM	WORD PARTS	DEFINITION
Erythrocytes		
anemia (an-NEE-mee-ah)	an- = without -emia = blood condition	A large group of conditions characterized by a reduction in the number of red blood cells or the amount of hemoglobin in the blood; results in less oxygen reaching the tissues.
aplastic anemia (a-PLAS-tik / an-NEE-mee-ah)	a- = without -plastic = pertaining to development an- = without -emia = blood condition	Severe form of anemia that develops as a consequence of loss of functioning red bone marrow. Results in a decrease in the number of all the formed elements. Treatment may eventually require a bone marrow transplant.
erythrocytosis (ee-RITH-row-sigh-toe-sis)	erythr/o = red -cytosis = more than normal number of cells	The condition of having too many red blood cells.
erythropenia (ee-RITH-row-pen-ee-ah)	erythr/o = red -penia = too few	The condition of having too few red blood cells.
hemolytic anemia (hee-moh-LIT-ik / an-NEE-mee-ah)	hem/o = blood -lytic = destruction an- = without -emia = blood condition	An anemia that develops as the result of the destruction of erythrocytes.
hemolytic reaction (hee-moh-LIT-ik)	hem/o = blood -lytic = destruction	The destruction of a patient's erythrocytes that occurs when receiving a transfusion of an incompatible blood type. Also called a *transfusion reaction.*
hypochromic anemia (hi-poe-CHROME-ik / an-NEE-mee-ah)	hypo- = insufficient chrom/o = color -ic = pertaining to an- = without -emia = blood condition	Anemia resulting from having insufficient hemoglobin in the erythrocytes. Named because the hemoglobin molecule is responsible for the dark red color of the erythrocytes.
iron-deficiency anemia	an- = without -emia = blood condition	Anemia resulting from not having sufficient iron to manufacture hemoglobin.
pernicious anemia (PA) (per-NISH-us / an-NEE-mee-ah)	an- = without -emia = blood condition	Anemia associated with insufficient absorption of vitamin B_{12} by the digestive system. Vitamin B_{12} is necessary for erythrocyte production.
polycythemia vera (pol-ee-sigh-THEE-mee-ah / VAIR-rah)	poly- = many cyt/o = cell hem/o = blood -ia = condition	Production of too many red blood cells by the bone marrow. Blood becomes too thick to easily flow through the blood vessels.
sickle cell anemia	an- = without -emia = blood condition	A genetic disorder in which erythrocytes take on an abnormal curved or "sickle" shape. These cells are fragile and are easily damaged, leading to a hemolytic anemia (see Figure 6.5 ■).

Pathology *(continued)*

TERM	WORD PARTS	DEFINITION

Normal red blood cells   **Sickled cells**

■ **Figure 6.5** Comparison of normal-shaped erythrocytes and the abnormal sickle shape noted in patients with sickle cell anemia.

TERM	WORD PARTS	DEFINITION
thalassemia (thal-ah-SEE-mee-ah)	-emia = blood condition	A genetic disorder in which the body is unable to make functioning hemoglobin, resulting in anemia.
Leukocytes		
leukemia (loo-KEE-mee-ah)	leuk/o = white -emia = blood condition	Cancer of the white blood cell–forming red bone marrow resulting in a large number of abnormal and immature white blood cells circulating in the blood.
leukocytosis (LOO-koh-sigh-toh-sis)	leuk/o = white -cytosis = more than normal number of cells	The condition of having too many white blood cells.
leukopenia (LOO-koh-pen-ee-ah)	leuk/o = white -penia = too few	The condition of having too few white blood cells.
Platelets		
thrombocytosis (throm-boh-sigh-TOH-sis)	thromb/o = clot -cytosis = more than normal number of cells	The condition of having too many platelets.
thrombopenia (THROM-boh-pen-ee-ah)	thromb/o = clot -penia = too few	The condition of having too few platelets.

Diagnostic Procedures

TERM	WORD PARTS	DEFINITION
Clinical Laboratory Tests		
blood culture and sensitivity (C&S)		Sample of blood is incubated in the laboratory to check for bacterial growth. If bacteria are present, they are identified and tested to determine which antibiotics they are sensitive to.
complete blood count (CBC)		Combination of blood tests including red blood cell count (RBC), white blood cell count (WBC), hemoglobin (Hgb), hematocrit (Hct), white blood cell differential, and platelet count.

Diagnostic Procedures *(continued)*

TERM	WORD PARTS	DEFINITION
erythrocyte sedimentation rate (ESR, sed rate) (eh-RITH-roh-sight / sed-ih-men-TAY-shun)	erythr/o = red -cyte = cell	Blood test to determine the rate at which mature red blood cells settle out of the blood after the addition of an anticoagulant. This is an indicator of the presence of an inflammatory disease.
hematocrit (HCT, Hct, crit) (hee-MAT-oh-krit)	hemat/o = blood -crit = separation of	Blood test to measure the volume of red blood cells (erythrocytes) within the total volume of blood.
hemoglobin (Hgb, hb) (hee-moh-GLOH-bin)	hem/o = blood -globin = protein	A blood test to measure the amount of hemoglobin present in a given volume of blood.
platelet count (PLAYT-let)		Blood test to determine the number of platelets in a given volume of blood.
prothrombin time (Pro time, PT) (proh-THROM-bin)	thromb/o = clot	A measure of the blood's coagulation abilities by measuring how long it takes for a clot to form after prothrombin has been activated.
red blood cell count (RBC)		Blood test to determine the number of erythrocytes in a volume of blood. A decrease in red blood cells may indicate anemia; an increase may indicate polycythemia.
red blood cell morphology	morph/o = shape -logy = study of	Examination of a specimen of blood for abnormalities in the shape (morphology) of the erythrocytes. Used to determine diseases like sickle cell anemia.
sequential multiple analyzer computer (SMAC)		Machine for doing multiple blood chemistry tests automatically.
white blood cell count (WBC)		Blood test to measure the number of leukocytes in a volume of blood. An increase may indicate the presence of infection or a disease such as leukemia. A decrease in white blood cells may be caused by radiation therapy or chemotherapy.
white blood cell differential (diff) (diff-er-EN-shal)		Blood test to determine the number of each variety of leukocytes.
Medical Procedures		
bone marrow aspiration (as-pih-RAY-shun)		Sample of bone marrow is removed by aspiration with a needle and examined for diseases such as leukemia or aplastic anemia.
phlebotomy (fleh-BOT-oh-me)	phleb/o = vein -otomy = cutting into	Incision into a vein in order to remove blood for a diagnostic test. Also called *venipuncture*.

■ **Figure 6.6** Phlebotomist using a needle to withdraw blood.

Therapeutic Procedures

TERM	WORD PARTS	DEFINITION
Medical Procedures		
autologous transfusion (aw-TALL-oh-gus / trans-FYOO-zhun)	auto- = self	Procedure for collecting and storing a patient's own blood several weeks prior to the actual need. It can then be used to replace blood lost during a surgical procedure.
blood transfusion (trans-FYOO-zhun)	trans- = across fus/o = pouring -ion = action	Artificial transfer of blood into the bloodstream.
	MED TERM TIP Before a patient receives a blood transfusion, the laboratory performs a **type and cross-match**. This test first double-checks the blood type of both the donor's and recipient's blood. Then a cross-match is performed. This process mixed together small samples of both bloods and observes the mixture for adverse reactions.	
bone marrow transplant (BMT)		Patient receives red bone marrow from a donor after the patient's own bone marrow has been destroyed by radiation or chemotherapy.
homologous transfusion (hoh-MALL-oh-gus / trans-FYOO-zhun)	homo- = same	Replacement of blood by transfusion of blood received from another person.
packed red cells		A transfusion in which most of the plasma, leukocytes, and platelets have been removed, leaving on erythrocytes.
plasmapheresis (plaz-mah-fah-REE-sis)	-apheresis = removal, carry away	Method of removing plasma from the body without depleting the formed elements. Whole blood is removed and the cells and plasma are separated. The cells are returned to the patient along with a donor plasma transfusion.
whole blood		Refers to the mixture of both plasma and formed elements.

Pharmacology

CLASSIFICATION	WORD PARTS	ACTION	EXAMPLES
anticoagulant (an-tih-koh-AG-yoo-lant)	anti- = against coagul/o = clotting	Substance that prevents blood clot formation. Commonly referred to as *blood thinners*.	heparin, HepLock; warfarin, Coumadin
antihemorrhagic (an-tih-hem-er-RAJ-ik)	anti- = against hem/o = blood -rrhagic = pertaining to abnormal flow	Substance that prevents or stops hemorrhaging; a *hemostatic agent*.	aminocaproic acid, Amicar; vitamin K
antiplatelet agents (an-tih-PLATE-let)	anti- = against	Substance that interferes with the action of platelets. Prolongs bleeding time. Used to prevent heart attacks and strokes.	clopidogrel, Plavix; ticlopidine, Ticlid

Pharmacology *(continued)*

CLASSIFICATION	WORD PARTS	ACTION	EXAMPLES
hematinic (hee-mah-TIN-ik)	hemat/o = blood -ic = pertaining to	Substance that increases the number of erythrocytes or the amount of hemoglobin in the blood.	epoetin alfa, Procrit; darbepoetin alfa, Aranesp
thrombolytic (throm-boh-LIT-ik)	thromb/o = clot -lytic = destruction	Term meaning able to dissolve existing blood clots.	alteplase, Activase; streptokinase, Streptase

Abbreviations

ALL	acute lymphocytic leukemia	**lymphs**	lymphocytes
AML	acute myelogenous leukemia	**monos**	monocytes
basos	basophils	**PA**	pernicious anemia
BMT	bone marrow transplant	**PCV**	packed cell volume
CBC	complete blood count	**PMN, polys**	polymorphonuclear neutrophil
CLL	chronic lymphocytic leukemia	**PT, pro-time**	prothrombin time
CML	chronic myelogenous leukemia		
diff	differential	**RBC**	red blood cell
eosins, eos	eosinophils	**Rh+**	Rh-positive
ESR, SR, sed rate	erythrocyte sedimentation rate	**Rh–**	Rh-negative
		segs	segmented neutrophils
HCT, Hct, crit	hematocrit	**SMAC**	sequential multiple analyzer computer
		WBC	white blood cell
Hgb, Hb, HGB	hemoglobin		

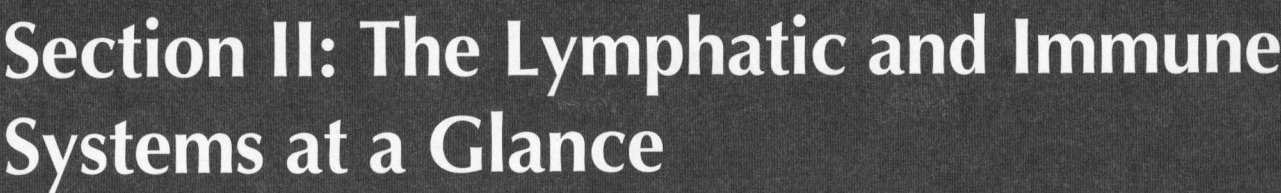

Section II: The Lymphatic and Immune Systems at a Glance

Function

The lymphatic system consists of a network of lymph vessels that pick up excess tissue fluid, cleanse it, and return it to the circulatory system. It also picks up fats that have been absorbed by the digestive system. The immune system fights disease and infections.

Organs

Here are the primary structures that comprise the lymphatic and immune system.

lymph nodes
lymphatic vessels
spleen
thymus gland
tonsils

Word Parts

Here are the most common word parts (with their meanings) used to build lymphatic and immune system terms. For a more comprehensive list, refer to the Terminology section of this chapter.

Combining Forms

adenoid/o	adenoids	nucle/o	nucleus
axill/o	axilla, underarm	path/o	disease
immun/o	protection	splen/o	spleen
inguin/o	groin region	thym/o	thymus gland
lymph/o	lymph	tonsill/o	tonsils
lymphaden/o	lymph node	tox/o	poison
lymphangi/o	lymph vessel		

Suffixes

-edema	swelling
-globulin	protein

The Lymphatic and Immune Systems Illustrated

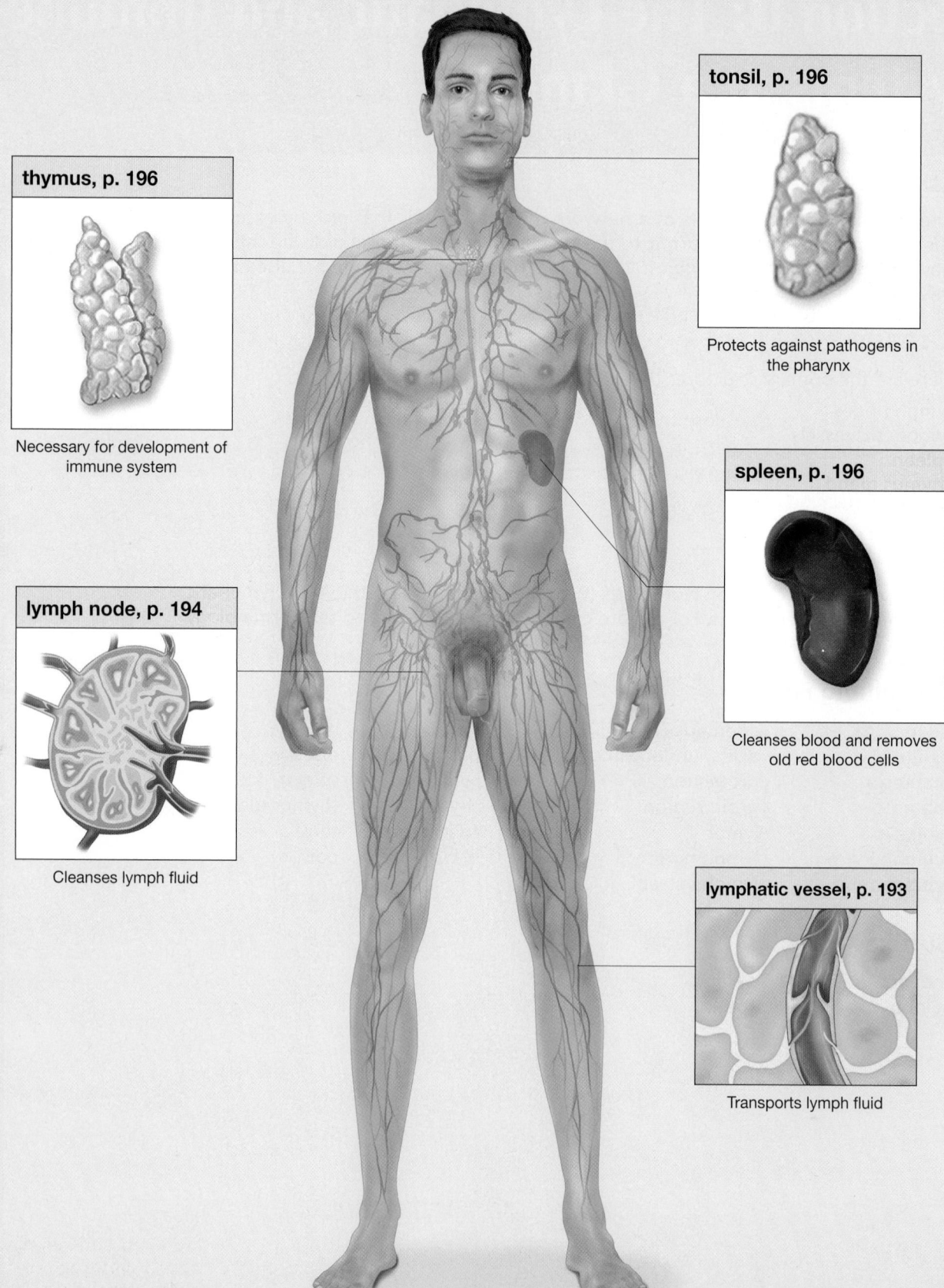

thymus, p. 196

Necessary for development of immune system

tonsil, p. 196

Protects against pathogens in the pharynx

spleen, p. 196

Cleanses blood and removes old red blood cells

lymph node, p. 194

Cleanses lymph fluid

lymphatic vessel, p. 193

Transports lymph fluid

Anatomy and Physiology of the Lymphatic and Immune Systems

lacteals (lack-TEE-als)
lymph (LIMF)
lymph nodes
lymphatic vessels (lim-FAT-ik)

spleen
thymus gland (THIGH-mus)
tonsils (TON-sulls)

The lymphatic system consists of a network of **lymphatic vessels, lymph nodes,** the **spleen,** the **thymus gland,** and the **tonsils.** These organs perform several quite diverse functions for the body. First, they collect excess tissue fluid throughout the body and return it to the circulatory system. The fluid, once inside a lymphatic vessel, is referred to as **lymph.** Lymph vessels located around the small intestines, called **lacteals,** are able to pick up absorbed fats for transport. Additionally, the lymphatic system works with the immune system to form the groups of cells, tissues, organs, and molecules that serve as the body's primary defense against the invasion of pathogens. These systems work together defending the body against foreign invaders and substances, as well as removing our own cells that have become diseased.

Lymphatic Vessels

lymphatic capillaries (CAP-ih-lair-eez)
lymphatic ducts
right lymphatic duct

thoracic duct
valves

The lymphatic vessels form an extensive network of ducts throughout the entire body. However, unlike the circulatory system, these vessels are not in a closed loop. Instead, they serve as one-way pipes conducting lymph from the tissues toward the thoracic cavity (see Figure 6.7 ■). These vessels begin as very small

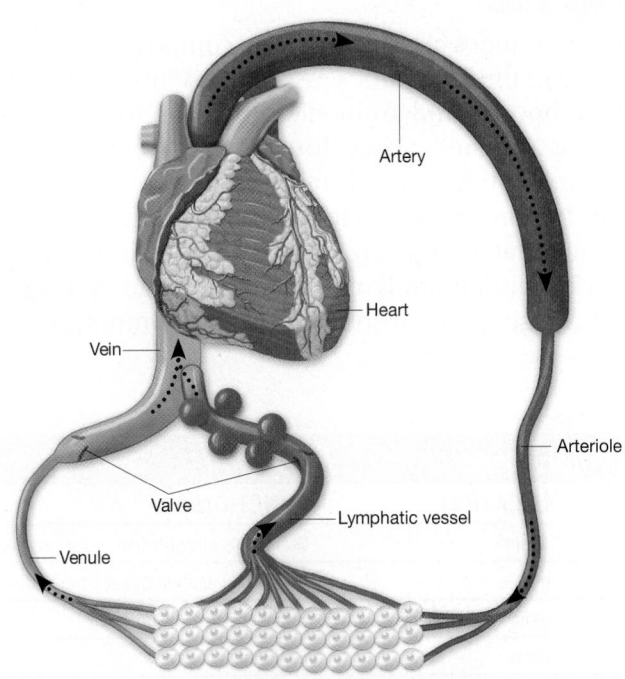

Artery

Heart

Vein

Arteriole

Valve

Lymphatic vessel

Venule

Cells in the body tissues

■ **Figure 6.7** Lymphatic vessels (green) pick up excess tissue fluid, purify it in lymph nodes, and return it to the circulatory system.

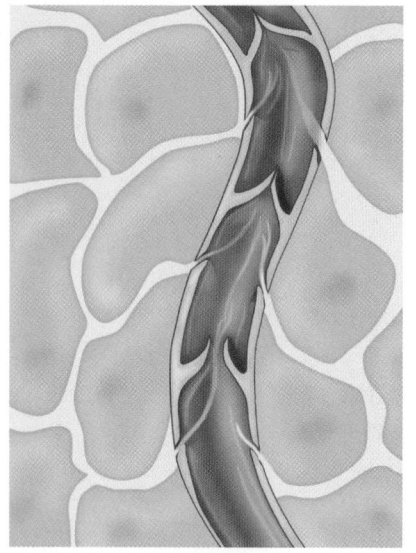
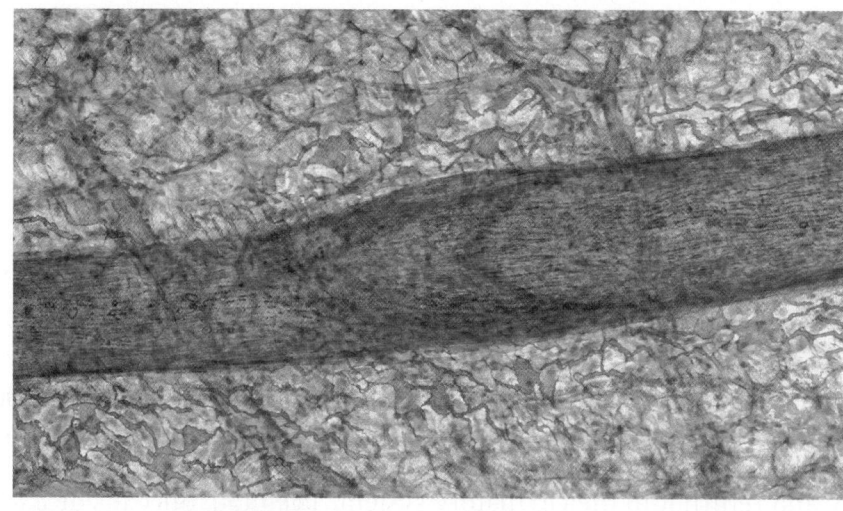

■ **Figure 6.8** (A) Lymphatic vessel with valves within tissue cells; (B) photomicrograph of lymphatic vessel with valve clearly visible. *(Michael Abbey/Photo Researchers, Inc.)*

lymphatic capillaries in the tissues. Excessive tissue fluid enters these capillaries to begin the trip back to the circulatory system. The capillaries merge into larger lymphatic vessels. This is a very low pressure system, so these vessels have **valves** along their length to ensure that lymph can only move forward toward the thoracic cavity (see Figure 6.8 ■). These vessels finally drain into one of two large **lymphatic ducts,** the **right lymphatic duct** or the **thoracic duct.** The smaller right lymphatic duct drains the right arm and the right side of the head, neck, and chest. This duct empties lymph into the right subclavian vein. The larger thoracic duct drains lymph from the rest of the body and empties into the left subclavian vein (see Figure 6.9 ■).

> **MED TERM TIP**
>
> The term *capillary* is also used to describe the minute blood vessels within the circulatory system. This is one of several general medical terms, such as valves, cilia, and hair, that are used in several systems.

Lymph Nodes

lymph glands

Lymph nodes are small organs composed of lymphatic tissue located along the route of the lymphatic vessels. These nodes, also referred to as **lymph glands,** house lymphocytes and antibodies and therefore work to remove pathogens and cell debris as lymph passes through them on its way back to the thoracic cavity (see Figure 6.10 ■). Lymph nodes also serve to trap and destroy cells from cancerous tumors. Although found throughout the body, lymph nodes are particularly concentrated in several regions. For example, lymph nodes concentrated in the neck region drain lymph from the head. See again Figure 6.9 and Table 6.2 ■ for a description of some of the most important sites for lymph nodes.

> **MED TERM TIP**
>
> In surgical procedures to remove a malignancy from an organ, such as a breast, the adjacent lymph nodes are also tested for cancer. If cancerous cells are found in the tested lymph nodes, the disease is said to have spread or *metastasized*. Tumor cells may then spread to other parts of the body by means of the lymphatic system.

Table 6.2	Sites for Lymph Nodes	
NAME	**LOCATION**	**FUNCTION**
axillary (AK-sih-lair-ee)	armpits	Drain arms and shoulder region; cancer cells from breasts may be present
cervical (SER-vih-kal)	neck	Drain head and neck; may be enlarged during upper respiratory infections
inguinal (ING-gwih-nal)	groin	Drain legs and lower pelvis
mediastinal (mee-dee-ass-TYE-nal)	chest	Drain chest cavity

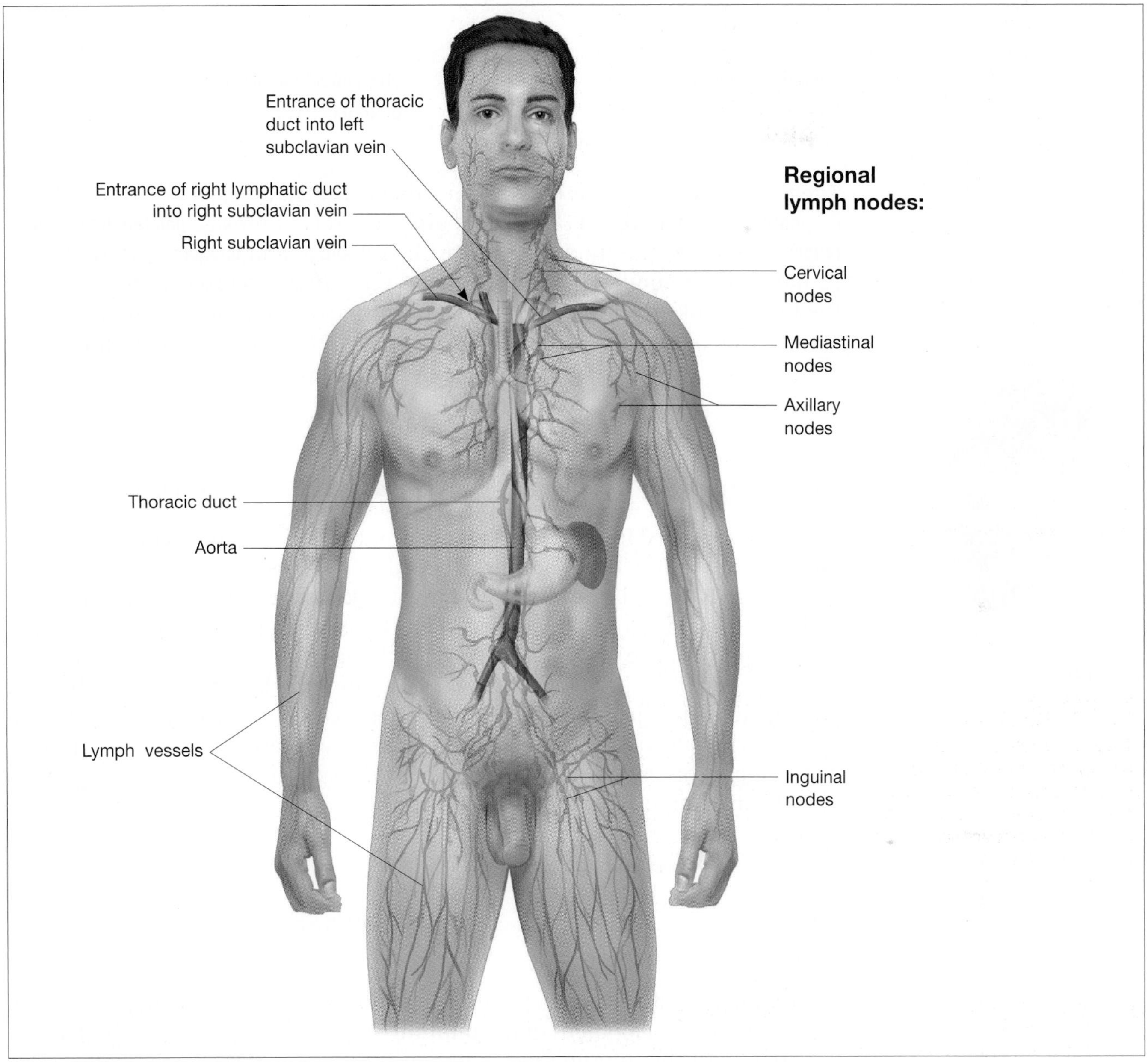

Entrance of thoracic
duct into left
subclavian vein

Entrance of right lymphatic duct
into right subclavian vein

Right subclavian vein

**Regional
lymph nodes:**

Cervical
nodes

Mediastinal
nodes

Axillary
nodes

Thoracic duct

Aorta

Lymph vessels

Inguinal
nodes

■ **Figure 6.9** Location of lymph vessels, lymphatic ducts, and areas of lymph node concentrations.

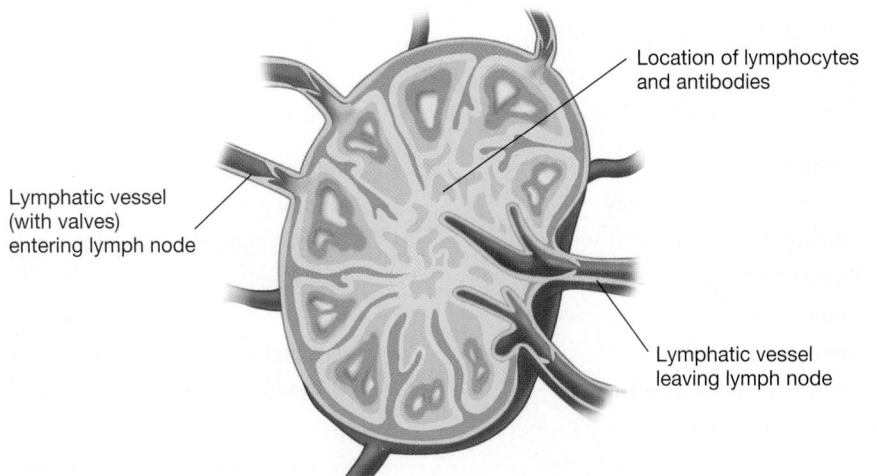

Location of lymphocytes
and antibodies

Lymphatic vessel
(with valves)
entering lymph node

Lymphatic vessel
leaving lymph node

■ **Figure 6.10** Structure of
a lymph node.

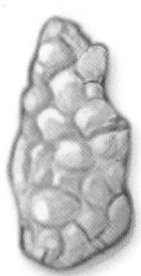

Figure 6.11 Shape of a tonsil.

Tonsils

adenoids (ADD-eh-noydz)

lingual tonsils (LING-gwal)

palatine tonsils (PAL-ah-tyne)

pharyngeal tonsils (fair-IN-jee-al)

pharynx (FAIR-inks)

The tonsils are collections of lymphatic tissue located on each side of the throat or **pharynx** (see Figure 6.11 ■). There are three sets of tonsils: **palatine tonsils, pharyngeal tonsils** (commonly referred to as the **adenoids**), and **lingual tonsils.** All tonsils contain a large number of leukocytes and act as filters to protect the body from the invasion of pathogens through the digestive or respiratory systems. Tonsils are not vital organs and can safely be removed if they become a continuous site of infection.

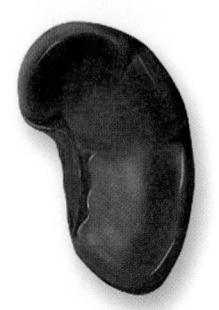

Figure 6.12 Shape of the spleen.

Spleen

blood sinuses

macrophages (MACK-roh-fayj-ez)

The spleen, located in the upper left quadrant of the abdomen, consists of lymphatic tissue that is highly infiltrated with blood vessels (see Figure 6.12 ■). These vessels spread out into slow-moving **blood sinuses.** The spleen filters out and destroys old red blood cells, recycles the iron, and also stores some of the blood supply for the body. Phagocytic **macrophages** line the blood sinuses in the spleen to engulf and remove pathogens. Because the blood is moving through the organ slowly, the macrophages have time to carefully identify pathogens and worn-out red blood cells. The spleen is also not a vital organ and can be removed due to injury or disease. However, without the spleen, a person's susceptibility to a bloodstream infection may be increased.

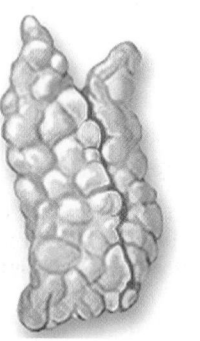

Figure 6.13 Shape of the thymus gland.

Thymus Gland

T cells

T lymphocytes

thymosin (thigh-MOH-sin)

The thymus gland, located in the upper portion of the mediastinum, is essential for the proper development of the immune system (see Figure 6.13 ■). It assists the body with the immune function and the development of antibodies. This organ's hormone, **thymosin,** changes lymphocytes to **T lymphocytes** (simply called **T cells**), which play an important role in the immune response. The thymus is active in the unborn child and throughout childhood until adolescence, when it begins to shrink in size.

Immunity

acquired immunity

active acquired immunity

bacteria (bak-TEE-ree-ah)

cancerous tumors

fungi (FUN-jee)

immune response

immunity (im-YOO-nih-tee)

immunizations (im-yoo-nih-ZAY-shuns)

natural immunity

passive acquired immunity

protozoans (proh-toh-ZOH-anz)

toxins

vaccinations (vak-sih-NAY-shuns)

viruses

Immunity is the body's ability to defend itself against pathogens, such as **bacteria, viruses, fungi, protozoans, toxins,** and **cancerous tumors.** Immunity comes in two forms: **natural immunity** and **acquired immunity.** Natural immunity, also called *innate immunity,* is not specific to a particular disease and does not require prior exposure to the pathogenic agent. A good example of natural immunity is the macrophage. These leukocytes are present throughout all the tissues of the body, but are concentrated in areas of high exposure to invading bacteria, like the lungs and digestive system. They are very active phagocytic cells, ingesting and digesting any pathogen they encounter (see Figure 6.14 ■).

Acquired immunity is the body's response to a specific pathogen and may be established either passively or actively. **Passive acquired immunity** results when a person receives protective substances produced by another human or animal. This may take the form of maternal antibodies crossing the placenta to a baby or an antitoxin or gamma globulin injection. **Active acquired immunity** develops following direct exposure to the pathogenic agent. The agent stimulates the body's **immune response,** a series of different mechanisms all geared to neutralize the agent. For example, a person typically can catch chickenpox only once because once the body has successfully fought the virus, it will be able to more quickly recognize and kill it in the future. **Immunizations** or **vaccinations** are special types of active acquired immunity. Instead of actually being exposed to the infectious agent and having the disease, a person is exposed to a modified or weakened pathogen that is still capable of stimulating the immune response but not actually causing the disease.

Immune Response

antibody (AN-tih-bod-ee)	**cell-mediated immunity**
antibody-mediated immunity	**cellular immunity**
antigen–antibody complex	**cytotoxic** (sigh-toh-TOK-sik)
antigens (AN-tih-jens)	**humoral immunity** (HYOO-mor-al)
B cells	**natural killer (NK) cells**
B lymphocytes	

Disease-causing agents are recognized as being foreign because they display proteins that are different from a person's own natural proteins. Those foreign proteins, called **antigens,** stimulate the immune response. The immune response consists of two distinct and different processes: **humoral immunity** (also called **antibody-mediated immunity**) and **cellular immunity** (also called **cell-mediated immunity**).

> **MED TERM TIP**
>
> The term *humoral* comes from the Latin word for "liquid." It is the old-fashioned term to refer to the fluids of the body.

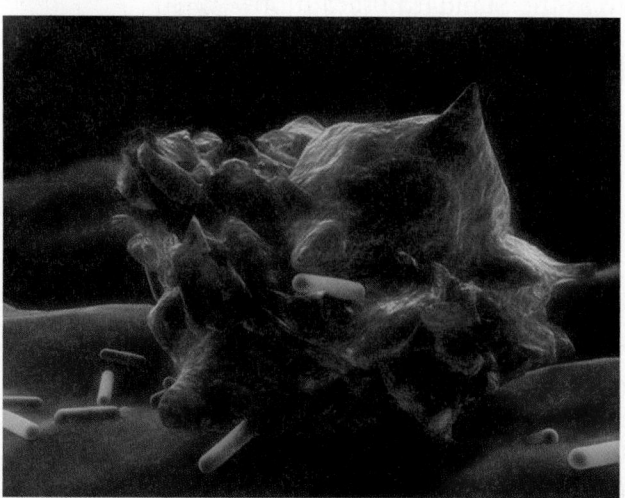

■ **Figure 6.14** Enhanced photomicrograph showing a macrophage (purple) attacking bacillus *Escherichia coli* (green). *(Sebastian Kaulitzki/ Shutterstock)*

Humoral immunity refers to the production of **B lymphocytes,** also called **B cells,** which respond to antigens by producing a protective protein, an **antibody.** Antibodies combine with the antigen to form an **antigen–antibody complex.** This complex either targets the foreign substance for phagocytosis or prevents the infectious agent from damaging healthy cells.

Cellular immunity involves the production of T cells and **natural killer** (NK) **cells.** These defense cells are **cytotoxic,** meaning that they physically attack and destroy pathogenic cells.

Standard Precautions

cross-infection	**reinfection**
nosocomial infection (no-so-KOH-mee-all)	**self-inoculation**
Occupational Safety and Health Administration (OSHA)	

Hospitals and other healthcare settings contain a large number of infective pathogens. Patients and healthcare workers are exposed to each other's pathogens and sometimes become infected. An infection acquired in this manner, as a result of hospital exposure, is referred to as a **nosocomial infection.** Nosocomial infections can spread in several ways. **Cross-infection** occurs when a person, either a patient or healthcare worker, acquires a pathogen from another patient or healthcare worker. **Reinfection** takes place when a patient becomes infected again with the same pathogen that originally brought him or her to the hospital. **Self-inoculation** occurs when a person becomes infected in a different part of the body by a pathogen from another part of his or her own body—such as intestinal bacteria spreading to the urethra.

With the appearance of the hepatitis B virus (HBV) in the mid-1960s and the human immunodeficiency virus (HIV) in the mid-1980s, the fight against spreading infections took on even greater significance. In 1987 the **Occupational Safety and Health Administration** (OSHA) issued mandatory guidelines to ensure that all employees at risk of exposure to body fluids are provided with personal protective equipment. These guidelines state that all human blood, tissue, and body fluids must be treated as if they were infected with HIV, HBV, or other bloodborne pathogens. These guidelines were expanded in 1992 and 1996 to encourage the fight against not just bloodborne pathogens, but all nosocomial infections spread by contact with blood, mucous membranes, nonintact skin, and all body fluids (including amniotic fluid, vaginal secretions, pleural fluid, cerebrospinal fluid, peritoneal fluid, pericardial fluid, and semen). These guidelines are commonly referred to as the Standard Precautions:

1. Wash hands before putting on and after removing gloves and before and after working with each patient or patient equipment.
2. Wear gloves when in contact with any body fluid, mucous membrane, or nonintact skin or if you have chapped hands, a rash, or open sores.
3. Wear a nonpermeable gown or apron during procedures that are likely to expose you to any body fluid, mucous membrane, or nonintact skin.
4. Wear a mask and protective equipment or a face shield when patients are coughing often or if body fluid droplets or splashes are likely.
5. Wear a facemask and eyewear that seal close to the face during procedures that cause body tissues to be vaporized.
6. Remove for proper cleaning any shared equipment—such as a thermometer, stethoscope, or blood pressure cuff—that has come into contact with body fluids, mucous membrane, or nonintact skin.

MED TERM TIP

Analyzing the word parts that make up the term *cytotoxic* gives you a quick idea of this cell's function.
- cyt/o = cell
- tox/o = poison
- -ic = pertaining to

MED TERM TIP

The simple act of thoroughly washing your hands is the most effective method of preventing the spread of infectious diseases.

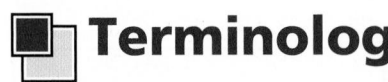 Terminology

Word Parts Used to Build Lymphatic and Immune System Terms

The following lists contain the combining forms, suffixes, and prefixes used to build terms in the remaining sections of this chapter.

Combining Forms

adenoid/o	adenoids
axill/o	axilla, underarm
cortic/o	outer region, cortex
immun/o	protection
inguin/o	groin

lymph/o	lymph
lymphaden/o	lymph node
lymphangi/o	lymph vessel
nucle/o	nucleus
path/o	disease

pneumon/o	lung
sarc/o	flesh
splen/o	spleen
thym/o	thymus gland
tonsill/o	tonsils

Suffixes

-al	pertaining to
-ar	pertaining to
-ary	pertaining to
-atic	pertaining to
-ectomy	surgical removal
-edema	swelling
-genic	producing

-globulin	protein
-gram	record
-graphy	process of recording
-ia	condition
-iasis	abnormal condition
-ic	pertaining to
-itis	inflammation

-logy	study of
-megaly	enlarged
-oma	tumor
-osis	abnormal condition
-pathy	disease
-therapy	treatment

Prefixes

anti-	against

auto-	self

mono-	one

Anatomical Terms

TERM	WORD PARTS	DEFINITION
axillary (AK-sih-lair-ee)	axill/o = axilla, underarm -ary = pertaining to	Pertaining to the underarm region.
immunoglobulins (im-yoo-noh-GLOB-yoo-linz)	immun/o = protection -globulin = protein	Antibodies secreted by the B cells. All antibodies are immunoglobulins and assist in protecting the body and its surfaces from the invasion of bacteria. For example, the immunoglobulin IgA in colostrum, the first milk from the mother, helps to protect the newborn from infection.
inguinal (ING-gwih-nal)	inguin/o = groin -al = pertaining to	Pertaining to the groin region.
lymphangial (lim-FAN-gee-al)	lymphangi/o = lymph vessel -al = pertaining to	Pertaining to lymph vessels.

Anatomical Terms (continued)

TERM	WORD PARTS	DEFINITION
lymphatic (lim-FAT-ik)	lymph/o = lymph -atic = pertaining to	Pertaining to lymph.
splenic (SPLEN-ik)	splen/o = spleen -ic = pertaining to	Pertaining to the spleen.
thymic (THIGH-mik)	thym/o = thymus gland -ic = pertaining to	Pertaining to the thymus gland.
tonsillar (ton-sih-lar)	tonsill/o = tonsils -ar = pertaining to	Pertaining to the tonsils.

Pathology

TERM	WORD PARTS	DEFINITION
Medical Specialties		
allergist (AL-er-jist)		A physician who specializes in testing for and treating allergies.
immunology (im-yoo-NALL-oh-jee)	immun/o = protection -logy = study of	A branch of medicine concerned with diagnosis and treatment of infectious diseases and other disorders of the immune system. Physician is an *immunologist.*
pathology (path-OL-oh-gee)	path/o = disease -logy = study of	A branch of medicine concerned with determining the underlying causes and development of diseases. Physician is an *immunologist.*
Signs and Symptoms		
hives		Appearance of wheals as part of an allergic reaction.
inflammation (in-flah-MA-shun)		The tissues' response to injury from pathogens or physical agents. Characterized by redness, pain, swelling, and feeling hot to touch.

> **MED TERM TIP**
>
> Word Watch: The terms *inflammation* and *inflammatory* are spelled with two *m*'s, while *inflame* and *inflamed* each have only one *m*. These may be the most commonly misspelled terms by medical terminology students.

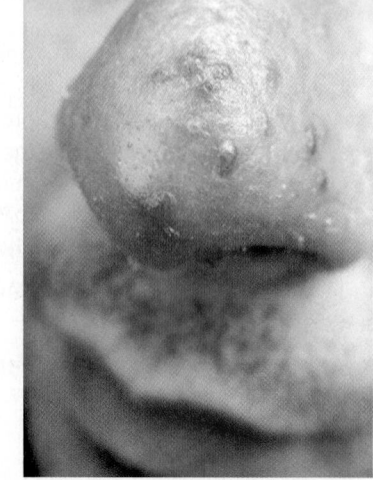

■ **Figure 6.15** Inflammation as illustrated by cellulitis of the nose. Note that the area is red and swollen. It is also painful and hot to touch.

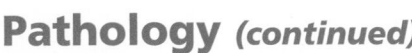

Pathology *(continued)*

TERM	WORD PARTS	DEFINITION
lymphedema (limf-eh-DEE-mah)	lymph/o = lymph -edema = swelling	Edema appearing in the extremities due to an obstruction of the lymph flow through the lymphatic vessels.
pathogenic (path-oh-JEN-ik)	path/o = disease -genic = producing	An adjective term to describe something—such as bacteria, viruses, or toxins—that produce disease.
splenomegaly (splee-noh-MEG-ah-lee)	splen/o = spleen -megaly = enlarged	An enlarged spleen.
urticaria (er-tih-KAY-ree-ah)		Severe itching associated with hives, usually linked to food allergy, stress, or drug reactions.
Allergic Reactions		
allergy (AL-er-jee)		Hypersensitivity to a common substance in the environment or to a medication. The substance causing the allergic reaction is called an *allergen.*
anaphylactic shock (an-ah-fih-LAK-tik)		Life-threatening condition resulting from a severe allergic reaction. Examples of instances that may trigger this reaction include bee stings, medications, or the ingestion of foods. Circulatory and respiratory problems occur, including respiratory distress, hypotension, edema, tachycardia, and convulsions. Also called **anaphylaxis.**
Lymphatic System		
adenoiditis (add-eh-noyd-EYE-tis)	adenoid/o = adenoids -itis = inflammation	Inflammation of the adenoids.
autoimmune disease	auto- = self	A disease resulting from the body's immune system attacking its own cells as if they were pathogens. Examples include systemic lupus erythematosus, rheumatoid arthritis, and multiple sclerosis.
elephantiasis (el-eh-fan-TYE-ah-sis)	-iasis = abnormal condition	Inflammation, obstruction, and destruction of the lymph vessels resulting in enlarged tissues due to edema.
Hodgkin's disease (HD) (HOJ-kins)		Also called *Hodgkin's lymphoma.* Cancer of the lymphatic cells found in concentration in the lymph nodes. Named after Thomas Hodgkin, a British physician, who first described it.
lymphadenitis (lim-fad-en-EYE-tis)	lymphaden/o = lymph node -itis = inflammation	Inflammation of the lymph nodes. Referred to as *swollen glands.*
lymphadenopathy (lim-fad-eh-NOP-ah-thee)	lymphaden/o = lymph node -pathy = disease	A general term for lymph node diseases.
lymphangioma (lim-fan-jee-OH-mah)	lymphangi/o = lymph vessel -oma = tumor	A tumor in a lymphatic vessel.

Pathology *(continued)*

TERM	WORD PARTS	DEFINITION
lymphoma (lim-FOH-mah)	lymph/o = lymph -oma = tumor	A tumor in lymphatic tissue.
mononucleosis (mono) (mon-oh-nook-lee-OH-sis)	mono- = one nucle/o = nucleus -osis = abnormal condition	Acute infectious disease with a large number of abnormal mononuclear lymphocytes. Caused by the Epstein–Barr virus. Abnormal liver function may occur.
non-Hodgkin's lymphoma (NHL)	lymph/o = lymph -oma = tumor	Cancer of the lymphatic tissues other than Hodgkin's lymphoma.

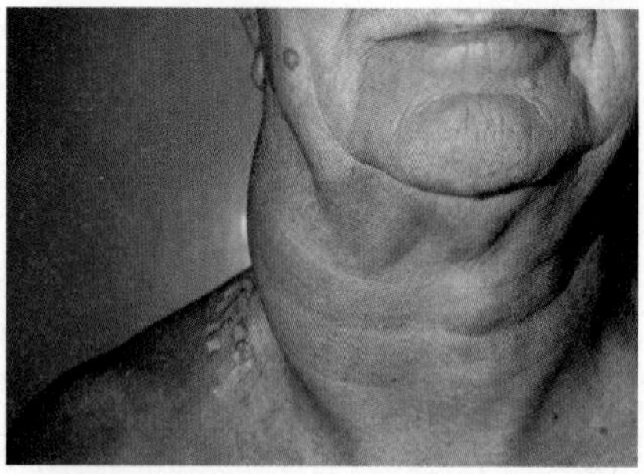

■ **Figure 6.16** Photo of the neck of a patient with non-Hodgkin's lymphoma showing the swelling associated with enlarged lymph nodes.

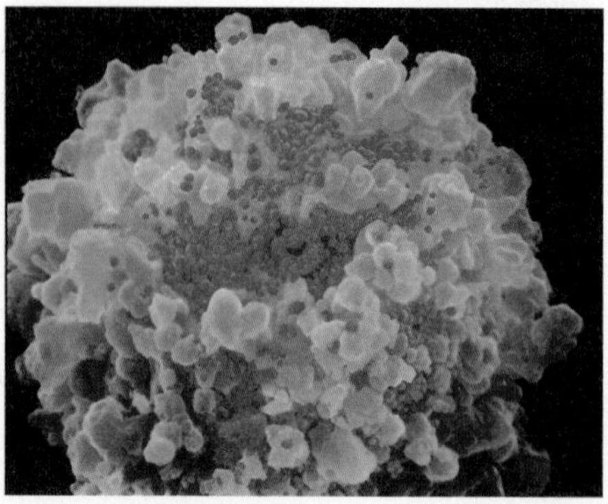

TERM	WORD PARTS	DEFINITION
thymoma (thigh-MOH-mah)	thym/o = thymus gland -oma = tumor	A tumor of the thymus gland.
tonsillitis (ton-sil-EYE-tis)	tonsill/o = tonsils -itis = inflammation	Inflammation of the tonsils.

Immune System

TERM	WORD PARTS	DEFINITION
acquired immunodeficiency syndrome (AIDS) (ac-quired / im-you-noh-dee-FIH-shen-see / SIN-drohm)	immun/o = protection	Disease involving a defect in the cell-mediated immunity system. A syndrome of opportunistic infections occurring in the final stages of infection with the human immunodeficiency virus (HIV). This virus attacks T4 lymphocytes and destroys them, reducing the person's ability to fight infection.
AIDS-related complex (ARC)		Early stage of AIDS. There is a positive test for the virus, but only mild symptoms of weight loss, fatigue, skin rash, and anorexia.
graft versus host disease (GVHD)		Serious complication of bone marrow transplant (graft). Immune cells from the donor bone marrow attack the recipient's (host's) tissues.
human immunodeficiency virus (HIV) (im-yoo-noh-dee-FIH-shen-see)	immun/o = protection	Virus that causes AIDS; also known as a **retrovirus**.

■ **Figure 6.17** Color-enhanced scanning electron micrograph of HIV virus (red) infecting T-helper cells (green). *(National Institute for Biological Standards and Control (U.K.)/Science Photo Library/Photo Researchers, Inc.)*

Pathology *(continued)*

TERM	WORD PARTS	DEFINITION
immunocompromised (im-you-noh-KOM-pro-mized)	immun/o = protection	Having an immune system that is unable to respond properly to pathogens. Also called *immunodeficiency disorder.*
Kaposi's sarcoma (KS) (KAP-oh-seez / sar-KOH-mah)	sarc/o = flesh -oma = tumor	Form of skin cancer frequently seen in patients with AIDS. It consists of brownish-purple papules that spread from the skin and metastasize to internal organs. Named for Moritz Kaposi, an Austrian dermatologist.
opportunistic infections		Infectious diseases associated with patients who have compromised immune systems and therefore a lowered resistance to infections and parasites. May be the result of HIV infection.
pneumocystis pneumonia (PCP) (noo-moh-SIS-tis / new-MOH-nee-ah)	pneumon/o = lung -ia = condition	Pneumonia common in patients with weakened immune systems, such as AIDS patients, caused by the *Pneumocystis jirovecii* fungus.
sarcoidosis (sar-koyd-OH-sis)	-osis = abnormal condition	Disease of unknown cause that forms fibrous lesions commonly appearing in the lymph nodes, liver, skin, lungs, spleen, eyes, and small bones of the hands and feet.
severe combined immunodeficiency syndrome (SCIDS)	immun/o = protection	Disease seen in children born with a non-functioning immune system. Often these children are forced to live in sealed sterile rooms.

Diagnostic Procedures

TERM	WORD PARTS	DEFINITION
Clinical Laboratory Tests		
enzyme-linked immunosorbent assay (ELISA) (EN-zym / LINK'T / im-yoo-noh-sor-bent / ASS-say)	immun/o = protection	Blood test for an antibody to the HIV virus. A positive test means that the person has been exposed to the virus. There may be a false-positive reading, and then the Western blot test would be used to verify the results.
Western blot		Test used as a backup to the ELISA blood test to detect the presence of the antibody to HIV (AIDS virus) in the blood.
Diagnostic Imaging		
lymphangiogram (lim-FAN-jee-oh-gram)	lymphangi/o = lymph vessel -gram = record	X-ray record of the lymphatic vessels produced by lymphangiography.
lymphangiography (lim-FAN-jee-oh-graf-ee)	lymphangi/o = lymph vessel -graphy = process of recording	X-ray taken of the lymph vessels after the injection of dye into the foot. The lymph flow through the chest is traced.

Diagnostic Procedures *(continued)*

TERM	WORD PARTS	DEFINITION
Additional Diagnostic Procedures		
Monospot		Blood test for infectious mononucleosis.
scratch test		Form of allergy testing in which the body is exposed to an allergen through a light scratch on the skin.

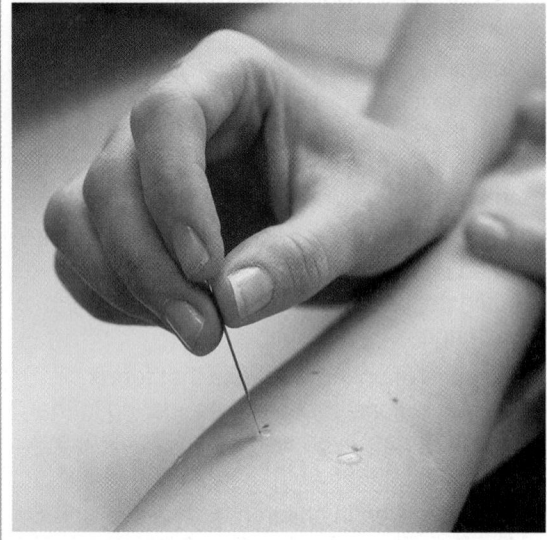
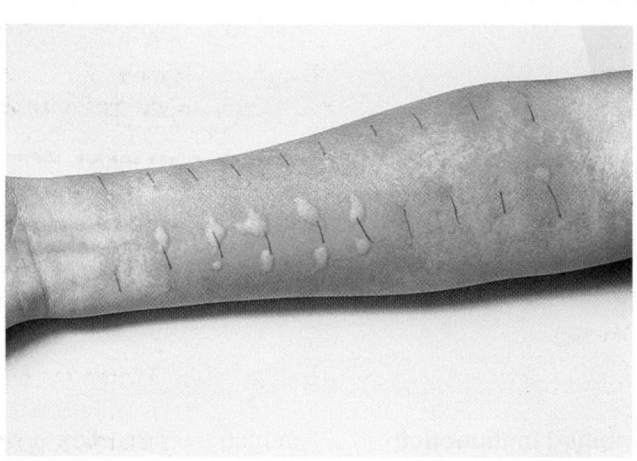

A

B

■ **Figure 6.18** (A) Scratch test; patient is exposed to allergens through a light scratch on the skin; (B) Positive scratch test results. Inflammation indicates person is allergic to that substance. *(A. James King-Holmes/ Science Photo Library/Photo Researchers, Inc. B. SUI/Photo Researchers, Inc.)*

Therapeutic Procedures

TERM	WORD PARTS	DEFINITION
Medical Procedures		
immunotherapy (IM-yoo-noh-thair-ah-pee)	immun/o = protection -therapy = treatment	Giving a patient an injection of immunoglobulins or antibodies in order to treat a disease. The antibodies may be produced by another person or animal, for example, antivenom for snake bites. More recent developments include treatments to boost the activity of the immune system, especially to treat cancer and AIDS.
vaccination (vak-sih-NAY-shun)		Exposure to a weakened pathogen that stimulates the immune response and antibody production in order to confer protection against the full-blown disease. Also called *immunization*.

Therapeutic Procedures *(continued)*

TERM	WORD PARTS	DEFINITION
Surgical Procedures		
adenoidectomy (add-eh-noyd-EK-toh-mee)	adenoid/o = adenoids -ectomy = surgical removal	Surgical removal of the adenoids.
lymphadenectomy (lim-fad-eh-NEK-toh-mee)	lymphaden/o = lymph node -ectomy = surgical removal	Removal of a lymph node. This is usually done to test for malignancy.
splenectomy (splee-NEK-toh-mee)	splen/o = spleen -ectomy = surgical removal	Surgical removal of the spleen.
thymectomy (thigh-MEK-toh-mee)	thym/o = thymus gland -ectomy = surgical removal	Surgical removal of the thymus gland.
tonsillectomy (ton-sih-LEK-toh-mee)	tonsill/o = tonsils -ectomy = surgical removal	Surgical removal of the tonsils.

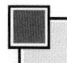

Pharmacology

CLASSIFICATION		ACTION	EXAMPLES
antihistamine (an-tih-HIST-ah-meen)	anti- = against	Blocks the effects of histamine released by the body during an allergic reaction.	cetirizine, Zyrtec; diphenhydramine, Benadryl
corticosteroids (core-tih-koh-STARE-royds)	cortic/o = outer region, cortex	A hormone produced by the adrenal cortex that has very strong anti-inflammatory properties. Particularly useful in treating autoimmune diseases.	prednisone; methylprednisolone, Solu-Medrol
immunosuppressants (im-yoo-noh-sue-PRESS-antz)	immun/o = protection	Blocks certain actions of the immune system. Required to prevent rejection of a transplanted organ.	mycophenolate mofetil, CellCept; cyclosporine, Neoral
protease inhibitor drugs (PROH-tee-ace)		Inhibits protease, an enzyme viruses need to reproduce.	indinavir, Crixivan; saquinavir, Fortovase
reverse transcriptase inhibitor drugs (trans-KRIP-tays)		Inhibits reverse transcriptase, an enzyme needed by viruses to reproduce.	lamivudine, Epivir; zidovudine, Retrovir

Abbreviations

AIDS	acquired immunodeficiency syndrome	**KS**	Kaposi's sarcoma
ARC	AIDS-related complex	**mono**	mononucleosis
ELISA	enzyme-linked immunosorbent assay	**NHL**	non-Hodgkin's lymphoma
GVHD	graft versus host disease	**NK**	natural killer cells
HD	Hodgkin's disease	**PCP**	pneumocystis pneumonia
HIV	human immunodeficiency virus	**SCIDS**	severe combined immunodeficiency syndrome
Ig	immunoglobulins (IgA, IgD, IgE, IgG, IgM)		

Chapter Review

Real-World Applications

Medical Record Analysis

This Discharge Summary contains 11 medical terms. Underline each term and write it in the list below the report. Then define each term. Note: Some terms are defined in other chapters; use your glossary-index to locate and define these terms.

Discharge Summary

Admitting Diagnosis:	Splenomegaly, weight loss, diarrhea, fatigue, chronic cough
Final Diagnosis:	Non-Hodgkin's lymphoma of spleen; splenectomy
History of Present Illness:	Patient is a 36-year-old businessman who was first seen in the office with complaints of feeling generally "run down," intermittent diarrhea, weight loss, and, more recently, a dry cough. He states he has been aware of these symptoms for approximately six months. Monospot and ELISA are both negative. In spite of a 35-pound weight loss, he has abdominal swelling and splenomegaly was detected. He was admitted to the hospital for further evaluation and treatment.
Summary of Hospital Course:	Full-body MRI confirmed splenomegaly and located a 3-cm encapsulated tumor in the spleen. Biopsies taken from the splenic tumor confirmed the diagnosis of non-Hodgkin's lymphoma. The patient underwent splenectomy for removal of the tumor.
Discharge Plans:	Patient was discharged home following recovery from the splenectomy. The abdominal swelling and diarrhea were resolved, but the dry cough persisted. He was referred to an oncologist for evaluation and surveillance for metastases.

	Term	Definition
1	_____	_____
2	_____	_____
3	_____	_____
4	_____	_____
5	_____	_____
6	_____	_____
7	_____	_____
8	_____	_____
9	_____	_____
10	_____	_____
11	_____	_____

Chart Note Transcription

The chart note below contains 10 phrases that can be reworded with a medical term that you learned in this chapter. Each phrase is identified with an underline. Determine the medical term and write your answers in the space provided.

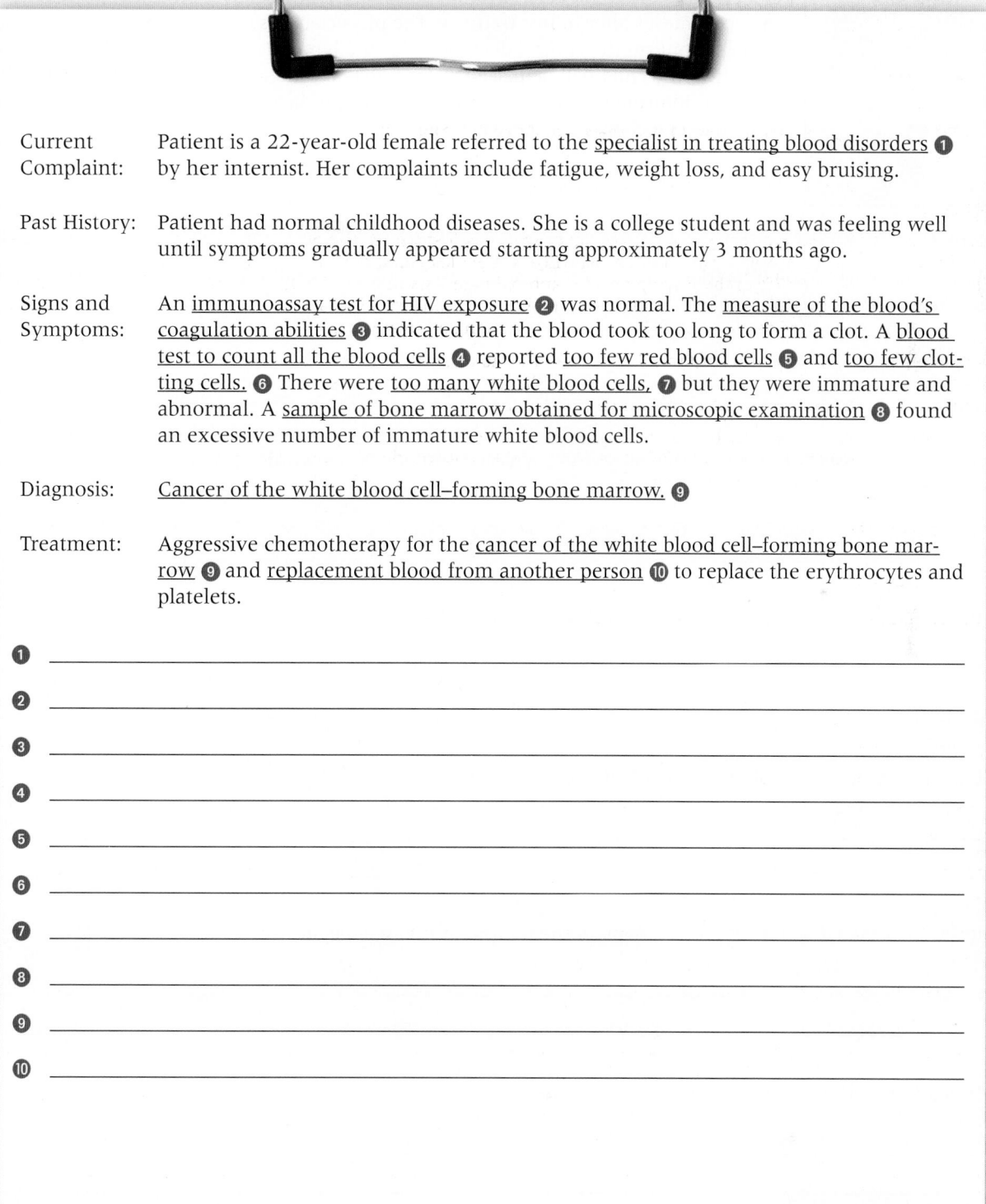

Current Complaint: Patient is a 22-year-old female referred to the <u>specialist in treating blood disorders</u> **1** by her internist. Her complaints include fatigue, weight loss, and easy bruising.

Past History: Patient had normal childhood diseases. She is a college student and was feeling well until symptoms gradually appeared starting approximately 3 months ago.

Signs and Symptoms: An <u>immunoassay test for HIV exposure</u> **2** was normal. The <u>measure of the blood's coagulation abilities</u> **3** indicated that the blood took too long to form a clot. A <u>blood test to count all the blood cells</u> **4** reported <u>too few red blood cells</u> **5** and <u>too few clotting cells.</u> **6** There were <u>too many white blood cells,</u> **7** but they were immature and abnormal. A <u>sample of bone marrow obtained for microscopic examination</u> **8** found an excessive number of immature white blood cells.

Diagnosis: <u>Cancer of the white blood cell–forming bone marrow.</u> **9**

Treatment: Aggressive chemotherapy for the <u>cancer of the white blood cell–forming bone marrow</u> **9** and <u>replacement blood from another person</u> **10** to replace the erythrocytes and platelets.

1 _____

2 _____

3 _____

4 _____

5 _____

6 _____

7 _____

8 _____

9 _____

10 _____

Case Study

Below is a case study presentation of a patient with a condition covered in this chapter. Read the case study and answer the questions below. Some questions will ask for information not included within this chapter. Use your text, a medical dictionary, or any other reference material you choose to answer these questions.

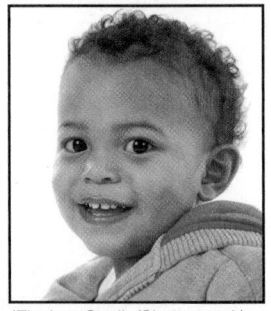

A 2-year-old boy is being seen by a hematologist. The child's symptoms include the sudden onset of high fevers, thrombopenia, epistaxis, gingival bleeding, petechiae, and ecchymoses after minor traumas. The physician has ordered a bone marrow aspiration to confirm the clinical diagnosis of acute lymphocytic leukemia. If the diagnosis is positive, the child will be placed immediately on intensive chemotherapy. The physician has informed the parents that treatment produces remission in 90% of children with ALL, especially those between the ages of 2 and 8.

(Flashon Studio/Shutterstock)

1. What pathological condition does the hematologist suspect? Look this condition up in a reference source and include a short description of it.

   _____

   _____

2. List and define each of the patient's presenting symptoms in your own words.

   _____

   _____

3. What diagnostic test did the physician perform? Describe it in your own words.

   _____

   _____

4. Explain the phrase "clinical diagnosis" in your own words.

   _____

   _____

5. If the suspected diagnosis is correct, explain the treatment that will begin.

   _____

   _____

6. What do you think the term "remission" means?

   _____

   _____

Practice Exercises

A. Complete the Statement

1. The study of the blood is called _____.

2. The organs of the lymphatic system other than lymphatic vessels and lymph nodes are the _____, _____, and _____.

3. The two lymph ducts are the _____ and _____.

4. The primary concentrations of lymph nodes are the _____, _____, _____, and _____ regions.

5. The process whereby cells ingest and destroy bacteria within the body is _____.

6. The formed elements of blood are the _____, _____, and _____.

7. The fluid portion of blood is called _____.

8. _____ immunity develops following direct exposure to a pathogen.

9. Humoral immunity is also referred to as _____ immunity.

10. The medical term for blood clotting is _____.

B. Suffix Practice

Use the following suffixes to create medical terms for the following definitions.

-penia	-globin	-cytosis	-cyte	–globulin

1. too few white (cells) _____

2. too few red (cells) _____

3. too few clotting (cells) _____

4. too few of all cells _____

5. increase in white cells _____

6. increase in red cells _____

7. increase in clotting cells _____

8. blood protein _____

9. immunity protein _____

10. red cell _____

11. white cell _____

12. lymph cell _____

C. Combining Form Practice

The combining form **splen**/o refers to the spleen. Use it to write a term that means:

1. enlargement of the spleen _____

2. surgical removal of the spleen _____

3. cutting into the spleen _____

The combining form **lymph**/o refers to the lymph. Use it to write a term that means:

4. lymph cells _____

5. tumor of the lymph system _____

The combining form **lymphaden**/o refers to the lymph nodes. Use it to write a term that means:

6. disease of a lymph gland _____

7. tumor of a lymph gland _____

8. inflammation of a lymph gland _____

The combining form **immun**/o refers to the immune system. Use it to write a term that means:

9. specialist in the study of the immune system _____

10. immune protein _____

11. study of the immune system _____

The combining form **hemat**/o refers to blood. Use it to write a term that means:

12. relating to the blood _____

13. blood tumor or mass _____

14. blood formation _____

The combining form **hem**/o refers to blood. Use it to write a term that means:

15. blood destruction _____

16. blood protein _____

D. What Does it Stand For?

1. basos _____

2. CBC _____

3. Hgb _____

4. PT _____

5. GVHD _____

6. RBC _____

7. PCV _____

8. ESR _____

9. diff _____

10. lymphs _____

E. Terminology Matching

Match each term to its definition.

1. _____ thalassemia   a. fluid portion of blood

2. _____ lacteals   b. disease in which blood does not clot

3. _____ A, B, AB, O   c. conditions with reduced number of RBCs

4. _____ plasma   d. mass of blood

5. _____ dyscrasia   e. blood type

6. _____ hematoma   f. blood-clotting protein

7. _____ anemia   g. type of anemia

8. _____ serum   h. general term for blood disorders

9. _____ hemophilia   i. lymph vessels around intestine

10. _____ fibrinogen   j. plasma with inactivated fibrinogen

F. What's the Abbreviation?

1. acquired immunodeficiency syndrome _____

2. AIDS-related complex _____

3. human immunodeficiency virus _____

4. acute lymphocytic leukemia _____

5. bone marrow transplant _____

6. mononucleosis _____

7. Kaposi's sarcoma _____

8. eosinophils _____

9. immunoglobulin _____

10. severe combined immunodeficiency syndrome _____

G. Define the Combining Form

	Combining Form	Example from Chapter
1. lymph node	_____	_____
2. clot	_____	_____
3. blood	_____	_____
4. tonsil	_____	_____
5. poison	_____	_____
6. eat/swallow	_____	_____
7. lymph vessel	_____	_____
8. disease	_____	_____
9. spleen	_____	_____
10. lymph	_____	_____

H. Fill in the Blank

Kaposi's sarcoma	mononucleosis	Hodgkin's disease	aplastic
polycythemia vera	anaphylactic shock	AIDS	pernicious
pneumocystis	HIV		

1. The condition characterized by the production of too many red blood cells is called _____ .

2. The Epstein–Barr virus is thought to be responsible for what infectious disease? _____ .

3. A life-threatening allergic reaction is _____ .

4. The virus responsible for causing AIDS is _____ .

5. A cancer that is seen frequently in AIDS patients is _____ .

6. An ELISA is used to test for _____ .

7. Malignant tumors concentrate in lymph nodes with this disease: _____ .

8. A type of pneumonia seen in AIDS patients is _____ pneumonia.

9. _____ anemia is a severe form of anemia caused by nonfunctioning red bone marrow.

10. _____ anemia is the result of a vitamin B_{12} deficiency.

I. Terminology Matching

Match each term to its definition.

1. _____ allergy

2. _____ nosocomial

3. _____ phagocytosis

4. _____ hives

5. _____ antibody

6. _____ antigen

7. _____ Hodgkin's disease

8. _____ sarcoidosis

9. _____ vaccination

10. _____ ELISA

a. seen in an allergic reaction

b. substance that stimulates antibody formation

c. a hypersensitivity reaction

d. engulfing

e. protective blood protein

f. a type of cancer

g. autoimmune disease

h. infection acquired in the hospital

i. blood test for AIDS

j. immunization

J. Pharmacology Challenge

Fill in the classification for each drug description, then match the brand name.

Drug Description	Classification	Brand Name
1. _____ inhibits enzyme needed for viral reproduction	_____	a. HepLock
2. _____ prevents blood clot formation	_____	b. Activase
3. _____ stops bleeding	_____	c. Solu-Medrol
4. _____ blocks effects of histamine	_____	d. Amicar
5. _____ prevents rejection of a transplanted organ	_____	e. Epivir
6. _____ dissolves existing blood clots	_____	f. CellCept
7. _____ increases number of erythrocytes	_____	g. Procrit
8. _____ strong anti-inflammatory properties	_____	h. Zyrtec
9. _____ interferes with action of platelets	_____	i. Plavix

K. Terminology Matching

Match each term to its definition.

1. _____ culture and sensitivity

2. _____ hematocrit

3. _____ complete blood count

4. _____ erythrocyte sedimentation rate

5. _____ prothrombin time

6. _____ white cell differential

7. _____ red cell morphology

a. measure of blood's clotting ability

b. counts number of each type of blood cell

c. examines cells for abnormal shape

d. checks blood for bacterial growth and best antibiotic to use

e. determines number of each type of white blood cell

f. measures percent of whole blood that is red blood cells

g. an indicator of the presence of an inflammatory condition

MEDICAL TERMINOLOGY INTERACTIVE

Medical Terminology Interactive is a premium online homework management system that includes a host of features to help you study. Registered users will find:

- Fun games and activities built within a virtual hospital
- Powerful tools that track and analyze your results—allowing you to create a personalized learning experience
- Videos, flashcards, and audio pronunciations to help enrich your progress
- Streaming video lesson presentations and self-paced learning modules

www.pearsonhighered.com/mti

Labeling Exercise

Image A

Write the labels for this figure on the numbered lines provided.

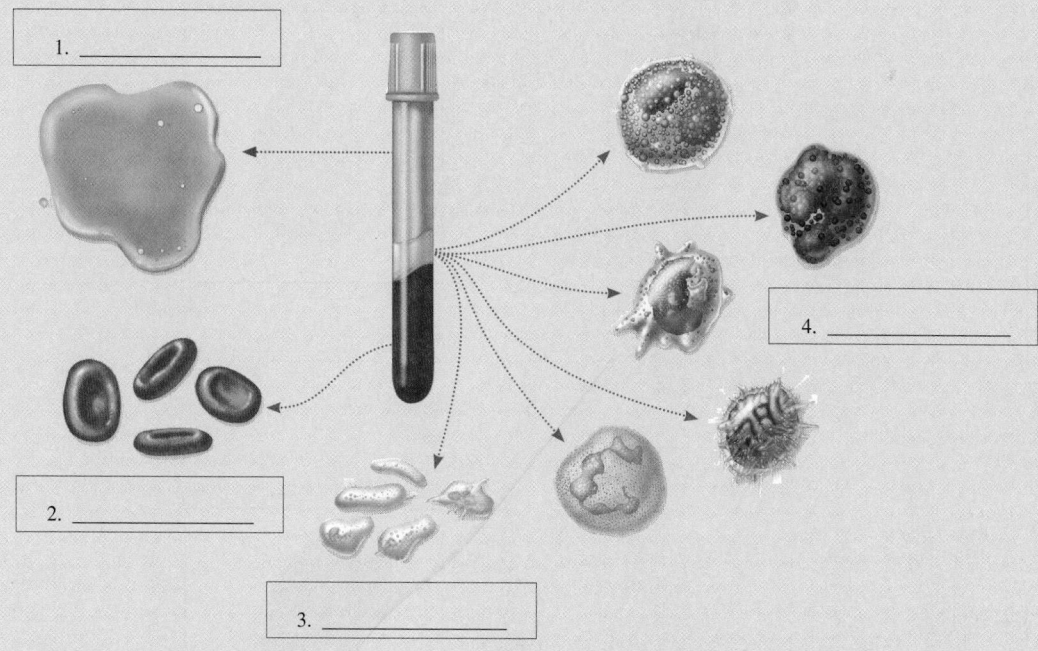

1. _____

2. _____

3. _____

4. _____

Image B

Write the labels for this figure on the numbered lines provided.

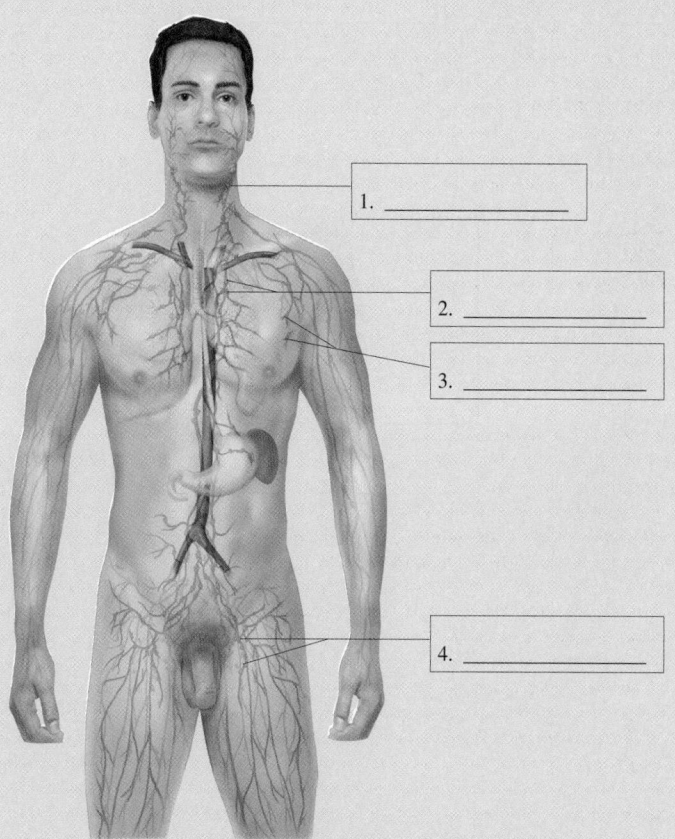

1. _____

2. _____

3. _____

4. _____

Image C

Write the labels for this figure on the numbered lines provided.

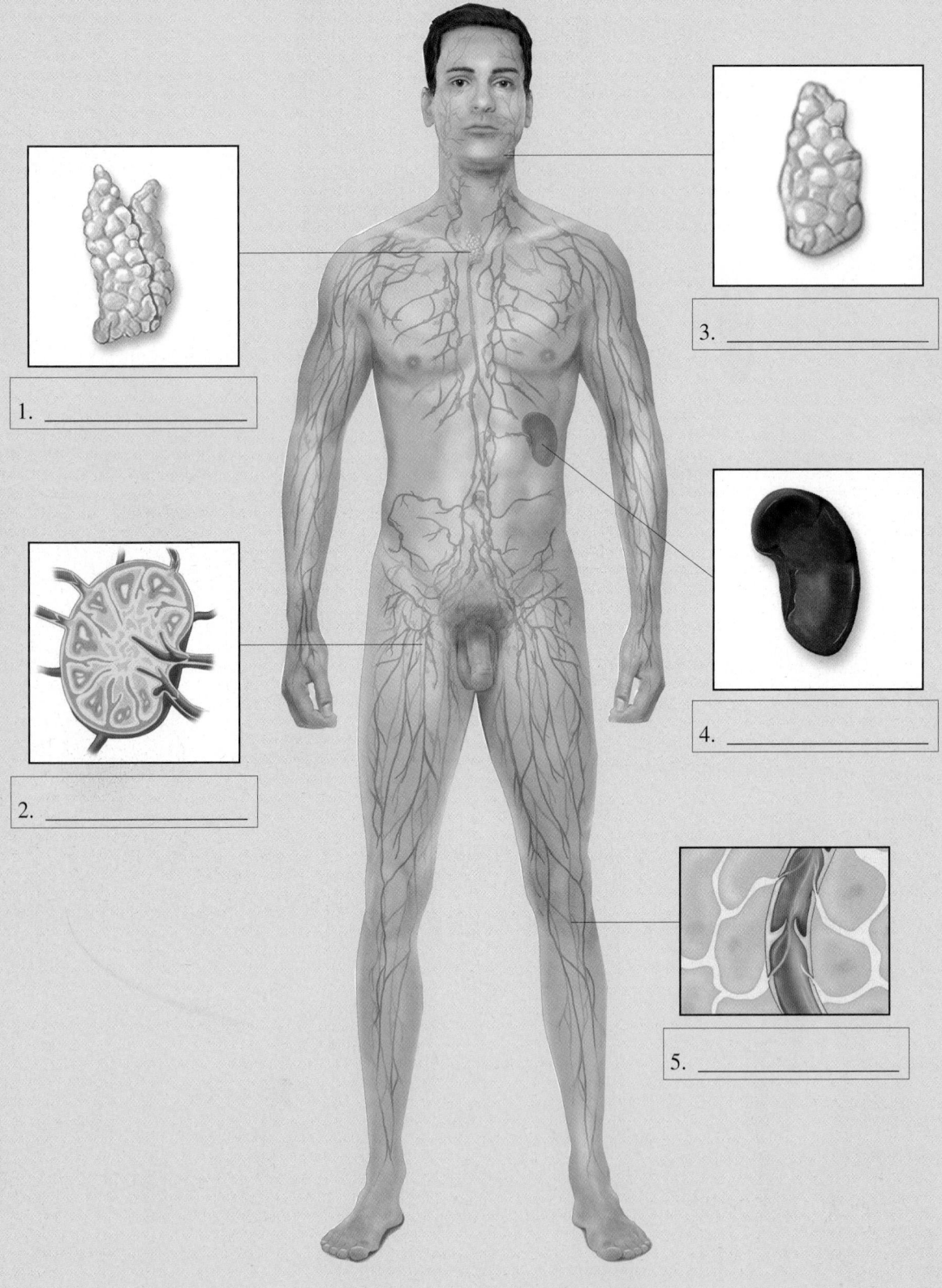

1. _____

2. _____

3. _____

4. _____

5. _____

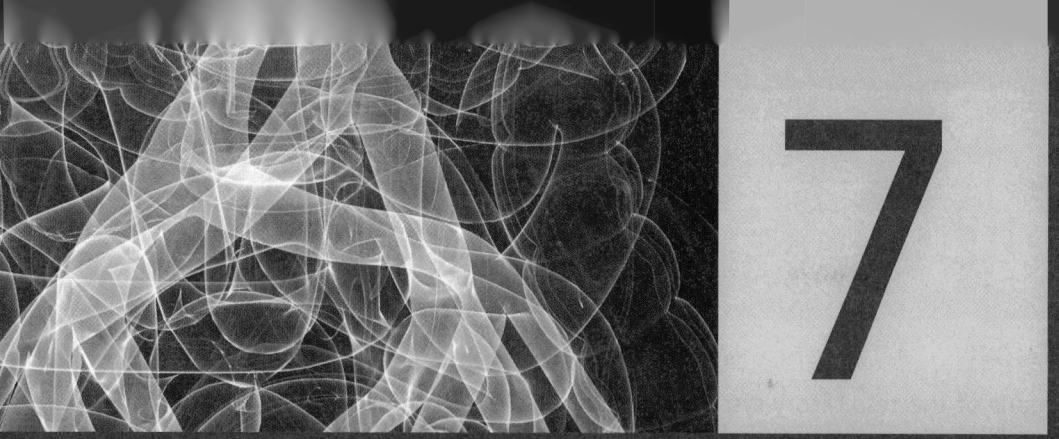

7

RESPIRATORY SYSTEM

Learning Objectives

Upon completion of this chapter, you will be able to

- Identify and define the combining forms and suffixes introduced in this chapter.

- Correctly spell and pronounce medical terms and major anatomical structures relating to the respiratory system.

- Locate and describe the major organs of the respiratory system and their functions.

- List and describe the lung volumes and capacities.

- Describe the process of respiration.

- Identify and define respiratory system anatomical terms.

- Identify and define selected respiratory system pathology terms.

- Identify and define selected respiratory system diagnostic procedures.

- Identify and define selected respiratory system therapeutic procedures.

- Identify and define selected medications relating to the respiratory system.

- Define selected abbreviations associated with the respiratory system.

Respiratory System at a Glance

Function

The organs of the respiratory system are responsible for bringing fresh air into the lungs, exchanging oxygen for carbon dioxide between the air sacs of the lungs and the blood stream, and exhaling the stale air.

Organs

Here are the primary structures that comprise the respiratory system.

nasal cavity **trachea**
pharynx **bronchial tubes**
larynx **lungs**

Word Parts

Here are the most common word parts (with their meanings) used to build respiratory system terms. For a more comprehensive list, refer to the Terminology section of this chapter.

Combining Forms

aer/o	air	orth/o	straight, upright
alveol/o	alveolus; air sac	ox/o, ox/i	oxygen
anthrac/o	coal	pharyng/o	pharynx
atel/o	incomplete	pleur/o	pleura
bronch/o	bronchus	pneum/o	lung, air
bronchi/o	bronchus	pneumon/o	lung, air
bronchiol/o	bronchiole	pulmon/o	lung
coni/o	dust	rhin/o	nose
diaphragmat/o	diaphragm	sept/o	wall
epiglott/o	epiglottis	sinus/o	sinus, cavity
laryng/o	larynx	spir/o	breathing
lob/o	lobe	trache/o	trachea, windpipe
nas/o	nose	tuss/o	cough
muc/o	mucus		

Suffixes

-capnia	carbon dioxide	-pnea	breathing
-osmia	smell	-ptysis	spitting
-phonia	voice	-spasm	involuntary muscle contraction
-plegia	paralysis	-thorax	chest

Respiratory System Illustrated

nasal cavity, p. 220

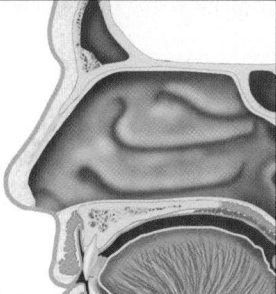

Cleanses, warms, and humidifies inhaled air

pharynx & larynx, p. 222

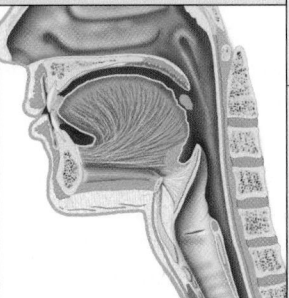

Carries air to the trachea through the voice box

bronchial tubes, p. 223

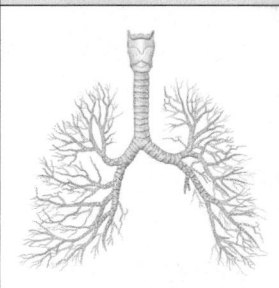

Air passageways inside the lung

trachea, p. 223

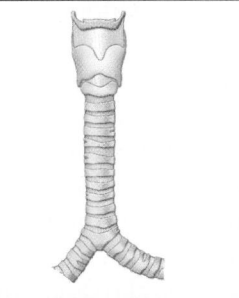

Transports air to and from lungs

lungs, p. 224

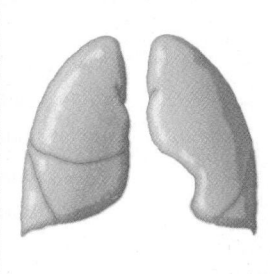

Site of gas exchange between air and blood

Anatomy and Physiology of the Respiratory System

bronchial tubes (BRONG-key-all)	**lungs**
carbon dioxide	**nasal cavity** (NAY-zl)
exhalation (eks-hah-LAY-shun)	**oxygen** (OK-sih-jen)
external respiration	**pharynx** (FAIR-inks)
inhalation (in-hah-LAY-shun)	**trachea** (TRAY-kee-ah)
internal respiration	**ventilation**
larynx (LAIR-inks)	

The organs of the respiratory system include the **nasal cavity, pharynx, larynx, trachea, bronchial tubes,** and **lungs.** These organs function together to perform the mechanical and, for the most part, unconscious mechanism of respiration. The cells of the body require the continuous delivery of oxygen and removal of carbon dioxide. The respiratory system works in conjunction with the cardiovascular system to deliver oxygen to all the cells of the body. The process of respiration must be continuous; interruption for even a few minutes can result in brain damage and/or death.

The process of respiration can be subdivided into three distinct parts: **ventilation, external respiration,** and **internal respiration.** Ventilation is the flow of air between the outside environment and the lungs. **Inhalation** is the flow of air into the lungs, and **exhalation** is the flow of air out of the lungs. Inhalation brings fresh **oxygen** (O_2) into the air sacs, while exhalation removes **carbon dioxide** (CO_2) from the body.

External respiration refers to the exchange of oxygen and carbon dioxide that takes place in the lungs. These gases diffuse in opposite directions between the air sacs of the lungs and the bloodstream. Oxygen enters the bloodstream from the air sacs to be delivered throughout the body. Carbon dioxide leaves the bloodstream and enters the air sacs to be exhaled from the body.

Internal respiration is the process of oxygen and carbon dioxide exchange at the cellular level when oxygen leaves the bloodstream and is delivered to the tissues. Oxygen is needed for the body cells' metabolism, all the physical and chemical changes within the body that are necessary for life. The by-product of metabolism is the formation of a waste product, carbon dioxide. The carbon dioxide enters the bloodstream from the tissues and is transported back to the lungs for disposal.

Nasal Cavity

cilia (SIL-ee-ah)	**nasal septum**
mucus (MYOO-kus)	**palate** (PAL-at)
mucous membrane	**paranasal sinuses** (pair-ah-NAY-zl)
nares (NAIR-eez)	

The process of ventilation begins with the nasal cavity. Air enters through two external openings in the nose called the **nares.** The nasal cavity is divided down the middle by the **nasal septum,** a cartilaginous plate. The **palate** in the roof of the mouth separates the nasal cavity above from the mouth below. The walls of the nasal cavity and the nasal septum are made up of flexible cartilage covered with **mucous membrane** (see Figure 7.1 ■). In fact, much of the respiratory tract

---

MED TERM TIP

The terms *inhalation* and *inspiration* (in- = inward + spir/o = breathing) can be used interchangeably. Similarly, the terms *exhalation* and *expiration* (ex- = outward + spir/o = breathing) are interchangeable.

MED TERM TIP

Anyone who has experienced a nosebleed, or *epistaxis*, is aware of the plentiful supply of blood vessels in the nose.

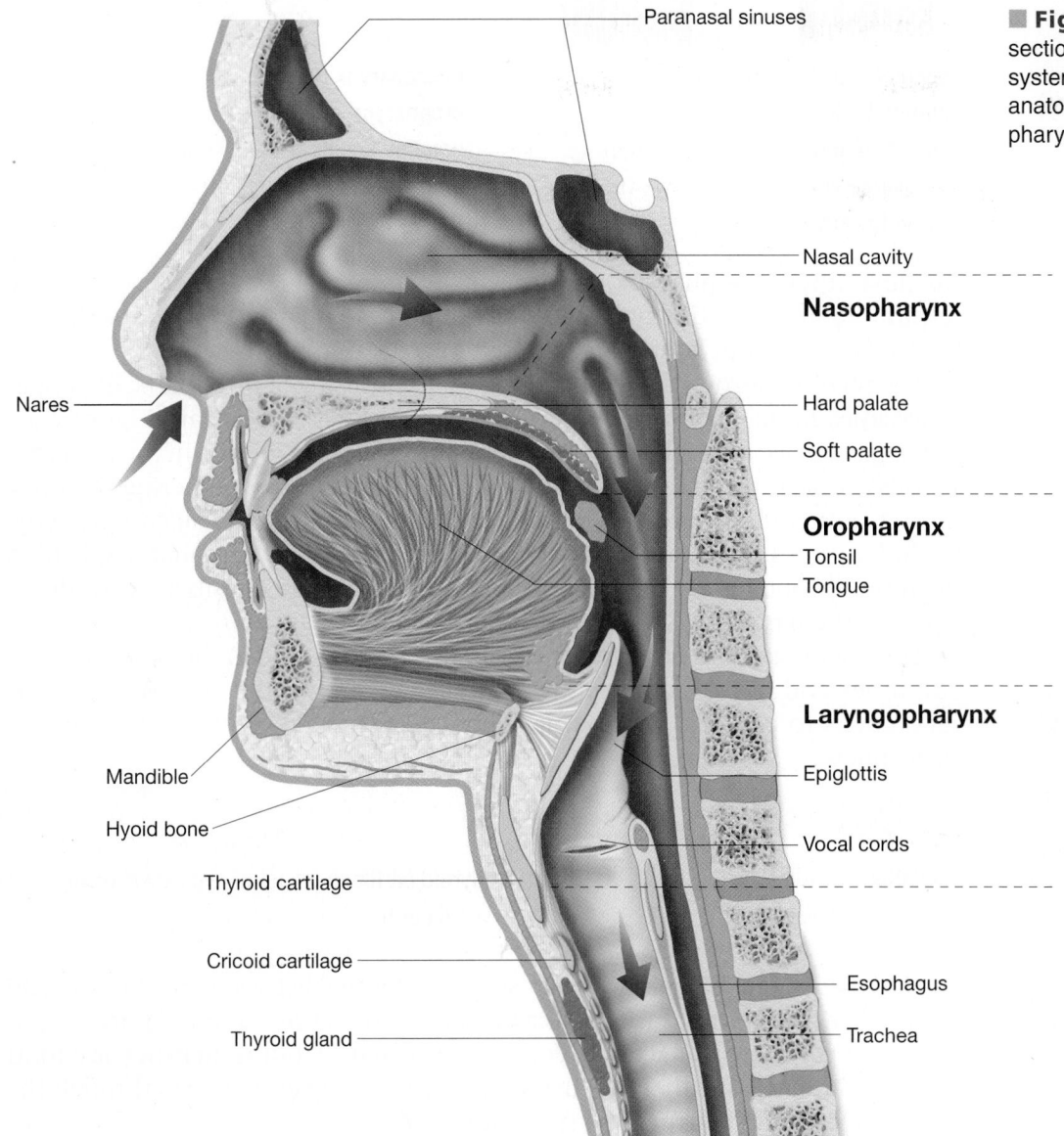

■ **Figure 7.1** Sagittal section of upper respiratory system illustrating the internal anatomy of the nasal cavity, pharynx, larynx, and trachea.

Paranasal sinuses

Nasal cavity

Nasopharynx

Hard palate

Soft palate

Oropharynx

Tonsil

Tongue

Laryngopharynx

Epiglottis

Vocal cords

Esophagus

Trachea

Nares

Mandible

Hyoid bone

Thyroid cartilage

Cricoid cartilage

Thyroid gland

is covered with mucous membrane, which secretes a sticky fluid, **mucus,** to help cleanse the air by trapping dust and bacteria. Since this membrane is also wet, it moisturizes inhaled air as it passes by the surface of the cavity. Very small hairs or **cilia** line the opening to the nose (as well as much of the airways), and filter out large dirt particles before they can enter the lungs. Capillaries in the mucous membranes warm inhaled air as it passes through the airways. Additionally, several **paranasal sinuses,** or air-filled cavities, are located within the facial bones. The sinuses act as an echo chamber during sound production and give resonance to the voice.

MED TERM TIP

Word Watch: The term *cilia* means hair, and there are other body systems that have cilia or cilia-like processes. For example, when discussing the eye, *cilia* means eyelashes.

Pharynx

adenoids (ADD-eh-noydz)	**nasopharynx** (nay-zoh-FAIR-inks)
auditory tube	**oropharynx** (or-oh-FAIR-inks)
eustachian tube (yoo-STAY-she-en)	**palatine tonsils** (PAL-ah-tine)
laryngopharynx (lair-ring-goh-FAIR-inks)	**pharyngeal tonsils** (fair-IN-jee-al)
lingual tonsils (LING-gwal)	

Air next enters the pharynx, also called the *throat*, which is used by both the respiratory and digestive systems. At the end of the pharynx, air enters the trachea while food and liquids are shunted into the esophagus.

The pharynx is roughly a 5-inch-long tube consisting of three parts: the upper **nasopharynx,** middle **oropharynx,** and lower **laryngopharynx** (see again Figure 7.1). Three pairs of tonsils (collections of lymphatic tissue) are located in the pharynx. Tonsils are strategically placed to help keep pathogens from entering the body through either the air breathed or food and liquid swallowed. The nasopharynx, behind the nose, contains the **adenoids** or **pharyngeal tonsils.** The oropharynx, behind the mouth, contains the **palatine tonsils** and the **lingual tonsils.** Tonsils are considered a part of the lymphatic system and are discussed in Chapter 6.

The opening of the **eustachian** or **auditory tube** is also found in the nasopharynx. The other end of this tube is in the middle ear. Each time you swallow, this tube opens to equalize air pressure between the middle ear and the outside atmosphere.

Larynx

epiglottis (ep-ih-GLOT-iss)	**thyroid cartilage** (THIGH-royd / CAR-tih-lij)
glottis (GLOT-iss)	**vocal cords**

The larynx, or *voice box*, is a muscular structure located between the pharynx and the trachea and contains the **vocal cords** (see again Figure 7.1 and Figure 7.2 ■). The vocal cords are not actually cordlike in structure, but rather they are folds of membranous tissue that produce sound by vibrating as air passes through the **glottis,** the opening between the two vocal cords.

A flap of cartilaginous tissue, the **epiglottis,** sits above the glottis and provides protection against food and liquid being inhaled into the lungs. The epiglottis covers the larynx and trachea during swallowing and shunts food and liquid from the pharynx into the esophagus. The walls of the larynx are composed of several cartilage plates held together with ligaments and muscles. One of these cartilages, the **thyroid cartilage,** forms what is known as the *Adam's apple.* The thyroid cartilage is generally larger in males than in females and helps to produce the deeper male voice.

MED TERM TIP

In the early 1970s it was common practice to remove the tonsils and adenoids in children suffering from repeated infections. However, it is now understood how important these organs are to remove pathogens from the air we breathe and the food we eat. Antibiotic treatment has also reduced the severity of infections.

MED TERM TIP

Stuttering may actually result from faulty neuromuscular control of the larynx. Some stutterers can sing or whisper without difficulty. Both singing and whispering involve movements of the larynx that differ from those required for regular speech.

MED TERM TIP

The term *Adam's apple* is thought to come from a fable that when Adam realized he had sinned in the Garden of Eden, he was unable to swallow the apple in his throat.

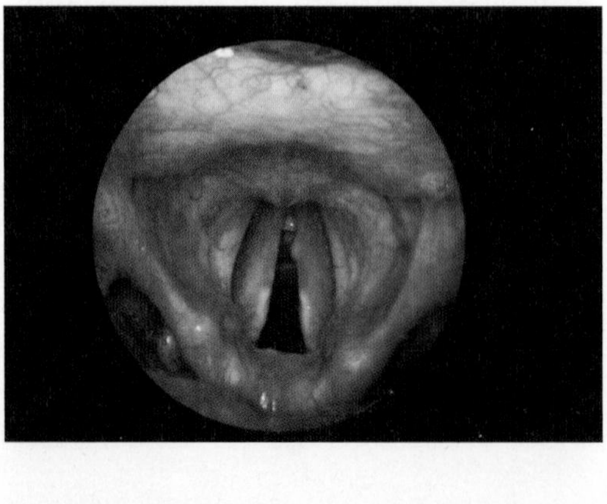

Figure 7.2 The vocal cords within the larynx, superior view from the pharynx. *(CNRI/Photo Researchers, Inc.)*

Trachea

The trachea, also called the *windpipe,* is the passageway for air that extends from the pharynx and larynx down to the main bronchi (see Figure 7.3 ■). Measuring approximately 4 inches in length, it is composed of smooth muscle and cartilage rings and is lined by mucous membrane and cilia. Therefore, it also assists in cleansing, warming, and moisturizing air as it travels to the lungs.

Bronchial Tubes

alveoli (al-VEE-oh-lye)
bronchioles (BRONG-key-ohlz)
bronchus (BRONG-kus)

pulmonary capillaries
respiratory membrane

The distal end of the trachea divides to form the left and right main (primary) bronchi. Each **bronchus** enters one of the lungs and branches repeatedly to form secondary and tertiary bronchi. Each branch becomes narrower until the narrowest branches, the **bronchioles,** are formed (see Figure 7.4 ■). Each bronchiole terminates in a small group of air sacs, called **alveoli.** Each lung has approximately 150 million alveoli. The walls of alveoli are elastic, giving them the ability to expand to hold air and then recoil to their original size. A network of **pulmonary capillaries** from the pulmonary blood vessels tightly encases each alveolus (see Figure 7.5 ■). In fact, the walls of the alveoli and capillaries are so tightly associated with each other they are referred to as a single unit, the **respiratory membrane.** The exchange of oxygen and carbon dioxide between the air within the alveolus and the blood inside the capillaries takes place across the respiratory membrane.

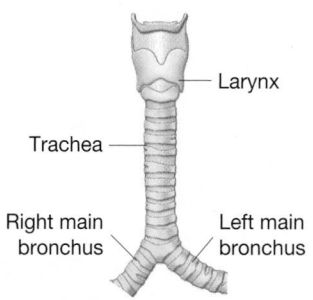

■ **Figure 7.3** Structure of the trachea, which extends from the larynx above to the main bronchi below.

MED TERM TIP

The respiratory system can be thought of as an upside-down tree and its branches. The trunk of the tree consists of the pharynx, larynx, and trachea. The trachea then divides into two branches, the bronchi. Each bronchus divides into smaller and smaller branches. In fact, this branching system of tubes is referred to as the *bronchial tree.*

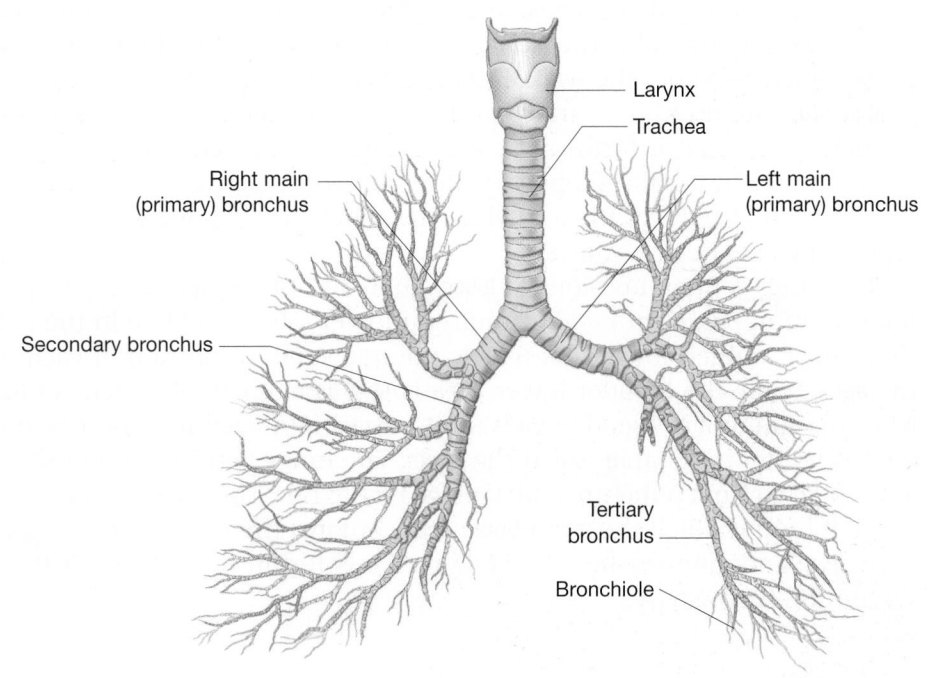

■ **Figure 7.4** The bronchial tree. Note how each main bronchus enters a lung and then branches into smaller and smaller primary bronchi, secondary bronchi, and bronchioles.

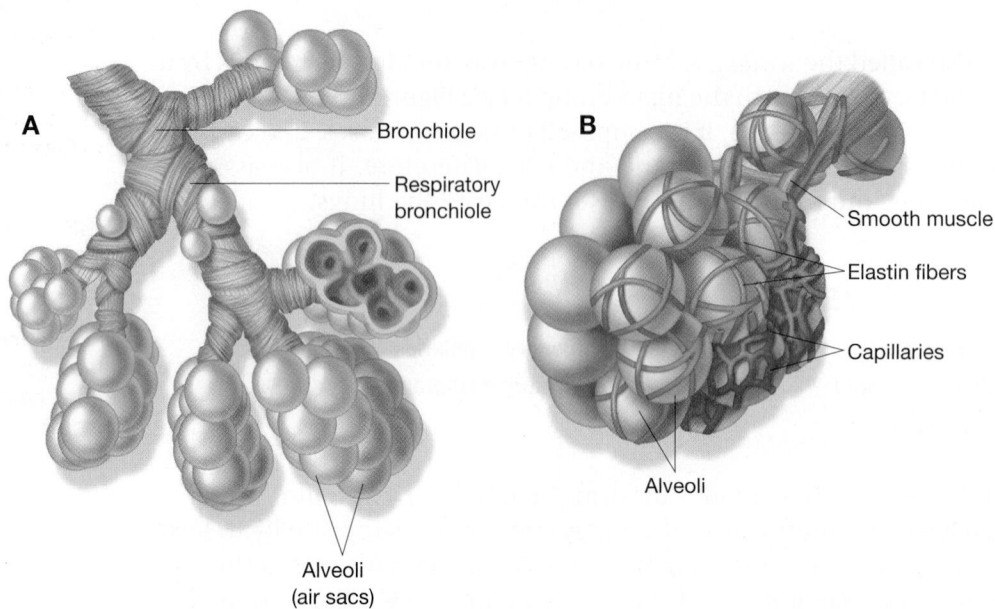

■ **Figure 7.5** (A) Each bronchiole terminates in an alveolar sac, a group of alveoli; (B) alveoli encased by network capillaries, forming the respiratory membrane.

Lungs

apex	**parietal pleura** (pah-RYE-eh-tal)
base	**pleura** (PLOO-rah)
hilum (HYE-lum)	**pleural cavity**
lobes	**serous fluid** (SEER-us)
mediastinum (mee-dee-ass-TYE-num)	**visceral pleura** (VISS-er-al)

Each lung is the total collection of the bronchi, bronchioles, and alveoli. They are spongy to the touch because they contain air. The lungs are protected by a double membrane called the **pleura.** The pleura's outer membrane is the **parietal pleura,** which also lines the wall of the chest cavity. The inner membrane, or **visceral pleura,** adheres to the surface of the lungs. The pleural membrane is folded in such a way that it forms a sac around each lung, referred to as the **pleural cavity.** There is normally slippery, watery **serous fluid** between the two layers of the pleura that reduces friction when the two layers rub together as the lungs repeatedly expand and contract.

The lungs contain divisions or **lobes.** There are three lobes in the larger right lung (right upper, right middle, and right lower lobes) and two in the left lung (left upper and left lower lobes). The pointed superior portion of each lung is the **apex,** while the broader lower area is the **base.** Entry of structures like the bronchi, pulmonary blood vessels, and nerves into each lung occurs along its medial border in an area called the **hilum.** The lungs within the thoracic cavity are protected from puncture and damage by the ribs. The area between the right and left lung is called the **mediastinum** and contains the heart, aorta, esophagus, thymus gland, and trachea. See Figure 7.6 ■ for an illustration of the lungs within the chest cavity.

MED TERM TIP

Some of the abnormal lung sounds heard with a stethoscope, such as crackling and rubbing, are made when the parietal and/or visceral pleura become inflamed and rub against one another.

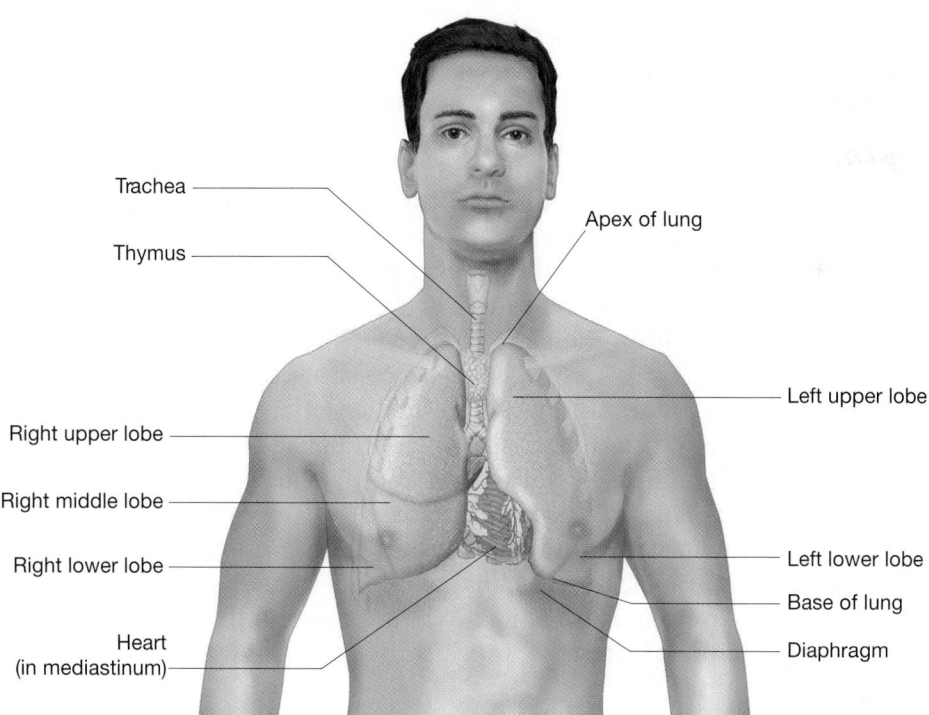

Trachea

Thymus

Apex of lung

Left upper lobe

Right upper lobe

Right middle lobe

Right lower lobe

Heart (in mediastinum)

Left lower lobe

Base of lung

Diaphragm

Lung Volumes and Capacities

pulmonary function test   **respiratory therapist**

For some types of medical conditions, like emphysema, it is important to measure the volume of air flowing in and out of the lungs to determine lung capacity. Lung volumes are measured by **respiratory therapists** to aid in determining the functioning level of the respiratory system. Collectively, these measurements are called **pulmonary function tests.** Table 7.1 ■ lists and defines the four lung volumes and four lung capacities.

Table 7.1	Lung Volumes and Capacities
TERM	**DEFINITION**
Tidal volume (TV)	The amount of air that enters the lungs in a single inhalation or leaves the lungs in a single exhalation of quiet breathing. In an adult this is normally 500 mL.*
Inspiratory reserve volume (IRV)	The amount of air that can be forcibly inhaled after a normal inspiration. Also called *complemental air;* generally measures around 3,000 mL.*
Expiratory reserve volume (ERV)	The amount of air that can be forcibly exhaled after a normal quiet exhalation. This is also called *supplemental air;* approximately 1,000 mL.*
Residual volume (RV)	The air remaining in the lungs after a forced exhalation; about 1,500 mL* in the adult.
Inspiratory capacity (IC)	The volume of air inhaled after a normal exhale.
Functional residual capacity (FRC)	The air that remains in the lungs after a normal exhalation has taken place.
Vital capacity (VC)	The total volume of air that can be exhaled after a maximum inhalation. This amount will be equal to the sum of TV, IRV, and ERV.
Total lung capacity (TLC)	The volume of air in the lungs after a maximal inhalation.

*There is a normal range for measurements of the volume of air exchanged. The numbers given are for the average measurement.

Respiratory Muscles

diaphragm   **intercostal muscles** (in-ter-COS-tal)

Air moves in and out of the lungs due to the difference between the atmospheric pressure and the pressure within the chest cavity. The **diaphragm,** the muscle separating the abdomen from the thoracic cavity, produces this difference in pressure. To do this, the diaphragm contracts and moves downward. This increase in thoracic cavity volume causes a decrease in pressure, or negative thoracic pressure, within the chest cavity. Air then flows into the lungs (inhalation) to equalize the pressure. The **intercostal muscles** between the ribs assist in inhalation by raising the rib cage to further enlarge the thoracic cavity. See Figure 7.7 ■ for an illustration of the role of the diaphragm in inhalation. Similarly, when the diaphragm and intercostal muscles relax, the thoracic cavity becomes smaller. This produces an increase in pressure within the cavity, or positive thoracic pressure, and air flows out of the lungs, resulting in exhalation. Therefore, a quiet, unforced exhalation is a passive process since it does not require any muscle contraction. When a forceful inhalation or exhalation is required, additional chest and neck muscles become active to create larger changes in thoracic pressure.

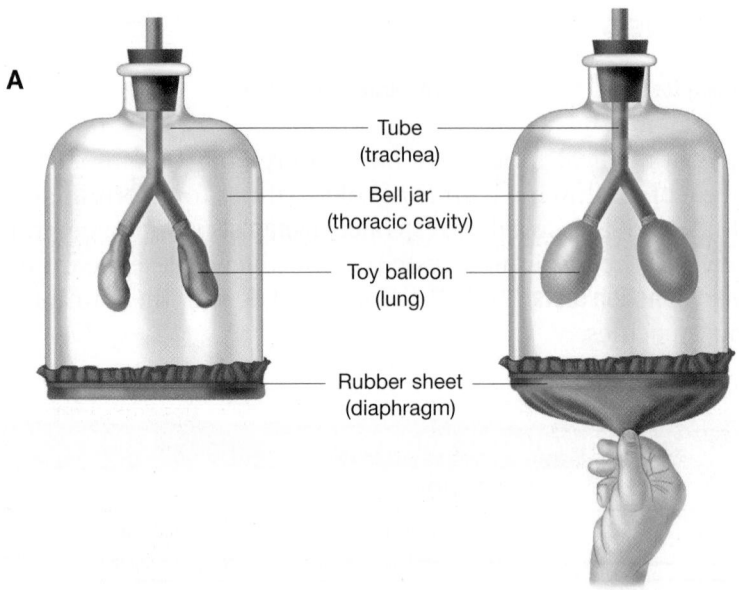

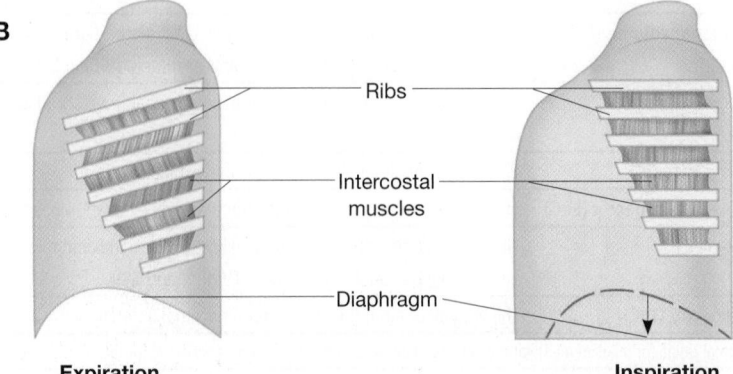

■ **Figure 7.7** (A) Bell jar apparatus demonstrating how downward movement of the diaphragm results in air flowing into the lungs; (B) action of the intercostal muscles lifts the ribs to assist the diaphragm in enlarging the volume of the thoracic cavity.

Respiratory Rate

vital signs

Respiratory rate (measured in breaths per minute) is one of our **vital signs** (VS), along with heart rate, temperature, and blood pressure. The respiratory rate is normally regulated by the level of CO_2 in the blood. When the CO_2 level is high, we breathe more rapidly to expel the excess. Likewise, when CO_2 levels drop, our respiratory rate will also drop.

When the respiratory rate falls outside the range of normal, it may indicate an illness or medical condition. For example, when a patient is running an elevated temperature and has shortness of breath (SOB) due to pneumonia, the respiratory rate may increase dramatically. Or a brain injury or some medications, such as those for pain, can cause a decrease in the respiratory rate. See Table 7.2 ■ for normal respiratory rate ranges for different age groups.

MED TERM TIP

Diaphragmatic breathing is taught to singers and public speakers. You can practice this type of breathing by allowing your abdomen to expand during inhalation and contract during exhalation while your shoulders remain motionless.

MED TERM TIP

When divers wish to hold their breath longer, they first hyperventilate (breath faster and deeper) in order to get rid of as much CO_2 as possible. This will hold off the urge to breathe longer, allowing a diver to stay submerged longer.

Table 7.2	Respiratory Rates for Different Age Groups
AGE	**RESPIRATIONS PER MINUTE**
Newborn	30–60
1-year-old	18–30
16-year-old	16–20
Adult	12–20

Terminology

Word Parts Used to Build Respiratory System Terms

The following lists contain the combining forms, suffixes, and prefixes used to build terms in the remaining sections of this chapter.

Combining Forms

aer/o	air	cyst/o	cyst, bladder	ox/o	oxygen
alveol/o	alveolus	cyt/o	cell	pharyng/o	pharynx
angi/o	vessel	diaphragmat/o	diaphragm	pleur/o	pleura
anthrac/o	coal	embol/o	plug	pneum/o	air
arteri/o	artery	epiglott/o	epiglottis	pneumon/o	lung
atel/o	incomplete	fibr/o	fibers	pulmon/o	lung
bi/o	life	hem/o	blood	py/o	pus
bronch/o	bronchus	hist/o	tissue	rhin/o	nose
bronchi/o	bronchus	laryng/o	larynx	sept/o	wall
bronchiol/o	bronchiole	lob/o	lobe	sinus/o	sinus
carcin/o	cancer	muc/o	mucus	somn/o	sleep
cardi/o	heart	nas/o	nose	spir/o	breathing
coni/o	dust	orth/o	straight	thorac/o	chest
cortic/o	outer region, cortex	ot/o	ear	trache/o	trachea
cyan/o	blue	ox/i	oxygen	tuss/o	cough

Suffixes

-al	pertaining to
-algia	pain
-ar	pertaining to
-ary	pertaining to
-capnia	carbon dioxide
-centesis	puncture to withdraw fluid
-dynia	pain
-eal	pertaining to
-ectasis	dilation
-ectomy	surgical removal
-emia	blood condition
-genic	produced by
-gram	record
-graphy	process of recording
-ia	condition

-ial	pertaining to
-ic	pertaining to
-ism	state of
-itis	inflammation
-logy	study of
-lytic	destruction
-meter	instrument to measure
-metry	process of measuring
-oma	tumor
-osis	abnormal condition
-osmia	smell
-ostomy	surgically create an opening
-otomy	cutting into
-phonia	voice

-plasm	formation
-plasty	surgical repair
-plegia	paralysis
-pnea	breathing
-ptysis	spitting
-rrhagia	abnormal flow condition
-rrhea	discharge
-scope	instrument for viewing
-scopy	process of visually examining
-spasm	involuntary muscle spasm
-stenosis	narrowing
-thorax	chest
-tic	pertaining to

Prefixes

a-	without
an-	without
anti-	against
brady-	slow
de-	without

dys-	abnormal, difficult
endo-	within
eu-	normal
hyper-	excessive

hypo-	insufficient
pan-	all
poly-	many
tachy-	fast

■ Anatomical Terms

TERM	WORD PARTS	DEFINITION
alveolar (al-VEE-oh-lar)	alveol/o = alveolus -ar = pertaining to	Pertaining to the alveoli.
bronchial (BRONG-ee-all)	bronch/o = bronchus -ial = pertaining to	Pertaining to a bronchus.
bronchiolar (brong-KEY-oh-lar)	bronchiol/o = bronchiole -ar = pertaining to	Pertaining to a bronchiole.
diaphragmatic (dye-ah-frag-MAT-ik)	diaphragmat/o = diaphragm -ic = pertaining to	Pertaining to the diaphragm.
epiglottic (ep-ih-GLOT-ik)	epiglott/o = epiglottis -ic = pertaining to	Pertaining to the epiglottis.
laryngeal (lair-in-GEE-all)	laryng/o = larynx -eal = pertaining to	Pertaining to the larynx.

■ Anatomical Terms *(continued)*

TERM	WORD PARTS	DEFINITION
nasal (NAY-zal)	nas/o = nose -al = pertaining to	Pertaining to the nose or nasal cavity.
pharyngeal (fair-in-GEE-all)	pharyng/o = pharynx -eal = pertaining to	Pertaining to the pharynx.
pleural (PLOO-ral)	pleur/o = pleura -al = pertaining to	Pertaining to the pleura.
pulmonary (PULL-mon-air-ee)	pulmon/o = lung -ary = pertaining to	Pertaining to the lung.
septal (SEP-tal)	sept/o = wall -al = pertaining to	Pertaining to the nasal septum.
thoracic (tho-RASS-ik)	thorac/o = chest -ic = pertaining to	Pertaining to the chest.
tracheal (TRAY-key-al)	trache/o = trachea -al = pertaining to	Pertaining to the trachea.

■ Pathology

TERM	WORD PARTS	DEFINITION
Medical Specialties		
internal medicine		Branch of medicine involving the diagnosis and treatment of diseases and conditions of internal organs such as the respiratory system. The physician is an *internist*.
otorhinolaryngology (ENT) (oh-toh-rye-noh-lair-in-GOL-oh-jee)	ot/o = ear rhin/o = nose laryng/o = larynx -logy = study of	Branch of medicine involving the diagnosis and treatment of conditions and diseases of the ear, nose, and throat region. The physician is an *otorhinolaryngologist*. This medical specialty may also be referred to as *otolaryngology*.
pulmonology (pull-mon-ALL-oh-jee)	pulmon/o = lung -logy = study of	Branch of medicine involved in the diagnosis and treatment of diseases and disorders of the respiratory system. Physician is a *pulmonologist*.
respiratory therapy	spir/o = breathing	Allied health specialty that assists patients with respiratory and cardiopulmonary disorders. Duties of a *respiratory therapist* include conducting pulmonary function tests, monitoring oxygen and carbon dioxide levels in the blood, administering breathing treatments, and ventilator management.
thoracic surgery (tho-RASS-ik)	thorac/o = chest -ic = pertaining to	Branch of medicine involving the diagnosis and treatment of conditions and diseases of the respiratory system by surgical means. Physician is a *thoracic surgeon*.

Pathology *(continued)*

TERM	WORD PARTS	DEFINITION
Signs and Symptoms		
anosmia (ah-NOZ-mee-ah)	an- = without -osmia = smell	Lack of the sense of smell.
anoxia (ah-NOK-see-ah)	an- = without ox/o = oxygen -ia = condition	Condition of receiving almost no oxygen from inhaled air.
aphonia (a-FOH-nee-ah)	a- = without -phonia = voice	Condition of being unable to produce sounds.
apnea (AP-nee-ah)	a- = without -pnea = breathing	Not breathing.
asphyxia (as-FIK-see-ah)	a- = without -ia = condition	Lack of oxygen that can lead to unconsciousness and death if not corrected immediately; also called *asphyxiation* or *suffocation*. Common causes include drowning, foreign body in the respiratory tract, poisoning, and electric shock.
aspiration (as-peer-RAY-shun)	spir/o = breathing	Refers to withdrawing fluid from a body cavity using suction. For example, using a long needle and syringe to withdraw fluid from the pleural cavity, or using a vacuum pump to remove phlegm from a patient's airways. Additionally, it refers to inhaling food, liquid, or a foreign object into the airways, which may lead to the development of pneumonia.
bradypnea (bray-DIP-nee-ah)	brady- = slow -pnea = breathing	Breathing too slowly; a low respiratory rate.
bronchiectasis (brong-key-EK-tah-sis)	bronchi/o = bronchus -ectasis = dilation	Dilated bronchus.
bronchospasm (BRONG-koh-spazm)	bronch/o = bronchus -spasm = involuntary muscle spasm	Involuntary muscle spasm of the smooth muscle in the wall of the bronchus.
Cheyne–Stokes respiration (CHAIN / STOHKS / res-pir-AY-shun)	spir/o = breathing	Abnormal breathing pattern in which there are long periods (10–60 seconds) of apnea followed by deeper, more rapid breathing. Named for John Cheyne, a Scottish physician, and Sir William Stokes, an Irish surgeon.
clubbing		Abnormal widening and thickening of the ends of the fingers and toes associated with chronic oxygen deficiency. Seen in patients with chronic respiratory conditions or circulatory problems.
crackles		Abnormal sound made during inspiration. Usually indicates the presence of fluid or mucus in the small airways. Also called *rales*.

Pathology *(continued)*

TERM	WORD PARTS	DEFINITION
cyanosis (sigh-ah-NO-sis)	cyan/o = blue -osis = abnormal condition	Refers to the bluish tint of skin that is receiving an insufficient amount of oxygen or circulation.
dysphonia (dis-FOH-nee-ah)	dys- = difficult, abnormal -phonia = voice	Condition of having difficulty producing sounds or producing abnormal sounds.
dyspnea (DISP-nee-ah)	dys- = abnormal, difficult -pnea = breathing	Term describing difficult or labored breathing.
epistaxis (ep-ih-STAKS-is)		Nosebleed.
eupnea (yoop-NEE-ah)	eu- = normal -pnea = breathing	Normal breathing and respiratory rate.
hemoptysis (hee-MOP-tih-sis)	hem/o = blood -ptysis = spitting	To cough up blood or blood-stained sputum.
hemothorax (hee-moh-THOH-raks)	hem/o = blood -thorax = chest	Presence of blood in the chest cavity.
hypercapnia (high-per-CAP-nee-ah)	hyper- = excessive -capnia = carbon dioxide	Condition of having excessive carbon dioxide in the body.
hyperpnea (high-per-NEE-ah)	hyper- = excessive -pnea = breathing	Taking deep breaths.
hyperventilation (HYE-per-vent-ill-a-shun)	hyper- = excessive	Breathing both too fast (tachypnea) and too deep (hyperpnea).
hypocapnia (high-poh-CAP-nee-ah)	hypo- = insufficient -capnia = carbon dioxide	An insufficient level of carbon dioxide in the body; a very serious problem because it is the presence of carbon dioxide that stimulates respiration, not the absence of oxygen. Therefore, a person with low carbon dioxide levels would respond with an increased respiratory rate.
hypopnea (high-POP-nee-ah)	hypo- = insufficient -pnea = breathing	Taking shallow breaths.
hypoventilation (HYE-poh-vent-ill-a-shun)	hypo- = insufficient	Breathing both too slow (bradypnea) and too shallow (hypopnea).
hypoxemia (high-pox-EE-mee-ah)	hypo- = insufficient ox/o = oxygen -emia = blood condition	Condition of having an insufficient amount of oxygen in the bloodstream.
hypoxia (high-POX-ee-ah)	hypo- = insufficient ox/o = oxygen -ia = condition	Condition of receiving an insufficient amount of oxygen from inhaled air.
laryngoplegia (lair-RING-goh-plee-gee-ah)	laryng/o = larynx -plegia = paralysis	Paralysis of the muscles controlling the larynx.

■ Pathology *(continued)*

TERM	WORD PARTS	DEFINITION
orthopnea (or-THOP-nee-ah)	orth/o = straight -pnea = breathing	Term describing dyspnea that is worsened by lying flat. The patient feels able to breath easier while sitting straight up; a common occurrence in those with pulmonary disease.
pansinusitis (pan-sigh-nus-EYE-tis)	pan- = all sinus/o = sinus -itis = inflammation	Inflammation of all the paranasal sinuses.
patent (PAY-tent)		Open or unblocked, such as a patent airway.
phlegm (FLEM)		Thick mucus secreted by the membranes lining the respiratory tract. When phlegm is coughed through the mouth, it is called *sputum*. Phlegm is examined for color, odor, and consistency and tested for the presence of bacteria, viruses, and fungi.
pleural rub (PLOO-ral)	pleur/o = pleura -al = pertaining to	Grating sound made when the two layers of the pleura rub together during respiration. It is caused when one of the surfaces becomes thicker as a result of inflammation or other disease conditions. This rub can be felt through the fingertips when placed on the chest wall or heard through a stethoscope.
pleurodynia (ploor-oh-DIN-ee-ah)	pleur/o = pleura -dynia = pain	Pleural pain.
pyothorax (pye-oh-THOH-raks)	py/o = pus -thorax = chest	Presence of pus in the chest cavity; indicates a bacterial infection.
rhinitis (rye-NYE-tis)	rhin/o = nose -itis = inflammation	Inflammation of the nasal cavity.
rhinorrhagia (rye-noh-RAH-jee-ah)	rhin/o = nose -rrhagia = abnormal flow condition	Rapid flow of blood from the nose.
rhinorrhea (rye-noh-REE-ah)	rhin/o = nose -rrhea = discharge	Discharge from the nose; commonly called a *runny nose.*
rhonchi (RONG-kigh)		Somewhat musical sound during expiration, often found in asthma or infection. Caused by spasms of the bronchial tubes. Also called *wheezing.*
shortness of breath (SOB)		Term used to indicate that a patient is having some difficulty breathing; also called *dyspnea*. The causes can range from mild SOB after exercise to SOB associated with heart disease.
sputum (SPEW-tum)		Mucus or phlegm coughed up from the lining of the respiratory tract.

MED TERM TIP

The term *sputum,* from the Latin word meaning "to spit," now refers to the material coughed up and spit out from the respiratory system.

Pathology *(continued)*

TERM	WORD PARTS	DEFINITION
stridor (STRIGH-dor)		Harsh, high-pitched, noisy breathing sound made when there is an obstruction of the bronchus or larynx. Found in conditions such as croup in children.
tachypnea (tak-ip-NEE-ah)	tachy- = fast -pnea = breathing	Breathing fast; a high respiratory rate.
thoracalgia (thor-ah-KAL-jee-ah)	thorac/o = chest -algia = pain	Chest pain. Does not refer to angina pectoris.
tracheostenosis (tray-kee-oh-steh-w-sis)	trache/o = trachea -stenosis = narrowing	Narrowing of the trachea.

Upper Respiratory System

TERM	WORD PARTS	DEFINITION
croup (KROOP)		Acute respiratory condition found in infants and children characterized by a barking type of cough or stridor.
diphtheria (dif-THEAR-ee-ah)	-ia = condition	Bacterial upper respiratory infection characterized by the formation of a thick membranous film across the throat and a high mortality rate. Rare now due to the DPT (diphtheria, pertussis, tetanus) vaccine.
laryngitis (lair-in-JYE-tis)	laryng/o = larynx -itis = inflammation	Inflammation of the larynx.
nasopharyngitis (nay-zoh-fair-in-JYE-tis)	nas/o = nose pharyng/o = pharynx -itis = inflammation	Inflammation of the nasal cavity and pharynx; commonly called the *common cold*.
pertussis (per-TUH-is)	tuss/o = cough	Commonly called *whooping cough*, due to the whoop sound made when coughing. An infectious bacterial disease of the upper respiratory system that children receive immunization against as part of their DPT shots.
pharyngitis (fair-in-JYE-tis)	pharyng/o = pharynx -itis = inflammation	Inflammation of the pharynx; commonly called a *sore throat*.
rhinomycosis (rye-noh-my-KOH-sis)	rhin/o = nose myc/o = fungus -osis = abnormal condition	Fungal infection of the nasal cavity.

Bronchial Tubes

TERM	WORD PARTS	DEFINITION
asthma (AZ-mah)		Disease caused by various conditions, like allergens, and resulting in constriction of the bronchial airways, dyspnea, coughing, and wheezing. Can cause violent spasms of the bronchi (bronchospasms) but is generally not a life-threatening condition. Medication can be very effective.

MED TERM TIP

The term *asthma*, from the Greek word meaning "panting," describes the breathing pattern of a person having an asthma attack.

Pathology *(continued)*

TERM	WORD PARTS	DEFINITION
bronchiectasis (brong-key-EK-tah-sis)	bronchi/o = bronchus -ectasis = dilation	Abnormal enlargement of bronchi; may be the result of a lung infection. This condition can be irreversible and result in destruction of the bronchial walls. Major symptoms include coughing up a large amount of purulent sputum, crackles, and hemoptysis.
bronchitis (brong-KIGH-tis)	bronch/o = bronchus -itis = inflammation	Inflammation of a bronchus.
bronchogenic carcinoma (brong-koh-JEN-ik / car-sin-OH-mah)	bronch/o = bronchus -genic = produced by carcin/o = cancer -oma = tumor	Malignant tumor originating in the bronchi. Usually associated with a history of cigarette smoking.

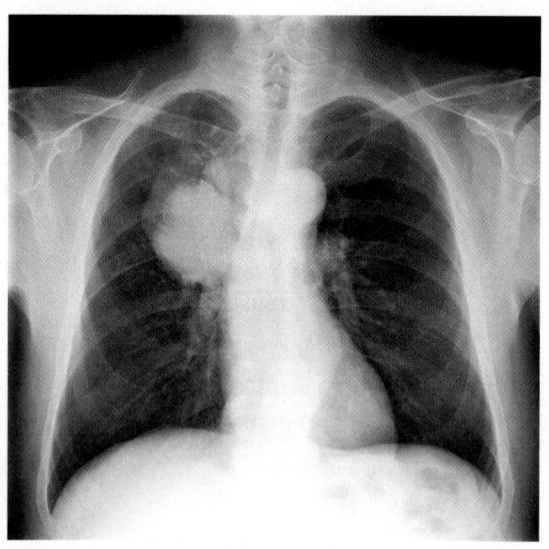

■ **Figure 7.8** Color-enhanced X-ray of large malignant tumor in the right lung. *(Du Cane Medical Imaging Ltd./Photo Researchers, Inc.)*

Lungs

adult respiratory distress syndrome (ARDS)	spir/o = breathing -al = pertaining to	Acute respiratory failure in adults characterized by tachypnea, dyspnea, cyanosis, tachycardia, and hypoxemia. May follow trauma, pneumonia, or septic infections. Also called *acute respiratory distress syndrome.*
anthracosis (an-thra-KOH-sis)	anthrac/o = coal -osis = abnormal condition	Type of pneumoconiosis that develops from the collection of coal dust in the lung. Also called *black lung* or *miner's lung.*
asbestosis (az-bes-TOH-sis)	-osis = abnormal condition	Type of pneumoconiosis that develops from collection of asbestos fibers in the lungs. May lead to the development of lung cancer.

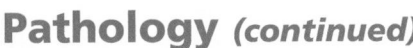

Pathology *(continued)*

TERM	WORD PARTS	DEFINITION
atelectasis (at-eh-LEK-tah-sis)	atel/o = incomplete -ectasis = dilation	Condition in which the alveoli in a portion of the lung collapse, preventing the respiratory exchange of oxygen and carbon dioxide. Can be caused by a variety of conditions, including pressure on the lung from a tumor or other object. Term also used to describe the failure of a newborn's lungs to expand.
chronic obstructive pulmonary disease (COPD) (PULL-mon-air-ee)	pulmon/o = lung -ary = pertaining to	Progressive, chronic, and usually irreversible group of conditions, like emphysema, in which the lungs have a diminished capacity for inspiration (inhalation) and expiration (exhalation). The person may have dyspnea upon exertion and a cough.
cystic fibrosis (CF) (SIS-tik / fye-BROH-sis)	cyst/o = cyst, bladder -ic = pertaining to fibr/o = fibers -osis = abnormal condition	Hereditary condition causing the exocrine glands to malfunction. The patient produces very thick mucus that causes severe congestion within the lungs and digestive system. Through more advanced treatment, many children are now living into adulthood with this disease. The term *cystic* in cystic fibrosis refers to cysts that form in the pancreas.
emphysema (em-fih-SEE-mah)		Pulmonary condition characterized by the destruction of the walls of the alveoli, resulting in fewer overexpanded air sacs. Can occur as a result of long-term heavy smoking. Air pollution also worsens this disease. The patient may not be able to breathe except in a sitting or standing position.
histoplasmosis (his-toh-plaz-MOH-sis)	hist/o = tissue -plasm = formation -osis = abnormal condition	Pulmonary infection caused by the fungus *Histoplasma capsulatum,* found in dust and in the droppings of pigeons and chickens. The translation of the name of this condition reflects the microscopic appearance of the fungus.
infant respiratory distress syndrome (IRDS)	spir/o = breathing	Lung condition most commonly found in premature infants that is characterized by tachypnea and respiratory grunting. The condition is caused by a lack of surfactant necessary to keep the lungs inflated. Also called *hyaline membrane disease* (HMD) and *respiratory distress syndrome of the newborn.*
influenza (in-floo-EN-za)		Viral infection of the respiratory system characterized by chills, fever, body aches, and fatigue. Commonly called the *flu.*
Legionnaire's disease (lee-jen-AYRZ)		Severe, often fatal bacterial infection characterized by pneumonia and liver and kidney damage. Named after people who came down with it at an American Legion convention in 1976.

Pathology *(continued)*

TERM	WORD PARTS	DEFINITION
Mycoplasma pneumonia (MY-koh-plaz-ma)	myc/o = fungus -plasm = formation	Less severe but longer lasting form of pneumonia caused by the *Mycoplasma pneumoniae* bacteria. Also called *walking pneumonia.* The translation of the name of this condition reflects the microscopic appearance of the bacteria.
pneumoconiosis (noo-moh-koh-nee-OH-sis)	pneum/o = lung coni/o = dust -osis = abnormal condition	Condition that is the result of inhaling environmental particles that become toxic. Can be the result of inhaling coal dust (anthracosis) or asbestos (asbestosis).
pneumocystis pneumonia (PCP) (noo-moh-SIS-tis / new-MOH-nee-ah)	pneum/o = lung cyst/o = cyst, bladder pneumon/o = lung -ia = condition	Pneumonia with a nonproductive cough, very little fever, and dyspnea caused by the fungus *Pneumocystis jirovecii.* An opportunistic infection often seen in those with weakened immune systems, such as AIDS patients.
pneumonia (new-MOH-nee-ah)	pneumon/o = lung -ia = condition	Inflammatory condition of the lung that can be caused by bacteria, viruses, fungi, and aspirated substances. Results in the filling of the alveoli and air spaces with fluid.
pulmonary edema (PULL-mon-air-ee / eh-DEE-mah)	pulmon/o = lung -ary = pertaining to	Condition in which lung tissue retains an excessive amount of fluid, especially in the alveoli. Results in dyspnea.
pulmonary embolism (PULL-mon-air-ee / EM-boh-lizm)	pulmon/o = lung -ary = pertaining to embol/o = plug -ism = state of	Obstruction of the pulmonary artery or one of its branches by an embolus (often a blood clot broken away from another area of the body). May cause an infarct in the lung tissue.
pulmonary fibrosis (fi-BROH-sis)	pulmon/o = lung -ary = pertaining to fibr/o = fibers -osis = abnormal condition	Formation of fibrous scar tissue in the lungs that leads to decreased ability to expand the lungs. May be caused by infections, pneumoconiosis, autoimmune diseases, and toxin exposure.
severe acute respiratory syndrome (SARS)	spir/o = breathing	Acute viral respiratory infection that begins like the flu but quickly progresses to severe dyspnea; high fatality rate. First appeared in China in 2003.
silicosis (sil-ih-KOH-sis)	-osis = abnormal condition	Type of pneumoconiosis that develops from the inhalation of silica (quartz) dust found in quarrying, glass works, sandblasting, and ceramics.
sleep apnea (AP-nee-ah)	a- = without -pnea = breathing	Condition in which breathing stops repeatedly during sleep long enough to cause a drop in oxygen levels in the blood.
sudden infant death syndrome (SIDS)		Unexpected and unexplained death of an apparently well infant under 1 year of age. The child suddenly stops breathing for unknown reasons.

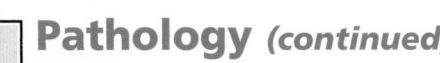

Pathology *(continued)*

TERM	WORD PARTS	DEFINITION
tuberculosis (TB) (too-ber-kyoo-LOH-sis)	-osis = abnormal condition	Infectious disease caused by the bacteria *Mycobacterium tuberculosis.* Most commonly affects the respiratory system and causes inflammation and calcification in the lungs. Tuberculosis incidence is on the increase and is seen in many patients with weakened immune systems. Multidrug-resistant tuberculosis is a particularly dangerous form of the disease because some bacteria have developed a resistance to the standard drug therapy.
Pleural Cavity		
empyema (em-pye-EE-mah)	py/o = pus	Pus with in the pleural space usually associated with a bacterial infection. Also called *pyothorax.*
pleural effusion (PLOO-ral / eh-FYOO-zhun)	pleur/o = pleura -al = pertaining to	Abnormal accumulation of fluid in the pleural cavity preventing the lungs from fully expanding. Physicians can detect the presence of fluid by tapping the chest (percussion) or listening with a stethoscope (auscultation).
pleurisy (PLOOR-ih-see)	pleur/o = pleura	Inflammation of the pleura characterized by sharp chest pain with each breath. Also called *pleuritis.*
pneumothorax (new-moh-THOH-raks)	pneum/o = air -thorax = chest	Collection of air or gas in the pleural cavity, which may result in collapse of the lung.

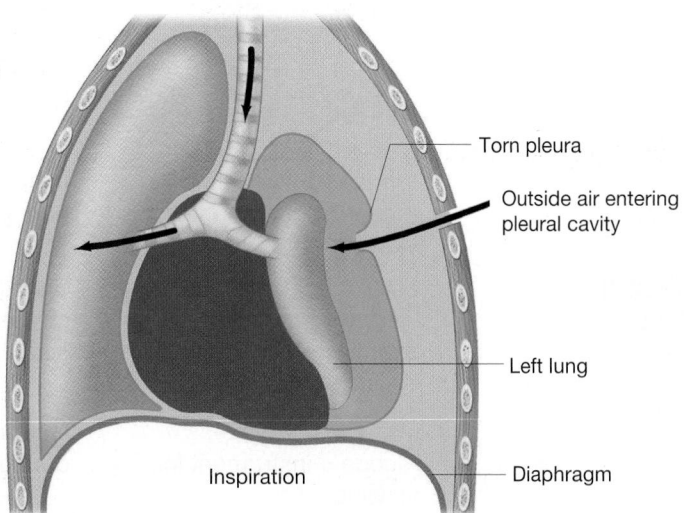

■ **Figure 7.9** Pneumothorax. Figure illustrates how puncture of thoracic wall and tearing of pleural membrane allows air into lung and results in collapsed lung.

Diagnostic Procedures

TERM	WORD PARTS	DEFINITION
Clinical Laboratory Tests		
arterial blood gases (ABGs) (ar-TEE-ree-al)	arteri/o = artery -al = pertaining to	Testing for the gases present in the blood. Generally used to assist in determining the levels of oxygen (O_2) and carbon dioxide (CO_2) in the blood.
sputum culture and sensitivity (C&S) (SPEW-tum)		Testing sputum by placing it on a culture medium and observing any bacterial growth. The specimen is then tested to determine antibiotic effectiveness.
sputum cytology (SPEW-tum / sigh-TALL-oh-jee)	cyt/o = cell -logy = study of	Examining sputum for malignant cells.
Diagnostic Imaging		
bronchogram (BRONG-koh-gram)	bronch/o = bronchus -gram = record	X-ray record of the bronchus produced by bronchography.
bronchography (brong-KOG-rah-fee)	bronch/o = bronchus -graphy = process of recording	X-ray of the lung after a radiopaque substance has been inserted into the trachea or bronchial tube. Resulting X-ray is called a *bronchogram.*
chest X-ray (CXR)		Taking a radiographic picture of the lungs and heart from the back and sides.
pulmonary angiography (PULL-mon-air-ee / an-jee-OG-rah-fee)	pulmon/o = lung -ary = pertaining to angi/o = vessel -graphy = process of recording	Injecting dye into a blood vessel for the purpose of taking an X-ray of the arteries and veins of the lungs.
ventilation-perfusion scan (per-FUSE-shun)		Nuclear medicine diagnostic test that is especially useful in identifying pulmonary emboli. Radioactive air is inhaled for the ventilation portion to determine if air is filling the entire lung. Radioactive intravenous injection shows if blood is flowing to all parts of the lung.
Endoscopic Procedures		
bronchoscope (BRONG-koh-scope)	bronch/o = bronchus -scope = instrument for viewing	Instrument used to view inside a bronchus during a *bronchoscopy.*
bronchoscopy (Bronch) (brong-KOSS-koh-pee)	bronch/o = bronchus -scopy = process of visually examining	Visual examination of the inside of the bronchi; uses an instrument called a *bronchoscope* (see Figure 7.10 ■).
laryngoscope (lair-RING-go-scope)	laryng/o = larynx -scope = instrument for viewing	Instrument used to view inside the larynx during a *laryngoscopy.*
laryngoscopy (lair-in-GOSS-koh-pee)	laryng/o = larynx -scopy = process of visually examining	Examination of the interior of the larynx with a lighted instrument called a *laryngoscope.*

Diagnostic Procedures *(continued)*

TERM	WORD PARTS	DEFINITION

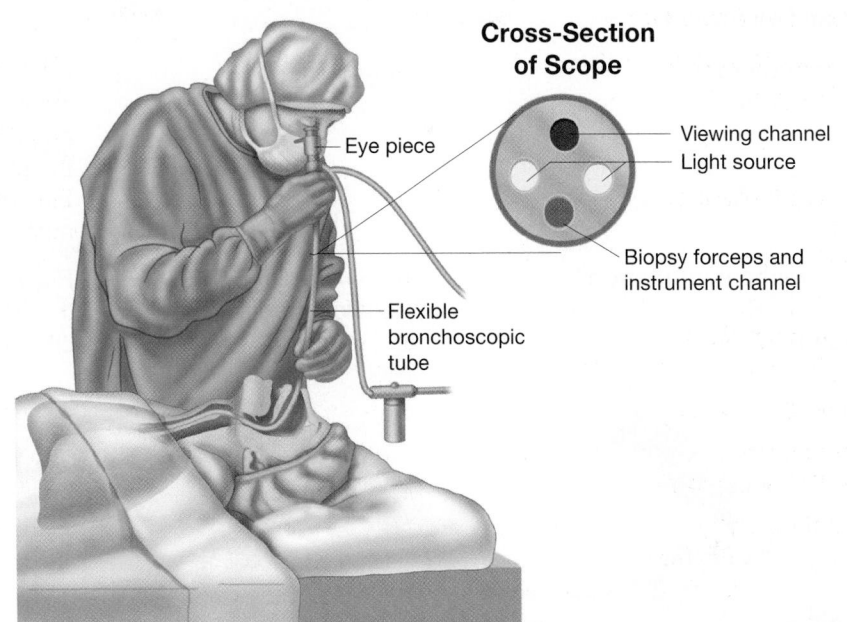

Cross-Section of Scope

Eye piece — Viewing channel — Light source — Biopsy forceps and instrument channel — Flexible bronchoscopic tube

■ **Figure 7.10** Bronchoscopy. Figure illustrates physician using a bronchoscope to inspect the patient's bronchial tubes. Advances in technology include using a videoscope, which projects the internal view of the bronchus onto a video screen.

Pulmonary Function Tests

TERM	WORD PARTS	DEFINITION
oximeter (ox-IM-eh-ter)	ox/i = oxygen -meter = instrument to measure	Instrument that measures the amount of oxygen in the bloodstream.
oximetry (ox-IM-eh-tree)	ox/i = oxygen -metry = process of measuring	Measures the oxygen level in the blood using a device, an *oximeter,* placed on the patient's fingertip or earlobe.
pulmonary function test (PFT) (PULL-mon-air-ee)	pulmon/o = lung -ary = pertaining to	Group of diagnostic tests that give information regarding air flow in and out of the lungs, lung volumes, and gas exchange between the lungs and bloodstream.
spirometer (spy-ROM-eh-ter)	spir/o = breathing -meter = instrument to measure	Instrument to measure lung capacity used for *spirometry.*
spirometry (spy-ROM-eh-tree)	spir/o = breathing -metry = process of measuring	Procedure to measure lung capacity using a *spirometer.*

Additional Diagnostic Procedures

TERM	WORD PARTS	DEFINITION
polysomnography (polly-som-NOG-rah-fee)	poly- = many somn/o = sleep -graphy = process of recording	Monitoring a patient while sleeping to identify sleep apnea. Also called *sleep apnea study.*
sweat test		Test for cystic fibrosis. Patients with this disease have an abnormally large amount of salt in their sweat.
tuberculin skin tests (TB test) (too-BER-kyoo-lin)		Applying the tuberculin purified protein derivative (PPD) under the surface of the skin to determine if the patient has been exposed to tuberculosis. Also called a *Mantoux test.*

■ Therapeutic Procedures

TERM	WORD PARTS	DEFINITION
Respiratory Therapy		
aerosol therapy (AIR-oh-sol)	aer/o = air	Medication suspended in a mist intended for inhalation. Delivered by a *nebulizer,* which provides the mist for a period of time while the patient breathes, or a *metered-dose inhaler* (MDI), which delivers a single puff of mist.
endotracheal intubation (en-doh-TRAY-kee-al / in-too-BAY-shun)	endo- = within trache/o = trachea -al = pertaining to	Placing of a tube through the mouth, through the glottis, and into the trachea to create a patent airway.

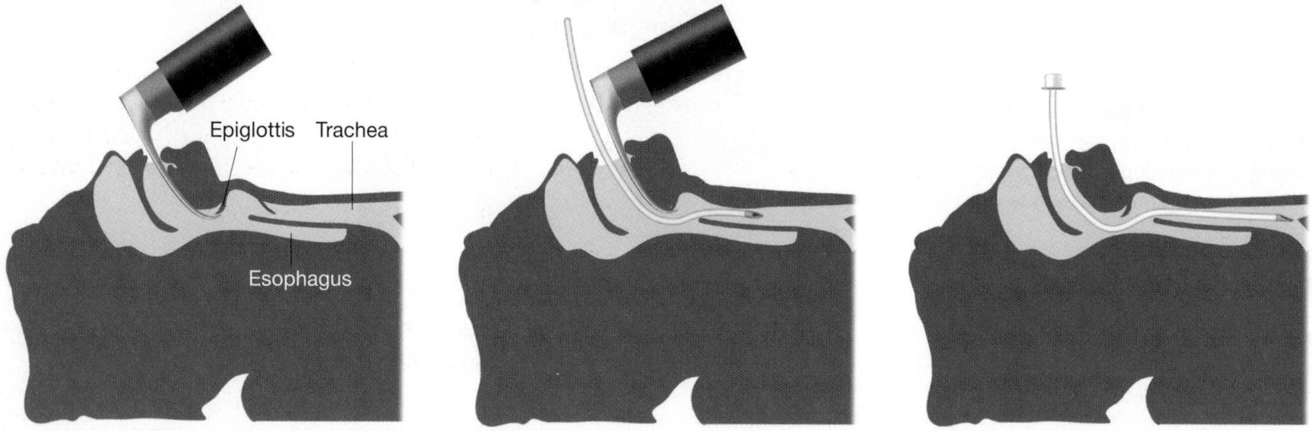

■ Figure 7.11 Endotracheal intubation. First, a lighted scope is used to identify the trachea from the esophagus. Next, the tube is placed through the pharynx and into the trachea. Finally, the scope is removed, leaving the tube in place.

TERM	WORD PARTS	DEFINITION
intermittent positive pressure breathing (IPPB)		Method for assisting patients in breathing using a mask connected to a machine that produces an increased positive thoracic pressure.
nasal cannula (CAN-you-lah)	nas/o = nose -al = pertaining to	Two-pronged plastic device for delivering oxygen into the nose; one prong is inserted into each naris.
postural drainage	-al = pertaining to	Drainage of secretions from the bronchi by placing the patient in a position that uses gravity to promote drainage. Used for the treatment of cystic fibrosis and bronchiectasis.
supplemental oxygen therapy	-al = pertaining to	Providing a patient with additional concentration of oxygen to improve oxygen levels in the bloodstream. Oxygen may be provided by a mask or nasal cannula.
ventilator (VENT-ih-later)		Machine that provides artificial ventilation for a patient unable to breathe on his or her own. Also called a *respirator.*

Therapeutic Procedures *(continued)*

TERM	WORD PARTS	DEFINITION
Surgical Procedures		
bronchoplasty (BRONG-koh-plas-tee)	bronch/o = bronchus -plasty = surgical repair	Surgical repair of a bronchus.
laryngectomy (lair-in-JEK-toh-mee)	laryng/o = larynx -ectomy = surgical removal	Surgical removal of the larynx.
laryngoplasty (lair-RING-goh-plas-tee)	laryng/o = larynx -plasty = surgical repair	Surgical repair of the larynx.
lobectomy (loh-BEK-toh-mee)	lob/o = lobe -ectomy = surgical removal	Surgical removal of a lobe of a lung.
pleurectomy (ploor-EK-toh-mee)	pleur/o = pleura -ectomy = surgical removal	Surgical removal of the pleura.
pleurocentesis (ploor-oh-sen-TEE-sis)	pleur/o = pleura -centesis = puncture to withdraw fluid	Procedure involving insertion of a needle into the pleura space to withdraw fluid; may be a treatment for excess fluid accumulating or to obtain fluid for diagnostic examination.
rhinoplasty (RYE-noh-plas-tee)	rhin/o = nose -plasty = surgical repair	Surgical repair of the nose.
thoracentesis (thor-ah-sen-TEE-sis)	thorac/o = chest -centesis = puncture to withdraw fluid	Surgical puncture of the chest wall for the removal of fluids. Also called *thoracocentesis.*

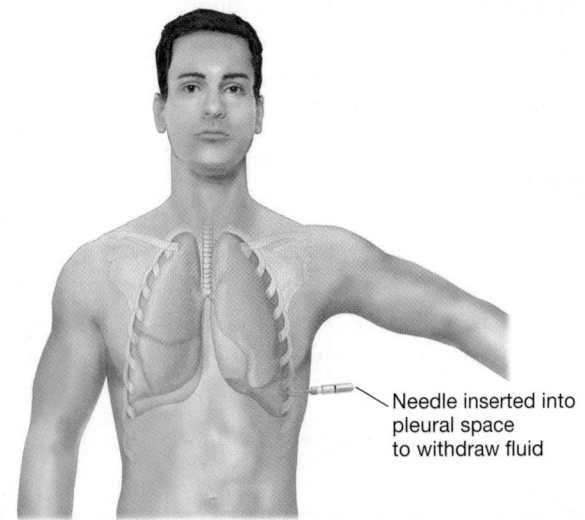

Needle inserted into
pleural space
to withdraw fluid

■ **Figure 7.12** Thoracentesis. A needle is inserted between the ribs to withdraw fluid from the pleural sac at the base of the left lung.

TERM	WORD PARTS	DEFINITION
thoracostomy (thor-ah-KOS-toh-mee)	thorac/o = chest -ostomy = surgically create an opening	Insertion of a tube into the chest cavity for the purpose of draining off fluid or air. Also called *chest tube.*
thoracotomy (thor-ah-KOT-oh-mee)	thorac/o = chest -otomy = cutting into	To cut into the chest cavity.

Therapeutic Procedures *(continued)*

TERM	WORD PARTS	DEFINITION
tracheotomy (tray-kee-OTT-oh-mee)	trache/o = trachea -otomy = cutting into	Surgical procedure often performed in an emergency that creates an opening directly into the trachea to allow the patient to breathe easier; also called *tracheostomy*.

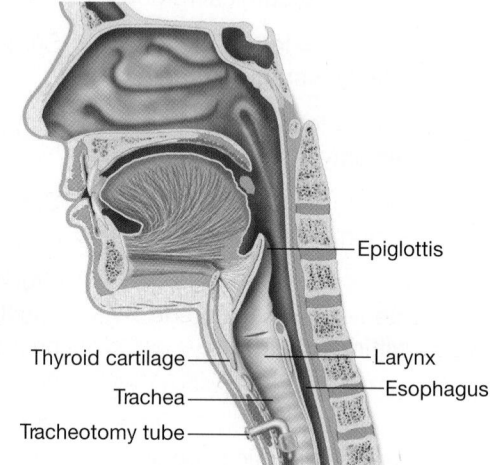

Figure 7.13 A tracheotomy tube in place, inserted through an opening in the front of the neck and anchored within the trachea.

(Labels: Epiglottis, Thyroid cartilage, Larynx, Esophagus, Trachea, Tracheotomy tube)

Additional Procedures

TERM	WORD PARTS	DEFINITION
cardiopulmonary resuscitation (CPR) (car-dee-oh-PULL-mon-air-ee / ree-suss-ih-TAY-shun)	cardi/o = heart pulmon/o = lung -ary = pertaining to	Emergency treatment provided by persons trained in CPR and given to patients when their respirations and heart stop. CPR provides oxygen to the brain, heart, and other vital organs until medical treatment can restore a normal heart and pulmonary function.
Heimlich maneuver (HYME-lik)		Technique for removing a foreign body from the trachea or pharynx by exerting diaphragmatic pressure. Named for Harry Heimlich, a U.S. thoracic surgeon.
percussion (per-KUH-shun)		Use of the fingertips to tap on a surface to determine the condition beneath the surface. Determined in part by the feel of the surface as it is tapped and the sound generated.

Pharmacology

CLASSIFICATION	WORD PARTS	ACTION	EXAMPLES
antibiotic (an-tih-bye-AW-tic)	anti- = against bi/o = life -tic = pertaining to	Kills bacteria causing respiratory infections.	ampicillin; amoxicillin, Amoxil; ciprofloxacin, Cipro
antihistamine (an-tih-HIST-ah-meen)	anti- = against	Blocks the effects of histamine that has been released by the body during an allergy attack.	fexofenadine, Allegra; loratadine, Claritin; diphenhydramine, Benadryl

Pharmacology *(continued)*

CLASSIFICATION	WORD PARTS	ACTION	EXAMPLES
antitussive (an-tih-TUSS-ive)	anti- = without tuss/o = cough	Relieves the urge to cough.	hydrocodon, Hycodan; dextromethorphan, Vicks Formula 44
bronchodilator (BRONG-koh-dye-late-or)	bronch/o = bronchus	Relaxes muscle spasms in bronchial tubes. Used to treat asthma.	albuterol, Proventil, Ventolin; theophyllin, Theo-Dur
corticosteroids (core-tih-koh-STAIR-ryods)	cortic/o = outer region, cortex	Reduces inflammation and swelling in the respiratory tract.	fluticasone, Flonase; mometasone, Nasonex; triamcinolone, Azmacort
decongestant (dee-kon-JES-tant)	de- = without	Reduces stuffiness and congestion throughout the respiratory system.	oxymetazoline, Afrin, Dristan, Sinex; pseudoephedrine, Drixoral, Sudafed
expectorant (ek-SPEK-toh-rant)		Improves the ability to cough up mucus from the respiratory tract.	guaifenesin, Robitussin, Mucinex
mucolytic (myoo-koh-LIT-ik)	muc/o = mucus -lytic = destruction	Liquefies mucus so it is easier to cough and clear it from the respiratory tract.	N-acetyl-cysteine, Mucomyst

Abbreviations

ABGs	arterial blood gases	**MDI**	metered-dose inhaler
ARDS	adult (or acute) respiratory distress syndrome	**O₂**	oxygen
		PCP	pneumocystis pneumonia
Bronch	bronchoscopy	**PFT**	pulmonary function test
CO₂	carbon dioxide	**PPD**	purified protein derivative
COPD	chronic obstructive pulmonary disease	**R**	respiration
CPR	cardiopulmonary resuscitation	**RA**	room air
C&S	culture and sensitivity	**RDS**	respiratory distress syndrome
CTA	clear to auscultation	**RLL**	right lower lobe
CXR	chest X-ray	**RML**	right middle lobe
DOE	dyspnea on exertion	**RRT**	registered respiratory therapist
DPT	diphtheria, pertussis, tetanus injection	**RV**	reserve volume
ENT	ear, nose, and throat	**RUL**	right upper lobe
ERV	expiratory reserve volume	**SARS**	severe acute respiratory syndrome
FRC	functional residual capacity	**SIDS**	sudden infant death syndrome
HMD	hyaline membrane disease	**SOB**	shortness of breath
IC	inspiratory capacity	**TB**	tuberculosis
IPPB	intermittent positive pressure breathing	**TLC**	total lung capacity
IRDS	infant respiratory distress syndrome	**TPR**	temperature, pulse, and respiration
IRV	inspiratory reserve volume	**TV**	tidal volume
LLL	left lower lobe	**URI**	upper respiratory infection
LUL	left upper lobe	**VC**	vital capacity

Chapter Review

Real-World Applications

Medical Record Analysis

This Pulmonology Consultation Report contains 12 medical terms. Underline each term and write it in the list below the report. Then define each term.

Pulmonology Consultation Report

Reason for Consultation:	Evaluation of increasingly severe asthma.
History of Present Illness:	Patient is a 10-year-old male who first presented to the Emergency Room with dyspnea, coughing, and wheezing at 7 years of age. Attacks are increasing in frequency, and there do not appear to be any precipitating factors such as exercise. No other family members are asthmatics.
Results of Physical Examination:	Patient is currently in the ER with marked dyspnea, cyanosis around the lips, prolonged expiration, and a hacking cough producing thick phlegm. Auscultation revealed rhonchi throughout lungs. ABGs indicate hypoxemia. Spirometry reveals moderately severe airway obstruction during expiration. This patient responded to Proventil and he is beginning to cough less and breathe with less effort.
Assessment:	Acute asthma attack with severe airway obstruction. There is no evidence of infection. In view of increasing severity and frequency of attacks, all his medications should be reevaluated for effectiveness and all attempts to identify precipitating factors should be made.
Recommendations:	Patient is to continue to use Proventil for relief of bronchospasms. Instructions for taking medications and controlling severity of asthma attacks were carefully reviewed with the patient and his family.

	Term	Definition
1	_____	_____
2	_____	_____
3	_____	_____
4	_____	_____
5	_____	_____
6	_____	_____
7	_____	_____
8	_____	_____
9	_____	_____
10	_____	_____
11	_____	_____
12	_____	_____

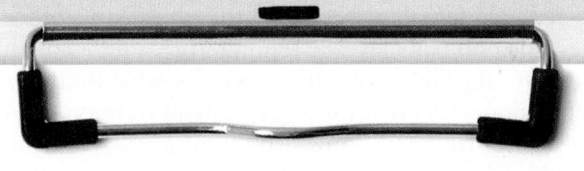

Chart Note Transcription

The chart note below contains 11 phrases that can be reworded with a medical term that you learned in this chapter. Each phrase is identified with an underline. Determine the medical term and write your answers in the space provided.

Current Complaint: A 43-year-old female was brought to the Emergency Room by her family. She complained of <u>painful and labored breathing,</u> ❶ <u>rapid breathing,</u> ❷ and fever. Symptoms began 3 days ago, but have become much worse during the past 12 hours.

Past History: Patient is a mother of three and a business executive. She has had no surgeries or previous serious illnesses.

Signs and Symptoms: Temperature is 103°F, respiratory rate is 20 breaths/minute, blood pressure is 165/98, and heart rate is 90 bpm. <u>A blood test to measure the levels of oxygen in the blood</u> ❸ indicates a marked <u>low level of oxygen in the blood.</u> ❹ The <u>process of listening to body sounds</u> ❺ of the lungs revealed <u>abnormal crackling sounds</u> ❻ over the left lower chest. She is producing large amounts of <u>pus-filled</u> ❼ <u>mucus coughed up from the respiratory tract</u> ❽ and a <u>chest X-ray</u> ❾ shows a large cloudy patch in the lower lobe of the left lung.

Diagnosis: Left lower lobe <u>inflammatory condition of the lungs caused by bacterial infection.</u> ❿

Treatment: Patient was started on intravenous antibiotics. She also required a <u>tube placed through the mouth to create an airway</u> ⓫ for 3 days.

❶ _____

❷ _____

❸ _____

❹ _____

❺ _____

❻ _____

❼ _____

❽ _____

❾ _____

❿ _____

⓫ _____

Case Study

Below is a case study presentation of a patient with a condition discussed in this chapter. Read the case study and answer the questions below. Some questions will ask for information not included within this chapter. Use your text, a medical dictionary, or any other reference material you choose to answer these questions.

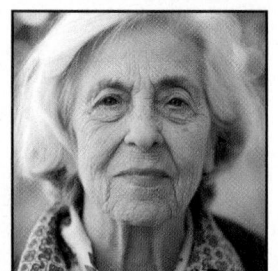

An 88-year-old female was seen in the physician's office complaining of dyspnea, dizziness, orthopnea, elevated temperature, and a cough. Lung auscultation revealed crackles over the right bronchus. CXR revealed fluid in the RUL. The patient was sent to the hospital with an admitting diagnosis of pneumonia. Vital signs upon admission were temperature 102°F, pulse 100 BPM and rapid, respirations 24 breaths/min and labored, blood pressure 180/110. She was treated with IV antibiotics and IPPB. She responded well to treatment and was released home to her family with oral antibiotics on the third day.

(© Francesco De Napoli/istockphoto.com)

1. What was this patient's admitting diagnosis? Look this condition up in a reference source and include a short description of it.

    _____

    _____

2. List and define each of the patient's presenting symptoms in your own words.

    _____

    _____

3. Define auscultation and CXR. Describe what each revealed in your own words.

    _____

    _____

4. What does the term "vital signs" mean? Describe this patient's vital signs.

    _____

    _____

5. Describe the treatments this patient received while in the hospital in your own words.

    _____

    _____

6. Explain the change in the patient's medication when she was discharged home.

    _____

    _____

Practice Exercises

A. Complete the Statement

1. The primary function of the respiratory system is _____.

2. The movement of air in and out of the lungs is called _____.

3. Define external respiration: _____.

4. Define internal respiration: _____.

5. The organs of the respiratory system are _____, _____,

   _____, _____, _____, and _____.

6. The passageway for food, liquids, and air is the _____.

7. The _____ helps to keep food out of the respiratory tract.

8. The function of the cilia in the nose is to _____.

9. The muscle that divides the thoracic cavity from the abdominal cavity is the _____.

10. The respiratory rate for an adult is _____ to _____ respirations per minute.

11. The respiratory rate for a newborn is _____ to _____ respirations per minute.

12. The right lung has _____ lobes; the left lung has _____ lobes.

13. The air sacs at the ends of the bronchial tree are called _____.

14. The term for the double membrane around the lungs is _____.

15. The nasal cavity is separated from the mouth by the _____.

16. The small branches of the bronchi are the _____.

B. Define the Suffix

	Definition	Example from Chapter
1. -ectasis	_____	_____
2. -capnia	_____	_____
3. -phonia	_____	_____
4. -thorax	_____	_____
5. -pnea	_____	_____
6. -ptysis	_____	_____
7. -osmia	_____	_____

C. Combining Form Practice

The combining form **rhin/o** refers to the nose. Use it to write a term that means:

1. inflammation of the nose _____

2. abnormal flow from the nose _____

3. discharge from the nose _____

4. surgical repair of the nose _____

The combining form **laryng/o** refers to the larynx or voice box. Use it to write a term that means:

5. inflammation of the larynx _____

6. spasm of the larynx _____

7. visual examination of the larynx _____

8. pertaining to the larynx _____

9. cutting into the larynx _____

10. removal of the larynx _____

11. surgical repair of the larynx _____

12. paralysis of the larynx _____

The combining form **bronch/o** refers to the bronchus. Use it to write a term that means:

13. pertaining to bronchus _____

14. inflammation of the bronchus _____

15. visually examine the interior of the bronchus _____

16. produced by bronchus _____

17. spasm of the bronchus _____

The combining form **thorac/o** refers to the chest. Use it to write a term that means:

18. surgical repair of the chest _____

19. cutting into the chest _____

20. chest pain _____

21. pertaining to chest _____

The combining form **trache/o** refers to the trachea. Use it to write a term that means:

22. cutting into the trachea _____

23. surgical repair of the trachea _____

24. narrowing of the trachea _____

25. pertaining to inside the trachea _____

26. inflammation of the trachea _____

D. Define the Combining Form

Definition	Example from Chapter

1. trache/o _____ _____

2. laryng/o _____ _____

3. bronch/o _____ _____

4. spir/o _____ _____

5. pneum/o _____ _____

6. rhin/o _____ _____

7. coni/o _____ _____

8. pleur/o _____ _____

9. epiglott/o _____ _____

10. alveol/o _____ _____

11. pulmon/o _____ _____

12. ox/o _____ _____

13. sinus/o _____ _____

14. lob/o _____ _____

15. nas/o _____ _____

E. Suffix Practice

The suffix -pnea means breathing. Use this suffix to write a medical term that means:

1. normal breathing _____

2. difficult or labored breathing _____

3. rapid breathing _____

4. can breathe only in an upright position _____

5. lack of breathing _____

F. Name That Term

1. the process of breathing in _____

2. spitting up of blood _____

3. blood clot in the pulmonary artery _____

4. inflammation of a sinus _____

5. sore throat _____

6. air in the pleural cavity _____

7. whooping cough _____

8. cutting into the pleura _____

9. pain in the pleural region _____

10. common cold _____

G. What's the Abbreviation?

1. upper respiratory infection _____

2. pulmonary function test _____

3. left lower lobe _____

4. oxygen _____

5. carbon dioxide _____

6. intermittent positive pressure breathing _____

7. chronic obstructive pulmonary disease _____

8. bronchoscopy _____

9. total lung capacity _____

10. tuberculosis _____

11. infant respiratory distress syndrome _____

H. What Does it Stand For?

1. CXR _____

2. TV _____

3. TPR _____

4. ABGs _____

5. DOE _____

6. RUL _____

7. SIDS _____

8. TLC _____

9. ARDS _____

10. MDI _____

11. CTA _____

12. SARS _____

I. Terminology Matching

Match each term to its definition.

1. _____ inhaling environmental particles   a. polysomnography

2. _____ whooping cough   b. Mantoux test

3. _____ may result in collapsed lung   c. oximetry

4. _____ test to identify sleep apnea   d. epistaxis

5. _____ respiratory tract mucus   e. pneumoconiosis

6. _____ sweat test   f. emphysema

7. _____ measures oxygen levels in blood   g. walking pneumonia

8. _____ *Mycoplasma* pneumonia   h. pneumothorax

9. _____ disease with overexpanded air sacs   i. empyema

10. _____ tuberculin test   j. phlegm

11. _____ nosebleed   k. pertussis

12. _____ pus in the pleural space   l. test for cystic fibrosis

J. Define the Term

1. total lung capacity _____

2. tidal volume _____

3. residual volume _____

K. Fill in the Blank

anthracosis	sputum cytology	cardiopulmonary resuscitation	patent
thoracentesis	respirator	ventilation-perfusion scan	rhonchi
supplemental oxygen	hyperventilation		

1. When the patient's breathing and heart stopped, the paramedics began _____.

2. The physician performed a _____ to remove fluid from the chest.

3. A _____ is also called a ventilator.

4. The patient received _____ through a nasal cannula.

5. An endotracheal intubation was performed to establish a _____ airway.

6. A _____ is a particularly useful test to identify a pulmonary embolus.

7. The result of the _____ was negative for cancer.

8. _____ involves tachypnea and hyperpnea.

9. _____ are wheezing lung sounds.

10. Miners are at risk of developing _____.

L. Pharmacology Challenge

Fill in the classification for each drug description, then match the brand name.

	Drug Description	Classification	Brand Name
1.	_____ Reduces stuffiness and congestion	_____	a. Hycodan
2.	_____ Relieves the urge to cough	_____	b. Flonase
3.	_____ Kills bacteria	_____	c. Cipro
4.	_____ Improves ability to cough up mucus	_____	d. Ventolin
5.	_____ Liquefies mucus	_____	e. Allegra
6.	_____ Relaxes bronchial muscle spasms	_____	f. Afrin
7.	_____ Blocks allergy attack	_____	g. Robitussin
8.	_____ Reduces inflammation and swelling	_____	h. Mucomyst

Labeling Exercise

Image A

Write the labels for this figure on the numbered lines provided.

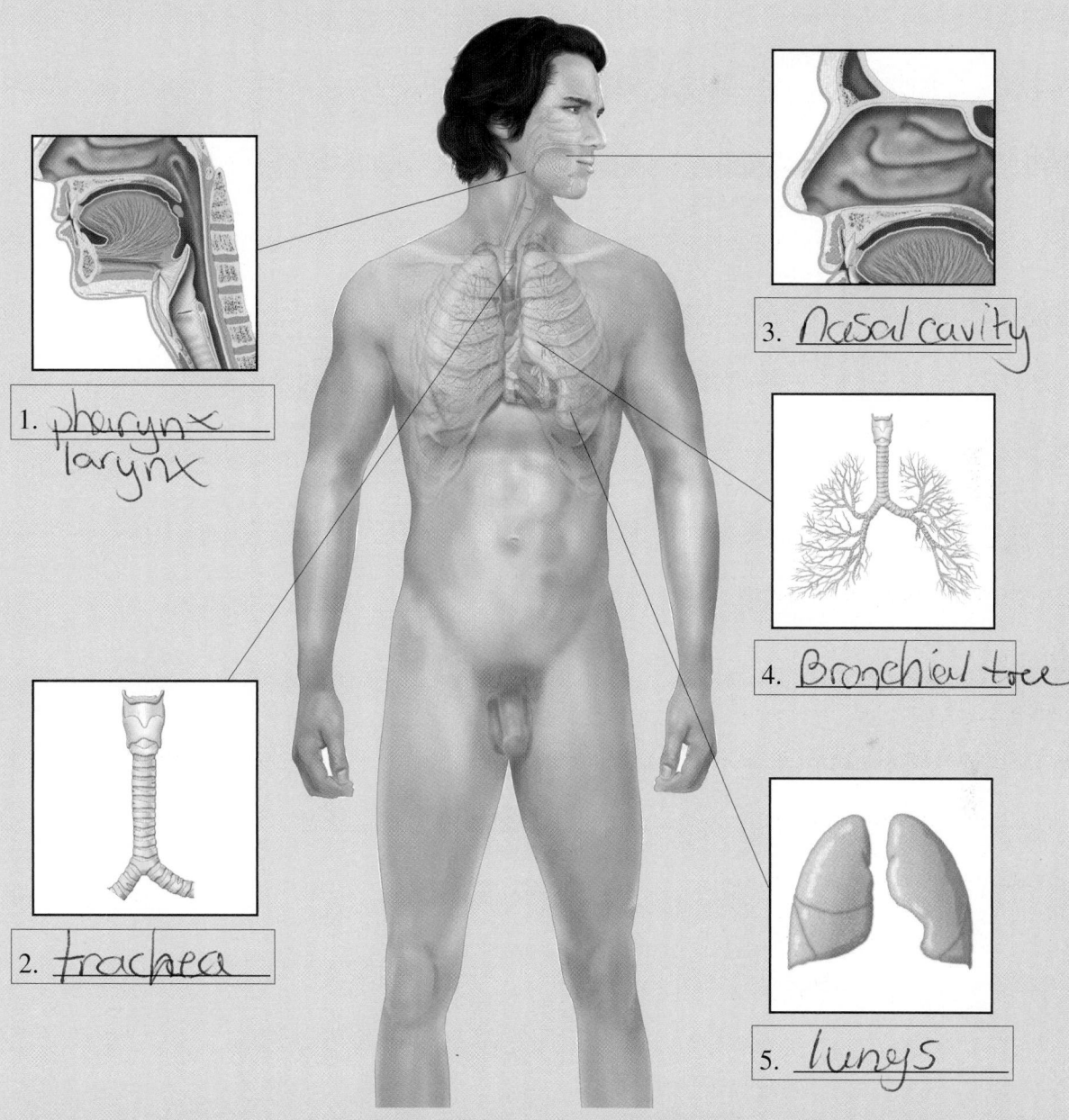

1. pharynx / larynx

2. trachea

3. Nasal cavity

4. Bronchial tree

5. lungs

MEDICAL TERMINOLOGY INTERACTIVE

Medical Terminology Interactive is a premium online homework management system that includes a host of features to help you study. Registered users will find:

- Fun games and activities built within a virtual hospital
- Powerful tools that track and analyze your results—allowing you to create a personalized learning experience
- Videos, flashcards, and audio pronunciations to help enrich your progress
- Streaming video lesson presentations and self-paced learning modules

www.pearsonhighered.com/mti

Image B

Write the labels for this figure on the numbered lines provided.

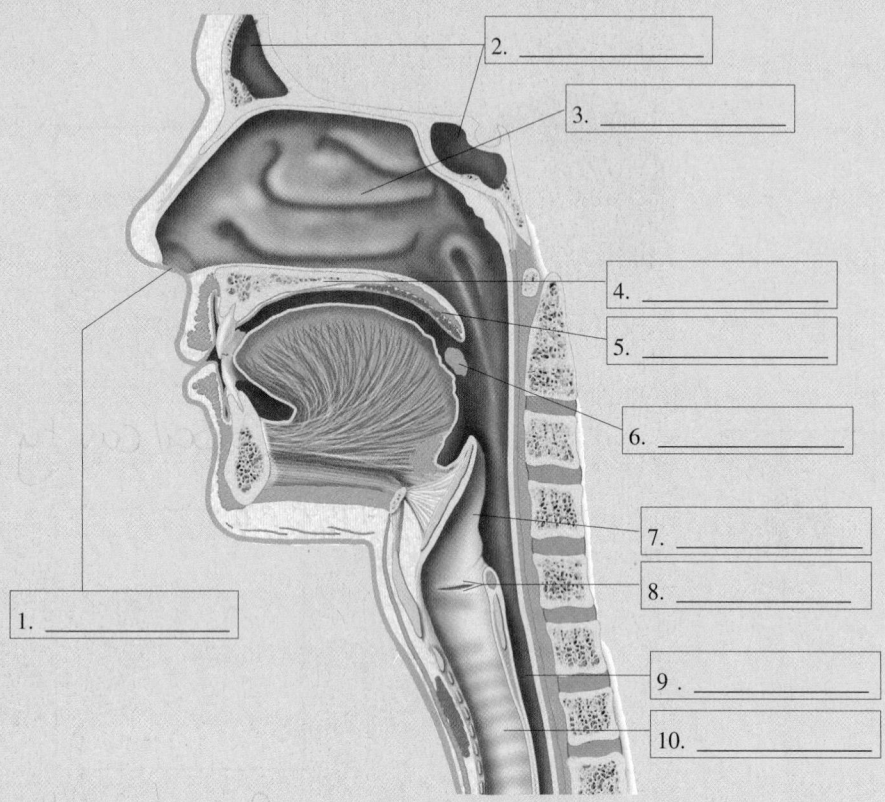

2. _____

3. _____

4. _____

5. _____

6. _____

7. _____

8. _____

1. _____

9. _____

10. _____

Image C

Write the labels for this figure on the numbered lines provided.

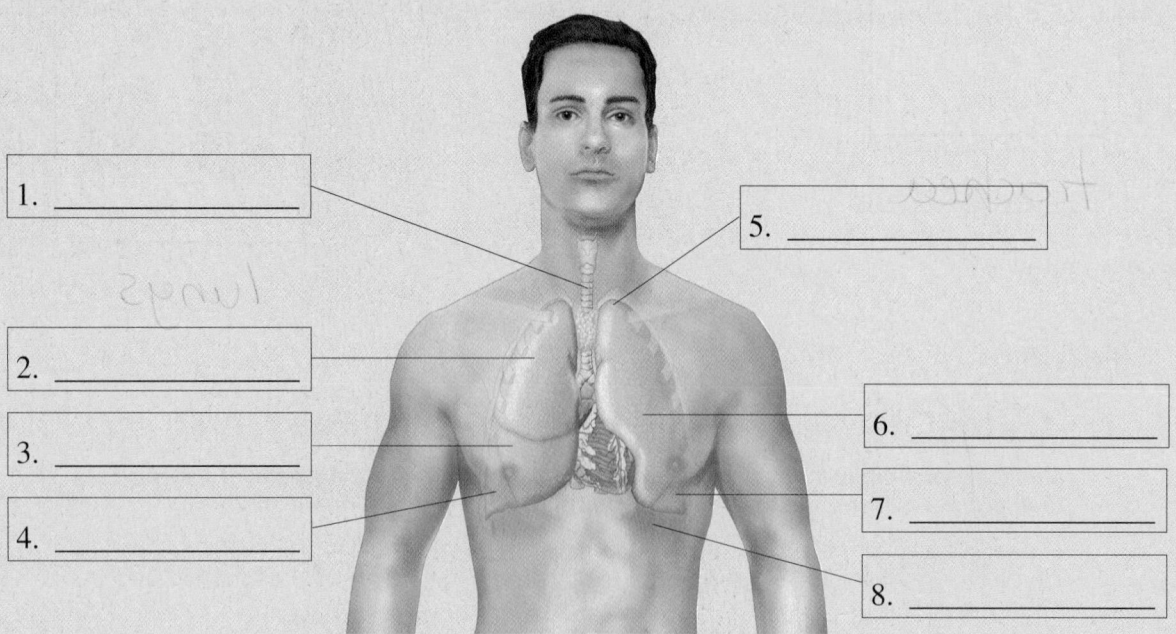

1. _____

5. _____

2. _____

6. _____

3. _____

7. _____

4. _____

8. _____

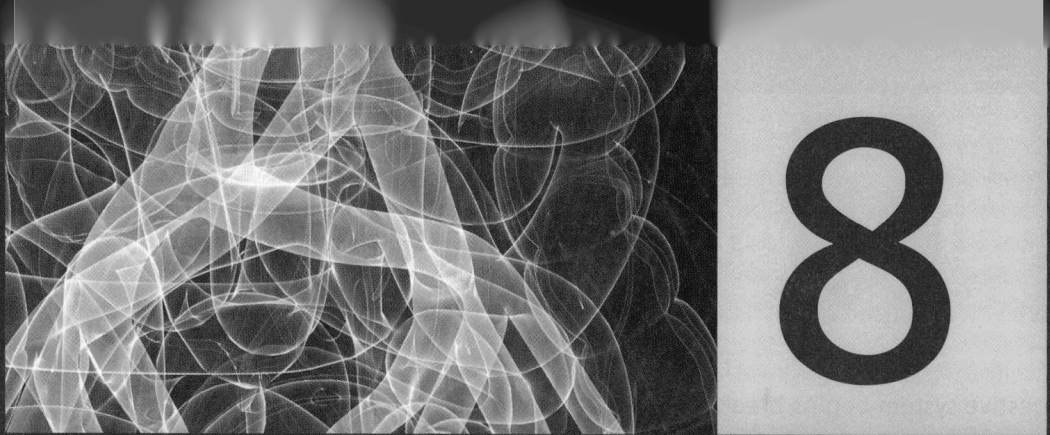

8

DIGESTIVE SYSTEM

Learning Objectives

Upon completion of this chapter, you will be able to

- Identify and define the combining forms and suffixes introduced in this chapter.

- Correctly spell and pronounce medical terms and major anatomical structures relating to the digestive system.

- Locate and describe the major organs of the digestive system and their functions.

- Describe the function of the accessory organs of the digestive system.

- Identify the shape and function of each type of tooth.

- Identify and define digestive system anatomical terms.

- Identify and define selected digestive system pathology terms.

- Identify and define selected digestive system diagnostic procedures.

- Identify and define selected digestive system therapeutic procedures.

- Identify and define selected medications relating to the digestive system.

- Define selected abbreviations associated with the digestive system.

Digestive System at a Glance

Function

The digestive system begins breaking down food through mechanical and chemical digestion. After being digested, nutrient molecules are absorbed into the body and enter the bloodstream; any food not digested or absorbed is eliminated as solid waste.

Organs

Here are the primary structures that comprise the digestive system.

colon	pancreas
esophagus	pharynx
gallbladder (GB)	salivary glands
liver	small intestine
oral cavity	stomach

Word Parts

Here are the most common word parts (with their meanings) used to build digestive system terms. For a more comprehensive list, refer to the Terminology section of this chapter.

Combining Forms

an/o	anus	gloss/o	tongue
append/o	appendix	hepat/o	liver
appendic/o	appendix	ile/o	ileum
bar/o	weight	jejun/o	jejunum
bucc/o	cheek	labi/o	lip
cec/o	cecum	lapar/o	abdomen
cholangi/o	bile duct	lingu/o	tongue
chol/e	bile, gall	lith/o	stone
cholecyst/o	gallbladder	odont/o	tooth
choledoch/o	common bile duct	or/o	mouth
cirrh/o	yellow	palat/o	palate
col/o	colon	pancreat/o	pancreas
colon/o	colon	pharyng/o	pharynx (throat)
dent/o	tooth	polyp/o	polyp
diverticul/o	pouch	proct/o	anus and rectum
duoden/o	duodenum	pylor/o	pylorus
enter/o	small intestine	pyr/o	fire
esophag/o	esophagus	rect/o	rectum
gastr/o	stomach	sialaden/o	salivary gland
gingiv/o	gums	sigmoid/o	sigmoid colon

Suffixes

-emesis	vomit	-pepsia	digestion
-istry	specialty of	-phagia	eat, swallow
-lithiasis	condition of stones	-prandial	pertaining to a meal
-orexia	appetite	-tripsy	surgical crushing

Digestive System Illustrated

salivary glands, p. 264

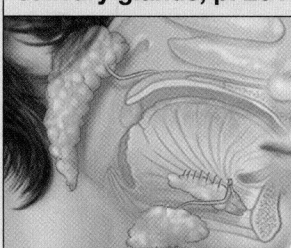

Produces saliva

oral cavity, p. 258

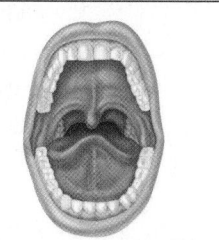

Ingests, chews, and swallows food

esophagus, p. 261

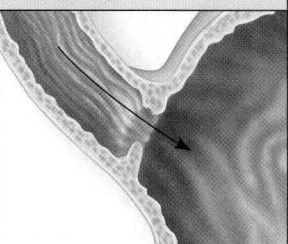

Transports food to the stomach

stomach, p. 262

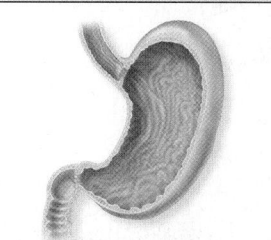

Secretes acid and mixes food to start digestion

pancreas, p. 265

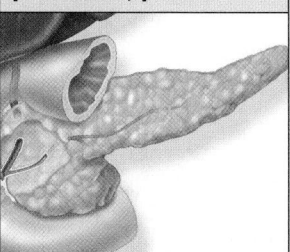

Secretes digestive enzymes and buffers

liver & gallbladder, p. 265

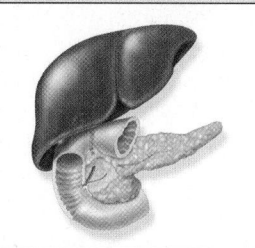

Produces and stores bile

small intestine, p. 262

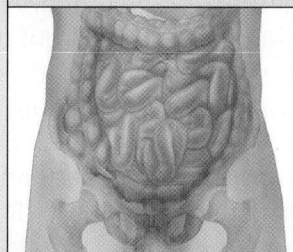

Digests and absorbs nutrients

colon, p. 263

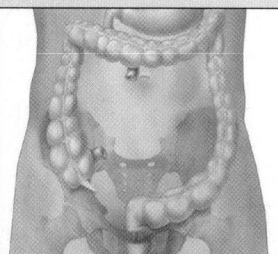

Reabsorbs water and stores feces

Anatomy and Physiology of the Digestive System

accessory organs	**gut**
alimentary canal (al-ih-MEN-tar-ree)	**liver**
colon (COH-lon)	**oral cavity**
esophagus (eh-SOFF-ah-gus)	**pancreas** (PAN-kree-ass)
gallbladder	**pharynx** (FAIR-inks)
gastrointestinal system	**salivary glands** (SAL-ih-vair-ee)
(gas-troh-in-TESS-tih-nal)	**small intestine**
gastrointestinal tract	**stomach** (STUM-ak)

MED TERM TIP

The term *alimentary* comes from the Latin term *alimentum* meaning "nourishment."

The digestive system, also known as the **gastrointestinal (GI) system,** includes approximately 30 feet of a continuous muscular tube called the **gut, alimentary canal,** or **gastrointestinal tract** that stretches between the mouth and the anus. Most of the organs in this system are actually different sections of this tube. In order, beginning at the mouth and continuing to the anus, these organs are the **oral cavity, pharynx, esophagus, stomach, small intestine, colon, rectum,** and **anus.** The **accessory organs** of digestion are those that participate in the digestion process, but are not part of the continuous alimentary canal. These organs, which are connected to the gut by a duct, are the **liver, pancreas, gallbladder,** and **salivary glands.**

The digestive system has three main functions: digesting food, absorbing nutrients, and eliminating waste. Digestion includes the physical and chemical breakdown of large food particles into simple nutrient molecules like glucose, triglycerides, and amino acids. These simple nutrient molecules are absorbed from the intestines and circulated throughout the body by the cardiovascular system. They are used for growth and repair of organs and tissues. Any food that cannot be digested or absorbed by the body is eliminated from the gastrointestinal system as a solid waste.

Oral Cavity

cheeks	**saliva** (suh-LYE-vah)
gingiva (JIN-jih-veh)	**taste buds**
gums	**teeth**
lips	**tongue**
palate (PAL-at)	**uvula** (YU-vyu-lah)

Digestion begins when food enters the mouth and is mechanically broken up by the chewing movements of the **teeth.** The muscular **tongue** moves the food within the mouth and mixes it with **saliva** (see Figure 8.1 ■). Saliva contains digestive enzymes to break down carbohydrates and slippery lubricants to make food easier to swallow. **Taste buds,** found on the surface of the tongue, can distinguish the bitter, sweet, sour, and salty flavors in our food. The roof of the oral cavity is known as the **palate** and is subdivided into the hard palate (the bony anterior portion) and the soft palate (the flexible posterior portion). Hanging down from the posterior edge of the soft palate is the **uvula.** The uvula serves two important functions. First, it has a role in speech production, and second, it is the location of the gag reflex. This reflex is stimulated when food enters the throat without swallowing (e.g., laughing with food in your mouth). It is important because swallowing also results in the epiglottis covering the larynx to prevent food from entering the lungs (see Figure 8.2 ■). The **cheeks** form the

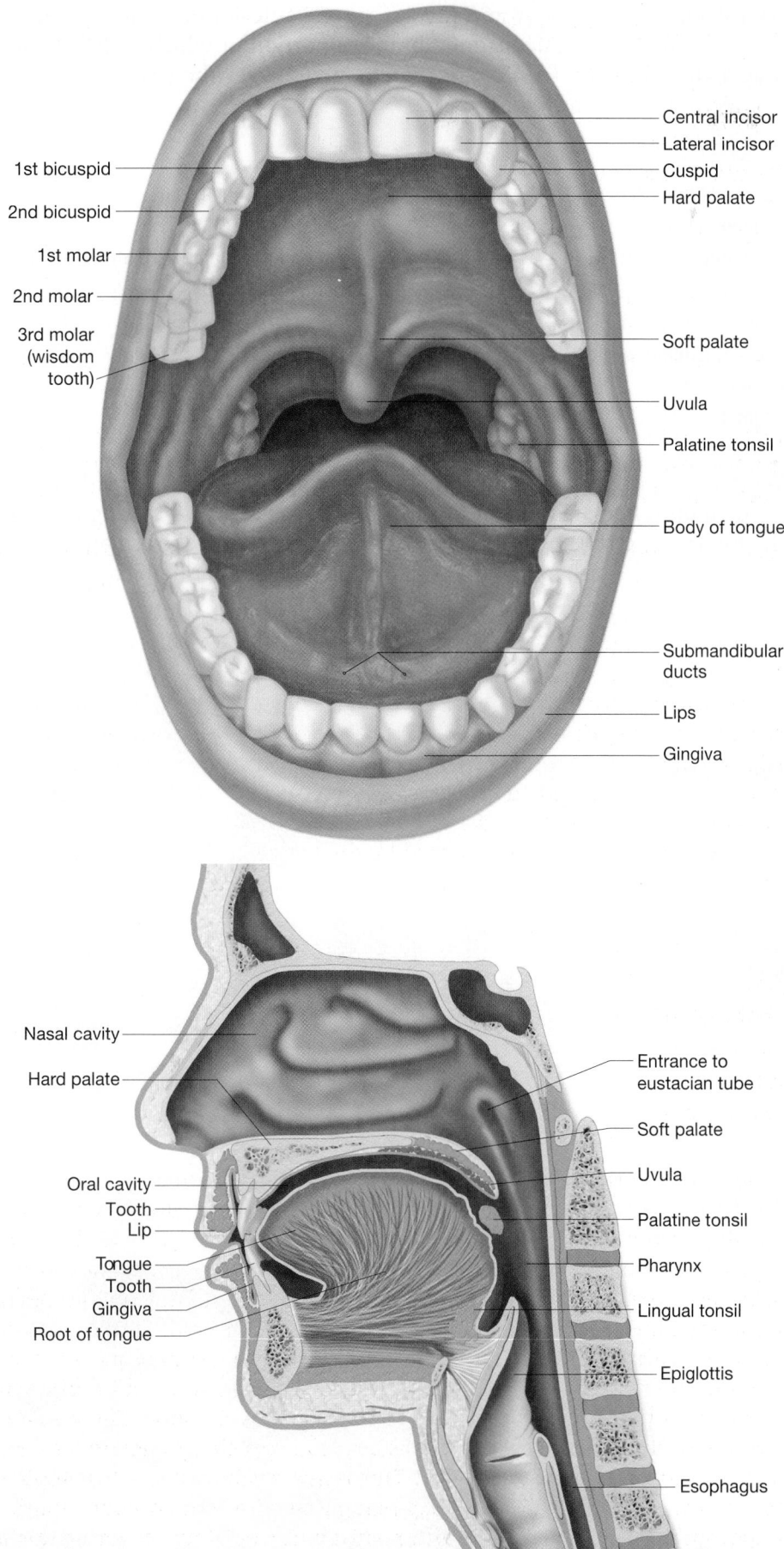

Central incisor
Lateral incisor
Cuspid
Hard palate

1st bicuspid
2nd bicuspid
1st molar
2nd molar
3rd molar (wisdom tooth)

Soft palate
Uvula
Palatine tonsil
Body of tongue
Submandibular ducts
Lips
Gingiva

Nasal cavity
Hard palate
Oral cavity
Tooth
Lip
Tongue
Tooth
Gingiva
Root of tongue

Entrance to eustacian tube
Soft palate
Uvula
Palatine tonsil
Pharynx
Lingual tonsil
Epiglottis
Esophagus
Trachea

■ **Figure 8.2**   Structures of the oral cavity, pharynx, and esophagus.

lateral walls of this cavity and the **lips** are the anterior opening. The entire oral cavity is lined with mucous membrane, a portion of which forms the **gums,** or **gingiva,** that combine with connective tissue to cover the jaw bone and seal off the teeth in their bony sockets.

Teeth

bicuspids (bye-CUSS-pids)	**incisors** (in-SIGH-zors)
canines (KAY-nines)	**molars** (MOH-lars)
cementum (see-MEN-tum)	**periodontal ligaments** (pair-ee-on-DON-tal)
crown	**permanent teeth**
cuspids (CUSS-pids)	**premolars** (pree-MOH-lars)
deciduous teeth (dee-SID-yoo-us)	**pulp cavity**
dentin (DEN-tin)	**root**
enamel	**root canal**

MED TERM TIP

There are three different molars, simply referred to as the first, second, or third molars. However, the third molar has a more common name, the wisdom tooth. Not every person ever forms all four wisdom teeth. Unfortunately, most people do not have enough room in their jaws for the third molars to properly erupt through the gum, a condition requiring surgical removal of the third molar, referred to as an *impacted wisdom tooth.*

Teeth are an important part of the first stage of digestion. The teeth in the front of the mouth bite, tear, or cut food into small pieces. These cutting teeth include the **cuspids** (or **canines**) and the **incisors** (see Figure 8.3 ■). The remaining posterior teeth grind and crush food into even finer pieces. These grinding teeth include the

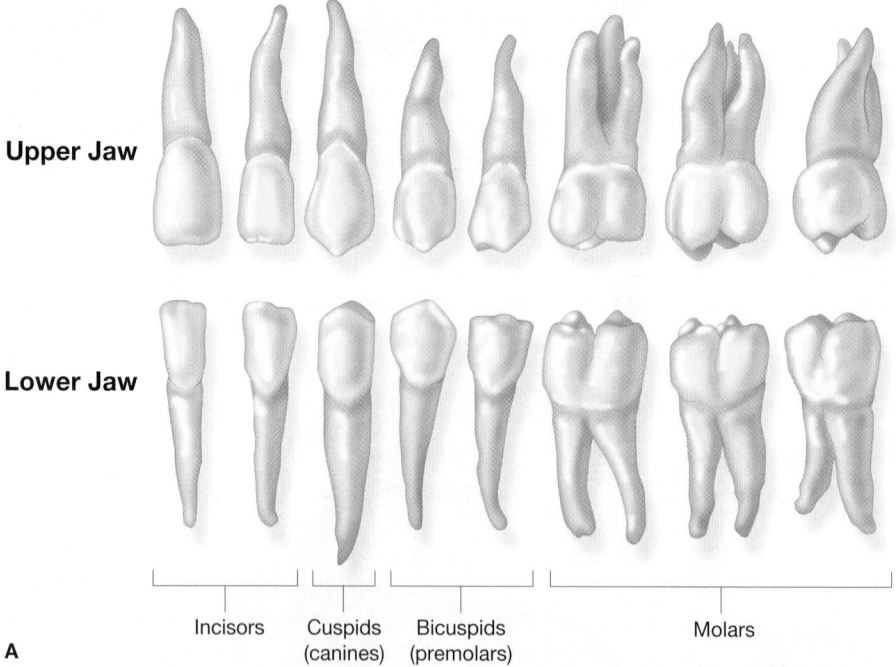

Upper Jaw

Lower Jaw

A

| Incisors | Cuspids (canines) | Bicuspids (premolars) | Molars |

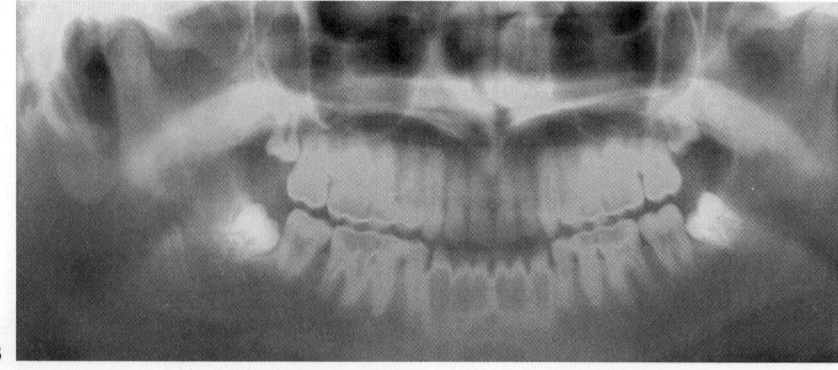

B

■ **Figure 8.3** (A) The name and shape of the adult teeth. These teeth represent those found in the right side of the mouth. Those of the left side would be a mirror image. The incisors and cuspids are cutting teeth. The bicuspids and molars are grinding teeth. (B) Color-enhanced X-ray of all teeth. Note the four wisdom teeth (third molars) that have not erupted. *(Photo Researchers, Inc.)*

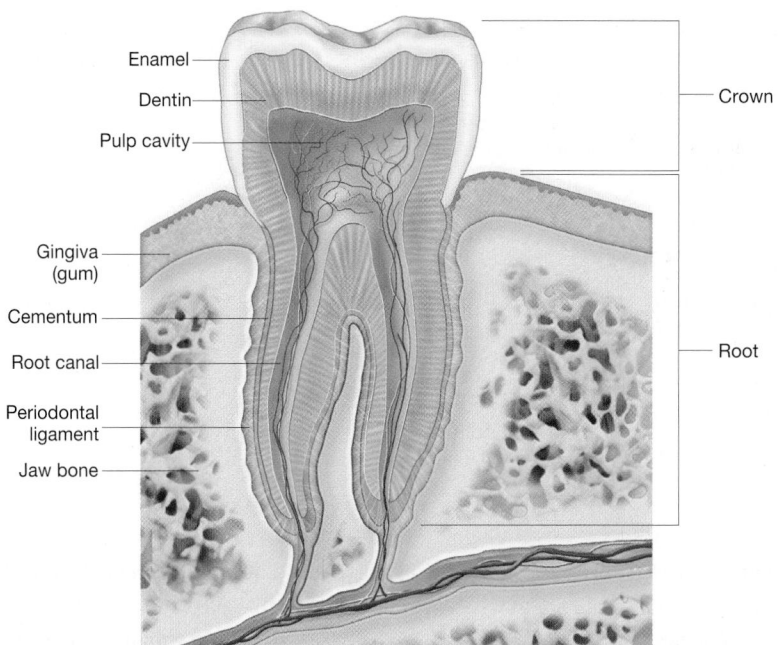

Enamel
Dentin
Pulp cavity

Crown

Gingiva (gum)
Cementum
Root canal
Periodontal ligament
Jaw bone

Root

Figure 8.4   An adult tooth, longitudinal view showing internal structures of the crown and root.

bicuspids (or **premolars**) and the **molars.** A tooth can be subdivided into the **crown** and the **root.** The crown is that part of the tooth visible above the gum line; the root is below the gum line. The root is anchored in the bony socket of the jaw by **cementum** and tiny **periodontal ligaments.** The crown of the tooth is covered by a layer of **enamel,** the hardest substance in the body. Under the enamel layer is **dentin,** the substance that makes up the main bulk of the tooth. The hollow interior of a tooth is called the **pulp cavity** in the crown and the **root canal** in the root. These cavities contain soft tissue made up of blood vessels, nerves, and lymph vessels (see Figure 8.4 ■).

Humans have two sets of teeth. The first set, often referred to as baby teeth, are **deciduous teeth.** There are 20 teeth in this set that erupt through the gums between the ages of 6 and 28 months. At approximately 6 years of age, these teeth begin to fall out and are replaced by the 32 **permanent teeth.** This replacement process continues until about 18–20 years of age.

Pharynx

epiglottis (ep-ih-GLOT-iss)   **laryngopharynx**
oropharynx

When food is swallowed, it enters the **oropharynx** and then the **laryngopharynx** (see again Figure 8.2). Remember from your study of the respiratory system in Chapter 7 that air is also traveling through these portions of the pharynx. The **epiglottis** is a cartilaginous flap that folds down to cover the larynx and trachea so that food is prevented from entering the respiratory tract and instead continues into the esophagus.

Esophagus

peristalsis (pair-ih-STALL-sis)

The esophagus is a muscular tube of about 10 inches long in adults. Food entering the esophagus is carried through the thoracic cavity and diaphragm and into the abdominal cavity where it enters the stomach (see Figure 8.5 ■). Food is propelled along the esophagus by wavelike muscular contractions called **peristalsis.** In fact, peristalsis works to push food through the entire gastrointestinal tract.

MED TERM TIP

The combining form *dent/o* means teeth. Hence we have terms such as dentist and dentistry. The combining form *odont/o* also means teeth and when combined with *orth/o*, which means straight, we have the specialty of *orthodontics*, or straightening teeth.

MED TERM TIP

It takes about 10 seconds for swallowed food to reach the stomach.

Figure 8.5 The stomach. Longitudinal view showing regions and internal structures.

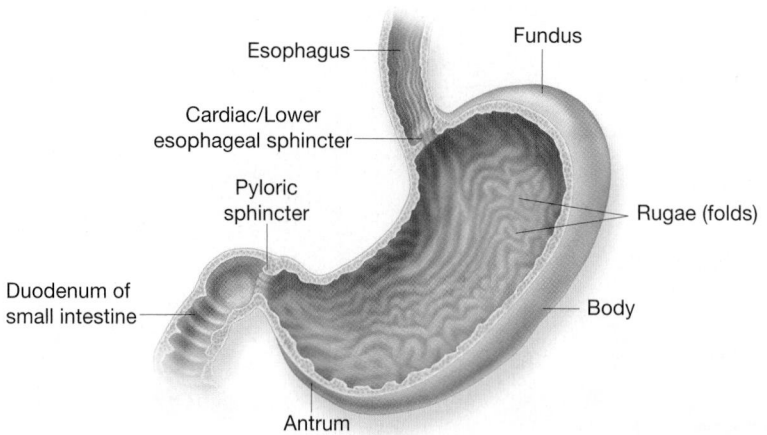

Esophagus

Fundus

Cardiac/Lower esophageal sphincter

Pyloric sphincter

Rugae (folds)

Duodenum of small intestine

Body

Antrum

Stomach

antrum (AN-trum)
body
cardiac sphincter (CAR-dee-ak / SFINGK-ter)
chyme (KIGHM)
fundus (FUN-dus)
hydrochloric acid

lower esophageal sphincter
  (eh-soff-ah-JEE-al / SFINGK-ter)
pyloric sphincter (pigh-LOR-ik / SFINGK-ter)
rugae (ROO-gay)
sphincters (SFINGK-ters)

The stomach, a J-shaped muscular organ that acts as a bag or sac to collect and churn food with digestive juices, is composed of three parts: the **fundus** or upper region, the **body** or main portion, and the **antrum** or lower region (see again Figure 8.5). The folds in the lining of the stomach are called **rugae.** When the stomach fills with food, the rugae stretch out and disappear. **Hydrochloric acid** (HCl) is secreted by glands in the mucous membrane lining of the stomach. Food mixes with hydrochloric acid and other gastric juices to form a liquid mixture called **chyme,** which then passes through the remaining portion of the digestive system.

Entry into and exit from the stomach is controlled by muscular valves called **sphincters.** These valves open and close to ensure that food can only move forward down the gut tube. The **cardiac sphincter,** named for its proximity to the heart, is located between the esophagus and the fundus; also called the **lower esophageal sphincter** (LES), it keeps food from flowing backward into the esophagus.

The antrum tapers off into the **pyloric sphincter,** which regulates the passage of food into the small intestine. Only a small amount of the chyme is allowed to enter the small intestine with each opening of the sphincter for two important reasons. First, the small intestine is much narrower than the stomach and cannot hold as much as the stomach can. Second, the chyme is highly acidic and must be thoroughly neutralized as it leaves the stomach.

MED TERM TIP

It is easier to remember the function of the pyloric sphincter when you note that *pylor/o* means "gatekeeper." This gatekeeper controls the forward movement of food. Sphincters are rings of muscle that can be opened and closed to control entry and exit from hollow organs like the stomach, colon, and bladder.

Small Intestine

duodenum
  (doo-oh-DEE-num / doo-OD-eh-num)
ileocecal valve (ill-ee-oh-SEE-kal)

ileum (ILL-ee-um)
jejunum (jee-JOO-num)

The small intestine, or small bowel, is the major site of digestion and absorption of nutrients from food. It is located between the pyloric sphincter and the colon (see Figure 8.6 ■). Because the small intestine is concerned with absorption of food products, an abnormality in this organ can cause malnutrition. The small intestine, with an average length of 20 feet, is the longest portion of the alimentary canal and has three sections: the **duodenum,** the **jejunum,** and the **ileum.**

MED TERM TIP

Word Watch: Be careful not to confuse the word root *ile/o* meaning "ileum," a portion of the small intestines, and *ili/o* meaning "ilium," a pelvic bone.

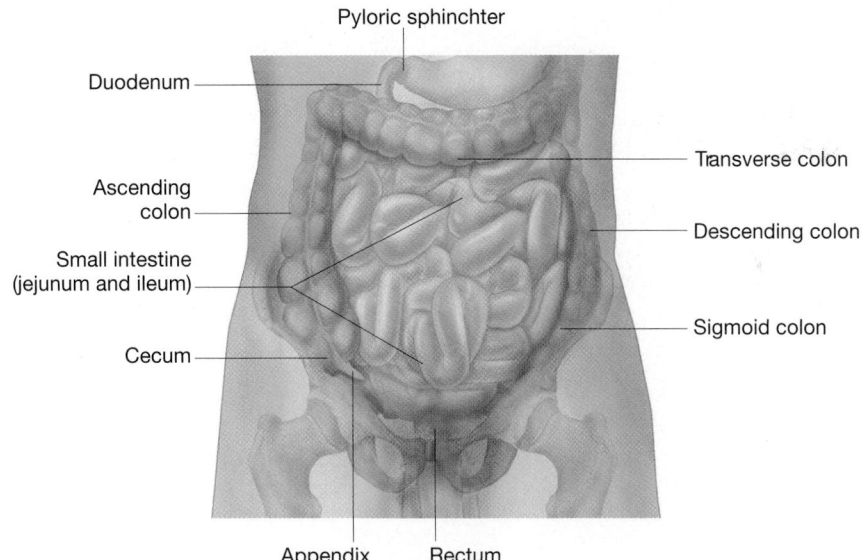

Pyloric sphinchter

Duodenum

Ascending colon

Small intestine (jejunum and ileum)

Cecum

Transverse colon

Descending colon

Sigmoid colon

Appendix   Rectum

■ Figure 8.6 The small intestine. Anterior view of the abdominopelvic cavity illustrating how the three sections of small intestine—duodenum, jejunum, and ileum—begin at the pyloric sphincter and end at the colon, but are not arranged in an orderly fashion.

- The duodenum extends from the pyloric sphincter to the jejunum, and is about 10–12 inches long. Digestion is completed in the duodenum after the liquid chyme from the stomach is mixed with digestive juices from the pancreas and gallbladder.
- The jejunum, or middle portion, extends from the duodenum to the ileum and is about 8 feet long.
- The ileum is the last portion of the small intestine and extends from the jejunum to the colon. At 12 feet in length, it is the longest portion of the small intestine. The ileum connects to the colon with a sphincter called the **ileocecal valve.**

Colon

anal sphincter (AY-nal / SFINGK-ter)	**feces** (FEE-seez)
anus (AY-nus)	**rectum** (REK-tum)
ascending colon	**sigmoid colon** (SIG-moyd)
cecum (SEE-kum)	**transverse colon**
defecation	**vermiform appendix** (VER-mih-form / ah-PEN-diks)
descending colon	

Fluid that remains after the complete digestion and absorption of nutrients in the small intestine enters the colon or large intestine (see Figure 8.7 ■). Most of this fluid is water that is reabsorbed into the body. The material that remains after absorption is solid waste called **feces** (or stool). This is the product evacuated in bowel movements (BM).

The colon is approximately 5 feet long and extends from the **cecum** to the **anus.** The cecum is a pouch or saclike area in the first 2–3 inches at the beginning of the colon. The **vermiform appendix** is a small worm-shaped outgrowth at the end of the cecum. The remaining colon consists of the **ascending colon, transverse colon, descending colon,** and **sigmoid colon.** The ascending colon on the right side extends from the cecum to the lower border of the liver. The transverse colon begins where the ascending colon leaves off and moves horizontally across the upper abdomen toward the spleen. The descending colon then travels down the left side of the body to where the sigmoid colon begins. The sigmoid colon curves in an S-shape back to the midline of the body and ends at the **rectum.** The rectum, where feces is stored, leads into the anus, which contains the **anal sphincter.** This sphincter consists of rings of voluntary and involuntary muscles to control the evacuation of feces or **defecation.**

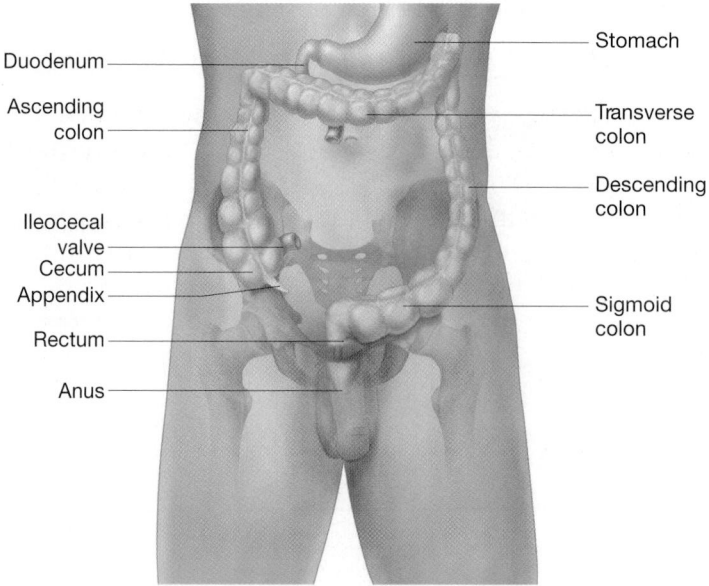

Figure 8.7 The regions of the colon beginning with the cecum and ending at the anus.

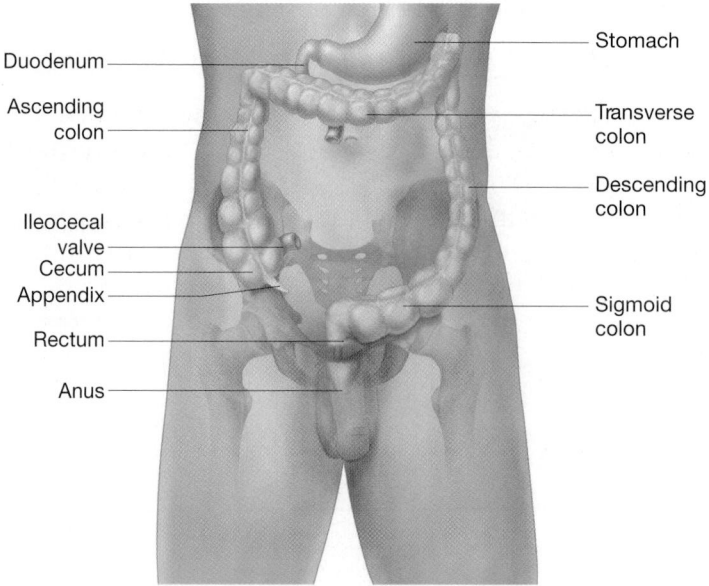

Duodenum

Ascending colon

Ileocecal valve
Cecum
Appendix
Rectum
Anus

Stomach

Transverse colon

Descending colon

Sigmoid colon

Accessory Organs of the Digestive System

As described earlier, the accessory organs of the digestive system are the salivary glands, the liver, the pancreas, and the gallbladder. In general, these organs function by producing much of the digestive fluids and enzymes necessary for the chemical breakdown of food. Each is attached to the gut tube by a duct.

Salivary Glands

amylase (AM-ill-ace)

bolus

parotid glands (pah-ROT-id)

sublingual glands (sub-LING-gwal)

submandibular glands
(sub-man-DIB-yoo-lar)

Salivary glands in the oral cavity produce saliva. This very watery and slick fluid allows food to be swallowed with less danger of choking. Saliva mixed with food in the mouth forms a **bolus,** chewed food that is ready to swallow. Saliva also contains the digestive enzyme **amylase** that begins the digestion of carbohydrates. There are three pairs of salivary glands. The **parotid glands** are in front of the ears, and the **submandibular glands** and **sublingual glands** are in the floor of the mouth (see Figure 8.8 ■).

Figure 8.8 The salivary glands, parotid, sublingual, and submandibular. This image shows the position of each gland and its duct emptying into the oral cavity.

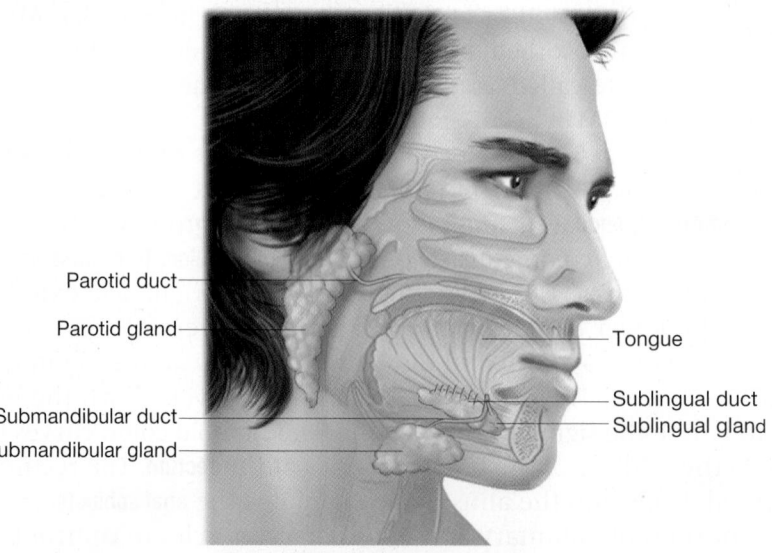

Parotid duct

Parotid gland

Submandibular duct
Submandibular gland

Tongue

Sublingual duct
Sublingual gland

Liver

bile (BYE-al)   **emulsification** (ee-mull-sih-fih-KAY-shun)

The liver, a large organ located in the right upper quadrant of the abdomen, has several functions including processing the nutrients absorbed by the intestines, detoxifying harmful substances in the body, and producing **bile** (see Figure 8.9 ■). Bile is important for the digestion of fats and lipids because it breaks up large fat globules into much smaller droplets, making them easier to digest in the watery environment inside the intestines. The process is called **emulsification.**

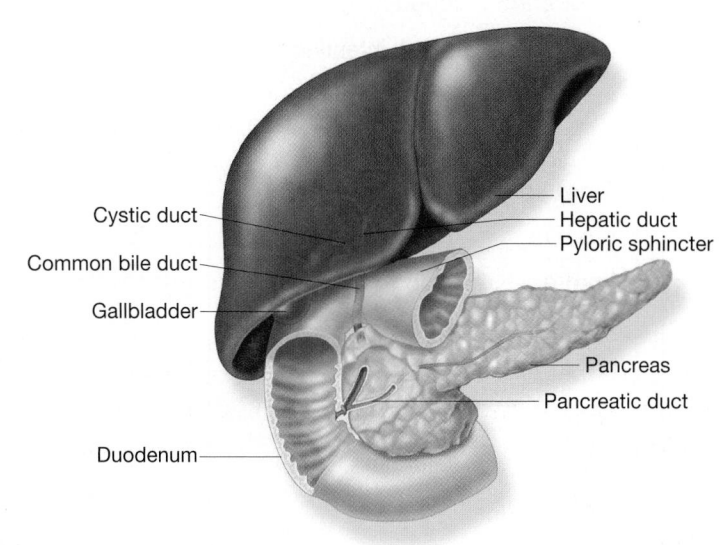

Cystic duct —
Common bile duct —
Gallbladder —
Duodenum —
— Liver
— Hepatic duct
— Pyloric sphincter
— Pancreas
— Pancreatic duct

■ **Figure 8.9** The accessory organs of the digestive system: the liver, gallbladder, and pancreas. Image shows the relationship of these three organs and their ducts to the duodenum.

Gallbladder

common bile duct   **cystic duct** (SIS-tik)
hepatic duct (hep-PAT-tik)

Bile produced by the liver is stored in the gallbladder (GB). As the liver produces bile, it travels down the **hepatic duct** and up the **cystic duct** into the gallbladder (see again Figure 8.9). In response to the presence of fat in the chyme, the muscular wall of the gallbladder contracts and sends bile back down the cystic duct and into the **common bile duct** (CBD), which carries bile to the duodenum where it is able to emulsify the fat in chyme.

Pancreas

buffers   **pancreatic duct** (pan-kree-AT-ik)
pancreatic enzymes (pan-kree-AT-ik / EN-zimes)

The pancreas, connected to the duodenum by the **pancreatic duct,** produces two important secretions for digestion: **buffers** and **pancreatic enzymes** (see again Figure 8.9). Buffers neutralize acidic chyme that has just left the stomach, and pancreatic enzymes chemically digest carbohydrates, fats, and proteins. The pancreas is also an endocrine gland that produces the hormones insulin and glucagon, which play a role in regulating the level of glucose in the blood and are discussed in further detail in Chapter 11.

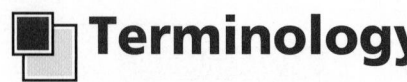 Terminology

Word Parts Used to Build Digestive System Terms

The following lists contain the combining forms, suffixes, and prefixes used to build terms in the remaining sections of this chapter.

Combining Forms

an/o	anus	diverticul/o	pouch	nas/o	nose
append/o	appendix	duoden/o	duodenum	odont/o	tooth
appendic/o	appendix	enter/o	small intestine	or/o	mouth
bar/o	weight	esophag/o	esophagus	orth/o	straight
bucc/o	cheek	gastr/o	stomach	palat/o	palate
carcin/o	cancer	gingiv/o	gums	pancreat/o	pancreas
cec/o	cecum	gloss/o	tongue	pharyng/o	pharynx
chol/e	bile	hem/o	blood	polyp/o	polyp
cholangi/o	bile duct	hemat/o	blood	proct/o	anus and rectum
cholecyst/o	gallbladder	hepat/o	liver	pylor/o	pylorus
choledoch/o	common bile duct	ile/o	ileum	pyr/o	fire
cirrh/o	yellow	jejun/o	jejunum	rect/o	rectum
col/o	colon	labi/o	lip	sialaden/o	salivary gland
colon/o	colon	lapar/o	abdomen	sigmoid/o	sigmoid colon
cutane/o	skin	lingu/o	tongue	ven/o	vein
dent/o	tooth	lith/o	stone		

Suffixes

-al	pertaining to	-itis	inflammation	-pexy	surgical fixation
-algia	pain	-lithiasis	condition of stones	-phagia	eating
-centesis	process of removing fluid	-logy	study of	-plasty	surgical repair
-eal	pertaining to	-oma	tumor	-plegia	paralysis
-ectomy	surgical removal	-orexia	appetite	-prandial	a meal
-emesis	vomiting	-osis	abnormal condition	-ptosis	drooping
-gram	record	-ostomy	create a new opening	-scope	instrument to view
-graphy	process of recording	-otomy	cutting into	-scopy	process of viewing
-ic	pertaining to	-ous	pertaining to	-tic	pertaining to
-istry	specialty of	-pepsia	digestion	-tripsy	surgical crushing

Prefixes

a-	without
an-	without
anti-	against
brady-	slow
dys-	abnormal
endo-	within

hyper-	excessive
hypo-	under
intra-	within
per-	through
peri-	around

poly-	many
post-	after
retro-	backwards
sub-	under
trans-	across

Anatomical Terms

TERM	WORD PARTS	DEFINITION
anal	an/o = anus -al = pertaining to	Pertaining to the anus. **MED TERM TIP** Word Watch: Be careful when using the combining form *an/o* meaning "anus" and the prefix *an* meaning "none."
buccal (BYOO-kal)	bucc/o = cheek -al = pertaining to	Pertaining to the cheeks.
buccolabial (BYOO-koh-labe-ee-all)	bucc/o = cheek labi/o = lip -al = pertaining to	Pertaining to the cheeks and lips.
cecal (SEE-kal)	cec/o = cecum -al = pertaining to	Pertaining to the cecum.
cholecystic (koh-lee-SIS-tik)	cholecyst/o = gallbladder -ic = pertaining to	Pertaining to the gallbladder.
colonic (koh-LON-ik)	colon/o = colon -ic = pertaining to	Pertaining to the colon.
colorectal (kohl-oh-REK-tall)	col/o = colon rect/o = rectum -al = pertaining to	Pertaining to the colon and rectum.
dental (DENT-all)	dent/o = tooth -al = pertaining to	Pertaining to the teeth.
duodenal (duo-DEN-all / do-ODD-in-all)	duoden/o = duodenum -al = pertaining to	Pertaining to the duodenum.
enteric (en-TARE-ik)	enter/o = small intestine -ic = pertaining to	Pertaining to the small intestine.
esophageal (eh-soff-ah-JEE-al)	esophag/o = esophagus -eal = pertaining to	Pertaining to the esophagus.
gastric (GAS-trik)	gastr/o = stomach -ic = pertaining to	Pertaining to the stomach.
gingival (JIN-jih-vul)	gingiv/o = gums -al = pertaining to	Pertaining to the gums.
glossal (GLOSS-all)	gloss/o = tongue -al = pertaining to	Pertaining to the tongue.

Anatomical Terms *(continued)*

TERM	WORD PARTS	DEFINITION
hepatic (hep-AT-ik)	hepat/o = liver -ic = pertaining to	Pertaining to the liver.
hypoglossal (high-poe-GLOSS-all)	hypo- = under gloss/o = tongue -al = pertaining to	Pertaining to under the tongue.
ileal (ILL-ee-all)	ile/o = ileum -al = pertaining to	Pertaining to the ileum.
jejunal (jih-JUNE-all)	jejun/o = jejunum -al = pertaining to	Pertaining to the jejunum.
nasogastric (nay-zoh-GAS-trik)	nas/o = nose gastr/o = stomach -ic = pertaining to	Pertaining to the nose and stomach.
oral (OR-ral)	or/o = mouth -al = pertaining to	Pertaining to the mouth.
pancreatic (pan-kree-AT-ik)	pancreat/o = pancreas -ic = pertaining to	Pertaining to the pancreas.
pharyngeal (fair-in-JEE-all)	pharyng/o = pharynx -eal = pertaining to	Pertaining to the pharynx.
pyloric (pie-LORE-ik)	pylor/o = pylorus -ic = pertaining to	Pertaining to the pylorus.
rectal (RECK-tall)	rect/o = rectum -al = pertaining to	Pertaining to the rectum.
sigmoidal (sig-MOYD-all)	sigmoid/o = sigmoid colon -al = pertaining to	Pertaining to the sigmoid colon.
sublingual (sub-LING-gwal)	sub- = under lingu/o = tongue -al = pertaining to	Pertaining to under the tongue.

Pathology

TERM	WORD PARTS	DEFINITION
Medical Specialties		
dentistry	dent/o = tooth -istry = specialty of	Branch of healthcare involved with the prevention, diagnosis, and treatment of conditions involving the teeth, jaw, and mouth. Practitioner is a *dentist*.
gastroenterology (gas-troh-en-ter-ALL-oh-jee)	gastr/o = stomach enter/o = small intestine -logy = study of	Branch of medicine involved in diagnosis and treatment of diseases and disorders of the digestive system. Physician is a *gastroenterologist*.
oral surgery	or/o = mouth -al = pertaining to	Branch of dentistry that uses surgical means to treat dental conditions. Specialist is an *oral surgeon*.

■ Pathology (continued)

TERM	WORD PARTS	DEFINITION
orthodontics (or-thoh-DON-tiks)	orth/o = straight odont/o = tooth -ic = pertaining to	Branch of dentistry concerned with correction of problems with tooth alignment. Specialist is an *orthodontist*.
periodontics (pair-ee-oh-DON-tiks)	peri- = around odont/o = tooth -ic = pertaining to	Branch of dentistry concerned with treating conditions involving the gums and tissues surrounding the teeth. Specialist is a *periodontist*.
proctology (prok-TOL-oh-jee)	proct/o = anus and rectum -logy = study of	Branch of medicine involved in diagnosis and treatment of diseases and disorders of the anus and rectum. Physician is a *proctologist*.
Signs and Symptoms		
anorexia (an-oh-REK-see-ah)	an- = without -orexia = appetite	General term meaning loss of appetite that may accompany other conditions. Also used to refer to *anorexia nervosa*, which is an eating disorder involving the refusal to eat.
aphagia (ah-FAY-jee-ah)	a- = without -phagia = eating	Being unable to swallow or eat.
ascites (ah-SIGH-teez)		Collection or accumulation of fluid in the peritoneal cavity.
bradypepsia (brad-ee-PEP-see-ah)	brady- = slow -pepsia = digestion	Having a slow digestive system.
cachexia (ka-KEK-see-ah)		Loss of weight and generalized wasting that occurs during a chronic disease.
cholecystalgia (koh-lee-sis-TAL-jee-ah)	cholecyst/o = gallbladder -algia = pain	Having gallbladder pain.
constipation (kon-stih-PAY-shun)		Experiencing difficulty in defecation or infrequent defecation.
dentalgia (dent-AL-gee-ah)	dent/o = tooth -algia = pain	Tooth pain.
diarrhea (dye-ah-REE-ah)		Passing of frequent, watery, or bloody bowel movements. Usually accompanies gastrointestinal (GI) disorders.
dysorexia (dis-oh-REKS-ee-ah)	dys- = abnormal -orexia = appetite	Abnormal appetite; usually a diminished appetite.
dyspepsia (dis-PEP-see-ah)	dys- = difficult -pepsia = digestion	"Upset stomach"; indigestion.
dysphagia (dis-FAY-jee-ah)	dys- = abnormal -phagia = eating	Having difficulty swallowing or eating.
emesis (EM-eh-sis)		Vomiting.
gastralgia (gas-TRAL-jee-ah)	gastr/o = stomach -algia = pain	Stomach pain.
hematemesis (hee-mah-TEM-eh-sis)	hemat/o = blood -emesis = vomiting	Vomiting blood.
hematochezia (he-mat-oh-KEY-zee-ah)	hemat/o = blood	Passing bright red blood in the stools.

Pathology *(continued)*

TERM	WORD PARTS	DEFINITION
hyperemesis (high-per-EM-eh-sis)	hyper- = excessive -emesis = vomiting	Excessive vomiting.
jaundice (JAWN-diss)		Yellow cast to the skin, mucous membranes, and the whites of the eyes caused by the deposit of bile pigment from too much bilirubin in the blood. Bilirubin is a waste product produced when worn-out red blood cells are broken down. May be a symptom of a disorder such as gallstones blocking the common bile duct or carcinoma of the liver. Also called *icterus*.
melena (me-LEE-nah)		Passage of dark tarry stools. Color is the result of digestive enzymes working on blood in the gastrointestinal tract.
nausea (NAW-see-ah)	**MED TERM TIP** The term *nausea* comes from the Greek word for "seasickness."	Urge to vomit.
obesity		Body weight that is above a healthy level. A person whose weight interferes with normal activity and body function has *morbid obesity.*
polyphagia (pall-ee-FAY-jee-ah)	poly- = many -phagia = eating	Excessive eating; eating too much.
postprandial (post-PRAN-dee-all)	post- = after -prandial = a meal	After a meal.
pyrosis (pie-ROW-sis)	pyr/o = fire -osis = abnormal condition	Pain and burning sensation usually caused by stomach acid splashing up into the esophagus. Commonly called *heartburn.*
regurgitation (ree-gur-jih-TAY-shun)		Return of fluids and solids from the stomach into the mouth.
Oral Cavity		
aphthous ulcers (AF-thus)		Painful ulcers in the mouth of unknown cause. Commonly called *canker sores.*
cleft lip (CLEFT)		Congenital anomaly in which the upper lip and jaw bone fail to fuse in the midline, leaving an open gap. Often seen along with a cleft palate. Corrected with surgery.
cleft palate (CLEFT / PAL-at)		Congenital anomaly in which the roof of the mouth has a split or fissure. Corrected with surgery.
dental caries (KAIR-eez)	dent/o = tooth -al = pertaining to	Gradual decay and disintegration of teeth caused by bacteria; may lead to abscessed teeth. Commonly called a *tooth cavity.*
gingivitis (jin-jih-VIGH-tis)	gingiv/o = gums -itis = inflammation	Inflammation of the gums.

■ Pathology *(continued)*

TERM	WORD PARTS	DEFINITION
herpes labialis (HER-peez / lay-bee-AL-iz)	labi/o = lip	Infection of the lip by the herpes simplex virus type 1 (HSV-1). Also called *fever blisters* or *cold sores.*
periodontal disease (pair-ee-oh-DON-tal)	peri- = around odont/o = tooth -al = pertaining to	Disease of the supporting structures of the teeth, including the gums and bones; the most common cause of tooth loss.
sialadenitis (sigh-al-add-eh-NIGH-tis)	sialaden/o = salivary gland -itis = inflammation	Inflammation of a salivary gland.
Pharynx and Esophagus		
esophageal varices (eh-soff-ah-JEE-al / VAIR-ih-seez)	esophag/o = esophagus -eal = pertaining to	Enlarged and swollen varicose veins in the lower end of the esophagus. If these rupture, serious hemorrhage results; often related to liver disease.
gastroesophageal reflux disease (GERD) (gas-troh-ee-sof-ah-GEE-all / REE-fluks)	gastr/o = stomach esophag/o = esophagus -eal = pertaining to	Acid from the stomach flows backward up into the esophagus causing inflammation and pain.
pharyngoplegia (fair-in-goh-PLEE-jee-ah)	pharyng/o = pharynx -plegia = paralysis	Paralysis of the throat muscles.
Stomach		
gastric carcinoma (GAS-trik / car-si-NOH-mah)	gastr/o = stomach -ic = pertaining to	Cancerous tumor in the stomach.
gastritis (gas-TRY-tis)	gastr/o = stomach -itis = inflammation	Stomach inflammation.
gastroenteritis (gas-troh-en-ter-EYE-tis)	gastr/o = stomach enter/o = small intestines -itis = inflammation	Inflammation of stomach and small intestine.
hiatal hernia (high-AY-tal / HER-nee-ah)	-al = pertaining to	Protrusion of the stomach through the diaphragm (also called a *diaphragmatocele*) and extending into the thoracic cavity; gastroesophageal reflux disease is a common symptom.

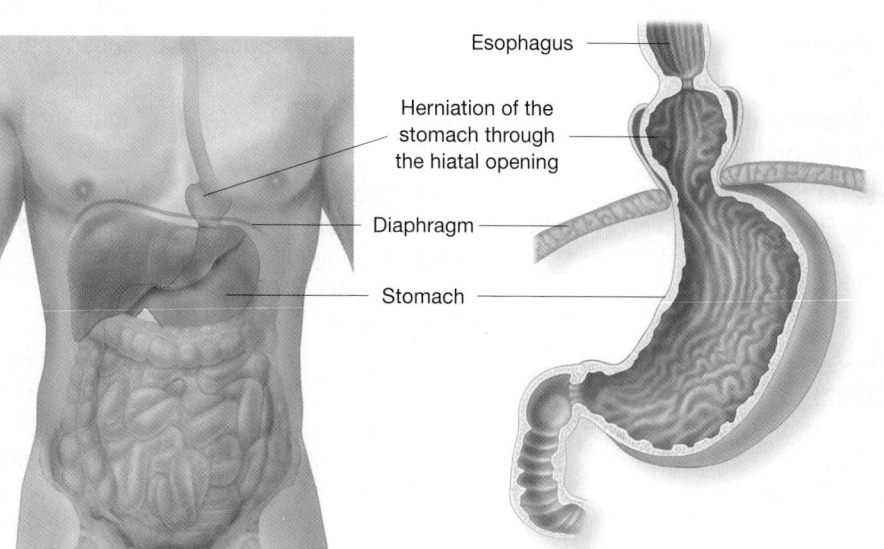

Esophagus

Herniation of the stomach through the hiatal opening

Diaphragm

Stomach

■ **Figure 8.10** A hiatal hernia or diaphragmatocele. A portion of the stomach protrudes through the diaphragm into the thoracic cavity.

Pathology *(continued)*

TERM	WORD PARTS	DEFINITION
peptic ulcer disease (PUD) (PEP-tik / ULL-sir)	-ic = pertaining to	Ulcer occurring in the lower portion of the esophagus, stomach, and/or duodenum; thought to be caused by the acid of gastric juices. Initial damage to the protective lining of the stomach may be caused by a *Helicobacter pylori* (*H. pylori*) bacterial infection. If the ulcer extends all the way through the wall of the stomach, it is called a *perforated ulcer,* which requires immediate surgery to repair.

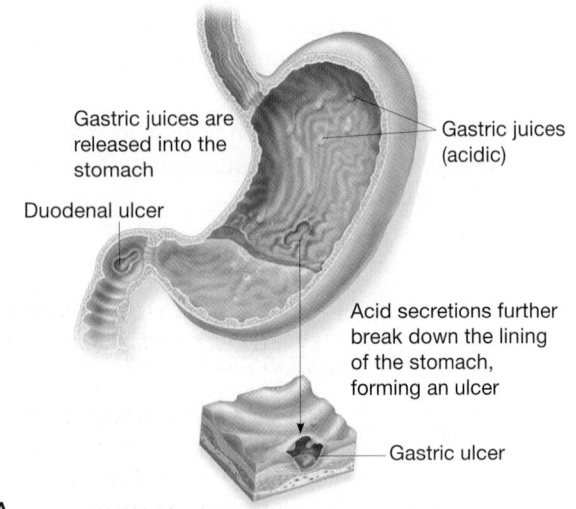

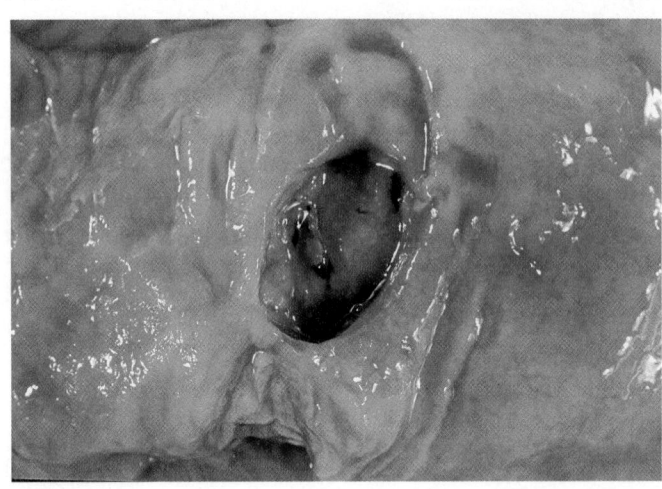

Gastric juices are released into the stomach

Duodenal ulcer

Gastric juices (acidic)

Acid secretions further break down the lining of the stomach, forming an ulcer

Gastric ulcer

A

B

■ **Figure 8.11**   (A) Figure illustrating the location and appearance of a peptic ulcer in both the stomach and the duodenum; (B) photomicrograph illustrating a gastric ulcer. *(Dr. E. Walker/Science Photo Library/Photo Researchers, Inc.)*

Small Intestine and Colon

TERM	WORD PARTS	DEFINITION
anal fistula (FIH-styoo-lah)	-al = pertaining to	Abnormal tube-like passage from the surface around the anal opening directly into the rectum.
appendicitis (ah-pen-dih-SIGH-tis)	appendic/o = appendix -itis = inflammation	Inflammation of the appendix; may require an *appendectomy.*
bowel incontinence (in-CON-tih-nence)		Inability to control defecation.
colorectal carcinoma (kohl-oh-REK-tall / car-ci-NOH-mah)	col/o = colon rect/o = rectum -al = pertaining to carcin/o = cancer -oma = tumor	Cancerous tumor along the length of the colon and rectum.
Crohn's disease (KROHNZ)		Form of chronic inflammatory bowel disease affecting primarily the ileum and/or colon. Also called *regional ileitis.* This autoimmune condition affects all the layers of the bowel wall and results in scarring and thickening of the gut wall.

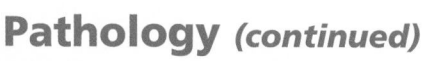

Pathology *(continued)*

TERM	WORD PARTS	DEFINITION
diverticulitis (dye-ver-tik-yoo-LYE-tis)	diverticul/o = pouch -itis = inflammation	Inflammation of a *diverticulum* (an out-pouching off the gut), especially in the colon. Inflammation often results when food becomes within the pouch.

Diverticulum

Infection in diverticulum

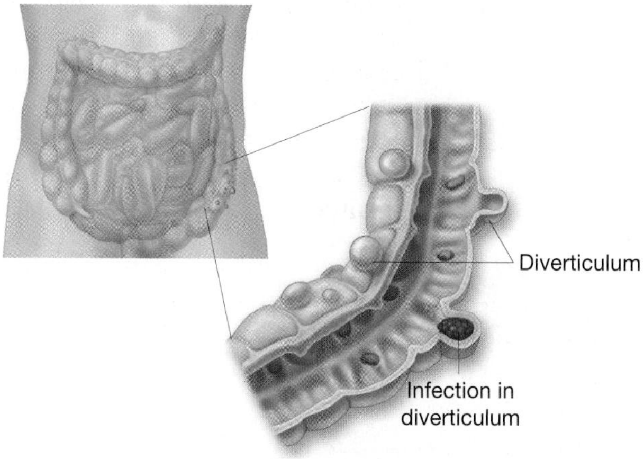

■ **Figure 8.12**   Diverticulosis. Figure illustrates external and internal appearance of diverticula.

TERM	WORD PARTS	DEFINITION
diverticulosis (dye-ver-tik-yoo-LOW-sis)	diverticul/o = pouch -osis = abnormal condition	Condition of having diverticula (outpouches off the gut). May lead to *diverticulitis* if one becomes inflamed.
dysentery (dis-in-TARE-ee)		Disease characterized by diarrhea, often with mucus and blood, severe abdominal pain, fever, and dehydration. Caused by ingesting food or water contaminated by chemicals, bacteria, protozoans, or parasites.
enteritis (en-ter-EYE-tis)	enter/o = small intestine -itis = inflammation	Inflammation of the small intestines.
hemorrhoids (HEM-oh-roydz)	hem/o = blood	Varicose veins in the rectum and anus.
ileus (ILL-ee-us)		Severe abdominal pain, inability to pass stools, vomiting, and abdominal distension as a result of an intestinal blockage. The blockage can be a physical block such as a tumor or the failure of bowel contents to move forward due to loss of peristalsis (a nonmechanical blockage). May require surgery to reverse the blockage.
inguinal hernia (ING-gwih-nal / HER-nee-ah)	-al = pertaining to	Hernia or protrusion of a loop of small intestines into the inguinal (groin) region through a weak spot in the abdominal muscle wall that develops into a hole. May become *incarcerated* or *strangulated* if the muscle tightens down around the loop of intestines and cuts off its blood flow. See Figure 8.13 ■.

Pathology *(continued)*

TERM	WORD PARTS	DEFINITION

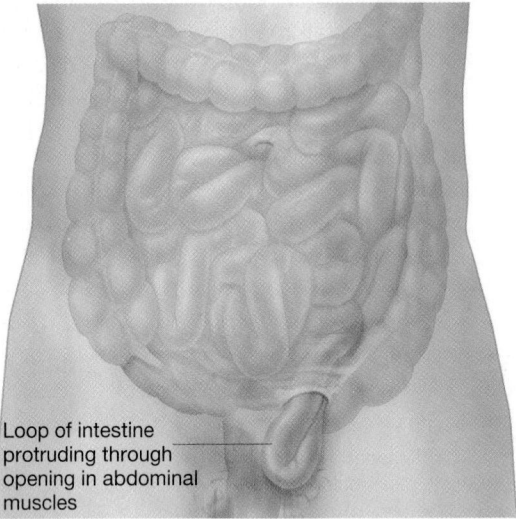

■ **Figure 8.13**   An inguinal hernia. A portion of the small intestine is protruding through the abdominal muscles into the groin region.

Loop of intestine protruding through opening in abdominal muscles

---

intussusception
(in-tuh-suh-SEP-shun)

Result of the intestine slipping or telescoping into another section of intestine just below it. More common in children.

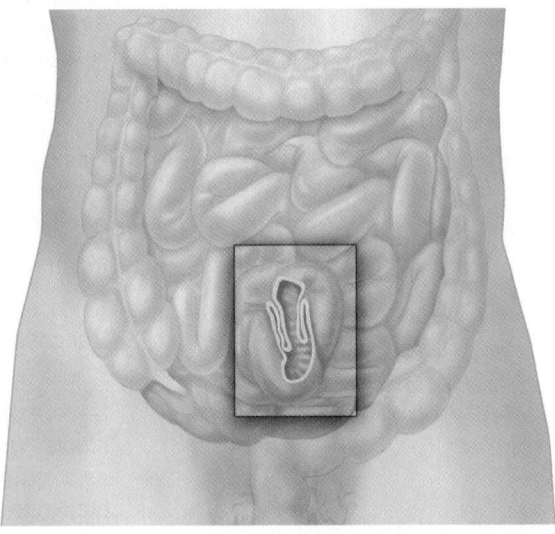

■ **Figure 8.14**   Intussusception. A short length of small intestine has telescoped into itself.

---

irritable bowel syndrome (IBS)

Disturbance in the functions of the intestine from unknown causes. Symptoms generally include abdominal discomfort and an alteration in bowel activity. Also called *spastic colon* or *functional bowel syndrome.*

---

polyposis
(pall-ee-POH-sis)

polyp/o = polyp
-osis = abnormal condition

Presence of small tumors, called **polyps,** containing a pedicle or stemlike attachment in the mucous membranes of the large intestine (colon); may be precancerous. See Figure 8.15 ■.

Pathology *(continued)*

TERM	WORD PARTS	DEFINITION

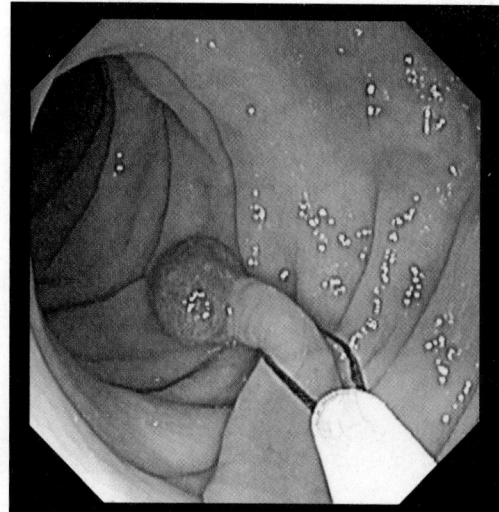

Figure 8.15 Endoscopic view of a polyp in the colon. Note the mushroom-like shape, an enlarged top growing at the end of a stem. It is being removed by means of a wire loop slipped over the polyp and then tightened to cut it off. *(David M. Martin, M.D./ Photo Researchers, Inc.)*

TERM	WORD PARTS	DEFINITION
proctoptosis (prok-top-TOH-sis)	proct/o = rectum and anus -ptosis = drooping	Prolapsed or drooping rectum.
ulcerative colitis (ULL-sir-ah-tiv / koh-LYE-tis)	col/o = colon -itis = inflammation	Chronic inflammatory condition resulting in numerous ulcers formed on the mucous membrane lining of the colon; the cause is unknown. Also known as *inflammatory bowel disease* (IBD).
volvulus (VOL-vyoo-lus)		Condition in which the bowel twists upon itself causing an obstruction; painful and requires immediate surgery.

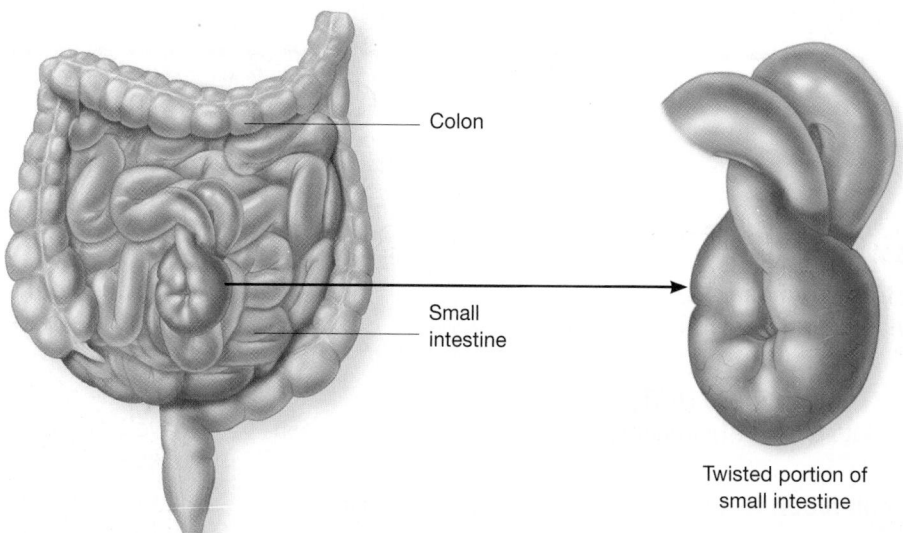

Colon

Small intestine

Twisted portion of small intestine

Figure 8.16 Volvulus. A length of small intestine has twisted around itself, cutting off blood circulation to the twisted loop.

Accessory Organs

TERM	WORD PARTS	DEFINITION
cholecystitis (koh-lee-sis-TYE-tis)	cholecyst/o = gallbladder -itis = inflammation	Inflammation of the gallbladder; most commonly caused by gallstones in the gallbladder or common bile duct that block the flow of bile.

Pathology *(continued)*

TERM	WORD PARTS	DEFINITION
cholelithiasis (koh-lee-lih-THIGH-ah-sis)	chol/e = bile -lithiasis = condition of stones	Presence of gallstones; may or may not cause symptoms such as *cholecystalgia*.

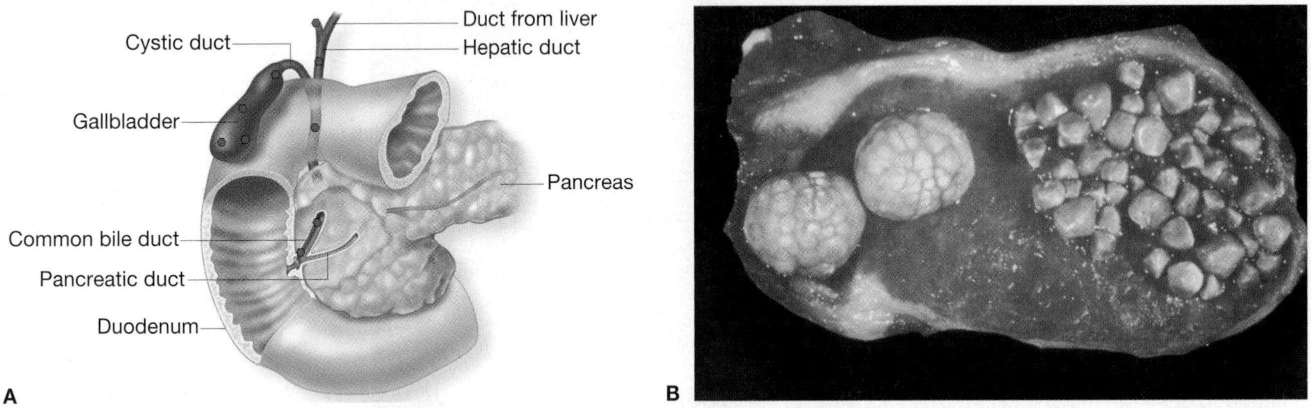

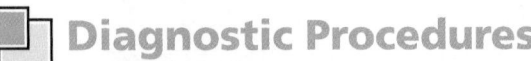

Cystic duct — Gallbladder — Common bile duct — Pancreatic duct — Duodenum — Duct from liver — Hepatic duct — Pancreas

A   B

■ **Figure 8.17**   (A) Common sites for cholelithiasis; (B) a gallbladder specimen with multiple gallstones *(Biophoto Associates/Photo Researchers, Inc.).*

TERM	WORD PARTS	DEFINITION
cirrhosis (sih-ROH-sis)	cirrh/o = yellow -osis = abnormal condition	Chronic disease of the liver associated with failure of the liver to function properly.
hepatitis (hep-ah-TYE-tis)	hepat/o = liver -itis = inflammation	Inflammation of the liver, usually due to a viral infection. Different viruses are transmitted by different routes, such as sexual contact or from exposure to blood or fecally contaminated water or food.
hepatoma (hep-ah-TOH-mah)	hepat/o = liver -oma = tumor	Liver tumor.
pancreatitis (pan-kree-ah-TYE-tis)	pancreat/o = pancreas -itis = inflammation	Inflammation of the pancreas.

Diagnostic Procedures

TERM	WORD PARTS	DEFINITION
Clinical Laboratory Tests		
alanine transaminase (ALT) (AL-ah-neen / trans-AM-in-nase)		Enzyme normally present in the blood. Blood levels are increased in persons with liver disease.
aspartate transaminase (AST) (ass-PAR-tate / trans-AM-in-nase)		Enzyme normally present in the blood. Blood levels are increased in persons with liver disease.
fecal occult blood test (FOBT) (uh-CULT)	-al = pertaining to	Laboratory test on the feces to determine if microscopic amounts of blood are present. Also called *hemoccult* or *stool guaiac*.
ova and parasites (O&P) (OH-vah / PAR-ah-sights)		Laboratory examination of feces with a microscope for the presence of parasites or their eggs.
serum bilirubin (SEE-rum / BILLY-rubin)		Blood test to determine the amount of the waste product bilirubin in the bloodstream. Elevated levels indicate liver disease.

Diagnostic Procedures *(continued)*

TERM	WORD PARTS	DEFINITION
stool culture		Laboratory test of feces to determine if any pathogenic bacteria are present.
Diagnostic Imaging		
bite-wing X-ray		X-ray taken with a part of the film holder held between the teeth and parallel to the teeth.
cholecystogram (koh-lee-SIS-toh-gram)	cholecyst/o = gallbladder -gram = record	X-ray image of the gallbladder.
intravenous cholecystography (in-trah-VEE-nus / koh-lee-sis-TOG-rah-fee)	intra- = within ven/o = vein -ous = pertaining to cholecyst/o = gallbladder -graphy = process of recording	Dye is administered intravenously to the patient allowing for X-ray visualization of the gallbladder and bile ducts.
lower gastrointestinal series (lower GI series)	gastr/o = stomach -al = pertaining to	X-ray image of the colon and rectum is taken after the administration of barium (a radiopaque dye) by enema. Also called a *barium enema (BE)*.

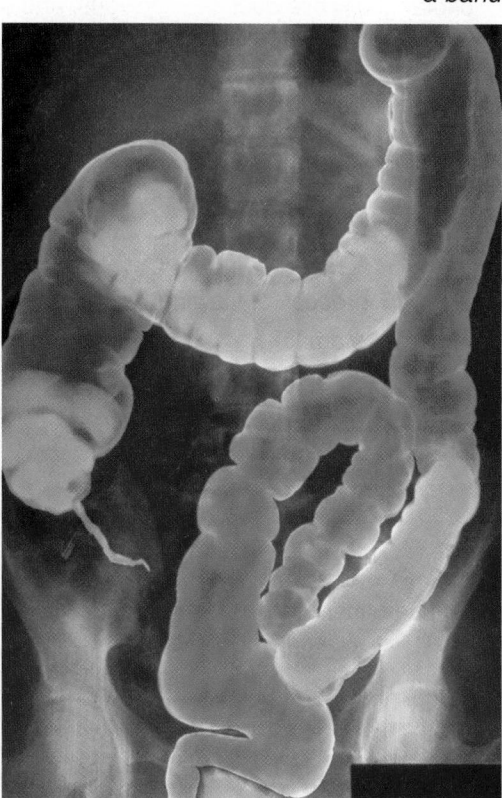

■ **Figure 8.18** Color-enhanced X-ray of the colon taken during a barium enema. *(CNRI/Science Photo Library/Photo Researchers, Inc.)*

percutaneous transhepatic cholangiography (PTC) (per-kyoo-TAY-nee-us / trans-heh-PAT-ik / koh-lan-jee-OG-rah-fee)	per- = through cutane/o = skin -ous = pertaining to trans- = across hepat/o = liver -ic = pertaining to cholangi/o = bile duct -graphy = process of recording	Procedure in which contrast medium is injected directly into the liver to visualize the bile ducts. Used to detect obstructions such as gallstones in the common bile duct.

Diagnostic Procedures *(continued)*

TERM	WORD PARTS	DEFINITION
upper gastrointestinal (UGI) series	gastr/o = stomach -al = pertaining to	Patient is administered a barium contrast material orally and then X-rays are taken to visualize the esophagus, stomach, and duodenum. Also called a *barium swallow*.

Endoscopic Procedures

TERM	WORD PARTS	DEFINITION
colonoscope (koh-LON-oh-scope)	colon/o = colon -scope = instrument to view	Instrument used to view the colon.
colonoscopy (koh-lon-OSS-koh-pee)	colon/o = colon -scopy = process of viewing	Flexible fiberscope called a *colonoscope* is passed through the anus, rectum, and colon; used to examine the upper portion of the colon. Polyps and small growths can be removed during this procedure (see again Figure 8.15).
endoscopic retrograde chol-angiopancreatography (ERCP) (en-doh-SKOP-ik / RET-roh-grayd / koh-lan-jee-oh-pan-kree-ah-TOG-rah-fee)	endo- = within -scopy = process of viewing -ic = pertaining to retro- = backwards cholangi/o = bile duct pancreat/o = pancreas -graphy = process of recording	Procedure using an endoscope to visually examine the hepatic duct, common bile duct, and pancreatic duct. First an endoscope is passed through the patient's mouth, esophagus, and stomach until it reaches the duodenum where the pancreatic and common bile ducts empty. Then a thin catheter is passed through the endoscope and into the ducts (in the retrograde direction). Contrast dye is then used to visualize these ducts on an X-ray.
esophagogastroduodenoscopy (EGD) (eh-soff-ah-go-gas-troh-duo-den-OS-koh-pee)	esophag/o = esophagus gastr/o = stomach duoden/o = duodenum -scopy = process of viewing	Use of a flexible fiberoptic endoscope to visually examine the esophagus, stomach, and beginning of the duodenum.
gastroscope (GAS-troh-scope)	gastr/o = stomach -scope = instrument to view	Instrument used to view inside the stomach.
gastroscopy (gas-TROS-koh-pee)	gastr/o = stomach -scopy = process of viewing	Procedure in which a flexible *gastroscope* is passed through the mouth and down the esophagus in order to visualize inside the stomach. Used to diagnose peptic ulcers and gastric carcinoma.
laparoscope (LAP-ah-roh-scope)	lapar/o = abdomen -scope = instrument to view	Instrument used to view inside the abdomen.
laparoscopy (lap-ar-OSS-koh-pee)	lapar/o = abdomen -scopy = process of viewing	*Laparoscope* is passed into the abdominal wall through a small incision. The abdominal cavity is then visually examined for tumors and other conditions with this lighted instrument. Also called *peritoneoscopy*.
sigmoidoscope (sig-MOYD-oh-scope)	sigmoid/o = sigmoid colon -scope = instrument to view	Instrument used to view inside the sigmoid colon.
sigmoidoscopy (sig-moid-OS-koh-pee)	sigmoid/o = sigmoid colon -scopy = process of viewing	Procedure using a flexible *sigmoidoscope* to visually examine the sigmoid colon. Commonly done to diagnose cancer and polyps.

Additional Diagnostic Procedures

TERM	WORD PARTS	DEFINITION
paracentesis (pair-ah-sin-TEE-sis)	-centesis = process of removing fluid	Insertion of a needle into the abdominal cavity to withdraw fluid. Tests to diagnose diseases may be conducted on the fluid.

Therapeutic Procedures

TERM	WORD PARTS	DEFINITION
Dental Procedures		
bridge		Dental appliance to replace missing teeth. It is attached to adjacent teeth for support.
crown		Artificial covering for a tooth that is created to replace the original enamel covering of the tooth.
denture (DEN-chur)	dent/o = tooth	Partial or complete set of artificial teeth that are set in plastic materials. Acts as a substitute for the natural teeth and related structures.
extraction	ex- = outward	Removing or "pulling" of teeth.
implant (IM-plant)		Prosthetic device placed in the jaw to which a tooth or denture may be anchored.
root canal	-al = pertaining to	Dental treatment involving the pulp cavity of the root of a tooth. Procedure is used to save a tooth that is badly infected or abscessed.
Medical Procedures		
gavage (guh-VAHZH)		Use of a nasogastric (NG) tube to place liquid nourishment directly into the stomach.
lavage (lah-VAHZH)		Use of a nasogastric (NG) tube to wash out the stomach. For example, after ingestion of dangerous substances.
nasogastric intubation (NG tube) (NAY-zo-gas-trik / in-two-BAY-shun)	nas/o = nose gastr/o = stomach -ic = pertaining to	Procedure in which a flexible catheter is inserted into the nose and down the esophagus to the stomach. May be used for feeding or to suction out stomach fluids.
total parenteral nutrition (TPN) (pair-in-TARE-all)	-al = pertaining to	Providing 100% of a patient's nutrition intravenously. Used when a patient is unable to eat.
Surgical Procedures		
anastomosis (ah-nas-toh-MOH-sis)		To surgically create a connection between two organs or vessels. For example, joining together two cut ends of the intestines after a section is removed.
appendectomy (ap-en-DEK-toh-mee)	append/o = appendix -ectomy = surgical removal	Surgical removal of the appendix.
bariatric surgery (bear-ee-AT-rik)	bar/o = weight	Group of surgical procedures such as stomach stapling and restrictive banding to reduce the size of the stomach. A treatment for morbid (extreme) obesity.
cholecystectomy (koh-lee-sis-TEK-toh-mee)	cholecyst/o = gallbladder -ectomy = surgical removal	Surgical removal of the gallbladder.
choledocholithotripsy (koh-led-oh-koh-LITH-oh-trip-see)	choledoch/o = common bile duct lith/o = stone -tripsy = surgical crushing	Crushing of a gallstone in the common bile duct.
colectomy (koh-LEK-toh-mee)	col/o = colon -ectomy = surgical removal	Surgical removal of the colon.

Therapeutic Procedures (continued)

TERM	WORD PARTS	DEFINITION
colostomy (koh-LOSS-toh-mee)	col/o = colon -ostomy = create a new opening	Surgical creation of an opening of some portion of the colon through the abdominal wall to the outside surface. Fecal material (stool) drains into a bag worn on the abdomen.

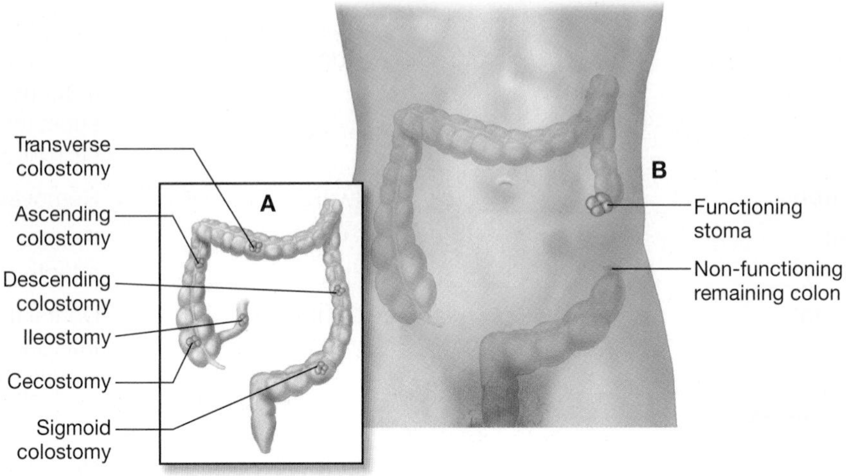

Transverse colostomy
Ascending colostomy
Descending colostomy
Ileostomy
Cecostomy
Sigmoid colostomy

A

B
Functioning stoma
Non-functioning remaining colon

■ **Figure 8.19**   (A) The colon illustrating various ostomy sites; (B) colostomy in the descending colon, illustrating functioning stoma and nonfunctioning distal sigmoid colon and rectum.

TERM	WORD PARTS	DEFINITION
diverticulectomy (dye-ver-tik-yoo-LEK-toh-mee)	diverticul/o = pouch -ectomy = surgical removal	Surgical removal of a diverticulum.
exploratory laparotomy (ek-SPLOR-ah-tor-ee / lap-ah-ROT-oh-mee)	lapar/o = abdomen -otomy = cutting into	Abdominal operation for the purpose of examining the abdominal organs and tissues for signs of disease or other abnormalities.
fistulectomy (fis-tyoo-LEK-toh-mee)	-ectomy = surgical removal	Removal of a fistula.
gastrectomy (gas-TREK-toh-mee)	gastr/o = stomach -ectomy = surgical removal	Surgical removal of the stomach.
gastric stapling	gastr/o = stomach -ic = pertaining to	Procedure that closes off a large section of the stomach with rows of staples. Results in a much smaller stomach to assist very obese patients to lose weight.
gastrostomy (gas-TROSS-toh-mee)	gastr/o = stomach -ostomy = create a new opening	Surgical procedure to create an opening in the stomach.
hemorrhoidectomy (hem-oh-royd-EK-toh-mee)	-ectomy = surgical removal	Surgical removal of hemorrhoids from the anorectal area.
hernioplasty (her-nee-oh-PLAS-tee)	-plasty = surgical repair	Surgical repair of a hernia. Also called *herniorrhaphy*.
ileostomy (ill-ee-OSS-toh-mee)	ile/o = ileum -ostomy = create a new opening	Surgical creation of an opening in the ileum.
laparoscopic cholecystectomy (lap-ar-oh-SKOP-ik / koh-lee-sis-TEK-toh-mee)	lapar/o = abdomen -scopy = process of viewing -ic = pertaining to cholecyst/o = gallbladder -ectomy = surgical removal	Surgical removal of the gallbladder through a very small abdominal incision with the assistance of a laparoscope.

Therapeutic Procedures *(continued)*

TERM	WORD PARTS	DEFINITION
laparotomy (lap-ah-ROT-oh-mee)	lapar/o = abdomen -otomy = cutting into	Surgical incision into the abdomen.
liver transplant		Transplant of a liver from a donor.
palatoplasty (pa-LOT-toh-plas-tee)	palat/o = palate -plasty = surgical repair	Surgical repair of the palate.
pharyngoplasty (fair-ING-oh-plas-tee)	pharyng/o = pharynx -plasty = surgical repair	Surgical repair of the throat.
proctopexy (PROK-toh-pek-see)	proct/o = rectum and anus -pexy = surgical fixation	Surgical fixation of the rectum and anus.

Pharmacology

CLASSIFICATION	WORD PARTS	ACTION	EXAMPLES
anorexiant (an-oh-REKS-ee-ant)	an- = without -orexia = appetite	Treats obesity by suppressing appetite.	phendimetrazine, Adipost, Obezine; phentermine, Zantryl, Adipex
antacid	anti- = against	Used to neutralize stomach acids.	calcium carbonate, Tums; aluminum hydroxide and magnesium hydroxide, Maalox, Mylanta
antidiarrheal (an-tee-dye-ah-REE-all)	anti- = against -al = pertaining to	Used to control diarrhea.	loperamide, Imodium; diphenoxylate and atropine, Lomotil; kaolin/pectin, Kaopectate
antiemetic (an-tye-ee-MEH-tik)	anti- = against -emesis = vomit -tic = pertaining to	Treats nausea, vomiting, and motion sickness.	prochlorperazine, Compazine; promethazine, Phenergan
H_2-receptor antagonist	anti- = against	Used to treat peptic ulcers and gastroesophageal reflux disease. When stimulated, H_2-receptors increase the production of stomach acid. Using an antagonist to block these receptors results in a low acid level in the stomach.	ranitidine, Zantac; cimetidine, Tagamet; famotidine, Pepcid
laxative **MED TERM TIP** The term *laxative* refers to a medication to stimulate a bowel movement; comes from the Latin term meaning "to relax."		Treats constipation by stimulating a bowel movement.	senosides, Senokot; psyllium, Metamucil
proton pump inhibitors		Used to treat peptic ulcers and gastroesophageal reflux disease. Blocks the stomach's ability to secrete acid.	esomeprazole, Nexium; omeprazole, Prilosec

Abbreviations

ac	before meals	**HDV**	hepatitis D virus
ALT	alanine transaminase	**HEV**	hepatitis E virus
AST	aspartate transaminase	**HSV-1**	herpes simplex virus type 1
Ba	barium	**IBD**	inflammatory bowel disease
BE	barium enema	**IBS**	irritable bowel syndrome
BM	bowel movement	**IVC**	intravenous cholangiography
BS	bowel sounds	**n&v**	nausea and vomiting
CBD	common bile duct	**NG**	nasogastric (tube)
EGD	esophagogastroduodenoscopy	**NPO**	nothing by mouth
ERCP	endoscopic retrograde cholangio-pancreatography	**O&P**	ova and parasites
		pc	after meals
FOBT	fecal occult blood test	**PO**	by mouth
GB	gallbladder	**pp**	postprandial
GERD	gastroesophageal reflux disease	**PTC**	percutaneous transhepatic cholangiography
GI	gastrointestinal		
HAV	hepatitis A virus	**PUD**	peptic ulcer disease
HBV	hepatitis B virus	**TPN**	total parenteral nutrition
HCl	hydrochloric acid	**UGI**	upper gastrointestinal series
HCV	hepatitis C virus		

Chapter Review

Real-World Applications

Medical Record Analysis

This Gastroenterology Consultation Report contains 12 medical terms. Underline each term and write it in the list below the report. Then define each term.

Gastroenterology Consultation Report

Reason for Consultation:
Evaluation of recurrent epigastric pain with anemia and melena.

History of Present Illness:
Patient is a 56-year-old male. He reports a long history of mild dyspepsia characterized by burning epigastric pain, especially when his stomach is empty. This pain has been relieved by over-the-counter antacids. Approximately two weeks ago, the pain became significantly worse and he noted that his stools were dark and tarry.

Results of Physical Examination:
CBC indicates anemia, and a fecal occult blood test is positive for blood. A blood test for *Helicobacter pylori* is positive. Gastroscopy located an ulcer in the lining of the stomach. This ulcer is 1.5 cm in diameter and deep. There is evidence of active bleeding from the ulcer.

Assessment:
Peptic ulcer disease.

Recommendations:
A gastrectomy to remove the ulcerated portion of stomach is indicated because the ulcer is already bleeding.

	Term	Definition
1	_____	_____
2	_____	_____
3	_____	_____
4	_____	_____
5	_____	_____
6	_____	_____
7	_____	_____
8	_____	_____
9	_____	_____
10	_____	_____
11	_____	_____
12	_____	_____

Chart Note Transcription

The chart note below contains 12 phrases that can be reworded with a medical term that you learned in this chapter. Each phrase is identified with an underline. Determine the medical term and write your answers in the space provided.

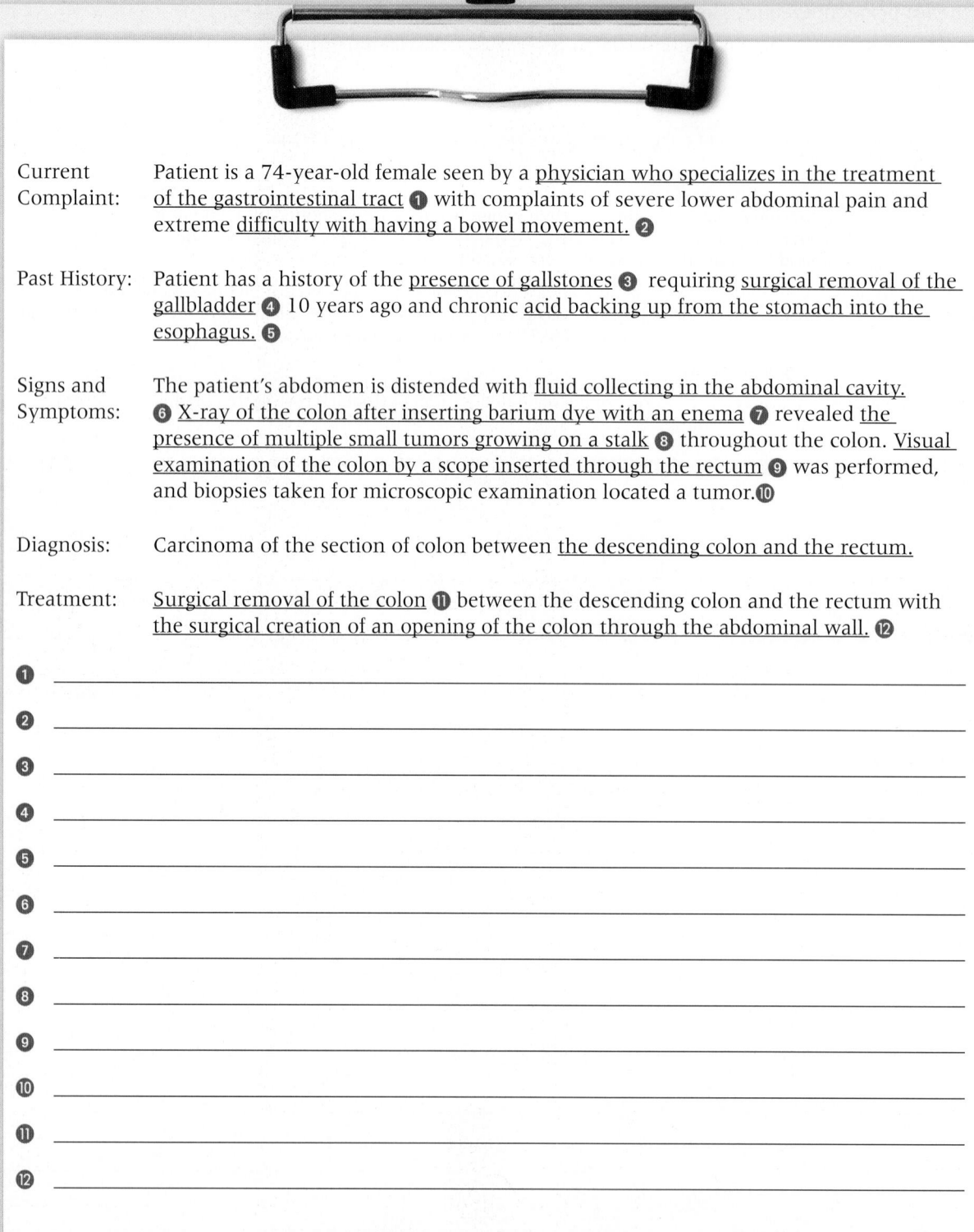

Current Complaint: Patient is a 74-year-old female seen by a <u>physician who specializes in the treatment of the gastrointestinal tract</u> ❶ with complaints of severe lower abdominal pain and extreme <u>difficulty with having a bowel movement.</u> ❷

Past History: Patient has a history of the <u>presence of gallstones</u> ❸ requiring <u>surgical removal of the gallbladder</u> ❹ 10 years ago and chronic <u>acid backing up from the stomach into the esophagus.</u> ❺

Signs and Symptoms: The patient's abdomen is distended with <u>fluid collecting in the abdominal cavity.</u> ❻ <u>X-ray of the colon after inserting barium dye with an enema</u> ❼ revealed <u>the presence of multiple small tumors growing on a stalk</u> ❽ throughout the colon. <u>Visual examination of the colon by a scope inserted through the rectum</u> ❾ was performed, and biopsies taken for microscopic examination located a tumor.❿

Diagnosis: Carcinoma of the section of colon between <u>the descending colon and the rectum.</u>

Treatment: <u>Surgical removal of the colon</u> ⓫ between the descending colon and the rectum with <u>the surgical creation of an opening of the colon through the abdominal wall.</u> ⓬

❶ _____

❷ _____

❸ _____

❹ _____

❺ _____

❻ _____

❼ _____

❽ _____

❾ _____

❿ _____

⓫ _____

⓬ _____

Case Study

Below is a case study presentation of a patient with a condition discussed in this chapter. Read the case study and answer the questions below. Some questions will ask for information not included within this chapter. Use your text, a medical dictionary, or any other reference material you choose to answer these questions.

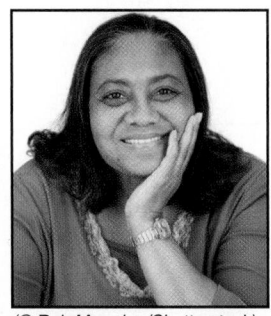

A 60-year-old obese female has come into the ER due to severe RUQ pain for the past 2 hours. Patient also reports increasing nausea but denies emesis. Patient states she has been told she has cholelithiasis by her family physician following a milder episode of this pain 2 years ago. In addition to severe pain, patient displays a moderate degree of scleral jaundice. Abdominal ultrasound identified acute cholecystitis and a large number of gallstones. Because of the jaundice a PTC was performed and confirmed choledocholithiasis. Patient was sent to surgery for laparoscopic cholecystectomy to remove the gallbladder and all gallstones. She recovered without incident.

(© Rob Marmion/Shutterstock)

1.   Define each of the patient's symptoms.

_____

_____

2.   The patient has severe RUQ pain. What organs are located in the RUQ?

_____

_____

3.   After reading the definition of jaundice, what is most likely causing this patient to have it?

_____

_____

4.   Describe the diagnostic imaging procedures this patient received.

_____

_____

5.   What is the difference between cholelithiasis and cholecystitis?

_____

_____

6.   The patient's gallbladder was removed laparoscopically. What does that mean?

_____

_____

Practice Exercises

A. Complete the Statement

1. The digestive system is also known as the _____ system.

2. The continuous muscular tube of the digestive system is called the _____ or _____ and stretches between the _____ and _____.

3. The accessory organs of the digestive system are the _____, _____, _____, and _____.

4. The three main functions of the digestive system are _____, _____, and _____.

5. The incisors are examples of _____ teeth and the molars are examples of _____ teeth.

6. Food is propelled through the gut by wavelike muscular contractions called _____.

7. Food in the stomach is mixed with _____ and other gastric juices to form a watery mixture called _____.

8. The three sections of small intestine in order are the _____, _____, and _____.

9. The S-shaped section of colon that curves back toward the rectum is called the _____ colon.

10. _____ produced by the liver is responsible for the _____ of fats. It is stored in the _____.

B. Combining Form Practice

The combining form **gastr/o** refers to the stomach. Use it to write a term that means:

1. inflammation of the stomach_____

2. study of the stomach and small intestines_____

3. removal of the stomach _____

4. visual exam of the stomach _____

5. stomach pain_____

6. enlargement of the stomach_____

7. cutting into the stomach_____

The combining form **esophag/o** refers to the esophagus. Use it to write a term that means:

8. inflammation of the esophagus _____

9. visual examination of the esophagus _____

10. surgical repair of the esophagus _____

11. pertaining to the esophagus _____

12. stretched-out esophagus _____

The combining form **proct/o** refers to the rectum and anus. Use it to write a term that means:

13. surgical fixation of the rectum and anus _____

14. drooping of the rectum and anus _____

15. inflammation of the rectum and anus _____

16. specialist in the study of the rectum and anus _____

The combining form **cholecyst/o** refers to the gallbladder. Use it to write a term that means:

17. removal of the gallbladder _____

18. condition of having gallbladder stones _____

19. gallbladder stone surgical crushing _____

20. gallbladder inflammation _____

The combining form **lapar/o** refers to the abdomen. Use it to write a term that means:

21. instrument to view inside the abdomen _____

22. cutting into the abdomen _____

23. visual examination of the abdomen _____

The combining form **hepat/o** refers to the liver. Use it to write a term that means:

24. liver tumor _____

25. enlargement of the liver _____

26. pertaining to the liver _____

27. inflammation of the liver _____

The combining form **pancreat/o** refers to the pancreas. Use it to write a term that means:

28. inflammation of the pancreas _____

29. pertaining to the pancreas _____

The combining form **col/o** refers to the colon. Use it to write a term that means:

30. create an opening in the colon _____

31. inflammation of the colon _____

C. Define the Combining Form

	Definition	Example from Chapter
1. esophag/o	_____	_____
2. hepat/o	_____	_____
3. ile/o	_____	_____
4. proct/o	_____	_____
5. gloss/o	_____	_____
6. labi/o	_____	_____
7. jejun/o	_____	_____
8. sigmoid/o	_____	_____
9. rect/o	_____	_____
10. gingiv/o	_____	_____
11. cholecyst/o	_____	_____
12. duoden/o	_____	_____
13. an/o	_____	_____
14. enter/o	_____	_____
15. dent/o	_____	_____

D. Suffix Practice

Use the following suffixes to create a medical term for the following definitions.

-orexia	-phagia	-pepsia	-prandial
-emesis	-lithiasis		

1. after meals _____

2. condition of having gallstones _____

3. no appetite _____

4. difficulty swallowing _____

5. vomiting blood _____

6. slow digestion _____

E. What Does it Stand For?

1. BM _____

2. UGI _____

3. BE _____

4. BS _____

5. n & v _____

6. O & P _____

7. PO _____

8. CBD _____

9. NPO _____

10. pp _____

F. Terminology Matching

Match each term to its definition.

1.	_____ dentures	a.	excess body weight
2.	_____ anorexia	b.	chronic liver disease
3.	_____ hematemesis	c.	heartburn
4.	_____ pyrosis	d.	small colon tumors
5.	_____ obesity	e.	fluid accumulation in abdominal cavity
6.	_____ constipation	f.	vomit blood
7.	_____ melena	g.	bowel twists on self
8.	_____ ascites	h.	set of artificial teeth
9.	_____ cirrhosis	i.	loss of appetite
10.	_____ spastic colon	j.	difficulty having BM
11.	_____ polyposis	k.	irritable bowel syndrome
12.	_____ volvulus	l.	black tarry stool
13.	_____ hiatal hernia	m.	yellow skin color
14.	_____ ulcerative colitis	n.	bloody diarrhea
15.	_____ dysentery	o.	diaphragmatocele
16.	_____ jaundice	p.	inflammatory bowel disease

G. What's the Abbreviation?

1. nasogastric _____

2. gastrointestinal _____

3. hepatitis B virus _____

4. fecal occult blood test _____

5. inflammatory bowel disease _____

6. herpes simplex virus type 1 _____

7. aspartate transaminase _____

8. after meals _____

9. peptic ulcer disease _____

10. gastroesophageal reflux disease _____

H. Define the Term

1. colonoscopy_____

2. bite wing X-ray_____

3. hematochezia _____

4. serum bilirubin_____

5. cachexia _____

6. lavage _____

7. hernioplasty _____

8. extraction _____

9. choledocholithotripsy _____

10. anastomosis_____

I. Fill in the Blank

colonoscopy	barium swallow	lower GI series
gastric stapling	colostomy	colectomy
total parenteral nutrition	choledocholithotripsy	liver biopsy
ileostomy	fecal occult blood test	intravenous cholecystography

1. Excising a small piece of hepatic tissue for microscopic examination is called a(n) _____.

2. When a surgeon performs a total or partial colectomy for cancer, she may have to create an opening on the surface of the skin for fecal matter to leave the body. This procedure is called a(n) _____.

3. Another name for an upper GI series is a(n) _____.

4. Mr. White has had a radiopaque material placed into his large bowel by means of an enema for the purpose of viewing his colon. This procedure is called a(n) _____.

5. A(n) _____ is the surgical removal of the colon.

6. Jessica has been on a red meat-free diet in preparation for a test of her feces for the presence of hidden blood. This test is called a(n) _____.

7. Dr. Mendez uses equipment to crush gallstones in the common bile duct. This procedure is called a(n) _____.

8. Mrs. Alcazar required _____ because she could not eat following her intestinal surgery.

9. Mr. Bright had a(n) _____ to treat his morbid obesity.

10. Visualizing the gallbladder and bile ducts by injecting a dye into the patient's arm is called a(n) _____.

11. Passing an instrument into the anus and rectum in order to see the colon is called a(n) _____.

12. Ms. Fayne suffers from Crohn's disease, which has necessitated the removal of much of her small intestine. She has had a surgical passage created for the external disposal of waste material from the ileum. This is called a(n) _____.

J. Terminology Matching

Match each term to its definition.

1. _____ dentures	a. tooth decay
2. _____ cementum	b. prosthetic device used to anchor a tooth
3. _____ root canal	c. inflammation of the gums
4. _____ crown	d. full set of artificial teeth
5. _____ bridge	e. portion of the tooth covered by enamel
6. _____ implant	f. replacement for missing teeth
7. _____ gingivitis	g. anchors root in bony socket of jaw
8. _____ dental caries	h. surgery on the tooth pulp

K. Pharmacology Challenge

Fill in the classification for each drug description, then match the brand name.

Drug Description	Classification	Brand Name
1. _____ Controls diarrhea	_____	a. Pepcid
2. _____ Blocks stomach's ability to secrete acid	_____	b. Obezine
3. _____ Treats motion sickness	_____	c. Metamucil
4. _____ Blocks acid-producing receptors	_____	d. Compazine
5. _____ Suppresses appetite	_____	e. Maalox
6. _____ Stimulates a bowel movement	_____	f. Imodium
7. _____ Neutralizes stomach acid	_____	g. Nexium

Labeling Exercise

Image A

Write the labels for this figure on the numbered lines provided.

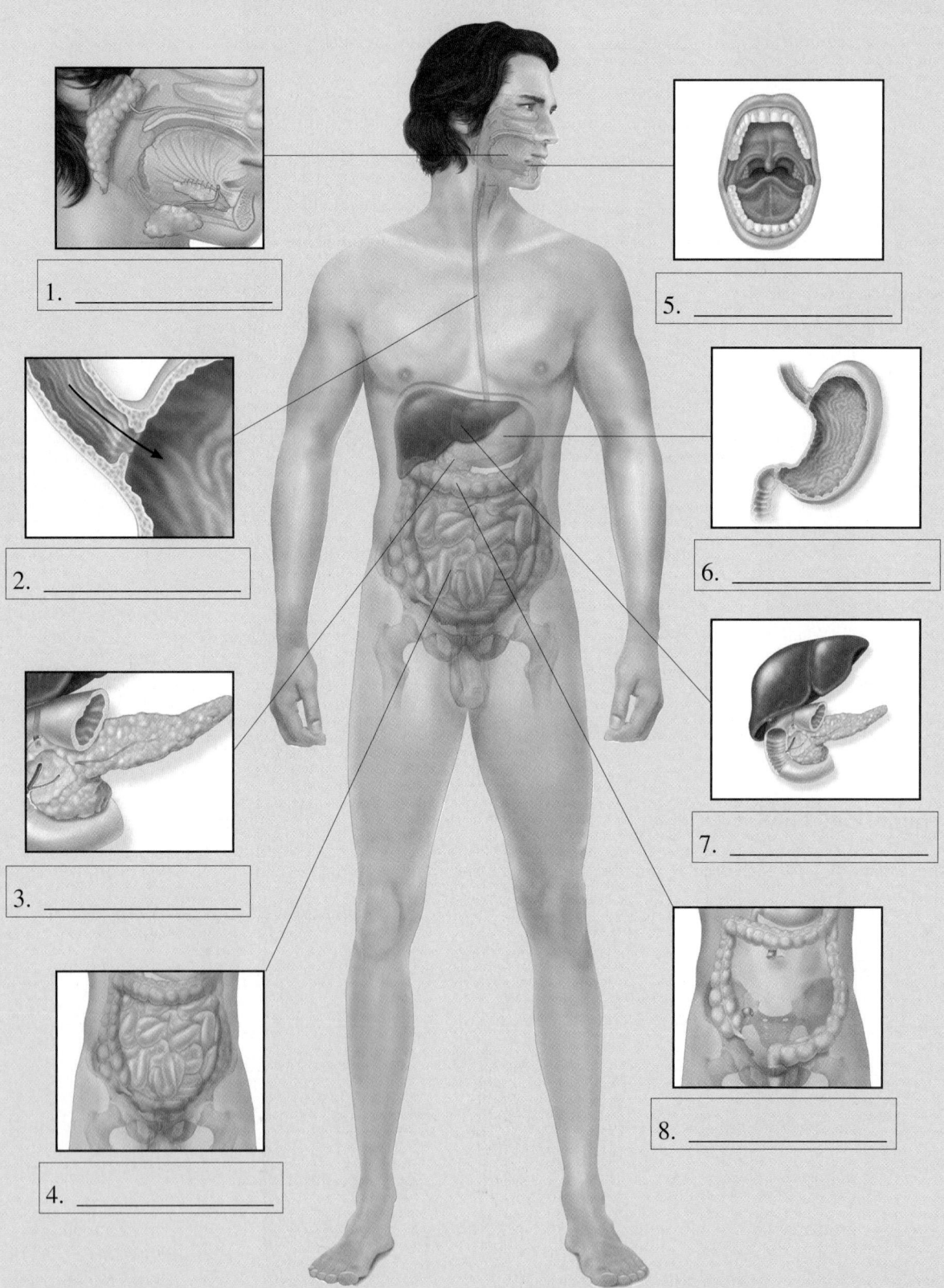

1. _____

2. _____

3. _____

4. _____

5. _____

6. _____

7. _____

8. _____

Image B

Write the labels for this figure on the numbered lines provided.

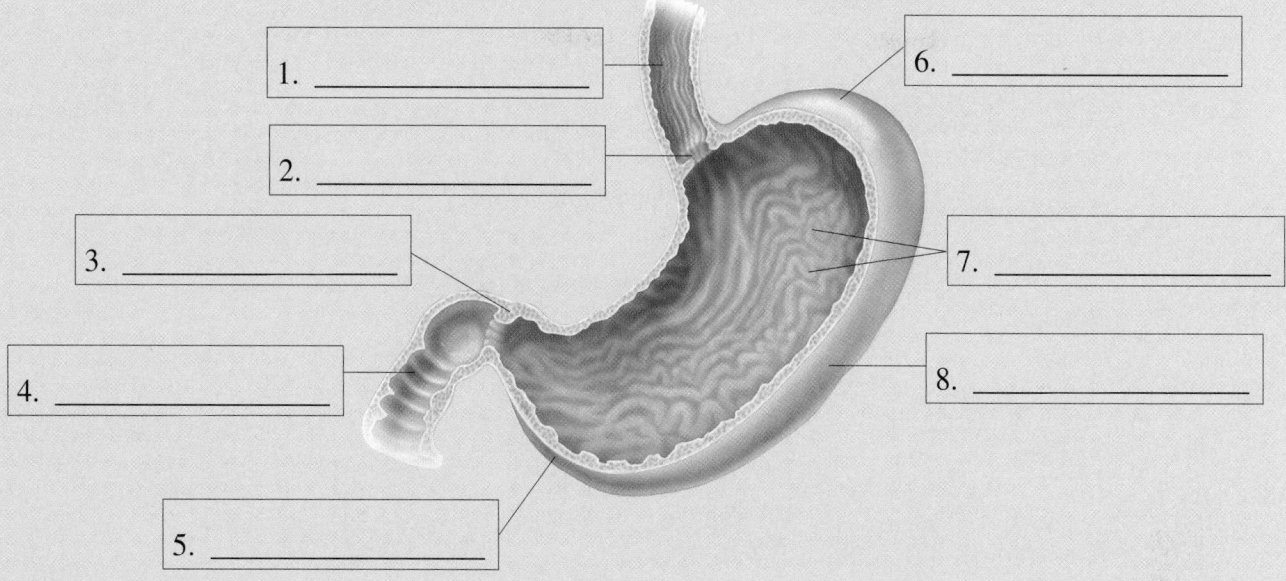

1. _____

2. _____

3. _____

4. _____

5. _____

6. _____

7. _____

8. _____

Image C

Write the labels for this figure on the numbered lines provided.

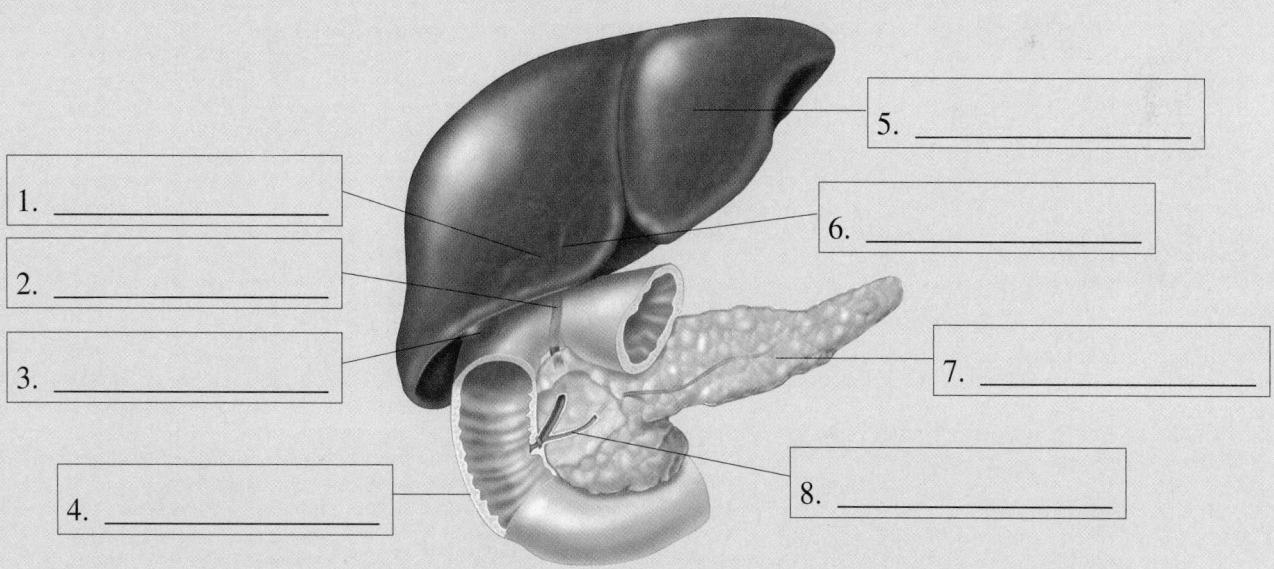

1. _____

2. _____

3. _____

4. _____

5. _____

6. _____

7. _____

8. _____

MEDICAL TERMINOLOGY INTERACTIVE

Medical Terminology Interactive is a premium online homework management system that includes a host of features to help you study. Registered users will find:

- Fun games and activities built within a virtual hospital
- Powerful tools that track and analyze your results—allowing you to create a personalized learning experience
- Videos, flashcards, and audio pronunciations to help enrich your progress
- Streaming video lesson presentations and self-paced learning modules

www.pearsonhighered.com/mti

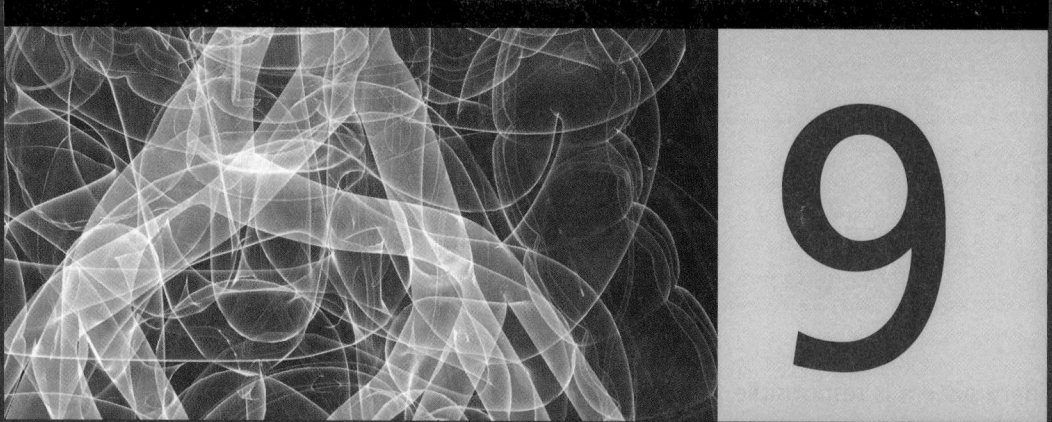

9

URINARY SYSTEM

Learning Objectives

Upon completion of this chapter, you will be able to

- Identify and define the combining forms and suffixes introduced in this chapter.

- Correctly spell and pronounce medical terms and major anatomical structures relating to the urinary system.

- Locate and describe the major organs of the urinary system and their functions.

- Describe the nephron and the mechanisms of urine production.

- Identify the characteristics of urine and a urinalysis.

- Identify and define urinary system anatomical terms.

- Identify and define selected urinary system pathology terms.

- Identify and define selected urinary system diagnostic procedures.

- Identify and define selected urinary system therapeutic procedures.

- Identify and define selected medications relating to the urinary system.

- Define selected abbreviations associated with the urinary system.

Urinary System at a Glance

Function

The urinary system is responsible for maintaining a stable internal environment for the body. In order to achieve this state, the urinary system removes waste products, adjusts water and electrolyte levels, and maintains the correct pH.

Organs

Here are the primary structures that comprise the urinary system.

kidneys　　　　　　　　　　**urethra**
ureters　　　　　　　　　　**urinary bladder**

Word Parts

Here are the most common word parts (with their meanings) used to build urinary system terms. For a more comprehensive list, refer to the Terminology section of this chapter.

Combining Forms

azot/o	nitrogenous waste	noct/i	night
bacteri/o	bacteria	olig/o	scanty
cyst/o	bladder, pouch	protein/o	protein
glomerul/o	glomerulus	pyel/o	renal pelvis
glycos/o	sugar, glucose	ren/o	kidney
keton/o	ketones	ureter/o	ureter
lith/o	stone	urethr/o	urethra
meat/o	meatus	urin/o	urine
nephr/o	kidney	ur/o	urine

Suffixes

-lith	stone
-lithiasis	condition of stones
-ptosis	drooping
-tripsy	surgical crushing
-uria	condition of the urine

Urinary System Illustrated

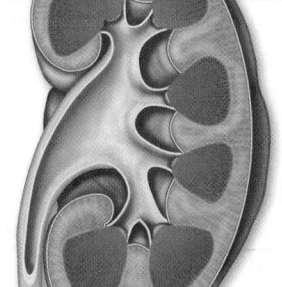

kidney, p. 298

Filters blood and produces urine

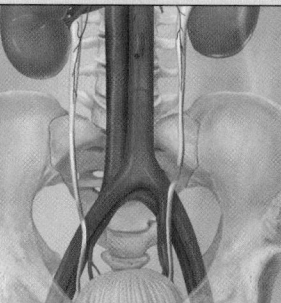

ureter, p. 299

Transports urine to the bladder

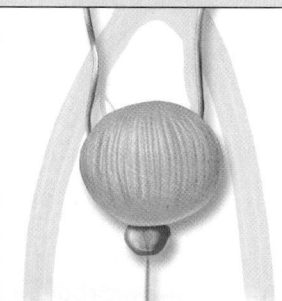

urinary bladder, p. 300

Stores urine

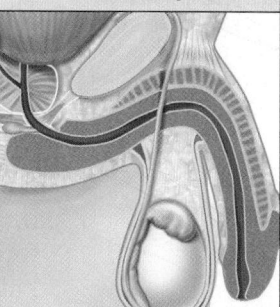

male urethra, p. 301

Transports urine to exterior

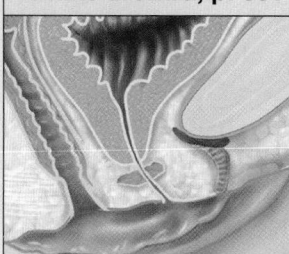

female urethra, p. 301

Transports urine to exterior

■ Anatomy and Physiology of the Urinary System

genitourinary system
  (jen-ih-toh-YOO-rih-nair-ee)
kidneys
nephrons (NEF-ronz)
uremia (yoo-REE-mee-ah)

ureters (YOO-reh-ters)
urethra (yoo-REE-thrah)
urinary bladder
  (YOO-rih-nair-ee)
urine (YOO-rin)

Think of the urinary system, sometimes referred to as the **genitourinary** (GU) **system,** as similar to a water filtration plant. Its main function is to filter and remove waste products from the blood. These waste materials result in the production and excretion of **urine** from the body.

The urinary system is one of the hardest working systems of the body. All the body's metabolic processes result in the production of waste products. These waste products are a natural part of life but quickly become toxic if they are allowed to build up in the blood, resulting in a condition called **uremia.** Waste products in the body are removed through a very complicated system of blood vessels and kidney tubules. The actual filtration of wastes from the blood takes place in millions of **nephrons,** which make up each of your two **kidneys.** As urine drains from each kidney, the **ureters** transport it to the **urinary bladder.** We are constantly producing urine, and our bladders can hold about one quart of this liquid. When the urinary bladder empties, urine moves from the bladder down the **urethra** to the outside of the body.

Kidneys

calyx (KAY-liks)
cortex (KOR-teks)
hilum (HIGH-lum)
medulla (meh-DULL-ah)
renal artery

renal papilla (pah-PILL-ah)
renal pelvis
renal pyramids
renal vein
retroperitoneal (ret-roh-pair-ih-toh-NEE-al)

The two kidneys are located in the lumbar region of the back above the waist on either side of the vertebral column. They are not inside the peritoneal sac, a location referred to as **retroperitoneal.** Each kidney has a concave or indented area on the edge toward the center that gives the kidney its bean shape. The center of this concave area is called the **hilum.** The hilum is where the **renal artery** enters and the **renal vein** leaves the kidney (see Figure 9.1 ■). The renal artery delivers the blood that is full of waste products to the kidney and the renal vein returns the now cleansed blood to the general circulation. The ureters also leave the kidneys at the hilum. The ureters are narrow tubes that lead from the kidneys to the bladder.

When a surgeon cuts into a kidney, several structures or areas are visible. The outer portion, called the **cortex,** is much like a shell for the kidney. The inner area is called the **medulla.** Within the medulla are a dozen or so triangular-shaped areas, the **renal pyramids,** which resemble their namesake, the Egyptian pyramids. The tip of each pyramid points inward toward the hilum. At its tip, called the **renal papilla,** each pyramid opens into a **calyx** (plural is *calyces*), which is continuous with the **renal pelvis.** The calyces and ultimately the renal pelvis collect urine as it is formed. The ureter for each kidney arises from the renal pelvis (see Figure 9.2 ■).

MED TERM TIP

The urinary system and the male reproductive system share some of the same organs, particularly the urethra. Hence the term *genitourinary* (GU) is sometimes used to describe the urinary system. The reproductive system is discussed in Chapter 10.

MED TERM TIP

From the time of early man, there has been an interest in urine. Drawings on cave walls and hieroglyphics in Egyptian pyramids reveal interest in urine as a means of determining the physical state of the body. Some of the first doctors, called *pisse prophets,* believed that examining the urine would help treat a patient. Now urologists treat disorders of the urinary tract in both men and women, as well as disorders of the male reproductive tract.

MED TERM TIP

At any one time, about 20% of your blood is being filtered by your kidneys. In this way, all your blood is cleansed every few minutes.

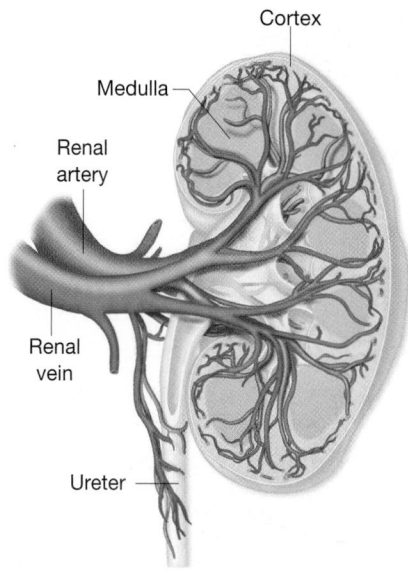

Figure 9.1 Kidney structure. Longitudinal section showing the renal artery entering and the renal vein and ureter exiting at the hilium of the kidney.

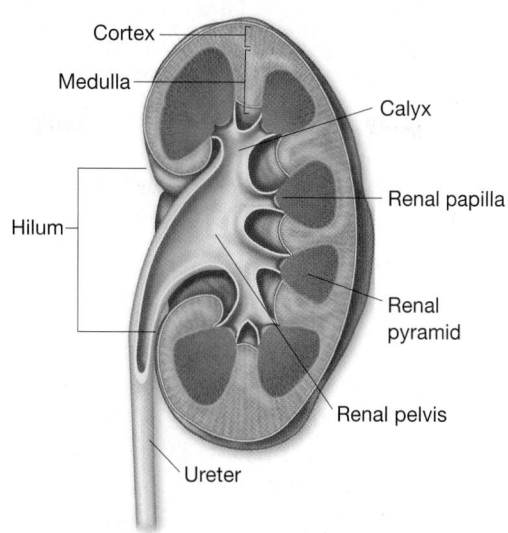

Figure 9.2 Longitudinal section of a kidney illustrating the internal structures.

Nephrons

afferent arteriole (AFF-er-ent)
Bowman's capsule
collecting tubule
distal convoluted tubule
　　(DISS-tall / con-voh-LOOT-ed)
efferent arteriole (EF-er-ent)
glomerular capsule (glom-AIR-yoo-lar)

glomerulus (glom-AIR-yoo-lus)
loop of Henle
nephron (NEF-ron)
nephron loop
proximal convoluted tubule
　　(PROK-sim-al / con-voh-LOOT-ed)
renal corpuscle (KOR-pus-ehl)

renal tubule

The functional or working unit of the kidney is the **nephron**. There are more than one million of these microscopic structures in each human kidney. Each nephron consists of the **renal corpuscle** and the **renal tubule** (see Figure 9.3 ■). The renal corpuscle is the blood-filtering portion of the nephron. It has a double-walled cuplike structure called the **glomerular capsule** (also known as **Bowman's capsule**) that encases a ball of capillaries called the **glomerulus**. An **afferent arteriole** carries blood to the glomerulus, and an **efferent arteriole** carries blood away from the glomerulus.

Water and substances that were removed from the bloodstream in the renal corpuscle flow into the renal tubules to finish the urine production process. This continuous tubule is divided into four sections: the **proximal convoluted tubule,** followed by the narrow **nephron loop** (also known as the **loop of Henle**), then the **distal convoluted tubule,** and finally the **collecting tubule.**

Ureters

As urine drains out of the renal pelvis it enters the ureter, which carries it down to the urinary bladder (see Figure 9.4 ■). Ureters are very narrow tubes measuring less than ¼-inch wide and 10–12 inches long that extend from the renal pelvis to the urinary bladder. Mucous membrane lines the ureters just as it lines most passages that open to the external environment.

MED TERM TIP

The kidney bean is so named because it resembles a kidney in shape. Each organ weighs 4–6 ounces, is 2–3 inches wide and approximately 1 inch thick, and is about the size of your fist. In most people the left kidney is slightly higher and larger than the right kidney. Functioning kidneys are necessary for life, but it is possible to live with only one functioning kidney.

MED TERM TIP

Afferent, meaning moving toward, and *efferent,* meaning moving away from, are terms used when discussing moving either toward or away from the central point in many systems. For example, there are afferent and efferent nerves in the nervous system.

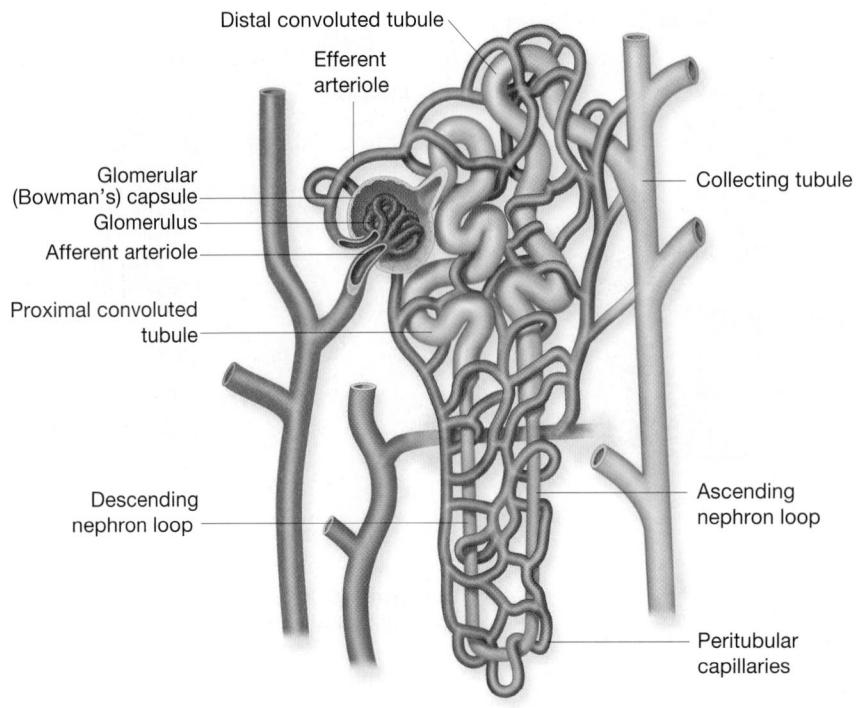

Figure 9.3 The structure of a nephron, illustrating the nephron structure in relation to the circulatory system.

Distal convoluted tubule

Efferent arteriole

Glomerular (Bowman's) capsule

Glomerulus

Afferent arteriole

Proximal convoluted tubule

Collecting tubule

Descending nephron loop

Ascending nephron loop

Peritubular capillaries

Urinary Bladder

external sphincter (SFINGK-ter)
internal sphincter

rugae (ROO-gay)
urination

The urinary bladder is an elastic muscular sac that lies in the base of the pelvis just behind the pubic symphysis (see Figure 9.5 ■). It is composed of three layers of smooth muscle tissue lined with mucous membrane containing **rugae** or folds that allow it to stretch. The bladder receives the urine directly from the ureters, stores it, and excretes it by **urination** through the urethra.

Generally, an adult bladder will hold 250 mL of urine. This amount then creates an urge to void or empty the bladder. Involuntary muscle action causes the bladder to contract and the **internal sphincter** to relax. The internal sphincter protects us from having our bladder empty at the wrong time. Voluntary action

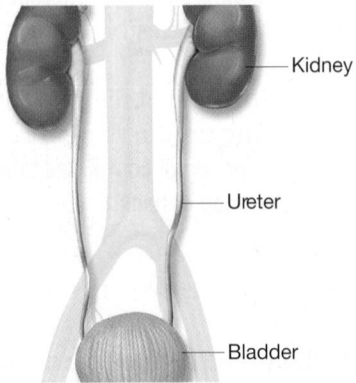

Kidney

Ureter

Bladder

Figure 9.4 The ureters extend from the kidneys to the urinary bladder.

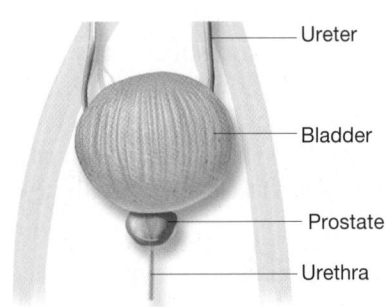

Ureter

Bladder

Prostate

Urethra

Figure 9.5 The structure of the urinary bladder. (Note the prostate gland.)

controls the **external sphincter,** which opens on demand to allow the intentional emptying of the bladder. The act of controlling the emptying of urine is developed sometime after a child is 2 years of age.

Urethra

urinary meatus (mee-AY-tus)

The urethra is a tubular canal that carries the flow of urine from the bladder to the outside of the body (see Figure 9.6 ■ for the male urethra). The external opening through which urine passes out of the body is called the **urinary meatus.** Mucous membrane also lines the urethra as it does other structures of the urinary system. This is one of the reasons that infection spreads up the urinary tract. The urethra is 1–2 inches long in the female and 8 inches long in the male. In a woman it functions only as the outlet for urine and is in front of the vagina. In the male, however, it has two functions: an outlet for urine and the passageway for semen to leave the body.

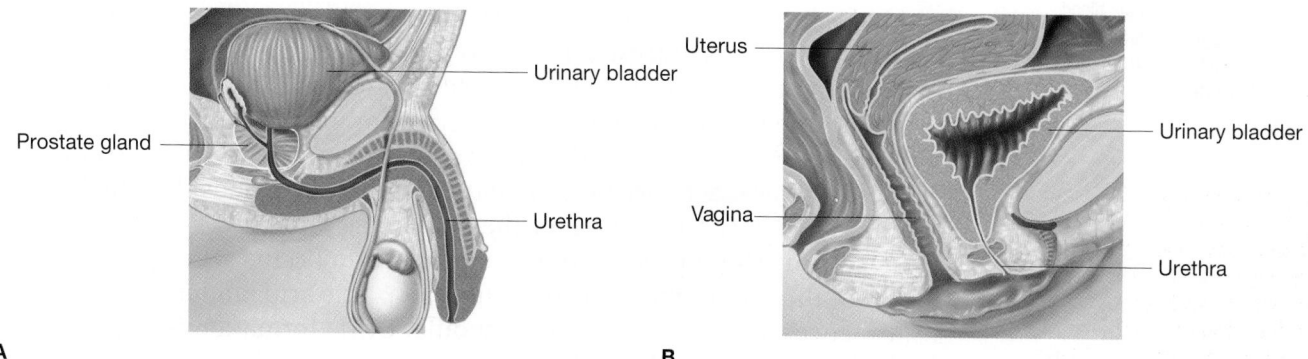

A   **B**

■ **Figure 9.6** (A) The male urethra extends from the urinary bladder in the floor of the pelvis through the penis to the urinary meatus; (B) the much shorter female urethra extends from the urinary bladder to the floor of the pelvis and exits just in front of the vaginal opening.

Role of Kidneys in Homeostasis

electrolytes (ee-LEK-troh-lites)   **homeostasis** (hoh-mee-oh-STAY-sis)

The kidneys are responsible for **homeostasis** or balance in the body. They continually adjust the chemical conditions in the body, allowing us to survive. Because of its interaction with the bloodstream and its ability to excrete substances from the body, the urinary system maintains the body's proper balance of water and chemicals. If the body is low on water, the kidneys conserve it, or in the opposite case, if there is excess water in the body, the kidneys excrete the excess. In adition to water, the kidneys regulate the level of **electrolytes**—small biologically important molecules such as sodium (Na^+), potassium (K^+), chloride (Cl), and bicarbonate (HCO_3^-). Finally, the kidneys play an important role in maintaining the correct pH range within the body, making sure we do not become too acidic or too alkaline. The kidneys accomplish these important tasks through the production of urine.

> **MED TERM TIP**
>
> Mucous membranes will carry infections up the urinary tract from the urinary meatus and urethra into the bladder and eventually up the ureters and the kidneys if not stopped. It is never wise to ignore a simple bladder infection or what is called *cystitis.*

Stages of Urine Production

filtration   **reabsorption**

glomerular filtrate   **secretion**

peritubular capillaries

As wastes and unnecessary substances are removed from the bloodstream by the nephrons, many desirable molecules are also removed initially. Waste products are eliminated from the body, but other substances such as water, electrolytes, and nutrients must be returned to the bloodstream. Urine, in its final form ready for elimination from the body, is the ultimate product of this entire process.

Urine production occurs in three stages: **filtration, reabsorption,** and **secretion.** Each of these steps is performed by a different section of the nephrons (see Figure 9.7 ■).

1. **Filtration.** The first stage is the filtering of particles, which occurs in the renal corpuscle. The pressure of blood flowing through the glomerulus forces material out of the bloodstream, through the wall of the glomerular capsule, and into the renal tubules. This fluid in the tubules is called the **glomerular filtrate** and consists of water, electrolytes, nutrients such as glucose and amino acids, wastes, and toxins.

2. **Reabsorption.** After filtration, the filtrate passes through the four sections of the tubule. As the filtrate moves along its twisted journey, most of the water and much of the electrolytes and nutrients are reabsorbed into the **peritubular capillaries,** a capillary bed that surrounds the renal tubules. They can then reenter the circulating blood.

3. **Secretion.** The final stage of urine production occurs when the special cells of the renal tubules secrete ammonia, uric acid, and other waste substances directly into the renal tubule. Urine formation is now finished; it passes into the collecting tubules, renal papilla, calyx, renal pelvis, and ultimately into the ureter.

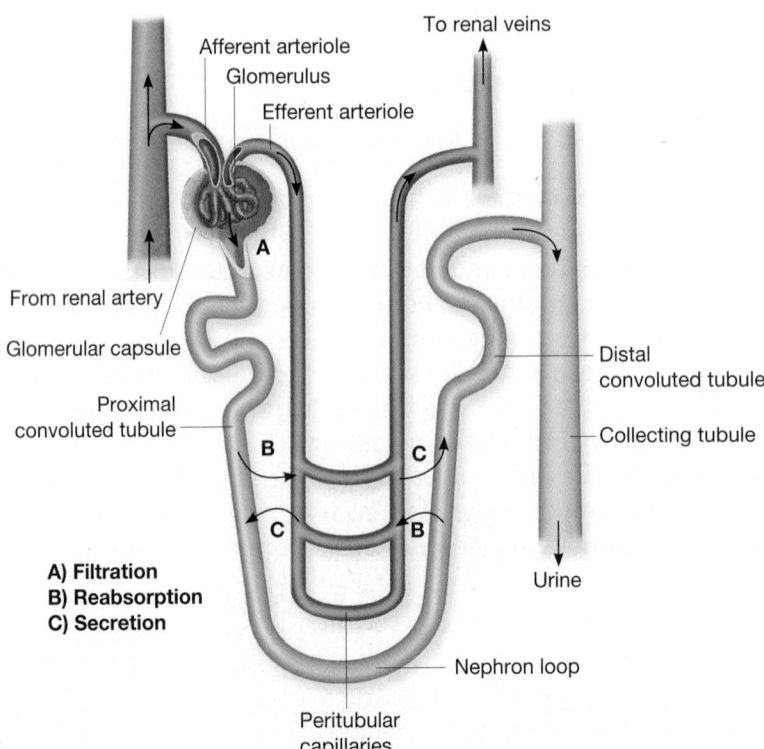

A) Filtration
B) Reabsorption
C) Secretion

The three
...duction:
...n, and

Urine

albumin (al-BEW-min)
nitrogenous wastes (nigh-TROJ-eh-nus)
specific gravity
urinalysis (yoo-rih-NAL-ih-sis)

Urine is normally straw-colored to clear, and sterile. Although it is 95% water, it also contains many dissolved substances, such as electrolytes, toxins, and **nitrogenous wastes,** the byproducts of muscle metabolism. At times the urine also contains substances that should not be there, such as glucose, blood, or **albumin,** a protein that should remain in the blood. This is the reason for performing a **urinalysis,** a physical and chemical analysis of urine, which gives medical personnel important information regarding disease processes occurring in a patient. Normally, during a 24-hour period the output of urine will be 1,000–2,000 mL, depending on the amount of fluid consumed and the general health of the person. Normal urine is acidic because this is one way our bodies dispose of excess acids. **Specific gravity** indicates the amount of dissolved substances in urine. The specific gravity of pure water is 1.000. The specific gravity of urine varies from 1.001 to 1.030. Highly concentrated urine has a higher specific gravity, while the specific gravity of very dilute urine is close to that of water. See Table 9.1 ■ for the normal values for urine testing and Table 9.2 ■ for abnormal findings.

MED TERM TIP

The color, odor, volume, and sugar content of urine have been examined for centuries. Color charts for urine were developed by 1140, and "taste testing" was common in the late seventeenth century. By the nineteenth century, urinalysis was a routine part of a physical examination.

Table 9.1	Values for Urinalysis Testing
ELEMENT	**NORMAL FINDINGS**
Color	Straw-colored, pale yellow to deep gold
Odor	Aromatic
Appearance	Clear
Specific gravity	1.001–1.030
pH	5.0–8.0
Protein	Negative to trace
Glucose	None
Ketones	None
Blood	Negative

Table 9.2	Abnormal Urinalysis Findings
ELEMENT	**IMPLICATIONS**
Color	Color varies depending on the patient's fluid intake and output or medication. Brown or black urine color indicates a serious disease process.
Odor	A fetid or foul odor may indicate infection. While a fruity odor may be found in diabetes mellitus, dehydration, or starvation. Other odors may be due to medication or foods.
Appearance	Cloudiness may mean that an infection is present.
Specific gravity	Concentrated urine has a higher specific gravity. Dilute urine, such as can be found with diabetes insipidus, acute tubular necrosis, or salt-restricted diets, has a lower specific gravity.
pH	A pH value below 7.0 (acidic) is common in urinary tract infections, metabolic or respiratory acidosis, diets high in fruits or vegetables, or administration of some drugs. A pH higher than 7.0 (basic or alkaline) is common in metabolic or respiratory alkalosis, fever, high-protein diets, and taking ascorbic acid.
Protein	Protein may indicate glomerulonephritis or preeclampsia in a pregnant woman.
Glucose	Small amounts of glucose may be present as the result of eating a high-carbohydrate meal, stress, pregnancy, and taking some medications, such as aspirin or corticosteroids. Higher levels may indicate poorly controlled diabetes, Cushing's syndrome, or infection.
Ketones	The presence of ketones may indicate poorly controlled diabetes, dehydration, starvation, or ingestion of large amounts of aspirin.
Blood	Blood may indicate glomerulonephritis, cancer of the urinary tract, some types of anemia, taking of some medications (such as blood thinners), arsenic poisoning, reactions to transfusion, trauma, burns, and convulsions.

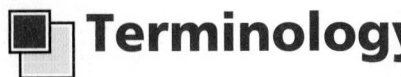 # Terminology

Word Parts Used to Build Urinary System Terms

The following lists contain the combining forms, suffixes, and prefixes used to build terms in the remaining sections of this chapter.

Combining Forms

azot/o	nitrogenous waste	**keton/o**	ketones	**py/o**	pus
bacteri/o	bacteria	**lith/o**	stone	**pyel/o**	renal pelvis
bi/o	life	**meat/o**	meatus	**ren/o**	kidney
carcin/o	cancer	**necr/o**	death	**ur/o**	urine
corpor/o	body	**nephr/o**	kidney	**ureter/o**	ureter
cyst/o	bladder, pouch	**neur/o**	nerve	**urethr/o**	urethra
glomerul/o	glomerulus	**noct/i**	night	**urin/o**	urine
glycos/o	sugar	**olig/o**	scanty	**ven/o**	vein
hem/o	blood	**peritone/o**	peritoneum		
hemat/o	blood	**protein/o**	protein		

Suffixes

-al	pertaining to	**-lithiasis**	condition of stones	**-pathy**	disease
-algia	pain	**-logist**	one who studies	**-pexy**	surgical fixation
-ar	pertaining to	**-logy**	study of	**-plasty**	surgical repair
-ary	pertaining to	**-lysis**	to destroy (to break down)	**-ptosis**	drooping
-cele	protrusion			**-rrhagia**	abnormal flow condition
-eal	pertaining to	**-malacia**	softening		
-ectasis	dilated	**-megaly**	enlarged	**-sclerosis**	hardening
-ectomy	surgical removal	**-meter**	instrument to measure	**-scope**	instrument to visually examine
-emia	blood condition				
-genic	produced by	**-oma**	tumor	**-scopy**	process of visually examining
-gram	record	**-ory**	pertaining to		
-graphy	process of recording	**-osis**	abnormal condition	**-stenosis**	narrowing
-ic	pertaining to	**-ostomy**	create a new opening	**-tic**	pertaining to
-itis	inflammation	**-otomy**	cutting into	**-tripsy**	surgical crushing
-lith	stone	**-ous**	pertaining to	**-uria**	urine condition

Prefixes

an-	without	**extra-**	outside of	**poly-**	many
anti-	against	**hydro-**	water	**retro-**	backward
dys-	abnormal, difficult	**intra-**	within		

Anatomical Terms

TERM	WORD PARTS	DEFINITION
cystic (SIS-tik)	cyst/o = bladder -ic = pertaining to	Pertaining to the bladder.
renal (REE-nal)	ren/o = kidney -al = pertaining to	Pertaining to the kidney.
ureteral (yoo-REE-ter-all)	ureter/o = ureter -al = pertaining to	Pertaining to the ureter.

> **MED TERM TIP**
> Word Watch: Be particularly careful when using the three very similar combining forms: *uter/o* meaning "uterus," *ureter/o* meaning "ureter," and *urethr/o* meaning "urethra."

TERM	WORD PARTS	DEFINITION
urethral (yoo-REE-thral)	urethr/o = urethra -al = pertaining to	Pertaining to the urethra.
urinary (yoo-rih-NAIR-ee)	urin/o = urine -ary = pertaining to	Pertaining to urine.

 ## Pathology

TERM	WORD PARTS	DEFINITION
Medical Specialties		
nephrology (neh-FROL-oh-jee)	nephr/o = kidney -logy = study of	Branch of medicine involved in diagnosis and treatment of diseases and disorders of the kidney. Physician is a *nephrologist*.
urology (yoo-RAL-oh-jee)	ur/o = urine -logy = study of	Branch of medicine involved in diagnosis and treatment of diseases and disorders of the urinary system (and male reproductive system). Physician is a *urologist*.
Signs and Symptoms		
anuria (an-YOO-ree-ah)	an- = without -uria = urine condition	Complete suppression of urine formed by the kidneys and a complete lack of urine excretion.
azotemia (a-zo-TEE-mee-ah)	azot/o = nitrogenous waste -emia = blood condition	Accumulation of nitrogenous waste in the bloodstream. Occurs when the kidney fails to filter these wastes from the blood.
bacteriuria (back-teer-ree-YOO-ree-ah)	bacteri/o = bacteria -uria = urine condition	Presence of bacteria in the urine.

Pathology *(continued)*

TERM	WORD PARTS	DEFINITION
calculus (KAL-kew-lus)		Stone formed within an organ by an accumulation of mineral salts. Found in the kidney, renal pelvis, ureters, bladder, or urethra. Plural is *calculi*.

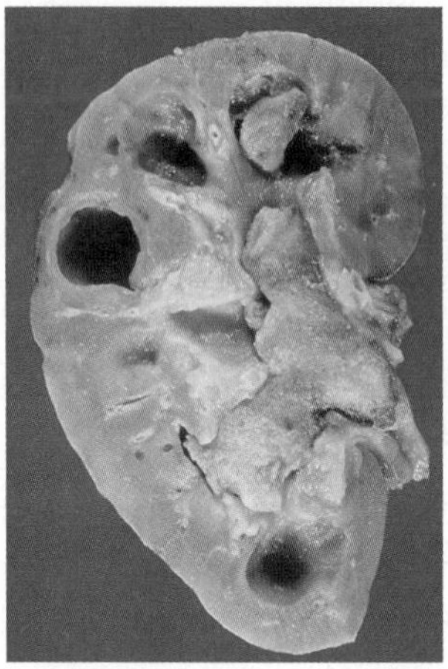

■ **Figure 9.8** Photograph of sectioned kidney specimen illustrating extensive renal calculi. *(Photo Researchers, Inc.)*

TERM	WORD PARTS	DEFINITION
cystalgia (sis-TAL-jee-ah)	cyst/o = bladder -algia = pain	Urinary bladder pain.

> **MED TERM TIP**
> Word Watch: Be careful using the combining forms *cyst/o* meaning "bladder" and *cyt/o* meaning "cell."

TERM	WORD PARTS	DEFINITION
cystolith (SIS-toh-lith)	cyst/o = bladder -lith = stone	Bladder stone.
cystorrhagia (sis-toh-RAH-jee-ah)	cyst/o = bladder -rrhagia = abnormal flow condition	Profuse bleeding from the urinary bladder.
diuresis (dye-yoo-REE-sis)		Increased formation and excretion of urine.
dysuria (dis-YOO-ree-ah)	dys- = abnormal, difficult -uria = urine condition	Difficult or painful urination.
enuresis (en-yoo-REE-sis)		Involuntary discharge of urine after the age by which bladder control should have been established. This usually occurs by the age of 5. *Nocturnal enuresis* refers to bed-wetting at night.
frequency		Greater-than-normal occurrence in the urge to urinate, without an increase in the total daily volume of urine. Frequency is an indication of inflammation of the bladder or urethra.
glycosuria (glye-kohs-YOO-ree-ah)	glycos/o = sugar -uria = urine condition	Presence of sugar in the urine.
hematuria (hee-mah-TOO-ree-ah)	hemat/o = blood -uria = urine condition	Presence of blood in the urine.

■ Pathology (continued)

TERM	WORD PARTS	DEFINITION
hesitancy		Decrease in the force of the urine stream, often with difficulty initiating the flow. It is often a symptom of a blockage along the urethra, such as an enlarged prostate gland.
ketonuria (key-tone-YOO-ree-ah)	keton/o = ketones -uria = urine condition	Presence of ketones in the urine. This occurs when the body burns fat instead of glucose for energy, such as in uncontrolled diabetes mellitus.
nephrolith (NEF-roh-lith)	nephr/o = kidney -lith = stone	Kidney stone.
nephromalacia (nef-roh-mah-LAY-she-ah)	nephr/o = kidney -malacia = softening	Kidney is abnormally soft.
nephromegaly (nef-roh-MEG-ah-lee)	nephr/o = kidney -megaly = enlarged	Kidney is enlarged.
nephrosclerosis (nef-roh-skleh-ROH-sis)	nephr/o = kidney -sclerosis = hardening	Kidney tissue has become hardened.
nocturia (nok-TOO-ree-ah)	noct/i = night -uria = urine condition	Having to urinate frequently during the night.
oliguria (ol-ig-YOO-ree-ah)	olig/o = scanty -uria = urine condition	Producing too little urine.
polyuria (pol-ee-YOO-ree-ah)	poly- = many -uria = urine condition	Producing an unusually large volume of urine.
proteinuria (pro-ten-YOO-ree-ah)	protein/o = protein -uria = urine condition	Presence of protein in the urine.
pyuria (pye-YOO-ree-ah)	py/o = pus -uria = urine condition	Presence of pus in the urine.
renal colic (KOL-ik)	ren/o = kidney -al = pertaining to -ic = pertaining to	Pain caused by a kidney stone. Can be an excruciating pain and generally requires medical treatment.
stricture (STRIK-chur)		Narrowing of a passageway in the urinary system.
uremia (yoo-REE-me-ah)	ur/o = urine -emia = blood condition	Accumulation of waste products (especially nitrogenous wastes) in the bloodstream. Associated with renal failure.
ureterectasis (yoo-ree-ter-EK-tah-sis)	ureter/o = ureter -ectasis = dilated	Ureter is stretched out or dilated.
ureterolith (yoo-REE-teh-roh-lith)	ureter/o = ureter -lith = stone	Stone in the ureter.
ureterostenosis (yoo-ree-ter-oh-sten-OH-sis)	ureter/o = ureter -stenosis = narrowing	Ureter has become narrow.
urethralgia (yoo-ree-THRAL-jee-ah)	urethr/o = urethra -algia = pain	Urethral pain.

■ Pathology *(continued)*

TERM	WORD PARTS	DEFINITION
urethrorrhagia (yoo-ree-throh-RAH-jee-ah)	urethr/o = urethra -rrhagia = abnormal flow condition	Profuse bleeding from the urethra.
urethrostenosis (yoo-ree-throh-steh-NOH-sis)	urethr/o = urethra -stenosis = narrowing	Urethra has become narrow.
urgency (ER-jen-see)		Feeling the need to urinate immediately.
urinary incontinence (in-CON-tin-ens)	urin/o = urine -ary = pertaining to	Involuntary release of urine. In some patients an indwelling catheter is inserted into the bladder for continuous urine drainage.

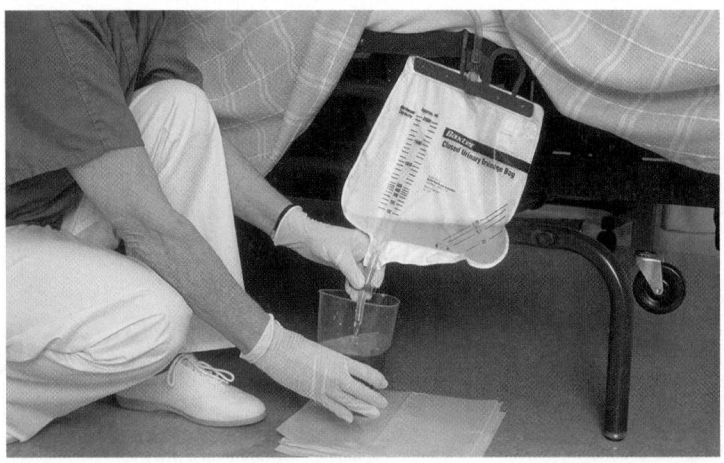

■ **Figure 9.9** Healthcare worker draining urine from a bladder catheter bag.

urinary retention	urin/o = urine -ary = pertaining to	Inability to fully empty the bladder, often indicates a blockage in the urethra.

Kidney

acute tubular necrosis (ATN) (ne-KROH-sis)	-ar = pertaining to necr/o = death -osis = abnormal condition	Damage to the renal tubules due to presence of toxins in the urine or to ischemia. Results in oliguria.
diabetic nephropathy (ne-FROH-path-ee)	-ic = pertaining to nephr/o = kidney -pathy = disease	Accumulation of damage to the glomerulus capillaries due to the chronic high blood sugars of diabetes mellitus.
glomerulonephritis (gloh-mair-yoo-loh-neh-FRYE-tis)	glomerul/o = glomerulus nephr/o = kidney -itis = inflammation	Inflammation of the kidney (primarily of the glomerulus). Since the glomerular membrane is inflamed, it becomes more permeable and will allow protein and blood cells to enter the filtrate. Results in protein in the urine (proteinuria) and hematuria.
hydronephrosis (high-droh-neh-FROH-sis)	hydro- = water nephr/o = kidney -osis = abnormal condition	Distention of the renal pelvis due to urine collecting in the kidney; often a result of the obstruction of a ureter.
nephritis (neh-FRYE-tis)	nephr/o = kidney -itis = inflammation	Kidney inflammation.

Pathology *(continued)*

TERM	WORD PARTS	DEFINITION
nephrolithiasis (nef-roh-lith-EE-a-sis)	nephr/o = kidney -lithiasis = condition of stones	Presence of calculi in the kidney. Usually begins with the solidification of salts present in the urine.
nephroma (neh-FROH-ma)	nephr/o = kidney -oma = tumor	Kidney tumor.
nephropathy (neh-FROP-ah-thee)	nephr/o = kidney -pathy = disease	General term describing the presence of kidney disease.
nephroptosis (nef-rop-TOH-sis)	nephr/o = kidney -ptosis = drooping	Downward displacement of the kidney out of its normal location; commonly called a *floating kidney.*
nephrotic syndrome (NS)	nephr/o = kidney -tic = pertaining to	Damage to the glomerulus resulting in protein appearing in the urine, proteinuria, and the corresponding decrease in protein in the bloodstream. Also called *nephrosis.*
polycystic kidneys (POL-ee-sis-tik)	poly- = many cyst/o = pouch -tic = pertaining to	Formation of multiple cysts within the kidney tissue. Results in the destruction of normal kidney tissue and uremia.

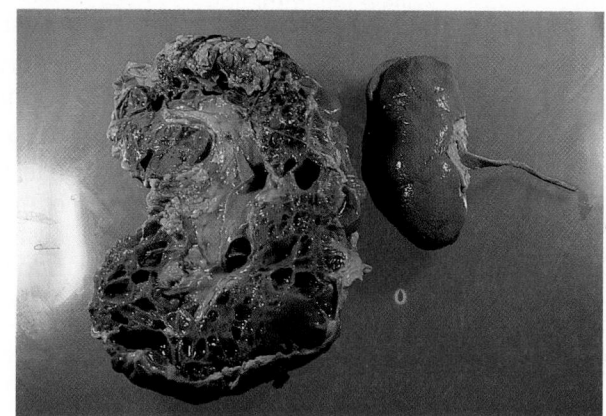

■ **Figure 9.10** Photograph of a polycystic kidney on the left compared to a normal kidney on the right. *(Simon Fraser/ Royal Victoria Infirmary, Newcastle/Science Photo Library/Photo Researchers, Inc.)*

TERM	WORD PARTS	DEFINITION
pyelitis (pye-eh-LYE-tis)	pyel/o = renal pelvis -itis = inflammation	Renal pelvis inflammation.
pyelonephritis (pye-eh-loh-neh-FRYE-tis)	pyel/o = renal pelvis nephr/o = kidney -itis = inflammation	Inflammation of the renal pelvis and the kidney. One of the most common types of kidney disease. It may be the result of a lower urinary tract infection that moved up to the kidney by way of the ureters. There may be large quantities of white blood cells and bacteria in the urine. Blood (hematuria) may even be present in the urine in this condition. Can occur with any untreated or persistent case of cystitis.
renal cell carcinoma	ren/o = kidney -al = pertaining to carcin/o = cancer -oma = tumor	Cancerous tumor that arises from kidney tubule cells.

◼ Pathology *(continued)*

TERM	WORD PARTS	DEFINITION
renal failure	ren/o = kidney -al = pertaining to	Inability of the kidneys to filter wastes from the blood resulting in uremia. May be acute or chronic. Major reason for a patient being placed on dialysis.
Wilm's tumor (VILMZ)		Malignant kidney tumor found most often in children.
Urinary Bladder		
bladder cancer		Cancerous tumor that arises from the cells lining the bladder; major sign is hematuria.
bladder neck obstruction (BNO)		Blockage of the bladder outlet. Often caused by an enlarged prostate gland in males.
cystitis (sis-TYE-tis)	cyst/o = bladder -itis = inflammation	Urinary bladder inflammation.
cystocele (SIS-toh-seel)	cyst/o = bladder -cele = protrusion	Hernia or protrusion of the urinary bladder into the wall of the vagina.
interstitial cystitis (in-ter-STISH-al / sis-TYE-tis)	-al = pertaining to cyst/o = bladder -itis = inflammation	Disease of unknown cause in which there is inflammation and irritation of the bladder. Most commonly seen in middle-aged women.
neurogenic bladder (noo-roh-JEN-ik)	neur/o = nerve -genic = produced by	Loss of nervous control that leads to retention; may be caused by spinal cord injury or multiple sclerosis.
urinary tract infection (UTI)	urin/o = urine -ary = pertaining to	Infection, usually from bacteria, of any organ of the urinary system. Most often begins with cystitis and may ascend into the ureters and kidneys. Most common in women because of their shorter urethra.

◼ Diagnostic Procedures

TERM	WORD PARTS	DEFINITION
Clinical Laboratory Tests		
blood urea nitrogen (BUN) (yoo-REE-ah / NIGH-troh-jen)		Blood test to measure kidney function by the level of nitrogenous waste (urea) that is in the blood.
clean catch specimen (CC)		Urine sample obtained after cleaning off the urinary opening and catching or collecting a urine sample in midstream (halfway through the urination process) to minimize contamination from the genitalia.

Diagnostic Procedures *(continued)*

TERM	WORD PARTS	DEFINITION
creatinine clearance (kree-AT-tih-neen)		Test of kidney function. Creatinine is a waste product cleared from the bloodstream by the kidneys. For this test, urine is collected for 24 hours, and the amount of creatinine in the urine is compared to the amount of creatinine that remains in the bloodstream.
urinalysis (U/A, UA) (yoo-rih-NAL-ih-sis)	urin/o = urine -lysis = to destroy (to break down)	Laboratory test consisting of the physical, chemical, and microscopic examination of urine.
urine culture and sensitivity (C&S)		Laboratory test of urine for bacterial infection. Attempt to grow bacteria on a culture medium in order to identify it and determine which antibiotics it is sensitive to.
urinometer (yoo-rin-OH-meter)	urin/o = urine -meter = instrument to measure	Instrument to measure the specific gravity of urine; part of a urinalysis.
Diagnostic Imaging		
cystogram (SIS-toh-gram)	cyst/o = bladder -gram = record	X-ray record of the urinary bladder.
cystography (sis-TOG-rah-fee)	cyst/o = bladder -graphy = process of recording	Process of instilling a contrast material or dye into the bladder by catheter to visualize the urinary bladder on X-ray.
excretory urography (EU) (EKS-kreh-tor-ee / yoo-ROG-rah-fee)	-ory = pertaining to ur/o = urine -graphy = process of recording	Injecting dye into the bloodstream and then taking an X-ray to trace the action of the kidney as it excretes the dye.
intravenous pyelography (IVP) (in-trah-VEE-nus / pye-eh-LOG-rah-fee)	intra- = within ven/o = vein -ous = pertaining to pyel/o = renal pelvis -graphy = process of recording	Diagnostic X-ray procedure in which a dye is injected into a vein and then X-rays are taken to visualize the renal pelvis as the dye is removed by the kidneys.
kidneys, ureters, bladder (KUB)		X-ray taken of the abdomen demonstrating the kidneys, ureters, and bladder without using any contrast dye. Also called a *flat-plate abdomen*.
nephrogram (NEH-fro-gram)	nephr/o = kidney -gram = record	X-ray record of the kidney.
pyelogram (PYE-eh-loh-gram)	pyel/o = renal pelvis -gram = record	X-ray record of the renal pelvis.

Diagnostic Procedures *(continued)*

TERM	WORD PARTS	DEFINITION
retrograde pyelography (RP) (RET-roh-grayd/ pye-eh-LOG-rah-fee)	retro- = backward pyel/o = renal pelvis -graphy = process of recording	Diagnostic X-ray procedure in which dye is inserted through the urethra to outline the bladder, ureters, and renal pelvis.

■ **Figure 9.11** Color-enhanced retrograde pyelogram X-ray. Radiopaque dye outlines urinary bladder, ureters, and renal pelvis. *(Clinique Ste. Catherine/CNRI/ Science Photo Library/Photo Researchers, Inc.)*

TERM	WORD PARTS	DEFINITION
voiding cystourethrography (VCUG) (sis-toh-yoo-ree-THROG-rah-fee)	cyst/o = bladder urethr/o = urethra -graphy = process of recording	X-ray taken to visualize the urethra while the patient is voiding after a contrast dye has been placed in the bladder.
Endoscopic Procedure		
cystoscope (SIS-toh-scope)	cyst/o = bladder -scope = instrument to visually examine	Instrument used to visually examine the inside of the urinary bladder.
cystoscopy (cysto) (sis-TOSS-koh-pee)	cyst/o = bladder -scopy = process of visually examining	Visual examination of the urinary bladder using an instrument called a *cystoscope*.
urethroscope (yoo-REE-throh-scope)	urethr/o = urethra -scope = instrument to visually examine	Instrument to visually examine the inside of the urethra.

Therapeutic Procedures

TERM	WORD PARTS	DEFINITION
Medical Treatments		
catheter (KATH-eh-ter)		Flexible tube inserted into the body for the purpose of moving fluids into or out of the body. Most commonly used to refer to a tube threaded through the urethra into the bladder to withdraw urine (see again Figure 9.9).
catheterization (cath) (kath-eh-ter-ih-ZAY-shun)		Insertion of a tube through the urethra and into the urinary bladder for the purpose of withdrawing urine or inserting dye.

Therapeutic Procedures *(continued)*

TERM	WORD PARTS	DEFINITION
extracorporeal shockwave litho-tripsy (ESWL) (eks-trah-cor-POR-ee-al / shockwave / LITH-oh-trip-see)	extra- = outside of corpor/o = body -eal = pertaining to lith/o = stone -tripsy = surgical crushing	Use of ultrasound waves to break up stones. Process does not require invasive surgery.

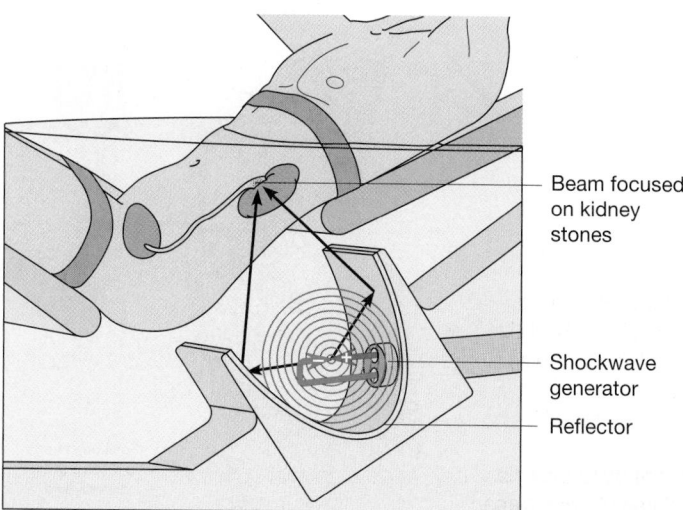

Beam focused
on kidney
stones

Shockwave
generator

Reflector

■ **Figure 9.12** Extracorporeal shockwave lithotripsy, a noninvasive procedure using high-frequency sound waves to shatter kidney stones.

hemodialysis (HD) (hee-moh-dye-AL-ih-sis)	hem/o = blood	Use of an artificial kidney machine that filters the blood of a person to remove waste products. Use of this technique in patients who have defective kidneys is lifesaving.

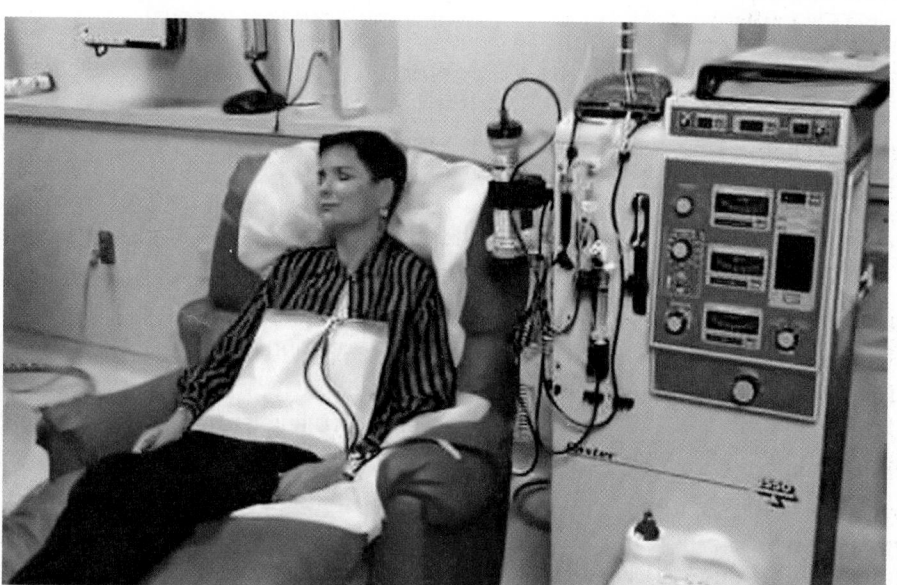

■ **Figure 9.13** Patient undergoing hemodialysis. Patient's blood passes through hemodialysis machine for cleansing and is then returned to her body.

Therapeutic Procedures *(continued)*

TERM	WORD PARTS	DEFINITION
peritoneal dialysis (pair-ih-TOH-nee-al / dye-AL-ih-sis)	peritone/o = peritoneum -eal = pertaining to	Removal of toxic waste substances from the body by placing warm chemically balanced solutions into the peritoneal cavity. Wastes are filtered out of the blood across the peritoneum. Used in treating renal failure and certain poisonings.

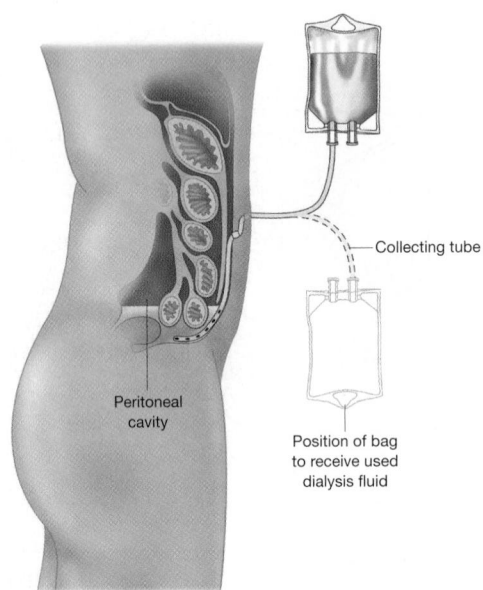

Collecting tube

Peritoneal cavity

Position of bag to receive used dialysis fluid

■ **Figure 9.14** Peritoneal dialysis. Chemically balanced solution is placed into the abdominal cavity to draw impurities out of the bloodstream. It is removed after several hours.

Surgical Treatments

TERM	WORD PARTS	DEFINITION
cystectomy (sis-TEK-toh-me)	cyst/o = bladder -ectomy = surgical removal	Surgical removal of the urinary bladder.
cystopexy (SIS-toh-pek-see)	cyst/o = bladder -pexy = surgical fixation	Surgical fixation of the urinary bladder.
cystoplasty (SIS-toh-plas-tee)	cyst/o = bladder -plasty = surgical repair	To repair the urinary bladder by surgical means.
cystostomy (sis-TOSS-toh-mee)	cyst/o = bladder -ostomy = create a new opening	To create a new opening into the urinary bladder through the abdominal wall.
cystotomy (sis-TOT-oh-mee)	cyst/o = bladder -otomy = cutting into	To cut into the urinary bladder.
lithotomy (lith-OT-oh-me)	lith/o = stone -otomy = cutting into	To cut into an organ for the purpose of removing a stone.
lithotripsy (LITH-oh-trip-see)	lith/o = stone -tripsy = surgical crushing	Destroying or crushing stones in the bladder or urethra.
meatotomy (mee-ah-TOT-oh-me)	meat/o = meatus -otomy = cutting into	To cut into the meatus in order to enlarge the opening of the urethra.
nephrectomy (ne-FREK-toh-mee)	nephr/o = kidney -ectomy = surgical removal	Surgical removal of a kidney.
nephrolithotomy (nef-roh-lith-OT-oh-mee)	nephr/o = kidney lith/o = stone -otomy = cutting into	To cut into the kidney in order to remove stones.

Therapeutic Procedures *(continued)*

TERM	WORD PARTS	DEFINITION
nephropexy (NEF-roh-pek-see)	nephr/o = kidney -pexy = surgical fixation	Surgical fixation of a kidney; to anchor it in its normal anatomical position.
nephrostomy (neh-FROS-toh-mee)	nephr/o = kidney -ostomy = create a new opening	To create a new opening into the kidney through the abdominal wall.
nephrotomy (neh-FROT-oh-mee)	nephr/o = kidney -otomy = cutting into	To cut into the kidney.
pyeloplasty (PIE-ah-loh-plas-tee)	pyel/o = renal pelvis -plasty = surgical repair	To repair the renal pelvis by surgical means.
renal transplant	ren/o = kidney -al = pertaining to	Surgical placement of a donor kidney.

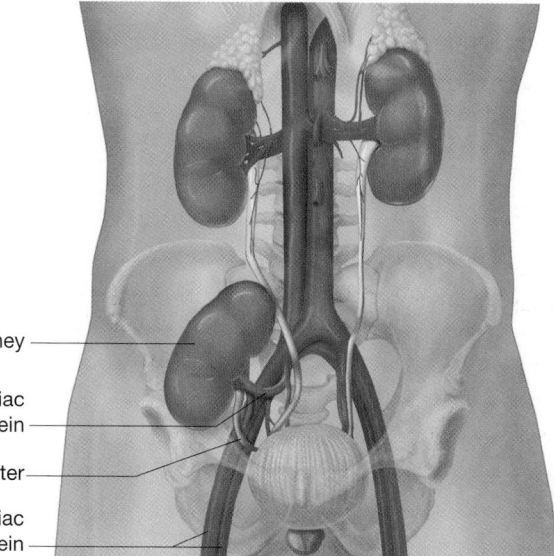

Transplanted kidney

Internal iliac artery and vein

Grafted ureter

External iliac artery and vein

■ **Figure 9.15** Figure illustrates location utilized for implantation of donor kidney.

Pharmacology

CLASSIFICATION	WORD PARTS	ACTION	EXAMPLES
antibiotic	anti- = against bi/o = life -tic = pertaining to	Used to treat bacterial infections of the urinary tract.	ciprofloxacin, Cipro; nitrofurantoin, Macrobid
antispasmodic (an-tye-spaz-MAH-dik)	anti- = against -ic = pertaining to	Medication to prevent or reduce bladder muscle spasms.	oxybutynin, Ditropan; neostigmine, Prostigmine
diuretic (dye-yoo-REH-tiks)	-tic = pertaining to	Medication that increases the volume of urine produced by the kidneys. Useful in the treatment of edema, kidney failure, heart failure, and hypertension.	furosemide, Lasix; spironolactone, Aldactone

Abbreviations

AGN	acute glomerulonephritis	**HD**	hemodialysis
ARF	acute renal failure	**H$_2$O**	water
ATN	acute tubular necrosis	**I&O**	intake and output
BNO	bladder neck obstruction	**IPD**	intermittent peritoneal dialysis
BUN	blood urea nitrogen	**IVP**	intravenous pyelogram
CAPD	continuous ambulatory peritoneal dialysis	**K$^+$**	potassium
cath	catheterization	**KUB**	kidney, ureter, bladder
CC	clean catch urine specimen	**mL**	milliliter
Cl$^-$	chloride	**Na$^+$**	sodium
CRF	chronic renal failure	**NS**	nephrotic syndrome
C&S	culture and sensitivity	**pH**	acidity or alkalinity of urine
cysto	cystoscopy	**RP**	retrograde pyelogram
ESRD	end-stage renal disease	**SG, sp. gr.**	specific gravity
ESWL	extracorporeal shockwave lithotripsy	**U/A, UA**	urinalysis
EU	excretory urography	**UC**	urine culture
GU	genitourinary	**UTI**	urinary tract infection
HCO$_3^-$	bicarbonate	**VCUG**	voiding cystourethrography

Chapter Review

Real-World Applications

Medical Record Analysis

This Discharge Summary contains 13 medical terms. Underline each term and write it in the list below the report. Then define each term.

Discharge Summary

Admitting Diagnosis:	Severe right side pain and hematuria.
Final Diagnosis:	Pyelonephritis right kidney, complicated by chronic cystitis.
History of Present Illness:	Patient has long history of frequent bladder infections, but denies any recent lower pelvic pain or dysuria. Earlier today he had rapid onset of severe right side pain and is unable to stand fully erect. His temperature was 101°F, and his skin was sweaty and flushed. He was admitted from the ER for further testing and diagnosis.
Summary of Hospital Course:	Clean catch urinalysis revealed gross hematuria and pyuria, but no albuminuria. A culture and sensitivity was ordered to identify the pathogen and an antibiotic was started. Cystoscopy showed evidence of chronic cystitis, bladder irritation, and a bladder neck obstruction. The obstruction appears to be congenital and the probable cause of the chronic cystitis. The patient was catheterized to ensure complete emptying of the bladder, and fluids were encouraged. Patient responded well to the antibiotic therapy and fluids, and his symptoms improved.
Discharge Plans:	Patient was discharged home after 3 days in the hospital. He was switched to an oral antibiotic for the pyelonephritis and chronic cystitis. A repeat urinalysis is scheduled for next week. After all inflammation is corrected, will repeat cystoscopy to reevaluate bladder neck obstruction.

	Term	Definition
1	_____	_____
2	_____	_____
3	_____	_____
4	_____	_____
5	_____	_____
6	_____	_____
7	_____	_____
8	_____	_____
9	_____	_____
10	_____	_____
11	_____	_____
12	_____	_____
13	_____	_____

Chart Note Transcription

The chart note below contains 11 phrases that can be reworded with a medical term that you learned in this chapter. Each phrase is identified with an underline. Determine the medical term and write your answers in the space provided.

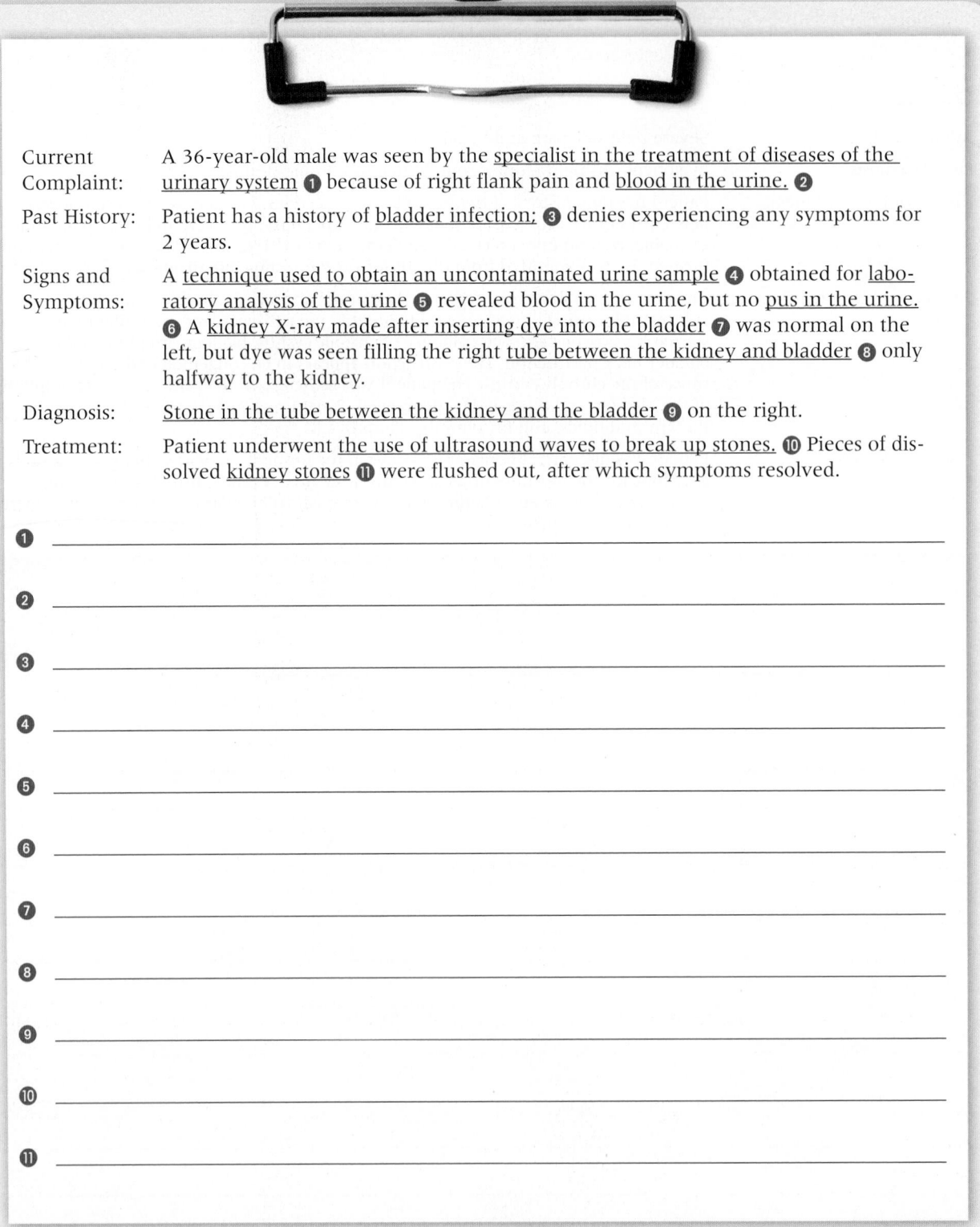

Current Complaint: A 36-year-old male was seen by the <u>specialist in the treatment of diseases of the urinary system</u> ❶ because of right flank pain and <u>blood in the urine.</u> ❷

Past History: Patient has a history of <u>bladder infection;</u> ❸ denies experiencing any symptoms for 2 years.

Signs and Symptoms: A <u>technique used to obtain an uncontaminated urine sample</u> ❹ obtained for <u>laboratory analysis of the urine</u> ❺ revealed blood in the urine, but no <u>pus in the urine.</u> ❻ A <u>kidney X-ray made after inserting dye into the bladder</u> ❼ was normal on the left, but dye was seen filling the right <u>tube between the kidney and bladder</u> ❽ only halfway to the kidney.

Diagnosis: <u>Stone in the tube between the kidney and the bladder</u> ❾ on the right.

Treatment: Patient underwent <u>the use of ultrasound waves to break up stones.</u> ❿ Pieces of dissolved <u>kidney stones</u> ⓫ were flushed out, after which symptoms resolved.

❶ _____

❷ _____

❸ _____

❹ _____

❺ _____

❻ _____

❼ _____

❽ _____

❾ _____

❿ _____

⓫ _____

Case Study

Below is a case study presentation of a patient with a condition discussed in this chapter. Read the case study and answer the questions below. Some questions will ask for information not included within this chapter. Use your text, a medical dictionary, or any other reference material you choose to answer these questions.

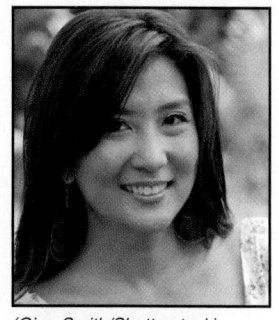

A 32-year-old female is seen in the urologist's office because of a fever, chills, and generalized fatigue. She also reported urgency, frequency, dysuria, and hematuria. In addition, she noticed that her urine was cloudy with a fishy odor. The physician ordered the following tests: a clean catch specimen for a U/A, a urine C&S, and a KUB. The U/A revealed pyuria, bacteriuria, and a slightly acidic pH. A common type of bacteria was grown in the culture. X-rays reveal acute pyelonephritis resulting from cystitis, which has spread up to the kidney from the bladder. The patient was placed on an antibiotic and encouraged to "push fluids" by drinking 2L of water a day.

(Gina Smith/Shutterstock)

Questions

1. This patient has two urinary system infections in different locations; name them. Which one caused the other and how?

    _____

    _____

2. List and define each of the patient's presenting symptoms in your own words.

    _____

    _____

3. What diagnostic tests did the urologist order? Describe them in your own words.

    _____

    _____

4. Explain the results of each diagnostic test in your own words.

    _____

    _____

5. What were the physician's treatment instructions for this patient? Explain the purpose of each treatment.

    _____

    _____

6. Describe the normal appearance of urine.

    _____

    _____

Practice Exercises

A. Complete the Statement

1. The functional or working units of the kidneys are the _____.

2. The three stages of urine production are _____, _____,

   and _____.

3. Na⁺, K⁺, and Cl⁻ are collectively known as _____.

4. The term that describes the location of the kidneys is _____.

5. The center of the concave side of the kidney is the _____.

6. The glomerular capsule surrounds the _____.

7. The tip of each renal pyramid opens into a(n) _____.

8. There are _____ ureters and _____ urethra.

9. Urination can also be referred to as _____ or _____.

10. A(n) _____ is the physical and chemical analysis of urine.

B. Combining Form Practice

The combining form **nephr/o** refers to the kidney. Use it to write a term that means:

1. surgical fixation of the kidney _____

2. X-ray record of the kidney _____

3. condition of kidney stones _____

4. removal of a kidney _____

5. inflammation of the kidney _____

6. kidney disease _____

7. hardening of the kidney _____

The combining form **cyst/o** refers to the urinary bladder. Use it to write a term that means:

8. inflammation of the bladder _____

9. abnormal flow condition from the bladder _____

10. surgical repair of the bladder _____

11. instrument to view inside the bladder _____

12. bladder pain _____

The combining form **pyel/o** refers to the renal pelvis. Use it to write a term that means:

13. surgical repair of the renal pelvis _____

14. inflammation of the renal pelvis _____

15. X-ray record of the renal pelvis _____

The combining form **ureter/o** refers to one or both of the ureters. Use it to write a term that means:

16. a ureteral stone _____

17. ureter dilation _____

18. ureter narrowing _____

The combining form **urethr/o** refers to the urethra. Use it to write a term that means:

19. urethra inflammation _____

20. instrument to view inside the urethra _____

C. Define the Combining Form

	Definition	Example from Chapter
1. ur/o		
2. meat/o		
3. cyst/o		
4. ren/o		
5. pyel/o		
6. glycos/o		
7. noct/i		
8. olig/o		
9. ureter/o		
10. glomerul/o		

D. Pharmacology Challenge

Fill in the classification for each drug description, then match the brand name.

	Drug Description	Classification	Brand Name
1.	_____ Reduces bladder muscle spasms	_____	a. Lasix
2.	_____ Treats bacterial infections	_____	b. Ditropan
3.	_____ Increases volume of urine produced	_____	c. Cipro

E. Define the Term

1. micturition _____

2. diuretic _____

3. renal colic _____

4. catheterization _____

5. pyelitis _____

6. glomerulonephritis _____

7. lithotomy _____

8. enuresis _____

9. meatotomy _____

10. diabetic nephropathy _____

11. urinalysis _____

12. hesitancy _____

F. Name That Term

1. absence of urine _____

2. blood in the urine _____

3. kidney stone _____

4. crushing a stone _____

5. inflammation of the urethra _____

6. pus in the urine _____

7. bacteria in the urine _____

8. painful urination _____

9. ketones in the urine _____

10. protein in the urine _____

11. (too) much urine _____

G. What's the Abbreviation?

1. potassium _____

2. sodium _____

3. urinalysis _____

4. blood urea nitrogen _____

5. specific gravity _____

6. intravenous pyelogram _____

7. bladder neck obstruction _____

8. intake and output _____

9. acute tubular necrosis _____

10. end stage renal disease _____

H. What Does it Stand For?

1. KUB _____

2. cath _____

3. cysto _____

4. GU _____

5. ESWL _____

6. UTI _____

7. UC _____

8. RP _____

9. ARF _____

10. BUN _____

11. CRF _____

12. H_2O _____

I. Terminology Matching

Match each term to its definition.

1. _____ Wilm's tumor	a.	kidney stones
2. _____ electrolytes	b.	feeling the need to urinate immediately
3. _____ nephrons	c.	childhood malignant kidney tumor
4. _____ nephron loop	d.	swelling of the kidney due to urine collecting in the renal pelvis
5. _____ calyx	e.	involuntary release of urine
6. _____ incontinence	f.	collects urine as it is produced
7. _____ hydronephrosis	g.	sodium and potassium
8. _____ urgency	h.	functional unit of the kidneys
9. _____ nephrolithiasis	i.	part of the renal tubule
10. _____ polycystic kidneys	j.	multiple cysts in the kidneys

J. Define the Suffix

	Definition	Example from Chapter
1. -ptosis	_____	_____
2. -uria	_____	_____
3. -lith	_____	_____
4. -tripsy	_____	_____
5. -lithiasis	_____	_____

K. Fill in the Blank

renal transplant	ureterectomy	intravenous pyelogram (IVP)
cystostomy	pyelolithectomy	nephropexy
renal biopsy	cystoscopy	urinary tract infection

1. Juan suffered from chronic renal failure. His sister, Maria, donated one of her normal kidneys to him, and he had a(n)

   _____.

2. Anesha's floating kidney needed surgical fixation. Her physician performed a surgical procedure known as

   _____.

3. Kenya's physician stated that she had a general infection that he referred to as a UTI. The full name for this infection is

   _____.

4. The surgeons operated on Robert to remove calculi from his renal pelvis. The name of this surgery is

   _____.

5. Charles had to have a small piece of his kidney tissue removed so that the physician could perform a microscopic evalua-

   tion. This procedure is called a(n) _____.

6. Naomi had to have one of her ureters removed due to a stricture. This procedure is called _____.

7. The physician had to create a temporary opening between Eric's bladder and his abdominal wall. This procedure is called

   _____.

8. Sally's bladder was visually examined using a special instrument. This procedure is called a(n) _____.

9. The doctors believe that Jacob has a tumor of the right kidney. They are going to do a test called a(n) _____

   that requires them to inject a radiopaque contrast medium intravenously so that they can see the kidney on X-ray.

Labeling Exercise

Image A

Write the labels for this figure on the numbered lines provided.

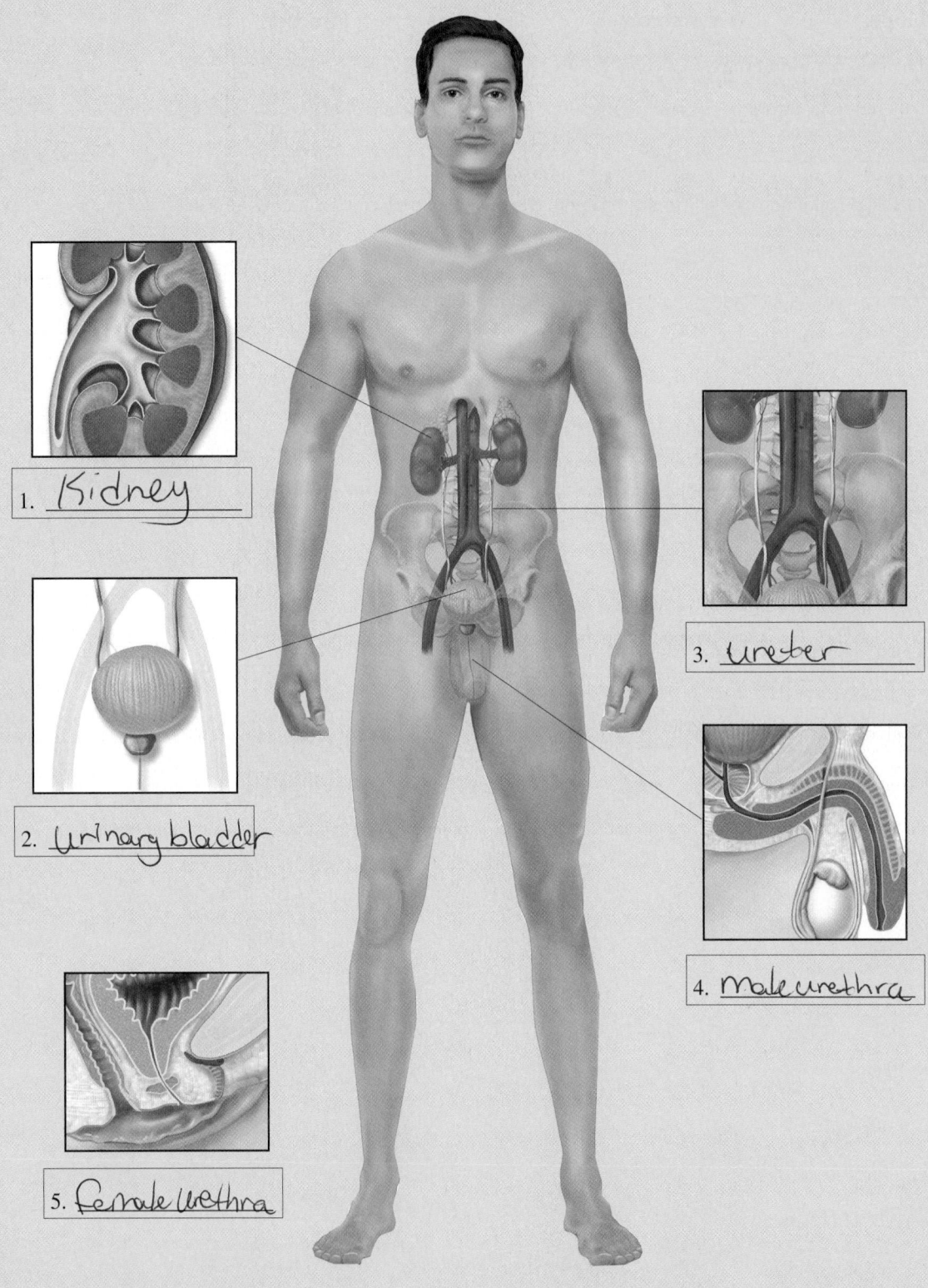

1. _Kidney_

2. _Urinary bladder_

3. _ureter_

4. _male urethra_

5. _female urethra_

Image B

Write the labels for this figure on the numbered lines provided.

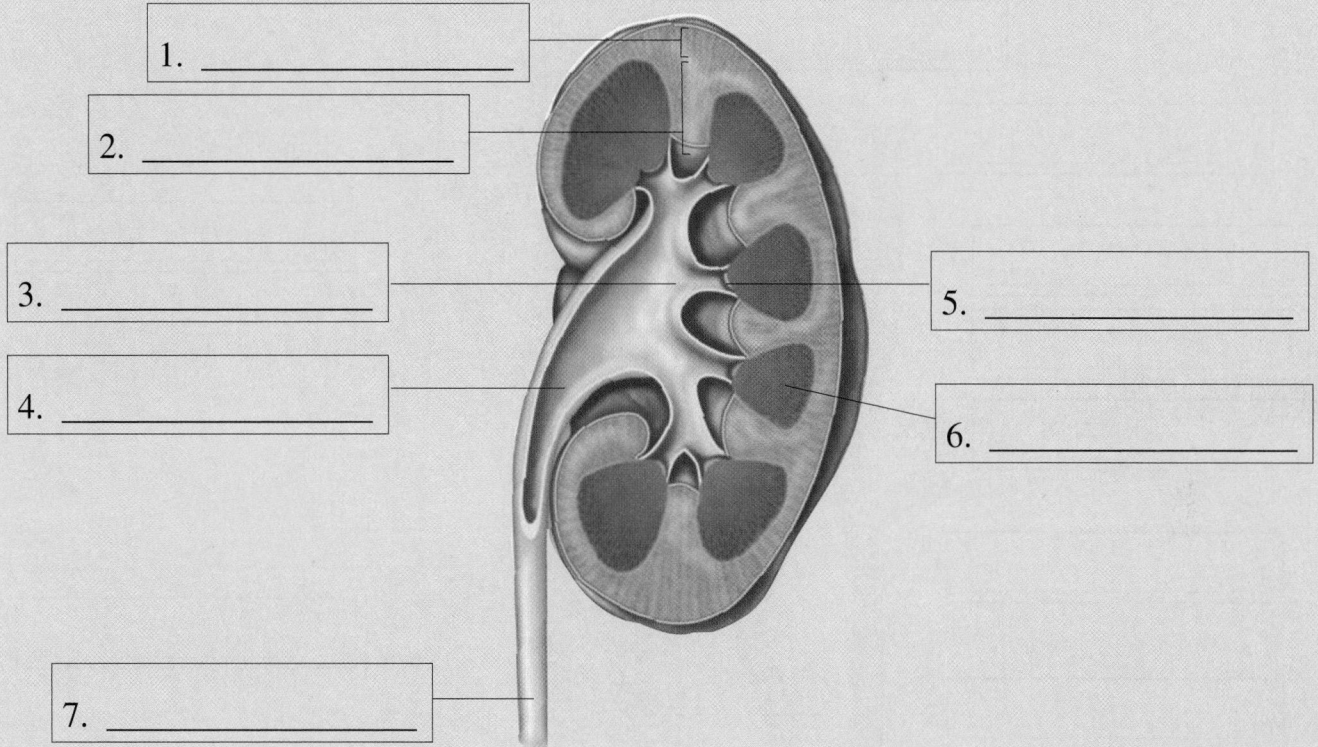

1. _____

2. _____

3. _____

4. _____

5. _____

6. _____

7. _____

Image C

Write the labels for this figure on the numbered lines provided.

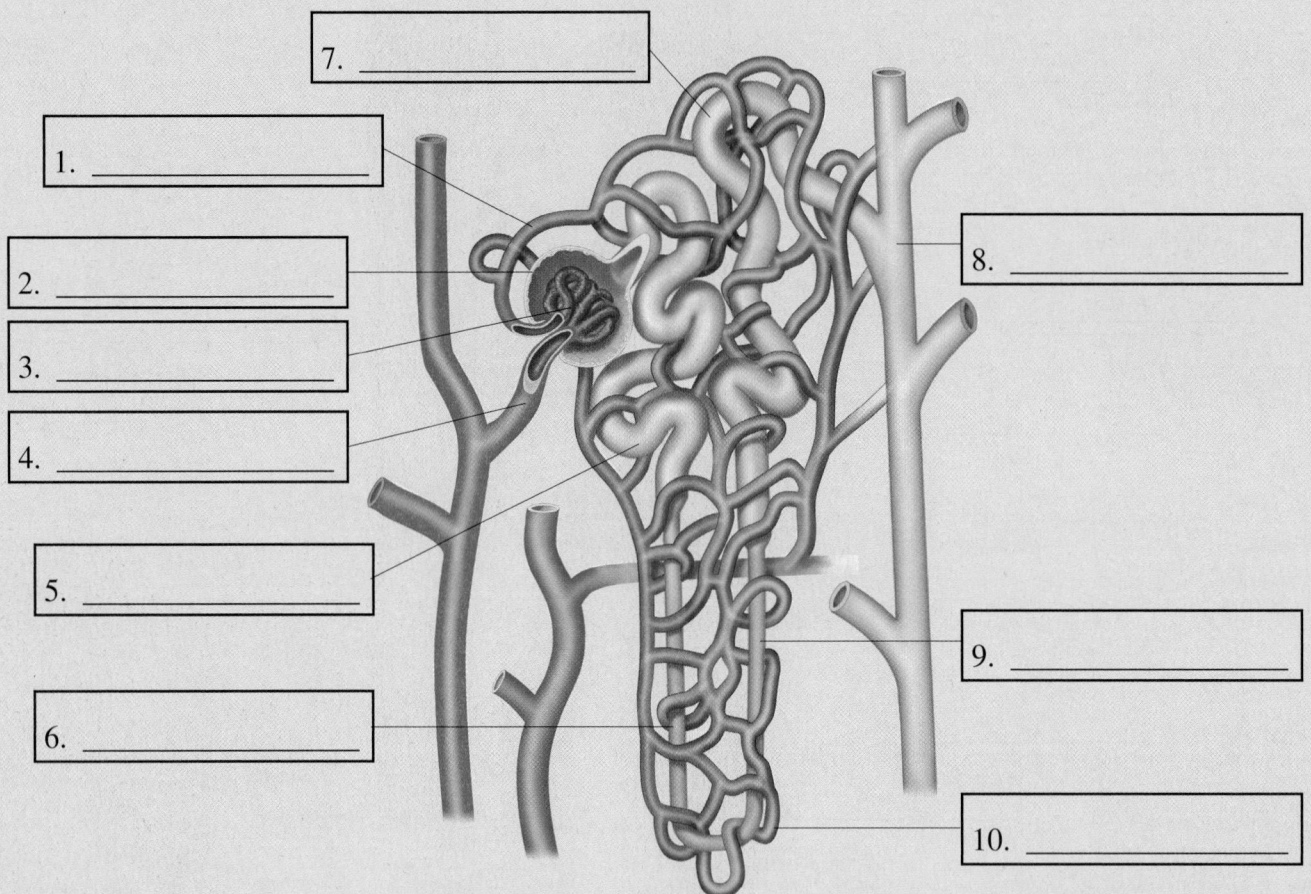

7. _____

1. _____

2. _____

3. _____

4. _____

5. _____

6. _____

8. _____

9. _____

10. _____

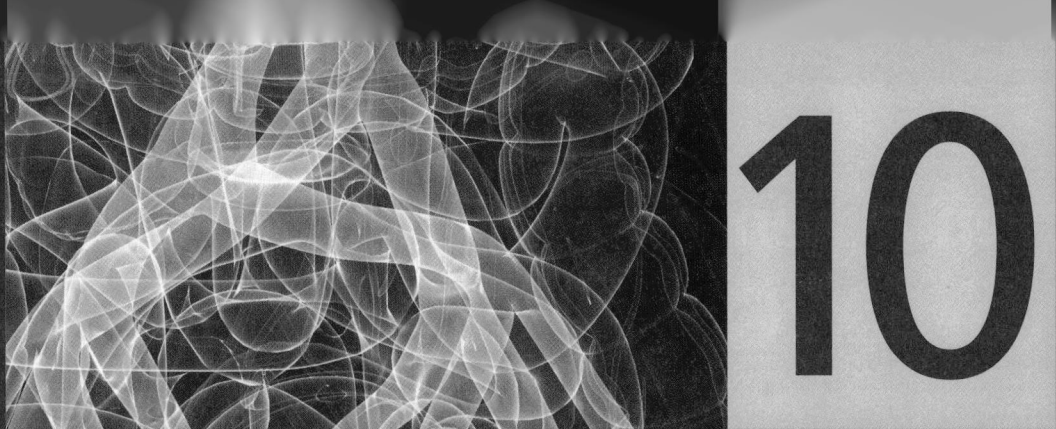

10

REPRODUCTIVE SYSTEM

Learning Objectives

Upon completion of this chapter, you will be able to

- Identify and define the combining forms and suffixes introduced in this chapter.

- Correctly spell and pronounce medical terms and major anatomical structures relating to the reproductive systems.

- Locate and describe the major organs of the reproductive systems and their functions.

- Use medical terms to describe circumstances relating to pregnancy.

- Identify the symptoms and origin of sexually transmitted diseases.

- Identify and define reproductive system anatomical terms.

- Identify and define selected reproductive system pathology terms.

- Identify and define selected reproductive system diagnostic procedures.

- Identify and define selected reproductive system therapeutic procedures.

- Identify and define selected medications relating to the reproductive systems.

- Define selected abbreviations associated with the reproductive systems.

Section I: Female Reproductive System at a Glance

Function

The female reproductive system produces ova (the female reproductive cells), provides a location for fertilization and growth of a baby, and secretes female sex hormones. In addition, the breasts produce milk to nourish the newborn.

Organs

Here are the primary structures that comprise the cardiovascular system.

breasts	uterus
uterine tubes	vagina
ovaries	vulva

Word Parts

Here are the most common word parts (with their meanings) used to build female reproductive system terms. For a more comprehensive list, refer to the Terminology section of this chapter.

Combining Forms

amni/o	amnion	men/o	menses, menstruation
cervic/o	neck, cervix		
chori/o	chorion	metr/o	uterus
colp/o	vagina	nat/o	birth
culd/o	cul-de-sac	o/o	egg
embry/o	embryo	oophor/o	ovary
episi/o	vulva	ovari/o	ovary
fet/o	fetus	perine/o	perineum
gynec/o	woman, female	salping/o	uterine tubes, uterine tubes
hymen/o	hymen		
hyster/o	uterus	uter/o	uterus
lact/o	milk	vagin/o	vagina
mamm/o	breast	vulv/o	vulva
mast/o	breast		

Suffixes

-arche	beginning
-cyesis	state of pregnancy
-gravida	pregnancy
-para	to bear (offspring)
-partum	childbirth
-salpinx	uterine tube
-tocia	labor, childbirth

Female Reproductive System Illustrated

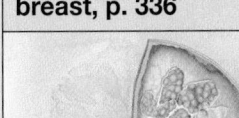
breast, p. 336

Produces milk

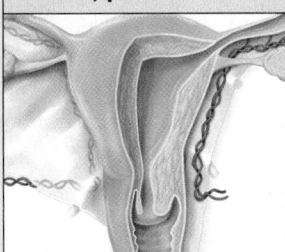
uterus, p. 334

Site of development of fetus

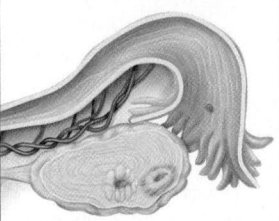
uterine tube, p. 333

Transports ovum to uterus

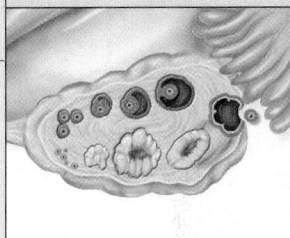
ovary, p. 332

Produces ova and secretes
estrogen and progesterone

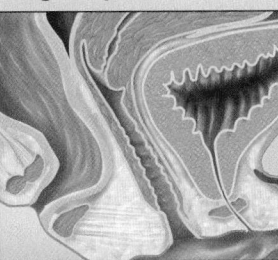
vagina, p. 335

Receives semen during
intercourse; birth canal

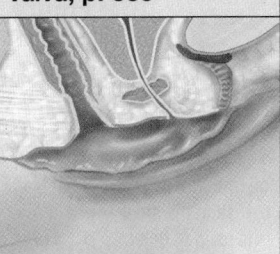
vulva, p. 335

Protects vaginal orifice
and urinary meatus

Anatomy and Physiology of the Female Reproductive System

breasts

fertilization

genitalia (jen-ih-TAY-lee-ah)

ova (OH-vah)

ovaries (OH-vah-reez)

pregnancy

sex hormones

uterine tubes (YOO-ter-in)

uterus (YOO-ter-us)

vagina (vah-JIGH-nah)

vulva (VULL-vah)

The female reproductive system plays many vital functions that ensure the continuation of the human race. First, it produces **ova,** the female reproductive cells. It then provides a place for **fertilization** to occur and for a baby to grow during **pregnancy.** The **breasts** provide nourishment for the newborn. Finally, this system secretes the female **sex hormones.**

This system consists of both internal and external **genitalia,** or reproductive organs (see Figure 10.1 ■). The internal genitalia are located in the pelvic cavity and consist of the **uterus,** two **ovaries,** two **uterine tubes,** and the **vagina,** which extends to the external surface of the body. The external genitalia are collectively referred to as the **vulva.**

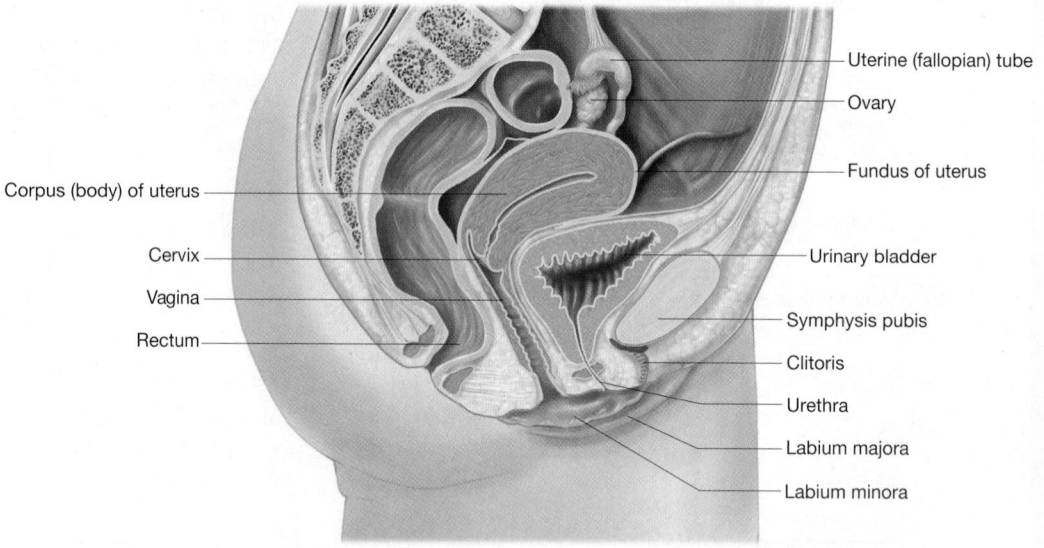

■ Figure 10.1   The female reproductive system, sagittal view showing organs of the system in relation to the urinary bladder and rectum.

MED TERM TIP

The singular for egg is *ovum.* The plural term for many eggs is *ova.* The term *ova* is not used exclusively when discussing the human reproductive system. For instance, testing the stool for ova and parasites is used to detect the presence of parasites or their ova in the digestive tract, a common cause for severe diarrhea. Ova are produced in the ovary by a process called *oogenesis* (*o/o* = egg and *-genesis* = produced).

Internal Genitalia

Ovaries

estrogen (ESS-troh-jen)

follicle stimulating hormone (FOLL-ih-kl)

luteinizing hormone (loo-teh-NIGH-zing)

ovulation (ov-yoo-LAY-shun)

progesterone (proh-JES-ter-ohn)

There are two ovaries, one located on each side of the uterus within the pelvic cavity (see again Figure 10.1). These are small almond-shaped glands that

produce ova (singular is *ovum*) and the female sex hormones (see Figure 10.2 ■). In humans approximately every 28 days hormones from the anterior pituitary, **follicle stimulating hormone** (FSH) and **luteinizing hormone** (LH), stimulate maturation of ovum and trigger **ovulation,** the process by which one ovary releases an ovum (see Figure 10.3 ■). The principal female sex hormones produced by the ovaries, **estrogen** and **progesterone,** stimulate the lining of the uterus to be prepared to receive a fertilized ovum. These hormones are also responsible for the female secondary sexual characteristics.

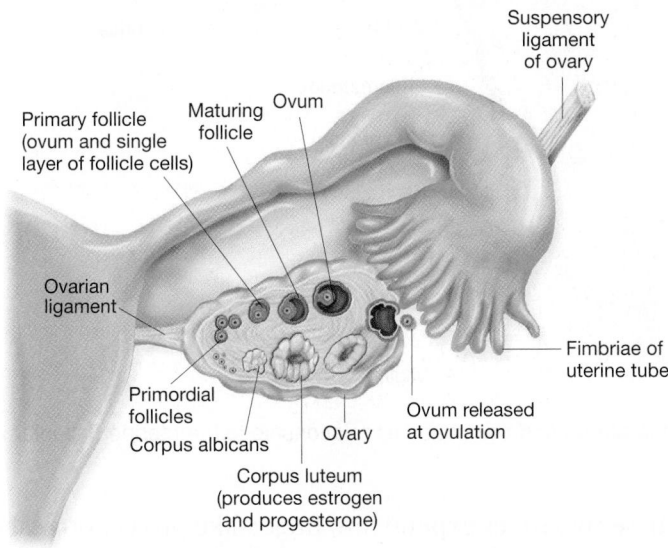

■ Figure 10.2 Structure of the ovary and uterine (fallopian) tube. Figure illustrates stages of ovum development and the relationship of the ovary to the uterine tube.

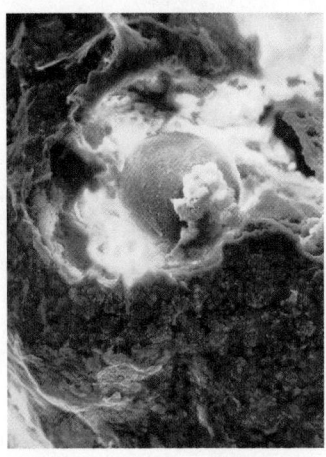

■ Figure 10.3 Color-enhanced scanning electron micrograph showing an ovum (pink) released by the ovary at ovulation surrounded by follicle (white) tissue. The external surface of the ovary is brown in this photo. *(P.M. Motta and J. Van Blekrom/Science Photo Library/Photo Researchers, Inc.)*

Uterine Tubes

conception (con-SEP-shun) **fimbriae** (FIM-bree-ay)
fallopian tubes (fah-LOH-pee-an) **oviducts** (OH-vih-ducts)

The uterine tubes, also called the **fallopian tubes** or **oviducts,** are approximately 5 1/2 inches long and run from the area around each ovary to either side of the upper portion of the uterus (see Figures 10.4 ■ and 10.5 ■). As they near the ovaries,

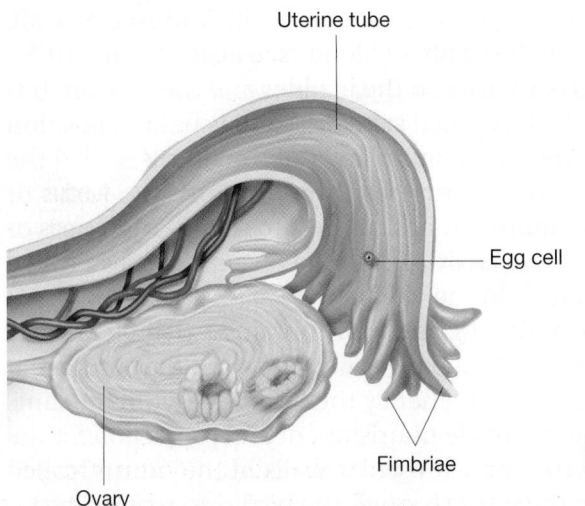

■ Figure 10.4 Uterine (fallopian) tube, showing released ovum within the uterine tube.

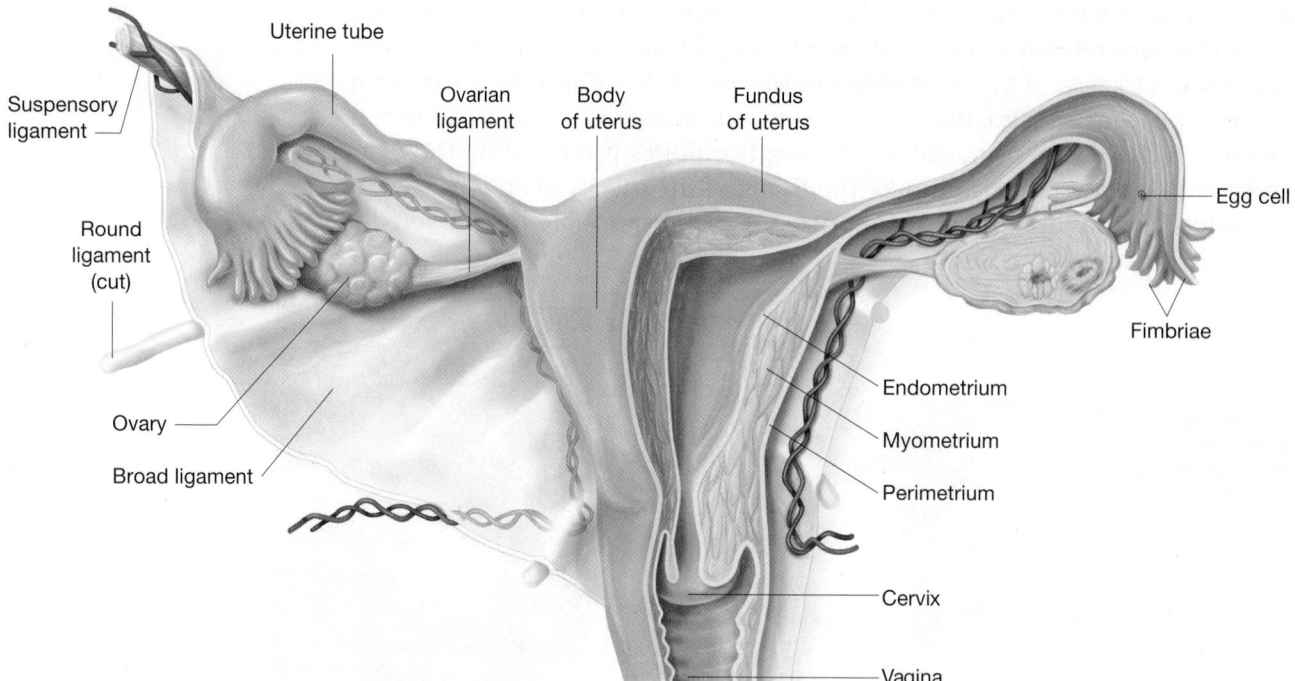

Suspensory ligament

Round ligament (cut)

Ovary

Broad ligament

Uterine tube

Ovarian ligament

Body of uterus

Fundus of uterus

Egg cell

Fimbriae

Endometrium

Myometrium

Perimetrium

Cervix

Vagina

■ **Figure 10.5**   The uterus. Cutaway view shows regions of the uterus and cervix and its relationship to the uterine (fallopian) tubes and vagina.

the unattached ends of these two tubes expand into finger-like projections called **fimbriae.** The fimbriae catch an ovum after ovulation and direct it into the uterine tube. The uterine tube can then propel the ovum from the ovary to the uterus so that it can implant. The meeting of the egg and sperm, called fertilization or **conception,** normally takes place within the upper one-half of the uterine tubes.

Uterus

anteflexion (an-tee-FLEK-shun)	**menopause** (MEN-oh-pawz)
cervix (SER-viks)	**menstrual period** (MEN-stroo-all)
corpus (KOR-pus)	**menstruation** (men-stroo-AY-shun)
endometrium (en-doh-MEE-tre-um)	**myometrium** (my-oh-MEE-tre-um)
fundus (FUN-dus)	**perimetrium** (pear-ee-MEE-tre-um)
menarche (men-AR-kee)	**puberty** (PEW-ber-tee)

The uterus is a hollow, pear-shaped organ that contains a thick muscular wall, a mucous membrane lining, and a rich supply of blood (see again Figure 10.5). It lies in the center of the pelvic cavity between the bladder and the rectum. It is normally bent slightly forward, which is called **anteflexion,** and is held in position by strong fibrous ligaments anchored in the outer layer of the uterus, called the **perimetrium** (see again Figure 10.1). The uterus has three sections: the **fundus** or upper portion, between where the uterine tubes connect to the uterus; **corpus** or body, which is the central portion; and **cervix** (Cx), or lower portion, also called the neck of the uterus, which opens into the vagina.

The inner layer, or **endometrium,** of the uterine wall contains a rich blood supply. The endometrium reacts to hormonal changes every month that prepare it to receive a fertilized ovum. In a normal pregnancy the fertilized ovum implants in the endometrium, which can then provide nourishment and protection for the developing fetus. Contractions of the thick muscular walls of the uterus, called the **myometrium,** assist in propelling the fetus through the birth canal at delivery.

If a pregnancy is not established, the endometrium is sloughed off, resulting in **menstruation** or the **menstrual period.** During a pregnancy, the lining of the uterus does not leave the body but remains to nourish the fetus. A girl's first menstrual period occurs during **puberty** (the sequence of events by which a child becomes a young adult capable of reproduction) and is called **menarche** (*men/o* = menstruation, *-arche* = beginning), while the ending of menstrual activity and childbearing years is called **menopause.** This generally occurs between the ages of 40 and 55.

MED TERM TIP

Word Watch: Be careful using the combining forms *uter/o* meaning "uterus" and *ureter/o* meaning "ureter."

Vagina

Bartholin's glands (BAR-toh-linz)
hymen (HIGH-men)
vaginal orifice (VAJ-ih-nal / OR-ih-fis)

The vagina is a muscular tube lined with mucous membrane that extends from the cervix of the uterus to the outside of the body (see Figure 10.6 ■). The vagina allows for the passage of the menstrual flow. In addition, during intercourse, it receives the male's penis and semen, which is the fluid containing sperm. The vagina also serves as the birth canal through which the baby passes during a normal vaginal birth.

The **hymen** is a thin membranous tissue that partially covers the external vaginal opening or **vaginal orifice.** This membrane is broken by the use of tampons, during physical activity, or during sexual intercourse. A pair of glands (called **Bartholin's glands**) are located on either side of the vaginal orifice and secrete mucus for lubrication during intercourse.

MED TERM TIP

Word Watch: Be careful using the combining forms *colp/o* meaning "vagina" and *culd/o* meaning "cul-de-sac (rectouterine pouch)."

Vulva

clitoris (KLIT-oh-ris)
erectile tissue (ee-REK-tile)
labia majora (LAY-bee-ah / mah-JOR-ah)
labia minora (LAY-bee-ah / min-NOR-ah)
perineum (pair-ih-NEE-um)
urinary meatus (YOO-rih-nair-ee / mee-AY-tus)

The vulva is a general term that refers to the group of structures that make up the female external genitalia. The **labia majora** and **labia minora** are folds of skin that serve as protection for the genitalia, the vaginal orifice, and the **urinary meatus** (see Figure 10.7 ■). Since the urinary tract and the reproductive organs are located in proximity to one another and each contains mucous membranes that can transport infection, there is a danger of infection entering the urinary tract. The

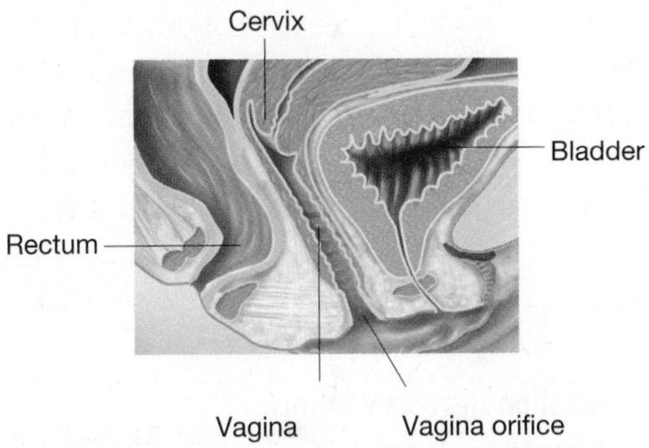

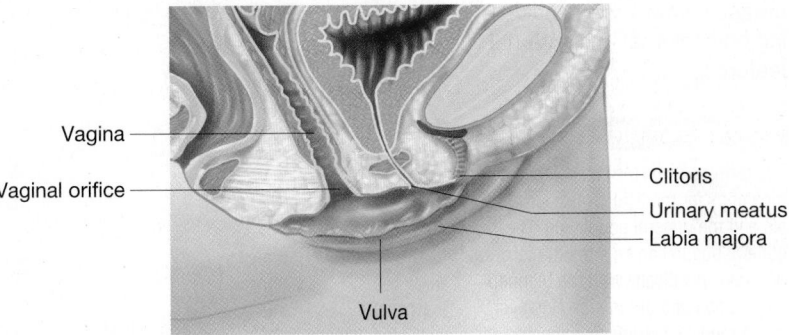

■ **Figure 10.6** The vagina, sagittal section showing the location of the vagina and its relationship to the cervix, uterus, rectum, and bladder.

■ **Figure 10.7** The vulva, sagittal section illustrating how the labia majora and labia minora cover and protect the vaginal orifice, clitoris, and urinary meatus.

clitoris is a small organ containing sensitive **erectile tissue** that is aroused during sexual stimulation and corresponds to the penis in the male. The region between the vaginal orifice and the anus is referred to as the **perineum.**

Breast

areola (ah-REE-oh-la)

lactation (lak-TAY-shun)

lactiferous ducts (lak-TIF-er-us)

lactiferous glands (lak-TIF-er-us)

mammary glands (MAM-ah-ree)

nipple

nurse

The breasts, or **mammary glands,** play a vital role in the reproductive process because they produce milk, a process called **lactation,** to nourish the newborn. The size of the breasts, which varies greatly from woman to woman, has no bearing on the ability to **nurse** or feed a baby. Milk is produced by the **lactiferous glands** and is carried to the **nipple** by the **lactiferous ducts** (see Figure 10.8 ■). The **areola** is the pigmented area around the nipple. As long as the breast is stimulated by the nursing infant, the breast will continue to secrete milk.

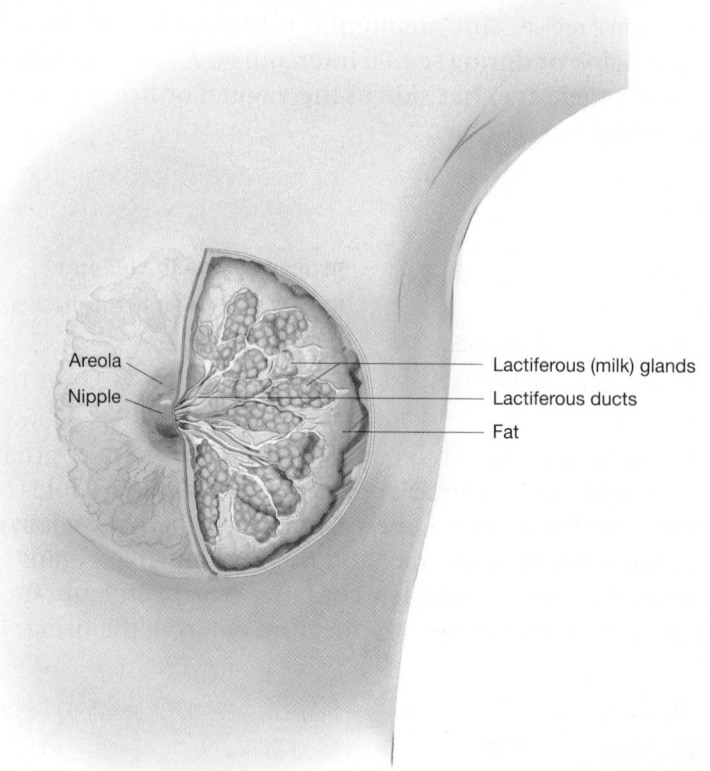

Areola

Nipple

Lactiferous (milk) glands

Lactiferous ducts

Fat

■ **Figure 10.8** The breast, cutaway view showing both internal and external features.

MID TERM TIP

The term *abortion* (AB) has different meanings for medical professionals and the general population. The general population equates the term *abortion* specifically with the planned termination of a pregnancy. However, to the medical community, abortion is a broader medical term meaning that a pregnancy has ended before a fetus is *viable,* meaning before it can live on its own.

Pregnancy

amnion (AM-nee-on)

amniotic fluid (am-nee-OT-ik)

chorion (KOR-ree-on)

embryo (EM-bree-oh)

fetus (FEE-tus)

gestation (jess-TAY-shun)

placenta (plah-SEN-tah)

premature

umbilical cord (um-BILL-ih-kal)

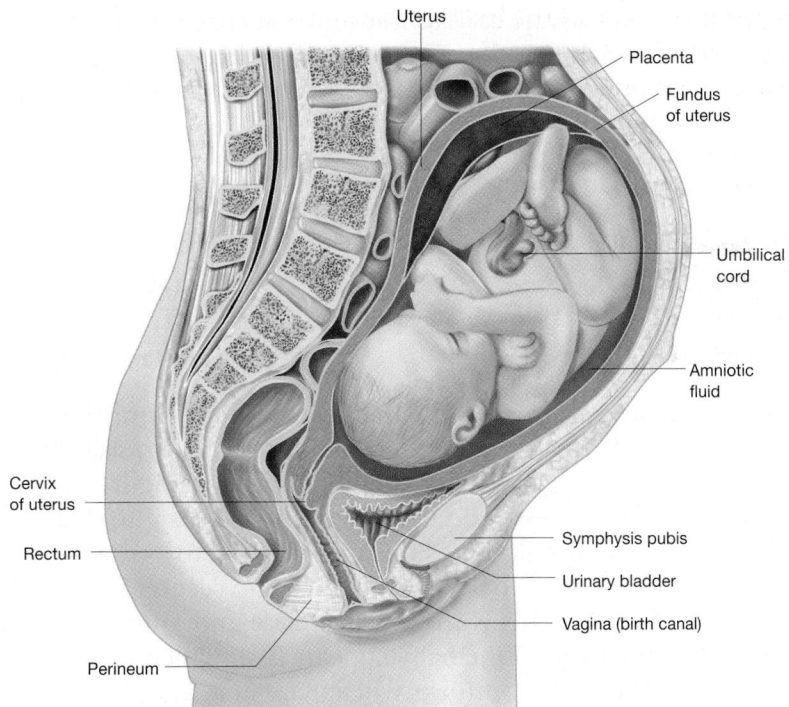

Uterus

Placenta

Fundus
of uterus

Umbilical
cord

Amniotic
fluid

Cervix
of uterus

Rectum

Symphysis pubis

Urinary bladder

Vagina (birth canal)

Perineum

■ **Figure 10.9** A full-term pregnancy. Image illustrates position of the fetus and the structures associated with pregnancy.

Pregnancy refers to the period of time during which a fetus grows and develops in its mother's uterus (see Figure 10.9 ■). The normal length of time for a pregnancy (**gestation**) is 40 weeks. If a baby is born before completing at least 37 weeks of gestation, it is considered **premature.**

During pregnancy the female body undergoes many changes. In fact, all of the body systems become involved in the development of a healthy infant. From the time the fertilized egg implants in the uterus until approximately the end of the eighth week, the infant is referred to as an **embryo** (see Figure 10.10 ■). During this period all the major organs and body systems are formed. Following the embryo stage and lasting until birth, the infant is called a **fetus** (see Figure 10.11 ■). During this time, the longest period of gestation, the organs mature and begin to function.

The fetus receives nourishment from its mother by way of the **placenta,** which is a spongy, blood-filled organ that forms in the uterus next to the fetus. The placenta is commonly referred to as the afterbirth. The fetus is attached to the

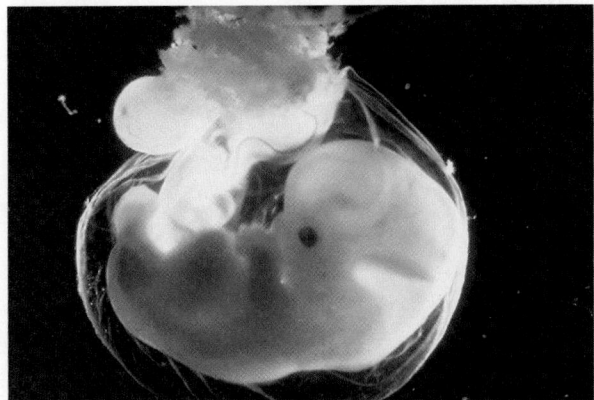

■ **Figure 10.10** Photograph illustrating the development of an embryo. *(Photo Researchers, Inc.)*

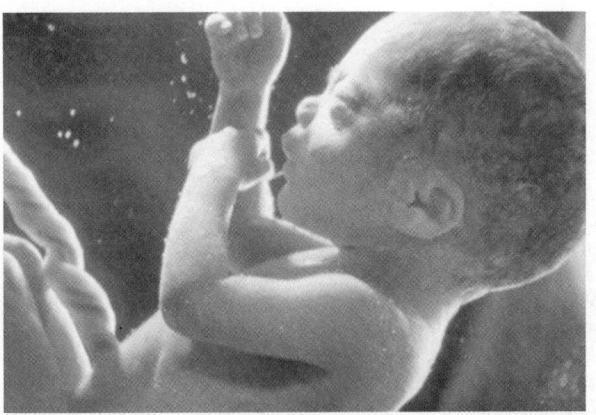

■ **Figure 10.11** Photograph illustrating the development of a fetus. *(Petit Format/Photo Researchers, Inc.)*

placenta by way of the **umbilical cord** and is surrounded by two membranous sacs, the **amnion** and the **chorion.** The amnion is the innermost sac, and it holds the **amniotic fluid** in which the fetus floats. The chorion is an outer, protective sac and also forms part of the placenta.

Labor and Delivery

breech presentation	**effacement** (eh-FACE-ment)
crowning	**expulsion stage** (ex-PULL-shun)
delivery	**labor**
dilation stage (dye-LAY-shun)	**placental stage** (plah-SEN-tal)

Labor is the actual process of expelling the fetus from the uterus and through the vagina. The first stage is referred to as the **dilation stage,** in which the uterine muscle contracts strongly to expel the fetus (see Figure 10.12A ■). During this process the fetus presses on the cervix and causes it to dilate or expand. As the cervix dilates, it also becomes thinner, referred to as **effacement.** When the cervix is completely dilated to 10 centimeters, the second stage of labor begins (see Figure 10.12B ■). This is the **expulsion stage** and ends with **delivery** of the baby. Generally, the head of the baby appears first, which is referred to as **crowning.** In some cases the baby's buttocks will appear first, and this is referred to as a **breech presentation** (see Figure 10.13 ■). The last stage of labor is the **placental stage** (see Figure 10.12C ■). Immediately after childbirth, the uterus continues to contract, causing the placenta to be expelled through the vagina.

A

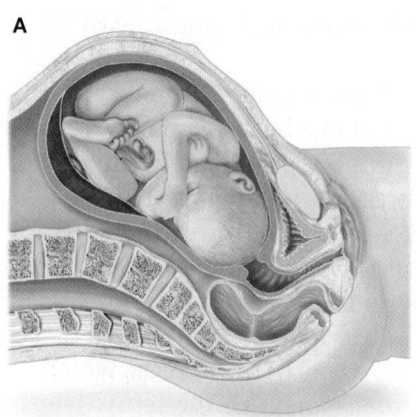

DILATION STAGE:
Uterine contractions dilate cervix

B

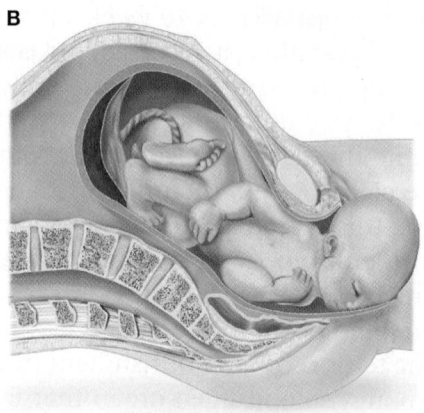

EXPULSION STAGE:
Birth of baby or expulsion

C

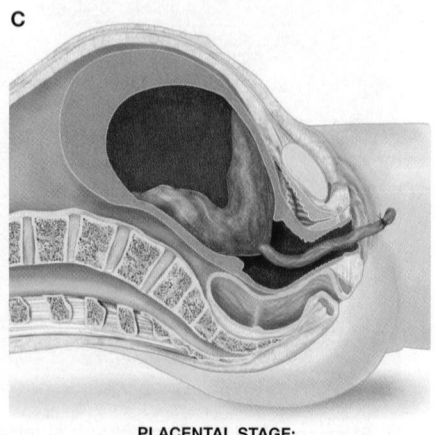

PLACENTAL STAGE:
Delivery of placenta

■ **Figure 10.12** The stages of labor and delivery. (A) During the dilation stage the cervix thins and dilates to 10 cm. (B) During the expulsion stage the infant is delivered. (C) During the placental stage the placenta is delivered.

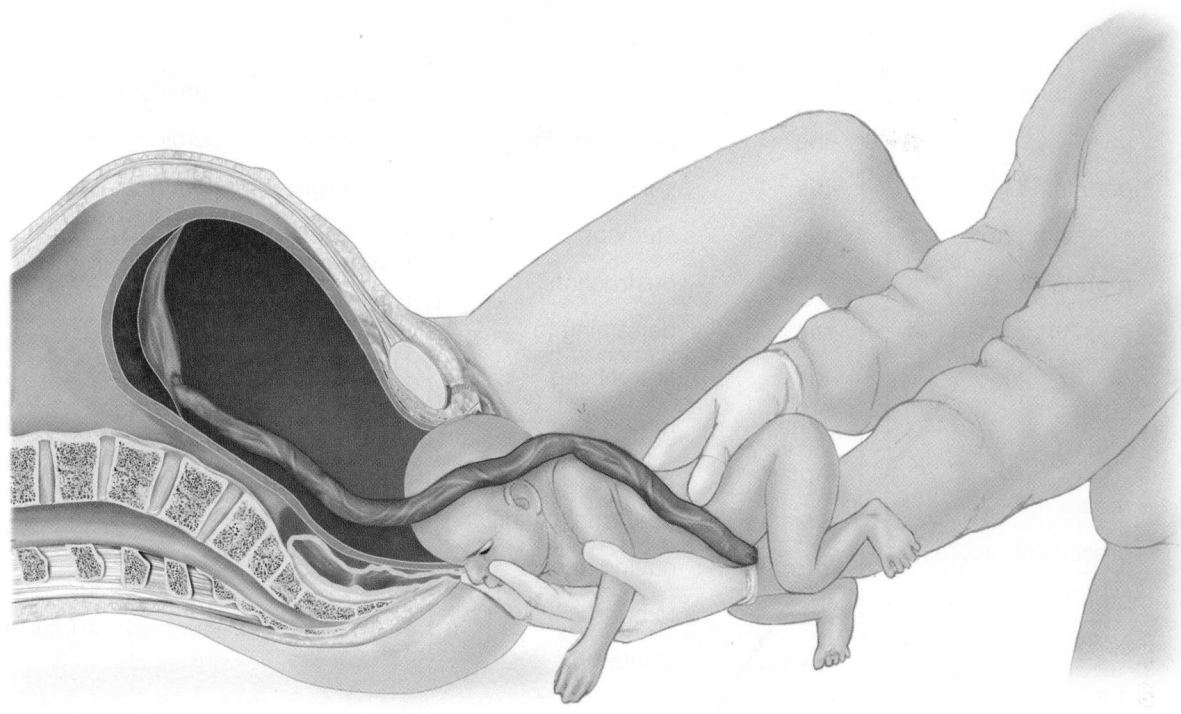

■ **Figure 10.13**   A breech birth. This image illustrates a newborn that has been delivered buttocks first.

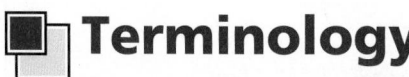 # Terminology

Word Parts Used to Build Female Reproductive System Terms

The following lists contain the combining forms, suffixes, and prefixes used to build terms in the remaining sections of this chapter.

Combining Forms

abdomin/o	abdomen	**hem/o**	blood	**or/o**	mouth
amni/o	amnion	**hemat/o**	blood	**ovari/o**	ovary
bi/o	life	**hymen/o**	hymen	**pelv/o**	pelvis
carcin/o	cancer	**hyster/o**	uterus	**perine/o**	perineum
cervic/o	cervix	**lact/o**	milk	**py/o**	pus
chori/o	chorion	**lapar/o**	abdomen	**rect/o**	rectum
colp/o	vagina	**later/o**	side	**salping/o**	uterine tube
culd/o	cul-de-sac	**mamm/o**	breast	**son/o**	sound
cyst/o	bladder, pouch	**mast/o**	breast	**tox/o**	poison
embry/o	embryo	**men/o**	menstruation	**uter/o**	uterus
episi/o	vulva	**metr/o**	uterus	**vagin/o**	vagina
fet/o	fetus	**nat/o**	birth	**vulv/o**	vulva
fibr/o	fibers	**olig/o**	scanty		
gynec/o	woman	**oophor/o**	ovary		

Suffixes

-al	pertaining to	**-ic**	pertaining to	**-pexy**	surgical fixation
-algia	pain	**-ine**	pertaining to	**-plasty**	surgical repair
-an	pertaining to	**-itis**	inflammation	**-rrhagia**	abnormal flow condition
-ary	pertaining to	**-logy**	study of		
-cele	protrusion	**-lytic**	destruction	**-rrhaphy**	suture
-centesis	puncture to withdraw fluid	**-nic**	pertaining to	**-rrhea**	discharge
		-oid	resembling	**-rrhexis**	rupture
-cyesis	pregnancy	**-oma**	tumor	**-salpinx**	uterine tube
-ectomy	surgical removal	**-opsy**	to view	**-scope**	instrument for viewing
-gram	record	**-osis**	abnormal condition		
-graphy	process of recording	**-otomy**	cutting into	**-scopy**	process of viewing
-gravida	pregnancy	**-para**	to bear	**-tic**	pertaining to
-ia	condition	**-partum**	childbirth	**-tocia**	labor and childbirth
-iasis	abnormal condition				

Prefixes

a-	without	**in-**	not	**post-**	after
ante-	before	**intra-**	inside	**pre-**	before
bi-	two	**multi-**	many	**primi-**	first
contra-	against	**neo-**	new	**pseudo-**	false
dys-	abnormal, difficult	**nulli-**	none	**ultra-**	beyond
endo-	within	**peri-**	around		

Anatomical Terms

TERM	WORD PARTS	DEFINITION
amniotic (am-nee-OT-ik)	amni/o = amnion -tic = pertaining to	Pertaining to the amnion.
cervical (SER-vih-kal)	cervic/o = cervix -al = pertaining to	Pertaining to the cervix.
chorionic (koh-ree-ON-ik)	chori/o = chorion -nic = pertaining to	Pertaining to the chorion.
embryonic (em-bree-ON-ik)	embry/o = embryo -nic = pertaining to	Pertaining to the embryo.
fetal (FEE-tall)	fet/o = fetus -al = pertaining to	Pertaining to the fetus.
lactic (LAK-tik)	lact/o = milk -ic = pertaining to	Pertaining to milk.
mammary (MAM-mah-ree)	mamm/o = breast -ary = pertaining to	Pertaining to the breast.

Anatomical Terms *(continued)*

TERM	WORD PARTS	DEFINITION
ovarian (oh-VAIR-ee-an)	ovari/o = ovary -an = pertaining to	Pertaining to the ovary.
perineal (per-ih-NEE-al)	perine/o = perineum -al = pertaining to	Pertaining to the perineum.
uterine (YOO-ter-in)	uter/o = uterus -ine = pertaining to	Pertaining to the uterus.
vaginal (VAJ-ih-nal)	vagin/o = vagina -al = pertaining to	Pertaining to the vagina.
vulvar (VUL-var)	vulv/o = vulva -ar = pertaining to	Pertaining to the vulva.

Pregnancy Terms

TERM	WORD PARTS	DEFINITION
antepartum (an-tee-PAR-tum)	ante- = before -partum = childbirth	Period of time before birth.
colostrum (kuh-LOS-trum)		Thin fluid first secreted by the breast after delivery. It does not contain much protein, but is rich in antibodies.
fraternal twins	-al = pertaining to	Twins that develop from two different ova fertilized by two different sperm. Although twins, these siblings do not have identical DNA.
identical twins	-al = pertaining to	Twins that develop from the splitting of one fertilized ovum. These siblings have identical DNA.
lactorrhea (lak-toh-REE-ah)	lact/o = milk -rrhea = flow	Discharge of milk from the breast.
meconium (meh-KOH-nee-um)		First bowel movement of a newborn. It is greenish-black in color and consists of mucus and bile.
multigravida (mull-tih-GRAV-ih-dah)	multi- = many -gravida = pregnancy	A woman who has been pregnant two or more times.
multipara (mull-TIP-ah-rah)	multi- = many -para = to bear	A woman who has given birth to a live infant two or more times.
neonate (NEE-oh-nayt)	neo- = new nat/o = birth	Term for a newborn baby.
nulligravida (null-ih-GRAV-ih-dah)	nulli- = none -gravida = pregnancy	A woman who has not been pregnant.
nullipara (null-IP-ah-rah)	nulli- = none -para = to bear	A woman who has not given birth to a live infant.
postpartum (post-PAR-tum)	post- = after -partum = childbirth	Period of time shortly after birth.
primigravida (prem-ih-GRAV-ih-dah)	primi- = first -gravida = pregnancy	A woman who is pregnant for the first time.
primipara (prem-IP-ah-rah)	primi- = first -para = to bear	A woman who has given birth to a live infant once.

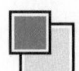 **Pathology**

TERM	WORD PARTS	DEFINITION
Medical Specialties		
gynecology (GYN) (gigh-neh-KOL-oh-jee)	gynec/o = woman -logy = study of	Branch of medicine specializing in the diagnosis and treatment of conditions of the female reproductive system. Physician is called a *gynecologist*.
neonatology (nee-oh-nay-TALL-oh-jee)	neo- = new nat/o = birth -logy = study of	Branch of medicine specializing in the diagnosis and treatment of conditions involving newborns. Physician is called a *neonatologist*.
obstetrics (OB) (ob-STET-riks)		Branch of medicine specializing in the diagnosis and treatment of women during pregnancy and childbirth, and immediately after childbirth. Physician is called an *obstetrician*.
Signs and Symptoms		
amenorrhea (ah-men-oh-REE-ah)	a- = without men/o = menstruation -rrhea = flow	Condition of having no menstrual flow.
amniorrhea (am-nee-oh-REE-ah)	amni/o = amnion -rrhea = flow	Flow of amniotic fluid when the amnion ruptures.
dysmenorrhea (dis-men-oh-REE-ah)	dys- = abnormal, painful men/o = menstruation -rrhea = flow	Condition of having abnormal or painful menstrual flow.
dystocia (dis-TOH-she-ah)	dys- = abnormal, difficult -tocia = labor and childbirth	Difficult labor and childbirth.
hematosalpinx (hee-mah-toh-SAL-pinks)	hemat/o = blood -salpinx = uterine tube	Presence of blood in a uterine tube.
mastalgia (mas-TAL-jee-ah)	mast/o = breast -algia = pain	Breast pain.
menorrhagia (men-oh-RAY-jee-ah)	men/o = menstruation -rrhagia = abnormal flow condition	Condition of having abnormally heavy menstrual flow during normal menstruation time.
metrorrhagia (meh-troh-RAY-jee-ah)	metr/o = uterus -rrhagia = abnormal flow condition	Term is used to describe uterine bleeding between menstrual periods.
metrorrhea (meh-troh-REE-ah)	metr/o = uterus -rrhea = discharge	Having a discharge (such as mucus or pus) from the uterus that is not the menstrual flow.
oligomenorrhea (ol-lih-goh-men-oh-REE-ah)	olig/o = scanty men/o = menstruation -rrhea = flow	Condition of having light menstrual flow.
Ovary		
oophoritis (oh-off-oh-RIGH-tis)	oophor/o = ovary -itis = inflammation	Inflammation of the ovary.

Pathology *(continued)*

TERM	WORD PARTS	DEFINITION
ovarian carcinoma (oh-VAY-ree-an / kar-sih-NOH-mah)	ovari/o = ovary -an = pertaining to carcin/o = cancer -oma = tumor	Cancer of the ovary.
ovarian cyst (oh-VAY-ree-an / SIST)	ovari/o = ovary -an = pertaining to	Cyst that develops within the ovary. These may be multiple cysts and may rupture, causing pain and bleeding.
Uterine Tubes		
pyosalpinx (pie-oh-SAL-pinks)	py/o = pus -salpinx = uterine tube	Presence of pus in a uterine tube.
salpingitis (sal-ping-JIGH-tis)	salping/o = uterine tube -itis = inflammation	Inflammation of the uterine tube.
Uterus		
cervical cancer (SER-vih-kal)	cervic/o = cervix -al = pertaining to	Malignant growth in the cervix. Some cases are caused by the *human papilloma virus* (HPV), a sexually transmitted virus for which there is now a vaccine. An especially difficult type of cancer to treat that causes 5% of the cancer deaths in women. Pap smear tests have helped to detect early cervical cancer.
endocervicitis (en-doh-ser-vih-SIGH-tis)	endo- = within cervic/o = cervix -itis = inflammation	Inflammation that occurs within the cervix.
endometrial cancer (en-doh-MEE-tree-al)	endo- = within metr/o = uterus -al = pertaining to	Cancer of the endometrial lining of the uterus.
endometritis (en-doh-meh-TRY-tis)	endo- = within metr/o = uterus -itis = inflammation	Inflammation of the endometrium (inner layer of the uterine wall)

> **MED TERM TIP**
>
> Word Watch: Be careful when using the combining form *metr/o* meaning "uterus" and the suffix *-metry* meaning "process of measuring."

fibroid tumor (FIGH-broyd / TOO-mor)	fibr/o = fibers -oid = resembling	Benign tumor or growth that contains fiber-like tissue. Uterine fibroid tumors are the most common tumors in women.

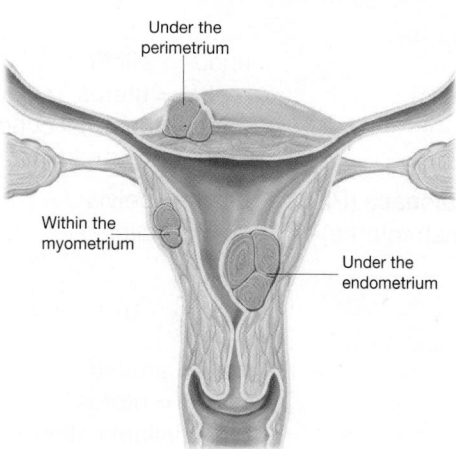

Figure 10.14   Common sites for the development of fibroid tumors.

▪ Pathology *(continued)*

TERM	WORD PARTS	DEFINITION
hysterorrhexis (hiss-ter-oh-REK-sis)	hyster/o = uterus -rrhexis = rupture	Rupture of the uterus; may occur during labor.
menometrorrhagia (men-oh-met-thro-RAY-jee-ah)	men/o = menstruation metr/o = uterus -rrhagia = abnormal flow condition	Excessive bleeding during the menstrual period and at intervals between menstrual periods.
premenstrual syndrome (PMS) (pre-MEN-stroo-al / SIN-drohm)	pre- = before men/o = menstruation -al = pertaining to	Symptoms that develop just prior to the onset of a menstrual period, which can include irritability, headache, tender breasts, and anxiety.
prolapsed uterus (pro-LAPS'D / YOO-ter-us)		Fallen uterus that can cause the cervix to protrude through the vaginal opening. Generally caused by weakened muscles from vaginal delivery or as the result of pelvic tumors pressing down.

Vagina

TERM	WORD PARTS	DEFINITION
candidiasis (kan-dih-DYE-ah-sis)	-iasis = abnormal condition	Yeast infection of the skin and mucous membranes that can result in white plaques on the tongue and vagina.

> **MED TERM TIP**
>
> The term *candida* comes from a Latin term meaning "dazzling white." Candida is the scientific name for yeast and refers to the very white discharge that is the hallmark of a yeast infection.

TERM	WORD PARTS	DEFINITION
cystocele (SIS-toh-seel)	cyst/o = bladder -cele = protrusion	Hernia or outpouching of the bladder that protrudes into the vagina. This may cause urinary frequency and urgency.
rectocele (REK-toh-seel)	rect/o = rectum -cele = protrusion	Protrusion or herniation of the rectum into the vagina.
toxic shock syndrome (TSS)	tox/o = poison -ic = pertaining to	Rare and sometimes fatal staphylococcus infection that generally occurs in menstruating women. Initial infection of the vagina is associated with prolonged wearing of a super-absorbent tampon.
vaginitis (vaj-ih-NIGH-tis)	vagin/o = vagina -itis = inflammation	Inflammation of the vagina.

Pelvic Cavity

TERM	WORD PARTS	DEFINITION
endometriosis (en-doh-mee-tree-OH-sis)	endo- = within metr/o = uterus -osis = abnormal condition	Abnormal condition of endometrium tissue appearing throughout the pelvis or on the abdominal wall. This tissue is normally found within the uterus.
pelvic inflammatory disease (PID) (PELL-vik / in-FLAM-mah-toh-ree)	pelv/o = pelvis -ic = pertaining to	Chronic or acute infection, usually bacterial, that has ascended through the female reproductive organs and out into the pelvic cavity. May result in scarring that interferes with fertility.
perimetritis (pair-ih-meh-TRY-tis)	peri- = around metr/o = uterus -itis = inflammation	Inflammation in the pelvic cavity around the outside of the uterus.

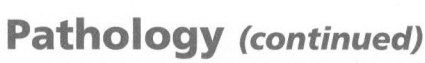 **Pathology** *(continued)*

TERM	WORD PARTS	DEFINITION
Breast		
breast cancer		Malignant tumor of the breast. Usually forms in the milk-producing gland tissue or the lining of the milk ducts (see Figure 10.15A ■).
fibrocystic breast disease (figh-bro-SIS-tik)	fibr/o = fibers cyst/o = pouch -ic = pertaining to	Benign cysts forming in the breast (see Figure 10.15B ■).

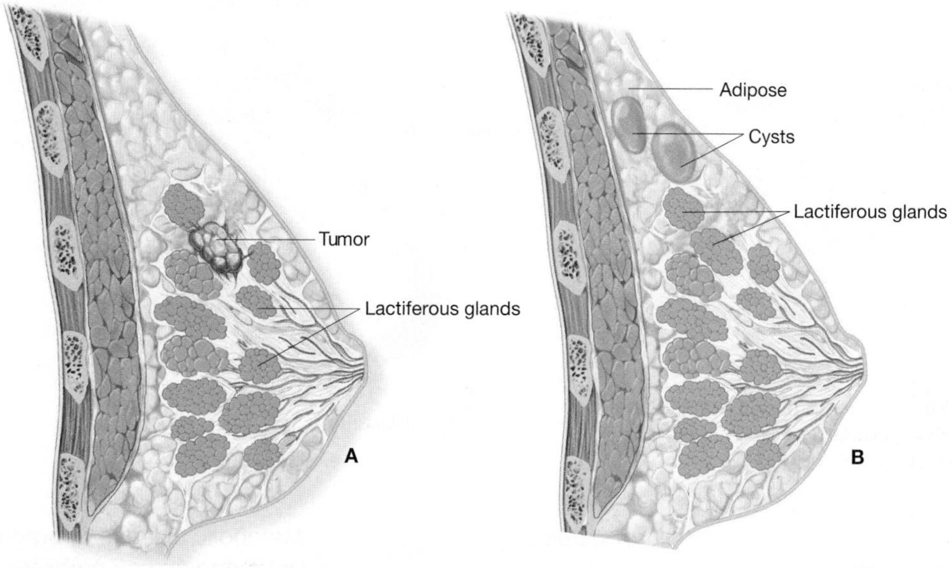

■ **Figure 10.15**   Comparison of breast cancer and fibrocystic disease. (A) Breast with a malignant tumor growing in the lactiferous gland and duct; (B) the location of a fibrocystic lump in the adipose tissue covering the breast.

TERM	WORD PARTS	DEFINITION
mastitis (mas-TYE-tis)	mast/o = breast -itis = inflammation	Inflammation of the breast.
Pregnancy		
abruptio placentae (ah-BRUP-tee-oh / plah-SEN-tee)		Emergency condition in which the placenta tears away from the uterine wall prior to delivery of the infant. Requires immediate delivery of the baby.
eclampsia (eh-KLAMP-see-ah)	-ia = condition	Further worsening of preeclampsia symptoms with the addition of seizures and coma; may occur between the 20th week of pregnancy and up to 6 weeks postpartum.
hemolytic disease of the newborn (HDN) (hee-moh-LIT-ik)	hem/o = blood -lytic = destruction	Condition developing in the baby when the mother's blood type is Rh-negative and the baby's blood is Rh-positive. Antibodies in the mother's blood enter the fetus's bloodstream through the placenta and destroy the fetus's red blood cells, causing anemia, jaundice, and enlargement of the spleen. Treatment is early diagnosis and blood transfusion. Also called *erythroblastosis fetalis.*

Pathology *(continued)*

TERM	WORD PARTS	DEFINITION
infertility	in- = not	Inability to produce children. Generally defined as no pregnancy after properly timed intercourse for 1 year.
placenta previa (plah-SEN-tah / PREE-vee-ah)		A placenta that is implanted in the lower portion of the uterus and, in turn, blocks the birth canal.

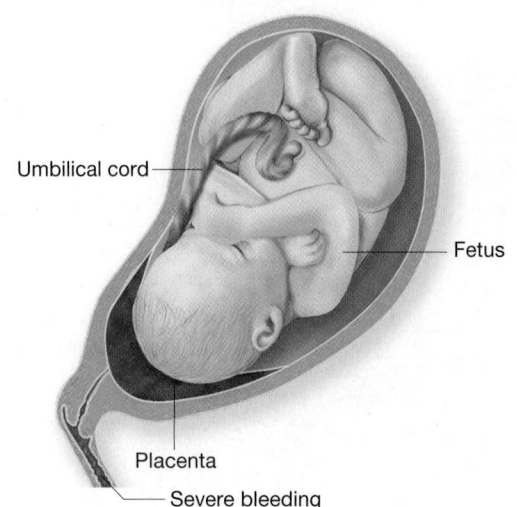

Umbilical cord

Fetus

Placenta

Severe bleeding

■ **Figure 10.16** Placenta previa, longitudinal section showing the placenta growing over the opening into the cervix.

TERM	WORD PARTS	DEFINITION
preeclampsia (pre-eh-KLAMP-see-ah)	pre- = before	Metabolic disease of pregnancy. If untreated, it may progress to eclampsia. Symptoms include hypertension, headaches, albumin in the urine, and edema. May occur between the 20th week of pregnancy and up to 6 weeks postpartum. Also called *toxemia.*
prolapsed umbilical cord (pro-LAPS'D / um-BILL-ih-kal)		When the umbilical cord of the baby is expelled first during delivery and is squeezed between the baby's head and the vaginal wall. This presents an emergency situation since the baby's circulation is compromised.
pseudocyesis (soo-doh-sigh-EE-sis)	pseudo- = false -cyesis = pregnancy	Condition in which the body reacts as if there is a pregnancy (especially hormonal changes), but there is no pregnancy.
salpingocyesis (sal-ping-goh-sigh-EE-sis)	salping/o = uterine tube -cyesis = pregnancy	Pregnancy that occurs in the uterine tube instead of in the uterus.
spontaneous abortion		Unplanned loss of a pregnancy due to the death of the embryo or fetus before the time it is viable, commonly referred to as a *miscarriage.*
stillbirth		Birth in which a viable-aged fetus dies shortly before or at the time of delivery.

Diagnostic Procedures

TERM	WORD PARTS	DEFINITION
Clinical Laboratory Tests		
Pap (Papanicolaou) **smear** (pap-ah-NIK-oh-low)		Test for the early detection of cancer of the cervix named after the developer of the test, George Papanicolaou, a Greek physician. A scraping of cells is removed from the cervix for examination under a microscope.
pregnancy test (PREG-nan-see)		Chemical test that can determine a pregnancy during the first few weeks. Can be performed in a physician's office or with a home-testing kit.
Diagnostic Imaging		
hysterosalpingography (HSG) (hiss-ter-oh-sal-pin-GOG-rah-fee)	hyster/o = uterus salping/o = uterine tube -graphy = process of recording	Taking of an X-ray after injecting radiopaque material into the uterus and uterine tubes.
mammogram (MAM-moh-gram)	mamm/o = breast -gram = record	X-ray record of the breast.
mammography (mam-OG-rah-fee)	mamm/o = breast -graphy = process of recording	X-ray to diagnose breast disease, especially breast cancer.
pelvic ultrasonography (PELL-vik / ull-trah-son-OG-rah-fee)	pelv/o = pelvis -ic = pertaining to ultra- = beyond son/o = sound -graphy = process of recording	Use of high-frequency sound waves to produce an image or photograph of an organ, such as the uterus, ovaries, or fetus.
Endoscopic Procedures		
colposcope (KOL-poh-scope)	colp/o = vagina -scope = instrument for viewing	Instrument used to view inside the vagina.
colposcopy (kol-POS-koh-pee)	colp/o = vagina -scopy = process of viewing	Examination of vagina using an instrument called a *colposcope.*
culdoscopy (kul-DOS-koh-pee)	culd/o = cul-de-sac -scopy = process of viewing	Examination of the female pelvic cavity, particularly behind the uterus, by introducing an endoscope through the wall of the vagina.
laparoscope (LAP-ah-row-scope)	lapar/o = abdomen -scope = instrument for viewing	Instrument used to view inside the abdomen.
laparoscopy (lap-ar-OS-koh-pee)	lapar/o = abdomen -scopy = process of viewing	Examination of the peritoneal cavity using an instrument called a *laparoscope.* The instrument is passed through a small incision made by the surgeon into the abdominopelvic cavity.

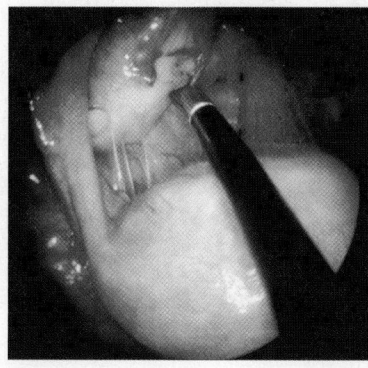

■ **Figure 10.17** Photograph taken during a laparoscopic procedure. The fundus of the uterus is visible below the probe, the ovary is at the tip of the probe, and the uterine tube extends along the left side of the photo. *(Southern Illinois University/ Photo Researchers, Inc.)*

Diagnostic Procedures *(continued)*

TERM	WORD PARTS	DEFINITION
Obstetrical Diagnostic Procedures		
amniocentesis (am-nee-oh-sen-TEE-sis)	amni/o = amnion -centesis = puncture to withdraw fluid	Puncturing of the amniotic sac using a needle and syringe for the purpose of withdrawing amniotic fluid for testing. Can assist in determining fetal maturity, development, and genetic disorders.
Apgar score (AP-gar)		Evaluation of a neonate's adjustment to the outside world. Observes color, heart rate, muscle tone, respiratory rate, and response to stimulus at 1 minute and 5 minutes after birth.
chorionic villus sampling (CVS) (kor-ree-ON-ik / vill-us)	chori/o = chorion -nic = pertaining to	Removal of a small piece of the chorion for genetic analysis. May be done at an earlier stage of pregnancy than amniocentesis.
fetal monitoring (FEE-tal)	fet/o = fetus -al = pertaining to	Using electronic equipment placed on the mother's abdomen or the fetus' scalp to check the fetal heart rate (FHR) and fetal heart tone (FHT) during labor. The normal heart rate of the fetus is rapid, ranging from 120 to 160 beats per minute. A drop in the fetal heart rate indicates the fetus is in distress.
Additional Diagnostic Procedures		
cervical biopsy (SER-vih-kal / BYE-op-see)	cervic/o = cervix -al = pertaining to bi/o = life -opsy = to view	Taking a sample of tissue from the cervix to test for the presence of cancer cells.
endometrial biopsy (EMB) (en-doh-MEE-tre-al BYE-op-see)	endo- = within metr/o = uterus -al = pertaining to bi/o = life -opsy = to view	Taking a sample of tissue from the lining of the uterus to test for abnormalities.
pelvic examination (PELL-vik)	pelv/o = pelvis -ic = pertaining to	Physical examination of the vagina and adjacent organs performed by a physician placing the fingers of one hand into the vagina. An instrument called a *speculum* is used to open the vagina.

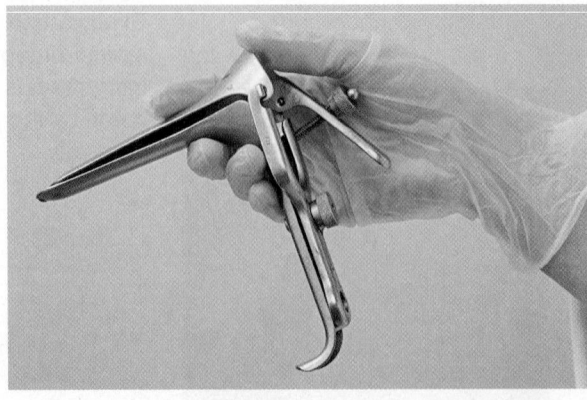

■ **Figure 10.18** A speculum used to hold the vagina open in order to visualize the cervix.

Therapeutic Procedures

TERM	WORD PARTS	DEFINITION
Medical Procedures		
barrier contraception (kon-trah-SEP-shun)	contra- = against	Prevention of a pregnancy using a device to prevent sperm from meeting an ovum. Examples include condoms, diaphragms, and cervical caps.
hormonal contraception	-al = pertaining to contra- = against	Use of hormones to block ovulation and prevent conception. May be in the form of a pill, a patch, an implant under the skin, or an injection.
intrauterine device (IUD) (in-trah-YOO-ter-in)	intra- = inside uter/o = uterus -ine = pertaining to	Device inserted into the uterus by a physician for the purpose of contraception.

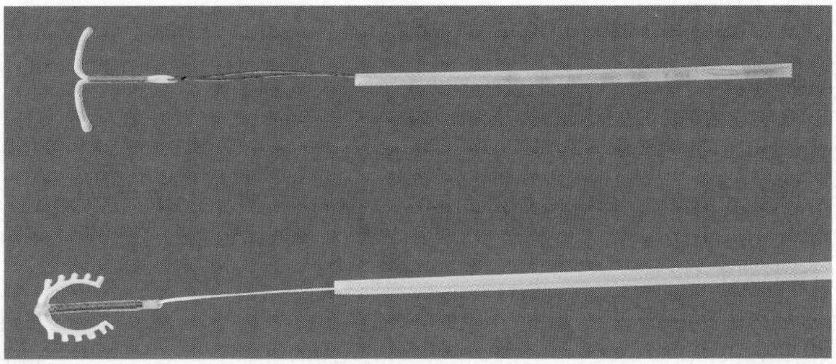

■ **Figure 10.19** Photographs illustrating the shape of two different intrauterine devices (IUDs). *(Jules Selmes and Debi Treloar/ Dorling Kindersley)*

TERM	WORD PARTS	DEFINITION
Surgical Procedures		
amniotomy (am-nee-OT-oh-mee)	amni/o = amnion -otomy = cutting into	Surgically cutting open the amnion; commonly referred to as "breaking the water."
cervicectomy (ser-vih-SEK-toh-mee)	cervic/o = cervix -ectomy = surgical removal	Surgical removal of the cervix.
cesarean section (CS, C-section) (see-SAYR-ee-an)		Surgical delivery of a baby through an incision into the abdominal and uterine walls. Legend has it that the Roman emperor, Julius Caesar, was the first person born by this method.
conization (kon-ih-ZAY-shun)		Surgical removal of a core of cervical tissue. Also refers to partial removal of the cervix.
dilation and curettage (D & C) (dye-LAY-shun / koo-reh-TAHZ)		Surgical procedure in which the opening of the cervix is dilated and the uterus is scraped or suctioned of its lining or tissue. Often performed after a spontaneous abortion and to stop excessive bleeding from other causes.
elective abortion		Legal termination of a pregnancy for non-medical reasons.
episiorrhaphy (eh-peez-ee-OR-ah-fee)	episi/o = vulva -rrhaphy = suture	To suture the perineum; procedure to repair an episiotomy postpartum. Note that the combining form *episi/o* is used even though the perineum is not part of the vulva.
episiotomy (eh-peez-ee-OT-oh-mee)	episi/o = vulva -otomy = cutting into	Surgical incision of the perineum to facilitate the delivery process. Can prevent an irregular tearing of tissue during birth. Note that the combining form *episi/o* is used even though the perineum is not part of the vulva.

Therapeutic Procedures *(continued)*

TERM	WORD PARTS	DEFINITION
hymenectomy (high-men-EK-toh-mee)	hymen/o = hymen -ectomy = surgical removal	Surgical removal of the hymen.
hysterectomy (hiss-ter-EK-toh-mee)	hyster/o = uterus -ectomy = surgical removal	Surgical removal of the uterus.
hysteropexy (HISS-ter-oh-pek-see)	hyster/o = uterus -pexy = surgical fixation	To surgically anchor the uterus to its proper location in the pelvic cavity; a treatment for a prolapsed uterus.
laparotomy (lap-ah-ROT-oh-mee)	lapar/o = abdomen -otomy = cutting into	To cut open the abdomen; performed in order to complete other surgical procedures inside the abdomen or performed during a C-section.
lumpectomy (lump-EK-toh-mee)	-ectomy = surgical removal	Removal of only a breast tumor and the tissue immediately surrounding it.
mammoplasty (MAM-moh-plas-tee)	mamm/o = breast -plasty = surgical repair	Surgical repair or reconstruction of the breast.
mastectomy (mass-TEK-toh-mee)	mast/o = breast -ectomy = surgical removal	Surgical removal of the breast.
oophorectomy (oh-off-oh-REK-toh-mee)	oophor/o = ovary -ectomy = surgical removal	Surgical removal of the ovary.
radical mastectomy (mast-EK-toh-mee)	-al = pertaining to mast/o = breast -ectomy = surgical removal	Surgical removal of the breast tissue plus chest muscles and axillary lymph nodes.
salpingectomy (sal-ping-JECK-toh-mee)	salping/o = uterine tube -ectomy = surgical removal	Surgical removal of the uterine tube.
simple mastectomy (mast-EK-toh-mee)	mast/o = breast -ectomy = surgical removal	Surgical removal of the breast tissue.
therapeutic abortion		Termination of a pregnancy for the health of the mother or another medical reason.
total abdominal hysterectomy— bilateral salpingo-oophorectomy (TAH-BSO) (hiss-ter-EK-toh-me / sal-ping-goh / oh-oh-foe-REK-toh-mee)	abdomin/o = abdomen -al = pertaining to hyster/o = uterus -ectomy = surgical removal bi- = two later/o = side -al = pertaining to salping/o = uterine tube oophor/o = ovary -ectomy = surgical removal	Removal of the entire uterus, cervix, both ovaries, and both uterine tubes.
tubal ligation (TOO-bal / lye-GAY-shun)	-al = pertaining to	Surgical tying off of the uterine tubes to prevent conception from taking place. Results in sterilization of the female.
vaginal hysterectomy (VAJ-ih-nal / hiss-ter-EK-toh-me)	vagin/o = vagina -al = pertaining to hyster/o = uterus -ectomy = surgical removal	Removal of the uterus through the vagina rather than through an abdominal incision.

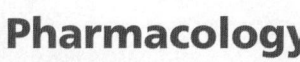

Pharmacology

CLASSIFICATION	WORD PARTS	ACTION	EXAMPLES
abortifacient (ah-bore-tih-FAY-shee-ent)		Medication that terminates a pregnancy.	mifepristone, Mifeprex; dino-prostone, Prostin E2
fertility drug		Medication that triggers ovulation. Also called *ovulation stimulant.*	clomiphene, Clomid; follitro-pin alfa, Gonal-F
hormone replacement therapy (HRT)		Menopause or the surgical loss of the ovaries results in the lack of estrogen production. Replacing this hormone may prevent some of the consequences of menopause, especially in younger women who have surgically lost their ovaries.	conjugated estrogens, Cenestin, Premarin
oral contraceptive pills (OCPs) (kon-trah-SEP-tive)	or/o = mouth -al = pertaining to contra- = against	Birth control medication that uses low doses of female hormones to prevent conception by blocking ovulation.	desogestrel/ethinyl estradiol, Ortho-Cept; ethinyl estradiol/norgestrel, Lo/Ovral
oxytocin (ox-ee-TOH-sin)		Oxytocin is a natural hormone that begins or improves uterine contractions during labor and delivery.	oxytocin, Pitocin, Syntocinon

Abbreviations

AB	abortion		**HPV**	human papilloma virus
AI	artificial insemination		**HRT**	hormone replacement therapy
BSE	breast self-examination		**HSG**	hysterosalpingography
CS, C-section	cesarean section		**IUD**	intrauterine device
			IVF	*in vitro* fertilization
CVS	chorionic villus sampling		**LBW**	low birth weight
Cx	cervix		**LH**	luteinizing hormone
D & C	dilation and curettage		**LMP**	last menstrual period
EDC	estimated date of confinement		**NB**	newborn
EMB	endometrial biopsy		**OB**	obstetrics
ERT	estrogen replacement therapy		**OCPs**	oral contraceptive pills
FEKG	fetal electrocardiogram		**PAP**	Papanicolaou test
FHR	fetal heart rate		**PI, para I**	first delivery
FHT	fetal heart tone		**PID**	pelvic inflammatory disease
FSH	follicle-stimulating hormone		**PMS**	premenstrual syndrome
FTND	full-term normal delivery		**TAH-BSO**	total abdominal hysterectomy–bilateral salpingo-oophorectomy
GI, grav I	first pregnancy		**TSS**	toxic shock syndrome
GYN, gyn	gynecology		**UC**	uterine contractions
HCG, hCG	human chorionic gonadotropin			
HDN	hemolytic disease of the newborn			

Section II: Male Reproductive System at a Glance

Function

Similar to the female reproductive system, the male reproductive system is responsible for producing sperm, the male reproductive cell, secreting the male sex hormones, and delivering sperm to the female reproductive tract.

Organs

Here are the primary structures that comprise the male reproductive system.

bulbourethral glands	**seminal vesicles**
epididymis	**testes**
penis	**vas deferens**
prostate gland	

Word Parts

Here are the most common word parts (with their meanings) used to build male reproductive system terms. For a more comprehensive list, refer to the Terminology section of this chapter.

Combining Forms

andr/o	male	orchid/o	testes
balan/o	glans penis	pen/o	penis
crypt/o	hidden	prostat/o	prostate
epididym/o	epididymis	spermat/o	sperm
genit/o	genitals	testicul/o	testes
orch/o	testes	vas/o	vas deferens
orchi/o	testes	vesicul/o	seminal vesicle

Suffixes

-cide	to kill
-spermia	condition of sperm

Male Reproductive System Illustrated

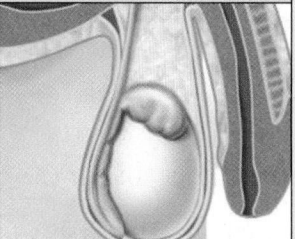

testes, p. 354

Produces sperm and secretes testosterone

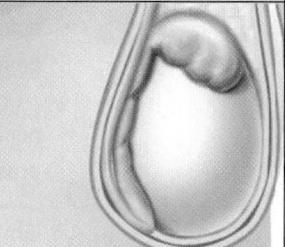

epididymis, p. 355

Stores sperm

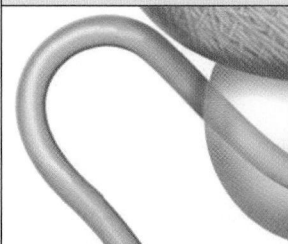

vas deferens, p. 356

Transports sperm to urethra

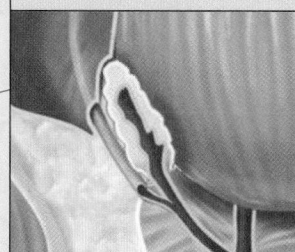

seminal vesicles, p. 356

Secretes fluid for semen

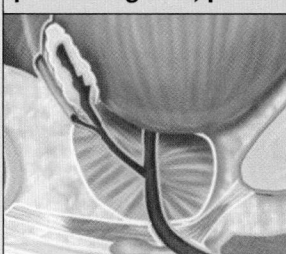

prostate gland, p. 356

Secretes fluid for semen

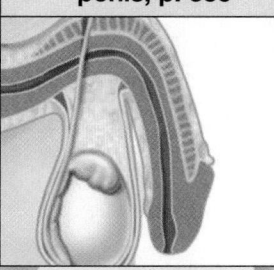

penis, p. 355

Delivers semen during intercourse

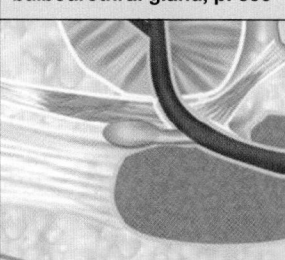

bulbourethral gland, p. 356

Secretes fluid for semen

Anatomy and Physiology of the Male Reproductive System

bulbourethral glands
    (buhl-boh-yoo-REE-thral)
epididymis (ep-ih-DID-ih-mis)
genitourinary system
    (jen-ih-toh-YOO-rih-nair-ee)
penis (PEE-nis)
prostate gland (PROSS-tayt)

semen (SEE-men)
seminal vesicles (SEM-ih-nal / VESS-ih-kls)
sex hormones
sperm
testes (TESS-teez)
vas deferens (VAS / DEF-er-enz)

The male reproductive system has two main functions. The first is to produce **sperm,** the male reproductive cell; the second is to secrete the male **sex hormones.** In the male, the major organs of reproduction are located outside the body: the **penis,** and the two **testes,** each with an **epididymis** (see Figure 10.20 ■). The penis contains the urethra, which carries both urine and **semen** to the outside of the body. For this reason, this system is sometimes referred to as the **genitourinary system** (GU).

The internal organs of reproduction include two **seminal vesicles,** two **vas deferens,** the **prostate gland,** and two **bulbourethral glands.**

External Organs of Reproduction

Testes

perineum
scrotum (SKROH-tum)
seminiferous tubules (sem-ih-NIF-er-us / TOO-byools)

spermatogenesis
    (sper-mat-oh-JEN-eh-sis)
testicles (test-IH-kles)
testosterone (tess-TOSS-ter-ohn)

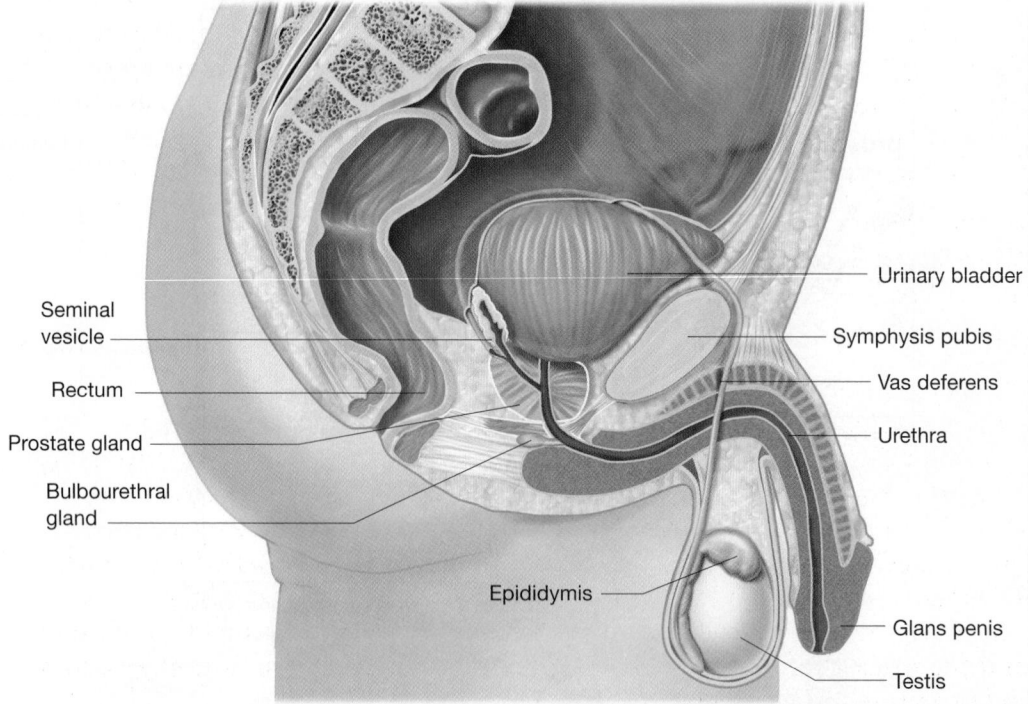

Seminal vesicle
Rectum
Prostate gland
Bulbourethral gland
Epididymis

Urinary bladder
Symphysis pubis
Vas deferens
Urethra
Glans penis
Testis

■ **Figure 10.20** The male reproductive system, sagittal section showing the organs of the system and their relation to the urinary bladder and rectum.

The testes (singular is *testis*) or **testicles** are oval in shape and are responsible for the production of sperm (see again Figure 10.20). This process, called **spermatogenesis,** takes place within the **seminiferous tubules** that make up the insides of the testes (see Figure 10.21 ■). The testes must be maintained at the proper temperature for the sperm to survive. This lower temperature level is achieved by the placement of the testes suspended in the **scrotum,** a sac outside the body. The **perineum** of the male is similar to that in the female and is the area between the scrotum and the anus. The male sex hormone **testosterone,** which is responsible for the development of the male reproductive organs, sperm, and secondary sex characteristics, is also produced by the testes.

MED TERM TIP

Spermatozoon and its plural form, *spermatozoa*, are other terms that mean "sperm." You have no doubt realized that there can be several terms with the same meaning in medical terminology. You must continue to remain flexible when working with these terms in your career. In some cases, one term will be more commonly used, depending on the type of medical specialty or even what part of the country you are in.

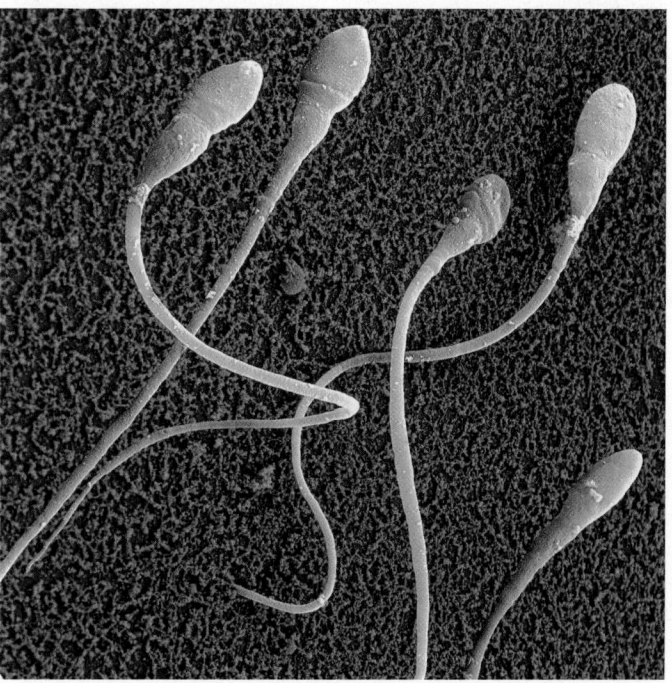

■ **Figure 10.21** Electron-micrograph of human sperm.

(Juergen Berger, Max-Planck Institute/ Science Photo Library/Photo Researchers, Inc.)

Epididymis

Each epididymis is a coiled tubule that lies on top of the testes within the scrotum (see again Figure 10.20). This elongated structure serves as the location for sperm maturation and storage until they are ready to be released into the vas deferens.

Penis

circumcision (ser-kum-SIH-zhun)

ejaculation (ee-jak-yoo-LAY-shun)

erectile tissue (ee-REK-tile)

glans penis (GLANS / PEE-nis)

prepuce (PREE-pyoos)

sphincter (SFINGK-ter)

urinary meatus (YOO-rih-nair-ee / me-AY-tus)

The penis is the male sex organ containing **erectile tissue** that is encased in skin (see again Figure 10.20). This organ delivers semen into the female vagina. The soft tip of the penis is referred to as the **glans penis.** It is protected by a covering called the **prepuce** or foreskin. It is this covering of skin that is removed during the procedure known as **circumcision.** The penis becomes erect during sexual stimulation, which allows it to be placed within the female for the **ejaculation** of semen. The male urethra extends from the urinary bladder to the external opening in the penis, the **urinary meatus,** and serves a dual function: the elimination of urine and the ejaculation of semen. During the ejaculation process, a **sphincter** closes to keep urine from escaping.

MED TERM TIP

During sexual intercourse, which is also referred to as *coitus*, the male can eject up to 100 million sperm cells. The adult male produces nearly 200 million sperm daily.

Internal Organs of Reproduction

Vas Deferens

spermatic cord (sper-MAT-ik)

Each vas deferens carries sperm from the epididymis up into the pelvic cavity. They travel up in front of the urinary bladder, over the top, and then back down the posterior side of the bladder to empty into the urethra (see again Figure 10.20). They, along with nerves, arteries, veins, and lymphatic vessels running between the pelvic cavity and the testes, form the **spermatic cord.**

Seminal Vesicles

The two seminal vesicles are small glands located at the base of the urinary bladder (see again Figure 10.20). These vesicles are connected to the vas deferens just before it empties into the urethra. The seminal vesicles secrete a glucose-rich fluid that nourishes the sperm. This liquid, along with the sperm, constitutes semen, the fluid that is eventually ejaculated during sexual intercourse.

Prostate Gland

The single prostate gland is located just below the urinary bladder (see again Figure 10.20). It surrounds the urethra and when enlarged can cause difficulty in urination. The prostate is important for the reproductive process since it secretes an alkaline fluid that assists in keeping the sperm alive by neutralizing the pH of the urethra and vagina.

Bulbourethral Glands

Cowper's glands (KOW-perz)

The bulbourethral glands, also known as **Cowper's glands,** are two small glands located on either side of the urethra just below the prostate (see again Figure 10.20). They produce a mucus-like lubricating fluid that joins with semen to become a part of the ejaculate.

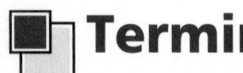

Terminology

Word Parts Used to Build Male Reproductive System Terms

The following lists contain the combining forms, suffixes, and prefixes used to build terms in the remaining sections of this chapter.

Combining Forms

andr/o	male		**olig/o**	scanty		**testicul/o**	testicle
balan/o	glans penis		**orch/o**	testes		**ur/o**	urine
carcin/o	cancer		**orchi/o**	testes		**urethr/o**	urethra
crypt/o	hidden		**orchid/o**	testes		**varic/o**	dilated vein
epididym/o	epididymis		**pen/o**	penis		**vas/o**	vas deferens
genit/o	genital		**prostat/o**	prostate gland		**vesicul/o**	seminal vesicle
hydr/o	water		**rect/o**	rectum			
immun/o	protection		**spermat/o**	sperm			

Suffixes

-al	pertaining to
-ar	pertaining to
-cele	protrusion
-cide	to kill
-ectomy	surgical removal
-gen	that which produces
-iasis	abnormal condition
-ic	pertaining to

-ile	pertaining to
-ism	state of
-itis	inflammation
-logy	study of
-lysis	destruction
-oid	resembling
-oma	tumor
-osis	abnormal condition

-ostomy	create a new opening
-otomy	cutting into
-pexy	surgical fixation
-plasia	growth
-plasty	surgical repair
-rrhea	discharge
-spermia	sperm condition

Prefixes

a-	without
an-	without
anti-	against

dys-	abnormal, difficult
epi-	upon

hyper-	excessive
hypo-	below

Anatomical Terms

TERM	WORD PARTS	DEFINITION
balanic (buh-LAN-ik)	balan/o = glans penis -ic = pertaining to	Pertaining to the glans penis.
epididymal (ep-ih-DID-ih-mal)	epididym/o = epididymis -al = pertaining to	Pertaining to the epididymis.
penile (PEE-nile)	pen/o = penis -ile = pertaining to	Pertaining to the penis.
prostatic (pross-TAT-ik)	prostat/o = prostate gland -ic = pertaining to	Pertaining to the prostate gland.
spermatic (sper-MAT-ik)	spermat/o = sperm -ic = pertaining to	Pertaining to sperm.
testicular (tes-TIK-yoo-lar)	testicul/o = testes -ar = pertaining to	Pertaining to the testes.
vasal (VAY-sal)	vas/o = vas deferens -al = pertaining to	Pertaining to the vas deferens.
vesicular (veh-SIC-yoo-lar)	vesicul/o = seminal vesicle -ar = pertaining to	Pertaining to the seminal vesicle.

MED TERM TIP

Word Watch: Be careful using the combining forms *vesic/o* meaning "bladder" and *vesicul/o* meaning "seminal vesicle."

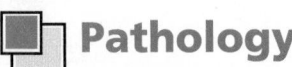

Pathology

TERM	WORD PARTS	DEFINITION
Medical Specialties		
urology (yoo-RAL-oh-jee)	ur/o = urine -logy = study of	Branch of medicine involved in diagnosis and treatment of diseases and disorders of the urinary system and male reproductive system. Physician is a *urologist*.
Signs and Symptoms		
aspermia (ah-SPER-mee-ah)	a- = without -spermia = sperm condition	Condition of having no sperm.
balanorrhea (bah-lah-noh-REE-ah)	balan/o = glans penis -rrhea = discharge	Discharge from the glans penis.
oligospermia (ol-ih-goh-SPER-mee-ah)	olig/o = scanty -spermia = sperm condition	Condition of having too few sperm, making the chances of fertilization very low.
spermatolysis (sper-mah-TOL-ih-sis)	spermat/o = sperm -lysis = destruction	Term that refers to anything that destroys sperm.
Testes		
anorchism (an-OR-kizm)	an- = without orch/o = testes -ism = condition	The absence of testes; may be congenital or as the result of an accident or surgery.
cryptorchidism (kript-OR-kid-izm)	crypt/o = hidden orchid/o = testes -ism = state of	Failure of the testes to descend into the scrotal sac before birth. Usually, the testes will descend before birth. A surgical procedure called orchidopexy may be required to bring the testes down into the scrotum permanently. Failure of the testes to descend could result in sterility in the male or an increased risk of testicular cancer.
hydrocele (HIGH-droh-seel)	hydr/o = water -cele = protrusion	Accumulation of fluid around the testes or along the spermatic cord. Common in infants.
sterility		Inability to father children due to a problem with spermatogenesis.
testicular carcinoma (kar-sih-NOH-mah)	testicul/o = testicle -ar = pertaining to carcin/o = cancer -oma = tumor	Cancer of one or both testicles; most common cancer in men under age 40.
testicular torsion	testicul/o = testicle -ar = pertaining to	Twisting of the spermatic cord.
varicocele (VAIR-ih-koh-seel)	varic/o = dilated vein -cele = protrusion	Enlargement of the veins of the spermatic cord that commonly occurs on the left side of adolescent males.
Epididymis		
epididymitis (ep-ih-did-ih-MYE-tis)	epididym/o = epididymis -itis = inflammation	Inflammation of the epididymis.
Prostate Gland		
benign prostatic hyperplasia (BPH) (bee-NINE / pross-TAT-ik / high-PER-troh-fee)	prostat/o = prostate gland -ic = pertaining to hyper- = excessive -plasia = growth	Noncancerous enlargement of the prostate gland commonly seen in males over age 50. Formerly called *benign prostatic hypertrophy*.

■ Pathology *(continued)*

TERM	WORD PARTS	DEFINITION
prostate cancer (PROSS-tayt)		Slow-growing cancer that affects a large number of males after age 50. The prostate-specific antigen (PSA) test is used to assist in early detection of this disease.
prostatitis (pross-tah-TYE-tis)	prostat/o = prostate gland -itis = inflammation	Inflammation of the prostate gland.
Penis		
balanitis (bal-ah-NYE-tis)	balan/o = glans penis -itis = inflammation	Inflammation of the glans penis.
epispadias (ep-ih-SPAY-dee-as)	epi- = upon	Congenital opening of the urethra on the dorsal surface of the penis.
erectile dysfunction (ED) (ee-REK-tile)	-ile = pertaining to dys- = abnormal, difficult	Inability to engage in sexual intercourse due to inability to maintain an erection. Also called *impotence*.
hypospadias (high-poh-SPAY-dee-as)	hypo- = below	Congenital opening of the male urethra on the underside of the penis.
phimosis (fih-MOH-sis)	-osis = abnormal condition	Narrowing of the foreskin over the glans penis resulting in difficulty with hygiene. This condition can lead to infection or difficulty with urination. The condition is treated with circumcision, the surgical removal of the foreskin.
priapism (pri-ah-pizm)	-ism = state of	A persistent and painful erection due to pathological causes, not sexual arousal.
Sexually Transmitted Diseases		
chancroid (SHANG-kroyd)	-oid = resembling	Highly infectious nonsyphilitic venereal ulcer.
chlamydia (klah-MID-ee-ah)		Bacterial infection causing genital inflammation in males and females. Can lead to pelvic inflammatory disease in females and eventual infertility.
genital herpes (JEN-ih-tal / HER-peez)	genit/o = genital -al = pertaining to	Spreading skin disease that can appear like a blister or vesicle on the genital region of males and females; may spread to other areas of the body. Caused by a sexually transmitted virus.

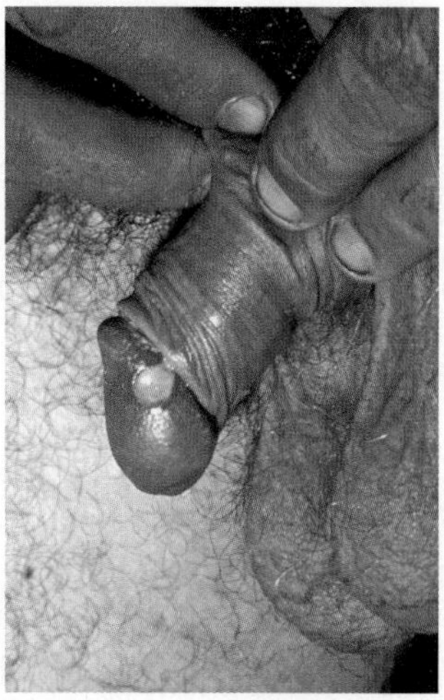

■ **Figure 10.22** Photograph showing a chancroid on the glans penis. *(Joe Miller/Centers for Disease Control)*

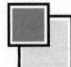 **Pathology** *(continued)*

TERM	WORD PARTS	DEFINITION
genital warts (JEN-ih-tal)	genit/o = genital -al = pertaining to	Growth of warts on the genitalia of both males and females that can lead to cancer of the cervix in females. Caused by the sexual transmission of the human papilloma virus (HPV).
gonorrhea (GC) (gon-oh-REE-ah)	-rrhea = discharge	Sexually transmitted bacterial infection of the mucous membranes of either sex. Can be passed on to an infant during the birth process.
human immunodeficiency virus (HIV)	immun/o = protection	Sexually transmitted virus that attacks the immune system.
sexually transmitted disease (STD)		Disease usually acquired as the result of sexual intercourse. Formerly referred to as *venereal disease* (VD).
syphilis (SIF-ih-lis)		Infectious, chronic, bacterial venereal disease that can involve any organ. May exist for years without symptoms, but is fatal if untreated. Treated with the antibiotic penicillin.
trichomoniasis (trik-oh-moh-NYE-ah-sis)	-iasis = abnormal condition	Genitourinary infection caused by a single-cell protist that is usually without symptoms (asymptomatic) in both males and females. In women the disease can produce itching and/or burning, a foul-smelling discharge, and result in vaginitis.

 Diagnostic Procedures

TERM	WORD PARTS	DEFINITION
Clinical Laboratory Tests		
prostate-specific antigen (PSA) (PROSS-tayt-specific / AN-tih-jen)	anti- = against -gen = that which produces	Blood test to screen for prostate cancer. Elevated blood levels of PSA are associated with prostate cancer.
semen analysis (SEE-men / ah-NAL-ih-sis)		Procedure used when performing a fertility workup to determine if the male is able to produce sperm. Semen is collected by the patient after abstaining from sexual intercourse for a period of 3–5 days. The sperm in the semen are analyzed for number, swimming strength, and shape. Also used to determine if a vasectomy has been successful. After a period of 6 weeks, no further sperm should be present in a sample from the patient.
Additional Diagnostic Procedures		
digital rectal exam (DRE) (DIJ-ih-tal / REK-tal)	rect/o = rectum -al = pertaining to	Manual examination for an enlarged prostate gland performed by palpating (feeling) the prostate gland through the wall of the rectum.

Therapeutic Procedures

TERM	WORD PARTS	DEFINITION
Surgical Procedures		
balanoplasty (BAL-ah-noh-plas-tee)	balan/o = glans penis -plasty = surgical repair	Surgical repair of the glans penis.
castration (kass-TRAY-shun)		Removal of the testicles in the male or the ovaries in the female.
circumcision (ser-kum-SIH-zhun)		Surgical removal of the end of the prepuce or foreskin of the penis. Generally performed on the newborn male at the request of the parents. The primary reason is for ease of hygiene. Circumcision is also a ritual practice in some religions.
epididymectomy (ep-ih-did-ih-MEK-toh-mee)	epididym/o = epididymis -ectomy = surgical removal	Surgical removal of the epididymis.
orchidectomy (or-kid-EK-toh-mee)	orchid/o = testes -ectomy = surgical removal	Surgical removal of one or both testes.
orchidopexy (OR-kid-oh-peck-see)	orchid/o = testes -pexy = surgical fixation	Surgical fixation to move undescended testes into the scrotum and to attach them to prevent retraction. Used to treat cryptorchidism.
orchiectomy (or-kee-EK-toh-mee)	orchi/o = testes -ectomy = surgical removal	Surgical removal of one or both testes.
orchiotomy (or-kee-OT-oh-mee)	orchi/o = testes -otomy = cutting into	To cut into the testes.
orchioplasty (OR-kee-oh-plas-tee)	orchi/o = testes -plasty = surgical repair	Surgical repair of testes.
prostatectomy (pross-tah-TEK-toh-mee)	prostat/o = prostate gland -ectomy = surgical removal	Surgical removal of the prostate gland.
sterilization (ster-ih-lih-ZAY-shun)		Process of rendering a male or female sterile or unable to conceive children.
transurethral resection of the prostate (TUR, TURP) (trans-yoo-REE-thrall / REE-sek-shun / PROSS-tayt)	trans- = across urethr/o = urethra -al = pertaining to	Surgical removal of the part of the prostate gland that is blocking urine flow by inserting a device through the urethra and removing prostate tissue.
vasectomy (vas-EK-toh-mee)	vas/o = vas deferens -ectomy = surgical removal	Removal of a segment or all of the vas deferens to prevent sperm from leaving the male body. Used for contraception purposes. See Figure 10.23 ▪.

> **MED TERM TIP**
>
> The vas deferens is the tubing that is severed during a procedure called a *vasectomy*. A vasectomy results in the sterilization of the male since the sperm are no longer able to travel into the urethra and out of the penis during sexual intercourse. The surgical procedure to reverse a vasectomy is a *vasovasostomy*. A new opening is created in order to reconnect one section of the vas deferens to another section of the vas deferens, thereby reestablishing an open tube for sperm to travel through.

Therapeutic Procedures (continued)

TERM	WORD PARTS	DEFINITION

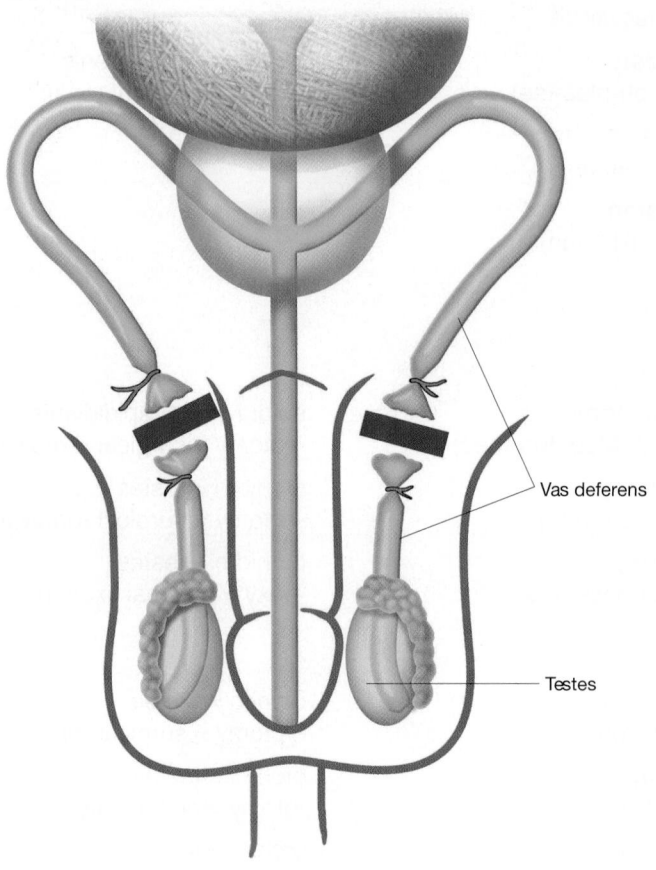

Vas deferens

Testes

Figure 10.23   A vasectomy, showing how each vas deferens is tied off in two places and then a section is removed from the middle. This prevents sperm from traveling through the vas deferens during ejaculation.

TERM	WORD PARTS	DEFINITION
vasovasostomy (vas-oh-vay-ZOS-toh-mee)	vas/o = vas deferens -ostomy = create a new opening	Surgical procedure to reconnect the vas deferens to reverse a vasectomy.

Pharmacology

CLASSIFICATION	WORD PARTS	ACTION	EXAMPLES
androgen therapy (AN-droh-jen)	andr/o = male -gen = that which produces	Replacement of male hormones to treat patients who produce insufficient hormone naturally.	testosterone cypionate, Andronate, depAndro
antiprostatic agents (an-tye-pross-TAT-ik)	anti- = against prostat/o = prostate gland -ic = pertaining to	Medication to treat early cases of benign prostatic hyperplasia. May prevent surgery for mild cases.	finasteride, Proscar; dutasteride, Avodart
erectile dysfunction agents (ee-REK-tile)	-ile = pertaining to dys- = abnormal, difficult	Medication that temporarily produces an erection in patients with erectile dysfunction.	sildenafil citrate, Viagra; tadalafil, Cialis
spermatocide (sper-mah-toh-LIT-ik)	spermat/o = sperm -cide = to kill	Destruction of sperm. One form of birth control is the use of spermatolytic creams.	octoxynol 9, Semicid, Ortho-Gynol

Abbreviations

BPH	benign prostatic hyperplasia	**RPR**	rapid plasma reagin (test for syphilis)
DRE	digital rectal exam	**SPP**	suprapubic prostatectomy
ED	erectile dysfunction	**STD**	sexually transmitted disease
GC	gonorrhea	**TUR**	transurethral resection
GU	genitourinary	**TURP**	transurethral resection of the prostate
PSA	prostate-specific antigen	**VD**	venereal disease

Chapter Review

Real-World Applications

Medical Record Analysis

This High-Risk Obstetrics Consultation Report contains 12 medical terms. Underline each term and write it in the list below the report. Then define each term.

High-Risk Obstetrics Consultation Report

Reason for Consultation:	High-risk pregnancy with late-term bleeding
History of Present Illness:	Patient is 23 years old. She is currently estimated to be at 175 days of gestation. Amniocentesis at 20 weeks shows a normally developing male fetus. She noticed a moderate degree of bleeding this morning but denies any cramping or pelvic pain. She immediately saw her obstetrician who referred her for high-risk evaluation.
Past Medical History:	This patient is multigravida but nullipara with three early miscarriages without obvious cause.
Results of Physical Examination:	Patient appears well nourished and abdominal girth appears consistent with length of gestation. Pelvic ultrasound indicates placenta previa with placenta almost completely overlying cervix. However, there is no evidence of abruptio placentae at this time. Fetal size estimate is consistent with 25 weeks of gestation. The fetal heartbeat is strong with a rate of 130 beats/minute.
Recommendations:	Fetus appears to be developing well and in no distress at this time. The placenta appears to be well attached on ultrasound, but the bleeding is cause for concern. With the extremely low position of the placenta, this patient is at very high risk for abruptio placentae. She will require C-section at onset of labor.

Term

1. _____   _____

2. _____   _____

3. _____   _____

4. _____   _____

5. _____   _____

6. _____   _____

7. _____   _____

8. _____   _____

9. _____   _____

10. _____   _____

11. _____   _____

12. _____   _____

Chart Note Transcription

The chart note below contains 10 phrases that can be reworded with a medical term that you learned in this chapter. Each phrase is identified with an underline. Determine the medical term and write your answers in the space provided.

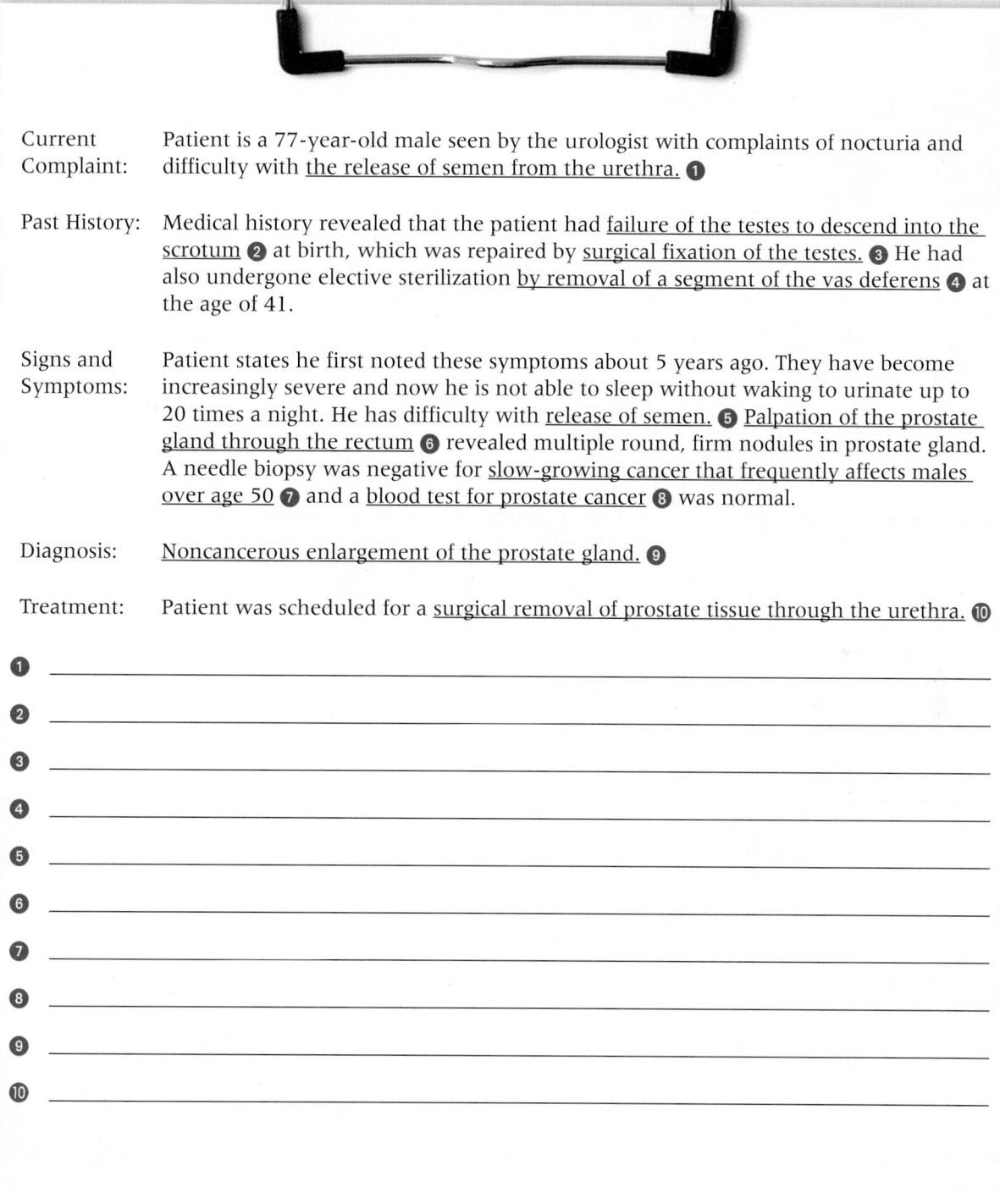

Current
Complaint: Patient is a 77-year-old male seen by the urologist with complaints of nocturia and difficulty with the release of semen from the urethra. ❶

Past History: Medical history revealed that the patient had failure of the testes to descend into the scrotum ❷ at birth, which was repaired by surgical fixation of the testes. ❸ He had also undergone elective sterilization by removal of a segment of the vas deferens ❹ at the age of 41.

Signs and
Symptoms: Patient states he first noted these symptoms about 5 years ago. They have become increasingly severe and now he is not able to sleep without waking to urinate up to 20 times a night. He has difficulty with release of semen. ❺ Palpation of the prostate gland through the rectum ❻ revealed multiple round, firm nodules in prostate gland. A needle biopsy was negative for slow-growing cancer that frequently affects males over age 50 ❼ and a blood test for prostate cancer ❽ was normal.

Diagnosis: Noncancerous enlargement of the prostate gland. ❾

Treatment: Patient was scheduled for a surgical removal of prostate tissue through the urethra. ❿

❶ _____

❷ _____

❸ _____

❹ _____

❺ _____

❻ _____

❼ _____

❽ _____

❾ _____

❿ _____

Case Study

Below is a case study presentation of a patient with a condition covered by this chapter. Read the case study and answer the questions below. Some questions will ask for information not included within this chapter. Use your text, a medical dictionary, or any other reference material you choose to answer these questions.

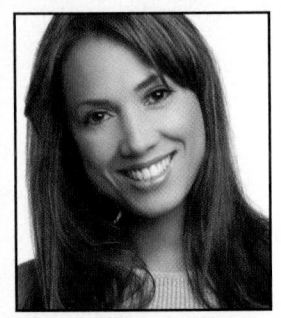

A 22-year-old female has come into the gynecologist's office complaining of fever, malaise, dysuria, and vaginal leukorrhea. Upon examination the physician observes fluid-filled vesicles on her cervix, vulva, and perineum. Several have ruptured into ulcers with marked erythema and edema. Palpation revealed painful and enlarged inguinal lymph nodes. She also has an extragenital lesion on her mouth. Her diagnosis is genital herpes.

(Jason Stitt/Shutterstock)

Questions

1. What pathological condition does this patient have? Look this condition up in a reference source and include a short description of it.

    _____

    _____

2. List and define each of the patient's presenting symptoms in your own words. Leukorrhea is a term you have not seen before. Can you give its meaning just from its word parts?

    _____

    _____

3. Describe the results of the physician's examination in your own words.

    _____

    _____

4. Explain what extragenital lesion means.

    _____

    _____

5. Explain what palpation means.

    _____

    _____

6. What is the potential effect of having this virus present in open genital lesions on the patient's future pregnancy and child birth?

    _____

    _____

Practice Exercises

A. Complete the Statement

1. The study of the female reproductive system is the medical specialty of _____.

2. A physician who specializes in the treatment of women is called a(n) _____.

3. The three stages of labor and delivery are the _____ stage, the _____ stage, and the _____ stage.

4. The time required for the development of a fetus is called _____.

5. The cessation of menstruation is called _____.

6. The female sex cell is a(n) _____.

7. The inner lining of the uterus is called the _____.

8. The organ in which the developing fetus resides is called the _____.

9. The tubes that extend from the outer edges of the uterus and assist in transporting the ova and sperm are called _____.

10. One of the longest terms used in medical terminology refers to the removal of the uterus, cervix, ovaries, and uterine tubes. This term is _____.

B. What Does it Stand For?

1. SPP _____

2. TUR _____

3. GU _____

4. BPH _____

5. DRE _____

6. PSA _____

C. Define the Term

1. spermatogenesis _____

2. hydrocele _____

3. transurethral resection of the prostate (TURP) _____

4. sterility _____

5. orchiectomy _____

6. vasectomy _____

7. castration _____

D. Combining Form Practice

The combining form **colp/o** refers to the vagina. Use it to write a term that means:

1. visual examination of the vagina _____

2. instrument used to examine the vagina _____

The combining form **cervic/o** refers to the cervix. Use it to write a term that means:

3. removal of the cervix _____

4. inflammation of the cervix _____

5. pertaining to the cervix _____

The combining form **hyster/o** also refers to the uterus. Use it to write a term that means:

6. surgical fixation of the uterus _____

7. removal of the uterus _____

8. rupture of the uterus _____

The combining form **oophor/o** refers to the ovaries. Use it to write a term that means:

9. inflammation of an ovary _____

10. removal of an ovary _____

The combining form **mamm/o** refers to the breasts. Use it to write a term that means:

11. pertaining to the breasts _____

12. record of breast _____

13. surgical repair of breast _____

The combining form **amni/o** refers to the amnion. Use it to write a term that means:

14. pertaining to the amnion _____

15. cutting into amnion _____

16. flow from amnion _____

E. What Does it Stand For?

1. Cx _____

2. LMP _____

3. FHR _____

4. PID _____

5. GYN _____

6. CS _____

7. NB _____

8. PMS _____

9. TSS _____

10. LBW _____

F. What's the Abbreviation?

1. first pregnancy _____

2. artificial insemination _____

3. uterine contractions _____

4. full-term normal delivery _____

5. intrauterine device _____

6. dilation and curettage _____

7. hormone replacement therapy _____

8. gynecology _____

9. abortion _____

10. oral contraception pills _____

G. Define the Combining Form

	Definition	Example from Chapter
1. **metr/o**	_____	_____
2. **hyster/o**	_____	_____
3. **gynec/o**	_____	_____
4. **episi/o**	_____	_____
5. **oophor/o**	_____	_____
6. **ovari/o**	_____	_____
7. **salping/o**	_____	_____
8. **men/o**	_____	_____
9. **vagin/o**	_____	_____
10. **mast/o**	_____	_____

H. Terminology Matching

Match each term to its definition.

1. _____ hemolytic disease of the newborn
2. _____ ovary
3. _____ vagina
4. _____ abruptio placentae
5. _____ placenta
6. _____ endometrium
7. _____ clitoris
8. _____ candidiasis
9. _____ Pap smear
10. _____ uterine tube
11. _____ dysmenorrhea
12. _____ breech presentation
13. _____ Apgar
14. _____ neonate
15. _____ eclampsia

a. seizures and coma during pregnancy
b. erythroblastosis fetalis
c. detached placenta
d. female erectile tissue
e. produces eggs
f. normal place for fertilization
g. buttocks first to appear in birth canal
h. birth canal
i. nourishes fetus
j. uterine lining
k. measures newborn's adjustment to outside world
l. test for cervical cancer
m. newborn
n. yeast infection
o. painful menstruation

I. Define the Suffix

	Definition	Example from Chapter
1. -tocia	_____	_____
2. -gravida	_____	_____
3. -arche	_____	_____
4. -cyesis	_____	_____
5. -partum	_____	_____
6. -para	_____	_____
7. -salpinx	_____	_____
8. -spermia	_____	_____

J. Fill in the Blank

premenstrual syndrome	stillbirth	conization	laparoscopy
D & C	puberty	endometriosis	eclampsia
fibroid tumor	cesarean section		

1. Kesha had a core of tissue from her cervix removed for testing. This is called _____ .

2. Joan delivered a baby that had died while still in the uterus. She had a(n) _____ .

3. Ashley has just started her first menstrual cycle. She is said to have entered _____ .

4. Kimberly is experiencing tender breasts, headaches, and some irritability just prior to her monthly menstrual cycle. This may be _____ .

5. Ana has been scheduled for an examination in which her physician will use an instrument to observe her abdominal cavity to rule out the diagnosis of severe endometriosis. The physician will insert the instrument through a small incision. This procedure is called a(n) _____ .

6. Lenora is scheduled to have a hysterectomy as a result of a long history of large benign growths in her uterus that have caused pain and bleeding. Lenora has a(n) _____ .

7. Tiffany's physician has recommended that she have a uterine scraping to stop excessive bleeding after a miscarriage. She will be scheduled for a(n) _____ .

8. Stacey is having frequent prenatal checkups to prevent the serious condition of pregnancy called _____ .

9. Marion has experienced painful menstrual periods as a result of the lining of her uterus being displaced into her pelvic cavity. This is called _____ .

10. Because her cervix was not dilating, Shataundra was informed that she will probably require a(n) _____ for her baby's delivery.

K. Complete the Statement

1. The male reproductive system is a combination of the _____ and _____ systems.

2. The male's external organs of reproduction consist of the _____, _____, and the _____ .

3. Another term for the prepuce is the _____ .

4. The organs responsible for developing the sperm cells are the _____ .

5. The glands of lubrication and fluid production at each side of the male urethra are the _____ .

6. The male sex hormone is _____ .

7. The area between the scrotum and the anus is called the _____ .

L. Terminology Matching

Match each term to its definition.

1. _____ gonorrhea

2. _____ genital herpes

3. _____ human immunodeficiency virus

4. _____ syphilis

5. _____ venereal disease

6. _____ genital warts

7. _____ chancroid

8. _____ chlamydia

9. _____ trichomoniasis

a. also called STD

b. caused by parasitic microorganism

c. treated with penicillin

d. caused by human papilloma virus

e. can pass to infant during birth

f. genitourinary infection

g. venereal ulcer

h. attacks the immune system

i. skin disease with vesicles

M. Combining Form Practice

The combining form **prostat/o** refers to the prostate. Use this to write a term that means:

1. removal of prostate _____

2. pertaining to the prostate _____

3. inflammation of the prostate _____

The combining form **orchi/o** refers to the testes. Use this to write a term that means:

4. removal of the testes _____

5. surgical repair of the testes _____

6. incision into the testes _____

The suffix **-spermia** refers to a sperm condition. Use this to write a term that means:

7. condition of being without sperm _____

8. condition of having too few (scanty) sperm _____

The combining form **spermat/o** refers to sperm. Use this to write a term that means:

9. sperm forming _____

10. sperm destruction _____

N. Pharmacology Challenge

Fill in the classification for each drug description, then match the brand name.

Drug Description	Classification	Brand Name
1. _____ replacement male hormone	_____	a. Pitocin
2. _____ improves uterine contractions	_____	b. Avodart
3. _____ treats early BPH	_____	c. Clomid
4. _____ blocks ovulation	_____	d. Semicid
5. _____ kills sperm	_____	e. Mifeprex
6. _____ produces an erection	_____	f. Andronate
7. _____ replaces estrogen	_____	g. Ortho-Cept
8. _____ terminates a pregnancy	_____	h. Viagra
9. _____ triggers ovulation	_____	i. Premarin

Labeling Exercise

Image A

Write the labels for this figure on the numbered lines provided.

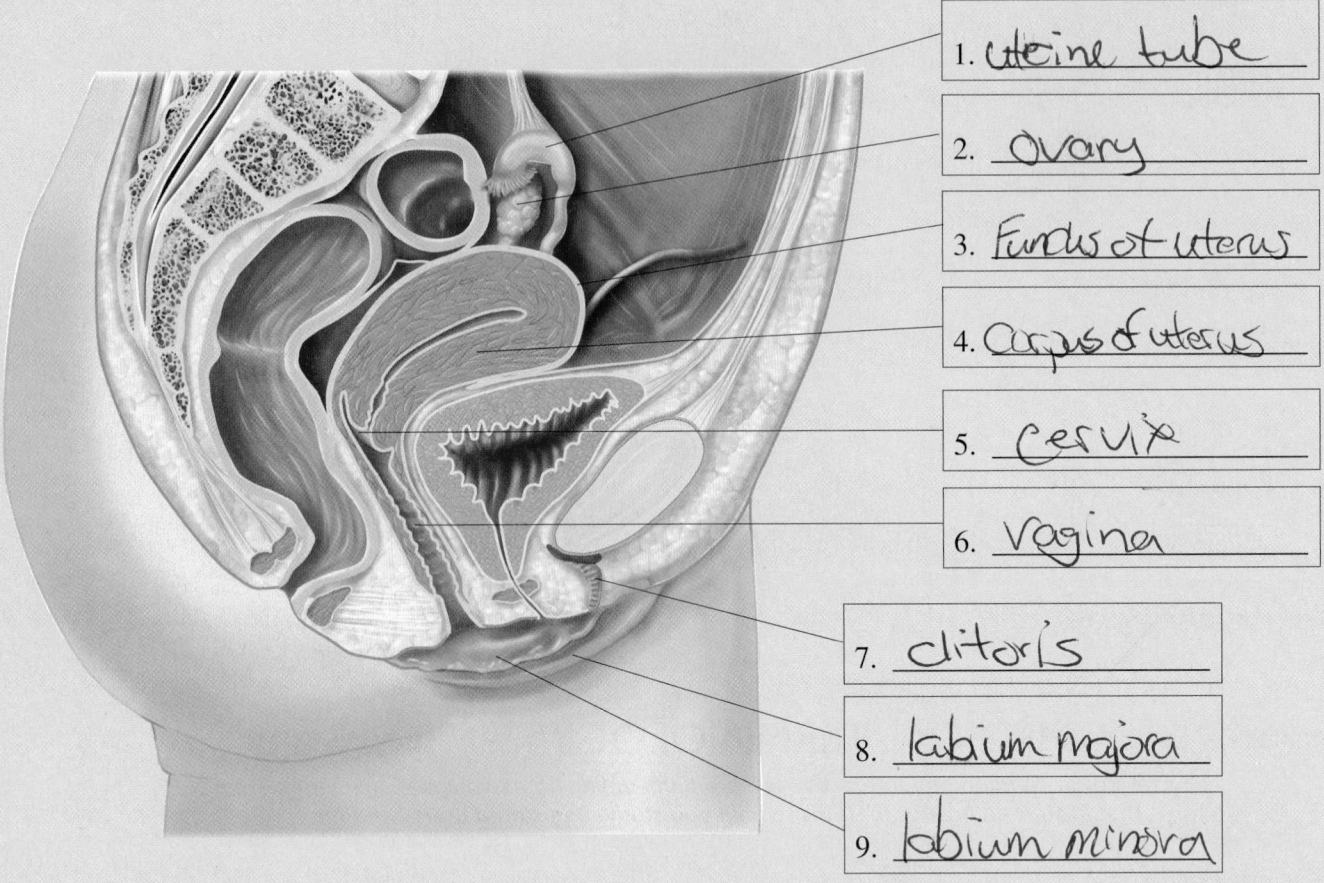

1. uterine tube
2. ovary
3. Fundus of uterus
4. Corpus of uterus
5. Cervix
6. vagina
7. clitoris
8. labium majora
9. labium minora

Write the labels for this figure on the numbered lines provided.

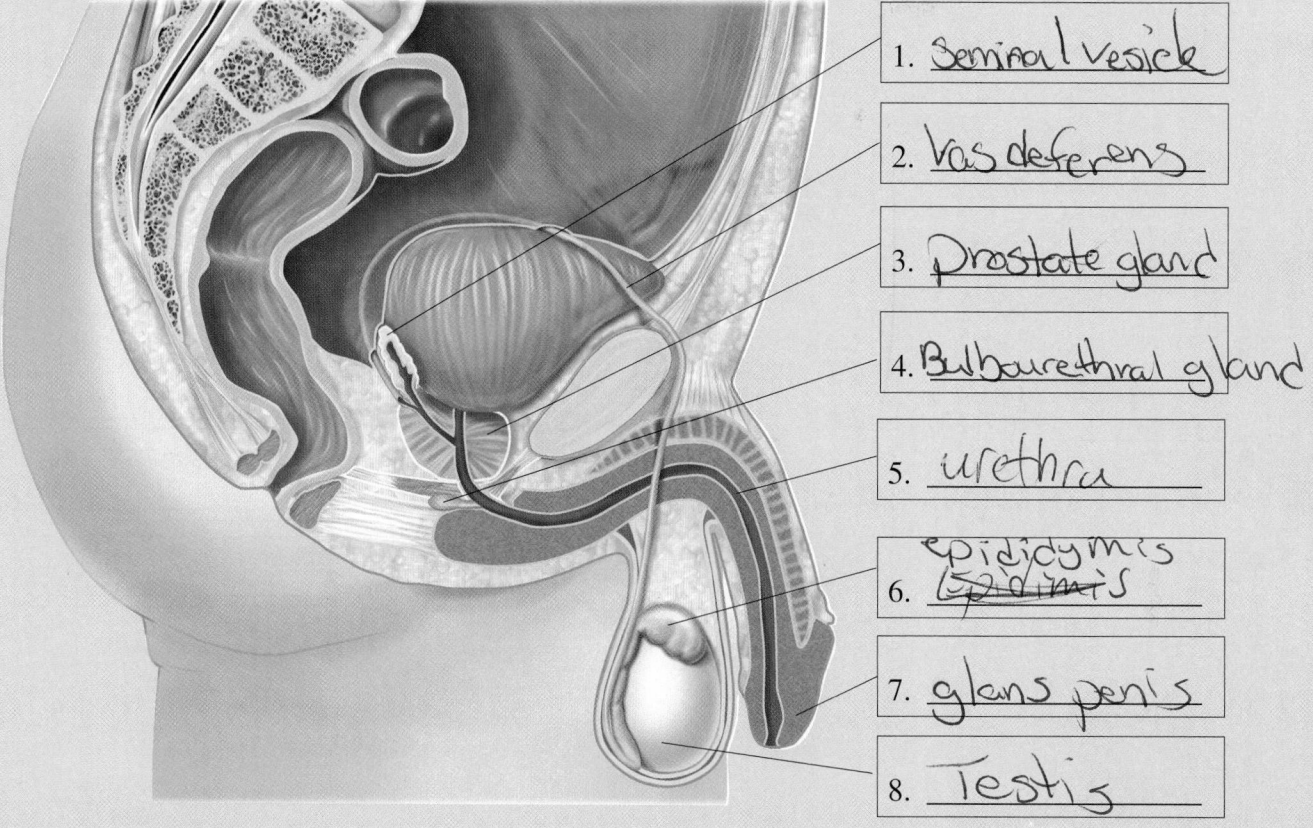

1. Seminal vesicle

2. Vas deferens

3. Prostate gland

4. Bulbourethral gland

5. urethra

6. epididymis ~~epidimis~~

7. glans penis

8. Testis

Image C

Write the labels for this figure on the numbered lines provided.

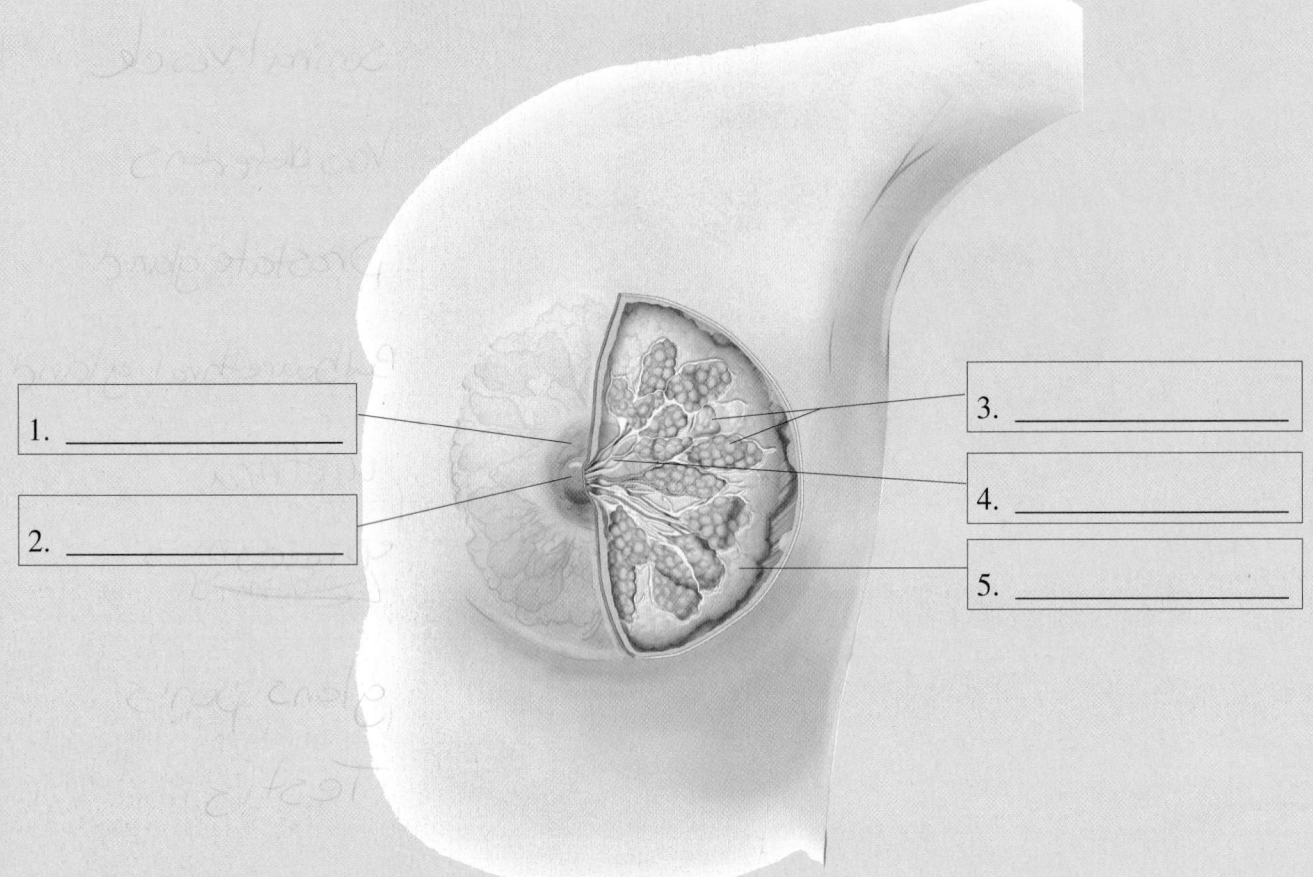

1. _____

2. _____

3. _____

4. _____

5. _____

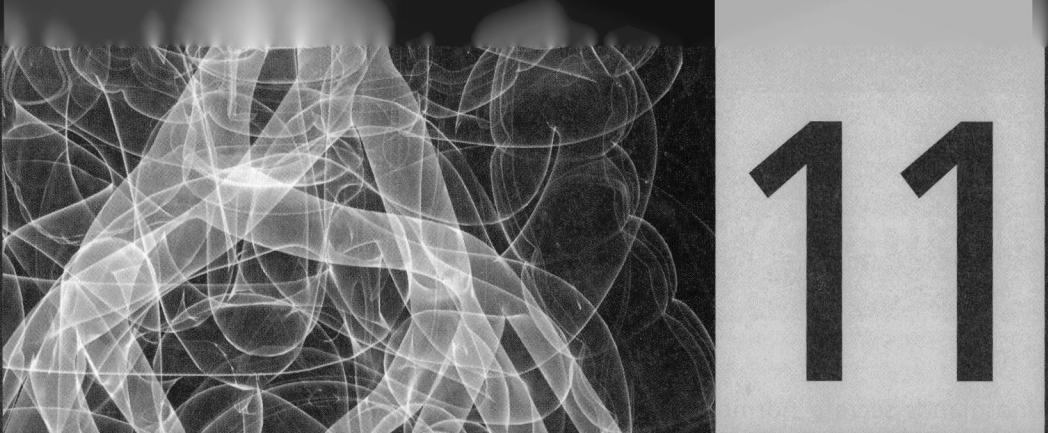

11

ENDOCRINE SYSTEM

Learning Objectives

Upon completion of this chapter, you will be able to

- Identify and define the combining forms and suffixes introduced in this chapter.
- Correctly spell and pronounce medical terms and major anatomical structures relating to the endocrine system.
- Locate and describe the major organs of the endocrine system and their functions.
- List the major hormones secreted by each endocrine gland and describe their functions.
- Identify and define endocrine system anatomical terms.
- Identify and define selected endocrine system pathology terms.
- Identify and define selected endocrine system diagnostic procedures.
- Identify and define selected endocrine system therapeutic procedures.
- Identify and define selected medications relating to the endocrine system.
- Define selected abbreviations associated with the endocrine system.

Endocrine System at a Glance

Function

Endocrine glands secrete hormones that regulate many body activities such as metabolic rate, water and mineral balance, immune system reactions, and sexual functioning.

Organs

Here are the primary structures that comprise the endocrine system.

adrenal glands	pituitary gland
ovaries	testes
pancreas (islets of Langerhans)	thymus gland
parathyroid glands	thyroid gland
pineal gland	

Word Parts

Here are the most common word parts used to build endocrine system terms. For a more comprehensive list, refer to the Terminology section of this chapter.

Combining Forms

acr/o	extremities	ket/o	ketones
adren/o	adrenal glands	mineral/o	minerals, electrolytes
adrenal/o	adrenal glands	natr/o	sodium
andr/o	male	ophthalm/o	eye
calc/o	calcium	ovari/o	ovary
crin/o	to secrete	pancreat/o	pancreas
estr/o	female	parathyroid/o	parathyroid gland
gluc/o	glucose	pineal/o	pineal gland
glyc/o	sugar	pituitar/o	pituitary gland
glycos/o	sugar	testicul/o	testes
gonad/o	sex glands	thym/o	thymus gland
home/o	sameness	thyr/o	thyroid gland
iod/o	iodine	thyroid/o	thyroid gland
kal/i	potassium	toxic/o	poison

Suffixes

-dipsia	thirst	-pressin	to press down
-prandial	relating to a meal	-tropin	to stimulate

Endocrine System Illustrated

pineal gland, p. 384

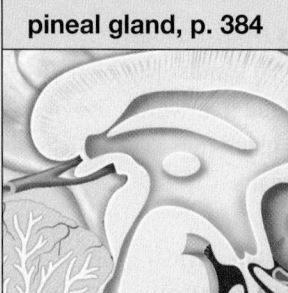

Regulates circadian rhythm

thyroid gland, p. 387
parathyroid glands, p. 384

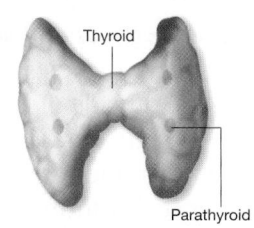

Thyroid

Parathyroid

Regulates metabolic rate
Regulate blood calcium level

adrenal glands, p. 382

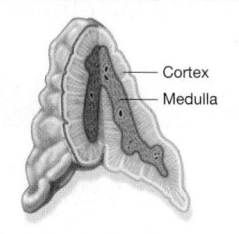

Cortex
Medulla

Regulate water and
electrolyte levels

pancreas, p. 383

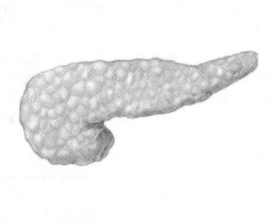

Regulates blood sugar levels

pituitary gland, p. 384

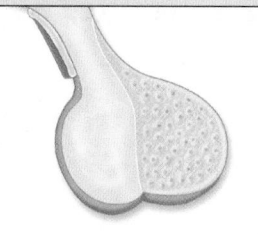

Regulates many other
endocrine glands

thymus gland, p. 387

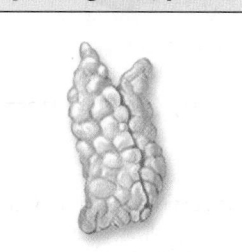

Development of
immune system

ovaries, p. 382

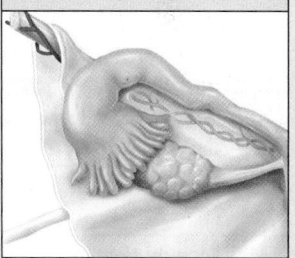

Regulate female
reproductive system

testes, p. 386

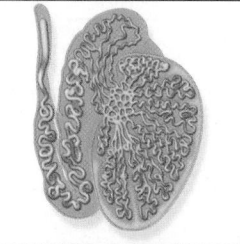

Regulate male
reproductive system

■ Anatomy and Physiology of the Endocrine System

adrenal glands (ad-REE-nal)	**pancreas** (PAN-kree-ass)
endocrine glands (EN-doh-krin)	**parathyroid glands** (pair-ah-THIGH-royd)
endocrine system	**pineal gland** (pih-NEAL)
exocrine glands (EKS-oh-krin)	**pituitary gland** (pih-TOO-ih-tair-ee)
glands	**target organs**
homeostasis (hoe-me-oh-STAY-sis)	**testes** (TESS-teez)
hormones (HOR-mohnz)	**thymus gland** (THIGH-mus)
ovaries (OH-vah-reez)	**thyroid gland** (THIGH-royd)

> **MED TERM TIP**
>
> The terms *endocrine* and *exocrine* were constructed to reflect the function of each type of gland. As glands, they both secrete, indicated by the combining form *crin/o*. The prefix *exo-*, meaning "external" or "outward," tells us that exocrine gland secretions are carried to the outside of the body or to a passageway connected to the outside of the body. However, the prefix *endo-*, meaning "within" or "internal," indicates that endocrine gland secretions are carried to other internal body structures by the bloodstream.

The **endocrine system** is a collection of **glands** that secrete **hormones** directly into the bloodstream. Hormones are chemicals that act on their **target organs** to either increase or decrease the target's activity level. In this way the endocrine system is instrumental in maintaining **homeostasis** (*home/o* = sameness; *-stasis* = standing still)—that is, adjusting the activity level of most of the tissues and organs of the body to maintain a stable internal environment.

The body actually has two distinct types of glands: **exocrine glands** and **endocrine glands.** Exocrine glands release their secretions into a duct that carries them to the outside of the body or to a passageway connected to the outside of the body. For example, sweat glands release sweat into a sweat duct that travels to the surface of the body. Endocrine glands, however, release hormones directly into the bloodstream. For example, the thyroid gland secretes its hormones directly into the bloodstream. Because endocrine glands have no ducts, they are also referred to as *ductless glands.*

The endocrine system consists of the following glands: two **adrenal glands,** two **ovaries** in the female, four **parathyroid glands,** the **pancreas,** the **pineal gland,** the **pituitary gland,** two **testes** in the male, the **thymus gland,** and the **thyroid gland.** The endocrine glands as a whole affect the functions of the entire body. Table 11.1 ■ presents a description of the endocrine glands, their hormones, and their functions.

Table 11.1   Endocrine Glands and Their Hormones

GLAND AND HORMONE	WORD PARTS	FUNCTION
Adrenal cortex	adren/o = adrenal gland -al = pertaining to	
Glucocorticoids such as cortisol	gluc/o = glucose cortic/o = outer portion	Regulates carbohydrate levels in the body.
Mineralocorticoids such as aldosterone	mineral/o = minerals, electrolytes cortic/o = outer portion	Regulates electrolytes and fluid volume in body.
Steroid sex hormones such as androgen	andr/o = male -gen = that which produces	Male sex hormones from adrenal cortex may be converted to estrogens in the bloodstream. Responsible for reproduction and secondary sexual characteristics.
Adrenal medulla	adren/o = adrenal gland -al = pertaining to	
Epinephrine (adrenaline)	epi- = above nephr/o = kidney -ine = pertaining to	Intensifies response during stress; "fight-or-flight" response.
Norepinephrine	epi- = above nephr/o = kidney -ine = pertaining to	Chiefly a vasoconstrictor.

Table 11.1	Endocrine Glands and Their Hormones (continued)	
GLAND AND HORMONE	**WORD PARTS**	**FUNCTION**
Ovaries		
Estrogen	estr/o = female -gen = that which produces	Stimulates development of secondary sex characteristics in females; regulates menstrual cycle.
Progesterone	pro- = before estr/o = female	Prepares for conditions of pregnancy.
Pancreas		
Glucagon		Stimulates liver to release glucose into the blood.
Insulin		Regulates and promotes entry of glucose into cells.
Parathyroid glands		
Parathyroid hormone (PTH)		Stimulates bone breakdown; regulates calcium level in the blood.
Pituitary anterior lobe		
Adrenocorticotropin hormone (ACTH)	adren/o = adrenal gland cortic/o = outer portion -tropin = to stimulate	Regulates function of adrenal cortex.
Gonadotropins	gonad/o = gonads -tropin = to stimulate	
Follicle-stimulating hormone (FSH)		Stimulates growth of eggs in female and sperm in males.
Luteinizing hormone (LH)		Regulates function of male and female gonads and plays a role in releasing ova in females.
Growth hormone (GH)		Stimulates growth of the body.
Melanocyte-stimulating hormone (MSH)	melan/o = black -cyte = cell	Stimulates pigment in skin.
Prolactin	pro- = before lact/o = milk	Stimulates milk production.
Thyroid-stimulating hormone (TSH)		Regulates function of thyroid gland.
Pituitary posterior lobe		
Antidiuretic hormone (ADH)	anti- = against -tic = pertaining to	Stimulates reabsorption of water by the kidneys.
Oxytocin		Stimulates uterine contractions and releases milk into ducts.
Testes		
Testosterone		Promotes sperm production and development of secondary sex characteristics in males.
Thymus		
Thymosin	thym/o = thymus gland	Promotes development of cells in immune system.
Thyroid gland		
Calcitonin (CT)		Stimulates deposition of calcium into bone.
Thyroxine (T_4)	thyr/o = thyroid gland -ine = pertaining to	Stimulates metabolism in cells.
Triiodothyronine (T_3)	tri- = three iod/o = iodine thyr/o = thyroid gland -ine = pertaining to	Stimulates metabolism in cells.

Adrenal Glands

adrenal cortex (KOR-tex)	**estrogen** (ESS-troh-jen)
adrenal medulla (meh-DOOL-lah)	**glucocorticoids** (gloo-koh-KOR-tih-koydz)
adrenaline (ah-DREN-ah-lin)	**mineralocorticoids**
aldosterone (al-DOSS-ter-ohn)	(min-er-al-oh-KOR-tih-koydz)
androgens (AN-druh-jenz)	**norepinephrine** (nor-ep-ih-NEF-rin)
corticosteroids (kor-tih-koh-STAIR-oydz)	**progesterone** (proh-JESS-ter-ohn)
cortisol (KOR-tih-sal)	**steroid sex hormones** (STAIR-oyd)
epinephrine (ep-ih-NEF-rin)	

The two adrenal glands are located above each of the kidneys (see Figure 11.1 ■). Each gland is composed of two sections: **adrenal cortex** and **adrenal medulla.**

The outer adrenal cortex manufactures several different families of hormones: **mineralocorticoids, glucocorticoids,** and **steroid sex hormones.** However, because they are all produced by the cortex, they are collectively referred to as **corticosteroids.** The mineralocorticoid hormone, **aldosterone,** regulates sodium (Na⁺) and potassium (K⁺) levels in the body. The glucocorticoid hormone, **cortisol,** regulates carbohydrates in the body. The adrenal cortex of both men and women secretes steroid sex hormones, **androgens** (which may be converted to **estrogen** once released into the bloodstream). These hormones regulate secondary sexual characteristics. All hormones secreted by the adrenal cortex are steroid hormones.

The inner adrenal medulla is responsible for secreting the hormones **epinephrine,** also called **adrenaline,** and **norepinephrine.** These hormones are critical during emergency situations because they increase blood pressure, heart rate, and respiration levels. This helps the body perform better during emergencies or otherwise stressful times.

> **MED TERM TIP**
>
> The term *cortex* is frequently used in anatomy to indicate the outer portion of an organ such as the adrenal gland or the kidney. The term *cortex* means "bark," as in the bark of a tree. The term *medulla* means "marrow." Because marrow is found in the inner cavity of bones, the term came to stand for the middle of an organ.

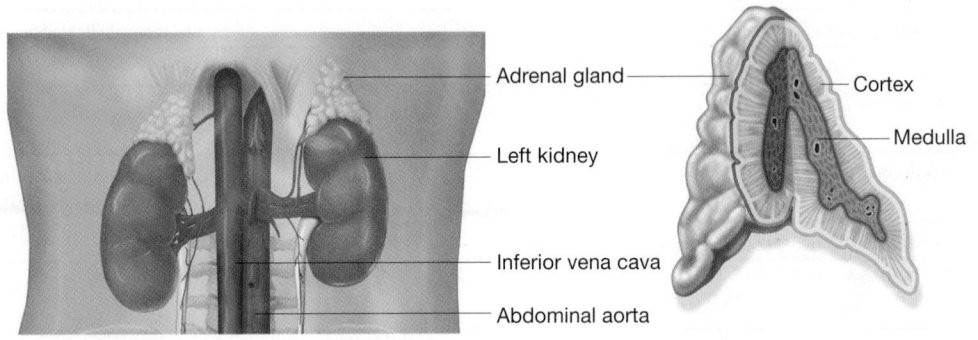

■ **Figure 11.1**   The adrenal glands. These glands sit on top of each kidney. Each adrenal is subdivided into an outer cortex and an inner medulla. Each region secretes different hormones.

- Adrenal gland
- Cortex
- Medulla
- Left kidney
- Inferior vena cava
- Abdominal aorta

Ovaries

estrogen	**menstrual cycle** (men-STROO-all)
gametes (gam-EATS)	**ova**
gonads (GOH-nadz)	**progesterone**

The two ovaries are located in the lower abdominopelvic cavity of the female (see Figure 11.2 ■). They are the female **gonads.** Gonads are organs that produce **gametes** or the reproductive sex cells. In the case of females, the gametes are the **ova.** Of importance to the endocrine system, the ovaries produce the female sex hormones, **estrogen** and **progesterone.** Estrogen is responsible for the appearance of the female sexual characteristics and regulation of the **menstrual cycle.** Progesterone helps to maintain a suitable uterine environment for pregnancy.

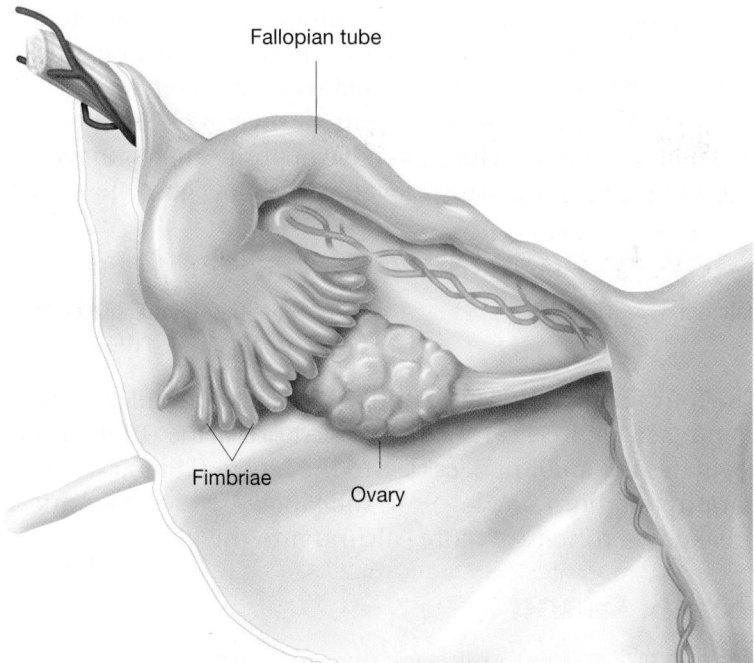

Figure 11.2
The ovaries. In addition to producing ova, the ovaries secrete the female sex hormones, estrogen and progesterone.

Fallopian tube

Fimbriae

Ovary

Pancreas

glucagon (GLOO-koh-gon)
insulin (IN-suh-lin)

islets of Langerhans
(EYE-lets / of / LAHNG-er-hahnz)

The pancreas is located along the lower curvature of the stomach (see Figure 11.3A ■). It is the only organ in the body that has both endocrine and exocrine functions. The exocrine portion of the pancreas releases digestive enzymes through a duct into the duodenum of the small intestine. The endocrine sections of the pancreas, **islets of Langerhans,** are named after Dr. Paul Langerhans, a German anatomist. The islets cells produce two different hormones: **insulin** and **glucagon** (see Figure 11.3B ■). Insulin, produced by beta (β) islet cells, stimulates the cells of the body to take in glucose from the bloodstream, lowering the body's blood sugar level. This occurs after a meal has been eaten and the carbohydrates are absorbed into the bloodstream. In this way the cells obtain the glucose they need for cellular respiration.

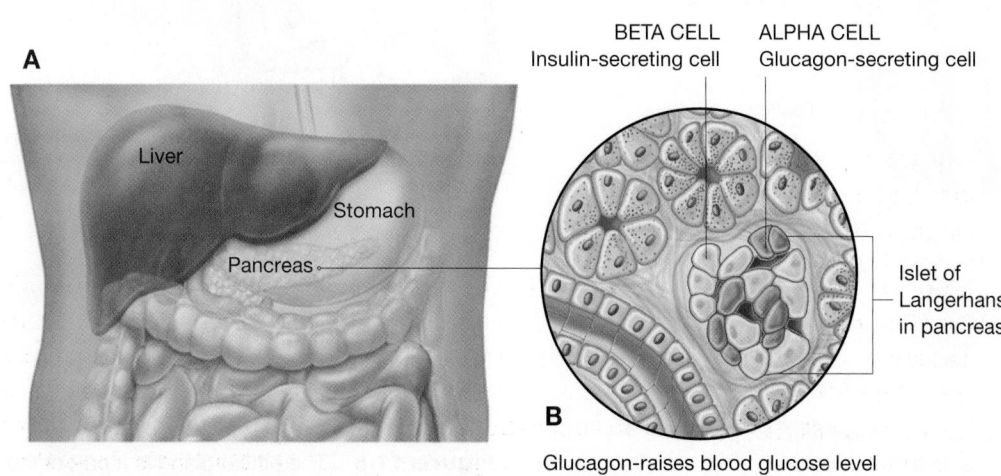

A

Liver

Stomach

Pancreas

BETA CELL
Insulin-secreting cell

ALPHA CELL
Glucagon-secreting cell

Islet of Langerhans in pancreas

B

Glucagon-raises blood glucose level
Insulin-lowers blood glucose level

Figure 11.3
The pancreas. This organ sits just below the stomach and is both an exocrine and an endocrine gland. The endocrine regions of the pancreas are called the islets of Langerhans and they secrete insulin and glucagon.

Another set of islet cells, the alpha (α) cells, secrete a different hormone, glucagon, which stimulates the liver to release glucose, thereby raising the blood glucose level. Glucagon is released when the body needs more sugar, such as at the beginning of strenuous activity or several hours after the last meal has been digested. Insulin and glucagon have opposite effects on blood sugar level. Insulin will reduce the blood sugar level, while glucagon will increase it.

Parathyroid Glands

calcium   **parathyroid hormone**
                                          (pair-ah-THIGH-royd / HOR-mohn)

The four tiny parathyroid glands are located on the dorsal surface of the thyroid gland (see Figure 11.4 ■). The **parathyroid hormone** (PTH) secreted by these glands regulates the amount of **calcium** in the blood. If blood calcium levels fall too low, parathyroid hormone levels in the blood are increased and will stimulate bone breakdown to release more calcium into the blood.

Pineal Gland

circadian rhythm (seer-KAY-dee-an)   **melatonin** (mel-ah-TOH-nin)
thalamus (THALL-mus)

The pineal gland is a small pine cone-shaped gland that is part of the **thalamus** region of the brain (see Figure 11.5 ■). The pineal gland secretes **melatonin,** a hormone not well understood, but that plays a role in regulating the body's **circadian rhythm.** This is the 24-hour clock that governs our periods of wakefulness and sleepiness.

Pituitary Gland

adrenocorticotropin hormone   **follicle-stimulating hormone**
    (ah-dree-noh-kor-tih-koh-TROH-pin)   (FOLL-ih-kl / STIM-yoo-lay-ting)
anterior lobe   **gonadotropins** (go-nad-oh-TROH-pins)
antidiuretic hormone   **growth hormone**
    (an-tye-dye-yoo-RET-ik)   **hypothalamus** (high-poh-THAL-ah-mus)

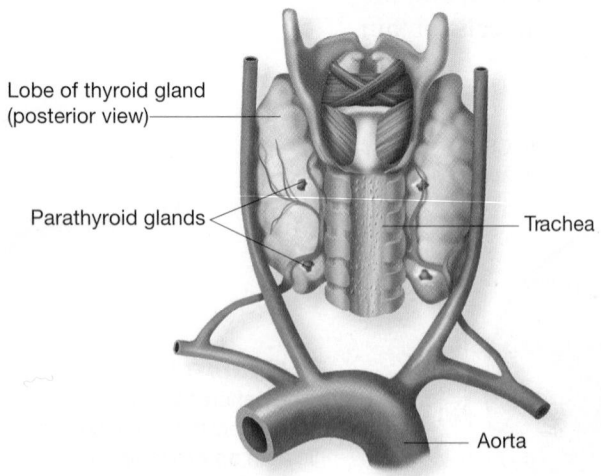

Lobe of thyroid gland
(posterior view)

Parathyroid glands

Trachea

Aorta

■ **Figure 11.4** The parathyroid glands. These four glands are located on the posterior side of the thyroid gland. They secrete parathyroid hormone.

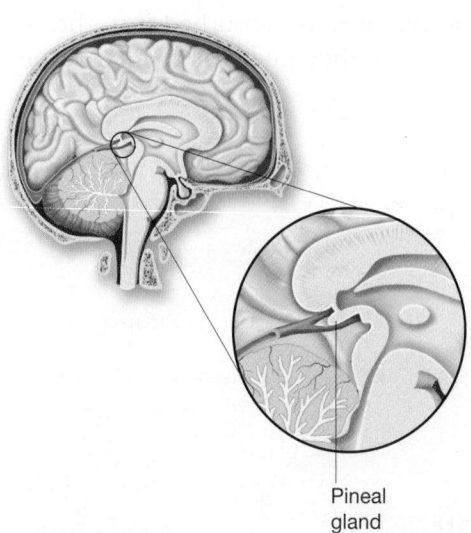

Pineal gland

■ **Figure 11.5** The pineal gland is a part of the thalamus region of the brain. It secretes melatonin.

luteinizing hormone (LOO-tee-in-eye-zing)

melanocyte-stimulating hormone

oxytocin (ok-see-TOH-sin)

posterior lobe

prolactin (proh-LAK-tin)

somatotropin (so-mat-oh-TROH-pin)

thyroid-stimulating hormone

The pituitary gland is located underneath the brain (see Figure 11.6 ■). The small marble-shaped gland is divided into an **anterior lobe** and a **posterior lobe.** Both lobes are controlled by the **hypothalamus,** a region of the brain active in regulating automatic body responses.

The anterior pituitary secretes several different hormones (see Figure 11.7 ■). **Growth hormone** (GH), also called **somatotropin,** promotes growth of the body by stimulating cells to rapidly increase in size and divide. **Thyroid-stimulating hormone** (TSH) regulates the function of the thyroid gland. **Adrenocorticotropin hormone** (ACTH) regulates the function of the adrenal cortex. **Prolactin** (PRL) stimulates milk production in the breast following pregnancy and birth. **Follicle-stimulating hormone** (FSH) and **luteinizing hormone** (LH) both exert their influence on the male and female gonads. Therefore, these two hormones together are referred to as the **gonadotropins.** Follicle-stimulating hormone is responsible for the development of ova in ovaries and sperm in testes. It also stimulates the ovary to secrete estrogen. Luteinizing hormone stimulates secretion of sex hormones in both males and females and plays a role in releasing ova in females. **Melanocyte-stimulating hormone** (MSH) stimulates melanocytes to produce more melanin, thereby darkening the skin.

The posterior pituitary secretes two hormones, **antidiuretic hormone** (ADH) and **oxytocin.** Antidiuretic hormone promotes water reabsorption by the kidney tubules. Oxytocin stimulates uterine contractions during labor and delivery, and after birth the release of milk from the mammary glands.

MED TERM TIP

The pituitary gland is sometimes referred to as the "master gland" because several of its secretions regulate other endocrine glands.

MED TERM TIP

Many people use the term *diabetes* to refer to diabetes mellitus (DM). But there is another type of diabetes, called *diabetes insipidus* (DI), that is a result of the inadequate secretion of the antidiuretic hormone (ADH) from the pituitary gland.

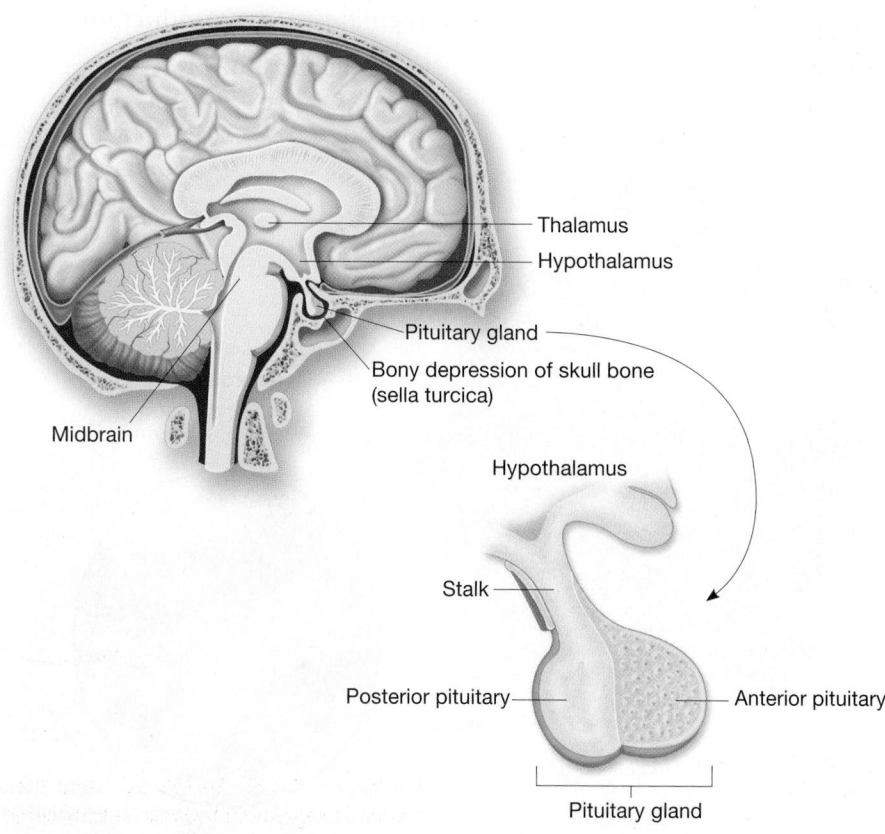

Thalamus

Hypothalamus

Pituitary gland

Bony depression of skull bone (sella turcica)

Midbrain

Hypothalamus

Stalk

Posterior pituitary

Anterior pituitary

Pituitary gland

■ **Figure 11.6**
The pituitary gland lies just underneath the brain. It is subdivided into anterior and posterior lobes. Each lobe secretes different hormones.

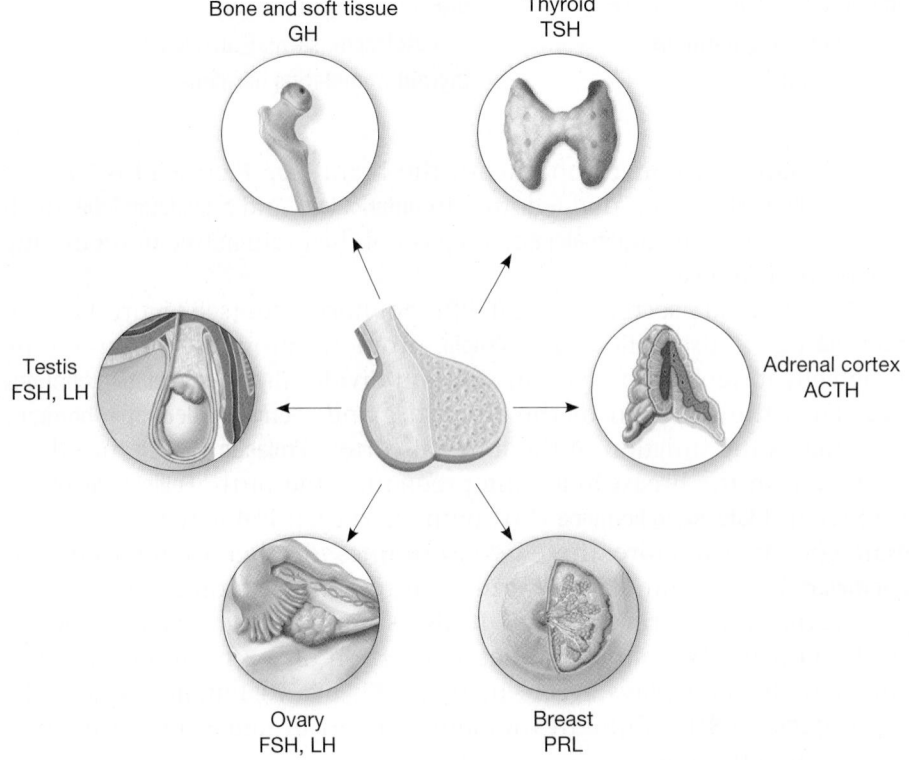

Bone and soft tissue
GH

Thyroid
TSH

Testis
FSH, LH

Adrenal cortex
ACTH

Ovary
FSH, LH

Breast
PRL

Testes

sperm   **testosterone** (tess-TOSS-ter-own)

The testes are two oval glands located in the scrotal sac of the male (see
Figure 11.8 ■). They are the male gonads, which produce the male gametes,
sperm, and the male sex hormone, **testosterone.** Testosterone produces the male
secondary sexual characteristics and regulates sperm production.

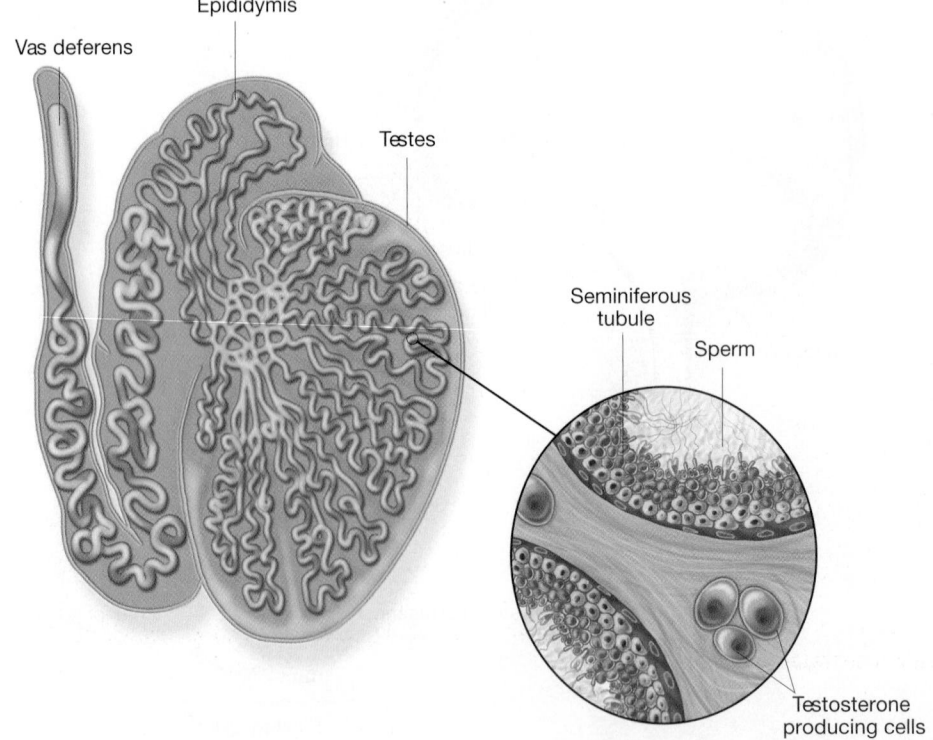

Vas deferens

Epididymis

Testes

Seminiferous
tubule

Sperm

Testosterone
producing cells

Thymus Gland

T cells   **thymosin** (thigh-MOH-sin)

In addition to its role as part of the immune system, the thymus is also one of the endocrine glands because it secretes the hormone **thymosin.** Thymosin, like the rest of the thymus gland, is important for proper development of the immune system. The thymus gland is located in the mediastinal cavity anterior and superior to the heart (see Figure 11.9 ■). The thymus is present at birth and grows to its largest size during puberty. At puberty it begins to shrink and eventually is replaced with connective and adipose tissue.

The most important function of the thymus is the development of the immune system in the newborn. It is essential to the growth and development of thymic lymphocytes or **T cells,** which are critical for the body's immune system.

Thyroid Gland

calcitonin (kal-sih-TOH-nin)   **triiodothyronine**
iodine (EYE-oh-dine)   (try-eye-oh-doh-THIGH-roh-neen)
thyroxine (thigh-ROKS-in)

The thyroid gland, which resembles a butterfly in shape, has right and left lobes (see Figure 11.10 ■). It is located on either side of the trachea and larynx. The thyroid cartilage, or Adam's apple, is located just above the thyroid gland. This gland produces the hormones **thyroxine** (T_4) and **triiodothyronine** (T_3). These hormones are produced in the thyroid gland from the mineral **iodine.** Thyroxine and triiodothyronine help to regulate the production of energy and heat in the body to adjust the body's metabolic rate.

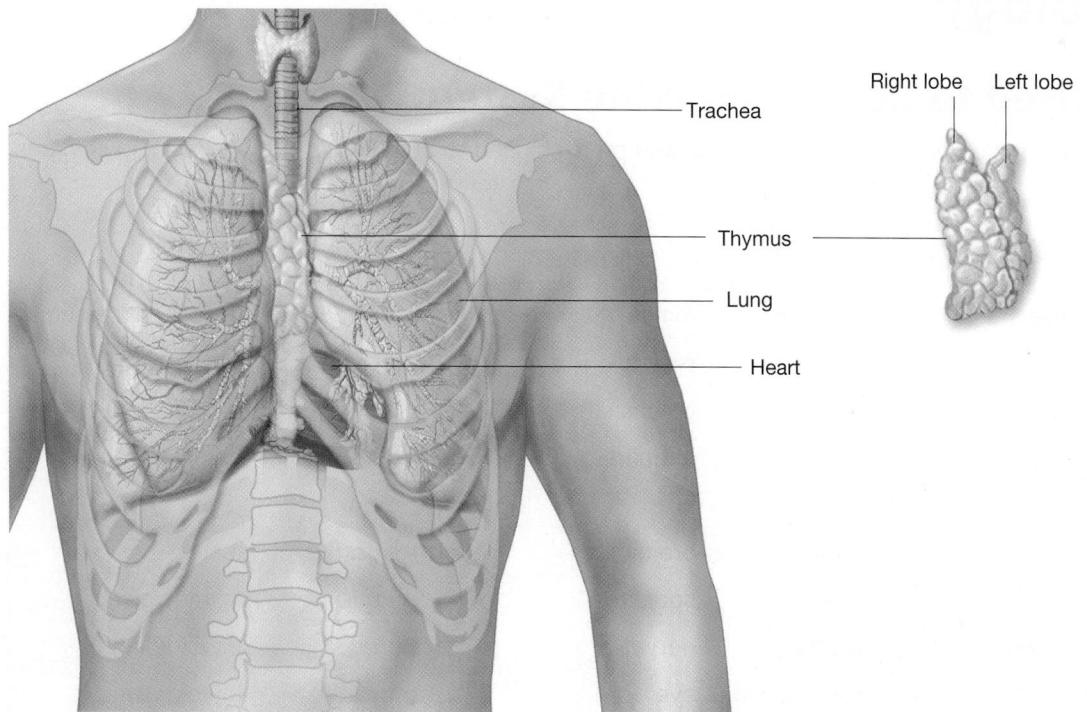

Right lobe   Left lobe

Trachea

Thymus

Lung

Heart

■ **Figure 11.9**   The thymus gland. This gland lies in the mediastinum of the thoracic cavity, just above the heart. It secretes thymosin.

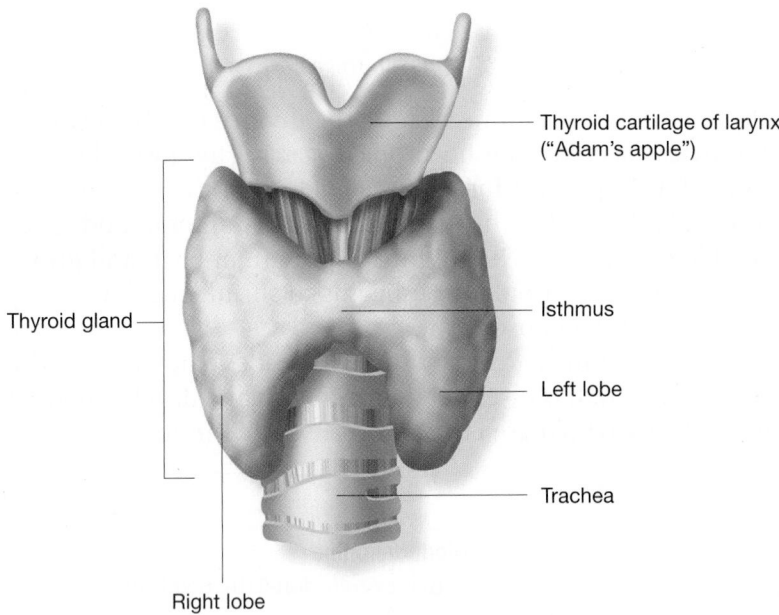

■ **Figure 11.10**   The thyroid gland is subdivided into two lobes, one on each side of the trachea.

Thyroid cartilage of larynx ("Adam's apple")

Isthmus

Thyroid gland

Left lobe

Trachea

Right lobe

MED TERM TIP

Iodine is found in many foods, including vegetables and seafood. It is also present in iodized salt, which is one of the best sources of iodine for people living in the Goiter Belt, composed of states located away from saltwater. A lack of iodine in the diet can lead to thyroid disorders, including *goiter*.

The thyroid gland also secretes **calcitonin** (CT) in response to hypercalcemia (too high blood calcium level). Its action is the opposite of parathyroid hormone and stimulates the increased deposition of calcium into bone, thereby lowering blood levels of calcium.

◼ Terminology

Word Parts Used to Build Endocrine System Terms

The following lists contain the combining forms, suffixes, and prefixes used to build terms in the remaining sections of this chapter.

Combining Forms

acr/o	extremities	**gynec/o**	female	**parathyroid/o**	parathyroid gland
aden/o	gland	**immun/o**	protection	**pineal/o**	pineal gland
adren/o	adrenal gland	**kal/i**	potassium	**pituitar/o**	pituitary gland
adrenal/o	adrenal gland	**lapar/o**	abdomen	**radi/o**	ray
calc/o	calcium	**lob/o**	lobe	**retin/o**	retina
carcin/o	cancer	**mast/o**	breast	**testicul/o**	testes
chem/o	drug	**natr/o**	sodium	**thym/o**	thymus gland
cortic/o	outer portion	**neur/o**	nerve	**thyr/o**	thyroid gland
crin/o	to secrete	**ophthalm/o**	eye	**thyroid/o**	thyroid gland
cyt/o	cell	**or/o**	mouth	**toxic/o**	poison
glyc/o	sugar	**ovari/o**	ovary	**vas/o**	vessel
glycos/o	sugar	**pancreat/o**	pancreas		

Suffixes

-al	pertaining to
-ary	pertaining to
-dipsia	thirst
-ectomy	surgical removal
-emia	blood condition
-emic	relating to a blood condition
-graphy	process of recording
-ia	condition

-ic	pertaining to
-ism	state of
-itis	inflammation
-logy	study of
-megaly	enlarged
-meter	instrument to measure
-oma	tumor
-osis	abnormal condition

-pathy	disease
-prandial	relating to a meal
-pressin	to press down
-scopy	procedure to visually examine
-tic	pertaining to
-uria	urine condition

Prefixes

anti-	against
endo-	within
ex-	outward

hyper-	excessive
hypo-	insufficient
pan-	all

poly-	many
post-	after

Anatomical Terms

TERM	WORD PARTS	DEFINITION
adrenal (ah-DREE-nall)	adren/o = adrenal gland -al = pertaining to	Pertaining to the adrenal glands.
ovarian (oh-VAIR-ee-an)	ovari/o = ovary -ian = pertaining to	Pertaining to the ovary.
pancreatic (pan-kree-AT-ik)	pancreat/o = pancreas -ic = pertaining to	Pertaining to the pancreas.
parathyroidal (pair-ah-THIGH-roy-dall)	parathyroid/o = parathyroid gland -al = pertaining to	Pertaining to the parathyroid gland.
pituitary (pih-TOO-ih-tair-ee)	pituitar/o = pituitary gland -ary = pertaining to	Pertaining to the pituitary gland.
testicular (tes-TIK-yoo-lar)	testicul/o = testes -ar = pertaining to	Pertaining to the testes.
thymic (THIGH-mik)	thym/o = thymus gland -ic = pertaining to	Pertaining to the thymus gland.
thyroidal (thigh-ROYD-all)	thyroid/o = thyroid gland -al = pertaining to	Pertaining to the thyroid gland.

Pathology

TERM	WORD PARTS	DEFINITION
Medical Specialties		
endocrinology (en-doh-krin-ALL-oh-jee)	endo- = within crin/o = to secrete -logy = study of	Branch of medicine involving diagnosis and treatment of conditions and diseases of endocrine glands. Physician is an *endocrinologist*.
Signs and Symptoms		
adrenomegaly (ad-ree-noh-MEG-ah-lee)	adren/o = adrenal gland -megaly = enlarged	Having one or both adrenal glands enlarged.
adrenopathy (ad-ren-OP-ah-thee)	adren/o = adrenal gland -pathy = disease	General term for adrenal gland disease.
edema (eh-DEE-mah)		Condition in which the body tissues contain excessive amounts of fluid.
endocrinopathy (en-doh-krin-OP-ah-thee)	endo- = within crin/o = to secrete -pathy = disease	General term for diseases of the endocrine system.
exophthalmos (eks-off-THAL-mohs)	ex- = outward ophthalm/o = eye	Condition in which the eyeballs protrude, such as in Graves' disease. This is generally caused by an overproduction of thyroid hormone.

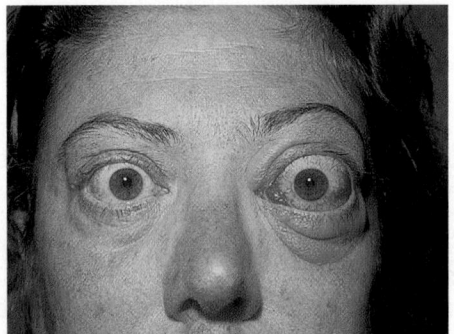

■ **Figure 11.11**
A photograph of a woman with exophthalmos. This condition is associated with hypersecretion of the thyroid gland. *(Custom Medical Stock Photo, Inc.)*

TERM	WORD PARTS	DEFINITION
glycosuria (glye-kohs-YOO-ree-ah)	glycos/o = sugar -uria = urine condition	Having a high level of sugar excreted in the urine.
gynecomastia (gigh-neh-koh-MAST-ee-ah)	gynec/o = female mast/o = breast -ia = condition	Development of breast tissue in males. May be a symptom of adrenal feminization.
hirsutism (HER-soot-izm)	-ism = state of	Condition of having an excessive amount of hair. Term generally used to describe females who have the adult male pattern of hair growth. Can be the result of a hormonal imbalance.
hypercalcemia (high-per-kal-SEE-mee-ah)	hyper- = excessive calc/o = calcium -emia = blood condition	Condition of having a high level of calcium in the blood; associated with hypersecretion of parathyroid hormone.
hyperglycemia (high-per-glye-SEE-mee-ah)	hyper- = excessive glyc/o = sugar -emia = blood condition	Condition of having a high level of sugar in the blood; associated with diabetes mellitus.

Pathology *(continued)*

TERM	WORD PARTS	DEFINITION
hyperkalemia (high-per-kal-EE-mee-ah)	hyper- = excessive kal/i = potassium -emia = blood condition	The condition of having a high level of potassium in the blood.
hypersecretion	hyper- = excessive	Excessive hormone production by an endocrine gland.
hypocalcemia (high-poh-kal-SEE-mee-ah)	hypo- = insufficient calc/o = calcium -emia = blood condition	The condition of having a low level of calcium in the blood; associated with hyposecretion of parathyroid hormone. Hypocalcemia may result in tetany.
hypoglycemia (high-poh-glye-SEE-mee-ah)	hypo- = insufficient glyc/o = sugar -emia = blood condition	Condition of having a low level of sugar in the blood.
hyponatremia (high-poh-nah-TREE-mee-ah)	hypo- = insufficient natr/o = sodium -emia = blood condition	Condition of having a low level of sodium in the blood.
hyposecretion	hypo- = insufficient	Deficient hormone production by an endocrine gland.
obesity (oh-BEE-sih-tee)		Having an abnormal amount of fat in the body.
polydipsia (pall-ee-DIP-see-ah)	poly- = many -dipsia = thirst	Excessive feeling of thirst.
polyuria (pall-ee-YOO-ree-ah)	poly- = many -uria = urine condition	Condition of producing an excessive amount of urine.
syndrome (SIN-drohm)		Group of symptoms and signs that, when combined, present a clinical picture of a disease or condition.
thyromegaly (thigh-roh-MEG-ah-lee)	thyr/o = thyroid gland -megaly = enlarged	Having an enlarged thyroid gland.
Adrenal Glands		
Addison's disease (AD-ih-sons)		Disease named for British physician Thomas Addison; results from a deficiency in adrenocortical hormones. There may be an increased pigmentation of the skin, generalized weakness, and weight loss.
adrenal feminization (ad-REE-nal / fem-ih-nigh-ZAY-shun)	adren/o = adrenal gland -al = pertaining to	Development of female secondary sexual characteristics (such as breasts) in a male. Often as a result of increased estrogen secretion by the adrenal cortex.
adrenal virilism (ad-REE-nal / VIR-ill-izm)	adren/o = adrenal gland -al = pertaining to -ism = state of	Development of male secondary sexual characteristics (such as deeper voice and facial hair) in a female. Often as a result of increased androgen secretion by the adrenal cortex.
adrenalitis (ad-ree-nal-EYE-tis)	adrenal/o = adrenal gland -itis = inflammation	Inflammation of one or both adrenal glands.

■ Pathology *(continued)*

TERM	WORD PARTS	DEFINITION
Cushing's syndrome (CUSH-ings / SIN-drohm)		Set of symptoms caused by excessive levels of cortisol due to high doses of corticosteroid drugs and adrenal tumors. The syndrome may present symptoms of weakness, edema, excess hair growth, skin discoloration, and osteoporosis.

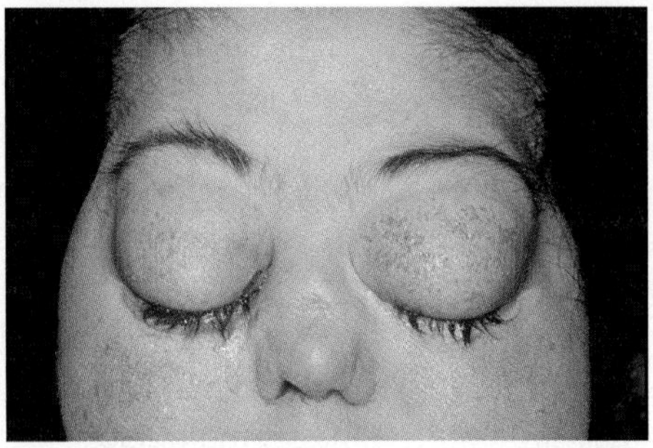

■ **Figure 11.12**   Cushing's syndrome. A photograph of a woman with the characteristic facial features of Cushing's syndrome. *(Biophoto Photo Associates/Photo Researchers, Inc.)*

TERM	WORD PARTS	DEFINITION
pheochromocytoma (fee-oh-kroh-moh-sigh-TOH-ma)	cyt/o = cell -oma = tumor	Usually benign tumor of the adrenal medulla that secretes epinephrine. Symptoms include anxiety, heart palpitations, dyspnea, profuse sweating, headache, and nausea.

Pancreas

TERM	WORD PARTS	DEFINITION
diabetes mellitus (DM) (dye-ah-BEE-teez / MELL-ih-tus)		Chronic disorder of carbohydrate metabolism resulting in hyperglycemia and glycosuria. There are two distinct forms of diabetes mellitus: *insulin-dependent diabetes mellitus* (IDDM) or *type 1,* and *non-insulin-dependent diabetes mellitus* (NIDDM) or *type 2.*
diabetic retinopathy (dye-ah-BET-ik / ret-in-OP-ah-thee)	-tic = pertaining to retin/o = retina -pathy = disease	Secondary complication of diabetes that affects the blood vessels of the retina, resulting in visual changes and even blindness.
insulin-dependent diabetes mellitus (IDDM) (dye-ah-BEE-teez / MELL-ih-tus)		Also called *type 1 diabetes mellitus.* It develops early in life when the pancreas stops insulin production. Patient must take daily insulin injections.
insulinoma (in-sue-lin-OH-mah)	-oma = tumor	Tumor of the islets of Langerhans cells of the pancreas that secretes an excessive amount of insulin.
ketoacidosis (KEE-toh-ass-ih-DOH-sis)	ket/o = ketones -osis = abnormal condition	Acidosis due to an excess of acidic ketone bodies (waste products). A serious condition requiring immediate treatment that can result in death for the diabetic patient if not reversed. Also called *diabetic acidosis.*
non-insulin-dependent diabetes mellitus (dye-ah-BEE-teez / MELL-ih-tus)		Also called *type 2 diabetes mellitus.* It typically develops later in life. The pancreas produces normal to high levels of insulin, but the cells fail to respond to it. Patients may take oral hypoglycemics to improve insulin function, or may eventually have to take insulin.
peripheral neuropathy (per-IF-eh-rall / new-ROP-ah-thee)	-al = pertaining to neur/o = nerve -pathy = disease	Damage to the nerves in the lower legs and hands as a result of diabetes mellitus. Symptoms include either extreme sensitivity or numbness and tingling.

Pathology *(continued)*

TERM	WORD PARTS	DEFINITION
Parathyroid Glands		
hyperparathyroidism (HIGH-per-pair-ah-THIGH-royd-izm)	hyper- = excessive parathyroid/o = parathyroid gland -ism = state of	Hypersecretion of parathyroid hormone; may result in hypercalcemia and Recklinghausen disease.
hypoparathyroidism (HIGH-poh-pair-ah-THIGH-royd-izm)	hypo- = insufficient parathyroid/o = parathyroid gland -ism = state of	Hyposecretion of parathyroid hormone; may result in hypocalcemia and tetany.
Recklinghausen disease (REK-ling-how-zenz)		Excessive production of parathyroid hormone resulting in degeneration of the bones.
tetany (TET-ah-nee)		Nerve irritability and painful muscle cramps resulting from hypocalcemia. Hypoparathyroidism is one cause of tetany.
Pituitary Gland		
acromegaly (ak-roh-MEG-ah-lee)	acr/o = extremities -megaly = enlarged	Chronic disease of adults that results in an elongation and enlargement of the bones of the head and extremities. There can also be mood changes. Due to an excessive amount of growth hormone in an adult.

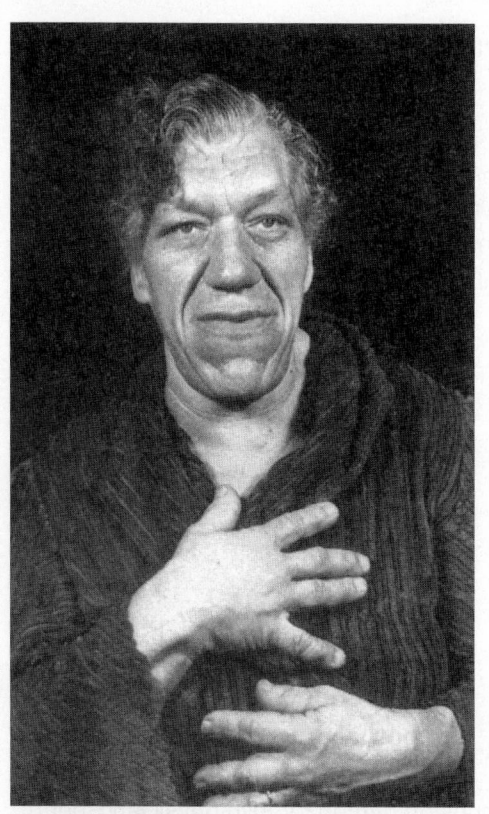

■ **Figure 11.13** Acromegaly. Photo of a woman illustrating the enlarged skull, jaw, and hands typical of acromegaly. *(Reprinted from American Journal of Medicine, Vol 20, Dr. William H. Daughaday, University of California/Irvine, ©1956. With permission from Excerpta Medica Inc.)*

diabetes insipidus (DI) (dye-ah-BEE-teez / in-SIP-ih-dus)		Disorder caused by the inadequate secretion of antidiuretic hormone by the posterior lobe of the pituitary gland. There may be polyuria and polydipsia.
dwarfism (DWARF-izm)	-ism = state of	Condition of being abnormally short in height. It may be the result of a hereditary condition or a lack of growth hormone.

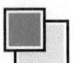 **Pathology** *(continued)*

TERM	WORD PARTS	DEFINITION
gigantism (JYE-gan-tizm)	-ism = state of	Excessive development of the body due to the overproduction of the growth hormone by the pituitary gland in a child or teenager. The opposite of *dwarfism*.
hyperpituitarism (HIGH-per-pih-TOO-ih-tuh-rizm)	hyper- = excessive pituitar/o = pituitary gland -ism = state of	Hypersecretion of one or more pituitary gland hormones.
hypopituitarism (HIGH-poh-pih-TOO-ih-tuh-rizm)	hypo- = insufficient pituitar/o = pituitary gland -ism = state of	Hyposecretion of one or more pituitary gland hormones.
panhypopituitarism (pan-high-poh-pih-TOO-ih-tair-izm)	pan- = all hypo- = insufficient pituitar/o = pituitary gland -ism = state of	Deficiency in all the hormones secreted by the pituitary gland. Often recognized because of problems with the glands regulated by the pituitary—adrenal cortex, thyroid, ovaries, and testes.
Thymus Gland		
thymitis (thigh-MY-tis)	thym/o = thymus gland -itis = inflammation	Inflammation of the thymus gland.
thymoma (thigh-MOH-mah)	thym/o = thymus gland -oma = tumor	A tumor in the thymus gland.
Thyroid Gland		
cretinism (KREE-tin-izm)	-ism = state of	Congenital condition in which a lack of thyroid hormones may result in arrested physical and mental development.
goiter (GOY-ter)		Enlargement of the thyroid gland.
Graves' disease		Condition named for Irish physician Robert Graves that results in overactivity of the thyroid gland and can cause a crisis situation. Symptoms include exophthalmos and goiter. A type of *hyperthyroidism*.
Hashimoto's thyroiditis (hash-ee-MOH-tohz / thigh-roy-DYE-tis)	thyroid/o = thyroid gland -itis = inflammation	Chronic autoimmune form of thyroiditis; results in hyposecretion of thyroid hormones.

■ **Figure 11.14**   Goiter. A photograph of a male with an extreme goiter or enlarged thyroid gland.

Pathology *(continued)*

TERM	WORD PARTS	DEFINITION
hyperthyroidism (hi-per-THIGH-royd-izm)	hyper- = excessive thyroid/o = thyroid gland -ism = state of	Hypersecretion of thyroid gland hormones.
hypothyroidism (high-poh-THIGH-royd-izm)	hypo- = insufficient thyroid/o = thyroid gland -ism = state of	Hyposecretion of thyroid gland hormones.
myxedema (miks-eh-DEE-mah)		Condition resulting from a hyposecretion of the thyroid gland in an adult. Symptoms can include anemia, slow speech, swollen facial features, edematous skin, drowsiness, and mental lethargy.
thyrotoxicosis (thigh-roh-toks-ih-KOH-sis)	thyr/o = thyroid gland toxic/o = poison -osis = abnormal condition	Condition resulting from marked overproduction of the thyroid gland. Symptoms include rapid heart action, tremors, enlarged thyroid gland, exophthalmos, and weight loss.
All Glands		
adenocarcinoma (ad-eh-no-car-sih-NO-mah)	aden/o = gland carcin/o = cancer -oma = tumor	Cancerous tumor in a gland that is capable of producing the hormones secreted by that gland. One cause of hypersecretion pathologies.

Diagnostic Procedures

TERM	WORD PARTS	DEFINITION
Clinical Laboratory Tests		
blood serum test		Blood test to measure the level of substances such as calcium, electrolytes, testosterone, insulin, and glucose. Used to assist in determining the function of various endocrine glands.
fasting blood sugar (FBS)		Blood test to measure the amount of sugar circulating throughout the body after a 12-hour fast.
glucose tolerance test (GTT) (GLOO-kohs)		Test to determine the blood sugar level. A measured dose of glucose is given to a patient either orally or intravenously. Blood samples are then drawn at certain intervals to determine the ability of the patient to use glucose. Used for diabetic patients to determine their insulin response to glucose.
protein-bound iodine test (PBI)		Blood test to measure the concentration of thyroxine (T_4) circulating in the bloodstream. The iodine becomes bound to the protein in the blood and can be measured. Useful in establishing thyroid function.

Diagnostic Procedures *(continued)*

TERM	WORD PARTS	DEFINITION
radioimmunoassay (RIA) (ray-dee-oh-im-yoo-noh-ASS-ay)	radi/o = ray immun/o = protection	Blood test that uses radioactively tagged hormones and antibodies to measure the quantity of hormone in the plasma.
thyroid function test (TFT) (THIGH-royd)		Blood test used to measure the levels of thyroxine, triiodothyronine, and thyroid-stimulating hormone in the bloodstream to assist in determining thyroid function.
total calcium		Blood test to measure the total amount of calcium to assist in detecting parathyroid and bone disorders.
two-hour postprandial glucose tolerance test (post-PRAN-dee-al)	post- = after -prandial = relating to a meal	Blood test to assist in evaluating glucose metabolism. The patient eats a high carbohydrate diet and then fasts overnight before the test. Then the blood sample is taken 2 hours after a meal.
Diagnostic Imaging		
thyroid echography (THIGH-royd / eh-KOG-rah-fee)	-graphy = process of recording	Ultrasound examination of the thyroid that can assist in distinguishing a thyroid nodule from a cyst.
thyroid scan (THIGH-royd)		Test in which radioactive iodine is administered that localizes in the thyroid gland. The gland can then be visualized with a scanning device to detect pathology such as tumors.

 # Therapeutic Procedures

TERM	WORD PARTS	DEFINITION
Medical Procedures		
chemical thyroidectomy (thigh-royd-EK-toh-mee)	chem/o = drug -al = pertaining to thyroid/o = thyroid gland -ectomy = surgical removal	Large dose of radioactive iodine is given in order to kill thyroid gland cells without having to actually do surgery.
glucometer	gluc/o = glucose -meter = instrument to measure	Device designed for a diabetic to use at home to measure the level of glucose in the bloodstream.
hormone replacement therapy		Artificial replacement of hormones in patients with hyposecretion disorders. May be oral pills, injections, or adhesive skin patches.
Surgical Procedures		
adrenalectomy (ad-ree-nal-EK-toh-mee)	adrenal/o = adrenal gland -ectomy = surgical removal	Surgical removal of one or both adrenal glands.
laparoscopic adrenalectomy (lap-row-SKOP-ik / ad-ree-nal-EK-toh-mee)	lapar/o = abdomen -scopy = procedure to visually examine -ic = pertaining to adren/o = adrenal gland -ectomy = surgical removal	Removal of the adrenal gland through a small incision in the abdomen and using endoscopic instruments.

Therapeutic Procedures *(continued)*

TERM	WORD PARTS	DEFINITION
lobectomy (lobe-EK-toh-mee)	lob/o = lobe -ectomy = surgical removal	Removal of a lobe from an organ. In this case, one lobe of the thyroid gland.
parathyroidectomy (pair-ah-thigh-royd-EK-toh-mee)	parathyroid/o = parathyroid gland -ectomy = surgical removal	Surgical removal of one or more of the parathyroid glands.
pinealectomy (PIN-ee-ah-LEK-toh-mee)	pineal/o = pineal gland -ectomy = surgical removal	Surgical removal of the pineal gland.
thymectomy (thigh-MEK-toh-mee)	thym/o = thymus gland -ectomy = surgical removal	Surgical removal of the thymus gland.
thyroidectomy (thigh-royd-EK-toh-mee)	thyroid/o = thyroid gland -ectomy = surgical removal	Surgical removal of the thyroid gland.

Pharmacology

CLASSIFICATION	WORD PARTS	ACTION	EXAMPLES
antithyroid agents	anti- = against	Medication given to block production of thyroid hormones in patients with hypersecretion disorders.	methimazole, Tapazole; propylthiouracil
corticosteroids (kor-tih-koh-STAIR-oydz)	cortic/o = outer portion	Although the function of these hormones in the body is to regulate carbohydrate metabolism, they also have a strong anti-inflammatory action. Therefore they are used to treat severe chronic inflammatory diseases such as rheumatoid arthritis. Long-term use of corticosteroids has adverse side effects such as osteoporosis and the symptoms of Cushing's disease. Also used to treat adrenal cortex hyposecretion disorders such as Addison's disease.	prednisone, Deltasone
human growth hormone therapy		Hormone replacement therapy with human growth hormone in order to stimulate skeletal growth. Used to treat children with abnormally short stature.	somatropin, Genotropin; somatrem, Protropin
insulin (IN-suh-lin)		Administered to replace insulin for type 1 diabetics or to treat severe type 2 diabetics.	human insulin, Humulin L
oral hypoglycemic agents (high-poh-glye-SEE-mik)	or/o = mouth -al = pertaining to hypo- = insufficient glyc/o = sugar -emic = relating to a blood condition	Medications taken by mouth that cause a decrease in blood sugar; not used for insulin-dependent patients.	metformin, Glucophage; glipizide, Glucotrol

Pharmacology *(continued)*

CLASSIFICATION	WORD PARTS	ACTION	EXAMPLES
thyroid replacement hormone		Hormone replacement therapy for patients with hypothyroidism or who have had a thyroidectomy.	levothyroxine, Levo-T; liothyronine, Cytomel
vasopressin (vaz-oh-PRESS-in)	vas/o = vessel -pressin = to press down	Given to control diabetes insipidus and promote reabsorption of water in the kidney tubules.	desmopressin acetate, Desmopressin; conivaptan, Vaprisol

 Abbreviations

α	alpha	**LH**	luteinizing hormone
ACTH	adrenocorticotropin hormone	**MSH**	melanocyte-stimulating hormone
ADH	antidiuretic hormone	**Na⁺**	sodium
β	beta	**NIDDM**	non-insulin-dependent diabetes mellitus
BMR	basal metabolic rate	**NPH**	neutral protamine Hagedorn (insulin)
CT	calcitonin	**PBI**	protein-bound iodine
DI	diabetes insipidus	**PRL**	prolactin
DM	diabetes mellitus	**PTH**	parathyroid hormone
FBS	fasting blood sugar	**RAI**	radioactive iodine
FSH	follicle-stimulating hormone	**RIA**	radioimmunoassay
GH	growth hormone	**T₃**	triiodothyronine
GTT	glucose tolerance test	**T₄**	thyroxine
IDDM	insulin-dependent diabetes mellitus	**TFT**	thyroid function test
K⁺	potassium	**TSH**	thyroid-stimulating hormone

Chapter Review

Real-World Applications

Medical Record Analysis

This Discharge Summary below contains 10 medical terms. Underline each term and write it in the list below the report. Then define each term.

Discharge Summary

Admitting Diagnosis:	Hyperglycemia, ketoacidosis, glycosuria
Final Diagnosis:	New-onset type 1 diabetes mellitus
History of Present Illness:	A 12-year-old female patient presented to her physician's office with a 2-month history of weight loss, fatigue, polyuria, and polydipsia. Her family history is significant for a grandfather, mother, and older brother with type 1 diabetes mellitus. The pediatrician found hyperglycemia with a fasting blood sugar and glycosuria with a urine dipstick. She is being admitted at this time for management of new-onset diabetes mellitus.
Summary of Hospital Course:	At the time of admission, the FBS was 300 mg/100 mL and she was in ketoacidosis. She rapidly improved after receiving insulin; her blood glucose level normalized. The next day a glucose tolerance test confirmed the diagnosis of diabetes mellitus. The patient was started on insulin injections. Patient and family were instructed on diabetes mellitus, insulin, diet, exercise, and long-term complications.
Discharge Plans:	Patient was discharged to home with her parents. Her parents are to check her blood glucose levels twice daily and call the office for insulin dosage. She is to return to the office in 2 weeks.

	Term	Definition
1	_____	_____
2	_____	_____
3	_____	_____
4	_____	_____
5	_____	_____
6	_____	_____
7	_____	_____
8	_____	_____
9	_____	_____
10	_____	_____

Chart Note Transcription

The chart note below contains 11 phrases that can be reworded with a medical term that you learned in this chapter. Each phrase is identified with an underline. Determine the medical term and write your answers in the space provided.

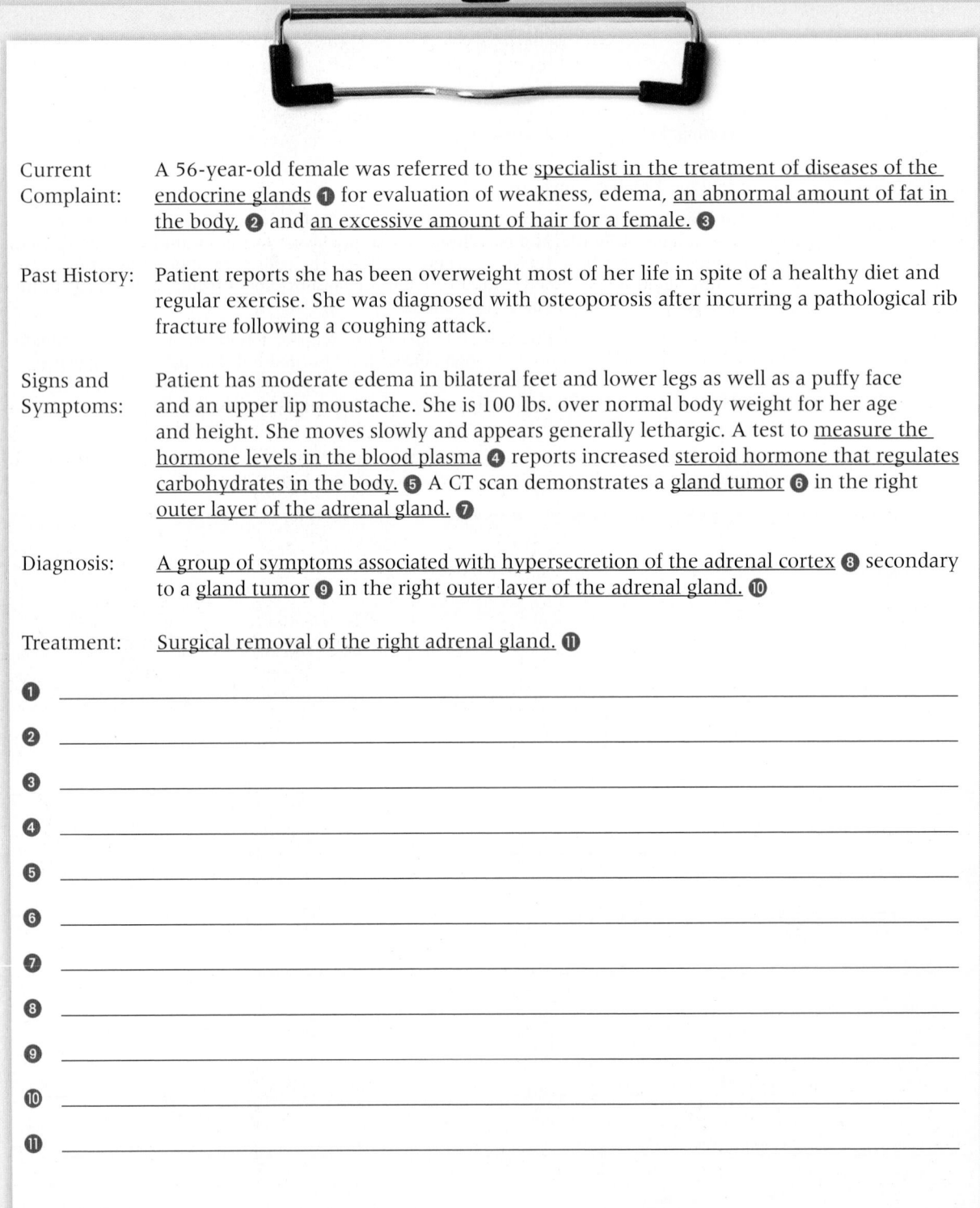

Current Complaint: A 56-year-old female was referred to the <u>specialist in the treatment of diseases of the endocrine glands</u> ❶ for evaluation of weakness, edema, <u>an abnormal amount of fat in the body,</u> ❷ and <u>an excessive amount of hair for a female.</u> ❸

Past History: Patient reports she has been overweight most of her life in spite of a healthy diet and regular exercise. She was diagnosed with osteoporosis after incurring a pathological rib fracture following a coughing attack.

Signs and Symptoms: Patient has moderate edema in bilateral feet and lower legs as well as a puffy face and an upper lip moustache. She is 100 lbs. over normal body weight for her age and height. She moves slowly and appears generally lethargic. A test to <u>measure the hormone levels in the blood plasma</u> ❹ reports increased <u>steroid hormone that regulates carbohydrates in the body.</u> ❺ A CT scan demonstrates a <u>gland tumor</u> ❻ in the right <u>outer layer of the adrenal gland.</u> ❼

Diagnosis: <u>A group of symptoms associated with hypersecretion of the adrenal cortex</u> ❽ secondary to a <u>gland tumor</u> ❾ in the right <u>outer layer of the adrenal gland.</u> ❿

Treatment: <u>Surgical removal of the right adrenal gland.</u> ⓫

❶ _____

❷ _____

❸ _____

❹ _____

❺ _____

❻ _____

❼ _____

❽ _____

❾ _____

❿ _____

⓫ _____

Case Study

Below is a case study presentation of a patient with a condition covered in this chapter. Read the case study and answer the questions below. Some questions will ask for information not included within this chapter. Use your text, a medical dictionary, or any other reference material you choose to answer these questions.

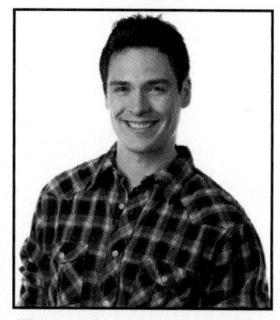

A 22-year-old college student was admitted to the emergency room after his friends called an ambulance when he passed out in a bar. He had become confused, developed slurred speech, and had difficulty walking after having only one beer to drink. In the ER he was noted to have diaphoresis, rapid respirations and pulse, and was disoriented. Upon examination, needle marks were found on his abdomen and outer thighs. The physician ordered blood serum tests that revealed hyperglycemia and ketoacidosis. Unknown to his friends, this young man has had diabetes mellitus since early childhood. The patient quickly recovered following an insulin injection.

(Flashon Studio/Shutterstock)

1. What pathological condition has this patient had since childhood? Look this condition up in a reference source and include a short description of it.

   _____

   _____

2. List and define each symptom noted in the ER in your own words.

   _____

   _____

3. What diagnostic test was performed? Describe it in your own words.

   _____

   _____

4. Explain the results of the test.

   _____

   _____

5. What specific type of diabetes does this young man probably have? Justify your answer.

   _____

   _____

6. Describe the other type of diabetes mellitus that this young man did not have.

   _____

   _____

Practice Exercises

A. Complete the Statement

1. The study of the endocrine system is called _____.

2. The master endocrine gland is the _____.

3. _____ is a general term for the sexual organs that produce gametes.

4. The term for the hormones produced by the outer portion of the adrenal cortex is _____.

5. The hormone produced by the testes is _____.

6. The two hormones produced by the ovaries are _____ and _____.

7. An inadequate supply of the hormone _____ causes diabetes insipidus.

8. The endocrine gland associated with the immune system is the _____.

9. The term for a protrusion of the eyeballs in Graves' disease is _____.

10. A general medical term for a hormone-secreting cancerous tumor is _____.

B. Combining Form Practice

The combining form **thyroid/o** refers to the thyroid. Use it to write a term that means:

1. removal of the thyroid _____

2. pertaining to the thyroid _____

3. state of excessive thyroid _____

The combining form **pancreat/o** refers to the pancreas. Use it to write a term that means:

4. pertaining to the pancreas _____

5. inflammation of the pancreas _____

6. removal of the pancreas _____

7. cutting into the pancreas _____

The combining form **adren/o** refers to the adrenal glands. Use it to write a term that means:

8. pertaining to the adrenal gland _____

9. enlargement of the adrenal glands _____

10. adrenal gland disease _____

The combining form **thym/o** refers to the thymus glands. Use it to write a term that means:

11. tumor of the thymus gland _____

12. removal of the thymus gland _____

13. pertaining to the thymus gland _____

14. inflammation of the thymus gland _____

C. Define the Combining Form

	Definition	Example from Chapter
1. natr/o	_____	_____
2. estr/o	_____	_____
3. pineal/o	_____	_____
4. pituitar/o	_____	_____
5. kal/i	_____	_____
6. calc/o	_____	_____
7. parathyroid/o	_____	_____
8. acr/o	_____	_____
9. glyc/o	_____	_____
10. gonad/o	_____	_____

D. Terminology Matching

Match the term to its definition.

1. _____ protein-bound iodine test

2. _____ fasting blood sugar

3. _____ radioimmunoassay

4. _____ thyroid scan

5. _____ 2-hour postprandial glucose tolerance test

6. _____ glucose tolerance test

a. measures levels of hormones in the blood

b. determines glucose metabolism after patient receives a measured dose of glucose

c. test of glucose metabolism 2 hours after eating a meal

d. measures blood sugar level after 12-hour fast

e. measures T4 concentration in the blood

f. uses radioactive iodine

E. What's the Abbreviation?

1. non-insulin-dependent diabetes mellitus _____

2. insulin-dependent diabetes mellitus _____

3. adrenocorticotropin hormone _____

4. parathyroid hormone _____

5. triiodothyronine _____

6. thyroid-stimulating hormone _____

7. fasting blood sugar _____

8. prolactin _____

F. Terminology Matching

Match each term to its definition.

1. _____ Cushing's disease   a. enlarged thyroid

2. _____ goiter   b. overactive adrenal cortex

3. _____ acromegaly   c. hyperthyroidism

4. _____ gigantism   d. underactive adrenal cortex

5. _____ cretinism   e. enlarged bones of head and extremities

6. _____ myxedema   f. may cause polyuria and polydipsia

7. _____ diabetes mellitus   g. an autoimmune disease

8. _____ diabetes insipidus   h. arrested physical and mental development

9. _____ Hashimoto's thyroiditis   i. disorder of carbohydrate metabolism

10. _____ Graves' disease   j. insufficient thyroid hormone in an adult

11. _____ Addison's disease   k. excessive growth hormone in a child

G. What Does it Stand For?

1. PBI _____

2. K^+ _____

3. T_4 _____

4. GTT _____

5. DM _____

6. BMR _____

7. Na^+ _____

8. ADH _____

H. Suffix Practice

Use the following suffixes to create medical terms for the following definitions.

-pressin	-uria	-tropin
-dipsia	-emia	-prandial

1. the presence of sugar or glucose in the urine _____

2. to press down a vessel _____

3. excessive urination _____

4. condition of excessive calcium in the blood _____

5. excessive thirst _____

6. stimulate adrenal cortex _____

7. after a meal _____

I. Define the Term

1. corticosteroid _____

2. hirsutism _____

3. tetany _____

4. diabetic retinopathy _____

5. hyperglycemia _____

6. hypoglycemia _____

7. adrenaline _____

8. insulin _____

9. thyrotoxicosis _____

10. hypersecretion _____

J. Fill in the Blank

insulinoma	ketoacidosis	pheochromocytoma
gynecomastia	panhypopituitarinism	Hashimoto's thyroiditis

1. The doctor found that Marsha's high level of insulin and hypoglycemia was caused by a(n) _____.

2. Kevin developed _____ as a result of his diabetes mellitus and required emergency treatment.

3. It was determined that Karen had _____ when doctors realized she had problems with her thyroid gland, adrenal cortex, and ovaries.

4. Luke's high epinephrine level was caused by a(n) _____.

5. When it was determined that Carl's thyroiditis was an autoimmune condition, it became obvious that he had _____.

6. Excessive sex hormones caused Jack to develop _____.

K. Pharmacology Challenge

Fill in the classification for each drug description, then match the brand name.

	Drug Description	**Classification**	**Brand Name**
1.	_____ strong anti-inflammatory	_____	a. genotropin
2.	_____ stimulates skeletal growth	_____	b. Desmopressin
3.	_____ treats type 1 diabetes mellitus	_____	c. Tapazole
4.	_____ blocks production of thyroid hormone	_____	d. glucophage
5.	_____ treats type 1 diabetes mellitus	_____	e. Deltasone
6.	_____ controls diabetes insipidus	_____	f. Humulin

MEDICAL TERMINOLOGY INTERACTIVE

Medical Terminology Interactive is a premium online homework management system that includes a host of features to help you study. Registered users will find:

- Fun games and activities built within a virtual hospital
- Powerful tools that track and analyze your results—allowing you to create a personalized learning experience
- Videos, flashcards, and audio pronunciations to help enrich your progress
- Streaming video lesson presentations and self-paced learning modules

www.pearsonhighered.com/mti

Labeling Exercise

Image A

Write the labels for this figure on the numbered lines provided.

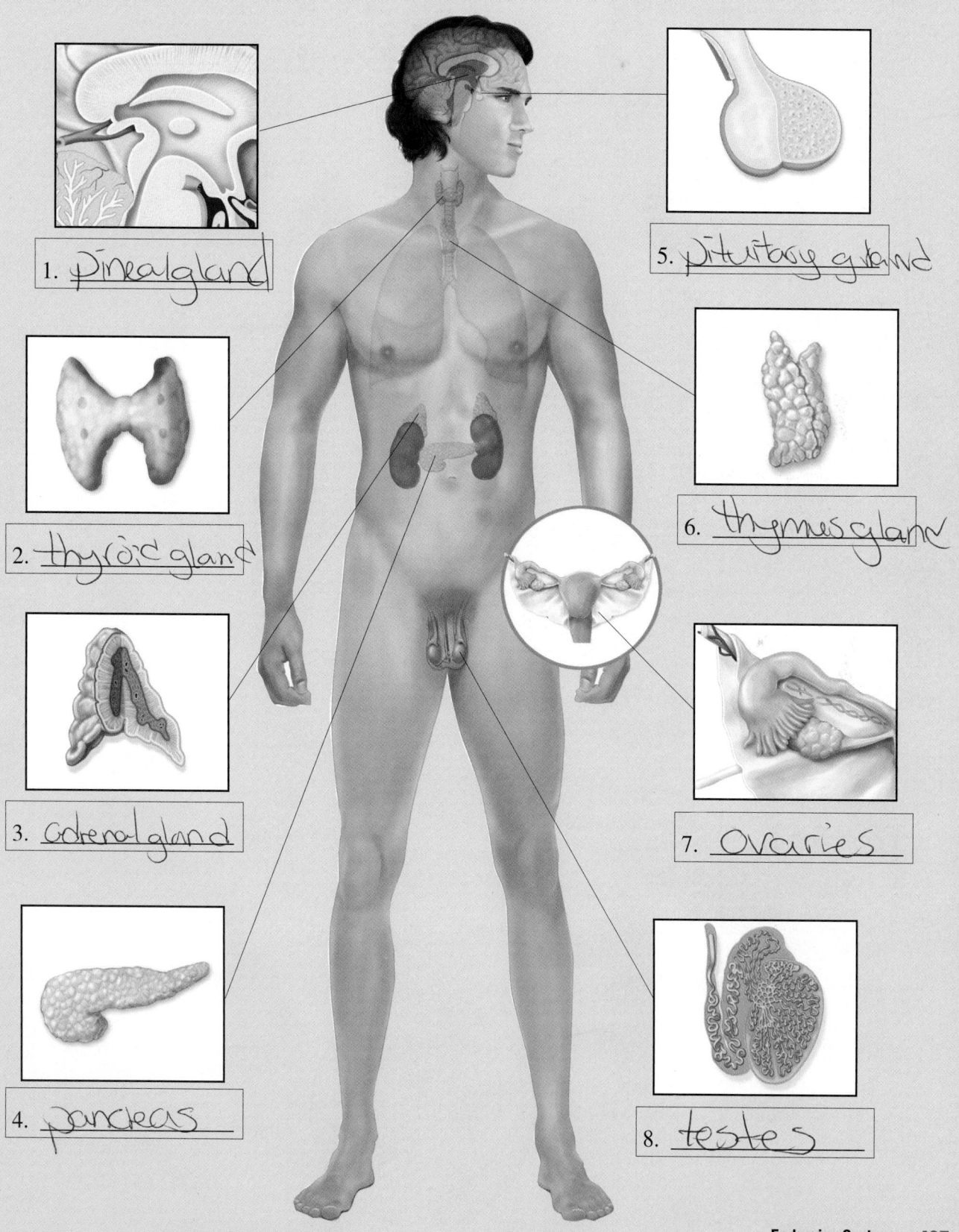

1. Pineal gland

2. thyroid gland

3. adrenal gland

4. pancreas

5. pituitary gland

6. thymus gland

7. Ovaries

8. testes

Image B

Write the labels for this figure on the numbered lines provided.

2. (target)_____

3. (hormone)_____

8. (target)_____

9. (hormone)_____

1. _____

4. (target)_____

5. (hormones)_____, _____

10. (target)_____

11. (hormone)_____

6. (target)_____

7. (hormones)_____, _____

12. (target)_____

13. (hormone)_____

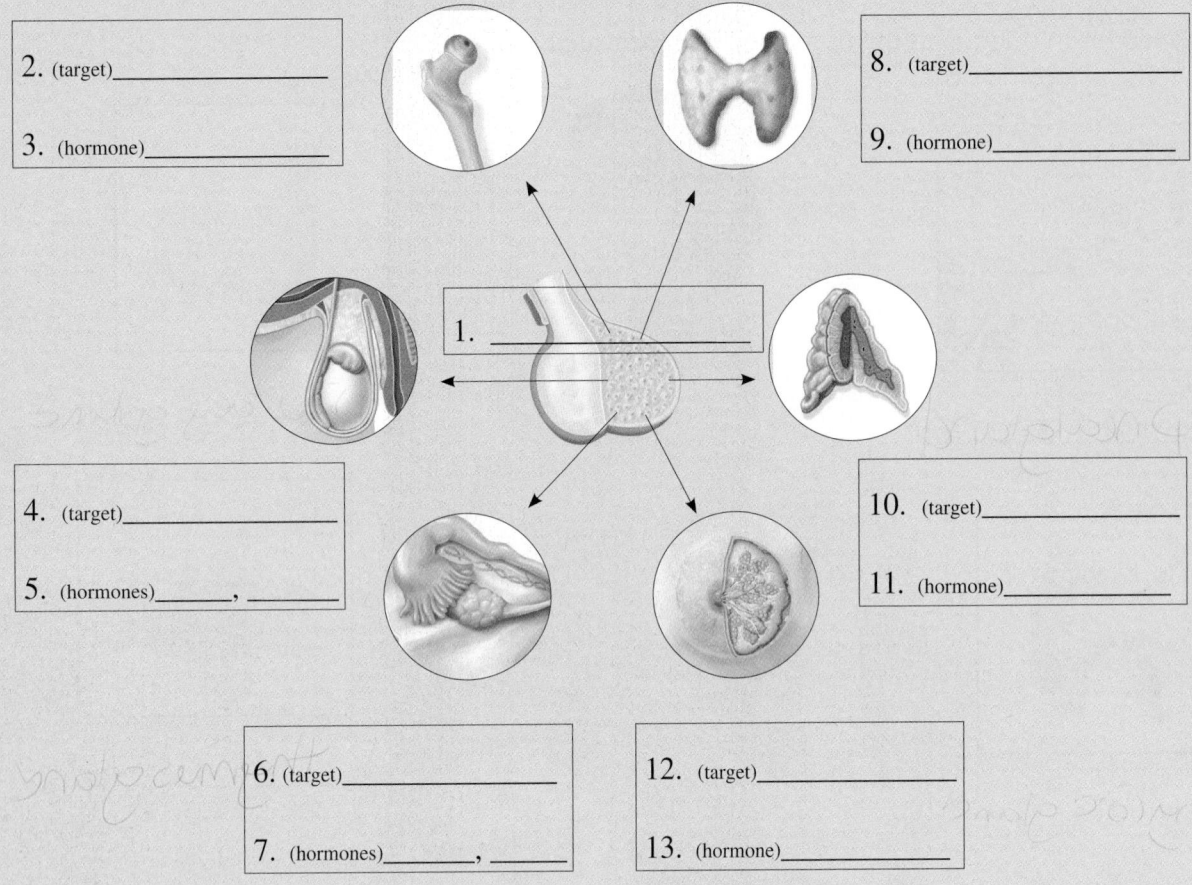

Image C

Write the labels for this figure on the numbered lines provided.

1. _____

2. _____

4. Insulin-secreting cell

_____

5. Glucagon-secreting cell

_____

3. _____

6. _____

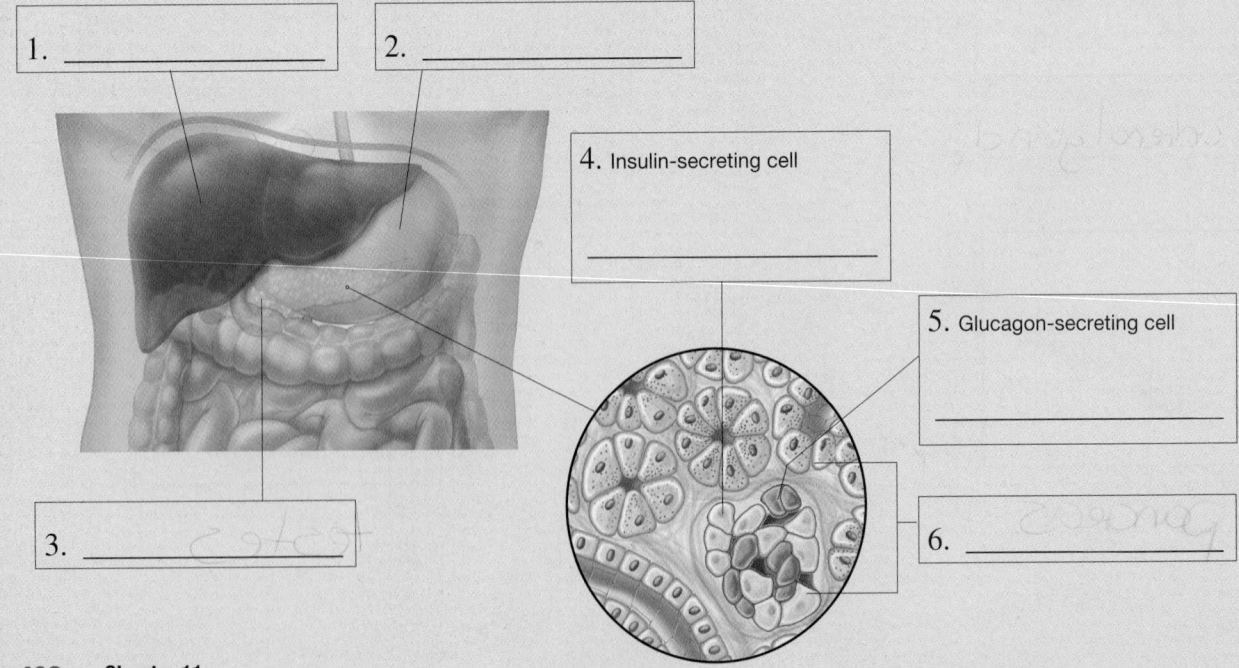

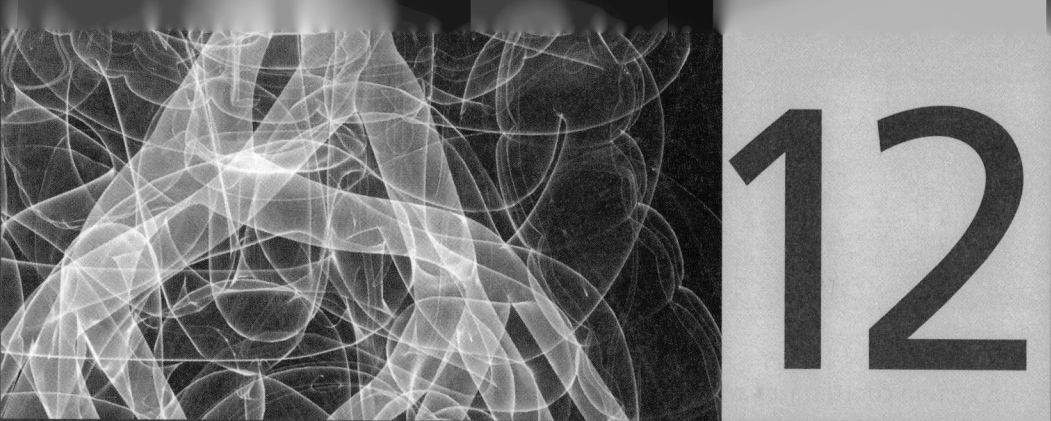

12

Learning Objectives

Upon completion of this chapter, you will be able to

- Identify and define the combining forms and suffixes introduced in this chapter.
- Correctly spell and pronounce medical terms and major anatomical structures relating to the nervous system.
- Locate and describe the major organs of the nervous system and their functions.
- Describe the components of a neuron.
- Distinguish between the central nervous system, peripheral nervous system, and autonomic nervous system.
- Identify and define nervous system anatomical terms.
- Identify and define selected nervous system pathology terms.
- Identify and define selected nervous system diagnostic procedures.
- Identify and define selected nervous system therapeutic procedures.
- Identify and define selected medications relating to the nervous system.
- Define selected abbreviations associated with the nervous system.

NERVOUS SYSTEM

Nervous System at a Glance

Function

The nervous system coordinates and controls body function. It receives sensory input, makes decisions, and then orders body responses.

Organs

Here are the primary structures that comprise the nervous system.

brain   spinal cord
nerves

Word Parts

Here are the most common word parts (with their meanings) used to build nervous system terms. For a more comprehensive list, refer to the Terminology section of this chapter.

Combining Forms

alges/o	sense of pain	mening/o	meninges
astr/o	star	meningi/o	meninges
cephal/o	head	myel/o	spinal cord
cerebell/o	cerebellum	neur/o	nerve
cerebr/o	cerebrum	poli/o	gray matter
clon/o	rapid contracting and relaxing	pont/o	pons
		radicul/o	nerve root
dur/o	dura mater	thalam/o	thalamus
encephal/o	brain	thec/o	sheath (meninges)
esthes/o	sensation, feeling	ton/o	tone
gli/o	glue	ventricul/o	brain ventricle
medull/o	medulla oblongata		

Suffixes

-paresis	weakness	-taxia	muscle coordination
-phasia	speech	-trophic	pertaining to development
-plegia	paralysis		

Nervous System Illustrated

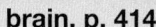
brain, p. 414

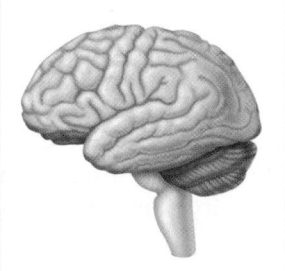

Coordinates body functions

spinal cord, p. 416

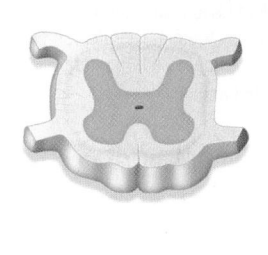

Transmits messages to and
from the brain

nerves, p. 418

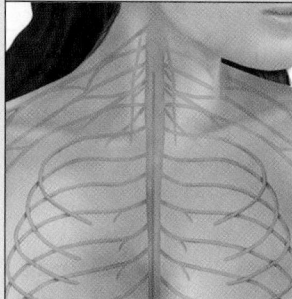

Transmit messages to and
from the central nervous
system

Anatomy and Physiology of the Nervous System

brain
central nervous system
cranial nerves (KRAY-nee-al)
glands
muscles

nerves
peripheral nervous system (per-IF-er-al)
sensory receptors
spinal cord
spinal nerves

The nervous system is responsible for coordinating all the activity of the body. To do this, it first receives information from both external and internal **sensory receptors** and then uses that information to adjust the activity of **muscles** and **glands** to match the needs of the body.

The nervous system can be subdivided into the **central nervous system** (CNS) and the **peripheral nervous system** (PNS). The central nervous system consists of the **brain** and **spinal cord.** Sensory information comes into the central nervous system, where it is processed. Motor messages then exit the central nervous system carrying commands to muscles and glands. The **nerves** of the peripheral nervous system are **cranial nerves** and **spinal nerves.** Sensory nerves carry information to the central nervous system, and motor nerves carry commands away from the central nervous system. All portions of the nervous system are composed of nervous tissue.

> **MED TERM TIP**
>
> Neuroglial tissue received its name as a result of its function. This tissue holds neurons together. Therefore, it was called *neuroglial*, a term literally meaning "nerve glue."

Nervous Tissue

axon (AK-son)
dendrites (DEN-drights)
myelin (MY-eh-lin)
nerve cell body
neuroglial cells (noo-ROH-glee-all)

neuron (NOO-ron)
neurotransmitter
    (noo-roh-TRANS-mit-ter)
synapse (sih-NAPSE)
synaptic cleft (sih-NAP-tik)

Nervous tissue consists of two basic types of cells: **neurons** and **neuroglial cells.** Neurons are individual nerve cells. These are the cells that are capable of conducting electrical impulses in response to a stimulus. Neurons have three basic parts: **dendrites,** a **nerve cell body,** and an **axon** (see Figure 12.1A ■). Dendrites are highly branched projections that receive impulses. The nerve cell body contains the nucleus and many of the other organelles of the cell (see Figure 12.1B ■). A neuron has only a single axon, a projection from the nerve cell body that conducts the electrical impulse toward its destination. The point at which the axon of one neuron meets the dendrite of the next neuron is called a **synapse.** Electrical impulses cannot pass directly across the gap between two neurons, called the **synaptic cleft.** They instead require the help of a chemical messenger, called a **neurotransmitter.**

A variety of neuroglial cells are found in nervous tissue. Each has a different support function for the neurons. For example, some neuroglial cells produce **myelin,** a fatty substance that acts as insulation for many axons so that they conduct electrical impulses faster. Neuroglial cells *do not* conduct electrical impulses.

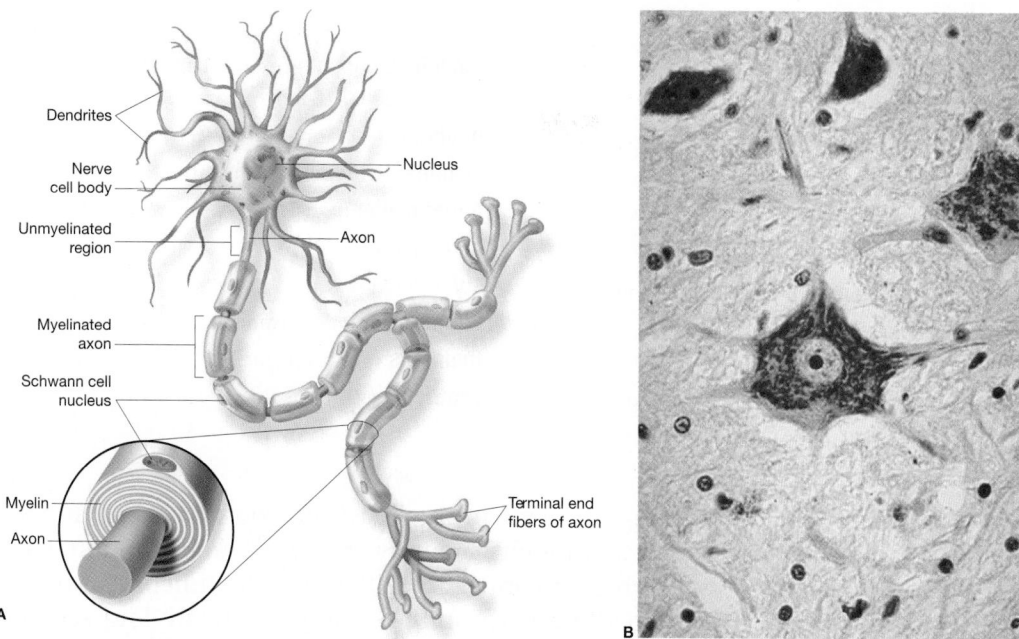

Figure 12.1 (A) The structure of a neuron, showing the dendrites, nerve cell body, and axon. (B) Photomicrograph of typical neuron showing the nerve cell body, nucleus, and dendrites.

Central Nervous System

gray matter

meninges (men-IN-jeez)

myelinated (MY-eh-lih-nayt-ed)

tract

white matter

Because the central nervous system is a combination of the brain and spinal cord, it is able to receive impulses from all over the body, process this information, and then respond with an action. This system consists of both **gray** and **white matter.** Gray matter is comprised of unsheathed or uncovered cell bodies and dendrites. White matter is **myelinated** nerve fibers (see Figure 12.2 ■). The myelin sheath makes the nervous tissue appear white. Bundles of nerve fibers interconnecting different parts of the central nervous system are called **tracts.** The central nervous system is encased and protected by three membranes known as the **meninges.**

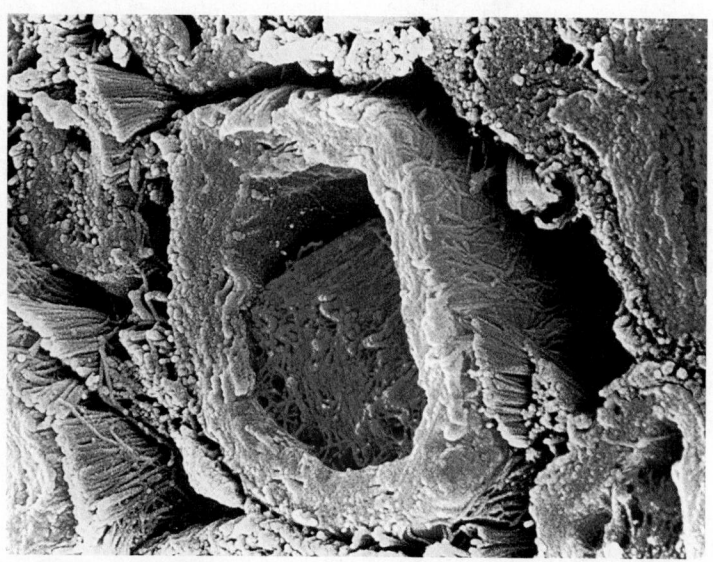

Figure 12.2 Electronmicrograph illustrating an axon (red) wrapped in its myelin sheath (blue). *(Quest/Science Photo Library/Photo Researchers, Inc.)*

The Brain

brain stem
cerebellum (ser-eh-BELL-um)
cerebral cortex (seh-REE-bral / KOR-teks)
cerebral hemisphere
cerebrospinal fluid (ser-eh-broh-SPY-nal)
cerebrum (SER-eh-brum)
diencephalon (dye-en-SEFF-ah-lon)
frontal lobe
gyri (JYE-rye)
hypothalamus (high-poh-THAL-ah-mus)

medulla oblongata (meh-DULL-ah / ob-long-GAH-tah)
midbrain
occipital lobe (ock-SIP-ih-tal)
parietal lobe (pah-RYE-eh-tal)
pons (PONZ)
sulci (SULL-kye)
temporal lobe (TEM-por-al)
thalamus (THAL-ah-mus)
ventricles (VEN-trik-lz)

The brain is one of the largest organs in the body and coordinates most body activities. It is the center for all thought, memory, judgment, and emotion. Each part of the brain is responsible for controlling different body functions, such as temperature regulation, blood pressure, and breathing. There are four sections to the brain: the **cerebrum, cerebellum, diencephalon,** and **brain stem** (see Figure 12.3 ■).

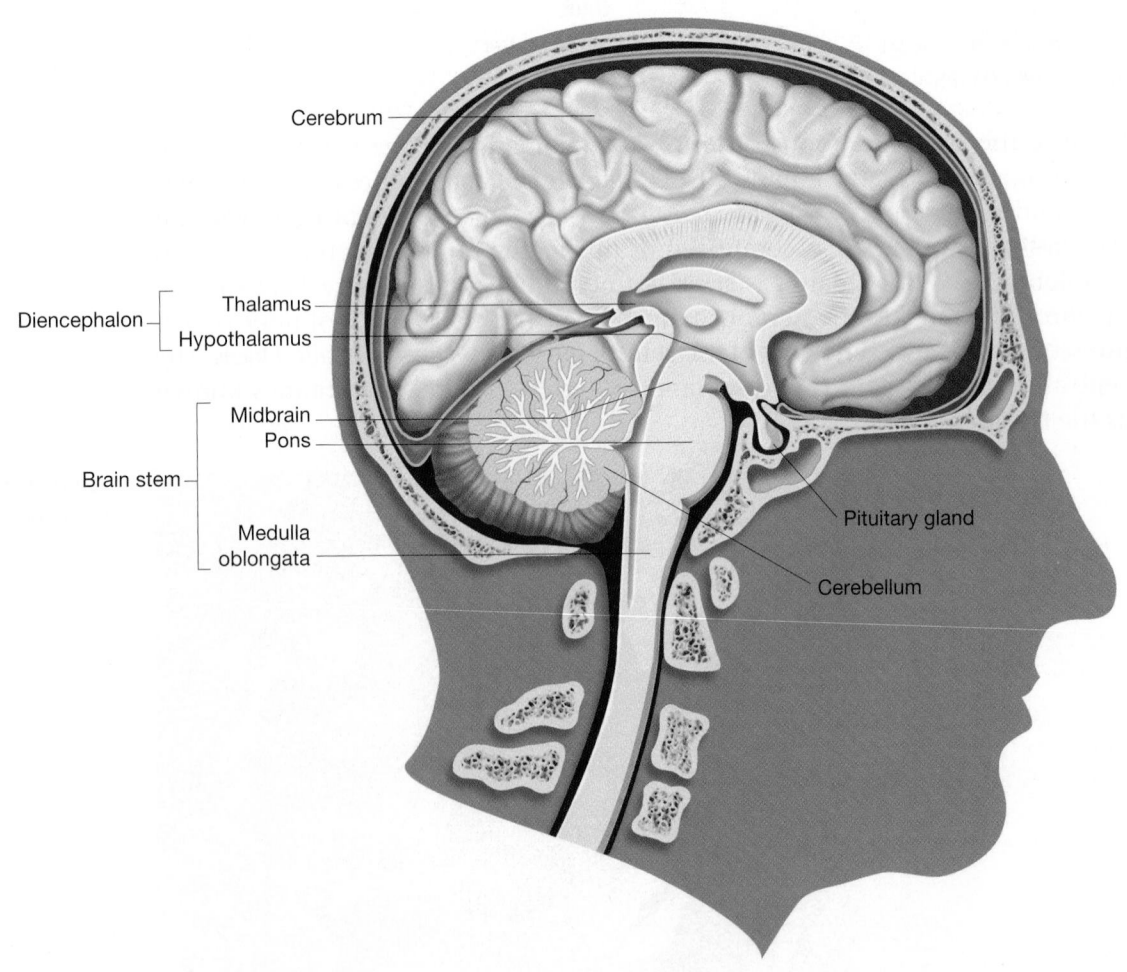

■ **Figure 12.3** The regions of the brain.

The largest section of the brain is the cerebrum. It is located in the upper portion of the brain and is the area that processes thoughts, judgment, memory, problem solving, and language. The outer layer of the cerebrum is the **cerebral cortex,** which is composed of folds of gray matter. The elevated portions of the cerebrum, or convolutions, are called **gyri** and are separated by fissures, or valleys, called **sulci.** The cerebrum is subdivided into left and right halves called **cerebral hemispheres.** Each hemisphere has four lobes. The lobes and their locations and functions are as follows (see Figure 12.4 ■):

1. **Frontal lobe:** Most anterior portion of the cerebrum; controls motor function, personality, and speech
2. **Parietal lobe:** Most superior portion of the cerebrum; receives and interprets nerve impulses from sensory receptors and interprets language
3. **Occipital lobe:** Most posterior portion of the cerebrum; controls vision
4. **Temporal lobe:** Left and right lateral portion of the cerebrum; controls hearing and smell

The diencephalon, located below the cerebrum, contains two of the most critical areas of the brain, the **thalamus** and the **hypothalamus.** The thalamus is composed of gray matter and acts as a center for relaying impulses from the eyes, ears, and skin to the cerebrum. Our pain perception is controlled by the thalamus. The hypothalamus located just below the thalamus controls body temperature, appetite, sleep, sexual desire, and emotions. The hypothalamus is actually responsible for controlling the autonomic nervous system, cardiovascular system, digestive system, and the release of hormones from the pituitary gland.

The cerebellum, the second largest portion of the brain, is located beneath the posterior part of the cerebrum. This part of the brain aids in coordinating voluntary body movements and maintaining balance and equilibrium. The cerebellum refines the muscular movement that is initiated in the cerebrum.

The final portion of the brain is the brain stem. This area has three components: **midbrain, pons,** and **medulla oblongata.** The midbrain acts as a pathway for

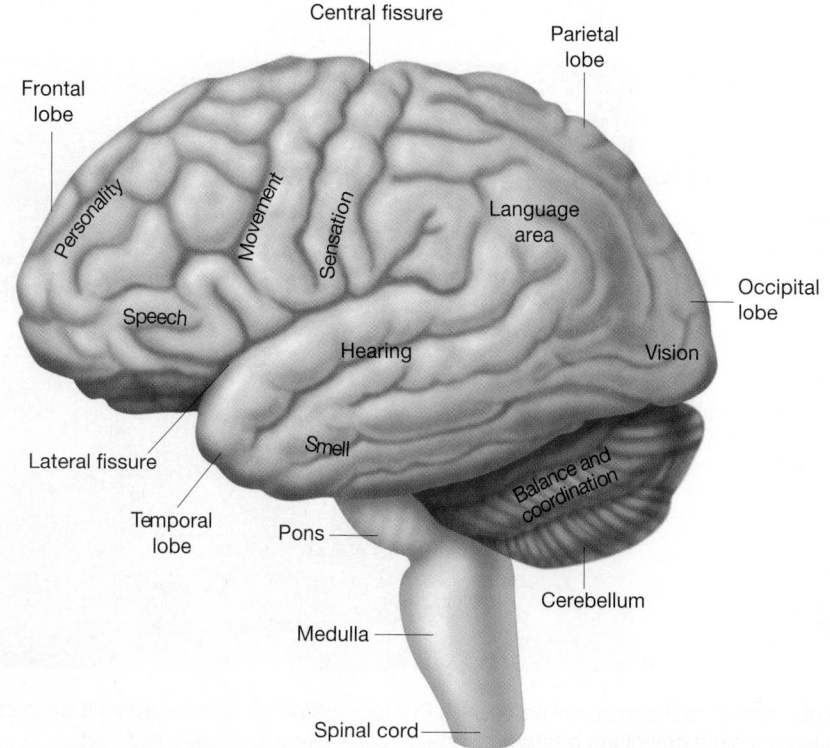

■ Figure 12.4 The functional regions of the cerebrum.

impulses to be conducted between the brain and the spinal cord. The pons—a term meaning bridge—connects the cerebellum to the rest of the brain. The medulla oblongata is the most inferior positioned portion of the brain; it connects the brain to the spinal cord. However, this vital area contains the centers that control respiration, heart rate, temperature, and blood pressure. Additionally, this is the site where nerve tracts cross from one side of the brain to control functions and movement on the other side of the body. In other words, with few exceptions, the left side of the brain controls the right side of the body and vice versa.

The brain has four interconnected cavities called **ventricles:** one in each cerebral hemisphere, one in the thalamus, and one in front of the cerebellum. These contain **cerebrospinal fluid** (CSF), which is the watery, clear fluid that provides protection from shock or sudden motion to the brain and spinal cord.

Spinal Cord

ascending tracts	**spinal cavity**
central canal	**vertebral canal**
descending tracts	**vertebral column**

The function of the spinal cord is to provide a pathway for impulses traveling to and from the brain. The spinal cord is actually a column of nervous tissue extending from the medulla oblongata of the brain down to the level of the second lumbar vertebra within the **vertebral column.** The 33 vertebrae of the backbone line up to form a continuous canal for the spinal cord called the **spinal cavity** or **vertebral canal** (see Figure 12.5 ■).

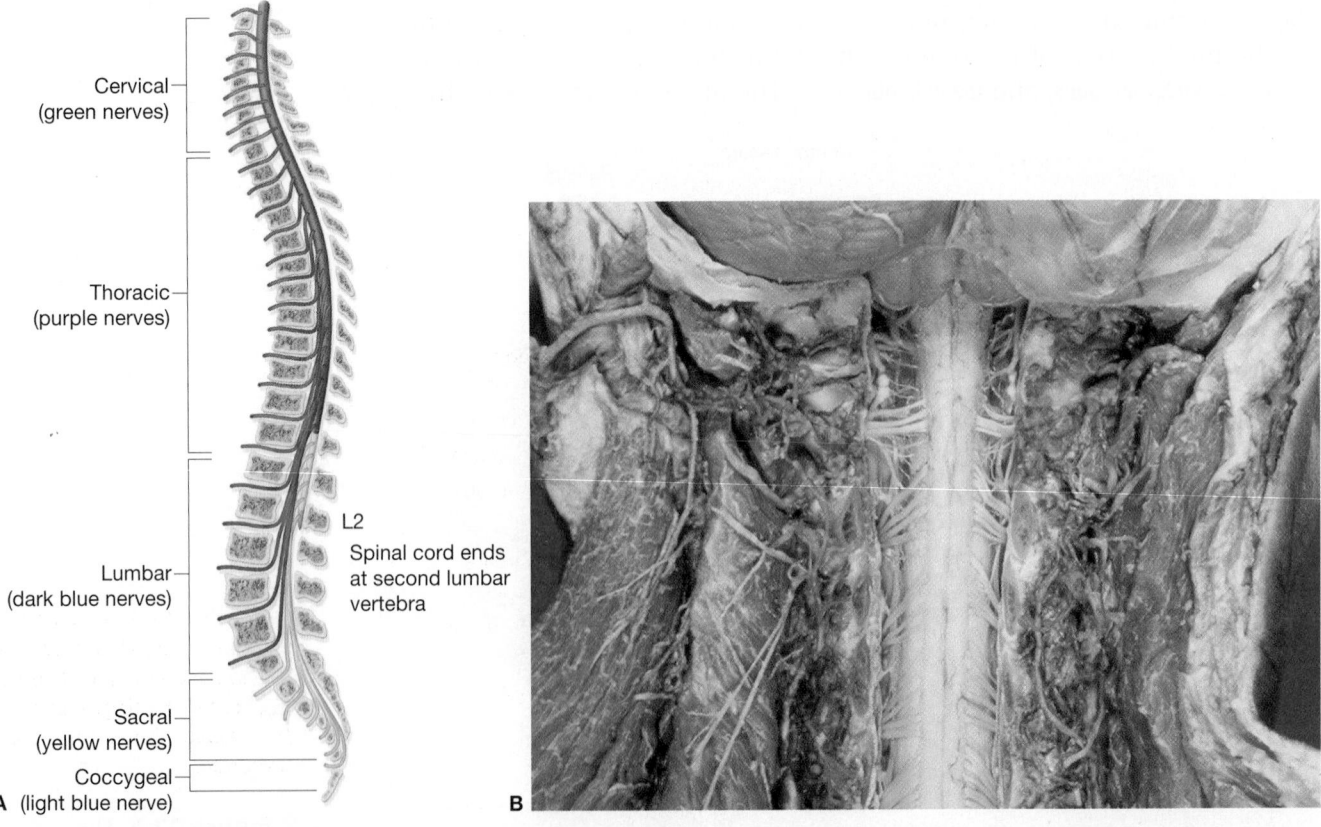

Cervical
(green nerves)

Thoracic
(purple nerves)

L2
Spinal cord ends
at second lumbar
vertebra

Lumbar
(dark blue nerves)

Sacral
(yellow nerves)

Coccygeal
A (light blue nerve)

B

■ **Figure 12.5** (A) The levels of the spinal cord and spinal nerves. (B) Photograph of the spinal cord as it descends from the brain. The spinal nerve roots are clearly visible branching off from the spinal cord. *(Photo Researchers, Inc.)*

Similar to the brain, the spinal cord is also protected by cerebrospinal fluid. It flows down the center of the spinal cord within the **central canal.** The inner core of the spinal cord consists of cell bodies and dendrites of peripheral nerves and therefore is gray matter. The outer portion of the spinal cord is myelinated white matter. The white matter is either **ascending tracts** carrying sensory information up to the brain or **descending tracts** carrying motor commands down from the brain to a peripheral nerve.

Meninges

arachnoid layer (ah-RAK-noyd) **subarachnoid space** (sub-ah-RAK-noyd)
dura mater (DOO-rah / MATE-er) **subdural space** (sub-DOO-ral)
pia mater (PEE-ah / MATE-er)

The meninges are three layers of connective tissue membranes surrounding the brain and spinal cord (see Figure 12.6 ■). Moving from external to internal, the meninges are:

1. **Dura mater:** Meaning *tough mother;* it forms a tough, fibrous sac around the central nervous system
2. **Subdural space:** Actual space between the dura mater and arachnoid layers
3. **Arachnoid layer:** Meaning *spiderlike;* it is a thin, delicate layer attached to the pia mater by weblike filaments
4. **Subarachnoid space:** Space between the arachnoid layer and the pia mater; it contains cerebrospinal fluid that cushions the brain from the outside
5. **Pia mater:** Meaning *soft mother;* it is the innermost membrane layer and is applied directly to the surface of the brain and spinal cord

> **MED TERM TIP**
>
> Certain disease processes attack the gray matter and the white matter of the central nervous system. For instance, *poliomyelitis* is a viral infection of the gray matter of the spinal cord. The combining term *poli/o* means "gray matter." This disease has almost been eradicated, due to the polio vaccine.

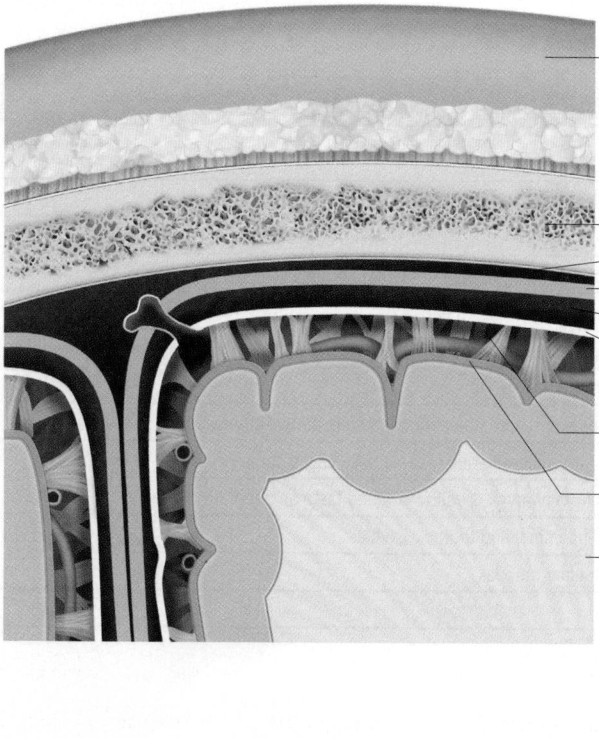

Skin

Bone of skull
Epidural space
Dura mater
Subdural space
Arachnoid layer

Subarachnoid space

Pia mater

Brain

■ **Figure 12.6** The meninges. This figure illustrates the location and structure of each layer of the meninges and their relationship to the skull and brain.

Peripheral Nervous System

afferent neurons (AFF-er-ent)

autonomic nervous system (aw-toh-NOM-ik)

efferent neurons (EFF-er-ent)

ganglion (GANG-lee-on)

motor neurons

nerve root

sensory neurons

somatic nerves

The peripheral nervous system (PNS) includes both the 12 pairs of cranial nerves and the 31 pairs of spinal nerves. A nerve is a group or bundle of axon fibers located outside the central nervous system that carries messages between the central nervous system and the various parts of the body. Whether a nerve is cranial or spinal is determined by where the nerve originates. Cranial nerves arise from the brain, mainly at the medulla oblongata. Spinal nerves split off from the spinal cord, and one pair (a left and a right) exits between each pair of vertebrae. The point where either type of nerve is attached to the central nervous system is called the **nerve root.** The names of most nerves reflect either the organ the nerve serves or the portion of the body the nerve is traveling through. The entire list of cranial nerves is found in Table 12.1 ■. Figure 12.7 ■ illustrates some of the major spinal nerves in the human body.

Although most nerves carry information to and from the central nervous system, individual neurons carry information in only one direction. **Afferent neurons,** also called **sensory neurons,** carry sensory information from a sensory receptor to the central nervous system. **Efferent neurons,** also called **motor neurons,** carry activity instructions from the central nervous system to muscles or glands out in the body (see Figure 12.8 ■). The nerve cell bodies of the neurons forming the nerve are grouped together in a knot-like mass, called a **ganglion,** located outside the central nervous system.

The nerves of the peripheral nervous system are subdivided into two divisions, the **autonomic nervous system** (ANS) and **somatic nerves,** each serving a different area of the body.

> **MED TERM TIP**
>
> Because nerve tracts cross from one side of the body to the other side of the brain, damage to one side of the brain results in symptoms appearing on the opposite side of the body. Since nerve cells that control the movement of the right side of the body are located in the left side of the medulla oblongata, a stroke that paralyzed the right side of the body would actually have occurred in the left side of the brain.

Table 12.1	Cranial Nerves	
NUMBER	**NAME**	**FUNCTION**
I	Olfactory	Transports impulses for sense of smell
II	Optic	Carries impulses for sense of sight
III	Oculomotor	Motor impulses for eye muscle movement and the pupil of the eye
IV	Trochlear	Controls superior oblique muscle of eye on each side
V	Trigeminal	Carries sensory facial impulses and controls muscles for chewing; branches into eyes, forehead, upper and lower jaw
VI	Abducens	Controls an eyeball muscle to turn eye to side
VII	Facial	Controls facial muscles for expression, salivation, and taste on two-thirds of tongue (anterior)
VIII	Vestibulocochlear	Responsible for impulses of equilibrium and hearing; also called auditory nerve
IX	Glossopharyngeal	Carries sensory impulses from pharynx (swallowing) and taste on one-third of tongue
X	Vagus	Supplies most organs in abdominal and thoracic cavities
XI	Accessory	Controls the neck and shoulder muscles
XII	Hypoglossal	Controls tongue muscles

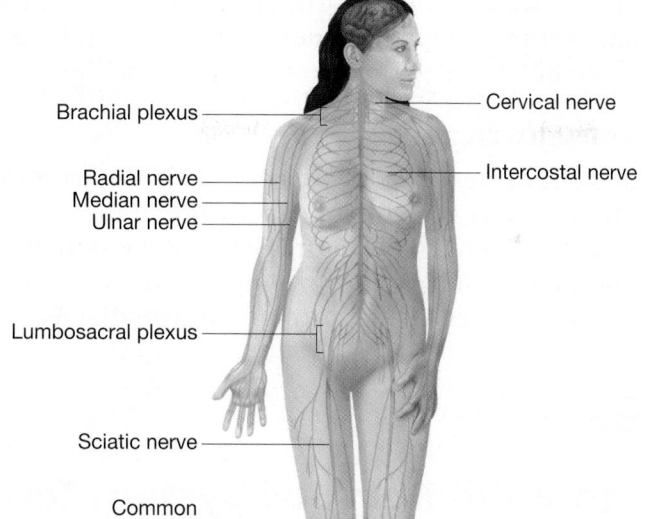

Brachial plexus

Radial nerve
Median nerve
Ulnar nerve

Lumbosacral plexus

Sciatic nerve

Common peroneal nerve

Cervical nerve

Intercostal nerve

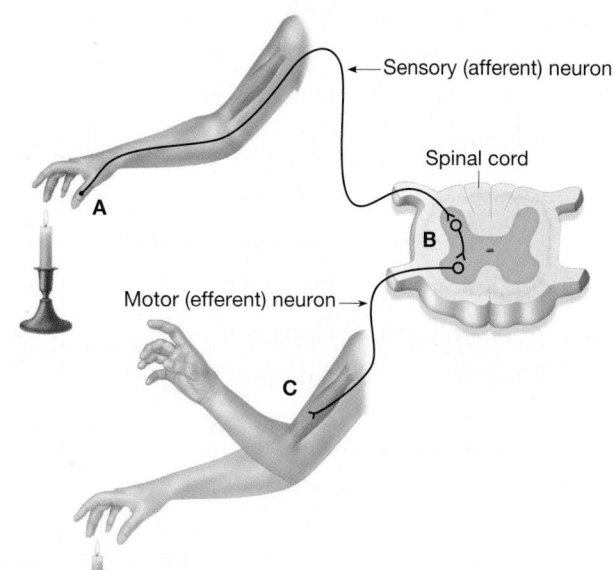

Sensory (afferent) neuron

Spinal cord

Motor (efferent) neuron

A

B

C

■ **Figure 12.8** The functional structure of the peripheral nervous system. (A) Afferent or sensory neurons carry sensory information to the spinal cord; (B) the spinal cord receives incoming sensory information and delivers motor messages; (C) efferent or motor neurons deliver motor commands to muscles and glands.

Autonomic Nervous System

parasympathetic branch
(pair-ah-sim-pah-THET-ik)

sympathetic branch (sim-pah-THET-ik)

The autonomic nervous system is involved with the control of involuntary or unconscious bodily functions. It may increase or decrease the activity of the smooth muscle found in viscera and blood vessels, cardiac muscle, and glands. The autonomic nervous system is divided into two branches: **sympathetic branch** and **parasympathetic branch.** The sympathetic nerves control the "fight or flight" reaction during times of stress and crisis. These nerves increase heart rate, dilate airways, increase blood pressure, inhibit digestion, and stimulate the production

of adrenaline during a crisis. The parasympathetic nerves serve as a counterbalance for the sympathetic nerves, the "rest and digest" reaction. Therefore, they cause heart rate to slow down, lower blood pressure, and stimulate digestion.

Somatic Nerves

Somatic nerves serve the skin and skeletal muscles and are mainly involved with the conscious and voluntary activities of the body. The large variety of sensory receptors found in the dermis layer of the skin use somatic nerves to send their information, such as touch, temperature, pressure, and pain, to the brain. These are also the nerves that carry motor commands to skeletal muscles.

 # Terminology

Word Parts Used to Build Nervous System Terms

The following lists contain the combining forms, suffixes, and prefixes used to build terms in the remaining sections of this chapter.

Combining Forms

alges/o	sense of pain	**encephal/o**	brain	**neur/o**	nerve
angi/o	vessel	**esthes/o**	sensation, feeling	**poli/o**	gray matter
arteri/o	artery	**gli/o**	glue	**pont/o**	pons
astr/o	star	**hemat/o**	blood	**radicul/o**	nerve root
cephal/o	head	**isch/o**	to hold back	**scler/o**	hard
cerebell/o	cerebellum	**later/o**	side	**spin/o**	spine
cerebr/o	cerebrum	**lumb/o**	low back	**thalam/o**	thalamus
clon/o	rapid contracting and relaxing	**medull/o**	medulla oblongata	**thec/o**	sheath
cyt/o	cell	**mening/o**	meninges	**tom/o**	to cut
dur/o	dura mater	**meningi/o**	meninges	**ton/o**	muscle tone
electr/o	electricity	**my/o**	muscle	**vascul/o**	blood vessel
		myel/o	spinal cord	**ventricul/o**	ventricle

Suffixes

-al	pertaining to	**-ia**	condition, state	**-pathy**	disease
-algia	pain	**-ic**	pertaining to	**-phasia**	speech
-ar	pertaining to	**-ine**	pertaining to	**-plasty**	surgical repair
-ary	pertaining to	**-itis**	inflammation	**-plegia**	paralysis
-asthenia	weakness	**-logy**	study of	**-rrhaphy**	suture
-cele	protrusion	**-nic**	pertaining to	**-taxia**	muscle coordination
-eal	pertaining to	**-oma**	tumor, swelling	**-tic**	pertaining to
-ectomy	surgical removal	**-osis**	abnormal condition	**-trophic**	pertaining to development
-gram	record	**-otomy**	cutting into		
-graphy	process of recording	**-paresis**	weakness		

Prefixes

a-	without	hemi-	half	poly-	many
an-	without	hydro-	water	quadri-	four
anti-	against	hyper-	excessive	semi-	partial
bi-	two	intra-	within	sub-	below
dys-	abnormal, difficult	mono-	one	un-	not
endo-	within	para-	abnormal, two like parts of a pair		
epi-	above				

Anatomical Terms

TERM	WORD PARTS	DEFINITION
cerebellar (ser-eh-BELL-ar)	cerebell/o = cerebellum -ar = pertaining to	Pertaining to the cerebellum.
cerebral (seh-REE-bral)	cerebr/o = cerebrum -al = pertaining to	Pertaining to the cerebrum.
cerebrospinal (ser-eh-broh-SPY-nal)	cerebr/o = cerebrum spin/o = spine -al = pertaining to	Pertaining to the cerebrum and spine.
encephalic (IN-seh-FAL-ik)	encephal/o = brain -ic = pertaining to	Pertaining to the brain.
intrathecal (in-tra-THEE-kal)	intra- = within thec/o = sheath -al = pertaining to	Pertaining to within the meninges, specifically the subdural or subarachnoid space.
medullary (MED-yoo-lair-ee)	medull/o = medulla oblongata -ary = pertaining to	Pertaining to the medulla oblongata.
myelonic (MY-eh-LON-ik)	myel/o = spinal cord -nic = pertaining to	Pertaining to the spinal cord.
meningeal (meh-NIN-jee-all)	mening/o = meninges -eal = pertaining to	Pertaining to the meninges.
neural (NOO-rall)	neur/o = nerve -al = pertaining to	Pertaining to nerves.
neuroglial (noo-RIG-lee-al)	neur/o = nerve gli/o = glue -al = pertaining to	Pertaining to the support cells, glial cells, of nerves.
pontine (pon-TEEN)	pont/o = pons -ine = pertaining to	Pertaining to the pons.
thalamic (tha-LAM-ik)	thalam/o = thalamus -ic = pertaining to	Pertaining to the thalamus.
ventricular (ven-TRIK-yoo-lar)	ventricul/o = ventricle -ar = pertaining to	Pertaining to the ventricles.

Pathology

TERM	WORD PARTS	DEFINITION
Medical Specialties		
anesthesiology (an-es-thee-zee-ol-oh-jee)	an- = without esthes/o = sensation, feeling -logy = study of	Branch of medicine specializing in all aspects of anesthesia, including for surgical procedures, resuscitation measures, and the management of acute and chronic pain. Physician is an *anesthesiologist.*
neurology (noo-rol-oh-jee)	neur/o = nerve -logy = study of	Branch of medicine concerned with diagnosis and treatment of diseases and conditions of the nervous system. Physician is a *neurologist.*
neurosurgery (noo-roh-SIR-jury)	neur/o = nerve	Branch of medicine concerned with treating conditions and diseases of the nervous systems by surgical means. Physician is a *neurosurgeon.*
Signs and Symptoms		
absence seizure		Type of epileptic seizure that lasts only a few seconds to half a minute, characterized by a loss of awareness and an absence of activity. It is also called a *petit mal seizure.*
analgesia (an-al-JEE-zee-ah)	an- = without alges/o = sense of pain -ia = state	Absence of pain.
anesthesia (an-ess-THEE-zee-ah)	an- = without esthes/o = feeling, sensations -ia = condition	Lack of feeling or sensation.
aphasia (ah-FAY-zee-ah)	a- = without -phasia = speech	Inability to communicate verbally or in writing due to damage of the speech or language centers in the brain.
ataxia (ah-TAK-see-ah)	a- = without -taxia = muscle coordination	Lack of muscle coordination.
aura (AW-ruh)		Sensations, such as seeing colors or smelling an unusual odor, that occur just prior to an epileptic seizure or migraine headache.
cephalalgia (seff-al-AL-jee-ah)	cephal/o = head -algia = pain	Headache.
coma (COH-mah)		Profound unconsciousness resulting from an illness or injury.
conscious (KON-shus)		Condition of being awake and aware of surroundings.
convulsion (kon-VULL-shun)		Severe involuntary muscle contractions and relaxations. These have a variety of causes, such as epilepsy, fever, and toxic conditions.

Pathology *(continued)*

TERM	WORD PARTS	DEFINITION
delirium (dee-LEER-ee-um)		Abnormal mental state characterized by confusion, disorientation, and agitation.
dementia (dee-MEN-she-ah)		Progressive impairment of intellectual function that interferes with performing activities of daily living. Patients have little awareness of their condition. Found in disorders such as Alzheimer's.
dysphasia (dis-FAY-zee-ah)	dys- = abnormal, difficult -phasia = speech	Difficulty communicating verbally or in writing due to damage of the speech or language centers in the brain.
focal seizure (FOE-kal)	-al = pertaining to	Localized seizure often affecting one limb.
hemiparesis (hem-ee-par-EE-sis)	hemi- = half -paresis = weakness	Weakness or loss of motion on one side of the body.
hemiplegia (hem-ee-PLEE-jee-ah)	hemi- = half -plegia = paralysis	Paralysis on only one side of the body.
hyperesthesia (high-per-ess-THEE-zee-ah)	hyper- = excessive esthes/o = feeling, sensations -ia = condition	Abnormally heightened sense of feeling, sense of pain, or sensitivity to touch.
monoparesis (mon-oh-pah-REE-sis)	mono- = one -paresis = weakness	Muscle weakness in one limb.
monoplegia (mon-oh-PLEE-jee-ah)	mono- = one -plegia = paralysis	Paralysis of one limb.
neuralgia (noo-RAL-jee-ah)	neur/o = nerve -algia = pain	Nerve pain.
palsy (PAWL-zee)		Temporary or permanent loss of the ability to control movement.
paralysis (pah-RAL-ih-sis)		Temporary or permanent loss of function or voluntary movement.
paraplegia (pair-ah-PLEE-jee-ah)	para- = two like parts of a pair -plegia = paralysis	Paralysis of the lower portion of the body and both legs.
paresthesia (par-es-THEE-zee-ah)	para- = abnormal esthes/o = sensation, feeling -ia = condition	Abnormal sensation such as burning or tingling.
quadriplegia (kwod-rih-PLEE-jee-ah)	quadri- = four -plegia = paralysis	Paralysis of all four limbs.
seizure (SEE-zyoor)		Sudden, uncontrollable onset of symptoms, such as in an epileptic seizure.
semiconscious (sem-ee-KON-shus)	semi- = partial	State of being aware of surroundings and responding to stimuli only part of the time.

Pathology *(continued)*

TERM	WORD PARTS	DEFINITION
syncope (SIN-koh-pee)		Fainting.
tonic-clonic seizure	ton/o = muscle tone clon/o = rapid contracting and relaxing -ic = pertaining to	Type of severe epileptic seizure characterized by a loss of consciousness and convulsions. The seizure alternates between strong continuous muscle spasms (tonic) and rhythmic muscle contraction and relaxation (clonic). It is also called a *grand mal seizure.*
tremor (TREM-or)		Involuntary repetitive alternating movement of a part of the body.
unconscious (un-KON-shus)	un- = not	State of being unaware of surroundings, with the inability to respond to stimuli.
Brain		
Alzheimer's disease (ALTS-high-merz)		Chronic, organic mental disorder consisting of dementia, which is more prevalent in adults after 65 years of age. Involves progressive disorientation, apathy, speech and gait disturbances, and loss of memory. Named for German neurologist Alois Alzheimer.
astrocytoma (ass-troh-sigh-TOH-mah)	astr/o = star cyt/o = cell -oma = tumor	Tumor of the brain or spinal cord composed of astrocytes, one type of neuroglial cells.
brain tumor		Intracranial mass, either benign or malignant. A benign tumor of the brain can still be fatal since it will grow and cause pressure on normal brain tissue.
cerebellitis (ser-eh-bell-EYE-tis)	cerebell/o = cerebellum -itis = inflammation	Inflammation of the cerebellum.

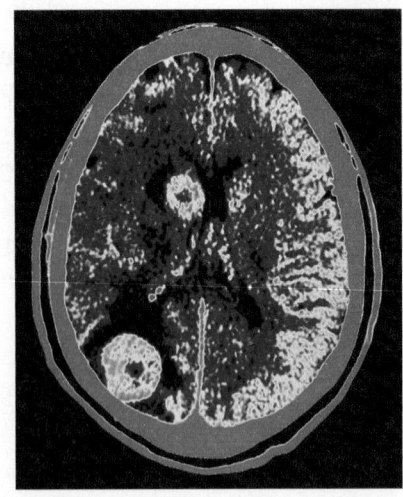

■ **Figure 12.9** Color-enhanced CT scan showing two malignant tumors in the brain. *(Scott Camazine/Photo Researchers, Inc.)*

Pathology *(continued)*

TERM	WORD PARTS	DEFINITION
cerebral aneurysm (AN-yoo-rizm)	cerebr/o = cerebrum -al = pertaining to	Localized abnormal dilation of a blood vessel, usually an artery; the result of a congenital defect or weakness in the wall of the vessel. A ruptured aneurysm is a common cause of a hemorrhagic cerebrovascular accident.

Figure 12.10 Common locations for cerebral artery aneurysms in the Circle of Willis.

cerebral contusion (kon-TOO-shun)	cerebr/o = cerebrum -al = pertaining to	Bruising of the brain from a blow or impact.
cerebral palsy (CP) (ser-REE-bral / PAWL-zee)	cerebr/o = cerebrum -al = pertaining to	Nonprogressive brain damage resulting from a defect, trauma, or oxygen deprivation at the time of birth.
cerebrovascular accident (CVA) (ser-eh-broh-VASS-kyoo-lar)	cerebr/o = cerebrum vascul/o = blood vessel -ar = pertaining to	Development of an infarct due to loss in the blood supply to an area of the brain. Blood flow can be interrupted by a ruptured blood vessel (hemorrhage), a floating clot (embolus), a stationary clot (thrombosis), or compression. The extent of damage depends on the size and location of the infarct and often includes dysphasia and hemiplegia. Commonly called a *stroke*.

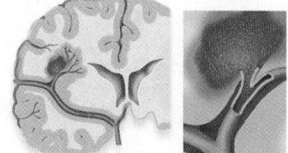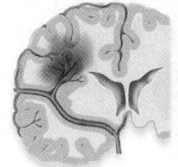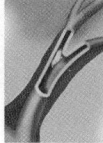

Cerebral hemorrhage: Cerebral artery ruptures and bleeds into brain tissue.

Cerebral embolism: Embolus from another area lodges in cerebral artery and blocks blood flow.

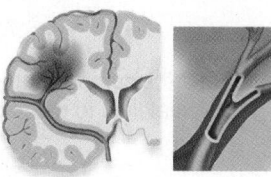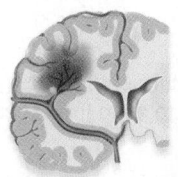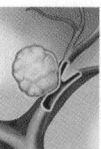

Figure 12.11 The four common causes for cerebrovascular accidents.

Cerebral thrombosis: Blood clot forms in cerebral artery and blocks blood flow.

Compression: Pressure from tumor squeezes adjacent blood vessel and blocks blood flow.

■ Pathology (continued)

TERM	WORD PARTS	DEFINITION
concussion (kon-KUSH-un)		Injury to the brain resulting from the brain being shaken inside the skull from a blow or impact. Symptoms vary and may include: headache, blurred vision, nausea or vomiting, dizziness, and balance problems. Also called *mild traumatic brain injury* (TBI).
encephalitis (en-seff-ah-LYE-tis)	encephal/o = brain -itis = inflammation	Inflammation of the brain.
epilepsy (EP-ih-lep-see)		Recurrent disorder of the brain in which seizures and loss of consciousness occur as a result of uncontrolled electrical activity of the neurons in the brain.
hydrocephalus (high-droh-SEFF-ah-lus)	hydro- = water cephal/o = head	Accumulation of cerebrospinal fluid within the ventricles of the brain, causing the head to be enlarged. It is treated by creating an artificial shunt for the fluid to leave the brain. If left untreated, it may lead to seizures and mental retardation.

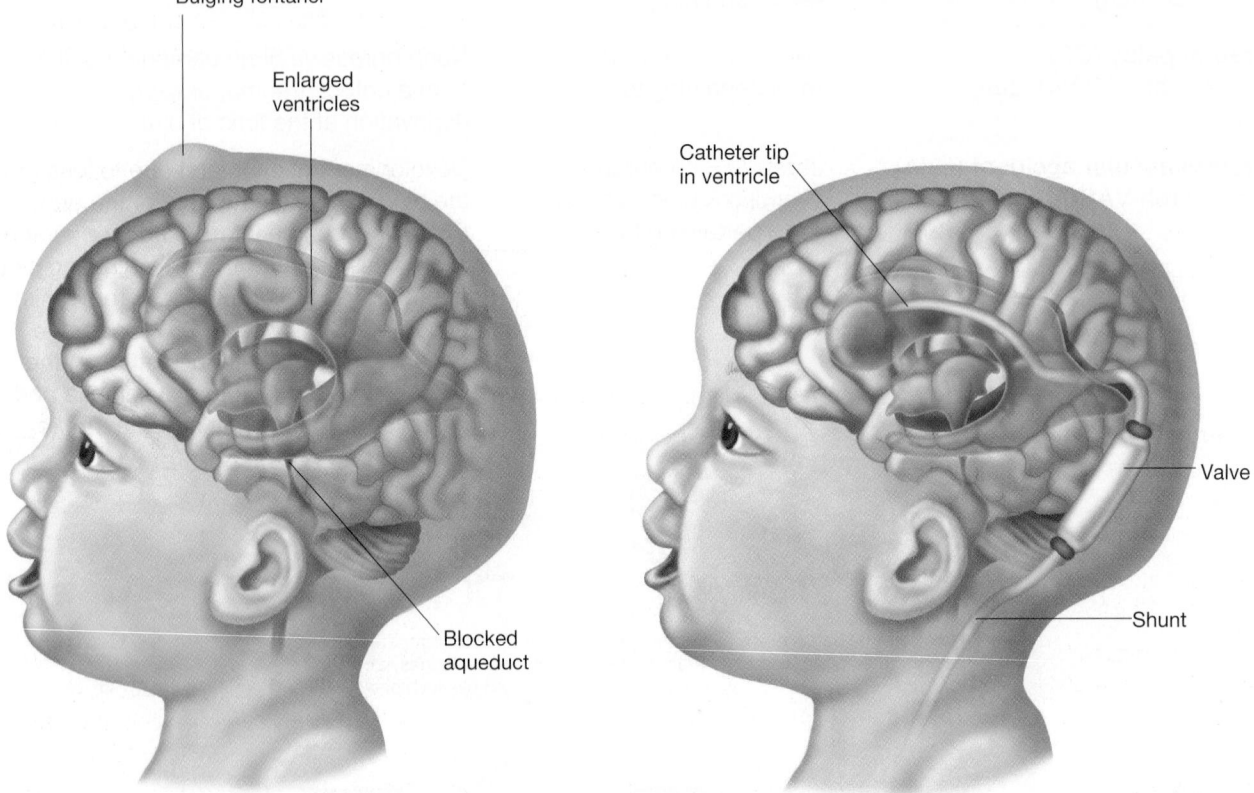

■ **Figure 12.12** Hydrocephalus. The figure on the left is a child with the enlarged ventricles of hydrocephalus. The figure on the right is the same child with a shunt to send the excess cerebrospinal fluid to the abdominal cavity.

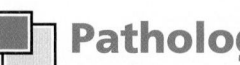

Pathology *(continued)*

TERM	WORD PARTS	DEFINITION
migraine (MY-grain)		Specific type of headache characterized by severe head pain, sensitivity to light, dizziness, and nausea.
Parkinson's disease (PARK-in-sons)		Chronic disorder of the nervous system with fine tremors, muscular weakness, rigidity, and a shuffling gait. Named for British physician Sir James Parkinson.
Reye syndrome (RISE / SIN-drohm)		Combination of symptoms first recognized by Australian pathologist R. D. K. Reye that includes acute encephalopathy and damage to various organs, especially the liver. This occurs in children under age 15 who have had a viral infection. It is also associated with taking aspirin. For this reason, it's not recommended for children to use aspirin.
transient ischemic attack (TIA) (TRAN-shent / iss-KEM-ik)	isch/o = to hold back hem/o = blood -ic = pertaining to	Temporary interference with blood supply to the brain, causing neurological symptoms such as dizziness, numbness, and hemiparesis. May eventually lead to a full-blown stroke (cerebrovascular accident).

Spinal Cord

TERM	WORD PARTS	DEFINITION
amyotrophic lateral sclerosis (ALS) (ah-my-oh-TROFF-ik / LAT-er-al / skleh-ROH-sis)	a- = without my/o = muscle -trophic = pertaining to development later/o = side -al = pertaining to scler/o = hard -osis = abnormal condition	Disease with muscular weakness and atrophy due to degeneration of motor neurons of the spinal cord. Also called *Lou Gehrig's disease,* after the New York Yankees baseball player who died from the disease.
meningocele (men-IN-goh-seel)	mening/o = meninges -cele = protrusion	Congenital condition in which the meninges protrude through an opening in the vertebral column (see Figure 12.13B ■). See *spina bifida.*
myelitis (my-eh-LYE-tis)	myel/o = spinal cord -itis = inflammation	Inflammation of the spinal cord.
myelomeningocele (my-eh-loh-meh-NIN-goh-seel)	myel/o = spinal cord mening/o = meninges -cele = protrusion	Congenital condition in which the meninges and spinal cord protrude through an opening in the vertebral column (see Figure 12.13C ■). See *spina bifida.*
poliomyelitis (poh-lee-oh-my-eh-lye-tis)	poli/o = gray matter myel/o = spinal cord -itis = inflammation	Viral inflammation of the gray matter of the spinal cord. Results in varying degrees of paralysis; may be mild and reversible or may be severe and permanent. This disease has been almost eliminated due to the discovery of a vaccine in the 1950s.

Pathology *(continued)*

TERM	WORD PARTS	DEFINITION
spina bifida (SPY-nah / BIFF-ih-dah)	spin/o = spine bi- = two	Congenital defect in the walls of the spinal canal in which the laminae of the vertebra do not meet or close (see Figure 12.13A ■). May result in a meningocele or a myelomeningocele—meninges or the spinal cord being pushed through the opening.

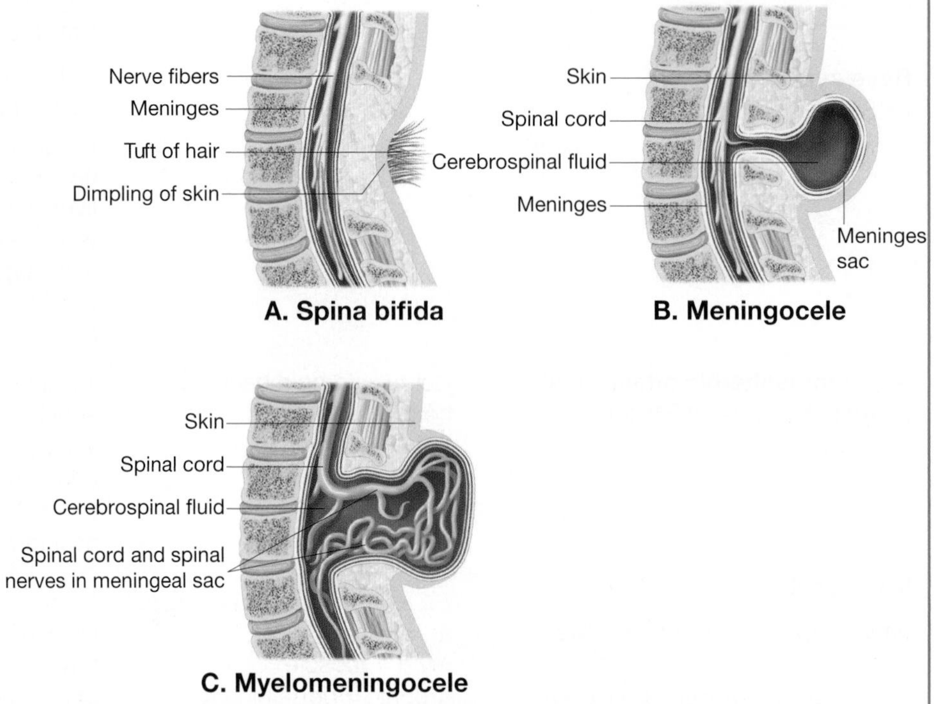

Nerve fibers
Meninges
Tuft of hair
Dimpling of skin

Skin
Spinal cord
Cerebrospinal fluid
Meninges

Meninges sac

A. Spina bifida

B. Meningocele

Skin
Spinal cord
Cerebrospinal fluid
Spinal cord and spinal nerves in meningeal sac

C. Myelomeningocele

■ **Figure 12.13** Spina bifida. (A) Spina bifica occulta; the vertebra is not complete, but there is no protrusion of nervous system structures. (B) Meningocele; the meninges sac protrudes through the opening in the vertebra. (C) Myelomeningocele; the meninges sac and spinal cord protrude through the opening in the vertebra.

TERM	WORD PARTS	DEFINITION
spinal cord injury (SCI)	spin/o = spine -al = pertaining to	Damage to the spinal cord as a result of trauma. Spinal cord may be bruised or completely severed.

Nerves

TERM	WORD PARTS	DEFINITION
Bell's palsy (BELLZ / PAWL-zee)		One-sided facial paralysis due to inflammation of the facial nerve, probably viral in nature. The patient cannot control salivation, tearing of the eyes, or expression, but most will eventually recover.
Guillain-Barré syndrome (GHEE-yan / bah-RAY)		Disease of the nervous system in which nerves lose their myelin covering. May be caused by an autoimmune reaction. Characterized by loss of sensation and/or muscle control starting in the legs. Symptoms then move toward the trunk and may even result in paralysis of the diaphragm.
multiple sclerosis (MS) (MULL-tih-pl / skleh-ROH-sis)	scler/o = hard -osis = abnormal condition	Inflammatory disease of the central nervous system in which there is extreme weakness and numbness due to loss of myelin insulation from nerves.
myasthenia gravis (my-ass-THEE-nee-ah / GRAV-iss)	my/o = muscle -asthenia = weakness	Disease with severe muscular weakness and fatigue due to insufficient neurotransmitter at a synapse.

Pathology *(continued)*

TERM	WORD PARTS	DEFINITION
neuroma (noo-ROH-mah)	neur/o = nerve -oma = tumor	Nerve tumor or tumor of the connective tissue sheath around a nerve.
neuropathy (noo-ROP-ah-thee)	neur/o = nerve -pathy = disease	General term for disease or damage to a nerve.
polyneuritis (pol-ee-noo-RYE-tis)	poly- = many neur/o = nerve -itis = inflammation	Inflammation of two or more nerves.
radiculitis (rah-dick-yoo-LYE-tis)	radicul/o = nerve root -itis = inflammation	Inflammation of a nerve root; may be caused by a herniated nucleus pulposus.
radiculopathy (rah-dick-yoo-LOP-ah-thee)	radicul/o = nerve root -pathy = disease	Refers to the condition that occurs when a herniated nucleus pulposus puts pressure on a nerve root. Symptoms include pain and numbness along the path of the affected nerve.
shingles (SHING-lz)		Eruption of painful blisters on the body along a nerve path. Thought to be caused by a *Herpes zoster* virus infection of the nerve root.

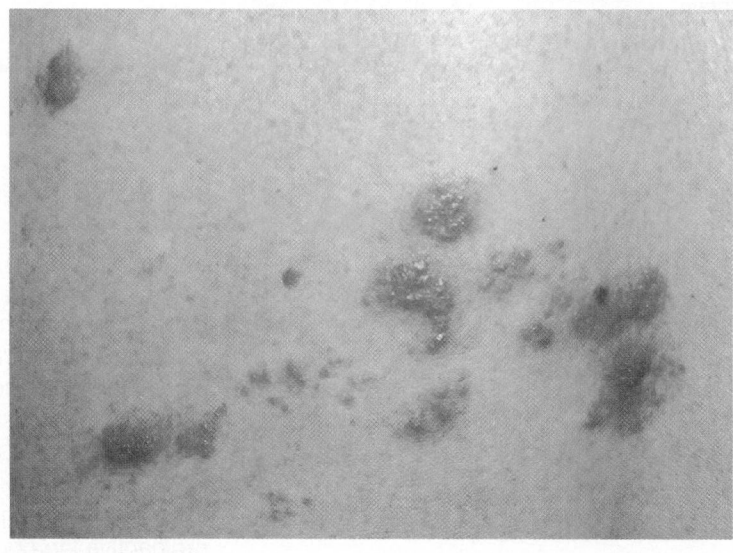

■ **Figure 12.14** Photograph of the skin eruptions associated with shingles. *(Stephen VanHorn/Shutterstock)*

Meninges

TERM	WORD PARTS	DEFINITION
epidural hematoma (ep-ih-DOO-ral / hee-mah-TOH-mah)	epi- = above dur/o = dura mater -al = pertaining to hemat/o = blood -oma = swelling	Mass of blood in the space outside the dura mater of the brain and spinal cord.
meningioma (meh-nin-jee-OH-mah)	meningi/o = meninges -oma = tumor	A tumor in the meninges.
meningitis (men-in-JYE-tis)	mening/o = meninges -itis = inflammation	Inflammation of the meninges around the brain or spinal cord caused by bacterial or viral infection. Symptoms include fever, headache, neck stiffness, lethargy, vomiting, irritability, and photophobia.

Pathology *(continued)*

TERM	WORD PARTS	DEFINITION
subdural hematoma (sub-DOO-ral / hee-mah-TOH-mah)	sub- = below dur/o = dura mater -al = pertaining to hemat/o = blood -oma = swelling	Mass of blood forming beneath the dura mater if the meninges are torn by trauma. May exert fatal pressure on the brain if the hematoma is not drained by surgery.

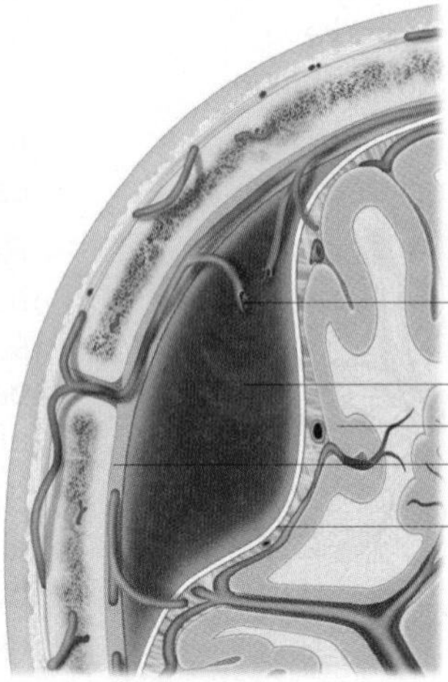

Torn cerebral vein
Subdural hematoma
Compressed brain tissue
Dura mater
Arachnoid layer

■ Figure 12.15 A subdural hematoma. A meningeal vein is ruptured and blood has accumulated in the subdural space, producing pressure on the brain.

Diagnostic Procedures

TERM	WORD PARTS	DEFINITION
Clinical Laboratory Tests		
cerebrospinal fluid analysis (ser-eh-broh-SPY-nal / an-NAL-ih-sis)	cerebr/o = cerebrum spin/o = spine -al = pertaining to	Laboratory examination of the clear, watery, colorless fluid from within the brain and spinal cord. Infections and the abnormal presence of blood can be detected in this test.
Diagnostic Imaging		
brain scan		Image of the brain taken after injection of radioactive isotopes into the circulation.
cerebral angiography (seh-REE-bral / an-jee-OG-rah-fee)	cerebr/o = cerebrum -al = pertaining to angi/o = vessel -graphy = process of recording	X-ray of the blood vessels of the brain after the injection of radiopaque dye.
echoencephalography (ek-oh-en-SEFF-ah-log-rah-fee)	encephal/o = brain -graphy = process of recording	Recording of the ultrasonic echoes of the brain. Useful in determining abnormal patterns of shifting in the brain.
myelogram (MY-eh-loh-gram)	myel/o = spinal cord -gram = record	X-ray record of the spinal cord.

MED TERM TIP

The combining form *myel/o* means "marrow" and is used for both the spinal cord and bone marrow. To the ancient Greek philosophers and physicians, the spinal cord appeared to be much like the marrow found in the medullary cavity of a long bone.

Diagnostic Procedures (continued)

TERM	WORD PARTS	DEFINITION
myelography (my-eh-LOG-rah-fee)	myel/o = spinal cord -graphy = process of recording	Injection of radiopaque dye into the spinal canal. An X-ray is then taken to examine the normal and abnormal outlines made by the dye.
positron emission tomography (PET) (PAHZ-ih-tron / ee-MISH-un / toh-MOG-rah-fee)	tom/o = to cut -graphy = process of recording	Image of the brain produced by measuring gamma rays emitted from the brain after injecting glucose tagged with positively charged isotopes. Measurement of glucose uptake by the brain tissue indicates how metabolically active the tissue is.

Additional Diagnostic Tests

TERM	WORD PARTS	DEFINITION
Babinski reflex (bah-BIN-skeez)		Reflex test developed by French neurologist Joseph Babinski to determine lesions and abnormalities in the nervous system. The Babinski reflex is present if the great toe extends instead of flexes when the lateral sole of the foot is stroked. The normal response to this stimulation is flexion of the toe.
electroencephalogram (EEG) (ee-lek-troh-en-SEFF-ah-loh-gram)	electr/o = electricity encephal/o = brain -gram = record	Record of the brain's electrical patterns.
electroencephalography (EEG) (ee-lek-troh-en-SEFF-ah-LOG-rah-fee)	electr/o = electricity encephal/o = brain -graphy = process of recording	Recording the electrical activity of the brain by placing electrodes at various positions on the scalp. Also used in sleep studies to determine if there is a normal pattern of activity during sleep.
lumbar puncture (LP) (LUM-bar / PUNK-chur)	lumb/o = low back -ar = pertaining to	Puncture with a needle into the lumbar area (usually the fourth intervertebral space) to withdraw fluid for examination and for the injection of anesthesia. Also called *spinal puncture* or *spinal tap.*

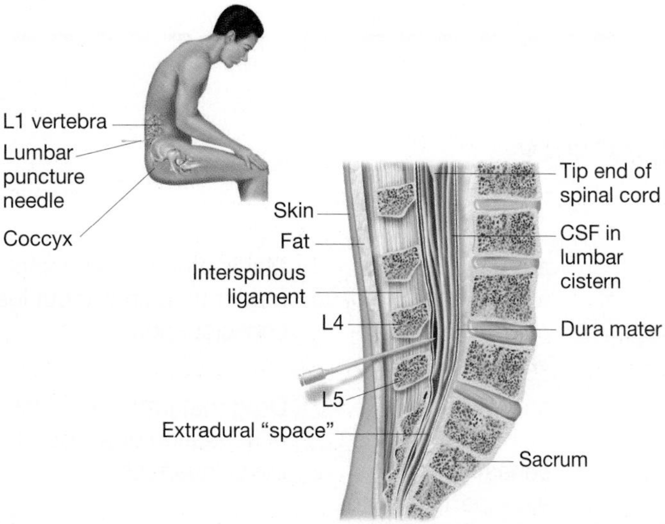

L1 vertebra
Lumbar puncture needle
Coccyx
Skin
Fat
Interspinous ligament
L4
Extradural "space"
L5
Tip end of spinal cord
CSF in lumbar cistern
Dura mater
Sacrum

Figure 12.16 A lumbar puncture. The needle is inserted between the lumbar vertebrae and into the spinal canal.

TERM	WORD PARTS	DEFINITION
nerve conduction velocity		Test that measures how fast an impulse travels along a nerve. Can pinpoint an area of nerve damage.

Therapeutic Procedures

TERM	WORD PARTS	DEFINITION
Medical Procedures		
nerve block		Injection of regional anesthetic to stop the passage of sensory or pain impulses along a nerve path.
Surgical Procedures		
carotid endarterectomy (kah-ROT-id / end-ar-ter-EK-toh-mee)	endo- = within arteri/o = artery -ectomy = surgical removal	Surgical procedure for removing an obstruction within the carotid artery, a major artery in the neck that carries oxygenated blood to the brain. Developed to prevent strokes, but is found to be useful only in severe stenosis with transient ischemic attack.
cerebrospinal fluid shunts (ser-eh-bro-SPY-nal)	cerebr/o = cerebrum spin/o = spine -al = pertaining to	Surgical procedure in which a bypass is created to drain cerebrospinal fluid. It is used to treat hydrocephalus by draining the excess cerebrospinal fluid from the brain and diverting it to the abdominal cavity.
laminectomy (lam-ih-NEK-toh-mee)	-ectomy = surgical removal	Removal of a portion of a vertebra, called the lamina, in order to relieve pressure on the spinal nerve.
neurectomy (noo-REK-toh-mee)	neur/o = nerve -ectomy = surgical removal	Surgical removal of a nerve.
neuroplasty (NOOR-oh-plas-tee)	neur/o = nerve -plasty = surgical repair	Surgical repair of a nerve.
neurorrhaphy (noo-ROR-ah-fee)	neur/o = nerve -rrhaphy = suture	To suture a nerve back together. Actually refers to suturing the connective tissue sheath around the nerve.
tractotomy (track-OT-oh-mee)	-otomy = cutting into	Surgical interruption of a nerve tract in the spinal cord. Used to treat intractable pain or muscle spasms.

Pharmacology

CLASSIFICATION	WORD PARTS	ACTION	EXAMPLES
analgesic (an-al-JEE-zik)	an- = without alges/o = sense of pain -ic = pertaining to	Medication to treat minor to moderate pain without loss of consciousness.	aspirin, Bayer, Ecotrin; acetaminophen, Tylenol; ibuprofen, Motrin
anesthetic (an-ess-THET-ik)	an- = without esthes/o = feeling, sensation -tic = pertaining to	Drug that produces a loss of sensation or a loss of consciousness.	lidocaine, Xylocaine; pentobarbital, Nembutal; propofol, Diprivan; procaine, Novocain

Pharmacology *(continued)*

CLASSIFICATION	WORD PARTS	ACTION	EXAMPLES
anticonvulsant (an-tye-kon-VULL-sant)	anti- = against	Substance that reduces the excitability of neurons and therefore prevents the uncontrolled neuron activity associated with seizures.	carbamazepine, Tegretol; phenobarbital, Nembutal
dopaminergic drugs (dope-ah-men-ER-gik)	-ic = pertaining to	Group of medications to treat Parkinson's disease by either replacing the dopamine that is lacking or increasing the strength of the dopamine that is present.	levodopa; L-dopa, Larodopa; levodopa/carbidopa, Sinemet
hypnotic (hip-NOT-tik)	-ic = pertaining to	Drug that promotes sleep.	secobarbital, Seconal; temazepam, Restoril
narcotic analgesic (nar-KOT-tik)	-ic = pertaining to an- = without alges/o = sense of pain -ic = pertaining to	Drug used to treat severe pain; has the potential to be habit forming if taken for a prolonged time. Also called *opiates*.	morphine, MS Contin; oxycodone, OxyContin; meperidine, Demerol
sedative (SED-ah-tiv)		Drug that has a relaxing or calming effect.	amobarbital, Amytal; butabarbital, Butisol

Abbreviations

ALS	amyotrophic lateral sclerosis	**HA**	headache
ANS	autonomic nervous system	**ICP**	intracranial pressure
CNS	central nervous system	**LP**	lumbar puncture
CP	cerebral palsy	**MS**	multiple sclerosis
CSF	cerebrospinal fluid	**PET**	positron emission tomography
CVA	cerebrovascular accident	**PNS**	peripheral nervous system
CVD	cerebrovascular disease	**SCI**	spinal cord injury
EEG	electroencephalogram, electroencephalography	**TBI**	traumatic brain injury
		TIA	transient ischemic attack

Chapter Review

Real-World Applications

Medical Record Analysis

This Discharge Summary contains 12 medical terms. Underline each term and write it in the list below the report. Then define each term.

Discharge Summary

Admitting Diagnosis:	Paraplegia following motorcycle accident.
Final Diagnosis:	Comminuted L2 fracture with epidural hematoma and spinal cord injury resulting in complete paraplegia at the L2 level.
History of Present Illness:	Patient is a 23-year-old male who was involved in a motorcycle accident. He was unconscious for 35 minutes but was fully aware of his surroundings upon regaining consciousness. He was immediately aware of total anesthesia and paralysis below the waist.
Summary of Hospital Course:	CT scan revealed extensive bone destruction at the fracture site and that the spinal cord was severed. Patient was unable to voluntarily contract any lower extremity muscles and was not able to feel touch or pinpricks. Lumbar laminectomy with spinal fusion was performed to stabilize the fracture and remove the epidural hematoma. The immediate postoperative recovery period proceeded normally. Patient began physical therapy and occupational therapy. After 2 months, X-rays indicated full healing of the spinal fusion and patient was transferred to a rehabilitation institute.
Discharge Plans:	Patient was transferred to a rehabilitation institute to continue intensive PT and OT.

	Term	Definition
1	_____	_____
2	_____	_____
3	_____	_____
4	_____	_____
5	_____	_____
6	_____	_____
7	_____	_____
8	_____	_____
9	_____	_____
10	_____	_____
11	_____	_____
12	_____	_____

Chart Note Transcription

The chart note below contains 11 phrases that can be reworded with a medical term that you learned in this chapter. Each phrase is identified with an underline. Determine the medical term and write your answers in the space provided.

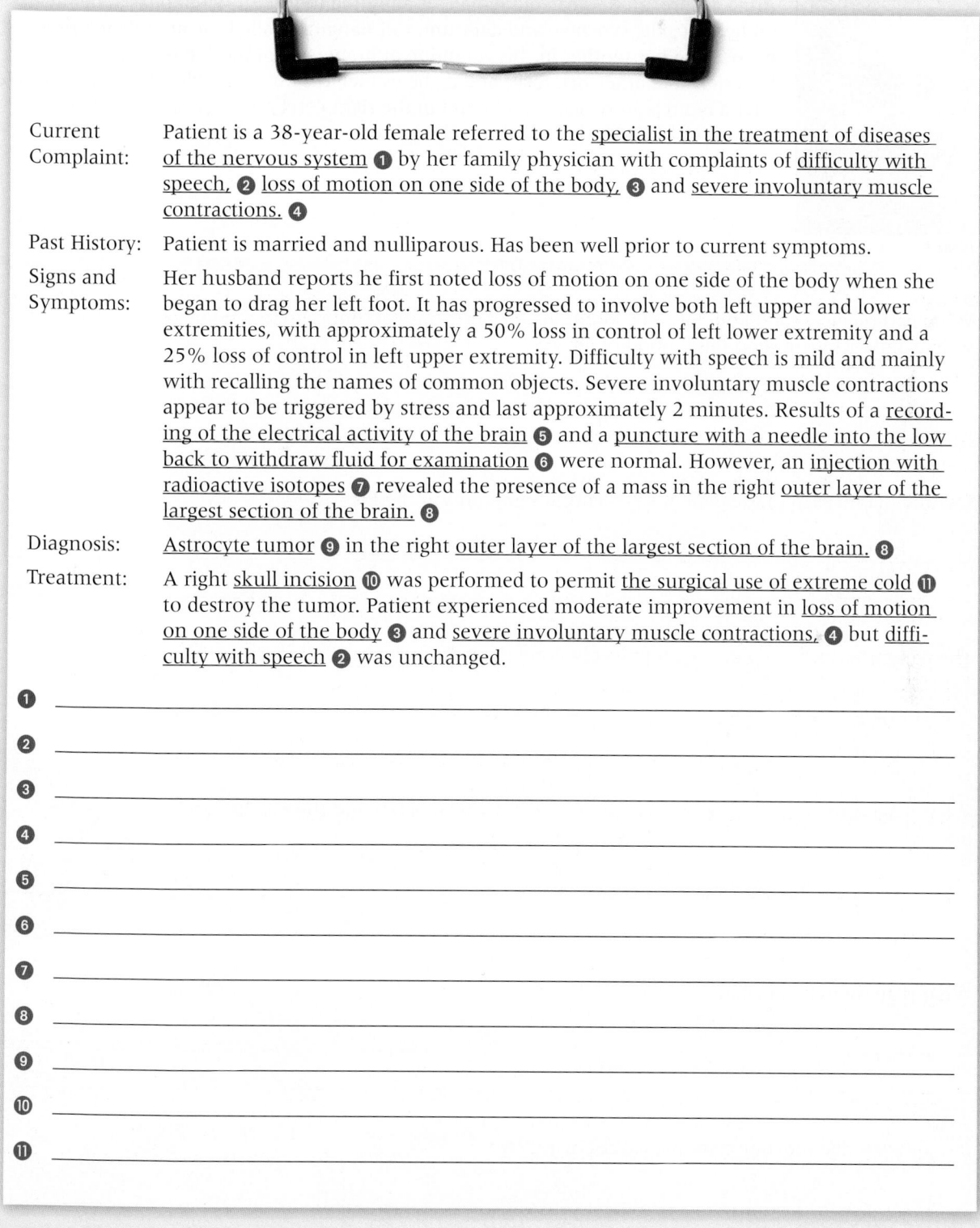

Current Complaint:	Patient is a 38-year-old female referred to the <u>specialist in the treatment of diseases of the nervous system</u> ❶ by her family physician with complaints of <u>difficulty with speech,</u> ❷ <u>loss of motion on one side of the body,</u> ❸ and <u>severe involuntary muscle contractions.</u> ❹
Past History:	Patient is married and nulliparous. Has been well prior to current symptoms.
Signs and Symptoms:	Her husband reports he first noted loss of motion on one side of the body when she began to drag her left foot. It has progressed to involve both left upper and lower extremities, with approximately a 50% loss in control of left lower extremity and a 25% loss of control in left upper extremity. Difficulty with speech is mild and mainly with recalling the names of common objects. Severe involuntary muscle contractions appear to be triggered by stress and last approximately 2 minutes. Results of a <u>recording of the electrical activity of the brain</u> ❺ and a <u>puncture with a needle into the low back to withdraw fluid for examination</u> ❻ were normal. However, an <u>injection with radioactive isotopes</u> ❼ revealed the presence of a mass in the right <u>outer layer of the largest section of the brain.</u> ❽
Diagnosis:	<u>Astrocyte tumor</u> ❾ in the right <u>outer layer of the largest section of the brain.</u> ❽
Treatment:	A right <u>skull incision</u> ❿ was performed to permit <u>the surgical use of extreme cold</u> ⓫ to destroy the tumor. Patient experienced moderate improvement in <u>loss of motion on one side of the body</u> ❸ and <u>severe involuntary muscle contractions,</u> ❹ but <u>difficulty with speech</u> ❷ was unchanged.

❶ _____

❷ _____

❸ _____

❹ _____

❺ _____

❻ _____

❼ _____

❽ _____

❾ _____

❿ _____

⓫ _____

Case Study

Below is a case study presentation of a patient with a condition covered in this chapter. Read the case study and answer the questions below. Some questions will ask for information not included within this chapter. Use your text, a medical dictionary, or any other reference material you choose to answer these questions.

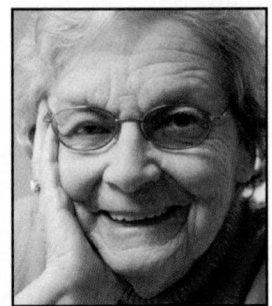

Anna Moore, an 83-year-old female, is admitted to the ER with aphasia, hemiparesis on her left side, syncope, and delirium. Her daughter called the ambulance after discovering her mother in this condition at home. Mrs. Moore has a history of hypertension, atherosclerosis, and diabetes mellitus. She was admitted to the hospital after a brain scan revealed an infarct in the right cerebral hemisphere leading to a diagnosis of CVA of the middle cerebral artery.

(iofoto/Shutterstock)

1. What pathological condition does Ms. Moore have? Look this condition up in a reference source and include a short description of it.

_____

_____

2. List and define each of the patient's presenting symptoms in the ER.

_____

_____

3. The patient has a history of three significant conditions. Describe each in your own words.

_____

_____

4. What diagnostic test did the physician perform? Describe this test and the results in your own words.

_____

_____

5. What is an infarct and what causes it?

_____

_____

6. List and describe the four common causes of a CVA.

_____

_____

Practice Exercises

A. Complete the Statement

1. The study of the nervous system is called _____.

2. The organs of the nervous system are the _____, _____, and _____.

3. The two divisions of the nervous system are the _____ and _____.

4. The neurons that carry impulses away from the brain and spinal cord are called _____ neurons.

5. The neurons that carry impulses to the brain and spinal cord are called _____ neurons.

6. The largest portion of the brain is the _____.

7. The second largest portion of the brain is the _____.

8. The occipital lobe controls _____.

9. The temporal lobe controls _____ and _____.

10. The two divisions of the autonomic nervous system are the _____ and _____.

B. Terminology Matching

Match each term to its definition.

1. _____ olfactory

2. _____ optic

3. _____ oculomotor

4. _____ trochlear

5. _____ trigeminal

6. _____ abducens

7. _____ facial

8. _____ vestibulocochlear

9. _____ glossopharyngeal

10. _____ vagus

11. _____ accessory

12. _____ hypoglossal

a. carries facial sensory impulses

b. turns eye to side

c. controls tongue muscles

d. controls eye muscles and pupils

e. swallowing

f. controls facial muscles

g. controls oblique eye muscles

h. smell

i. controls neck and shoulder muscles

j. hearing and equilibrium

k. vision

l. organs in lower body cavities

C. Combining Form Practice

The combining form **neur/o** refers to the nerve. Use it to write a term that means:

1. inflammation of the nerve _____

2. specialist in nerves _____

3. pain in the nerve _____

4. inflammation of many nerves _____

5. removal of a nerve _____

6. surgical repair of a nerve _____

7. nerve tumor _____

8. suture of a nerve _____

The combining form **mening/o** refers to the meninges or membranes. Use it to write a term that means:

9. inflammation of the meninges _____

10. protrusion of the meninges _____

11. protrusion of the spinal cord and the meninges _____

The combining form **encephal/o** refers to the brain. Use it to write a term that means:

12. X-ray record of the brain _____

13. disease of the brain _____

14. inflammation of the brain _____

15. protrusion of the brain _____

The combining form **cerebr/o** refers to the cerebrum. Use it to write a term that means:

16. pertaining to the cerebrum and spinal cord _____

17. pertaining to the cerebrum _____

D. What Does it Stand For?

1. TIA _____

2. MS _____

3. SCI _____

4. CNS _____

5. PNS _____

6. HA _____

7. CP _____

8. LP _____

9. ALS _____

E. Terminology Matching

Match each term to its definition.

1. _____ aura   a. loss of ability to control movement

2. _____ meningitis   b. sensations before a seizure

3. _____ coma   c. seizure with convulsions

4. _____ shingles   d. congenital hernia of meninges

5. _____ syncope   e. seizure without convulsion

6. _____ palsy   f. inflammation of meninges

7. _____ absence seizure   g. profound unconsciousness

8. _____ tonic-clonic seizure   h. *Herpes zoster* infection

9. _____ meningocele   i. fainting

F. What's the Abbreviation?

1. cerebrospinal fluid _____

2. cerebrovascular disease _____

3. electroencephalogram _____

4. intracranial pressure _____

5. positron emission tomography _____

6. cerebrovascular accident _____

7. subarachnoid hemorrhage _____

8. autonomic nervous system _____

G. Define the Procedures and Tests

1. myelography _____

2. cerebral angiography _____

3. Babinski's reflex _____

4. nerve conduction velocity _____

5. cerebrospinal fluid analysis _____

6. PET scan _____

7. echoencephalography _____

8. lumbar puncture _____

H. Define the Suffix

	Definition	Example from Chapter
1. -plegia		
2. -taxia		
3. -trophic		
4. -paresis		
5. -phasia		

I. Define the Combining Form

	Definition	Example from Chapter Term
1. mening/o		
2. encephal/o		
3. cerebell/o		
4. myel/o		
5. cephal/o		
6. thalam/o		
7. neur/o		
8. radicul/o		
9. cerebr/o		
10. pont/o		

J. Define the Term

1. astrocytoma _____

2. epilepsy _____

3. anesthesia _____

4. hemiparesis _____

5. neurosurgeon _____

6. analgesia _____

7. focal seizure _____

8. quadriplegia _____

9. subdural hematoma _____

10. intrathecal _____

K. Terminology Matching

Match each term to its definition.

1. _____ neurologist   a. sudden attack

2. _____ cerebrovascular accident   b. a type of severe headache

3. _____ concussion   c. loss of intellectual ability

4. _____ aphasia   d. physician who treats nervous problem

5. _____ migraine   e. stroke

6. _____ seizure   f. mild traumatic brain injury

7. _____ dementia   g. loss of ability to speak

8. _____ ataxia   h. congenital anomaly

9. _____ spina bifida   i. state of being unaware

10. _____ unconscious   j. lack of muscle coordination

L. Fill in the Blank

Parkinson's disease	transient ischemic attack	cerebral palsy	cerebrospinal fluid shunt
Bell's palsy	subdural hematoma	amyotrophic lateral sclerosis	nerve conduction velocity
delirium	cerebral aneurysm		

1. Dr. Martin noted that the 96-year-old patient suffered from _____ when she determined that he was confused, disoriented, and agitated.

2. Lucinda's _____ resulted in increasing muscle weakness as the motor neurons in her spinal cord degenerated.

3. The diagnosis of _____ was correct because the weakness affected only one side of Charles's face.

4. A cerebral angiogram was ordered because Dr. Larson suspected Mrs. Constantine had a(n) _____.

5. Roberta's symptoms included fine tremors, muscular weakness, rigidity, and a shuffling gait, leading to a diagnosis of _____.

6. Matthew's hydrocephalus required the placement of a(n) _____.

7. Because Mae's hemiparesis was temporary, the final diagnosis was _____.

8. Following the car accident, a CT scan showed a(n) _____ was putting pressure on the brain, necessitating immediate neurosurgery.

9. Birth trauma resulted in the newborn developing _____.

10. A(n) _____ test was performed in order to pinpoint the exact position of the nerve damage.

M. Pharmacology Challenge

Fill in the classification for each drug description, then match the brand name.

Drug Description	Classification	Brand Name
1. _____ produces loss of sensation	_____	a. L-Dopa
2. _____ treats Parkinson's disease	_____	b. Amytal
3. _____ promotes sleep	_____	c. OxyContin
4. _____ medication for mild pain	_____	d. Seconal
5. _____ produces a calming effect	_____	e. Xylocaine
6. _____ treats severe pain	_____	f. Tegretol
7. _____ treats seizures	_____	g. Motrin

Labeling Exercise

Image A

Write the labels for this figure on the numbered lines provided.

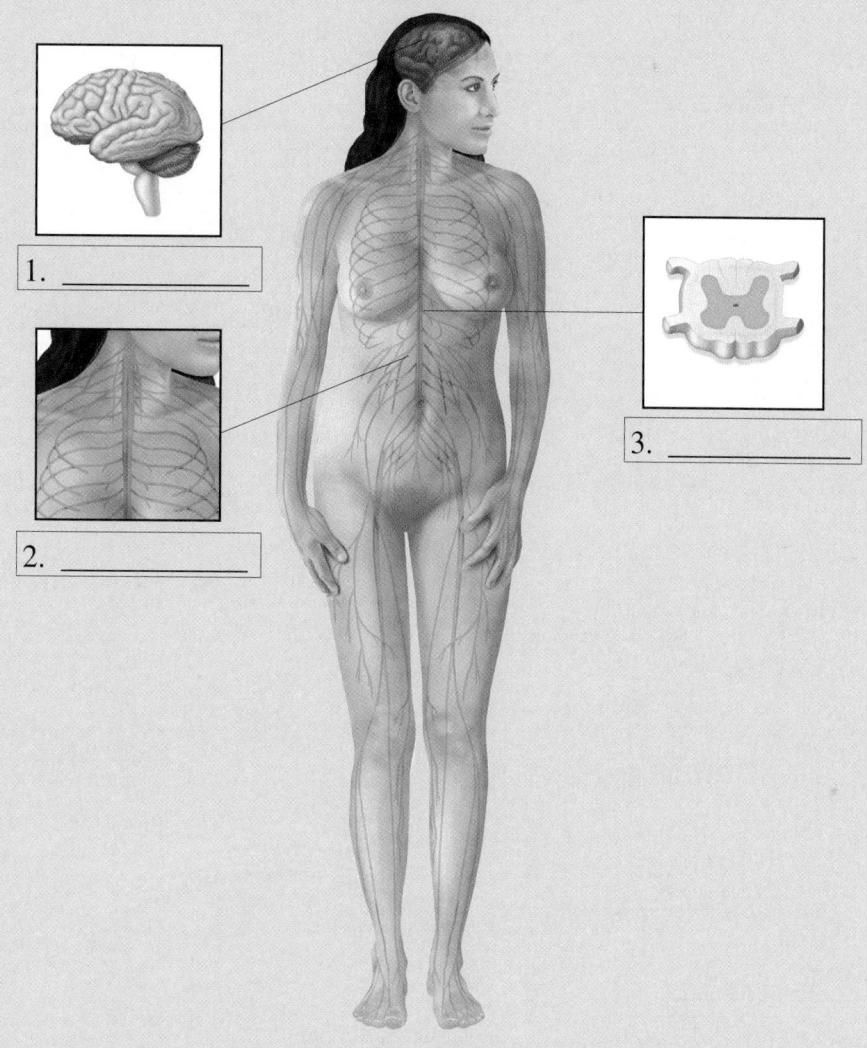

1. _____

2. _____

3. _____

MEDICAL TERMINOLOGY INTERACTIVE

Medical Terminology Interactive is a premium online homework management system that includes a host of features to help you study. Registered users will find:

- Fun games and activities built within a virtual hospital
- Powerful tools that track and analyze your results—allowing you to create a personalized learning experience
- Videos, flashcards, and audio pronunciations to help enrich your progress
- Streaming video lesson presentations and self-paced learning modules

www.pearsonhighered.com/mti

Image B

Write the labels for this figure on the numbered lines provided.

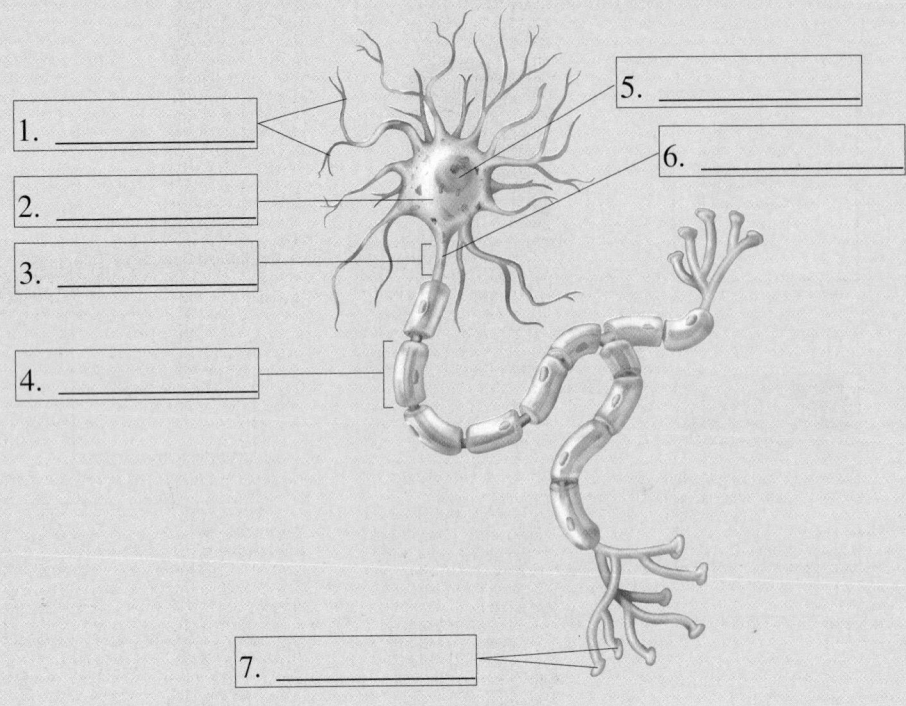

1. _____

2. _____

3. _____

4. _____

5. _____

6. _____

7. _____

Image C

Write the labels for this figure on the numbered lines provided.

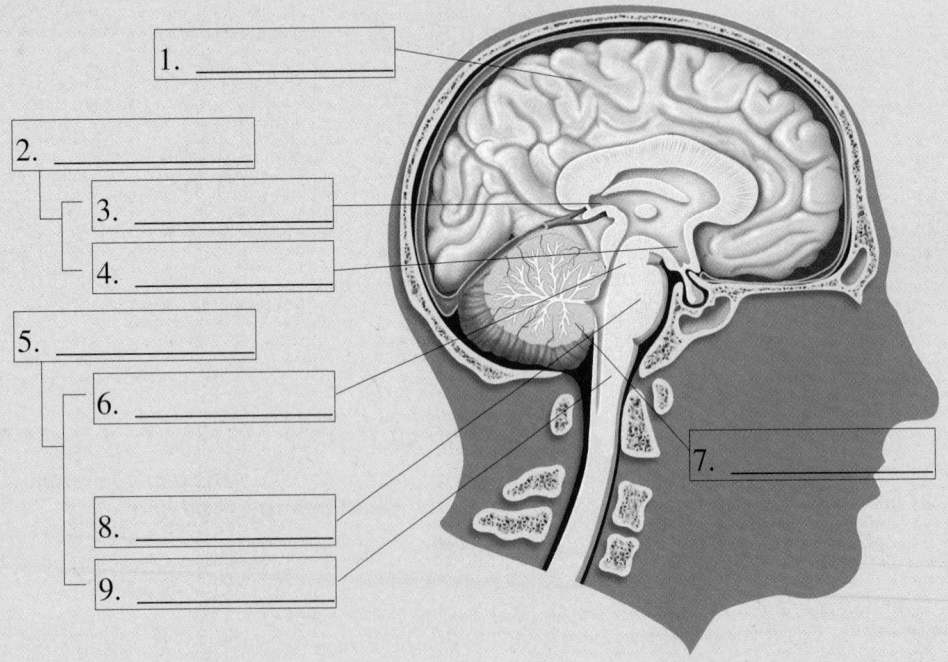

1. _____

2. _____

3. _____

4. _____

5. _____

6. _____

7. _____

8. _____

9. _____

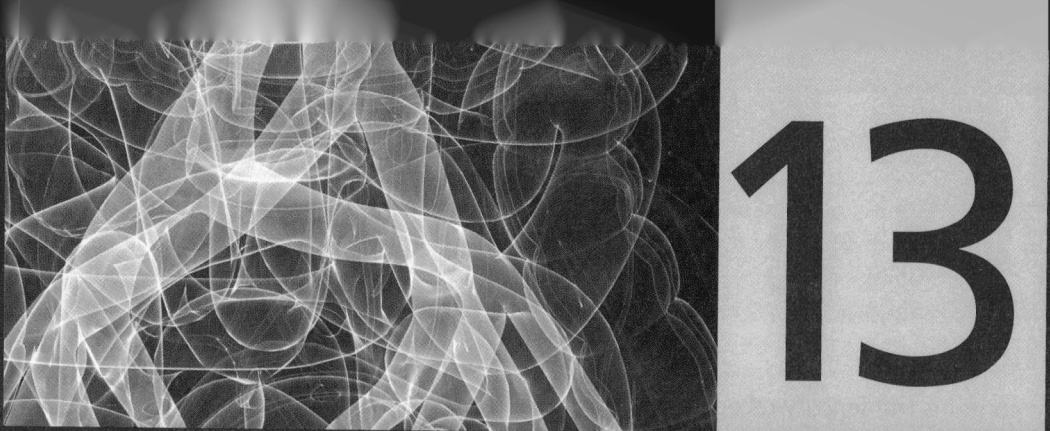

13

Learning Objectives

Upon completion of this chapter, you will be able to

- Identify and define the combining forms and suffixes introduced in this chapter.

- Correctly spell and pronounce medical terms and major anatomical structures relating to the eye and ear.

- Locate and describe the major structures of the eye and ear and their functions.

- Describe how we see.

- Describe the path of sound vibration.

- Identify and define eye and ear anatomical terms.

- Identify and define selected eye and ear pathology terms.

- Identify and define selected eye and ear diagnostic procedures.

- Identify and define selected eye and ear therapeutic procedures.

- Identify and define selected medications relating to the eye and ear.

- Define selected abbreviations associated with the eye and ear.

SPECIAL SENSES: THE EYE AND EAR

Section I: The Eye at a Glance

Function

The eye contains the sensory receptor cells for vision.

Structures

Here are the primary structures that comprise the eye.

choroid	eyelids
conjunctiva	lacrimal apparatus
eye muscles	retina
eyeball	sclera

Word Parts

Here are the most common word parts (with their meanings) used to build eye terms. For a more comprehensive list, refer to the Terminology section of this chapter.

Combining Forms

ambly/o	dull, dim	mi/o	lessening
aque/o	water	mydr/i	widening
blast/o	immature, embryonic	nyctal/o	night
blephar/o	eyelid	ocul/o	eye
chromat/o	color	ophthalm/o	eye
conjunctiv/o	conjunctiva	opt/o	eye, vision
corne/o	cornea	optic/o	eye, vision
cycl/o	ciliary muscle	papill/o	optic disk
dacry/o	tear, tear duct	phac/o	lens
dipl/o	double	phot/o	light
emmetr/o	correct, proper	presby/o	old age
glauc/o	gray	pupill/o	pupil
ir/o	iris	retin/o	retina
irid/o	iris	scler/o	sclera
kerat/o	cornea	stigmat/o	point
lacrim/o	tears	uve/o	choroid
macul/o	macula lutea	vitre/o	glassy

Suffixes

-ician	specialist	-opsia	vision condition
-metrist	specialist in measuring	-tropia	turned condition
-opia	vision condition		

The Eye Illustrated

retina, p. 449
contains sensory
receptors for sight

cornea, p. 448
admits light rays
into the eyeball

iris and pupil, p. 449
regulate amount of
light entering the
eyeball l

lens, p. 449
focuses light rays
onto the retina

choroid layer, p. 449
supplies blood to
eye structures

sclera, p. 448
tough, protective
outer layer of eyeball

Anatomy and Physiology of the Eye

conjunctiva (kon-JUNK-tih-vah)	**lacrimal apparatus** (LAK-rim-al)
eye muscles	**ophthalmology** (off-thal-MALL-oh-gee)
eyeball	**optic nerve** (OP-tik)
eyelids	

The study of the eye is known as **ophthalmology** (Ophth). The **eyeball** is the incredible organ of sight that transmits an external image by way of the nervous system—the **optic nerve**—to the brain. The brain then translates these sensory impulses into an image with computerlike accuracy.

In addition to the eyeball, several external structures play a role in vision. These are the **eye muscles, eyelids, conjunctiva,** and **lacrimal apparatus.**

The Eyeball

choroid (KOR-oyd)	**retina** (RET-in-ah)
sclera (SKLAIR-ah)	

The actual eyeball is composed of three layers: the **sclera,** the **choroid,** and the **retina.**

Sclera

cornea (COR-nee-ah)	**refracts**

The outer layer, the sclera, provides a tough protective coating for the inner structures of the eye. Another term for the sclera is the white of the eye.

The anterior portion of the sclera is called the **cornea** (see Figure 13.1 ■). This clear, transparent area of the sclera allows light to enter the interior of the eyeball. The cornea actually bends, or **refracts,** the light rays.

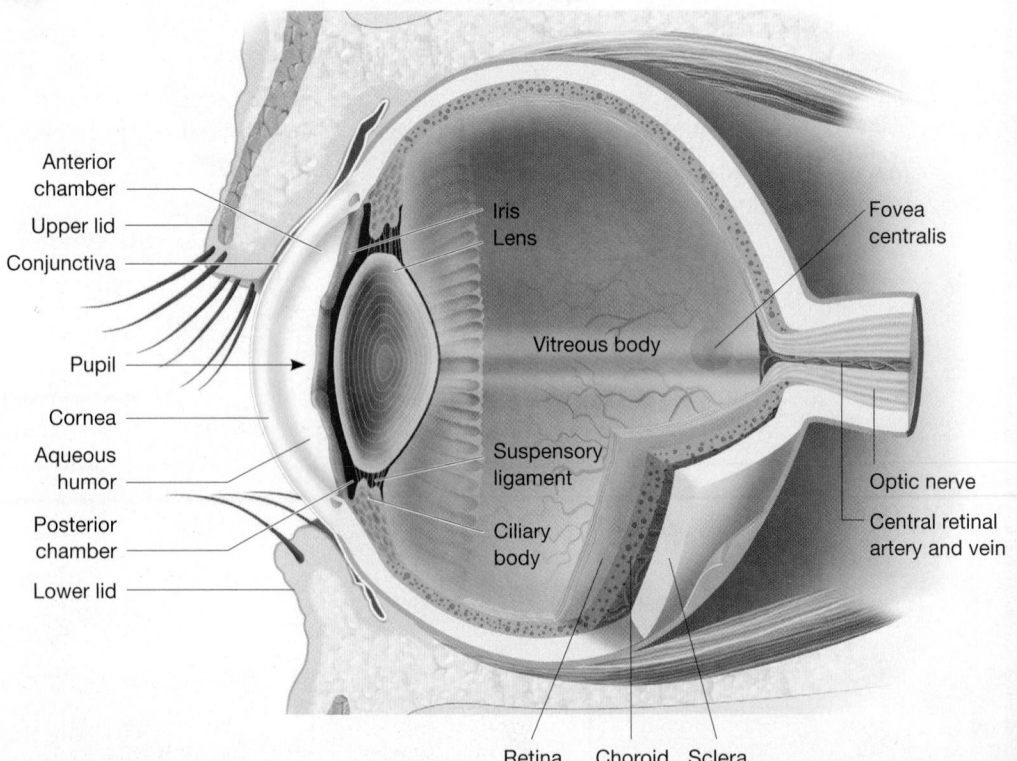

■ Figure 13.1
The internal structures of the eye.

Choroid

ciliary body (SIL-ee-ar-ee)   **iris**
lens   **pupil**

The second or middle layer of the eyeball is called the choroid. This opaque layer provides the blood supply for the eye.

    The anterior portion of the choroid layer consists of the **iris, pupil,** and **ciliary body** (see again Figure 13.1). The iris is the colored portion of the eye and contains smooth muscle. The pupil is the opening in the center of the iris that allows light rays to enter the eyeball. The iris muscle contracts or relaxes to change the size of the pupil, thereby controlling how much light enters the interior of the eyeball. Behind the iris is the **lens.** The lens is not actually part of the choroid layer, but it is attached to the muscular ciliary body. By pulling on the edge of the lens, these muscles change the shape of the lens so it can focus incoming light onto the retina.

> **MED TERM TIP**
>
> The function of the choroid, to provide the rest of the eyeball with blood, is responsible for an alternate name for this layer—*uvea.* The combining form *uve/o* means "vascular."

Retina

aqueous humor (AY-kwee-us)   **optic disk**
cones   **retinal blood vessels** (RET-in-al)
fovea centralis (FOH-vee-ah / sen-TRAH-lis) **rods**
macula lutea (MAK-yoo-lah / loo-TEE-ah)   **vitreous humor** (VIT-ree-us)

The third and innermost layer of the eyeball is the retina. It contains the sensory receptor cells (**rods** and **cones**) that respond to light rays. Rods are active in dim light and help us to see in gray tones. Cones are active only in bright light and are responsible for color vision. When the lens projects an image onto the retina, it strikes an area called the **macula lutea,** or yellow spot (see Figure 13.1). In the center of the macula lutea is a depression called the **fovea centralis,** meaning central pit. This pit contains a high concentration of sensory receptor cells and, therefore, is the point of clearest vision. Also visible on the retina is the **optic disk.** This is the point where the **retinal blood vessels** enter and exit the eyeball and where the optic nerve leaves the eyeball (see Figure 13.2 ■). There are no sensory receptor cells in the optic disk and therefore it causes a blind spot in each eye's field of vision. The interior spaces of the eyeball are not empty. The spaces between the cornea and lens are filled with **aqueous humor,** a watery fluid, and the large open area between the lens and retina contains **vitreous humor,** a semisolid gel.

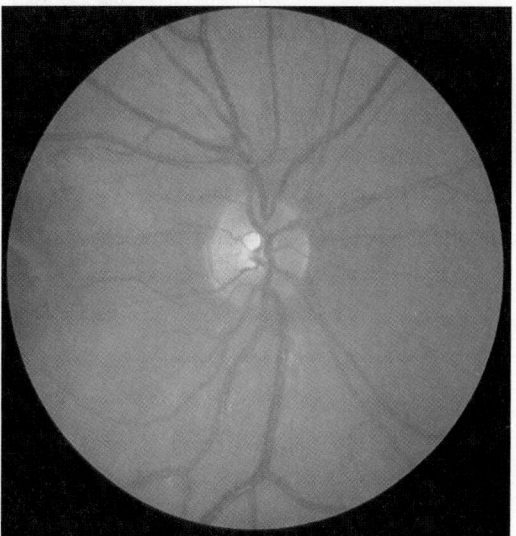

■ **Figure 13.2**
Photograph of the retina of the eye. The optic disk appears yellow and the retinal arteries radiate out from it.
(Photo Researchers, Inc.)

Muscles of the Eye

oblique muscles (oh-BLEEK)   **rectus muscles** (REK-tus)

Six muscles connect the actual eyeball to the skull (see Figure 13.3 ■). These muscles allow for change in the direction of each eye's sightline. In addition, they provide support for the eyeball in the eye socket. Children may be born with a weakness in some of these muscles and may require treatments such as eye exercises or even surgery to correct this problem commonly referred to as crossed eyes or *strabismus* (see Figure 13.4 ■). The muscles involved are the four **rectus** and two **oblique muscles.** Rectus muscles (meaning straight) pull the eye up, down, left, or right in a straight line. Oblique muscles are on an angle and produce diagonal eye movement.

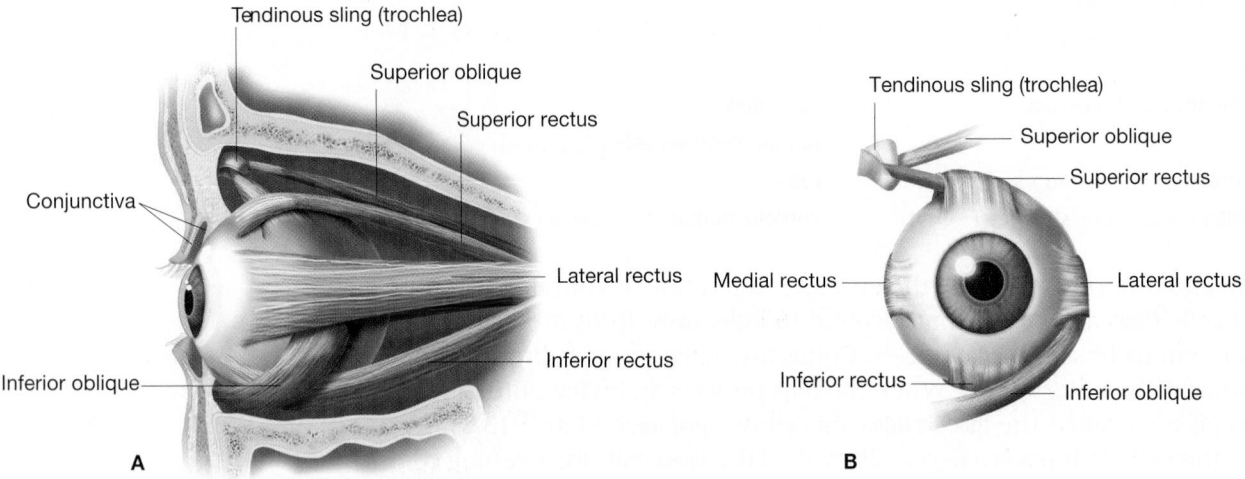

■ **Figure 13.3**   The arrangement of the external eye muscles: (A) lateral and (B) anterior views.

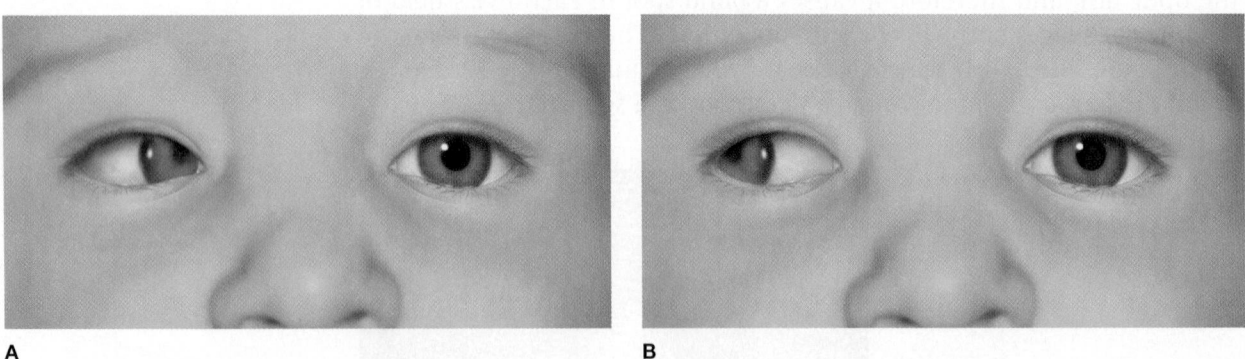

■ **Figure 13.4**   Examples of common forms of strabismus: (A) esotropia with the right eye turning inward and (B) exotropia with the right eye turning outward.

The Eyelids

cilia (SIL-ee-ah)　　　　　　　　　　　　　**eyelashes**
sebaceous glands (see-BAY-shus)

A pair of eyelids over each eyeball provides protection from foreign particles, injury from the sun and intense light, and trauma (see Figure 13.1). Both the upper and lower edges of the eyelids have **eyelashes** or **cilia** that protect the eye from foreign particles. In addition, **sebaceous glands** located in the eyelids secrete lubricating oil onto the eyeball.

Conjunctiva

mucous membrane

The conjunctiva of the eye is a **mucous membrane** lining. It forms a continuous covering on the underside of each eyelid and across the anterior surface of each eyeball (see again Figure 13.1). This serves as protection for the eye by sealing off the eyeball in the socket.

Lacrimal Apparatus

lacrimal ducts　　　　　　　　　　　　**lacrimal gland**
nasal cavity　　　　　　　　　　　　　　**nasolacrimal duct** (naz-oh-LAK-rim-al)
tears

The **lacrimal gland** is located under the outer upper corner of each eyelid. These glands produce **tears.** Tears serve the important function of washing and lubricating the anterior surface of the eyeball. **Lacrimal ducts** located in the inner corner of the eye socket then collect the tears and drain them into the **nasolacrimal duct.** This duct ultimately drains the tears into the **nasal cavity** (see Figure 13.5 ■).

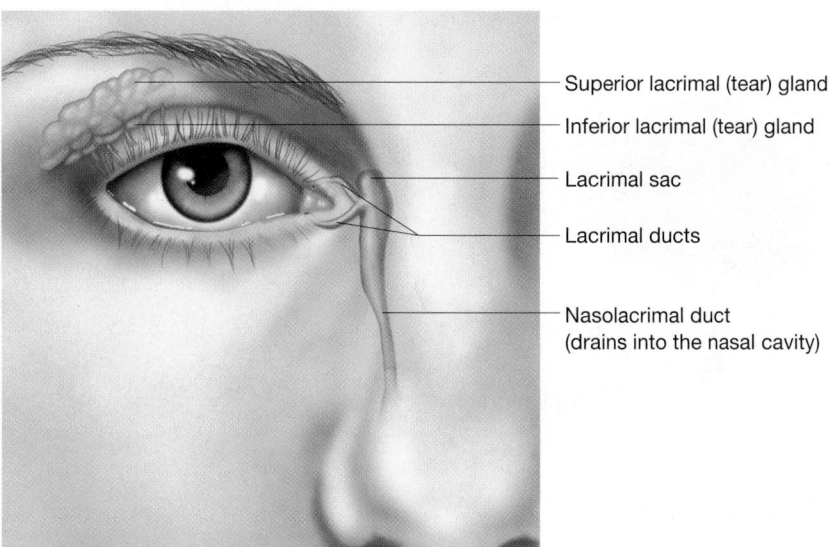

　　　　　　　— Superior lacrimal (tear) gland
　　　　　　　— Inferior lacrimal (tear) gland
　　　　　　　— Lacrimal sac
　　　　　　　— Lacrimal ducts
　　　　　　　— Nasolacrimal duct
　　　　　　　　(drains into the nasal cavity)

■ **Figure 13.5**
The structure of the lacrimal apparatus.

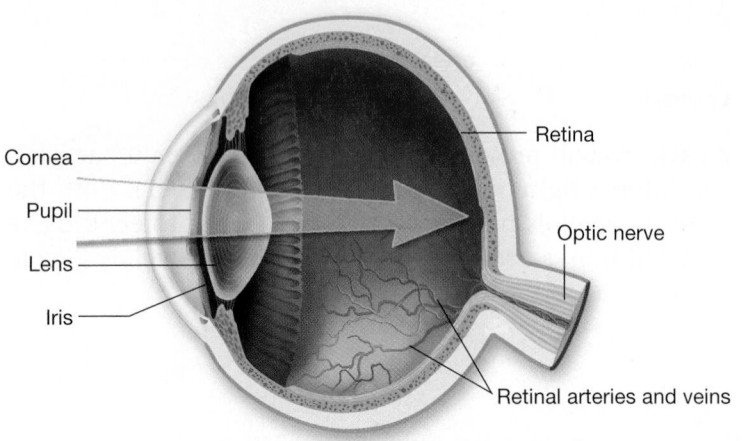

■ **Figure 13.6** The path of light through the cornea, iris, lens, and striking the retina.

How We See

When light rays strike the eye, they first pass through the cornea, pupil, aqueous humor, lens, and vitreous humor (see Figure 13.6 ■). They then strike the retina and stimulate the rods and cones. When the light rays hit the retina, an upside-down image is sent along nerve impulses to the optic nerve (see Figure 13.7 ■). The optic nerve transmits these impulses to the brain, where the upside-down image is translated into the right-side-up image we are looking at.

Vision requires proper functioning of four mechanisms:

1. Coordination of the external eye muscles so that both eyes move together.
2. The correct amount of light admitted by the pupil.
3. The correct focus of light on the retina by the lens.
4. The optic nerve transmitting sensory images to the brain.

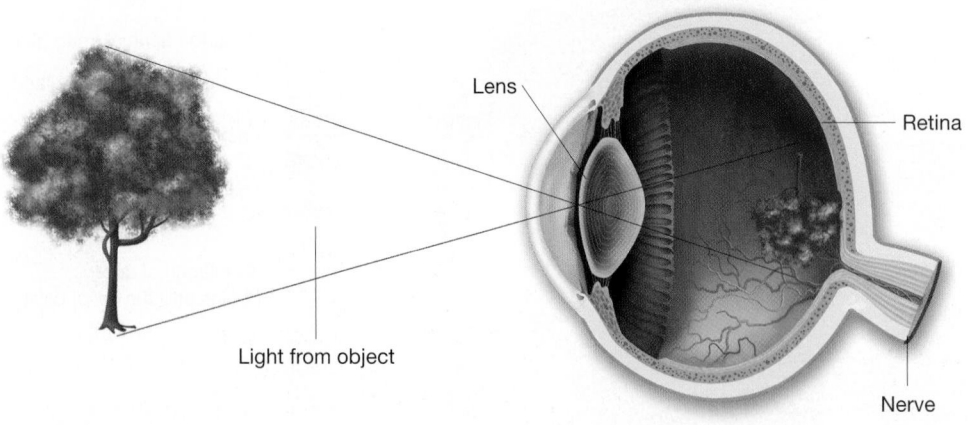

■ **Figure 13.7** The image formed on the retina is inverted. The brain rights the image as part of the interpretation process.

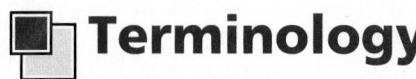 Terminology

Word Parts Used to Build Eye Terms

The following lists contain the combining forms, suffixes, and prefixes used to build terms in the remaining sections of this chapter.

Combining Forms

aden/o	gland	**emmetr/o**	correct, proper	**optic/o**	eye, vision
ambly/o	dull, dim	**esthes/o**	sensation, feeling	**papill/o**	optic disc
angi/o	vessel	**glauc/o**	gray	**phac/o**	lens
aque/o	water	**ir/o**	iris	**phot/o**	light
bi/o	life	**irid/o**	iris	**presby/o**	old age
blast/o	immature, embryonic	**kerat/o**	cornea	**pupill/o**	pupil
blephar/o	eyelid	**lacrim/o**	tears	**retin/o**	retina
chromat/o	color	**macul/o**	macula lutea	**scler/o**	sclera
conjuctiv/o	conjunctiva	**mi/o**	lessening	**stigmat/o**	point
corne/o	cornea	**myc/o**	fungus	**ton/o**	tone
cry/o	cold	**mydr/i**	widening	**uve/o**	choroid
cycl/o	ciliary body	**nyctal/o**	night	**vitre/o**	glassy
cyst/o	sac	**ocul/o**	eye	**xer/o**	dry
dacry/o	tears	**ophthalm/o**	eye		
dipl/o	double	**opt/o**	eye, vision		

Suffixes

-al	pertaining to	**-logist**	one who studies	**-pathy**	disease
-algia	pain	**-logy**	study of	**-pexy**	surgical fixation
-ar	pertaining to	**-malacia**	softening	**-phobia**	fear
-ary	pertaining to	**-meter**	instrument to measure	**-plasty**	surgical repair
-atic	pertaining to	**-metrist**	specialist in measuring	**-plegia**	paralysis
-ectomy	surgical removal			**-ptosis**	drooping
-edema	swelling	**-metry**	process of measuring	**-rrhagia**	abnormal flow condition
-graphy	process of recording	**-oma**	tumor		
-ia	condition	**-opia**	vision condition	**-scope**	instrument for viewing
-ic	pertaining to	**-opsia**	vision condition		
-ician	specialist	**-osis**	abnormal condition	**-scopy**	process of visually examining
-ism	state of	**-otomy**	cutting into	**-tic**	pertaining to
-itis	inflammation	**-ous**	pertaining to	**-tropia**	turned condition

Prefixes

a-	without		exo-	outward		intra-	within
an-	without		extra-	outside of		micro-	small
anti-	against		hemi-	half		mono-	one
de-	without		hyper-	excessive		myo-	to shut
eso-	inward						

Anatomical Terms

TERM	WORD PARTS	DEFINITION
aqueous (AK-wee-us)	aque/o = water -ous = pertaining to	Pertaining to water or being water-like.
conjunctival (kon-JUNK-tih-vall)	conjuctiv/o = conjunctiva -al = pertaining to	Pertaining to the conjunctiva.
corneal (KOR-nee-all)	corne/o = cornea -al = pertaining to	Pertaining to the cornea. **MED TERM TIP** Word Watch: Be careful using the combining forms *core/o* meaning "pupil" and *corne/o* meaning "cornea."
extraocular (EKS-truh-OK-yoo-lar)	extra- = outside of ocul/o = eye -ar = pertaining to	Pertaining to being outside the eyeball; for example, the extraocular eye muscles.
iridal (ir-id-al)	irid/o = iris -al = pertaining to	Pertaining to the iris.
lacrimal (LAK-rim-al)	lacrim/o = tears -al = pertaining to	Pertaining to tears.
macular (MACK-uoo-lar)	macul/o = macula lutea -ar = pertaining to	Pertaining to the macula lutea.
ocular (OCK-yoo-lar)	ocul/o = eye -ar = pertaining to	Pertaining to the eye.
intraocular (in-trah-OCK-yoo-lar)	intra- = within ocul/o = eye -ar = pertaining to	Pertaining to within the eye.
ophthalmic (off-THAL-mik)	ophthalm/o = eye -ic = pertaining to	Pertaining to the eye.
optic (OP-tik)	opt/o = eye, vision -ic = pertaining to	Pertaining to the eye or vision.
optical (OP-tih-kal)	optic/o = eye, vision -al = pertaining to	Pertaining to the eye or vision.
pupillary (PYOO-pih-lair-ee)	pupill/o = pupil -ary = pertaining to	Pertaining to the pupil.
retinal (RET-in-al)	retin/o = retina -al = pertaining to	Pertaining to the retina.
scleral (SKLAIR-all)	scler/o = sclera -al = pertaining to	Pertaining to the sclera.
uveal (YOO-vee-al)	uve/o = choroid -al = pertaining to	Pertaining to the choroid layer of the eye.
vitreous (VIT-ree-us)	vitre/o = glass -ous = pertaining to	Pertaining to the vitreous humor.

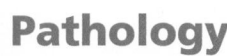 # Pathology

TERM	WORD PARTS	DEFINITION
Medical Specialties		
ophthalmologist (opf-thal-MOLL-oh-jist)	ophthalm/o = eye -logist = one who studies	Medical doctor who has specialized in the diagnosis and treatment of eye conditions and diseases.
ophthalmology (opf-thal-MOLL-oh-jee)	ophthalm/o = eye -logy = study of	Branch of medicine involving the diagnosis and treatment of conditions and diseases of the eye and surrounding structures.
optician (op-TISH-an)	opt/o = vision -ician = specialist	Person trained in grinding and fitting corrective lenses.
optometrist (op-TOM-eh-trist)	opt/o = vision -metrist = specialist in measuring	Doctor of optometry.
optometry (op-TOM-eh-tree)	opt/o = vision -metry = process of measuring	Medical profession specializing in examining the eyes, testing visual acuity, and prescribing corrective lenses.
Signs and Symptoms		
blepharoptosis (blef-ah-rop-TOH-sis)	blephar/o = eyelid -ptosis = drooping	Drooping eyelid.
cycloplegia (sigh-kloh-PLEE-jee-ah)	cycl/o = ciliary body -plegia = paralysis	Paralysis of the ciliary body. This affects changing the shape of the lens to bring images into focus.
diplopia (dip-LOH-pee-ah)	dipl/o = double -opia = vision condition	Condition of seeing double.
emmetropia (EM) (em-eh-TROH-pee-ah)	emmetr/o = correct, proper -opia = vision condition	State of normal vision.
iridoplegia (ir-id-oh-PLEE-jee-ah)	irid/o = iris -plegia = paralysis	Paralysis of the iris. This affects changing the size of the pupil to regulate the amount of light entering the eye.
nyctalopia (nik-tah-LOH-pee-ah)	nyctal/o = night -opia = vision condition	Difficulty seeing in dim light; also called *night-blindness*. Usually due to damaged rods.

> **MED TERM TIP**
> The simple translation of *nyctalopia* is "night vision." However, it is used to mean "night blindness."

TERM	WORD PARTS	DEFINITION
ophthalmalgia (off-thal-MAL-jee-ah)	ophthalm/o = eye -algia = pain	Eye pain.
ophthalmoplegia (off-thal-moh-PLEE-jee-ah)	ophthalm/o = eye -plegia = paralysis	Paralysis of one or more of the extraocular eye muscles.
ophthalmorrhagia (off-thal-moh-RAH-jee-ah)	ophthalm/o = eye -rrhagia = abnormal flow condition	Bleeding from the eye.
papilledema (pah-pill-eh-DEEM-ah)	papill/o = optic disc -edema = swelling	Swelling of the optic disk. Often as a result of increased intraocular pressure. Also called *choked disk*.

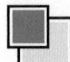 **Pathology** *(continued)*

TERM	WORD PARTS	DEFINITION
photophobia (foh-toh-FOH-bee-ah)	phot/o = light -phobia = fear	Although the term translates into *fear of light,* it actually means a strong sensitivity to bright light.
presbyopia (prez-bee-OH-pee-ah)	presby/o = old age -opia = vision condition	Visual loss due to old age, resulting in difficulty in focusing for near vision (such as reading).
scleromalacia (sklair-oh-mah-LAY-she-ah)	scler/o = sclera -malacia = softening	Softening of the sclera.
xerophthalmia (zee-ROP-thal-mee-ah)	xer/o = dry ophthalm/o = eye -ia = condition	Dry eyes.

Eyeball

TERM	WORD PARTS	DEFINITION
achromatopsia (ah-kroh-mah-TOP-see-ah)	a- = without chromat/o = color -opsia = vision condition	Condition of color blindness—unable to perceive one or more colors; more common in males.
amblyopia (am-blee-OH-pee-ah)	ambly/o = dull, dim -opia = vision condition	Loss of vision not as a result of eye pathology. Usually occurs in patients who see two images. In order to see only one image, the brain will no longer recognize the image being sent to it by one of the eyes. May occur if strabismus is not corrected. This condition is not treatable with a prescription lens. Commonly referred to as *lazy eye.*
astigmatism (Astigm) (ah-STIG-mah-tizm)	a- = without stigmat/o = point -ism = state of	Condition in which light rays are focused unevenly on the retina, causing a distorted image, due to an abnormal curvature of the cornea.
cataract (KAT-ah-rakt)		Damage to the lens causing it to become opaque or cloudy, resulting in diminished vision. Treatment is usually surgical removal of the cataract or replacement of the lens.

MED TERM TIP

The term *cataract* comes from the Latin word meaning "waterfall." This refers to how a person with a cataract sees the world—as if looking through a waterfall.

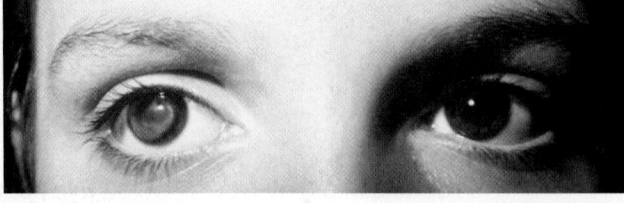

■ **Figure 13.8** Photograph of a person with a cataract in the right eye.

TERM	WORD PARTS	DEFINITION
corneal abrasion	corne/o = cornea -al = pertaining to	Scraping injury to the cornea. If it does not heal, it may develop into an ulcer.
glaucoma (glau-KOH-mah)	glauc/o = gray -oma = mass	Increase in intraocular pressure, which, if untreated, may result in atrophy (wasting away) of the optic nerve and blindness. Glaucoma is treated with medication and surgery. There is an increased risk of developing glaucoma in persons over age 60, of African ancestry, who have sustained a serious eye injury, and in anyone with a family history of diabetes or glaucoma.

Pathology *(continued)*

TERM	WORD PARTS	DEFINITION
hyperopia (high-per-OH-pee-ah)	hyper- = excessive -opia = vision condition	With this condition a person can see things in the distance but has trouble reading material at close range. Also known as *far-sightedness.* This condition is corrected with converging or biconvex lenses.

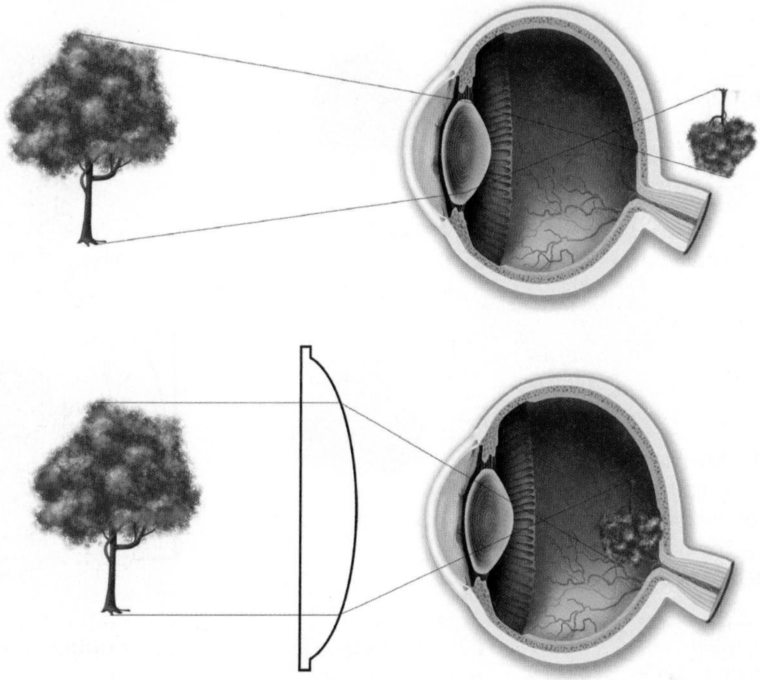

Hyperopia (farsightedness)

Corrected with biconvex lens

■ **Figure 13.9** Hyperopia (farsightedness). In the uncorrected top figure, the image would come into focus behind the retina, making the image on the retina blurry. The bottom image shows how a biconvex lens corrects this condition.

TERM	WORD PARTS	DEFINITION
iritis (eye-RYE-tis)	ir/o = iris -itis = inflammation	Inflammation of the iris.
keratitis (kair-ah-TYE-tis)	kerat/o = cornea -itis = inflammation	Inflammation of the cornea. **MED TERM TIP** Word Watch: Be careful using the combining form *kerat/o,* which means both "cornea" and "hard protein keratin."
legally blind		Describes a person who has severely impaired vision. Usually defined as having visual acuity of 20/200 that cannot be improved with corrective lenses or having a visual field of less than 20 degrees.
macular degeneration (MAK-yoo-lar)	macul/o = macula lutea -ar = pertaining to	Deterioration of the macular area of the retina of the eye. May be treated with laser surgery to destroy the blood vessels beneath the macula.
monochromatism (mon-oh-KROH-mah-tizm)	mono- = one chromat/o = color -ism = state of	Unable to perceive one color.

Pathology *(continued)*

TERM	WORD PARTS	DEFINITION
myopia (MY) (my-OH-pee-ah)	myo- = to shut -opia = vision condition	With this condition a person can see things close up but distance vision is blurred. Also known as *nearsightedness.* This condition is corrected with diverging or biconcave lenses. Named because persons with myopia often partially shut their eyes, squint, in order to see better.

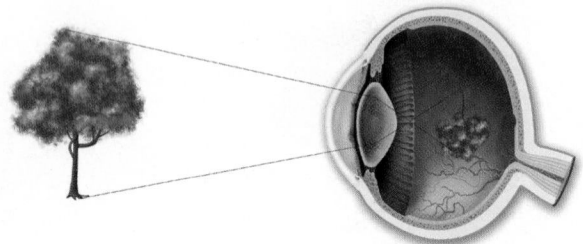

Myopia (nearsightedness)

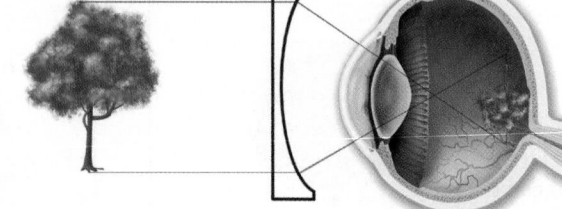

Corrected with biconcave lens

■ **Figure 13.10**   Myopia (nearsightedness). In the uncorrected top figure, the image comes into focus in front of the lens, making the image on the retina blurry. The bottom image shows how a biconcave lens corrects this condition.

TERM	WORD PARTS	DEFINITION
oculomycosis (ok-yoo-loh-my-KOH-sis)	ocul/o = eye myc/o = fungus -osis = abnormal condition	Fungus infection of the eye.
retinal detachment (RET-in-al)	retin/o = retina -al = pertaining to	Occurs when the retina becomes separated from the choroid layer. This separation seriously damages blood vessels and nerves, resulting in blindness. May be treated with surgical or medical procedures to stabilize the retina and prevent separation.
retinitis pigmentosa (ret-in-EYE-tis / pig-men-TOH-sah)	retin/o = retina -itis = inflammation	Progressive disease of the eye resulting in the retina becoming hard (sclerosed), pigmented (colored), and atrophying (wasting away). There is no known cure for this condition.
retinoblastoma (RET-in-noh-blast-OH-mah)	retin/o = retina blast/o = immature, embryonic -oma = tumor	Malignant eye tumor occurring in children, usually under the age of 3. Requires enucleation.
retinopathy (ret-in-OP-ah-thee)	retin/o = retina -pathy = disease	General term for disease affecting the retina.
scleritis (skler-EYE-tis)	scler/o = sclera -itis = inflammation	Inflammation of the sclera.

Pathology *(continued)*

TERM	WORD PARTS	DEFINITION
uveitis (yoo-vee-EYE-tis)	uve/o = choroid -itis = inflammation	Inflammation of the choroid layer.
Conjunctiva		
conjunctivitis (kon-junk-tih-VYE-tis)	conjuctiv/o = conjunctiva -itis = inflammation	Inflammation of the conjunctiva usually as the result of a bacterial infection. Commonly called pink eye.
pterygium (the-RIJ-ee-um)		Hypertrophied conjunctival tissue in the inner corner of the eye.
Eyelids		
blepharitis (blef-ah-RYE-tis)	blephar/o = eyelid -itis = inflammation	Inflammation of the eyelid.
hordeolum (hor-DEE-oh-lum)		Refers to a *stye* (or *sty*), a small purulent inflammatory infection of a sebaceous gland of the eyelid; treated with hot compresses and/or surgical incision.
Lacrimal Apparatus		
dacryoadenitis (dak-ree-oh-ad-eh-NYE-tis)	dacry/o = tears aden/o = gland -itis = inflammation	Inflammation of the lacrimal gland.
dacryocystitis (dak-ree-oh-sis-TYE-tis)	dacry/o = tears cyst/o = sac -itis = inflammation	Inflammation of the lacrimal sac.
Eye Muscles		
esotropia (ST) (ess-oh-TROH-pee-ah)	eso- = inward -tropia = turned condition	Inward turning of the eye; also called *cross-eyed.* An example of a form of strabismus (muscle weakness of the eye).
exotropia (XT) (eks-oh-TROH-pee-ah)	exo- = outward -tropia = turned condition	Outward turning of the eye; also called *wall-eyed.* Also an example of strabismus (muscle weakness of the eye).
strabismus (strah-BIZ-mus)		Eye muscle weakness commonly seen in children resulting in the eyes looking in different directions at the same time. May be corrected with glasses, eye exercises, and/or surgery.
Brain-Related Vision Pathologies		
hemianopia (hem-ee-ah-NOP-ee-ah)	hemi- = half a- = without -opia = vision condition	Loss of vision in half of the visual field. A stroke patient may suffer from this disorder.
nystagmus (niss-TAG-mus)		Jerky-appearing involuntary eye movements, usually left and right. Often an indication of brain injury.

Diagnostic Procedures

TERM	WORD PARTS	DEFINITION
Eye Examination Tests		
color vision tests		Use of polychromic (multicolored) charts to determine the ability of the patient to recognize color.

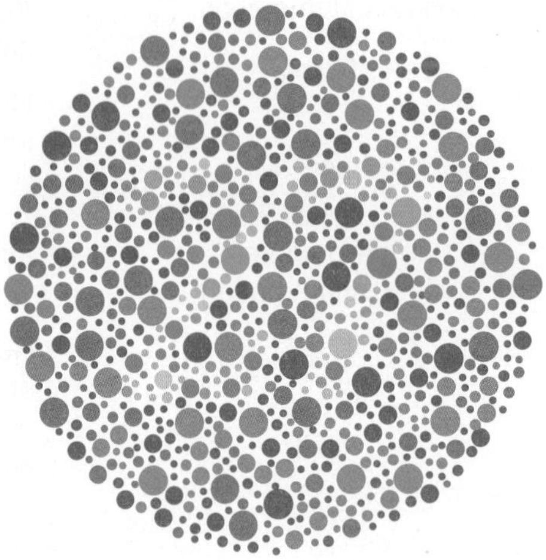

■ **Figure 13.11**   An example of color blindness test. A person with red-green color blindness would not be able to distinguish the green 27 from the surrounding red circles.

TERM	WORD PARTS	DEFINITION
fluorescein angiography (floo-oh-RESS-ee-in / an-jee-OG-rah-fee)	angi/o = vessel -graphy = process of recording	Process of injecting a dye (fluorescein) to observe the movement of blood and detect lesions in the macular area of the retina. Used to determine if there is a detachment of the retina.
fluorescein staining (floo-oh-RESS-ee-in)		Applying dye eye drops that are a bright green fluorescent color. Used to look for corneal abrasions or ulcers.
keratometer (KAIR-ah-toh-mee-ter)	kerat/o = cornea -meter = instrument to measure	An instrument used to measure the curvature of the cornea.
keratometry (kair-ah-TOM-eh-tree)	kerat/o = cornea -metry = process of measuring	Measurement of the curvature of the cornea using an instrument called a *keratometer*.
ophthalmoscope (off-THAL-moh-scope)	ophthalm/o = eye -scope = instrument for viewing	Instrument used to examine the inside of the eye through the pupil.
ophthalmoscopy (off-thal-MOSS-koh-pee)	ophthalm/o = eye -scopy = process of visually examining	Examination of the interior of the eyes using an instrument called an *ophthalmoscope* (see Figure 13.12 ■). The physician dilates the pupil in order to see the cornea, lens, and retina. Used to identify abnormalities in the blood vessels of the eye and some systemic diseases.

■ Diagnostic Procedures *(continued)*

TERM	WORD PARTS	DEFINITION

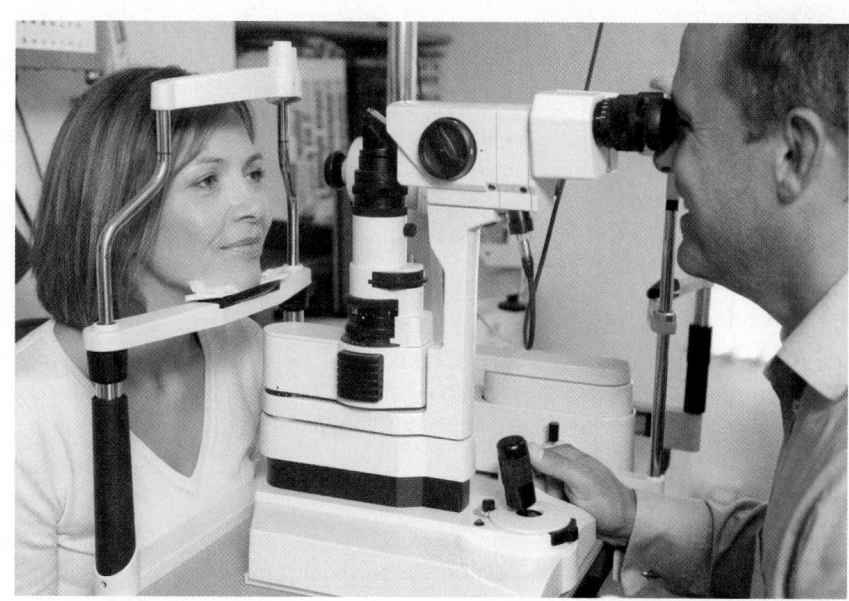

■ **Figure 13.12** Examination of the interior of the eye using an ophthalmoscope. *(Monkey Business Images/Shutterstock)*

TERM	WORD PARTS	DEFINITION
optometer (op-TOM-eh-ter)	opt/o = vision -meter = instrument to measure	Instrument used to measure how well the eye is able to focus images clearly on the retina.
refractive error test (ree-FRAK-tiv)		Vision test for a defect in the ability of the eye to accurately focus the image that is hitting it. Refractive errors result in myopia and hyperopia.
slit lamp microscopy	micro- = small -scopy = process of visually examining	Examining the posterior surface of the cornea.
Snellen chart (SNEL-enz)		Chart used for testing distance vision named for Dutch ophthalmologist Hermann Snellen. It contains letters of varying size and is administered from a distance of 20 feet. A person who can read at 20 feet what the average person can read at this distance is said to have 20/20 vision.
tonometry (tohn-OM-eh-tree)	ton/o = tone -metry = process of measuring	Measurement of the intraocular pressure of the eye using a *tonometer* to check for the condition of glaucoma. The physician places the tonometer lightly on the eyeball and a pressure measurement is taken. Generally part of a normal eye exam for adults.
visual acuity (VA) **test** (VIZH-oo-al / ah-KYOO-ih-tee)	-al = pertaining to	Measurement of the sharpness of a patient's vision. Usually, a Snellen chart is used for this test in which the patient identifies letters from a distance of 20 feet.

Therapeutic Procedures

TERMS	WORD PARTS	DEFINITION
Surgical Procedures		
blepharectomy (blef-ah-REK-toh-mee)	blephar/o = eyelid -ectomy = surgical removal	Surgical removal of the eyelid.
blepharoplasty (BLEF-ah-roh-plass-tee)	blephar/o = eyelid -plasty = surgical repair	Surgical repair of the eyelid. A common plastic surgery to correct blepharoptosis.
conjunctivoplasty (kon-junk-tih-VOH-plas-tee)	conjuctiv/o = conjunctiva -plasty = surgical repair	Surgical repair of the conjunctiva.
cryoextraction (cry-oh-eks-TRAK-shun)	cry/o = cold	Procedure in which cataract is lifted from the lens with an extremely cold probe.
cryoretinopexy (cry-oh-RET-ih-noh-pek-see)	cry/o = cold retin/o = retina -pexy = surgical fixation	Surgical fixation of the retina by using extreme cold.
enucleation (ee-new-klee-AH-shun)		Surgical removal of an eyeball.
iridectomy (ir-id-EK-toh-mee)	irid/o = iris -ectomy = surgical removal	Surgical removal of the iris.
iridosclerotomy (ir-ih-doh-skleh-ROT-oh-mee)	irid/o = iris scler/o = sclera -otomy = cutting into	To cut into the iris and sclera.
keratoplasty (KAIR-ah-toh-plass-tee)	kerat/o = cornea -plasty = surgical repair	Surgical repair of the cornea is the simple translation of this term that is utilized to mean corneal transplant.
laser-assisted in-situ keratomileusis (LASIK) (in-SIH-tyoo / kair-ah-toh-mih-LOO-sis)	kerat/o = cornea	Correction of myopia using laser surgery to remove corneal tissue.

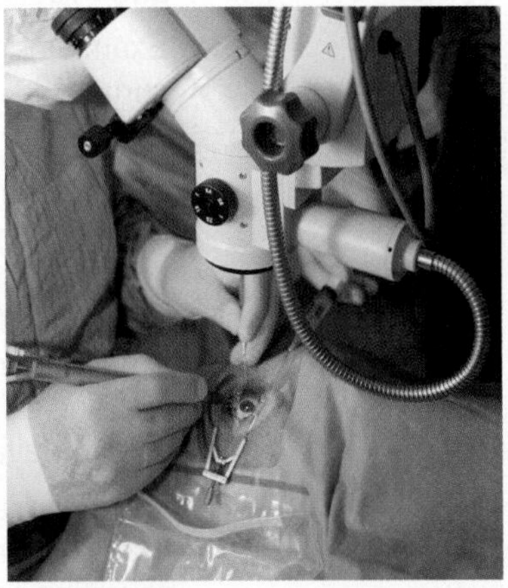

Figure 13.13 LASIK surgery uses a laser to reshape the cornea. *(mehmetcan/Shutterstock)*

TERMS	WORD PARTS	DEFINITION
laser photocoagulation (LAY-zer / foh-toh-koh-ag-yoo-LAY-shun)	phot/o = light	Use of a laser beam to destroy very small precise areas of the retina. May be used to treat retinal detachment or macular degeneration.
phacoemulsification (fak-oh-ee-mull-sih-fih-KAY-shun)	phac/o = lens	Use of high-frequency sound waves to emulsify (liquefy) a lens with a cataract, which is then aspirated (removed by suction) with a needle.
photorefractive keratectomy (PRK) (foh-toh-ree-FRAK-tiv / kair-ah-TEK-toh-mee)	phot/o = light kerat/o = cornea -ectomy = surgical removal	Use of a laser to reshape the cornea and correct errors of refraction.
prosthetic lens implant (pros-THET-ik)		Use of an artificial lens to replace the lens removed during cataract surgery.

Therapeutic Procedures *(continued)*

TERMS	WORD PARTS	DEFINITION
radial keratotomy (RK) (RAY-dee-all / kair-ah-TOT-oh-mee)	-al = pertaining to kerat/o = cornea -otomy = cutting into	Spokelike incisions around the cornea that result in it becoming flatter. A surgical treatment for myopia.
retinopexy (ret-ih-noh-PEX-ee)	retin/o = retina -pexy = surgical fixation	Surgical fixation of the retina. One treatment for a detaching retina.
scleral buckling (SKLAIR-al)	scler/o = sclera -al = pertaining to	Placing a band of silicone around the outside of the sclera that stabilizes a detaching retina.
sclerotomy (skleh-ROT-oh-mee)	scler/o = sclera -otomy = cutting into	To cut into the sclera.
strabotomy (strah-BOT-oh-mee)	-otomy = cutting into	Incision into the eye muscles in order to correct strabismus.

Pharmacology

CLASSIFICATION	WORD PARTS	ACTION	EXAMPLES
anesthetic ophthalmic solution (off-THAL-mik)	an- = without esthes/o = sensation, feeling -ic = pertaining to ophthalm/o = eye -ic = pertaining to	Eye drops for pain relief associated with eye infections, corneal abrasions, or surgery.	proparacain, Ak-Taine, Ocu-Caine; tetracaine, Opticaine, Pontocaine
antibiotic ophthalmic solution (off-THAL-mik)	anti- = against bi/o = life -ic = pertaining to ophthalm/o = eye -ic = pertaining to	Eye drops for the treatment of bacterial eye infections.	erythromycin, Del-Mycin, Ilotycin Ophthalmic
antiglaucoma medications (an-tye-glau-KOH-mah)	anti- = against glauc/o = gray -oma = mass	Group of drugs that reduce intraocular pressure by lowering the amount of aqueous humor in the eyeball. May achieve this by either reducing the production of aqueous humor or increasing its outflow.	timolol, Betimol, Timoptic; acetazolamide, Ak-Zol, Dazamide; prostaglandin analogs, Lumigan, Xalatan
artificial tears		Medications, many of them over the counter, to treat dry eyes.	buffered isotonic solutions, Akwa Tears, Refresh Plus, Moisture Eyes
miotic drops (my-OT-ik)	mi/o = lessening -tic = pertaining to	Any substance that causes the pupil to constrict. These medications may also be used to treat glaucoma.	physostigmine, Eserine Sulfate, Isopto Eserine; carbachol, Carbastat, Miostat
mydriatic drops (mid-ree-AT-ik)	mydr/i = widening -atic = pertaining to	Any substance that causes the pupil to dilate by paralyzing the iris and/or ciliary body muscles. Particularly useful during eye examinations and eye surgery.	atropine sulfate, Atropine-Care Ophthalmic, Atropisol Ophthalmic
ophthalmic decongestants	ophthalm/o = eye -ic = pertaining to de- = without	Over-the-counter medications that constrict the arterioles of the eye and reduce redness and itching of the conjunctiva.	tetrahydrozoline, Visine, Murine

Abbreviations

ARMD	age-related macular degeneration	**Ophth.**	ophthalmology
Astigm	astigmatism	**OS**	left eye
c.gl.	correction with glasses	**OU**	each eye/both eyes
D	diopter (lens strength)	**PERRLA**	pupils equal, round, react to light and accommodation
DVA	distance visual acuity		
ECCE	extracapsular cataract extraction	**PRK**	photorefractive keratectomy
EENT	eye, ear, nose, and throat	**REM**	rapid eye movement
EM	emmetropia	**s.gl.**	without correction or glasses
EOM	extraocular movement	**SMD**	senile macular degeneration
ICCE	intracapsular cataract extraction	**ST**	esotropia
IOP	intraocular pressure	**VA**	visual acuity
LASIK	laser-assisted in-situ keratomileusis	**VF**	visual field
OD	right eye	**XT**	exotropia

MED TERM TIP

The abbreviations for right eye (OD) and left eye (OS) are easy to remember when we know their origins. OD stands for *oculus* (eye) *dexter* (right). OS has its origin in *oculus* (eye) *sinister* (left). At one time in history it was considered to be sinister if a person looked at another from only the left side. Hence the term *oculus sinister* (OS) means left eye.

Section II: The Ear at a Glance

Function

The ear contains the sensory receptors for hearing and equilibrium (balance).

Structures

Here are the primary structures that comprise the ear.

auricle   **external ear**
inner ear   **middle ear**

Word Parts

Here are the most common word parts (with their meanings) used to build ear terms. For a more comprehensive list, refer to the Terminology section of this chapter.

Combining Forms

acous/o	hearing	myring/o	tympanic membrane (eardrum)
audi/o	hearing		
audit/o	hearing	ot/o	ear
aur/o	ear	salping/o	auditory tube (eustachian tube)
auricul/o	ear		
cerumin/o	cerumen	staped/o	stapes
cochle/o	cochlea	tympan/o	tympanic membrane (eardrum)
labyrinth/o	labyrinth (inner ear)		

Suffixes

-cusis	hearing
-otia	ear condition

The Ear Illustrated

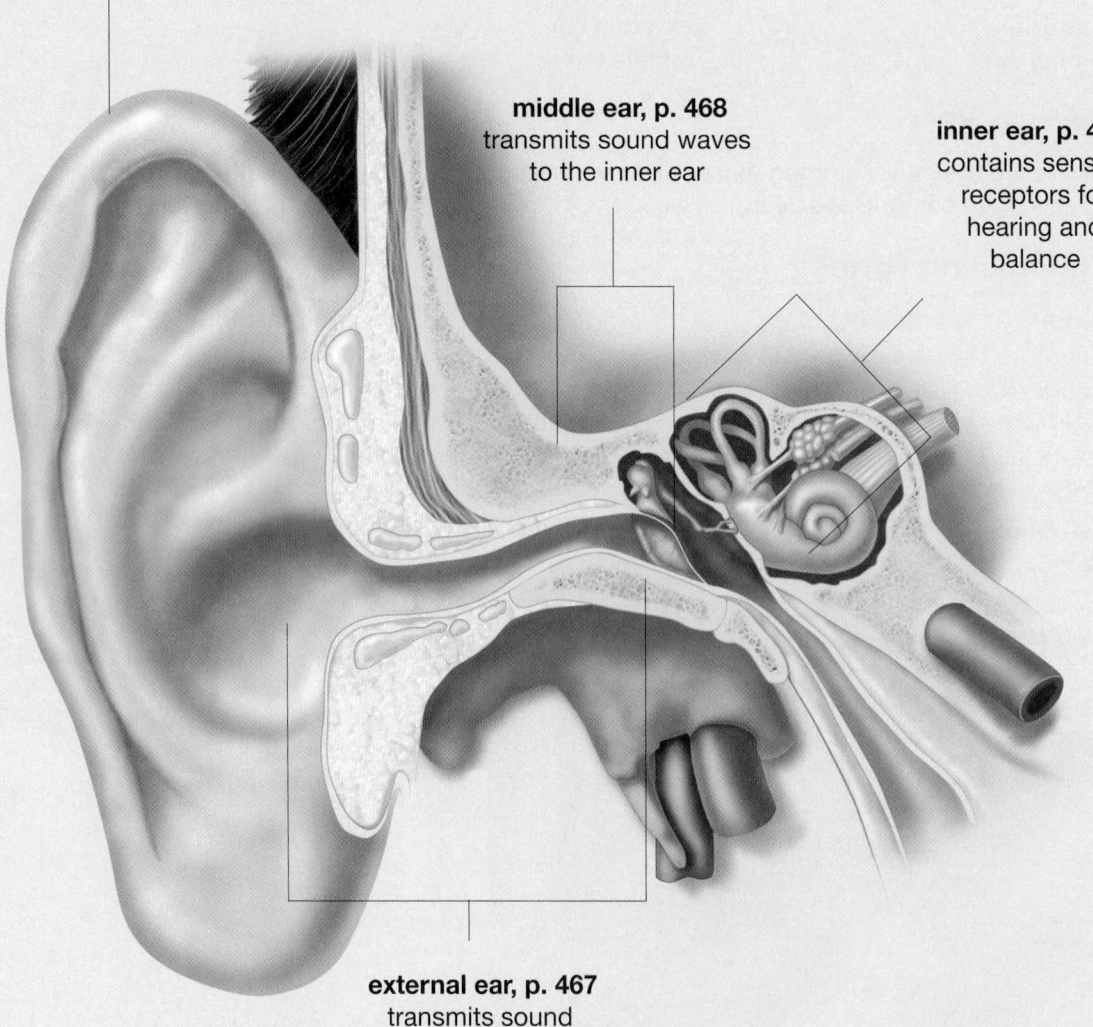

auricle, p. 467
directs sound waves into the ear canal

middle ear, p. 468
transmits sound waves to the inner ear

inner ear, p. 468
contains sensory receptors for hearing and balance

external ear, p. 467
transmits sound waves to the middle ear

Anatomy and Physiology of the Ear

audiology (aw-dee-OL-oh-jee)	**middle ear**
cochlear nerve (KOK-lee-ar)	**otology** (oh-TOL-oh-jee)
equilibrium (ee-kwih-LIB-ree-um)	**vestibular nerve** (ves-TIB-yoo-lar)
external ear	**vestibulocochlear nerve**
hearing	(ves-tib-yoo-loh-KOK-lee-ar)
inner ear	

The study of the ear is referred to as **otology** (Oto), and the study of hearing disorders is called **audiology.** While there is a large amount of overlap between these two areas, there are also examples of ear problems that do not affect hearing. The ear is responsible for two senses: **hearing** and **equilibrium,** or our sense of balance. Hearing and equilibrium sensory information is carried to the brain by cranial nerve VIII, the **vestibulocochlear nerve.** This nerve is divided into two major branches. The **cochlear nerve** carries hearing information, and the **vestibular nerve** carries equilibrium information.

The ear is subdivided into three areas: **external ear, middle ear,** and **inner ear.**

External Ear

auditory canal (AW-dih-tor-ee)	**pinna** (PIN-ah)
auricle (AW-rih-k'l)	**tympanic membrane** (tim-PAN-ik)
cerumen (seh-ROO-men)	
external auditory meatus	
(AW-dih-tor-ee / me-A-tus)	

The external ear consists of three parts: the **auricle,** the **auditory canal,** and the **tympanic membrane** (see Figure 13.14 ■). The auricle or **pinna** is what is commonly referred to as the *ear* because this is the only visible portion. The auricle with its

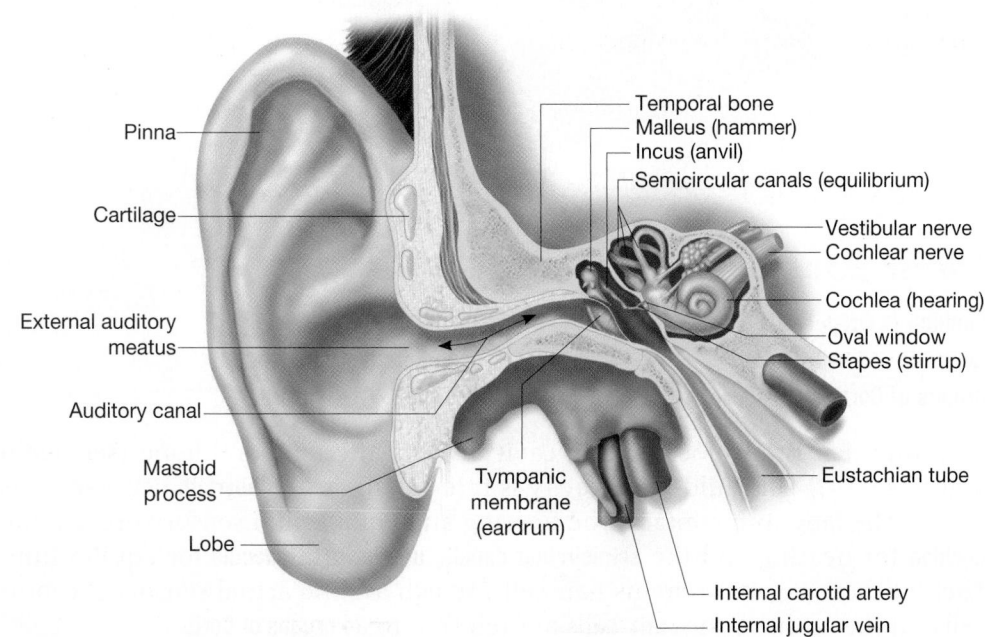

■ **Figure 13.14** The internal structures of the outer, middle, and inner ear.

MED TERM TIP

The term *tympanic membrane* comes from the Greek word for "drumhead." The tympanic membrane or eardrum vibrates to sound waves like a drum head.

earlobe has a unique shape in each person and functions like a funnel to capture sound waves as they go past the outer ear and channel them through the **external auditory meatus.** The sound then moves along the auditory canal and causes the tympanic membrane (eardrum) to vibrate. The tympanic membrane actually separates the external ear from the middle ear. Ear wax or **cerumen** is produced in oil glands in the auditory canal. This wax helps to protect and lubricate the ear. It is also just barely liquid at body temperature. This causes cerumen to slowly flow out of the auditory canal, carrying dirt and dust with it. Therefore, the auditory canal is self-cleaning.

Middle Ear

auditory tube (AW-dih-tor-ee)   **ossicles** (OSS-ih-kls)

eustachian tube (yoo-STAY-she-en)   **oval window**

incus (ING-kus)   **stapes** (STAY-peez)

malleus (MAL-ee-us)

MED TERM TIP

The three bones in the middle ear are referred to by terms that are similar to their shape. Thus, the malleus is called the hammer, the incus is the anvil, and the stapes is the stirrup (see Figure 13.15).

The middle ear is located in a small cavity in the temporal bone of the skull. This air-filled cavity contains three tiny bones called **ossicles** (see Figure 13.15 ■). These three bones, the **malleus, incus,** and **stapes,** are vital to the hearing process. They amplify the vibrations in the middle ear and transmit them to the inner ear from the malleus to the incus and finally to the stapes. The stapes, the last of the three ossicles, is attached to a very thin membrane that covers the opening to the inner ear called the **oval window.**

The **eustachian tube** or **auditory tube** connects the nasopharynx with the middle ear (see Figure 13.14). Each time you swallow the eustachian tube opens. This connection allows pressure to equalize between the middle ear cavity and the atmospheric pressure.

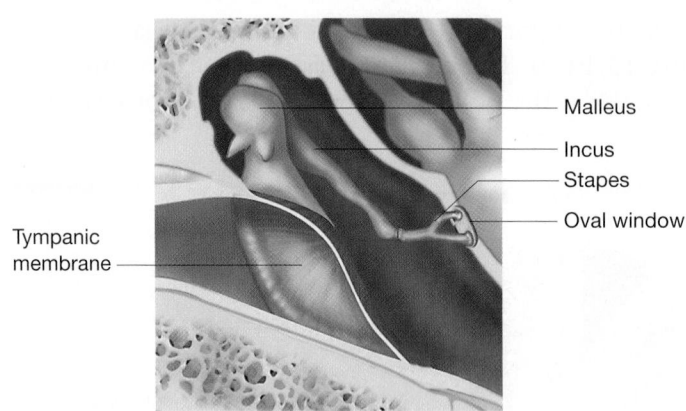

Malleus
Incus
Stapes
Oval window

Tympanic membrane

■ Figure 13.15 Closeup view of the ossicles within the middle ear. These three bones extend from the tympanic membrane to the oval window.

Inner Ear

cochlea (KOK-lee-ah)   **saccule** (SAK-yool)

labyrinth (LAB-ih-rinth)   **semicircular canals**

organs of Corti (KOR-tee)   **utricle** (YOO-trih-k'l)

MED TERM TIP

Frequently, children will twirl in circles and fall or stumble from dizziness when they stop. This is caused from a temporary imbalance in the inner ear.

The inner ear is also located in a cavity within the temporal bone (see again Figure 13.14). This fluid-filled cavity is referred to as the **labyrinth** because of its shape. The labyrinth contains the hearing and equilibrium sensory organs: the **cochlea** for hearing and the **semicircular canals, utricle,** and **saccule** for equilibrium. Each of these organs contains hair cells, which are the actual sensory receptor cells. In the cochlea, the hair cells are referred to as **organs of Corti.**

How We Hear

conductive hearing loss (kon-DUK-tiv)
sensorineural hearing loss (sen-soh-ree-NOO-ral)

Figure 13.16 ■ outlines the path of sound through the outer ear and middle ear and into the cochlea of the inner ear. Sound waves traveling down the external auditory canal strike the eardrum, causing it to vibrate. The ossicles conduct these vibrations across the middle ear from the eardrum to the oval window. Oval window movements initiate vibrations in the fluid that fills the cochlea. As the fluid vibrations strike a hair cell, they bend the small hairs and stimulate the nerve ending. The nerve ending then sends an electrical impulse to the brain on the cochlear portion of the vestibulocochlear nerve.

Hearing loss can be divided into two main categories: **conductive hearing loss** and **sensorineural hearing loss.** Conductive refers to disease or malformation of the outer or middle ear. All sound is weaker and muffled in conductive hearing loss since it is not conducted correctly to the inner ear. Sensorineural hearing loss is the result of damage or malformation of the inner ear (cochlea) or the cochlear nerve. In this hearing loss, some sounds are distorted and heard incorrectly. There can also be a combination of both conductive and sensorineural hearing loss.

MED TERM TIP

Hearing impairment is becoming a greater problem for the general population for several reasons. First, people are living longer. Hearing loss can accompany old age, and there are a greater number of people over 50 years of age requiring hearing assistance. In addition, sound technology has produced music quality that was never available before. However, listening to loud music either naturally or through earphones can cause gradual damage to the hearing mechanism.

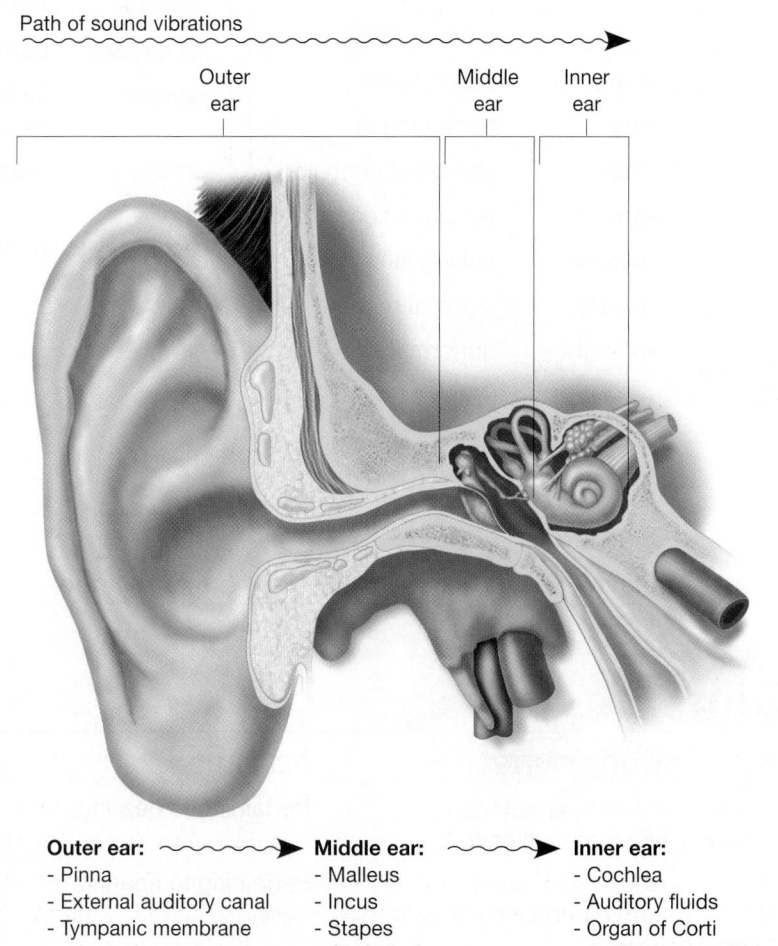

Path of sound vibrations

Outer ear   Middle ear   Inner ear

Outer ear:
- Pinna
- External auditory canal
- Tympanic membrane

Middle ear:
- Malleus
- Incus
- Stapes
- Oval window

Inner ear:
- Cochlea
- Auditory fluids
- Organ of Corti
- Auditory nerve fibers
- Cerebral cortex

■ **Figure 13.16** The path of sound waves through the outer, middle, and inner ear.

Terminology

Word Parts Used to Build Ear Terms

The following lists contain the combining forms, suffixes, and prefixes used to build terms in the remaining sections of this chapter.

Combining Forms

acous/o	hearing		**cochle/o**	cochlea		**presby/o**	old age
audi/o	hearing		**labyrinth/o**	labyrinth		**py/o**	pus
audit/o	hearing		**laryng/o**	larynx		**rhin/o**	nose
aur/o	ear		**myc/o**	fungus		**salping/o**	auditory tube
auricul/o	ear		**myring/o**	tympanic membrane		**staped/o**	stapes
bi/o	life		**neur/o**	nerve		**tympan/o**	tympanic membrane
cerumin/o	cerumen		**ot/o**	ear			

Suffixes

-al	pertaining to		**-meter**	instrument to measure		**-rrhea**	discharge
-algia	pain		**-metry**	process of measuring		**-rrhexis**	rupture
-ar	pertaining to		**-oma**	mass, tumor		**-sclerosis**	hardening
-cusis	hearing		**-ory**	pertaining to		**-scope**	instrument to visually examine
-ectomy	pertaining to		**-osis**	abnormal condition		**-scopy**	process of visually examining
-emesis	vomiting		**-otia**	ear condition			
-gram	record		**-otomy**	cutting into		**-tic**	pertaining to
-ic	pertaining to		**-plasty**	surgical repair			
-itis	inflammation		**-rrhagia**	abnormal flow			
-logy	study of						

Prefixes

an- = without		**bi-** = two		**micro-** = small	
anti- = against		**macro-** = large		**mono-** = one	

Anatomical Terms

TERM	WORD PARTS	DEFINITION
acoustic (ah-KOOS-tik)	acous/o = hearing -tic = pertaining to	Pertaining to hearing.
auditory (AW-dih-tor-ee)	audit/o = hearing -ory = pertaining to	Pertaining to hearing.

Anatomical Terms *(continued)*

TERM	WORD PARTS	DEFINITION
aural (AW-ral)	aur/o = ear -al = pertaining to	Pertaining to the ear. **MED TERM TIP** Word Watch: Be careful when using two terms that sound the same—*aural* meaning "pertaining to the ear" and *oral* meaning "pertaining to the mouth."
auricular (aw-RIK-cu-lar)	auricul/o = ear -ar = pertaining to	Pertaining to the ear.
binaural (bin-AW-rall)	bi- = two aur/o = ear -al = pertaining to	Pertaining to both ears.
cochlear (KOK-lee-ar)	cochle/o = cochlea -ar = pertaining to	Pertaining to the cochlea.
monaural (mon-AW-rall)	mono- = one aur/o = ear -al = pertaining to	Pertaining to one ear.
otic (OH-tik)	ot/o = ear -ic = pertaining to	Pertaining to the ear.
tympanic (tim-PAN-ik)	tympan/o = tympanic membrane -ic = pertaining to	Pertaining to the tympanic membrane.

Pathology

TERM	WORD PARTS	DEFINITION
Medical Specialties		
audiology (aw-dee-OL-oh-jee)	audi/o = hearing -logy = study of	Medical specialty involved with measuring hearing function and identifying hearing loss. Specialist is an *audiologist*.
otorhinolaryngology (ENT) (oh-toh-rye-noh-lair-in-GOL-oh-jee)	ot/o = ear rhin/o = nose laryng/o = larynx -logy = study of	Branch of medicine involving the diagnosis and treatment of conditions and diseases of the ear, nose, and throat. Also referred to as *ENT*. Physician is an *otorhinolaryngologist*.
Signs and Symptoms		
macrotia (mah-KROH-she-ah)	macro- = large -otia = ear condition	Condition of having abnormally large ears.
microtia (my-KROH-she-ah)	micro- = small -otia = ear condition	Condition of having abnormally small ears.
otalgia (oh-TAL-jee-ah)	ot/o = ear -algia = pain	Ear pain.
otopyorrhea (oh-toh-pye-oh-REE-ah)	ot/o = ear py/o = pus -rrhea = discharge	Discharge of pus from the ear.
otorrhagia (oh-toh-RAH-jee-ah)	ot/o = ear -rrhagia = abnormal flow	Bleeding from the ear.

Pathology *(continued)*

TERM	WORD PARTS	DEFINITION
presbycusis (pres-bih-KOO-sis)	presby/o = old age -cusis = hearing condition	Normal loss of hearing that can accompany the aging process.
residual hearing (rih-ZID-yoo-al)	-al = pertaining to	Amount of hearing that is still present after damage has occurred to the auditory mechanism.
tinnitus (tin-EYE-tus)		Ringing in the ears.
tympanorrhexis (tim-pan-oh-REK-sis)	tympan/o = tympanic membrane -rrhexis = rupture	Rupture of the tympanic membrane.
vertigo (VER-tih-goh)		Dizziness caused by the sensation that the room is spinning.
Hearing Loss		
anacusis (an-ah-KOO-sis)	an- = without -cusis = hearing	Total absence of hearing; inability to perceive sound. Also called *deafness.*
deafness		Inability to hear or having some degree of hearing impairment.
External Ear		
ceruminoma (seh-roo-men-oh-ma)	cerumin/o = cerumen -oma = mass	Excessive accumulation of ear wax resulting in a hard wax plug. Sound becomes muffled.
otitis externa (OE) (oh-TYE-tis / ex-TERN-ah)	ot/o = ear -itis = inflammation	External ear infection. May be caused by bacteria or fungus. Also called *otomycosis* and commonly referred to as *swimmer's ear.*
otomycosis (oh-toh-my-KOH-sis)	ot/o = ear myc/o = fungus -osis = abnormal condition	Fungal infection of the ear. One type of otitis externa.
Middle Ear		
myringitis (mir-ing-JYE-tis)	myring/o = tympanic membrane -itis = inflammation	Inflammation of the tympanic membrane.
otitis media (OM) (oh-TYE-tis / MEE-dee-ah)	ot/o = ear -itis = inflammation	Seen frequently in children; commonly referred to as a *middle ear infection.* Often preceded by an upper respiratory infection during which pathogens move from the pharynx to the middle ear via the eustachian tube. Fluid accumulates in the middle ear cavity. The fluid may be watery, *serous otitis media,* or full of pus, *purulent otitis media.*
otosclerosis (oh-toh-sklair-OH-sis)	ot/o = ear -sclerosis = hardening	Loss of mobility of the stapes bone, leading to progressive hearing loss.
salpingitis (sal-pin-JIH-tis)	salping/o = auditory tube -itis = inflammation	Inflammation of the auditory tube.

MED TERM TIP

Word Watch: Be careful using the combining form *salping/o,* which can mean either "Eustachian tube" or "fallopian tube."

TERM	WORD PARTS	DEFINITION
tympanitis (tim-pan-EYE-tis)	tympan/o = tympanic membrane -itis = inflammation	Inflammation of the tympanic membrane.

Pathology *(continued)*

TERM	WORD PARTS	DEFINITION
Inner Ear		
acoustic neuroma (ah-KOOS-tik / noor-OH-mah)	acous/o = hearing -tic = pertaining to neur/o = nerve -oma = tumor	Benign tumor of the eighth cranial nerve sheath. The pressure causes symptoms such as tinnitus, headache, dizziness, and progressive hearing loss.
labyrinthitis (lab-ih-rin-THIGH-tis)	labyrinth/o = labyrinth -itis = inflammation	May affect both the hearing and equilibrium portions of the inner ear. Also referred to as an *inner ear infection.*
Ménière's disease (may-nee-ARZ)		Abnormal condition within the labyrinth of the inner ear that can lead to a progressive loss of hearing. The symptoms are dizziness or vertigo, hearing loss, and tinnitus (ringing in the ears). Named for French physician Prosper Ménière.

Diagnostic Procedures

TERM	WORD PARTS	DEFINITION
Audiology Tests		
audiogram (AW-dee-oh-gram)	audi/o = hearing -gram = record	Graphic record that illustrates the results of audiometry.
audiometer (aw-dee-OM-eh-ter)	audi/o = hearing -meter = instrument to measure	Instrument to measure hearing.
audiometry (aw-dee-OM-eh-tree)	audi/o = hearing -metry = process of measuring	Test of hearing ability by determining the lowest and highest intensity (decibels) and frequencies (hertz) that a person can distinguish. The patient may sit in a sound-proof booth and receive sounds through earphones as the technician decreases the sound or lowers the tones.

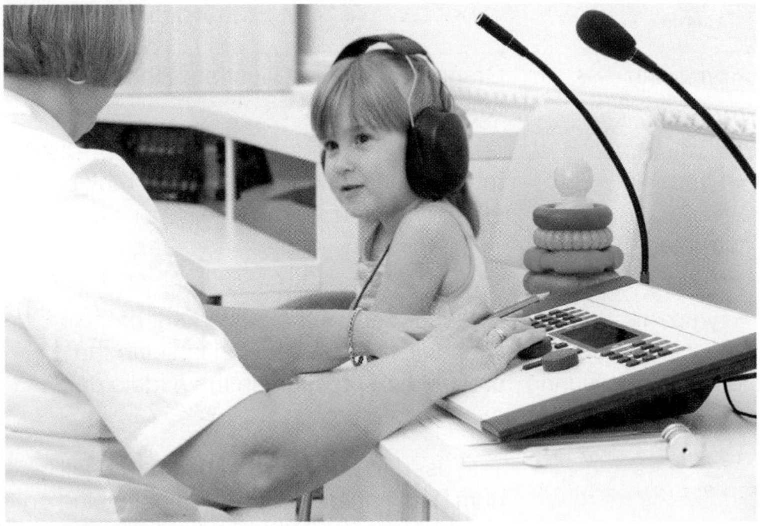

■ **Figure 13.17** Audiometry exam being administered to a young child who is wearing the ear phones through which sounds are given. *(Capifrutta/Shutterstock)*

decibel (dB) (DES-ih-bel)		Measures the intensity or loudness of a sound. Zero decibels is the quietest sound measured and 120 dB is the loudest sound commonly measured.

Diagnostic Procedures *(continued)*

TERM	WORD PARTS	DEFINITION
hertz (Hz)		Measurement of the frequency or pitch of sound. The lowest pitch on an audiogram is 250 Hz. The measurement can go as high as 8000 Hz, which is the highest pitch measured.
Rinne and Weber tuning-fork tests (RIN-eh)		Tests that assess both nerve and bone conduction of sound. The physician holds a tuning fork, an instrument that produces a constant pitch when it is struck, against or near the bones on the side of the head.
Otology Tests		
otoscope (OH-toh-scope)	ot/o = ear -scope = instrument to visually examine	Instrument to view inside the ear canal.
otoscopy (oh-TOSS-koh-pee)	ot/o = ear -scopy = process of visually examining	Examination of the ear canal, eardrum, and outer ear using an *otoscope*.

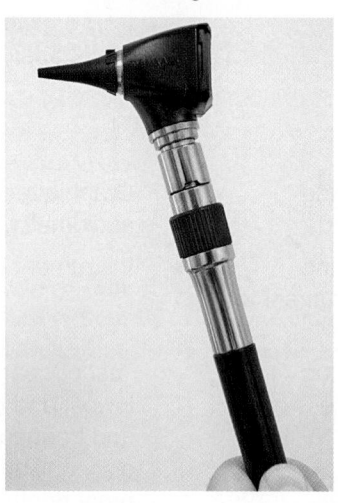

■ **Figure 13.18** An otoscope, used to visually examine the external auditory ear canal and tympanic membrane.

> **MED TERM TIP**
>
> Small children are prone to placing objects in their ears. In some cases, as with peas and beans, these become moist in the ear canal and swell, which makes removal difficult. *Otoscopy*, or the examination of the ear using an *otoscope*, can aid in identifying and removing the cause of hearing loss if it is due to foreign bodies.

TERM	WORD PARTS	DEFINITION
tympanogram (TIM-pah-no-gram)	tympan/o = tympanic membrane -gram = record	Graphic record that illustrates the results of tympanometry.
tympanometer (tim-pah-NOM-eh-ter)	tympan/o = tympanic membrane -meter = instrument to measure	Instrument used to measure the movement of the tympanic membrane.
tympanometry (tim-pah-NOM-eh-tree)	tympan/o = tympanic membrane -metry = process of measuring	Measurement of the movement of the tympanic membrane. Can indicate the presence of pressure in the middle ear.
Balance Tests		
falling test		Test used to observe balance and equilibrium. The patient is observed balancing on one foot, then with one foot in front of the other, and then walking forward with eyes open. The same test is conducted with the patient's eyes closed. Swaying and falling with the eyes closed can indicate an ear and equilibrium malfunction.

Therapeutic Procedures

TERM	WORD PARTS	DEFINITION
Audiology Procedures		

American Sign Language (ASL)

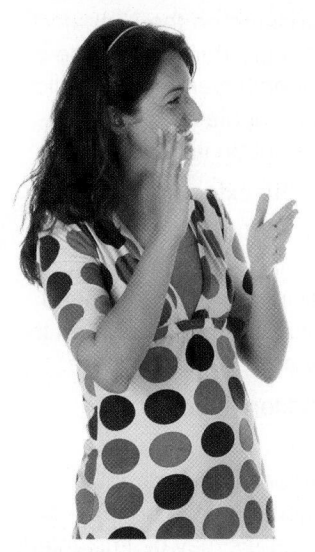 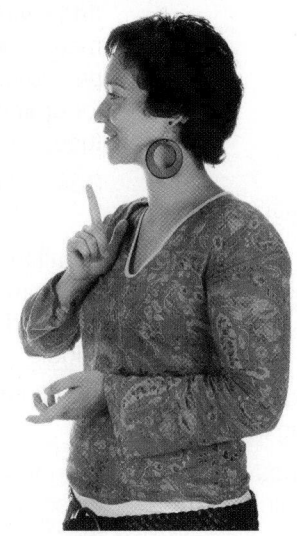

Nonverbal method of communicating in which the hands and fingers are used to indicate words and concepts. Used by both persons who are deaf and persons with speech impairments.

■ **Figure 13.19** Two women having a conversation using American Sign Language. *(Vladimir Mucibabic/ Shutterstock)*

TERM	WORD PARTS	DEFINITION
hearing aid		Apparatus or mechanical device used by persons with impaired hearing to amplify sound. Also called an *amplification device.*
Surgical Procedures		

cochlear implant
(KOK-lee-ar)

cochle/o = cochlea
-ar = pertaining to

Mechanical device surgically placed under the skin behind the outer ear (pinna) that converts sound signals into magnetic impulses to stimulate the auditory nerve. Can be beneficial for those with profound sensorineural hearing loss.

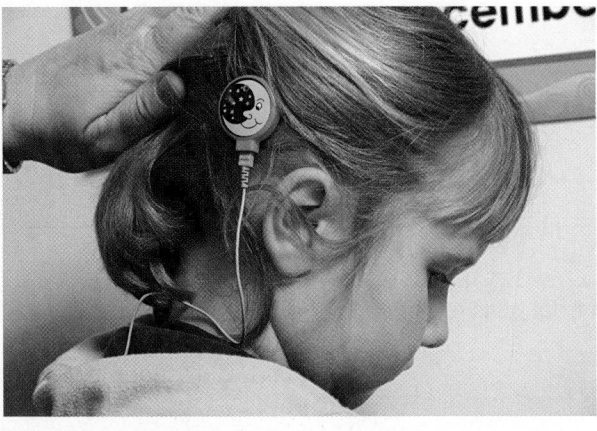

■ **Figure 13.20** Photograph of a child with a cochlear implant. This device sends electrical impulses directly to the brain.

TERM	WORD PARTS	DEFINITION
labyrinthectomy (lab-ih-rin-THEK-toh-mee)	labyrinth/o = labyrinth -ectomy = surgical removal	Surgical removal of the labyrinth.
labyrinthotomy (lab-ih-rinth-OT-oh-mee)	labyrinth/o = labyrinth -otomy = cutting into	To cut into the labyrinth.
myringectomy (mir-in-GEK-toh-mee)	myring/o = tympanic membrane -ectomy = surgical removal	Surgical removal of the tympanic membrane.
myringoplasty (mir-IN-goh-plass-tee)	myring/o = tympanic membrane -plasty = surgical repair	Surgical repair of the tympanic membrane.

Therapeutic Procedures *(continued)*

TERM	WORD PARTS	DEFINITION
myringotomy (mir-in-GOT-oh-mee)	myring/o = tympanic membrane -otomy = cutting into	Surgical puncture of the eardrum with removal of fluid and pus from the middle ear to eliminate a persistent ear infection and excessive pressure on the tympanic membrane. A pressure equalizing tube is placed in the tympanic membrane to allow for drainage of the middle ear cavity; this tube typically falls out on its own.
otoplasty (OH-toh-plas-tee)	ot/o = ear -plasty = surgical repair	Surgical repair of the external ear.
pressure equalizing tube (PE tube)		Small tube surgically placed in a child's eardrum to assist in drainage of trapped fluid and to equalize pressure between the middle ear cavity and the atmosphere.
salpingotomy (sal-pin-GOT-oh-mee)	salping/o = auditory tube -otomy = cutting into	To cut into the auditory tube.
stapedectomy (stay-pee-DEK-toh-mee)	staped/o = stapes -ectomy = pertaining to	Removal of the stapes bone to treat otosclerosis (hardening of the bone). A prosthesis or artificial stapes may be implanted.
tympanectomy (tim-pan-EK-toh-mee)	tympan/o = tympanic membrane -ectomy = surgical removal	Surgical removal of the tympanic membrane.
tympanoplasty (tim-pan-oh-PLASS-tee)	tympan/o = tympanic membrane -plasty = surgical repair	Surgical repair of the tympanic membrane.
tympanotomy (tim-pan-OT-oh-mee)	tympan/o = tympanic membrane -otomy = cutting into	To cut into the tympanic membrane.

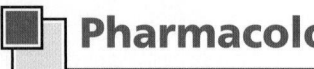 **Pharmacology**

CLASSIFICATION	WORD PARTS	ACTION	EXAMPLES
antibiotic otic solution (OH-tik)	anti- = against bi/o = life -tic = pertaining to ot/o = ear -ic = pertaining to	Eardrops to treat otitis externa.	Neomycin, polymyxin B and hydrocortisone solution, Otocort, Cortisporin, Otic Care
antiemetics (an-tye-ee-mit-tiks)	anti- = against -emesis = vomiting -tic = pertaining to	Medications effective in treating the nausea associated with vertigo.	meclizine, Antivert, Meni-D; prochlorperazine, Compazine
anti-inflammatory otic solution (OH-tik)	anti- = against -ory = pertaining to ot/o = ear -ic = pertaining to	Reduces inflammation, itching, and edema associated with otitis externa.	antipyrine and benzoaine, Allergan Ear Drops, A/B Otic
wax emulsifiers		Substances used to soften ear wax to prevent buildup within the external ear canal.	carbamide peroxide, Debrox Drops, Murine Ear Drops

Abbreviations

AD	right ear	**HEENT**	head, ears, eyes, nose, throat
AS	left ear	**Hz**	hertz
ASL	American Sign Language	**OM**	otitis media
AU	both ears	**Oto**	otology
BC	bone conduction	**PE tube**	pressure equalizing tube
dB	decibel	**PORP**	partial ossicular replacement prosthesis
EENT	eyes, ears, nose, throat	**SOM**	serous otitis media
ENT	ear, nose, and throat	**TORP**	total ossicular replacement prosthesis

Chapter Review

Real-World Applications

Medical Record Analysis

This Ophthalmology Consultation Report contains 11 medical terms. Underline each term and write it in the list below the report. Then define each term.

Ophthalmology Consultation Report

Reason for Consultation: Evaluation of progressive loss of vision in right eye.

History of Present Illness: Patient is a 79-year-old female who has noted gradual deterioration of vision and increasing photophobia during the past year, particularly in the right eye. She states that it feels like there is a film over her right eye. She denies any change in vision in her left eye. Patient has used corrective lenses her entire adult life for hyperopia.

Results of Physical Examination: Visual acuity test showed no change in this patient's long-standing hyperopia. The pupils react properly to light. Intraocular pressure is normal. Ophthalmoscopy after application of mydriatic drops revealed presence of large opaque cataract in lens of right eye. There is a very small cataract forming in the left eye. There is no evidence of retinopathy, macular degeneration, or keratitis.

Assessment: Diminished vision in right eye secondary to cataract.

Recommendations: Phacoemulsification of cataract followed by prosthetic lens implant.

	Term	Definition
1	_____	_____
2	_____	_____
3	_____	_____
4	_____	_____
5	_____	_____
6	_____	_____
7	_____	_____
8	_____	_____
9	_____	_____
10	_____	_____
11	_____	_____

Chart Note Transcription

The chart note below contains 10 phrases that can be reworded with a medical term that you learned in this chapter. Each phrase is identified with an underline. Determine the medical term and write your answers in the space provided.

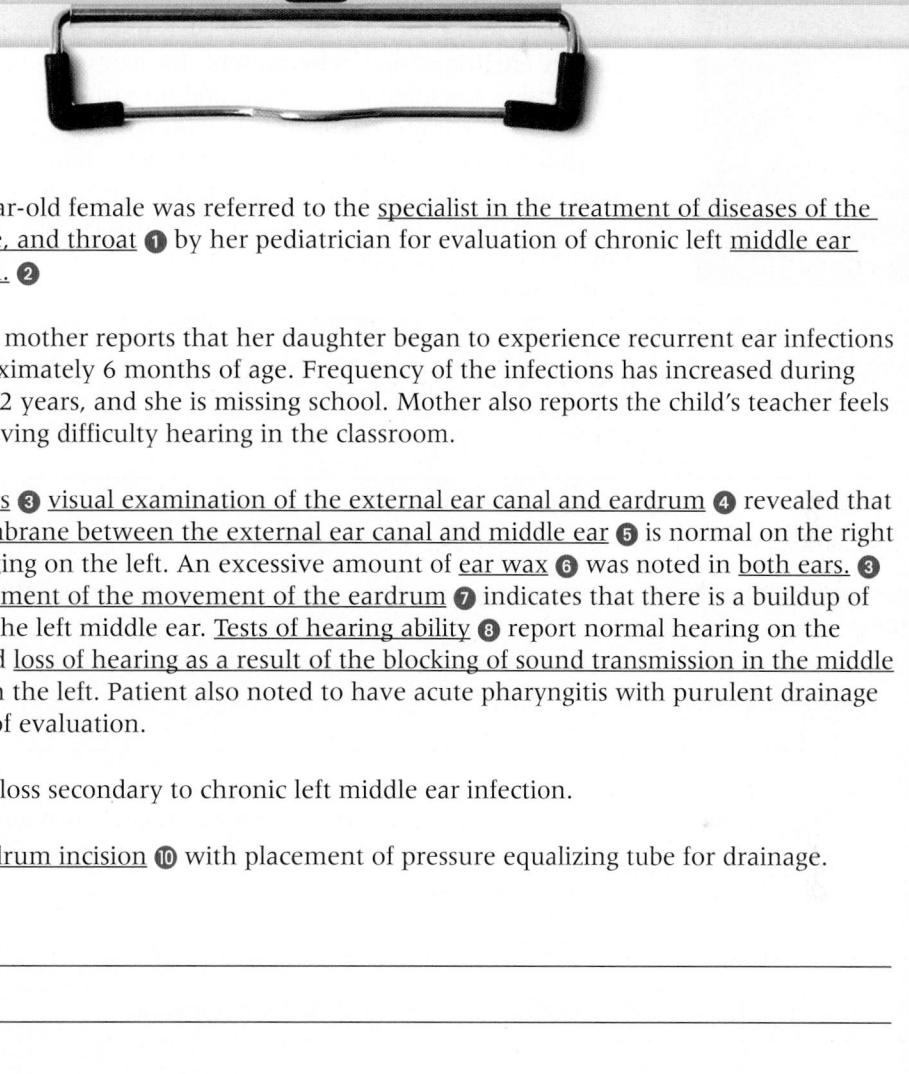

Current
Complaint:
An 8-year-old female was referred to the specialist in the treatment of diseases of the ear, nose, and throat ❶ by her pediatrician for evaluation of chronic left middle ear infection. ❷

Past History:
Patient's mother reports that her daughter began to experience recurrent ear infections at approximately 6 months of age. Frequency of the infections has increased during the past 2 years, and she is missing school. Mother also reports the child's teacher feels she is having difficulty hearing in the classroom.

Signs and
Symptoms:
Both ears ❸ visual examination of the external ear canal and eardrum ❹ revealed that the membrane between the external ear canal and middle ear ❺ is normal on the right and bulging on the left. An excessive amount of ear wax ❻ was noted in both ears. ❸ Measurement of the movement of the eardrum ❼ indicates that there is a buildup of fluid in the left middle ear. Tests of hearing ability ❽ report normal hearing on the right and loss of hearing as a result of the blocking of sound transmission in the middle ear ❾ on the left. Patient also noted to have acute pharyngitis with purulent drainage at time of evaluation.

Diagnosis:
Hearing loss secondary to chronic left middle ear infection.

Treatment:
Left eardrum incision ❿ with placement of pressure equalizing tube for drainage.

❶ _____

❷ _____

❸ _____

❹ _____

❺ _____

❻ _____

❼ _____

❽ _____

❾ _____

❿ _____

Case Study

Below is a case study presentation of a patient with a condition covered in this chapter. Read the case study and answer the questions below. Some questions will ask for information not included within this chapter. Use your text, a medical dictionary, or any other reference material you choose to answer these questions.

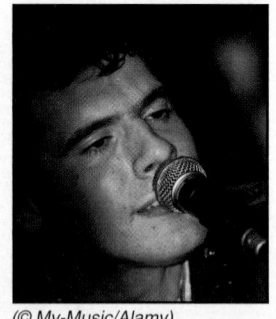

This 35-year-old male musician was seen in the EENT clinic complaining of a progressive hearing loss over the past 15 years. He is now unable to hear what is being said if there is any environmental noise present. He states that he has played with a group of musicians using amplified instruments and no earplugs for the past 20 years. External ear structures appear normal bilaterally with otoscopy. Tympanometry is normal bilaterally. Audiometry reveals diminished hearing bilaterally. Rinne and Weber tuning-fork tests indicate that the patient has a moderate amount of conductive hearing loss but rule out sensorineural hearing loss. Diagnosis is moderate bilateral conductive hearing loss as a result of prolonged exposure to loud noise. Patient is referred for evaluation for a hearing aid.

(© My-Music/Alamy)

1. Which type of hearing loss does this patient appear to have? Look this condition up in a reference source and include a short description of it.

    _____

    _____

2. Explain how the other type of hearing loss (the type ruled out by the Rinne and Weber tuning-fork tests) is different from what this patient has.

    _____

    _____

3. What diagnostic tests did the physician perform? Describe them in your own words.

    _____

    _____

4. Explain the difference between a hearing aid and a cochlear implant.

    _____

    _____

5. How do you think this patient could have avoided this hearing loss?

    _____

    _____

Practice Exercises

A. Complete the Statement

1. The study of the eye is _____.

2. Another term for eyelashes is _____.

3. The glands responsible for tears are called _____ glands.

4. The clear, transparent portion of the sclera is called the _____.

5. The innermost layer of the eye, which is composed of sensory receptors, is the _____.

6. The pupil of the eye is actually a hole in the _____.

7. The three bones in the middle ear are the _____, _____, and _____.

8. The study of the ear is called _____.

9. Another term for the eardrum is _____.

10. _____ is produced in the oil glands in the auditory canal.

11. The _____ tube connects the nasopharynx with the middle ear.

12. The _____ is responsible for conducting impulses from the ear to the brain.

B. Pharmacology Challenge

Fill in the classification for each drug description, then match the brand name.

Drug Description	Classification	Brand Name
1. _____ treats dry eyes	_____	a. Atropine-Care
2. _____ reduces intraocular pressure	_____	b. Allergan Ear Drops
3. _____ ear drops for ear infection	_____	c. Timoptic
4. _____ dilates pupil	_____	d. Opticaine
5. _____ treats nausea from vertigo	_____	e. Debrox Drops
6. _____ eye drops for bacterial infection	_____	f. Eserine Sulfate
7. _____ treats ear itching	_____	g. Antivert
8. _____ constricts pupil	_____	h. Refresh Plus
9. _____ softens cerumen	_____	i. Otocort
10. _____ eye drops for pain	_____	j. Del-Mycin

C. Combining Form Practice

The combining form **blephar/o** refers to the eyelid. Use it to write a term that means:

1. inflammation of the eyelid _____

2. surgical repair of the eyelid _____

3. drooping of the upper eyelid _____

The combining form **retin/o** refers to the retina. Use it to write a term that means:

4. a disease of the retina _____

5. surgical fixation of the retina _____

The combining form **ophthalm/o** refers to the eye. Use it to write a term that means:

6. the study of the eye _____

7. pertaining to the eye _____

8. an eye examination using a scope _____

The combining form **irid/o** refers to the iris. Use it to write a term that means:

9. iris paralysis _____

10. removal of the iris _____

The combining form **ot/o** refers to the ear. Write a word that means:

11. ear surgical repair _____

12. pus flow from the ear _____

13. pain in the ear _____

14. inflammation of the ear _____

The combining form **tympan/o** refers to the eardrum. Write a word that means:

15. eardrum rupture _____

16. eardrum incision _____

17. eardrum inflammation _____

The combining form **audi/o** refers to hearing. Write a word that means:

18. record of hearing _____

19. instrument to measure hearing _____

20. study of hearing _____

D. Name That Suffix

	Suffix	Example from Chapter
1. to turn		
2. vision		
3. inflammation of		
4. the study of		
5. cutting into		
6. surgical repair		
7. surgical fixation		
8. pain		
9. ear condition		
10. hearing		

E. Define the Combining Form

	Definition	Example from Chapter
1. dacry/o		
2. uve/o		
3. aque/o		
4. phot/o		
5. kerat/o		
6. vitre/o		
7. dipl/o		
8. glauc/o		
9. presby/o		
10. ambly/o		
11. aur/o		
12. staped/o		
13. acous/o		
14. salping/o		
15. myring/o		

F. Answer the Question

1. Describe the difference between conductive hearing loss and sensorineural hearing loss. _____

_____

2. List in order the eyeball structures light rays pass through: _____, _____,

_____, _____

3. Describe the role of the conjunctiva. _____

_____

4. List the ossicles and what they do. _____

_____

G. Terminology Matching

Match each term to its definition.

1. _____ emmetropia   a. opacity of the lens

2. _____ sclera   b. muscle regulating size of pupil

3. _____ cataract   c. nearsightedness

4. _____ conjunctiva   d. protective membrane of eye

5. _____ iris   e. blind spot

6. _____ xerophthalmia   f. involuntary movements of eye

7. _____ myopia   g. white of eye

8. _____ nystagmus   h. normal vision

9. _____ optic disk   i. dry eyes

10. _____ vitreous humor   j. material filling eyeball

H. What Does it Stand For?

1. Oto _____

2. OU _____

3. REM _____

4. Hz _____

5. SMD _____

6. PERRLA _____

7. IOP _____

8. dB _____

9. OD _____

10. VF _____

I. Terminology Matching

Match each term to its definition.

1. _____ myringotomy   a. removal of stapes bone

2. _____ tympanoplasty   b. reconstruction of eardrum

3. _____ otoplasty   c. surgical puncture of eardrum

4. _____ stapedectomy   d. change size of pinna

5. _____ anacusis   e. absence of hearing

6. _____ falling test   f. treats sensorineural hearing loss

7. _____ PE tube   g. tuning fork tests

8. _____ cochlear implant   h. swimmer's ear

9. _____ otitis externa   i. drains off fluid

10. _____ Rinne & Weber   j. balance test

J. What's the Abbreviation?

1. pressure equalizing tube _____

2. eye, ear, nose, and throat _____

3. bone conduction _____

4. both ears _____

5. otitis media _____

6. emmetropia _____

7. exotropia _____

8. left eye _____

9. extraocular movement _____

10. visual acuity _____

K. Fill in the Blank

emmetropia	tonometry	Ménière's disease
hyperopia	cataract	hordeolum
acoustic neuroma	strabismus	myopia
otorhinolaryngologist	presbycusis	
conjunctivitis	inner ear	

1. Cheri is having a regular eye checkup. The pressure reading test that the physician will do to detect glaucoma is

   _____.

2. Carlos's ophthalmologist tells him that he has normal vision. This is called _____.

3. Ana has been given an antibiotic eye ointment for pink eye. The medical term for this condition is _____.

4. Adrian is nearsighted and cannot read signs in the distance. This is called _____.

5. Ivan is scheduled to have surgery to have the opaque lens of his right eye removed. This condition is a(n)

   _____.

6. Roberto has developed a stye on the corner of his left eye. He has been told to treat it with hot compresses. This condition

   is called a(n) _____.

7. Judith has twin boys with crossed eyes that will require surgical correction. The medical term for this condition is

   _____.

8. Beth is farsighted and has difficulty reading textbooks. Her eyeglass correction will be for _____.

9. Grace was told by her physician that her hearing loss was a part of the aging process. The term for this is

   _____.

10. Stacey is having frequent middle ear infections and wishes to be treated by a specialist. She would go to a(n)

    _____.

11. Warren was told that his dizziness may be caused by a problem in the _____ area.

12. Shantel is suffering from an abnormal condition of the inner ear, vertigo, and tinnitus. She may have

    _____.

13. Keisha was told that her tumor of the eighth cranial nerve was benign, but she still experienced a hearing loss as a result

    of the tumor. This tumor is called a(n) _____.

L. Define the Term

1. amblyopia _____

2. diplopia _____

3. mydriatic _____

4. miotic _____

5. presbyopia _____

6. tinnitus _____

7. stapes _____

8. tympanometry _____

9. eustachian tube _____

10. labyrinth _____

11. audiogram _____

12. otitis media _____

MEDICAL TERMINOLOGY INTERACTIVE

Medical Terminology Interactive is a premium online homework management system that includes a host of features to help you study. Registered users will find:

- Fun games and activities built within a virtual hospital
- Powerful tools that track and analyze your results—allowing you to create a personalized learning experience
- Videos, flashcards, and audio pronunciations to help enrich your progress
- Streaming video lesson presentations and self-paced learning modules

www.pearsonhighered.com/mti

Labeling Exercise

Write the labels for this figure on the numbered lines provided.

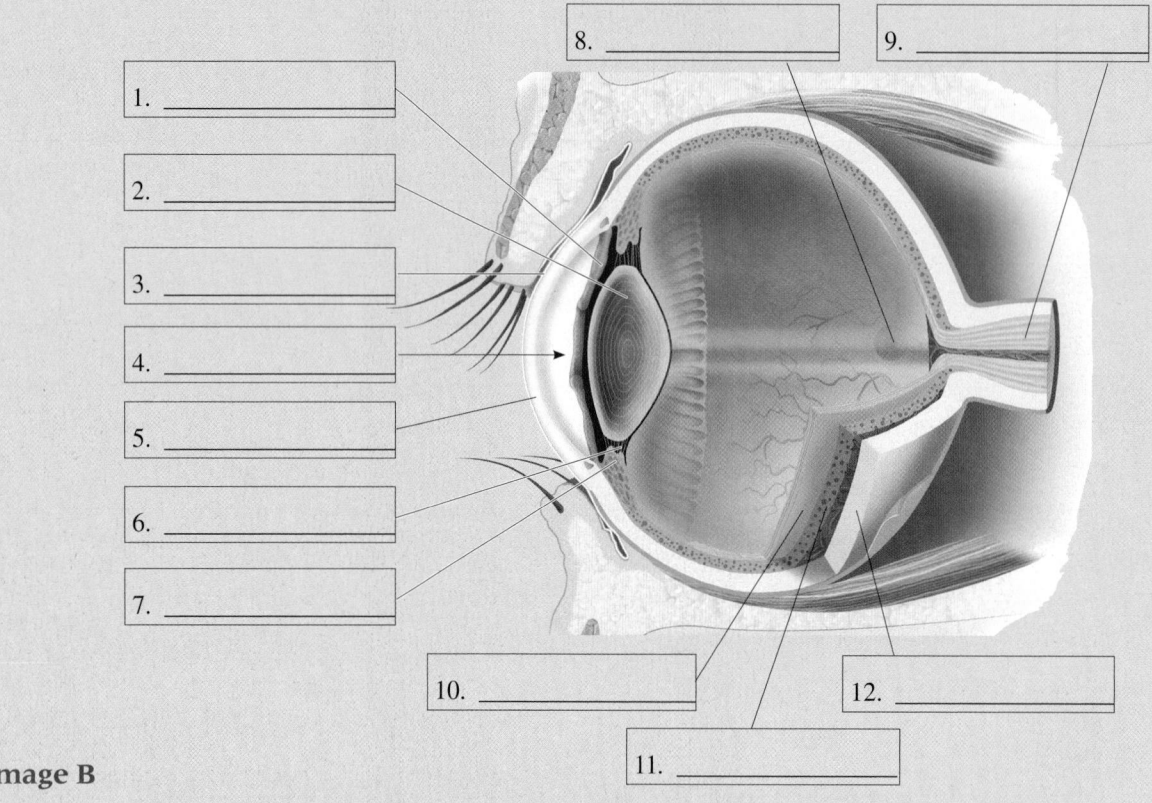

8. _____   9. _____

1. _____

2. _____

3. _____

4. _____

5. _____

6. _____

7. _____

10. _____   12. _____

11. _____

Image B

Write the labels for this figure on the numbered lines provided.

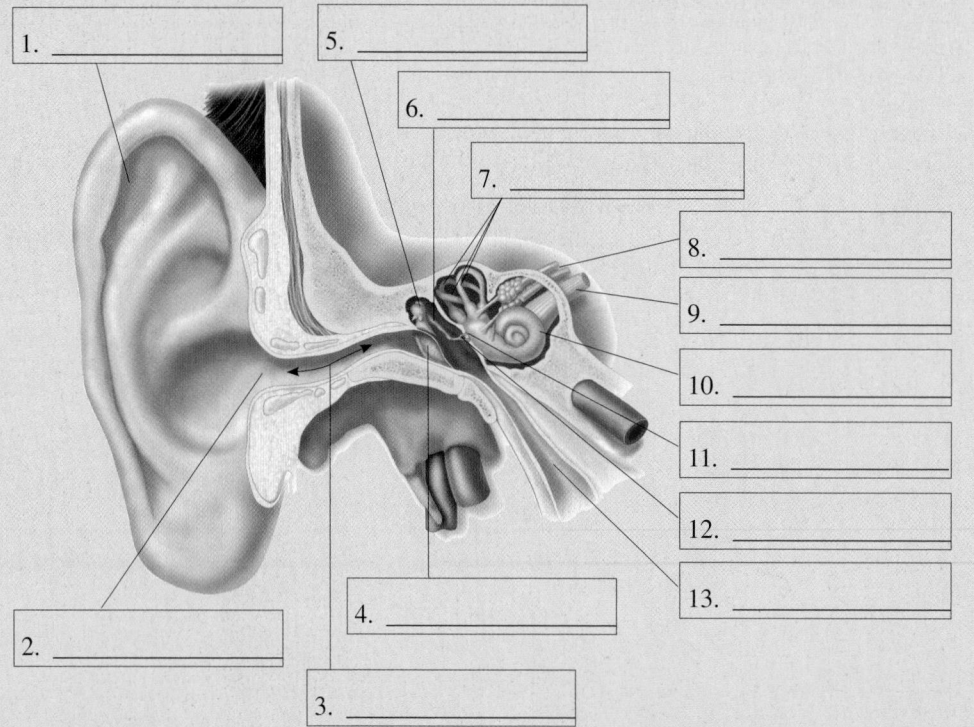

1. _____   5. _____

6. _____

7. _____

8. _____

9. _____

10. _____

11. _____

12. _____

13. _____

2. _____

4. _____

3. _____

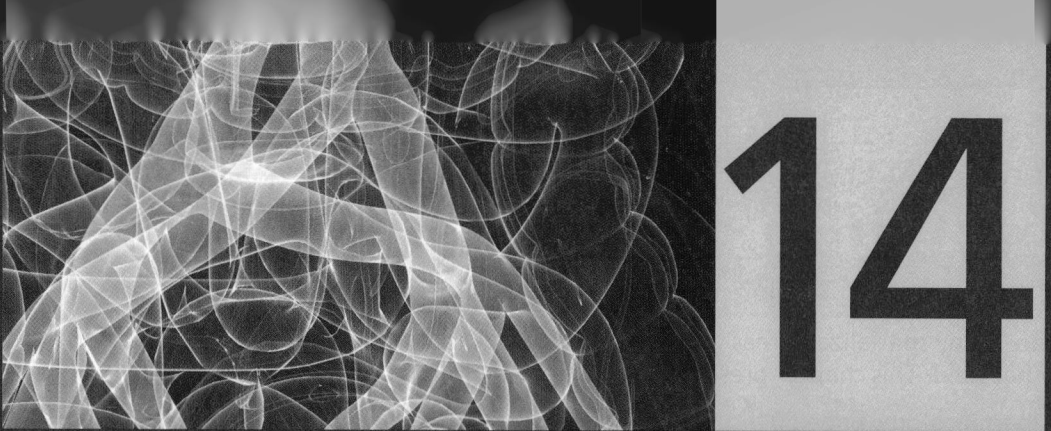

14

SPECIAL TOPICS

Learning Objectives

Upon completion of this chapter, you will be able to

- Identify and define the combining forms and suffixes introduced in this chapter.

- Correctly spell and pronounce medical terms relating to the medical fields introduced in this chapter.

- Describe pertinent information relating to pharmacology.

- Describe pertinent information relating to mental health.

- Describe pertinent information relating to diagnostic imaging.

- Describe pertinent information relating to rehabilitation services.

- Describe pertinent information relating to surgery.

- Describe pertinent information relating to oncology.

- Identify and define vocabulary terms relating to the topics.

- Identify and define selected pathology terms relating to the topics.

- Identify and define selected diagnostic procedures relating to the topics.

- Identify and define selected therapeutic procedures relating to the topics.

- Define selected abbreviations associated with the topics.

Introduction

There are many specialized areas within medicine, and each has medical terms relating to that field. This chapter presents medical terminology from six of these fields:

1. Pharmacology, page 501
2. Mental Health, page 510
3. Diagnostic Imaging, page 517
4. Rehabilitation Services, page 524
5. Surgery, page 530
6. Oncology, page 536

Section I: Pharmacology at a Glance

Word Parts

Here are the most common word parts (with their meanings) used to build pharmacy terms.

Combining Forms

aer/o	air	muscul/o	muscle
bucc/o	cheek	or/o	mouth
chem/o	drug	pharmac/o	drug
cutane/o	skin	rect/o	rectum
derm/o	skin	thec/o	sheath (meninges)
enter/o	intestine	topic/o	a specific area
hal/o	to breathe	toxic/o	poison
iatr/o	physician, medicine, treatment	vagin/o	vagina
		ven/o	vein
idi/o	distinctive		
lingu/o	tongue		

Suffixes

-al	pertaining to	-ical	pertaining to
-ary	pertaining to	-ist	specialist
-genic	produced by	-logy	study of
-ic	pertaining to	-phylaxis	protection

Prefixes

anti-	against	para-	near, beside
contra-	against	pro-	before
in-	inward	sub-	under
intra-	within	trans-	through

Pharmacology

pharmacology (far-ma-KALL-oh-jee)

Pharmacology is the study of the origin, characteristics, and effects of drugs. Drugs are obtained from many different sources. Some drugs, such as vitamins, are found naturally in the foods we eat. Others, such as hormones, are obtained from animals. Penicillin and some of the other antibiotics are developed from mold, which is a fungus. Plants have been the source of many of today's drugs. Many drugs, such as those used in chemotherapy, are synthetic, meaning they are developed by artificial means in a laboratory.

Drug Names

brand name

chemical name

generic name

nonproprietary name
  (non-prah-PRYE-ah-tair-ee)

pharmaceutical (far-mih-SOO-tih-kal)

pharmacist (FAR-mah-sist)

proprietary name
  (proh-PRYE-ah-tair-ee)

trademark

All drugs are chemicals. The **chemical name** describes the chemical formula or molecular structure of a particular drug. For example, the chemical name for ibuprofen, an over-the-counter pain medication, is 2-*p*-isobutylphenyl propionic acid. Just as in this case, chemical names are usually very long, so a shorter name is given to the drug. This name is the **generic** or **nonproprietary name,** and it is recognized and accepted as the official name for a drug.

Each drug has only one generic name, such as ibuprofen, and this name is not subject to copyright protection, so any **pharmaceutical** manufacturer may use it. However, the pharmaceutical company that originally developed the drug has exclusive rights to produce it for 17 years. After that time, any manufacturer may produce and sell the drug. When a company manufactures a drug for sale, it must choose a **brand name,** or **proprietary name** for its product. This is the company's **trademark** for the drug. For example, ibuprofen is known by several brand names, including Motrin™, Advil™, and Nuprin™. All three contain the same ibuprofen; they are just marketed by different pharmaceutical companies. (See Table 14.1 ■ for examples of different drug names.)

Generic drugs are usually priced lower than brand name drugs. A physician can indicate on the prescription if the **pharmacist** may substitute a generic drug for a brand name. The physician may prefer that a particular brand name drug be used if he or she believes it to be more effective than the generic drug.

> **MED TERM TIP**
>
> The terms *drug* and *medication* have the same meaning. However, the general public often uses the term *drug* to refer to a narcotic type of medication. The term can also mean illegal chemical substances. For purposes of medical terminology, use of the word *drug* means medication.

> **MED TERM TIP**
>
> Look for these word parts:
>
> chem/o = drug
> pharmac/o = drug
> -al = pertaining to
> -ary = pertaining to
> -ic = pertaining to
> -ical = pertaining to
> -ist = specialist
> -logy = study of

Table 14.1	Examples of Different Drug Names	
CHEMICAL NAME	**GENERIC NAME**	**BRAND NAMES**
2-*p*-isobutylphenyl propionic acid	Ibuprofen	Motrin™
		Advil™
		Nuprin™
Acetylsalicylic acid	Aspirin	Anacin™
		Bufferin™
		Excedrin™
S-2-[1-(methylamino) ethyl] benzenemethanol hydrochloride	Pseudoephedrine hydrochloride	Sudafed™
		Actifed™
		Nucofed™

Legal Classification of Drugs

controlled substances

Drug Enforcement Agency

over-the-counter drug

prescription (prih-SKRIP-shun)

prescription drug (prih-SKRIP-shun)

A **prescription drug** can only be ordered by licensed healthcare practitioners such as physicians, dentists, or physician assistants. These drugs must include the words "Caution: Federal law prohibits dispensing without prescription" on their labels. Antibiotics, such as penicillin, and heart medications, such as digoxin, are available only by prescription. A **prescription** is the written explanation to the pharmacist regarding the name of the medication, the dosage, and the times of administration. A licensed practitioner can also give a prescription order orally to a pharmacist.

A drug that does not require a prescription is referred to as an **over-the-counter** (OTC) **drug.** Many medications or drugs can be purchased without a prescription, for example, aspirin, antacids, and antidiarrheal medications. However, taking aspirin along with an anticoagulant, such as coumadin, can cause internal bleeding in some people, and OTC antacids interfere with the absorption of the prescription drug tetracycline into the body. It is better for the physician or pharmacist to advise the patient on the proper OTC drugs to use with prescription drugs.

Certain drugs are **controlled substances** if they have a potential for being addictive (habit forming) or can be abused. The **Drug Enforcement Agency** (DEA) enforces the control of these drugs. Some of the more commonly prescribed controlled substances are:

- butabarbital
- chloral hydrate
- codeine
- diazepam
- oxycontin
- morphine
- phenobarbital
- secobarbital

Controlled drugs are classified as Schedule I through Schedule V, indicating their potential for abuse. The differences between each schedule are listed in Table 14.2 ■.

MED TERM TIP

It is critical that patients receive the correct drug, but it is not possible to list or remember all the drug names. You must acquire the habit of looking up any drug name you do not recognize in the *Physician's Desk Reference (PDR)*. Every medical office or medical facility should have a copy of this book.

Table 14.2	Schedule for Controlled Substances
CLASSIFICATION	**MEANING**
Schedule I	Drugs with the highest potential for addiction and abuse. They are not accepted for medical use. Examples are heroin and LSD.
Schedule II	Drugs with a high potential for addiction and abuse accepted for medical use in the United States. Examples are codeine, cocaine, morphine, opium, and secobarbital.
Schedule III	Drugs with a moderate to low potential for addiction and abuse. Examples are butabarbital, anabolic steroids, and acetaminophen with codeine.
Schedule IV	Drugs with a lower potential for addiction and abuse than Schedule III drugs. Examples are chloral hydrate, phenobarbital, and diazepam.
Schedule V	Drugs with a low potential for addiction and abuse. An example is low-strength codeine combined with other drugs to suppress coughing.

How to Read a Prescription

A prescription is not difficult to read once you understand the symbols that are used. Symbols and abbreviations based on Latin and Greek words are used to save time for the physician. For example, the abbreviation po, meaning to be taken by mouth, comes from the Latin term *per os,* which means "by mouth."

See Figure 14.1 ■ for an example of a prescription. In this example, the prescribed medication (Rx) is Tagamet (a medication to reduce stomach acid) in the 800 milligram (mg) size. The instructions on the label are to say (Sig) to take 1 (ı–˙) by mouth (po) every (q) bedtime (hs). The pharmacist is to dispense (disp) 30 tablets (#30). The prescription concludes by informing the pharmacist to refill the prescription two times, and he or she may substitute with another medication. Each prescription must contain the date, physician's name, address, and Drug Enforcement Agency number as well as the patient's name and date of birth. The physician must also sign his or her name at the bottom of the prescription. A blank prescription cannot be handed to a patient.

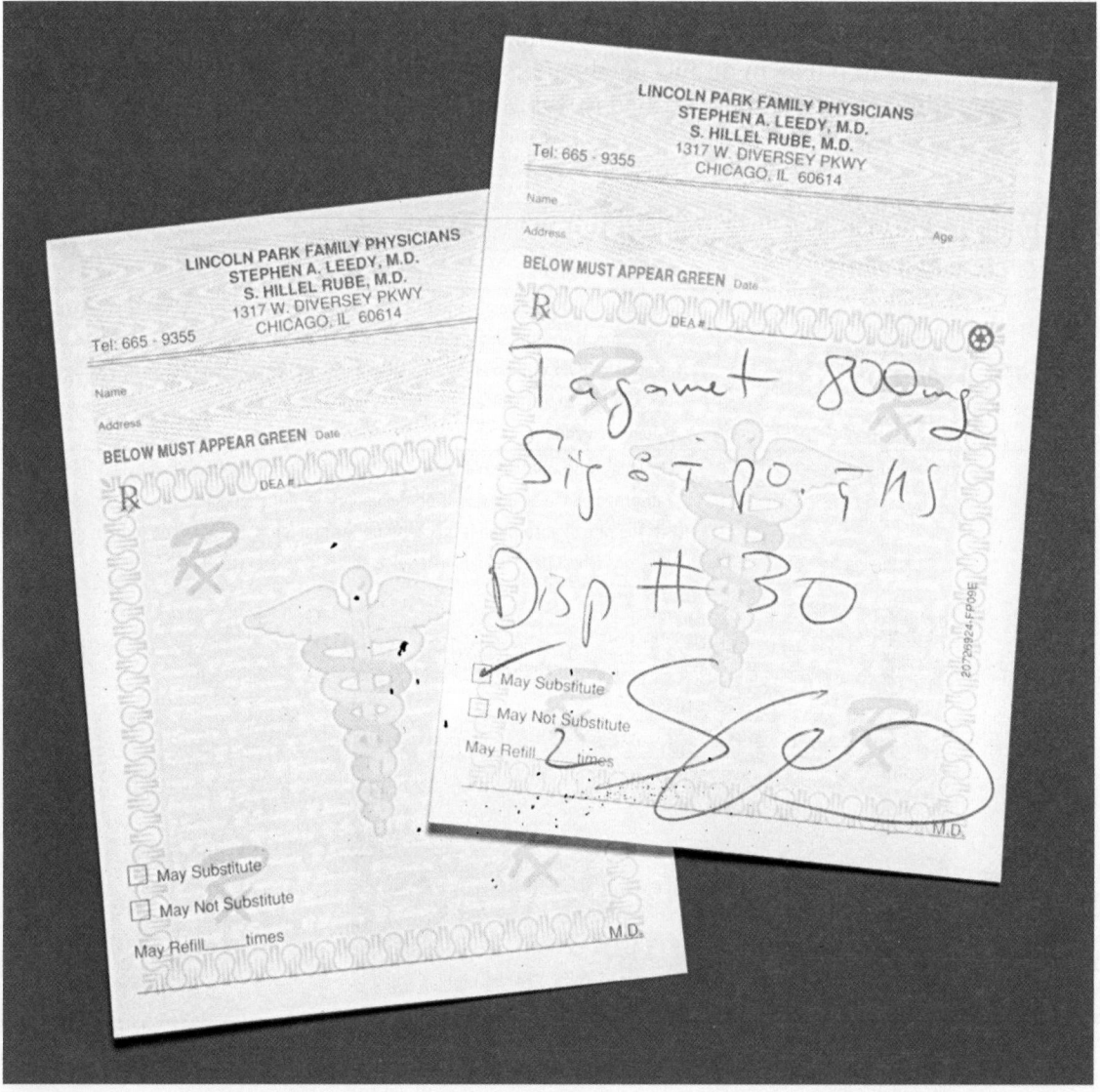

■ **Figure 14.1** A sample prescription written by a physician.

The physician's instruction to the patient will be placed on the label. The pharmacist will also include instructions about the medication and alert the patient to side effects that may need to be reported to the physician. In addition, any special instructions regarding the medication (i.e., take with meals, do not take along with dairy products) will also be supplied by the pharmacist.

Routes and Methods of Drug Administration

aerosol (AIR-oh-sol)

buccal (BUCK-al)

eardrops

eyedrops

inhalation (in-hah-LAY-shun)

oral (OR-al)

parenteral (par-EN-ter-al)

rectal (REK-tal)

sublingual (sub-LING-gwal)

suppositories (suh-POZ-ih-tor-ees)

topical (TOP-ih-kal)

transdermal (tranz-DER-mal)

vaginal (VAJ-in-al)

MED TERM TIP

Many abbreviations have multiple meanings, such as od, which can mean overdose (od) or right eye (OD), depending on whether the letters are lowercase or uppercase. Care must be taken when reading abbreviations since some may be written too quickly, making them difficult to decipher. Never create your own abbreviations. Some of the most common abbreviations are listed above.

The method by which a drug is introduced into the body is referred to as the *route of administration*. To be effective, drugs must be administered by a particular route. In some cases, there may be a variety of routes by which a drug can be administered. For instance, the female hormone estrogen can be administered orally in pill form or by a patch applied to the skin. The most common routes of administration are described in Table 14.3 ■.

Table 14.3	Common Routes of Drug Administration	
METHOD	**WORD PARTS**	**DESCRIPTION**
oral	or/o = mouth -al = pertaining to	Includes all drugs given by mouth. The advantages are ease of administration and a slow rate of absorption via the stomach and intestinal wall. The disadvantages include slowness of absorption and destruction of some chemical compounds by gastric juices. In addition, some medications, such as aspirin, can have a corrosive action on the stomach lining.
sublingual	sub- = under lingu/o = tongue -al = pertaining to	Includes drugs that are held under the tongue and not swallowed. The medication is absorbed by the blood vessels on the underside of the tongue as the saliva dissolves it. The rate of absorption is quicker than the oral route. Nitroglycerin to treat angina pectoris (chest pain) is administered by this route.
inhalation	in- = inward hal/o = to breathe	Includes drugs inhaled directly into the nose and mouth. **Aerosol** sprays are administered by this route (see Figure 14.3). ■

■ **Figure 14.2** Sublingual medication administration. Photograph of a male patient placing a nitroglycerine tablet under his tongue.

Table 14.3   Common Routes of Drug Administration (continued)

METHOD	WORD PARTS	DESCRIPTION

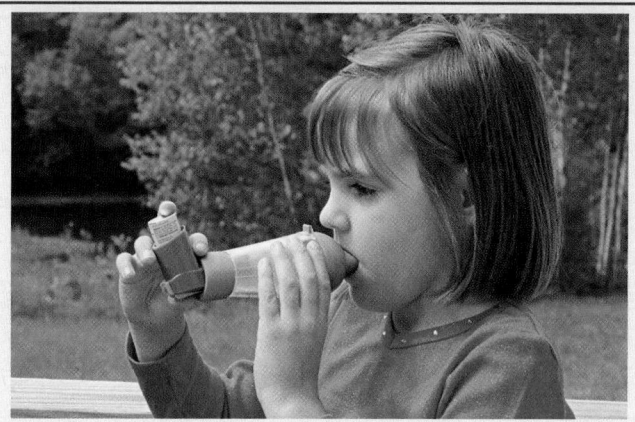

Figure 14.3 Inhalation medication administration. Photograph of a young girl using a metered-dose inhaler.

METHOD	WORD PARTS	DESCRIPTION
parenteral	para- = near, beside enter/o = intestine -al = pertaining to	An invasive method of administering drugs as it requires the skin to be punctured by a needle. The needle with syringe attached is introduced either under the skin or into a muscle, vein, or body cavity.
intracavitary (in-trah-KAV-ih-tair-ee)	intra- = within -ary = pertaining to	Injection into a body cavity such as the peritoneal and chest cavity.
intradermal (ID) (in-trah-DER-mal)	intra- = within derm/o = skin -al = pertaining to	Very shallow injection just under the top layer of skin. Commonly used in skin testing for allergies and tuberculosis testing.

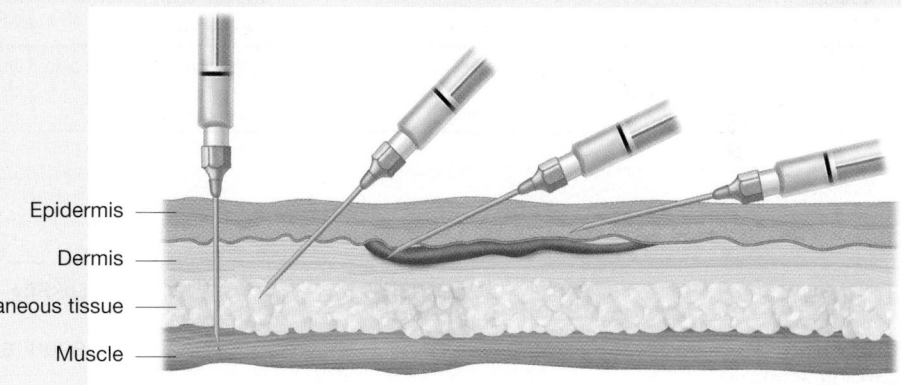

Intramuscular   Subcutaneous   Intravenous   Intradermal

Epidermis
Dermis
Subcutaneous tissue
Muscle

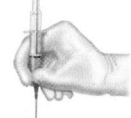 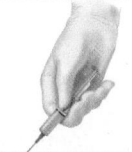 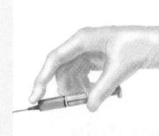

Intramuscular   Subcutaneous   Intravenous   Intradermal

Figure 14.4 Parenteral medication administration. The angle of needle insertion for four different types of parenteral injections.

METHOD	WORD PARTS	DESCRIPTION
intramuscular (IM) (in-trah-MUSS-kyoo-lar)	intra- = within muscul/o = muscle -ar = pertaining to	Injection directly into the muscle of the buttocks, thigh, or upper arm. Used when there is a large amount of medication or it is irritating (see again Figure 14.4).
intrathecal (in-trah-THEE-kal)	intra- = within thec/o = sheath (meninges) -al = pertaining to	Injection into the meningeal space surrounding the brain and spinal cord.

(Continued)

Table 14.3	Common Routes of Drug Administration (continued)	
METHOD	**WORD PARTS**	**DESCRIPTION**
intravenous (IV) (in-trah-VEE-nus)	intra- = within ven/o = vein -ous = pertaining to	Injection into the veins. This route may be set up to deliver medication very quickly or to deliver a continuous drip of medication (see again Figure 14.4).
subcutaneous (SC) (sub-kyoo-TAY-nee-us)	sub- = under cutane/o = skin -ous = pertaining to	Injection into the subcutaneous layer of the skin, usually the upper, outer arm or abdomen (see again Figure 14.4); for example, insulin injection.
transdermal	trans- = through derm/o = skin -al = pertaining to	Includes medications that coat the underside of a patch, which is applied to the skin where it is then absorbed. Examples include birth control patches, nicotine patches, and sea sickness patches.
rectal	rect/o = rectum -al = pertaining to	Includes medications introduced directly into the rectal cavity in the form of **suppositories** or solution. Drugs may have to be administered by this route if the patient is unable to take them by mouth due to nausea, vomiting, or surgery.
topical	topic/o = a specific area -al = pertaining to	Includes medications applied directly to the skin or mucous membranes. They are distributed in ointment, cream, or lotion form, and are used to treat skin infections and eruptions.
vaginal	vagin/o = vagina -al = pertaining to	Includes tablets and suppositories that may be inserted vaginally to treat vaginal yeast infections and other irritations.
eyedrops		Includes drops used during eye examinations to dilate the pupil of the eye for better examination of the interior of the eye. They are also placed into the eye to control eye pressure in glaucoma and treat infections.
eardrops		Includes drops placed directly into the ear canal for the purpose of relieving pain or treating infection.
buccal	bucc/o = cheek -al = pertaining to	Includes drugs that are placed under the lip or between the cheek and gum.

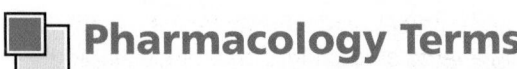

Pharmacology Terms

TERM	WORD PARTS	DEFINITION
addiction (ah-DICK-shun)		Acquired dependence on a drug.
additive		Sum of the action of two (or more) drugs given. In this case, the total strength of the medications is equal to the sum of the strength of each individual drug.
antidote (AN-tih-doht)	anti- = against	Substance that will neutralize poisons or their side effects.
broad spectrum		Ability of a drug to be effective against a wide range of microorganisms.
contraindication (kon-trah-in-dih-KAY-shun)	contra- = against	Condition in which a particular drug should not be used.
cumulative action		Action that occurs in the body when a drug is allowed to accumulate or stay in the body.

Pharmacology Terms (continued)

TERM	WORD PARTS	DEFINITION
drug interaction		Occurs when the effect of one drug is altered because it was taken at the same time as another drug.
drug tolerance		Decrease in susceptibility to a drug after continued use of the drug.
habituation (hah-bich-yoo-AY-shun)		Development of an emotional dependence on a drug due to repeated use.
iatrogenic (eye-ah-troh-JEN-ik)	iatr/o = medicine -genic = produced by	Usually an unfavorable response resulting from taking a medication.
idiosyncrasy (id-ee-oh-SIN-krah-see)	idi/o = distinctive	Unusual or abnormal response to a drug or food.
placebo (plah-SEE-boh)		Inactive, harmless substance used to satisfy a patient's desire for medication. This is also used in research when given to a control group of patients in a study in which another group receives a drug. The effect of the placebo versus the drug is then observed.
potentiation (poe-ten-chee-A-shun)		Giving a patient a second drug to boost (potentiate) the effect of another drug. The total strength of the drugs is greater than the sum of the strength of the individual drugs.
prophylaxis (proh-fih-LAK-sis)	pro- = before -phylaxis = protection	Prevention of disease. For example, an antibiotic can be used to prevent the occurrence of a disease.
side effect		Response to a drug other than the effect desired. Also called an *adverse reaction*.
tolerance (TAHL-er-ans)		Development of a capacity for withstanding a large amount of a substance, such as foods, drugs, or poison, without any adverse effect. A decreased sensitivity to further doses will develop.
toxicity (tok-SISS-ih-tee)	toxic/o = poison	Extent or degree to which a substance is poisonous.
unit dose		Drug dosage system that provides prepackaged, prelabeled, individual medications that are ready for immediate use by the patient.

Abbreviations

@	at		NPO	nothing by mouth
ā	before		NS	normal saline
ac	before meals		od	overdose
ad lib	as desired		oint	ointment
ante	before		OTC	over the counter
APAP	acetaminophen (Tylenol™)		oz	ounce
aq	aqueous (water)		p̄	after
ASA	aspirin		pc	after meals
bid	twice a day		PCA	patient-controlled administration
c̄	with		PDR	*Physician's Desk Reference*
cap(s)	capsule(s)		per	with
d	day		po	by mouth
d/c, DISC	discontinue		prn	as needed
DC, disc	discontinue		pt	patient
DEA	Drug Enforcement Agency		q	every
dil	dilute		qam	every morning
disp	dispense		qh	every hour
dtd	give of such a dose		qhs	at bedtime
Dx	diagnosis		qid	four times a day
et	and		qs	quantity sufficient
FDA	Federal Drug Administration		Rx	take
gm	gram		s̄	without
gr	grain		SC	subcutaneous
gt	drop		Sig	label as follows/directions
gtt	drops		sl	under the tongue
hs	at bedtime		sol	solution
ī	one		s̄s̄	one-half
ID	intradermal		stat	at once/immediately
īī	two		Subc, SubQ	subcutaneous
īīī	three		suppos, supp	suppository
IM	intramuscular		susp	suspension
inj	injection		syr	syrup
IU	international unit		T, tbsp	tablespoon
IV	intravenous		t, tsp	teaspoon
kg	kilogram		tab	tablet
L	liter		tid	three times a day
mcg	microgram		TO	telephone order
mEq	milliequivalent		top	apply topically
mg	milligram		u	unit
mL	milliliter		VO	verbal order
no sub	no substitute		wt	weight
noc	night		x	times
non rep	do not repeat			

Section II: Mental Health at a Glance

Word Parts

Here are the most common word parts (with their meanings) used to build mental health terms.

Combining Forms

amnes/o	forgetfulness		path/o	disease
anxi/o	fear, worry		ped/o	child
chondr/o	cartilage		pharmac/o	drug
compuls/o	drive, compel		phob/o	irrational fear
deluss/o	false belief		phren/o	mind
depress/o	to press down		psych/o	mind
electr/o	electricity		pyr/o	fire
factiti/o	artificial, contrived		schiz/o	split
hallucin/o	imagined perception		soci/o	society
klept/o	to steal		somat/o	body
ment/o	mind		somn/o	sleep
obsess/o	besieged by thoughts			

Suffixes

-al	pertaining to		-logist	one who studies
-ar	pertaining to		-logy	study of
-ia	state, condition		-mania	frenzy
-iatrist	physician		-orexia	appetite
-iatry	medical treatment		-ous	pertaining to
-ic	pertaining to		-philia	attracted to
-ism	state of		-therapy	treatment
-logical	pertaining to the study of		-tic	pertaining to

Prefixes

an-	without		dis-	apart
anti-	against		ex-	outward
auto-	self		hyper-	excessive
bi-	two		hypo-	below
de-	without		in-	not

Mental Health Disciplines

Psychology

abnormal psychology	**normal psychology**
clinical psychologist (sigh-KALL-oh-jist)	**psychology** (sigh-KALL-oh-jee)

> **MED TERM TIP**
>
> All social interactions pose some problems for some people. These problems are not necessarily abnormal. One means of judging if behavior is abnormal is to compare one person's behavior with others in the community. Also, if a person's behavior interferes with the activities of daily living, it is often considered abnormal.

Psychology is the study of human behavior and thought processes. This behavioral science is primarily concerned with understanding how human beings interact with their physical environment and with each other. Behavior can be divided into two categories: normal and abnormal. The study of **normal psychology** includes how the personality develops, how people handle stress, and the stages of mental development. In contrast, **abnormal psychology** studies and treats behaviors that are outside of normal and that are detrimental to the person or society. These maladaptive behaviors range from occasional difficulty coping with stress, to bizarre actions and beliefs, to total withdrawal. A **clinical psychologist,** though not a physician, is a specialist in evaluating and treating persons with mental and emotional disorders.

Psychiatry

psychiatric nurse (sigh-kee-AT-rik)	**psychiatrist** (sigh-KIGH-ah-trist)
psychiatric social worker	**psychiatry** (sigh-KIGH-ah-tree)

> **MED TERM TIP**
>
> Look for these word parts:
>
> psych/o = mind
> -iatrist = physician
> -iatry = medical treatment
> -logist = one who studies
> -logy = study of

Psychiatry is the branch of medicine that deals with the diagnosis, treatment, and prevention of mental disorders. A **psychiatrist** is a medical physician specializing in the care of patients with mental, emotional, and behavioral disorders. Other health professions also have specialty areas in caring for clients with mental illness. Good examples are **psychiatric nurses** and **psychiatric social workers.**

Pathology

The legal definition of mental disorder is "impaired judgment and lack of self-control." The guide for terminology and classifications relating to psychiatric disorders is the *Diagnostic and Statistical Manual of Mental Disorders, Fourth Edition* (Text Revision) (DSM-IV-TR™), which is published by the American Psychiatric Association (2004). The DSM organizes mental disorders into 14 major diagnostic categories of mental disorders.

> **MED TERM TIP**
>
> Mental disorders are sometimes more simply characterized by whether they are a *neurosis* or a *psychosis*. Neuroses are inappropriate coping mechanisms to handle stress, such as phobias and panic attacks. Psychoses involve extreme distortions of reality and disorganization of a person's thinking, including bizarre behaviors, hallucinations, and delusions. Schizophrenia is an example of a psychosis.

TERM	WORD PARTS	DEFINITION
Anxiety disorders	anxi/o = fear, worry	Characterized by persistent worry and apprehension.
panic attacks	-ic = pertaining to	Feeling of intense apprehension, terror, or sense of impending danger.
anxiety (ang-ZY-eh-tee)	anxi/o = fear, worry	Feeling of dread in the absence of a clearly identifiable stress trigger.
phobias (FOH-bee-ahs)	phob/o = irrational fear -ia = state, condition	Irrational fear, such as *arachnophobia*, or fear of spiders.

■ Pathology (continued)

TERM	WORD PARTS	DEFINITION
obsessive–compulsive disorder (OCD) (ob-SESS-iv / kom-PUHL-siv)	obsess/o = besieged by thoughts compuls/o = drive, compel	Performing repetitive rituals to reduce anxiety.
Cognitive disorders		Deterioration of mental functions due to temporary brain or permanent brain dysfunction.
dementia (dee-MEN-she-ah)	de- = without ment/o = mind -ia = state, condition	Progressive confusion and disorientation.
Alzheimer's disease (ALTS-high-merz)		Degenerative brain disorder with gradual loss of cognitive abilities.
Disorders diagnosed in infancy and childhood		Mental disorders associated with childhood; include:
mental retardation	ment/o = mind -al = pertaining to	Subaverage intellectual functioning.
attention-deficit/hyperactivity disorder (ADHD)	hyper- = excessive	Inattention and impulsive behavior.
autism (AW-tizm)	auto- = self -ism = state of	Condition involving deficits in social interaction, communication skills, and restricted patterns of behavior.
Dissociative disorders	dis- = apart soci/o = society	Disorders in which severe emotional conflict is so repressed that a split in the personality may occur or the person may lose memory.
amnesia (am-NEE-zee-ah)	amnes/o = forgetfulness -ia = state, condition	Loss of memory.
dissociative identity disorder		Having two or more distinct personalities.
Eating disorders		Abnormal behaviors related to eating; include:
anorexia nervosa (an-oh-REK-see-ah / ner-VOH-sah)	an- = without -orexia = appetite	Refusal to eat.

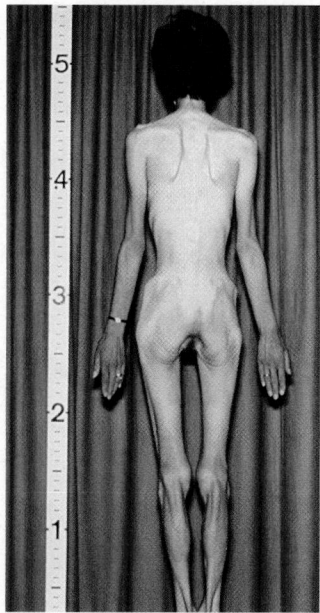

■ **Figure 14.5** Photograph of a young woman suffering from anorexia nervosa, posterior view. *(Custom Medical Stock Photo, Inc.)*

■ Pathology *(continued)*

TERM	WORD PARTS	DEFINITION
bulimia (boo-LIM-ee-ah)	-ia = state, condition	Binge eating and intentional vomiting.
Factitious disorders	factiti/o = artificial, contrived -ous = pertaining to	Intentionally feigning illness symptoms in order to gain attention.
malingering		Pretending to be ill or injured.
Impulse control disorders		Inability to resist an impulse to perform some act that is harmful to the individual or others; include:
kleptomania (klep-toh-MAY-nee-ah)	klept/o = to steal -mania = frenzy	Stealing.
pyromania (pie-roh-MAY-nee-ah)	pyr/o = fire -mania = frenzy	Setting fires.
explosive disorder	ex- = outward	Violent rages.
pathological gambling (path-ah-LOJ-ih-kal)	path/o = disease -logical = pertaining to the study of	Inability to stop gambling.
Mood disorders		Characterized by instability in mood; include:
major depression	depress/o = to press down	Feelings of hopelessness, helplessness, worthlessness; lack of pleasure in any activity; potential for suicide.
mania (MAY-nee-ah)	-mania = frenzy	Extreme elation.
bipolar disorder (BPD)	bi- = two -ar = pertaining to	Alternation between periods of deep depression and mania.

> **MED TERM TIP**
>
> The healthcare professional must take all threats of suicide from patients seriously. Psychologists tell us that there is no clear suicide type, which means that we cannot predict who will actually take his or her own life. Always tell the physician about any discussion a patient has concerning suicide. If you believe a patient is in danger of suicide, do not be afraid to ask, "Are you thinking about suicide?"

TERM	WORD PARTS	DEFINITION
Personality disorders		Inflexible or maladaptive behavior patterns that affect a person's ability to function in society; include:
paranoid personality disorder		Exaggerated feelings of persecution.
narcissistic personality disorder (nar-sis-SIST-ik)		Abnormal sense of self-importance.
antisocial personality disorder	anti- = against soci/o = society -al = pertaining to	Behaviors that are against legal or social norms.

Pathology *(continued)*

TERM	WORD PARTS	DEFINITION
passive aggressive personality		Indirect expression of hostility or anger.
Schizophrenia	schiz/o = split phren/o = mind -ia = state, condition	Mental disorders characterized by distortions of reality such as:
delusions (dee-LOO-zhuns)	deluss/o = false belief	A false belief held even in the face of contrary evidence.
hallucinations (hah-loo-sih-NAY-shuns)	hallucin/o = imagined perception	Perceiving something that is not there.
Sexual disorders		Disorders include aberrant sexual activity and sexual dysfunction; include:
pedophilia (pee-doh-FILL-ee-ah)	ped/o = child -philia = attracted to	Sexual interest in children.
masochism (MAS-oh-kizm)	-ism = state of	Gratification derived from being hurt or abused.
voyeurism (VOY-er-izm)	-ism = state of	Gratification derived from observing others engaged in sexual acts.
Sleeping disorders		Disorders relating to sleeping; include:
insomnia (in-SOM-nee-ah)	in- = not somn/o = sleep -ia = state, condition	Inability to sleep.
sleepwalking		Getting up and walking around unaware while sleeping.
Somatoform disorders	somat/o = body	Patient has physical symptoms for which no physical disease can be determined; include:
hypochondria (high-poh-KON-dree-ah)	hypo- = below chondr/o = cartilage -ia = state, condition	A preoccupation with health concerns. Named for the location of the liver and spleen, below the rib cartilage. The ancient Greeks thought these organs controlled mood.
conversion reaction		Anxiety is transformed into physical symptoms such as heart palpitations, paralysis, or blindness.
Substance-related disorders		Overindulgence or dependence on chemical substances including alcohol, illegal drugs, and prescription drugs.

Therapeutic Procedures

TERM	WORD PARTS	DEFINITION
Electroconvulsive therapy (ECT) (ee-lek-troh-kon-VULL-siv)	electr/o = electricity	Procedure occasionally used for cases of prolonged major depression. This controversial treatment involves placement of an electrode on one or both sides of the patient's head and a current is turned on briefly causing a convulsive seizure. A low level of voltage is used in modern electroconvulsive therapy, and the patient is administered a muscle relaxant and anesthesia. Advocates of this treatment state that it is a more effective way to treat severe depression than using drugs. It is not effective with disorders other than depression, such as schizophrenia and alcoholism.
Psychopharmacology (sigh-koh-far-mah-KALL-oh-jee)	psych/o = mind pharmac/o = drug -logy = study of	Study of the effects of drugs on the mind and particularly the use of drugs in treating mental disorders. The main classes of drugs for the treatment of mental disorders are:
antipsychotic drugs	anti- = against psych/o = mind -tic = pertaining to	Major tranquilizers include chlorpromazine (Thorazine™), haloperidol (Haldol™), clozapine (Clozaril™), and risperidone. These drugs have transformed the treatment of patients with psychoses and schizophrenia by reducing patient agitation and panic and shortening schizophrenic episodes. One of the side effects of these drugs is involuntary muscle movements, which approximately one-fourth of all adults who take the drugs develop.
antidepressant drugs	anti- = against depress/o = to press down	Classified as stimulants and alter the patient's mood by affecting levels of neurotransmitters in the brain. Antidepressants, such as serotonin norepinephrine reuptake inhibitors, are nonaddictive but they can produce unpleasant side effects such as dry mouth, weight gain, blurred vision, and nausea.
minor tranquilizers		Include Valium™ and Xanax™. These are also classified as central nervous system depressants and are prescribed for anxiety.
lithium		Special category of drug used successfully to calm patients who suffer from bipolar disorder (depression alternating with manic excitement).

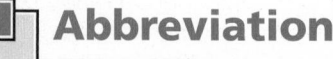 Therapeutic Procedures *(continued)*

TERM	WORD PARTS	DEFINITION
Psychotherapy (sigh-koh-THAIR-ah-pee)	psych/o = mind -therapy = treatment	A method of treating mental disorders by mental rather than chemical or physical means. It includes:
psychoanalysis	psych/o = mind	Method of obtaining a detailed account of the past and present emotional and mental experiences from the patient to determine the source of the problem and eliminate the effects. It is a system developed by Sigmund Freud that encourages the patient to discuss repressed, painful, or hidden experiences with the hope of eliminating or minimizing the problem.
humanistic psychotherapy	-tic = pertaining to psych/o = mind -therapy = treatment	Therapist does not delve into the patients' past when using these methods. Instead, it is believed that patients can learn how to use their own internal resources to deal with their problems. The therapist creates a therapeutic atmosphere, which builds patient self-esteem and encourages discussion of problems, thereby gaining insight in how to handle them. Also called *client-centered* or *nondirective psychotherapy.*
family and group psychotherapy	psych/o = mind -therapy = treatment	Often described as solution focused, the therapist places minimal emphasis on patient past history and strong emphasis on having patient state and discuss goals and then find a way to achieve them.

Abbreviations

AD	Alzheimer's disease	**ECT**	electroconvulsive therapy
ADD	attention-deficit disorder	**MA**	mental age
ADHD	attention-deficit/hyperactivity disorder	**MAO**	monoamine oxidase
BPD	bipolar disorder	**MMPI**	Minnesota Multiphasic Personality Inventory
CA	chronological age		
DSM	*Diagnostic and Statistical Manual of Mental Disorders*	**OCD**	obsessive–compulsive disorder
		SAD	seasonal affective disorder

Section III: Diagnostic Imaging at a Glance

Word Parts

Here are the most common word parts (with their meanings) used to build diagnostic imaging terms.

Combining Forms

anter/o	front	radi/o	ray (X-ray)
fluor/o	fluorescence, luminous	roentgen/o	X-ray
later/o	side	son/o	sound
nucle/o	nucleus	tom/o	to cut
poster/o	back		

Suffixes

-al	pertaining to	-logy	study of
-ar	pertaining to	-lucent	to shine through
-graphy	process of recording	-opaque	nontransparent
-ic	pertaining to	-scopy	process of visually examining
-ior	pertaining to		
-logist	one who studies		

Prefix

ultra-	beyond

Diagnostic Imaging

roentgenology (rent-gen-ALL-oh-jee)   **X-rays**

Diagnostic imaging is the medical specialty that uses a variety of methods to produce images of the internal structures of the body. These images are then used to diagnose disease. This area of medicine began as **roentgenology** (**roentgen/o** = X-ray; **-logy** = study of), named after German physicist Wilhelm Roentgen who discovered roentgen rays in 1895. This discovery, now commonly known as **X-rays,** revolutionized the diagnosis of disease.

Diagnostic Imaging Terms

TERM	WORD PARTS	DEFINITION
anteroposterior view (AP view)	anter/o = front poster/o = back -ior = pertaining to	Positioning the patient so that the X-rays pass through the body from the anterior side to the posterior side.
barium (Ba) (BAH-ree-um)		Soft metallic element from the earth used as a radiopaque X-ray dye.
film		Thin sheet of cellulose material coated with a light-sensitive substance that is used in taking photographs. There is a special photographic film that is sensitive to X-rays.
film badge		Badge containing film that is sensitive to X-rays. This is worn by all personnel in radiology to measure the amount of X-rays to which they are exposed.
lateral view	later/o = side -al = pertaining to	Positioning of the patient so that the side of the body faces the X-ray machine.
oblique view (oh-BLEEK)		Positioning of the patient so that the X-rays pass through the body on an angle.
posteroanterior view (PA view)	poster/o = back anter/o = front -ior = pertaining to	Positioning of the patient so that the X-rays pass through the body from the posterior side to the anterior side.
radiography (ray-dee-OG-rah-fee)	radi/o = X-ray -graphy = process of recording	Making of X-ray pictures.
radioisotope (ray-dee-oh-EYE-soh-tohp)	radi/o = X-ray	Radioactive form of an element.
radiologist (ray-dee-ALL-oh-jist)	radi/o = X-ray -logist = one who studies	Physician who uses images to diagnose abnormalities and radiant energy to treat various conditions such as cancer.
radiolucent (ray-dee-oh-LOO-cent)	radi/o = X-ray -lucent = to shine through	Structures that allow X-rays to pass through; expose the photographic plate and appear as black areas on the X-ray.
radiopaque (ray-dee-oh-PAYK)	radi/o = X-ray -opaque = nontransparent	Structures that are impenetrable to X-rays, appearing as a light area on the radiograph (X-ray).

Diagnostic Imaging Terms *(continued)*

TERM	WORD PARTS	DEFINITION
roentgen (RENT-gen)	roentgen/o = X-ray	Unit for describing an exposure dose of radiation.
scan		Recording on a photographic plate the emission of radioactive waves after a substance has been injected into the body.
shield		Device used to protect against radiation.
tagging		Attaching a radioactive material to a chemical, and tracing it as it moves through the body.
uptake		Absorption of radioactive material and medicines into an organ or tissue.
X-ray		High-energy wave that can penetrate most solid matter and present the image on photographic film.

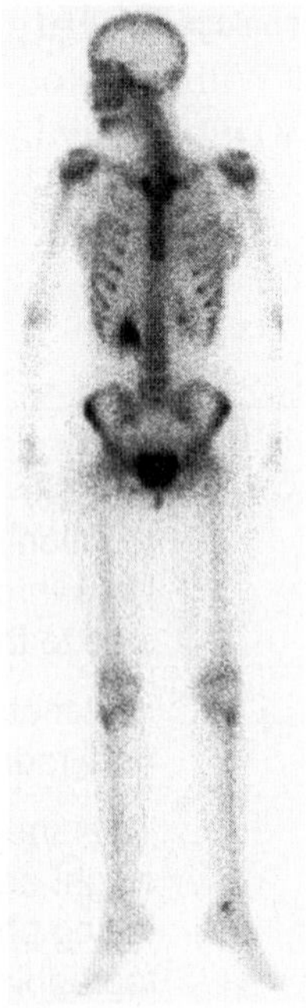

■ **Figure 14.6** Nuclear medicine. Bone scan produced after injection of a radioactive substance into the body. *(Getty Images, Inc/Photodisc)*

Diagnostic Imaging Procedures

TERM	WORD PARTS	DEFINITION
computed tomography scan (CT scan) (toh-MOG-rah-fee)	tom/o = to cut -graphy = process of recording	Imaging technique that is able to produce a cross-sectional view of the body. X-ray pictures are taken at multiple angles through the body. A computer then uses all these images to construct a composite cross-section. Refer back to Figure 12.9 in Chapter 12 for an example of a computed tomography scan showing a brain tumor.

Diagnostic Imaging Procedures *(continued)*

TERM	WORD PARTS	DEFINITION
contrast studies		Radiopaque substance is injected or swallowed. X-rays are then taken that will outline the body structure containing the radiopaque substance. For example, angiograms and myelograms.

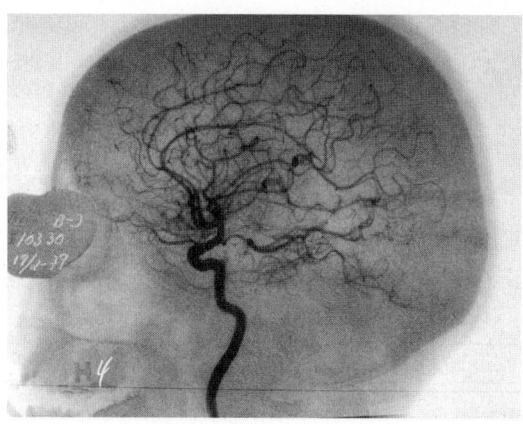

■ **Figure 14.7** Contrast study. X-ray of cerebral blood vessels taken after injection of a radiopaque substance into the bloodstream.

TERM	WORD PARTS	DEFINITION
Doppler ultrasonography	ultra- = beyond son/o = sound -graphy = process of recording	Use of ultrasound to record the velocity of blood flowing through blood vessels. Used to detect blood clots and blood vessel obstructions.
fluoroscopy (floo-or-OS-koh-pee)	fluor/o = luminous -scopy = process of visually examining	X-rays strike a fluorescing screen rather than a photographic plate, causing it to glow. The glowing screen changes from minute to minute; therefore movement, such as the heart beating or the digestive tract moving, can be seen.
magnetic resonance imaging (MRI) (REZ-oh-nence)	-ic = pertaining to	Use of electromagnetic energy to produce an image of soft tissues in any plane of the body. Atoms behave differently when placed in a strong magnetic field. When the body is exposed to this magnetic field the nuclei of the body's atoms emit radio-frequency signals that can be used to create an image.

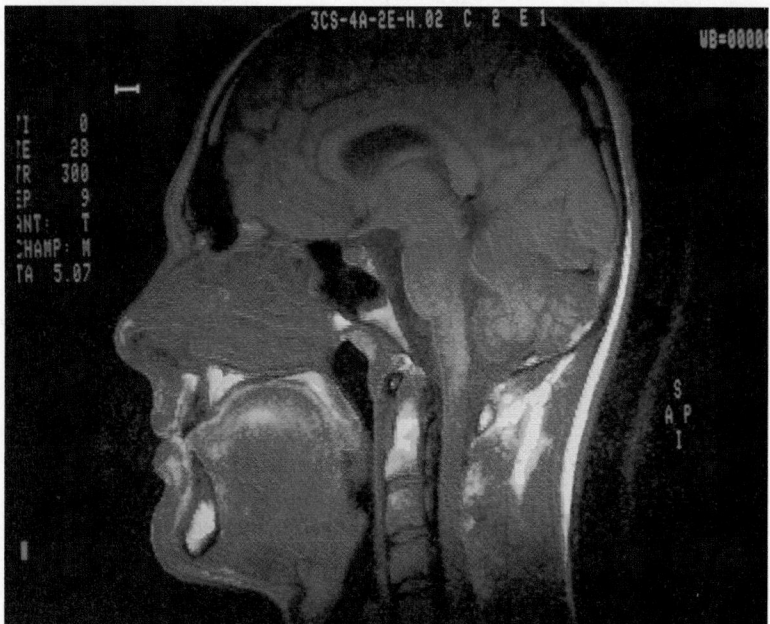

■ **Figure 14.8** Color-enhanced magnetic resonance image (MRI) showing a sagittal view of the head. *(Photo Researchers, Inc.)*

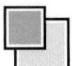

Diagnostic Imaging Procedures *(continued)*

TERM	WORD PARTS	DEFINITION
nuclear medicine	nucle/o = nucleus -ar = pertaining to	Use of radioactive substances to diagnose diseases. A radioactive substance known to accumulate in certain body tissues is injected or inhaled. After waiting for the substance to travel to the body area of interest, the radioactivity level is recorded. Commonly referred to as a *scan* (see again Figure 14.6). See Table 14.4 ■ for examples of the radioactive substances used in nuclear medicine.

Table 14.4	Substances Used to Visualize Various Body Organs in Nuclear Medicine
ORGAN	**SUBSTANCE**
bone	technetium (^{99m}Tc)–labeled phosphate
tumors	gallium (^{67}Ga)
lungs	xenon (^{133}Xe)
liver	technetium (^{99m}Tc)–labeled sulfur
heart	thallium (^{201}Tl)
thyroid	iodine (^{131}I)

TERM	WORD PARTS	DEFINITION
positron emission tomography (PET) (POS-ih-tron / eh-MIS-shun / toh-MOG-rah-fee)	tom/o = to cut -graphy = process of recording	Image is produced following the injection of radioactive glucose. The glucose will accumulate in areas of high metabolic activity. Therefore, this process will highlight areas that are consuming a large quantity of glucose. This may show an active area of the brain or a tumor.

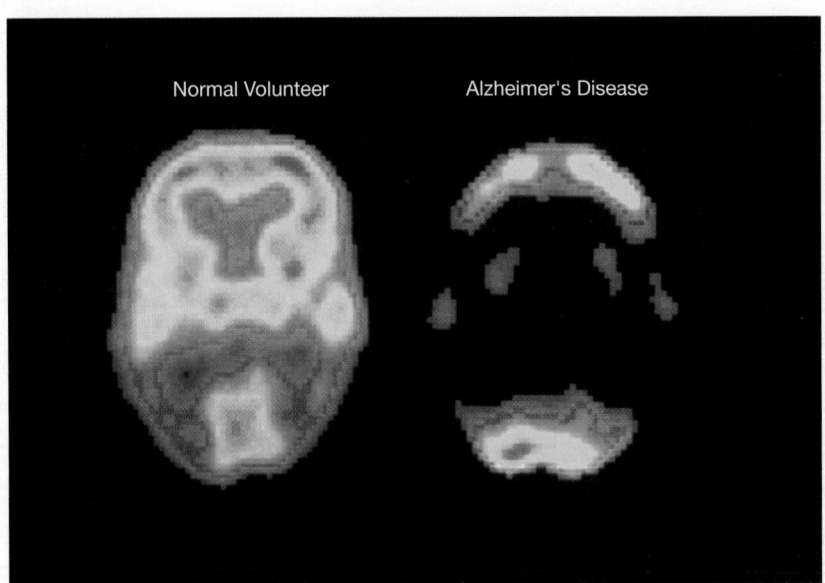

■ **Figure 14.9** Positron emission tomography (PET) image showing the difference in the metabolic activity of the brain of a person with Alzheimer's disease and that of a normal person. *(Science Source/Photo Researchers Inc.)*

TERM	WORD PARTS	DEFINITION
radiology (ray-dee-ALL-oh-jee)	radi/o = X-ray -logy = study of	Use of high-energy radiation, X-rays, to expose a photographic plate. The image is a black-and-white picture with radiopaque structures such as bone appearing white and radiolucent tissue such as muscles appearing dark.

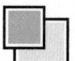

Diagnostic Imaging Procedures *(continued)*

TERM	WORD PARTS	DEFINITION
ultrasound (US) (ULL-trah-sound)	ultra- = beyond	Use of high-frequency sound waves to produce an image. Sound waves directed into the body from a transducer will bounce off internal structures and echo back to the transducer. The speed of the echo is dependent on the density of the tissue. A computer is able to correlate speed of echo with density and produce an image. Used to visualize internal organs, heart valves, and fetuses.

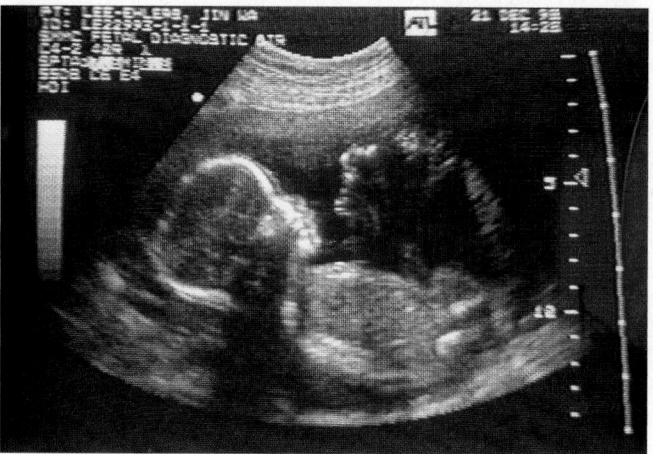

Figure 14.10 Ultrasound showing the outline of a fetus. *(Chad Ehlers/Stock Connection)*

Abbreviations

67^{Ga}	radioactive gallium		**DI**	diagnostic imaging
99m^{Tc}	radioactive technetium		**DSA**	digital subtraction angiography
131^{I}	radioactive iodine		**ERCP**	endoscopic retrograde cholangiopancreatography
201^{Tl}	radioactive thallium			
133^{Xe}	radioactive xenon		**Fx**	fracture
Angio	angiography		**GB**	gallbladder X-ray
AP	anteroposterior		**IVC**	intravenous cholangiogram
Ba	barium		**IVP**	intravenous pyelogram
BaE	barium enema		**KUB**	kidneys, ureters, bladder
CAT	computerized axial tomography		**LAT**	lateral
Ci	curie		**LGI**	lower gastrointestinal series
CT	computerized tomography		**LL**	left lateral
CXR	chest X-ray		**mA**	milliampere
decub	lying down		**mCi**	millicurie

Abbreviations *(continued)*

MRA	magnetic resonance angiography	**Ra**	radium
MRI	magnetic resonance imaging	**rad**	radiation-absorbed dose
NMR	nuclear magnetic resonance	**RL**	right lateral
PA	posteroanterior	**RRT**	registered radiologic technologist
PET	positron emission tomography		
PTC	percutaneous transhepatic cholangiography	**UGI**	upper gastrointestinal series
		US	ultrasound
R	roentgen		

Section IV: Rehabilitation Services at a Glance

Word Parts

Here are the most common word parts (with their meanings) used to build rehabilitation services terms.

Combining Forms

cry/o	cold	my/o	muscle
cutane/o	skin	orth/o	straight, correct
electr/o	electric current	phon/o	sound
erg/o	work	physic/o	body
habilitat/o	ability	prosthet/o	addition
hydr/o	water	therm/o	heat

Suffixes

-al	pertaining to	-ous	pertaining to
-graphy	process of recording	-phoresis	carrying
-ic	pertaining to	-therapy	treatment
-nomics	pertaining to laws	-tic	pertaining to

Prefixes

re-	again
trans-	across
ultra-	beyond

◼ Rehabilitation Services

occupational therapy   **physical therapy**

The goal of rehabilitation is to prevent disability and restore as much function as possible following disease, illness, or injury. Rehabilitation services include the healthcare specialties of **physical therapy** (PT) and **occupational therapy** (OT).

Physical Therapy

Physical therapy (PT) involves treating disorders using physical means and methods. Physical therapy personnel assess joint motion, muscle strength and endurance, function of heart and lungs, performance of activities required in daily living, and the ability to carry out other responsibilities. Physical therapy treatment includes gait training, therapeutic exercise, massage, joint and soft tissue mobilization, thermotherapy, cryotherapy, electrical stimulation, ultrasound, and hydrotherapy. These methods strengthen muscles, improve motion and circulation, reduce pain, and increase function.

Occupational Therapy

Occupational therapy (OT) assists patients to regain, develop, and improve skills that are important for independent functioning (activities of daily living). Occupational therapy personnel work with people who, because of illness, injury, or developmental or psychological impairments, require specialized training in skills that will enable them to lead independent, productive, and satisfying lives in regard to personal care, work, and leisure. Occupational therapists instruct patients in the use of adaptive equipment and techniques, body mechanics, and energy conservation. They also employ modalities such as heat, cold, and therapeutic exercise.

◼ Rehabilitation Services Terms

TERM	WORD PARTS	DEFINITION
activities of daily living (ADL)		Activities usually performed in the course of a normal day, such as eating, dressing, and washing.

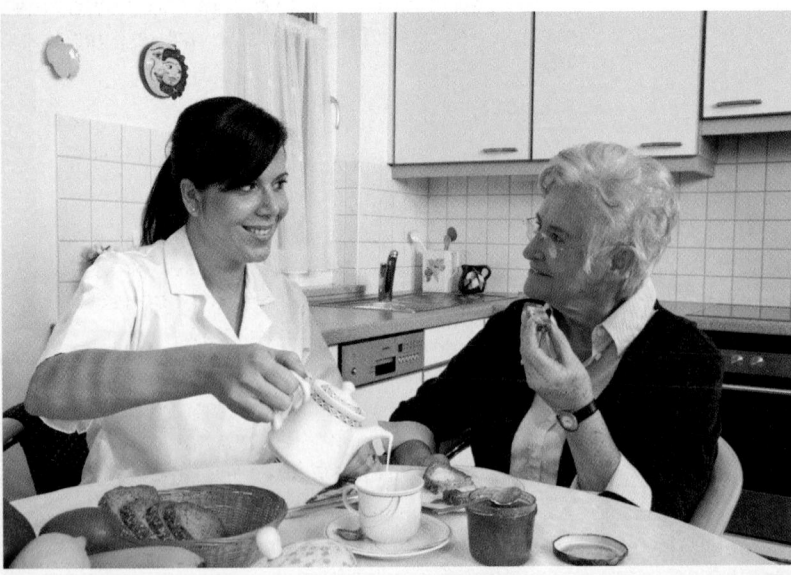

◼ **Figure 14.11** Photograph of an occupational therapist assisting a patient with learning independence in activities of daily living (ADLs). *(Gina Sanders/ Shutterstock)*

◼ Rehabilitation Services Terms *(continued)*

TERM	WORD PARTS	DEFINITION
adaptive equipment		Modification of equipment or devices to improve the function and independence of a person with a disability.

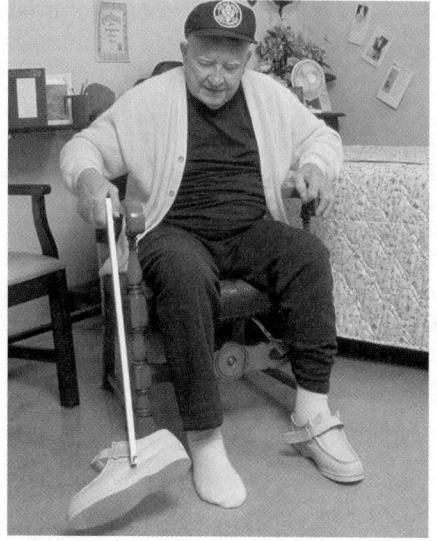 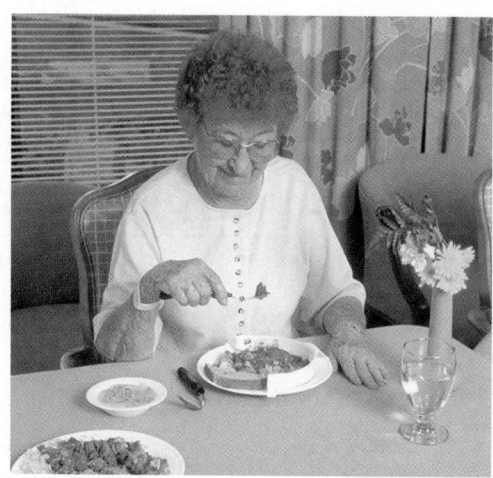

◼ **Figure 14.12** Using adaptive equipment: (A) male putting on shoe; (B) female eating one handed.

A   **B**

TERM	WORD PARTS	DEFINITION
body mechanics	-ic = pertaining to	Use of good posture and position while performing activities of daily living to prevent injury and stress on body parts.
ergonomics (er-goh-NOM-iks)	erg/o = work -nomics = pertaining to laws	Study of human work including how the requirements for performing work and the work environment affect the musculoskeletal and nervous systems.
fine motor skills		Use of precise and coordinated movements in such activities such as writing, buttoning, and cutting.
gait (GAYT)		Manner of walking.
gross motor skills		Use of large muscle groups that coordinate body movements such as walking, running, jumping, and balance.
lower extremity (LE)		Refers to one of the legs.
mobility		State of having normal movement of all body parts.
orthotics (or-THOT-iks)	orth/o = straight -tic = pertaining to	Use of equipment, such as splints and braces, to support a paralyzed muscle, promote a specific motion, or correct musculoskeletal deformities.
physical medicine	physic/o = body -al = pertaining to	Branch of medicine focused on restoring function. Primarily cares for patients with musculoskeletal and nervous system disorders. Physician is a *physiatrist*.
prosthetics (pros-THET-iks)	prosthet/o = addition -ic = pertaining to	Artificial devices, such as limbs and joints, that replace a missing body part.

■ Rehabilitation Services Terms *(continued)*

TERM	WORD PARTS	DEFINITION
range of motion (ROM)		Range of movement of a joint, from maximum flexion through maximum extension. It is measured as degrees of a circle.
rehabilitation	re- = again habilitat/o = ability	Process of treatment and exercise that can help a person with a disability attain maximum function and well-being.
upper extremity (UE)		Refers to one of the arms.

■ Therapeutic Procedures

TERM	WORD PARTS	DEFINITION
active exercises		Exercises that a patient performs without assistance.
active range of motion (AROM)		Range of motion for joints that a patient is able to perform without assistance from someone else.
active-resistive exercises		Exercises in which the patient works against resistance applied to a muscle, such as a weight. Used to increase strength.
cryotherapy (cry-oh-THAIR-ah-pee)	cry/o = cold -therapy = treatment	Using cold for therapeutic purposes.
debridement (day-breed-MON)		Removal of dead or damaged tissue from a wound. Commonly performed for burn therapy.
electromyography (EMG) (ee-LEK-troh-my-OG-rah-fee)	electr/o = electricity my/o = muscle -graphy = process of recording	The recording of a muscle's response to electrical stimulation. The graphic record produced is an *electromyogram*.
gait training		Assisting a patient to learn to walk again or how to use an assistive device to walk.

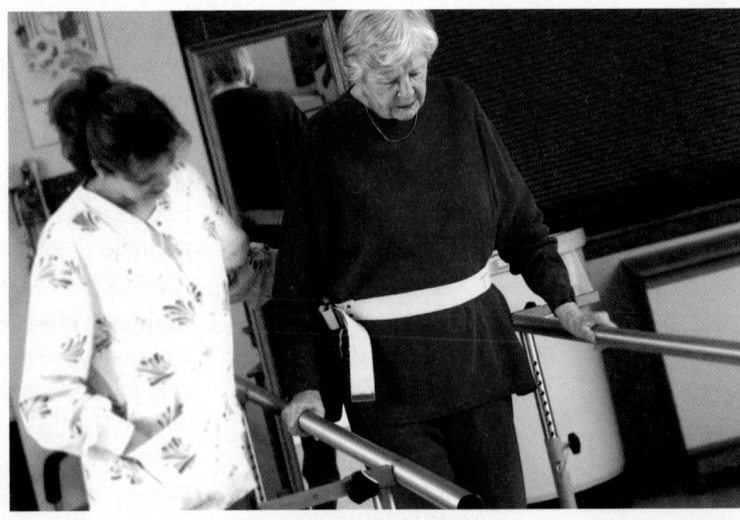

■ **Figure 14.13** Physical therapist assisting a patient to walk in the parallel bars.
(auremar/Shutterstock)

Therapeutic Procedures (continued)

TERM	WORD PARTS	DEFINITION
hydrotherapy (high-droh-THAIR-ah-pee)	hydr/o = water -therapy = treatment	Application of warm water as a therapeutic treatment. Can be done in baths, swimming pools, and whirlpools.
massage		Kneading or applying pressure by hands to a part of the patient's body to promote muscle relaxation and reduce tension.
mobilization		Treatments such as exercise and massage to restore movement to joints and soft tissue.
moist hot packs		Applying moist warmth to a body part to produce the slight dilation of blood vessels in the skin. Causes muscle relaxation in the deeper regions of the body and increases circulation, which aids healing.
nerve conduction velocity		Test to determine if nerves have been damaged by recording the rate at which an electrical impulse travels along a nerve. If the nerve is damaged, the velocity will be decreased.
pain control		Managing pain through a variety of means, including medications, biofeedback, and mechanical devices.
passive range of motion (PROM)		Therapist putting a patient's joints through available range of motion without assistance from the patient.
phonophoresis (foh-noh-foh-REE-sis)	phon/o = sound -phoresis = carrying	Use of ultrasound waves to introduce medication across the skin and into the subcutaneous tissues.
postural drainage with clapping	-al = pertaining to	Draining secretions from the bronchi or a lung cavity by having the patient lie so that gravity allows drainage to occur. Clapping is using the hand in a cupped position to perform percussion on the chest. Assists in loosening secretions and mucus.
therapeutic exercise (thair-ah-PEW-tik)	-ic = pertaining to	Exercise planned and carried out to achieve a specific physical benefit, such as improved range of motion, muscle strength, or cardiovascular function.
thermotherapy (ther-moh-THAIR-ah-pee)	therm/o = heat -therapy = treatment	Applying heat to the body for therapeutic purposes.
traction		Process of pulling or drawing, usually with a mechanical device. Used in treating orthopedic (bone and joint) problems and injuries.
transcutaneous electrical nerve stimulation (TENS) (tranz-kyoo-TAY-nee-us)	trans- = across cutane/o = skin -ous = pertaining to electr/o = electricity -al = pertaining to	Application of an electric current to a peripheral nerve to relieve pain.

Therapeutic Procedures *(continued)*

TERM	WORD PARTS	DEFINITION
ultrasound (US)	ultra- = beyond	Use of high-frequency sound waves to create heat in soft tissues under the skin. It is particularly useful for treating injuries to muscles, tendons, and ligaments, as well as muscle spasms.
whirlpool		Bath in which there are continuous jets of hot water reaching the body surfaces.

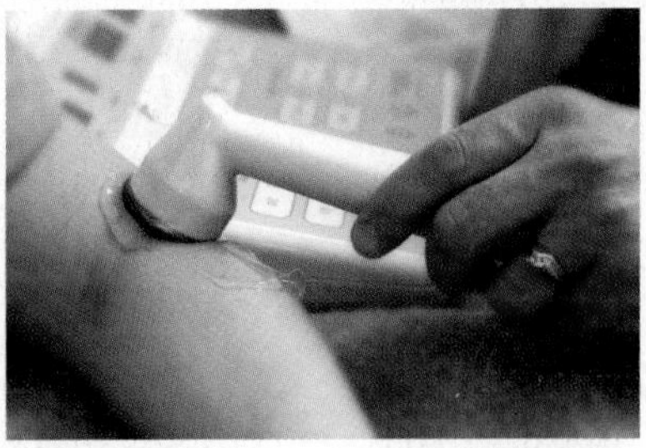

■ **Figure 14.14** Patient receiving ultrasound treatment to the left elbow. *(GWImages/Shutterstock)*

Abbreviations

AAROM	active assistive range of motion		**PROM**	passive range of motion
ADL	activities of daily living		**PT**	physical therapy
AROM	active range of motion		**ROM**	range of motion
EMG	electromyogram		**TENS**	transcutaneous electrical stimulation
e-stim	electrical stimulation		**UE**	upper extremity
LE	lower extremity		**US**	ultrasound
OT	occupational therapy			

Section V: Surgery at a Glance

Word Parts

Here are the most common word parts (with their meanings) used to build surgery terms.

Combining Forms

alges/o	pain	hem/o	blood
aspir/o	to breathe in	later/o	side
cis/o	to cut	lith/o	stone
cry/o	cold	recumb/o	to lie back
cutane/o	skin	sect/o	to cut
dilat/o	to widen	specul/o	to look at
electr/o	electricity	tenacul/o	to hold
esthes/o	sensation, feeling	topic/o	a specific area
hal/o	to breathe	ven/o	vein

Suffixes

-al	pertaining to	-otomy	to cut into
-ia	state, condition	-ous	pertaining to
-ic	pertaining to	-scopic	pertaining to visually examining
-ist	specialist		
-logist	one who studies	-stasis	standing still
-logy	study of	-stat	standing still

Prefixes

an-	without	peri-	around
dis-	apart	post-	after
endo-	within	pre-	before
in-	inward	re-	again
intra-	within	sub-	under

■ Surgery

operative report	surgery
surgeon	

Surgery is the branch of medicine dealing with operative procedures to correct deformities and defects, repair injuries, and diagnose and cure diseases. A **surgeon** is a physician who has completed additional training of 5 years or more in a surgical specialty area. These specialty areas include orthopedics; neurosurgery; gynecology; ophthalmology; urology; and thoracic, vascular, cardiac, plastic, and general surgery. The surgeon must complete an **operative report** for every procedure that he or she performs. This is a detailed description that includes:

- preoperative diagnosis
- indication for the procedure
- name of the procedure
- surgical techniques employed
- findings during surgery
- postoperative diagnosis
- name of the surgeon

This report also includes information pertaining to the patient such as name, address, age, patient number, and date of the procedure.

Surgical terminology includes terms related to anesthesiology, surgical instruments, surgical procedures, incisions, and suture materials. Specific surgical procedures are frequently named by using the combining form for the body part being operated on and adding a suffix that describes the procedure. For example, an incision into the chest is a *thoracotomy*, removal of the stomach is *gastrectomy*, and surgical repair of the skin is *dermatoplasty*. A list of the most frequently used surgical suffixes is found in Chapter 1 and common surgical procedures are defined in each system chapter.

Anesthesia

anesthesia (an-ess-THEE-zee-ah)	**local anesthesia**
anesthesiologist (an-es-thee-zee-OL-jist)	**nurse anesthetist** (ah-NES-the-tist)
general anesthesia	**regional anesthesia**
inhalation (in-hah-LAY-shun)	**subcutaneous** (sub-kyoo-TAY-nee-us)
intravenous (in-trah-VEE-nus)	**topical anesthesia**

An **anesthesiologist** is a physician who specializes in the practice of administering anesthetics. A **nurse anesthetist** is a registered nurse who has received additional training and education in the administration of anesthetic medications. **Anesthesia** results in the loss of feeling or sensation. The most common types of anesthesia are general, regional, local, and topical anesthesia (see Table 14.5 ■).

Surgical Instruments

Physicians have developed surgical instruments since the time of the early Egyptians. Instruments include surgical knives, saws, clamps, drills, and needles. Some of the more commonly used surgical instruments are listed in Table 14.6 ■ and are shown in Figure 14.15 ■.

Table 14.5	Types of Anesthesia	
TYPE	**WORD PARTS**	**DESCRIPTION**
general anesthesia (GA)	an- = without esthes/o = sensation, feeling -ia = state, condition	Produces a loss of consciousness including an absence of pain sensation. The patient's vital signs (VS)—heart rate, breathing rate, pulse, and blood pressure—are carefully monitored when using a general anesthetic.
intravenous (IV)	intra- = within ven/o = vein -ous = pertaining to	Route for administering general anesthesia via injection into a vein.
inhalation	in- = inward hal/o = to breath	Route for administering general anesthesia by breathing it in.
regional anesthesia	-al = pertaining to an- = without esthes/o = sensation, feeling -ia = state, condition	Also referred to as a nerve block. This anesthetic interrupts a patient's pain sensation in a particular region of the body, such as the arm. The anesthetic is injected near the nerve that will be blocked from sensation. The patient usually remains conscious.
local anesthesia	-al = pertaining to an- = without esthes/o = sensation, feeling -ia = state, condition	Produces a loss of sensation in one localized part of the body. The patient remains conscious.
subcutaneous	sub- = under cutane/o = skin -ous = pertaining to	Method of applying local anesthesia involving injecting the anesthetic under the skin. This type of anesthetic is used to deaden the skin prior to suturing a laceration.
topical	topic/o = a specific area -al = pertaining to	Method of applying local anesthesia involving placing a liquid or gel directly onto a specific area of skin. This type of anesthetic is used on the skin, the cornea, and the mucous membranes in dental work.

Table 14.6	Common Surgical Instruments	
INSTRUMENT	**WORD PARTS**	**USE**
aspirator (AS-pih-ray-tor)	aspir/o = to breathe in	Suctions fluid
clamp		Grasps tissue; controls bleeding
curette (kyoo-RET)		Scrapes and removes tissue
dilator (dye-LAY-tor)	dilat/o = to widen	Enlarges an opening by stretching
forceps (FOR-seps)		Grasps tissue
hemostat (HEE-moh-stat)	hem/o = blood -stat = standing still	Forceps to grasp blood vessel to control bleeding
probe		Explores tissue
scalpel		Cuts and separates tissue
speculum (SPEK-yoo-lum)	specul/o = to look at	Spreads apart walls of a cavity
tenaculum (the-NAK-yoo-lum)	tenacul/o = to hold	Long-handled clamp
trephine (treh-FINE)		Saw that removes disk-shaped piece of tissue or bone

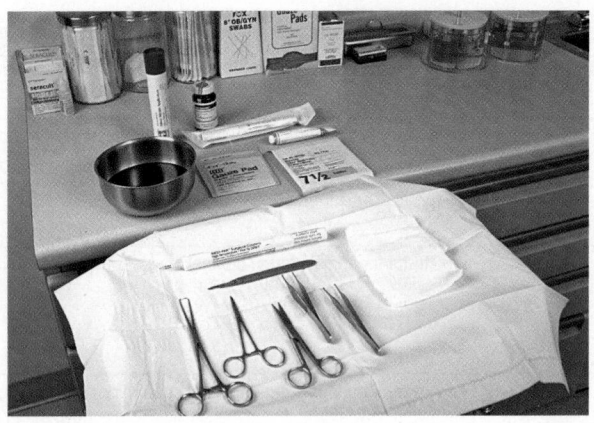

Figure 14.15 Surgical instruments prepared for a procedure.

Surgical Positions

Patients are placed in specific positions so the surgeon is able to reach the area that is to be operated on. Table 14.7 ■ describes and Figure 14.16 ■ illustrates some common surgical positions.

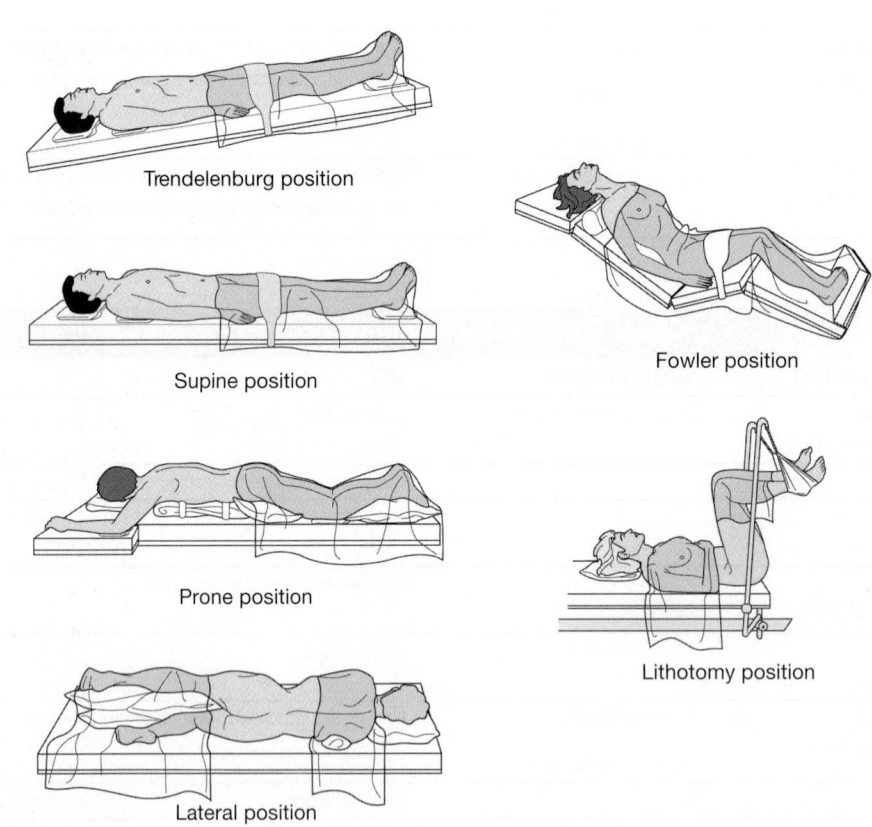

Trendelenburg position

Supine position

Fowler position

Prone position

Lithotomy position

Figure 14.16 Examples of common surgical positions.

Lateral position

Table 14.7	Common Surgical Positions	
POSITION	**WORD PARTS**	**DESCRIPTION**
Fowler		Sitting with back positioned at a 45° angle
lateral recumbent (ree-KUM-bent)	later/o = side -al = pertaining to recumb/o = to lie back	Lying on either the left or right side
lithotomy (lith-OT-oh-mee)	lith/o = tone -otomy = to cut into	Lying face up with hips and knees bent at 90° angles
prone (PROHN)		Lying horizontal and face down
supine (soo-PINE)		Lying horizontal and face up; also called dorsal recumbent
Trendelenburg (TREN-dee-len-berg)		Lying face up and on an incline with head lower than legs

Surgery Terms

TERM	WORD PARTS	DEFINITION
analgesic (an-al-JEE-zik)	an- = without alges/o = pain -ic = pertaining to	Medication to relieve pain.
anesthetic (an-ess-THET-ik)	an- = without esthes/o = sensation, feeling -ic = pertaining to	Medication to produce partial to complete loss of sensation.
cauterization (kaw-ter-ih-ZAY-shun)		Use of heat, cold, electricity, or chemicals to scar, burn, or cut tissues.
circulating nurse		Nurse who assists the surgeon and scrub nurse by providing needed materials during the procedure and by handling the surgical specimen. This person does not wear sterile clothing and may enter and leave the operating room during the procedure.
cryosurgery (cry-oh-SER-jer-ee)	cry/o = cold	Technique of exposing tissues to extreme cold to produce cell injury and destruction. Used in the treatment of malignant tumors or to control pain and bleeding.
day surgery		Type of outpatient surgery in which the patient is discharged on the same day he or she is admitted; also called *ambulatory surgery*.
dissection (dih-SEK-shun)	dis- = apart sect/o = to cut	Surgical cutting of parts for separation and study.
draping		Process of covering the patient with sterile cloths that allow only the operative site to be exposed to the surgeon.

Surgery Terms *(continued)*

TERM	WORD PARTS	DEFINITION
electrocautery (ee-lek-troh-KAW-ter-ee)	electr/o = electricity	Use of an electric current to stop bleeding by coagulating blood vessels.
endoscopic surgery (en-doh-SKOP-ik)	endo- = within -scopic = pertaining to visually examining	Use of a lighted instrument to examine the interior of a cavity.
hemostasis (hee-moh-STAY-sis)	hem/o = blood -stasis = standing still	Stopping the flow of blood using instruments, pressure, and/or medication.
intraoperative (in-trah-OP-er-ah-tiv)	intra- = within	Period of time during surgery.
laser surgery		Use of a controlled beam of light for cutting, hemostasis, or tissue destruction.
perioperative (per-ee-OP-er-ah-tiv)	peri- = around	Period of time that includes before, during, and after a surgical procedure.
postoperative (post-op) (post-OP-er-ah-tiv)	post- = after	Period of time immediately following the surgery.
preoperative (preop, pre-op) (pree-OP-er-ah-tiv)	pre- = before	Period of time preceding surgery.
resection (ree-SEK-shun)	re- = again sect/o = to cut	To surgically cut out or remove; excision.
scrub nurse		Surgical assistant who hands instruments to the surgeon. This person wears sterile clothing and maintains the sterile operative field.
suture material (SOO-cher)		Used to close a wound or incision. Examples are catgut, silk thread, or staples. They may or may not be removed when the wound heals, depending on the type of material that is used.

Abbreviations

D & C	dilation and curettage	**PARR**	postanesthetic recovery room
Endo	endoscopy	**preop, pre-op**	preoperative
EUA	exam under anesthesia		
GA	general anesthesia	**prep**	preparation, prepared
I & D	incision and drainage	**T & A**	tonsillectomy and adenoidectomy
MUA	manipulation under anesthesia	**TAH**	total abdominal hysterectomy
OR	operating room	**TURP**	transurethral resection of prostate

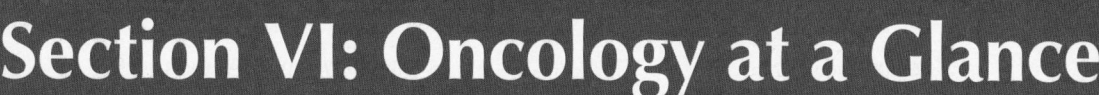

Section VI: Oncology at a Glance

Word Parts

Here are the most common word parts (with their meanings) used to build oncology terms.

Combining Forms

bi/o	life	miss/o	to send back
blast/o	primitive cell	morbid/o	ill
capsul/o	to box	mort/o	death
carcin/o	cancerous	mutat/o	to change
chem/o	drug	onc/o	tumor
cyt/o	cell	path/o	disease
immun/o	protection	radic/o	root
lapar/o	abdomen	radi/o	rays (X-rays)
laps/o	to slide back	tox/o	poison

Suffixes

-al	pertaining to	-oma	tumor
-gen	that which produces	-opsy	to view
-genic	producing	-otomy	to cut into
-logic	pertaining to studying	-plasia	growth, formation
-logist	one who studies	-plasm	growth, formation
-logy	study of	-therapy	treatment

Prefixes

en-	inward	neo-	new
hyper-	excessive	re-	again
in-	within		

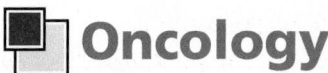

Oncology

benign (bee-NINE)
carcinoma (kar-sin-NOH-mah)
malignant (mah-LIG-nant)

oncology (ong-KALL-oh-jee)
protocol (PROH-toh-kall)
tumors

Oncology is the branch of medicine dealing with **tumors.** A tumor can be classified as **benign** or **malignant.** A benign tumor is one that is generally not progressive or recurring. Generally, a benign tumor will have the suffix *-oma* at the end of the term. However, a malignant tumor indicates that there is a cancerous growth present (see Figure 14.17 ■). These terms will usually have the word *carcinoma* added. The medical specialty of oncology primarily treats patients who have cancer.

The treatment for cancer can consist of a variety or a combination of treatments. The **protocol** (prot) for a particular patient will consist of the actual plan of care, including the medications, surgeries, and treatments such as chemotherapy and radiation therapy. Often, the entire healthcare team, including the physician, oncologist, radiologist, nurse, patient, and family, will assist in designing the treatment plan.

> **MED TERM TIP**
>
> Carcinoma or cancer (Ca) can affect almost every organ in the body. The medical term reflects the area of the body affected as well as the type of tumor cell. For example, there can be an esophageal carcinoma, gastric adenocarcinoma, or adenocarcinoma of the uterus.

Staging Tumors

grade
metastases (meh-TASS-tah-seez)

pathologist (path-ALL-oh-jist)
staging

The process of classifying tumors based on their degree of tissue invasion and the potential response to therapy is referred to as **staging.** The TNM staging system is frequently used, with the *T* referring to the tumor's size and invasion, the *N* referring to lymph node involvement, and the *M* referring to the presence of **metastases** (mets) of the tumor cells (see Figure 14.18 ■).

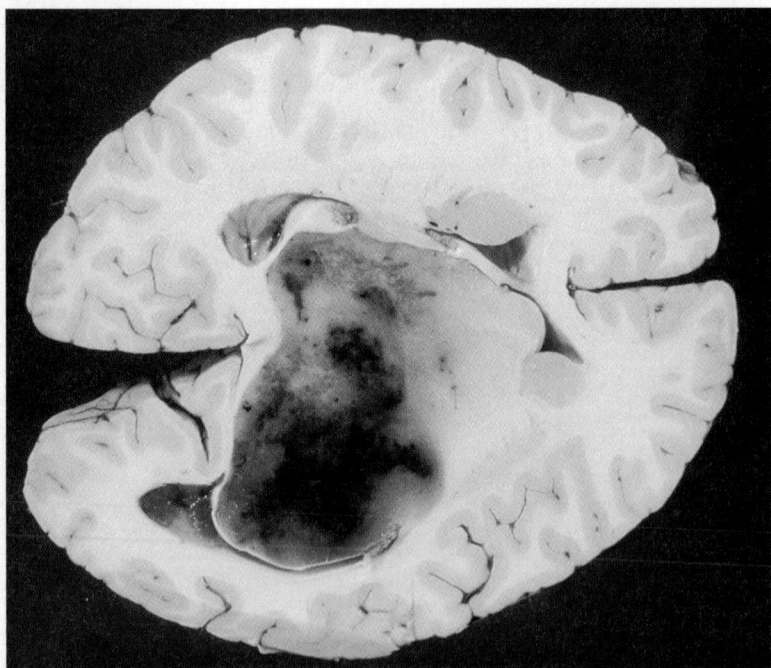

■ **Figure 14.17** Photograph of a brain specimen with a large malignant tumor. *(Biophoto Associates/Photo Researchers, Inc.)*

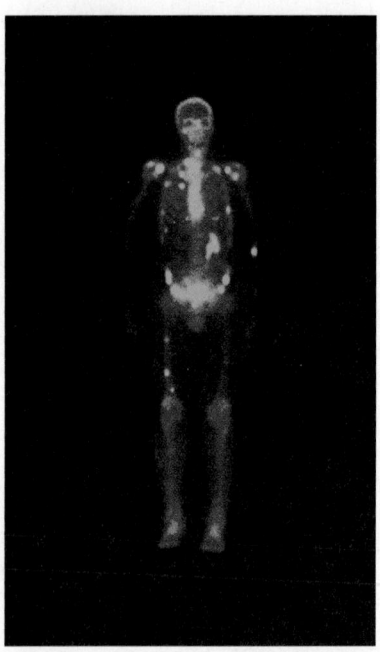

■ **Figure 14.18** Nuclear medicine bone scan showing metastatic tumors in the skeleton. *(Medical Body Scans/Photo Researchers, Inc.)*

In addition, a tumor can be graded from grade I through grade IV. The **grade** is based on the microscopic appearance of the tumor cells. The **pathologist** rates or grades the cells based on whether the tumor resembles the normal tissue. The classification system is illustrated in Table 14.8 ■. The cells in a grade I tumor are well differentiated, which makes it easier to treat than the more advanced grades.

Table 14.8	Tumor Grade Classification
GRADE	**MEANING**
GX	Grade cannot be determined
GI	Cells are well differentiated
GII	Cells are moderately differentiated
GIII	Cells are poorly differentiated
GIV	Cells are undifferentiated

Oncology Terms

TERM	WORD PARTS	DEFINITION
carcinogen (kar-SIN-oh-jen)	carcin/o = cancer -gen = that which produces	Substance or chemical agent that produces or increases the risk of developing cancer. For example, cigarette smoke and insecticides are considered to be carcinogens.

MED TERM TIP

The term *benign* comes from the Latin term *bene,* which means "kind or good." On the other hand, the term *malignant* comes from the Latin term *mal,* meaning "bad or malicious."

TERM	WORD PARTS	DEFINITION
carcinoma in situ (CIS) (kar-sin-NOH-mah)	carcin/o = cancer -oma = tumor	Malignant tumor whose cells have not spread beyond the original site.
encapsulated (en-CAP-soo-lay-ted)	en- = inward capsul/o = to box	Growth enclosed in a sheath of tissue that prevents tumor cells from invading surrounding tissue.
hyperplasia (high-per-PLAY-zee-ah)	hyper- = excessive -plasia = growth	Excessive development of normal cells within an organ.
invasive disease (in-VAY-siv)	in- = within	Tendency of a malignant tumor to spread to immediately surrounding tissue and organs.

Oncology Terms *(continued)*

TERM	WORD PARTS	DEFINITION
metastasis (mets) (meh-TASS-tah-sis)		Movement and spread of cancer cells from one part of the body to another. Metastases is plural.

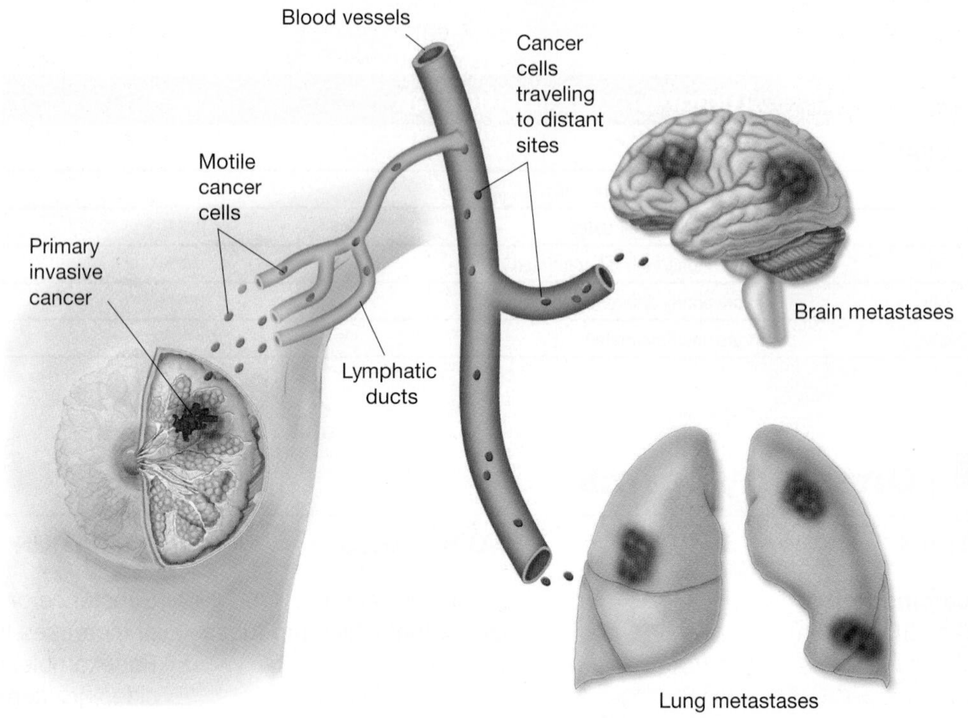

Blood vessels

Cancer cells traveling to distant sites

Motile cancer cells

Primary invasive cancer

Brain metastases

Lymphatic ducts

Lung metastases

■ **Figure 14.19** Illustration showing how the primary breast tumor metastasized through the lymphatic and blood vessels to secondary sites in the brain and lungs.

TERM	WORD PARTS	DEFINITION
morbidity (mor-BID-ih-tee)	morbid/o = ill	Number representing the sick persons in a particular population.
mortality (mor-TAL-ih-tee)	mort/o = death	Number representing the deaths in a particular population.
mutation (mew-TAY-shun)	mutat/o = to change	Change or transformation from the original.
neoplasm (NEE-oh-plazm)	neo- = new -plasm = growth	New and abnormal growth or tumor. These can be benign or malignant.
oncogenic (ong-koh-JEN-ik)	onc/o = tumor -genic = producing	Cancer causing.
primary site		Term used to designate where a malignant tumor first appeared.
relapse (REE-laps)	re- = again laps/o = to slide back	Return of disease symptoms after a period of improvement.
remission (rih-MISH-un)	re- = again miss/o = to send back	Period during which the symptoms of a disease or disorder leave. Can be temporary.

Diagnostic Procedures

TERM	WORD PARTS	DEFINITION
biopsy (bx) (BYE-op-see)	bi/o = life -opsy = to view	Excision of a small piece of tissue for microscopic examination to assist in determining a diagnosis.
cytologic testing (sigh-toh-LAH-jik)	cyt/o = cell -logic = pertaining to studying	Examination of cells to determine their structure and origin. Pap smears are considered a form of cytologic testing.
exploratory surgery		Surgery performed for the purpose of determining if cancer is present or if a known cancer has spread. Biopsies are generally performed.
staging laparotomy (lap-ah-ROT-oh-mee)	lapar/o = abdomen -otomy = to cut into	Surgical procedure in which the abdomen is entered to determine the extent and staging of a tumor.

Therapeutic Procedures

TERM	WORD PARTS	DEFINITION
chemotherapy (chemo) (kee-moh-THAIR-ah-pee)	chem/o = drug -therapy = treatment	Treating disease by using chemicals that have a toxic effect on the body, especially cancerous tissue.
hormone therapy		Treatment of cancer with natural hormones or with chemicals that produce hormone-like effects.
immunotherapy (im-yoo-noh-THAIR-ah-pee)	immun/o = protection -therapy = treatment	Strengthening the immune system to attack cancerous cells.
palliative therapy (PAL-ee-ah-tiv)		Treatment designed to reduce the intensity of painful symptoms, but does not produce a cure.
radiation therapy	radi/o = X-rays	Exposing tumors and surrounding tissues to X-rays, gamma rays, neutrons, protons, and other sources to kill cancer cells and shrink tumors.
radical surgery	radic/o = root -al = pertaining to	Extensive surgery to remove as much tissue associated with a tumor as possible.
radioactive implant (ray-dee-oh-AK-tiv)	radi/o = rays	Embedding a radioactive source directly into tissue to provide a highly localized radiation dosage to damage nearby cancerous cells. Also called *brachytherapy*.

Abbreviations

bx	biopsy	**mets**	metastases
Ca	cancer	**MTX**	methotrexate
chemo	chemotherapy	**prot**	protocol
CIS	carcinoma in situ	**st**	stage
5-FU	5-fluorouracil	**TNM**	tumor, nodes, metastases
GA	gallium		

Chapter Review

Real-World Applications

Chart Note Transcription

The chart note below contains 11 phrases that can be reworded with a medical term that you learned in this chapter. Each phrase is identified with an underline. Determine the medical term and write your answers in the space provided.

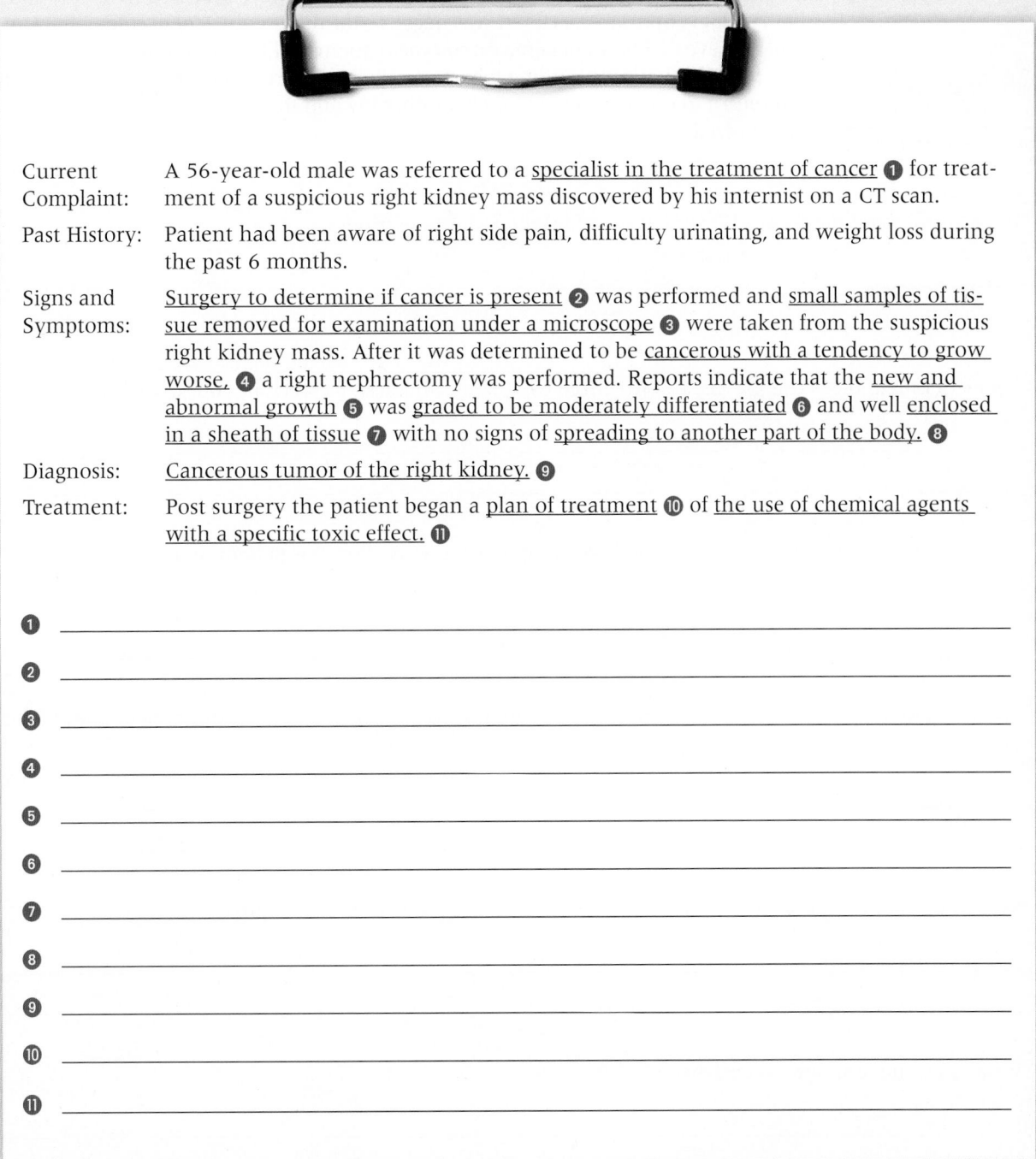

Current Complaint: A 56-year-old male was referred to a <u>specialist in the treatment of cancer</u> **1** for treatment of a suspicious right kidney mass discovered by his internist on a CT scan.

Past History: Patient had been aware of right side pain, difficulty urinating, and weight loss during the past 6 months.

Signs and Symptoms: <u>Surgery to determine if cancer is present</u> **2** was performed and <u>small samples of tissue removed for examination under a microscope</u> **3** were taken from the suspicious right kidney mass. After it was determined to be <u>cancerous with a tendency to grow worse,</u> **4** a right nephrectomy was performed. Reports indicate that the <u>new and abnormal growth</u> **5** was <u>graded to be moderately differentiated</u> **6** and well <u>enclosed in a sheath of tissue</u> **7** with no signs of <u>spreading to another part of the body.</u> **8**

Diagnosis: <u>Cancerous tumor of the right kidney.</u> **9**

Treatment: Post surgery the patient began a <u>plan of treatment</u> **10** of <u>the use of chemical agents with a specific toxic effect.</u> **11**

1 _____

2 _____

3 _____

4 _____

5 _____

6 _____

7 _____

8 _____

9 _____

10 _____

11 _____

Case Study

Below is a case study presentation of a patient with a condition covered by this chapter. Read the case study and answer the questions below. Some questions will ask for information not included within this chapter. Use your text, a medical dictionary, or any other reference material you choose to answer these questions.

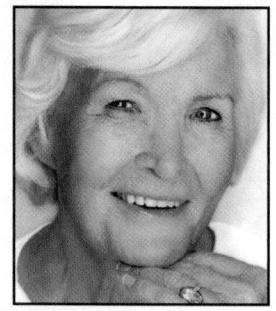

(Martina Ebel/Shuterstock)

Patient is a 72-year-old female complaining of increasing dyspnea with activity during the past 6 months. She now has a frequent harsh cough producing thick sputum and occasional hemoptysis. Patient is thin and short of stature. She is not SOB sitting in examination room. CT scan of the bronchial tree confirmed the presence of a mass in the right lung. Sputum was collected for sputum culture and sensitivity and sputum cytology. Sputum specimen was negative for the presence of bacteria. Sputum cytology revealed bronchogenic carcinoma. Patient will be referred to thoracic surgeon for consultation regarding lobectomy. Following recovery from this surgery she is to return to oncology clinic for chemotherapy and to determine if the tumor has metastasized.

1. What is this patient's diagnosis? Look it up and write a short description.

   _____

   _____

2. The patient had three complaints. List the three complaints and describe each in your own words.

   _____

   _____

3. Describe in your own words the diagnostic imaging procedure used on this patient and the results.

   _____

   _____

4. List and describe in your own words the clinical laboratory diagnostic test run on this patient and the results of each test.

   _____

   _____

5. What surgical procedure will this patient undergo? Describe it in your own words.

   _____

   _____

6. What does the term *metastasized* mean?

   _____

   _____

Practice Exercises

A. Complete the Statement

1. The reference book containing important information regarding medications is the _____.

2. A person specializing in the dispensing of medications is a _____.

3. The accepted official name for a drug is the _____ name.

4. The trade name for a drug is the _____ name.

5. What does the chemical name represent? _____

6. What federal agency enforces controls over the use of drugs causing dependency? _____

B. Drug Administration Practice

Name the route of drug administration for the following descriptions.

1. under the tongue _____

2. into the anus or rectum _____

3. applied to the skin _____

4. injected under the first layer of skin _____

5. injected into a muscle _____

6. injected into a vein _____

7. by mouth _____

C. Define the Term

1. idiosyncrasy _____

2. parenteral _____

3. placebo _____

4. toxicity _____

5. side effect _____

6. unit dose _____

7. habituation _____

8. antidote _____

9. contraindication _____

10. prophylaxis _____

D. What Does it Stand For?

1. gr _____

2. bid _____

3. tid _____

4. ad lib _____

5. prn _____

6. ante _____

7. OTC _____

8. gt _____

9. Sig _____

10. stat _____

11. mg _____

12. aq _____

13. noc _____

14. NPO _____

15. hs _____

16. IV _____

17. TO _____

18. gtt _____

19. pc _____

20. d/c _____

E. Prescription Practice

Write out the following prescription instructions in the space provided.

1. Pravachol, 20 mg, Sig. ī daily hs, 30, refill 3x, no sub. _____

2. Lanoxin, 0.125 mg, Sig. iii stat, then ii q AM, 100, refills prn. _____

3. Synthroid, 0.075 mg, Sig. ī daily, 100, refill x4. _____

4. Norvasc, 5 mg, ī q am, 60, refillable. _____

F. Terminology Matching

Match each term to its definition.

1. _____ cognitive disorder
2. _____ factitious disorder
3. _____ dissociative disorder
4. _____ eating disorder
5. _____ sleeping disorder
6. _____ mood disorder
7. _____ impulse control disorder
8. _____ somatoform disorder
9. _____ personality disorder
10. _____ sexual disorder
11. _____ anxiety disorder

a. hypochondria
b. kleptomania
c. masochism
d. narcissistic personality
e. insomnia
f. bipolar disease
g. panic attacks
h. amnesia
i. dementia
j. anorexia nervosa
k. malingering

G. Name the Treatment

Identify each mental health treatment from its description.

1. depressant drugs prescribed for anxiety _____

2. client-centered psychotherapy _____

3. drug used to calm patients with bipolar disorder _____

4. reduces patient agitation and panic and shortens schizophrenic episodes _____

5. obtains a detailed account of the past and present emotional and mental experiences _____

6. stimulants that alter the patient's mood by affecting neurotransmitter levels _____

H. Name the Anesthesia

Identify the type of anesthesia for each description.

1. produces loss of consciousness and absence of pain _____

2. produces loss of sensation in one localized part of the body _____

3. anesthetic applied directly onto a specific skin area _____

4. also referred to as a nerve block _____

I. Terminology Matching

Match thet term to its definition.

1. _____ ultrasound

2. _____ MRI

3. _____ Doppler US

4. _____ nuclear medicine scan

5. _____ CT scan

6. _____ contrast study

7. _____ fluoroscopy

8. _____ radiography

9. _____ PET scan

a. radiopaque substances used to outline hollow structures

b. records velocity of blood flowing through vessels

c. image created by electromagnetic energy

d. glowing screen shows movement

e. making an X-ray

f. multiple-angle X-rays compiled into a cross-section

g. uses radioactive substances

h. image of internal organs using sound waves

i. indicates metabolic activity

J. What Does it Stand For?

1. ROM _____

2. OT _____

3. ADL _____

4. LE _____

5. EMG _____

6. TENS _____

7. PT _____

8. PROM _____

9. e-stim _____

10. US _____

K. Name the Procedure Described

Identify the rehabilitation procedure described by each phrase.

1. kneading or applying pressure by hands _____

2. removal of dead and damaged tissue from a wound _____

3. using water for treatment purposes _____

4. drainage of secretions from the bronchi _____

5. exercises performed by a patient without resistance _____

6. medication introduced by ultrasound waves _____

7. use of cold for therapeutic purposes _____

8. pulling with a mechanical device _____

L. Terminology Matching

Match each term to its definition.

1. _____ forceps

2. _____ tenaculum

3. _____ Trendelenburg

4. _____ lithotomy

5. _____ curette

6. _____ aspirator

7. _____ supine

8. _____ probe

9. _____ scalpel

10. _____ lateral recumbent

a. scrapes and removes tissue

b. cuts and separates tissue

c. lying horizontal and face up

d. lying on either the left or right side

e. long-handled clamp

f. explores tissue

g. lying face up with hips and knees bent at 90° angle

h. grasps tissue

i. suctions fluid

j. lying face up on an incline, head lower than legs

M. What Does it Stand For?

1. MRI _____

2. Ba _____

3. AP _____

4. CT _____

5. RL _____

6. PA _____

7. LL _____

8. PET _____

9. UGI _____

10. KUB _____

N. Terminology Matching

Match each term to its definition.

1. _____ oncogenic

   a. examine cells to determine their structure and origin

2. _____ benign

   b. the plan for care for any individual patient

3. _____ encapsulated

   c. biopsy

4. _____ relapse

   d. growth that is not recurrent or progressive

5. _____ primary site

   e. placing a radioactive substance directly into the tissue

6. _____ protocol

   f. where the malignant tumor first appeared

7. _____ staging laparotomy

   g. growth is enclosed in a tissue sheath

8. _____ cytologic testing

   h. cancer causing

9. _____ radioactive implant

   i. abdominal surgery to determine extent of tumor

10. _____ bx

   j. return of disease symptoms

MEDICAL TERMINOLOGY INTERACTIVE

Medical Terminology Interactive is a premium online homework management system that includes a host of features to help you study. Registered users will find:

- Fun games and activities built within a virtual hospital
- Powerful tools that track and analyze your results—allowing you to create a personalized learning experience
- Videos, flashcards, and audio pronunciations to help enrich your progress
- Streaming video lesson presentations and self-paced learning modules

www.pearsonhighered.com/mti

Appendices

Appendix I
Word Parts Arranged Alphabetically and Defined

The word parts that have been presented in this textbook are summarized with their definitions for quick reference. Prefixes are listed first, followed by combining forms and suffixes.

Prefix	Definition	Prefix	Definition
a-	without, away from	intra-	inside, within
ab-	away from	macro-	large
ad-	toward	micro-	small
allo-	other, different from usual	mono-	one
an-	without	multi-	many
ante-	before, in front of	myo-	to shut
anti-	against	neo-	new
auto-	self	nulli-	none
bi-	two	pan-	all
brady-	slow	para-	abnormal, two like parts of a pair, beside, near
circum-	around		
contra-	against	per-	through
de-	without	peri-	around
dis-	apart	poly-	many
dys-	abnormal, difficult, painful	post-	after
e-	outward, without	pre-	before, in front of
en-	inward	primi-	first
endo-	inner, within	pro-	before
epi-	upon, over, above	pseudo-	false
eso-	inward	quadri-	four
eu-	normal, good	re-	again
ex-	external, outward	retro-	backward, behind
exo-	outward	semi-	partial, half
extra-	outside of	sub-	below, under
hemi-	half	supra-	above
hetero-	different	tachy-	fast, rapid
homo-	same	tetra-	four
hydro-	water	trans-	across, through
hyper-	excessive, over, above	tri-	three
hypo-	below, under	ultra-	beyond, excess
in-	inward, without, not, within	un-	not
inter-	among, between	xeno-	strange, foreign

Combining Form	Definition	Combining Form	Definition
abdomin/o	abdomen	aden/o	gland
acous/o	hearing	adenoid/o	adenoids
acr/o	extremities	adip/o	fat

Combining Form	Definition	Combining Form	Definition
adren/o	adrenal glands	cephal/o	head
adrenal/o	adrenal glands	cerebell/o	cerebellum
aer/o	air	cerebr/o	cerebrum
agglutin/o	clumping	cerumin/o	cerumen
albin/o	white	cervic/o	neck, cervix
alges/o	sense of pain	chem/o	chemical, drug
alveol/o	alveolus; air sac	chol/e	bile, gall
ambly/o	dull, dim	cholangi/o	bile duct
amnes/o	forgetfulness	cholecyst/o	gallbladder
amni/o	amnion	choledoch/o	common bile duct
an/o	anus	chondr/o	cartilage
andr/o	male	chori/o	chorion
angi/o	vessel	chrom/o	color
ankyl/o	stiff joint	chromat/o	color
anter/o	front	cirrh/o	yellow
anthrac/o	coal	cis/o	to cut
anxi/o	fear, worry	clavicul/o	clavicle
aort/o	aorta	clon/o	rapid contracting and relaxing
append/o	appendix	coagul/o	clotting
appendic/o	appendix	coccyg/o	coccyx
aque/o	water	cochle/o	cochlea
arteri/o	artery	col/o	colon
arthr/o	joint	colon/o	colon
articul/o	joint	colp/o	vagina
aspir/o	to breathe in	compuls/o	drive, compel
astr/o	star	coni/o	dust
atel/o	incomplete	conjunctiv/o	conjunctiva
ather/o	fatty substance	corne/o	cornea
atri/o	atrium	coron/o	heart
audi/o	hearing	corpor/o	body
audit/o	hearing	cortic/o	outer portion, cortex
aur/o	ear	cost/o	rib
auricul/o	ear	crani/o	skull
axill/o	axilla, underarm	crin/o	to secrete
azot/o	nitrogenous waste	crur/o	leg
bacteri/o	bacteria	cry/o	cold
balan/o	glans penis	crypt/o	hidden
bar/o	weight	culd/o	cul-de-sac
bas/o	base	cutane/o	skin
bi/o	life	cyan/o	blue
blast/o	immature, embryonic	cycl/o	ciliary body, ciliary muscle
blephar/o	eyelid	cyst/o	bladder, pouch, sac
brachi/o	arm	cyt/o	cell
bronch/o	bronchus	dacry/o	tear duct, tears
bronchi/o	bronchus	deluss/o	false belief
bronchiol/o	bronchiole	dent/o	tooth
bucc/o	cheek	depress/o	to press down
burs/o	bursa, sac	derm/o	skin
calc/o	calcium	dermat/o	skin
capsul/o	to box	diaphor/o	profuse sweating
carcin/o	cancer	diaphragmat/o	diaphragm
cardi/o	heart	dilat/o	to widen
carp/o	carpus, wrist	dipl/o	double
caud/o	tail	dist/o	away from
cec/o	cecum	diverticul/o	pouch

Combining Form	Definition	Combining Form	Definition
dors/o	back of body	hydr/o	water
duct/o	to bring	hymen/o	hymen
duoden/o	duodenum	hyster/o	uterus
dur/o	dura mater	iatr/o	physician, medicine, treatment
electr/o	electricity	ichthy/o	scaly, dry
embol/o	plug	idi/o	distinctive
embry/o	embryo	ile/o	ileum
emmetr/o	correct, proper	ili/o	ilium
encephal/o	brain	immun/o	immunity, protection
enter/o	small intestine	infer/o	below
eosin/o	rosy red	inguin/o	groin region
epididym/o	epididymis	iod/o	iodine
epiglott/o	epiglottis	ir/o	iris
episi/o	vulva	irid/o	iris
epitheli/o	epithelium	isch/o	to hold back
erg/o	work	ischi/o	ischium
erythr/o	red	jejun/o	jejunum
esophag/o	esophagus	kal/i	potassium
esthes/o	sensation, feeling	kerat/o	cornea, hard, horny
estr/o	female	ket/o	ketones
extens/o	to stretch out	keton/o	ketones
factiti/o	artificial, contrived	kinesi/o	movement
fasci/o	fibrous band	klept/o	to steal
femor/o	femur	kyph/o	hump
fet/o	fetus	labi/o	lip
fibr/o	fibers	labyrinth/o	labyrinth (inner ear)
fibrin/o	fibers, fibrous	lacrim/o	tears
fibul/o	fibula	lact/o	milk
flex/o	to bend	lamin/o	lamina, part of vertebra
fluor/o	fluorescence, luminous	lapar/o	abdomen
fus/o	pouring	laps/o	to slide back
gastr/o	stomach	laryng/o	larynx, voice box
genit/o	genitals	later/o	side
gingiv/o	gums	leuk/o	white
glauc/o	gray	lingu/o	tongue
gli/o	glue	lip/o	fat
glomerul/o	glomerulus	lith/o	stone
gloss/o	tongue	lob/o	lobe
gluc/o	glucose	lord/o	bent backwards
glute/o	buttock	lumb/o	loin, low back
glyc/o	sugar	lymph/o	lymph
glycos/o	sugar, glucose	lymphaden/o	lymph node
gonad/o	sex glands	lymphangi/o	lymph vessel
granul/o	granules	macul/o	macula lutea
gynec/o	female, woman	mamm/o	breast
habilitat/o	ability	mandibul/o	mandible
hal/o	to breathe	mast/o	breast
hallucin/o	imagined perception	maxill/o	maxilla
hem/o	blood	meat/o	meatus
hemat/o	blood	medi/o	middle
hepat/o	liver	medull/o	inner portion, medulla, oblongata
hidr/o	sweat		
hist/o	tissue	melan/o	black
home/o	sameness	men/o	menses, menstruation
humer/o	humerus	mening/o	meninges

Combining Form	Definition	Combining Form	Definition
meningi/o	meninges	parathyroid/o	parathyroid gland
ment/o	mind	patell/o	patella
metacarp/o	metacarpals	path/o	disease
metatars/o	metatarsals	pect/o	chest
metr/o	uterus	ped/o	child, foot
mi/o	lessening	pedicul/o	lice
mineral/o	minerals, electrolytes	pelv/o	pelvis
miss/o	to send back	pen/o	penis
morbid/o	ill	perine/o	perineum
morph/o	shape	peritone/o	peritoneum
mort/o	death	phac/o	lens
muc/o	mucus	phag/o	eat, swallow
muscul/o	muscles	phalang/o	phalanges
mutat/o	to change	pharmac/o	drug
my/o	muscle	pharyng/o	pharynx (throat)
myc/o	fungus	phleb/o	vein
mydr/i	widening	phob/o	irrational fear
myel/o	bone marrow, spinal cord	phon/o	sound
myocardi/o	heart muscle	phot/o	light
myos/o	muscle	phren/o	mind
myring/o	tympanic membrane (eardrum)	physic/o	body
		pineal/o	pineal gland
nas/o	nose	pituitar/o	pituitary gland
nat/o	birth	plant/o	sole of foot
natr/o	sodium	pleur/o	pleura
necr/o	death	pneum/o	lung, air
nephr/o	kidney	pneumon/o	lung, air
neur/o	nerve	pod/o	foot
neutr/o	neutral	poli/o	gray matter
noct/i	night	polyp/o	polyp
nucle/o	nucleus	pont/o	pons
nyctal/o	night	poster/o	back
o/o	egg	presby/o	old age
obsess/o	besieged by thoughts	proct/o	rectum and anus
ocul/o	eye	prostat/o	prostate gland
odont/o	tooth	prosthet/o	addition
olig/o	scanty	protein/o	protein
onc/o	tumor	proxim/o	near to
onych/o	nail	psych/o	mind
oophor/o	ovary	pub/o	genital region, pubis
ophthalm/o	eye	pulmon/o	lung
opt/o	eye, vision	pupill/o	pupil
optic/o	eye, vision	py/o	pus
or/o	mouth	pyel/o	renal pelvis
orch/o	testes	pylor/o	pylorus
orchi/o	testes	pyr/o	fire
orchid/o	testes	radi/o	radius, ray (X-ray)
orth/o	straight, correct, upright	radic/o	root
oste/o	bone	radicul/o	nerve root
ot/o	ear	rect/o	rectum
ovari/o	ovary	recumb/o	to lie back
ox/o, ox/i	oxygen	ren/o	kidney
palat/o	palate	retin/o	retina
pancreat/o	pancreas	rhin/o	nose
papill/o	optic disc	rhytid/o	wrinkle

Combining Form	Definition	Combining Form	Definition
roentgen/o	X-ray	thec/o	sheath (meninges)
rotat/o	to revolve	therm/o	heat
sacr/o	sacrum	thorac/o	chest, thorax
salping/o	auditory tube (eustachian tube), uterine tubes, fallopian tubes	thromb/o	clot
		thym/o	thymus gland
sanguin/o	blood	thyr/o	thyroid gland
sarc/o	flesh (muscular substance)	thyroid/o	thyroid gland
scapul/o	scapula	tibi/o	tibia
schiz/o	split	tom/o	to cut
scler/o	hard, sclera	ton/o	tone
scoli/o	crooked, bent	tonsill/o	tonsils
seb/o	oil	topic/o	a specific area
sect/o	to cut	tox/o	poison
sept/o	a wall	toxic/o	poison
septic/o	infection	trache/o	trachea, windpipe
sialaden/o	salivary gland	trich/o	hair
sigmoid/o	sigmoid colon	tuss/o	cough
sinus/o	sinus, cavity	tympan/o	tympanic membrane (eardrum)
soci/o	society		
somat/o	body	uln/o	ulna
somn/o	sleep	ungu/o	nail
son/o	sound	ur/o	urine
specul/o	to look at	ureter/o	ureter
spermat/o	sperm	urethr/o	urethra
sphygm/o	pulse	urin/o	urine
spin/o	spine	uter/o	uterus
spir/o	breathing	uve/o	choroid
splen/o	spleen	vagin/o	vagina
spondyl/o	vertebrae	valv/o	valve
staped/o	stapes	valvul/o	valve
stern/o	sternum	varic/o	dilated vein
steth/o	chest	vas/o	vas deferens, vessel, duct
stigmat/o	point	vascul/o	blood vessel
super/o	above	ven/o	vein
synov/o	synovial membrane	ventr/o	belly
synovi/o	synovial membrane	ventricul/o	brain ventricle, ventricle
system/o	systems	vers/o	to turn
tars/o	ankle, tarsus	vertebr/o	vertebra
ten/o	tendon	vesic/o	bladder
tenacul/o	to hold	vesicul/o	seminal vesicle
tend/o	tendon	viscer/o	internal organ
tendin/o	tendon	vitre/o	glassy
testicul/o	testes, testicle	vulv/o	vulva
thalam/o	thalamus	xer/o	dry

Suffix	Definition	Suffix	Definition
-ac	pertaining to	-asthenia	weakness
-al	pertaining to	-atic	pertaining to
-algia	pain	-blast	immature, embryonic
-an	pertaining to	-capnia	carbon dioxide
-apheresis	removal, carry away	-cele	hernia, protrusion
-ar	pertaining to	-centesis	puncture to withdraw fluid
-arche	beginning	-cide	to kill
-ary	pertaining to	-clasia	to surgically break

Suffix	Definition	Suffix	Definition
-crit	separation of	-manometer	instrument to measure pressure
-cusis	hearing		
-cyesis	state of pregnancy	-megaly	enlargement, large
-cyte	cell	-meter	instrument for measuring
-cytosis	more than the normal number of cells	-metrist	specialist in measuring
		-metry	process of measuring
-derma	skin condition	-nic	pertaining to
-desis	fuse, stabilize	-nomics	pertaining to laws
-dipsia	thirst	-oid	resembling
-dynia	pain	-ole	small
-eal	pertaining to	-oma	mass, tumor, swelling
-ectasis	dilation	-opaque	nontransparent
-ectomy	surgical removal	-opia	vision condition
-edema	swelling	-opsia	vision condition
-emesis	vomit	-opsy	view of
-emia	blood condition	-orexia	appetite
-gen	that which produces	-ory	pertaining to
-genesis	produces, generates	-ose	pertaining to
-genic	producing, produced by	-osis	abnormal condition
-globin	protein	-osmia	smell
-globulin	protein	-ostomy	surgically create an opening,
-gram	record or picture	-otia	ear condition
-graph	instrument for recording	-otomy	cutting into
-graphy	process of recording	-ous	pertaining to
-gravida	pregnancy	-para	to bear (offspring)
-ia	condition, state	-paresis	weakness
-iac	pertaining to	-partum	childbirth
-iasis	abnormal condition	-pathy	disease
-iatrist	physician	-penia	abnormal decrease, too few
-iatry	medical treatment	-pepsia	digestion
-ic	pertaining to	-pexy	surgical fixation
-ical	pertaining to	-phagia	eat, swallow
-ician	specialist	-phasia	speech
-ile	pertaining to	-phil	attracted to
-ine	pertaining to	-philia	attracted to
-ion	action, condition	-phobia	fear
-ior	pertaining to	-phonia	voice
-ism	state of	-phoresis	carrying
-ist	specialist	-phylaxis	protection
-istry	specialty of	-plasia	development, growth, formation
-itis	inflammation		
-kinesia	movement	-plasm	formation, development, growth
-listhesis	slipping		
-lith	stone	-plastic	pertaining to development
-lithiasis	condition of stones	-plasty	surgical repair
-logic	pertaining to studying	-plegia	paralysis
-logical	pertaining to the study of	-pnea	breathing
-logist	one who studies	-poiesis	formation
-logy	study of	-porosis	porous
-lucent	to shine through	-prandial	pertaining to a meal
-lysis	destruction	-pressin	to press down
-lytic	destruction	-ptosis	drooping
-malacia	abnormal softening	-ptysis	spitting
-mania	frenzy	-rrhage	abnormal flow, excessive

Suffix	Definition	Suffix	Definition
-rrhagia	abnormal flow condition	-taxia	muscle coordination
-rrhagic	pertaining to abnormal flow	-tension	pressure
-rrhaphy	suture	-therapy	treatment
-rrhea	discharge, flow	-thorax	chest
-rrhexis	rupture	-tic	pertaining to
-salpinx	uterine tube	-tocia	labor, childbirth
-sclerosis	hardening	-tome	instrument to cut
-scope	instrument for viewing	-tonia	tone
-scopic	pertaining to visually examining	-tonic	pertaining to tone
		-tripsy	surgical crushing
-scopy	process of visually examining	-trophic	pertaining to development
-spasm	involuntary muscle contraction	-trophy	nourishment, development
-spermia	condition of sperm	-tropia	turned condition
-stasis	standing still	-tropin	to stimulate
-stat	standing still	-ule	small
-stenosis	narrowing	-uria	condition of the urine

Appendix II
Word Parts Arranged Alphabetically by Definition

The definitions of the word parts that have been presented in this textbook are presented here and are arranged alphabetically. Prefixes are listed first, followed by combining forms and suffixes.

Definition	Prefix	Definition	Prefix
abnormal	dys-, para-	inside	intra-
above	hyper-, epi-, supra-	inward	en-, eso-, in-
across	trans-	large	macro-
after	post-	many	multi-, poly-
again	re-	near	para-
against	anti-, contra-	new	neo-
all	pan-	none	nulli-
among	inter-	normal	eu-
apart	dis-	not	in-, un-
around	circum-, peri-	one	mono-
away from	a-, ab-	other	allo-
backward	retro-	outside of	extra-
before	ante-, pre-, pro-	outward	ex-, exo-, e-
behind	retro-	over	epi-, hyper-
below	hypo-, sub-	painful	dys-
beside	para-	partial	semi-
between	inter-	same	homo-
beyond	ultra-	self	auto-
different from usual	allo-	to shut	myo-
different	hetero-	slow	brady-
difficult	dys-	small	micro-
excess	ultra-	strange	xeno-
excessive	hyper-	three	tri-
external	ex-	through	trans-, per-
false	pseudo-	toward	ad-
fast	tachy-	two	bi-
first	primi-	two like parts of a pair	para-
foreign	xeno-	under	hypo-, sub-
four	quadri-, tetra-	upon	epi-
good	eu-	water	hydro-
half	semi-, hemi-	within	endo-, in-, intra-
in front of	ante-, pre-	without	e-, a-, an-, de-, in-
inner	endo-		

Definition	Combining Form	Definition	Combining Form
abdomen	abdomin/o, lapar/o	air	aer/o, pneum/o, pneumon/o
ability	habilitat/o		
above	super/o	air sac	alveol/o
addition	prosthet/o	alveolus	alveol/o
adenoids	adenoid/o	amnion	amni/o
adrenal glands	adren/o, adrenal/o	ankle	tars/o

Definition	Combining Form	Definition	Combining Form
anus	an/o	cartilage	chondr/o
aorta	aort/o	cavity	sinus/o
appendix	append/o, appendic/o	cecum	cec/o
		cell	cyt/o
arm	brachi/o	cerebellum	cerebell/o
artery	arteri/o	cerebrum	cerebr/o
artificial	factiti/o	cerumen	cerumin/o
atrium	atri/o	cervix	cervic/o
auditory tube	salping/o	to change	mutat/o
away from	dist/o	cheek	bucc/o
axilla	axill/o	chemical	chem/o
back	poster/o	chest	pect/o, steth/o, thorac/o
back of body	dors/o		
bacteria	bacteri/o	child	ped/o
base	bas/o	chorion	chori/o
belly	ventr/o	choroid	uve/o
below	infer/o	ciliary body	cycl/o
to bend	flex/o	ciliary muscle	cycl/o
bent	scoli/o	clavicle	clavicul/o
bent backwards	lord/o	clot	thromb/o
besieged by thoughts	obsess/o	clotting	coagul/o
bile duct	cholangi/o	clumping	agglutin/o
bile	chol/e	coal	anthrac/o
birth	nat/o	coccyx	coccyg/o
black	melan/o	cochlea	cochle/o
bladder	vesic/o, cyst/o	cold	cry/o
blood	hem/o, hemat/o, sanguin/o	colon	col/o, colon/o
		color	chrom/o, chromat/o
blood vessel	vascul/o	common bile duct	choledoch/o
blue	cyan/o	compel	compuls/o
body	corpor/o, physic/o, somat/o	conjunctiva	conjunctiv/o
		contrived	factiti/o
bone	oste/o	cornea	corne/o, kerat/o
bone marrow	myel/o	correct	emmetr/o, orth/o
to box	capsul/o	cortex	cortic/o
brain	encephal/o	cough	tuss/o
brain ventricle	ventricul/o	crooked	scoli/o
breast	mamm/o, mast/o	cul-de-sac	culd/o
to breathe	hal/o	to cut	cis/o, sect/o, tom/o
to breathe in	aspir/o	death	mort/o, necr/o
breathing	spir/o	diaphragm	diaphragmat/o
to bring	duct/o	dilated vein	varic/o
bronchiole	bronchiol/o	dim	ambly/o
bronchus	bronch/o, bronchi/o	disease	path/o
bursa	burs/o	distinctive	idi/o
buttock	glute/o	double	dipl/o
calcium	calc/o	drive	compuls/o
cancer	carcin/o	drug	chem/o, pharmac/o
carpus	carp/o	dry	ichthy/o, xer/o

Definition	Combining Form	Definition	Combining Form
duct	vas/o	glassy	vitre/o
dull	ambly/o	glomerulus	glomerul/o
duodenum	duoden/o	glucose	glycos/o, gluc/o
dura mater	dur/o	glue	gli/o
dust	coni/o	granules	granul/o
ear	aur/o, auricul/o, ot/o	gray	glauc/o
		gray matter	poli/o
eardrum	myring/o, tympan/o	groin region	inguin/o
eat	phag/o	gums	gingiv/o
egg	o/o	hair	trich/o
electricity	electr/o	hard	kerat/o, scler/o
electrolytes	mineral/o	head	cephal/o
embryo	embry/o	hearing	audi/o, audit/o, acous/o
embryonic	blast/o		
epididymis	epididym/o	heart	cardi/o, coron/o
epiglottis	epiglott/o	heart muscle	myocardi/o
epithelium	epitheli/o	heat	therm/o
esophagus	esophag/o	hidden	crypt/o
eustachian tube	salping/o	to hold	tenacul/o
extremities	acr/o	to hold back	isch/o
eye	ocul/o, ophthalm/o, opt/o, optic/o	horny	kerat/o
		humerus	humer/o
eyelid	blephar/o	hump	kyph/o
fallopian tubes	salping/o	hymen	hymen/o
false belief	deluss/o	ileum	ile/o
fat	adip/o, lip/o	ilium	ili/o
fatty substance	ather/o	ill	morbid/o
fear	anxi/o	imagined perception	hallucin/o
feeling	esthes/o	immature	blast/o
female	estr/o, gynec/o	immunity	immun/o
femur	femor/o	incomplete	atel/o
fetus	fet/o	infection	septic/o
fibers	fibr/o, fibrin/o	inner portion	medull/o
fibrous	fibrin/o	internal organ	viscer/o
fibrous band	fasci/o	iodine	iod/o
fibula	fibul/o	iris	ir/o, irid/o
fire	pyr/o	irrational fear	phob/o
flesh (muscular substance)	sarc/o	ischium	ischi/o
fluorescence	fluor/o	jejunum	jejun/o
foot	ped/o, pod/o	joint	arthr/o, articul/o
forgetfulness	amnes/o	ketones	ket/o, keton/o
front	anter/o	kidney	nephr/o, ren/o
fungus	myc/o	labyrinth	labyrinth/o
gall	chol/e	inner ear	labyrinth/o
gallbladder	cholecyst/o	lamina	lamin/o
genital region	pub/o	larynx	laryng/o
genitals	genit/o	leg	crur/o
gland	aden/o	lens	phac/o
glans penis	balan/o	lessening	mi/o

Definition	Combining Form	Definition	Combining Form
lice	pedicul/o	nucleus	nucle/o
to lie back	recumb/o	oil	seb/o
life	bi/o	old age	presby/o
light	phot/o	outer portion	cortic/o
lip	labi/o	ovary	oophor/o, ovari/o
liver	hepat/o	oxygen	ox/o, ox/i
lobe	lob/o	palate	palat/o
loin	lumb/o	pancreas	pancreat/o
to look at	specul/o	parathyroid gland	parathyroid/o
low back	lumb/o	part of vertebra	lamin/o
luminous	fluor/o	patella	patell/o
lung	pulmon/o, pneum/o, pneumon/o	pelvis	pelv/o
		penis	pen/o
		perineum	perine/o
lymph	lymph/o	peritoneum	peritone/o
lymph node	lymphaden/o	phalanges	phalang/o
lymph vessel	lymphangi/o	pharynx	pharyng/o
macula lutea	macul/o	physician	iatr/o
male	andr/o	pineal gland	pineal/o
mandible	mandibul/o	pituitary gland	pituitar/o
maxilla	maxill/o	pleura	pleur/o
meatus	meat/o	plug	embol/o
medicine	iatr/o	point	stigmat/o
medulla oblongata	medull/o	poison	tox/o, toxic/o
meninges	mening/o, meningi/o, thec/o	polyp	polyp/o
		pons	pont/o
menses	men/o	potassium	kal/i
menstruation	men/o	pouch	diverticul/o, cyst/o
metacarpals	metacarp/o	pouring	fus/o
metatarsals	metatars/o	to press down	depress/o
middle	medi/o	profuse sweating	diaphor/o
milk	lact/o	proper	emmetr/o
mind	ment/o, phren/o, psych/o	prostate gland	prostat/o
		protection	immun/o
minerals	mineral/o	protein	protein/o
mouth	or/o	pubis	pub/o
movement	kinesi/o	pulse	sphygm/o
mucus	muc/o	pupil	pupill/o
muscle	my/o, myos/o, muscul/o	pus	py/o
		pylorus	pylor/o
nail	onych/o, ungu/o	radius	radi/o
near to	proxim/o	rapid contracting and relaxing	clon/o
neck	cervic/o		
nerve	neur/o	ray (X-ray)	radi/o
nerve root	radicul/o	rectum	rect/o
neutral	neutr/o	rectum and anus	proct/o
night	noct/l, nyctal/o	red	erythr/o
nitrogenous waste	azot/o	renal pelvis	pyel/o
nose	nas/o, rhin/o	retina	retin/o

Definition	Combining Form	Definition	Combining Form
to revolve	rotat/o	swallow	phag/o
rib	cost/o	sweat	hidr/o
root	radic/o	synovial membrane	synov/o, synovi/o
rosy red	eosin/o	systems	system/o
sac	burs/o, cyst/o	tail	caud/o
sacrum	sacr/o	tarsus	tars/o
salivary gland	sialaden/o	tear duct	dacry/o
sameness	home/o	tears	dacry/o, lacrim/o
scaly	ichthy/o	tendon	ten/o, tend/o, tendin/o
scanty	olig/o		
scapula	scapul/o	testes	orch/o, orchi/o, orchid/o, testicul/o
sclera	scler/o		
to secrete	crin/o	thalamus	thalam/o
seminal vesicle	vesicul/o	thorax	thorac/o
to send back	miss/o	throat	pharyng/o
sensation	esthes/o	thymus gland	thym/o
sense of pain	alges/o	thyroid gland	thyr/o, thyroid/o
sex glands	gonad/o	tibia	tibi/o
shape	morph/o	tissue	hist/o
sheath (meninges)	thec/o	tone	ton/o
side	later/o	tongue	gloss/o, lingu/o
sigmoid colon	sigmoid/o	tonsils	tonsill/o
sinus	sinus/o	tooth	dent/o, odont/o
skin	cutane/o, derm/o, dermat/o	trachea	trache/o
		treatment	iatr/o
skull	crani/o	tumor	onc/o
sleep	somn/o	to turn	vers/o
to slide back	laps/o	tympanic membrane	myring/o, tympan/o
small intestine	enter/o	ulna	uln/o
society	soci/o	underarm	axill/o
sodium	natr/o	upright	orth/o
sole of foot	plant/o	ureter	ureter/o
sound	phon/o, son/o	urethra	urethr/o
specific area	topic/o	urine	ur/o, urin/o
sperm	spermat/o	uterine tubes	salping/o
spinal cord	myel/o	uterus	hyster/o, metr/o, uter/o
spine	spin/o		
spleen	splen/o	vagina	colp/o, vagin/o
split	schiz/o	valve	valv/o, valvul/o
stapes	staped/o	vas deferens	vas/o
star	astr/o	vein	phleb/o, ven/o
to steal	klept/o	ventricle	ventricul/o
sternum	stern/o	vertebra	vertebr/o, spondyl/o
stiff joint	ankyl/o	vessel	angi/o, vas/o
stomach	gastr/o	vision	opt/o, optic/o
stone	lith/o	voice box	laryng/o
straight	orth/o	vulva	episi/o, vulv/o
to stretch out	extens/o	wall	sept/o
sugar	glyc/o, glycos/o	water	aque/o, hydr/o

Definition	Combining Form	Definition	Combining Form
weight	bar/o	work	erg/o
white	albin/o, leuk/o	worry	anxi/o
to widen	dilat/o	wrinkle	rhytid/o
widening	mydr/i	wrist	carp/o
windpipe	trache/o	X-ray	roentgen/o
woman	gynec/o	yellow	cirrh/o

Definition	Suffix	Definition	Suffix
abnormal condition	-iasis, -osis	fear	-phobia
abnormal decrease	-penia	flow	-rrhea
abnormal flow condition	-rrhagia	formation	-poiesis, -plasia, -plasm
abnormal flow	-rrhage		
abnormal flow (pertaining to)	-rrhagic	frenzy	-mania
		fuse	-desis
abnormal softening	-malacia	generates	-genesis
action	-ion	growth	-plasia, -plasm
appetite	-orexia	hardening	-sclerosis
attracted to	-phil, -philia	hearing	-cusis
to bear (offspring)	-para	hernia	-cele
beginning	-arche	immature	-blast
blood condition	-emia	inflammation	-itis
breathing	-pnea	pressure (instrument to measure)	-manometer
carbon dioxide	-capnia		
carry away	-apheresis	involuntary muscle contraction	-spasm
carrying	-phoresis		
cell	-cyte	to kill	-cide
chest	-thorax	labor	-tocia
childbirth	-partum, -tocia	large	-megaly
condition	-ion, -ia	laws (pertaining to)	-nomics
condition of sperm	-spermia	mass	-oma
condition of stones	-lithiasis	meal (pertaining to a)	-prandial
condition of the urine	-uria	measuring (instrument for)	-meter
cut (instrument to)	-tome	measuring (process of)	-metry
cutting into	-otomy	medical treatment	-iatry
destruction	-lytic, -lysis	more than the normal number of cells	-cytosis
development	-plasia, -trophy, -plasm		
		movement	-kinesia
development (pertaining to)	-plastic, -trophic	muscle coordination	-taxia
digestion	-pepsia	narrowing	-stenosis
dilation	-ectasis	nontransparent	-opaque
discharge	-rrhea	nourishment	-trophy
disease	-pathy	one who studies	-logist
drooping	-ptosis	pain	-algia, -dynia
ear condition	-otia	paralysis	-plegia
eat	-phagia	pertaining to	-ac, -al, -an, -ar, -ary, -atic, -eal, -ia, -iac, -ic, -ical, -ile, -ine, -ior, -nic, -ory, -ose, -ous, -tic
embryonic	-blast		
enlargement	-megaly		
excessive flow	-rrhage		
fallopian tube	-salpinx	physician	-iatrist

Definition	Suffix	Definition	Suffix
porous	-porosis	to stimulate	-tropin
pregnancy	-gravida	stone	-lith
pregnancy (state of)	-cyesis	studying (pertaining to)	-logic
pressure	-tension	study of	-logy
to press down	-pressin	study of (pertaining to the)	-logical
produced by	-genic	surgical fixation	-pexy
produces	-genesis	surgical removal	-ectomy
producing	-genic	surgical repair	-plasty
protection	-phylaxis	to surgically break	-clasia
protein	-globin, -globulin	surgically create an opening	-ostomy
protrusion	-cele	suture	-rrhaphy
puncture to withdraw fluid	-centesis	swallow	-phagia
record or picture	-gram	swelling	-edema, -oma
recording (instrument for)	-graph	that which produces	-gen
recording (process of)	-graphy	thirst	-dipsia
removal	-apheresis	tone	-tonia
resembling	-oid	tone (pertaining to)	-tonic
rupture	-rrhexis	too few	-penia
separation of	-crit	treatment	-therapy
to shine through	-lucent	tumor	-oma
skin condition	-derma	turned condition	-tropia
slipping	-listhesis	uterine tube	-salpinx
small	-ole, -ule	viewing (instrument for)	-scope
smell	-osmia	view of	-opsy
specialist	-ician, -ist	vision condition	-opia, -opsia
specialist in measuring	-metrist	visually examining (pertaining to)	-scopic
specialty of	-istry	visually examining (process of)	-scopy
speech	-phasia		
spitting	-ptysis	voice	-phonia
stabilize	-desis	vomit	-emesis
standing still	-stasis, -stat	weakness	-asthenia, -paresis
state	-ia		
state of	-ism		

Appendix III
Abbreviations

Abbreviation	Meaning	Abbreviation	Meaning
@	at	ASL	American Sign Language
5-FU	5-fluorouracil	AST	aspartate transaminase
^{67}Ga	radioactive gallium	Astigm	astigmatism
^{99m}Tc	radioactive technetium	ATN	acute tubular necrosis
^{131}I	radioactive iodine	AU	both ears
^{133}Xe	radioactive xenon	AV, A-V	atrioventricular
^{201}Tl	radioactive thallium	β	beta
α	alpha	Ba	barium
$\bar{a}$	before	BaE	barium enema
AAROM	active assistive range of motion	basos	basophils
		BBB	bundle branch block (L for left; R for right)
AB	abortion		
ABGs	arterial blood gases	BC	bone conduction
ac	before meals	BCC	basal cell carcinoma
ACTH	adrenocorticotropin hormone	BDT	bone density testing
ad lib	as desired	BE	barium enema, below elbow
AD	Alzheimer's disease, right ear	bid	twice a day
ADD	attention-deficit disorder	BK	below knee
ADH	antidiuretic hormone	BM	bowel movement
ADHD	attention-deficit/hyperactivity disorder	BMD	bone mineral density
		BMR	basal metabolic rate
ADL	activities of daily living	BMT	bone marrow transplant
AE	above elbow	BNO	bladder neck obstruction
AF	atrial fibrillation	BP	blood pressure
AGN	acute glomerulonephritis	BPD	bipolar disorder
AI	artificial insemination	BPH	benign prostatic hyperplasia
AIDS	acquired immunodeficiency syndrome	bpm	beats per minute
		Bronch	bronchoscopy
AK	above knee	BS	bowel sounds
ALL	acute lymphocytic leukemia	BSE	breast self-examination
ALS	amyotrophic lateral sclerosis	BUN	blood urea nitrogen
ALT	alanine transaminase	BX, bx	biopsy
AMI	acute myocardial infarction	$\bar{c}$	with
AML	acute myelogenous leukemia	C1, C2, etc.	first cervical vertebra, second cervical vertebra, etc.
Angio	angiography		
ANS	autonomic nervous system	Ca	calcium, cancer
ante	before	CA	chronological age
AP	anteroposterior	CABG	coronary artery bypass graft
APAP	acetaminophen (Tylenol™)	CAD	coronary artery disease
aq	aqueous (water)	cap(s)	capsule(s)
ARC	AIDS-related complex	CAPD	continuous ambulatory peritoneal dialysis
ARDS	adult (or acute) respiratory distress syndrome		
		CAT	computerized axial tomography
ARF	acute renal failure		
ARMD	age-related macular degeneration	cath	catheterization
		CBC	complete blood count
AROM	active range of motion	CBD	common bile duct
AS	arteriosclerosis, left ear	CC	cardiac catheterization, chief complaint, clean catch urine specimen
ASA	aspirin		
ASD	atrial septal defect		
ASHD	arteriosclerotic heart disease	CCU	coronary care unit

Abbreviation	Meaning	Abbreviation	Meaning
c.gl.	correction with glasses	DSM	*Diagnostic and Statistical Manual of Mental Disorders*
chemo	chemotherapy		
CHF	congestive heart failure	dtd	give of such a dose
Ci	curie	DTR	deep tendon reflex
CIS	carcinoma in situ	DVA	distance visual acuity
Cl⁻	chloride	DVT	deep vein thrombosis
CLL	chronic lymphocytic leukemia	Dx	diagnosis
CML	chronic myelogenous leukemia	DXA	dual-energy absorptiometry
		e-stim	electrical stimulation
CNS	central nervous system	ECC	extracorporeal circulation
CO_2	carbon dioxide	ECCE	extracapsular cataract extraction
CoA	coarctation of the aorta		
COPD	chronic obstructive pulmonary disease	ECG, EKG	electrocardiogram
		ECHO	echocardiogram
CP	cerebral palsy, chest pain	ECT	electroconvulsive therapy
CPK	creatine phosphokinase	ED	erectile dysfunction
CPR	cardiopulmonary resuscitation	EDC	estimated date of confinement
CRF	chronic renal failure		
C&S	culture and sensitivity	EEG	electroencephalogram, electroencephalography
CS, C-section	cesarean section		
CSD	congenital septal defect	EENT	eye, ear, nose, and throat
CSF	cerebrospinal fluid	EGD	esophagogastroduodenoscopy
CT	calcitonin, computerized tomography	ELISA	enzyme-linked immunosorbent assay
CTA	clear to auscultation	EM	emmetropia
CTS	carpal tunnel syndrome	EMB	endometrial biopsy
CV	cardiovascular	EMG	electromyogram
CVA	cerebrovascular accident	Endo	endoscopy
CVD	cerebrovascular disease	ENT	ear, nose, and throat
CVS	chorionic villus sampling	EOM	extraocular movement
Cx	cervix	eosins, eos	eosinophils
CXR	chest X-ray	ERCP	endoscopic retrograde cholangiopancreatography
cysto	cystoscopy		
d	day	ERT	estrogen replacement therapy
D	diopter (lens strength)	ERV	expiratory reserve volume
dB	decibel	ESR, SR, sed rate	erythrocyte sedimentation rate
D & C	dilation and curettage		
d/c, DISC	discontinue	ESRD	end-stage renal disease
DC, disc	discontinue	ESWL	extracorporeal shockwave lithotripsy
DEA	Drug Enforcement Agency		
decub	decubitus ulcer, lying down	et	and
Derm, derm	dermatology	EU	excretory urography
DI	diabetes insipidus, diagnostic imaging	EUA	exam under anesthesia
		FBS	fasting blood sugar
diff	differential	FDA	Federal Drug Administration
dil	dilute	FEKG	fetal electrocardiogram
disp	dispense	FHR	fetal heart rate
DJD	degenerative joint disease	FHT	fetal heart tone
DM	diabetes mellitus	FOBT	fecal occult blood test
DOE	dyspnea on exertion	FRC	functional residual capacity
DPT	diphtheria, pertussis, tetanus injection	FS	frozen section
		FSH	follicle-stimulating hormone
DRE	digital rectal exam	FTND	full-term normal delivery
DSA	digital subtraction angiography	FX, Fx	fracture
		GA	gallium, general anesthesia

Abbreviation	Meaning	Abbreviation	Meaning
GB	gallbladder, gallbladder X-ray	ICP	intracranial pressure
GC	gonorrhea	ICU	intensive care unit
GERD	gastroesophageal reflux disease	I&D	incision and drainage
GH	growth hormone	ID	intradermal
GI, grav I	first pregnancy	IDDM	insulin-dependent diabetes mellitus
GI	gastrointestinal	Ig	immunoglobulins (IgA, IgD, IgE, IgG, IgM)
gm	gram		
GOT	glutamic oxaloacetic transaminase	IM	intramuscular
gr	grain	inj	injection
gt	drop	I&O	intake and output
gtt	drops	IOP	intraocular pressure
GTT	glucose tolerance test	IPD	intermittent peritoneal dialysis
GU	genitourinary	IPPB	intermittent positive pressure breathing
GVHD	graft versus host disease		
GYN, gyn	gynecology	IRDS	infant respiratory distress syndrome
H_2O	water		
HA	headache	IRV	inspiratory reserve volume
HAV	hepatitis A virus	IU	international unit
HBV	hepatitis B virus	IUD	intrauterine device
HCG, hCG	human chorionic gonadotropin	IV	intravenous
		IVC	intravenous cholangiogram, intravenous cholangiography
HCl	hydrochloric acid	IVF	in vitro fertilization
HCO_3^-	bicarbonate	IVP	intravenous pyelogram
HCT, Hct, crit	hematocrit	JRA	juvenile rheumatoid arthritis
HCV	hepatitis C virus	K^+	potassium
HD	Hodgkin's disease, hemodialysis	kg	kilogram
		KS	Kaposi's sarcoma
HDN	hemolytic disease of the newborn	KUB	kidney, ureter, bladder
		L1, L2, etc.	first lumbar vertebra, second lumbar vertebra, etc.
HDV	hepatitis D virus		
HEENT	head, ears, eyes, nose, throat	L	liter
HEV	hepatitis E virus	LASIK	laser-assisted in-situ keratomileusis
Hgb, Hb, HGB	hemoglobin		
HIV	human immunodeficiency virus	LAT, lat	lateral
		LBW	low birth weight
HMD	hyaline membrane disease	LE	lower extremity
HNP	herniated nucleus pulposus	LGI	lower gastrointestinal series
HPV	human papilloma virus	LH	luteinizing hormone
HRT	hormone replacement therapy	LL	left lateral
hs	at bedtime	LLE	left lower extremity
HSG	hysterosalpingography	LLL	left lower lobe
HSV-1	herpes simplex virus type 1	LLQ	left lower quadrant
HSV	herpes simplex virus	LMP	last menstrual period
HTN	hypertension	LP	lumbar puncture
Hz	hertz	LUE	left upper extremity
ī	one	LUL	left upper lobe
īī	two	LUQ	left upper quadrant
īīī	three	LVAD	left ventricular assist device
IBD	inflammatory bowel disease	LVH	left ventricular hypertrophy
IBS	irritable bowel syndrome	lymphs	lymphocytes
IC	inspiratory capacity	MA	mental age
ICCE	intracapsular cataract extraction	mA	milliampere
		MAO	monoamine oxidase

Abbreviation	Meaning	Abbreviation	Meaning
mcg	microgram	OM	otitis media
mCi	millicurie	O&P	ova and parasites
MD	muscular dystrophy	Ophth.	ophthalmology
MDI	metered-dose inhaler	OR	operating room
mEq	milliequivalent	ORIF	open reduction–internal fixation
mets	metastases		
mg	milligram	Orth, ortho	orthopedics
MI	myocardial infarction, mitral insufficiency	OS	left eye
		OT	occupational therapy
mL	milliliter	OTC	over the counter
mm Hg	millimeters of mercury	Oto	otology
MM	malignant melanoma	OU	each eye/both eyes
MMPI	Minnesota Multiphasic Personality Inventory	oz	ounce
		$\bar{p}$	after
mono	mononucleosis	P	pulse
monos	monocytes	PA	pernicious anemia, posteroanterior
MR	mitral regurgitation		
MRA	magnetic resonance angiography	PAC	premature atrial contraction
		PAP	Papanicolaou test
MRI	magnetic resonance imaging	PARR	postanesthetic recovery room
MS	mitral stenosis, multiple sclerosis, musculoskeletal	PBI	protein-bound iodine
		pc	after meals
MSH	melanocyte-stimulating hormone	PCA	patient-controlled administration
MTX	methotrexate	PCP	pneumocystis pneumonia
MUA	manipulation under anesthesia	PCV	packed cell volume
		PDA	patent ductus arteriosus
MVP	mitral valve prolapse	PDR	*Physician's Desk Reference*
Na⁺	sodium	PE tube	pressure equalizing tube
NB	newborn	per	with
NG	nasogastric (tube)	PERRLA	pupils equal, round, react to light and accommodation
NHL	non-Hodgkin's lymphoma		
NIDDM	non-insulin-dependent diabetes mellitus	PET	positron emission tomography
		PFT	pulmonary function test
NK	natural killer cells	pH	acidity or alkalinity of urine
NMR	nuclear magnetic resonance	PI, para I	first delivery
no sub	no substitute	PID	pelvic inflammatory disease
noc	night	PMN, polys	polymorphonuclear neutrophil
non rep	do not repeat	PMS	premenstrual syndrome
NPH	neutral protamine Hagedorn (insulin)	PNS	peripheral nervous system
		PO, po	by mouth
NPO	nothing by mouth	PORP	partial ossicular replacement prosthesis
NS	nephrotic syndrome, normal saline		
		pp	postprandial
NSAID	nonsteroidal anti-inflammatory drug	PPD	purified protein derivative
		preop, pre-op	preoperative
n&v	nausea and vomiting	prep	preparation, prepared
O₂	oxygen	PRK	photorefractive keratectomy
OA	osteoarthritis	PRL	prolactin
OB	obstetrics	prn	as needed
OCD	obsessive–compulsive disorder	PROM	passive range of motion
OCPs	oral contraceptive pills	prot	protocol
od	overdose	PSA	prostate-specific antigen
OD	right eye	PT, pro-time	prothrombin time
oint	ointment	pt	patient

Abbreviation	Meaning	Abbreviation	Meaning
PT	physical therapy	SCIDS	severe combined immunodeficiency syndrome
PTC	percutaneous transhepatic cholangiography	segs	segmented neutrophils
PTCA	percutaneous transluminal coronary angioplasty	s.gl.	without correction or glasses
		SG, sp. gr.	specific gravity
PTH	parathyroid hormone	SG	skin graft
PUD	peptic ulcer disease	SIDS	sudden infant death syndrome
PVC	premature ventricular contraction	Sig	label as follows/directions
		SK	streptokinase
q	every	sl	under the tongue
qam	every morning	SLE	systemic lupus erythematosus
qh	every hour	SMAC	sequential multiple analyzer computer
qhs	at bedtime		
qid	four times a day	SMD	senile macular degeneration
qs	quantity sufficient	SOB	shortness of breath
R	respiration, roentgen	sol	solution
Ra	radium	SOM	serous otitis media
RA	rheumatoid arthritis, room air	SPP	suprapubic prostatectomy
rad	radiation-absorbed dose	ST	esotropia
RAI	radioactive iodine	st	stage
RBC	red blood cell	stat	at once/immediately
RDS	respiratory distress syndrome	STD	sexually transmitted disease
REM	rapid eye movement	STSG	split-thickness skin graft
Rh+	Rh-positive	Subc, SubQi	subcutaneous
Rh−	Rh-negative	subcu, SC, sc, subq	
RIA	radioimmunoassay		
RL	right lateral	suppos, supp	suppository
RLE	right lower extremity	susp	suspension
RLL	right lower lobe	syr	syrup
RLQ	right lower quadrant	T & A	tonsillectomy and adenoidectomy
RML	right middle lobe		
ROM	range of motion	T, tbsp	tablespoon
RP	retrograde pyelogram	t, tsp	teaspoon
RPR	rapid plasma reagin (test for syphilis)	T1, T2, etc.	first thoracic vertebra, second thoracic vertebra, etc.
RRT	registered radiologic technologist, registered respiratory therapist	T_3	triiodothyronine
		T_4	thyroxine
		tab	tablet
RUE	right upper extremity	TAH-BSO	total abdominal hysterectomy–bilateral salpingo-oophorectomy
RUL	right upper lobe		
RUQ	right upper quadrant		
RV	reserve volume	TAH	total abdominal hysterectomy
Rx	take	TB	tuberculosis
$\overline{s}$	without	TENS	transcutaneous electrical stimulation
$\overline{ss}$	one-half		
S1	first heart sound	TFT	thyroid function test
S2	second heart sound	THA	total hip arthroplasty
SA, S-A	sinoatrial	THR	total hip replacement
SAD	seasonal affective disorder	TIA	transient ischemic attack
SARS	severe acute respiratory syndrome	tid	three times a day
		TKA	total knee arthroplasty
SC	subcutaneous	TKR	total knee replacement
SCC	squamous cell carcinoma	TLC	total lung capacity
SCI	spinal cord injury	TNM	tumor, nodes, metastases

Abbreviation	Meaning	Abbreviation	Meaning
TO	telephone order	UE	upper extremity
top	apply topically	UGI	upper gastrointestinal series
TORP	total ossicular replacement prosthesis	URI	upper respiratory infection
tPA	tissue-type plasminogen activator	US	ultrasound
		UTI	urinary tract infection
TPN	total parenteral nutrition	UV	ultraviolet
TPR	temperature, pulse, and respiration	VA	visual acuity
		VC	vital capacity
TSH	thyroid-stimulating hormone	VCUG	voiding cystourethrography
TSS	toxic shock syndrome	VD	venereal disease
TUR	transurethral resection	VF	visual field
TURP	transurethral resection of the prostate	Vfib	ventricular fibrillation
		VO	verbal order
TV	tidal volume	VSD	ventricular septal defect
u	unit	VT	ventricular tachycardia
U/A, UA	urinalysis	WBC	white blood cell
UC	urine culture, uterine contractions	wt	weight
		x	times
		XT	exotropia

Chapter 1 Answers

Practice Exercises

A. 1. combining form 2. o 3. suffix 4. prefix
5. spelling 6. word root, combining vowel, prefix, suffix

B. 1. l 2. e 3. j 4. f 5. d 6. k 7. m 8. o 9. g 10. n 11. b
12. h 13. a 14. c 15. i

C. 1. surgical repair 2. narrowing 3. inflammation
4. pertaining to 5. pain 6. cutting into
7. enlargement 8. surgical removal of
9. excessive, abnormal flow 10. puncture to
remove fluid 11. record or picture 12. pertaining to 13. abnormal softening 14. state of
15. to suture 16. surgical creation of opening
17. surgical fixation 18. discharge or flow
19. process of visually examining 20. tumor, mass

D. 1. pulmonology 2. neuralgia or neurodynia
3. rhinorrhea 4. nephromalacia 5. cardiomegaly
6. gastrotomy 7. dermatitis 8. laryngectomy
9. arthroplasty 10. adenopathy

E. 1. intra-/endo- 2. macro- 3. pre-/ante- 4. peri-
5. neo- 6. a-/an-/de- 7. hemi-/semi- 8. dys-
9. supra-/ hyper- 10. hyper- 11. poly-/multi-
12. brady- 13. auto- 14. trans- 15. bi-

F. 1. tachy-, fast 2. pseudo-, false 3. hypo-, under/
below 4. inter-, among/between 5. eu-, normal/
good 6. post-, after 7. mono-, one 8. sub-,
below/under

G. 1. metastases 2. ova 3. diverticula 4. atria
5. di agnoses 6. vertebrae

H. 1. cardiology 2. gastrology 3. dermatology
4. ophthalmology 5. immunology 6. nephrology 7. hematology 8. gynecology 9. neurology
10. pathology

I. 1. cardiomalacia 2. gastrostomy 3. rhinoplasty
4. hypertrophy 5. pathology 6. adenoma
7. gastroenterology 8. otitis 9. hydrotherapy
10. carcinogen

J. 1. gland 2. cancer 3. heart 4. chemical 5. to cut
6. skin 7. small intestine 8. stomach 9. female
10. blood 11. water 12. immunity 13. voice box
14. disease 15. kidney 16. nerve 17. eye 18. ear
19. lung 20. nose

Chapter 2 Answers

Practice Exercises

A. 1. cells, tissues, organs, systems, body 2. cell
membrane, cytoplasm, nucleus 3. histology
4. epithelial 5. anatomical 6. right lower
7. cranial, spinal 8. nine 9. right iliac 10. pleural,
pericardial

B. 1. c 2. a 3. b

C. 1. epi-; above 2. peri-; around or about
3. hypo-; under or below 4. retro-; behind or
backward

D. 1. n 2. f 3. k 4. d 5. a 6. e 7. m 8. i 9. b 10. j 11. h
12. l 13. c 14. g

E. 1. MS 2. lat 3. RUQ 4. CV 5. GI 6. AP 7. OB
8. LLQ

F. 1. dorsal 2. thoracic 3. superior 4. caudal
5. visceral 6. lateral 7. distal 8. neural
9. pulmonology 10. muscular 11. ventral
12. anterior 13. cephalic 14. medial

G. 1. internal organ 2. back 3. abdomen 4. chest
5. middle 6. belly 7. front 8. tissues 9. epithelium
10. skull 11. cell 12. near to 13. head

H. 1. integumentary, d 2. cardiovascular, i
3. digestive, g 4. female reproductive, b
5. musculoskeletal (skeletal), a 6. respiratory, j
7. urinary, c 8. male reproductive, f 9. nervous, h
10. musculoskeletal (muscular), e

I. 1. cephalic 2. pubic 3. crural 4. gluteal
5. cervical 6. brachial 7. dorsum 8. thoracic

J. 1. a 2. c 3. f 4. e 5. a 6. d 7. b 8. e 9. c 10. b

K. 1. otorhinolaryngology 2. cardiology
3. gynecology 4. orthopedics
5. ophthalmology 6. urology
7. dermatology 8. gastroenterology

Labeling Exercises

A. 1. cephalic 2. cervical 3. thoracic 4. brachial
5. abdominal 6. pelvic 7. pubic 8. crural 9. trunk
10. vertebral 11. dorsum 12. gluteal

B. 1. frontal or coronal plane 2. sagittal or median
plane 3. transverse or horizontal plane

Chapter 3 Answers
Real World Applications

Medical Record Analysis

1. basal cell carcinoma—Cancerous tumor of the basal cell layer of the epidermis. A frequent type of skin cancer that rarely metastasizes or spreads. These cancers can arise on sun exposed skin.
2. lesions—A general term for a wound, injury, or abnormality.
3. biopsies—A piece of tissue is removed by syringe and needle, knife, punch, or brush to examine under a microscope. Used to aid in diagnosis.
4. excised—to surgically cut out.
5. pruritus—Severe itching.
6. anterior—Pertaining to the front side of the body.
7. erythema—Redness or flushing of the skin.
8. depigmentation—Loss of normal skin color or pigment.
9. epidermis—The superficial layer of the skin.
10. dermis—The middle layer of the skin.
11. dermatoplasty—Skin grafting; transplantation of skin.

Chart Note Transcription

1. ulcer 2. dermatologist 3. pruritus 4. erythema 5. pustules 6. dermis 7. necrosis 8. culture and sensitivity 9. cellulitis 10. debridement

Case Study

1. Systemic lupus erythematosus; another example is rheumatoid arthritis
2. Erythema—skin redness; photosensitivity—intolerance to strong light; alopecia—baldness; stiffness in joints
3. Exfoliative cytology and fungal scrapings—in both tests cells are scraped away from the skin and examined under a microscope in order to make a diagnosis; in order to make sure the rash was not caused by something else like a fungal infection
4. Internist—anti-inflammatory—to reduce pain, swelling, and stiffness in joints; dermatologist—corticosteroid cream to anti-inflammatory to reduce the red rash
5. Completing examinations and various diagnostic tests in order to collect information necessary for a diagnosis

Practice Exercises

A. 1. epidermis, dermis, subcutaneous layer 2. basal cell 3. adipose 4. dermis 5. keratin 6. melanin 7. corium 8. nail bed 9. sebaceous, sweat 10. apocrine

B. 1. cold 2. skin 3. profuse sweating 4. pus 5. blue 6. nail 7. fat 8. sweat 9. wrinkles 10. oil 11. hair 12. death
C. 1. redness involving superficial layer of skin 2. burn damage through epidermis and into dermis causing vesicles 3. burn damage to full thickness of epidermis and dermis
D. 1. e 2. f 3. i 4. j 5. a 6. c 7. l 8. g 9. k 10. h 11. d 12. b
E. 1. flat, discolored area 2. small solid raised spot less than 0.5 cm 3. fluid filled sac 4. crack-like lesion 5. raised spot containing pus 6. small, round swollen area 7. fluid-filled blister 8. open sore 9. firm, solid mass larger than 0.5 cm 10. torn or jagged wound
F. 1. dermatitis 2. dermatosis 3. dermatome 4. dermatologist 5. dermatoplasty 6. dermatology 7. melanoma 8. melanocyte 9. ichthyoderma 10. leukoderma 11. erythroderma 12. onychomalacia 13. paronychia 14. onychophagia 15. onychectomy
G. 1. h 2. i 3. j 4. e 5. c 6. a 7. f 8. g 9. b 10. d
H. 1. FS 2. I & D 3. ID 4. subq, subcu, SC, sc 5. UV 6. BX, bx
I. 1. culture and sensitivity 2. basal cell carcinoma 3. dermatology 4. skin graft 5. decubitus ulcer 6. malignant melanoma
J. 1. xeroderma 2. petechiae 3. tinea 4. scabies 5. paronychia 6. Kaposi's sarcoma 7. impetigo 8. keloid 9. exfoliative cytology 10. frozen section
K. 1. antifungal, f 2. antipruritic, d 3. antiparasitic, a 4. antiviral, c 5. corticosteroid cream, b 6. anesthetic, g 7. antibiotic, e

Labeling Exercise

A. 1. epidermis 2. dermis 3. subcutaneous layer 4. sweat gland 5. sweat duct 6. hair shaft 7. sebaceous gland 8. arrector pili muscle 9. sensory receptors
B. 1. epidermis 2. dermis 3. subcutaneous layer 4. sebaceous gland 5. arrector pili muscle 6. hair shaft 7. hair follicle 8. hair root 9. papilla
C. 1. free edge 2. lateral nail groove 3. lunula 4. nail bed 5. nail body 6. cuticle 7. nail root

Chapter 4 Answers
Real World Applications

Medical Record Analysis

1. osteoarthritis—Joint inflammation resulting in degeneration of the bones and joints, especially those bearing weight. Results in bone rubbing against bone; 2. bilateral—pertaining to both sides; 3. TKA—Surgical reconstruction of a knee joint by implanting a prosthetic knee joint. Also called *total*

knee replacement (TKR); 4. orthopedic surgeon—Physician that specializes in the diagnosis and treatment of conditions of the musculoskeletal system using surgical means; 5. CT scan—computed tomography scan—imaging technique that produces cross-sectional view of the body; 6. physical therapy—treats disorders using physical means and methods; includes joint motion and muscle strength; 7. ROM—range of movement of a joint, from maximum flexion through maximum extension; it is measure das degrees of a circle; 8. gait training—learning how to walk; 9. occupational therapy—assists patients to regain, develop, and improve skills that are important for independent functioning; 10. ADLs—activities of daily living

Chart Note Transcription

1. Colles' fracture (fx) 2. cast 3. fracture 4. orthopedist 5. osteoporosis 6. computerized axial tomography (CT or CAT scan) 7. flexion 8. extension 9. comminuted fracture (fx) 10. femur 11. total hip arthroplasty (THA)

Case Study

1. Rheumatoid arthritis; 2. Cartilage damage and crippling deformities; 3. Osteoarthritis; 4. Bone scan—radioactive dye is used to visualize the body; erythrocyte sedimentation rate—a blood test that can determine if a person has an inflammatory disease; 5. Anti-inflammatory medication to reduce inflammation and provide some pain relief; physical therapy—treatment using warm water and exercises to maintain the flexibility of the joints; 6. Acute—brief disease, also used to mean sudden and severe disease; Chronic—disease of a long duration

Practice Exercises

A. 1. axial, appendicular 2. smooth 3. frame, protect vital organs, work with muscles for movement, store minerals, red blood cell production 4. myoneural 5. short 6. periosteum 7. wrist 8. cancellous 9. synovial 10. skeletal, smooth, cardiac 11. foramen 12. diaphysis

B. 1. femoral 2. sternal 3. clavicular 4. coccygeal 5. maxillary 6. tibial 7. patellar 8. phalangeal 9. humeral 10. pubic

C. 1. osteocyte 2. osteoblast 3. osteoporosis 4. osteopathy 5. osteotomy 6. osteotome 7. osteomyelitis 8. osteomalacia 9. osteochondroma 10. myopathy 11. myoplasty 12. myorrhaphy 13. electromyogram 14. myasthenia 15. tenodynia 16. tenorrhaphy 17. arthrodesis 18. arthroplasty 19. arthrotomy 20. arthritis 21. arthrocentesis 22. arthralgia 23. chondrectomy 24. chondroma 25. chondromalacia

D. 1. -desis 2. -asthenia 3. -listhesis 4. -clasia 5. -kinesia 6. -porosis

E. 1. cervical, 7 2. thoracic, 12 3. lumbar, 5 4. sacrum, 1 (5 fused) 5. coccyx, 1 (3–5 fused)

F. 1. S = -scopy; visual examination of inside of a joint 2. P = inter-, S = -al; pertaining to between vertebrae 3. S = -malacia; softening of cartilage 4. S = -ectomy; surgical removal of disk 5. P = intra- S = -al; pertaining to inside the skull 6. P = sub-, -ar = pertaining to; pertaining to under the scapula

G. 1. lamina, part of vertebra 2. stiff joint 3. cartilage 4. vertebrae 5. muscle 6. straight 7. hump 8. tendon 9. bone marrow 10. joint

H. 1. IM 2. TKR 3. HNP 4. DTR 5. UE 6. L5 7. BDT 8. AK 9. fx/FX 10. NSAID

I. 1. medical doctor who treats musculoskeletal system 2. uses manipulation of vertebral column 3. specialty that treats disorders of feet 4. fitting of braces and splints 5. fabricates and fits artificial limbs

J. 1. e 2. d 3. b 4. c 5. a 6. h 7. g 8. f

K. 1. osteoporosis 2. rickets 3. lateral epicondylitis 4. herniated nucleus pulposus 5. osteogenic sarcoma 6. scoliosis 7. pseudotrophic muscular dystrophy 8. systemic lupus erythematosus 9. spondylolisthesis 10. carpal tunnel syndrome

L. 1. c 2. h 3. f 4. g 5. d 6. e 7. a 8. b

M. 1. patella 2. tarsals 3. clavicle 4. femur 5. phalanges 6. carpals 7. tibia 8. scapula 9. phalanges

N. 1. degenerative joint disease 2. electromyogram 3. first cervical vertebra 4. sixth thoracic vertebra 5. intramuscular 6. deep tendon reflexes 7. juvenile rheumatoid arthritis 8. left lower extremity 9. orthopedics 10. carpal tunnel syndrome

O. 1. surgical repair of cartilage 2. slow movement 3. porous bone 4. abnormal increase in lumbar spine curve (swayback) 5. lack of development/nourishment 6. bone marrow tumor 7. artificial substitute for a body part 8. cutting into skull 9. puncture of a joint to withdraw fluid 10. bursa inflammation

P. 1. nonsteroidal anti-inflammatory drugs, b 2. corticosteroids, e 3. skeletal muscle relaxants, a 4. bone reabsorption inhibitors, c 5. calcium supplements, d

Labeling Exercise

A. 1. skull 2. cervical vertebrae 3. sternum 4. ribs 5. thoracic vertebrae 6. lumbar vertebrae 7. ilium 8. pubis 9. ischium 10. femur 11. patella 12. tibia 13. fibula 14. tarsals 15. metatarsals 16. phalanges 17. maxilla 18. mandible 19. scapula 20. humerus 21. ulna 22. radius 23. sacrum 24. coccyx 25. carpals 26. metacarpals 27. phalanges

B. 1. proximal epiphysis 2. diaphysis 3. distal epiphysis 4. articular cartilage 5. epiphyseal line 6. spongy or cancellous bone 7. compact or cortical bone 8. medullary cavity

C. 1. periosteum 2. synovial membrane 3. articular cartilage 4. joint cavity 5. joint capsule

Chapter 5 Answers
Real World Applications

Medical Record Analysis

1. hypertension—Blood pressure above the normal range. 2. tachycardia—The condition of having a fast heart rate; typically more than 100 beats/minute while at rest. 3. congestive heart failure (CAD)—Pathological condition of the heart in which there is a reduced outflow of blood from the left side of the heart because the left ventricle myocardium has become too weak to efficiently pump blood. Results in weakness, breathlessness, and edema. 4. mitral valve prolapse—Condition in which the cusps or flaps of the heart valve are too loose and fail to shut tightly, allowing blood to flow backward through the valve when the heart chamber contracts. Most commonly occurs in the mitral valve, but may affect any of the heart valves. 5. palpitations—Pounding, racing heartbeats. 6. electrocardiography (EKG)—Process of recording the electrical activity of the heart. Useful in the diagnosis of abnormal cardiac rhythm and heart muscle (myocardium) damage. 7. cardiac enzymes—Blood test to determine the level of enzymes specific to heart muscles in the blood. An increase in the enzymes may indicate heart muscle damage such as a myocardial infarction. These enzymes include creatine phosphokinase (CPK), lactate dehydrogenase (LDH), and glutamic oxaloacetic transaminase (GOT). 8. echocardiography—Noninvasive diagnostic method using ultrasound to visualize internal cardiac structures. Cardiac valve activity can be evaluated using this method. 9. stress test—Method for evaluating cardiovascular fitness. The patient is placed on a treadmill or a bicycle and then subjected to steadily increasing levels of work. An EKG and oxygen levels are taken while the patient exercises. The test is stopped if abnormalities occur on the EKG. Also called an *exercise test* or a *treadmill test*. 10. angiocardiography—X-rays taken after the injection of an opaque material into a blood vessel. Can be performed on the aorta as an aortic angiogram, on the heart as an angiocardiogram, and on the brain as a cerebral angiogram. 11. coronary artery disease (CAD)—Insufficient blood supply to the heart muscle due to an obstruction of one or more coronary arteries. May be caused by atherosclerosis and may cause angina pectoris and myocardial infarction. 12. myocardial infarction—Condition caused by the partial or complete occlusion or closing of one or more of the coronary arteries. Symptoms include a squeezing pain or heavy pressure in the middle of the chest (angina pectoris). A delay in treatment could

result in death. Also referred to as a *heart attack*. 13. mitral valve replacement—Removal of a diseased heart valve and replacement with an artificial valve.

Chart Note Transcription

1. angina pectoris 2. bradycardia 3. hyper tension 4. myocardial infarction (MI) 5. electrocardiogram (EKG, ECG) 6. cardiac enzymes 7. coronary artery disease (CAD) 8. cardiac catheterization 9. stress test (treadmill test) 10. percutaneous transluminal coronary angioplasty (PTCA) 11. coronary artery bypass graft (CABG)

Case Study

1. Heart attack; condition caused by the partial or complete occlusion or closing of one or more of the coronary arteries. Symptoms include a squeezing pain or heavy pressure in the middle of the chest (angina pectoris). A delay in treatment could result in death. 2. The main complaint, the one the patient is most aware of or most anxious about. 3. Angina pectoris—Condition in which there is severe pain with a sensation of constriction around the heart; caused by a deficiency of oxygen to the heart muscle. 4. Nausea—feeling of need to vomit; dyspnea–difficulty breathing; diaphoresis–profuse sweating 5. Cardiac enzymes; angiocardiography; cardiac scan; electrocardiography; stress testing; cardiac catheterization; Holter monitor 6. Smokes; overweight; family history; sedentary lifestyle. He can stop smoking, lose weight, and become more active.

Practice Exercises

A. 1. cardiology 2. endocardium, myocardium, epicardium 3. sinoatrial node 4. away from 5. tricuspid, pulmonary, mitral (bicuspid), aortic 6. atria, ventricles 7. pulmonary 8. apex 9. septum 10. systole, diastole

B. 1. cardiac 2. cardiomyopathy 3. cardiomegaly 4. tachycardia 5. bradycardia 6. electrocardiogram 7. angiostenosis 8. angiitis 9. angiospasm 10. arterial 11. arteriosclerosis 12. arteriole

C. 1. endocarditis 2. epicarditis 3. myocarditis

D. 1. heart 2. valve 3. chest 4. artery 5. vein 6. vessel 7. ventricle 8. clot 9. atrium 10. fatty substance

E. 1. venous 2. cardiology 3. venogram 4. electro cardiography 5. hypertension 6. hypotension 7. valvoplasty 8. interventricular 9. atherectomy 10. arteriostenosis

F. 1. -tension 2. -stenosis 3. -manometer 4. -ule, -ole 5. -sclerosis

G. 1. f 2. h 3. d 4. g 5. b 6. i 7. a 8. c 9. e 10. j

H. 1. blood pressure 2. congestive heart failure 3. myocardial infarction 4. coronary care unit 5. premature ventricular contraction 6. cardiopulmonary resuscitation 7. coronary artery

disease 8. chest pain 9. electrocardiogram 10. first heart sound

I. 1. MVP 2. VSD 3. PTCA 4. Vfib 5. DVT 6. LDH 7. CoA 8. tPA 9. CV 10. ECC

J. 1. c 2. g 3. j 4. a 5. d 6. b 7. i 8. e 9. f 10. h

K. 1. thin flexible tube 2. an area of dead tissue 3. a blood clot 4. pounding heartbeat 5. back-flow 6. weakened and ballooning arterial wall 7. complete stoppage of heart activity 8. serious cardiac arrhythmia 9. heart attack 10. varicose veins in anal region

L. 1. murmur 2. defibrillation 3. hypertension 4. pacemaker 5. varicose veins 6. angina pectoris 7. CCU 8. MI 9. angiography 10. echocardiogram 11. Holter monitor 12. CHF

M. 1. antiarrhythmic, e 2. antilipidemic, g 3. cardiotonic, f 4. diuretic, h 5. anticoagulant, b 6. thrombolytic, a 7. vasodilator, d 8. calcium channel blocker, c

Labeling Exercise

A. 1. pulmonary arteries 2. vena cavae 3. right atrium 4. right ventricle 5. systemic veins 6. capillary bed lungs 7. pulmonary veins 8. aorta 9. left atrium 10. left ventricle 11. systemic arteries 12. systemic capillary beds

B. 1. superior vena cava 2. aorta 3. pulmonary trunk 4. pulmonary valve 5. right atrium 6. tricuspid valve 7. right ventricle 8. inferior vena cava 9. pulmonary artery 10. pulmonary vein 11. left atrium 12. aortic valve 13. mitral or bicuspid valve 14. left ventricle 15. endocardium 16. myocardium 17. pericardium

Chapter 6 Answers
Real World Applications

Medical Record Analysis

1. splenomegaly—An enlarged spleen.
2. non-Hodgkin's lymphoma—Cancer of the lymphatic tissues other than Hodgkin's lymphoma.
3. spleen—An organ located in the upper left quadrant of the abdomen. Consists of lymphatic tissue that is highly infiltrated with blood vessels. It filters out and destroys old red blood cells.
4. splenectomy—The surgical removal of the spleen.
5. Monospot—A blood test for infectious mononucleosis.
6. enzyme-linked immunosorbent assay (ELISA)—A blood test for an antibody to the AIDS virus. A positive test means that the person has been exposed to the virus. There may be a false-positive reading, and then the Western blot test would be used to verify the results.
7. Magnetic resonance imaging (MRI)—Medical imaging that uses radio-frequency radiation as its source of energy. It does not require the injection of contrast medium or exposure to ionizing radiation. The technique is useful for visualizing large blood vessels, the heart, the brain, and soft tissues
8. tumor—Abnormal growth of tissue that may be benign or malignant.
9. biopsy—A piece of tissue is removed by syringe and needle, knife, punch, or brush to examine under a microscope. Used to aid in diagnosis.
10. oncologist—A physician who specializes in the treatment of cancer.
11. metastases—The spreading of a cancerous tumor from its original site to different locations of the body.

Chart Note Transcription

1. hematologist 2. ELISA 3. prothrombin time 4. complete blood count (CBC) 5. erythropenia 6. thrombopenia 7. leukocytosis 8. bone marrow aspiration 9. leukemia 10. homologous transfusion

Case Study

1. Acute lymphocytic leukemia
2. High fever; thrombopenia—too few platelets; epistaxis—nose bleed; gingival bleeding—gums bleeding; petechiae—pinpoint bruises; ecchymoses—large black and blue bruises
3. Bone marrow aspiration—sample of bone marrow is removed by aspiration with a needle and examined for diseases.
4. A diagnosis based on the results of the physician's direct examination rather than based on other tests like x-rays and lab work
5. Chemotherapy—treating disease by using chemicals that have a toxic effect upon the body, especially cancerous tissue
6. Remission—a period during which the symptoms of a disease or disorder leave. Can be temporary.

Practice Exercises

A. 1. hematology 2. spleen, tonsils, thymus 3. thoracic duct, right lymphatic duct 4. axillary, cervical, mediastinal, inguinal 5. phagocytosis 6. erythrocytes (red blood cells), leukocytes (white blood cells), platelets (thrombocytes) 7. plasma 8. active acquired 9. antibody-mediated 10. hemostasis

B. 1. leukopenia 2. erythropenia 3. thrombopenia 4. pancytopenia 5. leukocytosis 6. erythrocytosis 7. thrombocytosis 8. hemoglobin 9. immunoglobulin 10. erythrocyte 11. leukocyte 12. lymphocyte

C.   1. splenomegaly 2. splenectomy
     3. splenotomy 4. lymphocytes 5. lymphoma
     6. lymphadenopathy 7. lymphadenoma
     8. lymphadenitis 9. immunologist 10. immu-
     noglobulin 11. immunology 12. hematic
     13. hematoma 14. hematopoiesis 15. hemo-
     lytic 16. hemoglobin
D.   1. basophil 2. complete blood count
     3. hemoglobin 4. prothrombin time 5. graft
     vs. host disease 6. red blood count/red blood
     cell 7. packed cell volume 8. erythrocyte
     sedimentation rate 9. differential
     10. lymphocyte
E.   1. g 2. i 3. e 4. a 5. h 6. d 7. c 8. j 9. b 10. f
F.   1. AIDS 2. ARC 3. HIV 4. ALL 5. BMT 6. mono
     7. KS 8. eosins, eos 9. IG 10. SCIDS
G.   1. lymphaden/o 2. thromb/o 3. sanguin/o,
     hem/o, hemat/o 4. tonsill/o 5. tox/o 6. phag/o
     7. lymphangi/o 8. path/o 9. splen/o
     10. lymph/o
H.   1. polycythemia vera 2. mononucleosis 3. ana-
     phylac tic shock 4. HIV 5. Kaposi's sarcoma
     6. AIDS 7. Hodgkin's disease 8. Pneumocystis
     9. aplastic 10. pernicious
I.   1. c 2. h 3. d 4. a 5. e 6. b 7. f 8. g 9. j 10. i
J.   1. reverse transcriptase inhibitor, e 2. anticoagu-
     lant, a 3. antihemorrhagic, d 4. antihistamine, h
     5. immunosuppresant, f 6. thrombolytic, b
     7. hematinic, g 8. corticosteroid, c 9. antiplate-
     let agent, i
K.   1. d 2. f 3. b 4. g 5. a 6. e 7. c

Labeling Exercise

A.   1. plasma 2. red blood cells or erythrocytes
     3. platelets or thrombocytes 4. white blood
     cells or leukocytes
B.   1. cervical nodes 2. mediastinal nodes 3. axillary
     nodes 4. inguinal nodes
C.   1. thymus gland 2. lymph node 3. tonsil
     4. spleen 5. lymphatic vessels

Chapter 7 Answers
Real World Applications

Medical Record Analysis

1.   asthma—Disease caused by various conditions,
     like allergens, and resulting in constriction of
     the bronchial airways, dyspnea, coughing, and
     wheezing. Can cause violent spasms of the
     bronchi (bronchospasms) but is generally not a
     life-threatening condition. Medication can be
     very effective.
2.   dyspnea—Term describing difficult or labored
     breathing.

3.   cyanosis—Refers to the bluish tint of skin that
     is receiving an insufficient amount of oxygen or
     circulation.
4.   expiration—To breath out; exhale or expiration
5.   phlegm—Thick mucus secreted by the mem-
     branes that line the respiratory tract. When
     phlegm is coughed through the mouth, it is
     called *sputum*. Phlegm is examined for color,
     odor, and consistency.
6.   auscultation—To listen to body sounds, usually
     using a stethoscope.
7.   rhonchi—Somewhat musical sound during
     expiration, often found in asthma or infection.
     Caused by spasms of the bronchial tubes. Also
     called *wheezing*.
8.   arterial blood gases (ABGs)—Testing for the
     gases present in the blood. Generally used to
     assist in determining the levels of oxygen (O_2)
     and carbon dioxide (CO_2) in the blood.
9.   hypoxemia—The condition of having an insuf-
     ficient amount of oxygen in the bloodstream.
10. spirometry—Procedure to measure lung capac-
     ity using a *spirometer*.
11. Proventil—Medication that elaxes muscle
     spasms in bronchial tubes. Used to treat asthma.
12. bronchospasms—An involuntary muscle
     spasm of the smooth muscle in the wall of the
     bronchus.

Chart Note Transcription

1. dyspnea 2. tachyp nea 3. arterial blood gases
(ABGs) 4. hypoxemia 5. auscultation 6. crackles
7. purulent 8. sputum 9. CXR 10. pneumonia
11. endotracheal intubation

Case Study

1.   Pneumonia
2.   dyspnea-difficulty breathing; dizziness;
     orthopnea-comfortable breathing only while
     sitting up; elevated temperature, cough
3.   Auscultation (listening to the body sounds)
     revealed crackles (abnormal sound); chest x-ray
     revealed fluid in the upper lobe of the right
     lung.
4.   A method of determining a patient's general
     health and heart and lung function by measur-
     ing pulse (100 BPM and rapid), respiratory rate
     (24 breaths/min and labored), temperature
     (102°F), and blood pressure (180/110)
5.   IV antibiotics—medicine to kill bacteria given
     into a vein; intermittent positive pressure
     breathing—method of assisting patients in
     breathing by using a machine that produces an
     increased pressure
6.   The IV antibiotics were changed to oral
     antibiotics—she started taking pills.

Practice Exercises

A. 1. exchange of O_2 and CO_2 2. ventilation
3. exchange of O_2 and CO_2 in the lungs
4. exchange of O_2 and CO_2 at cellular level
5. nasal cavity, pharynx, larynx, trachea, bronchial tubes, lungs 6. pharynx 7. epiglottis
8. filter out dust 9. diaphragm 10. 12–20
11. 30–60 12. 3; 2 13. alveoli 14. pleura
15. palate 16. bronchioles

B. 1. dilation 2. carbon dioxide 3. voice 4. chest
5. breathing 6. spitting 7. smell

C. 1. rhinitis 2. rhinorrhagia 3. rhinorrhea
4. rhinoplasty 5. laryngitis 6. laryngospasm
7. laryngoscopy 8. laryngeal 9. laryngotomy 10. laryngectomy 11. laryngoplasty
12. laryngoplegia 13. bronchial 14. bronchitis
15. bronchoscopy 16. bronchogenic 17. bronchospasm 18. thoracoplasty 19. thoracotomy
20. thoracalgia 21. thoracic 22. tracheotomy
23. tracheoplasty 24. tracheostenosis 25. endotracheal 26. tracheitis

D. 1. trachea or windpipe 2. larynx 3. bronchus
4. breathing 5. lung or air 6. nose 7. dust
8. pleura 9. epiglottis 10. alveolus or air sac
11. lung 12. oxygen 13. sinus 14. lobe 15. nose

E. 1. eupnea 2. dyspnea 3. tachypnea
4. orthopnea 5. apnea

F. 1. inhalation or inspiration 2. hemoptysis
3. pulmonary emboli 4. sinusitis 5. pharyngitis
6. pneumothorax 7. pertussis 8. pleurotomy
9. pleurodynia 10. nasopharyngitis

G. 1. URI 2. PFT 3. LLL 4. O_2 5. CO_2 6. IPPB 7. COPD
8. Bronch 9. TLC 10. TB 11. IRDS

H. 1. chest X-ray 2. tidal volume 3. temperature, pulse, respirations 4. arterial blood gases
5. dyspnea on exertion 6. right upper lobe
7. sudden infant death syndrome 8. total lung capacity 9. adult respiratory distress syndrome
10. metered dose inhaler 11. clear to auscultation 12. severe acute respiratory syndrome

I. 1. e 2. k 3. h 4. a 5. j 6. l 7. c 8. g 9. f 10. b 11. d
12. i

J. 1. volume of air in the lungs after a maximal inhalation or inspiration 2. amount of air entering lungs in a single inspiration or leaving air in single expiration of quiet breathing 3. air remaining in the lungs after a forced expiration

K. 1. cardiopulmonary resuscitation 2. thoracentesis 3. respirator 4. supplemental oxygen
5. patent 6. ventilation-perfusion scan 7. sputum cytology 8. hyperventilation 9. rhonchi
10. anthracosis

L. 1. decongestant, f 2. antitussive, a 3. antibiotic, c 4. expectorant, g 5. mucolytic, h 6. bronchodilator, d 7. antihistamine, e 8. corticosteroid, b

Labeling Exercise

A. 1. pharynx and larynx 2. trachea 3. nasal cavity
4. bronchial tubes 5. lungs

B. 1. nares 2. paranasal sinuses 3. nasal cavity
4. hard palate 5. soft palate 6. palatine tonsil
7. epiglottis 8. vocal cords 9. esophagus
10. trachea

C. 1. trachea 2. right upper lobe 3. right middle lobe 4. right lower lobe 5. apex of lung 6. left upper lobe 7. left lower lobe 8. diaphragm

Chapter 8 Answers
Real World Applications

Medical Record Analysis

1. epigastric—Pertaining to the area above the stomach.
2. anemia—A large group of conditions characterized by a reduction in the number of red blood cells or the amount of hemoglobin in the blood; results in less oxygen reaching the tissues.
3. melena—Passage of dark tarry stools. Color is the result of digestive enzymes working on blood in the gastrointestinal tract.
4. dyspepsia—An "upset stomach"
5. antacids—Medication to neutralize stomach acid
6. complete blood count (CBC)—A combination of blood tests including: red blood cell count, white blood cell count, hemoglobin, hematocrit, white blood cell differential, and platelet count.
7. fecal occult blood—Laboratory test on the feces to determine if microscopic amounts of blood are present. Also called *hemoccult* or *stool guaiac*.
8. *Helicobacter pylori*—A bacteria that may damage the lining of the stomach setting up the conditions for peptic ulcer disease to develop
9. gastroscopy—Procedure in which a flexible *gastroscope* is passed through the mouth and down the esophagus in order to visualize inside the stomach. Used to diagnose peptic ulcers and gastric carcinoma.
10. ulcer—An open sore or lesion in the skin or mucous membrane.
11. peptic ulcer disease—Ulcer occurring in the lower portion of the esophagus, stomach, and/or duodenum; thought to be caused by the acid of gastric juices. Initial damage to the protective lining of the stomach may be caused by a *Helicobacter pylori* (*H. pylori*) bacterial

infection. If the ulcer extends all the way through the wall of the stomach, it is called a *perforated ulcer* which requires immediate surgery to repair.

12. gastrectomy—surgical removal of the stomach

Chart Note Transcription

1. gastroenterologist 2. constipation 3. cholelithiasis 4. cholecystectomy 5. gastroesophageal reflux disease 6. ascites 7. lower gastrointestinal series 8. polyposis 9. colonoscopy 10. sigmoid colon 11. colectomy 12. colostomy

Case Study

1. severe RUQ pain-severe pain is located in the upper right corner of the abdomen; nausea-feeling the urge to vomit; emesis-vomiting; scleral jaundice-the whites of the eye have a yellowish cast to them
2. gallbladder, right kidney, majority of the liver, a small portion of the pancreas, portion of colon and small intestine
3. gallstones blocking the common bile duct so bile can't drain into the small intestine
4. abdominal ultrasound- The use of high frequency sound waves to produce an image of an organ, such as the uterus and ovaries or a fetus; percutaneous transhepatic cholangiography (PTC)- Procedure in which contrast medium is injected directly into the liver to visualize the bile ducts; used to detect obstructions such as gallstones in the common bile duct.
5. cholelithiasis is the condition of having gallstones present in the gallbladder, they may not be causing any symptoms; cholecystitis is the inflammation of the gallbladder that occurs when gallstones block the flow of bile out of the gallbladder
6. laparoscopic cholecystectomy- The gallbladder was removed through a very small abdominal incision with the assistance of a laparoscope.

Practice Exercises

A. 1. gastrointestinal 2. gut, alimentary canal, mouth, anus 3. salivary glands, liver, gallbladder, pancreas 4. digesting food, absorbing nutrients, eliminating waste 5. cutting, grinding 6. peristalsis 7. hydrochloric acid, chyme 8. duodenum, jejunum, ileum 9. sigmoid 10. bile, eumulsification, gallbladder
B. 1. gastritis 2. gastroenterology 3. gastrectomy 4. gastroscopy 5. gastralgia 6. gastromegaly 7. gastrotomy 8. esophagitis 9. esophagoscopy 10. esophagoplasty 11. esophageal

12. esophagectasis 13. proctopexy 14. proctoptosis 15. proctitis 16. proctologist 17. cholecystectomy 18. cholecystolithiasis 19. cholecystolithotripsy 20. cholecystitis 21. laparoscope 22. laparotomy 23. laparoscopy 24. hepatoma 25. hepatomegaly 26. hepatic 27. hepatitis 28. pancreatitis 29. pancreatic 30. colostomy 31. colitis

C. 1. esophagus 2. liver 3. ileum 4. anus and rectum 5. tongue 6. lip 7. jejunum 8. sigmoid colon 9. rectum 10. gum 11. gallbladder 12. duodenum 13. anus 14. small intestine 15. tooth

D. 1. postprandial 2. cholelithiasis 3. anorexia 4. dysphagia 5. hematemesis 6. bradypepsia

E. 1. bowel movement 2. upper gastrointestinal series 3. barium enema 4. bowel sounds 5. nausea and vomiting 6. ova and parasites 7. by mouth 8. common bile duct 9. nothing by mouth 10. postprandial

F. 1. h 2. i 3. f 4. c 5. a 6. j 7. l 8. e 9. b 10. k 11. d 12. g 13. o 14. p 15. n 16. m

G. 1. NG 2. GI 3. HBV 4. FOBT 5. IBD 6. HSV-1 7. AST 8. pc 9. PUD 10. GERD

H. 1. visual exam of the colon 2. tooth X-ray 3. bright red blood in the stools 4. blood test to determine amount of waste product in the bloodstream 5. weight loss and wasting from a chronic illness 6. use NG tube to wash out stomach 7. surgical repair of hernia 8. pulling teeth 9. surgical crushing of common bile duct stone 10. surgically create a connection between two organs

I. 1. liver biopsy 2. colostomy 3. barium swallow 4. lower GI series 5. colectomy 6. fecal occult blood test 7. choledocholithotripsy 8. total parenteral nutrition 9. gastric stapling 10. intravenous cholecystography 11. colonoscopy 12. ileostomy

J. 1. d 2. g 3. h 4. e 5. f 6. b 7. c 8. a

K. 1. antidiarrheal, f 2. proton pump inhibitor, g 3. antiemetic, d 4. H_2-receptor antagonist, a 5. anorexiant, b 6. laxative, c 7. antacid, e

Labeling Exercise

A. 1. salivary glands 2. esophagus 3. pancreas 4. small intestine 5. oral cavity 6. stomach 7. liver and gallbladder 8. colon

B. 1. esophagus 2. cardiac or lower esophageal sphincter 3. pyloric sphincter 4. duodenum 5. antrum 6. fundus of stomach 7. rugae 8. body of stomach

C. 1. cystic duct 2. common bile duct 3. gallbladder 4. duodenum 5. liver 6. hepatic duct 7. pancreas 8. pancreatic duct

Chapter 9 Answers
Real World Applications

Medical Record Analysis

1. hematuria—The presence of blood in the urine.
2. pyelonephritis—Inflammation of the renal pelvis and the kidney. One of the most common types of kidney disease. It may be the result of a lower urinary tract infection that moved up to the kidney by way of the ureters. There may be large quantities of white blood cells and bacteria in the urine. Blood (hematuria) may even be present in the urine in this condition. Can occur with any untreated or persistent case of cystitis.
3. chronic cystitis—Urinary bladder inflammation
4. dysuria—Difficult or painful urination
5. clean catch urinalysis—Laboratory test that consists of the physical, chemical, and microscopic examination of urine. Laboratory test that consists of the physical, chemical, and microscopic examination of urine.
6. pyuria—The presence of pus in the urine.
7. culture and sensitivity—Laboratory test of urine for bacterial infection. Attempt to grow bacteria on a culture medium in order to identify it and determine which antibiotics it is sensitive to.
8. pathogen—Anything, such as bacteria, viruses, fungi, or toxins, that may cause disease
9. antibiotic—Medication used to treat bacterial infections of the urinary tract.
10. cystoscopy—Visual examination of the urinary bladder using an instrument called a *cystoscope*.
11. bladder neck obstruction—Blockage of the bladder outlet. Often caused by an enlarged prostate gland in males.
12. congenital present from birth
13. catheterized—Insertion of a tube through the urethra and into the urinary bladder for the purpose of withdrawing urine or inserting dye.

Chart Note Transcription

1. urologist 2. hematuria 3. cystitis 4. clean-catch specimen 5. urinalysis (U/A, UA) 6. pyuria 7. retrograde pyelogram 8. ureter 9. ureterolith 10. extracorporeal shockwave lithotripsy (ESWL) 11. calculi

Case Study

1. Cystitis—Inflammation of the urinary bladder; pyelonephritis–Inflammation of the renal pelvis and the kidney. One of the most common types of kidney disease. It may be the result of a lower urinary tract infection that moved up to the kidney by way of the ureters. There may be large quantities of white blood cells and bacteria in the urine. Blood (hematuria) may even be present in the urine in this condition. Can occur with any untreated or persistent case of cystitis.
2. Fever; chills; fatigue; urgency—Feeling the need to urinate immediately; frequency—Urge to urinate more often than normal; dysuria—Difficult or painful urination; hematuria—Blood in the urine; cloudy urine with a fishy smell—Urine was not clear and smelled bad
3. Clean catch specimen—Urine sample obtained after cleaning off the urinary opening and catching or collecting a urine sample in midstream (halfway through the urination process) to minimize contamination from the genitalia.; U/A (urinalysis)—A physical, chemical, and microscopic examination of the urine; urine C&S (culture & sensitivity)—Test for the presence and identification of bacteria in the urine; KUB (kidney, ureters, and bladder)—An x-ray of the urinary organs
4. Pyuria—Pus in the urine; bacteriuria—Bacteria in the urine; acidic pH—Indicates a urinary tract infection; culture and sensitivity—Revealed a common type of bacteria; KUB—Pyelonephritis
5. antibiotic—To kill the bacteria; push fluids—To flush out the bladder.
6. Clear yellow to deep gold color, aromatic odor, specific gravity between 1.010–1.030, pH between 5.0–8.0, very little protein, no glucose, ketones, or blood

Practice Exercises

A. 1. nephrons 2. filtration, reabsorption, secretion 3. electrolytes 4. retroperitoneal 5. hilum 6. glomerulus 7. calyx 8. two, one 9. micturition, voiding 10. urinalysis

B. 1. nephropexy 2. nephrogram 3. nephrolithiasis 4. nephrectomy 5. nephritis 6. nephropathy 7. nephrosclerosis 8. cystitis 9. cystorrhagia 10. cystoplasty 11. cystoscope 12. cystalgia 13. pyeloplasty 14. pyelitis 15. pyelogram 16. ureterolith 17. ureterectasis 18. ureterostenosis 19. urethritis 20. urethroscope

C. 1. urine 2. meatus 3. urinary bladder 4. kidney 5. renal pelvis 6. sugar 7. night 8. scanty 9. ureter 10. glomerulus

D. 1. antispasmodic, b 2. antibiotic, c 3. diuretic, a

E. 1. urination, voiding 2. increases urine production 3. pain associated with kidney stone 4. inserting a tube through urethra into the bladder 5. inflammation of renal pelvis 6. inflammation of glomeruli in the kidney 7. cutting into an organ to remove stone 8. bedwetting 9. enlargement of urethral opening 10. damage to glomerulus secondary to diabetes mellitus 11. lab test of chemical

composition of urine 12. decrease in force of urine stream

F. 1. anuria 2. hematuria 3. calculus/nephrolith 4. lithotripsy 5. urethritis 6. pyuria 7. bacteriuria 8. dysuria 9. ketonuria 10. proteinuria 11. polyuria

G. 1. K+ 2. Na+ 3. UA 4. BUN 5. SG, sp.gr. 6. IVP 7. BNO 8. I & O 9. ATN 10. ESRD

H. 1. kidneys, ureters, bladder 2. catheter/catheterization 3. cystoscopy 4. genitourinary 5. extracorporeal shockwave lithotripsy 6. urinary tract infection 7. urine culture 8. retrograde pyelogram 9. acute renal failure 10. blood urea nitrogen 11. chronic renal failure 12. water

I. 1. c 2. g 3. h 4. i 5. f 6. e 7. d 8. b 9. a 10. j

J. 1. drooping 2. condition of the urine 3. stone 4. surgical crushing 5. condition of stones

K. 1. renal transplant 2. nephropexy 3. urinary tract infection 4. pyelolithectomy 5. renal biopsy 6. ureterectomy 7. cystostomy 8. cystoscopy 9. IVP

Labeling Exercise

A. 1. kidney 2. urinary bladder 3. ureter 4. male urethra 5. female urethra

B. 1. cortex 2. medulla 3. calyx 4. renal pelvis 5. renal papilla 6. renal pyramid 7. ureter

C. 1. efferent arteriole 2. glomerular (Bowman's) capsule 3. glomerulus 4. afferent arteriole 5. proximal convoluted tubule 6. descending nephron loop 7. distal convoluted tubule 8. collecting tubule 9. ascending nephron loop 10. peritubular capillaries

Chapter 10 Answers
Real World Applications

Medical Chart Analysis

1. gestation—The length of time of pregnancy, normally about 40 weeks.

2. amniocentesis—Puncturing of the amniotic sac using a needle and syringe for the purpose of withdrawing amniotic fluid for testing. Can assist in determining fetal maturity, development, and genetic disorders.

3. fetus—The unborn infant from approximately week 9 until birth.

4. obstetrician—Branch of medicine specializing in the diagnosis and treatment of women during pregnancy and childbirth, and immediately after childbirth. Physician is called an *obstetrician*.

5. multigravida—A woman who has not been pregnant.

6. nullipara—A woman who has not given birth to a live infant.

7. miscarriage—Unplanned loss of a pregnancy due to the death of the embryo or fetus before the time it is viable, also referred to as a *spontaneous abortion*.

8. pelvic ultrasound—Use of high frequency sound waves to produce an image or photograph of an organ, such as the uterus, ovaries, or fetus.

9. placenta previa—A placenta that is implanted in the lower portion of the uterus and, in turn, blocks the birth canal.

10. abruptio placentae—Emergency condition in which the placenta tears away from the uterine wall prior to delivery of the infant. Requires immediate delivery of the baby.

11. placenta—The organ than connects the fetus to the mothers uterus, supplies fetus with oxygen and nutrients.

12. C-section—Surgical delivery of a baby through an incision into the abdominal and uterine walls.

Chart Note Transcription

1. ejaculation 2. cryptorchidism 3. orchidopexy 4. vasectomy 5. ejaculation 6. digital rectal exam (DRE) 7. prostate cancer 8. prostate-specific antigen (PSA) 9. benign prostatic hyperplasia (BPH) 10. transurethral resection (TUR)

Case Study

1. Genital herpes.
2. Fever—she has a temperature; malaise–a feeling of general discomfort; dysuria–painful urination; vaginal leukorrhea–a white discharge or flow from the vagina
3. Vesicles—small fluid-filled blisters; ulcers–crater like erosions of the skin; erythema–redness; edema–swelling
4. An abnormality located on the body in some area outside of the genital region
5. To feel with your hands
6. There is a risk of passing the virus to the baby as it passes through the birth canal.

Practice Exercises

A. 1. gynecology 2. gynecologist 3. dilation, expulsion, placental 4. gestation 5. menopause 6. ovum 7. endometrium 8. uterus 9. uterine tubes 10. total abdominal hysterectomy–bilateral salpingo-oophorectomy

B. 1. suprapubic prostatectomy 2. transurethral resection 3. genitourinary 4. benign prostatic hyperplasia 5. digital rectal exam 6. prostate-specific antigen

C. 1. the formation of mature sperm 2. accumulation of fluid within the testes 3. surgical removal of the prostate gland by inserting a

device through the urethra and removing prostate tissue 4. inability to father children due to a problem with spermatogenesis 5. surgical removal of the testes 6. surgical removal of part or all of the vas deferens 7. Removal of the testicles in the male or the ovaries in the female.

D. 1. colposcopy 2. colposcope 3. cervicectomy 4. cervicitis 5. cervical 6. hysteropexy 7. hysterectomy 8. hysterorrhexis 9. oophoritis 10. oophorectomy 11. mammary 12. mammogram 13. mammoplasty 14. amniotic 15. amniotomy 16. amniorrhea

E. 1. cervix 2. last menstrual period 3. fetal heart rate 4. pelvic inflammatory disease 5. gynecology 6. cesarean section 7. newborn 8. premenstrual syndrome 9. toxic shock syndrome 10. low birth weight

F. 1. GI, grav I 2. AI 3. UC 4. FTND 5. IUD 6. D & C 7. HRT 8. gyn/GYN 9. AB 10. OCPs

G. 1. uterus 2. uterus 3. female 4. vulva 5. ovary 6. ovary 7. uterine tube 8. menstruation or menses 9. vagina 10. breast

H. 1. b 2. e 3. h 4. c 5. i 6. j 7. d 8. n 9. l 10. f 11. o 12. g 13. k 14. m 15. a

I. 1. labor, childbirth 2. pregnancy 3. beginning 4. pregnancy 5. childbirth 6. to bear (offspring) 7. uterine tube 8. sperm condition

J. 1. conization 2. stillbirth 3. puberty 4. premenstrual syndrome 5. laparoscopy 6. fibroid tumor 7. D & C 8. eclampsia 9. endometriosis 10. cesarean section

K. 1. urinary, reproductive 2. testes, epididymis, penis 3. foreskin 4. testes 5. bulbourethral glands 6. testosterone 7. perineum

L. 1. e 2. i 3. h 4. c 5. a 6. d 7. g 8. b 9. f

M. 1. prostatectomy 2. prostatic 3. prostatitis 4. orchiectomy 5. orchioplasty 6. orchiotomy 7. aspermia 8. oligospermia 9. spermatogenesis 10. spermatolysis

N. 1. androgen therapy, f 2. oxytocin, a 3. antiprostatic agent, b 4. birth control pills, g 5. spermatocide, d 6. erectile dysfunction agent, h 7. hormone replacement therapy, i 8. abortifacient, e 9. fertility drug, c

Labeling Exercise

A. 1. uterine tube 2. ovary 3. fundus of uterus 4. corpus (body) of uterus 5. cervix 6. vagina 7. clitoris 8. labium majora 9. labium minora

B. 1. seminal vesicle 2. vas deferens 3. prostate gland 4. bulbourethral gland 5. urethra 6. epididymis 7. glans penis 8. testis

C. 1. areola 2. nipple 3. lactiferous gland 4. lactiferous duct 5. fat

Chapter 11 Answers
Real World Applications

Medical Record Analysis

1. hyperglycemia—The condition of having a high level of sugar in the blood; associated with diabetes mellitus.
2. ketoacidosis—Acidosis due to an excess of acidic ketone bodies (waste products). A serious condition requiring immediate treatment that can result in death for the diabetic patient if not reversed. Also called *diabetic acidosis.*
3. glycosuria—Having a high level of sugar excreted in the urine.
4. type 1 diabetes mellitus—Also called *insulin-dependent diabetes mellitus.* It develops early in life when the pancreas stops insulin production. Patient must take daily insulin injections.
5. polyuria—The condition of producing and excessive amount of urine.
6. polydipsia—Excessive feeling of thirst.
7. fasting blood sugar–Blood test to measure the amount of sugar circulating throughout the body after a 12-hour fast.
8. insulin—Medication administered to replace insulin for type 1 diabetics or to treat severe type 2 diabetics.
9. glucose tolerance test—Test to determine the blood sugar level. A measured dose of glucose is given to a patient either orally or intravenously. Blood samples are then drawn at certain intervals to determine the ability of the patient to use glucose. Used for diabetic patients to determine their insulin response to glucose.
10. glucometer—A device that is designed for a diabetic to use at home to measure the level of glucose in the bloodstream.

Chart Note Transcription

1. endocrinologist 2. obesity 3. hirsutism 4. radio immunoassay (RIA) 5. cortisol 6. adenoma 7. adrenal cortex 8. Cushing's syndrome 9. adenoma 10. adrenal cortex 11. adrenalectomy

Case Study

1. Diabetes mellitus
2. Diaphoresis—Profuse sweating; rapid respirations—Breathing fast; rapid pulse—Fast heart rate; disorientation—Confused about his surroundings
3. Blood serum test—Lab test to measure the levels of different substances in the blood, used to determine the function of endocrine glands

4. Hyperglycemia—blood level of glucose is too high; ketoacidosis–an excessive amount of acidic ketone bodies in the body
5. Type 1, insulin-dependent, or juvenile diabetes mellitus because he has had it since childhood and he is taking insulin shots.
6. Type 2, non-insulin-dependent diabetes mellitus typically develops later in life. The pancreas produces normal to high levels of insulin, but the cells fail to respond to it. Patients may take oral hypoglycemic agents to improve insulin function, or may eventually have to take insulin.

Practice Exercises

A. 1. endocrinology 2. pituitary 3. gonads 4. corticosteroids 5. testosterone 6. estrogen, progesterone 7. antidiuretic hormone (ADH) 8. thymus gland 9. exophthalmos 10. adenocarcinoma
B. 1. thyroidectomy 2. thyroidal 3. hyperthyroidism 4. pancreatic 5. pancreatitis 6. pancreatectomy 7. pancreatotomy 8. adrenal 9. adrenomegaly 10. adrenopathy 11. thymoma 12. thymectomy 13. thymic 14. thymitis
C. 1. sodium 2. female 3. pineal gland 4. pituitary gland 5. potassium 6. calcium 7. parathyroid glands 8. extremities 9. sugar 10. sex glands
D. 1. e 2. d 3. a 4. f 5. c 6. b
E. 1. NIDDM 2. IDDM 3. ACTH 4. PTH 5. T_3 6. TSH 7. FBS 8. PRL
F. 1. b 2. a 3. e 4. k 5. h 6. j 7. i 8. f 9. g 10. c 11. d
G. 1. protein-bound iodine 2. potassium 3. thyroxine 4. glucose tolerance test 5. diabetes mellitus 6. basal metabolic rate 7. sodium 8. antidiuretic hormone
H. 1. glycosuria 2. vasopressin 3. polyuria 4. hypercalcemia 5. polydipsia 6. adrenocorticotropin 7. postprandial
I. 1. hormone obtained from cortex of adrenal gland 2. having excessive hair 3. a nerve condition characterized with spasms of extremities; can occur from imbalance of pH and calcium or disorder of parathyroid gland 4. disorder of the retina occurring with diabetes mellitus 5. increase in blood sugar level 6. decrease in blood sugar level 7. another term for epinephrine; produced by inner portion of adrenal gland 8. hormone produced by pancreas; essential for metabolism of blood sugar 9. toxic condition due to hyperactivity of thyroid gland 10. a condition resulting when the endocrine gland secretes more hormone than is needed by the body
J. 1. insulinoma 2. ketoacidosis 3. panhypopituitarinism 4. pheochromocytoma 5. Hashimoto's thyroiditis 6. gynecomastia

K. 1. corticosteroids, e 2. human growth hormone therapy, a 3. oral hypoglycemic agent, d 4. antithyroid agent, c 5. insulin, f 6. vasopressin, b

Labeling Exercise

A. 1. pineal gland 2. thyroid and parathyroid glands 3. adrenal glands 4. pancreas 5. pituitary gland 6. thymus gland 7. ovary 8. testis
B. 1. pituitary gland 2. bone and soft tissue 3. GH 4. testes 5. FSH, LH 6. ovary 7. FSH, LH 8. thyroid gland 9. TSH 10. adrenal cortex 11. ACTH 12. breast 13. PRL
C. 1. liver 2. stomach 3. pancreas 4. beta cell 5. alpha cell 6. islet of Langerhans

Chapter 12 Answers
Real World Applications

Medical Chart Analysis

1. paraplegia—Paralysis of the lower portion of the body and both legs.
2. comminuted fracture—Fracture in which the bone is shattered, splintered, or crushed into many small pieces or fragments.
3. epidural hematoma—Mass of blood in the space outside the dura mater of the brain and spinal cord.
4. spinal cord injury—Damage to the spinal cord as a result of trauma. Spinal cord may be bruised or completely severed.
5. unconscious—State of being unaware of surroundings, with the inability to respond to stimuli.
6. anesthesia—The lack of feeling or sensation.
7. paralysis—Temporary or permanent loss of function or voluntary movement.
8. computed tomography scan (CT scan)—An imaging technique that is able to produce a cross-sectional view of the body.
9. laminectomy—Removal of a portion of a vertebra, called the lamina, in order to relieve pressure on the spinal nerve.
10. spinal fusion—Surgical immobilization of adjacent vertebrae. This may be done for several reasons, including correction for a herniated disk.
11. physical therapy (PT)—treats disorders using physical means and methods; includes joint motion and muscle strength
12. occupational therapy (OT)—assists patients to regain, develop, and improve skills that are important for independent functioning

Chart Note Transcription

1. neurologist 2. dysphasia 3. hemiplegia 4. convulsions 5. electroencephalography (EEG) 6. lumbar puncture (LP) 7. brain scan 8. cerebral cortex 9. astrocytoma 10. craniotomy 11. cryosurgery

Case Study

1. Cerebrovascular Accident (CVA or stroke)
2. aphasia—Inability to speak; hemiparesis—Weakness on one side of the body; syncope—Fainting; delirium—Abnormal mental state with confusion, disorientation, and agitation
3. hypertension—High blood pressure; atherosclerosis—Hardening of arteries due to build up of yellow fatty substances; diabetes mellitus—Inability to make or use insulin properly to control blood sugar levels
4. brain scan—An image of the brain after injection of radioactive isotopes into the circulation; revealed an infarct in the right cerebral hemisphere
5. infarct—An area of tissue within an organ that undergoes necrosis (death) following the loss of its blood supply
6. hemorrhage—Ruptured blood vessel; thrombus—Stationary clot; embolus—Floating clot; compression—Pinching off a blood vessel

Practice Exercises

A. 1. neurology 2. brain, spinal cord, nerves 3. peripheral nervous system, central nervous system 4. efferent or motor 5. afferent or sensory 6. cerebrum 7. cerebellum 8. eyesight 9. hearing, smell 10. parasympathetic, sympathetic

B. 1. h 2. k 3. d 4. g 5. a 6. b 7. f 8. j 9. e 10. l 11. i 12. c

C. 1. neuritis 2. neurologist 3. neuralgia 4. polyneuritis 5. neurectomy 6. neuroplasty 7. neuroma 8. neurorrhaphy 9. meningitis 10. meningocele 11. myelomeningocele 12. encephalogram 13. encephalopathy 14. encephalitis 15. encephalocele 16. cerebrospinal 17. cerebral

D. 1. transient ischemic attack 2. multiple sclerosis 3. spinal cord injury 4. central nervous system 5. peripheral nervous system 6. headache 7. cerebral palsy 8. lumbar puncture 9. amyotrophic lateral sclerosis

E. 1. b 2. f 3. g 4. h 5. i 6. a 7. e 8. c 9. d

F. 1. CSF 2. CVD 3. EEG 4. ICP 5. PET 6. CVA 7. SAH 8. ANS

G. 1. injecting radiopaque dye into spinal canal to examine under X-ray the outlines made by the dye 2. X-ray of the blood vessels of the brain after the injection of radiopaque dye 3. reflex test on bottom of foot to detect lesion and abnormalities of nervous system 4. test that measures how fast an impulse travels along a nerve to pinpoint an area of nerve damage 5. laboratory examination of fluid taken from the brain and spinal cord 6. positron emission tomography to measure cerebral blood flow, blood volume, oxygen, and glucose uptake 7. recording the ultrasonic echoes of the brain 8. needle puncture into the spinal cavity to withdraw fluid

H. 1. paralysis 2. muscular coordination 3. pertaining to development 4. weakness 5. speech

I. 1. meninges 2. brain 3. cerebellum 4. spinal cord 5. head 6. thalamus 7. nerve 8. nerve root 9. cerebrum 10. pons

J. 1. tumor of astrocyte cells 2. seizure 3. without sensation 4. weakness of one-half of body 5. physician that treats nervous system with surgery 6. without sense of pain 7. localized seizure of one limb 8. paralysis of all four limbs 9. accumulation of blood in the subdural space 10. within the meninges

K. 1. d 2. e 3. f 4. g 5. b 6. a 7. c 8. j 9. h 10. i

L. 1. delirium 2. amyotrophic lateral sclerosis 3. Bell's palsy 4. cerebral aneurysm 5. Parkinson's disease 6. cerebrospinal fluid shunt 7. transient ischemic attack 8. subdural hematoma 9. cerebral palsy 10. nerve conduction velocity

M. 1. anesthetic, e 2. dopaminergic drugs, a 3. hypnotic, d 4. analgesic, g 5. sedative, b 6. narcotic analgesic, c 7. anticonvulsant, f

Labeling Exercise

A. 1. brain 2. spinal nerves 3. spinal cord

B. 1. dendrites 2. nerve cell body 3. unmyelinated region 4. myelinated axon 5. nucleus 6. axon 7. terminal end fibers

C. 1. cerebrum 2. diencephalon 3. thalamus 4. hypothalamus 5. brain stem 6. midbrain 7. cerebellum 8. pons 9. medulla oblongata

Chapter 13 Answers
Real World Applications

Medical Record Analysis

1. photophobia—Although the term translates into *fear of light*, it actually means a strong sensitivity to bright light.
2. hyperopia—With this condition a person can see things in the distance but has trouble reading material at close range. Also known as *farsightedness*. This condition is corrected with converging or biconvex lenses.

3. visual acuity test—Measurement of the sharpness of a patient's vision. Usually, a Snellen chart is used for this test in which the patient identifies letters from a distance of 20 feet.

4. intraocular—Pertaining to inside the eye.

5. ophthalmoscopy—Examination of the interior of the eyes using an instrument called an *ophthalmoscope*. The physician dilates the pupil in order to see the cornea, lens, and retina. Used to identify abnormalities in the blood vessels of the eye and some systemic diseases.

6. mydriatic drops—Any substance that causes the pupil to dilate by paralyzing the iris and/or ciliary body muscles. Particularly useful during eye examinations and eye surgery.

7. cataract—Damage to the lens causing it to become opaque or cloudy, resulting in diminished vision. Treatment is usually surgical removal of the cataract or replacement of the lens.

8. retinopathy—A general term for disease affecting the retina

9. macular degeneration—Deterioration of the macular area of the retina of the eye. May be treated with laser surgery to destroy the blood vessels beneath the macula.

10. phacoemulsification—Use of high-frequency sound waves to emulsify (liquefy) a lens with a cataract, which is then aspirated (removed by suction) with a needle.

11. prosthetic lens implant—The use of an artificial lens to replace the lens removed during cataract surgery.

Chart Note Transcription

1. otorhinolaryngologist (ENT) 2. otitis media (OM) 3. AU, binaural 4. otoscopy 5. tympanic membrane 6. cerumen 7. tympanometry 8. audiometric test 9. conductive hearing loss 10. my ringotomy

Case Study

1. conductive hearing loss results from disease or malformation of the outer or middle ear; all sound is weaker because it is not conducted correctly to the inner ear.

2. sensorineural hearing loss result of damage or malformation of the inner ear or the cochlear nerve

3. otoscopy examination of the auditory canal and middle ear; tympanometry measurement of the movement of the tympanic membrane; audiometry test for hearing ability; Rinne and Weber tuning-fork tests assess both the nerve and bone conduction of

4. Hearing aids or amplification devices amplify sound and will work best for conductive hearing loss; cochlear implant is a device that converts sound signals into magnetic impulses to stimulate the auditory nerve and is used to treat profound sensorineural hearing loss.

5. Protect his ears better during playing music by wearing earplugs

Practice Exercises

A. 1. ophthalmology 2. cilia 3. lacrimal 4. cornea 5. retina 6. iris 7. malleus, incus, stapes 8. otology 9. tympanic membrane 10. cerumen 11. eustachian or auditory 12. vestibulocochlear nerve

B. 1. artificial tears, h 2. antiglaucoma medication, c 3. antibiotic otic solution, i 4. mydriatic, a 5. antiemetic, g 6. antibiotic ophthalmic solution, j 7. anti-inflammatory otic solution, b 8. miotic, f 9. wax emulsifier, e 10. anesthetic ophthalmic solution, d

C. 1. blepharitis 2. blepharoplasty 3. blepharoptosis 4. retinopathy 5. retinopexy 6. ophthalmology 7. ophthalmic 8. ophthalmoscopy 9. iridoplegia 10. iridectomy 11. otoplasty 12. otopyorrhea 13. otalgia 14. otitis 15. tympanorrhexis 16. tympanotomy 17. tympanitis 18. audiogram 19. audiometer 20. audiology

D. 1. -tropia 2. -opia 3. -itis 4. -logy 5. -otomy 6. -plasty 7. -pexy 8. -algia 9. -otia 10. -cusis

E. 1. tear or tear duct 2. choroid 3. water 4. light 5. cornea 6. glassy 7. double 8. gray 9. old age 10. dull or dim 11. ear 12. stapes 13. hearing 14. eustachian or auditory tube 15. eardrum or tympanic membrane

F. 1. conductive—problem with outer or middle ear, muffles sound; sensorineural—damage of inner ear or nerve 2. cornea, pupil, lens, retina 3. mucous membrane that covers and protects front of eyeball 4. incus, malleus, stapes, vibrate to amplify and conduct sound waves from outer ear to inner ear

G. 1. h 2. g 3. a 4. d 5. b 6. i 7. c 8. f 9. e 10. j

H. 1. otology 2. both eyes 3. rapid eye movement 4. hertz 5. senile macular degeneration 6. pupils equal, round, react to light and accommodation 7. intraocular pressure 8. decibel 9. right eye 10. visual field

I. 1. c 2. b 3. d 4. a 5. e 6. j 7. i 8. f 9. h 10. g

J. 1. PE tube 2. EENT 3. BC 4. AU 5. OM 6. EM 7. XT 8. OS 9. EOM 10. VA

K. 1. tonometry 2. emmetropia 3. conjunctivitis 4. myopia 5. cataract 6. hordeolum 7. strabismus 8. hyperopia 9. presbycusis 10. otorhinolaryngologist 11. inner ear 12. Ménière's disease 13. acoustic neuroma

L. 1. dull/dim vision 2. double vision 3. enlarge or widen pupil 4. constrict pupil 5. diminished vision of old age 6. ringing in the ears 7. middle ear bone 8. measure movement in eardrum 9. auditory tube 10. inner ear 11. results of hearing test 12. middle ear infection

Labeling Exercise

A. 1. iris 2. lens 3. conjunctiva 4. pupil 5. cornea 6. suspensory ligaments 7. ciliary body 8. fovea centralis 9. optic nerve 10. retina 11. choroid 12. sclera

B. 1. pinna 2. external auditory meatus 3. auditory canal 4. tympanic membrane 5. malleus 6. incus 7. semicircular canals 8. vestibular nerve 9. cochlear nerve 10. cochlea 11. round window 12. stapes 13. Eustachian tube

Chapter 14 Answers
Real World Applications

Chart Note Transcription

1. oncologist 2. exploratory surgery 3. biopsies 4. malignant 5. neoplasm 6. Grade II 7. encapsulated 8. metastases 9. nephrocarcinoma 10. protocol 11. chemotherapy

Case Study

1. bronchogenic carcinoma lung cancer that begins in the bronchial tubes; 2. dyspnea difficulty breathing, cough producing thick sputum coughing up thick mucus material, hemoptysis coughing up blood; 3. computed tomography scan (CT scan)—An imaging technique that is able to produce a cross-sectional view of the body. X-ray pictures are taken at multiple angles through the body. A computer then uses all these images to construct a composite cross-section, scan revealed a mass in the right lung; 4. sputum culture and sensitivity testing sputum by placing it on a culture medium and observing any bacterial growth. The specimen is then tested to determine antibiotic effectiveness, there was no bacterial growth; sputum cytology examining sputum for malignant cells, cells were found that confirmed the presence of bronchogenic carcinoma; 5. lobectomy, removal of a lobe of the lung; 6. the tumor has spread to other areas of the body

Practice Exercises

A. 1. *Physician's Desk Reference* (PDR) 2. pharmacist 3. generic or nonproprietary 4. brand or proprietary 5. the chemical formula 6. Drug Enforcement Agency

B. 1. sublingual 2. rectal 3. topical 4. intradermal 5. intramuscular 6. intravenous 7. oral

C. 1. unusual or abnormal response to a drug 2. administration of a drug through a needle and syringe under the skin, or into a muscle, vein, or body cavity 3. harmless substance to satisfy patient's desire for medication 4. extent to which a substance is poisonous 5. response to drug other than the expected response 6. prepackaged and prelabeled method of medication distribution 7. emotional dependence on a drug 8. substance that neutralizes poisons 9. condition under which a particular drug should not be used 10. prevention of disease

D. 1. grain 2. two times a day 3. three times a day 4. as desired 5. as needed 6. before 7. over the counter 8. drop 9. label as follows/directions 10. immediately 11. milligram 12. aqueous 13. night 14. nothing by mouth 15. at bedtime 16. intravenous 17. telephone order 18. drops 19. after meals 20. discontinue

E. 1. Pravachol, 20 milligrams each, take one every day at bedtime, supply with 30, refill three times with no substitutions 2. Lanoxin, 0.125 milligram each, take three now and then 2 every morning, supply with 100 and may refill as needed 3. Synthroid, 0. 075 milligram each, take 1 every day, supply with 100 and may refill four times 4. Norvasc, 5 milligram each, take 1 every morning, supply with 60 and may refill

F. 1. i 2. k 3. h 4. j 5. e 6. f 7. b 8. a 9. d 10. c 11. g

G. 1. minor tranquilizers 2. humanistic psychotherapy 3. lithium 4. antipsychotic drugs 5. psychoanalysis 6. antidepressant drugs

H. 1. general anesthesia 2. local anesthesia 3. topical anesthesia 4. regional anesthesia

I. 1. h 2. c 3. b 4. g 5. f 6. a 7. d 8. e 9. i

J. 1. range of motion 2. occupational therapy 3. activities of daily living 4. lower extremity 5. electromyogram 6. transcutaneous electrical nerve stimulation 7. physical therapy 8. passive range of motion 9. electrical stimulation 10. ultrasound

K. 1. massage 2. debridement 3. hydrotherapy 4. postural drainage with clapping 5. active exercises 6. phonophoresis 7. cryotherapy 8. traction

L. 1. h 2. e 3. j 4. g 5. a 6. i 7. c 8. f 9. b 10. d

M. 1. magnetic resonance imaging 2. barium 3. anteroposterior 4. computerized tomography 5. right lateral 6. posteroanterior 7. left lateral 8. positron emission tomography 9. upper gastrointestinal series 10. kidneys, ureters, bladder

N. 1. h 2. d 3. g 4. j 5. f 6. b 7. i 8. a 9. e 10. c

A

Abbreviations, 11. *See also* individual subject headings

Abdomen
anatomical divisions of, 36t
clinical divisions of, 36t

abdominal, pertaining to abdomen, 33, 39

Abdominal aorta, 382f

Abdominal cavity, superior portion of abdominopelvic cavity, 34, 34f, 35t

Abdominal region, 33, 33f

Abdominopelvic cavity, ventral cavity consisting of abdominal and pelvic cavities; contains digestive, urinary, and reproductive organs, 34, 35, 36t

Abducens nerve, 418t

Abduction, directional term meaning to move away from median or middle line of body, 9, 116, 116f

Abnormal psychology, study and treatment of behaviors outside of normal and detrimental to person or society; these maladaptive behaviors range from occasional difficulty coping with stress, to bizarre actions and beliefs, to total withdrawal, 500

ABO system, major system of blood typing, 182

Abortifacient, medication that terminates a pregnancy, 351

Abortion (AB), 336

Abrasion, scraping away a portion of skin surface; performed to remove acne scars, tattoos, and scar tissue, 58

Abruptio placentae, emergency condition in which placenta tears away from uterine wall before twentieth week of pregnancy; requires immediate delivery of baby, 345

Abscess, a collection of pus in skin, 63

Absence seizure, type of epileptic seizure that lasts only a few seconds to half a minute, characterized by loss of awareness and absence of activity; also called *petit mal seizure,* 422

Acapnia, lack of carbon dioxide, 218

Accessory nerve, 418t

Accessory organs, accessory organs to digestive system consist of organs that are part of system, but not part of continuous tube from mouth to anus; accessory organs are liver, pancreas, gallbladder, and salivary glands, 258, 264–65

ACE inhibitor drugs, medication that produces vasodilation and decreases blood pressure, 163

Achromatopsia, condition of color blindness; more common in males, 456

Acidosis, excessive acidity of body fluids due to accumulation of acids, as in diabetic acidosis, 392

Acne, inflammatory disease of sebaceous glands and hair follicles resulting in papules and pustules, 63

Acne rosacea, hypertrophy of sebaceous glands causing thickened skin generally on nose, forehead, and cheeks, 63

Acne vulgaris, common form of acne occurring in adolescence from oversecretion of oil glands; characterized by papules, pustules, blackheads, and whiteheads, 63

Acoustic, pertaining to hearing, 470

Acoustic neuroma, benign tumor of eighth cranial nerve sheath, which can cause symptoms from pressure being exerted on tissues, 473

Acquired immunity, protective response of body to a specific pathogen, 197

Acquired immunodeficiency syndrome (AIDS), disease involving a defect in cell-mediated immunity system; syndrome of opportunistic infections occurring in final stages of infection with human immunodeficiency virus (HIV); virus attacks T_4 lymphocytes and destroys them, which reduces person's ability to fight infection, 66, 202

Acromegaly, chronic disease of adults resulting in elongation and enlargement of bones of head and extremities, 393, 393f

Action, type of movement a muscle produces, 115

Active acquired immunity, immunity developing after direct exposure to a pathogen, 196, 197

Active exercises, exercises that a patient performs without assistance, 516

Active range of motion (AROM), range of motion for joints that a patient is able to perform without assistance of someone else, 516

Active-resistive exercises, exercises in which patient will work against artificial resistance applied to a muscle, such as a weight; used to increase strength, 516

Activities of daily living (ADL), activities usually performed in course of a normal day, such as eating, dressing, and washing, 514, 514*f*

Acute care hospitals, hospitals that typically provide services to diagnose (laboratory, diagnostic imaging) and treat (surgery, medications, therapy) diseases for a short period of time; in addition, they usually provide emergency and obstetrical care; also called general hospital, 13

Acute respiratory distress syndrome, 234

Acute tubular necrosis (ATN), damage to renal tubules due to presence of toxins in urine or to ischemia; results in oliguria, 308

Adam's apple, 222, 388*f*

Adaptive equipment, equipment that has been structured to aid in mobility, eating, and managing other activities of daily living; equipment includes special walkers and spoons for stroke patient, 514, 515*f*

Addiction, acquired dependence on a drug, 496

Addison's disease, disease resulting from a deficiency in adrenocortical hormones; there may be an increased pigmentation of skin, generalized weakness, and weight loss, 391

Additive, sum of action of two (or more) drugs given; in this case, total strength of medications is equal to sum of strength of each individual drug, 496

Adduction, directional term meaning to move toward median or middle line of body, 9, 116*t*, 116*f*

Adenocarcinoma, malignant adenoma in a glandular organ, 395

Adenoidectomy, excision of adenoids, 205

Adenoiditis, inflammation of adenoid tissue, 201

Adenoids, another term for pharyngeal tonsils; tonsils are a collection of lymphatic tissue found in nasopharynx to combat microorganisms entering body through nose or mouth, 196, 222

Adhesion, scar tissue forming in fascia surrounding a muscle making it difficult to stretch muscle, 120

Adipose, type of connective tissue; also called fat; it stores energy and provides protective padding for underlying structures, 25

Adjective suffixes, 8

Adrenal, pertaining to adrenal gland, 389

Adrenal cortex, outer portion of adrenal glands; secretes several families of hormones: mineralocorticoids, glucocorticoids, and steroid sex hormones, 380*t*, 382, 382*f*

Adrenal feminization, development of female secondary sexual characteristics (such as breasts) in a male; often as a result of increased estrogen secretion by adrenal cortex, 391

Adrenal glands, pair of glands in endocrine system located just above each kidney; glands are composed of two sections, cortex and medulla, that function independently of each other; cortex secretes steroids, such as aldosterone, cortisol, androgens, estrogens, and progestins; medulla secretes epinephrine and norepinephrine; adrenal glands are regulated by adrenocorticotropin hormone, which is secreted by pituitary gland, 30*t*, 380, 382, 382*t*, 391

Adrenal medulla, inner portion of adrenal gland; secretes epinephrine and norepinephrine, 380*t*, 382, 382*f*

Adrenal virilism, development of male secondary sexual characteristics (such as deeper voice and facial hair) in a female; often as a result of increased androgen secretion by adrenal cortex, 391

Adrenalectomy, excision of adrenal gland, 396

Adrenaline, hormone produced by adrenal medulla; also known as epinephrine; some of its actions include increasing heart rate and force of contraction, bronchodilation, and relaxation of intestinal muscles, 380*t*, 382

Adrenalitis, inflammation of adrenal gland, 391

Adrenocorticotropin hormone (ACTH), hormone secreted by anterior pituitary; regulates function of adrenal gland cortex, 381*t*, 384, 385

Adrenomegaly, enlarged adrenal gland, 390

Adrenopathy, adrenal gland disease, 390

Adult respiratory distress syndrome (ARDS), acute respiratory failure in adults characterized by tachypnea, dyspnea, cyanosis, tachycardia, and hypoxemia, 234

Adverse reaction, 497

Aerosol, drugs inhaled directly into nose and mouth, 494, 494*t*

Aerosol therapy, medication suspended in mist intended to be inhaled; delivered by a *nebulizer,* which delivers mist for period of time while patient breathes, or a *metered dose inhaler* (MDI), which delivers a single puff of mist, 240

Afferent, 299

Afferent arteriole, arteriole that carries blood into glomerulus, 299, 300*f*, 302*f*

Afferent neurons, nerve that carries impulses to brain and spinal cord from skin and sense organs; also called sensory neurons, 418

Agglutinate, clumping together to form small clusters; platelets agglutinate to start clotting process, 182

Agranulocytes, nongranular leukocyte; this is one of two types of leukocytes found in plasma that are classified as either monocytes or lymphocytes, 181, 181*t*

AIDS-related complex (ARC), early stage of AIDS; there is a positive test for virus but only mild symptoms of weight loss, fatigue, skin rash, and anorexia, 202

Alanine transaminase (ALT), enzyme normally present in blood; blood levels are increased in persons with liver disease, 276

Albinism, condition in which person is not able to produce melanin; albino person has white hair and skin and pupils of eye are red, 63

Albumin, protein normally found circulating in bloodstream; it is abnormal for albumin to be in urine, 180, 303

Aldosterone, hormone produced by adrenal cortex; regulates levels of sodium and potassium in body and as a side effect volume of water lost in urine, 380*t*, 382

Alimentary canal, also known as gastrointestinal system or digestive system; system covers area between mouth and anus and includes 30 feet of intestinal tubing; has a wide range of functions; system serves to store and digest food, absorb nutrients, and eliminate waste; major organs of system are mouth, pharynx, esophagus, stomach, small intestine, colon, rectum, and anus, 258

Allergen, antigen capable of causing a hypersensitivity or allergy in body, 201

Allergist, physician who specializes in testing for and treating allergies, 200

Allergy, hypersensitivity to a substance in environment or medication, 201

Allograft, skin graft from one person to another; donor is usually a cadaver, 70

Alopecia, absence or loss of hair, especially of head, 69

Alveolar, pertaining to alveoli,

Alveoli, tiny air sacs at end of each bronchiole; alveoli are surrounded by capillary network; gas exchange takes place as oxygen and carbon dioxide diffuse across alveolar and capillary walls, 223, 224*f*

Alzheimer's disease (AD), chronic, organic mental disorder consisting of dementia that is more prevalent in adults between 40 and 60; involves progressive disorientation, apathy, speech and gait disturbances, and loss of memory, 424, 501

Amblyopia, loss of vision not as a result of eye pathology; usually occurs in patients who see two images; in order to see only one image, brain will no longer recognize image being sent to it by one of eyes; may occur if strabismus is not corrected; commonly referred to as lazy eye, 456

Ambulatory care center, facility that provides services that do not require overnight hospitalization; services range from simple surgeries, to diagnostic testing, to therapy; also called a surgical center or outpatient clinic, 13

Amenorrhea, absence of menstruation, which can be result of many factors, including pregnancy, menopause, and dieting, 342

American Sign Language (ASL), nonverbal method of communicating in which hands and fingers are used to indicate words and concepts; used by people who are deaf and speech impaired, 475, 475*f*

Amino acids, organic substances found in plasma, used by cells to build proteins, 180

Amnesia, loss of memory in which people forget their identity as a result of head injury or disorder, such as epilepsy, senility, and alcoholism; can be either temporary or permanent, 501

Amniocentesis, puncturing of amniotic sac using a needle and syringe for purpose of withdrawing amniotic fluid for testing; can assist in determining fetal maturity, development, and genetic disorders, 348

Amnion, inner of two membranous sacs surrouding fetus; amniotic sac contains amniotic fluid in which baby floats, 338, 340

Amniorrhea, discharge of amniotic fluid, 342

Amniotic, pertaining to amnion, 340

Amniotic fluid, fluid inside amniotic sac, 336, 337*f*, 338

Amniotomy, incision into amniotic sac, 349

Amplification device, 475

Amputation, partial or complete removal of a limb for a variety of reasons, including tumors, gangrene, intractable pain, crushing injury, or uncontrollable infection, 107

Amylase, digestive enzyme found in saliva that begins digestion of carbohydrates, 264

Amyotrophic lateral sclerosis (ALS), disease with muscular weakness and atrophy due to degeneration of motor neurons of spinal cord; also called *Lou Gehrig's disease,* after New York Yankees' baseball player who died from disease, 427

Anacusis, total absence of hearing; unable to perceive sound; also called *deafness,* 472

Anal, pertaining to anus, 267

Anal fistula, abnormal tubelike passage from surface around anal opening directly into rectum, 272

Anal sphincter, ring of muscle that controls anal opening, 263

Analgesia, reduction in perception of pain or sensation due to neurological condition or medication, 422

Analgesic, substance that relieves pain without loss of consciousness; may be either narcotic or non-narcotic; narcotic drugs are derived from opium poppy and act on brain to cause pain relief and drowsiness, 432, 523

Anaphylactic shock, life-threatening condition resulting from ingestion of food or medications that produce severe allergic response; circulatory and respiratory problems occur, including respiratory distress, hypotension, edema, tachycardia, and convulsions, 201

Anaphylaxis, severe reaction to antigen, 201

Anastomosis, creating a passageway or opening between two organs or vessels, 279

Anatomical position, used to describe positions and relationships of a structure in human body; for descriptive purposes assumption is always that person is in anatomical position; body is standing erect with arms at side of body, palms of hands facing forward, and eyes looking straight ahead; legs are parallel with feet and toes pointing forward, 31, 32f

Ancillary reports, report in patient's medical record from various treatments and therapies patient has received, such as rehabilitation, social services, respiratory therapy, or from dietician, 12

Androgen, class of steroid hormones secreted by adrenal cortex; these hormones, such as testosterone, produce a masculinizing effect, 380t, 382

Androgen therapy, replacement male hormones to treat patients who produce insufficient hormone naturally, 362

Anemia, reduction in number of red blood cells (RBCs) or amount of hemoglobin in blood; results in less oxygen reaching tissues, 186

Anesthesia, partial or complete loss of sensation with or without loss of consciousness as a result of drug, disease, or injury, 422, 520, 521t

Anesthesiologist, physician who has specialization in practice of administering anesthetics, 422, 520

Anesthesiologist's report, medical record document that relates details regarding drugs given to patient and patient's response to anesthesia and vital signs during surgery, 12

Anesthesiology, branch of medicine specializing in all aspects of anesthesia, including for surgical procedures, resuscitation measures, and management of acute and chronic pain; physician is *anesthesiologist*, 422

Anesthetic, substance that produces a lack of feeling that may be of local or general effect, depending on type of administration, 72, 432, 523

Anesthetic ophthalmic solution, eyedrops for pain relief associated with eye infections and corneal abrasions, 463

Aneurysm, weakness in wall of artery that results in localized widening of artery, 157, 157f

Aneurysmectomy, surgical removal of aneurysm, 162

Angiitis, inflammation of vessels, 153

Angina pectoris, severe chest pain with sensation of constriction around heart; caused by a deficiency of oxygen to heart muscle, 154, 155f

Angiogram, record of a vessel, 159

Angiography, process of taking X-ray of blood or lymphatic vessels after injection of a radiopaque substance, 159

Angioplasty, surgical repair of blood vessels, 163, 163f

Angiospasm, involuntary muscle contraction of a vessel, 153

Angiostenosis, narrowing of a vessel, 153

Anhidrosis, abnormal condition of no sweat, 58

Ankylosing spondylitis, inflammatory spinal condition that resembles rheumatoid arthritis; results in gradual stiffening and fusion of vertebrae; more common in men than women, 103

Anorchism, congenital absence of one or both testes, 358

Anorexia, loss of appetite that can accompany other conditions such as gastrointestinal (GI) upset, 269

Anorexia nervosa, type of eating disorder characterized by severe disturbance in body image and marked refusal to eat, 501, 501f

Anorexiant, substance that treats obesity by suppressing appetite, 281

Anosmia, loss of sense of smell, 230

Anoxia, lack of oxygen, 230

Antacid, substance that neutralizes acid in stomach, 281

Antagonistic pairs, pair of muscles arranged around a joint that produce opposite actions, 115, 116–18t

Anteflexion, while uterus is normally in this position, exaggeration of forward bend of uterus is abnormal; forward bend is near neck of uterus; position of cervix, or opening of uterus, remains normal, 334

Antepartum, before birth, 341

Anterior, directional term meaning near or on front or belly side of body, 34f, 37t

Anterior lobe, anterior portion of pituitary gland; secretes adrenocorticotropin hormone, follicle-stimulating hormone, growth hormone, luteinizing hormone, melanocyte-stimulating hormone, prolactin, and thyroid-stimulating hormone, 385

Anterior pituitary gland, 385f, 386f

Anterior tibial artery, 148f

Anterior tibial vein, 150f

Anteroposterior view (AP), positioning patient so that X-rays pass through body from anterior side to posterior side, 507

Anthracosis, type of pneumoconiosis that develops from collection of coal dust in lung; also called black lung or miner's lung, 234

Anti-inflammatory otic solution, reduces inflammation, itching, and edema associated with otitis externa, 476

Anti-virals, substance that weakens viral infection in body, often by interfering with virus's ability to replicate, 72

Antiarrhythmic, controls cardiac arrhythmias by altering nerve impulses within heart, 163

Antibiotic, substance that destroys or prohibits growth of microorganisms; used to treat bacterial infections; not found effective in treating viral infections; to be effective, it must be taken regularly for specified period, 72, 242, 315

Antibiotic ophthalmic solution, eyedrops for treatment of bacterial eye infections, 463

Antibiotic otic solution, eardrops to treat otitis externa, 476

Antibody, protein material produced in body as a response to invasion of foreign substance, 198

Antibody-mediated immunity, production of antibodies by B cells in response to an antigen; also called *humoral immunity*, 197

Anticoagulant, substance that prevents or delays clotting or coagulation of blood, 163, 189

Anticonvulsant, prevents or relieves convulsions; drugs such as phenobarbital reduce excessive stimulation in brain to control seizures and other symptoms of epilepsy, 433

Antidepressant drugs, medications classified as stimulants that alter patient's mood by affecting levels of neurotransmitters in brain, 504

Antidiarrheal, prevents or relieves diarrhea, 281

Antidiuretic hormone (ADH), hormone secreted by posterior pituitary; promotes water reabsorption by kidney tubules, 381t, 385

Antidote, substance that will neutralize poisons or their side effects, 496

Antiemetic, substance that controls nausea and vomiting, 281, 476

Antifungal, substance that kills fungi infecting skin, 72

Antigen, substance capable of inducing formation of antibody; antibody then intereacts with antigen in antigen–antibody reaction, 197

Antigen-antibody complex, combination of antigen with its specific antibody; increases susceptibility to phagocytosis and immunity, 197, 198

Antiglaucoma medications, group of drugs that reduce intraocular pressure by lowering amount of aqueous humor in eyeball; may achieve this by either reducing production of aqueous humor or increasing its outflow, 463

Antihemorrhagic, substance that prevents or stops hemorrhaging, 189

Antihistamine, substance that acts to control allergic symptoms by counteracting histamine, which exists naturally in body, and which is released in allergic reactions, 205, 242

Antilipidemic, substance that reduces amount of cholesterol and lipids in bloodstream; treats hyperlipidemia, 163

Antiparasitic, substance that kills mites or lice, 72

Antiplatelet agent, substance that interferes with action of platelets; prolongs bleeding time; commonly referred to as blood thinner; used to prevent heart attacks and strokes, 163, 189

Antiprostatic agents, medications to treat early cases of benign prostatic hypertrophy; may prevent surgery for mild cases, 362

Antipruritic, substance that reduces severe itching, 72

Antipsychotic drugs, major tranquilizer drugs that have transformed treatment of patients with psychoses and schizophrenia by reducing patient agitation and panic and shortening schizophrenic episodes, 504

Antiseptic, substance used to kill bacteria in skin cuts and wounds or at a surgical site, 72

Antisocial personality disorder, personality disorder in which patient engages in behaviors that are illegal or outside of social norms, 502

Antispasmodic, medication to prevent or reduce bladder muscle spasms, 315

Antithyroid agents, medication given to block production of thyroid hormones in patients with hypersecretion disorders, 397

Antitussive, substance that controls or relieves coughing; codeine is an ingredient in many prescription cough medicines that acts upon the brain to control coughing, 243

Antrum, tapered distal end of the stomach, 262, 262f

Anuria, complete suppression of urine formed by kidneys and complete lack of urine excretion, 305

Anus, terminal opening of digestive tube, 263, 264*f*

Anvil, 467*f,* 468

Anxiety, feeling of apprehension or worry, 500

Anxiety disorders, characterized by persistent worry and apprehension; includes panic attacks, anxiety, phobias, and obsessive-compulsive disorder, 500

Aorta, largest artery in body; located in mediastinum and carries oxygenated blood away from left side of heart, 35*t,* 140*f,* 141*f,* 142*f,* 144, 145*f,* 146*f,* 195*f,* 384*f*

Aortic, pertaining to aorta, 152

Aortic arch, 148*f*

Aortic semilunar valve, 144*f*

Aortic valve, semilunar valve between left ventricle of heart and aorta in heart; prevents blood from flowing backwards into ventricle, 142*f,* 143, 144*f,* 145*f*

Apex, directional term meaning tip or summit; an area of lungs and heart, 37*t,* 141, 141*f,* 145*f,* 224, 225*f*

Apgar score, evaluation of neonate's adjustment to outside world; observes color, heart rate, muscle tone, respiratory rate, and response to stimulus, 348

Aphagia, not eating, 269

Aphasia, inability to communicate through speech; often after effect of stroke (CVA), 422

Aphonia, no voice, 230

Aphthous ulcers, painful ulcers in mouth of unknown cause; commonly called *canker sores,* 270

Aplastic anemia, severe form of anemia that develops as consequence of loss of functioning red bone marrow; results in decrease in number of all formed elements; treatment may eventually require bone marrow transplant, 186

Apnea, condition of not breathing, 230

Apocrine gland, type of sweat gland that opens into hair follicles located in pubic, anal, and mammary areas; glands secrete substance that can produce odor when it comes into contact with bacteria on skin causing what is commonly referred to as body odor, 56

Appendectomy, surgical removal of appendix, 279

Appendicitis, inflammation of appendix, 272

Appendicular skeleton, appendicular skeleton consists of bones of upper and lower extremities, shoulder, and pelvis, 89, 92, 93*f*

Appendix, 36*t,* 263*f,* 264*f*

Aqueous, pertaining to water or being water-like, 454

Aqueous humor, watery fluid filling spaces between cornea and lens, 448*f,* 449

Arachnoid layer, delicate middle layer of meninges, 417, 417*f*

Areola, pigmented area around nipple of breast, 336, 336*f*

Arrector pili, small slip of smooth muscle attached to hairs; when this muscle contracts hair shaft stands up and results in "goose bumps," 53*f,* 55, 55*f*

Arrhythmia, irregularity in heartbeat or action, 154

Arterial, pertaining to artery, 152

Arterial anastomosis, surgical joining together of two arteries; performed if artery is severed or if damaged section of artery is removed, 162

Arterial blood gases (ABG), lab test that measures amount of oxygen, carbon dioxide, and nitrogen in blood, and pH, 238

Arteries, blood vessels that carry blood away from heart, 28*t,* 87*f,* 140, 147, 147*f* 148*f*

Arteriole, smallest branch of arteries; carries blood to capillaries, 147, 152, 193*f*

Arteriorrhexis, ruptured artery, 157

Arteriosclerosis (AS), condition with thickening, hardening, and loss of elasticity of walls of arteries, 157

Arthralgia, pain in a joint, 100

Arthrocentesis, removal of synovial fluid with needle from joint space, such as in knee, for examination, 107

Arthroclasia, surgically breaking loose a stiffened joint, 107

Arthrodesis, surgical fusion or stiffening of a joint to provide stability; sometimes done to relieve pain of arthritis, 107

Arthrogram, record of a joint, 106

Arthrography, visualization of joint by radiographic study after injection of contrast medium into joint space, 106

Arthroscope, instrument to view inside joint, 3, 106

Arthroscopic surgery, use of arthroscope to facilitate performing surgery on joint, 107

Arthroscopy, examination of interior of joint by entering joint with arthroscope; arthroscope contains small television camera allowing physician to view interior of joint on monitor during procedure, 107

Arthrotomy, surgically cutting into a joint, 97

Articular, pertaining to a joint, 98

Articular cartilage, layer of cartilage covering ends of bones forming synovial joint, 86, 87*f,* 96*f*

Articulation, another term for a joint, point where two bones meet, 95

Artificial tears, medications, many of them over-the-counter, to treat dry eyes, 463

Asbestosis, type of pneumoconiosis developing from collection of asbestos fibers in lungs; may lead to development of lung cancer, 234

Ascending colon, section of colon following cecum; ascends right side of abdomen, 263, 263*f,* 264*f*

Ascending tracts, nerve tracts carrying sensory information up spinal cord to brain, 417

Ascites, collection or accumulation of fluid in peritoneal cavity, 269

Aspartate transaminase (AST), enzyme normally present in blood; blood levels are increased in persons with liver disease, 276

Aspermia, lack of, or failure to ejaculate, sperm, 358

Asphyxia, lack of oxygen that can lead to unconsciousness and death if not corrected immediately; some common causes are drowning, foreign body in respiratory tract, poisoning, and electric shock, 230

Asphyxiation, 230

Aspiration, for respiratory system, refers to inhaling food, liquid, or a foreign object into airways; term also refers to withdrawing fluid from body cavity using suction, 230

Aspirator, surgical instrument used to suction fluids, 521*t*

Asthma, disease caused by various conditions, such as allergens, and resulting in constriction of bronchial airways and labored respirations; can cause violent spasms of the bronchi (bronchospasms) but is generally not a life-threatening condition; medication can be very effective, 233

Astigm, 456

Astigmatism (Astigm), condition in which light rays are focused unevenly on eye, which causes distorted image due to abnormal curvature of cornea, 456

Astrocytoma, tumor of brain or spinal cord composed of astrocytes, 424

Ataxia, having lack of muscle coordination as a result of disorder or disease, 422

Atelectasis, condition in which lung tissue collapses, which prevents respiratory exchange of oxygen and carbon dioxide; can be caused by a variety of conditions, including pressure upon lung from tumor or other object, 235

Atherectomy, excision of fatty substance, 162

Atheroma, tumor-like collection of fatty substances, 157

Atherosclerosis, most common form of arteriosclerosis; caused by formation of yellowish plaques of cholesterol buildup on inner walls of arteries, 158

Atherosclerotic plaque, 154*f*, 155*f*

Atonia, lack of tone, 120

Atresia, congenital lack of a normal body opening, 323

Atria, two upper chambers of heart; left atrium receives blood returning from lungs, and right atrium receives blood returning from body, 143

Atrial, pertaining to atrium, 152

Atrial septal defect (ASD), 155

Atrioventricular bundle, in heart, conducts electrical impulse from atrioventricular node into ventricles, 145, 146*f*

Atrioventricular node, this area at junction of right atrium and ventricle receives stimulus from sinoatrial node and sends impulse to ventricles through bundle of His, 145, 146*f*

Atrioventricular valve (AV, A-V), heart valves located between atrium and ventricle; includes tricuspid valve in right side of heart and bicuspid or mitral valve in left side of heart, 143

Atrophy, lack or loss of normal development, 120

Attention deficit-hyperactivity disorder (ADHD), type of mental disorder diagnosed in childhood characterized by poor attention and inability to control behavior; child may or may not be hyperactive, 501

Audiogram, chart that shows faintest sounds patient can hear during audiometry testing, 473

Audiologist, provides comprehensive array of services related to prevention, diagnosis, and treatment of hearing impairment and its associated communication disorders, 444–471

Audiology, study of hearing, 441–467, 471

Audiometer, instrument to measure hearing, 473

Audiometry, process of measuring hearing, 473, 473*f*

Auditory, pertaining to hearing, 470

Auditory canal, canal that leads from external opening of ear to eardrum, 467, 467*f*

Auditory tube, another name for eustachian tube connecting middle ear and pharynx, 222, 468

Aura, sensations, such as seeing colors or smelling unusual odor, that occur just prior to epileptic seizure or a migraine headache, 422

Aural, pertaining to ear, 471

Auricle, also called pinna; external ear; functions to capture sound waves as they go past outer ear, 467–68, 467*f*

Auricular, pertaining to ear, 471

Auscultation, listening to sounds within body by using stethoscope, 159

Autism, type of mental disorder diagnosed in childhood in which child exhibits extreme degree of withdrawal from all social contacts, 501

Autograft, skin graft from person's own body, 70, 70*f*

Autoimmune disease, disease resulting from he body's immune system attacking its own cells as if they were pathogens; examples include systemic lupus erythematosus, rheumatoid arthritis, and multiple sclerosis, 201

Autologous transfusion, procedure for collecting and storing patient's own blood several weeks prior to actual need; can then be used to replace blood lost during surgical procedure, 189

Autonomic nervous system (ANS), portion of nervous system consisting of nerves to internal organs that function involuntarily; regulates functions of glands (especially salivary, gastric, and sweat glands), adrenal medulla, heart, and smooth muscle tissue; system is divided into two parts: sympathetic and parasympathetic, 145, 418, 419–20

Axial skeleton, axial skeleton includes bones in head, spine, chest, and trunk, 89–91, 90*f*

Axillary, pertaining to armpit; there is a collection of lymph nodes in this area that drains each arm, 194*t*, 199*f*

Axon, single projection of a neuron that conducts impulse away from nerve cell body, 412, 413*f*

Azotemia, accumulation of nitrogenous waste in bloodstream; occurs when kidney fails to filter these wastes from blood, 305

B

B cells, common name for B lymphocytes, responds to foreign antigens by producing protective antibodies, 198

B lymphocytes, humoral immunity cells, which respond to foreign antigens by producing protective antibodies; simply referred to as *B cells,* 198

Babinski's reflex, reflex test to determine lesions and abnormalities in nervous system; Babinski reflex is present if great toe extends instead of flexes when lateral sole of foot is stroked; normal response to this stimulation would be flexion, or upward movement, of toe, 431

Bacteria, primitive, single-celled microorganisms that are present everywhere; some are capable of causing disease in humans, 197

Bacteriuria, bacteria in urine, 305

Balanic, pertaining to glans penis, 357

Balanitis, inflammation of skin covering glans penis, 359

Balanoplasty, surgical repair of glans penis, 361

Balanorrhea, discharge from glans penis, 358

Balloon angioplasty, 163*f*

Bariatric surgery, group of surgical procedures such as stomach stapling and restrictive banding to reduce size of stomach; treatment for morbid (extreme) obesity, 279

Barium (Ba), soft metallic element from earth used as radiopaque X-ray dye, 507

Barium enema (BE), 277, 277*f*

Barium swallow, 278

Barrier contraception, prevention of pregnancy using a device to prevent sperm from meeting ovum; examples include condoms, diaphragms, and cervical caps, 349

Bartholin's glands, glands located on either side of vaginal opening that secrete mucus for vaginal lubrication, 335

Basal cell carcinoma (BCC), tumor of basal cell layer of epidermis; frequent type of skin cancer that rarely metastasizes or spreads; these cancers can arise on sun-exposed skin, 63, 63*f*

Basal layer, deepest layer of epidermis; this living layer constantly multiplies and divides to supply cells to replace cells that are sloughed off skin surface, 53

Base, directional term meaning bottom or lower part, 37*t*, 224, 225*f*

Basilic vein, 150*f*

Basophil (Basos), granulocyte white blood cell that releases histamine and heparin in damaged tissues, 181*f*, 181*t*, 184

Bell jar apparatus, 226*f*

Bell's palsy, one-sided facial paralysis with unknown cause; person cannot control salivation, tearing of eyes, or expression; patient will eventually recover, 428

Benign, not cancerous; benign tumor is generally not progressive or recurring, 526

Benign prostatic hypertrophy (BPH), enlargement of prostate gland commonly seen in males over 50, 358

Beta blocker drugs, medication that treats hypertension and angina pectoris by lowering heart rate, 164

Biceps, arm muscle named for number of attachment points; *bi-* means two and biceps have two heads attached to bone, 115

Bicuspid valve, valve between left atrium and ventricle; prevents blood from flowing backwards into atrium; has two cusps or flaps; also called mitral valve, 143*f*, 145*f*

Bicuspids, premolar permanent teeth having two cusps or projections that assist in grinding food; humans have eight bicuspids, 260*f*, 261*f*

Bilateral, 471

Bile, substance produced by liver and stored in gallbladder; added to chyme in duodenum and functions to emulsify fats so they can be digested and absorbed; cholesterol is essential to bile production, 265

Bile duct, 265*f*, 276*f*

Bilirubin, waste product produced from destruction of worn-out red blood cells; disposed of by liver, 181

Binaural, referring to both ears, 471

Biopsy (Bx, bx), piece of tissue is removed by syringe and needle, knife, punch, or brush to examine under a microscope; used to aid in diagnosis, 70, 529

Bipolar disorder (BPD), mental disorder in which patient has alternating periods of depression and mania, 502

Bite-wing x-ray, x-ray taken with part of film holder held between teeth, and film held parallel to teeth, 277

Black lung, 234

Bladder, 354*f*

Bladder cancer, cancerous tumor that arises from cells lining bladder; major symptom is hematuria, 310

Bladder neck obstruction (BNO), blockage of bladder outlet into urethra, 310

Blepharectomy, excision of eyelid, 462

Blepharitis, inflammatory condition of eyelash follicles and glands of eyelids that results in swelling, redness, and crusts of dried mucus on lids; can be result of allergy or infection, 459

Blepharoplasty, surgical repair of eyelid, 462

Blepharoptosis, drooping eyelid, 455

Blood, major component of hematic system; consists of watery plasma, red blood cells, and white blood cells, 24*f*, 28*t*, 178–90, 181*f*, 303*t*
   abbreviations, 190
   ABO system, 182
   anatomical terms, 184
   anatomy and physiology, 180–83
   diagnostic procedures, 187–88
   erythrocytes, 180–81, 181*f*
   leukocytes, 181, 181*f*, 181*t*
   pathology, 184–87
   pharmacology, 189–190
   plasma, 180
   platelets, 182
   Rh factor, 183
   terminology, 183–88
   therapeutic procedures, 189
   typing, 182–83

Blood clot, hard collection of fibrin, blood cells, and tissue debris that is end result of hemostasis or blood clotting process, 184, 185*f*

Blood culture and sensitivity (C&S), sample of blood is incubated in laboratory to check for bacterial growth; if bacteria are present, they are identified and tested to determine which antibiotics they are sensitive to, 187

Blood poisoning, 185

Blood pressure (BP), measurement of pressure that is exerted by blood against walls of a blood vessel, 149

Blood serum test, blood test to measure level of substances such as calcium, electrolytes, testosterone, insulin, and glucose; used to assist in determining function of various endocrine glands, 395

Blood sinuses, spread-out blood vessels within spleen resulting in slow-moving blood flow, 196

Blood thinners, 189

Blood transfusion, artificial transfer of blood into bloodstream, 189

Blood tumor, 185

Blood typing, blood of one person is different from another's due to presence of antigens on surface of erythrocytes; major method of typing blood is ABO system and includes types A, B, O, and AB; other major method of typing blood is Rh factor, consisting of two types, Rh+ and Rh–, 182–83

Blood urea nitrogen (BUN), blood test to measure kidney function by level of nitrogenous waste, or urea, that is in blood, 310

Blood vessels, closed system of tubes that conducts blood throughout body; consists of arteries, veins, and capillaries, 140, 146–50, 528*f*

Body, (1) whole, living individual; sum of all cells, tissues, organs, and systems working together to sustain life; (2) main portion of organ such as stomach or uterus, 248

Body cavities, 34–35, 35*t*–36*t*

Body mechanics, use of good posture and position while performing activities of daily living to prevent injury and stress on body parts, 515

Body organization
   abbreviations, 41
   body, 31–38
   body cavities, 34–35
   body planes, 32–33
   body regions, 33
   cells, 24
   directional/positional terms, 35, 35*t*–36*t*, 37*f*, 37*t*–38*t*
   levels of, 24–31
   organs and systems, 27, 27*t*–31*t*
   terminology, 38–41
   tissues, 25, 26*f*

Body planes, 32–33

Body regions, 33

Bolus, chewed up morsel of food ready to be swallowed, 264

Bone, type of connective tissue and organ of musculoskeletal system; they provide support for body and serve as sites of muscle attachments, 25, 27*t*, 86–89
   adjective forms of names, 94
   marrow, 86
   projections and depressions, 88–89
   structure, 86–87

Bone graft, piece of bone taken from patient and used to replace removed bone or bony defect at another site, 107

Bone marrow, soft tissue found inside cavities in bones; produces blood cells, 86

Bone marrow aspiration, removing a sample of bone marrow by syringe for microscopic examination; useful for diagnosing such diseases as leukemia; for example, a proliferation (massive increase) of a white blood cells cloud confirm diagnosis of acute leukemia, 188

Bone marrow transplant (BMT), patient receives red bone marrow from donor after patient's own bone marrow has been destroyed by radiation or chemotherapy, 189

Bone reabsorption inhibitors, conditions resulting in weak and fragile bones, such as osteoporosis and Paget's disease, are improved by medications that reduce reabsorption of bones, 109

Bone scan, patient is given radioactive dye and then scanning equipment is used to visualize bones; is especially useful in observing progress of treatment for osteomyelitis and cancer metastases to bone, 106, 508*f*, 526*f*

Bowel incontinence, inability to control defecation, 272

Bowman's capsule, also called glomerular capsule; part of renal corpuscle; is a double-walled cuplike structure that encircles glomerulus; in filtration stage of urine production, waste products filtered from blood enter Bowman's capsule as glomerular filtrate, 299, 300*f*

Brachial, pertaining to the arm, 33, 39*f*

Brachial artery, 148*f*

Brachial Plexus, 419*f*

Brachial region, arm regions of the body, 33, 33*f*

Brachial vein, 150*f*

Brachiocephalic veins, 150*f*

Brachytherapy, 529

Bradycardia, abonormally slow heart rate, below 60 bpm, 153

Bradykinesia, slow movement, commonly seen with rigidity of Parkinson's disease, 120

Bradypepsia, slow digestion rate, 269

Bradypnea, slow breathing, 231

Brain, one of the largest organs in body and coordinates most body activities; is center for all thought, memory, judgment, and emotion; each part of brain is responsible for controlling different body functions, such as temperature regulation and breathing; four sections to brain are cerebrum, cerebellum, diencephalon, and brain stem, 25, 31*t*, 35*t*, 412, 414–16, 414*f*

Brain metastases, 528*f*

Brain scan, injection of radioactive isotopes into circulation to determine function and abnormality of brain, 430

Brain stem, this area of brain has three components: medulla oblongata, pons, and midbrain; brain stem is pathway for impulses to be conducted between brain and spinal cord; also contains centers that control respiration, heart rate, and blood pressure; in addition, twelve pairs of cranial nerves begin in brain stem, 414, 414*f*

Brain tumor, intracranial mass, either benign or malignant; benign tumor of brain can be fatal since it will grow and cause pressure on normal brain tissue; most malignant brain tumors in children are gliomas, 424, 424*f*

Brand name, name a pharmaceutical company chooses as trademark or market name for its drug; also called *proprietary* or *trade name,* 491

Breast cancer, malignant tumor of breast; usually forms in milk-producing gland tissue or lining of milk ducts, 345, 345*f*

Breasts, milk-producing glands to provide nutrition for newborn; also called *mammary gland,* 30*t,* 331*f,* 332, 336, 336*f*

Breech presentation, placement of fetus in which buttocks or feet are presented first for delivery rather than head, 338, 339*f*

Bridge, dental appliance attached to adjacent teeth for support to replace missing teeth, 279

Broad spectrum, ability of drug to be effective against a wide range of microorganisms, 496

Bronchial, pertaining to the bronchi, 228

Bronchial tree, 223*f*

Bronchial tube, organ of respiratory system that carries air into each lung, 29*t,* 219*f,* 220, 223

Bronchiectasis, results from dilation of bronchus or bronchi that can result from infection; this abnormal stretching can be irreversible and result in destruction of bronchial walls; major symptom is large amount of purulent (pus-filled) sputum; rales (bubbling chest sound) and hemoptysis may be present, 230, 234

Bronchiolar, pertaining to a bronchiole, 228

Bronchioles, narrowest air tubes in lungs; each bronchiole terminates in tiny air sacs called alveoli, 223, 224, 224*f*

Bronchitis, acute or chronic inflammation of lower respiratory tract that often occurs after other childhood infections such as measles, 234

Bronchodilator, dilates or opens bronchi (airways in lungs) to improve breathing, 243

Bronchogenic carcinoma, malignant lung tumor that originates in bronchi; usually associated with history of cigarette smoking, 234, 234*f*

Bronchogram, X-ray record of lungs and bronchial tubes, 238

Bronchography, process of taking X-ray of lung after radiopaque substance has been placed into trachea or bronchial tree, 238

Bronchoplasty, surgical repair of a bronchial defect, 241

Bronchoscope, instrument to view inside a bronchus, 238, 239f

Bronchoscopy (Bronch), using bronchoscope to visualize bronchi; instrument can also be used to obtain tissue for biopsy and to remove foreign objects, 238, 239f

Bronchospasm, involuntary muscle spasm in bronchi, 230

Bronchus, distal end of trachea splits into left and right main bronchi as it enters each lung; each main bronchus is subdivided into smaller branches; smallest bronchi are bronchioles; each bronchiole ends in tiny air sacs called alveoli, 223, 223f

Bruit, 144

Buccal, (1) pertaining to cheeks; (2) drugs that are placed under lip or between cheek and gum, 264, 494, 496t

Buccolabial, pertaining to cheeks and lips, 267

Buffers, chemicals that neutralize acid, particularly stomach acid, 265

Bulbourethral gland, also called *Cowper's gland*; these two small male reproductive system glands are located on either side of urethra just distal to prostate; secretion from these glands neutralizes acidity in urethra and vagina, 30t, 353f, 354, 354f, 356

Bulimia, eating disorder characterized by recurrent binge eating and then purging of food with laxatives and vomiting, 502

Bundle branch block (BBB), occurs when electrical impulse is blocked from travelling down bundle of His or bundle branches; results in ventricles beating at a different rate than atria; also called a *heart block,* 154

Bundle branches, part of conduction system of heart; electrical signal travels down interventricular septum, 145, 146f, 154

Bundle of His, bundle of His is located in interventricular septum; receives electrical impulse from atrioventricular node and distributes it through ventricular walls, causing them to contract simultaneously, 145, 146f, 154

Bunion, inflammation of bursa of the great toe, 105

Bunionectomy, removal of bursa at joint of great toe, 107

Burn, full-thickness burn exists when all layers are burned; also called *third-degree burn;* partial-thickness burn exists when first layer of skin, epidermis, is burned, and second layer of skin, dermis, is damaged; also called *second-degree burn; first-degree burn* damages only epidermis, 64, 64f

Bursa, saclike connective tissue structure found in some joints; protects moving parts from friction; some common bursa locations are elbow, knee, and shoulder joints, 96

Bursectomy, excision of a bursa, 108

Bursitis, inflammation of bursa between bony prominences and muscles or tendons; common in shoulder and knee, 96, 100

C

Cachexia, loss of weight and generalized wasting that occurs during a chronic disease, 269

Calcitonin (CT), hormone secreted by thyroid gland; stimulates deposition of calcium into bone, 381t, 388

Calcium (Ca⁺), inorganic substance found in plasma; is important for bones, muscles, and nerves, 180, 384

Calcium channel blocker drugs, medication that treats hypertension, angina pectoris, and congestive heart failure by causing heart to beat less forcefully and less often, 164

Calcium supplements, maintaining high blood levels of calcium in association with vitamin D helps maintain bone density and treats osteomalacia, osteoporosis, and rickets, 109

Calculus, stone formed within organ by accumulation of mineral salts; found in kidney, renal pelvis, bladder, or urethra; plural is *calculi,* 306, 306f

Callus, mass of bone tissue that forms at fracture site during its healing, 100

Calyx, duct that connects renal papilla to renal pelvis; urine flows from collecting tubule through calyx and into renal pelvis, 298, 299f

Cancellous bone, bony tissue found inside a bone; contains cavities that hold red bone marrow; also called *spongy bone,* 86, 87, 87f

Cancerous tumors, malignant growths in the body, 197

Candidiasis, yeastlike infection of skin and mucous membranes that can result in white plaques on tongue and vagina, 344

Canines, also called cuspid teeth or eyeteeth; permanent teeth located between incisors and biscuspids that assist in biting and cutting food; humans have four canine teeth, 260, 260f

Canker sores, 270

Capillaries, smallest blood or lymphatic vessels; blood capillaries are very thin to allow gas, nutrient, and waste exchange between blood and tissues; lymph capillaries collect lymph fluid from tissues and carry it to larger lymph vessels, 139f, 140, 149, 194, 224f

Capillary bed, network of capillaries found in a given tissue or organ, 149

Carbon dioxide (CO$_2$), waste product of cellular energy production; is removed from cells by blood and eliminated from body by lungs, 141, 220

Carbuncle, inflammation and infection of skin and hair follicle that may result from several untreated boils; most commonly found on neck, upper back, or head, 69

Carcinogen, substance or chemical agent that produces cancer or increases risk of developing it; for example, cigarette smoke and insecticides are considered to be carcinogens, 527

Carcinoma, new growth or malignant tumor that occurs in epithelial tissue; can spread to other organs through blood or direct extension from organ, 526

Carcinoma in situ (CIS), malignant tumor that has not extended beyond original site, 527

Cardiac, pertaining to the heart, 152

Cardiac arrest, when heart stops beating and circulation ceases, 154

Cardiac catheterization (CC), passage of thin tube (catheter) through arm vein and blood vessel leading into heart; done to detect abnormalities, to collect cardiac blood samples, and to determine pressure within cardiac area, 160

Cardiac enzymes, complex protein molecules found only in heart muscle; cardiac enzymes are taken by blood sample to determine amount of heart disease or damage, 159

Cardiac muscle, involuntary muscle found in heart, 25, 26f, 113, 113f, 114, 114f, 141

Cardiac scan, patient is given radioactive thallium intravenously and then scanning equipment is used to visualize heart; is especially useful in determining myocardial damage, 159

Cardiac sphincter, also called *lower esophageal sphincter*; prevents food and gastric juices from backing up into esophagus, 262, 262f

Cardiologist, physician specializing in treating diseases and conditions of cardiovascular system, 154

Cardiology, branch of medicine specializing in conditions of cardiovascular system, 28t, 152

Cardiomegaly, abnormally enlarged heart, 154

Cardiomyopathy, general term for disease of myocardium that may be caused by alcohol abuse, parasites, viral infection, and congestive heart failure, 155

Cardiopulmonary resuscitation (CPR), emergency treatment provided by persons trained in CPR and given to patients when their respirations and heart stop; provides oxygen to brain, heart, and other vital organs until medical treatment can restore a normal heart and pulmonary function, 161, 242

Cardiorrhexis, ruptured heart, 143

Cardiotonic, substance that strengthens the heart muscle, 164

Cardiovascular, pertaining to the heart and blood vessels, 39

Cardiovascular system (CV), system that transports blood to all areas of body; organs of cardiovascular system include heart and blood vessels (arteries, veins, and capillaries); also called *circulatory system,* 28t, 137–76
  abbreviations, 164–65
  anatomical terms, 152
  anatomy and physiology, 140–50
  diagnostic procedures, 159–60
  pathology, 152–58
  pharmacology, 163–64
  terminology, 151–60
  therapeutic procedures, 161–63

Cardioversion, 161

Carditis, 6

Carotid artery, 148f, 467f

Cardiovascular technician, healthcare professional trained to perform a variety of diagnostic and therapeutic procedures including electrocardiography, echocardiography, and exercise stress tests, 152

Carotid endarterectomy, surgical procedure for removing obstruction within carotid artery, major artery in neck that carries oxygenated blood to brain; developed to prevent strokes but found to be useful only in severe stenosis with TIA, 432

Carpal, pertaining to the wrist, 93f, 94

Carpal tunnel release, surgical cutting of ligament in wrist to relieve nerve pressure caused by carpal tunnel disease, which can be caused by repetitive motion such as typing, 122

Carpal tunnel syndrome (CTS), painful disorder of wrist and hand, induced by compression of median nerve as it passes under ligaments on palm side of wrist; symptoms include weakness, pain, burning, tingling, and aching in forearm, wrist, and hand, 121

Carpals, wrist bones in upper extremity, 92, 93f, 94, 94f, 98

Cartilage, strong, flexible connective tissue found in several locations in body, such as covering ends of bones in synovial joint, nasal septum, external ear, eustachian tube, larynx, trachea, bronchi, and intervertebral discs, 25, 86, 467f

Cartilaginous joints, joint that allows slight movement but holds bones firmly in place by solid piece of cartilage; public symphysis is an example of a cartilaginous joint; fetal skeleton is composed of cartilaginous tissue, 96

Cast, application of solid material to immobilize extremity or portion of body as a result of fracture, dislocation, or severe injury; is most often made of plaster of Paris, 109

Castration, excision of testicles in male or ovaries in female, 361

Cataract, diminished vision resulting from lens of eye becoming opaque or cloudy; treatment is usually surgical removal of cataract, 456, 456*f*

Cath, 312

Catheter (cath), flexible tube inserted into body for purpose of moving fluids into or out of body; in cardiovascular system used to place dye into blood vessels so they may be visualized on X-rays; in urinary system used to drain urine from bladder, 160, 308*f*, 312*f*

Catheterization, insertion of a tube through urethra and into urinary bladder for purpose of withdrawing urine or inserting dye, 312

Caudal, directional term meaning toward feet or tail, or below, 37*f*, 37*t*

Cauterization, destruction of tissue using electric current, caustic product, or hot iron, or by freezing, 71, 523

Cecal, pertaining to the cecum, 267

Cecum, first portion of colon; is a blind pouch off beginning of large intestine; appendix grows out of end of cecum, 263, 263*f*, 264*f*

Cell, basic unit of all living things; all tissues and organs in body are composed of cells; they perform survival functions such as reproduction, respiration, metabolism, and excretion; some cells also able to carry on specialized functions, such as contraction by muscle cells and electrical impulse transmission by nerve cells, 24

Cell membrane, outermost boundary of the cell, 24

Cell-mediated immunity, immunity resulting from activation of sensitized T lymphocytes; immune response causes antigens to be destroyed by direct action of cells; also called *cellular immunity,* 197

Cellular immunity, also called cell-mediated immunity; process results in production of T cells and natural killer, NK, cells that directly attach to foreign cells; immune response fights invasion by viruses, bacteria, fungi, and cancer, 185

Cellulitis, inflammation of cellular or connective tissues, 65

Cementum, anchors root of a tooth into socket of jaw, 260, 261, 261*f*

Central canal, canal that extends down length of spinal cord; contains cerebrospinal fluid, 417

Central fissure, 415*f*

Central nervous system (CNS), portion of nervous system consisting of brain and spinal cord; receives impulses from all over body, processes information, and then responds with action; consists of both gray and white matter, 413–17
brain, 414–16
meninges, 413, 417
spinal cord, 416–417

Centrifuge, 179*f*

Cephalalgia, a headache, 422

Cephalic, directional term meaning toward the head, or above, 37*t*, 39

Cephalic region, head region of the body, 33, 33*f*

Cephalic vein, 150*f*

Cerebellar, pertaining to cerebellum, 421

Cerebellitis, inflammation of cerebellum, 424

Cerebellum, second largest portion of brain, located beneath posterior portion of cerebrum; this part of brain aids in coordinating voluntary body movements and maintaining balance and equilibrium; is attached to brain stem by pons; cerebellum refines muscular movement that is initiated in cerebrum, 414, 414*f*, 415*f*

Cerebral, pertaining to the cerebrum, 421

Cerebral aneurysm, localized abnormal dilatation of blood vessel, usually artery; result of congenital defect or weakness in wall of vessel; ruptured aneurysm is a common cause for hemorrhagic CVA, 425, 425*f*

Cerebral angiography, x-ray of blood vessels of brain after injection of radiopaque dye, 430

Cerebral contusion, bruising of brain from blow or impact; symptoms last longer than 24 hours and include unconsciousness, dizziness, vomiting, unequal pupil size, and shock, 425

Cerebral cortex, outer layer of cerebrum; is composed of folds of gray matter called gyri, which are separated by sulci, 414, 415

Cerebral hemispheres, division of cerebrum into right and left halves, 415

Cerebral palsy (CP), group of disabilities caused by injury to brain either before or during birth or very early in infancy; most common permanent disability in childhood, 425

Cerebrospinal, pertaining to cerebrum and spine, 421

Cerebrospinal fluid (CSF), watery, clear fluid found in ventricles of brain; provides protection from shock or sudden motion to brain, 414, 416

Cerebrospinal fluid analysis, laboratory examination of clear, watery, colorless fluid from within brain and spinal cord; infections and abnormal presence of blood can be detected in this test, 430

Cerebrospinal fluid shunts, surgical procedure in which bypass is created to drain cerebrospinal fluid; used to treat hydrocephalus by draining excess cerebrospinal fluid from brain and diverting it to abdominal cavity, 432

Cerebrovascular accident (CVA), also called a *stroke;* development of infarct due to loss in blood supply to area of brain; blood flow can be interrupted by ruptured blood vessel (hemorrhage), floating clot (embolus), stationary clot (thrombosis), or compression; extent of damage depends on size and location of infarct and often includes speech problems and muscle paralysis, 425, 425*f*

Cerebrum, largest section of brain; located in upper portion and is area that possesses thoughts, judgment, memory, association skills, and ability to discriminate between items; outer layer of cerebrum is cerebral cortex, which is composed of folds of gray matter; elevated portions of cerebrum, or convolutions, are called gyri and are separated by fissures or sulci; cerebrum has both a left and right division or hemisphere, each with its own four lobes: frontal, parietal, occipital, and temporal, 414, 414*f*

Cerumen, also called ear wax; thick, waxy substance produced by oil glands in auditory canal; helps to protect and lubricate ear, 467, 468

Ceruminoma, hard accumulation of ear wax in ear canal, 472

Cervical, (1) pertaining to the neck; (2) pertaining to cervix, 98, 416*f*

Cervical biopsy, taking a sample of tissue from cervix to test for presence of cancer cells, 348

Cervical cancer, malignant growth in cervix; especially difficult type of cancer to treat, it causes 5% of cancer deaths in women; Pap tests have helped to detect early cervical cancer, 343

Cervical nerve, 419*f*

Cervical nodes, 194*t*, 195*f*

Cervical region, neck region of body, 33, 33*f*

Cervical vertebrae (C1, C2, etc.), seven vertebrae in neck region, 89, 91, 92*t*

Cervicectomy, excision of cervix, 349

Cervix (Cx), narrow, distal portion of uterus that joins to vagina, 332*f*, 334, 334*f*, 335*f*, 337*f*

Cesarean section (CS, C-section), surgical delivery of baby through incision into abdominal and uterine walls; legend has it that Roman emperor Julius Caesar was first person born by this method, 349

Chancroid, highly infectious nonsyphilitic venereal ulcer, 359, 359*f*

Cheeks, form lateral walls of oral cavity, 258, 260

Chemabrasion, abrasion using chemicals; also called a *chemical peel,* 71

Chemical name, name for a drug based on its chemical formula or molecular structure, 491, 491*t*

Chemical thyroidectomy, large dose of radioactive iodine is given in order to kill thyroid gland cells without having to actually do surgery, 396

Chemo, 529

Chemotherapy (chemo), treating disease by using chemicals that have a toxic effect on body, especially cancerous tissue, 529

Chest tube, 241

Chest x-ray (CXR), taking radiograhic picture of lungs and heart from back and sides, 228

Cheyne-Stokes respiration, abnormal breathing pattern in which there are long periods (10 to 60 seconds) of apnea followed by deeper, more rapid breathing, 230

Chicken pox, 68, 68*f*

Chiropractic, healthcare profession concerned with diagnosis and treatment of spine and musculoskeletal system with intention of affecting nervous system and improving health; healthcare practitioner is a *chiropractor,* 99

Chiropractor, 99

Chlamydia, parasitic microorganism causing genital infections in males and females; can lead to pelvic inflammatory disease in females and eventual infertility, 359

Choked disk, 455

Cholecystalgia, gallbladder pain, 269

Cholecystectomy, surgical excision of gallbladder; removal of gallbladder through laparoscope is newer procedure with fewer complications than more invasive abdominal surgery; laparoscope requires a small incision into abdominal cavity, 279

Cholecystic, pertaining to gallbladder, 267

Cholecystitis, inflammation of gallbladder, 275

Cholecystogram, dye given orally to patient is absorbed and enters gallbladder; X-ray is then taken, 275

Choledocholithotripsy, crushing of a gallstone in common bile duct, 279

Cholelithiasis, formation or presence of stones or calculi in gallbladder or common bile duct, 276, 276*f*

Chondrectomy, excision of cartilage, 108

Chondroma, cartilage tumor, 100

Chondromalacia, softening of cartilage, 100

Chondroplasty, surgical repair of cartilage, 108

Chordae tendineae, 135*f*

Chorion, outer of two membranous sacs surrounding fetus; helps to form placenta, 336, 339

Chorionic, pertaining to chorion, 340

Chorionic villus sampling (CVS), removal of small piece of chorion for genetic analysis; may be done at earlier stage of pregnancy than amniocentesis, 348

Choroid, middle layer of eyeball; this layer provides blood supply for eye, 448, 448f, 449

Choroid layer, 447f

Chronic obstructive pulmonary disease (COPD), progressive, chronic, and usually irreversible condition in which lungs have diminished capacity for inspiration (inhalation) and expiration (exhalation); person may have difficulty breathing on exertion (dyspnea) and a cough; also called *chronic obstructive lung disease (COLD)*, 235

Chyme, semisoft mixture of food and digestive fluids that pass from stomach into small intestines, 262

Cicatrix, a scar, 67

Cilia, term for eyelashes that protect eye from foreign particles or for nasal hairs that help filter dust and bacteria out of inhaled air, 221, 451

Ciliary body, intraocular eye muscles that change shape of the lens, 448f, 449

Circadian rhythm, 24-hour clock that governs our periods of wakefulness and sleepiness, 384

Circulating nurse, nurse who assists surgeon and scrub nurse by providing needed materials during procedure and by handling surgical specimen; person does not wear sterile clothing and may enter and leave operating room during procedure, 523

Circulatory system, system that transports blood to all areas of body; organs of circulatory system include heart and blood vessels (arteries, veins, and capillaries); also called *cardiovascular system,* 140, 140f

Circumcision, surgical removal of end of prepuce or foreskin of penis; generally performed on newborn male at request of parents; primary reason is for ease of hygiene; is also a ritual practice in some religions, 355, 361

Circumduction, movement in a circular direction from a central point, 118

Cirrhosis, chronic disease of the liver, 276

Clamp, surgical instrument used to grasp tissue and control bleeding, 521t

Clavicle, also called collar bone; bone of pectoral girdle, 92, 93f, 94, 94f, 94t

Clavicular, pertaining to clavicle or collar bone, 98

Clean catch specimen (CC), urine sample obtained after cleaning off urinary opening and catching or collecting a sample in midstream (halfway through urination process) to minimize contamination from genitalia, 310

Cleft lip, congenital anomaly in which upper lip fails to come together; often seen along with cleft palate; corrected with surgery, 270

Cleft palate, congenital anomaly in which roof of mouth has split or fissure; corrected with surgery, 270

clinical psychologist (PhD), diagnoses and treats mental disorders; specializes in using individual and group counseling to treat patients with mental and emotional disorders, 500

Clinical psychology, 500

Clitoris, small organ containing erectile tissue covered by labia minora; contains sensitive tissue aroused during sexual stimulation and is similar to penis in male, 332f, 335–36, 335f

Closed fracture, simple fracture with no open skin or wound, 100, 101f

Clubbing, abnormal widening and thickening of ends of fingers and toes associated with chronic oxygen deficiency; seen in patients with chronic respiratory conditions or circulatory problems, 230

Coagulate, convert liquid to gel or solid, as in blood coagulation, 185

Coarctation of the aorta (CoA), severe congenital narrowing of aorta, 158

Coccygeal, pertaining to coccyx or tailbone, 98, 416f

Coccyx, tailbone, four small fused vertebrae at distal end of vertebral column, 89, 90f, 91f, 92f, 92t

Cochlea, portion of labyrinth associated with hearing; is rolled in shape of snail shell; organs of Corti line cochlea, 467f, 468

Cochlear, pertaining to cochlea, 471

Cochlear implant, mechanical device surgically placed under skin behind outer ear (pinna); converts sound signals into magnetic impulses to stimulate auditory nerve; can be beneficial for those with profound sensorineural hearing loss, 475, 475f

Cochlear nerve, branch of vestibulocochlear nerve that carries hearing information to brain, 467, 467f

Cognitive disorders, deterioration of mental functions due to temporary brain or permanent brain dysfunction; includes dementia and Alzheimer's disease, 501

Coitus, 355

Cold sores, 271

Colectomy, surgical removal of colon, 279

Collagen fibers, fibers made up of insoluble fibrous protein present in connective tissue that forms flexible mat to protect skin and other parts of body, 54

Collecting tubule, portion of renal tubule, 299, 300f, 302f

Colles' fracture, specific type of wrist fracture, 101, 101f

Colon, also called *large intestine;* functions to reabsorb most of fluid in digested food; material that remains after water reabsorption is feces; sections of colon are cecum, ascending colon, transverse colon, descending colon, and sigmoid colon, 27t, 33t, 34t, 243f, 244, 249–50

Colonic, pertaining to colon, 267

Colonoscope, instrument to view inside colon, 278

Colonoscopy, flexible fiberscope passed through anus, rectum, and colon is used to examine upper portion of colon; polyps and small growths can be removed during procedure, 278

Color vision tests, use of polychromic (multicolored) charts to determine ability of patient to recognize color, 460, 460f

Colorectal, pertaining to colon and rectum, 267

Colorectal carcinoma, cancerous tumor along length of colon and rectum, 272

Colostomy, surgical creation of opening in some portion of colon through abdominal wall to outside surface; fecal material (stool) drains into bag worn on abdomen, 280, 280f

Colostrum, thin fluid first secreted by breast after delivery; does not contain much protein, but is rich in antibodies, 341

Colposcope, instrument to view inside vagina, 347

Colposcopy, visual examination of cervix and vagina using colposcope or instrument with magnifying lens, 347

Coma, profound unconsciousness resulting from illness or injury, 422

Combining form, word root plus combining vowel; is always written with a / between word root and combining vowel; for example, in combining form *cardi/o, cardi* is word root and */o* is combining vowel, 3–4

Combining vowel, vowel inserted between word parts that makes it possible to pronounce long medical terms; is usually the vowel *o,* 2, 3–4

Comedo, medical term for blackhead; is an accumulation of sebum in sebaceous gland that has become blackened, 58

Comminuted fracture, fracture in which bone is shattered, splintered, or crushed into many pieces or fragments; fracture is completely through bone, 101

Common bile duct (CBD), duct that carries bile from gallbladder to duodenum, 265–265f, 276f

Common iliac artery, 148f

Common iliac vein, 150f

Compact bone, hard exterior surface bone; also called *cortical bone,* 86, 87f, 96f

Complemental air, 225t

Complete blood count (CBC), blood test consisting of five tests; red blood cell count

(RBC), white blood count (WBC), hemoglobin (Hg), hematocrit (Hct), and white blood cell differential, 187

Compound fracture, open fracture in which skin has been broken through by fracture, 101, 101f

Compression fracture, fracture involving loss of height of vertebral body, 101

Computed tomography scan (CT scan, CAT), imaging technique able to produce cross-sectional view of body; X-ray pictures are taken at multiple angles through body and computer uses all images to construct composite cross-section, 508

Conception, fertilization of ovum by a sperm, 333, 334

Concussion, injury to brain resulting from blow or impact from object; can result in unconsciousness, dizziness, vomiting, unequal pupil size, and shock, 426

Conductive hearing loss, loss of hearing as a result of blocking of sound transmission in middle ear and outer ear, 469

Condyle, refers to rounded portion at end of a bone, 88, 88f

Cones, sensory receptors of retina that are active in bright light and see in color, 449

Confidentiality, 14

Congenital anomalies, 337

Congenital septal defect (CSD), defect, present at birth, in wall separating two chambers of heart; results in a mixture of oxygenated and deoxygenated blood being carried to surrounding tissues; there can be atrial septal defect (ASD) and ventricular septal defect (VSD), 155

Congestive heart failure (CHF), pathological condition of heart in which there is reduced outflow of blood from left side of heart; results in weakness, breathlessness, and edema, 155

Conization, surgical removal of core of cervical tissue; also refers to partial removal of cervix, 349

Conjunctiva, protective mucous membrane lining on underside of each eyelid and across anterior surface of each eyeball, 448, 448f, 450f, 451, 459

Conjunctival, pertaining to conjunctiva, 454

Conjunctivitis, also referred to as *pink eye* or inflammation of conjunctiva, 459

Conjunctivoplasty, surgical repair of conjunctiva, 459

Connective tissue, supporting and protecting tissue in body structures; examples are fat or adipose tissue, cartilage, and bone, 25, 26f

Conscious, condition of being awake and aware of surroundings, 422

Constipation, experiencing difficulty in defecation or infrequent defecation, 269

Consultation reports, document in patient's medical record; reports given by specialists who physician has requested to evaluate patient, 12

Contracture, abnormal shortening of muscle, making it difficult to stretch muscle, 120

Contraindication, condition in which particular drug should not be used, 496

Contrast studies, radiopaque substance is injected or swallowed; X-rays are then taken that outline body structure containing radiopaque substance, 509, 509f

Controlled substances, drugs that have potential for being addictive (habit forming) or can be abused, 492, 492t

Contusion, injury caused by blow to body; causes swelling, pain, and bruising; skin is not broken, 58

Conversion reaction, somatoform disorder in which patient unconsciously substitutes physical signs or symptoms for anxiety; most common physical signs or symptoms are blindness, deafness, and paralysis, 503

Convulsions, severe involuntary muscle contractions and relaxations; these have a variety of causes, such as epilepsy, fever, and toxic conditions, 399

Corium, living layer of skin located between epidermis and subcutaneous tissue; also referred to as *dermis,* it contains hair follicles, sweat glands, sebaceous glands, blood vessels, lymph vessels, nerve fibers, and muscle fibers, 54

Cornea, portion of sclera that is clear and transparent and allows light to enter interior of eye; also plays role in bending light rays, 447f, 448, 448f, 452f

Corneal, pertaining to cornea, 454

Corneal abrasion, scraping injury to cornea; if it does not heal, it may develop into ulcer, 456

Coronal plane, vertical plane that divides body into front (anterior or ventral) and back (posterior or dorsal) sections; also called *frontal plane,* 32f, 33

Coronal section, sectional view of body produced by cut along frontal plane; also called *frontal section,* 33

Coronary, pertaining to heart, 147, 152

Coronary arteries, group of three arteries that branch off aorta and carry blood to myocardium, 147, 147f

Coronary artery bypass graft (CABG), open-heart surgery in which blood vessel is grafted to route blood around point of constriction in diseased coronary artery, 162

Coronary artery disease (CAD), insufficient blood supply to heart muscle due to obstruction of one or more coronary arteries; may be caused by atherosclerosis and may cause angina pectoris and myocardial infarction, 155, 155f

Corpus, body or central portion of uterus, 332f, 334

Corpus (uterus), 332f

Corpus albicans, 333f

Corpus luteum, 333f

Cortex, outer layer of organ; in endocrine system, it refers to outer layer of adrenal glands; in urinary system, outer layer of kidney, 298, 299f, 382, 382f

Cortical, pertaining to cortex, 98

Cortical bone, hard exterior surface bone; also called *compact bone,* 86, 87f

Corticosteroid cream, powerful anti-inflammatory cream, 72

Corticosteroids, general term for group of hormones secreted by adrenal contex; they include mineralocorticoid hormones, glucocorticoid hormones, and steroid sex hormones; used as medication for its strong anti-inflammatory properties, 109, 205, 243, 382, 397

Cortisol, steroid hormone secreted by adrenal cortex; regulates carbohydrate metabolism, 382

Costal, pertaining to ribs, 98

Cowper's glands, also called *bulbourethral glands;* these two small male reproductive system glands are located on either side of urethra just distal to prostate; secretion from these glands neutralizes acidity in urethra and vagina, 356

Crackles, abnormal sound made during inspiration; usually indicates presesnce of fluid or mucus in small airways; also called *rales,* 230

Cranial, pertaining to skull, 39, 98

Cranial bones, 91t

Cranial cavity, dorsal body cavity; is within skull and contains brain, 34, 34f, 35t

Cranial nerves, nerves that arise from brain, 412, 418t

Craniotomy, incision into skull, 108

Cranium, skull; bones that form protective covering over brain, 89, 90f

Creatine phosphokinase (CPK), muscle enzyme found in skeletal muscle and cardiac muscle; blood test becomes elevated in disorders such as heart attack, muscular dystrophy, and other skeletal muscle pathologies, 122

Creatinine, waste product of muscle metabolism, 180

Creatinine clearance, test of kidney function; creatinine is waste product cleared from bloodstream by kidneys; for this test, urine is collected for 24 hours and amount of creatinine in urine is compared to amount of creatinine that remains in bloodstream, 311

Crepitation, sound of broken bones rubbing together, 100

Cretinism, congenital condition due to lack of thyroid that may result in arrested physical and mental development, 394

Crick in the neck, 121

Cricoid cartilage, 221f

Crohn's disease, form of chronic inflammatory bowel disease affecting ileum and/or colon; also called *regional ileitis,* 272

Cross infection, occurs when person, either patient or healthcare worker, acquires pathogen from another patient or healthcare worker, 198

Cross-eyed, 459

Cross-section, internal view of body produced by slice perpendicular to long axis of structure, 33

Croup, acute viral respiratory infection common in infants and young children and characterized by hoarse cough, 233

Crown, portion of tooth covered by enamel; also artificial covering for tooth created to replace original enamel, 261, 261f, 279

Crowning, when head of baby is visible through vaginal opening; a sign that birth is imminent, 338

Crural, pertaining to leg, 39

Crural region, lower extremity region of body, 33, 33f

Cryoextraction, procedure in which cataract is lifted from lens with extremely cold probe, 462

Cryoretinopexy, surgical fixation of retina by using extreme cold, 462

Cryosurgery, exposing tissues to extreme cold in order to destroy them; used in treating malignant tumors and to control pain and bleeding, 71, 523

Cryotherapy, using cold for therapeutic purposes, 516

Cryptorchidism, failure of testes to descend into scrotal sac before birth; generally, testes will descend before boy is 1 year old; surgical procedure called orchidopexy may be required to bring testes down into scrotum permanently; failure of testes to descend could result in sterility in male, 358

Culdoscopy, examination of female pelvic cavity by introducing endoscope through wall of vagina, 347

Culture and sensitivity (C&S), laboratory test in which colony of pathogens that have been removed from infected area are grown to identify pathogen and then determine its sensitivity to variety of antibiotics, 70, 187, 238, 311

Cumulative action, action that occurs in body when drug is allowed to accumulate or stay in body, 496

Curettage, removal of superficial skin lesions with curette (surgical instrument shaped like spoon) or scraper, 71

Curette, surgical instrument used to scrape and remove tissue, 521t

Cushing's syndrome, set of symptoms that result from hypersecretion of adrenal cortex; may be result of tumor of adrenal glands; syndrome may present symptoms of weakness, edema, excess hair growth, skin discoloration, and osteoporosis, 392, 392f

Cuspids, permanent teeth located between incisors and bicuspids that assist in biting and cutting food; humans have four cuspids; also called canine teeth or eyeteeth, 260, 260f

Cusps, leaflets or flaps of heart valve, 143

Cutaneous, pertaining to skin, 57

Cutaneous membrane, this is another term for skin, 52

Cuticle, thin skinlike layer overlapping base of nail, 55

Cyanosis, slightly bluish color of skin due to deficiency of oxygen and excess of carbon dioxide in blood; is caused by variety of disorders, ranging from chronic lung disease to congenital and chronic heart problems, 55, 58, 231

Cycloplegia, paralysis of ciliary body, 455

Cyst, fluid-filled sac under skin, 58, 58f

Cystalgia, bladder pain, 306

Cystectomy, excision of bladder, 314

Cystic, pertaining to bladder, 305

Cystic duct, duct leading from gallbladder to common bile duct; carries bile, 265, 265f, 276f

Cystic fibrosis (CF), hereditary condition causing exocrine glands to malfunction; patient produces very thick mucus that causes severe congestion within lungs and digestive system; through more advanced treatment, many children are now living into adulthood with this disease, 235

Cystitis, inflammation of bladder, 301, 310

Cystocele, hernia or outpouching of bladder that protrudes into vagina; may cause urinary frequency and urgency, 310, 344

Cystogram, record of bladder, 311

Cystography, process of instilling contrast material or dye into bladder by catheter to visualize urinary bladder on X-ray, 311

Cystolith, bladder stone, 306

Cystopexy, surgical fixation of bladder, 314

Cystoplasty, surgical repair of bladder, 314

Cystorrhagia, rapid bleeding from bladder, 306

Cystoscope, instrument used to visually examine bladder, 312

Cystoscopy (cysto), visual examination of urinary bladder using instrument called cystoscope, 312

Cystostomy, creation of opening through body wall and into bladder, 314

Cystotomy, incision into bladder, 314

Cytologic testing, examination of cells to determine structure and origin; pap smears are considered a form of cytologic testing, 529

Cytology, study of cells, 24, 39

Cytoplasm, watery internal environment of a cell, 24

Cytotoxic, pertaining to poisoning cells, 197, 198

D

Dacryoadenitis, inflammation of lacrimal gland, 459

Dacryocystitis, inflammation of tear sac, 459

Day surgery, type of outpatient surgery in which patient is discharged on same day he or she is admitted; also called ambulatory surgery, 523

Deafness, inability to hear or having some degree of hearing impairment, 472

Debridement, removal of foreign material and dead or damaged tissue from wound, 71, 516

Decibel (dB), measures intensity or loudness of sound; zero decibels is quietest sound measured and 120 dB is loudest sound commonly measured, 473

Deciduous teeth, 20 teeth that begin to erupt around age of 6 months; eventually pushed out by permanent teeth, 260, 261

Decongestant, substance that reduces nasal congestion and swelling, 243

Decubitus ulcer (decub), bedsore or pressure sore caused by pressure over bony prominences on body; caused by lack of blood flow, 65

Deep, directional term meaning away from surface of body, 37t

Deep tendon reflex (DTR), muscle contraction in response to stretch caused by striking muscle tendon with reflex hammer; test used to determine if muscles are responding properly, 122

Defecation, evacuation of feces from rectum, 263

Defibrillation, procedure that converts serious irregular heartbeats, such as fibrillation, by giving electric shocks to heart, 161, 161f

Delirium, state of mental confusion with lack of orientation to time and place, 423

Delivery, emergence of baby from birth canal, 338, 338f

Delusions, false belief held with conviction even in face of strong evidence to contrary, 503

Dementia, progressive impairment of intellectual function that interferes with performing activities of daily living; patients have little awareness of their condition; found in disorders such as Alzheimer's, 423, 521

Dendrite, branched process off a neuron that receives impulses and carries them to cell body, 412, 413f

Dental, pertaining to teeth 267

Dental caries, gradual decay and disintegration of teeth caused by bacteria that can result in inflamed tissue and abscessed teeth; commonly called a *tooth cavity*, 270

Dentalgia, tooth pain, 269

Dentin, main bulk of tooth; is covered by enamel, 260, 261, 261f

Dentist, practitioner of dentistry, 268

Dentistry, branch of healthcare involved with prevention, diagnosis, and treatment of conditions involving teeth, jaw, and mouth; dentistry is practiced by *dentist* or *oral surgeon*, 268

Denture, partial or complete set of artificial teeth that are set in plastic materials; substitute for natural teeth and related structures, 279

Deoxygenated, blood in veins that is low in oxygen content, 140

Depigmentation, loss of normal skin color or pigment, 59

Depression, downward movement, as in dropping shoulders, 88–89, 118t

Dermabrasion, abrasion or rubbing using wire brushes or sandpaper, 71

Dermal, pertaining to skin, 57

Dermatitis, inflammation of skin, 65

Dermatologist, physician specialized in diagnosis and treatment of diseases of integumentary system, 58

Dermatology (Derm, derm), branch of medicine specializing in conditions of integumentary system, 27t, 39, 58

Dermatome, instrument for cutting skin or thin transplants of skin, 70

Dermatoplasty, surgical repair of skin, 71, 520

Dermatosis, abnormal condition of skin, 65

Dermis, living layer of skin located between epidermis and subcutaneous tissue; also referred to as corium or *true skin;* contains hair follicles, sweat glands, sebaceous glands, blood vessels, lymph vessels, nerve fibers, and muscle fibers, 52, 53f, 54

Descending aorta, 145f

Descending colon, section of colon that descends left side of abdomen, 263, 263f, 264f

Descending tracts, nerve tracts carrying motor signals down spinal cord to muscles, 416, 417

Diabetes insipidus (DI), disorder caused by inadequate secretion of hormone by posterior lobe of pituitary gland; there may be polyuria and polydipsia; is more common in young, 385, 393

Diabetes mellitus (DM), serious disease in which pancreas fails to produce insulin or insulin does not work properly; consequently, patient has very high blood sugar; kidney will attempt to lower high blood sugar level by excreting excess sugar in urine, 385, 392

Diabetic acidosis, 392

Diabetic nephropathy, accumulation of damage to glomerulus capillaries due to chronic high blood sugars of diabetes mellitus, 308

Diabetic retinopathy, secondary complication of diabetes that affects blood vessels of retina, resulting in visual changes and even blindness, 392

Diagnostic and Statistical Manual of Mental Disorders, Fourth Edition (Test Revision) (DSM-IV-TR), 500

Diagnostic imaging (DI), 506–12
   abbreviations, 511–12
   procedures, 508–11
   vocabulary, 507–08

Diagnostic reports, found in patient's medical record, it consists of results of all diagnostic tests performed on patient, principally from lab and medical imaging (for example, X-ray and ultrasound), 12

Diaphoresis, excessive or profuse sweating, 59

Diaphragm, major muscle of inspiration; separates thoracic from abdominal cavity, 34, 34f, 141f, 225f, 226, 226f

Diaphragmatic, pertaining to diaphragm, 228

Diaphragmatocele, 271

Diaphysis, shaft portion of long bone, 86, 87f

Diarrhea, passing of frequent, watery bowel movements; usually accompanies gastrointestinal (GI) disorders, 269

Diastole, period of time during which heart chamber is relaxed, 144

Diastolic pressure, lower pressure within blood vessels during relaxation phase of heart beat, 149

Diencephalon, portion of brain that contains two of most critical areas of brain, thalamus and hypothalamus, 414, 414f

Digestive system, system that digests food and absorbs nutrients; organs include mouth, pharynx, esophagus, stomach, small and large intestines, liver, gallbladder, and anus; also called gastrointestinal system, 29t, 255–84, 257f
   abbreviations, 282
   accessory organs of, 264–65
   anatomical terms, 267–68
   anatomy and physiology, 258–65
   colon, 263, 264f
   diagnostic procedures, 276–78
   esophagus, 261–262f
   gallbladder, 265
   liver, 265, 265f
   oral cavity, 258, 259f, 260
   pancreas, 265
   pathology, 268–76
   pharmacology, 281
   pharynx, 261
   salivary glands, 264, 264f
   small intestine, 262–63
   stomach, 262
   teeth, 260–61
   terminology, 266–78
   therapeutic procedures, 279–89

Digital rectal exam (DRE), manual examination for enlarged prostate gland performed by palpating (feeling) prostate gland through wall of rectum, 360

Digital veins, 150f

Dilation and curettage (D&C), surgical procedure in which opening of cervix is dilated and uterus is scraped or suctioned of its lining or tissue; often performed after spontaneous abortion and to stop excessive bleeding from other causes, 349

Dilation stage, first stage of labor; begins with uterine contractions that press fetus against cervix causing it to dilate to 10 cm and become thin; thinning of cervix is called effacement, 338, 338f

Dilator, surgical instrument used to enlarge opening by stretching, 521t

Diphtheria, bacterial infection of respiratory system characterized by severe inflammation that can form membrane coating in upper respiratory tract that can cause marked difficulty breathing, 233

Diplopia, double vision, 455

Directional/positional terms, 35, 37f

Discharge summary, part of patient's medical record; a comprehensive outline of patient's entire hospital stay; includes condition at time of admission, admitting diagnosis, test results, treatments and patient's response, final diagnosis, and follow-up plans, 12

Dislocation, occurs when bones in joint are displaced from their normal alignment, 105

Disorders diagnosed in infancy and childhood, mental disorders associated with childhood; include mental retardation, attention deficit disorder, and autism, 501

Dissection, surgical cutting of parts for separation and study, 523

Dissociative disorders, disorders in which severe emotional conflict is so repressed that split in personality occurs; include amnesia and multiple personality disorder, 501

Dissociative identity disorder, having two or more distinct personalities, 501

Distal, directional term meaning located farthest from point of attachment to body, 37f, 37t, 39

Distal convoluted tubule, portion of renal tubule, 299, 300f, 302f

Diuresis, abnormal secretion of large amounts of urine, 306

Diuretic, substance that increases excretion of urine, which promotes loss of water and salt from body; can assist in lowering blood pressure; therefore, these drugs are used to treat hypertension; potassium in body may be depleted with continued use of diuretics; potassium-rich foods such as bananas, kiwi, and orange juice can help correct deficiency, 164, 315

Diverticulectomy, surgical removal of diverticulum, 280

Diverticulitis, inflammation of diverticulum or sac in intestinal tract, especially in colon, 273, 273f

Diverticulosis, abnormal condition of having diverticula (out pouches off gut), 273

Diverticulum, 273, 273f

Dopaminergic drugs, group of medications to treat Parkinson's disease by either replacing dopamine that is lacking or increasing strength of dopamine that is present, 433

Doppler ultrasonography, measurement of sound-wave echos as they bounce off tissues and organs to produce image; in cardiovascular system, used to measure velocity of blood moving through blood vessels to look for blood clots, 160, 501

Dorsal, directional term meaning near or on back or spinal cord side of body, 37f, 37t, 39

Dorsal cavities, 34, 34t, 35t

Dorsiflexion, backward bending, as of hand or foot, 116t, 117f

Dorsum, refers to posterior region of back of body, 33, 33f

Draping, process of covering patient with sterile cloths that allow only operative site to be exposed to surgeon, 523

Drug, 491
 administration, 494, 494t–96t
 classification, 492, 492t
 names, 491, 491t

Drug Enforcement Agency (DEA), government agency that enforces regulation of controlled substances, 492

Drug interaction, occurs when effect of one drug is altered because it was taken at same time as another drug, 497

Drug tolerance, decrease in susceptibility to drug after continued use of drug, 497

Dry gangrene, late stages of gangrene characterized by affected area becoming black and leathery, 65

Dual-energy absorptiometry (DXA), measurement of bone density using low dose X-ray for purpose of detecting osteoporosis, 106

Duchenne's muscular dystrophy, 121

Duodenal, pertaining to duodenum, 267

Duodenum, first section of small intestines; digestion is completed in duodenum after chyme mixes with digestive juices from pancreas and gallbladder, 262, 263f, 264f, 265f, 272f, 276f

Dura mater, term means tough mother; is fibrous outermost meninges layer that forms a tough protective layer, 417, 417f, 430f

Dwarfism, condition of being abnormally small; may be result of hereditary condition or endocrine dysfunction, 393

Dyscrasia, general term indicating presence of disease affecting blood, 185

Dysentery, disease characterized by diarrhea, often with mucus and blood, severe abdominal pain, fever, and dehydration, 273

Dyskinesia, difficult or painful movement, 120

Dysmenorrhea, painful cramping associated with menstruation, 342

Dysorexia, abnormal appetite, 269

Dyspepsia, indigestion, 269

Dysphagia, having difficulty eating, 269

Dysphasia, impairment of speech as a result of brain lesion, 423

Dysphonia, abnormal voice, 231

Dyspnea, difficult, labored breathing, 231, 232

Dystocia, abnormal or difficult labor and childbirth, 342

Dystonia, abnormal tone, 120

Dystrophy, 6

Dysuria, painful or difficult urination; a symptom in many disorders, such as cystitis, urethritis, enlarged prostate in male, and prolapsed uterus in female, 306

E

Ear, 31t, 465–77, 466f, 467f
 abbreviations, 477
 anatomical terms, 470–71
 anatomy and physiology, 467–69
 diagnostic procedures, 473–74
 external, 467–68, 467f
 hearing, 469, 469f
 inner, 468
 middle, 468
 pathology, 471–73
 pharmacology, 476
 terminology, 470–74
 therapeutic procedures, 475–76

Eardrops, substance placed directly into ear canal for purpose of relieving pain or treating infection, 494, 496

Eating disorders, abnormal behaviors related to eating; include anorexia nervosa and bulimia, 501

Ecchymosis, skin discoloration or bruise caused by blood collecting under skin, 59, 59f

Echocardiography (ECHO), noninvasive diagnostic method using ultrasound to visualize internal cardiac structures; cardiac valve activity can be evaluated using this method, 160

Echoencephalography, recording of ultrasonic echoes of brain; useful in determining abnormal patterns of shifting in brain, 430

Eclampsia, convulsive seizures and coma that can occur in woman between twentieth week of pregnancy and first week of postpartum; often associated with hypertension, 345

Ectopic pregnancy, 333

Eczema, superficial dermatitis accompanied by papules, vesicles, and crusting, 65

Edema, condition in which body tissues contain excessive amounts of fluid, 390

Effacement, thinning of cervix during labor, 338

Efferent, 299

Efferent arteriole, arteriole that carries blood away from glomerulus, 299, 300f, 302f

Efferent neurons, nerves that carry impulses away from brain and spinal cord to muscles and glands; also called *motor neurons,* 418, 419f

Egg cell, 333f, 334f

Ejaculation, impulse of forcing seminal fluid from male urethra, 355

Elastin fibers, 224f

Elbow, 88

Elective abortion, legal termination of pregnancy for nonmedical reasons, 349

Electrocardiogram (ECG, EKG), record of electrical activity of heart; useful in diagnosis of abnormal cardiac rhythm and heart muscle (myocardium) damage, 146f, 160

Electrocardiography, process of recording electrical activity of heart, 160

Electrocautery, to destroy tissue with electric current, 71, 524

Electroconvulsive therapy (ECT), procedure occasionally used for cases of prolonged major depression in which electrode is placed on one or both sides of patient's head and current is turned on briefly causing convulsive seizure; low level of voltage is used in modern ECT, and patient is administered a muscle relaxant and anesthesia; advocates of treatment state that it is a more effective way to treat severe depression than with use of drugs; is not effective with disorders other than depression, such as schizophrenia and alcoholism, 504

Electroencephalogram (EEG), record of brain's electrical activity, 431

Electroencephalography (EEG), recording electrical activity of brain by placing electrodes at various positions on scalp; also used in sleep studies to determine if there is a normal pattern of activity during sleep, 431

Electrolyte, chemical compound that separates into charged particles, or ionizes, in solution; sodium chloride (NaCl) and potassium (K) are examples of electrolytes, 301

Electromyogram (EMG), record of muscle electricity, 122, 516

Electromyography, recording of electrical patterns of muscle in order to diagnose diseases, 122, 516

Elephantiasis, inflammation, obstruction, and destruction of lymph vessels that results in enlarged tissues due to edema, 201

Elevation, muscle action that raises body part, as in shrugging the shoulders, 118t

Embolectomy, surgical removal of embolus or clot from a blood vessel, 162

Embolus, obstruction of blood vessel by blood clot that moves from another area, 153, 153f

Embryo, term to describe developing infant from fertilization until end of eighth week, 336, 337, 337f

Embryonic, pertaining to embryo, 340

Emesis, vomiting, usually with some force, 269

Emmetropia (EM), state of normal vision, 455

Emphysema, pulmonary condition that can occur as result of long-term heavy smoking; air pollution also worsens this disease; patient may not be able to breathe except in sitting or standing position, 235

Empyema, pus within pleural space, usually result of infection, 237

Emulsification, to make fats and lipids more soluble in water, 265

Enamel, hardest substance in body; covers outer surface of teeth, 260, 261, 261f

Encapsulated, growth enclosed in sheath of tissue that prevents tumor cells from invading surrounding tissue, 527

Encephalic, pertaining to brain, 421

Encephalitis, inflammation of brain due to disease factors such as rabies, influenza, measles, or smallpox, 426

Endarterectomy, removal of inside layer of an artery, 162

Endings
  plural, 10
  singular, 10

Endocarditis, inflammation of inner lining layer of heart; may be due to microorganisms or to abnormal immunological response, 142, 155

Endocardium, inner layer of heart, which is very smooth and lines chambers of heart, 142, 142f

Endocervicitis, inflammation of inner aspect of cervix, 343

Endocrine glands, glandular system that secretes hormones directly into bloodstream rather than into duct; endocrine glands are frequently referred to as ductless glands; endocrine system includes thyroid gland, adrenal glands, parathyroid glands, pituitary gland, pancreas (islets of Langerhans), testes, ovaries, and thymus gland, 380, 380t–381t

Endocrine system, body system consisting of glands that secrete hormones directly into blood stream; endocrine glands include adrenal glands, parathyroid glands, pancreas, pituitary gland, testes, ovaries, thymus gland, and thyroid gland, 30t, 377–98, 379f, 380
  abbreviations, 398
  adrenal glands, 382, 382f
  anatomical terms, 389
  anatomy and physiology, 380–88
  diagnostic procedures, 395–96
  ovaries, 382, 383f
  pancreas, 383–84, 383f
  parathyroid glands, 384
  pathology, 390–95
  pharmacology, 397–98
  pineal gland, 384
  pituitary gland, 384–85, 385f, 386f
  terminology, 388–96
  testes, 386, 386f
  therapeutic procedures, 396–97
  thymus gland, 387, 387f
  thyroid gland, 387–388, 388f

Endocrinologist, physician who specializes in treatment of endocrine glands, including diabetes, 390

Endocrinology, branch of medicine specializing in conditions of endocrine system, 30t, 39, 390

Endocrinopathy, disease of endocrine system, 390

Endometrial biopsy (EMB), taking sample of tissue from lining of uterus to test for abnormalities, 348

Endometrial cancer, cancer of endometrial lining of uterus, 343

Endometriosis, abnormal condition of endometrium tissue appearing throughout pelvis or on abdominal wall; this tissue is usually found within uterus, 344

Endometritis, inflammation of endometrial lining of uterus, 343

Endometrium, inner lining of uterus; contains rich blood supply and reacts to hormonal changes every month, which results in menstruation; during pregnancy, lining of uterus does not leave body but remains to nourish unborn child, 334, 334f

Endoscopic retrograde cholanglopancreatography (ERCP), using endoscope to X-ray bile and pancreatic ducts, 278

Endoscopic surgery, use of lighted instrument to examine interior of cavity, 524

Endothelium, 147f

Endotracheal intubation, placing tube through mouth to create airway, 240, 240f

Enteric, pertaining to small intestines, 267

Enteritis, inflammation of only small intestine, 273

Enucleated, loss of cell's nucleus, 180

Enucleation, surgical removal of an eyeball, 462

Enuresis, involuntary discharge of urine after age by which bladder control should have been established; usually occurs by age 5; also called bedwetting at night, 306

Enzyme-linked immunosorbent assay (ELISA), blood test for antibody to AIDS virus; positive test means that person has been exposed to virus; in case of false-positive reading, Western blot test would be used to verify results, 203

Eosinophils (eosins, eos), granulocyte white blood cells that destroy parasites and increase during allergic reactions, 181t

Epicardium, outer layer of heart; forms part of pericardium, 142

Epicondyle, projection located above or on condyle, 88, 88f

Epidermal, pertaining to upon skin, 57

Epidermis, superficial layer of skin; is composed of squamous epithelium cells; these are flat scalelike cells that are arranged in layers, called stratified squamous epithelium; many layers of epidermis create a barrier to infection; epidermis does not have a blood supply, so is dependent on deeper layers of skin for nourishment; however, deepest epidermis layer is called basal layer; these cells are alive and constantly dividing; older cells are pushed out toward surface by new cells forming beneath; during this process, they shrink and die, becoming filled with a protein called keratin; keratin-filled cells are sloughed off as dead cells, 52, 53, 53f, 54f

Epididymal, pertaining to epididymis, 357

Epididymectomy, surgical excision of epididymis, 361

Epididymis, coiled tubule that lies on top of testes within scrotum; this tube stores sperm as they are produced and turns into vas deferens, 30t, 353f, 354, 354f, 355, 358, 386f

Epididymitis, inflammation of epididymis causing pain and swelling in inguinal area, 358

Epidural hematoma, mass of blood in space outside dura mater of brain and spinal cord, 429

Epidural space, 417f

Epigastric, pertaining to above stomach; anatomical division of abdomen, middle section of upper row, 36t, 39

Epigastric region, 36t

Epiglottic, pertaining to epiglottis, 228

Epiglottis, flap of cartilage that covers larynx when person swallows; prevents food and drink from entering larynx and trachea, 221f, 222, 242f, 259f, 261

Epilepsy, recurrent disorder of brain in which convulsive seizures and loss of consciousness occur, 426

Epinephrine, hormone produced by adrenal medulla; also known as *adrenaline;* some of its actions include increased heart rate and force of contraction, bronchodilation, and relaxation of intestinal muscles, 380t, 382

Epiphyseal line, 87f

Epiphysis, wide ends of a long bone, 86

Episiorrhaphy, suture vulva, 349

Episiotomy, surgical incision of perineum to facilitate delivery process; can prevent irregular tearing of tissue during birth, 349

Epispadias, congenital opening of urethra on dorsal surface of penis, 359

Epistaxis, nosebleed, 220, 231

Epithelial tissue, tissue found throughout body as skin, outer covering of organs, and inner lining for tubular or hollow structures, 25, 26f

Epithelium, epithelial tissue composed of close-packed cells that form covering for and lining of body structures, 25

Equilibrium, sense of balance, 467, 467f

Erectile dysfunction (ED), inability to copulate due to inability to maintain erection; also called *impotence,* 359

Erectile dysfunction agents, medications that temporarily produce erection in patients with erectile dysfunction, 362

Erectile tissue, tissue with numerous blood vessels and nerve endings; becomes filled with blood and enlarges in size in response to sexual stimulation, 335, 336, 355

Ergonomics, study of human work including how requirements for performing work and work environment affect musculoskeletal and nervous system, 515

Erythema, redness or flushing of skin, 59

Erythroblastosis fetalis, 345

Erythrocyte sedimentation rate (ESR, sed rate), blood test to determine rate at which mature red blood cells settle out of blood after addition of anticoagulant; indicator of presence of inflammatory disease, 188

Erythrocytes, also called red blood cells or RBCs; cells that contain hemoglobin, an iron-containing pigment that binds oxygen in order to transport it to cells of body, 28t, 180–81, 181f, 186–87, 187f

Erythrocytosis, too many red cells, 186

Erythroderma, red skin, 59

Erythropenia, too few red cells, 186

Eschar, thick layer of dead tissue and tissue fluid that develops over deep burn area, 59

Esophageal, pertaining to esophagus, 267

Esophageal varices, enlarged and swollen varicose veins in lower end of esophagus; they can rupture and result in serious hemorrhage, 271

Esophagectasis, stretched out or dilated esophagus, 252

Esophagogastroduodenoscopy (EGD), use of flexible fiberoptic scope to visually examine esophagus, stomach, and beginning of duodenum, 278

Esophagus, tube that carries food from pharynx to stomach, 29t, 35t, 221f, 242f, 258, 259f, 261–62, 262f, 271

Esotropia, inward turning of eye; example of a form of strabismus (muscle weakness of eye), 450f, 459

Estrogen, one of hormones produced by ovaries; works with progesterone to control menstrual cycle and it responsible for producing secondary sexual characteristics, 332, 333, 380t, 381t, 382

Ethmoid bone, cranial bone, 89, 91t

Eupnea, normal breathing, 231

Eustachian tube, tube or canal that connects middle ear with nasopharynx and allows for balance of pressure between outer and middle ear; infection can travel via mucous membranes of eustachian tube, resulting in middle ear infections, 222, 467f, 468

Eversion, directional term meaning turning outward, 117t, 117f

Ewing's sarcoma, malignant growth found in shaft of long bones that spreads through periosteum; removal is treatment of choice, as tumor will metastasize or spread to other organs, 103

Excretory urography (EU), injection of dye into bloodstream followed by taking X-ray to trace action of kidney as it excretes dye, 311

Exfoliative cytology, scraping cells from tissue and then examining them under microscope, 70

Exhalation, to breathe air out of lungs; also called expiration, 220

Exocrine, 380

Exocrine glands, glands that secrete substances into a duct; examples include tears and tear ducts, 380

Exophthalmos, condition in which eyeballs protrude, such as in Graves' disease; generally caused by overproduction of thyroid hormone, 390, 390f

Exostosis, bone spur, 103

Exotropia, outward turning of eye; also an example of strabismus (muscle weakness of eye), 450f, 459

Expectorant, substance that assists in removal of secretions from bronchopulmonary membranes, 243

Expiration, 220, 226f

Expiratory reserve volume (ERV), amount of air that can be forcibly exhaled after normal quiet respiration; also called *supplemental air*, 225t

Exploratory laparotomy, abdominal operation for purpose of examining abdominal organs and tissues for signs of disease or other abnormalities, 280

Exploratory surgery, surgery performed for purpose of determining if there is cancer present or if known cancer has spread; biopsies are generally performed, 529

Explosive disorder, impulse control disorder in which patient is unable to control violent rages, 502

Expulsion stage, stage of labor and delivery during which baby is delivered, 338, 338f

Extension, movement that brings limb into or toward a straight condition, 116t, 116f

Extensor carpi, muscle named for its action, extension, 115

External auditory meatus, opening into external ear canal, 467, 467f, 468

External ear, outermost portion of ear; consists of auricle, auditory canal, and eardrum, 466f, 467–68, 472

External iliac artery, 148f, 315f

External iliac vein, 150f, 315f

External oblique, muscle named for direction of its fibers, on an oblique angle, 115

External respiration, exchange of oxygen and carbon dioxide that takes place in lungs, 220

External sphincter, ring of voluntary muscle that controls emptying of urine from bladder, 300, 301

Extracorporeal circulation (ECC), during open heart surgery, routing of blood to heart-lung machine so it can be oxygenated and pumped to rest of body, 161

Extracorporeal shockwave lithotripsy (ESWL), use of ultrasound waves to break up stones; process does not require surgery, 313f

Extraction, removing or pulling teeth, 279

Extraocular, pertaining to being outside eyeball, for example extraocular eye muscles, 454

Eye, 31t, 447f, 448f
   abbreviations, 464
   anatomical terms, 454
   anatomy and physiology, 448–52
   conjunctiva, 451

   diagnostic procedures, 460–61
   eyeball, 448–49
   eyelids, 448f, 451, 459
   lacrimal apparatus, 451, 451f
   muscles, 450
   pathology, 455–59
   pharmacology, 463
   retina, 449, 452f
   terminology, 453–61
   therapeutic procedures, 462–63
   vision, 452, 452f

Eye muscles, there are six muscles that connect eyeball to orbit cavity; muscles allow for rotation of eyeball, 450

Eyeball, eye by itself, without any appendages such as eye muscles or tear ducts, 448–49

Eyedrops, substance placed into eye to control eye pressure in glaucoma; also used during eye examinations to dilate pupil of eye for better examination of interior of eye, 494, 496

Eyelashes, along upper and lower edges of eyelids; protect eye from foreign particles; also called *cilia*, 451

Eyelids, upper and lower fold of skin that provides protection from foreign particles, injury from sun and intense light, and trauma; both upper and lower edges of eyelids have small hairs or cilia; in addition, sebaceous or oil glands are located in eyelids which secrete lubricating oil, 448f, 451, 459

F

Facial bones, skull bones that surround mouth, nose, and eyes; muscles for chewing are attached to facial bones, 89, 91f, 91t

Facial nerve, 418t

Factitious disorders, intentionally feigning illness symptoms in order to gain attention such as malingering, 502

Falling test, test used to observe balance and equilibrium; patient is observed balancing on one foot, then with one foot in front of the other, and then walking forward with eyes open; same test is conducted with patient's eyes closed; swaying and falling with eyes closed can indicate ear and equilibrium malfunction, 474

Fallopian tubes, organs in female reproductive system that transport eggs from ovary to uterus, 30t, 35t, 333, 334f

Family and group psychotherapy, form of psychological counseling in which therapist places minimal emphasis on patient past history and strong emphasis on having patient state and discuss goals and then find a way to achieve them, 505

Farsightedness, 457, 457f

Fascia, connective tissue that wraps muscles; it tapers at each end of a skeletal muscle to form tendons, 114

Fascial, pertaining to fascia, 119

Fasciitis, inflammation of fascia, 121

Fasciotomy, incision into fascia, 122

Fasting blood sugar (FBS), blood test to measure amount of sugar circulating throughout body after 12-hour fast, 395

Fats, lipid molecules transported throughout body dissolved in blood, 180

Fecal occult blood test (FOBT), laboratory test on feces to determine if microscopic amounts of blood are present; also called hemoccult or stool guaiac, 276

Feces, food that cannot be digested becomes waste product and is expelled or defecated as feces, 263

Federal Drug Administration (FDA), 498

Female reproductive system, system responsible for producing eggs for reproduction and provides place for growing baby; organs include ovaries, fallopian tubes, uterus, vagina, and mammary glands, 30t, 331f, 332f
　　abbreviations, 351
　　anatomical terms, 340–41
　　anatomy and physiology, 332–39
　　breast, 336
　　diagnostic procedures, 347–48
　　internal genitalia, 332–35
　　pathology, 342–46
　　pharmacology, 351
　　terminology, 339–48
　　therapeutic procedures, 349–50
　　vulva, 335–36

Female urethra, 301f

Femoral, pertaining to femur or thigh bone, 98

Femoral artery, 148f

Femoral vein, 150f

Femur, also called thigh bone; is a lower extremity bone, 85f, 88f, 92, 93f, 94, 95f, 95t

Fertility drug, medication that triggers ovulation; also called ovulation stimulant, 351

Fertilization, also called impregnation; fusion of ova and sperm to produce embryo, 332

Fetal, pertaining to fetus, 340

Fetal monitoring, using electronic equipment placed on mother's abdomen to check baby's heart rate and strength during labor, 348

Fetus, term to describe developing newborn from end of eighth week until birth, 336, 337, 337f

Fever blisters, 271

Fibrillation, abnormal quivering or contractions of heart fibers; when this occurs within fibers of ventricle of heart, arrest and death can occur; emergency equipment to defibrillate, or convert heart to a normal beat, is necessary, 156

Fibrin, whitish protein formed by action of thrombin and fibrinogen, which is basis for clotting of blood, 182

Fibrinogen, blood protein that is essential for clotting to take place, 180

Fibrinolysis, destruction of fibers, 173

Fibrinous, pertaining to being fibrous, 184

Fibrocystic breast disease, benign cysts forming in breast, 345, 345f

Fibroid tumor, benign tumor or growth that contains fiberlike tissue; uterine fibroid tumors are most common tumors in women, 343, 343f

Fibromyalgia, condition with widespread aching and pain in muscles and soft tissue, 121

Fibrous joints, joint that has almost no movement because ends of bones are joined together by thick fibrous tissue; sutures of skull are example, 95, 96

Fibula, one of the lower leg bones in lower extremity, 85f, 92, 93f, 94, 95f, 95t

Fibular, pertaining to fibula, a lower leg bone, 98

Fibular vein, 150f

Film, thin sheet of cellulose material coated with light-sensitive substance used in taking photographs; there is a special photographic film that is sensitive to X-rays, 507

Film badge, badge containing film that is sensitive to X-rays; is worn by all personnel in radiology to measure amount of X-rays to which they are exposed, 507

Filtration, first stage of urine production during which waste products are filtered from blood, 302, 302f

Fimbriae, fingerlike extensions on end of fallopian tubes; drape over each ovary in order to direct ovum into fallopian tube after it is expelled by ovary, 333, 333f, 334, 334f, 383f

Fine motor skills, use of precise and coordinated movements in such activities as writing, buttoning, and cutting, 515

First-degree burn, 64, 64f

Fissure, deep groove or slit-type opening, 59, 59f, 88, 89

Fistulectomy, excision of a fistula, 280

Fixation, procedure to stabilize fractured bone while it heals; external fixation includes casts, splints, and pins inserted through skin; internal fixation includes pins, plates, rods, screws, and wires that are applied during an open reduction, 109

Flat bone, type of bone with thin flattened shape; examples include scapula, ribs, and pelvic bones, 86, 87f

Flexion, act of bending or being bent, 116t, 116f

Flexor carpi, muscle named for its action, flexion, 115

Floating kidney, 309

Fluorescein angiography, process of injecting dye (fluorescein) to observe movement of blood for detecting lesions in macular area of retina; used to determine if there is detachment of retina, 460

Fluorescein staining, applying dye eyedrops that are bright green fluorescent color; used to look for corneal abrasions or ulcers, 460

Fluoroscopy, x-rays strike glowing screen which can change from minute to minute, therefore able to show movement such as digestive tract moving, 509

Flutter, arrhythmia in which atria beat too rapidly, but in regular pattern, 156

Focal seizure, localized epileptic seizure often affecting one limb, 423

Follicle-stimulating hormone (FSH), hormone secreted by anterior pituitary gland; stimulates growth of eggs in females and sperm in males, 381t, 384, 385

Foramen, passage or opening through bone for nerves and blood vessels, 88, 89

Forceps, surgical instrument used to grasp tissues, 521t

Formed elements, solid, cellular portion of blood; consists of erythrocytes, leukocytes, and platelets, 180

Fossa, shallow cavity or depression within or on surface of a bone, 88, 89

Fovea capitis, 88f

Fovea centralis, area of retina that has sharpest vision, 448f, 449

Fowler position, surgical position in which patient is sitting with back positioned at 45[[deg]] angle, 522f, 523t

Fracture (FX, Fx), injury to bone that causes it to break; named to describe type of damage to bone, 100–02

Fraternal twins, twins that develop from two different ova fertilized by two different sperm; although twins, these siblings do not have identical DNA, 341

Free edge, exposed edge of a nail that is trimmed when nails become too long, 55, 55f

Frequency, greater than normal occurrence in urge to urinate, without increase in total daily volume of urine; frequency is indication of inflammation of bladder or urethra, 306

Frontal bone, forehead bone of skull, 89, 91f, 91t

Frontal lobe, one of four cerebral hemisphere lobes; controls motor functions, 414, 415, 415f

Frontal plane, vertical plane that divides body into front (anterior or ventral) and back (posterior or dorsal) sections; also called *coronal plane,* 32, 32f, 33

Frontal section, sectional view of body produced by cut along frontal plane; also called *coronal section,* 32, 33

Frozen section (FS), thin piece of tissue is cut from frozen specimen for rapid examination under a microscope, 70

Full-term pregnancy, 337f

Functional bowel syndrome, 274

Functional residual capacity (FRC), air that remains in lungs after normal exhalation has taken place, 225t

Fundus, domed upper portion of organ such as stomach or uterus, 262, 262f

Fundus (uterus), 332f, 334, 334f, 337f

Fungal scrapings, scrapings, taken with curette or scraper, of tissue from lesions are placed on a growth medium and examined under a microscope to identify fungal growth, 70

Fungi, organisms found in Kingdom Fungi; some are capable of causing disease in humans, such as yeast infections or histoplasmosis, 196, 197

Funny bone, 88

Furuncle, staphylococcal skin abscess with redness, pain, and swelling; also called a *boil,* 69

G

Gait, manner of walking, 515

Gait training, assisting person to learn to walk again or how to use assistive device to walk, 516

Gallbladder (GB), small organ located just under liver; functions to store bile produced by liver; gallbladder releases bile into duodenum through common bile duct, 29t, 35t, 36t, 257f, 258, 265, 265f, 276f

Gametes, reproductive sex cells—ova and sperm, 382

Gamma globulin, protein component of blood containing antibodies that help to resist infection, 180

Ganglion, knotlike mass of nerve tissue located outside brain and spinal cord, 418

Ganglion cyst, cyst that forms on tendon sheath, usually on hand, wrist, or ankle, 121

Gangrene, necrosis of skin usually due to deficient blood supply, 65

Gastralgia, stomach pain, 269

Gastrectomy, surgical removal of stomach, 280

Gastric, pertaining to stomach, 267

Gastric carcinoma, cancerous tumor of stomach, 271

Gastric stapling, procedure that closes off large section of stomach with rows of staples; results in a much smaller stomach to assist very obese patients to lose weight, 280

Gastritis, inflammation of stomach that can result in pain, tenderness, nausea, and vomiting, 271

Gastroenteritis, inflammation of stomach and small intestines, 3, 271

Gastroenterologist, physician specialized in treating diseases and conditions of gastrointestinal tract, 268

Gastroenterology, branch of medicine specializing in conditions of gastrointestinal system, 29t, 40, 268

Gastroesophageal reflux disease (GERD), acid from stomach backs up into esophagus, causing inflammation and pain, 271

Gastrointestinal (GI), 29t

Gastrointestinal system (GI), system that digests food and absorbs nutrients; organs include mouth, pharynx, esophagus, stomach, small and large intestines, liver, gallbladder, and anus; also called digestive system, 258

Gastrointestinal tract, continuous tube that extends from mouth to anus; also called gut or alimentary canal, 258

Gastroscope, instrument to view inside stomach, 278

Gastroscopy, flexible gastroscope is passed through mouth and down esophagus in order to visualize inside stomach; used to diagnose peptic ulcers and gastric carcinoma, 278

Gastrostomy, surgical creation of gastric fistula or opening through abdominal wall; opening is used to place food into stomach when esophagus is not entirely open (esophageal stricture), 280

Gavage, using nasogastric tube to place liquid nourishment directly into stomach, 279

General anesthesia (GA), general anesthesia produces a loss of consciousness including absence of pain sensation; administered to patient by either intravenous or inhalation method; patient's vital signs are carefully monitored when using general anesthetic, 520, 521t

General hospital, hospitals that typically provide services to diagnose (laboratory, diagnostic imaging) and treat (surgery, medications, therapy) diseases for a short period of time; in addition, they usually provide emergency and obstetrical care; also called acute care hospital, 13

Generic name, recognized and accepted official name for a drug; each drug has only one generic name; this name is not subject to trademark, so any pharmaceutical manufacturer may use it; also called nonproprietary name, 491, 491t

Genital herpes, creeping skin disease that can appear like a blister or vesicle, caused by sexually transmitted virus, 359

Genital warts, growths and elevations of warts on genitalia of both males and females that can lead to cancer of cervix in females, 360

Genitalia, male and female reproductive organs, 332

Genitourinary system (GU), organs of the urinary system and female or male sexual organs, 298, 354

Gestation, length of time from conception to birth, generally nine months; calculated from first day of last menstrual period, with a range of from 259 days to 280 days, 336, 337

Gigantism, excessive development of body due to overproduction of growth hormone by pituitary gland; opposite of dwarfism, 394

Gingiva, tissue around teeth; also called gums, 258, 259f, 260, 261f

Gingival, pertaining to gums, 267

Gingivitis, inflammation of gums characterized by swelling, redness, and tendency to bleed, 270

Glands, organs of body that release secretions; exocrine glands, like sweat glands, release their secretions into ducts; endocrine glands, such as thyroid gland, release their hormones directly into blood stream, 380, 412
  adrenal, 30t
  apocrine, 56
  bulbourethral, 354, 356
  lymph, 194
  parathyroid, 30t
  pineal, 30t, 380, 384, 384f
  pituitary, 30t, 380, 384–85, 385f, 393–94, 414f
  prostate, 30t, 36t, 301f, 354, 354f, 356, 358–59
  salivary, 29t, 257f, 258, 264, 264f
  sebaceous, 27t, 52, 55, 55f
  sudoriferous, 56
  sweat, 27t, 52, 56
  thymus, 28t, 30t, 35t, 193, 196, 196f, 379f, 380, 381t, 387, 387f, 394
  thyroid, 30t, 221f, 379f, 380, 381t, 387–88, 388f, 394–95

Glans penis, larger and softer tip of penis; is protected by covering called prepuce or foreskin, 354f, 355

Glaucoma, increase in intraocular pressure that, if untreated, may result in atrophy (wasting away) of optic nerve and blindness; treated with medication and surger; there is increased risk of developing glaucoma in persons over 60 years of age, people of African ancestry, persons who have sustained serious eye injury, and anyone with family history of diabetes or glaucoma, 456

Globulins, one type of protein found dissolved in plasma, 180

Glomerular, 300f

Glomerular capsule, also called Bowman's capsule; part of renal corpuscle; is a double-walled cuplike structure that encircles glomerulus; in filtration stage of urine production, waste products filtered from blood enter Bowman's capsule as glomerular filtrate, 299, 300f, 302f

Glomerular filtrate, product of filtration stage of urine production; water, electrolytes, nutrients, wastes, and toxins that are filtered from blood passing through glomerulus; filtrate enters Bowman's capsule, 302

Glomerulonephritis, inflammation of kidney (primarily of glomerulus); since glomerular membrane is inflamed, it becomes more permeable and will allow protein and blood cells to enter filtrate; results in protein in urine (proteinuria) and hematuria, 308

Glomerulus, ball of capillaries encased by Bowman's capsule; in filtration stage of urine production, wastes filtered from blood leave glomerulus capillaries and enter Bowman's capsule, 299, 300f, 302f

Glossal, pertaining to tongue, 267

Glossopharyngeal nerve, 418t

Glottis, opening between vocal cords; air passes through glottis as it moves through larynx; changing tension of vocal cords changes size of opening, 222

Glucagon, hormone secreted by pancreas; stimulates liver to release glucose into blood, 359t, 361

Glucocorticoids, group of hormones secreted by adrenal cortex; regulate carbohydrate levels in body; cortisol is an example, 380t, 382

Glucose, form of sugar used by cells of body to make energy; transported to cells in blood, 180

Glucose tolerance test (GTT), test to determine blood sugar level; a measured dose of glucose is given to patient either orally or intravenously; blood samples are then drawn at certain intervals to determine ability of patient to utilize glucose; used for diabetic patients to determine their insulin response to glucose, 395

Glutamic oxaloacetic transaminase (GOT), 159

Gluteal, pertaining to buttocks, 40

Gluteal region, refers to buttock region of body, 33, 33f

Gluteus maximus, muscle named for its size and location; gluteus means rump area and maximus means large, 115

Glycosuria, presence of an excess of sugar in urine, 306, 390

Goiter, enlargement of thyroid gland, 394, 394f

Gonadotropins, common name for follicle-stimulating hormone and luteinizing hormone, 318t, 384, 385

Gonads, organs responsible for producing sex cells; female gonads are ovaries, and they produce ova; male gonads are testes, and they produce sperm, 382

Gonorrhea, sexually transmitted inflammation of mucous membranes of either sex; can be passed on to infant during birth process, 360

Grade, tumor can be graded from grade I through grade IV; grade is based on microscopic appearance of tumor cells; grade I tumor is well differentiated and is easier to treat than more advanced grades, 526, 527, 527t

Graft versus host disease (GVHD), serious complication of bone marrow transplant; immune cells from donor bone marrow (graft) attack recipient's (host's) tissues, 202

Grand mal seizure, 424

Granulocytes, granular polymorphonuclear leukocyte; there are three types: neutrophil, eosinophil, and basophil, 181, 181t

Graves' disease, condition, named for Robert Graves, an Irish physician, resulting in overactivity of thyroid gland and can result in crisis situation; also called hyperthyroidism, 394

Gray matter, tissue within central nervous system; consists of unsheathed or uncovered nerve cell bodies and dendrites, 413, 417

Great saphenous vein, 150f

Greenstick fracture, fracture in which there is incomplete break; one side of bone is broken and other side is bent; this type of fracture is commonly found in children due to their softer and more pliable bone structure, 102

Gross motor skills, use of large muscle groups that coordinate body movements such as walking, running, jumping, and balance, 515

Growth hormone (GH), hormone secreted by anterior pituitary that stimulates growth of body, 381t, 384, 385

Guillain-Barré syndrome, disease of nervous system in which nerves lose their myelin covering; may be caused by autoimmune reaction; characterized by loss of sensation and/or muscle control in arms and legs; symptoms then move toward trunk and may even result in paralysis of diaphragm, 428

Gums, tissue around teeth; also called gingiva, 258, 260

Gut, name for continuous muscular tube that stretches between mouth and anus; also called *alimentary canal,* 258

Gynecologist, physician specialized in treating conditions and diseases of female reproductive system, 342

Gynecology (GYN, gyn), branch of medicine specializing in conditions of female reproductive system, 30*t*, 40, 342

Gynecomastia, development of breast tissue in males; may be symptom of adrenal feminization, 390

Gyri, convoluted, elevated portions of cerebral cortex; they are separated by fissures or sulci; singular is gyrus, 414, 415

H

H₂-receptor antagonist, blocks production of stomach acids, 281

Habituation, development of emotional dependence on drug due to repeated use, 497

Hair, structure in integumentary system, 27*t*, 52, 53*f*, 54–55, 55*f*, 69

Hair follicle, cavities in dermis that contain hair root; hair grows longer from root, 54, 55, 55*f*

Hair root, deeper cells that divide to grow hair longer, 54, 55, 55*f*

Hair shaft, older keratinized cells that form most of length of a hair, 54, 55, 55*f*

Hallucinations, perception of object that is not there or event that has not happened; may be visual, auditory, olfactory, gustatory, or tactile, 503

Hammer, 467*f*, 468

Hand, 96*f*

Hard palate, 221*f*, 259*f*

Hashimoto's disease, chronic form of thyroiditis, named for Japanese surgeon, 394

Head, large ball-shaped end of a bone; may be separated from shaft of bone by area called neck, 88, 88*f*

Health Insurance Portability and Accountability Act (HIPAA), 14

Health maintenance organization (HMO), organization that contracts with group of physicians and other healthcare workers to provide care exclusively for its members; HMO pays healthcare workers prepaid fixed amount per member, called capitation, whether that member requires medical attention or not, 13

Healthcare settings, 13

Hearing, one of special senses; sound waves detected by ear, 467

Hearing aid, apparatus or mechanical device used by persons with impaired hearing to amplify sound; same as amplification device, 475

Hearing impairment, 469

Heart, organ of cardiovascular system that contracts to pump blood through blood vessels, 28*t*, 35*t*, 139*f*, 140, 141–46, 193*f*, 225*f*, 387*f*
  chambers, 143
  conduction system of, 145, 146*f*
  layers, 142
  valves, 143, 144*f*

Heart attack, 156

Heart transplantation, replacement of diseased or malfunctioning heart with donor's heart, 162

Heart valve prolapse, cusps or flaps of heart valve are too loose and fail to shut tightly, allowing blood to flow backwards through valve when heart chamber contracts; most commonly occurs in mitral valve, but may affect any of heart valves, 156

Heart valve stenosis, cusps or flaps of heart valve are too stiff; therefore, they are unable to open fully, making it difficult for blood to flow through, or to shut tightly, allowing blood to flow backwards; condition may affect any of heart valves, 156

Heartburn, 270

Heimlich maneuver, technique for removing foreign body or food from trachea or pharynx when it is choking a person; maneuver consists of applying pressure just under diaphragm to pop obstruction out, 242

Hematemesis, to vomit blood from gastrointestinal tract, often looks like coffee grounds, 269

Hematic, pertaining to blood, 40, 184

Hematic system, system that consists of plasma and blood cells—erythrocytes, leukocytes, and platelets; responsible for transporting oxygen, protecting against pathogens, and controlling bleeding, 28*t*

Hematinic, substance that increases number of erythrocytes or amount of hemoglobin in blood, 190

Hematochezia, passing bright red blood in stools, 269

Hematocrit (Hct, Hct, crit), blood test to measure volume of red blood cells (erythrocytes) within total volume of blood, 188

Hematologist, physician who specializes in treating diseases and conditions of blood, 184

Hematology, branch of medicine specializing in conditions of hematic system, 28*t*, 40, 184

Hematoma, swelling or mass of blood caused by break in vessel in organ or tissue, or beneath skin, 185

Hematopoiesis, process of forming blood, 180

Hematosalpinx, condition of having blood in fallopian tubes, 342

Hematuria, condition of blood in urine, 306

Hemianopia, loss of vision in half of visual field; stroke patient may suffer from this disorder, 459

Hemiparesis, weakness or loss of motion on one side of body, 423

Hemiplegia, paralysis on only one side of body, 423

Hemoccult, 276

Hemodialysis (HD), use of artificial kidney machine that filters blood of a person to remove waste products; use of this technique in patients who have defective kidneys is lifesaving, 313, 313f

Hemoglobin (Hgb, Hb, HGB), iron-containing pigment of red blood cells that carries oxygen from lungs to tissue, 180, 188

Hemolytic anemia, anemia that develops as result of excessive loss of erythrocytes, 186

Hemolytic disease of the newborn (HDN), condition in which antibodies in mother's blood enter fetus's blood and cause anemia, jaundice, edema, and enlargement of liver and spleen; also called *erythroblastosis fetalis,* 345

Hemolytic reaction, destruction of patient's erythrocytes that occurs when receiving transfusion of incompatible blood type; also called a *transfusion reaction,* 186

Hemophilia, hereditary blood disease in which there is a prolonged blood clotting time; is transmitted by sex-linked trait from females to males; appears almost exclusively in males, 185

Hemoptysis, coughing up blood or blood-stained sputum, 231

Hemorrhage, blood flow, escape of blood from a blood vessel, 185

Hemorrhoid, varicose veins in rectum, 158, 273

Hemorrhoidectomy, surgical excision of hemorrhoids from anorectal area, 280

Hemostasis, to stop bleeding or stagnation of circulating blood, 182, 524

Hemostat, surgical instrument used to grasp blood vessels to control bleeding, 521t

Hemostatic agent, 189

Hemothorax, condition of having blood in chest cavity, 231

Hepatic, pertaining to liver, 268

Hepatic duct, duct that leads from liver to common bile duct; transports bile, 265, 265f, 276f

Hepatic portal vein, 150f

Hepatitis, infectious, inflammatory disease of liver; hepatitis B and C types are spread by contact with blood and bodily fluids of infected person, 276

Hepatoma, liver tumor, 276

Herniated nucleus pulposus (HNP), rupture of fibrocartilage disk between two vertebrae; results in pressure on spinal nerve and causes pain, weakness, and nerve damage; also called a slipped disk, 104, 104f

Hernioplasty, surgical repair of a hernia; also called herniorrhaphy, 280

Herniorrhaphy, 280

Herpes labialis, infection of lip by herpes simplex virus type 1 (HSV-1); also called *fever blisters* or *cold sores,* 271

Herpes simplex virus (HSV), 65

Herpes zoster virus, 429

Hertz (Hz), measurement of frequency or pitch of sound; lowest pitch on audiogram is 250 Hz; measurement can go as high as 8000 Hz, which is highest pitch measured, 474

Hesitancy, decrease in force of urine stream, often with difficulty initiating flow; often a symptom of blockage along urethra, such as enlarged prostate gland, 307

Heterograft, skin graft from animal of another species (usually a pig) to a human; also called a *xenograft,* 71

Hiatal hernia, protrusion of stomach through diaphragm and extending into thoracic cavity; gastroesophageal reflux disease is a common symptom, 271, 271f

Hilum, controlled entry/exit point of an organ such as kidney or lung, 224, 298, 299f

Hipbone, 93f

Hirsutism, excessive hair growth over body, 59, 390

Histology, study of tissues, 25, 40

Histoplasma capsulatum, 235

Histoplasmosis, pulmonary disease caused by fungus found in dust in droppings of pigeons and chickens, 235

History and physical, medical record document written by admitting physician; details patient's history, results of physician's examination, initial diagnoses, and physician's plan of treatment, 11

Hives, appearance of wheals as part of allergic reaction, 62, 200

Hodgkin's disease (HD), also called Hodgkin's lymphoma; cancer of lymphatic cells found in concentration in lymph nodes, 201f

Hodgkin's lymphoma, 201, 202f

Holter monitor, portable ECG monitor worn by patient for a period of a few hours to a few days to assess heart and pulse activity as person goes through activities of daily living, 160

Home health care, agencies that provide nursing, therapy, personal care, or housekeeping services in patient's own home, 13

Homeostasis, steady state or state of balance within body; kidneys assist in maintaining this regulatory, steady state, 301, 380

Homologous transfusion, replacement of blood by transfusion of blood received from another person, 189

Hordeolum, a *stye* (or sty), a small purulent inflammatory infection of a sebaceous gland of eye, treated with hot compresses and surgical incision, 459

Horizontal plane, horizontal plane that divides body into upper (superior) and lower (inferior) sections; also called *transverse plane,* 32, 33

Hormonal contraception, use of hormones to block ovulation and prevent contraception; may be in pill form, patch or implant under skin, or injection, 349

Hormone, chemical substance secreted by endocrine gland; enters blood stream and is carried to target tissue; hormones work to control functioning of target tissue; given to replace loss of natural hormones or to treat disease by stimulating hormonal effects, 380

Hormone replacement therapy (HRT), artificial replacement of hormones in patient who is unable to produce sufficient hormones; example is estrogen replacement in menopausal women, 351, 396

Hormone therapy, treatment of cancer with natural hormones or with chemicals that produce hormonelike effects, 529

Hospice, organized group of healthcare workers who provide supportive treatment to dying patients and their families, 13

Human growth hormone therapy, therapy with human growth hormone in order to stimulate skeletal growth; used to treat children with abnormally short stature, 397

Human immunodeficiency virus (HIV), virus that causes AIDS; also known as a retrovirus, 202, 202*f,* 360

Human papilloma virus (HPV), 343

Humanistic psychotherapy, form of psychological counseling in which therapist does not delve into patients' past; it is believed that patients can learn how to use their own internal resources to deal with their problems, 505

Humeral, pertaining to humerus or upper arm bone, 98

Humerus, upper arm bone in upper extremity, 85*f,* 87*f,* 92, 93*f,* 94, 94*f,* 94*f*

Humoral immunity, immunity that responds to antigens, such as bacteria and foreign agents, by producing antibodies; also called *antibody-mediated immunity,* 197

Humpback, 104

Hunchback, 104

Hyaline membrane disease (HMD), 235

Hydrocele, accumulation of fluid within testes, 358

Hydrocephalus, accumulation of cerebrospinal fluid within ventricles of brain, causing head to be enlarged; treated by creating artificial shunt for fluid to leave brain, 426, 426*f*

Hydrochloric acid (HCl), acid secreted by stomach lining; aids in digestion, 262

Hydronephrosis, distention of pelvis due to urine collecting in kidney resulting from obstruction, 308

Hydrotherapy, using water for treatment purposes, 517

Hymen, thin membranous tissue that covers external vaginal opening or orifice; membrane is broken during first sexual encounter of female; can also be broken prematurely by use of tampons or during some sports activities, 335

Hymenectomy, surgical removal of hymen; performed when hymen tissue is particularly tough, 350

Hyoid bone, single, U-shaped bone suspended in neck between mandible and larynx; a point of attachment for swallowing and speech muscles, 89, 221*f*

Hypercalcemia, condition of having excessive amount of calcium in blood, 390

Hypercapnia, excessive carbon dioxide, 231

Hyperemesis, excessive vomiting, 270

Hyperemia, redness of skin caused by increased blood flow to skin, 59

Hyperesthesia, having excessive sensation, 423

Hyperglycemia, having excessive amount of glucose (sugar) in blood, 390

Hyperhidrosis, abnormal condition of excessive sweat, 59

Hyperkalemia, condition of having excessive amount of potassium in blood, 391

Hyperkinesia, excessive amount of movement, 120

Hyperlipidemia, condition of having too high a level of lipids such as cholesterol in bloodstream; risk factor for developing atherosclerosis and coronary artery disease, 185

Hyperopia, with this condition a person can see things in the distance but has trouble reading material at close vision; also known as *farsightedness,* 457, 457*f*

Hyperparathyroidism, state of excessive thyroid, 393

Hyperpigmentation, abnormal amount of pigmentation in skin, which is seen in diseases such as acromegaly and adrenal insufficiency, 59

Hyperpituitarism, state of excessive pituitary gland, 394

Hyperplasia, excessive development of normal cells within an organ, 527

Hyperpnea, excessive deep breathing, 231

Hypersecretion, excessive hormone production by endocrine gland, 391

Hypertension (HTN), high blood pressure, 158

Hyperthyroidism, condition resulting from overactivity of thyroid gland that can result in a crisis situation; also called *Graves' disease,* 394, 395

Hypertonia, excessive tone, 120

Hypertrophy, increase in bulk or size of a tissue or structure, 120

Hyperventilation, to breathe both fast (tachypnea) and deep (hyperpnea), 231

Hypnotic, substance used to produce sleep or hypnosis, 433

Hypocalcemia, condition of having a low calcium level in blood, 391

Hypochondria, somatoform disorder involving a preoccupation with health concerns, 503

Hypochondriac, term meaning *pertaining to under the cartilage,* 36t, 40

Hypochromic anemia, anemia resulting from having insufficient hemoglobin in erythrocytes; named because hemoglobin molecule is responsible for dark red color of erythrocytes, 186

Hypodermic, pertaining to under skin, 57

Hypodermis, deepest layer of skin; composed primarily of adipose, 54

Hypogastric, pertaining to below stomach; anatomical division of abdomen, middle section of bottom row, 36t

Hypogastric region, 36t

Hypoglossal, pertaining to under tongue, 268

Hypoglossal nerve, 418t

Hypoglycemia, condition of having low sugar level in blood, 391

Hypokinesia, insufficient movement, 120

Hyponatremia, condition of having low sodium level in blood, 391

Hypoparathyroidism, state of insufficient thyroid, 393

Hypopituitarism, state of insufficient pituitary gland, 394

Hypopnea, insufficient or shallow breathing, 231

Hyposecretion, deficient hormone production by an endocrine gland, 391

Hypospadias, congenital opening of male urethra on underside of penis, 359

Hypotension, low blood pressure, 158

Hypothalamus, portion of diencephalon that lies just below thalamus; controls body temperature, appetite, sleep, sexual desire, and emotions such as fear; also regulates release of hormones from pituitary gland and regulates parasympathetic and sympathetic nervous systems, 384, 385, 385f, 414, 414f, 415

Hypothyroidism, result of deficiency in secretion by thyroid gland; results in lowered basal metabolism rate with obesity, dry skin, slow pulse, low blood pressure, sluggishness, and goiter; treatment is replacement with synthetic thyroid hormone, 395

Hypotonia, insufficient tone, 120

Hypoventilation, to breathe both slow (bradypnea) and shallow (hypopnea), 231

Hypoxemia, deficiency of oxygen in blood, 231

Hypoxia, absence of oxygen in tissues, 231

Hysterectomy, removal of uterus, 350

Hysteropexy, surgical fixation of uterus, 350

Hysterorrhexis, rupture of uterus, 344

Hysterosalpingectomy, 9

Hysterosalpingography (HSG), process of taking X-ray of uterus and oviducts after radiopaque material is injected into organs, 347

I

Iatrogenic, usually unfavorable response that results from taking medication, 497

Ichthyoderma, dry and scaly skin condition, 59

Ichthyosis, condition in which skin becomes dry, scaly, and keratinized, 65

Identical twins, twins that develop from splitting of one fertilized ovum; these siblings have identical DNA, 341

Idiosyncrasy, unusual or abnormal response to drug or food, 497

Ileal, pertaining to ileum, 268

Ileocecal valve, sphincter between ileum and cecum, 262, 263, 264f

Ileostomy, surgical creation of passage through abdominal wall into ileum, 280, 280f

Ileum, third portion of small intestines; joins colon at cecum; ileum and cecum are separated by ileocecal valve, 10, 262–63, 263f

Ileus, severe abdominal pain, inability to pass stools, vomiting, and abdominal distention as a result of intestinal blockage; may require surgery to reverse blockage, 273

Iliac, pertaining to ilium; one of pelvic bones, 98

Ilium, one of three bones that form the os coxae or innominate bone of the pelvis, 10, 5f, 92, 94, 95f, 95t

Immune response, ability of lymphocytes to respond to specific antigens, 196, 197–98

Immunity, body's ability to defend itself against pathogens, 196–98

immune response, 196, 197–98

standard precautions, 198

Immunization, providing protection against communicable diseases by stimulating immune system to produce antibodies against that disease; children can now be immunized for: hepatitis B, diphtheria, tetanus, pertussis, tetanus, *Haemophilus influenzae* type b, polio, measles, mumps, rubella, and chickenpox; also called *vaccination,* 196, 197, 204

Immunocompromised, having immune system unable to respond properly to pathogens, 203

Immunodeficiency disorder, 203

Immunoglobulins (Ig), antibodies secreted by B cells; all antibodies are immunoglobulins; assist in protecting body and its surfaces from invasion of bacteria; for example, immunoglobulin IgA in colostrum, first milk from mother, helps to protect newborn from infection, 199

Immunologist, physician who specializes in treating infectious diseases and other disorders of immune system, 200

Immunology, branch of medicine specializing in conditions of lymphatic and immune systems, 28*t,* 200

Immunosuppressants, substances that block certain actions of immune system; required to prevent rejection of transplanted organ, 205

Immunotherapy, production or strengthening of patient's immune system in order to treat disease, 204, 529

Impacted fracture, fracture in which bone fragments are pushed into each other, 102

Impetigo, highly contagious staphylococcal skin infection, most commonly occurring on faces of children; begins as blisters that then rupture and dry into thick, yellow crust, 66, 66*f*

Implant, prosthetic device placed in jaw to which a tooth or denture may be anchored, 279

Implantable cardiovert-defibrillator, device implanted in heart that delivers electrical shock to restore normal heart rhythm; particularly useful for persons who experience ventricular fibrillation, 161

Impulse control disorders, inability to resist impulse to perform some act harmful to individual or others; includes kleptomania, pyromania, explosive disorder, and pathological gambling, 502

Incision and drainage (I&D), making incision to create opening for drainage of material such as pus, 71

Incisors, biting teeth in very front of mouth that function to cut food into smaller pieces; humans have eight incisors, 259*f,* 260, 260*f*

Incus, one of three ossicles of middle ea; also called *anvil,* 467*f,* 468, 468*f*

Infant respiratory distress syndrome (IRDS), lung condition most commonly found in premature infants characterized by tachypnea and respiratory grunting; also called *hyaline membrane disease* (HMD) and *respiratory distress syndrome of the newborn,* 235

Infarct, area of tissue within organ that undergoes necrosis (death) following loss of blood supply, 153

Inferior, directional term meaning toward feet or tail, or below, 34*f,* 37*t*

Inferior vena cava, branch of vena cava that drains blood from abdomen and lower body, 142*f,* 144, 145*f,* 150*f,* 157*f,* 382*f*

Infertility, inability to produce children; generally defined as no pregnancy after properly timed intercourse for one year, 346

Inflammation, tissue response to injury from pathogens or physical agents; characterized by redness, pain, swelling, and feeling hot to touch, 200, 200*f*

Inflammatory bowel disease (IBD), 275

Influenza, viral infection of respiratory system characterized by chills, fever, body aches, and fatigue; commonly called the *flu,* 235

Informed consent, medical record document, voluntarily signed by patient or responsible party, that clearly describes purpose, methods, procedures, benefits, and risks of diagnostic or treatment procedure, 12

Inguinal, pertaining to groin area; there is a collection of lymph nodes in this region that drain each leg, 194*t,* 199

Inguinal hernia, hernia or outpouching of intestines into inguinal region of body, 258, 258*f*

Inguinal nodes, 273, 274*f*

Inhalation, (1) to breathe air into lungs; also called *inspiration;* (2) to introduce drugs into body by inhaling them, 220, 494*t,* 495*f,* 520, 521*t*

Innate immunity, 197

Inner ear, innermost section of ear; contains cochlea, semicircular canals, saccule, and utricle, 466*f,* 467, 467*f,* 468, 469*f*

Inner ear infection, 473

Innominate bone, also called os coxae or hip bone; pelvis portion of lower extremity; consists of ilium, ischium, and pubis and unites with sacrum and coccyx to form pelvis, 92, 94

Insertion, attachment of skeletal muscle to more movable bone in joint, 115

Insomnia, sleeping disorder characterized by marked inability to fall asleep, 503

Inspiration, 220, 226*f*

Inspiratory capacity (IC), volume of air inhaled after normal exhale, 225*t*

Inspiratory reserve volume (IRV), air that can be forcibly inhaled after normal respiration has taken place; also called *complemental air,* 225*t*

Insulin, hormone secreted by pancreas; regulates level of sugar in blood stream; the more insulin present in blood, the lower blood sugar will be, 381*t,* 383, 397

Insulin-dependent diabetes mellitus (IDDM), also called type 1 diabetes mellitus; develops early in life when pancreas stops insulin production; persons with IDDM must take daily insulin injections, 392

Insulinoma, tumor of islets of Langerhans cells of pancreas that secretes excessive amount of insulin, 392

Integument, another term for skin, 52

Integumentary system, skin and its appendages including sweat glands, oil glands, hair, and nails; sense organs that allow us to respond to changes in temperature, pain, touch, and pressure are located in skin; largest organ in body, 27*t,* 52–82, 51*f*

    abbreviations, 72

    accessory organs, 54–55

    anatomical terms, 57

    anatomy and physiology of, 52–55

    diagnostic procedures, 70

    pathology, 58–69

    pharmacology, 72

    skin, 52–54

    terminology, 56–57

    therapeutic procedures, 70–71

Interatrial, pertaining to between atria, 152

Interatrial septum, wall or septum that divides left and right atria, 143

Intercostal muscles, muscles between ribs; when they contract, they raise ribs, which helps to enlarge thoracic cavity, 226

Intercostal nerve, 419*f*

Intermittent claudication, attacks of severe pain and lameness caused by ischemia of muscles, typically calf muscles; brought on by walking even very short distances, 120

Intermittent positive pressure breathing (IPPB), method for assisting patients to breathe using mask connected to a machine that produces increased pressure, 240

Internal genitalia, 332–35

Internal iliac artery, 148*f,* 315*f*

Internal iliac vein, 148*f,* 315*f*

Internal medicine, branch of medicine involving diagnosis and treatment of diseases and conditions of internal organs such as respiratory system; physician is *internist,* 229

Internal respiration, process of oxygen and carbon dioxide exchange at cellular level when oxygen leaves bloodstream and is delivered to tissues, 220

Internal sphincter, ring of involuntary muscle that keeps urine within bladder, 300

Internist, physician specialized in treating diseases and conditions of internal organs such as respiratory system, 229

Internodal pathway, 146*f*

Interstitial cystitis, disease of unknown cause in which there is inflammation and irritation of bladder; most commonly seen in middle-aged women, 310

Interventricular, pertaining to between ventricles, 152

Interventricular septum, wall or septum that divides left and right ventricles, 143, 145*f,* 146*f*

Intervertebral, pertaining to between vertebrae, 98

Intervertebral disk, fibrous cartilage cushion between vertebrae, 89, 91

Intracavitary, injection into body cavity such as peritoneal and chest cavity, 495*t*

Intracoronary artery stent, placing a stent within coronary artery to treat coronary ischemia due to atherosclerosis, 162

Intracranial, pertaining to inside skull, 98

Intradermal (ID), (1) pertaining to within skin; (2) injection of medication into skin, 57, 495*t*

Intramuscular (IM), injection of medication into muscle, 123, 495*t*

Intraocular, pertaining to within eye, 454

Intraoperative, period of time during operation, 524

Intrathecal, (1) pertaining to within meninges; (2) injection into meninges space surrounding brain and spinal cord, 421, 495*t*

Intrauterine device (IUD), device inserted into uterus by physician for purpose of contraception, 349, 349*f*

Intravenous (IV), injection into veins; this route can be set up so that there is continuous administration of medication, 496*t,* 520

Intravenous cholecystography, dye is administered intravenously to patient that allows for X-ray visualization of gallbladder, 277

Intravenous pyelogram (IVP), injecting contrast medium into vein and then taking X-ray to visualize renal pelvis, 316

Intussusception, intestinal condition in which one portion of intestine telescopes into adjacent portion causing obstruction and gangrene if untreated, 274, 274*f*

Invasive disease, tendency of malignant tumor to spread to immediately surrounding tissue and organs, 527

Inversion, directional term meaning turning inward or inside out, 117*t,* 117*f*

Involuntary muscles, muscles under control of subconscious regions of brain; smooth muscles found in internal organs and cardiac muscles are examples of involuntary muscle tissue, 113

Iodine, mineral required by thyroid to produce its hormones, 387

Iridal, pertaining to iris, 454

Iridectomy, excision of iris, 462

Iridoplegia, paralysis of iris, 455

Iridosclerotomy, incision into iris and sclera, 462

Iris, colored portion of eye; can dilate or constrict to change size of pupil and control amount of light entering interior of eye, 447f, 448f, 449, 452f

Iritis, inflammation of iris, 457

Iron-deficiency anemia, anemia resulting from having insufficient iron to manufacture hemoglobin, 186

Irregular bones, type of bone having irregular shape; vertebrae are irregular bones, 86, 87f

Irritable bowel syndrome (IBS), disturbance in functions of intestine from unknown causes; symptoms generally include abdominal discomfort and alteration in bowel activity; also called *functional bowel syndrome* or *spastic colon,* 274

Ischemia, localized and temporary deficiency of blood supply due to obstruction of circulation, 153

Ischial, pertaining to ischium, one of pelvic bones, 98

Ischium, one of three bones forming os coxae or innominate bone of pelvis, 85f, 92, 94, 95f, 95t

Islets of Langerhans, regions within pancreas that secrete insulin and glucagon, 383, 383f

Isthmus, 388f

J

Jaundice, yellow cast to skin, mucous membranes, and whites of eyes caused by deposit of bile pigment from too much bilirubin in blood; bilirubin is a waste product produced when worn-out red blood cells are broken down; may be symptom of disorders such as gallstones blocking common bile duct or carcinoma of liver, 270

Jaw bone, 261f

Jejunal, pertaining to jejunum, 268

Jejunostomy, 263

Jejunum, middle portion of small intestines; site of nutrient absorption, 262–63, 263f

Joint, point at which two bones meet; provides flexibility, 27t, 86, 95–96

Joint capsule, elastic capsule that encloses synovial joints, 95, 96

Jugular vein, 150f, 467f

K

Kaposi's sarcoma (KS), form of skin cancer frequently seen in acquired immunodeficiency syndrome (AIDS) patients; consists of brownish-purple papules that spread from skin and metastasize to internal organs, 66, 203

Keloid, formation of scar after injury or surgery resulting in raised, thickened red area, 66, 66f

Keratin, hard protein substance produced by body; found in hair and nails, and filling inside of epidermal cells, 53

Keratitis, inflammation of cornea, 457

Keratometer, instrument to measure cornea, 460

Keratometry, measurement of curvature of cornea using instrument called a keratometer, 460

Keratoplasty, surgical repair of cornea (corneal transplant), 462

Keratosis, overgrowth and thickening of epithelium, 66

Ketoacidosis, acidosis due to excess of ketone bodies (waste products); serious condition requiring immediate treatment and can result in death for diabetic patient if not reversed, 392t

Ketones, 303t

Ketonuria, ketones in urine, 307

Kidneys, two kidneys located in lumbar region of back behind parietal peritoneum; under muscles of back, just a little above waist; have concave or depressed area that gives them bean-shaped appearance; center of this concavity is called hilum, 29t, 35, 37t, 297f, 298–99, 299f, 300f, 301, 382f

Kidneys, ureters, bladder (KUB), x-ray taken of abdomen demonstrating kidneys, ureters, and bladder without using any contrast dye; also called flat-plate abdomen, 311

Kinesiology, study of movement, 120

Kleptomania, impulse control disorder in which patient is unable to refrain from stealing; items are often trivial and unneeded, 502

Kyphosis, abnormal increase in outward curvature of thoracic spine; also known as hunchback or humpback, 104, 104f

L

Labia majora, outer folds of skin that serves as protection for female external genitalia and urethral meatus, 335, 335f

Labia minora, inner folds of skin that serves as protection for female external genitalia and urethral meatus, 335, 335f

Labor, period of time beginning with uterine contractions and ending with birth of baby; there are three stages: dilation, expulsion, and placental stage, 338

Labor and delivery, 338–39

Labyrinth, term referring to inner ear; several fluid-filled cavities within temporal bone; labyrinth consists of cochlea, vestibule, and three semicircular canals; hair cells called organs of Corti line inner ear; hair cells change sound vibrations to electrical impulses and send impulses to brain via vestibulocochlear nerve, 468

Labyrinthectomy, excision of labyrinth, 475

Labyrinthitis, labyrinth inflammation, 473

Labyrinthotomy, incision in labyrinth, 475

Laceration, torn or jagged wound; incorrectly used to describe a cut, 66

Lacrimal, pertaining to tears, 454

Lacrimal apparatus, consists of lacrimal gland, lacrimal ducts, and nasolacrimal duct, 451, 459

Lacrimal bone, facial bone, 89, 91f, 91t

Lacrimal ducts, tear ducts located in inner corner of eye socket; collect tears and drain them into lacrimal sac, 451, 451f

Lacrimal gland, gland located in outer corner of each eyelid; washes anterior surface of eye with fluid called tears, 451, 451f

Lactate dehydrogenase **(LDH),** 159

Lactation, function of secreting milk after childbirth from breasts or mammary glands, 336

Lacteals, lymphatic vessels in intestines that serve to absorb fats from diet, 193

Lactic, pertaining to milk, 340

Lactiferous ducts, carry milk from milk-producing glands to nipple, 336, 336f

Lactiferous glands, milk-producing glands in breast, 336, 336f

Lactorrhea, discharge of milk, 341

Laminectomy, removal of portion of a vertebra in order to relieve pressure on spinal nerve, 108, 432

Laparoscope, instrument to view inside abdomen, 278, 347

Laparoscopic adrenalectomy, excision of adrenal gland through small incision in abdomen and using endoscopic instruments, 396

Laparoscopic cholecystectomy, excision of gallbladder using laparoscope, 280

Laparoscopy, instrument or scope is passed into abdominal wall through small incision; abdominal cavity is then examined for tumors and other conditions with this lighted instrument; also called *peritoneoscopy,* 278, 347, 347f

Laparotomy, incision into abdomen, 281, 350

Laryngeal, pertaining to larynx, 228

Laryngectomy, surgical removal of larynx; procedure is most frequently performed for excision of cancer, 241

Laryngitis, inflammation of larynx causing difficulty in speaking, 233

Laryngopharynx, inferior section of pharynx; lies at same level in neck as larynx; air has already entered larynx, therefore laryngopharynx carries food and drink to esophagus, 211f, 222, 261

Laryngoplasty, surgical repair of larynx, 241

Laryngoplegia, paralysis of voice box, 231

Laryngoscope, instrument to view larynx, 238

Laryngoscopy, examination of interior of larynx with lighted instrument called *laryngoscope,* 238

Larynx, also called *voice box;* respiratory system organ responsible for producing speech; located just below pharynx, 29t, 222, 223f,

Laser photocoagulation, use of laser beam to destroy very small precise areas of the retina; may be used to treat retinal detachment or macular degeneration, 462

Laser surgery, use of controlled beam of light for cutting, hemostasis, or tissue destruction, 524

Laser therapy, removal of skin lesions and birthmarks using laser beam that emits intense heat and power at a close range; laser converts frequencies of light into one small, powerful beam, 471

Laser-assisted in-situ keratomileusis (LASIK), correction of myopia using laser surgery to remove corneal tissue, 436, 462f

Lateral (lat), directional term meaning to the side, 37f, 37t

Lateral epicondylitis, inflammation of muscle attachment to lateral epicondyle of elbow; often caused by strongly gripping; commonly called tennis elbow, 121

Lateral fissure, 415f

Lateral recumbent position, lying on either left or right side, 522f, 523t

Lateral view, positioning patient so that side of body faces X-ray machine, 507

Lavage, using NG tube to wash out stomach, 279

Laxative, mild cathartic, 281

Lazy eye, 456

Left atrium, 140*f*, 142*f*, 145*f*, 146*f*

Left coronary artery, 147*f*

Left hypochondriac, anatomical division of abdomen, left side of upper row, 36*t*

Left iliac, anatomical division of abdomen, left side of upper row, 36*t*

Left lower quadrant (LLQ), clinical division of abdomen; contains portions of small and large intestines, left ovary and fallopian tube, and left ureter, 36*t*

Left lumbar, anatomical division of abdomen, left side of middle row, 36*t*

Left upper quadrant (LUQ), clinical division of abdomen; contains left lobe of liver, spleen, stomach, portion of pancreas, and portion of small and large intestines, 36*t*

Left ventricle, 140*f*, 142*f*, 145*f*

Legally blind, describes person who has severely impaired vision; usually defined as having visual acuity of 20/200, 457

Legionnaire's disease, severe, often fatal disease characterized by pneumonia and gastrointestinal symptoms; caused by gram-negative bacillus and named after people who came down with it at American Legion convention in 1976, 235

Lens, transparent structure behind pupil and iris; functions to bend light rays so they land on retina, 447*f*, 448*f*, 449, 452*f*

Lesion, general term for wound, injury, or abnormality, 60

Leukemia, cancer of WBC-forming bone marrow; results in large number of abnormal WBCs circulating in blood, 187

Leukocytes, also called *white blood cells* or WBCs; group of several different types of cells that provide protection against invasion of bacteria and other foreign material; able to leave bloodstream and search out foreign invaders (bacteria, virus, and toxins), where they perform phagocytosis, 28*t*, 178, 180, 181*t*, 181, 187

Leukocytosis, too many white cells, 187

Leukoderma, disappearance of pigment from skin in patches, causing milk-white appearance; also called *vitiligo,* 60

Leukopenia, too few white (cells), 187

Ligaments, very strong bands of connective tissue that bind bones together at a joint, 86

Ligation and stripping, surgical treatment for varicose veins; damaged vein is tied off (ligation) and removed (stripping), 163

Lingual tonsils, tonsils located on very posterior section of tongue as it joins with pharynx, 196, 222, 259*f*

Lipocytes, medical term for cells that contain fat molecules, 54

Lipoma, fatty tumor that generally does not metastasize, 60

Liposuction, removal of fat beneath skin by means of suction, 71

Lips, anterior opening of oral cavity, 258, 259*f*

Lithium, special category of drug used successfully to calm patients who suffer from bipolar disorder, 504

Lithotomy, surgical incision to remove kidney stones, 314

Lithotomy position, lying face up with hips and knees bent at 90[[deg]] angles, 522*f*, 523*t*

Lithotripsy, destroying or crushing kidney stones in bladder or urethra with device called lithotriptor, 314

Liver, large organ located in right upper quadrant of abdomen; serves many functions in body; its digestive system role includes producing bile, processing absorbed nutrients, and detoxifying harmful substances, 29*t*, 35*t*, 36*t*, 256, 257*f*, 258, 265, 265*f*

Liver transplant, transplant of a liver from a donor, 281

Lobe, ear, 467*f*

Lobectomy, surgical removal of a lobe from an organ, such as a lung; often treatment of choice for lung cancer; may also be removal of one lobe of thyroid gland, 241, 397

Lobes, subdivisions of organ such as lungs or brain, 224

Local anesthesia, substance that produces a loss of sensation in one localized part of body; patient remains conscious when this type of anesthetic is used; administered either topically or via subcutaneous route, 520, 521*t*

Long bone, type of bone longer than it is wide; examples include femur, humerus, and phalanges, 86, 87*f*

Long-term care facility, facility that provides long-term care for patients who need extra time to recover from illness or accident before they return home or for persons who can no longer care for themselves; also called a *nursing home,* 13

Longitudinal section, internal view of body produced by lengthwise slice along long axis of structure, 32, 33

Loop of Henle, portion of renal tubule, 299, 300*f*, 302*f*

Lordosis, abnormal increase in forward curvature of lumbar spine; also known as *swayback,* 104*f*, 105

Lower esophageal sphincter, also called cardiac sphincter; prevents food and gastric juices from backing up into esophagus, 262

Lower extremity (LE), the leg, 33, 94, 95f, 95t, 515

Lower gastrointestinal series (lower GI series), x-ray image of colon and rectum is taken after administration of barium by enema; also called *barium enema,* 277, 277f

Lumbar, pertaining to five low back vertebrae, 98

Lumbar puncture (LP), puncture with needle into lumbar area (usually fourth intervertebral space) to withdraw fluid for examination and for injection of anesthesia; also called *spinal puncture* or *spinal tap,* 431, 431f

Lumbar vertebrae, five vertebrae in low back region, 89, 91, 92t

Lumbosacral plexus, 419f

Lumen, space, cavity, or channel within tube or tubular organ or structure in body, 146, 147f

Lumpectomy, excision of only a breast tumor and tissue immediately surrounding it, 350

Lung metastases, 528f

Lung volumes/capacities, 225, 225t

Lungs, major organs of respiration; consist of air passageways, bronchi and bronchioles, and air sacs, alveoli; gas exchange takes place within alveoli, 29t, 36t, 140f, 218, 219f, 220, 224–25

Lunula, lighter-colored, half-moon region at base of a nail, 55

Luteinizing hormone (LH), hormone secreted by anterior pituitary; regulates function of male and female gonads and plays a role in releasing ova in females, 333, 381t, 385

Lymph, clear, transparent, colorless fluid found in lymphatic vessels and cisterna chyli, 193

Lymph glands, another name for *lymph nodes;* small organs composed of lymphatic tissue located along route of lymphatic vessels; remove impurities from lymph and manufacture lymphocytes and antibodies, 194

Lymph nodes, small organs in lymphatic system that filter bacteria and other foreign organisms from body fluids, 28t, 193f, 194, 194t, 195f

Lymphadenectomy, excision of the lymph node; this is usually done to test for malignancy, 205

Lymphadenitis, inflammation of lymph glands; referred to as swollen glands, 201

Lymphadenopathy, disease of lymph nodes, 201

Lymphangial, pertaining to lymph vessels, 199

Lymphangiogram, x-ray taken of lymph vessels after injection of dye; lymph flow through chest is traced, 203

Lymphangiography, process of taking X-ray of lymph vessels after injection of radiopaque material, 203

Lymphangioma, lymph vessel tumor, 199

Lymphatic, pertaining to lymph, 200

Lymphatic and immune system, 28t, 192f
    abbreviations, 205
    anatomical terms, 199–200
    anatomy and physiology, 193–98
    diagnostic procedures, 203–04
    immunity, 196–98
    lymph nodes, 194, 194t, 195f
    pathology, 200–03
    pharmacology, 205
    spleen, 196, 196f
    terminology, 199–200
    therapeutic procedures, 204–05
    thymus gland, 196, 196f
    tonsils, 196, 196f

Lymphatic capillaries, smallest lymph vessels; they collect excessive tissue fluid, 193, 194

Lymphatic ducts, two largest vessels in lymphatic system, right lymphatic duct and thoracic duct, 193, 194, 195f

Lymphatic system, system that helps body fight infection; organs include spleen, lymph vessels, and lymph nodes, 28t, 192f

Lymphatic vessels, extensive network of vessels throughout entire body; conduct lymph from tissue toward thoracic cavity, 28t, 193f, 193–94, 194f, 195f

Lymphedema, edema appearing in extremities due to obstruction of lymph flow through lymphatic vessels, 201

Lymphocytes (lymphs), agranulocyte white blood cell that provides protection through immune response, 181t, 195f

Lymphoma, tumor of lymphatic tissue, 202

M

Macrophage, phagocytic cells found in large quantities in lymph nodes; they engulf foreign particles, 196, 197f

Macrotia, abnormally large ears, 471

Macula lutea, images are projected onto area of retina, 449

Macular, pertaining to macula lutea, 454

Macular degeneration, deterioration of macular area of retina of eye; may be treated with laser surgery to destroy blood vessels beneath macula, 457

Macule, flat, discolored area flush with skin surface; example would be freckle or birthmark, 60, 60f

Magnetic resonance imaging (MRI), medical imaging that uses radio-frequency radiation as its source of energy; does not require injection of contrast medium or exposure to ionizing radiation; technique is useful for visualizing large blood vessels, heart, brain, and soft tissues, 104f, 509, 509f

Major depression, mood disorder characterized by marked loss of interest in usually enjoyable activities, disturbances in sleep and eating patterns, fatigue, suicidal thoughts, and feelings of hopelessness, worthlessness, and guilt, 502

Male reproductive system, system responsible for producing sperm for reproduction; organs include testes, vas deferens, urethra, prostate gland, and penis, 30t, 352–73, 353f, 354f
    abbreviations, 363
    anatomical terms, 356–57
    anatomy and physiology, 354–56
    bulbourethral glands, 356
    diagnostic procedures, 360
    epididymis, 355
    external organs of, 354–34
    internal organs of, 356
    pathology, 358–60
    penis, 354
    pharmacology, 362
    prostate gland, 356
    seminal vesicles, 356
    terminology, 356–57
    testes, 354–55
    therapeutic procedures, 361–62
    vas deferens, 356

Male urethra, 297f, 301f

Malignant, tumor that is cancerous; tumors are generally progressive and recurring, 526, 526f

Malignant melanoma (MM), malignant, darkly pigmented tumor or mole on skin, 66, 66f

Malingering, type of factitious disorder in which patient intentionally feigns illness for attention or secondary gain, 502

Malleus, one of three ossicles of middle ear; also called *hammer,* 467f, 468, 468f

Mammary, pertaining to breast, 340

Mammary glands, breasts; milk-producing glands to provide nutrition for newborn, 336

Mammogram, x-ray record of breast, 347

Mammography, process of X-raying breast, 347

Mammoplasty, surgical repair of breast, 350

Mandible, lower jawbone, 85f, 89, 91f, 91t, 221f

Mandibular, pertaining to mandible or lower jaw, 98

Mania, mood disorder characterized by extreme elation and euphoria; patient displays rapid speech, flight of ideas, decreased sleep, distractibility, grandiosity, and poor judgment, 502

Masochism, sexual disorder characterized by receiving sexual gratification from being hurt or abused, 503

Massage, kneading or applying pressure by hands to a part of patient's body to promote muscle relaxation and reduce tension, 517

Mastalgia, breast pain, 342

Mastectomy, excision of breast, 352

Mastitis, inflammation of breast, common during lactation but can occur at any age, 345

Mastoid process, 467f

Maxilla, upper jawbone, 89, 91f, 91t

Maxillary, pertaining to maxilla or upper jaw, 98

Meatotomy, surgical enlargement of urinary opening (meatus), 314

Meconium, substance that collects in intestines of fetus and becomes first stool of newborn, 341

Medial, directional term meaning to middle or near middle of body or structure, 37f, 37t

Median cubital vein, 150f

Median nerve, 419f

Median plane, when sagittal plane passes through middle of body, dividing it into equal right and left halves; also called *midsagittal plane,* 30, 32

Mediastinal, collection of lymph nodes located in mediastinum (central chest area) that drain chest, 194t, 195f

Mediastinum, central region of chest cavity; contains organs between lungs, including heart, aorta, esophagus, and trachea, 34, 35t, 141f, 224, 225f

Medical record, documents details of patient's hospital stay; each health care professional that has contact with patient in any capacity completes appropriate report of that contact and adds it to medical chart; this results in permanent physical record of patient's day-to-day condition, when and what services received, and response to treatment; also called a chart, 11–12

Medical terms, interpreting, 9–10
    pronunciation, 9–10
    spelling, 10

Medication, 491

Medulla, central area of an organ; in endocrine system refers to adrenal medulla; in urinary system, refers to inner portion of kidney, 298, 299f, 415f

Medulla oblongata, portion of brain stem that connects spinal cord with brain; contains respiratory, cardiac, and blood pressure control centers, 414, 414f, 415

Medullary, pertaining to medulla of organ like kidney or to medullla oblongata, 99

Medullary cavity, large open cavity that extends length of shaft of long bone; contains yellow bone marrow, 86, 87

Melanin, black color pigment in skin; helps to prevent sun's ultraviolet rays from entering body, 53, 54

Melanocyte-stimulating hormone (MSH), hormone secreted by anterior pituitary; stimulates pigment production in skin, 381*t*, 385

Melanocytes, special cells in basal layer of epidermis; they contain black pigment melanin that gives skin its color and protects against ultraviolet rays of sun, 53

Melanoma, also called *malignant melanoma;* dangerous form of skin cancer caused by overgrowth of melanin in melanocyte; may metastasize or spread; exposure to ultraviolet light is a risk factor for developing melanoma, 66, 66*f*

Melatonin, hormone secreted by pineal gland; plays a role in regulating body's circadian rhythm, 384

Melena, passage of dark tarry stools; color is result of digestive enzymes working on blood in stool, 270

Menarche, first menstrual period, 334, 335

Ménière's disease, abnormal condition within labyrinth of inner ear that can lead to progressive loss of hearing; symptoms are dizziness or vertigo, hearing loss, and tinnitus (ringing in ears), 473

Meningeal, pertaining to meninges, 421

Meninges, three connective tissue membrane layers that surround brain and spinal cord; three layers are dura mater, arachnoid layer, and pia mater; dura mater and arachnoid layer are separated by subdural space; arachnoid layer and pia mater are separated by subarachnoid space, 413, 417, 429

Meningioma, slow-growing tumor in meninges of brain, 429

Meningitis, inflammation of membranes of spinal cord and brain caused by microorganism, 429

Meningocele, congenital hernia in which meninges, or membranes, protrude through opening in spinal column or brain, 427, 428*f*

Menometrorrhagia, excessive bleeding during menstrual period and at intervals between menstrual periods, 344

Menopause, cessation or ending of menstrual activity; generally between ages of 40 and 55, 334, 335

Menorrhagia, excessive bleeding during menstrual period; can be either in total number of days or amount of blood or both, 342

Menstrual cycle, 28-day fertility cycle in women; includes ovulation and sloughing off endometrium if pregnancy does not occur, 382

Menstrual period, another name for menstrual cycle, 334, 335

Menstruation, loss of blood and tissue as endometrium is shed by uterus; flow exits body through cervix and vagina; flow occurs approximately every 28 days, 334, 335

Mental health, 499–05
  abbreviations, 505
  disciplines, 500
  pathology, 500–04
  psychiatry, 500
  psychology, 500
  therapeutic procedures, 504–05

Mental retardation, disorder characterized by diminished ability to process intellectual functions, 501

Metacarpal, pertaining to hand bones, 99

Metacarpals, hand bones in upper extremity, 92, 93*f*, 94, 94*t*

Metastacized, 194

Metastases (mets), spreading of cancerous tumor from original site to different locations of body; singular is metastasis, 526, 526*f*

Metastasis (mets), movement and spread of cancer cells from one part of body to another; metastases is plural, 528, 528*f*

Metastasize, when cancerous cells migrate away from tumor site; commonly move through lymphatic system and become trapped in lymph nodes, 194

Metatarsal, pertaining to foot bones, 99

Metatarsals, ankle bones in lower extremity, 92, 93*f*, 94, 95*f*, 95*t*

Metered dose inhaler (MDI), 240

Metrorrhagia, rapid (menstrual) blood flow from uterus, 342

Metrorrhea, discharge from uterus, 342

Microtia, abnormally small ears, 471

Micturition, another term for urination, 300

Midbrain, portion of brain stem, 385*f*, 414, 414*f*, 415

Middle ear, middle section of ear; contains ossicles, 466*f*, 467, 467*f*, 468, 468*f*

Middle ear infection, 472

Midline organs, 36*t*

Midsagittal plane, when sagittal plane passes through middle of body, dividing it into equal right and left halves, also called *median plane,* 32

Migraine, specific type of headache characterized by severe head pain, photophobia, vertigo, and nausea, 427

Miner's lung, 234

Mineralocorticoids, group of hormones secreted by adrenal cortex; regulate electrolytes and fluid volume in body; aldosterone is an example, 380*t*, 382

Minnesota Multiphasic Personality Inventory (MMPI), 505

Minor tranquilizers, medications that are central nervous system depressants and are prescribed for anxiety, 504

Miotic drops, substance that causes pupil to constrict, 463

Miscarriage, 346

Mitral valve, valve between left atrium and ventricle in heart; prevents blood from flowing backwards into atrium; also called bicuspid valve because it has two cusps or flaps, 142f, 143, 144f

Mobility, state of having normal movement of all body parts, 515

Mobilization, treatments such as exercise and massage to restore movement to joints and soft tissue, 517

Moist hot packs, applying moist warmth to body part to produce slight dilation of blood vessels in skin; causes muscle relaxation in deeper regions of body and increases circulation, which aids healing, 517

Molars, large somewhat flat-topped back teeth; function to grind food; humans have up to twelve molars, 260f, 261

Monoaural, referring to one ear, 471

Monochromatism, unable to perceive one color, 457

Monocytes (monos), agranulocyte white blood cell important for phagocytosis, 181t

Mononucleosis (Mono), acute infectious disease with large number of atypical lymphocytes; caused by Epstein–Barr virus; there may be abnormal liver function, 202

Monoparesis, weakness of one extremity, 423

Monoplegia, paralysis of one extremity, 423

Monospot, test of infectious mononucleosis in which there is nonspecific antibody called heterophile antibody, 204

Mood disorders, characterized by instability in mood; includes major depression, mania, and bipolar disorder, 502

Morbid obesity, 270

Morbidity, number that represents number of sick persons in particular population, 528

Mortality, number that represents number of deaths in particular population, 528

Motor neurons, nerves that carry activity instruction from CNS to muscles or glands out in body; also called efferent neurons, 114, 418, 419f

Mucolytic, substance that liquefies mucus so it is easier to cough and clear it from respiratory tract, 243

Mucous membrane, membrane that lines body passages that open directly to exterior of body, such as mouth and reproductive tract, and secretes thick substance, or mucus, 220–21

Mucus, sticky fluid secreted by mucous membrane lining of respiratory tract; assists in cleansing air by trapping dust and bacteria, 221

Multigravida, woman who has had more than one pregnancy, 341

Multipara, woman who has given birth to more than one child, 341

Multiple sclerosis (MS), inflammatory disease of central nervous system; rare in children; generally strikes adults between ages of 20 and 40; there is progressive weakness and numbness, 428

Murmur, abnormal heart sound as soft blowing sound or harsh click; may be soft and heard only with a stethoscope, or so loud it can be heard several feet away; also called a bruit, 153

Muscle actions, 115, 116t–17t

Muscle biopsy, removal of muscle tissue for pathological examination, 122

Muscle cells, 24f

Muscle tissue, tissue able to contract and shorten its length, thereby producing movement; muscle tissue may be under voluntary control (attached to bones) or involuntary control (heart and digestive organs), 25, 26f

Muscle tissue fibers, bundles of muscle tissue that form muscle, 25, 113

Muscle wasting, 120

Muscles, bundles of parallel muscle tissue fibers; as fibers contract (shorten in length) they pull whatever they are attached to closer togethe; may move two bones closer together or make opening narrowier; muscle contraction occurs when message is transmitted from brain through nervous system to muscles, 27t, 113, 412; see also Muscular system

Muscular, pertaining to muscles, 120

Muscular dystrophy (MD), inherited disease causing progressive muscle weakness and atrophy, 121

Muscular system, 111–135, 112f
   abbreviations, 123
   anatomical terms, 119
   anatomy and physiology, 113–18
   combining forms, 119
   diagnostic procedures, 122
   muscle types, 113
   pathology, 120–22
   pharmacology, 123
   suffixes, 119
   terminology, 119
   terminology for muscle actions, 115, 116t,118t
   treatment procedures, 122–23

Musculoskeletal system (MS) system providing support for body and produces movement; organs include: muscles, tendons, bones, joints, and cartilage; see Muscular system; Skeletal system

Mutation, change or transformation from original, 528

Myalgia, muscle pain, 120

Myasthenia, lack of muscle strength, 120

Myasthenia gravis, disorder causing loss of muscle strength and paralysis; autoimmune disease, 428

Mycoplasma pneumonia, less severe but longer lasting form of pneumonia caused by *Mycoplasma pneumoniae* bacteria; also called *walking pneumonia,* 236

Mydriatic drops, substance that causes pupil to dilate, 463

Myelin, tissue that wraps around many of nerve fibers; composed of fatty material and functions as insulator, 412, 413*f*, 414

Myelinated, nerve fibers covered with layer of myelin, 413

Myelitis, inflammation of spinal cord, 427

Myelogram, x-ray record of spinal cord following injection of meninges with radiopaque dye, 430

Myelography, injection of radiopaque dye into spinal canal; an X-ray is taken to examine normal and abnormal outlines made by dye, 106, 431

Myeloma, malignant neoplasm originating in plasma cells in bone, 103

Myelomeningocele, hernia composed of meninges and spinal cord, 427, 428*f*

Myelonic, pertaining to spinal cord, 421

Myocardial, pertaining to heart muscle, 119, 152

Myocardial infarction (MI), condition caused by partial or complete occlusion or closing of one or more of coronary arteries; symptoms include severe chest pain or heavy pressure in middle of chest; delay in treatment could result in death; also referred to as *MI* or *heart attack,* 142, 155, 155*f*, 156, 156*f*

Myocarditis, inflammation of heart muscle, 157

Myocardium, middle layer of muscle; thick and composed of cardiac muscle; layer produces heart contraction, 114, 142, 142*f*, 145*f*

Myometrium, middle muscle layer of uterus, 334, 334*f*

Myoneural junction, point at which nerve contacts muscle fiber, 114

Myopathy, any disease of muscles, 121

Myopia, with this condition person can see things that are close up but distance vision is blurred; also known as *nearsightedness,* 458, 458*f*

Myoplasty, surgical repair of muscle, 123

Myorrhaphy, suture a muscle, 123

Myorrhexis, muscle ruptured, 121

Myotonia, muscle tone, 120

Myringectomy, excision of eardrum, 475

Myringitis, eardrum inflammation, 472

Myringoplasty, surgical reconstruction of eardrum; also called *tympanoplasty,* 475

Myringotomy, surgical puncture of eardrum with removal of fluid and pus from middle ear, to eliminate persistent ear infection and excessive pressure on tympanic membrane; polyethylene tube is placed in tympanic membrane to allow for drainage of middle ear cavity, 476

Myxedema, condition resulting from hypofunction of thyroid gland; symptoms can include anemia, slow speech, enlarged tongue and facial features, edematous skin, drowsiness, and mental apathy, 395

N

Nail bed, connects nail body to connective tissue underneath, 55

Nail body, flat plate of keratin that forms most of nails, 55

Nail root, base of nail; nails grow longer from root, 55

Nails, structure in integumentary system, 27*t*, 55, 55*f*, 63

Narcissistic personality, personality disorder characterized by abnormal sense of self-importance, 502

Narcotic analgesic, drug used to treat severe pain; has potential to be habit forming if taken for prolonged time; also called opiates, 433

Nares, external openings of nose that open into nasal cavity, 220, 221*f*

Nasal, pertaining to nose, 229

Nasal bone, facial bone, 89, 91*f*, 91*t*

Nasal cannula, two-pronged plastic device for delivering oxygen into nose; one prong is inserted into each naris, 240

Nasal cavity, large cavity just behind external nose that receives outside air; covered with mucous membrane to cleanse air; nasal septum divides nasal cavity into left and right halves, 29*t*, 220–21*f*, 259*f*, 451

Nasal septum, flexible cartilage wall that divides nasal cavity into left and right halves; covered by mucous membrane, 220

Nasogastric (NG), pertaining to nose and stomach, 268

Nasogastric intubation (NG tube), flexible catheter is inserted into nose and down esophagus to stomach; may be used for feeding or to suction out stomach fluids, 279

Nasolacrimal duct, duct that collects tears from inner corner of eye socket and drains them into nasal cavity, 451, 451*f*

Nasopharyngitis, inflammation of nasal cavity and throat, 233

Nasopharynx, superior section of pharynx that receives air from nose, 221f, 222

Natural immunity, immunity not specific to particular disease and does not require prior exposure to pathogen; also called innate immunity, 197

Natural killer (NK) cells, t cells that can kill by entrapping foreign cells, tumor cells, and bacteria; also called T8 cells, 197, 198

Nausea, feeling of needing to vomit, 270

Nearsightedness, 458, 458f

Nebulizer, 240

Neck, narrow length of bone that connects ball of ball-and-socket joint to diaphysis of long bone, 88, 88f

Necrosis, dead tissue, 60

Neonate, term used to describe newborn infant during first four weeks of life, 341

Neonatologist, specialist in treatment of newborn, 342

Neonatology, study of newborn, 342

Neoplasm, abnormal growth of tissue that may be benign or malignant; also called a *tumor,* 528

Nephrectomy, excision of a kidney, 314

Nephritis, inflammation of kidney, 314

Nephrogram, x-ray of kidney, 311

Nephrolith, kidney stone, 307

Nephrolithiasis, presence of calculi in kidney, 309

Nephrolithotomy, incision into kidney to remove a stone, 314

Nephrologist, specialist in treatment of kidney disorders, 305

Nephrology, branch of medicine specializing in conditions of urinary system, 29t, 40, 305

Nephroma, kidney tumor, 309

Nephromalacia, softening of kidney, 307

Nephromegaly, enlarged kidney, 307

Nephron, functional or working unit of kidney that filters blood and produces urine; there are more than 1 million nephrons in adult kidney; each nephron consists of renal corpuscle and renal tubules, 298, 299, 300f

Nephropathy, kidney disease, 309

Nephropexy, surgical fixation of kidney, 315

Nephroptosis, drooping kidney, 309

Nephrosclerosis, hardening of kidney, 307

Nephrosis, abnormal condition (degeneration) of kidney, 309

Nephrostomy, creating new opening across body wall into kidney, 315

Nephrotic syndrome (NS), damage to glomerulus resulting in protein appearing in urine, proteinuria, and corresponding decrease in protein in bloodstream, 309

Nephrotomy, incision into kidney, 315

Nerve block, also referred to as regional anesthesia; this anesthetic interrupts patient's pain sensation in particular region of body; anesthetic is injected near nerve that will be blocked from sensation; patient usually remains conscious, 432, 521t

Nerve cell body, portion of nerve cell that includes nucleus, 412, 413f

Nerve cells, 24f

Nerve conduction velocity, test to determine if nerves have been damaged by recording rate at which electrical impulse travels along nerve; if nerve is damaged, velocity will be decreased, 431, 517

Nerve root, point where spinal or cranial nerve is attached to CNS, 418

Nerves, structures in nervous system that conduct electrical impulses from brain and spinal cord to muscles and other organs, 25, 31t, 411f, 412

Nervous system, system that coordinates all conscious and subconscious activities of body; organs include: brain, spinal cord, and nerves, 31t, 410–44, 411f
  abbreviations, 433
  anatomical terms, 421
  anatomy and physiology, 412–20
  central, 413–17
  diagnostic procedures, 430–31
  nervous tissue, 412
  pathology, 422–30
  peripheral, 418–20
  pharmacology, 432–33
  terminology, 420–21
  therapeutic procedures, 432

Nervous tissue, nervous tissue conducts electrical impulses to and from brain and rest of body, 25, 26f, 412

Neural, pertaining to nerves, 421

Neuralgia, nerve pain, 423

Neurectomy, excision of a nerve, 432

Neurogenic bladder, loss of nervous control that leads to retention; may be caused by spinal cord injury or multiple sclerosis, 310

Neuroglial, pertaining to support cells, glial cells, of nerves, 421

Neuroglial cells, cells that perform support functions for neurons, 412

Neurologist, physician who specializes in disorders of nervous system, 422

Neurology, branch of medicine specializing in conditions of nervous system, 31t, 422

Neuroma, nerve tumor, 429

Neuron, name for individual nerve cell; neurons group together to form nerves and other nervous tissue, 25, 412

Neuropathy, disease of nerves, 429

Neuroplasty, surgical repair of nerves, 432

Neurorrhaphy, suture a nerve, 432

Neurosurgery, branch of medicine specializing in surgery on nervous system, 31t, 422

Neurotransmitter, chemical messenger that carries electrical impulse across gap between two neurons, 412

Neutrophils, granulocyte white blood cells that are important for phagocytosis; also most numerous of leukocytes, 179f, 181f, 181t

Nevus, pigmented (colored) congenital skin blemish, birthmark, or mole; usually benign but may become cancerous, 60

Night-blindness, 455

Nipple, point at which milk is released from breast, 336, 336f

Nitrogenous wastes, waste products that contain nitrogen; products, such as ammonia and urea, are produced during protein metabolism, 303

Nocturia, excessive urination during night; may or may not be abnormal, 307

Nocturnal enuresis, 306

Nodule, solid, raised group of cells, 60, 60f

Non-Hodgkins's lymphoma (NHL), cancer of lymphatic tissues other than Hodgkin's lymphoma, 202

Non-insulin-dependent diabetes mellitus (NIDDM), also called type 2 diabetes mellitus; develops later in life when pancreas produces insufficient insulin; persons may take oral hypoglycemics to stimulate insulin secretion, or may eventually have to take insulin, 392, 398

Nonproprietary name, recognized and accepted official name for drug; each drug has only one generic name, which is not subject to trademark, so any pharmaceutical manufacturer may use it; also called *generic name,* 491

Nonsteroidal antiinflammatory drugs (NSAIDs), large group of drugs including aspirin and ibuprofen that provide mild pain relief and anti-inflammatory benefits for conditions such as arthritis, 109

Norepinephrine, hormone secreted by adrenal medulla; a strong vasoconstrictor, 380t, 382

Normal psychology, behaviors that include how personality develops, how people handle stress, and stages of mental development, 500

Nosocomial infection, infection acquired as result of hospital exposure, 198

Nuclear medicine, use of radioactive substances to diagnose diseases; radioactive substance known to accumulate in certain body tissues is injected or inhaled; after waiting for substance to travel to body area of interest radioactivity level is recorded; commonly referred to as a *scan,* 510

Nucleus, organelle of cell that contains DNA, 24, 413f

Nulligravida, woman who has never been pregnant, 341

Nullipara, woman who has never produced a viable baby, 341

Number prefixes, 6

Nurse, to breastfeed a baby, 336

Nurse anesthetist, registered nurse who has received additional training and education in administration of anesthetic medications, 520

Nurse's notes, medical record document that records patient's care throughout day; includes vital signs, treatment specifics, patient's response to treatment, and patient's condition, 12

Nursing home, facility that provides long-term care for patients who need extra time to recover from illness or accident before they return home or for persons who can no longer care for themselves; also called *long-term care facility,* 13

Nyctalopia, difficulty seeing in dim light; usually due to damaged rods, 455

Nystagmus, jerky-appearing involuntary eye movement, 459

O

Obesity, having abnormal amount of fat in body, 270, 391

Oblique fracture, fracture at angle to bone, 102, 102f

Oblique muscles, oblique means slanted; two of eye muscles are oblique muscles, 450, 450f

Oblique view, positioning patient so that X-rays pass through body on angle, 507

Obsessive-compulsive disorder (OCD), type of anxiety disorder in which person performs repetitive rituals in order to reduce anxiety, 501

Obstetrician, 342

Obstetrics (OB), branch of medicine that treats women during pregnancy and childbirth, and immediately after childbirth, 30t, 342

Occipital bone, cranial bone, 89, 91f, 91t

Occipital lobe, one of four cerebral hemisphere lobes; controls eyesight, 414, 415, 415f

Occupational Safety and Health Administration (OSHA), federal agency that issued mandatory guidelines to ensure that all employees at risk of exposure to body fluids are provided with personal protective equipment, 198

Occupational therapy (OT), assists patients to regain, develop, and improve skills that are important for independent functioning; occupational therapy personnel work with people who, because of illness, injury, developmental, or psychological impairments, require specialized training in skills that will enable them to lead independent, productive, and satisfying lives; occupational therapists instruct patients in use of adaptive equipment and techniques, body mechanics, and energy conservation; also employ modalities such as heat, cold, and therapeutic exercise, 514

Ocular, pertaining to eye, 454

Oculomotor nerve, 418*t*

Oculomycosis, condition of eye fungus, 458

Olfactory nerve, 418*t*

Oligomenorrhea, scanty menstrual flow, 342

Oligospermia, condition of having few sperm, 358

Oliguria, condition of scanty amount of urine, 307

Oncogenic, cancer causing, 528

Oncology, branch of medicine dealing with tumors, 525–30

    abbreviations, 530

    diagnostic procedures, 529

    staging tumors, 526–27, 527*t*

    therapeutic procedures, 529

    vocabulary, 527–28

Onychectomy, excision of a nail, 71

Onychia, infected nailbed, 69

Onychomalacia, softening of nails, 60

Onychomycosis, abnormal condition of nail fungus, 69

Onychophagia, nail biting, 69

Oophorectomy, removal of an ovary, 350

Oophoritis, inflammation of an ovary, 342

Open fracture, 101, 101*f*

Operative report, medical record report from surgeon detailing operation; includes pre- and postprocedure itself, and how patient tolerated procedure, 12, 520

Ophthalmalgia, eye pain, 455

Ophthalmic, pertaining to eyes, 454

Ophthalmic decongestants, over-the-counter medications that constrict arterioles of eye, reduce redness and itching of conjunctiva, 463

Ophthalmologist, physician specialized in treating conditions and diseases of eye, 455

Ophthalmology (Ophth), branch of medicine specializing in condition of eye, 31*t*, 448, 455

Ophthalmoplegia, paralysis of eye, 455

Ophthalmorrhagia, rapid bleeding from eye, 455

Ophthalmoscope, instrument to view inside eye, 460, 461*f*

Ophthalmoscopy, examination of interior of eyes using instrument called ophthalmoscope; physician will dilate pupil in order to see cornea, lens, and retina; identifies abnormalities in blood vessels of eye and some systemic diseases, 460

Opiates, 433

Opportunistic infections, infectious diseases associated with AIDS since they occur as a result of lowered immune system and resistance of body to infections and parasites, 203

Opposition, moves thumb away from palm; ability to move thumb into contact with other fingers, 118*t*

Optic, pertaining to eye, 454

Optic disk, area of retina associated with optic nerve; also called blind spot, 449

Optic nerve, second cranial nerve that carries impulses from retinas to brain, 418*t*, 448, 448*f*, 452*f*

Optical, pertaining to eye or vision, 454

Optician, grinds and fits prescription lenses and contacts as prescribed by physician or optometrist, 455

Optometer, instrument to measure vision, 461

Optometrist (OD), doctor of optometry; provides care for eyes including examining eyes for diseases, assessing visual acuity, prescribing corrective lenses and eye treatments, and educating patients, 455

Optometry, process of measuring vision, 455

Oral, (1) pertaining to mouth; (2) administration of medication through mouth, 268, 471, 494*t*

Oral cavity, the mouth, 29*t*, 257*f*, 258–61, 259*f*

Oral contraceptive pills (OCPs), birth control medication that uses low doses of female hormones to prevent conception by blocking ovulation, 351

Oral hypoglycemic agents, medication taken by mouth that causes decrease in blood sugar; not used for insulin-dependent patients; no proof that medication will prevent long-term complications of diabetes mellitus, 397

Oral surgeon, practitioner of oral surgery, 268

Oral surgery, branch of dentistry that uses surgical means to treat dental conditions; specialist is *oral surgeon*, 268

Orbit, 91*f*

Orchidectomy, excision of testes, 361

Orchidopexy, surgical fixation to move undescended testes into scrotum and attaching to prevent retraction, 358, 361

Orchiectomy, surgical removal of testes, 361

Orchioplasty, surgical repair of testes, 361

Orchiotomy, incision into testes, 361

Organs, group of different types of tissue coming together to perform special functions; for example, heart contains muscular fibers, nerve tissue, and blood vessels, 27–31, 27*t*–37*t*

Organs of Corti, sensory receptor hair cells lining cochlea; these cells change sound vibrations to electrical impulses and send impulses to brain via vestibulocochlear nerve, 468

Origin, attachment of skeletal muscle to less movable bone in joint, 115

Oropharynx, middle section of pharynx that receives food and drink from mouth, 221*f*, 222, 261

Orthodontic, pertaining to straight teeth, 261

Orthodontics, dental specialty concerned with straightening teeth, 269

Orthodontist, dental specialist in straightening teeth, 269

Orthopedic surgeon, 100

Orthopedic surgery, branch of medicine specializing in surgical treatments of musculoskeletal system, 27*t*, 100

Orthopedics (Ortho), branch of medicine specializing in diagnosis and treatment of conditions of musculoskeletal system, 27*t*, 100

Orthopedist, 100

Orthopnea, term to describe patient who needs to sit up straight in order to breathe comfortably, 232

Orthostatic hypotension, sudden drop in blood pressure person experiences when standing up suddenly, 153

Orthotics, use of equipment, such as splints and braces, to support paralyzed muscle, promote specific motion, or correct musculoskeletal deformities, 100, 515

Os coxae, also called innominate bone or hip bone; pelvis portion of lower extremity; consists of ilium, ischium, and pubis and unites with sacrum and coccyx to form pelvis, 92, 94, 95*t*

Osseous tissue, bony tissue; one of hardest tissues in body, 86

Ossicles, three small bones in middle ear; bones are incus, malleus, and stapes; ossicles amplify and conduct sound waves to inner ear, 468, 468*f*

Ossification, process of bone formation, 86

Ostealgia, bone pain, 100

Osteoarthritis (OA), noninflammatory type of arthritis resulting in degeneration of bones and joints, especially those bearing weight, 3, 105

Osteoblast, embryonic bone cell, 86

Osteochondroma, tumor composed of both cartilage and bony substance, 103

Osteoclasia, intentional breaking of bone in order to correct deformity, 108

Osteocyte, mature bone cells, 86

Osteogenic sarcoma, most common type of bone cancer; usually begins in osteocytes found at ends of long bones, 103

Osteomalacia, softening of bones caused by deficiency of phosphorus or calcium; is thought that in children cause is insufficient sunlight and vitamin D, 103

Osteomyelitis, inflammation of bone and bone marrow due to infection; can be difficult to treat, 100

Osteopathy, form of medicine that places great emphasis on musculoskeletal system and body system as a whole; manipulation is also used as part of treatment, 103

Osteoporosis, decrease in bone mass that results in thinning and weakening of bone with resulting fractures; bone becomes more porous, especially in spine and pelvis, 103

Osteotome, instrument to cut bone, 108

Osteotomy, incision into bone, 108

Otalgia, ear pain, 471

Otic, pertaining to ear, 471

Otitis externa (OE), external ear infection; most commonly caused by fungus; also called *otomycosis* and commonly referred to as *swimmer's ear,* 472

Otitis media (OM), commonly referred to as middle ear infection; seen frequently in children; often preceded by upper respiratory infection, 472

Otolaryngology, 229

Otologist, physician specialized in diagnosis and treatment of diseases of ear, 444

Otology (Oto), study of ear, 467

Otomycosis, fungal infection of ear, usually in auditory canal, 472

Otoplasty, corrective surgery to change size of external ear or pinna; surgery can either enlarge or lessen size of pinna, 476

Otopyorrhea, pus discharge from ear, 471

Otorhinolaryngologist, 219, 471

Otorhinolaryngology (ENT), branch of medicine that treats diseases of ears, nose, and throat; also referred to as *ENT,* 29*t*, 31*t*, 229, 471

Otorrhagia, bleeding from ear, 471

Otosclerosis, progressive hearing loss caused by immobility of stapes bone, 472

Otoscope, instrument to view inside ear, 474, 474*f*

Otoscopy, examination of ear canal, eardrum, and outer ear using otoscope; foreign material can be removed from ear canal with this procedure, 474

Outer ear, 469*f*

Outpatient clinic, facility that provides services not requiring overnight hospitalization; services range from simple surgeries to diagnostic testing to therapy; also called ambulatory care center or surgical center, 13

Ova, female sex cells or gametes produced in ovary; ovum fuses with sperm to produce embryo; singular is ovum, 332, 333*f*, 383

Ova and parasites (O&P), laboratory examination of feces with microscope for presence of parasites or their eggs, 276

Oval window, division between middle and inner ear, 468, 468*f*

Ovarian, pertaining to ovaries, 341

Ovarian carcinoma, cancer of ovary, 343

Ovarian cyst, sac that develops within ovary, 343

Ovaries, female gonads; two glands located on either side of lower abdominopelvic region of female; responsible for production of sex cells, ova, and hormones estrogen and progesterone, 30*t*, 35*t*, 36*t*, 332*f*, 332–33, 333*f*, 379*f*, 380, 381*t*, 382, 383*f*

Over-the-counter (OTC), drugs accessible in drugstores without prescription; also called *nonprescription drugs,* 492

Oviducts, tubes that carry ovum from ovary to uterus; also called fallopian tubes or uterine tubes, 333

Ovulation, release of an ovum from ovary, 333

Ovulation stimulant, 351

Oximeter, instrument to measure oxygen, 239

Oximetry, process of measuring oxygen, 239

Oxygen (O₂), gaseous element absorbed by blood from air sacs in lungs; necessary for cells to make energy, 140, 141, 220

Oxygenated, term for blood with a high oxygen level, 140

Oxytocin, hormone secreted by posterior pituitary; stimulates uterine contractions during labor and delivery, 351, 381*t*, 385

P

Pacemaker, another name for sinoatrial node of heart, 145, 146*f*

Pacemaker implantation, electrical device that substitutes for natural pacemaker of heart; controls beating of heart by series of rhythmic electrical impulses; external pacemaker has electrodes on outside of body; internal pacemaker has electrodes surgically implanted within chest wall, 161, 161*f*

Packed red cells, transfusion of only formed elements and without plasma, 189

Paget's disease, fairly common metabolic disease of bone from unknown causes; usually attacks middle-aged and elderly people and is characterized by bone destruction and deformity, 103

Pain control, managing pain through use of a variety of means, including medications, biofeedback, and mechanical devices, 517

Palate, roof of mouth; anterior portion is hard or bony, and posterior portion is soft or flexible, 220, 258

Palatine bone, facial bone, 89, 91*t*

Palatine tonsils, tonsils located in lateral wall of pharynx close to mouth, 196, 222, 259*f*

Palatoplasty, surgical repair of palate, 281

Palliative therapy, treatment designed to reduce intensity of painful symptoms, but not to produce a cure, 529

Pallor, abnormal paleness of skin, 60

Palpitations, pounding, racing heartbeat, 153

Palsy, temporary or permanent loss of ability to control movement, 423

Pancreas, organ in digestive system that produces digestive enzymes; also a gland in endocrine system that produces two hormones, insulin and glucagon, 29*t*, 30*t*, 35*t*, 36*t*, 257*f*, 258, 265, 265*f*, 276*f*, 379*f*, 380, 381*t*, 383–84, 383*f*

Pancreatic, pertaining to pancreas, 268, 389

Pancreatic duct, duct carrying pancreatic juices from pancreas to duodenum, 265, 265*f*

Pancreatic enzymes, digestive enzymes produced by pancreas and added to chyme in duodenum, 265

Pancreatitis, inflammation of pancreas, 276

Pancytopenia, too few of all types of blood cells, 185

Panhypopituitarism, deficiency in all hormones secreted by pituitary gland; often recognized because of problems with glands regulated by pituitary—adrenal cortex, thyroid, ovaries, and testes, 394

Panic attacks, type of anxiety disorder characterized by sudden onset of intense apprehension, fear, terror, or impending doom often accompanied by racing heart rate, 500

Pansinusitis, inflammation of all sinuses, 232

Pap (Papanicolaou) smear, test for early detection of cancer of cervix named after developer of test, George Papanicolaou, a Greek physician; a scraping of cells is removed from cervix for examination under a microscope, 347

Papilla, 55*f*

Papillary muscle, 135*f*

Papilledema, swelling of optic disk, often as a result of increased intraocular pressure; also called *choked disk,* 455

Papule, small, solid, circular raised spot on surface of skin, often as a result of inflammation in oil gland, 61, 61*f*

Paracentesis, insertion of needle into abdominal cavity to withdraw fluid; tests to diagnose disease may be conducted on fluid, 278

Paralysis, temporary or permanent loss of function or voluntary movement, 423

Paranasal sinuses, air-filled cavities within facial bones that open into nasal cavity; act as echo chamber during sound production, 221, 221*f*

Paranoid personality disorder, personality disorder characterized by exaggerated feelings of persecution, 502

Paraplegia, paralysis of lower portion of body and both legs, 423

Parasympathetic branch, branch of autonomic nervous system; serves as counterbalance for sympathetic nerves; therefore, it causes heart rate to slow down, lower blood pressure, constrict eye pupils, and increase digestion, 419

Parathyroid glands, four small glands located on back surface of thyroid gland; parathyroid hormone secreted by these glands regulates amount of calcium in blood, 30*t*, 378, 379*t*, 380, 381*t*, 384, 384*f*

Parathyroid hormone (PTH), hormone secreted by parathyroid glands; the more hormone, the higher the calcium level in blood and lower the level stored in bone; low hormone level will cause tetany, 381*t*, 384

Parenteral, route for introducing medication other than through gastrointestinal tract; most commonly involves injection into body through needle and syringe, 494, 495*t*

Parathyroidal, pertaining to parathyroid glands, 389

Parathyroidectomy, excision of one or more of parathyroid glands; performed to halt progress of hyperparathyroidism, 397

Parenteral administration of drugs, 495*t*

Paresthesia, abnormal sensation such as burning or tingling, 423

Parietal bone, cranial bone, 89, 91*f*, 91*t*

Parietal layer, outer pleural layer around lungs; lines inside of chest cavity, 34, 35

Parietal lobe, one of four cerebral hemisphere lobes; receives and interprets nerve impulses from sensory receptors, 414, 415, 415*f*

Parietal pericardium, outer layer of pericardium surrounding heart, 142

Parietal peritoneum, outer layer of serous membrane sac lining abdominopelvic cavity, 34, 35

Parietal pleura, outer layer of serous membrane sac lining thoracic cavity, 34, 35, 224

Parkinson's disease, chronic disorder of nervous system with fine tremors, muscular weakness, rigidity, and shuffling gait, 427

Paronychia, infection around nail, 69

Parotid duct, 264*f*

Parotid glands, pair of salivary glands located in front of ears, 264, 264*f*

Passive acquired immunity, immunity that results when person receives protective substances produced by another human or animal; may take form of maternal antibodies crossing placenta to baby or antitoxin injection, 196, 197

Passive aggressive personality, personality disorder in which person expresses feelings or anger or hostility through indirect or covert actions, 503

Passive aggressive disorder, 475

Passive range of motion (PROM), therapist putting patient's joints through full range of motion without assistance from patient, 517

Patella, also called *kneecap;* lower extremity bone, 85, 94, 95*f*, 95*t*

Patellar, pertaining to patella or kneecap, 99

Patent, open or unblocked, such as patent airway, 232

Patent ductus arteriosus (PDA), congenital heart anomaly in which opening between pulmonary artery and aorta fails to close at birth; condition requires surgery, 158

Pathogenic, pertaining to microscopic organisms, such as bacteria, capable of causing disease, 201

Pathogens, disease-bearing organisms, 52, 181

Pathologic fracture, fracture caused by diseased or weakened bone, 102

Pathological gambling, impulse control disorder in which patient is unable to control urge to gamble, 502

Pathologist, physician who specializes in evaluating specimens removed from living or dead patients, 527

Pathologist's report, medical record report given by pathologist who studies tissue removed from patient (for example: bone marrow, blood, or tissue biopsy), 12

Pathology, branch of medicine specializing in studying how disease affects body, 200

Pectoral girdle, consists of clavicle and scapula; functions to attach upper extremity to axial skeleton, 92, 93*f*, 94, 94*f*

Pediculosis, infestation with lice, 67

Pedophilia, sexual disorder characterized by having sexual interest in children, 503

Pelvic, pertaining to pelvis, 99

Pelvic cavity, inferior portion of abdominopelvic cavity, 34, 34*f*, 35*t*

Pelvic examination, physical examination of vagina and adjacent organs performed by physician placing fingers of one hand into vagina; visual examination is performed using speculum, 348

Pelvic girdle, consists of ilium, ischium, and pubis; functions to attach lower extremity to axial skeleton, 93*f*, 95*f*, 95*t*

Pelvic inflammatory disease (PID), any inflammation of female reproductive organs, generally bacterial in nature, 344

Pelvic region, lowest anterior region of trunk, 33, 34*f*

Pelvic ultrasonography, use of ultrasound waves to produce image or photograph of organ, such as uterus, ovaries, or fetus, 347

Pelvis, 96f

Penile, pertaining to penis, 357

Penis, male sex organ; composed of erectile tissue that becomes erect during sexual stimulation, allowing it to be placed within female vagina for ejaculation of semen; larger, soft tip is referred to as glans penis, 30t, 353f, 354, 355

Peptic ulcer disease (PUD), ulcer occurring in lower portion of esophagus, stomach, and duodenum and thought to be caused by acid of gastric juices, 272, 272f

Percussion, use of fingertips to tap body lightly and sharply; aids in determining size, position, and consistency of underlying body part, 242

Percutaneous diskectomy, thin catheter tube is inserted into intervertebral disk through skin and herniated or ruptured disk material is sucked out or a laser is used to vaporize it, 108

Percutaneous transhepatic cholangiography (PTC), contrast medium is injected directly into liver to visualize bile ducts; used to detect obstructions, 277

Percutaneous transluminal coronary angioplasty (PTCA), method for treating localized coronary artery narrowing; balloon catheter is inserted through skin into coronary artery and inflated to dilate narrow blood vessel, 163

Perforated ulcer, 272

Pericardial cavity, cavity formed by serous membrane sac surrounding heart, 34, 35, 35t

Pericarditis, inflammatory process or disease of pericardium, 10, 157

Pericardium, double-walled outer sac around heart; inner layer of pericardium is called epicardium, outer layer is heart itself; this sac contains pericardial fluid that reduces friction caused by heart beating, 141f, 142, 142f

Perimetritis, inflammation around uterus, 344

Perimetrium, outer layer of uterus, 334, 334f

Perineal, pertaining to perineum, 341

Perineum, in male, external region between scrotum and anus; in female, external region between vagina and anus, 335, 336, 337f, 354, 355

Periodontal disease, disease of supporting structures of teeth, including gums and bones, 271

Periodontal ligaments, small ligaments that anchor root of tooth in socket of jaw, 260, 261, 261f

Periodontics, branch of dentistry concerned with treating conditions involving gums and tissues surrounding teeth; specialist is a *periodontist,* 269

Periodontist, dental specialist in treating conditions involving gums and tissues surrounding teeth, 269

Perioperative, period of time that includes before, during, and after surgical procedure, 524

Periosteum, membrane that covers most bones; contains numerous nerves and lymphatic vessels, 86, 87f

Peripheral nervous system (PNS), portion of nervous system that contains cranial nerves and spinal nerves; these nerves are mainly responsible for voluntary muscle movement, smell, taste, sight, and hearing, 412, 418–20

Peripheral neuropathy, damage to nerves in lower legs and hands as a result of diabetes mellitus; symptoms include either extreme sensitivity or numbness and tingling, 392

Peripheral vascular disease (PVD), any abnormal condition affecting blood vessels outside heart; symptoms may include pain, pallor, numbness, and loss of circulation and pulses, 158

Peristalsis, wavelike muscular movements in wall of digestive system tube—esophagus, stomach, small intestines, and colon—that function to move food along tube, 261

Peritoneal, pertaining to peritoneum, 40

Peritoneal dialysis, removal of toxic waste substances from body by placing warm chemically balanced solutions into peritoneal cavity; used in treating renal failure and certain poisonings, 314, 314f

Peritoneoscopy, 278

Peritoneum, membranous sac that lines abdominal cavity and encases abdominopelvic organs; kidneys are exception since they lay outside peritoneum and alongside vertebral column, 34, 35

Peritubular capillaries, capillary bed surrounding renal tubules, 300f, 302, 302f

Permanent teeth, 32 permanent teeth begin to erupt at about age 6; generally complete by age sixteen, 260, 261

Pernicious anemia (PA), anemia associated with insufficient absorption of vitamin B$_{12}$ by digestive system, 186

Peroneal artery, 148f

Peroneal nerve, 419f

Personality disorders, inflexible or maladaptive behavior patterns that affect person's ability to function in society; includes paranoid personality disorder, narcissistic personality disorder, antisocial personality disorder, and passive aggressive personality, 502

Perspiration, another term for sweating, 56

Pertussis, contagious bacterial infection of larynx, trachea, and bronchi characterized by coughing attacks that end with whooping sound; also called *whooping cough,* 223

Petechiae, flat, pinpoint, purplish spots from bleeding under skin, 61, 61*f*

Petit mal seizure, 422

pH, 303*t*

Phacoemulsification, use of high-frequency sound waves to emulsify (liquefy) lens with cataract, which is then aspirated (removed by suction) with needle, 462

Phagocyte, neutrophil component of blood; has ability to ingest and destroy bacteria, 181

Phagocytosis, process of engulfing or ingesting material; several types of white blood cells function by engulfing bacteria, 181, 181*t*

Phalangeal, pertaining to phalanges or finger and toe bones, 99

Phalanges, finger bones in upper extremities and toe bones in lower extremities, 92, 92*f*, 94, 94*f*, 95*f*, 95*t*

Pharmaceutical, related to medications or pharmacies, 491

Pharmacist (RPh or PharmD), receives drug requests made by physicians, and gathers pertinent information that would affect dispensing of certain drugs, reviews patients' medications for drug interactions, provides healthcare workers with information regarding drugs, and educates public, 491

Pharmacology, study of origins, nature, properties, and effects of drugs on living organism, 490–98
   abbreviations, 498
   drug administration routes and methods, 494, 494–69*t*
   drug names, 491, 491*t*
   legal classification of drugs, 492, 492*t*
   prescription reading, 493–94
   vocabulary, 96–97

Pharyngeal, pertaining to pharynx, 229, 268

Pharyngeal tonsils, another term for *adenoids;* tonsils are collection of lymphatic tissue found in nasopharynx to combat microorganisms entering body through nose, 196, 222

Pharyngitis, inflammation of mucous membrane of pharynx, usually caused by viral or bacterial infection; commonly called *sore throat,* 233

Pharyngoplasty, surgical repair of pharynx, 281

Pharyngoplegia, paralysis of pharynx, 271

Pharynx, medical term for throat; passageway that conducts air from nasal cavity to trachea and also carries food and drink from mouth to esophagus; pharynx is divided into three sections: nasopharynx, oropharynx, and laryngopharynx, 29*t*, 196, 221*f*, 222, 258, 259*f*, 261, 271

Pheochromocytoma, usually benign tumor of adrenal medulla that secretes epinephrine; symptoms include anxiety, heart palpitations, dyspnea, profuse sweating, headache, and nausea, 392

Phimosis, narrowing of foreskin over glans penis that results in difficulty with hygiene; condition can lead to infection or difficulty with urination; treated with circumcision, surgical removal of foreskin, 359

Phlebitis, inflammation of a vein, 158

Phlebography, 149

Phlebotomist, 188, 188*f*

Phlebotomy, creating opening into vein to withdraw blood, 188, 188*f*

Phlegm, thick mucus secreted by membranes that line respiratory tract; when phlegm is coughed through mouth, is called *sputum;* phlegm is examined for color, odor, and consistency, 232

Phobias, type of anxiety disorder in which person has irrational fears; example is arachnophobia, fear of spiders, 500

Phonophoresis, use of ultrasound waves to introduce medication across skin into subcutaneous tissues, 517

Photophobia, strong sensitivity to bright light, 456

Photorefractive keratectomy (PRK), use of laser to reshape cornea to correct errors of refraction, 462

Photosensitivity, condition in which skin reacts abnormally when exposed to light such as ultraviolet rays of sun, 61

Physical medicine, use of natural methods, including physical therapy, to cure diseases and disorders, 515

Physical therapy (PT), treating disorders using physical means and methods; physical therapy personnel assess joint motion, muscle strength and endurance, function of heart and lungs, and performance of activities required in daily living, along with other responsibilities; physical therapy treatment includes gait training, therapeutic exercise, massage, joint and soft tissue mobilization, thermal and cryotherapy, electrical stimulation, ultrasound, and hydrotherapy; methods strengthen muscles, improve motion and circulation, reduce pain, and increase function, 514

Physician's offices, individual or groups of physicians providing diagnostic and treatment services in arivate office setting rather than hospital, 13

Physician's orders, medical record document that contains complete list of care, medications, tests, and treatments physician orders for patient, 12

Physician's progress notes, part of patient's medical record; physician's daily record of patient's condition, results of physician's examinations, summary of test results, updated assessment and diagnoses, and further plans for patient's care, 12

Physician's Desk Reference (PDR), 492

Pia mater, term means soft mother; this thin innermost meninges layer is applied directly to surface of brain, 417, 417f

Pineal gland, gland in endocrine system that produces hormone called melatonin, 30t, 297f, 397f, 380, 384, 384f

Pinealectomy, surgical removal of pineal gland, 397

Pinna, also called *auricle;* external ear, which functions to capture sound waves as they go past outer ear, 467, 467f

Pisse prophets, 298

Pituitary, pertaining to pituitary gland, 389

Pituitary anterior lobe, 381t

Pituitary gland, endocrine gland located behind optic nerve in brain; also called master gland since it controls functions of many other endocrine glands; is divided into two lobes: anterior and posterior; anterior pituitary gland secretes hormones that aid in controlling growth and stimulating thyroid gland, sexual glands, and adrenal cortex; posterior pituitary is responsible for antidiuretic hormone and oxytocin, 30t, 379f, 380, 384–86, 385f, 393, 414f

Pituitary posterior lobe, 381t

Placebo, inactive, harmless substance used to satisfy patient's desire for medication; also given to control groups of patients in research studies in which another group receives drug; effect of placebo versus drug is then observed, 497

Placenta, also called afterbirth; organ attached to uterine wall composed of maternal and fetal tissues; oxygen, nutrients, carbon dioxide, and wastes are exchanged between mother and baby through placenta; baby is attached to placenta by way of umbilical cord, 336, 337, 337f

Placenta previa, occurs when placenta is in lower portion of uterus and thus blocks birth canal, 346, 346f

Placental stage, third stage of labor, which takes place after delivery of infant; uterus resumes strong contractions and placenta detaches from uterine wall and is delivered through vagina, 338, 338f

Plantar flexion, bend sole of foot; point toes downward, 116, 116f

Plaque, yellow, fatty deposit of lipids in artery, 154, 154f, 155f

Plasma, liquid portion of blood containing 90% water; remaining 10% consists of plasma proteins (serum albumin, serum globulin, fibrinogen, and prothrombin), inorganic substances (calcium, potassium, and sodium), organic components (glucose, amino acids, cholesterol), and waste products (urea, uric acid, ammonia, and creatinine), 28t, 179f, 180

Plasma proteins, proteins that are found in plasma; includes serum albumin, serum globulin, fibrinogen, and prothrombin, 180

Plasmapheresis, method of removing plasma from body without depleting formed elements; whole blood is removed and cells and plasma are separated; cells are returned to patient along with donor plasma transfusion, 189

Plastic surgery, surgical specialty involved in repair, reconstruction, or improvement of body structures such as skin that are damaged, missing, or misshapen; physician is plastic surgeon, 58

Platelet count, blood test to determine number of platelets in given volume of blood, 188

Platelets, cells responsible for coagulation of blood; also called thrombocytes and contain no hemoglobin, 28t, 179f, 180, 182f

Pleura, protective double layer of serous membrane around lungs; parietal membrane is outer layer and visceral layer is inner membrane; secretes thin, watery fluid to reduce friction associated with lung movement, 34, 35, 224

Pleural, pertaining to pleura, 41

Pleural cavity, cavity formed by serous membrane sac surrounding lungs, 34, 35, 35t, 224

Pleural effusion, abnormal presence of fluid or gas in pleural cavity; physicians can detect presence of fluid by tapping chest (percussion) or listening with stethoscope (auscultation), 237

Pleural rub, grating sound made when two surfaces, such as pleural surfaces, rub together during respiration; caused when one of surfaces becomes thicker as result of inflammation or other disease conditions; rub can be felt through fingertips when placed on chest wall or heard through stethoscope, 232

Pleurectomy, excision of pleura, 241

Pleurisy, inflammation of pleura, 237

Pleuritis, 237

Pleurocentesis, puncture of pleura to withdraw fluid from thoracic cavity in order to diagnose disease, 241

Pleurodynia, pleural pain, 232

Plural endings, 10

Pneumoconiosis, condition resulting from inhaling environmental particles that become toxic, such as coal dust (anthracosis) or asbestos (asbestosis), 236

Pneumocystis pneumonia (PCP), Pneumonia with a nonproductive cough, very little fever, and dyspnea caused by fungus *Pneumocystis jirovecii;* opportunistic infection often seen in those with weakened immune systems, such as AIDS patients, 203, 236

Pneumonia, inflammatory condition of lung, which can be caused by bacterial and viral infections, diseases, and chemicals, 236

Pneumothorax, collection of air or gas in pleural cavity, which can result in collapse of lung, 237, 237*f*

Podiatrist, 100

Podiatry, healthcare profession specializing in diagnosis and treatment of disorders of feet and lower legs; healthcare professional is *podiatrist,* 100

Poliomyelitis, acute viral disease that causes inflammation of gray matter of spinal cord, resulting in paralysis in some cases; has been brought under almost total control through vaccinations, 427

Polyarteritis, inflammation of many arteries, 158

Polycystic kidneys, formation of multiple cysts within kidney tissue; results in destruction of normal kidney tissue and uremia, 309, 309*f*

Polycythemia vera, production of too many red blood cells in bone marrow, 186

Polydipsia, condition of having excessive amount of thirst, such as in diabetes, 391

Polymyositis, disease involving muscle inflammation and weakness from unknown cause, 121

Polyneuritis, inflammation of many nerves, 429

Polyp, small tumor with pedicle or stem attachment; commonly found in vascular organs such as nose, uterus, and rectum, 274, 275*f*

Polyphagia, to eat excessively, 270

Polyposis, small tumors that contain pedicle or footlike attachment in mucous membranes of large intestine (colon), 274, 275*f*

Polysomnography, monitoring a patient while sleeping to identify sleep apnea; also called *sleep apnea study,* 239

Polyuria, condition of having excessive urine production; can be a symptom of disease conditions such as diabetes, 307, 391

Pons, this portion of brain stem forms bridge between cerebellum and cerebrum; also where nerve fibers cross from one side of brain to control functions and movement on other side of brain, 414, 414*f,* 415, 415*f*

Pontine, pertaining to pons, 421

Popliteal artery, 148*f*

Popliteal vein, 150*f*

Positron emission tomography (PET), use of positive radionuclides to reconstruct brain sections; measurements can be taken of oxygen and glucose uptake, cerebral blood flow, and blood volume, 431, 510, 510*f*

Posterior, directional term meaning near or on back or spinal cord side of body, 37*f,* 37*t*

Posterior lobe, posterior portion of pituitary gland; secretes antidiuretic hormone and oxytocin, 385

Posterior pituitary gland, 384*f*

Posterior tibial artery, 148*f*

Posterior tibial vein, 150*f*

Posteroanterior (PA) view, positioning patient so that X-rays pass through body from back to front, 507

Postoperative, period of time immediately following surgery, 524

Postpartum, period immediately after delivery or childbirth, 341

Postprandial (PP), pertaining to after a meal, 270

Postural drainage, draining secretions from bronchi by placing patient in position that uses gravity to promote drainage; used for treatment of cystic fibrosis and bronchiectasis, and before lobectomy surgery, 240

Postural drainage with clapping, drainage of secretions from bronchi or a lung cavity by having patient lie so that gravity allows drainage to occur; clapping is using hand in cupped position to perform percussion on chest; assists in loosening secretions and mucus, 517

Potassium, inorganic substance found in plasma; important for bones and muscles, 180

Potentiation, giving patient second drug to boost (potentiate) effect of another drug; total strength of drugs is greater than sum of strength of individual drugs, 497

Preeclampsia, toxemia of pregnancy that, if untreated, can result in true eclampsia; symptoms include hypertension, headaches, albumin in urine, and edema, 346

Prefix, word part added in front of word root; frequently gives information about location of organ, number of parts or time (frequency); not all medical terms have prefix, 2, 3, 4–6

number, 6

Pregnancy, time from fertilization of ovum to birth of newborn, 314, 336–39

labor and delivery, 338–39

Pregnancy test, chemical test that can determine pregnancy during first few weeks; can be performed in physician's office or with home-testing kit, 347

Premature, infant born prior to 37 weeks of gestation, 337

Premenstrual syndrome (PMS), symptoms that develop just prior to onset of menstrual period, which can include irritability, headache, tender breasts, and anxiety, 344

Premolar, another term for bicuspid teeth, 260, 260f

Preoperative (preop, pre-op), period of time preceding surgery, 524

Prepatellar bursitis, 96

Prepuce, also called foreskin; protective covering over glans penis; this covering of skin is removed during circumcision, 355

Presbycusis, loss of hearing that can accompany aging process, 472

Presbyopia, visual loss due to old age, resulting in difficulty in focusing for near vision (such as reading), 456

Prescription, written explanation to pharmacist regarding name of medication, dosage, and times of administration, 492, 493, 493f

Prescription drug, drug that can only be ordered by licensed physician, dentist, or veterinarian, 492

Pressure equalizing tube (PE tube), small tube surgically placed in child's ear to assist in drainage of infection, 476

Priapism, persistent and painful erection due to pathological causes, not sexual arousal, 359

Primary site, designates where malignant tumor first appeared, 528

Primigravida, woman who has been pregnant once, 341

Primipara, woman who has given birth once, 341

Probe, surgical instrument used to explore tissue, 521t

Procedural suffixes, 8–9

Process, projection from surface of a bone, 88

Proctologist, specialist in rectum, 269

Proctology, branch of medicine specializing in conditions of lower gastrointestinal system, 29t, 269

Proctopexy, surgical fixation of rectum, 281

Proctoptosis, drooping rectum, 275

Progesterone, one of hormones produced by ovaries; works with estrogen to control menstrual cycle, 332, 333, 381t, 382

Prolactin (PRL), hormone secreted by anterior pituitary; stimulates milk production, 381t, 385

Prolapsed umbilical cord, when umbilical cord of baby is expelled first during delivery and is squeezed between baby's head and vaginal wall; presents emergency situation since baby's circulation is compromised, 346

Prolapsed uterus, fallen uterus that can cause cervix to protrude through vaginal opening; generally caused by weakened muscles from vaginal delivery or as result of pelvic tumors pressing down, 344

Pronation, to turn downward or backward, as with hand or foot, 118t, 119f

Prone, directional term meaning lying horizontally facing downward, 38f, 38t

Prone position, 522f, 523t

Pronunciation, of medical terms, 9–10

Prophylaxis, prevention of disease; for example, antibiotic can be used to prevent occurrence of disease, 497

Proprietary name, name a pharmaceutical company chooses as trademark or market name for its drug; also called *brand* or *trade name,* 491

Prostate cancer, slow-growing cancer that affects large number of males after age 50; PSA (prostate-specific antigen) test is used to assist in early detection of this disease, 357

Prostate gland, gland in male reproductive system that produces fluids that nourish sperm, 30t, 35t, 300f, 301f, 353f, 354, 354f, 356

Prostate-specific antigen (PSA), blood test to screen for prostate cancer; elevated blood levels of PSA associated with prostate cancer, 360

Prostatectomy, surgical removal of prostate gland, 361

Prostatic, pertaining to prostate gland, 357

Prostatitis, inflamed condition of prostate gland that may be result of infection, 359

Prosthesis, artificial device used as substitute for body part either congenitally missing or absent as result of accident or disease; for instance, artificial leg or hip prosthesis, 107

Prosthetic hip joint, 108f

Prosthetic lens implant, use of artificial lens to replace lens removed during cataract surgery, 462

Prosthetics, artificial devices, such as limbs and joints, that replace missing body part, 100, 515

Prosthetist, 100

Protease inhibitor drugs, medications that inhibit protease, enzyme viruses need to reproduce, 205

Protein-bound iodine test (PBI), blood test to measure concentration of thyroxine (T_4) circulating in blood stream; iodine becomes bound to protein in blood and can be measured; useful in establishing thyroid function, 395

Proteinuria, protein in urine, 307

Prothrombin, protein element within blood that interacts with calcium salts to form thrombin, 182

Prothrombin time (Pro time), measurement of time it takes for sample of blood to coagulate, 188

Protocol (prot), actual plan of care, including medications, surgeries, and treatments for care of patient; often, entire healthcare team, including physician, oncologist, radiologist, nurse, and patient, will assist in designing treatment plan, 526

Proton pump inhibitor, blocks stomach's ability to secrete acid; used to treat peptic ulcers and gastroesophageal reflux disease, 281

Protozoans, single-celled organisms that can infect body, 197

Proximal, directional term meaning located closest to point of attachment to body, 37f, 37t

Proximal convoluted tubule, portion of renal tubule, 299, 300f, 302f

Pruritus, severe itching, 61

Pseudocyesis, false pregnancy, 346

Pseudohypertrophic muscular dystrophy, one type of inherited muscular dystrophy in which muscle tissue is gradually replaced by fatty tissue, making muscle look strong, 121

Psoriasis, chronic inflammatory condition consisting of crusty papules forming patches with circular borders, 67, 67f

Psychiatric nurse, nurse with additional training in care of patients with mental, emotional, and behavioral disorders, 500

Psychiatric social work, social worker with additional training in care of patients with mental, emotional, or behavioral disorders, 500

Psychiatrist (MD or DO), physician with specialized training in diagnosing and treating mental disorders; prescribes medication and conducts counseling, 500

Psychiatry, branch of medicine that deals with the diagnosis, treatment, and prevention of mental disorders, 500

Psychoanalysis, method of obtaining a detailed account of past and present emotional and mental experiences from patient to determine source of problem and eliminate effects, 505

Psychology, study of human behavior and thought process; behavioral science is primarily concerned with understanding how human beings interact with their physical environment and with each other, 500

Psychopharmacology, study of effects of drugs on mind and particularly use of drugs in treating mental disorders; main classes of drugs for treatment of mental disorders are antipsychotic drugs, antidepressant drugs, minor tranquilizers, and lithium, 504

Psychotherapy, method of treating mental disorders by mental rather than chemical or physical means; includes psychoanalysis, humanistic therapies, and family and group therapy, 505

Pterygium, hypertrophied conjunctival tissue in inner corner of eye, 459

Puberty, beginning of menstruation and ability to reproduce; usually occurs around age 16, 335

Pubic, pertaining to pubis; one of pelvic bones, 99

Pubic region, genital region of body, 33, 33f

Pubis, one of three bones that form os coxae or innominate bone, 88, 89f, 94, 95f, 95t

Pulmonary, pertaining to lung, 229

Pulmonary angiography, injecting dye into blood vessel for purpose of taking X-ray of arteries and veins of lungs, 239

Pulmonary artery, large artery that carries deoxygenated blood from right ventricle to lung, 140f, 144, 145f

Pulmonary capillaries, network of capillaries in lungs that tightly encase each alveolus; site of gas exchange, 223

Pulmonary circulation, pulmonary circulation transports deoxygenated blood from right side of heart to lungs where oxygen and carbon dioxide are exchanged; then it carries oxygenated blood back to left side of heart, 140

Pulmonary edema, condition in which lung tissue retains excessive amount of fluid; results in labored breathing, 236

Pulmonary embolism, blood clot or air bubble in pulmonary artery or one of its branches, 236

Pulmonary fibrosis, formation of fibrous scar tissue in lungs, which leads to decreased ability to expand lungs; may be caused by infections, pneumoconiosis, autoimmune diseases, and toxin exposure, 236

Pulmonary function test (PFT), breathing equipment used to determine respiratory function and measure lung volumes and gas exchange, 225, 239

Pulmonary semilunar valve, 144f

Pulmonary trunk, 133f, 142f

Pulmonary valve, semilunar valve between right ventricle and pulmonary artery in heart; prevents blood from flowing backwards into ventricle, 142f, 143, 144f, 145f

Pulmonary vein, large vein that returns oxygenated blood from lungs to left atrium, 140f, 144, 145f

Pulmonologist, physician specialized in treating diseases and disorders of respiratory system, 229

Pulmonology, branch of medicine specializing in conditions of respiratory system, 29t

Pulp cavity, hollow interior of tooth; contains soft tissue made up of blood vessels, nerves, and lymph vessels, 260, 261, 261f

Pulse (P), expansion and contraction produced by blood as it moves through artery; pulse can be taken at several pulse points throughout body where artery is close to surface, 149

Pupil, hole in center of iris; size of pupil is changed by iris dilating or constricting, 447f, 448f, 449, 452f

Pupillary, pertaining to pupil, 454

Purified protein derivative (PPD), 239

Purkinje fibers, part of conduction system of heart; found in ventricular myocardium, 144, 146f

Purpura, hemorrhages into skin and mucous membranes, 61, 61f,

Purulent, pus-filled sputum, which can be result of infection, 61

Pustule, raised spot on skin containing pus, 62, 62f

Pyelitis, inflammation of renal pelvis, 309

Pyelogram, x-ray record of the pelvis after injection of radiopaque dye, 311

Pyelonephritis, inflammation of renal pelvis and kidney; one of most common types of kidney disease; may be result of lower urinary tract infection that moved up to kidney by way of ureters; may be large quantities of white blood cells and bacteria in urine, and blood (hematuria) may even be present in urine in this condition; can occur with any untreated or persistent case of cystitis, 309

Pyeloplasty, surgical repair of renal pelvis, 315

Pyloric, pertaining to pylorus, 268

Pyloric sphincter, sphincter at distal end of stomach; controls passage of food into duodenum, 262, 262f, 265f

Pyoderma, pus producing skin infection, 62

Pyosalpinx, condition of having pus in fallopian tubes, 343

Pyothorax, condition of having pus in chest cavity, 232, 237

Pyromania, impulse control disorder in which patient is unable to control impulse to start fires, 502

Pyrosis, heartburn, 270

Pyuria, presence of pus in urine, 307

Q

Quadriplegia, paralysis of all four extremities; same as tetraplegia, 423

R

Radial, pertaining to radius; lower arm bone, 99

Radial artery, 148f

Radial keratotomy, spokelike incisions around cornea that result in it becoming flatter; surgical treatment for myopia, 463

Radial nerve, 419f

Radial vein, 150f

Radiation therapy, use of X-rays to treat disease, especially cancer, 529

Radical mastectomy, surgical removal of breast tissue plus chest muscles and axillary lymph nodes, 350

Radical surgery, extensive surgery to remove as much tissue associated with tumor as possible, 529

Radiculitis, nerve root inflammation, 429

Radiculopathy, disease of nerve root, 429

Radioactive implant, embedding radioactive source directly into tissue to provide highly localized radiation dosage to damage nearby cancerous cells; also called *brachytherapy,* 529

Radiography, making of X-ray pictures, 100, 507

Radioimmunoassay (RIA), test used to measure levels of hormones in plasma of blood, 396

Radioisotope, radioactive form of element, 507

Radiologist, physician who practices diagnosis and treatment by use of radiant energy; responsible for interpreting X-ray films, 507

Radiology, branch of medicine that uses radioactive substances such as X-rays, isotopes, and radiation to prevent, diagnose, and treat diseases, 510

Radiolucent, structures that allow X-rays to pass through and expose photographic plate, making it appear as black area on X-ray, are termed radiolucent, 507

Radiopaque, structures impenetrable to X-rays, appearing as light area on radiograph (X-ray), 507

Radius, one of forearm bones in upper extermity, 92, 93f, 94, 94f

Range of motion (ROM), range of movement of a joint, from maximum flexion through maximum extension; measured as degrees of a circle, 516

Raynaud's phenomenon, periodic ischemic attacks affecting extremities of body, especially fingers, toes, ears, and nose; affected extremities become cyanotic and very painful; attacks are brought on by arterial constriction due to extreme cold or emotional stress, 158

Reabsorption, second phase of urine production; substances needed by body are reabsorbed as filtrate passes through kidney tubules, 302

Recklinghausen disease, excessive production of parathyroid hormone, which results in degeneration of bones, 393

Rectal, (1) pertaining to rectum; (2) substances introduced directly into rectal cavity in form of suppositories or solution; drugs may have to be administered by this route if patient is unable to take them by mouth due to nausea, vomiting, and surgery, 268, 494, 496t

Rectocele, protrusion or herniation of rectum into vagina, 344

Rectum, area at end of digestive tube for storage of feces that leads to anus, 258, 263, 263f, 264f, 332f, 335f, 337f, 354f

Rectus abdominis, muscle named for its location and direction of its fibers: rectus means straight and abdominis means abdominal, 115

Rectus muscles, rectus means straight; four of eye muscles are rectus muscles, 450, 450f

Red blood cell count (RBC), blood test to determine number of erythrocytes in volume of blood; decrease in red blood cells may indicate anemia; increase may indicate polycythemia, 188

Red blood cell morphology, examination of blood for abnormalities in shape (morphology) of erythrocytes; used to determine diseases like sickle-cell anemia, 188

Red blood cells (RBC), also called erythrocytes or RBCs; cells that contain hemoglobin and iron-containing pigment that binds oxygen in order to transport it to cells of body, 169f, 170

Red bone marrow, tissue that manufactures most of blood cells; found in cancellous bone cavities, 86, 87

Reduction, correcting a fracture by realigning bone fragments; *closed reduction* is doing this without entering body; *open reduction* is making surgical incision at site of fracture to do reduction, often necessary where there are bony fragments to be removed, 109

Refractive error test, eye examination performed by physician to determine and correct refractive errors in eye, 461

Refracts, bending of light rays as they enter eye, 448

Regional anesthesia, regional anesthesia is also referred to as nerve block; anesthetic interrupts patient's pain sensation in a particular region of body; anesthetic is injected near nerve that will be blocked from sensation; patient usually remains conscious, 520, 521t

Regional ileitis, 272

Regurgitation, to flow backwards; in cardiovascular system refers to blood flowing backwards through valve; in digestive system refers to food flowing backwards from stomach to mouth, 154, 270

Rehabilitation, process of treatment and exercise that can help person with disability attain maximum function and well-being, 516

Rehabilitation centers, facilities that provide intensive physical and occupational therapy; include inpatient and outpatient treatment, 13

Rehabilitation services, 513–18

    abbreviations, 518

    occupational therapy, 514

    physical therapy, 514

    therapeutic procedures, 516–18

    vocabulary, 514–16

Reinfection, infection that occurs when person becomes infected again with same pathogen that originally brought him or her to hospital, 198

Relapse, return of disease symptoms after period of improvement, 528

Remission, period during which symptoms of disease or disorder leave; can be temporary, 528

Renal, pertaining to kidney, 305

Renal artery, artery that originates from abdominal aorta and carries blood to nephrons of kidney, 148f, 298, 299f, 302f

Renal cell carcinoma, cancerous tumor that arises from kidney tubule cells, 309

Renal colic, pain caused by kidney stone, which can be excruciating and generally requires medical treatment, 307

Renal corpuscle, part of a nephron; double-walled cuplike structure called glomerular capsule or Bowman's capsule and contains capillary network called glomerulus; afferent arteriole carries blood to glomerulus and efferent arteriole carries blood away from glomerulus; filtration stage of urine production occurs in renal corpuscle as wastes are filtered from blood in glomerulus and enter Bowman's capsule, 299

Renal failure, inability of kidneys to filter wastes from blood resulting in uremia; may be acute or chronic; major reason for patient being placed on dialysis, 310

Renal papilla, tip of renal pyramid, 298, 299f

Renal pelvis, large collecting site for urine within kidney; collects urine from each calyx; urine leaves renal pelvis via ureter, 298, 299f

Renal pyramid, triangular-shaped region of renal medulla, 298, 299f

Renal transplant, surgical replacement with a donor kidney, 315, 315f

Renal tubule, network of tubes found in a nephron; consists of proximal convoluted tubule, loop of Henle, distal tubule, and collecting tubule; reabsorption and secretion stages of urine production occur within renal tubule; as glomerular filtrate passes through renal tubule, most of water and some of dissolved substances, such as amino acids and electrolytes, are reabsorbed; at same time, substances that are too large to filter into Bowman's capsule, such as urea, are secreted directly from bloodstream into renal tubule; filtrate that reaches collecting tubule becomes urine, 299

Renal vein, vein that carries blood away from kidneys, 150f, 298, 299f, 302f

Repetitive motion disorder, group of chronic disorders involving tendon, muscle, joint, and nerve damage, resulting from tissue being subjected to pressure, vibration, or repetitive movements for prolonged periods, 121

Reproductive system, 329–79

Resection, to surgically cut out; excision, 524

Residual hearing, amount of hearing that is still present after damage has occurred to auditory mechanism, 472

Residual volume (RV), air remaining in lungs after forced exhalation, 215t

Respirator, 240

Respiratory membrane, formed by tight association of walls of alveoli and capillaries; gas exchange between lungs and blood occurs across this membrane, 223, 224f

Respiratory muscles, 226

Respiratory rate, 277, 277t

Respiratory system, system that brings oxygen into lungs and expels carbon dioxide; organs include nose, pharynx, larynx, trachea, bronchial tubes, and lungs, 29t, 217–54, 218f

   abbreviations, 243

   anatomical terms, 228–29

   anatomy and physiology, 220–27

   bronchial tubes, 223–24

   diagnostic procedures, 238–39

   larynx, 222

   lung volumes/capacities, 225

   lungs, 224

   muscles, 226

   nasal cavity, 220–21

   pathology, 229–37

   pharmacology, 242–43

   pharynx, 222

   rate, 227

   terminology, 227–29

   therapeutic procedures, 240–42

   trachea, 223

Respiratory therapist (RT), allied health professional whose duties include conducting pulmonary function tests, monitoring oxygen and carbon dioxide levels in blood, and administering breathing treatments, 225, 229

Respiratory therapy, allied health specialty that assists patients with respiratory and cardiopulmonary disorders, 229

Retina, innermost layer of eye; contains visual receptors called rods and cones; rods and cones receive light impulses and transmit them to brain via optic nerve, 447f, 448, 448f, 449, 449f, 452f

Retinal, pertaining to retina, 454

Retinal arteries, 452f

Retinal blood vessels, blood vessels that supply oxygen to rods and cones of retina, 449

Retinal detachment, occurs when retina becomes separated from choroid layer; separation seriously damages blood vessels and nerves, resulting in blindness, 458

Retinal veins, 430f

Retinitis pigmentosa, progressive disease of eye resulting in retina becoming hard (sclerosed), pigmented (colored), and atrophied (wasting away); no known cure, 458

Retinoblastoma, malignant glioma of retina, 458

Retinopathy, retinal disease, 458

Retinopexy, surgical fixation of retina, 463

Retrograde pyelogram (RP), diagnostic X-ray in which dye is inserted through urethra to outline bladder, ureters, and renal pelvis, 312, 312f

Retroperitoneal, pertaining to behind peritoneum; used to describe position of kidneys, which is outside of peritoneal sac alongside spine, 35, 298

Retrovirus, 202

Reverse transcriptase inhibitor drugs, medication that inhibits reverse transcriptase, enzyme needed to viruses to reproduce, 205

Reye's syndrome, brain inflammation that occurs in children following viral infection, usually flu or chickenpox; characterized by vomiting and lethargy and may lead to coma and death, 427

Rh factor, antigen marker found on erythrocytes of persons with Rh+ blood, 182–83

Rh-negative (Rh-), person with Rh– blood type; person's RBCs do not have Rh marker and will make antibodies against Rh+ blood, 183

Rh-positive (Rh+), person with Rh+ blood type; person's RBCs have Rh marker, 183

Rheumatoid arthritis (RA), chronic form of arthritis with inflammation of joints, swelling, stiffness, pain, and changes in cartilage that can result in crippling deformities, 105, 105f

Rhinitis, inflammation of nose, 232

Rhinomycosis, condition of having fungal infection in nose, 232

Rhinoplasty, plastic surgery of nose, 233

Rhinorrhagia, rapid and excessive flow of blood from nose, 241

Rhinorrhea, watery discharge from nose, expecially with allergies or a cold, runny nose, 232

Rhonchi, somewhat musical sound during expiration, often found in asthma or infection, and caused by spasms of bronchial tubes; also called *wheezing*, 232

Rhytidectomy, surgical removal of excess skin to eliminate wrinkles; commonly referred to as a *facelift,* 71

Rib cage, also called chest cavity; formed by curved ribs extending from vertebral column around sides and attaching to sternum; ribs are part of axial skeleton, 89, 91, 92*f*

Ribs, 90*f,* 91*f*

Rickets, deficiency in calcium and vitamin D found in early childhood that results in bone deformities, especially bowed legs, 103

Right atrium, 140*f,* 142*f,* 145*f*

Right coronary artery, 147*f*

Right hypochondriac, anatomical division of abdomen; right upper row, 36*t*

Right iliac, anatomical division of abdomen; right lower row; also called *right inguinal,* 36*t*

Right lower quadrant (RLQ), clinical division of abdomen; contains portions of small and large intestines, right ovary and fallopian tube, appendix, right ureter, 36*t*

Right lumbar, anatomical division of abdomen, right middle row, 36*t*

Right lymphatic duct, one of two large lymphatic ducts drains right arm and right side of neck and chest; empties lymph into right subclavian vein, 194, 195

Right upper quadrant (RUQ), clinical division of abdomen; contains right lobe of liver, gallbladder, portion of pancreas, and portions of small and large intestine, 36*t*

Right ventricle, 140*f,* 142*f,* 145*f*

Rinne and Weber tuning-fork tests, physician holds tuning fork, instrument that produces constant pitch when it is struck against or near bones on side of head; these tests assess both nerve and bone conduction of sound, 474

Rods, sensory receptors of retina that are active in dim light and do not perceive color, 449

Roentgen (r), unit for describing exposure dose of radiation, 508

Roentgenology, X-rays, 507

Root, portion of tooth below gum line, 260, 261*f*

Root canal, dental treatment involving pulp cavity of root of tooth; procedure used to save tooth that is badly infected or abscessed, 260, 261, 261*f,* 279

Rotation, moving around a central axis, 118*t*

Rotator cuff injury, rotator cuff consists of joint capsule of shoulder joint reinforced by tendons from several shoulder muscles; at high risk for strain or tearing injuries, 112

Round window, 468*f*

Route of administration, 494

Rubella, contagious viral skin infection; commonly called *German measles,* 67

Rugae, prominent folds in mucosa of stomach; smooth out and almost disappear allowing stomach to expand when full of food; also found in urinary bladder, 262, 262*f,* 300

Rule of nines, 65*f*

S

Saccule, found in inner ear; plays role in equilibrium, 468

Sacral, pertaining to sacrum, 99

Sacrum, five fused vertebrae that form large flat bone in upper buttock region, 85*f,* 89, 90*f,* 92*t*

Sagittal plane, vertical plane that divides body into left and right sections, 32, 32*f*

Sagittal section, sectional view of body produced by cut along sagittal plane, 32

Saliva, watery fluid secreted into mouth from salivary glands; contains digestive enzymes that break down carbohydrates and lubricants that make it easier to swallow food, 258

Salivary glands, exocrine glands with ducts that open into mouth; produce saliva, which makes bolus of food easier to swallow and begins digestive process; there are three pairs of salivary glands: parotid, submandibular, and sublingual, 29*t,* 257*f,* 258, 264

Salpingectomy, excision of fallopian tubes, 350

Salpingitis, inflammation of fallopian tube or tubes; also, inflammation of eustachian tube, 343, 472

Salpingocyesis, tubal pregnancy, 346

Salpingotomy, incision into fallopian tubes, 476

Sanguinous, pertaining to blood, 184

Sarcoidosis, inflammatory disease of lymph system in which lesions may appear in liver, skin, lungs, lymph nodes, spleen, eyes, and small bones of hands and feet, 203

Scabies, contagious skin disease caused by egg-laying mite that causes intense itching; often seen in children, 67

Scalpel, surgical instrument used to cut and separate tissue, 521*t*

Scan, recording emission of radioactive waves on photographic plate after substance has been injected into body, 508

Scapula, also called shoulder blade; upper extremity bone, 92, 93*f,* 94, 94*f*

Scapular, pertaining to scapula or shoulder blade, 99

Schedule I, drugs with highest potential for addiction and abuse; not accepted for medical use; examples are heroin and LSD, 492*t*

Schedule II, drugs with high potential for addiction and abuse accepted for medical use in United States; examples are codeine, cocaine, morphine, opium, and secobarbital, 492*t*

Schedule III, drugs with moderate-to-low potential for addiction and abuse; examples are butabarbital, anabolic steroids, and acetaminophen with codeine, 492t

Schedule IV, drugs with lower potential for addiction and abuse than Schedule III drugs; examples are chloral hydrate, phenobarbital, and diazepam, 492t

Schedule V, drugs with low potential for addiction and abuse; example is low-strength codeine combined with other drugs to suppress coughing, 492t

Schizophrenia, mental disorders characterized by distortions of reality such as delusions and hallucinations, 503

Schwann cell, 413f

Sciatic nerve, 419f

Sclera, tough protective outer layer of eyeball; commonly referred to as white of eye, 447f, 448, 448f

Scleral, pertaining to sclera, 454

Scleral buckling, placing a band of silicone around outside of sclera to stabilize detaching retina, 463

Scleritis, inflammation of sclera, 458

Scleroderma, disorder in which skin becomes taut, thick, and leatherlike, 62

Scleromalacia, softening of sclera, 456

Sclerotomy, incision into sclera, 453

Scoliosis, abnormal lateral curvature of spine, 104f, 105

Scratch test, form of allergy testing in which body is exposed to allergen through light scratch in skin, 204, 204f

Scrotum, sac that serves as container for testes; sac, which is divided by septum, supports testicles and lies between legs and behind penis, 354, 355

Scrub nurse, surgical assistant who hands instruments to surgeon; person wears sterile clothing and maintains sterile operative field, 524

Sebaceous cyst, sac under skin filled with sebum or oil from sebaceous gland; can grow to large size and may need to be excised, 67

Sebaceous glands, also called oil glands; produce substance called sebum that lubricates skin surface, 27t, 50, 55, 55f, 451

Seborrhea, excessive discharge of sebum, 62

Sebum, thick, oily substance secreted by sebaceous glands that lubricates skin to prevent drying out; when sebum accumulates, it can cause congestion in sebaceous glands and whiteheads or pimples may form; when sebum becomes dark it is referred to as comedo or blackhead, 55

Second-degree burn, 64, 64f

Secretion, third phase of urine production; additional waste products are added to filtrate as it passes through kidney tubules, 302

Sedative, produces relaxation without causing sleep, 433

Seizure, sudden attack of severe muscular contractions associated with loss of consciousness; seen in grand mal epilepsy, 423

Self-innoculation, infection that occurs when person becomes infected in different part of body by pathogen from another part of his or her own body, such as intestinal bacteria spreading to urethra, 198

Semen, semen contains sperm and fluids secreted by male reproductive system glands; leaves body through urethra, 354

Semen analysis, procedure used when performing fertility workup to determine if male is able to produce sperm; semen is collected by patient afer abstaining from sexual intercourse for a period of three to five days; sperm in semen are analyzed for number, swimming strength, and shape; also used to determine if vasectomy has been successful; after a period of six weeks, no sperm should be present in sample from patient, 360

Semicircular canals, portion of labyrinth associated with balance and equilibrium, 467

Semiconscious, state of being aware of surroundings and responding to stimuli only part of time, 423

Semilunar valve, heart valves located between ventricles and great arteries leaving heart; pulmonary valve is located between right ventricle, and pulmonary artery and aortic valve are located between left ventricle and aorta, 143

Seminal vesicles, two male reproductive system glands located at base of bladder; secrete fluid that nourishes sperm into vas deferens; fluid plus sperm constitutes much of semen, 30t, 35t, 96f, 353f, 354, 356

Seminiferous tubules, network of coiled tubes that make up bulk of testes; sperm development takes place in walls of tubules and mature sperm are released into tubule in order to leave testes, 354, 355

Sensorineural hearing loss, type of hearing loss in which sound is conducted normally through external and middle ear but there is a defect in inner ear or with cochlear nerve, resulting in inability to hear; hearing aid may help, 469

Sensory neurons, nerves that carry sensory information from sensory receptors to brain; also called *afferent neurons,* 418, 419f

Sensory receptors, nerve fibers located directly under skin surface; these receptors detect temperature, pain, touch, and pressure; messages for these sensations are conveyed to brain and spinal cord from nerve endings in skin, 52, 53*f*, 412

Sepsis, 185

Septal, pertaining to nasal septum, 229

Septicemia, having bacteria in blood stream; commonly referred to as *blood poisoning*, 185

Sequential multiple analyzer computer (SMAC), machine for doing multiple blood chemistry tests automatically, 188

Serous fluid, watery secretion of serous membranes, 224

Serum, clear, sticky fluid that remains after blood has clotted, 180

Serum bilirubin, blood test to determine amount of waste product bilirubin in bloodstream; elevated levels indicate liver disease, 276

Serum lipoprotein level, laboratory test to measure amount of cholesterol and triglycerides in blood, 159

Severe acute respiratory syndrome (SARS), acute viral respiratory infection that begins like the flu but quickly progresses to severe dyspnea; high fatality rate; first appeared in China in 2003, 236

Severe combined immunodeficiency syndrome (SCIDS), disease seen in children born with nonfunctioning immune system; often forced to live in sealed sterile rooms, 203

Sex hormones, hormones secreted by gonads and adrenal cortex; estrogen and progesterone in females and testosterone in males, 332, 354

Sexual disorders, disorders include aberrant sexual activity and sexual dysfunction; includes pedophilia, masochism, voyeurism, low sex drive, and premature ejaculation, 503

Sexually transmitted disease (STD), disease usually acquired as result of sexual intercourse; formerly more commonly referred to as venereal disease, 360

Shield, protective device used to protect against radiation, 508

Shingles, eruption of vesicles along nerve, causing rash and pain; caused by same virus as chickenpox, 429, 429*f*

Short bone, type of bone that is roughly cube shaped; carpals are short bones, 86, 87

Shortness of breath (SOB), term used to indicate that patient is having some difficulty breathing; cause can range from mild SOB after exercise to SOB associated with heart disease, 232

Sialadenitis, inflammation of salivary gland, 271

Sickle cell anemia, severe, chronic, incurable disorder that results in anemia and causes joint pain, chronic weakness, and infections; more common in people of Mediterranean and African heritage; actual blood cell is crescent shaped, 186, 187*f*

Side effect, response to drug other than effect desired, 497

Sigmoid colon, final section of colon; follows S-shaped path and terminates in rectum, 263, 263*f*

Sigmoidal, pertaining to sigmoid colon, 268

Sigmoidoscope, instrument to view inside sigmoid colon, 278

Sigmoidoscopy, using flexible sigmoidoscope to visually examine sigmoid colon; commonly done to diagnose cancer and polyps, 278

Silicosis, form of respiratory disease resulting from inhalation of silica (quartz) dust; considered an occupational disease, 236

Simple fracture, 100

Simple mastectomy, surgical removal of breast tissue, 350

Singular endings, 10

Sinoatrial node (SA), also called pacemaker of heart; area of right atria that initiates electrical pulse that causes heart to contract, 145, 146*f*

Sinus, hollow cavity within bone, 88, 89

Skeletal, pertaining to skeleton, 119

Skeletal muscle, voluntary muscle attached to bones by tendon, 25, 113, 113*f*, 114, 114*f*

Skeletal muscle relaxant, produces relaxation of skeletal muscle, 112

Skeletal muscle tissue, 25

Skeletal system, 27*t*, 84–110, 85*f*
   abbreviations, 110
   anatomical terms, 98–99
   anatomy and physiology, 86–96
   appendicular skeleton, 89, 92–94, 93*f*
   axial skeleton, 89–92, 90*f*
   bones, 86–89
   diagnostic procedures, 106–107
   joints, 95–96
   pathology, 99–106
   pharmacology, 109
   terminlogy, 97–98
   therapeutic procedures, 107–109

Skeleton, bones forming framework for body; site for skeletal muscle attachments, 89
   appendicular, 89, 92–94, 93*f*
   axial, 89–92, 90*f*

Skin, major organ of integumentary system; forms barrier between external and internal environments, 27*t*, 50, 51*f*, 52–54, 53*f*, 395*f*

Skin graft (SG), transfer of skin from normal area to cover another site; used to treat burn victims and after some surgical procedures, 71

Skull, **84,** 85*f*, 91*f*, 91*t*, 96*f*, 417*f*

Sleep apnea, condition in which breathing stops repeatedly during sleep long enough to cause drop in oxygen levels in blood, 236

Sleep apnea study, 239

Sleeping disorder, any condition that interferes with sleep other than environmental noises; can include difficulty sleeping (insomnia), nightmares, night terrors, sleepwalking, and apnea, 503

Sleepwalking, sleeping disorder in which patient performs complex activities while asleep, 503

Slit lamp microscopy, in ophthalmology, examining posterior surface of cornea, 461

Small intestine, portion of digestive tube between stomach and colon, and major site of nutrient absorption; there are three sections: duodenum, jejunum, and ileum, 29*t*, 35*t*, 36*t*, 257*f*, 258, 262–63, 263*f*

Smooth muscle, involuntary muscle found in internal organs such as digestive organs or blood vessels, 25, 26*f*, 113, 113*f*, 114, 147*f*, 154*f*, 224*f*

Snellen chart, chart used for testing distance vision; contains letters of varying size and is administered from distance of 20 feet; person who can read at 20 feet what average person can read at that distance is said to have 20/20 vision, 461

Sodium (Na⁺), inorganic substance found in plasma, 180

Soft palate, 221*f*, 259*f*

Somatic nerves, nerves that serve skin and skeletal muscles and are mainly involved with conscious and voluntary activities of body, 418, 420

Somatoform disorders, patient has physical symptoms for which no physical disease can be determined; include hypochondria and conversion reaction, 503

Somatotropin, another name for growth hormone; hormone that promotes growth of body by stimulating cells to rapidly increase in size and divide, 385

Sound waves, 469*f*

Spasm, sudden, involuntary, strong muscle contraction, 120

Spastic colon, 274

Specialty senses, special sense organs perceive environmental conditions; eyes, ears, nose, and tongue contain special sense organs, 31

Specialty care hospitals, hospitals that provide care for very specific types of disease; example is psychiatric hospital, 13

Specific gravity (sp. grav.), characteristic of urine that indicates amount of dissolved substances in urine, 303

Speculum, surgical instrument used to spread apart walls of cavity, 348, 348*f*, 521*t*

Spelling, of medical terms, 10

Sperm, also called spermatozoon (plural is spermatozoa); male sex cell; one sperm fuses with ovum to produce a new being, 354, 355*f*, 386, 386*f*

Sperm cells, 24*f*

Spermatic, pertaining to sperm, 357

Spermatic cord, term for cordlike collection of structures that include vas deferens, arteries, veins, nerves, and lymph vessels; spermatic cord suspends testes within scrotum, 356

Spermatocide, substance that kills sperm, 362

Spermatogenesis, formation of mature sperm, 354

Spermatolysis, destruction of sperm, 358

Spermatozoon, 355

Sphenoid bone, cranial bone, 89, 91*f*, 91*t*

Sphincter, ring of muscle around tubular organ; can contract to control opening of tube, 262, 355

Sphygmomanometer, instrument for measuring blood pressure; also referred to as *blood pressure cuff,* 149, 159, 159*f*

Spina bifida, congenital defect in walls of spinal canal in which laminae of vertebra do not meet or close; results in membranes of spinal cord being pushed through opening; can also result in other defects, such as hydrocephalus, 105, 428*f*, 428

Spinal, pertaining to spine, 41

Spinal cavity, dorsal body cavity within spinal column that contains spinal cord, 34, 35*t*, 416

Spinal column, 92*t*

Spinal cord, spinal cord provides pathway for impulses traveling to and from brain; column of nerve fibers that extends from medulla oblongata of brain down to level of second lumbar vertebra, 25, 31*t*, 35*t*, 311*f*, 412, 415*f*, 416, 416*f*, 419*f*

Spinal cord injury (SCI), bruising or severing of spinal cord from blow to vertebral column resulting in muscle paralysis and sensory impairment below injury level, 428

Spinal fusion, surgical immobilization of adjacent vertebrae; may be done for several reasons, including correction for herniated disk, 108

Spinal nerves, nerves that arise from spinal cord, 412, 419*f*

Spinal puncture, 431, 431*f*

Spinal stenosis, narrowing of spinal canal causing pressure on cord and nerves, 105

Spinal tap, 431, 431*f*

Spiral fracture, fracture in S-shaped spiral; can be caused by twisting injury, 102

Spirometer, instrument consisting of container into which patient can exhale for purpose of measuring air capacity of lungs, 239

Spirometry, using device to measure breathing capacity of lungs, 239

Spleen, organ in lymphatic system that filters microorganisms and old red blood cells from blood, 28*t*, 35*t*, 36*t*, 192*f*, 193, 196, 196*f*

Splenectomy, excision of spleen, 205

Splenic, pertaining to spleen, 200

Splenomegaly, enlargement of spleen, 201

Split-thickness skin graft (STSG), 72

Spondylolisthesis, forward sliding of lumbar vertebra over vertebra below it, 105

Spondylosis, 105

Spongy bone, bony tissue found inside bone; contains cavities that hold red bone marrow; also called *cancellous bone,* 86, 87*f*

Spontaneous abortion, loss of fetus without any artificial aid; also called *miscarriage,* 346

Sprain, pain and disability caused by trauma to joint; ligament may be torn in severe sprains, 106

Sputum, mucus or phlegm coughed up from lining of respiratory tract; tested to determine what type of bacteria of virus is present as aid in selecting proper antibiotic treatment, 232

Sputum culture and sensitivity (C&S), testing sputum by placing it on culture medium and observing any bacterial growth; specimen is then tested to determine antibiotic effectiveness, 238

Sputum cytology, testing for malignant cells in sputum, 238

Squamous cell carcinoma (SCC), epidermal cancer that may go into deeper tissue but does not generally metastasize, 67

Staging, process of classifying tumors based on degree of tissue invasion and potential response to therapy; TNM staging system is frequently used; T refers to tumor's size and invasion, N refers to lymph node involvement, and M refers to presence of metastases of tumor cells, 526–27

Staging laparotomy, surgical procedure in which abdomen is entered to determine extent and staging of tumor, 529

Staging tumors, 526–27

Standard precautions, 198

Stapedectomy, removal of stapes bone to treat otosclerosis (hardening of bone); prosthesis or artificial stapes may be implanted, 476

Stapes, one of three ossicles of middle ear; attached to oval window leading to inner ear; also called *stirrup,* 467*f*, 468, 468*f*

Stent, stainless steel tube placed within blood vessel or duct to widen lumen, 162*f*, 163

Sterility, inability to father children due to problem with spermatogenesis, 358

Sterilization, process of rendering male or female sterile or unable to conceive children, 361

Sternal, pertaining to sternum or breast bone, 99

Sternocleidomastoid, muscle named for its attachments, sternum, clavicle, and mastoid process, 115

Sternum, also called *breast bone;* part of axial skeleton and anterior attachment for ribs, 85*f*, 89, 90*f*

Steroid sex hormones, class of hormones secreted by adrenal cortex; includes aldosterone, cortisol, androgens, estrogens, and progestins, 380*t*, 382

Stethoscope, instrument for listening to body sounds, such as chest, heart, or intestines, 159

Stillbirth, viable-aged fetus dies before or at time of delivery, 346

Stirrup, 467*f*, 468, 468*f*

Stomach, J-shaped muscular organ that acts as sac to collect, churn, digest, and store food; composed of three parts: fundus, body, and antrum; hydrochloric acid is secreted by glands in mucous membrane lining of stomach; food mixes with other gastric juices and hydrochloric acid to form semisoft mixture called chyme, which then passes into duodenum, 29*t*, 35*t*, 257*f*, 258, 271, 271*f*

Stool culture, laboratory test of feces to determine if there are any pathogenic bacteria present, 277

Stool guaiac, 276

Strabismus, eye muscle weakness resulting in each eye looking in different direction at same time; may be corrected with glasses, eye exercises, and/or surgery; also called *lazy eye* or *crossed eyes,* 450, 450*f*, 459

Strabotomy, incision into eye muscles in order to correct strabismus, 463

Strain, trauma to muscle from excessive stretching or pulling, 122

Stratified squamous epithelium, layers of flat or scalelike cells found in epidermis; *stratified* means multiple layers and *squamous* means flat, 53

Strawberry hemangioma, congenital collection of dilated blood vessels causing red birthmark that fades a few months after birth, 68, 68*f*

Stress fracture, slight fracture caused by repetitive low-impact forces, like running, rather than single forceful impact, 102

Stress testing, method for evaluating cardiovascular fitness; patient is placed on treadmill or bicycle and then subjected to steadily increasing levels of work; EKG and oxygen levels are taken while patient exercises, 160, 160*f*

Striated muscle, another name for skeletal muscle, referring to its striped appearance under microscope, 114, 114*f*

Stricture, narrowing of passageway in urinary system, 307

Stridor, harsh, high-pitched, noisy breathing sound made when there is obstruction of bronchus or larynx; found in conditions such as croup in children, 233

Stroke, 425

Stye (sty), 459

Subarachnoid space, space located between arachnoid layer and pia mater;contains cerebrospinal fluid, 417, 417*f*

Subcutaneous (SC, sc, sub-q, subcu), (1) pertaining to under skin; (2) injection of medication under skin, 54, 65, 495*f*, 495*t*, 521*t*, 521*t*

Subclavian artery, 148*f*

Subclavian vein, 150*f*, 195*f*

Subcutaneous layer, deepest layer of skin where fat is formed; layer of fatty tissue protects deeper tissues of body and acts as insulation for heat and cold, 52, 54*f*

Subdural hematoma, mass of blood forming beneath dura mater of brain, 430, 430*f*

Subdural space, space located between dura mater and arachnoid layer, 417, 417*f*

Sublingual (SL), (1) pertaining to under tongue; (2) administration of medicine by placing it under tongue, 268, 494, 494*t*, 494*f*

Sublingual duct, 264*f*

Sublingual glands, pair of salivary glands in floor of mouth, 264*f*

Subluxation, incomplete dislocation, joint alignment is disrupted, but ends of bones remain in contact, 106

Submandibular ducts, 259*f*, 264*f*

Submandibular glands, pair of salivary glands in floor of mouth, 264, 264*f*

subq, 52

Substance-related disorders, overindulgence or dependence on chemical substances including alcohol, illegal drugs, and prescription drugs, 503

Sudden infant death syndrome (SIDS), sudden, unexplained death of infant in which postmortem examination fails to determine cause of death, 236

Sudoriferous glands, typical sweat glands of skin, 56

Suffix, word part attached to end of word; frequently indicates condition, disease, or procedure; almost all medical terms have a suffix, 2, 3, 6–9

adjective, 8

procedural, 8–9

surgical, 8

Suffocation, 230

Sulci, also called *fissures;* grooves that separate gyri of cerebral cortex; singular is sulcus, 415

Superficial, directional term meaning toward surface of body, 37*t*

Superior, directional term meaning toward head, or above, 37*f*, 37*t*

Superior mesenteric vein, 150*f*

Superior vena cava, branch of vena cava that drains blood from chest and upper body, 142*f*, 145*f*, 150*f*

Supination, turn palm or foot upward, 118*t*, 118*f*

Supine, directional term meaning lying horizontally and facing upward, 38*f*, 38*t*

Supine position, 522*f*, 523*t*

Supplemental air, 225*t*

Supplemental oxygen therapy, providing patient with additional concentration of oxygen to improve oxygen levels in bloodstream; oxygen may be provided by mask or nasal cannula, 240

Suppositories (suppos), method for administering medication by placing it in substance that will melt after being placed in body cavity, usually rectally, and release medication, 494, 496*t*

Suppurative, containing or producing pus, 62

Surgeon, physician who has completed additional training of five years or more in surgical specialty area; specialty areas include orthopedics; neurosurgery; gynecology; ophthalmology; urology; and thoracic, vascular, cardiac, plastic, and general surgery, 520

Surgery, branch of medicine dealing with operative procedures to correct deformities and defects, repair injuries, and diagnose and cure diseases, 519–24

abbreviations, 524

anesthesia, 520,521*t*

surgical instruments, 520,521*t*

surgical positions, 522, 523*t*, 522*f*

vocabulary, 523–24

Surgical center, facility that provides services that range from simple surgeries to diagnostic testing to therapy and do not require overnight hospitalization; also called *ambulatory care center* or *outpatient clinic,* 13

Surgical instruments, 521*t*, 522*f*

Surgical positions, 522*f*, 523*t*

Surgical suffixes, 8

Suspensory ligament, 448*f*

Suture, 91*f*

Suture material, used to close wound or incision; examples are catgut, silk thread, or staples; may or may not be removed when wound heals, depending on type of material used, 524

Sweat duct, duct leading from sweat gland to surface of skin; carries sweat, 56

Sweat glands, glands that produce sweat, which assists body in maintaining its internal temperature by creating a cooling effect when it evaporates, 27*t*, 50, 52, 56

Sweat pore, surface opening of sweat duct, 56

Sweat test, test performed on sweat to determine level of chloride; there is an increase in skin chloride in disease cystic fibrosis, 239

Swimmer's ear, 472

Sympathetic branch, branch of autonomic nervous system; stimulates body in times of stress and crisis by increasing heart rate, dilating airways to allow for more oxygen, increasing blood pressure, inhibiting digestion, and stimulating production of adrenaline during crisis, 419

Symphysis pubis, 332*f*, 337*f*, 354*f*

Synapse, point at which axon of one neuron meets dendrite of next neuron, 412

Synaptic cleft, gap between two neurons, 412

Syncope, fainting, 424

Syndrome, group of symptoms and signs that when combined present clinical picture of disease or condition, 391

Synovectomy, excision of synovial membrane, 108

Synovial, pertaining to synovial membrane, 99

Synovial fluid, fluid secreted by synovial membrane in synovial joint; lubricates joint and reduces friction, 95, 96

Synovial joint, freely moving joint that is lubricated by synovial fluid, 95, 96, 96*f*

Synovial membrane, membrane that lines synovial joint; secretes lubricating fluid called *synovial fluid,* 95, 96

Synovitis, inflammation of synovial membrane, 100

Syphilis, infectious, chronic, venereal disease that can involve any organ; may exist for years without symptoms; treated with antibiotic pencillin, 360

System, several organs working in compatible manner to perform complex function or functions; examples include digestive system, cardiovascular system, and respiratory system, 27–31, 27*t*–31*t*

Systematic, pertaining to a system, 37

Systemic circulation, systematic circulation transports oxygenated blood from left side of heart to cells of body and then back to right side of heart, 140

Systemic lupus erythematosus (SLE), chronic disease of connective tissue that injures skin, joints, kidneys, nervous system, and mucous membranes; may produce characteristic butterfly rash across cheeks and nose, 68, 106

Systemic veins, 140*f*

Systole, period of time during which heart chamber is contracting, 144, 146*f*

Systolic pressure, maximum pressure within blood vessels during heart contraction, 149

T

T cells, lymphocytes active in cellular immunity, 196, 387

T lymphocytes, type of lymphocyte involved with producing cells that physically attack and destroy pathogens, 196

Tachycardia, abnormally fast heart rate, over 100 bpm, 154

Tachypnea, rapid breathing rate, 233

Tagging, attachment of radioactive material to chemical and tracing it as it moves through body, 508

Talipes, congenital deformity of foot; also referred to as *clubfoot,* 106

Target organs, organs that hormones act on to either increase or decrease organ's activity level, 380

Tarsal, pertaining to ankle, 99

Tarsals, ankle bones in lower extremity, 92, 93*f*, 94, 95*f*, 95*t*

Taste buds, found on surface of tongue; designed to detect bitter, sweet, sour, and salty flavors in our food, 258

Tears, fluid that washes and lubricates anterior surface of eyeball, 451

Teeth, structures in mouth that mechanically break up food into smaller pieces during chewing, 258, 260–61, 260*f*

Temporal bone, cranial bone, 89, 91*f*, 91*t*, 467*f*

Temporal lobe, one of four cerebral hemisphere lobes; controls hearing and smell, 414, 415, 415*f*

Tenaculum, long-handled clamp surgical instrument, 521*t*

Tendinitis, inflammation of tendon, 122

Tendinous, pertaining to tendon, 119

Tendons, strong connective tissue cords that attach skeletal muscles to bones, 25, 121

Tendoplasty, surgical repair of a tendon, 123

Tendotomy, incision into a tendon, 123

Tennis elbow, 121

Tenodesis, surgical procedure to stabilize a joint by anchoring down tendons of muscles that move joint, 123

Tenodynia, pain in tendon, 121

Tenoplasty, surgical repair of tendon, 123

Tenorrhaphy, suture a tendon, 123

Testes, male gonads; oval glands located in scrotum that produce sperm and male hormone, testosterone, 30t, 96f, 354–55, 354f, 358, 362f, 380, 381t, 386, 386f

Testicles, also called *testes* (singular is testis); oval-shaped organs responsible for development of sperm within seminiferous tubules; testes must be maintained at proper temperature for sperm to survive; lower temperature level is controlled by placement of scrotum outside body; hormone testosterone, which is responsible for growth and development of male reproductive organs, is also produced by testes, 354

Testicular, pertaining to testes, 357

Testicular carcinoma, cancer of one or both testicles, 358

Testicular torsion, twisting of spermatic cord, 358

Testis, 297f, 354f, 386f

Testosterone, male hormone produced in testes; responsible for growth and development of male reproductive organs, 354, 355, 381t, 386, 386f

Tetany, condition resulting from calcium deficiency in blood; characterized by muscle twitches, cramps, and spasms, 384, 393

Tetralogy of Fallot, combination of four congenital anomalies: pulmonary stenosis, interventricular septal defect, abnormal blood supply to aorta, and hypertrophy of right ventricle; needs immediate surgery to correct, 157

Thalamic, pertaining to thalamus, 421

Thalamus, portion of diencephalon; composed of gray matter and acts as center for relaying impulses from eyes, ears, and skin to cerebrum; pain perception is also controlled by thalamus, 384, 384f, 385f, 415

Thalassemia, genetic disorder in which person is unable to make functioning hemoglobin; results in anemia, 187

Therapeutic abortion, termination of pregnancy for health of mother, 350

Therapeutic exercise, exercise planned and carried out to achieve specific physical benefit, such as improved range of motion, muscle strength, or cardiovascular function, 517

Thermotherapy, applying heat to body for therapeutic purposes, 517

Third-degree burn, 64, 64f

Thoracalgia, chest pain, 233

Thoracentesis, surgical puncture of chest wall for removal of fluids, 241, 241f

Thoracic, pertaining to chest, 99, 299

Thoracic cavity, ventral body cavity in chest area containing lungs and heart, 34, 34f, 35t

Thoracic duct, largest lymph vessel; drains entire body except for right arm, chest wall, and both lungs; empties lymph into left subclavian vein, 193, 194, 195f

Thoracic region, chest region of body, 33, 33f

Thoracic surgeon, physician specialized in treating conditions and diseases of respiratory system by surgical teams, 229

Thoracic surgery, branch of medicine specializing in surgery on respiratory system and thoracic cavity, 29t, 229

Thoracic vertebrae (T1, T2, etc.), 12 vertebrae in chest region, 85f, 89, 92t

Thoracostomy, insertion of tube into chest for purpose of draining off fluid or air, 241

Thoracotomy, incision into chest, 241

Thrombin, clotting enzyme that converts fibrinogen to fibrin, 182

Thrombocytes, also called *platelets;* play critical part in blood-clotting process by agglutinating into small clusters and releasing thrombokinase, 182, 184

Thrombocytosis, too many clotting cells (platelets), 187

Thrombolytic, able to dissolve existing blood clots, 164

Thrombolytic therapy, drugs, such as streptokinase or tissue-type plasminogen activator, are injected into blood vessel to dissolve clots and restore blood flow, 162

Thrombopenia, too few clotting (cells), 187

Thrombophlebitis, inflammation of vein that results in formation of blood clots within vein, 158

Thromboplastin, substance released by platelets; reacts with prothrombin to form thrombin, 182

Thrombus, blood clot, 154

Thymectomy, removal of thymus gland, 205, 397

Thymic, pertaining to thymus gland, 200, 389

Thymitis, inflammation of thymus gland, 394

Thymoma, malignant tumor of thymus gland, 202, 394

Thymosin, hormone secreted by thymus gland; causes lymphocytes to change into T lymphocytes, 196, 381t, 387

Thymus gland, endocrine gland located in upper mediastinum that assists body with immune function and development of antibodies; as part of immune response it secretes hormone, thymosin, that changes lymphocytes to T cells, 28t, 30t, 35t, 192f, 193, 196, 196f, 214f, 379f, 380, 381t, 387, 387f

Thyroid cartilage, piece of cartilage associated with larynx; commonly called Adam's apple and is larger in males, 221f, 222

Thyroid echography, ultrasound examination of thyroid that can assist in distinguishing thyroid nodule from cyst, 396

Thyroid function test (TFT), blood tests used to measure levels of T_3, T_4, and TSH in blood stream to assist in determining thyroid function, 396

Thyroid gland, endocrine gland located on either side of trachea; shape resembles butterfly with large left and right lobe connected by narrow isthmus; gland produces hormones thyroxine (also known as T_4 and triiodothyronine (also known as T_3), 30*t*, 221*f*, 379*f*, 380, 381*t*, 387–88, 388*f*

Thyroid replacement hormone, given to replace thyroid in patients with hypothyroidism or who have had thyroidectomy, 398

Thyroid replacement therapy, 398

Thyroid scan, test in which radioactive element is administered that localizes in thyroid gland; gland can then be visualized with scanning device to detect pathology such as tumors, 396

Thyroid-stimulating hormone (TSH), hormone secreted by anterior pituitary; regulates function of thyroid gland, 381*t*, 385

Thyroidal, pertaining to thyroid gland, 389

Thyroidectomy, removal of entire thyroid or portion (partial thyroidectomy) to treat variety of conditions, including nodes, cancer, and hyperthyroidism, 397

Thyromegaly, enlarged thyroid, 391

Thyrotoxicosis, condition that results from overproduction of thyroid glands; symptoms include rapid heart action, tremors, enlarged thyroid gland, exophthalmos, and weight loss, 395

Thyroxine (T_4), hormone produced by thyroid gland; also known as T_4 and requires iodine for production; hormone regulates level of cell metabolism; the greater the level of hormone in the bloodstream, the higher cell metabolism will be, 381*t*, 387

Tibia, also called *shin bone;* lower extremity bone, 92, 93*f*, 95, 95*f*, 95*t*

Tibial, pertaining to tibia or shin bone, 99

Tidal volume (TV), amount of air that enters lungs in single inhalation or leaves lungs in single exhalation of quiet breathing, 225*t*

Tinea, fungal skin disease resulting in itching, scaling lesions, 68

Tinea capitis, fungal infection of scalp; commonly called *ringworm,* 68

Tinea pedis, fungal infection of foot; commonly called *athlete's foot,* 68

Tinnitus, ringing in ears, 472

Tissues, formed when cells of same type are grouped to perform one activity; for example, nerve cells combine to form nerve fibers; there are four types: nerve, muscle, epithelial, and connective, 25

connective, 25

epithelial, pertaining to epithelium, 25

muscle, 25

nervous, 25

Tolerance, development of capacity for withstanding large amount of substance, such as foods, drugs, or poison, without any adverse effect; decreased sensitivity to further doses will develop, 497

Tongue, muscular organ in floor of mouth; works to move food around inside mouth and is also necessary for speech, 221*f*, 258, 264*f*

Tonic-clonic seizure, type of severe epileptic seizure characterized by loss of consciousness and convulsions; seizure alternates between strong continuous muscle spasms (tonic) and rhythmic muscle contraction and relaxation (clonic); also called *grand mal seizure,* 424

Tonometry, measurement of intraocular pressure of eye using tonometer to check for condition of glaucoma; after local anesthetic is applied, physician places tonometer lightly upon eyeball and pressure measurement is taken; generally part of normal eye exam for adults, 461

Tonsillar, pertaining to tonsils, 200

Tonsillectomy, surgical removal of tonsils, 205

Tonsillitis, inflammation of tonsils, 202

Tonsils, collections of lymphatic tissue located in pharynx to combat microorganisms entering body through nose or mouth; include pharyngeal tonsils, palatine tonsils, and lingual tonsils, 28*t*, 192*f*, 193, 196, 196*f*

Tooth cavity, 270

Topical, applied directly to skin or mucous membranes; distributed in ointment, cream, or lotion form; used to treat skin infections and eruptions, 494, 496*t*

Topical anesthesia, topical anesthesia is applied using either liquid or gel placed directly onto specific area; patient remains conscious; this type of anesthetic is used on skin, cornea, and mucous membranes in dental work, 520, 521*t*

Torticollis, severe neck spasms pulling head to one side; commonly called *wryneck* or *crick in the neck,* 121

Total abdominal hysterectomy - bilateral salpingo-oophorectomy (TAH-BSO), removal of entire uterus, cervix, both ovaries, and both fallopian tubes, 350

Total calcium, blood test to measure total amount of calcium to assist in detecting parathyroid and bone disorders, 396

Total hip arthroplasty (THA), surgical reconstruction of hip by implanting prosthetic or artificial hip joint; also called *total hip replacement,* 108

Total hip replacement (THR), 108

Total knee arthroplasty (TKA), surgical reconstruction of knee joint by implanting prosthetic knee joint; also called *total knee replacement,* 108

Total knee replacement (TKR), **108**

Total lung capacity (TLC), volume of air in lungs after maximal inhalation, 225*t*

Total parenteral nutrition (TPN), providing 100% of patient's nutrition intravenously; used when patient is unable to eat, 279

Toxemia, 346

Toxic shock syndrome (TSS), rare and sometimes fatal staphylococcus infection that generally occurs in menstruating women, 344

Toxicity, extent or degree to which substance is poisonous, 497

Toxins, substances poisonous to body; many are filtered out of blood by kidney, 197

Tracheal, pertaining to trachea, 229

Trachea, also called *windpipe;* conducts air from larynx down to main bronchi in chest, 29*t*, 35*t*, 218, 219*f*, 220, 221*f*, 223, 223*f*, 225*f*, 384*f*, 387*f*, 388*f*

Tracheostenosis, narrowing and stenosis of lumen or opening into trachea, 233

Tracheostomy, surgical procedure used to make opening in trachea to create airway; tracheostomy tube can be inserted to keep opening patent, 242, 242*f*

Tracheotomy, surgical incision into trachea to provide airway, 242, 242*f*

Tract, bundle of fibers located within central nervous system, 413

Traction, process of pulling or drawing, usually with mechanical device; used in treating orthopedic (bone and joint) problems and injuries, 109, 517

Tractotomy, incision into spinal cord tract, 432

Trademark, pharmaceutical company's brand name for drug, 491

Transcutaneous electrical nerve stimulation (TENS), application of mild electrical stimulation to skin via electrodes placed over painful area, causing interference with transmission of painful stimuli; can be used in pain management to interfere with normal pain mechanism, 517

Transdermal, route of drug administration; medication coats underside of patch applied to skin; medication is then absorbed across skin, 494, 496

Transfusion reaction, 186

Transient ischemic attack (TIA), temporary interference with blood supply to brain, causing neurological symptoms such as dizziness, numbness, and hemiparesis; may lead
eventually to full-blown stroke (CVA), 427

Transurethral resection of the prostate (TUR, TURP), surgical removal of prostate gland by inserting device through urethra and removing prostate tissue, 361

Transverse colon, section of colon that crosses upper abdomen from right side of body to left, 263, 263*f*

Transverse fracture, complete fracture straight across bone at right angles to long axis of bone, 102, 102*f*

Transverse plane, horizontal plane that divides body into upper (superior) and lower (inferior) sections; also called *horizontal plane,* 32, 32*f*

Transverse section, sectional view of body produced by cut along transverse plane, 32

Treadmill test, 160, 160*f*

Tremor, involuntary quivering movement of a part of body, 424

Trendelenburg position, surgical position in which patient is lying face up and on incline with head lower than legs, 522*f*, 523*t*

Trephine, surgical saw used to remove disk-shaped piece of tissue, 521*t*

Trichomoniasis, genitourinary infection usually without symptoms (asymptomatic) in both males and females; in women disease can produce itching and/or burning and foul-smelling discharge, and can result in vaginitis, 360

Trichomycosis, abnormal condition of hair fungus, 69

Tricuspid valve, valve between right atrium and ventricle of heart; prevents blood from flowing backwards into atrium; has three cusps or flaps, 142*f*, 143, 145*f*, 145*f*

Trigeminal nerve, 418*t*

Triiodothyronine (T₃), hormone produced by thyroid gland known as T_3 that requires iodine for its production; hormone regulates level of cell metabolism; the greater the level of hormone in blood stream, the higher cell metabolism will be, 381*t*, 387

Trochanter, large blunt process that provides attachment for tendons and muscles, 88, 88*f*

Trochlear nerve, 418*t*

Trunk, torso region of body, 33, 33*f*

Tubal ligation, surgical tying off of fallopian tubes to prevent conception from taking place; results in sterilization of female, 350

Tubal pregnancy, 333

Tubercle, small, rounded process that provides attachment for tendons and muscles, 88

Tuberculin skin tests (TB test), applying chemical agent (Tine or Mantoux tests) under surface of skin to determine if patient has been exposed to tuberculosis, 239

Tuberculosis (TB), infectious disease caused by tubercle bacillus, *Myocobacterium tuberculosis;* most commonly affects respiratory system and causes inflammation and calcification of system; tuberculosis is again on uprise and is seen in many patients who have AIDS, 237

Tuberosity, large, rounded process that provides attachment to tendons and muscles, 83

Tumor, abnormal growth of tissue that may be benign or malignant; also called *neoplasm,* 526, 528

Two-hour postprandial glucose tolerance test, blood test to assist in evaluating glucose metabolism; patient eats high-carbohydrate diet and fasts overnight before test; blood sample is then taken two hours after meal, 396

Tympanectomy, excision of eardrum, 472

Tympanic, pertaining to eardrum, 471

Tympanic membrane, also called eardrum; as sound moves along auditory canal, it strikes tympanic membrane causing it to vibrate; this conducts sound wave into middle ear, 467, 467*f*

Tympanitis, eardrum inflammation, 472

Tympanogram, graphic record that illustrates results ofs tympanometry, 474

Tympanometer, instrument to measure eardrum, 474

Tympanometry, measurement of movement of tympanic membrane; can indicate presence of pressure in middle ear, 474

Tympanoplasty, another term for surgical reconstruction of eardrum; also called *myringoplasty,* 476

Tympanorrhexis, ruptured eardrum, 472

Tympanotomy, incision into eardrum, 476

Type A blood, one of ABO blood types; person with type A markers on his or her RBCs; type A blood will make anti-B antibodies, 182

Type AB blood, one of ABO blood types; person with both type A and type B markers on his or her RBCs; since it has both markers, it will not make antibodies against either A or B blood, 182

Type B blood, one of ABO blood types; person with type B markers on his or her RBCs; type B blood will make anti-A antibodies, 182

Type O blood, one of ABO blood types; person with no markers on his or her RBCs; type O blood will not react with anti-A or anti-B antibodies; therefore, is considered universal donor, 182

Type and cross-match, lab test performed before person receives blood transfusion; double checks blood type of both donor's and recipient's blood, 189

U

Ulcer, open sore or lesion in skin or mucous membrane, 62, 62*f*

Ulcerative colitis, ulceration of unknown origin of mucous membranes of colon; also known as *inflammatory bowel disease* (IBD), 275

Ulna, one of forearm bones in upper extremity, 92, 93*f*, 94, 94*f*

Ulnar, pertaining to ulna, one of lower arm bones, 99

Ulnar artery, 148*f*

Ulnar nerve, 419*f*

Ulnar vein, 150*f*

Ultrasound (US), use of high-frequency sound waves to create heat in soft tissues under skin; particularly useful for treating injuries to muscles, tendons, and ligaments, as well as muscle spasms; in radiology, ultrasound waves can be used to outline shapes of tissues, organs, and fetus, 511, 511*f*, 518

Ultraviolet (UV), 72

Umbilical, anatomical division of abdomen; middle section of middle row, 36*t*

Umbilical cord, cord extending from baby's umbilicus (navel) to placenta; contains blood vessels that carry oxygen and nutrients from mother to baby and carbon dioxide and wastes from baby to mother, 336, 337*f*, 338

Unconscious, condition or state of being unaware of surroundings with inability to respond to stimuli, 424

Ungual, 57

Unit dose, drug dosage system that provides prepackaged, prelabeled, individual medications ready for immediate use by the patient, 497

Universal donor, type O blood is considered universal donor; since it has no markers on RBC surface, it will not trigger reaction with anti-A or anti-B antibodies, 182

Universal recipient, person with type AB blood has no antibodies against other blood types and therefore, in emergency, can receive any type of blood, 182

Upper extremity (UE), the arm, 31, 92, 93*f*, 94, 94*f*, 516

Upper gastrointestinal (UGI) series, administering barium contrast material orally and then taking X-ray to visualize esophagus, stomach, and duodenum, 278

Uptake, absorption of radioactive material and medicines into organ or tissue, 508

Urea, waste product of protein metabolism; diffuses through tissues in lymph and is returned to circulatory system for transport to kidneys, 180

Uremia, excess of urea and other nitrogenous waste in blood, 298, 307, 307

Ureteral, pertaining to ureter, 305

Ureterectasis, dilation of ureter, 307

Ureterolith, a calculus in ureter, 307

Ureterostenosis, narrowing of ureter, 307

Ureters, organs in urinary system that transport urine from kidney to bladder, 29t, 35t, 36t, 297f, 298, 299f, 300f

Urethra, tube that leads from urinary bladder to outside of body; in male it is also used by reproductive system to release semen, 29t, 35t, 297f, 298, 300f, 301, 301f, 332f, 354f

Urethral, pertaining to urethra, 305

Urethralgia, urethral pain, 307

Urethrorrhagia, rapid bleeding from urethra, 308

Urethroscope, instrument to view inside urethra, 312

Urethrostenosis, narrowing of urethra, 308

Urgency, feeling need to urinate immediately, 308

Urinalysis (U/A, UA), laboratory test consisting of physical, chemical, and microscopic examination of urine, 303, 303t, 311

Urinary, pertaining to urine, 305

Urinary bladder, organ in the urinary system that stores urine, 29t, 35t, 297f, 298, 300–01, 300f, 301f, 310f, 332f, 337f, 354f

Urinary incontinence, involuntary release of urine; in some patients indwelling catheter is inserted into bladder for continuous urine drainage, 308

Urinary meatus, external opening of urethra, 301, 301f, 335, 335f, 355

Urinary retention, inability to fully empty bladder, often indicates blockage in urethra, 308

Urinary system, system that filters wastes from blood and excretes waste products in form of urine; organs include kidneys, ureters, urinary bladder, and urethra, 29t, 295–328, 297f

    abbreviations, 316

    anatomical terms, 315

    anatomy and physiology, 292–303

    diagnostic procedures, 310–12

    homeostasis, kidneys and, 301

    kidneys, 298–99

    pathology, 305–10

    pharmacology, 315

    terminology, 304–05

    therapeutic procedures, 312–15

    ureters, 299

    urethra, 301

    urinary bladder, 300–301

    urinary production stages, 302

    urine, 303

Urinary tract infection (UTI), infection, usually from bacteria such as *E. coli*, of any organ of urinary system; most often begins with cystitis and may ascend into ureters and kidneys; most common in women because of shorter urethra, 310

Urination, release of urine from urinary bladder, 310

Urine, fluid that remains in urinary system following three stages of urine production: filtration, reabsorption, and secretion, 298, 302, 302f,

    production, 302, 302f

Urine culture and sensitivity (C&S), laboratory test of urine for bacterial infection; attempt to grow bacteria on culture medium in order to identify it and determine which antibiotics it is sensitive to, 311

Urinometer, instrument to measure urine, 311

Urologist, physician specialized in treating conditions and diseases of urinary system and male reproductive system, 305, 358

Urology, branch of medicine specializing in conditions of urinary system and male reproductive system, 29t, 30t, 305

Urticaria, hives, skin eruption of pale reddish wheals (circular elevations of skin) with severe itching; usually associated with food allergy, stress, or drug reactions, 62, 201

Uterine, pertaining to uterus, 341

Uterine tubes, tubes that carry ovum from ovary to uterus; also called *fallopian tubes* or *oviducts*, 333, 343

Uterus, also called *womb;* internal organ of female reproductive system; hollow, pear-shaped organ is located in lower pelvic cavity between urinary bladder and rectum; uterus receives fertilized ovum and becomes implanted in uterine wall, which provides nourishment and protection for developing fetus; divided into three regions: fundus, corpus, and cervix, 30t, 35t, 301f, 331f, 332, 334–35, 334f

Utricle, found in inner ear; plays role in equilibrium, 468

Uveal, pertaining to choroid layer of eye, 454

Uveitis, inflammation of uvea of eye, 459

Uvula, structure that hangs down from posterior edge of soft palate, helps in production of speech, and is location of gag reflex, 258, 259f

V

Vaccination, providing protection against communicable diseases by stimulating immune system to produce antibodies against that disease; children can now be immunized for: hepatitis B, diphtheria, tetanus, pertussis, *Haemophilus influenzae* type b, polio, measles, mumps, rubella, and chickenpox; also called *immunization*, 196, 197, 204

Vagina, organ in female reproductive system that receives penis and semen, 30*t*, 35*t*, 301*f*, 332, 332*f*, 334*f*, 335, 335*f*, 337*f*, 344

Vaginal, (1) pertaining to vagina; (2) tablets and suppositories inserted vaginally and used to treat vaginal yeast infections and other irritations, 341, 494, 496*t*

Vaginal hysterectomy, removal of uterus through vagina rather than through abdominal incision, 350

Vaginal orifice, external vaginal opening; may be covered by hymen, 335, 335*f*

Vaginitis, inflammation of vagina, 344

Vagus nerve, 418*t*

Valve replacement, excision of diseased heart valve and replacement with artificial valve, 163

Valves, flaplike structures found within tubular organs such as lymph vessels, veins, and heart; function to prevent backflow of fluid, 193, 194, 194*f,*

Valvoplasty, surgical repair of valve, 163

Valvular, pertaining to valve, 152

Valvulitis, inflammation of valve, 157

Varicella, contagious viral skin infection; commonly called *chickenpox*, 68, 68*f*

Varicocele, enlargement of veins of spermatic cord, which commonly occurs on left side of adolescent males; seldom needs treatment, 358

Varicose veins, swollen and distended veins, usually in legs, 158

Vas deferens, also called ductus deferens; vas deferens is long, straight tube that carries sperm from epididymis up into pelvic cavity, where it continues around bladder and empties into urethra; one component, along with nerves and blood vessels, of spermatic cord, 30*t*, 35*t*, 96*f*, 354, 354*f*, 356, 362*f*, 386*f*

Vasal, pertaining to vas deferens, 357

Vascular, pertaining to vessels, 152

Vasectomy, removal of segment or all of vas deferens to prevent sperm from leaving male body; used for contraception purposes, 361, 362*f*

Vasoconstrictor, contracts smooth muscle in walls of blood vessels; raises blood pressure, 164

Vasodilator, produces relaxation of blood vessels to lower blood pressure, 164

Vasopressin, substance given to control diabetes insipidus and promote reabsorption of water in kidney tubules, 398

Vasovasostomy, creation of new opening between two sections of vas deferens; used to reverse vasectomy, 362

Vegetation, 155

Veins, blood vessels of cardiovascular system that carry blood toward heart, 28*t*, 53*f*, 139*f*, 140, 142*f*, 147*f*, 149, 193*f*

Vena cava, 140*f*

Venereal disease (VD), 360

Venipuncture, 188

Venogram, 143

Venous, pertaining to vein, 152

Ventilation, movement of air in and out of lungs, 220

Ventilation-perfusion scan, nuclear medicine diagnostic test especially useful in identifying pulmonary emboli; radioactive air is inhaled for ventilation portion to determine if air is filling entire lung; radioactive intravenous injection shows whether blood is flowing to all parts of lung, 238

Ventilator, machine that provides artificial ventilation for patient unable to breath on his or her own; also called *respirator*, 240

Ventral, directional term meaning near or on front or belly side of body, 34*f*, 37*t*

Ventral cavities, 35*t*

Ventricles, two lower chambers of heart that receive blood from atria and pump it back out of heart; left ventricle pumps blood to body, and right ventricle pumps blood to lungs; also fluid-filled spaces within cerebrum; contain cerebrospinal fluid, which is watery, clear fluid that provides protection from shock or sudden motion to brain, 142, 414, 416

Ventricular, pertaining to ventricle, 152

Ventricular septal defect (VSD), 155

Venules, smallest veins; receive deoxygenated blood leaving capillaries, 149, 152, 192*f*

Vermiform appendix, small outgrowth at end of cecum; function or purpose is unknown, 263

Verruca, warts; benign neoplasm (tumor) caused by virus; has rough surface that is removed by chemicals and/or laser therapy, 68

Vertebrae, 90*f*

Vertebral, pertaining to vertebrae, 41

Vertebral canal, bony canal through vertebrae that contains spinal cord, 416

Vertebral column, part of axial skeleton; a column of 26 vertebrae that forms backbone and protects spinal cord; divided into five sections: cervical, thoracic, and lumbar vertebrae, sacrum, and coccyx; also called *spinal column*, 89, 91, 92*f*, 92*t*, 416

Vertebral region, spinal column region of body, 33, 33*f*

Vertigo, dizziness, 472

Vesicle, small, fluid-filled raised spot on skin, 62, 62*f*

Vesicular, pertaining to seminal vesicle, 357

Vestibular nerve, branch of vestibulocochlear nerve responsible for sending equilibrium information to brain, 467, 467*f*

Vestibulocochlear nerve, eighth cranial nerve; responsible for hearing and balance, 418*t*, 467

Viruses, group of infectious particles that cause disease, 197

Viscera, name for internal organs of body, such as lungs, stomach, and liver, 34, 35

Visceral, pertaining to viscera or internal organs, 41

Visceral layer, inner pleural layer; adheres to surface of lung, 34, 35

Visceral muscle, muscle found in walls of internal organs such as stomach, 114, 114*f*

Visceral pericardium, inner layer of pericardium surrounding heart, 142

Visceral peritoneum, inner layer of serous membrane sac encasing abdominopelvic viscera, 34, 35

Visceral pleura, inner layer of serous membrane sac encasing thoracic viscera, 34, 35, 224

Vision, 452

Visual acuity (VA) test, measurement of sharpness of patient's vision; usually, a Snellen chart is used for this test and patient identifies letters from distance of 20 feet, 461

Vital capacity (VC), total volume of air that can be exhaled after maximum inhalation; amount will be equal to sum of tidal volume, inspiratory reserve volume, and expiratory reserve volume, 225*t*

Vital signs (VS), respiration, pulse, temperature, skin color, blood pressure, and reaction of pupils; signs of condition of body functions, 227

Vitamin D therapy, maintaining high blood levels of calcium in association with vitamin D helps maintain bone density and treats osteomalacia, osteoporosis, and rickets, 109

Vitiligo, disappearance of pigment from skin in patches, causing a milk-white appearance; also called *leukoderma,* 69

Vitreous, pertaining to vitreous humor, 454

Vitreous body, 448*f*

Vitreous humor, transparent jellylike substance inside eyeball, 449

Vocal cords, structures within larynx that vibrate to produce sound and speech, 221*f*, 222, 222*f*

Voiding, another term for urination, 300

Voiding cystourethrography (VCUG), x-ray taken to visualize urethra while patient is voiding after contrast dye has been placed in bladder, 312

Voluntary muscles, muscles that person can consciously choose to contract; skeletal muscles of arm and leg are examples, 113

Volvulus, condition in which bowel twists upon itself and causes painful obstruction that requires immediate surgery, 275, 275*f*

Vomer bone, facial bone, 89, 91*t*

von Recklinghausen's disease, 393

Voyeurism, sexual disorder characterized by receiving sexual gratification from observing others engaged in sexual acts, 503

Vulva, general term meaning external female genitalia; consists of Bartholin's glands, labia major, labia minora, and clitoris, 30*t*, 331*f*, 332, 335, 335*f*

Vulvar, pertaining to vulva, 341

W

Walking pneumonia, 236

Wall-eyed, 459

Warts, 68

Wax emulsifiers, substances used to soften ear wax to prevent buildup within external ear canal, 476

Western blot, test used as backup to ELISA blood test to detect presence of antibody to HIV (AIDS virus) in blood, 203

Wet gangrene, area of gangrene becoming infected by pus-producing bacteria, 69

Wheal, small, round raised area on skin that may be accompanied by itching, 63, 63*f*

Whiplash, 105

Whirlpool, bath in which there are continuous jets of hot water reaching body surfaces, 518

White blood cell count (WBC), blood test to measure number of leukocytes in volume of blood; increase may indicate presence of infection or disease such as leukemia; decrease in WBCs is caused by X-ray therapy and chemotherapy, 188

White blood cell differential (diff), blood test to determine the number of each variety of leukocyte, 188

White blood cells (WBC), blood cells that provide protection against invasion of bacteria and other foreign material, 24*f*, 180

White matter, tissue in central nervous system; consists of myelinated nerve fibers, 413, 414

Whole blood, refers to mixture of both plasma and formed elements, 179*f*, 189

Whooping cough, 233

Wilm's tumor, malignant kidney tumor found most often in children, 310

Windpipe, 223
Wisdom teeth, 216
Womb, 334
Word building, 9
Word root, foundation of medical term that
provides basic meaning of word; in general,
word root will indicate body system or part of
body being discussed; word may have more
than one word root, 2, 3
Wryneck, 121

X

X-rays, high-energy wave that can penetrate
most solid matter and present image on
photographic film, 507, 508
Xenograft, skin graft from animal of another
species (usually pig); also called *heterograft,* 71

Xeroderma, dry skin, 63
Xerophthalmia, dry eyes, 456

Y

Yellow bone marrow, yellow bone marrow is
located mainly in center of diaphysis of long
bones; contains mainly fat cells, 86, 87, 87*f*

Z

Zygomatic bone, facial bone, 89, 91, 91*f*, 91*t*

MAP PAGES

66

RUSSIA

SWEDEN FINLAND

ESTONIA

LATVIA

64

EUROPE AND
COUNTRY INDEX
ON ENDPAPER

UKRAINE

SLOVAK REP.

MOLDOVA

HUNGARY

ROMANIA

CROATIA

BOS. &
HERZ.

SERB.
& MONT.

MAC.

BULG.

GREECE

KAZAKHSTAN

68

MONGOLIA

74

70

NORTH
KOREA

JAPAN

72

100 **88**

TURKEY

GEORGIA

ARM. AZER.

TURKMENISTAN

UZBEKISTAN

KYRGYZSTAN

65

96

103

SYRIA

IRAQ

TAJIK.

91

AFGHAN.

CHINA

SOUTH
KOREA

76

144

106

JORDAN

IRAN

92

PAKISTAN

NEPAL

90

69

TAIWAN

Tropic of Cancer

LIBYA

EGYPT

KUWAIT

QATAR

U.A.E.

OMAN

94

54

INDIA

BANG.

BURMA

86

LAOS

PACIFIC
OCEAN

134

CHAD

SUDAN

SAUDI
ARABIA

98

ERITREA

YEMEN

SRI
LANKA

78

THAILAND

CAMB.

VIETNAM

80

PHILIPPINES

133

120

DJIBOUTI

ETHIOPIA

SOMALI
REP.

95

CENTRAL
AFRICAN
REP.

118

UGANDA

KENYA

84

87

MALAYSIA

82

CONGO

(DEM. REP. OF THE)

RWANDA

BURUNDI

TANZANIA

121

INDONESIA

132

PAPUA
NEW GUINEA

133

ANGOLA

121

ZAMBIA

MALAWI

79

E. TIMOR

124

126

133

133

133

MOZAMBIQUE

MADAGASCAR

121

INDIAN
OCEAN

121

Equator

International Dateline

NAMIBIA

ZIMBABWE

BOTSWANA

126

133

Tropic of Capricorn

SWAZILAND

AUSTRALIA

SOUTH
AFRICA

LESOTHO

128

130

NEW
ZEALAND

131

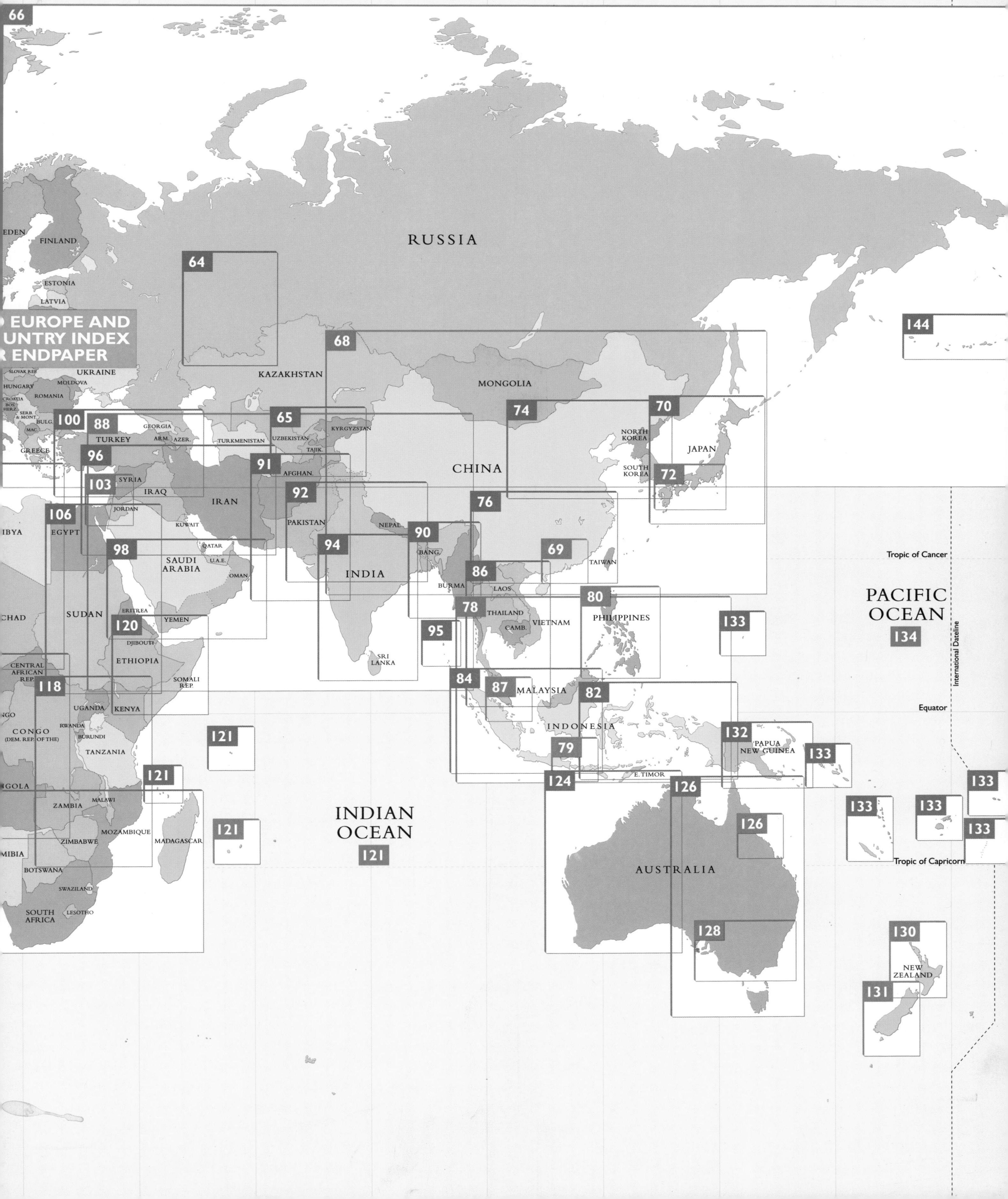

OXFORD

ATLAS OF THE WORLD

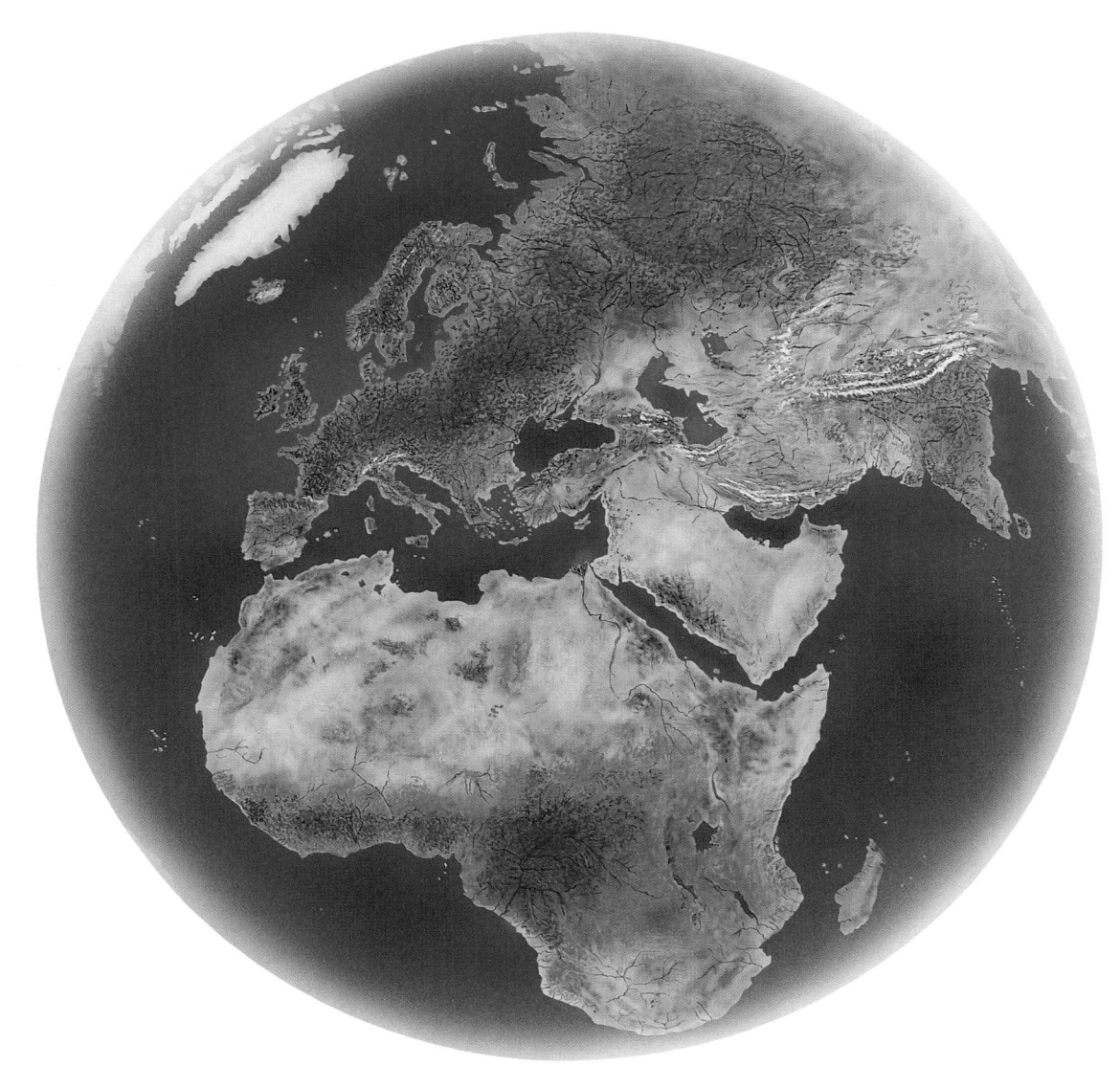

TWELFTH EDITION

ACKNOWLEDGEMENTS

IMAGES OF EARTH (PAGES IX–XXIV)
All satellite images in this section courtesy
of NPA Group Limited, Edenbridge, Kent
(www.satmaps.com)

THE GAZETTEER OF NATIONS
TEXT Keith Lye

INTRODUCTION TO WORLD GEOGRAPHY
PICTURE ACKNOWLEDGEMENTS
Alamy /*Peter Bowater* 36
Corbis /*Jay Dickman* 47 (bottom left),
/*Royalty-Free* 27, 32, 35, /*Vince Streano* 39,
/*Liba Taylor* 42, /*David Turnley* 47 (bottom right)
NASA/GSFC 22 (bottom left and right),
/*Cathy Clerbaux, NCAR Atmospheric Chemistry
Division* 21 (bottom right)
NOAO/AURA/NSF/Todd Boroson 2
NPA Group 9, 13, 18, 48, /*Image provided by
the USGS EROS Data Center Satellite Systems
Branch* 23
Science Photo Library /*Earth Satellite
Corporation* 20

STAR CHARTS
Wil Tirion

CARTOGRAPHY BY PHILIP'S

CITY MAPS
PAGE 11, DUBLIN: The town plan of Dublin
is based on Ordnance Survey Ireland by
permission of the Government Permit
Number 7735. © Ordnance Survey Ireland
and Government of Ireland.

Ordnance Survey®   PAGE 11, EDINBURGH,
and PAGE 15, LONDON:
This product includes mapping data licensed
from Ordnance Survey® with the permission
of the Controller of Her Majesty's Stationery
Office. © Crown copyright 2004. All rights
reserved. Licence number 100011710.

VECTOR DATA: Courtesy of Gräfe and Unser
Verlag GmbH, München, Germany (city
center maps of Bangkok, Beijing, Cape Town,
Jerusalem, Mexico City, Moscow, Singapore,
Sydney, Tokyo and Washington D.C.)

Copyright © 2004 Philip's

Philip's, a division of
Octopus Publishing Group Limited,
2–4 Heron Quays, London E14 4JP

Published in North America by
Oxford University Press, Inc.
198 Madison Avenue,
New York, NY 10016

www.oup.com/us/atlas

OXFORD   Oxford is a registered trademark
UNIVERSITY PRESS   of Oxford University Press

*Library of Congress Cataloging-in-Publication Data
available*

ISBN 0–19–522147–8

Printing (last digit): 9 8 7 6 5 4 3 2 1

Printed in Spain

FOREWORD

AN AUTHORITATIVE AND SERIOUS REFERENCE WORK, the Oxford *Atlas of the World* is one of the finest atlases available anywhere in the world. The atlas incorporates computer-derived maps which have been produced using the very latest in digital cartographic techniques.

The Oxford *Atlas of the World* has been devised with the help of a panel of specialist geography consultants from the United Kingdom and the United States, whose specialties range from the history of cartography, urban and social geography, epidemiology, and the European Union to biogeography and applied geomorphology. The result of their valuable input can be seen in the wealth of maps and data contained in the "*Introduction to World Geography*" section of this atlas.

Country names are shown in conventional English form and are those that are in common usage. They are the forms used by publications such as *Newsweek* and *The Washington Post,* and by the BBC and the British Foreign Office. Alternative country names appear in brackets on the maps where space permits – for example, Burma (Myanmar) – and are cross-referenced in the index, for example, Côte d'Ivoire = Ivory Coast.

HOW TO USE THE ATLAS
The atlas is divided into a number of sections which are explained below.

WORLD STATISTICS AND IMAGES OF EARTH
World statistics on topics such as area and population for every country in the world, and physical dimensions – including the largest islands, lakes and seas, the highest mountains and the longest rivers, by continent. Also included in this section is a listing of the world's largest cities by population, arranged in country alphabetical order. This section is followed by a beautifully illustrated satellite section showing 16 of the world's major regions and cities in the Americas, Europe, Africa, Asia, and Australasia.

THE GAZETTEER OF NATIONS
A comprehensive A–Z reference providing concise profiles of every country's geography, climate, history, politics, and economy, together with ready-reference tables, and illustrated with flags and locator maps.

INTRODUCTION TO WORLD GEOGRAPHY
A richly informative section comprising 48 pages of maps, charts, graphs, and diagrams which explain key themes about the world in which we live. The topics covered include the Solar System, oceans, climate, the environment, energy, and trade. Explanatory text on each spread describes the patterns shown by the data.

CITY MAPS
A detailed selection of maps for 67 urban areas around the world. These are useful for planning trips abroad as well as for comparative studies of cities worldwide. Also included is a 7-page index to the city maps.

WORLD MAPS
An outstanding collection of 176 pages of distinctive Philip's cartography. The highly acclaimed physical world maps combine relief shading with layer-colored contours to give a striking visual picture of the Earth's surface. Roads, railroads, canals, and airports are accurately depicted on the maps, and towns and cities are clearly marked. More information on the key features employed in the construction and presentation of the maps is given on the facing page.

GEOGRAPHICAL GLOSSARY, REGIONS IN THE NEWS, AND INDEX
The 75,000-name index to the world maps includes geographical features as well as towns and cities, with both latitude/longitude and letter/figure grid references. Preceding the index is a list of geographical terms from various foreign languages that may be found in the place names on the maps and also in the index, together with their meanings. Finally, completing the Atlas is a selection of detailed, up-to-date maps highlighting regions around the world that are currently in the news, such as Iraq, Afghanistan, the Near East, Kashmir, and the latest expansion of the European Union.

SPECIALIST GEOGRAPHY CONSULTANTS

THE EDITORS are grateful to the following people for acting as specialist geography consultants on the "*Introduction to World Geography*" front section:
Professor D. Brunsden Kings College, University of London, UK
Dr C. Clarke Oxford University, UK
Professor P. Haggett University of Bristol, UK
Professor M-L. Hsu University of Minnesota, Minnesota, USA
Professor K. McLachlan Geopolitical and International Boundaries Research Centre, School of Oriental and African Studies, University of London, UK

Professor M. Monmonier Syracuse University, New York, USA
Professor M. J. Tooley University of St Andrews, UK
Dr T. Unwin Royal Holloway, University of London, UK

THE EDITORS would also like to thank:
Keith Lye
Robin Scagell
Dr I. S. Evans Durham University, UK
Dr Andrew Tatham The Royal Geographical Society

WORLD MAPS

The reference maps which form the main body of this atlas have been prepared in accordance with the highest standards of international cartography to provide an accurate and detailed representation of the Earth. The scales and projections used have been carefully chosen to give balanced coverage of the world, while emphasizing the most densely populated and economically significant regions. A hallmark of Philip's mapping is the use of hill shading and relief coloring to create a graphic impression of landforms: this makes the maps exceptionally easy to read. However, knowledge of the key features employed in the construction and presentation of the maps will enable the reader to derive the fullest benefit from the atlas.

MAP SEQUENCE

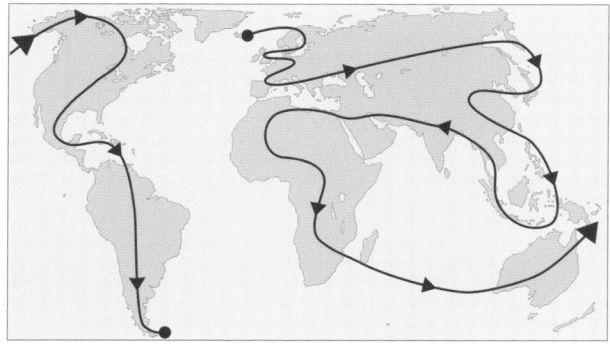

The atlas covers the Earth continent by continent: first Europe; then its land neighbor Asia (mapped north before south, in a clockwise sequence), then Africa, Australia and Oceania, North America, and South America. This is the classic arrangement adopted by most cartographers since the 16th century. For each continent, there are maps at a variety of scales. First, physical relief and political maps of the whole continent; then a series of larger-scale maps of the regions within the continent, each followed, where required, by still larger-scale maps of the most important and densely populated areas. The governing principle is that by turning the pages of the atlas, the reader moves steadily from north to south through each continent, with each map overlapping its neighbors.

MAP PRESENTATION

With very few exceptions (for example, for the Arctic and Antarctic), the maps are drawn with north at the top, regardless of whether they are presented upright or sideways on the page. In the borders will be found the map title; a locator diagram showing the area covered; continuation arrows showing the page numbers for maps of adjacent areas; the scale; the projection used; the degrees of latitude and longitude; and the letters and figures used in the index for locating place names and geographical features. Physical relief maps also have a height reference panel identifying the colors used for each layer of contouring.

MAP SYMBOLS

Each map contains a vast amount of detail which can only be conveyed clearly and accurately by the use of symbols. Points and circles of varying sizes locate and identify the relative importance of towns and cities; different styles of type are employed for administrative, geographical, and regional place names to aid identification. A variety of pictorial symbols denote landforms such as glaciers, marshes, and coral reefs, and man-made structures including roads, railroads, airports, and canals. International borders are shown by red lines. Where neighboring countries are in dispute, for example in parts of the Middle East, the maps show the *de facto* boundary between nations, regardless of the legal or historical situation. The

symbols are explained on the first page of the World Maps section of the atlas.

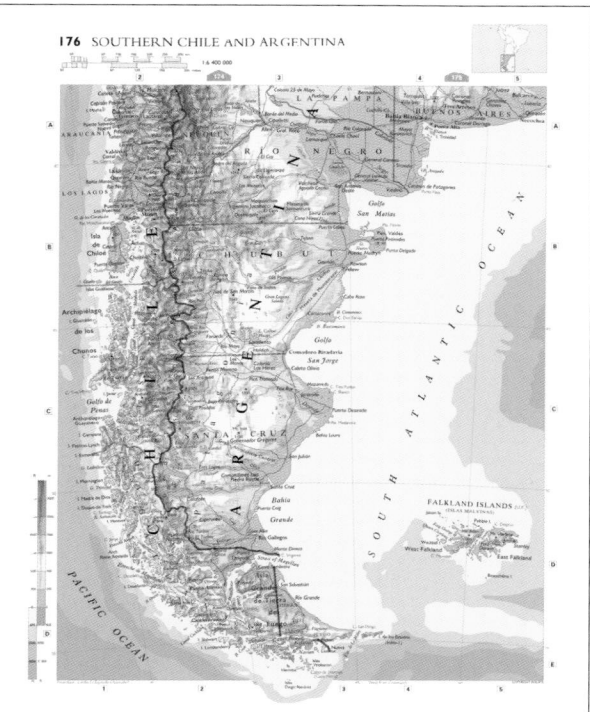

MAP SCALES

1:16 000 000
1 inch = 252 statute miles

The scale of each map is given in the numerical form known as the "representative fraction." The first figure is always one, signifying one unit of distance on the map; the second figure, usually in millions, is the number by which the map unit must be multiplied to give the equivalent distance on the Earth's surface. Calculations can easily be made in centimeters and kilometers, by dividing the Earth units figure by 100 000 (i.e. deleting the last five 0s). Thus 1:1 000 000 means 1 cm = 10 km. The calculation for inches and miles is more laborious, but 1 000 000 divided by 63 360 (the number of inches in a mile) shows that 1:1 000 000 means approximately 1 inch = 16 miles. The table below provides distance equivalents for scales down to 1:50 000 000.

LARGE SCALE		
1:1 000 000	1 cm = 10 km	1 inch = 16 miles
1:2 500 000	1 cm = 25 km	1 inch = 39.5 miles
1:5 000 000	1 cm = 50 km	1 inch = 79 miles
1:6 000 000	1 cm = 60 km	1 inch = 95 miles
1:8 000 000	1 cm = 80 km	1 inch = 126 miles
1:10 000 000	1 cm = 100 km	1 inch = 158 miles
1:15 000 000	1 cm = 150 km	1 inch = 237 miles
1:20 000 000	1 cm = 200 km	1 inch = 316 miles
1:50 000 000	1 cm = 500 km	1 inch = 790 miles
SMALL SCALE		

MEASURING DISTANCES

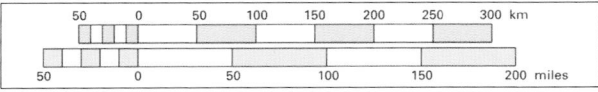

Although each map is accompanied by a scale bar, distances cannot always be measured with confidence because of the distortions involved in portraying the curved surface of the Earth on a flat page. As a general rule, the larger the map scale, the more accurate and reliable will be the distance measured. On small-scale maps such as those of the world and of entire continents, measurement may only be accurate along the "standard parallels," or central axes, and should not be attempted without considering the map projection.

MAP PROJECTIONS

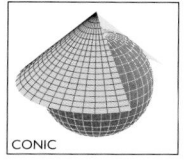 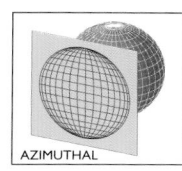 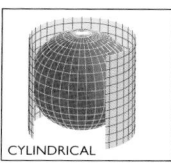

Unlike a globe, no flat map can give a true scale representation of the world in terms of area, shape, and position of every region. Each of the numerous systems that have been devised for projecting the curved surface of the Earth on to a flat page involves the sacrifice of accuracy in one or more of these elements. The variations in shape and position of land masses such as Alaska, Greenland and Australia, for example, can be quite dramatic when different projections are compared.

For this atlas, the guiding principle has been to select projections that involve the least distortion of size and distance. The projection used for each map is noted in the border. Most fall into one of three categories – conic, azimuthal, or cylindrical – whose basic concepts are shown above. Each involves plotting the forms of the Earth's surface on a grid of latitude and longitude lines, which may be shown as parallels, curves, or radiating spokes.

LATITUDE AND LONGITUDE

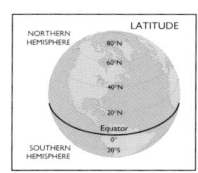 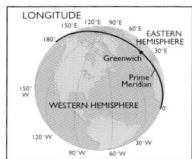 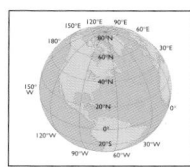

Accurate positioning of individual points on the Earth's surface is made possible by reference to the geometrical system of latitude and longitude. Latitude parallels are drawn west–east around the Earth and numbered by degrees north and south of the Equator, which is designated 0° of latitude. Longitude meridians are drawn north–south and numbered by degrees east and west of the prime meridian, 0° of longitude, which passes through Greenwich in England. By referring to these co-ordinates and their subdivisions of minutes (1/60th of a degree) and seconds (1/60th of a minute), any place on Earth can be located to within a few hundred yards. Latitude and longitude are indicated by blue lines on the maps; they are straight or curved according to the projection employed. Reference to these lines is the easiest way of determining the relative positions of places on different maps, and for plotting compass directions.

NAME FORMS

For ease of reference, both English and local name forms appear in the atlas. Oceans, seas, and countries are shown in English throughout the atlas; country names may be abbreviated to their commonly accepted form (e.g. Germany, not The Federal Republic of Germany). Conventional English forms are also used for place names on the smaller-scale maps of the continents. However, local name forms are used on all large-scale and regional maps, with the English form given in brackets only for important cities – the large-scale map of Russia and Central Asia thus shows Moskva (Moscow). For countries which do not use a Roman script, place names have been transcribed according to the systems adopted by the British and US Geographic Names Authorities. For China, the Pin Yin system has been used, with some more widely known forms appearing in brackets, as with Beijing (Peking). Both English and local names appear in the index, the English form being cross-referenced to the local form.

CONTENTS

WORLD STATISTICS

COUNTRIES VI
CITIES VII
PHYSICAL DIMENSIONS VIII

IMAGES OF EARTH

VANCOUVER, CANADA IX
LOS ANGELES, USA X
NEW YORK, USA XI
RIVER AMAZON, BRAZIL XII
SANTIAGO, CHILE XIII
LONDON, UK XIV
IJSSELMEER, NETHERLANDS XV
NAPLES, ITALY XVI
STRAIT OF GIBRALTAR XVII
CAIRO, EGYPT XVIII
WESTERN CAPE, SOUTH AFRICA XIX
TEHRAN, IRAN XX
KARACHI, PAKISTAN XXI
TOKYO, JAPAN XXII
SYDNEY, AUSTRALIA XXIII
CHRISTCHURCH,
    NEW ZEALAND XXIV

THE GAZETTEER OF NATIONS

AN A–Z GAZETTEER OF
    COUNTRIES 1–32

INTRODUCTION TO WORLD GEOGRAPHY

THE UNIVERSE 2–3
THE SOLAR SYSTEM 4–5
TIME AND MOTION 6–7
OCEANS 8–9
GEOLOGY 10–11
LANDFORMS 12–13
ATMOSPHERE AND WEATHER 14–15
CLIMATE 16–17
WATER AND VEGETATION 18–19
THE NATURAL
    ENVIRONMENT 20–21
PEOPLE AND THE
    ENVIRONMENT 22–23
POPULATION 24–25
CITIES 26–27
THE HUMAN FAMILY 28–29
CONFLICT AND
    COOPERATION 30–31
AGRICULTURE 32–33
ENERGY 34–35
MINERALS 36–37
MANUFACTURING 38–39
TRADE 40–41
HEALTH 42–43
WEALTH 44–45
STANDARDS OF LIVING 46–47

CITY MAPS

AMSTERDAM 2
ATHENS 2
ATLANTA 3
BAGHDAD 3
BANGKOK 3
BARCELONA 4
BEIJING 4
BERLIN 5
BOSTON 6
BRUSSELS 6
BUDAPEST 7
BUENOS AIRES 7
CAIRO 7
CALCUTTA (KOLKATA) 8
CANTON 8
CAPE TOWN 8
CHICAGO 9
COPENHAGEN 10
DELHI 10
DUBLIN 11
EDINBURGH 11
HELSINKI 12
HONG KONG 12
ISTANBUL 12
JAKARTA 13
JERUSALEM 13
JOHANNESBURG 13
KARACHI 14
LAGOS 14
LISBON 14
LONDON 15
LOS ANGELES 16
LIMA 16
MADRID 17
MANILA 17
MELBOURNE 17
MEXICO CITY 18
MIAMI 18
MILAN 18
MONTREAL 19
MOSCOW 19
MUMBAI 20
MUNICH 20
NEW YORK 21
OSAKA 22
OSLO 22
PARIS 23
PRAGUE 24
RIO DE JANEIRO 24
ROME 25
SAN FRANCISCO 25
ST PETERSBURG 26
SANTIAGO 26
SÃO PAULO 26
SEOUL 26
SHANGHAI 27
SINGAPORE 27
STOCKHOLM 28
SYDNEY 28
TOKYO 29
TEHRAN 30
TIANJIN 30
TORONTO 30
VIENNA 31
WARSAW 31
WASHINGTON 32
WELLINGTON 32

INDEX TO CITY MAPS

33–39

WORLD MAPS

THE WORLD

MAP SYMBOLS 1

THE WORLD: PHYSICAL 2–3
1:76 000 000

THE WORLD: POLITICAL 4–5
1:76 000 000

ARCTIC OCEAN 6
1:28 000 000

ANTARCTICA 7
1:28 000 000

ATLANTIC OCEAN 8
1:41 000 000

ISLANDS OF THE
    ATLANTIC 9
BERMUDA 1:400 000
NEW PROVIDENCE ISLAND 1:400 000
MADEIRA 1:800 000
AZORES 1:1 600 000
CANARY ISLANDS 1:1 600 000
FALKLAND ISLANDS 1:6 400 000
ASCENSION ISLAND 1:400 000
ST HELENA 1:400 000
CAPE VERDE ISLANDS 1:8 000 000

GREENLAND 10
1:10 000 000

ICELAND 11
1:2 000 000

EUROPE

EUROPE: PHYSICAL 12
1:16 000 000

EUROPE: POLITICAL 13
1:16 000 000

SCANDINAVIA 14–15
1:4 000 000
ICELAND 1:4 000 000

DENMARK AND
    SOUTHERN SWEDEN 16–17
1:2 000 000

SOUTHERN NORWAY 18
1:2 000 000

BRITISH ISLES 19
1:4 000 000

ENGLAND AND WALES 20–21
1:1 600 000

SCOTLAND 22
1:1 600 000

IRELAND 23
1:1 600 000

NETHERLANDS, BELGIUM
    AND LUXEMBOURG 24
1:2 000 000

FRANCE 25
1:4 000 000

NORTHERN FRANCE 26–27
1:2 000 000

SOUTHERN FRANCE 28–29
1:2 000 000

GERMANY 30–31
1:2 000 000

SWITZERLAND 32–33
1:800 000

AUSTRIA, CZECH
    REPUBLIC AND
    SLOVAK REPUBLIC 34–35
1:2 000 000

CENTRAL EUROPE 36–37
1:4 000 000

MEDITERRANEAN
    ISLANDS 38–39
IBIZA, MAJORCA, MINORCA 1:800 000
MALTA 1:400 000
CORFU 1:800 000
RHODES 1:800 000
LEVKAS, ZANTE, CEPHALONIA 1:800 000
CRETE 1:1 000 000
CYPRUS 1:1 000 000

EASTERN SPAIN 40–41
1:2 000 000

WESTERN SPAIN AND
    PORTUGAL 42–43
1:2 000 000

NORTHERN ITALY,
    SLOVENIA AND
    CROATIA 44–45
1:2 000 000

SOUTHERN ITALY 46–47
1:2 000 000

SOUTHERN GREECE AND
    WESTERN TURKEY 48–49
1:2 000 000

SERBIA AND MONTENEGRO,
    BULGARIA AND
    NORTHERN GREECE 50–51
1:2 000 000

HUNGARY, ROMANIA AND
    THE LOWER DANUBE 52–53
1:2 000 000

POLAND AND THE
    SOUTHERN BALTIC 54–55
1:2 000 000

EASTERN EUROPE AND
    TURKEY 56–57
1:8 000 000

BALTIC STATES,
    BELARUS
    AND UKRAINE 58–59
1:4 000 000

THE VOLGA BASIN
    AND THE CAUCASUS 60–61
1:4 000 000

ASIA

ASIA: PHYSICAL   62
1:40 000 000

ASIA: POLITICAL   63
1:40 000 000

SOUTHERN URALS   64
1:4 000 000

CENTRAL ASIA   65
1:4 000 000

RUSSIA
AND CENTRAL ASIA   66–67
1:16 000 000

CHINA
AND THE FAR EAST   68–69
1:12 000 000
HONG KONG AND MACAU 1:800 000

JAPAN   70–71
1:4 000 000
RYUKYU ISLANDS 1:4 000 000

SOUTHERN JAPAN   72–73
1:2 000 000

NORTHERN CHINA
AND KOREA   74–75
1:4 800 000

SOUTHERN CHINA   76–77
1:4 800 000

INDONESIA AND THE
PHILIPPINES   78–79
1:10 000 000
JAVA AND MADURA 1:6 000 000
BALI 1:1 600 000

PHILIPPINES   80–81
1:3 200 000

EASTERN INDONESIA   82–83
1:5 600 000

WESTERN INDONESIA   84–85
1:5 600 000

MAINLAND SOUTHEAST
ASIA   86–87
1:4 800 000
KO PHUKET 1:800 000
KO SAMUI 1:800 000
PINANG 1:800 000
SINGAPORE 1:800 000

SOUTHERN ASIA AND
THE MIDDLE EAST   88–89
1:14 000 000

BANGLADESH,
NORTHEASTERN INDIA
AND BURMA   90
1:4 800 000

AFGHANISTAN
AND PAKISTAN   91
1:5 600 000

NORTHERN INDIA
AND NEPAL   92–93
1:4 800 000

SOUTHERN INDIA AND
SRI LANKA   94–95
1:4 800 000

LAKSHADWEEP ISLANDS 1:4 800 000
ANDAMAN AND
NICOBAR ISLANDS 1:4 800 000

THE MIDDLE EAST   96–97
1:5 600 000

SOUTHERN ARABIAN
PENINSULA   98–99
1:5 600 000

TURKEY AND
TRANSCAUCASIA   100–101
1:4 000 000

ARABIA AND THE HORN
OF AFRICA   102
1:12 000 000

THE NEAR EAST   103
1:2 000 000

AFRICA

AFRICA: PHYSICAL   104
1:33 600 000

AFRICA: POLITICAL   105
1:33 600 000

THE NILE VALLEY   106–107
1:6 400 000
THE NILE DELTA 1:3 200 000

CENTRAL NORTH
AFRICA   108–109
1:6 400 000

NORTHWEST AFRICA   110–111
1:6 400 000

WEST AFRICA   112–113
1:6 400 000

CENTRAL AFRICA   114–115
1:6 400 000
SÃO TOMÉ AND PRÍNCIPE 1:6 400 000

SOUTHERN AFRICA   116–117
1:6 400 000
MADAGASCAR 1:6 400 000

EAST AFRICA   118–119
1:6 400 000

THE HORN OF AFRICA   120
1:6 400 000

INDIAN OCEAN   121
1:40 000 000
COMOROS 1:6 400 000
SEYCHELLES 1:2 000 000
RÉUNION 1:2 000 000
MAURITIUS 1:2 000 000

AUSTRALIA AND OCEANIA

AUSTRALIA AND OCEANIA:
PHYSICAL
AND POLITICAL   122–123
1:16 000 000

WESTERN AUSTRALIA   124–125
1:6 400 000

EASTERN AUSTRALIA   126–127
1:6 400 000
WHITSUNDAY GROUP 1:2 000 000
TASMANIA 1:6 400 000

SOUTHEAST
AUSTRALIA   128–129
1:3 200 000

NEW ZEALAND –
NORTH ISLAND   130
1:2 800 000

NEW ZEALAND –
SOUTH ISLAND   131
1:2 800 000
CHATHAM ISLANDS 1:2 800 000

PAPUA NEW GUINEA   132
1:5 200 000

ISLANDS OF THE
SOUTHWEST PACIFIC   133
1:4 000 000
FIJI 1:4 000 000
VANUATU 1:4 000 000
SOLOMON ISLANDS 1:4 000 000
TONGA 1:4 000 000
GUAM 1:4 000 000
TAHITI AND MOOREA 1:4 000 000
SAMOAN ISLANDS 1:4 000 000
NEW CALEDONIA 1:4 000 000

PACIFIC OCEAN   134–135
1:43 200 000

NORTH AMERICA

NORTH AMERICA:
PHYSICAL   136
1:28 000 000

NORTH AMERICA:
POLITICAL   137
1:28 000 000

CANADA   138–139
1:12 000 000
ALASKA 1:24 000 000

EASTERN CANADA   140–141
1:5 600 000

WESTERN CANADA   142–143
1:5 600 000

ALASKA   144
1:8 000 000

HAWAII   145
1:2 000 000
OAHU 1:500 000

UNITED STATES   146–147
1:9 600 000
HAWAII 1:8 000 000

EASTERN
UNITED STATES   148–149
1:4 800 000

NORTHEASTERN
UNITED STATES   150–151
1:2 000 000

SOUTHEASTERN
UNITED STATES   152–153
1:2 000 000

MIDDLE UNITED STATES   154–155
1:4 800 000

CHICAGO AND
THE MIDWEST   156–157
1:2 000 000

WESTERN
UNITED STATES   158–159
1:4 800 000

CENTRAL AND SOUTHERN
CALIFORNIA AND WESTERN
WASHINGTON   160–161
1:2 000 000

MEXICO   162–163
1:6 400 000

CENTRAL AMERICA AND
THE WEST INDIES   164–165
1:6 400 000
JAMAICA 1:2 400 000
GUADELOUPE 1:1 600 000
MARTINIQUE 1:1 600 000
PUERTO RICO 1:2 400 000
VIRGIN ISLANDS 1:1 600 000
ST LUCIA 1:800 000
BARBADOS 1:800 000

SOUTH AMERICA

SOUTH AMERICA:
PHYSICAL   166
1:28 000 000

SOUTH AMERICA:
POLITICAL   167
1:28 000 000

SOUTH AMERICA –
NORTHWEST   168–169
1:6 400 000
TRINIDAD AND TOBAGO 1:2 000 000

EASTERN BRAZIL   170–171
1:6 400 000

SOUTH AMERICA –
WEST   172–173
1:6 400 000
GALAPAGOS ISLANDS 1:3 200 000
EASTER ISLAND 1:400 000

CENTRAL
SOUTH AMERICA   174–175
1:6 400 000

SOUTHERN CHILE AND
ARGENTINA   176
1:6 400 000

GEOGRAPHICAL
GLOSSARY   177–178

INDEX TO WORLD
MAPS   179–304

WORLD: REGIONS
IN THE NEWS   305

World Statistics: Countries

This alphabetical list includes the principal countries and territories of the world. If a territory is not completely independent, the country it is associated with is named. The area figures give the total area of land, inland water, and ice. The population figures are 2003 estimates where available. The annual income is the Gross Domestic Product per capita† in US dollars. The figures are the latest available, usually 2002 estimates.

Country/Territory	Area km² Thousands	Area miles² Thousands	Population Thousands	Capital	Annual Income US $
Afghanistan	652	252	28,717	Kabul	700
Albania	28.7	11.1	3,582	Tirana	4,400
Algeria	2,382	920	32,819	Algiers	5,400
American Samoa (US)	0.20	0.08	70	Pago Pago	8,000
Andorra	0.47	0.18	69	Andorra La Vella	19,000
Angola	1,247	481	10,766	Luanda	1,700
Anguilla (UK)	0.10	0.04	13	The Valley	8,600
Antigua & Barbuda	0.44	0.17	68	St John's	11,000
Argentina	2,780	1,074	38,741	Buenos Aires	10,500
Armenia	29.8	11.5	3,326	Yerevan	3,600
Aruba (Netherlands)	0.19	0.07	71	Oranjestad	28,000
Australia	7,741	2,989	19,732	Canberra	26,900
Austria	83.9	32.4	8,188	Vienna	27,900
Azerbaijan	86.6	33.4	7,831	Baku	3,700
Azores (Portugal)	2.2	0.86	236	Ponta Delgada	15,000
Bahamas	13.9	5.4	297	Nassau	15,300
Bahrain	0.69	0.27	667	Manama	15,100
Bangladesh	144	55.6	138,448	Dhaka	1,800
Barbados	0.43	0.17	277	Bridgetown	15,000
Belarus	208	80.2	10,322	Minsk	8,700
Belgium	30.5	11.8	10,289	Brussels	29,200
Belize	23.0	8.9	266	Belmopan	4,900
Benin	113	43.5	7,041	Porto-Novo	1,100
Bermuda (UK)	0.05	0.02	64	Hamilton	35,200
Bhutan	47.0	18.1	2,140	Thimphu	1,300
Bolivia	1,099	424	8,586	La Paz/Sucre	2,500
Bosnia-Herzegovina	51.2	19.8	3,989	Sarajevo	1,900
Botswana	582	225	1,573	Gaborone	8,500
Brazil	8,514	3,287	182,033	Brasília	7,600
Brunei	5.8	2.2	358	Bandar Seri Begawan	18,600
Bulgaria	111	42.8	7,538	Sofia	6,500
Burkina Faso	274	106	13,228	Ouagadougou	1,100
Burma (= Myanmar)	677	261	42,511	Rangoon	1,700
Burundi	27.8	10.7	6,096	Bujumbura	500
Cambodia	181	69.9	13,125	Phnom Penh	1,600
Cameroon	475	184	15,746	Yaoundé	1,700
Canada	9,971	3,850	32,207	Ottawa	29,300
Canary Is. (Spain)	7.2	2.8	1,682	Las Palmas/Santa Cruz	19,900
Cape Verde Is.	4.0	1.6	412	Praia	1,400
Cayman Is. (UK)	0.26	0.10	42	George Town	35,000
Central African Republic	623	241	3,684	Bangui	1,200
Chad	1,284	496	9,253	Ndjaména	1,000
Chile	757	292	15,665	Santiago	10,100
China	9,597	3,705	1,286,975	Beijing	4,700
Colombia	1,139	440	41,662	Bogotá	6,100
Comoros	2.2	0.86	633	Moroni	700
Congo	342	132	2,954	Brazzaville	900
Congo (Dem. Rep. of the)	2,345	905	56,625	Kinshasa	600
Cook Is. (NZ)	0.24	0.09	21	Avarua	5,000
Costa Rica	51.1	19.7	3,896	San José	8,300
Croatia	56.5	21.8	4,422	Zagreb	9,800
Cuba	111	42.8	11,263	Havana	2,700
Cyprus	9.3	3.6	772	Nicosia	13,200
Czech Republic	78.9	30.5	10,249	Prague	15,300
Denmark	43.1	16.6	5,384	Copenhagen	28,900
Djibouti	23.2	9.0	457	Djibouti	1,300
Dominica	0.75	0.29	70	Roseau	5,400
Dominican Republic	48.5	18.7	8,716	Santo Domingo	6,300
East Timor	14.9	5.7	998	Dili	500
Ecuador	284	109	13,710	Quito	3,200
Egypt	1,001	387	74,719	Cairo	4,000
El Salvador	21.0	8.1	6,470	San Salvador	4,600
Equatorial Guinea	28.1	10.8	510	Malabo	2,700
Eritrea	118	45.4	4,362	Asmara	700
Estonia	45.1	17.4	1,409	Tallinn	11,000
Ethiopia	1,104	426	66,558	Addis Ababa	700
Færoe Is. (Denmark)	1.4	0.54	46	Tórshavn	22,000
Fiji Islands	18.3	7.1	869	Suva	5,600
Finland	338	131	5,191	Helsinki	25,800
France	552	213	60,181	Paris	26,000
French Guiana (France)	90.0	34.7	187	Cayenne	14,400
French Polynesia (France)	4.0	1.5	262	Papeete	5,000
Gabon	268	103	1,322	Libreville	6,500
Gambia, The	11.3	4.4	1,501	Banjul	1,800
Gaza Strip (OPT)*	0.36	0.14	1,275	–	600
Georgia	69.7	26.9	4,934	Tbilisi	3,200
Germany	357	138	82,398	Berlin	26,200
Ghana	239	92.1	20,468	Accra	2,000
Gibraltar (UK)	0.006	0.002	28	Gibraltar Town	17,500
Greece	132	50.9	10,666	Athens	19,100
Greenland (Denmark)	2,176	840	56	Nuuk (Godthåb)	20,000
Grenada	0.34	0.13	89	St George's	5,000
Guadeloupe (France)	1.7	0.66	440	Basse-Terre	9,000
Guam (US)	0.55	0.21	164	Agana	21,000
Guatemala	109	42.0	13,909	Guatemala City	3,900
Guinea	246	94.9	9,030	Conakry	2,100
Guinea-Bissau	36.1	13.9	1,361	Bissau	700
Guyana	215	83.0	702	Georgetown	3,800
Haiti	27.8	10.7	7,528	Port-au-Prince	1,400
Honduras	112	43.3	6,670	Tegucigalpa	2,500
Hong Kong (China)	1.1	0.42	7,394	–	27,200
Hungary	93.0	35.9	10,045	Budapest	13,300
Iceland	103	39.8	281	Reykjavik	30,200
India	3,287	1,269	1,049,700	New Delhi	2,600
Indonesia	1,905	735	234,893	Jakarta	3,100
Iran	1,648	636	68,279	Tehran	6,800
Iraq	438	169	24,683	Baghdad	2,400
Ireland	70.3	27.1	3,924	Dublin	29,300
Israel	20.6	8.0	6,117	Jerusalem	19,500
Italy	301	116	57,998	Rome	25,100
Ivory Coast (= Côte d'Ivoire)	322	125	16,962	Yamoussoukro	1,400
Jamaica	11.0	4.2	2,696	Kingston	3,800
Japan	378	146	127,214	Tokyo	28,700
Jordan	89.3	34.5	5,460	Amman	4,300
Kazakhstan	2,725	1,052	16,764	Astana	7,200
Kenya	580	224	31,639	Nairobi	1,100
Kiribati	0.73	0.28	99	Tarawa	800
Korea, North	121	46.5	22,466	Pyŏngyang	1,000
Korea, South	99.3	38.3	48,289	Seoul	19,600
Kuwait	17.8	6.9	2,183	Kuwait City	17,500
Kyrgyzstan	200	77.2	4,893	Bishkek	2,900
Laos	237	91.4	5,922	Vientiane	1,800
Latvia	64.6	24.9	2,349	Riga	8,900
Lebanon	10.4	4.0	3,728	Beirut	4,800
Lesotho	30.4	11.7	1,862	Maseru	2,700
Liberia	111	43.0	3,317	Monrovia	1,000
Libya	1,760	679	5,499	Tripoli	6,200
Liechtenstein	0.16	0.06	33	Vaduz	25,000
Lithuania	65.2	25.2	3,593	Vilnius	8,400
Luxembourg	2.6	1.0	454	Luxembourg	48,900
Macau (China)	0.02	0.007	470	–	18,500
Macedonia (FYROM)	25.7	9.9	2,063	Skopje	5,100
Madagascar	587	227	16,980	Antananarivo	800
Madeira (Portugal)	0.78	0.30	241	Funchal	22,700
Malawi	118	45.7	11,651	Lilongwe	600
Malaysia	330	127	23,093	Kuala Lumpur/Putrajaya	8,800
Maldives	0.30	0.12	330	Malé	3,900
Mali	1,240	479	11,626	Bamako	900
Malta	0.32	0.12	400	Valletta	17,200
Marshall Is.	0.18	0.07	56	Majuro	1,600
Martinique (France)	1.1	0.43	426	Fort-de-France	10,700
Mauritania	1,026	396	2,913	Nouakchott	1,700
Mauritius	2.0	0.79	1,210	Port Louis	10,100
Mayotte (France)	0.37	0.14	178	Mamoundzou	600
Mexico	1,958	756	104,908	Mexico City	8,900
Micronesia, Fed. States of	0.70	0.27	108	Palikir	2,000
Moldova	33.9	13.1	4,440	Chişinău	2,600
Monaco	0.001	0.0004	32	Monaco	27,000
Mongolia	1,567	605	2,712	Ulan Bator	1,900
Montserrat (UK)	0.10	0.04	9	Plymouth	3,400
Morocco	447	172	31,689	Rabat	3,900
Mozambique	802	309	17,479	Maputo	1,100
Namibia	824	318	1,927	Windhoek	6,900
Nauru	0.02	0.008	13	Yaren District	5,000
Nepal	147	56.8	26,470	Katmandu	1,400
Netherlands	41.5	16.0	16,151	Amsterdam/The Hague	27,200
Netherlands Antilles (Neths)	0.80	0.31	216	Willemstad	11,400
New Caledonia (France)	18.6	7.2	211	Nouméa	14,000
New Zealand	271	104	3,951	Wellington	20,100
Nicaragua	130	50.2	5,129	Managua	2,200
Niger	1,267	489	11,059	Niamey	800
Nigeria	924	357	133,882	Abuja	900
Northern Mariana Is. (US)	0.46	0.18	80	Saipan	12,500
Norway	324	125	4,546	Oslo	33,000
Oman	310	119	2,807	Muscat	8,300
Pakistan	796	307	150,695	Islamabad	2,000
Palau	0.46	0.18	20	Koror	9,000
Panama	75.5	29.2	2,961	Panamá	6,200
Papua New Guinea	463	179	5,296	Port Moresby	2,100
Paraguay	407	157	6,037	Asunción	4,300
Peru	1,285	496	28,410	Lima	5,000
Philippines	300	116	84,620	Manila	4,600
Poland	323	125	38,623	Warsaw	9,700
Portugal	88.8	34.3	10,102	Lisbon	19,400
Puerto Rico (US)	8.9	3.4	3,886	San Juan	11,100
Qatar	11.0	4.2	817	Doha	20,100
Réunion (France)	2.5	0.97	755	St-Denis	5,600
Romania	238	92.0	22,272	Bucharest	7,600
Russia	17,075	6,593	144,526	Moscow	9,700
Rwanda	26.3	10.2	7,810	Kigali	1,200
St Kitts & Nevis	0.26	0.10	39	Basseterre	8,800
St Lucia	0.54	0.21	162	Castries	5,400
St Vincent & Grenadines	0.39	0.15	117	Kingstown	2,900
Samoa	2.8	1.1	178	Apia	5,600
San Marino	0.06	0.02	28	San Marino	34,600
São Tomé & Príncipe	0.96	0.37	176	São Tomé	1,200
Saudi Arabia	2,150	830	24,294	Riyadh	11,400
Senegal	197	76.0	10,580	Dakar	1,500
Serbia & Montenegro	102	39.4	10,656	Belgrade	2,200
Seychelles	0.46	0.18	80	Victoria	7,800
Sierra Leone	71.7	27.7	5,733	Freetown	500
Singapore	0.68	0.26	4,609	Singapore	25,200
Slovak Republic	49.0	18.9	5,430	Bratislava	12,400
Slovenia	20.3	7.8	1,936	Ljubljana	19,200
Solomon Is.	28.9	11.2	509	Honiara	1,700
Somalia	638	246	8,025	Mogadishu	600
South Africa	1,221	471	42,769	C. Town/Pretoria/Bloem.	10,000
Spain	498	192	40,217	Madrid	21,200
Sri Lanka	65.6	25.3	19,742	Colombo	3,700
Sudan	2,506	967	38,114	Khartoum	1,400
Suriname	163	63.0	435	Paramaribo	3,400
Swaziland	17.4	6.7	1,161	Mbabane	4,800
Sweden	450	174	8,878	Stockholm	26,000
Switzerland	41.3	15.9	7,319	Bern	32,000
Syria	185	71.5	17,586	Damascus	3,700
Taiwan	36.0	13.9	22,603	Taipei	18,000
Tajikistan	143	55.3	6,864	Dushanbe	1,300
Tanzania	945	365	35,922	Dodoma	600
Thailand	513	198	64,265	Bangkok	7,000
Togo	56.8	21.9	5,429	Lomé	1,400
Tonga	0.65	0.25	108	Nuku'alofa	2,200
Trinidad & Tobago	5.1	2.0	1,104	Port of Spain	10,000
Tunisia	164	63.2	9,925	Tunis	6,800
Turkey	775	299	68,109	Ankara	7,300
Turkmenistan	488	188	4,776	Ashkhabad	6,700
Turks & Caicos Is. (UK)	0.43	0.17	19	Cockburn Town	9,600
Tuvalu	0.03	0.01	11	Fongafale	1,100
Uganda	241	93.1	25,633	Kampala	1,200
Ukraine	604	233	48,055	Kiev	4,500
United Arab Emirates	83.6	32.3	2,485	Abu Dhabi	22,100
United Kingdom	242	93.4	60,095	London	25,500
United States of America	9,629	3,718	290,343	Washington, DC	36,300
Uruguay	175	67.6	3,413	Montevideo	7,900
Uzbekistan	447	173	25,982	Tashkent	2,600
Vanuatu	12.2	4.7	199	Port-Vila	2,900
Vatican City	0.0004	0.0002	1	Vatican City	N/A
Venezuela	912	352	24,655	Caracas	5,400
Vietnam	332	128	81,625	Hanoi	2,300
Virgin Is. (UK)	0.15	0.06	22	Road Town	16,000
Virgin Is. (US)	0.35	0.13	125	Charlotte Amalie	19,000
Wallis & Futuna Is. (France)	0.20	0.08	16	Mata-Utu	2,000
West Bank (OPT)*	5.9	2.3	2,237	–	800
Western Sahara	266	103	262	El Aaiún	N/A
Yemen	528	204	19,350	Sana	800
Zambia	753	291	10,307	Lusaka	800
Zimbabwe	391	151	12,577	Harare	2,100

*OPT = Occupied Palestinian Territory N/A = Not available

† Gross Domestic Product per capita has been measured using the purchasing power parity method. This enables comparisons to be made between countries through their purchasing power (in US dollars), showing real price levels of goods and services rather than using currency exchange rates.

This list shows the principal cities with more than 750,000 inhabitants. The figures are taken from the most recent census or estimate available, usually 2000, and as far as possible are the population of the metropolitan area or urban agglomeration (for example, greater New York, Mexico, or Paris). All the figures are in thousands. Local name forms have been used for the smaller cities (for example, Thessaloniki).

AFGHANISTAN
Kabul — 2,602
ALGERIA
Algiers — 1,722
ANGOLA
Luanda — 2,697
ARGENTINA
Buenos Aires — 12,024
Córdoba — 1,368
Rosario — 1,279
Mendoza — 934
San Miguel de Tucumán — 792
ARMENIA
Yerevan — 1,407
AUSTRALIA
Sydney — 4,086
Melbourne — 3,466
Brisbane — 1,627
Perth — 1,381
Adelaide — 1,096
AUSTRIA
Vienna — 1,807
AZERBAIJAN
Baku — 1,792
BANGLADESH
Dhaka — 12,519
Chittagong — 3,651
Khulna — 1,442
Rajshahi — 1,035
BELARUS
Minsk — 1,717
BELGIUM
Brussels — 964
BOLIVIA
La Paz — 1,487
Santa Cruz — 1,035
Cochabamba — 797
BRAZIL
São Paulo — 17,962
Rio de Janeiro — 10,652
Belo Horizonte — 4,224
Pôrto Alegre — 3,757
Recife — 3,346
Salvador — 3,238
Fortaleza — 3,066
Curitiba — 2,562
Brasília — 2,051
Campinas — 1,434
Belém — 1,658
Manaus — 1,467
Santos — 1,270
Goiânia — 1,117
São José dos Campos — 972
São Luís — 968
Maceió — 886
Teresina — 848
Campo Grande — 821
Natal — 806
BULGARIA
Sofia — 1,187
BURKINA FASO
Ouagadougou — 831
BURMA (MYANMAR)
Rangoon — 4,393
Mandalay — 770
CAMBODIA
Phnom Penh — 1,070
CAMEROON
Douala — 1,642
Yaoundé — 1,420
CANADA
Toronto — 4,881
Montréal — 3,511
Vancouver — 2,079
Ottawa — 1,107
Calgary — 972
Edmonton — 957
CHILE
Santiago — 5,467
CHINA
Shanghai — 12,887
Beijing — 10,839
Tianjin — 9,156
Hong Kong — 6,860
Wuhan — 5,169
Chongqing — 4,900
Shenyang — 4,828
Guangzhou — 3,893
Chengdu — 3,294
Xi'an — 3,123
Changchun — 3,093
Harbin — 2,928
Nanjing — 2,740
Zibo — 2,675
Dalian — 2,628
Jinan — 2,568
Guiyang — 2,533
Linyi — 2,498
Taiyuan — 2,415
Qingdao — 2,316
Zhengzhou — 2,070
Zaozhuang — 2,048
Liupanshui — 2,023
Handan — 1,996
Jinxi — 1,821
Lu'an — 1,818
Hangzhou — 1,780
Tianmen — 1,779
Changsha — 1,775
Wanxian — 1,759
Lanzhou — 1,730
Nanchang — 1,722
Kunming — 1,701
Yantai — 1,681
Tangshan — 1,671
Xuzhou — 1,636
Xiantao — 1,614
Shijiazhuang — 1,603
Heze — 1,600
Yancheng — 1,562
Yulin — 1,558
Xinghua — 1,556
Tai'an — 1,503
Pingxiang — 1,502
Anshan — 1,453
Luoyang — 1,451
Jilin — 1,435
Qiqihar — 1,435
Suining (Sichuan) — 1,428
Ürümqi — 1,415
Fushun — 1,413
Fuzhou — 1,397
Neijiang — 1,393
Changde — 1,374
Zhanjiang — 1,368
Huainan — 1,354
Yiyang — 1,343
Xintai — 1,325
Baotou — 1,319
Dongguan — 1,319
Nanning — 1,311
Weifang — 1,287
Wenzhou — 1,269
Hefei — 1,242
Huaian — 1,232
Yueyang — 1,213
Suqian — 1,189
Tianshui — 1,187
Suzhou — 1,183
Shantou — 1,176
Ningbo — 1,173
Yuzhou — 1,173
Datong — 1,165
Jingmen — 1,153
Leshan — 1,137
Shenzhen — 1,131
Wuxi — 1,127
Xiaoshan — 1,124
Zaoyang — 1,121
Yixing — 1,108
Yongzhou — 1,097
Chifeng — 1,087
Huzhou — 1,077
Daqing — 1,076
Zigong — 1,072
Mianyang — 1,065
Nanchong — 1,055
Fuyu — 1,025
Jining (Shandong) — 1,019
Hohhot — 978
Xinyi (Guangdong) — 973
Benxi — 957
Jixi — 949
Liuzhou — 928
Xiangxiang — 908
Yichun (Heilongjiang) — 904
Xianyang — 896
Linqing — 891
Changzhou — 886
Zhangjiagang — 886
Zhangjiakou — 880
Jiamusi — 874
Yichun (Jiangxi) — 871
Zhaotong — 851
Yuyao — 848
Jinzhou — 834
Xuanzhou — 823
Huaibei — 814
Xinyu — 808
Mudanjiang — 801
Hengyang — 799
Jiaxing — 791
Anshun — 789
Fuxin — 785
Tongliao — 785
Hunjiang — 772
Kaifeng — 769
COLOMBIA
Bogotá — 6,771
Medellín — 2,866
Cali — 2,233
Barranquilla — 1,683
Bucaramanga — 937
Cartagena — 845
Cúcuta — 772
CONGO
Brazzaville — 1,306
CONGO (DEM. REP.)
Kinshasa — 5,054
Lubumbashi — 965
Mbuji-Mayi — 806
COSTA RICA
San José — 961
CROATIA
Zagreb — 1,067
CUBA
Havana — 2,256
CZECH REPUBLIC
Prague — 1,203
DENMARK
Copenhagen — 1,332
DOMINICAN REPUBLIC
Santo Domingo — 2,563
Santiago de los Caballeros — 804
ECUADOR
Guayaquil — 2,118
Quito — 1,616
EGYPT
Cairo — 9,462
Alexandria — 3,506
Shubrâ el Kheima — 937
EL SALVADOR
San Salvador — 1,341
ETHIOPIA
Addis Ababa — 2,645
FINLAND
Helsinki — 937
FRANCE
Paris — 9,630
Lyons — 1,353
Marseilles — 1,290
Lille — 991
Nice — 889
Toulouse — 761
Bordeaux — 754
GEORGIA
Tbilisi — 1,406
GERMANY
Berlin — 3,387
Hamburg — 1,705
Munich — 1,195
Cologne — 963
GHANA
Accra — 1,868
GREECE
Athens — 3,116
Thessaloniki — 789
GUATEMALA
Guatemala — 3,242
GUINEA
Conakry — 1,232
HAITI
Port-au-Prince — 1,769
HONDURAS
Tegucigalpa — 949
HUNGARY
Budapest — 1,819
INDIA
Mumbai (Bombay) — 16,086
Kolkata (Calcutta) — 13,058
Delhi — 12,441
Chennai (Madras) — 6,353
Bangalore — 5,567
Hyderabad — 5,445
Ahmedabad — 4,427
Pune (Poona) — 3,655
Surat — 2,699
Kanpur — 2,641
Jaipur — 2,259
Lucknow — 2,221
Nagpur — 2,089
Patna — 1,658
Indore — 1,597
Vadodara — 1,465
Bhopal — 1,425
Coimbatore — 1,420
Ludhiana — 1,368
Cochin (Kochi) — 1,340
Visakhapatnam — 1,309
Agra — 1,293
Varanasi — 1,199
Madurai — 1,187
Meerut — 1,143
Nashik — 1,117
Jabalpur — 1,100
Jamshedpur — 1,081
Asansol — 1,065
Bhilainagar-Durg — 1,049
Dhanbad — 1,046
Allahabad — 1,035
Faridabad — 1,018
Vijayawada — 999
Rajkot — 974
Amritsar — 955
Srinagar — 954
Ghaziabad — 928
Trivandrum — 885
Calicut (Kozhikode) — 875
Aurangabad — 868
Gwalior — 855
Solapur — 853
Ranchi — 844
Tiruchchirapalli — 837
Jodhpur — 833
Guwahati — 797
Chandigarh — 791
Hubli-Dharwad — 776
Mysore — 776
INDONESIA
Jakarta — 11,018
Bandung — 3,409
Surabaya — 2,461
Medan — 1,879
Palembang — 1,422
Ujung Pandang — 1,051
Bandar Lampung — 915
Malang — 787
Semarang — 787
Tegal — 762
Bogor — 761
IRAN
Tehran — 6,979
Mashhad — 1,990
Esfahan — 1,381
Tabriz — 1,274
Karaj — 1,200
Shiraz — 1,124
Qom — 888
Ahvaz — 871
Bakhtaran — 771
IRAQ
Baghdad — 4,865
Basra — 1,338
Mosul — 1,131
Irbil — 840
IRELAND
Dublin — 985
ISRAEL
Tel Aviv-Yafo — 2,001
ITALY
Rome — 2,649
Milan — 1,183
Naples — 993
Turin — 857
IVORY COAST
Abidjan — 3,790
JAPAN
Tokyo — 12,064
Yokohama — 6,427
Osaka — 2,599
Nagoya — 2,172
Sapporo — 1,922
Kobe — 1,493
Kyoto — 1,468
Fukuoka — 1,341
Kawasaki — 1,250
Hiroshima — 1,126
Kitakyushu — 1,011
Sendai — 1,008
Chiba — 887
Sakai — 792
JORDAN
Amman — 1,148
KAZAKHSTAN
Almaty — 1,130
KENYA
Nairobi — 2,233
KOREA, NORTH
Pyŏngyang — 3,124
Hamhung — 821
KOREA, SOUTH
Seoul — 9,888
Pusan — 3,830
Inch'on — 2,884
Taegu — 2,675
Taejŏn — 1,522
Kwangju — 1,379
Sŏngnam — 1,353
Ulsan — 1,340
Ansan — 984
Puch'on — 900
Suwŏn — 876
P'ohang — 790
KUWAIT
Kuwait — 879
LATVIA
Riga — 811
LEBANON
Beirut — 2,070
LIBYA
Tripoli — 1,733
Benghazi — 829
MADAGASCAR
Antananarivo — 1,603
MALAYSIA
Kuala Lumpur — 1,379
MALI
Bamako — 1,114
MEXICO
Mexico City — 18,066
Guadalajara — 3,697
Monterrey — 3,267
Puebla — 1,888
Toluca — 1,455
Tijuana — 1,297
León — 1,293
Ciudad Juárez — 1,239
Torreón — 1,012
San Luis Potosí — 857
Mérida — 849
Querétaro — 798
Mexicali — 771
Culiacán — 750
MONGOLIA
Ulan Bator — 764
MOROCCO
Casablanca — 3,357
Rabat — 1,616
Fès — 907
Marrakesh — 822
MOZAMBIQUE
Maputo — 1,094
NEPAL
Katmandu — 1,176
NETHERLANDS
Amsterdam — 1,105
Rotterdam — 1,078
NEW ZEALAND
Auckland — 1,102
NICARAGUA
Managua — 1,009
NIGER
Niamey — 775
NIGERIA
Lagos — 8,665
Ibadan — 1,549
Ogbomosho — 809
NORWAY
Oslo — 779
PAKISTAN
Karachi — 10,032
Lahore — 5,452
Faisalabad — 2,142
Rawalpindi — 1,521
Gujranwala — 1,325
Multan — 1,263
Hyderabad — 1,221
Peshawar — 1,066
Islamabad — 791
PANAMA
Panamá — 1,173
PARAGUAY
Asunción — 1,262
PERU
Lima — 7,443
PHILIPPINES
Manila — 9,950
Davao — 1,146
POLAND
Warsaw — 1,626
Lódz — 815
PORTUGAL
Lisbon — 3,861
Porto — 1,940
PUERTO RICO
San Juan — 2,217
ROMANIA
Bucharest — 2,001
RUSSIA
Moscow — 8,367
Saint Petersburg — 4,635
Nizhniy Novgorod — 1,332
Novosibirsk — 1,321
Yekaterinburg — 1,218
Omsk — 1,174
Samara — 1,132
Ufa — 1,102
Kazan — 1,063
Chelyabinsk — 1,045
Perm — 1,014
Rostov — 1,012
Volgograd — 1,000
Voronezh — 918
Saratov — 881
Ulyanovsk — 864
Krasnoyarsk — 840
Togliatti — 771
SAUDI ARABIA
Riyadh — 3,180
Jedda — 1,490
Mecca — 770
SENEGAL
Dakar — 2,078
SERBIA AND MONTENEGRO
Belgrade — 1,673
SIERRA LEONE
Freetown — 822
SINGAPORE
Singapore — 4,131
SOMALIA
Mogadishu — 1,162
SOUTH AFRICA
Johannesburg — 2,950
Cape Town — 2,930
Durban — 2,391
Pretoria — 1,590
Port Elizabeth — 1,006
SPAIN
Madrid — 3,017
Barcelona — 1,527
SUDAN
Khartoum — 2,742
SWEDEN
Stockholm — 1,612
Gothenburg — 778
SWITZERLAND
Zürich — 939
SYRIA
Aleppo — 2,229
Damascus — 2,144
Homs — 811
TAIWAN
Taipei — 2,550
Kaohsiung — 1,463
T'aichung — 950
TANZANIA
Dar es Salaam — 2,115
THAILAND
Bangkok — 7,372
TUNISIA
Tunis — 1,892
TURKEY
Istanbul — 8,953
Ankara — 3,203
Izmir — 2,250
Bursa — 1,184
Adana — 1,133
Gaziantep — 862
Konya — 761
UGANDA
Kampala — 1,213
UKRAINE
Kiev — 2,621
Kharkov — 1,521
Dnepropetrovsk — 1,122
Donetsk — 1,065
Odessa — 1,027
Zaporozhye — 863
Lvov — 794
UNITED ARAB EMIRATES
Abu Dhabi — 928
Dubai — 886
UNITED KINGDOM
London — 8,089
Birmingham — 2,373
Manchester — 2,353
Liverpool — 852
Glasgow — 832
UNITED STATES OF AMERICA
New York — 17,800
Los Angeles — 11,789
Chicago — 8,308
Philadelphia — 5,149
Miami — 4,919
Dallas–Fort Worth — 4,146
Boston — 4,032
Washington — 3,934
Detroit — 3,903
Houston — 3,823
Atlanta — 3,500
San Francisco — 3,229
Phoenix — 2,907
Seattle — 2,712
San Diego — 2,674
Minneapolis–St Paul — 2,389
St Louis — 2,078
Baltimore — 2,076
Tampa–St Petersburg — 2,062
Denver — 1,985
Cleveland — 1,787
Pittsburgh — 1,753
Portland — 1,583
San Jose — 1,538
San Bernardino — 1,507
Cincinnati — 1,503
Norfolk–Virginia Beach — 1,394
Sacramento — 1,393
Kansas City — 1,362
San Antonio — 1,328
Las Vegas — 1,314
Milwaukee — 1,309
Indianapolis — 1,219
Providence — 1,175
Orlando — 1,157
Columbus — 1,133
New Orleans — 1,009
Buffalo — 977
Memphis — 972
Austin — 902
Stamford — 889
Salt Lake City — 888
Jacksonville — 882
Louisville — 864
Hartford — 852
Richmond — 819
Charlotte — 759
URUGUAY
Montevideo — 1,324
UZBEKISTAN
Tashkent — 2,148
VENEZUELA
Caracas — 3,153
Maracaibo — 1,901
Valencia — 1,893
Maracay — 1,100
Ciudad Guayana — 966
Barquisimeto — 923
VIETNAM
Ho Chi Minh City — 4,619
Hanoi — 3,751
Haiphong — 1,676
YEMEN
Sana' — 1,327
ZAMBIA
Lusaka — 1,653
ZIMBABWE
Harare — 1,791
Bulawayo — 824

WORLD STATISTICS: PHYSICAL DIMENSIONS

Each topic list is divided into continents and within a continent the items are listed in order of size. The bottom part of many of the lists is selective in order to give examples from as many different countries as possible. The order of the continents is the same as in the atlas, beginning with Europe and ending with South America. The figures are rounded as appropriate.

World, Continents, Oceans

	km²	miles²	%
The World	509,450,000	196,672,000	–
Land	149,450,000	57,688,000	29.3
Water	360,000,000	138,984,000	70.7
Asia	44,500,000	17,177,000	29.8
Africa	30,302,000	11,697,000	20.3
North America	24,241,000	9,357,000	16.2
South America	17,793,000	6,868,000	11.9
Antarctica	14,100,000	5,443,000	9.4
Europe	9,957,000	3,843,000	6.7
Australia & Oceania	8,557,000	3,303,000	5.7
Pacific Ocean	179,679,000	69,356,000	49.9
Atlantic Ocean	92,373,000	35,657,000	25.7
Indian Ocean	73,917,000	28,532,000	20.5
Arctic Ocean	14,090,000	5,439,000	3.9

Ocean Depths

Atlantic Ocean

	m	ft
Puerto Rico (Milwaukee) Deep	9,220	30,249
Cayman Trench	7,680	25,197
Gulf of Mexico	5,203	17,070
Mediterranean Sea	5,121	16,801
Black Sea	2,211	7,254
North Sea	660	2,165

Indian Ocean

	m	ft
Java Trench	7,450	24,442
Red Sea	2,635	8,454

Pacific Ocean

	m	ft
Mariana Trench	11,022	36,161
Tonga Trench	10,882	35,702
Japan Trench	10,554	34,626
Kuril Trench	10,542	34,587

Arctic Ocean

	m	ft
Molloy Deep	5,608	18,399

Mountains

Europe

		m	ft
Elbrus	Russia	5,642	18,510
Mont Blanc	France/Italy	4,807	15,771
Monte Rosa	Italy/Switzerland	4,634	15,203
Dom	Switzerland	4,545	14,911
Liskamm	Switzerland	4,527	14,852
Weisshorn	Switzerland	4,505	14,780
Taschorn	Switzerland	4,490	14,730
Matterhorn/Cervino	Italy/Switzerland	4,478	14,691
Mont Maudit	France/Italy	4,465	14,649
Dent Blanche	Switzerland	4,356	14,291
Nadelhorn	Switzerland	4,327	14,196
Grandes Jorasses	France/Italy	4,208	13,806
Jungfrau	Switzerland	4,158	13,642
Grossglockner	Austria	3,797	12,457
Mulhacén	Spain	3,478	11,411
Zugspitze	Germany	2,962	9,718
Olympus	Greece	2,917	9,570
Triglav	Slovenia	2,863	9,393
Gerlachovka	Slovak Republic	2,655	8,711
Galdhöpiggen	Norway	2,468	8,100
Kebnekaise	Sweden	2,117	6,946
Ben Nevis	UK	1,343	4,406

Asia

		m	ft
Everest	China/Nepal	8,850	29,035
K2 (Godwin Austen)	China/Kashmir	8,611	28,251
Kanchenjunga	India/Nepal	8,598	28,208
Lhotse	China/Nepal	8,516	27,939
Makalu	China/Nepal	8,481	27,824
Cho Oyu	China/Nepal	8,201	26,906
Dhaulagiri	Nepal	8,172	26,811
Manaslu	Nepal	8,156	26,758
Nanga Parbat	Kashmir	8,126	26,660
Annapurna	Nepal	8,078	26,502
Gasherbrum	China/Kashmir	8,068	26,469
Broad Peak	China/Kashmir	8,051	26,414
Xixabangma	China	8,012	26,286
Kangbachen	India/Nepal	7,902	25,925
Trivor	Pakistan	7,720	25,328
Pik Kommunizma	Tajikistan	7,495	24,590
Demavend	Iran	5,604	18,386
Ararat	Turkey	5,165	16,945
Gunong Kinabalu	Malaysia (Borneo)	4,101	13,455
Fuji-San	Japan	3,776	12,388

Africa

		m	ft
Kilimanjaro	Tanzania	5,895	19,340
Mt Kenya	Kenya	5,199	17,057
Ruwenzori (Margherita)	Ug./Congo (D.R.)	5,109	16,762
Ras Dashan	Ethiopia	4,620	15,157
Meru	Tanzania	4,565	14,977
Karisimbi	Rwanda/Congo (D.R.)	4,507	14,787
Mt Elgon	Kenya/Uganda	4,321	14,176
Batu	Ethiopia	4,307	14,130
Toubkal	Morocco	4,165	13,665
Mt Cameroon	Cameroon	4,070	13,353

Oceania

		m	ft
Puncak Jaya	Indonesia	5,029	16,499
Puncak Trikora	Indonesia	4,750	15,584
Puncak Mandala	Indonesia	4,702	15,427
Mt Wilhelm	Papua New Guinea	4,508	14,790
Mauna Kea	USA (Hawaii)	4,205	13,796
Mauna Loa	USA (Hawaii)	4,169	13,681
Aoraki Mt Cook	New Zealand	3,753	12,313
Mt Kosciuszko	Australia	2,230	7,316

North America

		m	ft
Mt McKinley (Denali)	USA (Alaska)	6,194	20,321
Mt Logan	Canada	5,959	19,551
Pico de Orizaba	Mexico	5,610	18,405
Mt St Elias	USA/Canada	5,489	18,008
Popocatepetl	Mexico	5,452	17,887
Mt Foraker	USA (Alaska)	5,304	17,401
Ixtaccihuatl	Mexico	5,286	17,342
Lucania	Canada	5,227	17,149
Mt Steele	Canada	5,073	16,644
Mt Bona	USA (Alaska)	5,005	16,420
Mt Whitney	USA	4,418	14,495
Tajumulco	Guatemala	4,220	13,845
Chirripó Grande	Costa Rica	3,837	12,589
Pico Duarte	Dominican Rep.	3,175	10,417

South America

		m	ft
Aconcagua	Argentina	6,962	22,841
Bonete	Argentina	6,872	22,546
Ojos del Salado	Argentina/Chile	6,863	22,516
Pissis	Argentina	6,779	22,241
Mercedario	Argentina/Chile	6,770	22,211
Huascaran	Peru	6,768	22,204
Llullaillaco	Argentina/Chile	6,723	22,057
Nudo de Cachi	Argentina	6,720	22,047
Yerupaja	Peru	6,632	21,758
Sajama	Bolivia	6,542	21,463
Chimborazo	Ecuador	6,267	20,561
Pico Colon	Colombia	5,800	19,029
Pico Bolivar	Venezuela	5,007	16,427

Antarctica

		m	ft
Vinson Massif		4,897	16,066
Mt Kirkpatrick		4,528	14,855

Rivers

Europe

		km	miles
Volga	Caspian Sea	3,700	2,300
Danube	Black Sea	2,850	1,770
Ural	Caspian Sea	2,535	1,575
Dnepr (Dnipro)	Black Sea	2,285	1,420
Kama	Volga	2,030	1,260
Don	Black Sea	1,990	1,240
Petchora	Arctic Ocean	1,790	1,110
Oka	Volga	1,480	920
Dnister (Dniester)	Black Sea	1,400	870
Vyatka	Kama	1,370	850
Rhine	North Sea	1,320	820
N. Dvina	Arctic Ocean	1,290	800
Elbe	North Sea	1,145	710

Asia

		km	miles
Yangtze	Pacific Ocean	6,380	3,960
Yenisey–Angara	Arctic Ocean	5,550	3,445
Huang He	Pacific Ocean	5,464	3,395
Ob–Irtysh	Arctic Ocean	5,410	3,360
Mekong	Pacific Ocean	4,500	2,795
Amur	Pacific Ocean	4,400	2,730
Lena	Arctic Ocean	4,400	2,730
Irtysh	Ob	4,250	2,640
Yenisey	Arctic Ocean	4,090	2,540
Ob	Arctic Ocean	3,680	2,285
Indus	Indian Ocean	3,100	1,925
Brahmaputra	Indian Ocean	2,900	1,800
Syrdarya	Aral Sea	2,860	1,775
Salween	Indian Ocean	2,800	1,740
Euphrates	Indian Ocean	2,700	1,675
Amudarya	Aral Sea	2,540	1,575

Africa

		km	miles
Nile	Mediterranean	6,670	4,140
Congo	Atlantic Ocean	4,670	2,900
Niger	Atlantic Ocean	4,180	2,595
Zambezi	Indian Ocean	3,540	2,200
Oubangi/Uele	Congo (D.R.)	2,250	1,400
Kasai	Congo (D.R.)	1,950	1,210
Shaballe	Indian Ocean	1,930	1,200
Orange	Atlantic Ocean	1,860	1,155
Cubango	Okavango Delta	1,800	1,120
Limpopo	Indian Ocean	1,600	995
Senegal	Atlantic Ocean	1,600	995

Australia

		km	miles
Murray–Darling	Southern Ocean	3,750	2,330
Darling	Murray	3,070	1,905
Murray	Southern Ocean	2,575	1,600
Murrumbidgee	Murray	1,690	1,050

North America

		km	miles
Mississippi–Missouri	Gulf of Mexico	6,020	3,740
Mackenzie	Arctic Ocean	4,240	2,630
Mississippi	Gulf of Mexico	3,780	2,350
Missouri	Mississippi	3,780	2,350
Yukon	Pacific Ocean	3,185	1,980
Rio Grande	Gulf of Mexico	3,030	1,880
Arkansas	Mississippi	2,340	1,450
Colorado	Pacific Ocean	2,330	1,445
Red	Mississippi	2,040	1,270
Columbia	Pacific Ocean	1,950	1,210
Saskatchewan	Lake Winnipeg	1,940	1,205

South America

		km	miles
Amazon	Atlantic Ocean	6,450	4,010
Paraná–Plate	Atlantic Ocean	4,500	2,800
Purus	Amazon	3,350	2,080
Madeira	Amazon	3,200	1,990
São Francisco	Atlantic Ocean	2,900	1,800
Paraná	Plate	2,800	1,740
Tocantins	Atlantic Ocean	2,750	1,710
Paraguay	Paraná	2,550	1,580
Orinoco	Atlantic Ocean	2,500	1,550
Pilcomayo	Paraná	2,500	1,550
Araguaia	Tocantins	2,250	1,400

Lakes

Europe

		km²	miles²
Lake Ladoga	Russia	17,700	6,800
Lake Onega	Russia	9,700	3,700
Saimaa system	Finland	8,000	3,100
Vänern	Sweden	5,500	2,100

Asia

		km²	miles²
Caspian Sea	Asia	371,800	143,550
Lake Baykal	Russia	30,500	11,780
Aral Sea	Kazakhstan/Uzbekistan	28,687	11,086
Tonlé Sap	Cambodia	20,000	7,700
Lake Balqash	Kazakhstan	18,500	7,100

Africa

		km²	miles²
Lake Victoria	East Africa	68,000	26,000
Lake Tanganyika	Central Africa	33,000	13,000
Lake Malawi/Nyasa	East Africa	29,600	11,430
Lake Chad	Central Africa	25,000	9,700
Lake Turkana	Ethiopia/Kenya	8,500	3,300
Lake Volta	Ghana	8,500	3,300

Australia

		km²	miles²
Lake Eyre	Australia	8,900	3,400
Lake Torrens	Australia	5,800	2,200
Lake Gairdner	Australia	4,800	1,900

North America

		km²	miles²
Lake Superior	Canada/USA	82,350	31,800
Lake Huron	Canada/USA	59,600	23,010
Lake Michigan	USA	58,000	22,400
Great Bear Lake	Canada	31,800	12,280
Great Slave Lake	Canada	28,500	11,000
Lake Erie	Canada/USA	25,700	9,900
Lake Winnipeg	Canada	24,400	9,400
Lake Ontario	Canada/USA	19,500	7,500
Lake Nicaragua	Nicaragua	8,200	3,200

South America

		km²	miles²
Lake Titicaca	Bolivia/Peru	8,300	3,200
Lake Poopo	Bolivia	2,800	1,100

Islands

Europe

		km²	miles²
Great Britain	UK	229,880	88,700
Iceland	Atlantic Ocean	103,000	39,800
Ireland	Ireland/UK	84,400	32,600
Novaya Zemlya (N.)	Russia	48,200	18,600
Sicily	Italy	25,500	9,800
Corsica	France	8,700	3,400

Asia

		km²	miles²
Borneo	Southeast Asia	744,360	287,400
Sumatra	Indonesia	473,600	182,860
Honshu	Japan	230,500	88,980
Sulawesi (Celebes)	Indonesia	189,000	73,000
Java	Indonesia	126,700	48,900
Luzon	Philippines	104,700	40,400
Hokkaido	Japan	78,400	30,300

Africa

		km²	miles²
Madagascar	Indian Ocean	587,040	226,660
Socotra	Indian Ocean	3,600	1,400
Réunion	Indian Ocean	2,500	965

Oceania

		km²	miles²
New Guinea	Indonesia/Papua NG	821,030	317,000
New Zealand (S.)	Pacific Ocean	150,500	58,100
New Zealand (N.)	Pacific Ocean	114,700	44,300
Tasmania	Australia	67,800	26,200
Hawaii	Pacific Ocean	10,450	4,000

North America

		km²	miles²
Greenland	Atlantic Ocean	2,175,600	839,800
Baffin Is.	Canada	508,000	196,100
Victoria Is.	Canada	212,200	81,900
Ellesmere Is.	Canada	212,000	81,800
Cuba	Caribbean Sea	110,860	42,800
Hispaniola	Dominican Rep./Haiti	76,200	29,400
Jamaica	Caribbean Sea	11,400	4,400
Puerto Rico	Atlantic Ocean	8,900	3,400

South America

		km²	miles²
Tierra del Fuego	Argentina/Chile	47,000	18,100
Falkland Is. (E.)	Atlantic Ocean	6,800	2,600

IMAGES OF EARTH

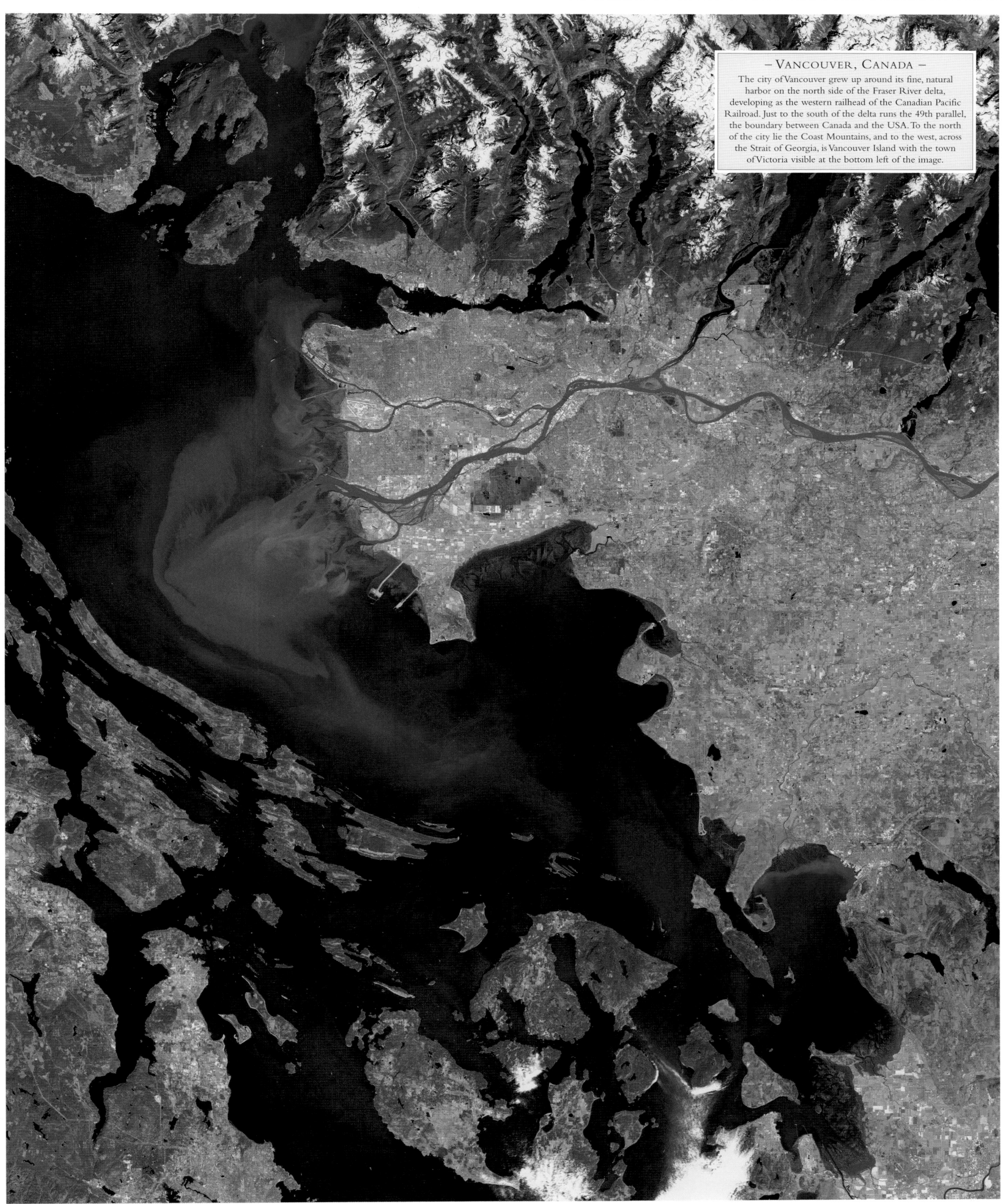

- VANCOUVER, CANADA -

The city of Vancouver grew up around its fine, natural harbor on the north side of the Fraser River delta, developing as the western railhead of the Canadian Pacific Railroad. Just to the south of the delta runs the 49th parallel, the boundary between Canada and the USA. To the north of the city lie the Coast Mountains, and to the west, across the Strait of Georgia, is Vancouver Island with the town of Victoria visible at the bottom left of the image.

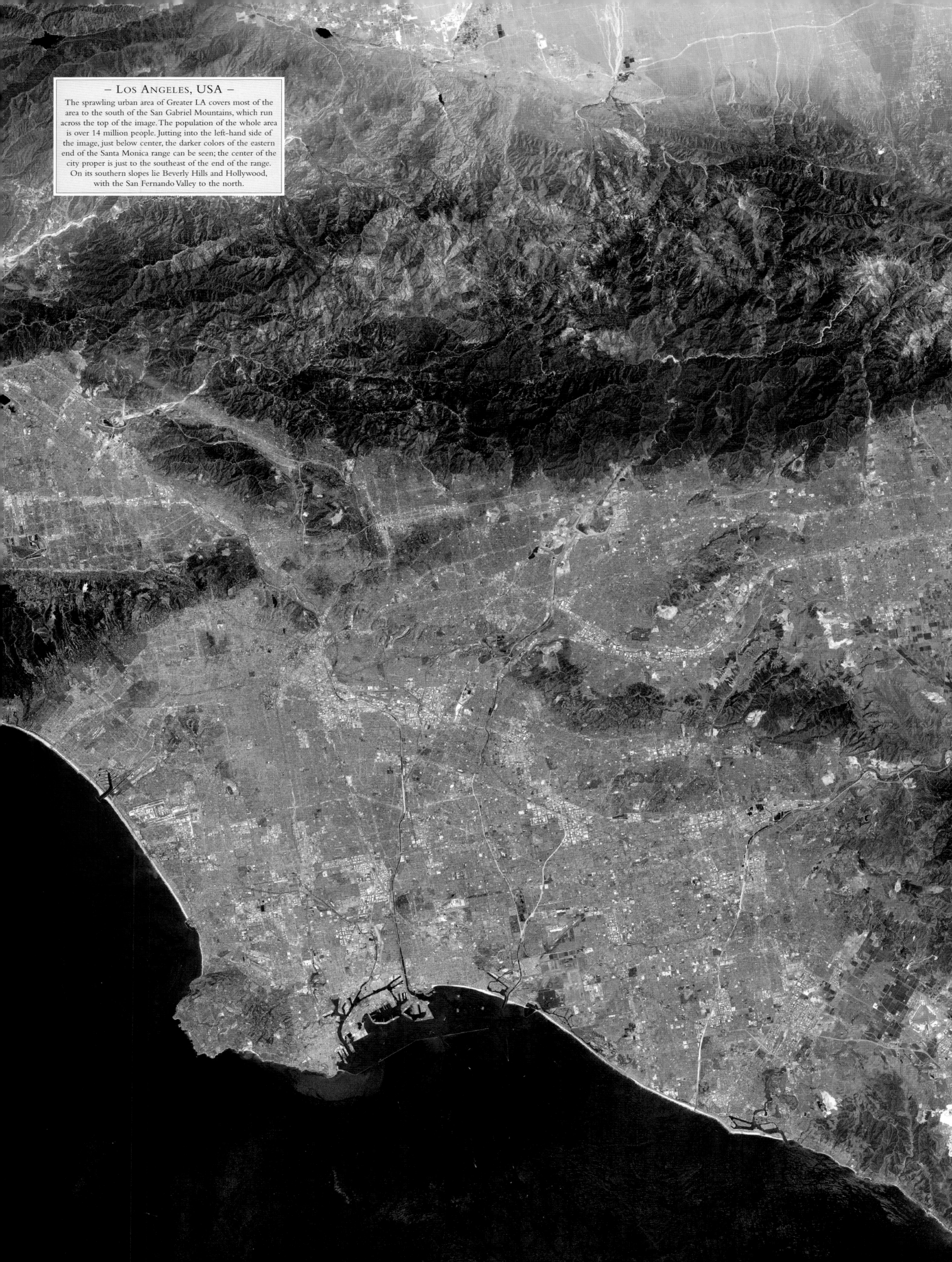

— LOS ANGELES, USA —

The sprawling urban area of Greater LA covers most of the
area to the south of the San Gabriel Mountains, which run
across the top of the image. The population of the whole area
is over 14 million people. Jutting into the left-hand side of
the image, just below center, the darker colors of the eastern
end of the Santa Monica range can be seen; the center of the
city proper is just to the southeast of the end of the range.
On its southern slopes lie Beverly Hills and Hollywood,
with the San Fernando Valley to the north.

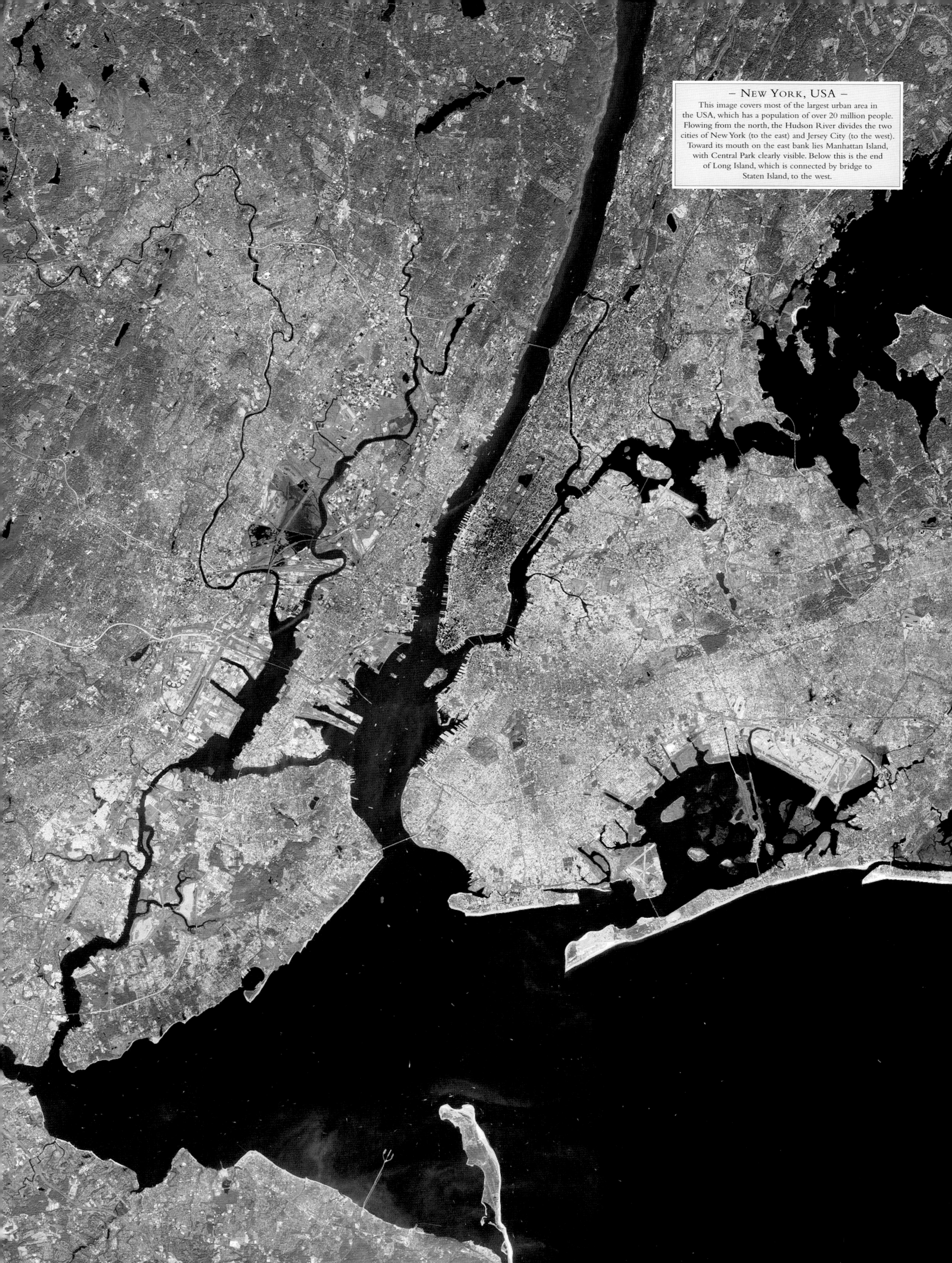

– New York, USA –

This image covers most of the largest urban area in
the USA, which has a population of over 20 million people.
Flowing from the north, the Hudson River divides the two
cities of New York (to the east) and Jersey City (to the west).
Toward its mouth on the east bank lies Manhattan Island,
with Central Park clearly visible. Below this is the end
of Long Island, which is connected by bridge to
Staten Island, to the west.

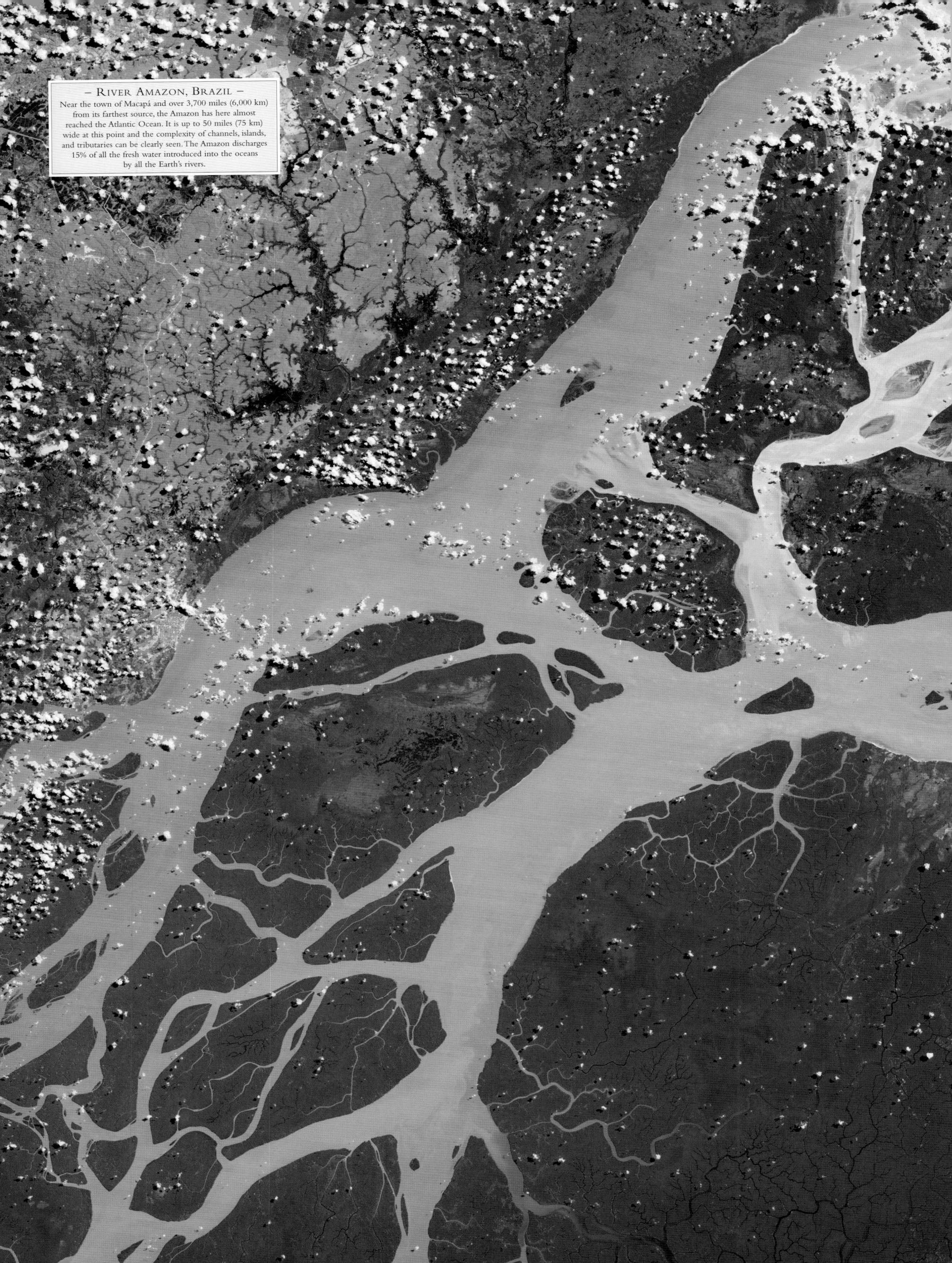

Near the town of Macapá and over 3,700 miles (6,000 km)
from its farthest source, the Amazon has here almost
reached the Atlantic Ocean. It is up to 50 miles (75 km)
wide at this point and the complexity of channels, islands,
and tributaries can be clearly seen. The Amazon discharges
15% of all the fresh water introduced into the oceans
by all the Earth's rivers.

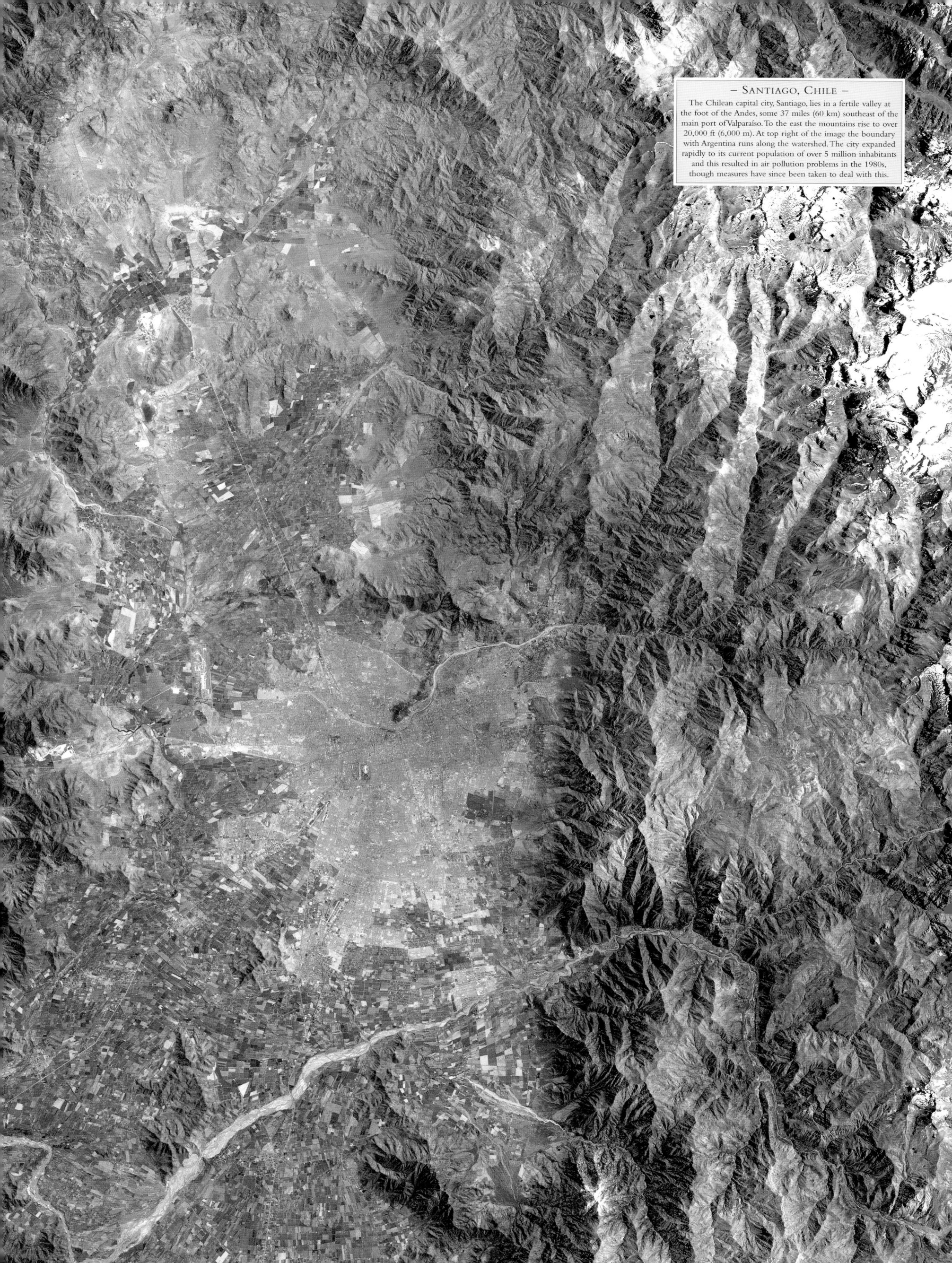

— SANTIAGO, CHILE —

The Chilean capital city, Santiago, lies in a fertile valley at the foot of the Andes, some 37 miles (60 km) southeast of the main port of Valparaíso. To the east the mountains rise to over 20,000 ft (6,000 m). At top right of the image the boundary with Argentina runs along the watershed. The city expanded rapidly to its current population of over 5 million inhabitants and this resulted in air pollution problems in the 1980s, though measures have since been taken to deal with this.

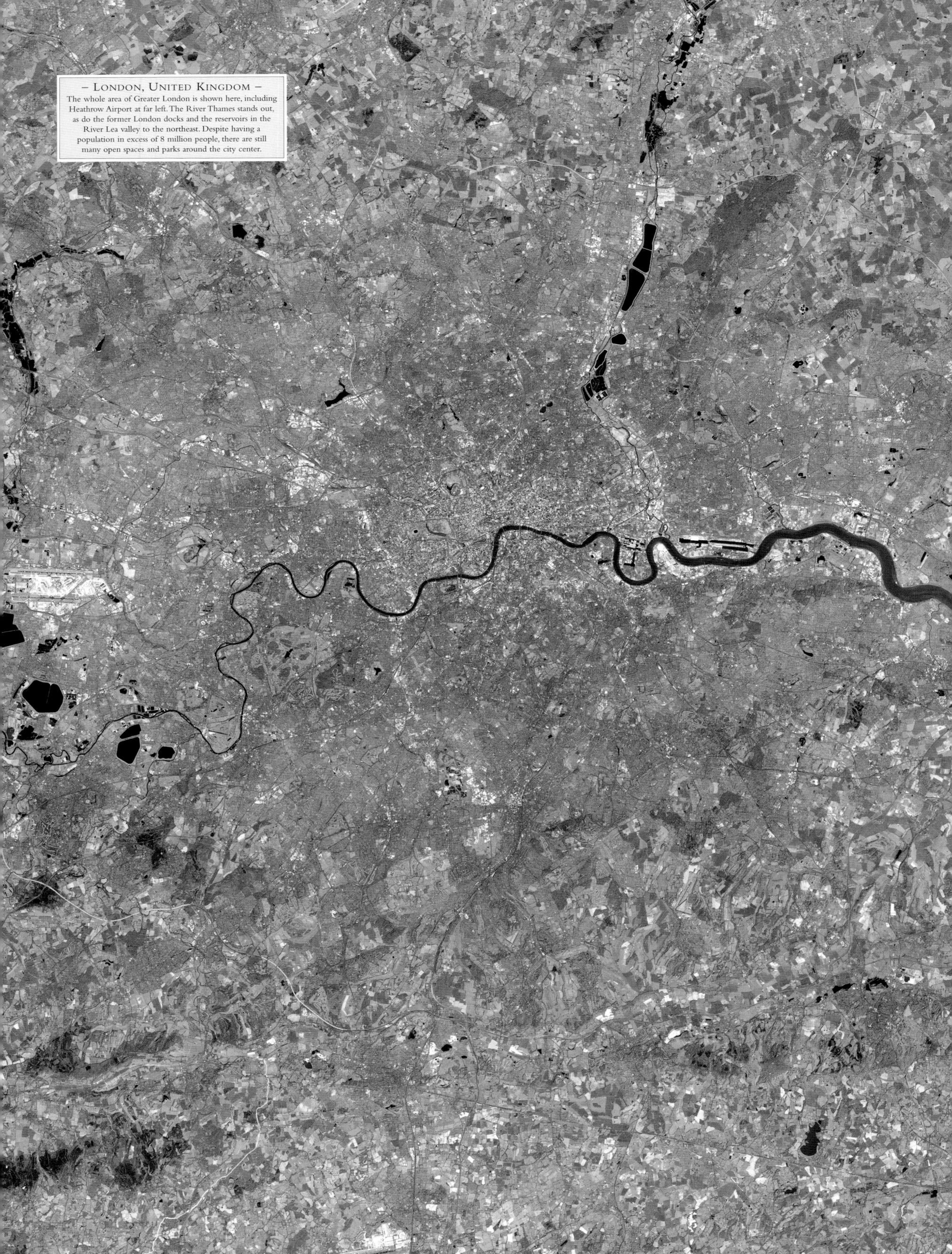

– LONDON, UNITED KINGDOM –
The whole area of Greater London is shown here, including
Heathrow Airport at far left. The River Thames stands out,
as do the former London docks and the reservoirs in the
River Lea valley to the northeast. Despite having a
population in excess of 8 million people, there are still
many open spaces and parks around the city center.

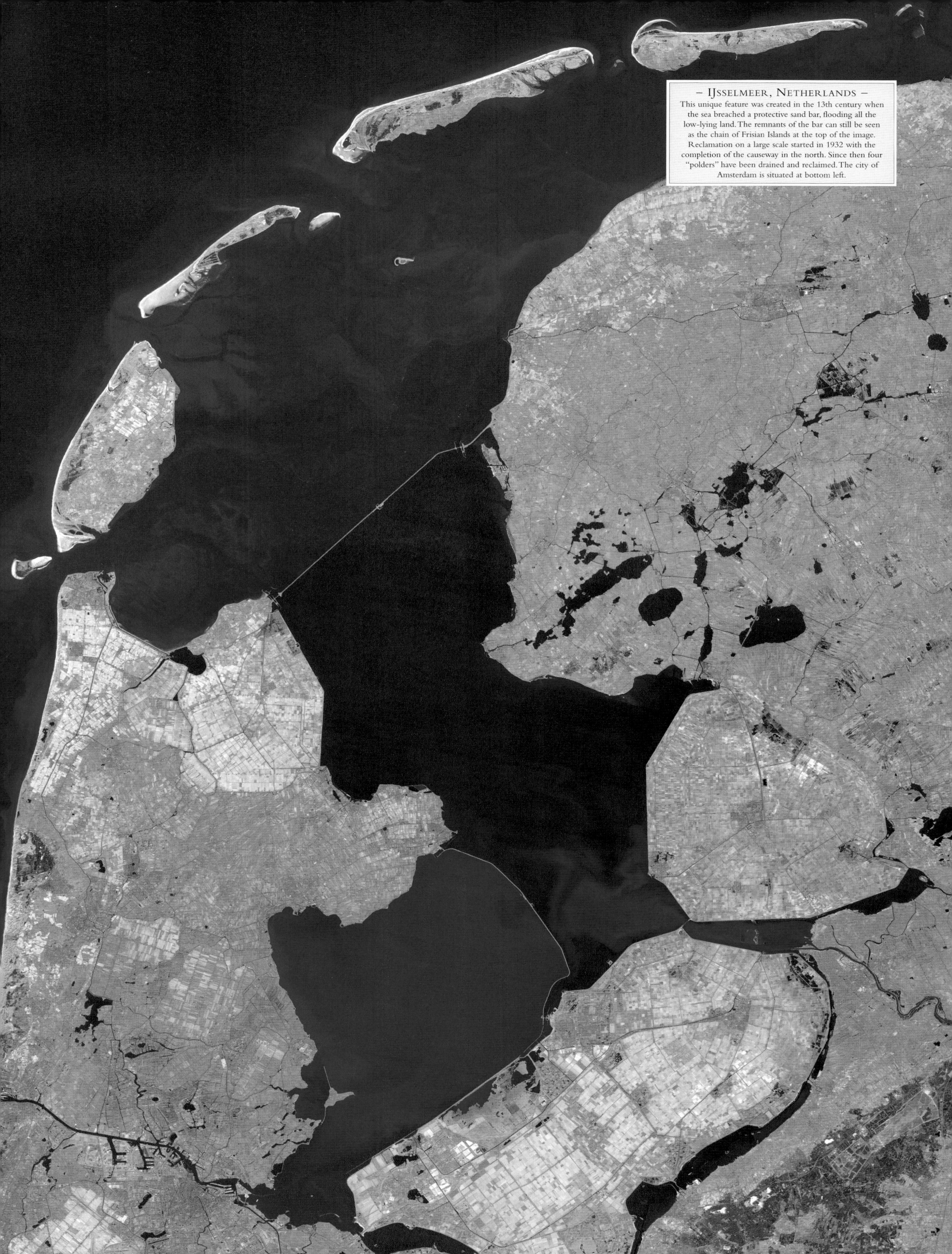

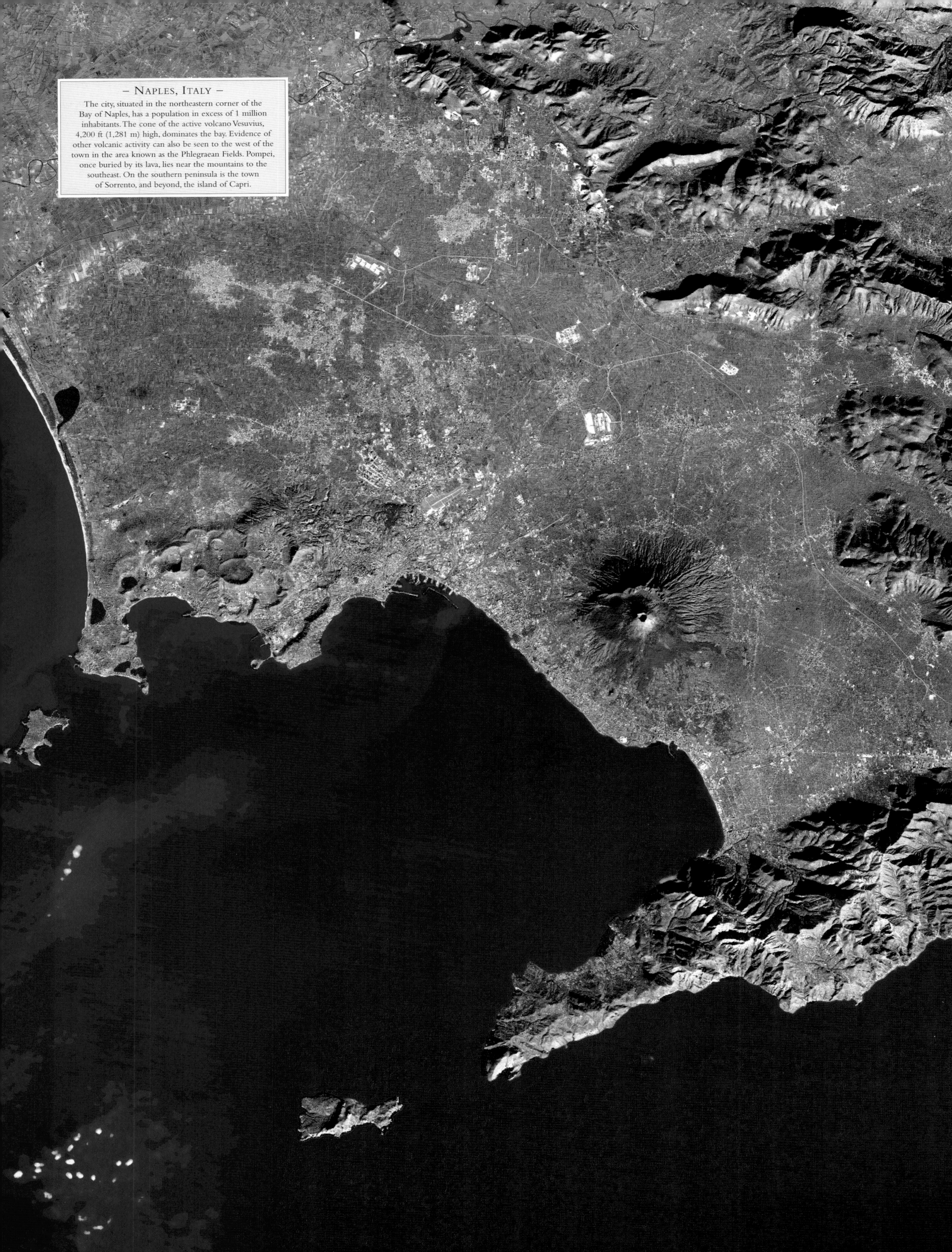

— NAPLES, ITALY —

The city, situated in the northeastern corner of the
Bay of Naples, has a population in excess of 1 million
inhabitants. The cone of the active volcano Vesuvius,
4,200 ft (1,281 m) high, dominates the bay. Evidence of
other volcanic activity can also be seen to the west of the
town in the area known as the Phlegraean Fields. Pompei,
once buried by its lava, lies near the mountains to the
southeast. On the southern peninsula is the town
of Sorrento, and beyond, the island of Capri.

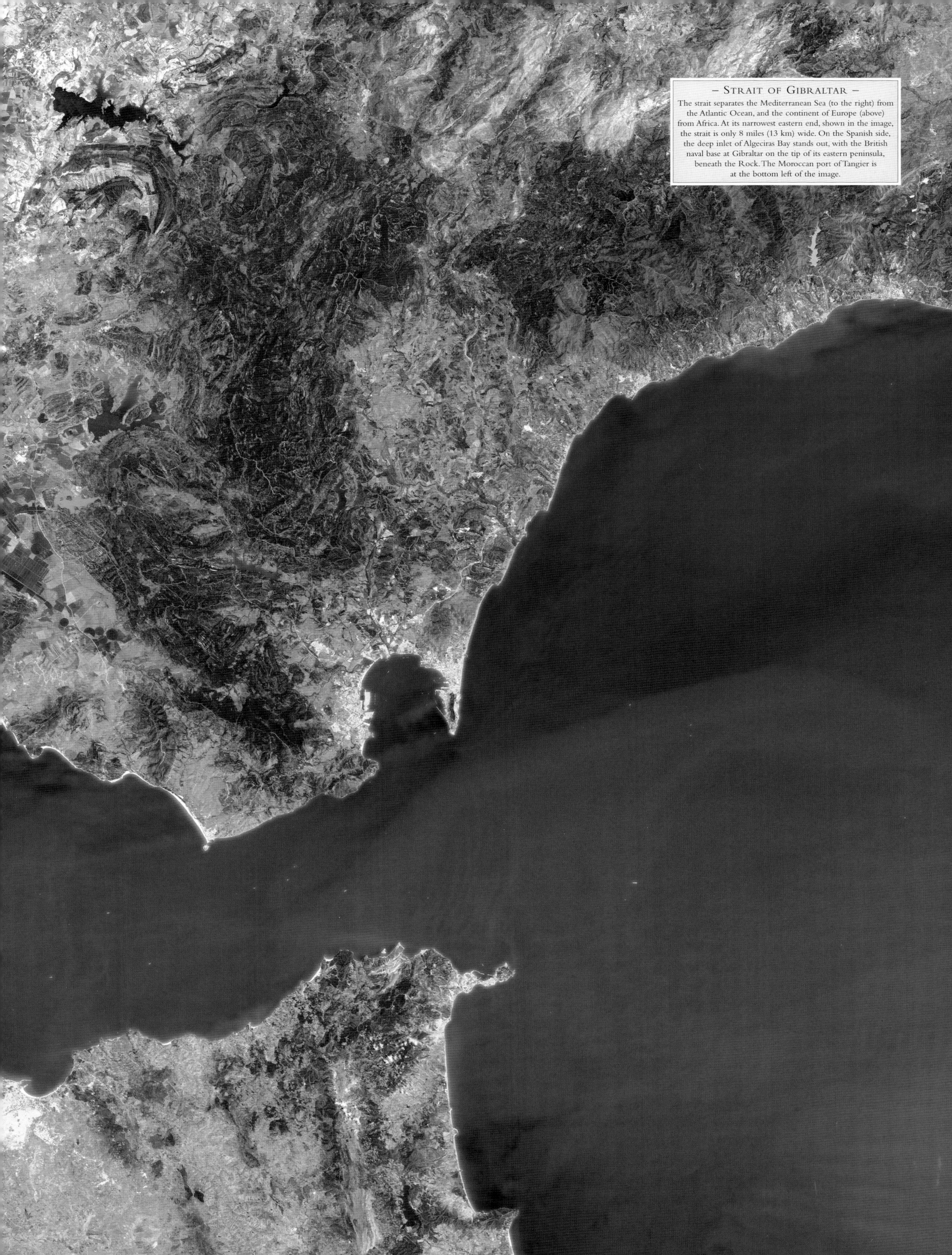

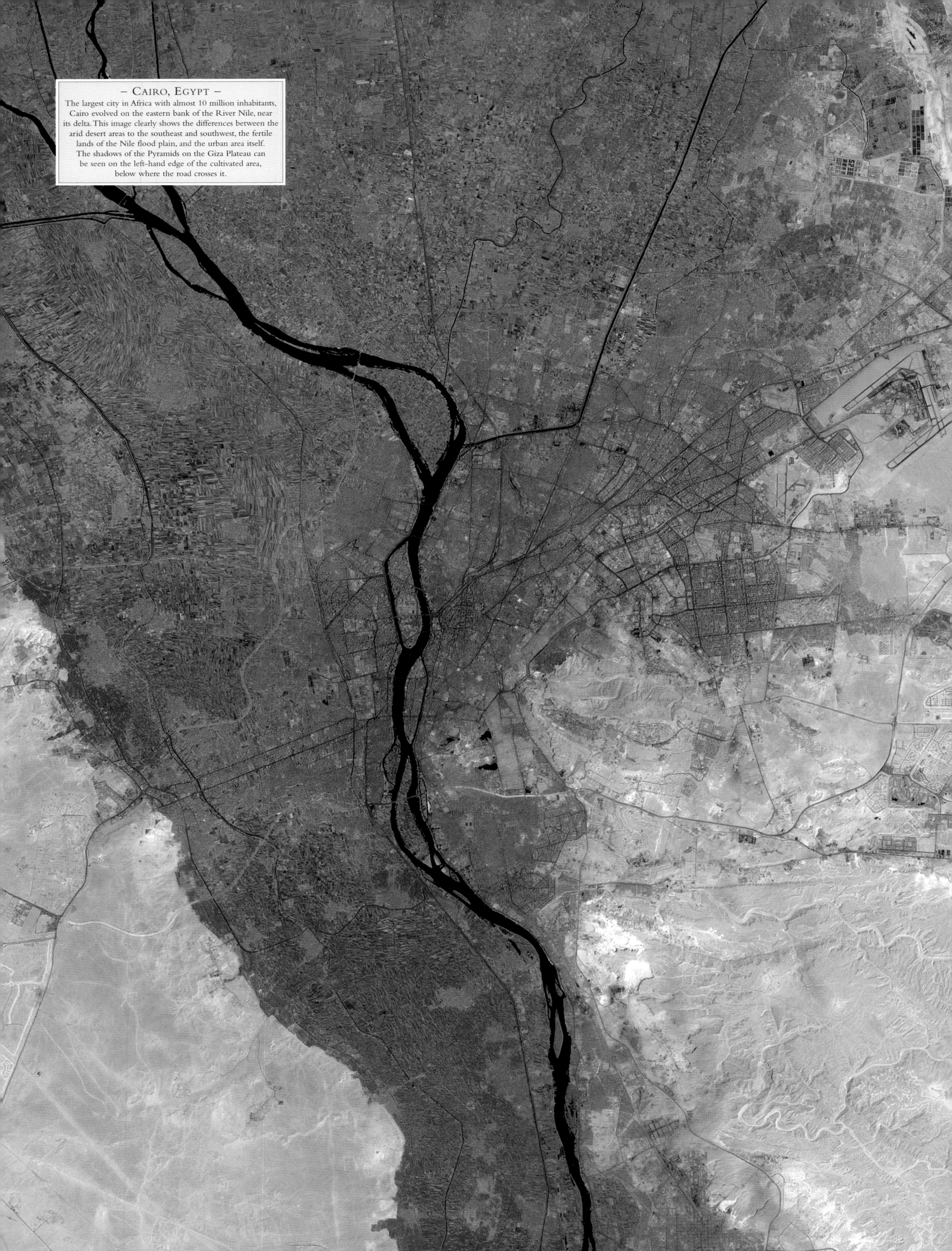

— CAIRO, EGYPT —

The largest city in Africa with almost 10 million inhabitants, Cairo evolved on the eastern bank of the River Nile, near its delta. This image clearly shows the differences between the arid desert areas to the southeast and southwest, the fertile lands of the Nile flood plain, and the urban area itself. The shadows of the Pyramids on the Giza Plateau can be seen on the left-hand edge of the cultivated area, below where the road crosses it.

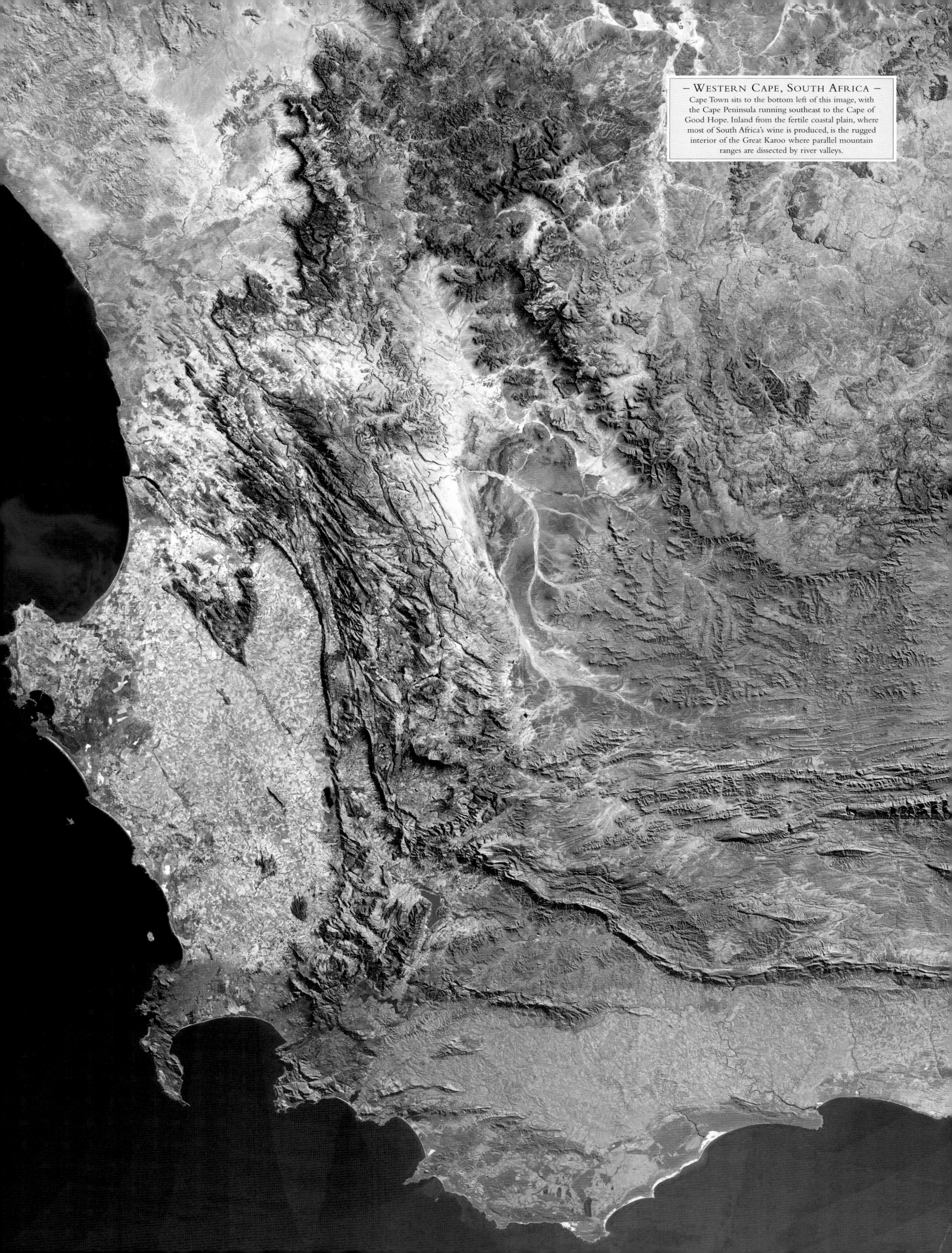

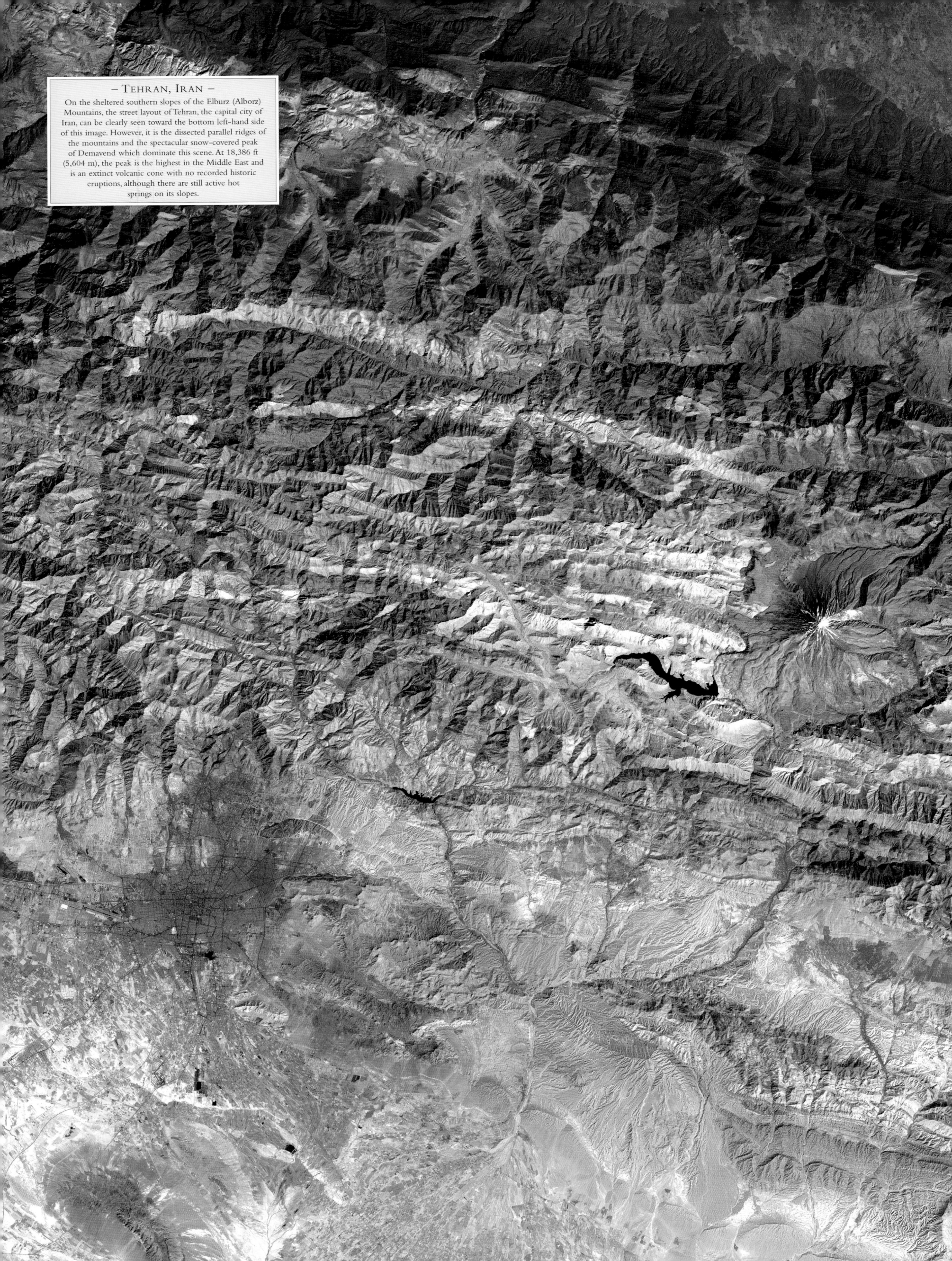

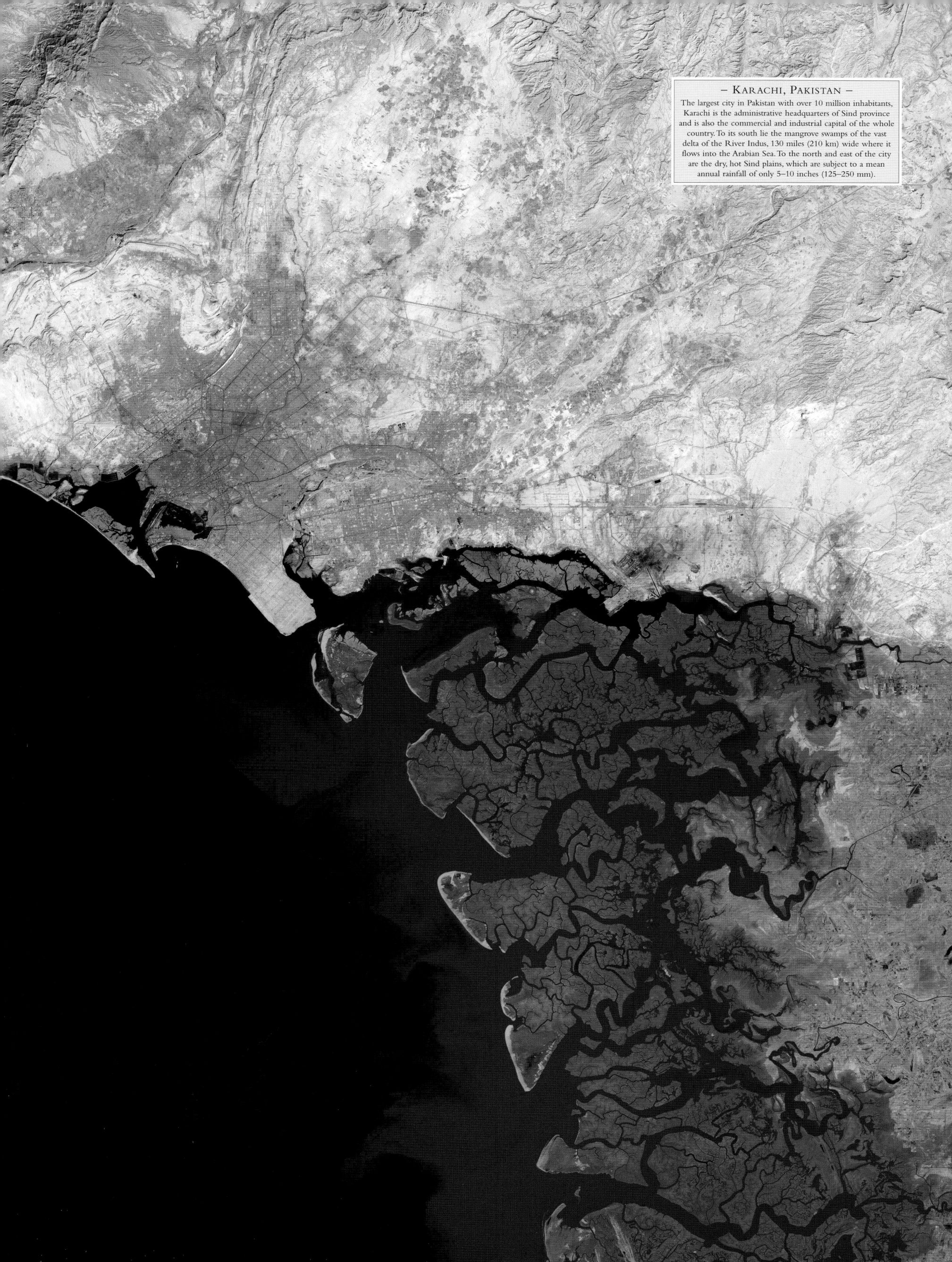

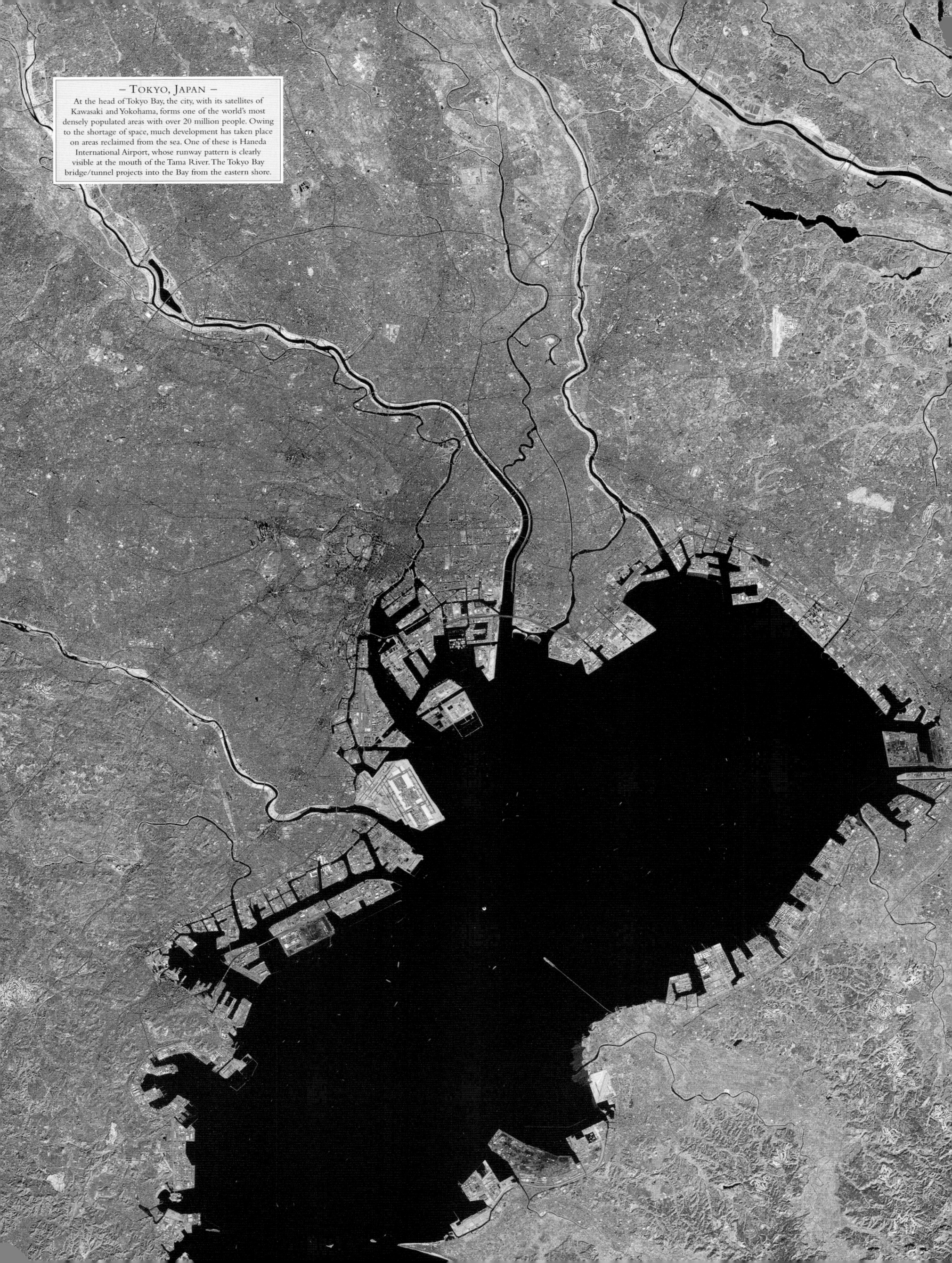

— TOKYO, JAPAN —

At the head of Tokyo Bay, the city, with its satellites of
Kawasaki and Yokohama, forms one of the world's most
densely populated areas with over 20 million people. Owing
to the shortage of space, much development has taken place
on areas reclaimed from the sea. One of these is Haneda
International Airport, whose runway pattern is clearly
visible at the mouth of the Tama River. The Tokyo Bay
bridge/tunnel projects into the Bay from the eastern shore.

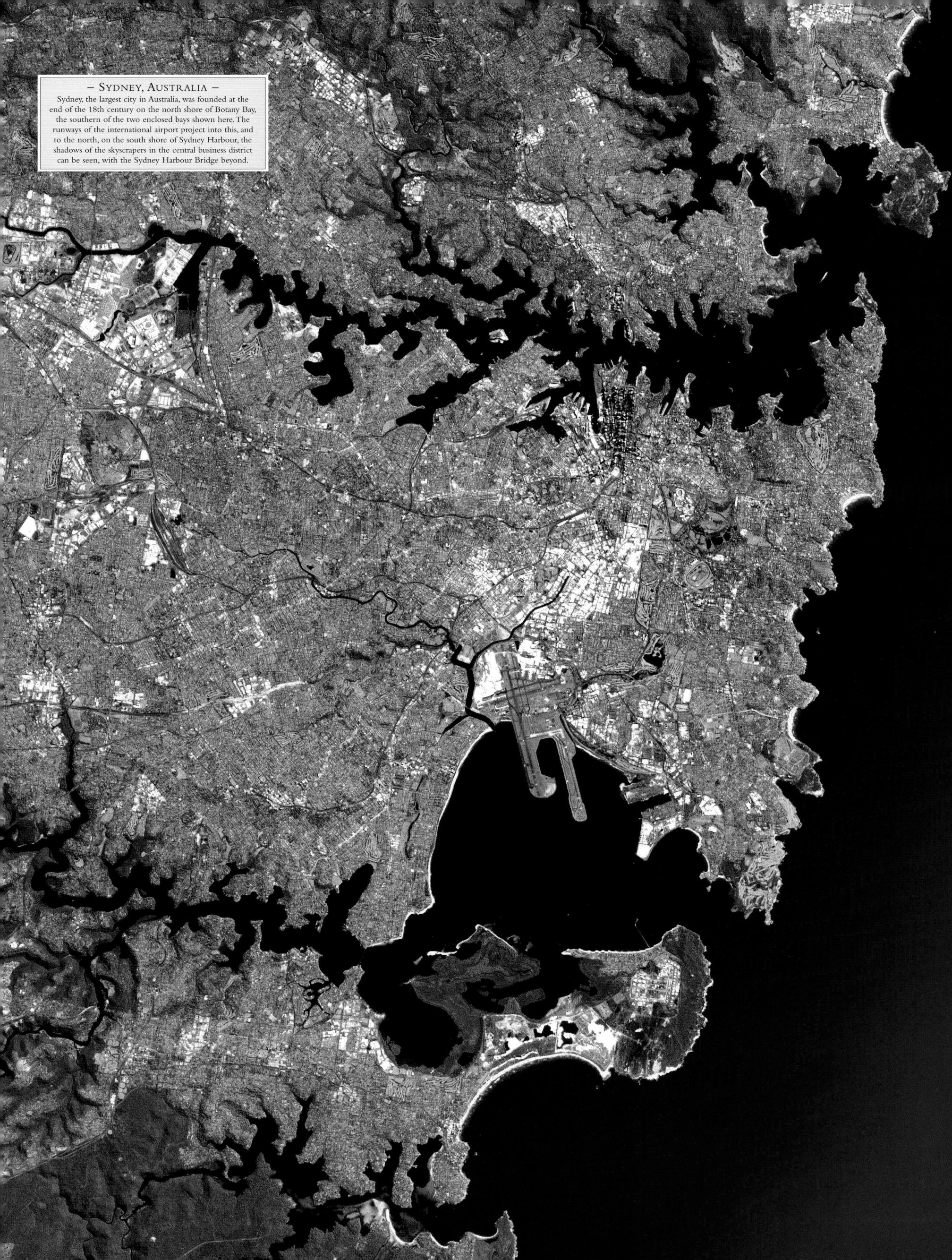

— SYDNEY, AUSTRALIA —

Sydney, the largest city in Australia, was founded at the
end of the 18th century on the north shore of Botany Bay,
the southern of the two enclosed bays shown here. The
runways of the international airport project into this, and
to the north, on the south shore of Sydney Harbour, the
shadows of the skyscrapers in the central business district
can be seen, with the Sydney Harbour Bridge beyond.

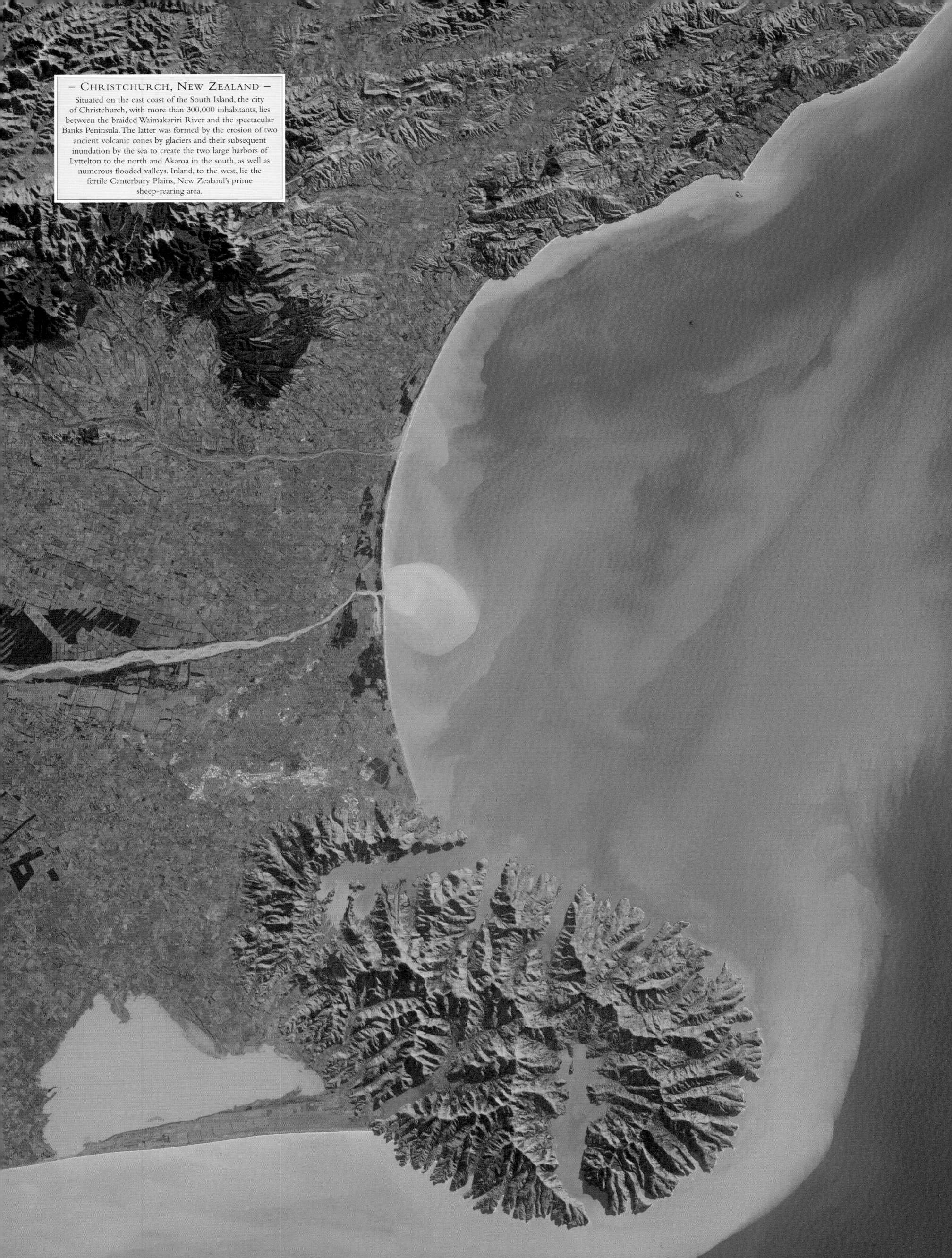

THE GAZETTEER OF NATIONS

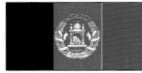

AFGHANISTAN

GEOGRAPHY The Republic of Afghanistan is a landlocked, mountainous country in southern Asia. The central highlands reach a height of more than 22,966 ft [7,000 m] in the east and make up nearly three-quarters of Afghanistan. The main range is the Hindu Kush, which is cut by deep, fertile valleys.

In winter, northerly winds bring cold, snowy weather to the mountains, but summers are hot and dry.

POLITICS & ECONOMY The modern history of Afghanistan began in 1747, when the various tribes in the area united for the first time. In the 19th century, Russia and Britain struggled for control of the country. Following Britain's withdrawal in 1919, Afghanistan became fully independent. Soviet troops invaded Afghanistan in 1979 to support a socialist regime in Kabul, but they withdrew in 1989. By the early 21st century, a group called the Taliban ("Islamic students") controlled 90% of the country. In 2001, following the refusal of the Taliban government to hand over the terrorist leader Osama bin Laden, an international force invaded Afghanistan. In 2002, a coalition government was set up under Hamid Karzai. A draft constitution was approved in 2004, but periodic conflict has dogged economic recovery.

Afghanistan is a poor country and more than 60% of its people are farmers or nomadic herders. Natural gas is produced, together with some coal, copper, gold, precious stones and salt.

AREA 251,772 SQ MI [652,090 SQ KM] **POPULATION** 28,717,000
CAPITAL (POPULATION) KABUL (1,565,000)
GOVERNMENT TRANSITIONAL **ETHNIC GROUPS** PASHTUN
(PATHAN) 44%, TAJIK 25%, HAZARA 10%, UZBEK 8%, OTHERS 13%
LANGUAGES PASHTU, DARI/PERSIAN (BOTH OFFICIAL), UZBEK
RELIGIONS ISLAM (SUNNI MUSLIM 84%, SHI'ITE MUSLIM 15%), OTHERS 1%
CURRENCY AFGHANI = 100 PULS

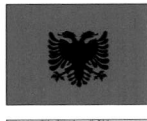

ALBANIA

GEOGRAPHY The Republic of Albania lies in the Balkan peninsula, facing the Adriatic Sea. About 70% of the land is mountainous, but most Albanians live in the west on the coastal lowlands.

The coastal areas of Albania experience a typical Mediterranean climate, with fairly dry, sunny summers and cool, moist winters. The mountains have a severe climate, with heavy winter snowfalls.

POLITICS & ECONOMY Albania is one of Europe's poorest nations. A former Communist country, Albania adopted a multi-party system in the early 1990s. The change proved difficult. But after elections in 1997, a socialist government committed to a market system took office. In 2001, the stability of the region was threatened when Albanian-speaking Kosovars and Macedonians, many of whom favored the creation of a greater Albania, fought with government forces in northwestern Macedonia.

In 2001, agriculture employed more than 60% of the people. Since 1991, private ownership of land has been encouraged, replacing the former state farm and collective system. Albania has some minerals. Chromite, copper and nickel are exported.

AREA 11,100 SQ MI [28,748 SQ KM] **POPULATION** 3,582,000
CAPITAL (POPULATION) TIRANA (300,000) **GOVERNMENT** MULTIPARTY
REPUBLIC **ETHNIC GROUPS** ALBANIAN 95%, GREEK 3%, MACEDONIAN,
VLACHS, GYPSY **LANGUAGES** ALBANIAN (OFFICIAL) **RELIGIONS** MANY
PEOPLE SAY THEY ARE NON-BELIEVERS; OF THE BELIEVERS, 70% FOLLOW ISLAM
AND 30% FOLLOW CHRISTIANITY (ORTHODOX 20%, ROMAN CATHOLIC 10%)
CURRENCY LEK = 100 QINDARS

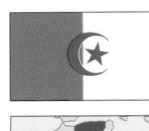

ALGERIA

GEOGRAPHY The People's Democratic Republic of Algeria is Africa's second largest country after Sudan. Most Algerians live in the north, on the fertile coastal plains and hill country bordering the Mediterranean Sea. Four-fifths of Algeria is in the Sahara. The coast has a Mediterranean climate, but the arid Sahara is hot by day and cool at night.

POLITICS & ECONOMY France ruled Algeria from 1830 until 1962, when the socialist FLN (National Liberation Front) formed a one-party government. Following the recognition of opposition parties in 1989, a Muslim group, the FIS (Islamic Salvation Front), won an election in 1991. The FLN canceled the elections and civil conflict broke out. About 100,000 people were killed

in the 1990s. In 1999, following the withdrawal of the other candidates who alleged fraud, Abdelaziz Bouteflika, who was assumed to be favored by the army, was elected president. Though Bouteflika's peace offensive reduced the violence, sporadic conflict continued. Bouteflika was re-elected in 2004.

Algeria is a developing country, whose chief resources are oil and natural gas, which were discovered in the Sahara in 1956. The natural gas reserves are among the world's largest, and gas and oil account for 90% of Algeria's exports. Cement, iron and steel, textiles, and vehicles are manufactured. Barley, citrus fruits, dates, potatoes, and wheat are the major crops.

AREA 919,590 SQ MI [2,381,741 SQ KM] **POPULATION** 32,819,000
CAPITAL (POPULATION) ALGIERS (2,562,000)
GOVERNMENT SOCIALIST REPUBLIC **ETHNIC GROUPS** ARAB-BERBER 99%
LANGUAGES ARABIC AND BERBER (OFFICIAL), FRENCH **RELIGIONS** SUNNI
MUSLIM 99% **CURRENCY** ALGERIAN DINAR = 100 CENTIMES

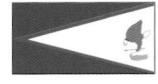

AMERICAN SAMOA

An "unincorporated territory" of the United States, American Samoa lies in the south-central Pacific Ocean.

AREA 77 SQ MI [199 SQ KM]
POPULATION 70,000 **CAPITAL** PAGO PAGO

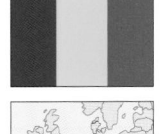

ANDORRA

A mini-state situated in the Pyrenees Mountains, Andorra is a co-principality whose main activity is tourism. Most Andorrans live in the six valleys (the Valls) that drain into the River Valira.

AREA 181 SQ MI [468 SQ KM]
POPULATION 69,000 **CAPITAL** ANDORRA LA VELLA

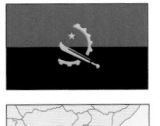

ANGOLA

GEOGRAPHY The Republic of Angola is a large country in southwestern Africa. Much of the country is part of the plateau that forms most of southern Africa, with a narrow coastal plain in the west.

Angola has a tropical climate, with temperatures of over 68°F [20°C] throughout the year, though the highest areas are cooler. The coast is dry, but the rainfall increases to the north and east.

POLITICS & ECONOMY Bantu-speaking people settled in Angola in the 13th century and later founded large kingdoms, such as the Kongo and Mbundu. Portugal controlled the coastal slave trade from the 17th century and extended their control inland in the 19th century. Angola became independent from Portugal in 1975, after which rival nationalist groups struggled for power. Despite a ceasefire in the mid-1990s, conflict finally ended in 2002, when the rebel leader, Jonas Savimbi, was killed in action and his successors negotiated peace.

Angola is a developing country, where 70% of the people are poor farmers. The main food crops are cassava and maize. Coffee is exported. Angola has important oil reserves and oil is exported. Angola also produces diamonds and has reserves of copper, manganese, and phosphates.

AREA 481,351 SQ MI [1,246,700 SQ KM] **POPULATION** 10,766,000
CAPITAL (POPULATION) LUANDA (2,500,000)
GOVERNMENT MULTIPARTY REPUBLIC
ETHNIC GROUPS OVIMBUNDU 37%, KIMBUNDU 25%, BAKONGO 13%,
OTHERS 25% **LANGUAGES** PORTUGUESE (OFFICIAL), MANY OTHERS
RELIGIONS TRADITIONAL BELIEFS 47%, ROMAN CATHOLIC 38%,
PROTESTANT 15%
CURRENCY KWANZA = 100 LWEI

ANGUILLA

Formerly part of St Kitts and Nevis, Anguilla, the most northerly of the Leeward Islands, became a British dependency (now a British overseas territory) in 1980. The main source of revenue is now tourism, although lobster still accounts for half the island's exports.

AREA 37 SQ MI [96 SQ KM]
POPULATION 13,000 **CAPITAL** THE VALLEY

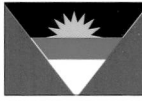

ANTIGUA & BARBUDA

A former British dependency in the Caribbean, Antigua and Barbuda became independent in 1981. Tourism is the main industry, though sugar is an important product.

AREA 171 SQ MI [442 SQ KM]
POPULATION 68,000 **CAPITAL** ST JOHN'S

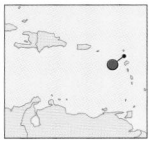
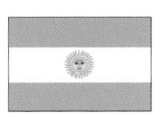

ARGENTINA

GEOGRAPHY The Argentine Republic is South America's second largest and the world's eighth largest country. The high Andes range in the west contains Mount Aconcagua, the highest peak in the Americas. In southern Argentina, the Andes Mountains overlook Patagonia, a plateau region. In east-central Argentina lies a fertile plain called the pampas.

The climate varies from subtropical in the north to temperate in the south. Rainfall is abundant in the northeast but lower to the west and south. Patagonia is largely desert.

POLITICS & ECONOMY The earliest people were American Indians, but 86% of the people are now of European ancestry. Spain took control in the 16th century and ruled until 1816. Argentina later suffered from instability and periods of military rule. In 1982, Argentina's military regime invaded the Falkland (Malvinas) Islands, but Britain regained the territory later that year. Civilian rule was restored in 1983 and, in 1994, Argentina adopted a new constitution.

The World Bank classifies Argentina as an "upper-middle-income" developing country. About 90% of the people live in urban areas. Manufactures include food products, cars, electrical equipment, and textiles. Oil is the chief natural resource and the chief farm products are beef, maize, and wheat. Oil is exported, together with meat, wheat, maize, vegetable oils, hides and skins, and wool. In 1991, Argentina, Brazil, Paraguay, and Uruguay set up an alliance, Mercosur, aimed at creating a common market. However, in late 2001, a severe economic crisis threatened anarchy, though, by late 2003, there were signs of recovery.

AREA 1,073,512 SQ MI [2,780,400 SQ KM] **POPULATION** 38,741,000
CAPITAL (POPULATION) BUENOS AIRES (2,965,000)
GOVERNMENT FEDERAL REPUBLIC **ETHNIC GROUPS** EUROPEAN 97%,
MESTIZO, AMERINDIAN **LANGUAGES** SPANISH (OFFICIAL)
RELIGIONS ROMAN CATHOLIC 92%, PROTESTANT 2%,
JEWISH 2%, OTHERS **CURRENCY** ARGENTINE PESO = 10,000 AUSTRALS

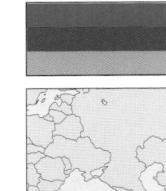

ARMENIA

GEOGRAPHY The Republic of Armenia is a landlocked country in southwestern Asia. Most of Armenia consists of a rugged plateau, crisscrossed by long faults (cracks). Movements along the faults cause earthquakes. The highest point is Mount Aragats, at 13,419 ft [4,090 m] above sea level.

The height of the land, which averages 4,920 ft [1,500 m] above sea level gives rise to severe winters and cool summers. The highest peaks are snow-capped, but the total yearly rainfall is generally low.

POLITICS & ECONOMY In 1920, Armenia became a Communist republic and, in 1922, it became, with Azerbaijan and Georgia, part of the Transcaucasian Republic within the Soviet Union. But the three territories became separate Soviet Socialist Republics in 1936. After the breakup of the Soviet Union in 1991, Armenia became an independent republic. Fighting broke out over Nagorno-Karabakh, an area enclosed by Azerbaijan where the majority of the people are Armenians. In 1992, Armenia occupied the territory between it and Nagorno-Karabakh. A ceasefire agreed in 1994 left Armenia in control of about 20% of Azerbaijan's land area. Talks aimed at settling the dispute failed in 2001.

The World Bank classifies Armenia as a "lower-middle-income" economy. The conflict has badly damaged the economy, but the government has encouraged free enterprise, selling farmland and government-owned businesses.

AREA 11,506 SQ MI [29,800 SQ KM] **POPULATION** 3,326,000
CAPITAL (POPULATION) YEREVAN (1,249,000)
GOVERNMENT MULTIPARTY REPUBLIC **ETHNIC GROUPS** ARMENIAN 93%,
RUSSIAN 2%, AZERI 1%, OTHERS (MOSTLY KURDS) 4%
LANGUAGES ARMENIAN (OFFICIAL) **RELIGIONS** ARMENIAN APOSTOLIC 94%
CURRENCY DRAM = 100 COUMA

NOTE: This alphabetical list includes the principal countries and territories of the world. The area figures give the total area of land, inland water, and ice. The population figures are 2003 estimates where available. The capital city population is for the "city proper" (rather than its urban agglomeration) where available, using the latest census or estimate.

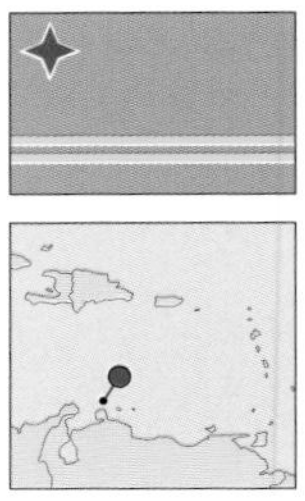

ARUBA

Formerly part of the Netherlands Antilles, Aruba (the most western of the Lesser Antilles) became a separate self-governing Dutch territory in 1986.

AREA 75 sq mi [193 sq km]
POPULATION 71,000 **CAPITAL** Oranjestad

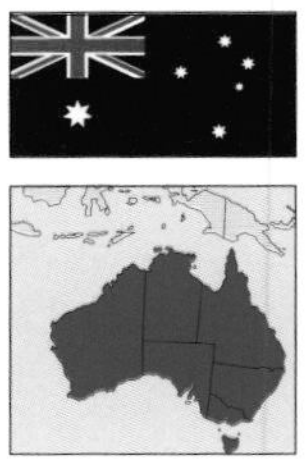

AUSTRALIA

GEOGRAPHY The Commonwealth of Australia, the world's sixth largest country, is also a continent. Australia is the flattest of the continents and the main highland area is in the east. Here the Great Dividing Range separates the eastern coastal plains from the Central Plains. This range extends from the Cape York Peninsula to Victoria in the far south. The longest rivers, the Murray and Darling, drain the southeastern part of the Central Plains. The Western Plateau makes up two-thirds of Australia. A few mountain ranges break the monotony of the generally flat landscape.

Only 10% of Australia has an average yearly rainfall of more than 39 in [1,000 mm]. These areas include the tropical north, where Darwin is situated, the northeast coast, and the southeast, where Sydney is located. The interior is dry, and water is quickly evaporated in the heat.

POLITICS & ECONOMY The Aboriginal people of Australia entered the continent from Southeast Asia more than 50,000 years ago. The first European explorers were Dutch in the 17th century, but they did not settle. In 1770, the British Captain Cook explored the east coast and, in 1788, the first British settlement was established for convicts on the site of what is now Sydney. Australia has strong ties with the British Isles. But in the last 50 years, people from other parts of Europe and, most recently, from Asia have settled in Australia. Ties with Britain were also weakened by Britain's membership of the European Union. Many Australians believe that they should become more involved with the nations of eastern Asia and the Americas rather than with Europe. In 1999, Australians voted to retain the country's status as a monarchy by a vote of about 55% to 45%. In 2003, Australian troops joined the coalition force led by the United States in invading Iraq and overthrowing Saddam Hussein.

Australia is a prosperous country. Crops can be grown on only 6% of the land, but dry pasture covers another 58%. Yet the country remains a major producer and exporter of farm products, particularly cattle, wheat, and wool. Grapes grown for wine-making are also important. The country is a major producer of minerals, including bauxite, coal, copper, diamonds, gold, iron ore, manganese, nickel, silver, tin, tungsten, and zinc. Australia also produces oil and natural gas. Metals, minerals and farm products account for the bulk of exports. Australia's imports are mostly manufactured goods, especially machinery, though industry is now important, especially the manufacture of consumer goods.

AREA 2,988,885 sq mi [7,741,220 sq km] **POPULATION** 19,732,000 **CAPITAL (POPULATION)** Canberra (309,000) **GOVERNMENT** Federal constitutional monarchy **ETHNIC GROUPS** Caucasian 92%, Asian 7%, Aboriginal 1% **LANGUAGES** English (official) **RELIGIONS** Roman Catholic 26%, Anglican 26%, other Christian 24%, non-Christian 24% **CURRENCY** Australian dollar = 100 cents

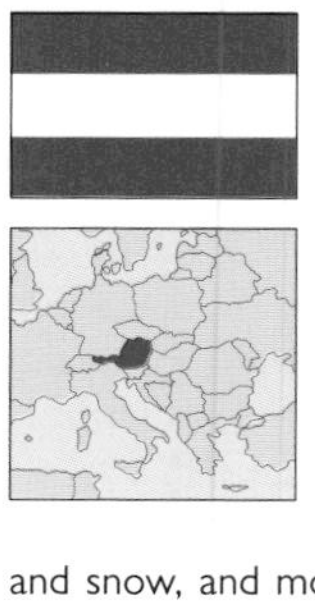

AUSTRIA

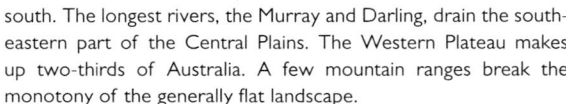

GEOGRAPHY Austria is a landlocked country in Europe. Northern Austria contains the valley of the River Danube, which flows from Germany to the Black Sea, and the Vienna basin. Southern Austria contains ranges of the Alps, their highest point at Grossglockner, 12,457 ft [3,797 m] above sea level.

The climate is influenced by westerly and easterly winds. Moist westerly winds bring rain and snow, and moderate temperatures. Dry easterly winds bring cold weather in winter and hot weather in summer.

POLITICS & ECONOMY Formerly part of the monarchy of Austria-Hungary, which collapsed in 1918, Austria was annexed by Germany in 1938. After World War II, the Allies partitioned and occupied the country. In 1955, Austria became a neutral federal republic. It joined the European Union on January 1, 1995, but was a focus of controversy when, in 2000, a coalition government was formed by the right-wing People's Party and the extreme right-wing Freedom Party. The Freedom Party lost much of its support in 2002, but it remained part of the ruling coalition.

Austria has a highly developed economy, with plenty of hydroelectric power and some oil, gas and coal reserves. The country's leading economic activity is manufacturing metals and metal products. Crops are grown on 18% of the land, and another 24% is pasture. Dairy and livestock farming are the leading activities. Major crops include barley, potatoes, rye, sugar beet, and wheat. Tourism is a major activity in this scenic country.

AREA 32,378 sq mi [83,859 sq km] **POPULATION** 8,188,000 **CAPITAL (POPULATION)** Vienna (1,560,000) **GOVERNMENT** Federal republic **ETHNIC GROUPS** Austrian 90%, Croatian, Slovene, others **LANGUAGES** German (official) **RELIGIONS** Roman Catholic 78%, Protestant 5%, Islam and others 17% **CURRENCY** Euro = 100 cents

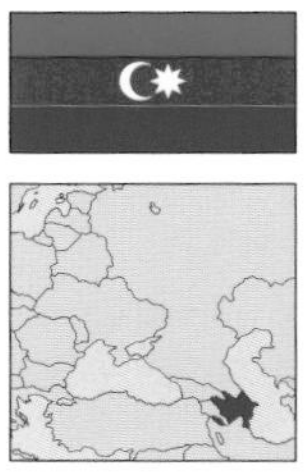

AZERBAIJAN

GEOGRAPHY The Azerbaijani Republic is a country in the southwest of Asia, facing the Caspian Sea to the east. It includes an area called the Naxçivan Autonomous Republic, which is completely cut off from the rest of Azerbaijan by Armenian territory. The Caucasus Mountains border Russia in the north.

Azerbaijan has hot summers and cool winters. The plains are fairly dry, but the mountains are rainy.

POLITICS & ECONOMY After the Russian Revolution of 1917, attempts were made to form a Transcaucasian Federation made up of Armenia, Azerbaijan and Georgia. When this failed, Azerbaijanis set up an independent state. But Russian forces occupied the area in 1920. In 1922, the Communists set up a Transcaucasian Republic consisting of Armenia, Azerbaijan and Georgia under Russian control. In 1936, the three areas became separate Soviet Socialist Republics within the Soviet Union. In 1991, following the breakup of the Soviet Union, Azerbaijan became an independent nation. After independence, the country's economic progress was slow, partly because of the conflict with Armenia over the enclave of Nagorno-Karabakh, a region in Azerbaijan where the majority of people are Armenians. A ceasefire in 1994 left Armenia in control of about 20% of Azerbaijan's area, including Nagorno-Karabakh. Attempts to resolve the problem failed in 2001.

In the mid-1990s, the World Bank classified Azerbaijan as a "lower-middle-income" economy. Yet by the late 1990s, the enormous oil reserves in the Baku area, on the Caspian Sea and in the sea itself, held out great promise for the future. Oil extraction and manufacturing, including oil refining and the production of chemicals, machinery and textiles, are now the most valuable activities.

AREA 33,436 sq mi [86,600 sq km] **POPULATION** 7,831,000 **CAPITAL (POPULATION)** Baku (1,792,000) **GOVERNMENT** Federal multiparty republic **ETHNIC GROUPS** Azeri 90%, Dagestani 3%, Russian, Armenian, others **LANGUAGES** Azerbaijani (official), Russian, Armenian **RELIGIONS** Islam 93%, Russian Orthodox 2%, Armenian Orthodox 2% **CURRENCY** Azerbaijani manat = 100 gopik

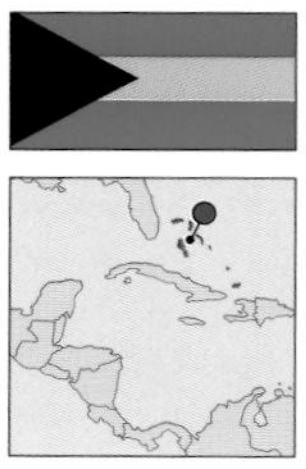

BAHAMAS

A coral-limestone archipelago off the coast of Florida, the Bahamas became independent from Britain in 1973, and has since developed strong ties with the United States. Tourism and banking are major activities.

AREA 5,358 sq mi [13,878 sq km]
POPULATION 297,000 **CAPITAL** Nassau

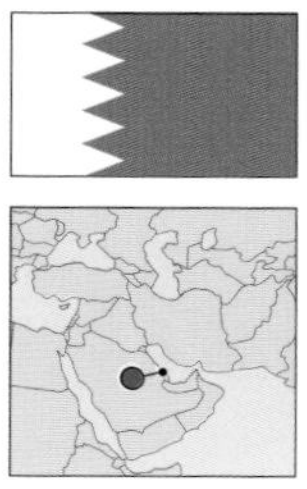

BAHRAIN

The Kingdom of Bahrain, an island nation in the Persian Gulf, became independent from the UK in 1971. Oil accounts for 80% of its exports.

AREA 268 sq mi [694 sq km]
POPULATION 667,000 **CAPITAL** Manama

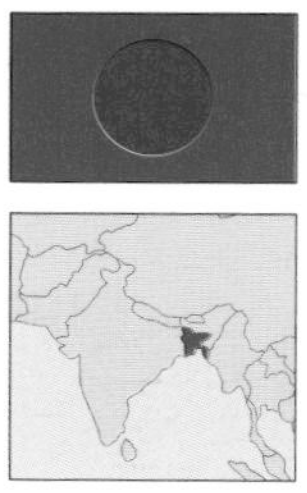

BANGLADESH

GEOGRAPHY The People's Republic of Bangladesh is one of the world's most densely populated countries. Apart from hilly regions in the far northeast and southeast, most of the land is flat and covered by fertile alluvium spread over the land by the Ganges, Brahmaputra and Meghna rivers. These rivers overflow when they are swollen by the annual monsoon rains. Floods also occur along the coast, 357 mi [575 km] long, when cyclones (hurricanes) drive seawater inland. Bangladesh has a tropical monsoon climate. Dry northerly winds blow in winter, but, in summer, moist winds from the south bring monsoon rains. Heavy monsoon rains cause floods. In 1998, about two-thirds of the entire country was submerged, causing great suffering.

POLITICS & ECONOMY In 1947, British India was partitioned between the mainly Hindu India and the Muslim Pakistan. Pakistan consisted of two parts, West and East Pakistan, which were separated by about 1,000 mi [1,600 km] of Indian territory. Differences developed between West and East Pakistan. In 1971, the East Pakistanis rebelled. After a nine-month civil war, they declared East Pakistan to be a separate nation named Bangladesh.

Bangladesh is one of the world's poorest countries. Its economy depends mainly on agriculture, which employs over half the population. Bangladesh is the world's fourth largest producer of rice.

AREA 55,598 sq mi [143,998 sq km] **POPULATION** 138,448,000 **CAPITAL (POPULATION)** Dhaka (3,839,000) **GOVERNMENT** Multiparty republic **ETHNIC GROUPS** Bengali 98%, tribal groups **LANGUAGES** Bengali (official), English **RELIGIONS** Islam 83%, Hinduism 16% **CURRENCY** Taka = 100 paisas

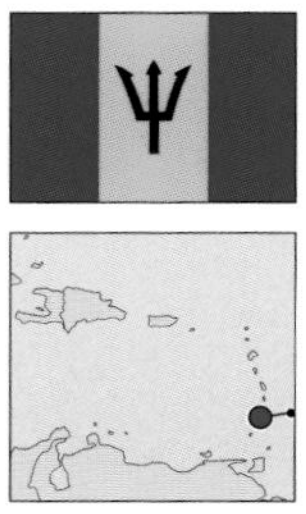

BARBADOS

The most easterly Caribbean country, Barbados became independent from the UK in 1960. A densely populated island, Barbados is prosperous by comparison with most Caribbean countries.

AREA 166 sq mi [430 sq km]
POPULATION 277,000 **CAPITAL** Bridgetown

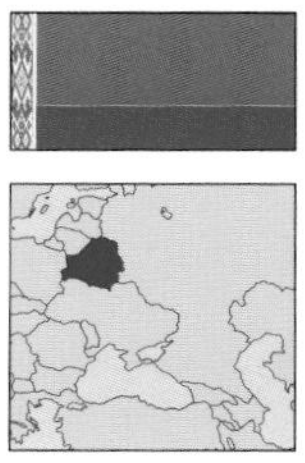

BELARUS

GEOGRAPHY The Republic of Belarus is a landlocked country in Eastern Europe. The land is low-lying and mostly flat. In the south, much of the land is marshy and this area contains Europe's largest marsh and peat bog, the Pripet Marshes. The climate is affected by both the moderating influence of the Baltic Sea and continental conditions to the east. The winters are cold and the summers warm.

POLITICS & ECONOMY In 1918, Belarus (White Russia) became an independent republic, but Russia invaded the country and, in 1919, a Communist state was set up. In 1922, Belarus became a founder republic of the Soviet Union. In 1991, Belarus again became an independent republic, though Belarus continued to support reunification with Russia. In 1998, Belarus and Russia set up a "union state," with plans to have a common currency, a customs union, and common foreign and defense policies. But any surrender of sovereignty was not expected. In 2003, the Russian President Vladimir Putin agreed to deepen ties with Belarus, but also stated that he did not wish to create anything like the Soviet Union.

The World Bank classifies Belarus as an "upper-middle-income" economy. Like other former republics of the Soviet Union, it faces many problems in turning from Communism to a free-market economy.

AREA 80,154 sq mi [207,600 sq km] **POPULATION** 10,322,000 **CAPITAL (POPULATION)** Minsk (1,677,000) **GOVERNMENT** Multiparty republic **ETHNIC GROUPS** Belarusian 81%, Russian 11%, Polish, Ukrainian, others **LANGUAGES** Belarusian, Russian (both official) **RELIGIONS** Eastern Orthodox 80%, others 20% **CURRENCY** Belarusian rouble = 100 kopecks

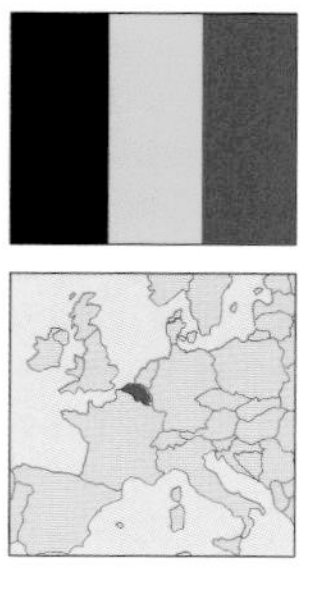

BELGIUM

GEOGRAPHY The Kingdom of Belgium is a densely populated country in western Europe. Behind the coastline on the North Sea, which is 39 mi [63 km] long, lie its coastal plains. Central Belgium consists of low plateaux and the only highland region is the Ardennes in the southeast.

Belgium has a cool, temperate climate. Moist winds from the Atlantic Ocean bring fairly heavy rain, especially in the Ardennes. In January and February much snow falls on the Ardennes.

POLITICS & ECONOMY In 1815, Belgium and the Netherlands united as the "low countries," but Belgium became independent in 1830. Belgium's economy was weakened by the two World

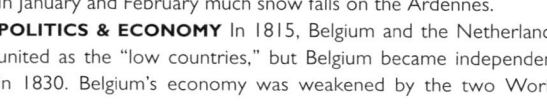

Wars, but, from 1945, the country recovered quickly, first through collaboration with the Netherlands and Luxembourg, which formed a customs union called Benelux, and later through its membership of the European Union.

A central political problem in Belgium has been the tension between the Dutch-speaking Flemings and the French-speaking Walloons. In the 1970s, the government divided the country into three economic regions: Dutch-speaking Flanders, French-speaking Wallonia and bilingual Brussels. In 1993, Belgium adopted a federal constitution, with each region having its own parliament. Elections under this system were held in 1995, 1999, and 2003.

Belgium is a major trading nation, with a highly developed economy. Most of the materials needed for manufacturing are imported. Its main products include chemicals, processed food and steel. The textile industry is important. It has existed since medieval times in the Belgian province of Flanders. In 2002, the parliament voted to phase out the use of nuclear energy by 2025.

Agriculture employs only 2% of the people, but Belgian farmers produce most of the food needed by the people. Barley and wheat are the chief crops, followed by flax, hops, potatoes and sugar beet, but the most valuable activities are dairy farming and livestock rearing.

AREA 11,787 SQ MI [30,528 SQ KM]
POPULATION 10,289,000
CAPITAL (POPULATION) BRUSSELS (136,000)
GOVERNMENT FEDERAL CONSTITUTIONAL MONARCHY
ETHNIC GROUPS BELGIAN 89% (FLEMING 58%, WALLOON 31%), OTHERS 11% **LANGUAGES** DUTCH, FRENCH, GERMAN (ALL OFFICIAL)
RELIGIONS ROMAN CATHOLIC 75%, OTHERS 25%
CURRENCY EURO = 100 CENTS

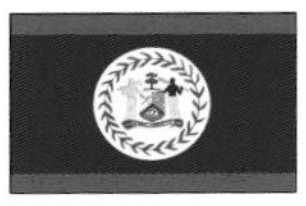
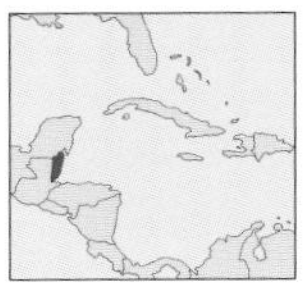

BELIZE

GEOGRAPHY Behind the southern coastal plain, the land rises to the Maya Mountains, which reach 3,674 ft [1,120 m] at Victoria Peak. The north is mostly low-lying and swampy. Temperatures are high all year round, while the average annual rainfall ranges from 51 in [1,300 mm] in the north to over 150 in [3,800 mm] in the south. Hurricanes sometimes occur. One in 2001 killed 22 people and left 12,000 homeless.

POLITICS & ECONOMY From 1862, Belize (then called British Honduras) was a British colony. Full independence was achieved in 1981, but Guatemala, which had claimed the area since the early 19th century, opposed Belize's independence and British troops remained to prevent a possible invasion. In 1983, Guatemala reduced its claim to the southern fifth of Belize. Improved relations in the early 1990s led Guatemala to recognize Belize's independence and, in 1992, Britain agreed to withdraw its troops from the country.

The World Bank classifies Belize as a "lower-middle-income" developing country. Its economy is based on agriculture and sugarcane is the chief commercial crop and export. Other crops include bananas, beans, citrus fruits, maize, and rice. Forestry, fishing, and tourism are other important activities.

AREA 8,867 SQ MI [22,966 SQ KM] **POPULATION** 266,000
CAPITAL (POPULATION) BELMOPAN (8,000)
GOVERNMENT CONSTITUTIONAL MONARCHY **ETHNIC GROUPS** MESTIZO 49%, CREOLE 25%, MAYAN INDIAN 11%, GARIFUNA 6%, OTHERS 9%
LANGUAGES ENGLISH (OFFICIAL), SPANISH, CREOLE
RELIGIONS ROMAN CATHOLIC 50%, PROTESTANT 27%, OTHERS
CURRENCY BELIZEAN DOLLAR = 100 CENTS

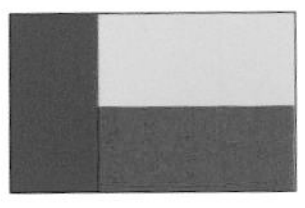
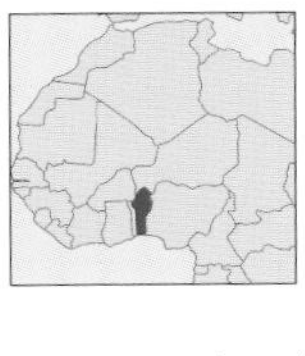

BENIN

GEOGRAPHY The Republic of Benin is one of Africa's smallest countries. It extends north–south for about 390 mi [620 km]. Lagoons line the short coastline, and the country has no natural harbors.

Benin has a hot, wet climate. The average annual temperature on the coast is about 77°F [25°C], and the average rainfall is about 52 in [1,330 mm]. The inland plains are wetter than the coast.

POLITICS & ECONOMY After slavery was ended in the 19th century, the French began to gain influence in the area. Benin became self-governing in 1958 and fully independent in 1960. After much instability and many changes of government, a military group took over in 1972. The country, renamed Benin in 1975, became a one-party socialist state. Socialism was abandoned in 1989. Multiparty elections were held in the 1990s and the early 2000s.

Benin is a poor developing country. About 70% of the people earn their living by farming, though many remain at subsistence level. The chief exports include cotton, petroleum, and palm products. Cocoa, coffee, groundnuts (peanuts), tobacco, and shea nuts are also grown for export.

AREA 43,483 SQ MI [112,622 SQ KM] **POPULATION** 7,041,000
CAPITAL (POPULATION) PORTO-NOVO (233,000)
GOVERNMENT MULTIPARTY REPUBLIC **ETHNIC GROUPS** FON, ADJA, BARIBA, YORUBA, FULANI **LANGUAGES** FRENCH (OFFICIAL), FON, ADJA, YORUBA
RELIGIONS TRADITIONAL BELIEFS 50%, CHRISTIANITY 30%, ISLAM 20%
CURRENCY CFA FRANC = 100 CENTIMES

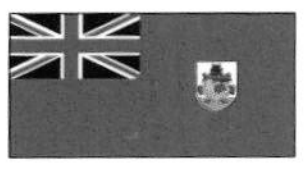
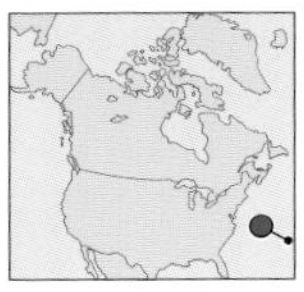

BERMUDA

A group of about 150 small islands situated 570 mi [920 km] east of the USA. Bermuda remains Britain's oldest overseas territory, but it has a long tradition of self-government.

AREA 21 SQ MI [53 SQ KM]
POPULATION 64,000 **CAPITAL** HAMILTON

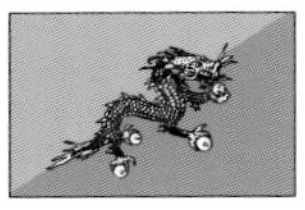
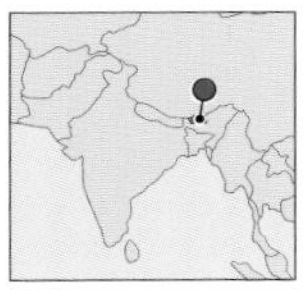

BHUTAN

GEOGRAPHY A mountainous, isolated Himalayan country located between India and Tibet. The climate is similar to that of Nepal, being dependent on altitude and affected by monsoonal winds.

POLITICS & ECONOMY The monarch of Bhutan is head of both state and government and this predominantly Buddhist country remains, even in the Asian context, both conservative and poor. Bhutan is the world's most "rural" country, with about 87% of the population dependent on agriculture and only 7% living in towns.

AREA 18,147 SQ MI [47,000 SQ KM] **POPULATION** 2,140,000
CAPITAL (POPULATION) THIMPHU (35,000)
GOVERNMENT CONSTITUTIONAL MONARCHY **ETHNIC GROUPS** BHUTANESE 50%, NEPALESE 35% **LANGUAGES** DZONGKHA (OFFICIAL) **RELIGIONS** BUDDHISM 75%, HINDUISM 25% **CURRENCY** NGULTRUM = 100 CHETRUM

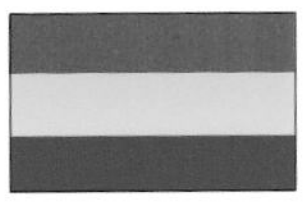
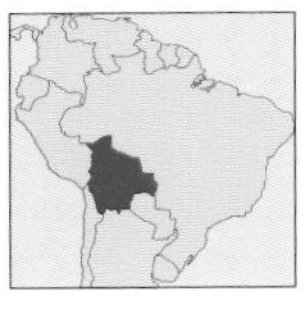

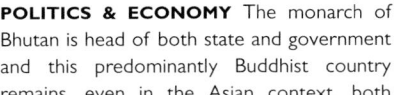

BOLIVIA

GEOGRAPHY The Republic of Bolivia is a landlocked country which straddles the Andes Mountains in central South America. The Andes rise to a height of 21,464 ft [6,542 m] at Nevado Sajama in the west.

About 40% of Bolivians live on a high plateau called the Altiplano in the Andean region, while the sparsely populated east is essentially a vast lowland plain.

The Bolivian climate is greatly affected by altitude, with the Andean peaks permanently snow-covered, and the eastern plains remaining hot and humid.

POLITICS & ECONOMY American Indians have lived in Bolivia for at least 10,000 years. The main groups today are the Aymara and Quechua people.

In the last 50 years, Bolivia, an independent country since 1825, has been ruled by a succession of civilian and military governments, which violated human rights. Constitutional government was restored in 1982. From the 1980s, Bolivia has pursued economic reforms and free-market policies.

Bolivia is one of the poorest countries in South America. It has several natural resources, including tin, silver and natural gas, but the chief activity is agriculture, which employs 47% of the people. Coca, which is used to make cocaine, is exported illegally. In 2002–3, the production of coca plummeted, causing much social unrest and ethnic tensions. The government hoped that oil and gas would soon replace coca as the chief export.

AREA 424,162 SQ MI [1,098,581 SQ KM] **POPULATION** 8,586,000
CAPITAL (POPULATION) LA PAZ (SEAT OF GOVERNMENT, 940,000); SUCRE (LEGAL CAPITAL/SEAT OF JUDICIARY, 177,000)
GOVERNMENT MULTIPARTY REPUBLIC **ETHNIC GROUPS** MESTIZO 30%, QUECHUA 30%, AYMARA 25%, WHITE 15% **LANGUAGES** SPANISH, AYMARA, QUECHUA (ALL OFFICIAL) **RELIGIONS** ROMAN CATHOLIC 95%
CURRENCY BOLIVIANO = 100 CENTAVOS

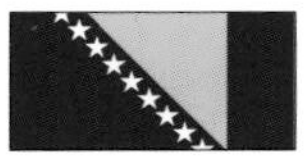
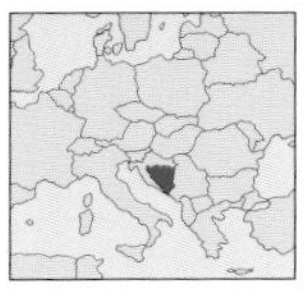

BOSNIA-HERZEGOVINA

GEOGRAPHY The Republic of Bosnia-Herzegovina is one of the five republics to emerge from the former Federal People's Republic of Yugoslavia. Much of the country is mountainous or hilly, with an arid limestone plateau in the southwest. The River Sava, which forms most of the northern border with Croatia, is a tributary of the River Danube. Because of the country's odd shape, the coastline is limited to a short stretch of 13 mi [20 km] on the Adriatic coast.

A Mediterranean climate, with dry, sunny summers and moist, mild winters, prevails only near the coast. Inland, the weather is more severe, with hot, dry summers and bitterly cold, snowy winters.

POLITICS & ECONOMY In 1918, Bosnia-Herzegovina became part of the Kingdom of the Serbs, Croats and Slovenes, which was renamed Yugoslavia in 1929. Germany occupied the area during World War II (1939–45). From 1945, Communist governments ruled Yugoslavia as a federation containing six republics, one of which was Bosnia-Herzegovina. In the 1980s, the country faced problems as Communist policies proved unsuccessful and differences arose between ethnic groups.

In 1990, free elections were held in Bosnia-Herzegovina and the non-Communists won a majority. A Muslim, Alija Izetbegovic, was elected president. In 1991, Croatia and Slovenia, other parts of the former Yugoslavia, declared themselves independent. In 1992, Bosnia-Herzegovina held a vote on independence. Most Bosnian Serbs boycotted the vote, while the Muslims and Bosnian Croats voted in favor. Many Bosnian Serbs, opposed to independence, started a war against the non-Serbs. They soon occupied more than two-thirds of the land. The Bosnian Serbs were accused of "ethnic cleansing" – that is, the killing or expulsion of other ethnic groups from Serb-occupied areas. The war was later extended when Croat forces seized other parts of the country.

In 1995, the conflict was resolved. Under an agreement, the country's boundaries were maintained, but the territory was divided into two self-governing provinces, one Bosnian-Serb and the other Muslim-Croat, under a central unified government. At first, the country's future seemed uncertain. But, by 2004, its main problems were economic rather than political.

The economy of Bosnia-Herzegovina, the least developed of the six republics of the former Yugoslavia apart from Macedonia, was shattered by the war in the early 1990s. Before the war, manufactures were the main exports, including electrical, machinery and transport equipment, and textiles. Farm products include fruits, maize, tobacco, vegetables, and wheat, but food has to be imported.

AREA 19,767 SQ MI [51,197 SQ KM] **POPULATION** 3,989,000
CAPITAL (POPULATION) SARAJEVO (529,000)
GOVERNMENT FEDERAL REPUBLIC **ETHNIC GROUPS** BOSNIAN 48%, SERB 37%, CROAT 14% **LANGUAGES** BOSNIAN, SERBIAN, CROATIAN
RELIGIONS ISLAM 40%, SERBIAN ORTHODOX 31%, ROMAN CATHOLIC 15%, OTHERS 14% **CURRENCY** CONVERTIBLE MARKA = 100 CONVERTIBLE PFENNIGA

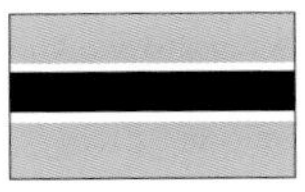
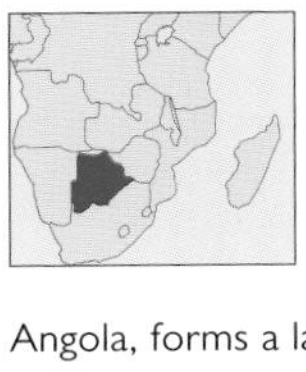

BOTSWANA

GEOGRAPHY The Republic of Botswana is a landlocked country in southern Africa. The Kalahari, a semidesert area covered mostly by grasses and thorn scrub, covers much of the country. Most of the south has no permanent streams. But large depressions in the north are inland drainage basins. In one of them, the Okavango River, which rises in Angola, forms a large, swampy delta.

Temperatures are high in the summer months (October to April), but the winter months are much cooler. In winter, nighttime temperatures sometimes drop below freezing point. The average annual rainfall ranges from over 16 in [400 mm] in the east to less than 8 in [200 mm] in the southwest.

POLITICS & ECONOMY The earliest inhabitants of the region were the San, who are also called Bushmen. They had a nomadic way of life, hunting wild animals and collecting wild plant foods.

Britain ruled the area as the Bechuanaland Protectorate between 1885 and 1966. When the country became independent, it was renamed Botswana. Since then, the country has been a stable, multiparty democracy. However, a major setback occurred in the early 21st century, when health officials announced that around 25% of the people were infected with HIV/AIDS. In 1966, Botswana was extremely poor, depending on meat and live cattle for its exports. But the discovery of minerals, including coal, cobalt, copper, diamonds and nickel, has boosted the economy. About 17% of the people now depend on agriculture, raising cattle and growing crops. Industries include the processing of farm products.

AREA 224,606 sq mi [581,730 sq km] **POPULATION** 1,573,000
CAPITAL (POPULATION) Gaborone (186,000)
GOVERNMENT Multiparty republic **ETHNIC GROUPS** Tswana (or Setswana) 79%, Kalanga 11%, Basarwa 3%, others
LANGUAGES English (official), Setswana **RELIGIONS** Traditional beliefs 85%, Christianity 15% **CURRENCY** Pula = 100 thebe

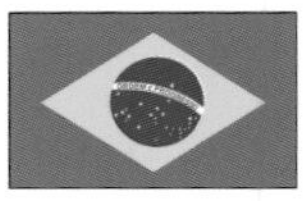
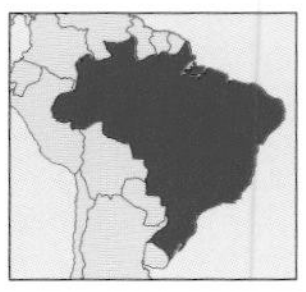

BRAZIL

GEOGRAPHY The Federative Republic of Brazil is the world's fifth largest country. It contains three main regions. The Amazon basin in the north covers more than half of Brazil. The Amazon, the world's second longest river, has a far greater volume than any other river. The second region, the northeast, consists of a coastal plain and the *sertão*, which is the name for the inland plateaux and hill country. The main river in this region is the São Francisco.

The third region is made up of the plateaux in the southeast. This region, which covers about a quarter of the country, is the most developed and densely populated part of Brazil. Its main river is the Paraná, which flows south through Argentina.

Manaus has high temperatures all through the year. The rainfall is heavy, though the period from June to September is drier than the rest of the year. The capital, Brasília, and the city Rio de Janeiro also have tropical climates, with much more marked dry seasons than Manaus. The far south has a temperate climate. The northeastern interior is the driest region, with an average annual rainfall of only 10 in [250 mm] in places. The rainfall is also unreliable and severe droughts are common in this region.

POLITICS & ECONOMY The Portuguese explorer Pedro Alvarez Cabral claimed Brazil for Portugal in 1500. With Spain occupied in western South America, the Portuguese began to develop their colony, which was more than 90 times as big as Portugal. To do this, they enslaved many local Amerindian people and introduced about 4 million African slaves. Brazil declared itself an independent empire in 1822 and a republic in 1889. From the 1930s, Brazil faced periods of military rule and widespread corruption. Civilian rule was restored in 1985. Brazil adopted a new constitution in 1988.

The United Nations has described Brazil as a "Rapidly Industrializing Country," or RIC. Its total volume of production is one of the largest in the world. But many people, including poor farmers and residents of the *favelas* (city slums), do not share in the country's fast economic growth. Widespread poverty, together with high inflation and unemployment led to the election as president of left-winger Luiz Inácio Lula da Silva (popularly known as "Lula") in 2002. In office, he adopted a pragmatic approach to Brazil's many problems, but his popularity continued.

Industry is the most important economic sector. Brazil is among the world's top producers of bauxite, chrome, diamonds, gold, iron ore, manganese and tin. It is also a major manufacturing country. Its products include aircraft, cars, chemicals, processed food, including raw sugar, iron and steel, paper and textiles.

Brazil is one of the world's leading farming countries and agriculture employs 22% of the people. Coffee is a major export. Other leading products include bananas, citrus fruits, cocoa, maize, rice, soybeans, and sugarcane. Brazil is also the top producer of eggs, meat, and milk in South America.

Forestry is a major industry, though many people fear that the exploitation of the rain forests, with 1.5% to 4% of Brazil's forest being destroyed every year, is a disaster for the entire world.

AREA 3,287,338 sq mi [8,514,215 sq km] **POPULATION** 182,033,000
CAPITAL (POPULATION) Brasília (2,016,000)
GOVERNMENT Federal republic
ETHNIC GROUPS White 55%, Mulatto 38%, Black 6%, others 1% **LANGUAGES** Portuguese (official)
RELIGIONS Roman Catholic 80%
CURRENCY Real = 100 centavos

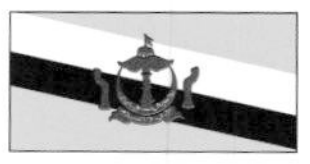
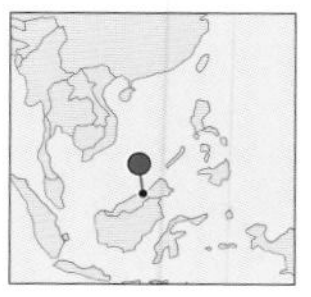

BRUNEI

The Islamic Sultanate of Brunei, a British protectorate until 1984, lies on the north coast of Borneo. The climate is tropical and rain forests cover large areas. Brunei is a prosperous country because of its oil and natural gas production, and the Sultan is said to be among the world's richest men.

AREA 2,226 sq mi [5,765 sq km] **POPULATION** 358,000
CAPITAL (POPULATION) Bandar Seri Begawan (50,000)

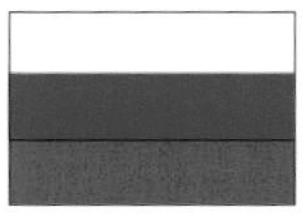
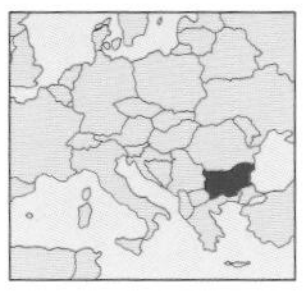

BULGARIA

GEOGRAPHY The Republic of Bulgaria is a country in the Balkan peninsula, facing the Black Sea in the east. The heart of Bulgaria is mountainous. The main ranges are the Balkan Mountains in the center and the Rhodope (or Rhodopi) Mountains in the south.

Summers are hot and winters are cold, though seldom severe. The rainfall is moderate.

POLITICS & ECONOMY Ottoman Turks ruled Bulgaria from 1396 and ethnic Turks still form a sizable minority in the country. In 1879, Bulgaria became a monarchy, and in 1908 it became fully independent. Bulgaria was an ally of Germany in World War I (1914–18) and again in World War II (1939–45). In 1944, Soviet troops invaded Bulgaria and, after the war, the monarchy was abolished and the country became a Communist ally of the Soviet Union. In the late 1980s, reforms in the Soviet Union led Bulgaria's government to introduce a multiparty system in 1990. A non-Communist government was elected in 1991, the first free elections in 44 years. Throughout the 1990s, Bulgaria faced many problems. In 2001, a coalition led by the former King Siméon, who had left Bulgaria in 1948, won the elections. Siméon became prime minister. In 2004, Bulgaria became a member of the North Atlantic Treaty Organization.

According to the World Bank, Bulgaria in the 1990s was a "lower-middle-income" developing country. Bulgaria has some deposits of minerals, including brown coal, manganese, and iron ore. But manufacturing is the leading activity, though, in the early 1990s, much of its industrial plant was out of date. Leading products include chemicals, processed foods, metal products, machinery, and textiles. Manufactures are the leading exports.

AREA 42,823 sq mi [110,912 sq km] **POPULATION** 7,538,000
CAPITAL (POPULATION) Sofia (1,139,000) **GOVERNMENT** Multiparty republic **ETHNIC GROUPS** Bulgarian 84%, Turkish 9%, Gypsy 5%, Macedonian, Armenian, others **LANGUAGES** Bulgarian (official), Turkish **RELIGIONS** Bulgarian Orthodox 83%, Islam 12%, Roman Catholic 2%, others **CURRENCY** Lev = 100 stotinki

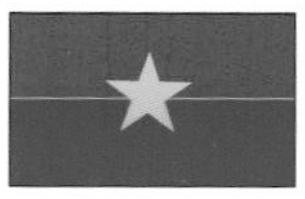
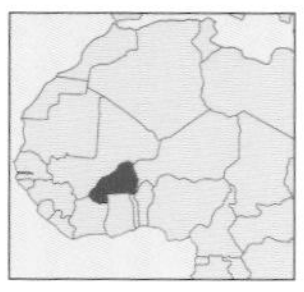

BURKINA FASO

GEOGRAPHY The Democratic People's Republic of Burkina Faso is a landlocked country, a little larger than the United Kingdom, in West Africa. But Burkina Faso has only one-sixth of the population of the UK. The country consists of a plateau, between about 650 ft and 2,300 ft [300 m to 700 m] above sea level. The plateau is cut by several rivers.

The capital city, Ouagadougou, in central Burkina Faso, has high temperatures throughout the year. Most of the rain falls between May and September, but the rainfall is erratic and droughts are common.

POLITICS & ECONOMY The people of Burkina Faso are divided into two main groups. The Voltaic group includes the Mossi, who form the largest single group, and the Bobo. The French conquered the Mossi capital of Ouagadougou in 1897 and they made the area a protectorate. In 1919, the area became a French colony called Upper Volta. After independence in 1960, Upper Volta became a one-party state. But it was unstable – military groups seized power several times and political killings took place. In 1984, the country's name was changed to Burkina Faso. In 1991 and 1998, the former military leader, Captain Blaise Compaoré, was elected president, but the military continued to play an important part in the government.

Burkina Faso is one of the world's 20 poorest countries and has become very dependent on foreign aid. Most of Burkina Faso is dry with thin soils. The country's main food crops are beans, maize, millet, rice, and sorghum. Cotton, groundnuts, and shea nuts, whose seeds produce a fat used to make cooking oil and soap, are grown for sale abroad. Livestock are also an important export.

The country has few resources and manufacturing is on a small scale. There are some deposits of manganese, zinc, lead, and nickel in the north of the country, but there is not yet a good enough transport system there. Many young men seek jobs abroad in Ghana and Ivory Coast. The money they send home to their families is important to the country's economy.

AREA 105,791 sq mi [274,000 sq km] **POPULATION** 13,228,000
CAPITAL (POPULATION) Ouagadougou (637,000)
GOVERNMENT Multiparty republic **ETHNIC GROUPS** Mossi 40%, Gurunsi, Senufo, Lobi, Bobo, Mande, Fulani **LANGUAGES** French (official), Mossi, Fulani **RELIGIONS** Islam 50%, traditional beliefs 40%, Christianity 10% **CURRENCY** CFA franc = 100 centimes

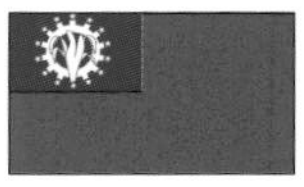
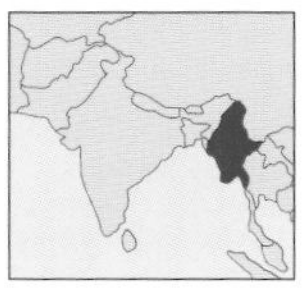

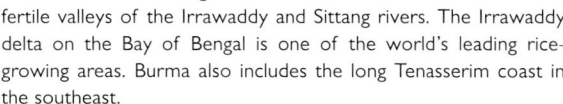

BURMA (MYANMAR)

GEOGRAPHY The Union of Burma is now officially known as the Union of Myanmar; its name was changed in 1989. Mountains border the country in the east and west, with the highest mountains in the north. Burma's highest mountain is Hkakabo Razi, which is 19,294 ft [5,881 m] high. Between these ranges is central Burma, which contains the fertile valleys of the Irrawaddy and Sittang rivers. The Irrawaddy delta on the Bay of Bengal is one of the world's leading rice-growing areas. Burma also includes the long Tenasserim coast in the southeast.

Burma has a tropical monsoon climate. There are three seasons. The rainy season runs from late May to mid-October. A cool, dry season follows, between late October and the middle part of February. The hot season lasts from late February to mid-May, though temperatures remain high during the humid rainy season.

POLITICS & ECONOMY Many groups settled in Burma in ancient times. Some, called the hill peoples, live in remote mountain areas where they have retained their own cultures. The ancestors of the country's main ethnic group today, the Burmese, arrived in the 9th century AD.

Britain conquered Burma in the 19th century and made it a province of British India. But, in 1937, the British granted Burma limited self-government. Japan conquered Burma in 1942, but the Japanese were driven out in 1945. Burma became a fully independent country in 1948.

Revolts by Communists and various hill people led to instability in the 1950s. In 1962, Burma became a military dictatorship and, in 1974, a one-party state. Attempts to control minority liberation movements and the opium trade led to repressive rule. The National League for Democracy led by Aung San Suu Kyi won the elections in 1990, but the military continued their repressive rule throughout the 1990s, earning Burma the reputation for having one of the world's worst human rights records. Its admission to ASEAN (Association of Southeast Asian Nations) in 1997 may have implied regional recognition of the regime. However, the European Union continued to voice its concerns over human rights abuses. The opposition leader Aung San Suu Kyi was released in 2002, but she was soon placed under "protective custody."

Agriculture is the main activity, employing 66% of the people. The chief crop is rice. Maize, pulses, oilseeds, and sugarcane are other major products. Forestry is important. Teak and rice together make up about two-thirds of the total value of the exports. Burma has many mineral resources, though they are mostly undeveloped, but the country is famous for its precious stones, especially rubies. Manufacturing is mostly on a small scale.

AREA 261,227 sq mi [676,578 sq km] **POPULATION** 42,511,000
CAPITAL (POPULATION) Rangoon (2,513,000) **GOVERNMENT** Military regime **ETHNIC GROUPS** Burman 68%, Shan 9%, Karen 7%, Rakhine 4%, Chinese, Indian, Mon **LANGUAGES** Burmese (official); minority ethnic groups have their own languages **RELIGIONS** Buddhism 89%, Christianity, Islam **CURRENCY** Kyat = 100 pyas

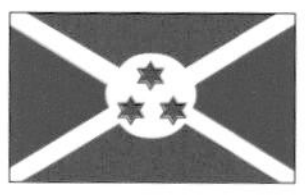
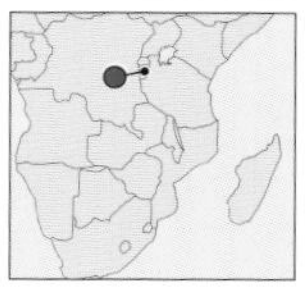

BURUNDI

GEOGRAPHY The Republic of Burundi is the fifth smallest country in mainland Africa. It is also the second most densely populated after its northern neighbor, Rwanda. Part of the Great African Rift Valley, which runs throughout eastern Africa into southwestern Asia, lies in western Burundi. It includes part of Lake Tanganyika.

Bujumbura, the capital city, lies on the shore of Lake Tanganyika. It has a warm climate. A dry season occurs from June to September, but the other months are fairly rainy. The mountains and plateaux to the east are cooler and wetter, but the rainfall generally decreases to the east.

POLITICS & ECONOMY The Twa, a pygmy people, were the first known inhabitants of Burundi. About 1,000 years ago, the Hutu, a people who speak a Bantu language, gradually began to settle the area, pushing the Twa into remote areas.

From the 15th century, the Tutsi, a cattle-owning people from the northeast, gradually took over the country. The Hutu, though greatly outnumbering the Tutsi, were forced to serve the Tutsi overlords.

Germany conquered the area that is now Burundi and Rwanda in the late 1890s. The area, called Ruanda-Urundi, was taken by Belgium during World War I (1914–18). In 1961, the people of Urundi voted to become a monarchy, while the people of Ruanda voted to become a republic. The two territories became fully independent as Burundi and Rwanda in 1962. After 1962, the rivalries between the Hutu and Tutsi led to periodic outbreaks of

fighting. The Tutsi monarchy was ended in 1966 and Burundi became a republic. Instability continued with coups and massacres as Tutsis and Hutus fought against each other. Following a power-sharing agreement in 2001, further conflict threatened the holding of elections in 2004.

Burundi is one of the world's ten poorest countries. About 93% of the people are farmers who live mostly at subsistence level. The main food crops are beans, cassava, maize, and sweet potatoes. Cattle, goats, and sheep are raised, and fishing is also important. However, Burundi has to import food.

AREA 10,747 sq mi [27,834 sq km] **POPULATION** 6,096,000
CAPITAL (POPULATION) Bujumbura (235,000)
GOVERNMENT Republic **ETHNIC GROUPS** Hutu 85%, Tutsi 14%, Twa (Pygmy) 1% **LANGUAGES** French and Kirundi (both official)
RELIGIONS Roman Catholic 62%, traditional beliefs 23%, Islam 10%, Protestant 5% **CURRENCY** Burundi franc = 100 centimes

CAMBODIA

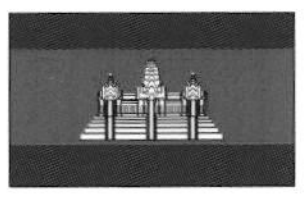
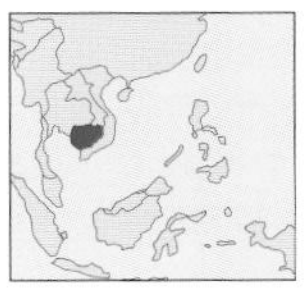

GEOGRAPHY The Kingdom of Cambodia is a country in Southeast Asia. Low mountains border the country except in the southeast. But most of Cambodia consists of plains drained by the River Mekong, which enters Cambodia from Laos in the north and exits through Vietnam in the southeast. The northwest contains Tonlé Sap (or Great Lake). In the dry season, this lake drains into the River Mekong. But in the wet season, the level of the Mekong rises and water flows in the opposite direction from the river into Tonlé Sap – the lake then becomes the largest freshwater lake in Asia.

Cambodia has a tropical monsoon climate, with high temperatures throughout the year. The dry season, when winds blow from the north or northeast, runs from November to April. During the rainy season (May to October), moist winds blow from the south or southeast. The high humidity and heat often make conditions unpleasant. Rainfall is heaviest near the coast, and rather lower inland.

POLITICS & ECONOMY From 802 to 1432, the Khmer people ruled a great empire, which reached its peak in the 12th century. The Khmer capital was at Angkor. The Hindu stone temples built there and at nearby Angkor Wat form the world's largest group of religious buildings. France ruled the country between 1863 and 1954, when the country became an independent monarchy. But the monarchy was abolished in 1970 and Cambodia became a republic.

In 1970, US and South Vietnamese troops entered Cambodia but left after destroying North Vietnamese Communist camps in the east. The country became involved in the Vietnamese War, and then in a civil war as Cambodian Communists of the Khmer Rouge organization fought for power. The Khmer Rouge took over Cambodia in 1975 and launched a reign of terror in which between 1 million and 2.5 million people were killed. In 1979, Vietnamese and Cambodian troops overthrew the Khmer Rouge government. But fighting continued between factions. Vietnam withdrew in 1989, and in 1991 Prince Sihanouk was recognized as head of state. Elections were held in May 1993, and in September 1993 the monarchy was restored. Sihanouk again became king. In 1997, the prime minister, Prince Norodom Ranariddh, was deposed, so ending four years of democratic rule. Further elections were held in 1998 and, in 2001, the government set up courts to try leaders of the Khmer Rouge.

Cambodia is a poor country whose economy has been wrecked by war. Until the 1970s, the country's farmers produced most of the food needed by the people. But by 1986, it was only able to supply 80% of its needs. Farming is the main activity and rice, rubber, and maize are major products. Manufacturing is almost non-existent, apart from rubber processing and a few factories producing items for sale in Cambodia.

AREA 69,898 sq mi [181,035 sq km] **POPULATION** 13,125,000
CAPITAL (POPULATION) Phnom Penh (1,000,000) **GOVERNMENT** Constitutional monarchy **ETHNIC GROUPS** Khmer 90%, Vietnamese 5%, Chinese 1%, others **LANGUAGES** Khmer (official), French, English
RELIGIONS Buddhism 95%, others 5% **CURRENCY** Riel = 100 sen

CAMEROON

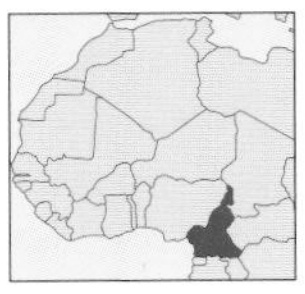

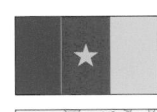

GEOGRAPHY The Republic of Cameroon in West Africa got its name from the Portuguese word *camarões*, or prawns. This name was used by Portuguese explorers who fished for prawns along the coast. Behind the narrow coastal plains on the Gulf of Guinea, the land rises to a series of plateaux, with a mountainous region in the southwest where the volcano Mount Cameroon is situated. In the north, the land slopes down toward the Lake Chad basin.

The rainfall is heavy, especially in the highlands. The rainiest months near the coast are June to September. The rainfall decreases to the north and the far north has a hot, dry climate. Temperatures are high on the coast, whereas the inland plateaux are cooler.

POLITICS & ECONOMY Germany lost Cameroon during World War I (1914–18). The country was then divided into two parts, one ruled by Britain and the other by France. In 1960, French Cameroon became the independent Cameroon Republic. In 1961, after a vote in British Cameroon, part of the territory joined the Cameroon Republic to become the Federal Republic of Cameroon. The other part joined Nigeria. In 1972, Cameroon became a unitary state called the United Republic of Cameroon. It adopted the name Republic of Cameroon in 1984, but the country had two official languages. In 1995, partly to placate English-speaking people, Cameroon became the 52nd member of the Commonwealth.

Like most countries in tropical Africa, Cameroon's economy is based on agriculture, which employs 74% of the people. The chief food crops include cassava, maize, millet, sweet potatoes, and yams. The country also has plantations to produce such crops as cocoa and coffee for export.

Cameroon is fortunate in having some oil, the country's chief export, and bauxite. Although Cameroon has few manufacturing and processing industries, its mineral exports and its self-sufficiency in food production make it one of the better-off countries in tropical Africa.

AREA 183,568 sq mi [475,442 sq km] **POPULATION** 15,746,000
CAPITAL (POPULATION) Yaoundé (649,000) **GOVERNMENT** Multiparty republic **ETHNIC GROUPS** Cameroon Highlanders 31%, Bantu 27%, Kirdi 11%, Fulani 10%, others **LANGUAGES** French and English (both official) **RELIGIONS** Christianity 40%, traditional beliefs 40%, Islam 20% **CURRENCY** CFA franc = 100 centimes

CANADA

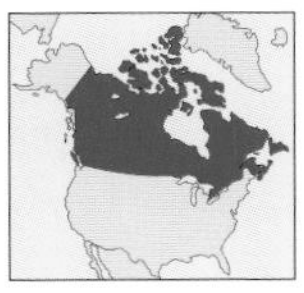

GEOGRAPHY Canada is the world's second largest country after Russia. It is thinly populated, however, with much of the land too cold or too mountainous for human settlement. Most Canadians live within 186 mi [300 km] of the southern border.

Western Canada is rugged. It includes the Pacific ranges and the mighty Rocky Mountains. East of the Rockies are the interior plains. In the north lie the bleak Arctic islands, while to the south lie the densely populated lowlands around lakes Erie and Ontario and in the St Lawrence River valley.

Canada has a cold climate. In winter, temperatures fall below freezing point throughout most of Canada. But the southwestern coast has a relatively mild climate. Along the Arctic Circle, mean temperatures are below freezing for seven months a year.

Western and southeastern Canada experience high rainfall, but the prairies are dry with 10 in to 20 in [250 mm to 500 mm] of rain every year.

POLITICS & ECONOMY Canada's first people, the ancestors of the Native Americans, or Indians, arrived in North America from Asia around 40,000 years ago. Later arrivals were the Inuit (Eskimos), who also came from Asia. Europeans reached the Canadian coast in 1497 and a race began between Britain and France for control of the territory.

France gained an initial advantage, and the French founded Québec in 1608. But the British later occupied eastern Canada. In 1867, Britain passed the British North America Act, which set up the Dominion of Canada, which was made up of Québec, Ontario, Nova Scotia, and New Brunswick. Other areas were added, the last being Newfoundland in 1949. Canada fought alongside Britain in both World Wars and many Canadians feel close ties with Britain. Canada is a constitutional monarchy, and the British monarch is Canada's head of state.

Rivalries between French- and English-speaking Canadians continue. In 1995, Québeckers voted against a move to make Québec a sovereign state. The majority was less than 1% and this issue seems unlikely to disappear. Another problem concerns the rights of the Aboriginal minorities, who would like to have more say in the running of their own affairs. To this end, in 1999, Canada created a new territory called Nunavut for the Inuit population in the north. Nunavut covers approximately 64% of what was formerly the eastern part of Northwest Territories.

Canada is a highly developed and prosperous country. Although farmland covers only 8% of the country, Canadian farms are highly productive. Canada is one of the world's leading producers of barley, wheat, meat, and milk. Forestry and fishing are other important industries. It is rich in natural resources, especially oil and natural gas, and is a major exporter of minerals. The country also produces copper, gold, iron ore, uranium, and zinc. Manufacturing is highly developed, especially in the cities where 79% of the people live. Canada has many factories that process farm and mineral products. It also produces cars, chemicals, electronic goods, machinery, paper, and timber products.

AREA 3,849,653 sq mi [9,970,610 sq km] **POPULATION** 32,207,000
CAPITAL (POPULATION) Ottawa (774,000)
GOVERNMENT Federal multiparty constitutional monarchy
ETHNIC GROUPS British origin 28%, French origin 23%, other European 15%, Amerindian/Inuit 2%, others
LANGUAGES English and French (both official)
RELIGIONS Roman Catholic 46%, Protestant 36%, Judaism, Islam, Hinduism **CURRENCY** Canadian dollar = 100 cents

CAPE VERDE

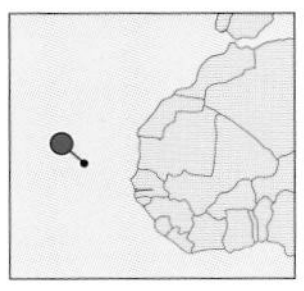

Cape Verde consists of ten large and five small islands, and is situated 350 mi [560 km] west of Dakar in Senegal. The islands have a tropical climate, with high temperatures all year round. Cape Verde became independent from Portugal in 1975 and is rated as a "low-income" developing country by the World Bank.

AREA 1,557 sq mi [4,033 sq km]
POPULATION 412,000 **CAPITAL** Praia

CAYMAN ISLANDS

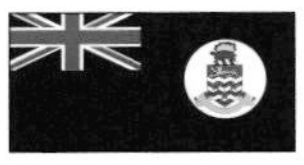
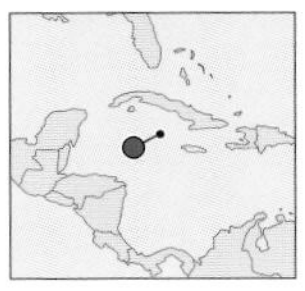

The Cayman Islands are an overseas territory of the UK, consisting of three low-lying islands. Financial services are the main economic activity and the islands offer a secret tax haven to many companies and banks.

AREA 102 sq mi [264 sq km]
POPULATION 42,000 **CAPITAL** George Town

CENTRAL AFRICAN REPUBLIC

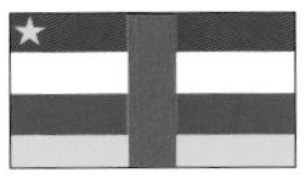
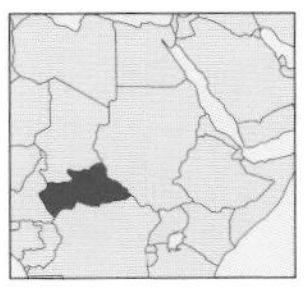

GEOGRAPHY The Central African Republic is a remote, landlocked country in the heart of Africa. It consists mostly of a plateau lying between 1,970 ft and 2,620 ft [600 m to 800 m] above sea level. The Ubangi drains the south, while the Chari (or Shari) River flows from the north to the Lake Chad basin. The climate is warm throughout the year, while the annual average rainfall in the capital Bangui totals 62 in [1,574 mm]. The north is drier, with an average annual rainfall of about 31 in [800 mm].

POLITICS & ECONOMY France set up an outpost at Bangui in 1899 and ruled the country as a colony from 1894. Known as Ubangi-Shari, the country was ruled by France as part of French Equatorial Africa until it gained independence in 1960.

Central African Republic became a one-party state in 1962, but army officers seized power in 1966. The head of the army, Jean-Bedel Bokassa, made himself emperor in 1976. The country was renamed the Central African Empire, but after a brutal reign, the tyrannical Bokassa was overthrown in a military coup in 1979. The country again became a republic.

The country adopted a new, multiparty constitution in 1991. Multiparty elections were held in 1993 and 1998. However, an army uprising began in 2002, culminating in the overthrow by a military coup of the elected President Patassé in 2003. He was succeeded by General François Bezize.

The World Bank classifies Central African Republic as a "low-income" developing country. Over 80% of the people are farmers, and most of them produce little more than they need to feed their families. The main crops are bananas, maize, manioc, millet, and yams. Coffee, cotton, timber, and tobacco are produced for export, mainly on commercial plantations. The country's development has been impeded by its remote position, its poor transport system and its untrained work force. The country depends heavily on aid, especially from France.

AREA 240,534 sq mi [622,984 sq km] **POPULATION** 3,684,000
CAPITAL (POPULATION) Bangui (553,000) **GOVERNMENT** Multiparty republic **ETHNIC GROUPS** Baya 33%, Banda 27%, Mandjia 13%, Sara 10%, Mboum 7%, Mbaka 4%, others **LANGUAGES** French (official), Sangho **RELIGIONS** Traditional beliefs 35%, Protestant 25%, Roman Catholic 25%, Islam 15% **CURRENCY** CFA franc = 100 centimes

CHAD

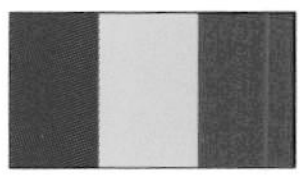

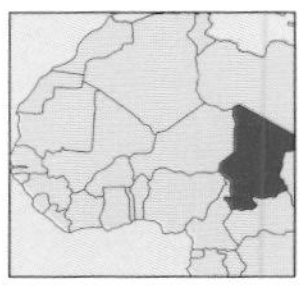

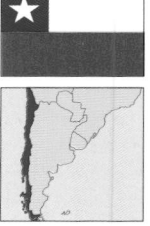

GEOGRAPHY The Republic of Chad is a landlocked country in north-central Africa. It is Africa's fifth largest country and is over twice the size of France, the country which once ruled it as a colony.

Ndjamena in central Chad has a hot, tropical climate, with a marked dry season from November to April. The south of the country is wetter, with an average yearly rainfall of around 39 in [1,000 mm]. The burning-hot desert in the north has an average yearly rainfall of less than 5 in [130 mm].

POLITICS & ECONOMY Chad straddles two worlds. The north is populated by Muslim Arab and Berber peoples, while black Africans, who follow traditional beliefs or who have converted to Christianity, live in the south. French explorers were active in the area in the late 19th century. France made Chad a colony in 1902.

Since becoming independent in 1960, Chad has been hit by ethnic conflict. The 1970s were marked by civil war and coups. Chad and Libya were in dispute over the northern Aozou Strip but, in 1994, the International Court of Justice ruled against Libya's claim over the area. A new constitution was adopted in 1997, but rebellions and conflict in several areas marred the country's progress.

Hit by drought and civil war, Chad is one of the world's poorest countries. Farming, fishing and livestock raising employ 83% of the people. Groundnuts, millet, rice and sorghum are major food crops in the south, but the chief export crop is cotton. Chad has few manufacturing industries, but its oil reserves hold out hope for development. The production of oil began in 2003.

AREA 495,752 sq mi [1,284,000 sq km] **POPULATION** 9,253,000 **CAPITAL (POPULATION)** Ndjamena (530,000) **GOVERNMENT** Multiparty republic **ETHNIC GROUPS** 200 distinct groups: mostly Muslim in the north and center; mostly Christian or animist in the south **LANGUAGES** French and Arabic (both official), many others **RELIGIONS** Islam 51%, Christianity 35%, animist 7% **CURRENCY** CFA franc = 100 centimes

CHILE

GEOGRAPHY The Republic of Chile stretches about 2,650 mi [4,260 km] from north to south, although the maximum east–west distance is only about 267 mi [430 km]. The high Andes Mountains form Chile's eastern borders with Argentina and Bolivia. To the west are basins and valleys, with coastal uplands overlooking the shore. Most people live in the central valley, where Santiago is situated.

Santiago has a Mediterranean climate, with hot, dry summers from November to March and mild, moist winters from April to October. The Atacama Desert in the north is one of the world's driest places, while southern Chile is cold and stormy.

POLITICS & ECONOMY Amerindian people reached the southern tip of South America 8,000 years ago. In 1520, Portuguese navigator Ferdinand Magellan was the first European to sight Chile. The country became a Spanish colony in the 1540s. Chile became independent in 1818. During a war (1879–83), it gained mineral-rich areas from Peru and Bolivia.

In 1970, Salvador Allende became the first Communist leader to be elected democratically. He was overthrown in 1973 by army officers, who were supported by the CIA. General Augusto Pinochet then ruled as a dictator. A new constitution was introduced in 1981 and elections were held in 1989. In 2000, a socialist, Ricardo Lagos, was elected president. Pinochet, who had been charged with presiding over acts of torture, was found to be too ill to stand trial in 2001.

The World Bank classifies Chile as a "lower-middle-income" developing country. Mining is important, especially copper production. Minerals dominate exports. The most valuable activity is manufacturing; products include processed foods, metals, iron and steel, transport equipment, and textiles. The chief crop is wheat, while beans, fruits, maize, and livestock products are also important. Chile's fishing industry is one of the world's largest.

AREA 292,133 sq mi [756,626 sq km] **POPULATION** 15,665,000 **CAPITAL (POPULATION)** Santiago (4,789,000) **GOVERNMENT** Multiparty republic **ETHNIC GROUPS** Mestizo 95%, Amerindian 3% **LANGUAGES** Spanish (official) **RELIGIONS** Roman Catholic 89%, Protestant 11% **CURRENCY** Chilean peso = 100 centavos

CHINA

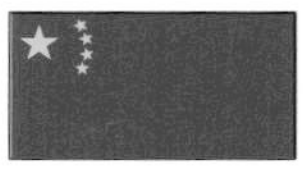

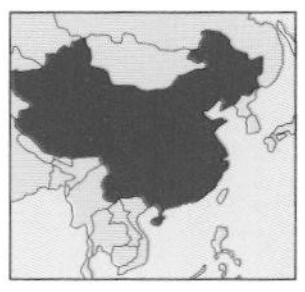

GEOGRAPHY The People's Republic of China is the world's third largest country. Most people live in the east – on the coastal plains or in the fertile valleys of the Huang He (Hwang Ho or Yellow River), the Chang Jiang (Yangtze Kiang), which is Asia's longest river at 3,960 mi [6,380 km], and the Xi Jiang (Si Kiang). Western China is thinly populated. It includes the bleak Tibetan plateau which is bounded by the Himalaya, the world's highest mountain range. Other ranges include the Kunlun Shan, the Altun Shan and the Tian Shan. Deserts include the Gobi Desert along the Mongolian border and the Taklimakan Desert in the far west.

Beijing has cold winters and warm summers with moderate rainfall. To the south, Shanghai has milder winters and more rain. The southeast has a wet, subtropical climate, but the west has a severe climate. Lhasa has very cold winters and a low rainfall.

POLITICS & ECONOMY China is one of the world's oldest civilizations, going back 3,500 years. Under the Han dynasty (202 BC to AD 220), the Chinese empire was as large as the Roman empire. Mongols conquered China in the 13th century, but Chinese rule was restored in 1368. The Manchu people of Mongolia ruled the country from 1644 to 1912, when the country became a republic.

War with Japan (1937–45) was followed by civil war between the nationalists and the Communists. The Communists triumphed in 1949, setting up the People's Republic of China. In the 1980s, following the death of the revolutionary leader Mao Zedong (Mao Tse-tung) in 1976, China encouraged formerly forbidden policies, namely private enterprise and foreign investment. But the Communist leaders have not permitted political freedom. Opponents are still harshly treated, while attempts to negotiate some degree of autonomy for Tibet have been rejected.

China's economy has expanded greatly since the 1970s, with many Communist policies being abandoned. Foreign investors have help to set up many new industries in the east. Between 1989 and 2002, the economy grew by an average of 9.3% per year. With its cheap labor, trained managers and engineers, China has overtaken Japan to become the fourth largest exporter to the United States. It has benefited from the return of Hong Kong in 1997 and its admission to the World Trade Organization (WTO) in 2001. China would also like to regain the prosperous island of Taiwan, also a member of the WTO, but this seems unlikely in the near future. In 2004, the government announced plans to slow down economic growth by diverting resources to the rural poor, who had become relatively disadvantaged by the economic boom.

Despite its recent success, China remains a poor country. In the late 1990s, agriculture still employed nearly half of the people, although only 10% of the land is farmed. Products include rice, sweet potatoes, tea and wheat, and many fruits and vegetables. Livestock farming, especially pig rearing, is important. Resources include coal, iron ore, and other metals. Manufactures include cement, chemicals, fertilizers, machinery, telecommunications and recording equipment, and textiles. China is now a major producer of consumer goods, including air-conditioners, cameras, hard-disk drives and computer monitors, refrigerators, television sets, and washing machines.

AREA 3,705,387 sq mi [9,596,961 sq km] **POPULATION** 1,286,975,000 **CAPITAL (POPULATION)** Beijing (7,362,000) **GOVERNMENT** Single-party Communist republic **ETHNIC GROUPS** Han Chinese 92%, many others **LANGUAGES** Mandarin Chinese (official) **RELIGIONS** Atheist (official) **CURRENCY** Renminbi yuan = 10 jiao = 100 fen

COLOMBIA

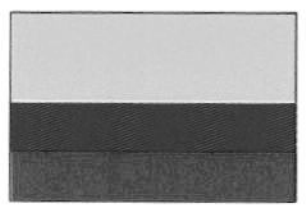

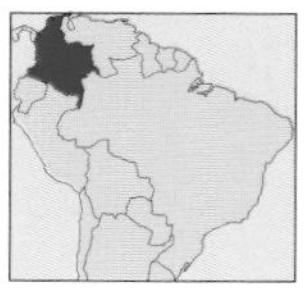

GEOGRAPHY The Republic of Colombia, in northeastern South America, is the only country in the continent to have coastlines on both the Pacific and the Caribbean Sea. Colombia also contains the northernmost ranges of the Andes Mountains.

There is a tropical climate in the lowlands, but the altitude greatly affects the climate of the Andes. The capital, Bogotá, which stands on a plateau in the eastern Andes at about 9,200 ft [2,800 m] above sea level, has mild temperatures throughout the year. The rainfall is heavy, especially on the Pacific coast.

POLITICS & ECONOMY Amerindian people have lived in Colombia for thousands of years. But today, only a small proportion of the people are of unmixed Amerindian ancestry. Mestizos (people of mixed white and Amerindian ancestry) form the largest group, followed by whites and mulattos (people of mixed European and African ancestry).

Spaniards opened up the area in the early 16th century. They set up a territory known as the Vice-royalty of the New Kingdom of Granada, including Colombia, Ecuador, Panama, and Venezuela. In 1819, the area became independent, but Ecuador and Venezuela soon split away, followed by Panama in 1903. Instability has marked its recent history. Political rivalries led to civil wars in 1899–1902 and 1949–57, when a coalition government was formed. The coalition ended in 1986 when the Liberal Party was elected. Colombia faces economic and security problems, notably combating left-wing guerrillas and right-wing paramilitaries, while controlling a large illicit drug industry. In the early 2000s, the US provided aid to help Colombia fight drug-trafficking. Colombia exports oil, coffee, and chemicals.

AREA 439,735 sq mi [1,138,914 sq km] **POPULATION** 41,662,000 **CAPITAL (POPULATION)** Bogotá (6,545,000) **GOVERNMENT** Multiparty republic **ETHNIC GROUPS** Mestizo 58%, White 20%, Mulatto 14%, Black 4% **LANGUAGES** Spanish (official) **RELIGIONS** Roman Catholic 90% **CURRENCY** Colombian peso = 100 centavos

COMOROS

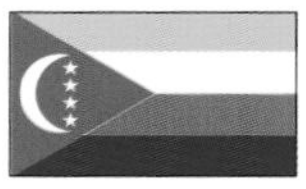

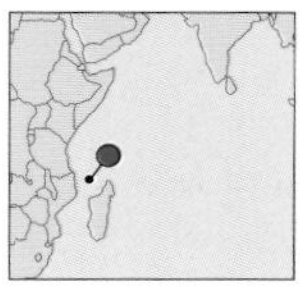

The Federal Islamic Republic of the Comoros consists of three large islands and some smaller ones, lying at the north end of the Mozambique Channel in the Indian Ocean. The country became independent from France in 1974, but the people on a fourth island, Mayotte, voted to remain French. In 1997, secessionists on the island of Anjouan, who favored a return to French rule, defeated forces from Grand Comore and, in 1998, they voted overwhelmingly to break away from the Comoros. Most people are subsistence farmers, although cash crops such as coconuts, coffee, cocoa, and spices are also produced. The main exports are cloves, perfume oils, and vanilla.

AREA 863 sq mi [2,235 sq km] **POPULATION** 633,000 **CAPITAL** Moroni

CONGO

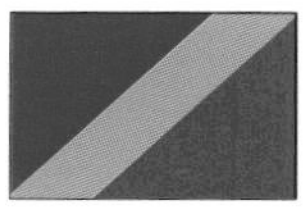

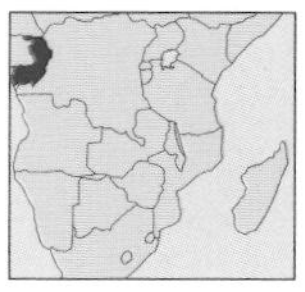

GEOGRAPHY The Republic of Congo is a country on the River Congo in west-central Africa. The Equator runs through the center of the country. Congo has a narrow coastal plain on which its main port, Pointe Noire, stands. Behind the plain are uplands through which the River Niari has carved a fertile valley. Central Congo consists of high plains. The north contains large swampy areas in the valleys of the tributaries of the River Congo.

Congo has a hot, wet equatorial climate. Brazzaville has a dry season between June and September. The coast is drier and cooler than the rest of Congo, because of the cold offshore Benguela ocean current.

POLITICS & ECONOMY Part of the huge Kongo kingdom between the 15th and 18th centuries, the coast of the Congo later became a center of the European slave trade. The area came under French protection in 1880. It was later governed as part of a larger region called French Equatorial Africa. The country remained under French control until 1960.

Congo became a one-party state in 1964 and a military group took over the government in 1968. In 1970, Congo declared itself a Communist country, though it continued to seek aid from Western countries. The government officially abandoned its Communist policies in 1990. Multiparty elections were held in 1992, but the elected president, Pascal Lissouba, was overthrown in 1997 by former president Denis Sassou-Nguesso. Civil war again occurred in January 1999, but peace was restored. In 2002, Sassou-Nguesso was elected president.

The World Bank classifies Congo as a "lower-middle-income" developing country. Agriculture is the most important activity, employing more than 60% of the people. But many farmers produce little more than they need to feed their families. Major food crops include bananas, cassava, maize, and rice, while the leading cash crops are coffee and cocoa. Congo's main exports are oil (which makes up 90% of the total) and timber. Manufacturing is relatively unimportant at the moment, still hampered by poor transport links, but it is gradually being developed.

AREA 132,046 sq mi [342,000 sq km] **POPULATION** 2,954,000 **CAPITAL (POPULATION)** Brazzaville (938,000) **GOVERNMENT** Military regime **ETHNIC GROUPS** Kongo 48%, Sangha 20%, Teke 17%, M'bochi 12% **LANGUAGES** French (official), many others **RELIGIONS** Christianity 50%, animist 48%, Islam 2% **CURRENCY** CFA franc = 100 centimes

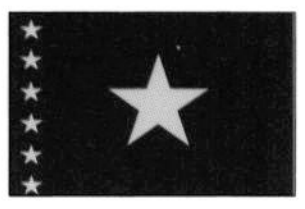

CONGO (DEM. REP. OF THE)

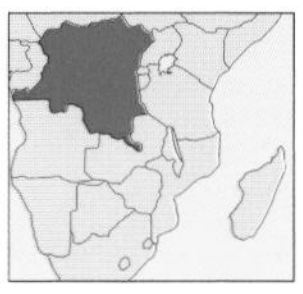

GEOGRAPHY The Democratic Republic of the Congo, formerly known as Zaïre, is the world's 12th largest country. Much of the country lies within the drainage basin of the huge River Congo. The river reaches the sea along the country's coastline, which is 25 mi [40 km] long. Mountains rise in the east, where the country's borders run through lakes Tanganyika, Kivu, Edward, and Albert. The equatorial region has high temperatures and heavy rainfall throughout the year.

POLITICS & ECONOMY Pygmies were the first inhabitants of the region, with Portuguese navigators not reaching the coast until 1482, but the interior was not explored until the late 19th century. In 1885, the country, called Congo Free State, became the personal property of King Léopold II of Belgium. In 1908, the country became a Belgian colony.

The Belgian Congo became independent in 1960 and was renamed Zaïre in 1971. Ethnic rivalries caused instability until 1965, when the country became a one-party state, ruled by President Mobutu. The government allowed the formation of political parties in 1990, but elections were repeatedly postponed. In 1996, fighting broke out in eastern Zaïre, as the Tutsi–Hutu conflict in Burundi and Rwanda spilled over. The rebel leader Laurent Kabila took power in 1997, ousting Mobutu and renaming the country. A rebellion against Kabila broke out in 1998. Rwanda and Uganda supported the rebels, while Angola, Chad, Namibia and Zimbabwe assisted Kabila. A peace treaty was signed in 1999, but fighting continued. Kabila was assassinated in 2001. His son, Major-General Joseph Kabila, who became president, worked to end a war which, by early 2003, had claimed over 2 million lives. But unrest continued and a failed coup occurred in March 2004.

The World Bank classifies the Democratic Republic of the Congo as a "low-income" developing country, despite its reserves of copper, the main export, and other minerals. Agriculture, mainly at subsistence level, employs 63% of the people.

AREA 905,350 SQ MI [2,344,858 SQ KM] **POPULATION** 56,625,000
CAPITAL (POPULATION) KINSHASA (4,665,000)
GOVERNMENT SINGLE-PARTY REPUBLIC
ETHNIC GROUPS OVER 200; THE LARGEST ARE MONGO, LUBA, KONGO, MANGBETU-AZANDE
LANGUAGES FRENCH (OFFICIAL), TRIBAL LANGUAGES
RELIGIONS ROMAN CATHOLIC 50%, PROTESTANT 20%, ISLAM 10%, OTHERS
CURRENCY CONGOLESE FRANC = 100 CENTIMES

COSTA RICA

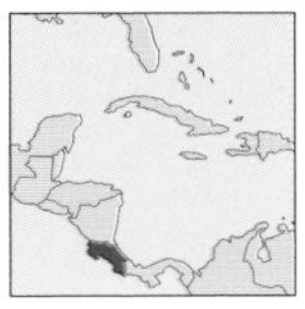

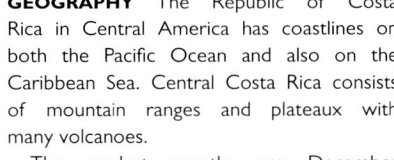

GEOGRAPHY The Republic of Costa Rica in Central America has coastlines on both the Pacific Ocean and also on the Caribbean Sea. Central Costa Rica consists of mountain ranges and plateaux with many volcanoes.

The coolest months are December and January. The northeast trade winds bring heavy rain to the Caribbean coast. There is less rainfall in the highlands and on the Pacific coastlands.

POLITICS & ECONOMY Christopher Columbus reached the Caribbean coast in 1502 and rumors of treasure soon attracted many Spaniards to settle in the country. Spain ruled the country until 1821, when Spain's Central American colonies broke away to join Mexico in 1822. In 1823, the Central American states broke with Mexico and set up the Central American Federation. Later, this large union broke up and Costa Rica became fully independent in 1838.

From the late 19th century, Costa Rica experienced a number of revolutions, with periods of dictatorship and periods of democracy. In 1948, following a revolt, the armed forces were abolished. Since 1948, Costa Rica has enjoyed a long period of stable democracy, which many in Latin America admire and envy.

Costa Rica is classified by the World Bank as a "lower-middle-income" developing country and one of the most prosperous countries in Central America. There are high educational standards and a high average life expectancy (about 74 years for men and 79 years for women). Agriculture employs 19% of the people. Costa Rica's natural resources include its forests, but it lacks minerals apart from some bauxite and manganese. Manufacturing is increasing. The United States is Costa Rica's main trading partner. Tourism is a fast-growing industry.

AREA 19,730 SQ MI [51,100 SQ KM] **POPULATION** 3,896,000 **CAPITAL (POPULATION)** SAN JOSÉ (337,000) **GOVERNMENT** MULTIPARTY REPUBLIC **ETHNIC GROUPS** WHITE (INCLUDING MESTIZO) 94%, BLACK 3%, AMERINDIAN 1%, CHINESE 1%, OTHERS **LANGUAGES** SPANISH (OFFICIAL), ENGLISH **RELIGIONS** ROMAN CATHOLIC 76%, EVANGELICAL 14% **CURRENCY** COSTA RICAN COLÓN = 100 CÉNTIMOS

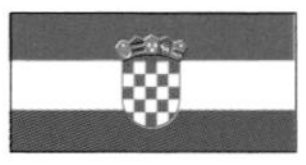

CROATIA

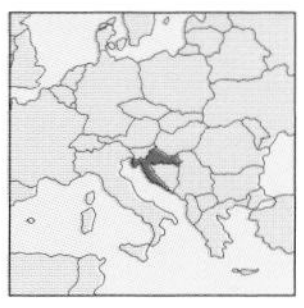

GEOGRAPHY The Republic of Croatia was one of the six republics that made up the former Communist country of Yugoslavia until it became independent in 1991. The region bordering the Adriatic Sea is called Dalmatia. It includes the coastal ranges, which contain large areas of bare limestone. Most of the rest of the country consists of the fertile Pannonian plains.

The coastal area has a typical Mediterranean climate, with hot, dry summers and mild, moist winters. Inland, the climate becomes more continental. Winters are cold, while temperatures often soar to 100°F [38°C] in the summer months.

POLITICS & ECONOMY Slav people settled in the area around 1,400 years ago. In 803, Croatia became part of the Holy Roman empire and the Croats soon adopted Christianity. Croatia was an independent kingdom in the 10th and 11th centuries. In 1102, the king of Hungary also became king of Croatia, creating a union that lasted 800 years. In 1526, part of Croatia came under the Turkish Ottoman empire, while the rest came under the Austrian Habsburgs.

After Austria–Hungary was defeated in World War I (1914–18), Croatia became part of the new Kingdom of the Serbs, Croats, and Slovenes. This kingdom was renamed Yugoslavia in 1929. Germany occupied Yugoslavia during World War II (1939–45). Croatia was proclaimed independent, but it was really ruled by the invaders.

After the war, Communists took power with Josip Broz Tito as the country's leader. Despite ethnic differences between the people, Tito held Yugoslavia together until his death in 1980. In the 1980s, economic and ethnic problems, including a deterioration in relations with Serbia, threatened stability. In the 1990s, Yugoslavia split into five nations, one of which was Croatia, which declared itself independent in 1991.

After Serbia supplied arms to Serbs living in Croatia, war broke out between the two republics, causing great damage. Croatia lost more than 30% of its territory. But in 1992, the United Nations sent a peacekeeping force to Croatia, which effectively ended the war with Serbia.

In 1992, when war broke out in Bosnia-Herzegovina, Bosnian Croats occupied parts of the country. But in 1994, Croatia helped to end Croat–Muslim conflict in Bosnia-Herzegovina and, in 1995, after retaking some areas occupied by Serbs, it helped to draw up the Dayton Peace Accord, ending the civil war. The wars in the early 1990s disrupted the economy. But in the early 21st century, stability, which is so vital to the valuable tourist industry, seemed to be returning, although early accession to European Union membership was ruled out in 2003. Manufactures are Croatia's main exports.

AREA 21,829 SQ MI [56,538 SQ KM] **POPULATION** 4,422,000 **CAPITAL (POPULATION)** ZAGREB (779,000) **GOVERNMENT** MULTIPARTY REPUBLIC **ETHNIC GROUPS** CROAT 90%, SERB 5%, OTHERS **LANGUAGES** CROATIAN 96% **RELIGIONS** ROMAN CATHOLIC 88%, ORTHODOX 4%, ISLAM 1%, OTHERS **CURRENCY** KUNA = 100 LIPAS

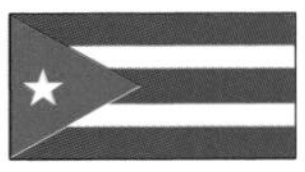

CUBA

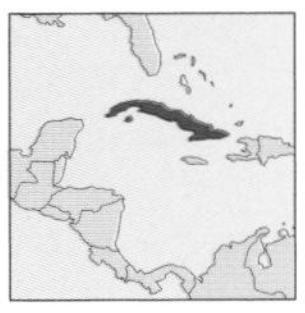

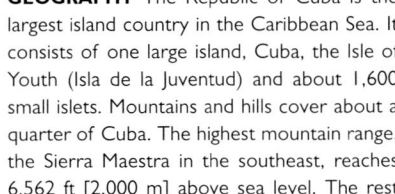

GEOGRAPHY The Republic of Cuba is the largest island country in the Caribbean Sea. It consists of one large island, Cuba, the Isle of Youth (Isla de la Juventud) and about 1,600 small islets. Mountains and hills cover about a quarter of Cuba. The highest mountain range, the Sierra Maestra in the southeast, reaches 6,562 ft [2,000 m] above sea level. The rest of the land consists of gently rolling country or coastal plains, crossed by fertile valleys carved by the short, mostly shallow and narrow rivers.

Cuba lies in the tropics. But sea breezes moderate the temperature, warming the land in winter and cooling it in summer.

POLITICS & ECONOMY Christopher Columbus discovered the island in 1492 and Spaniards began to settle there from 1511. Spanish rule ended in 1898, when the United States defeated Spain in the Spanish–American War. American influence in Cuba remained strong until 1959, when revolutionary forces under Fidel Castro overthrew the dictatorial government of Fulgencio Batista.

The United States opposed Castro's policies, when he turned to the Soviet Union for assistance. In 1961, Cuban exiles attempting an invasion were defeated. In 1962, the US learned that nuclear missile bases armed by the Soviet Union had been established in Cuba. The US ordered the Soviet Union to remove the missiles and bases and, after a few days, when many people feared that a world war might break out, the Soviet Union agreed to the American demands.

Cuba's relations with the Soviet Union remained strong until 1991, when the Soviet Union was broken up. The loss of Soviet aid greatly damaged Cuba's economy, but Castro maintained his left-wing policies. In 2000, the United States lifted its food embargo on Cuba, but Cuba again came under fire in 2003 following the arrests of 78 opponents of the regime.

The government runs Cuba's economy and owns 70% of the farmland. Agriculture is important and sugar is the chief export, followed by refined nickel ore. Other exports include cigars, citrus fruits, fish, medical products and rum.

Before 1959, US companies owned most of Cuba's manufacturing industries. But under Fidel Castro, they became government property. After the collapse of Communist governments in the Soviet Union and its allies, Cuba worked to increase its trade with Latin America and China.

AREA 42,803 SQ MI [110,861 SQ KM] **POPULATION** 11,263,000
CAPITAL (POPULATION) HAVANA (2,192,000)
GOVERNMENT SOCIALIST REPUBLIC
ETHNIC GROUPS MULATTO 51%, WHITE 37%, BLACK 11%
LANGUAGES SPANISH (OFFICIAL) **RELIGIONS** CHRISTIANITY
CURRENCY CUBAN PESO = 100 CENTAVOS

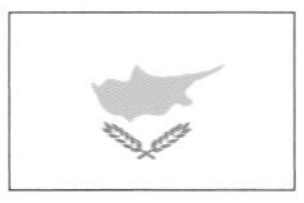

CYPRUS

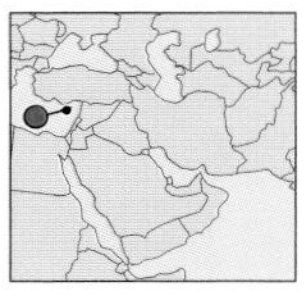

GEOGRAPHY The Republic of Cyprus is an island nation in the northeastern Mediterranean Sea. Geographers regard it as part of Asia, but it resembles southern Europe in many ways. Its scenic mountain ranges include the southern Troodos Mountains, which reach 6,401 ft [1,951 m] at Mount Olympus, and the Kyrenia range in the north. Between them lies the Mesaoria plain. The climate is Mediterranean, with typically hot, dry summers and mild, moist winters. But the island's proximity to southwestern Asia gives it a hotter climate than places in the western Mediterranean.

POLITICS & ECONOMY Greeks settled on Cyprus around 3,200 years ago. From AD 330, the island was part of the Byzantine empire. In the 1570s, Cyprus became part of the Turkish Ottoman empire. Turkish rule continued until 1878 when Cyprus was leased to Britain. Britain annexed the island in 1914 and proclaimed it a colony in 1925.

In the 1950s, Greek Cypriots, who made up four-fifths of the population, began a campaign for *enosis* (union) with Greece. Their leader was the Greek Orthodox Archbishop Makarios. A secret guerrilla force called EOKA attacked the British, who exiled Makarios. Cyprus became an independent country in 1960, although Britain retained two military bases. Independent Cyprus had a constitution which provided for power-sharing between the Greek and Turkish Cypriots. But the constitution proved unworkable and fighting broke out between the two communities. In 1964, the United Nations sent in a peacekeeping force, but communal clashes recurred in 1967.

In 1974, Cypriot forces led by Greek officers overthrew Makarios. This led Turkey to invade northern Cyprus, a territory occupying about 40% of the island. Many Greek Cypriots fled from the north, which, in 1979, was proclaimed the Turkish Republic of Northern Cyprus. The only country to recognize this state was Turkey. The United Nations regarded Cyprus as a single unit under the Greek-Cypriot government in the south. In 2002, the European Union invited Cyprus to become a member in 2004. In April 2004, the people voted on a UN plan to reunify the island. The Turkish-Cypriots voted in favor, but the Greek-Cypriots voted against. Hence, only the south was admitted to EU membership on May 1, 2004.

Cyprus got its name from the Greek word *kypros*, meaning copper. But little copper remains and the chief minerals today are asbestos and chromium. However, the most valuable activity in Cyprus is tourism. Manufactures include cement, clothes, footwear, tiles and wine.

In the early 1990s. the United Nations reclassified Cyprus as a developed rather than a developing country, reflecting the rapid economic progress in the south. But the north lagged far behind the prosperous Greek-Cypriot south.

AREA 3,572 sq mi [9,251 sq km] **POPULATION** 772,000
CAPITAL (POPULATION) Nicosia (198,000)
GOVERNMENT Multiparty republic **ETHNIC GROUPS** Greek Cypriot 77%, Turkish Cypriot 18%, others **LANGUAGES** Greek and Turkish (both official), English **RELIGIONS** Greek Orthodox 78%, Islam 18%
CURRENCY Cypriot pound = 100 cents

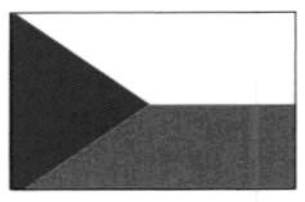

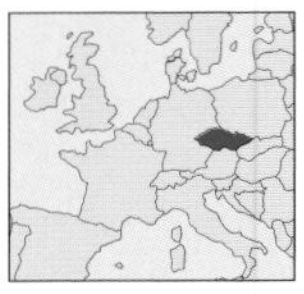

CZECH REPUBLIC

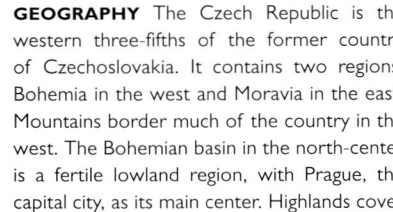

GEOGRAPHY The Czech Republic is the western three-fifths of the former country of Czechoslovakia. It contains two regions: Bohemia in the west and Moravia in the east. Mountains border much of the country in the west. The Bohemian basin in the north-center is a fertile lowland region, with Prague, the capital city, as its main center. Highlands cover much of the center of the country, with lowlands in the southeast.

The climate is influenced by its landlocked position in east-central Europe. Prague has warm, sunny summers and cold winters. The average rainfall is moderate, with 20 in to 30 in [500 mm to 750 mm] every year in lowland areas.

POLITICS & ECONOMY After World War I (1914–18), Czechoslovakia was created. Germany seized the country in World War II (1939–45). In 1948, Communist leaders took power and Czechoslovakia was allied to the Soviet Union. When democratic reforms were introduced in the Soviet Union in the late 1980s, the Czechs also demanded reforms. Free elections were held in 1990, but differences between the Czechs and Slovaks led to the partitioning of the country on January 1, 1993. The Czech Republic became a member of NATO in 1999. In 2003, 77% of Czechs voted in favor of their country becoming a member of the European Union. This took place on May 1, 2004.

Under Communist rule the Czech Republic became one of the most industrialized parts of Eastern Europe. The country has deposits of coal, uranium, iron ore, magnesite, tin, and zinc. Manufacturing employs about 29% of the Czech Republic's entire work force. Farming is also important. Under Communism, the government owned the land, but private ownership is now being restored. The country was admitted into the OECD in 1995.

AREA 30,450 sq mi [78,866 sq km] **POPULATION** 10,249,000
CAPITAL (POPULATION) Prague (1,193,000)
GOVERNMENT Multiparty republic **ETHNIC GROUPS** Czech 81%, Moravian 13%, Slovak 3%, Polish, German, Silesian, Gypsy, Hungarian, Ukrainian **LANGUAGES** Czech (official) **RELIGIONS** Atheist 40%, Roman Catholic 39%, Protestant 4%, Orthodox 3%, others
CURRENCY Czech koruna = 100 haler

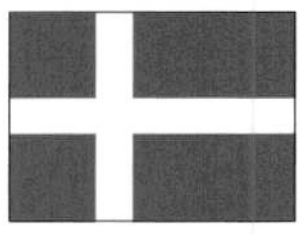

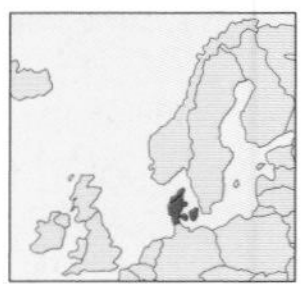

DENMARK

GEOGRAPHY The Kingdom of Denmark is the smallest country in Scandinavia. It consists of a peninsula, called Jutland (or Jylland), which is joined to Germany, and more than 400 islands, 89 of which are inhabited. The land is flat and mostly covered by rocks dropped there by huge ice sheets during the last Ice Age. The highest point in Denmark is on Jutland. It is only 568 ft [173 m] above sea level. Denmark has a mild, moist climate, except during cold spells in winter when The Sound between Sjælland and Sweden may freeze over.

POLITICS & ECONOMY Danish Vikings terrorized much of Western Europe for about 300 years after AD 800. In the late 14th century, Denmark formed a union with Norway and Sweden (which included Finland). Sweden broke away in 1523, while Denmark lost Norway to Sweden in 1814. After 1945, Denmark became a member of the North Atlantic Treaty Organization. It joined the European Union in 1973, though it did not adopt the euro in 2000. The Danes enjoy a high standard of living, but the country's welfare programs are extremely costly.

Denmark has some oil and gas and the economy is highly developed. Manufacturing employs about 16% of the people. Products include furniture, processed food, machinery, television sets, and textiles. Farms cover about three-quarters of the land. Farming employs only 3% of the people, but it is highly scientific. Meat and dairy farming are the chief activities.

AREA 16,639 sq mi [43,094 sq km] **POPULATION** 5,384,000
CAPITAL (POPULATION) Copenhagen (499,000) **GOVERNMENT** Parliamentary monarchy **ETHNIC GROUPS** Scandinavian, Inuit, Færoese **LANGUAGES** Danish (official), English, Færoese **RELIGIONS** Evangelical Lutheran 95% **CURRENCY** Danish krone = 100 øre

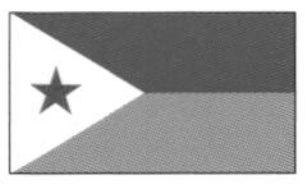

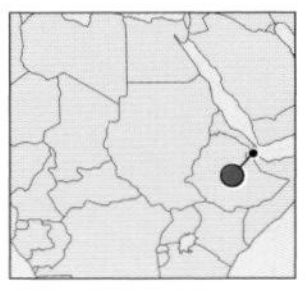

DJIBOUTI

GEOGRAPHY The Republic of Djibouti in eastern Africa occupies a strategic position where the Red Sea meets the Gulf of Aden. Djibouti has one of the world's hottest and driest climates.

POLITICS & ECONOMY France set up a territory called French Somaliland in 1888. Its capital, Djibouti, became important when a railroad was built to Addis Ababa and Djibouti became the main outlet for Ethiopian trade. In 1967, France renamed the dependency the French Territory of the Afars and Issas, but it was renamed Djibouti on independence in 1977. It became a one-party state in 1981, but a new constitution (1992) permitted four parties which had to maintain a balance between the country's ethnic groups. Conflict between the Afars and Issas flared up in 1992 and 1993, but a peace agreement was signed in 1994.

Djibouti is a poor country. Its economy is based largely on the revenue it gets from its port and the railroad to Addis Ababa.

AREA 8,958 sq mi [23,200 sq km] **POPULATION** 457,000
CAPITAL (POPULATION) Djibouti (317,000) **GOVERNMENT** Multiparty republic **ETHNIC GROUPS** Somali 60%, Afar 35% **LANGUAGES** Arabic and French (both official) **RELIGIONS** Islam 94%, Christianity 6%
CURRENCY Djiboutian franc = 100 centimes

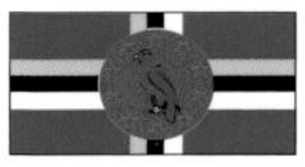

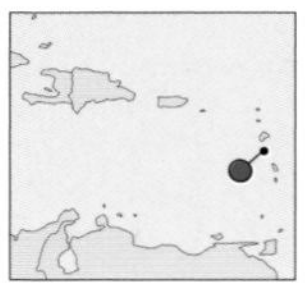

DOMINICA

The Commonwealth of Dominica, a former British colony, became independent in 1978. The island has a mountainous spine and less than 10% of the land is cultivated. But agriculture employs 18% of the people. The manufacture of coconut-based soap is important, while tourism and mining are other economic activities.

AREA 290 sq mi [751 sq km] **POPULATION** 70,000 **CAPITAL** Roseau

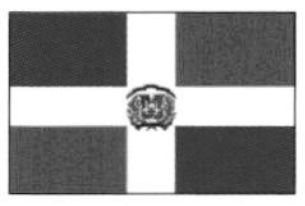

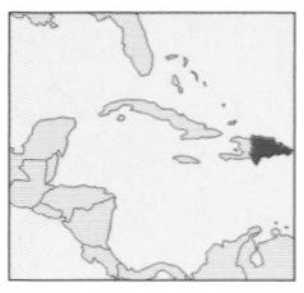

DOMINICAN REPUBLIC

GEOGRAPHY Second largest of the Caribbean nations in both area and population, the Dominican Republic shares the island of Hispaniola with Haiti, with the Dominican Republic occupying the eastern two-thirds. The country is mountainous, and the generally hot and humid climate eases with altitude.

POLITICS & ECONOMY In 1492, Christopher Columbus landed on Hispaniola and Spaniards soon settled the island, followed by the French who occupied the western third of the island (which is now Haiti). The island was held by Haitians from 1822 until 1844, when the Dominican Republic was established. Civil war broke out in 1966 but US intervention ended the conflict. Since 1966, the young democracy has survived violent elections under the watchful eye of the United States.

The Dominican Republic is a developing country and agriculture is the chief activity. Sugarcane, rice, bananas, and cocoa are leading crops. Food processing is also important and some ferronickel is produced.

AREA 18,730 sq mi [48,511 sq km] **POPULATION** 8,716,000
CAPITAL (POPULATION) Santo Domingo (2,061,000)
GOVERNMENT Multiparty republic **ETHNIC GROUPS** Mulatto 73%, White 16%, Black 11% **LANGUAGES** Spanish (official) **RELIGIONS** Roman Catholic 95% **CURRENCY** Dominican peso = 100 centavos

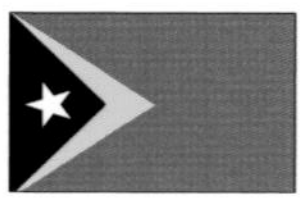

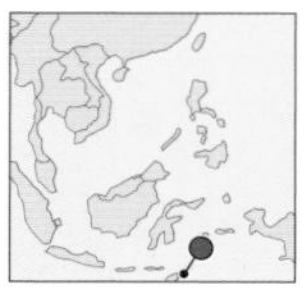

EAST TIMOR

The Republic of East Timor became fully independent and the world's newest country on May 20, 2002. The land is mainly rugged. Temperatures are generally high and the rainfall is moderate. Portugal ruled the area from the late 19th century, when it was called Portuguese Timor. Portugal withdrew in 1975 and Indonesia seized the area. Guerrilla activity mounted under Indonesian rule and, in 1999, the people voted for independence. Agriculture is the main activity. East Timor is heavily dependent on foreign aid. Offshore oil and natural gas deposits hold out hope for the future, though the ownership of some of the oilfields is disputed with Australia.

AREA 5,743 sq mi [14,874 sq km] **POPULATION** 998,000 **CAPITAL** Dili

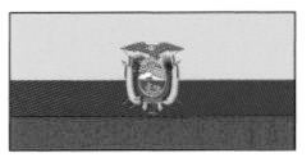

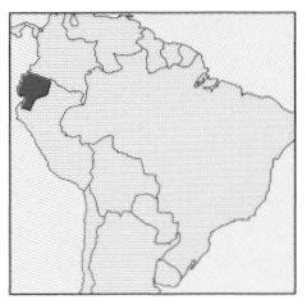

ECUADOR

GEOGRAPHY The Republic of Ecuador straddles the Equator on the west coast of South America. Three ranges of the high Andes Mountains form the backbone of the country. Between the towering, snow-capped peaks of the mountains, some of which are volcanoes, lie a series of high plateaux, or basins. Nearly half of Ecuador's population lives on these plateaux.

The climate in Ecuador depends on the height above sea level. Though the coastline is cooled by the cold Peruvian Current, temperatures are between 73°F and 77°F [23°C to 25°C] all through the year. In Quito, at 8,200 ft [2,500 m] above sea level, temperatures are 57°F to 59°F [14°C to 15°C], though the city is just south of the Equator.

POLITICS & ECONOMY The Inca people of Peru conquered much of what is now Ecuador in the late 15th century. They introduced their language, Quechua, which is widely spoken today. Spanish forces defeated the Incas in 1533 and took control of Ecuador. The country became independent in 1822, following the defeat of a Spanish force in a battle near Quito.

In the 19th and 20th centuries, Ecuador suffered from political instability, while successive governments failed to tackle the country's social and economic problems. A war with Peru in 1941 led to a loss of territory. Disputes continued until 1995, but a border agreement was signed in January 1998. Economic crises in the early 21st century led the government to abolish the sucre, its official currency, and replace it with the US dollar.

The World Bank classifies Ecuador as a "lower-middle-income" developing country. Agriculture employs 30% of the people and bananas, cocoa, and coffee are all important crops. Fishing, forestry, mining, and manufacturing are other activities.

AREA 109,483 sq mi [283,561 sq km] **POPULATION** 13,710,000
CAPITAL (POPULATION) Quito (1,648,000)
GOVERNMENT Multiparty republic
ETHNIC GROUPS Mestizo (mixed White/Amerindian) 65%, Amerindian 25%, White 7%, Black 3%
LANGUAGES Spanish (official), Quechua
RELIGIONS Roman Catholic 95%
CURRENCY US dollar = 100 cents

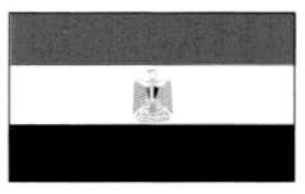

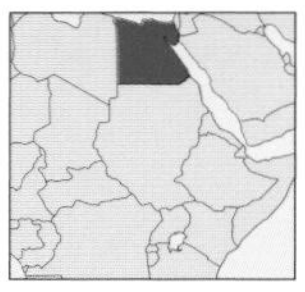

EGYPT

GEOGRAPHY The Arab Republic of Egypt is Africa's second largest country by population after Nigeria, though it ranks 13th in area. Most of Egypt is desert. Almost all the people live either in the Nile Valley and its fertile delta or along the Suez Canal, the artificial waterway between the Mediterranean and Red seas. This canal shortens the sea journey between the United Kingdom and India by 6,027 mi [9,700 km]. Recent attempts have been made to irrigate parts of the western desert and thus redistribute the rapidly growing Egyptian population into previously uninhabited regions.

Apart from the Nile Valley, Egypt has three other main regions. The Western and Eastern deserts are parts of the Sahara. The Sinai peninsula (Es Sina), to the east of the Suez Canal, is a mountainous desert region, geographically within Asia. It contains Egypt's highest peak, Gebel Katherina (8,650 ft [2,637 m]); few people live in this area.

Egypt is a dry country. The low rainfall occurs, if at all, in winter and the country is one of the sunniest places on Earth.

POLITICS & ECONOMY Ancient Egypt, which was founded about 5,000 years ago, was one of the great early civilizations. Throughout the country, pyramids, temples and richly decorated tombs are memorials to its great achievements.

After Ancient Egypt declined, the country came under successive foreign rulers. Arabs occupied Egypt in AD 639–42. They introduced the Arabic language and Islam. Their influence was so great that most Egyptians now regard themselves as Arabs.

Egypt came under British rule in 1882, but it gained partial independence in 1922, becoming a monarchy. The monarchy was abolished in 1952, when Egypt became a republic. The creation of Israel in 1948 led Egypt into a series of wars in 1948–9, 1956, 1967, and 1973. Since the late 1970s, Egypt has sought for peace. In 1979, Egypt signed a peace treaty with Israel and regained the Sinai region which it had lost in a war in 1967. Extremists opposed contacts with Israel and, in 1981, President Sadat, who had signed the treaty, was assassinated.

While Egypt plays a major part in Arab affairs, most of its people are poor. Some Islamic fundamentalists, who dislike Western influences on their way of life, have resorted to violence. In the

1990s, attacks on foreign visitors caused a decline in the valuable tourist industry, as also did the events of September 11, 2001, and the subsequent "war against terrorism." In 1999, Hosni Mubarak, president since 1981, was himself attacked by extremists, but he was re-elected to a fourth term in office.

Egypt is Africa's second most industrialized country after South Africa, but most people are poor. Oil and textiles are the main exports.

AREA 386,659 sq mi [1,001,449 sq km] **POPULATION** 74,719,000
CAPITAL (POPULATION) Cairo (6,801,000)
GOVERNMENT Republic
ETHNIC GROUPS Egyptians/Bedouins/Berbers 99%
LANGUAGES Arabic (official), French, English
RELIGIONS Islam (mainly Sunni Muslim) 94%, Christianity (mainly Coptic Christian) and others 6%
CURRENCY Egyptian pound = 100 piastres

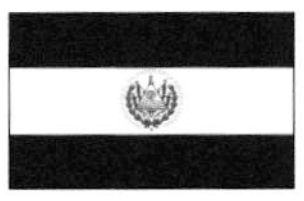

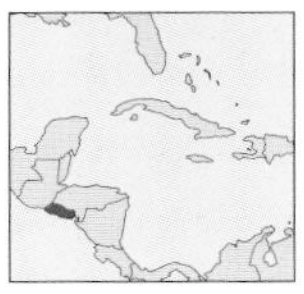

EL SALVADOR

GEOGRAPHY The Republic of El Salvador is the only country in Central America which does not have a coast on the Caribbean Sea. El Salvador has a narrow coastal plain along the Pacific Ocean. Behind the coastal plain, the coastal range is a zone of rugged mountains, including volcanoes, which overlooks a densely populated inland plateau. Beyond the plateau, the land rises to the sparsely populated interior highlands. The coast has a hot, tropical climate. Inland the climate is moderated by the altitude. Rain falls on practically every afternoon between May and October.

POLITICS & ECONOMY Amerindians have lived in El Salvador for thousands of years. The ruins of Mayan pyramids built between AD 100 and 1000 are still found in the western part of the country. Spanish soldiers conquered the area in 1524 and 1525, and Spain ruled until 1821. In 1823, all the Central American countries, except for Panama, set up a Central American Federation. But El Salvador withdrew in 1840 and declared its independence in 1841. El Salvador suffered from instability throughout the 19th century. The 20th century saw a more stable government, but from 1931 military dictatorships alternated with elected governments.

The country remained poor. In the 1970s, protesters demanded that the government introduce reforms to help the poor. Kidnappings and murders committed by left- and right-wing groups caused instability. A civil war broke out in 1979 between the US-backed government forces and left-wing guerrillas. In 12 years, more than 750,000 people died and many were made homeless. A ceasefire was agreed in 1992 and democratic elections were held in 1993, 1999, and 2003. By 2003, the economy had shown signs of recovery, but the World Bank still classifies El Salvador as a "lower-middle-income" economy.

About three-quarters of the country is farmed. Coffee, grown in the highlands, is the main export, followed by sugar and cotton, which grow on the coastal lowlands. Fishing for lobsters and shrimps is important, but manufacturing is on a small scale.

AREA 8,124 sq mi [21,041 sq km] **POPULATION** 6,470,000
CAPITAL (POPULATION) San Salvador (473,000)
GOVERNMENT Republic **ETHNIC GROUPS** Mestizo (mixed White and Amerindian) 90%, White 9%, Amerindian 1%
LANGUAGES Spanish (official) **RELIGIONS** Roman Catholic 83%
CURRENCY US dollar = 100 cents

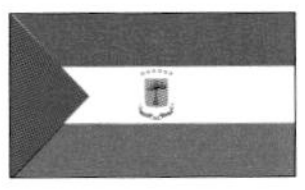

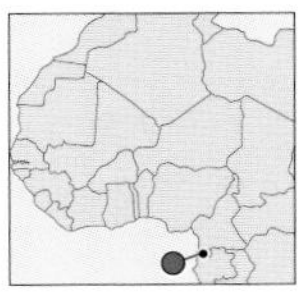

EQUATORIAL GUINEA

GEOGRAPHY The Republic of Equatorial Guinea is a small republic in west-central Africa. It consists of a mainland territory which makes up 90% of the land area, called Rio Muni, between Cameroon and Gabon, and five offshore islands in the Bight of Bonny, the largest of which is Bioko. The island of Annobon lies 350 mi [560 km] southwest of Rio Muni. Rio Muni consists mainly of hills and plateaux behind the coastal plains.

The climate is hot and humid. Bioko is mountainous, with the land rising to 9,869 ft [3,008 m], and hence it is particularly rainy. However, there is a marked dry season between the months of December and February. Mainland Rio Muni has a similar climate, though the rainfall diminishes inland.

POLITICS & ECONOMY Portuguese navigators reached the area in 1471. In 1778, Portugal granted Bioko, together with rights over Rio Muni, to Spain.

In 1959, Spain made Bioko and Rio Muni provinces of overseas Spain and, in 1963, it gave the provinces a degree of self-government. Equatorial Guinea became independent in 1968.

The first president of Equatorial Guinea, Francisco Macias Nguema, proved to be a tyrant. He was overthrown in 1979 and a group of officers, led by Lieutenant-Colonel Teodoro Obiang Nguema Mbasogo, set up a Supreme Military Council to rule the country. In 1991, the people voted to set up a multiparty democracy. Elections were held in the 1990s, but accusations of human rights abuses continued.

Agriculture employs more than half of the people and the most valuable crop is coffee. Oil has been produced since 1966 and, by 2002, it accounted for about 60% of the country's gross national product.

AREA 10,830 sq mi [28,051 sq km] **POPULATION** 510,000
CAPITAL (POPULATION) Malabo (30,000) **GOVERNMENT** Multiparty republic (transitional) **ETHNIC GROUPS** Bubi (on Bioko), Fang (in Rio Muni) **LANGUAGES** Spanish and French (both official)
RELIGIONS Christianity **CURRENCY** CFA franc = 100 centimes

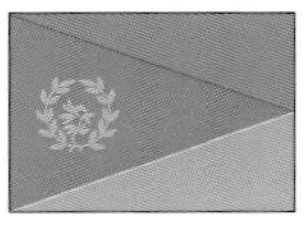

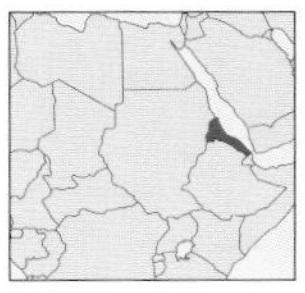

ERITREA

GEOGRAPHY The State of Eritrea consists of a hot, dry coastal plain facing the Red Sea, with a fairly mountainous area in the center. Most people live in the cooler highland area.

POLITICS & ECONOMY From the 1st century AD, Eritrea was part of the ancient Kingdom of Axum, which adopted Christianity in the 4th century AD. It began to decline in the 7th century. The Ottoman Turks took over the area in the 16th century and it became an Italian colony in the 1880s. The Italians were driven out in 1941 and, in 1952, it became part of Ethiopia.

A guerrilla struggle launched in 1961 ended in 1993, when Eritrea became independent. Economic recovery was hampered by conflict with Yemen over three islands in the Red Sea. In 1988–9, clashes occurred along the border with Ethiopia. A peace agreement was signed in 2000, but arguments again broke out in 2003 over the proposed redrawing of the boundaries.

The main economic activities are farming and livestock rearing. The few manufacturing industries are based mainly in Asmara.

AREA 45,405 sq mi [117,600 sq km] **POPULATION** 4,362,000
CAPITAL (POPULATION) Asmara (358,000) **GOVERNMENT** Transitional government **ETHNIC GROUPS** Tigrinya 50%, Tigre and Kunama 40%, Afar 4%, Saho 3%, others **LANGUAGES** Afar, Arabic, Tigre and Kunama, Tigrinya **RELIGIONS** Islam, Coptic Christian, Roman Catholic **CURRENCY** Nakfa = 100 cents

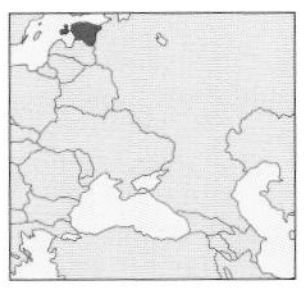

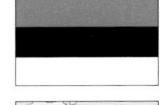

ESTONIA

GEOGRAPHY The Republic of Estonia is the smallest of the three states on the Baltic Sea, which were formerly part of the Soviet Union, but which became independent in the early 1990s. Estonia consists of a generally flat plain which was covered by ice sheets during the Ice Age. The land is strewn with moraine (rocks deposited by the ice).

The country is dotted with more than 1,500 small lakes. The large Lake Peipus (Chudskoye Ozero) and the River Narva together make up much of Estonia's eastern border with Russia. Estonia also has more than 800 islands, which together make up about a tenth of the country. The largest island is Saaremaa (Sarema). Despite its northerly position, Estonia has a fairly mild climate because of the moderating effects of the sea.

POLITICS & ECONOMY The ancestors of the Estonians, who are related to the Finns, settled in the area several thousand years ago. German crusaders, known as the Teutonic Knights, introduced Christianity in the early 13th century. By the 16th century, German noblemen owned much of the land in Estonia. In 1561, Sweden took the northern part of the country and Poland the south. From 1625, Sweden controlled the entire country until Sweden handed it over to Russia in 1721.

Estonian nationalists campaigned for their independence from around the mid-19th century. Finally, Estonia was proclaimed independent in 1918. In 1919, the government began to break up the large estates and distribute land among the peasants.

In 1939, Germany and the Soviet Union agreed to take over parts of Eastern Europe. In 1940, Soviet forces occupied Estonia, but they were driven out by the Germans in 1941. Soviet troops returned in 1944 and Estonia became one of the 15 Soviet Socialist Republics of the Soviet Union. The Estonians strongly opposed Soviet rule. Many of them were deported to Siberia.

Political changes in the Soviet Union in the late 1980s led to renewed demands for freedom. In 1990, the Estonian government declared the country independent and, finally, the Soviet Union recognized this act in September 1991, shortly before the Soviet Union was dissolved. Estonia adopted a new constitution in 1992, when multiparty elections were held for a new national assembly. In 1993, Estonia negotiated an agreement with Russia to withdraw its troops.

Under Soviet rule, Estonia was the most prosperous of the three Baltic states. Since 1988, Estonia has worked to restructure its economy. Turning increasingly to the West, it became a member of both the North Atlantic Treaty Organization and the European Union in 2004. Estonia's resources include oil shale and its forests. Industries produce fertilizers, processed food, machinery, petrochemical products, wood products, and textiles. Agriculture and fishing are also important activities.

AREA 17,413 sq mi [45,100 sq km] **POPULATION** 1,409,000
CAPITAL (POPULATION) Tallinn (418,000) **GOVERNMENT** Multiparty republic **ETHNIC GROUPS** Estonian 65%, Russian 28%, Ukrainian 3%, Belarusian 2%, Finnish 1% **LANGUAGES** Estonian (official), Russian
RELIGIONS Lutheran, Russian and Estonian Orthodox, Methodist, Baptist, Roman Catholic **CURRENCY** Estonian kroon = 100 senti

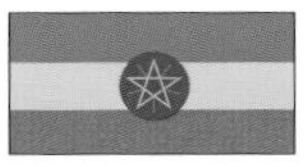

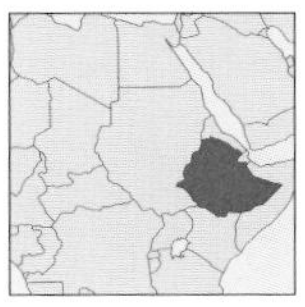

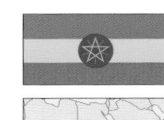

ETHIOPIA

GEOGRAPHY Ethiopia is a landlocked country in northeastern Africa. The land is mainly mountainous, though there are extensive plains in the east, bordering southern Eritrea, and in the south, bordering Somalia. The highlands are divided into two blocks by an arm of the Great Rift Valley which runs throughout eastern Africa. North of the Rift Valley, the land is especially rugged, rising to 15,157 ft [4,620 m] at Ras Dashen. Southeast of Ras Dashen is Lake Tana, source of the River Abay (Blue Nile).

The climate in Ethiopia is greatly affected by the altitude. Addis Ababa, at 8,000 ft [2,450 m], has an average yearly temperature of 68°F [20°C]. The rainfall is generally more than 39 in [1,000 mm]. But the lowlands bordering the Eritrean coast are hot.

POLITICS & ECONOMY Ethiopia was the home of an ancient monarchy, which became Christian in the 4th century. In the 7th century, Muslims gained control of the lowlands, but Christianity survived in the highlands. Ethiopia resisted attempts to colonize it, but Italy invaded the country in 1935. The Italians were driven out in 1941 during World War II.

In 1952, Eritrea, on the Red Sea coast, was federated with Ethiopia. But in 1961, Eritrean nationalists demanded their freedom and began a struggle that ended in their independence in 1993. Clashes along the border with Eritrea occurred in 1998 and 1999, but a peace agreement was signed in 2000, though a disagreement arose in 2003 about the status of Badme, the village where the conflict began. Some Ethiopian minorities would like self-government and, in 1995, the country was divided into nine provinces, each with its own regional assembly.

Ethiopia is one of the world's poorest countries, particularly in the 1970s and 1980s when it was plagued by civil war and famine caused partly by long droughts. Many richer countries have sent aid (money and food) to help the Ethiopian people. Agriculture remains the leading activity.

AREA 426,370 sq mi [1,104,300 sq km] **POPULATION** 66,558,000
CAPITAL (POPULATION) Addis Ababa (2,424,000) **GOVERNMENT** Federation of nine provinces **ETHNIC GROUPS** Oromo 40%, Amhara and Tigre 32%, Sidamo 9%, Shankella 6%, Somali 6%, others
LANGUAGES Amharic (official), many others **RELIGIONS** Islam 47%, Ethiopian Orthodox 40%, traditional beliefs 12%
CURRENCY Birr = 100 cents

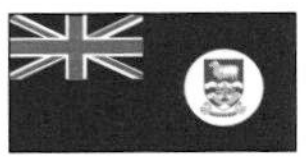

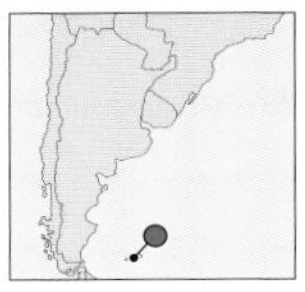

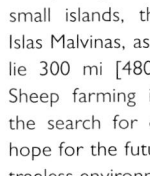

FALKLAND ISLANDS

Comprising two main islands and over 200 small islands, the Falkland Islands (or the Islas Malvinas, as they are called in Argentina) lie 300 mi [480 km] from South America. Sheep farming is the main activity, though the search for oil and diamonds holds out hope for the future of this harsh and virtually treeless environment.

AREA 4,700 sq mi [12,173 sq km] **POPULATION** 3,000
CAPITAL (POPULATION) Stanley (1,600)

FÆROE ISLANDS

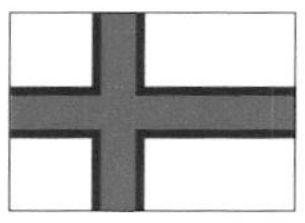

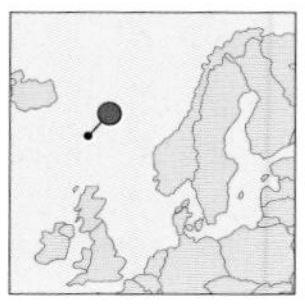

The Færoe Islands are a group of 18 volcanic islands and some reefs in the North Atlantic Ocean. The islands have been Danish since the 1380s, but they became largely self-governing in 1948. In 1998, the government of the Færoes announced its intention to become independent of Denmark.

AREA 540 sq mi [1,399 sq km]
POPULATION 46,000 **CAPITAL** Tórshavn

FIJI ISLANDS

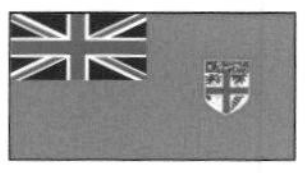

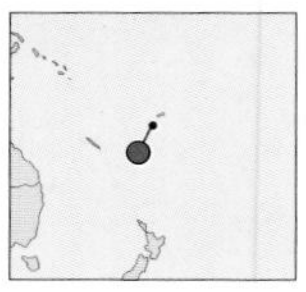

The Fiji Islands (the official name of Fiji since 1998) is a republic consisting of more than 800 Melanesian islands, the biggest being Viti Levu and Vanua Levu. The climate is tropical. A former British colony, Fiji became independent in 1970. Its recent history has been marred by efforts by ethnic Fijians to impose their rule, stopping members of the ethnic Indian community from holding senior cabinet posts. This action provoked international criticism.

AREA 7,056 sq mi [18,274 sq km] **POPULATION** 869,000 **CAPITAL** Suva

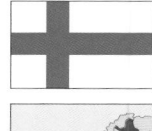

FINLAND

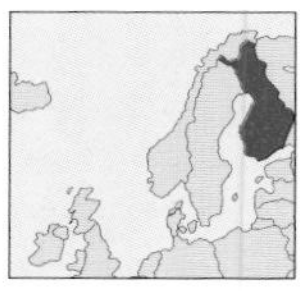

GEOGRAPHY The Republic of Finland is a beautiful country in northern Europe. In the south, behind the coastal lowlands where most Finns live, lies a region of sparkling lakes worn out by ice sheets in the Ice Age. The thinly populated northern uplands cover about two-fifths of the country.

Helsinki, the capital city, has warm summers, but the average temperatures between the months of December and March are below freezing point. Snow covers the land in winter. The north has less precipitation than the south, but it is much colder.

POLITICS & ECONOMY Between 1150 and 1809, Finland was under Swedish rule. The close links between the countries continue today. Swedish remains an official language in Finland and many towns have Swedish as well as Finnish names.

In 1809, Finland became a grand duchy of the Russian empire. It finally declared itself independent in 1917, after the Russian Revolution and the collapse of the Russian empire. But during World War II (1939–45), the Soviet Union declared war on Finland and took part of Finland's territory. Finland allied itself with Germany, but it lost more land to the Soviet Union at the end of the war.

After World War II, Finland became a neutral country and negotiated peace treaties with the Soviet Union. Finland also strengthened its relations with other northern European countries and became an associate member of the European Free Trade Association (EFTA) in 1961. Finland became a full member of EFTA in 1986, but in 1992, along with most of its fellow EFTA members, it applied for membership of the European Union, which it finally achieved on January 1, 1995. On January 1, 2002, the euro became Finland's sole official unit of currency.

Forests are Finland's most valuable resource, and forestry accounts for about 35% of the country's exports. The chief manufactures are wood products, pulp, and paper. Since World War II, Finland has set up many other industries, producing such things as machinery and transport equipment. Its economy has expanded rapidly, but there has been a large increase in the number of unemployed people.

AREA 130,558 sq mi [338,145 sq km] **POPULATION** 5,191,000
CAPITAL (POPULATION) Helsinki (549,000)
GOVERNMENT Multiparty republic **ETHNIC GROUPS** Finnish 93%, Swedish 6% **LANGUAGES** Finnish and Swedish (both official)
RELIGIONS Evangelical Lutheran 89% **CURRENCY** Euro = 100 cents

FRANCE

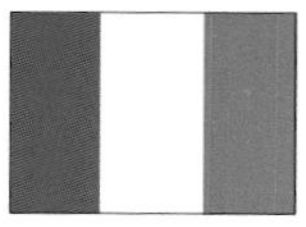

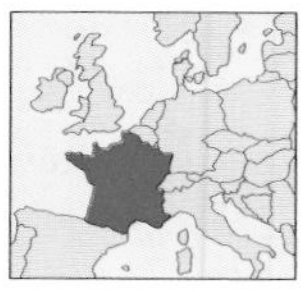

GEOGRAPHY The Republic of France is the largest country in Western Europe. The scenery is extremely varied. The Vosges Mountains overlook the Rhine valley in the northeast, the Jura Mountains and the Alps form the borders with Switzerland and Italy in the southeast, while the Pyrenees straddle France's border with Spain. The only large highland area entirely within France is the Massif Central between the Rhône-Saône valley and the basin of Aquitaine in southern France.

Brittany (Bretagne) and Normandy (Normande) form a scenic hill region. Fertile lowlands cover most of northern France, including the densely populated Paris basin. Another major lowland area, the Aquitanian basin, is in the southwest, while the Rhône-Saône valley and the Mediterranean lowlands are in the southeast.

The climate of France varies from west to east and from north to south. The west comes under the moderating influence of the Atlantic Ocean, giving generally mild weather. To the east, summers are warmer and winters colder. The climate also becomes warmer as one travels from north to south. The Mediterranean Sea coast has hot, dry summers and mild, moist winters. The Alps, Jura and Pyrenees mountains have snowy winters. Winter sports centers are found in all three areas. Large glaciers occupy high valleys in the Alps.

POLITICS & ECONOMY The Romans conquered France (then called Gaul) in the 50s BC. Roman rule began to decline in the fifth century AD and, in 486, the Frankish realm (as France was called) became independent under a Christian king, Clovis. In 800, Charlemagne, who had been king since 768, became emperor of the Romans. He extended France's boundaries, but, in 843, his empire was divided into three parts and the area of France contracted. After the Norman invasion of England in 1066, large areas of France came under English rule, but this was finally ended in 1453.

France later became a powerful monarchy. But the French Revolution (1789–99) ended absolute rule by French kings. In 1799, Napoleon Bonaparte took power and fought a series of brilliant military campaigns before his final defeat in 1815. The monarchy was restored until 1848, when the Second Republic was founded. In 1852, Napoleon's nephew became Napoleon III, but the Third Republic was established in 1875. France was the scene of much fighting during World War I (1914–18) and World War II (1939–45), causing great loss of life and much damage to the economy.

In 1946, France adopted a new constitution, establishing the Fourth Republic. But political instability and costly colonial wars slowed France's post-war recovery. In 1958, Charles de Gaulle was elected president and he introduced a new constitution, giving the president extra powers and inaugurating the Fifth Republic.

Since the 1960s, France has made rapid economic progress, becoming one of the most prosperous nations in the European Union. But France's government faced a number of problems, including unemployment, pollution and the growing number of elderly people, who find it difficult to live when inflation rates are high. One social problem concerns the presence in France of large numbers of immigrants from Africa and southern Europe, many of whom live in poor areas.

A socialist government was elected in 1997 and, in 2002, the euro, the single European currency, became France's sole official unit of currency. However, in 2002, center-right parties defeated the socialists. France has a long record of independence in foreign affairs and, in 2003, it angered the United States and some of its European allies by opposing the invasion of Iraq.

France is one of the world's most developed countries. Its natural resources include its fertile soil, together with deposits of bauxite, coal, iron ore, oil and natural gas, and potash. France is also one of the world's top manufacturing nations, and it has often innovated in bold and imaginative ways. The TGV and hypermarkets are typical examples. Paris is a world center of fashion industries, but France has many other industrial towns and cities. Major manufactures include aircraft, cars, chemicals, electronic and metal products, machinery, processed food, steel and textiles.

Agriculture employs about 2% of the people, but France is the largest producer of farm products in Western Europe, producing most of the food it needs. Wheat is the leading crop and livestock farming is of major importance. Fishing and forestry are leading industries, while tourism is a major activity.

AREA 212,934 sq mi [551,500 sq km] **POPULATION** 60,181,000
CAPITAL (POPULATION) Paris (2,152,000) **GOVERNMENT** Multiparty republic **ETHNIC GROUPS** Celtic, Latin, Arab, Teutonic, Slavic
LANGUAGES French (official) **RELIGIONS** Roman Catholic 85%, Islam 8%, others **CURRENCY** Euro = 100 cents

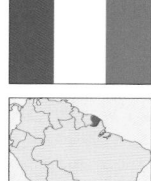

FRENCH GUIANA

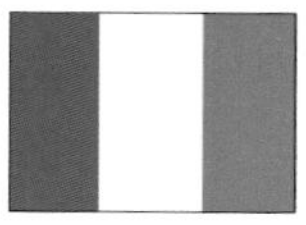

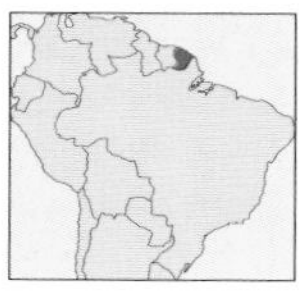

GEOGRAPHY French Guiana is the smallest country in mainland South America. The coastal plain is swampy in places, but some dry areas are cultivated. Inland lies a plateau, with the low Tumachumac Mountains in the south. Most of the rivers run north toward the Atlantic Ocean.

French Guiana has a hot, equatorial climate, with high temperatures throughout the year. The rainfall is heavy, especially between December and June, but it is dry between August and October. The northeast trade winds blow constantly across the country.

POLITICS & ECONOMY The first people to live in what is now French Guiana were Amerindians. Today, only a few of them survive in the interior. The first Europeans to explore the coast arrived in 1500, and they were followed by adventurers seeking El Dorado, the mythical city of gold. Cayenne was founded in 1637 by a group of French merchants. The area became a French colony in the late 17th century.

France used the colony as a penal settlement for political prisoners from the times of the French Revolution in the 1790s. From the 1850s to 1945, the country became notorious as a place where prisoners were harshly treated. Many of them died, unable to survive in the tropical conditions.

In 1946, French Guiana became an overseas department of France, and in 1974 it also became an administrative region. An independence movement developed in the 1980s, but most people want to retain their links with France and continue to obtain financial aid to develop their territory.

Although it has rich forest and mineral resources, such as bauxite (aluminum ore), French Guiana is a developing country. It depends greatly on France for money to run its services and the government is the country's biggest employer. Since 1968, Kourou in French Guiana, the European Space Agency's rocket-launching site, has earned money for France by sending communications satellites into space.

AREA 34,749 sq mi [90,000 sq km] **POPULATION** 187,000
CAPITAL (POPULATION) Cayenne (51,000) **GOVERNMENT** Overseas department of France **ETHNIC GROUPS** Black or Mulatto 66%, East Indian/Chinese and Amerindian 12%, White 12%, others 10%
LANGUAGES French (official) **RELIGIONS** Roman Catholic
CURRENCY Euro = 100 cents

FRENCH POLYNESIA

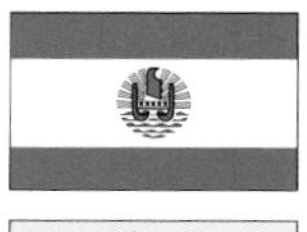

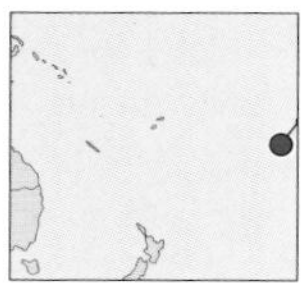

French Polynesia consists of 130 islands, scattered over 1.5 million sq mi [4 million sq km] of the Pacific Ocean. Tribal chiefs in the area agreed to a French protectorate in 1843. They gained increased autonomy in 1984, but the links with France ensure a high standard of living.

AREA 1,544 sq mi [4,000 sq km]
POPULATION 262,000 **CAPITAL** Papeete

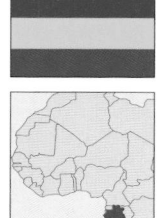

GABON

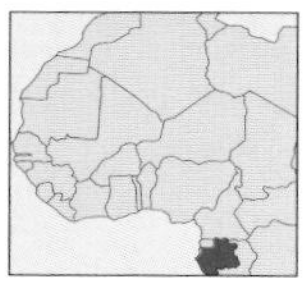

GEOGRAPHY The Gabonese Republic lies on the Equator in west-central Africa. In area, it is a little larger than the United Kingdom, with a coastline 500 mi [800 km] long. Behind the narrow, partly lagoon-lined coastal plain, the land rises to hills, plateaux and mountains divided by deep valleys carved by the River Ogooué and its tributaries.

Most of Gabon has an equatorial climate, with high temperatures and humidity throughout the year. The rainfall is heavy and the skies are often cloudy.

POLITICS & ECONOMY Gabon became a French colony in the 1880s, but it achieved full independence in 1960. In 1964, an attempted coup was put down when French troops intervened and crushed the revolt. In 1967, Bernard-Albert Bongo, who later renamed himself El Hadj Omar Bongo, became president. He declared Gabon a one-party state in 1968. Opposition parties were legalized in 1991, but Bongo was re-elected president in 1993. In 2003, the constitution was changed, enabling Bongo to stand as president as many times as he wished.

Gabon's natural resources include its forests, oil and gas deposits, manganese, and uranium. Its mineral deposits make it one of Africa's better-off countries. But agriculture still employs two-fifths of the people and many farmers produce little more than they need to support their families.

AREA 103,347 sq mi [267,668 sq km] **POPULATION** 1,322,000
CAPITAL (POPULATION) Libreville (362,000)
GOVERNMENT Multiparty republic
ETHNIC GROUPS Four major Bantu tribes: Fang, Bapounou, Nzebi and Obamba **LANGUAGES** French (official), Fang, Myene, Nzebi, Bapounou/Eschira, Bandjabi
RELIGIONS Christianity 75%, animist, Islam
CURRENCY CFA franc = 100 centimes

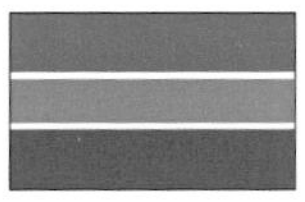
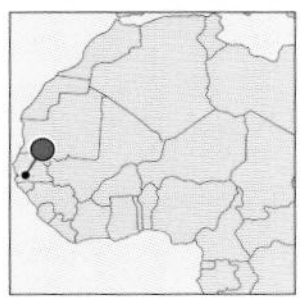

GAMBIA, THE

GEOGRAPHY The Republic of The Gambia is the smallest country in mainland Africa. It consists of a narrow strip of land bordering the River Gambia. The Gambia is almost entirely enclosed by Senegal, except along the short Atlantic coastline.

The Gambia has hot and humid summers, but the winter temperatures (November to May) drop to around 61°F [16°C]. In the summer, moist southwesterlies bring rain, which is heaviest on the coast.

POLITICS & ECONOMY English traders bought rights to trade on the River Gambia in 1588, and in 1664 the English established a settlement on an island in the river estuary. In 1765, the British founded Senegambia, which included parts of The Gambia and Senegal. In 1783, Britain handed this colony over to France. In the 19th century, Britain and France discussed the exchange of The Gambia for some other French territory, but an agreement was reached and Britain made The Gambia a British colony in 1888.

The Gambia achieved independence in 1965 and it became a republic in 1970. Relations between the English-speaking Gambians and the French-speaking Senegalese are a major political issue. In 1981, an attempted coup in The Gambia was put down with the help of Senegalese troops. In 1982, The Gambia and Senegal set up a defense alliance, called the Confederation of Senegambia. But this alliance was dissolved in 1989. In 1994, a military group overthrew the president, Sir Dawda Jawara, who fled into exile. Captain Yahya Jammeh, who took power, was elected president in 1996 and re-elected in 2001.

Agriculture employs more than 50% of the people. The main food crops include cassava, millet, and sorghum, but groundnuts and groundnut products are the chief exports. Tourism is a growing industry.

AREA 4,361 sq mi [11,295 sq km] **POPULATION** 1,501,000
CAPITAL (POPULATION) Banjul (42,000)
GOVERNMENT Military regime
ETHNIC GROUPS Mandinka 42%, Fula 18%, Wolof 16%, Jola 10%, Serahuli 9%, others
LANGUAGES English (official), Mandinka, Wolof, Fula
RELIGIONS Islam 90%, Christianity 9%, traditional beliefs 1%
CURRENCY Dalasi = 100 butut

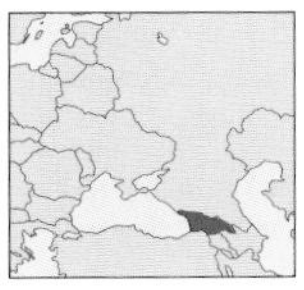

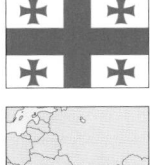

GEORGIA

GEOGRAPHY Georgia is a country on the borders of Europe and Asia, facing the Black Sea. The land is rugged with the Caucasus Mountains forming its northern border. The highest mountain in this range, Mount Elbrus (18,481 ft [5,633 m]), lies over the border with Russia.border in Russia.

The Black Sea plains have hot summers and mild winters. The rainfall is heavy, though inland areas are drier.

POLITICS & ECONOMY The first Georgian state was set up nearly 2,500 years ago. But for much of its history, the area was ruled by various conquerors. Christianity was introduced in AD 330. Georgia freed itself of foreign rule in the 11th and 12th centuries, but Mongol armies attacked in the 13th century. From the 16th to the 18th centuries, Iran and the Turkish Ottoman empire struggled for control of the area, and in the late 18th century Georgia sought the protection of Russia and, by the early 19th century, Georgia was part of the Russian empire. After the Russian Revolution of 1917, Georgia declared its independence, but Russia invaded, making the country part of the Soviet regime. Georgia declared itself independent in 1991. It became a separate country when the Soviet Union was dissolved in December 1991.

Georgia contains three regions containing minority peoples: Abkhazia in the northwest, South Ossetia in north-central Georgia, and Adjaria (also spelled Adzharia) in the southwest. Civil war broke out in South Ossetia in the early 1990s, while fierce fighting continued in Abkhazia until the late 1990s. In 2000, Georgia agreed to recognize Adjaria's autonomy in the country's constitution. In 2002, Russian and Georgian troops attacked Chechen rebels in Pankisi Gorge in northeastern Georgia. The USA also alleged that terrorists from Afghanistan and elsewhere were hiding in the area. In 2004, civil war threatened when Adjaria unsuccessfully challenged the authority of President Mikhail Saakashvili.

Georgia is a developing country. Agriculture is important. Major products include barley, citrus fruits, grapes for wine-making, maize, tea, tobacco, and vegetables. Food processing and silk and perfume-making are other important activities. Sheep and cattle are reared.

AREA 26,911 sq mi [69,700 sq km] **POPULATION** 4,934,000
CAPITAL (POPULATION) Tbilisi (1,268,000)
GOVERNMENT Multiparty republic **ETHNIC GROUPS** Georgian 70%, Armenian 8%, Russian 6%, Azeri 6%, Ossetian 3%, Greek 2%, Abkhaz 2%, others 3% **LANGUAGES** Georgian (official), Russian
RELIGIONS Georgian Orthodox 65%, Islam 11%, Russian Orthodox 10%, Armenian Apostolic 8%
CURRENCY Lari = 100 tetri

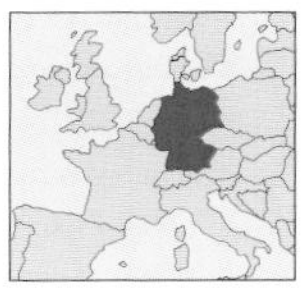

GERMANY

GEOGRAPHY The Federal Republic of Germany is the fourth largest country in Western Europe, after France, Spain and Sweden. The North German plain borders the North Sea in the northwest and the Baltic Sea in the northeast. Major rivers draining the plain include the Weser, Elbe and Oder.

The central highlands include the Harz Mountains, the Thuringian Forest (Thüringer Wald), the Ore Mountains (Erzgebirge), and the Bohemian Forest (Böhmerwald) on the Czech border. The Bavarian Alps in the south contain Germany's highest peak, Zugspitze, at 9,721 ft [2,963 m] above sea level. The Black Forest (Schwarzwald) in the southwest overlooks the River Rhine. Northwestern Germany has a mild climate, but the Baltic coasts are cooler. To the south, the climate becomes more continental, especially in the highlands. The precipitation is greatest on the uplands, with snow in winter.

POLITICS & ECONOMY Germany and its allies were defeated in World War I (1914–18) and the country became a republic. Adolf Hitler came to power in 1933 and ruled as a dictator. His order to invade Poland led to the start of World War II (1939–45), which ended with Germany in ruins.

In 1945, Germany was divided into four military zones. In 1949, the American, British and French zones were amalgamated to form the Federal Republic of Germany (West Germany), while the Soviet zone became the German Democratic Republic (East Germany), a Communist state. Berlin, which had also been partitioned, became a divided city. West Berlin was part of West Germany, while East Berlin became the capital of East Germany. Bonn was the capital of West Germany.

Tension between East and West mounted during the Cold War, but West Germany rebuilt its economy quickly. In East Germany, the recovery was less rapid. In the late 1980s, reforms in the Soviet Union led to unrest in East Germany. Free elections were held in East Germany in 1990 and, on October 3, 1990, Germany was reunited.

The united Germany adopted West Germany's official name, the Federal Republic of Germany. In the 1990s, the government faced many problems, especially those arising from the re-structuring of the economy of the former East Germany. In 1999, the parliament moved from Bonn to the reconstructed Reichstag building in Berlin. In 2003, Germany opposed the invasion of Iraq, incurring criticism from the United States.

West Germany's "economic miracle" after World War II was greatly helped by foreign aid. Today, Germany is one of the world's top economic powers. Manufacturing is the mainstay of the economy and manufactured goods are the chief exports. Cars and other vehicles, cement, chemicals, computers, electrical equipment, processed food, machinery, scientific instruments. ships, steel, textiles, and tools are manufactured. Germany has some coal, potash, and rock salt deposits, but it imports many industrial raw materials. Germany also imports food. Leading products include fruits, grapes for wine-making, potatoes, sugar beet, and vegetables. Livestock include beef and dairy cattle.

AREA 137,846 sq mi [357,022 sq km] **POPULATION** 82,398,000
CAPITAL (POPULATION) Berlin (3,387,000)
GOVERNMENT Federal multiparty republic **ETHNIC GROUPS** German 92%, Turkish 3%, Serbo-Croatian, Italian, Greek, Polish, Spanish
LANGUAGES German (official) **RELIGIONS** Protestant (mainly Lutheran) 34%, Roman Catholic 34%, Islam 4%, others
CURRENCY Euro = 100 cents

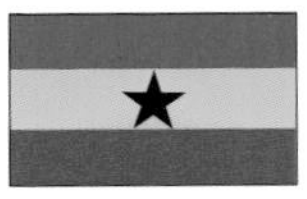
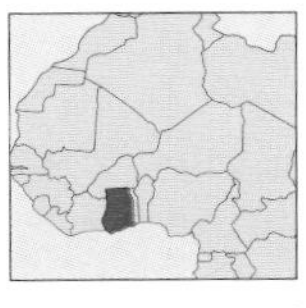

GHANA

GEOGRAPHY The Republic of Ghana faces the Gulf of Guinea in West Africa. This hot country, just north of the Equator, was formerly called the Gold Coast. Behind the thickly populated southern coastal plains, which are lined with lagoons, lies a plateau region in the southwest.

Accra has a hot, tropical climate. Rain occurs all through the year, though Accra is drier than areas inland.

POLITICS & ECONOMY Portuguese explorers reached the area in 1471 and named it the Gold Coast. The area became a center of the slave trade in the 17th century. The slave trade was ended in the 1860s and, gradually, the British took control of the area. After independence in 1957, attempts were made to develop the economy by creating large state-owned manufacturing industries. But debt and corruption, together with falls in the price of cocoa, the chief export, caused economic problems. This led to instability and frequent coups. In 1981, power was invested in a Provisional National Defense Council, led by Flight-Lieutenant Jerry Rawlings.

The government steadied the economy and introduced several new policies, including the relaxation of government controls. In 1992, the government introduced a new constitution, which allowed for multiparty elections. Rawlings was elected president in 1992 and 1996, but he retired in 2002. He was succeeded as president by John Ageykum Kufuor. The World Bank classifies Ghana as a "low-income" developing country. Most people are poor and farming employs 55% of the population.

AREA 92,098 sq mi [238,533 sq km] **POPULATION** 20,468,000
CAPITAL (POPULATION) Accra (949,000) **GOVERNMENT** Republic
ETHNIC GROUPS Akan 44%, Moshi-Dagomba 16%, Ewe 13%, Ga 8%, Gurma 3%, Yoruba 1% **LANGUAGES** English (official), Akan, Moshi-Dagomba, Ewe, Ga **RELIGIONS** Christianity 63%, traditional beliefs 21%, Islam 16% **CURRENCY** Cedi = 100 pesewas

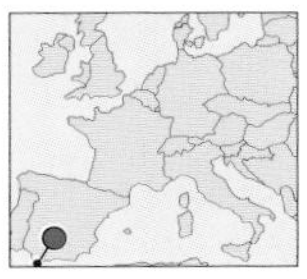

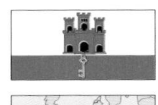

GIBRALTAR

Gibraltar occupies a strategic position on the south coast of Spain where the Mediterranean meets the Atlantic. It was recognized as a British possession in 1713 and, despite Spanish claims, its population has consistently voted to retain its contacts with Britain.

AREA 2.3 sq mi [6 sq km]
POPULATION 28,000 **CAPITAL** Gibraltar Town

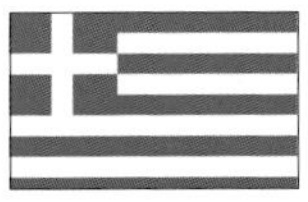
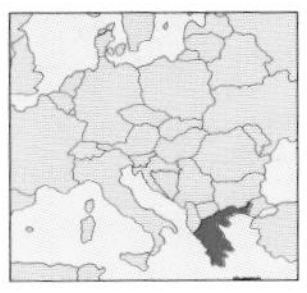

GREECE

GEOGRAPHY The Hellenic Republic, as Greece is officially called, is a rugged country situated at the southern end of the Balkan peninsula. Olympus, at 9,570 ft [2,917 m] is the highest peak. Islands make up about a fifth of the land.

Low-lying areas in Greece have mild, moist winters and hot, dry summers. The east coast has more than 2,700 hours of sunshine a year and only about half of the rainfall of the west. The mountains have a much more severe climate, with snow on the higher slopes in winter.

POLITICS & ECONOMY Around 2,500 years ago, Greece became the birthplace of Western civilization and Ancient Greek ruins and art still attract millions of tourists to the country. The first civilization, the Minoan, was centered on Crete. It flourished between about 3000 and 1400 BC. Following the end of the related Mycaenean period on the mainland (1580–1100 BC), a "dark age" lasted until about 800 BC. But from 750 BC, Greeks became rich traders and the city-state of Athens reached its peak in 461–431 BC. Greece became a Roman province in 146 BC and, in AD 365, it became part of the Byzantine Empire.

The Byzantine empire fell to the Turks in 1453. But Greece became an independent monarchy in 1830. After World War II (1939–45), when Germany ruled Greece, a civil war broke out between Greek Communists and nationalists. It ended in 1949 and a military dictatorship seized power in 1967. The monarchy was abolished in 1973 and democracy was restored in 1974. Greece joined the European Community (now the European Union) in 1981 and, on January 1, 2002, the euro became the sole unit of currency in Greece.

Greece is one of the EU's less economically developed members. Manufactured products include processed food, cement, chemicals, metal products, textiles, and tobacco. Greece also mines lignite (brown coal), bauxite, and chromite. Farmland covers about a third of the country and grazing land another 40%. Crops include barley, grapes for wine-making, dried fruits, olives, potatoes, sugar beet, and wheat. Livestock farming is also important. Greece's beaches and ancient ruins make the country a major tourist destination.

AREA 50,949 sq mi [131,957 sq km] **POPULATION** 10,666,000
CAPITAL (POPULATION) Athens (772,000)
GOVERNMENT Multiparty republic **ETHNIC GROUPS** Greek 98%
LANGUAGES Greek (official) **RELIGIONS** Greek Orthodox 98%
CURRENCY Euro = 100 cents

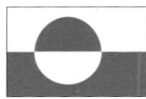

GREENLAND

Greenland is the world's largest island. Settlements are confined to the coast, because an ice sheet covers four-fifths of the land. Greenland became a Danish possession in 1380. Full internal self-government was granted in 1981 and, in 1997, Danish place names were superseded by Inuit forms. However, Greenland remains heavily dependent on Danish subsidies.

AREA 838,999 SQ MI [2,175,600 SQ KM] **POPULATION** 56,000
CAPITAL (POPULATION) NUUK (GODTHÅB) (14,000)

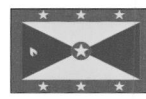

GRENADA

The most southerly of the Windward Islands in the Caribbean Sea, Grenada became independent from the UK in 1974. A military group seized power in 1983, when the prime minister was killed. US troops intervened and restored order and constitutional government.

AREA 133 SQ MI [344 SQ KM]
POPULATION 89,000 **CAPITAL** ST GEORGE'S

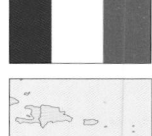

GUADELOUPE

Guadeloupe is a French overseas department which includes seven Caribbean islands, the largest of which is Basse-Terre. French aid has helped to maintain a reasonable standard of living for the people.

AREA 658 SQ MI [1,705 SQ KM]
POPULATION 440,000 **CAPITAL** BASSE-TERRE

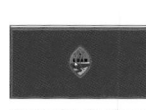

GUAM

Guam, a strategically important "unincorporated territory" of the USA, is the largest of the Mariana Islands in the Pacific Ocean. It is composed of a coralline limestone plateau.

AREA 212 SQ MI [549 SQ KM]
POPULATION 164,000 **CAPITAL** AGANA

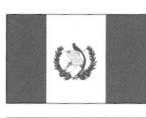

GUATEMALA

GEOGRAPHY The Republic of Guatemala in Central America contains a thickly populated mountain region, with fertile soils. The mountains, which run in an east–west direction, contain many volcanoes, some of which are active. Volcanic eruptions and earthquakes are common in the highlands. South of the mountains lie the thinly populated Pacific coastlands, while a large inland plain occupies the north.

The lowlands of Guatemala are not hot and rainy, but the central highlands are cooler and drier. Guatemala City has a pleasant, warm climate with a dry season between November and April.

POLITICS & ECONOMY Much of what is now Guatemala was part of the Maya empire which thrived between AD 300 and 900. Spain ruled the area from the 1520s until 1821. In 1823, Guatemala joined the Central American Federation. But it became fully independent in 1839. Instability and periodic violence have marred its progress since independence.

Guatemala has a long-standing claim over Belize, but this was reduced in 1983 to the southern fifth of the country. Violence became widespread in Guatemala from the early 1960s, because of the conflict between left-wing groups, including many Amerindians, and government forces. A peace accord was signed in 1996, ending a war that had lasted 36 years and claimed perhaps 200,000 lives.

Guatemala is ranked as a "lower-middle-income" economy. Agriculture employs 56% of the population. Coffee, sugar, bananas, and beef are exported and the spice cardamom and cotton are also important. Maize is the main food crop.

AREA 42,042 SQ MI [108,889 SQ KM] **POPULATION** 13,909,000
CAPITAL (POPULATION) GUATEMALA CITY (1,007,000)
GOVERNMENT REPUBLIC **ETHNIC GROUPS** LADINO (MIXED HISPANIC AND AMERINDIAN) 55%, AMERINDIAN 43%, OTHERS 2%
LANGUAGES SPANISH (OFFICIAL), AMERINDIAN LANGUAGES
RELIGIONS CHRISTIANITY, INDIGENOUS MAYAN BELIEFS
CURRENCY US DOLLAR; QUETZAL = 100 CENTAVOS

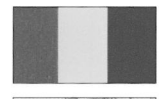

GUINEA

GEOGRAPHY The Republic of Guinea faces the Atlantic Ocean in West Africa. A flat, swampy plain borders the coast. Behind this plain, the land rises to a plateau region called Fouta Djalon. The Upper Niger plains, named after one of Africa's longest rivers, the Niger, which rises there, are in the northeast.

Guinea has a tropical climate and Conakry, on the coast, has heavy rains between May and November. This is also the coolest period in the year. During the dry season, hot, dry harmattan winds blow southwestward from the Sahara Desert.

POLITICS & ECONOMY Guinea came under the influence of several medieval African states, including Ancient Ghana and Ancient Mali. France began to control the area in the late 19th century. Guinea became independent in 1958. Its leaders pursued socialist policies but resorted to repressive measures to hold on to power. A military regime under Lansana Conté took over in 1984, but a multiparty system was restored in 1992. Conté was elected president in 1993 and re-elected in 1998 and 2002. From the late 1990s, Guinea was drawn into the conflicts taking place in Liberia and Sierra Leone.

Guinea is a "low-income" developing country. Its resources include bauxite (aluminum ore), diamonds, gold, iron ore, and uranium. Bauxite and alumina (processed bauxite) account for more than half of the exports. Agriculture employs 78% of the people, but most farmers are poor. Manufactures include alumina, processed food, and textiles.

AREA 94,925 SQ MI [245,857 SQ KM] **POPULATION** 9,030,000
CAPITAL (POPULATION) CONAKRY (1,508,000)
GOVERNMENT MULTIPARTY REPUBLIC
ETHNIC GROUPS PEUHL 40%, MALINKE 30%, SOUSSOU 20%, OTHERS 10% **LANGUAGES** FRENCH (OFFICIAL)
RELIGIONS ISLAM 85%, CHRISTIANITY 8%, TRADITIONAL BELIEFS 7%
CURRENCY GUINEAN FRANC = 100 CAURIS

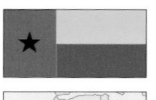

GUINEA-BISSAU

GEOGRAPHY The Republic of Guinea-Bissau, formerly known as Portuguese Guinea, is a small country in West Africa. The land is mostly low-lying, with a broad, swampy coastal plain and many flat offshore islands, including the Bijagós Archipelago.

The country has a tropical climate, with one dry season (December to May) and a rainy season from June to November.

POLITICS & ECONOMY Portuguese explorers reached Guinea-Bissau in 1446 and the area became a center of the slave trade. From 1836, Portugal administered Guinea-Bissau with the Cape Verde Islands but, in 1879, the territories were separated. Guinea-Bissau became a separate colony called Portuguese Guinea. But economic development in the colony was slow.

In 1956, African nationalists in Portuguese Guinea and Cape Verde founded the African Party for the Independence of Guinea and Cape Verde (PAIGC). Because Portugal seemed determined to hang on to its overseas territories, the PAIGC began a guerrilla war in 1963. By 1968, it held two-thirds of the country. In 1972, a rebel National Assembly, elected by the people in the PAIGC-controlled area, voted to make the country independent as Guinea-Bissau.

In 1974, newly independent Guinea-Bissau faced many problems arising from its under-developed economy and its lack of trained people to work in the administration. One objective of the leaders of Guinea-Bissau was to unite their country with Cape Verde. But, in 1980, army leaders overthrew Guinea-Bissau's government. The Revolutionary Council, which took over, opposed unification with Cape Verde. Guinea-Bissau ceased to be a one-party state in 1991 and multiparty elections were held in 1994. Civil war broke out in 1998 and a military coup occurred in May 1999. In elections in 1999 and 2000, Kumba Ialá was elected president, but he was removed in a coup in 2003.

Guinea-Bissau is a poor country. Agriculture employs 77% of the people, but most farming is at subsistence level. Major crops include beans, coconuts, groundnuts, maize, and rice.

AREA 13,948 SQ MI [36,125 SQ KM] **POPULATION** 1,361,000
CAPITAL (POPULATION) BISSAU (200,000)
GOVERNMENT "INTERIM" GOVERNMENT
ETHNIC GROUPS BALANTA 30%, FULA 20%, MANJACA 14%, MANDINGA 13%, PAPEL 7% **LANGUAGES** PORTUGUESE (OFFICIAL), CRIOULO
RELIGIONS TRADITIONAL BELIEFS 50%, ISLAM 45%, CHRISTIANITY 5%
CURRENCY CFA FRANC = 100 CENTIMES

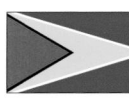

GUYANA

GEOGRAPHY The Cooperative Republic of Guyana is a country facing the Atlantic Ocean in northeastern South America. The coastal plain is flat and much of it is below sea level.

The climate is hot and humid, though the interior highlands are cooler than the coast. The rainfall is heavy, occurring on more than 200 days a year.

POLITICS & ECONOMY Britain gained control of the area in 1814 and ruled British Guiana until it became independent as Guyana in 1966. A black lawyer, Forbes Burnham, was the first prime minister. Under a new constitution adopted in 1980, the president's powers were increased. Burnham became president and served in this post until he died in 1985. He was succeeded by Hugh Desmond Hoyte, who was defeated in 1993 by an ethnic Indian, Cheddi Jagan. Jagan died in 1997 and was succeeded by his wife, Janet. In 1999, Bharat Jagdeo was elected president. He was re-elected in 2001.

Guyana is a poor country. Its resources include gold, bauxite (aluminum ore) and other minerals, forests, and fertile soils. Sugarcane and rice are leading crops. Guyana has potential for producing hydroelectricity from its many rivers.

AREA 83,000 SQ MI [214,969 SQ KM] **POPULATION** 702,000
CAPITAL (POPULATION) GEORGETOWN (150,000)
GOVERNMENT MULTIPARTY REPUBLIC
ETHNIC GROUPS EAST INDIAN 50%, BLACK 36%, AMERINDIAN 7%, OTHERS **LANGUAGES** ENGLISH (OFFICIAL), CREOLE, HINDI, URDU
RELIGIONS CHRISTIANITY 50%, HINDUISM 35%, ISLAM 10%, OTHERS
CURRENCY GUYANESE DOLLAR = 100 CENTS

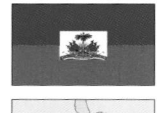

HAITI

GEOGRAPHY The Republic of Haiti occupies the western third of Hispaniola in the Caribbean. The land is mainly mountainous. The climate is hot and humid, though the northern highlands, with about 79 in [200 mm], have more than twice as much rainfall as the southern coast.

POLITICS & ECONOMY Visited by Christopher Columbus in 1492, Haiti was later developed by the French. The African slaves revolted in 1791 and the country became independent in 1804.

Since independence, Haiti has suffered from instability, violence and dictatorial rule. Elections in 1990 returned Jean-Bertrand Aristide as president, but he was overthrown in 1991. Following US intervention, he returned in 1994. In 1995, René Préval was elected president, but Aristide was again elected president in 2000 but, in 2004, he was forced to flee the country after massive public protests. Agriculture employs more than half of the people. Cocoa, coffee, and sugarcane are grown.

AREA 10,714 SQ MI [27,750 SQ KM] **POPULATION** 7,528,000
CAPITAL (POPULATION) PORT-AU-PRINCE (917,000)
GOVERNMENT MULTIPARTY REPUBLIC **ETHNIC GROUPS** BLACK 95%, MULATTO/WHITE 5% **LANGUAGES** FRENCH AND CREOLE (BOTH OFFICIAL)
RELIGIONS ROMAN CATHOLIC 80%, VOODOO
CURRENCY GOURDE = 100 CENTIMES

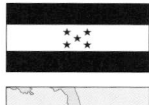

HONDURAS

GEOGRAPHY The Republic of Honduras is the second largest country in Central America. The northern coast on the Caribbean Sea extends more than 373 mi [600 km], but the Pacific coast in the southeast is only about 50 mi [80 km] long. Honduras has a tropical climate, but the highlands are cooler. The rainiest months are between May and November. Hurricanes often hit the north coast. Hurricane Mitch in 1998 caused the worst destruction in modern times.

POLITICS & ECONOMY Western Honduras was part of the Maya empire which flourished between AD 300 and 900. Christopher Columbus claimed the area for Spain in 1502 and Spain ruled from 1625 until 1821. Honduras became part of the Central American Federation but withdrew in 1838.

In the 1890s, American companies developed plantations to grow bananas. They soon became the country's chief source of income and Honduras became known as a "banana republic." But instability slowed economic progress. In 1969, Honduras fought a short "Soccer War" with El Salvador. The war was sparked off by the treatment of fans in a World Cup soccer series, though the real reason was that Salvadoreans in Honduras had been forced to give

up land. Since 1980, civilian governments have ruled Honduras, but the military remain influential.

Honduras is a developing country. Its few resources include silver, lead and zinc. Agriculture is the main activity. Bananas and coffee are exported and maize is the chief food crop. Honduras is one of Central America's least industrialized countries. Products include processed food, textiles, and wood products.

AREA 43,277 SQ MI [112,088 SQ KM] **POPULATION** 6,670,000
CAPITAL (POPULATION) TEGUCIGALPA (850,000)
GOVERNMENT REPUBLIC **ETHNIC GROUPS** MESTIZO 90%, AMERINDIAN 7%, BLACK (INCLUDING BLACK CARIB) 2%, WHITE 1% **LANGUAGES** SPANISH (OFFICIAL), AMERINDIAN DIALECTS **RELIGIONS** ROMAN CATHOLIC 97%
CURRENCY HONDURAN LEMPIRA = 100 CENTAVOS

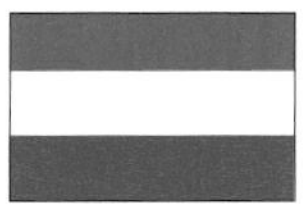

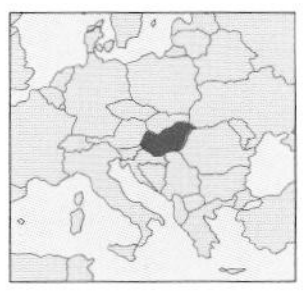

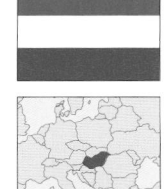

HUNGARY

GEOGRAPHY The Hungarian Republic is a landlocked country in central Europe. The land is mostly low-lying and drained by the Danube (Duna) and its tributary, the Tisza. Most of the land east of the Danube belongs to a region called the Great Plain (Nagyalföld), which covers about half of Hungary.

Hungary lies far from the moderating influence of the sea. As a result, summers are warmer and sunnier, and the winters colder than in Western Europe.

POLITICS & ECONOMY Hungary entered World War II (1939–45) in 1941, as an ally of Germany, but the Germans occupied the country in 1944. The Soviet Union invaded Hungary in 1944 and, in 1946, the country became a republic. The Communists gradually took over the government, taking complete control in 1949. From 1949, Hungary was an ally of the Soviet Union. In 1956, Soviet troops crushed an anti-Communist revolt. But in the 1980s, reforms in the Soviet Union led to the growth of anti-Communist groups in Hungary. In 1989, Hungary adopted a new constitution making it a multiparty state. Elections held in 1990 led to a victory for the non-Communist Democratic Forum. In 2002, the Hungarian Socialist Party, in alliance with the liberal Free Democrats, won a majority in parliament. In 2004, Hungary became a member of both the North Atlantic Treaty Organization and the European Union.

Before World War II, Hungary's economy was based mainly on agriculture. But the Communists set up many manufacturing industries. The new factories were owned by the government, as also was most of the land. However, from the late 1980s, the government has worked to increase private ownership. This change of policy caused many problems, including inflation and high rates of unemployment. Manufacturing is the chief activity. Major products include aluminum, chemicals, and electrical and electronic goods.

AREA 35,920 SQ MI [93,032 SQ KM] **POPULATION** 10,045,000
CAPITAL (POPULATION) BUDAPEST (1,825,000)
GOVERNMENT MULTIPARTY REPUBLIC
ETHNIC GROUPS MAGYAR 90%, GYPSY, GERMAN, SERB, ROMANIAN, SLOVAK **LANGUAGES** HUNGARIAN (OFFICIAL)
RELIGIONS ROMAN CATHOLIC 68%, CALVINIST 20%, LUTHERAN 5%, OTHERS **CURRENCY** FORINT = 100 FILLÉR

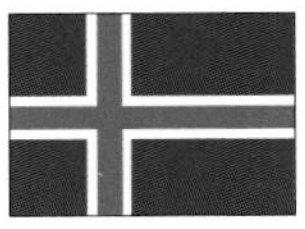

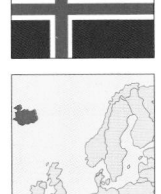

ICELAND

GEOGRAPHY The Republic of Iceland, in the North Atlantic Ocean, is closer to Greenland than Scotland. Iceland sits astride the Mid-Atlantic Ridge. It is slowly getting wider as the ocean is being stretched apart by continental drift.

Iceland has around 200 volcanoes, and eruptions are frequent. An eruption under the Vatnajökull ice cap in 1996 created a subglacial lake which subsequently burst, causing severe flooding. Geysers and hot springs are other common volcanic features. Ice caps and glaciers cover about an eighth of the land. The only habitable regions are the coastal lowlands.

Although it lies far to the north, Iceland's climate is moderated by the warm waters of the Gulf Stream. The port of Reykjavik is ice-free all the year round.

POLITICS & ECONOMY Norwegian Vikings colonized Iceland in AD 874, and in 930 the settlers founded the world's oldest parliament, the Althing.

Iceland united with Norway in 1262. But when Norway united with Denmark in 1380, Iceland came under Danish rule. Iceland became a self-governing kingdom, united with Denmark, in 1918. It became a fully independent republic in 1944, following a referendum in which 97% of the people voted to break their country's ties with Denmark.

Iceland has played an important part in European affairs and is a member of the North Atlantic Treaty Organization. Conflict with Britain over fishing rights have occurred since Iceland extended its territorial waters in the 1970s. Other fishing disputes with Norway, Russia and others continued in the 1990s.

Iceland has few resources besides the fishing grounds which surround it. Fishing and fish processing are major industries which dominate Iceland's overseas trade. Barely 1% of the land is used to grow crops, mainly root vegetables and fodder for livestock, but 23% of the country is used for grazing sheep and cattle. Vegetables and fruits are grown in greenhouses heated by water from hot springs.

AREA 39,768 SQ MI [103,000 SQ KM] **POPULATION** 281,000
CAPITAL (POPULATION) REYKJAVIK (108,000)
GOVERNMENT MULTIPARTY REPUBLIC
ETHNIC GROUPS ICELANDIC 97%, DANISH 1%
LANGUAGES ICELANDIC (OFFICIAL) **RELIGIONS** EVANGELICAL LUTHERAN 87%, OTHER PROTESTANT 4%, ROMAN CATHOLIC 2%, OTHERS
CURRENCY ICELANDIC KRÓNA = 100 AURAR

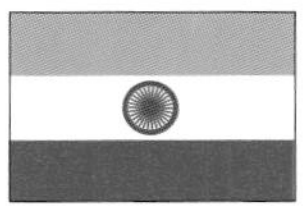

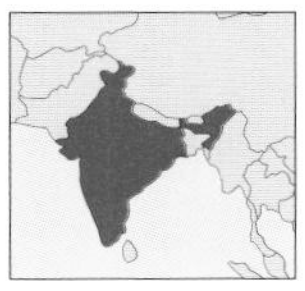

INDIA

GEOGRAPHY The Republic of India is the world's seventh largest country. In population, it ranks second only to China. The north is mountainous, with mountains and foothills of the Himalayan range. Rivers, such as the Brahmaputra and Ganges (Ganga), rise in the Himalaya and flow across the fertile northern plains. Southern India consists of a large plateau, called the Deccan. The Deccan is bordered by two mountain ranges, the Western Ghats and the Eastern Ghats.

India has three main seasons. The cool season runs from October to February. The hot season runs from March to June. The rainy monsoon season starts in the middle of June and continues into September. Delhi has a moderate rainfall, with about 25 in [640 mm] a year. The southwestern coast and the northeast have far more rain. Darjeeling in the northeast has an average annual rainfall of 120 in [3,040 mm]. But parts of the Thar Desert in the northwest have only 2 in [50 mm] of rain per year.

POLITICS & ECONOMY In southern India, most of the people are descendants of the dark-skinned Dravidians, who were among India's earliest people. Most northerners are descendants of lighter-skinned Aryans who arrived around 3,500 years ago.

India was the birthplace of several major religions, including Hinduism, Buddhism and Sikhism. Islam was introduced from about AD 1000. The Muslim Mughal empire was founded in 1526. From the 17th century, Britain began to gain influence. From 1858 to 1947, India was ruled as part of the British empire. An independence movement began after the Sepoy Rebellion (1857–9) and, in 1885, the Indian National Congress was formed. In 1920, Mohandas K. Gandhi became its leader and it soon became a mass movement. When independence was finally achieved in 1947, British India was divided into modern India and Muslim Pakistan. Partition was marred by mass slaughter as Hindus and Sikhs fled from Pakistan, and Indian Muslims poured into Pakistan. In the ensuing disputes, some 1 million people were killed.

Although India has 15 major languages and hundreds of minor ones, together with many religions, the country remains the world's largest democracy. It has faced many problems, especially with Pakistan, over the disputed territory of Jammu and Kashmir. Two wars in 1965 and 1972 failed to alter greatly the 1948 ceasefire lines. In the late 1980s, Kashmiri nationalists in the Indian-controlled area waged a campaign, demanding either integration into Pakistan or independence. India sent in troops and accused Pakistan of intervention. In the 1990s, Pakistani-backed guerrillas fought to break India's hold on the Srinigar valley, Kashmir's most populous region. The tense situation was further aggravated by the testing of nuclear devices by both India and Pakistan in 1998. In 2003–4, India and Pakistan launched a series of peace moves, raising hopes of an agreement, though conflict continued on the ground.

The World Bank classifies India as a "low-income" developing country. To boost the economy, the right-wing coalition government, led by the Hindu Bharatiya Janata Party, introduced free-enterprise policies in the 1990s. But the victory in 2004 of a left-wing coalition, led by the Congress Party, led to fears that economic reform might be halted.

Agriculture employs 64% of the people. Crops include rice, wheat, millet, sorghum, peas, and beans. India has more cattle than any other country. Milk is produced, but Hindus do not eat beef. Resources include coal, iron ore, and oil. Manufacturing has expanded greatly since 1947. Iron and steel, machinery, refined petroleum, textiles, and transport equipment are major products.

AREA 1,269,212 SQ MI [3,287,263 SQ KM] **POPULATION** 1,049,700,000
CAPITAL (POPULATION) NEW DELHI (295,000)
GOVERNMENT MULTIPARTY FEDERAL REPUBLIC
ETHNIC GROUPS INDO-ARYAN (CAUCASOID) 72%, DRAVIDIAN (ABORIGINAL) 25%, OTHERS (MAINLY MONGOLOID) 3%
LANGUAGES HINDI, ENGLISH, TELUGU, BENGALI, MARATHI, TAMIL, URDU, GUJARATI, MALAYALAM, KANNADA, ORIYA, PUNJABI, ASSAMESE, KASHMIRI, SINDHI AND SANSKRIT ARE ALL OFFICIAL LANGUAGES
RELIGIONS HINDUISM 82%, ISLAM 12%, CHRISTIANITY 2%, SIKHISM 2%, BUDDHISM AND OTHERS **CURRENCY** INDIAN RUPEE = 100 PAISA

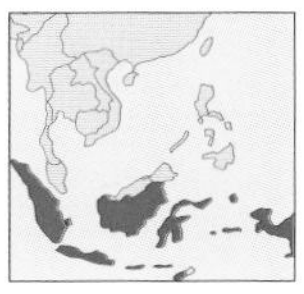

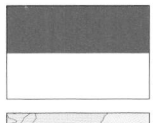

INDONESIA

GEOGRAPHY The Republic of Indonesia is an island nation in Southeast Asia. In all, Indonesia contains about 13,600 islands, less than 6,000 of which are inhabited. Three-quarters of the country is made up of five main areas: the islands of Sumatra, Java and Sulawesi (Celebes), together with Kalimantan (southern Borneo) and Irian Jaya (western New Guinea). The islands are generally mountainous and volcanic. The larger islands have extensive coastal lowlands. The climate is hot and humid, with a high rainfall. Only Java and the Sunda Islands have relatively dry seasons.

POLITICS & ECONOMY Indonesia is the world's most populous Muslim nation, though Islam was introduced as recently as the 15th century. The Dutch became active in the area in the early 17th century and Indonesia became a Dutch colony in 1799. After a long struggle, the Netherlands recognized Indonesia's independence in 1949. The economy has expanded, but ethnic and religious conflict have slowed down economic progress. In the early 21st century, Indonesia was facing many problems, arising from widespread corruption in the government and the army. Separatists were operating in Aceh province in northern Sumatra and in West Papua (formerly Irian Jaya), Christian-Muslim clashes led to loss of life in the Moluccas, and East (formerly Portuguese) Timor became an independent country in May 2002. In October 2002, terrorists bombed a night club in Bali. killing more than 180 people. Another suicide bombing took place in Jakarta in 2004.

Indonesia is a developing country. Its resources include oil, natural gas, tin and other minerals, its fertile volcanic soils, and its forests. Oil and gas are major exports. Timber, textiles, rubber, coffee, and tea are also exported. The principal food crop is rice. Manufacturing is increasing, particularly on Java.

AREA 735,354 SQ MI [1,904,569 SQ KM] **POPULATION** 234,893,000
CAPITAL (POPULATION) JAKARTA (9,374,000)
GOVERNMENT MULTIPARTY REPUBLIC
ETHNIC GROUPS JAVANESE 45%, SUNDANESE 14%, MADURESE 7%, COASTAL MALAYS 7%, APPROXIMATELY 300 OTHERS
LANGUAGES BAHASA INDONESIAN (OFFICIAL), MANY OTHERS
RELIGIONS ISLAM 88%, ROMAN CATHOLIC 3%, HINDUISM 2%, BUDDHISM 1%
CURRENCY INDONESIAN RUPIAH = 100 SEN

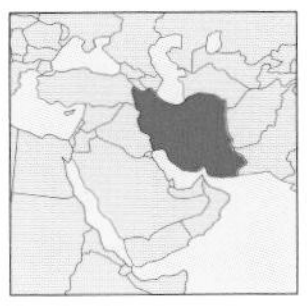

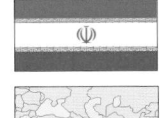

IRAN

GEOGRAPHY The Republic of Iran contains a barren central plateau which covers about half of the country. It includes the Dasht-e-Kavir (Great Salt Desert) and the Dasht-e-Lut (Great Sand Desert). The Elburz Mountains north of the plateau contain Iran's highest peak, Damavand, while narrow lowlands lie between the mountains and the Caspian Sea. West of the plateau are the Zagros Mountains, beyond which the land descends to the plains bordering the Persian Gulf.

Much of Iran has a severe, dry climate, with hot summers and cold winters. In Tehran, rain falls on only about 30 days in the year and the annual temperature range is more than 45°F [25°C]. The climate in the lowlands, however, is generally milder.

POLITICS & ECONOMY Iran was called Persia until 1935. The empire of Ancient Persia flourished between 550 and 350 BC, when it fell to Alexander the Great. Islam was introduced in AD 641.

Britain and Russia competed for influence in the area in the 19th century, and in the early 20th century the British began to develop the country's oil resources. In 1925, the Pahlavi family took power.

Reza Khan became shah (king) and worked to modernize the country. The Pahlavi dynasty was ended in 1979 when a religious leader, Ayatollah Ruhollah Khomeini, made Iran an Islamic republic. In 1980–8, Iran and Iraq fought a war over disputed borders. Khomeini died in 1989, but his fundamentalist views and anti-Western attitudes continued to dominate politics. In 1997, Mohammad Khatami, a liberal, was elected president, but conservative clerics made actual reform difficult. In 2003–4, Iran was in dispute with the international community over its nuclear energy program.

Iran's prosperity is based on its oil production and oil accounts for 95% of the country's exports. However, the economy was severely damaged by the Iran–Iraq war in the 1980s. Oil revenues have been used to develop a growing manufacturing sector. Agriculture is important even though farms cover only a tenth of the land. The main crops are wheat and barley. Livestock farming and fishing are other important activities, although Iran has to import much of the food it needs.

AREA 636,368 SQ MI [1,648,195 SQ KM] **POPULATION** 68,279,000
CAPITAL (POPULATION) TEHRAN (7,723,000)
GOVERNMENT ISLAMIC REPUBLIC **ETHNIC GROUPS** PERSIAN 51%, AZERI 24%, GILAKI AND MAZANDARANI 8%, KURD 7%, ARAB 3%, LUR 2%, BALUCHI 2%, TURKMEN 2% **LANGUAGES** PERSIAN 58%, TURKIC 26%, KURDISH **RELIGIONS** ISLAM (SHI'ITE MUSLIM 89%)
CURRENCY IRANIAN RIAL = 100 DINARS

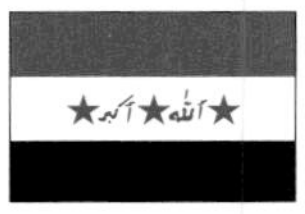
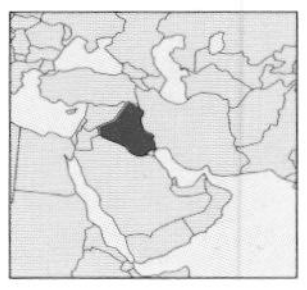

IRAQ

GEOGRAPHY The Republic of Iraq is a southwest Asian country at the head of the Persian Gulf. Rolling deserts cover western and southwestern Iraq, with part of the Zagros Mountains in the northeast, where farming can be practised without irrigation. The northern plains, across which flow the rivers Euphrates (Nahr al Furat) and Tigris (Nahr Dijlah), are dry. But the southern plains, including Mesopotamia, and the delta of the Shatt al Arab, the river formed south of Al Qurnah by the combined Euphrates and Tigris, contain irrigated farmland, together with marshes.

The climate of Iraq ranges from temperate in the north to subtropical in the south. Baghdad, in central Iraq, has cool winters, with occasional frosts, and hot summers. The rainfall is generally low.

POLITICS & ECONOMY Mesopotamia was the home of several great civilizations, including Sumer, Babylon and Assyria. It later became part of the Persian empire. Islam was introduced in AD 637 and Baghdad became the brilliant capital of the powerful Arab empire. But Mesopotamia declined after the Mongols invaded it in 1258. From 1534, Mesopotamia became part of the Turkish Ottoman empire. Britain invaded the area in 1916. In 1921, Britain renamed the country Iraq and set up an Arab monarchy. Iraq finally became independent in 1932.

By the 1950s, oil dominated Iraq's economy. In 1952, Iraq agreed to take 50% of the profits of the foreign oil companies. This revenue enabled the government to pay for welfare services and development projects. But many Iraqis felt that they should benefit more from their oil. Since 1958, when army officers killed the king and made Iraq a republic, Iraq has undergone turbulent times. In the 1960s, the Kurds, who live in northern Iraq and also in Iran, Turkey, Syria and Armenia, asked for self-rule. The government rejected their demands and war broke out. A peace treaty was signed in 1975, but conflict has continued.

In 1979, Saddam Hussein became Iraq's president. Under his leadership, Iraq invaded Iran in 1980, starting an eight-year war. Iraqi Kurds supported Iran and the Iraqi government attacked Kurdish villages with poison gas. In 1990, Iraqi troops occupied Kuwait, but an international force drove them out in 1991. Since 1991, Iraqi troops have attacked Shi'ite Marsh Arabs and Kurds. In 1998, Iraq's failure to permit UN inspectors, charged with disposing of Iraq's deadliest weapons, access to suspect sites led to the Western bombardment of Iraqi military sites. Another major offensive occurred in February 2001. In 2002 and 2003, pressure mounted on Iraq to dispose of its alleged weapons of mass destruction. In March 2003, a coalition force, headed by the United States, invaded Iraq. However, continuing conflict, even after the capture of Saddam Hussein in December 2003, put the planned transition to a democratic government in jeopardy.

Civil war, war damage in 1991 and 2003, UN sanctions and mismanagement have all contributed to economic chaos. Oil remains Iraq's main resource, but a UN trade embargo in 1990 halted oil exports. Farmland, including pasture, covers about a fifth of the land. Products include barley, cotton, dates, fruit, livestock, wheat, and wool, but Iraq still has to import food. Industries include oil refining and the manufacture of petrochemicals and consumer goods.

AREA 169,234 SQ MI [438,317 SQ KM] **POPULATION** 24,683,000
CAPITAL (POPULATION) BAGHDAD (5,605,000)
GOVERNMENT REPUBLIC **ETHNIC GROUPS** ARAB 77%, KURDISH 19%, ASSYRIAN AND OTHERS **LANGUAGES** ARABIC (OFFICIAL), KURDISH (OFFICIAL IN KURDISH AREAS), ASSYRIAN, ARMENIAN **RELIGIONS** ISLAM 97%, CHRISTIANITY AND OTHERS **CURRENCY** NEW IRAQI DINAR

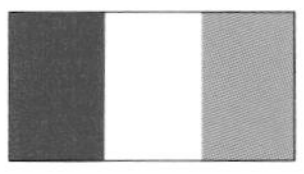
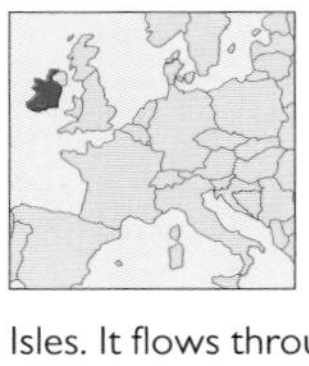

IRELAND

GEOGRAPHY The Republic of Ireland occupies five-sixths of the island of Ireland. The country consists of a large lowland region surrounded by a broken rim of low mountains. The uplands include the Mountains of Kerry where Carrauntoohill, Ireland's highest peak at 3,415 ft [1,041 m], is situated. The River Shannon is the longest in the British Isles. It flows through three large lakes, loughs Allen, Ree, and Derg.

Ireland has a mild, rainy climate influenced by the warm Gulf Stream current, whose effects are greatest in the west. However, Dublin in the east is cooler than places on the west coast.

POLITICS & ECONOMY In 1801, the Act of Union created the United Kingdom of Great Britain and Ireland. But Irish discontent intensified in the 1840s when a potato blight caused a famine in which a million people died and nearly a million emigrated. Britain was blamed for not having done enough to help. In 1916, an uprising in Dublin was crushed, but between 1919 and 1922 civil war occurred. In 1922, the Irish Free State was created as a Dominion in the British Commonwealth. But Northern Ireland remained part of the UK.

Ireland became a republic in 1949. Since then, Irish governments have sought to develop the economy, and it was for this reason that Ireland joined the European Community in 1973. In 1998, Ireland took part in the negotiations to produce a constitutional settlement in Northern Ireland. As part of the agreement, Ireland agreed to give up its constitutional claim on Northern Ireland. But the agreement proved difficult to implement.

Major farm products in Ireland include barley, cattle and dairy products, pigs, potatoes, poultry, sheep, sugar beet, and wheat, while fishing provides another valuable source of food. Farming is now profitable, aided by European Union grants, but manufacturing is the leading economic sector. Many factories produce food and beverages. Chemicals and pharmaceuticals, electronic equipment, machinery, paper, and textiles are also important.

AREA 27,132 SQ MI [70,273 SQ KM] **POPULATION** 3,924,000
CAPITAL (POPULATION) DUBLIN (482,000)
GOVERNMENT MULTIPARTY REPUBLIC **ETHNIC GROUPS** IRISH 94%
LANGUAGES IRISH (GAELIC) AND ENGLISH (BOTH OFFICIAL)
RELIGIONS ROMAN CATHOLIC 92%, PROTESTANT 3%
CURRENCY EURO = 100 CENTS

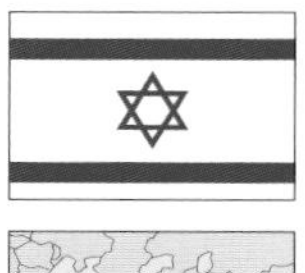
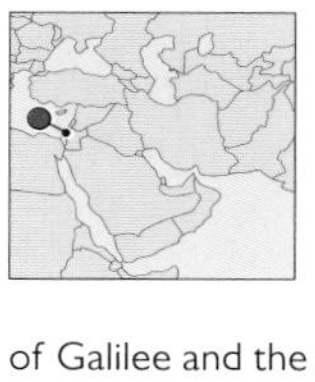

ISRAEL

GEOGRAPHY The State of Israel is a small country in the eastern Mediterranean. It includes a fertile coastal plain, where Israel's main industrial cities, Haifa (Hefa) and Tel Aviv-Jaffa are situated. Inland lie the Judaeo-Galilean highlands, which run from northern Israel to the northern tip of the Negev Desert. To the east lies part of the Great Rift Valley which contains the River Jordan, the Sea of Galilee and the Dead Sea. Summers are hot and dry. Winters on the coast are mild and moist, but the rainfall decreases from west to east and from north to south.

POLITICS & ECONOMY Israel is part of a region called Palestine. Some Jews have always lived in the area, though most modern Israelis are descendants of immigrants who began to settle there from the 1880s. Britain ruled Palestine from 1917. Large numbers of Jews escaping Nazi persecution arrived in the 1930s, provoking an Arab uprising against British rule. In 1947, the UN agreed to partition Palestine into an Arab and a Jewish state. Fighting broke out after Arabs rejected the plan. The State of Israel came into being in May 1948, but fighting continued into 1949. Other Arab-Israeli wars in 1956, 1967 and 1973 led to land gains for Israel.

In 1978, Israel signed a treaty with Egypt which led to the return of the occupied Sinai peninsula to Egypt in 1979. But conflict continued between Israel and the PLO (Palestine Liberation Organization). In 1993, the PLO and Israel agreed to establish Palestinian self-rule in two areas: the occupied Gaza Strip, and in the town of Jericho in the occupied West Bank. The agreement was extended in 1995 to include more than 30% of the West Bank. Israel's prime minister, Yitzhak Rabin, was assassinated in 1995. In 1996, his successor, Simon Peres, was defeated by the right-wing Benjamin Netanyahu, under whom the peace process stalled. In 1999, the left-wing Ehud Barak defeated Netanyahu and revived the peace process. But, following violence between the Palestinians and Israeli forces, Barak resigned. In 2001, Barak was defeated by the right-wing Ariel Sharon, who adopted a hardline policy against the Palestinians. In 2003, after Sharon won re-election, the United States exerted pressure on him to agree to the setting up of a Palestinian state.

Israel's most valuable activity is manufacturing and the country's products include chemicals, electronic equipment, fertilizers, military equipment, plastics, processed food, scientific instruments, and textiles. Fruits and vegetables are leading exports.

AREA 7,954 SQ MI [20,600 SQ KM] **POPULATION** 6,117,000
CAPITAL (POPULATION) JERUSALEM (685,000)
GOVERNMENT MULTIPARTY REPUBLIC **ETHNIC GROUPS** JEWISH 80%, ARAB AND OTHERS 20% **LANGUAGES** HEBREW AND ARABIC (BOTH OFFICIAL)
RELIGIONS JUDAISM 80%, ISLAM (MOSTLY SUNNI) 14%, CHRISTIANITY 2%, DRUZE AND OTHERS 2% **CURRENCY** NEW ISRAELI SHEKEL = 100 AGORAT

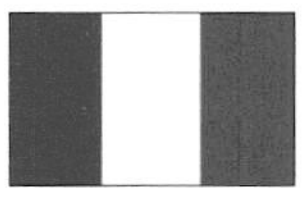
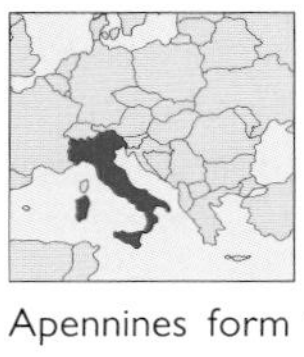

ITALY

GEOGRAPHY The Republic of Italy is famous for its history and traditions, its art and culture, and its beautiful scenery. Northern Italy is bordered in the north by the high Alps, with their many climbing and skiing resorts. The Alps overlook the northern plains – Italy's most fertile and densely populated region – drained by the River Po. The rugged Apennines form the backbone of southern Italy. Bordering the range are scenic hilly areas and coastal plains. Southern Italy contains a string of volcanoes, stretching from Vesuvius, through the Lipari Islands, to Etna on Sicily, the largest Mediterranean island. Northern Italy has cold, often snowy, winters, but the summer months are warm and sunny, with brief summer thunderstorms. Rainfall is abundant. The south has mild, moist winters and warm, dry summers.

POLITICS & ECONOMY Magnificent ruins throughout Italy testify to the glories of the ancient Roman Empire, which was founded, according to legend, in 753 BC. It reached its peak in the AD 100s. It finally collapsed in the 400s, although the Eastern Roman empire, also called the Byzantine empire, survived for another 1,000 years.

In the Middle Ages, Italy was split into many tiny states. These states made a great contribution to the revival of art and learning, called the Renaissance, in the 14th to 16th centuries. Beautiful cities, such as Florence (Firenze) and Venice (Venézia), testify to the artistic achievements of this period.

Italy finally became a united kingdom in 1861, although the Papal Territories (a large area ruled by the Roman Catholic Church) was not added until 1870. The Pope and his successors disputed the takeover of the Papal Territories. The dispute was finally resolved in 1929, when the Vatican City was set up in Rome as a fully independent state.

Italy fought in World War I (1914–18) alongside the Allies – Britain, France and Russia. In 1922, the dictator Benito Mussolini, leader of the Fascist party, took power. Under Mussolini, Italy conquered Ethiopia. During World War II (1939–45), Italy at first fought on Germany's side against the Allies. But in late 1943, Italy declared war on Germany. Italy became a republic in 1946. It has played an important part in European affairs. It was a founder member of the North Atlantic Treaty Organization (NATO) in 1949 and also of what has now become the European Union in 1958.

After the setting up of the European Union, Italy's economy developed quickly. But the country faced many problems. For example, much of the economic development was in the north. This forced many people to leave the poor south to find jobs in the north or abroad. Social problems, corruption at high levels of society, and a succession of weak coalition governments all contributed to instability. Elections in 1996 were won by the left-wing Olive Tree alliance led by Romano Prodi, who was replaced in 1998 by an ex-Communist, Massimo d'Alema, who tried but failed to introduce a two-party system. In 2001, a center-right coalition won a substantial majority in parliament and its leader, media tycoon Silvio Berlusconi, became prime minister.

Only 50 years ago, Italy was a mainly agricultural society. But today it is a leading industrial power. It lacks mineral resources, and imports most of the raw materials used in industry. Manufactures include textiles and clothing, processed food, machinery, cars, and chemicals. The chief industrial region is in the northwest.

Farmland covers around 42% of the land, pasture 17%, and forest and woodland 22%. Major crops include citrus fruits, grapes which are used to make wine, olive oil, sugar beet, and vegetables. Livestock farming is important, though meat is imported.

AREA 116,339 sq mi [301,318 sq km] **POPULATION** 57,998,000
CAPITAL (POPULATION) Rome (2,460,000)
GOVERNMENT Multiparty republic **ETHNIC GROUPS** Italian 94%, German, French, Albanian, Slovene, Greek **LANGUAGES** Italian (official), German, French, Slovene **RELIGIONS** Predominantly Roman Catholic **CURRENCY** Euro = 100 cents

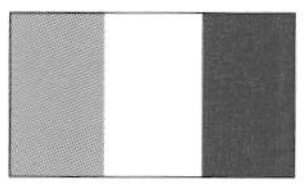

IVORY COAST

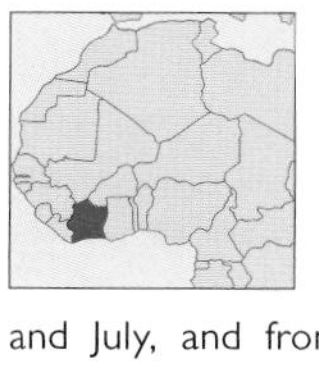

GEOGRAPHY The Republic of the Ivory Coast, in West Africa, is officially known as Côte d'Ivoire. The southeast coast is bordered by sand bars that enclose lagoons. The southwest coast is lined by rocky cliffs.

Ivory Coast has a hot and humid tropical climate, with high temperatures all year. The south has two rainy seasons: between May and July, and from October to November. Inland, the rainfall decreases and the north has one dry and one rainy season.

POLITICS & ECONOMY From 1895, Ivory Coast was governed as part of French West Africa, a massive union which also included what are now Benin, Burkina Faso, Guinea, Mali, Mauritania, Niger, and Senegal. In 1946, Ivory Coast became a territory in the French Union.

Ivory Coast became fully independent in 1960. Its first president, Félix Houphouët-Boigny, became the longest serving head of state in Africa with an uninterrupted period in office which ended with his death in 1993. Houphouët-Boigny, a pro-Western leader, made Ivory Coast a one-party state. In 1983, the National Assembly voted to make Yamoussoukro, the president's birthplace, the new capital. In 1999, a military coup occurred, but civilian rule was restored in 2000, when Laurent Gbagbo was elected president. An army rebellion began in September 2002. It continued into 2003 when a power-sharing coalition was set up, including members from rebel groups.

Agriculture employs about half of the people, and farm products make up nearly half the value of the exports. Manufacturing has grown in importance since 1960; products include fertilizers, processed food, refined oil, textiles, and timber.

AREA 124,503 sq mi [322,463 sq km] **POPULATION** 16,962,000
CAPITAL (POPULATION) Yamoussoukro (107,000)
GOVERNMENT Multiparty republic **ETHNIC GROUPS** Akan 42%, Voltaiques 18%, Northern Mandes 16%, Krous 11%, Southern Mandes 10% **LANGUAGES** French (official), many native dialects
RELIGIONS Islam 40%, Christianity 30%, traditional beliefs 30%
CURRENCY CFA franc = 100 centimes

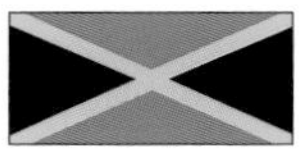

JAMAICA

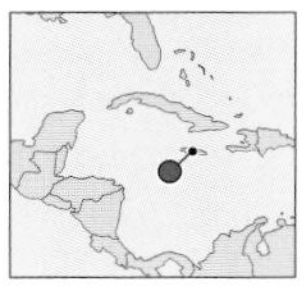

GEOGRAPHY Third largest of the Caribbean islands, half of Jamaica lies above 1,000 ft [300 m] and moist southeast trade winds bring rain to the central mountain range.

The "cockpit country" in the northwest of the island is an inaccessible limestone area of steep broken ridges and isolated basins.

POLITICS & ECONOMY Britain took Jamaica from Spain in the 17th century, and the island did not gain its independence until 1962. Some economic progress was made by the socialist government in the 1980s, but migration and unemployment remain high. Farming is the leading activity and sugarcane is the main crop, though bauxite production provides much of the country's income. Jamaica has some industries and tourism is a major industry.

AREA 4,244 sq mi [10,991 sq km] **POPULATION** 2,696,000
CAPITAL (POPULATION) Kingston (104,000)
GOVERNMENT Constitutional monarchy
ETHNIC GROUPS Black 91%, Mixed 7%, East Indian 1%
LANGUAGES English (official), patois English
RELIGIONS Protestant 61%, Roman Catholic 4%
CURRENCY Jamaican dollar = 100 cents

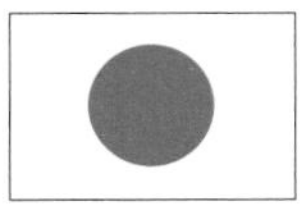

JAPAN

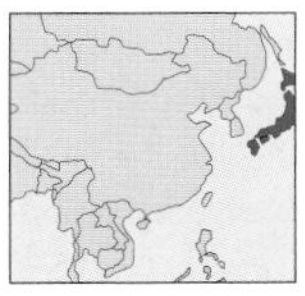

GEOGRAPHY Japan's four largest islands – Honshu, Hokkaido, Kyushu and Shikoku – make up 98% of the country. But Japan contains thousands of small islands. The four largest islands are mainly mountainous, while many of the small islands are the tips of volcanoes. Japan has more than 150 volcanoes, about 60 of which are active. Volcanic eruptions, earthquakes and tsunamis (destructive sea waves triggered by underwater earthquakes and eruptions) are common because the islands lie in an unstable part of our planet, where continental plates are always on the move. One powerful recent earthquake killed more than 5,000 people in Kobe in 1995.

The climate of Japan varies greatly from north to south. Hokkaido in the north has cold, snowy winters. At Sapporo, temperatures below 4°F [–20°C] have been recorded between December and March. But summers are warm, with temperatures sometimes exceeding 86°F [30°C]. Rain falls throughout the year, though Hokkaido is one of the driest parts of Japan. Tokyo has higher rainfall and temperatures, while the southern islands of Shikoku and Kyushu have warm temperate climates. Summers are long and hot. Winters are cold.

POLITICS & ECONOMY In the late 19th century, Japan began a program of modernization. Under its new imperial leaders, it began to look for lands to conquer. In 1894–5, it fought a war with China and, in 1904–5, it defeated Russia. Soon its overseas empire included Korea and Taiwan. In 1930, Japan invaded Manchuria (northeast China) and, in 1937, it began a war against China. In 1941, Japan launched an attack on the US base at Pearl Harbor in Hawaii. This drew both Japan and the United States into World War II.

Japan surrendered in 1945 when the Americans dropped atomic bombs on two cities, Hiroshima and Nagasaki. The United States occupied Japan until 1952. During this period, Japan adopted a democratic constitution. The emperor, who had previously been regarded as a god, became a constitutional monarch. Power was vested in the prime minister and cabinet, who are chosen from the Diet (elected parliament).

From the 1960s, Japan experienced many changes as the country rapidly built up new industries. By the early 1990s, Japan had become the world's second richest economic power after the US. But economic success has brought problems. For example, the rapid growth of cities has led to housing shortages and pollution. Another problem is that the proportion of people over 65 years of age is steadily increasing.

Japan has the world's second highest gross domestic product (GDP) after the United States. [The GDP is the total value of all goods and services produced in a country in one year.] The most important sector of the economy is industry. Yet Japan has to import most of the raw materials and fuels it needs for its industries. Its success is based on its use of the latest technology, its skilled and hard-working labor force, its vigorous export policies and its comparatively small government spending on defense. Manufactures dominate its exports, which include machinery, electrical and electronic equipment, vehicles and transport equipment, iron and steel, chemicals, textiles and ships. However, from the late 1990s, Japan experienced an economic slowdown, which merged in a recession in the early 21st century.

Japan is one of the world's top fishing nations and fish is an important source of protein. Because the land is so rugged, only 15% of the country can be farmed. Yet Japan produces about 70% of the food it needs. Rice is the chief crop, taking up about half of the total farmland. Other major products include fruits, sugar beet, tea, and vegetables. Livestock farming has increased since the 1950s.

AREA 145,880 sq mi [377,829 sq km] **POPULATION** 127,214,000
CAPITAL (POPULATION) Tokyo (8,130,000)
GOVERNMENT Constitutional monarchy
ETHNIC GROUPS Japanese 99%, Chinese, Korean, Brazilian and others
LANGUAGES Japanese (official) **RELIGIONS** Shintoism and Buddhism 84% (most Japanese consider themselves to be both Shinto and Buddhist), others **CURRENCY** Yen = 100 sen

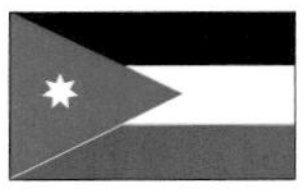

JORDAN

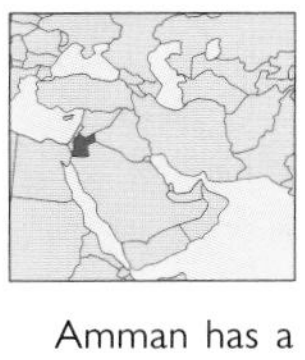

GEOGRAPHY The Hashemite Kingdom of Jordan is an Arab country in southwestern Asia. The Great Rift Valley in the west contains the River Jordan and the Dead Sea, which Jordan shares with Israel. East of the Rift Valley is the Transjordan plateau, where most Jordanians live. To the east and south lie vast areas of desert.

Amman has a much lower rainfall and longer dry season than the Mediterranean lands to the west. The Transjordan plateau, on which Amman stands, is a transition zone between the Mediterranean climate zone and the desert climate to the east.

POLITICS & ECONOMY In 1921, Britain created a territory called Transjordan east of the River Jordan. In 1923, Transjordan became self-governing, but Britain retained control of its defenses, finances, and foreign affairs. This territory became fully independent as Jordan in 1946. Jordan has suffered from instability arising from the Arab–Israeli conflict since the creation of the State of Israel in 1948. After the first Arab–Israeli War in 1948–9, Jordan acquired East Jerusalem and a fertile area called the West Bank. In 1967, Israel occupied this area. In Jordan, the presence of Palestinian refugees led to civil war in 1970–1.

In 1974, Arab leaders declared that the PLO (Palestine Liberation Organization) was the sole representative of the Palestinian people. In 1988, King Hussein of Jordan renounced Jordan's claims to the West Bank and passed responsibility for it to the PLO. Opposition parties were legalized in 1991 and elections were held in 1993. In October 1994, Jordan and Israel signed a peace treaty, ending a state of war that had lasted more than 40 years. Jordan's King Hussein commanded respect for his role in Middle Eastern affairs until his death in 1999. He was succeeded by his eldest son, who became Abdullah II. As king, he continued Jordan's efforts to further the Israel–Palestinian peace process. He also supported the US-declared war on terrorism.

Jordan lacks natural resources, apart from phosphates and potash, and the economy depends substantially on aid. The World Bank classifies Jordan as a "lower-middle-income" developing country. Because of the dry climate, less than 6% of the land is farmed or used as pasture. Jordan has an oil refinery and manufactures include cement, pharmaceuticals, processed food, fertilizers, and textiles.

AREA 34,495 sq mi [89,342 sq km] **POPULATION** 5,460,000
CAPITAL (POPULATION) Amman (1,253,000)
GOVERNMENT Constitutional monarchy **ETHNIC GROUPS** Arab 98%, of which Palestinians make up roughly half **LANGUAGES** Arabic (official) **RELIGIONS** Islam (mostly Sunni) 94%, Christianity (mostly Greek Orthodox) 6% **CURRENCY** Jordanian dinar = 1,000 fils

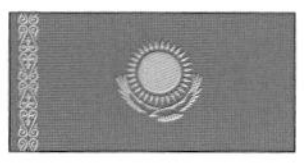

KAZAKHSTAN

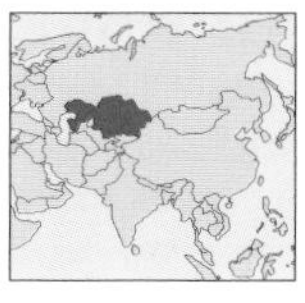

GEOGRAPHY Kazakhstan is a large country in west-central Asia. In the west, the Caspian Sea lowlands include the Karagiye depression, which reaches 433 ft [132 m] below sea level. The lowlands extend eastward through the Aral Sea area. The north contains high plains, but the highest land is along the eastern and southern borders. These areas include parts of the Altai and Tian Shan mountain ranges. Eastern Kazakhstan contains several freshwater lakes, the largest of which is Lake Balkhash. The water in the rivers has been used for irrigation, causing ecological problems. For example, the Aral Sea, deprived of water, shrank from 25,830 sq mi [66,900 sq km] in 1960 to 12,989 sq mi [33,642 sq km] in 1993. Large areas are now barren desert.

Kazakhstan lies far from the moderating influence of the oceans and it has an extreme climate. Winters are cold and snow covers the land for about 100 days at Almaty. The rainfall is generally low.

POLITICS & ECONOMY After the Russian Revolution of 1917, many Kazakhs wanted to make their country independent. But the Communists prevailed and in 1936 Kazakhstan became a republic of the Soviet Union, called the Kazakh Soviet Socialist Republic. During World War II and also after the war, the Soviet government moved many people from the west into Kazakhstan. From the 1950s, people were encouraged to work on a "Virgin Lands" project, which involved bringing large areas of grassland under cultivation.

Reforms in the Soviet Union in the 1980s led to its breakup in December 1991. Kazakhstan maintained contacts with Russia through the Commonwealth of Independent States (CIS). In 1997, the government moved its capital from Almaty to Aqmola (later renamed Astana), a town in the Russian-dominated north. It hoped that this would bring some Kazakh identity to the area. In the early 21st century, Kazakhstan's economy was in better shape than any other of the Central Asian ex-Soviet republics. However, its President Nursultan Nazarbaev was criticized for cracking down on political dissent and independent newspapers.

The World Bank classifies Kazakhstan as a "lower-middle-income" developing country. Livestock farming, especially sheep and cattle, is an important activity, and major crops include barley, cotton, rice and wheat. The country is rich in mineral resources, including coal and oil reserves, together with bauxite, copper, lead, tungsten, and zinc. Manufactures include chemicals, food products, machinery, and textiles. Oil is exported via a pipeline through Russia; however, to reduce dependence on Russia, Kazakhstan signed an agreement in 1997 to build a new pipeline to China. Other exports include metals, chemicals, grain, wool, and meat.

AREA 1,052,084 sq mi [2,724,900 sq km] **POPULATION** 16,764,000
CAPITAL (POPULATION) Astana (322,000) **GOVERNMENT** Multiparty republic **ETHNIC GROUPS** Kazakh 53%, Russian 30%, Ukrainian 4%, German 2%, Uzbek 2% **LANGUAGES** Kazakh (official); Russian, the former official language, is widely spoken **RELIGIONS** Islam 47%, Russian Orthodox 44% **CURRENCY** Tenge = 100 tiyn

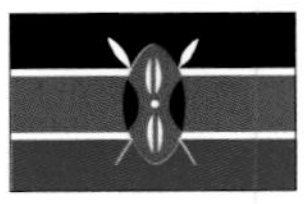
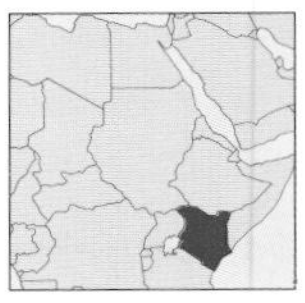

KENYA

GEOGRAPHY The Republic of Kenya is a country in East Africa which straddles the Equator. Behind the narrow coastal plain on the Indian Ocean, the land rises to high plains and highlands, broken by volcanic mountains, including Mount Kenya, the country's highest peak at 17,057 ft [5,199 m]. Crossing the country is an arm of the Great Rift Valley, on the floor of which are several lakes, including Baringo, Magadi, Naivasha, Nakuru and, on the northern frontier, Lake Turkana (formerly Lake Rudolf).

Mombasa on the coast is hot and humid. But inland, the climate is moderated by the height of the land. As a result, Nairobi, in the thickly populated southwestern highlands, has summer temperatures which are 18°F [10°C] lower than Mombasa. Nights can be cool, but temperatures do not fall below freezing. Nairobi's main rainy season is from April to May, with "little rains" in November and December. However, only about 15% of the country has a reliable rainfall of 31 in [800 mm].

POLITICS & ECONOMY The Kenyan coast has been a trading center for more than 2,000 years. Britain took over the coast in 1895 and soon extended its influence inland. In the 1950s, a secret movement, called Mau Mau, launched an armed struggle against British rule. Although Mau Mau was eventually defeated, Kenya became independent in 1963.

Many Kenyans felt that Kenya should have a strong central government, and Kenya was a one-party state for much of the time since 1963. But democracy was restored in the early 1990s and elections were held in 1992, 1997, and 2002. In 1999, Kenya, with Tanzania and Uganda, set up an East African Community, which aimed to create a customs union, a common market, a monetary union, and, ultimately, a political union.

According to the United Nations, Kenya is a "low-income" developing country. Agriculture employs about 80% of the people, but many Kenyans are subsistence farmers, growing little more than they need to support their families. The chief food crop is maize. The main cash crops and leading exports are coffee and tea. Manufactures include chemicals, leather and footwear, processed food, petroleum products, and textiles.

AREA 224,080 sq mi [580,367 sq km] **POPULATION** 31,639,000
CAPITAL (POPULATION) Nairobi (2,143,000)
GOVERNMENT Multiparty republic **ETHNIC GROUPS** Kikuyu 22%, Luhya 14%, Luo 13%, Kalenjin 12%, Kamba 11%, others
LANGUAGES Kiswahili and English (both official)
RELIGIONS Protestant 45%, Roman Catholic 33%, traditional beliefs 10%, Islam 10% **CURRENCY** Kenyan shilling = 100 cents

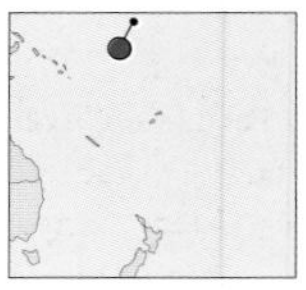

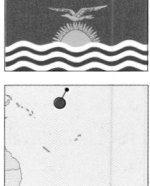

KIRIBATI

The Republic of Kiribati comprises three groups of corall atolls scattered over about 2 million sq mi [5 million sq km]. Kiribati straddles the equator and temperatures are high and the rainfall is abundant.

Formerly part of the British Gilbert and Ellice Islands, Kiribati became independent in 1979. The main export is copra and the country depends heavily on foreign aid.

AREA 280 sq mi [726 sq km] **POPULATION** 99,000 **CAPITAL** Tarawa

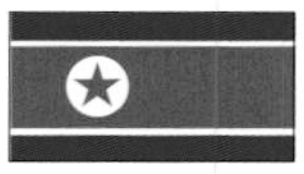
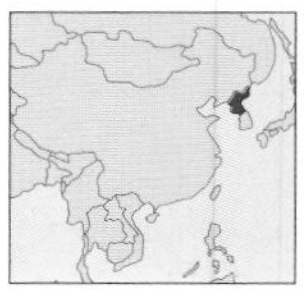

KOREA, NORTH

GEOGRAPHY The Democratic People's Republic of Korea occupies the northern part of the Korean peninsula which extends south from northeastern China. Mountains form the heart of the country, with the highest peak, Paektu-san, reaching 9,003 ft [2,744 m] on the northern border.

North Korea has a fairly severe climate, with bitterly cold winters when winds blow from across central Asia, bringing snow and freezing conditions. In summer, moist winds from the oceans bring rain.

POLITICS & ECONOMY North Korea was created in 1945, when the peninsula, which had been a Japanese colony since 1910, was divided into two parts. Soviet forces occupied the north, with US forces in the south. Soviet occupation led to a Communist government being established in 1948 under the leadership of Kim Il Sung. He initiated a Stalinist regime in which he assumed the role of dictator, and a personality cult developed around him. He was to become the world's most durable Communist leader.

The Korean War began in June 1950 when North Korean troops invaded the south. North Korea, aided by China and the Soviet Union, fought with South Korea, which was supported by troops from the United States and other UN members. The war ended in July 1953. An armistice was signed but no permanent peace treaty was agreed. The end of the Cold War in the late 1990s eased the situation. North and South Korea joined the United Nations in 1991 and they made several agreements, including one in which they agreed not to use force against each other. However, North Korea remained as isolated as ever.

In 1993, North Korea began a new international crisis by announcing that it was withdrawing from the Nuclear Non-Proliferation Treaty. This led to suspicions that North Korea, which had signed the Treaty in 1985, was developing its own nuclear weapons. Kim Il Sung, who had ruled as a virtual dictator from 1948 until his death in 1994, was succeeded by his son, Kim Jong Il. In the early 2000s, attempts were made to reconcile the two Koreas, though the prospect of reunification seemed remote. In 2003, North Korea's relations with the United States deteriorated sharply when the US accused North Korea of developing nuclear weapons.

North Korea's resources include coal, copper, iron ore, lead, tin tungsten and zinc. Under Communism, the country developed heavy, state-owned industries. Manufactures include chemicals, iron and steel, machinery, processed food, and textiles. Agriculture employs 32% of the people and rice is the chief crop. Economic mismanagement and successive floods in 1995 and 1996, and a drought in 1997, caused severe famine.

AREA 46,540 sq mi [120,538 sq km] **POPULATION** 22,466,000
CAPITAL (POPULATION) Pyŏngyang (2,725,000)
GOVERNMENT Single-party people's republic
ETHNIC GROUPS Korean 99%
LANGUAGES Korean (official)
RELIGIONS Buddhism and Confucianism
CURRENCY North Korean won = 100 chon

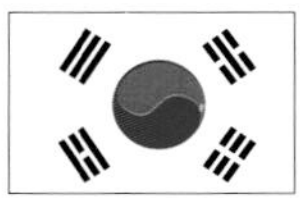
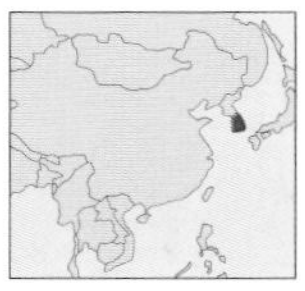

KOREA, SOUTH

GEOGRAPHY The Republic of Korea, as South Korea is officially known, occupies the southern part of the Korean peninsula. Mountains cover much of the country. The southern and western coasts are major farming regions. Many islands are found along the west and south coasts. The largest of these is Cheju-do, which contains South Korea's highest peak, Halla-San, which rises to 6,398 ft [1,950 m].

Like North Korea, South Korea is chilled in winter by cold, dry winds blowing from central Asia. Snow often covers the mountains in the east. The summers are hot and wet, especially in July and August.

POLITICS & ECONOMY After Japan's defeat in World War II (1939–45), North Korea was occupied by troops from the Soviet Union, while South Korea was occupied by United States forces. Attempts to reunify Korea failed and, in 1948, a National Assembly was elected in South Korea. This Assembly created the Republic of Korea, while North Korea became a Communist state. North Korean troops invaded the South in June 1950, sparking off the Korean War (1950–3).

In the 1950s, South Korea had a weak economy, which had been further damaged by the destruction caused by the Korean War. From the 1960s to the 1980s, South Korean governments worked to industrialize the economy. The governments were dominated by military leaders, who often used authoritarian methods and flouted human rights. In 1987, a new constitution was approved, enabling presidential elections to be held every five years. In 1991, South and North Korea became members of the United Nations and they signed agreements, including one in which they agreed not to use force against each other. Tensions continued, though hopes were raised when negotiations between the two countries took place in the early 21st century.

The World Bank classifies South Korea as an "upper-middle-income" developing country. It is also one of the world's fastest growing industrial economies. The country's resources include coal and tungsten, and its main manufactures are processed food and textiles. Since partition, heavy industries have been built up, making chemicals, fertilizers, iron and steel, and ships. South Korea has also developed the production of such things as computers, cars, and television sets. But, in late 1997, the expansion of the economy was halted by a market crash which affected many of the booming economies of eastern Asia. However, South Korea recovered faster than any other country in the region.

Farming remains important in South Korea. Rice is the chief crop, together with fruits, grains and vegetables, while fishing provides a major source of protein.

AREA 38,327 sq mi [99,268 sq km] **POPULATION** 48,289,000
CAPITAL (POPULATION) Seoul (10,231,000)
GOVERNMENT Multiparty republic **ETHNIC GROUPS** Korean 99%
LANGUAGES Korean (official) **RELIGIONS** No affiliation 46%, Christianity 26%, Buddhism 26%, Confucianism 1%
CURRENCY South Korean won = 100 chon

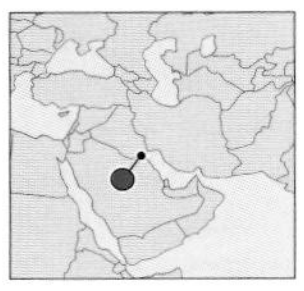

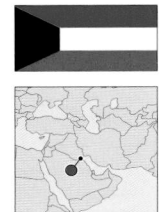

KUWAIT

The State of Kuwait at the north end of the Persian Gulf is an emirate (ruled by an emir or amir). The land is low-lying and largely desert. Summer temperatures are high but winters are cooler. The rainfall is low.

POLITICS & ECONOMY British influence began in 1775 and, in 1899, the local ruler concluded a treaty with Britain, agreeing to support British interests in return for British protection. Kuwait became independent in 1961. Its revenue from its oil exports made it highly prosperous. Iraq invaded Kuwait in 1990 and much damage was inflicted in 1991 when Kuwait was liberated by a coalition force. In the 1990s, reforms were introduced to make the country more democratic and raise the status of women. However, conservative Islamists, who opposed the reforms, won elections in 2003.

AREA 6,880 sq mi [17,818 sq km] **POPULATION** 2,183,000
CAPITAL (POPULATION) Kuwait City (29,000)

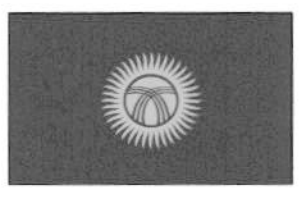
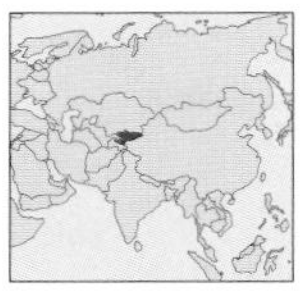

KYRGYZSTAN

GEOGRAPHY The Republic of Kyrgyzstan is a landlocked country between China, Tajikistan, Uzbekistan and Kazakhstan. The country is mountainous, with spectacular scenery. The highest mountain, Pik Pobedy in the Tian Shan range, reaches 24,406 ft [7,439 m] in the east. The lowlands have warm summers and cold winters. But January temperatures in the mountains plummet to –18°F [–28°C]. Kyrgyzstan has a low annual rainfall.

POLITICS & ECONOMY In 1876, Kyrgyzstan became a province of Russia and Russian settlement in the area began. In 1916, Russia crushed a rebellion among the Kyrgyz, and many subsequently fled to China. In 1922, the area became an autonomous oblast (self-governing region) of the newly formed Soviet Union but, in 1936, it became one of the Soviet Socialist Republics. Under Communist rule, local customs and religious worship were suppressed, but education and health services were greatly improved.

In 1991, Kyrgyzstan became an independent country following the breakup of the Soviet Union. The Communist party was dissolved, but the country maintained ties with Russia through an organization called the Commonwealth of Independent States. Kyrgyzstan adopted a new constitution in 1994 and parliamentary elections were held in 1995. In the early 21st century, many people were alarmed when Islamic guerrillas sought to set up an Islamic state in the Fergana valley, where Kyrgyzstan borders Tajikistan and Uzbekistan.

In the early 1990s, when Kyrgyzstan was working to reform its economy, the World Bank classified it as a "lower-middle-income" developing country. Agriculture, especially livestock rearing, is the chief activity. The chief products include cotton, eggs, fruits, grain, tobacco, vegetables, and wool. But food must be imported. Industries are mainly concentrated around the capital Bishkek.

AREA 77,181 sq mi [199,900 sq km] **POPULATION** 4,893,000
CAPITAL (POPULATION) Bishkek (753,000) **GOVERNMENT** Multiparty republic **ETHNIC GROUPS** Kyrgyz 65%, Russian 13%, Uzbek 13%
LANGUAGES Kyrgyz and Russian (both official) **RELIGIONS** Islam 75%, Russian Orthodox 20% **CURRENCY** Som = 100 tyiyn

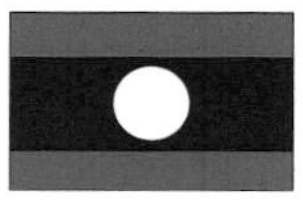
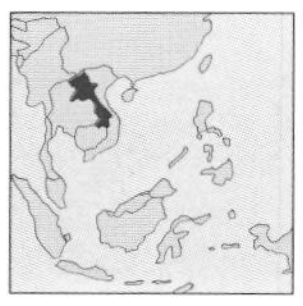

LAOS

GEOGRAPHY The Lao People's Democratic Republic is a landlocked country in Southeast Asia. Mountains and plateaux cover much of the country. Most people live on the plains bordering the River Mekong and its tributaries. This river, one of Asia's longest, forms much of the country's northwestern and south-western borders.

Laos has a tropical monsoon climate.

Winters are dry and sunny, with winds blowing in from the northeast. The temperatures rise until April, when the wind directions are reversed and moist southwesterly winds reach Laos, heralding the start of the wet monsoon season.

POLITICS & ECONOMY France made Laos a protectorate in the late 19th century and ruled it as part of French Indochina, a region which also included Cambodia and Vietnam. Laos became a member of the French Union in 1948 and an independent kingdom in 1954.

After independence, Laos suffered from instability caused by a long power struggle between royalist government forces and a pro-Communist group called the Pathet Lao. A civil war broke out in 1960 and continued into the 1970s. The Pathet Lao took control in 1975 and the king abdicated. Laos then came under the influence of Communist Vietnam, which had used Laos as a supply base during the Vietnam War (1957–75). From the early 1980s, the economy deteriorated and opposition appeared when bombings occurred in Vientiane in 2000. They were attributed to rebels in the minority Hmong tribe or to politicians who wanted faster economic reforms.

Laos is one of the world's poorest countries. Agriculture employs about 76% of the people, compared with 7% in industry and 17% in services. Rice is the main crop, and timber and coffee are both exported. But the most valuable export is electricity, which is produced at hydroelectric power stations on the River Mekong and is exported to Thailand. Laos also produces opium.

AREA 91,428 SQ MI [236,800 SQ KM] **POPULATION** 5,922,000
CAPITAL (POPULATION) VIENTIANE (528,000)
GOVERNMENT SINGLE-PARTY REPUBLIC
ETHNIC GROUPS LAO LOUM 68%, LAO THEUNG 22%, LAO SOUNG 9%
LANGUAGES LAO (OFFICIAL), FRENCH, ENGLISH **RELIGIONS** BUDDHISM 60%, TRADITIONAL BELIEFS AND OTHERS 40% **CURRENCY** KIP = 100 AT

LATVIA

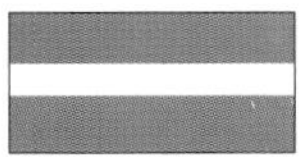
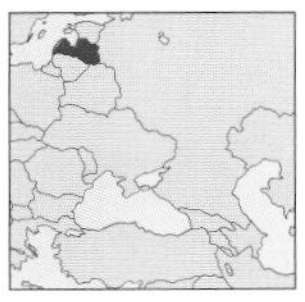

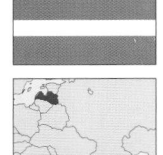

GEOGRAPHY The Republic of Latvia is one of three states on the southeastern corner of the Baltic Sea which were ruled as parts of the Soviet Union between 1940 and 1991. Latvia consists mainly of flat plains separated by low hills, composed of moraine (ice-worn rocks).

Riga has warm summers, but the winter months (from December to March) are subzero. In the winter, the sea often freezes over. The rainfall is moderate and it occurs throughout the year, with light snow in winter.

POLITICS & ECONOMY In 1800, Russia was in control of Latvia, but Latvians declared their independence after World War I. In 1940, under a German-Soviet pact, Soviet troops occupied Latvia, but they were driven out by the Germans in 1941. Soviet troops returned in 1944 and Latvia became part of the Soviet Union. Under Soviet rule, many Russian immigrants settled in Latvia and many Latvians feared that the Russians would become the dominant ethnic group.

In the late 1980s, when reforms were being introduced in the Soviet Union, Latvia's government ended absolute Communist rule and made Latvian the official language. In 1990, it declared the country to be independent, an act which was finally recognized by the Soviet Union in September 1991.

Latvia held its first free elections to its parliament (the Saeima) in 1993. Voting was limited only to citizens of Latvia on June 17, 1940, and their descendants. This meant that about 34% of Latvian residents were unable to vote. In 1994, Latvia restricted the naturalization of non-Latvians, including many Russian settlers, who were not allowed to vote or own land. However, in 1998, the government agreed that all children born since independence should have automatic citizenship. Its cultivation of closer ties to the West was realized in 2004 when Latvia was admitted to membership of both the North Atlantic Treaty Organization and the European Union.

The World Bank classifies Latvia as a "lower-middle-income" country and, in the 1990s, it faced many problems in turning its economy into a free-market system. Products include electronic goods, farm machinery, fertilizers, processed food, plastics, radios, and vehicles. Latvia produces only about a tenth of the electricity it needs. It imports the rest from Belarus, Russia, and Ukraine.

AREA 24,942 SQ MI [64,600 SQ KM] **POPULATION** 2,349,000
CAPITAL (POPULATION) RIGA (793,000)
GOVERNMENT MULTIPARTY REPUBLIC
ETHNIC GROUPS LATVIAN 58%, RUSSIAN 30%, BELARUSIAN, UKRAINIAN, POLISH, LITHUANIAN **LANGUAGES** LATVIAN (OFFICIAL), LITHUANIAN, RUSSIAN **RELIGIONS** LUTHERAN, ROMAN CATHOLIC, RUSSIAN ORTHODOX
CURRENCY LATVIAN LAT = 10 SANTIMI

LEBANON

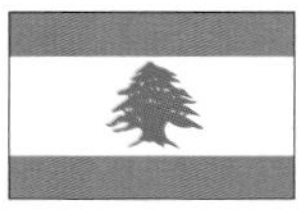
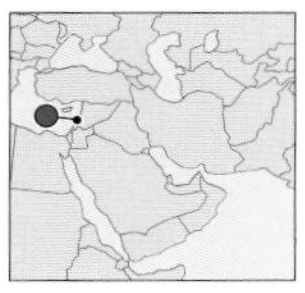

GEOGRAPHY The Republic of Lebanon is a country on the eastern shores of the Mediterranean Sea. Behind the coastal plain are the rugged Lebanon Mountains (Jabal Lubnan), which rise to 10,131 ft [3,088 m]. Another range, the Anti-Lebanon Mountains (Al Jabal Ash Sharqi), form the eastern border with Syria. Between the two ranges is the Bekaa (Beqaa) Valley, a fertile farming region.

The Lebanese coast has the hot, dry summers and mild, wet winters that are typical of many Mediterranean lands. Inland, onshore winds bring heavy rain to the western slopes of the mountains in the winter months, with snow at the higher altitudes.

POLITICS & ECONOMY Lebanon was ruled by Turkey from 1516 until World War I. France ruled the country from 1923, but Lebanon became independent in 1946. After independence, the Muslims and Christians agreed to share power, and Lebanon made rapid economic progress. But from the late 1950s, development was slowed by periodic conflict between Sunni and Shia Muslims, Druze and Christians. The situation was further complicated by the presence of Palestinian refugees who used bases in Lebanon to attack Israel.

In 1975, civil war broke out as private armies representing the many factions struggled for power. This led to intervention by Israel in the south and Syria in the north. UN peacekeeping forces arrived in 1978, but bombings, assassinations, and kidnappings became almost everyday events in the 1980s. From 1991, Lebanon enjoyed an uneasy peace. But, Israel continued to occupy an area in the south. In the 1990s, Israel launched several attacks on pro-Iranian Hezbollah guerrillas in Lebanon, but all Israeli troops were withdrawn in May 2000.

Lebanon's civil war almost destroyed valuable trade and financial services that had been Lebanon's chief source of income, together with tourism. Manufacturing, formerly a major activity, was badly hit.

AREA 4,015 SQ MI [10,400 SQ KM] **POPULATION** 3,728,000
CAPITAL (POPULATION) BEIRUT (1,148,000)
GOVERNMENT MULTIPARTY REPUBLIC **ETHNIC GROUPS** ARAB 95%, ARMENIAN 4%, OTHERS **LANGUAGES** ARABIC (OFFICIAL), FRENCH, ENGLISH, ARMENIAN **RELIGIONS** ISLAM 70%, CHRISTIANITY 30%
CURRENCY LEBANESE POUND = 100 PIASTRES

LESOTHO

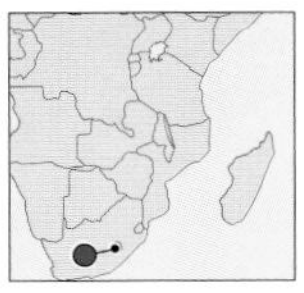

GEOGRAPHY The Kingdom of Lesotho is a landlocked country, completely enclosed by South Africa. The land is mountainous, rising to 11,424 ft [3,482 m] on the northeastern border. The Drakensberg range covers most of the country.

The climate of Lesotho is greatly affected by the altitude, because most of the country lies above 4,921 ft [1,500 m]. Summers are warm but winters are cold. The rainfall averages about 28 in [700 mm].

POLITICS & ECONOMY The Basotho nation was founded in the 1820s by King Moshoeshoe I, who united various groups fleeing from tribal wars in southern Africa. Britain made the area a protectorate in 1868 and, in 1871, placed it under the British Cape Colony in South Africa. But in 1884, Basutoland, as the area was called, was reconstituted as a British protectorate, where whites were not allowed to own land.

The country finally became independent in 1966 as the Kingdom of Lesotho, with Moshoeshoe II, great-grandson of Moshoeshoe I, as its king. Since independence, Lesotho has suffered instability. The military seized power in 1986 and stripped Moshoeshoe II of his powers in 1990, installing his son, Letsie III, as monarch. After elections in 1993, Moshoeshoe II was restored to office in 1995. But after his death in a car crash in 1996, Letsie III again became king. In 1998, an army revolt, following an election in which the ruling party won 79 out of the 80 seats, caused much damage to the economy, despite the intervention of a South African force. Lesotho also faces a health crisis. By 2003, an estimated 31% of all adults were infected with the HIV virus.

Lesotho is a "low-income" developing country. It lacks natural resources. Agriculture, mainly at subsistence level, light manufacturing and money sent home by Basotho working abroad are the main sources of income.

AREA 11,720 SQ MI [30,355 SQ KM] **POPULATION** 1,862,000
CAPITAL (POPULATION) MASERU (109,000)
GOVERNMENT CONSTITUTIONAL MONARCHY
ETHNIC GROUPS SOTHO 99% **LANGUAGES** SESOTHO AND ENGLISH (BOTH OFFICIAL) **RELIGIONS** CHRISTIANITY 80%, TRADITIONAL BELIEFS 20%
CURRENCY LOTI = 100 LISENTE

LIBERIA

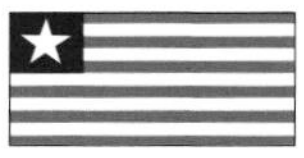
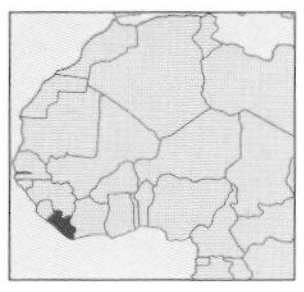

GEOGRAPHY The Republic of Liberia is a country in West Africa. Behind the coastline, 311 mi [500 km] long, lies a narrow coastal plain. Beyond, the land rises to a plateau region, with the highest land along the border with Guinea. Liberia has a tropical climate with high temperatures and high humidity all through the year. The rainfall is abundant all year round, but there is a particularly wet period from June to November. The rainfall generally increases from east to west.

POLITICS & ECONOMY In the late 18th century, some white Americans in the United States wanted to help freed black slaves to return to Africa. In 1816, they set up the American Colonization Society, which bought land in what is now Liberia.

In 1822, the Society landed former slaves at a settlement on the coast which they named Monrovia. In 1847, Liberia became a fully independent republic with a constitution much like that of the United States. For many years, the Americo-Liberians controlled the country's government. US influence remained strong and the American Firestone Company, which ran Liberia's rubber plantations, was especially influential. Foreign companies were also involved in exploiting Liberia's mineral resources, including its huge iron-ore deposits.

In 1980, a military group composed of people from the local population killed the Americo-Liberian president, William R. Tolbert. An army sergeant, Samuel K. Doe, was made president of Liberia. Elections held in 1985 resulted in victory for Doe. From 1989, the country was plunged into civil war between various ethnic groups. Doe was assassinated in 1990 and the struggle with rebel groups continued. West African peacekeeping forces arrived in Liberia and, in 1995, a ceasefire was agreed. A council of state, composed of former warlords, was set up and, in 1997, one of the warlords, Charles Taylor, was elected president. A ceasefire followed in 1998, but unrest continued. Another ceasefire was declared in 2003. Soon afterward, Taylor resigned and went into exile.

Liberia's civil war devastated its economy. Three out of every four people depend on agriculture, though many of them grow little more than they need to feed their families. Major food crops include cassava, rice, and sugarcane, while rubber, cocoa, and coffee are exported. But the most valuable export is iron ore.

Liberia also obtains revenue from its "flag of convenience," which is used by about one-sixth of the world's commercial shipping, exploiting low taxes.

AREA 43,000 SQ MI [111,369 SQ KM] **POPULATION** 3,317,000
CAPITAL (POPULATION) MONROVIA (421,000)
GOVERNMENT MULTIPARTY REPUBLIC **ETHNIC GROUPS** INDIGENOUS AFRICAN TRIBES 95% (INCLUDING KPELLE, BASSA, GREBO, GIO, KRU, MANO)
LANGUAGES ENGLISH (OFFICIAL), ETHNIC LANGUAGES
RELIGIONS CHRISTIANITY 40%, ISLAM 20%, TRADITIONAL BELIEFS AND OTHERS 40% **CURRENCY** LIBERIAN DOLLAR = 100 CENTS

LIBYA

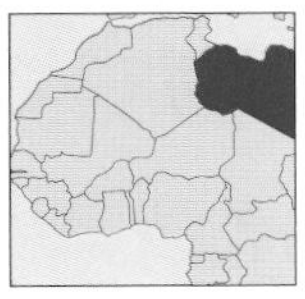

GEOGRAPHY The Socialist People's Libyan Arab Jamahiriya, as Libya is officially called, is a large country in North Africa. Most people live on the coastal plains in the northeast and northwest. The Sahara, the world's largest desert which occupies 95% of Libya, reaches the Mediterranean coast along the Gulf of Sidra (Khalij Surt).

The coastal plains in the northeast and northwest have Mediterranean climates, with hot, dry summers and mild, sometimes wet winters. Inland, the average yearly rainfall drops to 4 in [100 mm] or less.

POLITICS & ECONOMY Italy took over Libya in 1911, but lost it during World War II. Britain and France jointly ruled Libya until 1951, when the country became an independent kingdom.

In 1969, a military group headed by Colonel Muammar Gaddafi deposed the king and set up a military government. Under Gaddafi, the government took control of the economy and used money from oil exports to finance welfare services and development projects. Gaddafi was criticized for supporting terrorist groups around the world, and Libya became isolated from the mid-1980s. In 1998, he tried to restore Libya's reputation by surrendering for trial two Libyans suspected of planting a bomb on a PanAm plane which exploded over the Scottish town of Lockerbie in 1988. In 2001, one of the Libyans was found guilty and the other acquitted of the bombing. In 2003, Libya announced that it would pay compensation to victims of the bombing. In 2004, in a further attempt to lose its pariah status in international affairs, Libya declared that it was ending the production of all weapons of mass destruction, a move welcomed by Western nations.

The discovery of oil and natural gas in 1959 led to a transformation of Libya's economy. This formerly poor country soon became Africa's richest in terms of its per capita income. But it remains a developing country, because oil accounts for nearly all its export revenues. Agriculture is important, although Libya imports food. Crops include barley, citrus fruits, dates, olives, potatoes, and wheat, while cattle, sheep, and poultry are raised. Libya has oil refineries and petrochemical plants. Other manufactures include cement and steel.

AREA 679,358 SQ MI [1,759,540 SQ KM] **POPULATION** 5,499,000 **CAPITAL (POPULATION)** TRIPOLI (1,500,000) **GOVERNMENT** SINGLE-PARTY SOCIALIST STATE **ETHNIC GROUPS** LIBYAN ARAB AND BERBER 97% **LANGUAGES** ARABIC (OFFICIAL), BERBER **RELIGIONS** ISLAM (SUNNI MUSLIM) 97% **CURRENCY** LIBYAN DINAR = 1,000 DIRHAMS

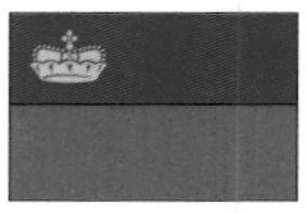

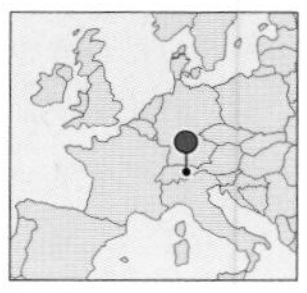

LIECHTENSTEIN

The tiny Principality of Liechtenstein is sandwiched between Switzerland and Austria. The River Rhine flows along its western border, while Alpine peaks rise in the east and south. The climate is relatively mild. Since 1924, Liechtenstein has been in a customs union with Switzerland. Taxation is low and the country is a haven for foreign companies. In 2003, the people voted to give their head of state, Prince Hans Adam II, sovereign powers. However, he later announced that he planned to retire from politics and hand over to his heir, Prince Alois, although Hans Adam II would remain head of state.

AREA 62 SQ MI [160 SQ KM] **POPULATION** 33,000 **CAPITAL** VADUZ

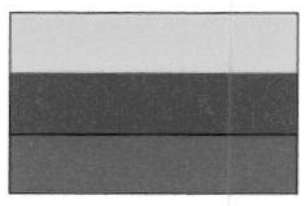

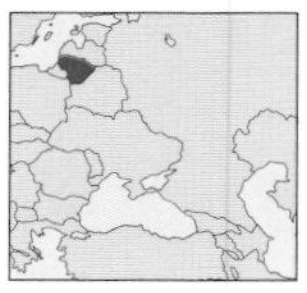

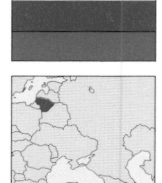

LITHUANIA

GEOGRAPHY The Republic of Lithuania is the southernmost of the three Baltic states which were ruled as part of the Soviet Union between 1940 and 1991. Much of the land is flat or gently rolling, with the highest land in the southeast.

Winters are cold and summers warm. The annual rainfall in the west is about 25 in [630 mm]. Eastern areas are drier.

POLITICS & ECONOMY The Lithuanian people were united into a single nation in the 12th century, and later joined a union with Poland. In 1795, Lithuania came under Russian rule. After World War I (1914–18), Lithuania declared itself independent, and in 1920 it signed a peace treaty with the Russians, though Poland held Vilnius until 1939. In 1940, the Soviet Union occupied Lithuania, but the Germans invaded in 1941. Soviet forces returned in 1944, and Lithuania was integrated into the Soviet Union. In 1988, when the Soviet Union was introducing reforms, the Lithuanians demanded independence. Their language is one of the oldest in the world, and the country was always the most homogenous of the Baltic states, staunchly Catholic and resistant of attempts to suppress their culture. Pro-independence groups won the national elections in 1990 and, in 1991, the Soviet Union recognized Lithuania's independence.

Since 1991, Lithuania has sought to reform its economy and introduce a private enterprise system. Lithuania has also drawn closer to the West and, in 2004, it became a member of both the North Atlantic Treaty Organization and the European Union.

The World Bank classifies Lithuania as a "lower-middle-income" developing country. Lithuania lacks natural resources, but manufacturing, based on imported materials, is the most valuable activity.

AREA 25,174 SQ MI [65,200 SQ KM] **POPULATION** 3,593,000
CAPITAL (POPULATION) VILNIUS (578,000)
GOVERNMENT MULTIPARTY REPUBLIC
ETHNIC GROUPS LITHUANIAN 80%, RUSSIAN 9%, POLISH 7%, BELARUSIAN 2% **LANGUAGES** LITHUANIAN (OFFICIAL), RUSSIAN, POLISH
RELIGIONS MAINLY ROMAN CATHOLIC **CURRENCY** LITAS = 100 CENTAI

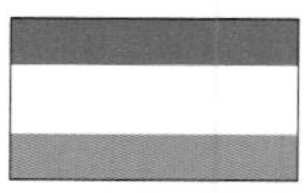

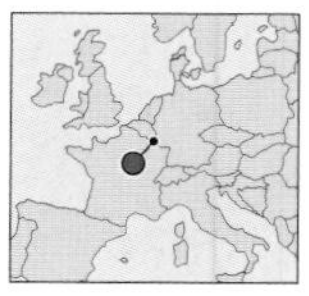

LUXEMBOURG

GEOGRAPHY The Grand Duchy of Luxembourg is one of the smallest and oldest countries in Europe. The north belongs to an upland region which includes the Ardenne in Belgium and Luxembourg, and the Eifel highlands in Germany.

Luxembourg has a temperate climate. The south has warm summers and falls, when grapes ripen in sheltered southeastern valleys. Winters are sometimes severe, especially in upland areas.

POLITICS & ECONOMY Germany occupied Luxembourg in World Wars I and II. In 1944–5, northern Luxembourg was the scene of the famous Battle of the Bulge. In 1948, Luxembourg joined Belgium and the Netherlands in a union called Benelux and, in the 1950s, it was one of the six founders of what is now the European Union. Luxembourg has played a major role in Europe. Its capital contains the headquarters of several international agencies, including the European Coal and Steel Community and the European Court of Justice. The city is also a major financial center.

Luxembourg has iron-ore reserves and is a major steel producer. It also has many high-technology industries, producing electronic goods and computers. Steel and other manufactures, including chemicals, rubber products, glass and aluminum, dominate the country's exports. Other major activities include tourism and financial services.

AREA 998 SQ MI [2,586 SQ KM] **POPULATION** 454,000
CAPITAL (POPULATION) LUXEMBOURG (77,000)
GOVERNMENT CONSTITUTIONAL MONARCHY (GRAND DUCHY)
ETHNIC GROUPS LUXEMBOURGER 71%, PORTUGUESE, ITALIAN, FRENCH, BELGIAN, SLAVS **LANGUAGES** LUXEMBOURGISH (OFFICIAL), FRENCH, GERMAN **RELIGIONS** ROMAN CATHOLIC 87%, OTHERS 13%
CURRENCY EURO = 100 CENTS

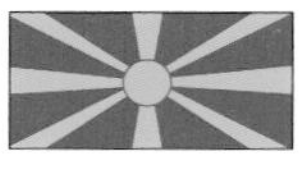

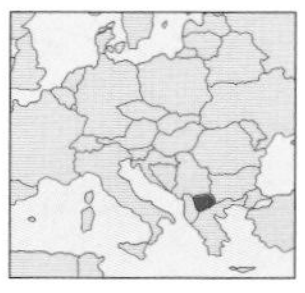

MACEDONIA (FYROM)

GEOGRAPHY The Republic of Macedonia is a country in southeastern Europe, which was once one of the six republics that made up the former Federal People's Republic of Yugoslavia. This landlocked country is largely mountainous or hilly. Macedonia has hot summers, though highland areas are cooler. Winters are cold and snowfalls are often heavy. The climate is fairly continental in character and rain occurs throughout the year.

POLITICS & ECONOMY Until the 20th century, Macedonia's history was closely tied to a larger area, also called Macedonia, which included parts of northern Greece and southwestern Bulgaria. This region reached its peak in power at the time of Philip II (382–336 BC) and his son Alexander the Great (336–323 BC). After Alexander's death, his empire was split up and it gradually declined. The area became a Roman province in the 140s BC and part of the Byzantine Empire from AD 395. In the 6th century, Slavs from eastern Europe settled in the area, followed by the Bulgars from central Asia in the 9th century. The Byzantine Empire regained control in 1018, but Serbia took Macedonia in the early 14th century. In 1371, the Ottoman Turks conquered the area and ruled it for more than 500 years. In 1913, at the end of the Balkan Wars, the area was divided between Serbia, Bulgaria and Greece. At the end of World War I, Serbian Macedonia became part of the Kingdom of the Serbs. Croats and Slovenes, which was renamed Yugoslavia in 1929. After World War II, Yugoslavia became a Communist country under ex-partisan leader Josip Broz Tito.

Tito died in 1980 and, in the early 1990s, the country broke up into five separate republics. Macedonia declared its independence in September 1991. Greece objected to this territory using the name Macedonia, which it considered to be a Greek name. It also objected to a symbol on Macedonia's flag and a reference in the constitution to the desire to reunite the three parts of the old Macedonia.

Macedonia adopted a new clause in its constitution rejecting any Macedonian claims on Greek territory and, in 1993, the United Nations accepted the new republic as a member under the name of The Former Yugoslav Republic of Macedonia (FYROM).

By the end of 1993, all the countries of the EU, except Greece, were establishing diplomatic relations with the FYROM. In 1995, Greece lifted its trade ban, when Macedonia agreed to redesign its flag and remove territorial claims from its constitution. In 2001, fighting along the Kosovo border spilled over into northwestern Macedonia. It was attributed to nationalists who want to create a Great Albania, including part of Macedonia. The uprising ended when the Macedonian government gave its Albanian-speakers increased rights.

The World Bank describes Macedonia as a "lower-middle-income" developing country. Manufactures dominate the country's exports. Macedonia mines coal, but imports all its oil and natural gas. The country is self-sufficient in its basic food needs.

AREA 9,928 SQ MI [25,713 SQ KM] **POPULATION** 2,063,000
CAPITAL (POPULATION) SKOPJE (430,000) **GOVERNMENT** MULTIPARTY REPUBLIC **ETHNIC GROUPS** MACEDONIAN 64%, ALBANIAN 25%, TURKISH 4%, ROMANIAN 3%, SERB 2% **LANGUAGES** MACEDONIAN AND ALBANIAN (OFFICIAL) **RELIGIONS** MACEDONIAN ORTHODOX 70%, ISLAM 29%
CURRENCY MACEDONIAN DENAR = 100 PARAS

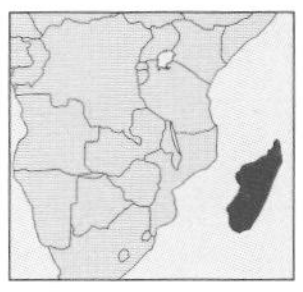

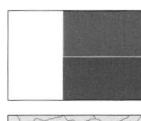

MADAGASCAR

GEOGRAPHY The Democratic Republic of Madagascar, in southeastern Africa, is an island nation, which has a larger area than France. Behind the narrow coastal plains in the east lies a highland zone, mostly between 2,000 ft and 4,000 ft [610 m to 1,220 m] above sea level. Broad plains border the Mozambique Channel in the west.

Temperatures in the highlands are moderated by the altitude. The winters (from April to September) are dry, but heavy rains occur in summer. The eastern coastlands are warm and humid. The west is drier and the south and southwest are hot and dry.

POLITICS & ECONOMY People from Southeast Asia began to settle on Madagascar around 2,000 years ago. Subsequent influxes from Africa and Arabia added to the island's diverse heritage, culture and language.

French troops defeated a Malagasy army in 1895 and Madagascar became a French colony. In 1960, it achieved full independence as the Malagasy Republic. In 1972, army officers seized control and, in 1975, under the leadership of Lieutenant-Commander Didier Ratsiraka, the country was renamed Madagascar. Parliamentary elections were held in 1977, but Ratsiraka remained president of a one-party socialist state. In 2002, the country came close to civil war when Ratsiraka and his opponent, Marc Ravalomanana, both claimed victory in presidential elections. Ravalomanana was eventually recognized as president and Ratsiraka went into exile.

Madagascar is one of the world's poorest countries. The land has been badly eroded because of the cutting down of the forests and overgrazing of the grasslands. Farming, fishing, and forestry employ about 80% of the people. The country's food crops include bananas, cassava, rice, and sweet potatoes. Coffee is the leading export.

AREA 226,657 SQ MI [587,041 SQ KM] **POPULATION** 16,980,000
CAPITAL (POPULATION) ANTANANARIVO (1,250,000)
GOVERNMENT REPUBLIC **ETHNIC GROUPS** MERINA, BETSIMISARAKA, BETSILEO, TSIMIHETY, SAKALAVA AND OTHERS
LANGUAGES MALAGASY AND FRENCH (BOTH OFFICIAL)
RELIGIONS TRADITIONAL BELIEFS 52%, CHRISTIANITY 41%, ISLAM 7%
CURRENCY MALAGASY FRANC = 100 CENTIMES

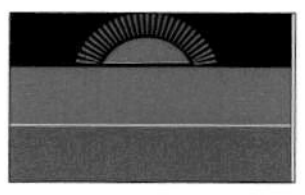

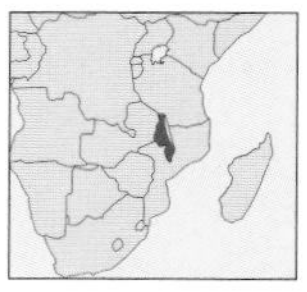

MALAWI

GEOGRAPHY The Republic of Malawi includes part of Lake Malawi, which is drained by the River Shire, a tributary of the River Zambezi. The land is mostly mountainous. The highest peak, Mulanje, reaches 9,843 ft [3,000 m] in the southeast.

While the low-lying areas of Malawi are hot and humid all year round, the uplands have a pleasant climate. Lilongwe, at about 3,609 ft [1,100 m] above sea level, has a warm and sunny climate. Frosts sometimes occur in July and August, in the middle of the long dry season.

POLITICS & ECONOMY Malawi, then called Nyasaland, became a British protectorate in 1891. In 1953, Britain established the Federation of Rhodesia and Nyasaland, which also included what are now Zambia and Zimbabwe. Black African opposition, led in Nyasaland by Dr Hastings Kamuzu Banda, led to the dissolution of the federation in 1963. In 1964, Nyasaland became independent as Malawi, with Banda as prime minister. Banda became president when the country became a republic in 1966 and, in 1971, he was made president for life. Banda ruled autocratically through the only party, the Malawi Congress Party. A multiparty system was restored in 1993. Banda and his party were defeated in elections in 1993. Bakili Muluzi became president and was re-elected in 1999. In 2004, Muluzi's nominee, Bingu wa Mutharika, was elected president.

Malawi is one of the world's poorest countries. More than 80% of the people are farmers, but many grow little more than they need to feed their families.

AREA 45,747 SQ MI [118,484 SQ KM] **POPULATION** 11,651,000
CAPITAL (POPULATION) LILONGWE (440,000)
GOVERNMENT MULTIPARTY REPUBLIC
ETHNIC GROUPS CHEWA, NYANJA, TONGA, TUMBUKA, LOMWE, YAO, NGONI AND OTHERS
LANGUAGES CHICHEWA AND ENGLISH (BOTH OFFICIAL)
RELIGIONS PROTESTANT 55%, ROMAN CATHOLIC 20%, ISLAM 20%
CURRENCY MALAWIAN KWACHA = 100 TAMBALA

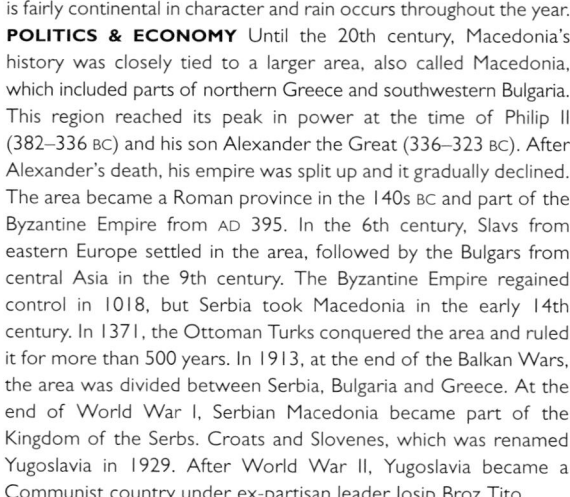

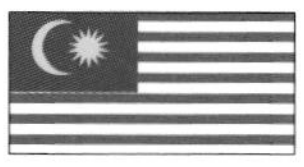

MALAYSIA

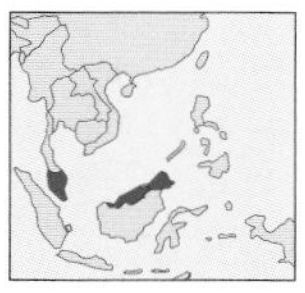

GEOGRAPHY The Federation of Malaysia consists of two main parts. Peninsular Malaysia, which is joined to mainland Asia, contains about 80% of the population. The other main regions, Sabah and Sarawak, are in northern Borneo, an island which Malaysia shares with Indonesia. Behind the coastal lowlands, the interior is mountainous.

Malaysia has a hot equatorial climate. The temperatures are high all through the year, though the mountains are much cooler than the lowland areas. The rainfall is heavy throughout the year.

POLITICS & ECONOMY Around 1,200 years ago, Indian traders introduced Hinduism and Buddhism into the Malay peninsula, while Arabs introduced Islam in the 15th century. Portuguese traders reached Melaka in 1509, but the Dutch took over in 1641. Britain became established in the area in 1786.

Japan occupied the area during World War II (1939–45), but the area reverted to British rule in 1945. In the 1940s and 1950s, Communist guerrillas battled unsuccessfully for power. Malaya (Peninsular Malaysia) became independent in 1957. Malaysia was created in 1963, when Malaya, Singapore, Sabah and Sarawak agreed to unite, but Singapore withdrew in 1965.

From 1981, under the leadership of Dr Mahathir bin Mohamad, Malaysia achieved rapid economic progress. However, together with other countries in eastern Asia, it experienced an economic recession in 1997. In response to the crisis, the government ordered the repatriation of many temporary foreign workers and initiated a series of austerity measures aimed at restoring confidence and avoiding the chronic debt problems affecting some other Asian countries. Mahathir bin Mohamad retired in 2003 and was succeeded as prime minister by Abdullah Ahmad Bud.

The World Bank classifies Malaysia as an "upper-middle-income" developing country. Palm oil, rubber, and tin are major products. Manufactures include cars, chemicals, a wide range of electronic goods, plastics, textiles, rubber, and wood products.

AREA 127,320 sq mi [329,758 sq km] **POPULATION** 23,093,000
CAPITAL (POPULATION) Kuala Lumpur (1,145,000); Putrajaya (administrative capital awaiting completion)
GOVERNMENT Federal constitutional monarchy
ETHNIC GROUPS Malay and other indigenous groups 58%, Chinese 24%, Indian 8%, others **LANGUAGES** Malay (official), Chinese, English **RELIGIONS** Islam, Buddhism, Daoism, Hinduism, Christianity, Sikhism **CURRENCY** Ringgit = 100 cents

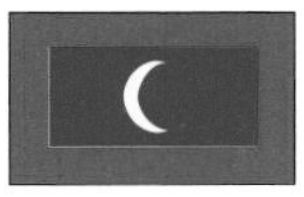

MALDIVES

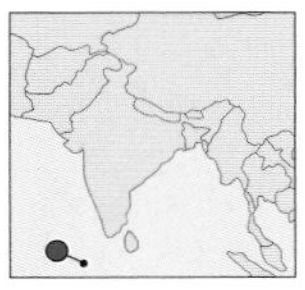

The Republic of the Maldives consists of about 1,200 low-lying coral islands, south of India. The highest point is 79 ft [24 m], but most of the land is only 6 ft [1.8 m] above sea level. The islands became a British territory in 1887 and independence was achieved in 1965. Tourism and fishing are the main industries.

AREA 115 sq mi [298 sq km] **POPULATION** 330,000 **CAPITAL** Malé

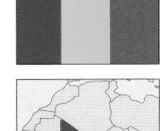

MALI

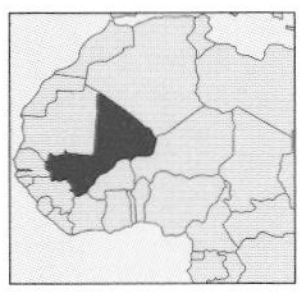

GEOGRAPHY The Republic of Mali is a landlocked country in northern Africa. The land is generally flat, with the highest land in the north. Northern Mali is hot and practically rainless. The south has enough rain for farming.

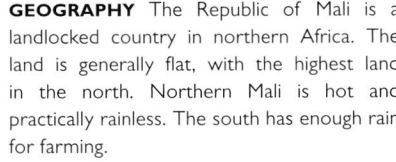

POLITICS & ECONOMY Between the 4th and 16th centuries, Mali was part of three African empires – ancient Ghana, ancient Mali, and Songhay. However, after 1591, when Songhay was defeated by Morocco, the area was divided into small kingdoms. France ruled the area, then known as French Sudan, from 1893 until the country became independent as Mali in 1960.

The first socialist government was overthrown in 1968 by an army group led by Moussa Traoré, but he was ousted in 1991. Multiparty democracy was restored in 1992 and Alpha Oumar Konaré was elected president. Konaré stood down in 2002 and Ahmadou Toure, who had restored democracy in 1992, was elected president.

Mali is one of the world's poorest countries and 70% of the land is desert or semidesert. Only about 2% of the land is used for growing crops, while 25% is used for grazing animals. Despite this, agriculture employs nearly 80% of the people, many of whom subsist by nomadic livestock rearing.

AREA 478,838 sq mi [1,240,192 sq km] **POPULATION** 11,626,000
CAPITAL (POPULATION) Bamako (1,016,000)
GOVERNMENT Multiparty republic **ETHNIC GROUPS** Mande 50% (Bambara, Malinke, Soninke), Peul 17%, Voltaic 12%, Songhai 6%, Tuareg and Moor 10%, others **LANGUAGES** French (official), many African languages **RELIGIONS** Islam 90%, traditional beliefs 9%, Christianity 1% **CURRENCY** CFA franc = 100 centimes

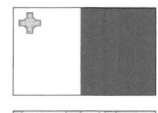

MALTA

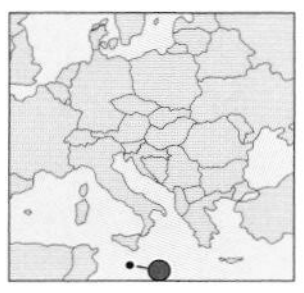

GEOGRAPHY The Republic of Malta consists of two main islands, Malta and Gozo, a third, much smaller island called Comino lying between the two large islands and two islets. The climate is typically Mediterranean, with hot, dry summers and mild, moist winters.

POLITICS & ECONOMY Malta has fascinating Stone and Bronze age remains. The islands later came under Phoenician, Greek, Carthaginian, Roman and Arab rule. In about 1090, Malta came under the Norman kings of Sicily and, from 1530, the Knights Hospitallers (also called the Knights of St John of Jerusalem). France took the islands in 1798, but the British drove them out in 1800. British rule was officially recognized in 1815.

During World War I (1914–18), Malta was an important naval base. In World War II (1939–45), Italian and German aircraft bombed the islands. In recognition of the islanders' bravery, the British King George VI awarded the George Cross to Malta in 1942. In 1953, Malta became a base for NATO (North Atlantic Treaty Organization). Malta became independent in 1964 and a republic in 1974. In 1979, Malta ceased to be a British military base and all British forces withdrew. Malta was declared a neutral country in the 1980s. It became a member of the European Union on May 1, 2004.

The World Bank classifies Malta as an "upper-middle-income" developing country. It lacks natural resources, and most people work in the former naval dockyards, which are now used for commercial shipbuilding and repair, in manufacturing industries and in the tourist industry.

Manufactures include chemicals, processed food, and chemicals. Farming is difficult, because of the rocky soils. Crops include barley, fruits, potatoes, and wheat. Malta also has a small fishing industry.

AREA 122 sq mi [316 sq km] **POPULATION** 400,000
CAPITAL (POPULATION) Valletta (9,000) **GOVERNMENT** Multiparty republic **ETHNIC GROUPS** Maltese 96%, British 2% **LANGUAGES** Maltese and English (both official) **RELIGIONS** Roman Catholic 98% **CURRENCY** Maltese lira = 100 cents

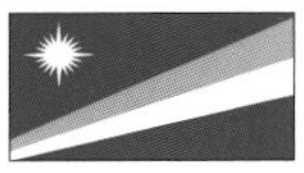

MARSHALL ISLANDS

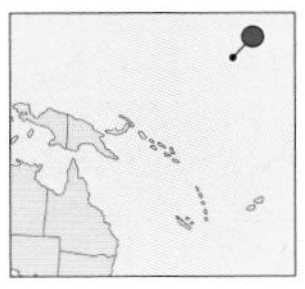

The Republic of the Marshall Islands, a former US territory, became fully independent in 1991. This island nation, lying north of Kiribati in a region known as Micronesia, is heavily dependent on US aid. The main activities are agriculture and tourism.

AREA 70 sq mi [181 sq km]
POPULATION 56,000 **CAPITAL** Majuro

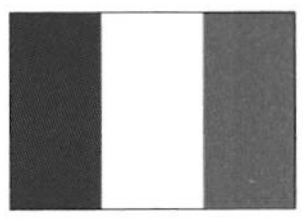

MARTINIQUE

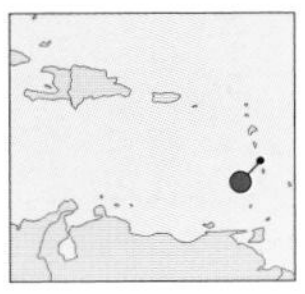

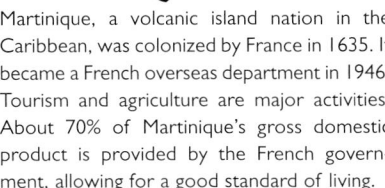

Martinique, a volcanic island nation in the Caribbean, was colonized by France in 1635. It became a French overseas department in 1946. Tourism and agriculture are major activities. About 70% of Martinique's gross domestic product is provided by the French government, allowing for a good standard of living.

AREA 425 sq mi [1,102 sq km]
POPULATION 426,000 **CAPITAL** Fort-de-France

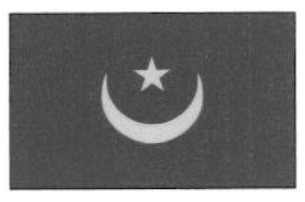

MAURITANIA

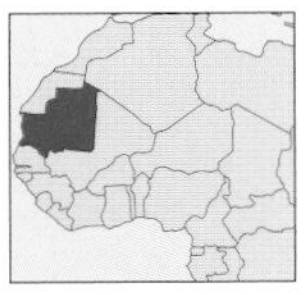

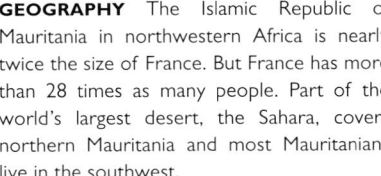

GEOGRAPHY The Islamic Republic of Mauritania in northwestern Africa is nearly twice the size of France. But France has more than 28 times as many people. Part of the world's largest desert, the Sahara, covers northern Mauritania and most Mauritanians live in the southwest.

The amount of rainfall and the length of the rainy season increase from north to south. Much of the land is desert, with dry northeast and easterly winds throughout the year. But southwesterly winds bring summer rain to the south.

POLITICS & ECONOMY Originally part of the great African empires of Ghana and Mali, France set up a protectorate in Mauritania in 1903, attempting to exploit the trade in gum arabic. The country became a territory of French West Africa and a French colony in 1920. French West Africa was a huge territory, which included present-day Benin, Burkina Faso, Guinea, Ivory Coast, Mali, Niger and Senegal, as well as Mauritania. In 1958, Mauritania became a self-governing territory in the French Union and it became fully independent in 1960.

In 1976, Spain withdrew from Spanish (now Western) Sahara, a territory bordering Mauritania to the north. Morocco occupied the northern two-thirds of this territory, while Mauritania took the rest. But Saharan guerrillas belonging to POLISARIO (the Popular Front for the Liberation of Saharan Territories) began an armed struggle for independence. In 1979, Mauritania withdrew from the southern part of Western Sahara, which was then occupied by Morocco. Democracy was restored after a new constitution was adopted in 1991. In 2003, the government cracked down on Islamic militants and other critics of the government.

The World Bank classifies Mauritania as a "low-income" developing country. Agriculture employs 38% of the people. Some are herders who move around with herds of cattle and sheep, though recent droughts forced many farmers to seek aid in the cities.

AREA 395,953 sq mi [1,025,520 sq km] **POPULATION** 2,913,000
CAPITAL (POPULATION) Nouakchott (735,000)
GOVERNMENT Multiparty Islamic republic
ETHNIC GROUPS Mixed Moor/Black 40%, Moor 30%, Black 30%
LANGUAGES Arabic and Wolof (both official), French
RELIGIONS Islam
CURRENCY Ouguiya = 5 khoums

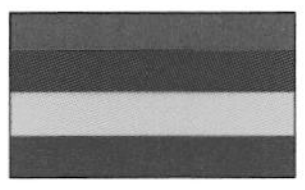

MAURITIUS

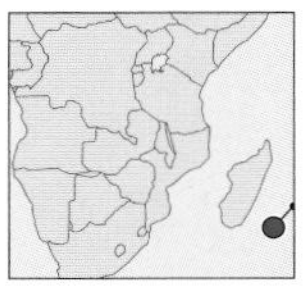

The Republic of Mauritius, an Indian Ocean nation lying east of Madagascar, was previously ruled by France and Britain until it achieved independence in 1968. It became a republic in 1992. Sugar production is in decline but tourism is vital to the economy.

AREA 788 sq mi [2,040 sq km]
POPULATION 1,210,000 **CAPITAL** Port Louis

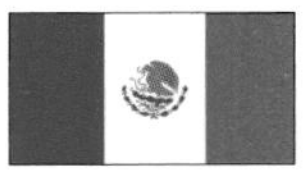

MEXICO

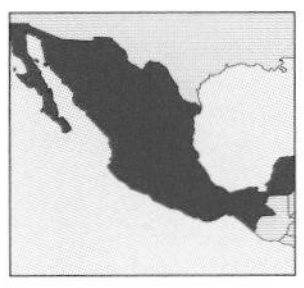

GEOGRAPHY The United Mexican States, as Mexico is officially named, is the world's most populous Spanish-speaking country. Much of the land is mountainous, although most people live on the central plateau. Mexico contains two large peninsulas, Lower (or Baja) California in the northwest and the flat Yucatán peninsula in the southeast.

The climate varies according to the altitude. The resort of Acapulco on the southwest coast has a dry and sunny climate. Mexico City, at about 7,546 ft [2,300 m] above sea level, is much cooler. Most rain occurs between June and September. The rainfall decreases north of Mexico City and northern Mexico is mainly arid.

POLITICS & ECONOMY In the mid-19th century, Mexico lost land to the United States, and between 1910 and 1921 violent revolutions created chaos.

Reforms were introduced in the 1920s and, in 1929, the Institutional Revolutionary Party (PRI) was formed. The PRI ruled Mexico effectively as a one-party state until it was finally defeated in 2001. The new president, Vicente Fox, faced many problems, including unemployment and rapid urbanization especially around Mexico City, demands for indigenous rights by Amerindian groups, and illegal emigration to the United States.

The World Bank classifies Mexico as an "upper-middle-income" developing country. Agriculture is important. Food crops include beans, maize, rice and wheat, while cash crops include coffee, cotton, fruits and vegetables. Beef cattle, dairy cattle and other livestock are raised and fishing is also important.

But oil and oil products are the chief exports, while manufacturing is the most valuable activity. Mexico is the world's leading silver producer, and it also mines copper, gold, lead, zinc, and other minerals. Many factories near the northern border assemble goods, such as car parts and electrical products, for US companies. These factories are called *maquiladoras*. Hope for the future lies in increasing economic cooperation with the USA and Canada

through NAFTA (North American Free Trade Association), which came into being on January 1, 1994.

AREA 756,061 sq mi [1,958,201 sq km] **POPULATION** 104,908,000
CAPITAL (POPULATION) Mexico City (8,236,000)
GOVERNMENT Federal republic
ETHNIC GROUPS Mestizo 60%, Amerindian 30%, White 9%
LANGUAGES Spanish (official)
RELIGIONS Roman Catholic 90%, Protestant 6%
CURRENCY Mexican peso = 100 centavos

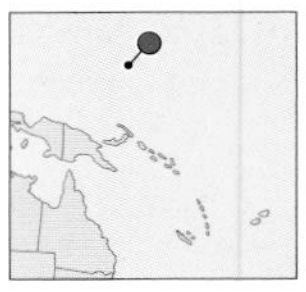

MICRONESIA

The Federated States of Micronesia, a former US territory covering a vast area in the western Pacific Ocean, became fully independent in 1991. The main export is copra. Fishing and tourism are also important.

AREA 271 sq mi [702 sq km]
POPULATION 108,000 **CAPITAL** Palikir

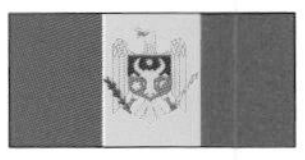

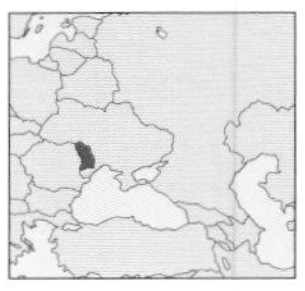

MOLDOVA

GEOGRAPHY The Republic of Moldova is a small country sandwiched between Ukraine and Romania. It was formerly one of the 15 republics that made up the Soviet Union. Much of the land is hilly and the highest areas are near the center of the country.

Moldova has a moderately continental climate, with warm summers and fairly cold winters when temperatures dip below freezing point. Most of the rain comes in the warmer months.

POLITICS & ECONOMY In the 14th century, the Moldavians formed a state called Moldavia. It included part of Romania and Bessarabia (now the modern country of Moldova). The Ottoman Turks took the area in the 16th century, but in 1812 Russia took over Bessarabia. In 1861, Moldavia and Walachia united to form Romania. Russia retook southern Bessarabia in 1878.

After World War I (1914–18), all of Bessarabia was returned to Romania, but the Soviet Union did not recognize this act. From 1944, the Moldovan Soviet Socialist Republic was part of the Soviet Union.

In 1989, the Moldovans asserted their independence and ethnicity by making Romanian the official language and, at the end of 1991, Moldova became an independent country. In 1992, fighting occurred between Moldovans and Russians in Trans-Dniester, a mainly Russian-speaking area east of the River Dniester. The first multiparty elections were held in 1994, when a proposal to unite with Romania was rejected. Economic problems made the government unpopular and, in 2001, Moldova became the first former Soviet state to return the Communist party to power in a general election. The new government adopted many Russification policies, proclaiming Russian an official language.

In terms of its GNP per capita, Moldova is Europe's poorest country. Agriculture is the leading activity and products include fruits, maize, tobacco, and wine. Moldova has few natural resources and it imports materials and fuels for its industries. Light industries, such as food processing and factories making household appliances, are increasing.

AREA 13,070 sq mi [33,851 sq km] **POPULATION** 4,440,000
CAPITAL (POPULATION) Chişinău (658,000)
GOVERNMENT Multiparty republic
ETHNIC GROUPS Moldovan/Romanian 65%, Ukrainian 14%, Russian 13%, others
LANGUAGES Moldovan/Romanian and Russian (official)
RELIGIONS Eastern Orthodox 98%
CURRENCY Moldovan leu = 100 bani

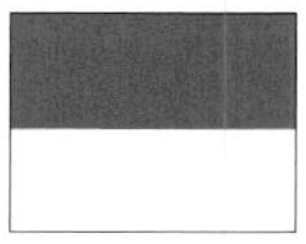

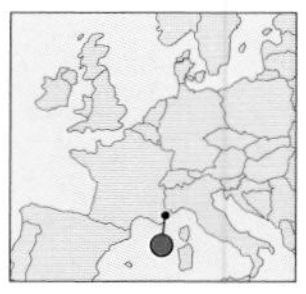

MONACO

The tiny Principality of Monaco consists of a narrow strip of coastline and a rocky peninsula on the French Riviera. Its considerable wealth is derived largely from banking, finance, gambling, and tourism. Monaco's citizens do not pay any state tax. Its attractions include the Monte Carlo casino and such sporting events as the Monte Carlo Rally and the Monaco Grand Prix.

AREA 0.4 sq mi [1 sq km] **POPULATION** 32,000 **CAPITAL** Monaco

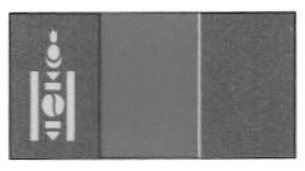

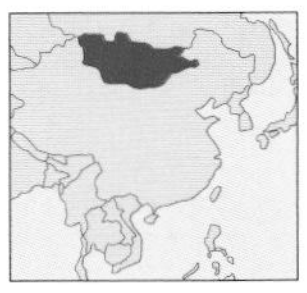

MONGOLIA

GEOGRAPHY The State of Mongolia is the world's largest landlocked country. It consists mainly of high plateaux, with the Gobi Desert in the southeast.

Ulan Bator lies on the northern edge of a desert plateau. It has bitterly cold winters. Summer temperatures are moderated by the altitude.

POLITICS & ECONOMY In the 13th century, Genghis Khan united the Mongolian peoples and built up a great empire. Under his grandson, Kublai Khan, the Mongol empire extended from Korea and China to eastern Europe and present-day Iraq.

The Mongol empire broke up in the late 14th century. In the early 17th century, Inner Mongolia came under Chinese control, and by the late 17th century Outer Mongolia had become a Chinese province. In 1911, the Mongolians drove the Chinese out of Outer Mongolia and made the area a Buddhist kingdom. But in 1924, under Russian influence, the Communist Mongolian People's Republic was set up. From the 1950s, Mongolia supported the Soviet Union in its disputes with China. In 1990, the people demonstrated for more freedom, and free elections in June 1990 resulted in victory for the Mongolian People's Revolutionary Party, which was composed of Communists. Communist rule ended in 1996, when the Democratic Union coalition won power. But the Communists regained power in 2000, though they were expected to continue free-market policies.

The World Bank classifies Mongolia as a "lower-middle-income" developing country. Most people were once nomads, who moved around with their herds of sheep, cattle, goats, and horses. Under Communist rule, most people were moved into permanent homes on government-owned farms. But livestock and animal products remain leading exports. The Communists also developed industry, especially the mining of coal, copper, gold, molybdenum, tin and tungsten, and manufacturing. Minerals and fuels now account for around half of Mongolia's exports.

AREA 604,826 sq mi [1,566,500 sq km] **POPULATION** 2,712,000
CAPITAL (POPULATION) Ulan Bator (760,000)
GOVERNMENT Multiparty republic **ETHNIC GROUPS** Khalkha Mongol 85%, Kazakh 6% **LANGUAGES** Khalkha Mongolian (official), Turkic, Russian **RELIGIONS** Tibetan Buddhist Lamaism 96%
CURRENCY Tugrik = 100 möngös

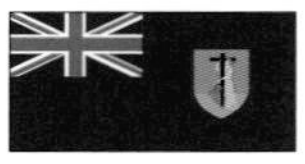

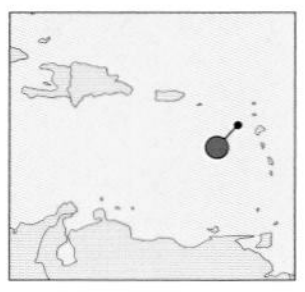

MONTSERRAT

Monserrat is a British overseas territory in the Caribbean Sea. The climate is tropical and hurricanes often cause much damage. Intermittent eruptions of the Soufrière Hills volcano between 1995 and 1998, and again in 2003, led to the emigration of many people and the virtual destruction of Plymouth, the capital, in the south.

AREA 39 sq mi [102 sq km] **POPULATION** 9,000 (prior to the volcanic activity) **CAPITAL** Plymouth

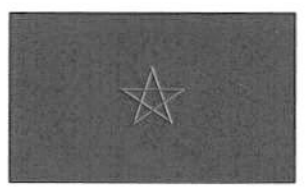

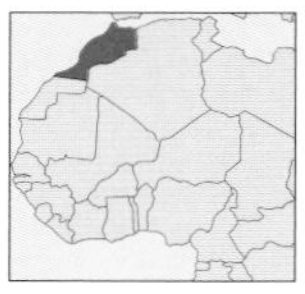

MOROCCO

GEOGRAPHY The Kingdom of Morocco lies in northwestern Africa. Its name comes from the Arabic Maghreb-el-Aksa, meaning "the farthest west." Behind the western coastal plain the land rises to a broad plateau and ranges of the Atlas Mountains. The High (Haut) Atlas contains the highest peak, Djebel Toubkal, at 13,665 ft [4,165 m]. East of the mountains, the land descends to the Sahara. The Canaries Current cools the Atlantic coast. Inland, summers are hot and dry. Winters are mild, with moderate rainfall. Snow often falls on the High Atlas Mountains.

POLITICS & ECONOMY The original people of Morocco were the Berbers. But in the 680s, Arab invaders introduced Islam and the Arabic language. By the early 20th century, France and Spain controlled Morocco, which became an independent kingdom in 1956. Although Morocco is a constitutional monarchy, King Hassan II ruled the country in a generally authoritarian way from the time of his accession to the throne in 1961 to his death in 1999. His son and successor, Mohamed VI, faced several problems, including the future of Western Sahara, which Hassan II had claimed for Morocco. In 2003, Morocco faced another problem when Islamic suicide bombers blew up a hotel in Casablanca.

Morocco is classified as a "lower-middle-income" developing country. It is the world's third largest producer of phosphate rock, which is used to make fertilizer. One of the reasons why Morocco wants to keep Western Sahara is that it, too, has large phosphate reserves. Farming employs 34% of Moroccans. Chief crops include barley, beans, citrus fruits, maize, olives, sugar beet, and wheat. Processed phosphates are exported, but most of Morocco's manufactures are for home consumption. Fishing and tourism are also important.

AREA 172,413 sq mi [446,550 sq km] **POPULATION** 31,689,000
CAPITAL (POPULATION) Rabat (1,220,000)
GOVERNMENT Constitutional monarchy
ETHNIC GROUPS Arab-Berber 99%
LANGUAGES Arabic (official), Berber dialects, French
RELIGIONS Islam 99% **CURRENCY** Moroccan dirham = 100 centimes

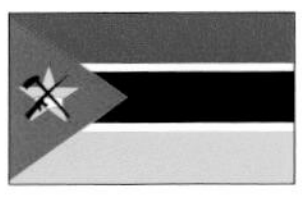

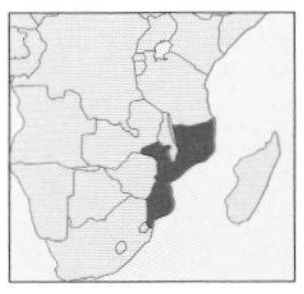

MOZAMBIQUE

GEOGRAPHY The Republic of Mozambique borders the Indian Ocean in southeastern Africa. The coastal plains are narrow in the north but broaden in the south. Inland lie plateaux and hills, which make up another two-fifths of Mozambique.

Mozambique has a mostly tropical climate. The capital Maputo, which lies outside the tropics, has hot and humid summers, though the winters are mild and fairly dry.

POLITICS & ECONOMY In 1885, when the European powers divided Africa, Mozambique was recognized as a Portuguese colony. But black African opposition to European rule gradually increased. In 1961, the Front for the Liberation of Mozambique (FRELIMO) was founded to oppose Portuguese rule. In 1964, FRELIMO launched a guerrilla war, which continued for ten years. Mozambique became independent in 1975.

After independence, Mozambique became a one-party state. Its government aided African nationalists in Rhodesia (now Zimbabwe) and South Africa. But the white governments of these countries helped an opposition group, the Mozambique National Resistance Movement (RENAMO) to lead an armed struggle against Mozambique's government. Civil war, combined with droughts, caused much suffering in the 1980s. In 1989, FRELIMO declared that it had dropped its Communist policies and ended one-party rule. The war ended in 1992 and multiparty elections in 1994 heralded more stable conditions. In 1995 Mozambique became the 53rd member of the Commonwealth.

In the early 1990s, the UN rated Mozambique as one of the world's poorest countries. The second half of the 1990s saw a surge in economic growth, but huge floods in 2000 and 2001 proved to be a major setback. About 80% of the people are poor and agriculture is the main activity. Crops include cassava, cotton, maize, rice, and tea.

AREA 309,494 sq mi [801,590 sq km] **POPULATION** 17,479,000
CAPITAL (POPULATION) Maputo (1,015,000)
GOVERNMENT Multiparty republic **ETHNIC GROUPS** Indigenous tribal groups (Shangaan, Chokwe, Manyika, Sena, Makua, others) 99%
LANGUAGES Portuguese (official), many others
RELIGIONS Traditional beliefs 50%, Christianity 30%, Islam 20%
CURRENCY Metical = 100 centavos

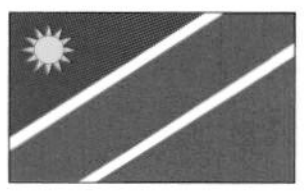

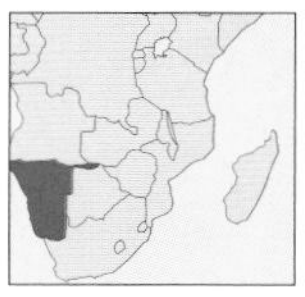

NAMIBIA

GEOGRAPHY The Republic of Namibia was formerly ruled by South Africa, which called it South West Africa. The country became independent in 1990. The coastal region contains the arid Namib Desert, which is virtually uninhabited. Inland is a central plateau, bordered by a rugged spine of mountains stretching north–south. Eastern Namibia contains part of the Kalahari Desert, a semidesert area which extends into Botswana. Namibia is a warm and arid country. Lying at 5,500 ft [1,700 m] above sea level, Windhoek has an average annual rainfall of about 15 in [370 mm], often occurring during thunderstorms in the hot summer months.

POLITICS & ECONOMY During World War I, South African troops defeated the Germans who ruled what is now Namibia. After World War II, many people challenged South Africa's right to govern the territory and a civil war began in the 1960s between African guerrillas and South African troops. A ceasefire was agreed in 1989 and Namibia became independent in 1990. In the 1990s, the government pursued a policy of "national reconciliation." An enclave on the coast, called Walvis Bay (Walvisbaai), remained part of South Africa until 1994, when it was transferred to Namibia. In 1999, a secessionist group staged

an unsuccessful uprising in the Caprivi Strip. In 2003–4, the government announced that it planned to speed up land reform by transferring farmland from white to black Namibians.

Namibia has reserves of diamonds, uranium, zinc, and copper. Minerals make up 80% of the exports, though agriculture employs about 40% of the people. Sea fishing is important, but overfishing has reduced the yields of the fishing fleet. The country has few industries, but tourism is expanding.

AREA 318,259 sq mi [824,292 sq km] **POPULATION** 1,927,000
CAPITAL (POPULATION) Windhoek (147,000)
GOVERNMENT Multiparty republic **ETHNIC GROUPS** Ovambo 50%, Kavango 9%, Herero 7%, Damara 7%, White 6%, Nama 5%
LANGUAGES English (official), Afrikaans, German, indigenous dialects **RELIGIONS** Christianity 90% (Lutheran 51%)
CURRENCY Namibian dollar = 100 cents

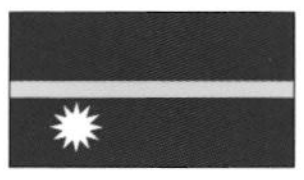

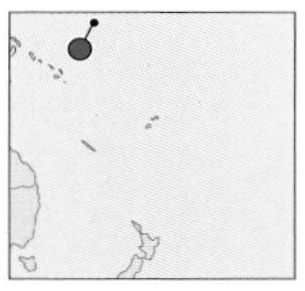

NAURU

Nauru is the world's smallest republic, located in the western Pacific Ocean, close to the equator. Independent since 1968, Nauru's prosperity is based on phosphate mining, but the reserves are running out.

AREA 8 sq mi [21 sq km]
POPULATION 13,000 **CAPITAL** Yaren

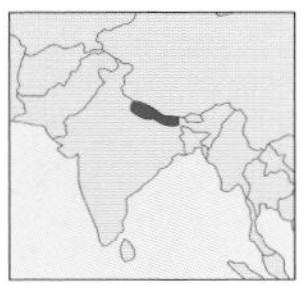

NEPAL

GEOGRAPHY Over three-quarters of Nepal lies in the Himalayan region, culminating in the world's highest peak (Mount Everest, or Chomolongma in Nepali) at 29,035 ft [8,850 m]. As a result, climatic conditions vary widely according to the altitude.

POLITICS & ECONOMY Nepal was united in the late 18th century, although its complex topography has ensured that it remains a diverse patchwork of peoples. From the mid-19th century to 1951, power was held by the royal Rana family. Attempts to introduce a democratic system in the 1950s failed. The first democratic elections in 32 years were held in 1991, but, by the early 21st century, Nepal faced many problems, including an uprising by Maoist guerrillas. In 2003, a brief ceasefire was agreed, but fighting continued in 2004. In 2001, King Birendra and other royal family members were shot dead by Crown Prince Dipendra in a family dispute.

Agriculture remains the chief activity in this overwhelmingly rural country and the government is heavily dependent on aid. Tourism, centered around the high Himalaya, grows in importance each year, although Nepal was closed to foreigners until 1951. There are also ambitious plans to exploit the hydroelectric potential offered by the ferocious Himalayan rivers.

AREA 56,827 sq mi [147,181 sq km] **POPULATION** 26,470,000
CAPITAL (POPULATION) Katmandu (695,000)
GOVERNMENT Constitutional monarchy **ETHNIC GROUPS** Brahman, Chetri, Newar, Gurung, Magar, Tamang, Sherpa and others
LANGUAGES Nepali (official), local languages
RELIGIONS Hinduism 86%, Buddhism 8%, Islam 4%
CURRENCY Nepalese rupee = 100 paisa

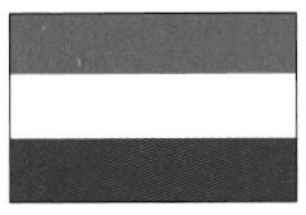

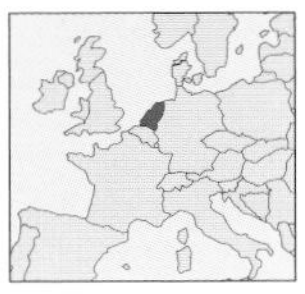

NETHERLANDS

GEOGRAPHY The Netherlands lies at the western end of the North European Plain, which extends to the Ural Mountains in Russia. Except for the far southeastern corner, the Netherlands is flat and about 40% lies below sea level at high tide. To prevent flooding, the Dutch have built dykes (sea walls) to hold back the waves. Large areas which were once under the sea, but which have been reclaimed, are called polders. Because of its position on the North Sea, the Netherlands has a temperate climate, with mild, rainy winters.

POLITICS & ECONOMY Before the 16th century, the area that is now the Netherlands was under a succession of foreign rulers, including the Romans, the Germanic Franks, the French and the Spanish. The Dutch declared their independence from Spain in 1581 and their status was finally recognized by Spain in 1648. In the 17th century, the Dutch built up a great overseas empire, especially in Southeast Asia. But in the early 18th century, the Dutch lost control of the seas to England.

France controlled the Netherlands from 1795 to 1813. In 1815, the Netherlands, then containing Belgium and Luxembourg, became an independent kingdom. Belgium broke away in 1830 and Luxembourg followed in 1890.

The Netherlands was neutral in World War I (1914–18), but was occupied by Germany in World War II (1939–45). After the war, the Netherlands Indies became independent as Indonesia. The Netherlands became active in West European affairs. With Belgium and Luxembourg, it formed a customs union called Benelux in 1948. In 1949, it joined NATO (the North Atlantic Treaty Organization), and the European Coal and Steel Community (ECSC) in 1953. In 1957, it became a founder member of the European Economic Community (now the European Union) and, in 2002, it adopted the euro as its sole unit of currency. In 2002, an anti-immigration group made sweeping gains in national elections. It joined a coalition government, which collapsed later that year. The group's vote collapsed in new elections in 2003.

The Netherlands is a highly industrialized country and industry and commerce are the most valuable activities. Its resources include natural gas, some oil, salt and china clay. But the Netherlands imports many of the materials needed by its industries and it is, therefore, a major trading country. Industrial products are wide-ranging, including aircraft, chemicals, electronic equipment, machinery, textiles, and vehicles. Agriculture employs only 5% of the people, but scientific methods are used and yields are high. Dairy farming is the leading farming activity. Major products include barley, flowers and bulbs, potatoes, sugar beet, and wheat.

AREA 16,033 sq mi [41,526 sq km] **POPULATION** 16,151,000
CAPITAL (POPULATION) Amsterdam (729,000); The Hague (seat of government, 440,000)
GOVERNMENT Constitutional monarchy
ETHNIC GROUPS Dutch 83%, Indonesian, Turkish, Moroccan and others **LANGUAGES** Dutch (official), Frisian
RELIGIONS Roman Catholic 31%, Protestant 21%, Islam 4%, others
CURRENCY Euro = 100 cents

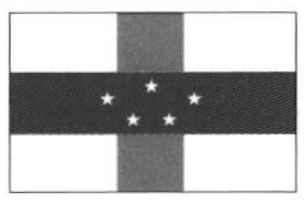

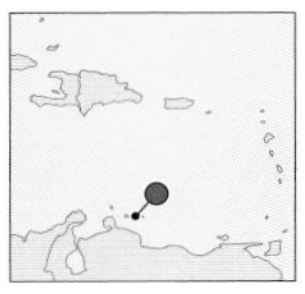

NETHERLANDS ANTILLES

The Netherlands Antilles consists of two different island groups; one off the coast of Venezuela, and the other at the northern end of the Leeward Islands, some 500 mi [800 km] away. They remain a self-governing Dutch territory. The island of Aruba was once part of the territory, but it broke away in 1986. Oil refining and tourism are important activities.

AREA 309 sq mi [800 sq km] **POPULATION** 216,000 **CAPITAL** Willemstad

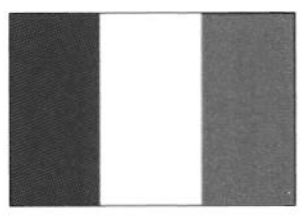

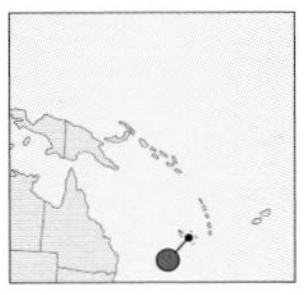

NEW CALEDONIA

New Caledonia is the most southerly of the Melanesian countries in the Pacific. A French possession since 1853 and an Overseas Territory since 1958. In 1998, France announced an agreement with local Melanesians that a vote on independence would be postponed until 2014. The country is rich in mineral resources, especially nickel.

AREA 7,172 sq mi [18,575 sq km] **POPULATION** 211,000 **CAPITAL** Nouméa

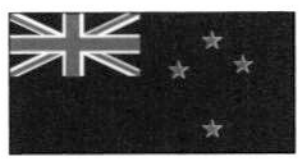

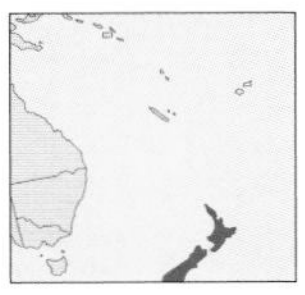

NEW ZEALAND

GEOGRAPHY New Zealand lies about 994 mi [1,600 km] southeast of Australia. It consists of two main islands and several other small ones. Much of North Island is volcanic. Active volcanoes include Ngauruhoe and Ruapehu. Hot springs and geysers are common, and steam from the ground is used to produce electricity. The Southern Alps, which contain the country's highest peak Aoraki Mount Cook at 12,313 ft [3,753 m], form the backbone of South Island. The island also has some large, fertile plains.

Auckland in the north has a warm, humid climate throughout the year. Wellington has cooler summers, while in Dunedin, in the southeast, temperatures sometimes dip below freezing in winter. The rainfall is heaviest on the western highlands.

POLITICS & ECONOMY Evidence suggests that early Maori settlers arrived in New Zealand more than 1,000 years ago. The Dutch navigator Abel Tasman reached New Zealand in 1642, but his discovery was not followed up. In 1769, the British Captain James Cook rediscovered the islands. In the early 19th century, British settlers arrived and, in 1840, under the Treaty of Waitangi, Britain took possession of the islands. From the 1870s, the Maoris were gradually integrated into colonial society.

In 1907, New Zealand became a self-governing dominion in the British Commonwealth. The country's economy developed quickly and the people became increasingly prosperous. However, after Britain joined the European Economic Community in 1973, New Zealand's exports to Britain shrank and the country had to reassess its economic and defense strategies and seek new markets. The world recession led the government to cut back on welfare spending in the 1990s. The preservation of Maori culture and Maori rights are also major issues. Ties with Britain have been gradually reduced. In 2003, the parliament voted to end the right of legal appeal to the Privy Council in London, one of New Zealand's last ties with its imperial past.

New Zealand's economy has traditionally depended on agriculture, but manufacturing now employs twice as many people as agriculture. Meat and dairy products are the most valuable farm products. Sheep rearing has declined as the area under cattle, deer, and vines has increased. Crops include barley, fruits, potatoes, other vegetables, and wheat. Fishing is also important.

AREA 104,453 sq mi [270,534 sq km] **POPULATION** 3,951,000
CAPITAL (POPULATION) Wellington (167,000)
GOVERNMENT Constitutional monarchy
ETHNIC GROUPS New Zealand European 74%, New Zealand Maori 10%, Polynesian 4% **LANGUAGES** English and Maori (both official) **RELIGIONS** Anglican 24%, Presbyterian 18%, Roman Catholic 15%, others
CURRENCY New Zealand dollar = 100 cents

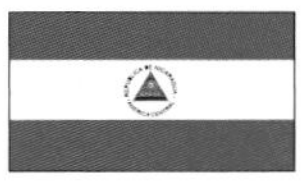

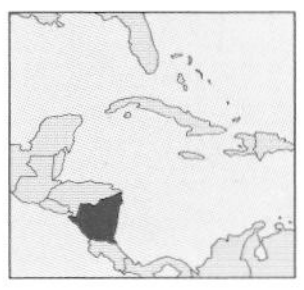

NICARAGUA

GEOGRAPHY The Republic of Nicaragua is a large country in Central America. In the east is a broad plain bordering the Caribbean Sea. The plain is drained by rivers that flow from the Central Highlands. The fertile western Pacific region contains about 40 volcanoes, many of which are active, and earthquakes are common.

Nicaragua has a tropical climate. Managua is hot throughout the year and there is a marked rainy season from May to October. In October 1998, Hurricane Mitch caused great devastation in Nicaragua. The Central Highlands and Caribbean region are cooler and wetter. The wettest region is the humid Caribbean plain.

POLITICS & ECONOMY In 1502, Christopher Columbus claimed the area for Spain, which ruled Nicaragua until 1821. By the early 20th century, the United States had considerable influence in the country and, in 1912, US forces entered Nicaragua to protect US interests. From 1927 to 1933, rebels under General Augusto César Sandino, tried to drive US forces out of the country. In 1933, US marines set up a Nicaraguan army, the National Guard, to help to defeat the rebels. Its leader, Anastasio Somoza Garcia, had Sandino murdered in 1934 and, from 1937, Somoza ruled as a dictator.

In the mid-1970s, many people began to protest against Somoza's rule. Many joined a guerrilla force, called the Sandinista National Liberation Front, named after General Sandino. The rebels defeated the Somoza regime in 1979. In the 1980s, the US-supported forces, called the "Contras," launched a campaign against the Sandinista government. The US government opposed the Sandinista regime, under Daniel José Ortega Saavedra, claiming that it was a Communist dictatorship. A coalition, the National Opposition Union, defeated the Sandinistas in elections in 1990. In 1996 and again in 2001, the Sandinista candidate Daniel Ortega was defeated in presidential elections.

In the early 1990s, Nicaragua faced many problems in rebuilding its shattered economy. Agriculture is the main activity, employing nearly half of the people. Coffee, cotton, sugar, and bananas are grown for export, while rice is the main food crop.

AREA 50,193 sq mi [130,000 sq km] **POPULATION** 5,129,000
CAPITAL (POPULATION) Managua (1,107,000)
GOVERNMENT Multiparty republic
ETHNIC GROUPS Mestizo 69%, White 17%, Black 9%, Amerindian 5%
LANGUAGES Spanish (official)
RELIGIONS Roman Catholic 85%, Protestant
CURRENCY Córdoba oro (gold córdoba) = 100 centavos

NIGER

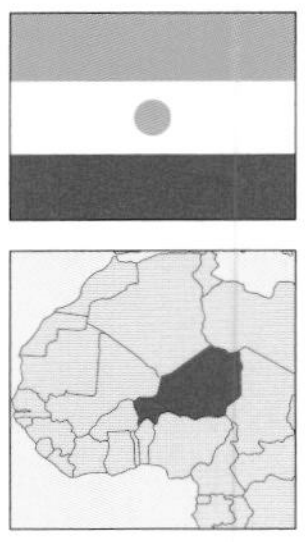

GEOGRAPHY The Republic of Niger is a landlocked nation in north-central Africa. The northern plateaux lie in the Sahara Desert, while Central Niger contains the rugged Aïr Mountains. The most fertile, densely populated region is the Niger valley in the southwest.

Niger has a tropical climate and the south has a rainy season between June and September. The north is practically rainless.

POLITICS & ECONOMY Since independence in 1960, Niger, a French territory from 1900, has suffered severe droughts. Food shortages and the collapse of the traditional nomadic way of life of some of Niger's people have caused political instability. After a period of military rule, a multiparty constitution was adopted in 1992, but the military again seized power in 1996. Later that year, the coup leader, Colonel Ibrahim Barre Mainassara, was elected president. He was assassinated in 1999, but parliamentary rule was rapidly restored and Tandja Mamadou was elected president later in the year.

Niger's chief resource is uranium and the country is the fourth largest producer. In 2003, accusations that Niger supplied uranium to Iraq for its nuclear program proved to be baseless. Some tin and tungsten are also mined, though other mineral reserves are largely untouched. Despite its resources, Niger is one of the world's poorest countries. Farming employs 76% of the people, but only 3% of the land can be used for crops and 8% for grazing.

AREA 489,189 sq mi [1,267,000 sq km] **POPULATION** 11,059,000
CAPITAL (POPULATION) Niamey (732,000)
GOVERNMENT Multiparty republic **ETHNIC GROUPS** Hausa 56%, Djerma 22%, Tuareg 8%, Fula 8%, others **LANGUAGES** French (official), Hausa, Djerma **RELIGIONS** Islam 80%, indigenous beliefs, Christianity **CURRENCY** CFA franc = 100 centimes

NIGERIA

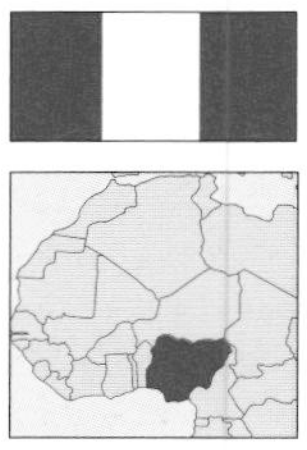

GEOGRAPHY The Federal Republic of Nigeria is the most populous nation in Africa. The country's main rivers are the Niger and Benue, which meet in central Nigeria. North of the two river valleys are high plains and plateaux. The Lake Chad basin is in the northeast, with the Sokoto plains in the northwest. The south contains hilly uplands and plains. The south has a hot, rainy climate. The north is drier and often hotter than the south.

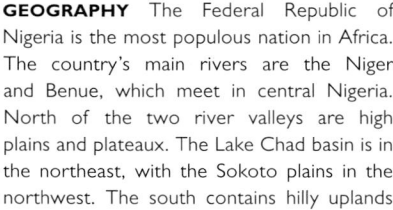

POLITICS & ECONOMY Nigeria has a long artistic tradition. Major cultures include the Nok (500 BC to AD 200), the Ife, a major Yoruba culture which developed about 1,000 years ago, and the Benin (15th to 17th centuries). Britain gradually extended its influence over the area in the second half of the 19th century.

Nigeria became independent in 1960 and a federal republic in 1963. A federal constitution dividing the country into regions was necessary because Nigeria contains more than 250 ethnic and linguistic groups, as well as several religious ones. Local rivalries have long been a threat to national unity, and six new states were created in 1996 in an attempt to overcome this. Civil war occurred between 1967 and 1970, when the people of the southeast attempted unsuccessfully to secede during the Biafran War. Between 1960 and 1998, Nigeria had only nine years of civilian government.

In 1998–9, civilian rule was restored. A former general, Olusegun Obasanjo, was elected president and he was re-elected in 2003. His government faced many problems, including religious clashes in the north, where several states adopted *sharia* (Islamic law). In 2004, the government declared that it had put down an uprising in the northeast aimed at creating a Muslim state.

Nigeria is a developing country with great potential. Its chief natural resource is oil, which accounts for most of its exports. Agriculture employs 43% of the people and the country is a major producer of cocoa, palm oil and palm kernels, groundnuts (peanuts), and rubber. Industry is increasing and manufactures include cement, chemicals, fertilizers, textiles, and timber.

AREA 356,667 sq mi [923,768 sq km] **POPULATION** 133,882,000
CAPITAL (POPULATION) Abuja (339,000)
GOVERNMENT Federal multiparty republic
ETHNIC GROUPS Hausa and Fulani 29%, Yoruba 21%, Ibo (or Igbo) 18%, Ijaw 10%, Kanuri 4%, many others
LANGUAGES English (official), Hausa, Yoruba, Ibo
RELIGIONS Islam 50%, Christianity 40%, traditional beliefs 10%
CURRENCY Naira = 100 kobo

NORTHERN MARIANA ISLANDS

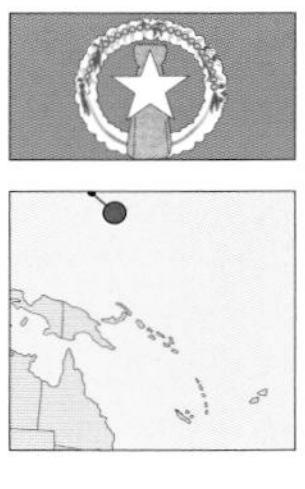

The Commonwealth of the Northern Mariana Islands contains 16 mountainous islands north of Guam in the western Pacific Ocean. In a 1975 plebiscite, the islanders voted for Commonwealth status in union with the United States and, in 1986, they were granted US citizenship.

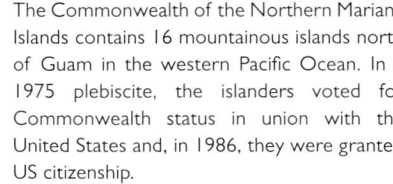

AREA 179 sq mi [464 sq km] **POPULATION** 80,000 **CAPITAL** Saipan

NORWAY

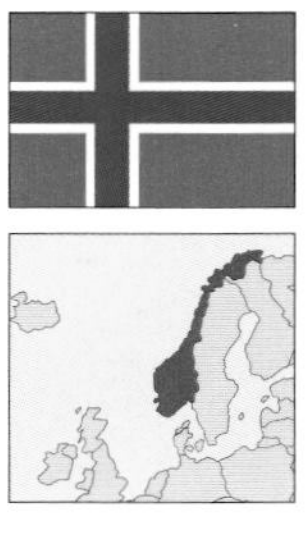

GEOGRAPHY The Kingdom of Norway forms the western part of the rugged Scandinavian peninsula. The deep inlets along the highly indented coastline were worn out by glaciers during the Ice Age. The warm North Atlantic Drift off the coast of Norway moderates the climate, with mild winters and cool summers. Nearly all the ports are ice-free throughout the year. Inland, winters are colder and snow cover lasts for at least three months a year.

POLITICS & ECONOMY Between about AD 800 and 1100, Norwegian Vikings ravaged western Europe. In 1380, Norway was united with Denmark. But in 1814, Denmark handed Norway over to Sweden, though it kept Norway's colonies – Greenland, Iceland, and the Færoe Islands. Norway briefly became independent, but Swedish forces defeated the Norwegians and Norway had to accept Sweden's king as its ruler. The union with Sweden ended in 1903.

Germany occupied Norway during World War II (1939–45). Norway recovered quickly after the war and it now has one of the world's highest standards of living. In 1960, Norway and six other countries formed the European Free Trade Association (EFTA). In 1994, the Norwegians voted against joining the European Union.

Norway's chief resources and exports are oil and natural gas which come from wells under the North Sea. Farmland covers only 3% of the land. Dairy farming and meat production are important, but Norway has to import food. Norway has many industries powered by cheap hydroelectricity.

AREA 125,049 sq mi [323,877 sq km] **POPULATION** 4,546,000
CAPITAL (POPULATION) Oslo (513,000)
GOVERNMENT Constitutional monarchy
ETHNIC GROUPS Norwegian 97%
LANGUAGES Norwegian (official)
RELIGIONS Evangelical Lutheran 86%
CURRENCY Norwegian krone = 100 ore

OMAN

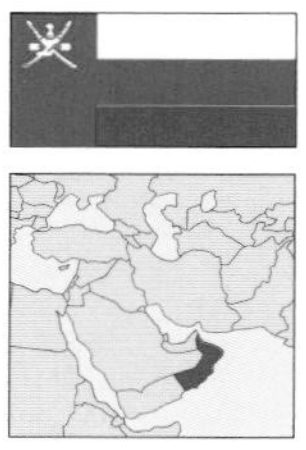

GEOGRAPHY The Sultanate of Oman occupies the southeastern corner of the Arabian peninsula. It also includes the tip of the Musandam peninsula, overlooking the strategic Strait of Hormuz.

Oman has a hot tropical climate. In Muscat, temperatures may reach 117°F [47°C] in the summer months.

POLITICS & ECONOMY British influence in Oman dates back to the end of the 18th century, but the country became fully independent in 1971. Since then, using revenue from oil, which was discovered in 1964, the absolute ruler, Qaboos ibn Said, and his government have sought to modernize the country. In 2000, Oman held its first direct elections to its consultative parliament. Unusually for the Gulf region, two women were returned.

The World Bank classifies Oman as an "upper-middle-income" country. Oil accounts for the bulk of the exports, while huge natural gas deposits were discovered in 1991. However, agriculture remains important. Major crops include alfalfa, bananas, coconuts, dates, limes, tobacco, vegetables, and wheat. Some cattle are raised and fishing, especially for sardines, is important. But Oman still has to import food.

AREA 119,498 sq mi [309,500 sq km] **POPULATION** 2,807,000
CAPITAL (POPULATION) Muscat (41,000)
GOVERNMENT Monarchy with consultative council
ETHNIC GROUPS Arab, Baluchi, Indian, Pakistani
LANGUAGES Arabic (official), Baluchi, English
RELIGIONS Islam (mainly Ibadhi), Hinduism
CURRENCY Omani rial = 100 baizas

PAKISTAN

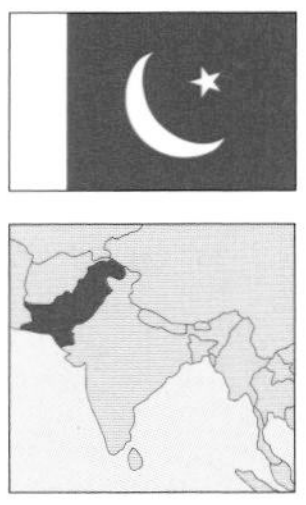

GEOGRAPHY The Islamic Republic of Pakistan contains high mountains, fertile plains and rocky deserts. The Karakoram range, which contains K2, the world's second highest peak, lies in the northern part of Jammu and Kashmir, which is occupied by Pakistan but claimed by India. Other mountains rise in the west. Plains, drained by the River Indus and its tributaries, occupy much of eastern Pakistan. Arid areas include the Thar Desert and the Baluchistan plateau. Most of Pakistan has hot summers and mild winters, though the mountains have cold winters. The rainfall is generally sparse.

POLITICS & ECONOMY Pakistan was the site of the Indus Valley civilization which developed about 4,500 years ago. But Pakistan's modern history dates from 1947, when British India was divided into India and Pakistan. Muslim Pakistan was divided into two parts: East and West Pakistan, but East Pakistan broke away in 1971 to become Bangladesh. In 1948–9, 1965 and 1971, Pakistan and India clashed over Kashmir. In 1998, Pakistan responded in kind to India's nuclear weapon tests but, in 2003–4, Pakistan and India raised hopes of a settlement in Kashmir.

Pakistan has been subject to several periods of military rule, but elections in 1988 led to Benazir Bhutto becoming prime minister. She was removed from office in 1990, but she returned as prime minister between 1993 and 1996. In 1997, Narwaz Sharif was elected prime minister, but a military coup in 1999 brought General Pervez Musharraf to power. In 2001, Pakistan supported the Western assault on Taliban forces in Afghanistan. In 2002, voters agreed to extend Musharraf's term in office by five years. In 2004, the government's moves toward democratization and its support for the international coalition against terrorism led the Commonwealth to restore Pakistan as a member.

According to the World Bank, Pakistan is a "low-income" developing country. The economy is based on farming or rearing goats and sheep. Agriculture employs nearly half the people. Major crops include cotton, fruits, rice, sugarcane, and wheat.

AREA 307,372 sq mi [796,095 sq km] **POPULATION** 150,695,000
CAPITAL (POPULATION) Islamabad (529,000)
GOVERNMENT Military regime **ETHNIC GROUPS** Punjabi, Sindhi, Pashtun (Pathan), Baluchi, Muhajir
LANGUAGES Urdu (official), many others
RELIGIONS Islam 97%, Christianity, Hinduism
CURRENCY Pakistani rupee = 100 paisa

PALAU

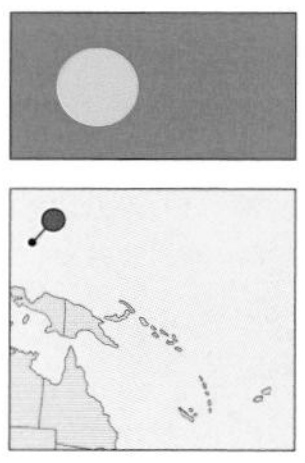

The Republic of Palau became fully independent in 1994, after the USA refused to accede to a 1979 referendum that declared this island nation a nuclear-free zone. In December 1994 Palau joined the United Nations. The economy relies heavily on US aid, tourism, fishing and subsistence agriculture. The main crops include cassava, coconuts, and copra.

AREA 177 sq mi [459 sq km] **POPULATION** 20,000 **CAPITAL** Koror

PANAMA

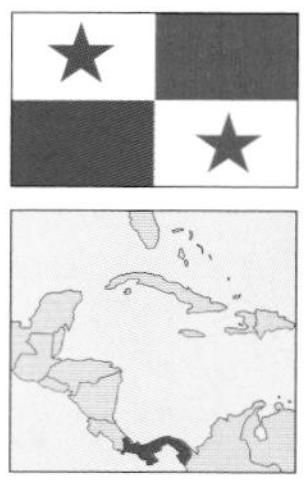

GEOGRAPHY The Republic of Panama forms an isthmus linking Central America to South America. The Panama Canal, which is 50.7 mi [81.6 km] long, cuts across the isthmus. It has made the country a major transport center.

Panama has a tropical climate. Temperatures are high, though the mountains are much cooler than the coastal plains. The main rainy season is between May and December.

POLITICS & ECONOMY Christopher Columbus landed in Panama in 1502 and Spain soon took the area. In 1821, Panama became independent from Spain and a province of Colombia.

In 1903, Colombia refused a request by the United States to build a canal. Panama then revolted against Colombia, and became independent. The United States then began to build the canal, which was opened in 1914. The United States administered the Panama Canal Zone, a strip of land along the canal. But many Panamanians resented US influence and, in 1979, the Canal Zone was returned to Panama. Control of the canal itself was handed over by the USA to Panama on December 31, 1999.

Panama's government has changed many times since independence, and there have been periods of military dictatorships. In 1983, General Manuel Antonio Noriega became Panama's leader. In 1988, two US grand juries in Florida indicted

Noriega on charges of drug trafficking. In 1989, Noriega was apparently defeated in a presidential election, but the government declared the election invalid. After the killing of a US marine, US troops entered Panama and arrested Noriega, who was convicted by a Miami court of drug offences in 1992. However, Panama held national elections in 1994. In 1999, Mireya Moscoso became Panama's first woman president. In 2003–4, she was criticized for failing to curb corruption and provide more jobs.

The World Bank classifies Panama as a "lower-middle-income" developing country. The Panama Canal is an important source of revenue and it generates many jobs in commerce, trade, manufacturing, and transport. Away from the Canal, the main activity is agriculture, which employs 18% of the people.

AREA 29,157 sq mi [75,517 sq km] **POPULATION** 2,961,000 **CAPITAL (POPULATION)** Panamá (484,000) **GOVERNMENT** Multiparty republic **ETHNIC GROUPS** Mestizo 70%, Black and Mulatto 14%, White 10%, Amerindian 6% **LANGUAGES** Spanish (official), English **RELIGIONS** Roman Catholic 85%, Protestant 15% **CURRENCY** US dollar; Balboa = 100 centésimos

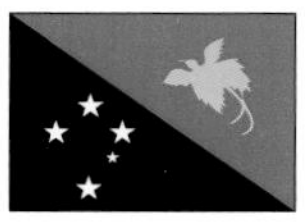
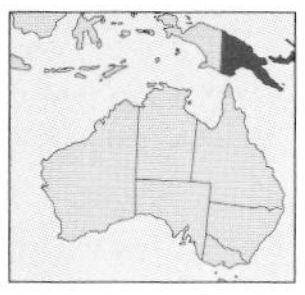

PAPUA NEW GUINEA

GEOGRAPHY Papua New Guinea is an independent country in the Pacific Ocean, north of Australia. It is part of a Pacific island region called Melanesia. Papua New Guinea includes the eastern part of New Guinea, the Bismarck Archipelago, the northern Solomon Islands, the D'Entrecasteaux Islands and the Louisiade Archipelago. The land is largely mountainous.

Papua New Guinea has a tropical climate, with high temperatures throughout the year. Most of the rain occurs during the monsoon season (from December to April), when the northwesterly winds blow. Winds blow from the southeast during the dry season.

POLITICS & ECONOMY The Dutch took western New Guinea (now part of Indonesia) in 1828, but it was not until 1884 that Germany took northeastern New Guinea and Britain took the southeast. In 1906, Britain handed the southeast over to Australia. It then became known as the Territory of Papua. When World War I broke out in 1914, Australia took German New Guinea and, in 1921, the League of Nations gave Australia a mandate to rule the area, which was named the Territory of New Guinea.

Japan invaded New Guinea in 1942, but the Allies reconquered the area in 1944. In 1949, Papua and New Guinea were combined into the Territory of Papua and New Guinea. Papua New Guinea became fully independent in 1975.

Since independence, the government has worked to develop its mineral reserves. One of the most valuable mines was on Bougainville, in the northern Solomon Islands. But the people of Bougainville demanded a larger share in the profits of the mine. Conflict broke out, the mine was closed and the Bougainville Revolutionary Army proclaimed the island independent. But their attempted secession was not recognized internationally. A final peace settlement, giving the island local autonomy, was agreed in 2001.

The World Bank classifies Papua New Guinea as a "lower-middle-income" developing country. Agriculture employs three out of every four people, many of whom produce little more than they need to feed their families. Minerals, notably copper and gold, are the most valuable exports.

AREA 178,703 sq mi [462,840 sq km] **POPULATION** 5,296,000 **CAPITAL (POPULATION)** Port Moresby (193,000) **GOVERNMENT** Constitutional monarchy **ETHNIC GROUPS** Papuan, Melanesian, Micronesian **LANGUAGES** English (official), Melanesian Pidgin; more than 700 indigenous languages **RELIGIONS** Traditional beliefs 34%, Roman Catholic 22%, Lutheran 16% **CURRENCY** Kina = 100 toea

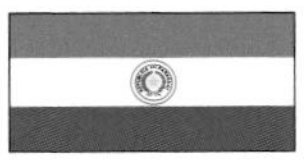
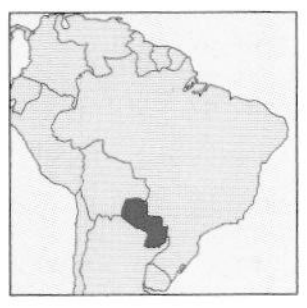

PARAGUAY

GEOGRAPHY The Republic of Paraguay is a landlocked country and rivers, notably the Paraná, Pilcomayo (Brazo Sur) and Paraguay, form most of its borders. A flat region called the Gran Chaco lies in the northwest, while the southeast contains plains, hills and plateaux. Northern Paraguay lies in the tropics, while the south is subtropical. Most of the country has a warm, humid climate.

POLITICS & ECONOMY In 1776, Paraguay became part of a large colony called the Vice-royalty of La Plata, with Buenos Aires as the capital. Paraguayans opposed this move and the country declared its independence in 1811.

For many years, Paraguay was torn by internal strife and conflict with its neighbors. A war against Brazil, Argentina, and Uruguay (1865–70) led to the deaths of more than half of Paraguay's population, and a great loss of territory.

General Alfredo Stroessner took power in 1954 and ruled as a dictator. His government imprisoned many opponents. Stroessner was overthrown in 1989. However, the return of democracy in the 1990s and 2000s often seemed precarious because of rivalries between politicians and army leaders, together with economic problems arising partly from the severe problems experienced in neighboring Argentina and Brazil.

The World Bank classifies Paraguay as a "lower-middle-income" developing country. Farming and forestry are important. Paraguay produces hydroelectricity and exports power to its neighbors.

AREA 157,047 sq mi [406,752 sq km] **POPULATION** 6,037,000 **CAPITAL (POPULATION)** Asunción (547,000) **GOVERNMENT** Multiparty republic **ETHNIC GROUPS** Mestizo 95% **LANGUAGES** Spanish and Guaraní (both official) **RELIGIONS** Roman Catholic 90%, Protestant **CURRENCY** Guaraní = 100 céntimos

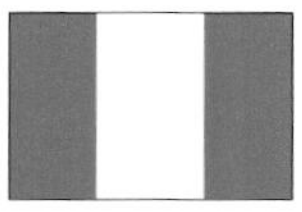
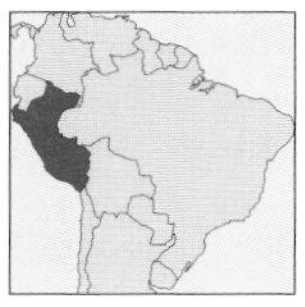

PERU

GEOGRAPHY The Republic of Peru lies in the tropics in western South America. A narrow coastal plain borders the Pacific Ocean in the west. Inland are ranges of the Andes Mountains, which rise to 22,205 ft [6,768 m] at Mount Huascarán, an extinct volcano. East of the Andes lies the Amazon basin.

Lima, on the coastal plain, has an arid climate. The coastal region is chilled by the cold, offshore Humboldt Current. The rainfall increases inland and many mountains in the high Andes are snow-capped.

POLITICS & ECONOMY Spanish conquistadors conquered Peru in the 1530s. In 1820, an Argentinian, José de San Martín, led an army into Peru and declared it independent. But Spain still held large areas. In 1823, the Venezuelan Simon Bolívar led another army into Peru and, in 1824, one of his generals defeated the Spaniards at Ayacucho. The Spaniards surrendered in 1826. Peru suffered much instability throughout the 19th century.

Instability continued in the 20th century. In 1980, when civilian rule was restored, a left-wing group called the Sendero Luminoso, or the "Shining Path," began guerrilla warfare against the government. In 1990, Alberto Fujimori, son of Japanese immigrants, became president. In 1992, he suspended the constitution and dismissed the legislature. The guerrilla leader, Abimael Guzmán, was arrested in 1992, but instability continued. Following his victory in disputed presidential elections in 2000, Fujimori resigned and sought sanctuary in Japan. In 2001, Alejandro Toledo became the first Peruvian of Amerindian descent to be elected president. He faced many problems, including, in 2003, a resurgence in activity by the Shining Path guerrillas.

The World Bank classifies Peru as a "lower-middle-income" developing country. Major food crops include beans, maize, potatoes, and rice. Fish products are exported, but the most valuable export is copper. Peru also produces lead, silver, zinc, and iron ore.

AREA 496,222 sq mi [1,285,216 sq km] **POPULATION** 28,410,000 **CAPITAL (POPULATION)** Lima (5,681,000) **GOVERNMENT** Transitional republic **ETHNIC GROUPS** Amerindian 45%, Mestizo 37%, White 15% **LANGUAGES** Spanish and Quechua (both official), Aymara, other Amazonian languages **RELIGIONS** Roman Catholic 90% **CURRENCY** New sol = 100 centavos

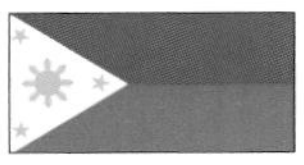
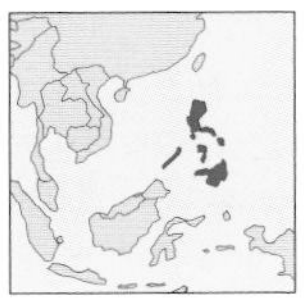

PHILIPPINES

GEOGRAPHY The Republic of the Philippines is an island country in southeastern Asia. It includes about 7,100 islands, of which 2,770 are named and about 1,000 are inhabited. Luzon and Mindanao, the two largest islands, make up more than two-thirds of the country. The land is mainly mountainous.

The country has a hot tropical climate. The dry season runs from December to April. The rest of the year is wet. Much of the rainfall comes from the typhoons which periodically strike the east coast.

POLITICS & ECONOMY The first European to reach the Philippines was the Portuguese navigator Ferdinand Magellan in 1521. Spanish explorers claimed the region in 1565 when they established a settlement on Cebu. The Spaniards ruled the country until 1898, when the United States took over at the end of the Spanish–American War. Japan invaded the Philippines in 1941, but US forces returned in 1944. The country became fully independent as the Republic of the Philippines in 1946.

Since independence, the country's problems have included armed uprisings by left-wing guerrillas demanding land reform, and Muslim separatist groups, crime, corruption and unemployment. The dominant figure in recent times was Ferdinand Marcos, who ruled in a dictatorial manner from 1965 to 1986. His successors were Corazon Aquino (1986–92), Fidel Ramos (1992–8), and Joseph Estrada, who resigned following accusations of corruption. He was succeeded by Vice-President Gloria Arroyo. In 2003, her government had to put down a military rebellion as well as combating Muslim terrorists and Islamic separatists.

The Philippines is a developing country which has a "lower-middle-income" economy. Agriculture employs 33% of the people. The main foods are rice and maize, while such crops as bananas, cocoa, coconuts, coffee, sugarcane, and tobacco are all grown commercially. Manufacturing now plays an increasingly important role in the economy.

AREA 115,830 sq mi [300,000 sq km] **POPULATION** 84,620,000 **CAPITAL (POPULATION)** Manila (1,581,000) **GOVERNMENT** Multiparty republic **ETHNIC GROUPS** Christian Malay 92%, Muslim Malay 4%, Chinese and others **LANGUAGES** Filipino (Tagalog) and English (both official), Spanish, many others **RELIGIONS** Roman Catholic 83%, Protestant 9%, Islam 5% **CURRENCY** Philippine peso = 100 centavos

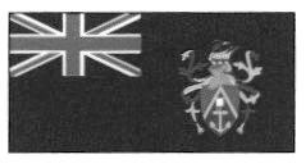
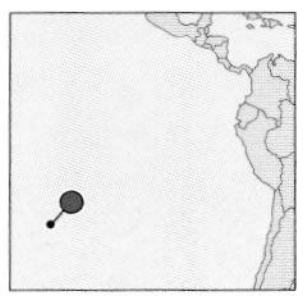

PITCAIRN

Pitcairn Island is a British overseas territory in the Pacific Ocean. Its inhabitants are descendants of the original settlers – nine mutineers from HMS *Bounty* and 18 Tahitians who arrived in 1790.

AREA 21 sq mi [55 sq km] **POPULATION** 50 **CAPITAL** Adamstown

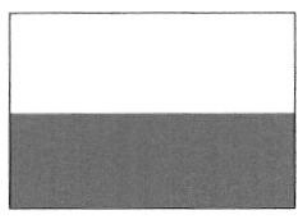
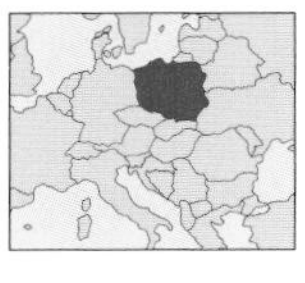

POLAND

GEOGRAPHY The Republic of Poland faces the Baltic Sea and, behind its lagoon-fringed coast, lies a broad plain. A plateau lies in the southeast, while the Sudeten Highlands straddle part of the border with the Czech Republic. Part of the Carpathian Range (the Tatra) lies in the southeast.

Poland's climate is influenced by its position in Europe. Warm, moist air masses come from the west, while cold air masses come from the north and east. Summers are warm, but winters are cold and snowy.

POLITICS & ECONOMY Poland's boundaries have changed several times in the last 200 years, partly as a result of its geographical location between the powers of Germany and Russia. It disappeared from the map in the late 18th century, when a Polish state called the Grand Duchy of Warsaw was set up. But in 1815, the country was partitioned, between Austria, Prussia and Russia. Poland became independent in 1918, but in 1939 it was divided between Germany and the Soviet Union. The country again became independent in 1945, when it lost land to Russia but gained some from Germany. Communists took power in 1948, but opposition mounted and eventually became focused through an organization called Solidarity.

Solidarity was led by a trade unionist, Lech Walesa. A coalition government was formed between Solidarity and the Communists in 1989. In 1990, the Communist party was dissolved and Walesa became president. But Walesa faced many problems in turning Poland toward a market economy. In presidential elections in 1995, Walesa was defeated by ex-Communist Aleksander Kwasniewski. However, Kwasniewski continued to follow westward-looking policies and he was re-elected president in 2000. Poland joined the North Atlantic Treaty Organization in 1999 and, on May 1, 2004, it became a member of the European Union.

Poland has large reserves of coal and deposits of various minerals which are used in its factories. Manufactures include chemicals, processed food, machinery, ships, steel, and textiles.

AREA 124,807 sq mi [323,250 sq km] **POPULATION** 38,623,000 **CAPITAL (POPULATION)** Warsaw (1,615,000) **GOVERNMENT** Multiparty republic **ETHNIC GROUPS** Polish 97%, Belarusian, Ukrainian, German **LANGUAGES** Polish (official) **RELIGIONS** Roman Catholic 95%, Eastern Orthodox **CURRENCY** Zloty = 100 groszy

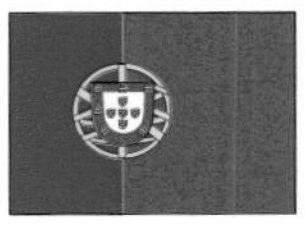
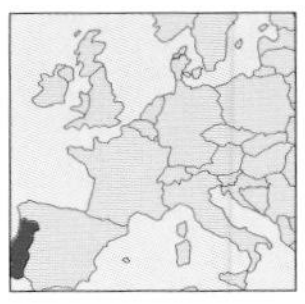

PORTUGAL

GEOGRAPHY The Republic of Portugal is the most westerly of Europe's mainland countries. The land rises from the coastal plains on the Atlantic Ocean to the western edge of the huge plateau, or Meseta, which occupies most of the Iberian peninsula. The climate is moderated by winds blowing from the Atlantic Ocean. Summers are cooler and winters are milder than in other Mediterranean lands. Portugal also contains two autonomous regions, the Azores and Madeira island groups.

POLITICS & ECONOMY Portugal became a separate country, independent of Spain, in 1143. In the 15th century, Portugal led the "Age of European Exploration." This led to the growth of a large Portuguese empire, with colonies in Africa, Asia and, most valuable of all, Brazil in South America. Portuguese power began to decline in the 16th century and, between 1580 and 1640, Portugal was ruled by Spain. Portugal lost Brazil in 1822 and, in 1910, Portugal became a republic. Instability hampered progress and army officers seized power in 1926. In 1928, they chose Antonio de Salazar to be minister of finance. He became prime minister in 1932 and ruled as a dictator from 1933.

Salazar ruled until 1968, but his successor, Marcello Caetano, was overthrown in 1974 by a group of army officers. The new government made most of Portugal's remaining colonies independent. Free elections were held in 1978. Portugal joined the European Community (now the European Union) in 1986 and, on January 1, 2002, the euro replaced the escudo as Portugal's sole official unit of currency.

Agriculture and fishing were the mainstays of the economy until the mid-20th century, when manufacturing became the most valuable activity. The timber industry received a major setback in 2003 when forest fires caused enormous damage.

AREA 34,285 SQ MI [88,797 SQ KM] **POPULATION** 10,102,000
CAPITAL (POPULATION) LISBON (663,000)
GOVERNMENT MULTIPARTY REPUBLIC **ETHNIC GROUPS** PORTUGUESE 99%
LANGUAGES PORTUGUESE (OFFICIAL) **RELIGIONS** ROMAN CATHOLIC 94%, PROTESTANT **CURRENCY** EURO = 100 CENTS

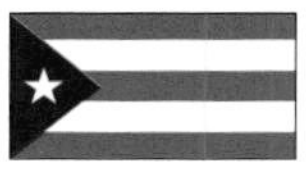
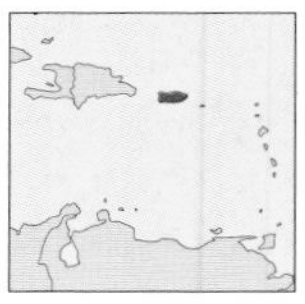

PUERTO RICO

The Commonwealth of Puerto Rico, a mainly mountainous island, is the easternmost of the Greater Antilles chain. The climate is hot and wet. Puerto Rico is a dependent territory of the USA and the people are US citizens. In 1998, 50.2% of the population voted in a referendum on possible statehood to maintain the status quo.

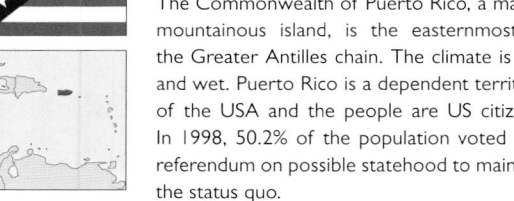

Puerto Rico is the most industrialized country in the Caribbean. Tax exemptions attract US companies to the island and manufacturing is expanding. The chief exports are chemicals and chemical products, machinery, and food.

AREA 3,427 SQ MI [8,875 SQ KM] **POPULATION** 3,886,000
CAPITAL (POPULATION) SAN JUAN (422,000)

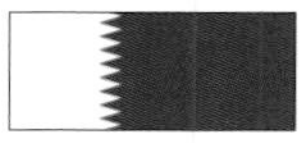
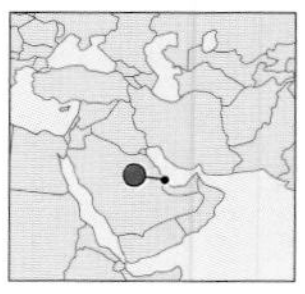

QATAR

The State of Qatar occupies a low, barren peninsula that extends northward from the Arabian peninsula into the Persian Gulf. The climate is hot and dry. Qatar became a British protectorate in 1916, but it became fully independent in 1971. Oil, first discovered in 1939, is the mainstay of the economy of this prosperous nation.

AREA 4,247 SQ MI [11,000 SQ KM] **POPULATION** 817,000 **CAPITAL** DOHA

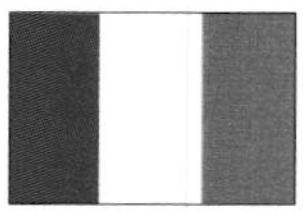
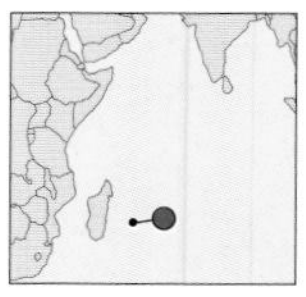

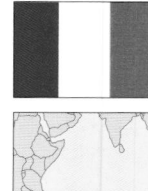

RÉUNION

Réunion is a French overseas department in the Indian Ocean. The land is mainly mountainous, though the lowlands are intensely cultivated. Sugar and sugar products are the main exports, but French aid, given to the island in return for its use as a military base, is important to the economy.

AREA 969 SQ MI [2,510 SQ KM]
POPULATION 755,000 **CAPITAL** ST-DENIS

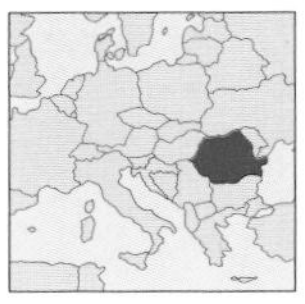

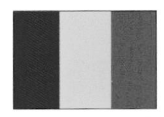

ROMANIA

GEOGRAPHY Romania is a country on the Black Sea in eastern Europe. Eastern and southern Romania form part of the Danube river basin. The delta region, near the mouths of the Danube, where the river flows into the Black Sea, is one of Europe's finest wetlands. The southern part of the coast contains several resorts. The heart of the country is called Transylvania. It is ringed in the east, south and west by scenic mountains which are part of the Carpathian mountain system. Romania has hot summers and cold winters. The rainfall is heaviest in spring and early summer.

POLITICS & ECONOMY From the late 18th century, the Turkish empire began to break up. The modern history of Romania began in 1861 when Walachia and Moldavia united. After World War I (1914–18), Romania, which had fought on the side of the victorious Allies, obtained large areas, including Transylvania, where most people were Romanians. This almost doubled the country's size and population. In 1939, Romania lost territory to Bulgaria, Hungary and the Soviet Union. Romania fought alongside Germany in World War II, and Soviet troops occupied the country in 1944. Hungary returned northern Transylvania to Romania in 1945, but Bulgaria and the Soviet Union kept former Romanian territory. In 1947, Romania officially became a Communist country.

In 1990, Romania held its first free elections since the end of World War II. The National Salvation Front, led by Ion Iliescu and containing many former Communist leaders, won a large majority. A new constitution, approved in 1991, made the country a democratic republic. Elections held under this constitution in 1992 again resulted in victory for Ion Iliescu, whose party was renamed the Party of Social Democracy (PDSR) in 1993. But the government faced many problems. In 1996, the center-right Democratic Convention defeated the PDSR, led by Emil Constantinescu, who became president. But Iliescu was re-elected president in 2000. Romania's desire to establish good relations with the West were rewarded when it became a member of the North Atlantic Treaty Organization in 2004.

According to the World Bank, Romania is a "lower-middle-income" economy. Under Communist rule, industry, including mining and manufacturing, became more important than agriculture.

AREA 92,043 SQ MI [238,391 SQ KM] **POPULATION** 22,272,000
CAPITAL (POPULATION) BUCHAREST (2,016,000)
GOVERNMENT MULTIPARTY REPUBLIC
ETHNIC GROUPS ROMANIAN 89%, HUNGARIAN 7%, ROMA 2%, UKRAINIAN **LANGUAGES** ROMANIAN (OFFICIAL), HUNGARIAN, GERMAN **RELIGIONS** EASTERN ORTHODOX 87%, PROTESTANT 7%, ROMAN CATHOLIC 5% **CURRENCY** LEU = 100 BANI

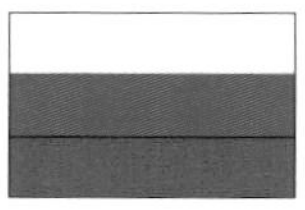
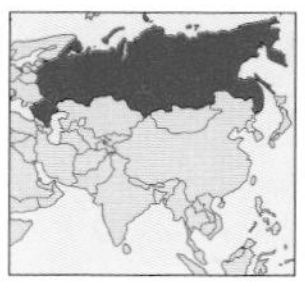

RUSSIA

GEOGRAPHY Russia is the world's largest country. About 25% lies west of the Ural Mountains in European Russia, where 80% of the population lives. It is mostly flat or undulating, but the land rises to the Caucasus Mountains in the south, where Russia's highest peak, Elbrus, at 18,481 ft [5,633 m], is found. Asian Russia, or Siberia, contains vast plains and plateaux, with mountains in the east and south. The Kamchatka peninsula in the far east has many active volcanoes. Russia contains many of the world's longest rivers, including the Yenisey-Angara and the Ob-Irtysh. It also includes part of the world's largest inland body of water, the Caspian Sea, and Lake Baikal, the world's deepest lake.

Moscow has a continental climate with cold and snowy winters and warm summers. Siberia has a harsher, drier climate.

POLITICS & ECONOMY In the 9th century AD, a state called Kievan Rus was formed by a group of people called the East Slavs. Kiev, now capital of Ukraine, became a major trading center, but, in 1237, Mongol armies conquered Russia and destroyed Kiev. Russia was part of the Mongol empire until the late 15th century. Under Mongol rule, Moscow became the leading Russian city.

In the 16th century, Moscow's grand prince was retitled "tsar." The first tsar, Ivan the Terrible, expanded Russian territory. In 1613, after a period of civil war, Michael Romanov became tsar, founding a dynasty which ruled until 1917. In the early 18th century, Tsar Peter the Great began to westernize Russia and, by 1812, when Napoleon failed to conquer the country, Russia was a major European power. But during the 19th century, many Russians demanded reforms and discontent was widespread.

In World War I (1914–18), the Russian people suffered great hardships and, in 1917, Tsar Nicholas II was forced to abdicate. In November 1917, the Bolsheviks seized power under Vladimir Lenin. In 1922, the Bolsheviks set up a new nation, the Union of Soviet Socialist Republics (also called the USSR or the Soviet Union).

From 1924, Joseph Stalin introduced a socialist economic program, suppressing all opposition. In 1939, the Soviet Union and Germany signed a non-aggression pact, but Germany invaded the Soviet Union in 1941. Soviet forces pushed the Germans back, occupying eastern Europe. They reached Berlin in May 1945. From the late 1940s, tension between the Soviet Union and its allies and Western nations developed into a "Cold War." This continued until 1991, when the Soviet Union was dissolved.

The Soviet Union collapsed because of the failure of its economic policies. From 1991, President Boris Yeltsin introduced democratic and economic reforms. Yeltsin retired in 1999 and, in 2000, was succeeded by Vladimir Putin. Putin has sought to develop increasing contacts with the West. He was re-elected by a landslide majority in 2004 and he supported the US-declared "war on terrorism," though he opposed the war on Iraq in 2003. But he was unable to halt the ongoing conflict in Chechenia, which claimed the lives of more than 4,500 Russian soldiers in 1999–2002. This conflict reveals that Russia's sheer size and ethnic diversity makes national unity difficult to achieve.

Russia's economy was thrown into disarray after the collapse of the Soviet Union, and in the early 1990s the World Bank described Russia as a "lower-middle-income" economy. Russia was admitted to the Council of Europe in 1997, essentially to discourage instability in the Caucasus. More significantly still, Boris Yeltsin was invited to attend the G7 summit in Denver in 1997. The summit became known as "the Summit of the Eight" and it appeared that Russia will now be included in future meetings of the world's most powerful economies. Industry is the most valuable activity, though, under Communist rule, manufacturing was less efficient than in the West, and the emphasis was on heavy industry. Today, light industries producing consumer goods are becoming important. Russia's adundant resources include oil and natural gas, coal, timber, metal ores, and hydroelectric power.

Most farmland is still government-owned or run as collectives. Russia is a major producer of farm products, though it imports grains. Major crops include barley, flax, fruits, oats, rye, potatoes, sugar beet, sunflower seeds, vegetables, and wheat.

AREA 6,592,812 SQ MI [17,075,400 SQ KM] **POPULATION** 144,526,000
CAPITAL (POPULATION) MOSCOW (8,297,000) **GOVERNMENT** FEDERAL MULTIPARTY REPUBLIC **ETHNIC GROUPS** RUSSIAN 82%, TATAR 4%, UKRAINIAN 3%, CHUVASH 1%, MORE THAN 100 OTHERS
LANGUAGES RUSSIAN (OFFICIAL), MANY OTHERS
RELIGIONS MAINLY RUSSIAN ORTHODOX, ISLAM, JUDAISM
CURRENCY RUSSIAN RUBLE = 100 KOPEKS

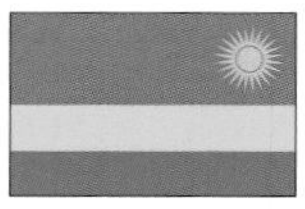
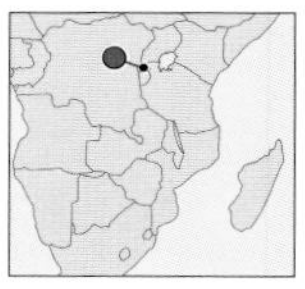

RWANDA

GEOGRAPHY The Republic of Rwanda is a small, landlocked country in east-central Africa. Lake Kivu and the River Ruzizi in the Great African Rift Valley form the country's western border.

Kigali stands on the central plateau of Rwanda. Here, temperatures are moderated by the altitude. The rainfall is abundant, but much heavier rain falls on the western mountains.

POLITICS & ECONOMY Germany conquered the area, called Ruanda-Urundi, in the 1890s. However, Belgium occupied the region during World War I (1914–18) and ruled it until 1961, when the people of Ruanda voted for their country to become a republic, called Rwanda. This decision followed a rebellion by the majority Hutu people against the Tutsi monarchy. About 150,000 deaths resulted from this conflict. Many Tutsis fled to Uganda, where they formed a rebel army. Burundi became independent as a monarchy, though it became a republic in 1966. Relations between Hutus and Tutsis continued to cause friction. Civil war broke out in 1994 and in 1996 the conflict spilled over into Congo (then Zaïre). Paul Kagame, Rwanda's effective leader since 1994, was elected president in 2000. His aim was to create unity.

According to the World Bank, Rwanda is a "low-income" developing country. Most people are poor farmers. Food crops include bananas, beans, cassava and sorghum. Some cattle are raised.

AREA 10,169 SQ MI [26,338 SQ KM] **POPULATION** 7,810,000
CAPITAL (POPULATION) KIGALI (234,000)
GOVERNMENT REPUBLIC **ETHNIC GROUPS** HUTU 84%, TUTSI 15%, TWA 1% **LANGUAGES** FRENCH, ENGLISH AND KINYARWANDA (ALL OFFICIAL) **RELIGIONS** ROMAN CATHOLIC 57%, PROTESTANT 26%, ADVENTIST 11%, ISLAM 5% **CURRENCY** RWANDAN FRANC = 100 CENTIMES

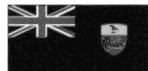

ST HELENA

St Helena, which became a British colony in 1834, is an isolated volcanic island in the south Atlantic Ocean. Now a British overseas territory, it is also the administrative center of Ascension and Tristan da Cunha.

AREA 47 SQ MI [122 SQ KM]

POPULATION 5,000 **CAPITAL** JAMESTOWN

ST KITTS AND NEVIS

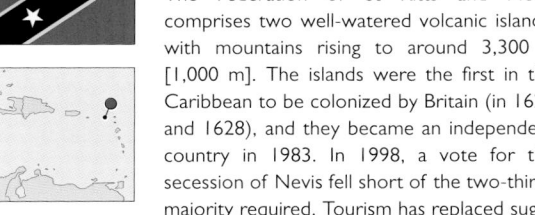

The Federation of St Kitts and Nevis comprises two well-watered volcanic islands, with mountains rising to around 3,300 ft [1,000 m]. The islands were the first in the Caribbean to be colonized by Britain (in 1623 and 1628), and they became an independent country in 1983. In 1998, a vote for the secession of Nevis fell short of the two-thirds majority required. Tourism has replaced sugar as the principal earner.

AREA 101 SQ MI [261 SQ KM] **POPULATION** 39,000

CAPITAL (POPULATION) BASSETERRE (12,000)

ST LUCIA

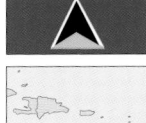

St Lucia, which became independent from Britain in 1979, is a mountainous, forested island of extinct volcanoes. It exports bananas and coconuts, and now attracts many tourists.

AREA 208 SQ MI [539 SQ KM]

POPULATION 162,000 **CAPITAL** CASTRIES

ST VINCENT AND THE GRENADINES

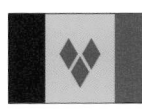

St Vincent and the Grenadines achieved its independence from Britain in 1979. Tourism is growing, but the territory is less prosperous than its neighbors.

AREA 150 SQ MI [388 SQ KM]

POPULATION 117,000 **CAPITAL** KINGSTOWN

SAMOA

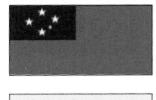

The Independent State of Samoa (formerly Western Samoa) comprises two islands in the South Pacific Ocean. Governed by New Zealand from 1920, the territory became independent in 1962. Exports include coconut cream and beer.

AREA 1,093 SQ MI [2,831 SQ KM]

POPULATION 178,000 **CAPITAL** APIA

SAN MARINO

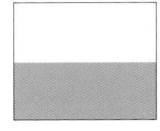

San Marino in northern Italy has been independent since 885 and a republic since the 14th century. It is the world's oldest republic. It has a friendship and cooperation treaty with Italy dating back to 1862. The state is governed by an elected council and has its own legal system. It has no armed forces and the police are "hired" from the Italian constabulary. The chief occupations are tourism, limestone quarrying, textiles, and wine-making.

AREA 24 SQ MI [61 SQ KM] **POPULATION** 28,000 **CAPITAL** SAN MARINO

SÃO TOMÉ AND PRÍNCIPE

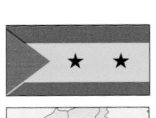

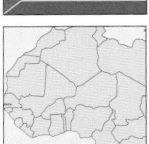

The Democratic Republic of São Tomé and Príncipe, a mountainous island territory west of Gabon, became a Portuguese colony in 1522. Following independence in 1975, the islands became a one-party Marxist state, but multiparty elections were held in 1991.

AREA 372 SQ MI [964 SQ KM] **POPULATION** 176,000 **CAPITAL** SÃO TOMÉ

SAUDI ARABIA

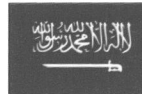

GEOGRAPHY The Kingdom of Saudi Arabia occupies about three-quarters of the Arabian peninsula in southwest Asia. Deserts cover most of the land. Mountains border the Red Sea plains in the west. In the north is the sandy Nafud Desert (An Nafud). In the south is the Rub' al Khali (the "Empty Quarter"), one of the world's bleakest deserts.

Saudi Arabia has a hot, dry climate. In the summer months, the temperatures in Riyadh often exceed 104°F [40°C], though the nights are cool.

POLITICS & ECONOMY Saudi Arabia contains the two holiest places in Islam – Mecca (or Makka), the birthplace of the Prophet Muhammad in AD 570, and Medina (Al Madinah) where Muhammad went in 622. These places are visited by many pilgrims.

Saudi Arabia was poor until the oil industry began to operate on the eastern plains in 1933. Oil revenues have been used to develop the country and Saudi Arabia has given aid to poorer Arab nations. The monarch has supreme authority and Saudi Arabia has no formal constitution. In the first Gulf War (1980–8), Saudi Arabia supported Iraq against Iran. But when Iraq invaded Kuwait in 1990, it joined the international alliance to drive Iraq's forces out of Kuwait in 1991. In 2001, relations with the US became strained after the terrorist attacks on September 11, 2001, partly because many alleged terrorists were Saudi nationals. Saudi Arabia denounced the attacks and, in 2004, a bombing occurred in Riyadh and the government cracked down on al Qaida suspects.

Saudi Arabia has about 25% of the world's known oil reserves and oil products make up about 90% of its exports. Agriculture remains important. Irrigation and desalination schemes have increased crop production.

AREA 829,995 SQ MI [2,149,690 SQ KM] **POPULATION** 24,294,000

CAPITAL (POPULATION) RIYADH (3,000,000)

GOVERNMENT ABSOLUTE MONARCHY WITH CONSULTATIVE ASSEMBLY

ETHNIC GROUPS ARAB 90%, AFRO-ASIAN 10%

LANGUAGES ARABIC (OFFICIAL)

RELIGIONS ISLAM 100%

CURRENCY SAUDI RIYAL = 100 HALALAS

SENEGAL

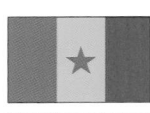

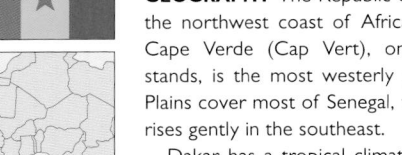

GEOGRAPHY The Republic of Senegal is on the northwest coast of Africa. The volcanic Cape Verde (Cap Vert), on which Dakar stands, is the most westerly point in Africa. Plains cover most of Senegal, though the land rises gently in the southeast.

Dakar has a tropical climate, with a short rainy season between July and October.

POLITICS & ECONOMY In 1882, Senegal became a French colony, and from 1895 it was ruled as part of French West Africa, the capital of which, Dakar, developed as a major port and city.

In 1959, Senegal joined French Sudan (now Mali) to form the Federation of Mali. But Senegal withdrew in 1960 and became the separate Republic of Senegal. Its first president, Léopold Sédar Senghor, served until 1981, when he was succeeded by Abdou Diouf. However, in 2000, Diouf was defeated in elections by Abdoulaye Wade. In 2003, conflict occurred in Casamance region in the south, where separatists wanted independence.

Senegal and The Gambia have always enjoyed close relations despite their differing French and British traditions. In 1981, Senegalese troops put down an attempted coup in The Gambia and, in 1982, the two countries set up a defense alliance, called the Confederation of Senegambia. But this confederation was dissolved in 1989.

According to the World Bank, Senegal is a "lower-middle-income" developing country. It was badly hit in the 1960s and 1970s by droughts, which caused starvation. Agriculture still employs 81% of the population though many farmers produce little more than they need to feed their families. Food crops include groundnuts, millet, and rice. Phosphates are the country's chief resource, but Senegal also refines oil which it imports from Gabon and Nigeria. Dakar is a busy port and has many industries.

AREA 75,954 SQ MI [196,722 SQ KM] **POPULATION** 10,580,000

CAPITAL (POPULATION) DAKAR (880,000)

GOVERNMENT MULTIPARTY REPUBLIC

ETHNIC GROUPS WOLOF 44%, PULAR 24%, SERER 15%

LANGUAGES FRENCH (OFFICIAL), TRIBAL LANGUAGES

RELIGIONS ISLAM 94%, CHRISTIANITY (MAINLY ROMAN CATHOLIC) 5%, TRADITIONAL BELIEFS 1%

CURRENCY CFA FRANC = 100 CENTIMES

SERBIA AND MONTENEGRO

GEOGRAPHY Serbia and Montenegro are two of the six republics which made up the country of Yugoslavia until it broke up in the early 1990s. From the early 1990s, Serbia and Montenegro were known as the Federal Republic of Yugoslavia. But, in 2003, the two republics became semi-independent and adopted the name of the Union of Serbia and Montenegro.

Behind the coastline on the Adriatic Sea lies an upland region, including the Dinaric Alps and part of the Balkan Mountains. The Pannonian plains, which are drained by the River Danube, are in the north. The coast has a Mediterranean climate. The interior highlands have bitterly cold winters and cool summers. The wettest season is the summer, but there is also plenty of sunshine.

POLITICS & ECONOMY People who became known as the South Slavs began to move into the region around 1,500 years ago. Each group, including the Serbs and Croats, founded its own state. But, by the 15th century, foreign countries controlled the region. Serbia and Montenegro were under the Turkish Ottoman empire.

In the 19th century, many Slavs worked for independence and Slavic unity. In 1914, Austria–Hungary declared war on Serbia, blaming it for the assassination of Archduke Francis Ferdinand of Austria–Hungary. This led to World War I and the defeat of Austria–Hungary. In 1918, the South Slavs united in the Kingdom of the Serbs, Croats and Slovenes, which consisted of Bosnia-Herzegovina, Croatia, Dalmatia, Montenegro, Serbia and Slovenia. The country was renamed Yugoslavia in 1929. Germany occupied Yugoslavia during World War II, but partisans, including a Communist force led by Josip Broz Tito, fought the invaders.

From 1945, the Communists controlled the country, which was called the Federal People's Republic of Yugoslavia. But after Tito's death in 1980, the country faced many problems. In 1990, non-Communist parties were permitted and non-Communists won majorities in elections in all but Serbia and Montenegro, where Socialists (former Communists) won control. Yugoslavia split apart in 1991–2 with Bosnia-Herzegovina, Croatia, Macedonia and Slovenia proclaiming their independence. The two remaining republics of Serbia and Montenegro became the new Yugoslavia.

Fighting broke out in Croatia and Bosnia-Herzegovina as rival groups struggled for power. In 1992, the United Nations withdrew recognition of Yugoslavia because of its failure to halt atrocities committed by Serbs living in Croatia and Bosnia. In 1995, Yugoslavia was involved in the talks that led to the Dayton Peace Accord, which brought peace to Bosnia-Herzegovina. But the issue of Yugoslav repression of minorities flared up again in 1998 in Kosovo, a province where the majority are ethnic Albanians. In response to Serb ethnic cleansing, NATO forces began an offensive against Yugoslavia. A Serb withdrawal was agreed in June 1999. Many Montenegrins wanted to secede and set up their own nation separate from Serbia. In 2003, Serbia and Montenegro set up a loose union, giving both republics semi-independence, and the name Yugoslavia passed into history. Montenegro agreed not to secede from this union for at least three years.

Under Communist rule, manufacturing became increasingly important in Yugoslavia. But in the early 1990s, the World Bank described what is now Serbia and Montenegro as a "lower-middle-income" economy. Resources include bauxite, coal, copper and other metals, oil and natural gas. Manufactures, which form the main exports, include aluminum, machinery, plastics, steel, textiles, and vehicles. Farming remains important. Crops include fruits, maize, potatoes, tobacco, and wheat. Cattle, pigs, and sheep are raised.

AREA 39,449 SQ MI [102,173 SQ KM] **POPULATION** 10,656,000

CAPITAL (POPULATION) BELGRADE (1,594,000)

GOVERNMENT FEDERAL REPUBLIC

ETHNIC GROUPS SERB 62%, ALBANIAN 17%, MONTENEGRIN 5%, HUNGARIAN 3%, OTHERS

LANGUAGES SERBIAN (OFFICIAL), ALBANIAN

RELIGIONS ORTHODOX 65%, ISLAM 19%, ROMAN CATHOLIC 4%, OTHERS

CURRENCY NEW DINAR = 100 PARAS

SEYCHELLES

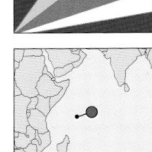

The Republic of Seychelles in the western Indian Ocean achieved independence from Britain in 1976. Coconuts are the main cash crop, and fishing and tourism are important to the country's economy.

AREA 176 SQ MI [455 SQ KM]

POPULATION 80,000 **CAPITAL** VICTORIA

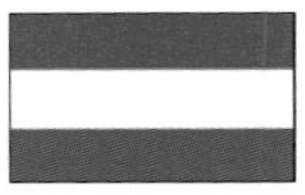
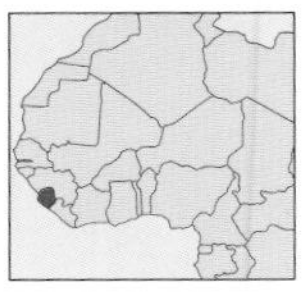

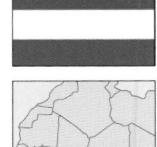

SIERRA LEONE

GEOGRAPHY The Republic of Sierra Leone in West Africa is about the same size as the Republic of Ireland. The coast contains several deep estuaries in the north, with lagoons in the south. The most prominent feature is the mountainous Freetown (or Sierra Leone) peninsula.

Sierra Leone has a tropical climate, with heavy rainfall between April and November.

POLITICS & ECONOMY A former British territory, Sierra Leone became independent in 1961 and a republic in 1971. It became a one-party state in 1978, but, in 1991, the people voted for the restoration of democracy. The military seized power in 1992 and a civil war caused much destruction in 1994–5. Elections in 1996 were followed by another military coup. In 1998, the West African Peace Force restored the deposed President Ahmed Tejan Kabbah. In 1999, a peace agreement followed further conflict. As part of this agreement, Foday Sankoh, one of the rebel leaders, became vice-president. However, he was arrested in 2000 and charged with war crimes. Conflict resumed, but another ceasefire was agreed. In 2004, President Kabbah declared a successful end to disarmament in Sierra Leone.

The World Bank classifies Sierra Leone as a "low-income" developing country Agriculture employs 60% of the people, though farming is mostly at subsistence level. The chief exports are minerals, including diamonds, bauxite, and rutile (titanium ore). The country has few manufacturing industries.

AREA 27,699 SQ MI [71,740 SQ KM] **POPULATION** 5,733,000
CAPITAL (POPULATION) FREETOWN (470,000)
GOVERNMENT SINGLE-PARTY REPUBLIC **ETHNIC GROUPS** NATIVE AFRICAN TRIBES 90% **LANGUAGES** ENGLISH (OFFICIAL), MENDE, TEMNE, KRIO
RELIGIONS ISLAM 60%, TRADITIONAL BELIEFS 30%, CHRISTIANITY 10%
CURRENCY LEONE = 100 CENTS

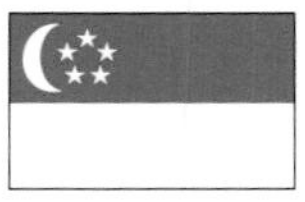
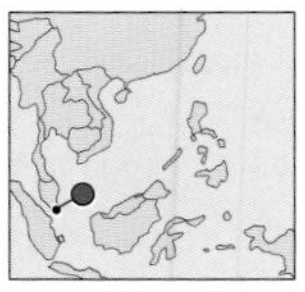

SINGAPORE

GEOGRAPHY The Republic of Singapore is an island country at the southern tip of the Malay peninsula. It consists of the large Singapore Island and 58 small islands, 20 of which are inhabited. Singapore has a hot, humid climate. Temperatures are high and rainfall is heavy throughout the year.

POLITICS & ECONOMY In 1819, Sir Thomas Stamford Raffles (1781–1826), agent of the British East India Company, made a treaty with the Sultan of Johor allowing the British to build a settlement on Singapore Island. Singapore soon became the leading British trading center in Southeast Asia and it later became a naval base. Japanese forces seized the island in 1942, but British rule was restored in 1945.

In 1963, Singapore became part of the Federation of Malaysia, which also included Malaya and the territories of Sabah and Sarawak on Borneo. In 1965, Singapore broke away and became independent.

The People's Action Party (PAP) has ruled Singapore since 1959. Its leader, Lee Kuan Yew, served as prime minister from 1959 until 1990, when he resigned and was succeeded by Goh Chok Tong. Under the PAP, the economy has expanded rapidly, though some considered its rule rather dictatorial. However, in 2004, Singapore began to relax some of its strict laws on public behavior.

The World Bank classifies Singapore as a "high-income" economy. A skilled work force has created a fast-growing economy, but the recession in 1997–8 was a setback. Trade and finance are leading activities. Manufactures include electronic products, machinery, scientific instruments, textiles, and ships. Singapore has a large oil refinery. Petroleum products and manufactures are the main exports.

AREA 264 SQ MI [683 SQ KM] **POPULATION** 4,609,000
CAPITAL (POPULATION) SINGAPORE CITY (3,894,000)
GOVERNMENT MULTIPARTY REPUBLIC
ETHNIC GROUPS CHINESE 77%, MALAY 14%, INDIAN 8%
LANGUAGES CHINESE, MALAY, TAMIL AND ENGLISH (ALL OFFICIAL)
RELIGIONS BUDDHISM, ISLAM, CHRISTIANITY, HINDUISM
CURRENCY SINGAPORE DOLLAR = 100 CENTS

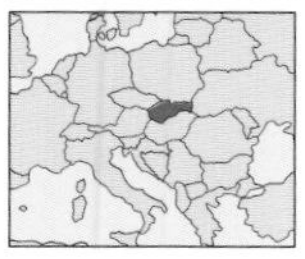

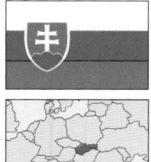

SLOVAK REPUBLIC

GEOGRAPHY The Slovak Republic is a predominantly mountainous country, consisting of part of the Carpathian range. The highest peak is Gerlachovka in the Tatra Mountains, which reaches 8,711 ft [2,655 m]. The south is a fertile lowland.

The Slovak Republic has cold winters and warm summers. Kosice, in the east, has average temperatures ranging from 27°F [–3°C] in January to 68°F [20°C] in July. The highland areas are much colder. Snow or rain falls throughout the year. Kosice has an average annual rainfall of 24 in [600 mm], the wettest months being July and August.

POLITICS & ECONOMY Slavic peoples settled in the region in the 5th century AD. They were subsequently conquered by Hungary, beginning a millennium of Hungarian rule and suppression of Slovak culture.

In 1867, Hungary and Austria united to form Austria–Hungary, of which the present-day Slovak Republic was a part. Austria–Hungary collapsed at the end of World War I (1914–18). The Czech and Slovak people then united to form a new nation, Czechoslovakia. But Czech domination led to resentment by many Slovaks. In 1939, the Slovak Republic declared itself independent, but Germany occupied the country. At the end of World War II, the Slovak Republic again became part of Czechoslovakia.

The Communist party took control in 1948. In the 1960s, many people sought reform, but they were crushed by the Russians. In the late 1980s, demands for democracy mounted and a non-Communist government took office in 1990. Elections in 1992 led to victory for the Movement for a Democratic Slovakia headed by a former Communist and nationalist, Vladimir Meciar, and the independent Slovak Republic came into existence on January 1, 1993.

Independence raised national aspirations among Slovakia's Magyar-speaking community, but relations with Hungary deteriorated when the Magyars felt that administrative changes under-represented them politically. The government also made Slovak the only official language. The government's autocratic rule and human rights record provoked international criticism. In 1998, Meciar's party was defeated and Mikulas Dzurinda replaced Meciar as prime minister. The government continued to strengthen its ties with the West and, in 2004, it became a member of both the North Atlantic Treaty Organization and the European Union.

Before 1948, the Slovak Republic's economy was based on farming, but Communist governments developed manufacturing industries, producing such things as chemicals, machinery, steel, and weapons. Since the late 1980s, many state-run businesses have been handed over to private owners.

AREA 18,924 SQ MI [49,012 SQ KM] **POPULATION** 5,430,000
CAPITAL (POPULATION) BRATISLAVA (449,000)
GOVERNMENT MULTIPARTY REPUBLIC
ETHNIC GROUPS SLOVAK 86%, HUNGARIAN 11%
LANGUAGES SLOVAK (OFFICIAL), HUNGARIAN
RELIGIONS ROMAN CATHOLIC 60%, PROTESTANT 8%, ORTHODOX 4%, OTHERS **CURRENCY** SLOVAK KORUNA = 100 HALIEROV

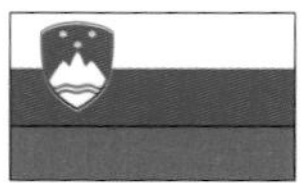
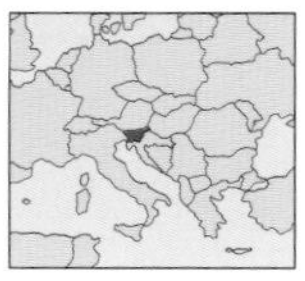

SLOVENIA

GEOGRAPHY The Republic of Slovenia was one of the six republics which made up the former Yugoslavia. Much of the land is mountainous, rising to 9,393 ft [2,863 m] at Mount Triglav in the Julian Alps (Julijske Alpe) in the northwest. Central Slovenia contains the limestone Karst region. The Postojna caves near Ljubljana are among the largest in Europe.

The coast has a mild Mediterranean climate, but inland the climate is more continental. The mountains are snow-capped in winter.

POLITICS & ECONOMY In the last 2,000 years, the Slovene people have been independent as a nation for less than 50 years. The Austrian Habsburgs ruled over the region from the 13th century until World War I. Slovenia became part of the Kingdom of the Serbs, Croats, and Slovenes (later called Yugoslavia) in 1918. During World War II, Slovenia was invaded and partitioned between Italy, Germany and Hungary, but, after the war, Slovenia again became part of Yugoslavia.

From the late 1960s, some Slovenes demanded independence, but the central government opposed the breakup of the country. In 1990, when Communist governments had collapsed throughout Eastern Europe, elections were held and a non-Communist coalition government was set up. Slovenia then declared itself independent. This led to fighting between Slovenes and the federal army, but Slovenia did not become a battlefield like other parts of the former Yugoslavia. The European Community recognized Slovenia's independence in 1992. The electors returned a coalition led by the Liberal Democrats in 1992, 1996, and 2000. In 2004, it achieved two of its major objectives in becoming a member of both the North Atlantic Treaty Organization and the European Union.

The reform of the formerly state-run economy caused problems for Slovenia. However, it has enjoyed considerable economic progress, with one of Europe's fastest growing economies. In 1992, the World Bank classified Slovenia's economy as "upper-middle-income."

Manufacturing is the leading activity and manufactures are the main exports. Manufactures include chemicals, machinery and transport equipment, metal goods, and textiles. Slovenia mines some iron ore, lead, lignite, and mercury. Agriculture and forestry employ 10% of the people. Fruits, maize, potatoes, and wheat are major crops, and many farmers raise animals.

AREA 7,821 SQ MI [20,256 SQ KM] **POPULATION** 1,936,000
CAPITAL (POPULATION) LJUBLJANA (264,000)
GOVERNMENT MULTIPARTY REPUBLIC
ETHNIC GROUPS SLOVENE 92%, CROAT 1%, SERB, HUNGARIAN, BOSNIAK
LANGUAGES SLOVENIAN (OFFICIAL), SERBO-CROATIAN
RELIGIONS MAINLY ROMAN CATHOLIC
CURRENCY TOLAR = 100 STOTIN

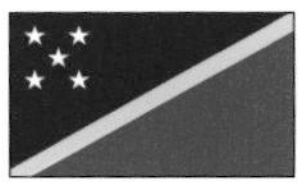
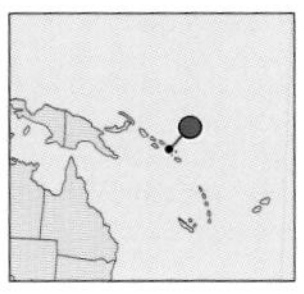

SOLOMON ISLANDS

The Solomon Islands, a chain of mainly volcanic islands in the Pacific Ocean, were a British territory between 1893 and 1978. The chain extends for some 1,400 mi [2,250 km]. They were the scene of fierce fighting during World War II. Most people are Melanesians, and the islands have a young population profile, with half the people aged under 20. Fish, coconuts and cocoa are leading products, though development is hampered by mountainous, forested terrain.

AREA 11,157 SQ MI [28,896 SQ KM] **POPULATION** 509,000
CAPITAL (POPULATION) HONIARA (49,000)

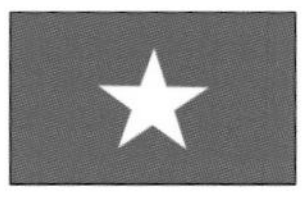
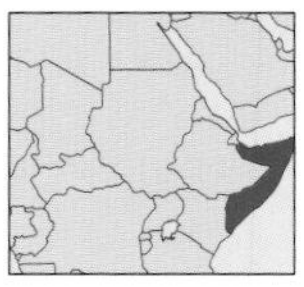

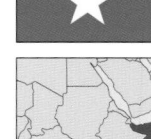

SOMALIA

GEOGRAPHY The Somali Democratic Republic, or Somalia, is in a region known as the "Horn of Africa." It is more than twice the size of Italy, the country which once ruled the southern part of Somalia. The most mountainous part of the country is in the north, behind the narrow coastal plains that border the Gulf of Aden.

Rainfall is light throughout Somalia. The wettest regions are the south and the northern mountains, but droughts often occur. Temperatures are high on the low plateaux and plains.

POLITICS & ECONOMY European powers became interested in the Horn of Africa in the 19th century. In 1884, Britain made the northern part of what is now Somalia a protectorate, while Italy took the south in 1905. The new boundaries divided the Somalis into five areas: the two Somalilands, Djibouti (which was taken by France in the 1880s), Ethiopia and Kenya. Since then, many Somalis have wanted to create a Greater Somalia. Italy invaded British Somaliland in 1940, but was defeated in 1941. Britain ruled both Somalilands until 1950, when the United Nations asked Italy to take over the former Italian Somaliland for ten years. In 1960, the two Somalilands became independent in a united Somalia.

Somalia has faced many problems. Economic difficulties led a military group to seize power in 1969. In the 1970s, Somalia supported an uprising of Somali-speaking people in the Ogaden region of Ethiopia. But, in 1988, Somalia and Ethiopia signed a peace treaty. In the 1990s, Somalia gradually broke apart. In 1991, the people in what was once British Somaliland set up the "Somaliland Republic," but it failed to get international recognition. The northeast, called Puntland, also seceded, while the south was riven by clan warfare. US troops sent into the south by the UN in 1993 were forced to withdraw in 1994 and clan fighting continued. A three-year transitional government set up in 2000 failed to bring peace and, in 2004, further talks took place in Kenya, following the calling of a truce between the rival clans.

Somalia is a developing country, whose economy has been shattered by drought, floods and war. Many Somalis are nomads who raise livestock. Live animals, meat, and hides and skins are exported, followed by bananas grown in the wetter south. Other crops include citrus fruits, cotton, maize, and sugarcane. Mining and manufacturing are relatively unimportant in the economy.

AREA 246,199 SQ MI [637,657 SQ KM] **POPULATION** 8,025,000
CAPITAL (POPULATION) MOGADISHU (900,000) **GOVERNMENT** SINGLE-PARTY REPUBLIC, MILITARY DOMINATED **ETHNIC GROUPS** SOMALI 85%, BANTU, ARAB **LANGUAGES** SOMALI (OFFICIAL), ARABIC **RELIGIONS** ISLAM (SUNNI MUSLIM) **CURRENCY** SOMALI SHILLING = 100 CENTS

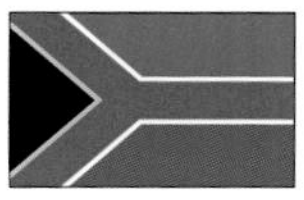

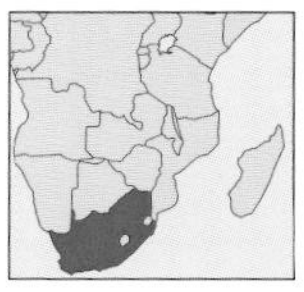

SOUTH AFRICA

GEOGRAPHY The Republic of South Africa is made up largely of the southern part of the huge plateau which makes up most of southern Africa. The highest peaks are in the Drakensberg range, which is formed by the uplifted rim of the plateau. The coastal plains include part of the Namib Desert in the northwest. Most of South Africa has a mild, sunny climate. Much of the coastal strip, including Cape Town, has warm, dry summers and mild, rainy winters. Inland, large areas are arid.

POLITICS & ECONOMY Early inhabitants in South Africa were the Khoisan. In the last 2,000 years, Bantu-speaking people moved into the area. Their descendants include the Zulu, Xhosa, Sotho, and Tswana. The Dutch founded a settlement at the Cape in 1652, but Britain took over in the early 19th century, making the area a colony. The Dutch, called Boers or Afrikaners, resented British rule and moved inland. Rivalry between the groups led to Anglo-Boer Wars in 1880–1 and 1899–1902.

In 1910, the country was united as the Union of South Africa. In 1948, the National Party won power and introduced a policy known as apartheid, under which non-whites had no votes and their human rights were strictly limited. In 1990, Nelson Mandela, leader of the African National Congress (ANC), was released from prison. Multi-racial elections were held in 1994 and Mandela became president. After Mandela's retirement in 1999, his successor, Thabo Mbeki, led the ANC to victory in national elections. In 2004, the ANC won again by a landslide. Taking almost 70% of the vote, it was far ahead of its nearest rival, the Democratic Alliance, which polled only 13%. However, the government faced massive problems of poverty and under-development, and maintaining national unity. South Africa also faces a major health crisis, with about 11% of its people infected with the HIV virus. It has the greatest number of infected people in the world, estimated by the UN in 2003 to be around 5 million.

South Africa is Africa's most developed country. However, most of the black people are poor, with low standards of living. Natural resources include diamonds, gold, and many other metals. Mining and manufacturing are the most valuable activities.

AREA 471,442 SQ MI [1,221,037 SQ KM] **POPULATION** 42,769,000
CAPITAL (POPULATION) CAPE TOWN (LEGISLATIVE, 855,000); PRETORIA (ADMINISTRATIVE, 692,000); BLOEMFONTEIN (JUDICIARY, 350,000)
GOVERNMENT MULTIPARTY REPUBLIC **ETHNIC GROUPS** BLACK 76%, WHITE 13%, COLORED 9%, ASIAN 2% **LANGUAGES** AFRIKAANS, ENGLISH, NDEBELE, PEDI, SOTHO, SWAZI, TSONGA, TSWANA, VENDA, XHOSA AND ZULU (ALL OFFICIAL) **RELIGIONS** CHRISTIANITY 68%, ISLAM 2%, HINDUISM 1% **CURRENCY** RAND = 100 CENTS

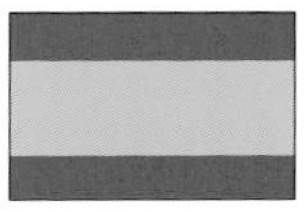

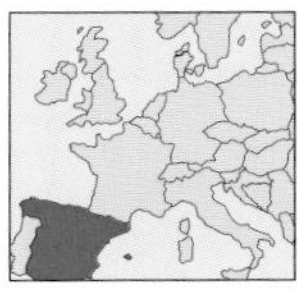

SPAIN

GEOGRAPHY The Kingdom of Spain is the second largest country in Western Europe after France. It shares the Iberian peninsula with Portugal. A large plateau, called the Meseta, covers most of Spain. Much of the Meseta is flat, but it is crossed by several mountain ranges, called sierras.

The northern highlands include the Cantabrian Mountains (Cordillera Cantabrica) and the high Pyrenees, which form Spain's border with France. But Mulhacén, the highest peak on the Spanish mainland, is in the Sierra Nevada in the southeast. Spain also contains fertile coastal plains. Other major lowlands are the Ebro river basin in the northeast and the Guadalquivir river basin in the southwest. Spain also includes the Balearic Islands in the Mediterranean Sea and the Canary Islands off the northwest coast of Africa.

The Meseta has a continental climate, with hot summers and cold winters, when temperatures often fall below freezing point. Snow frequently covers the mountain ranges on the Meseta. The Mediterranean coasts have hot, dry summers and mild winters.

POLITICS & ECONOMY In the 16th century, Spain became a world power. At its peak, it controlled much of Central and South America, parts of Africa and the Philippines in Asia. Spain began to decline in the late 16th century. Its sea power was destroyed by a British fleet in the Battle of Trafalgar (1805). By the 20th century, it was a poor country.

Spain became a republic in 1931, but the republicans were defeated in the Spanish Civil War (1936–9). General Francisco Franco (1892–1975) became the country's dictator, though, technically, it was a monarchy. When Franco died, the monarchy was restored. Prince Juan Carlos became king.

Spain has several groups with their own languages and cultures. Some of these people want to run their own regional affairs. In the northern Basque region, some nationalists have waged a terrorist campaign. A truce in 1998 was ended in 1999 when talks failed to produce results. In 2003, Spain's Supreme Court voted to ban Batasuna, the Basque separatist party.

Since the 1970s, regional parliaments with a considerable degree of autonomy have been set up in the Basque Country (called Euskadi in the indigenous language and Pais Vasco in Spanish), in Catalonia in the northeast, and in Galicia in the northwest. In March 2004, train bombings killed about 200 people in Madrid. But this was the work of al Qaida, not of Basque separatists. Following the bombings, the opposition socialists swept to power in national elections.

The revival of Spain's economy, which was shattered by the Civil War, began in the 1950s and 1960s, especially through the growth of tourism and manufacturing. Since the 1950s, Spain has changed from a poor country, dependent on agriculture, to a fairly prosperous industrial nation.

By 2001, agriculture employed 6% of the people, as compared with industry at 18%, and services, including tourism, at 76%. Arable and grazing land make up about two-thirds of Spain, while forest covers most of the rest of the land. Major crops include barley, citrus fruits, grapes for wine-making, olives, potatoes, and wheat. Apart from some high-grade iron ore in the north, Spain lacks natural resources. But it has many manufacturing industries. Products include cars, chemicals, clothing, electronics, processed food, metal goods, steel, and textiles.

AREA 192,103 SQ MI [497,548 SQ KM] **POPULATION** 40,217,000
CAPITAL (POPULATION) MADRID (2,939,000)
GOVERNMENT CONSTITUTIONAL MONARCHY
ETHNIC GROUPS COMPOSITE OF MEDITERRANEAN AND NORDIC TYPES
LANGUAGES CASTILIAN SPANISH (OFFICIAL) 74%, CATALAN 17%, GALICIAN 7%, BASQUE 2%
RELIGIONS ROMAN CATHOLIC 94%, OTHERS
CURRENCY EURO = 100 CENTS

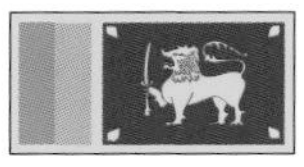

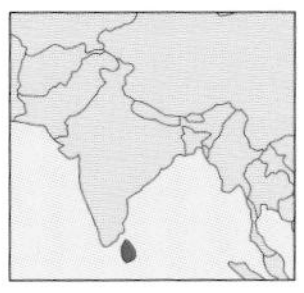

SRI LANKA

GEOGRAPHY The Democratic Socialist Republic of Sri Lanka is an island nation, separated from the southeast coast of India by the Palk Strait. The land is mostly low-lying, but a mountain region dominates the south-central part of the country.

The western part of Sri Lanka has a wet equatorial climate. Temperatures are high and the rainfall is heavy. Eastern Sri Lanka is drier than the west of the country.

POLITICS & ECONOMY From the early 16th century, Ceylon (as Sri Lanka was then known) was ruled successively by the Portuguese, Dutch and British. Independence was achieved in 1948 and the country was renamed Sri Lanka in 1972.

After independence, rivalries between the two main ethnic groups, the Sinhalese and Tamils, marred progress. In the 1950s, the government made Sinhala the official language. Following protests, the prime minister made provisions for Tamil to be used in some areas. In 1959, the prime minister was assassinated by a Sinhalese extremist and he was succeeded by Sirimavo Bandanaraike, the world's first woman prime minister.

Conflict between Tamils and Sinhalese continued in the 1970s and 1980s. In 1987, India helped to engineer a ceasefire. Indian troops arrived to enforce the agreement, but withdrew in 1990 after failing to subdue the main guerrilla group, the Tamil Tigers, who wanted to set up an independent Tamil homeland in northern Sri Lanka. In 1993, the country's president was assassinated by a suspected Tamil separatist. Offensives against the Tamil Tigers continued until hopes of peace were raised in 2002, with the signing of a ceasefire. But a power struggle broke out in 2003 between President Chandrika Kumaratunga and the prime minister, whom she accused of being soft in the peace talks. In a snap election in 2004, the president's United People's Freedom Alliance became the largest party in parliament. The peace process appeared stalled.

Sri Lanka is classed as a "low-income" economy. Agriculture employs about 33% of the people. Coconuts, rubber, and tea are exported, but rice is the main food crop. Factories process farm products and manufacture textiles.

AREA 25,332 SQ MI [65,610 SQ KM] **POPULATION** 19,742,000
CAPITAL (POPULATION) COLOMBO (642,000)
GOVERNMENT MULTIPARTY REPUBLIC
ETHNIC GROUPS SINHALESE 74%, TAMIL 18%, MOOR 7%
LANGUAGES SINHALA AND TAMIL (BOTH OFFICIAL)
RELIGIONS BUDDHISM 70%, HINDUISM 15%, CHRISTIANITY 8%, ISLAM 7%
CURRENCY SRI LANKAN RUPEE = 100 CENTS

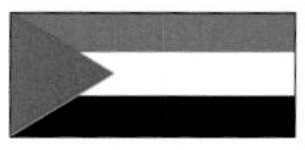

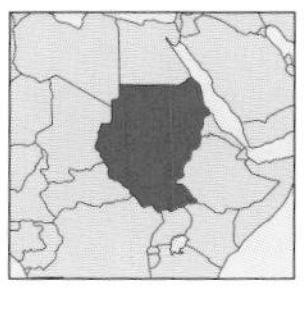

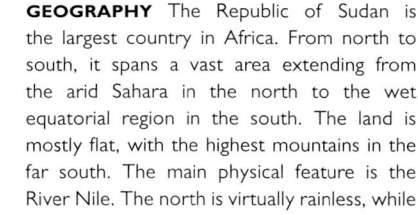

SUDAN

GEOGRAPHY The Republic of Sudan is the largest country in Africa. From north to south, it spans a vast area extending from the arid Sahara in the north to the wet equatorial region in the south. The land is mostly flat, with the highest mountains in the far south. The main physical feature is the River Nile. The north is virtually rainless, while the south has a wet equatorial climate.

POLITICS & ECONOMY In the 19th century, Egypt gradually took over Sudan. In 1881, a Muslim religious teacher, the Mahdi ("divinely appointed guide"), led an uprising. Britain and Egypt put the rebellion down in 1898. In 1899, they agreed to rule Sudan jointly as a condominium. After independence in 1952, the black Africans in the south, who were either Christians or followers of traditional religions, feared domination by the Muslim north. They objected to Arabic becoming the sole official language and, in 1964, civil war broke out. The war ended in 1972, when the south was granted regional self-government.

In 1983, the announcement that Islamic law would apply throughout Sudan sparked off further resistance from the rebel Sudan People's Liberation Army (SPLA) in the south. In 1998, Sudan's government announced that it accepted the idea of a referendum in the south. By 2004, talks that had started in 2002 held out hopes of peace. However, in 2004, conflict flared up in the western region of Darfur, where militias supported by government troops were accused of atrocities against the local people. Thousands of refugees fled into Chad.

Sudan is classed as a "low-income" developing country. Agriculture employs 60% of the people and cotton is the chief crop. Minerals include oil, the most valuable export, chromium, gold, and gypsum. Manufacturing is concerned mainly with processing local products.

AREA 967,494 SQ MI [2,505,813 SQ KM] **POPULATION** 38,114,000
CAPITAL (POPULATION) KHARTOUM (947,000)
GOVERNMENT MILITARY REGIME **ETHNIC GROUPS** BLACK 52%, ARAB 39%, BEJA 6%, OTHERS **LANGUAGES** ARABIC (OFFICIAL), NUBIAN, TA BEDAWIE **RELIGIONS** ISLAM 70%, TRADITIONAL BELIEFS 25%
CURRENCY SUDANESE DINAR = 10 SUDANESE POUNDS

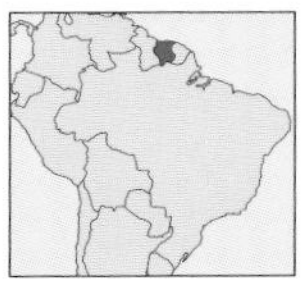

SURINAME

GEOGRAPHY The Republic of Suriname is sandwiched between French Guiana and Guyana in northeastern South America. The narrow coastal plain was once swampy, but it has been drained and now consists mainly of farmland. Inland lie hills and low mountains, which rise to 4,199 ft [1,280 m].

Suriname has a hot, wet and humid climate. Temperatures are high throughout the year.

POLITICS & ECONOMY In 1667, the British handed Suriname to the Dutch in return for New Amsterdam, an area that is now the state of New York. Slave revolts and Dutch neglect hampered development. In the early 19th century, Britain and the Netherlands disputed the ownership of the area. The British gave up their claims in 1813. Slavery was abolished in 1863 and, soon afterward, Indian and Indonesian laborers were introduced to work on the plantations. Suriname became fully independent in 1975, but the economy was weakened when thousands of skilled people emigrated from Suriname to the Netherlands. Following a coup in 1980, Suriname was ruled by a military dictator, Dési Bouterse. The adoption of a new constitution led to the restoration of democracy in 1988, though another military coup occurred in 1990. Elections were held in 1996, but instability, deteriorating relations with the Netherlands and economic problems continued. In 1999, Bouterse was convicted in absentia in the Netherlands of having led a cocaine-trafficking ring during and after his tenure in office.

The World Bank classifies Suriname as an "upper-middle-income" developing country. Its economy is based on mining and metal processing. Suriname is a leading producer of bauxite, from which the metal aluminum is made.

AREA 63,037 SQ MI [163,265 SQ KM] **POPULATION** 435,000
CAPITAL (POPULATION) PARAMARIBO (216,000)
GOVERNMENT MULTIPARTY REPUBLIC
ETHNIC GROUPS HINDUSTANI/EAST INDIAN 37%, CREOLE (MIXED WHITE AND BLACK) 31%, JAVANESE 15%, BLACK 10%, AMERINDIAN 2%, CHINESE 2%, OTHERS **LANGUAGES** DUTCH (OFFICIAL), SRANANG TONGA
RELIGIONS HINDUISM 27%, PROTESTANT 25%, ROMAN CATHOLIC 23%, ISLAM 20% **CURRENCY** SURINAMESE GUILDER = 100 CENTS

SWAZILAND

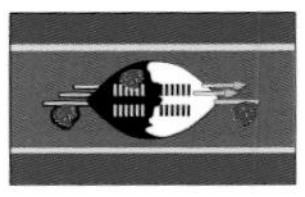
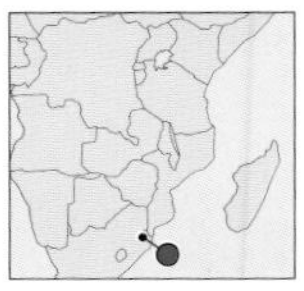

GEOGRAPHY The Kingdom of Swaziland is a small, landlocked country in southern Africa. The country has four regions which run north–south. In the west, the Highveld, with an average height of 3,950 ft [1,200 m], makes up 30% of Swaziland. The Middleveld, between 1,150 ft and 3,280 ft [350 m to 1,000 m], covers 28% of the country. The Lowveld, with an average height of 886 ft [270 m], covers another 33%. Finally, the Lebombo Mountains reach 2,600 ft [800 m] along the eastern border. The Lowveld is almost tropical, with average temperatures of 72°F [22°C] and low rainfall. The altitude moderates the climate in the west.

POLITICS & ECONOMY In 1894, Britain and the Boers of South Africa agreed to put Swaziland under the control of the South African Republic (the Transvaal). But at the end of the Anglo–Boer War (1899–1902), Britain took control of the country. In 1968, when Swaziland became fully independent as a constitutional monarchy, the head of state was King Sobhuza II. Sobhuza died in 1982 and was succeeded by one of his sons, Prince Makhosetive, who, in 1986, was installed as King Mswati III. Elections in 1993 and 1998, in which political parties were banned, failed to satisfy protesters who opposed the absolute monarchy. But Mswati continued to rule by decree. In 2003, he announced that democracy was not suitable for the Swazi people.

The World Bank classifies Swaziland as a "lower-middle-income" developing country. Agriculture employs 50% of the people, and farm products and processed foods, including soft drink concentrates, sugar, wood pulp, citrus fruits and canned fruit, are the leading exports. Many farmers live at subsistence level. Swaziland is heavily dependent on South Africa and the two countries are linked through a customs union. Swaziland shares two major problems with South Africa – the widespread poverty and the high incidence of HIV/AIDS.

AREA 6,704 SQ MI [17,364 SQ KM] **POPULATION** 1,161,000
CAPITAL (POPULATION) MBABANE (38,000)
GOVERNMENT MONARCHY **ETHNIC GROUPS** AFRICAN 97%, EUROPEAN 3% **LANGUAGES** SISWATI AND ENGLISH (BOTH OFFICIAL)
RELIGIONS ZIONIST (A MIX OF CHRISTIANITY AND TRADITIONAL BELIEFS) 40%, ROMAN CATHOLIC 20%, ISLAM 10% **CURRENCY** LILANGENI = 100 CENTS

SWEDEN

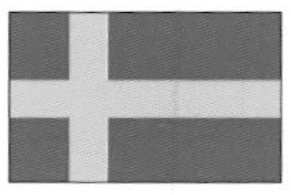
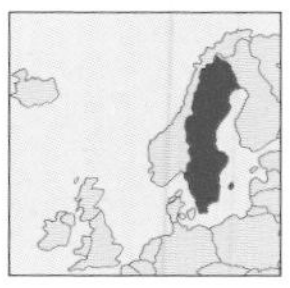

GEOGRAPHY The Kingdom of Sweden is the largest of the countries of Scandinavia in both area and population. It shares the Scandinavian peninsula with Norway. The western part of the country, along the border with Norway, is mountainous. The highest point is Kebnekaise, which reaches 6,946 ft [2,117 m] in the northwest.

The climate of Sweden becomes more severe from south to north. Stockholm has cold winters and cool summers. The far south is much milder.

POLITICS & ECONOMY Swedish Vikings plundered areas to the south and east between the 9th and 11th centuries. Sweden, Denmark and Norway were united in 1397, but Sweden regained its independence in 1523. In 1809, Sweden lost Finland to Russia, but, in 1814, it gained Norway from Denmark. The union between Sweden and Norway was dissolved in 1905. Sweden was neutral in World Wars I and II. Since 1945, Sweden has become a prosperous country. In 1995, it joined the European Union. However, many people were sceptical about the advantages of EU membership and Sweden did not adopt the euro, the single EU currency, in 1999.

Sweden has wide-ranging welfare services. But many people are concerned about the high cost of these services and the high taxes they must pay. In 1991, the Social Democrats, who had built up the welfare state, were defeated. They were re-elected in 1994. In 2003, the government held a referendum on replacing the country's currency with the EU's unit of currency, the euro, but the electorate rejected the proposal.

Sweden is a highly developed industrial country. Major products include steel and steel goods. Steel is used in the engineering industry to manufacture aircraft, cars, machinery, and ships. Sweden has some of the world's richest iron ore deposits. They are located near Kiruna in the far north. But most of this ore is exported, and Sweden imports most of the materials needed by its industries. Sweden also has a major forestry industry. Development of hydroelectricity has made up for the lack of oil and coal. In 1996, a decision was taken to decommission all of Sweden's nuclear power stations. This is said to be one of the boldest and most expensive environmental pledges ever made by a government.

AREA 173,731 SQ MI [449,964 SQ KM] **POPULATION** 8,878,000
CAPITAL (POPULATION) STOCKHOLM (744,000)
GOVERNMENT CONSTITUTIONAL MONARCHY **ETHNIC GROUPS** SWEDISH 91%, FINNISH, SAMI **LANGUAGES** SWEDISH (OFFICIAL), FINNISH, SAMI
RELIGIONS LUTHERAN 87%, ROMAN CATHOLIC, ORTHODOX
CURRENCY SWEDISH KRONA = 100 ÖRE

SWITZERLAND

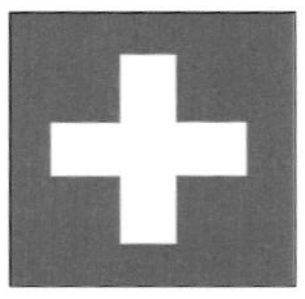
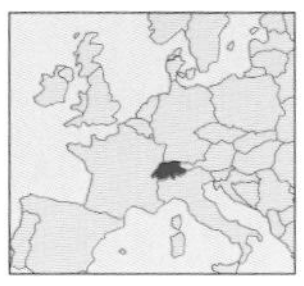

GEOGRAPHY The Swiss Confederation is a landlocked country in Western Europe. Much of the land is mountainous. The Jura Mountains lie along Switzerland's western border with France, while the Swiss Alps make up about 60% of the country in the south and east. Four-fifths of the people of Switzerland live on the fertile Swiss plateau, which contains most of Switzerland's large cities.

The climate of Switzerland varies greatly according to the height of the land. The plateau region has a central European climate with warm summers, but cold and snowy winters. Rain occurs all through the year. The rainiest months are in summer.

POLITICS & ECONOMY In 1291, three small cantons (states) united to defend their freedom against the Habsburg rulers of the Holy Roman Empire. They were Schwyz, Uri and Unterwalden, and they called the confederation they formed "Switzerland." Switzerland expanded and, in the 14th century, defeated Austria in three wars of independence. After a defeat by the French in 1515, the Swiss adopted a policy of neutrality, which they still follow. In 1815, the Congress of Vienna expanded Switzerland to 22 cantons and guaranteed its neutrality. Switzerland's 23rd canton, Jura, was created in 1979 from part of Bern. Neutrality combined with the vigor and independence of its people have made Switzerland prosperous. In 1993 and again in 2001, the Swiss people voted against starting negotiations to join the European Union. However, in 2002, the Swiss voted by a narrow majority to join the United Nations.

Although lacking in natural resources, Switzerland is a wealthy, industrialized country. Many workers are highly skilled. Major products include chemicals, electrical equipment, machinery and machine tools, precision instruments, processed food, watches and textiles. Farmers produce about three-fifths of the country's food – the rest is imported. Livestock raising, especially dairy farming, is the chief agricultural activity. Crops include fruits, potatoes, and wheat. Tourism and banking are also important. Swiss banks attract investors from all over the world.

AREA 15,940 SQ MI [41,284 SQ KM] **POPULATION** 7,319,000
CAPITAL (POPULATION) BERN (124,000) **GOVERNMENT** FEDERAL REPUBLIC **ETHNIC GROUPS** GERMAN 65%, FRENCH 18%, ITALIAN 10%, ROMANSCH 1%, OTHERS **LANGUAGES** FRENCH, GERMAN, ITALIAN AND ROMANSCH (ALL OFFICIAL) **RELIGIONS** ROMAN CATHOLIC 46%, PROTESTANT 40% **CURRENCY** SWISS FRANC = 100 CENTIMES

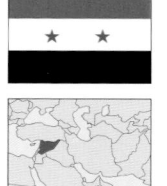

SYRIA

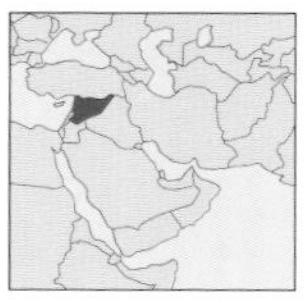

GEOGRAPHY The Syrian Arab Republic is a country in southwestern Asia. The narrow coastal plain is overlooked by a low mountain range which runs north–south. Another range, the Jabal ash Sharqi, runs along the border with Lebanon. South of this range is the Golan Heights, which Israel has occupied since 1967.

The coast has a Mediterranean climate, with dry, warm summers and wet, mild winters. The low mountains cut off Damascus from the sea. It has less rainfall than the coastal areas. To the east, the land becomes drier.

POLITICS & ECONOMY After the collapse of the Turkish Ottoman empire in World War I, Syria was ruled by France. Since independence in 1946, Syria has been involved in the Arab–Israeli wars and, in 1967, it lost a strategic border area, the Golan Heights, to Israel. In 1970, Lieutenant-General Hafez al-Assad took power, establishing a stable but repressive regime. In 1999, Syria had talks with Israel concerning the future of the Golan Heights. These talks formed part of an attempt to establish a peace settlement for the entire east Mediterranean region. Following the death of Assad in 2000, his son, Bashar Assad, succeeded him.

The World Bank classifies Syria as a "lower-middle-income" developing country. But it has great potential for development. Its main resources are oil, hydroelectricity from the dam at Lake Assad, and fertile land. Oil is the main export; farm products, textiles and phosphates are also important. Agriculture employs about 29% of the work force.

AREA 71,498 SQ MI [185,180 SQ KM] **POPULATION** 17,586,000
CAPITAL (POPULATION) DAMASCUS (1,394,000)
GOVERNMENT MULTIPARTY REPUBLIC **ETHNIC GROUPS** ARAB 90%, KURDISH, ARMENIAN, OTHERS **LANGUAGES** ARABIC (OFFICIAL), KURDISH, ARMENIAN **RELIGIONS** SUNNI MUSLIM 74%, OTHER ISLAM 16%
CURRENCY SYRIAN POUND = 100 PIASTRES

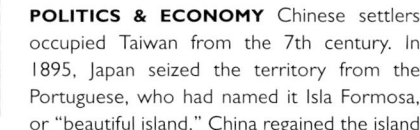

TAIWAN

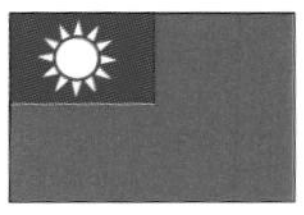
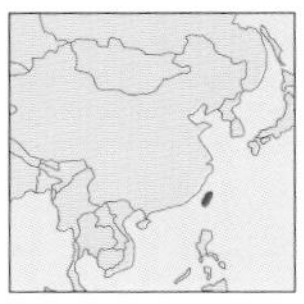

GEOGRAPHY High mountain ranges run down the length of the island, with dense forest in many areas. The climate is warm, moist and suitable for agriculture.

POLITICS & ECONOMY Chinese settlers occupied Taiwan from the 7th century. In 1895, Japan seized the territory from the Portuguese, who had named it Isla Formosa, or "beautiful island." China regained the island after World War II. In 1949, it became the refuge of the Nationalists who had been driven out of China by the Communists. They set up the Republic of China, which, with US help, began to expand its economy. Today, it produces a wide range of manufactured goods.

In the early 21st century, the Taiwanese declared full nationhood for Taiwan. But the government of mainland China threatened to attack the territory if it did not accept the fact that it was a self-governing province of China. But reunification seemed a remote prospect.

AREA 13,900 SQ MI [36,000 SQ KM] **POPULATION** 22,603,000
CAPITAL (POPULATION) TAIPEI (2,634,000)
GOVERNMENT UNITARY MULTIPARTY REPUBLIC
ETHNIC GROUPS TAIWANESE 84%, MAINLAND CHINESE 14%
LANGUAGES MANDARIN CHINESE (OFFICIAL), MIN, HAKKA
RELIGIONS BUDDHISM, TAOISM, CONFUCIANISM
CURRENCY NEW TAIWAN DOLLAR = 100 CENTS

TAJIKISTAN

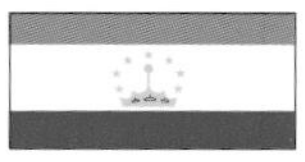
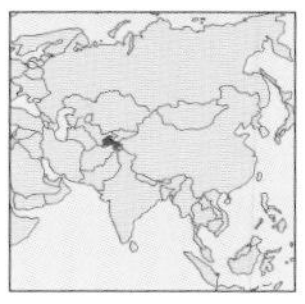

GEOGRAPHY The Republic of Tajikistan is one of the five central Asian republics that formed part of the former Soviet Union. Only 7% of the land is below 3,280 ft [1,000 m], while almost all of eastern Tajikistan is above 9,840 ft [3,000 m]. The highest point is Communism Peak (Pik Kommunizma), which reaches 24,590 ft [7,495 m]. The main ranges are the westward extension of the Tian Shan Range in the north and the snow-capped Pamirs in the southeast. Earthquakes are common throughout the country. The climate is continental, with hot, dry summers in the lower valleys and bitterly cold winters, especially in the mountains.

POLITICS & ECONOMY Russia conquered parts of Tajikistan in the late 19th century and, by 1920, Russia took complete control. In 1924, Tajikistan became part of the Uzbek Soviet Socialist Republic, but, in 1929, it was expanded, taking in some areas populated by Uzbeks, becoming the Tajik Soviet Socialist Republic.

While the Soviet Union began to introduce reforms during the 1980s, many Tajiks demanded freedom. In 1989, the Tajik government made Tajik the official language instead of Russian and, in 1990, it stated that its local laws overruled Soviet laws. Tajikistan became fully independent in 1991, following the breakup of the Soviet Union. In 1992, civil war broke out between the government, which was run by former Communists, and an alliance of democrats and Islamic forces. A ceasefire was agreed in 1996 and, in 1997, opposition leaders were brought into the government. Presidential elections were held in 1999. In 2003, changes to the constitution enabled Emomali Rakhmanov, Tajikistan's president since 1994, to serve two more seven-year terms in office after elections in 2006.

The World Bank classifies Tajikistan as a "low-income" developing country. Agriculture, mainly on irrigated land, is the main activity and cotton is the chief crop. Other crops include fruits, grains, and vegetables. The country has large hydroelectric power resources and it produces aluminum.

AREA 55,521 SQ MI [143,100 SQ KM] **POPULATION** 6,864,000
CAPITAL (POPULATION) DUSHANBE (529,000)
GOVERNMENT TRANSITIONAL DEMOCRACY
ETHNIC GROUPS TAJIK 65%, UZBEK 25%, RUSSIAN
LANGUAGES TAJIK (OFFICIAL), RUSSIAN
RELIGIONS ISLAM (SUNNI MUSLIM 85%)
CURRENCY SOMONI = 100 DIRAMS

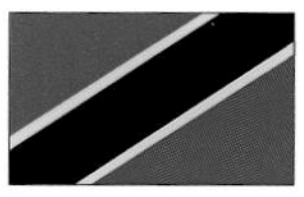
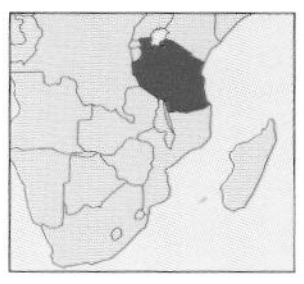

TANZANIA

GEOGRAPHY The United Republic of Tanzania consists of the former mainland country of Tanganyika and the island nation of Zanzibar, which also includes the island of Pemba. Behind a narrow coastal plain, most of Tanzania is a plateau, which is broken by arms of the Great African Rift Valley. In the west, this valley contains lakes Nyasa and Tanganyika. The highest peak is Kilimanjaro, Africa's tallest mountain.

The coast has a hot and humid climate, with the greatest rainfall in April and May. The inland plateaux and mountains are cooler and less humid.

POLITICS & ECONOMY Mainland Tanganyika became a German territory in the 1880s, while Zanzibar and Pemba became a British protectorate in 1890. Following Germany's defeat in World War I, Britain took over Tanganyika, which remained a British territory until its independence in 1961. In 1964, Tanganyika and Zanzibar united to form the United Republic of Tanzania. The country's president, Julius Nyerere, pursued socialist policies of self-help (*ujamaa*) and egalitarianism. Many of its social reforms were successful, though the country failed to make economic progress. Nyerere resigned as president in 1985, although he retained much influence until his death in 1999. His successors, Ali Hassan Mwinyi and, from 1995, Benjamin Mkapa, introduced more liberal economic policies.

Tanzania is one of the world's poorest countries. Crops are grown on only 4.2% of the land, yet agriculture employs 80% of the people. Food crops include bananas, cassava, maize, millet, and rice.

AREA 364,899 sq mi [945,090 sq km] **POPULATION** 35,922,000
CAPITAL (POPULATION) Dodoma (204,000)
GOVERNMENT Multiparty republic
ETHNIC GROUPS Native African 99% (of which 95% are Bantu consisting of more than 130 tribes)
LANGUAGES Swahili (Kiswahili) and English (both official)
RELIGIONS Islam 35% (99% in Zanzibar), traditional beliefs 35%, Christianity 30%
CURRENCY Tanzanian shilling = 100 cents

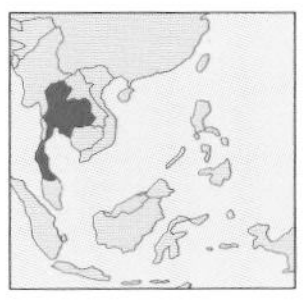

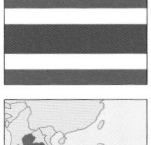

THAILAND

GEOGRAPHY The Kingdom of Thailand is one of the ten countries in Southeast Asia. The highest land is in the north, where Doi Inthanon, the highest peak, reaches 8,514 ft [2,595 m]. The Khorat plateau, in the north-east, makes up about 30% of the country and is the most heavily populated part of Thailand. In the south, Thailand shares the finger-like Malay peninsula with Burma and Malaysia.

Thailand has a tropical climate. Monsoon winds from the southwest bring heavy rains between the months of May and October. The rainfall in Bangkok is lower than in many other parts of Southeast Asia, because mountains shelter the central plains from the rain-bearing winds.

POLITICS & ECONOMY The first Thai state was set up in the 13th century. By 1350, it included most of what is now Thailand. European contact began in the early 16th century. But, in the late 17th century, the Thais, fearing interference in their affairs, forced all Europeans to leave. This policy continued for 150 years. In 1782, a Thai General, Chao Phraya Chakkri, became king, founding a dynasty which continues today. The country became known as Siam, and Bangkok became its capital. From the mid-19th century, contacts with the West were restored. In World War I, Siam supported the Allies against Germany and Austria-Hungary. But in 1941, the country was conquered by Japan and became its ally. However, after the end of World War II, it became an ally of the United States.

After 1967, when Thailand became a member of ASEAN (Association of Southeast Asian Nations), its economy expanded rapidly, especially in manufacturing and service industries. However, in 1997, it suffered a recession along with other eastern Asian economies. Thailand's political stability was disturbed in 2003, when several suspected Islamic militants were arrested. In 2004, more than 100 people died in clashes between Muslims and the police in southern Thailand.

Agriculture employs about two-fifths of the people and it remains an important sector of the economy. Rice is the chief crop. Cassava, cotton, maize, rubber, sugarcane, and tobacco are also grown. Tin and some other minerals are produced, but the chief exports are manufactures and food products. Tourism is another major source of income.

AREA 198,114 sq mi [513,115 sq km] **POPULATION** 64,265,000
CAPITAL (POPULATION) Bangkok (6,320,000)
GOVERNMENT Constitutional monarchy
ETHNIC GROUPS Thai 75%, Chinese 14%, others 11%
LANGUAGES Thai (official), English, ethnic and regional dialects
RELIGIONS Buddhism 95%, Islam, Christianity
CURRENCY Baht = 100 satang

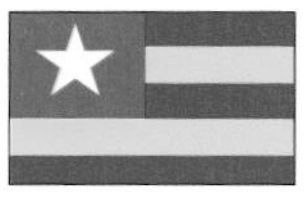
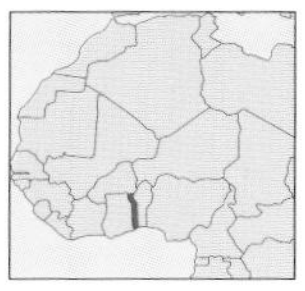

TOGO

GEOGRAPHY The Republic of Togo is a long, narrow country in West Africa. From north to south, it extends about 311 mi [500 km]. Its coastline on the Gulf of Guinea is only 40 mi [64 km] long and it is only 90 mi [145 km] at its widest point.

Togo has high temperatures all through the year. The main wet season is from March to July, with a minor wet season in October and November.

POLITICS & ECONOMY Togo became a German protectorate in 1884 but, in 1919, Britain took over the western third of the territory, while France took over the eastern two-thirds. In 1956, the people of British Togoland voted to join Ghana, while French Togoland became an independent republic in 1960.

A military regime took power in 1963. In 1967, General Gnassingbe Eyadema became head of state and suspended the constitution. Under a new constitution adopted in 1992, multiparty elections were held in 1994. However, in 1998, paramilitary policies stopped the count in the presidential elections when it became clear that Eyadema had been defeated. As a result, the leading opposition parties boycotted the elections in 1999 and 2002.

Togo is a poor, developing country. Farming employs 67% of the people and major food crops include cassava, maize, millet, and yams. The leading export is phosphate rock, which is used to make fertilizers.

AREA 21,925 sq mi [56,785 sq km] **POPULATION** 5,429,000
CAPITAL (POPULATION) Lomé (658,000)
GOVERNMENT Multiparty republic **ETHNIC GROUPS** Native African 99% (largest tribes are Ewe, Mina and Kabre) **LANGUAGES** French (official), African languages **RELIGIONS** Traditional beliefs 51%, Christianity 29%, Islam 20% **CURRENCY** CFA franc = 100 centimes

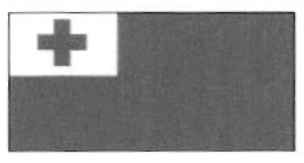
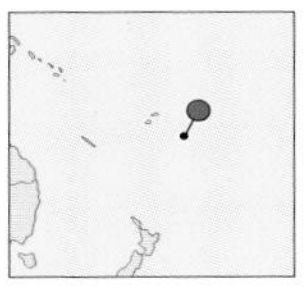

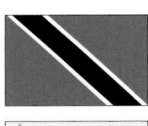

TONGA

The Kingdom of Tonga, a former British protectorate, became independent in 1970. Situated in the South Pacific Ocean, it contains more than 170 islands, 36 of which are inhabited. Agriculture is the main activity; coconuts, copra, fruits, and fish are leading products.

AREA 251 sq mi [650 sq km] **POPULATION** 108,000 **CAPITAL** Nuku'alofa

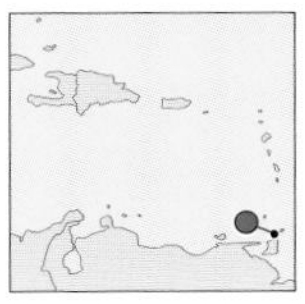

TRINIDAD AND TOBAGO

The Republic of Trinidad and Tobago became independent from Britain in 1962. These tropical islands, populated by people of African, Asian (mainly Indian) and European origin, are hilly and forested, though there are some fertile plains. Oil production is the mainstay of the economy.

AREA 1,981 sq mi [5,130 sq km]
POPULATION 1,104,000 **CAPITAL** Port-of-Spain

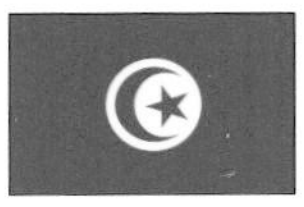
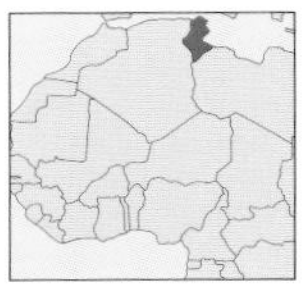

TUNISIA

GEOGRAPHY The Republic of Tunisia is the smallest country in North Africa. The mountains in the north are an eastward and comparatively low extension of the Atlas Mountains. To the north and east of the mountains lie fertile plains, especially between Sfax, Tunis and Bizerte. In the south, low-lying regions contain a vast salt pan, called the Chott Djerid, and part of the Sahara Desert.

Northern Tunisia has a Mediterranean climate, with dry, sunny summers, and mild winters with a moderate rainfall. The average yearly rainfall decreases toward the south.

POLITICS & ECONOMY In 1881, France established a protectorate over Tunisia and ruled the country until 1956. The new parliament abolished the monarchy and declared Tunisia to be a republic in 1957, with the nationalist leader, Habib Bourguiba, as president. His government introduced many reforms, including votes for women, but various problems arose, including unemployment among the middle class and fears that Western values introduced by tourists might undermine Muslim values. In 1987, the prime minister Zine el Abidine Ben Ali removed Bourguiba and succeeded him as president. In 2002, the bombing of a synagogue on Djerba, believed to be the work of al Qaida, led to a major crackdown on dissidents.

The World Bank classifies Tunisia as a "middle-income" developing country. The main resources and chief exports are phosphates and oil. Most industries are concerned with food processing. Agriculture employs 21% of the people; major crops being barley, dates, grapes, olives, and wheat. Fishing is important, as is tourism.

AREA 63,170 sq mi [163,610 sq km] **POPULATION** 9,925,000
CAPITAL (POPULATION) Tunis (702,000) **GOVERNMENT** Multiparty republic **ETHNIC GROUPS** Arab 98%, European 1% **LANGUAGES** Arabic (official), French **RELIGIONS** Islam 98%, Christianity 1%, others **CURRENCY** Tunisian dinar = 1,000 millimes

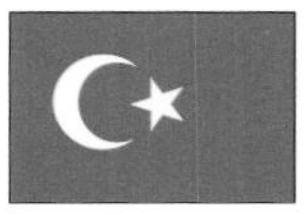
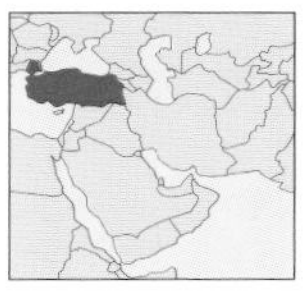

TURKEY

GEOGRAPHY The Republic of Turkey lies in two continents. European Turkey, also called Thrace, lies west of a waterway linking the Mediterranean and Black seas. Most of Asian Turkey consists of plateaux and mountains, which rise to 16,945 ft [5,165 m] at Mount Ararat (Agri Dagi) near the border with Armenia. Earthquakes are common. Central Turkey has a dry climate, with hot, sunny summers and cold winters. The west has a Mediterranean climate, but the Black Sea coast has cooler summers.

POLITICS & ECONOMY In AD 330, the Roman empire moved its capital to Byzantium, which it renamed Constantinople. Constantinople became capital of the East Roman (or Byzantine) empire in 395. Muslim Seljuk Turks from central Asia invaded Anatolia in the 11th century. In the 14th century, another group of Turks, the Ottomans, conquered the area. In 1453, the Ottoman Turks took Constantinople, which they called Istanbul. The Ottomans built up a vast empire which finally collapsed during World War I (1914–18). Turkey became a republic in 1923. Its leader, Mustafa Kemal, or Atatürk ("father of the Turks") began to modernize and secularize the country.

Since the 1940s, Turkey has sought to strengthen its ties with Western powers. It joined NATO (North Atlantic Treaty Organization) in 1951 and it applied to join the European Economic Community in 1987. But Turkey's conflict with Greece, together with its invasion of northern Cyprus in 1974, have led many Europeans to treat Turkey's aspirations with caution. Political instability, military coups, conflict with Kurdish nationalists in eastern Turkey and concern about the country's record on human rights are other problems. Turkey has enjoyed democracy since 1983, though, in 1998, the government banned the Islamist Welfare Party, which it accused of violating secular principles. In 1999, the Muslim Virtue Party (successor to Islamist Welfare Party) lost ground. The largest numbers of parliamentary seats were won by the ruling Democratic Left Party and the far-right National Action Party. However, in the elections in 2002, the moderate Islamic Justice and Development Party (AKP) won 362 of the 500 seats in parliament, while none of the parties in the former ruling coalition won 10% of the vote. In 2003, Turkey opened its airspace to American aircraft during the Iraq war. Turkey hopes to join the European Union and, in 2003–4, it supported attempts to reunify Cyprus prior to that island's admission to the EU.

The World Bank classifies Turkey as a "lower-middle-income" developing country. Agriculture employs 40% of the people, and barley, cotton, fruits, maize, tobacco, and wheat are major crops. Livestock farming is important and wool is a leading product. Turkey produces chromium, but manufacturing is the chief activity. Manufactures include processed farm products and textiles, cars, fertilizers, iron and steel, machinery, metal products, and paper products.

AREA 299,156 sq mi [774,815 sq km] **POPULATION** 68,109,000
CAPITAL (POPULATION) Ankara (2,984,000)
GOVERNMENT Multiparty republic **ETHNIC GROUPS** Turkish 80%, Kurdish 20% **LANGUAGES** Turkish (official), Kurdish, Arabic
RELIGIONS Islam (mainly Sunni Muslim) 99%
CURRENCY Turkish lira = 100 kurus

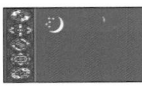

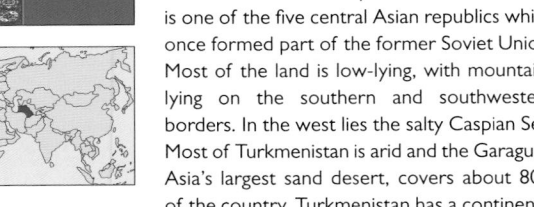

TURKMENISTAN

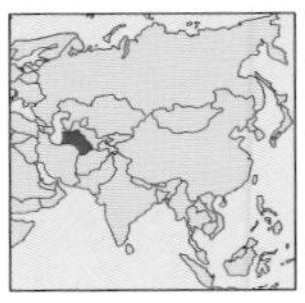

GEOGRAPHY The Republic of Turkmenistan is one of the five central Asian republics which once formed part of the former Soviet Union. Most of the land is low-lying, with mountains lying on the southern and southwestern borders. In the west lies the salty Caspian Sea. Most of Turkmenistan is arid and the Garagum, Asia's largest sand desert, covers about 80% of the country. Turkmenistan has a continental climate, with average annual rainfall varying from 3 in [80 mm] in the desert to 12 in [300 mm] in the mountains. Summer months are hot, but winter temperatures drop well below freezing point.

POLITICS & ECONOMY Just over 1,000 years ago, Turkic people settled in the lands east of the Caspian Sea and the name "Turkmen" comes from this time. Mongol armies conquered the area in the 13th century and Islam was introduced in the 14th century. Russia took over the area in the 1870s and 1880s. After the Russian Revolution of 1917, the area came under Communist rule and, in 1924, it became the Turkmen Soviet Socialist Republic. The Communists strictly controlled all aspects of life and discouraged religion. But they improved such services as education, health, housing, and transport.

In the 1980s, when the Soviet Union began to introduce reforms, the Turkmen began to demand more freedom. In 1990, the Turkmen government stated that its laws overruled Soviet laws. In 1991, Turkmenistan became fully independent after the breakup of the Soviet Union. But the country kept ties with Russia through the Commonwealth of Independent States (CIS).

In 1992, Turkmenistan adopted a new constitution, allowing for the setting up of political parties, providing that they were not ethnic or religious in character. But, effectively, Turkmenistan remained a one-party state and, in 1992, Saparmurad Niyazov, the former Communist and now Democratic Party leader, was the only candidate. In 1994, a referendum prolonged Niyazov's term of office to 2002, while, in 1999, the parliament declared him president for life. In 2002, Niyazov survived an attempt on his life.

Faced with many economic problems, Turkmenistan began to look south rather than to the CIS for support. As part of this policy, it joined the Economic Cooperation Organization which had been set up in 1985 by Iran, Pakistan and Turkey. In 1996, the completion of a rail link from Turkmenistan to the Iranian coast was seen as a highly significant step for the future economic development of Central Asia.

Turkmenistan's chief resources are oil and natural gas, but the main activity is agriculture, with cotton, grown on irrigated land, as the main crop. Grain and vegetables are also important. Manufactures include cement, glass, petrochemicals, and textiles.

AREA 188,455 SQ MI [488,100 SQ KM] **POPULATION** 4,776,000
CAPITAL (POPULATION) ASHKHABAD (521,000) **GOVERNMENT** SINGLE-PARTY REPUBLIC **ETHNIC GROUPS** TURKMEN 85%, UZBEK 5%, RUSSIAN 4%
LANGUAGES TURKMEN (OFFICIAL), RUSSIAN, UZBEK **RELIGIONS** ISLAM 89%, EASTERN ORTHODOX 9% **CURRENCY** TURKMEN MANAT = 100 TENESI

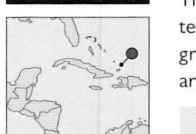

TURKS AND CAICOS ISLANDS

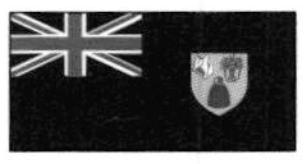
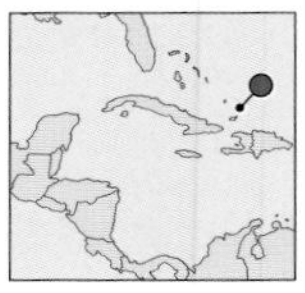

The Turks and Caicos Islands, a British territory in the Caribbean since 1776, are a group of about 30 islands. Fishing and tourism are major activities.

AREA 166 SQ MI [430 SQ KM]
POPULATION 19,000 **CAPITAL** COCKBURN TOWN

TUVALU

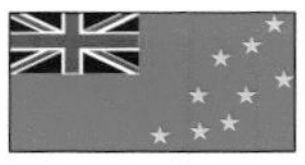
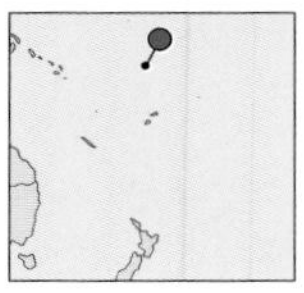

Tuvalu, formerly called the Ellice Islands, was a British territory from the 1890s until it became independent in 1978. It consists of nine low-lying coral atolls in the southern Pacific Ocean. Copra is the chief export.

AREA 10 SQ MI [26 SQ KM]
POPULATION 11,000 **CAPITAL** FONGAFALE

UGANDA

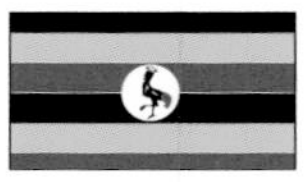
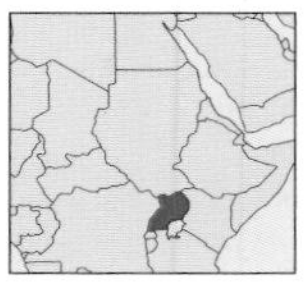

GEOGRAPHY The Republic of Uganda is a landlocked country on the East African plateau. It contains part of Lake Victoria, Africa's largest lake and a source of the River Nile, which occupies a shallow depression in the plateau.

The equator runs through Uganda and the country is warm throughout the year, though the high altitude moderates the temperature. The wettest regions are the lands to the north of Lake Victoria, where Kampala is situated, and the western mountains, especially the high Ruwenzori range.

POLITICS & ECONOMY Little is known of the early history of Uganda. When Europeans first reached the area in the 19th century, many of the people were organized in kingdoms, the most powerful of which was Buganda, the home of the Baganda people. Britain took over the country between 1894 and 1914, and ruled it until independence in 1962.

In 1967, Uganda became a republic and Buganda's Kabaka (king), Sir Edward Mutesa II, was made president. But tensions between the Kabaka and the prime minister, Apollo Milton Obote, led to the dismissal of the Kabaka in 1966. Obote also abolished the traditional kingdoms, including Buganda. Obote was overthrown in 1971 by an army group led by General Idi Amin Dada. Amin ruled as a dictator. He forced most of the Asians who lived in Uganda to leave the country and had many of his opponents killed.

In 1978, a border dispute between Uganda and Tanzania led Tanzanian troops to enter Uganda. With help from Ugandan opponents of Amin, they overthrew Amin's government. In 1980, Obote led his party to victory in national elections. But after charges of fraud, Obote's opponents began guerrilla warfare. A military group overthrew Obote in 1985, though strife continued until 1986, when Yoweri Museveni's National Resistance Movement seized power. In 1993, Museveni restored the traditional kingdoms, including Buganda where a new Kabaka was crowned. Museveni held elections in 1994 but political parties were not allowed. Museveni was elected president in 1996 and 2001. In 2003, the president announced that multiparty democracy would be restored, but he gave no date for the change.

The strife since the 1960s has greatly damaged the economy, but the economy grew during a period of stability in the 1990s. The situation worsened when Uganda intervened militarily in Congo (then Zaïre) in 1998. Agriculture dominates the economy, employing 80% of the people. The chief export is coffee.

AREA 93,065 SQ MI [241,038 SQ KM] **POPULATION** 25,633,000
CAPITAL (POPULATION) KAMPALA (774,000)
GOVERNMENT REPUBLIC IN TRANSITION
ETHNIC GROUPS BAGANDA 17%, ANKOLE 8%, BASOGO 8%, ITESO 8%, BAKIGA 7%, LANGI 6%, RWANDA 6%, BAGISU 5%, ACHOLI 4%, LUGBARA 4% AND OTHERS
LANGUAGES ENGLISH AND SWAHILI (BOTH OFFICIAL), GANDA
RELIGIONS ROMAN CATHOLIC 33%, PROTESTANT 33%, TRADITIONAL BELIEFS 18%, ISLAM 16%
CURRENCY UGANDAN SHILLING = 100 CENTS

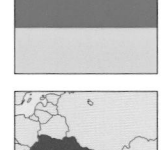

UKRAINE

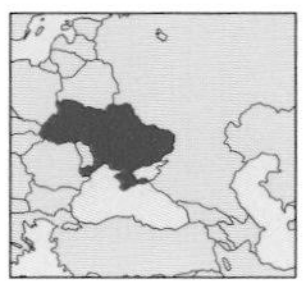

GEOGRAPHY Ukraine is the second largest country in Europe after Russia. It was formerly part of the Soviet Union, which split apart in 1991. This mostly flat country faces the Black Sea in the south. The Crimean peninsula includes a highland region overlooking Yalta. Ukraine has warm summers, but the winters are cold, becoming more severe from west to east. In the summer, the east of the country is often warmer than the west. The heaviest rainfall occurs in the summer.

POLITICS & ECONOMY Kiev was the original capital of the early Slavic civilization known as Kievan Rus. In the 17th and 18th centuries, parts of Ukraine came under Polish and Russian rule. But Russia gained most of Ukraine in the late 18th century. In 1918, Ukraine became independent, but in 1922 it became part of the Soviet Union. Millions of people died in the 1930s as a result of Soviet policies, while millions more died during the Nazi occupation (1941–4).

In the 1980s, Ukrainian people demanded more say over their affairs. The country became independent in 1991. Leonid Kuchma, who became president in 1994, came under fire in the early 2000s for maladministration and for his alleged involvement in the murder of a journalist. In 2003, Ukraine's Supreme Court ruled that Kuchma could not be prosecuted for crimes committed while in office and the Constitutional Court ruled that he could stand for a third term as president.

The World Bank classifies Ukraine as a "lower-middle-income" economy. Agriculture is important. Crops include wheat and sugar beet, which are the major exports, together with barley, maize, potatoes, sunflowers, and tobacco. Livestock rearing and fishing are also important industries.

Manufacturing is the chief economic activity. Major manufactures include iron and steel, machinery, and vehicles. Ukraine has large coalfields. The country imports oil and natural gas, but it has hydroelectric and nuclear power stations. In 1986, an accident at the Chernobyl (Chornobyl) nuclear power plant caused widespread nuclear radiation. The plant was finally closed in 2001.

AREA 233,089 SQ MI [603,700 SQ KM] **POPULATION** 48,055,000
CAPITAL (POPULATION) KIEV (2,590,000)
GOVERNMENT MULTIPARTY REPUBLIC
ETHNIC GROUPS UKRAINIAN 78%, RUSSIAN 17%, BELARUSIAN, MOLDOVAN, BULGARIAN, HUNGARIAN, POLISH
LANGUAGES UKRAINIAN (OFFICIAL), RUSSIAN
RELIGIONS MOSTLY UKRAINIAN ORTHODOX
CURRENCY HRYVNIA = 100 KOPIYKAS

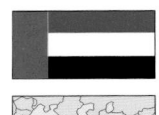

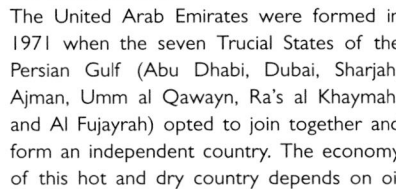

UNITED ARAB EMIRATES

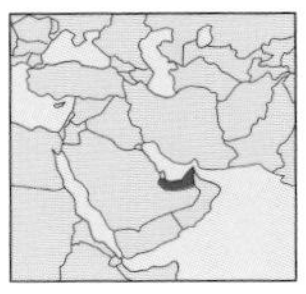

The United Arab Emirates were formed in 1971 when the seven Trucial States of the Persian Gulf (Abu Dhabi, Dubai, Sharjah, Ajman, Umm al Qawayn, Ra's al Khaymah, and Al Fujayrah) opted to join together and form an independent country. The economy of this hot and dry country depends on oil production, and oil revenues give the United Arab Emirates one of the highest per capita GNPs in Asia.

AREA 32,278 SQ MI [83,600 SQ KM] **POPULATION** 2,485,000
CAPITAL (POPULATION) ABU DHABI (363,000)

UNITED KINGDOM

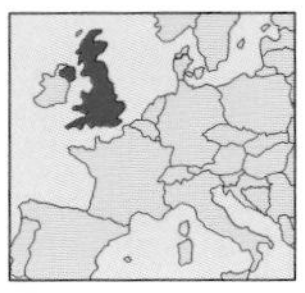

GEOGRAPHY The United Kingdom (or UK) is a union of four countries. Three of them – England, Scotland and Wales – make up Great Britain. The fourth country is Northern Ireland. The Isle of Man and the Channel Islands, including Jersey and Guernsey, are not part of the UK. They are self-governing British dependencies.

The land is highly varied. Much of Scotland and Wales is mountainous, and the highest peak is Scotland's Ben Nevis at 4,406 ft [1,343 m]. England has some highland areas, including the Cumbrian Mountains (or Lake District) and the Pennine range in the north. But England also has large areas of fertile lowland. Northern Ireland is also a mixture of lowlands and uplands. It contains the UK's largest lake, Lough Neagh.

The UK has a mild climate, influenced by the warm Gulf Stream which flows across the Atlantic from the Gulf of Mexico, then past the British Isles. Moist winds from the southwest bring rain, but the rainfall decreases from west to east. Winds from the east and north bring cold weather in winter.

POLITICS & ECONOMY In ancient times, Britain was invaded by many peoples, including Iberians, Celts, Romans, Angles, Saxons, Jutes, Norsemen, Danes, and Normans, who arrived in 1066. The evolution of the United Kingdom spanned hundreds of years. The Normans finally overcame Welsh resistance in 1282, when King Edward I annexed Wales and united it with England. Union with Scotland was achieved by the Act of Union of 1707. This created a country known as the United Kingdom of Great Britain.

Ireland came under Norman rule in the 11th century, and much of its later history was concerned with a struggle against English domination. In 1801, Ireland became part of the United Kingdom of Great Britain and Ireland. But in 1921, southern Ireland broke away to become the Irish Free State. Most of the people in the Irish Free State were Roman Catholics. In Northern Ireland, where the majority of the people were Protestants, most people wanted to remain citizens of the United Kingdom. As a result, the country's official name changed to the United Kingdom of Great Britain and Northern Ireland.

The modern history of the UK began in the 18th century when the British empire began to develop, despite the loss in 1783 of its 13 North American colonies which became the core of the modern United States. The other major event occurred in the late 18th century, when the UK became the first country to industrialize its economy.

The British empire broke up after World War II (1939–45), though the UK still administers many small, mainly island, territories around the world. The empire was transformed into the Commonwealth of Nations, a free association of independent countries which numbered 54 in 2001.

The UK has retained an important world role. For example, in 2001, it played a prominent role in creating a broad alliance to counter international terrorism following the attacks on the United

States. It was also a prominent member of the coalition force which invaded Iraq in 2003. However, the UK has recognized that its economic future lies within Europe. It became a member of the European Economic Community (now the European Union) in 1973. In the early 21st century, most people accepted the importance of the EU to the UK's economic future. But some feared a loss of British identity should the EU ever evolve into a political federation.

The UK is a major industrial and trading nation. It lacks natural resources apart from coal, iron ore, oil and natural gas, and has to import most of the materials it needs for its industries. The UK also has to import food, because it produces only about two-thirds of the food it needs. In the first half of the 20th century, Britain was a major exporter of cars, ships, steel, and textiles. But many industries have suffered from competition from other countries, with lower labor costs. Today, industries have to use high-technology in order to compete on the world market.

The UK is one of the world's most urbanized countries, and agriculture employs only 1% of the people. Production is high because of the use of scientific methods and modern machinery. However, in the early 21st century, especially following the outbreak of foot-and-mouth disease in 2001, questions were raised about the future of rural industries. Major crops include barley, potatoes, sugar beet, and wheat. Sheep are the leading livestock, but beef and dairy cattle, pigs, and poultry are also important. Fishing is another major activity and the UK is one of the largest fishing countries in the EU. Important catches include cod, haddock, plaice, and mackerel.

Service industries play a major part in the UK's economy. Financial and insurance services bring in much-needed foreign exchange, while tourism has become a major earner.

AREA 93,381 sq mi [241,857 sq km] **POPULATION** 60,095,000
CAPITAL (POPULATION) London (8,089,000)
GOVERNMENT Constitutional monarchy
ETHNIC GROUPS English 82%, Scottish 10%, Irish 2%, Welsh 2%, Ulster 2%, West Indian, Indian, Pakistani and others **LANGUAGES** English (official), Welsh, Gaelic
RELIGIONS Christianity (Anglican, Roman Catholic, Presbyterian, Methodist), Islam, Sikhism, Hinduism, Judaism
CURRENCY Pound sterling = 100 pence

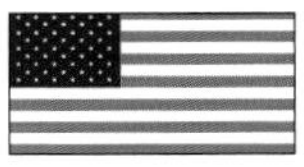

UNITED STATES OF AMERICA

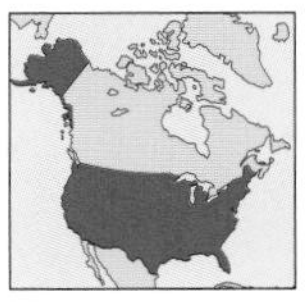

GEOGRAPHY The United States of America is the world's fourth largest country in area and the third largest in population. It contains 50 states, 48 of which lie between Canada and Mexico, plus Alaska in northwestern North America, and Hawaii, a group of volcanic islands in the North Pacific Ocean. Densely populated coastal plains lie to the east and south of the Appalachian Mountains. The central lowlands drained by the Mississippi–Missouri rivers stretch from the Appalachians to the Rocky Mountains in the west. The Pacific region contains fertile valleys, separated by mountain ranges.

The climate varies greatly, ranging from the Arctic cold of Alaska to the intense heat of Death Valley, a bleak desert in California. Of the 48 states between Canada and Mexico, winters are cold and snowy in the north, but mild in the south, a region which is often called the "Sun Belt."

POLITICS & ECONOMY The first people in North America, the ancestors of the Native Americans (or American Indians) arrived perhaps 40,000 years ago from Asia. Although Vikings probably reached North America 1,000 years ago, European exploration proper did not begin until the late 15th century.

The first Europeans to settle in large numbers were the British, who founded settlements on the eastern coast in the early 17th century. British rule ended in the War of ndependence (1775–83). The country expanded in 1803 when a vast territory in the south and west was acquired through the Louisiana Purchase, while the border with Mexico was fixed in the mid-19th century. The Civil War (1861–5) ended slavery and the serious threat that the nation might split into two parts. In the late 19th century, the West was opened up, while immigrants flooded in from Europe and elsewhere.

During the late 19th and early 20th centuries, industrialization led to the United States becoming the world's leading economic superpower and a pioneer in science and technology. It took on the mantle of the champion of Western democracy and, following the breakup of the former Soviet Union, it became the world's only superpower. But the attacks on the country on September 11, 2001, revealed its vulnerability to terrorists and rogue states. The response was vigorous. In 2001, it attacked the Taliban government in Afghanistan, which was protecting al Qaida terrorists. Then, in 2003, it led a coalition force to invade Iraq and overthrow the repressive regime of Saddam Hussein. However, it met with considerable resistance even after the capture of Saddam Hussein in December 2003.

The United States has the world's largest economy in terms of the total value of its production. Although agriculture employs only about 2% of the people, farming is highly mechanized and scientific, and the United States leads the world in farm production. Major products include beef and dairy cattle, together with such crops as cotton, fruits, groundnuts, maize, potatoes, soybeans, tobacco, and wheat.

The country's natural resources include oil, natural gas, and coal. There are also a wide range of metal ores which are used in manufacturing industries, together with timber, especially from the forests of the Pacific northwest. Manufacturing is the single most important activity, employing about 14% of the population. Major products include vehicles, food products, chemicals, machinery, printed goods, metal products, and scientific instruments. California is now the leading manufacturing state. Many southern states, petroleum rich and climatically favored, have also become highly prosperous in recent years.

AREA 3,717,792 sq mi [9,629,091 sq km] **POPULATION** 290,343,000
CAPITAL (POPULATION) Washington, DC (572,000)
GOVERNMENT Federal republic
ETHNIC GROUPS White 77%, African American 13%, Asian 4%, Amerindian 2%, others **LANGUAGES** English (official), Spanish, more than 30 others **RELIGIONS** Protestant 56%, Roman Catholic 28%, Islam 2%, Judaism 2%
CURRENCY US dollar = 100 cents

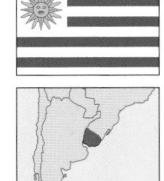

URUGUAY

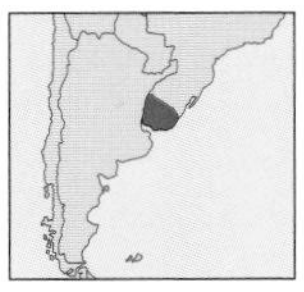

GEOGRAPHY Uruguay is South America's second smallest independent country after Suriname. The land consists mainly of flat plains and hills. The River Uruguay, which forms the country's western border, flows into the Río de la Plata, a large estuary which leads into the South Atlantic Ocean.

Uruguay has a mild climate, with rain in every month, though droughts sometimes occur. Summers are pleasantly warm, especially near the coast. The weather remains relatively mild throughout the winter.

POLITICS & ECONOMY In 1726, Spanish settlers founded Montevideo in order to halt the Portuguese gaining influence in the area. By the late 18th century, Spaniards had settled in most of the country. Uruguay became part of a colony called the Vice-royalty of La Plata, which also included Argentina, Paraguay, and parts of Bolivia, Brazil, and Chile. In 1820 Brazil annexed Uruguay, ending Spanish rule. In 1825, Uruguayans, supported by Argentina, began a struggle for independence. Finally, in 1828, Brazil and Argentina recognized Uruguay as an independent republic. Social and economic developments were slow in the 19th century, but, from 1903, Uruguay became stable and democratic.

From the 1950s, economic problems caused unrest. Terrorist groups, notably the Tupumaros, carried out murders and kidnappings. The army crushed the Tupamaros in 1972, but the army took over the government in 1973. Military rule continued until 1984 when elections were held. In the early 21st century, Uruguay faced many economic problems, many of which were the result of the economic crisis in its neighbor, Argentina, and its imposition of banking controls.

The World Bank classifies Uruguay as an "upper-middle-income" developing country. Agriculture employs only 4% of the people, but farm products, notably hides and leather goods, beef and wool, are the leading exports, while the leading manufacturing industries process farm products. The main crops include maize, potatoes, wheat, and sugar beet. Uruguay depends largely on hydroelectric power for energy and exports electricity to Argentina.

AREA 67,574 sq mi [175,016 sq km] **POPULATION** 3,413,000
CAPITAL (POPULATION) Montevideo (1,303,000)
GOVERNMENT Multiparty republic
ETHNIC GROUPS White 88%, Mestizo 8%, Mulatto or Black 4%
LANGUAGES Spanish (official)
RELIGIONS Roman Catholic 66%, Protestant 2%, Judaism 1%
CURRENCY Uruguayan peso = 100 centésimos

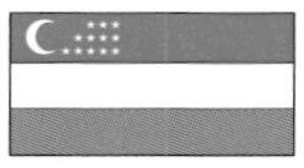

UZBEKISTAN

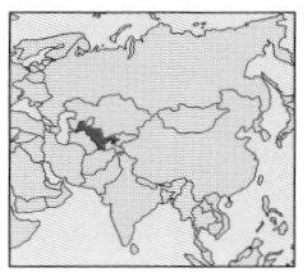

GEOGRAPHY The Republic of Uzbekistan is one of the five republics in Central Asia which were once part of the Soviet Union. Plains cover most of western Uzbekistan, with highlands in the east. The main rivers, the Amu (or Amu Darya) and Syr (or Syr Darya), drain into the Aral Sea. So much water has been taken from these rivers to irrigate the land that the Aral Sea has now shrunk to about a quarter of its size in 1960. The dried-up lake area has become desert, like much of the rest of the country. Uzbekistan has a continental climate with cold winters and hot summers. The west is extremely arid, with an average annual rainfall of about 8 in [200 mm].

POLITICS & ECONOMY Russia took the area in the 19th century. After the Russian Revolution of 1917, the Communists took over and, in 1924, they set up the Uzbek Soviet Socialist Republic. Under Communism, all aspects of Uzbek life were controlled and religious worship was discouraged. But education, health, housing and transport were improved. In the late 1980s, the people demanded more freedom and, in 1990, the government stated that its laws overruled those of the Soviet Union. Uzbekistan became independent in 1991 when the Soviet Union broke up, but it retained links with Russia through the Commonwealth of Independent States. Islam Karimov, leader of the People's Democratic Party (formerly the Communist Party), was elected president in December 1991. In 1992–3, many opposition leaders were arrested because the government said that they threatened national stability. In 1994–5, the PDP was victorious in national elections and, in 1995, a referendum extended Karimov's term in office until 2000, when he was again re-elected. In 2001, Karimov declared his support for the United States in combating terrorist bases in Afghanistan. But, in 2004, the United States criticized Uzbekistan for its suppression of democracy and human rights abuses.

The World Bank classifies Uzbekistan as a "lower-middle-income" developing country and the government still controls most economic activity. The country produces coal, copper, gold, oil, and natural gas.

AREA 172,741 sq mi [447,400 sq km] **POPULATION** 25,982,000
CAPITAL (POPULATION) Tashkent (2,143,000)
GOVERNMENT Socialist republic **ETHNIC GROUPS** Uzbek 80%, Russian 5%, Tajik 5%, Kazakh 3%, Tatar 2%, Kara-Kalpak 2%
LANGUAGES Uzbek (official), Russian **RELIGIONS** Islam 88%, Eastern Orthodox 9% **CURRENCY** Uzbekistani sum = 100 tiyin

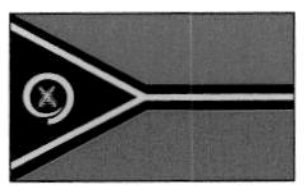

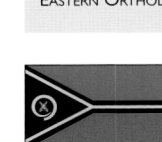

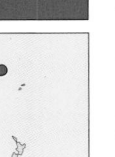

VANUATU

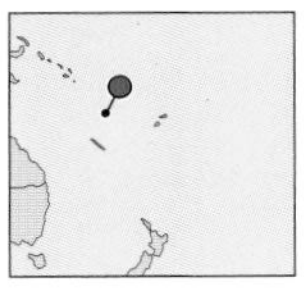

The Republic of Vanuatu, formerly the Anglo-French Condominium of the New Hebrides, became independent in 1980. It consists of a chain of 80 islands in the South Pacific Ocean. Its economy is based on agriculture and it exports copra, beef and veal, timber, and cocoa.

AREA 4,706 sq mi [12,189 sq km]
POPULATION 199,000 **CAPITAL** Port-Vila

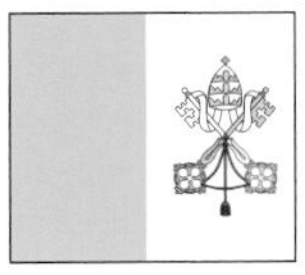

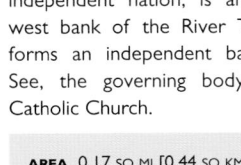

VATICAN CITY

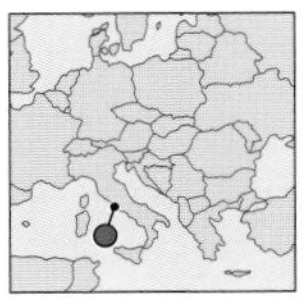

Vatican City State, the world's smallest independent nation, is an enclave on the west bank of the River Tiber in Rome. It forms an independent base for the Holy See, the governing body of the Roman Catholic Church.

AREA 0.17 sq mi [0.44 sq km]
POPULATION 1,000

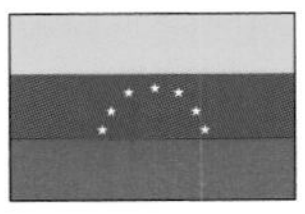

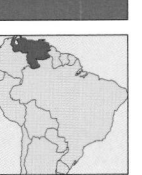

VENEZUELA

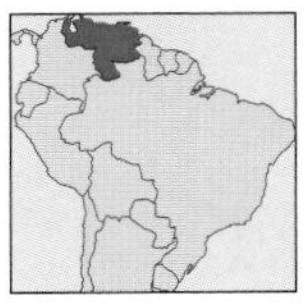

GEOGRAPHY The Bolivarian Republic of Venezuela, in northern South America, contains the Maracaibo lowlands around the oil-rich Lake Maracaibo in the west. Andean ranges enclose the lowlands and extend across most of northern Venezuela. The Orinoco river basin, containing tropical grasslands called *llanos*, lies between the northern highlands and the Guiana Highlands in the southeast. The Orinoco is Venezuela's longest river.

Venezuela has a tropical climate. Temperatures are high

throughout the year on the lowlands, though the mountains are much cooler. The rainfall is heaviest in the mountains. But much of the country has a marked dry season between December and April.

POLITICS & ECONOMY In the early 19th century, Venezuelans, such as Simón Bolívar and Francisco de Miranda, began a struggle against Spanish rule. Venezuela declared its independence in 1811. But it only became truly independent in 1821, when the Spanish were defeated in a battle near Valencia.

The development of Venezuela in the 19th and the first half of the 20th centuries was marred by instability, violence and periods of harsh dictatorial rule. But Venezuela has had elected governments since 1958. The country has greatly benefited from its oil resources which were first exploited in 1917. In 1960, Venezuela helped to form OPEC (the Organization of Petroleum Exporting Countries) and, in 1976, the government of Venezuela took control of the entire oil industry. In 1999, Hugo Chavez, who had staged an unsuccessful coup in 1992, was elected president. Chavez survived an attempted coup in April 2002 and a crippling general strike staged by his opponents between December 2002 and February 2003.

The World Bank classifies Venezuela as an "upper-middle-income" developing country. Oil accounts for 80% of the exports. Other exports include bauxite and aluminum, iron ore, and farm products. Agriculture employs 9% of people and cattle ranching is important; dairy cattle and poultry are also raised. Major crops include bananas, cassava, citrus fruits, coffee, and rice. The chief industry is petroleum refining. Other manufactures include aluminum, cement, processed food, steel, and textiles.

AREA 352,143 SQ MI [912,050 SQ KM] **POPULATION** 24,655,000
CAPITAL (POPULATION) CARACAS (1,823,000) **GOVERNMENT** FEDERAL REPUBLIC **ETHNIC GROUPS** SPANISH, ITALIAN, PORTUGUESE, ARAB, GERMAN, AFRICAN, INDIGENOUS PEOPLE **LANGUAGES** SPANISH (OFFICIAL), INDIGENOUS DIALECTS **RELIGIONS** ROMAN CATHOLIC 96%
CURRENCY BOLÍVAR = 100 CÉNTIMOS

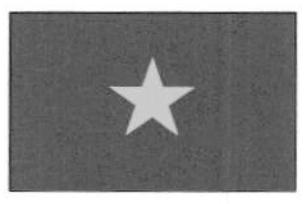
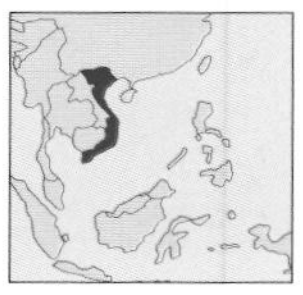

VIETNAM

GEOGRAPHY The Socialist Republic of Vietnam occupies an S-shaped strip of land facing the South China Sea in Southeast Asia. The coastal plains include two densely populated, fertile delta regions: the Red (Hong) delta facing the Gulf of Tonkin in the north, and the Mekong delta in the south.

Vietnam has a tropical climate, though the driest months of January to March are a little cooler than the wet, hot summer months, when monsoon winds blow from the southwest. Typhoons (cyclones or hurricanes) sometimes hit the coast, causing extensive flooding and much damage.

POLITICS & ECONOMY China dominated Vietnam for a thousand years before AD 939, when a Vietnamese state was founded. The French took over the area between the 1850s and 1880s. They ruled Vietnam as part of French Indochina, which also included Cambodia and Laos.

Japan conquered Vietnam during World War II (1939–45). In 1946, war broke out between a nationalist group, called the Vietminh, and the French colonial government. France withdrew in 1954 and Vietnam was divided into a Communist North Vietnam, led by the Vietminh leader, Ho Chi Minh, and a non-Communist South.

A force called the Viet Cong rebelled against South Vietnam's government in 1957 and a war began, which gradually increased in intensity. The United States aided the South, but after it withdrew in 1975, South Vietnam surrendered. In 1976, the united Vietnam became a Socialist Republic.

Vietnamese troops intervened in Cambodia in 1978 to defeat the Communist Khmer Rouge government, but it withdrew its troops in 1989. In the 1990s, Vietnam began to introduce reforms. In 1995, the United States opened an embassy in Hanoi and, in 2000, a major trade pact was agreed by the countries.

The World Bank classifies Vietnam as a "low-income" developing country and agriculture employs 67% of the population. The main food crop is rice. The country also produces chromium, oil (which was discovered off the south coast in 1986), phosphates, and tin.

AREA 128,065 SQ MI [331,689 SQ KM] **POPULATION** 81,625,000
CAPITAL (POPULATION) HANOI (1,074,000)
GOVERNMENT SOCIALIST REPUBLIC
ETHNIC GROUPS VIETNAMESE 87%, CHINESE, HMONG, THAI, KHMER, CHAM, MOUNTAIN GROUPS **LANGUAGES** VIETNAMESE (OFFICIAL), ENGLISH, CHINESE **RELIGIONS** BUDDHISM, CHRISTIANITY, INDIGENOUS BELIEFS
CURRENCY DONG = 10 HAO = 100 XU

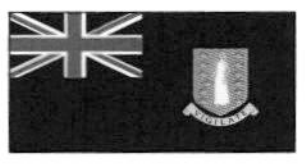
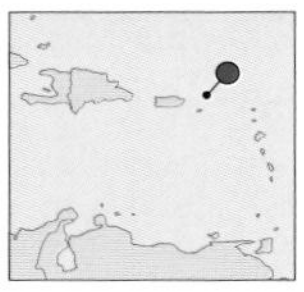

VIRGIN ISLANDS, BRITISH

The British Virgin Islands, the most northerly of the Lesser Antilles, are a British overseas territory, with a substantial measure of self-government.

AREA 58 SQ MI [151 SQ KM]
POPULATION 22,000 **CAPITAL** ROAD TOWN

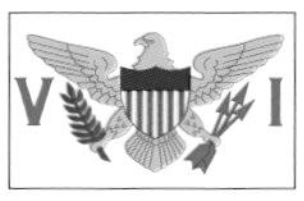
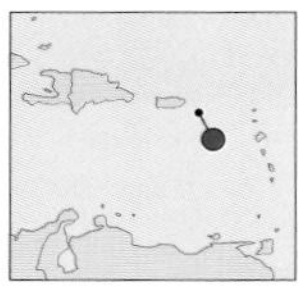

VIRGIN ISLANDS, US

The Virgin Islands of the United States, a group of three islands and 65 small islets, are a self-governing US territory. Purchased from Denmark in 1917, its residents are US citizens and they elect a non-voting delegate to the US House of Representatives.

AREA 134 SQ MI [347 SQ KM]
POPULATION 125,000 **CAPITAL** CHARLOTTE AMALIE

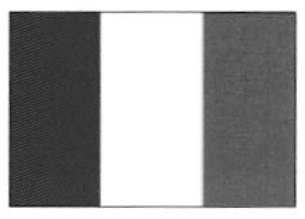
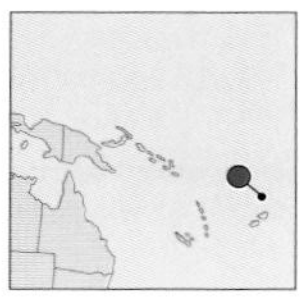

WALLIS AND FUTUNA

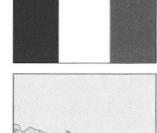

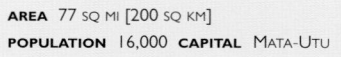

Wallis and Futuna, in the South Pacific Ocean, is the smallest and the poorest of France's overseas territories. French aid remains vital to an economy based on subsistence agriculture.

AREA 77 SQ MI [200 SQ KM]
POPULATION 16,000 **CAPITAL** MATA-UTU

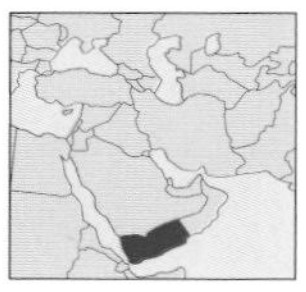

YEMEN

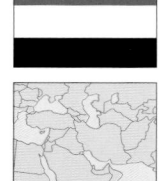

GEOGRAPHY The Republic of Yemen faces the Red Sea and the Gulf of Aden in the southwestern corner of the Arabian peninsula. Behind the narrow coastal plain along the Red Sea, the land rises to a mountain region called High Yemen. The climate ranges from hot and often humid conditions on the coast to the cooler highlands. Most of the country is arid. The south coasts are particularly hot and humid.

POLITICS & ECONOMY After World War I, northern Yemen, which had been ruled by Turkey, began to evolve into a separate state from the south, where Britain was in control. Britain withdrew in 1967 and a left-wing government took power in the south. In North Yemen, the monarchy was abolished in 1962 and the country became a republic.

Clashes occurred between the traditionalist Yemen Arab Republic in the north and the formerly British Marxist People's Democratic Republic of Yemen but, in 1990, the two Yemens merged to form a single country. Further conflict occurred in 1994, when southern secessionist forces were defeated. In 1998 and 1999, militants in the Aden-Abyan Islamic army sought to destabilize the country. In 2000, suicide bombers, thought to be part of the al Qaida network, steered a craft into a US destroyer in Aden harbor, killing 17 sailors, while, in 2002, three American missionaries were shot in a hospital in the south.

The World Bank classifies Yemen as a "low-income" developing country. Agriculture employs up to 50% of the people. Herders raise sheep and other animals, while farmers grow such crops as barley, fruits, wheat, and vegetables in highland valleys and around oases. Cash crops include coffee and cotton.

Imported oil is refined at Aden and petroleum extraction began in the northwest in the 1980s. Handicrafts, leather goods, and textiles are manufactured. Remittances from Yemenis abroad are a major source of revenue.

AREA 203,848 SQ MI [527,968 SQ KM] **POPULATION** 19,350,000
CAPITAL (POPULATION) SANA' (954,000) **GOVERNMENT** MULTIPARTY REPUBLIC **ETHNIC GROUPS** PREDOMINANTLY ARAB **LANGUAGES** ARABIC (OFFICIAL) **RELIGIONS** ISLAM **CURRENCY** YEMENI RIAL = 100 FILS

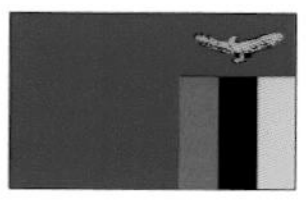
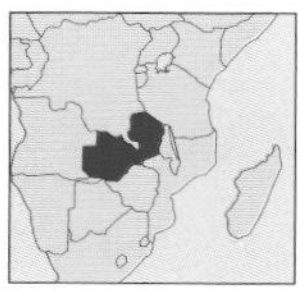

ZAMBIA

GEOGRAPHY The Republic of Zambia is a landlocked country in southern Africa. Zambia lies on the plateau that makes up most of southern Africa. Much of the land is between 2,950 ft and 4,920 ft [900 m to 1,500 m] above sea level. The Muchinga Mountains in the northeast rise above this flat land. Lakes include Bangweulu, which is entirely within Zambia, together with parts of lakes Mweru and Tanganyika in the north. Zambia lies in the tropics, but temperatures are moderated by the altitude.

POLITICS & ECONOMY European contact with Zambia began in the 19th century, when the explorer David Livingstone crossed the River Zambezi. In the 1890s, the British South Africa Company, set up by Cecil Rhodes (1853–1902), the British financier and statesman, made treaties with local chiefs and gradually took over the area. In 1911, the Company named the area Northern Rhodesia. In 1924, Britain took over the government of the country.

In 1953, Britain formed a federation of Northern Rhodesia, Southern Rhodesia (now Zimbabwe), and Nyasaland (now Malawi). Because of African opposition, the federation was dissolved in 1963 and Northern Rhodesia became independent as Zambia in 1964. Kenneth Kaunda became president and one-party rule was introduced in 1972. However, a new constitution was adopted in 1990 and, in 1991, Kaunda's party was defeated and Frederick Chiluba became president. Chiluba was re-elected in 1996. Chiluba stood down in 2001 and his party's candidate, Levy Mwanawasa, was elected president.

Copper, the main resource, accounted for 55% of the exports in 2001. Zambia also produces cobalt, lead, zinc, and gemstones. Agriculture employs 69% of the people, as compared with 4% in industry and mining. Food crops include cassava, fruits and vegetables, maize, millet, and sorghum, while cash crops include coffee, sugarcane, and tobacco.

AREA 290,586 SQ MI [752,618 SQ KM] **POPULATION** 10,307,000
CAPITAL (POPULATION) LUSAKA (1,270,000)
GOVERNMENT MULTIPARTY REPUBLIC **ETHNIC GROUPS** NATIVE AFRICAN (BEMBA, TONGA, MARAVI/NYANJA) **LANGUAGES** ENGLISH (OFFICIAL), BEMBA, KAONDA, NYANJA AND ABOUT 70 OTHERS **RELIGIONS** CHRISTIANITY 70%, ISLAM, HINDUISM **CURRENCY** ZAMBIAN KWACHA = 100 NGWEE

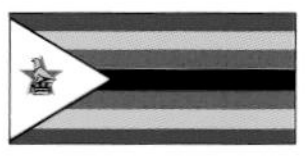
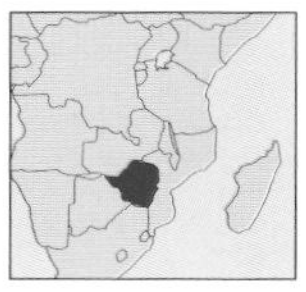

ZIMBABWE

GEOGRAPHY The Republic of Zimbabwe is a landlocked country in southern Africa. Most of the country lies on a high plateau between the Zambezi and Limpopo rivers between 2,950 ft and 4,920 ft [900 m to 1,500 m] above sea level. From October to March, the weather is hot and wet, but in the winter, daily temperatures can vary greatly.

POLITICS & ECONOMY The Shona people became dominant in the region about 1,000 years ago. The British South Africa Company, under the statesman Cecil Rhodes (1853–1902), occupied the area in the 1890s, after obtaining mineral rights from local chiefs. The area was named Rhodesia and later Southern Rhodesia. It became a self-governing British colony in 1923. Between 1953 and 1963, Southern and Northern Rhodesia (now Zambia) were joined to Nyasaland (Malawi) in the Central African Federation.

In 1965, the European government of Southern Rhodesia (then called Rhodesia) declared their country independent but Britain refused to accept this. Finally, after a civil war, the country became legally independent in 1980, though rivalries between the Shona and Ndebele people threatened stability. Order was restored when the Shona prime minister, Robert Mugabe, brought his Ndebele rivals into his government. In 1987, Mugabe became the country's executive president and, in 1991, the government renounced its Marxist ideology. Mugabe was re-elected president in 1990 and 1996. During the late 1990s, Mugabe threatened to seize white-owned farms without paying compensation to the owners. Despite international pressure, landless "war veterans" began to occupy white farms. The situation worsened in the early 2000s, resulting in violence and murder. In 2002, Mugabe was re-elected president amid accusations of electoral irregularities. The Commonwealth suspended Zimbabwe's membership for 12 months. However, in 2003, violence against Mugabe's opponents continued and, in 2004, the European Union renewed its sanctions against the country.

The World Bank classifies Zimbabwe as a "low-income" developing country. The country has valuable mineral resources and mining accounts for a fifth of the country's exports. Agriculture employs 26% of working people. Maize is the chief food crop, while cash crops include cotton, sugar, and tobacco. Cattle ranching is another important activity.

AREA 150,871 SQ MI [390,757 SQ KM] **POPULATION** 12,577,000
CAPITAL (POPULATION) HARARE (1,189,000)
GOVERNMENT MULTIPARTY REPUBLIC **ETHNIC GROUPS** SHONA 82%, NDEBELE 14%, OTHER AFRICAN GROUPS 2%, MIXED AND ASIAN 1%
LANGUAGES ENGLISH (OFFICIAL), SHONA, NDEBELE
RELIGIONS CHRISTIANITY, TRADITIONAL BELIEFS
CURRENCY ZIMBABWEAN DOLLAR = 100 CENTS

INTRODUCTION TO WORLD GEOGRAPHY

The Universe	2	Water and Vegetation	18	Agriculture	32
The Solar System	4	The Natural Environment	20	Energy	34
Time and Motion	6	People		Minerals	36
Oceans	8	and the Environment	22	Manufacturing	38
Geology	10	Population	24	Trade	40
Landforms	12	Cities	26	Health	42
Atmosphere and Weather	14	The Human Family	28	Wealth	44
Climate	16	Conflict and Cooperation	30	Standards of Living	46

THE UNIVERSE

For more information:
4 Orbits of the planets
Planetary data

About 13.7 billion years ago, time and space began with the most colossal explosion in cosmic history: the so-called "Big Bang" that is believed to have initiated the Universe. According to current theory, in the first millionth of a second of its existence it expanded from a dimensionless point of infinite mass and density into a fireball about 19 billion miles across – and it has been expanding ever since.

It took almost a million years for the primal fireball to cool enough for atoms to form. They were mostly hydrogen, still the most abundant material in the Universe. But the new matter was not evenly distributed around the young Universe, and a few billion years later atoms in relatively dense regions began to cling together under the influence of gravity, forming distinct masses of gas separated by vast expanses of empty space. To begin with, these first proto-galaxies were dark places: the Universe had cooled. But gravitational attraction continued, condensing matter into coherent lumps inside the galactic gas clouds. About 3 billion years later, some of these masses had contracted so much that internal pressure produced the high temperatures necessary to bring about nuclear fusion: the first stars were born.

There were several generations of stars, each feeding on the wreckage of its extinct predecessors as well as the original galactic gas swirls. With each new generation, progressively larger atoms were forged in stellar furnaces and the galaxy's range of elements, once restricted to hydrogen, grew larger. About 9 billion years after the Big Bang, a star formed on the outskirts of our galaxy with enough matter left over to create a retinue of planets. Nearly 5 billion years after that, human beings evolved.

The Sun is one of more than 100 billion stars in the home galaxy alone. Our galaxy, in turn, forms part of a local group of approximately 30 similar structures, some much larger than our own; there are at least 100 billion other galaxies in the Universe as a whole. The most distant ever observed, a highly energetic galactic core designated as quasar RD J030117+002025, lies about 13 billion light-years away.

LIFE OF A STAR

For most of its existence, a star produces energy by the nuclear fusion of hydrogen into helium at its core. The duration of this hydrogen-burning period – known as the *main sequence* – depends on the star's mass; the greater the mass, the higher the core temperatures and the sooner the star's supply of hydrogen is exhausted. Dim, dwarf stars consume their hydrogen slowly, eking it out over 1,000 billion years or more. The Sun, like other stars of its mass, should spend about 10 billion years on the main sequence; since it was formed less than 5 billion years ago, it still has half its life left.

Once all a star's core hydrogen has been fused into helium, nuclear activity moves outward into layers of unconsumed hydrogen. For a time, energy production sharply increases: the star grows hotter and expands enormously, turning into a so-called red giant. Its energy output will increase a thousandfold, and it will swell to a hundred times its present diameter.

After a few hundred million years, helium in the core will become sufficiently compressed to initiate a new cycle of nuclear fusion: from helium to carbon. The star will contract somewhat, before beginning its last expansion, in the Sun's case engulfing the Earth and perhaps Mars. In this bloated condition, the Sun's outer layers will break off into space, leaving a tiny inner core, mainly of carbon, that shrinks progressively under the force of its own gravity: dwarf stars can attain a density more than 10,000 times that of normal matter, with crushing surface gravities to match. Gradually, the nuclear fires will die down, and the Sun will reach its terminal stage: a black dwarf, emitting insignificant amounts of energy.

Black holes
However, stars more massive than the Sun may undergo another transformation. The additional mass allows gravitational collapse to continue indefinitely: eventually, all the star's remaining matter shrinks to a point, and its density approaches infinity – a state that will not permit even subatomic structures to survive.

The star has become a *black hole*: an anomalous "singularity" in the fabric of space and time. Although vast coruscations of radiation will be emitted by any matter falling into its grasp, the singularity itself has an escape velocity that exceeds the speed of light, and nothing can ever be released from it. Within the boundaries of the black hole, the laws of physics are suspended, but no physicist can ever observe the extraordinary events that may occur.

GALACTIC STRUCTURES

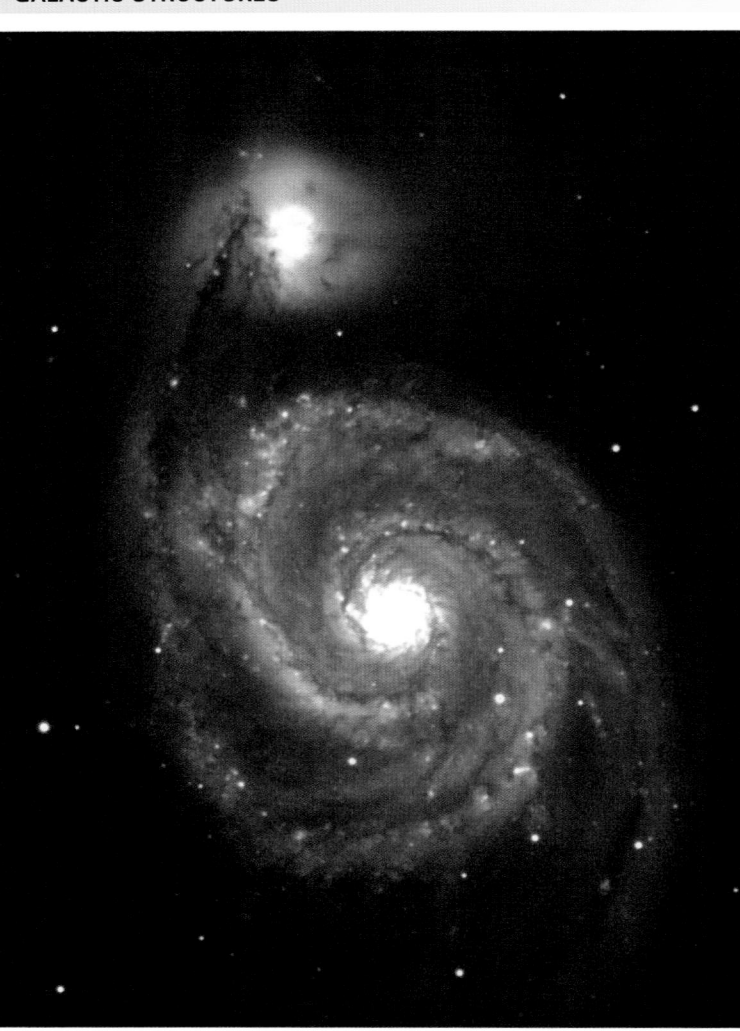

Many of the Universe's 100 billion galaxies show clear structural patterns, originally classified by the American astronomer Edwin Hubble in 1925. Spiral galaxies like our own have a central, almost spherical bulge and a surrounding disk composed of spiral arms. Barred spirals have a central bar of stars across the nucleus, with spiral arms trailing from the ends of the bar. Elliptical galaxies have a uniform appearance, ranging from a flattened disk to a near sphere. Most galaxies, however, have no obvious structure at all. Galaxies also vary enormously in size, from dwarf galaxies only 2,000 light-years across to great assemblies of stars 80 or more times larger.

▲ M51, the Whirlpool Nebula, comprises the large spiral galaxy NGC5194 and its smaller, barred companion NGC5195. M51 was the first astronomical object in which a spiral structure was identified, in 1845. Although smaller and less massive than our own Galaxy, M51 is much brighter, due to recent star formation.

THE HOME GALAXY

The Sun and its planets are located in one of the spiral arms of the Galaxy, a little less than 28,000 light-years from the galactic center and orbiting around it in a period of 200 million years. The center is invisible from the Earth, masked by vast, light-absorbing clouds of interstellar dust.

The Galaxy is probably around 12 billion years old and, like other spiral galaxies, has three distinct regions. The central bulge is about 30,000 light-years in diameter. The disk in which the Sun is located is not much more than 1,000 light-years thick, but approximately 100,000 light-years from end to end. Around the Galaxy is the halo, a spherical zone 300,000 light-years across, studded with globular star clusters and sprinkled with individual suns.

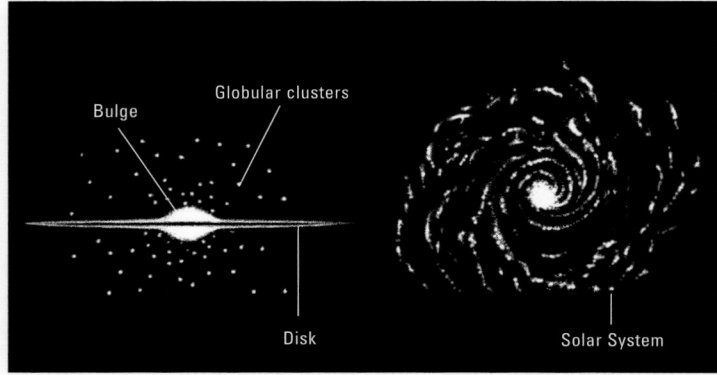

THE END OF THE UNIVERSE

The likely fate of the Universe is disputed. One theory (*top of diagram, below*) dictates that the expansion begun at the time of the Big Bang will continue "indefinitely," with aging galaxies moving further and further apart in an immense, dark graveyard.

Alternatively, gravity may overcome the expansion (*bottom of diagram*). Galaxies will fall back together until everything is again concentrated at a single point, followed by a new Big Bang and a new expansion, in an endlessly repeated cycle.

The first theory is supported by the amount of visible matter in the Universe; the second theory assumes that there is enough dark material in the Universe to bring about the gravitational collapse.

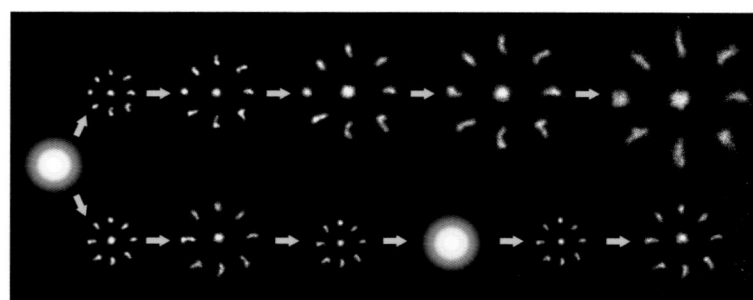

THE NEAREST STARS

The 22 nearest stars, excluding the Sun, with their distance from Earth in light-years*

Proxima Centauri	4.25	UV Ceti A	8.7	Epsilon Indi	11.2
Alpha Centauri A	4.3	UV Ceti B	8.7	Groombridge 34A	11.2
Alpha Centauri B	4.3	Ross 154	9.4	Groombridge 34B	11.2
Barnard's Star	6.0	Ross 248	10.3	L789-6	11.2
Wolf 359	7.8	Epsilon Eridani	10.7	Procyon A	11.4
Lalande 21185	8.3	Ross 128	10.9	Procyon B	11.4
Sirius A	8.7	61 Cygni A	11.1		
Sirius B	8.7	61 Cygni B	11.1		

Many of the nearest stars, like Alpha Centauri A and B, are double stars, orbiting about their common center of gravity and to all intents and purposes equidistant from Earth. Many of them are dim objects, with no name other than the designation given to them by the astronomers who first investigated them. However, they include Sirius, the brightest star in the sky, and Procyon, the seventh brightest. Both are far larger than the Sun; of the nearest stars, only Epsilon Eridani is similar in size and luminosity.

* A light-year equals approximately 5,900 billion miles

STAR CHARTS

NORTHERN HEAVENS

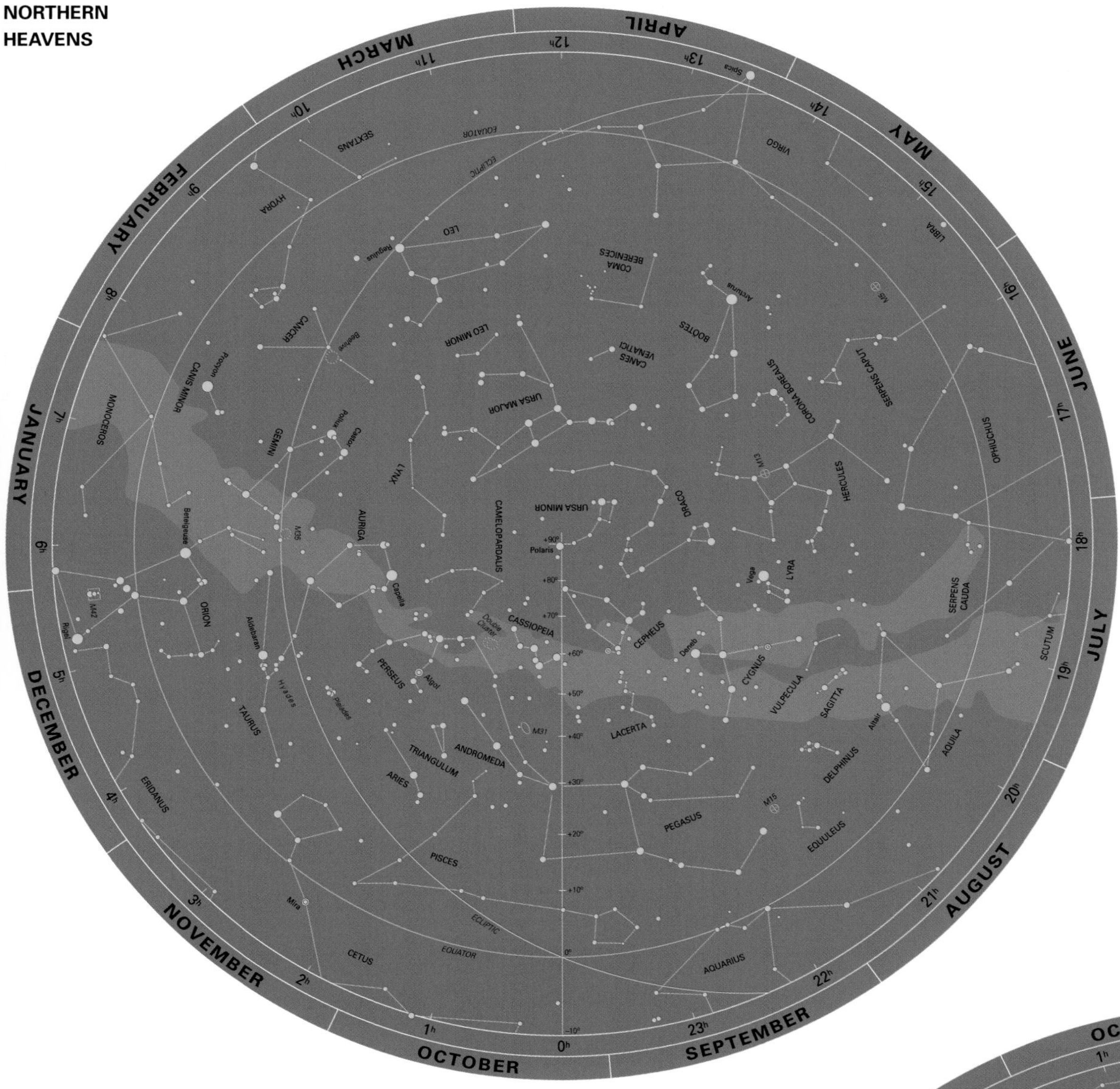

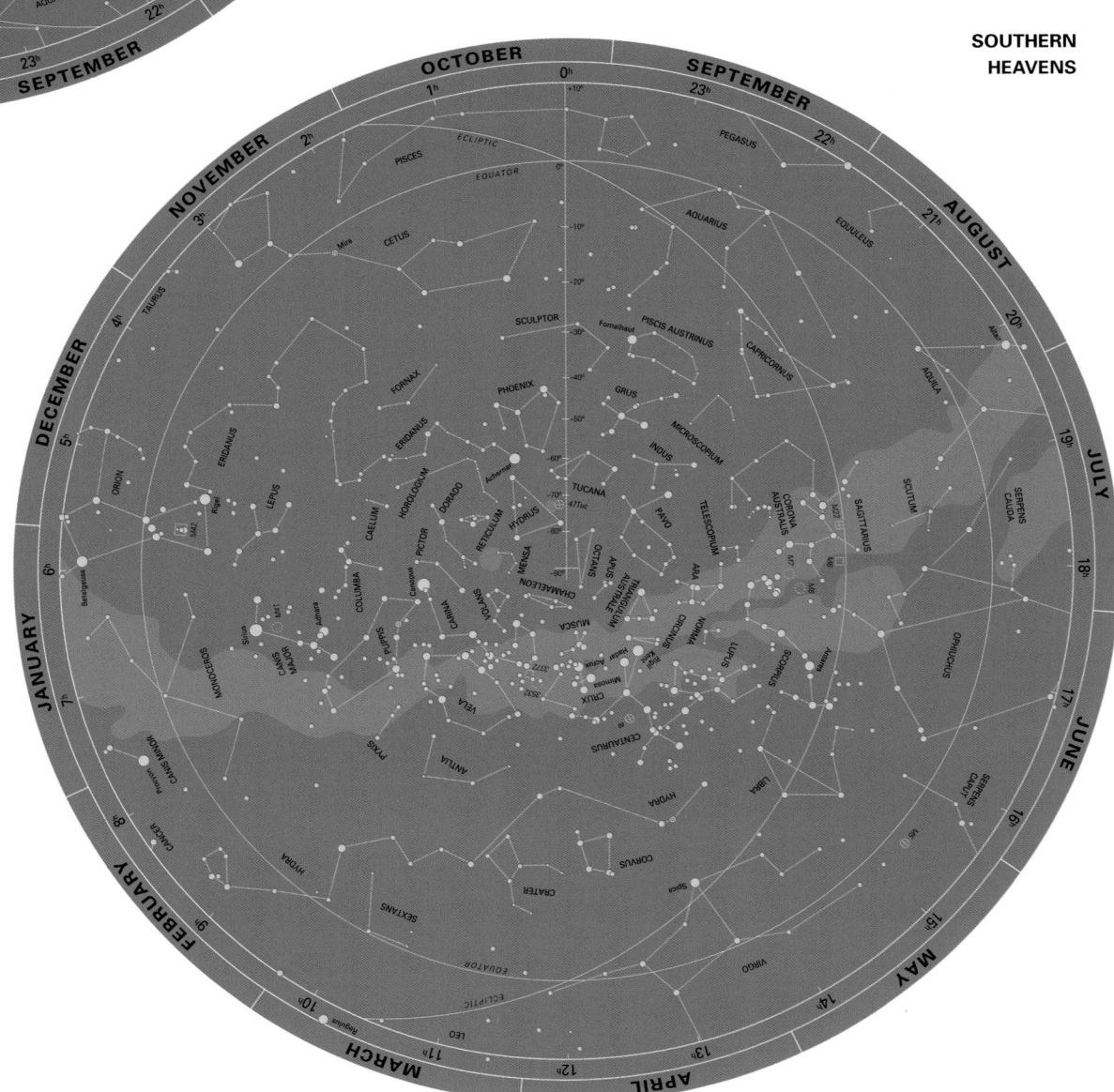

THE CONSTELLATIONS
The constellations and their English names

Andromeda	Andromeda	Lacerta	Lizard
Antlia	Air Pump	Leo	Lion
Apus	Bird of Paradise	Leo Minor	Little Lion
Aquarius	Water Carrier	Lepus	Hare
Aquila	Eagle	Libra	Scales
Ara	Altar	Lupus	Wolf
Aries	Ram	Lynx	Lynx
Auriga	Charioteer	Lyra	Lyre
Boötes	Herdsman	Mensa	Table
Caelum	Chisel	Microscopium	Microscope
Camelopardalis	Giraffe	Monoceros	Unicorn
Cancer	Crab	Musca	Fly
Canes Venatici	Hunting Dogs	Norma	Level
Canis Major	Great Dog	Octans	Octant
Canis Minor	Little Dog	Ophiuchus	Serpent Bearer
Capricornus	Goat	Orion	Orion
Carina	Keel	Pavo	Peacock
Cassiopeia	Cassiopeia	Pegasus	Winged Horse
Centaurus	Centaur	Perseus	Perseus
Cepheus	Cepheus	Phoenix	Phoenix
Cetus	Whale	Pictor	Easel
Chamaeleon	Chameleon	Pisces	Fishes
Circinus	Compasses	Piscis Austrinus	Southern Fish
Columba	Dove	Puppis	Ship's Stern
Coma Berenices	Berenice's Hair	Pyxis	Mariner's Compass
Corona Australis	Southern Crown	Reticulum	Net
Corona Borealis	Northern Crown	Sagitta	Arrow
Corvus	Crow	Sagittarius	Archer
Crater	Cup	Scorpius	Scorpion
Crux	Southern Cross	Sculptor	Sculptor
Cygnus	Swan	Scutum	Shield
Delphinus	Dolphin	Serpens	Serpent
Dorado	Swordfish	Sextans	Sextant
Draco	Dragon	Taurus	Bull
Equuleus	Little Horse	Telescopium	Telescope
Eridanus	Eridanus	Triangulum	Triangle
Fornax	Furnace	Triangulum Australe	Southern Triangle
Gemini	Twins	Tucana	Toucan
Grus	Crane	Ursa Major	Great Bear
Hercules	Hercules	Ursa Minor	Little Bear
Horologium	Clock	Vela	Sails
Hydra	Water Snake	Virgo	Virgin
Hydrus	Sea Serpent	Volans	Flying Fish
Indus	Indian	Vulpecula	Fox

SOUTHERN HEAVENS

Star charts are drawn as projections of a vast, hollow sphere with the observer in the middle. Each circle on this page represents slightly more than one hemisphere, centered on the north and south celestial poles respectively – projections of the Earth's poles in the heavens. At the present era, the north pole is marked by the star Polaris; the south pole has no such convenient reference point.

Astronomical coordinates are normally given in terms of "Right Ascension" for longitude and "Declination" for latitude or altitude. Since the stars appear to rotate around the Earth once every 24 hours, Right Ascension is measured eastward – counterclockwise – in hours and minutes and is marked around the edge of the map. One hour is equivalent to 15 angular degrees; zero on the scale is the point at which the Sun crosses the celestial equator at the spring equinox, known to astronomers as the "First Point of Aries." Unlike the Sun, stars always rise and set at the same point on the horizon. Declination measures (in degrees) a star's angular distance above or below the celestial equator and is marked on the vertical line.

Using the maps
First choose the one for your hemisphere and hold it with the month at the bottom. The stars in the lower part of the map are then due south (or north, in the southern hemisphere) at about 1 AM local time, not allowing for summer or daylight saving time. Their exact position above the horizon depends on your latitude. The closer to the Equator you live, the higher in the sky these stars will appear. Some additional stars from the map for the other hemisphere will be visible in the lower sky.

Stars near the top of the map will be below the opposite horizon at this date and time, but will be visible at other times of the night and year. The sky appears to move counterclockwise around the celestial pole during the course of the day (clockwise in the southern hemisphere), so the same stars will be visible at 11 PM a month earlier.

STAR MAGNITUDES
Apparent visual magnitudes

The magnitude scale of star brightnesses is developed from the system used by the Ancient Greeks in which the brightest stars were first magnitude and the faintest visible to the naked eye were sixth. Today the scale has a mathematical basis and extends, at the brightest end, through to negative magnitudes.

The Milky Way is shown in light blue on these charts.

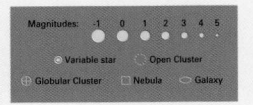

Magnitudes: -1 0 1 2 3 4 5

○ Variable star ○ Open Cluster
⊕ Globular Cluster ▭ Nebula ○ Galaxy

3

THE SOLAR SYSTEM

For more information:
2 The Home Galaxy
6 The seasons
  Day and night
7 The Moon

Lying 28,000 light-years from the center of one of billions of galaxies that comprise the observable Universe, our Solar System contains nine planets and their moons, innumerable asteroids and comets, and a miscellany of dust and gas, all tethered by the immense gravitational field of the Sun, the middling-sized star whose thermonuclear furnaces provide them all with heat and light.

The Solar System was formed about 4,600 million years ago, when a spinning cloud of gas, mostly hydrogen but seeded with other heavier elements, condensed enough to ignite a nuclear reaction and create a star. The Sun still accounts for almost 99.9% of the system's total mass.

By composition as well as distance, the planetary array divides quite neatly in two: an inner system of four small, solid planets, including the Earth, and an outer system, from Jupiter to Neptune, of four much larger planets composed of lighter materials, such as gas, liquid, and ice. Between the two groups lies a scattering of rocky asteroids, numbering perhaps as many as 45,000. These may be debris left over from the formation of the inner Solar System. The outermost planet, Pluto, may simply be the largest of a number of bodies composed of rock and ice orbiting beyond Neptune, similarly left over from the formation of the outer Solar System.

Much of the early history of science is the story of people trying to make sense of the errant points of light that were all they knew of the planets. Now, men have themselves stood on the Earth's Moon, space probes have landed on Mars and Venus, and orbiting radars have mapped far distant landscapes with astonishing accuracy, transforming our knowledge of our celestial environment.

In the 1980s, the Voyager space probes skimmed all four major planets of the outer Solar System, bringing new revelations with each close approach. And in July 2004, the Cassini-Huygens spacecraft will begin a detailed four-year tour of Saturn, its moons (in particular Titan), and its rings. Only Pluto, inscrutably distant in an orbit that takes it 50 times the Earth's distance from the Sun, remains unvisited by our messengers.

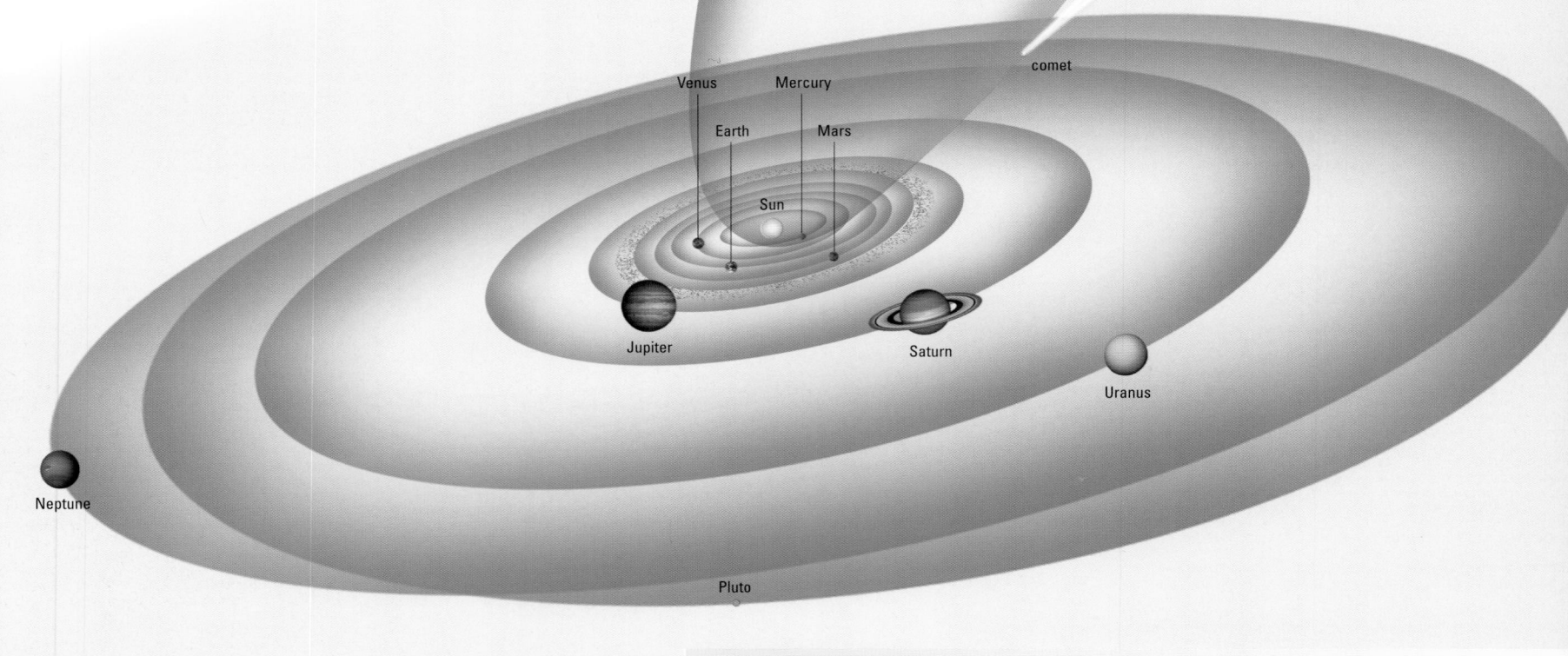

ORBITS OF THE PLANETS

The diagram above (*not drawn to scale*) shows the Solar System from the viewpoint of an observer a few light-hours distant in the direction of the constellation Hercules. Seen from such a position, above the plane of the ecliptic, all the planets revolve about the Sun in a counterclockwise direction. The perspective view exaggerates the elliptical form of all the planetary orbits: only Pluto and Mercury follow paths that deviate noticeably from circularity.

Near perihelion – its closest approach to the Sun – Pluto actually passes inside the orbit of Neptune, an event that last occurred in 1983. Pluto did not regain its station as the Sun's outermost planet until February 1999. In fact, Pluto comes closer to the Sun than Neptune for only a relatively brief 15-year period in the course of its 247.7-year orbit. The tilt of their respective orbits means that Neptune and Pluto will never collide with each other.

PLANETARY DATA

	Mean distance from Sun (million miles)	Mass (Earth = 1)	Period of orbit (Earth days/years)	Period of rotation (Earth days)	Equatorial diameter (miles)	Average density (water = 1)	Surface gravity (Earth = 1)	Escape velocity (miles/sec)	Number of known satellites
Sun	–	332,946	–	25.4	865,000	1.41	27.9	383.7	–
Mercury	36.0	0.055	87.97d	58.67	3,031	5.44	0.38	2.64	0
Venus	67.2	0.815	224.7d	243.00	7,521	5.25	0.90	6.44	0
Earth	93.0	1.0	365.3d	1.00	7,926	5.52	1.00	6.95	1
Mars	141.6	0.11	687.0d	1.028	4,222	3.94	0.38	3.13	2
Jupiter	483.4	317.9	11.86y	0.411	89,405	1.33	2.64	37.03	63
Saturn	886.7	95.2	29.46y	0.427	74,898	0.71	1.16	22.12	31
Uranus	1,783.3	14.6	84.01y	0.748	31,763	1.27	0.79	13.11	27
Neptune	2,794.3	17.2	164.8y	0.710	31,403	1.77	0.98	15.29	13
Pluto	3,666.1	0.002	247.7y	6.39	1,444	2.02	0.06	0.75	1

Planetary days are given in sidereal time – that is, with respect to the stars rather than the Sun. Most of the information in the table was confirmed by spacecraft and often obtained from photographs and other data transmitted back to the Earth.

In the case of Pluto, however, only Earthbound observations have been made, and no spacecraft will encounter it until well into the 21st century. Given the planet's small size and great distance, figures for its diameter and rotation period have only recently been confirmed.

Pluto is not massive enough to account for the perturbations in the orbits of Uranus and Neptune that led to its discovery in 1930, but it is now widely believed that these perturbations can be explained away as observational errors made by the earlier observers.

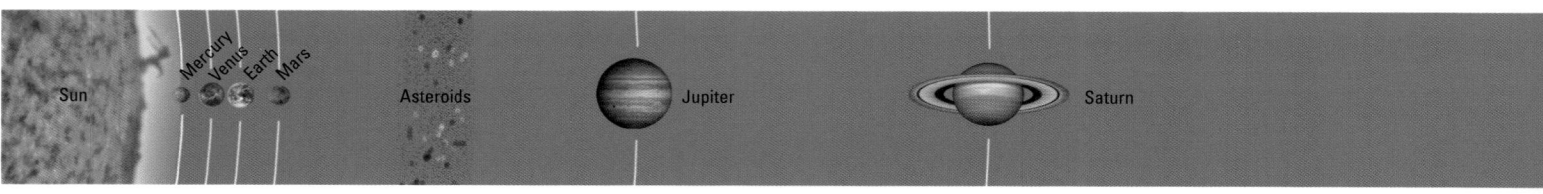

THE PLANETS

Mercury is the closest planet to the Sun and hence the fastest-moving. It is very hot, with a cratered, wrinkled surface very similar to that of Earth's Moon. It is small and has no gravity, hence there is no significant atmosphere.

Venus has much the same physical dimensions as Earth. Its dense atmosphere is composed of 97% carbon dioxide resulting in a runaway greenhouse effect that makes the Venusian surface, at 890°F, the hottest of all the planets in the Solar System. Radar mapping shows the land to be relatively level, with volcanic regions whose sulfurous discharges explain the sulfuric-acid rains reported by soft-landing space probes before they succumbed to Venus' fierce climate.

Earth seen from space is easily the most beautiful of the inner planets; it is also, and more objectively, the largest, as well as the only home of known life. Living things are the main reason why the Earth is able to retain a substantial proportion of corrosive and highly reactive oxygen in its atmosphere, a state of affairs that contradicts the laws of chemical equilibrium; the oxygen in turn supports the life that constantly regenerates it.

Mars, smaller and cooler than the Earth, is nevertheless the most likely planet other than Earth where life may have formed, though whether life could thrive in its current cold, dry and thin atmosphere is doubtful. The ice caps are mainly frozen carbon dioxide, though data from NASA's probe Mars Odyssey, launched in 2001, suggests that vast reservoirs of water ice may lie a few centimeters beneath the surface over much of the planet. But the surface itself is a dustbowl, where occasional storms whirl dust high into the atmosphere.

Jupiter masses almost three times as much as all the other planets combined; had it scooped up rather more matter during its formation, it might have evolved into a small companion star for the Sun. The planet is mostly gas, under intense pressure in the lower atmosphere above a core of fiercely compressed hydrogen and helium. The upper layers form strikingly-colored rotating belts, the outward sign of the intense storms created by Jupiter's rapid diurnal rotation. Close approaches by spacecraft have shown an orbiting ring system and discovered several previously unknown moons: Jupiter has at least 63 moons, though many are extremely small.

Saturn is structurally similar to Jupiter, rotating fast enough to produce an obvious bulge at its equator. It is composed of 89% hydrogen and 11% helium, and has wind velocities in the outer atmosphere of 1,600 feet per second. Ever since the invention of the telescope, however, Saturn's rings have been the feature that has attracted most observers. Voyager probes in 1980 and 1981 sent back detailed pictures that showed them to be composed of thousands of separate ringlets, each in turn made up of tiny icy particles.

Uranus was unknown to the ancients. Although it is faintly visible to the naked eye, it was not discovered until 1781. Its interior is largely water, with an atmosphere of hydrogen, helium and some methane, which gives the planet its blue-green color. Observations in 1977 suggested the presence of a faint ring system, amply confirmed when Voyager 2 swung past the planet in 1986.

Neptune is always more than 2.5 billion miles from Earth, and despite its diameter of over 31,000 miles, it can only be seen by telescope. Its discovery in 1846 was the result of mathematical predictions by astronomers seeking to explain irregularities in the orbit of Uranus, but until Voyager 2 closed with the planet in 1989, very little was known of it. Like Uranus, it has a ring system; recent observations have revealed a total of 13 moons.

Pluto is the most mysterious of the solar planets, if only because even the most powerful telescopes can scarcely resolve it from a point of light to a disk. It was discovered as recently as 1930, as the result of perturbations in the orbits of the two then outermost planets. Its small size, as well as its eccentric and highly tilted orbit, has led to suggestions that it is a former satellite of Neptune, somehow liberated from its primary. In 1978 Pluto was found to have a moon of its own, Charon, apparently half the size of Pluto itself.

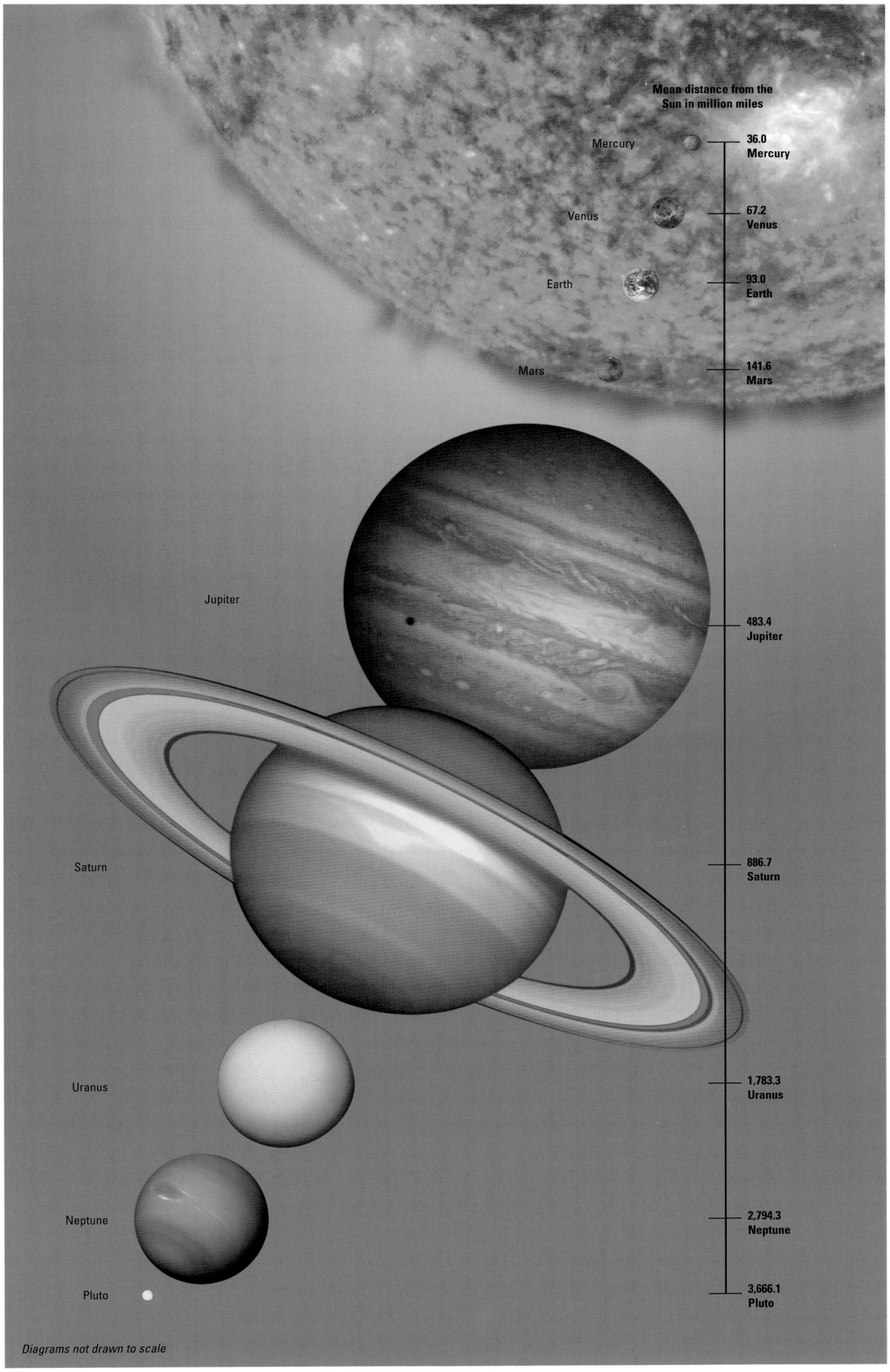

Mean distance from the Sun in million miles

Mercury — 36.0 Mercury

Venus — 67.2 Venus

Earth — 93.0 Earth

Mars — 141.6 Mars

Jupiter — 483.4 Jupiter

Saturn — 886.7 Saturn

Uranus — 1,783.3 Uranus

Neptune — 2,794.3 Neptune

Pluto — 3,666.1 Pluto

Diagrams not drawn to scale

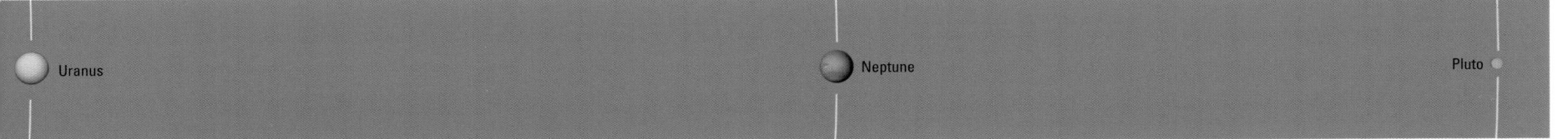

Uranus   Neptune   Pluto

TIME AND MOTION

For more information:

4 Orbits of the planets

9 Ocean currents

14 Circulation of the air

16 Climate

The basic unit of time measurement is the day, that is, one rotation of the Earth on its axis. Our present calendar is based on the solar year of 365.24 days, the time taken by the Earth to orbit the Sun.

Calendars based on the movements of the Sun and Moon have been used since ancient times. The average length of the year, according to the Julian Calendar introduced by Julius Caesar, was about 11 minutes too long. The cumulative error was rectified in 1582 by the Gregorian

Calendar, when Pope Gregory XIII decreed that the day following October 4 was October 15, and in that century years did not count as leap years unless they were divisible by 400. England finally adopted the reformed calendar in 1752, when it was 11 days behind the European mainland.

The rotation of the Earth on its axis causes day and night. Because the Earth rotates through 360° every 24 hours, the world is divided into 24 time zones centered on lines of longitude at 15° longitude.

The tilt of the Earth's axis, which is also called the "obliquity of the ecliptic," accounts for the seasons which are so familiar in the middle latitudes. However, geological evidence shows that, over long periods of time, climates change, and the advances and retreats of the ice during the Pleistocene Ice Age may have been caused by regular variations in the Earth's tilt, its orbit around the Sun, and changes in the season when it is closest to the Sun (perihelion).

THE SEASONS

Seasons occur because the Earth's axis is tilted at an angle of approximately 23½°. When the northern hemisphere is tilted to a maximum extent toward the Sun, on June 21, the Sun is overhead at the Tropic of Cancer (latitude 23½° North). This is midsummer, or the summer solstice, in the northern hemisphere.

On September 22 or 23, the Sun is overhead at the Equator, and day and night are of equal length throughout the world. This is the fall, or autumnal, equinox in the northern hemisphere.

On December 21 or 22, the Sun is overhead at the Tropic of Capricorn (23½° South), the winter solstice in the northern hemisphere. The overhead Sun then tracks north until, on March 21, it is overhead at the Equator. This is the spring, or vernal, equinox in the northern hemisphere.

In the southern hemisphere, the seasons are the reverse of those in the north.

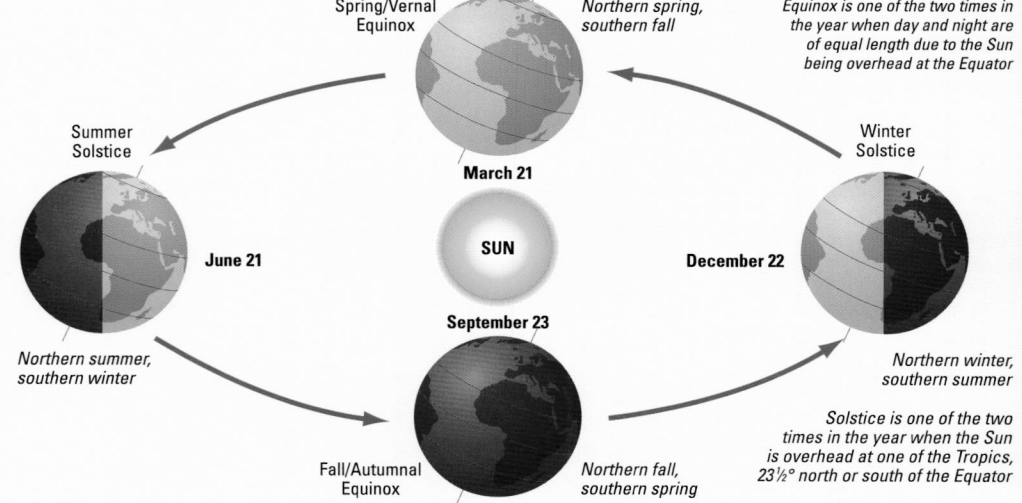

DAY AND NIGHT

The Sun appears to rise in the east, reach its highest point at noon, and then set in the west, to be followed by night. In reality, it is not the Sun that is moving but the Earth rotating from west to east. The moment when the Sun's upper limb first appears above the horizon is termed sunrise; the moment when the Sun's upper limb disappears below the horizon is sunset.

At the summer solstice in the northern hemisphere (June 21), the Arctic has total daylight and the Antarctic total darkness. The opposite occurs at the winter solstice (December 21 or 22). At the Equator, the length of day and night are almost equal all year.

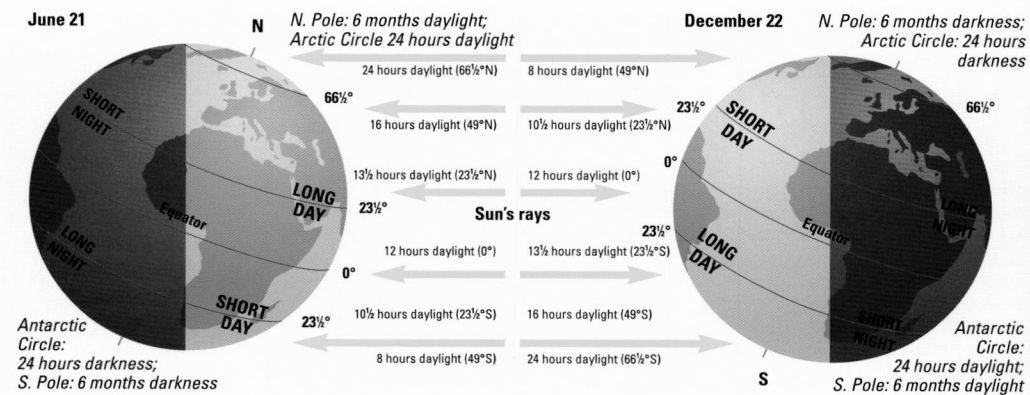

EARTH DATA

Aphelion (maximum distance from Sun):	94,452,780 miles	**Length of year:**	365 days, 5 hours, 48 minutes, 46 seconds of mean solar time	**Polar circumference:**	24,860 miles
Perihelion (minimum distance from Sun):	91,342,080 miles			**Equatorial diameter:**	7,926 miles
		Superficial area:	197,000,000 sq miles	**Polar diameter:**	7,900 miles
Angle of tilt (obliquity of the ecliptic):	23° 27′ 08″	**Land surface:**	57,500,000 sq miles (29.2%)	**Equatorial radius:**	3,964 miles
				Polar radius:	3,950 miles
Length of year – solar tropical (equinox to equinox):	365.24 days	**Water surface:**	139,500,000 sq miles (70.8%)	**Volume of the Earth:**	$260,000 \times 10^6$ cu miles
		Equatorial circumference:	23,903 miles	**Mass of the Earth:**	6.5×10^{21} tons

SUNRISE AND SUNSET

The term "equinox" comes from the Latin for "equal night." At the spring and fall equinoxes, the Sun is vertically overhead at midday at the Equator and all places on Earth have 12 hours of darkness and 12 hours of daylight. The graphs showing sunrise and sunset show that these occasions occur on March 21 and on September 22 or 23. The graphs also show that, because the Sun remains high in the sky at the Equator throughout the year, the length of day and night there remains roughly the same throughout the year, with sunrise around 6 AM and sunset around 6 PM.

The further north or south one travels, the greater the difference between the number of hours of daylight and darkness. For example, the graph (right) shows that at latitude 60°N sunrise varies from just after 9 AM in midwinter (on December 22 or 23) to about 2.30 AM in midsummer (around the summer solstice on June 21). By contrast, the second graph (far right) shows that sunset at latitude 60°N occurs at about 2.45 PM in midwinter and 9.20 PM in midsummer.

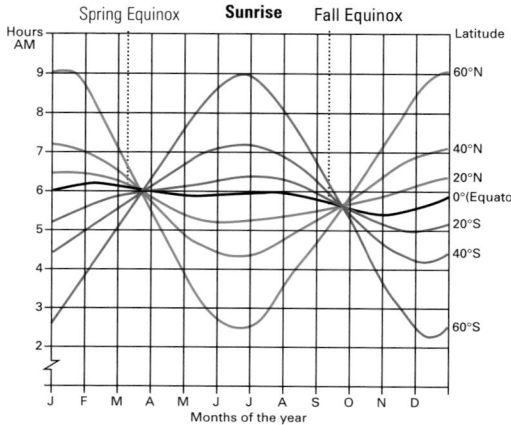

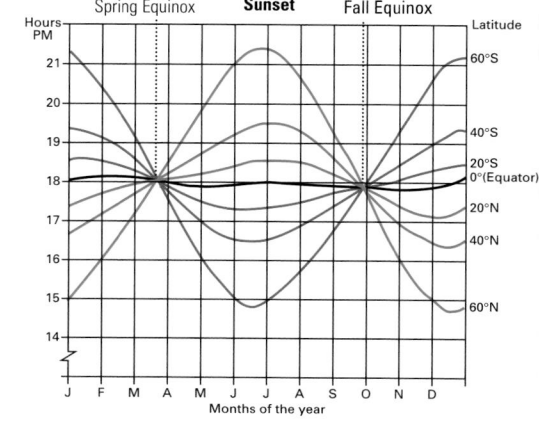

THE MOON

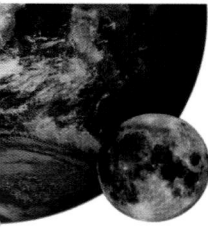

The Moon rotates more slowly than the Earth, making one complete turn on its axis in just over 27 days. Since this corresponds to its period of revolution around the Earth, the Moon always presents the same hemisphere or face to us, and we never see "the dark side." The interval between one full Moon and the next (and between new Moons) is about 29½ days – a lunar month. The apparent changes in the shape of the Moon are caused by its changing position in relation to the Earth; like the planets, it produces no light of its own and shines only by reflecting the rays of the Sun.

PHASES OF THE MOON

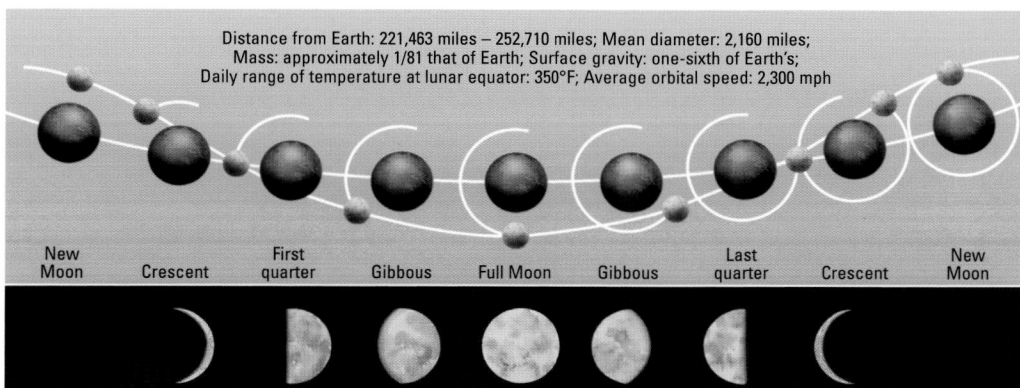

Distance from Earth: 221,463 miles – 252,710 miles; Mean diameter: 2,160 miles; Mass: approximately 1/81 that of Earth; Surface gravity: one-sixth of Earth's; Daily range of temperature at lunar equator: 350°F; Average orbital speed: 2,300 mph

New Moon | Crescent | First quarter | Gibbous | Full Moon | Gibbous | Last quarter | Crescent | New Moon

MOON DATA

Distance from Earth
The Moon orbits at a mean distance of 238,731 miles, at an average speed of 2,300 mph in relation to the Earth.

Size and mass
The average diameter of the Moon is 2,160 miles. It is 400 times smaller than the Sun but is about 400 times closer to the Earth, so we see them as the same size. The Moon has a mass of $7,975 \times 10^{19}$ tons, with a density 3.344 times that of water.

Visibility
Only 59% of the Moon's surface is directly visible from Earth. Reflected light takes 1.25 seconds to reach Earth – compared to 8 minutes 27.3 seconds for light to reach us from the Sun.

Temperature
With the Sun overhead, the temperature on the lunar equator can reach 243°F. At night it can sink to −261°F.

ECLIPSES

When the Moon passes between the Sun and the Earth it causes a partial eclipse of the Sun (1) if the Earth passes through the Moon's outer shadow (P), or a total eclipse (2) if the inner cone shadow crosses the Earth's surface. In a lunar eclipse, the Earth's shadow crosses the Moon and, again, provides either a partial or total eclipse.

Eclipses of the Sun and the Moon do not occur every month because of the 5° difference between the plane of the Moon's orbit and the plane in which the Earth moves. In the 1990s, only 14 lunar eclipses were possible – for example, seven partial and seven total. Each was visible only from certain, and variable, parts of the world. The same period witnessed 13 solar eclipses – six partial (or annular) and seven total.

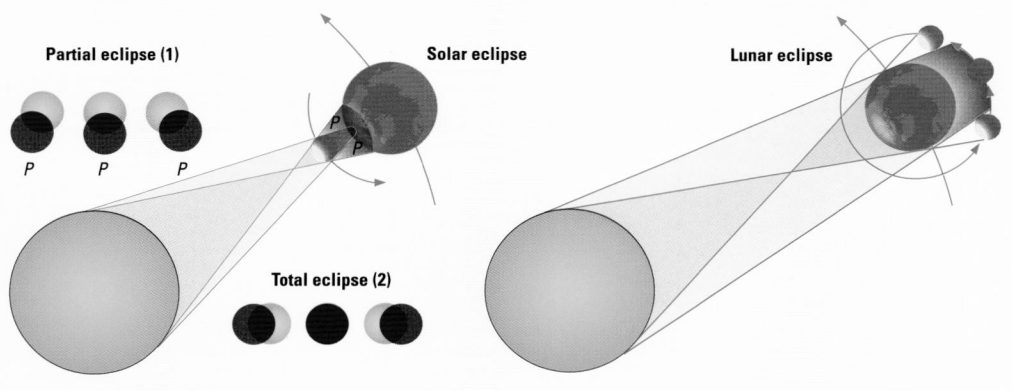

Partial eclipse (1) | Solar eclipse | Lunar eclipse
Total eclipse (2)

TIDES

The daily rise and fall of the ocean's tides are the result of the gravitational pull of the Moon and that of the Sun, though the effect of the latter is not as strong as that of the Moon. This effect is greatest on the hemisphere facing the Moon and causes a tidal "bulge." When the Sun, Earth, and Moon are in line, Spring tides occur: high tide reaches the highest values, and low tide falls to low levels. When lunar and solar forces are least coincidental with the Sun and Moon at an angle (near the Moon's first and third quarters), Neap tides occur, which have a small tidal range.

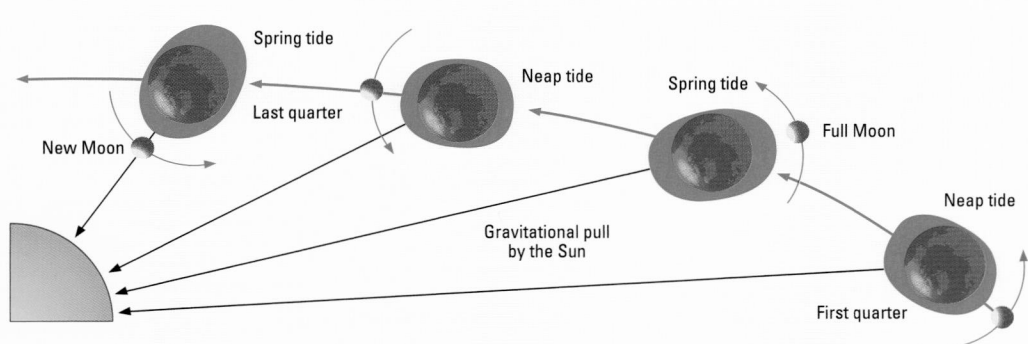

Spring tide | Neap tide | Spring tide | Full Moon | Last quarter | New Moon | Neap tide | Gravitational pull by the Sun | First quarter

TIME ZONES

The Earth rotates through 360° in 24 hours, and so moves 15° every hour. The world is divided into 24 standard time zones, each centered on lines of longitude at 15° intervals. At the center of the first zone is the Prime meridian or Greenwich meridian. All places to the west of Greenwich are one hour behind for every 15° of longitude; places to the east are ahead by one hour for every 15°.

International Date Line
When it is 12 noon at the Greenwich meridian, 180° east it is midnight of the same day – while 180° west the day is just beginning. To overcome this, the International Date Line was established, approximately following the 180° meridian. Thus, if you were to travel eastward from Japan (140°E) to Samoa (170°W), you would pass from Sunday night into Sunday morning.

10   Hours slow or fast of UT or Coordinated Universal Time

Zones using UT (GMT)

Zones slow of UT (GMT)

International boundaries

Zones fast of UT (GMT)

Half-hour zones

Time zone boundaries

International Date Line

Actual Solar Time when time at Greenwich is 12:00 (noon)

Note: Certain of the above time zones are affected by the incidence of "Summer Time" in countries where it is adopted.

Projection: Mercator

OCEANS

For more information:
7 Tides
10 Plate tectonics
14 Atmosphere
18 Hydrological cycle
   Water distribution
19 Watersheds
23 Water pollution
41 World shipping

The last 40 years have been described as the "Space Age," but another exciting and perhaps even more important area of discovery, proceeding at the same time, has been the exploration of the oceans which cover more than 70% of our planet. Studies of the ocean floor and oceanic islands have revealed features that help to explain how continents move, and how the movements are related to earthquakes and volcanic activity.

Manned submersibles have established that life exists even in the deepest trenches, where the pressure reaches 1,000 atmospheres, the equivalent of the force of six and a half tons bearing down on every square inch. Further exploration in the pitch-black environment of the ocean ridges has revealed strange forms of marine life around scalding hot vents. The creatures include giant tubeworms, blind shrimps, and bacteria, some of which are genetically very different from any other known life forms. In 1996, an analysis of one microorganism revealed that at least half of its 1,700 or so genes were hitherto unknown. This environment, which is based on chemicals, not sunlight, may resemble the places where life on Earth first began.

Another vital area of contemporary research concerns the interactions between the oceans and the atmosphere, as exemplified in the El Niño–Southern Oscillation (ENSO) cycle, and the bearing that these have on climatic change (see below).

Most geographers divide the world's ocean waters into four areas: the Pacific, Atlantic, Indian, and Arctic oceans. The most active zone in the oceans is the sunlit upper layer, where the water is moved around by wind-blown currents. It is the home of most sea life and acts as a membrane through which the ocean breathes,

LIFE IN THE OCEANS

An imaginary profile of the typical coastal and oceanic zones is shown, with a selection of the life forms that might occur in the waters off the Pacific Coast of Central America. The animals illustrated are not drawn to scale as the range of sizes is too great. Most marine life is confined to the first 650 feet, the upper sunlit (photic) zone, where sunlight can still penetrate. Plant and animal plankton, the basis of life in the oceans, occur in great quantities in all zones.

In the pelagic environment (open sea), vertical gradients, including those of light, temperature and salinity, determine the distribution of organisms. From the tidal zone at the coastline, the continental shelf, geologically still part of the continental land mass, drops gently to about 650 feet – the sunlit zone. At the end of the shelf, the seabed falls away in the steeper angle of the continental slope. The subsequent descent to the deep-ocean floor, known as the continental rise, is more gentle, with gradients between 1 in 100 and 1 in 700 until the abyssal plains and hills between 8,000 and 19,500 feet below the surface.

The deep-sea floor contains seamounts, some of which are capped by coral reefs, ocean ridges – the longest mountain chains on Earth – and deep-ocean trenches, especially in the Pacific Ocean where six trenches reach depths of more than 33,000 feet, including the Mariana Trench at 36,161 feet deep.

Each of these zones contains a distinctive community of species adapted to the different conditions of salinity, temperature, and light intensity. Indeed, a few organisms have been found even in the abyssal darkness of the great ocean trenches.

absorbing great quantities of carbon dioxide and partly exchanging it for oxygen.

As the depth increases, so light fades and temperatures fall until just before 3,000 feet where there is a marked temperature change at the thermocline, the boundary between the warm surface zone and the cold deep zone. Below the thermocline, slow currents are caused by density differences between bodies of water with varying temperatures and salinity.

ATOLL BUILDING

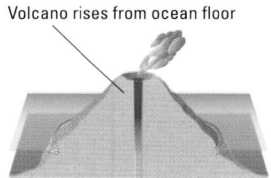

Volcano rises from ocean floor

Fringing reef

Extinct, eroding volcanic island

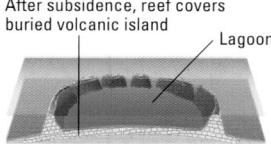

After subsidence, reef covers buried volcanic island

Lagoon

A coral atoll usually begins existence as a bare volcanic peak, thrusting above the surface of the ocean. A colony of coral – organisms with calcium carbonate skeletons – forms itself in the shallow water around the peak. The volcano is eroded and slowly sinks, leaving the coral forming a ring of hard limestone around its remnant. In time, the barrier reef of an atoll is all that remains.

EL NIÑO PHENOMENON

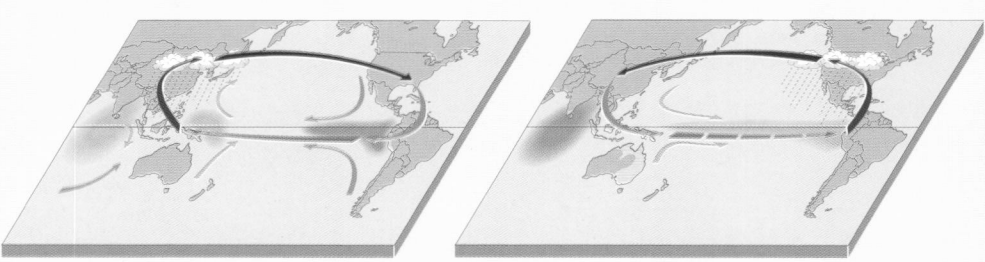

Normal year – Walker Circulation Cell

El Niño event

The importance of the ocean–atmosphere interaction is nowhere more dramatically demonstrated than in the El Niño phenomenon of the southern Pacific Ocean. Under normal conditions, called La Niña, cold, nutrient-rich water rises to the surface and spreads westward. In the western Pacific, sea surface temperatures reach 82°F or more and warm air rises, creating a low-pressure air system and causing heavy rains. The rising air spreads out and some of it descends over South America and the eastern Pacific, creating a high-pressure air system from which winds blow westward. This rotating system is called a Walker Circulation Cell.

An El Niño event is characterized by a reversal of currents. The upwelling of cold water off South America is greatly reduced and surface water temperatures rise, causing a drastic reduction in fish life. The heaviest rainfall is over the eastern Pacific, while Southeast Asia is drier than usual.

During an intense El Niño, the effects of the current and wind reversals affect the weather

around the world. In 1982–3, the monsoon rainfall was reduced in Australia and Southeast Asia, while in 1983–4 a severe drought occurred in the Sahel, south of the Sahara, and also in southern Africa. The southeast coast of the United States suffered storms and heavy rainfall, and even Europe experienced changes in weather patterns, possibly as a result of consequent changes in the course of the jet stream.

Scientists have found evidence that the frequency of the El Niño event, which normally occurs every three to seven years, and lasts between 12–18 months, may have increased in recent years. Another intense El Niño occurred in 1997–8, with resultant freak weather conditions across the entire Pacific region.

We do not fully understand the causes of the El Niño event, though some researchers are investigating possible connections between major volcanic eruptions in the tropical Pacific region, the ENSO cycle, and atmospheric circulation.

Crab
Seaweed — SEA LEVEL
Jellyfish
Green turtle
Anchovy
Dolphin
— SUNLIT ZONE 650 feet
Marlin
Snake eel
Bonito
Blue Whale
— TWILIGHT ZONE 3,000 feet
Phytoplankton and zooplankton
Lantern fish
Ray
Sperm whale
Deep-sea squid
— DARK ZONE 19,500 feet
Anglerfish
Halosaur
Sea cucumber
Sponge
— TRENCH ZONE 33,000 feet
Isopod

OCEAN CURRENTS

JANUARY CURRENTS AND TEMPERATURES
(Northern Hemisphere: winter)

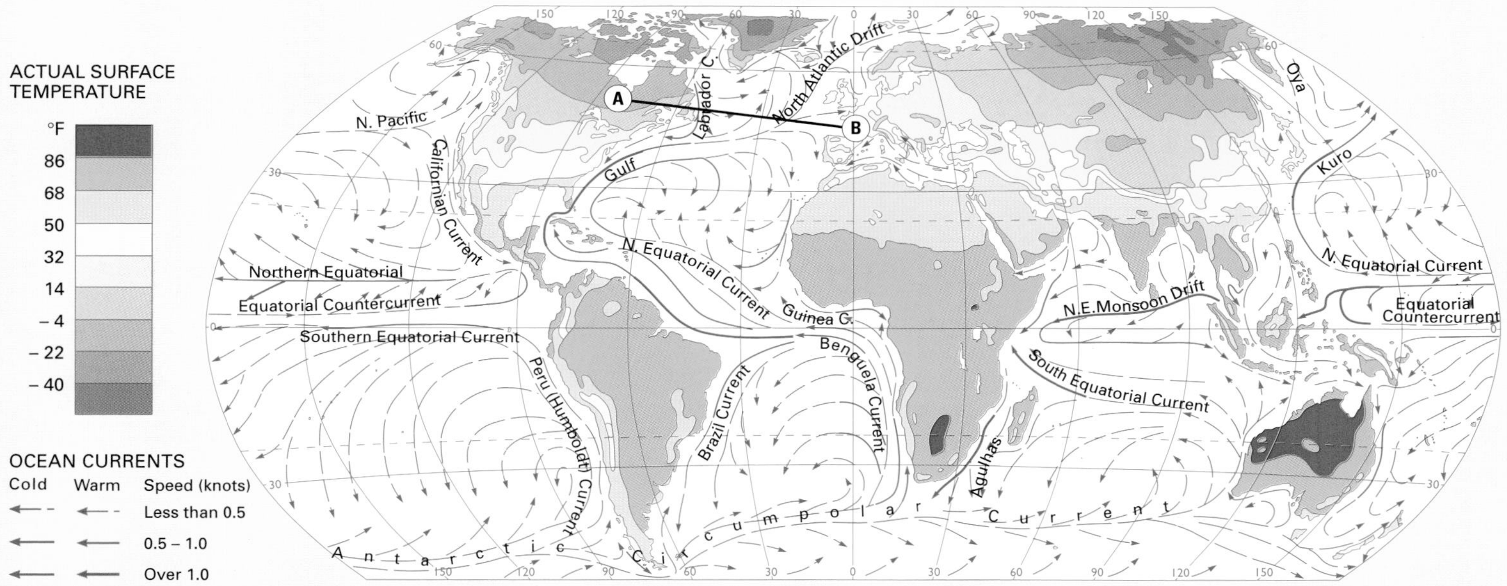

ACTUAL SURFACE
TEMPERATURE

°F
86
68
50
32
14
– 4
– 22
– 40

OCEAN CURRENTS
Cold   Warm   Speed (knots)
←-   ←-   Less than 0.5
←   ←   0.5 – 1.0
←   ←   Over 1.0

A ——————————— B   Location of the Atlantic Ocean profile shown bottom left

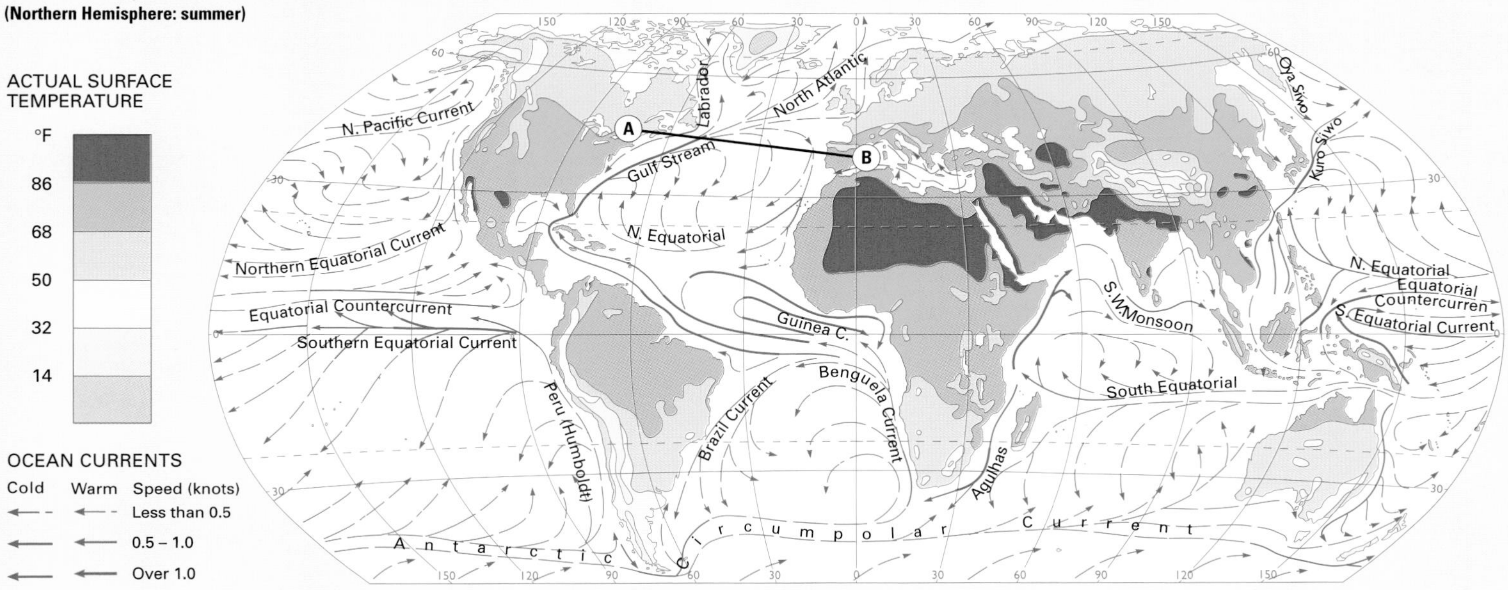

Moving immense quantities of energy as well as billions of tons of water every hour, the ocean currents are a vital part of the great heat engine that drives the Earth's climate. They themselves are produced by a twofold mechanism. At the surface, winds push huge masses of water before them; in the deep ocean, below an abrupt temperature gradient that separates the churning surface waters from the still depths, density variations cause slow vertical movements.

Coriolis effect
The pattern of circulation of the great surface currents is determined by the displacement known as the *Coriolis effect*. As the Earth turns, the vast mass of ocean water is deflected to one side. The deflection is most obvious near the Equator, where the Earth's surface is spinning eastward at 1,000 mph; currents moving poleward are curved clockwise in the northern hemisphere and counterclockwise in the southern hemisphere.

Ocean currents
The result is a system of spinning circles known as "gyres." Warm currents move constantly from the Equator toward the poles, while cold water moves in the reverse direction. In this way, ocean currents act like a thermostat, helping to regulate temperatures around the world.

Depending on the annual movements of the prevailing wind belts, some currents on or near the Equator may reverse their direction in the course of the year, a variation on which Asia's monsoon rains depend and whose occasional failure has brought disaster to millions of people.

JULY CURRENTS AND TEMPERATURES
(Northern Hemisphere: summer)

ACTUAL SURFACE
TEMPERATURE

°F
86
68
50
32
14

OCEAN CURRENTS
Cold   Warm   Speed (knots)
←-   ←-   Less than 0.5
←   ←   0.5 – 1.0
←   ←   Over 1.0

TOPOGRAPHY OF THE OCEAN FLOOR

Profile of the Atlantic Ocean

The deep-ocean floor was once believed to be flat, but sonar readings have shown that it is no more uniform than the surface of the continents. The profile (*below*) shows some of the features on the Atlantic Ocean floor between Massachusetts in North America and Gibraltar (*for location of profile, see maps above*).

Around the continents are shallow continental shelves composed of rocks that are less dense than the underlying oceanic crust. The continents end at the top of the steep continental slope, which descends to the abyss via the continental rise, made up of sediments washed down from the continental shelves.

The abyss contains large plains overlain by oozes but broken by volcanic seamounts and guyots (flat-topped seamounts), a few of which reach the surface as islands. The Mid-Atlantic Ridge contains a rift valley where new crustal rock is being formed as the plates on either side move apart.

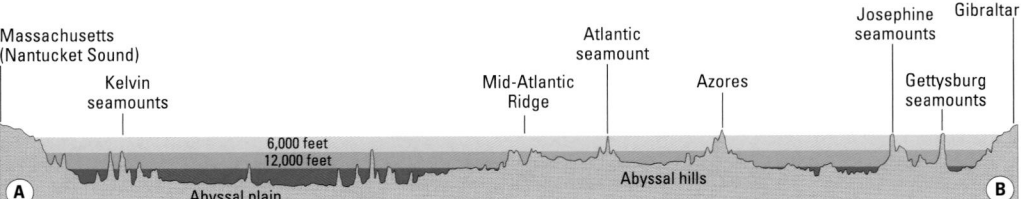

Massachusetts
(Nantucket Sound)
Kelvin seamounts
6,000 feet
12,000 feet
Abyssal plain
Mid-Atlantic Ridge
Atlantic seamount
Azores
Abyssal hills
Josephine seamounts
Gettysburg seamounts
Gibraltar
A   B

Topography of the ocean floor around Australia

In the image on the right, land areas are shown in gray, with shaded relief. The colors represent sea depths, with red representing the shallowest areas, through yellow and green to dark blue (the deepest).

The data for the sea topography are from the Seasat radar satellite. The deep blue area in the upper left is the Java Trench, which forms the boundary between the Indian-Australian plate and the Eurasian plate. In the top right, the New Guinea trench, which has a maximum depth of 29,865 feet, forms the border of the Indian-Australian and Pacific plates. Alongside the trenches are volcanic islands formed from magma, created as the edge of the Indian-Australian plate is subducted and melted.

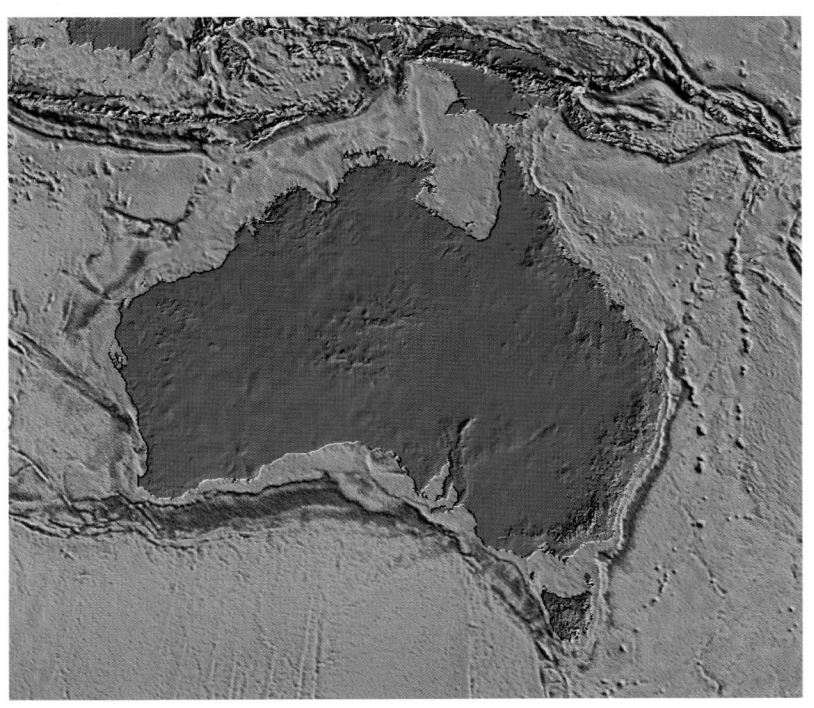

GEOLOGY OF THE EARTH

For more information:

12 Types of rock
   Mountain building
13 Surface processes
21 The carbon cycle
36 Minerals

Every year, earthquakes and volcanic eruptions cause much destruction throughout the world. Such phenomena were once thought to be unconnected, but since the late 1960s, scientists have understood that these events are surface manifestations of the tremendous forces operating in the Earth's interior that are slowly but constantly changing the face of our planet.

The Earth is divided into three zones. The crust, a brittle, low-density zone, overlies the dense mantle. Separating the crust from the mantle is a distinct boundary called the Mohorovičić (or Moho) discontinuity. Enclosed by the mantle is the Earth's core, which consists mainly of iron and nickel.

Temperatures inside the Earth range from about 1,600°F in the upper mantle to perhaps 9,000°F in the core. Heat creates convection currents in a semimolten part of the mantle called the asthenosphere. Above the asthenosphere is the lithosphere, a solid layer about 40 miles thick, consisting of the crust and part of the mantle. The lithosphere is divided into rigid plates, moved around by the currents in the asthenosphere, a process named plate tectonics.

The Earth was formed around 4.6 billion years ago. Lighter elements floated towards the surface, where they formed crustal rocks. The oldest rocks so far discovered are about 4 billion years old, while the oldest fossils occur in rocks formed around 3.5 billion years ago. An explosion of life occurred at the start of the Cambrian period, 570 million years ago. The fossil record since the start of the Cambrian has enabled scientists to piece together the story of life on Earth.

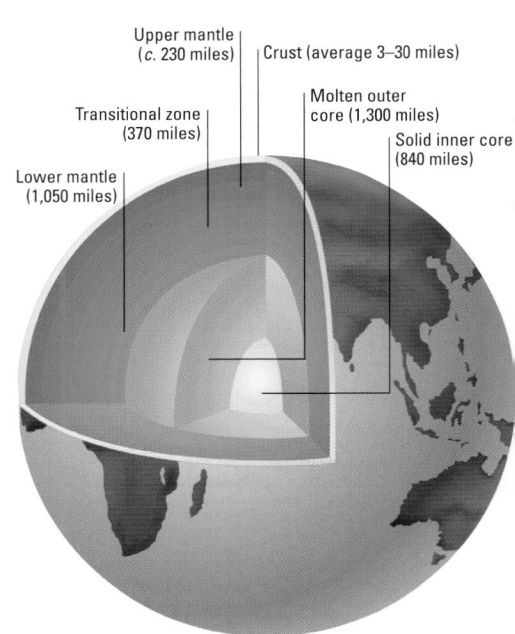

Upper mantle (c. 230 miles) — Crust (average 3–30 miles)
Transitional zone (370 miles) — Molten outer core (1,300 miles)
Lower mantle (1,050 miles) — Solid inner core (840 miles)

CONTINENTAL DRIFT

— Trench
— Rift
New ocean floor
— Zones of slippage

In 1915, Alfred Wegener produced a series of world maps proposing that, around 200 million years ago, the continents had been joined together in a supercontinent that he called Pangaea. This land mass started to break up about 180 million years ago and the parts drifted to their present positions. In the 1950s and 1960s, evidence from studies of the ocean floor suggested that the low-density continents rest on huge slow-moving plates. The arrows on the present-day world map (*below*) show that the continents are still on the move.

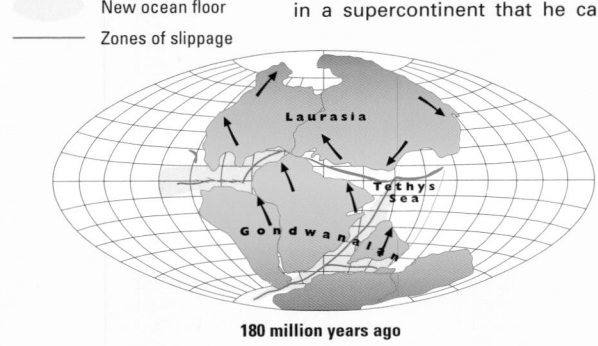

180 million years ago

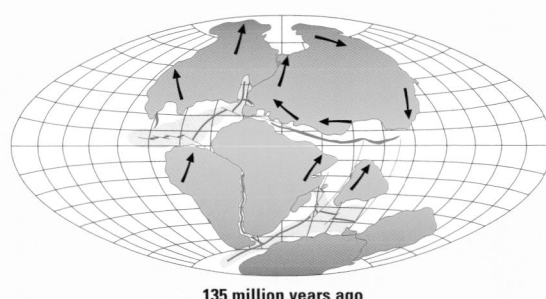

135 million years ago

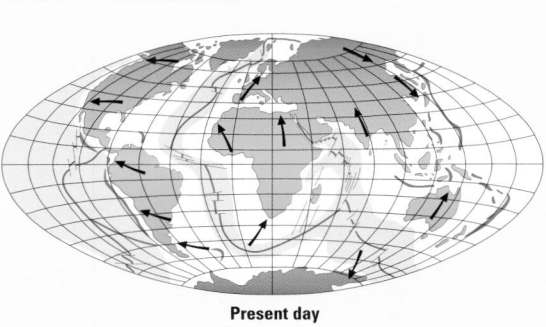

Present day

DISTRIBUTION OF VOLCANOES

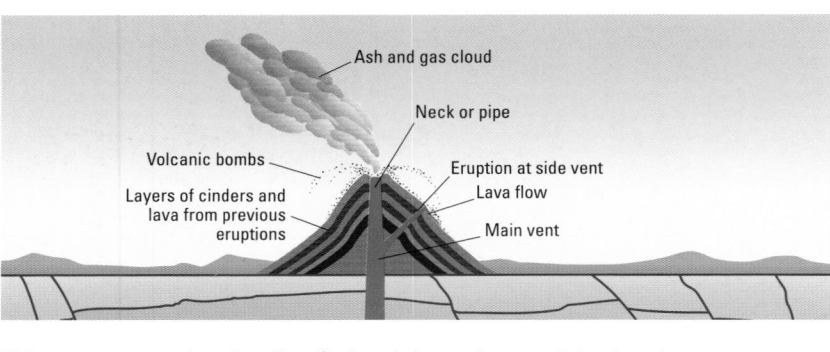

Ash and gas cloud
Neck or pipe
Volcanic bombs
Eruption at side vent
Lava flow
Layers of cinders and lava from previous eruptions
Main vent

Volcanoes occur when hot liquefied rock beneath the Earth's crust is pushed up by pressure to the surface as molten lava. There are some 550 known active volcanoes, around 20 of which are erupting at any one time.

• Submarine volcanoes
▲ Land volcanoes active since 1700
— Boundaries of tectonic plates

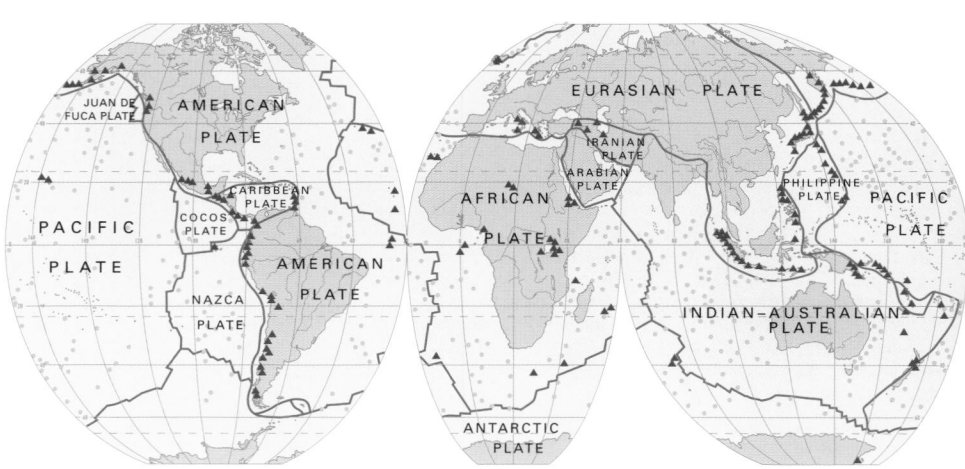

PLATE TECTONICS

The huge ridges that run through the oceans represent boundaries between plates. Here plates are diverging and molten magma from the mantle rises along a central rift valley to form new crustal rock. These ocean ridges, which are active zones where earthquakes and volcanic eruptions are common, are called constructive plate margins. Destructive plate margins, which occur when two plates converge, are marked by deep-ocean trenches as one plate is forced under the other. The descending plate is melted to produce the magma that fuels volcanoes alongside the trenches. Movements of descending plates are often sudden, triggering earthquakes in overlying continental areas.

Sea-floor spreading in the Atlantic Ocean and plate collision

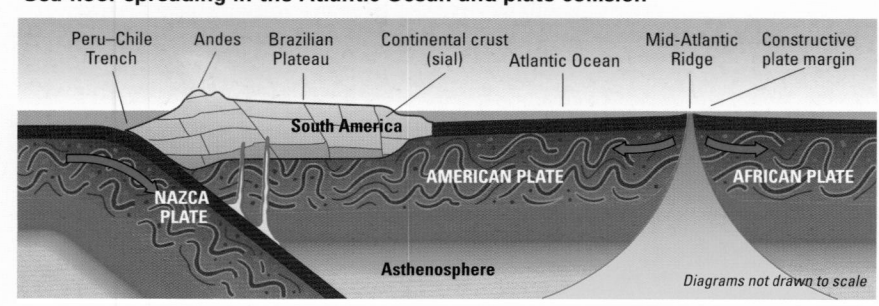

Peru–Chile Trench / Andes / Brazilian Plateau / Continental crust (sial) / Atlantic Ocean / Mid-Atlantic Ridge / Constructive plate margin
South America
NAZCA PLATE / AMERICAN PLATE / AFRICAN PLATE
Asthenosphere / Diagrams not drawn to scale

Sea-floor spreading in the Indian Ocean and continental plate collision

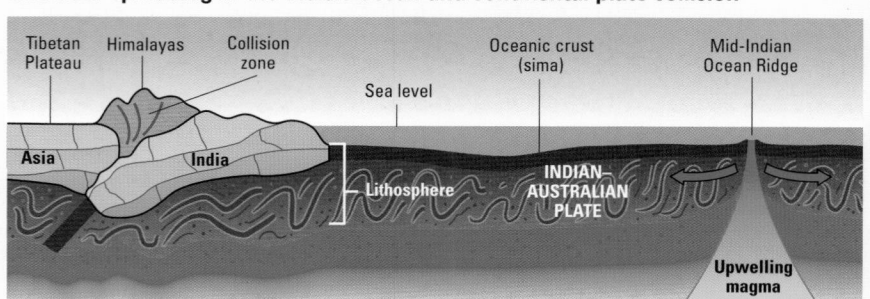

Tibetan Plateau / Himalayas / Collision zone / Oceanic crust (sima) / Mid-Indian Ocean Ridge
Sea level
Asia / India / Lithosphere / INDIAN–AUSTRALIAN PLATE
Upwelling magma

GEOLOGICAL TIME

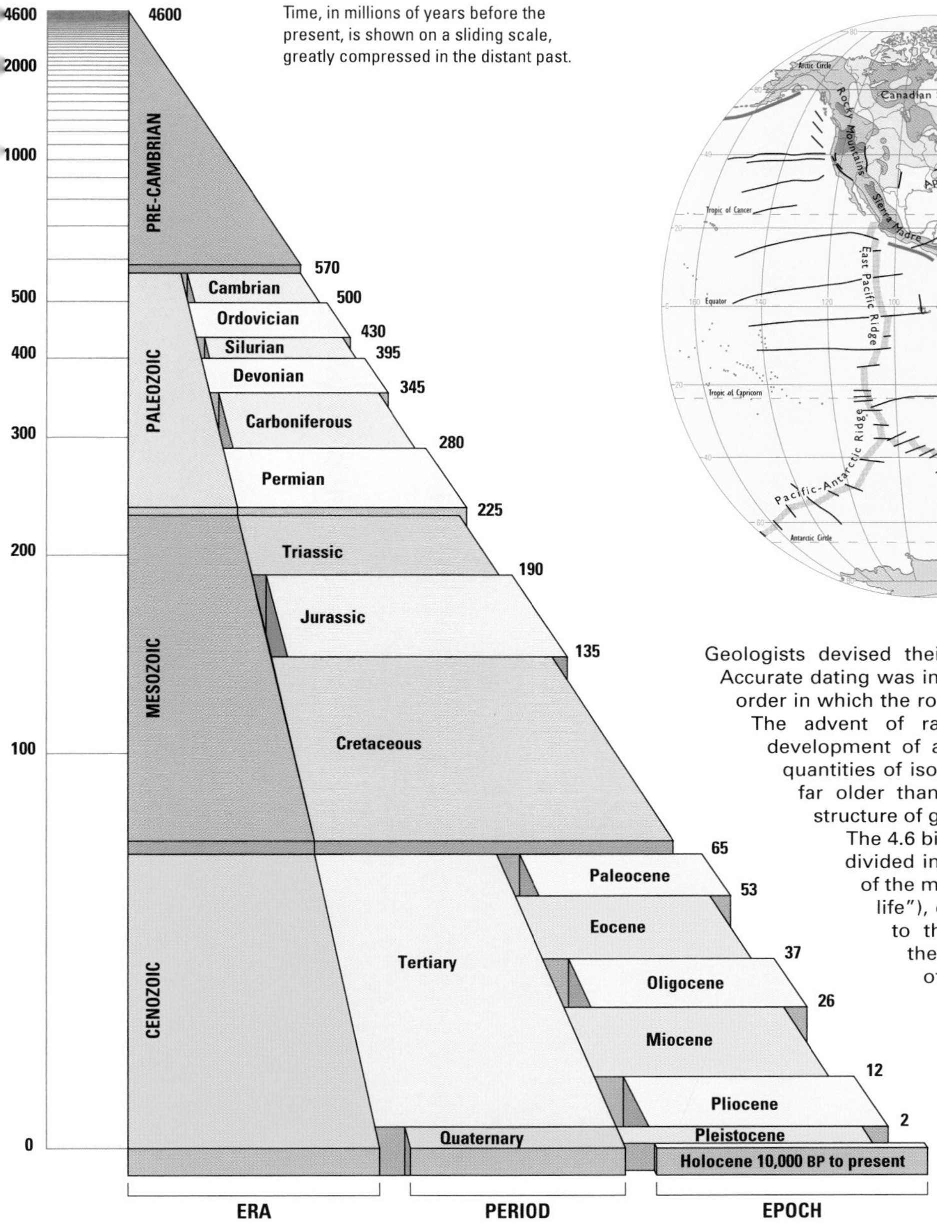

Time, in millions of years before the present, is shown on a sliding scale, greatly compressed in the distant past.

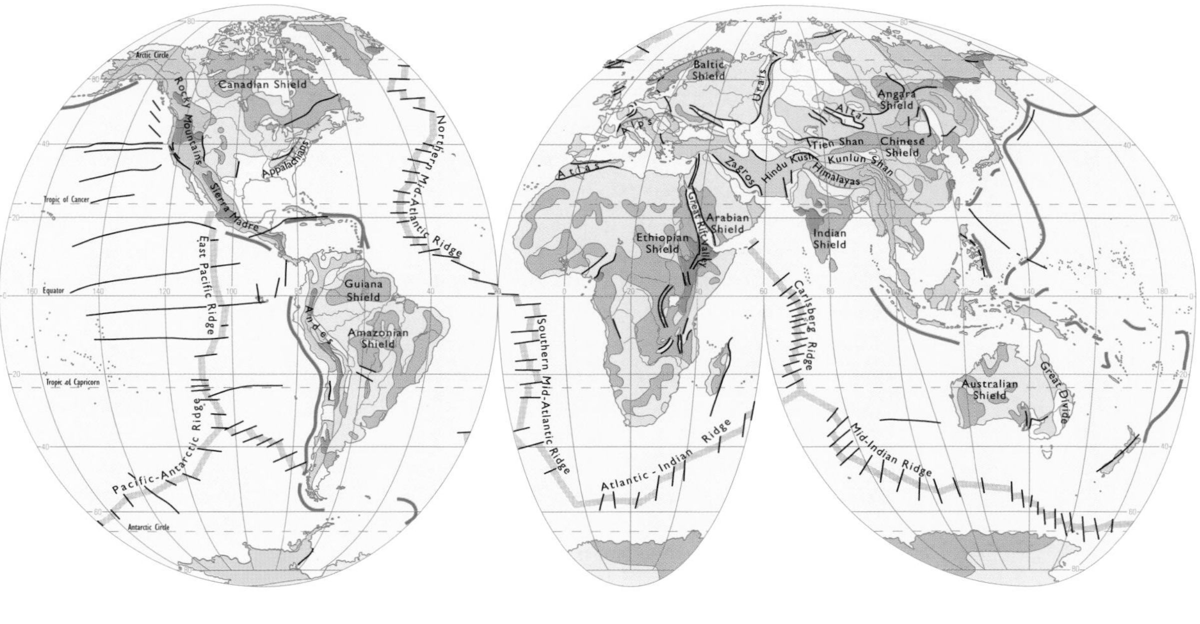

Scale (left axis, millions of years): 4600, 2000, 1000, 500, 400, 300, 200, 100, 0

Eras / Periods / Epochs:

- PRE-CAMBRIAN — 4600
- Cambrian — 570
- Ordovician — 500
- Silurian — 430
- Devonian — 395
- Carboniferous — 345
- Permian — 280
- PALEOZOIC
- Triassic — 225
- Jurassic — 190
- Cretaceous — 135
- MESOZOIC
- Paleocene — 65
- Eocene — 53
- Oligocene — 37
- Miocene — 26
- Pliocene — 12
- Tertiary
- Pleistocene — 2
- Quaternary
- Holocene 10,000 BP to present
- CENOZOIC

ERA | PERIOD | EPOCH

Geologists devised their timescale on the basis of relative, not calendar, ages. Accurate dating was impossible and estimates were often bitterly disputed, but the order in which the rocks were formed could be deduced from careful observation. The advent of radioactive dating – culminating in the 1950s with the development of a mass spectrometer capable of accurately measuring tiny quantities of isotopes – appears to have settled the arguments. The Earth is far older than geologists first imagined, but their painstakingly-created structure of geological time has withstood the advent of high technology.

The 4.6 billion (4,600 million) years since the formation of the Earth are divided into four great eras, further split into periods and, in the case of the most recent era, epochs. The present era is the Cenozoic ("new life"), extending backward through "middle life" and "ancient life" to the Pre-Cambrian, named after the Latin word for Wales, the location of some of the earliest known fossils. Most of the Earth's geological history is encompassed by the Pre-Cambrian: though traces of ancient life have since been found, it was largely the proliferation of fossils from the beginning of the Paleozoic era onward, some 570 million years ago, which first allowed precise subdivisions to be made.

Like the Cambrian, most are named after regions exemplifying a period's geology. Others – such as the Carboniferous ("coal-bearing") or the Cretaceous ("chalk-bearing") – are more directly descriptive.

Legend:
- Pre-Cambrian shields
- Sedimentary cover on Pre-Cambrian shields
- Paleozoic (Caledonian and Hercynian) folding
- Sedimentary cover on Paleozoic folding
- Mesozoic folding
- Sedimentary cover on Mesozoic folding
- Cenozoic (Alpine) folding
- Sedimentary cover on Cenozoic folding
- Intensive Mesozoic and Cenozoic vulcanism
- Principal faults
- Oceanic marginal troughs
- Midoceanic ridges
- Overthrust faults

EARTHQUAKES

Earthquake magnitude is usually rated according to either the Richter or the Modified Mercalli scale, both devised by seismologists in the 1930s. The Richter scale measures absolute earthquake power with mathematical precision: each step upward represents a tenfold increase in the amplitude of the shockwave. Theoretically, there is no upper limit, but the largest earthquakes measured have been rated at between 8.8 and 8.9. The 12-point Mercalli scale, based on observed effects, is often more meaningful, ranging from I (earthquakes noticed only by seismographs) to XII (total destruction); intermediate points include V (people awakened at night; unstable objects overturned), VII (collapse of ordinary buildings; chimneys and monuments fall), and IX (conspicuous cracks in ground; serious damage to reservoirs).

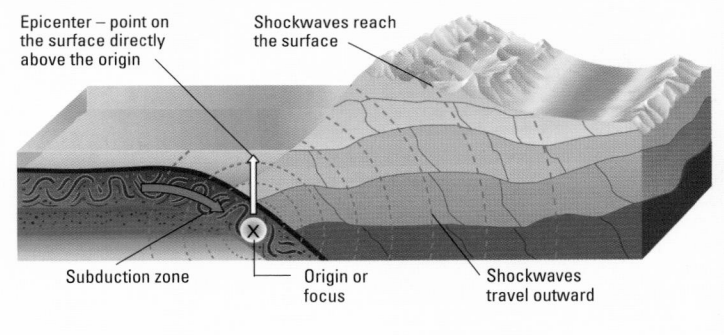

Epicenter – point on the surface directly above the origin

Shockwaves reach the surface

Subduction zone

Origin or focus

Shockwaves travel outward

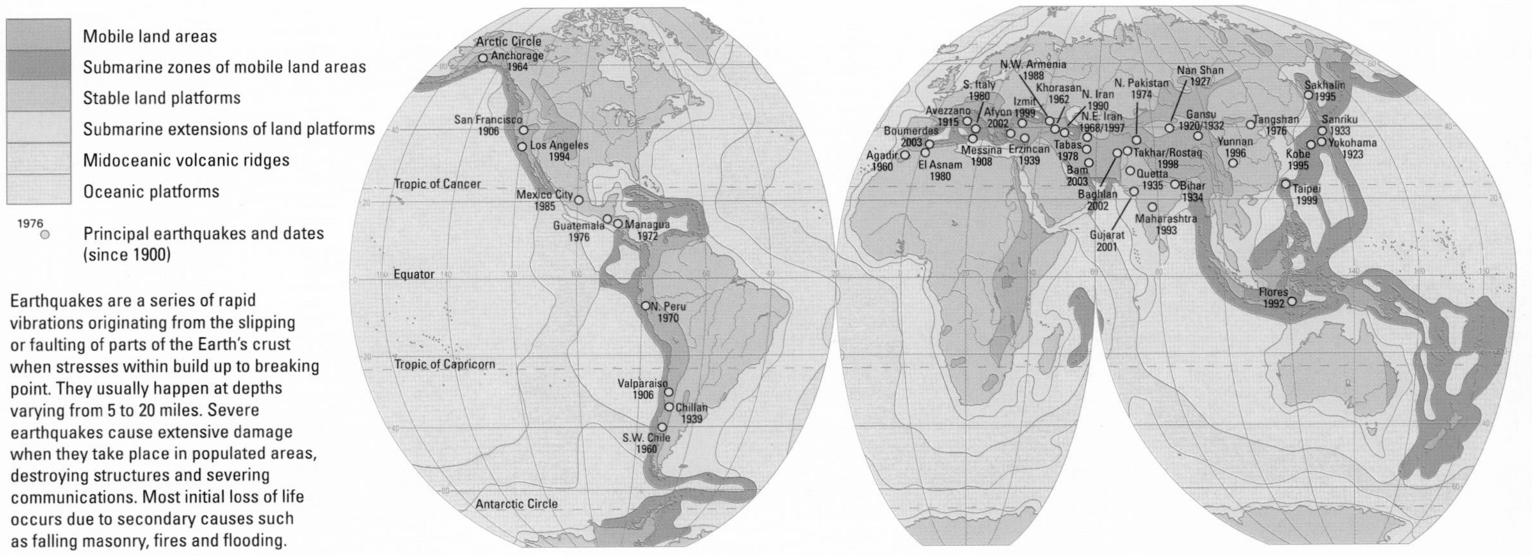

Legend:
- Mobile land areas
- Submarine zones of mobile land areas
- Stable land platforms
- Submarine extensions of land platforms
- Midoceanic volcanic ridges
- Oceanic platforms

1976 — Principal earthquakes and dates (since 1900)

Earthquakes are a series of rapid vibrations originating from the slipping or faulting of parts of the Earth's crust when stresses within build up to breaking point. They usually happen at depths varying from 5 to 20 miles. Severe earthquakes cause extensive damage when they take place in populated areas, destroying structures and severing communications. Most initial loss of life occurs due to secondary causes such as falling masonry, fires and flooding.

Notable Earthquakes Since 1900

Year	Location	Mag.	Deaths
1906	San Francisco, USA	8.3	3,000
1906	Valparaiso, Chile	8.6	22,000
1908	Messina, Italy	7.5	83,000
1915	Avezzano, Italy	7.5	30,000
1920	Gansu (Kansu), China	8.6	180,000
1923	Yokohama, Japan	8.3	143,000
1927	Nan Shan, China	8.3	200,000
1932	Gansu (Kansu), China	7.6	70,000
1933	Sanriku, Japan	8.9	2,990
1934	Bihar, India/Nepal	8.4	10,700
1935	Quetta, India*	7.5	60,000
1939	Chillan, Chile	8.3	28,000
1939	Erzincan, Turkey	7.9	30,000
1960	S. W. Chile	9.5	2,200
1960	Agadir, Morocco	5.8	12,000
1962	Khorasan, Iran	7.1	12,230
1964	Anchorage, USA	9.2	125
1968	N. E. Iran	7.4	12,000
1970	N. Peru	7.8	70,000
1972	Managua, Nicaragua	6.2	5,000
1974	N. Pakistan	6.3	5,200
1976	Guatemala	7.5	22,500
1976	Tangshan, China	8.2	255,000
1978	Tabas, Iran	7.7	25,000
1980	El Asnam, Algeria	7.3	20,000
1980	S. Italy	7.2	4,800
1985	Mexico City, Mexico	8.1	4,200
1988	N.W. Armenia	6.8	55,000
1990	N. Iran	7.7	36,000
1992	Flores, Indonesia	6.8	1,895
1993	Maharashtra, India	6.4	30,000
1994	Los Angeles, USA	6.6	51
1995	Kobe, Japan	7.2	5,000
1995	Sakhalin Is., Russia	7.5	1,000
1996	Yunnan, China	7.0	240
1997	N. E. Iran	7.1	2,400
1998	Takhar, Afghanistan	6.1	4,200
1998	Rostaq, Afghanistan	7.0	5,000
1999	Izmit, Turkey	7.4	15,000
1999	Taipei, Taiwan	7.6	1,700
2001	Gujarat, India	7.7	14,000
2002	Afyon, Turkey	6.5	44
2002	Baghlan, Afghanistan	6.1	1,000
2003	Boumerdes, Algeria	6.8	2,200
2003	Bam, Iran	6.6	30,000

The most devastating quake ever was at Shaanxi (Shenshi) province, central China, on January 3, 1556, when an estimated 830,000 people were killed.

* now Pakistan

LANDFORMS

For more information:

8 Oceans
10 The Earth's structure
   Plate tectonics
   Volcanoes
11 Geological time
18 Hydrological cycle
37 Structural regions

The theory of plate tectonics has offered new insights into how the Earth works, elucidating mysteries concerning continental drift, volcanic eruptions and earthquakes. It has also contributed to our understanding of how collisions between plates can squeeze up layers of sediments on seabeds, forming fold mountain ranges, such as the Himalayas.

Yet even as mountains rise, natural forces are wearing them away. In hot, dry climates, mechanical weathering (a result of rapid temperature changes) causes the outer layers of rocks to peel away, while, in cold mountain regions, boulders are prised apart when water freezes in cracks in rocks. Chemical weathering is responsible for hollowing out limestone caves and decomposing granites.

Climatic conditions have a great bearing on the principal agent of erosion in any particular area. Running water is most important in moist temperate regions. In cold regions, ice is the major agent of erosion, and in many mountain ranges, U-shaped valleys are evidence of the erosive power of valley glaciers.

Ice sheets molded much of the Earth's surface during the Ice Ages, the most recent of which, in the northern hemisphere, ended only 10,000 years ago. Polar climates also shape the scenery of the periglacial areas that border bodies of ice. Such areas are subject to constant freeze-thaw action, which creates such features as pingos (domed mounds).

Climatic change has also affected many of the landforms in hot deserts, which were shaped by running water at a time when the deserts enjoyed much wetter climates. However, the major agent of erosion in deserts today is wind-blown sand, which erodes rock strata to form mushroom-shaped rocks and caves.

The surface of the Earth is under constant assault from tectonic processes and the agents of erosion. The products of erosion, fragments of rock such as sand, are deposited to form sedimentary rocks. Metamorphic rocks are created when igneous or sedimentary rocks are buried and metamorphosed by heat and pressure. Eventually the rocks are recycled to form magma, which rises upward to start the rock cycle all over again.

THE ROCK CYCLE

James Hutton first proposed the rock cycle in the late 1700s after he observed the slow but steady effects of erosion.

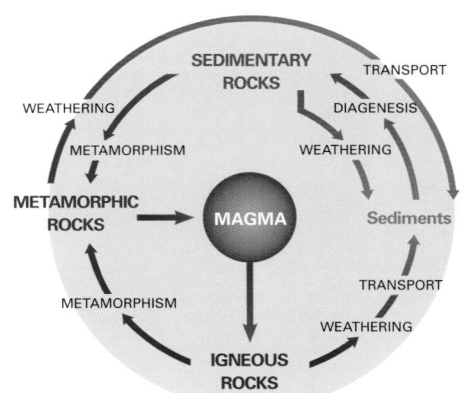

Rocks are divided into three types, according to the way in which they are formed:

Igneous rocks, including granite and basalt, are formed when magma cools inside the Earth's crust or on the surface.

Metamorphic rocks, such as slate, marble and quartzite, are formed below the Earth's surface by the compression or baking of existing rocks.

Sedimentary rocks, like sandstone and limestone, are formed on the surface of the Earth from the remains of living organisms and eroded fragments of older rocks.

MOUNTAIN BUILDING

Mountains are formed when pressures on the Earth's crust caused by continental drift become so intense that the surface buckles or cracks. This happens where oceanic crust is subducted by continental crust or, more dramatically, where two tectonic plates collide: the Rockies, Andes, Alps, Urals, and Himalayas resulted from such impacts. These are known as fold mountains because they were formed by the compression of the rocks. The Himalayas were formed from the folded former sediments of the Tethys Sea, which was trapped in the collision zone between the Indian-Australian and Eurasian plates.

The other main mountain-building processes occur when the crust fractures to create faults, allowing rock to be forced upward in large blocks, or when the pressure of magma within the crust forces the surface to bulge into a dome, or erupts to form a volcano.

Large mountain ranges may reveal a combination of these features. The Alps, for example, have been compressed so violently that the folds are fragmented by numerous faults and intrusions of molten igneous rock.

Over millions of years, even the greatest mountain ranges can be reduced by the agents of erosion (especially rivers) to a low, rugged landscape known as a peneplain.

Types of faults: Faults occur where the crust is being stretched or compressed so violently that the rock strata break in a horizontal or vertical movement. They are classified by the direction in which the blocks of rock have moved. A normal fault results when a vertical movement causes the surface to break apart; compression causes a reverse fault. Horizontal movement causes shearing, known as a strike-slip fault. When the rock breaks in two places, the central block may be pushed up in a horst fault, or sink (creating a rift valley) in a graben fault.

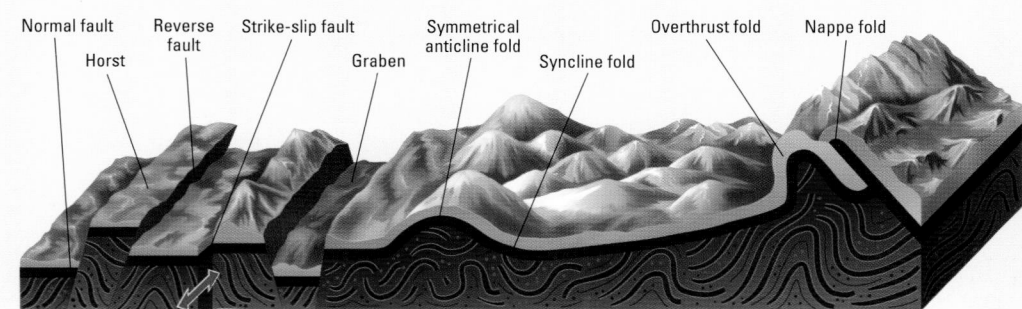

Types of fold: Folds occur when rock strata are squeezed and compressed. They are common, therefore, at destructive plate margins and where plates have collided, forcing the rocks to buckle into mountain ranges. Geographers give different names to the degrees of fold that result from continuing pressure on the rock. A simple fold may be symmetric, with even slopes on either side, but as the pressure builds up, one slope becomes steeper and the fold becomes asymmetric. Later, the ridge or "anticline" at the top of the fold may slide over the lower ground or "syncline" to form a recumbent fold. Eventually, the rock strata may break under the pressure to form an overthrust and finally a nappe fold.

CONTINENTAL GLACIATION

Many landforms in the northern hemisphere were shaped by ice sheets and meltwater during the Pleistocene Ice Age, which began about 2 million years ago. During the Ice Age, the ice sheets periodically advanced and retreated. The first map (*below left*) shows the ice cover at its greatest extent about 200,000 years BP (before the present), when it covered about 30% of the land surface, as compared with 10% today. About 18,000 years BP, the ice covered most of Canada and extended as far south as the Bristol Channel in England. Around the ice sheets, land areas experienced periglacial conditions.

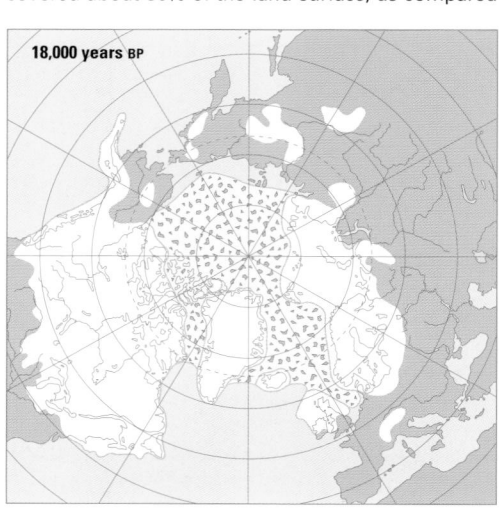

200,000 years BP

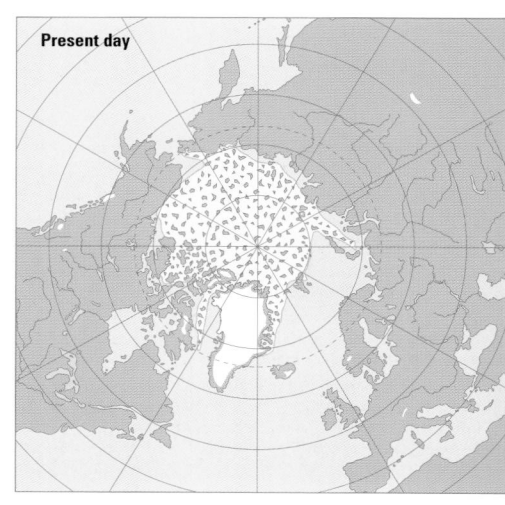

18,000 years BP

Present day

NATURAL LANDFORMS

Natural landforms reflect the influence of plate tectonics, through mountain-building and the generation of new rocks from the Earth's interior, together with the agents of erosion – running water, ice, winds, and coastal waves. Over millions of years, mountains are gradually eroded, with the eroded material redistributed, usually at lower levels. The resultant landforms reflect the major forces that have been at work, as well as the underlying geology, the climatic conditions, which often vary over time, and the vegetation cover. The study of these processes and the landforms they create is called geomorphology. The stylized diagram (*below*) shows some major natural landforms found in the mid-latitudes.

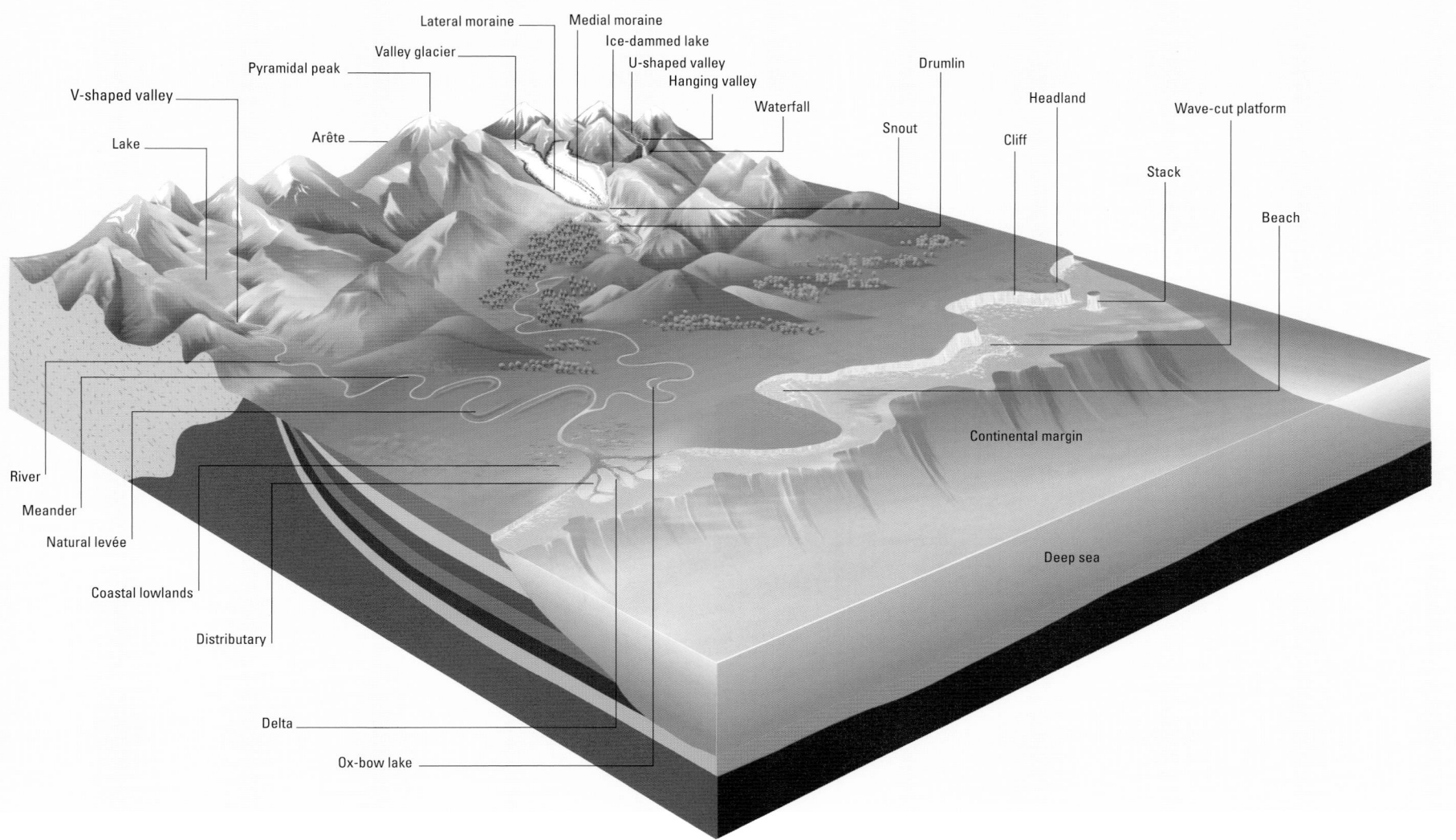

Labels:
V-shaped valley, Lake, Pyramidal peak, Arête, Valley glacier, Lateral moraine, Medial moraine, Ice-dammed lake, U-shaped valley, Hanging valley, Waterfall, Snout, Drumlin, Headland, Cliff, Stack, Wave-cut platform, Beach, River, Meander, Natural levée, Coastal lowlands, Distributary, Delta, Ox-bow lake, Continental margin, Deep sea

SURFACE PROCESSES

Catastrophic changes to landforms are caused periodically by such phenomena as avalanches, landslides and volcanic eruptions, but most of the processes that shape the Earth's surface operate extremely slowly in human terms.

Chemical weathering is at its greatest in warm, humid regions, while mechanical weathering (the physical breakup of rocks) predominates in cold mountain or hot desert regions. The most familiar type of chemical weathering is caused by the reaction of rainwater containing dissolved carbon dioxide on limestone; this leads to the creation of labyrinthine cave networks dissolved by groundwater. Mechanical weathering includes frost action, while in hot deserts, rapid temperature changes cause the outer layers of rocks to expand and contract until they crack and peel away, a process called exfoliation.

Running water is probably the world's leading agent of erosion and transportation. The energy of a river depends on several factors, including its velocity and volume, and its erosive power is at its peak when it is in full flood, sweeping soil, pebbles and even boulders along its course, cutting downward into the bedrock or widening its valley.

Sea waves also exert tremendous erosive power during storms, when they hurl pebbles and large rocks against the shore, undercutting cliffs and hollowing out caves. Headlands are often attacked on both sides, forming caves, then a natural arch and eventually an isolated stack.

Glacier ice forms in mountain hollows, called cirques, and spills out to form valley glaciers, which transport rocks shattered by frost action. As a glacier moves, rocks embedded in the base and sides scrape away bedrock, eroding steepsided, flat-bottomed, U-shaped valleys. Evidence of past glaciation in mountain regions includes cirques, knife-edged ridges, or arêtes, and pyramidal peaks, or horns.

DESERT LANDFORMS

Deserts are defined as places with an average annual precipitation of 10 inches [250 mm] per year, though places with a higher rainfall and a high evaporation rate may also qualify as deserts.

The three types of desert landforms are known by their Arabic names, a reflection of the fact that the Sahara in North Africa is the world's largest desert. Sand desert, called *erg*, covers about one-fifth of the world's deserts. The rest is divided between *hammada* (areas of bare rock) and *reg* (broad plains covered by loose gravel or pebbles).

The shapes of dunes in sand deserts reflect the character of local winds. Where winds are constant in direction, the sand often piles up in crescent-shaped dunes, called *barchans*. Barchans are constantly on the move and their forward march, unless halted by vegetation, may overwhelm settlements at oases. *Seif* dunes, named after the Arabic word for "sword," are long ridges of sand that lie parallel to the direction of the wind, but where winds are variable, the sand sheets are often featureless.

Wind-blown sand is an effective agent of erosion, but because of the weight of sand grains, this type of erosion is confined to within approximately 7 feet [2 meters] of the land surface, creating caves and mushroom-shaped rocks.

In assessing desert landforms, it is important to remember that other processes were at work in the past when the climate was very different from today. For example, cave paintings suggest that the Sahara had a much wetter climate after the end of the Ice Age and only began to dry up after about 5000 BC. However, human action, including overgrazing and the cutting down of trees for firewood, can turn a grassland region into desert – a process known as desertification.

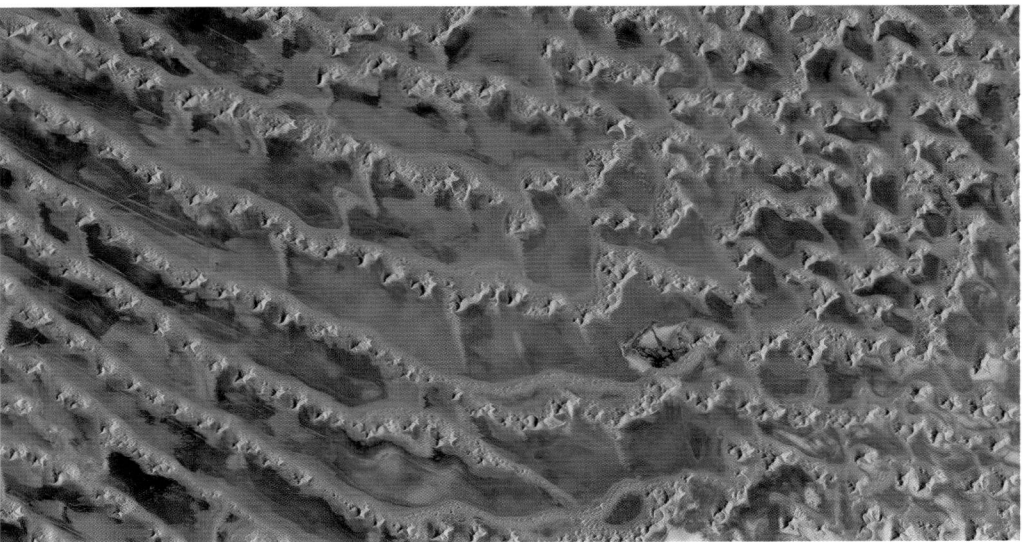

◄ This false-color satellite image of part of the Rub' al Khali, or "Empty Quarter," in Saudi Arabia shows part of the world's largest sand sea (*erg*), which covers almost 232,000 sq miles [600,000 sq km]. Showing many different types of sand dune, the image enhances the difference in color between the dune sand and the interdune areas, which have a higher clay composition. The blue "eye" is a partially flooded clay basin (*playa*).

THE ATMOSPHERE

For more information:
- 9 Ocean currents
- 17 Beaufort wind scale
  Climate change
  Monsoon
- 21 Solar energy
  Greenhouse effect
- 22 Greenhouse power
- 23 Acid rain

The atmosphere is a meteor shield, a radiation deflector, a thermal blanket, and a source of chemical energy for the Earth's diverse life forms. Five-sixths of its mass is in the lowest layer, the troposphere, which ranges in thickness from 11–6 miles between the Equator and the poles. Powered by the Sun, the air is always on the move, flowing generally from high- to low-pressure areas. The troposphere is the layer where virtually all weather phenomena, including clouds, precipitation and winds, occur. Above the troposphere is the stratosphere, which contains the important ozone layer and extends to about 30 miles above the Earth's surface. Beyond 60 miles, atmospheric density is lower than most laboratory vacuums.

CIRCULATION OF THE AIR

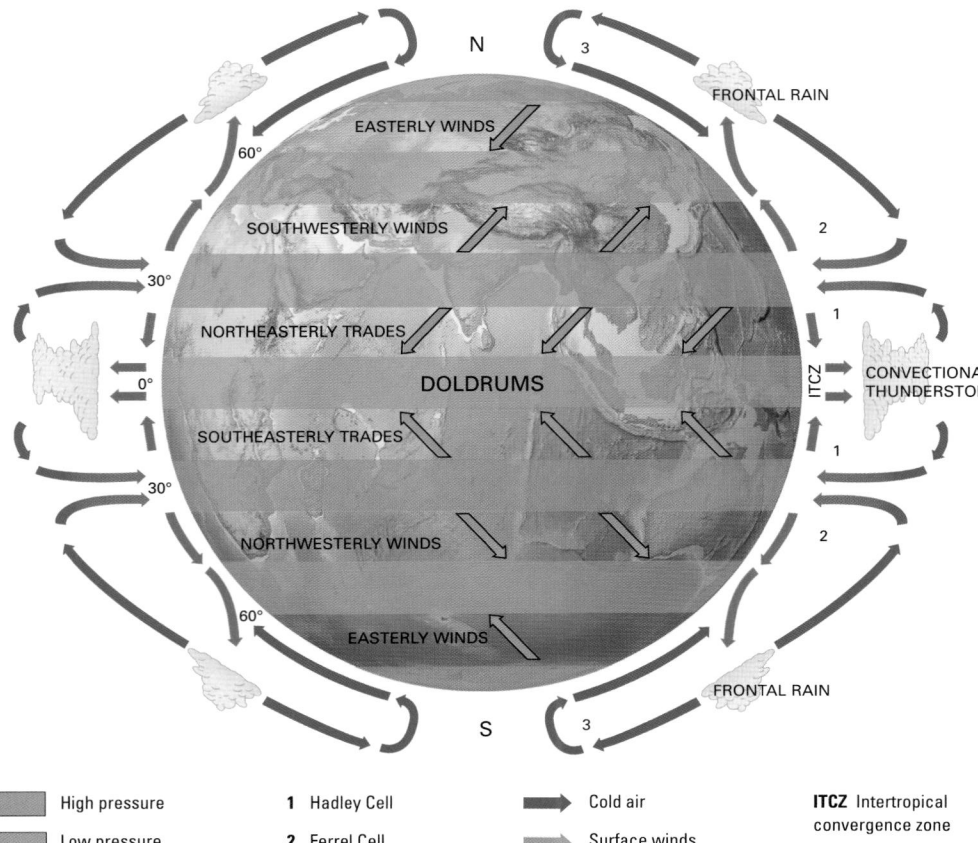

High pressure	1 Hadley Cell
Low pressure	2 Ferrel Cell
Warm air	3 Polar Cell

Cold air	**ITCZ** Intertropical
Surface winds	convergence zone
Clouds	

STRUCTURE OF THE ATMOSPHERE

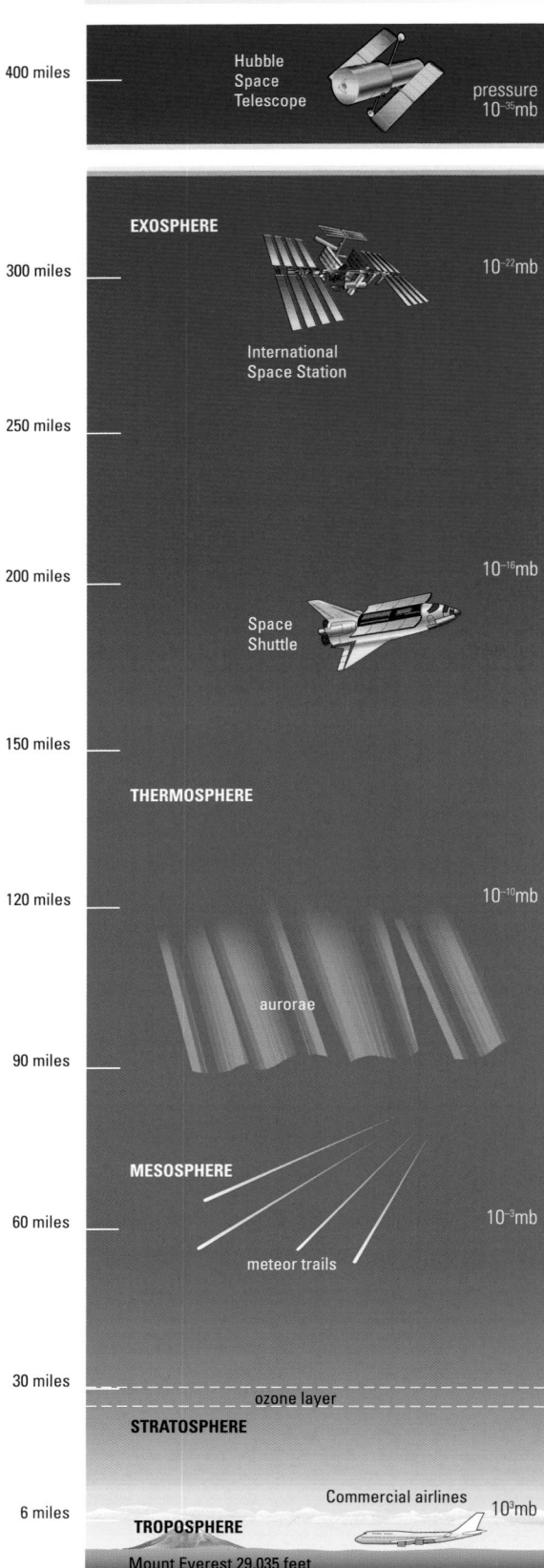

FRONTAL SYSTEMS

Depressions, or cyclones, form along the polar front where dense polar easterlies meet warm subtropical westerlies. Depressions occur when warm air flows into waves in the polar front, while cold air flows in behind it, creating rotating air systems that bring changeable weather.

Along the warm front (the boundary on the ground between the warm and cold air), the warm air flows upward over the cold air, producing a sequence of clouds that help forecasters to predict a depression's advance. Along the cold front, the advancing cold air forces warm air to rise steeply. Towering cumulonimbus clouds form in the rising air.

When the cold front overtakes the warm front, the warm air is pushed above ground level to form an occluded front. Cloud and rain persist along occlusions until temperatures equalize, the air mixes, and the depression dies out.

Depressions with these distinctive features are known as "frontal." The diagram below shows a cross-section through a depression and the associated cloud types and weather conditions that may be experienced.

CHEMICAL COMPOSITION

Gaseous composition of the principal atmospheric layers

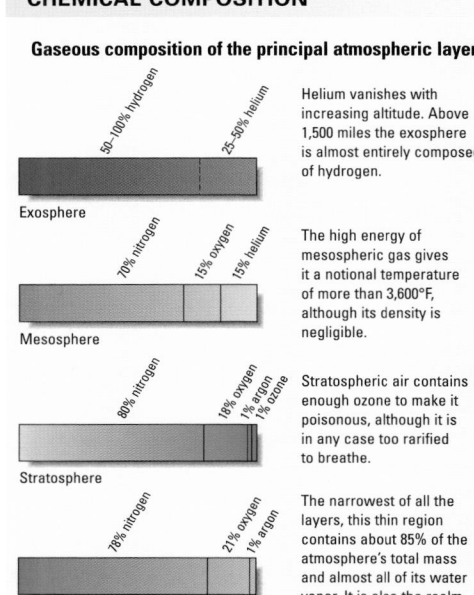

Helium vanishes with increasing altitude. Above 1,500 miles the exosphere is almost entirely composed of hydrogen.

The high energy of mesospheric gas gives it a notional temperature of more than 3,600°F, although its density is negligible.

Stratospheric air contains enough ozone to make it poisonous, although it is in any case too rarified to breathe.

The narrowest of all the layers, this thin region contains about 85% of the atmosphere's total mass and almost all of its water vapor. It is also the realm of the Earth's weather.

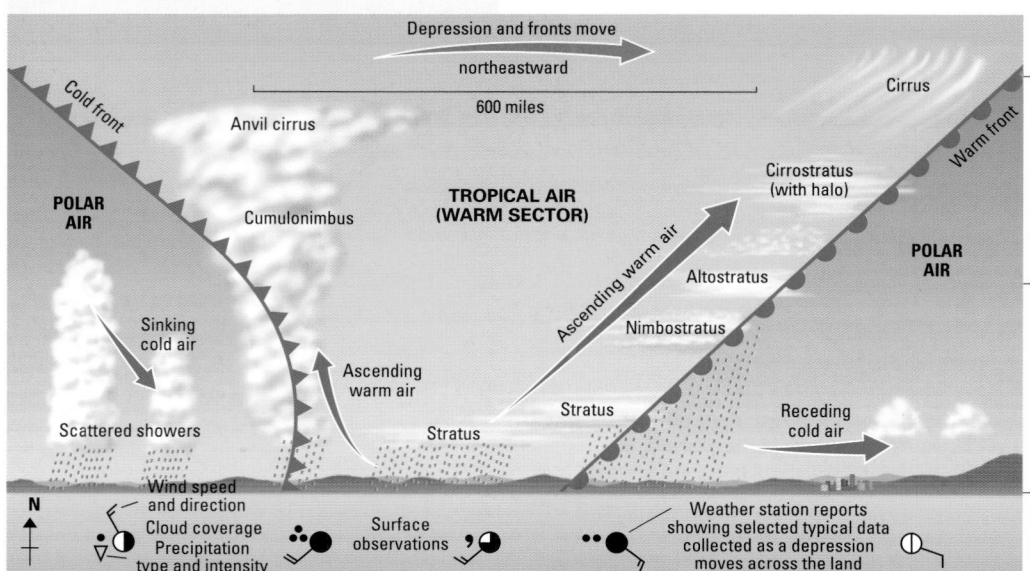

AIR MASSES

Air masses are bodies of air whose characteristics are broadly the same over a large area. Around the Equator, where the Sun's heat creates relatively high surface temperatures, warm air rises to create a zone of low pressure called the doldrums. The air cools and finally spreads out toward the poles. Around latitudes 30° north and south, the air sinks back to the surface, becoming warmer as it descends and creating zones of high pressure called the horse latitudes.

The high- and low-pressure zones are both areas of comparative calm, but between them lie the prevailing trade wind belts. Air also flows north and south from the high-pressure horse latitudes and these airflows meet up with cold, dense air flowing from the poles along the polar front.

This basic circulatory system is complicated by the Coriolis effect, brought about by the spinning Earth. Because of the Coriolis effect, the prevailing winds do not flow directly north–south but are deflected to the right in the northern hemisphere and to the left in the southern. Along the polar front, depressions form where the polar easterlies meet the westerlies.

The first classification of clouds was developed by a London chemist, Luke Howard, in 1803, and it was later modified by the World Meteorological Organization. The main types are divided into three groups according to their altitude, and into subgroups according to their shape, which vary from hairlike filaments (cirrus), heaps or piles (cumulus), and layers (stratus). Each cloud carries some kind of message, though not always a clear one, to weather forecasters.

CLASSIFICATION OF CLOUDS

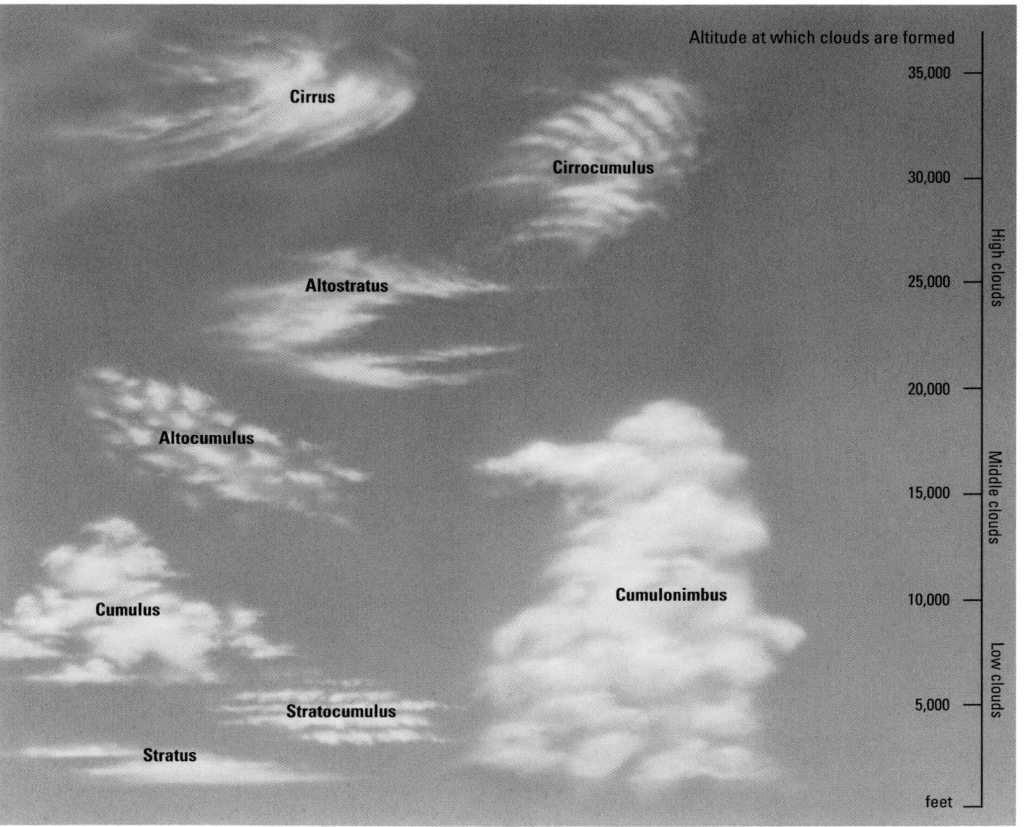

Altitude at which clouds are formed

Clouds form when damp, usually rising, air is cooled. Thus they form when a wind rises to cross hills or mountains; when a mass of air rises over, or is pushed up by, another mass of denser air; or when local heating of the ground causes convection currents.

The types of clouds are classified according to altitude as high, middle, or low. The high ones, composed of ice crystals, are cirrus, cirrostratus, and cirrocumulus.

The middle clouds are altostratus – a gray or bluish striated, fibrous or uniform sheet producing light drizzle – and altocumulus, a thicker and fluffier version of cirrocumulus.

Low clouds include nimbostratus, a dark gray layer that brings rain or snow; cumulus, a detached heap, dark at the base; stratus, which forms dull, overcast skies at low levels; and stratocumulus, which consists of fluffy grayish-white layers.

Cumulonimbus, associated with storms and rains, heavy and dense with a flat base and a high, fluffy outline, can be tall enough to occupy middle as well as low altitudes.

PRESSURE AND SURFACE WINDS

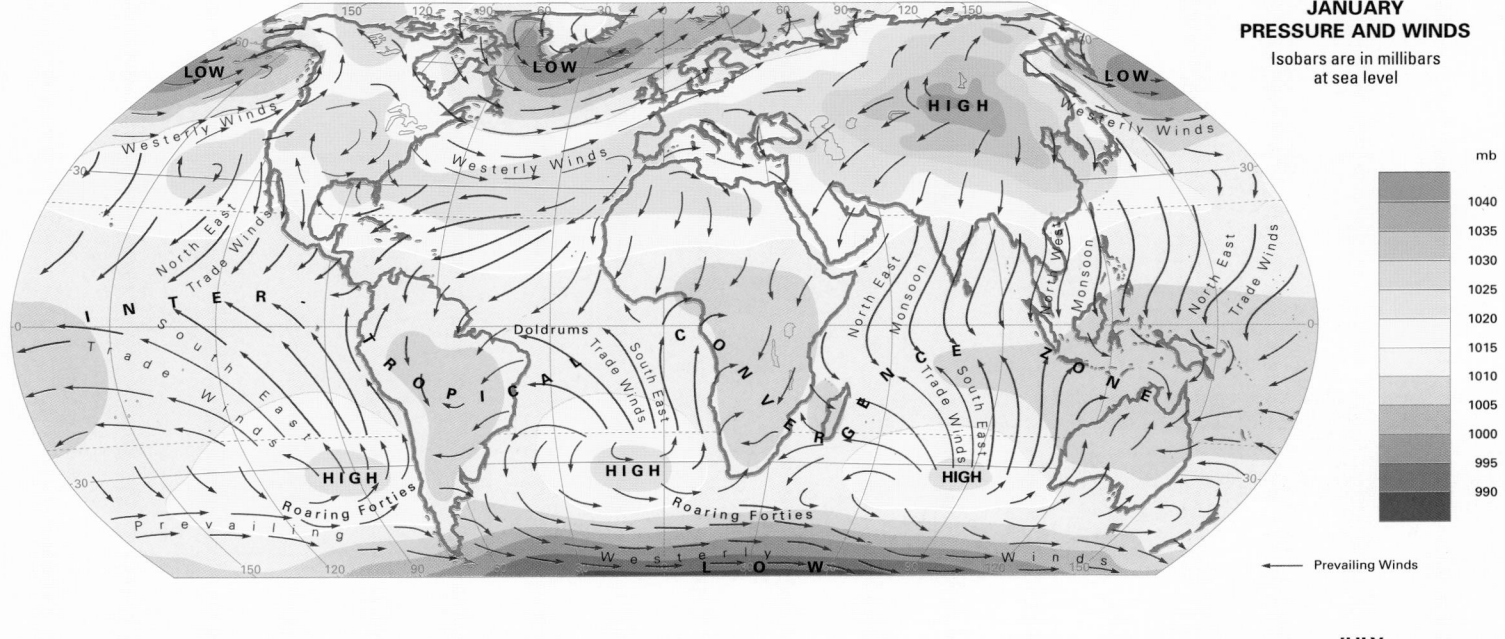

JANUARY PRESSURE AND WINDS

Isobars are in millibars at sea level

mb
1040
1035
1030
1025
1020
1015
1010
1005
1000
995
990

← Prevailing Winds

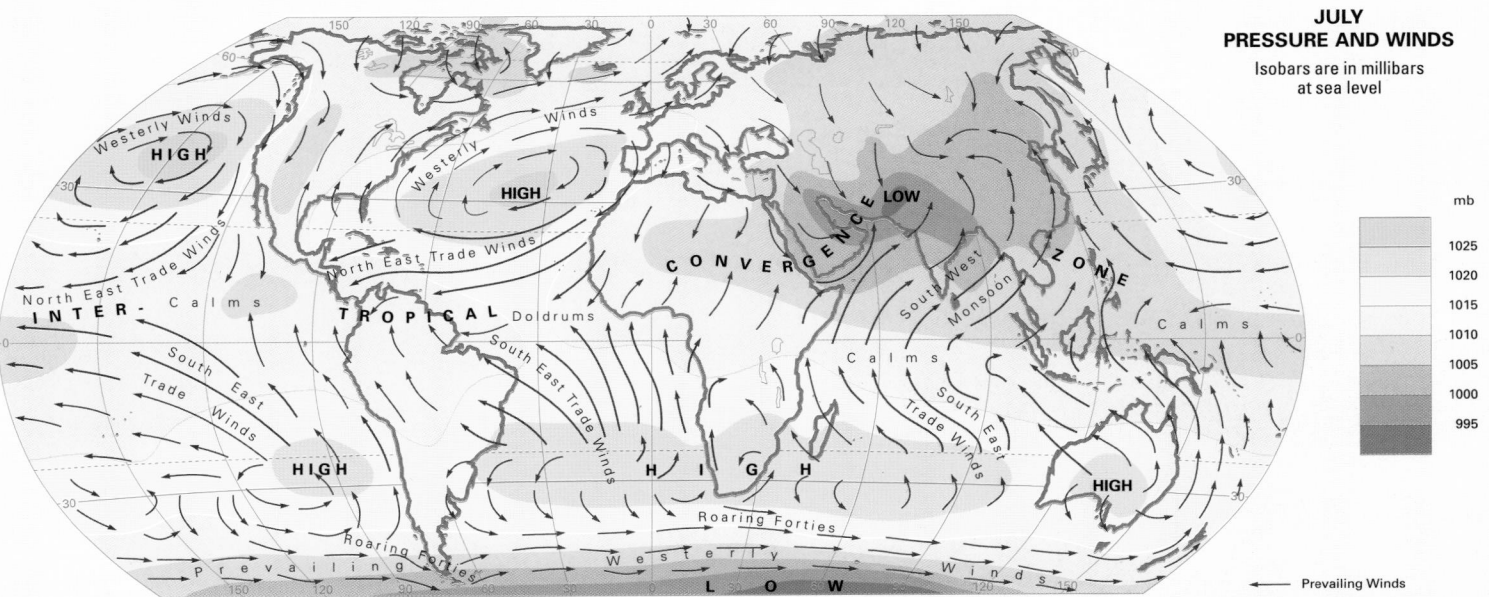

JULY PRESSURE AND WINDS

Isobars are in millibars at sea level

mb
1025
1020
1015
1010
1005
1000
995

← Prevailing Winds

CLIMATE RECORDS

Pressure and winds

Highest barometric pressure:
Agata, Siberia, 1,083.8 mb at altitude 862 ft [262 m], December 31, 1968.

Lowest barometric pressure:
Typhoon Tip, 300 mi [480 km] west of Guam, Pacific Ocean, 870 mb, October 12, 1979.

Highest recorded wind speed:
Mt Washington, New Hampshire, USA, 231 mph [371 km/h], April 12, 1934. This is three times as strong as hurricane force on the Beaufort Scale.

Windiest place:
Commonwealth Bay, George V Coast, Antarctica, where gales frequently reach over 200 mph [320 km/h].

Worst recorded storm:
Bangladesh (then East Pakistan) cyclone*, November 13, 1970 – over 300,000 dead or missing. The 1991 cyclone, Bangladesh's and the world's second worst in terms of loss of life, killed an estimated 138,000 people.

Worst recorded tornado:
Missouri/Illinois/Indiana, USA, March 18, 1925 – 792 deaths. The tornado was only 300 yds [275 m] wide.

* Tropical cyclones are known as hurricanes in Central and North America, as typhoons in the Far East, and as willy-willies in northern Australia.

CLIMATE

For more information:
9 Ocean currents
14 Circulation of the air
15 Classification of clouds
    Pressure and winds
18 Hydrological cycle
19 Natural vegetation
21 Greenhouse effect
22 Global warming

Weather is the day-to-day or hour-to-hour condition of the air, while climate is weather in the long term – the seasonal pattern of hot and cold, wet and dry, averaged over a long period.

Most classifications of climate are based on a system developed in the early 19th century by Vladimir Köppen, a Russian meteorologist. Using a code based on letters and a classification centered on two main features, temperature and precipitation, he identified five main climatic types: tropical (A), dry (B), warm temperate (C), cold temperate (D), and polar (E). A highland mountain climate (H) was added later to account for the variety of altitudinal climatic zones on high mountains. Each

of these main regions was then further subdivided.

Latitude is a major factor in determining climate, but other factors add to the complexity. These include the differential heating of land and sea, the distance from the sea, the effect of mountains on winds, and the influence of ocean currents. For example, New York City, Naples, and the Gobi Desert share almost the same latitude, but their climates are very different.

During the last Ice Age, the Earth underwent alternating cold periods, called glacials, separated by warm interglacials. The Milankovich theory suggests such cycles may be caused by variations in the Earth's path around the Sun, changing

from almost circular to elliptical every 95,000 years, and variations in the Earth's tilt from 21.5° to 24.5° every 42,000 years. Another factor is that the Earth is now closest to the Sun in the middle of winter in the northern hemisphere and furthest away in summer. But 12,000 years ago, at the height of the last glacial period, the northern winter fell with the Sun at its most distant.

Studies of these cycles suggest that we are now in an interglacial with a new glacial period on the way. However, scientists believe that global warming, largely a result of burning fossil fuels and deforestation, may be occurring much faster than the great, slow cycles of the Solar System.

Tropical rainy climates
All mean monthly temperatures above 64°F.

Af	Rain forest climate
Am	Monsoon climate
Aw	Savanna climate

Dry climates
Low rainfall combined with a wide range of temperatures

| BS | Steppe climate |
| BW | Desert climate |

Warm temperate rainy climates
The mean temperature is below 64°F but above 26°F and that of the warmest month is over 50°F.

Cw	Dry winter climate
Cs	Dry summer climate
Cf	Climate with no dry season

Cold temperate rainy climates
The mean temperature of the coldest month is below 26°F but that of the warmest month is still over 50°F.

| Dw | Dry winter climate |
| Df | Climate with no dry season |

Polar climates
The mean temperature of the warmest month is below 50°F, giving permanently frozen subsoil.

| ET | Tundra climate |

The mean temperature of the warmest month is below 32°F, giving permanent ice and snow.

| EF | Polar climate |

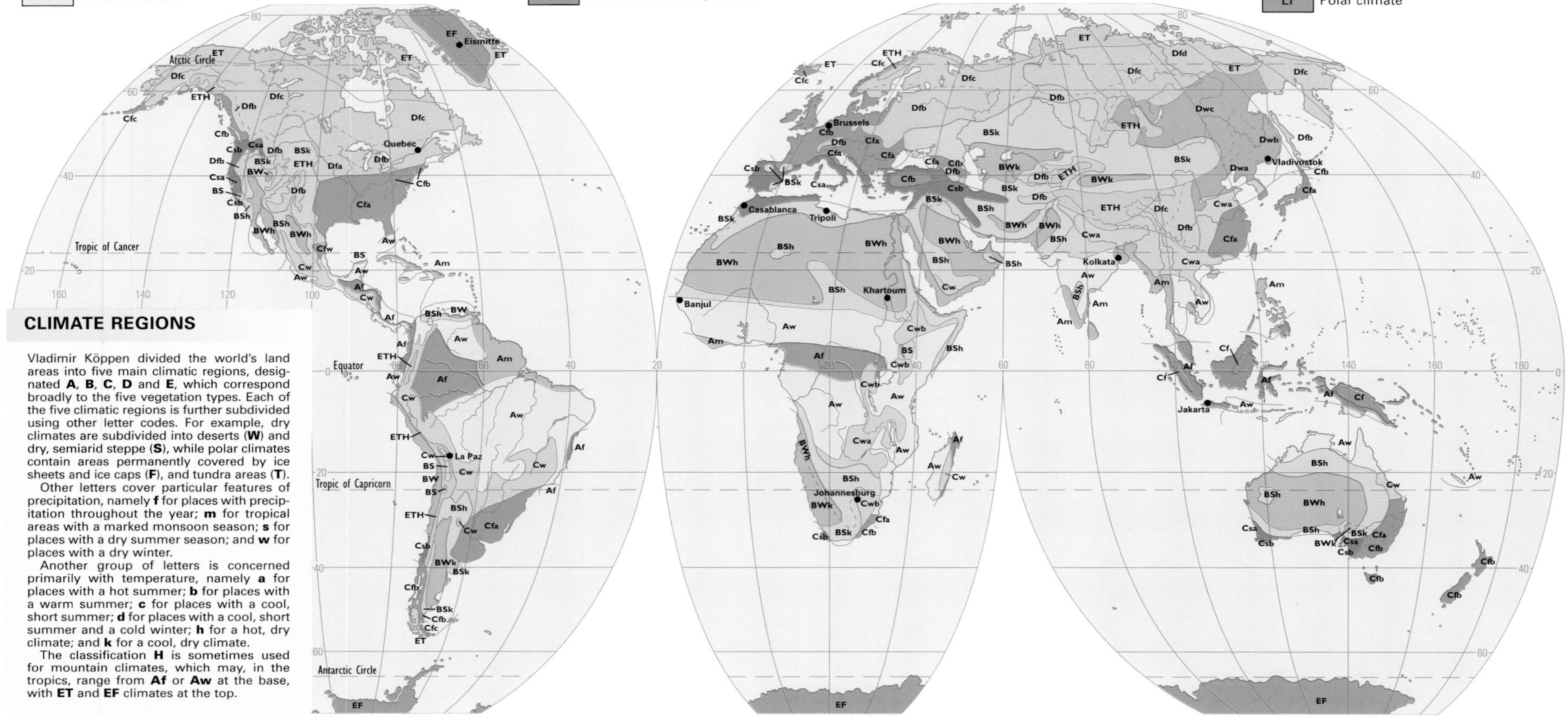

CLIMATE REGIONS

Vladimir Köppen divided the world's land areas into five main climatic regions, designated **A, B, C, D** and **E**, which correspond broadly to the five vegetation types. Each of the five climatic regions is further subdivided using other letter codes. For example, dry climates are subdivided into deserts (**W**) and dry, semiarid steppe (**S**), while polar climates contain areas permanently covered by ice sheets and ice caps (**F**), and tundra areas (**T**).

Other letters cover particular features of precipitation, namely **f** for places with precipitation throughout the year; **m** for tropical areas with a marked monsoon season; **s** for places with a dry summer season; and **w** for places with a dry winter.

Another group of letters is concerned primarily with temperature, namely **a** for places with a hot summer; **b** for places with a warm summer; **c** for places with a cool, short summer; **d** for places with a cool, short summer and a cold winter; **h** for a hot, dry climate; and **k** for a cool, dry climate.

The classification **H** is sometimes used for mountain climates, which may, in the tropics, range from **Af** or **Aw** at the base, with **ET** and **EF** climates at the top.

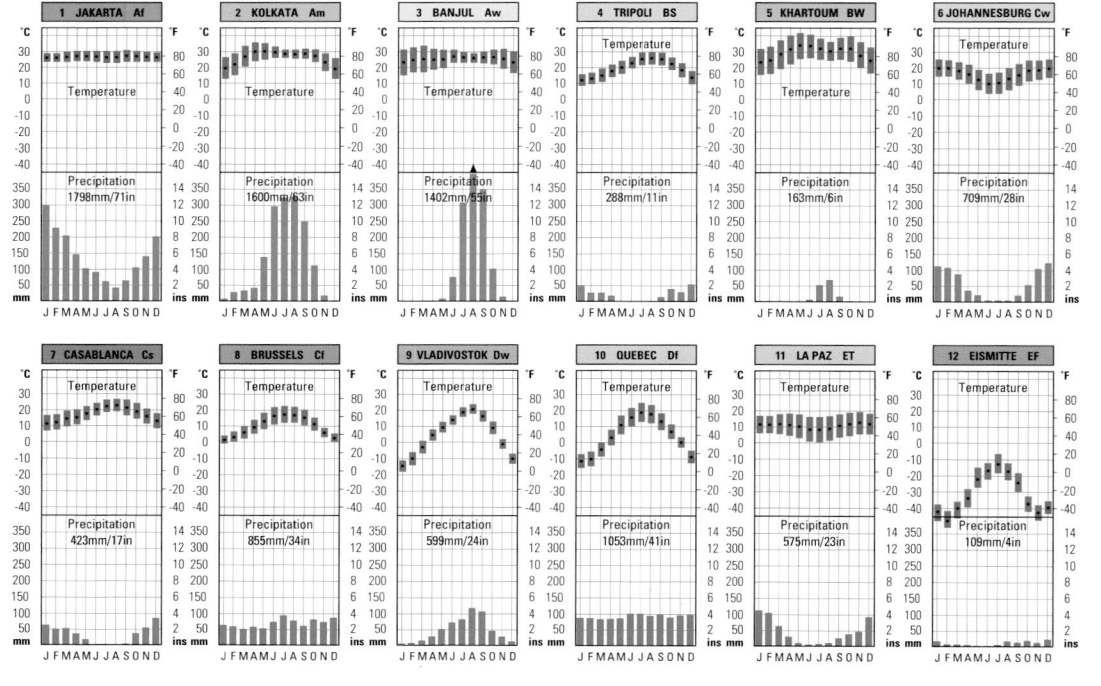

CLIMATE AND WEATHER TERMS

Anticyclone: area of high pressure with light winds and generally quiet weather.
Absolute humidity: amount of water vapor contained in a given volume of air.
Cloud cover: amount of cloud in the sky; measured in oktas (from 1–8), with 0 clear, and 8 total cover.
Condensation: the conversion of water vapor, or moisture in the air, into liquid.
Cyclone: violent storm resulting from counterclockwise rotation of winds in the northern hemisphere and clockwise in the southern: called hurricane in North America, typhoon in the Far East.
Depression: area of low pressure. The pressure gradient is toward the center.
Dew: water droplets condensed out of the air after the ground has cooled at night.
Dew point: temperature at which air becomes saturated (reaches a relative humidity of 100%) at a constant pressure.
Drizzle: precipitation where drops are less than 0.02 inches [0.5 mm] in diameter.
Evaporation: conversion of water from liquid into vapor or moisture in the air.
Front: the dividing line between two air masses.
Frost: dew that has frozen when the air temperature falls below freezing point.
Hail: frozen rain; small balls of ice, often falling during thunderstorms.

Hoar frost: formed on objects when the dew point is below freezing point.
Humidity: amount of moisture in the air.
Isobar: cartographic line connecting places of equal atmospheric pressure.
Isotherm: cartographic line connecting places of equal temperature.
Lightning: massive electrical discharge released in thunderstorm from cloud to cloud or cloud to ground, the result of the top becoming positively charged and the bottom negatively charged.
Precipitation: measurable rain, snow, sleet or hail.
Prevailing wind: most common direction of wind at a given location.
Rain: precipitation of liquid particles with diameter larger than 0.02 inches [0.5 mm].
Relative humidity: amount of water vapor contained in a given volume of air at a given temperature.
Snow: formed when water vapor condenses below freezing point.
Thunder: sound produced by the rapid expansion of air heated by lightning.
Tornado: severe funnel-shaped storm that twists as hot air spins vertically (waterspout at sea).
Whirlwind: rapidly rotating column of air, only a few feet across, made visible by dust.

CLIMATE CHANGE

Human factors, such as the emission of greenhouse gases through the burning of fossil fuels and deforestation, have contributed to global warming. The histogram (*below*) shows in blue the average global temperatures from 1860 to 1996. The red line is a 10-year running average. Overall, there is an upward trend, particularly so since the 1970s, when global warming became a matter of concern in scientific circles. The large year-to-year changes indicate the Earth's natural climatic variability and the influence of such factors as major volcanic eruptions.

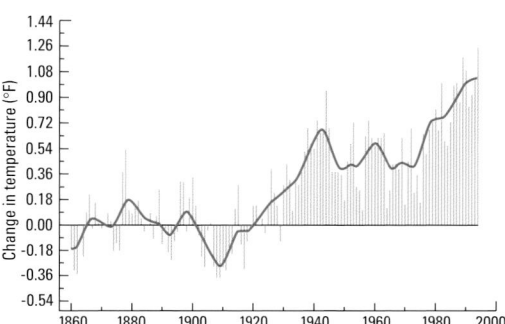

Data from the Hadley Center for Climate Research and Prediction

BEAUFORT WIND SCALE

Named after Admiral Sir Francis Beaufort, the 19th-century British naval officer who devised it, the Beaufort Scale assesses wind speed according to its effects. It was originally designed as an aid for sailors, but has since been adapted for use on the land. It is used internationally.

Scale	Wind speed mph	km/h	Effect
0	0–1	0–1	**Calm** Smoke rises vertically
1	1–3	1–5	**Light air** Wind direction shown only by smoke drift
2	4–7	6–11	**Light breeze** Wind felt on face; leaves rustle; vanes moved by wind
3	8–12	12–19	**Gentle breeze** Leaves and small twigs in constant motion; wind extends small flag
4	13–18	20–28	**Moderate** Raises dust and loose paper; small branches move
5	19–24	29–38	**Fresh** Small trees in leaf sway; crested wavelets on inland waters
6	25–31	39–49	**Strong** Large branches move; difficult to use umbrellas; overhead wires whistle
7	32–38	50–61	**Near gale** Whole trees in motion; difficult to walk against wind
8	39–46	62–74	**Gale** Twigs break from trees; walking very difficult
9	47–54	75–88	**Strong gale** Slight structural damage
10	55–63	89–102	**Storm** Trees uprooted; serious structural damage
11	64–72	103–117	**Violent storm** Widespread damage
12	73+	118+	**Hurricane**

THE MONSOON

Monsoon is the term given to the seasonal reversal of wind direction, most noticeably in Southeast Asia. It results from a combination of factors: the extreme heating and cooling of large land masses in relation to the less marked changes in temperature of the adjacent seas; the northward movement of the Intertropical Convergence Zone (ITCZ); and the effect of the Himalayas on the circulation of the air.

In March, winds blow outward from the mainland. But as the Sun and the ITCZ move northward, the land is intensely heated, and a low-pressure system develops. The southeast trade winds change direction and are sucked into the interior to become southwesterlies, bringing heavy rain. By November, the Sun and the ITCZ have again moved south and the wind directions are again reversed. Cool winds blow from the Asian interior to the sea, losing any moisture on the Himalayas before descending to the coast.

TEMPERATURE

Average temperature in January

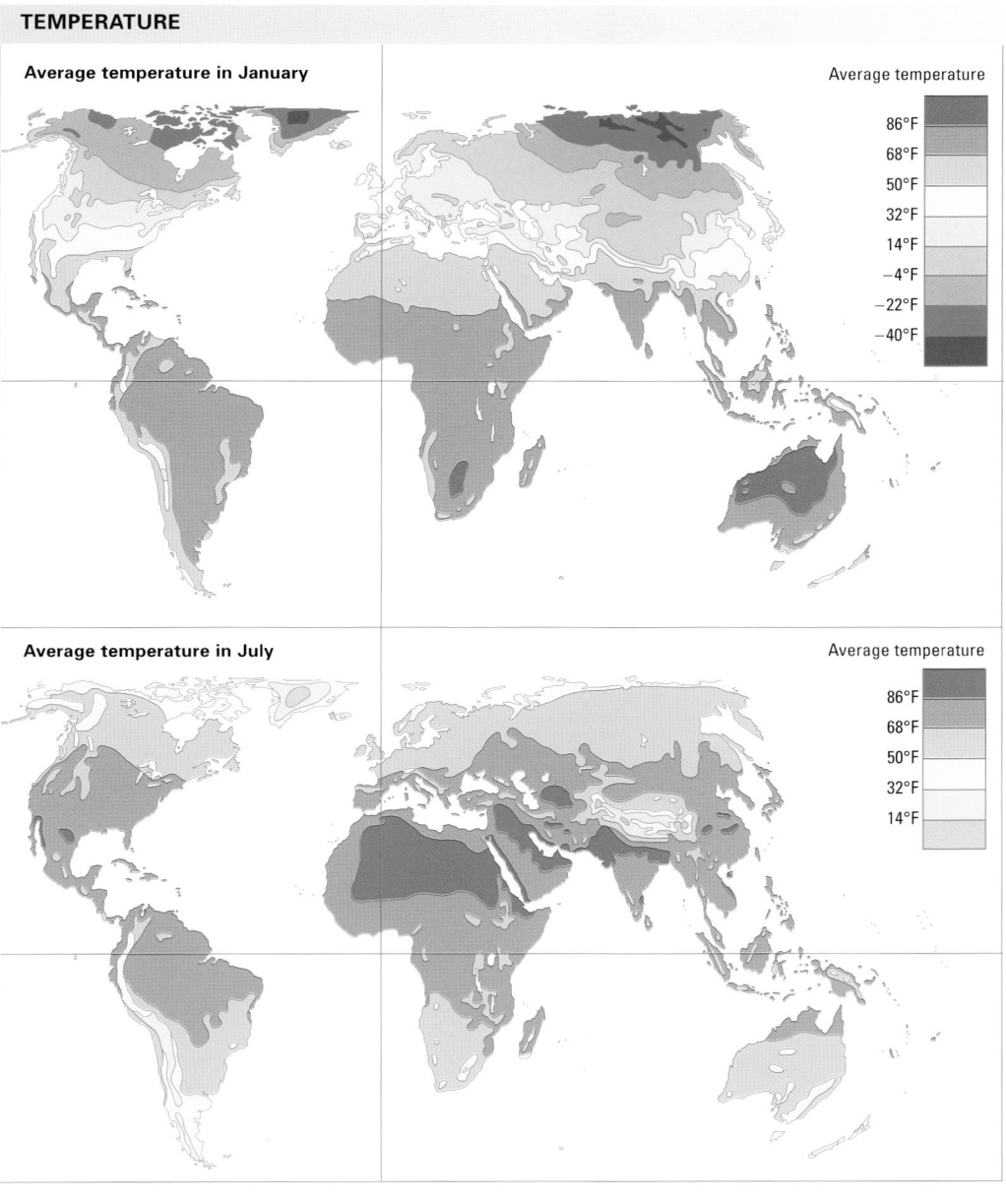

Average temperature

- 86°F
- 68°F
- 50°F
- 32°F
- 14°F
- –4°F
- –22°F
- –40°F

Average temperature in July

Average temperature

- 86°F
- 68°F
- 50°F
- 32°F
- 14°F

PRECIPITATION (RAINFALL AND SNOW)

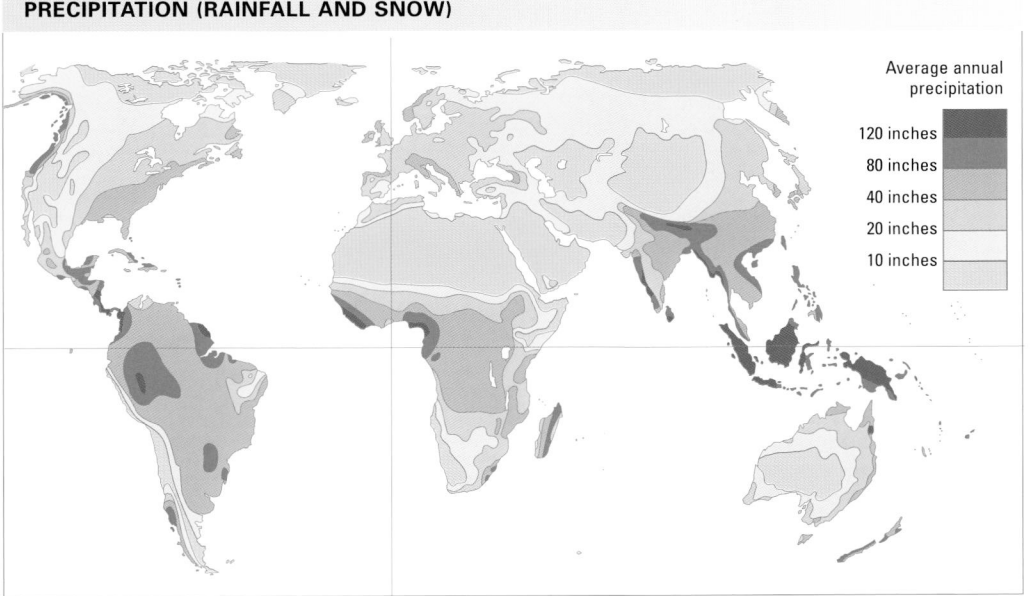

Average annual precipitation

- 120 inches
- 80 inches
- 40 inches
- 20 inches
- 10 inches

CLIMATE RECORDS

TEMPERATURE

Highest recorded temperature:
Al Aziziyah, Libya, 136.4°F [58°C], September 13, 1922.

Highest mean annual temperature:
Dallol, Ethiopia, 94°F [34.4°C], 1960–6.

Longest heatwave:
Marble Bar, W. Australia, 162 days over 100°F [38°C], October 23, 1923, to April 7, 1924.

Lowest recorded temperature (outside poles):
Verkhoyansk, Siberia, –90°F [–68°C], February 6, 1933. Verkhoyansk also registered the greatest annual range of temperature: –94°F to 98°F [–70°C to 37°C].

Lowest mean annual temperature:
Polus Nedostupnosti, Pole of Cold, Antarctica, –72°F [–57.8°C].

PRECIPITATION

Driest place:
Calama, N. Chile: no recorded rainfall in 400 years to 1971.

Wettest place (average):
Tututendo, Colombia: mean annual rainfall 463.4 inches [11,770 mm].

Wettest place (12 months):
Cherrapunji, Meghalaya, N.E. India, 1,040 inches [26,470 mm], August 1860 to August 1861. Cherrapunji also holds the record for rainfall in one month: 115 inches [2,930 mm], July 1861. (*See maps below.*)

Wettest place (24 hours):
Cilaos, Réunion, Indian Ocean, 73.6 inches [1,870 mm], March 15–16, 1952.

Heaviest hailstones:
Gopalganj, Bangladesh, up to 2.25 lb [1.02 kg], April 14, 1986 (killed 92 people).

Heaviest snowfall (continuous):
Bessans, Savoie, France, 68 inches [1,730 mm] in 19 hours, April 5–6, 1969.

Heaviest snowfall (season/year):
Paradise Ranger Station, Mt Rainier, Washington, USA, 1,224.5 inches [31,102 mm], February 19, 1971, to February 18, 1972.

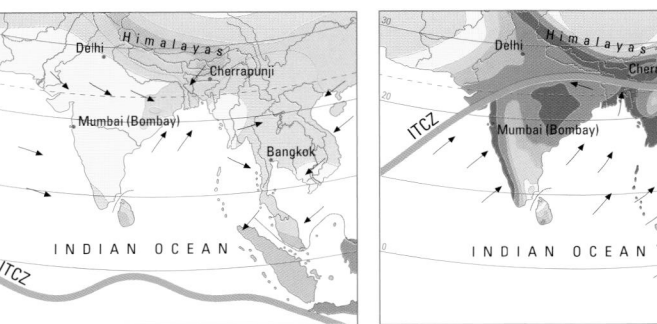

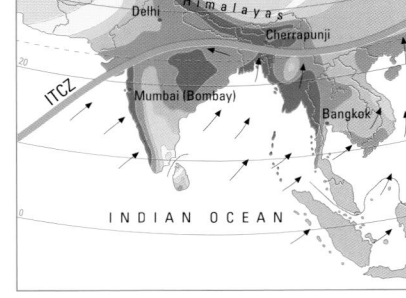

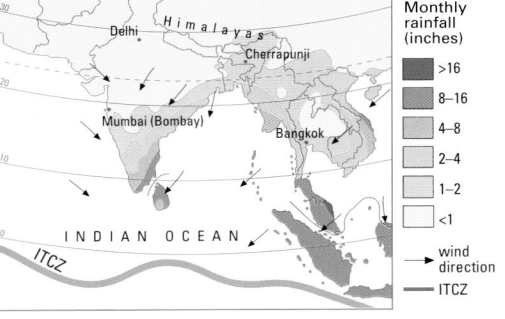

Monthly rainfall (inches)
- >16
- 8–16
- 4–8
- 2–4
- 1–2
- <1

→ wind direction
— ITCZ

March – Start of the hot, dry season. The ITCZ is over the southern Indian Ocean.

July – The rainy season. The ITCZ has migrated northward; winds blow onshore.

November – The ITCZ has returned south. The offshore winds are cool and dry.

WATER AND VEGETATION

For more information:
16 Climate regions
17 Precipitation
20 Biodiversity
23 Water pollution
    Deforestation

Without the hydrological cycle, by which water is constantly recycled between the oceans, the atmosphere and the land, the continents would be barren. Precipitation enables plants to grow and soils to form, creating the world's natural vegetation regions and the ecosystems that support animal life.

Running water also plays a major role in shaping landforms. Yet in many parts of the world, people do not have safe water to drink and suffer from diseases caused by water-borne organisms and pollution. In 2002, an estimated 1 billion people lacked access to safe water and 2.6 billion people lacked basic sanitation.

Experts argue that world demand for water is increasing at about twice the rate of population growth. It is predicted that, by 2025, half the world's population will face water shortages. This could lead to conflict and even boundary wars – 300 major rivers cross national frontiers and access to their water is likely to be disputed.

THE HYDROLOGICAL CYCLE

The world's water balance is regulated by the constant recycling of water between the oceans, the atmosphere and the land. The movement of water between these three reservoirs is known as the *hydrological cycle*. The oceans play a vital role in the hydrological cycle: 74% of the total precipitation falls over the oceans and 84% of the total evaporation comes from the oceans. Water vapor in the atmosphere circulates around the planet, transporting energy as well as the water itself. When the vapor cools, it falls as rain or snow. The whole cycle is driven by the Sun.

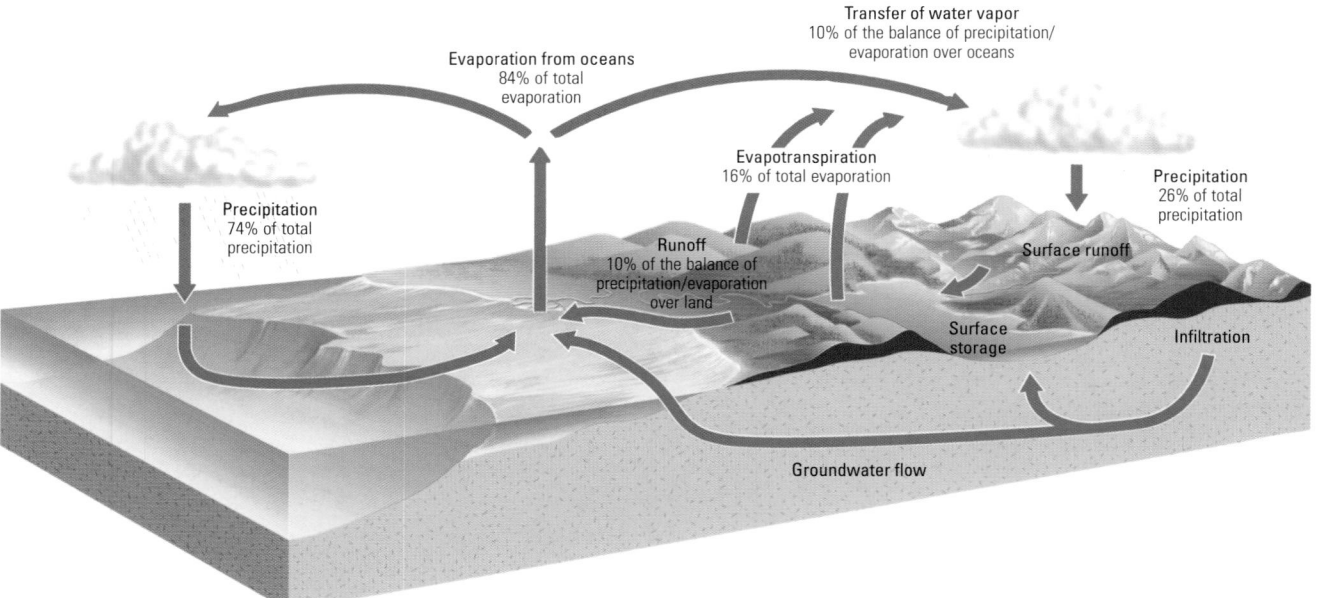

WATER DISTRIBUTION

The distribution of planetary water, by percentage. Oceans and ice caps together account for more than 99% of the total; the breakdown of the remainder is estimated.

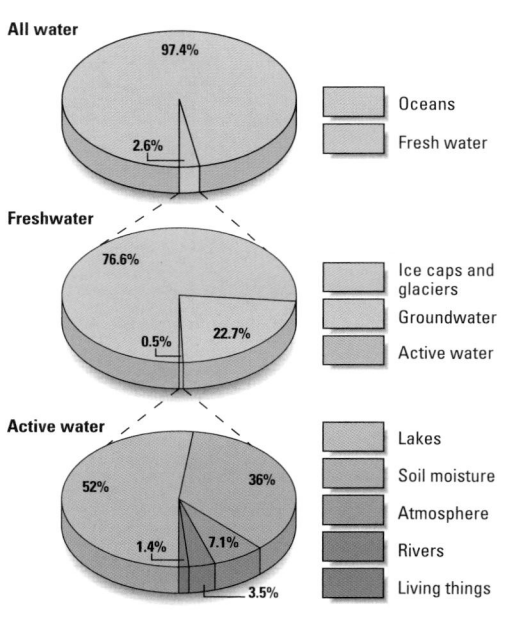

Almost all the world's water is 3,000 million years old, and all of it cycles endlessly through the hydrosphere, though at different rates. Water vapor circulates over days, even hours; deep-ocean water circulates over millennia; and ice-cap water remains solid for millions of years.

ANNUAL SEDIMENT YIELD

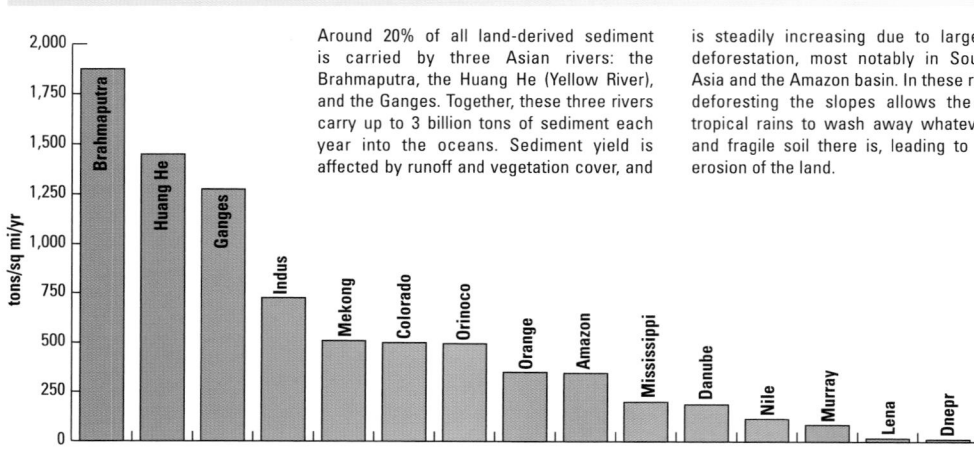

Around 20% of all land-derived sediment is carried by three Asian rivers: the Brahmaputra, the Huang He (Yellow River), and the Ganges. Together, these three rivers carry up to 3 billion tons of sediment each year into the oceans. Sediment yield is affected by runoff and vegetation cover, and is steadily increasing due to large-scale deforestation, most notably in Southeast Asia and the Amazon basin. In these regions, deforesting the slopes allows the heavy tropical rains to wash away whatever thin and fragile soil there is, leading to severe erosion of the land.

WATER RUNOFF

Annual freshwater runoff by continent in cubic miles

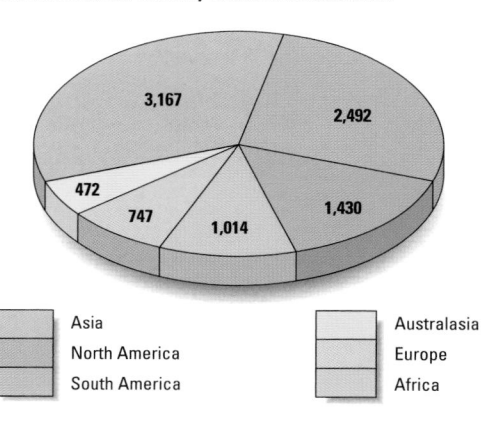

► The River Amazon is the world's second-longest river (after the River Nile), draining the vast rain forest basin of northern South America. The Amazon carries by far the greatest volume of water of any river in the world: the average rate of discharge is approximately 3,355,000 cu ft [95,000 cu m] per second, nearly three times as much as its nearest rival, the Congo. The flow is so great that its silt discolors the water up to 125 miles [200 km] into the Atlantic. At approximately 2.7 million sq miles [7 million sq km], the Amazon basin comprises nearly 40% of the whole of South America.

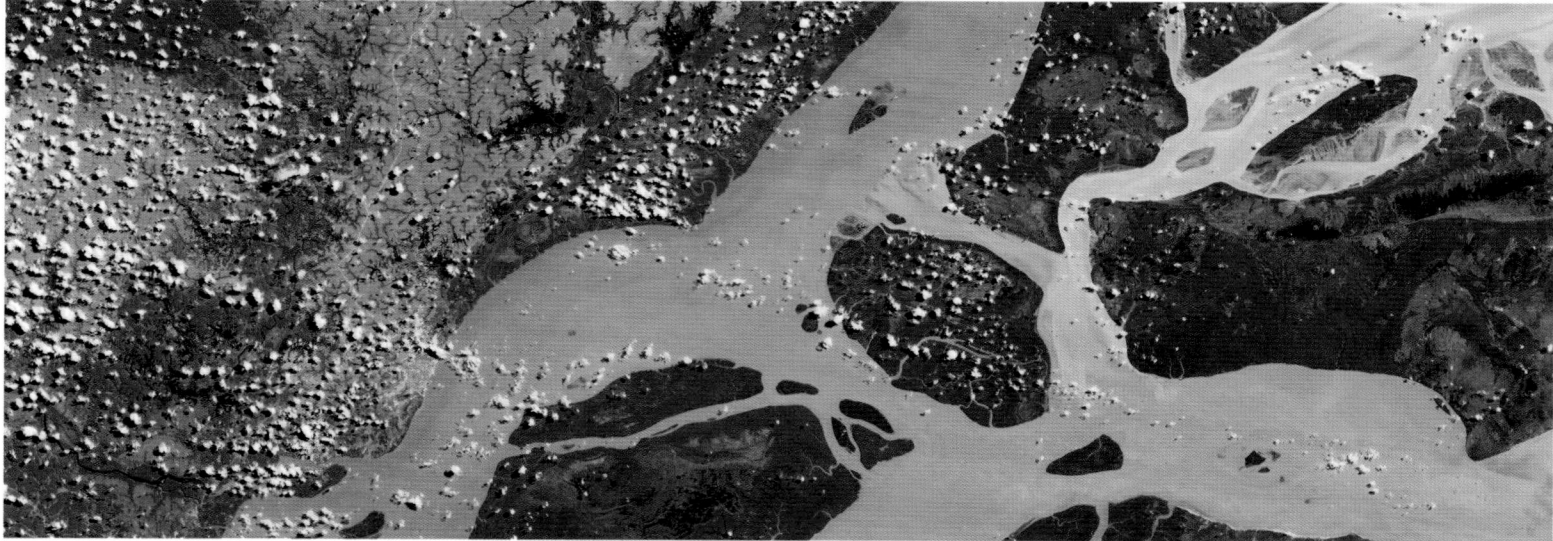

18

WATERSHEDS

The map below shows the world's major rivers, with the ranking of the 20 longest rivers shown in square brackets after their name, led by the Nile [1] and the Amazon [2].

The map shows the direction of freshwater flow on a continental scale, whereas the water runoff chart on the facing page indicates the quantities involved annually.

The rate of runoff varies seasonally and is affected by the surface vegetation and climate. Most of the world's major rivers discharge into the Atlantic Ocean.

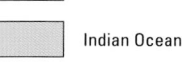

Where the rivers run

	Pacific Ocean
	Indian Ocean
	Arctic Ocean
	Atlantic Ocean
	Caribbean Sea– Gulf of Mexico
	Mediterranean Sea
	Inland basins, ice caps and deserts

NATURAL VEGETATION

The map below illustrates the natural "climax vegetation" of a region, as dictated by its climate and topography. In most cases, human agricultural activity has drastically altered the pattern of the vegetation. Western Europe, for example, lost most of its broadleaf forests many centuries ago, while elsewhere irrigation has turned some natural semideserts into productive land. The various vegetation regions support different kinds of animals and wildlife, and, in an undisturbed state, they are highly developed biological communities, or "biomes."

The blue line on the map represents the northern limit of tree growth, and the red lines indicate the northern and southern limits of palm growth.

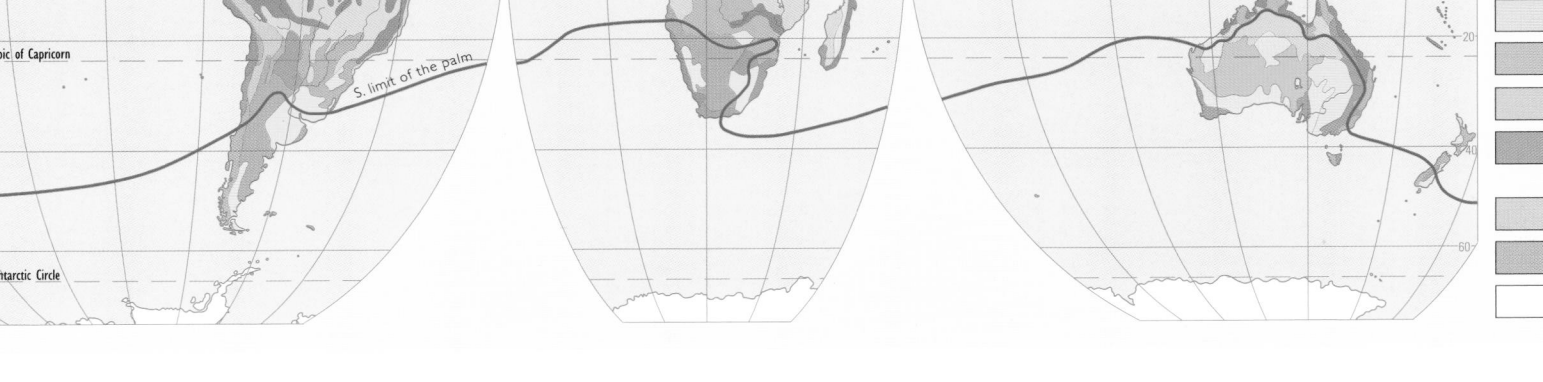

- Tropical rain forest
- Subtropical and temperate rain forest
- Monsoon woodland and open jungle
- Subtropical and temperate woodland, scrub, and bush
- Tropical savanna, with low trees and bush
- Tropical savanna and grasslands
- Dry semidesert, with shrub and grass
- Desert shrub
- Desert
- Dry steppe and shrub
- Temperate grasslands, prairie, and steppe
- Mediterranean hardwood forest and scrub
- Temperate deciduous forest and meadow
- Temperate deciduous and coniferous forest
- Northern coniferous forest (taïga)
- Mountainous forest, mainly coniferous
- High plateau steppe and tundra
- Arctic tundra
- Polar and mountainous ice desert

THE NATURAL ENVIRONMENT

For more information:

8 Oceans
14 Atmosphere
19 Natural vegetation
22 Carbon dioxide
   Greenhouse power
   Global warming
23 Acid rain
   Desertification
   Deforestation
   Water pollution

Recent discoveries of life forms in some of the world's most hostile environments, such as around the black smokers along the ocean ridges, prepared the way for the announcement by NASA scientists in 1996 that they had found microfossils in a Martian meteorite. But other scientists were sceptical, believing them to be natural mineral structures and not evidence of extraterrestrial life.

Until further evidence is available, the Earth remains the only planet where we know for sure that life exists. According to the fossil record, life on Earth appeared at least 3,500 million years ago. Since then, it has evolved from its primitive beginnings to its modern biodiversity, including millions of plants, animals and micro-organisms. Living organisms have not only adapted to the environ-ment, but they have also changed their environment to suit themselves. For example, the Earth's early atmosphere contained little oxygen, but the emergence of multicelled, oxygen-producing algae, around 2,000 million years ago, led to the creation of an oxygen-rich atmosphere. This enabled land animals to populate the ancient continents.

The amount of the greenhouse-gas carbon dioxide in the atmosphere would steadily increase from its present 0.03% were it not for plants. Without them, the Earth's atmos-phere would, in a few million years, be similar to that of Venus, where surface temperatures reach 890°F. The Earth has evolved into a complex control system, sensing and reacting to changes and tending always to maintain the balance it has achieved.

Much discussion has centered on how that balance changes. Only recently, scientists were suggesting that we may be living in an interglacial stage of the Pleistocene Ice Age. Since the 1980s, however, predictions of future climate patterns have concentrated more on global warming, caused by pollution that has led to an increase in greenhouse gases in the atmosphere. Interference in the natural cycles that control the environment may have consequences that are hard to predict.

Furthermore, we are currently experienc-ing a period of mass extinction of species, causing a rapid reduction in our planet's biodiversity. In 2002, a report by the Inter-national Union for the Conservation of Nature listed 11,167 organisms facing extinction. This was 121 more than in 2000.

THREATENED MAMMALS

The map shows the percentage of mammal species classified as threatened in 2002. Many scientists believe we are currently experiencing a period of mass extinction of species, rivaling five other periods in the past half a billion years. Among the most threatened mammals today are elephants, primates, and rhinoceroses.

Over 50%
25 – 50%
10 – 25%
5 – 10%
Under 5%
No data available

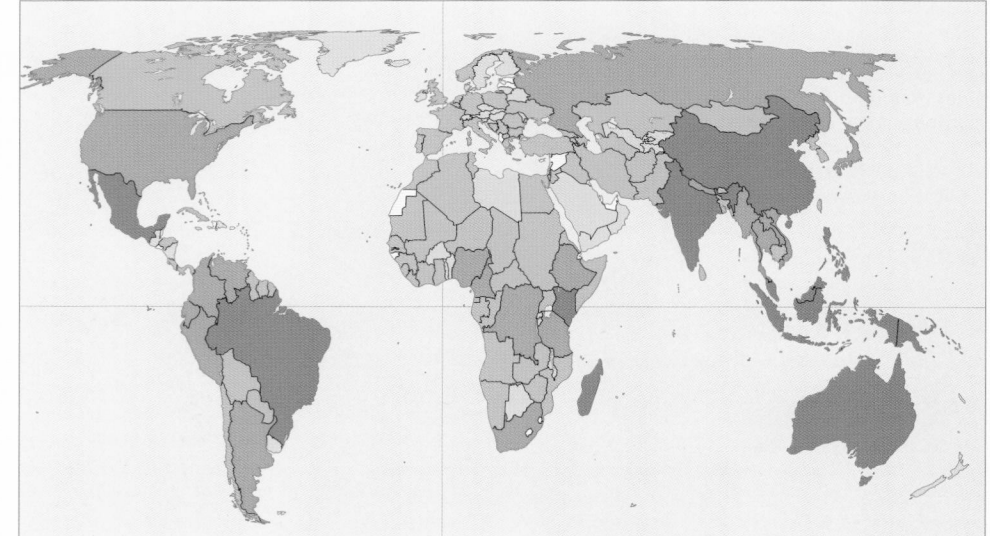

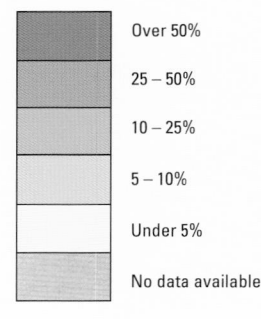

BIODIVERSITY IN CALIFORNIA, USA

This false-color satellite image of central California shows San Francisco lying just below the entrance to San Francisco Bay, with Oakland on the far side and San Jose to the southeast. California, nick-named the Golden State, is the third largest state in the United States and the most populous.

Due to its varied terrain and climate, California has a wide range of diverse habitats within a relatively small area. East of the forested Coast Ranges (the gray and red areas just inland from the bay) lies the fertile Central Valley, which appears as a red-and-blue checkerboard. In the northwest and southwest of the state (*not shown here*) lie parts of the Basin and Range region, much of which is desert. It includes Death Valley, which contains the country's lowest point on land, at 282 feet below sea level.

Natural vegetation
Forests cover about 40% of California and they include bristlecone pines, thought to be the oldest living things on Earth, together with coastal red-woods, the world's tallest trees. Wildlife is still abundant, though some species, such as the rare California condor, are on the endangered list.

The state has achieved much to protect its biodiversity. It contains eight of the 56 national parks in the United States. Two of them, Death Valley and Joshua Tree, were designated national parks as recently as 1994, as part of a conservation measure, including the protection of large areas of wilderness in the deserts.

California has vast resources and, were it a separate nation, it would rank among the world's ten most productive in terms of the total value of its goods and services. This means that, like the United States as a whole, it has resources, which many developing countries lack, to finance conservation measures. For example, the World Conservation Union reported in 1996 that 8% of mammals were threatened in the United States, as compared with 32% in the Philippines and 44% in Madagascar, two countries where habitat destruction has been proceeding on a large scale.

THE EARTH'S ENERGY BALANCE

Apart from a modest quantity of internal heat from its molten core, the Earth receives all of its energy from the Sun. If the planet is to remain at a constant temperature, it must reradiate exactly as much energy as it receives. Even a minute surplus would lead to a warmer Earth, a deficit to a cooler one. The temperature at which thermal equilibrium is reached depends on many factors, including the relative brightness of the Earth (its index of reflectivity, called the "albedo") and the heat-trapping capacity of the atmosphere (the "greenhouse effect").

Most of the Sun's energy arrives in the form of short-wave radiation. Some of the energy is reflected straight back into space, while some is absorbed by the atmosphere or by the Earth itself. Absorbed energy heats the Earth and its atmosphere alike, but since its temperature is much lower than that of the Sun, the outgoing energy is emitted at longer infrared wavelengths.

The diagram (*right*) shows short-wave radiation in yellow, with long-wave radiation in orange.

THE GREENHOUSE EFFECT

Constituting less than 1% of the atmosphere, the natural greenhouse gases (water vapor, carbon dioxide, methane, nitrous oxide, and ozone) have a disproportionate effect on the Earth's climate, and even its habitability. Like the glass panes in a greenhouse, the gases are transparent to most incoming short-wave radiation, which passes freely to heat the planet beneath. But when the warmed Earth retransmits that energy, in the form of longer-wave infrared radiation, the gases function as an opaque shield, preventing some of it from escaping, so that the planetary surface (like the interior of a greenhouse) stays relatively hot.

Over the last 150 years, there has been a gradual increase in the levels of greenhouse gases (with the exception of water vapor, which remains a constant in the system). Current predictions suggest that there could be a further rise of 2.5–8°F by the year 2100. A serious reduction in the greenhouse gases would be just as damaging, though. A total absence of carbon dioxide, for example, would leave the planet with a temperature roughly 60°F colder than it is at present.

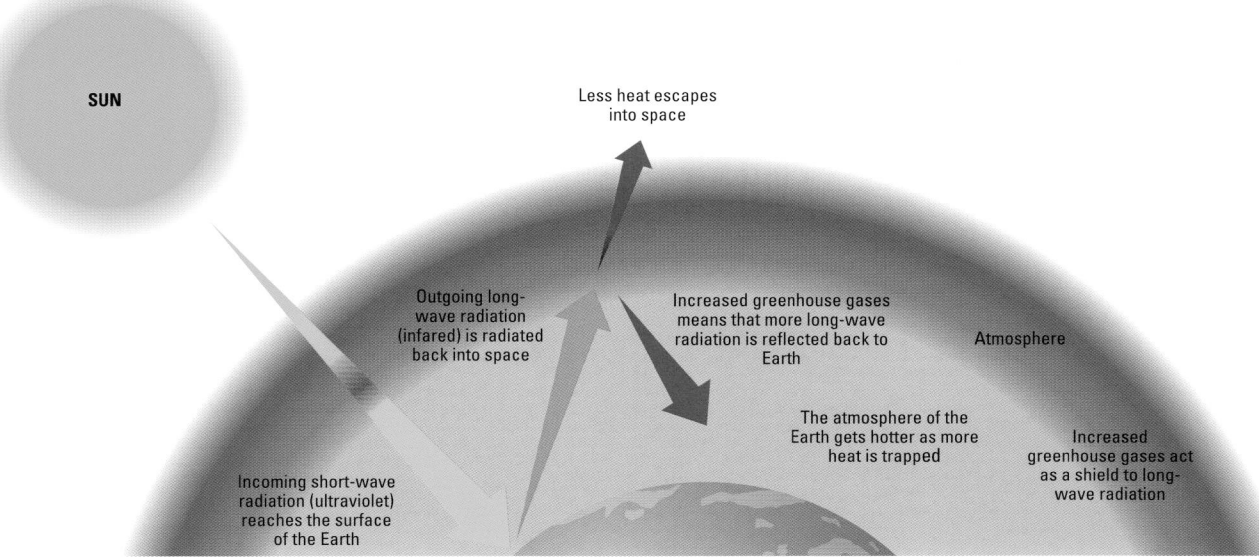

23% reflected by the cloud layer

25% absorbed by the atmosphere

21% diffuse radiation, some scattered back into space

3% absorbed by the clouds

Atmosphere

24% reaches the Earth's surface

Clouds

4% reflected from Earth's surface

SUN

Less heat escapes into space

Outgoing long-wave radiation (infared) is radiated back into space

Increased greenhouse gases means that more long-wave radiation is reflected back to Earth

Atmosphere

The atmosphere of the Earth gets hotter as more heat is trapped

Increased greenhouse gases act as a shield to long-wave radiation

Incoming short-wave radiation (ultraviolet) reaches the surface of the Earth

THE CARBON CYCLE

The Earth has a huge supply of carbon, only a small quantity of which is in the form of carbon dioxide. Of that, around 98% is dissolved in the sea; the fraction circulating in the air amounts to only 340 parts per million of the atmosphere, where its capacity as a greenhouse gas is the key regulator of the planetary temperature.

Living things, however, circulate carbon. Plants absorb carbon dioxide from the atmosphere and the carbon is then returned to circulation when the plants die, or is passed up the food chain to the herbivores, and then to the carnivores that feed on them. As organisms at each of these trophic levels

die, they decay, releasing the carbon, which then combines once more with the oxygen released during life. However, a small proportion of carbon is removed almost permanently, buried beneath mud on land or at sea, sinking as dead matter to the ocean floor. In time, it is slowly compressed into sedimentary rocks, such as limestone and chalk.

The carbon cycle has continued for a very long time. However, human beings have found a way to release fixed carbon at a faster rate than existing global systems can recirculate it. It has taken only a few human generations to deplete the fossil fuels that represent many millions of years of carbon accumulation.

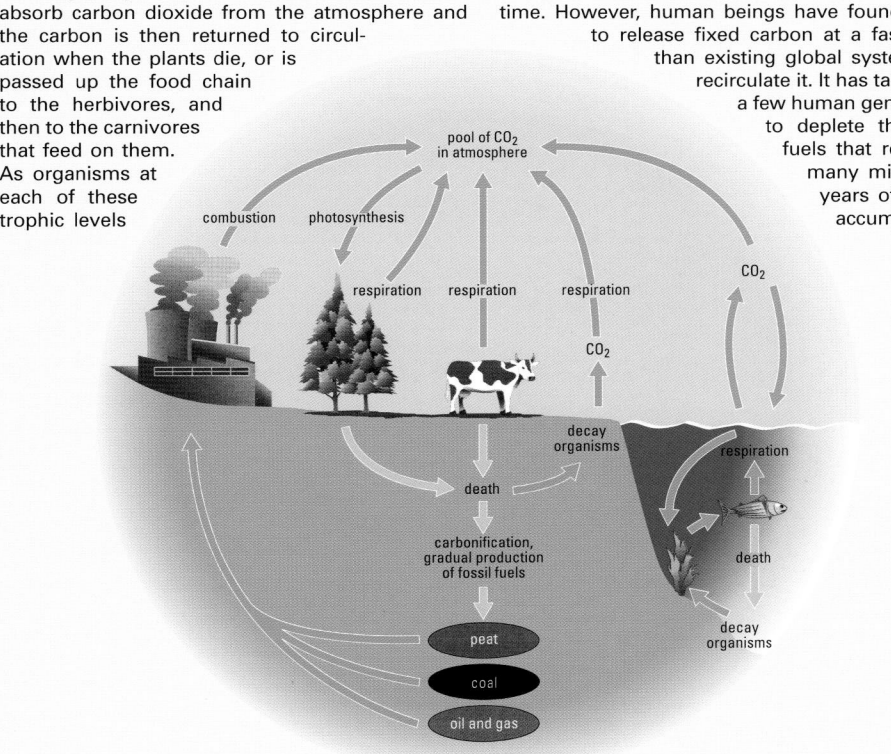

pool of CO₂ in atmosphere

combustion photosynthesis

respiration respiration respiration

CO₂

CO₂

decay organisms

respiration

death

death

carbonification, gradual production of fossil fuels

decay organisms

peat

coal

oil and gas

CARBON MONOXIDE CONCENTRATION

A colorless, odorless and poisonous gas, carbon monoxide (CO) is formed during the incomplete combustion of fossil fuels, occurring, for example, in coal gas and the exhaust fumes of cars. It is a major air pollutant and is now regulated by many world nations. The images below show the seasonal amounts and geographical sources of atmospheric carbon monoxide in the spring and summer months. Progressively higher levels of carbon monoxide are shown in green, yellow, orange, and red, while the blue areas have little or no atmospheric carbon monoxide.

Carbon monoxide can remain in the atmosphere for up to several months and can affect air quality in regions that are a long way from the original source of the pollution emissions.

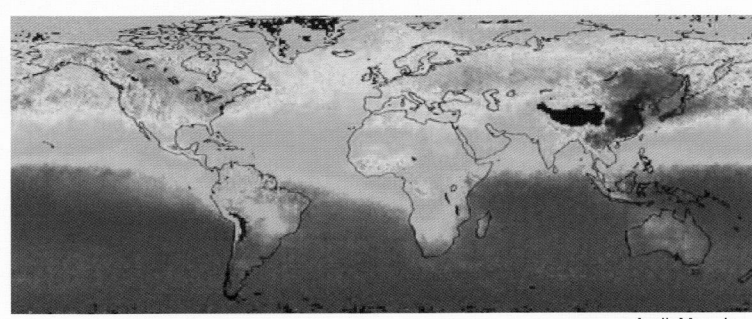

April, May, June

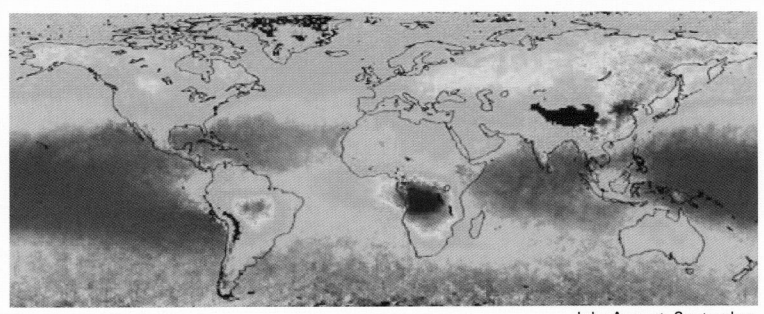

July, August, September

Carbon monoxide concentration (parts per billion by volume)

0   50   100   150   200   >250   no data

21

PEOPLE AND THE ENVIRONMENT

For more information:
8 Oceans
14 Atmosphere
16 Climate
21 Greenhouse effect
26 Urban pollution

In 1996, the Intergovernmental Panel on Climate Change issued a report stating that "The balance of evidence suggests a discernible human influence on global climate through emissions of carbon dioxide and other greenhouse gases." The report acknowledged that average global temperatures had risen by about 0.9°F since the mid-19th century, though there were still reasons for caution on attributing this entirely to actions taken by humans.

Human interference with nature is nothing new, at least since people turned from hunting and gathering to agriculture more than 10,000 years ago. At first, human actions seemed to have no ill effects because the systems that regulate the global environment were able to absorb damage. But from the late 18th century, the Industrial Revolution and the population explosion have caused massive pollution that threatens to overwhelm the Earth's ability to cope.

The 20th century experienced many disasters, including the dumping of industrial wastes in rivers and seas, accidents at nuclear power stations, and the creation of acid rain through the release of sulfur dioxides and nitrous oxides by the burning of fossil fuels. The release of greenhouse gases are held to be the main reason for global warming, while CFCs (chlorofluorocarbons) have damaged the ozone layer in the stratosphere, the planet's screen against ultraviolet radiation.

In December 1998, an international conference in Kyoto, Japan, reached an agreement to reduce the emission of greenhouse gases by 5.2% by 2012. But, in the early 21st century, the United States, which produces about a third of all emissions, opposed the Kyoto protocol.

Global warming will lead to melting ice sheets and the flooding of fertile coastal plains. Computer models suggest that it might affect ocean currents so that northwestern Europe, which owes its mild climate to the Gulf Stream, could expect bitterly cold winters. Some models have also suggested that cloud cover could increase, reflecting more solar energy back into space and thus start a new Ice Age.

In many tropical areas, deforestation is making productive land barren, while in the dry grasslands bordering deserts, the removal of plant cover is causing desertification. But human ingenuity can respond to this crisis in planet management.

GLOBAL WARMING

High atmospheric concentrations of heat-absorbing gases appear to be causing a rise in average temperatures worldwide – up to 3°F [1.5°C] by the year 2020, according to some estimates. Global warming is likely to bring about a rise in sea levels that may flood some of the world's densely populated coastal areas.

Evidence of global warming is attributed mainly to the "greenhouse effect," caused by the emission of certain gases, notably carbon dioxide, into the atmosphere (*see page 21*). Despite international action to control emissions of some greenhouse gases, carbon dioxide levels are still rising.

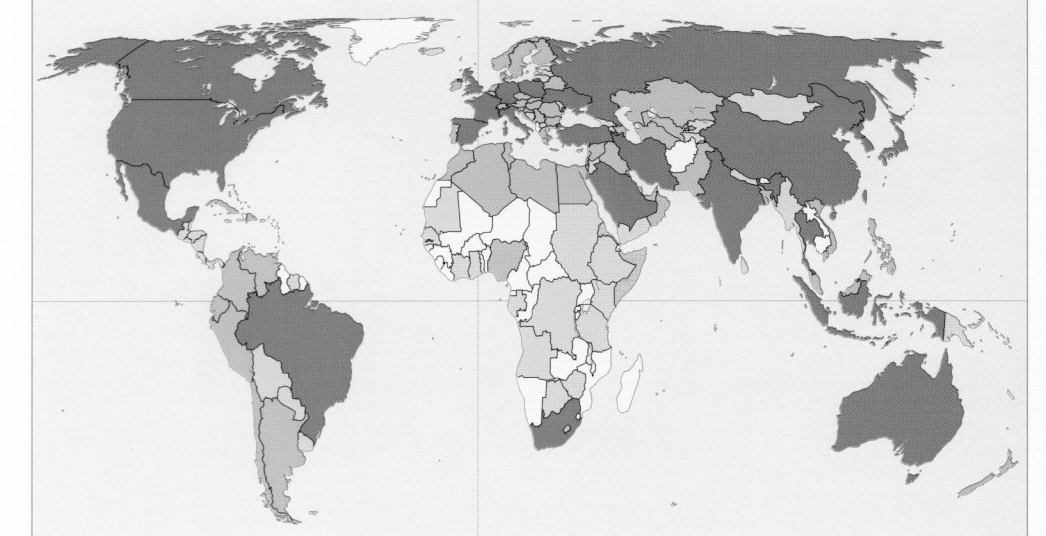

Carbon dioxide emissions in tons (latest available year)

- Over 50 million
- 5 – 50 million
- 0.5 – 5 million
- Under 0.5 million
- No data available

GREENHOUSE POWER

Relative contributions to the "greenhouse effect" by the major heat-absorbing gases in the atmosphere
The chart combines greenhouse potency and volume. Carbon dioxide has a greenhouse potential of only 1, but its concentration of 350 parts per million makes it predominate. CFC 12, with 25,000 times the absorption capacity of CO_2, is present only as 0.00044 ppm.

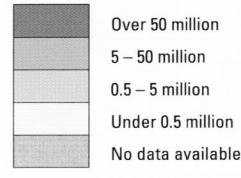

- Carbon dioxide (CO_2)
- Ozone
- Methane
- Nitrous oxide
- CFC 12
- CFC 11

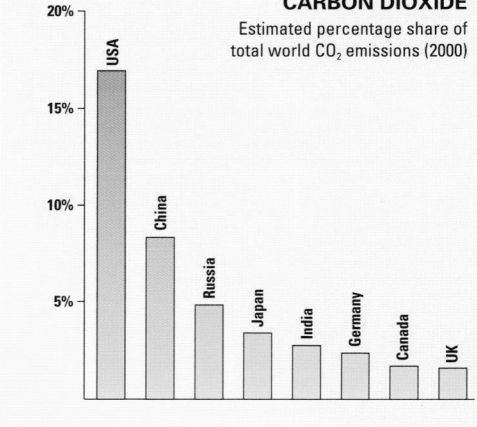

CARBON DIOXIDE
Estimated percentage share of total world CO_2 emissions (2000)

USA, China, Russia, Japan, India, Germany, Canada, UK

TEMPERATURE RISE
The rise in average temperatures caused by carbon dioxide and other greenhouse gases, assuming present trends continue (1960–2020)

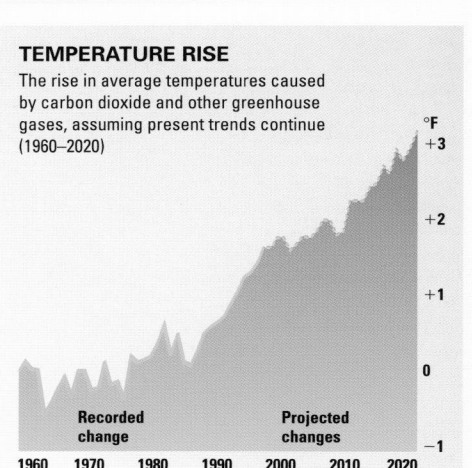

Recorded change — Projected changes

1960 1970 1980 1990 2000 2010 2020

THE THINNING OZONE LAYER

Total atmospheric ozone concentration in the southern and northern hemispheres (Dobson Units, 2000)
In 1985, scientists working in Antarctica discovered a thinning of the ozone layer, commonly known as an "ozone hole." This caused immediate alarm because the ozone layer absorbs most of the Sun's dangerous ultraviolet radiation, which is believed to cause an increase in skin cancer, cataracts, and damage to the immune system.

Since 1985, ozone depletion has increased and, by 2002, the ozone hole over the South Pole was estimated to be three times as large as the USA. The false-color images (*right*) show the total atmospheric ozone concentration in the southern hemisphere (in September 2000) and the northern hemisphere (in March 2000) with the ozone hole clearly identifiable at the centre. The data is from the Tiros weather satellite. The colors represent the ozone concentration in Dobson Units (DU).

Scientists agree that ozone depletion is caused by CFCs, a group of manufactured chemicals used in air-conditioning systems and refrigerators. In a 1987 treaty most industrial nations agreed to phase out CFCs and a complete ban on most CFCs was agreed after the end of 1995. However, scientists believe that the chemicals will remain in the atmosphere for 50 to 100 years. As a result, ozone depletion will continue for many years.

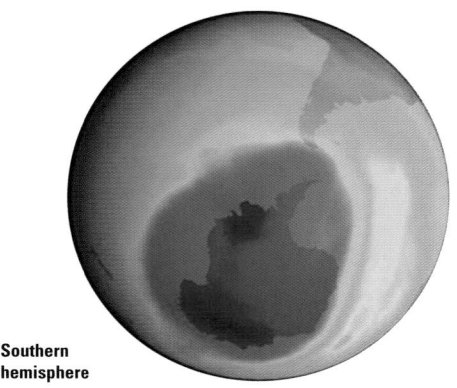

Southern hemisphere

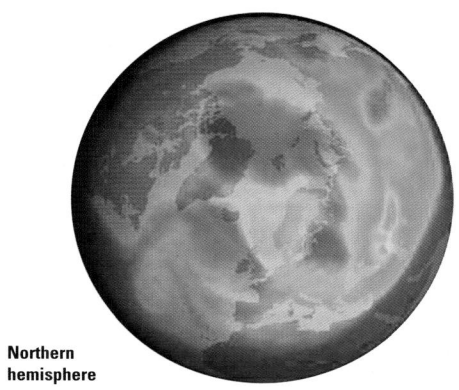

Northern hemisphere

WORLD POLLUTION

Acid rain and sources of acidic emissions (latest available year)
Acid rain is caused by high levels of sulfur and nitrogen in the atmosphere. They combine with water vapor and oxygen to form acids (H_2SO_4 and HNO_3) which fall as precipitation.

- Regions where sulfur and nitrogen oxides are released in high concentrations, mainly from fossil fuel combustion

- Major cities with high levels of air pollution (including nitrogen and sulfur emissions)

Areas of heavy acid deposition
pH numbers indicate acidity, decreasing from a neutral 7. Normal rain, slightly acid from dissolved carbon dioxide, never exceeds a pH of 5.6.

- pH less than 4.0 (most acidic)
- pH 4.0 to 4.5
- pH 4.5 to 5.0
- Areas where acid rain is a potential problem

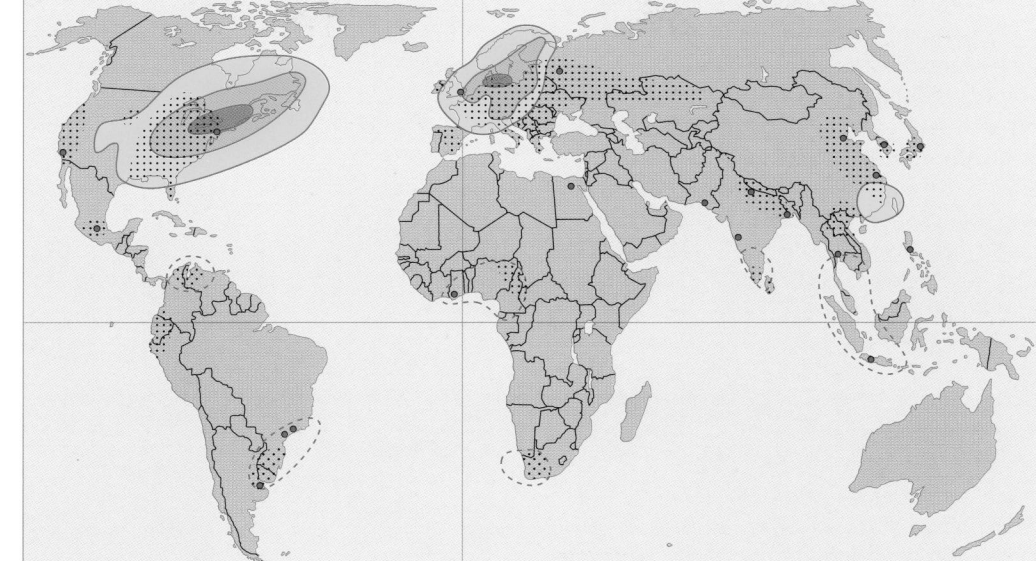

WATER POLLUTION

- Severely polluted sea areas and lakes
- Polluted sea areas and lakes
- Areas of frequent oil pollution by shipping
- Major oil tanker spills
- Major oil rig blow outs
- Offshore dumpsites for industrial and municipal waste
- Severely polluted rivers and estuaries

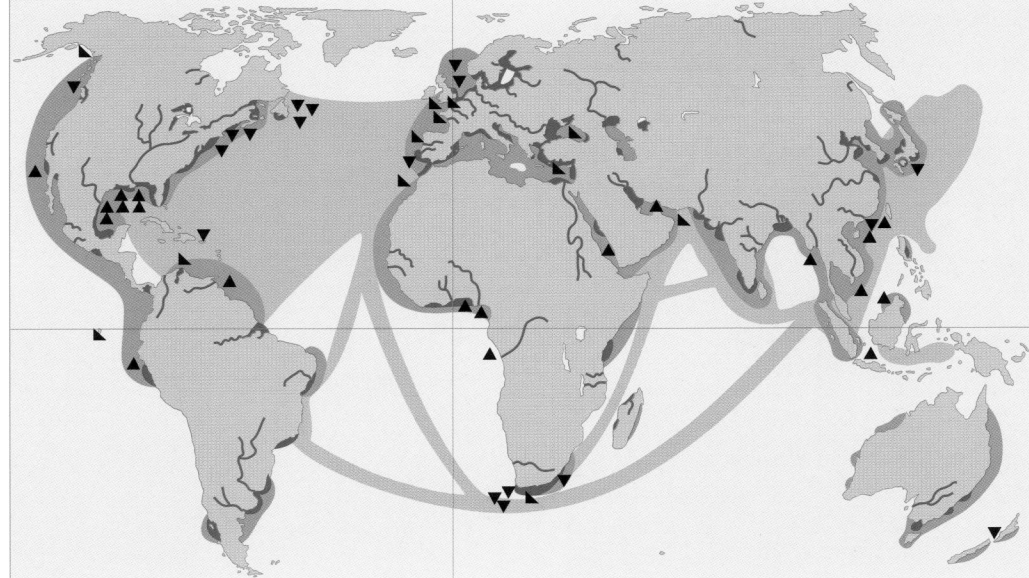

In December 2002, oil slicks from the 77,000-ton *Prestige* tanker, which broke up off Spain, caused environmental damage to the north coast of Spain and, in 2003, to the southwest coast of France. This was a small incident by comparison with some earlier events, such as the collision between the *Atlantic Empress* and the *Aegean Captain* in July 1979. This was the worst tanker incident ever, polluting the Caribbean with 1,890,000 barrels of crude oil.

Oil spills, however, declined in the 1980s, from a peak of 750,000 tons in 1979 to less than 50,000 tons in 1990. The most notorious spill of that period – when the *Exxon Valdez* ran aground in Prince William Sound, Alaska, in March 1989 – released only 267,000 barrels, a relatively small amount when compared with the 2,500,000 barrels spilled during the Gulf War of 1991. Oil spillage, poisoned rivers, and domestic sewage have in recent years badly contaminated parts of the oceans.

DESERTIFICATION

- Existing deserts
- Areas with a high risk of desertification
- Areas with a moderate risk of desertification
- Former areas of rain forest
- Existing rain forest

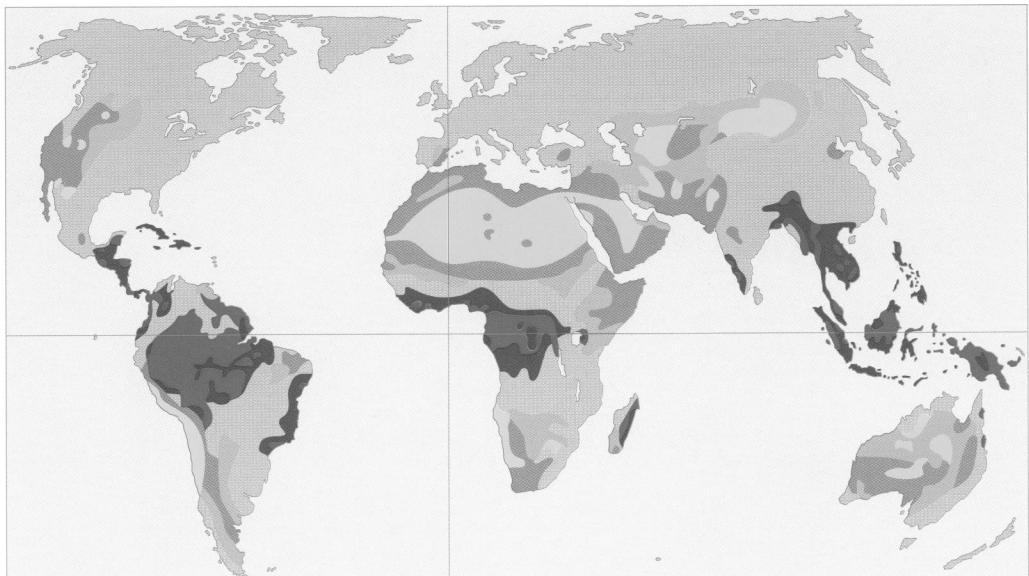

DEFORESTATION

Bolivia has over 100,000 sq miles [250,000 sq km] of dry tropical forest, home to animals such as jaguars and ocelots. It is, however, being cleared at a rate of over 2% per annum. This false-color image shows an area that has been almost completely cleared. The darkest areas are remnants of the original forest, some retained as wind breaks between newly created arable fields, growing such crops as soybeans.

Where deforestation occurs, there is an immediate danger that the vital topsoil will be eroded by wind or by rain. Proposals to clear large regions of the Amazonian rain forests, which play a key role in maintaining the Earth's oxygen balance, could cause an environmental catastrophe.

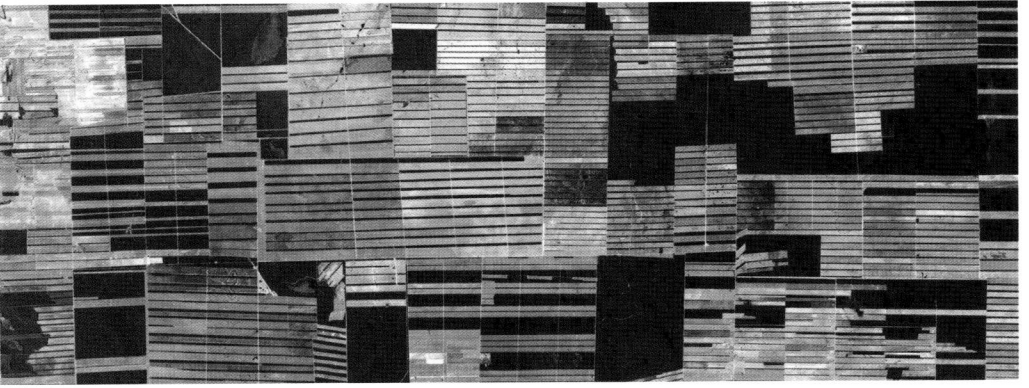

ANTARCTICA

The vast Antarctic ice sheet, containing some 70% of the Earth's fresh water, plays a crucial role in the circulation of the atmosphere and oceans, and hence the Earth's climate. The frozen southern continent is also the last remaining wilderness – the largest area to remain free from human colonization.

Various countries have pressed territorial claims over sections of Antarctica, spurred in recent years by its known and suspected mineral wealth: enough iron ore to supply the world at present levels for 200 years, large oil reserves and, probably, the biggest coal deposits on Earth.

The 1961 Antarctic Treaty set aside the area for peaceful uses only, guaranteeing freedom of scientific investigation, banning waste disposal and nuclear testing, and suspending the issue of territorial rights. By 1990, the original 12 signatories had grown to 25; a further 15 nations were granted observer status in subsequent deliberations.

In July 1991, a new accord banned all mineral exploration for a further 50 years. The ban can only be rescinded if all the present signatories, plus a majority of any future adherents, agree.

While the treaty has always lacked a formal mechanism for enforcement, it is firmly underwritten by public concern generated by the efforts of environmental pressure groups such as Greenpeace, which have campaigned vigorously to have Antarctica declared a "World Park."

However, from the mid-1990s, the continent appeared to be under threat from global warming, which some scientists believe was the cause of the breakup of ice shelves along the Antarctic peninsula. Rising temperatures have also disturbed the breeding patterns of Adelie penguins.

23

POPULATION

For more information:

26 Urbanization of the Earth

Urban population

27 Largest cities

33 Food and population

44 Wealth and population

In 8000 BC, following the development of agriculture, the world had an estimated population of 8 million and by AD 1000 it was about 300 million. The onset of the Industrial Revolution in the late 18th century led to a population explosion. The 1,000 million mark was passed by 1850, it doubled by the 1920s, and doubled again to 4,000 million by 1975.

In the 1990s, demographers estimated that the world's population, which passed the 6 billion mark in 1999, would reach 8.9 billion by 2050 and only level out in 2200, at a peak of around 11 billion. However, in the early 21st century, after the rate of population growth had shown signs of decline, the Institute for Applied Systems Analysis suggested that the world's population might peak at about 9 billion in 2070. Whatever the global projections, everyone agreed that the greatest population growth would be in the developing countries.

The developing world includes what the World Bank (2001) describes as low-income economies (average per capita GNP of US $420), lower-middle-income economies (average per capita GNP of US $1,200) and upper-middle-income economies (average per capita GNP of US $4,870). Most developing countries are in Africa, Asia, and Latin America. The developed world, made up of high-income, industrialized economies (average per capita GNP of US $26,440), contains Australasia, most of Europe and North America, and Japan.

In developing countries, a high proportion of the population is young and so these countries face high expenditure on health and education. In developed countries, the population pyramids are becoming top-heavy, with increasingly aging populations.

LARGEST NATIONS

The world's most populous nations, in millions (2003 est.)

1.	China	1,287
2.	India	1,050
3.	USA	290
4.	Indonesia	235
5.	Brazil	182
6.	Pakistan	151
7.	Russia	145
8.	Bangladesh	138
9.	Nigeria	134
10.	Japan	127
11.	Mexico	105
12.	Philippines	85
13.	Germany	82
14.	Vietnam	82
15.	Egypt	75
16.	Iran	68
17.	Turkey	68
18.	Ethiopia	67
19.	Thailand	64
20.	France	60
21.	UK	60
22.	Italy	58
23.	Congo (Dem.Rep.)	57
24.	South Korea	48
25.	Ukraine	48

MOST CROWDED NATIONS

Population per square mile (2003 est.)

1.	Monaco	80,000
2.	Singapore	17,727
3.	Vatican City	5,000
4.	Malta	3,333
5.	Maldives	2,750
6.	Bahrain	2,470
7.	Bangladesh	2,490
8.	Nauru	1,625
9.	Barbados	1,629
10.	Taiwan	1,626

LEAST CROWDED NATIONS

Population per square mile (2003 est.)

1.	Mongolia	4.5
2.	Namibia	6.1
3.	Australia	6.6
4.	Suriname	6.9
5.	Iceland	7.1
6.	Botswana	7.0
7.	Mauritania	7.4
8.	Libya	8.1
9.	Canada	8.4
10.	Guyana	8.5

POPULATION DENSITY

The places marked on the map reflect the size of the urban agglomerations and conurbations, rather than the actual city limits. San Francisco itself, for example, has an official population of less than a million people.

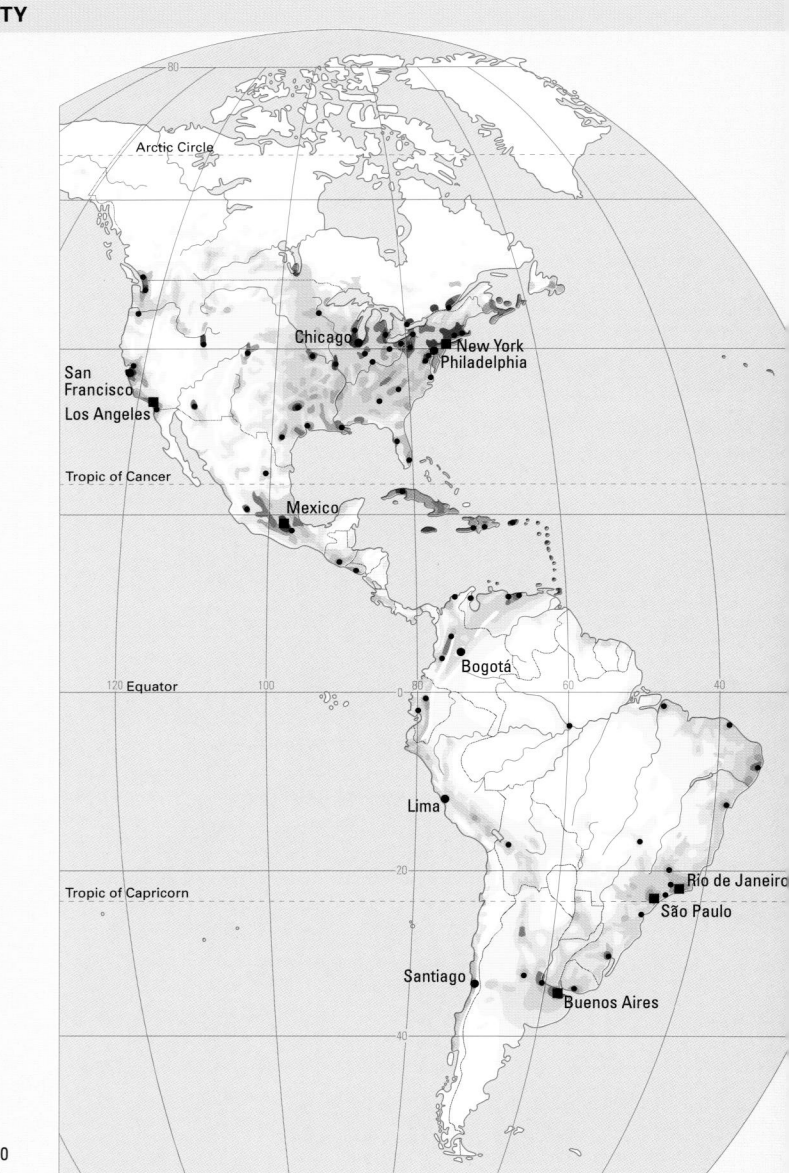

Inhabitants per square mile

- Over 500
- 250 – 500
- 125 – 250
- 65 – 125
- 15 – 65
- 8 – 15
- 3 – 8
- Under 3

Urban population

- ■ Over 10,000,000
- ● 5,000,000 – 10,000,000
- • 1,000,000 – 5,000,000

POPULATION CHANGE 1990–2000

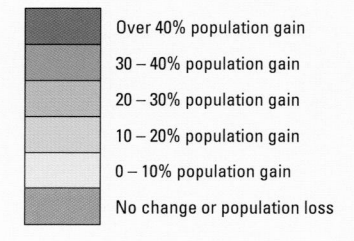

The population change for the years 1990–2000

- Over 40% population gain
- 30 – 40% population gain
- 20 – 30% population gain
- 10 – 20% population gain
- 0 – 10% population gain
- No change or population loss

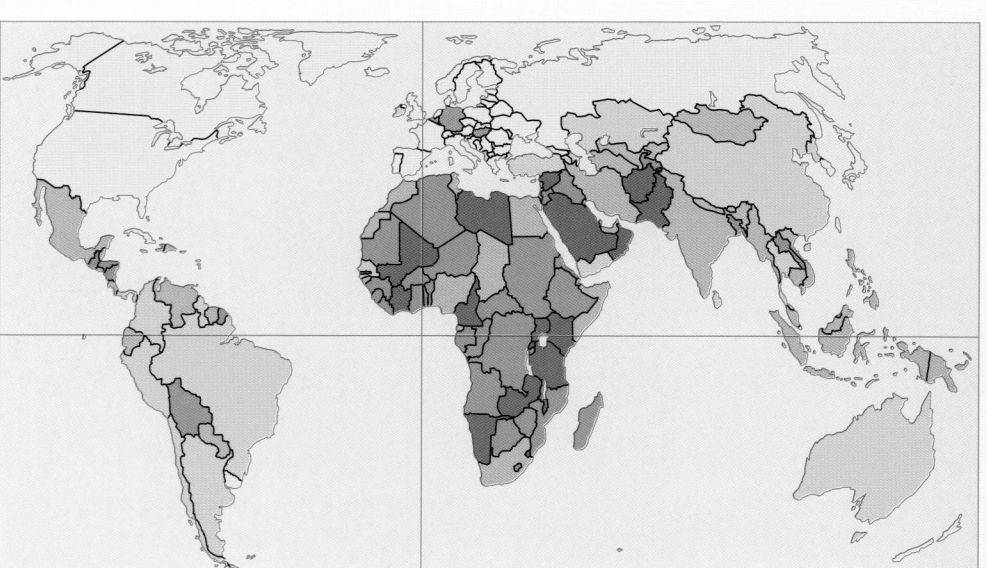

Top 5 countries		Bottom 5 countries	
Kuwait	+75.9%	Belgium	–0.1%
Namibia	+62.5%	Hungary	–0.2%
Afghanistan	+60.1%	Grenada	–2.4%
Mali	+55.5%	German	–3.2%
Tanzania	+54.6%	Tonga	–3.2%

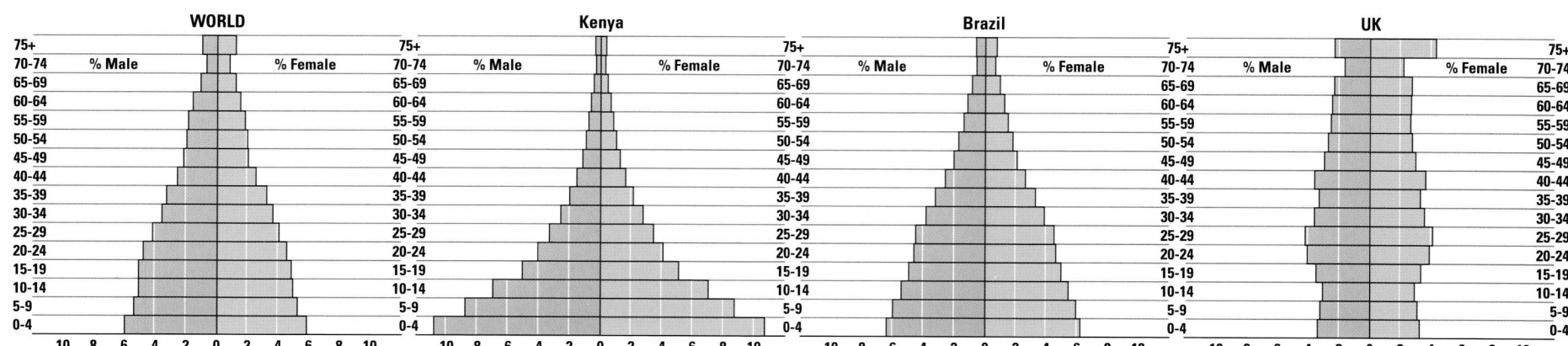

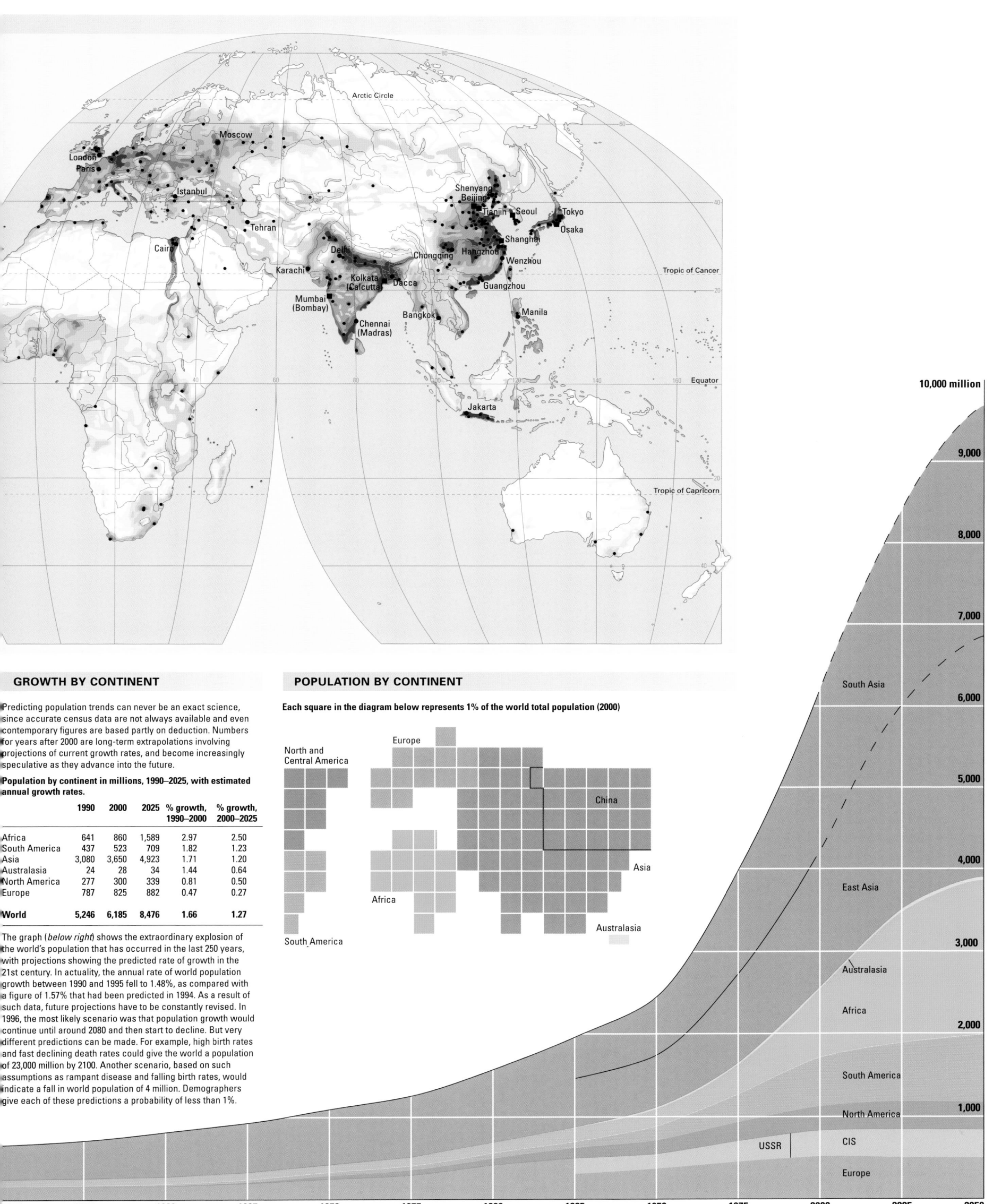

GROWTH BY CONTINENT

Predicting population trends can never be an exact science, since accurate census data are not always available and even contemporary figures are based partly on deduction. Numbers for years after 2000 are long-term extrapolations involving projections of current growth rates, and become increasingly speculative as they advance into the future.

Population by continent in millions, 1990–2025, with estimated annual growth rates.

	1990	2000	2025	% growth, 1990–2000	% growth, 2000–2025
Africa	641	860	1,589	2.97	2.50
South America	437	523	709	1.82	1.23
Asia	3,080	3,650	4,923	1.71	1.20
Australasia	24	28	34	1.44	0.64
North America	277	300	339	0.81	0.50
Europe	787	825	882	0.47	0.27
World	**5,246**	**6,185**	**8,476**	**1.66**	**1.27**

The graph (*below right*) shows the extraordinary explosion of the world's population that has occurred in the last 250 years, with projections showing the predicted rate of growth in the 21st century. In actuality, the annual rate of world population growth between 1990 and 1995 fell to 1.48%, as compared with a figure of 1.57% that had been predicted in 1994. As a result of such data, future projections have to be constantly revised. In 1996, the most likely scenario was that population growth would continue until around 2080 and then start to decline. But very different predictions can be made. For example, high birth rates and fast declining death rates could give the world a population of 23,000 million by 2100. Another scenario, based on such assumptions as rampant disease and falling birth rates, would indicate a fall in world population of 4 million. Demographers give each of these predictions a probability of less than 1%.

POPULATION BY CONTINENT

Each square in the diagram below represents 1% of the world total population (2000)

CITIES

For more information:

18 Water distribution
24 Population density
41 The great ports

Following the development of agriculture more than 10,000 years ago, people began to live in farming villages. Around 5,500 years ago, the world's first cities appeared in the lower Tigris and Euphrates valleys in Mesopotamia. Cities were founded in Ancient Egypt around 5,000 years ago and in China around 3,600 years ago. By contrast with the villages, most people in the early cities were not engaged in farming. Instead, they worked in craft industries, in government services, in religion, and in trade. The cities became centers of early civilizations and, through trade, their influence spread far and wide. However, they were dependent on the surrounding farming communities for their food and other materials.

In 1750, prior to the start of the Industrial Revolution, barely 3% of the world's population lived in urban areas. By 1850, London and Paris had more than a million people, and, by 1900, 14% of the world's population lived in cities. By 1950, the world had 83 cities with more than a million people, and

by 1996 there were 280; by 2015, experts predict there will be more than 500. New York City was the only city with a population in excess of 10 million in 1950; by 2015, experts predict there will be 27 such cities worldwide, the majority located in the developing world.

However, predictions have to be constantly revised in light of new data. For example, in the late 1990s, demographers calculated that urban areas then accounted for 50% of the world's population. But after much lower census figures emerged for many cities in the early 21st century, the estimated date by which half of the world's population would be living in cities was pushed back to 2007.

Urbanization is greatest in industrialized countries. For example, in 2000, 77.2% of the people in the United States lived in urban areas. However, in low-income countries, which contained nearly 60% of the world's population in the late 1990s, only 28% lived in urban areas.

The rapid rate of urbanization has created

many social problems, especially in cities that have been unable to provide enough jobs and services for the new arrivals. Many of the new city dwellers come from rural areas and take time to adjust to urban life and employment possibilities.

A typical city in a developing country contains millions of people living, often illegally, in shanty towns (or "informal settlements"), while thousands live on the streets. Yet many of these shanty towns are healthier than the industrial cities of 19th-century Europe and North America. Indeed, surveys have shown that migrants to cities in developing countries are less likely to face poverty than they are in rural areas, while benefiting from greater access to healthcare services and education.

Modern cities face many problems today, including pollution, crime, and unemployment. Yet, given competent central and local government, they are capable of generating the wealth they need to solve them, as well as making a major contribution to the nation's economy.

URBAN POPULATION

Percentage of total population living in towns and cities (2000)

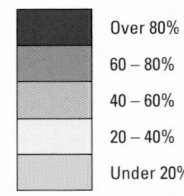

	Over 80%
	60 – 80%
	40 – 60%
	20 – 40%
	Under 20%

Most urbanized		Least urbanized	
Belgium	97%	Rwanda	6%
W. Sahara	96%	Bhutan	7%
Singapore	93%	East Timor	7%
UAE	93%	Burundi	9%
Iceland	93%	Nepal	11%

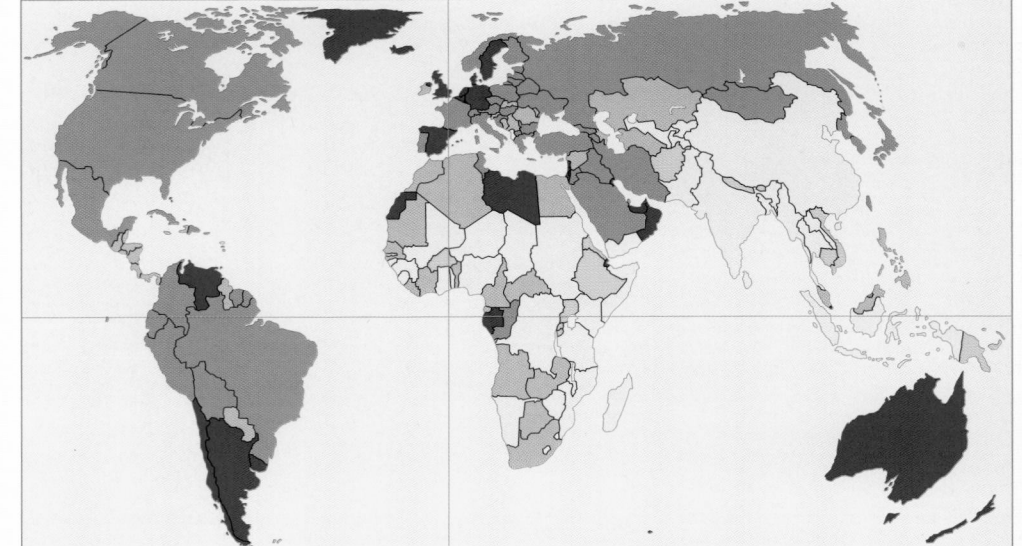

THE URBANIZATION OF THE EARTH

City-building, 1850–2000; each white spot represents a city of at least 1 million inhabitants

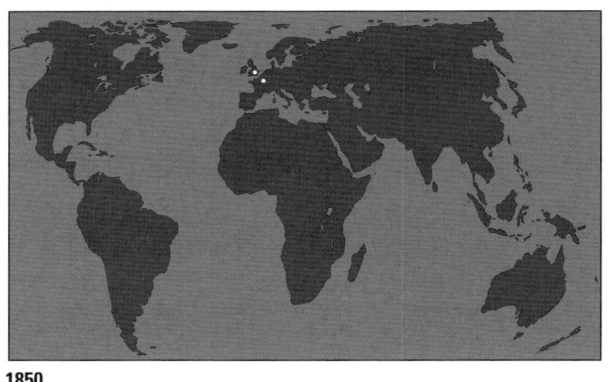

1850

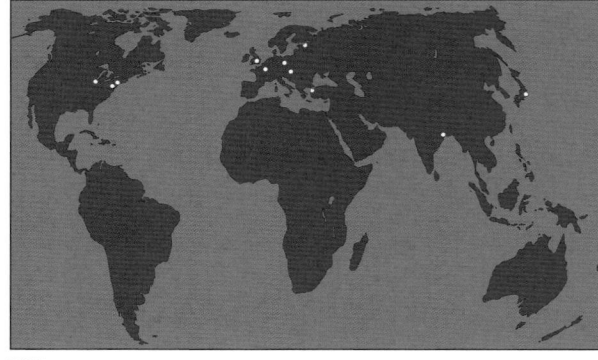

1900

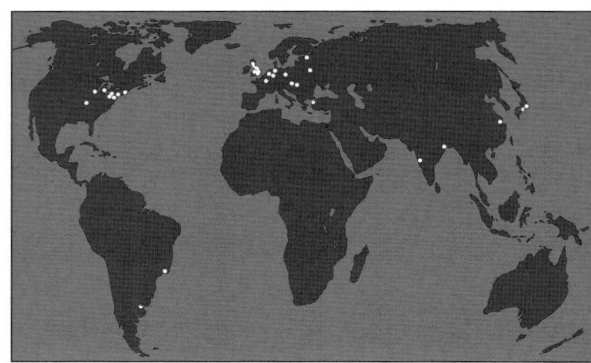

1925

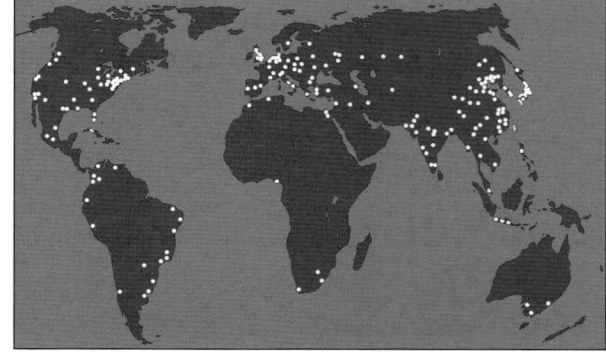

1950

1975

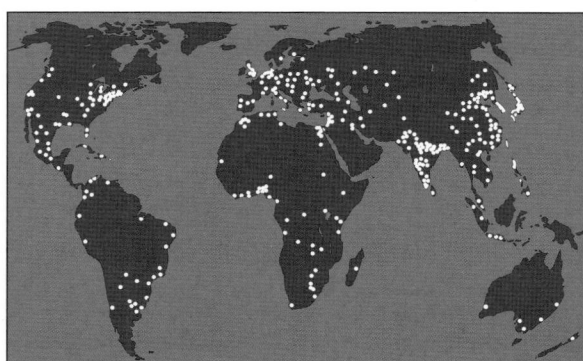

2000

EXPANDING CITIES

These graphs show the projected growth of some of the world's megacities between 1950 and 2015. New York City, the world's largest city in 1950, reached a peak in 1970, but it has since experienced periods of negative growth. London's population also declined between 1970 and 1985, before resuming a modest rate of increase.

In both cases, the divergence from world trends is explained in part by counting methods. Each lies at the center of a great agglomeration, and definitions of the "city limits" may vary over time. Also, in developing countries, many areas around the megacities, which are counted as urban, are in fact rural in character.

The rates of city population growth in developing countries have also often been over-estimated. For example, it was once predicted that Kolkata (Calcutta) would have a population of 40 million by the late 1990s. The reason why many estimates have proven incorrect is partly explained by a new trend, namely that rapid urban growth is now greatest, in some regions, in the smaller cities. For example, the main expansion in West Bengal is no longer in Kolkata (Calcutta), but in a rash of small cities across the state.

The growth of some of the world's largest cities in millions, 1950–2015
Comparisons of city populations over time are problematic due to changes in the definition of the city limits. These figures attempt to take such changes into consideration. The figure for London is the metropolitan region.

█ 1950 █ 2015

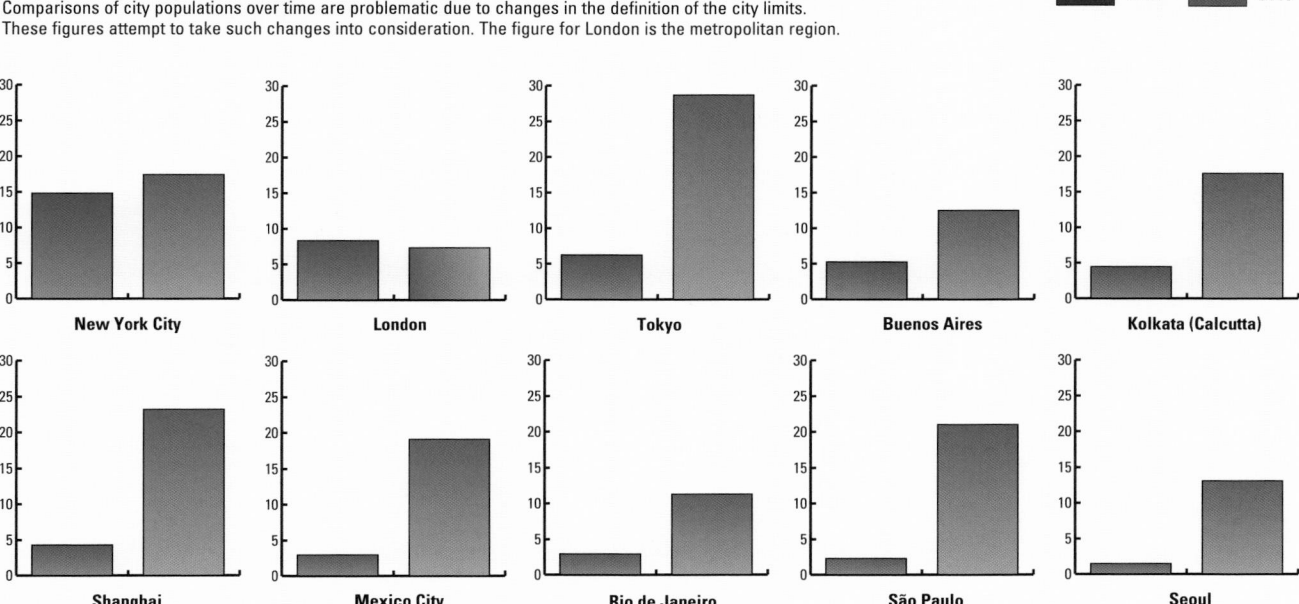

New York City | London | Tokyo | Buenos Aires | Kolkata (Calcutta)
Shanghai | Mexico City | Rio de Janeiro | São Paulo | Seoul

CITIES IN DANGER

In mid-2002, a "brown haze," stretching 2 mi [3 km] high, covered much of southern Asia. Caused mainly by the burning of coal and biomass, it caused respiratory diseases and many deaths. Alarm concerning urban air pollution had been expressed much earlier, but controls since the 1980s had proved difficult to enforce and expensive to introduce.

Those cities taking part in the United Nation's Global Environment Monitoring System frequently show dangerous levels of pollutants, ranging from soot to sulfur dioxide and photochemical smog. Air in the majority of cities without such sampling equipment is likely to be at least as bad. Traffic, a major source of air pollution worldwide, loses Thailand's work force 44 working days each year.

URBAN HOUSING NEEDS

Urbanization in most developing countries has been proceeding so rapidly that local governments have been unable to provide the necessary services and housing to meet demand.

In some cities, many people make their homes in squatter settlements, which are frequently without power, water and sanitation. Yet these communities are often a dynamic part of the city's economy, while their inhabitants sometimes take the initiative in setting up their own local government and self-help associations.

Some of the world's richest cities also have a homeless underclass, although calculating the numbers of people involved is problematic. Yet it is the case that homelessness and unemployment are currently affecting an increasing number of people in the developed world.

LARGEST CITIES

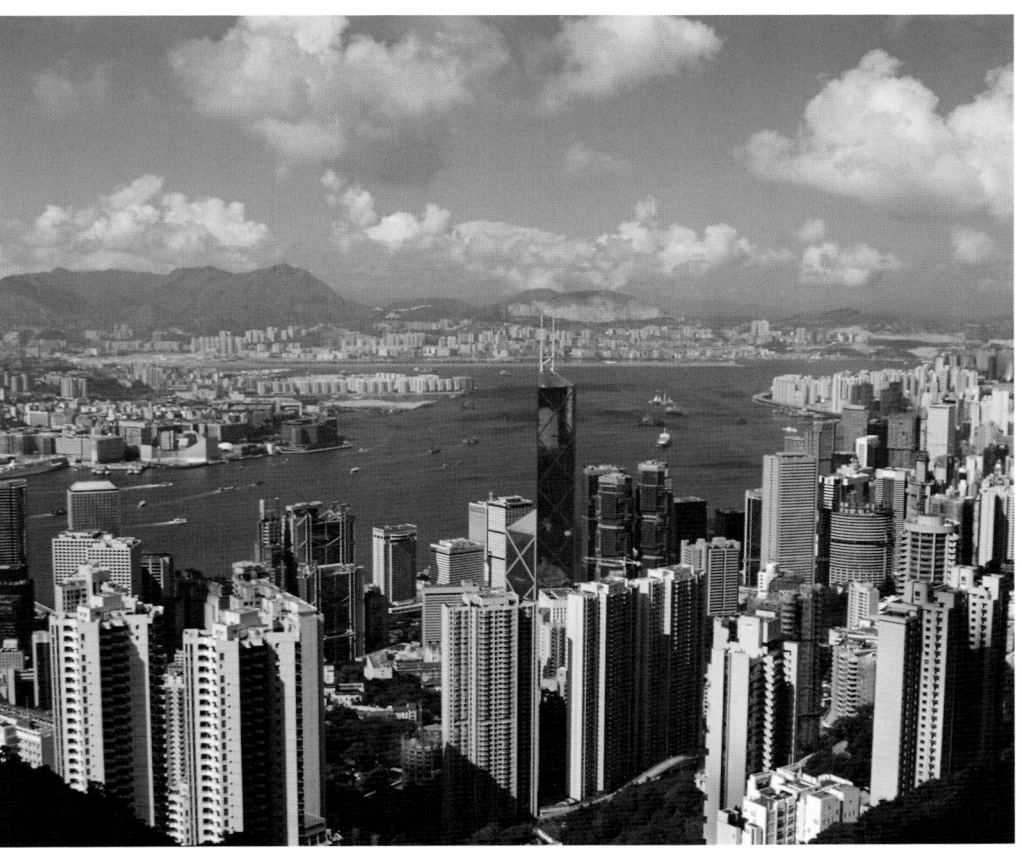

◄ The business district of Hong Kong City is located on the northern shore of Hong Kong Island. The cluster of modern high-rise buildings reflects the financial success of this tiny region, which has one of the strongest economies in Asia.

Early in the 21st century for the first time in history, the majority of the world's population will live in cities. Below is a list of all the cities with more than 10 million inhabitants, based on estimates for the year 2015.

1.	Tokyo–Yokohama	28.7
2.	Mumbai (Bombay)	27.4
3.	Lagos	24.1
4.	Shanghai	23.2
5.	Jakarta	21.5
6.	São Paulo	21.0
7.	Karachi	20.6
8.	Beijing	19.6
9.	Dhaka	19.2
10.	Mexico City	19.1
11.	Kolkata (Calcutta)	17.6
12.	Delhi	17.5
13.	New York City	17.4
14.	Tianjin	17.1
15.	Manila	14.9
16.	Cairo	14.7
17.	Los Angeles	14.5
18.	Seoul	13.1
19.	Buenos Aires	12.5
20.	Istanbul	12.1
21.	Rio de Janeiro	11.3
22.	Lahore	10.9
23.	Hyderabad	10.6
24.	Bangkok	10.4
25.	Osaka	10.2
26.	Lima	10.1
27.	Tehran	10.0

The city populations above are based on urban agglomerations rather than legal city limits. In some cases, where two adjacent cities have merged into one concentration, such as Tokyo–Yokohama, they have been regarded as a single unit.

URBAN ADVANTAGES

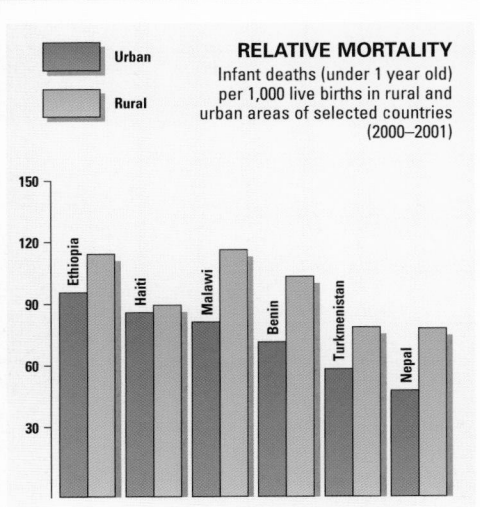

█ Urban █ Rural
RELATIVE MORTALITY
Infant deaths (under 1 year old) per 1,000 live births in rural and urban areas of selected countries (2000–2001)

Ethiopia, Haiti, Malawi, Benin, Turkmenistan, Nepal

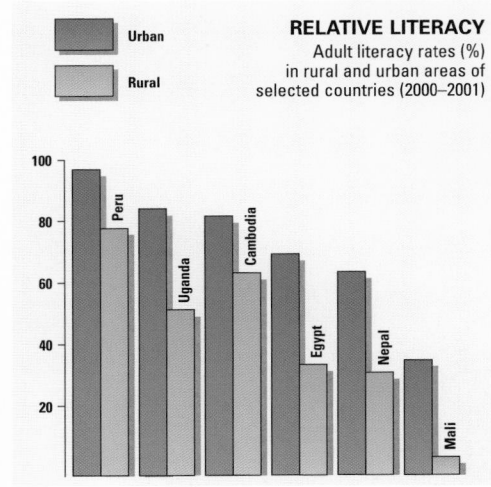

█ Urban █ Rural
RELATIVE LITERACY
Adult literacy rates (%) in rural and urban areas of selected countries (2000–2001)

Peru, Uganda, Cambodia, Egypt, Nepal, Mali

Despite overcrowding and poor housing, living standards in the developing world's cities are almost invariably better than in the surrounding countryside. Resources – financial, material and administrative – are concentrated in the towns, which are usually also the centers of political activity and pressure. Governments – frequently unstable, and rarely established on a solid democratic base – are usually more responsive to urban discontent than to rural misery.

In many developing countries, especially in Africa, food prices are kept artificially low, thus appeasing the underemployed urban masses at the expense of agricultural development.

This imbalance encourages further cityward migration, helping to account for the astonishing rate of post-1950 urbanization and putting great strain on the ability of many nations to provide even modest improvements for their people.

THE HUMAN FAMILY

For more information:
24 Population density
30 The world's refugees
War since 1945
31 United Nations
International
organizations

Racial, language and religious differences have led to appalling acts of inhumanity throughout history. Yet, strictly speaking, all human beings belong to one species, *Homo sapiens*, which has no subspecies. The differences between the three racial types which most people identify – Caucasoid, Mongoloid, and Negroid – reflect not so much evolutionary differences as long periods of separation.

Migration has recently mingled the various groups to an unprecedented extent, and most nations now have some degree of racial mixing. For example, the USA has often been called a melting pot, because of the large numbers of people from various

geographical locations which make up the population. The country has no official language but, until recently, English was spoken by the vast majority of the people. But in recent years, some of the immigrants from Mexico, Cuba, and other parts of Latin America have not learned English and speak only Spanish. This development disturbs those Americans who believe that the use of English binds the nation together, and several states have passed laws stating that English is their only official language.

Language is fundamental to human culture. Because definitions of languages vary, estimates of the total number range from 3,000 to 6,000, although most are

spoken by only a few people. Chinese is spoken by more people as a first language than any other, while English ranks second, but English is the leading international language, because so many people speak it as their second tongue.

Like language, religion encourages cohesion in single human groups and it satisfies a deep human need by assigning people a place in a divinely ordered world. Religion is a way in which a culture can express its individuality. For example, the rise of Islamic fundamentalism in the late 20th century was partly an expression of resentment that secular Western values were being imposed on Muslims.

WORLD MIGRATION

The greatest voluntary migration was the colonization of North America by 30–35 million European settlers during the 19th century. The greatest forced migration involved 9–11 million Africans taken as slaves to America between 1550 and 1860. The migrations shown on the map below are mostly international, as population

movements within borders are not usually recorded. Many of the statistics are necessarily estimates as so many refugees and migrant workers enter countries illegally and unrecorded. Emigrants may have a variety of motives for leaving, thus making it difficult to distinguish between voluntary and involuntary migrations.

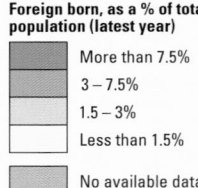
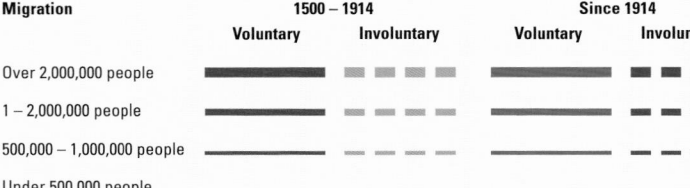

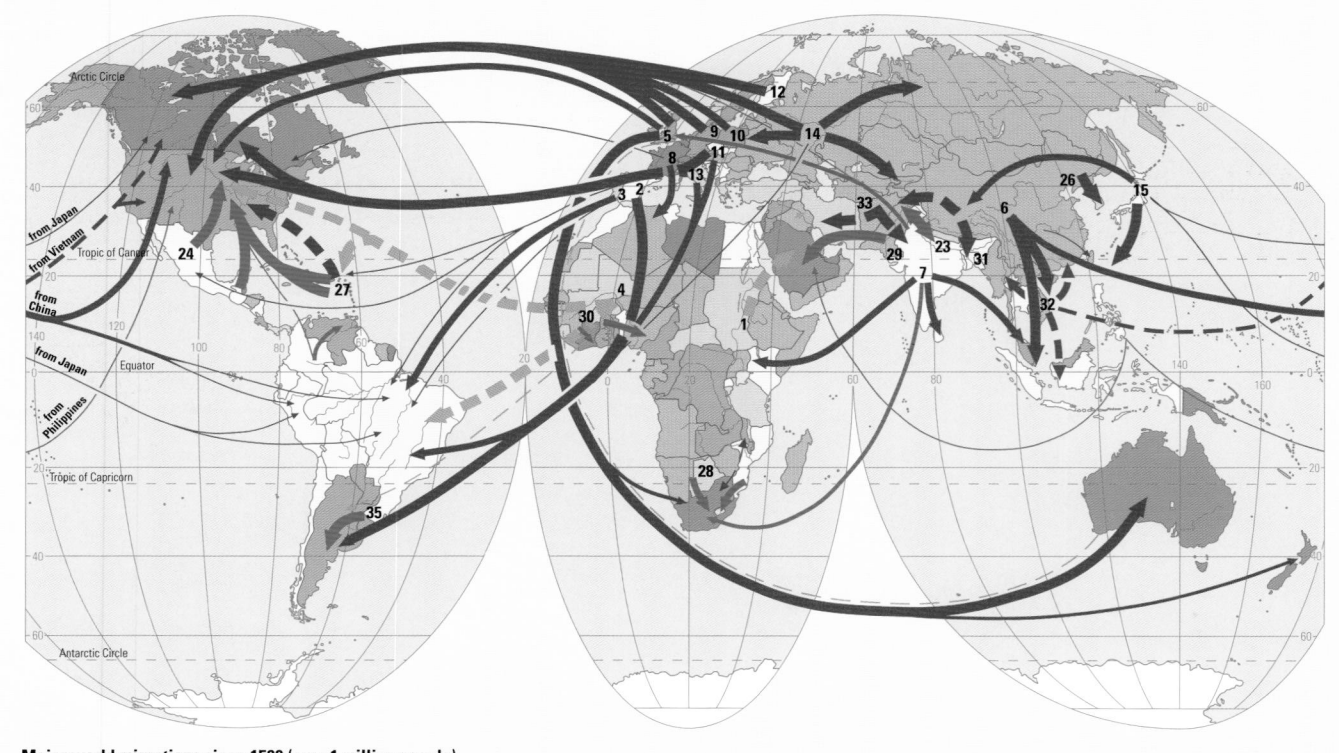

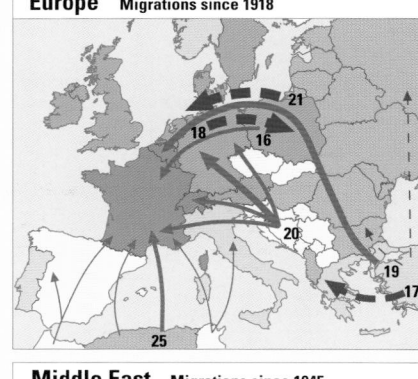

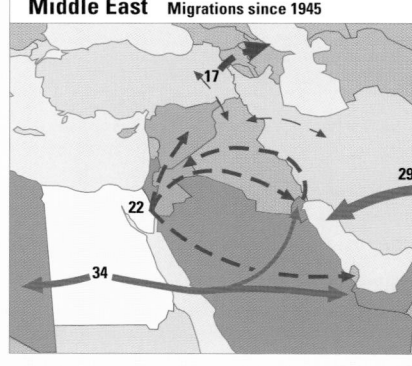

Major world migrations since 1500 (over 1 million people)

1. North and East African slaves to Arabia (4.3m)	1500–1900
2. Spanish to South and Central America (2.3m)	1530–1914
3. Portuguese to Brazil (1.4m)	1530–1914
4. West African slaves to South America (4.6m)	1550–1860
to Caribbean (4m)	1580–1860
to North/Central America (1m)	1650–1820
5. British and Irish to North America (13.5m)	1620–1914
to Australasia and South Africa (3m)	1790–1914
6. Chinese to South-east Asia (22m)	1820–1914
to North America (1m)	1880–1914
7. Indian migrant workers (3m)	1850–1914
8. French to North Africa (1.5m)	1850–1914
9. Germans to North America (5m)	1850–1914
10. Poles to North America (3.6m)	1850–1914
11. Austro-Hungarians to North America (3.2m)	1850–1914
to Western Europe (3.4m)	1850–1914
to South America (1.8m)	1850–1914
12. Scandinavians to North America (2.7m)	1850–1914
13. Italians to North America (5m)	1860–1914
to South America (3.7m)	1860–1914
14. Russians to North America (2.2m)	1880–1914
to Western Europe (2.2m)	1880–1914
to Siberia (6m)	1880–1914
to Central Asia (4m)	1880–1914
15. Japanese to Eastern Asia, Southeast Asia and America (8m)	1900–1914
16. Poles to Western Europe (1m)	1920–1940
17. Greeks and Armenians from Turkey (1.6m)	1922–1923
18. European Jews to extermination camps (5m)	1940–1944
19. Turks to Western Europe (1.9m)	1940–
20. Yugoslavs to Western Europe (2m)	1940–
21. Germans to Western Europe (9.8m)	1945–1947
22. Palestinian refugees (2m)	1947–
23. Indian and Pakistani refugees (15m)	1947
24. Mexicans to North America (9m)	1950–
25. North Africans to Western Europe (1.1m)	1950–
26. Korean refugees (5m)	1950–1954
27. Latin Americans and West Indians to North America (4.7m)	1960–
28. Migrant workers to South Africa (1.5m)	1960–
29. Indians and Pakistanis to The Gulf (2.4m)	1970–
30. Migrant workers to Nigeria and Ivory Coast (3m)	1970–
31. Bangladeshi and Pakistani refugees (2m)	1972
32. Vietnamese and Cambodian refugees (1.5m)	1975–
33. Afghan refugees (6.1m)	1979–
34. Egyptians to The Gulf and Libya (2.9m)	1980–
35. Migrant workers to Argentina (2m)	1980–
36. Mozambique refugees (1.7m)	1985–
37. Yugoslav/Balkan refugees (1.7m)	1992–
38. Rwanda/Burundi refugees (2.6m)	1994–

BUILDING THE USA

US Immigration, 1920 and 2000

For decades the USA was the magnet that attracted millions of immigrants, notably from Central and Eastern Europe, the flow peaking in the early years of the 20th century. By the mid-1990s the proportion of immigrants had increased again to pre-World War II rates, reaching almost 10% by 2000. However, the balance of origin had swung from Europe to Latin America and Asia, as the graphs indicate.

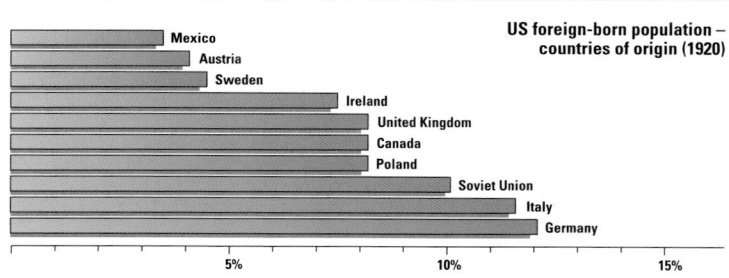

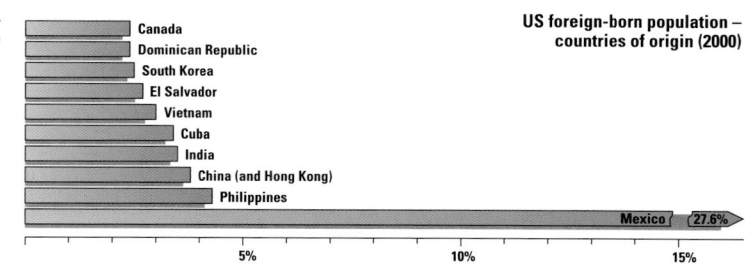

COPYRIGHT PHILIP'S

PREDOMINANT LANGUAGES

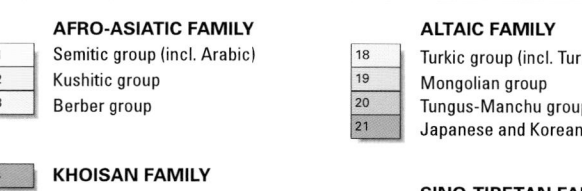

INDO-EUROPEAN FAMILY

1	Balto-Slavic group (incl. Russian, Ukrainian)
2	Germanic group (incl. English, German)
3	Celtic group
4	Greek
5	Albanian
6	Iranian group
7	Armenian
8	Romance group (incl. Spanish, Portuguese, French, Italian)
9	Indo-Aryan group (incl. Hindi, Bengali, Urdu, Punjabi, Marathi)
10	**CAUCASIAN FAMILY**

AFRO-ASIATIC FAMILY

11	Semitic group (incl. Arabic)
12	Kushitic group
13	Berber group
14	**KHOISAN FAMILY**
15	**NIGER-CONGO FAMILY**
16	**NILO-SAHARAN FAMILY**
17	**URALIC FAMILY**

ALTAIC FAMILY

18	Turkic group (incl. Turkish)
19	Mongolian group
20	Tungus-Manchu group
21	Japanese and Korean

SINO-TIBETAN FAMILY

22	Sinitic (Chinese) languages (incl. Mandarin, Wu, Yue)
23	Tibetic-Burmic languages
24	**TAI FAMILY**

AUSTRO-ASIATIC FAMILY

25	Mon-Khmer group
26	Munda group
27	Vietnamese
28	**DRAVIDIAN FAMILY** (incl. Telugu, Tamil)
29	**AUSTRONESIAN FAMILY** (incl. Malay-Indonesian, Javanese)
30	**OTHER LANGUAGES**

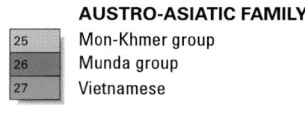

First-language speakers, in millions (1999)

Mandarin Chinese	885m
Spanish	332m
English	322m
Bengali	189m
Hindi	182m
Portuguese	170m
Russian	170m
Japanese	125m
German	98m
Wu Chinese	77m
Javanese	76m
Korean	75m
French	72m
Vietnamese	68m
Yue Chinese	66m
Marathi	65m
Tamil	63m
Turkish	59m
Urdu	58m

Languages form a kind of tree of development, splitting from a few ancient proto-tongues into branches that have grown apart and further divided with the passage of time. English and Hindi, for example, both belong to the great Indo-European family, although the relationship is only apparent after much analysis and comparison with non-Indo-European languages such as Chinese or Arabic. Hindi is part of the Indo-Aryan subgroup, whereas English is a member of Indo-European's Germanic branch. French, another Indo-European tongue, traces its descent through the Latin, or Romance, branch. A few languages – Basque is one example – have no apparent links with any other, living or dead. Most modern languages, of course, have acquired enormous quantities of vocabulary from each other.

DISTRIBUTION OF LIVING LANGUAGES

The figures refer to the number of languages currently in use in the regions shown

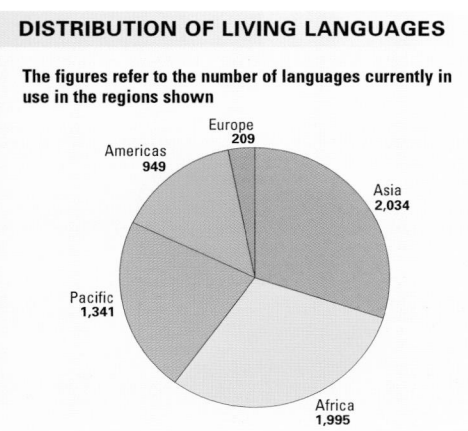

- Europe **209**
- Americas **949**
- Asia **2,034**
- Pacific **1,341**
- Africa **1,995**

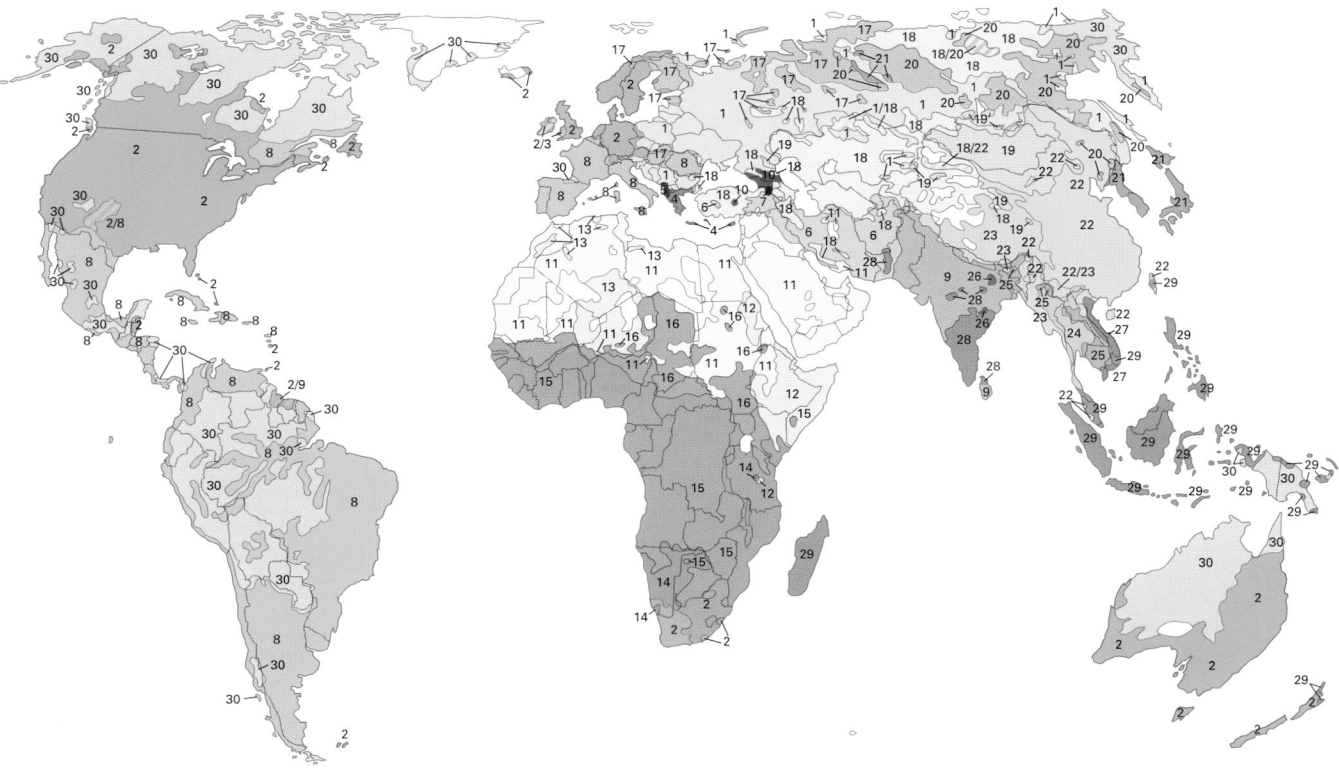

PREDOMINANT RELIGIONS

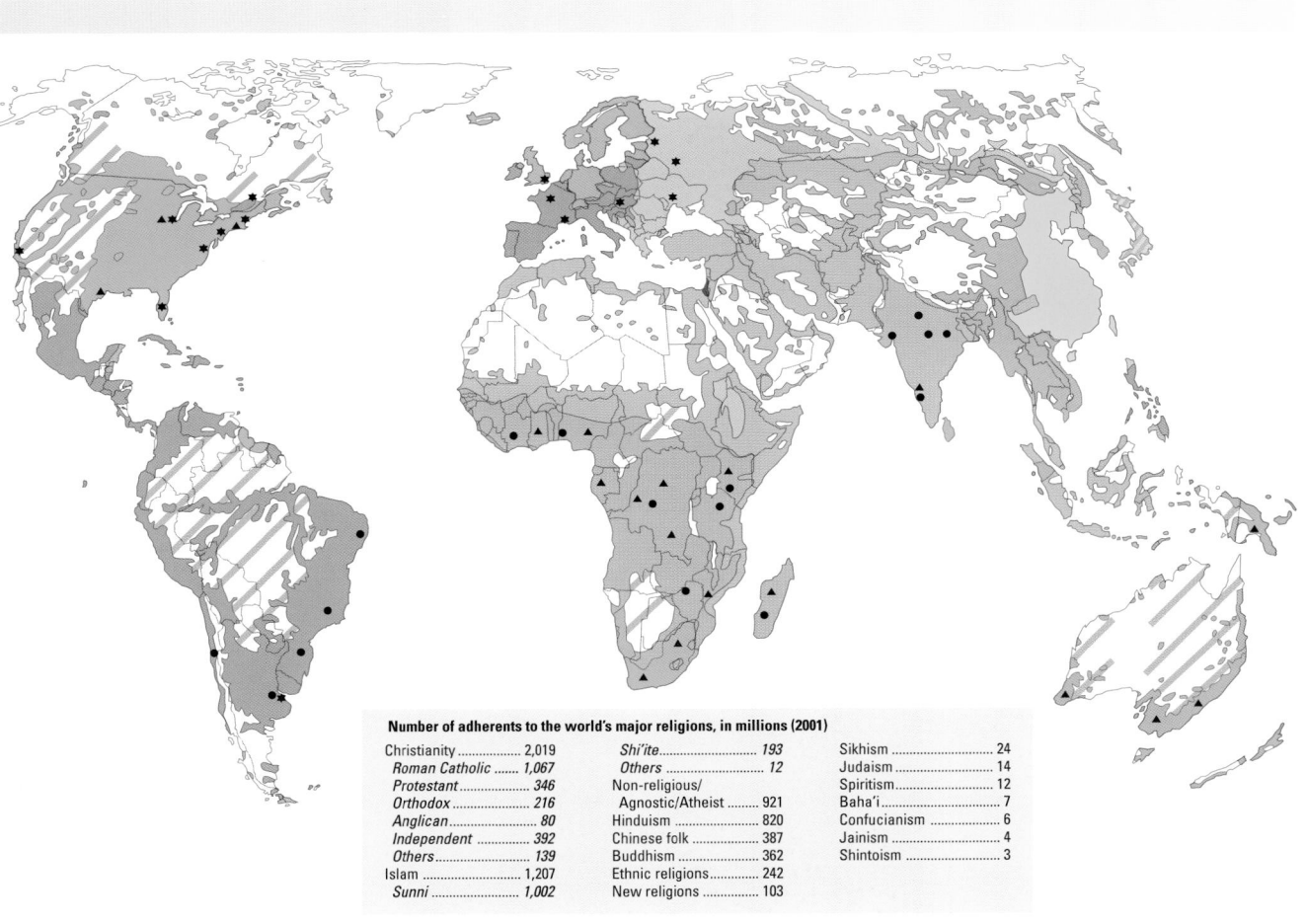

- Roman Catholicism
- Orthodox and other Eastern Churches
- Protestantism
- Sunni Islam
- Shia Islam
- Buddhism
- Hinduism
- Confucianism
- Judaism
- Shintoism
- Tribal Religions

Religions are not as easily mapped as the physical contours of the land. Divisions are often blurred and frequently overlapping: most nations include people of many different faiths – or no faith at all. Some religions, like Islam and Christianity, have proselytes worldwide; others, like Hinduism and Confucianism, are restricted to a particular area, though modern migrations have taken some Indians and Chinese very far from their cultural origins. It is also difficult to show the degree to which religion controls daily life: Christian Western Europe, for example, is now far less dominated by its religion than are the Islamic nations of the Middle East. Similarly, figures for the major faiths' adherents make no distinction between nominal believers enrolled at birth and those for whom religion is a vital part of their existence.

Number of adherents to the world's major religions, in millions (2001)

Christianity	2,019	*Shi'ite*	193	Sikhism	24
Roman Catholic	1,067	*Others*	12	Judaism	14
Protestant	346	Non-religious/		Spiritism	12
Orthodox	216	Agnostic/Atheist	921	Baha'i	7
Anglican	80	Hinduism	820	Confucianism	6
Independent	392	Chinese folk	387	Jainism	4
Others	139	Buddhism	362	Shintoism	3
Islam	1,207	Ethnic religions	242		
Sunni	1,002	New religions	103		

CONFLICT AND COOPERATION

For more information:

28 Migration

29 Religion

The 20th century witnessed two world wars, followed by a Cold War which several times threatened to erupt into a third world war, fought with nuclear weapons. The Cold War was marked by a great number of conflicts. Some were colonial wars, as the empires of the first half of the century fell apart, some were border wars, and some were civil wars. All the wars have caused great suffering among civilians, many of whom were forced to join the ranks of the world's refugees.

In the late 1980s, many people hoped that the end of the Cold War, following the collapse of Communist regimes in the former Soviet Union and Eastern Europe, would herald a new era of international stability. Instead, old ethnic and religious antagonisms surfaced in many areas, leading to civil war in such places as Chechenia, in Russia, and the former Yugoslavia. Nationalist rivalries, suppressed under Communist rule, replaced ideological factors as the major cause of conflict.

War is a very human activity, with no real equivalent in any other species. Yet humans also function well when they cooperate. Evolution has made this so. Hunter-gatherers in cooperative bands were far more effective than animals that prowled. Agriculture, urbanization, and industrialization all depend on the ability of humans to cooperate.

The creation of the United Nations in 1945 held out hope that the world's nations, tired of war, would have the means to control humanity's aggressive instincts. Although the UN lacks the power to halt conflicts, it has often helped to achieve negotiation. Economic pressures have led to another kind of cooperation, resulting in the creation of common markets and economic unions, such as ASEAN in Southeast Asia, the European Union, and NAFTA in North America.

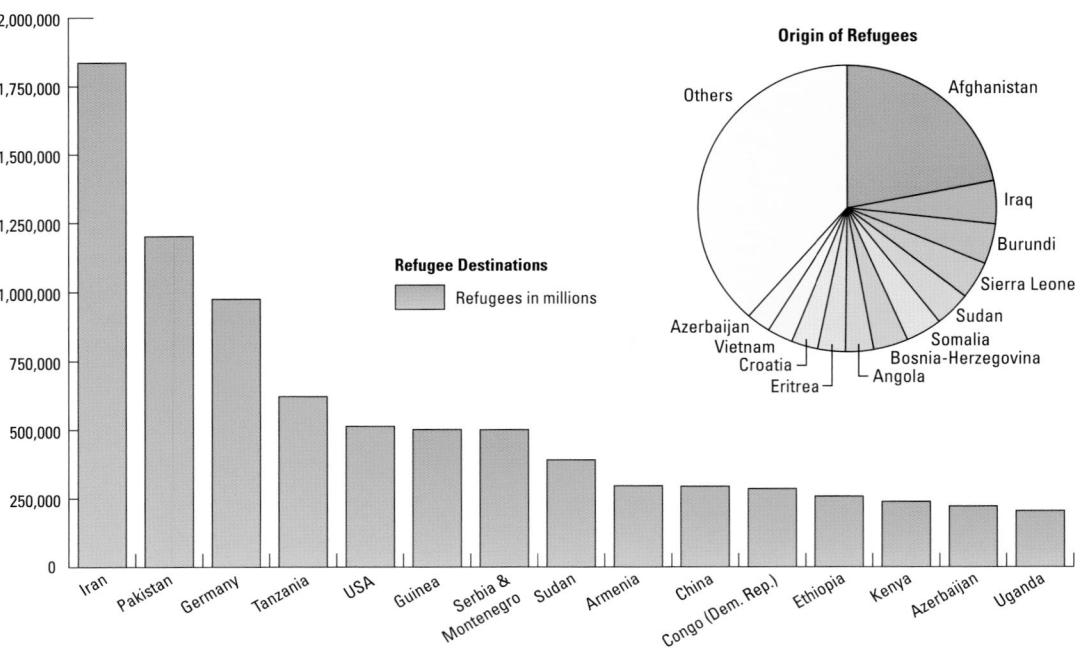

Origin of Refugees

Refugee Destinations — Refugees in millions

THE WORLD'S REFUGEES

Refugees by host nation (bar chart, left) and by nation of origin (pie chart, left) (2000). The source is the United Nations High Commission for Refugees (UNHCR). The 3.2 million Palestinian refugees living in Jordan, Syria, Lebanon, Gaza, and the West Bank fall under the mandate of United Nations Relief and Works Agency (UNRWA) and are not included on the graphs.

The pie chart shows the origins of the world's refugees, while the bar chart below shows their destinations. According to the United Nations High Commission for Refugees (UNHCR) in 2000 there were 12.1 million refugees. However, the UNHCR definition of a refugee, "a person who has left or remains outside their own country because they have a well-founded fear of persecution, or because their safety is threatened by events seriously disturbing public order," does not include people who are in a refugee-like situation but who have not been formally recognized. In 2000, there were a further 5.3 million people who were internally displaced, and a total "population of concern" 21.1 million people, worldwide.

All but a few who cross international boundaries seek asylum in neighboring countries, which are often the least equipped to deal with them. Lacking any rights or power, they frequently become an unwelcome burden to their hosts. Usually, the best any refugee can hope for is rudimentary food and shelter in temporary camps. Many Palestinians have been forced to live in camps since 1948.

WAR SINCE 1945

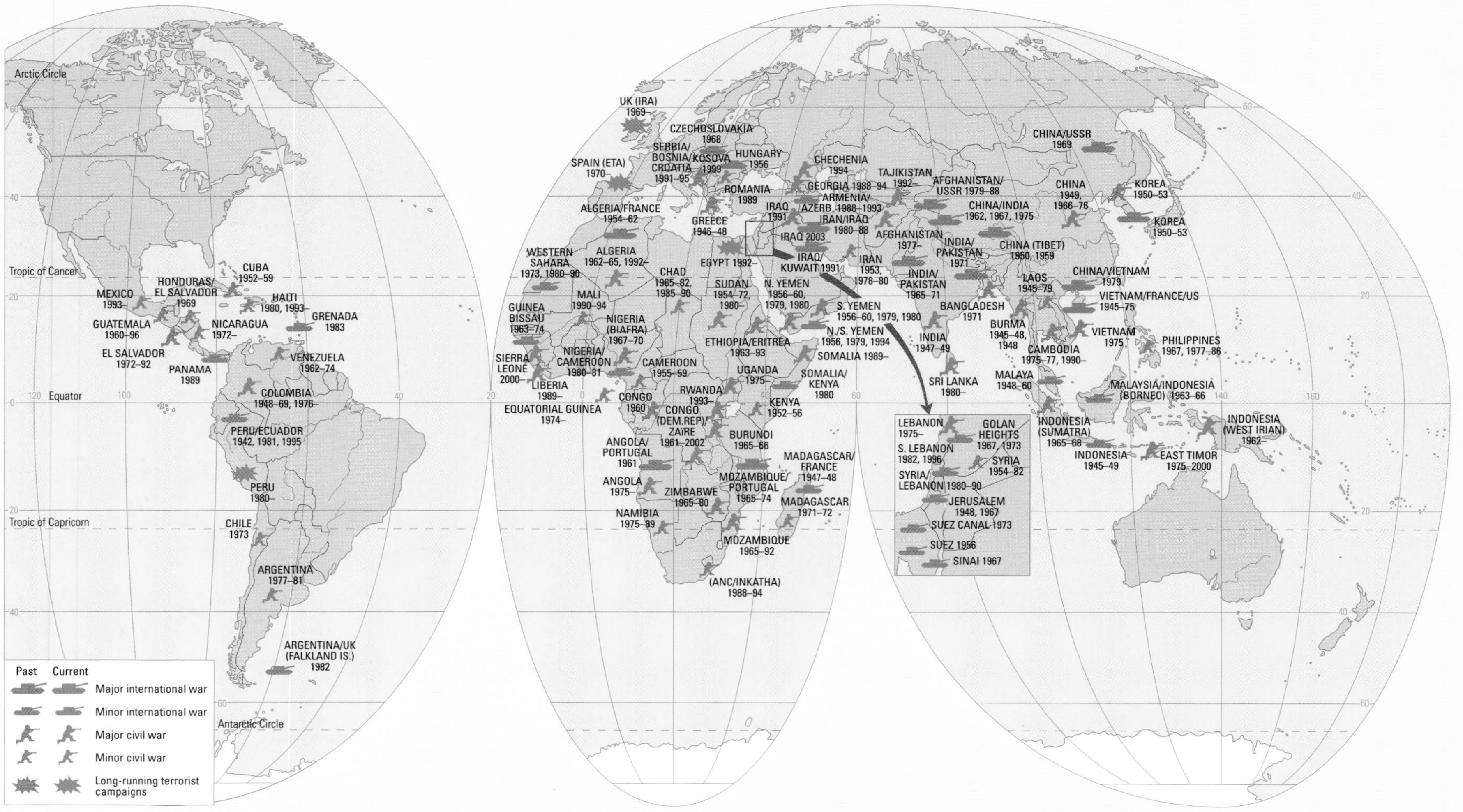

Past	Current	
		Major international war
		Minor international war
		Major civil war
		Minor civil war
		Long-running terrorist campaigns

INTERNATIONAL ORGANIZATIONS

OAS Organization of American States (formed in 1948). It aims to promote social and economic cooperation between countries in the developed North America and developing Latin America.

EFTA European Free Trade Organization (founded 1960). Since Austria, Finland, Portugal, and Sweden left to join the EU, it has four members: Iceland, Liechtenstein, Norway, and Switzerland.

EU European Union (evolved from the European Community in 1993). Cyprus, the Czech Republic, Estonia, Hungary, Latvia, Lithuania, Malta, Poland, the Slovak Republic, and Slovenia joined the EU in May 2004. The other 15 members of the EU are Austria, Belgium, Denmark, Finland, France, Germany, Greece, Ireland, Italy, Luxembourg, Netherlands, Portugal, Spain, Sweden, and the UK – together they aim to integrate economies, coordinate social developments and bring about political union. Bulgaria and Romania are expected to join in 2007.

AU The African Union was set up in 2002, taking over from the Organization of African Unity (1963). It has 53 members. Working languages are Arabic, English, French, and Portuguese.

COLOMBO PLAN (formed in 1951) Its 25 members aim to promote economic and social development in Asia and the Pacific.

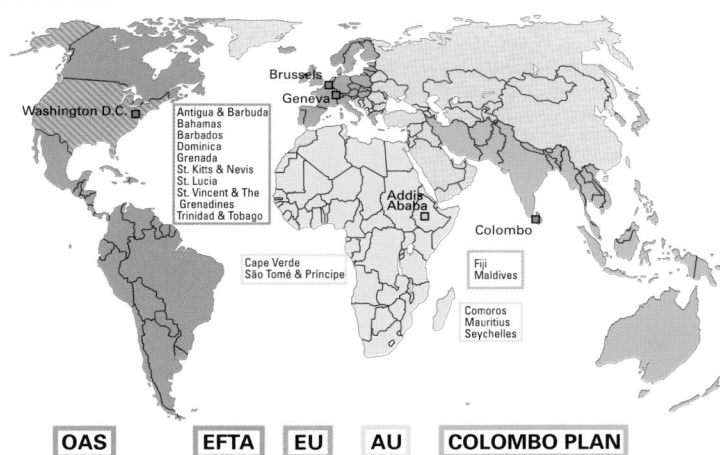

| OAS | EFTA | EU | AU | COLOMBO PLAN |

G8 Group of eight leading industrialized nations, comprising Canada, France, Germany, Italy, Japan, Russia, the UK, and the USA. Periodic meetings are held to discuss major world issues, such as world recessions.

OECD Organization for Economic Cooperation and Development (formed in 1961). It comprises 30 major free-market economies. The "G8" is its "inner group" of leading industrial nations, comprising Canada, France, Germany, Italy, Japan, Russia, the UK, and the USA.

ACP African-Caribbean-Pacific (formed in 1963). Members enjoy economic ties with the EU.

OPEC Organization of Petroleum Exporting Countries (formed in 1960). It controls about three-quarters of the world's oil supply. Gabon formally withdrew from OPEC in August 1996.

CIS The Commonwealth of Independent States (formed in 1991) comprises the countries of the former Soviet Union except for Estonia, Latvia, and Lithuania.

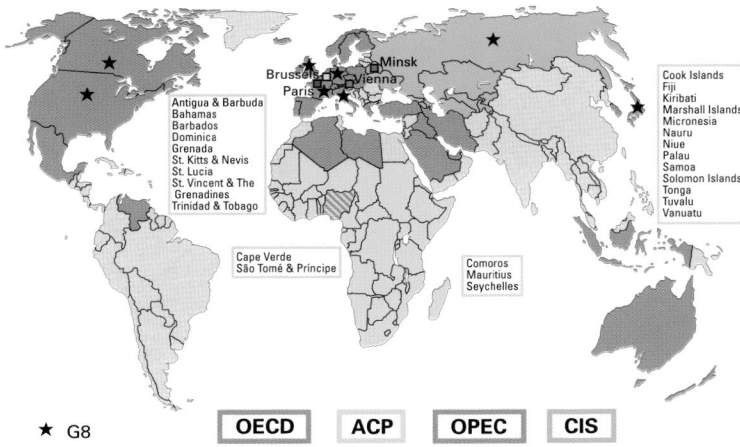

| ★ G8 | OECD | ACP | OPEC | CIS |

NATO North Atlantic Treaty Organization (formed in 1949). It continues despite the winding up of the Warsaw Pact in 1991. Bulgaria, Estonia, Latvia, Lithuania, Romania, the Slovak Republic, and Slovenia became members in 2004.

LAIA The Latin American Integration Association (formed in 1980) superceded the Latin American Free Trade Association formed in 1961. Its aim is to promote freer regional trade.

ARAB LEAGUE (1945) Aims to promote economic, social, political, and military cooperation. There are 22 member nations.

COMMONWEALTH The Commonwealth of Nations evolved from the British Empire. Pakistan was suspended in 1999, but reinstated in 2004. Zimbabwe was suspended in 2002 and, in response to its continued suspension, Zimbabwe left the Commonwealth in December 2003. It now comprises 16 Queen's realms, 31 republics and 6 indigenous monarchies, giving a total of 53 member states.

ASEAN Association of Southeast Asian Nations (formed in 1967). Cambodia joined in 1999.

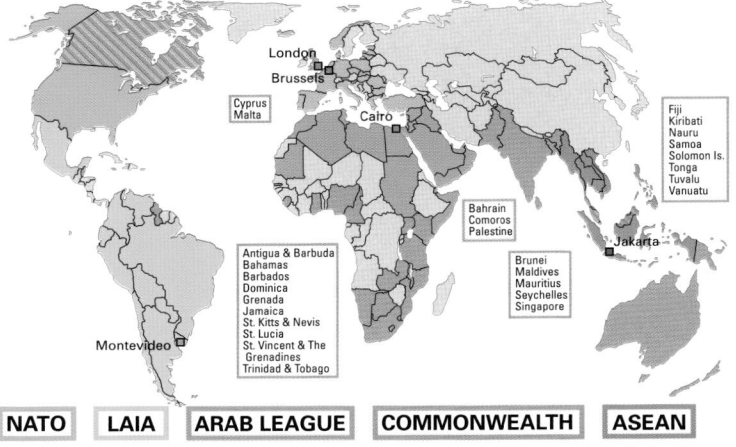

| NATO | LAIA | ARAB LEAGUE | COMMONWEALTH | ASEAN |

UNITED NATIONS

The United Nations Organization was born as World War II drew to its conclusion. Six years of strife had strengthened the world's desire for peace, but an effective international organization was needed to help achieve it. That body would replace the League of Nations which, since its inception in 1920, had failed to curb the aggression of at least some of its member nations. At the United Nations Conference on International Organization held in San Francisco, the United Nations Charter was drawn up. Ratified by the Security Council and signed by the 51 original members, it came into effect on October 24, 1945.

The Charter set out the aims of the organization: to maintain peace and security, and develop friendly relations between nations; to achieve international cooperation in solving economic, social, cultural, and humanitarian problems; to promote respect for human rights and fundamental freedoms; and to harmonize the activities of nations in order to achieve these common goals.

The United Nations has five principal organs:

The General Assembly The forum at which member nations discuss moral and political issues affecting world development, peace and security meets annually in September, under a newly-elected President whose tenure lasts one year. Any member can bring business to the agenda, and each member nation has one vote.

The Security Council A legislative and executive body, the Security Council is the primary instrument for establishing and maintaining international peace by attempting to settle disputes between nations. It has the power to dispatch UN forces, and member nations undertake to provide armed forces, assistance and facilities. The Security Council has ten temporary members elected by the General Assembly for two-year terms, and five permanent members – China, France, Russia, the UK, and the USA.

The Economic and Social Council By far the largest United Nations executive, the Council operates as a conduit between the General Assembly and the many United Nations agencies it instructs to implement Assembly decisions, and whose work it coordinates. The Council also commissions studies on economic conditions, collects data and makes recommendations to the Assembly.

The Secretariat This is the staff of the United Nations, and its task is to administer the policies and programs of the UN and its organs, and assist and advise the Head of the Secretariat, the Secretary-General – a full-time, non-political appointment made by the General Assembly.

The Trusteeship Council This no longer administers any of the original 11 trust territories as they are all now independent.

The International Court of Justice (the World Court) The World Court is the judicial organ of the United Nations. It deals only with United Nations disputes and all members are subject to its jurisdiction. There are 15 judges, elected for nine-year terms by the General Assembly and the Security Council.

The social and humanitarian operations of the UN include:

United Nations Development Program (UNDP) Plans and funds projects to help developing countries make better use of their resources.

United Nations International Childrens' Fund (UNICEF) Created at the General Assembly's first session in 1945 to help children in the aftermath of World War II, it now provides basic health care and aid worldwide.

Food and Agriculture Organization (FAO) Aims to raise living standards and nutrition levels in rural areas by improving food production and distribution.

United Nations Educational, Scientific and Cultural Organization (UNESCO) Promotes international cooperation through broader and better education.

World Health Organization (WHO) Promotes and provides for better health care, public and environmental health and medical research.

United Nations agencies are involved in many aspects of international trade, safety and security:

International Maritime Organization (IMO) Promotes unity amongst merchant shipping, especially in regard to safety, marine pollution, and standardization.

International Labor Organization (ILO) Seeks to improve labor conditions and promote productive employment to raise living standards.

World Meteorological Organization (WMO) Promotes cooperation in weather observation, reporting and forecasting.

World Trade Organization (WTO) On January 1, 1995, the WTO replaced GATT. It advocates a common code of conduct and its aim is the liberalization of world trade.

Disarmament Commission Considers and makes recommendations to the General Assembly on disarmament issues.

International Atomic Energy Agency (IAEA) Fosters development of peaceful uses for nuclear energy and establishes safety standards.

The World Bank comprises three United Nations agencies:

International Monetary Fund (IMF) Cultivates international monetary cooperation and the expansion of trade.

International Bank for Reconstruction and Development (IBRD) Provides funds and technical assistance to developing countries.

International Finance Corporation (IFC) Encourages the growth of productive private enterprise in less developed countries.

Membership There are two independent states which are not members of the UN – Taiwan and Vatican City. Official languages are Chinese, English, French, Russian, Spanish, and Arabic.

Funding The UN regular budget for 2002 was US $1.3 billion. Contributions are assessed by the members' ability to pay, with the maximum 22% of the total (USA's share), the minimum 0.01%. The EU pays over 37% of the budget.

Peacekeeping The UN has been involved in 54 peacekeeping operations worldwide since 1948.

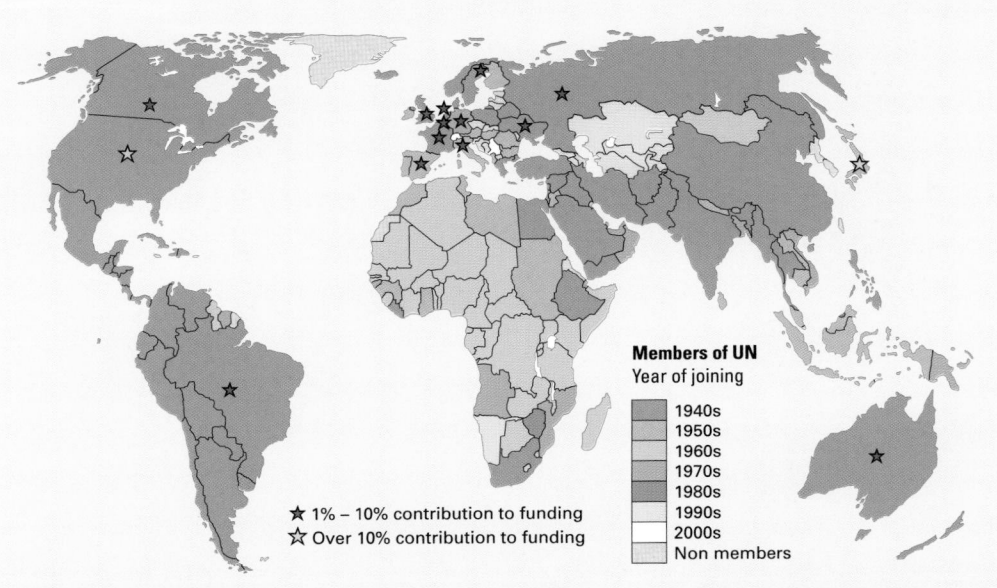

Members of UN
Year of joining

1940s
1950s
1960s
1970s
1980s
1990s
2000s
Non members

★ 1% – 10% contribution to funding
☆ Over 10% contribution to funding

AGRICULTURE

For more information:

16 Climate regions
17 Temperature and precipitation
18 Water distribution
19 Natural vegetation
38 Division of employment

When harvests are bad and world grain reserves fall, an old debate is revived, namely whether the population explosion will cause major food crises in the 21st century. Experts estimate that 3 billion tons of cereals will be needed to feed the world's population in 25 years' time, as compared with 1.9 billion tons at present. To expand food production to this extent, some argue, will place great strain on the environment.

Other experts, however, argue that there should be no food crises. World grain production tripled between 1950 and 1990, largely as a result of the Green Revolution, during which genetically improved, high-yield varieties of maize, rice, and wheat, the world's three leading staple crops, were developed.

These new varieties have helped many developing countries achieve food surpluses and prevent widespread starvation. Some people, however, oppose the use of genet-ically modified crops. In 2002, with severe droughts causing widespread starvation, Zambia and Zimbabwe both refused large maize donations from the USA because they might be genetically modified.

The only region of the world which seems likely to suffer food shortages in the 21st century is sub-Saharan Africa, where in the late 1990s the average daily calorie intake was 6% less than what was needed and where the population is expected to double in 20 years. Improved land management and a huge increase in global trade, especially in food distribution, is necessary if sub-Saharan Africans are not to go hungry.

The development of agriculture more than 10,000 years ago transformed human existence more than any other major advance. By supporting larger populations, it led to the growth of early civilizations and later it sustained people in the industrial cities that sprang up in the 19th century.

Today, agricultural production varies a great deal between the developed world, where it is highly mechanized and employs few people, such as 2% of the work force in the United States, and the developing world, such as sub-Saharan Africa, where it employs 66% of the work force. Many Africans are engaged in subsistence farming, providing the basic needs of their families but not contributing to the national economy. Much of Africa also suffers from economic mismanagement, as well as civil war and corruption.

Political problems have also affected food production in other parts of the world. The former USSR had much excellent farmland, but the failure of the collectives and state farms to maintain sufficiently high levels of production helped to bring about the collapse of Communism.

Farmers are under pressure not only to maintain high levels of production but also to increase them. However, the cultivation of marginal areas is one of the prime causes of soil erosion and desertification.

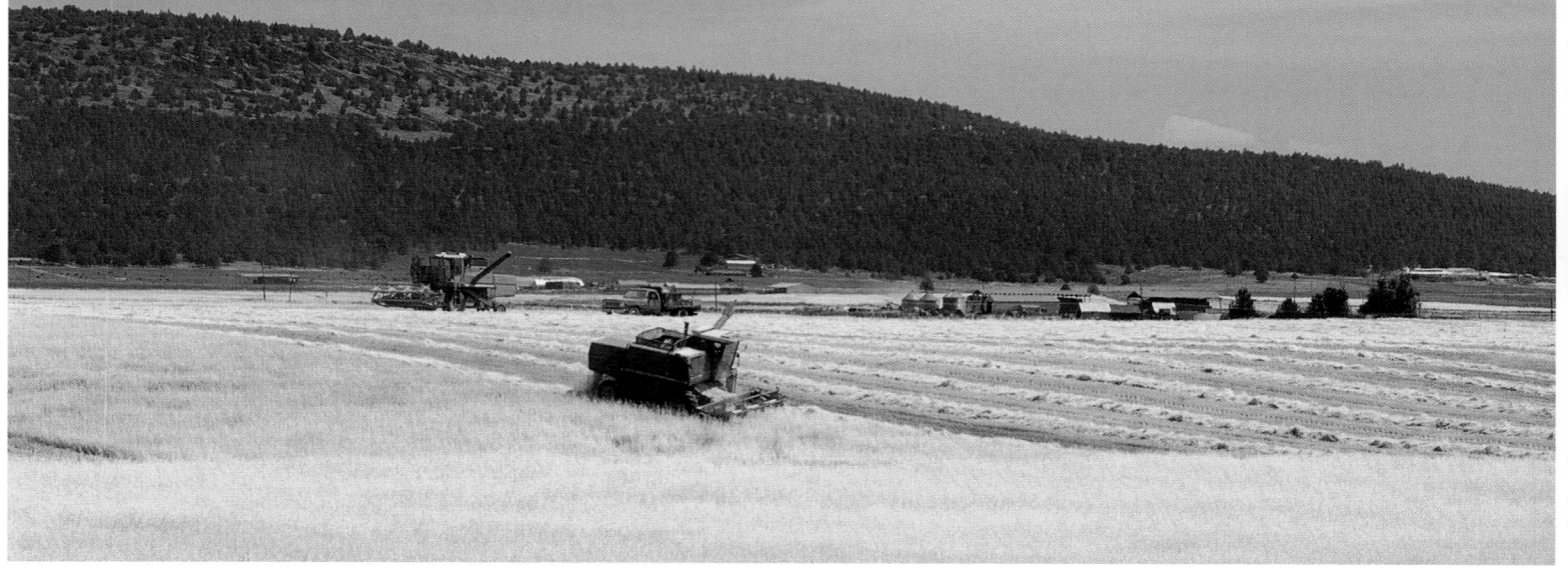

► The wheat harvest – photographed in Oregon, USA. Wheat, corn, rye, oats, and barley are grown in temperate regions, whereas rice, millet, sorghum, and maize require more tropical climates. Cereal cultivation was the basis of early civilizations, and, with the development of high-yielding strains, remains the world's most important food source today.

LAND USE

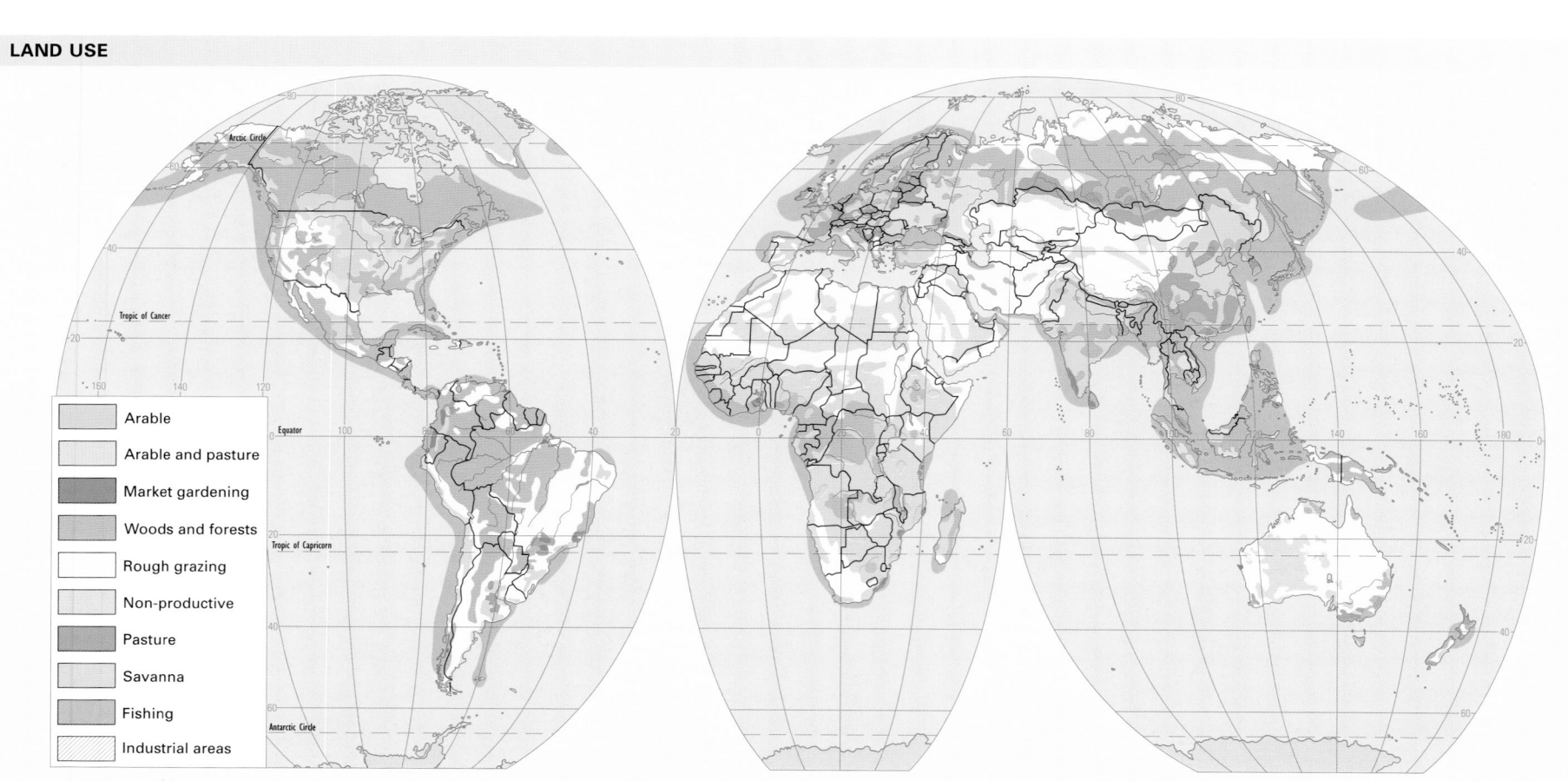

Arable

Arable and pasture

Market gardening

Woods and forests

Rough grazing

Non-productive

Pasture

Savanna

Fishing

Industrial areas

STAPLE CROPS

Wheat: Grown in a range of climates, with most varieties – including the highest-quality bread wheats – requiring temperate conditions. Mainly used in baking, it is also used for pasta and breakfast cereals.

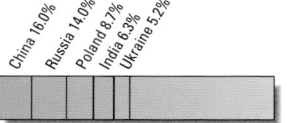

World total (2000): 576,317,000 tons

Maize: Originating in the New World and still an important human food in Africa and Latin America, in the developed world it is processed into breakfast cereals, oil, starches, and adhesives. It is also used for animal feed.

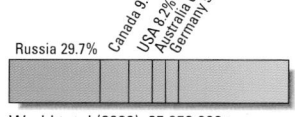

World total (2000): 590,791,000 tons

Oats: Most widely used to feed livestock, but eaten by humans as oatmeal or porridge. Oats have a beneficial effect on the cardiovascular system, and human consumption is likely to increase.

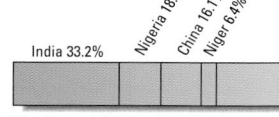

World total (2000): 25,953,000 tons

Millet: The name covers a number of small-grained cereals, members of the grass family with a short growing season. Used to produce flour, meal and animal feed, and fermented to make beer, especially in Africa.

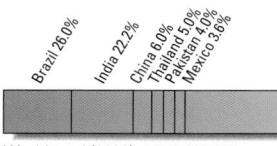

World total (2000): 27,255,000 tons

Rice: Thrives on the high humidity and temperatures of the Far East, where it is the traditional staple food of half the human race. Usually grown standing in water, rice responds well to continuous cultivation, with three or four crops annually.

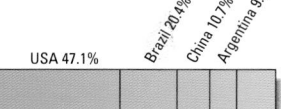

World total (2000): 598,852,000 tons

Potatoes: The most important of the edible tubers, potatoes grow in well-watered, temperate areas. Though weight for weight less nutritious than grain, they are a human staple as well as an important animal feed.

World total (2000): 311,288,000 tons

Soya: Beans from soya bushes (soybeans) are very high (30–40%) in protein. Most are processed into oil and proprietary protein foods. Consumption since 1950 has tripled, mainly due to the health-conscious developed world.

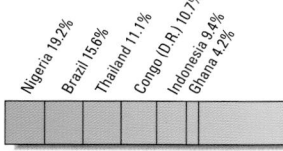

World total (2000): 161,993,000 tons

Cassava: A tropical shrub that needs high rainfall (over 125 inches annually) and a 10–30 month growing season to produce its large, edible tubers. Used as flour by humans, as cattle feed and in industrial starches.

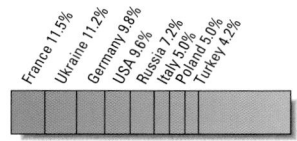

World total (2000): 172,737,000 tons

SUGARS

Sugarcane: Confined to tropical regions, cane sugar accounts for the bulk of international trade in sugar. Most is produced as a foodstuff, but some countries, notably Brazil and South Africa, distil sugar cane to make motor fuels.

World total (2000): 1,278,093,000 tons

Sugar beet: Closely related to the beetroot, sugar beet's yield after processing is indistinguishable from cane sugar. It is replacing sugarcane imports in Europe, to the detriment of the developing countries that rely on it as a major cash crop.

World total (2000): 244,780,000 tons

CEREALS & TUBERS

Cereals: These are grasses with starchy, edible seeds; every important civilization has depended on them as a source of food. The major cereal grains contain about 10% protein and 75% carbohydrate. Grain contributes more than any other group of foods to the energy and protein content of the human diet.

Starchy tuber crops or root crops: Second in importance after cereals as staple foods; easily cultivated, they provide high yields for little effort.

FOOD & POPULATION

Comparison of food production and population by continent
The left column indicates the % of world food production and the right shows population in proportion.

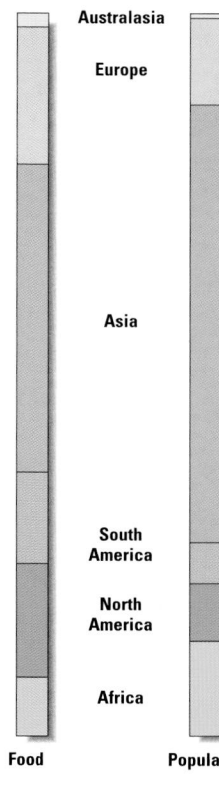

Food | Population

AGRICULTURAL POPULATION

Percentage of the total population dependent on agriculture for their livelihood (2000)

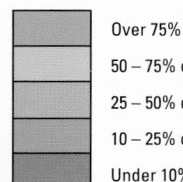

Over 75% dependent
50 – 75% dependent
25 – 50% dependent
10 – 25% dependent
Under 10% dependent

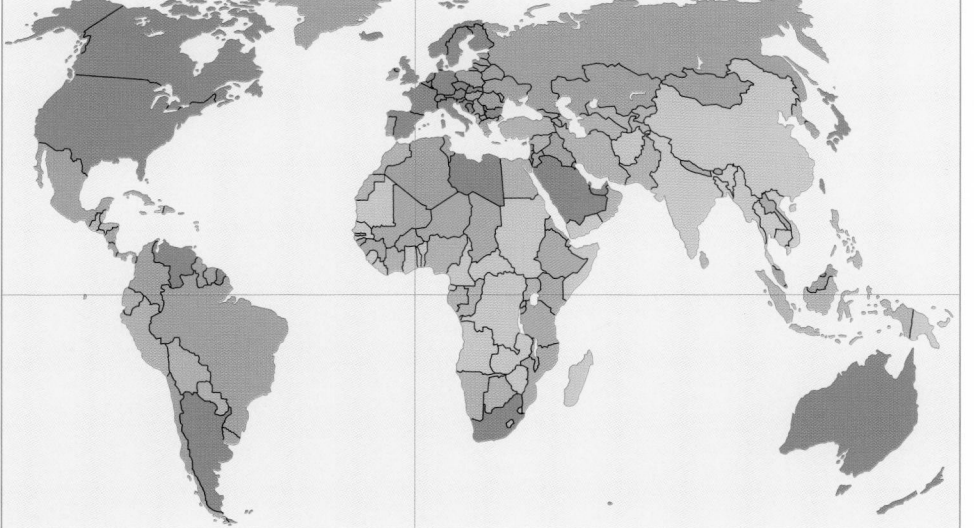

Top 5 countries		Bottom 5 countries	
Bhutan	93.7%	Singapore	0.1%
Nepal	93.0%	Brunei	0.7%
Burkina Faso	92.3%	Bahrain	1.0%
Burundi	90.4%	Kuwait	1.1%
Rwanda	90.3%	Qatar	1.3%

ANIMAL PRODUCTS

Traditionally, food animals subsisted on land unsuitable for cultivation, supporting agricultural production with their fertilizing dung. But free-ranging animals grow slowly and yield less meat than those more intensively reared; the demands of urban markets in the developed world have encouraged the growth of factory-like production methods.

A large proportion of staple crops, especially cereals, are fed to animals – an inefficient way to produce protein, but one likely to continue as long as people value meat and dairy products in their diet.

Cheese: Least perishable of all dairy products, cheese is milk fermented with selected bacterial strains to produce a foodstuff with a potentially immense range of flavors and textures. The vast majority of cheeses are made from cow's milk, although sheep and goat cheeses are highly prized.

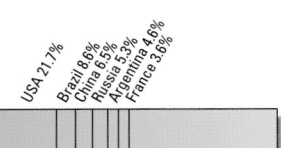

World total (2000): 16,045,000 tons

Beef and Veal: Most beef and veal is reared for home markets, and the top five producers are also the biggest consumers. The United States produces nearly a quarter of the world's beef and eats even more.

World total (2000): 57,170,000 tons

Milk: Many human groups, including most Asians, find raw milk indigestible after infancy, and it is often only the starting point for other dairy products such as butter, cheese, and yoghurt. Most world production comes from cows, but sheep's milk and goats' milk are also important.

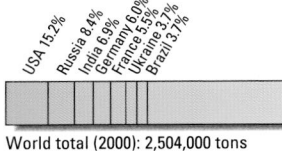

World total (2000): 2,504,000 tons

Butter: A traditional source of vitamin A as well as calories, butter has lost much popularity in the developed world for health reasons, although it remains a valuable food. Most butter from India, the world's largest producer, is clarified into ghee, which has religious as well as nutritional importance.

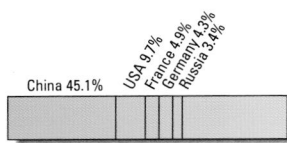

World total (2000): 7,049,000 tons

Pork: Although pork is forbidden to many millions, notably Muslims, on religious grounds, more is produced than any other meat in the world, mainly because it is the cheapest. It accounts for about 90% of China's meat output, although the per capita meat consumption is relatively low.

World total (2000): 90,909,000 tons

CRISIS IN AFRICA

Each year 40 million people, almost half of whom are children, die from starvation and related diseases. In 2000, 600 million people worldwide were estimated to be suffering from malnutrition. Africa suffers from more natural disasters than any other continent; pests such as locusts destroy crops, and tropical storms and floods ruin harvests. Famines periodically affect parts of Africa causing widespread hardship, even though enough food is produced worldwide to feed everyone.

A major phenomenon that affects the weather over tropical and subtropical regions areas around the world is called El Niño *(see page 8)*. It occurs when there is unusual warming in the tropical eastern Pacific Ocean, causing changes in the wind and pressure systems. Normal years are called La Niña. El Niño years included 1973–4, 1982–3, 1986–7, 1992, 1997–8, and 2002.

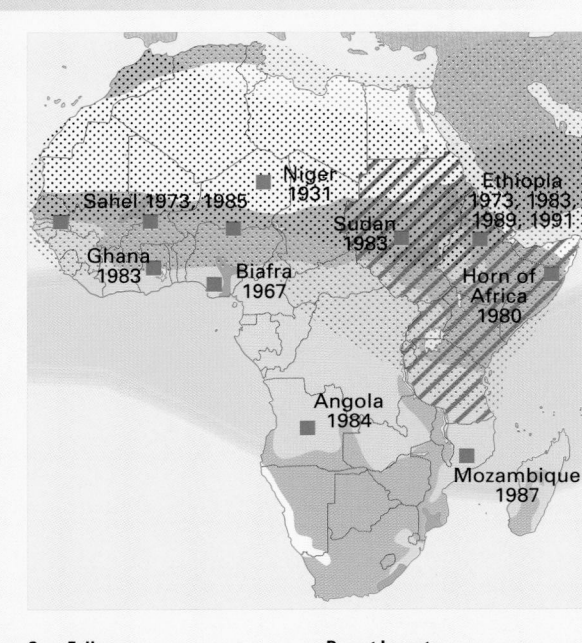

	Ocean areas affected by El Niño and La Niña temperature fluctuations
	Countries affected by 4 years of continuous drought, 1996–2000
	Areas liable to flood

Crop Failure
	Areas liable to periodic crop failure
	Areas where crop failures are rare
	Desert

Desert Locusts
	Areas liable to invasions by desert locusts
	Areas affected by 1993 swarm of desert locusts
■	Major famines since 1900 (with dates)

ENERGY

For more information:
21 The carbon cycle
22 Global warming
   Carbon dioxide
   Greenhouse power
23 Water pollution
36 Minerals
41 World shipping

Every year, the world's energy consumption is about the equivalent of what would come from burning 9 billion tons of oil (9,000 MtOe) – a 20-fold increase since 1850. Two-fifths of this total actually comes from burning oil and most of the rest comes from coal and natural gas.

The oil crises in the 1970s precipitated concern over dependence on finite fossil fuels as the primary source of energy, and growing environmental awareness has added impetus to the search for alternative energy resources. Fossil fuel combustion damages the environment through the release of gases and particulate matter, but two other major sources of energy, hydroelectricity and nuclear power, are also controversial. Hydroelectricity production involves flooding large areas to create reservoirs, while nuclear power stations generate dangerous radioactive wastes and can cause major disasters. Significantly, by 2002, five European countries – Belgium, Germany, the Netherlands, Spain, and Sweden – had plans to phase out the use of nuclear energy.

Alternative energy resources may soon provide a much larger proportion of the world's energy consumption. Solar and wind energy may become important in such countries as China and India, while tidal, wave and geothermal energy all have potential in appropriate areas. Experts calculate that solar power could, in theory, supply between five and ten times the present electricity supply of developing countries.

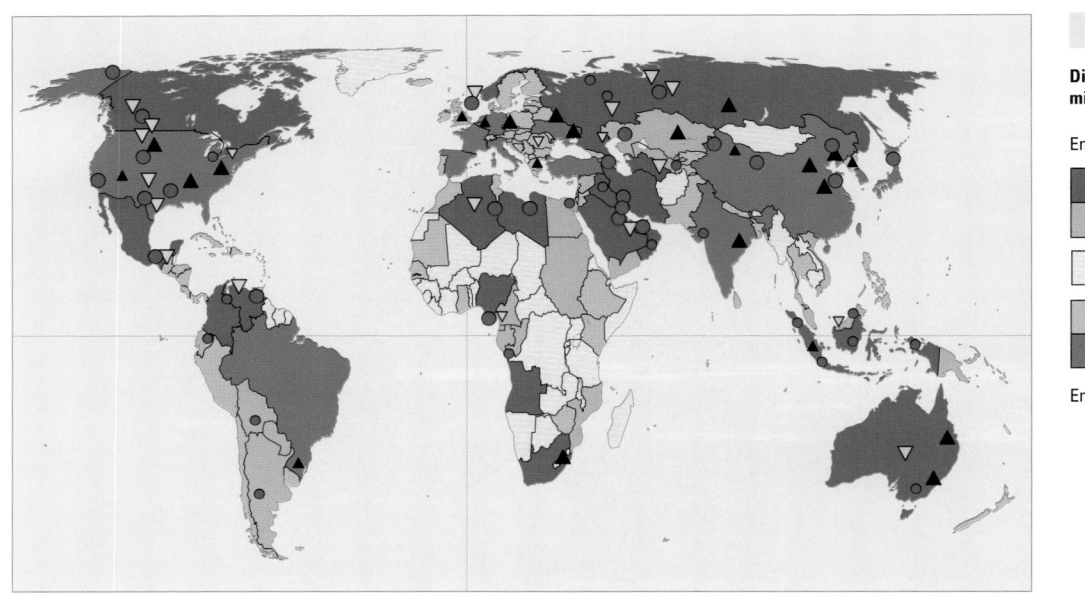

ENERGY BALANCE

Difference between energy production and consumption in millions of tons of oil equivalent (MtOe) (2000)

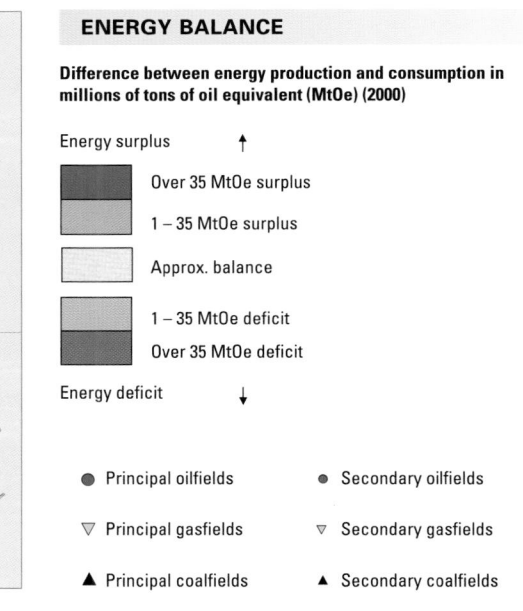

Energy surplus ↑

Over 35 MtOe surplus
1 – 35 MtOe surplus
Approx. balance
1 – 35 MtOe deficit
Over 35 MtOe deficit

Energy deficit ↓

● Principal oilfields   ● Secondary oilfields
▽ Principal gasfields   ▽ Secondary gasfields
▲ Principal coalfields   ▲ Secondary coalfields

ENERGY CONSUMPTION

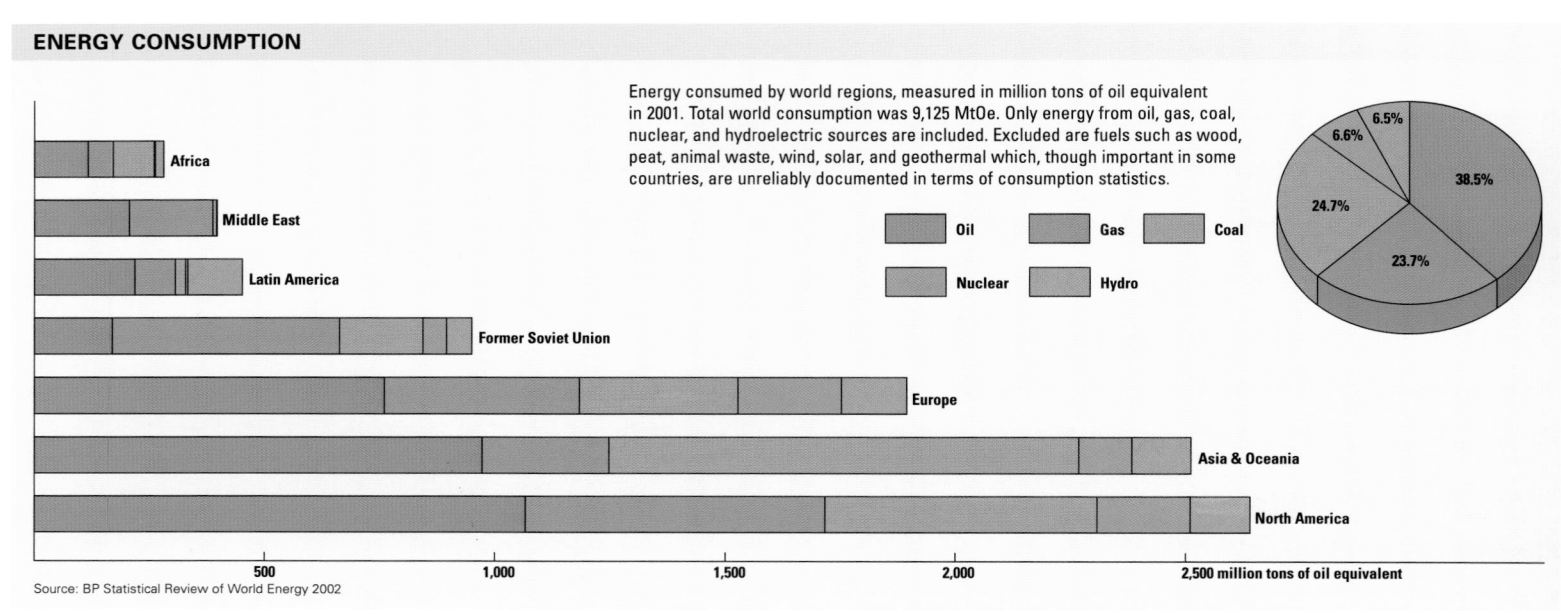

Energy consumed by world regions, measured in million tons of oil equivalent in 2001. Total world consumption was 9,125 MtOe. Only energy from oil, gas, coal, nuclear, and hydroelectric sources are included. Excluded are fuels such as wood, peat, animal waste, wind, solar, and geothermal which, though important in some countries, are unreliably documented in terms of consumption statistics.

Oil   Gas   Coal   Nuclear   Hydro

6.5%
6.6%
24.7%
38.5%
23.7%

Africa
Middle East
Latin America
Former Soviet Union
Europe
Asia & Oceania
North America

500   1,000   1,500   2,000   2,500 million tons of oil equivalent

Source: BP Statistical Review of World Energy 2002

ENERGY PRODUCTION

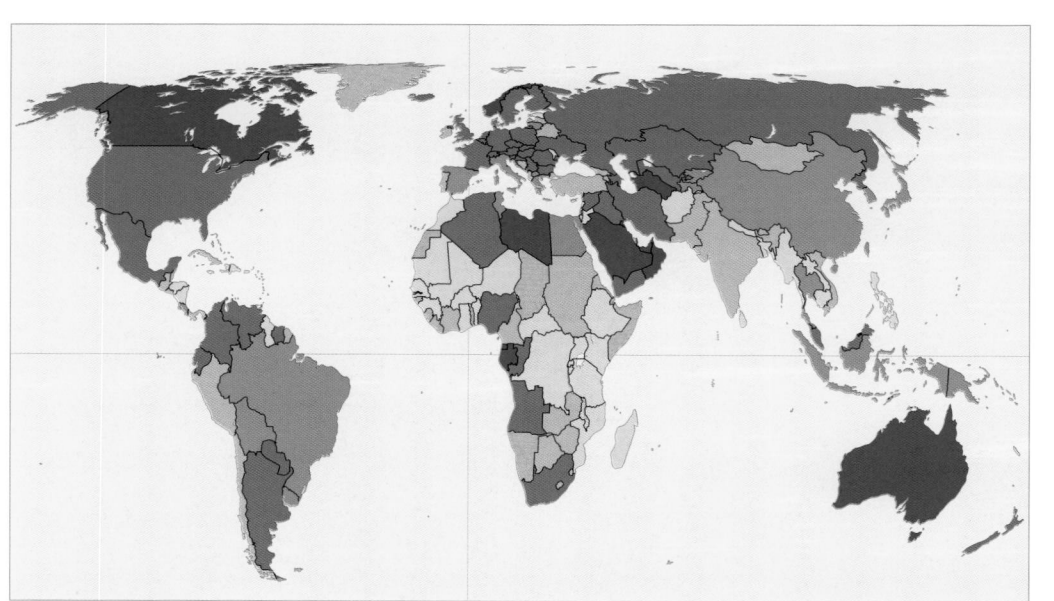

Energy production in tons of oil equivalent per capita (2000)

Over 10
1 – 10
0.5 – 1
0.1 – 0.5
Under 0.1
No data available

In developing countries traditional fuels are still very important. These so-called biomass fuels include wood, charcoal and dried dung. The pie chart (*right*) highlights the importance of biomass in terms of energy consumption in Nigeria. Collecting fuelwood can be a time-consuming task, sometimes taking all day.

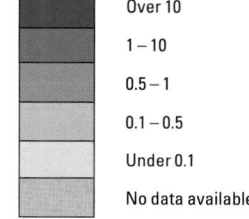

Nigeria

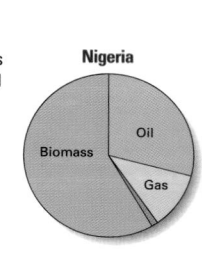

Biomass   Oil   Gas

OIL MOVEMENTS

Major world movements of oil in millions of tons (2001)

1.	Middle East to Asia (not China or Japan)	316.7
2.	Middle East to Japan	208.8
3.	Former Soviet Union to Europe	181.2
4.	Middle East to Europe	176.2
5.	Middle East to USA	138.0
6.	South and Central America to USA	126.3
7.	North Africa to Europe	96.9
8.	Canada to USA	88.0
9.	Mexico to USA	70.8
10.	West Africa to USA	68.1
11.	Europe to USA	46.2
12.	Middle East to Africa	41.0
13.	West Africa to Asia (not China or Japan)	36.9
14.	West Africa to Europe	34.9
15.	Middle East to China	34.2
16.	Asia (not China) to Japan	34.2

Total world imports   **2,159,300,000 tons**

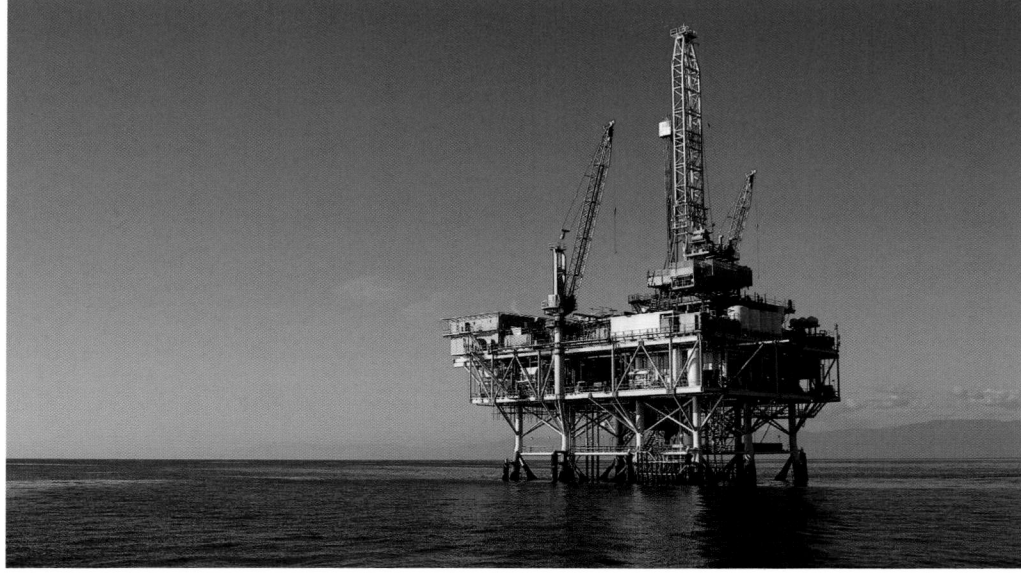

◄ With many of the world's onshore oilfields reaching their maturity, exploration and production in ever-deeper ocean waters is taking place to try to satisfy demand. The current deepest production well is in 6,004 ft [1,829 m] of water, offshore of Brazil. However, exploration wells off the coasts of Angola and Nigeria are already being drilled in water 8,000 ft [2,438 m] deep, and it is believed that wells in 10,000 ft [3,048 m] of water will soon be developed.

ENERGY RESERVES

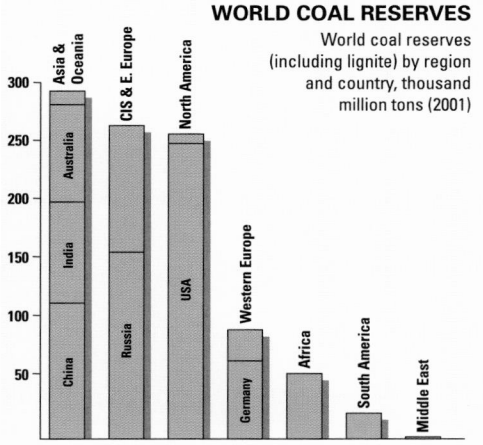

WORLD COAL RESERVES
World coal reserves (including lignite) by region and country, thousand million tons (2001)

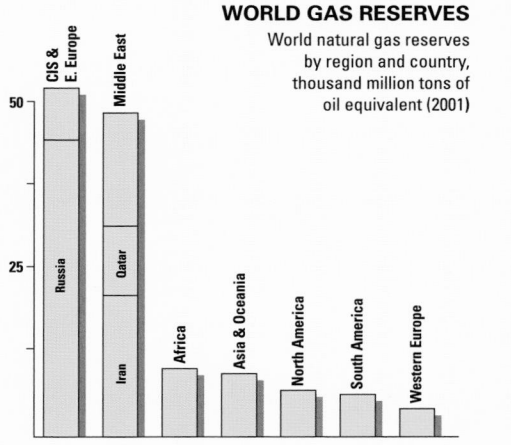

WORLD GAS RESERVES
World natural gas reserves by region and country, thousand million tons of oil equivalent (2001)

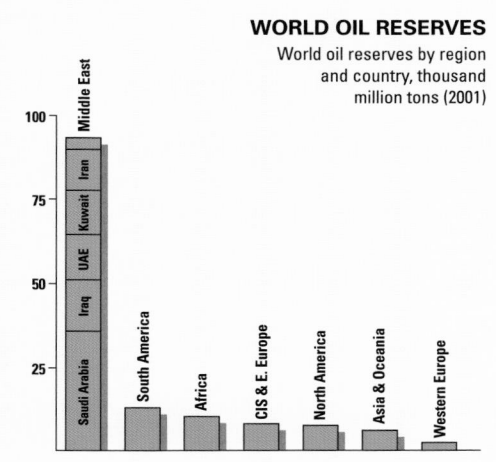

WORLD OIL RESERVES
World oil reserves by region and country, thousand million tons (2001)

NUCLEAR POWER

Major producers by percentage of world total (2000) and by percentage of domestic electricity generation (1999)

Country	% of world total production	Country	% of nuclear as proportion of domestic electricity
1. USA	30.5%	1. Lithuania	76.1%
2. France	15.7%	2. France	75.1%
3. Japan	12.6%	3. Belgium	58.2%
4. Germany	6.7%	4. Slovak Rep.	47.5%
5. Russia	4.6%	5. Sweden	44.2%
6. South Korea	4.1%	6. Ukraine	41.6%
7. UK	3.8%	7. Bulgaria	41.4%
8. Canada	2.9%	8. South Korea	39.1%
9. Ukraine	2.8%	9. Hungary	38.1%
= Sweden	2.8%	10. Slovenia	35.9%

Although the 1980s were a bad time for the nuclear power industry (major projects ran over budget and fears of long-term environmental damage were heavily reinforced by the 1986 disaster at Chernobyl), the industry picked up in the early 1990s. Whilst the number of reactors is still increasing, however, orders for new plants have shrunk. In 1997, the Swedish government began to decommission the country's 12 nuclear power plants.

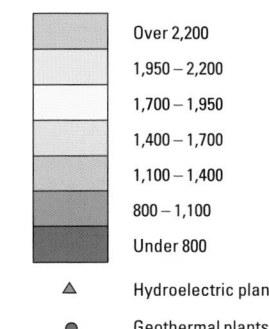

RENEWABLE ENERGY

Average annual solar irradiance in kWh/m², with selected major hydroelectric and geothermal power stations

	Over 2,200
	1,950 – 2,200
	1,700 – 1,950
	1,400 – 1,700
	1,100 – 1,400
	800 – 1,100
	Under 800
△	Hydroelectric plants
●	Geothermal plants

HYDROELECTRICITY

Major producers by percentage of world total (2000) and by percentage of domestic electricity generation (1999)

Country	% of world total production	Country	% of hydroelectric as proportion of domestic electricity
1. Canada	13.1%	1. Bhutan	99.9%
2. USA	12.0%	2. Paraguay	99.8%
3. Brazil	11.1%	= Zambia	99.8%
4. China	8.5%	4. Norway	99.1%
5. Russia	6.1%	5. Ethiopia	98.1%
6. Norway	4.6%	6. Congo (Rep. Dem.)	97.9%
7. Japan	3.3%	7. Tajikistan	97.8%
8. India	3.1%	8. Cameroon	97.3%
9. France	2.8%	9. Albania	97.2%
10. Sweden	2.7%	= Laos	97.2%

Countries heavily reliant on hydroelectricity are usually small and non-industrial: a high proportion of hydroelectric power more often reflects a modest energy budget than vast hydroelectric resources. The USA, for instance, produces only 8.5% of its power requirements from hydroelectricity; yet that 8.5% amounts to more than three times the hydropower generated by most of Africa.

ALTERNATIVE ENERGY RESOURCES

Solar: Each year the Sun bestows upon the Earth almost a million times as much energy as is locked up in all the planet's oil reserves, but only an insignificant fraction is trapped and used commercially. In a few installations around the world, mirrors focus the Sun's rays on to boilers, whose steam generates electricity by spinning turbines.

Wind: Caused by uneven heating of the Earth, winds are themselves a form of solar energy. Windmills have been long used for wind power; recent models, often arranged in banks on wind-swept high ground or off coastlines, usually generate electricity. Wind-power figures are given in the table (*right*) – it is the world's fastest growing energy source. In 2002, Germany, the USA, Spain, and Denmark produced nearly 16,000 MW.

Tidal: The energy from tides is potentially enormous, although only a few installations have so far been built to exploit it. In theory at least, waves and currents could also provide almost unimaginable power, and the thermal differences in the ocean depths are another huge well

of potential energy. But work on extracting it is still at the experimental stage.

Geothermal: The Earth's temperature rises by 1°F for every 50 feet descent, with much steeper temperature gradients in geologically active areas. El Salvador, for example, produces 39% of its electricity from geothermal power stations, whilst the USA is the world's leading producer. Some of the oldest and most successful applications are in Iceland, where 86% of all households are heated by geothermal energy.

Biomass: The oldest of human fuels ranges from animal dung, still burned in cooking fires in much of North Africa and elsewhere, to sugarcane plantations feeding high-technology distilleries to produce ethanol for motor-vehicle engines. In Brazil and South Africa, plant ethanol provides up to 25% of motor fuel. Throughout the developing world, most biomass energy comes from firewood: although accurate figures are impossible to obtain, it may yield as much as 10% of the world's total energy consumption.

WIND POWER

World wind energy generating capacity, in megawatts

1980	10
1982	90
1984	600
1986	1,270
1988	1,580
1989	1,730
1990	1,930
1991	2,170
1992	2,510
1993	3,050
1994	3,710
1995	4,820
1996	6,115
1997	7,630
1998	9,600

Wind power is the fastest growing source of energy. Between 1998 and 2002, world production more than doubled.

MINERALS

For more information:

10 Geology
39 Patterns of production
41 World shipping

The use of metals played a vital part in the evolving technologies of early peoples. Copper first came into use around 10,000 years ago, bronze about 5,000 years ago, and iron 3,300 years ago. In the early stages of the Industrial Revolution, the location of coal, iron ore, and water power usually determined the location of new industries. But due to continuing improvements in transport, including oil pipelines, industries can now be located almost anywhere.

Minerals are distributed unevenly and some industrial countries, lacking their own mineral resources, import most of the raw materials they need. Some imports come from mineral-rich countries, such as Australia, but others come from developing countries, especially in Africa and South America. Most developing countries export unprocessed ores, losing out on the higher revenues gained from exporting metals.

Most minerals come from land deposits, because undersea deposits, with the exception of oil reserves under the continental shelves, have been inaccessible. But shortages of terrestrial minerals may one day encourage exploitation of the ocean floor.

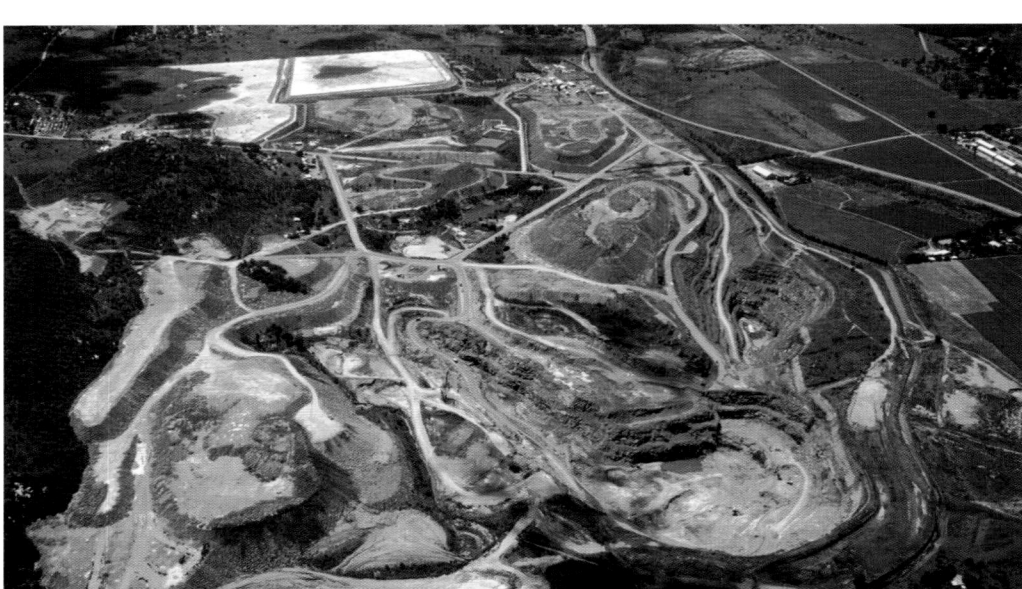

► An aerial view of gold mine excavations in Zimbabwe, for extraction both above and below ground. Once a major producer of gold, Zimbabwe's gold mining industry has greatly declined in recent years as a result of political and social unrest.

URANIUM

Uranium was first discovered by the German chemist Martin Klaproth in 1789. In its pure state, uranium is an immensely heavy, white metal. But although spent uranium is employed as a projectile in anti-missile cannons, where its mass ensures a lethal punch, its main use is as a fuel in nuclear reactors, and in nuclear weaponry.

Uranium is very scarce: the main source is the rare ore pitchblende, which itself contains only 0.2% uranium oxide. This blackish, lustrous ore occurs in quartz veins. Only a minute fraction of that is the radioactive U^{235} isotope, though so-called breeder reactors can transmute the more common U^{238} into highly radioactive plutonium.

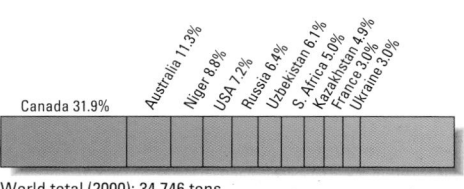

World total (2000): 34,746 tons

DIAMOND

Most of the world's diamond is found in kimberlite, or "blue ground," a basic peridotite rock; erosion may wash the diamond from its kimberlite matrix and deposit it with sand or gravel on river beds. Only a small proportion of the world's diamond, the most flawless, is cut into gemstones – "diamonds"; most are used in industry, where the material's remarkable hardness and abrasion resistance finds a use in cutting tools, drills, and dies. Australia produced 31.6% of the world's total in 2000. The other main producers are the Democratic Republic of the Congo (24.7%), Russia (20%), South Africa (10.5%), and Botswana (8.5%). Natural diamonds now account for less than 10% of all industrial diamond output. Synthetic diamond production in centres such as Ireland, Japan, Russia, and the USA far exceeds it.

METALS

* Figures for aluminum are for refined metal; all other figures refer to ore production

The world's leading producers of aluminum ore (bauxite) in 2000 were as follows:

1. Australia 38.6%
2. Guinea 11.8%
3. Brazil 10.4%
4. Jamaica 8.8%
5. China 6.3%
6. India 4.9%
7. Venezuela 3.5%
8. Suriname 3.1%
9. Russia 3.1%
10. Guyana 2.6%

The figures shown above are in stark contrast to the figures showing aluminum production (*see above right*). Australia, for example, produces 38.6% of the world's bauxite but only 5.9% of aluminum. Guinea and Jamaica account for over 20% of the bauxite mined but have no smelters and export virtually all of it to countries like the USA and Canada.

Aluminum: Produced mainly from its oxide, bauxite, which yields 25% of its weight in aluminum. The cost of refining and production is often too high for producer-countries to bear, so bauxite is largely exported. Lightweight and corrosion resistant, aluminum alloys are widely used in aircraft, vehicles, cans, and packaging.

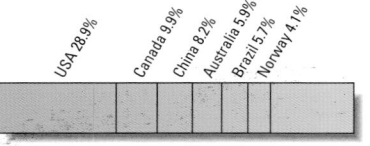

World total (2000): 23,900,000 tons *

Lead: A soft metal, obtained mainly from galena (lead sulfide), which occurs in veins associated with iron, zinc, and silver sulfides. Its use in vehicle batteries accounts for the USA's prime consumer status; lead is also made into sheeting and piping. Its use as an additive to paints and petrol is decreasing.

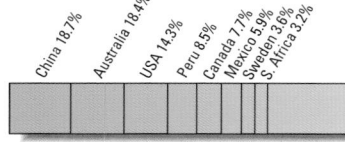

World total (2000): 2,980,000 tons *

Tin: Soft, pliable and non-toxic, used to coat "tin" (tin-plated steel) cans, in the manufacture of foils and in alloys. The principal tin-bearing mineral is cassiterite (SnO_2), found in ore formed from molten rock. Producers and refiners were hit by a price collapse in 1991.

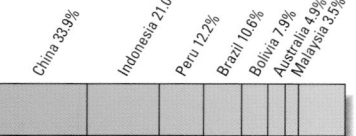

World total (2000): 200,000 tons *

Gold: Regarded for centuries as the most valuable metal in the world and used to make coins, gold is still recognized as the monetary standard. A soft metal, it is alloyed to make jewelry; the electronics industry values its corrosion resistance and conductivity.

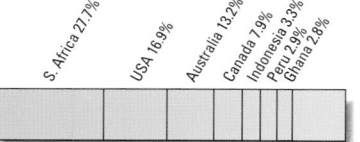

World total (2000): 2,445 tons *

Copper: Derived from low-yielding sulfide ores, copper is an important export for several developing countries. An excellent conductor of heat and electricity, it forms part of most electrical items, and is used in the manufacture of brass and bronze. Major importers include Japan and Germany.

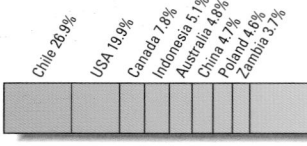

World total (2000): 12,900,000 tons *

Mercury: The only metal that is liquid at normal temperatures, most is derived from its sulfide, cinnabar, found only in small quantities in volcanic areas. Apart from its value in thermometers and other instruments, most mercury production is used in anti-fungal and anti-fouling preparations, and to make detonators.

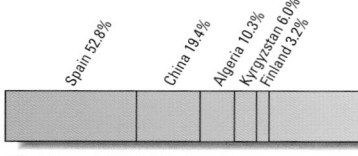

World total (2000): 1,800 tons *

Zinc: Often found in association with lead ores, zinc is highly resistant to corrosion, and about 40% of the refined metal is used to plate sheet steel, particularly vehicle bodies – a process known as galvanizing. Zinc is also used in dry batteries, paints, and dyes.

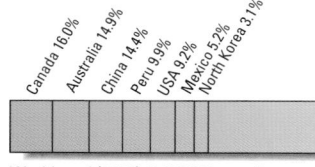

World total (2000): 8,000,000 tons *

Silver: Most silver comes from ores mined and processed for other metals (including lead and copper). Pure or alloyed with harder metals, it is used for jewelry and ornaments. Industrial use includes dentistry, electronics, photography, and as a chemical catalyst.

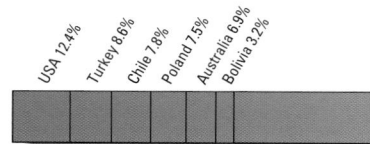

World total (2000): 17,900 tons *

DISTRIBUTION OF MINERALS

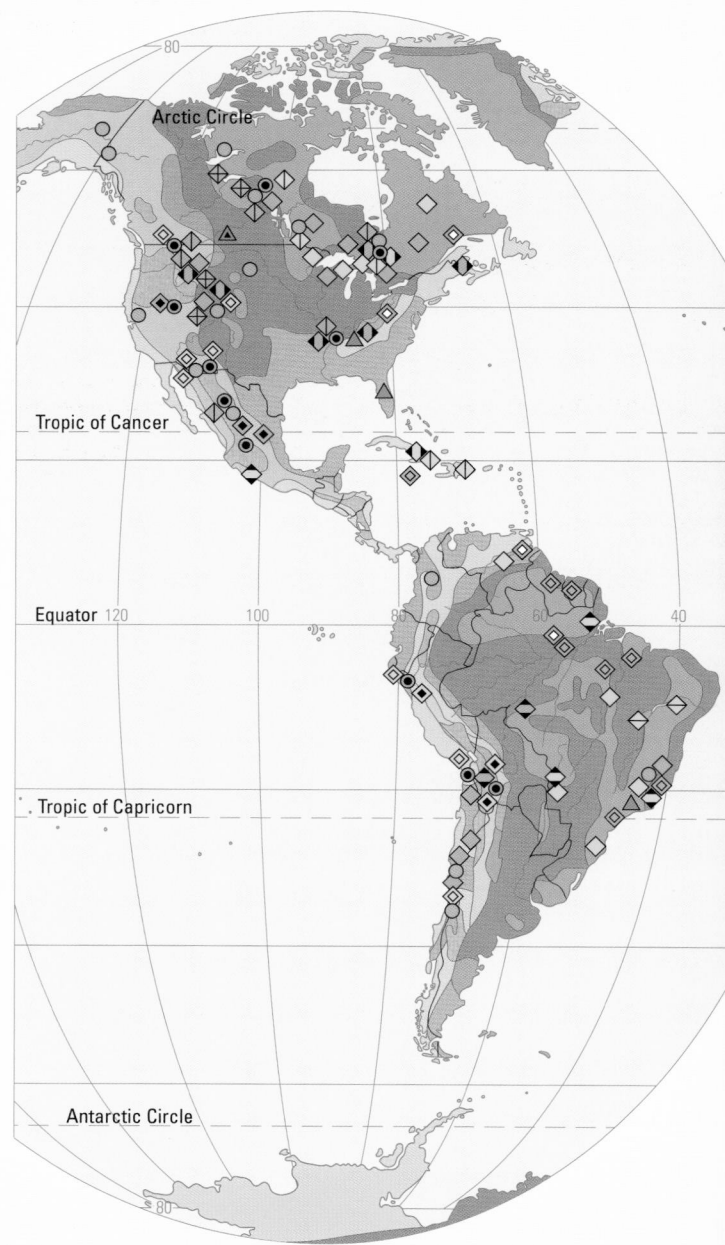

IRON ORE

Ever since the art of high-temperature smelting was discovered, some time in the second millennium BC, iron has been by far the most important metal known to man. The earliest iron plows transformed primitive agriculture and led to the first human population explosion, while iron weapons – or the lack of them – ensured the rise or fall of entire cultures.

Widely distributed around the world, iron ores usually contain 25–60% iron; blast furnaces process the raw product into pig-iron, which is then alloyed with carbon and other minerals to produce steels of various qualities. From the time of the Industrial Revolution, steel has been almost literally the backbone of modern civilization, the prime structural material on which all else is built.

Iron smelting usually developed close to the sources of ore and, later, to the coalfields that fueled the furnaces. Today, most ore comes from a few richly-endowed locations where large-scale mining is possible.

Iron and steel plants are generally built at coastal sites so that giant ore carriers, which account for a sizable proportion of the world's merchant fleet, can easily discharge their cargoes.

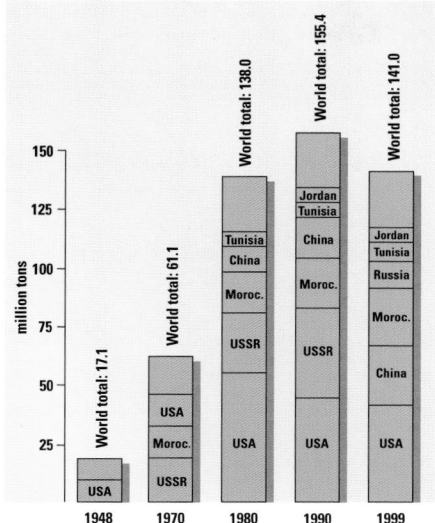

World production of phosphates in millions of tons (1999): Phosphate production is vital to the economies of several small countries. Nauru, for example, is heavily dependent on phosphate exports – the island has one of the world's richest deposits. In 1999, 500,000 tons were mined, employing 1,000 people. In Togo, earnings from phosphate exports have superseded all agricultural exports.

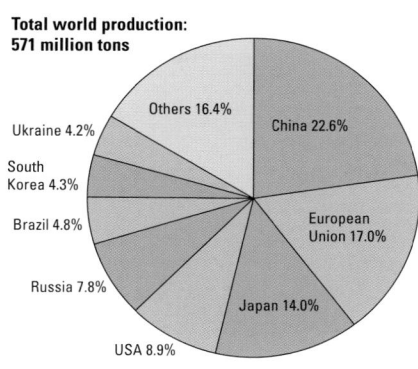

World production of pig-iron (2000): All countries with an annual output of more than 1 million tons are shown

Total world production: 571 million tons

- China 22.6%
- European Union 17.0%
- Japan 14.0%
- USA 8.9%
- Russia 7.8%
- Brazil 4.8%
- South Korea 4.3%
- Ukraine 4.2%
- Others 16.4%

Chromium: Most of the world's chromium production is alloyed with iron and other metals to produce steels with various different properties. Combined with iron, nickel, cobalt, and tungsten, chromium produces an exceptionally hard steel, resistant to heat; chrome steels are used for many household items where utility must be matched with appearance – cutlery, for example. Chromium is also used in the production of refractory bricks, and its salts for tanning and dyeing leather and cloth.

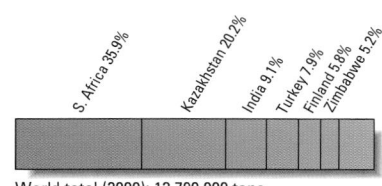

S. Africa 35.9% · Kazakhstan 20.2% · India 9.1% · Turkey 7.9% · Finland 5.8% · Zimbabwe 5.2%

World total (2000): 13,700,000 tons

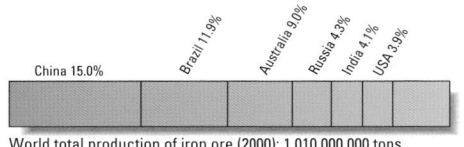

China 15.0% · Brazil 11.9% · Australia 9.0% · Russia 4.3% · India 4.1% · USA 3.9%

World total production of iron ore (2000): 1,010,000,000 tons

Percentage of total world phosphate production (1999)

1. USA	28.8%	7. Brazil	2.9%
2. China	17.8%	8. Israel	2.9%
3. Morocco	17.0%	9. South Africa	2.1%
4. Russia	7.9%	10. Syria	1.5%
5. Tunisia	5.7%	11. Senegal	1.3%
6. Jordan	4.3%	12. India	1.2%

Manganese: In its pure state, manganese is a hard, brittle metal. Alloyed with chrome, iron, and nickel, it produces abrasion-resistant steels; manganese-aluminum alloys are light but tough. Found in batteries and inks, manganese is also used in glass production. Manganese ores are frequently found in the same location as sedimentary iron ores. Pyrolusite (MnO_2) and psilomelane are the main economically-exploitable sources.

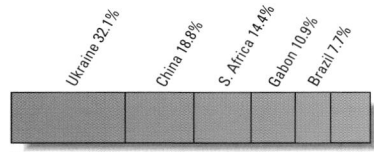

Ukraine 32.1% · China 18.8% · S. Africa 14.4% · Gabon 10.9% · Brazil 7.7%

World total (2000): 7,450,000 tons (metal content)

Nickel: Combined with chrome and iron, nickel produces stainless and high-strength steels; similar alloys go to make magnets and electrical heating elements. Nickel combined with copper is widely used to make coins; cupro-nickel alloy is very resistant to corrosion. Its ores yield only modest quantities of nickel – 0.5% to 3% – but also contain copper, iron, and small amounts of precious metals. Japan, USA, UK, Germany, and France are the principal importers.

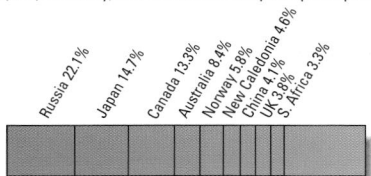

Russia 22.1% · Japan 14.7% · Canada 13.3% · Australia 8.4% · Norway 5.6% · New Caledonia 4.6% · China 3.9% · UK 3.6% · S. Africa 3.3%

World total (2000): 1,230,000 tons

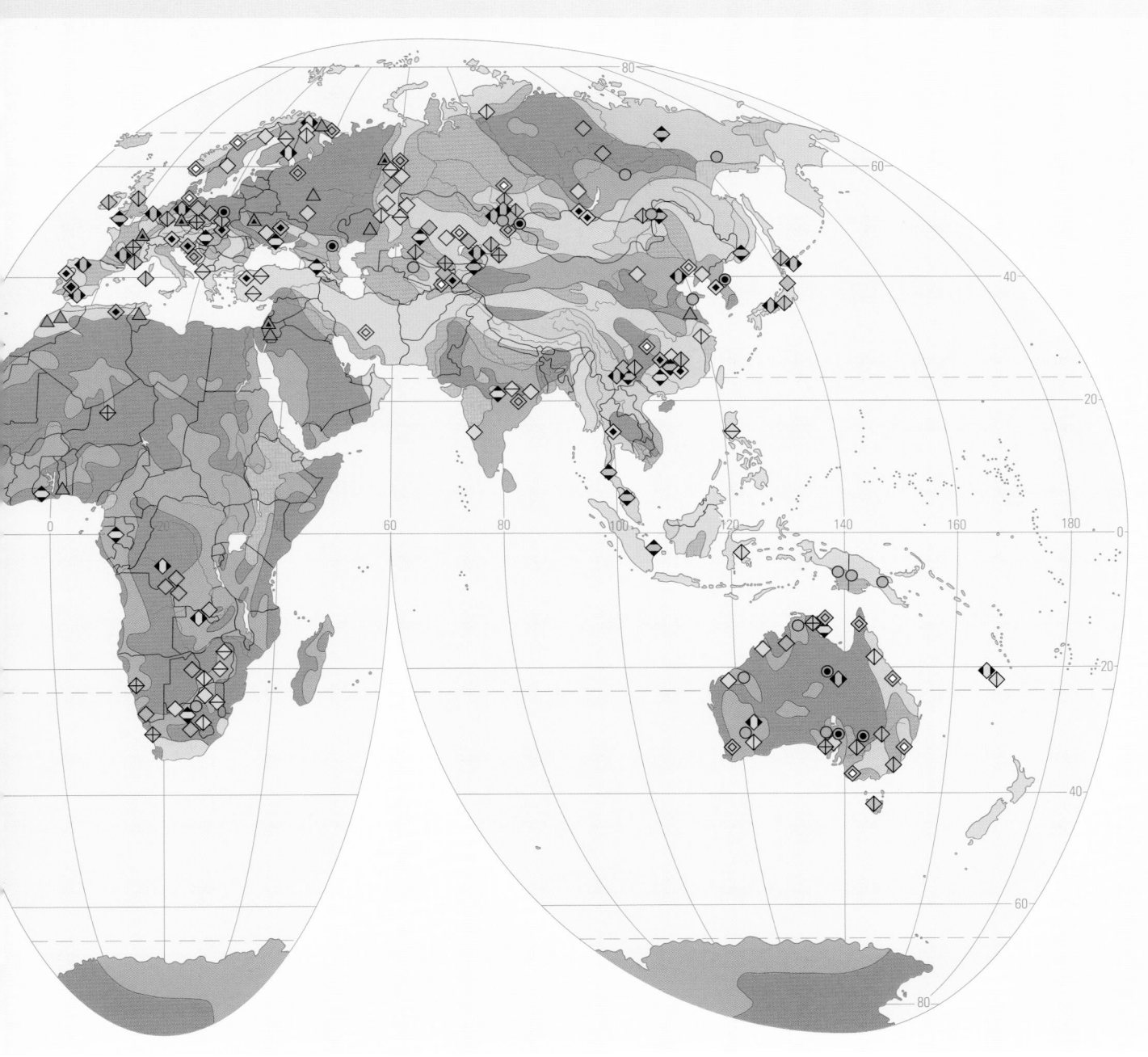

STRUCTURAL REGIONS

- Pre-Cambrian shields
- Sedimentary cover on Pre-Cambrian shields
- Paleozoic (Caledonian and Hercynian) folding
- Sedimentary cover on Paleozoic folding
- Mesozoic folding
- Sedimentary cover on Mesozoic folding
- Cenozoic (Alpine) folding
- Sedimentary cover on Cenozoic folding
- Intensive Mesozoic and Cenozoic vulcanism

DISTRIBUTION

Iron and ferroalloys
- Chrome
- Cobalt
- Iron ore
- Manganese
- Molybdenum
- Nickel ore
- Tungsten

Non-ferrous metals
- Bauxite (Aluminum)
- Copper
- Lead
- Mercury
- Tin
- Zinc
- Uranium

Precious metals and stones
- Diamonds
- Gold
- Silver

Fertilizers
- Phosphates
- Potash

MANUFACTURING

For more information:
18 Water distribution
32 Land use
36 Minerals
37 Iron and ferroalloys
40 Major exports
   Traded products

The Industrial Revolution which began in Britain in the late 18th century, represented a major technological advance in the evolution of human society. It enabled a group of countries to become prosperous by replacing expensive human labor with increasingly sophisticated machinery. In economic terms, manufacturing is the transformation of raw materials, energy, labor, and machines into finished goods, which have a higher value than the various elements used in production.

The economies of countries can be compared by reference to their per capita Gross National Products (or per capita GNPs), namely, the total value of goods and services produced in a country in a year, divided by the population.

The industrialized, or developed, countries accounted for 15% of the world's population in 2000 with an average per capita GNP of more than US $25,000. On the other hand, low-income developing countries, with small industrial sectors, accounted for 34% of the world's population. Their per capita GNPs are less than $755, with some as low as $200.

Kenya, with its low-income economy, had a per capita GNP in 2000 of US $350. Agriculture employs 19% of the people, industry 18%, and services 64%. The main industries are the processing of agricultural imports and import substitution (making such necessities as cement, footwear, and textiles). Heavy industry plays only a small part. By contrast, Germany had a per capita GNP in 2000 of $25,120. Agriculture employs only 2% of the population, with 30% in industry and 68% in services. Germany's industrial sector differs greatly from Kenya's, with its emphasis on vehicles, machinery, chemicals, and electronics.

Since the 1970s, some former developing countries in eastern Asia achieved rapid economic growth through industrialization. Despite setbacks in the late 1990s, they demonstrated that a developing industrial sector can transform an economy, which starts off with certain advantages, such as low labor costs. But economic success also depends on such factors as education to provide skills, and regulations that attract foreign investors. China, whose economy grew by more than 9% per year between 1989 and 2002, satisfies many of these criteria, though its record on human rights leaves much to be desired.

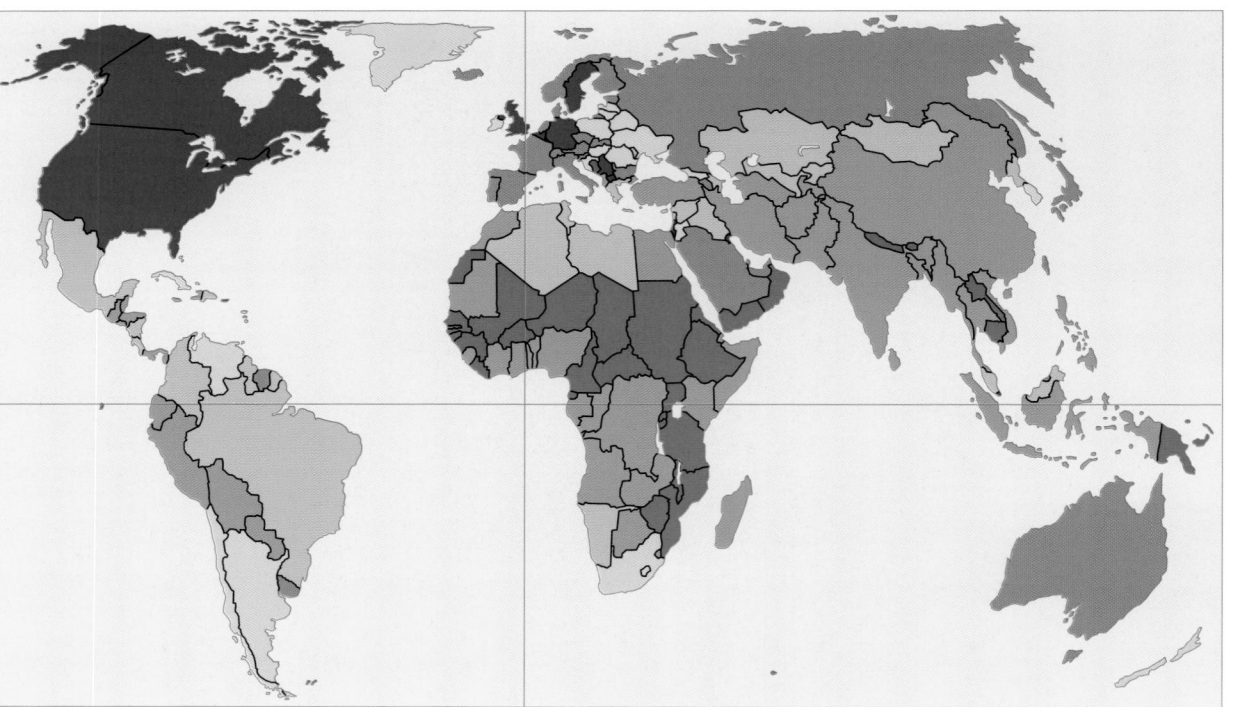

EMPLOYMENT

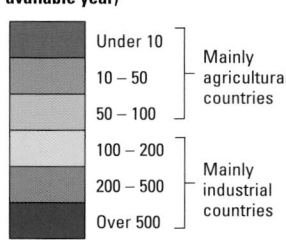

The number of workers employed in manufacturing for every 100 workers engaged in agriculture (latest available year)

Under 10	
10 – 50	Mainly agricultural countries
50 – 100	
100 – 200	
200 – 500	Mainly industrial countries
Over 500	

Selected countries (latest available year)

Singapore	8,860
UK	1,270
Belgium	820
Germany	800
Kuwait	767
Bahrain	660
USA	657
Israel	633

DIVISION OF EMPLOYMENT

Distribution of workers between agriculture, industry and services, selected countries (latest available year)

The six countries selected illustrate the usual stages of economic development, from dependence on agriculture through industrial growth to the expansion of the service sector.

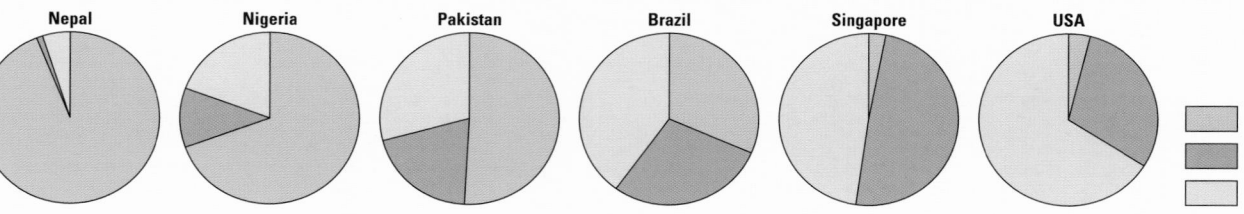

Nepal   Nigeria   Pakistan   Brazil   Singapore   USA

- Agriculture
- Industry
- Services

THE WORK FORCE

Percentages of men and women between 15 and 64 in employment, selected countries (latest available year)

The figures include employees and the self-employed, who in developing countries are often subsistence farmers. People in full-time education are excluded. Because of the population age structure in developing countries, the employed population has to support a far larger number of non-workers than its industrial equivalent. For example, more than 52% of Kenya's people are under 15, an age group that makes up less than a tenth of the UK population.

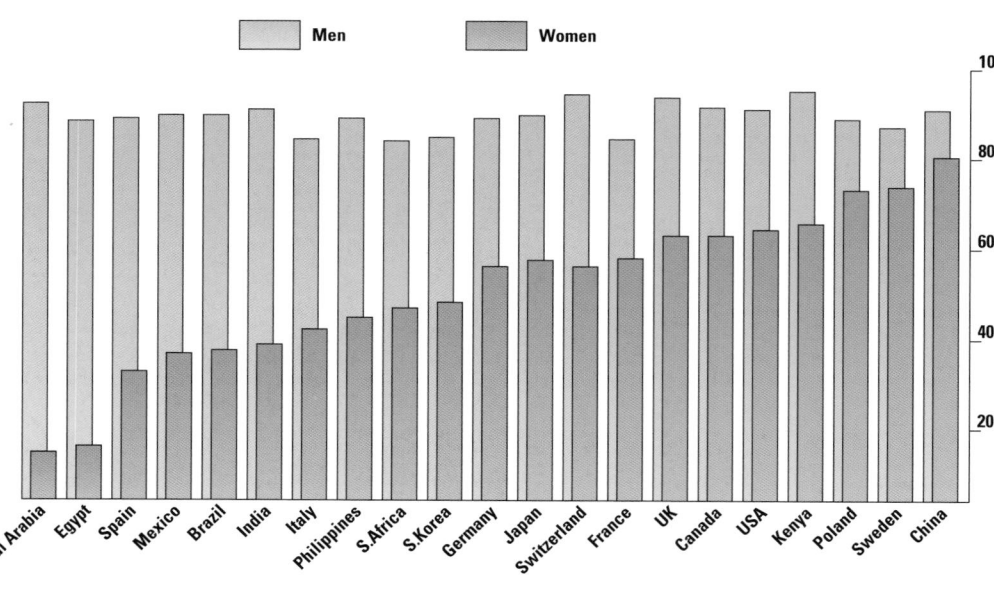

Men   Women

WEALTH CREATION

The Gross National Income (GNI) of the world's largest economies, US $ million (2001)

1.	USA	9,900,724	21.	Austria	194,463
2.	Japan	4,574,164	22.	Hong Kong	176,157
3.	Germany	1,947,951	23.	Turkey	168,335
4.	UK	1,451,442	24.	Denmark	166,345
5.	France	1,377,389	25.	Poland	163,907
6.	China	1,130,984	26.	Norway	160,577
7.	Italy	1,123,478	27.	Saudi Arabia	149,932
8.	Canada	661,881	28.	Indonesia	144,731
9.	Spain	586,874	29.	South Africa	125,486
10.	Mexico	550,456	30.	Greece	124,553
11.	Brazil	528,503	31.	Finland	124,171
12.	India	474,323	32.	Thailand	120,871
13.	South Korea	447,698	33.	Venezuela	117,169
14.	Netherlands	385,401	34.	Iran	112,855
15.	Australia	383,291	35.	Portugal	109,156
16.	Switzerland	266,503	36.	Israel	104,128
17.	Argentina	260,994	37.	Egypt	99,406
18.	Russia	253,413	38.	Singapore	99,404
19.	Belgium	239,779	39.	Ireland	88,385
20.	Sweden	225,894	40.	Malaysia	86,510

INDUSTRIAL OUTPUT

Industrial output (mining, manufacturing, construction, energy, and water production), US $ billion (latest available year)

1.	Japan	1,941	21.	Sweden	73
2.	USA	1,808	22.	Saudi Arabia	67
3.	Germany	780	=	Thailand	67
4.	France	415	24.	Mexico	65
5.	UK	354	25.	Turkey	51
6.	Italy	337	26.	Denmark	50
7.	China	335	27.	Finland	46
8.	Brazil	255	=	Poland	46
9.	South Korea	196	29.	Norway	44
10.	Spain	187	30.	Malaysia	37
11.	Canada	174	=	Portugal	37
12.	Russia	131	32.	Ukraine	34
13.	Netherlands	107	33.	Greece	33
14.	Australia	98	34.	Singapore	30
15.	Switzerland	96	35.	Venezuela	29
16.	India	94	=	Israel	29
17.	Argentina	87	37.	Chile	24
18.	Belgium	83	=	Colombia	24
=	Indonesia	83	=	Hong Kong	24
20.	Austria	79	=	Philippines	24

INDUSTRY AND TRADE

Manufactured goods (including machinery and transport) as a percentage of total exports (1999)

- Over 75%
- 50 – 75%
- 25 – 50%
- 10 – 25%
- Under 10%

Countries most dependent on the export of manufactured goods

Malta	91%
Bangladesh	90%
China	90%
Japan	88%
South Korea	83%
Luxembourg	83%
Pakistan	83%

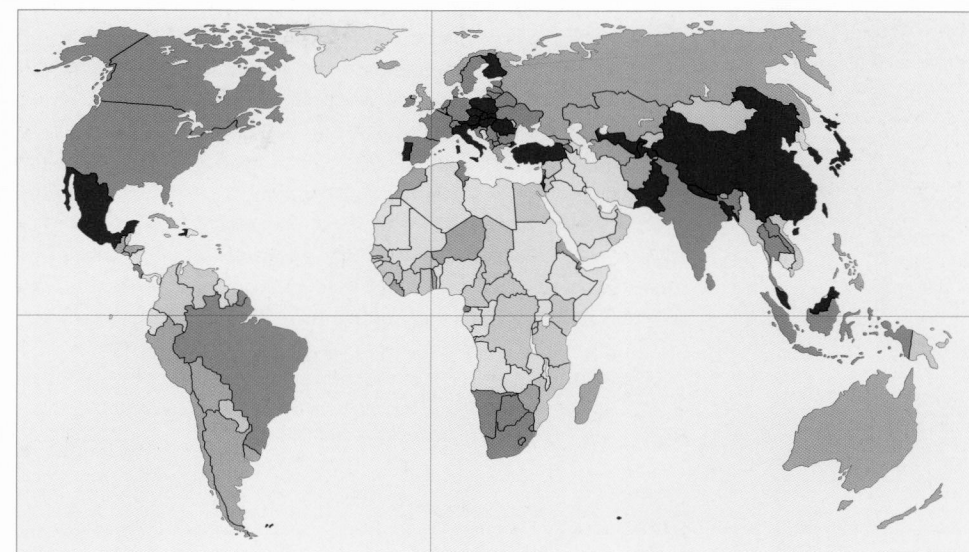

PATTERNS OF PRODUCTION

Breakdown of industrial output by value, selected countries (latest available year)

	Food & agric. products	Textiles & clothing	Machinery & transport	Chemicals	Other
Algeria	26%	20%	11%	1%	41%
Argentina	24%	10%	16%	12%	37%
Australia	18%	7%	21%	8%	45%
Austria	17%	8%	25%	6%	43%
Belgium	19%	8%	23%	13%	36%
Brazil	15%	12%	24%	9%	40%
Burkina Faso	62%	18%	2%	1%	17%
Canada	15%	7%	25%	9%	44%
Denmark	22%	6%	23%	10%	39%
Egypt	20%	27%	13%	10%	31%
Finland	13%	6%	24%	7%	50%
France	18%	7%	33%	9%	33%
Germany	12%	5%	38%	10%	36%
Greece	20%	22%	14%	7%	38%
Hungary	6%	11%	37%	11%	35%
India	11%	16%	26%	15%	32%
Indonesia	23%	11%	10%	10%	47%
Iran	13%	22%	22%	7%	36%
Ireland	28%	7%	20%	15%	28%
Israel	13%	10%	28%	8%	42%
Italy	7%	13%	32%	10%	38%
Japan	10%	6%	38%	10%	37%
Kenya	35%	12%	14%	9%	29%
Malaysia	21%	5%	23%	14%	37%
Mexico	24%	12%	14%	12%	39%
Netherlands	19%	4%	28%	11%	38%
New Zealand	26%	10%	16%	6%	43%
Norway	21%	3%	26%	7%	44%
Pakistan	34%	21%	8%	12%	25%
Philippines	40%	7%	7%	10%	35%
Poland	15%	16%	30%	6%	33%
Portugal	17%	22%	16%	8%	38%
Singapore	6%	5%	46%	8%	36%
South Africa	14%	8%	17%	11%	49%
South Korea	15%	17%	24%	9%	35%
Spain	17%	9%	22%	9%	43%
Sweden	10%	2%	35%	8%	44%
Thailand	30%	17%	14%	6%	33%
Turkey	20%	14%	15%	8%	43%
UK	14%	6%	32%	11%	36%
USA	12%	5%	35%	10%	38%
Venezuela	23%	8%	9%	11%	49%

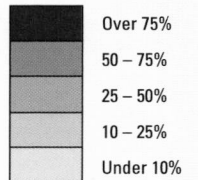

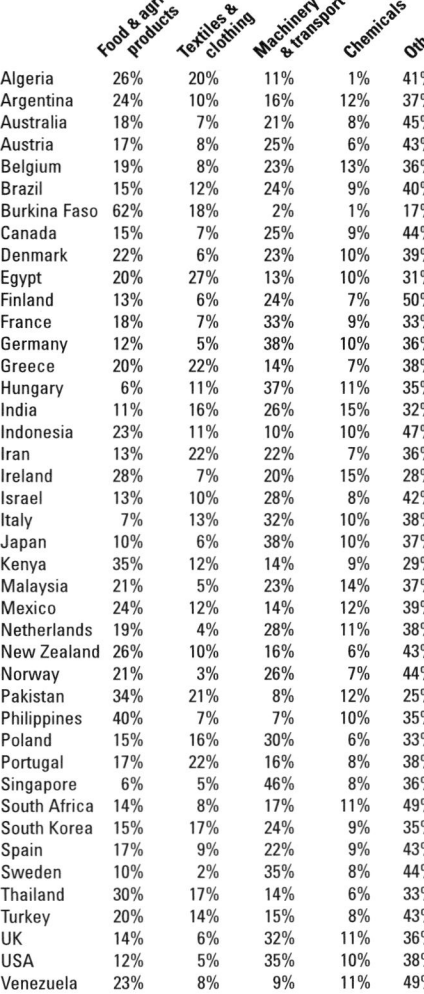

◄ This photograph shows a cement-manufacturing plant in Riverside, California, USA. Cement production figures are often an indicator of the relative prosperity of a country, since they show the construction of roads, dams and other infrastructure projects (*see the graph below*).

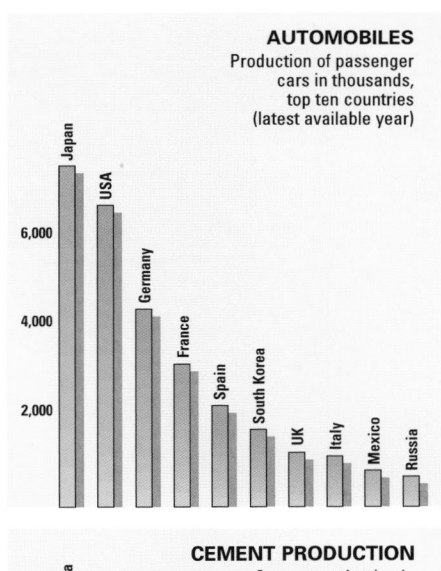

AUTOMOBILES
Production of passenger cars in thousands, top ten countries (latest available year)

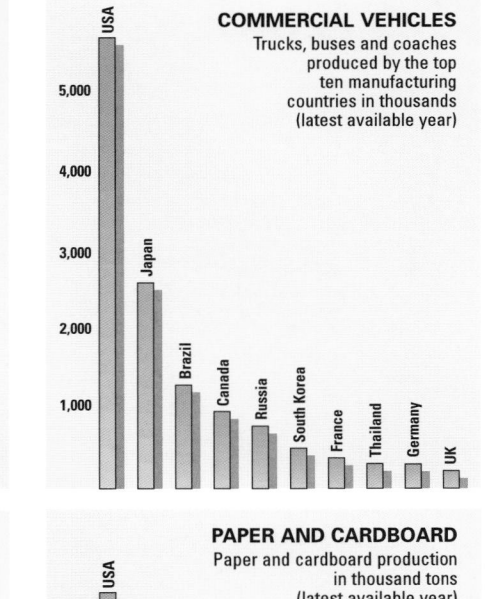

COMMERCIAL VEHICLES
Trucks, buses and coaches produced by the top ten manufacturing countries in thousands (latest available year)

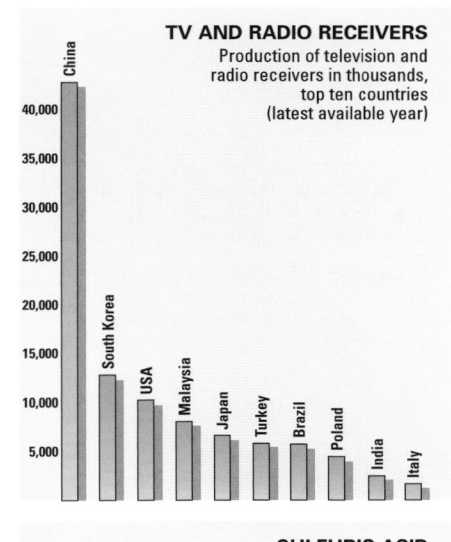

TV AND RADIO RECEIVERS
Production of television and radio receivers in thousands, top ten countries (latest available year)

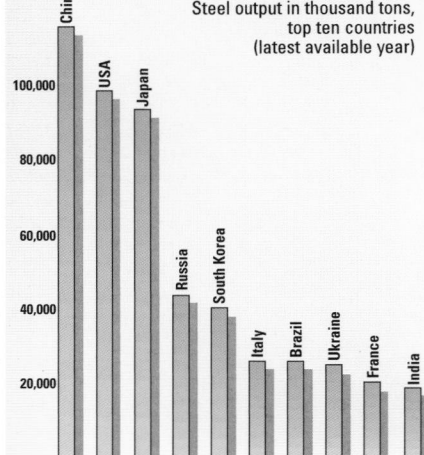

STEEL PRODUCTION
Steel output in thousand tons, top ten countries (latest available year)

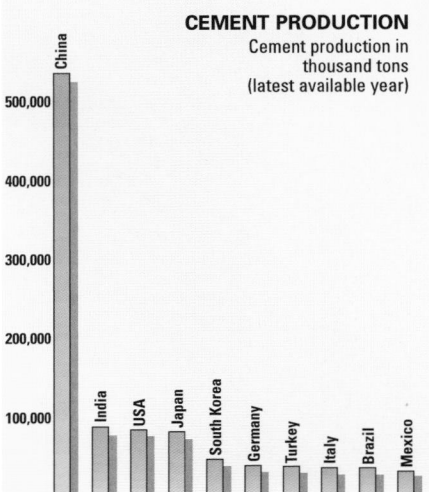

CEMENT PRODUCTION
Cement production in thousand tons (latest available year)

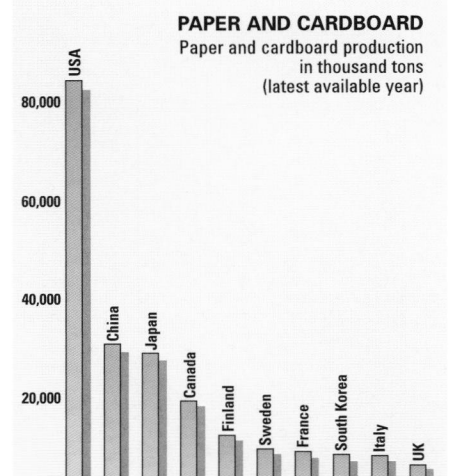

PAPER AND CARDBOARD
Paper and cardboard production in thousand tons (latest available year)

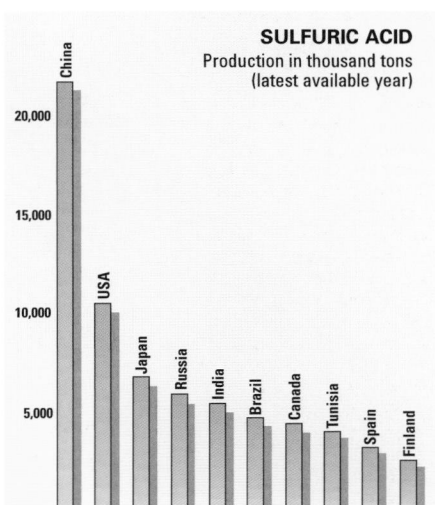

SULFURIC ACID
Production in thousand tons (latest available year)

TRADE

For more information:

31 International organizations
35 Movements of oil
36 Minerals
38 Wealth creation
39 Industry and trade
45 Air travel and tourism
   Inflation

Trade played a vital role in the growth of early civilizations and it was later a spur to European exploration and colonization. The colonial powers grew rich by exporting cheap manufactures, such as clothing and footwear, while obtaining primary products from their colonies.

From the late 19th century to the early 1950s, as transport technology improved, primary products, especially oil in the later stages of this period, dominated world trade. However, since that time, manufactures have become the chief commodities in world trade, which is dominated by the industrialized countries. Nearly half of all world trade flows between the developed market economies of the European Union, the United States and Japan, although a number of Asian economies, notably China, Malaysia, Singapore, South Korea, Taiwan, and Thailand, increased their share in the 1990s.

China's remarkable economic growth meant that, by 2002, it had overtaken Japan to become the fourth biggest exporter to the United States. China's low production costs, especially its cheap labor, was estimated to be one-twentieth of those of Japan, making its high-quality exports highly competitive in price. Growth in world trade is regarded as a sign of economic health, as is a favorable balance of trade (or trade surplus) in any country.

WORLD TRADE

Percentage share of total world exports by value (2000)

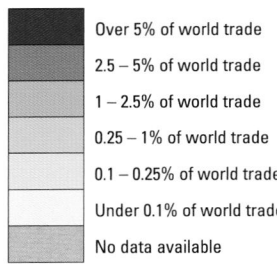

- Over 5% of world trade
- 2.5 – 5% of world trade
- 1 – 2.5% of world trade
- 0.25 – 1% of world trade
- 0.1 – 0.25% of world trade
- Under 0.1% of world trade
- No data available

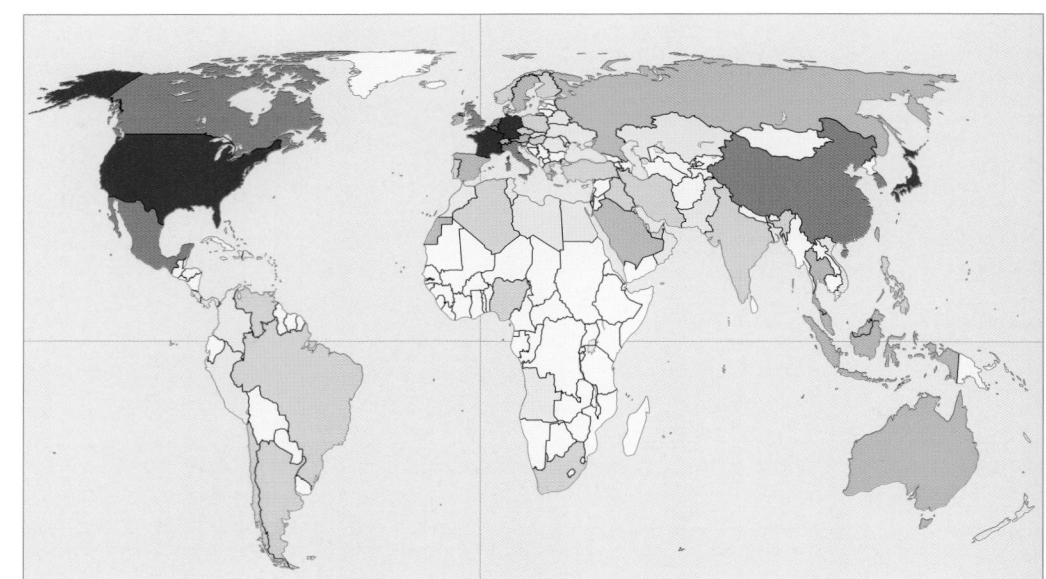

International trade is dominated by a handful of powerful maritime nations. The members of "G8" (Canada, France, Germany, Italy, Japan, Russia, the United Kingdom, and the United States) account for more than half the total. The majority of nations contribute less than a quarter of 1% to the worldwide total of exports. The countries of the European Union account for 35%, whereas the Pacific Rim nations account for over 50%.

DEPENDENCE ON TRADE

Exports as a percentage of GDP (2001)

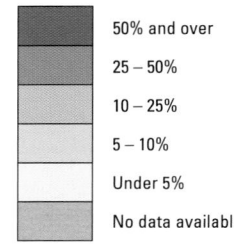

- 50% and over
- 25 – 50%
- 10 – 25%
- 5 – 10%
- Under 5%
- No data available

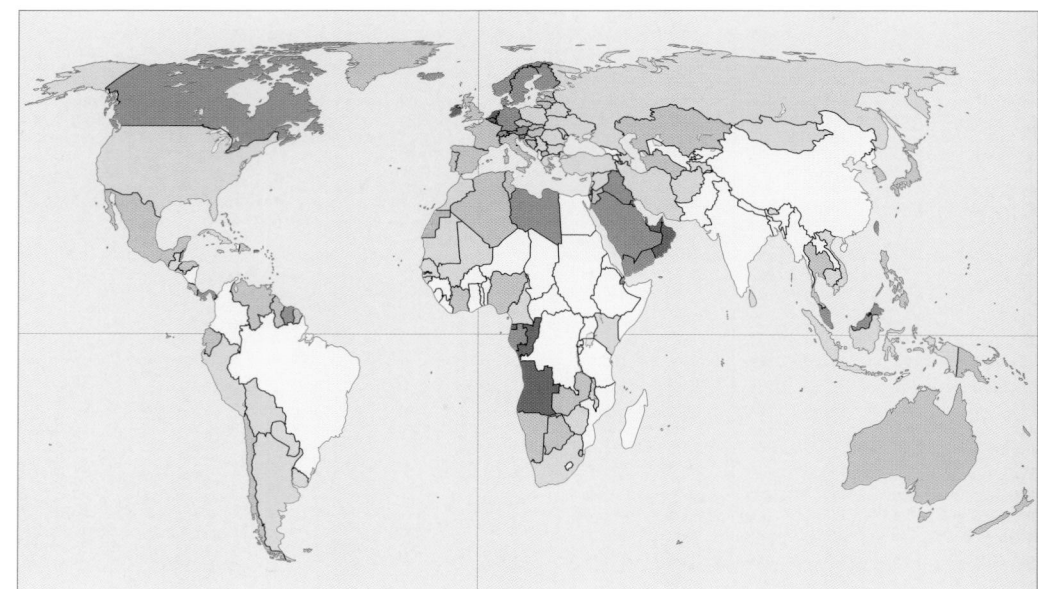

The character of world trade has changed a great deal in the last 50 years or so. While many developing countries still remain heavily dependent on exporting mineral ores, fossil fuels or farm products, such as coffee or cocoa, world trade is now dominated by manufactured goods. Since the 1980s, high-tech products, such as computer equipment, telecommunications gear and transistors, have become increasingly important.

TRADED PRODUCTS

Major manufactures traded by value, in millions of US $ (2000)

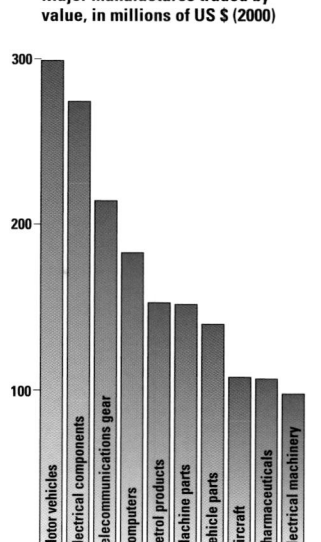

MAJOR EXPORTS

Leading manufactured items and their exporters (2000)

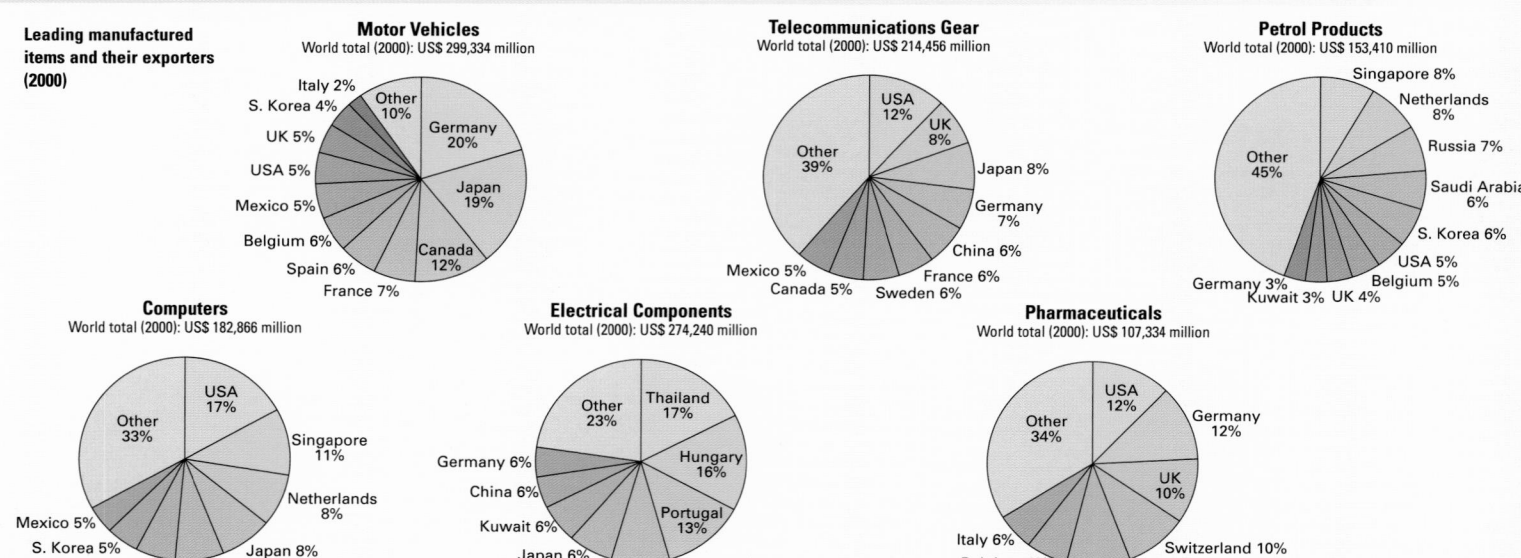

40

WORLD SHIPPING

While ocean passenger traffic is relatively modest nowadays, sea transport still carries most of the world's trade. Oil and bulk carriers make up the majority of the world fleet, although the general cargo category is the fastest growing. Two innovations have revolutionized sea transport. The first is the development of the roll-on/roll-off (Ro-Ro) method where lorries or even trains loaded with freight are driven straight on to the ship, thus saving time. The second is containerization in which goods are packed into containers (the dimensions of which are fixed) at the factory, driven to the port, and loaded on board by specialist machinery.

Almost 30% of world shipping today sails under a "flag of convenience," whereby owners take advantage of low taxes by registering their vessels in a foreign country the ships will never see, notably Panama and Liberia.

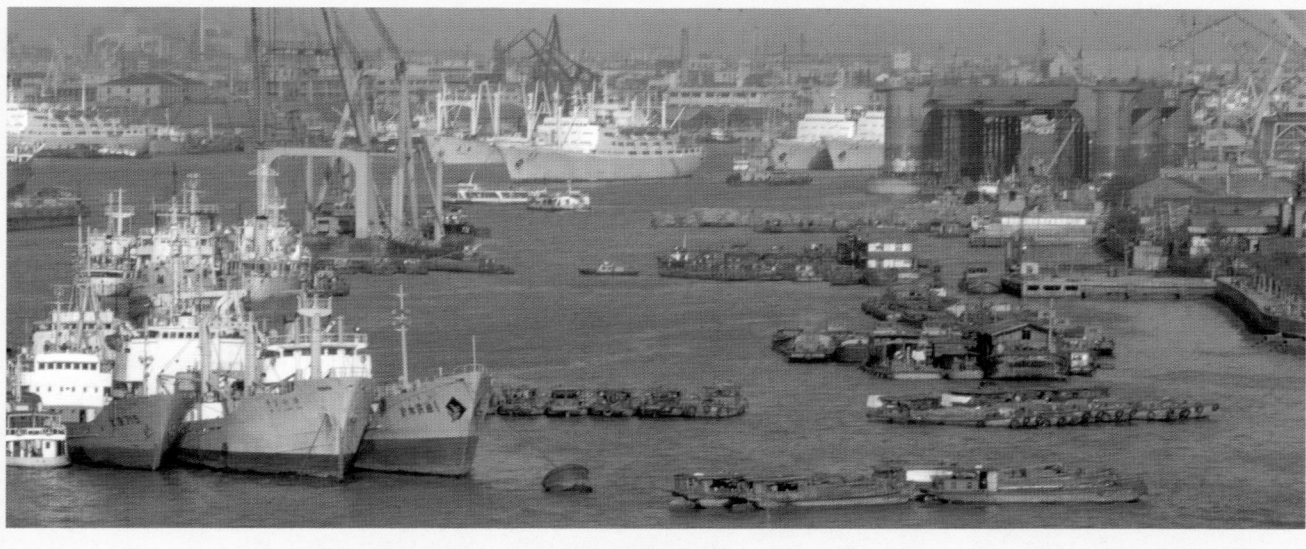

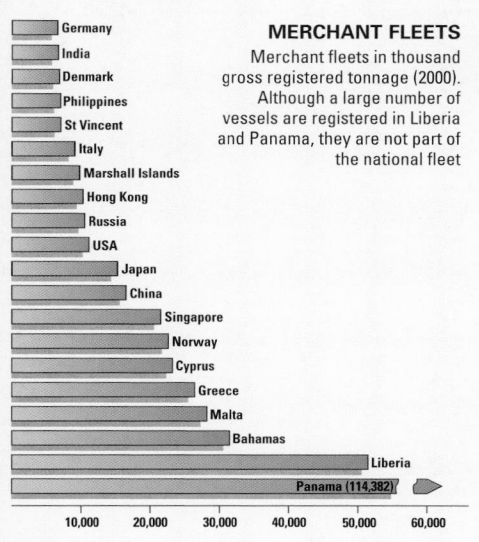

MERCHANT FLEETS

Merchant fleets in thousand gross registered tonnage (2000). Although a large number of vessels are registered in Liberia and Panama, they are not part of the national fleet

THE GREAT PORTS

Total cargo traffic, in million tons (2000)

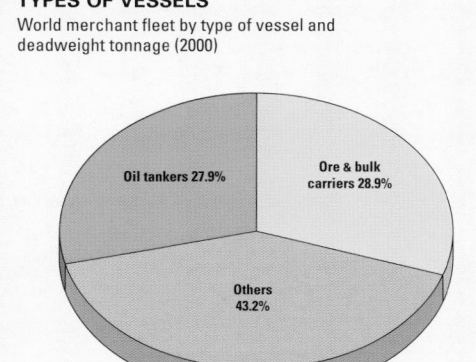

TYPES OF VESSELS

World merchant fleet by type of vessel and deadweight tonnage (2000)

Oil tankers 27.9%
Ore & bulk carriers 28.9%
Others 43.2%

▲ Shanghai is the largest port in China, lying on the Yangtze River, which is navigable for over 600 miles [1,000 km]. In this image more modern shipping can be seen alongside smaller traditional craft, which are used to trans-ship cargoes to smaller ports.

TRADE IN PRIMARY PRODUCTS

Primary products (excluding fuels, metals, and minerals) as a percentage of total export value (2000)

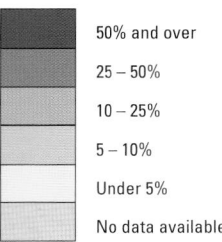

- 50% and over
- 25 – 50%
- 10 – 25%
- 5 – 10%
- Under 5%
- No data available

Primary products are raw materials or partly processed products that form the basis for manufacturing. They are the necessary requirements of industries and include agricultural products, minerals and timber, as well as many semimanufactured goods such as cotton, which has been spun but not woven, wood pulp or flour. Many developed countries have few natural resources and rely on imports for the majority of their primary products. The countries of Southeast Asia export hardwoods to the rest of the world, while many South American countries are heavily dependent on coffee exports.

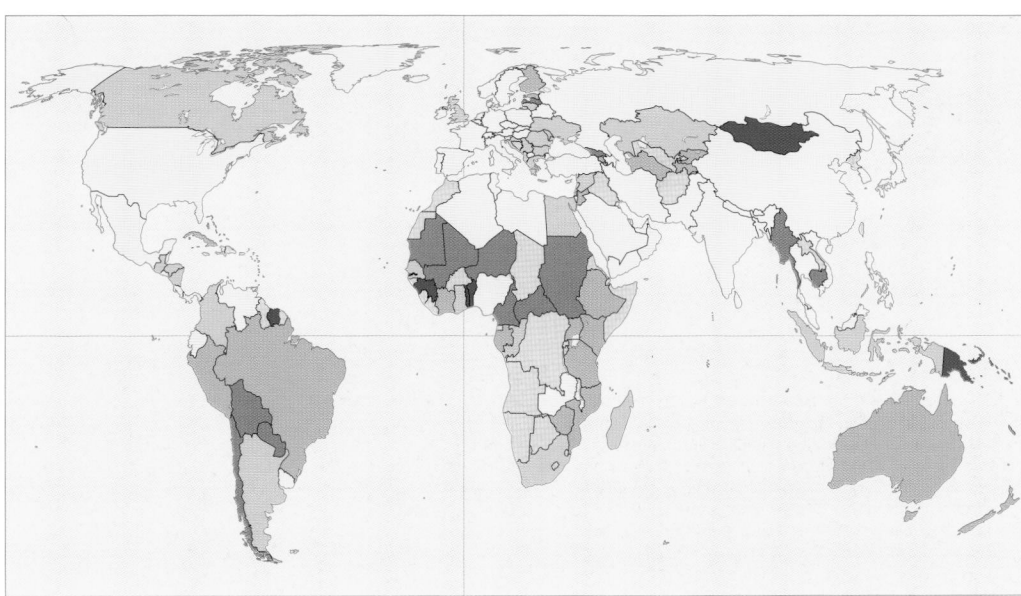

BALANCE OF TRADE

Value of exports in proportion to the value of imports (2000)

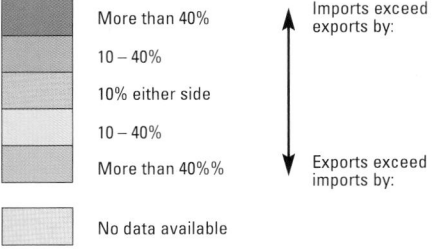

- More than 40%
- 10 – 40%
- 10% either side
- 10 – 40%
- More than 40%%

Imports exceed exports by:

Exports exceed imports by:

No data available

The total world trade balance should amount to zero, since exports must equal imports on a global scale. In practice, though, at least US $100 billion in exports go unrecorded, leaving the world with an apparent deficit and many countries in a better position than public accounting reveals. However, a favorable trade balance is not necessarily a sign of prosperity: many poorer countries must maintain a high surplus in order to service debts, and do so by restricting imports below the levels needed to sustain successful economies.

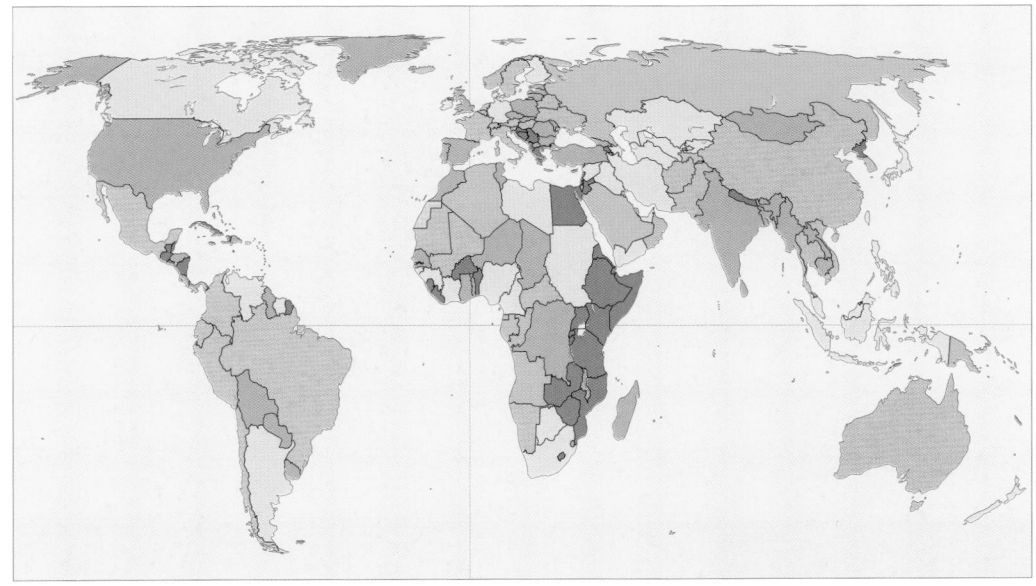

41

HEALTH

For more information:

18 Water distribution
27 Urban pollution
   Urban advantages
33 Crisis in Africa
   Food and population
47 Distribution of
   spending

Until the late 1990s, when the full extent of the AIDS crisis emerged, average life expectancies at birth were rising almost everywhere. By 2000, they ranged from 78 years in high income economies to 47 in sub-Saharan Africa. These figures represented an enormous advance on the situation in 1880, when citizens of Berlin had an estimated life expectancy of 30 years.

The ravages of AIDS have been greatest in southern Africa. One of the worst affected countries is Botswana, where nearly 40% of the adult population were thought to be infected by 2002. In Botswana, life expectancies were expected to fall to 27 years in 2010 instead of an original estimate of 74 years. However, in much of the world, average life expectancies are still increasing. The rises are attributed to improvements in agriculture and, hence, nutrition, as well as health education, improved sanitation and the quality of drinking water, together with advances in medicine.

Besides AIDS, the people of the developing world are subject to another affliction – malnutrition. The map below shows that in most of Africa, Asia, and Latin America, the average daily calorie supply per person is so low as to cause malnutrition. Malnutrition is a serious condition – among pregnant women it causes high rates of child mortality.

Deficiency diseases occur when people do not have a balanced diet. Protein deficiency causes stunting and kwashiorkor, which can be fatal, especially among young children, while vitamin deficiencies cause such illnesses as beri beri, pellagra, scurvy, and rickets. Iron deficiency causes anaemia, while a lack of iodine causes mental retardation.

Infectious diseases, in association with deficient diets, continue to affect people in developing countries. Around the turn of the century, a WHO report stated that infectious diseases cause over 16 million deaths a year. Most of the victims are young and otherwise fit people in developing countries. The major killers are AIDS, cholera, dysentery, malaria, measles, pneumonia, respiratory infections, tuberculosis, and typhoid.

Infectious diseases are much less important as causes of death in developed countries, where cancer and circulatory diseases, such as atherosclerosis and hypertension, which cause strokes and heart attacks, are the most common causes of fatality. Because these diseases tend to kill older people, they are relatively less important in the developing countries where people have shorter lifespans.

Harmful habits are also generally practiced more by the rich than the poor. For example, smoking is an important cause of death in developed countries, while high alcohol consumption has bad effects on health.

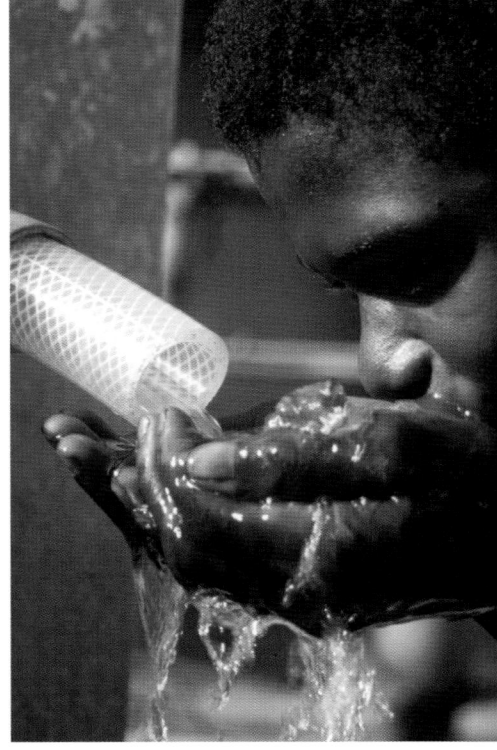

▲ Almost 17% of the world's population does not have access to safe water (the diagram at the bottom left-hand corner of this page shows how this breaks down by continent). This places a huge strain on the millions of mainly women and children who have to walk, collect and carry drinkable water in order to survive. UNICEF is dedicated to help improve this situation and to react swiftly in the case of emergencies such as civil war, as with the case of this man in Liberia.

FOOD CONSUMPTION

Average daily food intake in calories per person (2000)

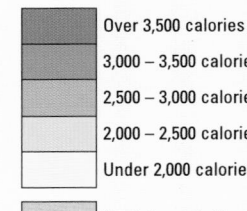

- Over 3,500 calories
- 3,000 – 3,500 calories
- 2,500 – 3,000 calories
- 2,000 – 2,500 calories
- Under 2,000 calories
- No data available

The daily food intake rated adequate by the World Health Organization is between 2,300 and 2,500 calories per day. Approximately 6 million children under the age of 5 years die of starvation each year, the vast majority in Africa. In 2000, the FAO estimated that 840 million people were undernourished, contrasting sharply with the overconsumption of food in some Western cultures.

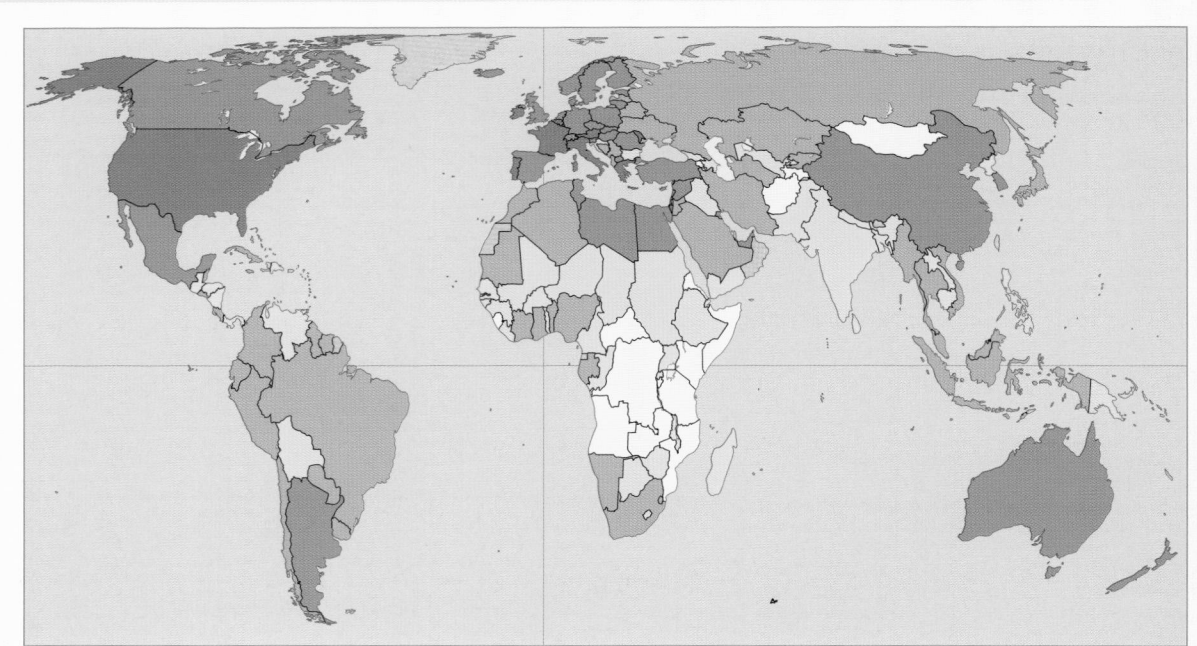

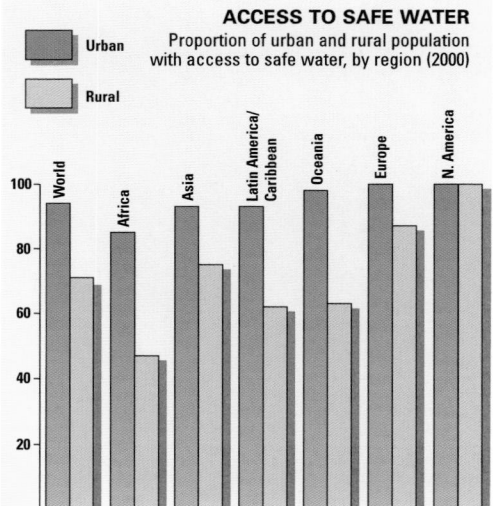

ACCESS TO SAFE WATER
Proportion of urban and rural population with access to safe water, by region (2000)
Urban / Rural
World, Africa, Asia, Latin America/Caribbean, Oceania, Europe, N. America

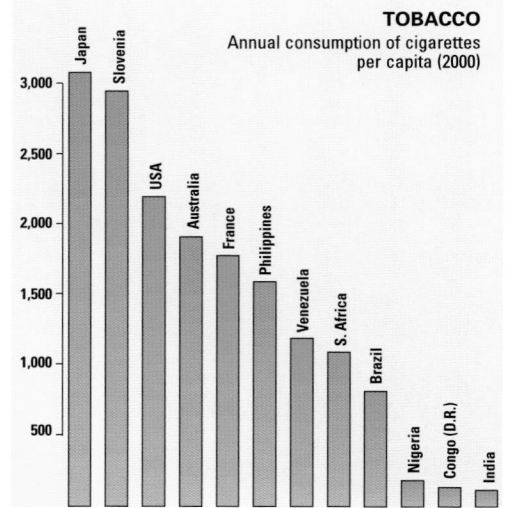

TOBACCO
Annual consumption of cigarettes per capita (2000)
Japan, Slovenia, USA, Australia, France, Philippines, Venezuela, S. Africa, Brazil, Nigeria, Congo (D.R.), India

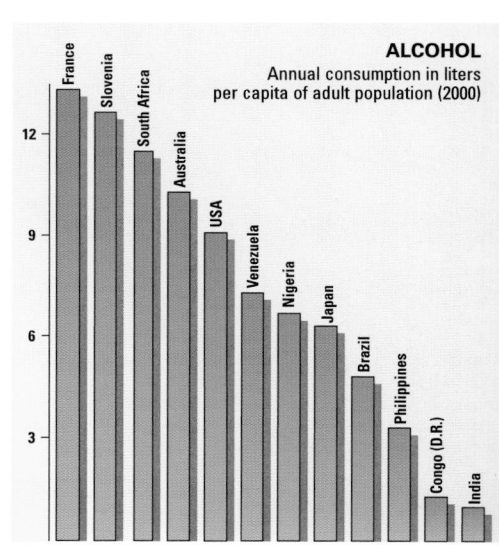

ALCOHOL
Annual consumption in liters per capita of adult population (2000)
France, Slovenia, South Africa, Australia, USA, Venezuela, Nigeria, Japan, Brazil, Philippines, Congo (D.R.), India

INFANT MORTALITY

Number of babies who died under the age of one, per 1,000 births (2000)

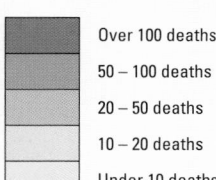

- Over 100 deaths
- 50 – 100 deaths
- 20 – 50 deaths
- 10 – 20 deaths
- Under 10 deaths

Highest infant mortality

Afghanistan	137 deaths
Western Sahara	134 deaths
Malawi	131 deaths

Lowest infant mortality

Iceland	5 deaths
Finland	4 deaths
Japan	4 deaths

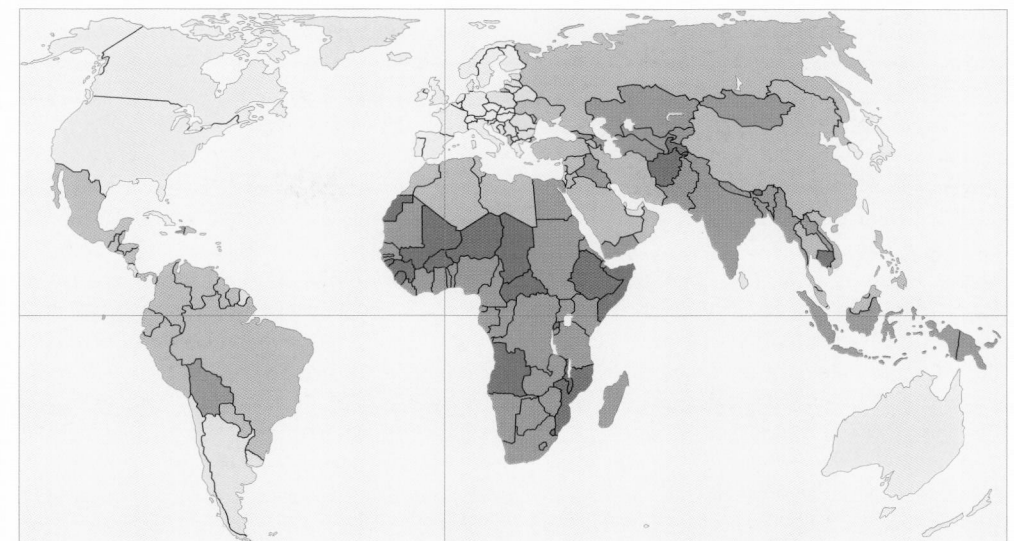

THE AIDS CRISIS

The Acquired Immune Deficiency Syndrome (AIDS) was first identified in 1981 when American doctors found otherwise healthy young men succumbing to rare infections. By 1984 the cause had been traced to the Human Immunodeficiency Virus (HIV), which can remain dormant for many years and perhaps indefinitely: only half of those known to carry the virus in 1981 had developed AIDS ten years later.

In Western countries in the 1990s, most AIDS deaths were among male homosexuals or needle-sharing drug-users. However, the disease is spreading fastest among heterosexual men and women, which is its usual vector in the developing world where most of its victims live.

In 2002, 25 million people had already died of AIDS and another 42 million were infected with the HIV virus. Around 30 million of them live in Africa. In some southern African countries, more than a third of the population carries the virus. In South Africa, which has the largest number of HIV infections, about 6 million people were expected to die of the disease between 2002 and 2012.

AIDS also has other serious consequences. A report by UNAIDS and UNICEF stated that the number of children orphaned by AIDS rose threefold between 1996 and 2002, reaching an all-time high of 13.4 million.

AIDS
Cases reported in 1999

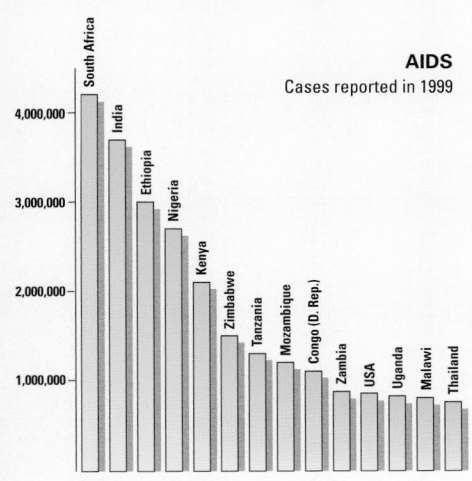

MEDICAL PROVISION

Doctors per 100,000 population, selected countries (2000)

Although the ratio of people to doctors gives a good approximation of a country's health provision, it is not an absolute indicator. Raw numbers may mask inefficiency and other weaknesses: the high proportion of physicians in Hungary, for example, has not prevented infant mortality rates more than twice as high as in the United Kingdom.

The definition of a doctor also varies from nation to nation. As well as registered medical practitioners, it may include trained medical assistants – an especially important category in developing countries, where they provide many of the same services as fully qualified physicians, including simple operations.

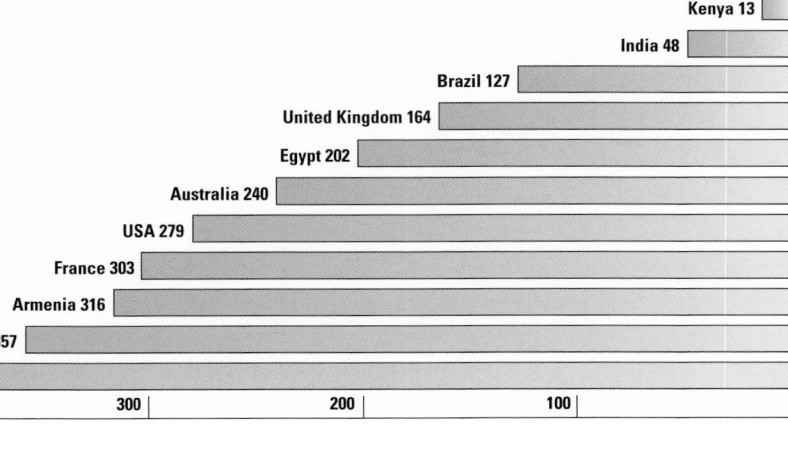

CAUSES OF DEATH

- Accidents, poisoning, and violence
- Respiratory and digestive diseases
- Nervous and circulatory diseases
- Metabolic disorders
- Cancers
- Infectious and parasitic diseases

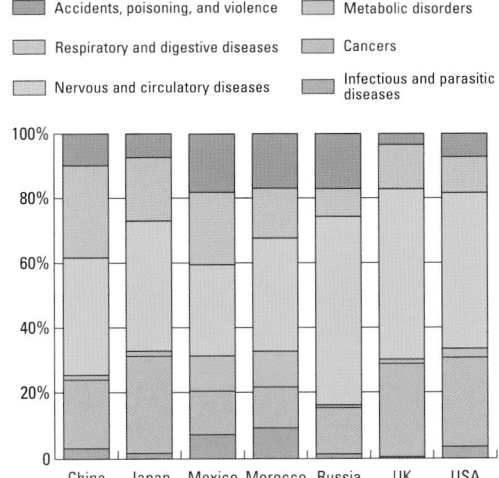

EXPENDITURE ON HEALTH

Public health expenditure per capita, in US $ (latest available year)

Countries with the highest spending		Countries with the lowest spending	
USA	$4,271	Mozambique	$8
Switzerland	$3,857	Tanzania	$8
Norway	$3,182	Sierra Leone	$8
Denmark	$2,785	Indonesia	$8
Luxembourg	$2,731	Chad	$7
Iceland	$2,701	Laos	$6
Germany	$2,697	Niger	$5
France	$2,288	Madagascar	$5
Japan	$2,243	Burundi	$5
Netherlands	$2,173	Ethiopia	$4

The allocation of limited funds for health care in developing countries is rarely evenly spread – the quality of treatment can vary enormously from place to place within the same country. Urban dwellers tend to have much better access to health provisions than those living in rural areas.

SANITATION
Percentage of population with access to sanitation services, selected countries (latest available year)

- Urban
- Rural

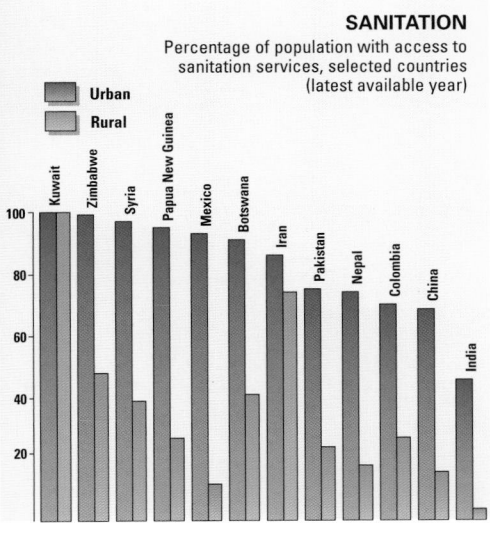

MALARIA
Cases of malaria per 100,000 people exposed to malaria-infected environments, selected countries* (latest available year)

*data not available for Africa where 80% of malaria cases occur

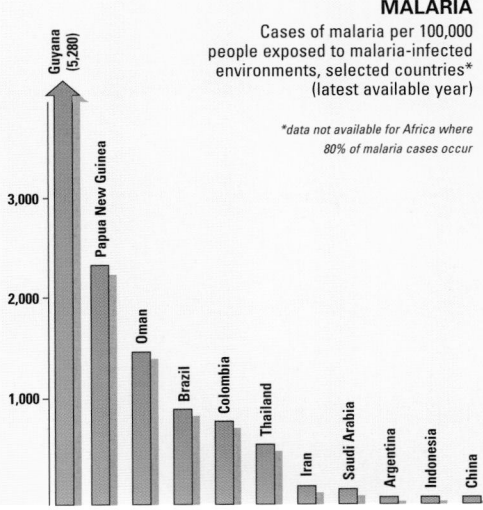

CIRCULATORY DISEASE IN EUROPE

Diseases of the circulatory system per 100,000 people (latest available year)

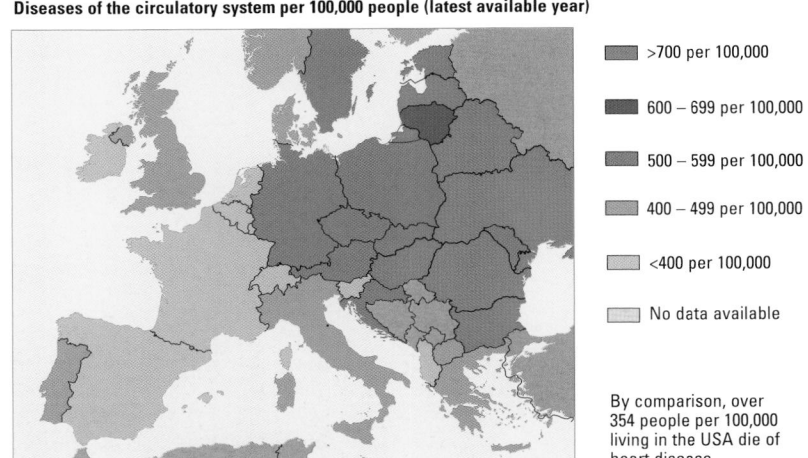

- >700 per 100,000
- 600 – 699 per 100,000
- 500 – 599 per 100,000
- 400 – 499 per 100,000
- <400 per 100,000
- No data available

By comparison, over 354 people per 100,000 living in the USA die of heart disease.

WEALTH

For more information:

38 Wealth creation
39 Industrial output
40 World trade
   Major exports
41 Balance of trade
47 Distribution of
   spending

Perhaps the most glaring differences in the world today are those between the rich and the poor. The World Bank divides countries into three main groups based on average economic production expressed in terms of per capita GNP (Gross National Product). They are the low-income economies, including most African countries and much of Asia; the middle-income economies, including most of Latin America and most of the former USSR; and the high-income economies of Canada, the United States, Western Europe, Japan, and Australia.

Per capita GNPs are a measure of the total goods and services produced by a country divided by the population, and then converted into US dollars at official exchange rates. They are useful indicators of a country's prosperity, though, like all statistics, they must be treated with care. For example, the prices for goods and services in China are far cheaper than they are in the United States. China's per capita GNP in 2000 was $840 (as compared with $34,100 in the USA), but the PPP (Purchasing Power Parity) estimate of China's per capita GNP was considerably higher at $3,920. Another problem with per capita GNPs is that they are averages, which often conceal wide internal variations.

The pattern of poverty varies from region to region. In Latin America, much progress has been made through industrialization, though startling inequalities still exist between rich and poor. China and other countries in eastern Asia, including South Korea and Taiwan, have followed Japan's example in pursuing export-led industrial policies. The success of China's Special Economic Zones, where foreign investment is encouraged, has led to a huge rise in China's per capita GNP.

Solutions to poverty in Africa are much harder to find because of its high population growth, civil wars, natural disasters and high inflation rates. Although Africa receives more aid than any other continent, aid is only a partial solution. Much aid has been wasted on overambitious projects, in the servicing of huge national debts, or lost by inexperienced or corrupt governments. One initiative in some African countries has been to improve the infrastructure and develop tourism, creating employment and providing much-needed foreign currency. But tourism alone cannot solve the problems of under-development.

The International Monetary Fund and the World Bank argue that real economic progress in Africa will be achieved only when African countries create market-friendly economies that encourage trade through export-led manufacturing, while at the same time strictly controlling public spending on welfare, the civil service, and other areas.

CONTINENTAL SHARES

Shares of population and of wealth (GNP) by continent

These generalized continental figures show the startling difference between rich and poor, but mask the successes or failures of individual countries. Japan, for example, with less than 4% of Asia's population, produces almost 70% of the continent's output. Within countries, the difference between rich and poor can also be startling. In Brazil, for example, the richest 20% of the population own 60% of the wealth.

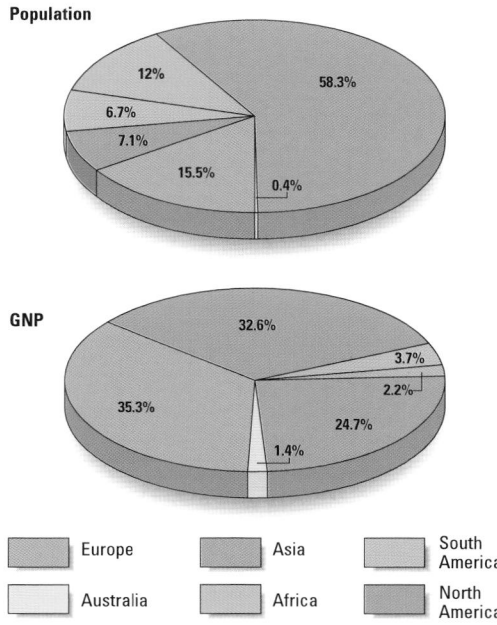

Population

GNP

Europe · Asia · South America · Australia · Africa · North America

LEVELS OF INCOME

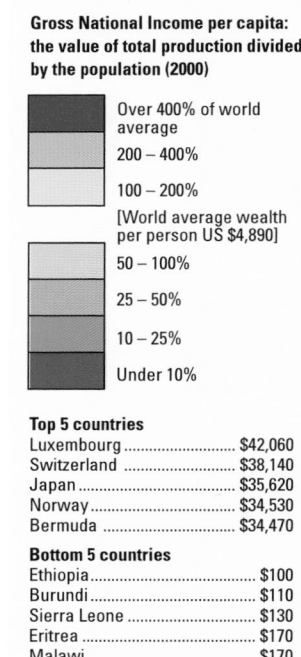

Gross National Income per capita: the value of total production divided by the population (2000)

- Over 400% of world average
- 200 – 400%
- 100 – 200%

[World average wealth per person US $4,890]

- 50 – 100%
- 25 – 50%
- 10 – 25%
- Under 10%

Top 5 countries

Luxembourg	$42,060
Switzerland	$38,140
Japan	$35,620
Norway	$34,530
Bermuda	$34,470

Bottom 5 countries

Ethiopia	$100
Burundi	$110
Sierra Leone	$130
Eritrea	$170
Malawi	$170

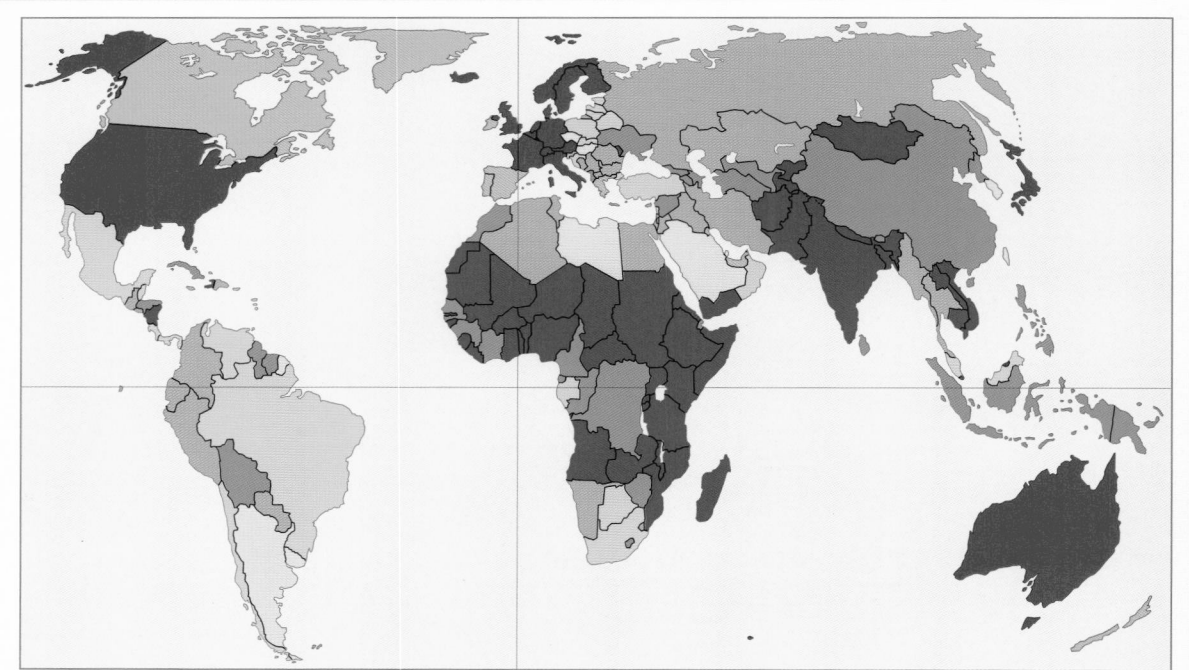

INDICATORS

The gap between the world's rich and poor is now so great that it is difficult to illustrate on a single graph. Within each income group (as defined by the World Bank), however, comparisons have some meaning. The wealth gap in many developing countries, though, is wide, with a small, rich class and a large, impoverished majority, while many high-income countries contain an underclass of unemployed and homeless people.

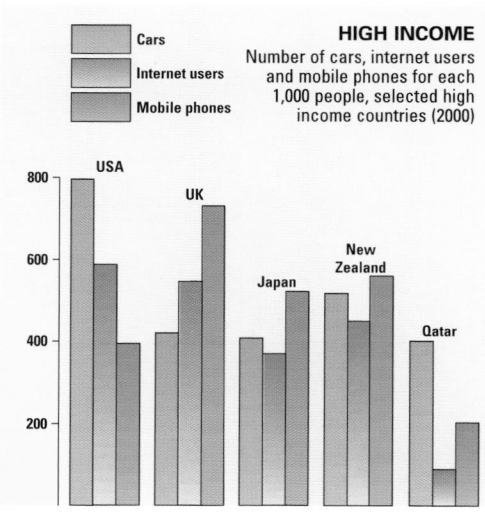

HIGH INCOME

Cars · Internet users · Mobile phones

Number of cars, internet users and mobile phones for each 1,000 people, selected high income countries (2000)

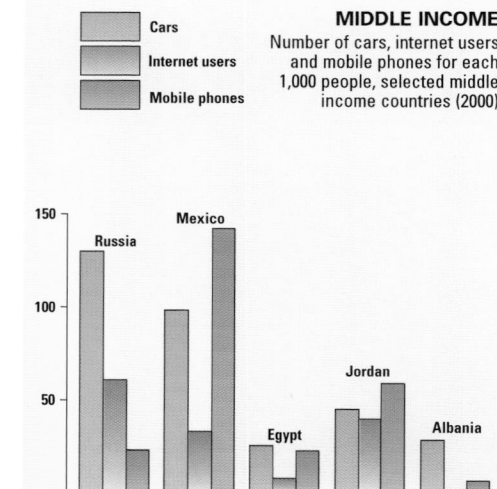

MIDDLE INCOME

Cars · Internet users · Mobile phones

Number of cars, internet users and mobile phones for each 1,000 people, selected middle income countries (2000)

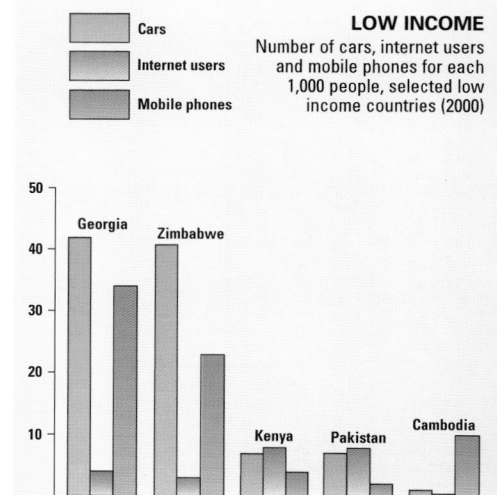

LOW INCOME

Cars · Internet users · Mobile phones

Number of cars, internet users and mobile phones for each 1,000 people, selected low income countries (2000)

STATE FINANCE

Inflation rates (*shown on the map, right*) are an indication of a country's financial stability and, usually, of its prosperity. Annual inflation rates above 20% are usually marked by slow or even negative growth of the GNP. Above 50%, it becomes hyperinflation and an economy is left reeling.

In the late 1980s and early 1990s, many high-income countries had to contend with annual inflation rates of 10% or more, while Japan, the growth leader, had an average inflation rate of just 1.3% between 1985 and 1994.

Market-friendly policies, including low taxes and state spending, liberal trade policies and a warm welcome for foreign investors, are major factors in countries that have enjoyed rapid economic growth in the decades since 1980. For example, the setting up of Special Economic Zones in eastern China has led to a spectacular rise in that country's per capita GNP.

Other successful countries include South Korea and Singapore, although an Asian market crash in 1997 temporarily halted the dramatic economic expansion of these countries.

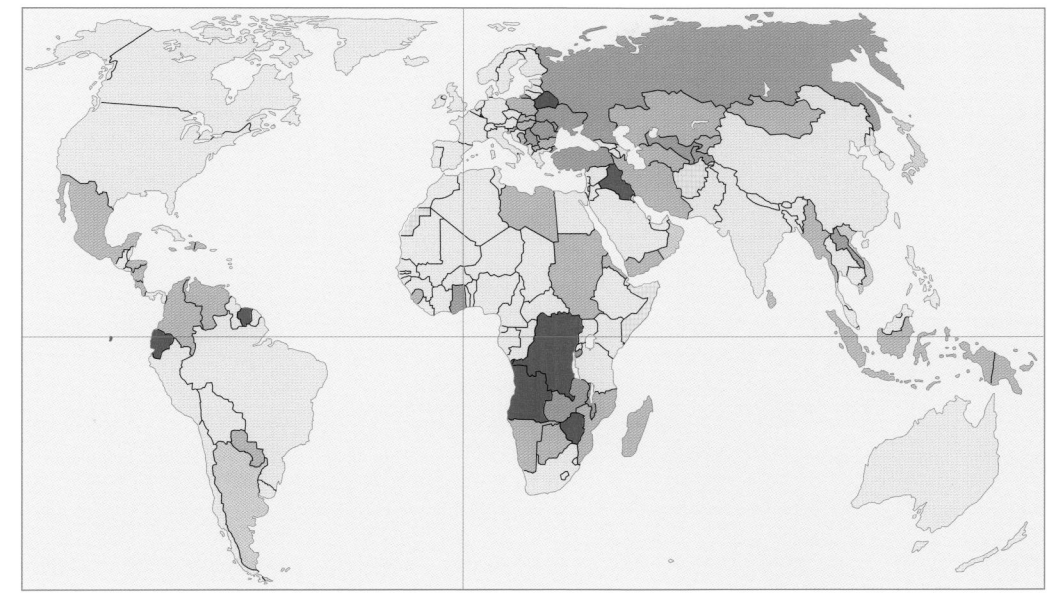

INFLATION

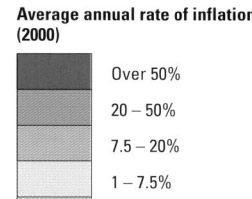

Average annual rate of inflation (2000)

- Over 50%
- 20 – 50%
- 7.5 – 20%
- 1 – 7.5%
- Negative inflation
- No data available

Highest average inflation
Congo (Dem. Rep.) 1,423%
Angola 740%
Turkmenistan 407%

Lowest average inflation
Antigua and Barbuda .... −11.5%
Argentina* .... −3.1%
Bahrain .... −0.1%

* During 2002, Argentina experienced a sharp rise in inflation which is not reflected on this map.

GROWTH IN GNI

GNI per capita annual growth rate (1998–9)

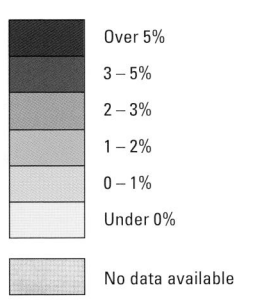

- Over 5%
- 3 – 5%
- 2 – 3%
- 1 – 2%
- 0 – 1%
- Under 0%
- No data available

Countries with highest growth rates
Equatorial Guinea 15.0%
Mozambique 10.0%
Palau 10.0%
South Korea 10.0%
Guinea-Bissau 9.5%

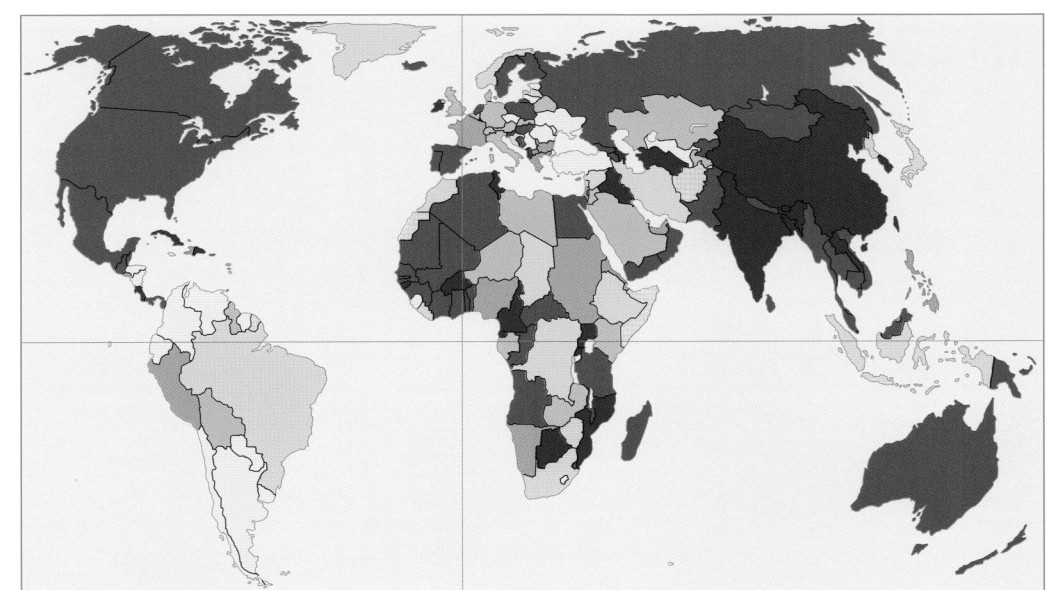

WORLD AIR TRAVEL

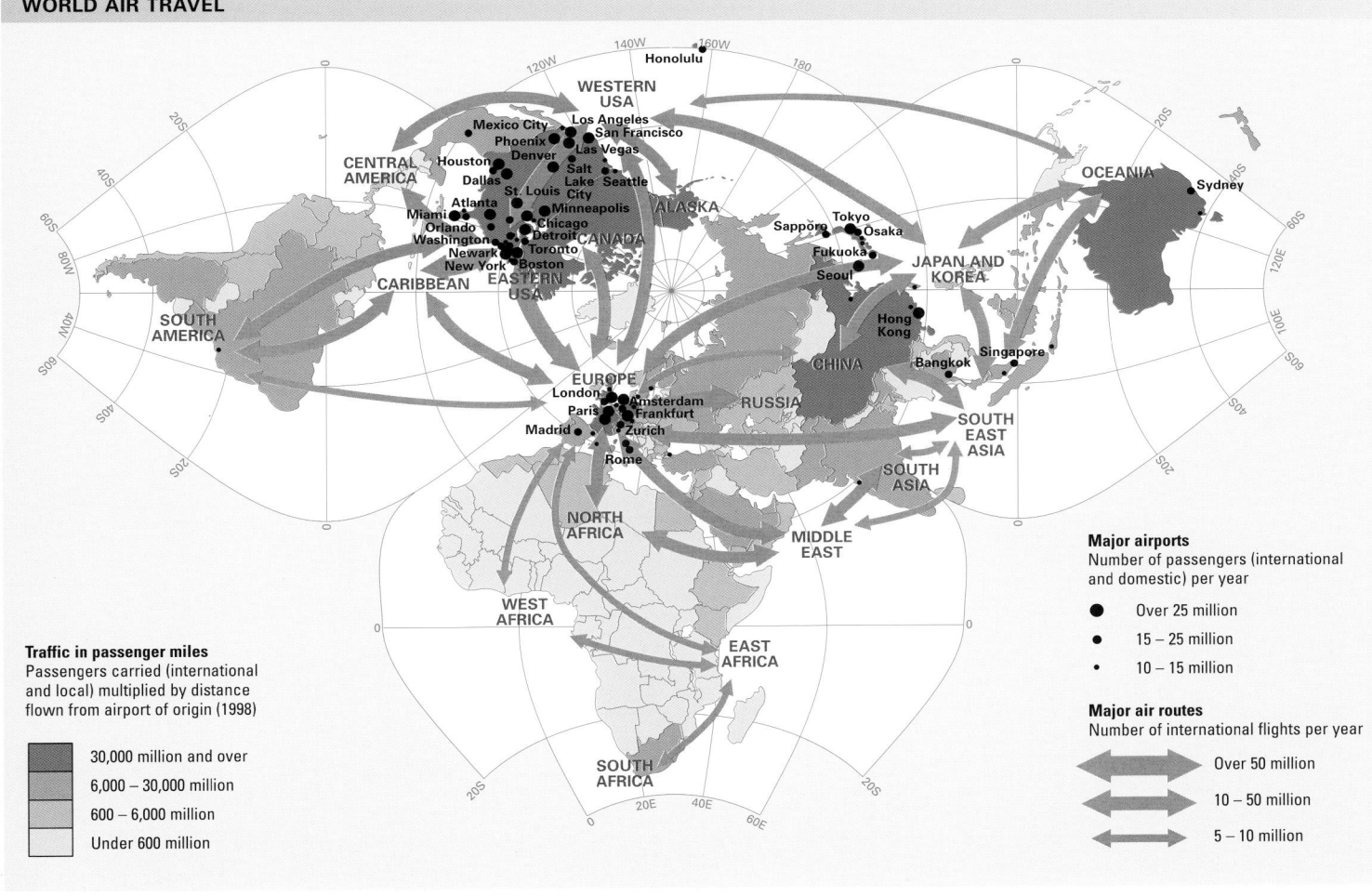

Traffic in passenger miles
Passengers carried (international and local) multiplied by distance flown from airport of origin (1998)

- 30,000 million and over
- 6,000 – 30,000 million
- 600 – 6,000 million
- Under 600 million

Major airports
Number of passengers (international and domestic) per year

- ● Over 25 million
- ● 15 – 25 million
- · 10 – 15 million

Major air routes
Number of international flights per year

- Over 50 million
- 10 – 50 million
- 5 – 10 million

Leisure and tourism is the world's second largest industry in terms of revenue generated. Small economies in attractive areas are often completely dominated by tourism: in some Caribbean islands, tourist spending provides over 90% of the total income and is the biggest foreign exchange earner. In cash terms, the USA is the world leader: its 2000 earnings exceeded US $82 billion, though that sum amounted to approximately 0.9% of its total GDP. Of the 51 million visitors to the USA, 29% came from Canada and 20% from Mexico. Germany spends the most on overseas tourism; this amounts to over US $50,000 million. The next biggest spenders are the USA, Japan, and the UK.

The world's busiest airport in terms of total number of passengers is Atlanta (76.9 million passengers in 2002); the busiest international airport is London's Heathrow.

WORLD'S BUSIEST AIRPORTS
Total passengers in millions (2002)

1.	Atlanta Hartsfield Intl. (ATL)	76.9
2.	Chicago O'Hare Intl. (ORD)	66.6
3.	London Heathrow (LHR)	63.3
4.	Tokyo Haneda (HND)	61.1
5.	Los Angeles Intl. (LAX)	56.2
6.	Dallas/Fort Worth Intl. (DFW)	52.8
7.	Frankfurt Intl. (FRA)	48.5
8.	Paris Charles de Gaulle (CDG)	48.4
9.	Amsterdam Schiphol (AMS)	40.7
10.	Denver Intl. (DEN)	35.7

STANDARDS OF LIVING

For more information:
18 Water supply
24 Population density
26 Urban population
27 Urban advantages
30 World's refugees
   War since 1945
38 Employment
   The work force
43 Infant mortality
44 Wealth

Wealth is a basic factor in determining standards of living. Everywhere, the rich have more of everything, including higher average life expectancies, while the poor have to spend most of their income on basic human needs, such as food and clothing. Yet poverty and wealth are relative terms: slum dwellers living on social security in an industrial society feel their poverty acutely, but have far more resources than an average African living in a rural area.

In 1990 the United Nations Development Program published its first Human Development Index (HDI), an attempt to construct a comparative scale by which a simplified form of well-being might be measured. The HDI, expressed as a value between 0 and 0.999, combines figures for life expectancy and literacy with a wealth scale, based on Purchasing Power Parity.

The world's countries are divided into three groups, those with a high HDI (0.800 and above); those with a medium HDI (0.500 to 0.799); and those with a low HDI (below 0.500). In 2002, Norway was top in the world rankings and Sierra Leone was bottom. In fact, of the 36 countries with a low HDI, 29 were from Africa, six from Asia, plus Haiti from the Caribbean. Besides having low per capita GNPs, the

average life expectancy in these countries was 59 years, while the adult literacy rate was 58%. By comparison, the average life expectancy at birth in countries in the high HDI group was 78 years, while the literacy rate was 98%.

Comparisons between countries with similar per capita GNPs reveal the effects of government actions. For example, the World Bank classifies both India and China as low-income economies, but India's HDI at 0.577 is much lower than that of China, at 0.726. This reflects not only China's economic progress in the 1980s and 1990s, but also differences in average life expectancies (63 years in India and 70 years in China), and adult literacy rates (52% in India and 82% in China).

Disparities in standards of living exist not only between countries but also between individuals, groups and regions within countries. For example, income distribution figures for 1995 show that, in the United States, the poorest 20% of households received less than 4% of the income.

Other contrasts exist in developing countries between rural communities, where incomes are low and basic services are often in short supply, and urban areas, where even those living in slums are

generally better off than their rural neighbours. Other striking differences exist between men and women. For example, while adult literacy rates for men and women living in developed countries are more or less the same, large differences exist in many developing countries. In 2001, in countries in the lowest HDI category, only 64% of women were literate, as compared with 73% of men.

Female education is a factor in population control, especially as women's fertility rates appear to fall in direct proportion to the amount of secondary education they receive. This point was acknowledged in 1994 by the UN Population Fund, which defined four main objectives relating to women and population control: the reduction of maternal, infant, and child mortality; better education, especially for girls; universal access to reproductive health services; and gender equality.

Statistical analysis presents many problems of interpretation, especially when trying to define such intangible factors as a sense of well-being. For example, education helps create wealth; but are rich countries wealthy because their people are well educated, or are they well educated because they are rich?

HUMAN DEVELOPMENT INDEX

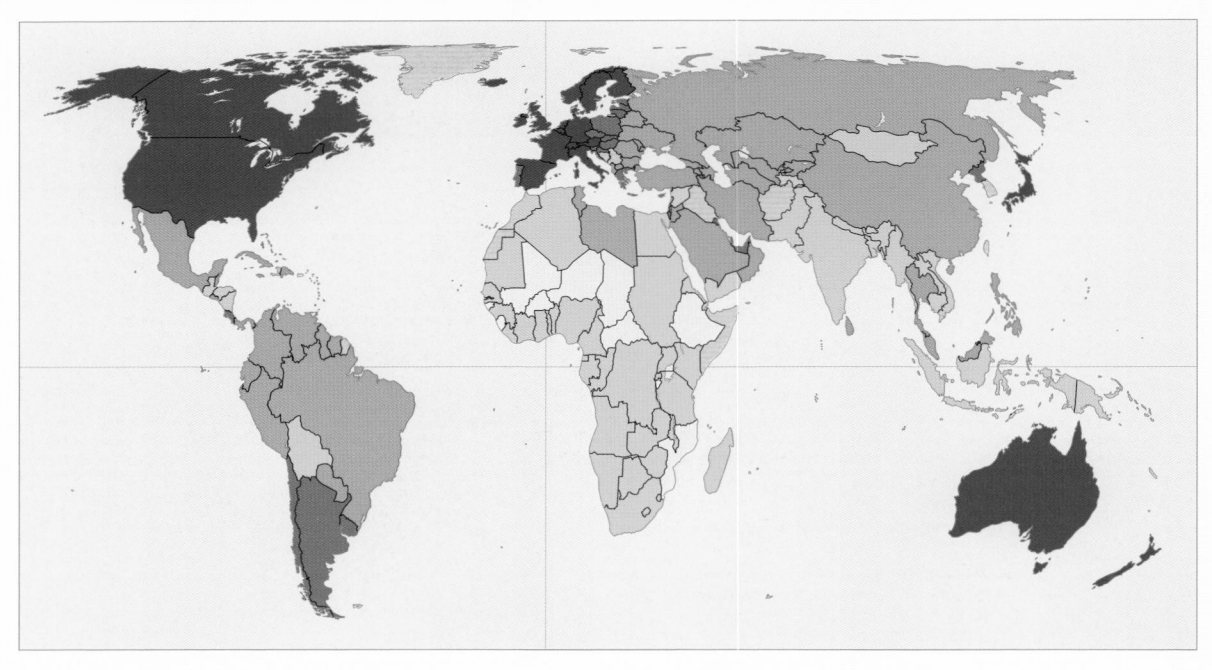

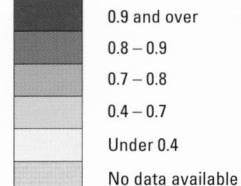

The Human Development Index (HDI), calculated by the UN Development Program (UNDP), gives a value to countries using indicators of life expectancy, education, and standards of living in 2000. Higher values show more developed countries.

- 0.9 and over
- 0.8 – 0.9
- 0.7 – 0.8
- 0.4 – 0.7
- Under 0.4
- No data available

Highest values
Norway 0.942
Sweden 0.941
Canada 0.940
USA 0.939
Belgium 0.939

Lowest values
Sierra Leone 0.275
Niger.. 0.277
Burundi 0.313
Mozambique................................. 0.322
Burkina Faso 0.325

EDUCATION

The developing countries made great efforts in the 1970s and 1980s to bring at least a basic education to their people. In all but the poorest nations, primary school enrolments rose above 60%. However, figures often include teenagers or young adults, and there are still 300 million children worldwide who receive no schooling at all. A lack of resources has restricted the development of secondary and higher education. Most primary school education is free in the poorer countries, but fees are often paid for secondary and higher education, thus heightening the differences between rich and poor.

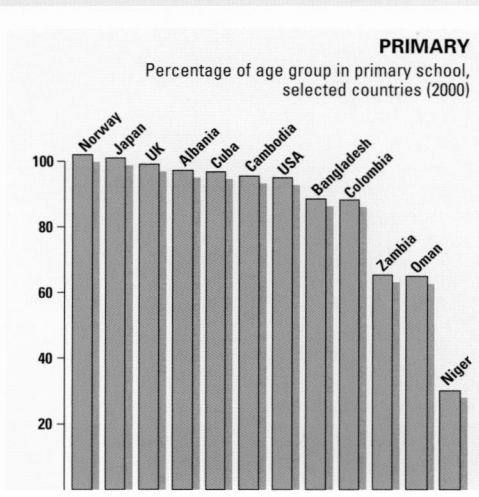

PRIMARY
Percentage of age group in primary school, selected countries (2000)

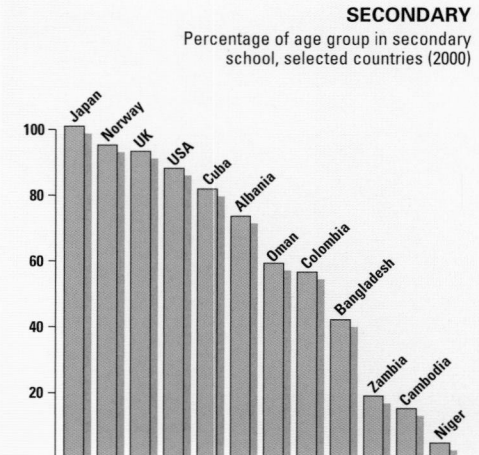

SECONDARY
Percentage of age group in secondary school, selected countries (2000)

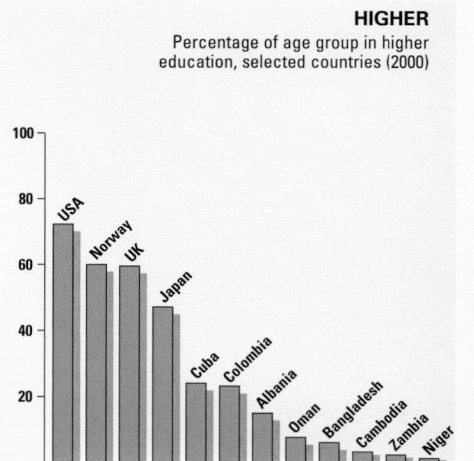

HIGHER
Percentage of age group in higher education, selected countries (2000)

DISTRIBUTION OF SPENDING

Percentage share of household spending (latest available year)

A high proportion of the average income of households in developing nations is spent on basic needs such as food and clothing. In most Western countries food and clothing account for less than 25% of expenditure.

Legend:
- Food
- Medicine & Education
- Clothing
- Transport
- Energy & Housing
- Other

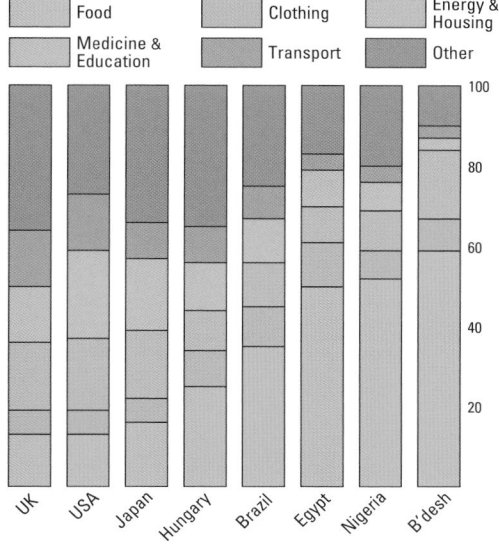

(UK, USA, Japan, Hungary, Brazil, Egypt, Nigeria, B'desh)

STANDARDS OF LIVING IN THE USA BY RACE, AGE, AND RELIGION

A comparison of measures of income and education, by selected characteristics (2001–2)

Median income per household (US $), by age and region

15–24 years	28,196
25–34 years	45,086
35–44 years	53,320
45–54 years	58,045
55–64 years	45,864
65 years and over	23,118
Northeast	45,716
Midwest	43,834
South	38,904
West	45,687

Per capita income (US $), by race and Hispanic origin of householder

ALL RACES	22,851
White	24,127
Black	14,953
Asian and Pacific Is.	24,277
Hispanic (any race)	13,003

The poorest 20% of households received just 3.6% of the income, whereas the richest 20% received 48.2%.

Percentage of persons aged 25 and over who have completed High School, by race or origin

ALL RACES	1975	62.5
	2001	84.1
White	1975	64.5
	2001	84.4
Black	1975	42.5
	2001	78.7
Hispanic	1975	37.9
	2001	57.0

FERTILITY AND EDUCATION

Fertility rates compared with female education, selected countries (1995–2000)

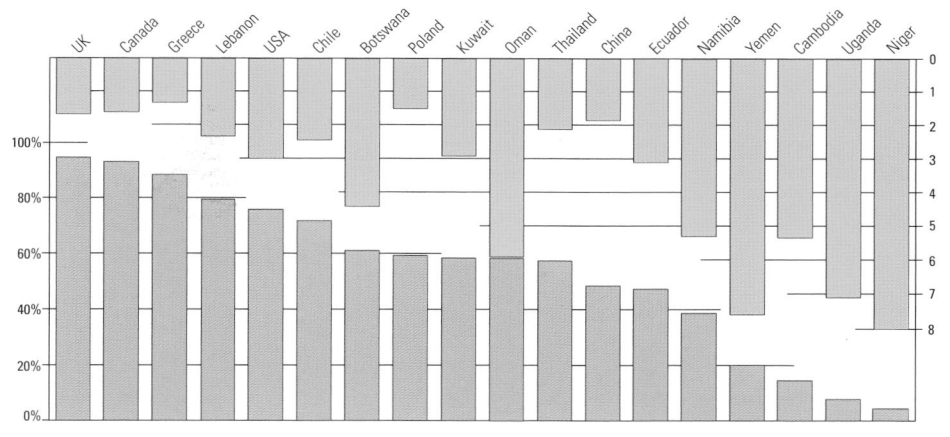

(UK, Canada, Greece, Lebanon, USA, Chile, Botswana, Poland, Kuwait, Oman, Thailand, China, Ecuador, Namibia, Yemen, Cambodia, Uganda, Niger)

Legend:
- Fertility rate: average number of children borne per woman
- Percentage of females aged 12–17 in secondary education

Access to secondary education is closely linked to low fertility rates in developed countries. By contrast, in many developing countries, women's lives are dominated by agriculture, or they lack access to secondary and higher education for cultural reasons, as in Muslim countries. Such disparities are reflected in women's parliamentary representation which is only one-seventh that of men, despite the emergence of such figures as Mrs Indira Gandhi, India's former prime minister. Female wages are also, on average, only two-thirds of those of men.

GENDER DEVELOPMENT INDEX

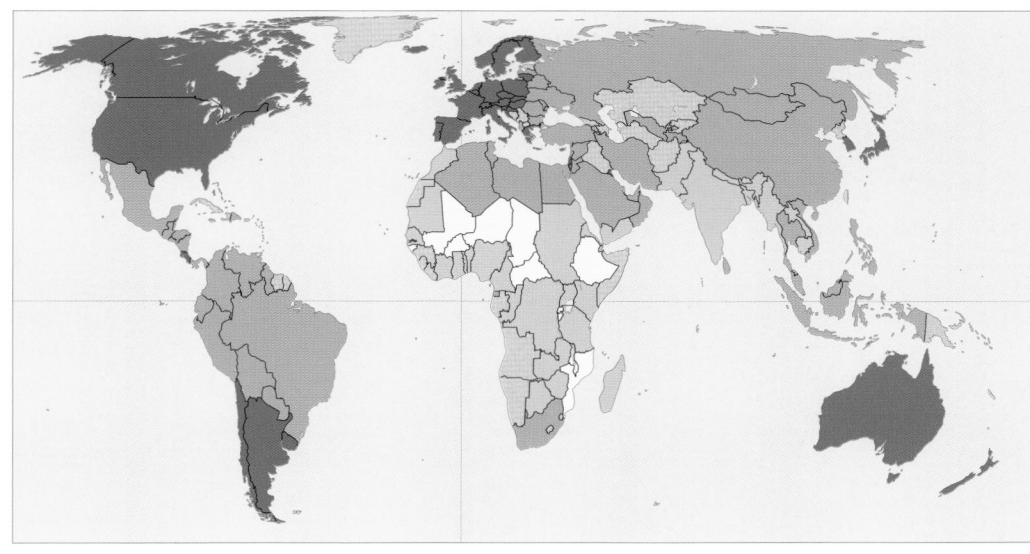

The Gender Development Index (GDI) shows economic and social differences between men and women by using various UNDP indicators (2002). Countries with higher values of GDI have more equality between men and women.

Legend:
- 0.8 and over
- 0.6 – 0.8
- 0.4 – 0.6
- Under 0.4
- No data available

Highest values

Norway	0.941
Australia	0.938
Canada	0.938
USA	0.937

Lowest values

Niger	0.263
Burundi	0.306
Mozambique	0.307
Burkina Faso	0.312

REGIONAL INEQUALITY IN ITALY

The southern part of Italy, known as the *Mezzogiorno*, has been described as one of the poorest parts of the European Union. It is identifiable on the map (*right*) as all the regions with a GDP per capita of less than US $12,000 (including the two islands of Sicily and Sardinia), plus Abruzzi whose capital is L'Aquila.

The *Mezzogiorno* region suffers from a lack of energy resources, minerals, industry, commerce, services and skilled labor. As a result, standards of living in the region are well below the rest of Italy. Employment is predominantly agricultural and small-scale.

The north of Italy accounts for 60% of the population but 80% of the GDP, whereas the *Mezzogiorno* accounts for 40% of the population and only 20% of the GDP. Manpower surpluses in the south led to emigration to other parts of Europe and the Americas.

It has also led, especially in the last 50 years, to inter-regional migration from the islands and the southern mainland to the north. The main regions attracting migrants are the northwest (the prosperous Liguria–Piedmont–Lombardy triangle, with its great industrial cities of Genoa, Milan, and Turin) and the Venetia region in the northeast.

As a result, the north has experienced much higher population growth rates than the rest of Italy.

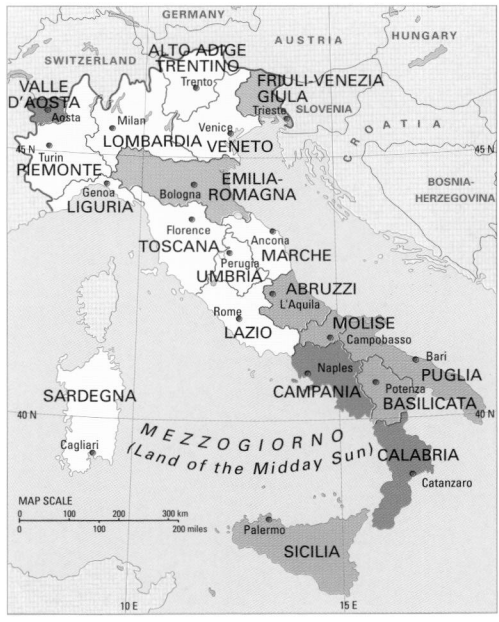

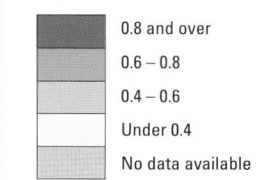

Gross Domestic Product (GDP) per capita in Italy, by region (1999)

Legend:
- Over US $20,000
- $16,000 – $19,999
- $12,000 – $15,999
- $8,000 – $11,999
- Under $8,000

The average GNI (Gross National Income) per capita for Italy was US $20,170. By comparison, the GNI for the UK was $23,590; for the USA $31,910; and for the EU $22,250.

The number of inhabitants per doctor, another social indicator, varies from less than 500 in the northwest of Italy to over 800 in the far south (the *Mezzogiorno*), with a national average of 607.

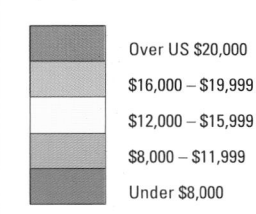

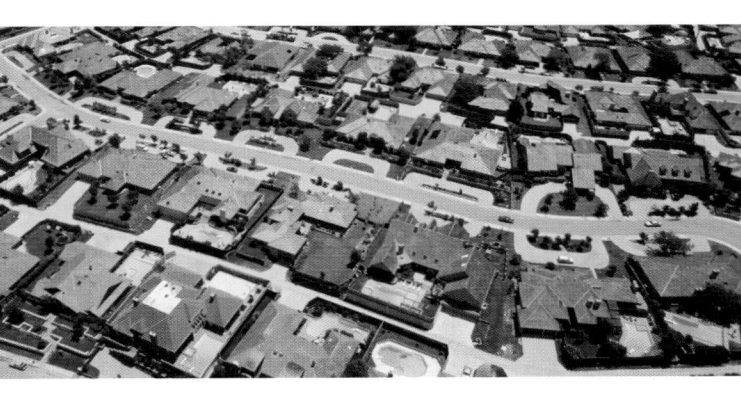

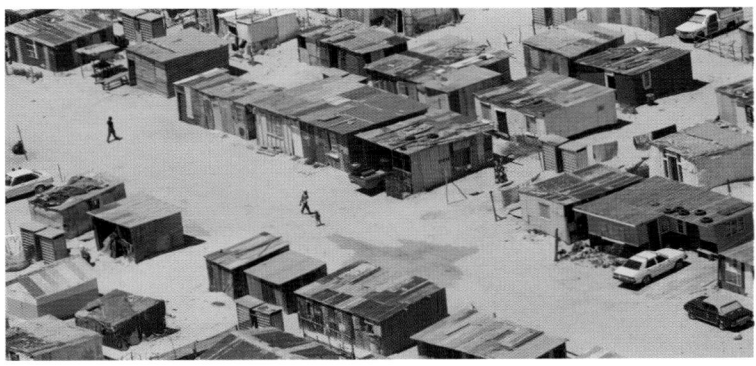

◄ These two images illustrate the reality of suburban life for people at either end of the economic scale. On the far left is part of a huge area of "tract housing" in California, where large houses of a similar design are laid out by a developer, complete with gardens, drives, and swimming pools. On the right is a much more haphazard arrangement of home-built, rudimentary shelters, many without sanitation and most with no electricity in Crossroads Township, outside Cape Town in South Africa.

47

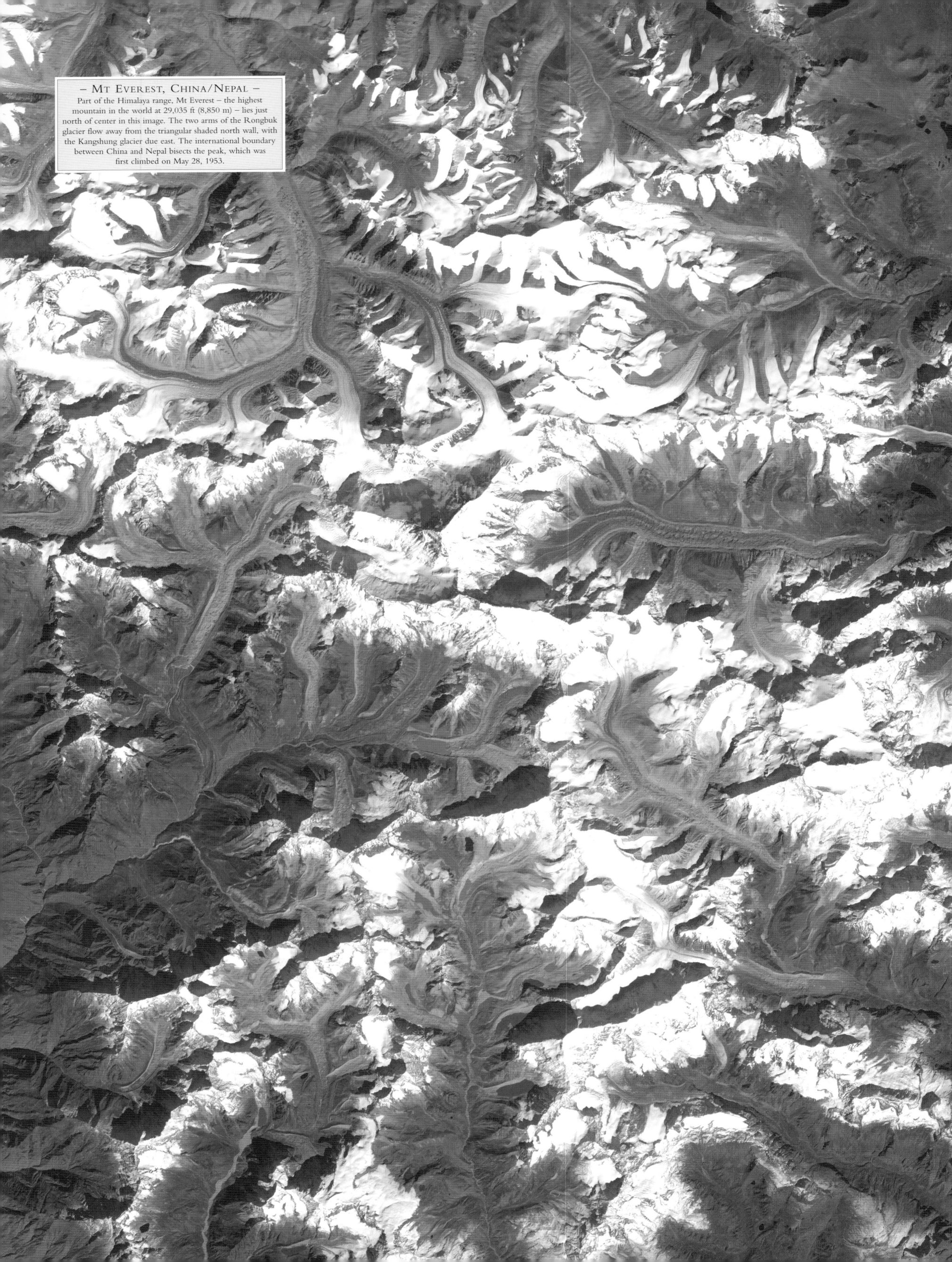

– MT EVEREST, CHINA/NEPAL –

Part of the Himalaya range, Mt Everest – the highest mountain in the world at 29,035 ft (8,850 m) – lies just north of center in this image. The two arms of the Rongbuk glacier flow away from the triangular shaded north wall, with the Kangshung glacier due east. The international boundary between China and Nepal bisects the peak, which was first climbed on May 28, 1953.

CITY MAPS

Amsterdam	2	Copenhagen	10	Manila	17	St Petersburg	26
Athens	2	Delhi	10	Melbourne	17	Santiago	26
Atlanta	3	Dublin	11	Mexico City	18	São Paulo	26
Baghdad	3	Edinburgh	11	Miami	18	Seoul	26
Bangkok	3	Helsinki	12	Milan	18	Shanghai	27
Barcelona	4	Hong Kong	12	Montréal	19	Singapore	27
Beijing	4	Istanbul	12	Moscow	19	Stockholm	28
Berlin	5	Jakarta	13	Mumbai	20	Sydney	28
Boston	6	Jerusalem	13	Munich	20	Tokyo	29
Brussels	6	Johannesburg	13	New York	21	Tehran	30
Budapest	7	Karachi	14	Osaka	22	Tianjin	30
Buenos Aires	7	Lagos	14	Oslo	22	Toronto	30
Cairo	7	Lisbon	14	Paris	23	Vienna	31
Calcutta (Kolkata)	8	London	15	Prague	24	Warsaw	31
Canton	8	Los Angeles	16	Rio de Janeiro	24	Washington	32
Cape Town	8	Lima	16	Rome	25	Wellington	32
Chicago	9	Madrid	17	San Francisco	25	Index	33–39

CITY MAPS

Motorway, freeway, expressway with toll – with road number	A10	**Primary road** – with road number dual carriageway single carriageway	14 / 14	**Principal station**	Estación del Norte
Motorway, freeway, expressway – with European road number	E51	**Secondary road** – with road number dual carriageway single carriageway	96 / 96	**Height above sea level (m)**	705 ▲
Road junction	○	**Other road**		**Airport**	✈
Under construction	= = =			**Airfield**	⊕
Tunnel	)---(	**Ferry**		**Central area coverage**	
		Railroad		**Urban area**	
				Woodlands and parks	

CENTRAL AREA MAPS

Motorway, freeway, expressway		**Limited access/ pedestrian road**		**Abbey, cathedral**	†
Through route		**Parking** (Europe only)	Ⓟ	**Church of interest**	†
Secondary road		**Railroad**		**Synagogue**	✡
Dual carriageway		**Rail/bus station**		**Shrine, temple**	⛩
Other road		**Underground, metro station**	Ⓜ Ⓤ Ⓢ Ⓣ	**Mosque**	☪
Tunnel	)---(	**Cable car**	+---+	**Public building**	▢
				Tourist information	ℹ
				Place of interest	Palace

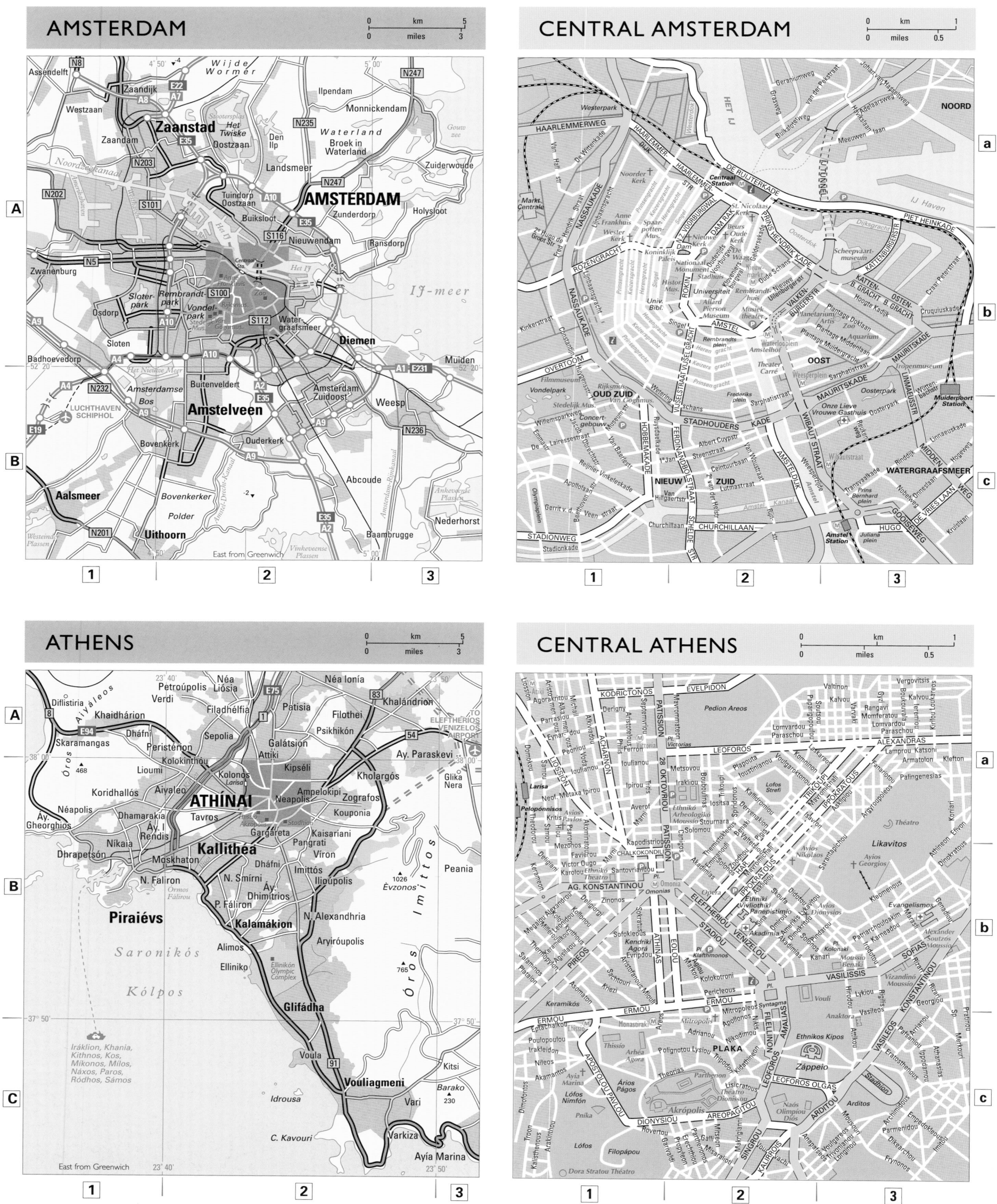

AMSTERDAM

CENTRAL AMSTERDAM

ATHENS

CENTRAL ATHENS

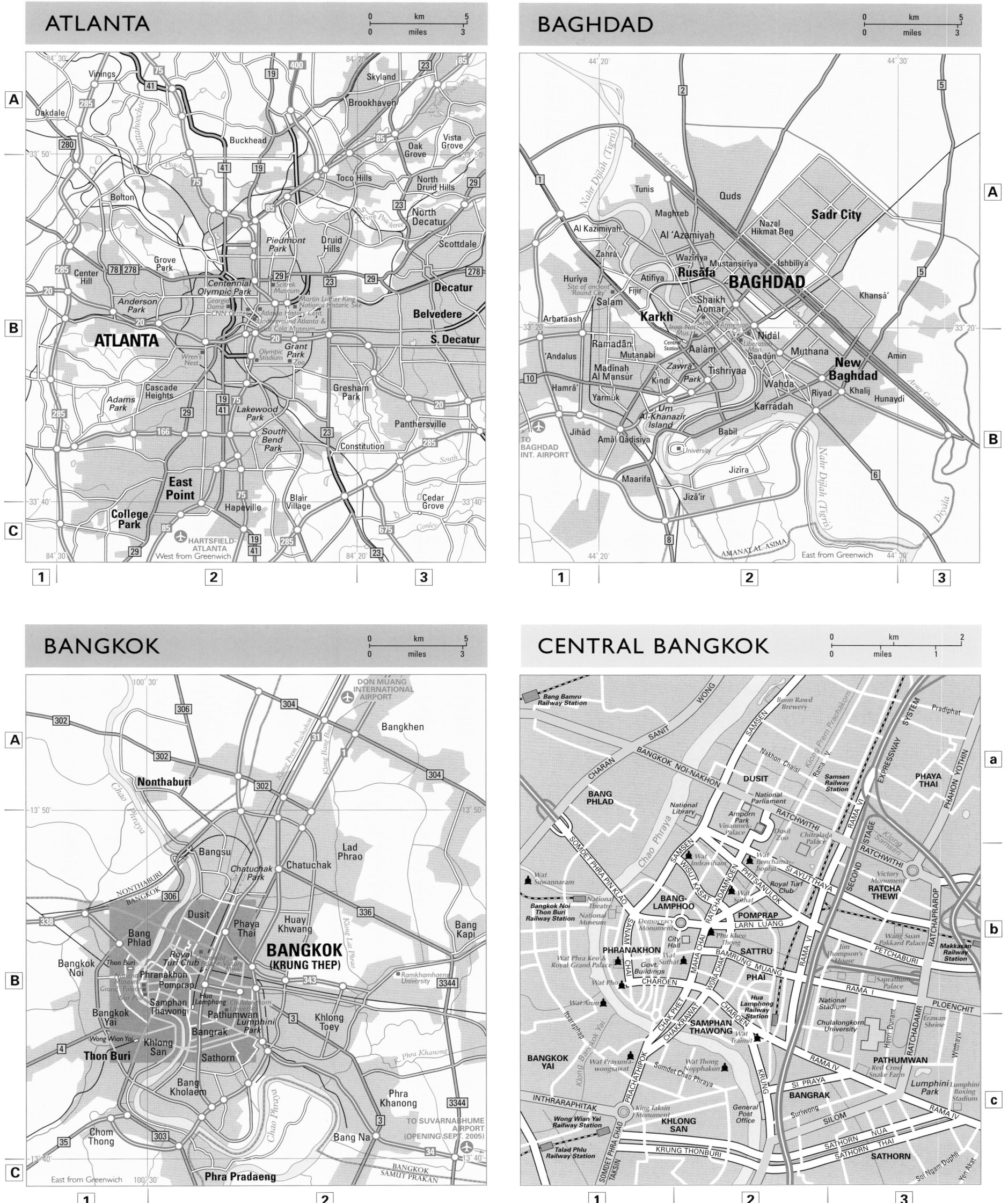

ATLANTA

BAGHDAD

BANGKOK

CENTRAL BANGKOK

COPYRIGHT PHILIP'S

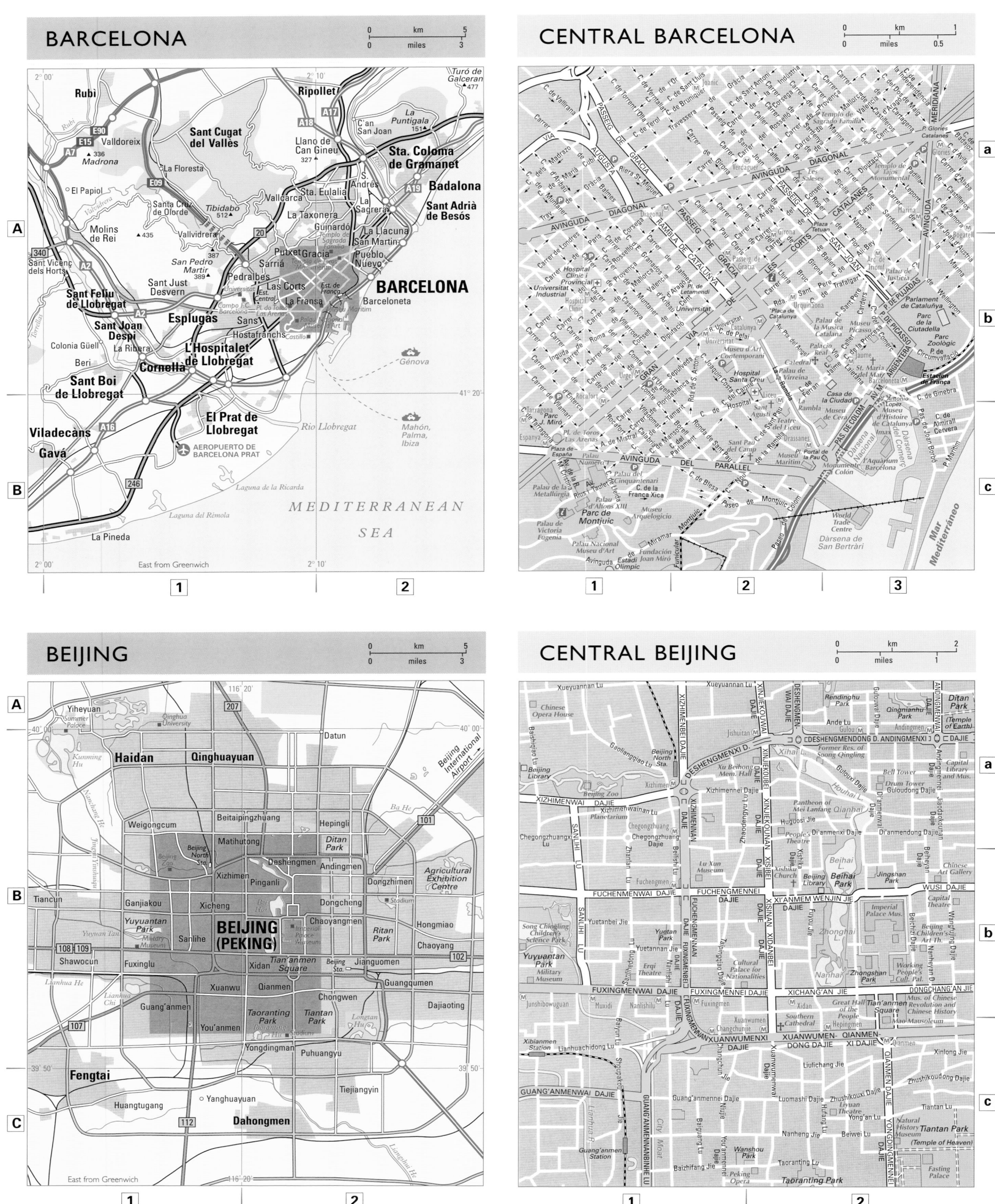

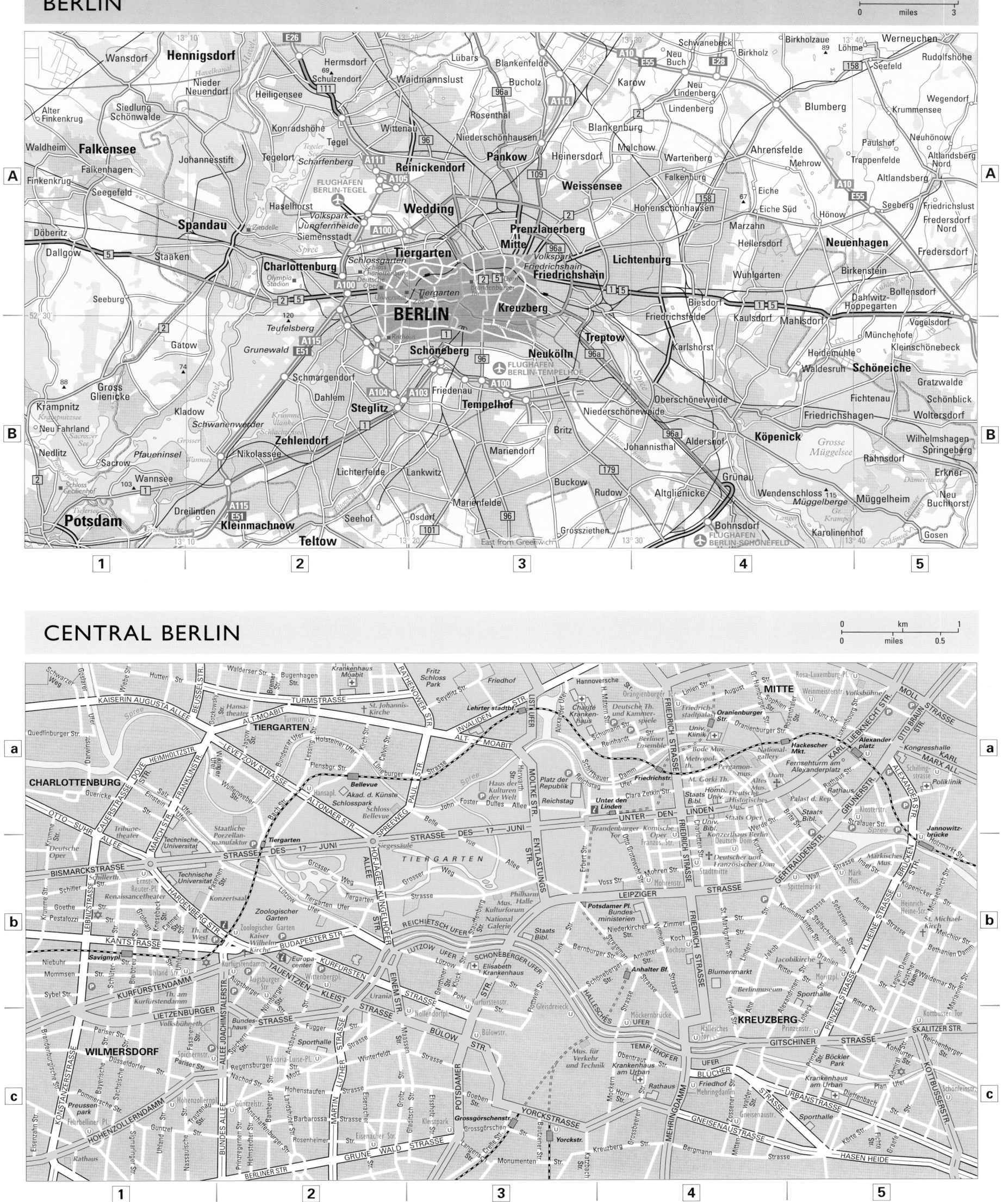

BOSTON

km 0 — 5
miles 0 — 3

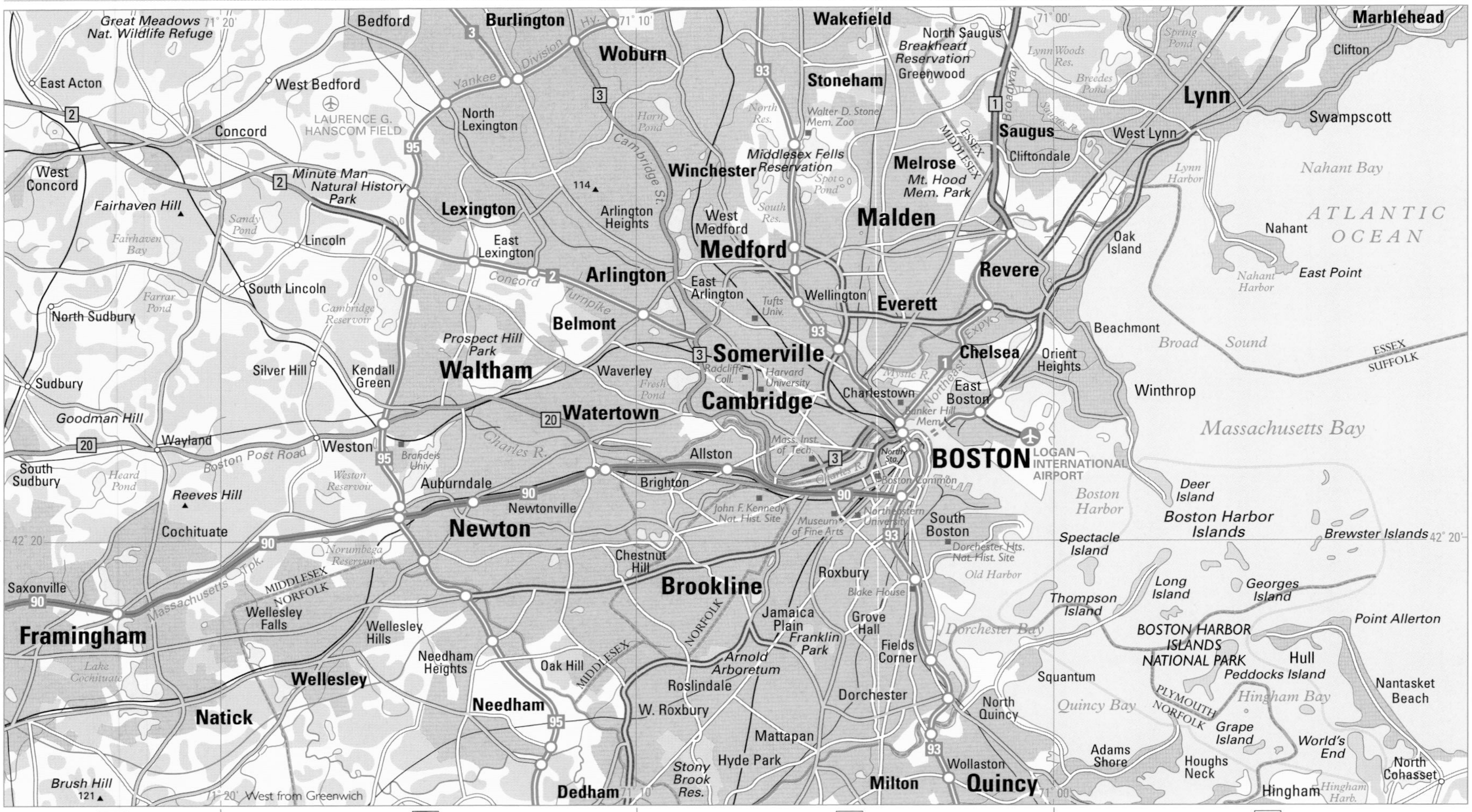

Great Meadows
Nat. Wildlife Refuge
East Acton
West Bedford
Bedford
Burlington
Woburn
Wakefield
Marblehead
West Concord
Concord
LAURENCE G. HANSCOM FIELD
North Lexington
Stoneham
North Saugus
Breakheart Reservation
Greenwood
Clifton
Lynn
Swampscott
West Concord
Minute Man Natural History Park
Lexington
East Lexington
Arlington Heights
Winchester
West Medford
Melrose
Mt. Hood Mem. Park
Saugus
West Lynn
Fairhaven Hill
Fairhaven Bay
Lincoln
South Lincoln
Belmont
Medford
East Arlington
Wellington
Malden
Revere
Nahant
Nahant Bay
ATLANTIC OCEAN
East Point
North Sudbury
Sudbury
Silver Hill
Kendall Green
Waverley
Fresh Pond
Somerville
Radcliffe Coll.
Harvard University
Charlestown
Chelsea
East Boston
Orient Heights
Beachmont
Winthrop
Broad Sound
ESSEX SUFFOLK
Goodman Hill
Wayland
Weston
Brandeis Univ.
Auburndale
Watertown
Cambridge
Mass. Inst. of Tech.
BOSTON
LOGAN INTERNATIONAL AIRPORT
Massachusetts Bay
South Sudbury
Heard Pond
Cochituate
Western Reservoir
Norumbega Reservation
Newton
Newtonville
Brighton
Allston
Boston Univ.
South Boston
Boston Common
Deer Island
Boston Harbor
Spectacle Island
Saxonville
Wellesley Falls
Wellesley Hills
Chestnut Hill
Brookline
Jamaica Plain
Roxbury
Franklin Park
Grove Hall
Fields Corner
Dorchester Bay
Old Harbor
Thompson Island
Long Island
Georges Island
Boston Harbor Islands
Brewster Islands
Point Allerton
Framingham
Natick
Wellesley
Needham Heights
Oak Hill
Needham
Arnold Arboretum
Roslindale
W. Roxbury
Dorchester
North Quincy
Squantum
Quincy Bay
BOSTON HARBOR ISLANDS NATIONAL PARK
Peddocks Island
Hull
Nantasket Beach
Brush Hill
Mattapan
Hyde Park
Stony Brook Res.
Dedham
Milton
Quincy
Wollaston
Adams Shore
Houghs Neck
World's End
Hingham
North Cohasset

West from Greenwich

1   2   3   4

BRUSSELS

km 0 — 5
miles 0 — 3

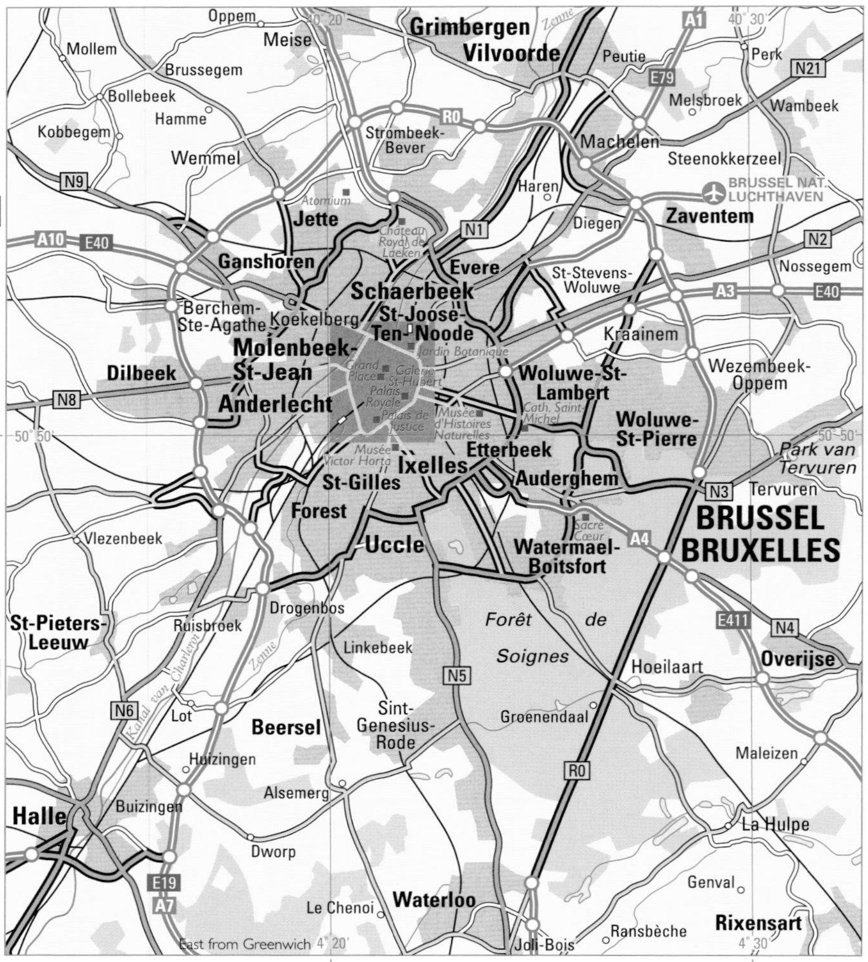

Oppem
Meise
Grimbergen
Vilvoorde
Mollem
Brussegem
Bollebeek
Kobbegem
Wemmel
Strombeek-Bever
Peutie
Perk
Melsbroek
Wambeek
Hamme
Jette
Haren
Machelen
Steenokkerzeel
BRUSSEL NAT. LUCHTHAVEN
Ganshoren
Evere
Diegen
Zaventem
Berchem-Ste-Agathe
Koekelberg
Schaerbeek
St-Joost-Ten-Noode
St-Stevens-Woluwe
Nossegem
Molenbeek-St-Jean
Woluwe-St-Lambert
Kraainem
Wezembeek-Oppem
Dilbeek
Anderlecht
Ixelles
Etterbeek
Woluwe-St-Pierre
Auderghem
Park van Tervuren
St-Gilles
Forest
Uccle
Watermael-Boitsfort
BRUSSEL BRUXELLES
St-Pieters-Leeuw
Drogenbos
Forêt de Soignes
Ruisbroek
Linkebeek
Hoeilaart
Overijse
Vlezenbeek
Beersel
Sint-Genesius-Rode
Groenendaal
Halle
Buizingen
Horizingen
Alsemberg
Dworp
La Hulpe
Waterloo
Le Chenoi
Genval
Ransbèche
Joli-Bois
Rixensart

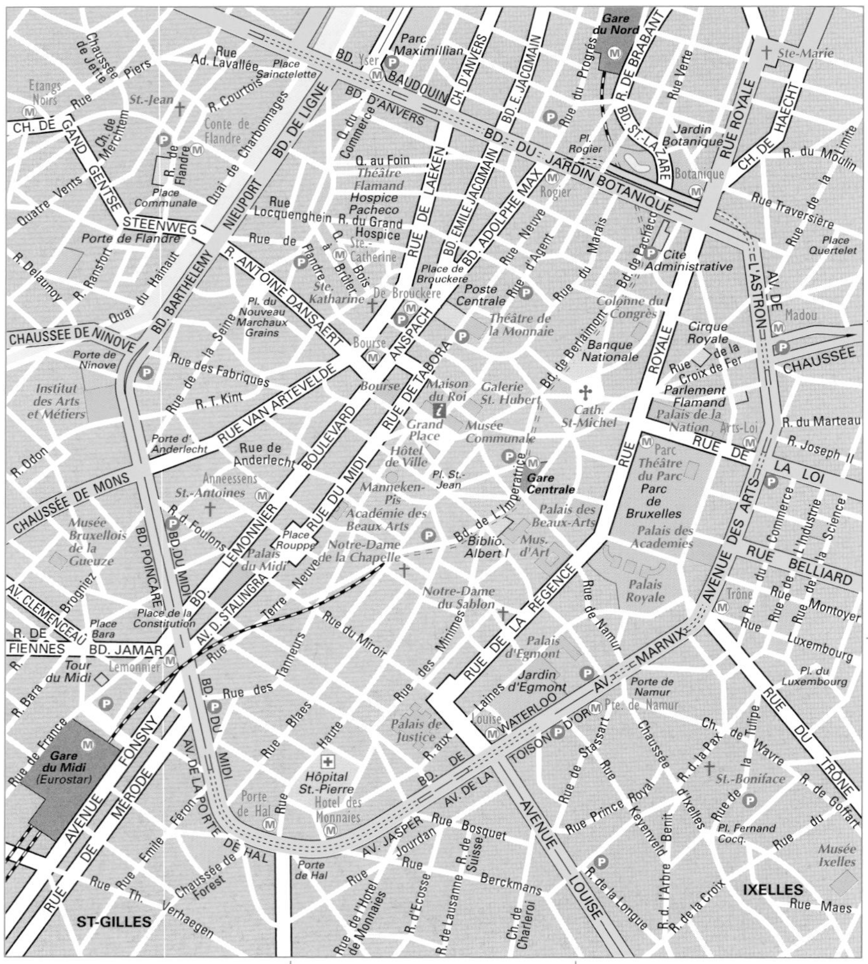

East from Greenwich

1   2   3

CENTRAL BRUSSELS

km 0 — 1
miles 0 — 0.5

Gare du Nord
Ste-Marie
Jardin Botanique
Parc Maximilien
BD. BAUDOUIN
Gare Centrale
Parc de Bruxelles
Palais de la Nation
Manneken-Pis
Notre-Dame du Sablon
Palais de Justice
Gare du Midi (Eurostar)
ST-GILLES
IXELLES
Porte de Hal

a   b   c

1   2   3

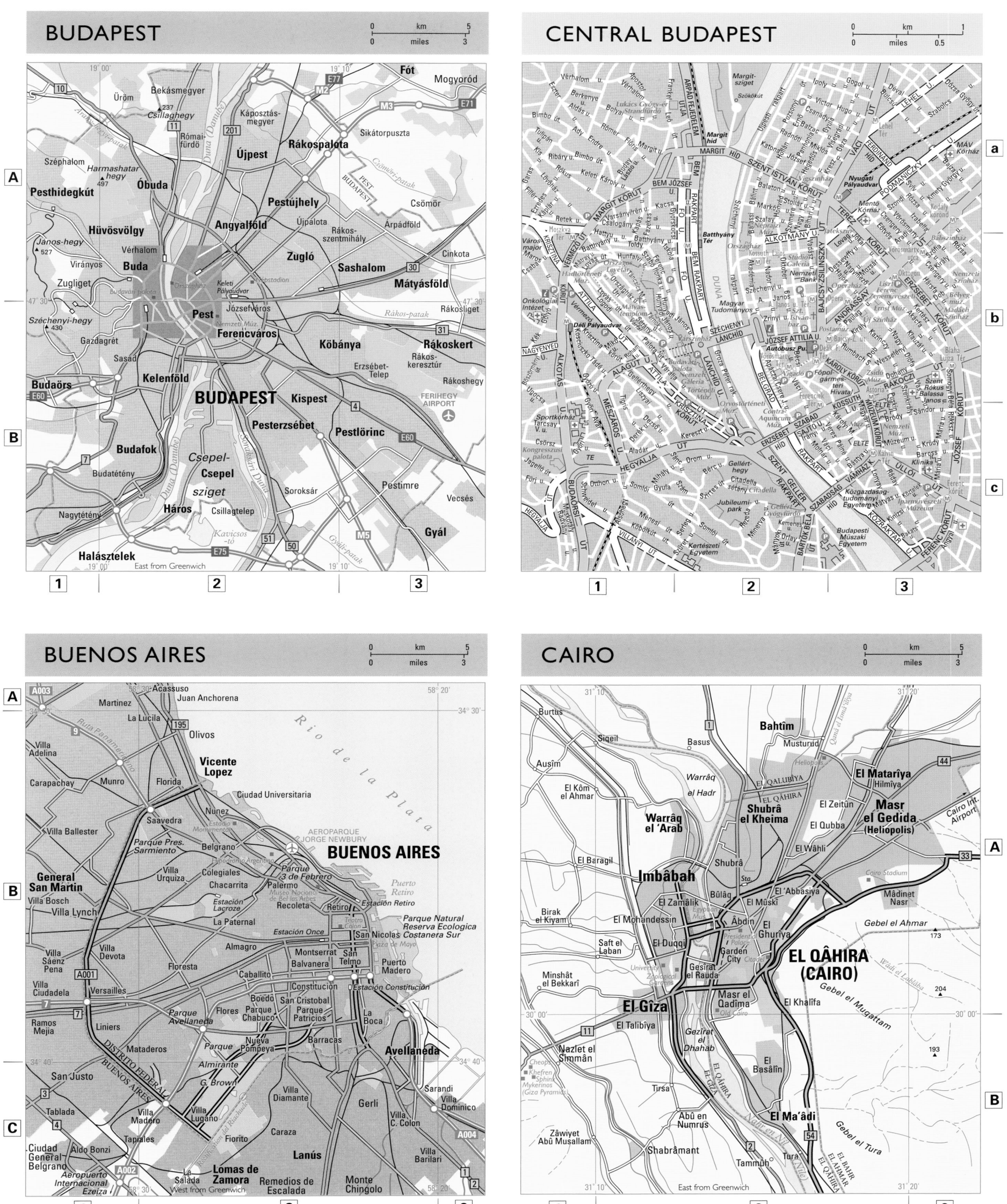

CALCUTTA (KOLKATA)

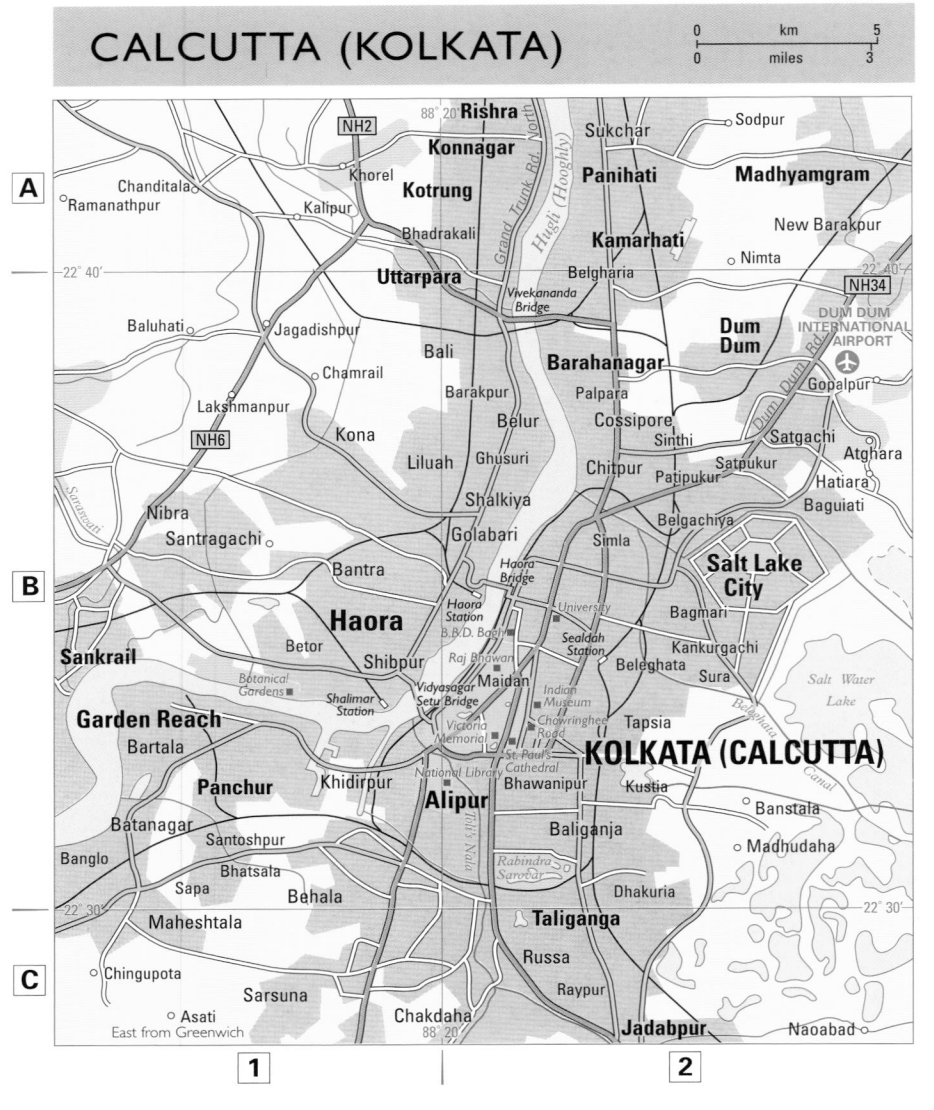

CANTON

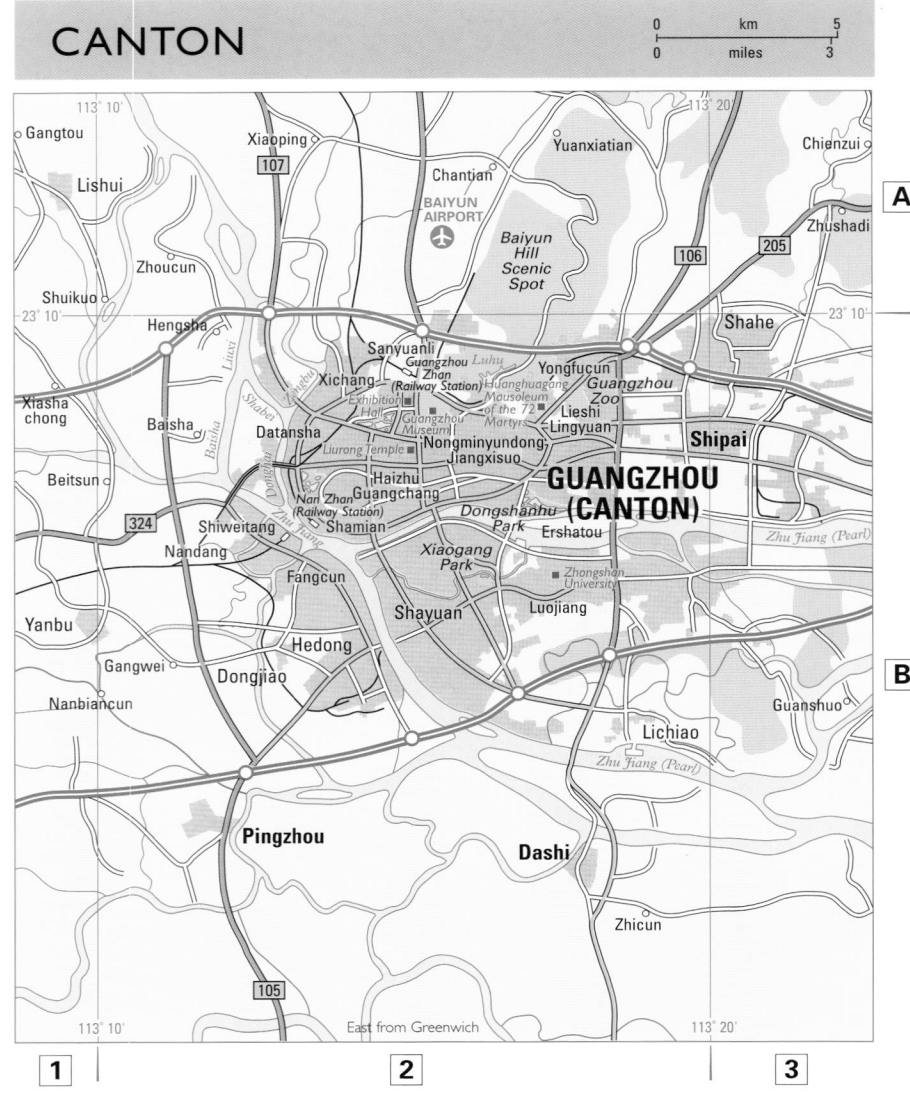

CAPE TOWN

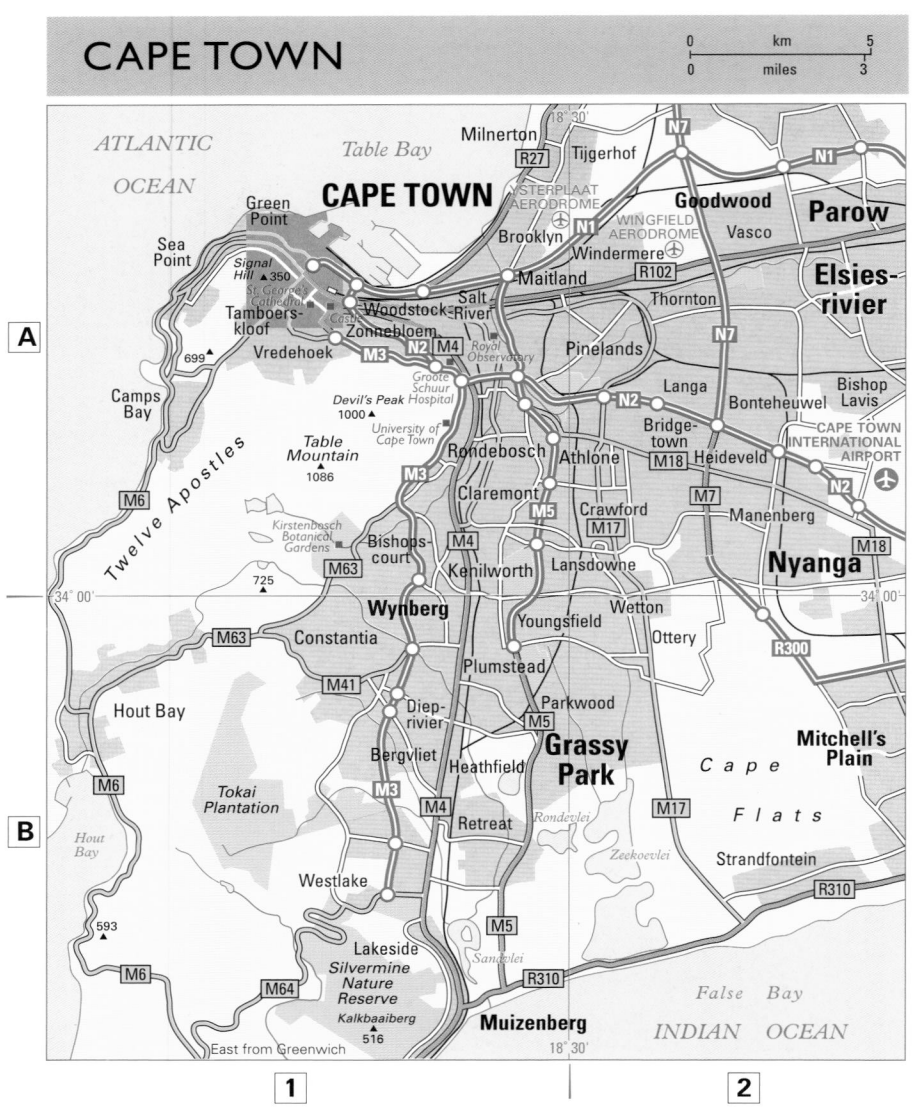

CENTRAL CAPE TOWN

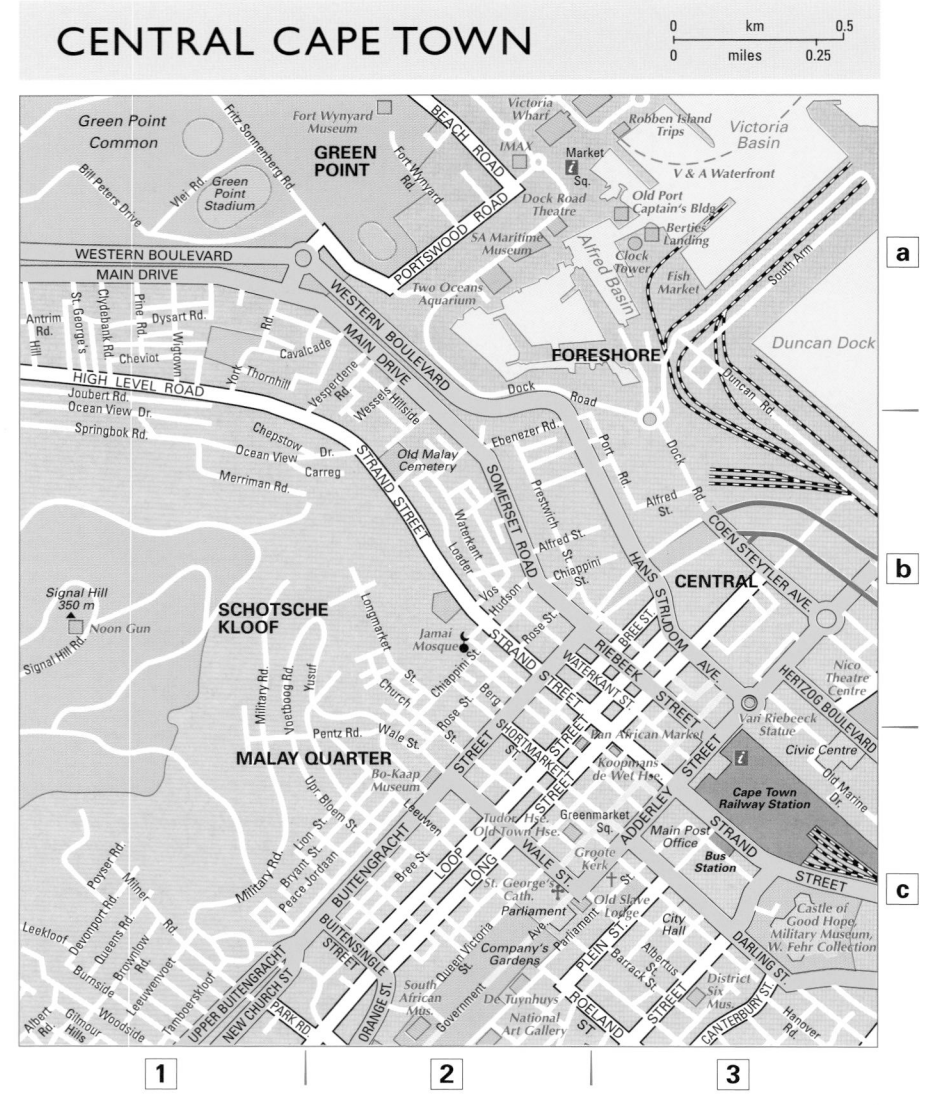

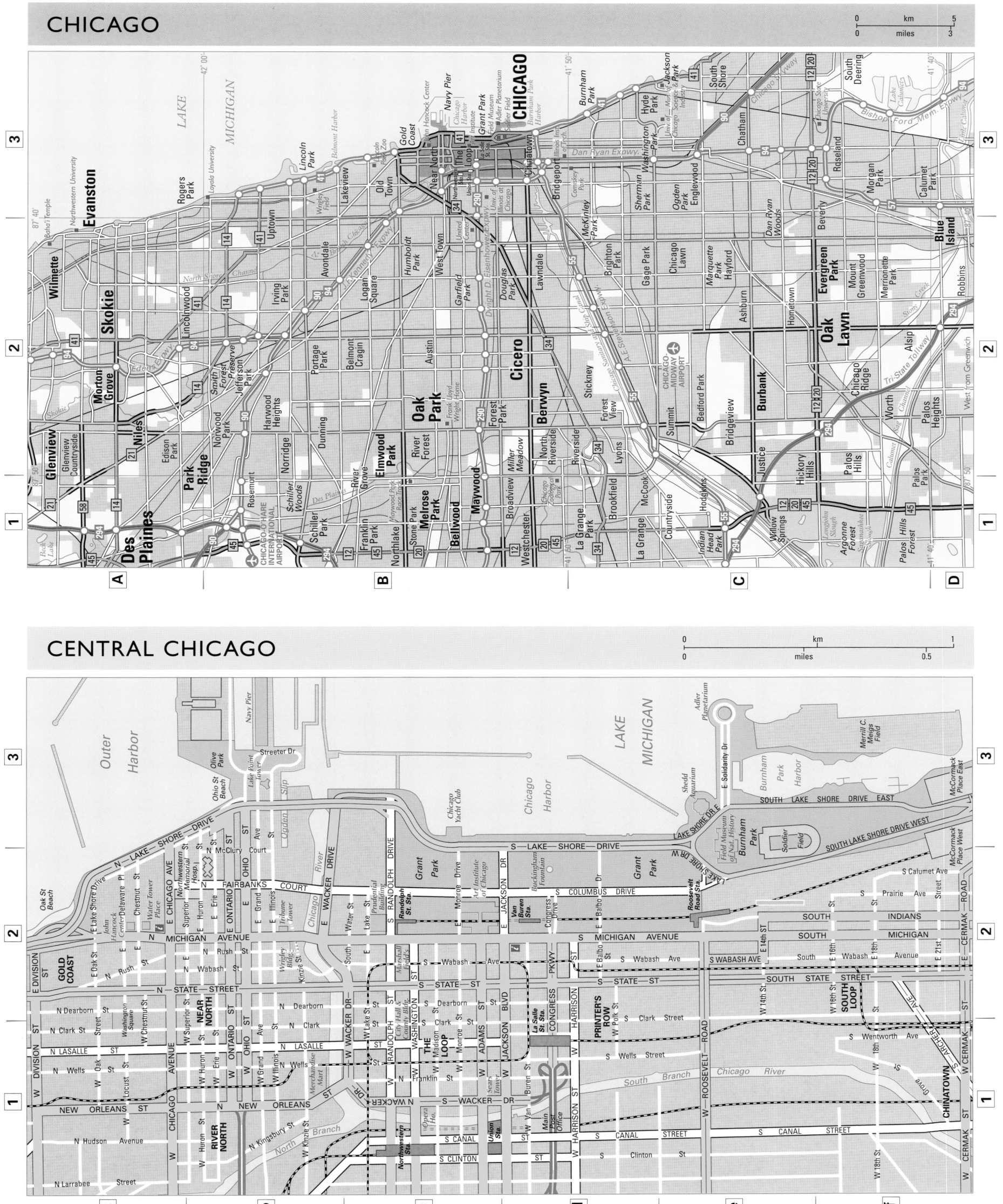

CHICAGO

0 km 5
0 miles 3

CENTRAL CHICAGO

0 km 1
0 miles 0.5

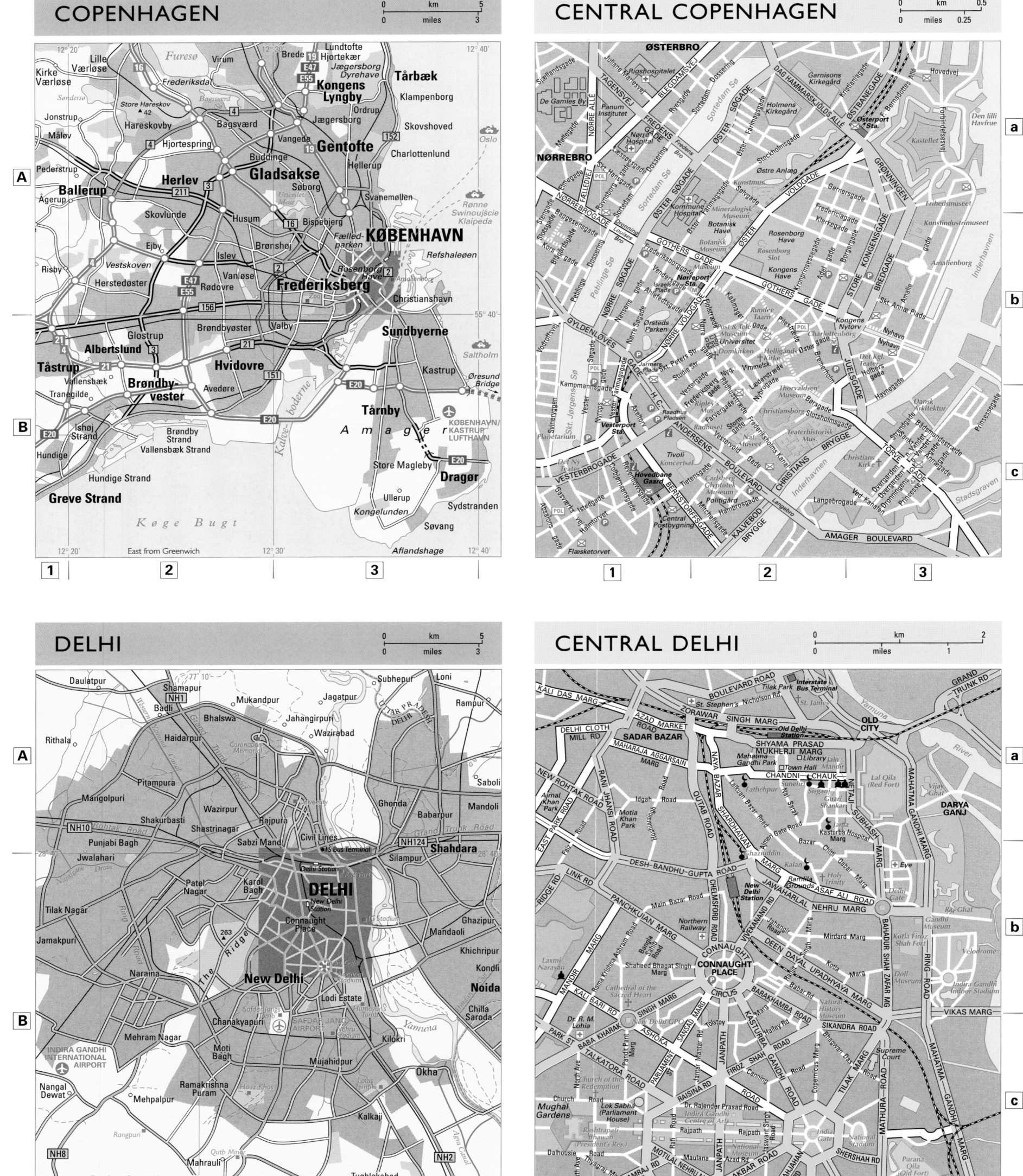

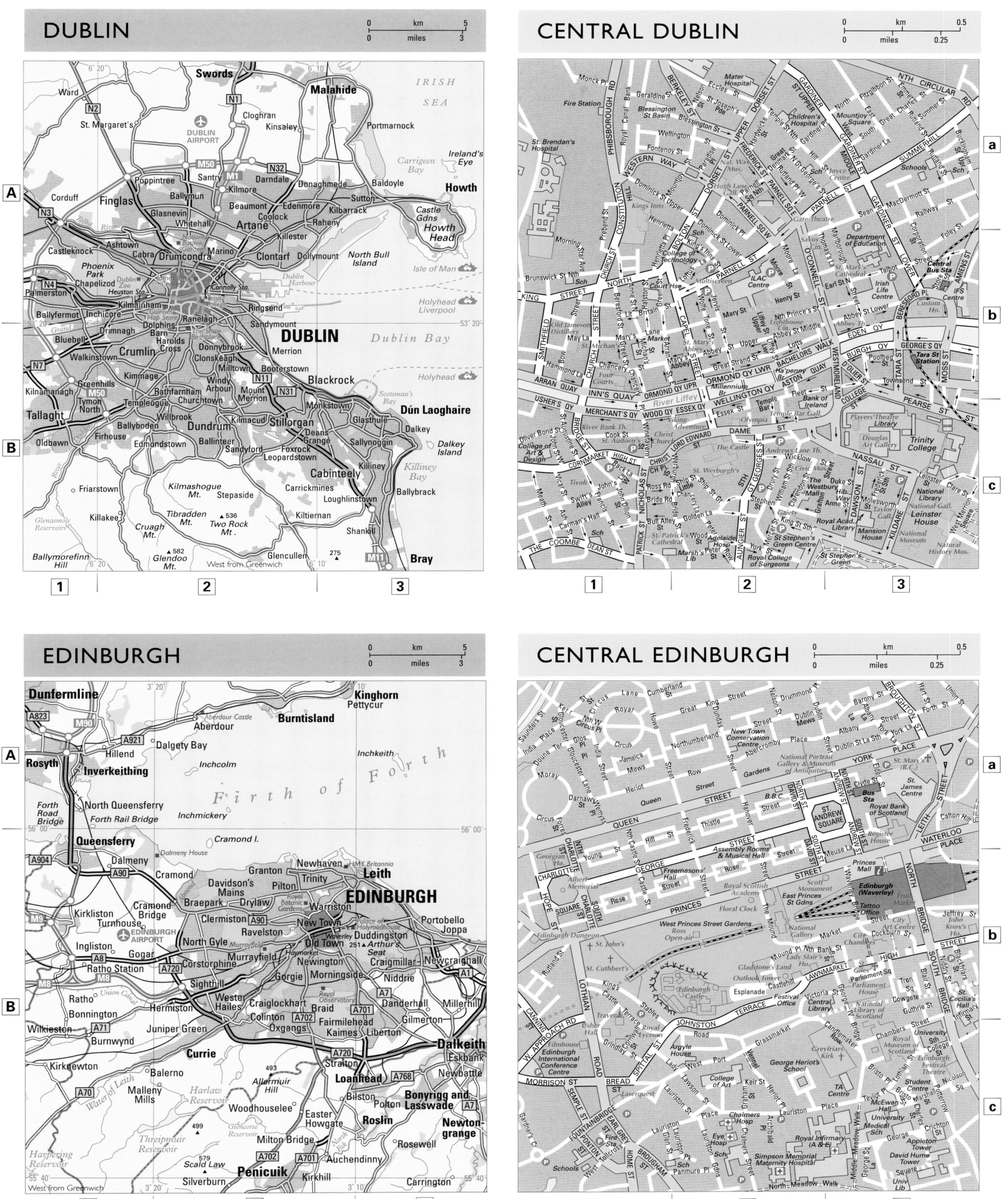

DUBLIN

km 5 / miles 3

CENTRAL DUBLIN

km 0.5 / miles 0.25

EDINBURGH

km 5 / miles 3

CENTRAL EDINBURGH

km 0.5 / miles 0.25

HELSINKI

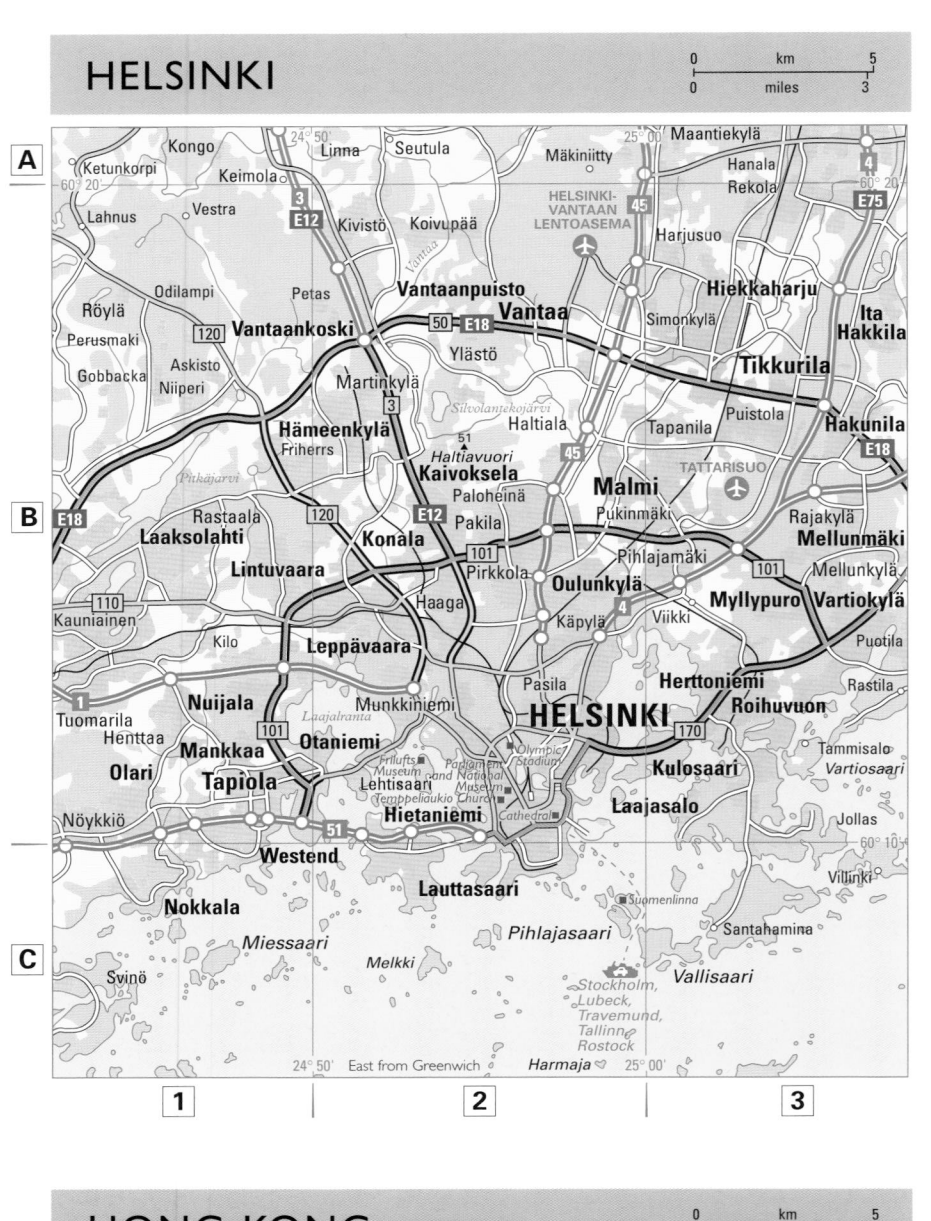

ISTANBUL

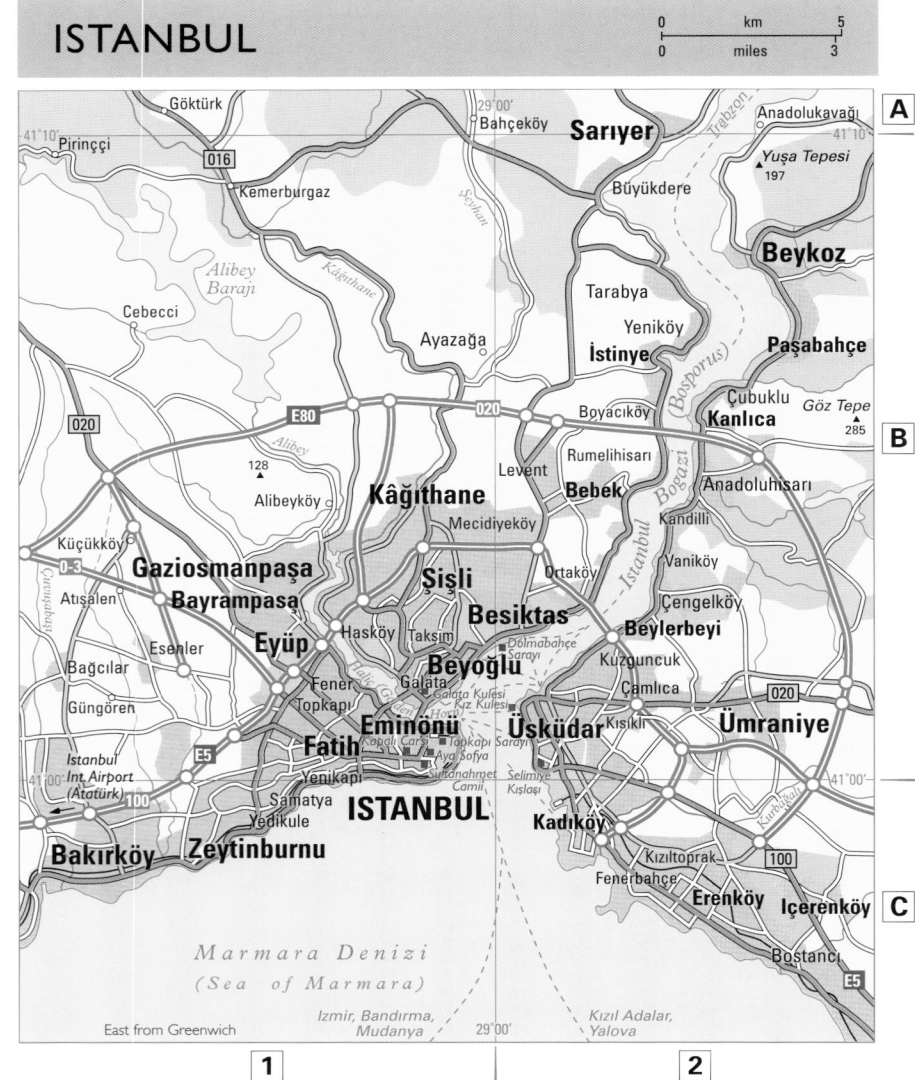

HONG KONG

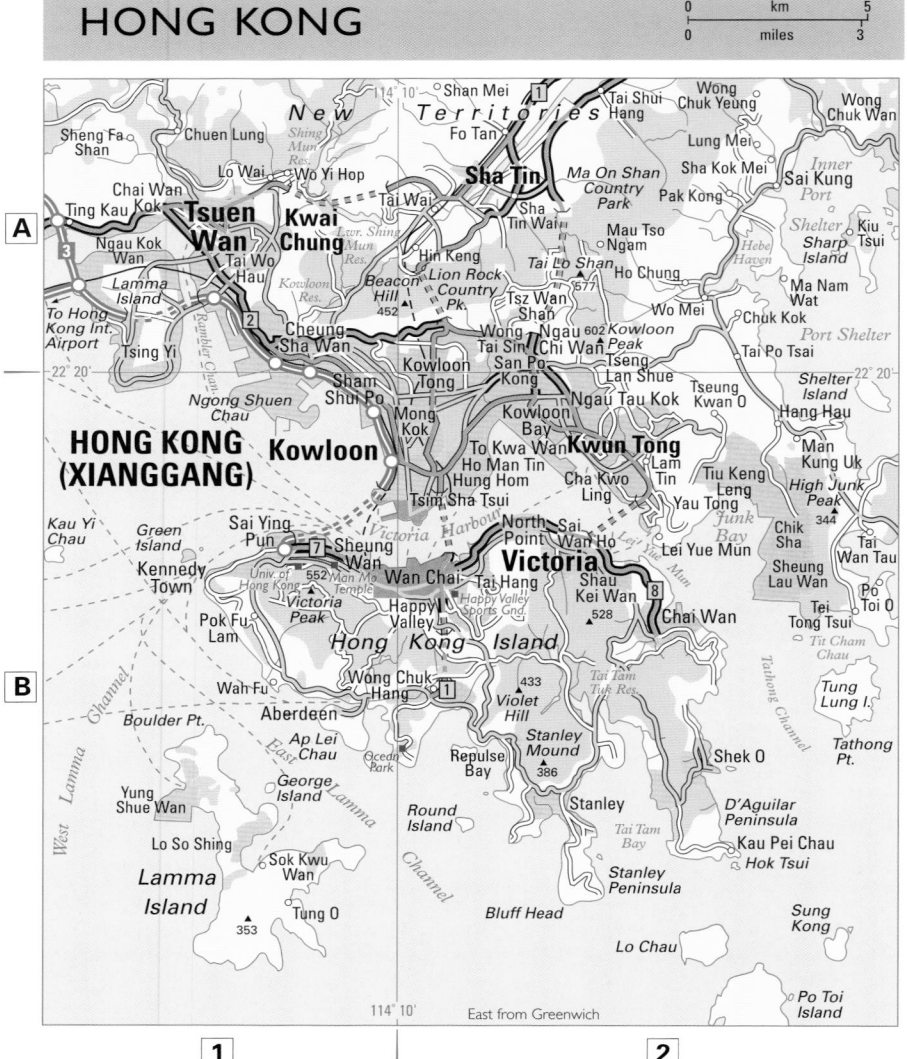

CENTRAL HONG KONG

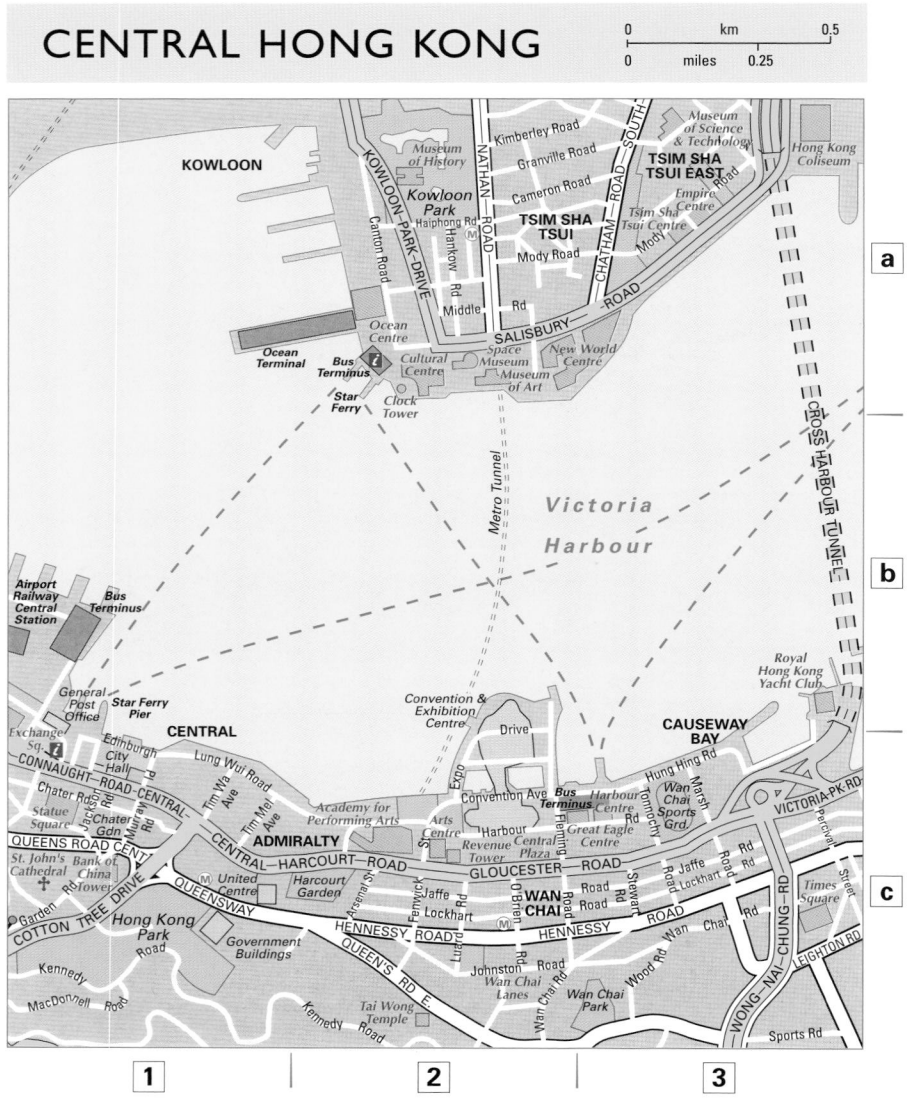

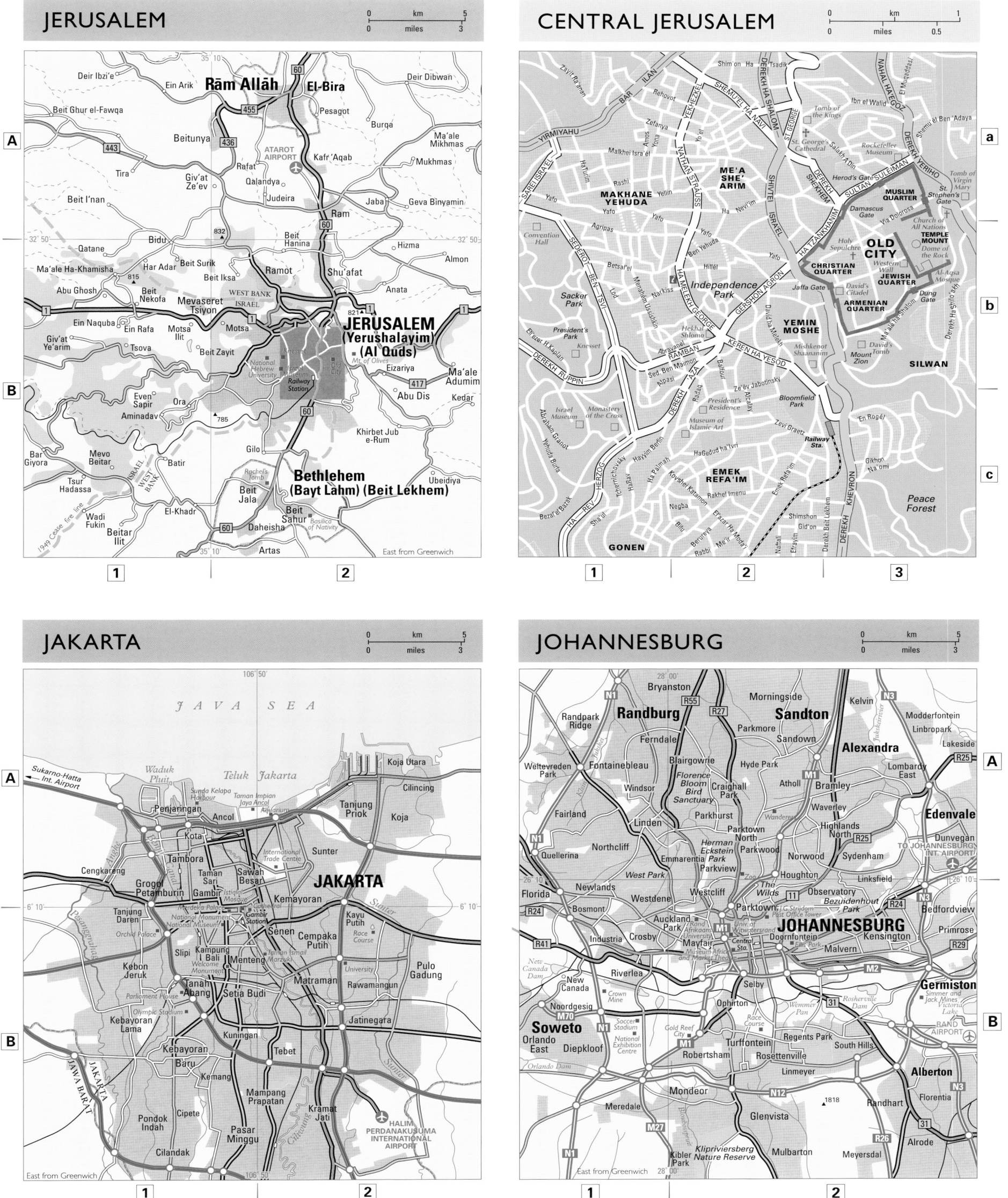

JERUSALEM

km 0—5
miles 0—3

Deir Ibzi'e
Ein Arik
Rām Allāh **El-Bira**
Deir Dibwan
Beit Ghur el-Fawqa
Beitunya
Pesagot
Burqa
Ma'ale Mikhmas
Beit I'nan
Beit Ghur el-Fawqa
Tira
Giv'at Ze'ev
Rafat
Qalandya
Judeira
Jaba
Geva Binyamin
Mukhmas
ATAROT AIRPORT
Kafr 'Aqab
Ram
Qatane
Bidu
Har Adar
Beit Surik
Beit Iksa
Beit Hanina
Hizma
Almon
Ma'ale Ha-Khamisha
Ramot
Shu'afat
Abu Ghosh
Beit Nekofa
Mevaseret Tsiyon
WEST BANK ISRAEL
Anata
Ein Naquba
Ein Rafa
Motsa Ilit
Motsa
JERUSALEM (Yerushalayim) (Al Quds)
Giv'at Ye'arim
Tsova
Beit Zayit
Mt of Olives
Eizariya
Ma'ale Adumim
Even Sapir
Ora
Aminadav
National Hebrew University
Jerusalem Railway Station
Abu Dis
Kedar
Bar Giyora
Mevo Beitar
Batir
Gilo
Khirbet Jub e-Rum
Tsur Hadassa
Bethlehem (Bayt Lahm) (Beit Lekhem)
Ubeidiya
Wadi Fukin
Beitar Ilit
El-Khadr
Beit Jala
Rachel's Tomb
Beit Sahur
Basilica of Nativity
Daheisha
Artas
East from Greenwich

CENTRAL JERUSALEM

km 0—1
miles 0—0.5

YIRMIYAHU
MAKHANE YEHUDA
ME'A SHE'ARIM
Tomb of the Kings
St. George's Cathedral
Rockefeller Museum
Herod's Gate
MUSLIM QUARTER
St. Stephen's Gate
Damascus Gate
Church of All Nations
Convention Hall
Holy Sepulchre
OLD CITY
TEMPLE MOUNT
Dome of the Rock
CHRISTIAN QUARTER
Western Wall
Al-Aqsa Mosque
Sacker Park
Independence Park
Jaffa Gate
David's Citadel
JEWISH QUARTER
President's Park
Knesset
ARMENIAN QUARTER
Dung Gate
Hekhal Shlomo
YEMIN MOSHE
David's Tomb
Mishkenot Shaananim
Mount Zion
SILWAN
Israel Museum
Monastery of the Cross
President's Residence
Bloomfield Park
En Rogel
Museum of Islamic Art
Railway Sta.
Peace Forest
EMEK REFA'IM
Gikhon Na'omi
GONEN

JAKARTA

km 0—5
miles 0—3

JAVA SEA
Waduk Pluit
Teluk Jakarta
Koja Utara
Sukarno-Hatta Int. Airport
Sunda Kelapa Harbour
Taman Impian Jaya Ancol
Cilincing
Penjaringan
Ancol
Aquarium
Tanjung Priok
Kota
Koja
Cengkareng
Tambora
Sunter
Groggol Petamburin
Taman Sari
Sawah Besar
International Trade Centre
Kemayoran
Tanjung Daren
Gambir
Istiqlal Mosque
JAKARTA
Kayu Putih
Merdeka Palace
National Monument
Gambir Station
Cempaka Putih
Race Course
Kebon Jeruk
Slipi
Kampung Bali
Welcome Monument
Senen
Orchid Palace
National Museum
Menteng
Taman Ismail Marzuki
Pulo Gadung
Parliament House
Tanah Abang
University
Rawamangun
Olympic Stadium
Kebayoran Lama
Setia Budi
Matraman
Jatinegara
Kebayoran Baru
Kuningan
Kemang
Tebet
Pondok Indah
Mampang Prapatan
Cipete
Kramat Jati
Pasar Minggu
HALIM PERDANAKUSUMA INTERNATIONAL AIRPORT
Cilandak
East from Greenwich
JAKARTA BARAT
JAWA BARAT

JOHANNESBURG

km 0—5
miles 0—3

Bryanston
Morningside
Kelvin
Randpark Ridge
Randburg
Sandton
Modderfontein
Linbropark
Ferndale
Parkmore
Sandown
Alexandra
Lakeside
Weltevreden Park
Fontainebleau
Blairgowrie
Hyde Park
Atholl
Bramley
Lombardy East
Windsor
Florence Bloom Bird Sanctuary
Craighall Park
Waverley
Fairland
Parkhurst
Parktown North
Highlands North
Sydenham
Edenvale
Quellerina
Northcliff
Herman Eckstein Park
Parkwood
Norwood
TO JOHANNESBURG INT. AIRPORT
Dunvegan
Linden
Emmarentia Park
Parkview
Zoo
Houghton
Linksfield
Florida
Newlands
Westdene
Westcliff
The Wilds
Observatory
Bedfordview
Bosmont
Parktown
T.G. Strijdom Post Office Tower
Bezuidenhout Park
Auckland Park
Univ. of Witwatersrand
Doornfontein
JOHANNESBURG
Kensington
Primrose
Industria
Crosby
Mayfair
Central Sta.
Ellis Park
Malvern
Museum Africa and Market Theatre
New Canada Dam
Riverlea
Selby
Germiston
Simmer and Jack Mines
Victoria Lake
Noordgesig
New Canada
Ophirton
Rosherville Dam
Crown Mine
Wemmer Pan
Soweto
Gold Reef City
Soccer Stadium
Turffontein
Regents Park
South Hills
RAND AIRPORT
Orlando East
Diepkloof
National Exhibition Centre
Robertsham
Rosettenville
Linmeyer
Alberton
Orlando Dam
Mondeor
Florentia
Meredale
Glenvista
Randhart
Klipriviersberg Nature Reserve
Kibler Park
Mulbarton
Meyersdal
Alrode
East from Greenwich

KARACHI

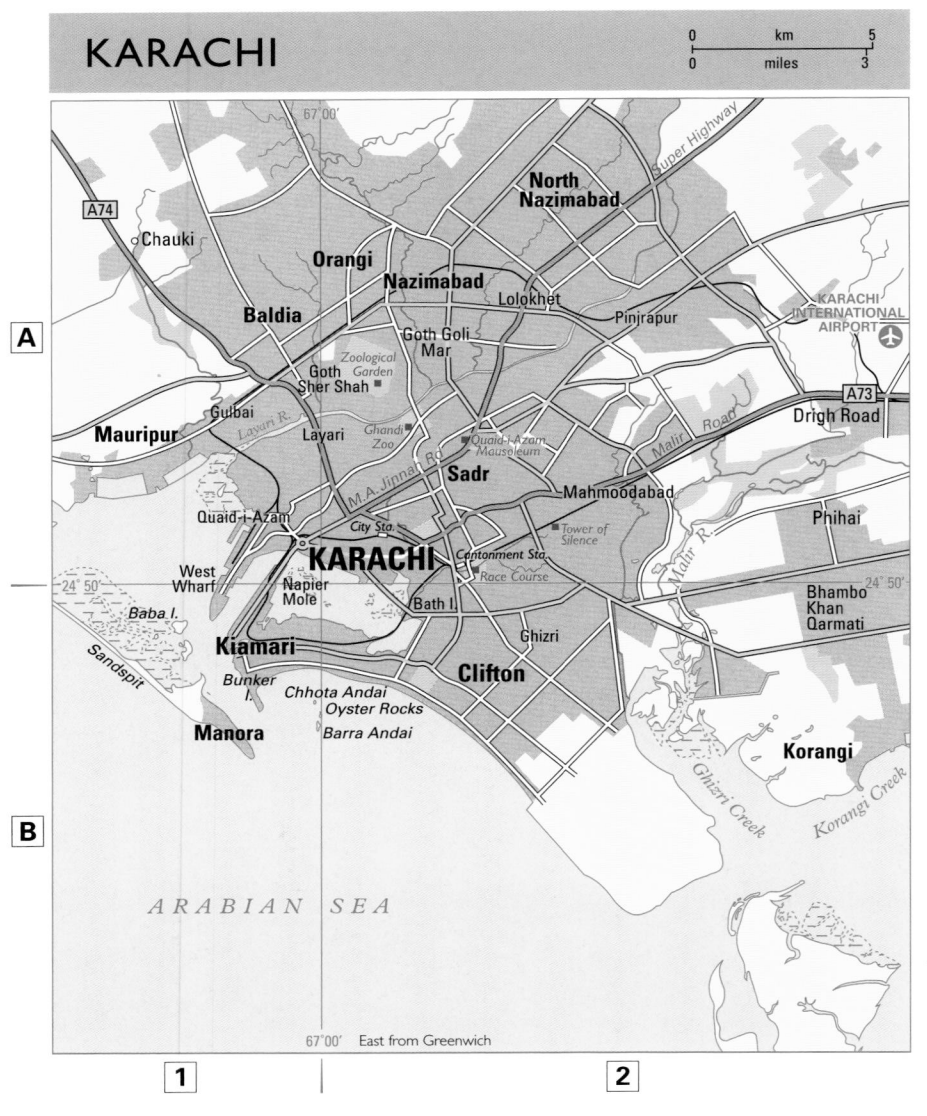

LAGOS

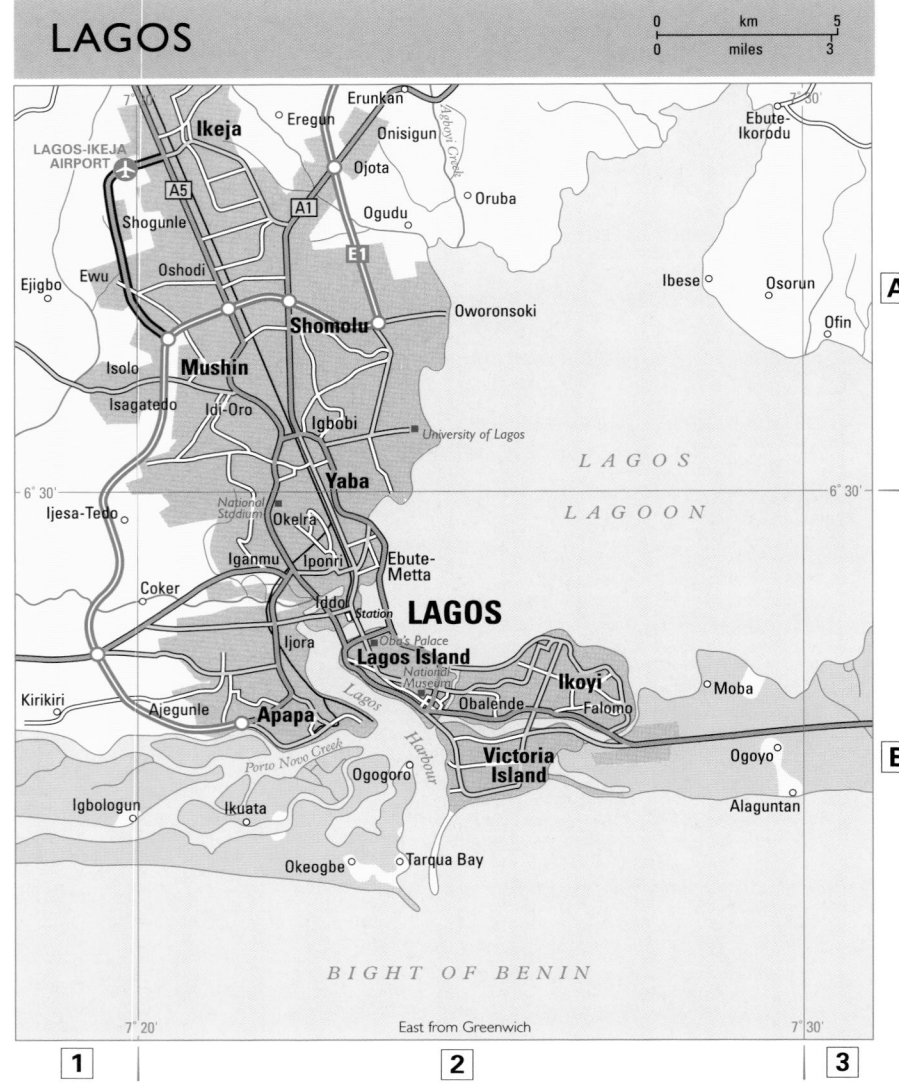

LISBON

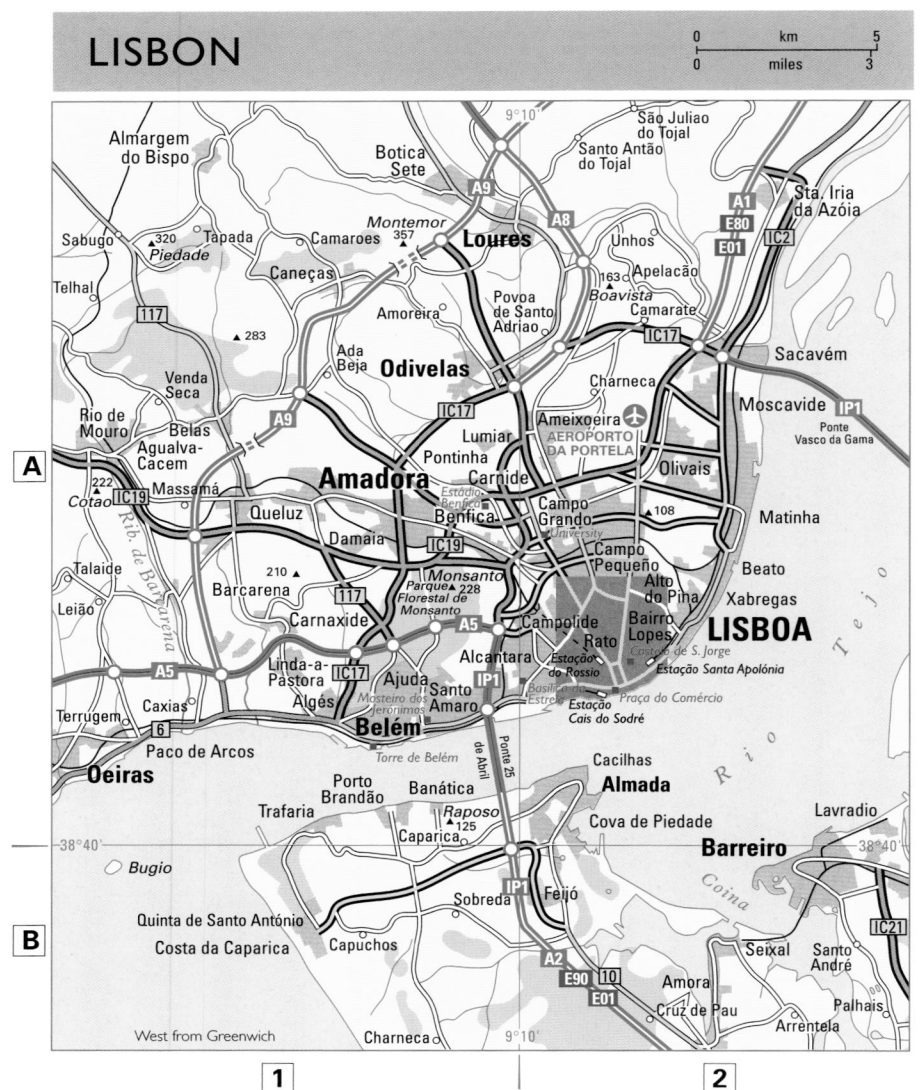

CENTRAL LISBON

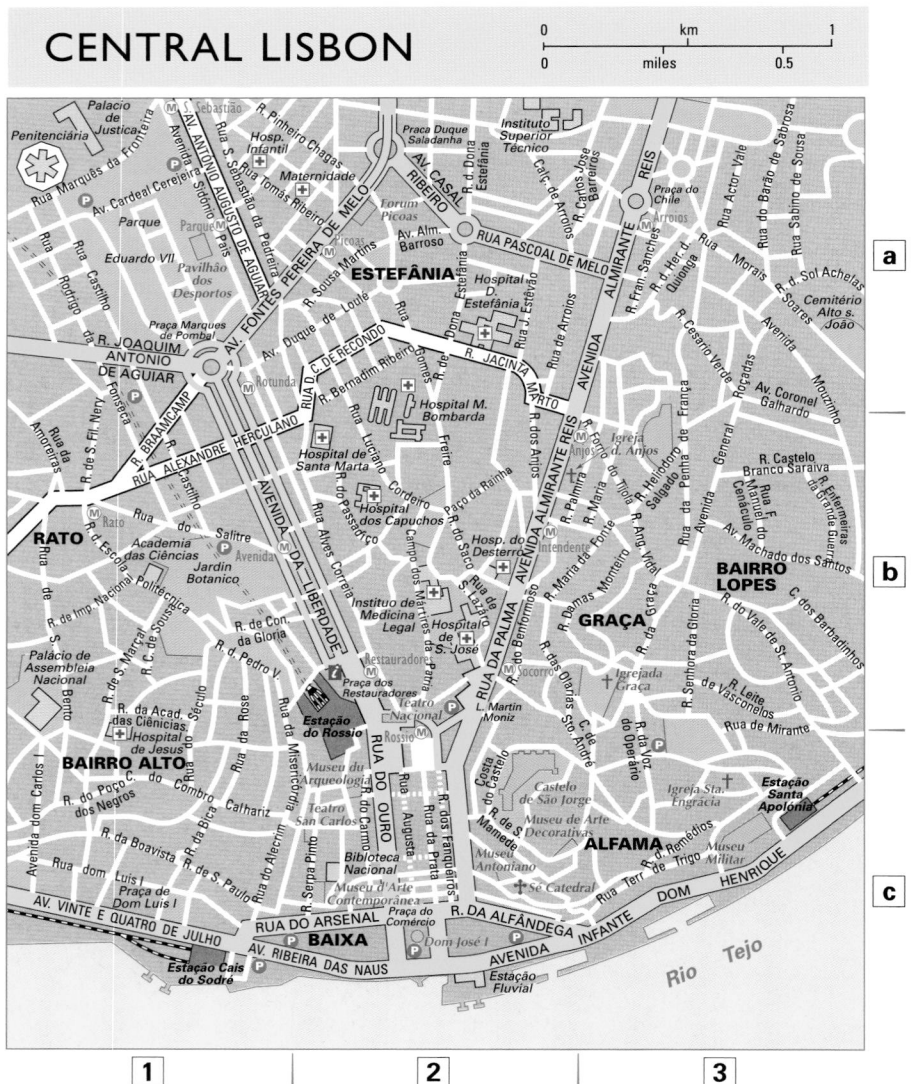

LONDON

km 0 — 5
miles 0 — 3

Northwood, Stanmore, Barnet, Finchley, Colney Hatch, Wood Green, Noel Park, Waltham Forest, Woodford, Stansted Airport, Woodford Bridge, GREATER LONDON, Hainault, Havering-atte-Bower, Harold Hill

Hatch End, Burnt Oak, Colindale, Hendon, Mill Hill, Muswell Hill, Hornsey, Tottenham, Walthamstow, Clayhall, Barkingside, Collier Row, Gidea Park, Gallows Corner, Romford

Pinner Green, Harrow Weald, Belmont, Queensbury, Church End, East End, Highgate, Haringey, Hornchurch, Elm Park, Rush Green

Ruislip Common, Eastcote, Pinner, Wealdstone, HARROW, Greenhill, Kenton, Hampstead Garden Suburb, Golders Green, Finsbury Park, Stoke Newington, Clapton, Lea Bridge, Hackney Wick, Stratford, Upton, Manor Park, Becontree, Heath

Ickenham, South Ruislip, Rayners Lane, West Harrow, Harrow on the Hill, Roxeth, Harrow School Rugby Gd., Kenwood House, Hampstead Heath, Tufnell Park, Highbury, Hometon, Bethnal Green, Bow, West Ham, A406, A13, Barking, Dagenham, South Hornchurch, Rainham

A — A

Cowley, Yeading, Greenford, Perivale, A40, Kensal Green, Dollis Hill, Cricklewood, Willesden Green, Gospel Oak, Kentish Town, Camden, Islington, Dalston, Shoreditch, Whitechapel, Poplar, Canning Town, London City Airport, North Woolwich, Creekmouth, Beckton, Wennington, River Thames, Thamesmead

West Drayton, HILLINGDON, EALING, Acton, Notting Hill, Paddington, Holborn, City, TOWER HAMLETS, NEWHAM, Docklands, Millennium Dome

53°10′, Osterley Park, Brentford, Chiswick, Turnham Green, Shepherd's Bush, Hyde Park, WESTMINSTER, Southwark, Bermondsey, Rotherhithe, Wapping, Limehouse, Isle of Dogs, A102, Abbey Wood, Belvedere, Erith, KENT, ESSEX

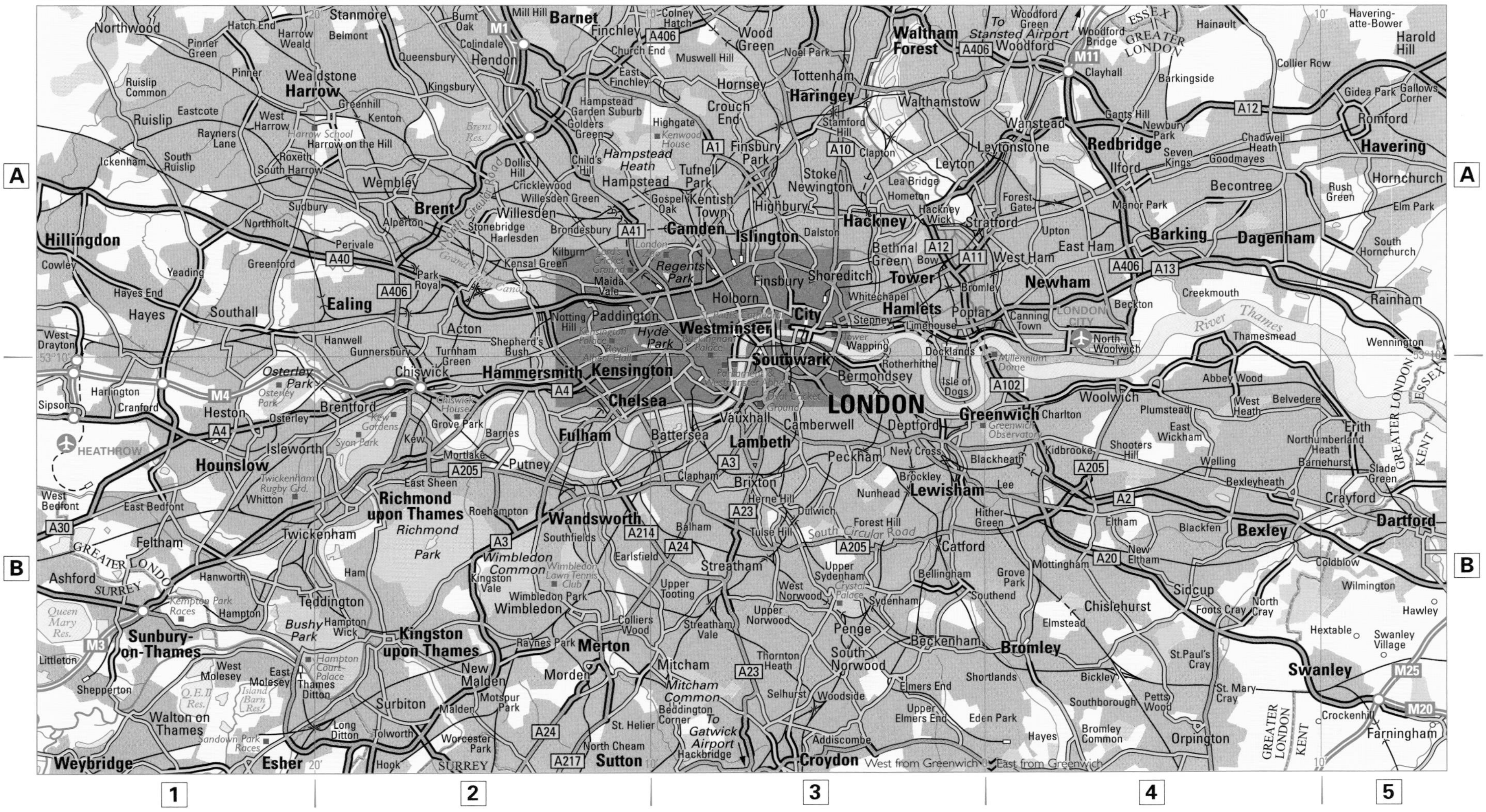

HEATHROW, M4, Osterley, Heston, Isleworth, HAMMERSMITH, KENSINGTON, CHELSEA, Fulham, Battersea, Vauxhall, Camberwell, LONDON, Deptford, GREENWICH, Charlton, Woolwich, Plumstead, East Wickham, Welling, Bexleyheath, Crayford, Dartford

Harlington, Cranford, Hounslow, Syon Park, Kew Gardens, Barnes, Putney, LAMBETH, Peckham, New Cross, Blackheath, Kidbrooke, Shooters Hill, Northumberland Heath, A30, A4, HOUNSLOW, Twickenham, Richmond upon Thames, Mortlake, Brixton, Herne Hill, Dulwich, Lee, Eltham, Blackfen, BEXLEY, DARTFORD

West Bedfont, East Bedfont, Whitton, East Sheen, Roehampton, Southfields, Clapham, A3, Streatham, South Norwood, Catford, Grove Park, Mottingham, Sidcup, North Cray, Coldblow, Wilmington

B — B

Ashford, GREATER LONDON, SURREY, Teddington, Richmond Park, Wimbledon Common, Kingston Vale, WANDSWORTH, A214, A24, Balham, Upper Tooting, Streatham Vale, A205, Upper Sydenham, Crystal Palace, Sydenham, Bellingham, Southend, Grove Park, Chislehurst, Foots Cray, North Cray, Hawley, Hextable, Swanley Village

Kempton Park Races, Hampton, Ham, Wimbledon, Colliers Wood, Thornton Heath, Penge, Beckenham, Shortlands, Bickley, St. Paul's Cray, Swanley, M25, M20

Sunbury-on-Thames, Q.E.II Res., West Molesey, East Molesey, Thames Ditton, New Malden, MERTON, Mitcham Common, Beddington Corner, Selhurst, Woodside, Elmers End, Eden Park, Bromley Common, Orpington, GREATER LONDON, KENT, M25, M20, Farningham

Weybridge, Walton on Thames, Shepperton, Sandown Park Races, Esher, Hook, Long Ditton, Surbiton, Tolworth, Worcester Park, Morden, MITCHAM, St. Helier, North Cheam, SUTTON, Hackbridge, Addiscombe, CROYDON, West from Greenwich, East from Greenwich, Crockenhill

Kingston upon Thames, A3, A24, A217, A23

1 2 3 4 5

CENTRAL LONDON

km 0 — 2
miles 0 — 1

KENSAL RISE, ST. JOHN'S WOOD, King's Cross, PENTONVILLE RD, HOXTON, SHOREDITCH

West Kilburn, Queen's Park, MAIDA VALE, Lord's Cricket Ground, Regent's Park, London Zoo, Euston, St. Pancras, King's Cross Thameslink, Angel, CITY ROAD, Old Street, Worship Street, EASTERN RD

a — a

WESTBOURNE GREEN, Edgware Road, Marylebone, Madame Tussaud's, Regent's Park, BLOOMSBURY, Russell Sq., CLERKENWELL, Farringdon, Barbican, Moorgate, Liverpool St., Whitechapel Art Gall.

PADDINGTON, Marble Arch, OXFORD STREET, SOHO, HOLBORN, British Museum, Mus. of St. Barts, London Wall, CITY, Bishopsgate, Leadenhall St., Fenchurch St.

BAYSWATER, Lancaster Gate, HYDE PARK, The Ring, Piccadilly Circus, Charing Cross, STRAND, FLEET ST., LUDGATE HILL, Bank, Cannon St., Monument

b — b

NOTTING HILL, NOTTING HILL GATE, KENSINGTON GARDENS, Serpentine, PARK LANE, MAYFAIR, ST. JAMES'S, National Gallery, BFI London IMAX, Tate Modern, SOUTHWARK, London Bridge, River Thames, The Design Museum

Holland Park, KENSINGTON, Kensington Palace, Serpentine Gallery, Apsley House & Wellington Mus., St. James's Palace, Green Park, Buckingham Palace, Waterloo East, Waterloo International, London Dungeon, HMS Belfast

KENSINGTON, Commonwealth Institute, KNIGHTSBRIDGE, CONSTITUTION HILL, Westminster, Houses of Parliament, Westminster Abbey, County Hall, London Eye, BOROUGH, NEWINGTON, BERMONDSEY

c — c

Olympia Exhibition Halls, Imperial Coll. Science, Nat. History & Geological Mus., BROMPTON, Victoria, Victoria Coach Stn., BELGRAVIA, Tate Britain, LAMBETH, Elephant & Castle, WALWORTH, OLD KENT ROAD

WEST KENSINGTON, Hammersmith Cemetery, SOUTH KENSINGTON, FULHAM, PIMLICO, KENNINGTON, The Oval Cricket Gd., CHELSEA, Chelsea Embankment, River Thames

1 2 3 4 5

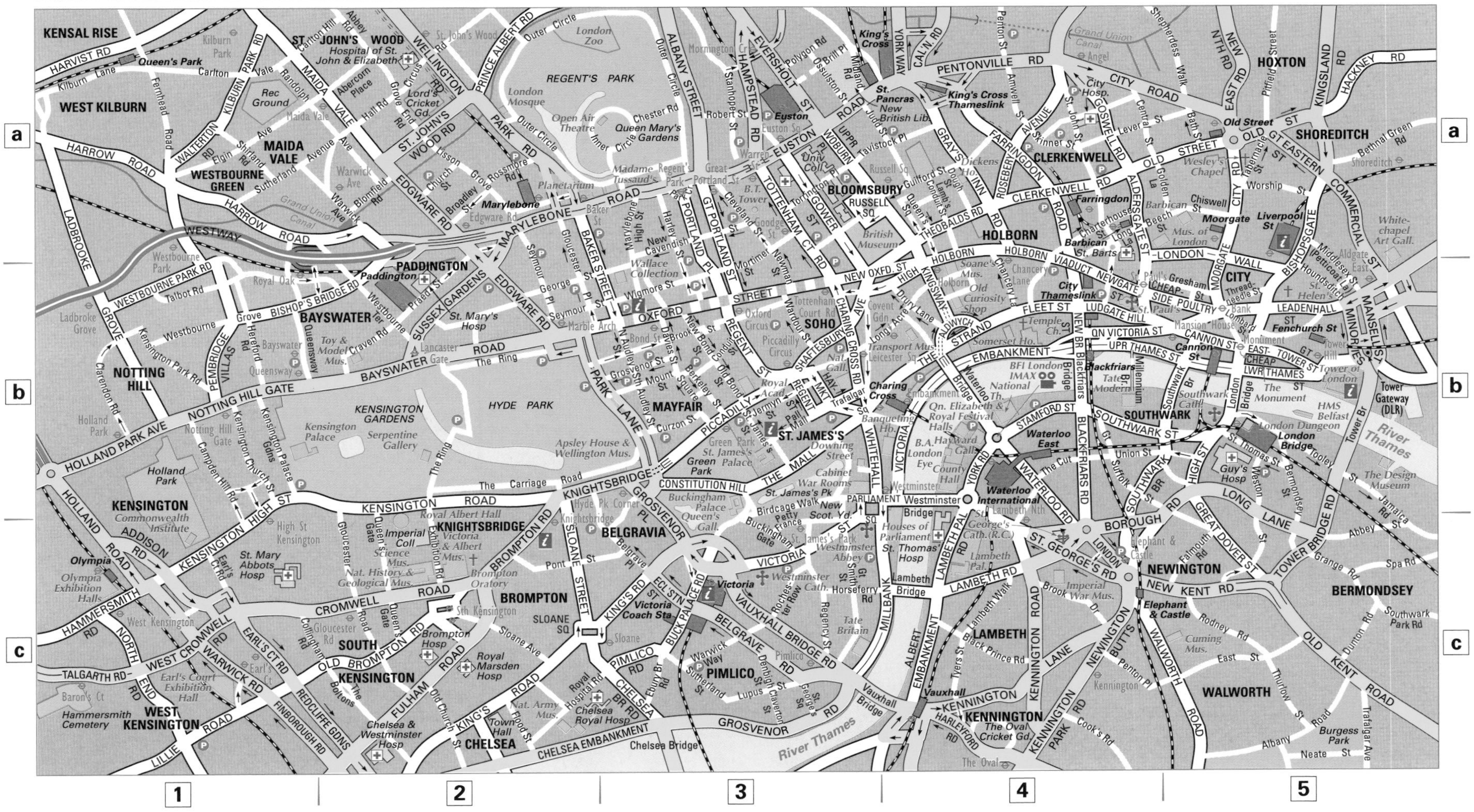

COPYRIGHT PHILIP'S

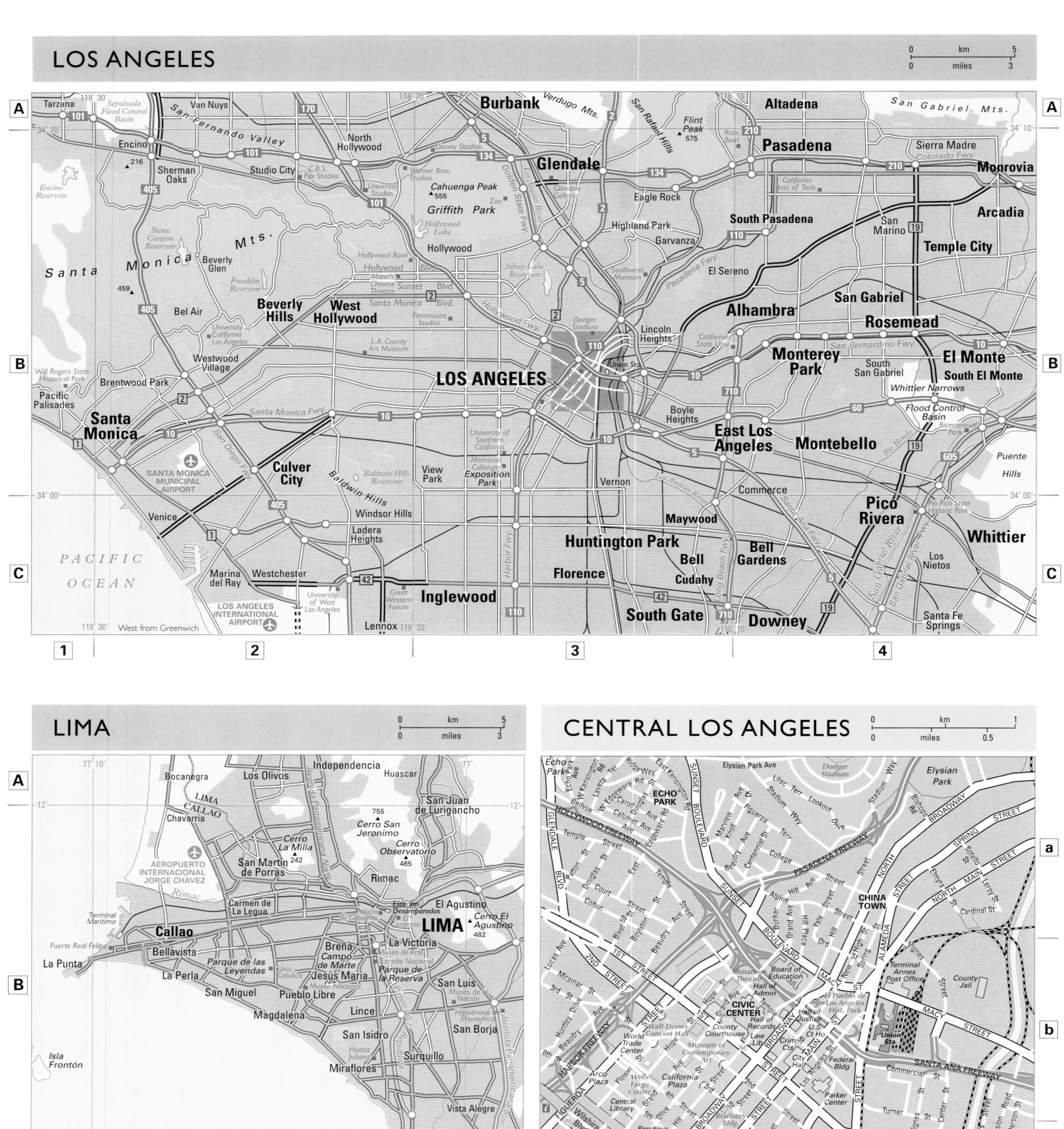

LOS ANGELES

LIMA

CENTRAL LOS ANGELES

COPYRIGHT PHILIP'S

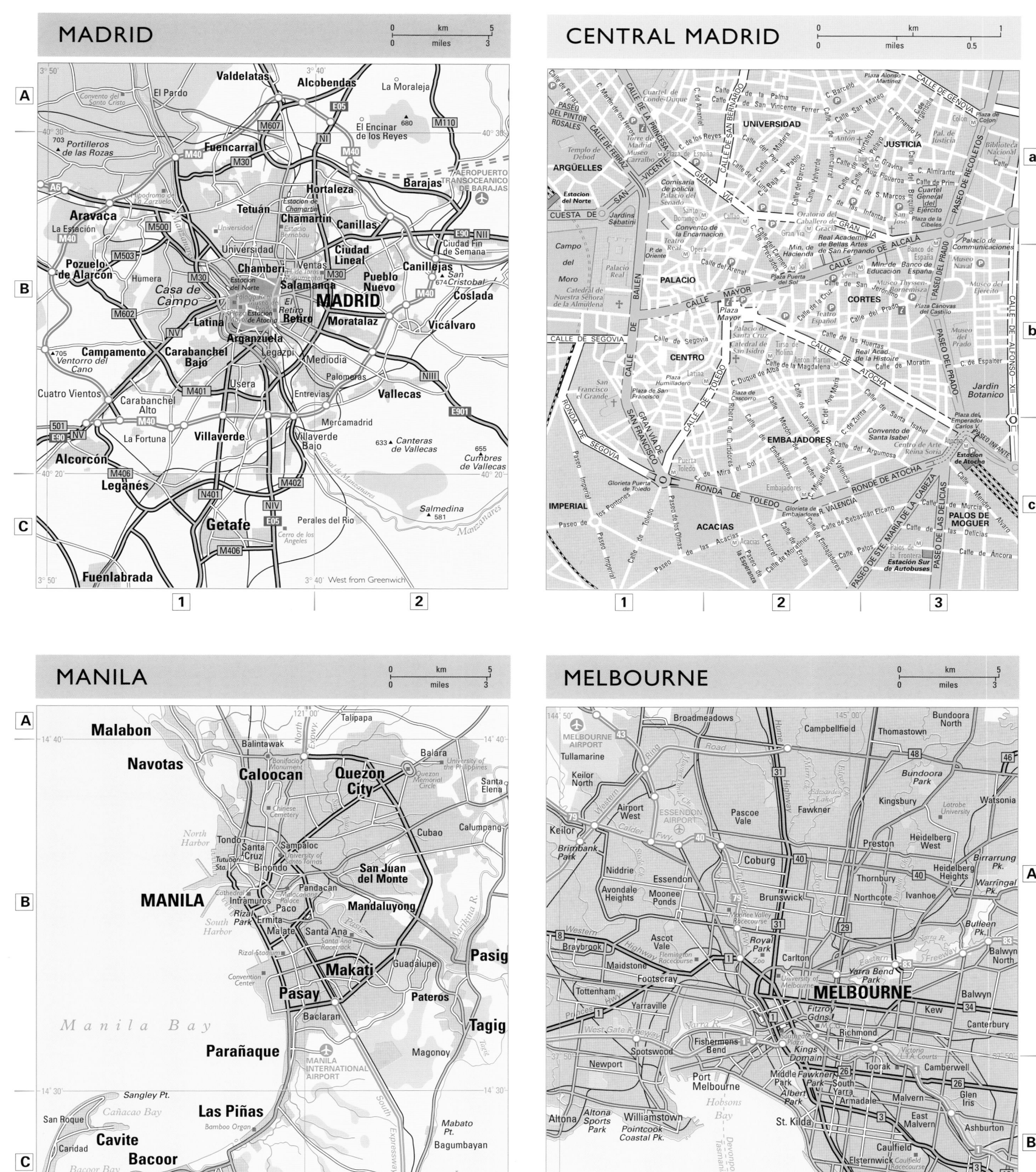

MADRID

km 5
miles 3

A — Valdelatas — Alcobendas — La Moraleja
El Pardo — Convento del Santo Cristo
703 Portilleros de las Rozas
Fuencarral — El Encinar de los Reyes — 680
M607 — M30 — M110 — NI
M40
B — Aravaca — La Estación — Hortaleza — Barajas — AEROPUERTO TRANSOCEANICO DE BARAJAS
Tetuán — Estación de Chamartin
Chamartin — Canillas
Pozuelo de Alarcón — Universidad — Ciudad Lineal — Ciudad Fin de Semana
Humera — Chamberi — San Cristobal — 674
Casa de Campo — Salamanca — MADRID — Canillejas
Latina — El Retiro — Pueblo Nuevo — Coslada
705 Ventorro del Cano — Arganzuela — Moratalaz — Vicálvaro
Campamento — Carabanchel Bajo — Legazpi — Mediodia
Cuatro Vientos — Carabanchel Alto — Usera — Palomeras — Entrevias — Vallecas
501 — La Fortuna — Villaverde — Mercamadrid — Canteras de Vallecas — 633 — Cumbres de Vallecas — 655
Alcorcón — Villaverde Bajo — Salmedina — 581
Leganés — Getafe — Perales del Rio
C — Cerro de los Angeles
Fuenlabrada — West from Greenwich

1 — 2

CENTRAL MADRID

km 1
miles 0.5

ARGÜELLES — UNIVERSIDAD — JUSTICIA
Estación del Norte — GRAN VIA
CUESTA DE — PALACIO — CORTES
Campo del Moro — Palacio Real — CENTRO — EMBAJADORES — PALOS DE MOGUER
IMPERIAL — ACACIAS

1 — 2 — 3

MANILA

km 5
miles 3

A — Malabon — Talipapa
Balintawak — Balara
Navotas — Bonifacio Monument — University of the Philippines
Caloocan — Quezon City — Quezon Memorial Circle — Santa Elena
North Harbor — Chinese Cemetery — Cubao — Calumpang
Tondo — Santa Cruz — Sampaloc — University of Santo Tomas
Binondo — Pandacan — San Juan del Monte
B — MANILA — Intramuros — Malacanang Palace — Paco — Mandaluyong
South Harbor — Rizal Park — Ermita — Santa Ana — Pasig
Cathedral — Malate — Santa Ana Racetrack
Rizal Stadium — Makati — Guadalupe — Pateros
Convention Center — Pasay — Baclaran — Tagig
Parañaque — Magonoy
Sangley Pt. — MANILA INTERNATIONAL AIRPORT
San Roque — Cañacao Bay — Las Piñas — Mabato Pt. — Bagumbayan
Caridad — Bamboo Organ
C — Cavite — Bacoor — Sucat
Binacayan — Bacoor Bay — Zapote — Bule — Laguna de Bay
Kawit — East from Greenwich

Manila Bay

1 — 2

MELBOURNE

km 5
miles 3

Broadmeadows — Campbellfield — Thomastown — Bundoora North
MELBOURNE AIRPORT — Tullamarine — Keilor North
Keilor — Airport West — Pascoe Vale — Fawkner — Kingsbury — Latrobe University — Watsonia
Brimbank Park — Niddrie — Essendon — Coburg — Preston — Heidelberg West — Birrarrung Pk.
Avondale Heights — Moonee Ponds — Brunswick — Thornbury — Northcote — Ivanhoe — Warringal Pk.
A — Maidstone — Ascot Vale — Royal Park Zoo — Carlton — Yarra Bend Park — Bulleen Pk. — Balwyn North
Braybrook — Footscray — University of Melbourne — MELBOURNE — Kew
Tottenham — Yarraville — Fitzroy Gdns. — Richmond — Canterbury
Newport — Spotswood — Kings Domain — Toorak — Camberwell
Port Melbourne — Middle Park — Fawkner Park — South Yarra — Malvern — Glen Iris
Altona — Williamstown — Albert Park — St. Kilda — Armadale — East Malvern — Ashburton
Altona Sports Park — Pointcook Coastal Pk. — Hobsons Bay — Caulfield — Caulfield Racecourse
B — Elwood — Elsternwick — Carnegie
Port Phillip Bay — Glenhuntly — Oakleigh
Brighton — Ormond — East from Greenwich

1 — 2

MEXICO CITY

km
0 — 5
miles
0 — 3

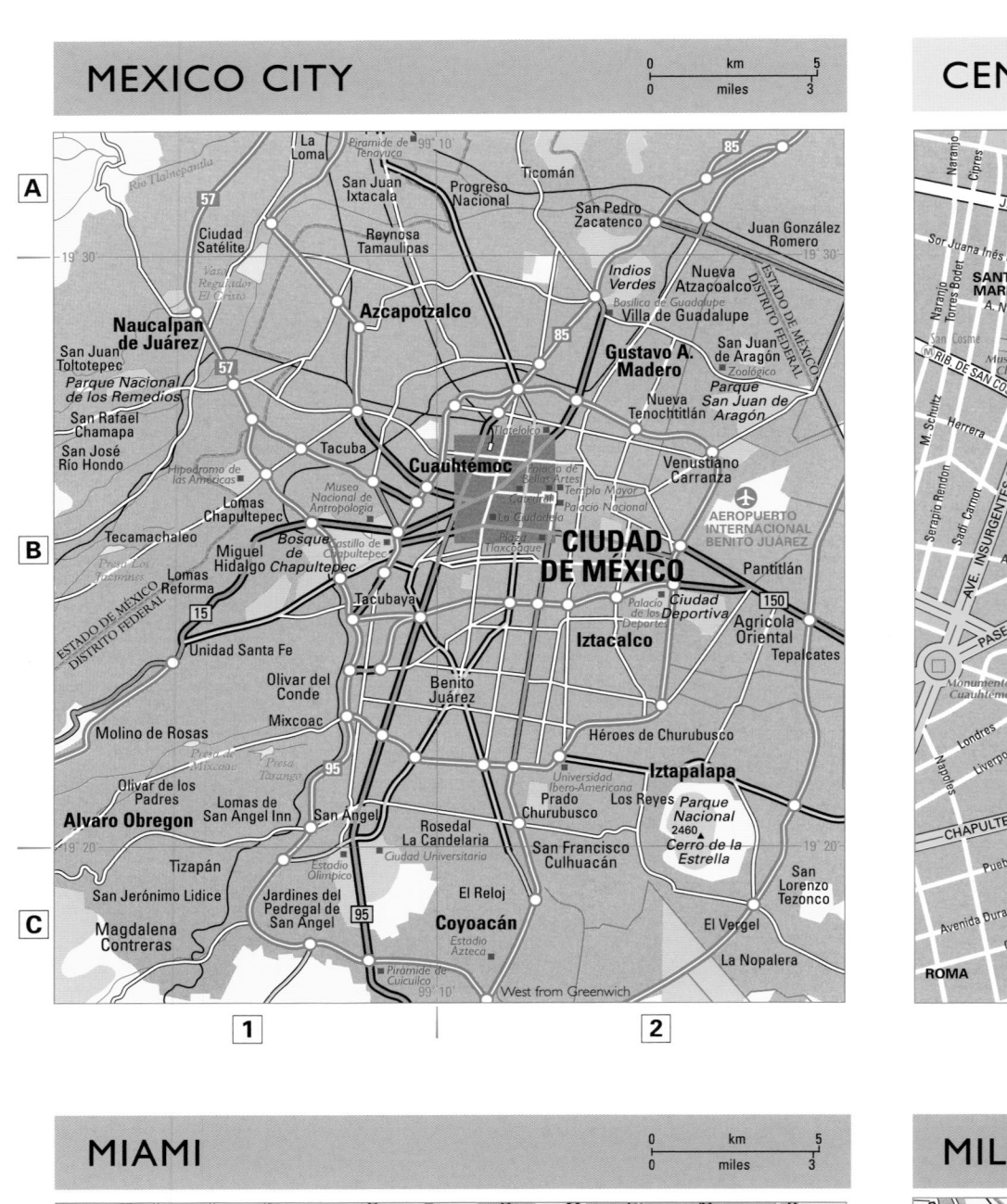

CENTRAL MEXICO CITY

km
0 — 1
miles
0 — 0.5

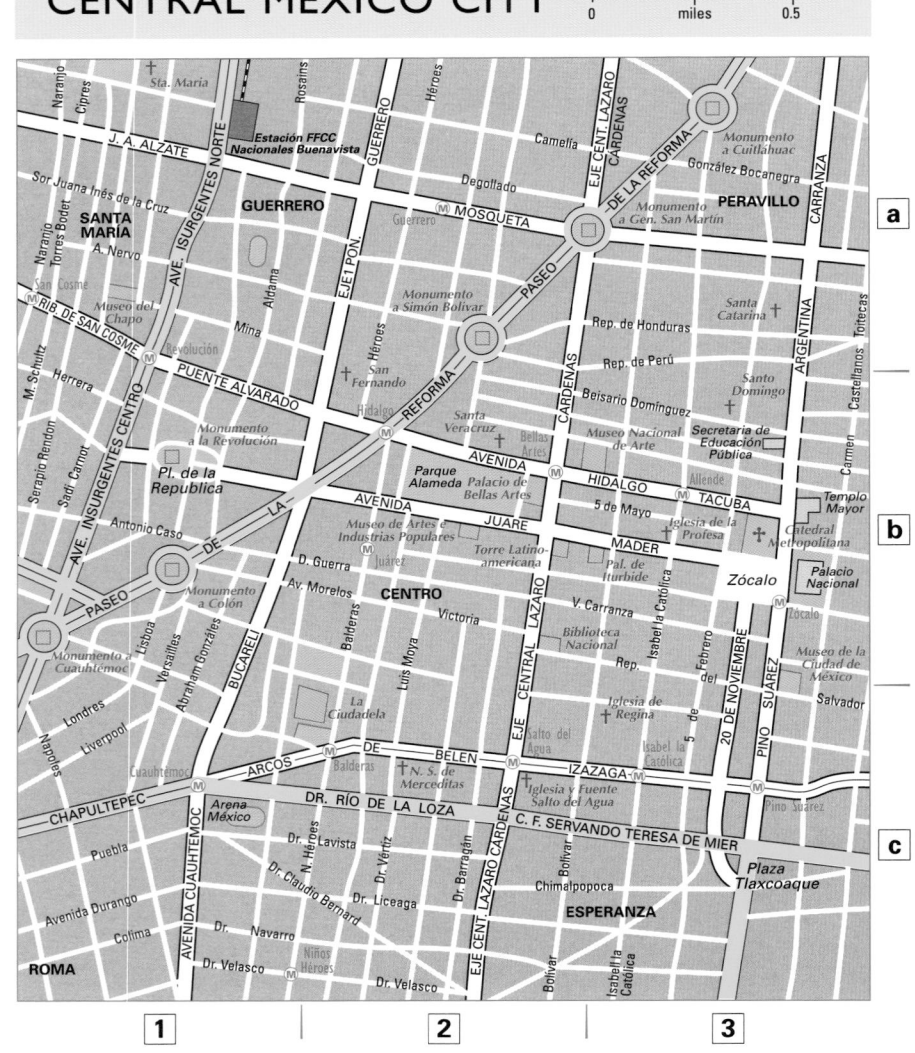

MIAMI

km
0 — 5
miles
0 — 3

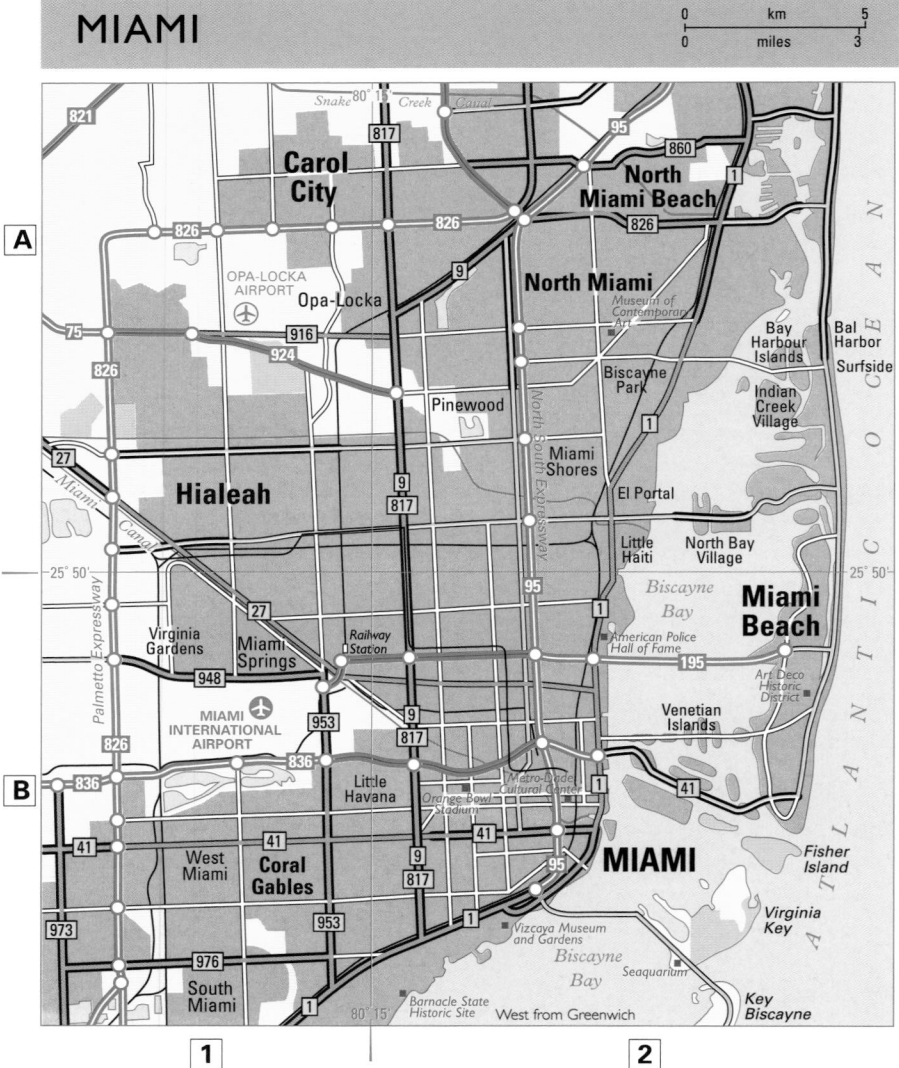

MILAN

km
0 — 5
miles
0 — 3

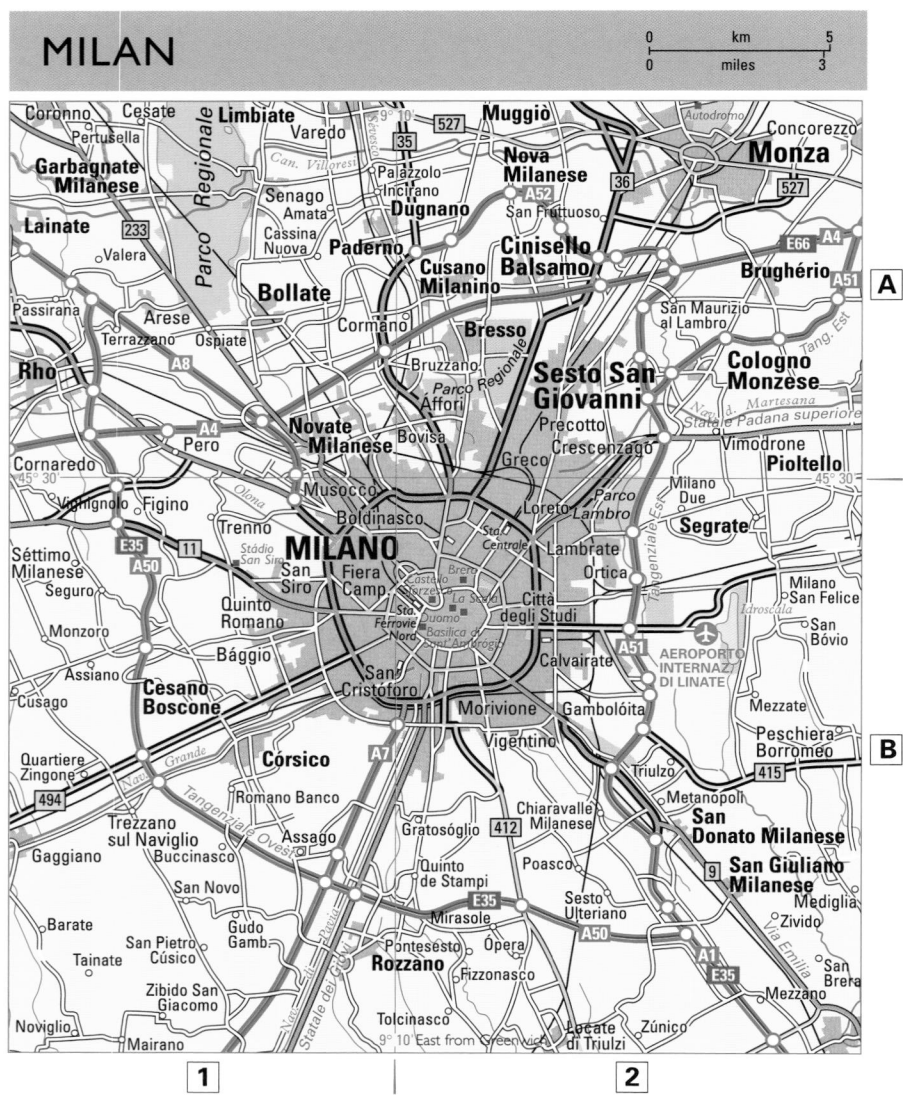

MOSCOW

km 5 / miles 3

Novonikolyskoye, Mitino, Putilkovo, Bratsevo, Degunino, Khimki-Khovrino, Vladykino, Babushkin, 157▲, Medvezhiy Ozyora, Medvezhiy Ozyora, Almazova, Pekhra-Pokrovskoye

Krasnogorsk, Chernyovo, Penyagino, Tushino, Nikolskiy, Petrovsko-Razumovskoye, Timiryazev Park, Dzerzhinskiy Park, Ostankino, Abramtsevo, Vostochnyy, 140▲, Balashikha, Novaya

Golyevo, Pavshino, Myakinino, Strogino, Pokrovsko-Sresnevo, Petrovskiy Park, Frunze, Sokolniki Park, Bogorodskoye, Galyanovo, Gorenki, Pekhra-Yakovievskaya

Arkhangelskoye, Troitse-Lykovo, Sokolniki, Dzerzhinskiy, Izmaylovo, Vishnyaki, Nikolskoye

Zakharkovo, Rublovo, Tatarovo, Cherepkovo, Mnevniki, Khorosovo, Yaroslav Station, Leningrad Station, Kazan Station, Sverdlov, Izmayloskiy Park, 150▲, Saltykovka

MOSKVA, Leportovo

Razdory, Krasno-Presnenskaya, Bauman, Kursk Station, Novogireyevo, Reutov, Kutsino

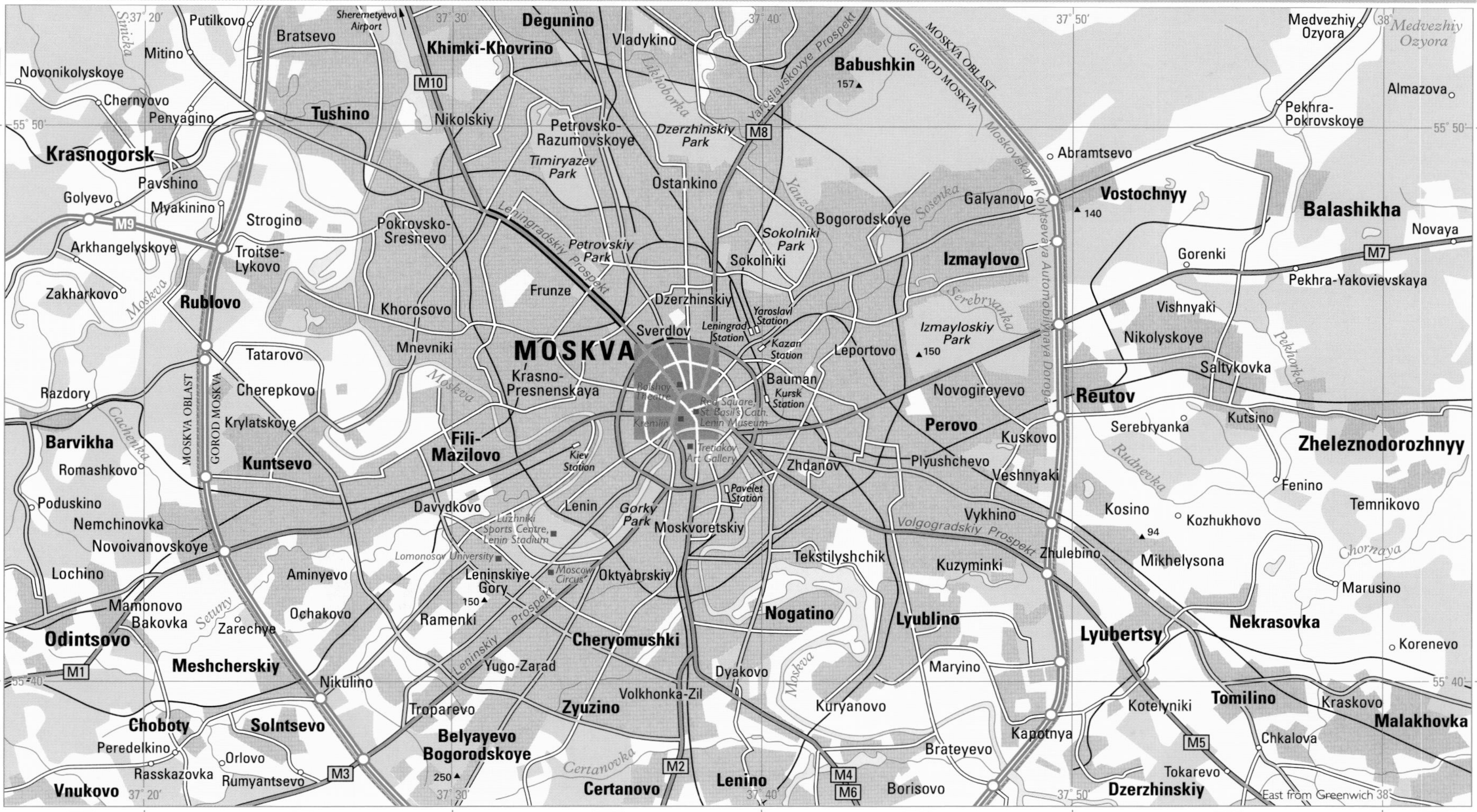

Barvikha, Krylatskoye, Fili-Mazilovo, Kuntsevo, Zhdanov, Perovo, Kuskovo, Plyushchevo, Veshnyaki, Serebryanka, Zheleznodorozhnyy

Romashkovo, Poduskino, Nemchinovka, Davdkovo, Lenin, Gorky Park, Moskvoretskiy, Pavelet Station, Vykhino, Kosino, Fenino, Temnikovo

Novoivanovskoye, Aminyevo, Lomonosov University, Moscow Circus, Oktyabrskiy, Tekstilyshchik, Kuzyminki, 94▲, Kozhukhovo, Marusino

Lochino, Mamonovo, Bakovka, Zarechye, Ochakovo, Leninskiye Gory, 150▲, Ramenki, Korenevo

Odintsovo, Meshcherskiy, Nikulino, Yugo-Zarad, Cheryomushki, Nogatino, Lyublino, Lyubertsy, Nekrasovka

Choboty, Solntsevo, Troparevo, Zyuzino, Dyakovo, Maryino, Tomilino, Kraskovo

Peredelkino, Orlovo, Belyayevo Bogorodskoye, 250▲, Volkhonka-Zil, Kuryanovo, Kotelniki, Malakhovka

Vnukovo, Rasskazovka, Rumyantsevo, Certanovo, Lenino, Borisovo, Brateyevo, Kapotnya, Dzerzhinskiy, Chkalova

East from Greenwich

1 2 3 4 5 6
A B C

MONTRÉAL

km 5 / miles 3

Île Jésus, Rivière-des-Prairies, Pointe-Aux-Trembles, Boucherville, Montréal Est, Laval, Vimont, St-Vincent-de-Paul, Montréal Nord, Anjou, Boucherville, Bélanger, St-Léonard, Laval, Sault-au-Récollet, St-Michel, Longue-Pointe, Île de Boucherville, Ahuntsic, Rosemont, Parc Maisonneuve, Jardin Botanique, Stade Olympique, Maisonneuve, Cartierville, Hochelaga, MONTRÉAL, Parc Lafontaine, Île Ste-Hélène, St-Laurent, Outremont, Mont-Royal, Parc Hélène de Champlain, Longueuil, St-Lambert, St-Hubert, Westmount, Greenfield Park, Lemoyne, Hampstead, Notre-Dame-de-Grâce, Côte-St-Luc, St-Pierre, Préville, Montréal Ouest, Verdun, Île des Soeurs, Brossard, Lachine, Lasalle, Île aux Herons, La Prairie, Kahnawake, Ste-Catherine, Candiac

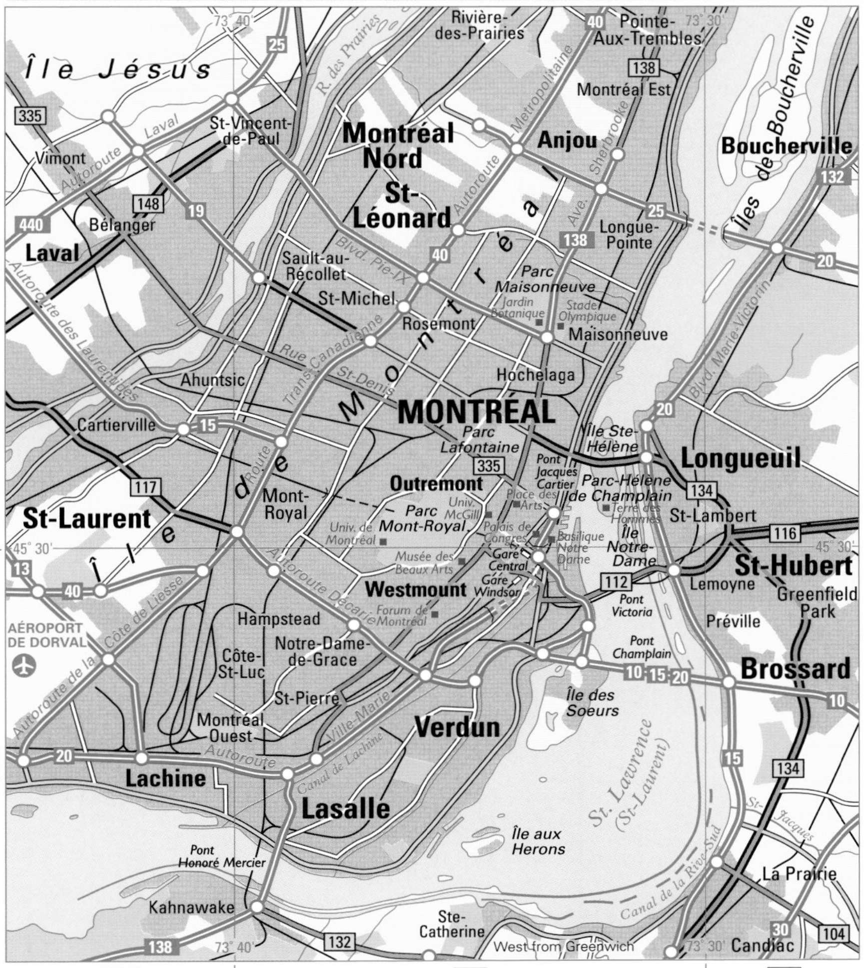

AÉROPORT DE DORVAL

West from Greenwich

1 2 3
A B

CENTRAL MOSCOW

km 1 / miles 0.5

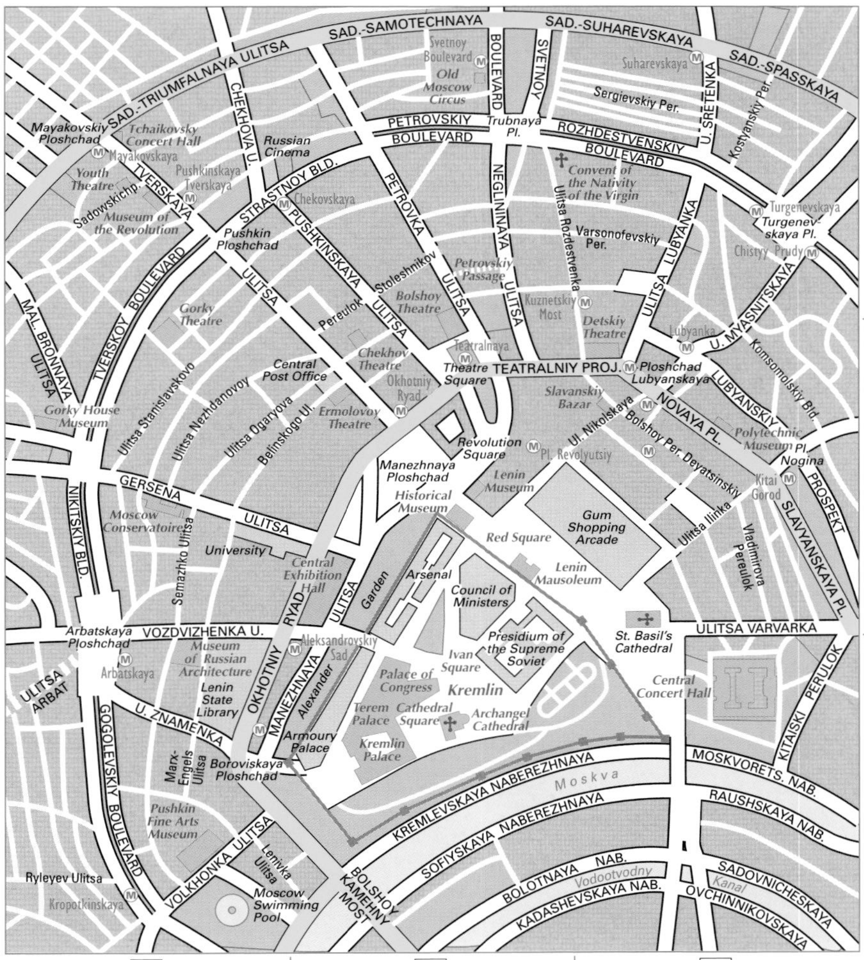

SAD-SAMOTECHNAYA, SAD-SUHAREVSKAYA, SAD-SPASSKAYA, Mayakovsky Ploshchad, Tchaikovsky Concert Hall, Russian Cinema, Svetnoy Boulevard, Old Moscow Circus, Sergievsky Per., Youth Theatre, Pushkinskaya, Petrovsky Bld., Convent of the Nativity of the Virgin, Museum of the Revolution, Pushkin Ploshchad, Bolshoi Theatre, Turgenevskaya Pl., Gorky Theatre, Chekhov Theatre, Kuznetsky Most, Detskiy Mir, TEATRALNIY PROJ., Ploshchad Lubyanskaya, Gorky House Museum, Ermolovay Theatre, Revolution Square, Slavanskiy Bazar, University, Manezhnaya Ploshchad, Lenin Museum, Polytechnic Museum Pl., Moscow Conservatoire, Central Exhibition Hall, Historical Museum, Gum Shopping Arcade, Red Square, Lenin Mausoleum, Arbatskaya Ploshchad, VOZDVIZHENKA U., Museum of Russian Architecture, Arsenal, Council of Ministers, St Basil's Cathedral, Central Concert Hall, ULITSA VARVARKA, Lenin State Library, Terem Palace, Kremlin, Archangel Cathedral, ULITSA ARBAT, Armoury Palace, Palace of Congress, Kremlin Palace, Presidium of the Supreme Soviet, Marx-Engels Ploshchad, Pushkin Fine Arts Museum, KREMLEVSKAYA NABEREZHNAYA, Moskva, SOFIYSKAYA NABEREZHNAYA, RAUSHSKAYA NAB., Ryleyev Ulitsa, Moscow Swimming Pool, BOLOTNAYA NAB., SADOVNICHESKAYA, OVCHINNIKOVSKAYA

1 2 3
a b c

MUMBAI

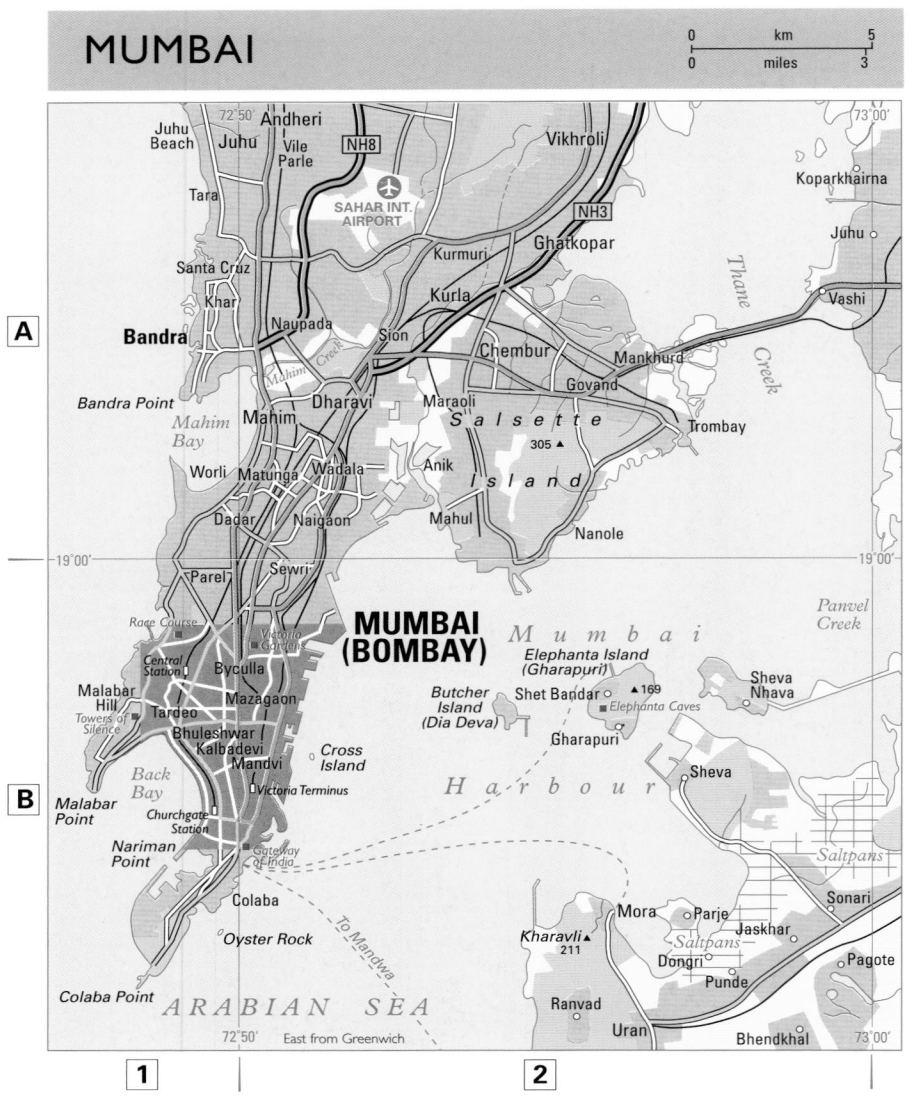

CENTRAL MUMBAI

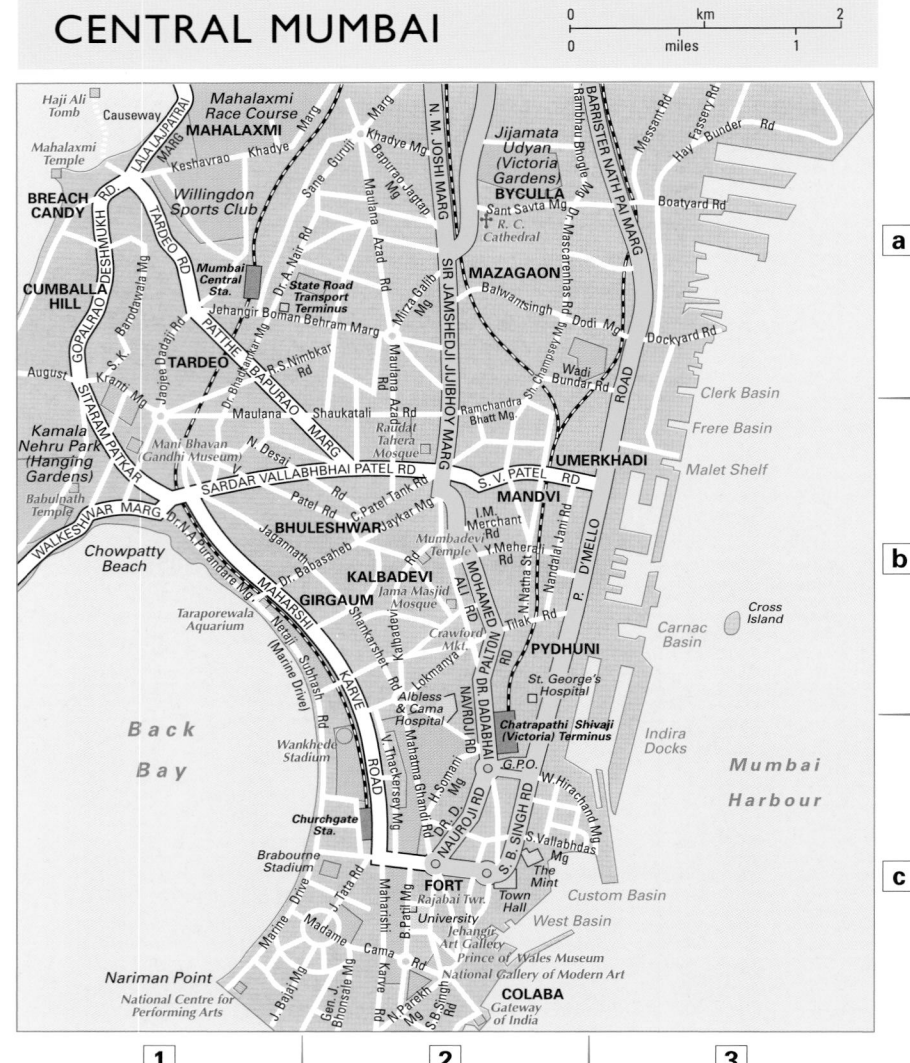

MUNICH

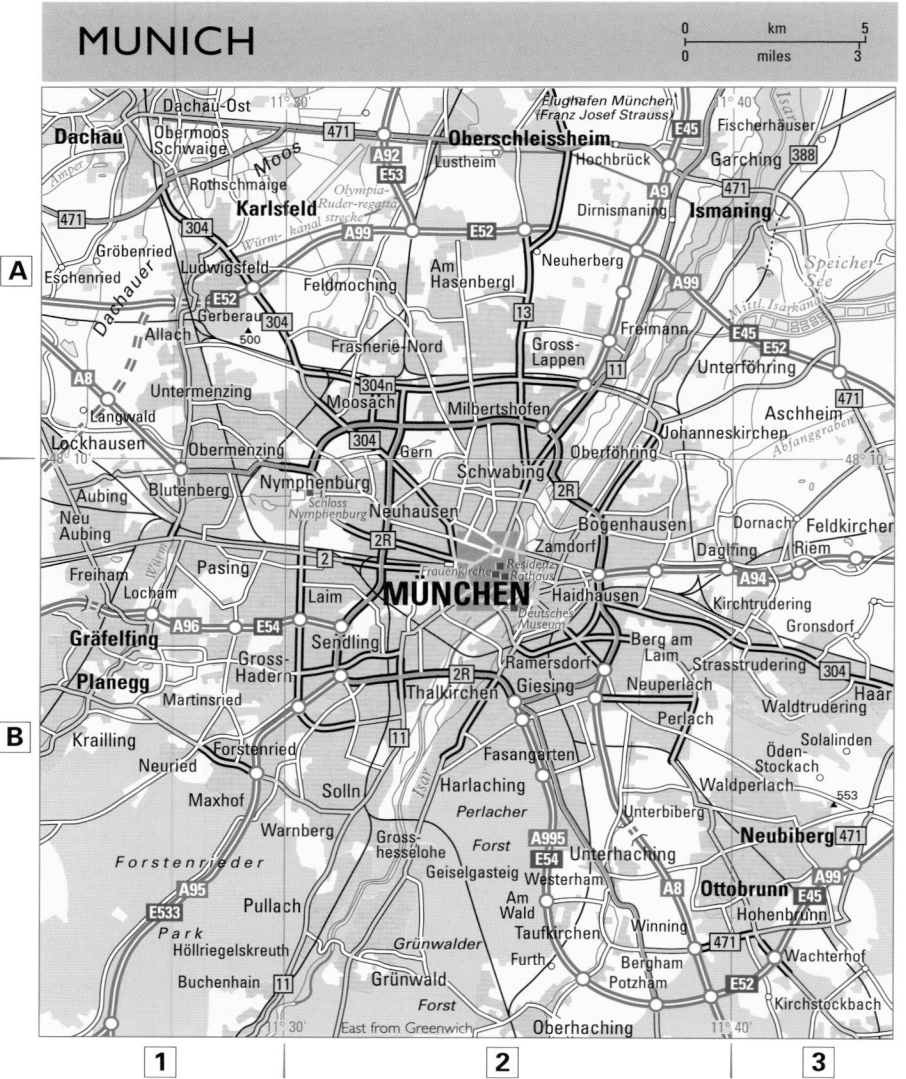

CENTRAL MUNICH

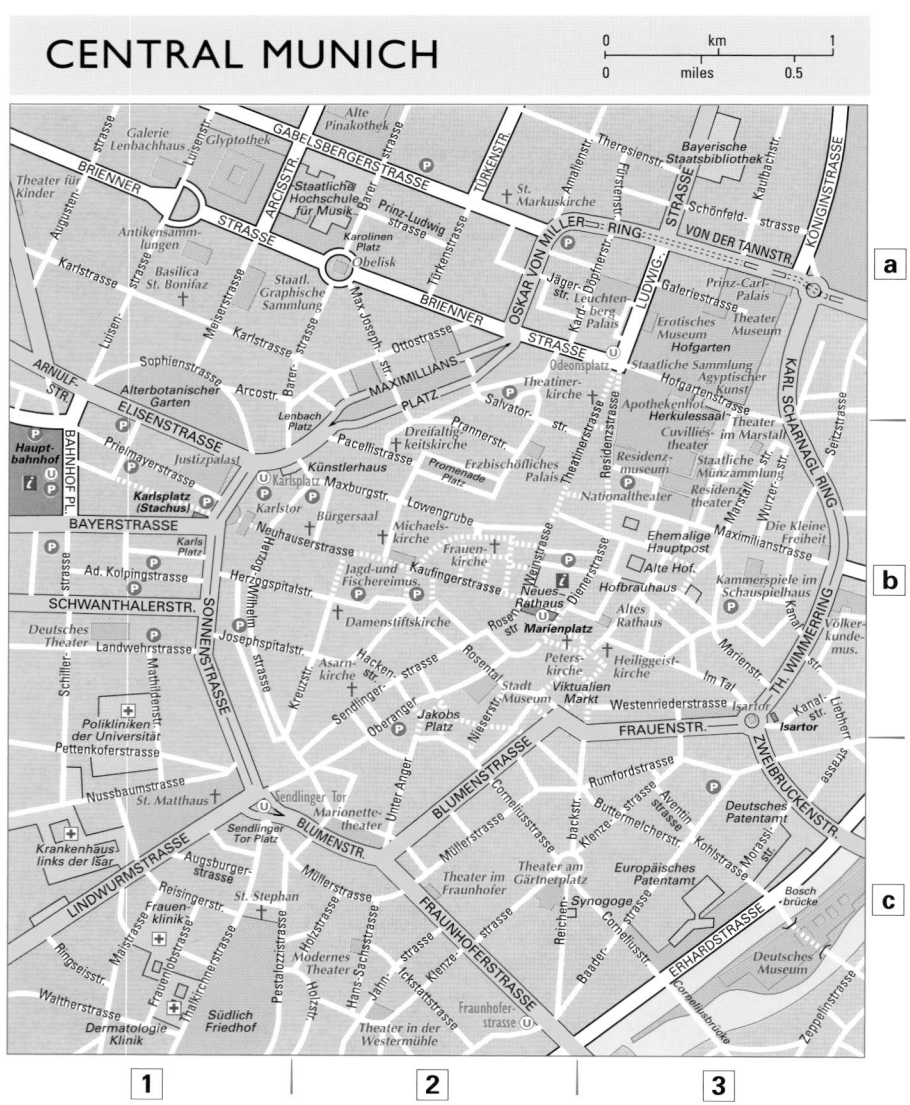

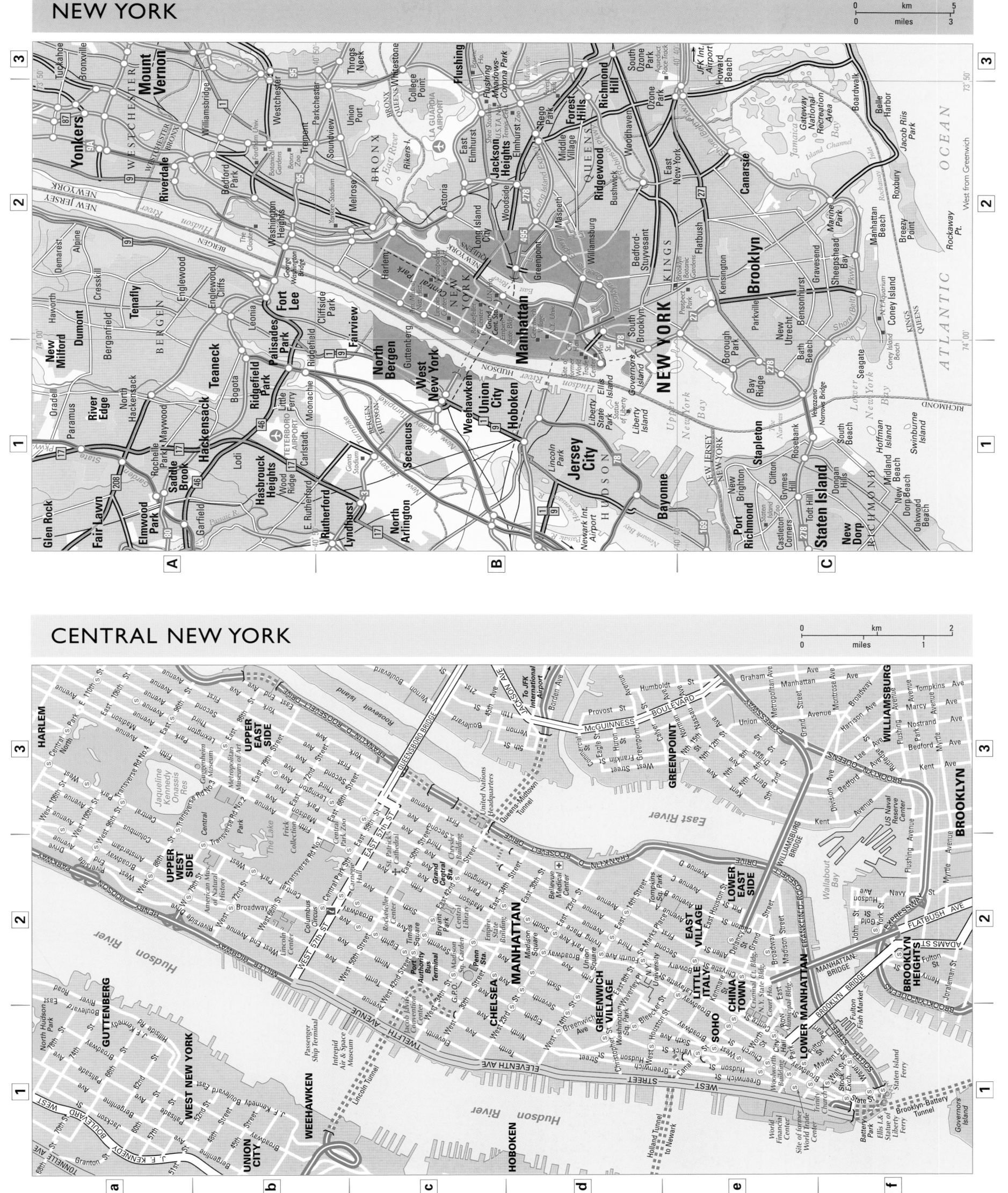

NEW YORK

CENTRAL NEW YORK

COPYRIGHT PHILIP'S

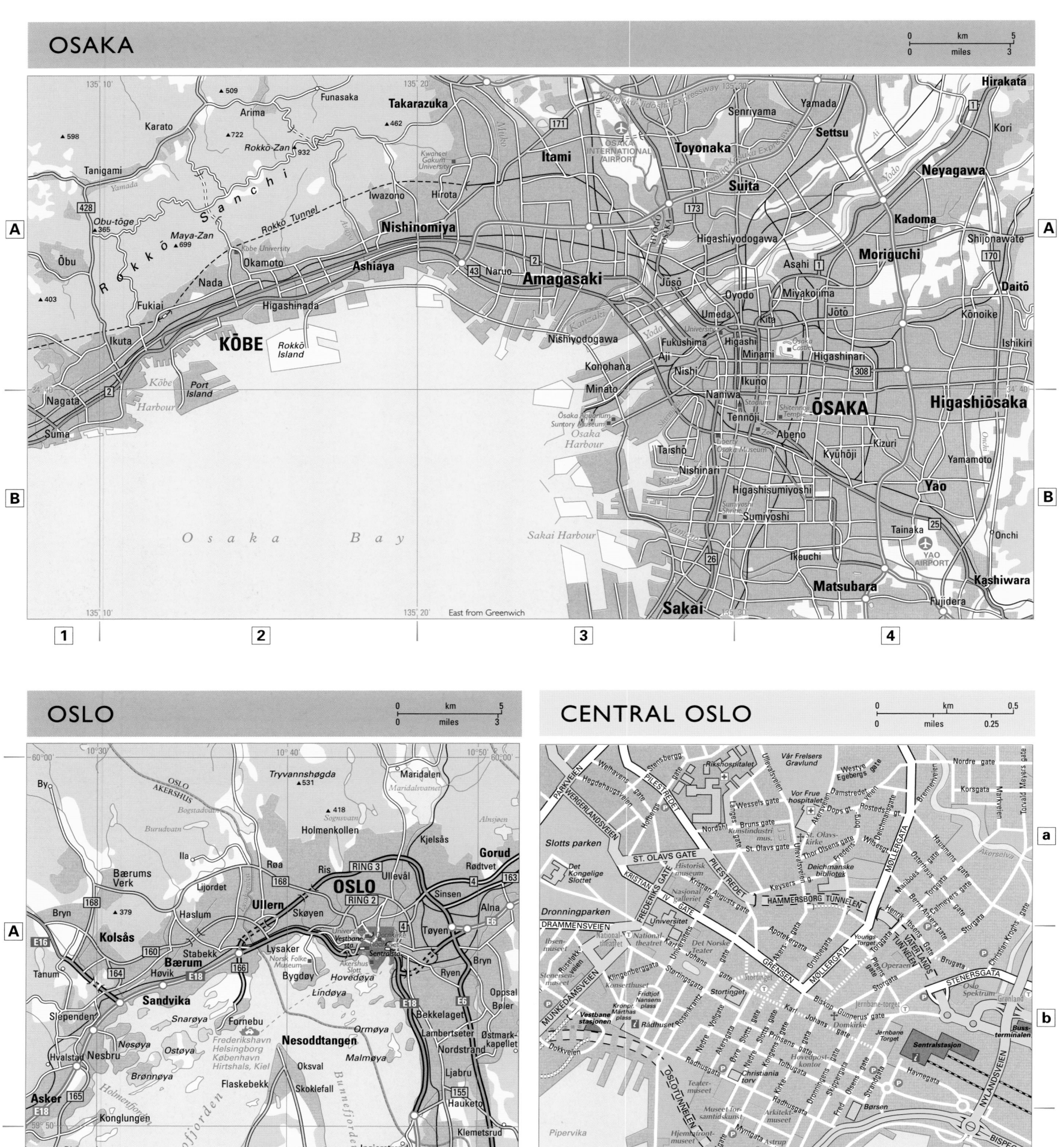

PARIS

km 0 — 5
miles 0 — 3

Carrières-sous-Poissy · Achères · Maisons-Laffitte · Argenteuil · Gennevilliers · Villeneuve-la-Garenne · St-Denis · Stains · Parc de la Courneuve · Le Blanc-Mesnil · Aulnay-sous-Bois · Sevran · Tremblay-en-France · Villeparisis

Sartrouville · Houilles · Bezons · Bois-Colombes · La Courneuve · Le Bourget · Drancy · Livry-Gargan · Vaujours · Coubron · Courtry · Villevaudé

Poissy · Mesnil-le-Roi · St-Germain · Carrières-sous-Bois · Colombes · Asnières · Clichy · St-Ouen · Aubervilliers · Bobigny · Pantin · Les Pavillons-sous-Bois · Clichy-sous-Bois · Montfermeil · Claye-Souilly

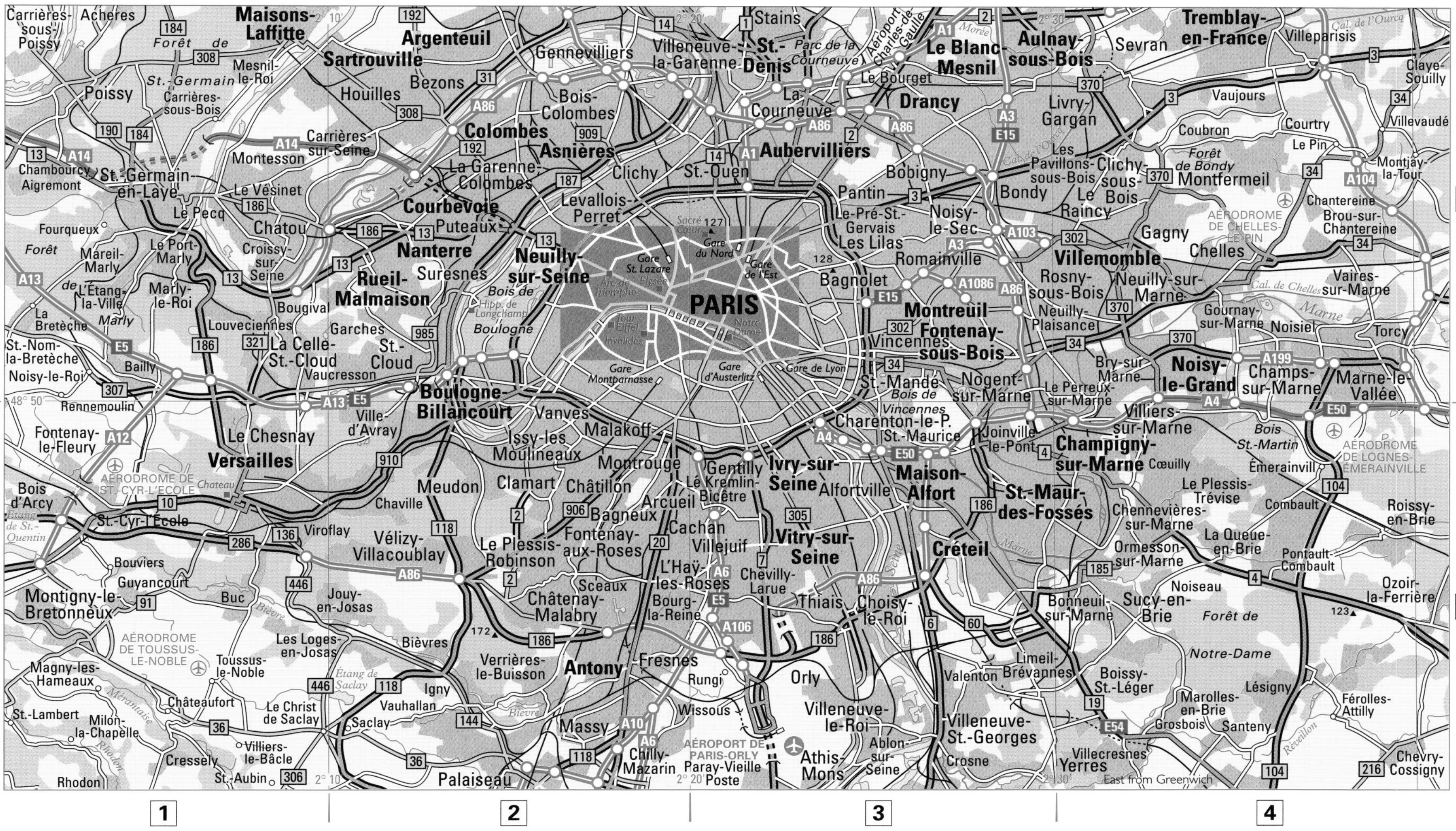

Chambourcy · St-Germain-en-Laye · Aigremont · Le Vésinet · La Garenne-Colombes · Courbevoie · Puteaux · Levallois-Perret · Sacré · Pré-St-Gervais · Les Lilas · Romainville · Gagny · Chanteraine · Brou-sur-Chantereine

Fourqueux · Mareil-Marly · Le Pecq · Chatou · Croissy-sur-Seine · Nanterre · Neuilly-sur-Seine · Noisy-le-Sec · Villemomble · Chelles

Marly-le-Roi · Rueil-Malmaison · Suresnes · Bois de Boulogne · PARIS · Montreuil · Vincennes · Rosny-sous-Bois · Neuilly-sur-Marne · Vaires-sur-Marne

Louveciennes · Garches · St-Cloud · Vaucresson · Fontenay-sous-Bois · Nogent-sur-Marne · Le Perreux-sur-Marne · Noisy-le-Grand · Champs-sur-Marne · Marne-la-Vallée

Versailles · Le Chesnay · Ville d'Avray · Boulogne-Billancourt · Vanves · Issy-les-Moulineaux · Malakoff · Montrouge · Gentilly · Le Kremlin-Bicêtre · Ivry-sur-Seine · Maisons-Alfort · St-Maur-des-Fossés · Champigny-sur-Marne

Meudon · Clamart · Châtillon · Arcueil · Cachan · Villejuif · Vitry-sur-Seine · Créteil · Sucy-en-Brie

Vélizy-Villacoublay · Viroflay · Le Plessis-Robinson · Fontenay-aux-Roses · Sceaux · Bourg-la-Reine · L'Haÿ-les-Roses · Chevilly-Larue · Thiais · Choisy-le-Roi · Bonneuil-sur-Marne · Boissy-St-Léger

Antony · Fresnes · Rungis · Orly · Valenton · Brévannes · Limeil

Massy · Chilly-Mazarin · Wissous · Athis-Mons · Ablon-sur-Seine · Crosne · Yerres

Palaiseau · Paray-Vieille-Poste · Villeneuve-le-Roi · Villeneuve-St-Georges

CENTRAL PARIS

km 0 — 1
miles 0 — 0.5

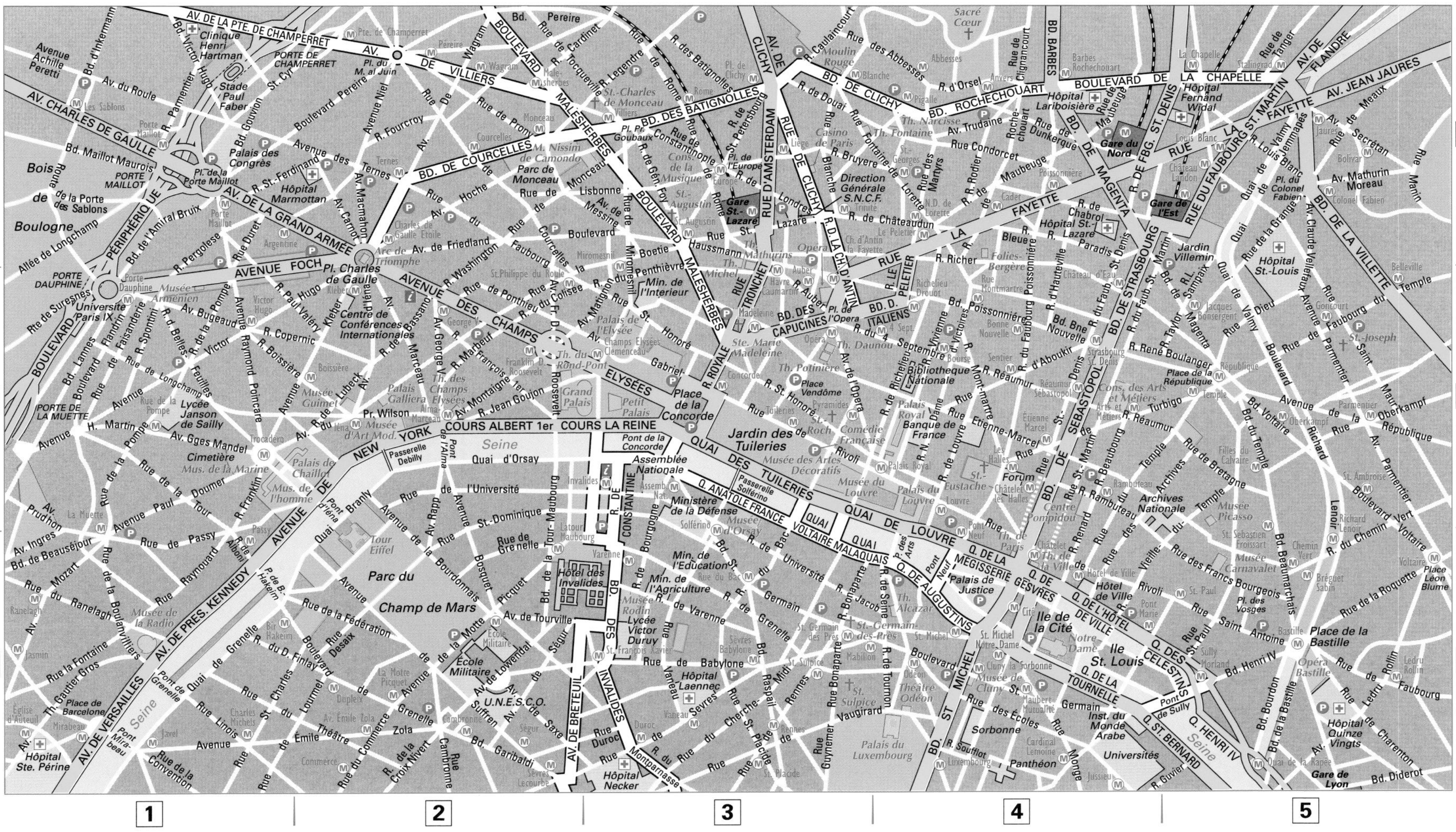

COPYRIGHT PHILIP'S

PRAGUE

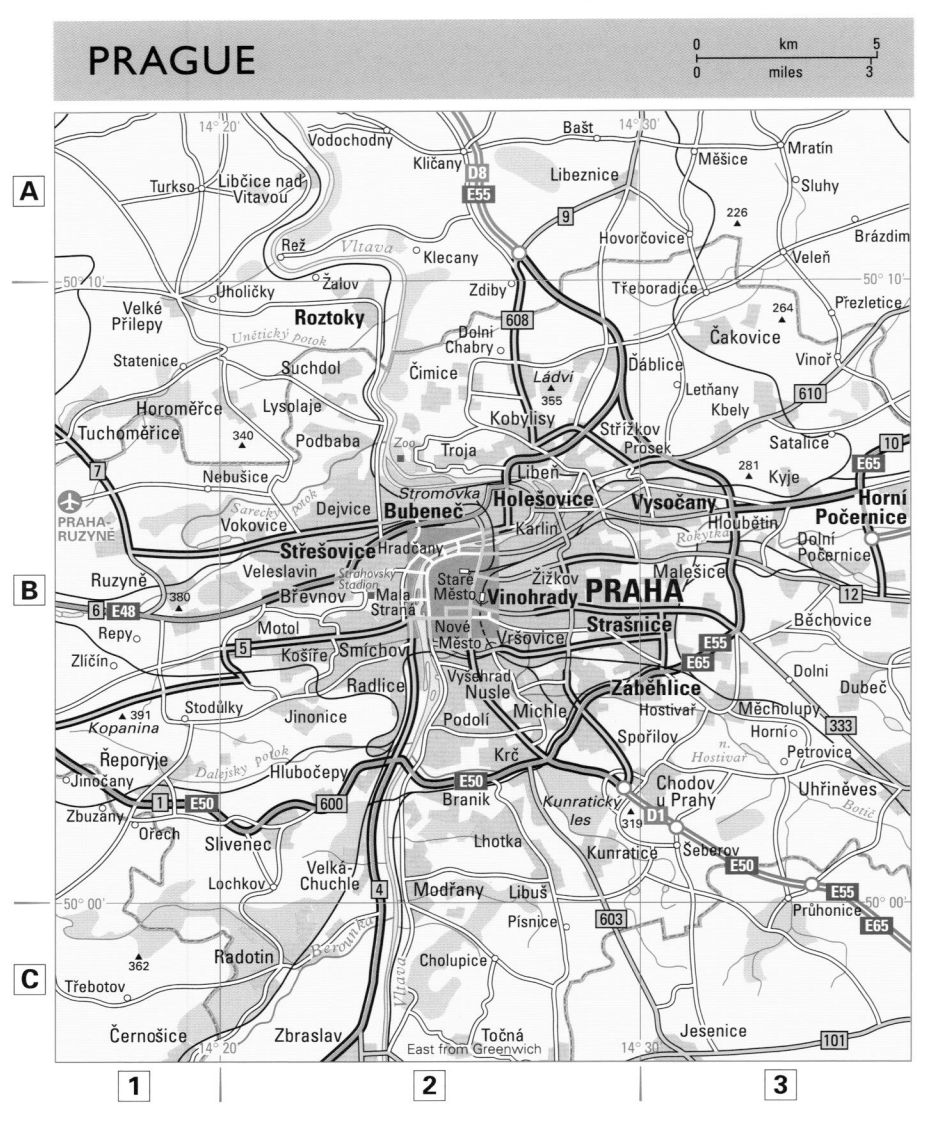

CENTRAL PRAGUE

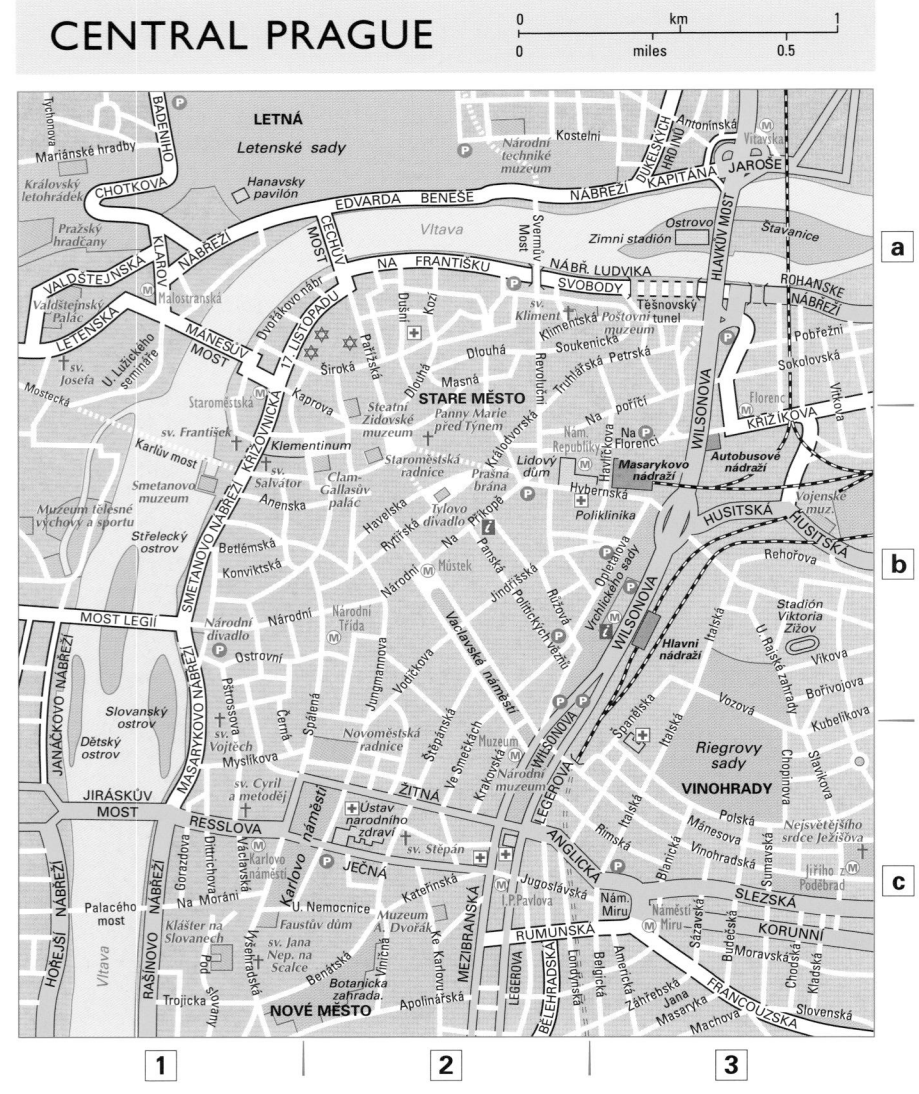

RIO DE JANEIRO

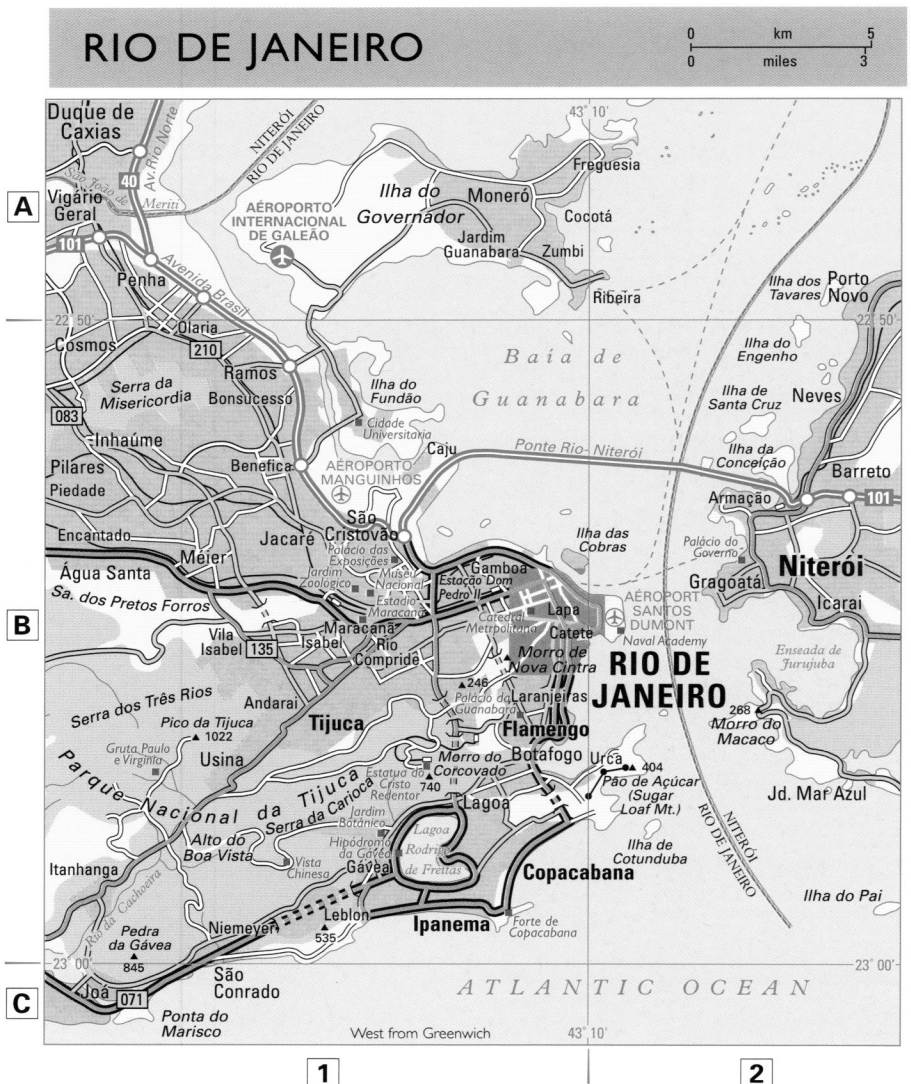

CENTRAL RIO DE JANEIRO

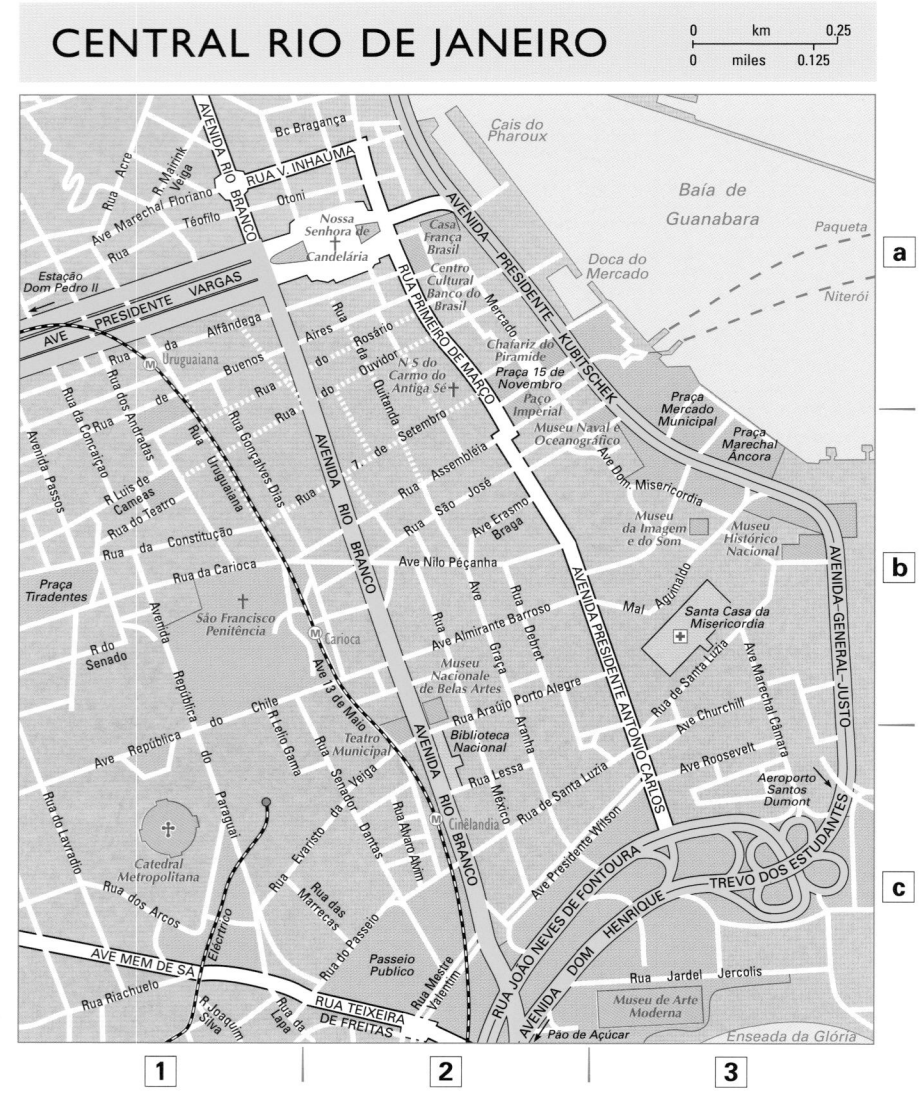

ROME

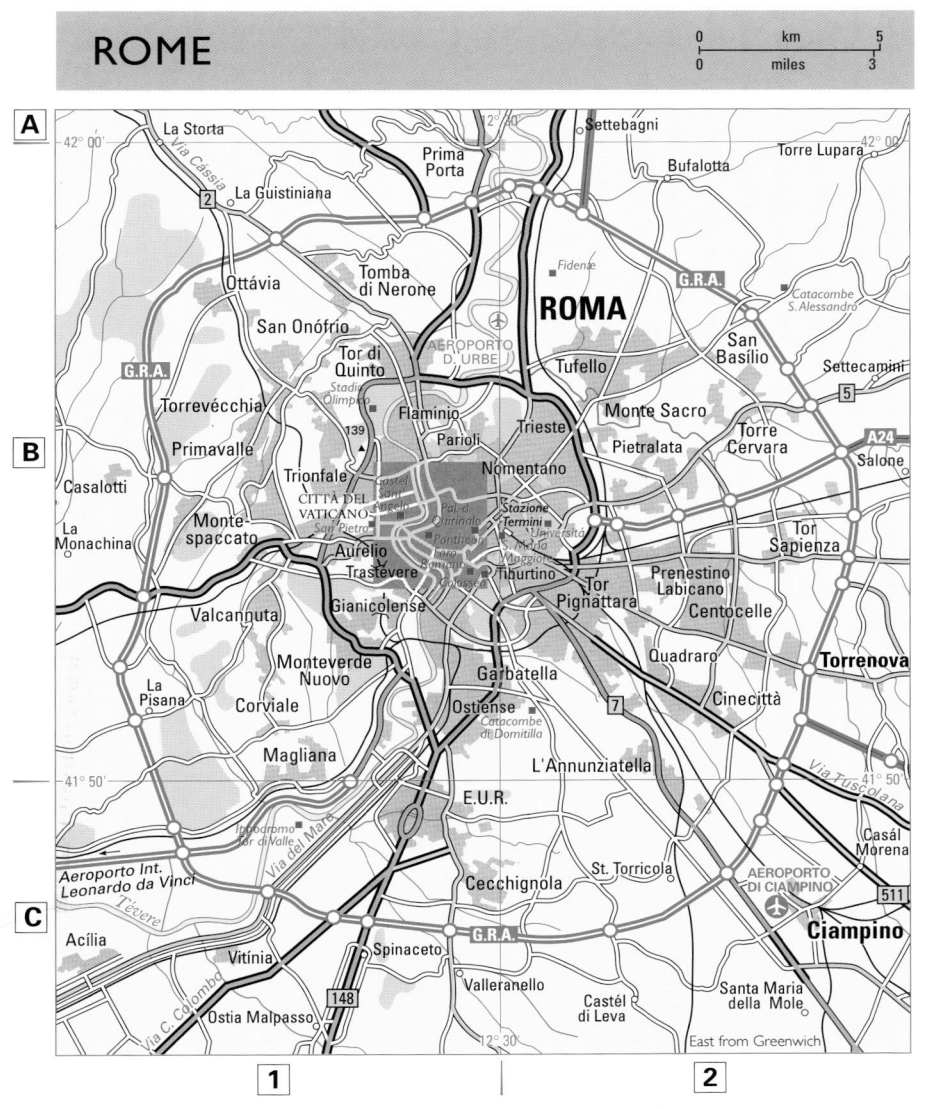

CENTRAL ROME

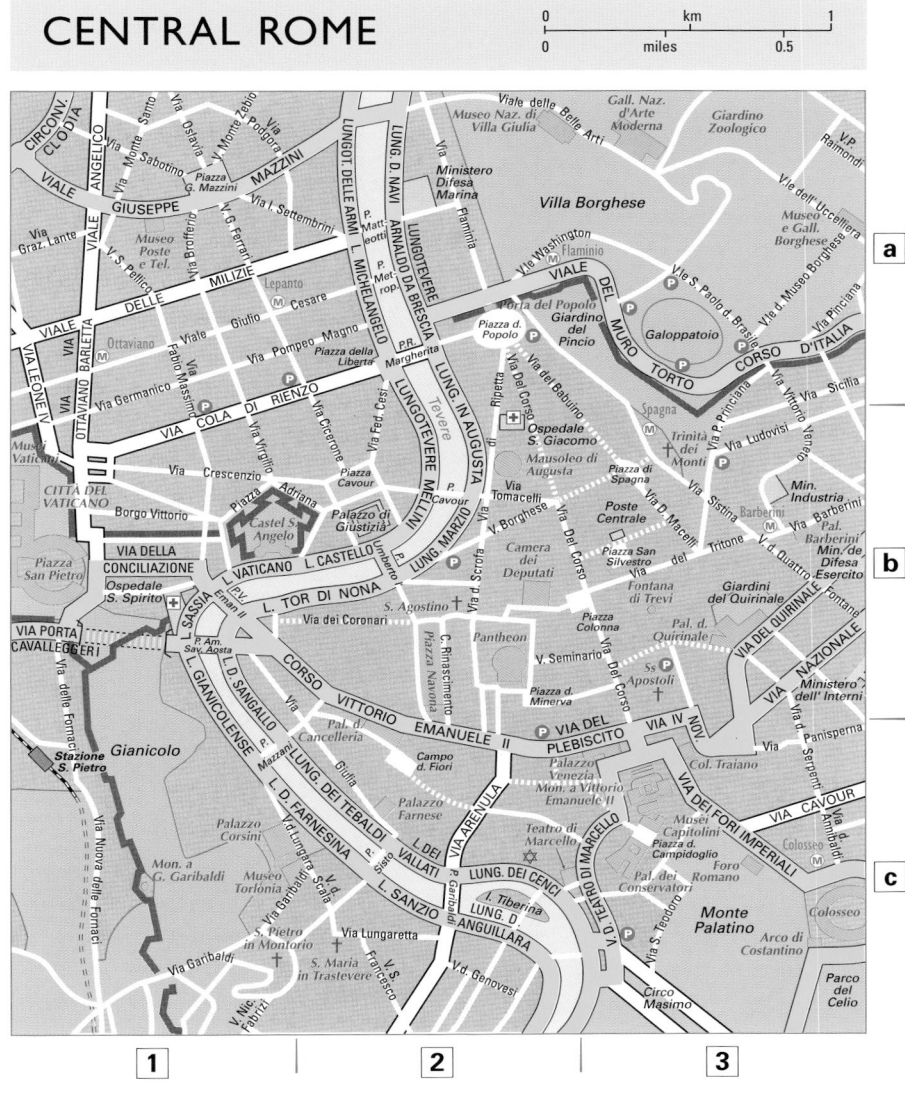

SAN FRANCISCO

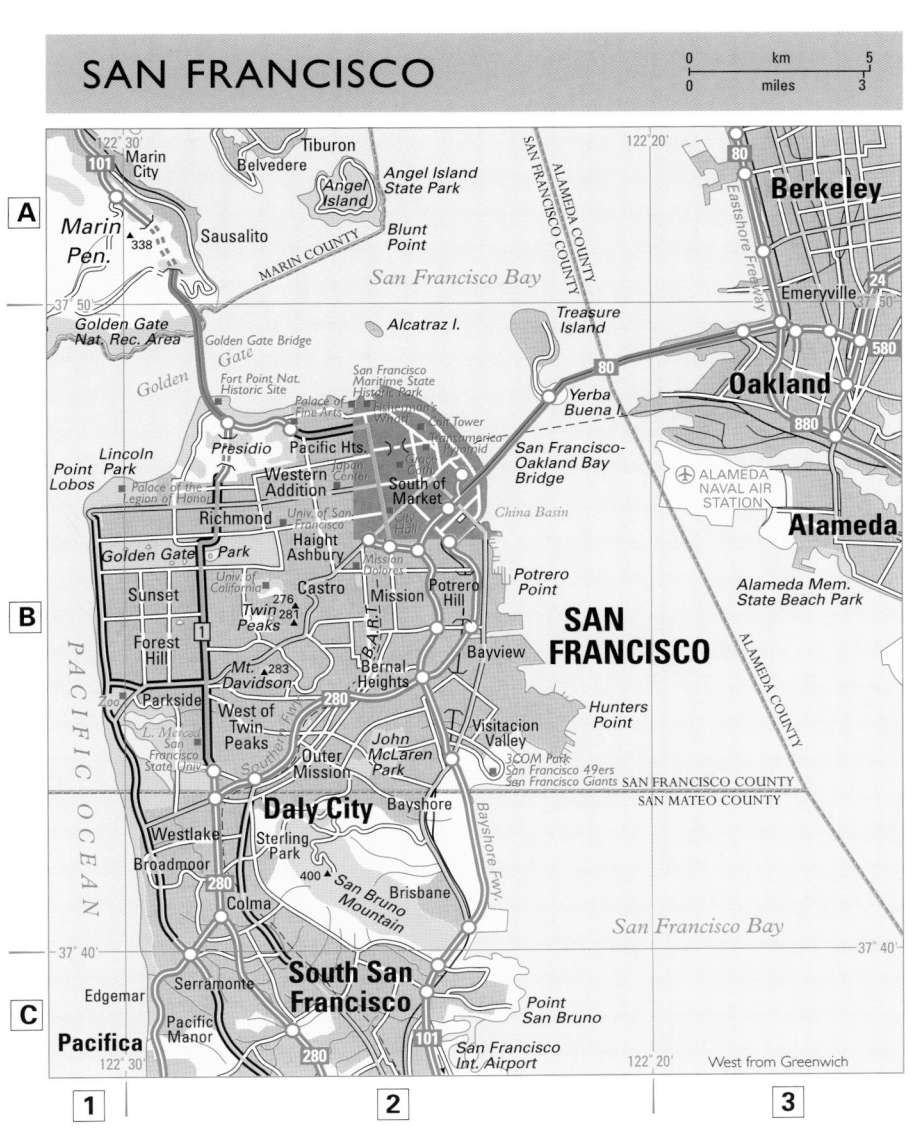

CENTRAL SAN FRANCISCO

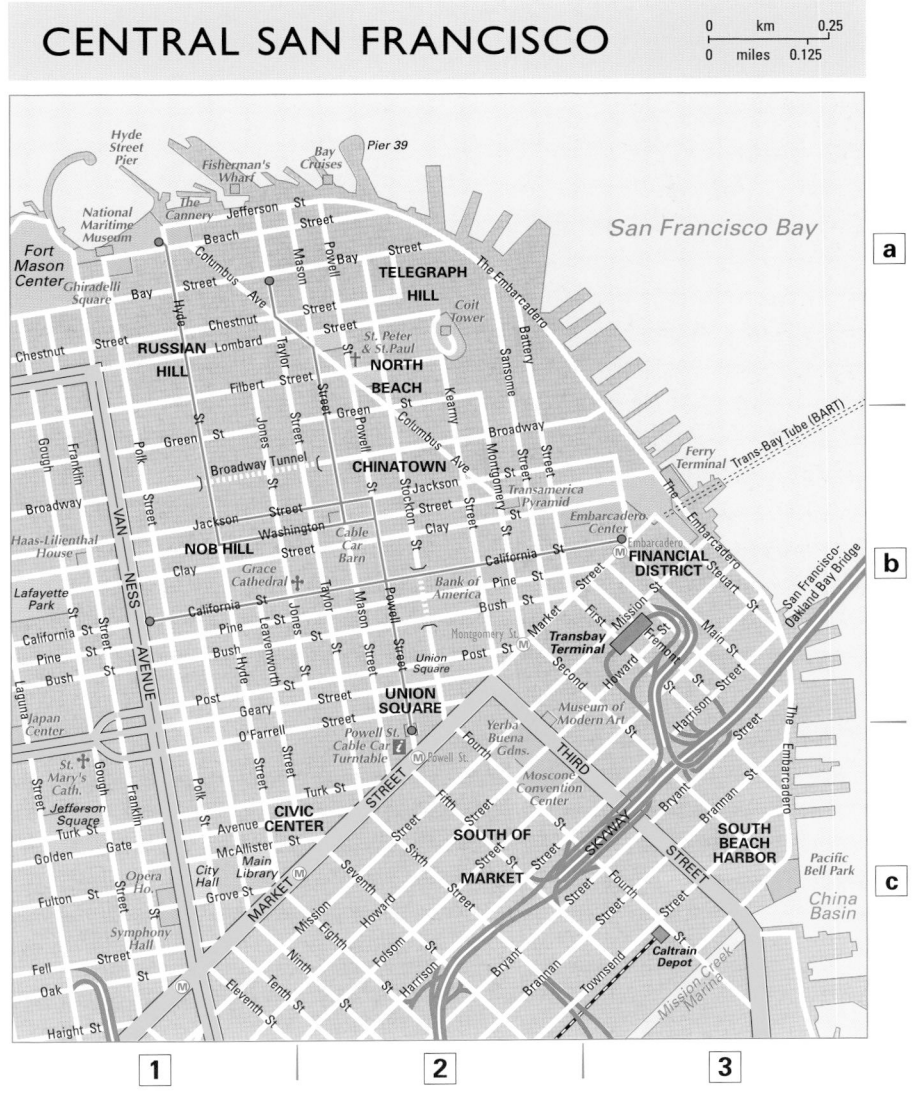

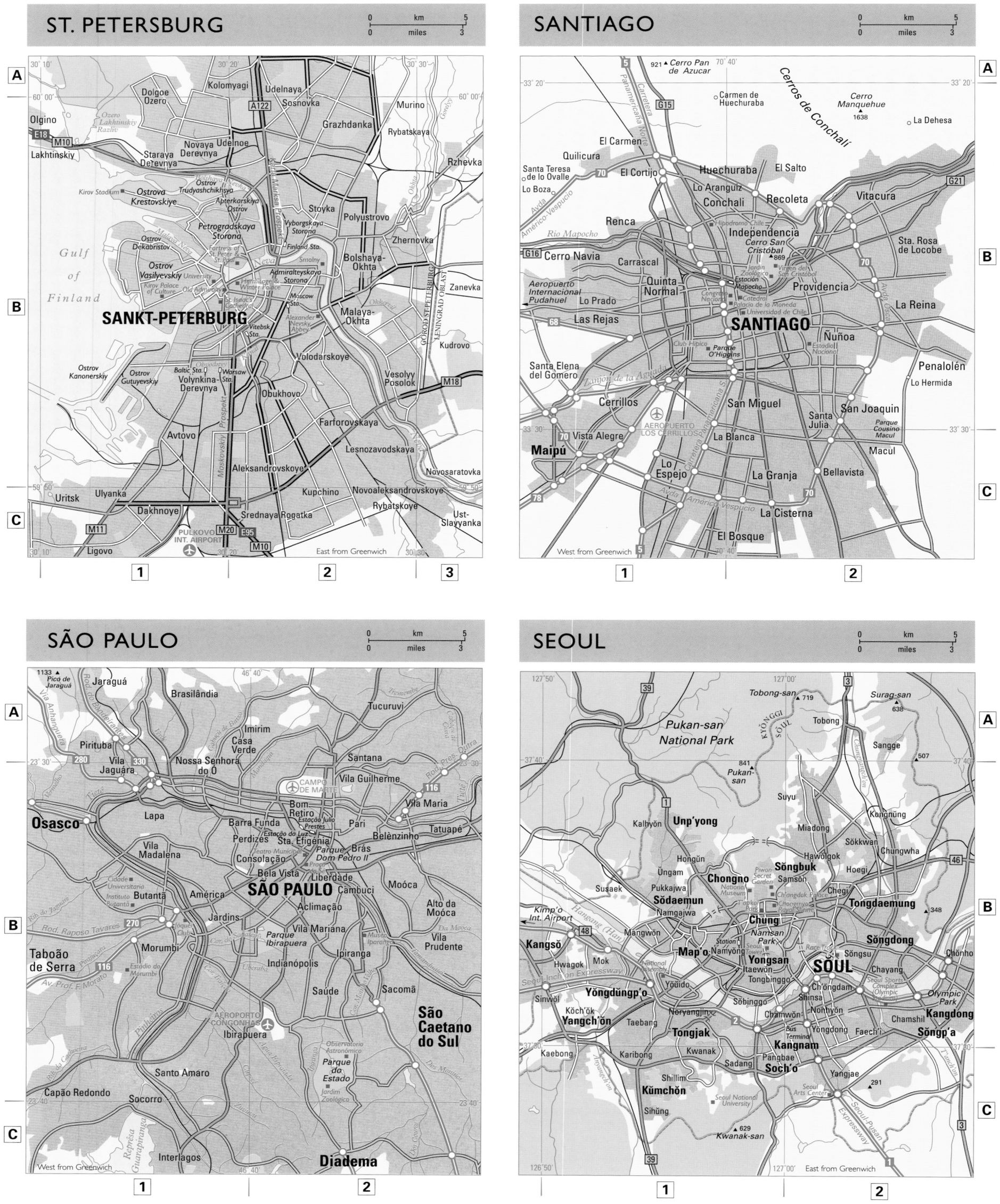

SHANGHAI

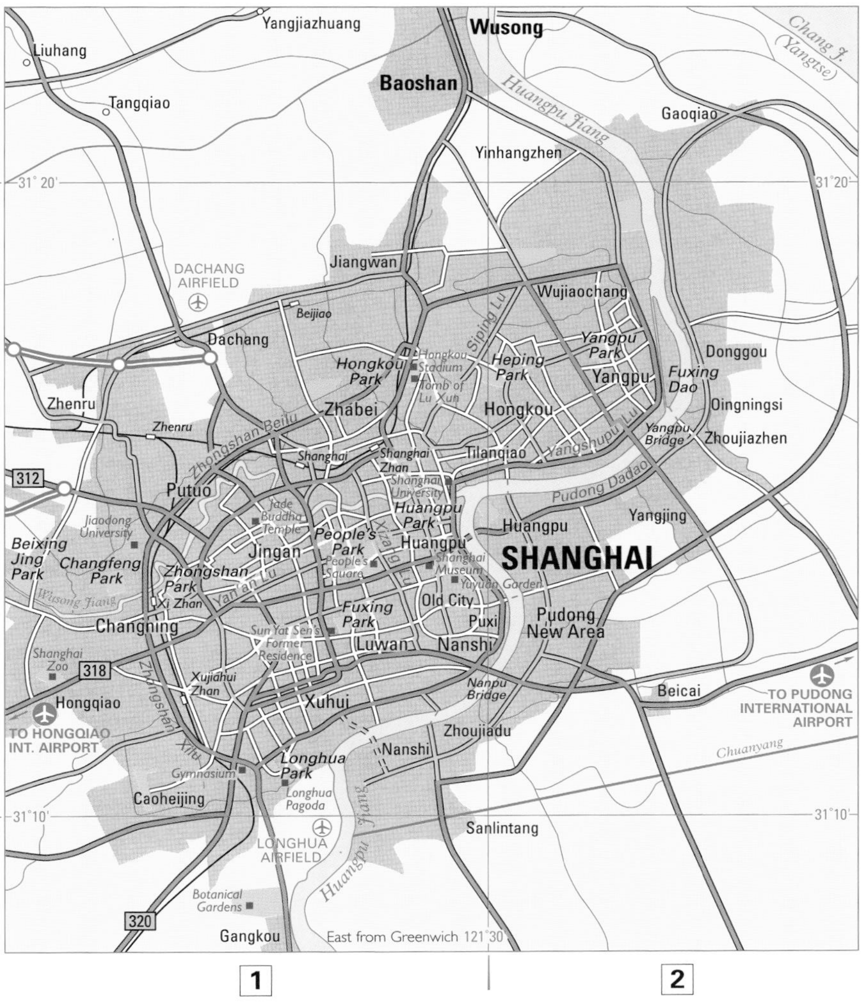

km 5
miles 3

A

Liuhang
Tangqiao
Yangjiazhuang
Wusong
Baoshan
Yinhangzhen
Gaoqiao
31° 20'
Dachang
AIRFIELD
Jiangwan
Wujiaochang
Beijiao
Zhenru
Dachang
Hongkou
Stadium
Heping
Park
Yangpu
Park
Yangpu
Fuxing
Dao
Donggou
Jiaotong
University
Zhenru
Zhenru
Hongkou
Park
Zhabei
Tomb of
Lu Xun
Hongkou
Oingningsi
Zhoujiazhen
Yangpu
Bridge
Putuo
Jade
Buddha
Temple
Shanghai
Shanghai
Zhan
Shanghai
Pudong Dadao
Huangpu
Yangjing
312
B
People's
Park
People's
Square
Yuyuan
Garden
Huangpu
Beixing
Jing
Park
Changfeng
Park
Jingan
Zhongshan
Park
Shanghai
Museum
Old City
Huangpu
Changning
Former
Residence
Fuxing
Park
Puxi
Pudong
New Area
Shanghai
Zoo
Xujiahui
Zhan
Sun Yat-Sen
Former
Residence
Luwan
Nanshi
Nanpu
Bridge
Beicai
TO HONGQIAO
INT. AIRPORT
318
Hongqiao
Xuhui
Gymnasium
Zhoujiadu
Chuanyang
TO PUDONG
INTERNATIONAL
AIRPORT
31° 10'
Caoheijing
Longhua
Park
Longhua
Pagoda
Nanshi
Sanlintang
31° 10'
C
LONGHUA
AIRFIELD
Botanical
Gardens
Huangpu Jiang
Chang J.
(Yangtse)
Huangpu Jiang
320
Gangkou
East from Greenwich 121° 30'

1 **2**

CENTRAL SINGAPORE

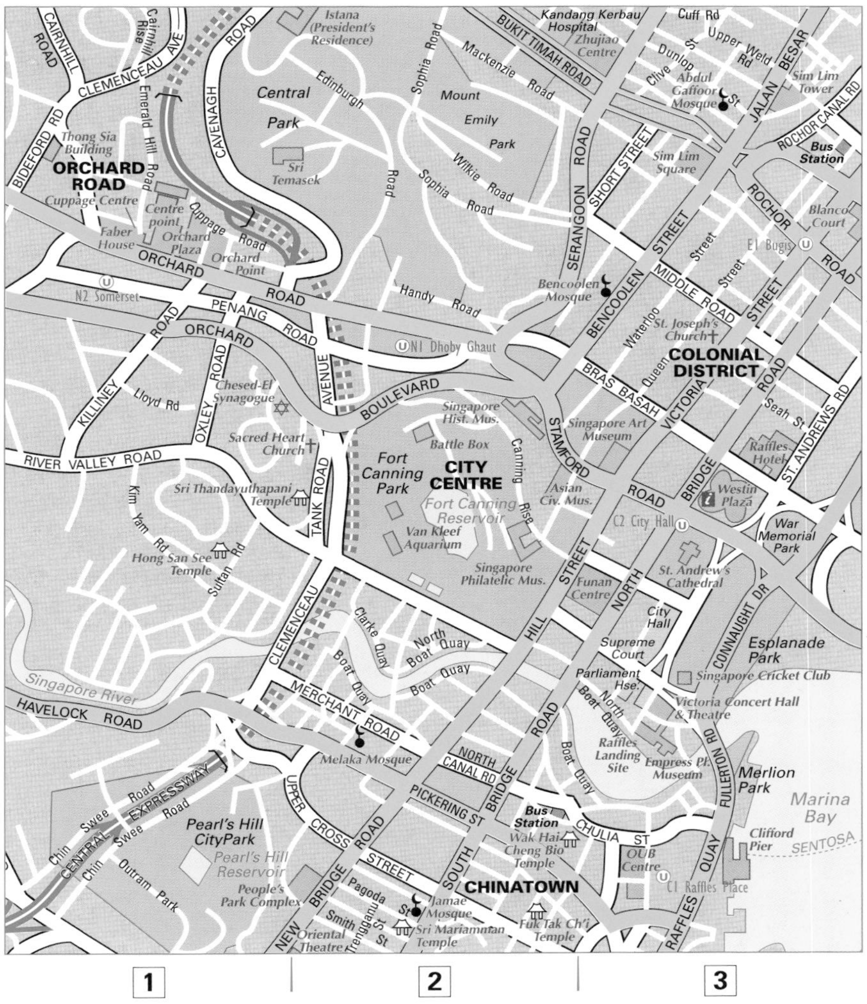

km 1
miles 0.5

CAIRNHILL ROAD
CLEMENCEAU AVE
ROAD
Istana
(President's
Residence)
Kandang Kerbau
Hospital
Zhujiao
Centre
Upper
Cuff Rd
BIDEFORD RD
Central
Park
Edinburgh
Emerald
Hill
Sri
Temasck
Mount
Emily
Park
Sophia
Road
Wilkie
Road
Mackenzie
Road
Sophia
Road
SERANGOON
SHORT STREET
ROCHOR
Sim Lim
Square
Blanco
Court
Upper
Abdul
Gafoor
Mosque
JALAN BESAR
Sim Lim
Tower
ROCHOR CANAL RD
a
**ORCHARD
ROAD**
Thong Sia
Building
Cuppage Centre
Faber
House
Centre
point,
Orchard
Plaza
Orchard
Point
ORCHARD
N2 Somerset
ROAD
PENANG
ROAD
Handy
Road
NI Dhoby Ghaut
ROAD
Bencoolen
Mosque
BENCOOLEN
MIDDLE ROAD
STREET
St. Joseph's
Church
Bus
Station
E Bugis
**COLONIAL
DISTRICT**
KILLNEY
ROAD
OXLEY
Lloyd Rd
Chesed-El
Synagogue
ORCHARD
BOULEVARD
Sacred Heart
Church
AVENUE
Singapore
Hist. Mus.
Battle Box
STAMFORD
VICTORIA
Singapore Art
Museum
Seah St
Raffles
Hotel
ST. ANDREW'S RD
b
RIVER VALLEY ROAD
Sri Thandayuthapani
Temple
Fort
Canning
Park
Asian
Civ. Mus.
**CITY
CENTRE**
Fort Canning
Reservoir
Van Kleef
Aquarium
TANK ROAD
Hong San See
Temple
Sultan
Mosque
Singapore
Philatelic Mus.
Hunan
Centre
BRIDGE
Westin
Plaza
C2 City Hall
War
Memorial
Park
CLEMENCEAU
Charu
Quay
Boat
Quay
Supreme
Court
City Hall
St. Andrew's
Cathedral
CONNAUGHT DR
c
MERCHANT
ROAD
Boat
Quay
Parliament
Hse.
Singapore River
HAVELOCK ROAD
Melaka Mosque
NORTH
CANAL
ROAD
PICKERING ST
SOUTH
Victoria Concert Hall
& Theatre
Singapore Cricket Club
Empress Pl.
Museum
Merlion
Park
Marina
Bay
Swee
Road
Swee
Rd
Pearl's Hill
City Park
Pearl's Hill
Reservoir
Chin
Chin
Durum Park
UPPER CROSS ROAD
CENTRAL
NEW BRIDGE ROAD
SOUTH BRIDGE ROAD
Pagoda
St
Jamae
Mosque
Sri Mariamman
Temple
Bus
Station
Wak Hai
Cheng Bio
Temple
Clifford
Pier
C1 Raffles Place
RAFFLES QUAY
OUB
Centre
Raffles
Landing
Site
OHIA ST
SENTOSA
People's
Park Complex
Oriental
Theatre
Smith
St
Yin Tak Ch'i
Temple
CHINATOWN

1 **2** **3**

SINGAPORE

km 10
miles 6

103° 40'
103° 50'
104° 00'
**Johor
Bahru**
Sembawang
Selat Johor
Malaya
Kranji
Ind. Est.
Woodlands
New Town
Chong
Pang
Yishun
New Town
Punggol
Point
Pulau
Tekong
Kechil
**Pulau
Tekong**
MALAYSIA
SINGAPORE
A
Lim
Chu
Kang
Sarimbun
Res.
Sarimbun
85
Sungai
Kadut
Ind. Est.
Zoological
Gardens
Seletar
Reservoir
Nee Soon
SELETAR
AIRPORT
Jalan
Kayu
Punggol
Pulau
Serangoon
Pulau Ubin
Serangoon
Harbour
Tg. Ladang
Pulau
Tekong
Kechil
Loyang
Ind. Est.
Changi
A
Murai
Res.
Ama
Keng
Choa Chu
Kang
Poyan
Res.
Bukit
Panjang
Nature Reserve
Bukit
Panjang
Upper Peirce
Reservoir
Seletar
Hills
Serangoon
Pasir Ris
CHANGI
INTERNATIONAL
AIRPORT
Bulim
132
Bt. Panjang
Bukit Timah
Nature Reserve
162
MacRitchie
Reservoir
**Ang Mo
Kio**
**Chia
Keng**
Tampines
Yan Kit
Choa Chu
Kang
88
Bukit Batok
Nature Parks
106
Air View
Park
Paya
Lebar
PAYA LEBAR
AIRPORT
Bedok
Reservoir
Tanah Merah
Golf Course
Nanyang
University
Chinese &
Japanese
Gardens
Jurong
Town
Raffles
Park
Pan-Island Expy.
Paya
Lebar
Tai
Seng
Simei
1° 20'N
Jurong
Bt. Peropok
62
Maryland
Victoria
Park
University
of Singapore
Botanic
Gardens
Duncan
**Toa
Payoh**
**Geylang
Serai**
Geylang
Chai Chee
Bedok
Frankel
1° 20'N
Tuas
Jurong
Industrial
Estate
Clementi
Holland
Village
Queenstown
Katong
East Coast
Park
Kg Tanjong
Penjuru
Pandan
Res.
Pasir
Panjang
Buona
Vista
Park
**Telok
Blangah**
Mt. Fabour
105
St Andrew's
Cathedral
City Hall
National Stadium
Kallang
Park
East Coast Pkwy.
B
Pulau
Pesek
Pulau
Merlimau
Pulau
Seraya
Pulau Ayer
Chawan
Pulau Ayer
Merbau
Pulau
Sakra
Selat Jurong
Selat Pandan
Selat Sinki
Pulau
Bukum
Cable
Car
World Trade
Centre
P. Brani
Sentosa
Thian Hock Keng
SINGAPORE
Straits of Singapore
B
103° 40'
103° 50'
East from Greenwich
104° 00'

1 **2** **3** **4**

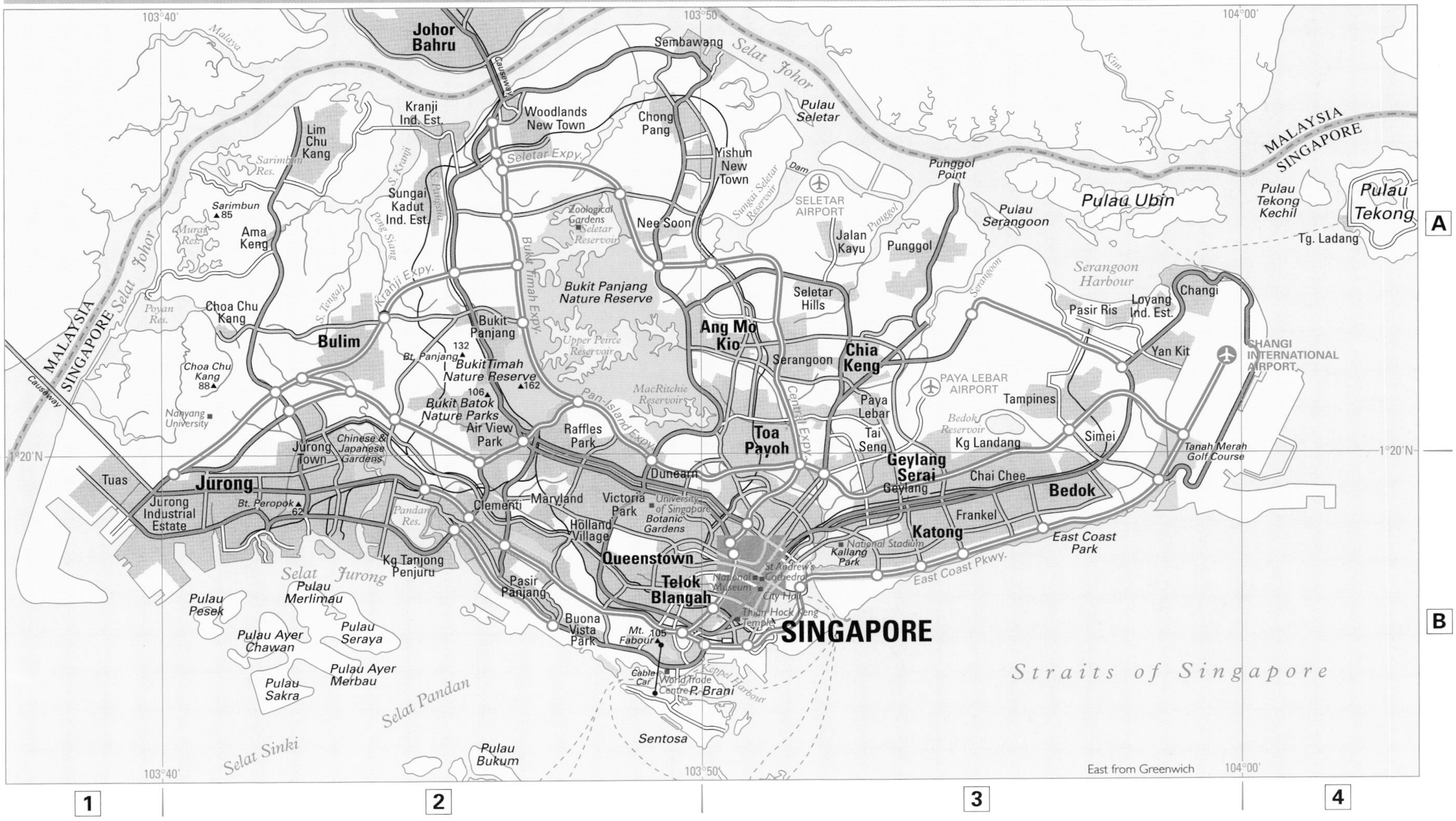

COPYRIGHT PHILIP'S

STOCKHOLM

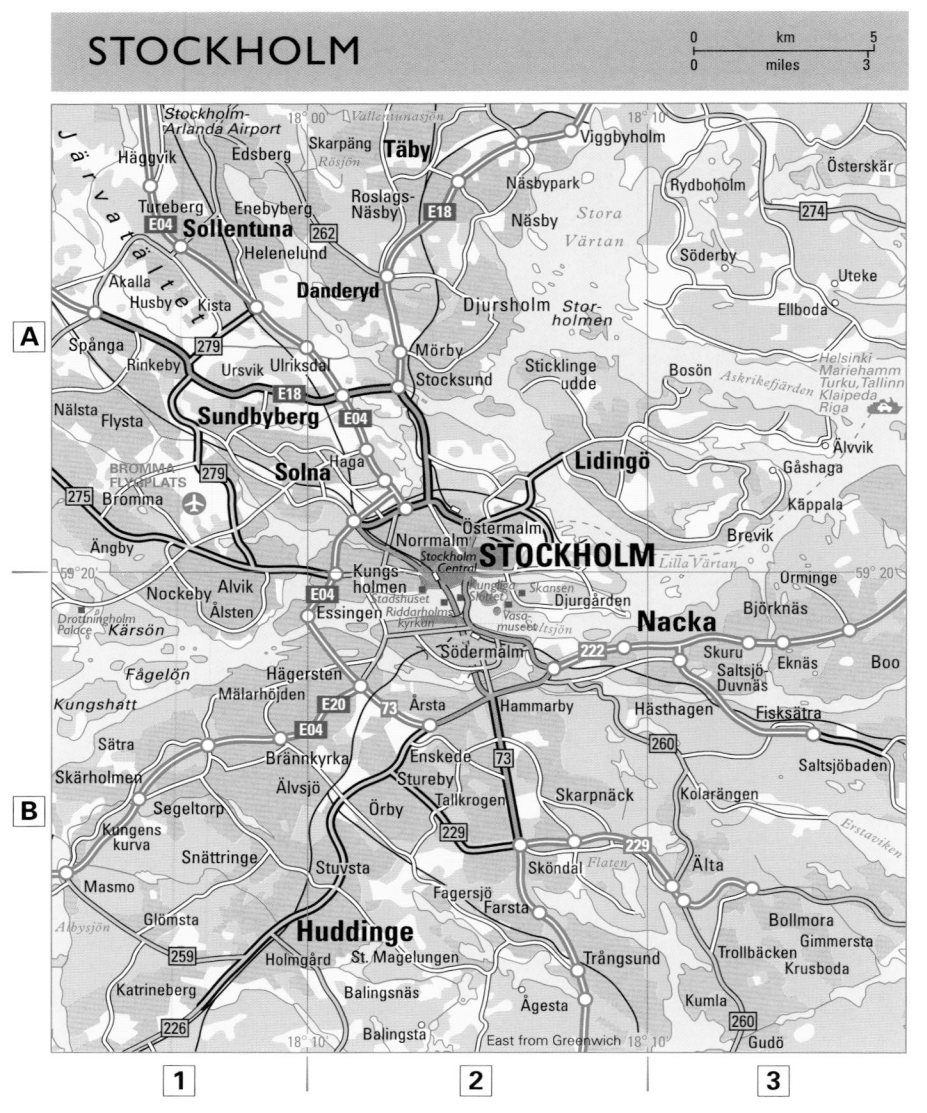

CENTRAL STOCKHOLM

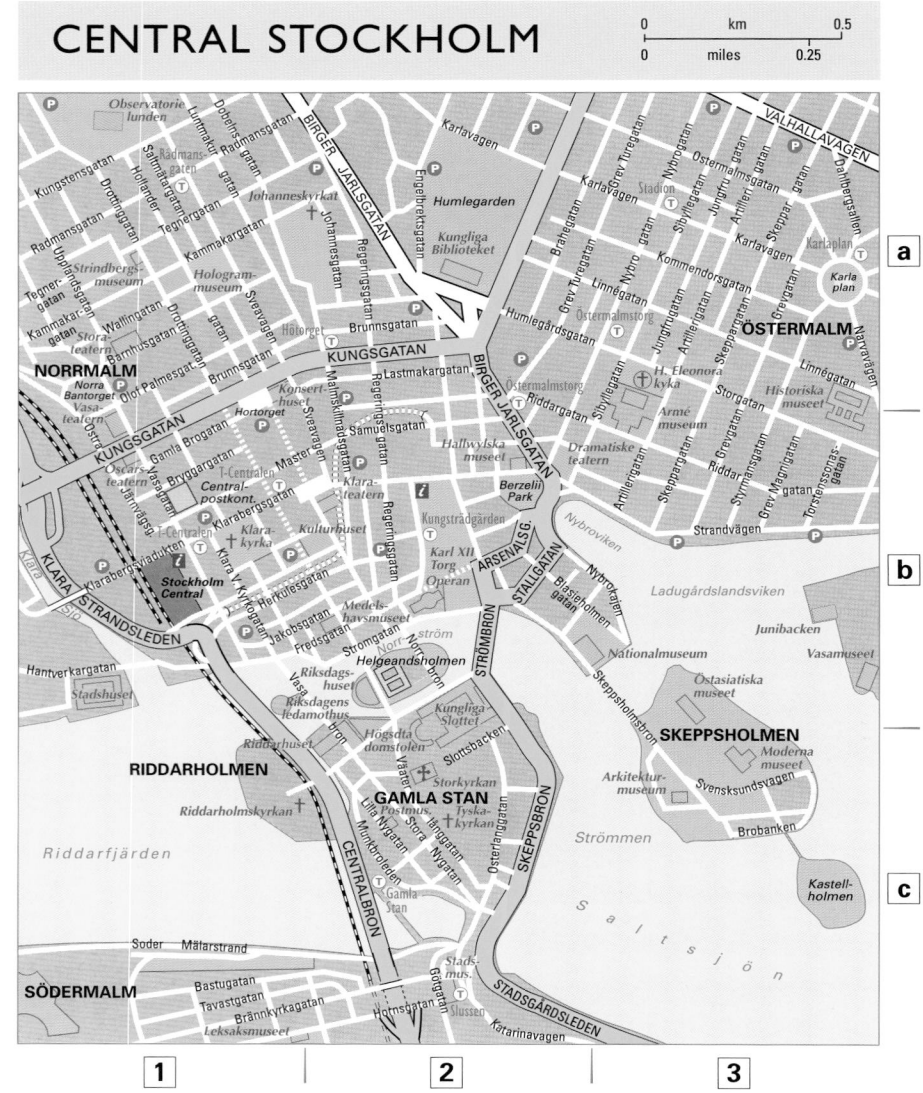

SYDNEY

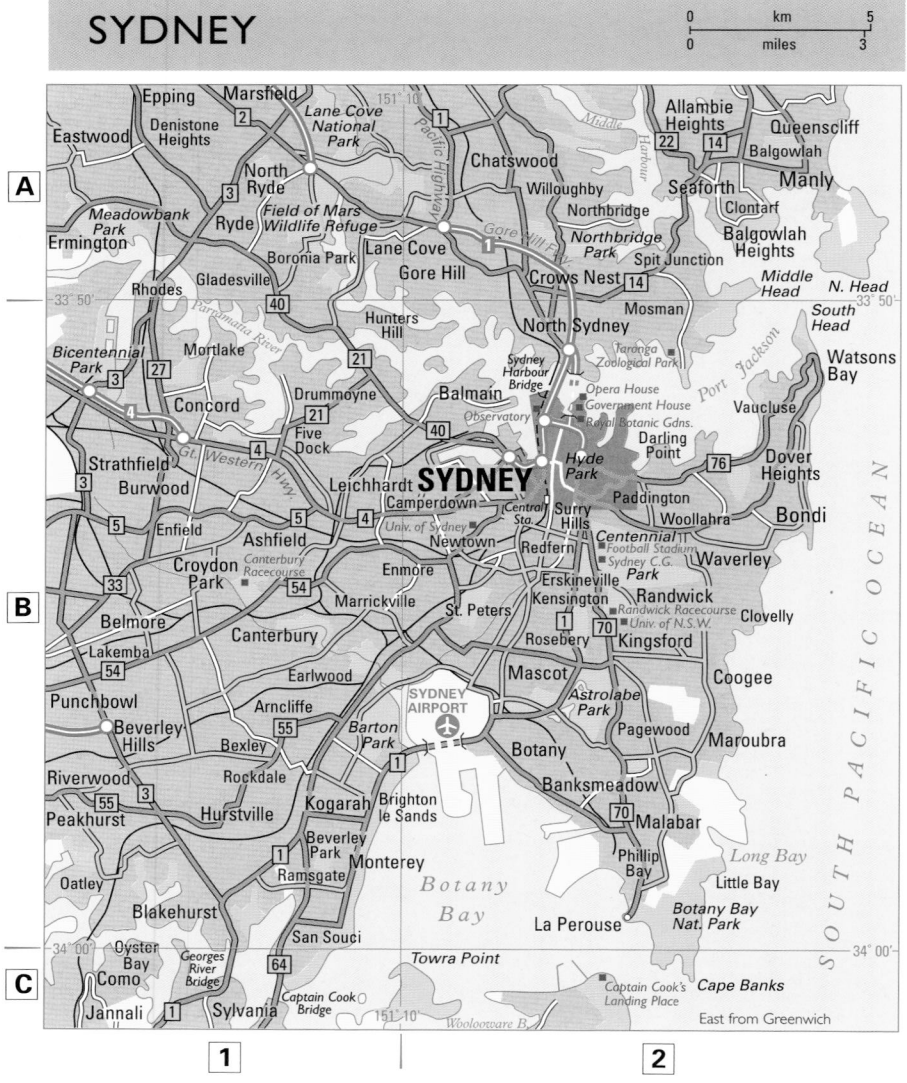

CENTRAL SYDNEY

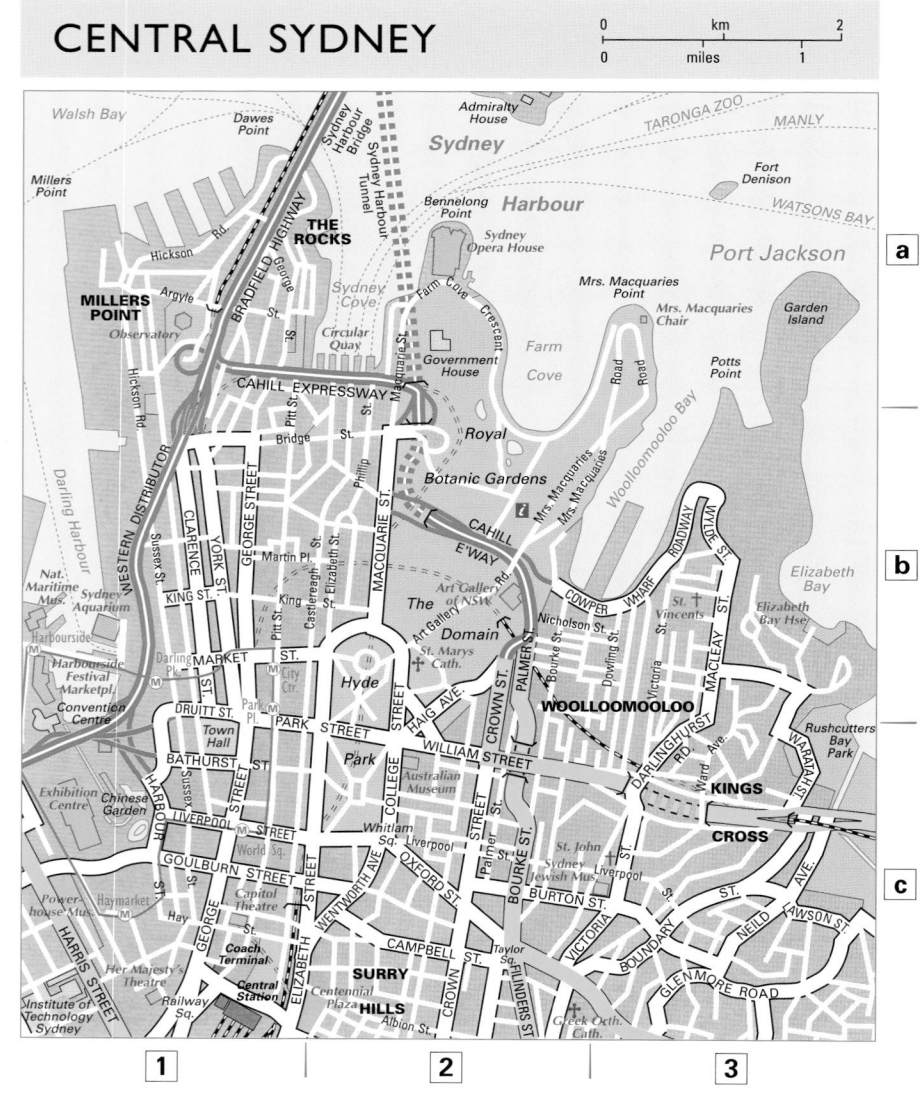

TOKYO

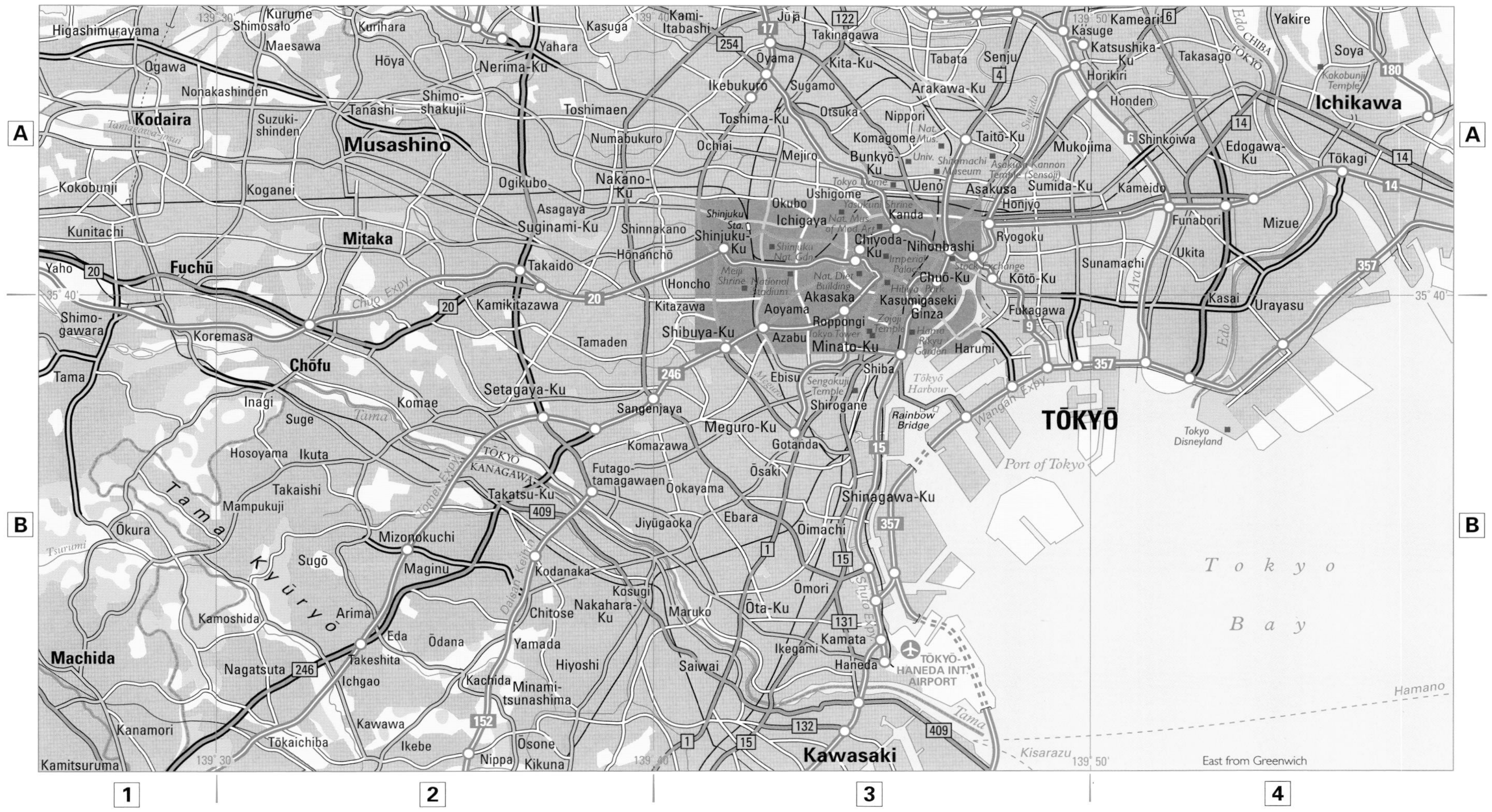

km 5
miles 3

A
Higashimurayama Kurume Shimosato Kurihara Kasuga Jūjō Takinagawa Kameari Yakire Soya
Ogawa Shimosshakujii Maesawa Yahara Kita-ku Senju Kasuge Katsushika-Ku Takasago Ichikawa
Kodaira Hōya Nerima-Ku Ōyama Tabata Horikiri Honden Kokubunji Temple
Nonakashinden Ikebukuro Sugamo Nippori Mukojima Edogawa-Ku Tōkagi
Suzuki-shinden Tanashi Shimo-shakujii Toshimaen Toshima-Ku Otsuka Komagome Taito-Ku Sumida-Ku Kameido Funabori
Kokubunji Ogikubo Nakano-Ku Mejiro Bunkyō-Ku Asakusa Honjyo Mizue
Koganei Asagaya Suginami-Ku Shinnakano Shinjuku Kanda Nihonbashi Ryogoku
Musashino Mitaka Shinjuku-Ku Chiyoda-Ku Kōtō-Ku
Kunitachi Honanchō Akasaka Kasumigaseki Ginza Sunamachi Urayasu
Fuchū Takaido Kamikitazawa Kitazawa Aoyama Roppongi Minato-Ku Fukagawa Kasai
Yaho Shimo-gawara Honcho Shibuya-Ku Azabu Shiba Harumi
Chōfu Setagaya-Ku Ebisu Shirogane Rainbow Bridge TŌKYŌ
Inagi Suge Komae Sangenjaya Meguro-Ku Sengokuji Temple Tokyo Disneyland
Koremasa Tama Futago-tamagawaen Komazawa Shirogane Port of Tokyo

B
Hosoyama Ikuta Takaishi Takatsu-Ku Jiyūgaoka Gotanda Shinagawa-Ku
Mampukuji Mizonokuchi Ookayama Ebara Ōsaki
Okura Sugō Maginu Kodanaka Ōimachi Tokyo Bay
Kamoshida Arima Chitose Nakahara-Ku Kosugi Maruko Ōta-Ku Omori
Machida Eda Ōdana Yamada Ōmori
Nagatsuta Takeshita Minami-tsunashima Hiyoshi Saiwai Ikegami Kamata
Ichigao Kawawa Haneda TOKYO-HANEDA INT AIRPORT
Kanamori Kachida Hamano
Kamitsuruma Tōkaichiba Osone Nippa Kikuna Kawasaki Kisarazu East from Greenwich

1 2 3 4

CENTRAL TOKYO

km 1
miles 0.5

a
OME-KAIDŌ ŌKUBO OKUBO-DORI OKUBO-DORI AKIHABARA ASAKUSABASHI
SHINJUKU-KU SHOKUAN-DORI Akihabara Station Akihabara
Sumitomo Bldg. ICHIGAYA KUDANKITA Nicolai-do Church YASUKUNI-DORI
Shinjuku Central Park Hanazono-jinja Shrine Yasukuni-jinja Shrine JIMBOCHO KANDA KODENMACHO
Tokyo City Hall Shinjuku Sta. YOTSUYA Science Technology Museum MARUNOUCHI
Shinjuku-sanchome Budokan Kitano-maru Park KANDAHEISEI
KŌEN-DORI MEIJI-DORI YASUKUNI-DORI Nat. Mus. of Modern Art NIHONBASHI
Minami-shinjuku Station SANBANCHO Fukiage Imperial Garden Stock Exchange
YAMATE-DORI Yoyogi Sta. Shinjuku-National Garden East Garden Tokyo Station CHŪŌ-KU

b
Sangūbashi Sta Meiji Shrine Treasurehouse Sendagaya Sta. CHIYODA-KU Imperial Palace MARUNOUCHI
Sword Museum Shinanomachi Sta. Yotsuya Sta. St. Ignatius National Theatre Outer Garden NIHONBASHI
Meiji Shrine Inner Garden National Stadium Jingū Inner Garden Suntory Art Museum
Meiji-jingū Shrine Jingū Baseball Stadium Akasaka Palace National Diet Building Government Buildings Bridgestone Mus. of Art
Yoyogi Park Togū Memorial Hall Jingū Outer Garden AOYAMA-DORI Hibiya Park KASUMIGASEKI GINZA
Yoyoji-hachiman Sta. Gaienmae Nogi-jinja Shrine AKASAKA Nissei Theatre Kabuki-za Theatre

c
INOKASHIRA-DORI Harajuku Sta. Oriental Bazaar AOYAMA Sony Centre TSUKIJI
Kanze No Play Theatre Meiji-jingū-mae Aoyama Cemetery TORANOMON Reinanzaka Church SHIMBASHI St. Luke's Int Hospital
YAMATE-DORI OMOTESANDO Nezu Art Museum Tokyo Tower Central Wholesale Market
SHIBUYA-KU Omotesandō ROPPONGI Shiba Park Tsukiji Hongan-ji Temple
Shibuya Sta. EXPRESSWAY No. 3 SHIBUYASEN MINATO-KU Zōjoji Temple Hama Rikyū Garden
DŌGEN-ZAKA KOMAZAWA-DORI AZABU SHIBA Hamamatsucho Station Haneda Airport HARUMI

1 2 3 4 5

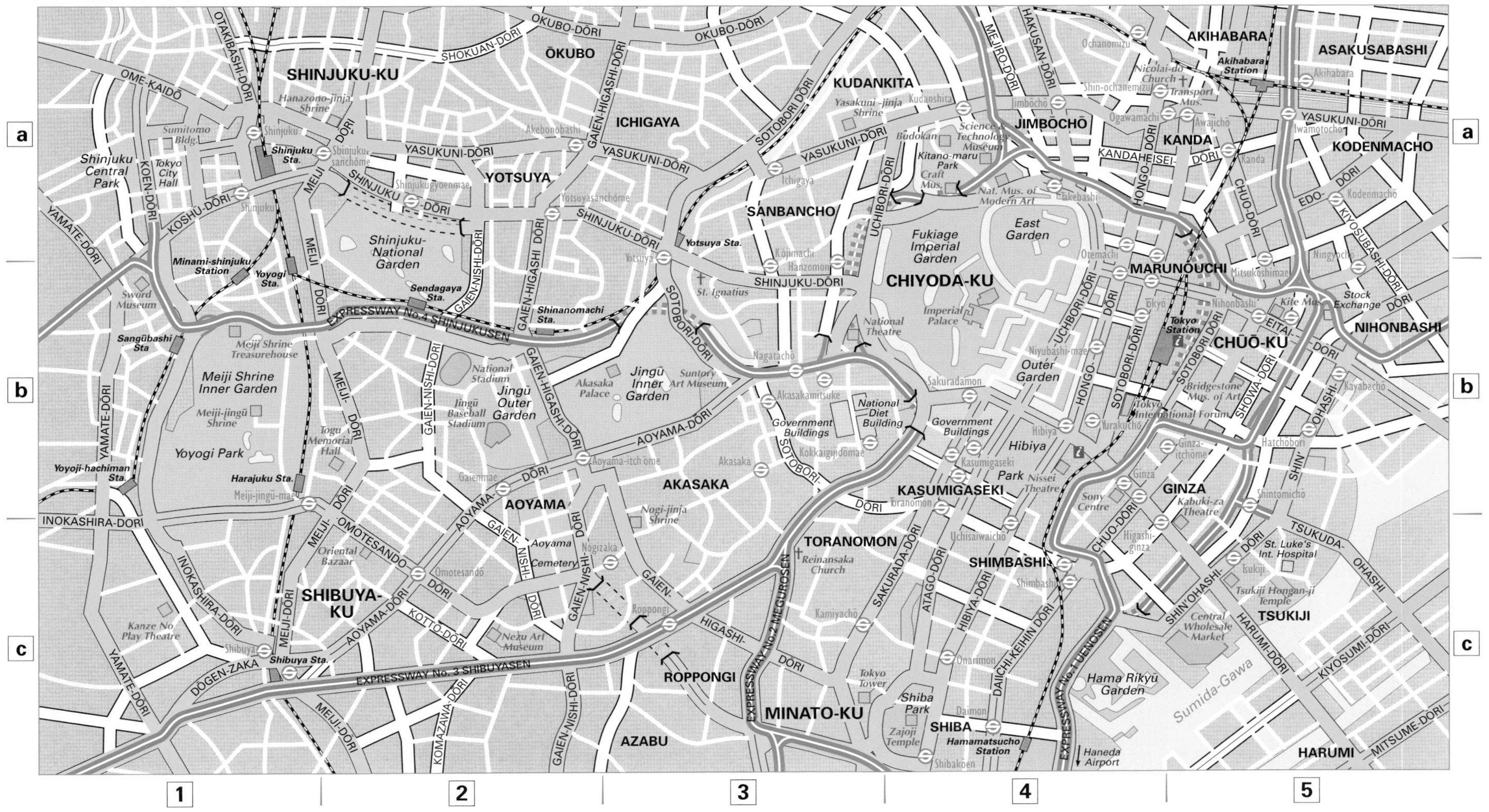

COPYRIGHT PHILIP'S

TEHRAN

km 0 — 5
miles 0 — 3

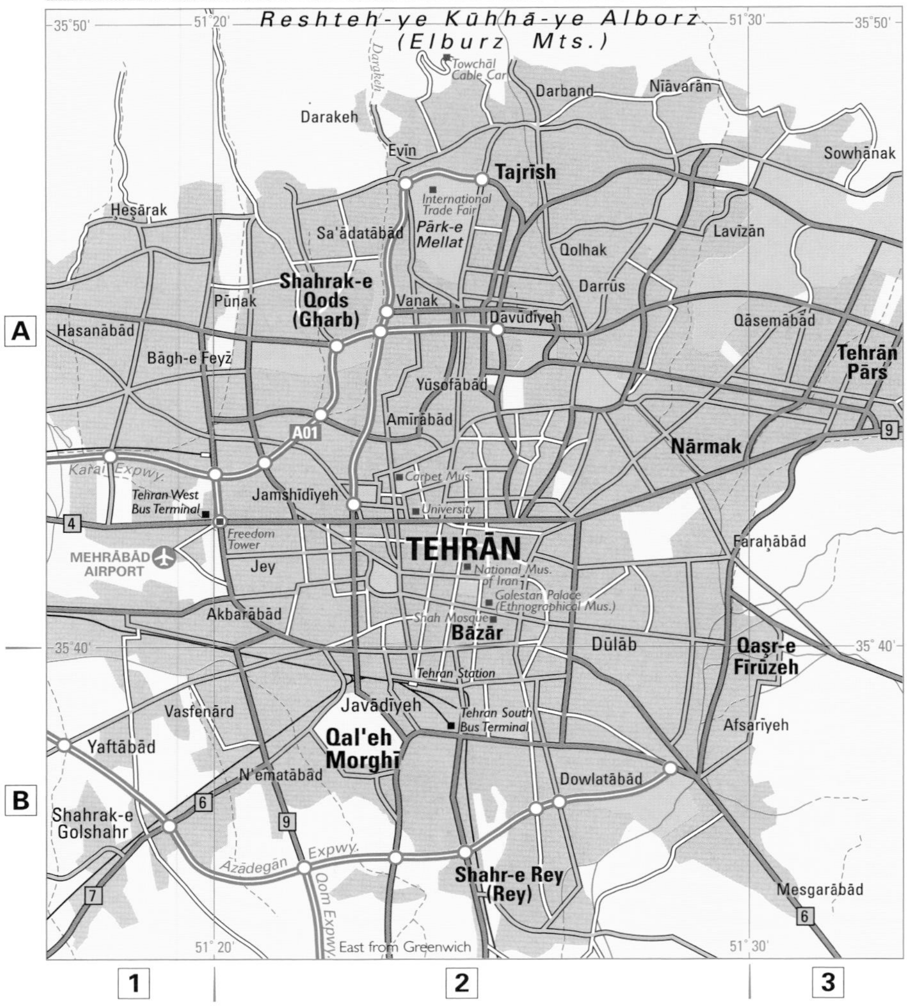

Reshteh-ye Kūhhā-ye Alborz
(Elburz Mts.)

Towchāl Cable Car
Darband · Niāvarān
Darakeh
Evin
Darband
Tajrīsh
Sa'ādatābād · Pārk-e Mellat
Qolhak · Sowhānak
Lavizān
Heşārak
Pūnak · Shahrak-e Qods (Gharb) · Vanak · Davūdiyeh · Darrūs · Qāsemābād
Hasanābād
Bāgh-e Feyż
Amirabād
Yūsofābād · Tehrān Pārs
A01
Jamshīdiyeh · Carpet Mus. · University · Nārmak
Tehran West Bus Terminal · Freedom Tower
MEHRĀBĀD AIRPORT
Jey · Farāhābād
TEHRĀN
National Mus. of Iran · Golestan Palace (Ethnographical Mus.)
Akbarābād · Shah Mosque · Bāzār
Dūlāb · Qaşr-e Fīrūzeh
Tehran Station
Vasfenārd · Javādiyeh · Tehran South Bus Terminal
Yaftābād · Qal'eh Morghī · Afsariyeh
N'ematābād · Dowlatābād
Shahrak-e Golshahr · Āzādegān Expwy. · Shahr-e Rey (Rey) · Mesgarābād
Qom Expwy.
East from Greenwich

TIANJIN

km 0 — 5
miles 0 — 3

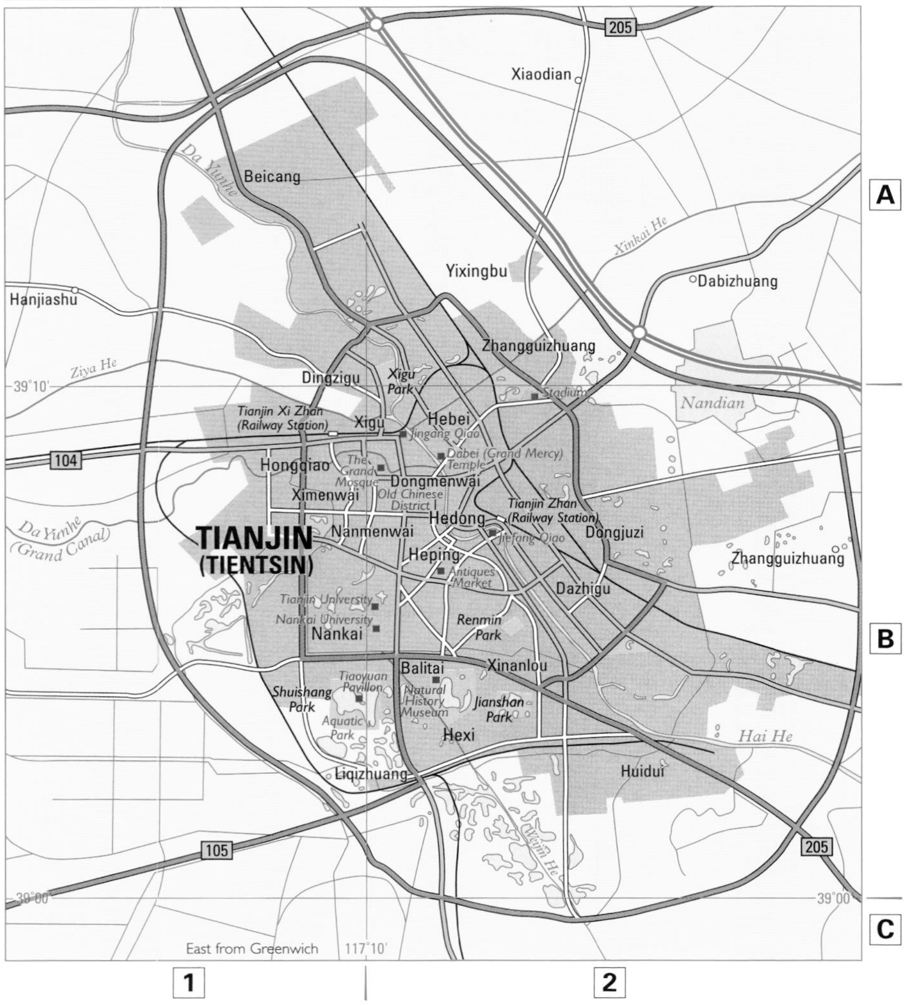

205
Xiaodian
Beicang
Da Yunhe
Hanjiashu · Yixingbu · Dabizhuang
Ziya He · Nandian
Dingzigu · Xigu Park · Zhangguizhuang
Tianjin Xi Zhan (Railway Station) · Xigu · Hebei
104
Honggiao · Ximenwai · Old Chinese District I · Dabei (Grand Mercy) Temple · Tianjin Zhan (Railway Station)
Da Yunhe (Grand Canal)
Nanmenwai · Hedong · Dongjuzi
Dongmenwai · Zhangguizhuang
Heping · Dazhigu
Tianjin University · Antiques Market
Nankai University · Nankai · Renmin Park · Xinanlou
Shuishang Park · Tiaoyuan Pavilion · Balitai · Natural History Museum · Jianshan Park
Aquatic Park · Hexi
Liqizhuang · Huidui · Hai He
105 · 205
East from Greenwich 117°10'

TORONTO

km 0 — 5
miles 0 — 3

Fairport
407 · Thornhill · East Don · Markham · Metro Toronto Zoo · West Rouge · Rouge Hill
Concord · Newtonbrook · Brown · Port Union
Woodbridge · Pine Grove · Edgeley · Willowdale · Agincourt · Malvern · Highland Creek
Fisherville · York University · Northmount · 404 · 401
Humber Summit · Black Creek Pioneer Village · North York · Lansing · Woodburn · West Hill
Beaumonte Heights · York Mills · Wexford · Bendale · Scarborough
Thistletown · Armour Heights · 401 · Cliffside
Kipling Heights · Downsview · DOWNSVIEW AIRPORT · Don Mills · Wilket Creek Park · Danforth
Rexdale · Humberlea · Lawrence Heights · Ontario Science Centre · Thorncliffe
Malton · Weston · Leaside · East York · Demonia Park · Birch Cliff
Woodbine Race Track · Mount Dennis · Forest Hill · Casa Loma · Kew Gardens
TORONTO INTERNATIONAL AIRPORT (LESTER B. PEARSON) · Humber Valley Village · York · Riverdale Park
Hanlon · Lambton Mills · Swansea · University of Toronto · City Hall · Parliament Buildings
Etobicoke · Islington · Kingsway · High Park · CN Tower & SkyDome · Old Fort York · Union Sta. · TORONTO
Markland Wood · Humber Bay · Parkdale · Exhibition Place · TORONTO CITY CENTRE AIRPORT
Burnhamthorpe · Summerville · Ontario Place · Island Park · Toronto Harbour
Mimico · Toronto Islands · Gibraltar Point · LAKE ONTARIO
New Toronto
Cooksville · Mississauga · Long Branch
West from Greenwich

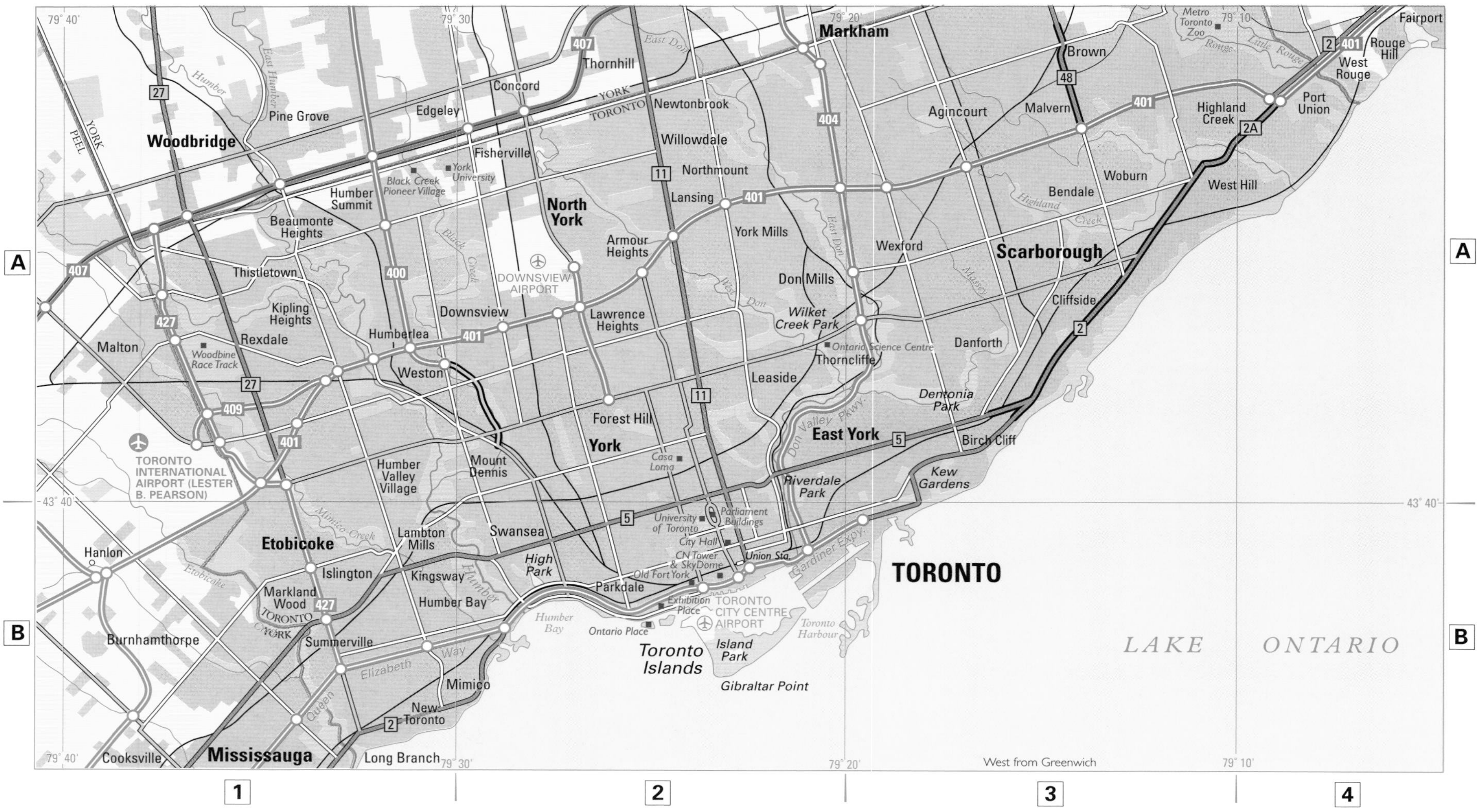

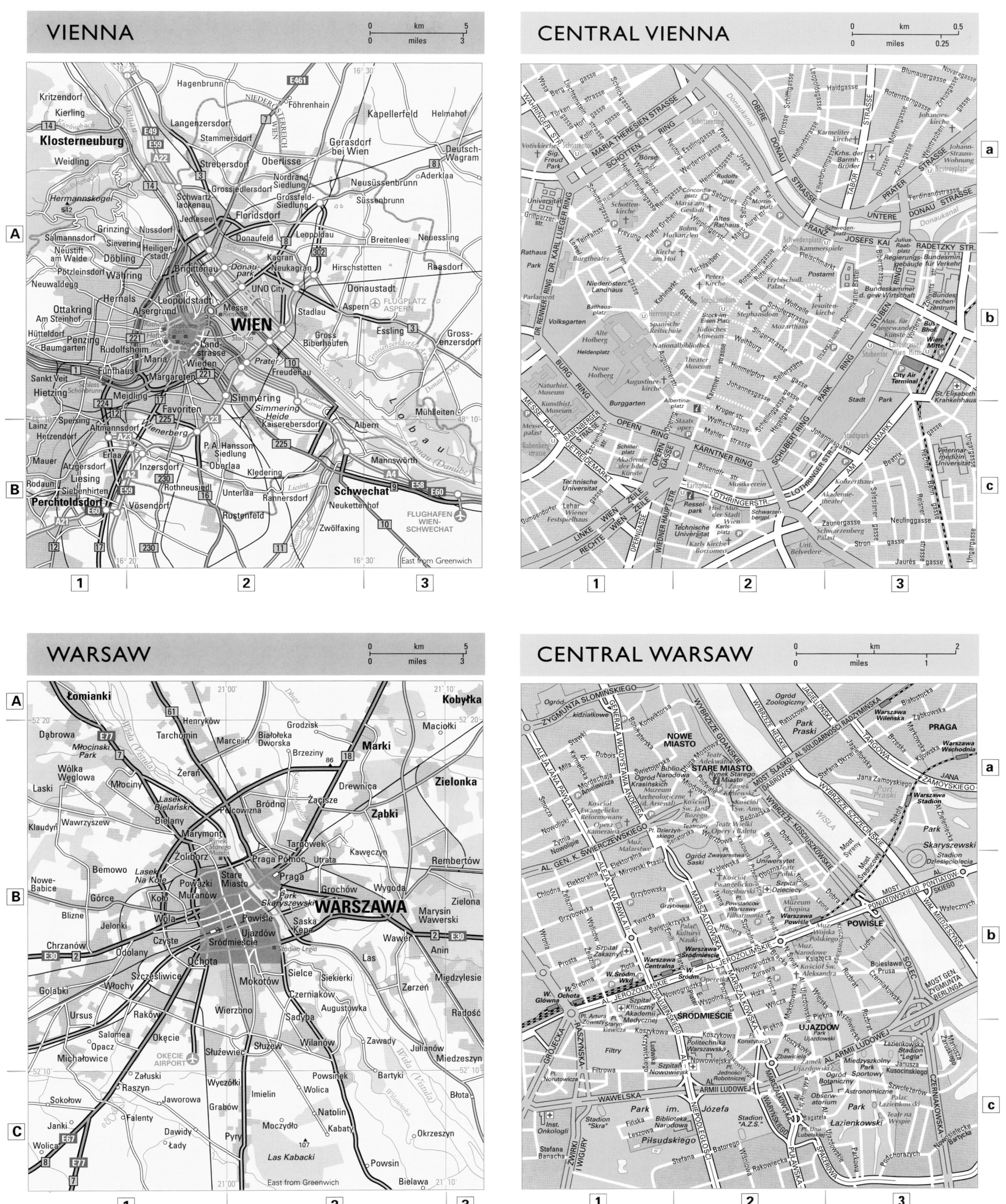

WASHINGTON

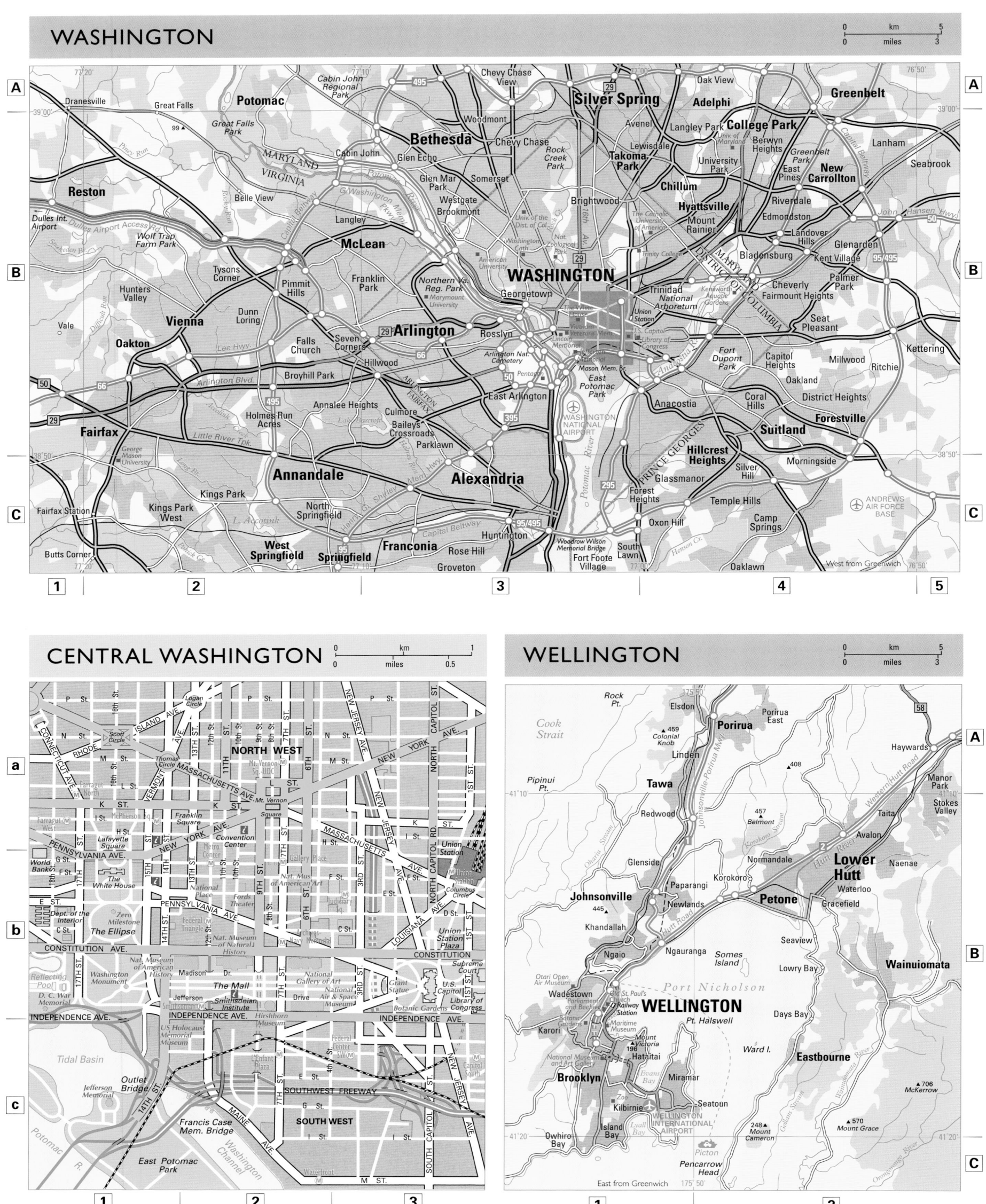

CENTRAL WASHINGTON

WELLINGTON

INDEX TO CITY MAPS

The index contains the names of all the principal places and features shown on the City Maps. Each name is followed by an additional entry in italics giving the name of the City Map within which it is located.

The number in bold type which follows each name refers to the number of the City Map page where that feature or place will be found.

The letter and figure which are immediately after the page number give the grid square on the map within which the feature or place is situated. The letter represents the latitude and the figure the longitude. Upper case letters refer to the City Maps, lower case letters to the Central Area Maps. The full geographic reference is provided in the border of the City Maps.

The location given is the centre of the city, suburb or feature and is not necessarily the name. Rivers, canals and roads are indexed to their name. Rivers carry the symbol → after their name.

An explanation of the alphabetical order rules and a list of the abbreviations used are to be found at the beginning of the World Map Index.

A

Aalām, *Baghdad* **3** B2
Aalsmeer, *Amsterdam* **2** B1
Abbey Wood, *London* **15** B4
Abcoude, *Amsterdam* **2** B2
Âbdin, *Cairo* **7** A2
Abeno, *Osaka* **22** B4
Aberdeen, *Hong Kong* **12** B2
Aberdour, *Edinburgh* **11** A2
Aberdour Castle, *Edinburgh* **11** A2
Abfanggraben →, *Munich* **20** A3
Ablon-sur-Seine, *Paris* **23** B3
Abramtsevo, *Moscow* **19** B4
Abu Dis, *Jerusalem* **13** B2
Abû en Numrus, *Cairo* **7** B2
Abu Ghosh, *Jerusalem* **13** B1
Acacias, *Madrid* **17** c2
Acassuso, *Buenos Aires* **7** A1
Accotink Cr. →, *Washington* **32** B2
Acheres, *Paris* **23** A1
Acília, *Rome* **25** C1
Aclimação, *São Paulo* **26** B2
Acton, *London* **15** A2
Açúcar, Pão de, *Rio de Janeiro* **24** B2
Ada Beja, *Lisbon* **14** A1
Adams Park, *Atlanta* **3** B2
Adams Shore, *Boston* **6** B4
Addiscombe, *London* **15** B3
Adelphi, *Washington* **32** A4
Aderklaa, *Vienna* **31** A3
Admiralteyskaya Storona, *St. Petersburg* **26** B2
Áffori, *Milan* **18** A2
Aflandshage, *Copenhagen* **10** B3
Afsarīyeh, *Tehran* **30** B2
Agboyi Cr. →, *Lagos* **14** A2
Ågerup, *Copenhagen* **10** A1
Ågesta, *Stockholm* **28** B2
Agincourt, *Toronto* **30** A3
Agora, Arhéa, *Athens* **2** c1
Agra Canal, *Delhi* **10** B2
Agricola Oriental, *Mexico City* **18** B2
Agua Espraiada →, *São Paulo* **26** B2
Agualva-Cacem, *Lisbon* **14** A1
Agustino, Cerro El, *Lima* **16** B2
Ahrensfelde, *Berlin* **5** A4
Ahuntsic, *Montreal* **19** A1
Ai →, *Osaka* **22** A4
Aigremont, *Paris* **23** A1
Air View Park, *Singapore* **27** A2
Airport West, *Melbourne* **17** A1
Aiyaleo, *Athens* **2** B2
Aiyáleos, Óros, *Athens* **2** B1
Ajegunle, *Lagos* **14** B2
Aji, *Osaka* **22** A3
Ajuda, *Lisbon* **14** A1
Akalla, *Stockholm* **28** A1
Akasaka, *Tokyo* **29** b3
Akbarābād, *Tehran* **30** A2
Akershus Slott, *Oslo* **22** A3
Akihabara, *Tokyo* **29** a5
Akrópolis, *Athens* **2** c2
Al 'Azamiyah, *Baghdad* **3** A2
Al Quds = Jerusalem, *Jerusalem* **13** B2
Alaguntan, *Lagos* **14** B2
Alameda, *San Francisco* **25** B3
Alameda, Parque, *Mexico City* **18** b2
Alameda Memorial State Beach Park, *San Francisco* **25** B3
Albern, *Vienna* **31** B2
Albert Park, *Melbourne* **17** B1
Alberton, *Johannesburg* **13** B2
Albertslund, *Copenhagen* **10** B2
Albysjön, *Stockholm* **28** B1
Alcantara, *Lisbon* **14** A1
Alcatraz I., *San Francisco* **25** B2
Alcobendas, *Madrid* **17** A2
Alcorcón, *Madrid* **17** B1
Aldershof, *Berlin* **5** B4
Aldo Bonzi, *Buenos Aires* **7** C1
Aleksandrovskoye, *St. Petersburg* **26** B2
Alexander Nevsky Abbey, *St. Petersburg* **26** B2
Alexander Soutzos Moussío, *Athens* **2** b3
Alexandra, *Johannesburg* **13** A2
Alexandra, *Singapore* **27** B2
Alexandria, *Washington* **32** C3
Alfama, *Lisbon* **14** c3
Alfortville, *Paris* **23** B3
Algés, *Lisbon* **14** A1
Alhambra, *Los Angeles* **16** B4
Alibey →, *Istanbul* **12** B1
Alibey Barajı, *Istanbul* **12** B1
Alibeyköy, *Istanbul* **12** B1
Alimos, *Athens* **2** B2
Alipur, *Calcutta* **8** B1
Allach, *Munich* **20** A1
Allambie Heights, *Sydney* **28** A2
Allard Pierson Museum, *Amsterdam* **2** b2
Allermuir Hill, *Edinburgh* **11** B2
Allerton, Pt., *Boston* **6** B4
Allston, *Boston* **6** A3
Almada, *Lisbon* **14** A2
Almagro, *Buenos Aires* **7** B2
Almargem do Bispo, *Lisbon* **14** A1
Almazovo, *Moscow* **19** A6
Almirante G. Brown, Parque, *Buenos Aires* **7** C2
Almon, *Jerusalem* **13** B2
Almond →, *Edinburgh* **11** B2
Alnabru, *Oslo* **22** A4
Alnsjøen, *Oslo* **22** A4
Alperton, *London* **15** A2
Alpine, *New York* **21** A2
Alrode, *Johannesburg* **13** B2
Alsemerg, *Brussels* **6** B1
Alsergrund, *Vienna* **31** A2
Alsip, *Chicago* **9** C2
Ålsten, *Stockholm* **28** B1
Älta, *Stockholm* **28** B3
Altadena, *Los Angeles* **16** A4
Alte-Donau →, *Vienna* **31** A2
Alte Hofburg, *Vienna* **31** b1
Alter Finkenkrug, *Berlin* **5** A1
Altes Rathaus, *Munich* **20** b3
Altglienicke, *Berlin* **5** B4
Altlandsberg, *Berlin* **5** A5
Altlandsberg Nord, *Berlin* **5** A5
Altmannsdorf, *Vienna* **31** B1
Alto da Moóca, *São Paulo* **26** B2
Alto do Pina, *Lisbon* **14** A2
Altona, *Melbourne* **17** B1
Alvaro Obregon, *Mexico City* **18** B1
Alvik, *Stockholm* **28** B1
Älvsjo, *Stockholm* **28** B2
Älvvik, *Stockholm* **28** A3
Am Hasenbergl, *Munich* **20** A2
Am Steinhof, *Vienna* **31** A1
Am Wald, *Munich* **20** B2
Ama Keng, *Singapore* **27** A2
Amadora, *Lisbon* **14** A1
Amagasaki, *Osaka* **22** A3
Amager, *Copenhagen* **10** B3
Amāl Qādisiya, *Baghdad* **3** B2
Amalienborg, *Copenhagen* **10** b3
Amata, *Milan* **18** A1
Ameixoeira, *Lisbon* **14** A2
América, *São Paulo* **26** B1
Amin, *Baghdad* **3** B2
Aminadov, *Jerusalem* **13** B1
Aminyevo, *Moscow* **19** B2
Amīrābād, *Tehran* **30** A2
Amora, *Lisbon* **14** B2
Amoreira, *Lisbon* **14** A1
Ampelokipi, *Athens* **2** B2
Amper →, *Munich* **20** A1
Amstel, *Amsterdam* **2** b2
Amstel →, *Amsterdam* **2** c2
Amstel-Drecht-Kanaal, *Amsterdam* **2** B2
Amstel Station, *Amsterdam* **2** c3
Amstelhof, *Amsterdam* **2** b2
Amstelveen, *Amsterdam* **2** B2
Amsterdam, *Amsterdam* **2** A2
Amsterdam-Rijnkanaal, *Amsterdam* **2** B3
Amsterdam Zoo, *Amsterdam* **2** b3
Amsterdam Zuidoost, *Amsterdam* **2** B2
Amsterdamse Bos, *Amsterdam* **2** B1
Anacostia, *Washington* **32** B4
Anadoluhisarı, *Istanbul* **12** B2
Anadolukavağı, *Istanbul* **12** A2
Anata, *Jerusalem* **13** B2
Ancol, *Jakarta* **13** A1
'Andalus, *Baghdad* **3** B1
Andarai, *Rio de Janeiro* **24** B1
Anderlecht, *Brussels* **6** A1
Anderson Park, *Atlanta* **3** B2
Andingmen, *Beijing* **4** B2
Andrews Air Force Base, *Washington* **32** C4
Ang Mo Kio, *Singapore* **27** A3
Ängby, *Stockholm* **28** A1
Angel I., *San Francisco* **25** A2
Angel Island State Park, *San Francisco* **25** A2
Angke, Kali →, *Jakarta* **13** A1
Angyalföld, *Budapest* **7** A2
Anik, *Mumbai* **20** A2
Anin, *Warsaw* **31** B2
Anjou, *Montreal* **19** A2
Annalee Heights, *Washington* **32** B2
Annandale, *Washington* **32** C2
Anne Frankhuis, *Amsterdam* **2** a1
Antony, *Paris* **23** B2
Anyangch'on, *Seoul* **26** C1
Aoyama, *Tokyo* **29** b2
Ap Lei Chau, *Hong Kong* **12** B1
Apapa, *Lagos* **14** B2
Apelacão, *Lisbon* **14** A2
Apterkarskiy Ostrov, *St. Petersburg* **26** B2
Ar Kazimiyah, *Baghdad* **3** B1
Ara →, *Tokyo* **29** A4
Arakawa-Ku, *Tokyo* **29** A3
Arany-hegyi-patak →, *Budapest* **7** A2
Aravaca, *Madrid* **17** B1
Arbataash, *Baghdad* **3** A1
Arc de Triomphe, *Paris* **23** a2
Arcadia, *Los Angeles* **16** B4
Arceuil, *Paris* **23** B2
Arco Plaza, *Los Angeles* **16** b1
Arese, *Milan* **18** A1
Arganzuela, *Madrid* **17** B1
Argenteuil, *Paris* **23** A2
Argonne Forest, *Chicago* **9** C1
Argüelles, *Madrid* **17** a1
Arima, *Osaka* **22** A2
Arima, *Tokyo* **29** B2
Ários Págos, *Athens* **2** c1
Arkhangelyskoye, *Moscow* **19** B1
Arlington, *Boston* **6** A2
Arlington, *Washington* **32** B3
Arlington Heights, *Boston* **6** A2
Arlington Nat. Cemetery, *Washington* **32** B3
Armação, *Rio de Janeiro* **24** B2
Armadale, *Melbourne* **17** B2
Armenian Quarter, *Jerusalem* **13** b3
Armour Heights, *Toronto* **30** A2
Arncliffe, *Sydney* **28** B1
Arnold Arboretum, *Boston* **6** B3
Árpádföld, *Budapest* **7** A3
Arrentela, *Lisbon* **14** B2
Årsta, *Stockholm* **28** B2
Art Institute, *Chicago* **9** c2
Artane, *Dublin* **11** A2
Artas, *Jerusalem* **13** B2
Arthur's Seat, *Edinburgh* **11** B3
Aryiróupolis, *Athens* **2** B2
Asagaya, *Tokyo* **29** A2
Asahi, *Osaka* **22** A4
Asakusa, *Tokyo* **29** A3
Asakusabashi, *Tokyo* **29** a5
Asati, *Calcutta* **8** C1
Aschheim, *Munich* **20** A3
Ascot Vale, *Melbourne* **17** A1
Ashburn, *Chicago* **9** C2
Ashburton, *Melbourne* **17** B2
Ashfield, *Sydney* **28** B1
Ashford, *London* **15** B1
Ashiya, *Osaka* **22** A2
Ashiya →, *Osaka* **22** A2
Ashtown, *Dublin* **11** A2
Askisto, *Helsinki* **12** B1
Askrikefjärden, *Stockholm* **28** A3
Asnières, *Paris* **23** A2
Aspern, *Vienna* **31** A2
Aspern, Flugplatz, *Vienna* **31** A3
Assago, *Milan* **18** B1
Assemblée Nationale, *Paris* **23** b3
Assendelft, *Amsterdam* **2** A1
Assiano, *Milan* **18** B1
Astoria, *New York* **21** B2
Astrolabe Park, *Sydney* **28** B2
Atarot Airport, *Jerusalem* **13** A2
Atghara, *Calcutta* **8** B2
Athens = Athínai, *Athens* **2** B2
Athínai, *Athens* **2** B2
Athis-Mons, *Paris* **23** B3
Athlone, *Cape Town* **8** A2
Atholl, *Johannesburg* **13** A2
Atīfīya, *Baghdad* **3** A2
Atişalen, *Istanbul* **12** B1
Atlanta, *Atlanta* **3** B2
Atlanta History Center, *Atlanta* **3** B2
Atomium, *Brussels* **6** A2
Attiki, *Athens* **2** A2
Atzgersdorf, *Vienna* **31** B1
Aubervilliers, *Paris* **23** A3
Aubing, *Munich* **20** B1
Auburndale, *Boston* **6** A2
Aucherdinny, *Edinburgh* **11** B2
Auckland Park, *Johannesburg* **13** B2
Auderghem, *Brussels* **6** B2
Augusta, Mausoleo di, *Rome* **25** b2
Augustówka, *Warsaw* **31** B2
Aulnay-sous-Bois, *Paris* **23** A3
Aurelio, *Rome* **25** B1
Ausîm, *Cairo* **7** A1
Austerlitz, Gare d', *Paris* **23** A3
Austin, *Chicago* **9** B2
Avalon, *Wellington* **32** B2
Avedøre, *Copenhagen* **10** B2
Avellaneda, *Buenos Aires* **7** C2
Avenel, *Washington* **32** B4
Avondale, *Chicago* **9** B2
Avondale Heights, *Melbourne* **17** A1
Avtovo, *St. Petersburg* **26** B1
Ayazağa, *Istanbul* **12** B1
Ayer Chawan, P., *Singapore* **27** B2
Ayer Merbau, P., *Singapore* **27** B2
Ayía Marina, *Athens* **2** C3
Ayía Paraskevi, *Athens* **2** A2
Áyios Dhimitrios, *Athens* **2** B2
Áyios Ioánnis Rendis, *Athens* **2** B1
Azabu, *Tokyo* **29** c3
Azcapotzalco, *Mexico City* **18** B1
Azteca, Estadia, *Mexico City* **18** C2
Azucar, Cerro Pan de, *Santiago* **26** A1

B

Baambrugge, *Amsterdam* **2** B2
Baba I., *Karachi* **14** B1
Babarpur, *Delhi* **10** A2
Babushkin, *Moscow* **19** A4
Back B., *Mumbai* **20** B1
Baclaran, *Manila* **17** B2
Bacoor, *Manila* **17** C1
Bacoor B., *Manila* **17** C1
Badalona, *Barcelona* **4** A2
Badhoevedorp, *Amsterdam* **2** A1
Badli, *Delhi* **10** A1
Bærum, *Oslo* **22** A2
Bağcılar, *Istanbul* **12** B1
Bággio, *Milan* **18** B1
Bāgh-e-Feyz, *Tehran* **30** A1
Baghdād, *Baghdad* **3** A2
Bagmari, *Calcutta* **8** B2
Bagneux, *Paris* **23** B2
Bagnolet, *Paris* **23** A3
Bagsværd, *Copenhagen* **10** A2
Bagsværd Sø, *Copenhagen* **10** A2
Baguiati, *Calcutta* **8** B2
Bagumbayan, *Manila* **17** C2
Bahçeköy, *Istanbul* **12** A1
Bahtîm, *Cairo* **7** A2
Baileys Crossroads, *Washington* **32** B3
Bailly, *Paris* **23** A1
Bairro Alto, *Lisbon* **14** c1
Bairro Lopes, *Lisbon* **14** b3
Baisha, *Canton* **8** B2
Baisha →, *Canton* **8** B2
Baixa, *Lisbon* **14** c2
Baiyun Airport, *Canton* **8** A2
Baiyun Hill Scenic Spot, *Canton* **8** B2
Bakırköy, *Istanbul* **12** C1
Bakovka, *Moscow* **19** B2
Bal Harbor, *Miami* **18** A2
Balara, *Manila* **17** B2
Balashikha, *Moscow* **19** B5
Baldia, *Karachi* **14** A1
Baldoyle, *Dublin* **11** A3
Baldwin Hills, *Los Angeles* **16** B2
Baldwin Hills Res., *Los Angeles* **16** B2
Balgowlah, *Sydney* **28** A2
Balgowlah Heights, *Sydney* **28** A2
Balham, *London* **15** B3
Bali, *Calcutta* **8** B1
Baliganja, *Calcutta* **8** B2
Balingsnäs, *Stockholm* **28** B2
Balingsta, *Stockholm* **28** B2
Balintawak, *Manila* **17** B1
Balitai, *Tianjin* **30** B2
Ballerup, *Copenhagen* **10** A2
Ballinteer, *Dublin* **11** B2
Ballyboden, *Dublin* **11** B2
Ballybrack, *Dublin* **11** B3
Ballyfermot, *Dublin* **11** A1
Ballymorefinn Hill, *Dublin* **11** B1
Ballymun, *Dublin* **11** A2
Balmain, *Sydney* **28** B2
Baluhati, *Calcutta* **8** B1
Balvanera, *Buenos Aires* **7** B2
Balwyn, *Melbourne* **17** A2
Balwyn North, *Melbourne* **17** A2
Banática, *Lisbon* **14** A1
Banco do Brasil, Centro Cultural, *Rio de Janeiro* **24** a2
Bandra, *Mumbai* **20** A1
Bandra Pt., *Mumbai* **20** A1
Bang Kapi, *Bangkok* **3** B2
Bang Kholaem, *Bangkok* **3** A2
Bang Na, *Bangkok* **3** B2
Bang Phlad, *Bangkok* **3** a1
Bangkhen, *Bangkok* **3** A2
Bangkok = Krung Thep, *Bangkok* **3** B2
Bangkok Noi, *Bangkok* **3** B1
Bangkok Yai, *Bangkok* **3** B1
Banglamphoo, *Bangkok* **3** b2
Banglo, *Calcutta* **8** B1
Bangrak, *Bangkok* **3** B2
Bangsu, *Bangkok* **3** B2
Bank, *London* **15** b5
Bank of America, *San Francisco* **25** b2
Bank of China Tower, *Hong Kong* **12** c1
Banks, C., *Sydney* **28** C2
Banksmeadow, *Sydney* **28** B2
Banstala, *Calcutta* **8** B2
Bantra, *Calcutta* **8** B1
Baoshan, *Shanghai* **27** A1
Bar Giyora, *Jerusalem* **13** B1
Barahanagar, *Calcutta* **8** B2
Barajas, *Madrid* **17** B2
Barajas, Aeropuerto Transoceanico de, *Madrid* **17** B2
Barakpur, *Calcutta* **8** A2
Barberini, Palazzo, *Rome* **25** b3
Barbican, *London* **15** a4
Barcarena, *Lisbon* **14** A1
Barcarena, Rib. de →, *Lisbon* **14** A1
Barcelona, *Barcelona* **4** A2
Barcelona-Prat, Aeropuerta de, *Barcelona* **4** B1
Barceloneta, *Barcelona* **4** A2
Barking, *London* **15** A4
Barkingside, *London* **15** A4
Barnes, *London* **15** B2
Barnet, *London* **15** A2
Barra Andai, *Karachi* **14** B2
Barra Funda, *São Paulo* **26** B2
Barracas, *Buenos Aires* **7** B2
Barranco, *Lima* **16** B2
Barreiro, *Lisbon* **14** B2
Barreto, *Rio de Janeiro* **24** B2
Bartala, *Calcutta* **8** B1
Barton Park, *Sydney* **28** B1
Bartyki, *Warsaw* **31** C2
Barvikha, *Moscow* **19** B1
Bastille, Place de la, *Paris* **23** c5
Basus, *Cairo* **7** A2
Batanagar, *Calcutta* **8** B1
Bath Beach, *New York* **21** C1
Bath I., *Karachi* **14** B2
Batir, *Jerusalem* **13** B1
Batok, Bukit, *Singapore* **27** A2
Battersea, *London* **15** B3
Battery Park, *New York* **21** f1
Bauman, *Moscow* **19** B4
Baumgarten, *Vienna* **31** A1
Bay Harbour Islands, *Miami* **18** A2
Bay Ridge, *New York* **21** C1
Bayonne, *New York* **21** B1
Bayshore, *San Francisco* **25** B3
Bayswater, *London* **15** b2
Bayt Lahm = Bethlehem, *Jerusalem* **13** B2
Bayview, *San Francisco* **25** B2
Bāzār, *Tehran* **30** A2
Beachmont, *Boston* **6** A4
Beacon Hill, *Hong Kong* **12** A2
Beato, *Lisbon* **14** A2
Beaumont, *Dublin* **11** A2
Beaumonte Heights, *Toronto* **30** A1
Bebek, *Istanbul* **12** B2
Běchovice, *Prague* **24** B3
Beck L., *Chicago* **9** A1
Beckenham, *London* **15** B3
Beckton, *London* **15** A4
Becontree, *London* **15** A4
Beddington Corner, *London* **15** B3
Bedford, *Boston* **6** A2
Bedford Park, *Chicago* **9** C2
Bedford Park, *New York* **21** A2
Bedford Stuyvesant, *New York* **21** B2
Bedford View, *Johannesburg* **13** B2
Bedok, *Singapore* **27** B3
Bedok, Res., *Singapore* **27** A3
Beersel, *Brussels* **6** B1
Behala, *Calcutta* **8** B1
Bei Hai, *Beijing* **4** B2
Beicai, *Shanghai* **27** B2
Beicang, *Tianjin* **30** A1
Beihai Park, *Beijing* **4** b2
Beijing, *Beijing* **4** B1
Beit Ghur el-Fawqa, *Jerusalem* **13** A1
Beit Hanina, *Jerusalem* **13** B2
Beit Iksa, *Jerusalem* **13** B2
Beit I'nan, *Jerusalem* **13** A1
Beit Jala, *Jerusalem* **13** B2
Beit Lekhem = Bethlehem, *Jerusalem* **13** B2
Beit Nekofa, *Jerusalem* **13** B1
Beit Sahur, *Jerusalem* **13** B2
Beit Surik, *Jerusalem* **13** B1
Beit Zayit, *Jerusalem* **13** B1
Beitaipingzhuan, *Beijing* **4** B1
Beitar Ilit, *Jerusalem* **13** B1
Beitsun, *Canton* **8** B2
Beitunya, *Jerusalem* **13** A2
Beixing Jing Park, *Shanghai* **27** B1
Békásmegyer, *Budapest* **7** A2
Bekkelaget, *Oslo* **22** A3
Bel Air, *Los Angeles* **16** B2
Bela Vista, *São Paulo* **26** B2
Bélanger, *Montreal* **19** A1
Belas, *Lisbon* **14** A1
Belas Artes, Museu Nacionale de, *Rio de Janeiro* **24** b2
Beleghata, *Calcutta* **8** B2
Belém, *Lisbon* **14** A1
Belém, Torre de, *Lisbon* **14** A1
Belènzinho, *São Paulo* **26** B2
Belgachiya, *Calcutta* **8** B2
Belgharia, *Calcutta* **8** B2
Belgrano, *Buenos Aires* **7** B2
Belgravia, *London* **15** c3
Bell, *Los Angeles* **16** C3
Bell Gardens, *Los Angeles* **16** C4
Bell Tower, *Beijing* **4** a2
Bellavista, *Lima* **16** B2
Bellavista, *Santiago* **26** C2
Belle Harbor, *New York* **21** C2
Belle View, *Washington* **32** B2
Bellevue, Schloss, *Berlin* **5** a2
Bellingham, *London* **15** B3
Bellwood, *Chicago* **9** B1
Belmont, *Boston* **6** A2
Belmont, *London* **15** A2
Belmont, *Wellington* **32** B2
Belmont Harbor, *Chicago* **9** B3
Belmore, *Sydney* **28** B1
Belur, *Calcutta* **8** B2
Belvedere, *Atlanta* **3** B3
Belvedere, *London* **15** B4
Belvedere, *San Francisco* **25** A2
Belyayevo Bogorodskoye, *Moscow* **19** C3
Bemowo, *Warsaw* **31** B1
Benaki, Moussío, *Athens* **2** b3
Bendale, *Toronto* **30** A3
Bendkhal, *Mumbai* **20** B2
Benefica, *Rio de Janeiro* **24** B1
Benfica, *Lisbon* **14** A1
Benito Juárez, *Mexico City* **18** B2
Benito Juárez, Aeropuerto Int., *Mexico City* **18** B2
Bensonhurst, *New York* **21** C2
Berchem-Sainte-Agathe, *Brussels* **6** A1
Berg am Laim, *Munich* **20** B2
Bergenfield, *New York* **21** A2
Bergham, *Munich* **20** B2
Bergvliet, *Cape Town* **8** B1
Beri, *Barcelona* **4** A1
Berkeley, *San Francisco* **25** A3
Berlin, *Berlin* **5** A3
Bermondsey, *London* **15** B3
Bernabeu, Estadio, *Madrid* **17** B1
Bernal Heights, *San Francisco* **25** B2
Berwyn, *Chicago* **9** B2
Berwyn Heights, *Washington* **32** B4
Besiktas, *Istanbul* **12** B2
Besós →, *Barcelona* **4** A2
Bethesda, *Washington* **32** B3
Bethlehem, *Jerusalem* **13** B2
Bethnal Green, *London* **15** A3
Betor, *Calcutta* **8** B1
Beurs, *Amsterdam* **2** b2
Beverley Hills, *Sydney* **28** B1
Beverley Park, *Sydney* **28** B1
Beverly, *Chicago* **9** C3
Beverly Glen, *Los Angeles* **16** B2
Beverly Hills, *Los Angeles* **16** B2
Bexley, *London* **15** B4
Bexley, *Sydney* **28** B1
Bexleyheath, *London* **15** B4
Beykoz, *Istanbul* **12** B2
Beylerbeyi, *Istanbul* **12** B2
Beyoğlu, *Istanbul* **12** B1
Bezons, *Paris* **23** A2
Bezuidenhout Park, *Johannesburg* **13** B2
Bhadrakali, *Calcutta* **8** A2
Bhalswa, *Delhi* **10** A2
Bhambo Khan Qarmati, *Karachi* **14** B2
Bhatsala, *Calcutta* **8** B1
Bhawanipur, *Calcutta* **8** B2
Bhuleshwar, *Mumbai* **20** b2
Białołeka Dworska, *Warsaw* **31** B2
Biblioteca Nacional, *Rio de Janeiro* **24** c2
Bicentennial Park, *Sydney* **28** B1
Bickley, *London* **15** B4
Bidu, *Jerusalem* **13** B1
Bielany, *Warsaw* **31** B1
Bielawa, *Warsaw* **31** C2
Biesdorf, *Berlin* **5** A4
Bièvre →, *Paris* **23** B1
Bièvres, *Paris* **23** B2
Bilston, *Edinburgh* **11** B2
Binacayan, *Manila* **17** C1
Binondo, *Manila* **17** B1
Birak el Kiyam, *Cairo* **7** A1
Birch Cliff, *Toronto* **30** A3
Birkenstein, *Berlin* **5** A5
Birkholz, *Berlin* **5** A4
Birkholzaue, *Berlin* **5** A4
Birrarrung Park, *Melbourne* **17** A2
Biscayne Bay, *Miami* **18** B2
Biscayne Park, *Miami* **18** A2
Bishop Lavis, *Cape Town* **8** A2
Bishopscourt, *Cape Town* **8** A1
Bispebjerg, *Copenhagen* **10** A3
Biwon Secret Garden, *Seoul* **26** B1
Björknas, *Stockholm* **28** B3
Black Cr. →, *Toronto* **30** A2
Blackfen, *London* **15** B4
Blackheath, *London* **15** B4
Blackrock, *Dublin* **11** B2
Bladensburg, *Washington* **32** B4
Blair Village, *Atlanta* **3** C2
Blairgowrie, *Johannesburg* **13** A2
Blakehurst, *Sydney* **28** B1
Blakstad, *Oslo* **22** B1
Blankenburg, *Berlin* **5** A3
Blankenfelde, *Berlin* **5** A3
Blizne, *Warsaw* **31** B1
Bloomsbury, *London* **15** a3
Błota, *Warsaw* **31** C3
Blue Island, *Chicago* **9** C2
Bluebell, *Dublin* **11** B1
Bluff Hd., *Hong Kong* **12** B2
Blumberg, *Berlin* **5** A4
Blunt Pt., *San Francisco* **25** A2
Blutenberg, *Munich* **20** B1
Blylaget, *Oslo* **22** B3
Bo-Kaap Museum, *Cape Town* **8** c2
Boa Vista, Alto do, *Rio de Janeiro* **24** B1
Boardwalk, *New York* **21** C3
Boavista, *Lisbon* **14** A2
Bobigny, *Paris* **23** A3
Bocanegra, *Lima* **16** A2
Boedo, *Buenos Aires* **7** B2
Bogenhausen, *Munich* **20** B2
Bogorodskoye, *Moscow* **19** B4
Bogota, *New York* **21** A1
Bogstadvatnet, *Oslo* **22** A2
Bohnsdorf, *Berlin* **5** B4
Bois-Colombes, *Paris* **23** A2
Bois-d'Arcy, *Paris* **23** B1
Boissy-St.-Léger, *Paris* **23** B4
Boldinasco, *Milan* **18** B1
Bøler, *Oslo* **22** A4
Bollate, *Milan* **18** A1
Bollebeek, *Brussels* **6** A1
Bollensdorf, *Berlin* **5** A5
Bollmora, *Stockholm* **28** B3
Bolshaya-Okhta, *St. Petersburg* **26** B2
Bolton, *Atlanta* **3** B2
Bom Retiro, *São Paulo* **26** B2
Bombay = Mumbai, *Mumbai* **20** B2
Bondi, *Sydney* **28** B2
Bondy, *Paris* **23** A3
Bondy, Forêt de, *Paris* **23** A4
Bonifacio Monument, *Manila* **17** B1
Bonneuil-sur-Marne, *Paris* **23** B4
Bonnington, *Edinburgh* **11** B1
Bonnyrig and Lasswade, *Edinburgh* **11** B3
Bonsucesso, *Rio de Janeiro* **24** B1
Bonteheuwel, *Cape Town* **8** A2
Boo, *Stockholm* **28** A3
Booterstown, *Dublin* **11** B2
Borisovo, *Moscow* **19** C4
Borle, *Mumbai* **20** A2
Boronia Park, *Sydney* **28** A1
Borough Park, *New York* **21** C2
Bosmont, *Johannesburg* **13** B1
Bosön, *Stockholm* **28** A3
Bosporus = Istanbul Boğazi, *Istanbul* **12** B2
Bostancı, *Istanbul* **12** C2
Boston Harbor, *Boston* **6** A4
Boston Harbor Islands, *Boston* **6** A4
Botafogo, *Rio de Janeiro* **24** B1
Botanisk Have, *Copenhagen* **10** b2
Botany, *Sydney* **28** B2
Botany B., *Sydney* **28** B2
Botany Bay Nat. Park, *Sydney* **28** B2
Botič →, *Prague* **24** B3
Botica Sete, *Lisbon* **14** A1
Boucherville, *Montreal* **19** A3
Boucherville, Îs. de, *Montreal* **19** A3
Bougival, *Paris* **23** A1
Boulder Pt., *Hong Kong* **12** B1
Boulogne, Bois de, *Paris* **23** A2
Boulogne-Billancourt, *Paris* **23** A2
Bourg-la-Reine, *Paris* **23** B2
Bouviers, *Paris* **23** B1
Bovenkerk, *Amsterdam* **2** B2
Bovenkerker Polder, *Amsterdam* **2** B2
Bovisa, *Milan* **18** A2
Bow, *London* **15** A3
Bowery, *New York* **21** e2
Boyacıköy, *Istanbul* **12** B2
Boyle Heights, *Los Angeles* **16** B3
Bradbury Building, *Los Angeles* **16** b2
Braepark, *Edinburgh* **11** B2
Braid, *Edinburgh* **11** B2
Bramley, *Johannesburg* **13** A2
Brandenburger Tor, *Berlin* **5** A3
Brani, P., *Singapore* **27** B3
Branik, *Prague* **24** B2
Brännkyrka, *Stockholm* **28** B2
Brás, *São Paulo* **26** B2
Brasilândia, *São Paulo* **26** A1
Brateyevo, *Moscow* **19** C4
Bratsevo, *Moscow* **19** A2
Bray, *Dublin* **11** B3
Braybrook, *Melbourne* **17** A1
Brázdim, *Prague* **24** A3
Breach Candy, *Mumbai* **20** a1
Breakheart Reservation, *Boston* **6** A3
Brede, *Copenhagen* **10** A3
Breeds Pond, *Boston* **6** A4
Breezy Point, *New York* **21** C2
Breitenlee, *Vienna* **31** A3
Breña, *Lima* **16** B2
Brent, *London* **15** A2
Brent Res., *London* **15** A2
Brentford, *London* **15** B2
Brentwood Park, *Los Angeles* **16** B2
Brera, *Milan* **18** B2
Bresso, *Milan* **18** A2
Brevik, *Stockholm* **28** A3
Břevnov, *Prague* **24** B2
Brewster Is., *Boston* **6** A4
Bridgeport, *Chicago* **9** B3
Bridgetown, *Cape Town* **8** A2
Bridgeview, *Chicago* **9** C2
Brighton, *Boston* **6** A3
Brighton, *Melbourne* **17** B1
Brighton le Sands, *Sydney* **28** B1
Brighton Park, *Chicago* **9** C2
Brightwood, *Washington* **32** B3
Brigittenau, *Vienna* **31** A2
Brimbank Park, *Melbourne* **17** A1
Brisbane, *San Francisco* **25** B2
British Museum, *London* **15** a3
Britz, *Berlin* **5** B3
Brixton, *London* **15** B3
Broad Sd., *Boston* **6** A4
Broadmeadows, *Melbourne* **17** A1
Broadmoor, *San Francisco* **25** B2
Broadview, *Chicago* **9** B1
Broadway, *New York* **21** e1
Brockley, *London* **15** B3
Bródno, *Warsaw* **31** B2
Bródnowski, Kanal, *Warsaw* **31** B2
Broek in Waterland, *Amsterdam* **2** A2
Bromley, *London* **15** B4
Bromley Common, *London* **15** B4
Bromma, *Stockholm* **28** A1
Bromma flygplats, *Stockholm* **28** A1
Brompton, *London* **15** c2
Brøndby Strand, *Copenhagen* **10** B2
Brøndbyøster, *Copenhagen* **10** B2
Brøndbyvester, *Copenhagen* **10** B2

Brondesbury, *London* 15 A2
Brønnøya, *Oslo* 22 A2
Brønshøj, *Copenhagen* 10 A2
Bronxville, *New York* 21 A3
Brookfield, *Chicago* 9 C1
Brookhaven, *Atlanta* 3 A2
Brookline, *Boston* 6 B3
Brooklyn, *Cape Town* 8 A1
Brooklyn, *New York* 21 C2
Brooklyn, *Wellington* 32 B1
Brooklyn Bridge, *New York* 21 f2
Brookmont, *Washington* 32 B3
Brossard, *Montreal* 19 B3
Brou-sur-Chantereine, *Paris* 23 A4
Brown, *Toronto* 30 A3
Broyhill Park, *Washington* 32 B2
Brughério, *Milan* 18 A2
Brunswick, *Melbourne* 17 A1
Brush Hill, *Boston* 6 B1
Brussegem, *Brussels* 6 A1
Brussel Nat. Luchthaven, *Brussels* 6 A2
Brussels = Bruxelles, *Brussels* 6 A2
Bruxelles, *Brussels* 6 A2
Bruzzano, *Milan* 18 A2
Bry-sur-Marne, *Paris* 23 A4
Bryanston, *Johannesburg* 13 A1
Bryn, *Oslo* 22 A1
Brzeziny, *Warsaw* 31 B2
Bubeneč, *Prague* 24 B2
Buc, *Paris* 23 B1
Buchenhain, *Munich* 20 B1
Buchholz, *Berlin* 5 A3
Buckhead, *Atlanta* 3 A2
Buckingham Palace, *London* 15 b3
Buckow, *Berlin* 5 B3
Buda, *Budapest* 7 A2
Budafok, *Budapest* 7 B2
Budaörs, *Budapest* 7 B1
Budapest, *Budapest* 7 B2
Budatétény, *Budapest* 7 B2
Budavaripalota, *Budapest* 7 b2
Buddinge, *Copenhagen* 10 A3
Budokan, *Tokyo* 29 a4
Buena Vista, *San Francisco* 25 B2
Buenos Aires, *Buenos Aires* 7 B2
Bufalotta, *Rome* 25 B2
Bugio, *Lisbon* 14 B1
Buiksloot, *Amsterdam* 2 A2
Buitenveldert, *Amsterdam* 2 B2
Buizingen, *Brussels* 6 B1
Bukit Panjang Nature Reserve, *Singapore* 27 A2
Bukit Timah Nature Reserve, *Singapore* 27 A2
Bukum, P., *Singapore* 27 B2
Bûlâq, *Cairo* 7 A2
Bule, *Manila* 17 C2
Bulim, *Singapore* 27 A2
Bullen Park, *Melbourne* 17 A2
Bundoora North, *Melbourne* 17 A2
Bundoora Park, *Melbourne* 17 A2
Bunker I., *Karachi* 14 B1
Bunkyo-Ku, *Tokyo* 29 A3
Bunnefjorden, *Oslo* 22 A3
Buona Vista Park, *Singapore* 27 B2
Burbank, *Chicago* 9 C2
Burbank, *Los Angeles* 16 A3
Burlington, *Boston* 6 A2
Burnham Park, *Chicago* 9 c2
Burnham Park Harbor, *Chicago* 9 B3
Burnhamthorpe, *Toronto* 30 B1
Burnt Oak, *London* 15 A2
Burntisland, *Edinburgh* 11 A2
Burnwynd, *Edinburgh* 11 B1
Burqa, *Jerusalem* 13 A2
Burtus, *Cairo* 7 A1
Burudvatn, *Oslo* 22 A2
Burwood, *Sydney* 28 B1
Bushwick, *New York* 21 B2
Bushy Park, *London* 15 B1
Butantã, *São Paulo* 26 B1
Butcher I., *Mumbai* 20 B2
Butts Corner, *Washington* 32 C2
Büyükdere, *Istanbul* 12 B2
Byculla, *Mumbai* 20 B2
Bygdøy, *Oslo* 22 A3

C

C.N. Tower, *Toronto* 30 B2
Cabaçu de Cima →, *São Paulo* 26 A2
Caballito, *Buenos Aires* 7 B2
Cabin John, *Washington* 32 B2
Cabin John Regional Park, *Washington* 32 A2
Cabinteely, *Dublin* 11 B3
Cabra, *Dublin* 11 A2
Cabuçú de Baixo →, *São Paulo* 26 A1
Cachan, *Paris* 23 B2
Cachenka →, *Moscow* 19 B1
Cachoeira, Rib. da →, *São Paulo* 26 B1
Cacilhas, *Lisbon* 14 A2
Cahuenga Pk., *Los Angeles* 16 B3
Cairo = El Qâhira, *Cairo* 7 A2
Caju, *Rio de Janeiro* 24 B1
Čakovice, *Prague* 24 B3
Calcutta = Kolkata, *Calcutta* 8 B2
California Inst. of Tech., *Los Angeles* 16 B4
California Plaza, *Los Angeles* 16 b1
California State Univ., *Los Angeles* 16 B3
Callao, *Lima* 16 B2
Caloocan, *Manila* 17 B1
Calumet Park, *Chicago* 9 C3
Calumet Sag Channel →, *Chicago* 9 C2
Calumpang, *Manila* 17 B2
Calvairate, *Milan* 18 B2
Camarate, *Lisbon* 14 A2
Camaroes, *Lisbon* 14 A1
Camberwell, *London* 15 B3
Camberwell, *Melbourne* 17 B2
Cambridge, *Boston* 6 A3
Cambridge Res., *Boston* 6 A2
Cambuci, *São Paulo* 26 B2
Camden, *London* 15 A3
Cameron, Mt., *Wellington* 32 B2
Çamlıca, *Istanbul* 12 B2
Camp Springs, *Washington* 32 C4
Campamento, *Madrid* 17 B1
Campbellfield, *Melbourne* 17 A1
Camperdown, *Sydney* 28 B2
Campidoglio, *Rome* 25 c3
Campo, Casa de, *Madrid* 17 B1
Campo F.C. Barcelona, *Barcelona* 4 A1
Campo Grando, *Lisbon* 14 A2
Campo Pequeño, *Lisbon* 14 A2
Campolide, *Lisbon* 14 A2
Camps Bay, *Cape Town* 8 A1
C'an San Joan, *Barcelona* 4 A2
Cañacao B., *Manila* 17 C1
Canarsie, *New York* 21 C2
Cancelleria, Palazzo dei, *Rome* 25 c2
Candiac, *Montreal* 19 B3
Caneças, *Lisbon* 14 A1
Canillas, *Madrid* 17 B2
Canillejas, *Madrid* 17 B2
Canning Town, *London* 15 A4
Canteras de Vallecas, *Madrid* 17 B2
Canterbury, *Melbourne* 17 A2
Canterbury, *Sydney* 28 B1
Canton = Guangzhou, *Canton* 8 B2
Caoheijing, *Shanghai* 27 B1
Capão Redondo, *São Paulo* 26 B1
Caparica, *Lisbon* 14 A2
Caparica, Costa da, *Lisbon* 14 B1
Cape Flats, *Cape Town* 8 B2
Cape Town, *Cape Town* 8 A1
Cape Town International Airport, *Cape Town* 8 A2
Capitol Heights, *Washington* 32 B4
Capitol Hill, *Washington* 32 B4
Capitolini, Musei, *Rome* 25 c3
Captain Cook Bridge, *Sydney* 28 C1
Captain Cook Landing Place Park, *Sydney* 28 C2
Capuchos, *Lisbon* 14 B1
Carabanchel Alto, *Madrid* 17 B1
Carabanchel Bajo, *Madrid* 17 B1
Carapachay, *Buenos Aires* 7 B1
Caraza, *Buenos Aires* 7 C2
Caridad, *Manila* 17 C1
Carioca, Sa. da, *Rio de Janeiro* 24 B1
Carlstadt, *New York* 21 A1
Carlton, *Melbourne* 17 A1
Carmen de Huechuraba, *Santiago* 26 B1
Carmen de la Legua, *Lima* 16 B2
Carnaxide, *Lisbon* 14 A1
Carnegie, *Melbourne* 17 B2
Carnegie Hall, *New York* 21 c2
Carnide, *Lisbon* 14 A1
Carol City, *Miami* 18 A1
Carrascal, *Santiago* 26 B1
Carrickmines, *Dublin* 11 B3
Carrières-sous-Bois, *Paris* 23 A1
Carrières-sous-Poissy, *Paris* 23 A1
Carrières-sur-Seine, *Paris* 23 A2
Carrigeen Bay, *Dublin* 11 A3
Cartierville, *Montreal* 19 A1
Casa Verde, *São Paulo* 26 A1
Casál Morena, *Rome* 25 C2
Casalotti, *Rome* 25 B1
Cascade Heights, *Atlanta* 3 B2
Castél di Leva, *Rome* 25 C2
Castel Sant'Angelo, *Rome* 25 B1
Castle, *Dublin* 11 c2
Castle, *Edinburgh* 11 b2
Castle of Good Hope, *Cape Town* 8 c3
Castleknock, *Dublin* 11 A1
Castleton Corners, *New York* 21 C1
Catedral Metropolitana, *Mexico City* 18 b3
Catedral Metropolitana, *Rio de Janeiro* 24 c1
Catete, *Rio de Janeiro* 24 B1
Catford, *London* 15 B3
Caulfield, *Melbourne* 17 B2
Causeway Bay, *Hong Kong* 12 c3
Cavite, *Manila* 17 C1
Caxias, *Lisbon* 14 A1
Cebeccı, *Istanbul* 12 B1
Cecchignola, *Rome* 25 C2
Cecilienhof, Schloss, *Berlin* 5 B1
Cedar Grove, *Atlanta* 3 C3
Cempaka Putih, *Jakarta* 13 B2
Çengelköy, *Istanbul* 12 B2
Cengkareng, *Jakarta* 13 A1
Centennial Park, *Sydney* 28 B2
Center Hill, *Atlanta* 3 B2
Centocelle, *Rome* 25 B2
Centraal Station, *Amsterdam* 2 a2
Central Park, *New York* 21 B2
Cerillos, *Santiago* 26 B1
Cerro de la Estrella, *Mexico City* 18 B2
Cerro de los Angeles, *Madrid* 17 C1
Cerro Navia, *Santiago* 26 B1
Certanovka →, *Moscow* 19 C3
Certanovo, *Moscow* 19 C3
Cesano Boscone, *Milan* 18 B1
Cesate, *Milan* 18 A1
Cha Kwo Ling, *Hong Kong* 12 B2
Chacarrita, *Buenos Aires* 7 B2
Chadwell Heath, *London* 15 A4
Chai Chee, *Singapore* 27 B3
Chai Wan, *Hong Kong* 12 B2
Chai Wan Kok, *Hong Kong* 12 A1
Chaillot, Palais de, *Paris* 23 b2
Chakdaha, *Calcutta* 8 C1
Chamartin, *Madrid* 17 B1
Chamberi, *Madrid* 17 B1
Chambourcy, *Paris* 23 A1
Champ de Mars, Parc du, *Paris* 23 c2
Champigny-sur-Marne, *Paris* 23 B4
Champlain, Pont, *Montreal* 19 B2
Champs Elysées, Avenue des, *Paris* 23 b2
Champs-sur-Marne, *Paris* 23 A4
Chamrail, *Calcutta* 8 B1
Chamshil, *Seoul* 26 B2
Chamwŏn, *Seoul* 26 B2
Chanakyapuri, *Delhi* 10 B2
Chanditala, *Calcutta* 8 A1
Changfeng Park, *Shanghai* 27 B1
Changi, *Singapore* 27 A3
Changi Int. Airport, *Singapore* 27 A3
Changning, *Shanghai* 27 B1
Chantereine, *Paris* 23 A4
Chantian, *Canton* 8 A2
Chao Phraya →, *Bangkok* 3 B2
Chaoyang, *Beijing* 4 B2
Chaoyangmen, *Beijing* 4 B2
Chapelizod, *Dublin* 11 A1
Chapultepec, Bosque de, *Mexico City* 18 B1
Chapultepec, Castillo de, *Mexico City* 18 B1
Charenton-le-Pont, *Paris* 23 B3
Charing Cross, *London* 15 b4
Charleroi, Kanal de →, *Brussels* 6 B1
Charles Bridge, *Prague* 24 b1
Charles Square, *Prague* 24 c1
Charlestown, *Boston* 6 A3
Charlottenburg, *Berlin* 5 A2
Charlottenburg, Schloss, *Berlin* 5 A2
Charlottenlund, *Copenhagen* 10 A3
Charlton, *London* 15 B4
Charneca, *Lisbon* 14 A2
Charneca, *Lisbon* 14 B1
Châteaufort, *Paris* 23 B1
Châtenay-Malabry, *Paris* 23 B2
Chatham, *Chicago* 9 C3
Châtillon, *Paris* 23 B2
Chatou, *Paris* 23 A1
Chatpur, *Calcutta* 8 B2
Chatswood, *Sydney* 28 A2
Chatuchak, *Bangkok* 3 B2
Chatuchak Park, *Bangkok* 3 B2
Chauki, *Karachi* 14 A1
Chavarria, *Lima* 16 B2
Chaville, *Paris* 23 B2
Chayang, *Seoul* 26 B2
Chegi, *Seoul* 26 B2
Chelles, *Paris* 23 A4
Chelles, Canal de, *Paris* 23 A4
Chells-le-Pin, Aérodrome, *Paris* 23 A4
Chelsea, *Boston* 6 A3
Chelsea, *London* 15 B2
Chelsea, *New York* 21 c1
Chembur, *Mumbai* 20 A2
Chennevières-sur-Marne, *Paris* 23 B4
Cheops, *Cairo* 7 B1
Cherepkovo, *Moscow* 19 B2
Chernyovo, *Moscow* 19 A1
Cheryomushki, *Moscow* 19 B3
Chestnut Hill, *Boston* 6 B2
Cheung Sha Wan, *Hong Kong* 12 A1
Cheverly, *Washington* 32 B4
Chevilly-Larue, *Paris* 23 B3
Chevry-Cossigny, *Paris* 23 B4
Chevy Chase, *Washington* 32 B3
Chevy Chase View, *Washington* 32 A3
Chia Keng, *Singapore* 27 A3
Chiaravalle Milanese, *Milan* 18 B2
Chicago, *Chicago* 9 B3
Chicago Harbor, *Chicago* 9 B3
Chicago Lawn, *Chicago* 9 C2
Chicago-Midway Airport, *Chicago* 9 C2
Chicago-O'Hare Int. Airport, *Chicago* 9 B1
Chicago Ridge, *Chicago* 9 C2
Chicago Sanitary and Ship Canal, *Chicago* 9 C2
Chienzui, *Canton* 8 A3
Chik Sha, *Hong Kong* 12 B2
Child's Hill, *London* 15 A2
Chilla Saroda, *Delhi* 10 B2
Chillum, *Washington* 32 B4
Chilly-Mazarin, *Paris* 23 B2
Chinatown, *Los Angeles* 16 a3
Chinatown, *New York* 21 e2
Chinatown, *San Francisco* 25 b2
Chinatown, *Singapore* 27 c2
Chingupota, *Calcutta* 8 C1
Chislehurst, *London* 15 B4
Chiswick, *London* 15 B2
Chiswick House, *London* 15 B2
Chitose, *Tokyo* 29 B2
Chitralada Palace, *Bangkok* 3 B2
Chiyoda-Ku, *Tokyo* 29 b4
Chkalova, *Moscow* 19 C5
Choa Chu Kang, *Singapore* 27 A2
Choboty, *Moscow* 19 C2
Chodov u Prahy, *Prague* 24 B3
Chōfu, *Tokyo* 29 B2
Choisy-le-Roi, *Paris* 23 B3
Cholupice, *Prague* 24 C2
Chom Thong, *Bangkok* 3 B1
Chong Pang, *Singapore* 27 A2
Ch'ŏngdam, *Seoul* 26 B2
Chongmyo Royal Shrine, *Seoul* 26 B1
Chongno, *Seoul* 26 B1
Chongwen, *Beijing* 4 B2
Chŏnho, *Seoul* 26 B2
Chopin, Muzeum, *Warsaw* 31 b2
Chornaya →, *Moscow* 19 B6
Chorrillos, *Lima* 16 C2
Chowpatty Beach, *Mumbai* 20 b1
Christian Quarter, *Jerusalem* 13 b3
Christiansborg, *Copenhagen* 10 c2
Christianshavn, *Copenhagen* 10 A3
Chrysler Building, *New York* 21 c2
Chrzanów, *Warsaw* 31 B1
Chuen Lung, *Hong Kong* 12 A1
Chuk Kok, *Hong Kong* 12 A2
Chulalongkom Univ., *Bangkok* 3 B2
Chung, *Seoul* 26 B1
Chunghwa, *Seoul* 26 B2
Chungnangch'on →, *Seoul* 26 B1
Chūō-Ku, *Tokyo* 29 b5
Church End, *London* 15 A2
Churchtown, *Dublin* 11 B2
Ciampino, *Rome* 25 C2
Ciampino, Aeroporto di, *Rome* 25 C2
Cicero, *Chicago* 9 B2
Cilandak, *Jakarta* 13 B1
Cilincing, *Jakarta* 13 A2
Ciliwung →, *Jakarta* 13 B2
Čimice, *Prague* 24 B2
Cinecittà, *Rome* 25 B2
Cinisello Bálsamo, *Milan* 18 A2
Cinkota, *Budapest* 7 A3
Cipete, *Jakarta* 13 B1
Citadella, *Budapest* 7 c2
Citta degli Studi, *Milan* 18 B2
Città del Vaticano, *Rome* 25 B1
City, *London* 15 A3
City Hall, *New York* 21 e1
Ciudad Deportiva, *Mexico City* 18 B2
Ciudad Fin de Semana, *Madrid* 17 B2
Ciudad General Belgrano, *Buenos Aires* 7 C1
Ciudad Lineál, *Madrid* 17 B2
Ciudad Satélite, *Mexico City* 18 A1
Ciudad Universitaria, *Buenos Aires* 7 B2
Ciudad Universitaria, *Mexico City* 18 C1
Ciutadella, Parc de la, *Barcelona* 4 b3
Civic Center, *Los Angeles* 16 b2
Clamart, *Paris* 23 B2
Clapham, *London* 15 B3
Clapton, *London* 15 A3
Claremont, *Cape Town* 8 A1
Clayhall, *London* 15 A4
Clerkenwell, *London* 15 a4
Clermiston, *Edinburgh* 11 B2
Clichy, *Paris* 23 A2
Clichy-sous-Bois, *Paris* 23 A4
Cliffside, *Toronto* 30 A3
Cliffside Park, *New York* 21 B2
Clifton, *Boston* 6 A4
Clifton, *Karachi* 14 B2
Clifton, *New York* 21 C1
Cliftondale, *Boston* 6 A3
Cloghran, *Dublin* 11 A2
Clonskeagh, *Dublin* 11 B2
Clontarf, *Dublin* 11 A2
Clontarf, *Sydney* 28 A2
Clovelly, *Sydney* 28 B2
Cobras, I. das, *Rio de Janeiro* 24 B2
Coburg, *Melbourne* 17 A1
Cochituate, *Boston* 6 A1
Cochituate, L., *Boston* 6 B1
Cocotá, *Rio de Janeiro* 24 A1
Cœuilly, *Paris* 23 B4
Coina, *Lisbon* 14 B2
Coit Tower, *San Francisco* 25 a2
Coker, *Lagos* 14 B2
Colaba, *Mumbai* 20 B1
Colaba Pt., *Mumbai* 20 B1
Colegiales, *Buenos Aires* 7 B2
Colindale, *London* 15 A2
Colinton, *Edinburgh* 11 B2
College Park, *Atlanta* 3 C2
College Park, *Washington* 32 B4
College Point, *New York* 21 B2
Collégien, *Paris* 23 A4
Collier Row, *London* 15 A4
Colliers Wood, *London* 15 B2
Colma, *San Francisco* 25 B2
Colney Hatch, *London* 15 A3
Cologno Monzese, *Milan* 18 A2
Colombes, *Paris* 23 A2
Colón, Monumente, *Barcelona* 4 c3
Colon, Plaza de, *Madrid* 17 a3
Colonia Güell, *Barcelona* 4 A1
Colonial Knob, *Wellington* 32 A1
Colosseo, *Rome* 25 c3
Columbus Circus, *New York* 21 b2
Combault, *Paris* 23 B4
Comércio, Praça do, *Lisbon* 14 A2
Commerce, *Los Angeles* 16 B4
Como, *Sydney* 28 C1
Company's Gardens, *Cape Town* 8 c2
Conceição, I. da, *Rio de Janeiro* 24 B2
Concertgebouw, *Amsterdam* 2 c1
Conchali, *Santiago* 26 B2
Concord, *Boston* 6 A1
Concord, *Sydney* 28 B1
Concord, *Toronto* 30 A2
Concorde, Place de la, *Paris* 23 b3
Concorezzo, *Milan* 18 A2
Coney Island, *New York* 21 C2
Congonhas, Aéroporto, *São Paulo* 26 B2
Connaught Place, *Delhi* 10 B2
Conservatori, Palazzo dei, *Rome* 25 c3
Consolação, *São Paulo* 26 B2
Constantia, *Cape Town* 8 B1
Constitución, *Buenos Aires* 7 B2
Constitution, *Atlanta* 3 B2
Convention and Exhibition Centre, *Hong Kong* 12 b2
Coogee, *Sydney* 28 B2
Cook Str., *Wellington* 32 A1
Cooksville, *Toronto* 30 B1
Coolock, *Dublin* 11 A2
Copacabana, *Rio de Janeiro* 24 B1
Copenhagen = København, *Copenhagen* 10 A2
Coral Gables, *Miami* 18 B2
Coral Hills, *Washington* 32 B4
Corcovado, Morro do, *Rio de Janeiro* 24 B1
Corduff, *Dublin* 11 A1
Cormano, *Milan* 18 A2
Cornaredo, *Milan* 18 A1
Córsico, *Milan* 18 B1
Corsini, Palazzo, *Rome* 25 c1
Corviale, *Rome* 25 B1
Coslada, *Madrid* 17 B2
Cossigny, *Paris* 23 B4
Cossipore, *Calcutta* 8 B2
Costantino, Arco di, *Rome* 25 c3
Costorphine, *Edinburgh* 11 B2
Cotao, *Lisbon* 14 A1
Côte St.-Luc, *Montreal* 19 B2
Cotunduba, I. de, *Rio de Janeiro* 24 B2
Coubron, *Paris* 23 A4
Countryside, *Chicago* 9 C1
Courbevoie, *Paris* 23 A2
Courtry, *Paris* 23 A4
Covent Garden, *London* 15 b4
Cowgate, *Edinburgh* 11 b3
Cowley, *London* 15 A1
Coyoacán, *Mexico City* 18 B2
Cragin, *Chicago* 9 B2
Craighall Park, *Johannesburg* 13 A2
Craiglockhart, *Edinburgh* 11 B2
Craigmillar, *Edinburgh* 11 B3
Cramond, *Edinburgh* 11 B2
Cramond Bridge, *Edinburgh* 11 B1
Cramond I., *Edinburgh* 11 B2
Cranford, *London* 15 B1
Crawford, *Cape Town* 8 A2
Crayford, *London* 15 B5
Creekmouth, *London* 15 A4
Crescenzago, *Milan* 18 A2
Cressely, *Paris* 23 B1
Cresskill, *New York* 21 A2
Creteil, *Paris* 23 B3
Cricklewood, *London* 15 A2
Cristo Redentor, Estatua do, *Rio de Janeiro* 24 B1
Crockenhill, *London* 15 B4
Croissy-Beaubourg, *Paris* 23 B4
Croissy-sur-Seine, *Paris* 23 A1
Crosby, *Johannesburg* 13 B1
Crosne, *Paris* 23 B3
Cross I., *Mumbai* 20 B2
Crouch End, *London* 15 A3
Crown Mine, *Johannesburg* 13 B1
Crows Nest, *Sydney* 28 A2
Croydon, *London* 15 B3
Croydon Park, *Sydney* 28 B1
Cruagh Mt., *Dublin* 11 B2
Crumlin, *Dublin* 11 B2
Cruz de Pau, *Lisbon* 14 B2
Crystal Palace, *London* 15 B3
Csepel, *Budapest* 7 B2
Csepelsziget, *Budapest* 7 B2
Csillaghegy, *Budapest* 7 A2
Csillagtelep, *Budapest* 7 B2
Csömör, *Budapest* 7 A3
Csömöri-patak →, *Budapest* 7 A3
Cuatro Vientos, *Madrid* 17 B1
Cuauhtémoc, *Mexico City* 18 B2
Cubao, *Manila* 17 B2
Çubuklu, *Istanbul* 12 B2
Cudahy, *Los Angeles* 16 C3
Cuicuilco, Pirámido de, *Mexico City* 18 C1
Culver City, *Los Angeles* 16 B2
Cumballa Hill, *Mumbai* 20 a1
Cumbres de Vallecas, *Madrid* 17 B2
Cupecé, *São Paulo* 26 B1
Currie, *Edinburgh* 11 B2
Cusago, *Milan* 18 B1
Cusano Milanino, *Milan* 18 A2
Custom House, *Dublin* 11 b3
Çuvuşabaşi →, *Istanbul* 12 B1
Czernriaków, *Warsaw* 31 B2
Czyste, *Warsaw* 31 B1

D

Da Moóca →, *São Paulo* 26 B2
Da Yunhe →, *Tianjin* 30 A1
Dabizhuang, *Tianjin* 30 A2
Ďablice, *Prague* 24 B2
Dąbrowa, *Warsaw* 31 B1
Dachang, *Shanghai* 27 B1
Dachang Airfield, *Shanghai* 27 B1
Dachau-Ost, *Munich* 20 A1
Dachauer Moos, *Munich* 20 A1
Dadar, *Mumbai* 20 A1
Dagenham, *London* 15 A4
Daglfing, *Munich* 20 B2
Daheisha, *Jerusalem* 13 B2
Dahlem, *Berlin* 5 B2
Dahlwitz-Hoppegarten, *Berlin* 5 A5
Dahongmen, *Beijing* 4 C2
Daitō, *Osaka* 22 A4
Dajiaoting, *Beijing* 4 B2
Dakhnoye, *St. Petersburg* 26 C1
Dalejsky potok →, *Prague* 24 B2
Dalgety Bay, *Edinburgh* 11 A1
Dalkeith, *Edinburgh* 11 B3
Dalkey, *Dublin* 11 B3
Dalkey Island, *Dublin* 11 B3
Dallgow, *Berlin* 5 A1
Dalmeny, *Edinburgh* 11 B1
Dalston, *London* 15 A3
Daly City, *San Francisco* 25 B2
Dam, *Amsterdam* 2 b2
Dam Rak, *Amsterdam* 2 a2
Damaia, *Lisbon* 14 A1
Dämeritzsee, *Berlin* 5 B5
Dan Ryan Woods, *Chicago* 9 C2
Danderhall, *Edinburgh* 11 B3
Danderyd, *Stockholm* 28 A2
Danforth, *Toronto* 30 A3
Darakeh, *Tehran* 30 A2
Darband, *Tehran* 30 A2
Darling Harbour, *Sydney* 28 b1
Darling Point, *Sydney* 28 B2
Darndale, *Dublin* 11 A2
Darrūs, *Tehran* 30 A2
Dartford, *London* 15 B5
Darya Ganj, *Delhi* 1 a3
Dashi, *Canton* 8 B2
Datansha, *Canton* 8 B2
Datun, *Beijing* 4 B2
Daulatpur, *Delhi* 10 A1
David's Citadel, *Jerusalem* 13 b3
David's Tomb, *Jerusalem* 13 b3
Davidson, Mt., *San Francisco* 25 B2
Davidson's Mains, *Edinburgh* 11 B2
Dāvūdiyeh, *Tehran* 30 A2
Davydkovo, *Moscow* 19 B2
Dawidy, *Warsaw* 31 C1
Days Bay, *Wellington* 32 B2
Dazhigu, *Tianjin* 30 B2
De Waag, *Amsterdam* 2 b2
Decatur, *Atlanta* 3 B3
Dedham, *Boston* 6 B2
Deer I., *Boston* 6 A4
Degunino, *Moscow* 19 A3
Deir Dibwan, *Jerusalem* 13 A2
Deir Ibzi'e, *Jerusalem* 13 A1
Dejvice, *Prague* 24 B2
Dekabristov, Ostrov, *St. Petersburg* 26 B1
Delhi, *Delhi* 10 B2
Delhi Gate, *Delhi* 1 b3
Demarest, *New York* 21 A2
Den Ilp, *Amsterdam* 2 A2
Denistone Heights, *Sydney* 28 A1
Dentonia Park, *Toronto* 30 A3
Deptford, *London* 15 B3
Deputati, Camera dei, *Rome* 25 b2
Des Plaines, *Chicago* 9 A1
Des Plaines →, *Chicago* 9 B1
Deshengmen, *Beijing* 4 B2
Deutsch-Wagram, *Vienna* 31 A3
Deutsche Oper, *Berlin* 5 A2
Deutscher Museum, *Munich* 20 B2
Devil's Peak, *Cape Town* 8 A1
Dháfni, *Athens* 2 B2
Dhakuria, *Calcutta* 8 B2
Dhamarakia, *Athens* 2 B1
Dharavi, *Mumbai* 20 A2
Dhrapersón, *Athens* 2 B1
Diadema, *São Paulo* 26 C2
Diegen, *Brussels* 6 A2
Diemen, *Amsterdam* 2 A2
Diepkloof, *Johannesburg* 13 B1
Dieprivier, *Cape Town* 8 B1
Difficult Run →, *Washington* 32 B2
Dilbeek, *Brussels* 6 A1
Dinzigu, *Tianjin* 30 A1
Dirnismaning, *Munich* 20 A2
District Heights, *Washington* 32 B4
Ditan Park, *Beijing* 4 a2
Diyāla →, *Baghdad* 3 B3
Djursholm, *Stockholm* 28 A2
Döberitz, *Berlin* 5 A1
Döbling, *Vienna* 31 A2
Docklands, *London* 15 A3
Dodder, R. →, *Dublin* 11 B1
Dodger Stadium, *Los Angeles* 16 B3
Dolgoe Ozero, *St. Petersburg* 26 A1
Doll Museum, *Delhi* 1 b3
Dollis Hill, *London* 15 A2
Dollymount, *Dublin* 11 A2
Dolni, *Prague* 24 B3
Dolni Chabry, *Prague* 24 B2
Dolni Počernice, *Prague* 24 B3
Dolphins Barn, *Dublin* 11 B2
Dom Pedro II, Parque, *São Paulo* 26 B2
Domain, The, *Sydney* 28 b2
Dome of the Rock, *Jerusalem* 13 b3
Don Mills, *Toronto* 30 A2
Don Muang Int. Airport, *Bangkok* 3 A2
Donaghmede, *Dublin* 11 A3
Donau-Oder Kanal, *Vienna* 31 A3
Donaufeld, *Vienna* 31 A2
Donaupark, *Vienna* 31 A2
Donaustadt, *Vienna* 31 A2
Dongan Hills, *New York* 21 C1
Dongcheng, *Beijing* 4 B2
Donggou, *Shanghai* 27 B2
Dongjiao, *Canton* 8 B2
Dongjuzi, *Tianjin* 30 B2
Dongmenwai, *Tianjin* 30 B2
Dongri, *Mumbai* 20 B2
Dongshanhu Park, *Canton* 8 B2
Dongzhimen, *Beijing* 4 B2
Donnybrook, *Dublin* 11 B2
Doornfontein, *Johannesburg* 13 B2
Dorchester, *Boston* 6 B3
Dorchester B., *Boston* 6 B3
Dornach, *Munich* 20 B3
Dorval, Aéroport de, *Montreal* 19 B1
Dos Couros →, *São Paulo* 26 C2
Dos Moninos →, *São Paulo* 26 C2
Douglas Park, *Chicago* 9 B2
Dover Heights, *Sydney* 28 B2
Dowlatābād, *Tehran* 30 B2
Downey, *Los Angeles* 16 C4
Downsview, *Toronto* 30 A1
Dragør, *Copenhagen* 10 B3
Drancy, *Paris* 23 A3
Dranesville, *Washington* 32 A1
Dreilinden, *Berlin* 5 B2
Drewnica, *Warsaw* 31 B2
Drigh Road, *Karachi* 14 A2
Drimnagh, *Dublin* 11 B2
Drogenbos, *Brussels* 6 B1
Druid Hills, *Atlanta* 3 B2
Drum Towwer, *Beijing* 4 a2
Drumcondra, *Dublin* 11 A2
Drummoyne, *Sydney* 28 B1
Drylaw, *Edinburgh* 11 B2
Dubeč, *Prague* 24 B3
Dublin, *Dublin* 11 A2
Dublin Airport, *Dublin* 11 A2
Dublin Bay, *Dublin* 11 B3
Dublin Harbour, *Dublin* 11 A2
Duddingston, *Edinburgh* 11 B3
Dugnano, *Milan* 18 A2
Dūlāb, *Tehran* 30 B2
Dulwich, *London* 15 B3
Dum Dum, *Calcutta* 8 B2
Dum Dum Int. Airport, *Calcutta* 8 B2
Dumont, *New York* 21 A2
Dún Laoghaire, *Dublin* 11 B3
Duna →, *Budapest* 7 A2
Duncan Dock, *Cape Town* 8 a3
Dundrum, *Dublin* 11 B2
Dunearn, *Singapore* 27 B2
Dunfermline, *Edinburgh* 11 A1
Dunn Loring, *Washington* 32 B2
Dunning, *Chicago* 9 B2
Dunvegan, *Johannesburg* 13 A2
Duomo, *Milan* 18 B2
Duque de Caxias, *Rio de Janeiro* 24 A1
Dusit, *Bangkok* 3 B2
Dusit Zoo, *Bangkok* 3 a2
Dworp, *Brussels* 6 B1
Dyakovo, *Moscow* 19 B3
Dzerzhinskiy, *Moscow* 19 C5
Dzerzhinskiy, *Moscow* 19 B3
Dzerzhinskiy Park, *Moscow* 19 B3

E

Eagle Rock, *Los Angeles* 16 B3
Ealing, *London* 15 A2
Earl's Court, *London* 15 c1
Earlsfield, *London* 15 B2
Earlwood, *Sydney* 28 B1
East Acton, *Boston* 6 A1
East Arlington, *Boston* 6 A3
East Arlington, *Washington* 32 B3
East Bedfont, *London* 15 B1
East Boston, *Boston* 6 A3
East Don →, *Toronto* 30 A2
East Elmhurst, *New York* 21 B2
East Finchley, *London* 15 A2
East Ham, *London* 15 A4
East Humber →, *Toronto* 30 A1
East Lamma Channel, *Hong Kong* 12 B1
East Lexington, *Boston* 6 A2
East Los Angeles, *Los Angeles* 16 B3
East Molesey, *London* 15 B1
East New York, *New York* 21 B2
East Pines, *Washington* 32 B4
East Point, *Atlanta* 3 B2
East Potomac Park, *Washington* 32 B3
East Pt., *Boston* 6 A4
East River →, *New York* 21 B2
East Rutherford, *New York* 21 A1
East Sheen, *London* 15 B2
East Village, *New York* 21 e2
East Wickham, *London* 15 B4
East York, *Toronto* 30 A2
Eastbourne, *Wellington* 32 B2
Eastcote, *London* 15 A1
Easter Howgate, *Edinburgh* 11 B2
Eastwood, *Sydney* 28 A1
Ebara, *Tokyo* 29 B3
Ebisu, *Tokyo* 29 B3
Ebute-Ikorodu, *Lagos* 14 A2
Ebute-Metta, *Lagos* 14 B2
Echo Park, *Los Angeles* 16 a1
Eda, *Tokyo* 29 B2
Edendale, *Johannesburg* 13 A2
Edenmore, *Dublin* 11 A2
Edgars Cr. →, *Melbourne* 17 A1
Edgeley, *Toronto* 30 A1
Edgemar, *San Francisco* 25 C2
Edinburgh, *Edinburgh* 11 B2
Edison Park, *Chicago* 9 A2
Edmondston, *Washington* 32 B4
Edmondstown, *Dublin* 11 B2
Edo →, *Tokyo* 29 B4
Edogawa-Ku, *Tokyo* 29 A4
Edsberg, *Stockholm* 28 A1
Edwards L., *Melbourne* 17 A1
Eiche, *Berlin* 5 A4
Eiche Sud, *Berlin* 5 A4
Eiffel, Tour, *Paris* 23 A2
Ein Arik, *Jerusalem* 13 A1
Ein Naquba, *Jerusalem* 13 B1
Ein Rafa, *Jerusalem* 13 B1
Eizariya, *Jerusalem* 13 B2
Ejby, *Copenhagen* 10 A2
Ejigbo, *Lagos* 14 A1
Ekeberg, *Oslo* 22 A3
Eknäs, *Stockholm* 28 B3
El 'Abbasiya, *Cairo* 7 A2
El Agustino, *Lima* 16 B2
El Baragil, *Cairo* 7 A1
El Basâlîn, *Cairo* 7 B2
El-Bira, *Jerusalem* 13 A2
El Bosque, *Santiago* 26 C2
El Carmen, *Santiago* 26 B1
El Cortijo, *Santiago* 26 B1
El Duqqi, *Cairo* 7 A2
El Encinar de los Reyes, *Madrid* 17 A2
El Ghurîya, *Cairo* 7 A2
El Gîza, *Cairo* 7 A2
El-Khadr, *Jerusalem* 13 B1
El Khalîfa, *Cairo* 7 A2
El Kôm el Ahmar, *Cairo* 7 A2
El Ma'âdi, *Cairo* 7 B2
El Matarîya, *Cairo* 7 A2
El Mohandessin, *Cairo* 7 A2
El Monte, *Los Angeles* 16 B4
El Mûskî, *Cairo* 7 A2
El Pardo, *Madrid* 17 A1
El Portal, *Miami* 18 A2
El Prat de Llobregat, *Barcelona* 4 B1
El Pueblo de L.A. Historic Park, *Los Angeles* 16 b2
El Qâhira, *Cairo* 7 A2
El Qubba, *Cairo* 7 A2
El Reloj, *Mexico City* 18 C2
El Retiro, *Madrid* 17 B1
El Salto, *Santiago* 26 B2
El Sereno, *Los Angeles* 16 B3
El Talibîya, *Cairo* 7 B2
El Vergel, *Mexico City* 18 C2
El Wâhli, *Cairo* 7 A2
El Zamâlik, *Cairo* 7 A2
El Zeitûn, *Cairo* 7 A2
Elephanta Caves, *Mumbai* 20 B2
Elephanta I., *Mumbai* 20 B2
Ellboda, *Stockholm* 28 A3
Ellinikón, *Athens* 2 B2
Ellinikón Olympic Complex, *Athens* 2 B2
Ellis I., *New York* 21 B1
Elm Park, *London* 15 A5
Elmers End, *London* 15 B3
Elmhurst, *New York* 21 B2
Elmstead, *London* 15 B4
Elmwood Park, *Chicago* 9 B2
Elmwood Park, *New York* 21 A1
Elsdon, *Wellington* 32 A1
Elsiesrivier, *Cape Town* 8 A2
Elsternwick, *Melbourne* 17 B2
Eltham, *London* 15 B4
Elwood, *Melbourne* 17 B1
Élysée, *Paris* 23 A2
Elysian Park, *Los Angeles* 16 a3
Embajadores, *Madrid* 17 c2
Embarcadero Center, *San Francisco* 25 b3
Emek Refa'im, *Jerusalem* 13 c2
Émerainville, *Paris* 23 B4
Emeryville, *San Francisco* 25 A3
Eminönü, *Istanbul* 12 B1
Emmarentia, *Johannesburg* 13 A2
Empire State Building, *New York* 21 c2
Encantado, *Rio de Janeiro* 24 B1
Encino, *Los Angeles* 16 B2
Encino Res., *Los Angeles* 16 B1
Enebyberg, *Stockholm* 28 A1
Enfield, *Sydney* 28 B1
Engenho, I. do, *Rio de Janeiro* 24 B2
Englewood, *Chicago* 9 C3
Englewood, *New York* 21 A2
Englewood Cliffs, *New York* 21 A2
Enmore, *Sydney* 28 B2
Enskede, *Stockholm* 28 B2
Entrevias, *Madrid* 17 B1
Epping, *Sydney* 28 A1
Erawan Shrine, *Bangkok* 3 c3
Eregun, *Lagos* 14 A2
Erenköy, *Istanbul* 12 C2
Erith, *London* 15 B5
Erlaa, *Vienna* 31 B1
Ermington, *Sydney* 28 A1
Ermita, *Manila* 17 B1
Ershatou, *Canton* 8 B2
Erskineville, *Sydney* 28 B2
Erunkan, *Lagos* 14 A2
Erzsébet-Telep, *Budapest* 7 B3
Eschenried, *Munich* 20 A1
Esenler, *Istanbul* 12 B1
Esher, *London* 15 B1
Eskbank, *Edinburgh* 11 B3
Esperanza, *Mexico City* 18 c3
Esplanade Park, *Singapore* 27 c3
Esplugas, *Barcelona* 4 A1
Esposizione Univ. di Roma (E.U.R.), *Rome* 25 C1
Essendon, *Melbourne* 17 A1
Essendon Airport, *Melbourne* 17 A1
Essingen, *Stockholm* 28 B1
Essling, *Vienna* 31 A3
Est, Gare de l', *Paris* 23 a5
Estadio Maracanã, *Rio de Janeiro* 24 B1
Estado, Parque do, *São Paulo* 26 B2
Estefânia, *Lisbon* 14 a2
Estrela, Basilica da, *Lisbon* 14 A2
Ethnikó Arheologiko Moussío, *Athens* 2 a2
Etobicoke, *Toronto* 30 B1
Etobicoke Cr. →, *Toronto* 30 B1
Etterbeek, *Brussels* 6 B2
Euston, *London* 15 a3
Evanston, *Chicago* 9 A2
Even Sapir, *Jerusalem* 13 B1
Evere, *Brussels* 6 A2
Everett, *Boston* 6 A3
Evergreen Park, *Chicago* 9 C2
Evīn, *Tehran* 30 A2
Évzonos, *Athens* 2 B2
Ewu, *Lagos* 14 A1
Exchange Square, *Hong Kong* 12 c1
Exposições, Palácio das, *Rio de Janeiro* 24 B1
Eyüp, *Istanbul* 12 B1

F

Fabour, Mt., *Singapore* 27 B2
Faechi, *Seoul* 26 B2
Fælledparken, *Copenhagen* 10 A3
Fågelön, *Stockholm* 28 B1
Fagersjö, *Stockholm* 28 B2
Fair Lawn, *New York* 21 A1
Fairfax, *Washington* 32 B2
Fairfax Station, *Washington* 32 C2
Fairhaven Bay, *Boston* 6 A1
Fairhaven Hill, *Boston* 6 A1
Fairland, *Johannesburg* 13 A1
Fairmilehead, *Edinburgh* 11 B2
Fairmount Heights, *Washington* 32 B4
Fairport, *Toronto* 30 A4
Fairview, *New York* 21 B2
Falenty, *Warsaw* 31 C1
Fálirou, Órmos, *Athens* 2 B2
Falkenburg, *Berlin* 5 A4
Falkenhagen, *Berlin* 5 A1
Falkensee, *Berlin* 5 A1
Falls Church, *Washington* 32 B2
Falomo, *Lagos* 14 B2
False Bay, *Cape Town* 8 B2
Fangcun, *Canton* 8 B2
Faraḥābād, *Tehran* 30 A2
Farforovskaya, *St. Petersburg* 26 B2
Farningham, *London* 15 B5
Farrar Pond, *Boston* 6 A1
Farsta, *Stockholm* 28 B2
Fasanerie-Nord, *Munich* 20 A2
Fasangarten, *Munich* 20 B2
Fasting Palace, *Beijing* 4 c2
Fatih, *Istanbul* 12 B1
Favoriten, *Vienna* 31 B2

Fawkner, Melbourne 17 A1
Fawkner Park, Melbourne 17 B1
Feijó, Lisbon 14 B2
Feldkirchen, Munich 20 B3
Feldmoching, Munich 20 A2
Feltham, London 15 B1
Fener, Istanbul 12 B1
Fenerbahçe, Istanbul 12 C2
Fengtai, Beijing 4 C1
Fenino, Moscow 19 B5
Ferencváros, Budapest 7 B2
Ferihegyi Airport, Budapest 7 B3
Ferndale, Johannesburg 13 A2
Férolles-Attilly, Paris 23 B4
Fichtenau, Berlin 5 B5
Fields Corner, Boston 6 B3
Fiera Camp, Milan 18 B1
Fifth Avenue, New York 21 b3
Figino, Milan 18 B1
Fijir, Baghdad 3 A2
Filadhélfia, Athens 2 A2
Fili-Mazilovo, Moscow 19 B2
Filothei, Athens 2 A2
Finchley, London 15 A2
Finglas, Dublin 11 A2
Finsbury, London 15 A3
Finsbury Park, London 15 A3
Fiorito, Buenos Aires 7 C2
Firhouse, Dublin 11 B2
Fischerhäuser, Munich 20 A3
Fisher Island, Miami 18 B2
Fishermans Bend, Melbourne 17 A1
Fisherman's Wharf, San Francisco 25 a1
Fisherville, Toronto 30 A2
Fisksätra, Stockholm 28 B3
Fitzroy Gardens, Melbourne 17 A1
Five Dock, Sydney 28 B1
Fjellstrand, Oslo 22 B2
Flamengo, Rio de Janeiro 24 B1
Flaminio, Rome 25 B1
Flaskebekk, Oslo 22 A2
Flatbush, New York 21 C2
Flaten, Stockholm 28 B2
Flemington Racecourse, Melbourne 17 A1
Flint Pk., Los Angeles 16 B3
Florence, Los Angeles 16 C3
Florence Bloom Bird Sanctuary, Johannesburg 13 A2
Florentia, Johannesburg 13 B2
Flores, Buenos Aires 7 B2
Floresta, Buenos Aires 7 B2
Florida, Buenos Aires 7 B2
Florida, Johannesburg 13 B1
Floridsdorf, Vienna 31 A2
Flushing, New York 21 B3
Flushing Meadows Corona Park, New York 21 B2
Flysta, Stockholm 28 A1
Fo Tan, Hong Kong 12 A2
Föhrenhain, Vienna 31 A2
Fontainebleau, Johannesburg 13 A1
Fontenay-aux-Roses, Paris 23 B2
Fontenay-le-Fleury, Paris 23 B1
Fontenay-sous-Bois, Paris 23 A3
Foots Cray, London 15 B4
Footscray, Melbourne 17 A1
Foreshore, Cape Town 8 a3
Forest, Brussels 6 B1
Forest Gate, London 15 A4
Forest Heights, Washington 32 C3
Forest Hill, London 15 B3
Forest Hill, Toronto 30 A2
Forest Hills, New York 21 B2
Forest Park, Chicago 9 B2
Forest View, Chicago 9 C2
Forestville, Washington 32 B4
Fornebu, Oslo 22 A2
Fornebu Airport, Oslo 22 A2
Foro Romano, Rome 25 c3
Forstenried, Munich 20 B1
Forstenrieder Park, Munich 20 B1
Fort, Mumbai 20 c2
Fort Canning Park, Singapore 27 b2
Fort Dupont Park, Washington 32 B4
Fort Foote Village, Washington 32 C3
Fort Lee, New York 21 A2
Fort Mason Center, San Francisco 25 a1
Forth, Firth of, Edinburgh 11 A2
Forth Rail Bridge, Edinburgh 11 A1
Forth Road Bridge, Edinburgh 11 A1
Fót, Budapest 7 A3
Fourqueux, Paris 23 A1
Foxrock, Dublin 11 B2
Framingham, Boston 6 B1
Franconia, Washington 32 C3
Frankel, Singapore 27 B3
Franklin Park, Boston 6 B3
Franklin Park, Chicago 9 B1
Franklin Park, Washington 32 B3
Franklin Res., Los Angeles 16 B2
Frauenkirche, Munich 20 b2
Frederiksberg, Copenhagen 10 A3
Frederiksdal, Copenhagen 10 A2
Fredersdorf, Berlin 5 A5
Freguesia, Rio de Janeiro 24 A1
Freidrichshain, Volkspark, Berlin 5 A3
Freiham, Munich 20 B1
Freimann, Munich 20 A2
Fresh Pond, Boston 6 A3
Fresnes, Paris 23 B2
Freudenau, Vienna 31 A2
Friarstown, Dublin 11 B1
Frick Collection, New York 21 b3
Friedenau, Berlin 5 B3
Friedrichsfelde, Berlin 5 B4
Friedrichshagen, Berlin 5 B4
Friedrichshain, Berlin 5 A3
Friedrichslust, Berlin 5 A5
Friherrs, Helsinki 12 B1
Frontón, I., Lima 16 B1
Frunze, Moscow 19 B3
Fuchū, Tokyo 29 A1
Fuencarral, Madrid 17 B1
Fuenlabrada, Madrid 17 C1
Fujidera, Osaka 22 B4
Fukagawa, Tokyo 29 B3
Fukiage Imperial Garden, Tokyo 29 a4
Fukiai, Osaka 22 A2
Fukushima, Osaka 22 A3
Fulham, London 15 B2
Funabori, Tokyo 29 A4
Funasaka, Osaka 22 A2
Fundão, I. do, Rio de Janeiro 24 B1
Fünfhaus, Vienna 31 A2
Furesø, Copenhagen 10 A2
Furth, Munich 20 B2
Futago-tamagawaen, Tokyo 29 B2
Fuxing Dao, Shanghai 27 B2
Fuxing Park, Shanghai 27 B1
Fuxinglu, Beijing 4 B1

G

Gage Park, Chicago 9 C2
Gagny, Paris 23 A4
Galata, Istanbul 12 B1
Galátsion, Athens 2 A2
Galeão, Aéroporto Int. de, Rio de Janeiro 24 A1
Galyanovo, Moscow 19 B4
Gambir, Jakarta 13 A1
Gamboa, Rio de Janeiro 24 B1
Gambolóita, Milan 18 B2
Gamla Stan , Stockholm 28 c2
Gamlebyen, Oslo 22 A3
Gangtou, Canton 8 A1
Gangwei, Canton 8 B2
Ganjiakou, Beijing 4 B1
Ganshoren, Brussels 6 A1
Gants Hill, London 15 A4
Gaoqiao, Shanghai 27 A2
Garbagnate Milanese, Milan 18 A1
Garbatella, Rome 25 B2
Garches, Paris 23 A2
Garching, Munich 20 A3
Garden City, Cairo 7 A2
Garden Reach, Calcutta 8 B1
Garder, Oslo 22 B2
Garfield, New York 21 A1
Garfield Park, Chicago 9 B2
Gargareta, Athens 2 B2
Garvanza, Los Angeles 16 B3
Gåshaga, Stockholm 28 A3
Gateway National Recreation Area, New York 21 C2
Gateway of India, Mumbai 20 B2
Gatow, Berlin 5 B1
Gávea, Rio de Janeiro 24 B1
Gávea, Pedra da, Rio de Janeiro 24 B1
Gazdagrét, Budapest 7 B1
Gebel el Ahmar, Cairo 7 A2
Gebel el Muqattam, Cairo 7 A2
Gebel el Tura, Cairo 7 B2
Geiselgasteig, Munich 20 B2
General San Martin, Buenos Aires 7 B1
Gennevilliers, Paris 23 A2
Gentilly, Paris 23 B3
Gentofte, Copenhagen 10 A3
Genval, Brussels 6 B2
George I., Hong Kong 12 B1
Georges I., Boston 6 B4
Georges River Bridge, Sydney 28 C1
Georgetown, Washington 32 B3
Georgia Dome, Atlanta 3 B2
Gerasdorf bei Wien, Vienna 31 A2
Gerberau, Munich 20 A1
Gerli, Buenos Aires 7 C2
Germiston, Johannesburg 13 B2
Gern, Munich 20 B2
Gesîrat el Rauda, Cairo 7 A2
Getafe, Madrid 17 C1
Geva Binyamin, Jerusalem 13 A2
Geylang Serai, Singapore 27 B3
Gezîrat el Dhahab, Cairo 7 B2
Gharapuri, Mumbai 20 B2
Ghatkopar, Mumbai 20 A2
Ghazipur, Delhi 10 B2
Ghizri, Karachi 14 B2
Ghizri Cr. →, Karachi 14 B2
Ghonda, Delhi 10 A2
Ghusuri, Calcutta 8 B2
Gianicolense, Rome 25 B1
Gianicolo, Rome 25 c1
Gibraltar Pt., Toronto 30 B2
Gidea Park, London 15 A5
Giesing, Munich 20 B2
Gilmerton, Edinburgh 11 B3
Gilo, Jerusalem 13 B2
Gimmersta, Stockholm 28 B3
Ginza, Tokyo 29 b5
Girgaum, Mumbai 20 b2
Giv'at Ye'arim, Jerusalem 13 B1
Giv'at Ze'ev, Jerusalem 13 A2
Giza Pyramids = Pyramids, Cairo 7 B1
Gjersjøen, Oslo 22 B3
Gladesville, Sydney 28 B1
Gladsakse, Copenhagen 10 A2
Glasnevin, Dublin 11 A2
Glassmanor, Washington 32 C3
Glasthule, Dublin 11 B3
Glen Iris, Melbourne 17 B2
Glen Mar Park, Washington 32 B3
Glen Rock, New York 21 A1
Glenarden, Washington 32 B4
Glenasmole Reservoirs, Dublin 11 B1
Glencorse Res., Edinburgh 11 B2
Glencullen, Dublin 11 B2
Glendale, Los Angeles 16 B3
Glendoo Mt., Dublin 11 B2
Glenhuntly, Melbourne 17 B2
Glenside, Wellington 32 B1
Glenview, Chicago 9 A2
Glenview Countryside, Chicago 9 A2
Glenvista, Johannesburg 13 B2
Glifádha, Athens 2 B2
Glömsta, Stockholm 28 B1
Glostrup, Copenhagen 10 B2
Gogar, Edinburgh 11 B2
Göktürk, Istanbul 12 A1
Golabari, Calcutta 8 B2
Golabki, Warsaw 31 B1
Gold Coast, Chicago 9 a2
Golden Gate, San Francisco 25 B2
Golden Gate Bridge, San Francisco 25 B2
Golden Gate Park, San Francisco 25 B2
Golden Horn, Istanbul 12 B1
Golders Green, London 15 A2
Gollans Stream →, Wellington 32 B2
Golyevo, Moscow 19 B1
Goodman Hill, Boston 6 A1
Goodmayes, London 15 A4
Goodwood, Cape Town 8 A2
Gopalpur, Calcutta 8 B2
Górce, Warsaw 31 B1
Gore Hill, Sydney 28 A2
Gorelyy →, St. Petersburg 26 A3
Gorenki, Moscow 19 B5
Gorgie, Edinburgh 11 B2
Gorky Park, Moscow 19 B3
Gosen, Berlin 5 B5
Gosener kanal, Berlin 5 B5
Gospel Oak, London 15 A3
Gotanda, Tokyo 29 B3
Goth Goli Mar, Karachi 14 A2
Goth Sher Shah, Karachi 14 A1
Gournay-sur-Marne, Paris 23 A4
Governador, I. do, Rio de Janeiro 24 A1
Governor's I., New York 21 B1
Graben, Vienna 31 b2
Grabów, Warsaw 31 C1
Graça, Lisbon 14 b3
Grace, Mt., Wellington 32 B2
Grace Cathedral, San Francisco 25 b1
Gracefield, Wellington 32 B2
Gracia, Barcelona 4 A2
Gräfelfing, Munich 20 B1
Gragoatá, Rio de Janeiro 24 B2
Grand Central Station, New York 21 c2
Grand Union Canal, London 15 A2
Grande Place, Brussels 6 b2
Grant Park, Atlanta 3 B2
Grant Park, Chicago 9 c2
Granton, Edinburgh 11 B2
Grape I., Boston 6 B4
Grassy Park, Cape Town 8 B2
Gratosóglio, Milan 18 B2
Gratzwalde, Berlin 5 B5
Gravesend, New York 21 C2
Grazhdanka, St. Petersburg 26 B2
Great Falls, Washington 32 B2
Great Falls Park, Washington 32 B2
Great Hall of the People, Beijing 4 b2
Great Meadows National Wildlife Refuge, Boston 6 A1
Greco, Milan 18 A2
Green I., Hong Kong 12 B1
Green Point, Cape Town 8 A1
Greenbelt, Washington 32 A4
Greenbelt Park, Washington 32 B4
Greenfield Park, Montreal 19 B3
Greenford, London 15 A1
Greenhill, London 15 A2
Greenhills, Dublin 11 B1
Greenmarket Square, Cape Town 8 c2
Greenpoint, New York 21 B2
Greenwich, London 15 B3
Greenwich Observatory, London 15 B3
Greenwich Village, New York 21 B2
Greenwood, Boston 6 A3
Grefsen, Oslo 22 A3
Gresham Park, Atlanta 3 B2
Greve Strand, Copenhagen 10 B1
Greyfriars Kirk, Edinburgh 11 c2
Griebnitzsee, Berlin 5 B1
Griffen Park, Los Angeles 16 B3
Grimbergen, Brussels 6 A2
Grinzing, Vienna 31 A2
Gröbenried, Munich 20 A1
Grochów, Warsaw 31 B2
Grodzisk, Warsaw 31 B2
Groenendaal, Brussels 6 B2
Grogol Petamburin, Jakarta 13 A1
Gronsdorf, Munich 20 B3
Grorud, Oslo 22 A4
Gross Glienicke, Berlin 5 B1
Gross-Hadern, Munich 20 B1
Gross-Lappen, Munich 20 A2
Grosse Krampe, Berlin 5 B5
Grosse Müggelsee, Berlin 5 B4
Grossenzersdorf, Vienna 31 A3
Grossenzersdorfer Arm →, Vienna 31 A3
Grosser Biberhaufen, Vienna 31 A2
Grosser Wannsee, Berlin 5 B2
Grossfeld-Siedlung, Vienna 31 A2
Grosshesselohe, Munich 20 B2
Grossjedlersdorf, Vienna 31 A2
Grossziethen, Berlin 5 B3
Grove Hall, Boston 6 B3
Grove Park, Atlanta 3 B2
Grove Park, London 15 B4
Grove Park, London 15 B2
Groveton, Washington 32 C3
Grünau, Berlin 5 B4
Grunewald, Berlin 5 B2
Grünwald, Munich 20 B2
Grünwalder Forst, Munich 20 B2
Grymes Hill, New York 21 C1
Guadalupe, Manila 17 B2
Guadalupe, Basilica de, Mexico City 18 B2
Guanabara, B. de, Rio de Janeiro 24 B1
Guanabara, Jardim, Rio de Janeiro 24 A1
Guanabara, Palácio da, Rio de Janeiro 24 B1
Guang'anmen, Beijing 4 B1
Guangqumen, Beijing 4 B2
Guangzhou, Canton 8 B2
Guanshuo, Canton 8 B3
Gudö, Stockholm 28 B3
Güell, Parque de, Barcelona 4 A2
Guerrero, Mexico City 18 a1
Guggenheim Museum, New York 21 b3
Guinardó, Barcelona 4 A2
Gulbai, Karachi 14 A1
Güngören, Istanbul 12 B1
Gunnersbury, London 15 B2
Gustavo A. Madero, Mexico City 18 B2
Guttenberg, New York 21 B1
Gutuyevskiy, Ostrov, St. Petersburg 26 B1
Guyancourt, Paris 23 B1
Gyál, Budapest 7 B3
Gyáli-patak →, Budapest 7 B2

H

Haaga, Helsinki 12 B2
Haar, Munich 20 B3
Hackbridge, London 15 B3
Hackensack, New York 21 A1
Hackensack →, New York 21 B1
Hackney, London 15 A3
Hackney Wick, London 15 A3
Haga, Stockholm 28 A2
Hagenbrunn, Vienna 31 A2
Hägersten, Stockholm 28 B1
Häggvik, Stockholm 28 A1
Hai He →, Tianjin 30 B2
Haidan, Beijing 4 B1
Haidarpur, Delhi 10 A1
Haidhausen, Munich 20 B2
Haight-Ashbury, San Francisco 25 B2
Hainault, London 15 A4
Haizhu Guangchang, Canton 8 B2
Hakunila, Helsinki 12 B3
Halásztelek, Budapest 7 B1
Haliç = Golden Horn, Istanbul 12 B1
Halim Perdanakusuma International Airport, Jakarta 13 B2
Halle, Brussels 6 B1
Haltiala, Helsinki 12 B2
Haltiavuori, Helsinki 12 B2
Ham, London 15 B2
Hämeenkylä, Helsinki 12 B1
Hammarby, Stockholm 28 B2
Hamme, Brussels 6 A1
Hammersmith, London 15 B2
Hampstead, London 15 A2
Hampstead, Montreal 19 B2
Hampstead Garden Suburb, London 15 A2
Hampstead Heath, London 15 A2
Hampton, London 15 B1
Hampton Court Palace, London 15 B1
Hampton Wick, London 15 B2
Hamrā', Baghdad 3 B1
Hanala, Helsinki 12 A3
Haneda, Tokyo 29 B3
Hang Hau, Hong Kong 12 B2
Hanging Gardens, Mumbai 20 b1
Hanjiashu, Tianjin 30 A1
Hanlon, Toronto 30 B1
Hanwell, London 15 A1
Hanworth, London 15 B1
Haora, Calcutta 8 B1
Hapeville, Atlanta 3 C2
Happy Valley, Hong Kong 12 B2
Har Adar, Jerusalem 13 B1
Haren, Brussels 6 A2
Hareskovby, Copenhagen 10 A2
Haringey, London 15 A3
Harjusuo, Helsinki 12 B3
Harlaching, Munich 20 B2
Harlaw Res., Edinburgh 11 B2
Harlem, New York 21 B2
Harlesden, London 15 A2
Harlington, London 15 B1
Harmaja, Helsinki 12 C2
Harmashatar hegy, Budapest 7 A2
Harolds Cross, Dublin 11 B2
Háros, Budapest 7 B2
Harperrig Reservoir, Edinburgh 11 B1
Harrow, London 15 A1
Harrow on the Hill, London 15 A1
Harrow School, London 15 A1
Harrow Weald, London 15 A1
Hartsfield-Atlanta International Airport, Atlanta 3 C2
Harumi, Tokyo 29 c5
Harvard Univ., Boston 6 A3
Harwood Heights, Chicago 9 B2
Hasanābād, Tehran 30 A1
Hasbrouck Heights, New York 21 A1
Haselhorst, Berlin 5 A2
Hasköy, Istanbul 12 B1
Hasle, Oslo 22 B2
Haslum, Oslo 22 A2
Hästhagen, Stockholm 28 B2
Hataitai, Wellington 32 B1
Hatch End, London 15 A1
Hatiara, Calcutta 8 B2
Hauketo, Oslo 22 A3
Havel →, Berlin 5 A2
Havelkanal, Berlin 5 A2
Havering, London 15 A5
Havering-atte-Bower, London 15 A5
Hawŏlgok, Seoul 26 B2
Haworth, New York 21 A2
Hayes, London 15 B4
Hayes, London 15 A1
Hayes End, London 15 A1
Hayford, Chicago 9 C2
Haywards, Wellington 32 A2
Heard Pond, Boston 6 A1
Heathfield, Cape Town 8 B1
Heathrow Airport, London 15 B1
Hebe Haven, Hong Kong 12 A2
Hebei, Tianjin 30 B2
Hedong, Canton 8 B2
Hedong, Tianjin 30 B2
Heidelberg Heights, Melbourne 17 A2
Heidelberg West, Melbourne 17 A2
Heidemühle, Berlin 5 B5
Heideveld, Cape Town 8 A2
Heiligensee, Berlin 5 A2
Heiligenstadt, Vienna 31 A2
Heinersdorf, Berlin 5 A3
Heldenplatz, Vienna 31 b1
Hélène Champlain, Parc, Montreal 19 A2
Helenelund, Stockholm 28 A1
Heliopolis = Masr el Gedida, Cairo 7 A2
Hellersdorf, Berlin 5 A4
Hellerup, Copenhagen 10 A3
Helmahof, Vienna 31 A3
Helsingfors = Helsinki, Helsinki 12 B2
Helsinki, Helsinki 12 B2
Helsinki Airport, Helsinki 12 B2
Hendon, London 15 A2
Hengsha, Canton 8 B2
Hennigsdorf, Berlin 5 A2
Henryków, Warsaw 31 B1
Henson Cr. →, Washington 32 C4
Henttaa, Helsinki 12 B1
Heping, Tianjin 30 B2
Heping Park, Shanghai 27 B2
Hepingli, Beijing 4 B2
Herlev, Copenhagen 10 A2
Herman Eckstein Park, Johannesburg 13 A2
Hermannskogel, Vienna 31 A1
Hermiston, Edinburgh 11 B2
Hermitage and Winter Palace, St. Petersburg 26 B1
Hermsdorf, Berlin 5 A2
Hernals, Vienna 31 A2
Herne Hill, London 15 B3
Héroes de Churubusco, Mexico City 18 B2
Herons, Î. aux, Montreal 19 B2
Herstedøster, Copenhagen 10 A2
Herttoniemi, Helsinki 12 B3
Ḥeşārak, Tehran 30 A1
Heston, London 15 B1
Hetzendorf, Vienna 31 B1
Hexi, Tianjin 30 B2
Hextable, London 15 B5
Hialeah, Miami 18 A1
Hickory Hills, Chicago 9 C2
Hiekkaharju, Helsinki 12 B3
Hietaniemi, Helsinki 12 B2
Hietzing, Vienna 31 A1
Higashi, Osaka 22 A4
Higashimurayama, Tokyo 29 A1
Higashinada, Osaka 22 A2
Higashinari, Osaka 22 A4
Higashiōsaka, Osaka 22 B4
Higashisumiyoshi, Osaka 22 B4
Higashiyodogawa, Osaka 22 A3
High Park, Toronto 30 B2
Highbury, London 15 A3
Highgate, London 15 A3
Highland Cr. →, Toronto 30 A3
Highland Creek, Toronto 30 A3
Highland Park, Los Angeles 16 B3
Highlands North, Johannesburg 13 A2
Hillcrest Heights, Washington 32 C4
Hillend, Edinburgh 11 A1
Hillingdon, London 15 A1
Hillwood, Washington 32 B3
Hilmîya, Cairo 7 A2
Hin Keng, Hong Kong 12 A2
Hingham, Boston 6 B4
Hingham B., Boston 6 B4
Hingham Harbor, Boston 6 B4
Hirakata, Osaka 22 A4
Hirota, Osaka 22 A3
Hirschstetten, Vienna 31 A2
Histórico Nacional, Museu, Rio de Janeiro 24 b3
Hither Green, London 15 B3
Hiyoshi, Tokyo 29 B2
Hizma, Jerusalem 13 B2
Hjortekær, Copenhagen 10 A3
Hjortespring, Copenhagen 10 A2
Hlubočepy, Prague 24 B2
Ho Chung, Hong Kong 12 A2
Ho Man Tin, Hong Kong 12 B2
Hoboken, New York 21 B1
Hobsons B., Melbourne 17 B1
Hochbrück, Munich 20 A2
Hochelaga, Montreal 19 A2
Hodgkins, Chicago 9 C1
Hoegi, Seoul 26 B2
Hoeilaart, Brussels 6 B2
Hofberg, Vienna 31 A2
Hoffman I., New York 21 C1
Hofgarten, Munich 20 a3
Högsdtadomstolen, Stockholm 28 c2
Hohenbrunn, Munich 20 B3
Hohenschönhausen, Berlin 5 A4
Holborn, London 15 a4
Holešovice, Prague 24 B2
Holland Village, Singapore 27 B2
Höllriegelskreuth, Munich 20 B1
Hollywood, Los Angeles 16 B3
Holmenkollen, Oslo 22 A3
Holmes Run Acres, Washington 32 B2
Holmgård, Stockholm 28 B1
Holysloot, Amsterdam 2 A3
Homerton, London 15 A3
Hometown, Chicago 9 C2
Hōnanchō, Tokyo 29 A2
Honcho, Tokyo 29 A3
Honden, Tokyo 29 A4
Hondo, Rio →, Los Angeles 16 B4
Hong Kong, Hong Kong 12 B1
Hong Kong, Univ. of, Hong Kong 12 B1
Hong Kong I., Hong Kong 12 B2
Hong Kong Park, Hong Kong 12 c1
Hongkou, Shanghai 27 B1
Hongkou Park, Shanghai 27 B1
Hongmiao, Beijing 4 B2
Hongqiao, Shanghai 27 B1
Hongqiao, Tianjin 30 B1
Hongqiao Airport, Shanghai 27 B1
Hongŭn, Seoul 26 B1
Honjyo, Tokyo 29 A3
Honoré Mercier, Pont, Montreal 19 B1
Hönow, Berlin 5 A4
Hooghly = Hugli →, Calcutta 8 A2
Hook, London 15 B2
Horikiri, Tokyo 29 A4
Horn Pond, Boston 6 A2
Hornchurch, London 15 A5
Horni, Prague 24 B3
Horni Počernice, Prague 24 B3
Hornsey, London 15 A3
Horoměřice, Prague 24 B1
Hortaleza, Madrid 17 B2
Hosoyama, Tokyo 29 B2
Hostafranchs, Barcelona 4 A1
Hostivař, Prague 24 B3
Hôtel des Invalides, Paris 23 c2
Houbětin, Prague 24 B3
Houghs Neck, Boston 6 B4
Houghton, Johannesburg 13 B2
Houilles, Paris 23 A2
Hounslow, London 15 B1
Houses of Parliament, London 15 c3
Hout Bay, Cape Town 8 B1
Hove Å →, Copenhagen 10 A1
Hovedøya, Oslo 22 A3
Høvik, Oslo 22 A2
Hovorčovice, Prague 24 A3
Howard Beach, New York 21 C2
Howth, Dublin 11 A3
Howth Head, Dublin 11 A3
Hoxton, London 15 a5
Hōya, Tokyo 29 A2
Hradčany, Prague 24 B2
Huanghuagang Mausoleum of the 72 Martyrs, Canton 8 B2
Huangpu, Shanghai 27 B2
Huangpu Jiang →, Shanghai 27 B1
Huangpu Park, Shanghai 27 B1
Huangtugang, Beijing 4 C1
Huascar, Lima 16 A2
Huay Khwang, Bangkok 3 B2
Huddinge, Stockholm 28 B2
Hudson →, New York 21 A2
Huechuraba, Santiago 26 B1
Huertas de San Beltran, Barcelona 4 A1
Hugli →, Calcutta 8 A2
Huidui, Tianjin 30 B2
Huizingen, Brussels 6 B1
Hull, Boston 6 B4
Humber →, Toronto 30 A1
Humber B., Toronto 30 B2
Humber Bay, Toronto 30 B2
Humber Summit, Toronto 30 A1
Humber Valley Village, Toronto 30 A1
Humberlea, Toronto 30 A1
Humboldt Park, Chicago 9 B2
Humera, Madrid 17 B1
Hunaydī, Baghdad 3 B2
Hundige, Copenhagen 10 B1
Hundige Strand, Copenhagen 10 B2
Hung Hom, Hong Kong 12 B2
Hunters Hill, Sydney 28 B1
Hunters Pt., San Francisco 25 B2
Hunters Valley, Washington 32 B2
Huntington, Washington 32 C3
Huntington Park, Los Angeles 16 C3
Hurīya, Baghdad 3 A1
Hurstville, Sydney 28 B1
Husby, Stockholm 28 A1
Husum, Copenhagen 10 A2
Hutt R. →, Wellington 32 B2
Hütteldorf, Vienna 31 A1
Hüvösvölgy, Budapest 7 A2
Hvalstad, Oslo 22 A1
Hvalstrand, Oslo 22 A2
Hvidovre, Copenhagen 10 B2
Hwagok, Seoul 26 B1
Hyattsville, Washington 32 B4
Hyde Park, Boston 6 B3
Hyde Park, Chicago 9 C3
Hyde Park, Johannesburg 13 A2
Hyde Park, London 15 A2
Hyde Park, Sydney 28 B2

I

Ibese, Lagos 14 A2
Ibirapuera, São Paulo 26 B1
Ibirapuera, Parque, São Paulo 26 B2
Icarai, Rio de Janeiro 24 B2
Içerenköy, Istanbul 12 C2
Ichgao, Tokyo 29 B2
Ichigaya, Tokyo 29 a3
Ichikawa, Tokyo 29 A4
Ickenham, London 15 A1
Iddo, Lagos 14 B2
Idi-Oro, Lagos 14 A2
Iganmu, Lagos 14 B2
Igbobi, Lagos 14 A2
Igbologun, Lagos 14 B1
Igny, Paris 23 B2
IJ, Het →, Amsterdam 2 A2
IJ-meer, Amsterdam 2 A3
Ijesa-Tedo, Lagos 14 B1
Ijora, Lagos 14 B2
IJtunnel, Amsterdam 2 a3
Ikebe, Tokyo 29 B2
Ikebukuro, Tokyo 29 A3
Ikegami, Tokyo 29 B3
Ikeja, Lagos 14 A2
Ikeuchi, Osaka 22 B4
Ikoyi, Lagos 14 B2
Ikuata, Lagos 14 B2
Ikuno, Osaka 22 A4
Ikuta, Osaka 22 A2
Ikuta, Tokyo 29 B2
Ila, Oslo 22 A2
Ilford, London 15 A4
Ilioúpolis, Athens 2 B2
Ilpendam, Amsterdam 2 A2
Ilsós →, Athens 2 B2
Imagem e do Som, Museu da, Rio de Janeiro 24 b3
Imbâbah, Cairo 7 A2
Imielin, Warsaw 31 C2
Imirim, São Paulo 26 A2
Imittós, Athens 2 B2
Imittoś, Óros, Athens 2 B2
Imperial Palace Museum, Beijing 4 b2
Inagi, Tokyo 29 B2
Inchcolm, Edinburgh 11 A2
Inchicore, Dublin 11 A1
Inchkeith, Edinburgh 11 A3
Inchmickery, Edinburgh 11 A2
Incirano, Milan 18 A1
Independencia, Lima 16 A2
Independencia, Santiago 26 B2
India Gate, Delhi 1 c2
Indian Creek Village, Miami 18 A2
Indian Head Park, Chicago 9 C1
Indianópolis, São Paulo 26 B2
Indios Verdes, Mexico City 18 B2
Indira Gandhi International Airport, Delhi 10 B1
Industria, Johannesburg 13 B1
Ingierstrand, Oslo 22 B3
Inglewood, Los Angeles 16 C3
Ingliston, Edinburgh 11 B1
Inhaúme, Rio de Janeiro 24 B1
Inner Port Shelter, Hong Kong 12 A2
Interlagos, São Paulo 26 C1
Intramuros, Manila 17 B1
Invalides, Paris 23 A2
Inverkeithing, Edinburgh 11 A1
Inzersdorf, Vienna 31 B2
Ipanema, Rio de Janeiro 24 B1
Ipiranga, São Paulo 26 B2
Ipiranga →, São Paulo 26 B2
Iponri, Lagos 14 B2
Ireland's Eye, Dublin 11 A3
Irving Park, Chicago 9 B2
Isabel, Rio de Janeiro 24 B1
Isagatedo, Lagos 14 A1
Isar →, Munich 20 A3
Ishbīlīya, Baghdad 3 A2
Ishikiri, Osaka 22 A4
Ishøj Strand, Copenhagen 10 B2
Island Bay, Wellington 32 B1
Island Park, Toronto 30 B2
Isle of Dogs, London 15 B3
Islev, Copenhagen 10 A2
Isleworth, London 15 B2
Islington, London 15 A3
Islington, Toronto 30 B1
Ismaning, Munich 20 A3
Ismayloskiy Park, Moscow 19 B4
Isolo, Lagos 14 A1
Issy-les-Moulineaux, Paris 23 B2
Istanbul, Istanbul 12 C1
Istanbul Boğazi, Istanbul 12 B2
Istinye, Istanbul 12 B2
Itä Hakkila, Helsinki 12 B3
Itaewŏn, Seoul 26 B1
Itahanga, Rio de Janeiro 24 B1
Itami, Osaka 22 A3
Ivanhoe, Melbourne 17 A2
Ivry-sur-Seine, Paris 23 B3
Iwazono, Osaka 22 A2
Ixelles, Brussels 6 B2
Izmaylovo, Moscow 19 B4
Iztacalco, Mexico City 18 B2
Iztapalapa, Mexico City 18 B2

J

Jaba, Jerusalem 13 A2
Jababpur, Calcutta 8 C2
Jacaré, Rio de Janeiro 24 B1
Jackson Heights, New York 21 B2
Jackson Park, Chicago 9 C3
Jacques Cartier, Montreal 19 A3
Jacques Cartier, Pont, Montreal 19 A2
Jade Buddha Temple, Shanghai 27 B1
Jægersborg, Copenhagen 10 A3
Jægersborg Dyrehave, Copenhagen 10 A3
Jagadishpur, Calcutta 8 B1
Jagatpur, Delhi 10 A2
Jaguaré, Rib. do →, São Paulo 26 B1
Jahangirpur, Delhi 10 A2
Jakarta, Jakarta 13 A2
Jakarta, Teluk, Jakarta 13 A1
Jalan Kayu, Singapore 27 A3
Jamaica B., New York 21 C3
Jamaica Plain, Boston 6 B3
Jamakpuri, Delhi 10 B1
Jamshīdīyeh, Tehran 30 A2
Janki, Warsaw 31 C1
Jannali, Sydney 28 C1
Japan Center, San Francisco 25 c1
Jaraguá, São Paulo 26 A1
Jaraguá, Pico de, São Paulo 26 A1
Jardim Paulista, São Paulo 26 B1
Jardin Botanique, Brussels 6 a3
Järvatältet, Stockholm 28 A1
Jaskhar, Mumbai 20 B2
Jatinegara, Jakarta 13 B2
Javādīyeh, Tehran 30 B2
Jaworowa, Warsaw 31 C1
Jedlesee, Vienna 31 A2
Jefferson Memorial, Washington 32 c1
Jefferson Park, Chicago 9 B2
Jelonki, Warsaw 31 B1
Jerónimos, Mosteiro dos, Lisbon 14 A1
Jersey City, New York 21 B1
Jerusalem, Jerusalem 13 B2
Jésus, Î., Montreal 19 A1
Jesús Maria, Lima 16 B2
Jette, Brussels 6 A1
Jewish Quarter, Jerusalem 13 b3
Jey, Tehran 30 B2
Jianguomen, Beijing 4 B2
Jiangwan, Shanghai 27 B1
Jianshan Park, Tianjin 30 B2
Jihād, Baghdad 3 B1
Jim Thompson's House, Bangkok 3 b3
Jimbōchō, Tokyo 29 a4
Jingan, Shanghai 27 B1
Jingu Outer Garden, Tokyo 29 b2
Jinočany, Prague 24 B1
Jinonice, Prague 24 B2
Jiyūgaoka, Tokyo 29 B3
Jizā'ir, Baghdad 3 B2
Jizīra, Baghdad 3 B2
Johannesburg, Johannesburg 13 B2
Johanneskirchen, Munich 20 A2
Johannesstift, Berlin 5 A2
Johannisthal, Berlin 5 B4
John Hancock Center, Chicago 9 a2
John McLaren Park, San Francisco 25 B2
Johnsonville, Wellington 32 B1
Joinville-le-Pont, Paris 23 B3
Joli-Bois, Brussels 6 B2
Jollas, Helsinki 12 B3
Jonstrup, Copenhagen 10 A2
Joppa, Edinburgh 11 B3
Jorge Chavez, Aeropuerto Int., Lima 16 B2
Jorge Newbury, Aeroparque, Buenos Aires 7 B2
Jósefa Piłsudskiego Park, Warsaw 31 B1
Jōtō, Osaka 22 A4
Jouy-en-Josas, Paris 23 B2
Juan Anchorena, Buenos Aires 7 A2
Juan González Romero, Mexico City 18 A2
Judeira, Jerusalem 13 A2
Juhu, Mumbai 20 A2
Jūjā, Tokyo 29 A3
Jukskeirivier →, Johannesburg 13 A2
Julianów, Warsaw 31 B2
Jungfernheide, Volkspark, Berlin 5 A2
Jungfernsee, Berlin 5 B1
Juniper Green, Edinburgh 11 B2
Junk B., Hong Kong 12 B2
Jurong, Singapore 27 B2
Jurong, Selat, Singapore 27 B2
Jurong Industrial Estate, Singapore 27 B1
Jurujuba, Enseada de, Rio de Janeiro 24 B2
Jūsō, Osaka 22 A3
Justice, Chicago 9 C2
Justicia, Madrid 17 a3
Jwalahari, Delhi 10 B1

K

Kabaty, Warsaw 31 C2
Kadıköy, Istanbul 12 C2
Kadoma, Osaka 22 A4
Kaebong, Seoul 26 C1
Kafr 'Aqab, Jerusalem 13 A2
Kâğıthane, Istanbul 12 B1
Kâğıthane →, Istanbul 12 B1
Kagran, Vienna 31 A2
Kahnawake, Montreal 19 B1
Kaimes, Edinburgh 11 B2
Kaisariani, Athens 2 B2
Kaiser Wilhelm Kirche, Berlin 5 b2
Kaiserebersdorf, Vienna 31 B2
Kaivoksela, Helsinki 12 B2
Kalamákion, Athens 2 B2
Kalbadevi, Mumbai 20 b2
Kalhyŏn, Seoul 26 B1
Kalipur, Calcutta 8 A1
Kalkaji, Delhi 10 B2
Kallithéa, Athens 2 B2
Kalveboderne, Copenhagen 10 B3
Kamarhati, Calcutta 8 A2
Kamata, Tokyo 29 B3
Kameari, Tokyo 29 A4
Kameido, Tokyo 29 A4
Kami-Itabashi, Tokyo 29 A3
Kamikitazawa, Tokyo 29 B2
Kamitsuruma, Tokyo 29 B1
Kamoshida, Tokyo 29 B2
Kampong Landang, Singapore 27 A3
Kampong Tanjong Penjuru, Singapore 27 B2
Kampung Bali, Jakarta 13 B1
Kanamori, Tokyo 29 B1
Kanda, Tokyo 29 a5
Kandilli, Istanbul 12 B2
Kangdong, Seoul 26 B2
Kangnam, Seoul 26 B1
Kangsŏ, Seoul 26 B1
Kankurgachi, Calcutta 8 B2
Kanlıca, Istanbul 12 B2
Kanonerskiy, Ostrov, St. Petersburg 26 B1
Kanzaki →, Osaka 22 A3

Kapellerfeld, *Vienna* 31 A2
Káposztásmegyer, *Budapest* 7 A2
Kapotnya, *Moscow* 19 C4
Käppala, *Stockholm* 28 A3
Käpylä, *Helsinki* 12 B2
Karachi, *Karachi* 14 A2
Karachi Int. Airport, *Karachi* 14 A2
Karato, *Osaka* 22 A2
Karibong, *Seoul* 26 C1
Karkh, *Baghdad* 3 A2
Karlin, *Prague* 24 B2
Karlsfeld, *Munich* 20 A1
Karlshorst, *Berlin* 5 B4
Karlsplatz, *Munich* 20 b1
Karntner Strasse, *Vienna* 31 b2
Karol Bagh, *Delhi* 10 B2
Karolinenhof, *Berlin* 5 B4
Karori, *Wellington* 32 B1
Karow, *Berlin* 5 A3
Karrādah, *Baghdad* 3 B2
Kärsön, *Stockholm* 28 B1
Kasai, *Tokyo* 29 B4
Kashiwara, *Osaka* 22 B4
Kastellet, *Copenhagen* 10 a3
Kastrup, *Copenhagen* 10 B3
Kastrup Lufthavn, *Copenhagen* 10 B3
Kasuga, *Tokyo* 29 A2
Kasuge, *Tokyo* 29 A3
Kasumigaseki, *Tokyo* 29 b4
Katong, *Singapore* 27 B3
Katrineberg, *Stockholm* 28 B1
Katsushika-Ku, *Tokyo* 29 A4
Kau Pei Chau, *Hong Kong* 12 B2
Kau Yi Chau, *Hong Kong* 12 B1
Kaulsdorf, *Berlin* 5 B4
Kauniainen, *Helsinki* 12 B1
Kawasaki, *Tokyo* 29 B3
Kawawa, *Tokyo* 29 B2
Kawęczyn, *Warsaw* 31 B2
Kayu Putih, *Jakarta* 13 B2
Kbely, *Prague* 24 B3
Kebayoran Baru, *Jakarta* 13 B1
Kebayoran Lama, *Jakarta* 13 B1
Kebon Jeruk, *Jakarta* 13 B1
Kedar, *Jerusalem* 13 B2
Keilor, *Melbourne* 17 A1
Keilor North, *Melbourne* 17 A1
Keimola, *Helsinki* 12 A1
Kelenföld, *Budapest* 7 B2
Kelvin, *Johannesburg* 13 A2
Kemang, *Jakarta* 13 B1
Kemayoran, *Jakarta* 13 B2
Kemerburgaz, *Istanbul* 12 B1
Kempton Park Races, *London* 15 B1
Kendall Green, *Boston* 6 A2
Kenilworth, *Cape Town* 8 A1
Kennedy Town, *Hong Kong* 12 B1
Kennington, *London* 15 c4
Kensal Green, *London* 15 A2
Kensal Rise, *London* 15 a1
Kensington, *Johannesburg* 13 B2
Kensington, *London* 15 B2
Kensington, *New York* 21 C2
Kensington, *Sydney* 28 B2
Kensington Palace, *London* 15 A2
Kent Village, *Washington* 32 B4
Kentish Town, *London* 15 A3
Kenton, *London* 15 A2
Kenwood House, *London* 15 A3
Kepa, *Warsaw* 31 B2
Keppel Harbour, *Singapore* 27 B2
Keramíkos, *Athens* 2 b1
Kettering, *Washington* 32 B5
Kew, *London* 15 B2
Kew, *Melbourne* 17 A2
Kew Gardens, *London* 15 B2
Kew Gardens, *Toronto* 30 B3
Key Biscayne, *Miami* 18 B2
Khaidhárion, *Athens* 2 A1
Khalándrion, *Athens* 2 A2
Khalīj, *Baghdad* 3 B2
Khandallah, *Wellington* 32 B1
Khansā', *Baghdad* 3 A2
Kharavli, *Mumbai* 20 B2
Khefren, *Cairo* 7 B1
Khichripur, *Delhi* 10 B2
Khidirpur, *Calcutta* 8 B1
Khimki-Khovrino, *Moscow* 19 A3
Khirbet Jub e-Rum, *Jerusalem* 13 B2
Khlong San, *Bangkok* 3 B2
Khlong Toey, *Bangkok* 3 B2
Kholargós, *Athens* 2 B2
Khorel, *Calcutta* 8 A1
Khorosovo, *Moscow* 19 B2
Kiamari, *Karachi* 14 B1
Kierling, *Vienna* 31 A1
Kierlingbach →, *Vienna* 31 A1
Kifisós →, *Athens* 2 B2
Kikuna, *Tokyo* 29 B2
Kilbarrack, *Dublin* 11 A3
Kilbirnie, *Wellington* 32 B1
Kilburn, *London* 15 A2
Killakee, *Dublin* 11 B2
Killester, *Dublin* 11 A2
Killiney, *Dublin* 11 B3
Killiney Bay, *Dublin* 11 B3
Kilmacud, *Dublin* 11 B2
Kilmainham, *Dublin* 11 A2
Kilmashogue Mt., *Dublin* 11 B2
Kilmore, *Dublin* 11 A2
Kilnamanagh, *Dublin* 11 B1
Kilo, *Helsinki* 12 B1
Kilokri, *Delhi* 10 B2
Kiltiernan, *Dublin* 11 B2
Kimmage, *Dublin* 11 B2
Kindi, *Baghdad* 3 B2
Kinghorn, *Edinburgh* 11 A2
King's Cross, *London* 15 a4
Kings Cross, *Sydney* 28 c3
Kings Domain, *Melbourne* 17 A1
Kings Park, *Washington* 32 C2
Kings Park West, *Washington* 32 C2
Kingsbury, *London* 15 A2
Kingsbury, *Melbourne* 17 A2
Kingsford, *Sydney* 28 B2
Kingston upon Thames, *London* 15 B2
Kingston Vale, *London* 15 B2
Kingsway, *Toronto* 30 B1
Kinsaley, *Dublin* 11 A2
Kipling Heights, *Toronto* 30 A1
Kipséli, *Athens* 2 B2
Kirchstockbach, *Munich* 20 B3
Kirchtrudering, *Munich* 20 B3
Kirikiri, *Lagos* 14 B1
Kirke Værløse, *Copenhagen* 10 A1
Kirkhill, *Edinburgh* 11 B2
Kirkliston, *Edinburgh* 11 B1
Kirknewton, *Edinburgh* 11 B1
Kirov Palace of Culture, *St. Petersburg* 26 B1
Kısıklı, *Istanbul* 12 B2
Kispest, *Budapest* 7 B2
Kista, *Stockholm* 28 A1
Kita, *Osaka* 22 A4
Kita-Ku, *Tokyo* 29 A3
Kitazawa, *Tokyo* 29 B3
Kiu Tsiu, *Hong Kong* 12 A2
Kivistö, *Helsinki* 12 B2
Kızıltoprak, *Istanbul* 12 C2
Kizu →, *Osaka* 22 B3
Kizuri, *Osaka* 22 B4
Kjelsås, *Oslo* 22 A3
Kladow, *Berlin* 5 B1
Klampenborg, *Copenhagen* 10 A3
Klaudyń, *Warsaw* 31 B1
Klecany, *Prague* 24 A2
Kledering, *Vienna* 31 B2
Klein Jukskei →, *Johannesburg* 13 A1
Kleinmachnow, *Berlin* 5 B2
Kleinschönebeck, *Berlin* 5 B5
Klemetsrud, *Oslo* 22 A4
Kličany, *Prague* 24 A2
Klipriviersberg Nature Reserve, *Johannesburg* 13 B2
Klosterneuburg, *Vienna* 31 A1
Knesset, *Jerusalem* 13 b1
Knightsbridge, *London* 15 c2
Köbánya, *Budapest* 7 B2
Kobbegem, *Brussels* 6 A1
Kōbe, *Osaka* 22 A2
Kōbe Harbour, *Osaka* 22 B2
København, *Copenhagen* 10 A2
Kobylisy, *Prague* 24 B2
Kobyłka, *Warsaw* 31 A3
Kŏch'ŏk, *Seoul* 26 B1
Kodaira, *Tokyo* 29 A1
Kodanaka, *Tokyo* 29 B2
Kodenmacho, *Tokyo* 29 a5
Koekelberg, *Brussels* 6 A1
Koganei, *Tokyo* 29 A2
Kogarah, *Sydney* 28 B1
Køge Bugt, *Copenhagen* 10 B2
Koivupää, *Helsinki* 12 B2
Koja, *Jakarta* 13 A2
Koja Utara, *Jakarta* 13 A2
Kokobunji, *Tokyo* 29 A1
Kokobunji-Temple, *Tokyo* 29 A4
Kolarängen, *Stockholm* 28 B3
Kolbotn, *Oslo* 22 B3
Kolkata, *Calcutta* 8 B2
Koło, *Warsaw* 31 B1
Kolokinthóu, *Athens* 2 B2
Kolomyagi, *St. Petersburg* 26 A1
Kolónos, *Athens* 2 B2
Kolsås, *Oslo* 22 A2
Komae, *Tokyo* 29 B2
Komagome, *Tokyo* 29 A3
Komazawa, *Tokyo* 29 B3
Kona, *Calcutta* 8 B1
Konala, *Helsinki* 12 B2
Kondli, *Delhi* 10 B2
Kongelige Slottet, *Oslo* 22 a1
Kongelunden, *Copenhagen* 10 B3
Kongens Lyngby, *Copenhagen* 10 A3
Kongnŭng, *Seoul* 26 B2
Kongo, *Helsinki* 12 A1
Koninklijk Paleis, *Amsterdam* 2 b2
Konnagar, *Calcutta* 8 A2
Konohana, *Osaka* 22 A3
Kōnoike, *Osaka* 22 A4
Konradshöhe, *Berlin* 5 A2
Kopanina, *Prague* 24 B1
Koparkhairna, *Mumbai* 20 A2
Köpenick, *Berlin* 5 B4
Korangi, *Karachi* 14 B2
Koremasa, *Tokyo* 29 B1
Korenevo, *Moscow* 19 B6
Kori, *Osaka* 22 A4
Koridhallós, *Athens* 2 B1
Korokoro, *Wellington* 32 B2
Korokoro Stream →, *Wellington* 32 B2
Kosino, *Moscow* 19 B5
Kosugi, *Tokyo* 29 B2
Kota, *Jakarta* 13 A1
Kotelyniki, *Moscow* 19 C5
Kōtō-Ku, *Tokyo* 29 A3
Kotrung, *Calcutta* 8 A2
Kouponia, *Athens* 2 B2
Kowloon, *Hong Kong* 12 B1
Kowloon Park, *Hong Kong* 12 a2
Kowloon Peak, *Hong Kong* 12 A2
Kowloon Res., *Hong Kong* 12 A1
Kowloon Tong, *Hong Kong* 12 A2
Kozhukhovo, *Moscow* 19 B5
Kraainem, *Brussels* 6 A2
Krailling, *Munich* 20 B1
Krampnitz, *Berlin* 5 B1
Krampnitzsee, *Berlin* 5 B1
Kranji, Sungei →, *Singapore* 27 A2
Kranji Industrial Estate, *Singapore* 27 A2
Kraskovo, *Moscow* 19 C5
Krasno-Presnenskaya, *Moscow* 19 B3
Krasnogorsk, *Moscow* 19 B1
Krč, *Prague* 24 B2
Krestovskiye, Ostrov, *St. Petersburg* 26 B1
Kreuzberg, *Berlin* 5 A3
Kritzendorf, *Vienna* 31 A1
Krumme Lanke, *Berlin* 5 B2
Krummensee, *Berlin* 5 A5
Krung Thep, *Bangkok* 3 B2
Krusboda, *Stockholm* 28 B3
Krylatskoye, *Moscow* 19 B2
Küçükköy, *Istanbul* 12 B1
Kudankita, *Tokyo* 29 a3
Kudrovo, *St. Petersburg* 26 B3
Kulosaari, *Helsinki* 12 B3
Kulturforum, *Berlin* 5 b3
Kultury i Nauki, Palac, *Warsaw* 31 b2
Kŭmch'ŏn, *Seoul* 26 C1
Kumla, *Stockholm* 28 B3
Kungens kurva, *Stockholm* 28 B1
Kungliga Slottet, *Stockholm* 28 b2
Kungshatt, *Stockholm* 28 B1
Kungsholmen, *Stockholm* 28 A2
Kuningan, *Jakarta* 13 B1
Kunitachi, *Tokyo* 29 A1
Kunming Hu, *Beijing* 4 B1
Kunratice, *Prague* 24 B2
Kunsthistorischesmuseum, *Vienna* 31 b1
Kuntsevo, *Moscow* 19 B2
Kupchino, *St. Petersburg* 26 B2
Kurbağalı →, *Istanbul* 12 C2
Kurihara, *Tokyo* 29 A2
Kurla, *Mumbai* 20 A2
Kurmuri, *Mumbai* 20 A2
Kurume, *Tokyo* 29 A2
Kuryanovo, *Moscow* 19 C4
Kuskovo, *Moscow* 19 B4
Kustia, *Calcutta* 8 B2
Kutsino, *Moscow* 19 B5
Kuzguncuk, *Istanbul* 12 B2
Kuzyminki, *Moscow* 19 B4
Kwai Chung, *Hong Kong* 12 A1
Kwanak, *Seoul* 26 C1
Kwanak-san, *Seoul* 26 C1
Kyje, *Prague* 24 B3
Kyūhōji, *Osaka* 22 B4

L

La Blanca, *Santiago* 26 C2
La Boca, *Buenos Aires* 7 B2
La Bretèche, *Paris* 23 A1
La Campiña, *Lima* 16 C2
La Celle-St.-Cloud, *Paris* 23 A1
La Ciudadela, *Mexico City* 18 c2
La Courneuve, *Paris* 23 A3
La Dehesa, *Santiago* 26 B2
La Encantada, *Lima* 16 C2
La Estación, *Madrid* 17 B1
La Floresta, *Barcelona* 4 A1
La Fortuna, *Madrid* 17 B1
La Fransa, *Barcelona* 4 A1
La Garenne-Colombes, *Paris* 23 A2
La Giustiniana, *Rome* 25 B1
La Grange, *Chicago* 9 C1
La Grange Park, *Chicago* 9 C1
La Granja, *Santiago* 26 C2
La Guardia Airport, *New York* 21 B2
La Hulpe, *Brussels* 6 B2
La Llacuna, *Barcelona* 4 A2
La Loma, *Mexico City* 18 A1
La Lucila, *Buenos Aires* 7 B2
La Maladrerie, *Paris* 23 A1
La Milla, Cerro, *Lima* 16 B2
La Monachina, *Rome* 25 B1
La Moraleja, *Madrid* 17 A2
La Nopalera, *Mexico City* 18 C2
La Paternal, *Buenos Aires* 7 B2
La Perla, *Lima* 16 B2
La Perouse, *Sydney* 28 B2
La Pineda, *Barcelona* 4 B1
La Pisana, *Rome* 25 B1
La Prairie, *Montreal* 19 B3
La Punta, *Lima* 16 B1
La Puntigala, *Barcelona* 4 A2
La Queue-en-Brie, *Paris* 23 B4
La Reina, *Santiago* 26 B2
La Ribera, *Barcelona* 4 A1
La Sagrera, *Barcelona* 4 A2
La Salada, *Buenos Aires* 7 C2
La Scala, *Milan* 18 B2
La Storta, *Rome* 25 A1
La Taxonera, *Barcelona* 4 A2
La Victoria, *Lima* 16 B2
Laajalahti, *Helsinki* 12 B1
Laajasalo, *Helsinki* 12 B3
Laaksolahti, *Helsinki* 12 B1
Lablâba, W. el →, *Cairo* 7 A2
Lac Cisterna, *Santiago* 26 C2
Lachine, *Montreal* 19 B1
Lad Phrao, *Bangkok* 3 B2
Ladera Heights, *Los Angeles* 16 C2
Ládvi, *Prague* 24 B2
Łady, *Warsaw* 31 C1
Lafontaine, Parc, *Montreal* 19 A2
Lagoa, *Rio de Janeiro* 24 B1
Lagos, *Lagos* 14 B2
Lagos Harbour, *Lagos* 14 B2
Lagos-Ikeja Airport, *Lagos* 14 A1
Lagos Island, *Lagos* 14 B2
Lagos Lagoon, *Lagos* 14 B2
Laguna de B., *Manila* 17 C2
Laim, *Munich* 20 B2
Lainate, *Milan* 18 A1
Lainz, *Vienna* 31 B1
Lakemba, *Sydney* 28 B1
Lakeside, *Cape Town* 8 B1
Lakeside, *Johannesburg* 13 A2
Lakeview, *Chicago* 9 B3
Lakewood Park, *Atlanta* 3 B2
Lakhtinskiy, *St. Petersburg* 26 B1
Lakhtinskiy Razliv, Oz., *St. Petersburg* 26 B1
Lakshmanpur, *Calcutta* 8 B1
Lal Qila, *Delhi* 1 a3
Lam Tin, *Hong Kong* 12 B2
Lambert, *Oslo* 22 A3
Lambeth, *London* 15 B3
Lambrate, *Milan* 18 B2
Lambro, Parco, *Milan* 18 B2
Lambton Mills, *Toronto* 30 B1
Lamma I., *Hong Kong* 12 B1
Landover Hills, *Washington* 32 B4
Landsmeer, *Amsterdam* 2 A2
Landstrasse, *Vienna* 31 A2
Landwehr kanal, *Berlin* 5 B3
Lane Cove, *Sydney* 28 A1
Lane Cove National Park, *Sydney* 28 A1
Langa, *Cape Town* 8 A2
Langenzersdorf, *Vienna* 31 A2
Langer See, *Berlin* 5 B4
Langley, *Washington* 32 B2
Langley Park, *Washington* 32 B4
Langwald, *Munich* 20 A1
Lanham, *Washington* 32 B4
Lankwitz, *Berlin* 5 B3
L'Annunziatella, *Rome* 25 C2
Lansdowne, *Cape Town* 8 A2
Lansing, *Toronto* 30 A2
Lanús, *Buenos Aires* 7 C2
Lapa, *Rio de Janeiro* 24 B1
Laranjeiras, *Rio de Janeiro* 24 B1
Larísa Sta., *Athens* 2 a1
Las, *Warsaw* 31 B2
Las Corts, *Barcelona* 4 A1
Las Kabacki, *Warsaw* 31 C2
Las Pinas, *Manila* 17 C1
Las Rejas, *Santiago* 26 B1
Lasalle, *Montreal* 19 B2
Lasek Bielański, *Warsaw* 31 B1
Lasek Na Kole, *Warsaw* 31 B1
Laski, *Warsaw* 31 B1
Latina, *Madrid* 17 B1
Laurence G. Hanscom Field, *Boston* 6 A2
Lauttasaari, *Helsinki* 12 C2
Laval, *Montreal* 19 A1
Lavīzān, *Tehran* 30 A2
Lavradio, *Lisbon* 14 A2
Lawndale, *Chicago* 9 B2
Lawrence Heights, *Toronto* 30 A2
Layari, *Karachi* 14 A2
Layari →, *Karachi* 14 A1
Lazare, Gare St., *Paris* 23 a3
Łazienkowski, Palac, *Warsaw* 31 c3
Łazienkowski Park, *Warsaw* 31 B2
Le Blanc-Mesnil, *Paris* 23 A3
Le Bourget, *Paris* 23 A3
Le Chenoi, *Brussels* 6 B2
Le Chesnay, *Paris* 23 B1
Le Christ de Saclay, *Paris* 23 B2
Le Kremlin-Bicêtre, *Paris* 23 B3
Le Mesnil-le-Roi, *Paris* 23 A1
Le Pecq, *Paris* 23 A1
Le Perreux, *Paris* 23 A3
Le Pin, *Paris* 23 A4
Le Plessis-Robinson, *Paris* 23 B2
Le Plessis-Trévise, *Paris* 23 B4
Le Port-Marly, *Paris* 23 A1
Le Pré-St.-Gervais, *Paris* 23 A3
Le Raincy, *Paris* 23 A4
Le Vésinet, *Paris* 23 A1
Lea Bridge, *London* 15 A3
Leaside, *Toronto* 30 A2
Leblon, *Rio de Janeiro* 24 B1
Lee, *London* 15 B4
Leganés, *Madrid* 17 C1
Legazpi, *Madrid* 17 B1
Lehtisaari, *Helsinki* 12 B2
Lei Yue Mun, *Hong Kong* 12 B2
Leião, *Lisbon* 14 A1
Leicester Square, *London* 15 b3
Leichhardt, *Sydney* 28 B1
Leith, *Edinburgh* 11 B3
Lemoyne, *Montreal* 19 B3
Lenin, *Moscow* 19 B3
Lenino, *Moscow* 19 C3
Leninskiye Gory, *Moscow* 19 B3
Lennox, *Los Angeles* 16 C2
Leonia, *New York* 21 A2
Leopardstown, *Dublin* 11 B2
Leopoldau, *Vienna* 31 A2
Leopoldstadt, *Vienna* 31 A2
Leportovo, *Moscow* 19 B4
Leppävaara, *Helsinki* 12 B1
Les Lilas, *Paris* 23 A3
Les Loges-en-Josas, *Paris* 23 B1
Les Pavillons-sous-Bois, *Paris* 23 A4
Lésigny, *Paris* 23 B4
Lesnozavodskaya, *St. Petersburg* 26 B2
L'Étang-la-Ville, *Paris* 23 A1
Letná, *Prague* 24 a1
Letňany, *Prague* 24 B3
Levallois-Perret, *Paris* 23 A2
Levent, *Istanbul* 12 B2
Lewisdale, *Washington* 32 B4
Lewisham, *London* 15 B3
Lexington, *Boston* 6 A2
Leyton, *London* 15 A3
Leytonstone, *London* 15 A4
L'Hay-les-Roses, *Paris* 23 B3
L'Hospitalet de Llobregat, *Barcelona* 4 A1
Lhotka, *Prague* 24 B2
Liangshui He →, *Beijing* 4 C2
Lianhua Chi, *Beijing* 4 B1
Lianhua He →, *Beijing* 4 B1
Libčice nad Vitavou, *Prague* 24 A2
Libeň, *Prague* 24 B2
Liberdade, *São Paulo* 26 B2
Liberdade, Ave da, *Lisbon* 14 b1
Liberton, *Edinburgh* 11 B3
Liberty I., *New York* 21 B1
Liberty State Park, *New York* 21 B1
Libeznice, *Prague* 24 A2
Library of Congress, *Washington* 32 c3
Libuš, *Prague* 24 B2
Lichiao, *Canton* 8 B2
Lichtenburg, *Berlin* 5 A4
Lichterfelde, *Berlin* 5 B2
Lidingö, *Stockholm* 28 A2
Lieshi Lingyuan, *Canton* 8 B2
Liesing, *Vienna* 31 B1
Liesing →, *Vienna* 31 B2
Liffey, R. →, *Dublin* 11 A1
Ligovo, *St. Petersburg* 26 C1
Lijordet, *Oslo* 22 A2
Likavitos, *Athens* 2 b3
Likhoborka →, *Moscow* 19 A3
Lilla Värtan, *Stockholm* 28 A3
Lille Værløse, *Copenhagen* 10 A2
Liluah, *Calcutta* 8 B1
Lim Chu Kang, *Singapore* 27 A2
Lima, *Lima* 16 B2
Limbiate, *Milan* 18 A1
Limehouse, *London* 15 A3
Limeil-Brévannes, *Paris* 23 B3
Linate, Aeroporto Internazionale di, *Milan* 18 B2
Linbropark, *Johannesburg* 13 A2
Lincoln, *Boston* 6 A2
Lincoln Center, *New York* 21 b2
Lincoln Heights, *Los Angeles* 16 B3
Lincoln Park, *Chicago* 9 B3
Lincoln Park, *New York* 21 B1
Lincoln Park, *San Francisco* 25 B1
Lincolnwood, *Chicago* 9 A2
Linda-a-Pastora, *Lisbon* 14 A1
Linden, *Johannesburg* 13 A2
Linden, *Wellington* 32 A1
Lindenberg, *Berlin* 5 A4
Lindøya, *Oslo* 22 A3
Liniers, *Buenos Aires* 7 B1
Linkebeek, *Brussels* 6 B2
Linksfield, *Johannesburg* 13 A2
Linmeyer, *Johannesburg* 13 B2
Linna, *Helsinki* 12 A2
Lintuvaara, *Helsinki* 12 B1
Lion Rock Country Park, *Hong Kong* 12 A2
Lioúmi, *Athens* 2 B2
Liqizhuang, *Tianjin* 30 B2
Lisboa, *Lisbon* 14 A2
Lisbon = Lisboa, *Lisbon* 14 A2
Lishui, *Canton* 8 A1
Little B., *Sydney* 28 B2
Little Calumet →, *Chicago* 9 D3
Little Ferry, *New York* 21 A1
Little Italy, *New York* 21 e2
Little Mermaid, *Copenhagen* 10 a3
Little Rouge →, *Toronto* 30 A4
Little Tokyo, *Los Angeles* 16 c2
Liuhang, *Shanghai* 27 A1
Liurong Temple, *Canton* 8 B2
Liuxi →, *Canton* 8 B2
Liverpool Street, *London* 15 a5
Livry-Gargan, *Paris* 23 A4
Ljan, *Oslo* 22 A3
Llano de Can Gineu, *Barcelona* 4 A2
Llobregat →, *Barcelona* 4 A1
Lo Aranguiz, *Santiago* 26 B2
Lo Boza, *Santiago* 26 B1
Lo Chau, *Hong Kong* 12 B2
Lo Espejo, *Santiago* 26 C1
Lo Hermida, *Santiago* 26 B2
Lo Prado, *Santiago* 26 B1
Lo So Shing, *Hong Kong* 12 B1
Lo Wai, *Hong Kong* 12 A1
Loanhead, *Edinburgh* 11 B3
Lobau, *Vienna* 31 A3
Lobos, Pt., *San Francisco* 25 B1
Locham, *Munich* 20 B1
Lochino, *Moscow* 19 B1
Lochkov, *Prague* 24 B2
Lockhausen, *Munich* 20 A1
Lodi, *New York* 21 A1
Lodi Estate, *Delhi* 10 B2
Logan Int. Airport, *Boston* 6 A4
Logan Square, *Chicago* 9 B2
Lognes-Émerainville, Aérodrome de, *Paris* 23 B4
Löhme, *Berlin* 5 A5
Lolokhet, *Karachi* 14 A2
Lomas Chapultepec, *Mexico City* 18 B1
Lomas de San Angel Inn, *Mexico City* 18 B1
Lomas de Zamora, *Buenos Aires* 7 C2
Lombardy East, *Johannesburg* 13 A2
Łomianki, *Warsaw* 31 A1
Lomus Reforma, *Mexico City* 18 B1
London, *London* 15 A3
London Bridge, *London* 15 b5
London City Airport, *London* 15 A4
London Zoo, *London* 15 A3
Long B., *Sydney* 28 B2
Long Branch, *Toronto* 30 B1
Long Brook →, *Washington* 32 C2
Long Ditton, *London* 15 B2
Long I., *Boston* 6 B4
Long Island City, *New York* 21 B2
Long Street, *Cape Town* 8 c2
Longchamp, Hippodrôme de, *Paris* 23 A2
Longhua Pagoda, *Shanghai* 27 B1
Longhua Park, *Shanghai* 27 B1
Longjohn Slough, *Chicago* 9 C1
Longtan Hu →, *Beijing* 4 B2
Longue-Pointe, *Montreal* 19 A2
Longueuil, *Montreal* 19 A3
Loni, *Delhi* 10 A2
Loop, The, *Chicago* 9 c1
Lord's Cricket Ground, *London* 15 A2
Loreto, *Milan* 18 B2
Los Angeles Int. Airport, *Los Angeles* 16 C2
Los Cerrillos, Aeropuerto, *Santiago* 26 B1
Los Nietos, *Los Angeles* 16 C4
Los Olivos, *Lima* 16 A2
Los Reyes, *Mexico City* 18 B2
Lot, *Brussels* 6 B1
Loughlinstown, *Dublin* 11 B3
Loures, *Lisbon* 14 A1
Louveciennes, *Paris* 23 A1
Louvre, Musée du, *Paris* 23 b4
Louvre, Palais du, *Paris* 23 b4
Lower East Side, *New York* 21 e2
Lower Hutt, *Wellington* 32 B2
Lower Manhattan, *New York* 21 e1
Lower New York B., *New York* 21 C1
Lower Shing Mun Res., *Hong Kong* 12 A1
Lowry Bay, *Wellington* 32 B2
Lu Xun Museum, *Beijing* 4 b1
Lübars, *Berlin* 5 A3
Ludwigsfeld, *Munich* 20 A1
Luhu, *Canton* 8 B2
Lumiar, *Lisbon* 14 A2
Lumphini Park, *Bangkok* 3 B2
Lundtofte, *Copenhagen* 10 A3
Lung Mei, *Hong Kong* 12 A2
Luojiang, *Canton* 8 B2
Lustheim, *Munich* 20 A2
Luwan, *Shanghai* 27 B1
Luxembourg, Palais du, *Paris* 23 c4
Luzhniki Sports Centre, *Moscow* 19 B3
Lyndhurst, *New York* 21 B1
Lynn, *Boston* 6 A4
Lynn Harbor, *Boston* 6 A4
Lynn Woods Res., *Boston* 6 A3
Lyon, Gare de, *Paris* 23 c5
Lyons, *Chicago* 9 C2
Lysaker, *Oslo* 22 A2
Lysakerselva →, *Oslo* 22 A2
Lysolaje, *Prague* 24 B2
Lyubertsy, *Moscow* 19 B5
Lyublino, *Moscow* 19 B4

M

Ma Nam Wat, *Hong Kong* 12 A2
Ma On Shan Country Park, *Hong Kong* 12 A2
Ma'ale Adumim, *Jerusalem* 13 B2
Ma'ale Ha Khamisha, *Jerusalem* 13 B1
Ma'ale Mikhmas, *Jerusalem* 13 A2
Maantiekylä, *Helsinki* 12 A3
Maarifa, *Baghdad* 3 B2
Mabato Pt., *Manila* 17 C2
Macaco, Morro do, *Rio de Janeiro* 24 B2
McCook, *Chicago* 9 C2
Machelen, *Brussels* 6 A2
Machida, *Tokyo* 29 B1
Maciołki, *Warsaw* 31 B2
McKerrow, *Wellington* 32 B2
McKinley Park, *Chicago* 9 C2
Mclean, *Washington* 32 B2
Macopocho, R. →, *Santiago* 26 B1
MacRitchie Res., *Singapore* 27 A2
Macul, *Santiago* 26 C2
Madame Tussaud's, *London* 15 a3
Madhudaha, *Calcutta* 8 B2
Madhyamgram, *Calcutta* 8 A2
Madīnah Al Mansūr, *Baghdad* 3 B2
Mâdinet Nasr, *Cairo* 7 A2
Madison Avenue, *New York* 21 c2
Madison Square, *New York* 21 d2
Madrid, *Madrid* 17 B1
Madrona, *Barcelona* 4 A1
Maesawa, *Tokyo* 29 A2
Magdalena, *Lima* 16 B2
Magdalena Contreras, *Mexico City* 18 C1
Maghreb, *Baghdad* 3 A2
Maginu, *Tokyo* 29 B2
Magliana, *Rome* 25 B1
Magny-les-Hameaux, *Paris* 23 B1
Magonoy, *Manila* 17 B2
Mahalaxmi, *Mumbai* 20 a1
Maheshtala, *Calcutta* 8 C1
Mahim, *Mumbai* 20 A2
Mahim B., *Mumbai* 20 A1
Mahlsdorf, *Berlin* 5 A4
Mahmoodabad, *Karachi* 14 A2
Mahrauli, *Delhi* 10 B1
Mahul, *Mumbai* 20 A2
Maida Vale, *London* 15 a1
Maidstone, *Melbourne* 17 A1
Maipú, *Santiago* 26 C1
Maisonneuve, Parc, *Montreal* 19 A2
Maisons-Alfort, *Paris* 23 B3
Maisons-Laffitte, *Paris* 23 A1
Maissoneuve, *Montreal* 19 A2
Maitland, *Cape Town* 8 A1
Makati, *Manila* 17 B2
Mäkiniitty, *Helsinki* 12 A2
Mala Straná, *Prague* 24 B2
Malabar, *Mumbai* 20 B1
Malabar, *Sydney* 28 B2
Malabar Hill, *Mumbai* 20 B1
Malabar Pt., *Mumbai* 20 B1
Malabon, *Manila* 17 B1
Malacañang Palace, *Manila* 17 B1
Malahide, *Dublin* 11 A3
Malakhovka, *Moscow* 19 C6
Malakoff, *Paris* 23 B2
Mälarhöjaen, *Stockholm* 28 B1
Malate, *Manila* 17 B1
Malay Quarter, *Cape Town* 8 c2
Malaya Neva, *St. Petersburg* 26 B1
Malaya-Okhta, *St. Petersburg* 26 B2
Malchow, *Berlin* 5 A3
Malden, *Boston* 6 A3
Malden, *London* 15 B2
Maleizen, *Brussels* 6 B3
Malešice, *Prague* 24 B3
Malir →, *Karachi* 14 B2
Mall, The, *Washington* 32 b2
Malleny Mills, *Edinburgh* 11 B2
Malmi, *Helsinki* 12 B2
Malmøya, *Oslo* 22 A3
Måløv, *Copenhagen* 10 A2
Malpasso, Ost., *Rome* 25 C1
Malton, *Toronto* 30 A1
Malvern, *Johannesburg* 13 B2
Malvern, *Melbourne* 17 B2
Malvern, *Toronto* 30 A3
Mamonovo, *Moscow* 19 B2
Mampang Prapatan, *Jakarta* 13 B1
Mampukuji, *Tokyo* 29 B2
Man Budrukh, *Mumbai* 20 A2
Man Khurd, *Mumbai* 20 A2
Mandaluyong, *Manila* 17 B2
Mandaoli, *Delhi* 10 B2
Mandaqui →, *São Paulo* 26 A2
Mandoli, *Delhi* 10 A2
Mandvi, *Mumbai* 20 B2
Manenberg, *Cape Town* 8 A2
Mang Kung Uk, *Hong Kong* 12 B2
Mangolpuri, *Delhi* 10 A1
Manguinhos, Aéroporto, *Rio de Janeiro* 24 B1
Mangwŏn, *Seoul* 26 B1
Manhattan, *New York* 21 B2
Manhattan Beach, *New York* 21 C2
Manila, *Manila* 17 B1
Manila B., *Manila* 17 B1
Manila Int. Airport, *Manila* 17 B2
Mankkaa, *Helsinki* 12 B1
Manly, *Sydney* 28 A2
Mannswörth, *Vienna* 31 B3
Manor Park, *London* 15 A4
Manor Park, *Wellington* 32 A2
Manora, *Karachi* 14 B1
Manquehue, Cerro, *Santiago* 26 B2
Manzanares, Canal de, *Madrid* 17 C2
Mao Mausoleum, *Beijing* 4 c2
Map'o, *Seoul* 26 B1
Maracanã, *Rio de Janeiro* 24 B1
Maraoli, *Mumbai* 20 A2
Marblehead, *Boston* 6 A4
Marcelin, *Warsaw* 31 B1
Mareil-Marly, *Paris* 23 A1
Margareten, *Vienna* 31 A2
Maria, *Vienna* 31 A2
Maridalen, *Oslo* 22 A3
Maridalsvatnet, *Oslo* 22 A3
Mariendorf, *Berlin* 5 B3
Marienfelde, *Berlin* 5 B3
Marienplatz, *Munich* 20 b2
Marikina →, *Manila* 17 B2
Marin City, *San Francisco* 25 A1
Marin Headlands State Park, *San Francisco* 25 A2
Marin Pen., *San Francisco* 25 A1
Marina del Rey, *Los Angeles* 16 C2
Marine Drive, *Mumbai* 20 b1
Marino, *Dublin* 11 A2
Maritim, Museu, *Barcelona* 4 c2
Markham, *Toronto* 30 A2
Marki, *Warsaw* 31 B2
Markland Wood, *Toronto* 30 B1
Marly, Forêt de, *Paris* 23 A1
Marly-le-Roi, *Paris* 23 A1
Marne →, *Paris* 23 B3
Marne-la-Vallée, *Paris* 23 A4
Marolles-en-Brie, *Paris* 23 B4
Maroubra, *Sydney* 28 B2
Marquette Park, *Chicago* 9 C2
Marrickville, *Sydney* 28 B1
Marsfield, *Sydney* 28 A1
Marshall Field's, *Chicago* 9 c2
Marte, Campo de, *São Paulo* 26 B2
Martesana, Navíglio della, *Milan* 18 A2
Martin Luther King National Historic Site, *Atlanta* 3 B2
Martinez, *Buenos Aires* 7 A1
Martinkylä, *Helsinki* 12 B2
Martinsried, *Munich* 20 B1
Maruko, *Tokyo* 29 B3
Marunouchi, *Tokyo* 29 b4
Marusino, *Moscow* 19 B5
Maryino, *Moscow* 19 B4
Maryland, *Singapore* 27 B2
Marylebone, *London* 15 A2
Marymont, *Warsaw* 31 B1
Marysin Wawerski, *Warsaw* 31 B2
Marzahn, *Berlin* 5 A4
Mascot, *Sydney* 28 B2
Masmo, *Stockholm* 28 B1
Maspeth, *New York* 21 B2
Masr el Gedida, *Cairo* 7 A2
Masr el Qadîma, *Cairo* 7 A2
Massachusetts B., *Boston* 6 A4
Massachusett's Inst. of Tech., *Boston* 6 A3
Massamá, *Lisbon* 14 A1
Massey →, *Toronto* 30 A3
Massy, *Paris* 23 B2
Matihutong, *Beijing* 4 B1
Matinha, *Lisbon* 14 A2
Matramam, *Jakarta* 13 B2
Matsubara, *Osaka* 22 B4
Mattapan, *Boston* 6 B3
Mátyásföld, *Budapest* 7 A3
Mátyástemplom, *Budapest* 7 b1
Mau Tso Ngam, *Hong Kong* 12 A2
Mauer, *Vienna* 31 B1
Mauripur, *Karachi* 14 A1
Maxhof, *Munich* 20 B1
Maya-Zan, *Osaka* 22 A2
Mayfair, *Johannesburg* 13 B2
Mayfair, *London* 15 b3
Mayor, Plaza, *Madrid* 17 b2
Maywood, *Chicago* 9 B1
Maywood, *Los Angeles* 16 C3
Maywood, *New York* 21 A1
Mazagaon, *Mumbai* 20 a2
Me'a She' Arim, *Jerusalem* 13 a2
Meadowbank Park, *Sydney* 28 A1
Měcholupy, *Prague* 24 B3
Měčice, *Prague* 24 A3
Mecidiyeköy, *Istanbul* 12 B2
Medford, *Boston* 6 A3
Mediodia, *Madrid* 17 B2
Medvezhiy Ozyora, *Moscow* 19 A5
Meguro →, *Tokyo* 29 B3
Meguro-Ku, *Tokyo* 29 B3
Mehpalpur, *Delhi* 10 B1
Mehrābād Airport, *Tehran* 30 A1
Mehram Nagar, *Delhi* 10 B1
Mehrow, *Berlin* 5 A4
Mei Lanfang, *Beijing* 4 a2
Meidling, *Vienna* 31 A2
Méier, *Rio de Janeiro* 24 B1
Meiji Shrine, *Tokyo* 29 b1
Meise, *Brussels* 6 A1
Mejiro, *Tokyo* 29 A3
Melbourne, *Melbourne* 17 A1
Melbourne Airport, *Melbourne* 17 A1
Melkki, *Helsinki* 12 C2
Mellunkylä, *Helsinki* 12 B3
Mellunmäki, *Helsinki* 12 B3
Melrose, *Boston* 6 A3
Melrose, *New York* 21 B2
Melrose Park, *Chicago* 9 B1
Melsbroek, *Brussels* 6 A2
Menteng, *Jakarta* 13 B1
Mérantaise →, *Paris* 23 B1
Mercamadrid, *Madrid* 17 B2
Merced, L., *San Francisco* 25 B2
Meredale, *Johannesburg* 13 B1
Merlimau, P., *Singapore* 27 B2
Merri Cr. →, *Melbourne* 17 A1
Merrion, *Dublin* 11 B2
Merrionette Park, *Chicago* 9 C2
Merton, *London* 15 B2
Mesgarābād, *Tehran* 30 B3
Meshcherskiy, *Moscow* 19 B2
Messe, *Vienna* 31 A2
Messe-palast, *Vienna* 31 c1
Metanópoli, *Milan* 18 B2
Metropolitan Museum of Art, *New York* 21 b3
Meudon, *Paris* 23 B2
Mevaseret Tsiyon, *Jerusalem* 13 B1
Mevo Beitar, *Jerusalem* 13 B1
México, Ciudad de, *Mexico City* 18 B1
Meyersdal, *Johannesburg* 13 B2
Mezzano, *Milan* 18 B2
Mezzate, *Milan* 18 B2
Miadong, *Seoul* 26 B2
Miami, *Miami* 18 B2
Miami Beach, *Miami* 18 B2
Miami Canal →, *Miami* 18 A1
Miami Int. Airport, *Miami* 18 B1
Miami Shores, *Miami* 18 A2
Miami Springs, *Miami* 18 B1
Miasto, *Warsaw* 31 B2
Michałowice, *Warsaw* 31 B1
Michigan Avenue, *Chicago* 9 b2
Michle, *Prague* 24 B2
Middle Harbour, *Sydney* 28 A2
Middle Hd., *Sydney* 28 A2
Middle Park, *Melbourne* 17 B1
Middle Village, *New York* 21 B2
Middlesex Fells Reservation, *Boston* 6 A3
Midi, Gare du, *Brussels* 6 c1
Midland Beach, *New York* 21 C1
Miedzeszyn, *Warsaw* 31 B3
Międzylesie, *Warsaw* 31 B3
Miessaari, *Helsinki* 12 C1
Miguel Hidalgo, *Mexico City* 18 B1
Mikhelysona, *Moscow* 19 B5
Milano, *Milan* 18 B1
Milano Due, *Milan* 18 B2
Milano San Felice, *Milan* 18 B2
Milbertshofen, *Munich* 20 A2
Mill Hill, *London* 15 A2
Millennium Dome, *London* 15 A4
Miller Meadow, *Chicago* 9 B2
Millerhill, *Edinburgh* 11 B3
Millers Point, *Sydney* 28 a1
Milltown, *Dublin* 11 B2
Millwood, *Washington* 32 B4
Milnerton, *Cape Town* 8 A1
Milon-la-Chapelle, *Paris* 23 B1
Milton, *Boston* 6 B3
Milton Bridge, *Edinburgh* 11 B2
Mimico, *Toronto* 30 B2
Minami, *Osaka* 22 A4
Minamitsunashima, *Tokyo* 29 B2
Minato, *Osaka* 22 B3
Minato-Ku, *Tokyo* 29 c3
Minshât el Bekkarî, *Cairo* 7 A1
Minute Man Nat. Hist. Park, *Boston* 6 A2
Miraflores, *Lima* 16 B2
Miramar, *Wellington* 32 B1
Misericordia, Sa. da, *Rio de Janeiro* 24 B1
Mission, *San Francisco* 25 B2
Mississauga, *Toronto* 30 B1
Mitaka, *Tokyo* 29 A2
Mitcham, *London* 15 B2
Mitcham Common, *London* 15 B3
Mitchell's Plain, *Cape Town* 8 B2
Mitino, *Moscow* 19 A2
Mitte, *Berlin* 5 A3
Mittel Isarkanal →, *Munich* 20 A3
Mixcoac, *Mexico City* 18 B1
Mixcoac, Presa de, *Mexico City* 18 B1
Miyakojima, *Osaka* 22 A4
Mizonokuchi, *Tokyo* 29 B2
Mizue, *Tokyo* 29 A4
Młocinski Park, *Warsaw* 31 B1
Młociny, *Warsaw* 31 B1
Mnevniki, *Moscow* 19 B2
Moba, *Lagos* 14 B2
Moczydło, *Warsaw* 31 C2
Modderfontein, *Johannesburg* 13 A2
Modřany, *Prague* 24 B2
Mogyoród, *Budapest* 7 A3
Moinho Velho, Cor. →, *São Paulo* 26 B2
Mok, *Seoul* 26 B1
Mokotów, *Warsaw* 31 B2
Molenbeek-Saint-Jean, *Brussels* 6 A1
Molino de Rosas, *Mexico City* 18 B1
Mollem, *Brussels* 6 A1
Mollins de Rey, *Barcelona* 4 A1
Mondeor, *Johannesburg* 13 B2
Moneda, Palacio de la, *Santiago* 26 B2
Moneró, *Rio de Janeiro* 24 A1
Mong Kok, *Hong Kong* 12 B2
Monkstown, *Dublin* 11 B3
Monnickendam, *Amsterdam* 2 A3
Monrovia, *Los Angeles* 16 B4
Monsanto, *Lisbon* 14 A1
Monsanto, Parque Florestal de, *Lisbon* 14 A1
Mont Royal, *Montreal* 19 A2
Mont-Royal, Parc, *Montreal* 19 A2
Montana de Montjuich, *Barcelona* 4 A1
Monte Chingolo, *Buenos Aires* 7 C2
Monte Palatino, *Rome* 25 c3
Montebello, *Los Angeles* 16 B4
Montemor, *Lisbon* 14 A1
Monterey Park, *Los Angeles* 16 B4
Montespaccato, *Rome* 25 B1
Montesson, *Paris* 23 A1

Monteverde Nuovo, *Rome* 25 B1
Montfermeil, *Paris* 23 A4
Montigny-le-Bretonneux, *Paris* 23 B1
Montjay-la-Tour, *Paris* 23 A4
Montjuic, Parc de, *Barcelona* 4 c1
Montparnasse, Gare, *Paris* 23 A2
Montréal, *Montreal* 19 A2
Montréal, Î. de, *Montreal* 19 A2
Montréal, Univ. de, *Montreal* 19 B2
Montréal Est, *Montreal* 19 A2
Montréal Nord, *Montreal* 19 A2
Montréal Ouest, *Montreal* 19 B1
Montreuil, *Paris* 23 A3
Montrouge, *Paris* 23 B2
Montserrat, *Buenos Aires* 7 B2
Monza, *Milan* 18 A2
Monzoro, *Milan* 18 B1
Moóca, *São Paulo* 26 B2
Moonachie, *New York* 21 B1
Moonee Ponds, *Melbourne* 17 A1
Moonee Valley Racecourse, *Melbourne* 17 A1
Moosach, *Munich* 20 A2
Mora, *Mumbai* 20 B2
Moratalaz, *Madrid* 17 B2
Mörby, *Stockholm* 28 A2
Morden, *London* 15 B2
Morée →, *Paris* 23 A3
Morgan Park, *Chicago* 9 C3
Moriguchi, *Osaka* 22 A4
Morivione, *Milan* 18 B2
Morningside, *Edinburgh* 11 B2
Morningside, *Johannesburg* 13 A2
Morningside, *Washington* 32 C4
Morro Solar, Cerro, *Lima* 16 C2
Mortlake, *London* 15 B2
Mortlake, *Sydney* 28 B1
Morton Grove, *Chicago* 9 A2
Morumbi, *São Paulo* 26 B1
Moscavide, *Lisbon* 14 A2
Moscow = Moskva, *Moscow* 19 B3
Moskhaton, *Athens* 2 B2
Moskva, *Moscow* 19 B3
Moskva →, *Moscow* 19 B2
Moskvoretskiy, *Moscow* 19 B3
Mosman, *Sydney* 28 A2
Móstoles, *Madrid* 17 C1
Moti Bagh, *Delhi* 10 B2
Motol, *Prague* 24 B1
Motsa, *Jerusalem* 13 B2
Motsa Ilit, *Jerusalem* 13 B1
Motspur Park, *London* 15 B2
Mottingham, *London* 15 B4
Moulin Rouge, *Paris* 23 a3
Mount Dennis, *Toronto* 30 A2
Mount Greenwood, *Chicago* 9 C2
Mount Hood Memorial Park, *Boston* 6 A3
Mount Merrion, *Dublin* 11 B2
Mount Rainier, *Washington* 32 B4
Mount Vernon, *New York* 21 A3
Mount Vernon Square, *Washington* 32 a2
Mount Zion, *Jerusalem* 13 b3
Mozarthaus, *Vienna* 31 b2
Müggelberge, *Berlin* 5 B4
Müggelheim, *Berlin* 5 B5
Muggiò, *Milan* 18 A2
Mughal Gardens, *Delhi* 1 c1
Mühleiten, *Vienna* 31 A3
Mühlenfliess →, *Berlin* 5 A5
Muiden, *Amsterdam* 2 A3
Muiderpoort Station, *Amsterdam* 2 b3
Muizenberg, *Cape Town* 8 B1
Mujahidpur, *Delhi* 10 B2
Mukandpur, *Delhi* 10 A2
Mukhmas, *Jerusalem* 13 A2
Muko →, *Osaka* 22 A3
Mukojima, *Tokyo* 29 A3
Mulbarton, *Johannesburg* 13 B2
Mumbai, *Mumbai* 20 B2
Mumbai Harbour, *Mumbai* 20 B2
Münchehofe, *Berlin* 5 B5
München, *Munich* 20 B2
Munich = München, *Munich* 20 B2
Munkkiniemi, *Helsinki* 12 B2
Munro, *Buenos Aires* 7 B1
Murai Res., *Singapore* 27 A2
Muranów, *Warsaw* 31 B1
Murino, *St. Petersburg* 26 B2
Murrayfield, *Edinburgh* 11 B2
Musashino, *Tokyo* 29 A2
Museu Nacional, *Rio de Janeiro* 24 B1
Mushin, *Lagos* 14 A2
Musiektheater, *Amsterdam* 2 b2
Muslim Quarter, *Jerusalem* 13 a3
Musocco, *Milan* 18 B1
Mustansiriya, *Baghdad* 3 A2
Musturud, *Cairo* 7 A2
Muswell Hill, *London* 15 A3
Mutanabi, *Baghdad* 3 B2
Muthana, *Baghdad* 3 B2
Myakinino, *Moscow* 19 B2
Mykerinos, *Cairo* 7 B1
Myllypuro, *Helsinki* 12 B3

N

Nacka, *Stockholm* 28 B3
Nada, *Osaka* 22 A2
Naenae, *Wellington* 32 B2
Nærsnes, *Oslo* 22 B1
Nagata, *Osaka* 22 B1
Nagatsuta, *Tokyo* 29 B2
Nagytétény, *Budapest* 7 B1
Nahant, *Boston* 6 A4
Nahant B., *Boston* 6 A4
Nahant Harbor, *Boston* 6 A4
Nahr Dijlah →, *Baghdad* 3 B2
Najafgarh Drain →, *Delhi* 10 B1
Nakahara-Ku, *Tokyo* 29 B2
Nakano-Ku, *Tokyo* 29 A2
Namgajwa, *Seoul* 26 B1
Namsan Park, *Seoul* 26 B1
Namyŏng, *Seoul* 26 B1
Nanbiancun, *Canton* 8 B1
Nanchang He →, *Beijing* 4 B1
Nandang, *Canton* 8 B2
Nandian, *Tianjin* 30 A2
Nangal Dewat, *Delhi* 10 B1
Naniwa, *Osaka* 22 B3
Nankai, *Tianjin* 30 B1
Nanmenwai, *Tianjin* 30 B2
Nanole, *Mumbai* 20 A2
Nanpu Bridge, *Shanghai* 27 B2
Nanshi, *Shanghai* 27 B1
Nantasket Beach, *Boston* 6 B4
Nanterre, *Paris* 23 A2
Naoabad, *Calcutta* 8 C2
Napier Mole, *Karachi* 14 B1
Naraina, *Delhi* 10 B1
Nariman Point, *Mumbai* 20 c1
Nariman Pt., *Mumbai* 20 B1
Nārmak, *Tehran* 30 A2
Naruo, *Osaka* 22 A3
Näsby, *Stockholm* 28 A2
Näsbypark, *Stockholm* 28 A2
Nathan Road, *Hong Kong* 12 a2
Natick, *Boston* 6 B2
National Maritime Museum, *San Francisco* 25 a1
National Museum, *Bangkok* 3 b1
Nationalmuseum, *Stockholm* 28 b2
Natolin, *Warsaw* 31 C2
Naturhistorischesmuseum, *Vienna* 31 b1
Naucalpan de Juárez, *Mexico City* 18 B1
Naupada, *Mumbai* 20 A2
Navíglio di Pavia, *Milan* 18 B1
Navíglio Grande, *Milan* 18 B1
Navona, Piazza, *Rome* 25 b2
Navotas, *Manila* 17 B1
Navy Pier, *Chicago* 9 b3
Nazal Hikmat Beg, *Baghdad* 3 A2
Nazimabad, *Karachi* 14 A2
Nazlet el Simmân, *Cairo* 7 B1
Néa Alexandhria, *Athens* 2 B2
Néa Faliron, *Athens* 2 B1
Néa Ionía, *Athens* 2 A2
Néa Liósia, *Athens* 2 A2
Néa Smírni, *Athens* 2 B2
Neapolis, *Athens* 2 B2
Near North, *Chicago* 9 b2
Nebušice, *Prague* 24 B1
Nederhorst, *Amsterdam* 2 B3
Nedlitz, *Berlin* 5 B1
Nee Soon, *Singapore* 27 A2
Needham Heights, *Boston* 6 B2
Nekrasovka, *Moscow* 19 B5
N'ematābād, *Tehran* 30 B2
Nemchinovka, *Moscow* 19 B1
Nemzeti Muz, *Budapest* 7 c3
Neponsit, *New York* 21 C2
Nerima-Ku, *Tokyo* 29 A3
Nesodden, *Oslo* 22 B3
Nesoddtangen, *Oslo* 22 A3
Nesøya, *Oslo* 22 A2
Neu Aubing, *Munich* 20 B1
Neu Buch, *Berlin* 5 A4
Neu Buchhorst, *Berlin* 5 B5
Neu Fahrland, *Berlin* 5 B1
Neu Lindenberg, *Berlin* 5 A4
Neubiberg, *Munich* 20 B3
Neue Hofburg, *Vienna* 31 b1
Neuenhagen, *Berlin* 5 A4
Neuessling, *Vienna* 31 A3
Neuhausen, *Munich* 20 B2
Neuherberg, *Munich* 20 A2
Neuhönow, *Berlin* 5 A5
Neuilly-Plaisance, *Paris* 23 A4
Neuilly-sur-Marne, *Paris* 23 A4
Neuilly-sur-Seine, *Paris* 23 A2
Neukagran, *Vienna* 31 A2
Neukettenhof, *Vienna* 31 B2
Neukölln, *Berlin* 5 B3
Neuperlach, *Munich* 20 B2
Neuried, *Munich* 20 B1
Neustift am Walde, *Vienna* 31 A1
Neusüssenbrunn, *Vienna* 31 A2
Neuwaldegg, *Vienna* 31 A1
Neva →, *St. Petersburg* 26 B2
Neves, *Rio de Janeiro* 24 B2
New Baghdād, *Baghdad* 3 B2
New Barakpur, *Calcutta* 8 A2
New Brighton, *New York* 21 C1
New Canada, *Johannesburg* 13 B1
New Canada Dam, *Johannesburg* 13 B1
New Carrollton, *Washington* 32 B4
New Cross, *London* 15 B3
New Delhi, *Delhi* 10 B2
New Dorp, *New York* 21 C1
New Dorp Beach, *New York* 21 C1
New Malden, *London* 15 B2
New Milford, *New York* 21 A1
New Territories, *Hong Kong* 12 A1
New Toronto, *Toronto* 30 B1
New Town, *Edinburgh* 11 B2
New Utrecht, *New York* 21 C2
Newark B., *New York* 21 B1
Newbattle, *Edinburgh* 11 B3
Newbury Park, *London* 15 A4
Newcraighall, *Edinburgh* 11 B3
Newham, *London* 15 A4
Newhaven, *Edinburgh* 11 B2
Newington, *Edinburgh* 11 B2
Newington, *London* 15 c5
Newlands, *Johannesburg* 13 B1
Newlands, *Wellington* 32 B1
Newport, *Melbourne* 17 B1
Newton, *Boston* 6 B2
Newtonbrook, *Toronto* 30 A2
Newtongrange, *Edinburgh* 11 B3
Newtonville, *Boston* 6 A2
Newtown, *Sydney* 28 B2
Neyagawa, *Osaka* 22 A4
Ngaio, *Wellington* 32 B1
Ngau Chi Wan, *Hong Kong* 12 A2
Ngau Tau Kok, *Hong Kong* 12 B2
Ngauranga, *Wellington* 32 B1
Ngong Shuen Chau, *Hong Kong* 12 B1
Ngua Kok Wan, *Hong Kong* 12 A1
Nīāvarān, *Tehran* 30 A2
Nibra, *Calcutta* 8 B1
Nidāl, *Baghdad* 3 B2
Niddrie, *Edinburgh* 11 B3
Niddrie, *Melbourne* 17 A1
Nieder Neuendorf, *Berlin* 5 A2
Niederschöneweide, *Berlin* 5 B3
Niederschönhausen, *Berlin* 5 A3
Niemeyer, *Rio de Janeiro* 24 B1
Nieuw Zuid, *Amsterdam* 2 c2
Nieuwe Kerk, *Amsterdam* 2 b2
Nieuwendam, *Amsterdam* 2 A2
Nihonbashi, *Tokyo* 29 b5
Niipperi, *Helsinki* 12 B1
Níkaia, *Athens* 2 B1
Nikolassee, *Berlin* 5 B2
Nikolskiy, *Moscow* 19 B2
Nikolyskoye, *Moscow* 19 B5
Nikulino, *Moscow* 19 B2
Nil, Nahr en →, *Cairo* 7 B2
Nile = Nil, Nahr en →, *Cairo* 7 B2
Niles, *Chicago* 9 A2
Nimta, *Calcutta* 8 A2
Ningyuan, *Tianjin* 30 B2
Nippa, *Tokyo* 29 B2
Nippori, *Tokyo* 29 A3
Nishi, *Osaka* 22 A3
Nishinari, *Osaka* 22 B3
Nishiyodogawa, *Osaka* 22 A3
Niterói, *Rio de Janeiro* 24 B2
Nob Hill, *San Francisco* 25 b1
Nockeby, *Stockholm* 28 B1
Noel Park, *London* 15 A3
Nogatino, *Moscow* 19 B4
Nogent-sur-Marne, *Paris* 23 A3
Noida, *Delhi* 10 B2
Noiseau, *Paris* 23 B4
Noisiel, *Paris* 23 A4
Noisy-le-Grand, *Paris* 23 A4
Noisy-le-Roi, *Paris* 23 A1
Noisy-le-Sec, *Paris* 23 A3
Nokkala, *Helsinki* 12 C1
Nomentano, *Rome* 25 B2
Nonakashinden, *Tokyo* 29 A2
Nongminyundong Jiangxisuo, *Canton* 8 B2
Nonhyŏn, *Seoul* 26 B2
Nonthaburi, *Bangkok* 3 A1
Noon Gun, *Cape Town* 8 b1
Noorder Kerk, *Amsterdam* 2 a1
Noordgesig, *Johannesburg* 13 B1
Noordzeekanaal, *Amsterdam* 2 A1
Nord, Gare du, *Paris* 23 a4
Nordrand-Siedlung, *Vienna* 31 A2
Nordstrand, *Oslo* 22 A3
Normandale, *Wellington* 32 B2
Nørrebro, *Copenhagen* 10 a1
Norridge, *Chicago* 9 B2
Norrmalm, *Stockholm* 28 a1
North Arlington, *New York* 21 B1
North Bay Village, *Miami* 18 A2
North Bergen, *New York* 21 B1
North Branch Chicago River →, *Chicago* 9 B2
North Bull Island, *Dublin* 11 A3
North Cambridge, *Boston* 6 A3
North Cheam, *London* 15 B2
North Cohasset, *Boston* 6 B4
North Cray, *London* 15 B4
North Decatur, *Atlanta* 3 B3
North Druid Hills, *Atlanta* 3 B3
North Esk →, *Edinburgh* 11 B2
North Gyle, *Edinburgh* 11 B2
North Hackensack, *New York* 21 A1
North Harbor, *Manila* 17 B1
North Hd., *Sydney* 28 A2
North Hollywood, *Los Angeles* 16 B2
North Lexington, *Boston* 6 A2
North Miami, *Miami* 18 A2
North Miami Beach, *Miami* 18 A2
North Nazimabad, *Karachi* 14 A2
North Pt., *Hong Kong* 12 B2
North Queensferry, *Edinburgh* 11 A1
North Quincy, *Boston* 6 B3
North Res., *Boston* 6 A3
North Riverside, *Chicago* 9 B2
North Saugus, *Boston* 6 A3
North Shore Channel →, *Chicago* 9 B2
North Springfield, *Washington* 32 C2
North Sudbury, *Boston* 6 A1
North Sydney, *Sydney* 28 B2
North Woolwich, *London* 15 A4
North York, *Toronto* 30 A2
Northbridge, *Sydney* 28 A2
Northbridge Park, *Sydney* 28 A2
Northcliff, *Johannesburg* 13 A1
Northcote, *Melbourne* 17 A2
Northlake, *Chicago* 9 B1
Northmount, *Toronto* 30 A2
Northolt, *London* 15 A1
Northumberland Heath, *London* 15 B5
Northwood, *London* 15 A1
Norumbega Res., *Boston* 6 B2
Norwood, *Johannesburg* 13 A2
Norwood Park, *Chicago* 9 B2
Noryangjin, *Seoul* 26 B1
Nossa Senhora de Candelária, *Rio de Janeiro* 24 a2
Nossa Senhora do Ó, *São Paulo* 26 B1
Nossegem, *Brussels* 6 A3
Notre-Dame, *Paris* 23 c4
Notre-Dame, Bois, *Paris* 23 B4
Notre-Dame-de-Grace, *Montreal* 19 B2
Notting Hill, *London* 15 b1
Nova Milanese, *Milan* 18 A2
Novate Milanese, *Milan* 18 A1
Novaya Derevnya, *St. Petersburg* 26 A1
Nové Město, *Prague* 24 B2
Novoaleksandrovskoye, *St. Petersburg* 26 B2
Novogireyevo, *Moscow* 19 B4
Novoivanovskoye, *Moscow* 19 B1
Novonikolyskoye, *Moscow* 19 A1
Novosaratovka, *St. Petersburg* 26 B3
Nowe-Babice, *Warsaw* 31 B1
Nöykkiö, *Helsinki* 12 B1
Nueva Atzacoalco, *Mexico City* 18 B2
Nueva Pompeya, *Buenos Aires* 7 C2
Nueva Tenochtitlán, *Mexico City* 18 B2
Nuijala, *Helsinki* 12 B1
Numabukuro, *Tokyo* 29 A2
Nunez, *Buenos Aires* 7 B2
Nunhead, *London* 15 B3
Ñuñoa, *Santiago* 26 B2
Nusle, *Prague* 24 B2
Nussdorf, *Vienna* 31 A2
Nyanga, *Cape Town* 8 A2
Nymphenburg, *Munich* 20 B2
Nymphenburg, Schloss, *Munich* 20 B2

O

Oak Grove, *Atlanta* 3 A3
Oak Island, *Boston* 6 A4
Oak Lawn, *Chicago* 9 C2
Oak Park, *Chicago* 9 B2
Oak View, *Washington* 32 A4
Oakdale, *Atlanta* 3 A2
Oakland, *San Francisco* 25 B3
Oakland, *Washington* 32 B4
Oaklawn, *Washington* 32 C4
Oakleigh, *Melbourne* 17 B2
Oakton, *Washington* 32 B2
Oakwood Beach, *New York* 21 C1
Oatley, *Sydney* 28 B1
Obalende, *Lagos* 14 B2
Oba's Palace, *Lagos* 14 B2
Oberföhring, *Munich* 20 B2
Oberhaching, *Munich* 20 B2
Oberlaa, *Vienna* 31 B2
Oberlisse, *Vienna* 31 A2
Obermenzing, *Munich* 20 A1
Obermoos Schwaige, *Munich* 20 A1
Oberschleissheim, *Munich* 20 A2
Oberschöneweide, *Berlin* 5 B4
Observatory, *Johannesburg* 13 B2
Observatory, *Sydney* 28 a1
Ōbu, *Osaka* 22 A1
Obu-tōge, *Osaka* 22 A1
Óbuda, *Budapest* 7 A2
Obukhovo, *St. Petersburg* 26 B2
Obvodnyy Kanal, *St. Petersburg* 26 B1
Ocean Park, *Hong Kong* 12 B2
Ochakovo, *Moscow* 19 B2
Ochota, *Warsaw* 31 B1
O'Connell Street, *Dublin* 11 b2
Ōdana, *Tokyo* 29 B2
Öden-Stockach, *Munich* 20 B3
Odilampi, *Helsinki* 12 B1
Odintsovo, *Moscow* 19 B1
Odivelas, *Lisbon* 14 A1
Odolany, *Warsaw* 31 B1
Oeiras, *Lisbon* 14 A1
Ofin, *Lagos* 14 A3
Ogawa, *Tokyo* 29 A1
Ogden Park, *Chicago* 9 C2
Ogikubo, *Tokyo* 29 A2
Ogogoro, *Lagos* 14 B2
Ogoyo, *Lagos* 14 B2
Ogudu, *Lagos* 14 A2
Ohariu Stream →, *Wellington* 32 B1
O'Higgins, Parque, *Santiago* 26 B2
Ōimachi, *Tokyo* 29 B3
Ojota, *Lagos* 14 A2
Okamoto, *Osaka* 22 A2
Okęcie, *Warsaw* 31 B1
Okęcie Airport, *Warsaw* 31 B1
Okelra, *Lagos* 14 B2
Okeogbe, *Lagos* 14 B2
Okha, *Delhi* 10 B2
Okhta →, *St. Petersburg* 26 B2
Okkervil →, *St. Petersburg* 26 B2
Okrzeszyn, *Warsaw* 31 C2
Oksval, *Oslo* 22 A3
Oktyabrskiy, *Moscow* 19 B3
Ōkubo, *Tokyo* 29 a2
Ōkura, *Tokyo* 29 B1
Olari, *Helsinki* 12 B1
Olaria, *Rio de Janeiro* 24 B1
Old Admiralty, *St. Petersburg* 26 B1
Old City, *Delhi* 1 a3
Old City, *Jerusalem* 13 b3
Old City, *Shanghai* 27 B1
Old Fort = Purana Qila, *Delhi* 1 c3
Old Harbor, *Boston* 6 B3
Old Town, *Chicago* 9 B3
Old Town, *Edinburgh* 11 B2
Oldbawn, *Dublin* 11 B1
Olgino, *St. Petersburg* 26 A1
Olimpico, Estadio, *Mexico City* 18 C1
Olivais, *Lisbon* 14 A2
Olivar de los Padres, *Mexico City* 18 B1
Olivar del Conde, *Mexico City* 18 B1
Olivos, *Buenos Aires* 7 B2
Olona →, *Milan* 18 B1
Olympia, *London* 15 c1
Olympic Stadium, *Helsinki* 12 B2
Olympique, Stade, *Montreal* 19 A2
Omonias, Pl., *Athens* 2 b1
Ōmori, *Tokyo* 29 B3
Onchi, *Osaka* 22 B4
Onchi →, *Osaka* 22 B4
Onisigun, *Lagos* 14 A2
Ōokayama, *Tokyo* 29 B3
Oosterpark, *Amsterdam* 2 b3
Oostzaan, *Amsterdam* 2 A2
Opa-Locka, *Miami* 18 A1
Opa-Locka Airport, *Miami* 18 A1
Opacz, *Warsaw* 31 B1
Opera House, *Sydney* 28 a2
Ophirton, *Johannesburg* 13 B2
Oppegård, *Oslo* 22 B3
Oppem, *Brussels* 6 A1
Oppsal, *Oslo* 22 A4
Ora, *Jerusalem* 13 B1
Oradell, *New York* 21 A1
Orange Bowl Stadium, *Miami* 18 B2
Orangi, *Karachi* 14 A2
Orchard Road, *Singapore* 27 a1
Ordrup, *Copenhagen* 10 A3
Orech, *Prague* 24 B1
Øresund, *Copenhagen* 10 A3
Orient Heights, *Boston* 6 A4
Orlando Dam, *Johannesburg* 13 B1
Orlando East, *Johannesburg* 13 B1
Orlovo, *Moscow* 19 C2
Orly, *Paris* 23 B3
Ormesson-sur-Marne, *Paris* 23 B4
Ormond, *Melbourne* 17 B2
Ormøya, *Oslo* 22 A3
Orpington, *London* 15 B4
Orsay, Musée d', *Paris* 23 b3
Országház, *Budapest* 7 b2
Országos Levéltár, *Budapest* 7 b1
Ortaköy, *Istanbul* 12 B2
Ortica, *Milan* 18 B2
Oruba, *Lagos* 14 A2
Orvostörteneti Múz., *Budapest* 7 c2
Ōsaka, *Osaka* 22 B4
Osaka B., *Osaka* 22 B2
Osaka Castle, *Osaka* 22 A4
Osaka Harbour, *Osaka* 22 B3
Osaka International Airport, *Osaka* 22 A3
Ōsaki, *Tokyo* 29 B3
Osasco, *São Paulo* 26 B1
Osdorf, *Berlin* 5 B3
Osdorp, *Amsterdam* 2 A1
Oshodi, *Lagos* 14 A2
Oslo, *Oslo* 22 A3
Oslofjorden, *Oslo* 22 B2
Ōsone, *Tokyo* 29 B2
Osorun, *Lagos* 14 A2
Ospiate, *Milan* 18 A1
Ostankino, *Moscow* 19 B3
Östasiatiskamuséet, *Stockholm* 28 b3
Österalm, *Stockholm* 28 a3
Østerbro, *Copenhagen* 10 a1
Osterley, *London* 15 B1
Osterley Park, *London* 15 B1
Östermalm, *Stockholm* 28 A2
Österskär, *Stockholm* 28 A3
Ostiense, *Rome* 25 B1
Østmarkkapellet, *Oslo* 22 A4
Østøya, *Oslo* 22 A2
Østre Aker, *Oslo* 22 A3
Ōta-Ku, *Tokyo* 29 B3
Otaniemi, *Helsinki* 12 B1
Otari Open Air Museum, *Wellington* 32 B1
Otsuka, *Tokyo* 29 A3
Ottakring, *Vienna* 31 A1
Ottávia, *Rome* 25 B1
Ottery, *Cape Town* 8 B2
Ottobrunn, *Munich* 20 B3
Oud Zuid, *Amsterdam* 2 b1
Oude Kerk, *Amsterdam* 2 b2
Ouderkerk, *Amsterdam* 2 B2
Oulunkylä, *Helsinki* 12 B2
Ourcq, Canal de l', *Paris* 23 A3
Outer Mission, *San Francisco* 25 B2
Outremont, *Montreal* 19 A2
Overijse, *Brussels* 6 B3
Owhiro Bay, *Wellington* 32 C1
Oworonsoki, *Lagos* 14 A2
Oxford Street, *London* 15 b3
Oxgangs, *Edinburgh* 11 B2
Oxon Hill, *Washington* 32 C4
Oyodo, *Osaka* 22 A3
Oyster B., *Sydney* 28 C1
Oyster Rock, *Mumbai* 20 B1
Oyster Rocks, *Karachi* 14 B2
Ozoir-la-Ferrière, *Paris* 23 B4
Ozone Park, *New York* 21 B2

P

Pacific Heights, *San Francisco* 25 B2
Pacific Manor, *San Francisco* 25 C2
Pacific Palisades, *Los Angeles* 16 B1
Pacifica, *San Francisco* 25 C2
Paco, *Manila* 17 B1
Paco de Arcos, *Lisbon* 14 A1
Paco Imperial, *Rio de Janeiro* 24 a2
Paddington, *London* 15 b2
Paddington, *Sydney* 28 B2
Paderno, *Milan* 18 A1
Pagewood, *Sydney* 28 B2
Pagote, *Mumbai* 20 B2
Pai, I. do, *Rio de Janeiro* 24 B2
Pak Kong, *Hong Kong* 12 A2
Pakila, *Helsinki* 12 B2
Palacio de Bellas Artes, *Mexico City* 18 b2
Palacio de Communicaciones, *Madrid* 17 a3
Palacio Nacional, *Mexico City* 18 b3
Palacio Real, *Barcelona* 4 b3
Palacio Real, *Madrid* 17 b1
Palaión Fáliron, *Athens* 2 B2
Palais de Justice, *Brussels* 6 c2
Palais Royal, *Paris* 23 b4
Palais Royale, *Brussels* 6 b3
Palaiseau, *Paris* 23 B2
Palau Nacional Museu d'Art, *Barcelona* 4 c1
Palazzolo, *Milan* 18 A1
Palermo, *Buenos Aires* 7 B2
Palhais, *Lisbon* 14 B2
Palisades Park, *New York* 21 A1
Palmer Park, *Washington* 32 B4
Palmerston, *Dublin* 11 A1
Paloheinä, *Helsinki* 12 B2
Palomeras, *Madrid* 17 B2
Palos Heights, *Chicago* 9 D2
Palos Hills, *Chicago* 9 C2
Palos Hills Forest, *Chicago* 9 C1
Palos Park, *Chicago* 9 C1
Palpara, *Calcutta* 8 B2
Panchur, *Calcutta* 8 B1
Pandacan, *Manila* 17 B2
Pandan, Selat, *Singapore* 27 B2
Pandan Res., *Singapore* 27 B2
Panepistimio, *Athens* 2 b2
Pangbae, *Seoul* 26 C1
Pangrati, *Athens* 2 B2
Pangsua, Sungei →, *Singapore* 27 A2
Panihati, *Calcutta* 8 A2
Panjang, Bukit, *Singapore* 27 A2
Panje, *Mumbai* 20 B2
Panke →, *Berlin* 5 A3
Pankow, *Berlin* 5 A3
Panthéon, *Paris* 23 c4
Pantheon, *Rome* 25 b2
Pantin, *Paris* 23 A3
Pantitlán, *Mexico City* 18 B2
Panvel Cr. →, *Mumbai* 20 B2
Paparangi, *Wellington* 32 B1
Papiol, *Barcelona* 4 A1
Paramus, *New York* 21 A1
Paranaque, *Manila* 17 B1
Paray-Vieille-Poste, *Paris* 23 B3
Parco Regionale, *Milan* 18 A1
Parel, *Mumbai* 20 B1
Pari, *São Paulo* 26 B2
Parioli, *Rome* 25 B1
Paris, *Paris* 23 A3
Paris-Orly, Aéroport de, *Paris* 23 B3
Pārk-e Mellat, *Tehran* 30 A2
Park Ridge, *Chicago* 9 A1
Park Royal, *London* 15 A2
Parkchester, *New York* 21 B2
Parkdale, *Toronto* 30 B2
Parkhurst, *Johannesburg* 13 A2
Parklawn, *Washington* 32 B3
Parkmore, *Johannesburg* 13 A2
Parkside, *San Francisco* 25 B2
Parktown, *Johannesburg* 13 B2
Parktown North, *Johannesburg* 13 A2
Parkview, *Johannesburg* 13 A2
Parkville, *New York* 21 C2
Parkwood, *Cape Town* 8 B1
Parkwood, *Johannesburg* 13 A2
Parow, *Cape Town* 8 A2
Parque Chabuco, *Buenos Aires* 7 B2
Parque Patricios, *Buenos Aires* 7 B2
Parramatta →, *Sydney* 28 A1
Parthenon, *Athens* 2 c2
Paşabahçe, *Istanbul* 12 B2
Pasadena, *Los Angeles* 16 B4
Pasar Minggu, *Jakarta* 13 B1
Pasay, *Manila* 17 B1
Pascoe Vale, *Melbourne* 17 A1
Paseo de la Reforma, *Mexico City* 18 b2
Pasig, *Manila* 17 B2
Pasig →, *Manila* 17 B2
Pasila, *Helsinki* 12 B2
Pasing, *Munich* 20 B1
Pasir Panjang, *Singapore* 27 B2
Pasir Ris, *Singapore* 27 A3
Passaic →, *New York* 21 B1
Passirana, *Milan* 18 A1
Patel Nagar, *Delhi* 10 B1
Pateros, *Manila* 17 B2
Pathersville, *Atlanta* 3 B3
Pathumwan, *Bangkok* 3 B2
Patipukur, *Calcutta* 8 B2
Patisia, *Athens* 2 A2
Paulo E. Virginia, Gruta, *Rio de Janeiro* 24 B1
Paulshof, *Berlin* 5 A5
Pavshino, *Moscow* 19 B1
Paya Lebar, *Singapore* 27 A3
Peachtree →, *Atlanta* 3 B2
Peakhurst, *Sydney* 28 B1
Peania, *Athens* 2 B3
Peckham, *London* 15 B3
Peddocks I., *Boston* 6 B4
Pederstrup, *Copenhagen* 10 A2
Pedralbes, *Barcelona* 4 A1
Pedregal de San Angel, Jardines del, *Mexico City* 18 C1
Pekhorka →, *Moscow* 19 C6
Pekhra-Pokrovskoye, *Moscow* 19 A5
Pekhra-Yakovievskaya, *Moscow* 19 B5
Peking = Beijing, *Beijing* 4 B1
Pelcowizna, *Warsaw* 31 B2
Pelopónnisos Sta., *Athens* 2 a1
Penalolén, *Santiago* 26 B2
Pencarrow Hd., *Wellington* 32 C2
Peng Siang →, *Singapore* 27 A2
Penge, *London* 15 B3
Penha, *Rio de Janeiro* 24 A1
Penicuik, *Edinburgh* 11 B2
Penjaringan, *Jakarta* 13 A1
Penn Station, *New York* 21 c2
Pennsylvania Avenue, *Washington* 32 b1
Pentland Hills, *Edinburgh* 11 B1
Penyagino, *Moscow* 19 A2
Penzing, *Vienna* 31 A1
People's Park, *Shanghai* 27 B1
People's Square, *Shanghai* 27 B1
Perales del Rio, *Madrid* 17 C2
Peravillo, *Mexico City* 18 a3
Perchtoldsdorf, *Vienna* 31 B1
Perdizes, *São Paulo* 26 B2
Peredelkino, *Moscow* 19 C2
Pergamon Museum, *Berlin* 5 a4
Peristérion, *Athens* 2 A2
Perivale, *London* 15 A2
Perk, *Brussels* 6 A2
Perlach, *Munich* 20 B2
Perlacher Forst, *Munich* 20 B2
Pero, *Milan* 18 A1
Peropok, Bukit, *Singapore* 27 B2
Perovo, *Moscow* 19 B4
Pershing Square, *Los Angeles* 16 c1
Pertusella, *Milan* 18 A1
Pesagot, *Jerusalem* 13 A2
Pesanggrahag, Kali →, *Jakarta* 13 B1
Peschiera Borromeo, *Milan* 18 B2
Pesek, P., *Singapore* 27 B2
Pest, *Budapest* 7 B2
Pesterzsébet, *Budapest* 7 B2
Pesthidegkút, *Budapest* 7 A1
Pestimre, *Budapest* 7 B3
Pestlörinc, *Budapest* 7 B3
Pestújhely, *Budapest* 7 A2
Petas, *Helsinki* 12 B2
Petone, *Wellington* 32 B2
Petrogradskaya Storona, *St. Petersburg* 26 B2
Petroúpolis, *Athens* 2 A2
Petrovice, *Prague* 24 B3
Petrovskiy Park, *Moscow* 19 B3
Petrovsko-Razumovskoye, *Moscow* 19 B3
Pettycur, *Edinburgh* 11 A2
Peutie, *Brussels* 6 A2
Pfaueninsel, *Berlin* 5 B1
Phaya Thai, *Bangkok* 3 B2
Phihai, *Karachi* 14 A2
Phillip B., *Sydney* 28 B2
Phoenix Park, *Dublin* 11 A2
Phra Khanong, *Bangkok* 3 B2
Phra Pradaeng, *Bangkok* 3 C2
Phranakhon, *Bangkok* 3 B1
Picasso, Museu, *Barcelona* 4 c2
Piccadilly, *London* 15 b3
Pico Rivera, *Los Angeles* 16 C4
Piedade, *Lisbon* 14 A1
Piedade, *Rio de Janeiro* 24 B1
Piedade, Cova da, *Lisbon* 14 A2
Piedmont Park, *Atlanta* 3 B2
Pietralata, *Rome* 25 B2
Pihlajamäki, *Helsinki* 12 B2
Pihlajasaari, *Helsinki* 12 C2
Pilares, *Rio de Janeiro* 24 B1
Pilton, *Edinburgh* 11 B2
Pimlico, *London* 15 c3
Pimmit Hills, *Washington* 32 B2
Pine Grove, *Toronto* 30 A1
Pinewood, *Miami* 18 A2
Piney Run →, *Washington* 32 B2
Pinganli, *Beijing* 4 B2
Pingzhou, *Canton* 8 B2
Pinheiros →, *São Paulo* 26 B1
Pinjrapur, *Karachi* 14 A2
Pinner, *London* 15 A1
Pinner Green, *London* 15 A1
Pioltello, *Milan* 18 A2
Pipinui Pt., *Wellington* 32 A1
Piraévs, *Athens* 2 B1
Pirajuçara →, *São Paulo* 26 B1
Pirinççi, *Istanbul* 12 B1
Pirituba, *São Paulo* 26 A1
Pirkkola, *Helsinki* 12 B2
Písnice, *Prague* 24 C2
Pitampura, *Delhi* 10 A1
Pitkäjärvi, *Helsinki* 12 B1
Planegg, *Munich* 20 B1
Plumstead, *Cape Town* 8 B1
Plumstead, *London* 15 B4
Plyushchevo, *Moscow* 19 B4
Pníka, *Athens* 2 c1
Po Toi I., *Hong Kong* 12 B2
Po Toi O, *Hong Kong* 12 B2
Poasco, *Milan* 18 B2
Podbaba, *Prague* 24 B2
Podoli, *Prague* 24 B2
Poduskino, *Moscow* 19 B1
Pointe-Aux-Trembles, *Montreal* 19 A2
Poissy, *Paris* 23 A1
Pok Fu Lam, *Hong Kong* 12 B1
Pokrovsko-Sresnevo, *Moscow* 19 B2
Polton, *Edinburgh* 11 B3
Polyustrovo, *St. Petersburg* 26 B2
Pompidou, Centre, *Paris* 23 b4
Pomprap, *Bangkok* 3 B2
Pondok Indah, *Jakarta* 13 B1
Ponta do Marisco, *Rio de Janeiro* 24 C1
Pontault-Combault, *Paris* 23 B4
Pontinha, *Lisbon* 14 A1
Poplar, *London* 15 A3
Popolo, Porta del, *Rome* 25 a2
Poppintree, *Dublin* 11 A2
Porirua, *Wellington* 32 A2
Porirua East, *Wellington* 32 A2
Port I., *Osaka* 22 A2
Port Melbourne, *Melbourne* 17 B1
Port Nicholson, *Wellington* 32 B2
Port Philip Bay, *Melbourne* 17 B1
Port Richmond, *New York* 21 C1
Port Shelter, *Hong Kong* 12 A2
Port Union, *Toronto* 30 A4
Portage Park, *Chicago* 9 B2
Portal de la Pau, Pl., *Barcelona* 4 c2
Portela, Aeroporto da, *Lisbon* 14 A2
Portmarnock, *Dublin* 11 A3
Porto Brandão, *Lisbon* 14 A1
Porto Novo, *Rio de Janeiro* 24 A2
Porto Novo Cr. →, *Lagos* 14 B2
Portobello, *Edinburgh* 11 B3
Portrero, *San Francisco* 25 B3
Potomac, *Washington* 32 A2
Potomac →, *Washington* 32 B3
Potrero Pt., *San Francisco* 25 B2
Potsdam, *Berlin* 5 B1
Potsdamer Platz, *Berlin* 5 b3
Potzham, *Munich* 20 B2
Pötzleinsdorf, *Vienna* 31 A1
Povoa de Santo Adriao, *Lisbon* 14 A2
Powązki, *Warsaw* 31 B1
Powiśle, *Warsaw* 31 B2
Powsin, *Warsaw* 31 C2
Powsinek, *Warsaw* 31 C2
Poyan Res., *Singapore* 27 A2
Pozuelo de Alarcon, *Madrid* 17 B1
Prado, Museo del, *Madrid* 17 b3
Prado Churubusco, *Mexico City* 18 B2
Praga, *Warsaw* 31 B2
Prague = Praha, *Prague* 24 B2
Praha, *Prague* 24 B2
Praha-Ruzyně Airport, *Prague* 24 B1
Praires, R. des →, *Montreal* 19 A2
Prater, *Vienna* 31 A2
Precotto, *Milan* 18 A2
Prenestino Labicano, *Rome* 25 B2
Prenzlauerberg, *Berlin* 5 A3
Preston, *Melbourne* 17 A1
Pretos Forros, Sa. dos, *Rio de Janeiro* 24 B1
Préville, *Montreal* 19 B3
Přezletice, *Prague* 24 B3
Prima Porta, *Rome* 25 B1
Primavalle, *Rome* 25 B1
Primrose, *Johannesburg* 13 B2
Princes Street, *Edinburgh* 11 b2
Printer's Row, *Chicago* 9 d2
Progreso Nacional, *Mexico City* 18 A2
Prosek, *Prague* 24 B3
Prospect Hill Park, *Boston* 6 A2
Providencia, *Santiago* 26 B2
Prudential Building, *Chicago* 9 c2
Průhonice, *Prague* 24 C3
Psikhikón, *Athens* 2 A2
Pudong New Area, *Shanghai* 27 B2
Pueblo Libre, *Lima* 16 B2
Pueblo Nuevo, *Barcelona* 4 A2
Pueblo Nuevo, *Madrid* 17 B2
Puerta del Sol, Plaza, *Madrid* 17 b2
Puerto Madero, *Buenos Aires* 7 B2
Puerto Retiro, *Buenos Aires* 7 B2
Puhuangyu, *Beijing* 4 B2
Puistola, *Helsinki* 12 B3
Pukan-san, *Seoul* 26 B1
Pukinmäki, *Helsinki* 12 B2
Pukkajwa, *Seoul* 26 B1
Pulkovo Int. Airport, *St. Petersburg* 26 C1
Pullach, *Munich* 20 B1
Pulo Gadung, *Jakarta* 13 B2
Pūnak, *Tehran* 30 A2
Punchbowl, *Sydney* 28 B1
Punde, *Mumbai* 20 B2
Punggol, *Singapore* 27 A3
Punggol, Sungei →, *Singapore* 27 A3
Punggol Pt., *Singapore* 27 A3
Punjabi Bagh, *Delhi* 10 A1
Puotila, *Helsinki* 12 B3
Purana Qila, *Delhi* 1 c3
Puteaux, *Paris* 23 A2
Putilkovo, *Moscow* 19 A2
Putney, *London* 15 B2
Putuo, *Shanghai* 27 B1
Putxet, *Barcelona* 4 A1
Puxi, *Shanghai* 27 B1
Pydhuni, *Mumbai* 20 b2
Pyramids, *Cairo* 7 B1
Pyry, *Warsaw* 31 C1

Q

Qalandya, *Jerusalem* 13 A2
Qal'eh Morghī, *Tehran* 30 B2
Qanâ el Ismâ'ilîya, *Cairo* 7 A2
Qāsemābād, *Tehran* 30 A3
Qasr-e Firūzeh, *Tehran* 30 B3
Qatane, *Jerusalem* 13 B1
Qianmen, *Beijing* 4 B2
Qinghuayuan, *Beijing* 4 B1
Qingningsi, *Shanghai* 27 B2
Qolhak, *Tehran* 30 A2
Quadraro, *Rome* 25 B2
Quaid-i-Azam, *Karachi* 14 A1
Quartiere Zingone, *Milan* 18 B1
Quds, *Baghdad* 3 A2
Queen Mary Res., *London* 15 B1
Queen Street, *Edinburgh* 11 a1
Queensbury, *London* 15 A2
Queenscliffe, *Sydney* 28 A2
Queensferry, *Edinburgh* 11 B1
Queenstown, *Singapore* 27 B2
Quellerina, *Johannesburg* 13 A1
Queluz, *Lisbon* 14 A1
Quezon City, *Manila* 17 B2
Quezon Memorial Circle, *Manila* 17 B2
Quilicura, *Santiago* 26 B1
Quincy, *Boston* 6 B3
Quincy B., *Boston* 6 B4
Quinta Normal, *Santiago* 26 B1
Quinto de Stampi, *Milan* 18 B2
Quinto Romano, *Milan* 18 B1
Quirinale, *Rome* 25 B1
Quirinale, Palazzo dei, *Rome* 25 b3

R

Raasdorf, *Vienna* 31 A3
Rådhuset, *Oslo* 22 A3
Radlice, *Prague* 24 B2
Radość, *Warsaw* 31 B3
Radotin, *Prague* 24 C2
Rafat, *Jerusalem* 13 A2
Raffles Hotel, *Singapore* 27 b3
Raffles Park, *Singapore* 27 B2
Raheny, *Dublin* 11 A3
Rahnsdorf, *Berlin* 5 B5
Rainham, *London* 15 A5
Raj Ghat, *Delhi* 1 b3
Rajakylä, *Helsinki* 12 B3
Rajpath, *Delhi* 1 c2
Rajpura, *Delhi* 10 A2
Rákos-patak →, *Budapest* 7 B3
Rákoshegy, *Budapest* 7 B3
Rákoskeresztúr, *Budapest* 7 B3

Rákoskert, *Budapest* 7 B3
Rákosliget, *Budapest* 7 B3
Rákospalota, *Budapest* 7 A2
Rákosszentmihály, *Budapest* 7 A2
Raków, *Warsaw* 31 B1
Ram, *Jerusalem* 13 A2
Rām Allāh, *Jerusalem* 13 A2
Ramadān, *Baghdad* 3 B2
Ramakrishna Puram, *Delhi* 10 B1
Ramanathpur, *Calcutta* 8 A1
Rambla, La, *Barcelona* 4 b2
Rambler Channel, *Hong Kong* 12 A1
Ramenki, *Moscow* 19 B2
Ramersdorf, *Munich* 20 B2
Ramos, *Rio de Janeiro* 24 B1
Ramos Mejia, *Buenos Aires* 7 B1
Ramot, *Jerusalem* 13 B2
Rampur, *Delhi* 10 A2
Ramsgate, *Sydney* 28 B1
Rand Afrikaans Univ., *Johannesburg* 13 B2
Rand Airport, *Johannesburg* 13 B2
Randburg, *Johannesburg* 13 A1
Randhart, *Johannesburg* 13 B2
Randpark Ridge, *Johannesburg* 13 A1
Randwick, *Sydney* 28 B2
Ranelagh, *Dublin* 11 A2
Rannersdorf, *Vienna* 31 B2
Ransbèche, *Brussels* 6 B2
Ransdorp, *Amsterdam* 2 A2
Ranvad, *Mumbai* 20 B2
Raposo, *Lisbon* 14 A1
Rashtrapati Bhawan, *Delhi* 1 c1
Rasskazovka, *Moscow* 19 C2
Rastaala, *Helsinki* 12 B1
Rastila, *Helsinki* 12 B3
Raszyn, *Warsaw* 31 C1
Ratcha Thewi, *Bangkok* 3 b3
Rathfarnham, *Dublin* 11 B2
Ratho, *Edinburgh* 11 B1
Ratho Station, *Edinburgh* 11 B1
Rato, *Lisbon* 14 A2
Ravelston, *Edinburgh* 11 B2
Rawamangun, *Jakarta* 13 B2
Rayners Lane, *London* 15 A1
Raynes Park, *London* 15 B2
Raypur, *Calcutta* 8 C2
Razdory, *Moscow* 19 B1
Real Felipe, Fuerte, *Lima* 16 B2
Recoleta, *Buenos Aires* 7 B2
Recoleta, *Santiago* 26 B2
Red Fort = Lal Qila, *Delhi* 1 a3
Redbridge, *London* 15 A4
Redfern, *Sydney* 28 B2
Redwood, *Wellington* 32 B1
Reeves Hill, *Boston* 6 A1
Refshaleøen, *Copenhagen* 10 A3
Regents Park, *Johannesburg* 13 B2
Regent's Park, *London* 15 a2
Rego Park, *New York* 21 B2
Reichstag, *Berlin* 5 a3
Reina Sofia, Centro de Arte, *Madrid* 17 c3
Reinickendorf, *Berlin* 5 A3
Rekola, *Helsinki* 12 B3
Rembertów, *Warsaw* 31 B2
Rembrandthuis, *Amsterdam* 2 b2
Rembrandtpark, *Amsterdam* 2 A2
Rembrandtsplein, *Amsterdam* 2 b2
Remedios, Parque Nacional de los, *Mexico City* 18 B1
Remedios de Escalada, *Buenos Aires* 7 C2
Rémola, Laguna del, *Barcelona* 4 B1
Renca, *Santiago* 26 B1
Renmin Park, *Tianjin* 30 B2
Rennemoulin, *Paris* 23 A1
Řeporyje, *Prague* 24 B1
Republica, Plaza de la, *Mexico City* 18 b1
République, Place de la, *Paris* 23 b5
Repulse Bay, *Hong Kong* 12 B2
Repy, *Prague* 24 B1
Residenz, *Munich* 20 B2
Residenzmuseum, *Munich* 20 b3
Reston, *Washington* 32 B2
Retiro, *Buenos Aires* 7 B2
Retiro, *Madrid* 17 B1
Retreat, *Cape Town* 8 B1
Reutov, *Moscow* 19 B5
Réveillon →, *Paris* 23 B4
Revere, *Boston* 6 A3
Rexdale, *Toronto* 30 A1
Reynosa Tamaulipas, *Mexico City* 18 A1
Rho, *Milan* 18 A1
Rhodes, *Sydney* 28 A1
Rhodon, *Paris* 23 B1
Rhodon →, *Paris* 23 B1
Ribeira, *Rio de Janeiro* 24 A1
Ricarda, Laguna de la, *Barcelona* 4 B1
Richmond, *Melbourne* 17 A2
Richmond, *San Francisco* 25 B2
Richmond Hill, *New York* 21 B2
Richmond Park, *London* 15 B2
Richmond upon Thames, *London* 15 B2
Riddarholmen, *Stockholm* 28 c1
Riddarhuset, *Stockholm* 28 c2
Ridgefield, *New York* 21 B1
Ridgefield Park, *New York* 21 A1
Ridgewood, *New York* 21 B2
Riem, *Munich* 20 B3
Rijksmuseum, *Amsterdam* 2 b1
Rikers I., *New York* 21 B2
Riksdagensledamothus, *Stockholm* 28 b2
Riksdagshuset, *Stockholm* 28 b2
Rimac, *Lima* 16 B2
Ringsend, *Dublin* 11 A2
Rinkeby, *Stockholm* 28 A1
Rio Compride, *Rio de Janeiro* 24 B1
Rio de Janeiro, *Rio de Janeiro* 24 B1
Rio de la Plata, *Buenos Aires* 7 B2
Rio de Mouro, *Lisbon* 14 A1
Ripollet, *Barcelona* 4 A1
Ris, *Oslo* 22 A3
Risby, *Copenhagen* 10 A1
Rishra, *Calcutta* 8 A2
Ritchie, *Washington* 32 B4
Rithala, *Delhi* 10 A1
Rive Sud, Canal de la, *Montreal* 19 B2
River Edge, *New York* 21 A1
River Forest, *Chicago* 9 B2
River Grove, *Chicago* 9 B1
Riverdale, *New York* 21 A2
Riverdale, *Washington* 32 B4
Riverdale Park, *Toronto* 30 A2
Riverlea, *Johannesburg* 13 B1
Riverside, *Chicago* 9 C2
Riverwood, *Sydney* 28 B1
Rivière-des-Praires, *Montreal* 19 A2
Rixensart, *Brussels* 6 B3
Riyad, *Baghdad* 3 B2
Rizal Park, *Manila* 17 B1
Rizal Stadium, *Manila* 17 B1
Røa, *Oslo* 22 A2
Robbins, *Chicago* 9 D2
Robertsham, *Johannesburg* 13 B2
Rochelle Park, *New York* 21 A1
Rock Cr. →, *Washington* 32 B3
Rock Creek Park, *Washington* 32 B3
Rock Pt., *Wellington* 32 A1
Rockaway Pt., *New York* 21 C2
Rockdale, *Sydney* 28 B1
Rockefeller Center, *New York* 21 c2
Rodaon, *Vienna* 31 B1
Rødovre, *Copenhagen* 10 A2
Rodrigo de Freitas, L., *Rio de Janeiro* 24 B1
Roehampton, *London* 15 B2
Rogers Park, *Chicago* 9 A2
Roihuvuori, *Helsinki* 12 B3
Roissy-en-Brie, *Paris* 23 B4
Rokin, *Amsterdam* 2 b2
Rokkō I., *Osaka* 22 A2
Rokkō Sanchi, *Osaka* 22 A2
Rokkō-Zan, *Osaka* 22 A2
Rokytka →, *Prague* 24 B3
Roma, *Rome* 25 B1
Római-Fürdö, *Budapest* 7 A2
Romainville, *Paris* 23 A3
Romano Banco, *Milan* 18 B1
Romashkovo, *Moscow* 19 B1
Rome = Roma, *Rome* 25 B1
Romford, *London* 15 A5
Rondebosch, *Cape Town* 8 A1
Roppongi, *Tokyo* 29 c3
Rose Hill, *Washington* 32 C3
Rosebank, *New York* 21 C1
Rosebery, *Sydney* 28 B2
Rosedal La Candelaria, *Mexico City* 18 B2
Roseland, *Chicago* 9 C3
Rosemead, *Los Angeles* 16 B4
Rosemont, *Montreal* 19 A2
Rosenborg Have, *Copenhagen* 10 A3
Rosenthal, *Berlin* 5 A3
Rosettenville, *Johannesburg* 13 B2
Rosewell, *Edinburgh* 11 B3
Rosherville Dam, *Johannesburg* 13 B2
Rösjön, *Stockholm* 28 A2
Roslags-Näsby, *Stockholm* 28 A2
Roslin, *Edinburgh* 11 B3
Roslindale, *Boston* 6 B3
Rosny-sous-Bois, *Paris* 23 A4
Rosslyn, *Washington* 32 B3
Rosyth, *Edinburgh* 11 A1
Rotherhithe, *London* 15 B3
Rothneusiedl, *Vienna* 31 B2
Rothschmaige, *Munich* 20 A1
Rouge Hill, *Toronto* 30 A4
Round I., *Hong Kong* 12 B2
Roxbury, *Boston* 6 B3
Roxeth, *London* 15 A1
Royal Botanic Garden, *Edinburgh* 11 B2
Royal Botanic Gardens, *Sydney* 28 b2
Royal Grand Palace, *Bangkok* 3 b1
Royal Observatory, *Edinburgh* 11 B2
Royal Park, *Melbourne* 17 A1
Royal Turf Club, *Bangkok* 3 b2
Röylä, *Helsinki* 12 B1
Rozas, Portilleros de las, *Madrid* 17 B1
Roztoky, *Prague* 24 B2
Rozzano, *Milan* 18 B1
Rubi →, *Barcelona* 4 A1
Rublovo, *Moscow* 19 B2
Rudnevka →, *Moscow* 19 B5
Rudolfsheim, *Vienna* 31 A2
Rudolfshöhe, *Berlin* 5 A5
Rudow, *Berlin* 5 B3
Rueil-Malmaison, *Paris* 23 A2
Ruisbroek, *Brussels* 6 B1
Ruislip, *London* 15 A1
Rumelihisarı, *Istanbul* 12 B2
Rumyantsevo, *Moscow* 19 C2
Rungis, *Paris* 23 B3
Rusāfa, *Baghdad* 3 A2
Rush Green, *London* 15 A5
Russa, *Calcutta* 8 C2
Russian Hill, *San Francisco* 25 a1
Rustenfeld, *Vienna* 31 B2
Rutherford, *New York* 21 B1
Ruzyně, *Prague* 24 B1
Rybatskaya, *St. Petersburg* 26 B2
Rydboholm, *Stockholm* 28 A3
Ryde, *Sydney* 28 A1
Rynek, *Warsaw* 31 a2
Ryogoku, *Tokyo* 29 A3
Rzhevka, *St. Petersburg* 26 B3

S

Sa'ādatābād, *Tehran* 30 A2
Saadūn, *Baghdad* 3 B2
Saavedra, *Buenos Aires* 7 B2
Saboli, *Delhi* 10 A2
Sabugo, *Lisbon* 14 A1
Sabzi Mand, *Delhi* 10 A2
Sacavém, *Lisbon* 14 A2
Saclay, *Paris* 23 B2
Saclay, Étang de, *Paris* 23 B1
Sacomã, *São Paulo* 26 B2
Sacré Cœur, *Paris* 23 a4
Sacrow, *Berlin* 5 B1
Sacrower See, *Berlin* 5 B1
Sadang, *Seoul* 26 C1
Sadar Bazar, *Delhi* 1 a1
Saddle Brook, *New York* 21 A1
Sadr, *Karachi* 14 A2
Sadr City, *Baghdad* 3 A2
Sadyba, *Warsaw* 31 B2
Saft el Laban, *Cairo* 7 A2
Saganashkee Slough, *Chicago* 9 C1
Sagene, *Oslo* 22 A3
Sagrada Família, Templo de, *Barcelona* 4 A2
Sagrado Familia, Templo de, *Barcelona* 4 a2
Sahar Int. Airport, *Mumbai* 20 A2
Sai Kung, *Hong Kong* 12 A2
Sai Wan Ho, *Hong Kong* 12 B2
Sai Ying Pun, *Hong Kong* 12 B1
St.-Aubin, *Paris* 23 B1
St.-Cloud, *Paris* 23 A2
St.-Cyr-l'École, *Paris* 23 B1
St.-Cyr-l'École, Aérodrome de, *Paris* 23 B1
St.-Denis, *Paris* 23 A3
St.-Germain, Forêt de, *Paris* 23 A1
St.-Germain-en-Laye, *Paris* 23 A1
St. Giles Cathedral, *Edinburgh* 11 b2
St-Gilles, *Brussels* 6 B2
St. Helier, *London* 15 B2
St.-Hubert, *Montreal* 19 B3
St. Hubert, Galerie, *Brussels* 6 b2
St. Isaac's Cathedral, *St. Petersburg* 26 B1
St. Jacques →, *Montreal* 19 B3
St. James's, *London* 15 b3
St. John's Cathedral, *Hong Kong* 12 c1
St-Joose-Ten-Noode, *Brussels* 6 A2
St. Kilda, *Melbourne* 17 B1
St. Lambert, *Montreal* 19 A3
St.-Lambert, *Paris* 23 B1
St.-Laurent, *Montreal* 19 A1
St. Lawrence →, *Montreal* 19 B2
St.-Lazare, Gare, *Paris* 23 A2
St.-Léonard, *Montreal* 19 A2
St. Magelungen, *Stockholm* 28 B2
St.-Mandé, *Paris* 23 A3
St. Margaret's, *Dublin* 11 A2
St.-Martin, Bois, *Paris* 23 B4
St. Mary Cray, *London* 15 B4
St.-Maur-des-Fossés, *Paris* 23 B3
St.-Maurice, *Paris* 23 B3
St.-Michel, *Montreal* 19 A2
St. Nikolaus-Kirken, *Prague* 24 B2
St.-Ouen, *Paris* 23 A3
St. Patrick's Cathedral, *Dublin* 11 c1
St. Patrick's Cathedral, *New York* 21 c2
St. Paul's Cathedral, *London* 15 b4
St. Paul's Cray, *London* 15 B4
St. Peters, *Sydney* 28 B2
St. Petersburg = Sankt Peterburg, *St. Petersburg* 26 B1
St.-Pierre, *Montreal* 19 B2
St-Pieters-Leeuw, *Brussels* 6 B1
St.-Quentin, Étang de, *Paris* 23 B1
St. Stephen's Green, *Dublin* 11 c3
St-Stevens-Woluwe, *Brussels* 6 A2
St.-Vincent-de-Paul, *Montreal* 19 A2
Ste.-Catherine, *Montreal* 19 B2
Ste.-Hélène, Î., *Montreal* 19 A2
Saiwai, *Tokyo* 29 B3
Sakai, *Osaka* 22 B3
Sakai Harbour, *Osaka* 22 B3
Sakra, P., *Singapore* 27 B2
Salam, *Baghdad* 3 A2
Salamanca, *Madrid* 17 B1
Sâllynoggin, *Dublin* 11 B3
Salmannsdorf, *Vienna* 31 A1
Salmedina, *Madrid* 17 C2
Salomea, *Warsaw* 31 B1
Salsette I., *Mumbai* 20 A2
Salt Lake City, *Calcutta* 8 B2
Salt River, *Cape Town* 8 A1
Salt Water L., *Calcutta* 8 B2
Saltsjö-Duvnäs, *Stockholm* 28 B3
Saltykovka, *Moscow* 19 B5
Samatya, *Istanbul* 12 C1
Sampaloc, *Manila* 17 B1
Samphan Thawong, *Bangkok* 3 B2
Samsŏn, *Seoul* 26 B2
San Andrés, *Barcelona* 4 A2
San Angel, *Mexico City* 18 B1
San Angelo, Castel, *Rome* 25 b1
San Basilio, *Rome* 25 B2
San Borja, *Lima* 16 B3
San Bóvio, *Milan* 18 B2
San Bruno, Pt., *San Francisco* 25 C2
San Bruno Mt., *San Francisco* 25 B2
San Cristobal, *Buenos Aires* 7 B2
San Cristobal, *Madrid* 17 B2
San Cristóbal, Cerro, *Santiago* 26 B2
San Cristoforo, *Milan* 18 B1
San Donato Milanese, *Milan* 18 B2
San Francisco, *San Francisco* 25 B2
San Francisco B., *San Francisco* 25 B3
San Francisco Culhuacán, *Mexico City* 18 C2
San Fruttuoso, *Milan* 18 A2
San Gabriel, *Los Angeles* 16 B4
San Giuliano Milanese, *Milan* 18 B2
San Isidro, *Lima* 16 B2
San Jerónimo Lidice, *Mexico City* 18 C1
San Joaquin, *Santiago* 26 B2
San José Rio Hondo, *Mexico City* 18 B1
San Juan →, *Manila* 17 B2
San Juan de Aragón, *Mexico City* 18 B2
San Juan de Aragón, Parque, *Mexico City* 18 B2
San Juan de Lurigancho, *Lima* 16 A2
San Juan del Monte, *Manila* 17 B2
San Juan Ixtacala, *Mexico City* 18 A1
San Juan Toltotepec, *Mexico City* 18 B1
San Just Desvern, *Barcelona* 4 A1
San Justo, *Buenos Aires* 7 C1
San Lorenzo Tezonco, *Mexico City* 18 C2
San Luis, *Lima* 16 B2
San Marino, *Los Angeles* 16 B4
San Martin, *Barcelona* 4 A2
San Martin de Porras, *Lima* 16 B2
San Miguel, *Lima* 16 B2
San Miguel, *Santiago* 26 B2
San Nicolas, *Buenos Aires* 7 B2
San Onófrio, *Rome* 25 B1
San Pedro Martir, *Barcelona* 4 A1
San Pedro Zacatenco, *Mexico City* 18 A2
San Pietro, Piazza, *Rome* 25 b1
San Po Kong, *Hong Kong* 12 A2
San Rafael Chamapa, *Mexico City* 18 B1
San Rafael Hills, *Los Angeles* 16 A3
San Roque, *Manila* 17 B2
San Siro, *Milan* 18 B1
San Souci, *Sydney* 28 B1
San Telmo, *Buenos Aires* 7 B2
San Vicenc dels Horts, *Barcelona* 4 A1
Sanbancho, *Tokyo* 29 a3
Sandown, *Johannesburg* 13 A2
Sandown Park Races, *London* 15 B1
Sandton, *Johannesburg* 13 A2
Sandvika, *Oslo* 22 A2
Sandy Pond, *Boston* 6 A2
Sandyford, *Dublin* 11 B2
Sandymount, *Dublin* 11 B2
Sangenjaya, *Tokyo* 29 B2
Sangge, *Seoul* 26 B2
Sangley Pt., *Manila* 17 C1
Sankrail, *Calcutta* 8 B1
Sankt Peterburg, *St. Petersburg* 26 B1
Sankt Veit, *Vienna* 31 A1
Sanlihe, *Beijing* 4 B1
Sanlintang, *Shanghai* 27 C1
Sans, *Barcelona* 4 A1
Sant Agusti, *Barcelona* 4 c2
Sant Ambrogio, Basilica di, *Milan* 18 B2
Sant Boi de Llobregat, *Barcelona* 4 A1
Sant Cugat, *Barcelona* 4 A1
Sant Feliu de Llobregat, *Barcelona* 4 A1
Sant Joan Despi, *Barcelona* 4 A1
Sant Maria del Mar, *Barcelona* 4 b3
Sant Pau del Camp, *Barcelona* 4 c2
Santa Ana, *Manila* 17 B2
Santa Coloma de Gramanet, *Barcelona* 4 A2
Santa Cruz, *Manila* 17 B1
Santa Cruz, *Mumbai* 20 A1
Santa Cruz, I. de, *Rio de Janeiro* 24 B2
Santa Cruz de Olorde, *Barcelona* 4 A1
Santa Efigénia, *São Paulo* 26 B2
Santa Elena, *Manila* 17 B2
Santa Elena del Gomero, *Santiago* 26 B1
Santa Eulalia, *Barcelona* 4 A2
Santa Fe Springs, *Los Angeles* 16 C4
Santa Iria da Azóia, *Lisbon* 14 A2
Santa Julia, *Santiago* 26 C2
Santa Maria, *Mexico City* 18 a1
Santa Monica, *Los Angeles* 16 B2
Santa Monica Mts., *Los Angeles* 16 B2
Santa Rosa De Locobe, *Santiago* 26 B2
Santa Teresa de la Ovalle, *Santiago* 26 B1
Santahamina, *Helsinki* 12 C3
Santana, *São Paulo* 26 A2
Santeny, *Paris* 23 B4
Santiago, *Santiago* 26 B2
Santiago de Surco, *Lima* 16 B2
Santo Amaro, *Lisbon* 14 A1
Santo Amaro, *São Paulo* 26 B1
Santo Andre, *Lisbon* 14 B2
Santo Antão do Tojal, *Lisbon* 14 A2
Santo António, Qta. de, *Lisbon* 14 B1
Santo Tomas, Univ. of, *Manila* 17 B1
Santos Dumont, Aéroport, *Rio de Janeiro* 24 B2
Santoshpur, *Calcutta* 8 B1
Santragachi, *Calcutta* 8 B1
Santry, *Dublin* 11 A2
Sanyuanli, *Canton* 8 B2
São Caetano do Sul, *São Paulo* 26 B2
São Conrado, *Rio de Janeiro* 24 C1
São Cristovão, *Rio de Janeiro* 24 B1
São Francisco Penitência, *Rio de Janeiro* 24 b1
São Jorge, Castelo de, *Lisbon* 14 A2
São Juliao do Tojal, *Lisbon* 14 A2
São Paulo, *São Paulo* 26 B2
Sapa, *Calcutta* 8 B1
Sapateiro, Cor. do →, *São Paulo* 26 B1
Sarandi, *Buenos Aires* 7 C2
Saraswati →, *Calcutta* 8 A1
Sarecky potok →, *Prague* 24 B2
Sarimbun, *Singapore* 27 A2
Sarimbun Res., *Singapore* 27 A2
Sarıyer, *Istanbul* 12 A2
Saronikós Kólpos, *Athens* 2 B1
Sarriá, *Barcelona* 4 A1
Sarsuna, *Calcutta* 8 C1
Sartrouville, *Paris* 23 A2
Sasad, *Budapest* 7 B2
Sashalom, *Budapest* 7 A3
Saska, *Warsaw* 31 B2
Satalice, *Prague* 24 B3
Satgachi, *Calcutta* 8 B2
Sathorn, *Bangkok* 3 B2
Satpukur, *Calcutta* 8 B2
Sätra, *Stockholm* 28 B1
Sattru Pha, *Bangkok* 3 b2
Saúde, *São Paulo* 26 B2
Saugus, *Boston* 6 A3
Saugus →, *Boston* 6 A3
Sault-au-Récollet, *Montreal* 19 A2
Sausalito, *San Francisco* 25 A2
Sawah Besar, *Jakarta* 13 A1
Saxonville, *Boston* 6 B1
Scald Law, *Edinburgh* 11 B2
Scarborough, *Toronto* 30 A3
Sceaux, *Paris* 23 B2
Schaerbeek, *Brussels* 6 A2
Scharfenberg, *Berlin* 5 A2
Scheepvartmuseum, *Amsterdam* 2 b3
Schiller Park, *Chicago* 9 B1
Schiller Woods, *Chicago* 9 B1
Schiphol, Luchthaven, *Amsterdam* 2 B1
Schlachtensee, *Berlin* 5 B2
Schlossgarten, *Berlin* 5 A2
Schmargendorf, *Berlin* 5 B2
Schönblick, *Berlin* 5 B5
Schönbrunn, Schloss, *Vienna* 31 A1
Schöneberg, *Berlin* 5 B3
Schöneiche, *Berlin* 5 B5
Schönwalde, *Berlin* 5 A1
Schotschekloof, *Cape Town* 8 b1
Schulzendorf, *Berlin* 5 A2
Schwabing, *Munich* 20 B2
Schwanebeck, *Berlin* 5 A4
Schwanenwerder, *Berlin* 5 B2
Schwarzlackenau, *Vienna* 31 A2
Schwechat, *Vienna* 31 B2
Scitrek Museum, *Atlanta* 3 B2
Scott Monument, *Edinburgh* 11 b2
Scottdale, *Atlanta* 3 B3
Sea Point, *Cape Town* 8 A1
Seabrook, *Washington* 32 B5
Seacliff, *San Francisco* 25 B2
Seaforth, *Sydney* 28 A2
Seagate, *New York* 21 C1
Sears Tower, *Chicago* 9 c1
Seat Pleasant, *Washington* 32 B4
Seaview, *Wellington* 32 B2
Šeberov, *Prague* 24 B3
Secaucus, *New York* 21 B1
Seddinsee, *Berlin* 5 B5
Seeberg, *Berlin* 5 A5
Seeburg, *Berlin* 5 A1
Seefeld, *Berlin* 5 A5
Seegefeld, *Berlin* 5 A1
Seehof, *Berlin* 5 B2
Segeltorp, *Stockholm* 28 B1
Segrate, *Milan* 18 B2
Seguro, *Milan* 18 B1
Seine →, *Paris* 23 B3
Seixal, *Lisbon* 14 B2
Selby, *Johannesburg* 13 B2
Seletar, P., *Singapore* 27 A3
Seletar Hills, *Singapore* 27 A3
Seletar Res., *Singapore* 27 A2
Selhurst, *London* 15 B3
Sembawang, *Singapore* 27 A2
Senago, *Milan* 18 A1
Sendinger Tor Platz, *Munich* 20 c1
Sendling, *Munich* 20 B2
Senju, *Tokyo* 29 A3
Senriyama, *Osaka* 22 A4
Sentosa, P., *Singapore* 27 B2
Seoul = Sŏul, *Seoul* 26 B2
Seoul National Univ., *Seoul* 26 C1
Seoul Tower, *Seoul* 26 B1
Sepolia, *Athens* 2 A2
Sepulveda Flood Control Basin, *Los Angeles* 16 A2
Serangoon, *Singapore* 27 A3
Serangoon, P., *Singapore* 27 A3
Serangoon, Sungei →, *Singapore* 27 A3
Serangoon Harbour, *Singapore* 27 A3
Seraya, P., *Singapore* 27 B2
Serebryanka, *Moscow* 19 B5
Serebryanka →, *Moscow* 19 B4
Serramonte, *San Francisco* 25 C2
Sesto San Giovanni, *Milan* 18 A2
Sesto Ulteriano, *Milan* 18 B2
Setagaya-Ku, *Tokyo* 29 B2
Seter, *Oslo* 22 A3
Setia Budi, *Jakarta* 13 B1
Settebagni, *Rome* 25 A2
Settecamini, *Rome* 25 B2
Séttimo Milanese, *Milan* 18 B1
Settsu, *Osaka* 22 A4
Setuny →, *Moscow* 19 B2
Seutula, *Helsinki* 12 A2
Seven Corners, *Washington* 32 B3
Seven Kings, *London* 15 A4
Sévesco →, *Milan* 18 A1
Sevran, *Paris* 23 A4
Sewri, *Mumbai* 20 B2
Sforzesso, Castello, *Milan* 18 B2
Sha Kok Mei, *Hong Kong* 12 A2
Sha Tin, *Hong Kong* 12 A2
Sha Tin Wai, *Hong Kong* 12 A2
Shabrâmant, *Cairo* 7 B2
Shahdara, *Delhi* 10 A2
Shahe, *Canton* 8 B2
Shahr-e Rey, *Tehran* 30 B2
Shahrak-e Golshahr, *Tehran* 30 B1
Shahrak-e Qods, *Tehran* 30 A2
Shaikh Aomar, *Baghdad* 3 A2
Shakurbasti, *Delhi* 10 A1
Shalkiya, *Calcutta* 8 B2
Sham Shui Po, *Hong Kong* 12 B1
Shamapur, *Delhi* 10 A1
Shamian, *Canton* 8 B2
Shan Mei, *Hong Kong* 12 A2
Shanghai, *Shanghai* 27 B2
Shankill, *Dublin* 11 B3
Sharp I., *Hong Kong* 12 A2
Shastrinagar, *Delhi* 10 A2
Shau Kei Wan, *Hong Kong* 12 B2
Shawocun, *Beijing* 4 B1
Shayuan, *Canton* 8 B2
Sheepshead Bay, *New York* 21 C2
Shek O, *Hong Kong* 12 B2
Shelter I., *Hong Kong* 12 B2
Sheng Fa Shan, *Hong Kong* 12 A1
Shepherds Bush, *London* 15 A2
Shepperton, *London* 15 B1
Sherman Oaks, *Los Angeles* 16 B2
Sherman Park, *Chicago* 9 C2
Shet Bandar, *Mumbai* 20 B2
Sheung Lau Wan, *Hong Kong* 12 B2
Sheung Wan, *Hong Kong* 12 B1
Sheva, *Mumbai* 20 B2
Sheva Nhava, *Mumbai* 20 B2
Shiba, *Tokyo* 29 c4
Shibpur, *Calcutta* 8 B1
Shibuya-Ku, *Tokyo* 29 c1
Shijōnawate, *Osaka* 22 A4
Shillim, *Seoul* 26 C1
Shimogawara, *Tokyo* 29 B1
Shimosalo, *Tokyo* 29 A2
Shimoshakujii, *Tokyo* 29 A2
Shinagawa-Ku, *Tokyo* 29 B3
Shing Mun Res., *Hong Kong* 12 A1
Shinjuku-Ku, *Tokyo* 29 a1
Shinjuku National Garden, *Tokyo* 29 a2
Shinkoiwa, *Tokyo* 29 A4
Shinnakano, *Tokyo* 29 A3
Shinsa, *Seoul* 26 B2
Shipai, *Canton* 8 B3
Shirinashi →, *Osaka* 22 B3
Shirogane, *Tokyo* 29 B3
Shiweitang, *Canton* 8 B2
Shogunle, *Lagos* 14 A2
Shomolu, *Lagos* 14 A2
Shooters Hill, *London* 15 B4
Shoreditch, *London* 15 a5
Shortlands, *London* 15 B4
Shu' afat, *Jerusalem* 13 B2
Shubrâ, *Cairo* 7 A2
Shubrâ el Kheima, *Cairo* 7 A2
Shuikuo, *Canton* 8 A2
Shuishang Park, *Tianjin* 30 B1
Sidcup, *London* 15 B4
Siebenhirten, *Vienna* 31 B1
Siedlung, *Berlin* 5 A1
Siekierki, *Warsaw* 31 B2
Sielce, *Warsaw* 31 B2
Siemensstadt, *Berlin* 5 A2
Sierra Madre, *Los Angeles* 16 B4
Sievering, *Vienna* 31 A2
Sighthill, *Edinburgh* 11 B2
Signal Hill, *Cape Town* 8 A1
Sihŭng, *Seoul* 26 C1
Sikátorpuszta, *Budapest* 7 A3
Silampur, *Delhi* 10 B2
Silver Hill, *Boston* 6 A2
Silver Hill, *Washington* 32 C4
Silver Spring, *Washington* 32 A3
Silvermine Nature Reserve, *Cape Town* 8 B1
Silvolantekojärvi, *Helsinki* 12 B2
Simei, *Singapore* 27 A3
Simla, *Calcutta* 8 B2
Simmering, *Vienna* 31 A2
Simmering Heide, *Vienna* 31 A2
Simonkylä, *Helsinki* 12 B3
Singapore, *Singapore* 27 B3
Singapore, Univ. of, *Singapore* 27 B2
Sinicka →, *Moscow* 19 A1
Sinki, Selat, *Singapore* 27 B2
Sint-Genesius-Rode, *Brussels* 6 B2
Sinwŏl, *Seoul* 26 B1
Sion, *Mumbai* 20 A2
Sipson, *London* 15 B1
Siqeil, *Cairo* 7 A1
Şişli, *Istanbul* 12 B1
Skansen, *Stockholm* 28 B2
Skärholmen, *Stockholm* 28 B1
Skarpäng, *Stockholm* 28 A2
Skarpnäck, *Stockholm* 28 B2
Skaryszewski Park, *Warsaw* 31 B2
Skeppsholmen, *Stockholm* 28 c3
Skokie, *Chicago* 9 A2
Skokie →, *Chicago* 9 A2
Skoklefall, *Oslo* 22 A3
Sköndal, *Stockholm* 28 B2
Skovlunde, *Copenhagen* 10 A2
Skovshoved, *Copenhagen* 10 A3
Skuru, *Stockholm* 28 B3
Skyland, *Atlanta* 3 A3
Slade Green, *London* 15 B5
Slemmestad, *Oslo* 22 B1
Slependen, *Oslo* 22 A2
Slipi, *Jakarta* 13 B1
Slivenec, *Prague* 24 B2
Sloten, *Amsterdam* 2 A1
Sloterpark, *Amsterdam* 2 A1
Sluhy, *Prague* 24 A3
Służew, *Warsaw* 31 B2
Służewiec, *Warsaw* 31 B2
Smíchov, *Prague* 24 B2
Smith Forest Preserve, *Chicago* 9 B2
Smithsonian Institute, *Washington* 32 b2
Smolny, *St. Petersburg* 26 B2
Snake Creek Canal →, *Miami* 18 A2
Snarøya, *Oslo* 22 A2
Snättringe, *Stockholm* 28 B1
Sŏbinggo, *Seoul* 26 B1
Søborg, *Copenhagen* 10 A2
Sobreda, *Lisbon* 14 B1
Soch'o, *Seoul* 26 C1
Sŏdaemun, *Seoul* 26 B1
Söderby, *Stockholm* 28 A3
Södermalm, *Stockholm* 28 B2
Sodpur, *Calcutta* 8 A2
Soeurs, Î. des, *Montreal* 19 B2
Sognsvatn, *Oslo* 22 A3
Soho, *London* 15 b3
Soho, *New York* 21 e1
Soignes, Forêt de, *Brussels* 6 B2
Sok Kwu Wan, *Hong Kong* 12 B1
Sŏkkwan, *Seoul* 26 B2
Sokolniki, *Moscow* 19 B4
Sokolniki Park, *Moscow* 19 B4
Sokołów, *Warsaw* 31 C1
Solalinden, *Munich* 20 B3
Soldier Field, *Chicago* 9 e3
Sollentuna, *Stockholm* 28 A1
Solln, *Munich* 20 B2
Solna, *Stockholm* 28 A1
Solntsevo, *Moscow* 19 C2
Somerset, *Washington* 32 B3
Somerville, *Boston* 6 A3
Somes Is., *Wellington* 32 B2
Sonari, *Mumbai* 20 B2
Søndersø, *Copenhagen* 10 A2
Sŏngbuk, *Seoul* 26 B2
Sŏngdong, *Seoul* 26 B2
Sŏngp'a, *Seoul* 26 B2
Sŏngsu, *Seoul* 26 B2
Soong Qingling, Former Res. of, *Beijing* 4 a2
Soroksár, *Budapest* 7 B2
Soroksari Duna →, *Budapest* 7 B2
Sosenka →, *Moscow* 19 B4
Sosnovka, *St. Petersburg* 26 B2
Sŏul, *Seoul* 26 B2
Soundview, *New York* 21 B2
South Beach, *New York* 21 C1
South Beach Harbor, *San Francisco* 25 c3
South Bend Park, *Atlanta* 3 B2
South Boston, *Boston* 6 A3
South Brooklyn, *New York* 21 B2
South Decatur, *Atlanta* 3 B3
South Deering, *Chicago* 9 C3
South El Monte, *Los Angeles* 16 B4
South Gate, *Los Angeles* 16 C3
South Harbor, *Manila* 17 B1
South Harrow, *London* 15 A1
South Hd., *Sydney* 28 B2
South Hills, *Johannesburg* 13 B2
South Hornchurch, *London* 15 A5
South Kensington, *London* 15 c2
South Lawn, *Washington* 32 C3
South Lincoln, *Boston* 6 A2
South Miami, *Miami* 18 B1
South Norwood, *London* 15 B3
South of Market, *San Francisco* 25 B2
South Ozone Park, *New York* 21 B3
South Pasadena, *Los Angeles* 16 B4
South Res., *Boston* 6 A3
South Ruislip, *London* 15 A1
South San Francisco, *San Francisco* 25 C2
South San Gabriel, *Los Angeles* 16 B4
South Shore, *Chicago* 9 C3
South Sudbury, *Boston* 6 A1
Southall, *London* 15 A1
Southborough, *London* 15 B4
Southend, *London* 15 B3
Southfields, *London* 15 B2
Southwark, *London* 15 B3
Søvang, *Copenhagen* 10 B3
Soweto, *Johannesburg* 13 B1
Sowhānak, *Tehran* 30 A3
Soya, *Tokyo* 29 A4
Spandau, *Berlin* 5 A1
Spånga, *Stockholm* 28 A1
Spanische Reitschule, *Vienna* 31 b1
Spectacle I., *Boston* 6 A4
Speicher-See, *Munich* 20 A3
Speising, *Vienna* 31 B1
Sphinx, *Cairo* 7 B1
Spinaceto, *Rome* 25 C1
Spit Junction, *Sydney* 28 A2
Spořilov, *Prague* 24 B3
Spot Pond, *Boston* 6 A3
Spotswood, *Melbourne* 17 B1
Spree →, *Berlin* 5 A2
Spring Pond, *Boston* 6 A4
Springeberg, *Berlin* 5 B5
Springfield, *Washington* 32 C2
Squantum, *Boston* 6 B3
Srednaya Rogatka, *St. Petersburg* 26 C2
Śródmieście, *Warsaw* 31 B2
Staaken, *Berlin* 5 A1
Stabekk, *Oslo* 22 A2
Stadhion, *Athens* 2 c3
Stadhuis, *Amsterdam* 2 b2
Stadlau, *Vienna* 31 A2
Stadshuset, *Stockholm* 28 b1
Stains, *Paris* 23 A3
Stamford Hill, *London* 15 A3
Stammersdorf, *Vienna* 31 A2
Stanley, *Hong Kong* 12 B2
Stanley Mound, *Hong Kong* 12 B2
Stanley Pen., *Hong Kong* 12 B2
Stanmore, *London* 15 A2
Stapleton, *New York* 21 C1
Star Ferry, *Hong Kong* 12 a2
Staraya Derevnya, *St. Petersburg* 26 B1
Stare, *Warsaw* 31 B2
Staré Město, *Prague* 24 B2
Starego Miasto, *Warsaw* 31 a2
Staten Island Zoo, *New York* 21 C1
Statenice, *Prague* 24 B1
Statue Square, *Hong Kong* 12 c1
Stedelijk Museum, *Amsterdam* 2 c1
Steele Creek, *Melbourne* 17 A1
Steenokkerzeel, *Brussels* 6 A2
Steglitz, *Berlin* 5 B2
Stepaside, *Dublin* 11 B2
Stephansdom, *Vienna* 31 b2
Stepney, *London* 15 A3
Sterling Park, *San Francisco* 25 B2
Sticklinge udde, *Stockholm* 28 A2
Stickney, *Chicago* 9 C2
Stillorgan, *Dublin* 11 B2
Stockholm, *Stockholm* 28 B2
Stocksund, *Stockholm* 28 A2
Stodůlky, *Prague* 24 B1
Stoke Newington, *London* 15 A3
Stokes Valley, *Wellington* 32 B2
Stone Canyon Res., *Los Angeles* 16 B2
Stone Park, *Chicago* 9 B1
Stonebridge, *London* 15 A2
Stoneham, *Boston* 6 A3
Stony Brook Res., *Boston* 6 B3
Stora Värtan, *Stockholm* 28 A2
Store Hareskov, *Copenhagen* 10 A2
Store Magleby, *Copenhagen* 10 B3
Storholmen, *Stockholm* 28 A2
Stoyka, *St. Petersburg* 26 B2
Straiton, *Edinburgh* 11 B3
Strand, *London* 15 b4
Strandfontein, *Cape Town* 8 B2
Strašnice, *Prague* 24 B2
Strasstrudering, *Munich* 20 B3
Stratford, *London* 15 A4
Strathfield, *Sydney* 28 B1
Streatham, *London* 15 B3
Streatham Vale, *London* 15 B3
Strebersdorf, *Vienna* 31 A2
Střešovice, *Prague* 24 B2
Střížkov, *Prague* 24 B2
Strogino, *Moscow* 19 B2
Strombeek-Bever, *Brussels* 6 A2
Stromovka, *Prague* 24 B2
Studio City, *Los Angeles* 16 B2
Stureby, *Stockholm* 28 B2
Stuvsta, *Stockholm* 28 B2
Subhepur, *Delhi* 10 A2
Sucat, *Manila* 17 C2
Suchdol, *Prague* 24 B2
Sucy-en-Brie, *Paris* 23 B4
Sudbury, *Boston* 6 A1
Sugamo, *Tokyo* 29 A3
Sugar Loaf Mt. = Açúcar, Pão de, *Rio de Janeiro* 24 B2
Suge, *Tokyo* 29 B2
Suginami-Ku, *Tokyo* 29 A2
Sugō, *Tokyo* 29 B2
Suita, *Osaka* 22 A4
Suitland, *Washington* 32 B4
Sukchar, *Calcutta* 8 A2
Suma, *Osaka* 22 B1
Sumida →, *Tokyo* 29 A3
Sumida-Ku, *Tokyo* 29 A3
Sumiyoshi, *Osaka* 22 B4
Summerville, *Toronto* 30 B1
Summit, *Chicago* 9 C2
Sunamachi, *Tokyo* 29 A4
Sunbury-on-Thames, *London* 15 B1
Sundbyberg, *Stockholm* 28 A1
Sundbyerne, *Copenhagen* 10 B3
Sung Kong, *Hong Kong* 12 B2
Sungei Kadut Industrial Estate, *Singapore* 27 A2
Sungei Selatar Res., *Singapore* 27 A3
Sunter, *Jakarta* 13 A2
Sunter, Kali →, *Jakarta* 13 B2
Suomenlinna, *Helsinki* 12 C2
Supreme Court, *Washington* 32 b3
Sura, *Calcutta* 8 B2
Surag-san, *Seoul* 26 A2
Surbiton, *London* 15 B2
Suresnes, *Paris* 23 A2
Surfside, *Miami* 18 A2
Surquillo, *Lima* 16 B2
Surrey Hills, *Sydney* 28 B2
Susaek, *Seoul* 26 B1
Süssenbrunn, *Vienna* 31 A2
Sutton, *Dublin* 11 A3
Sutton, *London* 15 B2
Suyu, *Seoul* 26 B2
Suzukishinden, *Tokyo* 29 A2
Svanemøllen, *Copenhagen* 10 A3
Sverdlov, *Moscow* 19 B3
Svestad, *Oslo* 22 B2
Svinö, *Helsinki* 12 C1
Swampscott, *Boston* 6 A4
Swanley, *London* 15 B4
Swansea, *Toronto* 30 B2
Swinburne I., *New York* 21 C1
Swords, *Dublin* 11 A2
Sydenham, *Johannesburg* 13 A2
Sydney, *Sydney* 28 B2
Sydney, Univ. of, *Sydney* 28 B2
Sydney Airport, *Sydney* 28 B2
Sydney Harbour Bridge, *Sydney* 28 B2
Sydstranden, *Copenhagen* 10 B3
Sylvania, *Sydney* 28 C1
Syntagma, Pl., *Athens* 2 b3
Syon Park, *London* 15 B2
Szczęsliwice, *Warsaw* 31 B1
Széchnenyi-hegy, *Budapest* 7 B1
Szent Istvánbaz, *Budapest* 7 b2
Széphalom, *Budapest* 7 A1

T

Tabata, *Tokyo* 29 A3
Tablada, *Buenos Aires* 7 C1
Table Bay, *Cape Town* 8 A1
Table Mountain, *Cape Town* 8 A1
Taboão da Serra, *São Paulo* 26 B1
Täby, *Stockholm* 28 A2
Tacuba, *Mexico City* 18 B1
Tacubaya, *Mexico City* 18 B1
Taebang, *Seoul* 26 B1
Tagig, *Manila* 17 B2
Tagig →, *Manila* 17 B2
Tai Hang, *Hong Kong* 12 B2
Tai Lo Shan, *Hong Kong* 12 A2
Tai Po Tsai, *Hong Kong* 12 A2
Tai Seng, *Singapore* 27 A3
Tai Shui Hang, *Hong Kong* 12 A2
Tai Tam B., *Hong Kong* 12 B2
Tai Tam Tuk Res., *Hong Kong* 12 B2

Tai Wai, *Hong Kong* 12 A1
Tai Wan Tau, *Hong Kong* 12 B2
Tai Wo Hau, *Hong Kong* 12 A1
Tainaka, *Osaka* 22 B4
Taishō, *Osaka* 22 B3
Taita, *Wellington* 32 B2
Tajrīsh, *Tehran* 30 A2
Takaido, *Tokyo* 29 A2
Takaishi, *Tokyo* 29 B2
Takarazuka, *Osaka* 22 A2
Takasago, *Tokyo* 29 A4
Takatsu-Ku, *Tokyo* 29 B2
Takeshita, *Tokyo* 29 B2
Takinegawa, *Tokyo* 29 A3
Takoma Park, *Washington* 32 B3
Taksim, *Istanbul* 12 B1
Talaide, *Lisbon* 14 A1
Taliganga, *Calcutta* 8 B2
Talipapa, *Manila* 17 A2
Tallaght, *Dublin* 11 B1
Tallkrogen, *Stockholm* 28 B2
Tama, *Tokyo* 29 B1
Tama →, *Tokyo* 29 B2
Tama Kyūryō, *Tokyo* 29 B2
Tamaden, *Tokyo* 29 B2
Tamagawa-josui →, *Tokyo* 29 A1
Taman Sari, *Jakarta* 13 A1
Tamanduateí →, *São Paulo* 26 B2
Tamboerskloof, *Cape Town* 8 A1
Tambora, *Jakarta* 13 A1
Tammisalo, *Helsinki* 12 B3
Tammūh, *Cairo* 7 B2
Tampines, *Singapore* 27 A3
Tanah Abang, *Jakarta* 13 B1
Tanigami, *Osaka* 22 A2
Tanjung Duren, *Jakarta* 13 B1
Tanjung Priok, *Jakarta* 13 A2
Tanum, *Oslo* 22 A1
Taoranting Park, *Beijing* 4 c2
Tapada, *Lisbon* 14 A1
Tapanila, *Helsinki* 12 B3
Tapiales, *Buenos Aires* 7 C1
Tapiola, *Helsinki* 12 B1
Tapsia, *Calcutta* 8 B2
Tara, *Mumbai* 20 A1
Tarabya, *Istanbul* 12 B2
Tarango, Presa, *Mexico City* 18 B1
Tårbæk, *Copenhagen* 10 A3
Tarchomin, *Warsaw* 31 B1
Tardeo, *Mumbai* 20 B1
Targówek, *Warsaw* 31 B2
Tårnby, *Copenhagen* 10 B3
Tarqua Bay, *Lagos* 14 B2
Tåstrup, *Copenhagen* 10 B1
Tatarovo, *Moscow* 19 B2
Tathong Channel,
Hong Kong 12 B2
Tathong Pt., *Hong Kong* 12 B2
Tatuapé, *São Paulo* 26 B2
Taufkirchen, *Munich* 20 B2
Tavares, I. dos,
Rio de Janeiro 24 A2
Távros, *Athens* 2 B2
Tawa, *Wellington* 32 A1
Teaneck, *New York* 21 A1
Teatro Municipal,
Rio de Janeiro 24 c2
Tebet, *Jakarta* 13 B2
Tecamachalco, *Mexico City* 18 B1
Teddington, *London* 15 B1
Tegel, *Berlin* 5 A2
Tegel, Flughafen, *Berlin* 5 A2
Tegeler See, *Berlin* 5 A2
Tegelort, *Berlin* 5 A2
Tehrān, *Tehran* 30 A2
Tehrān Pārs, *Tehran* 30 A3
Tei Tong Tsui, *Hong Kong* 12 B2
Tejo, Rio →, *Lisbon* 14 A2
Telegraph Hill, *San Francisco* 25 a2
Telhal, *Lisbon* 14 A1
Telok Blangah, *Singapore* 27 B2
Teltow, *Berlin* 5 B2
Teltow kanal, *Berlin* 5 B3
Temnikovo, *Moscow* 19 B6
Tempelhof, *Berlin* 5 B3
Tempelhof, Flughafen, *Berlin* 5 B3
Temple City, *Los Angeles* 16 B4
Temple Hills Park,
Washington 32 C4
Temple Mount, *Jerusalem* 13 b3
Templeogue, *Dublin* 11 B2
Templo Mayor, *Mexico City* 18 b3
Tenafly, *New York* 21 A2
Tenayuca, Piramide de,
Mexico City 18 A1
Tengah →, *Singapore* 27 A2
Tennoji, *Osaka* 22 B4
Tepalcates, *Mexico City* 18 B2
Terrazzano, *Milan* 18 A1
Terrugem, *Lisbon* 14 A1
Tervuren, *Brussels* 6 B3
Tervuren, Park van, *Brussels* 6 B3
Tetuán, *Madrid* 17 B1
Teufelsberg, *Berlin* 5 B2
Tévere →, *Rome* 25 B1
Thalkirchen, *Munich* 20 B2
Thames →, *London* 15 A4
Thames Ditton, *London* 15 B1
Thamesmead, *London* 15 A4
Thana Cr. →, *Mumbai* 20 A2
The Loop, *Chicago* 9 B3
The Ridge, *Delhi* 10 B2
The Wilds, *Johannesburg* 13 B2
Theater Carré, *Amsterdam* 2 b2
Théatro Dionissou, *Athens* 2 c2
Thiais, *Paris* 23 B3
Thissio, *Athens* 2 c1
Thistletown, *Toronto* 30 A1
Thomastown, *Melbourne* 17 A2
Thompson I., *Boston* 6 B4
Thon Buri, *Bangkok* 3 B1
Thornbury, *Melbourne* 17 A2
Thorncliffe, *Toronto* 30 A2
Thornhill, *Toronto* 30 A2
Thornton, *Cape Town* 8 A2
Thornton Heath, *London* 15 B3
Threipmuir Res., *Edinburgh* 11 B2
Throgs Neck, *New York* 21 B3
Thyssen Bornemisza, Museo,
Madrid 17 b3
Tian'anmen Square, *Beijing* 4 B2
Tiancun, *Beijing* 4 B1
Tianjin, *Tianjin* 30 B1
Tiantan Park, *Beijing* 4 c2
Tibidabo, *Barcelona* 4 A1
Tibradden Mt., *Dublin* 11 B2
Tiburon, *San Francisco* 25 A2
Tiburtino, *Rome* 25 B2
Ticomán, *Mexico City* 18 A2
Tiefersee, *Berlin* 5 B1
Tiejiangyin, *Beijing* 4 C2
Tientsin = Tianjin, *Tianjin* 30 B1
Tiergarten, *Berlin* 5 A3
Tietê →, *São Paulo* 26 B2
Tigerhof, *Cape Town* 8 A2
Tigris = Nahr Dijlah →,
Baghdad 3 B2
Tijuca, *Rio de Janeiro* 24 B1
Tijuca, Parque Nacional da,
Rio de Janeiro 24 B1
Tijuca, Pico da,
Rio de Janeiro 24 B1
Tikkurila, *Helsinki* 12 B3
Tilak Nagar, *Delhi* 10 B1
Tilanqiao, *Shanghai* 27 B1
Timah, Bukit, *Singapore* 27 A2
Times Square, *New York* 21 c2
Timiryazev Park, *Moscow* 19 B3
Ting Kau, *Hong Kong* 12 A1
Tira, *Jerusalem* 13 A1
Tirsa, *Cairo* 7 B2
Tishrīyaa, *Baghdad* 3 B2
Tiu Keng Leng, *Hong Kong* 12 B2
Tivoli, *Copenhagen* 10 a3
Tizapán, *Mexico City* 18 C1
Tlalnepantla →, *Mexico City* 18 A1
To Kwai Wan, *Hong Kong* 12 B2
Toa Payoh, *Singapore* 27 A3
Tobong, *Seoul* 26 B2
Tobong-san, *Seoul* 26 A2
Točná, *Prague* 24 C2
Toco Hills, *Atlanta* 3 B2
Todt Hill, *New York* 21 C1
Tōkagi, *Tokyo* 29 A4
Tokai Plantation, *Cape Town* 8 B1
Tōkaichiba, *Tokyo* 29 B2
Tokarevo, *Moscow* 19 C5
Tōkyō, *Tokyo* 29 B3
Tokyo B., *Tokyo* 29 B4
Tokyo-Haneda Int. Airport,
Tokyo 29 B3
Tokyo Harbour, *Tokyo* 29 B3
Tolka R. →, *Dublin* 11 A1
Tolworth, *London* 15 B2
Tomb of Lu Xun, *Shanghai* 27 B1
Tomb of the Kings, *Jerusalem* 13 a2
Tomba di Nerone, *Rome* 25 B1
Tomilino, *Moscow* 19 C5
Tondo, *Manila* 17 B1
Tongbinggo, *Seoul* 26 B1
Tongjak, *Seoul* 26 B1
Tongmaemung, *Seoul* 26 B2
Tongqiao, *Shanghai* 27 A1
Toorak, *Melbourne* 17 B2
Topkapı, *Istanbul* 12 B1
Tor di Quinto, *Rome* 25 B1
Tor Pignattara, *Rome* 25 B2
Tor Sapienza, *Rome* 25 B2
Toranomon, *Tokyo* 29 c3
Torcy, *Paris* 23 A4
Toronto, *Toronto* 30 B3
Toronto, Univ. of, *Toronto* 30 B2
Toronto Harbour, *Toronto* 30 B2
Toronto I., *Toronto* 30 B2
Toronto Int. Airport,
Toronto 30 A1
Toros Las Arenas, Pl. de,
Barcelona 4 c1
Toros Monumental, Templo
de, *Barcelona* 4 a3
Torre Latino-americana,
Mexico City 18 b2
Torre Lupara, *Rome* 25 B2
Torre Nova, *Rome* 25 B2
Torrellas →, *Barcelona* 4 A1
Torrevécchia, *Rome* 25 B1
Toshima-Ku, *Tokyo* 29 A3
Toshimaen, *Tokyo* 29 A2
Tottenham, *London* 15 A3
Tottenham, *Melbourne* 17 A1
Tour Eiffel, *Paris* 23 c2
Toussus-le-Noble, *Paris* 23 B1
Toussus-le-Noble,
Aérodrome de, *Paris* 23 B1
Tower Bridge, *London* 15 b5
Tower Hamlets, *London* 15 A3
Tower of London, *London* 15 b5
Towra Pt., *Sydney* 28 C2
Tøyen, *Oslo* 22 A3
Toyonaka, *Osaka* 22 A3
Trafalgar Square, *London* 15 b3
Trafaria, *Lisbon* 14 A1
Traição, Cor. →, *São Paulo* 26 B2
Tranegilde, *Copenhagen* 10 B2
Trångsund, *Stockholm* 28 B2
Transamerica Pyramid,
San Francisco 25 b2
Transbay Terminal,
San Francisco 25 b3
Trappenfelde, *Berlin* 5 A4
Trastévere, *Rome* 25 B1
Treasure I., *San Francisco* 25 B2
Třeboradice, *Prague* 24 B3
Třebotov, *Prague* 24 C1
Tremblay-en-France, *Paris* 23 A4
Tremembé →, *São Paulo* 26 A2
Tremont, *New York* 21 A2
Trenno, *Milan* 18 B1
Treptow, *Berlin* 5 B3
Três Rios, Sa. dos,
Rio de Janeiro 24 B1
Trevi, Fontana di, *Rome* 25 b3
Trezzano sul Navíglio, *Milan* 18 B1
Tribune Tower, *Chicago* 9 b2
Trieste, *Rome* 25 B2
Trinidad, *Washington* 32 B4
Trinity, *Edinburgh* 11 B2
Trinity College, *Dublin* 11 c3
Trionfale, *Rome* 25 B1
Triulzo, *Milan* 18 B2
Trocadero, *Paris* 23 b1
Troitse-Lykovo, *Moscow* 19 B2
Troja, *Prague* 24 B2
Trollbäcken, *Stockholm* 28 B3
Trombay, *Mumbai* 20 A2
Troparevo, *Moscow* 19 C2
Tropenmuseum, *Amsterdam* 2 b3
Trudyashchikhsya, Ostrov,
St. Petersburg 26 B1
Tryvasshøgda, *Oslo* 22 A3
Tseng Lan Shue, *Hong Kong* 12 A2
Tsim Sha Tsui, *Hong Kong* 12 a2
Tsing Yi, *Hong Kong* 12 A1
Tsova, *Jerusalem* 13 B1
Tsuen Wan, *Hong Kong* 12 A1
Tsukiji, *Tokyo* 29 c5
Tsur Hadassa, *Jerusalem* 13 B1
Tsurumi →, *Tokyo* 29 B3
Tsz Wan Shan, *Hong Kong* 12 A2
Tuas, *Singapore* 27 B1
Tuchoměřice, *Prague* 24 B1
Tuckahoe, *New York* 21 A3
Tucuruvi, *São Paulo* 26 A2
Tufello, *Rome* 25 B2
Tufnell Park, *London* 15 A3
Tughlakabad, *Delhi* 10 B2
Tuileries, Jardin des, *Paris* 23 b3
Tuindorp Oostzaan,
Amsterdam 2 A2
Tullamarine, *Melbourne* 17 A1
Tulse Hill, *London* 15 B3
Tung Lung I., *Hong Kong* 12 B2
Tung O, *Hong Kong* 12 B1
Tunis, *Baghdad* 3 A2
Tuomarila, *Helsinki* 12 B1
Tureberg, *Stockholm* 28 A1
Turffontein, *Johannesburg* 13 B2
Turkso, *Prague* 24 A1
Turnham Green, *London* 15 B2
Turnhouse, *Edinburgh* 11 B1
Tuscolana, Via, *Rome* 25 B2
Tushino, *Moscow* 19 A2
Twelve Apostles, *Cape Town* 8 A1
Twickenham, *London* 15 B1
Twickenham Rugby Ground,
London 15 B1
Twin Peaks, *San Francisco* 25 B2
Two Rock Mt., *Dublin* 11 B2
Tymon North, *Dublin* 11 B1
Tysons Corner, *Washington* 32 B2

U

U.S. Capitol, *Washington* 32 b3
Ubeidiya, *Jerusalem* 13 B2
Uberaba →, *São Paulo* 26 B2
Ubin, P., *Singapore* 27 A3
Uccle, *Brussels* 6 B2
Udelnaya, *St. Petersburg* 26 A2
Udelnoe, *St. Petersburg* 26 B1
Udlding, *Munich* 20 A1
Ueno, *Tokyo* 29 A3
Ŭholičky, *Prague* 24 B1
Uhřiněves, *Prague* 24 B3
Uithoorn, *Amsterdam* 2 B1
Újpalota, *Budapest* 7 A2
Újpest, *Budapest* 7 A2
Ukita, *Tokyo* 29 A4
Ullerup, *Copenhagen* 10 B3
Ullevål, *Oslo* 22 A3
Ulriksdal, *Stockholm* 28 A1
Ulyanka, *St. Petersburg* 26 B1
Um Al-Khanazir Island,
Baghdad 3 B2
Umeda, *Osaka* 22 A3
Umerkhadi, *Mumbai* 20 b2
Ümraniye, *Istanbul* 12 B2
Underground Atlanta,
Atlanta 3 B2
Unětický potok →, *Prague* 24 B2
Ŭngam, *Seoul* 26 B1
Unhos, *Lisbon* 14 A2
Unidad Santa Fe,
Mexico City 18 B1
Union City, *New York* 21 B1
Union Port, *New York* 21 B2
Union Square, *New York* 21 d2
Union Square, *San Francisco* 25 b2
Union Station, *Washington* 32 b3
United Nations H.Q.,
New York 21 c3
Universidad, *Madrid* 17 B1
Universidad de Chile,
Santiago 26 B2
University Park, *Washington* 32 B4
Unp'yong, *Seoul* 26 B1
Unter den Linden, *Berlin* 5 a4
Unterbiberg, *Munich* 20 B2
Unterföhring, *Munich* 20 A3
Unterhaching, *Munich* 20 B2
Unterlaa, *Vienna* 31 B2
Untermenzing, *Munich* 20 A1
Upper East Side, *New York* 21 b3
Upper Elmers End, *London* 15 B3
Upper New York B.,
New York 21 C1
Upper Norwood, *London* 15 B3
Upper Peirce Res., *Singapore* 27 A2
Upper Sydenham, *London* 15 B3
Upper Tooting, *London* 15 B3
Upper West Side, *New York* 21 a2
Upton, *London* 15 A4
Uptown, *Chicago* 9 B2
Uran, *Mumbai* 20 B2
Urayasu, *Tokyo* 29 B4
Urbe, Aeroporto d', *Rome* 25 B2
Urca, *Rio de Janeiro* 24 B2
Uritsk, *St. Petersburg* 26 C1
Üröm, *Budapest* 7 A2
Ursus, *Warsaw* 31 B1
Ursvik, *Stockholm* 28 A1
Usera, *Madrid* 17 B1
Ushigome, *Tokyo* 29 A3
Usina, *Rio de Janeiro* 24 B1
Üsküdar, *Istanbul* 12 B2
Ust-Slavyanka, *St. Petersburg* 26 C3
Uteke, *Stockholm* 28 A3
Utrata, *Warsaw* 31 B2
Uttarpara, *Calcutta* 8 B1
Utterslev Mose, *Copenhagen* 10 A2

V

Vadaul, *Mumbai* 20 A2
Vaires-sur-Marne, *Paris* 23 A4
Valby, *Copenhagen* 10 B2
Valcannuta, *Rome* 25 B1
Valdelatas, *Madrid* 17 A1
Vale, *Washington* 32 B1
Valenton, *Paris* 23 B3
Valera, *Milan* 18 A1
Vallcarca, *Barcelona* 4 A1
Valldoreix, *Barcelona* 4 A1
Vallecas, *Madrid* 17 B2
Vallensbæk, *Copenhagen* 10 B1
Vallensbæk Strand,
Copenhagen 10 B2
Vallentunasjön, *Stockholm* 28 A2
Valleranello, *Rome* 25 C1
Vallisaari, *Helsinki* 12 C3
Vallvidrera, *Barcelona* 4 A1
Vallvidrera →, *Barcelona* 4 A1
Van Goghmuseum,
Amsterdam 2 c1
Vanak, *Tehran* 30 A2
Vangede, *Copenhagen* 10 A3
Vaniköy, *Istanbul* 12 B2
Vanløse, *Copenhagen* 10 A2
Vantaa, *Helsinki* 12 B2
Vantaa →, *Helsinki* 12 B2
Vantaankoski, *Helsinki* 12 B2
Vantaanpuisto, *Helsinki* 12 B2
Vanves, *Paris* 23 B2
Varedo, *Milan* 18 A1
Varkiza, *Athens* 2 C2
Varszínház, *Budapest* 7 b2
Vartiokylä, *Helsinki* 12 B3
Vartiosaari, *Helsinki* 12 B3
Vasamuseet, *Stockholm* 28 b3
Vasco, *Cape Town* 8 A2
Vasfanārd, *Tehran* 30 B2
Vashi, *Mumbai* 20 A2
Vasilyevskiy, Ostrov,
St. Petersburg 26 B1
Vaso Regulador El Cristo,
Mexico City 18 B1
Vaucluse, *Sydney* 28 B2
Vaucresson, *Paris* 23 A1
Vauhallan, *Paris* 23 B2
Vaujours, *Paris* 23 A4
Vauxhall, *London* 15 c4
Vecsés, *Budapest* 7 B3
Veleň, *Prague* 24 A3
Veleslavin, *Prague* 24 B2
Vélizy-Villacoublay, *Paris* 23 B2
Velka-Chuchle, *Prague* 24 B2
Velké Přílepy, *Prague* 24 B1
Venda Seca, *Lisbon* 14 A1
Venetian Islands, *Miami* 18 B2
Venezia, Palazzo, *Rome* 25 c2
Venice, *Los Angeles* 16 C2
Ventas, *Madrid* 17 B1
Ventorro del Cano, *Madrid* 17 B1
Venustiano Carranza,
Mexico City 18 B2
Verde →, *São Paulo* 26 A1
Verdi, *Athens* 2 A2
Verdun, *Montreal* 19 B2
Vérhalom, *Budapest* 7 A2
Vermelho →, *São Paulo* 26 B1
Vernon, *Los Angeles* 16 B3
Verrières-le-Buisson, *Paris* 23 B2
Versailles, *Buenos Aires* 7 B1
Versailles, *Paris* 23 B1
Veshnyaki, *Moscow* 19 B4
Vesolyy Posolok,
St. Petersburg 26 B2
Vestra, *Helsinki* 12 B1
Vestskoven, *Copenhagen* 10 A2
Vicálvaro, *Madrid* 17 B2
Vicente Lopez, *Buenos Aires* 7 B2
Victoria, *Hong Kong* 12 B2
Victoria, *London* 15 c3
Victoria, Mt., *Wellington* 32 B1
Victoria, Pont, *Montreal* 19 B2
Victoria and Albert
Waterfront, *Cape Town* 8 a1
Victoria Gardens, *Mumbai* 20 B2
Victoria Harbour,
Hong Kong 12 B1
Victoria Island, *Lagos* 14 B2
Victoria L., *Johannesburg* 13 B2
Victoria Lawn Tennis Courts,
Melbourne 17 B2
Victoria Park, *Singapore* 27 B2
Victoria Peak, *Hong Kong* 12 B1
Victoria Wharf, *Cape Town* 8 a2
Vienna = Wien, *Vienna* 31 A2
Vienna, *Washington* 32 B2
View Park, *Los Angeles* 16 B3
Vigário Geral, *Rio de Janeiro* 24 A1
Vigentino, *Milan* 18 B2
Viggbyholm, *Stockholm* 28 A2
Vighignolo, *Milan* 18 B1
Viikki, *Helsinki* 12 B3
Vikhroli, *Mumbai* 20 A2
Vila Guilherme, *São Paulo* 26 B2
Vila Isabel, *Rio de Janeiro* 24 B1
Vila Jaguára, *São Paulo* 26 B1
Vila Madalena, *São Paulo* 26 B1
Vila Maria, *São Paulo* 26 B2
Vila Mariana, *São Paulo* 26 B2
Vila Prudente, *São Paulo* 26 B2
Viladecans, *Barcelona* 4 B1
Vile Parle, *Mumbai* 20 A2
Villa Adelina, *Buenos Aires* 7 B1
Villa Ballester, *Buenos Aires* 7 B1
Villa Barilari, *Buenos Aires* 7 C2
Villa Borghese, *Rome* 25 a3
Villa Bosch, *Buenos Aires* 7 B1
Villa C. Colon, *Buenos Aires* 7 C2
Villa Ciudadela,
Buenos Aires 7 B1
Villa de Guadalupe,
Mexico City 18 B2
Villa Devoto, *Buenos Aires* 7 B1
Villa Diamante, *Buenos Aires* 7 C2
Villa Dominico, *Buenos Aires* 7 C3
Villa Lugano, *Buenos Aires* 7 C1
Villa Lynch, *Buenos Aires* 7 B1
Villa Madero, *Buenos Aires* 7 C1
Villa Sáenz Pena,
Buenos Aires 7 B1
Villa Urquiza, *Buenos Aires* 7 B2
Villaverde, *Madrid* 17 B1
Villaverde Bajo, *Madrid* 17 B1
Ville-d'Avray, *Paris* 23 B2
Villecresnes, *Paris* 23 B4
Villejuif, *Paris* 23 B3
Villemomble, *Paris* 23 A4
Villeneuve-la-Garenne, *Paris* 23 A2
Villeneuve-le-Roi, *Paris* 23 B3
Villeneuve-St.-Georges, *Paris* 23 B3
Villeparisis, *Paris* 23 A4
Villevaudé, *Paris* 23 A4
Villiers-le-Bâcle, *Paris* 23 B1
Villiers-sur-Marne, *Paris* 23 B4
Villinki, *Helsinki* 12 C3
Villoresi, Canale, *Milan* 18 A1
Vilvoorde, *Brussels* 6 A2
Vimodrone, *Milan* 18 A2
Vimont, *Montreal* 19 A1
Vinanmek Palace, *Bangkok* 3 a2
Vincennes, *Paris* 23 A3
Vincennes, Bois de, *Paris* 23 B3
Vinings, *Atlanta* 3 A2
Vinohrady, *Prague* 24 c3
Vinoř, *Prague* 24 B3
Violet Hill, *Hong Kong* 12 B2
Virányos, *Budapest* 7 A1
Virgen del San Cristóbal,
Santiago 26 B2
Virginia Gardens, *Miami* 18 B1
Virginia Key, *Miami* 18 B2
Viroflay, *Paris* 23 B2
Víron, *Athens* 2 B2
Virum, *Copenhagen* 10 A2
Vishnyaki, *Moscow* 19 B5
Visitacion Valley,
San Francisco 25 B2
Vista Alegre, *Lima* 14 B3
Vista Alegre, *Santiago* 26 C1
Vista Grove, *Atlanta* 3 A3
Vitacura, *Santiago* 26 B2
Vitinia, *Rome* 25 C1
Vitry-sur-Seine, *Paris* 23 B3
Vizandinó, Moussío, *Athens* 2 b3
Vladykino, *Moscow* 19 A3
Vlezenbeek, *Brussels* 6 B1
Vltava →, *Prague* 24 B2
Vnukovo, *Moscow* 19 C1
Vokovice, *Prague* 24 B2
Volgelsdorf, *Berlin* 5 A5
Volkhonka-Zil, *Moscow* 19 C3
Vollen, *Oslo* 22 B1
Volodarskoye, *St. Petersburg* 26 B1
Volynkina-Derevnya,
St. Petersburg 26 B1
Vondelpark, *Amsterdam* 2 A2
Vösendorf, *Vienna* 31 B2
Vostochnyy, *Moscow* 19 B5
Voula, *Athens* 2 C2
Vouliagmeni, *Athens* 2 C2
Vredehoek, *Cape Town* 8 A1
Vršovice, *Prague* 24 B2
Vyborgskaya Storona,
St. Petersburg 26 B2
Vykhino, *Moscow* 19 B4
Vyšehrad, *Prague* 24 B2

W

Wachterhof, *Munich* 20 B3
Wadala, *Mumbai* 20 A2
Wadestown, *Wellington* 32 B1
Wadi Fukin, *Jerusalem* 13 B1
Wah Fu, *Hong Kong* 12 B1
Wahda, *Baghdad* 3 B2
Währing, *Vienna* 31 A2
Waidmannslust, *Berlin* 5 A3
Wainuiomata, *Wellington* 32 B2
Wainuiomata R. →,
Wellington 32 B2
Wakefield, *Boston* 6 A3
Waldesruh, *Berlin* 5 B4
Waldperlach, *Munich* 20 B3
Waldtrudering, *Munich* 20 B3
Walkinstown, *Dublin* 11 B1
Wall Street, *New York* 21 f1
Walt Disney Concert Hall,
Los Angeles 16 b1
Waltham, *Boston* 6 A2
Waltham Forest, *London* 15 A3
Walthamstow, *London* 15 A3
Walton on Thames, *London* 15 B1
Wambeek, *Brussels* 6 A3
Wan Chai, *Hong Kong* 12 B2
Wan Chai Lanes, *Hong Kong* 12 c2
Wandsworth, *London* 15 B2
Wankhede Stadium, *Mumbai* 20 c2
Wannsee, *Berlin* 5 B1
Wansdorf, *Berlin* 5 A1
Wanstead, *London* 15 A4
Wapping, *London* 15 A3
Ward, *Dublin* 11 A1
Ward I., *Wellington* 32 B2
Warnberg, *Munich* 20 B2
Warrâq el 'Arab, *Cairo* 7 A2
Warrâq el Hadr, *Cairo* 7 A2
Warringen Park, *Melbourne* 17 A2
Warriston, *Edinburgh* 11 B2
Warsaw = Warszawa,
Warsaw 31 B2
Warszawa, *Warsaw* 31 B2
Wartenberg, *Berlin* 5 A4
Washington, *Washington* 32 B3
Washington Heights,
New York 21 A2
Washington Monument,
Washington 32 b1
Washington Nat. Airport,
Washington 32 B3
Washington Park, *Chicago* 9 C3
Wat Arun, *Bangkok* 3 b1
Wat Pho, *Bangkok* 3 b1
Wat Phra Keo, *Bangkok* 3 b1
Wat Traimit, *Bangkok* 3 c2
Water of Leith, *Edinburgh* 11 B1
Water Tower Place, *Chicago* 9 a2
Watergraafsmeer,
Amsterdam 2 A2
Waterland, *Amsterdam* 2 A2
Waterloo, *Brussels* 6 B2
Waterloo, *Wellington* 32 B2
Waterloo International,
London 15 b4
Watermael-Boitsfort,
Brussels 6 B2
Watertown, *Boston* 6 A2
Watsonia, *Melbourne* 17 A2
Waverley, *Boston* 6 A2
Waverley, *Johannesburg* 13 A2
Waverley, *Sydney* 28 B2
Waverley Station, *Edinburgh* 11 b3
Wawer, *Warsaw* 31 B2
Wawrzyszew, *Warsaw* 31 B1
Wayland, *Boston* 6 A1
Wazirabad, *Delhi* 10 A2
Wazirīya, *Baghdad* 3 A2
Wazirpur, *Delhi* 10 A2
Wealdstone, *London* 15 A1
Wedding, *Berlin* 5 A3
Weehawken, *New York* 21 B1
Weesp, *Amsterdam* 2 B3
Weidling, *Vienna* 31 A1
Weidlingbach, *Vienna* 31 A1
Weigongcun, *Beijing* 4 B1
Weijing He →, *Tianjin* 30 B2
Weissensee, *Berlin* 5 A3
Wellesley, *Boston* 6 B2
Wellesley Falls, *Boston* 6 B2
Wellesley Hills, *Boston* 6 B2
Welling, *London* 15 B4
Wellington, *Boston* 6 A3
Wellington, *Wellington* 32 B1
Wells Fargo Center,
Los Angeles 16 b1
Weltevreden Park,
Johannesburg 13 A1
Wembley, *London* 15 A2
Wemmel, *Brussels* 6 A1
Wemmer Pan, *Johannesburg* 13 B2
Wenceslas Square, *Prague* 24 b2
Wendenschloss, *Berlin* 5 B4
Wenhuagong, *Tianjin* 30 B2
Wennington, *London* 15 A5
Werneuchen, *Berlin* 5 A5
West Bedford, *Boston* 6 A2
West Concord, *Boston* 6 A1
West Don →, *Toronto* 30 A2
West Drayton, *London* 15 A1
West Ham, *London* 15 A4
West Harrow, *London* 15 A1
West Heath, *London* 15 B4
West Hill, *Toronto* 30 A3
West Hollywood,
Los Angeles 16 B2
West Kensington, *London* 15 c1
West Kilburn, *London* 15 a1
West Lamma Channel,
Hong Kong 12 B1
West Lynn, *Boston* 6 A4
West Medford, *Boston* 6 A3
West Miami, *Miami* 18 B1
West Molesey, *London* 15 B1
West New York, *New York* 21 B1
West of Twin Peaks,
San Francisco 25 B2
West Park, *Johannesburg* 13 A1
West Rouge, *Toronto* 30 A4
West Roxbury, *Boston* 6 B3
West Springfield, *Washington* 32 C2
West Town, *Chicago* 9 B2
West Wharf, *Karachi* 14 B1
Westbourne Green, *London* 15 a1
Westchester, *Chicago* 9 B1
Westchester, *Los Angeles* 16 C2
Westchester, *New York* 21 A2
Westcliff, *Johannesburg* 13 B2
Westdene, *Johannesburg* 13 B1
Westend, *Helsinki* 12 C1
Wester Hailes, *Edinburgh* 11 B2
Westerham, *Munich* 20 B2
Western Addition,
San Francisco 25 B2
Western Wall, *Jerusalem* 13 b3
Westgate, *Washington* 32 B3
Westlake, *Cape Town* 8 B1
Westlake, *San Francisco* 25 B2
Westminster, *London* 15 A3
Westmount, *Montreal* 19 B2
Weston, *Boston* 6 A2
Weston, *Toronto* 30 A1
Weston Res., *Boston* 6 A2
Westwood Village,
Los Angeles 16 B2
Westzaan, *Amsterdam* 2 A1
Wetton, *Cape Town* 8 B2
Wexford, *Toronto* 30 A3
Weybridge, *London* 15 B1
Wezembeek-Oppem,
Brussels 6 A2
White House, The,
Washington 32 b1
Whitechapel, *London* 15 A3
Whitehall, *Dublin* 11 A2
Whitehall, *London* 15 b3
Whittier, *Los Angeles* 16 C4
Whitton, *London* 15 B1
Wieden, *Vienna* 31 A2
Wien, *Vienna* 31 A2
Wien-Schwechat, Flughafen,
Vienna 31 B3
Wienerberg, *Vienna* 31 B2
Wierzbno, *Warsaw* 31 B2
Wijde Wormer, *Amsterdam* 2 A2
Wilanów, *Warsaw* 31 B2
Wilanówka →, *Warsaw* 31 C2
Wilhelmshagen, *Berlin* 5 B5
Wilket Creek Park, *Toronto* 30 A2
Wilkieston, *Edinburgh* 11 B1
Willbrook, *Dublin* 11 B2
Willesden, *London* 15 A2
Willesden Green, *London* 15 A2
Williamsbridge, *New York* 21 A2
Williamsburg, *New York* 21 B2
Williamstown, *Melbourne* 17 B1
Willoughby, *Sydney* 28 A2
Willow Springs, *Chicago* 9 C1
Willowdale, *Toronto* 30 A2
Wilmersdorf, *Berlin* 5 c1
Wilmette, *Chicago* 9 A2
Wilmington, *London* 15 B5
Wilshire Boulevard,
Los Angeles 16 c1
Wimbledon, *London* 15 B2
Wimbledon Common,
London 15 B2
Wimbledon Park, *London* 15 B2
Wimbledon Tennis Ground,
London 15 B2
Winchester, *Boston* 6 A3
Windermere, *Cape Town* 8 A2
Windsor, *Johannesburg* 13 A1
Windsor Hills, *Los Angeles* 16 C2
Windy Arbour, *Dublin* 11 B2
Winning, *Munich* 20 B2
Winthrop, *Boston* 6 A4
Wissous, *Paris* 23 B2
Wittenau, *Berlin* 5 A2
Witwatersrand, Univ. of,
Johannesburg 13 B2
Włochy, *Warsaw* 31 B1
Wo Mei, *Hong Kong* 12 A2
Wo Yi Hop, *Hong Kong* 12 A1
Woburn, *Boston* 6 A3
Woburn, *Toronto* 30 A3
Woduk Pluit, *Jakarta* 13 A1
Wola, *Warsaw* 31 B1
Wolf Trap Farm Park,
Washington 32 B2
Wolica, *Warsaw* 31 C2
Wolica, *Warsaw* 31 C1
Wólka Węglowa, *Warsaw* 31 B1
Wollaston, *Boston* 6 B3
Woltersdorf, *Berlin* 5 B5
Woluwe-Saint-Lambert,
Brussels 6 A2
Woluwe-Saint-Pierre,
Brussels 6 A2
Wong Chuk Hang,
Hong Kong 12 B2
Wong Chuk Wan,
Hong Kong 12 A2
Wong Chuk Yeung,
Hong Kong 12 A2
Wong Tai Sin, *Hong Kong* 12 A2
Wood Green, *London* 15 A3
Wood Ridge, *New York* 21 A1
Woodbridge, *Toronto* 30 A1
Woodford, *London* 15 A4
Woodford Bridge, *London* 15 A4
Woodford Green, *London* 15 A4
Woodhaven, *New York* 21 B2
Woodhouselee, *Edinburgh* 11 B2
Woodlands New Town,
Singapore 27 A2
Woodmont, *Washington* 32 B3
Woodside, *London* 15 B3
Woodside, *New York* 21 B2
Woodstock, *Cape Town* 8 A1
Woollahra, *Sydney* 28 B2
Woolloomooloo, *Sydney* 28 b2
Woolooware B., *Sydney* 28 C1
Woolwich, *London* 15 B4
Woolworth Building,
New York 21 e1
World Trade Center, site of
former, *New York* 21 B1
World's End, *Boston* 6 B4
Worli, *Mumbai* 20 A1
Worth, *Chicago* 9 C2
Wren's Nest, *Atlanta* 3 B2
Wrigley Building, *Chicago* 9 b2
Wuhlgarten, *Berlin* 5 A4
Wujiaochang, *Shanghai* 27 B2
Würm →, *Munich* 20 B1
Würm-kanal, *Munich* 20 A1
Wusong, *Shanghai* 27 A1
Wyczółki, *Warsaw* 31 C1
Wygoda, *Warsaw* 31 B2
Wynberg, *Cape Town* 8 B1

X

Xabregas, *Lisbon* 14 A2
Xianggang = Hong Kong,
Hong Kong 12 B1
Xiaodian, *Tianjin* 30 A2
Xiaogang Park, *Canton* 8 B2
Xiaoping, *Canton* 8 A2
Xiasha chong, *Canton* 8 B2
Xichang, *Canton* 8 B1
Xicheng, *Beijing* 4 B1
Xidan, *Beijing* 4 B1
Xigu Park, *Tianjin* 30 A2
Xiguoan, *Tianjin* 30 A1
Ximenwai, *Tianjin* 30 B1
Xinanlou, *Tianjin* 30 B2
Xinkai He →, *Tianjin* 30 A2
Xizhimen, *Beijing* 4 B1
Xu Beihong Mem. Hall,
Beijing 4 a1
Xuanwu, *Beijing* 4 B1
Xuhui, *Shanghai* 27 B1

Y

Yaba, *Lagos* 14 A2
Yaftābād, *Tehran* 30 B1
Yahara, *Tokyo* 29 A2
Yaho, *Tokyo* 29 A1
Yakire, *Tokyo* 29 A4
Yamada, *Osaka* 22 A4
Yamada, *Tokyo* 29 B2
Yamamoto, *Osaka* 22 B4
Yamato →, *Osaka* 22 B3
Yamuna →, *Delhi* 10 B2
Yan Kit, *Singapore* 27 A3
Yanbu, *Canton* 8 B1
Yangch'ŏn, *Seoul* 26 B1
Yanghuayuan, *Beijing* 4 C1
Yangjae, *Seoul* 26 C2
Yangjiazhuang, *Shanghai* 27 A1
Yangpu, *Shanghai* 27 B2
Yangpu Park, *Shanghai* 27 B2
Yao, *Osaka* 22 B4
Yao Airport, *Osaka* 22 B4
Yarmūk, *Baghdad* 3 B1
Yarra →, *Melbourne* 17 A1
Yarra Bend Park, *Melbourne* 17 A2
Yarraville, *Melbourne* 17 A1
Yau Tong, *Hong Kong* 12 B2
Yauza →, *Moscow* 19 A4
Yeading, *London* 15 A1
Yedikule, *Istanbul* 12 C1
Yemin Moshe, *Jerusalem* 13 b2
Yenikapı, *Istanbul* 12 B1
Yeniköy, *Istanbul* 12 B2
Yerba Buena Gardens,
San Francisco 25 c2
Yerba Buena I.,
San Francisco 25 B2
Yerres, *Paris* 23 B4
Yerushalayim = Jerusalem,
Jerusalem 13 B2
Yiheyuan, *Beijing* 4 A1
Yinhangzhen, *Shanghai* 27 A2
Yishun New Town, *Singapore* 27 A3
Yixingbu, *Tianjin* 30 A2
Ylästö, *Helsinki* 12 B2
Yodo →, *Osaka* 22 A4
Yongdingman, *Beijing* 4 B2
Yŏngdong, *Seoul* 26 B2
Yŏngdŭngp'o, *Seoul* 26 B1
Yongfucun, *Canton* 8 B2
Yongjing, *Shanghai* 27 B2
Yongsan, *Seoul* 26 B1
Yonkers, *New York* 21 A2
York, *Toronto* 30 A2
York Mills, *Toronto* 30 A2
Yotsuya, *Tokyo* 29 a2
You'anmen, *Beijing* 4 B1
Yŏŭido, *Seoul* 26 B1
Youndsfield, *Cape Town* 8 B1
Yuanxiatian, *Canton* 8 A2
Yugo-Zarad, *Moscow* 19 B3
Yung Shue Wan, *Hong Kong* 12 B1
Yūsofābād, *Tehran* 30 A2
Yuyuantan Park, *Beijing* 4 b2

Z

Zaandam, *Amsterdam* 2 A1
Zaandijk, *Amsterdam* 2 A1
Zaanstad, *Amsterdam* 2 A1
Záběhlice, *Prague* 24 B2
Ząbki, *Warsaw* 31 B2
Zacisze, *Warsaw* 31 B2
Zahrā, *Baghdad* 3 A1
Zakharkovo, *Moscow* 19 B1
Žalov, *Prague* 24 A2
Załuski, *Warsaw* 31 C1
Zamdorf, *Munich* 20 B2
Zamek Królewski, *Warsaw* 31 a2
Zamek Ujazdowski, *Warsaw* 31 c3
Zanevka, *St. Petersburg* 26 B3
Zapote, *Manila* 17 C1
Záppeio, *Athens* 2 c2
Zarechye, *Moscow* 19 B2
Zaventem, *Brussels* 6 A2
Zawady, *Warsaw* 31 B2
Zāwiyet Abû Musallam,
Cairo 7 B1
Zawrā' Park, *Baghdad* 3 B2
Zbraslav, *Prague* 24 C2
Zbuzany, *Prague* 24 B1
Zdiby, *Prague* 24 A2
Zeekoevlei, *Cape Town* 8 B2
Zehlendorf, *Berlin* 5 B2
Zenne →, *Brussels* 6 B1
Zeraň, *Warsaw* 31 B1
Zerzeń, *Warsaw* 31 B2
Zeytinburnu, *Istanbul* 12 C1
Zhabei, *Shanghai* 27 B1
Zhangguizhuang, *Tianjin* 30 B2
Zhdanov, *Moscow* 19 B4
Zheleznodorozhnyy, *Moscow* 19 B6
Zhenru, *Shanghai* 27 B1
Zhernovka, *St. Petersburg* 26 B2
Zhicun, *Canton* 8 B2
Zhongshan Park, *Beijing* 4 b2
Zhongshan Park, *Shanghai* 27 B1
Zhoucun, *Canton* 8 A2
Zhoujiadu, *Shanghai* 27 B1
Zhoujiazhen, *Shanghai* 27 B1
Zhu Jiang →, *Canton* 8 B3
Zhulebino, *Moscow* 19 B5
Zhushadi, *Canton* 8 A3
Zielona, *Warsaw* 31 B3
Zielonka, *Warsaw* 31 B2
Ziya He →, *Tianjin* 30 A1
Žižkov, *Prague* 24 B2
Zličín, *Prague* 24 B1
Zócalo, *Mexico City* 18 b3
Zografos, *Athens* 2 B2
Zoliborz, *Warsaw* 31 B1
Zonnenbloem, *Cape Town* 8 A1
Zoo, *Beijing* 4 a1
Zugliget, *Budapest* 7 B1
Zugló, *Budapest* 7 A2
Zuiderwoude, *Amsterdam* 2 A3
Zumbi, *Rio de Janeiro* 24 A1
Zunderdorp, *Amsterdam* 2 A2
Zuvuvu →, *São Paulo* 26 C1
Zwanenburg, *Amsterdam* 2 A1
Zwölfaxing, *Vienna* 31 B2
Zyuzino, *Moscow* 19 C3

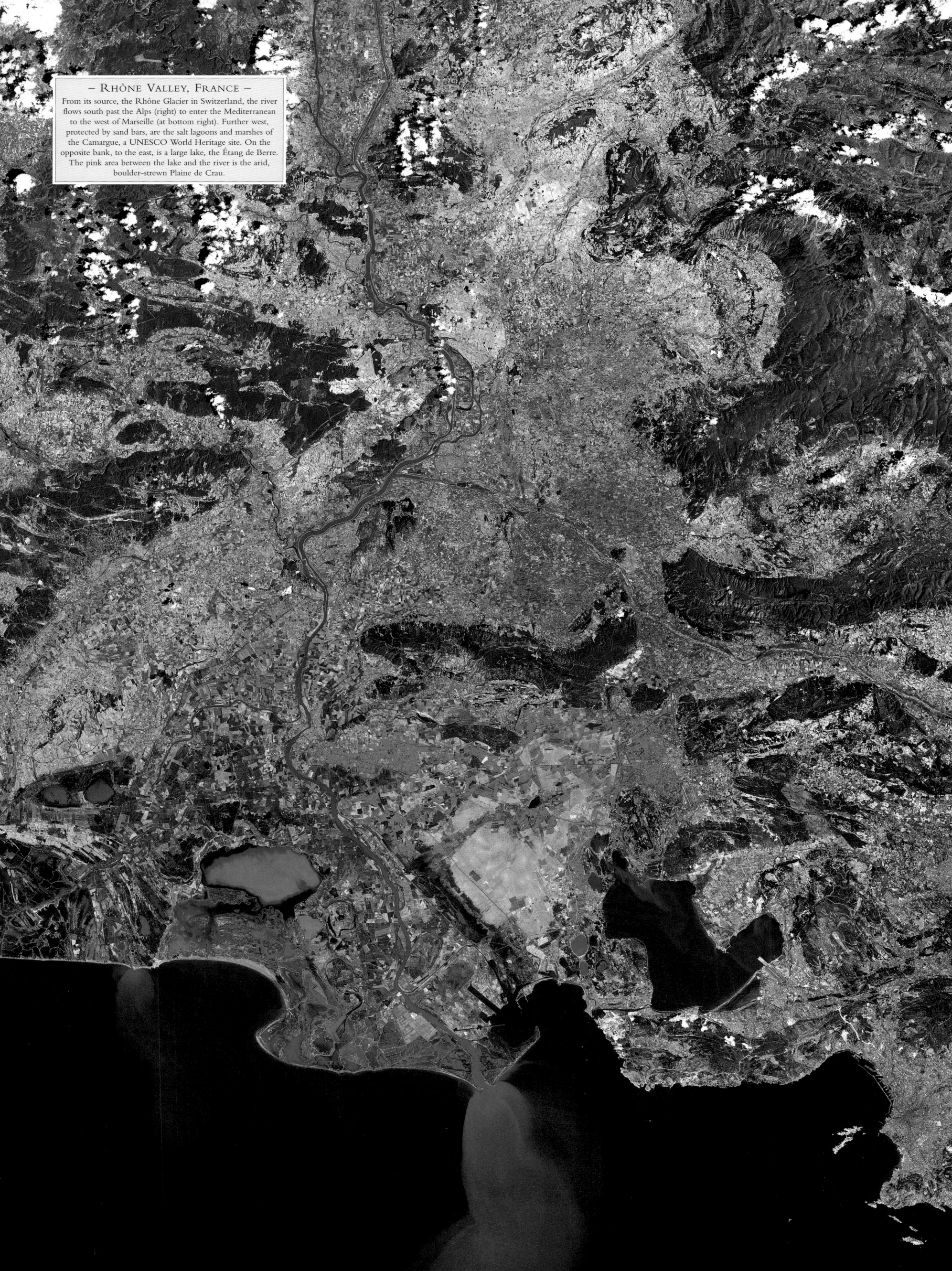

From its source, the Rhône Glacier in Switzerland, the river
flows south past the Alps (right) to enter the Mediterranean
to the west of Marseille (at bottom right). Further west,
protected by sand bars, are the salt lagoons and marshes of
the Camargue, a UNESCO World Heritage site. On the
opposite bank, to the east, is a large lake, the Étang de Berre.
The pink area between the lake and the river is the arid,
boulder-strewn Plaine de Crau.

WORLD MAPS

SETTLEMENTS

▣ **PARIS**   ◉ **Rotterdam**   ◉ **Livorno**   ◉ **Brugge**   ⊙ Exeter   ○ *Torremolinos*   ○ *Oberammergau*   ○ *Thira*

Settlement symbols and type styles vary according to the scale of each map and indicate the importance
of towns on the map rather than specific population figures

• *Vaduz*   Capital cities have red infills   ∴   Ruins or archaeological sites

⬠   Urban agglomerations   Wells in desert

ADMINISTRATION

——— International boundaries   ·········· Internal boundaries   **PERU**   Country names

- - - - International boundaries   ⬡ National parks   KENT   Administrative
(undefined or disputed)   *SNOWDONIA*   area names

International boundaries show the *de facto* situation where there are rival claims to territory

COMMUNICATIONS

═══ Motorways, freeways   ——— Principal railways   LHR ✈   Principal airports
and expressways   (and location identifier)

——— Principal roads   - - - Railways   ✈   Other airports
under construction

——— Other roads   ——— Other railways   ·········   Principal canals

⊣-·-⊢ Road tunnels   ⊣-·-⊢ Railway tunnels   ⋈   Passes

PHYSICAL FEATURES

——— Perennial streams   ⬭ Intermittent lakes   ▲ 8850   Elevations in metres

- ᴧ ᴧ - Intermittent streams   ⬭ Swamps and marshes   ▼ 8500   Sea depths in metres

⬭ Perennial lakes   ⬭ Permanent ice   *1134*   Height of lake surface
and glaciers   above sea level in metres

ELEVATION AND DEPTH TINTS

Height of land above sea level   Land below sea level   Depth of sea

in metres   6000 4000 3000 2000 1500 1000 400 200   0

                                                                                      6000 12 000 15 000 18 000 24 000   in feet

in feet   18 000 12 000 9000 6000 4500 3000 1200 600

                                                          0   200   2000   4000   5000   6000   8000   in metres

Some of the maps have different contours to highlight and clarify the principal relief features

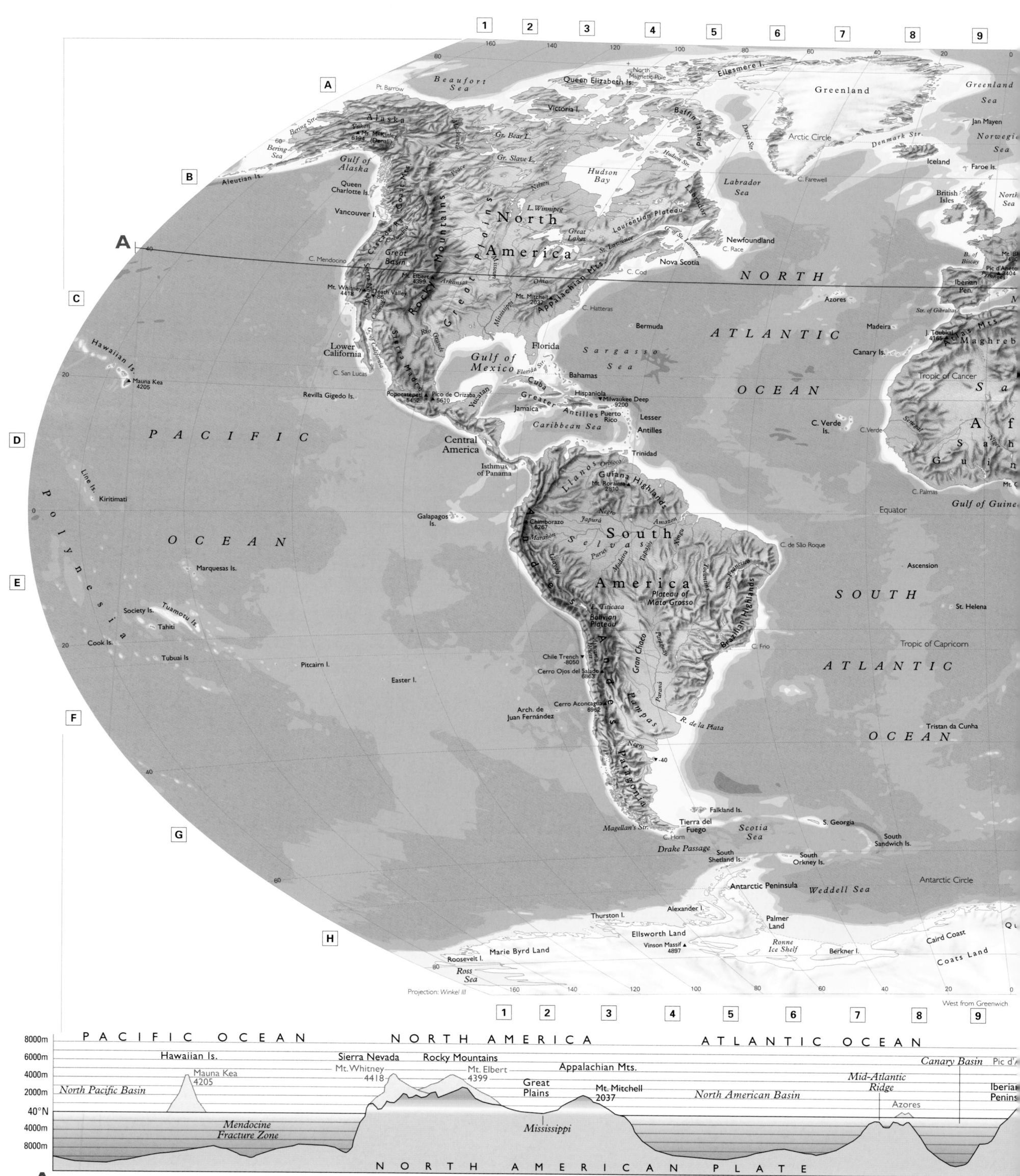

A

B

A

C

D

E

F

G

H

1 2 3 4 5 6 7 8 9

Beaufort Sea

Pt. Barrow

Alaska

Mt. McKinley (Denali) 6194

Bering Str.

Bering Sea

Aleutian Is.

Gulf of Alaska

Queen Charlotte Is.

Vancouver

Yukon

Mackenzie

Peace

Queen Elizabeth Is.

North Magnetic Pole

Victoria I.

Gr. Bear L.

Gr. Slave L.

Ellesmere I.

Greenland

Greenland Sea

Jan Mayen

Norwegian Sea

Baffin Island

Davis Str.

Arctic Circle

Denmark Str.

Iceland

Faroe Is.

British Isles

North Sea

Hudson Bay

Nelson

Hudson Str.

Labrador

Labrador Sea

Denmark Str.

C. Farewell

L. Winnipeg

North America

Great Plains

Great Lakes

Laurentian Plateau

St. Lawrence

G. of St. Lawrence

Newfoundland

C. Race

Nova Scotia

B. of Biscay

Mt. B

Pic d'Aneto 2404

Iberian Pen.

Rocky Mountains

Cascade Range

Columbia

C. Mendocino

Mt. Elbert 4399

Mt. Whitney 4418

Death Valley

Great Basin

Sierra Nevada

Arkansas

Missouri

Mississippi

Ohio

Mt. Mitchell 2037

Appalachian Mts.

C. Cod

C. Hatteras

NORTH

ATLANTIC

OCEAN

Azores

Madeira

Canary Is.

Maghreb

Atlas Mts. 4165

J. Toubkal

Str. of Gibraltar

Hawaiian Is.

Mauna Kea 4205

Lower California

C. San Lucas

Rio Grande

G. of California

Sierra Madre

Revilla Gigedo Is.

Popocatépetl 5452

Pico de Orizaba 5610

Yucatán

Gulf of Mexico

Florida

Florida Str.

Cuba

Bahamas

Greater Antilles

Hispaniola

Jamaica

Puerto Rico

Milwaukee Deep -9200

Lesser Antilles

Sargasso Sea

Bermuda

Tropic of Cancer

Sahara

C. Verde Is.

C. Verde

Af ri ca

Sahel

Senegal

Guin

Mt.

PACIFIC

OCEAN

Caribbean Sea

Trinidad

Central America

Isthmus of Panama

Llanos

Orinoco

Mt. Roraima 2810

Guiana Highlands

C. Palmas

Gulf of Guine

Equator

Polynesia

Line Is.

Kiritimati

Galapagos Is.

Chimborazo 6267

Negro

Marañón

Japurá

Amazon

Purus

Madeira

Tapajós

Xingu

Tocantins

C. de São Roque

Ascension

Marquesas Is.

South America

Selvas

Plateau of Mato Grosso

Brazilian Highlands

SOUTH

St. Helena

Society Is.

Tahiti

Tuamotu Is.

L. Titicaca

Bolivian Plateau

Andes

Gran Chaco

Paraná

C. Frio

Tropic of Capricorn

Cook Is.

Tubuai Is.

Pitcairn I.

Easter I.

Chile Trench -8050

Cerro Ojos del Salado 6863

Cerro Aconcagua 6960

Pampas

R. de la Plata

ATLANTIC

Tristan da Cunha

Arch. de Juan Fernández

Negro

Patagonia

-40

OCEAN

Falkland Is.

Tierra del Fuego

C. Horn

Magellan's Str.

Scotia Sea

S. Georgia

South Sandwich Is.

Drake Passage

South Shetland Is.

South Orkney Is.

Antarctic Circle

Antarctic Peninsula

Weddell Sea

Thurston I.

Alexander I.

Palmer Land

Caird Coast

Coats Land

Ross Sea

Roosevelt I.

Marie Byrd Land

Ellsworth Land

Vinson Massif 4897

Ronne Ice Shelf

Berkner I.

80

60

40

20

160 140 120 100 80 60 40 20

Projection: Winkel III

West from Greenwich

1 2 3 4 5 6 7 8 9

8000m	P A C I F I C O C E A N	N O R T H A M E R I C A	A T L A N T I C O C E A N	

6000m

Hawaiian Is.

Sierra Nevada

Rocky Mountains

Canary Basin

Pic d'

4000m

Mauna Kea 4205

Mt. Whitney 4418

Mt. Elbert 4399

Appalachian Mts.

Mid-Atlantic Ridge

Iberia

2000m

North Pacific Basin

Great Plains

Mt. Mitchell 2037

North American Basin

Azores

Iberian Penins

40°N

Mendocine Fracture Zone

Mississippi

4000m

8000m

N O R T H   A M E R I C A N   P L A T E

A

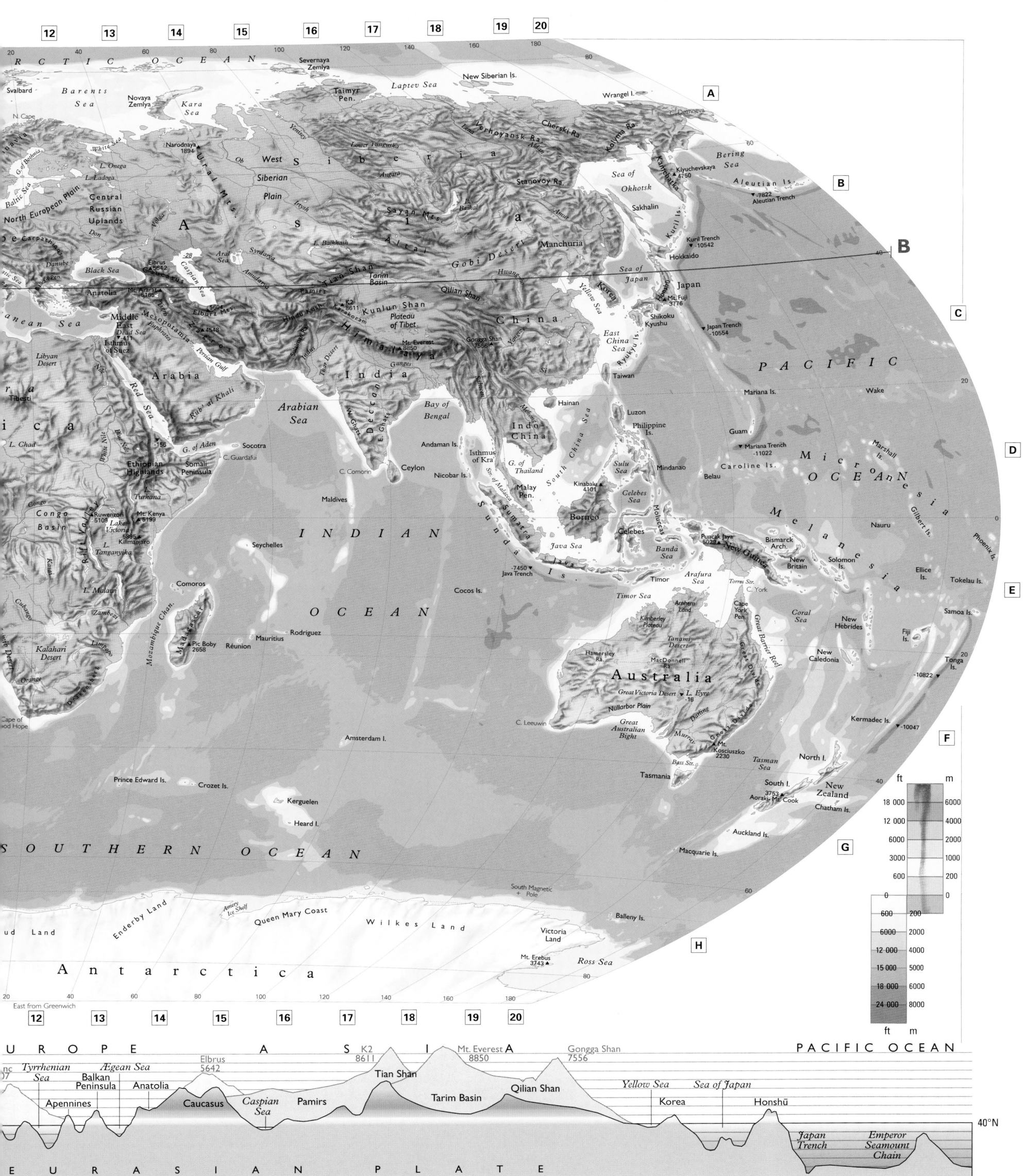

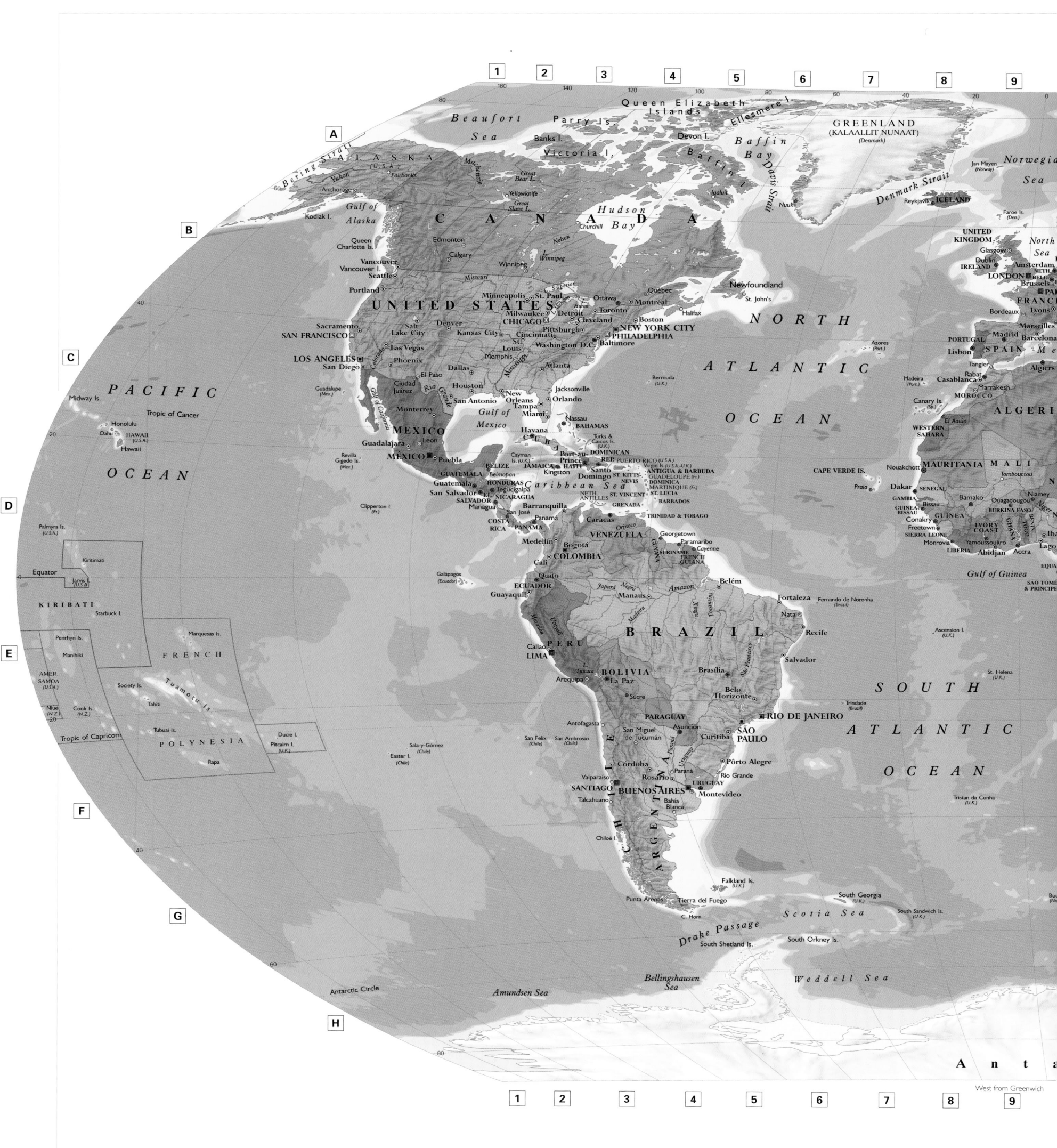

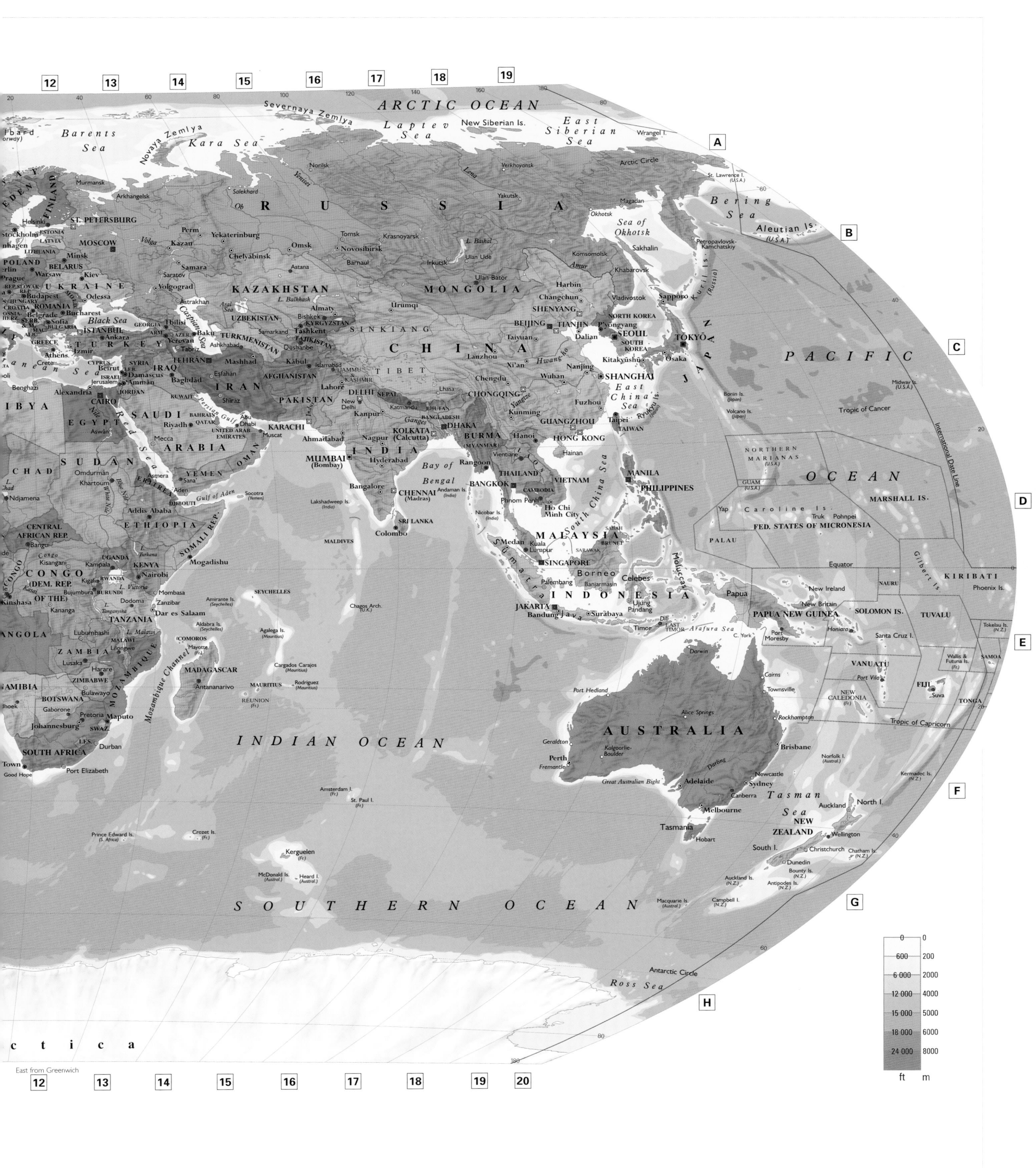

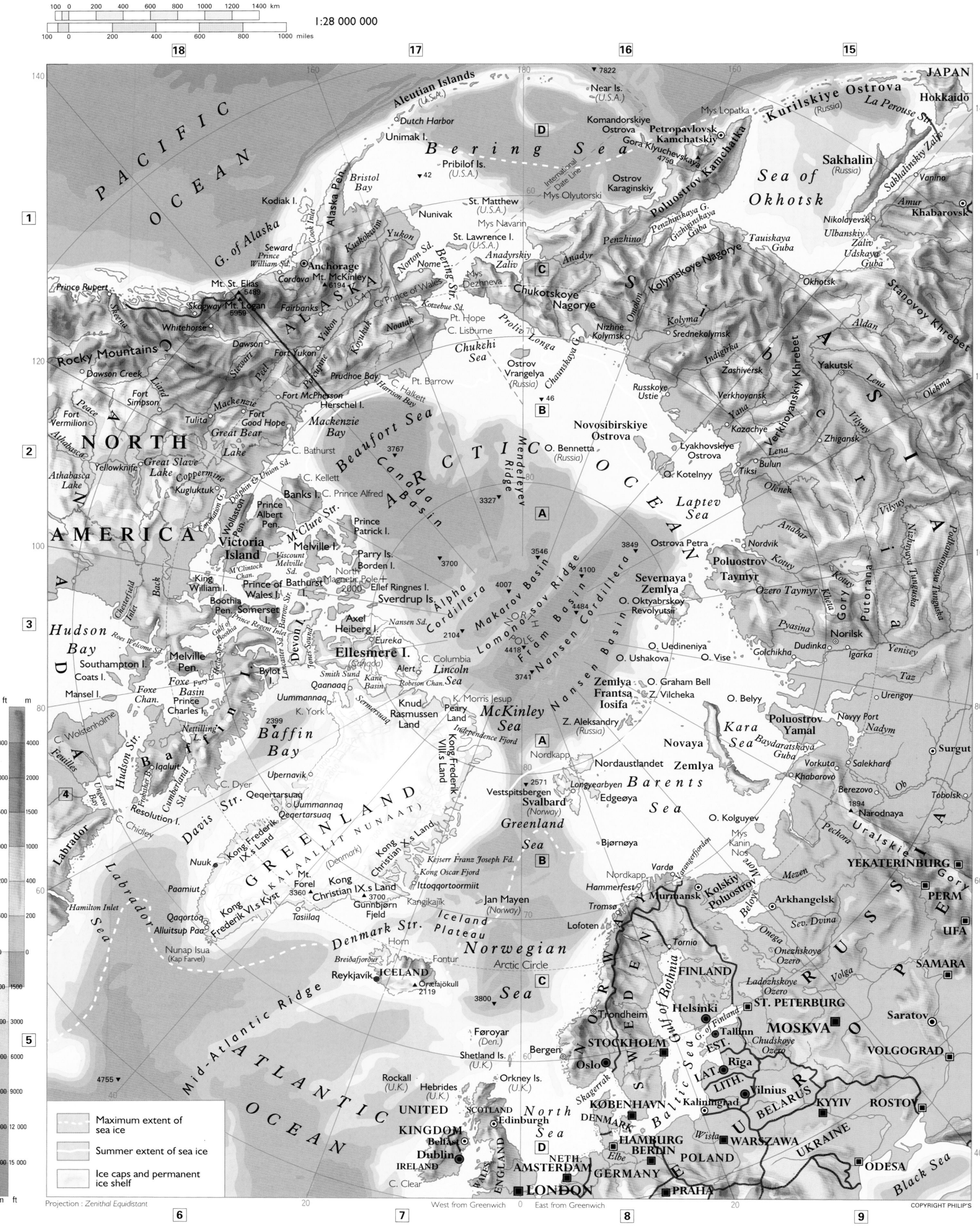

Projection : Zenithal Equidistant

COPYRIGHT PHILIP'S

	Maximum extent of sea ice
	Summer extent of sea ice
	Ice caps and permanent ice shelf

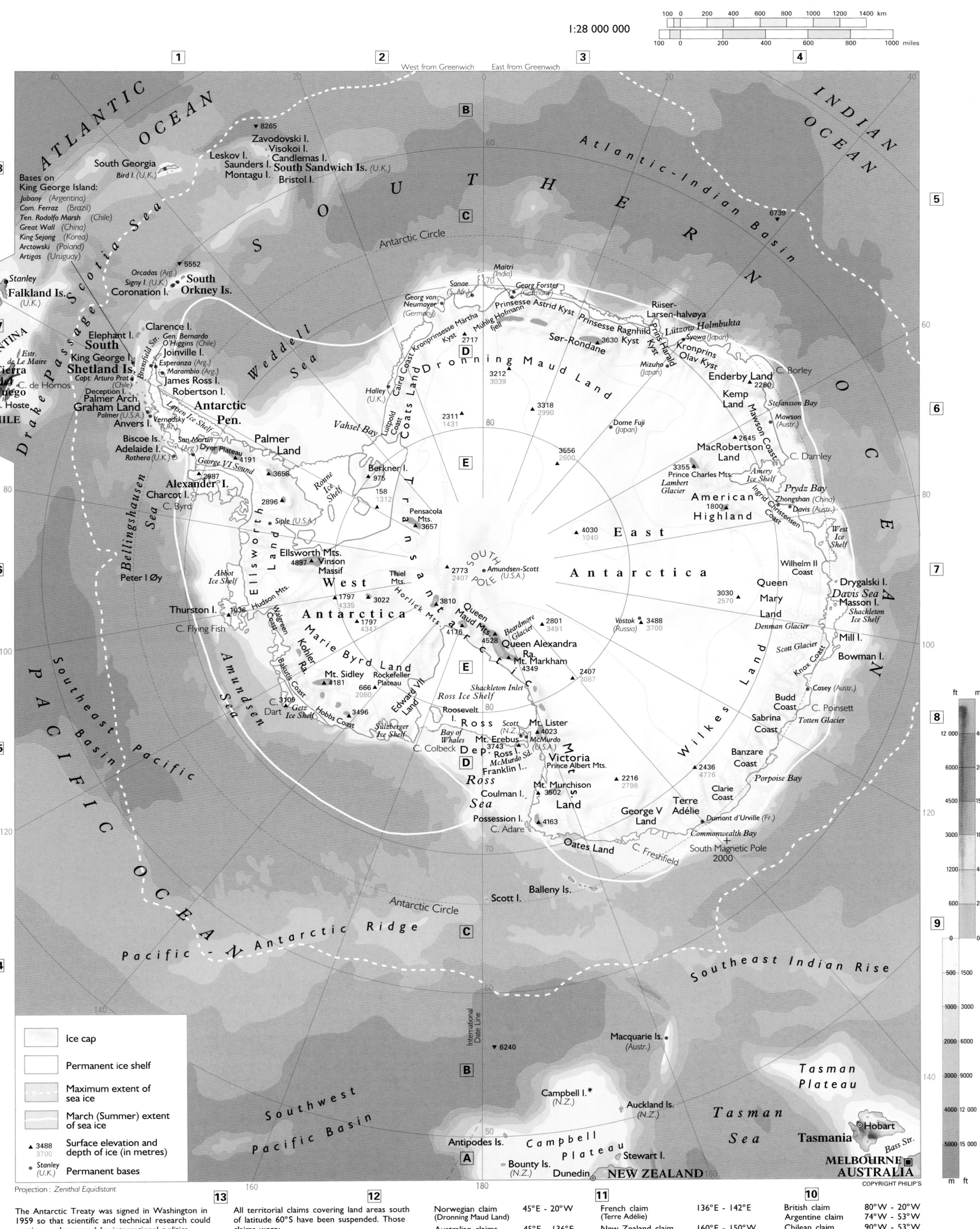

1:28 000 000

| 100 | 0 | 200 | 400 | 600 | 800 | 1000 | 1200 | 1400 km |
| 100 | 0 | 200 | 400 | 600 | 800 | 1000 miles |

West from Greenwich   East from Greenwich

ATLANTIC OCEAN

INDIAN OCEAN

SOUTHERN

Atlantic-Indian Basin

▼8265
Zavodovski I.
Visokoi I.
Leskov I. Candlemas I.
Saunders I.
South Sandwich Is. (U.K.)
Montagu I.
Bristol I.

South Georgia
Bird I. (U.K.)

Bases on
King George Island:
Jubany (Argentina)
Com. Ferraz (Brazil)
Ten. Rodolfo Marsh (Chile)
Great Wall (China)
King Sejong (Korea)
Arctowski (Poland)
Artigas (Uruguay)

Antarctic Circle

Maitri (India)
Sanae (S. Afr.)
Georg von Neumayer (Germany)
Georg Forster (Germany)

Riiser-Larsen-halvøya
Lützow Holmbukta

Stanley
Falkland Is.
(U.K.)

Orcadas (Arg.) ▼5552
Signy I. (U.K.)
Coronation I.
South Orkney Is.

Prinsesse Astrid Kyst
Prinsesse Ragnhild Kyst
Sør-Rondane

Kronprins Olav Kyst
Syowa (Japan)

Prins Harald Kyst
Mizuho (Japan)

Kronprinsesse Martha
Kyst

Mühlig Hofmann fjell

3630 Kyst

Kronprins

6739

ARGENTINA

Estr. de Le Maire
Tierra del Fuego
C. de Hornos
Hoste
CHILE

Clarence I.
Elephant I.
Gen. Bernardo O'Higgins (Chile)
South Shetland Is.
King George I.
Capt. Arturo Prat (Chile)
Deception I.
Palmer Arch.
Graham Land
Palmer (U.S.A.)
Anvers I.
Vernadsky (U.K.)

Joinville I.
Esperanza (Arg.)
Marambio (Arg.)
James Ross I.
Robertson I.

Halley (U.K.)

2717
Caird Coast
Dronning Maud Land
3212
3039

3318
2990

Enderby Land
C. Borley
2280

Dome Fuji (Japan)

Mawson (Austr.)
Kemp Land
Stefansson Bay

Weddell Sea

Larsen Ice Shelf
San Martin (Arg.)
Dyer Plateau
Palmer Land

Biscoe Is.
Adelaide I.
Rothera (U.K.)

Vahsel Bay
Berkner I.
2311
1431

3556
2600

MacRobertson Land

2645
C. Damley

Amery Ice Shelf
3355
Prince Charles Mts.
Lambert Glacier

American

Zhongshan (China)
Prydz Bay

George VI Sound
4191
Alexander I.
2987
Charcot I.
2896
C. Byrd
Siple (U.S.A.)

Ronne Ice Shelf
975
158
1312

Pensacola Mts.
3657

Highland
1800
2570

Davis (Austr.)

West Ice Shelf

Abbot Ice Shelf

Ellsworth Mts.
4897 Vinson Massif
1797
4335

Thiel Mts.
3022

3810
4116

2773
2407

Amundsen-Scott (U.S.A.)
SOUTH POLE

East Antarctica

4030
1040

3030
2570

Wilhelm II Coast

Queen Mary Land

Drygalski I.
Davis Sea
Masson I.
Shackleton Ice Shelf

Peter I Øy

Thurston I.
1936

Hudson Mts.
Walgreen Coast
West Antarctica
1797
4347

Horlick Mts.
Queen Maud Mts.
4528
Beardmore Glacier

2801
3491

Queen Alexandra Ra.
Mt. Markham
4349

Vostok (Russia)
3488
3700

2407
3087

Mill I.
Bowman I.

Denman Glacier
Scott Glacier
Knox Coast

C. Flying Fish

Marie Byrd Land
Kohler Ra.
Bakutis Coast

Mt. Sidley
4181
Rockefeller Plateau
666
2080

Casey (Austr.)
Totten Glacier
C. Poinsett

Budd Coast
Sabrina Coast

Bellingshausen Sea

Amundsen Sea

C. 3109
Dart
Getz Ice Shelf
Hobbs Coast
3496

Ross Ice Shelf

Shackleton Inlet

Edward VII Land
Roosevelt I.

Sulzberger Ice Shelf

Banzare Coast

Southeast Pacific Basin

Pacific

Bay of Whales
C. Colbeck
Ross I.
McMurdo Sd.
Franklin I.

Ross Dep.
Scott (N.Z.)
McMurdo (U.S.A.)
Mt. Lister
4023
Mt. Erebus
3743

Victoria

2436
4776
Clarie Coast

Porpoise Bay

Prince Albert Mts.
2216
2798

Wilkes Land

Coulman I.
Mt. Murchison
3502
Land

George V Land
Terre Adélie

Dumont d'Urville (Fr.)

PACIFIC OCEAN

Ross Sea

Possession I.
C. Adare
4163

Commonwealth Bay
South Magnetic Pole
2000
Oates Land
C. Freshfield

Antarctic Circle

Balleny Is.

Scott I.

Pacific-Antarctic Ridge

Southeast Indian Rise

International Date Line

▼6240

Macquarie Is. (Austr.)

ft   m
12 000   4000
6000   2000
4500   1500
3000   1000
1200   400
600   200

Southwest Pacific Basin

Campbell I. (N.Z.)

Tasman Plateau

Tasman Sea

Hobart

Antipodes Is.

Campbell Plateau

Stewart I.

Bounty Is. (N.Z.)
Dunedin
NEW ZEALAND

Tasmania

Bass Str.

MELBOURNE
AUSTRALIA
COPYRIGHT PHILIP'S

m   ft
0   0
500   1500
1000   3000
2000   6000
3000   9000
4000   12 000
5000   15 000
m   ft

Legend:
- Ice cap
- Permanent ice shelf
- Maximum extent of sea ice
- March (Summer) extent of sea ice
- ▲ 3488 / 3700 Surface elevation and depth of ice (in metres)
- • Stanley (U.K.) Permanent bases

Projection: Zenithal Equidistant

The Antarctic Treaty was signed in Washington in 1959 so that scientific and technical research could continue unhampered by international politics.

All territorial claims covering land areas south of latitude 60°S have been suspended. Those claims were:

Norwegian claim (Dronning Maud Land)	45°E - 20°W	
Australian claims	45°E - 136°E / 142°E - 160°E	
French claim (Terre Adélie)	136°E - 142°E	
New Zealand claim (Ross Dependency)	160°E - 150°W	
British claim	80°W - 20°W	
Argentine claim	74°W - 53°W	
Chilean claim	90°W - 53°W	

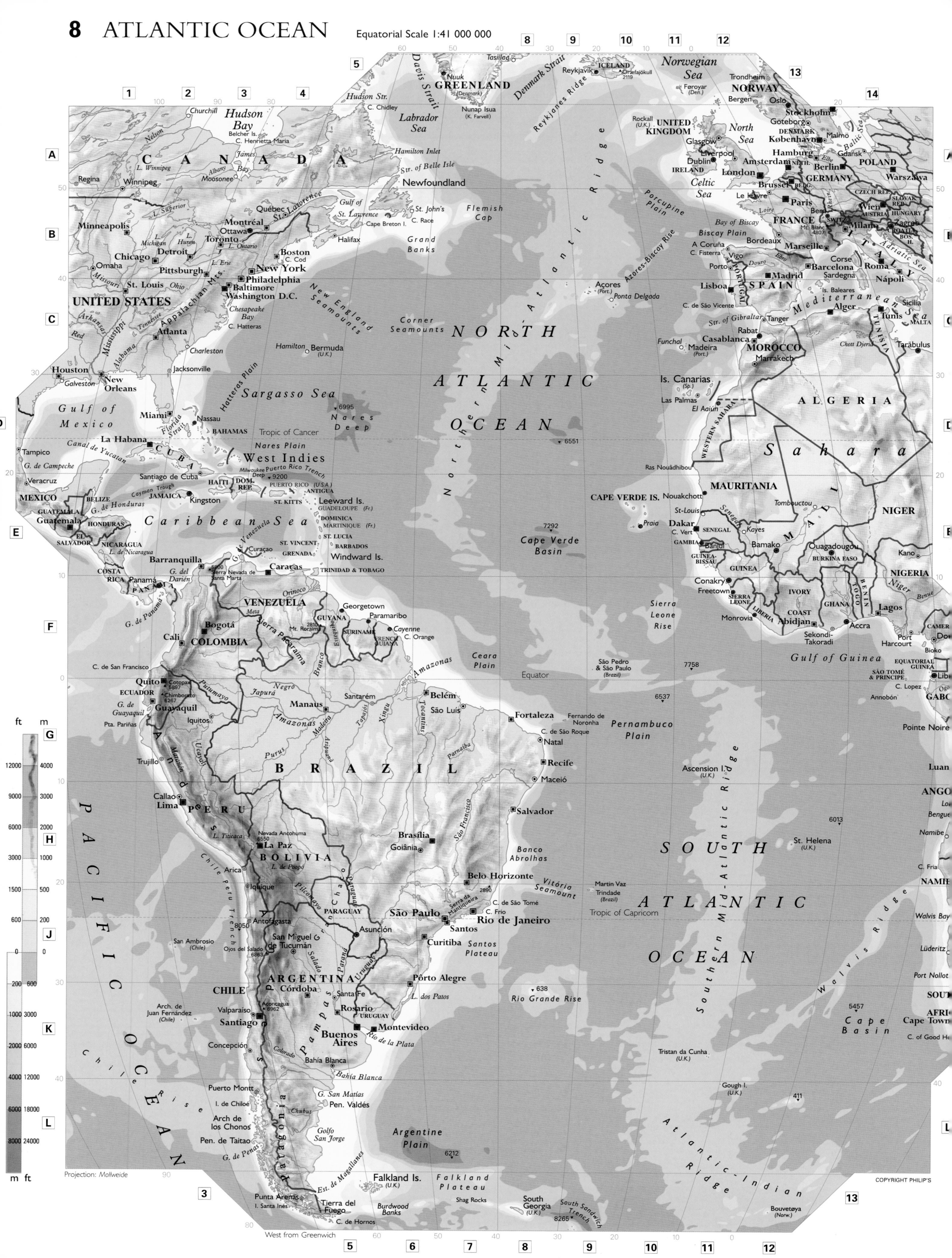

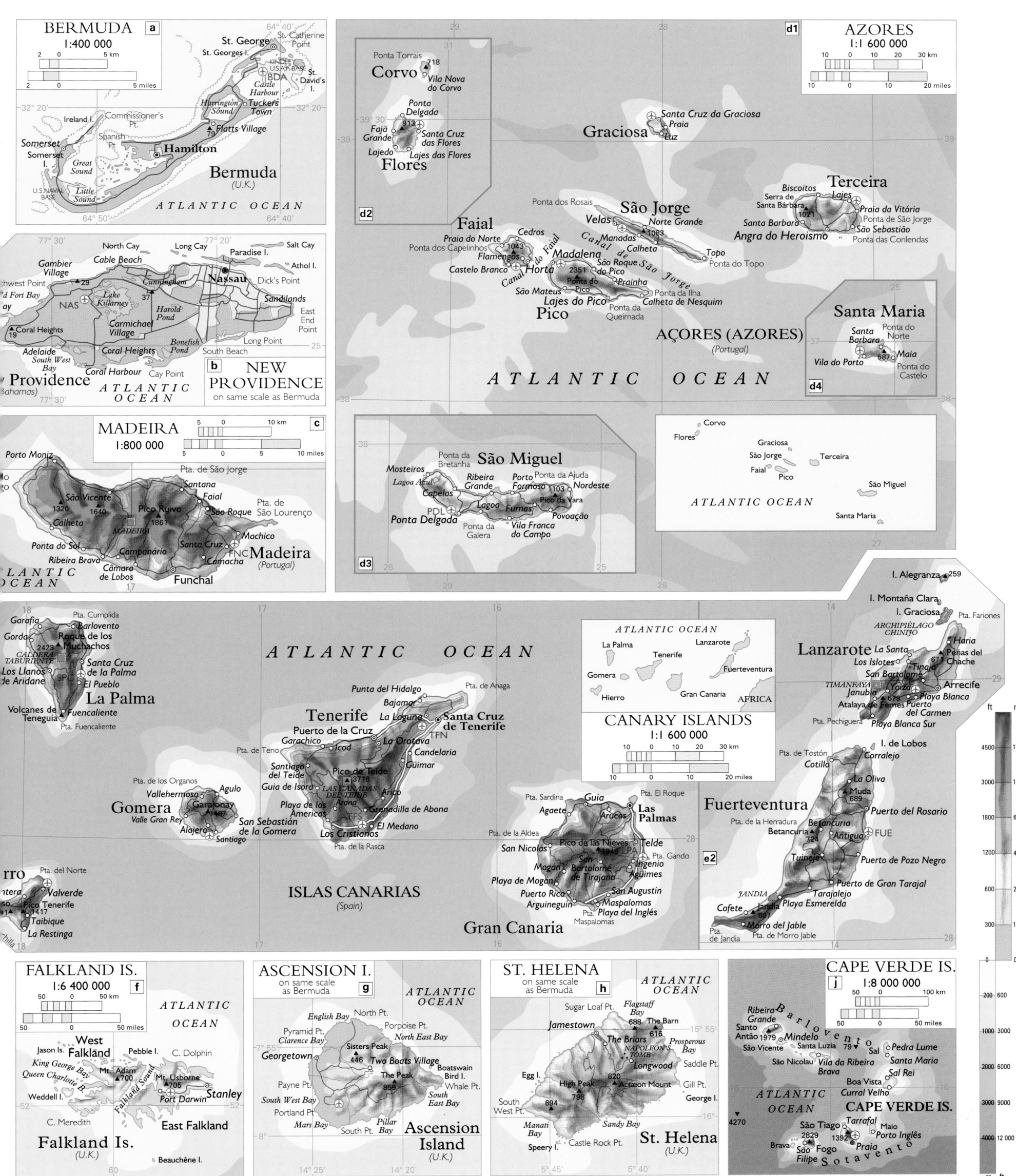

BERMUDA [a]
1:400 000

ATLANTIC OCEAN

St. George
St. Georges I.
St. Catherine Point
KINDLEY
U.S.A. BASE
BDA
St. David's I.
Castle Harbour
Tuckers Town
Harrington Sound
Flatts Village
79
Hamilton
Commissioner's Pt.
Ireland I.
Somerset
Somerset I.
Spanish Pt.
Great Sound
Little Sound
U.S. NAVAL BASE
BERMUDA (U.K.)

[b] NEW PROVIDENCE
on same scale as Bermuda

North Cay
Long Cay
Paradise I.
Salt Cay
Cable Beach
Gambier Village
Athol I.
Dick's Point
Nassau
Cunningham
37
Lake Killarney
NAS
29
Harold Pond
Sandilands
East End Point
Coral Heights
19
Carmichael Village
Bonefish Pond
Long Point
Adelaide
South West Bay
Coral Heights
Cay Point
South Beach
Coral Harbour
Providence
ATLANTIC OCEAN
Bahamas

MADEIRA [c]
1:800 000

Porto Moniz
Pta. de São Jorge
São Vicente
1320
Santana
Faial
1640
Pico Ruivo
1861
Calheta
São Roque
MADEIRA
Pta. de São Lourenço
Ponta do Sol
Santa Cruz
Machico
Ribeira Brava
Campanário
Câmara de Lobos
Camacha
FNC Madeira (Portugal)
Funchal
ATLANTIC OCEAN

CORVO / FLORES
Ponta Torrais
718
Corvo
Vila Nova do Corvo
Ponta Delgada
913
Fajã Grande
Santa Cruz das Flores
Lajedo
Lajes das Flores
Flores
[d2]

Ponta dos Rosais
Cedros
Velas
Norte Grande
Faial
Ponta do Norte
1043
Manadas
1083
Calheta
Ponta dos Capelinhos
Flamengos
Madalena
2351
São Roque do Pico
Topo
Castelo Branco
Horta
Ponta do Pico
Ponta do Topo
São Mateus
Prainha
Lajes do Pico
Ponta da Ilha
Calheta de Nesquim
Ponta da Queimada
Pico
Ponta da Ilha

GRACIOSA / TERCEIRA
Santa Cruz da Graciosa
Praia
Graciosa
Luz
Biscoitos
Lajes
Serra de Santa Bárbara
1021
Terceira
Praia da Vitória
Ponta de São Jorge
Santa Barbara
São Sebastião
Angra do Heroismo
Ponta das Conlendas
São Jorge
Canal de São Jorge

AÇORES (AZORES)
(Portugal)

ATLANTIC OCEAN

AZORES [d1]
1:1 600 000

SANTA MARIA [d4]
Santa Barbara
Ponta do Norte
587
Maia
Vila do Porto
Ponta do Castelo

SÃO MIGUEL [d3]
Ponta da Bretanha
Mosteiros
Ribeira Grande
Porto Formoso
Ponta da Ajuda
Nordeste
Lagoa Azul
Capelas
1103
Pico da Vara
PDL
Lagoa
Furnas
Ponta Delgada
Povoação
Ponta da Galera
Vila Franca do Campo

Corvo
Flores
Graciosa
São Jorge
Terceira
Faial
Pico
São Miguel
Santa Maria
ATLANTIC OCEAN

La Palma / Tenerife / Gomera / Hierro
ATLANTIC OCEAN

Pta. Cumplida
Garafia
Barlovento
Gorda
Roque de los Muchachos
2423
CALDERA TABURIENTE
Santa Cruz de la Palma
Los Llanos de Aridane
SPC
El Pueblo
La Palma
Volcanes de Teneguia
Fuencaliente
Pta. Fuencaliente

Punta del Hidalgo
Bajamar
Pta. de Anaga
La Laguna
Tenerife
Santa Cruz de Tenerife
Puerto de la Cruz
TFN
Garachico
La Orotava
Icod
Candelaria
Pta. de Teno
Santiago del Teide
Pico de Teide
3718
Güimar
Guia de Isora
LAS CAÑADAS DEL TEIDE
Arico
Pta. de los Organos
Agulo
Vallehermoso
Playa de las Américas
Granadilla de Abona
Gomera
Garajonay
1487
San Sebastián de la Gomera
El Medano
Valle Gran Rey
Alajero
Los Cristianos
Pta. de la Rasca
Santiago

rro
Pta. del Norte
Valverde
Pico Tenerife
1417
Taibique
La Restinga

ISLAS CANARIAS
(Spain)
Gran Canaria

CANARY ISLANDS
1:1 600 000
ATLANTIC OCEAN
La Palma
Lanzarote
Tenerife
Gomera
Fuerteventura
Hierro
Gran Canaria
AFRICA

Gran Canaria
Pta. Sardina
Guia
Pta. El Roque
Agaete
Arucas
Las Palmas
San Nicolás
Pico de las Nieves
1949
Telde
LPA
Pta. Gando
San Mogán
San Bartolomé de Tirajana
Ingenio
Agüimes
Playa de Mogán
Puerto Rico
San Augustín
Arguineguín
Maspalomas
Playa del Inglés
Maspalomas

Lanzarote / Fuerteventura
I. Alegranza
259
I. Montaña Clara
I. Graciosa
Pta. Fariones
ARCHIPIÉLAGO CHINIJO
La Santa
Haria
Peñas del Chache
67
Lanzarote
Los Islotes
Tinajo
San Bartolomé
TIMANFAYA
Yaiza
Arrecife
Janubio
679
Atalaya de Femes
Playa Blanca
Pta. Pechiguera
Puerto del Carmen
Playa Blanca Sur
Pta. de Tostón
I. de Lobos
Cotillo
Corralejo
La Oliva
Muda
689
Fuerteventura
Puerto del Rosario
Pta. de la Herradura
Betancuria
Betancuria
724
Antigua
FUE
Tuineje
Puerto de Pozo Negro
Puerto de Gran Tarajal
JANDIA
Tarajalejo
Cofete
Jandia
897
Playa Esmeralda
Pta. de Jandia
Morro del Jable
Pta. de Morro Jable

FALKLAND IS. [f]
1:6 400 000
ATLANTIC OCEAN
West Falkland
Jason Is.
Pebble I.
C. Dolphin
King George Bay
Mt. Adam
700
Queen Charlotte B.
Mt. Usborne
705
Stanley
Weddell I.
Port Darwin
Falkland Sound
East Falkland
C. Meredith
Falkland Is. (U.K.)
Beauchêne I.

ASCENSION I. [g]
on same scale as Bermuda
ATLANTIC OCEAN
English Bay
North Pt.
Pyramid Pt.
Clarence Bay
Porpoise Pt.
North East Bay
Georgetown
Sisters Peak
446
Two Boats Village
Boatswain Bird I.
Payne Pt.
The Peak
859
Whale Pt.
South West Bay
South East Bay
Portland Pt.
Mars Bay
Pillar Bay
South Pt.
Ascension Island (U.K.)

ST. HELENA [h]
on same scale as Bermuda
ATLANTIC OCEAN
Sugar Loaf Pt.
Flagstaff Bay
688
The Barn
616
Jamestown
The Briars
NAPOLEON'S TOMB
Prosperous Bay
Longwood
Saddle Pt.
Egg I.
820
Actaeon Mount
Gill Pt.
High Peak
George I.
694
798
South West Pt.
Manati Bay
Sandy Bay
Speery I.
Castle Rock Pt.
St. Helena (U.K.)

West from Greenwich

CAPE VERDE IS. [j]
1:8 000 000
Ribeira Grande
Santo Antão
1979
Mindelo
Barlovento
São Vicente
Santa Luzia
79
Sal
Pedra Lume
São Nicolau
Vila da Ribeira Brava
Santa Maria
Sal Rei
Boa Vista
Curral Velho
ATLANTIC OCEAN
CAPE VERDE IS.
São Tiago
Tarrafal
2829
1392
Maio
Porto Inglés
Brava
São Fogo
Praia
Filipe
4270
Sotavento

COPYRIGHT PHILIP'S

ft m
4500 1500
3000 1000
1800 600
1200 400
600 200
300 100
0
200 600
1000 3000
2000 6000
3000 9000
4000 12 000
m ft

1:10 000 000

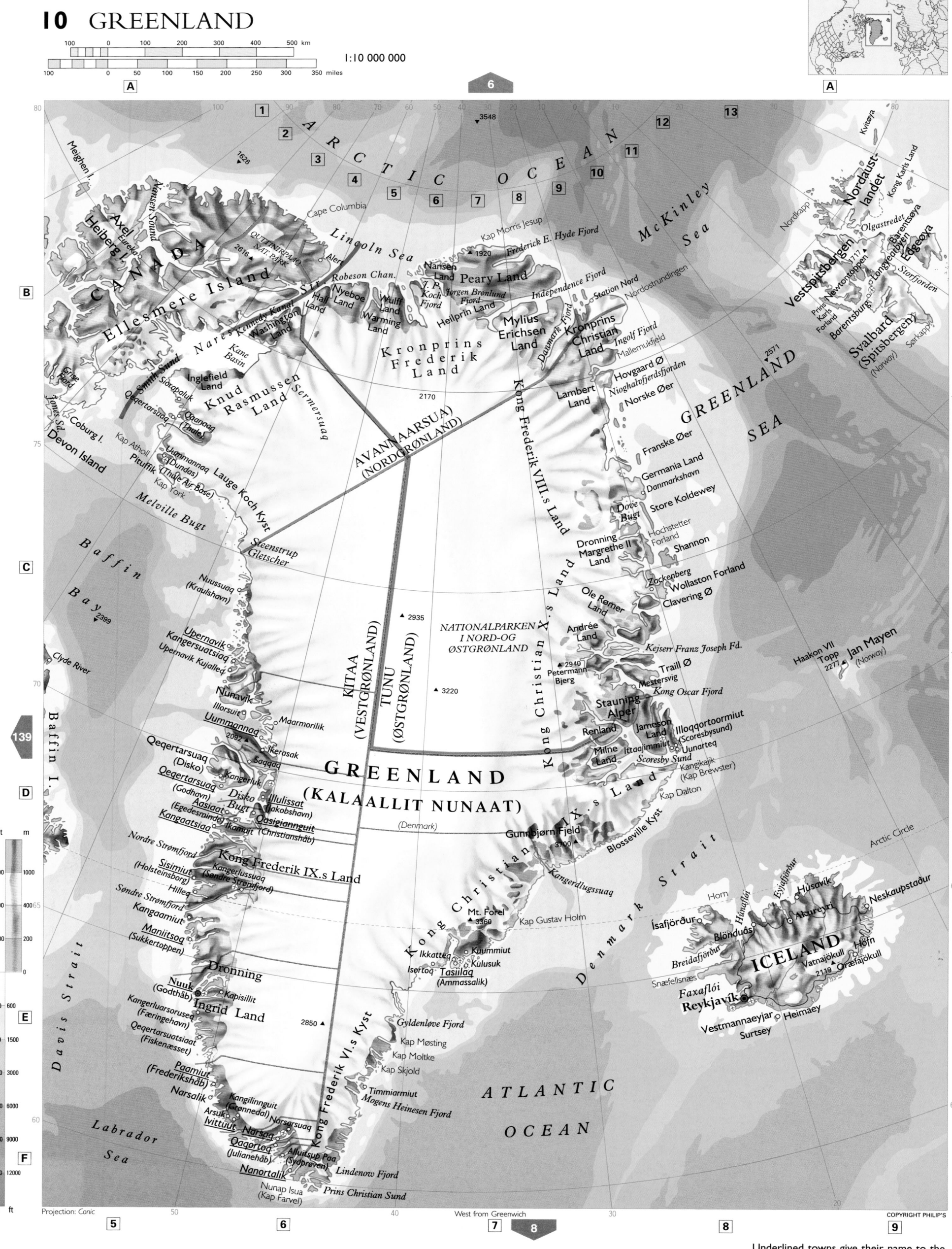

6

139

A R C T I C   O C E A N

CANADA

Ellesmere Island

Axel Heiberg I.

Meighen I.

Nansen Sound

Eureka

QUTTINIRPAAQ NAT. PARK

2616

1626

Cape Columbia

Alert

Lincoln Sea

Nares Strait

Kennedy Kanal

Robeson Chan.

Hall Land

Nyeboe Land

Wulff Land

Warming Land

Nansen Land

J. P. Koch Fjord

Jørgen Brønlund Fjord

Hellprin Land

Peary Land

3548

1920

Frederick E. Hyde Fjord

Independence Fjord

Station Nord

Nordostrundingen

McKinley Sea

Nordkapp

Nordaust-landet

Kong Karls Land

Kvitøya

Vestspitsbergen

Svalbard (Spitsbergen) (Norway)

Prins Karls Forland

Barentsøya

Edgeøya

Storfjorden

Sørkapp

Olgastretet

Longyearbyen

Barentsøya

Smith Sund

Siorapaluk

Qeqertarsuaq

Inglefield Land

Knud Rasmussen Land

Washington Land

Kane Basin

Sermersuaq

Kronprins Frederik Land

2170

Mylius Erichsen Land

Danmark Fjord

Kronprins Christian Land

Ingolf Fjord

Mallemukfjeld

GREENLAND SEA

Hovgaard Ø

Nioghalbfjordsfjorden

Lambert Land

Norske Øer

Franske Øer

Germania Land

Danmarkshavn

Store Koldewey

Dove Bugt

Hochstetter Forland

Dronning Margrethe II Land

Shannon

Zackenberg

Wollaston Forland

Clavering Ø

Andrée Land

Kong Christian X.s Land

Kejserr Franz Joseph Fd.

Traill Ø

Mestersvig

Kong Oscar Fjord

Stauning Alper

Jameson Land

Renland

Milne Land

Ittaqqimiit

Illoqqortoormiut (Scoresbysund)

Uunarteq

Scoresby Sund

Kangikajik (Kap Brewster)

Kap Dalton

Haakon VII Topp 2277

Jan Mayen (Norway)

2571

2935

2940

3220

2092

Petermann Bjerg

NATIONALPARKEN I NORD-OG ØSTGRØNLAND

AVANNAARSUA) (NORDGRØNLAND)

Coburg I.

Devon Island

Jones Sd.

Kap Atholl

Pituffik (Thule Air Base)

Uummannaq (Dundas)

Kap York

Qaanaaq (Thule)

Lauge Koch Kyst

Melville Bugt

Steenstrup Gletscher

Baffin Bay

2399

Clyde River

Nuussuaq (Kraulshavn)

Upernavik

Kangersuatsiaq

Upernavik Kujalleq

Nunavik

Illorsuit

Uummannaq

Maarmorilik

Ikerasak

Saqqaq

Qeqertarsuaq (Disko)

Disko

Kangerluk

Disko Bugt

Illulissat (Jakobshavn)

Aasiaat (Egedesminde)

Qasigiannguit (Christianshåb)

Qeqertarsuaq (Godhavn)

Kangaatsiaq

Ikamiut

Nordre Strømfjord

KITAA (VESTGRØNLAND)

TUNU (ØSTGRØNLAND)

GREENLAND (KALAALLIT NUNAAT)

(Denmark)

Gunnbjørn Fjeld 3700

Blosseville Kyst

Arctic Circle

Kong Frederik IX.s Land

Kangerlussuaq

Sisimiut (Holsteinsborg)

Kangerlussuaq (Søndre Strømfjord)

H/lle0

Søndre Strømfjord

Kangaamiut

Maniitsoq (Sukkertoppen)

Nuuk (Godthåb)

Kapisillit

Kangerluarsoruseq (Færingehavn)

Qeqertarsuatsiaat (Fiskenæsset)

Paamiut (Frederikshåb)

Narsalik

Dronning Ingrid Land

2850

Baffin I.

Davis Strait

Kong Christian IX.s Land

Kangerdlugssuaq

Mt. Forel 3360

Kap Gustav Holm

Ikkatteq

Isortoq

Kuummiut

Kulusuk

Tasiilaq (Ammassalik)

Denmark Strait

Horn

Hornafjörður

Ísafjörður

Breidafjörður

Snæfellsnæs

Faxaflói

Reykjavík

Húsavík

Akureyri

Neskaupstaður

Blönduós

Vatnajökull

Hofn

2119

Öræfajökull

ICELAND

Vestmannaeyjar

Heimaey

Surtsey

Gyldenløve Fjord

Kap Møsting

Kap Moltke

Kap Skjold

Timmiarmiut

Mogens Heinesen Fjord

ATLANTIC OCEAN

Kong Frederik VI.s Kyst

Arsuk

Kangilinnguit (Grønnedal)

Ivittuut

Narsaq

Qaqortoq (Julianehåb)

Narsarsuaq

Alluitsup Paa (Sydprøven)

Nanortalik

Nunap Isua (Kap Farvel)

Lindenow Fjord

Prins Christian Sund

Labrador Sea

Projection: Conic

West from Greenwich

COPYRIGHT PHILIP'S

Underlined towns give their name to the administrative area in which they stand.

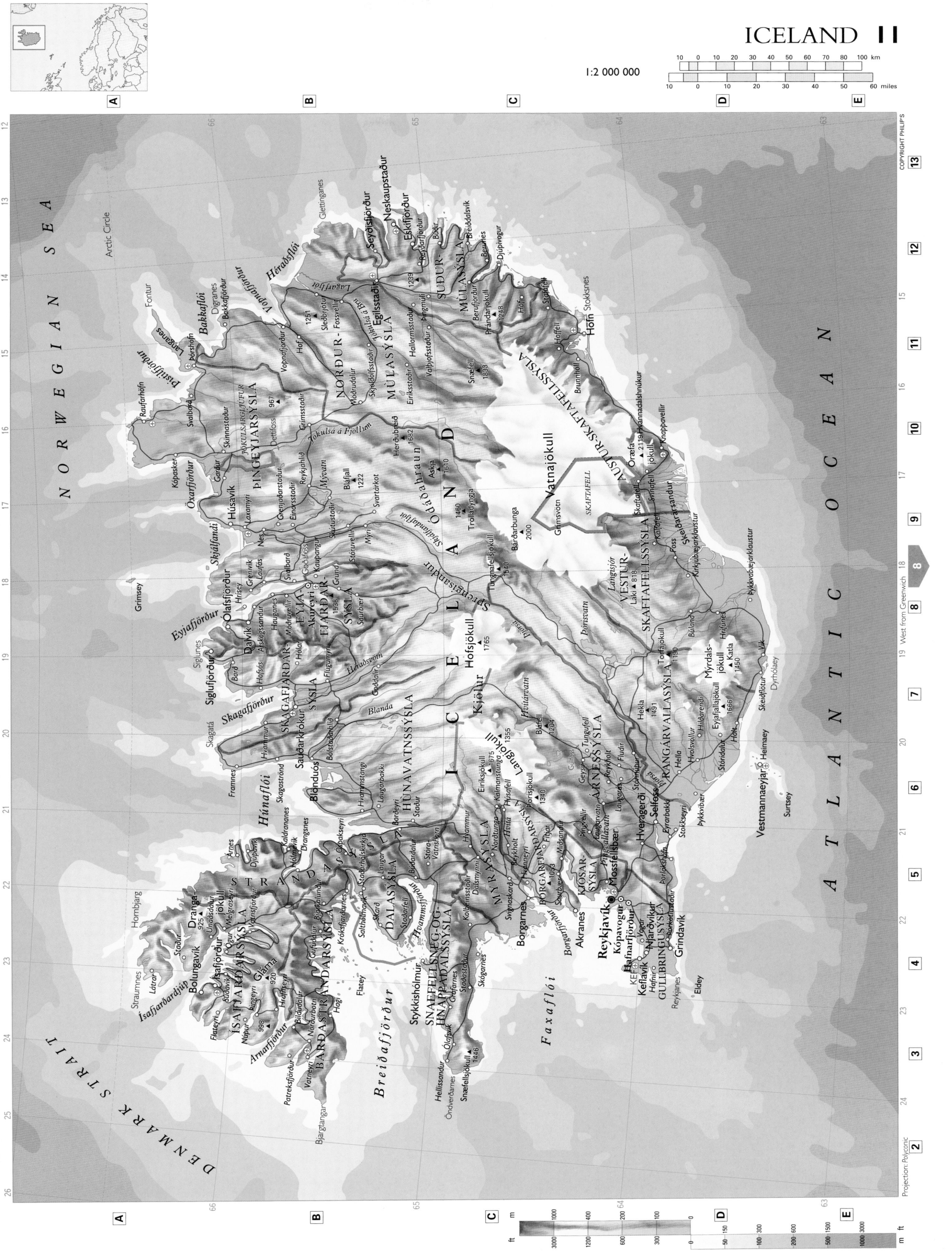

1:2 000 000

10 0 10 20 30 40 50 60 70 80 100 km
10 0 10 20 30 40 50 60 miles

COPYRIGHT PHILIP'S

Projection: Polyconic

NORWEGIAN SEA

DENMARK STRAIT

ATLANTIC OCEAN

ICELAND

Arctic Circle

West from Greenwich

1:16 000 000

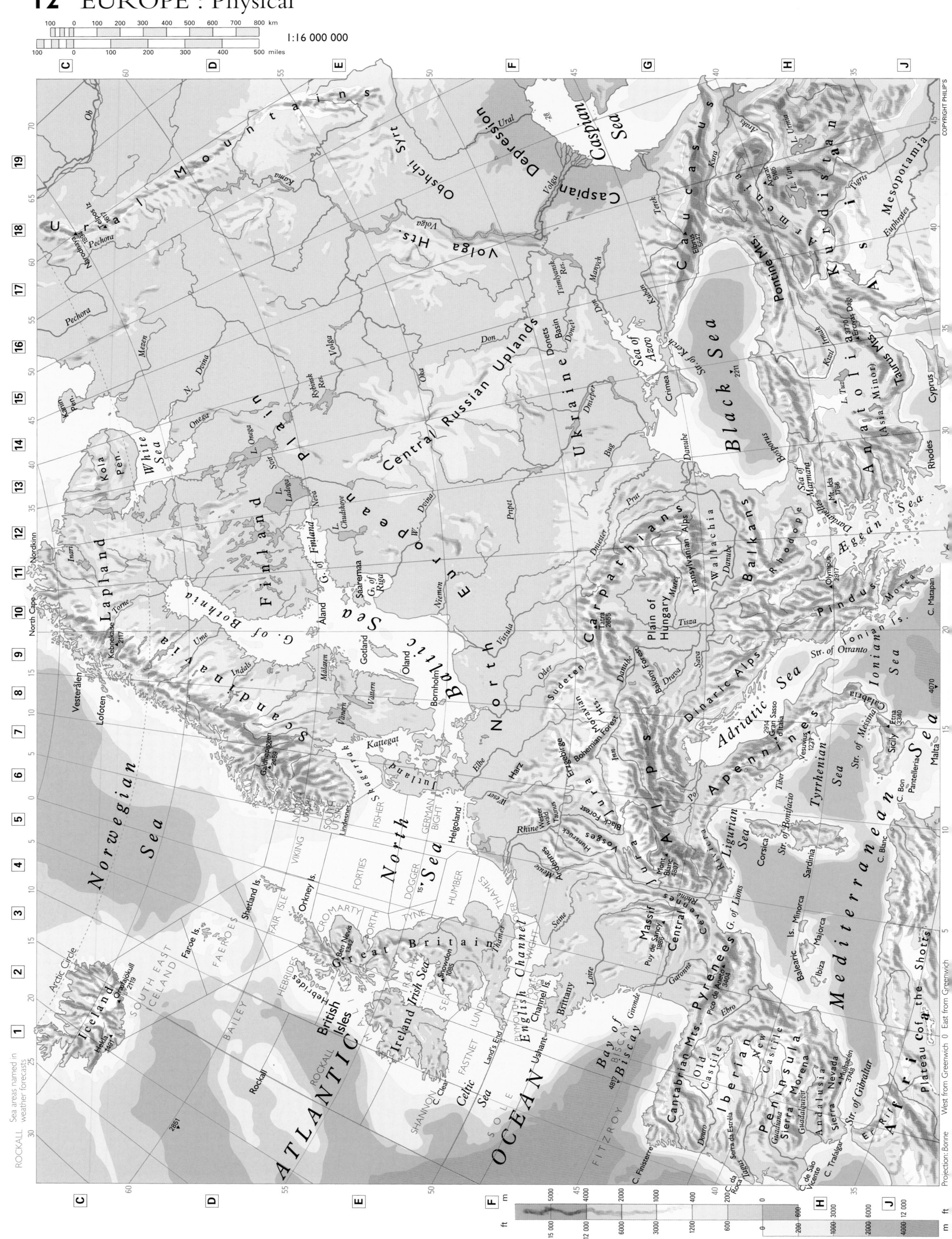

Projection: Bonne

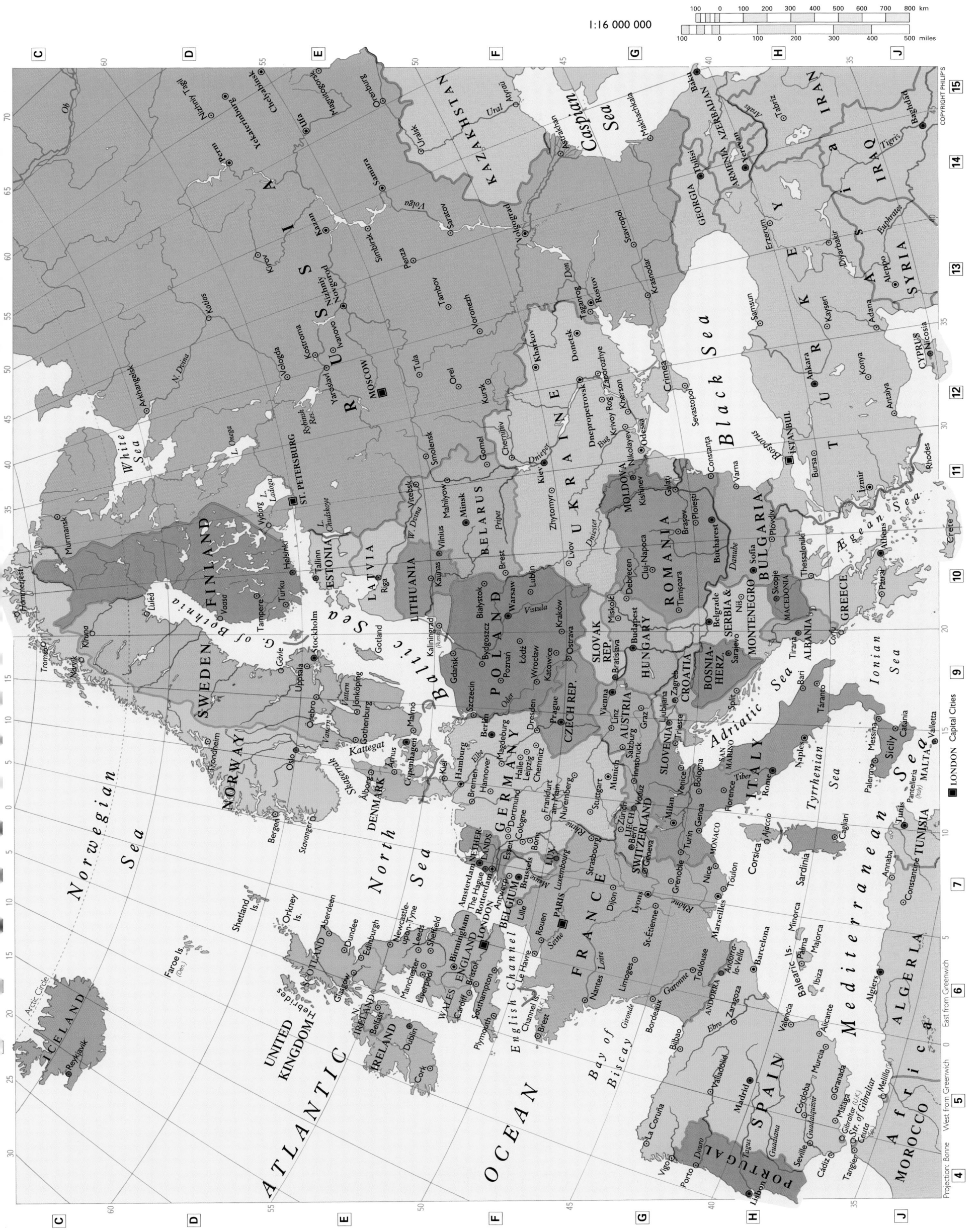

■ LONDON Capital Cities

Projection: Bonne

East from Greenwich

West from Greenwich

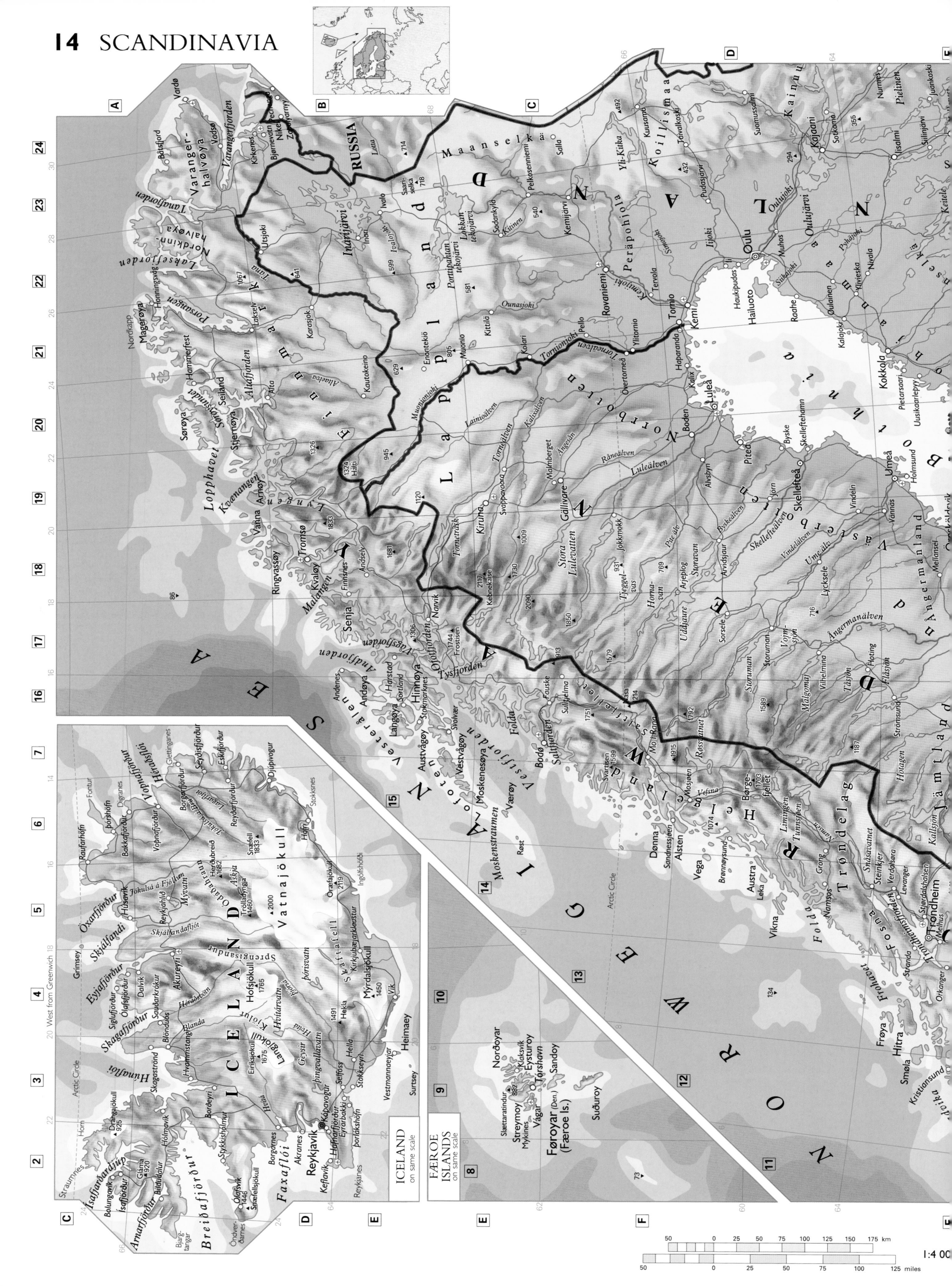

ICELAND
on same scale

FÆROE
ISLANDS
on same scale

1:4 00

50   0   25   50   75   100   125   150   175 km

50   0   25   50   75   100   125 miles

SCANDINAVIA

Countries and regions: FINLAND, ESTONIA, LATVIA, LITHUANIA, RUSSIA, BELARUS, POLAND, GERMANY, DENMARK, NORWAY, SWEDEN

Seas and gulfs: Gulf of Finland, Gulf of Riga, Gulf of Bothnia, BALTIC SEA, Kattegat, Skagerrak, Ålands hav

Major cities: Helsinki (Helsingfors), Tallinn, Riga, Vilnius, STOCKHOLM, Oslo, Göteborg (Gothenburg), KØBENHAVN (Copenhagen), Malmö, Kaliningrad (Russia), Gdańsk, Gdynia

Regions of Sweden: Uppland, Västmanland, Södermanland, Dalarna, Värmland, Dalsland, Bohuslän, Västergötland, Östergötland, Halland, Skåne, Blekinge, Småland, Gotland, Öland

Projection: Conic with two standard parallels

East from Greenwich

COPYRIGHT PHILIP'S

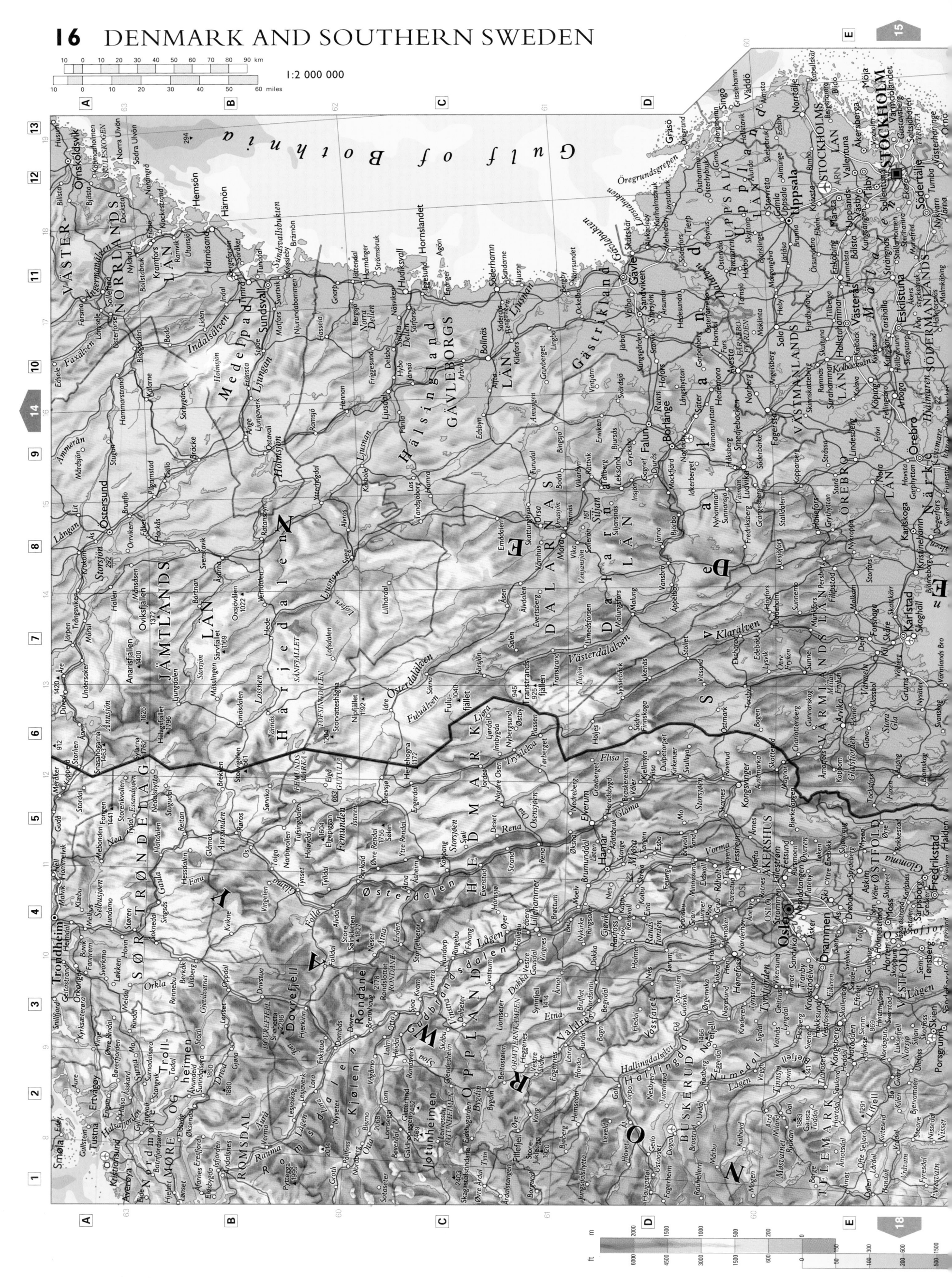

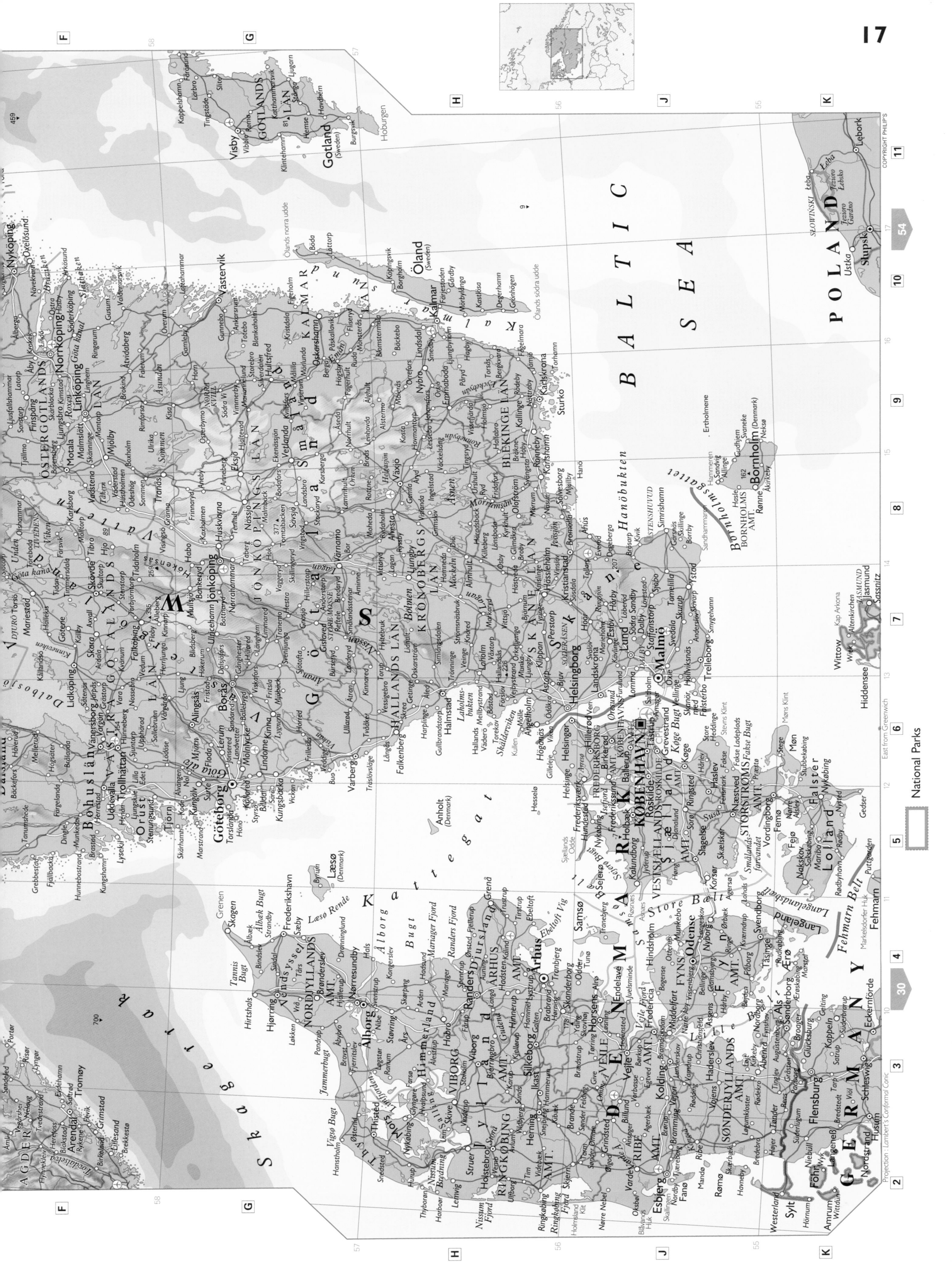

1:2 000 000

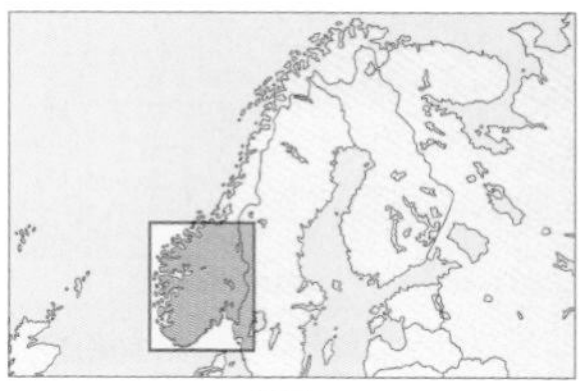

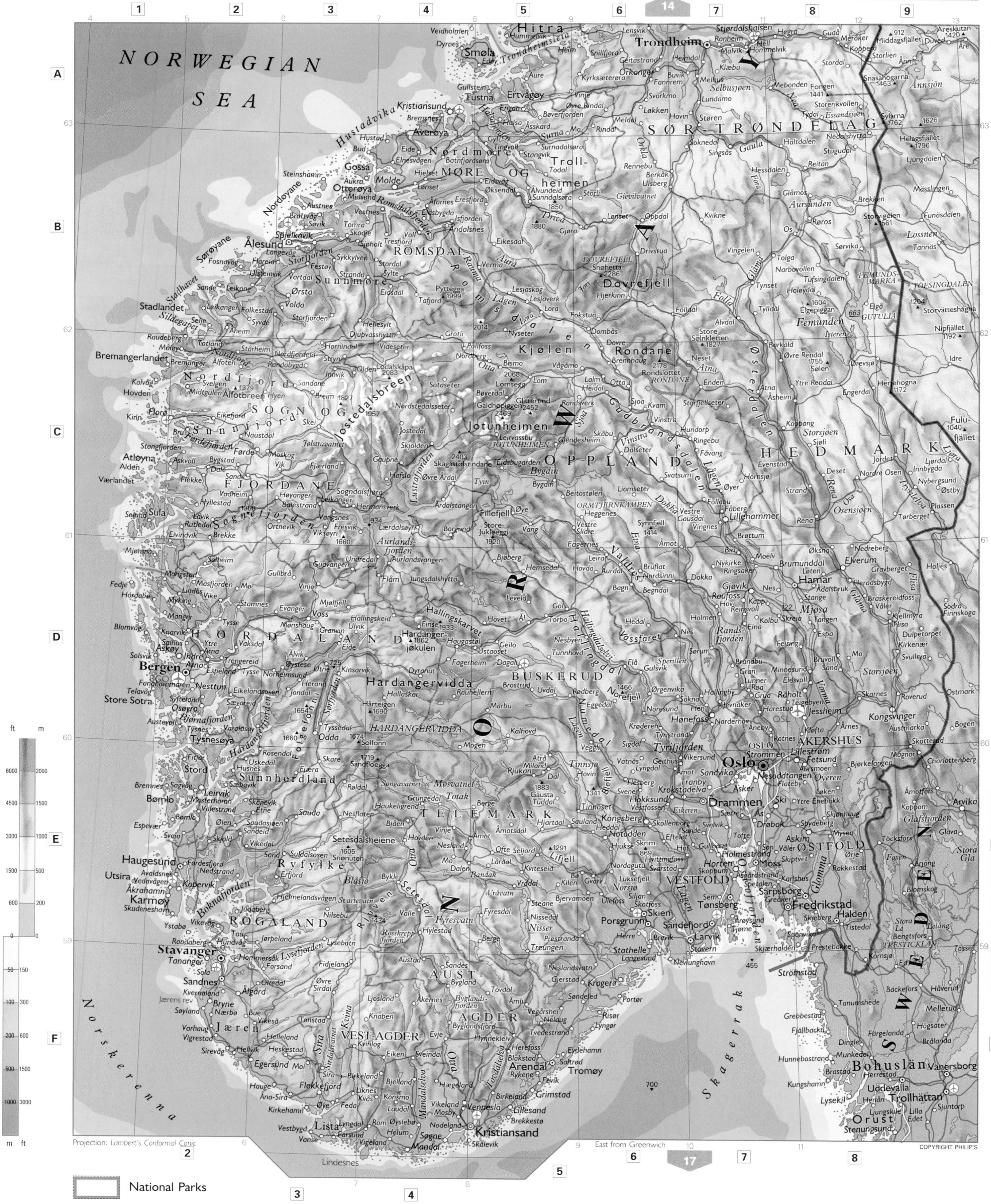

NORWEGIAN SEA

SØR TRØNDELAG

MØRE OG ROMSDAL

HEDMARK

OPPLAND

SOGN OG FJORDANE

HORDALAND

BUSKERUD

TELEMARK

ROGALAND

AUST-AGDER

VEST-AGDER

VESTFOLD

ØSTFOLD

AKERSHUS

SWEDEN

Trondheim
Ålesund
Molde
Kristiansund
Bergen
Stavanger
Sandnes
Haugesund
Oslo
Drammen
Skien
Porsgrunn
Larvik
Tønsberg
Sandefjord
Sarpsborg
Fredrikstad
Halden
Kongsvinger
Hamar
Lillehammer
Gjøvik
Kristiansand
Arendal

Jotunheimen
Dovrefjell
Hardangervidda
Rondane
Femunden
Mjøsa
Sognefjorden
Hardangerfjorden
Boknafjorden
Skagerrak

Galdhøpiggen 2452
Glittertind 2469
Snøhetta 2286

Projection: Lambert's Conformal Conic

East from Greenwich

COPYRIGHT PHILIP'S

National Parks

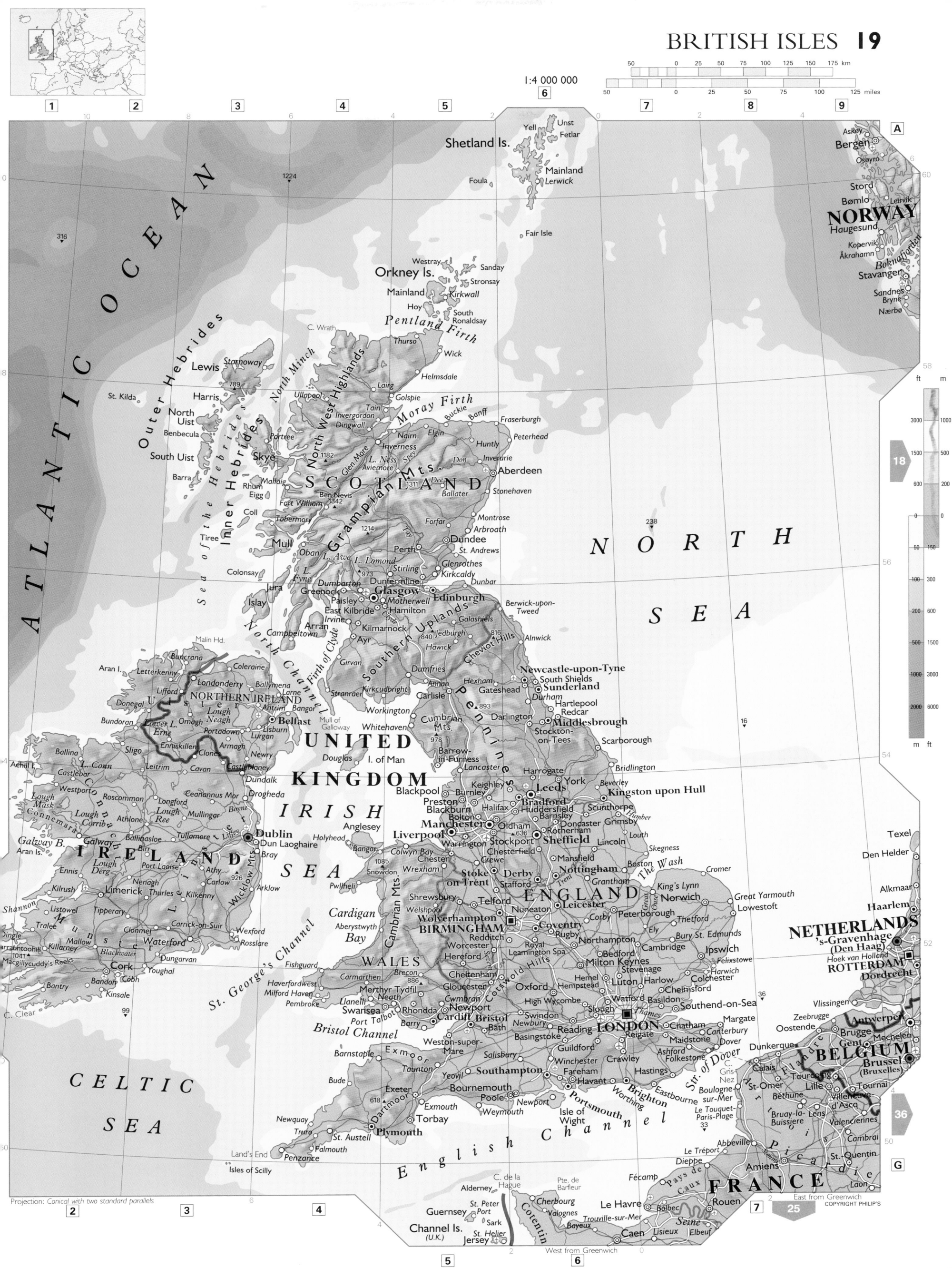

1:4 000 000

50   25   0   25   50   75   100   125   150   175 km
50   0   25   50   75   100   125 miles

NORWAY

Bergen
Oșøyro
Stord
Bømlo
Haugesund
Kopervik
Åkrahamn
Stavanger
Sandnes
Bryne
Nærbø
Boknafjorden
Askøy
Leirvik

Shetland Is.
Yell
Unst
Fetlar
Foula
Mainland
Lerwick

Fair Isle

ATLANTIC OCEAN

1224

316

Orkney Is.
Westray
Sanday
Stronsay
Mainland
Kirkwall
Hoy
South
Ronaldsay

C. Wrath
Pentland Firth
Thurso
Wick

Lewis
Stornoway
789
Harris
St. Kilda
North
Uist
Benbecula
South Uist
Barra

Outer Hebrides
North Minch
Ullapool
Lairg
Helmsdale
Golspie
Tain
Invergordon
Dingwall
Inverness
Nairn
Elgin
Buckie
Banff
Fraserburgh
Peterhead
Huntly
Inverurie
Aberdeen

Moray Firth

Skye
1182
Portree
Mallaig
Rhum
Eigg
Coll
Tiree
Tobermory
Mull
Colonsay

Sea of the Hebrides
Inner Hebrides

SCOTLAND
Ben Nevis
1342
Fort William
Glen More
Aviemore
L. Ness
Spey
1311
Dee
Ballater
Stonehaven

Grampian Mts.
1214
Perth
Forfar
Arbroath
Montrose

Oban
L. Awe
L. Lomond
Stirling
Dundee
St. Andrews
973
Glenrothes
Kirkcaldy
Dunfermline
Dunbar

Jura
Islay
Campbeltown
Arran
Greenock
Paisley
Dumbarton
Glasgow
Motherwell
East Kilbride
Hamilton
Irvine
Kilmarnock
Ayr
Edinburgh
Berwick-upon-Tweed
Galashiels
840
Jedburgh
Hawick
816
Cheviot Hills
Alnwick

Southern Uplands
Girvan
Dumfries
Annan

Malin Hd.
Buncrana
Coleraine
Ballymena
Larne
Antrim
Bangor
Stranraer
Kirkcudbright
Workington

North Channel
Firth of Clyde
Mull of
Galloway
Whitehaven
Carlisle
Hexham
Gateshead
Durham
Newcastle-upon-Tyne
South Shields
Sunderland
Hartlepool
Redcar
Middlesbrough
Stockton-
on-Tees
Darlington
893

Aran I.
Letterkenny
Lifford
Donegal
Londonderry
NORTHERN IRELAND
Ulster
Omagh
Lower L.
Erne
Enniskillen
Lough
Neagh
Lisburn
Lurgan
Portadown
Armagh
Newry
Belfast
Clones
Castleblaney

Bundoran
Ballina
Sligo
Leitrim
Cavan

Achill I.
Castlebar
L. Conn
Westport
Roscommon
Longford
Mullingar
Ceanannus Mor

Connemara
Lough
Mask
Lough
Corrib
Galway
Athlone
Lough
Ree
Tullamore
Boyne
Drogheda
Dundalk

Cumbrian
Mts.
978
Barrow-
in-Furness
Lancaster
Harrogate
Scarborough
Bridlington

I. of Man
Douglas

UNITED
KINGDOM

IRISH
SEA

ENGLAND

Pennines
York
Beverley
Kingston upon Hull

Galway B.
Aran Is.
Ennis
Limerick

IRELAND
Lough
Derg
Nenagh
Thurles
Roscommon
Athy
Carlow
Kilkenny

Dublin
Dun Laoghaire
Bray

Holyhead
Anglesey
Bangor
Colwyn Bay
1085
Snowdon
Wrexham

Blackpool
Preston
Blackburn
Bolton
Burnley
Halifax
Huddersfield
Barnsley

Liverpool
Warrington
Stockport
Manchester
Oldham
636
Rotherham
Sheffield
Doncaster
Scunthorpe
Grimsby
Louth

Humber

Skegness

Chester
Crewe
926
Wicklow Mts.
Arklow

Cambrian Mts.

Chesterfield
Mansfield
Nottingham
Boston
The Wash
Cromer

Stoke
on Trent
Derby
Stafford
Telford
Shrewsbury
Welshpool
Grantham
Trent
King's Lynn
Great Yarmouth
Lowestoft
Norwich

Listowel
Tralee
Killarney
1041
Macgillycuddy's Reeks
Mallow
Cork
Cobh
Kinsale

Cardigan
Bay
Aberystwyth
Pwllheli

WALES
886
Brecon

BIRMINGHAM
Wolverhampton
Nuneaton
Leicester
Coventry
Redditch
Royal
Leamington Spa
Rugby
Corby
Peterborough
Ely
Thetford
Bury St. Edmunds
Ipswich
Felixstowe
Harwich
Colchester
Chelmsford

Worcester
Hereford
Cotswold Hills
Northampton
Bedford
Milton Keynes
Cambridge

Texel
Den Helder
Alkmaar
Haarlem
NETHERLANDS
's-Gravenhage
(Den Haag)
Hoek van Holland
ROTTERDAM
Dordrecht

Waterford
Dungarvan
Youghal

Carmarthen
Merthyr Tydfil
Neath
Llanelli
Swansea
Port Talbot
Rhondda
Cwmbran
Newport
Cardiff
Barry

Cheltenham
Gloucester

Oxford
Hemel
Hempstead
High Wycombe
Luton
Stevenage
Harlow
Watford
Slough
LONDON
Reading
Newbury
Swindon
Basingstoke
Guildford

Vlissingen
Zeebrugge
Oostende
Brugge
Gent
Mechelen
Antwerpen
BELGIUM
Brussel
(Bruxelles)

Haverfordwest
Milford Haven
Pembroke
Fishguard

Bristol Channel
Weston-super-
Mare
Barnstaple
618
Exmoor
Bude
Newquay
Truro
St. Austell
Penzance
Land's End
Isles of Scilly
99

Bath
Bristol
Newport

Salisbury
Yeovil
Taunton
Dorchester
Exeter
Dartmoor
Torbay
Plymouth

Winchester
Southampton
Bournemouth
Poole
Portsmouth
Isle of
Wight
Newport
Weymouth

Fareham
Havant
Worthing
Brighton
Eastbourne
Hastings
Crawley
Reigate
Maidstone
Chatham
Southend-on-Sea
Thames
Margate
Canterbury
Dover
Folkestone
Ashford
Str. of Dover

Dunkerque
Calais
St-Omer
Boulogne-
sur-Mer
Gris-
Nez
C.
Le Touquet-
Paris-Plage
33

Flandre
Lille
Roubaix
Tourcoing
Villeneuve
d'Ascq
Bruay-la-
Buissière
Lens
Béthune
Valenciennes
Cambrai
St. Quentin

CELTIC
SEA

C. Clear

St. George's Channel

NORTH
SEA

238

16

English Channel

Alderney
C. de la
Hague
Pte. de
Barfleur
Cherbourg
Valognes
Cotentin
Guernsey
St. Peter
Port
Sark
Channel Is.
(U.K.)
St. Helier
Jersey

Abbeville
Le Tréport
Dieppe
Fécamp
Pays de
Caux
Bolbec
Le Havre
Trouville-sur-Mer
Bayeux
Caen
Lisieux
Elbeuf
Rouen
Seine
Amiens
Picardie
Laon
FRANCE

East from Greenwich
COPYRIGHT PHILIP'S
West from Greenwich

Projection: Conical with two standard parallels

ft   m
3000   1000
1500   500
600   200
0
50   150
100   300
200   600
500   1500
1000   3000
2000   6000
m   ft

18
36
25

1:1 600 000

10 0 10 20 30 40 50 60 70 80 km
10 0 10 20 30 40 50 miles

Key to English unitary authorities on map

25 HARTLEPOOL
26 DARLINGTON
27 STOCKTON-ON-TEES
28 MIDDLESBROUGH
29 REDCAR AND CLEVELAND
30 BLACKPOOL
31 BLACKBURN WITH DARWEN
32 HALTON
33 WARRINGTON
34 KINGSTON UPON HULL
35 NORTH EAST LINCOLNSHIRE
36 STOKE-ON-TRENT
37 TELFORD AND WREKIN
38 DERBY CITY
39 CITY OF NOTTINGHAM
40 LEICESTER CITY
41 RUTLAND
42 PETERBOROUGH
43 MILTON KEYNES
44 LUTON
45 NORTH SOMERSET
46 CITY OF BRISTOL
47 BATH AND NORTH EAST SOMERSET
48 SWINDON
49 READING
50 WOKINGHAM
51 WINDSOR AND MAIDENHEAD
52 SLOUGH
53 BRACKNELL FOREST
54 THURROCK
55 SOUTHEND-ON-SEA
56 MEDWAY
57 PLYMOUTH
58 TORBAY
59 POOLE
60 BOURNEMOUTH
61 SOUTHAMPTON
62 PORTSMOUTH
63 BRIGHTON AND HOVE

Key to Welsh unitary authorities on map

15 SWANSEA
16 NEATH PORT TALBOT
17 BRIDGEND
18 RHONDDA CYNON TAFF
19 MERTHYR TYDFIL
20 BLAENAU GWENT
21 CAERPHILLY
22 TORFAEN
23 CARDIFF
24 NEWPORT

NORTH SEA

IRISH SEA

North Channel

SCOTLAND

NORTHERN IRELAND

ISLE OF MAN

The Wash

NORTHUMBERLAND
CUMBRIA
DURHAM
LANCASHIRE
NORTH YORKSHIRE
EAST RIDING OF YORKSHIRE
LINCOLNSHIRE
CHESHIRE
STAFFORDSHIRE
DERBY
NOTTS

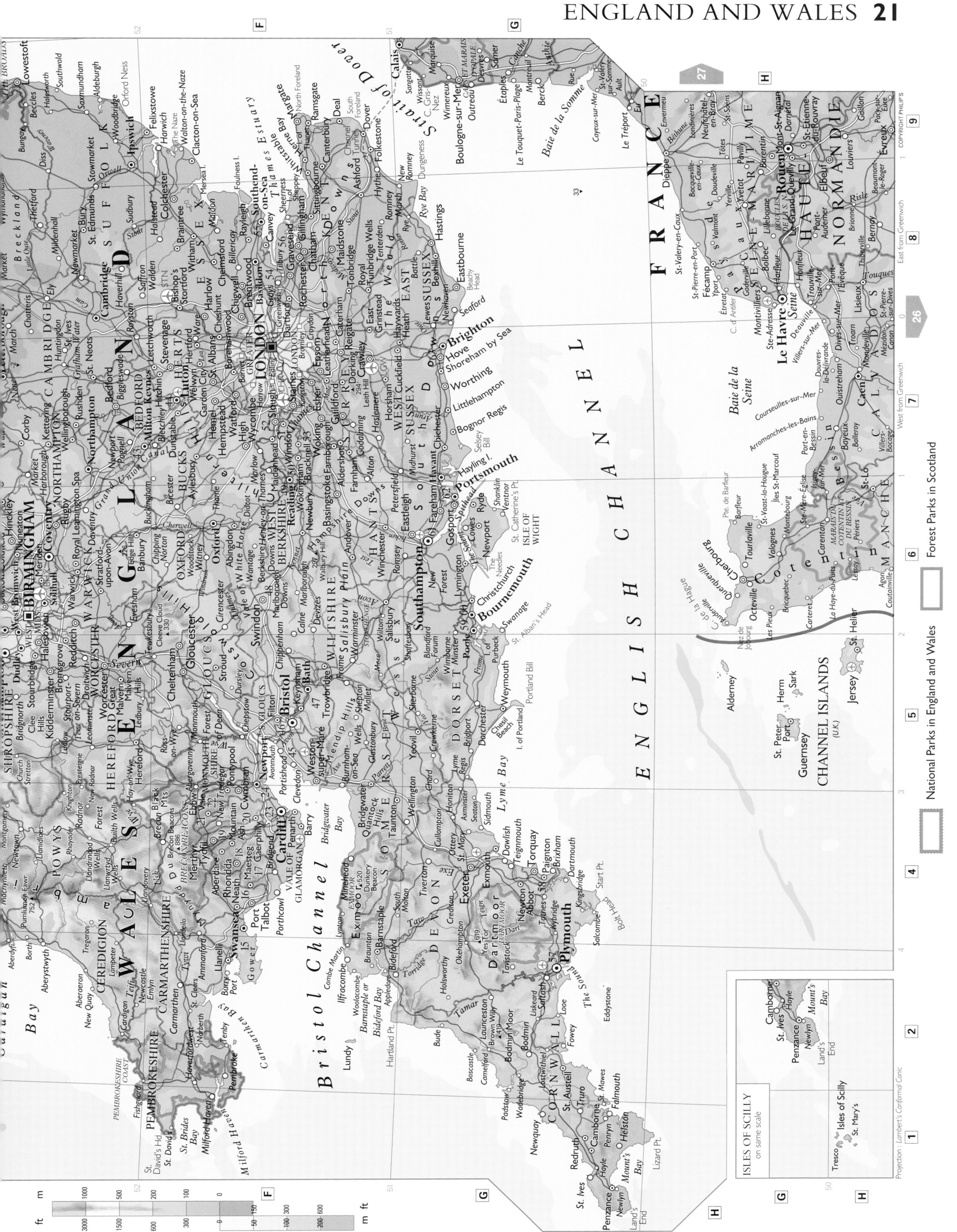

National Parks in England and Wales

Forest Parks in Scotland

Projection: Lambert's Conformal Conic

1:1 600 000

Key to Scottish unitary authorities on map
1 CITY OF ABERDEEN 8 EAST RENFREWSHIRE
2 DUNDEE CITY 9 NORTH LANARKSHIRE
3 WEST DUNBARTONSHIRE 10 FALKIRK
4 EAST DUNBARTONSHIRE 11 CLACKMANNANSHIRE
5 CITY OF GLASGOW 12 WEST LOTHIAN
6 INVERCLYDE 13 CITY OF EDINBURGH
7 RENFREWSHIRE 14 MIDLOTHIAN

ORKNEY IS. on same scale

ORKNEY
Kirkwall
Stromness
Scapa Flow
Hoy
Thurso
John o' Groats
Duncansby Head
Sinclair's Bay
Pentland Firth
North Ronaldsay
Papa Westray
Westray
Sanday
Eday
Rousay
Shapinsay
Stronsay
St. Mary's
Burray
South Ronaldsay

WESTERN ISLES
OUTER HEBRIDES
Lewis
Stornoway
Harris
North Uist
Benbecula
South Uist
Barra
Castlebay
Butt of Lewis
Broad Bay

Sutherland
Caithness
C. Wrath
Durness
Thurso
Wick
Reay Forest
Ben Hope
Dounreay
Halkirk
Helmsdale
Brora
Golspie
Dornoch
Tain
Lairg

HIGHLAND
Inverness
Loch Ness
Fort Augustus
Fort William
Ben Nevis
Glen Coe
Skye
Cuillin Hills
Portree
Kyle of Lochalsh
Mallaig
Ullapool
Dingwall
Nairn
Forres
Elgin

MORAY
Buckie
Lossiemouth
Keith
Huntly
Dufftown

ABERDEENSHIRE
Aberdeen
Peterhead
Fraserburgh
Ellon
Inverurie
Alford
Banchory
Stonehaven
Buchan
Cairngorm Mts.
CAIRNGORMS
Grampian Mountains
Braemar
Ballater
Aviemore

ANGUS
Forfar
Montrose
Brechin
Arbroath
Carnoustie

PERTH AND KINROSS
Perth
Pitlochry
Blairgowrie
Aberfeldy
Crieff
Dunkeld
Loch Tay
Ben Lawers

SCOTLAND

STIRLING
Stirling
Callander
Loch Lomond
TROSSACHS
Dunblane

FIFE
St. Andrews
Cupar
Glenrothes
Kirkcaldy
Leven
Dunfermline
Dundee
Firth of Tay

Dundee

ARGYLL AND BUTE
Oban
Lochgilphead
Inveraray
Dunoon
Rothesay
Campbeltown
Mull
Iona
Tiree
Coll
Islay
Jura
Colonsay
Oronsay
Tobermory
Bowmore
Port Ellen
Mull of Kintyre

Firth of Clyde
Arran
Goat Fell
Brodick

NORTH AYRSHIRE
Ardrossan
Saltcoats
Irvine
Kilwinning
Largs

Greenock
Gourock
Paisley
Glasgow
Clydebank
Dumbarton
Hamilton
East Kilbride
Motherwell
Coatbridge
Airdrie
Cumbernauld
Falkirk
Alloa

SOUTH AYRSHIRE
Ayr
Prestwick
Troon
Kilmarnock
Cumnock
Maybole
Girvan
Ailsa Craig

EAST AYRSHIRE

SOUTH LANARKSHIRE
Lanark
Biggar
Carluke
Wishaw
Strathaven

EDINBURGH
Leith
Musselburgh
Dalkeith
Penicuik
Bonnyrigg
Livingston
Bo'ness
Grangemouth
Dunbar
North Berwick
Haddington
EAST LOTHIAN

SCOTTISH BORDERS
Galashiels
Melrose
Kelso
Jedburgh
Hawick
Peebles
Selkirk
Coldstream
Duns

Berwick-upon-Tweed
Eyemouth

DUMFRIES & GALLOWAY
Dumfries
Stranraer
Newton Stewart
Castle Douglas
Kirkcudbright
Wigtown
Lockerbie
Moffat
Annan
Gretna
Langholm
Whithorn
Portpatrick

Galloway
Solway Firth

ENGLAND
Newcastle-upon-Tyne
Carlisle
Gateshead
Penrith
Workington
Whitehaven
Maryport
Keswick
CUMBRIA
NORTHUMBERLAND
DURHAM
Alnwick
Morpeth
Hexham
Haltwhistle
Hadrian's Wall
The Cheviot
Cheviot Hills
Bishop Auckland

NORTH SEA

ATLANTIC OCEAN

NORTH CHANNEL

NORTHERN IRELAND
Belfast
Bangor
Larne
Carrickfergus
Donaghadee
Newtownards

SHETLAND IS. on same scale

SHETLAND
Lerwick
Scalloway
Muckle Flugga
Unst
Yell
Fetlar
Whalsay
Bressay
Sumburgh Hd.
Foula
Papa Stour
St. Magnus Bay
Sullom Voe
Walls
West Burra

Forest Parks in Scotland

Projection: Lambert's Conformal Conic

1:1 600 000

10 0 10 20 30 40 50 60 70 80 km
10 0 10 20 30 40 50 miles

SCOTLAND
Kintyre
Mull of Oa
Brodick
Arran
Campbeltown
Mull of Kintyre
Ailsa Craig
Firth of Clyde

A T L A N T I C   O C E A N

Inishtrahull
Malin Hd.
Tory I.
Sheep Haven
Lough Swilly
Fanad Hd.
Mulroy B.
Malin Pen.
Carndonagh
Giants Causeway
Rathlin I.
Mts of Antrim
Fair Hd.
Rathmullan
L. Ryan
Horn Hd.
Bloody Foreland
Inishowen Pen.
Moville
Portstewart
Portrush
Ballycastle
Ballymoney
554
GLENARIFF
Trostan
Garron Pt.
Cairnryan
Stranraer
Portpatrick
269

Inishfree B.
Gweedore
Errigal
752
The Rosses
Aran I.
Crohy Hd.
Derryveagh Mts.
GLENVEAGH
683
Rathmelton
L. Foyle
Londonderry
LONDONDERRY
Buncrana
Coleraine
Limavady
Roe
Bann
ANTRIM
Ballymena
Larne

Gweebarra B.
Dawros Hd.
DONEGAL
Letterkenny
Glenties
Lifford
Strabane
Sion Mills
Newtownstewart
Sawel Mt.
683
Spertin Mts.
Magherafelt
Randalstown
Ballyclare
NORTHERN
Moneymore
Cookstown
Antrim
Carrickfergus
Belfast L.
Bangor
Donaghadee

Loughros More B.
Rossan Pt.
601
Slieve League
St. John's Pt.
Killybegs
Donegal
Lavagh More
676
U l s t e r
TYRONE
Omagh
Coalisland
Dungannon
Newtownabbey
Belfast
Comber
Newtownards
DOWN
Ards Pen.
Portaferry

Donegal Bay
Ballyshannon
Bundoran
Erne
Lower L. Erne
Castlederg
Derg
Enniskillen
FERMANAGH
Upper L. Erne
Dromore
Irvinestown
Blackwater
Craigavon
Lurgan
Portadown
Lagan
Banbridge
Tandragee
Lisburn
Saintfield
Ballynahinch
Downpatrick
Ballyquintin Pt.

Broad Haven
Erris Hd.
Mullet Pen.
Inishkea North
Inishkea South
Blacksod Bay
Belmullet
Killala B.
380
Killala
Ballina
Sligo Bay
Sligo
Dromore West
544
SLIGO
Collooney
Ballymote
L. Arrow
L. Allen
LEITRIM
Leitrim
Belturbet
Clones
Monaghan
MONAGHAN
Castleblaney
Cootehill
ARMAGH
Middletown
Keady
Armagh
Monaghan
Newry
577
Slieve Gullion
852
Slieve Donard
Mourne Mts.
Warrenpoint
Newcastle
Dundrum B.
Greenore
Kilkeel
Carlingford L.
St. John's Pt.
Dundrum

Achill Hd.
672
Achill I.
Clare I.
Clew Bay
Corraun Pen.
Newport
L. Conn
806
Nephin
Swinford
Charlestown
Boyle
Carrick-on-Shannon
CAVAN
L. Gowna
L. Sheelin
Cavan
Carrickmacross
Kingscourt
LOUTH
Ardee
Dunleer
Dundalk
Louth
Dundalk Bay
Clogher Hd.

Inishturk
Killary Harbour
Inishbofin
Inishshark
MAYO
765
Croagh Patrick
Mweelrea
819
Westport
Castlebar
Knock
Ballyhaunis
Claremorris
Ballinrobe
ROSCOMMON
Castlerea
Ballaghaderreen
L. Gara
Roscommon
LONGFORD
Longford
Granard
Castlepollard
Oldcastle
Ceanannus Mor (Kells)
Blackwater
MEATH
Drogheda
Balbriggan

C o n n a c h t
Connemara
CONNEMARA
Clifden
Slyne Hd.
Oughterard
Lough Mask
Lough Corrib
GALWAY
Tuam
Athenry
Ballinasloe
Loughrea
I R E L A N D
Roscommon
Athlone
WESTMEATH
Moate
Mullingar
Athboy
Trim
L e i n s t e r
Royal Canal
Maynooth
Swords
Malahide
Lambay I.
DUBLIN
Dublin
Howth Hd.
Dun Laoghaire

Bertraghboy B.
Slyne Hd.
Galway
Galway Bay
Black Hd.
Aran Is.
Inishmore
Inishmaan
Inisheer
BURREN
Cliffs of Moher
Hags Hd.
Liscannor Bay
Mal Bay
Mutton I.
368
Gort
Slieve Aughty
Portumna
Birr
CLARE
Ennistimon
Tulla
Ennis
Lough Derg
Shannon
OFFALY
Tullamore
Clara
Daingean
Edenderry
Grand Canal
Bog of Allen
Droichead Nua
KILDARE
Naas
Clondalkin
Bray
Greystones
123

Loop Hd.
Kilkee
Kilrush
Shannon Airport
Sixmilebridge
Limerick
694
Keeper Hill
Nenagh
Templemore
Thurles
TIPPERARY
Mountmellick
Port Laoise
Mountrath
LAOIS
Durrow
Athy
Carlow
Tullow
Muine Bheag
Shillelagh
WICKLOW
754
Wicklow
926
Lugnaquillia
Rathdrum
Wicklow Hd.

Mouth of the Shannon
Ballybunion
Foynes
Rathkeale
LIMERICK
Newcastle West
Listowel
Feale
Golden Vale
Tipperary
Cashel
Slievenamon
722
Carrick-on-Suir
Clonmel
Kilkenny
KILKENNY
Callan
796
Mt. Leinster
WEXFORD
Enniscorthy
Gorey
Arklow

Kerry Hd.
Tralee B.
Brandon B.
953
Brandon Mt.
Dingle
Slieve Mish
853
KERRY
Killarney
Killorglin
1041
Carrauntoohil
Macgillycuddy's Reeks
KILLARNEY
707
Boggeragh Mts
646
CORK
Macroom
Blarney
Cork
Mallow
Buttevant
Kanturk
Newmarket
Mitchelstown
Fermoy
Blackwater
WATERFORD
796
Knockmealdown Mts.
792
Comeragh Mts.
Waterford
Tramore
Dungarvan
Dungarvan Harbour
New Ross
Wexford
Rosslare
Rosslare Harbour
Greenore Pt.
Carnsore Pt.

Smerwick Harbour
Great Blasket I.
Dunmore Hd.
Inishvickillane
Valencia I.
Puffin I.
Great Skellig
Ballinskelligs B.
Cahersiveen
Kenmare
Kenmare River
Caha Mts.
707
Glengarriff
686
Bantry
Bantry Bay
Dunmanus B.
Skull
Mizen Hd.
Long I.
Baltimore
Sherkin I.
Clear I.
C. Clear
Fastnet Rock
Dunmanway
Bandon
Clonakilty
Clonakilty B.
Galley Hd.
Kinsale
Old Head of Kinsale
Cork Harbour
Crosshaven
Cobh
Passage West
Youghal
Youghal B.
Midleton

St. George's Channel
I R I S H   S E A

St. David's Hd.
St. David's
St. Brides Bay
115
WALES

C E L T I C   S E A

Projection: Lambert's Conformal Conic
West from Greenwich
COPYRIGHT PHILIP'S

ft	m
	1500 — 500
600 — 200
300 — 100
0 — 0
50 — 150
100 — 300
200 — 600
500 — 1500
1000 — 3000
2000 — 6000
m	ft

☐ National Parks

1:2 000 000

NORTH SEA

UNITED KINGDOM

NETHERLANDS

BELGIUM

LUXEMBOURG

GERMANY

FRANCE

National Parks

Underlined towns give their name to the administrative area in which they stand.

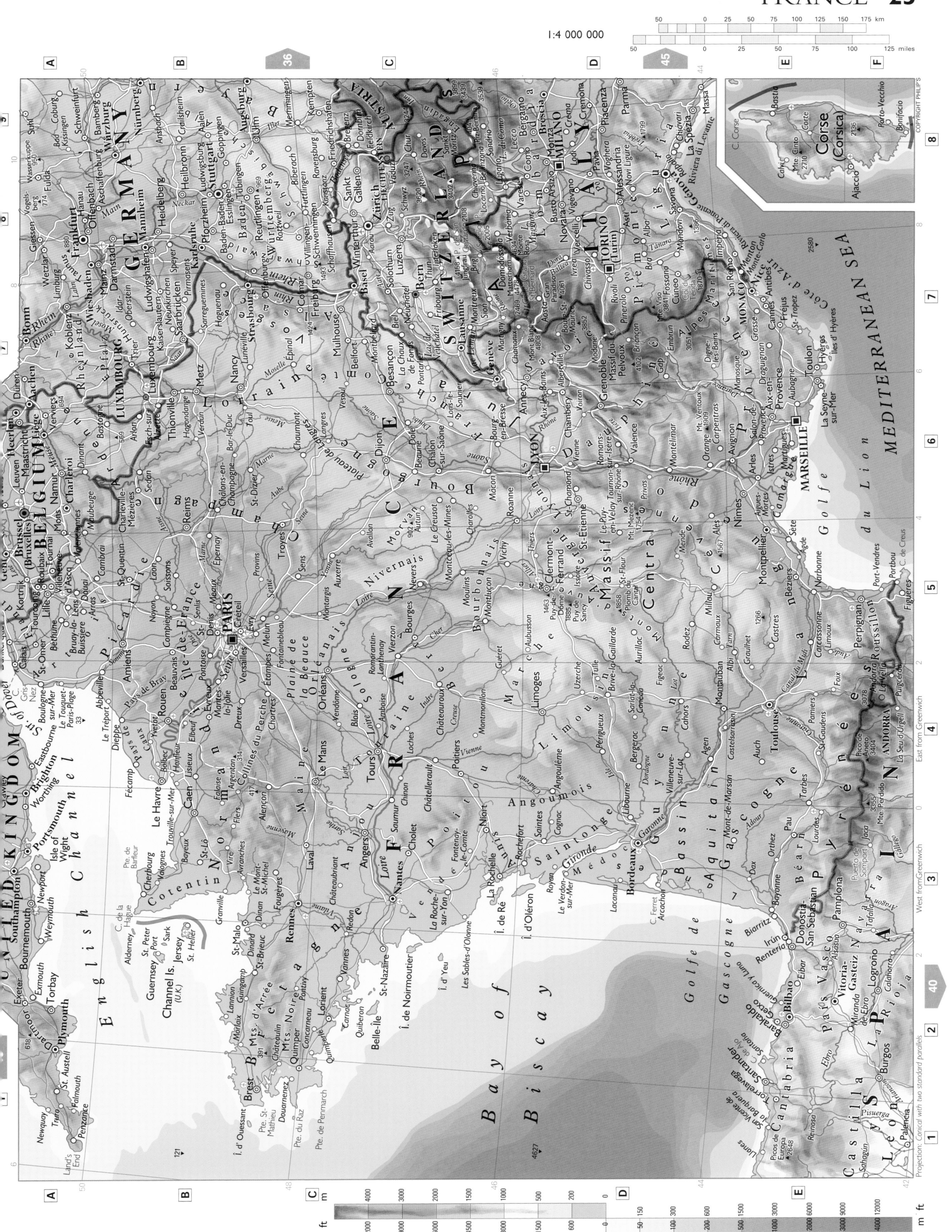

1:4 000 000

Corse
(Corsica)

MEDITERRANEAN SEA

GERMANY

BELGIUM

LUXEMBOURG

SWITZERLAND

ITALY

UNITED KINGDOM

FRANCE

SPAIN

ANDORRA

MONACO

AUSTRIA

Bay of Biscay

English Channel

Golfe de Gascogne

PARIS

Projection: Conical with two standard parallels

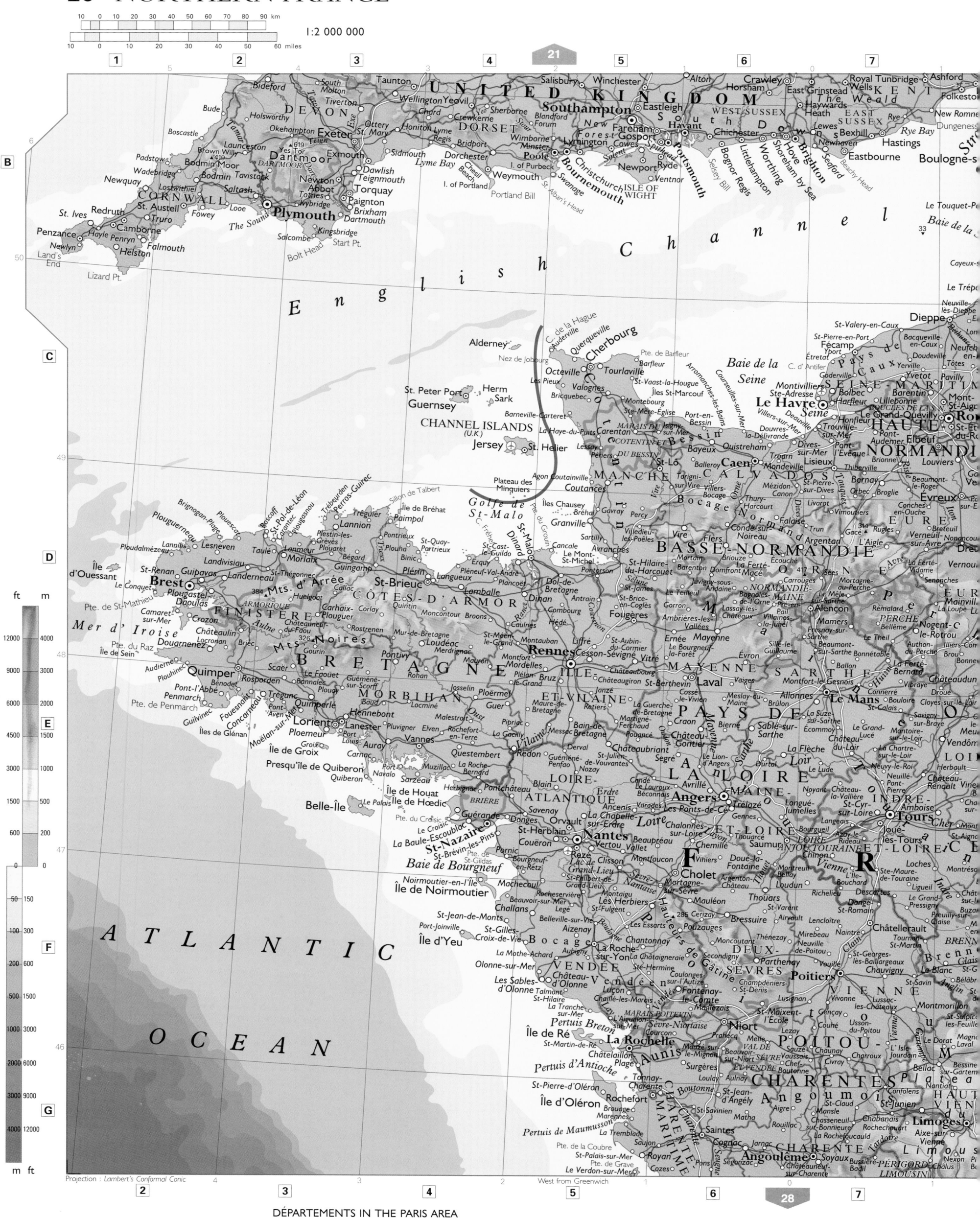

1:2 000 000

DÉPARTEMENTS IN THE PARIS AREA
1 Ville de Paris   3 Val-de-Marne
2 Seine-St-Denis   4 Hauts-de-Seine

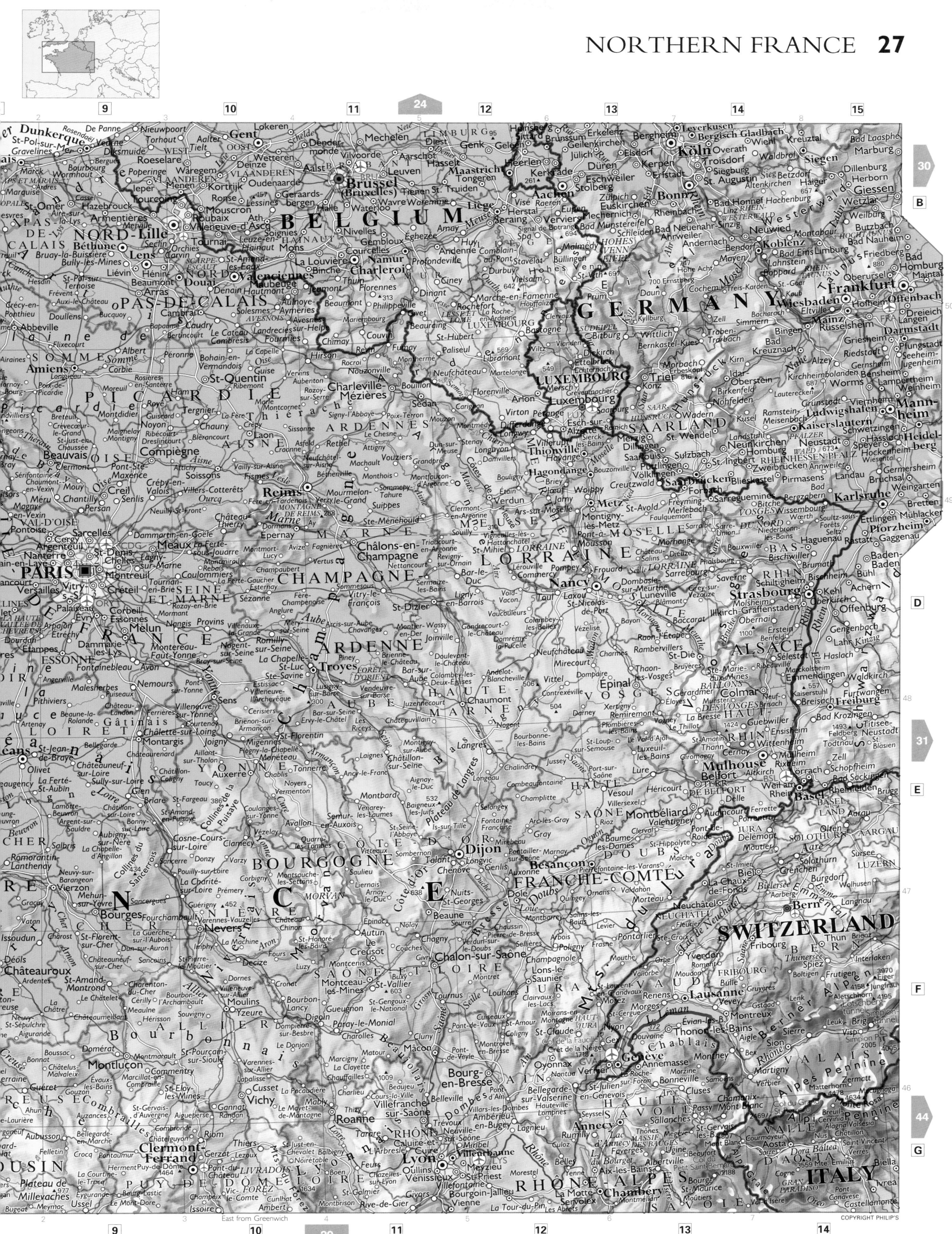

underlined towns give their name to the
administrative area in which they stand.

National Parks

Regional Nature Parks in France

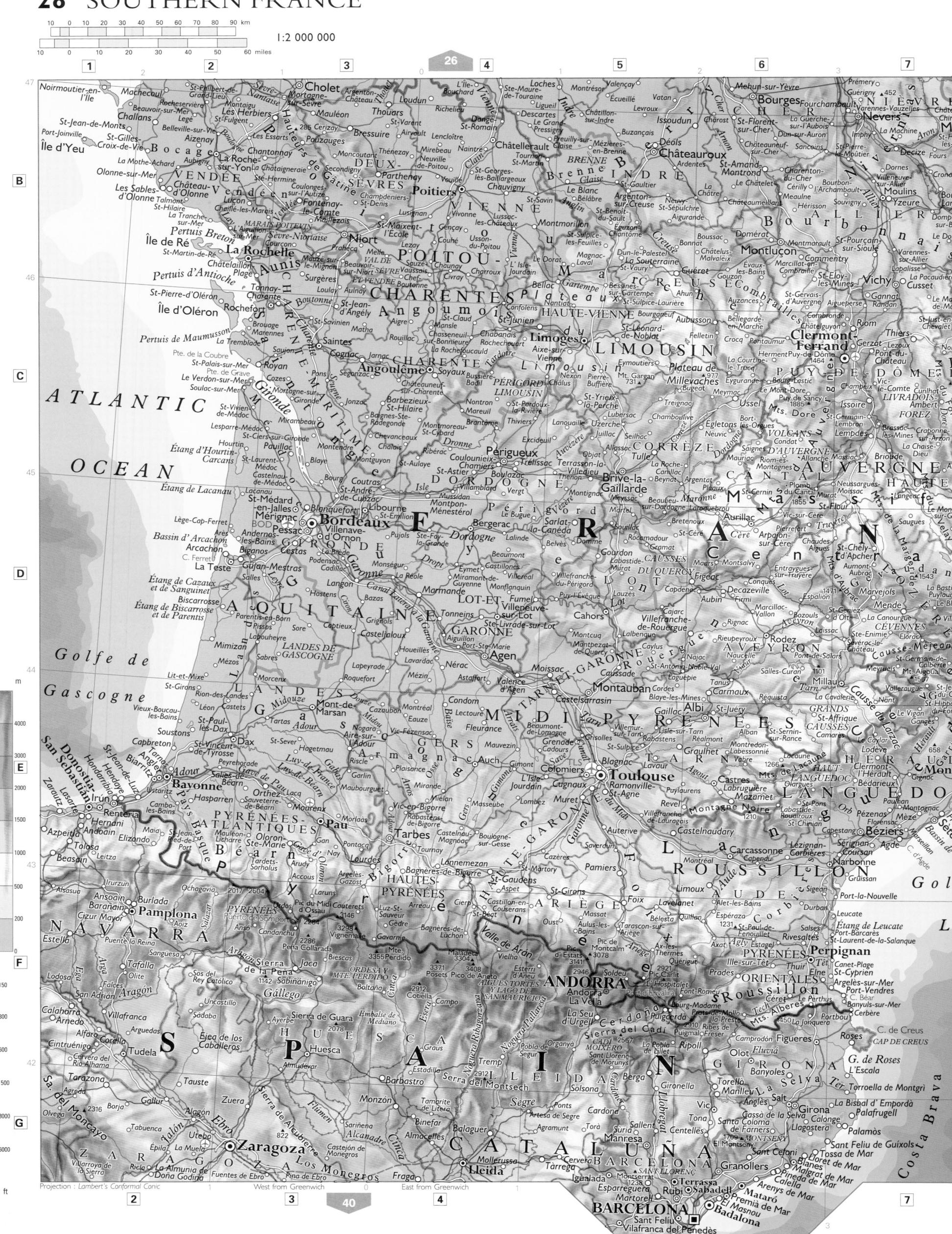

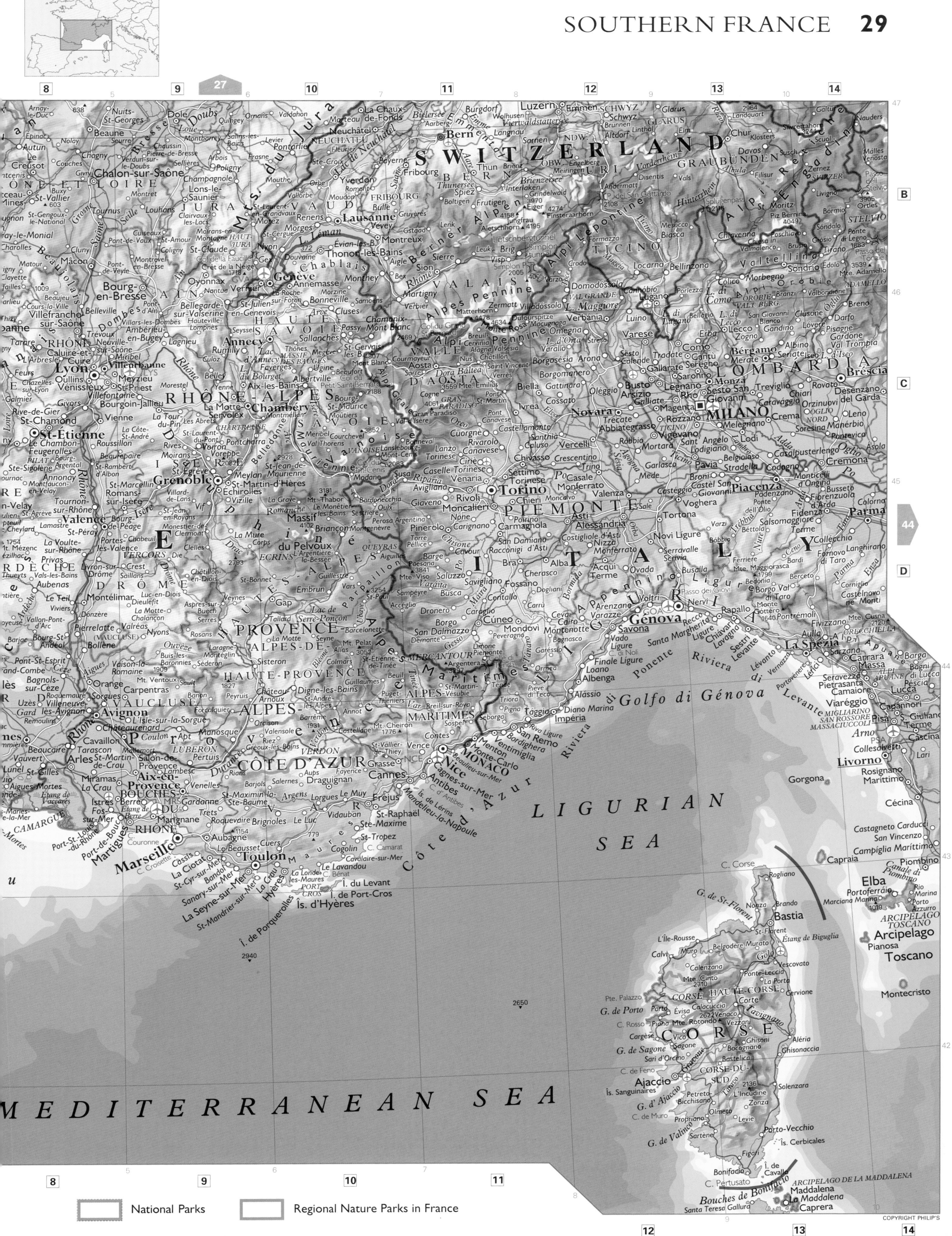

National Parks   Regional Nature Parks in France

COPYRIGHT PHILIP'S

1:2 000 000

km 10 0 10 20 30 40 50 60 70 80 90 km

miles 10 0 10 20 30 40 50 60 miles

NORTH SEA

BALTIC SEA

DENMARK

POLAND

GERMANY

NETHERLANDS

SCHLESWIG-HOLSTEIN

MECKLENBURG-VORPOMMERN

BRANDENBURG

SACHSEN-ANHALT

SACHSEN

THÜRINGEN

NIEDERSACHSEN

NORDRHEIN-WESTFALEN

HESSEN

BERLIN

HAMBURG

Bremen

Hannover

Rostock

Schwerin

Magdeburg

Leipzig

Dresden

Kiel

Flensburg

Lübeck

Potsdam

Erfurt

Kassel

Dortmund

Essen

Düsseldorf

Köln

Bonn

Rügen

Usedom

Oder

Elbe

Weser

Rhein

Ems

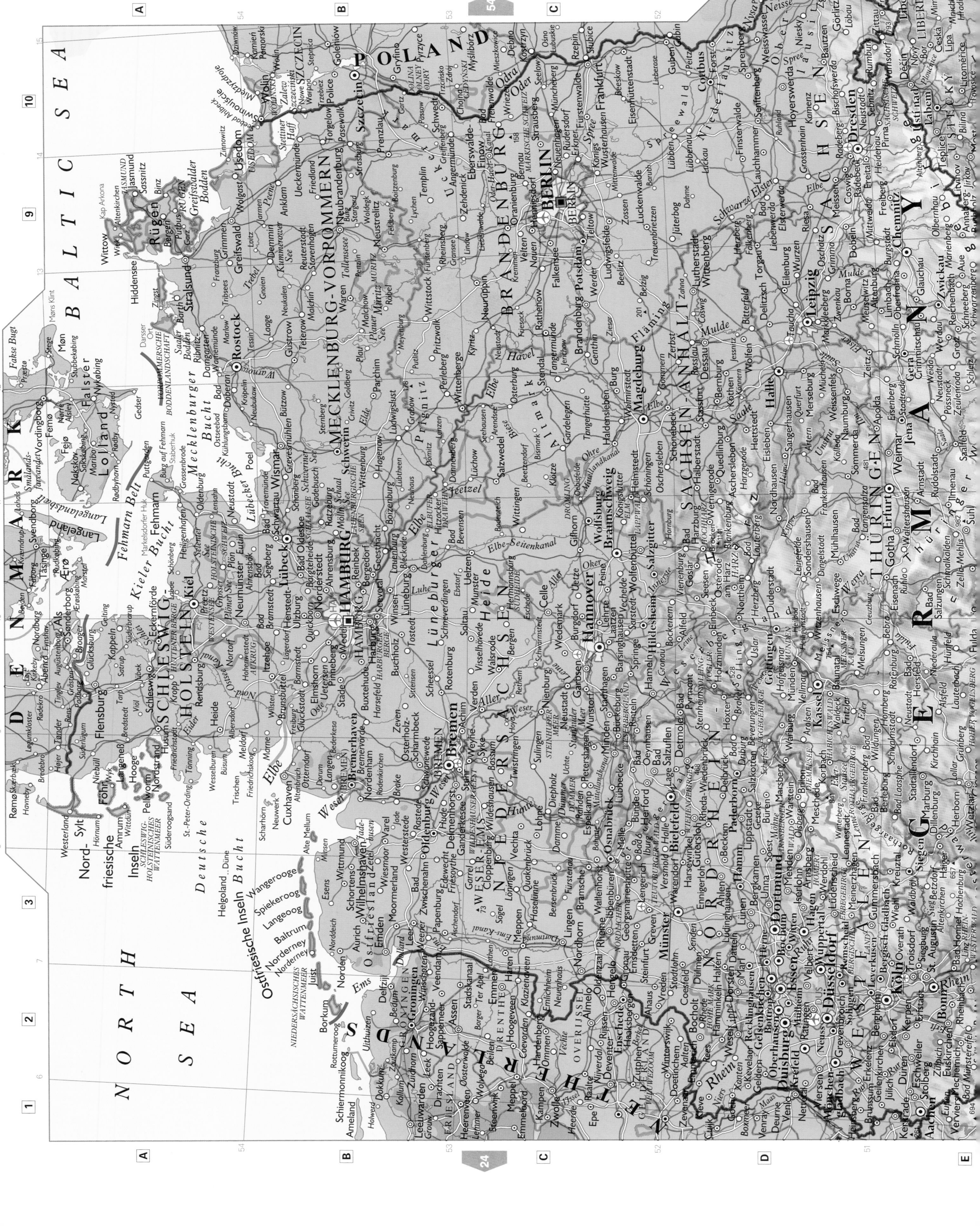

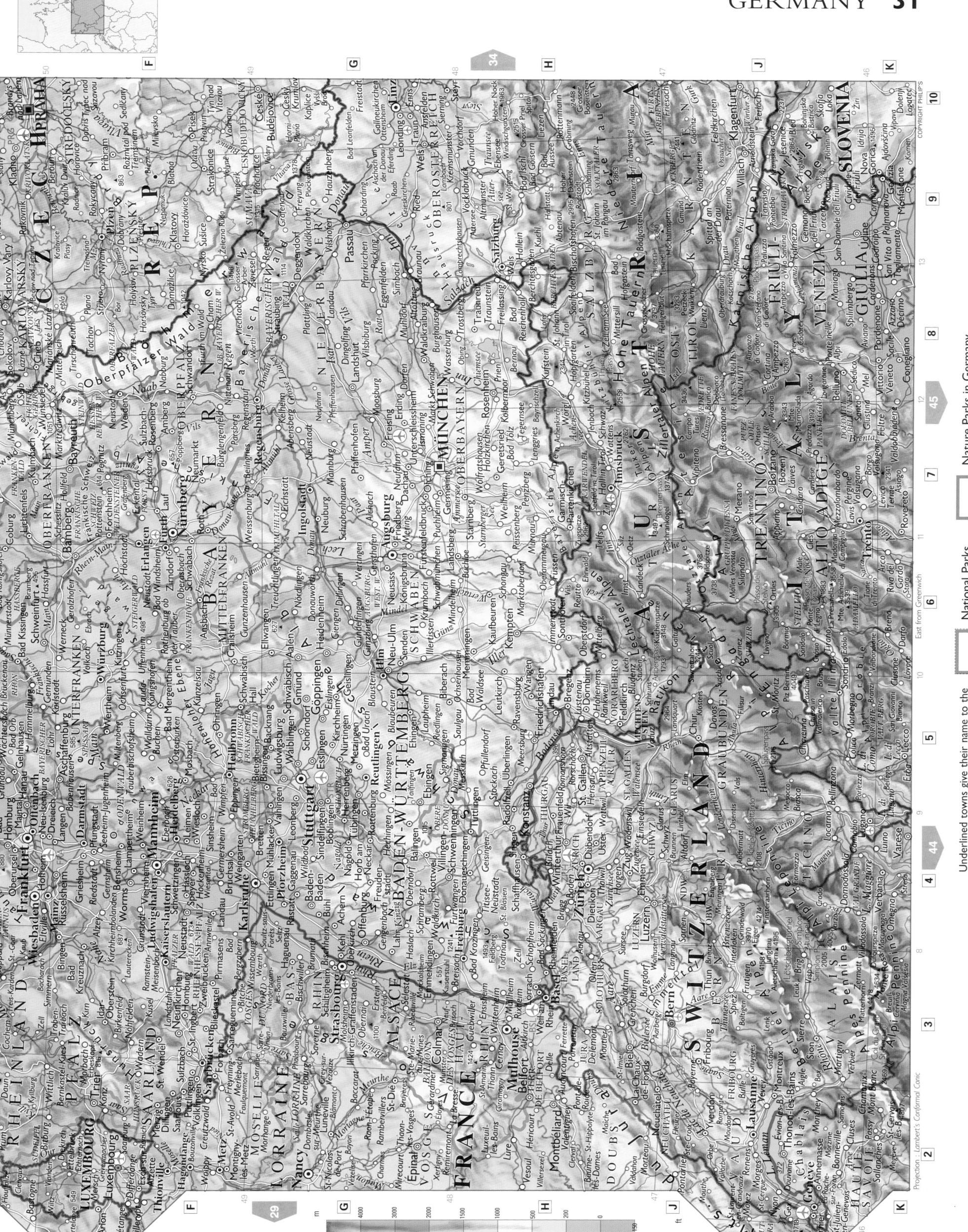

East from Greenwich

Projection : Lambert's Conformal Conic

Underlined towns give their name to the
administrative area in which they stand.

National Parks

Nature Parks in Germany

1:800 000

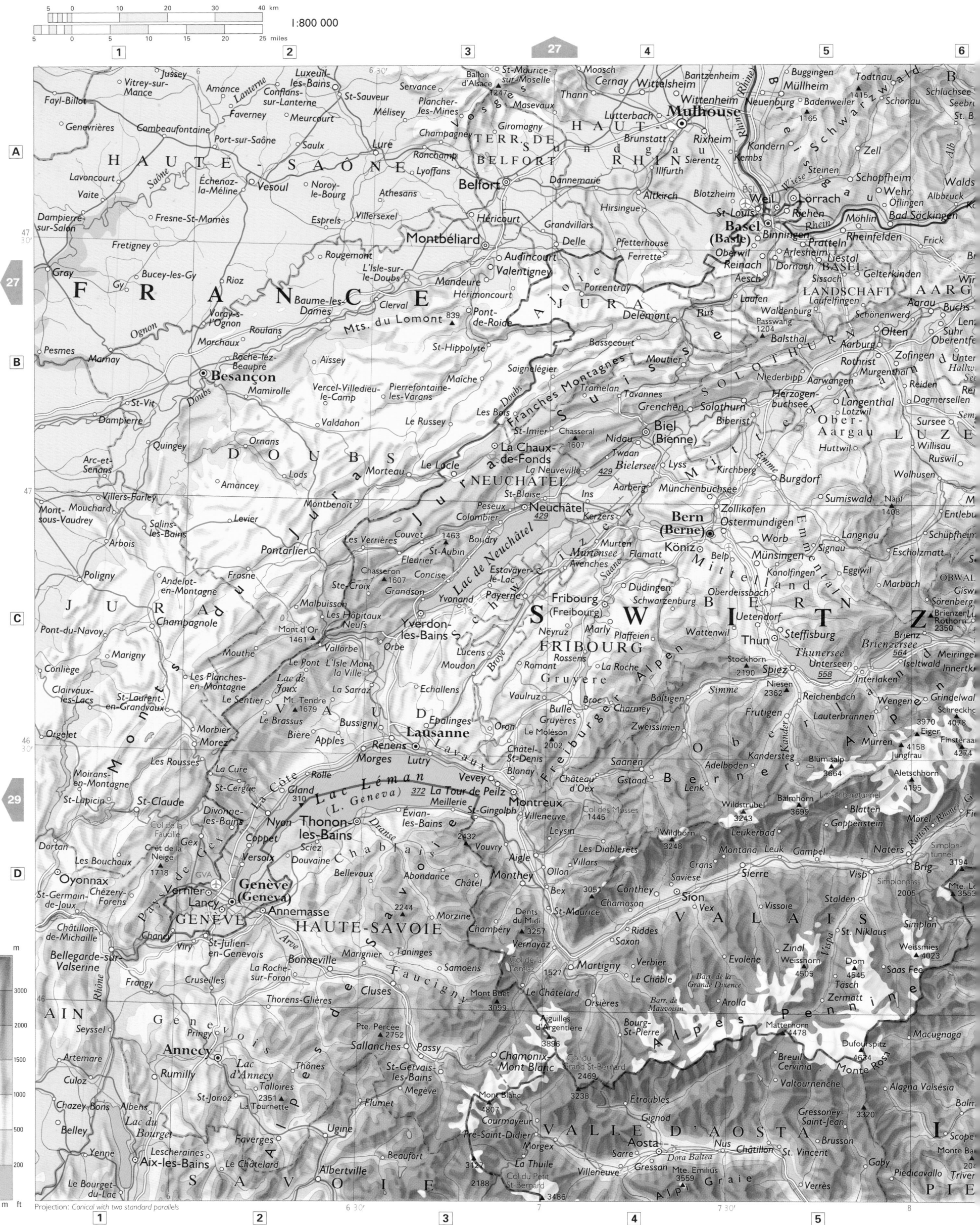

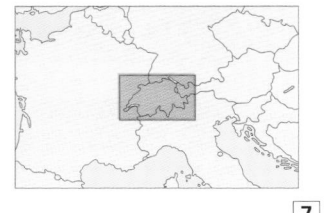

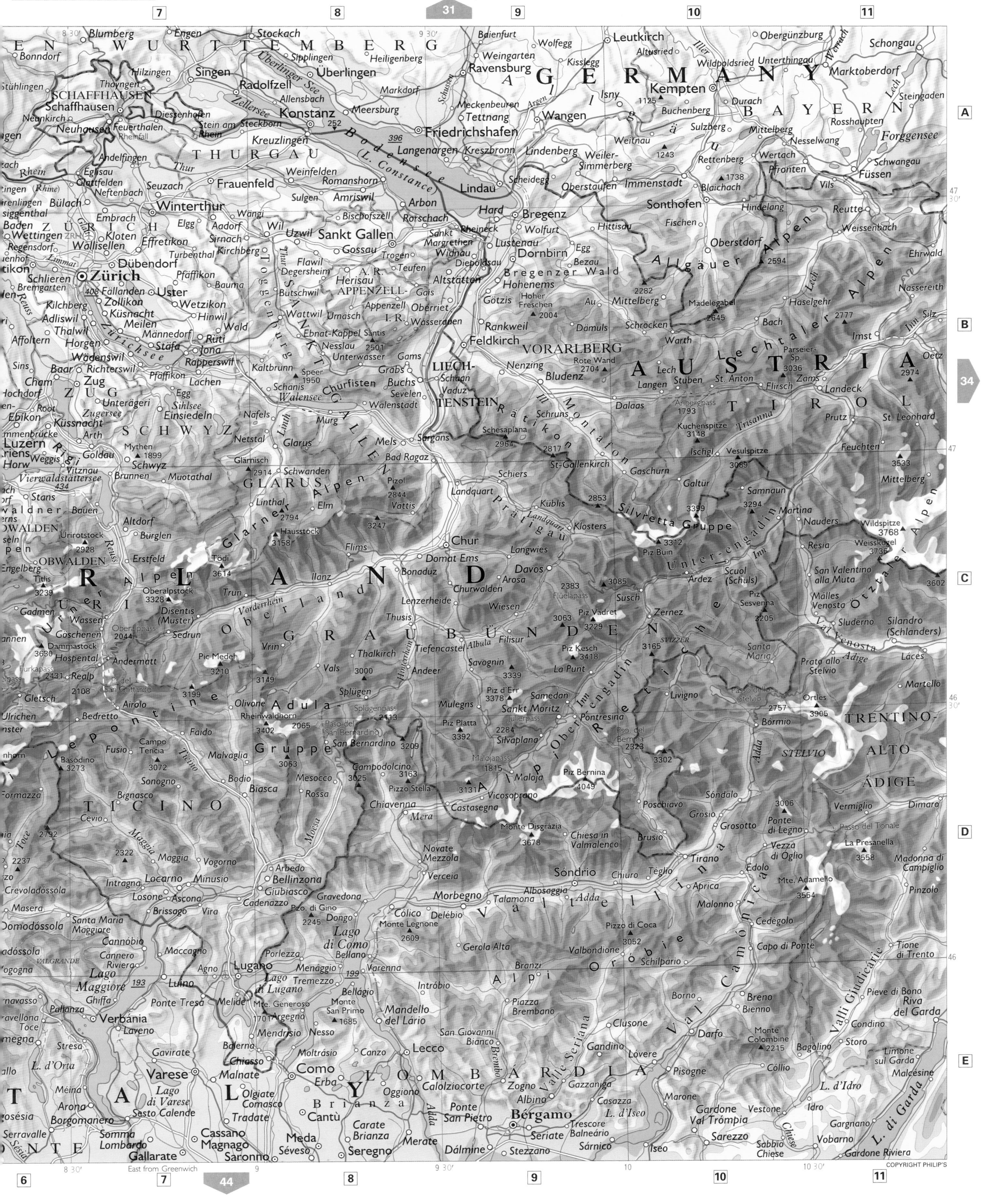

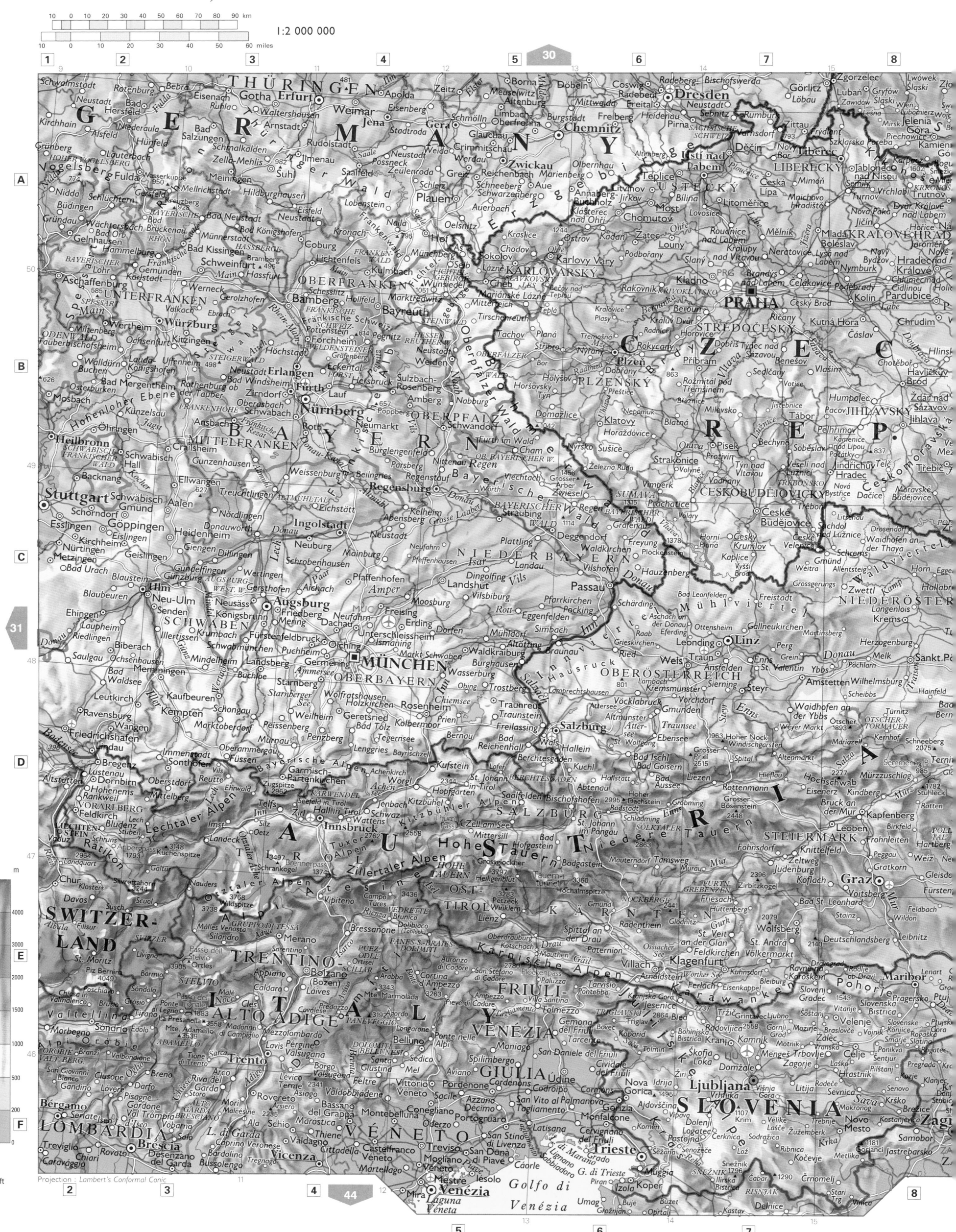

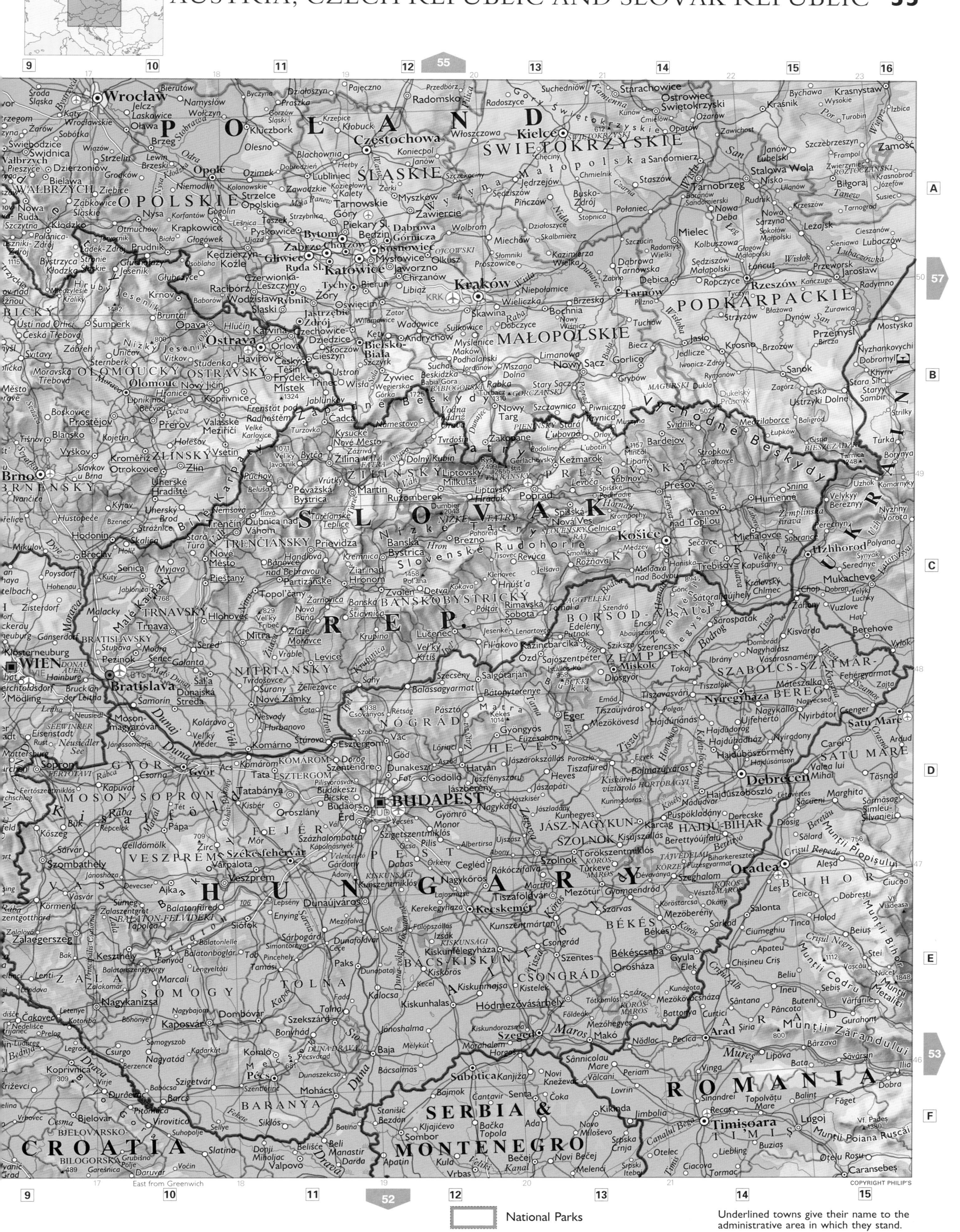

National Parks

Underlined towns give their name to the administrative area in which they stand.

East from Greenwich

COPYRIGHT PHILIP'S

1:4 000 000

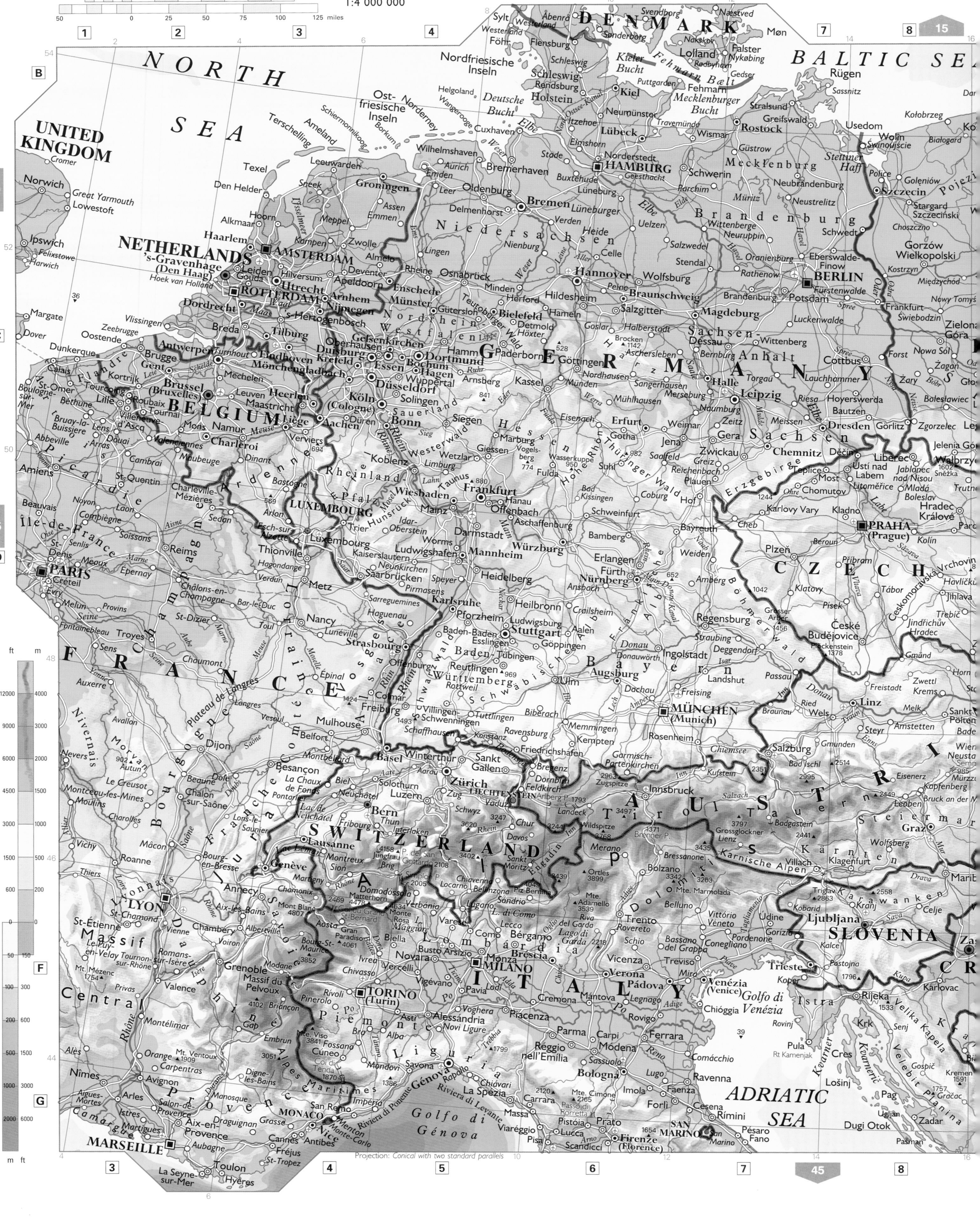
NORTH SEA
BALTIC SEA
ADRIATIC SEA
UNITED KINGDOM
NETHERLANDS
BELGIUM
LUXEMBOURG
FRANCE
GERMANY
DENMARK
CZECH
AUSTRIA
SWITZERLAND
LIECHTENSTEIN
ITALY
SLOVENIA
MONACO
SAN MARINO
AMSTERDAM
's-Gravenhage (Den Haag)
ROTTERDAM
Brussel (Bruxelles)
LUXEMBOURG
PARIS
HAMBURG
BERLIN
PRAHA (Prague)
MÜNCHEN (Munich)
Zürich
Bern
Genève
LYON
MARSEILLE
MILANO
TORINO (Turin)
Venézia (Venice)
Firenze (Florence)
Ljubljana
Frankfurt
Stuttgart
Köln (Cologne)
Düsseldorf
Dortmund
Hannover
Bremen
Leipzig
Dresden
Nürnberg
Strasbourg
Basel
Innsbruck
Salzburg
Linz
Graz
Trieste
Génova
Golfo di Génova
Golfo di Venézia
Projection: Conical with two standard parallels

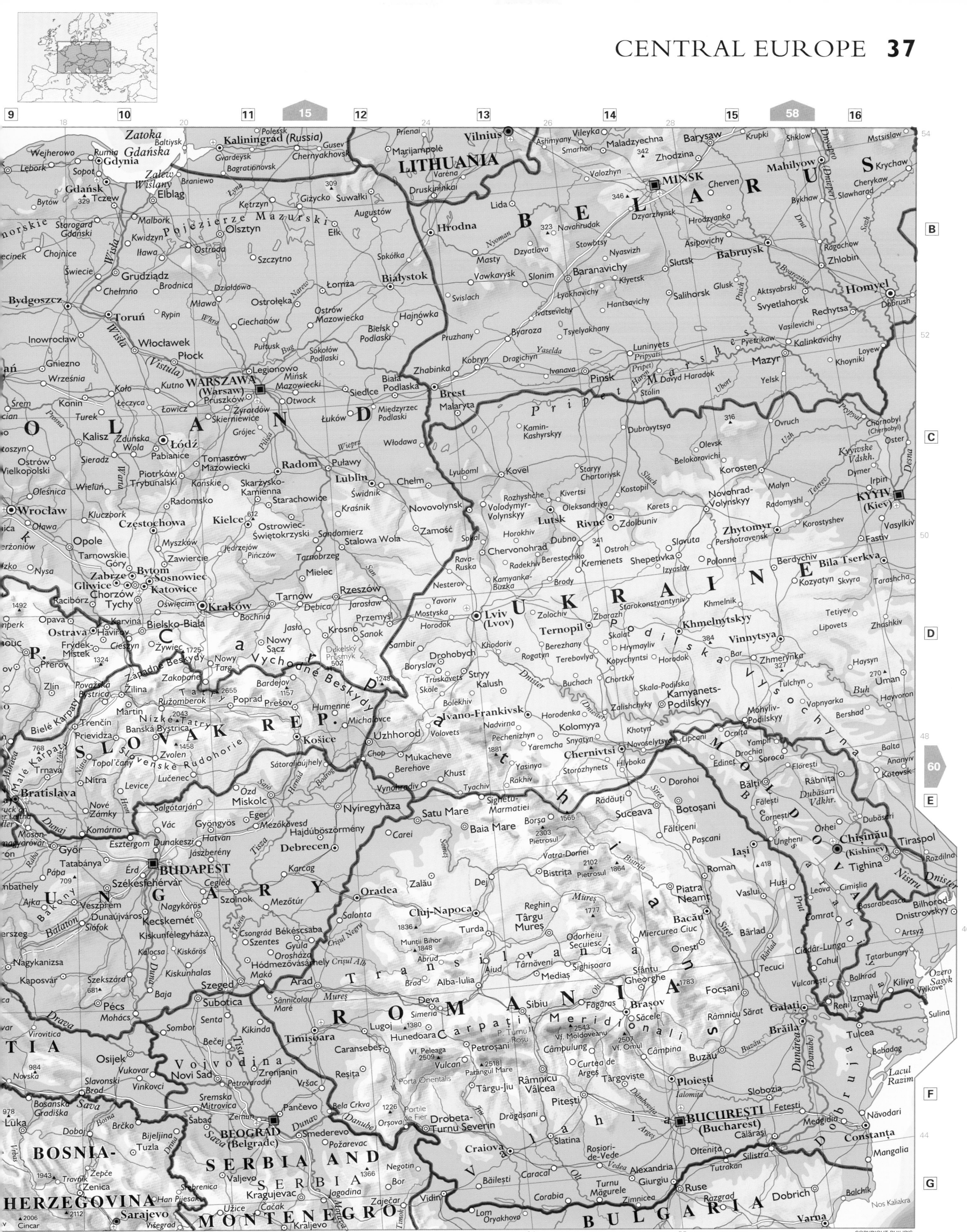

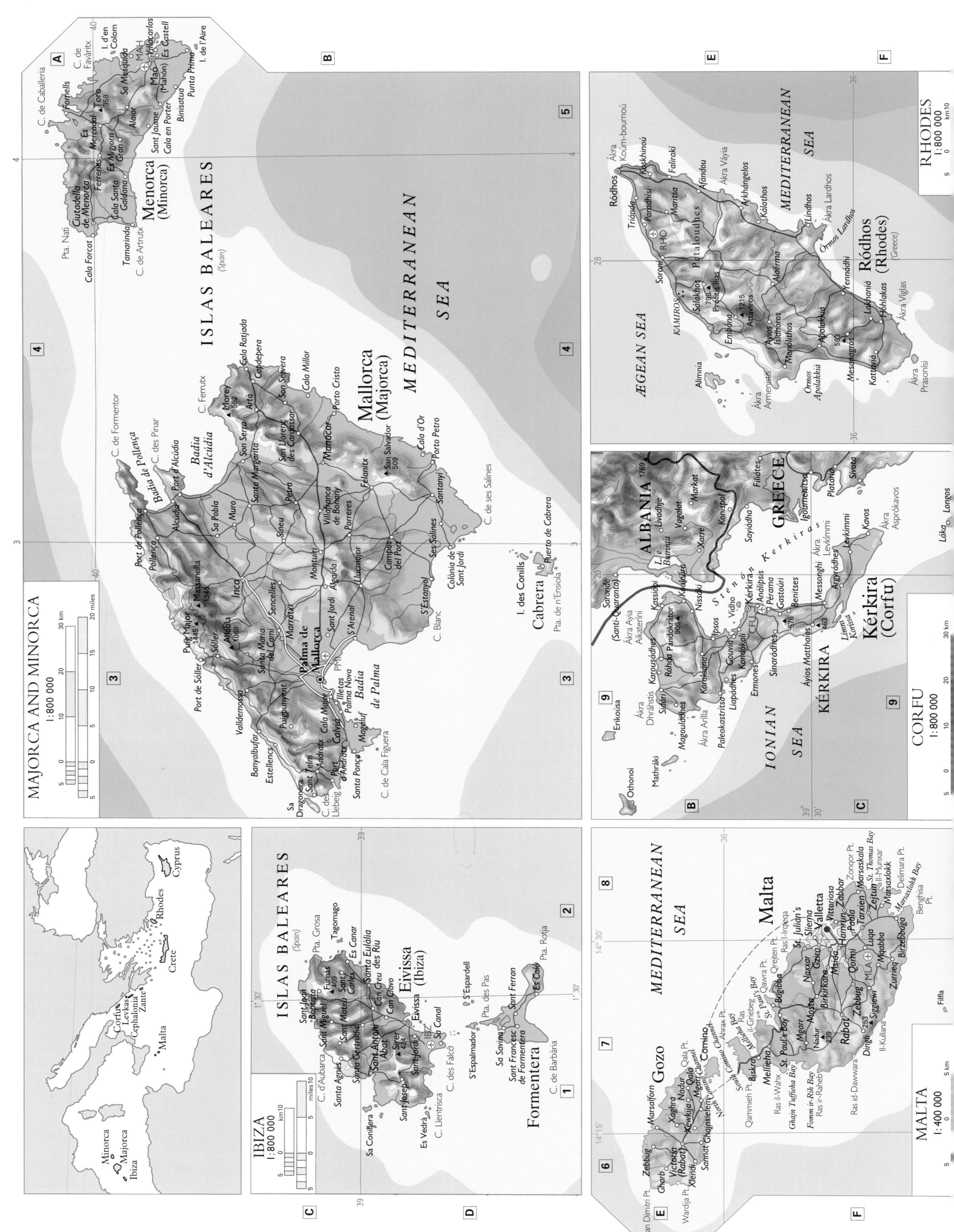

MAJORCA AND MINORCA
1:800 000

Menorca (Minorca)

C. de Caballería
Pta. Nati
Ciutadella de Menorca
C. de Artrux
Tamarinda
Cala Forcat
Ferreríes
Cala Santa Galdana
Es Migjorn Gran
Es Mercadal
Toro ▲ 358
Alaior
I. d'en Colom
I. de Favàritx
Sa Mesquida
MAÓ
Maó (Mahón)
Cala en Porter
Binisafúa
Villacarlos
Es Castell
Punta Prima
I. de l'Aire
Sant Jaume
C. de Favàritx

Mallorca (Majorca)

ISLAS BALEARES
(Spain)

C. de Formentor
Pollença
Port de Pollença
C. des Pinar
Badia de Pollença
C. de Formentor
Puig Major ▲ 1445
▲ 1068
Sóller
Port de Sóller
Valldemossa
Banyalbufar
Estellencs
Puigpunyent
Andratx
Port d'Andratx
Sant Telm
Santa Ponça
Magaluf
Palma Nova
Illetas
Calvià
Cala Major
C. de Cala Figuera
Sa Dragonera
C. des Llebeig
Alaró
Santa Maria del Camí
Alfàbia ▲ 1340
Massanella
Inca
Binissalem
Sencelles
Marràtxi
Sant Jordi
Palma de Mallorca
PMI
Badia de Palma
S'Arenal
Alcúdia
Port d'Alcúdia
Badia d'Alcúdia
Muro
Sa Pobla
Santa Margarita
Son Serra
Cala Millor
Son Servera
Capdepera
Cala Ratjada
Artà
Morey ▲ 562
C. Ferrutx
Petra
Sineu
Son Llorenç des Cardassar
Son Serra
Porto Cristo
Manacor
Vilafranca de Bonany
Porreres
Felanitx
San Salvador ▲ 509
Cala d'Or
Porto Petro
Santanyí
C. de ses Salines
Campos del Port
Colònia de Sant Jordi
Ses Salines
Algaida
Llucmajor
Montuïri
S'Estanyol
C. Blanc

Cabrera

I. des Conills
Puerto de Cabrera
Pta. de n'Ensiola
Colònia de Sant Jordi

MEDITERRANEAN SEA

IBIZA
1:800 000

ISLAS BALEARES
(Spain)

Pta. Grosa
Es Canar
Tagomago
Santa Eulalia del Riu
Sant Miquel
Sant Joan Baptista
Portinatx
Sant Mateu
Sant Antoni Abat
Sant Carles
Sant Rafel
Santa Gertrudis
Can Creu des Riu
Can Clavo
▲ 409 Furnàs
Siren ▲ 424
Sant Jordi
Eivissa (Ibiza)
IBZ
Sa Canal
C. d'Aubarca
Santa Agnès
Sant Josep
Sant Jordi
C. Llentrisca
Es Vedrà
Sa Conillera
S'Espardell
Pta. des Pas
S'Espalmador
Sa Savina
Sant Francesc de Formentera
Es Caló
Sant Ferran
Pta. Rotja
C. de Barbària
C. des Falcó

Formentera

Rhodes

Ákra Koúm-boumoú
Ródhos (Rhodes)
(Greece)
Maskhinoú
Faliraki
Afándou
Ákra Vávia
Arkhángelos
Ákra Lardhos
Líndhos
Ákra Lardhos
Pennádhi
Lakhaniá
Hóhlakas
Ákra Víglas
Ákra Prasonísi
Mesanagrós ▲ 563
Kattaviá
Ormos Apolakkiá
Alimnía
Ákra Armenísti
▲ 1215 Atáviros
▲ 798 Profítis Ilías
Embóna
Áyios Isídhoros
Monólithos
Sálakos
KÁMIROS
Soroní
RHO
Petaloudhes
Triánda
Kremastí
Paradhísi

AEGEAN SEA

MEDITERRANEAN SEA

Corfu

ALBANIA ▲ 1769
GREECE
Sarandë
L. Butrinti
Konispol
Livadhje
Vagalat
Markat
Karré
Sayiádha
Filiátes
Platariá
Igoumenítsa
Síviota
Sidhári
Róhda
Kassiópi
Kalámi
Ákra Ekateríni
Ákra Ayia
Karousádhes
Magouládhes
Ákra Dhrástis
Ákra Afílla
Paleokastrítsa
Áyios Matthaíos
Ermones
Liapádhes
Gardíki
Kondókali
Ípsos
Róhda Pandokrátor ▲ 906
Kérkira (Corfu)
(Greece)
KÉRKIRA
Kérkira
CFU
Gouviá
Pérama
Benítses
Gastoúri
Kanóni
Vidho
Nissáki
Sinés
Andípsis
Messonghí
Moraḯtika
Ayiós ▲ 576
Dhéka ▲ 463
Ágyiáddhes
Límni Korissía
Ákra Levkímmi
Levkímmi
Kávos
Ákra Asprókavos
Erikoúsa
Othonoí
Mathráki

IONIAN SEA

Láka
Longós

Malta

MEDITERRANEAN SEA

San Dimitri Pt.
Marsalforn
Żebbuġ
Xagħra
Xewkija
Victoria (Rabat)
Gharb
Xlendi
Nadur
Qala
Sannat Għajnsielem
Mġarr
Wardija Pt.
Comino
Cominotto
Ras il-Qala
Santa Marija Bay
North Comino Channel
South Comino Channel
Ħondoq ir-Rummien
Ramla Bay
Ras il-Wahx
Ghajn Tuffieha Bay
Fomm ir-Rih Bay
Ras ir-Raheb
Mellieħa
Anchor Bay
St. Paul's Bay
Xemxija
Mġarr
Mosta
Naxxar
Qormi
Birkirkara
Ħamrun
Msida
Valletta
Sliema
St. Julian's
Gżira
Floriana
Vittoriosa
Paola
Tarxien
Żabbar
Marsaskala
St. Thomas Bay
Żejtun
Marsaxlokk
Birżebbuġa
Delimara Pt.
Benghisa Pt.
Ras id-Dawwara
Luqa
MLA
Siġġiewi
Żurrieq
Mqabba
Qrendi
Żebbug
Dingli
▲ 253
Rabat
Mdina
Mtarfa
Attard
Dingli Cliffs
Il-Kullana
Nadur ▲ 239
Baħrija
Bidnija
Mġarr
Mġiebaħ Bay
Ġnejna Bay
Ras il-Griebeg
Għar Lapsi
Filfla

Gozo

Malta

Valletta

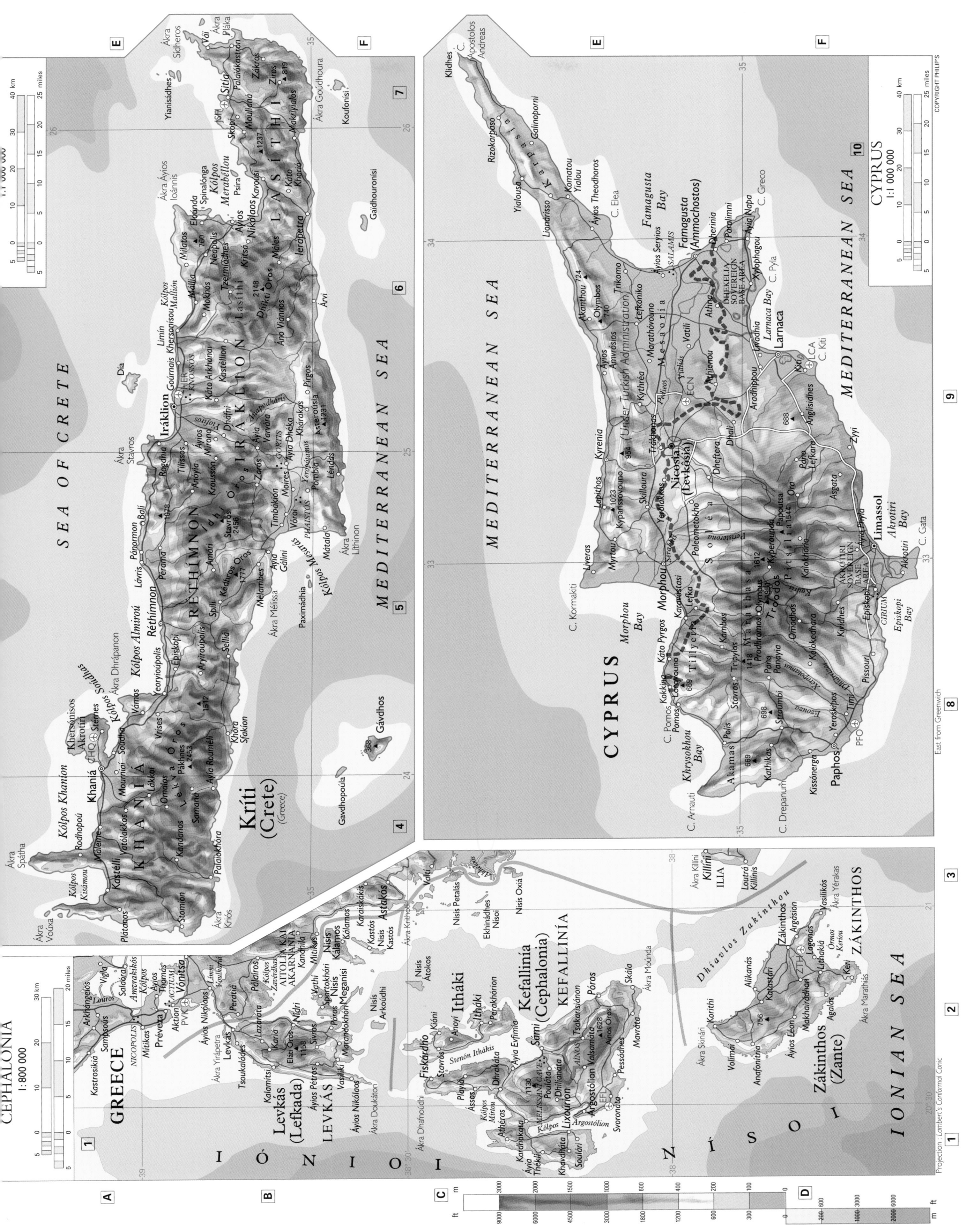

CEPHALONIA
1:800 000

Kríti (Crete)
(Greece)

CYPRUS
1:1 000 000

SEA OF CRETE

MEDITERRANEAN SEA

MEDITERRANEAN SEA

MEDITERRANEAN SEA

GREECE

CYPRUS

IONIAN SEA

I Ó N I O I   N Í S O I

Levkás (Lefkada)
LEVKÁS

Kefallinía (Cephalonia)
KEFALLINÍA

Zákinthos (Zante)
ZÁKINTHOS

KHANIÁ

RÉTHIMNON

IRÁKLION

LASÍTHI

East from Greenwich

Projection: Lambert's Conformal Conic

COPYRIGHT PHILIP'S

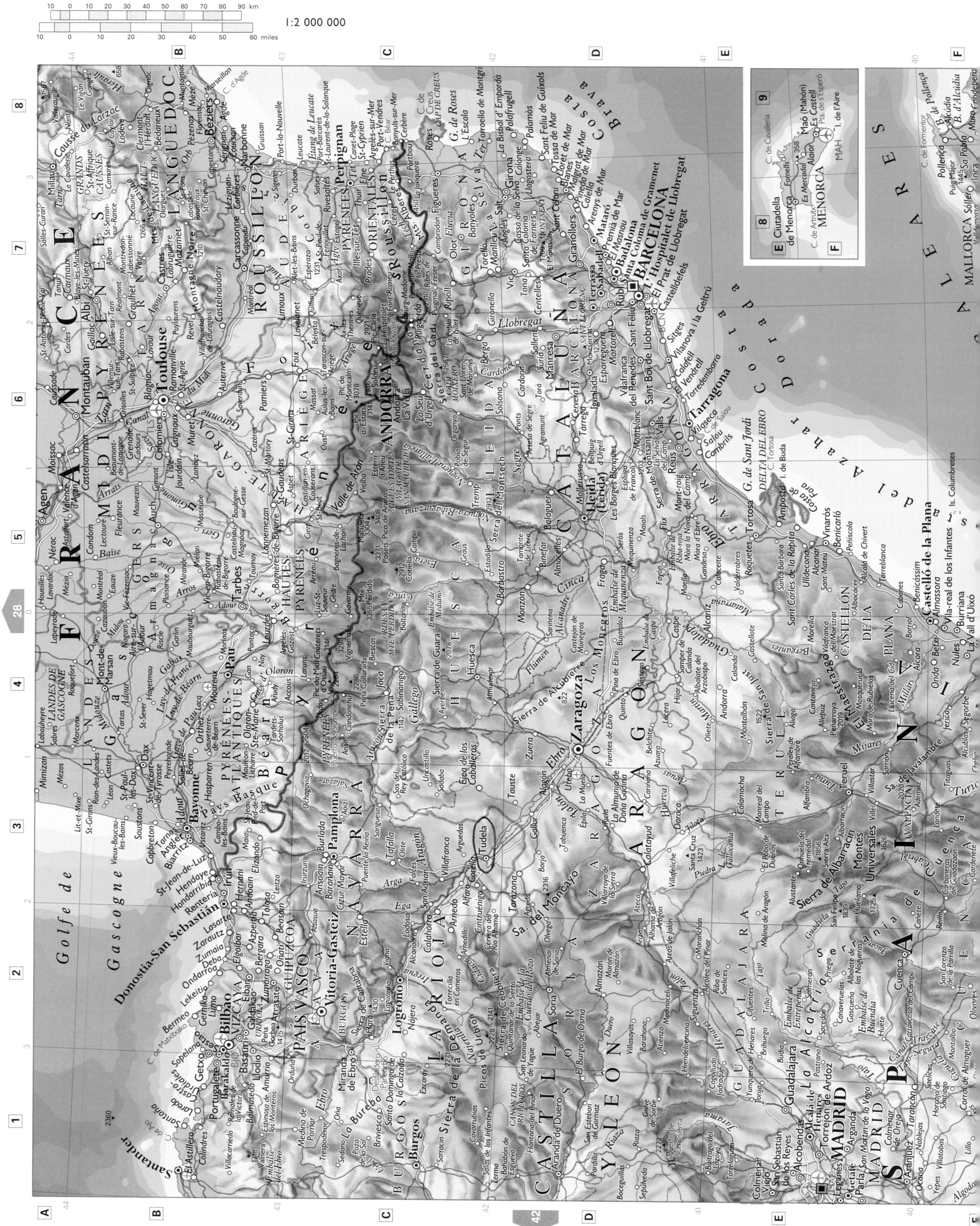

1:2 000 000

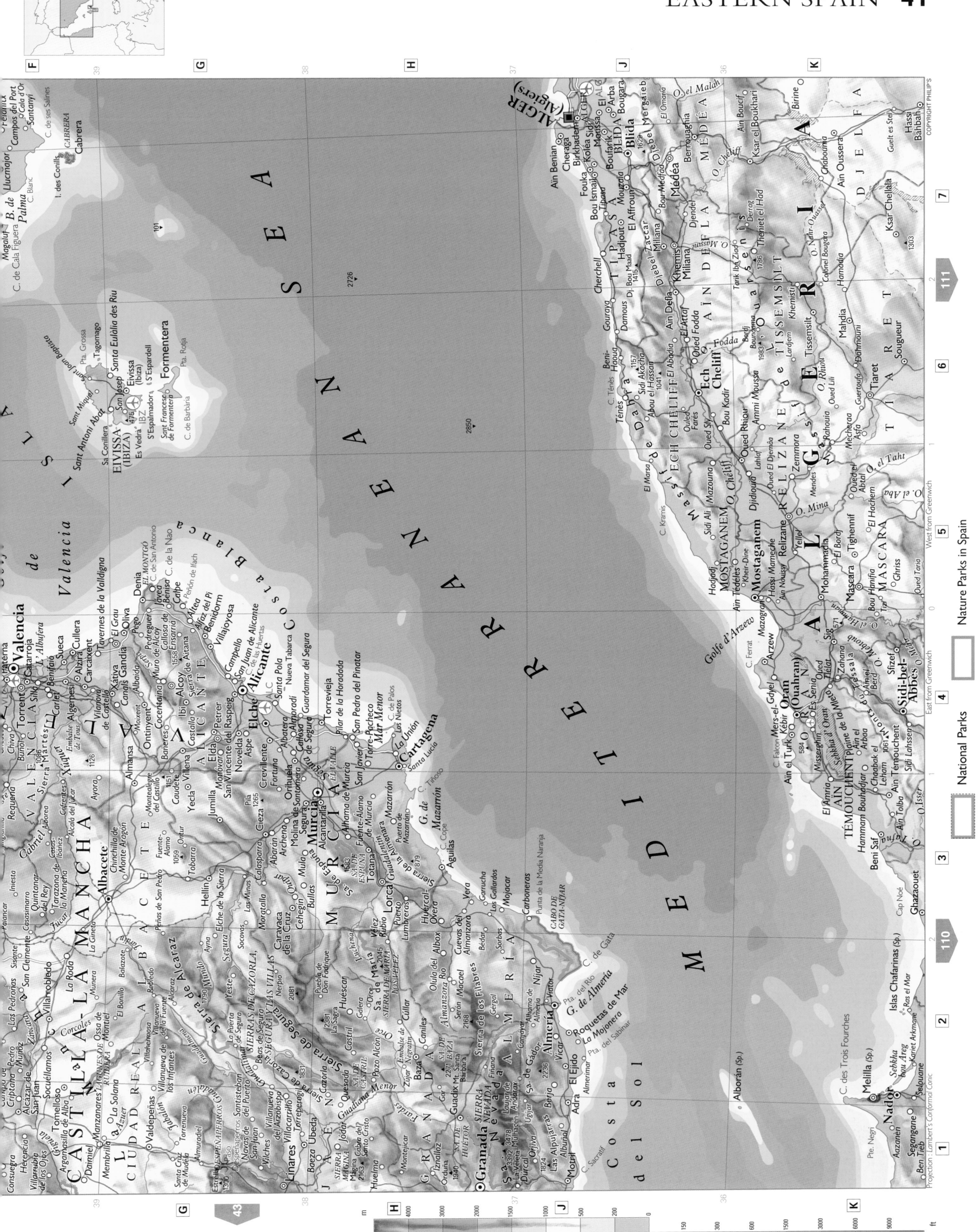

National Parks   Nature Parks in Spain

West from Greenwich   0   East from Greenwich

Projection: Lambert's Conformal Conic

m   ft

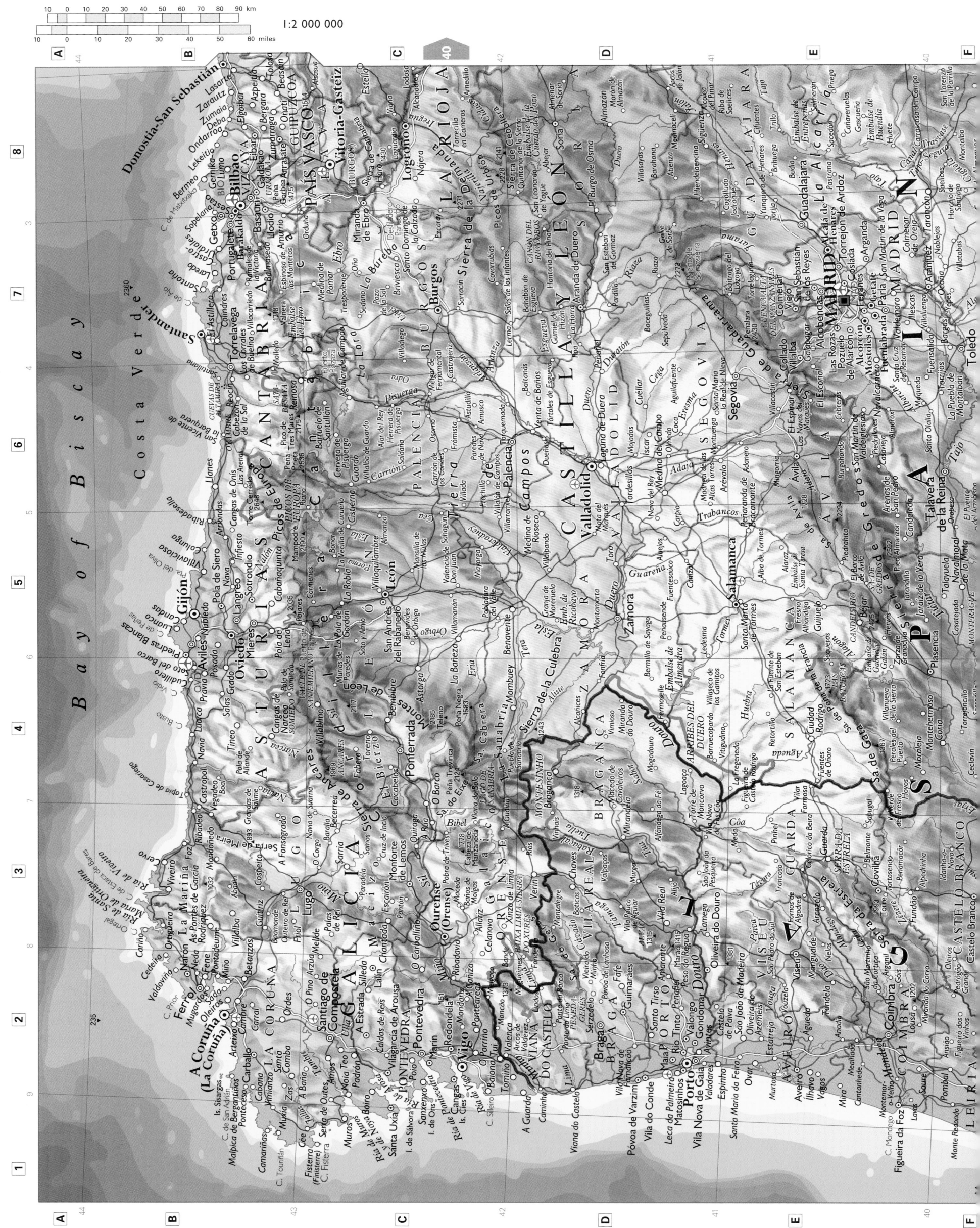

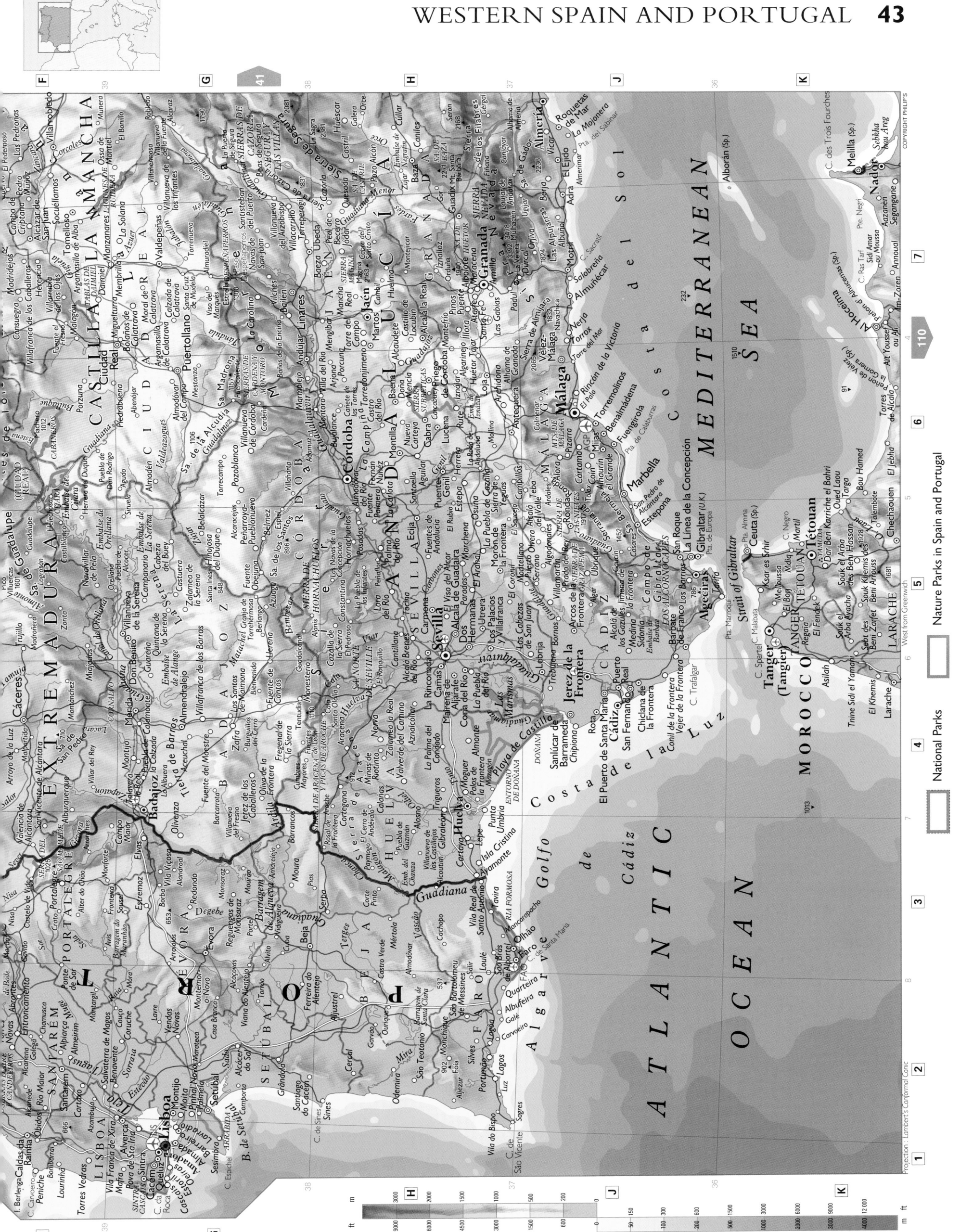

ATLANTIC OCEAN

MEDITERRANEAN SEA

MOROCCO

PORTUGAL

CASTILLA-LA MANCHA

EXTREMADURA

National Parks

Nature Parks in Spain and Portugal

Projection : Lambert's Conformal Conic

West from Greenwich

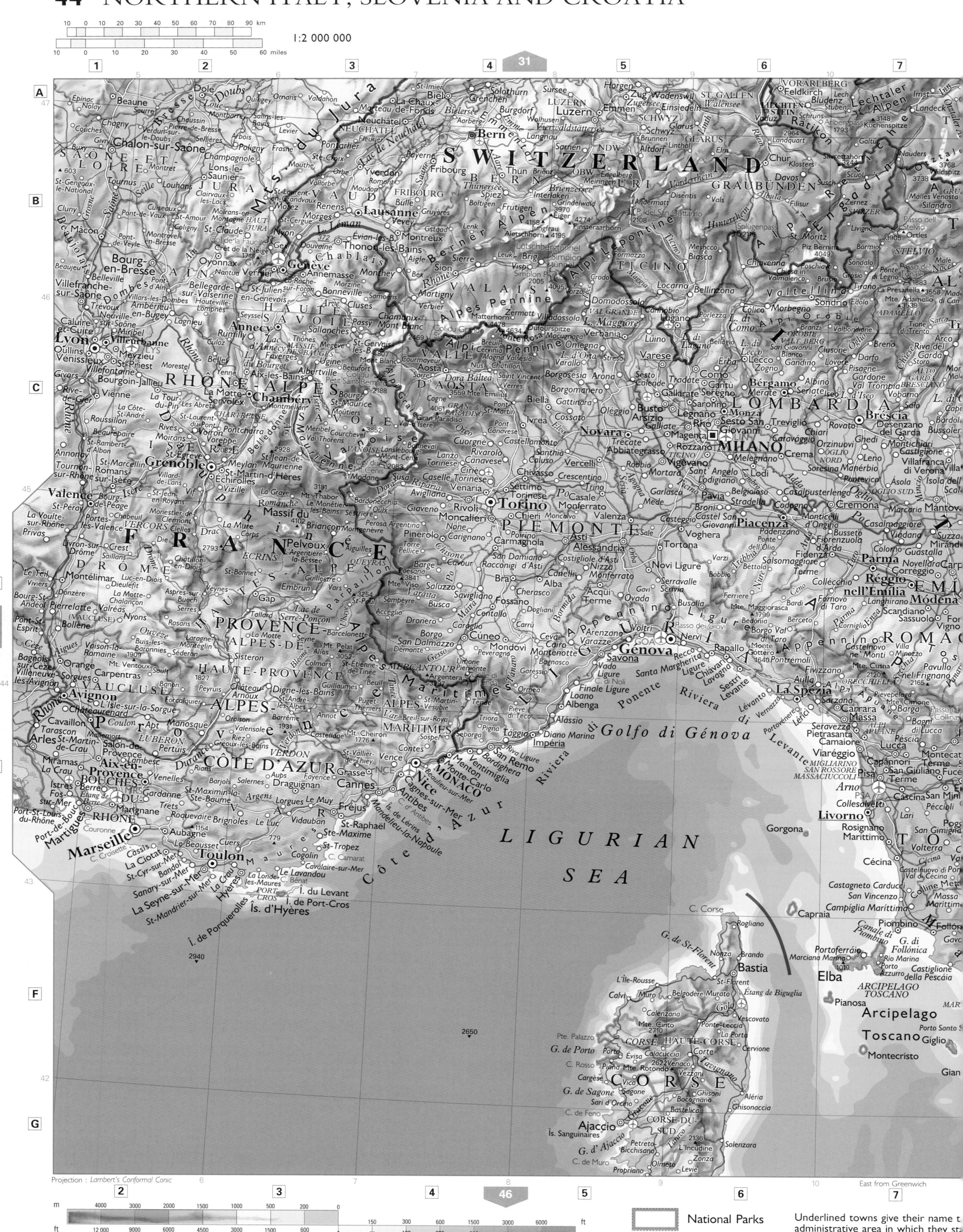

1:2 000 000

National Parks

Underlined towns give their name t
administrative area in which they sta

Projection : Lambert's Conformal Conic

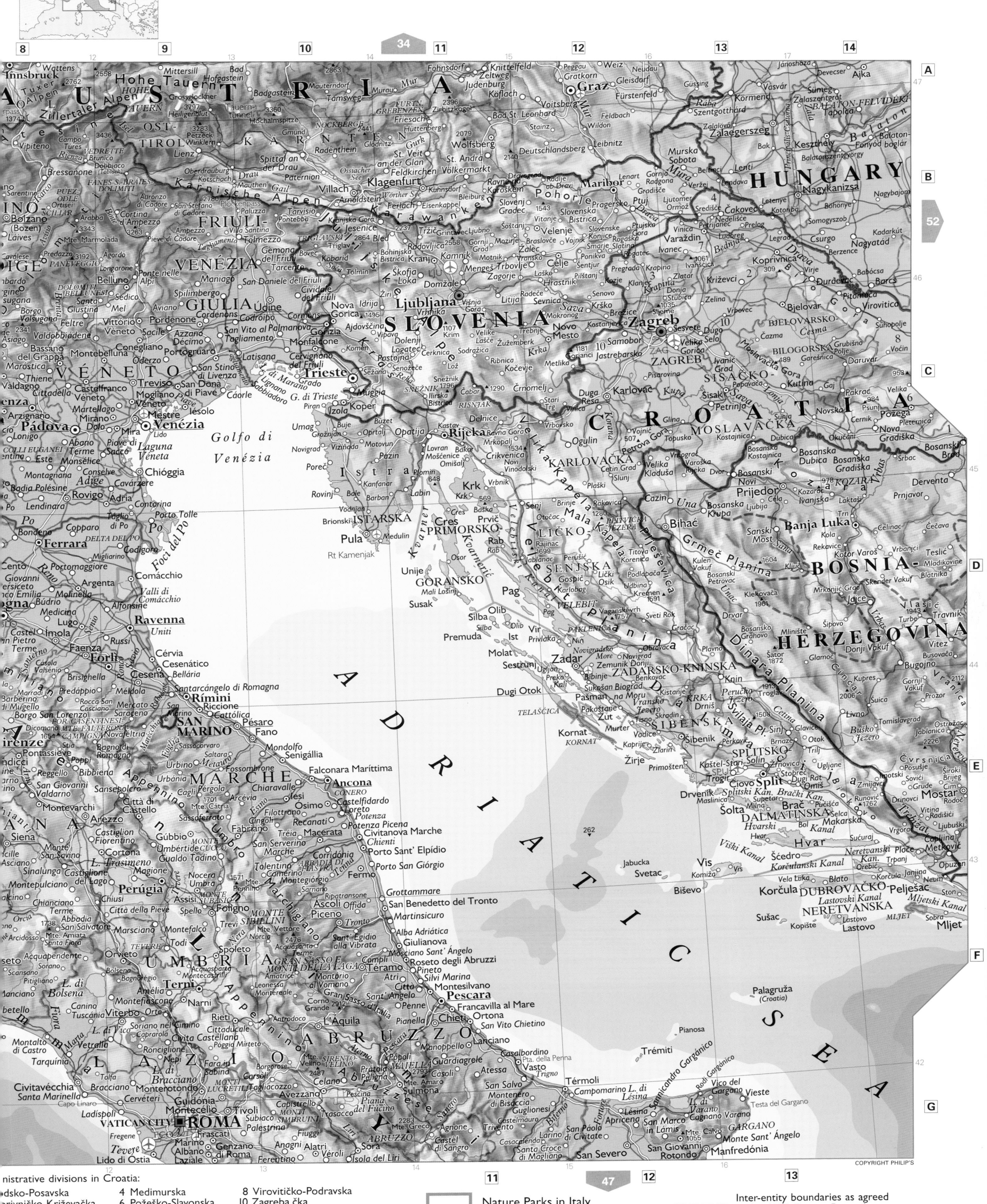

nistrative divisions in Croatia:

dsko-Posavska	4 Medimurska
rivničko-Križevačka	6 Požeško-Slavonska
pinsko-Zagorska	7 Varaždinska

8 Virovitičko-Podravska
10 Zagreba čka

☐ Nature Parks in Italy

– – – Inter-entity boundaries as agreed
at the 1995 Dayton Peace Agreement

1:2 000 000

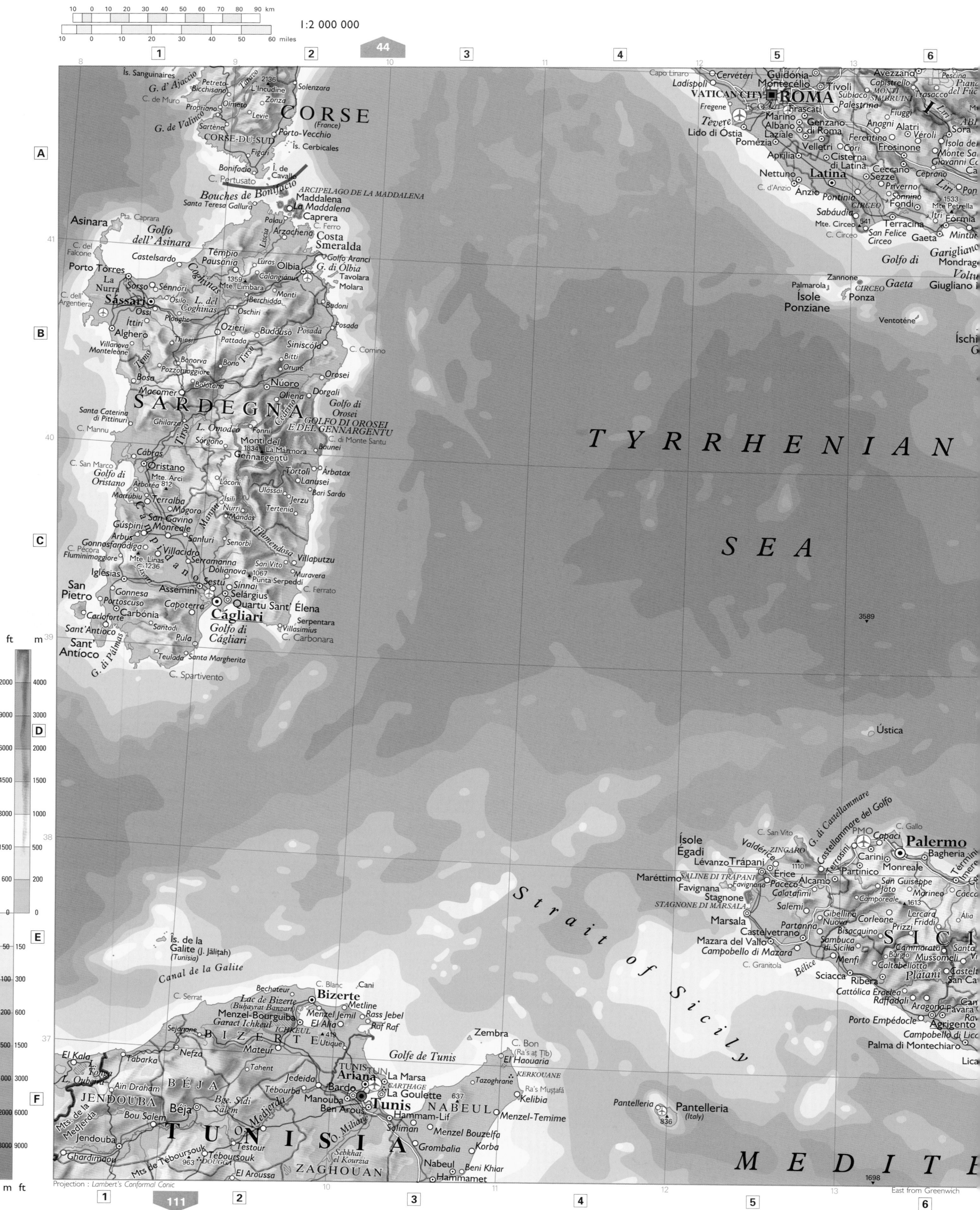

Projection : Lambert's Conformal Conic

East from Greenwich

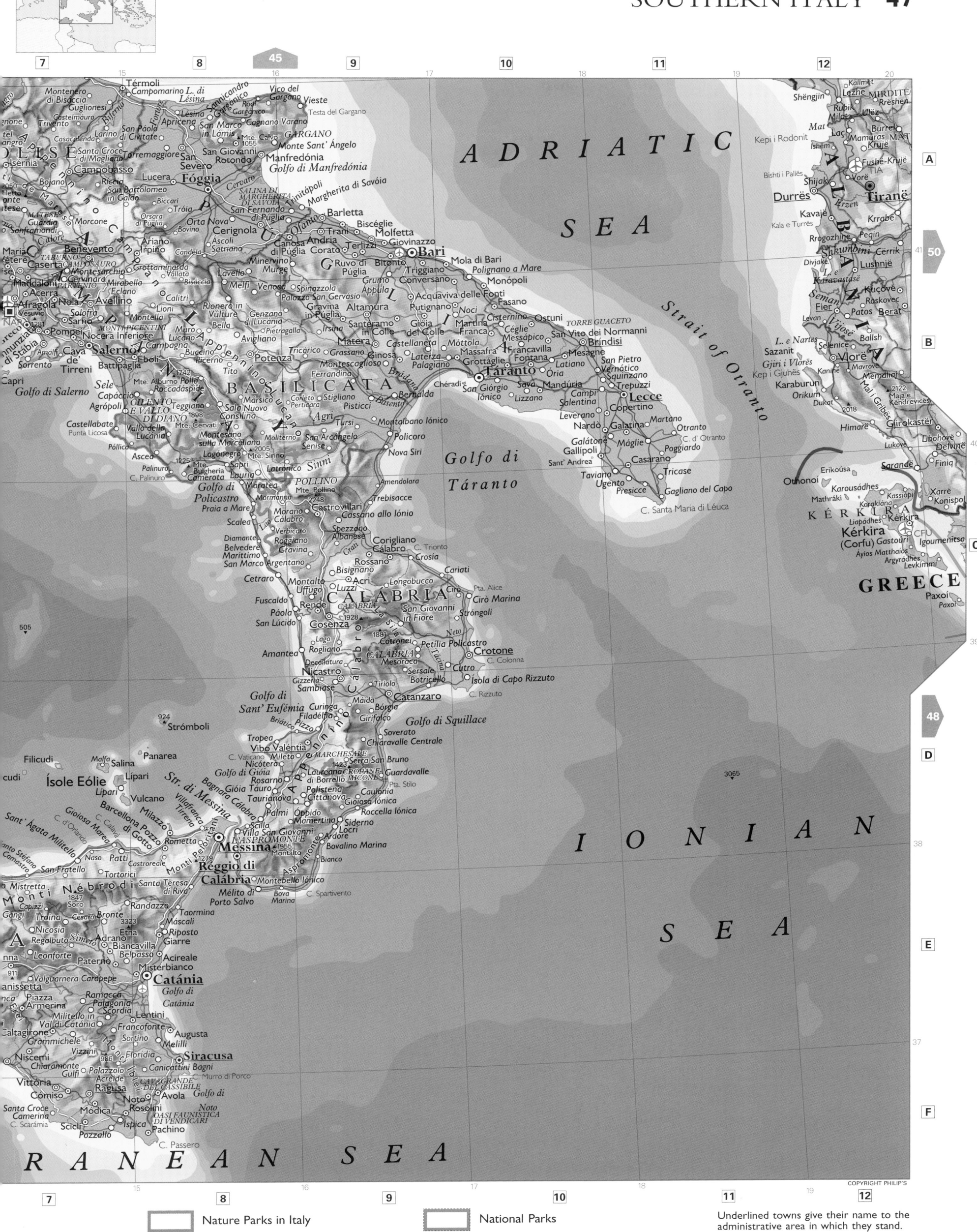

7   8   9   10   11   12

15   16   17   18   19   20

ADRIATIC SEA

Térmoli
Campomarino
Montenero di Bisáccia
Guglionesi
Castelmauro
Trivento
Larino
San Páolo di Civitate
Guardia Sanframondi
Bojano
Campobasso
Isernia
Benevento
Caserta
Avellino
Salerno
Golfo di Salerno
Capri
Golfo di Policastro

L. di Lésina
Sannicandro Garganico
Apricena
San Severo
San Marco in Lámis
San Giovanni Rotondo
Monte Sant' Ángelo
Manfredónia
Golfo di Manfredónia
Lucera
Fóggia
Cerignola
Barletta
Andria
Bari
Mola di Bari
Polignano a Mare
Monópoli
Fasano
Ostuni
Brindisi
Lecce

Vico del Gargano
Vieste
Testa del Gargano
GARGANO

Vieste

Potenza
BASILICATA
Matera
TARANTO
Golfo di Táranto
Crotone
CALABRIA
Catanzaro
Golfo di Squillace
Cosenza
Vibo Valéntia
Nicastro
Reggio di Calábria
Messina
Ísole Eólie
Strómboli
Panarea
Lípari
Vulcano
Catánia
Golfo di Catánia
Siracusa
Ragusa

IONIAN SEA

MEDITERRANEAN SEA

ALBANIA
Tiranë
Durrës
Vlorë
Gjirokastër
Sarandë

KÉRKIRA
Kérkira (Corfu)
GREECE
Paxoí

Strait of Otranto

50

48

A
B
C
D
E
F

39
40
41
38
37

Nature Parks in Italy   National Parks

Underlined towns give their name to the administrative area in which they stand.

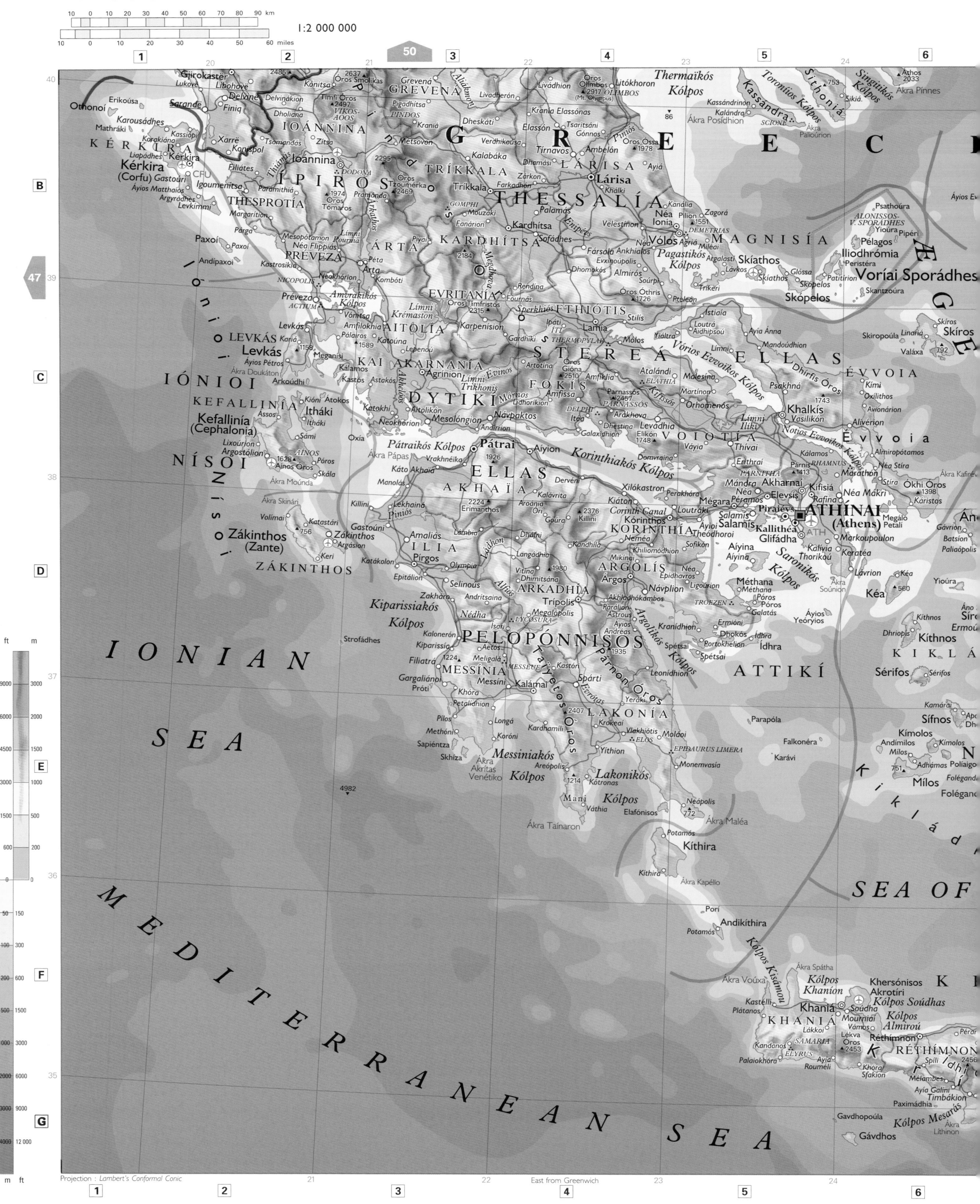

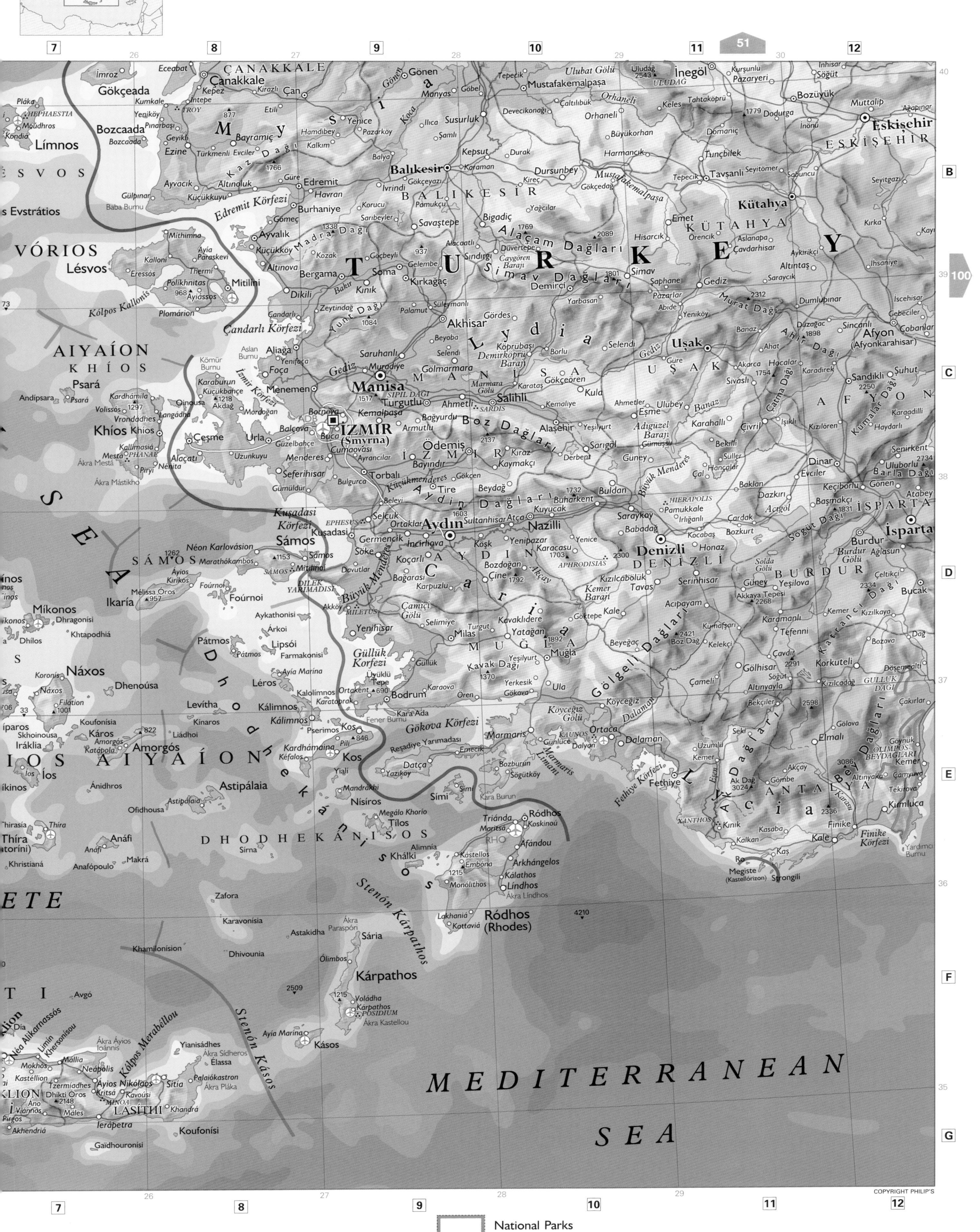

National Parks

1:2 000 000

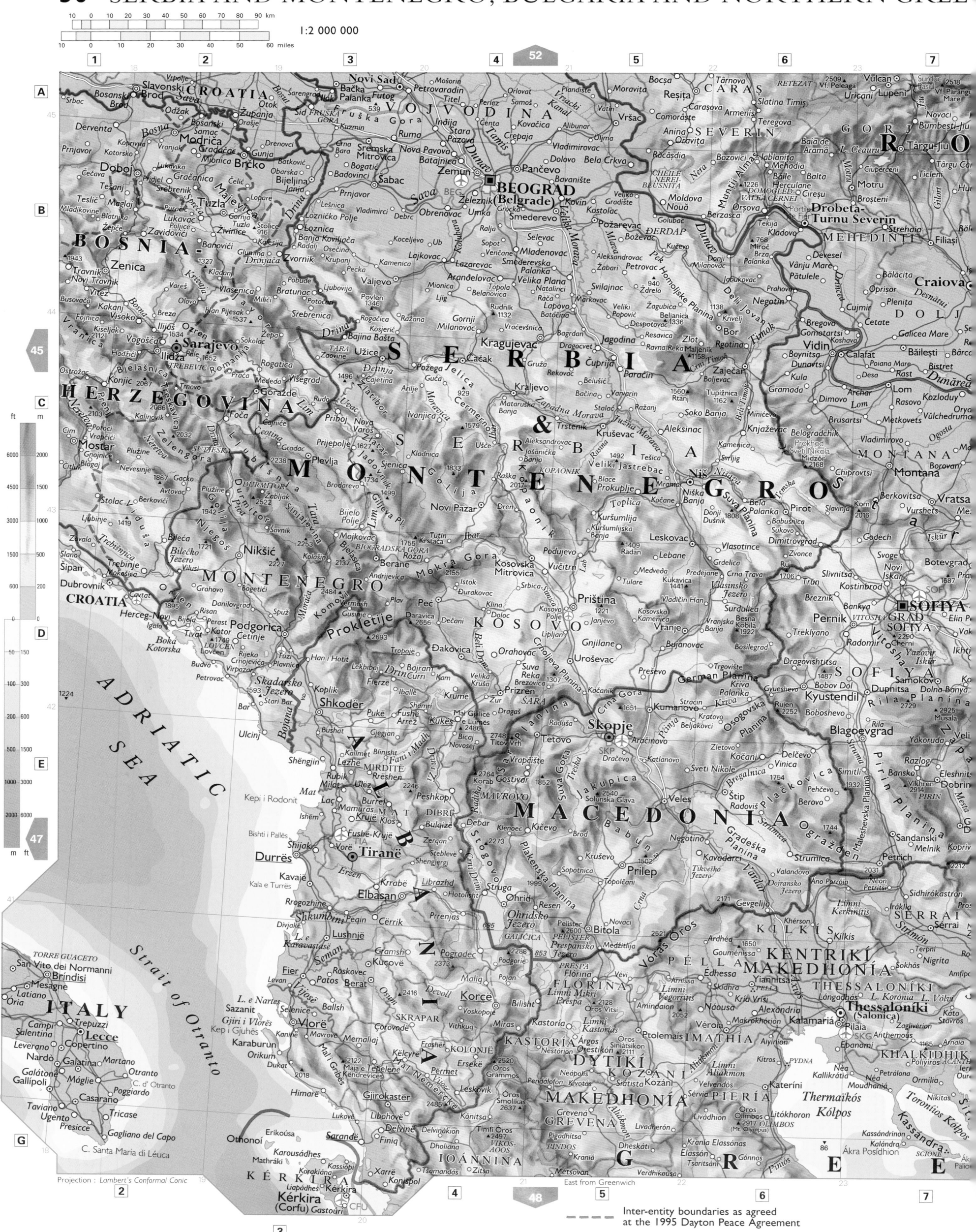

Projection : Lambert's Conformal Conic

East from Greenwich

Inter-entity boundaries as agreed
at the 1995 Dayton Peace Agreement

BLACK SEA

TURKEY

BULGARIA

ROMANIA

ANATOLIKÍ MAKEDHONÍA

KAÍ THRAKÍ

RODHOPI

THRÁCE

TEKİRDAĞ

KIRKLARELİ

KOCAELİ

Marmara Denizi (Sea of Marmara)

Thrakikón Pélagos

BUCUREŞTI (Bucharest)

Ploieşti · Buzău · Brăila · Galaţi · Constanţa · Varna · Burgas · Plovdiv · Pleven · Ruse · Dobrich · Edirne · İSTANBUL · Bursa

National Parks

Underlined towns give their name to the administrative area in which they stand.

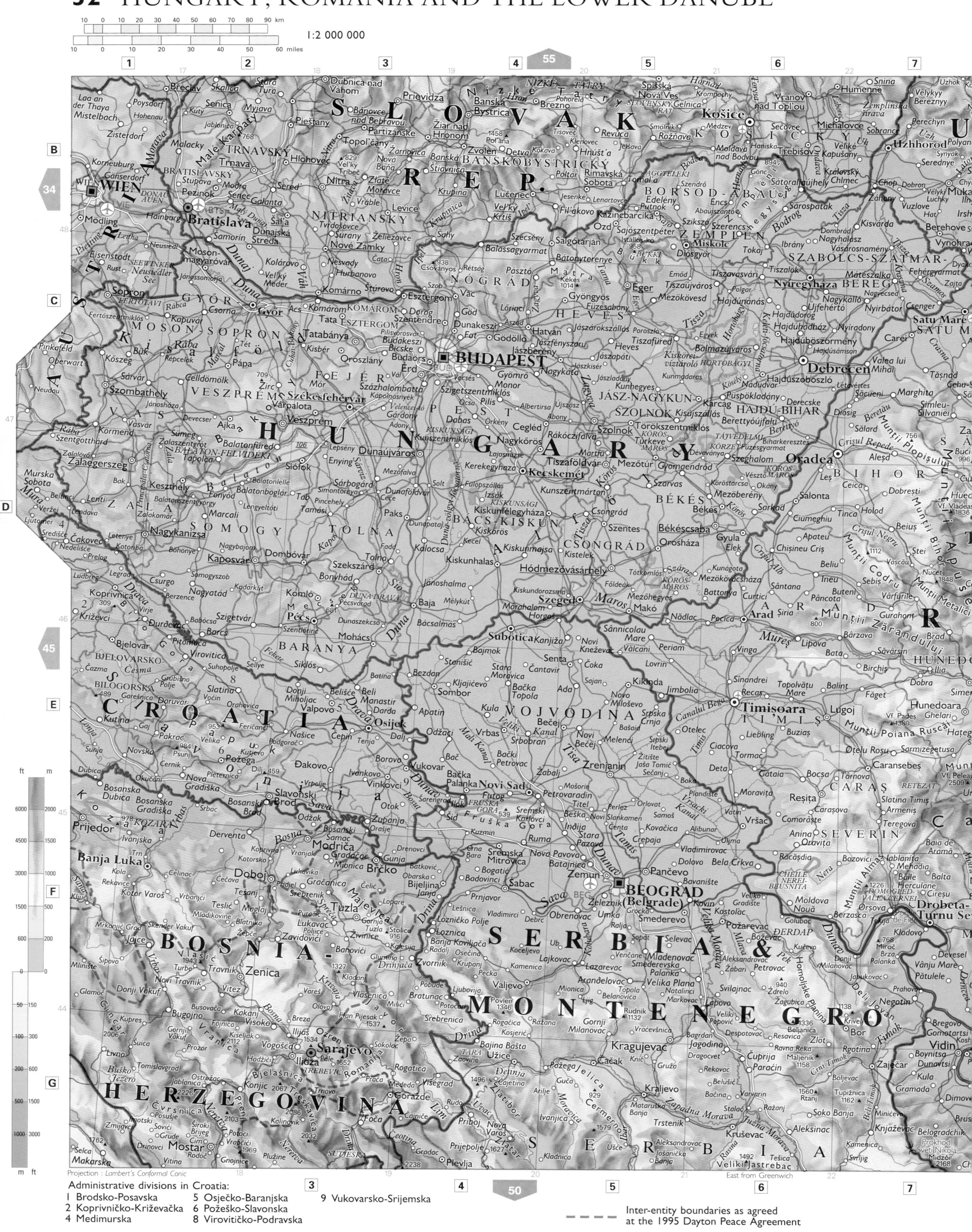

1:2 000 000

Projection : Lambert's Conformal Conic

Administrative divisions in Croatia:
1 Brodsko-Posavska   5 Osječko-Baranjska   9 Vukovarsko-Srijemska
2 Koprivničko-Križevačka   6 Požeško-Slavonska
4 Medimurska   8 Virovitičko-Podravska

East from Greenwich

– – – – – Inter-entity boundaries as agreed
at the 1995 Dayton Peace Agreement

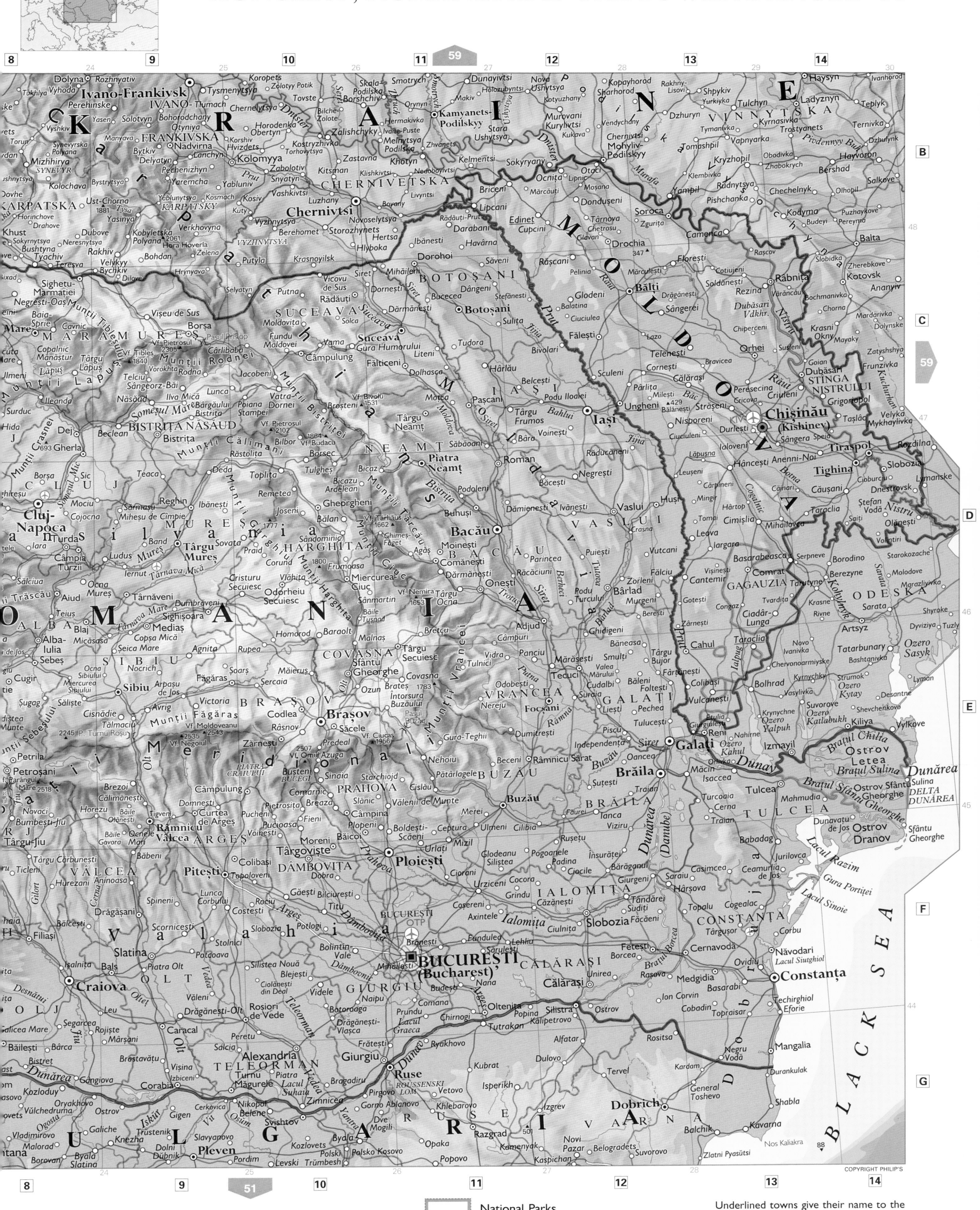

National Parks

Underlined towns give their name to the
administrative area in which they stand.

COPYRIGHT PHILIP'S

1:2 000 000

Underlined towns give their name to the administrative area in which they stand.

National Parks

Projection : Lambert's Conformal Conic

East from Greenwich

COPYRIGHT PHILIP'S

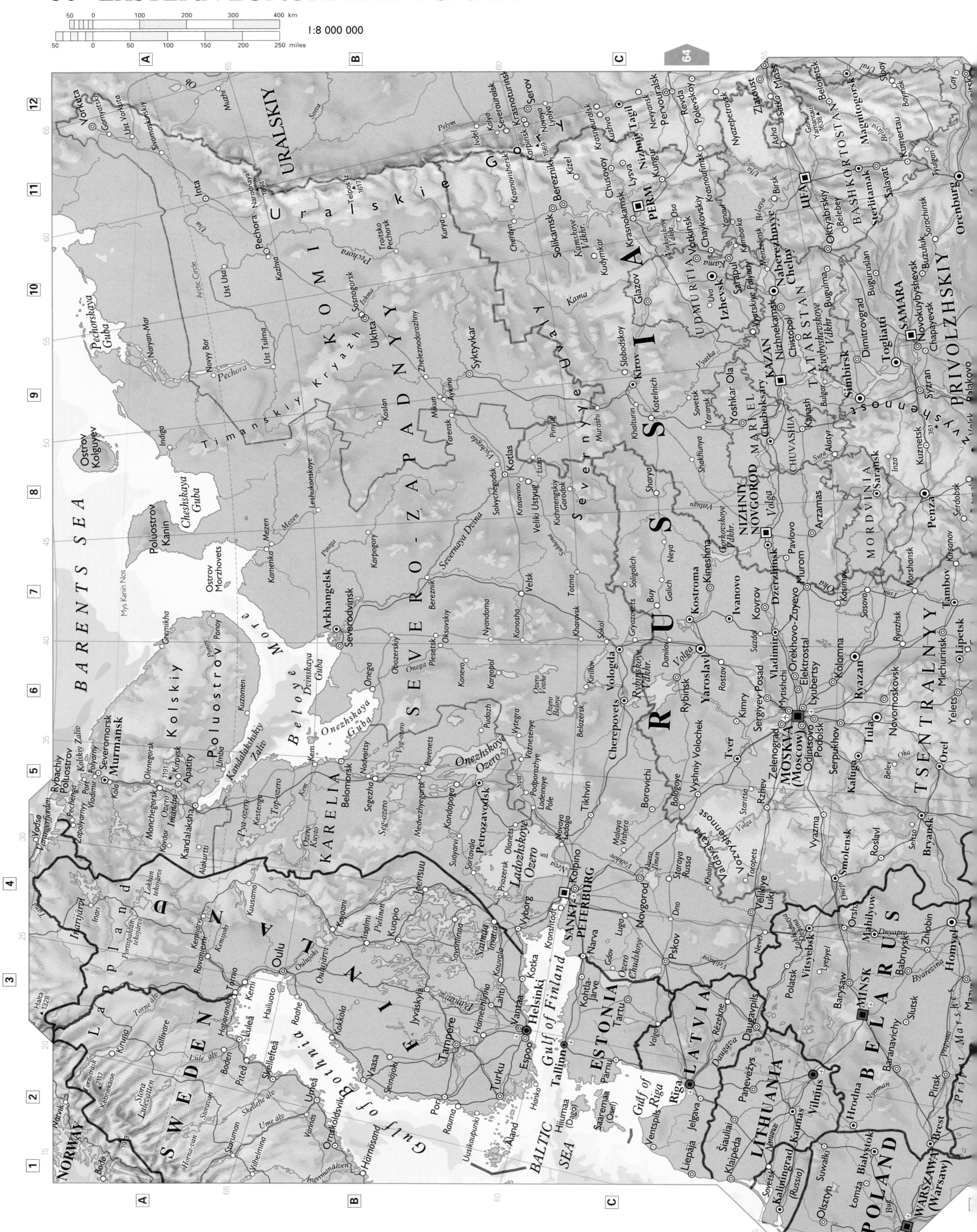

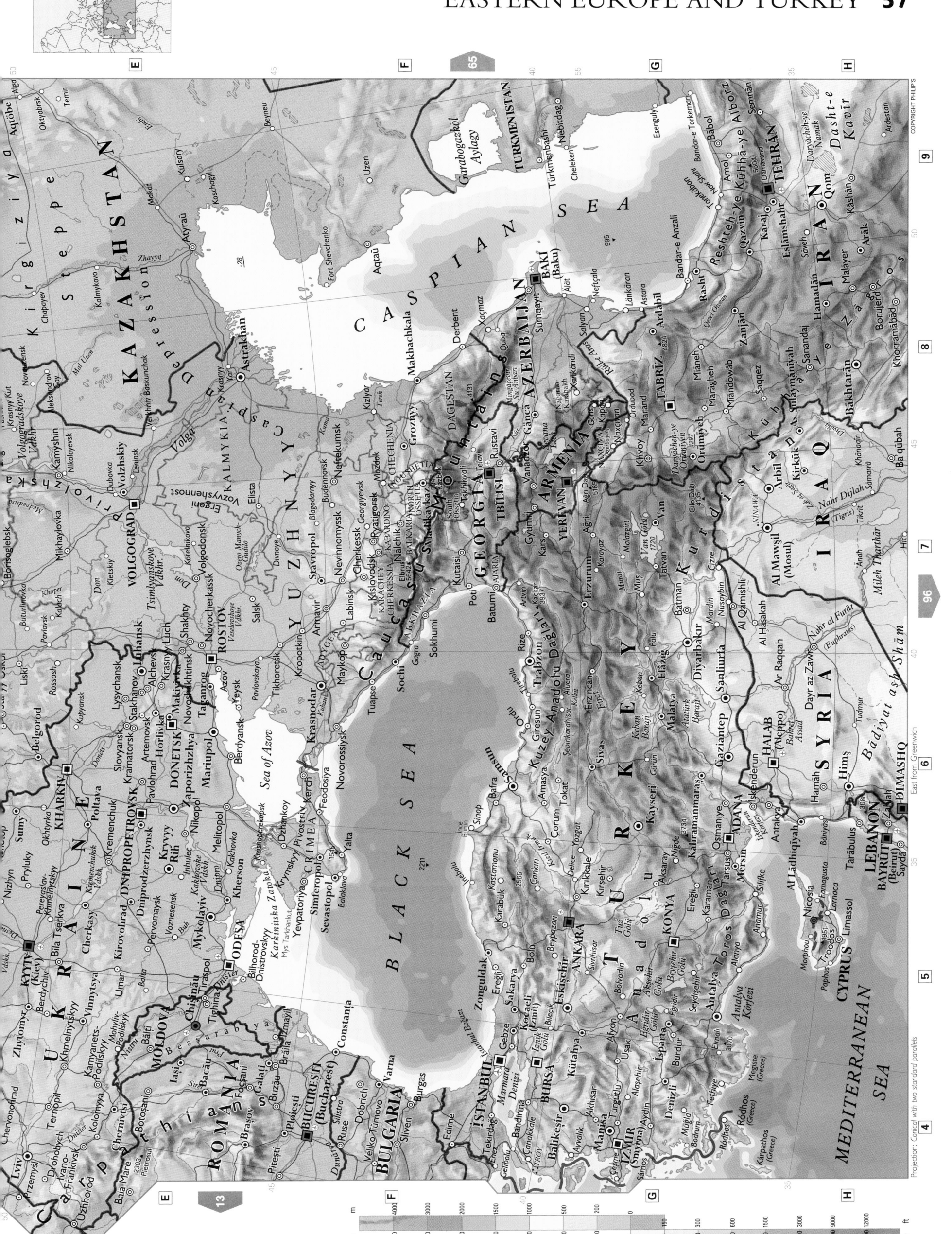

Projection: Conical with two standard parallels

East from Greenwich

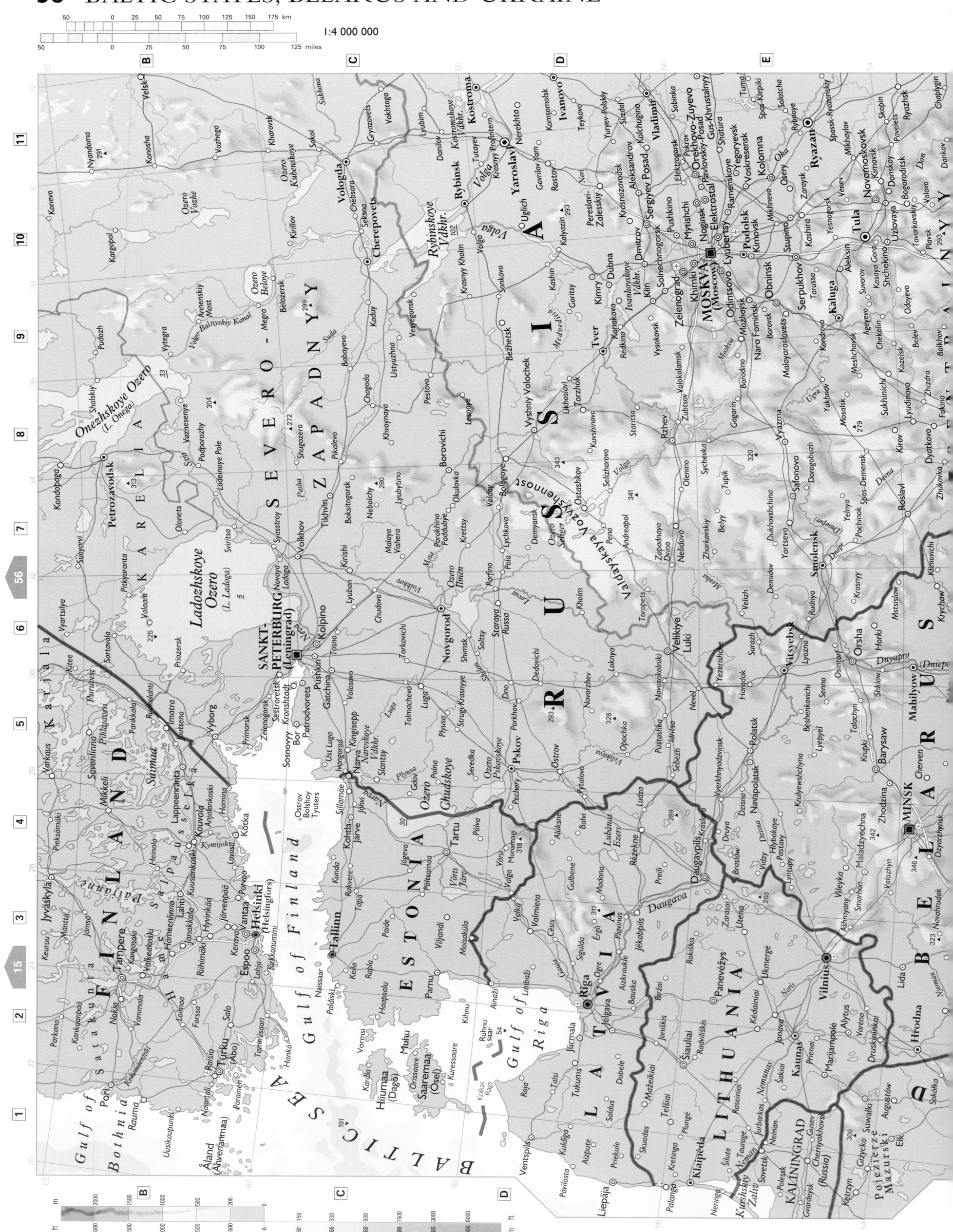

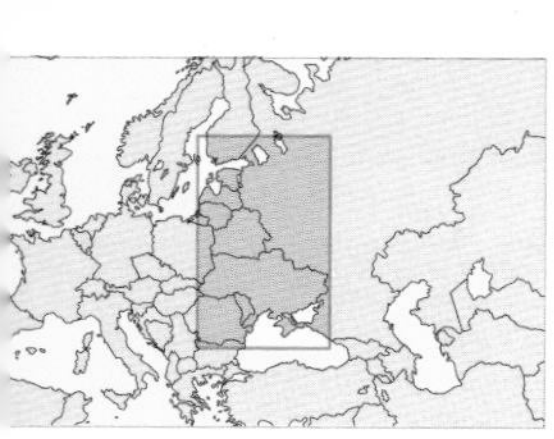

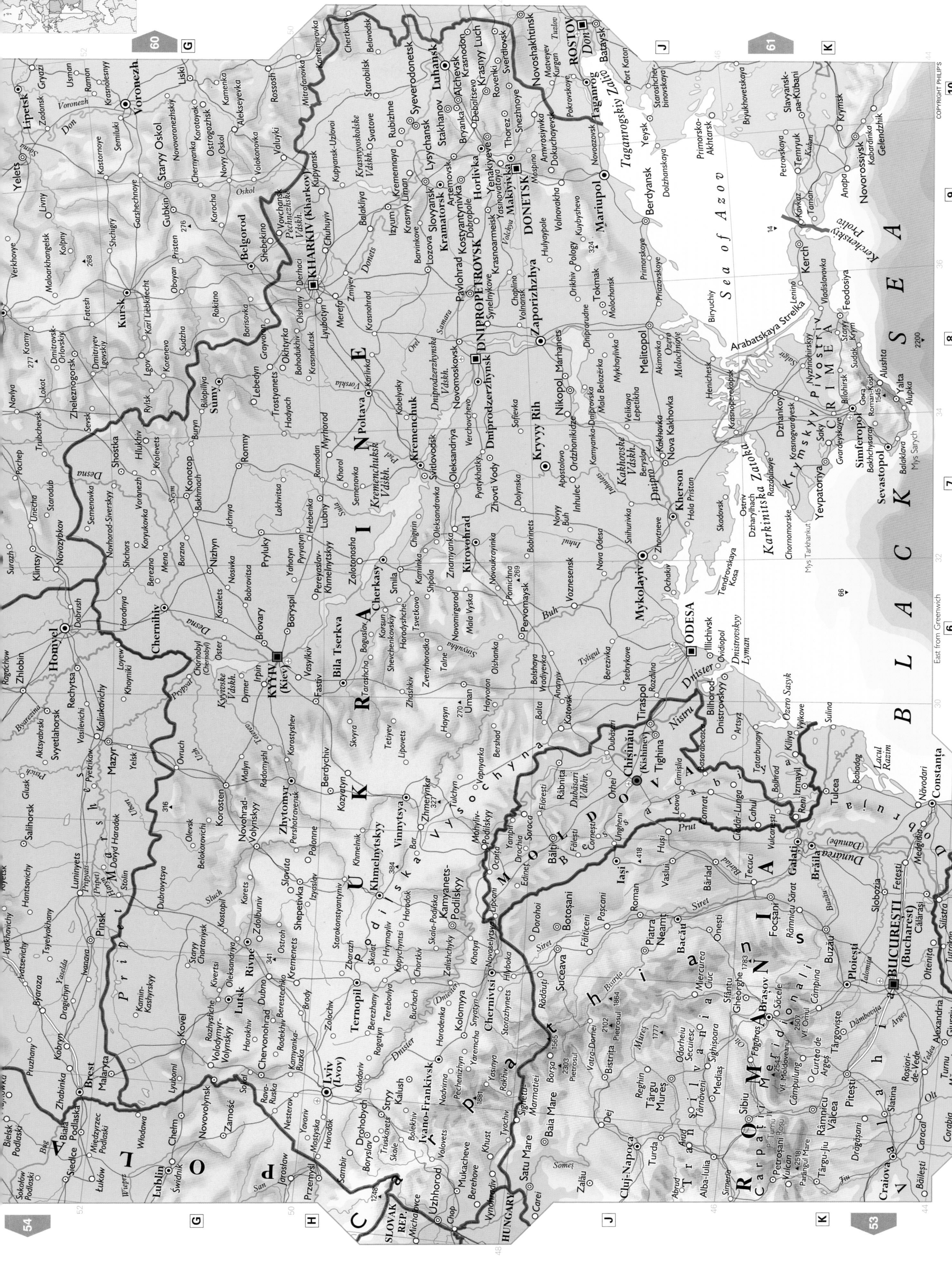
UKRAINE
MOLDOVA
ROMANIA
POLAND
BULGARIA
SLOVAK REP.
HUNGARY
BLACK SEA
Sea of Azov
KYYIV (Kiev)
KHARKIV (Kharkov)
DNIPROPETROVSK
DONETSK
ODESA
ROSTOV
Chişinău (Kishinev)
BUCUREŞTI (Bucharest)
Lviv (Lvov)
Homyel
Voronezh
Zaporizhzhya
Kryvyy Rih
Mykolayiv
Kherson
Simferopol
Sevastopol
Luhansk
Mariupol
Poltava
Kremenchuk
Cherkasy
Kirovohrad
Vinnytsya
Zhytomyr
Chernihiv
Sumy
Kursk
Belgorod
Constanţa
Galaţi
Brăila
Iaşi
Cluj-Napoca
Craiova
Ploieşti
Brest
Pinsk
Rivne
Lutsk
Ternopil
Chernivtsi
Lublin
Dnister
Prut
Desna
Pripyat
Crimea
Carpathians
Projection: Conical with two standard parallels
East from Greenwich
COPYRIGHT PHILIP'S

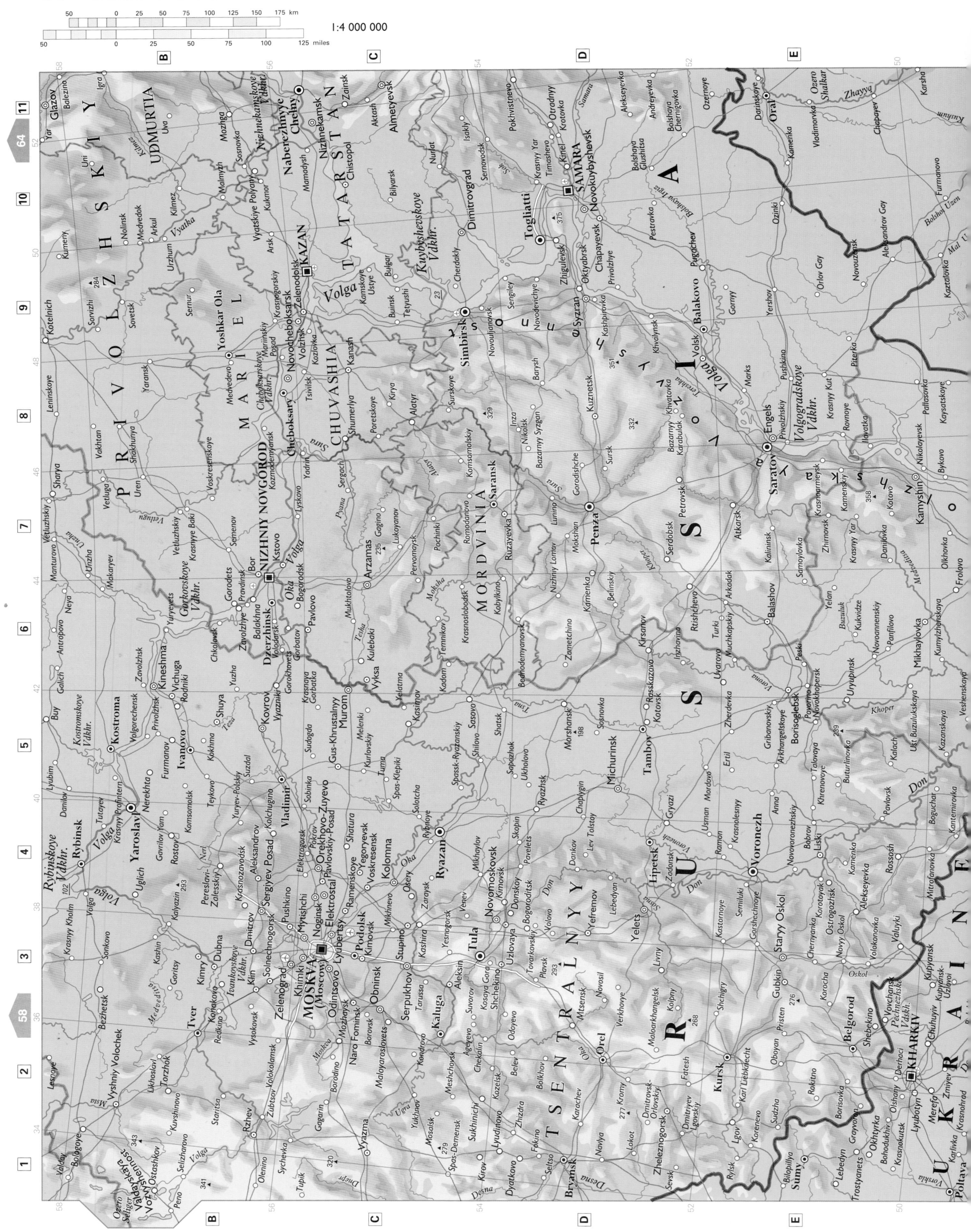

50   0   25   50   75   100 125 150 175 km

1:4 000 000

50   0   25   50   75   100 125 miles

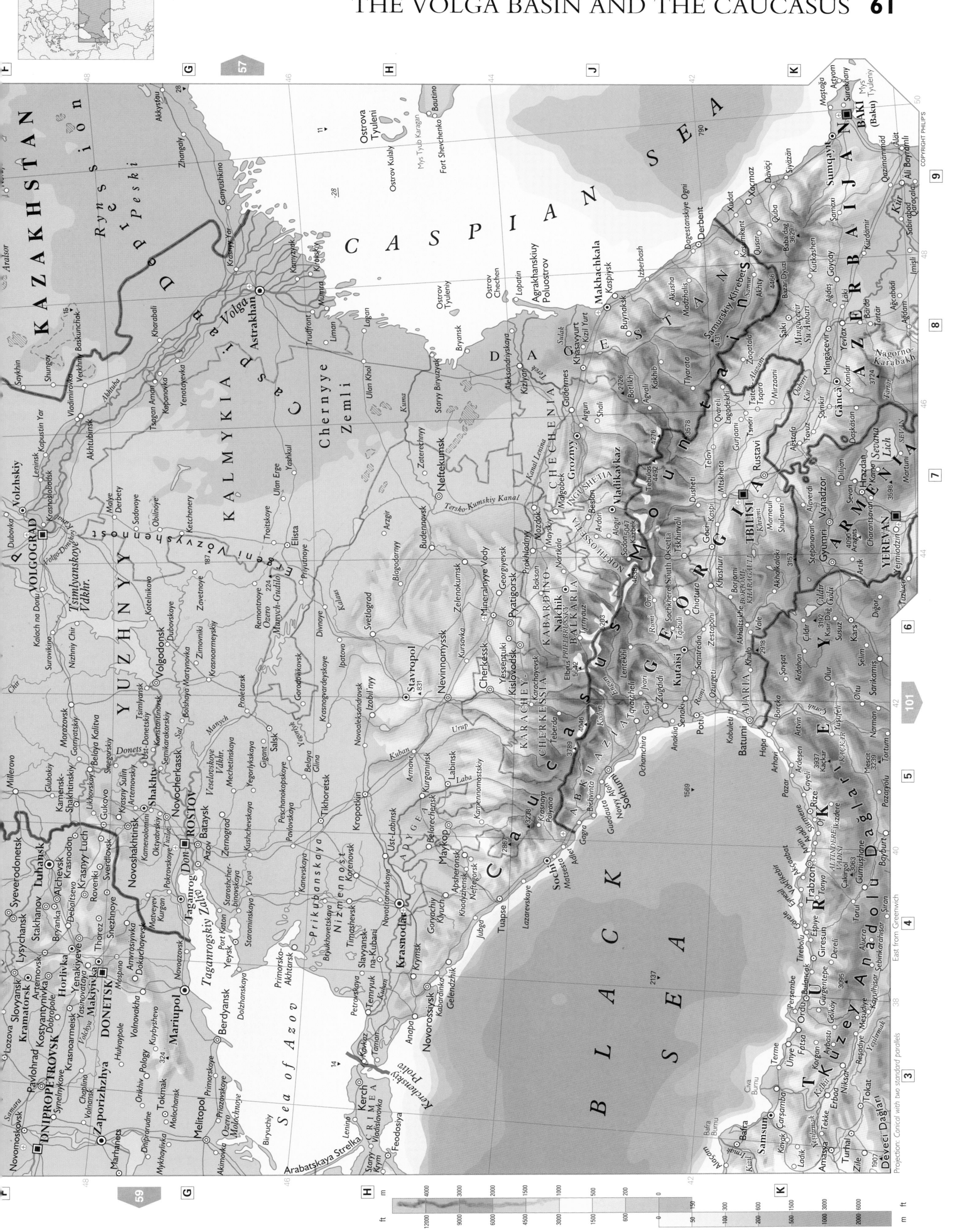

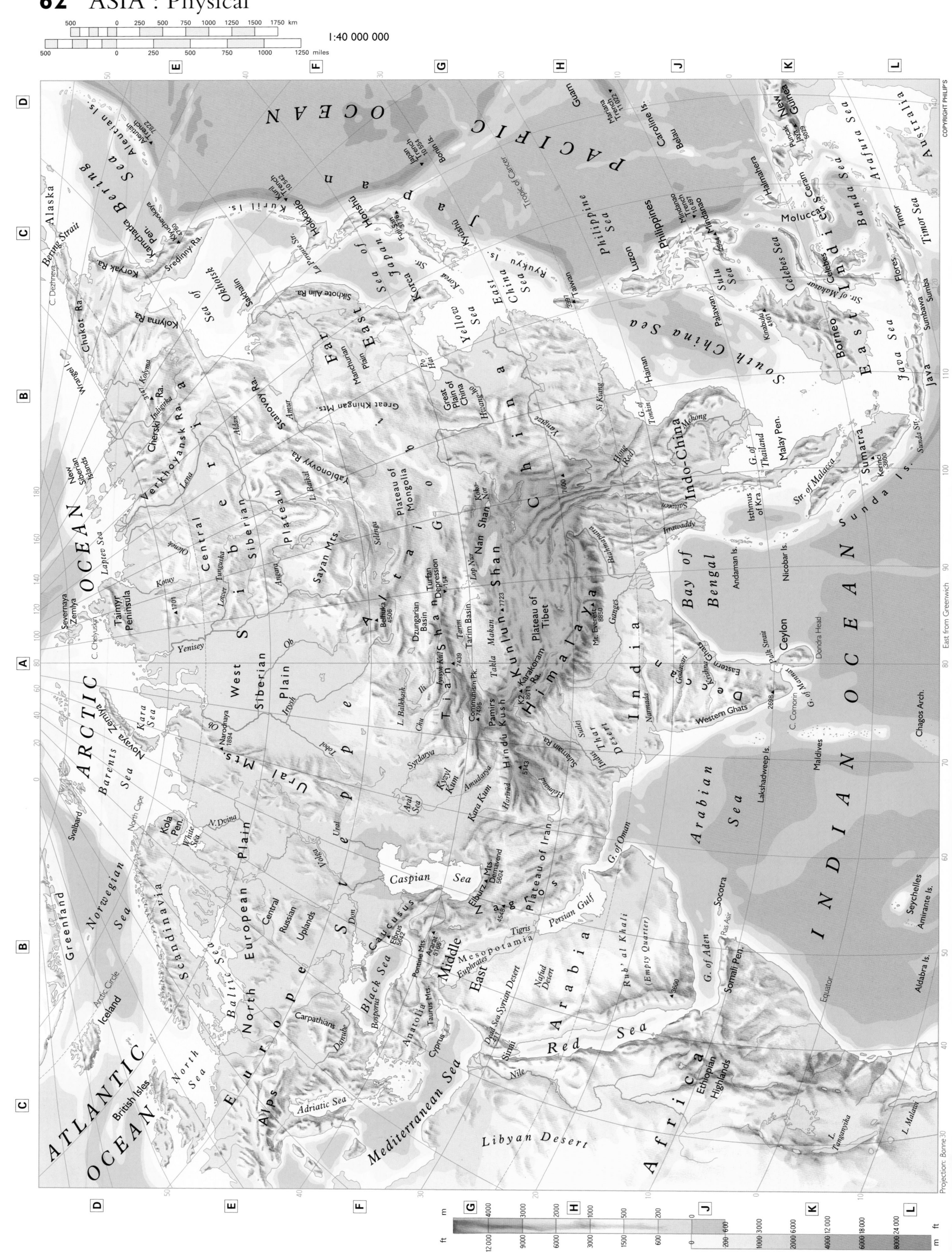

1:40 000 000

COPYRIGHT PHILIP'S

Projection: Bonne

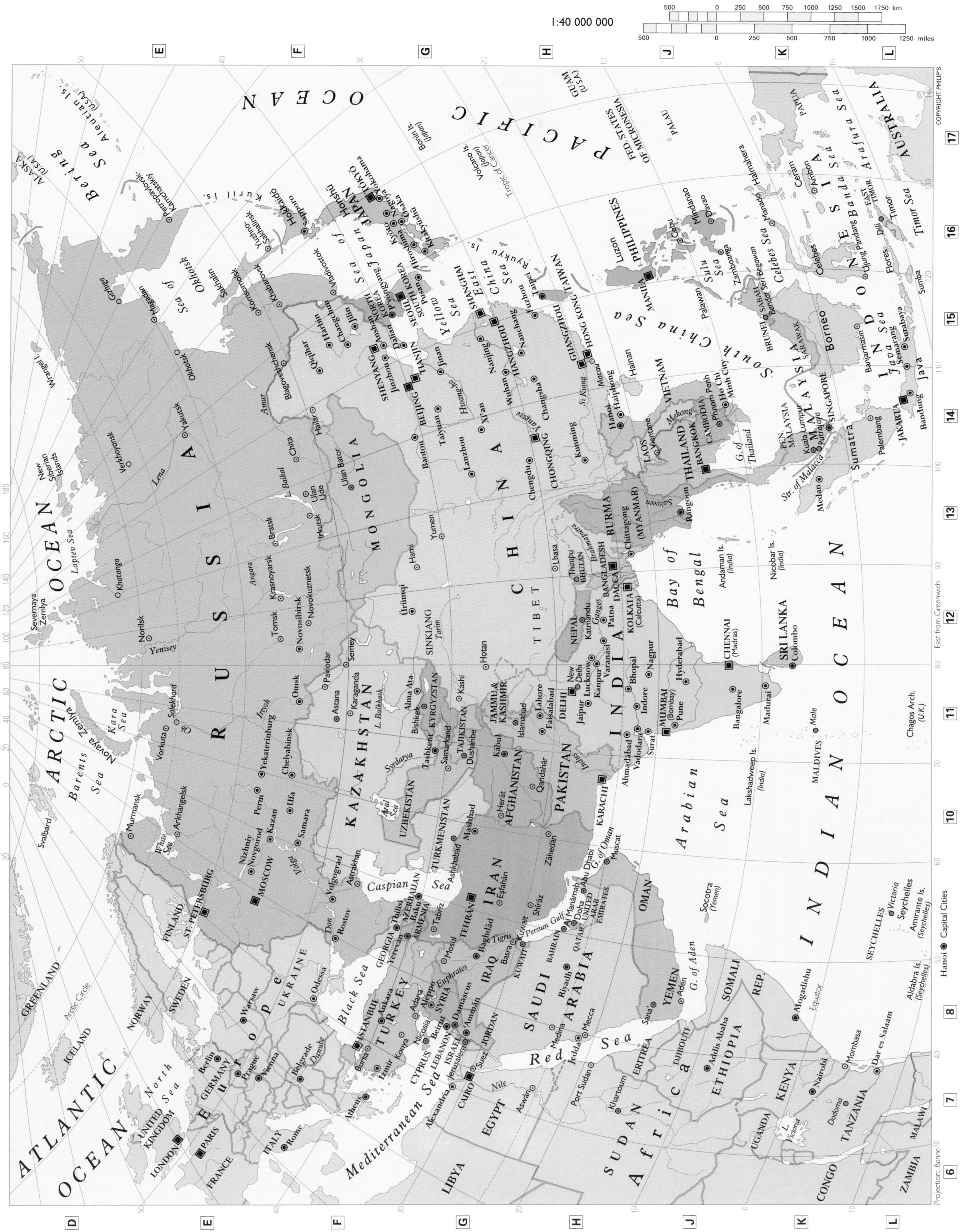

1:40 000 000

COPYRIGHT PHILIP'S

East from Greenwich

Projection: Bonne

Hanoi □ Capital Cities

50 25 0 25 50 75 100 125 150 175 km
50 0 25 50 75 100 125 miles

1:4 000 000

| 1 | 2 | 3 | 4 | 5 | 56 | 6 | 7 | 8 | 9 |

KOMI

Severnyye Uvaly

RUSSIA

Pinyug · Kazhim · Veslyana · Vishera · Gora Denezhkin Kamen 1493 · Kalya · Lozva

Murashi · Krasnoye · Nagorsk · Kay · Gayny · Kama · Cherdyn · Krasnovishersk · Pokrovsk-Uralskiy · 1065 · Severouralsk · Volchansk

Kirov · Slobodskoy · Belaya Kholunitsa · Peskovka · Chernaya Kholunitsa · Kosa · Kosa · Borovsk · 255 · Solikamsk · Usolye · Berezniki · 937 · Gora Konzhakovskiy Kamen 1569 · Karpinsk · Serov · Pelym

Yurya · Vyatka · Kirs · Kudymkar · Pozhva · Kamskoye Vdkhr. · Aleksandrovsk · Kizel · Gubakha 993 · Kachkanar · Lobva · Novaya Lyalya · Verkhoturye · Sosva

Khalturin · Novovyatsk · Zuyevka · Falenki · Yar · 337 · Chermoz · Dobryanka · Usva · Gremyachinsk · Pashiya · Verkhnyaya Tura · Krasnouralsk · Bolotovskoye

Kirovo-Chepetsk · Kumeny · Glazov · Vereshchagino · Krasnokamsk · Nytva · Ocher · Chusovaya · Chusovoy · Lysva · Kushva · Nizhnyaya Salda · Turinsk

Sorvizhi · 284 · Balezino · Kez · **PERM** · Sylva · 482 · **Nizhniy Tagil** 746 · Verkhnyaya Salda · Alapayevsk · Irbit · Nitsa

UDMURTIA · Igra · Zura · Kungur · Verkhniy Tagil · Nevyansk · Rezh · Artemovskiy · Troitskiy

MARI EL · Sovetsk · Nolinsk · Medvedok · Arkul · Kilmez · Uni · Yakshur Bodya · Votkinsk · Osa · 452 · Kuzino · Pervouralsk · Asbest · Sukhoy Log · Pyshma · Talitsa

Yoshkar Ola · Yaransk · Urzhum · Sernur · Kilmez · Uva · Izhevsk · Votkinskoye Vdkhr. · Achit · Nizhniye Sergi · Revda · **YEKATERINBURG** · Bogdanovich · Kamyshlov

Medvedevo · Sovetsk · Malmyzh · Mozhga · Chaykovskiy · Krasnoufimsk · Chernushka · Oktyabrskiy · Mikhaylovski · 678 · Polevskoy · Beloyarskiy · **Kamensk Uralskiy** · Dalmatovo

Mariinskiy Posad · Krasnogorskiy · Arsk · Sosnovka · Vyatskiye Polyany · Nizhnekamskoye Vdkhr. · Kambarka · Yanaul · Neftekamsk · Nyazepetrovsk · Verkhniy Ufaley · Sysert · Kataysk · Shadrinsk

Volzhsk · Zelenodolsk · Kukmor · Sarapul · Kama · 517 · Kasli · Techa

KAZAN · Mamadysh · Yelabuga · Menzelinsk · Belaya · Birsk · Krashyy Klyuch · Verkhniye Kigi · Kusa · Kyshtym · Argayash · Miass

Kozlovka · Kamskoye Ustye · **Naberezhnyye Chelny** · Nizhnekamsk · Ik · Dyurtyuli · Ufa · Karabash · **CHELYABINSK** · Kopeysk · Shchuchye · Shumikha

TATARSTAN · Chistopol · Zainsk · Aktash · Kushnarenkovo · Blagoveshchensk · Minyar · Yuryuzan · Satka · Berdyaush · **Zlatoust** · Miass · Novosineglazovskiy · Korkino

Buinsk · Tetyushi · Bilyarsk · Almetyevsk · Asha · Katav Ivanovsk · Bakal · 1406 · Chebarkul · Yemanzhelinsk

Bulgar · Kuybyshevskoye Vdkhr. · 23 · Leninogorsk · Bugulma · Tuymazy · **UFA** · Iglino · Chishmy · Gora Iremel 1582 · Yuzhnouralsk · Uvelskiy

Simbirsk · Cherdakly · Nurlat · Oktyabrskiy · Uchaly · Plast · Oktyabrskoye · Uy

Novoulyanovsk · Dimitrovgrad · Isakly · Belebey · 420 · Davlekanovo · Gora Yamantau 1638 · Tirlyanskiy · Stepnoye · **Troitsk**

Sengiley · 383 · Rayevskiy · Krasnousolskiy · Beloretsk · Verkhneuralsk · Buskul · Toguzak · Komsomolets

Novodevichye · Togliatti · Krasnyy Yar · Sernovodsk · Priyutovo · **BASHKORTOSTAN** · Petrovskoye · Verkhniy Avzyan 1118 · **Magnitogorsk** · Varna

Zhigulevsk · 375 · Timashevo · Bug'uruslan · Abdulino · **Sterlitamak** · Ishimbay · 1039 · 452 · Kartaly · Rudnyy

Oktyabrsk · Kinel · Otradnyy · Krotovka · Ponomarevka · 481 · Salavat · Verkhniy Avzyan · Sibay · 758 · Kizilskoye · Tobol

Syzran · **SAMARA** · Novokuybyshevsk · Meleuz · 659 · Baymak · Ordzhonikidze · Lisakovsk

Kashpirovka · Chapayevsk · Buzuluk · Grachevka · Kumertau · Submar · Bredy · Zhetiqara

PRIVOLZHSKIY · Pestravka · Alekseyevka · Totskoye · Sorochinsk · Bulanovo · Tyulgan · Chernyy Otrog · Iriklinskoye Vdkhr. · 414 · Zhailma

Pugachev · Bolshaya Glushitsa · Andreyevka · 405 · Obshchi · Syrt · Orenburg · Saraktash · Krasnoyarskiy · Yelizavetinka · Ozërnyy

Ozinki · Ozernoye · Novo-Sergiyevskiy · Perevolotskiy · **Ural** · Pervomayskiy · Energetik · Adamovka · Svetlyy

Darinskoye · Burli · Ilek · Krasnyy Kholm · Kuvandyk · Gay · Novoorsk · 418 · Kumak · Ozërnyy

Oral · Zhayyq · Kamenka · Aksay · Sol Iletsk · Iriklinskiy · Mednogorsk · **Orsk** · Yasnyy · Dombarovskiy

Novotroitsk · Chingirlau · Ilek · Akbulak · Martuk · Leninskoye 509 · Aktasty

Vladimirovka · Ozero Shalkar · Shalkar · Ureya · Bolshaya Khobda · Novoalekseyevka · Alga · Khromtau · Qarabutak · Turgayskaya Stolovaya Strana

KAZAKHSTAN · Chapayev · Dzhambeyty · **Aqtöbe** · Novorossiyskoye · Zhabasak

Kirgiziya Steppe · Furmanovo · Karsha · Karatobe · Oktyabrsk · Irtis

Mugodzhary

G

ft m
3000 1000
1500 500
600 200
50
0 0

1:4 000 000

50 0 25 50 75 100 125 150 175 km
50 0 25 50 75 100 125 miles

COPYRIGHT PHILIP'S

Projection: Conical with two standard parallels

East from Greenwich

K A Z A K H S T A N

K Y R G Y Z S T A N

U Z B E K I S T A N

T A J I K I S T A N

T U R K M E N I S T A N

A F G H A N I S T A N

C H I N A

XINJIANG UYGUR ZIZHIQU

ALMATY (Alma Ata)

Bishkek (Frunze)

TOSHKENT (Tashkent)

Dushanbe

Shymkent (Chimkent)

Taraz (Dzhambul)

Qyzylorda

Samarqand

Bukhoro

Qarshi

Nawoiy

Jizzakh

Namangan

Andijon

Farghona

Quqon (Kokand)

Khujand

Osh

Kashi (Kashgar)

Shache (Yarkand)

Mazar-e Sharif

Balkh

Qonduz

Termiz

Nurata Tizmasi

Peski Taukum

K y z y l K u m

Peski Muyunkum

Qaratau (Karatau)

Kirghiz Range

Talas Ala Too

Küngöy Ala Too

Terskey Ala Too

Ysyk-Köl (Issyk-Kul) 1609

Fergana Range

Moldo Too

Alai Range

Turkestan Range

Khrebet Zeravshanskiy

Khrebet Gissarskiy

Gorno-Badakhshan

Pamir

Sarykolskiy Khrebet

Zaalayskiy Khrebet

Pik Lenina 7134

Pik Revolyutsii 6974

Hindu Kush

Karakoram Range

Kunlun Shan

Syrdarya

Amudarya

Balqash Köl

Ozero Aydarkul

Step Sharidara

Dolina Farghonskaya

Mingteke Daban (Mintaka Pass)

Khunjerab Pass

Kongur Shan 7719

Muztagh-Ata 7546

6300

Chärjew (Chardzhou)

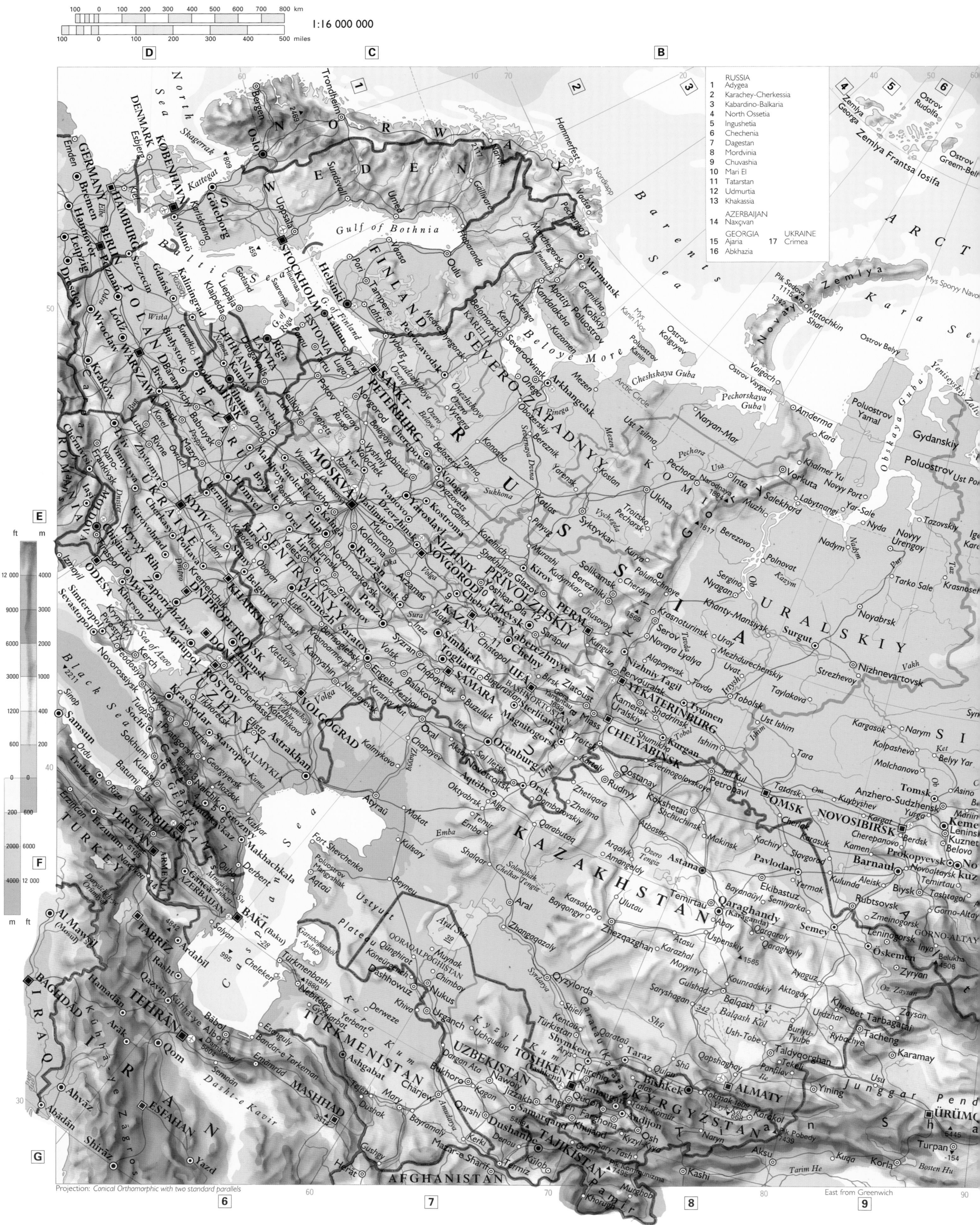

100 0 100 200 300 400 500 600 700 800 km

100 0 100 200 300 400 500 miles

1:16 000 000

Projection: Conical Orthomorphic with two standard parallels

East from Greenwich

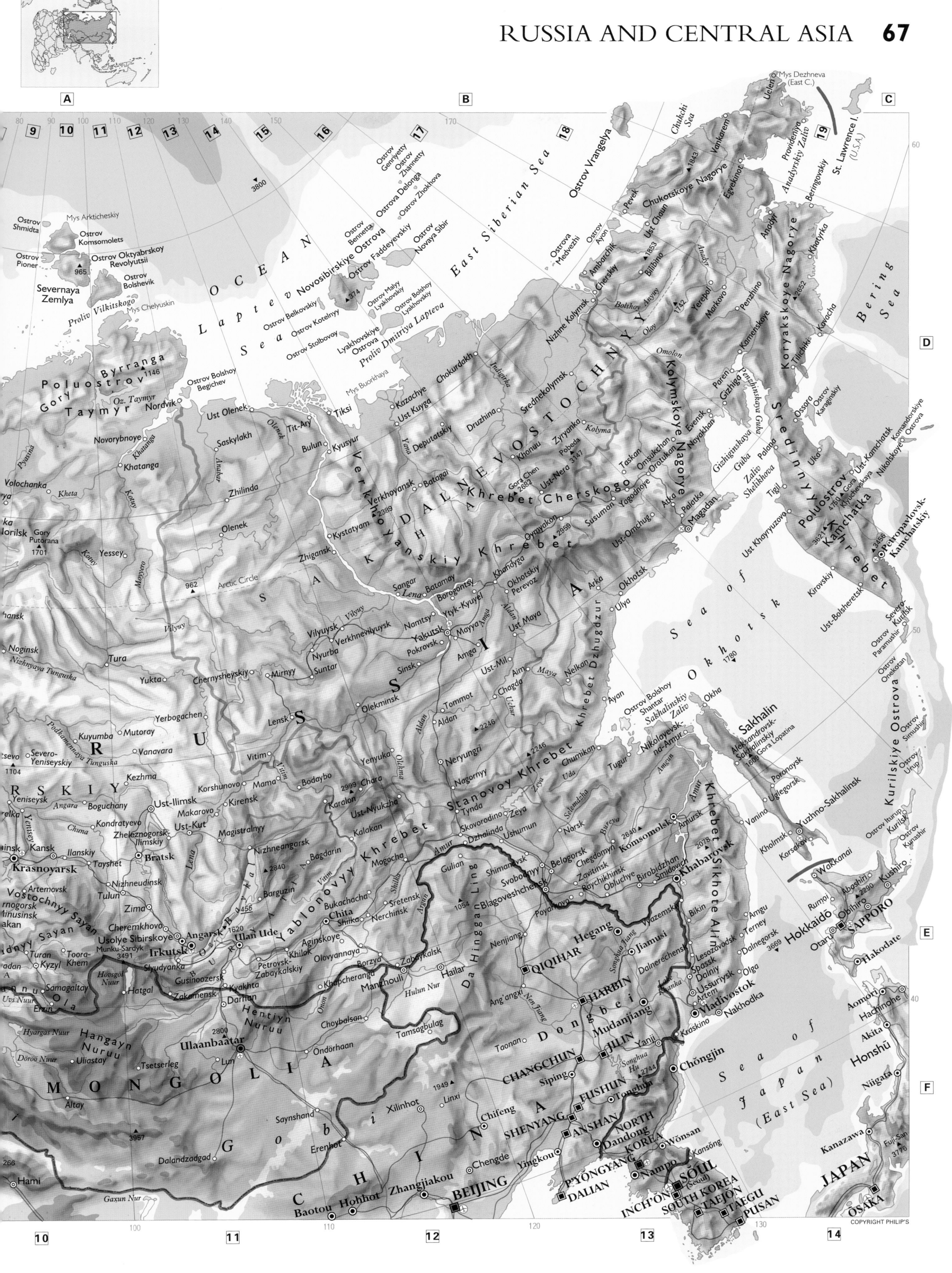

A B C

9 10 11 12 13 14 15 16 17 18 19

D

E

F

10 100 11 110 12 120 13 14 130

COPYRIGHT PHILIP'S

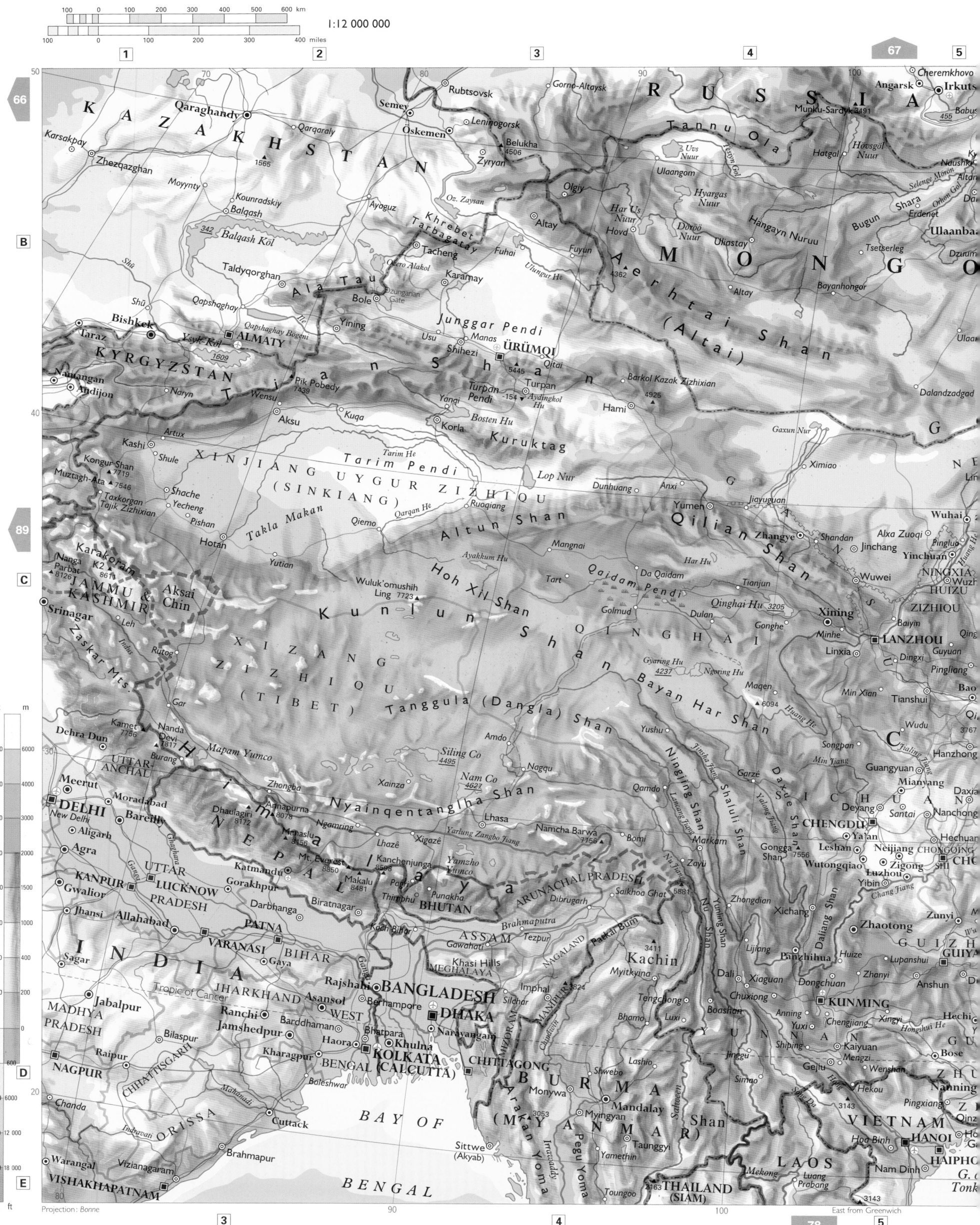

Projection: Bonne

East from Greenwich

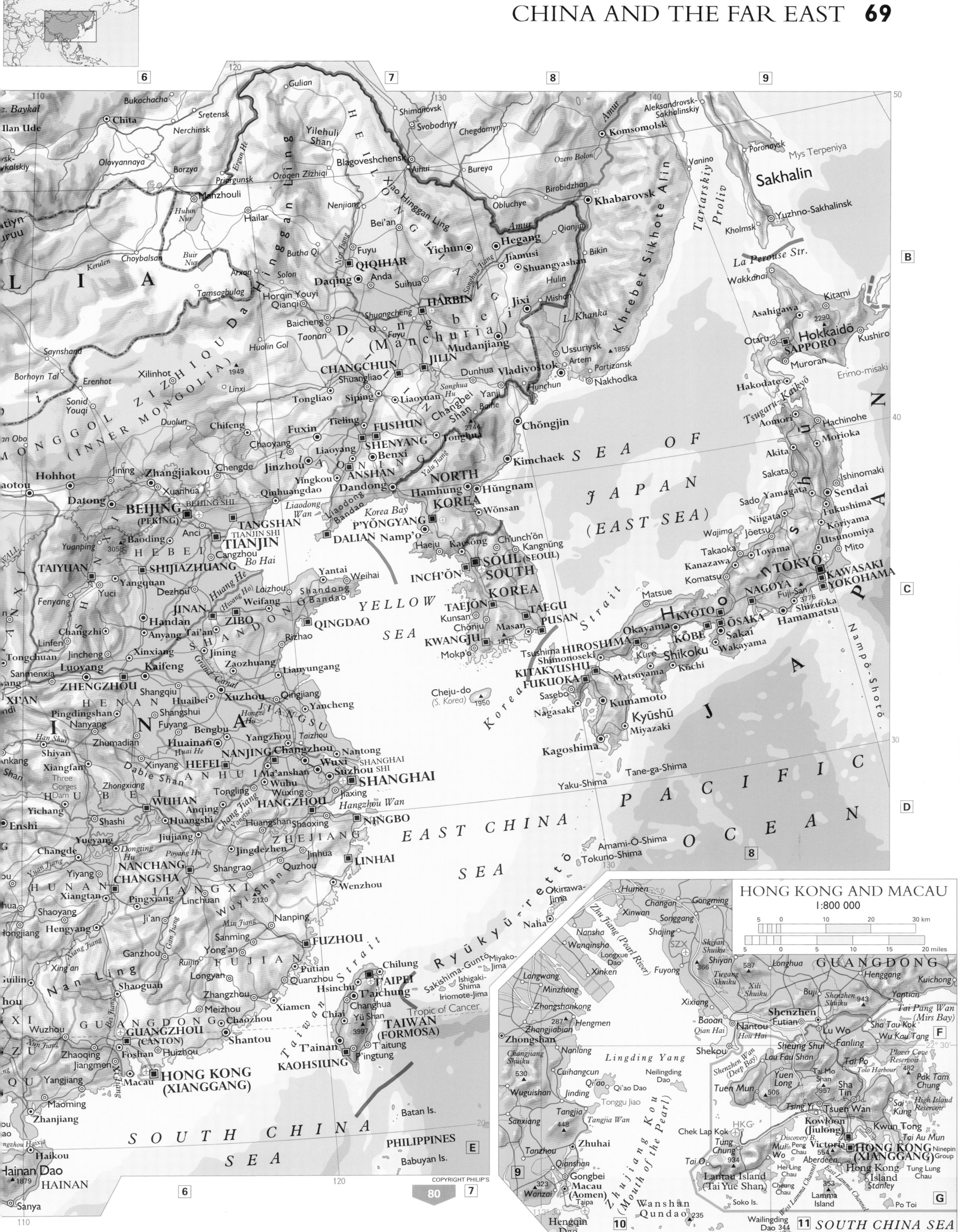

HONG KONG AND MACAU
1:800 000

SOUTH CHINA SEA

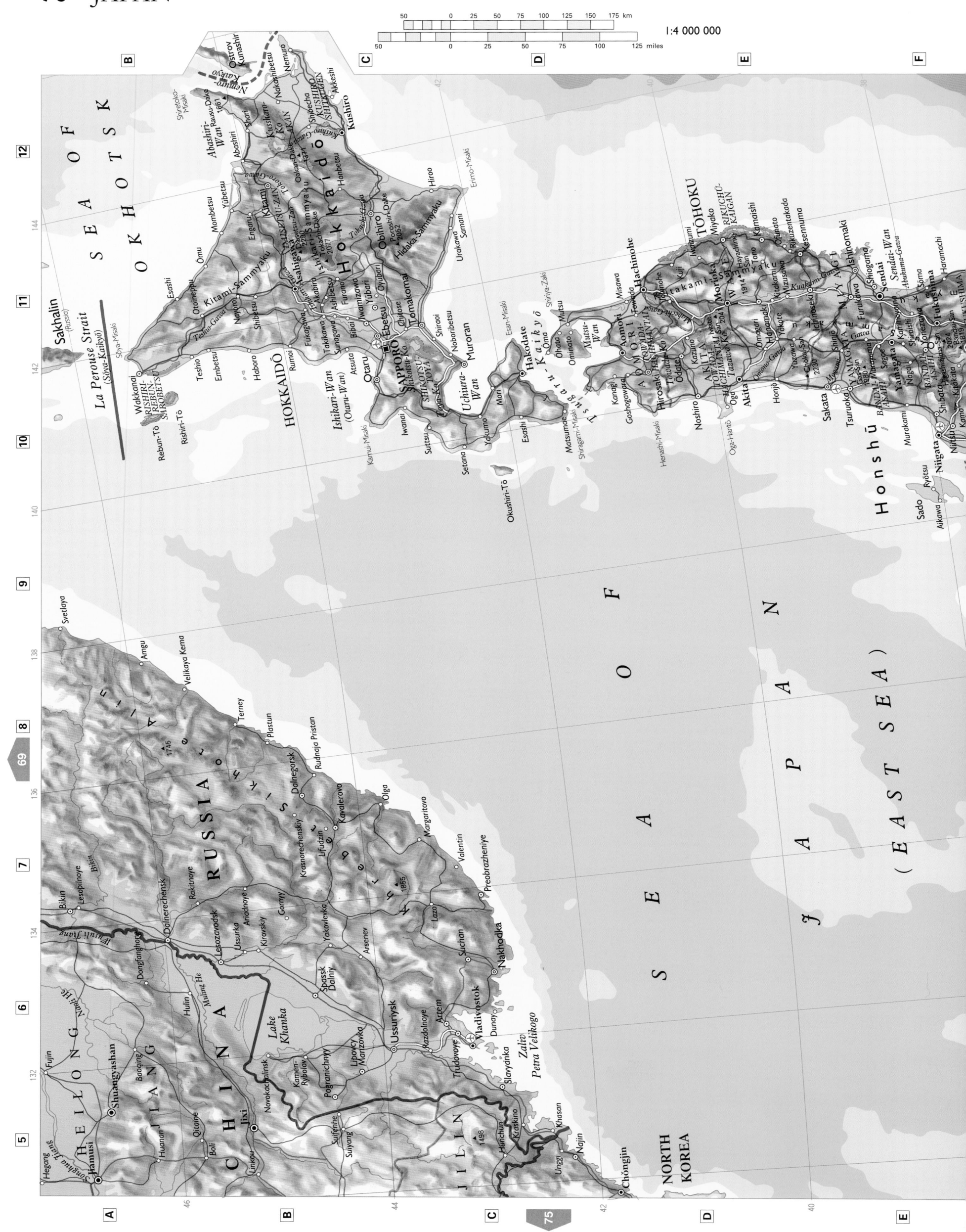

50 0 25 50 75 100 125 150 175 km
50 0 25 50 75 100 125 miles

1:4 000 000

SEA OF OKHOTSK

Sakhalin (Rossiya)

La Perouse Strait (Soya-Kaikyō)

HOKKAIDŌ

Ostrov Kunashir

Nemuro Kaikyō

SAPPORO

Hakodate

Tsugaru-Kaikyō

RUSSIA

S i k h o t e - A l i n

Svetlaya

Amgu

Terney

Plastun

Dalnegorsk

Olga

Kavalerovo

Preobrazheniye

Valentin

Nakhodka

Vladivostok

Ussuriysk

Lake Khanka

CHINA

HEILONGJIANG

JILIN

NORTH KOREA

Chŏngjin

Zaliv Petra Velikogo

SEA OF JAPAN (EAST SEA)

TŌHOKU

Honshū

AOMORI

AKITA

Aomori

Hachinohe

Akita

Sendai

Niigata

Sado

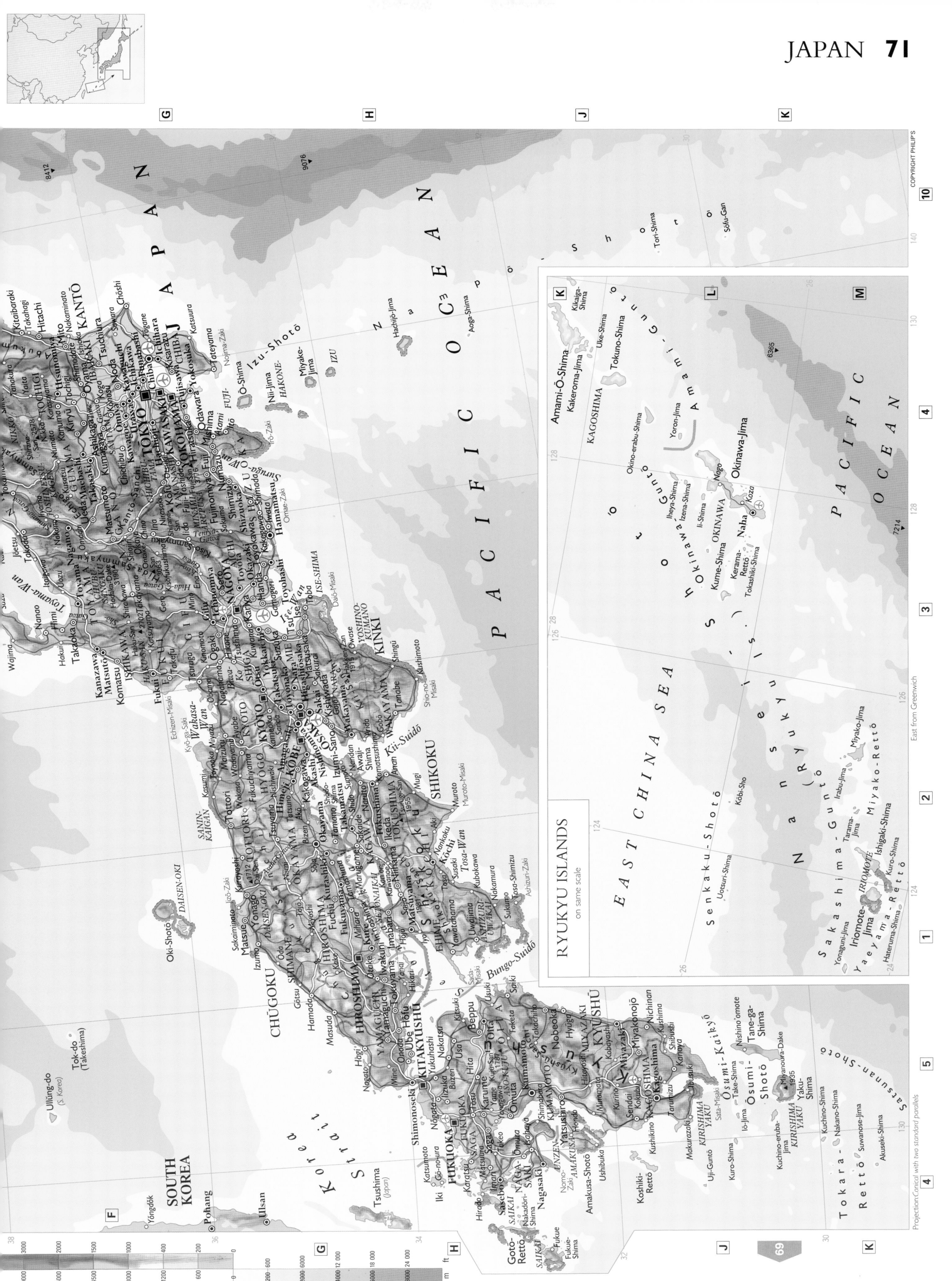

RYUKYU ISLANDS
on same scale

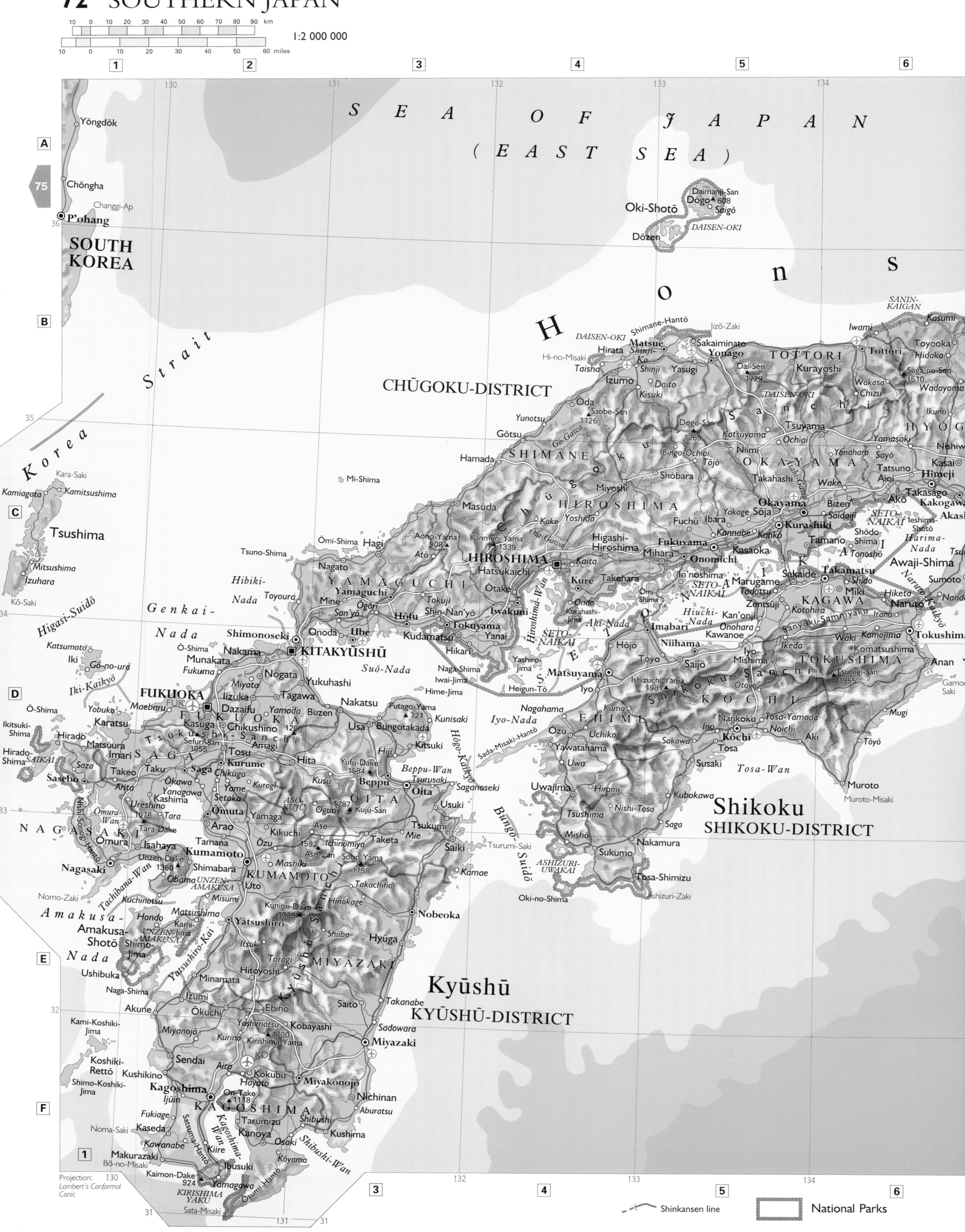

1:2 000 000

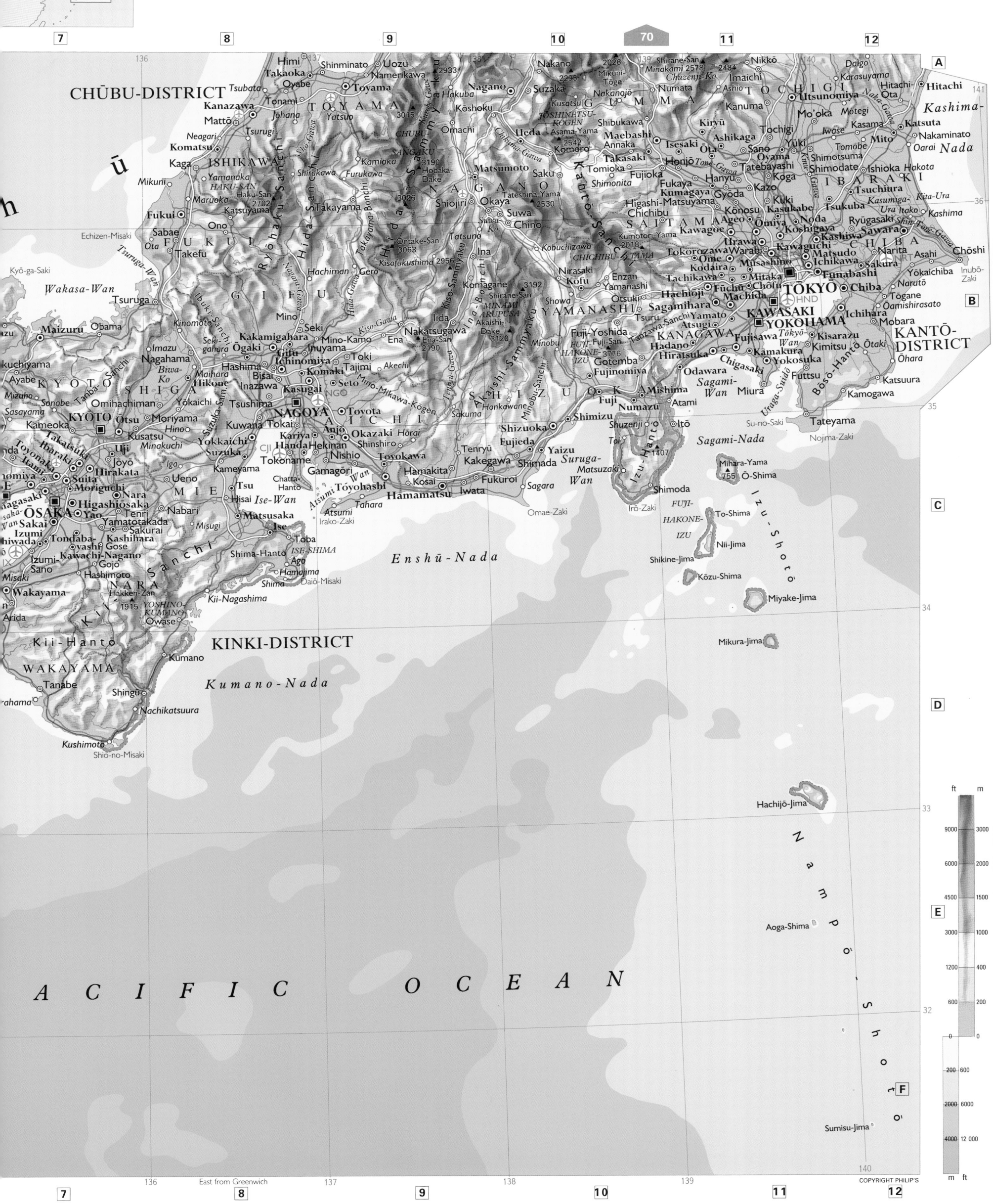

CHŪBU-DISTRICT

Himi
Takaoka
Shinminato
Uozu
Namerikawa
Nakano
Nikkō
Daigo
Karasuyama
Hitachi-Ota
Hitachi
Kashima-Nada

Tsubata
Toyama
TOYAMA
2933
Hakuba
Nagano
Suzaka
Minakami 2578
Imaichi

Kanazawa
Oyabe
Tonami
Yatsuo
Koshoku
Ueda
Asama-Yama
Numata
Chuzenji-Ko
Utsunomiya
Kanuma
TOCHIGI

Mattō
Johana
Tsurugi
Omachi
Kusatsu
YOSHINETSU-KOGEN
Shibukawa
Kiryū
Mo'oka
Kasama
Katsuta

Neagari
Kaga
Shirakawa
Kamioka
Ina
Maebashi
Annaka
Ashikaga
Sano
Oyama
Mito
Nakaminato
Oarai Nada

Komatsu
ISHIKAWA
Furukawa
Matsumoto
Saku
Tomioka
Takasaki
Honjō
Isesaki
Ōta
Tatebayashi
Koga
IBARAKI
Tsuchiura
Kashima

Fukui
FUKUI
Takayama
Shiojiri
Okaya
Suwa
Chino
SAITAMA
Kawagoe
Omiya
Noda
Kasukabe
Tsukuba
Itako

Osaka
NAGOYA
Toyota
Hamamatsu
TOKYO
KAWASAKI
YOKOHAMA
Chiba

NAGOYA

A C I F I C   O C E A N

KINKI-DISTRICT

Kumano-Nada

Enshū-Nada

Kii-Hantō

WAKAYAMA

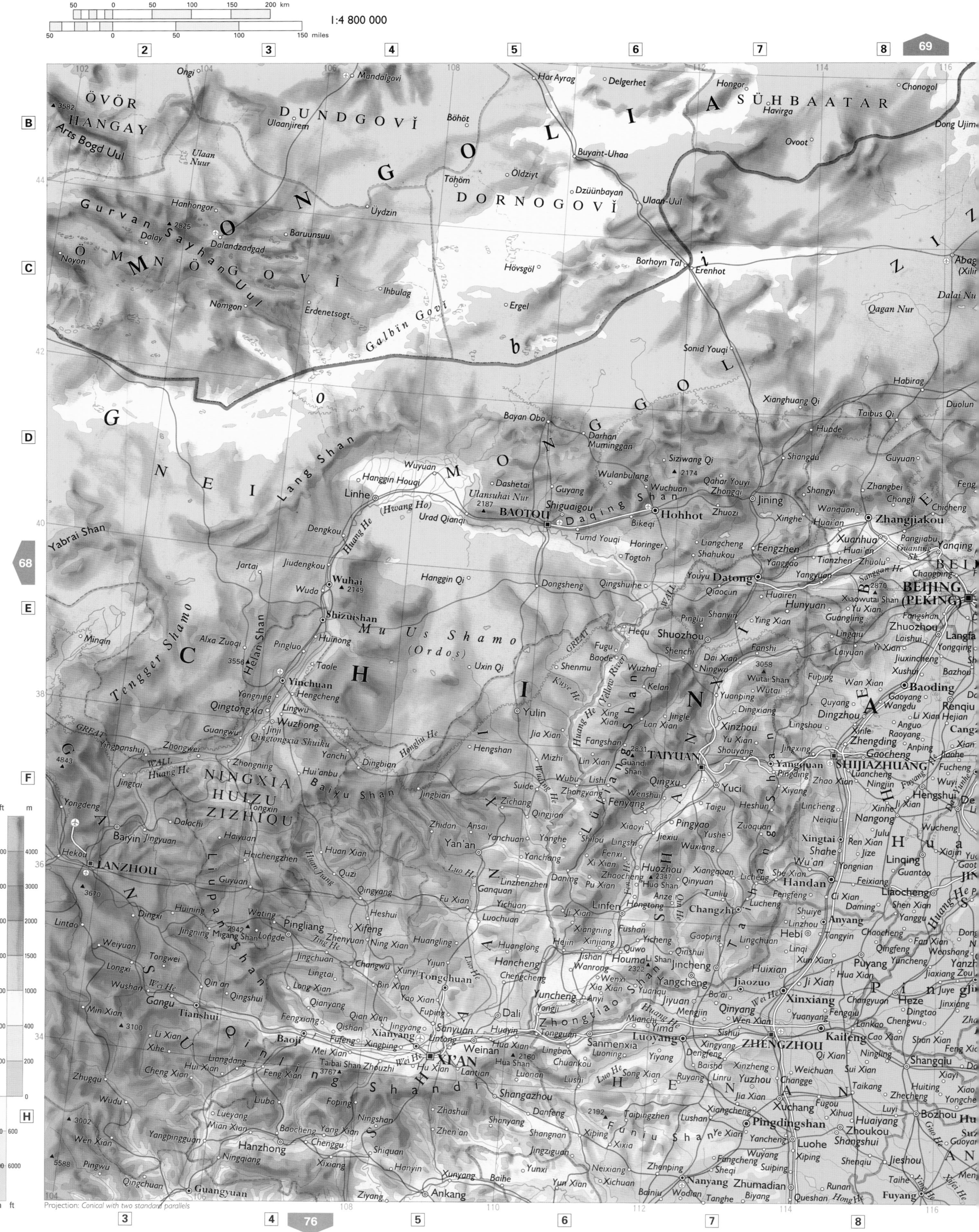

50 0 50 100 150 200 km
50 0 50 100 150 miles
1:4 800 000

68

Projection: Conical with two standard parallels

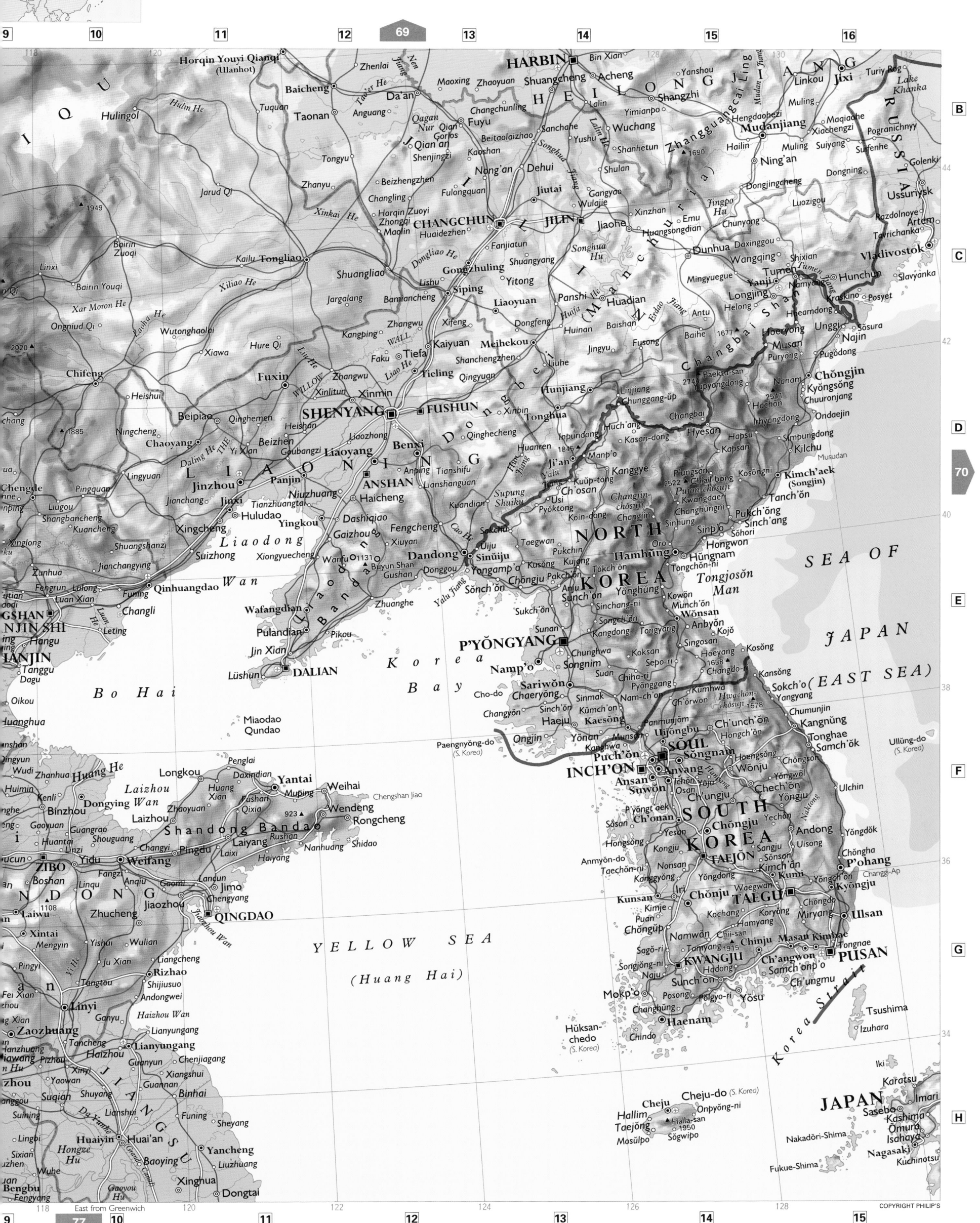

HARBIN

HEILONGJIANG

B

Horqin Youyi Qianqi
(Ulanhot)

Zhenlai
Maoxing Zhaoyuan Shuangcheng Acheng
Bin Xian
Yanshou
Linkou Jixi
Turiy Rog
Lake Khanka

Baicheng
Da'an
Tuquan
Taonan
Anguang
Fuyu
Changchunling
Yimianpo
Shangzhi
Muling
Hengdaohezi
Mudanjiang
Maqiaohe
Xiachengzi
Pogranichnyy

Hulingol
Hulin He

Nen Jiang

Taoer He

Qagan Nur Qian Gorlos
Beitaolaizhao
Sanchahe
Yushu
Wuchang
Shanhetun
Hailin
Suiyang

RUSSIA

Qian'an
Shenjingzi
Kaoshan
Songhua
Shulan
Ning'an
Dongning
Surfenhe
Golenki

Jarud Qi
Tongyu
Beizhengzhen
Changling
Dehui
Gangyao
Wulajie

Dongjingcheng
Luozigou

Razdolnoye
Ussuriysk

44

Xinkai He
Nong'an
Fulongquan

Horqin Zuoyi Zhongqi Maolin
Huaidezhen

CHANGCHUN
Jiutai

JILIN
Jiaohe
Xinzhan
Emu
Huangsongdian
Chunyang

Dunhua Daxinggou
Wangqing
Shixian
Mingyuegou

Yanji
Tumen
Hunchun

Vladivostok
Slavyanka

C

Jarud Qi

Tongliao

Kailu

Shuangliao
Lishu

Gongzhuling
Yitong

Dongliao He
Shuangyang
Panshi

Songhua Hu
Huadian

Longjing
Helong
Antu
Kraskino
Posyet

Xar Moron He
Jargalang
Bamiancheng
Siping
Liaoyuan
Xifeng
Dongfeng
Huinan
Baishan

Erdao Jiang

Puryong

Hoeryong
Namyang

Yongamdong

Sösura

42

Chifeng
Heishui

Kangping
Zhangwu

Meihekou
Huajia
Jingyu
Fusong

Baihe
1677

Musan
Pugdong
Najin

Beipiao
Qinghemen

Faku
Tiefa

Kaiyuan
Shanchengzhen
Liuhe
Hunjiang

Changbai
Hyesan
Paekdu-san
2744

Nanam
Chŏngjin
Kyŏngsŏng
Chuuronjang

D

Bairin Zuoqi
1949

Xinlitun

Tieling
Qingyuan

Linjiang
Chunggang-ŭp

Hŭch'ang
2541
Hŭchŏn
Nhyangdong
Ondaejin

70

Xiawa

Fuxin

Xinmin

Tonghua
Xinbin

Inpundong
Kasan-dong

Kilchu

Huren Qi

2020

Linxi
Qi

Chengle
nne

Chaoyang

1885

Ningcheng

SHENYANG
Heishan

FUSHUN

Donabei Dongbei

Hun Jiang
Huanren
1846

Ji'an
Manp'o

P'ungsan
2522 Chail-bong
Pujŏn-chŏsuji

Kosŏngni

Kanggye
Kŭup-tong

Ch'osan
Usi
Pyŏktong

Koin-dong

Changjin-chŏsuji
Changjin

Kimch'aek
(Songjin)

Tanch'ŏn

Musudan

Guangde

Pingquan
Liugou

Liaozhong

Qinghecheng

Changbai Shan

Hamhŭng

E

Shangbancheng
Kuancheng

Jinzhou
Beizhen
Goubangzi

Liaoyang
Benxi

Anping
Tianshifu
Lianshanguan

Kuandian

Koin-dong

Pyŏngyang
Sinŭng

Sinp'o
Sŏhori

Hongwon

Tongjosŏn Man

SEA OF

Jianchang
Jinxi

Tianzhuangtai
ANSHAN

Haicheng

Supung Shuiku

Taegwan

Pukch'in

Pukch'ŏng

Sinch'ang

Chengde

Jinzhou
Panjin

Niuzhuang

Sakchu
Ŭiju

Pyŏktong

Tŏkch'ŏn

Oro

Hŭngnam

SEA OF

40

Daling He

Yi Xian

Yingkou
Dashiqiao

Fengcheng
Xiuyan

Cao He

Dandong **Sinŭiju**
Yongamp'o

Kusŏng
Chŏngju Pakch'ŏn
Anju

Sunan

Tŏkch'ŏn

Tongch'ŏn-ni

Yŏnghŭng

KOREA

JAPAN

Xingcheng
Suizhong

Huludao
Gaizhou

Gushan

Donggou

Yalu Jiang
Sŏnch'ŏn

Amju
Sunch'ŏn

Sinchang-ni
Songch'ŏn

Wŏnsan

Munch'ŏn
Anbyŏn

E

Zunhua
Fengrun
Luan Xian

Qinhuangdao
Wafangdian

Wanfu 1131

Zhuanghe

Bryun Shan

Yŏngbyŏn

Tongnae

Sukch'ŏn

Sinanju

Tongyang
Kangdong
Yangdŏk

Koksan

Kowŏn

Munch'ŏn

GSHAN

NJIN SHI
Hangu

Changli
Leting

Liaodong Bandao

Pikou

Pulandian

Korea Bay

P'YŎNGYANG
Chunghwa

Namp'o
Songnim

Suan
Chiha-ri
Sepo-ri

Pyŏnggang

Hoeyang
1638

Changdo-ri
Kansŏng

Sokch'o
Yangyang

(**EAST SEA**)

38

IANJIN
Tanggu

Jin Xian

Lüshun
DALIAN

Cho-do
Chaeryŏng

Sariwŏn

Sinmak
Kŭmch'ŏn

Nam-ch'ŏn

Ch'ŏrwon
Kumhwa

Hyan-hon chŏsuji
1678

Chumunjin

Tanggu
Dagu
Oikou

Bo Hai

Miaodao
Qundao

Changyŏn
Ongjin

Haeju
Kaesŏng

Panmunjŏm
Uijŏngbu

Yangyang
Ch'unch'ŏn
Hongch'ŏn

Kangnŭng

Huanghua

Paengnyŏng-do
(S. Korea)

Yŏnan
Kanghwa

SŎUL Sŏngnam
Tonghae Samch'ŏk

INCH'ŏN **Puch'ŏn**
Anyang

Tchon-yaju
 Hongsŏng

Ullŭng-do
(S. Korea)

F

Jingyun
Wudi

Binzhou

Longkou
Penglai

Daxindian

Fushan

Chengshan Jiao

Ansan
Suwŏn

Osan
Ch'unju

Wŏnju

P'yŏng-t'aek
Ch'onan

Sŏsan

Yongwŏl
Chŏngsŏn

Ulchin

Zhanhua

Huang He

Laizhou Wan

Laizhou Wan

Huang Xian

Zhaoyuan

Yantai
Muping

Weihai

923

Wendeng

Chŏnju

SOUTH

Yŏngju

Dongying

Dongying Wan

Shouguang
Guangrao

Changyi

Laizhou
Pingdu

Laixi

Nanhuang
Shidao

Rongcheng

P'yŏng-t'aek

Ch'onan

Hongsŏng

Chŏngju

Kongju

Taejŏn

KOREA
Yech'ŏn

Sangju

Andong

Yŏngdŏk

Linzi
Huantai

Zibo
Boshan

Linqu
Anqiu

Gaomi

Jiaozhou
Chengyang

Jimo

Haiyang

Anmyŏn-do

Taech'ŏn-ni

Nonsan

Yŏngdong

Kimch'ŏn
Kumi

Taegu

Chŏngdo

P'ohang

Changgi-Ap

36

ZIBO

Laiwu

1108

Zhucheng

Jiaozhou Wan

QINGDAO

Kanggyŏng

Iri

Yesan

Kongju
Chŏngŭp

Puan

Puyŏ

Kimje

Nonsan

Yŏngdong

Koryŏng
Hamyang

Kochang

CHŎNJU

Miryang

Ulsan

Yŏngch'ŏn
Kyŏngju

NDONG

Xintai
Mengyin

Yishui
Wulian

Liangcheng

Pingyi

Kunsan

Sago-ri

Namwŏn
Chiri-san
1915

Chinju
Masan Kimhae

Tongnae

Ji Xian
Fei Xian

Rizhao
Shijiusuo

Andongwei

Sunch'ŏn

Songjong-ni

Tanyang

KWANGJU
Hddong

Ch'angwon
Samch'onp'o

PUSAN

YELLOW SEA

Xian

Linyi

Tangtou

Ganyu

Haizhou Wan

Songjiong-ni
Naju

Posong

Polgyo-ri

Yŏsu

Ch'ungmu

Korea Strait

Tsushima

G

Zaozhuang
Tancheng

Pizhou
Xinyi

Lianyungang

Haizhou

Guanyun

Chenjiagang

Hŭksan-chedo
(S. Korea)

Mokp'o

Chindo

Changhŭng
Haenam

Izuhara

34

Yaowan

Shuyang

Xiangshui

Binhai

Guannan

JIANGSU

Sixian
zhen

Suqian

Hongze Hu

Lianshui

Funing

Sheyang

Cheju Cheju-do (S. Korea)
Hallim Onpyŏng-ni

Iki
Karatsu

JAPAN
Sasebo
Imari

H

Lingbi

Bengbu
Fengyang

Grand Canal

Huai'an
Baoying

Yancheng

Liuzhuang

Taejŏng

Hallim
Mosulpo

Halla-san
1950
Sŏgwipo

Nakadōri-Shima

Ōmura
Isahaya

Kashima

Nagasaki
Kuchinotsu

Fukue-Shima

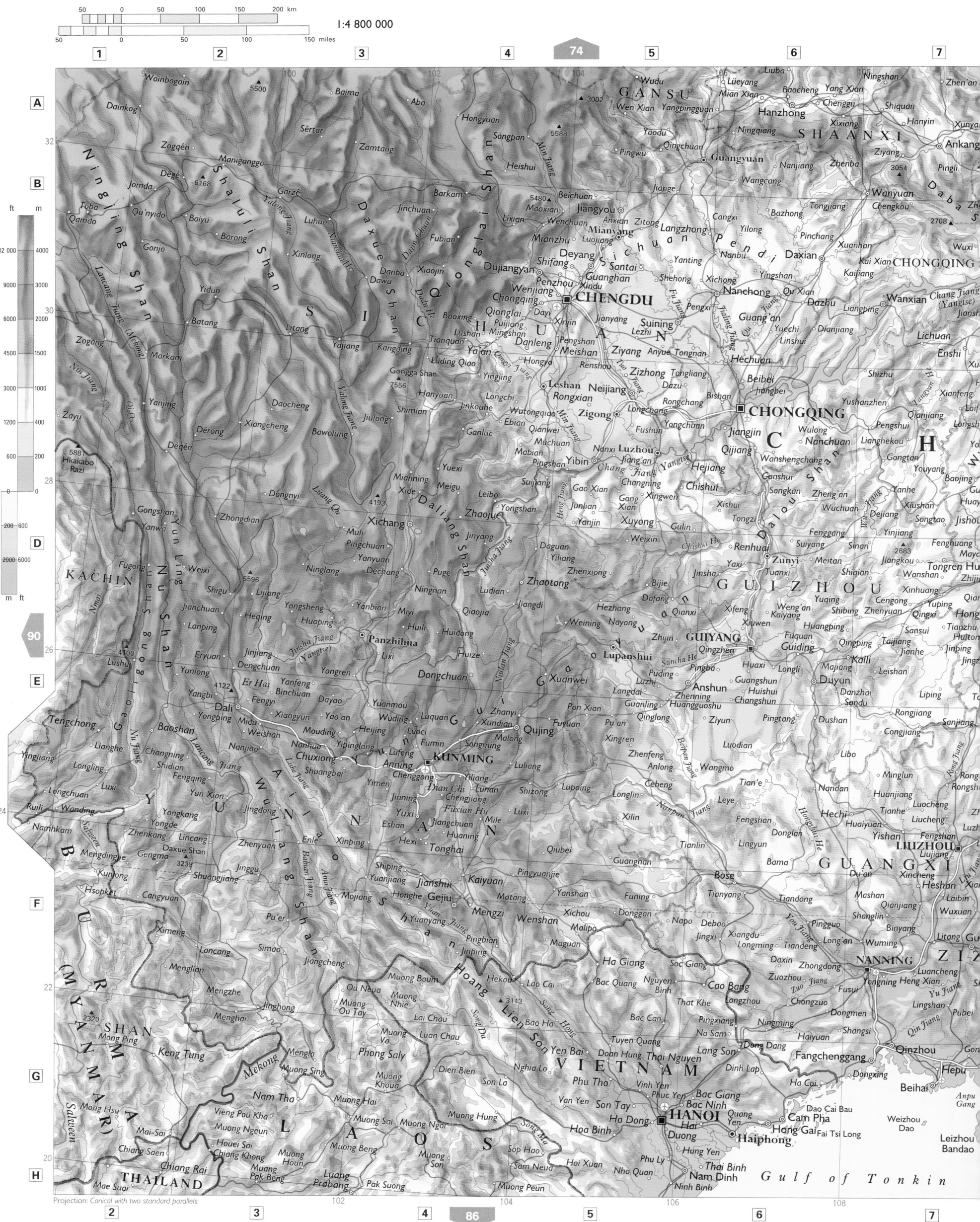

Projection: Conical with two standard parallels

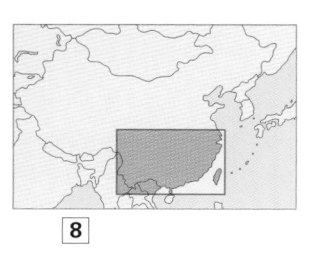

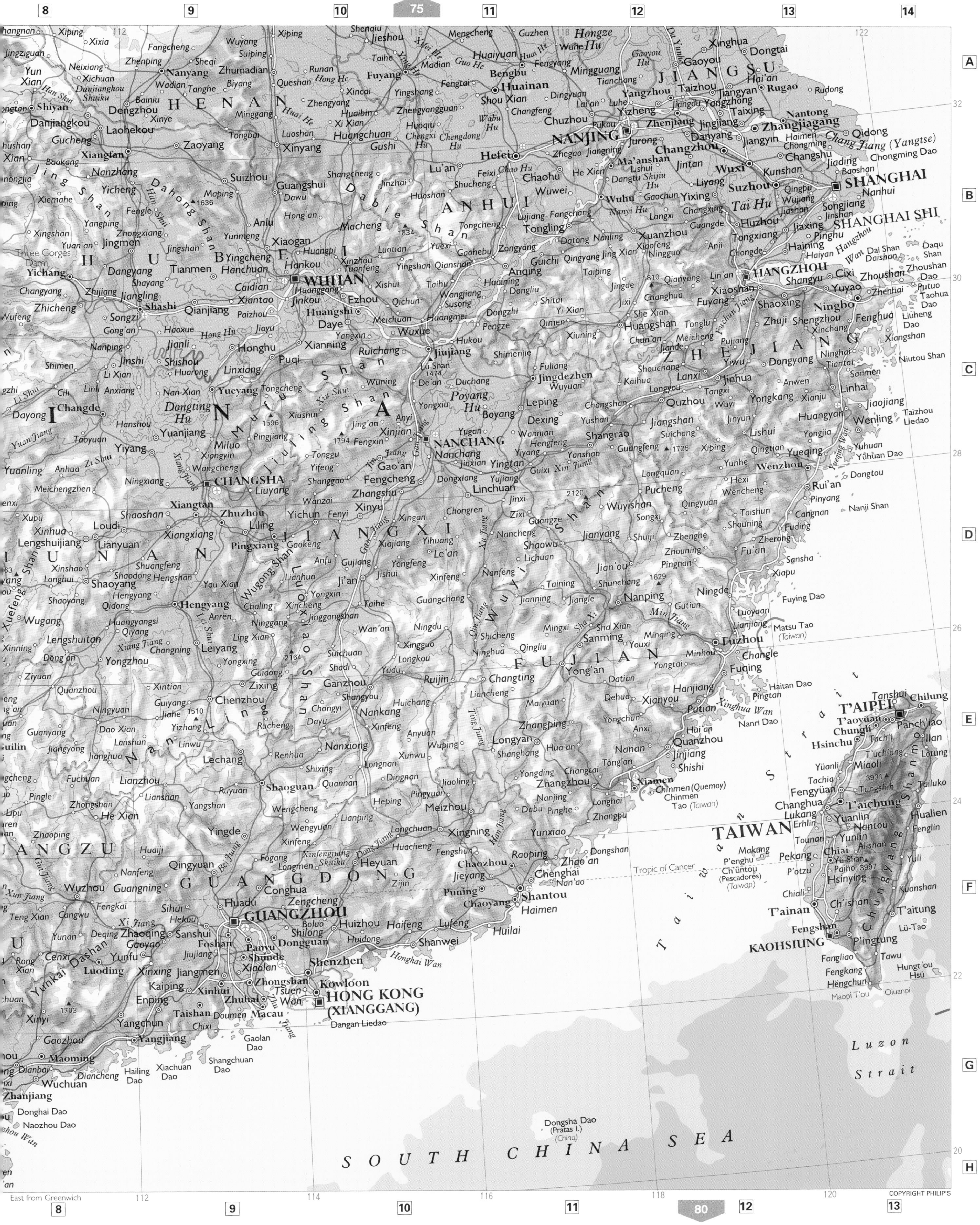

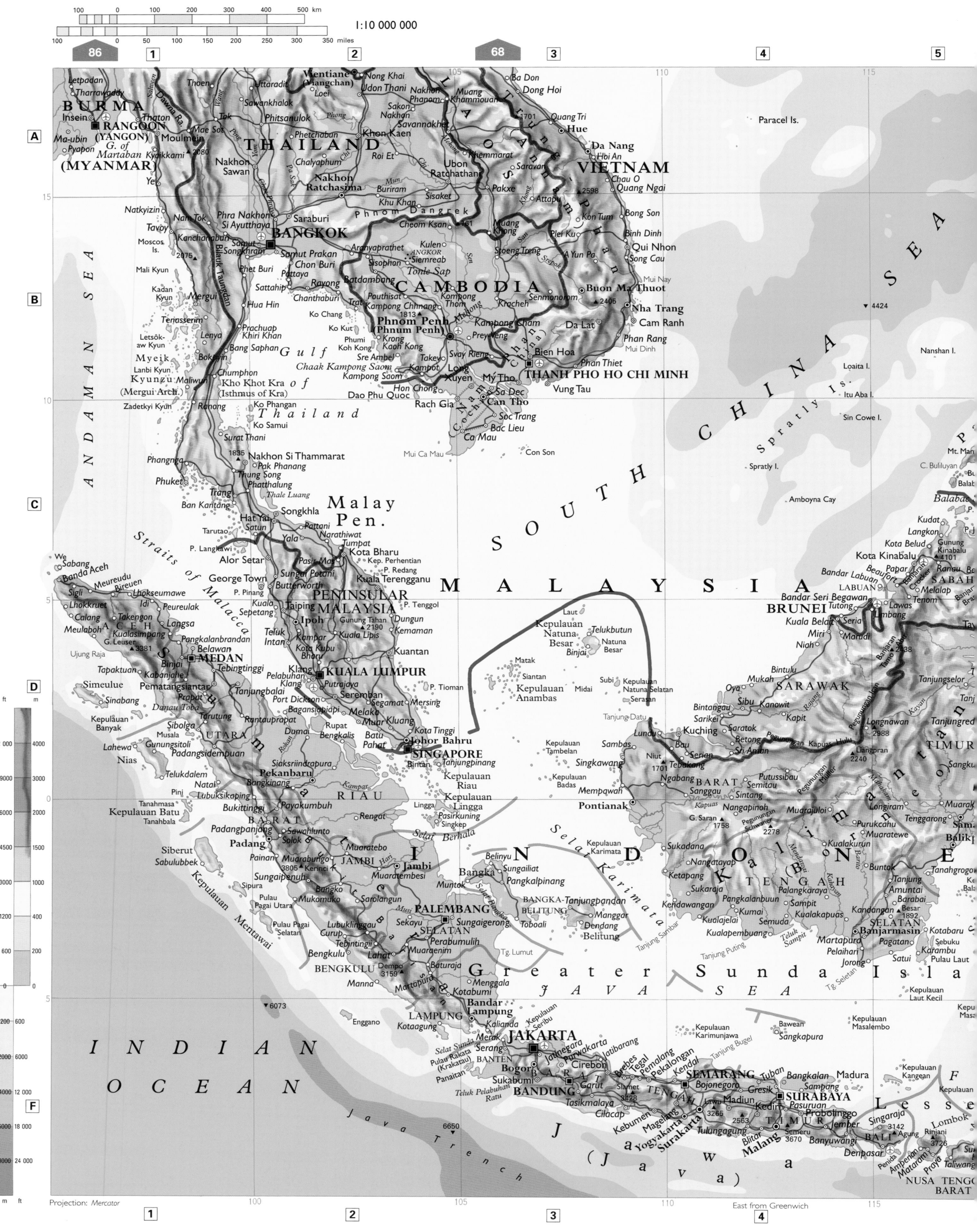

JAVA AND MADURA
1:6 000 000

50   0   50   100   150   200   250   300 km
50   0   50   100   150   200 miles

BALI
1:1 600 000

10   0   10   20   30 km
10   0   10   20 miles

PACIFIC OCEAN

INDIAN OCEAN

CELEBES SEA

CELEBES SEA

ARAFURA SEA

BANDA SEA

Major labels

MANILA, Quezon City, Luzon, Cebu, Bacolod, Iloilo, Davao, General Santos, Zamboanga, Mindanao, Cagayan de Oro, Manado, Gorontalo, Sulawesi (Celebes), Halmahera, Ternate, Tidore, Buru, Seram (Ceram), Ambon, Papua, Pegunungan Maoke, Pegunungan Van Rees, Jayapura, Sentani, PAPUA NEW GUINEA, Merauke, EAST TIMOR, Flores, Sumba, NUSA TENGGARA TIMUR, Kupang

JAKARTA, Bogor, BANDUNG, SEMARANG, SURABAYA, Surakarta, Yogyakarta, Malang, Madura, Jawa, Bali, Denpasar, Lombok, Mataram, Singaraja

COPYRIGHT PHILIP'S

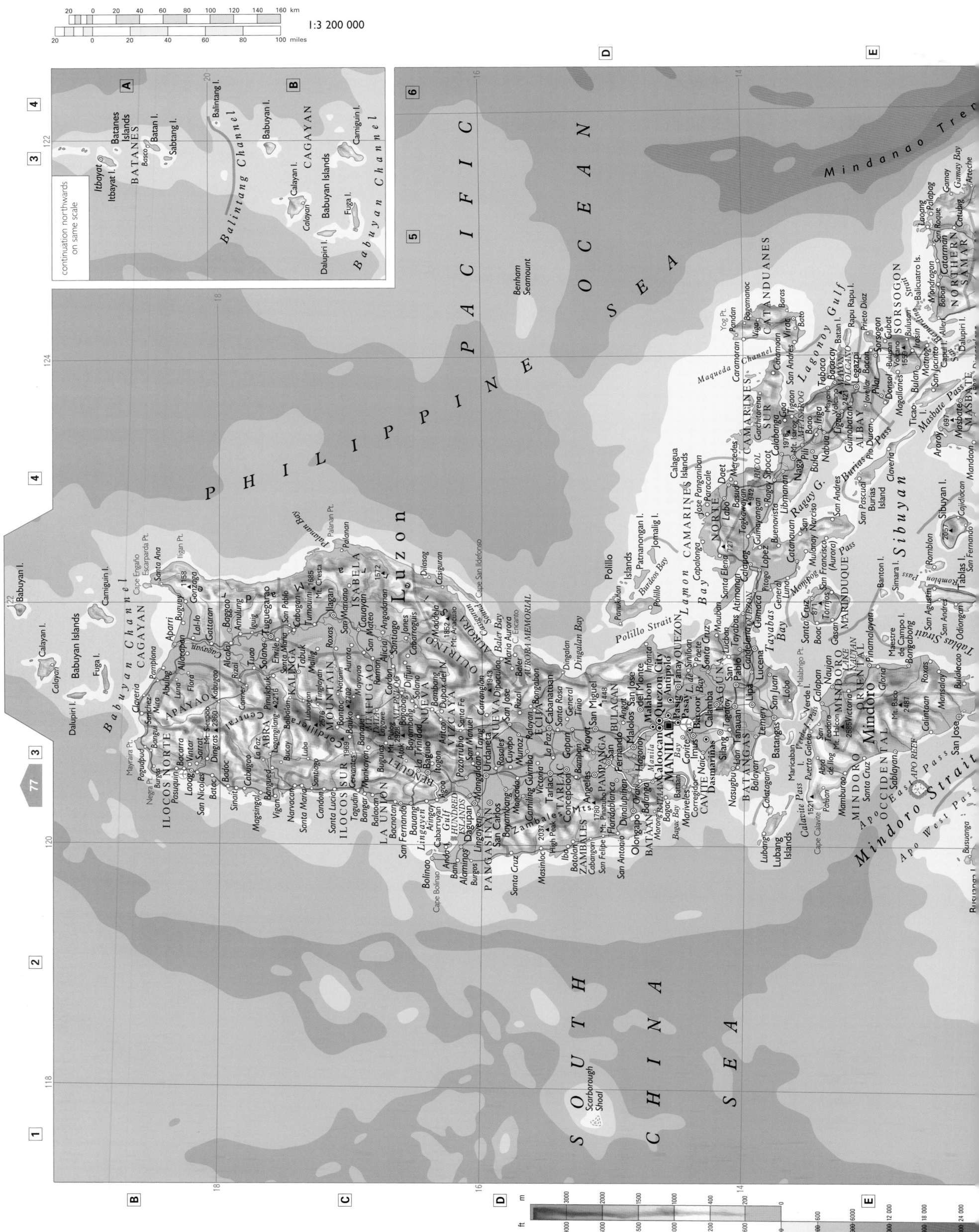

20 0 20 40 60 80 100 120 140 160 km

1:3 200 000

20 0 20 40 60 80 100 miles

continuation northwards
on same scale

Inset (top left)

Itbayat I.
Itbayat I.
Batanes Islands
BATANES
Bosco
Batan I.
Sabtang I.
Balintang I.
Babuyan I.
CAGAYAN
Camiguin I.
Calayan I.
Babuyan Islands
Fuga I.
Dalupiri I.
Coloyon
Balintang Channel
Babuyan Channel

Main map

PHILIPPINE PACIFIC OCEAN SEA

Benham Seamount

Mindanao Trench

SOUTH CHINA SEA

Scarborough Shoal

Luzon

Babuyan I.
Camiguin I.
Babuyan Islands
Calayan I.
Fuga I.
Dalupiri I.
Coloyon
Babuyan Channel

CAGAYAN
Aparri
Cape Engaño
Cape Escarparda Pt.
Iligan Pt.
Santa Ana
Palanan Pt.
Palanan
Palanan Bay
Casiguran
Cape San Ildefonso
ISABELA
AURORA MEMORIAL
AURORA
Baler Bay
Maria Aurora
Baler
Dingalan
Dingalan Bay

Polillo
Polillo Islands
Polillo Strait
Penukian I.
Patnanongan I.
Jomalig I.
Burdeos Bay

LAMON
Lamon Bay

CAMARINES Islands
Calagua Islands
Maqueda Channel
Caramoan
CAMARINES NORTE
Daet
Paracale
Mercedes
Jose Panganiban
Labo
Basud
BICOL
Naga
Pili
Iriga
Buhi
Libnanan
CAMARINES SUR
Lagonoy Gulf
San Andres
Virac
CATANDUANES
Bagamanoc
Baras
Bato

ALBAY
MT. MAYON
VOLCANO
Legazpi
Sorsogon
SORSOGON
Bulusan Volcano
Gubat
Bulan
Irosin
Matnog

NORTHERN SAMAR
Laoang
Palapag
Catarman
Catubig

MASBATE
Masbate

Sibuyan
Romblon
Tablas I.
Tablas Strait
Simara I.
Banton I.

MINDORO ORIENTAL
Mt. Halcon
Calapan
Naujan
Pinamalayan
Bongabong
Roxas
Mansalay
Bulalacao

MINDORO OCCIDENTAL
Mamburao
Sablayan
San Jose

APO REEF
Apo I.
East Pass
West Pass
Mindoro Strait
Apo West Trench

Lubang
Lubang Islands

Depth/Elevation scale

m ft
3000 9000
2000 6000
1500 4500
1000 3000
400 1200
200 600
0 0
-200 -600
-4000 -12000
-6000 -18000
-8000 -24000

EASTERN SAMAR
SOUTHERN LEYTE
LEYTE
BILIRAN
SURIGAO DEL NORTE
SURIGAO DEL SUR
AGUSAN DEL NORTE
AGUSAN DEL SUR
DAVAO ORIENTAL
DAVAO
DAVAO DEL SUR
CEBU
CENTRAL CEBU
BOHOL
SIQUIJOR
NEGROS ORIENTAL
NEGROS OCCIDENTAL
PANAY
CAPIZ
ANTIQUE
ILOILO
GUIMARAS
MISAMIS ORIENTAL
MISAMIS OCCIDENTAL
CAMIGUIN
BUKIDNON
LANAO DEL NORTE
LANAO DEL SUR
ZAMBOANGA
ZAMBOANGA DEL NORTE
ZAMBOANGA DEL SUR
MAGUINDANAO
SULTAN KUDARAT
NORTH COTABATO
COTABATO
SOUTH COTABATO
SARANGANI

PALAWAN
Puerto Princesa
Brooke's Point
Narra
Quezon
Aborlan

Mindanao
Davao
General Santos
Zamboanga
Cagayan de Oro
Iligan
Butuan
Surigao
Marawi City

Bacolod
Iloilo
Cebu
Tacloban
Ormoc

Bohol Sea
Camotes Sea
Visayan Sea
Sibuyan Sea
Tañon Strait
Leyte Gulf
Surigao Strait
Dinagat I.
Siargao I.
Bucas Grande I.
Homonhon I.
Panaon I.
Camiguin

SULU SEA
CELEBES SEA
Moro Gulf
Illana Bay
Sibuguey Bay
Panguil Bay
Dumanguilas Bay
Sarangani Bay
Davao Gulf

Basilan I.
Basilan Group
Pilas Group
Samales Group
Jolo
Jolo Group
SULU
Tapul Group
Pata I.
Siasi
TAWI-TAWI
Tawi-tawi Group
Bongao
Sibutu Group
Sibutu Passage
Sibutu Strait

Cuyo Islands
Quiniluban Group
Cagayan Is.
Cagayan Sulu I.
San Miguel Islands
Tubbataha Reefs

Palawan Passage
Balabac Strait
Balabac I.
Bugsuk I.
Cape Buliluyan
C. Melville

MALAYSIA
SABAH
BORNEO
Sandakan
Turtle Islands
Telok Labuk

Pulau Miangas (Indonesia)
Sarangani Islands

Mt. Apo 2954
Mt. Kitanglad
Mt. Kinabalian

Projection: Lambert Conformal Conic

1:5 600 000

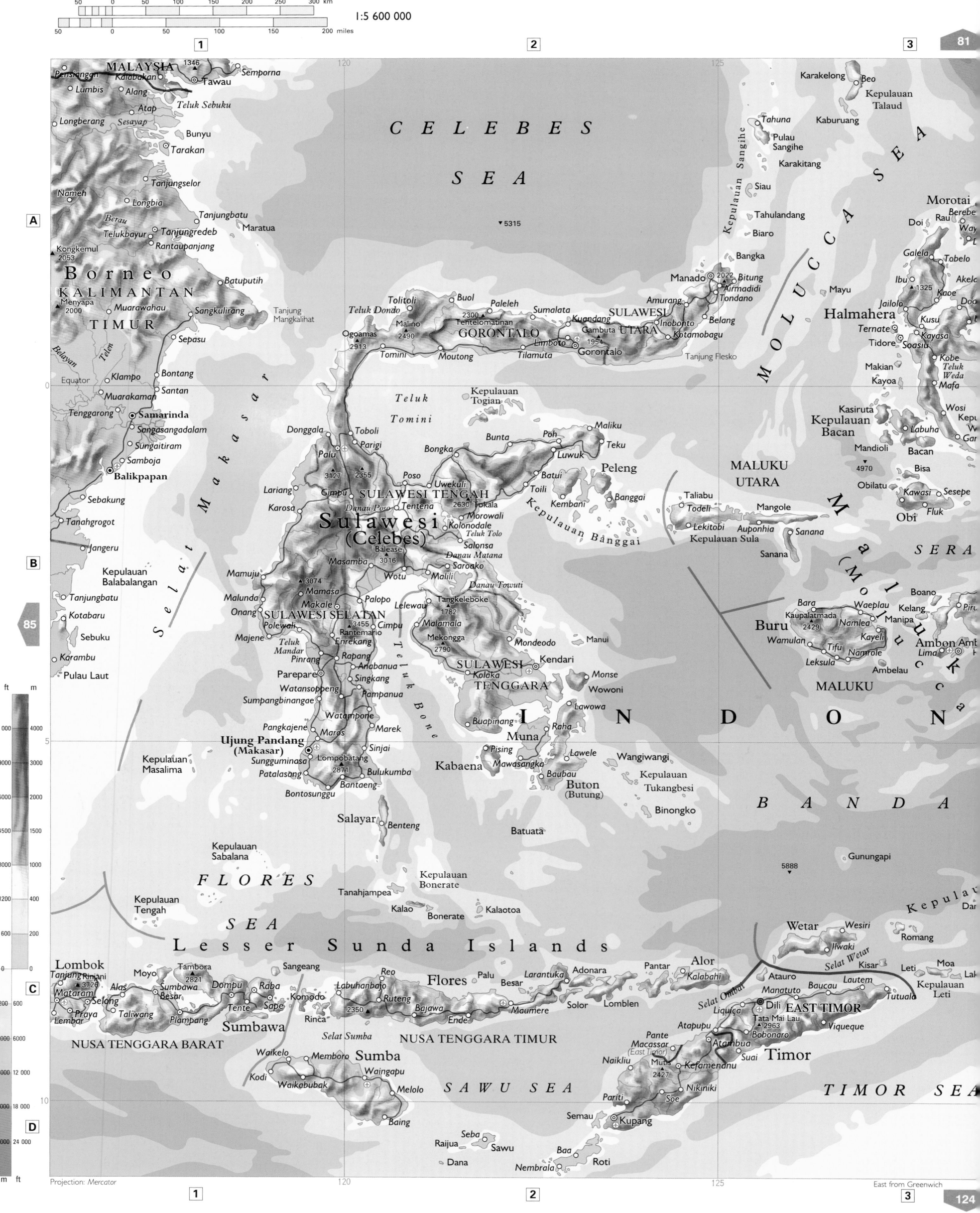

MALAYSIA
Pensiangan
Lumbis
Longberang
Nameh
Berau
Telukbayur
Kongkemul
2053

Kalabakan
Alang
Atap
Sesayap
Bunyu
Tarakan
Tanjungselor
Longbia
Tanjungbatu
Rantaupanjang
Batuputih

1346
Tawau
Semporna
Teluk Sebuku

Maratua
Tanjung
Mangkalihat

CELEBES SEA

▼5315

Karakelong
Beo
Kepulauan
Talaud
Kaburuang

Kepulauan Sangihe
Tahuna
Pulau
Sangihe
Karakitang

Siau
Tahulandang
Biaro
Bangka

Morotai
Doi
Rau
Berebe
Way
L
Galela
Tobelo
Ibu
1325
Akelo
Kaoe
Doo

Borneo
KALIMANTAN
TIMUR
Menyapa
2000
Muarawahau
Sangkulirang
Sepasu

Tolitoli
Teluk Dondo
Ogoamas
2913
Tomini
Buol
Paleleh
Malino
2490
2300
Tentelomatinan
Moutong
Tilamuta

Sumalata
Kuandang
GORONTALO
Limboto
Gorontalo
1954

Inobonto
SULAWESI
Amurang
UTARA
Kotamobagu
Belang

Manado
2022
Bitung
Airmadidi
Tondano

Mayu
Tanjung Flesko

Halmahera
Jailolo
Ternate
Tidore
Soasiu
Kusu
Kayasa
Kobe
Makian
Teluk
Kayoa
Weda
Mafa

Wosi
Kepu
Wo
Gar

Equator
Klampo
Bontang
Santan
Muarakaman
Tenggarong
Samarinda
Sangasangadalam
Sungaitiram
Samboja
Balikpapan

Teluk Tomini
Donggala
Toboli
Parigi
Palu
3127
2355
Poso
Danau Poso
Tentena
Uwekuli
Bongka
Bunta
Poh
Batui
Toili
Luwuk
Teku
Maliku

Kepulauan
Togian

Peleng
Kembani
Banggai

MALUKU
UTARA
4970
Mandioli
Obilatu

Kasiruta
Kepulauan
Bacan
Bacan
Bisa

Kawasi
Sesepe
Fluk
Obi

Sulawesi
(Celebes)
Balease
3016
Masamba
Wotu
Malili
Soroako
Danau Matana
Danau Towuti

Taliabu
Lekitobi
Todeli
Auponhia
Sanana
Mangole
Kepulauan Sula
Sanana

S E R A

Sebakung
Tanahgrogot
Jangeru
Kepulauan
Balabalangan
Tanjungbatu
Kotabaru
Sebuku
Karambu
Pulau Laut

Lariang
Gimpu
Karosa
SULAWESI TENGAH
Tokala
2630
Morowali
Kolonodale
Salonsa
Teluk Tolo
Saroako

Mamuju
3074
Mamasa
Palopo
Tangkeleboke
1782
Malamala
Mekongga
2790

Boano
Bara
Kaupalatmada
2429
Waeplau
Namlea
Manipa
Kelang
Piru

Malunda
Onang
Makale
SULAWESI SELATAN
Lelewau
Mondeodo

Buru
Wamulan
Tifu
Kayeli
Namrole
Leksula
Ambelau

Ambon
Lima

Majene
Polewali
3455
Cimpu
Rantemario
Enrekang
Rapang
Anabanua
Singkang
Rampanua
SULAWESI
Kolaka
TENGGARA
Kendari
Monse
Wowoni

MALUKU
M A L U C A

Teluk
Mandar
Pinrang
Parepare
Watansoppeng
Sumpangbinangae
Watamporie
Pangkajene
Maros
Marek

Buapinang
Raha
Lawowa

I N D O N

Teluk Bone
Ujung Pandang
(Makasar)
Sungguminasa
Patalasang
Lompobatang
2871
Sinjai
Bulukumba
Bantaeng
Bontosunggu

Pising
Mawasangka
Baubau
Lawele
Buton
(Butung)
Binongko

Wangiwangi
Kepulauan
Tukangbesi

B A N D A

Muna
Kabaena

Salayar
Benteng

Batuata

Kepulauan
Sabalana
Kepulauan
Masalima
Salima

Kepulauan
Bonerate
Tanahjampea
Kalao
Bonerate
Kalaotoa

Gunungapi
5888
▼

F L O R E S
Kepulauan
Tengah

S E A
L e s s e r   S u n d a   I s l a n d s

Wetar
Wesiri
Ilwaki
Romang

Kepulau
Dar

Lombok
Tanjung
Mataram
3726
Selong
Praya
Lembar

Moyo
Tambora
2821
Sumbawa
Besar
Alas
Selong
Taliwang

Dompu
Raba
Sape
Reo
Labuhanbajo
2350
Flores
Ruteng
Bajawa
Ende

Sangeang
Palu
Besar
Larantuka
Adonara
Pantar
Alor
Kalabahi
Solor
Lomblen

Atauro
Selat Wetar
Kisar
Leti
Moa
Lak

Manatuto
Baucau
Lautem
Tutuala
Kepulauan
Leti

Rinjani
Selat Sumba
Sumbawa
Komodo
Rinca
Tente
Plampang

NUSA TENGGARA BARAT
NUSA TENGGARA TIMUR
Maumere
Ataupupu
Liquiça
Dili
EAST TIMOR
Pante
Macassar
(East Timor)
Bobonaro
2963
Tata Mai Lau
Viqueque

Selat Ombai
Timor

Waikelo
Memboro
Sumba
Kodi
Waikabubak
Waingapu
Melolo

Naikliu
Mutis
2427
Kefamenanu
Nikiniki
Soe
Atambua
Suai

Baing

S A W U   S E A
Semau
Pariti
Kupang

TIMOR   SEA

Raijua
Sawu
Seba
Baa
Nembrala
Dana
Roti

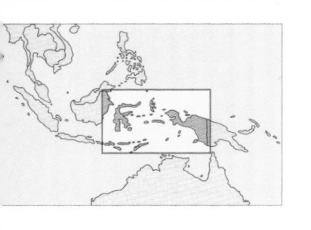

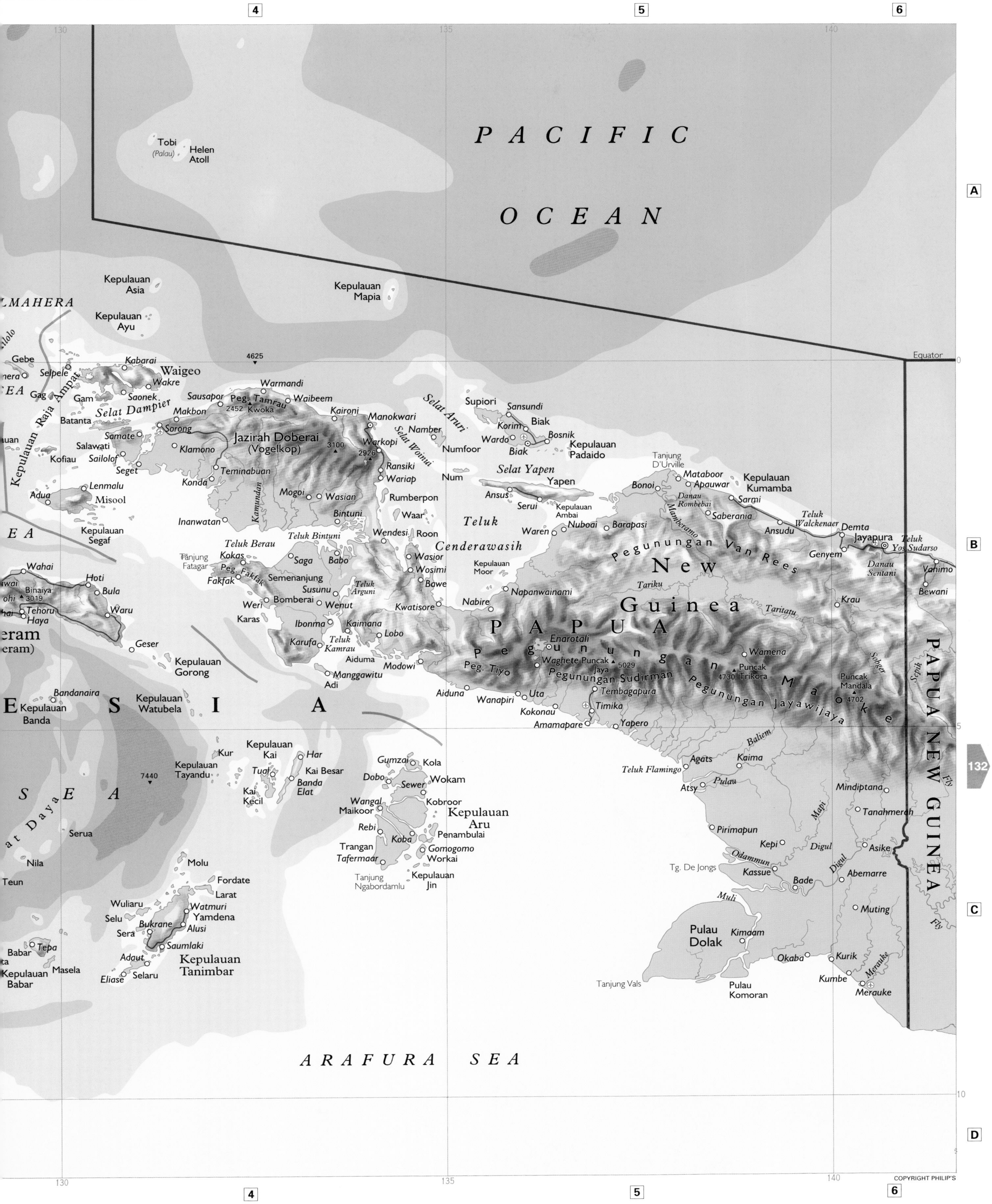

130

135

140

PACIFIC

OCEAN

Equator 0

A

Tobi
(Palau)
Helen
Atoll

Kepulauan
Asia

Kepulauan
Mapia

Kepulauan
Ayu

ILMAHERA

Gebe

4625

Kabarai

Selpele

nera

Gam

Waigeo

Wakre

Warmandi

Waibeem

SEA

Gag

Batanta

Selat Dampier

Makbon

Sausapor

Peg. Tamrau

2452 Kwoka

Kaironi

Manokwari

Supiori

Sansundi

Korim

Biak

Selat Aruri

Bosnik

ua

Salawati

Samate

Sorong

Klamono

Jazirah Doberai
(Vogelkop)

3100

Warkopi

2926

Namber

Warda

Biak

Selat Wonni

Kepulauan
Padaido

Kofiau

Sailolof

Seget

Teminabuan

Ransiki

Wariap

Num

Numfoor

Selat Yapen

Tanjung
D'Urville

Mataboor

Apauwar

Kepulauan
Kumamba

Sarmi

Lenmalu

Konda

Mogoi

Wasian

Rumberpon

Ansus

Serui

Yapen

Bonoi

Danau
Rombebai

Saberania

Teluk
Walckenaer

Ansudu

Demta

Adua

Misool

Inanwatan

Bintuni

Waar

Roon

Teluk

Waren

Kepulauan
Ambai

Nuboai

Barapasi

Pegunungan Van Rees

Genyem

Jayapura

Yos Sudarso

Kepulauan
Segaf

Teluk Berau

Saga

Babo

Wendesi

Cenderawasih

Kepulauan
Moor

Napanwainami

New

Danau
Sentani

Vahimo

Tanjung
Fatagar

Kokas

Semenanjung

Wasior

Wosimi

Tariku

Guinea

Bewani

Wahai

Hoti

Peg. Fakfak

Saga

Susunu

Bowe

Nabire

Krau

SEA

Binaiya
3019

Bula

Fakfak

Werl

Wenut

Kwatisore

PAPUA

Taritatu

ohi

Tehoru

Waru

Bomberai

Ibonma

Kaimana

Lobo

Enarotali

Pegunungan

Wamena

eram

Haya

Karas

Karufa

Teluk
Kamrau

Aiduma

Modowi

Waghete

Puncak
Jaya

5029

Puncak
Trikora

Puncak
Mandala

4730

4702

(eram)

Geser

Adi

Manggawitu

Peg. Tiyo

Pegunungan Sudirman

Pegunungan Jayawijaya

Sobger

Bandanaira

Kepulauan
Gorong

Aiduna

Wanapiri

Uta

Tembagapura

Timika

Sepik

E Kepulauan
Banda

ESIA

Kepulauan
Watubela

A

Amamapare

Kokonau

Yapero

Baliem

Kur

Kepulauan
Kai

Har

Gumzai

Kola

Agats

Kaima

Kepulauan
Tayandu

Tual

Kai Besar

Dobo

Wokam

Teluk Flamingo

Pulau

Mindiptana

7440

Kai
Kecil

Banda
Elat

Sewer

Kobroor

Atsy

Tanahmerah

SEA

SEA

Wangal

Maikoor

Kepulauan
Aru

Penambulai

Pirimapun

Kepi

Digul

Asike

at Daya

Rebi

Koba

Gomogomo

Tg. De Jongs

Odammun

Kassue

Bade

Abemarre

Serua

Trangan

Tafermaar

Workai

Muli

Muting

Nila

Molu

Tanjung
Ngabordamlu

Kepulauan
Jin

Kimaam

Kurik

Teun

Fordate

Larat

Pulau
Dolak

Okaba

Merauke

Wuliaru

Watmuri

Yamdena

Kumbe

Selu

Bukrane

Alusi

Sera

Tepa

Saumlaki

Kepulauan
Tanimbar

Tanjung Vals

Pulau
Komoran

Babar

ta

Adaut

Selaru

Eliase

Selaru

Kepulauan
Babar

Masela

ARAFURA SEA

B

132

C

D

COPYRIGHT PHILIP'S

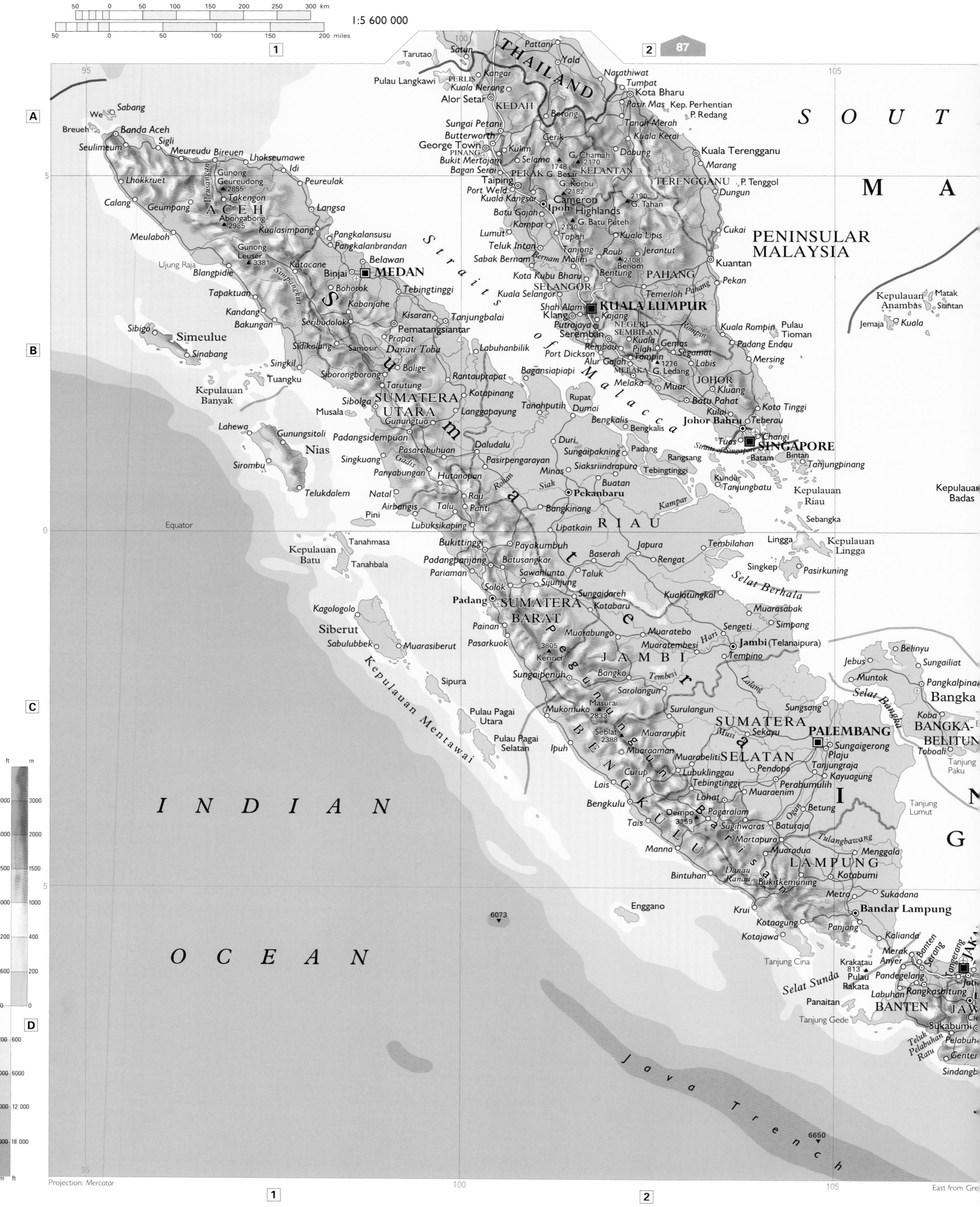

50   0   50   100   150   200   250   300 km

50   0   50   100   150   200 miles

1:5 600 000

1

2 **87**

Projection: Mercator

East from Gre

Map labels

THAILAND

SOUT
M A

PENINSULAR
MALAYSIA

Tarutao
Satun
Pattani
Yala
Narathiwat
Tumpat
Kota Bharu
Pasir Mas
Kep. Perhentian
P. Redang
Pulau Langkawi
PERLIS
Kuala Nerang
Kangar
Alor Setar
KEDAH
Betong
Tanah Merah
Kuala Krai
Kuala Terengganu
Marang
We
Sabang
Breueh
Banda Aceh
Sigli
Meureudu
Bireuen
Lhokseumawe
Idi
Butterworth
George Town
PINANG
Bukit Mertajam
Bagan Serai
Kulim
Selama
Gerik
Dabung
G. Chamah
2170
KELANTAN
TERENGGANU
P. Tenggol
Dungun
Seulimeum
Lhokkruet
Calang
Gunong
Geureudong
2855
Takengon
Peureulak
Langsa
Taiping
Port Weld
Kuala Kangsar
G. Korbu
2182
Ipoh
Cameron
Highlands
2130
G. Tahan
2190
Cukai
Geumpang
ACEH
Abongabong
2985
Kualasimpang
Pangkalansusu
Pangkalanbrandan
Batu Gajah
Kampar
G. Batu Puteh
Tapah
Kuala Lipis
Jerantut
Meulaboh
Gunong
Leuser
3381
Kutacane
Belawan
Lumut
Teluk Intan
Tanjong
Malim
Raub
Benom
2108
Bentung
PAHANG
Kuantan
Pekan
Ujung Raja
Blangpidie
Binjai
Bohorok
MEDAN
Sabak Bernam
Kota Kubu Bharu
Temerloh
Pahang
Kandang
Bakungan
Seribudolok
Kabanjahe
Tebingtinggi
Kisaran
Tanjungbalai
Kuala Selangor
SELANGOR
Shah Alam
Klang
KUALA LUMPUR
Kajang
Putrajaya
Temerloh
Kuala Rompin
Padang Endau
Pulau
Tioman
Tapaktuan
Sibigo
Simeulue
Sinabang
Singkil
Tuangku
Sidikalang
Samosir
Prapat
Danau Toba
Balige
Pematangsiantar
Labuhanbilik
Bagansiapiapi
Port Dickson
Alur Gajah
Rembau
Seremban
NEGERI
SEMBILAN
Kuala
Pilah
Tampin
Gemas
Segamat
Labis
G. Ledang
1276
JOHOR
Mersing
Kepulauan
Banyak
Lahewa
Gunungsitoli
Nias
Sirombu
Telukdalem
Musala
Sibolga
Siborongborong
Tarutung
SUMATERA
UTARA
Gunungtua
Padangsidempuan
Pasarsibuhuan
Gadis
Singkuang
Panyabungan
Hutanopan
Daludalu
Pasirpengarayan
Rokan
Siak
Rantauprapat
Kotapinang
Langgapayung
Tanahputih
Dumai
Bengkalis
Bengkalis
Duri
Rupat
Sungaipakning
Padang
Rangsang
Strait of Singapore
Tuas
Changi
SINGAPORE
Batam
Bintan
Tanjungpinang
Kundur
Tanjungbatu
Kepulauan
Riau
Kepulauan
Badas
Natal
Airbangis
Pini
Talu
Panti
Rau
Lubuksikaping
Bangkinang
Minas
Siaksriindrapura
Tebingtinggi
Buatan
PEKANBARU
RIAU
Kampar
Sebangka
Kepulauan
Banyak
Kepulauan
Batu
Tanahmasa
Tanahbala
Bukittinggi
Payakumbuh
Batusangkar
Baserah
Japura
Rengat
Tembilahan
Lingga
Kepulauan
Lingga
Singkep
Pasirkuning
Selat Berhala
Padangpanjang
Sawahlunto
Taluk
Pariaman
Solok
Sijunjung
Sungaidareh
Kotabaru
Kualatungkal
Muarasabak
Kagologolo
Kerinci
3805
Padang
SUMATERA
BARAT
Painan
Pasarkuok
Muarabungo
Muaratebo
Sengeti
Simpang
JAMBI
Hari
JAMBI (Telanaipura)
Tempino
Siberut
Sabulubbek
Muarasiberut
Sipura
Muaratembesi
Bangko
Tembesi
Sarolangun
Sungaipenuh
Jebus
Belinyu
Sungailiat
Muntok
Pangkalpinang
Bangka
Kepulauan
Mentawai
Pulau Pagai
Utara
Pulau Pagai
Selatan
Ipuh
Mukomuko
Masurai
2833
Seblat
2388
Muaraman
Muararupit
Surulangun
Muarabeliti
Lubuklinggau
Musi
Sekayu
SUMATERA
SELATAN
PALEMBANG
Sungaigerong
Plaju
Koba
Toboali
BANGKA-
BELITUN
Tanjung
Paku
Selat Bangka
Curup
Lais
Tebingtinggi
Pendopo
Tanjungraja
Kayuagung
Perabumulih
Muaraenim
Lahat
Bengkulu
Dempo
3159
Pagaralam
Sugihwaras
Baturaja
Betung
Ogan
I
G
Tanjung
Lumut
Tais
BENGKULU
Manna
Martapura
Muaradua
Tulangbawang
Menggala
LAMPUNG
Kotabumi
Metro
Sukadana
Bintuhan
Danau
Ranau
Bukitkemuning
Panjang
BANDAR LAMPUNG
Enggano
Krui
Kotaagung
Kotajawa
Kalianda
Merak
Anyer
Banten
Serang
Tangerang
JAK
Tanjung Cina
Krakatau
813
Pulau
Rakata
Selat Sunda
Pandegelang
Rangkasbitung
BANTEN
Panaitan
Labuhan
Jati
JAW
Tanjung Gede
Sukabumi
Teluk
Pelabuhan
Ratu
Pelabuhan
Ratu
Genter
Sindangb

6073

6650

INDIAN

OCEAN

Java Trench

Straits of Malacca

Strait of Malacca

Equator

ft   m
9000 3000
6000 2000
4500 1500
3000 1000
1200 400
600   200
0   0
0   0
200   600
2000 6000
4000 12 000
6000 18 000
m ft

95
100
105

A
B
C
D

1
2

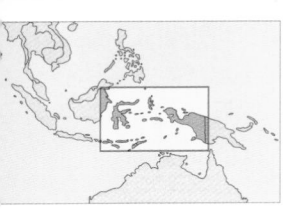

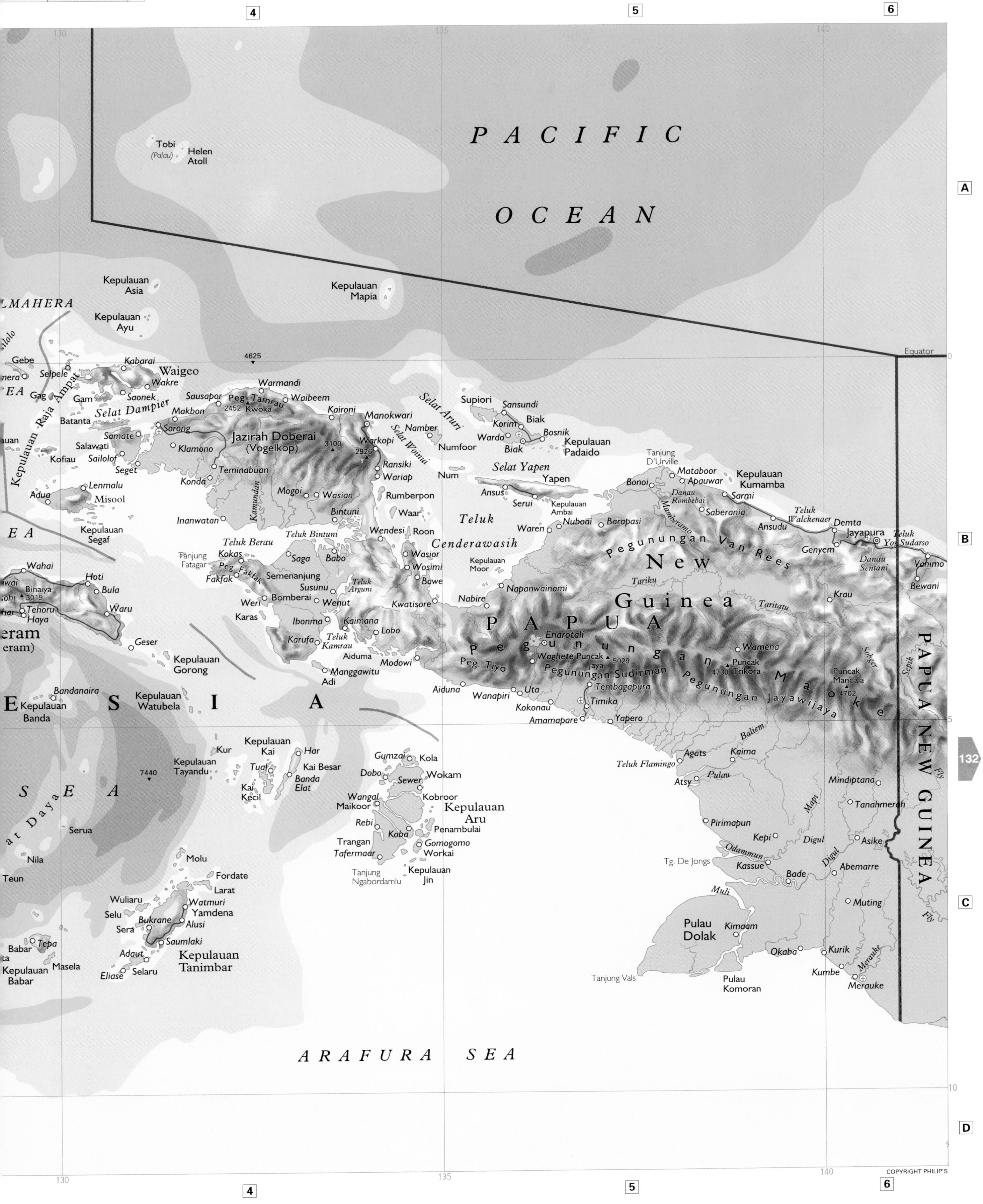

PACIFIC

OCEAN

Tobi
(Palau)
Helen
Atoll

Kepulauan
Asia

Kepulauan
Mapia

Kepulauan
Ayu

LMAHERA

Kepulauan
Raja Ampat

Gebe

Selpele
EA

Kabarai

4625 ▼

Waigeo
Wakre

Warmandi

Gam
Gag

Selat Dampier

Saonek

Sausapor
Makbon

Peg. Tamrau
2452 Kwoka
Waibeem
Kaironi
Manokwari

Supiori
Sansundi

Namber
Korim
Biak
Biak
Bosnik

Batanta

Sorong

Samate

Klamono
Jazirah Doberai
(Vogelkop)
3100 ▲
Warkopi
2926 ▲

Wardo
Numfoor
Num
Biak

Kepulauan
Padaido

Tanjung
D'Urville

Salawati

Kofiau

Sailolof

Seget

Konda
Teminabuan

Ransiki
Wariap

Selat Yapen
Yapen

Bonoi

Mataboor
Apauwar

Kepulauan
Kumamba

Danau
Rombebai

Sarmi

Adua

Lenmalu

Misool

Kepulauan
Segaf

Mogoi

Inanwatan

Wasian
Bintuni

Teluk Berau
Tanjung
Fatagar

Teluk Bintuni

Rumberpon

Waar

Wendesi
Roon

Ansus
Serui

Teluk

Waren

Kepulauan
Ambai
Nuboai

Barapasi

Saberania

Ansudu

Teluk
Walckenaer

Demta
Jayapura
Yos Sudarso

Genyem

Teluk

Pegunungan Van Rees

Krau

Danau
Sentani

Vohimo

Bewani

Wahai
Hoti

Binaiya
3019 ▲
Bula

Peg.
Kokas
Faktak

Saga
Babo

Semenanjung
Susunu

Wasior
Wosimi

Cenderawasih

Nabire

Napanwainami

New
Guinea

Tariku

Tarita

Taritatu

eram
Tehoru
Haya
Waru

Geser

Kepulauan
Gorong

Weri
Bomberai

Fakfak
Faktak

Wenut

Ibonma

Karas

Kaimana

Teluk
Arguni

Bawe

Kepulauan
Moor

Kwatisore

Kokonau

PAPUA

Pegunungan

Waghete
Puncak
Jaya

Enarotali
5029

Puncak
Trikora
4730

Wamena

Puncak
Mandala
4702

Schger

Bandanaira

Kepulauan
Banda

Kepulauan
Watubela

A

Karufa

Teluk
Kamrau

Lobo

Aiduma
Manggawitu
Adi

Modowi

Aiduna

Peg. Tiyo

Wanapiri

Uta

Timika

Tembagapura

Pegunungan Sudirman

Pegunungan Jayawijaya

Baliem

Kaima

Mindiptana

Kur

Kepulauan
Kai

Har

Kepulauan
Tayandu

7440 ▼

Tual

Kai Besar
Banda
Elat

Kai
Kecil

Gumzai

Dobo
Sewer

Kola

Wokam

Amamapare

Yapero

Agats

Teluk Flamingo

Pulau

Atsy

Mapi

Digul

Tanahmerah

Molu

Wangal
Maikoor

Rebi

Kobroor

Kepulauan
Aru

Koba
Penambulai

Trangan
Tafermaar

Gomogomo
Workai

Pirimapun

Kepi

Digul

Asike

Abemarre

Fordate
Larat

Tanjung
Ngabordamlu

Kepulauan
Jin

Tg. De Jongs

Odammun

Kassue

Bade

Muting

Wuliaru

Selu

Watmuri
Yamdena

Muli

Kimaam

Kurik

Sera
Bukrane
Alusi

Kepulauan
Tanimbar

Pulau
Dolak

Okaba

Kumbe

Merauke

Teba

Adaut
Saumlaki

Babar

Eliase
Selaru

Kepulauan
Babar
Masela

Tanjung Vals

Pulau
Komoran

ARAFURA   SEA

Equator

PAPUA NEW GUINEA

132

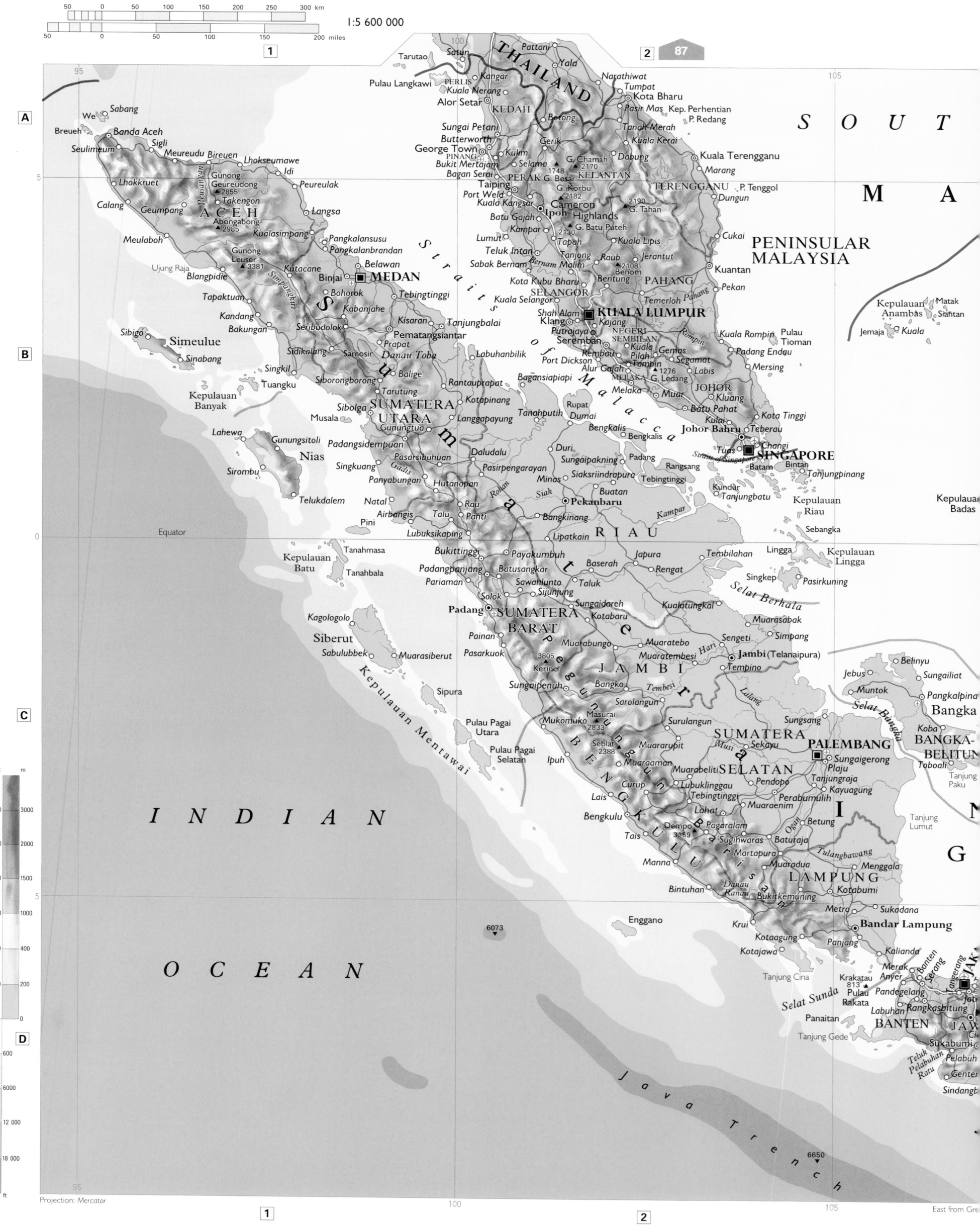

1:5 600 000

50 0 50 100 150 200 250 300 km
50 0 50 100 150 200 miles

Projection: Mercator

East from Gr

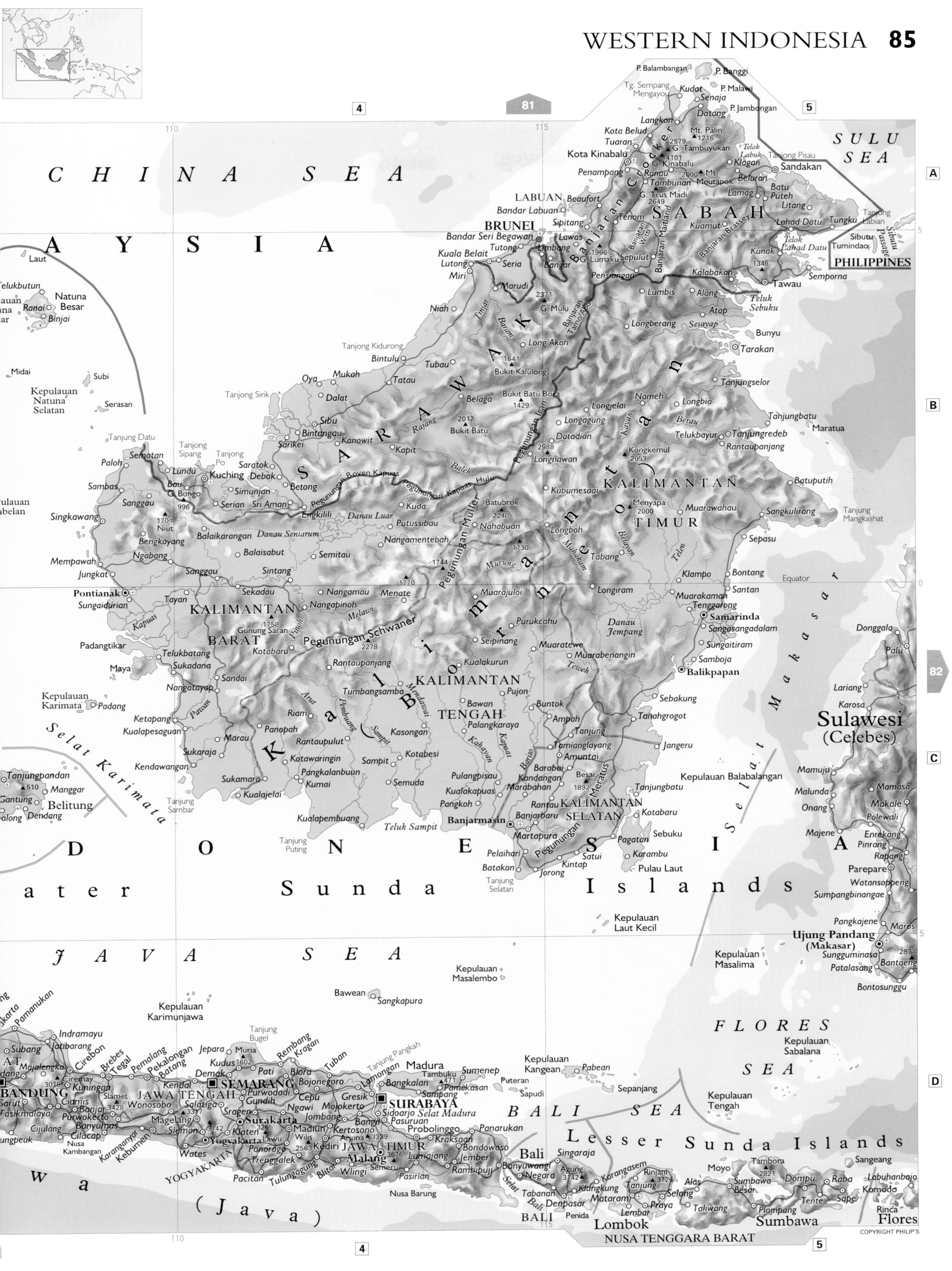

CHINA SEA

SULU SEA

MA LAYSIA

Laut

Natuna Besar
Ranai
Binjai

Midai

Kepulauan Natuna Selatan

Subi
Serasan

LABUAN
Bandar Labuan

BRUNEI
Bandar Seri Begawan
Kuala Belait
Lutong
Miri

P. Balambangan   P. Banggi
Tg. Sempang Mengayau   Kudat   P. Malawi
Langkon   Senaja   P. Jambongan
Datong

Kota Belud   Mt. Palin
Tuaran   G. Tambuyukon   1216
2579
Kota Kinabalu   G. Kinabalu   Klagan   Sandakan
Penampang   4101   Mt. Meutapok
Ranau   2000
Beaufort   Tambunan   Lamag
G. Trus Madi   Batu Puteh   Lahad Datu
Sipitang   2649   Kuamut   Tungku   Tanjong Labian
Lawas   Kunak   Sibutu Passage
Umbang   1966   Kalabakan   Tumindao
Bangar   Lumaku   Sapulut   Tawau   Semporna
Seria   Pensiangan   1346
Marudi   Lumbis   Alang

SABAH
Telok Labuk
Beluran

PHILIPPINES

SARAWAK

Niah   2371   Atap   Bunyu
G. Mulu   Longberang   Sesayap   Tarakan
Bintulu   Tubau   1641   Long Akah   Teluk Sebuku
Tanjong Kidurong   Bukit Kalulong   Longjelai   Nameh   Longbia
Oya   Mukah   Tatau   Bukit Batu Bora   Tanjungselor
Tanjong Sirik   Belaga   1429   Longagung   Berau   Tanjungbatu
Dalat   2012   Datadian   Telukbayur   Tanjungredeb   Maratua
Sibu   Bukit Batu   2988   Longnawan   Rantaupanjang
Bintangau   Kanowit   Kapit   Kubumesaai   Kongkemul   Batuputih
Sarikei   Baleh   2053
Tanjong Sipang   Boven Kapuas   Hulu   Menyapa   Tanjung Mangkalihat
Tanjung Datu   Saratok   Pegunungan Kapuas   Batubrok   2000   Muarawahau   Sangkulirang
Tanjong Po   Sri Aman   2240   KALIMANTAN   Sepasu
Sematan   Lundu   Engkilili   Kuda   Nahabuan   TIMUR   Sangasangadalam
Paloh   Debak   Putussibau   Longboh   Tabang   Samboja
Kuching   Betong   Danau Luar   1730
Sambas   Bau   Simunjan   Nangamentebah   1744   Muhakam   Klampo
Bungo   996   Serian   Danau Sentarum   Murung   Bontang
Singkawang   Balaikarangan   Semitau   1770   Longiram   Equator
1701   Balaisabut   Sintang   Muarajuloi   Muarakaman   Santan
Niut   Bengkayang   Nangamau   Samarinda   Donggala
Ngabang   Menate   Purukcahu   Sungaitiram   Palu

KALIMANTAN
BARAT

Pontianak
Sungaidurian
Tayan
Sekadau
Nangapinoh
Melawi
Seipinang
Danau Jempang
Tenggarong

Padangtikar
Kapuas
Gunung Saran   1758
Kotabaru
Pegunungan Schwaner   2278
Muaratewe
Muarabenangin
Teweh
Balikpapan

Maya
Telukbatang
Sukadana
Rantaupanjang
KALIMANTAN
TENGAH
Buntok
Sebakung

Nangatayap
Sandai
Riam   Arut
Tumbangsamba   Pujon
Bawan
Ampah
Tanahgrogot

Kepulauan Karimata
Padang
Ketapang
Kualapesaguan   Panopah   Pembuang   Mendawai   Kasongan
Palangkaraya   Tamianglayang   Sulawesi (Celebes)

Marau   Rantaupulut   Sampit   Kotabesi   Amuntai   Jangeru   Mamuju
Sukaraja   Katawaringin   Barabai   Kepulauan Balabalangan   Malunda
Kendawangan   Sukamara   Kumai   Semuda   Pulangpisau   Kandangan   Onang   Mamasa
Kualajelai   Pangkalanbuun   Kualakapuas   Besar   Makale
Tanjungpandan   510   Marabahan   1892   Tanjungbatu   Majene   Enrekang
Manggar   Kualapembuang   Pangkoh   Meratus   Kotabaru   Pinrang
Gantung   Belitung   Teluk Sampit   Banjarmasin   Banjarbaru   KALIMANTAN   Polewali   Rajang
Dendang   Tanjung Puting   Martapura   SELATAN   Parepare

Selat Karimata

Tanjung Sambar
Tanjung Selatan

INDONESIA
Sunda   Islands

Pelaihari   Pegunungan   Watansoppeng
Batakan   Satui   Kintap   Pulau Laut   Sumpangbinangae
Jorong   Karambu   Pangkajene
Maros

Ujung Pandang (Makasar)
Sungguminasa   2871
Bantaeng
Patalassang
Bontosunggu

JAVA SEA

Kepulauan Laut Kecil

Kepulauan Masalembo
Bawean   Sangkapura

Kepulauan Karimunjawa

Kepulauan Laut Kecil

Kepulauan Masalima

FLORES
Kepulauan Sabalana
SEA

Tanjung Bugel
Muria
Kepulauan Kangean   Pabean
Jepara   1602   Rembang   Tuban   Kangean   Puteran
Pamanukan   Pekalongan   Kudus   Kragan   Tanjung Pangkah   Sepanjang   Kepulauan Tengah
Indramayu   Batang   Pati   Blora   Lamongan   Madura   Sapudi
Jotibarang   Brebes   Pemalang   Demak   Bojonegoro   Tambuku   Sumenep
Subang   Cirebon   Tegal   Slamet   Kendal   Purwodadi   Cepu   471   Bangkalan   Pamekasan
Majalengka   3078   SEMARANG   Gundih   Ngawi   Gresik   Selat Madura
BANDUNG   Kuningan   JAWA TENGAH   Salatiga   Madiun   3265   Jombang   SURABAYA   BALI
Ciremay   Purwodadi   Sragen   Mojokerto   Sidoarjo   SEA
Garut   Ciamis   Banjar   Wonosobo   3317   Surakarta   Kertosono   Pasuruan
Tasikmalaya   Purwokerto   3428   Sleman   Lawu   Kediri   Bangil   Probolinggo   Panarukan   Lesser Sunda Islands
Cilacap   Magelang   3142   Yogyakarta   Aruna   3339   Kraksan   Bondowoso
Kambangan   Kebumen   Wates   Ponorogo   2563   Wilis   Lumajang   Jember   Bali   Singaraja
Banyumas   Karanganyar   YOGYAKARTA   Trenggalek   Blitar   3676   Rambipuji   Sangeang
Nusa Barung   Pacitan   Tulungagung   Wlingi   Semeru   Pasirian   Karangasem   Rinjani   Tambora
Agung   3724   2821
(Java)   Banyuwangi   3142   Dompu   Raba
Negara   Klungkung   Moyo
Tabanan   Tanjung   Selong   Sumbawa   Besar   Tente   Sape
NUSA TENGGARA BARAT   Mataram   Lembar   Plampang   Komodo
Penida   Denpasar   Praya   Taliwang
Lombok   Sumbawa   Rinca
BALI   Flores

JAVA SEA

ater   Sunda   Islands

J A V A   S E A

W a   (J a v a)

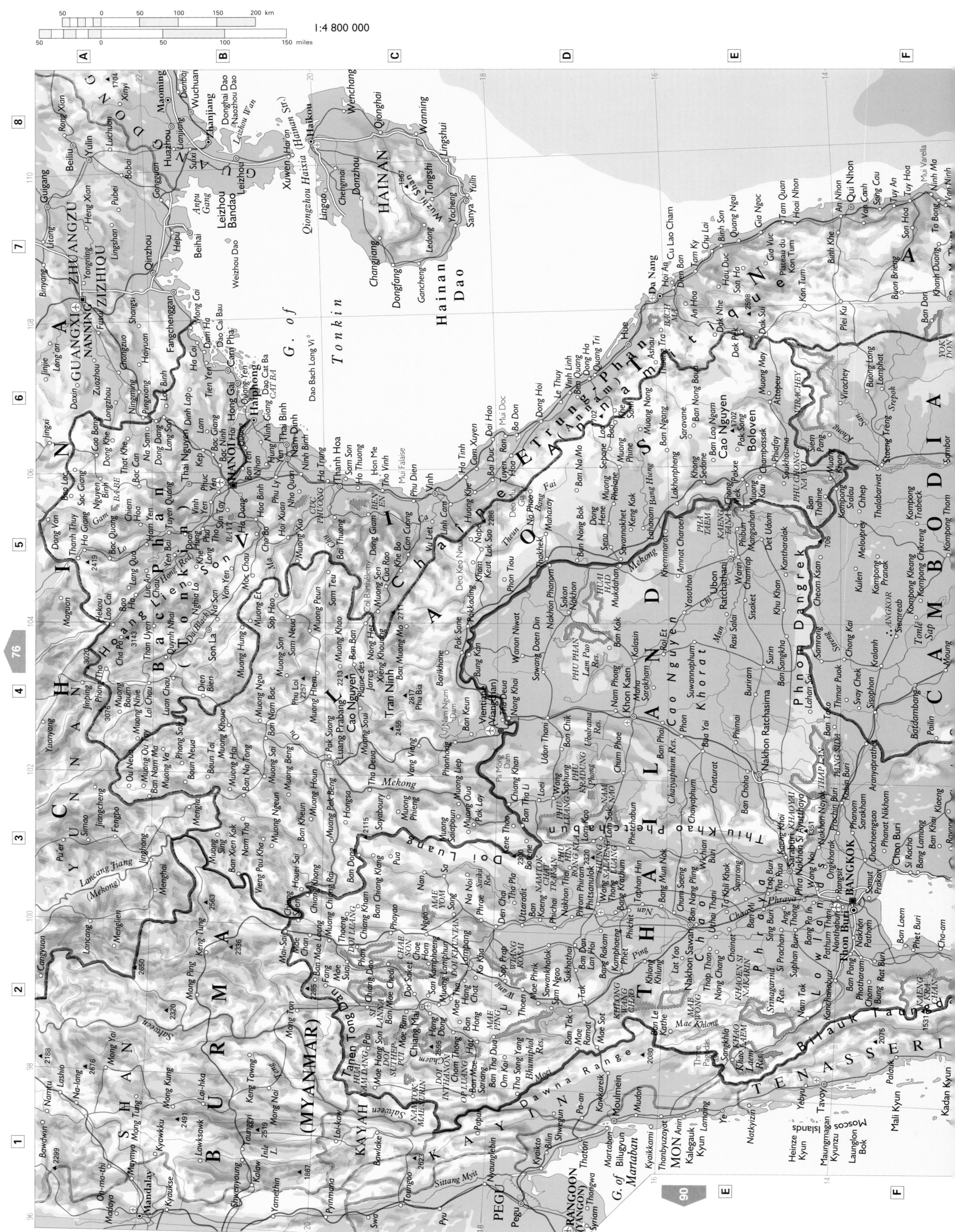

1:4 800 000

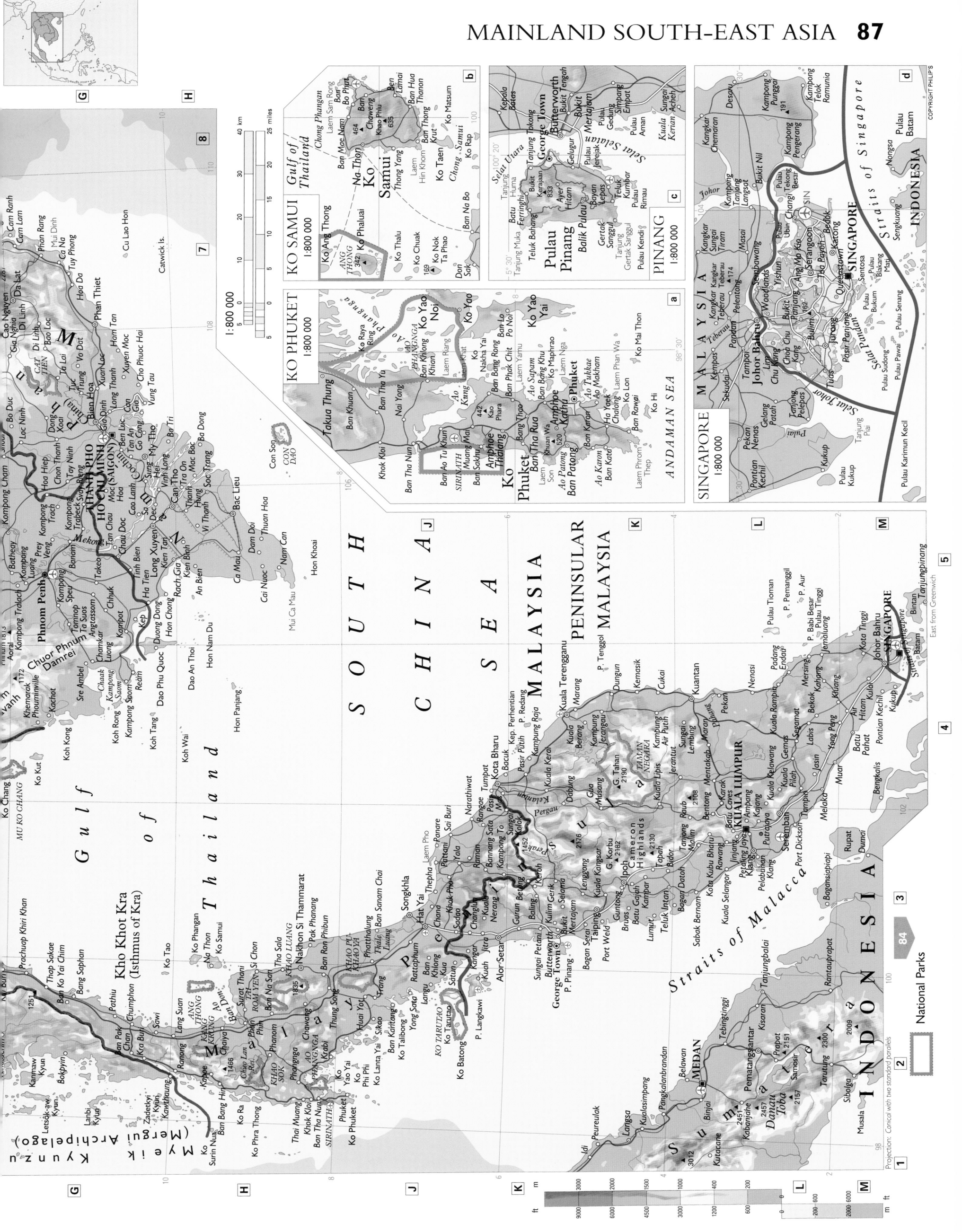

COPYRIGHT PHILIP'S

b

Gulf of Thailand

KO SAMUI
1:800 000

Chong Phangan
Laem Sam Rong
Ban Bo Phut
464
Ko Phangan
Chaweng
Ban Mae Nam
635
Na-Thon
Khao Phu
Ban Hua Thanon
Ko Matsum
Ko
Ban Thong Yang
Samui
Laem Thong Yang
Ko Taen
Chong Samui
Ko Rap

ANG THONG
342
Ko Ang Thong
Ko Phaluai

a

KO PHUKET
1:800 000

Takua Thung
Ban Khoai
Ko Raya
Rang
AO
PHANGNGA
Ban Tha Yu
Ban Khlong
Khian
Laem Riang
Ko Yao
Noi
Ko Yao
Yai
Ko Yao
Ban Lo
Noi
Ban Bang Rong
Ko Maphrao
Ko Nakha Yai
Nakha
Ban Phok Chit
Ko Mai Thon
Khok Kloi
Ban Tha Nun
AO
Kang
Ban Bang Khu
Laem Yamu
Ban Phan Wa
Ao Supam
Ao Po
Ko
Amphoe
Thalang
442
520
Ko
Phara
Ao Tukkae
Ao Makham
Ban Ao Tu Khun
Muang Mai
SIRINATH
Sakun
Ban Tha Rua
Amphoe
Kathu
Ko Karon
Ao Yon
Ko Lon
Ko Hi
Khok Bang
Bang Thao
Ko
Ban Karon
Ban Rawai
Ko Phuket
Phuket
Laem
Laem Phromthep
Ban Patong
Son
Ao Patong
Ao Karon
Ban Kata
Ha Yaek
Ao Makham
ANDAMAN SEA

c

George Town
Butterworth
Bukit Tengah
Kepala Betas
Bukit Mertajam
Pulau Aman
Gedung
Simpang Empat
Kuala Kerian Acheh
Tanjung Tokong
Pulau Pinang
Batu Feringghi
Teluk Bahang
Huma
833
Kampong
Bukit
Ayer Hitam
Gelugur
Selat Selatan
Sungai Kluang
Teluk Kumbar
Pulau Rimau
Balik Pulau
Gertak Sanggul
Tanjung Bungah
Bayan Lepas
Pulau Jerejak

PINANG
1:800 000
5° 30'   100° 20'

Pulau Pinang

d

Straits of Singapore
Kampong Punggai
Kampong Telok Ramunia
Desaru
Kangkar Chemaran
Nongsa
Pulau Batam
INDONESIA
Kampong Pengerang
Kampong
191
Johor
Kuala Sungai
Pulau Ubin
SIN
Kangkar
Tebrau
Tanjung Langsat
Pasir Gudang
Bukit Panjang
SINGAPORE
174
Changi
162
Bedok
Serangoon
Ang Mo Kio
Bukit Timah
Ubin
Jurong
Singapore
Queenstown
Sentosa
Pulau Blakang Mati
Pulau Bukum
Pulau Senang

MALAYSIA
Johor Bahru
Tanjung Piai
Pasir Panjang
Selat Johor
Pulau Sudong
Pulau Pawai

SINGAPORE
1:800 000

G   **H**   1:800 000

40 km
30   25 miles
20
10   15
5

8

7

M   U   A   N   G
CAT   TIEN
Cao Nguyen
Cam Ranh
Cam Lam
Phan Rang
Mui Dinh
Ca Na
Phan Thiet
Phan Ri
Cu Lao Hon
Tuy Phong
Ga Nghia
Di Linh
Da Lat
Ta Lai
Vo Dat
Ham Tan
Ban Tan
Catwick Is.
Tuc Trung
Cho Phuoc Hai
Xuan Loc
Long Thanh
Hoa Hiep
Xuan
Long
Thanh
Bo Duc
Loc Ninh
Bien Hoa
HO CHI MINH
THANH PHO
(SAIGON)
Tay Ninh
Chon Thanh
Go Dau
Go Cong
Hoa
Cho Moi
My Tho
Ben Luc
Tan An
Ba Dong
Long An
Tra On
Vung Tau
Con Son
CON DAO
Soc Trang
Bac Lieu
Ca Mau
Cha Doc
Hon Khoai
Mui Ca Mau
Nam Can

SOUTH
CHINA
SEA

J

Khemarak
1172
Phnom 813
Phnom Penh
Kampong Tralach
Kampong Cham
Prey Veng
Svay Rieng
1466

Gulf
of
Thailand

Ko Chang
MU KO CHANG
Ko Kut
Koh Kong
Kampot
Kep
Ha Tien
Kampong Trach
Rach Gia
Duong Dong
Dao Phu Quoc
Hon Chong
Kien Luong
An Bien
Hon Panjang
Dao An Thoi
Ko Tang
Ko Rong
Ko Wai

Kho Khot Kra
(Isthmus of Kra)

K

Prachuap Khiri Khan
1251
Thap Sakae
Bang Saphan
Ko Ra
Chumphon
Lang Suan
Ko Phangan
Na-Thon
Ko Samui
Ko Tao

NAKHON SI
THAMMARAT
Surat Thani
Pak Phanang
Thung Song
Huai Yot
Trang
Phatthalung
Songkhla
Hat Yai
Sadao
Yala
Narathiwat
Pattani
Betong

P   e   n   i   n   s   u   l   a   r

M   A   L   A   Y   S   I   A

Kota Bharu
Tumpat
Pasir Mas
Rantau Panjang
Kuala Krai
Kuala Terengganu
Marang
Dungun
Kemasik
Cukai
Kuantan
Pekan
KUALA LUMPUR
Klang
Port Swettenham
Seremban
Melaka
Muar
Batu Pahat
Pontian Kechil
Kukup

P   E   N   I   N   S   U   L   A   R

M   A   L   A   Y   S   I   A

George Town
Butterworth
P. Pinang
Bagan Serai
Taiping
Ipoh
Cameron Highlands
2182
2130
Tapah
Teluk Intan
Lumut

Straits of Malacca

Pulau Tioman
P. Pemanggil
P. Aur
P. Babi Besar
Pulau Tinggi

SINGAPORE
Johor Bahru
Singapore
Pulau Batam
Bintan
Tanjungpinang

I   N   D   O   N   E   S   I   A

S   u   m   a   t   e   r   a

MEDAN
Belawan
Tebingtinggi
Pematangsiantar
Prapat
Danau Toba
2151
2457
3012

East from Greenwich

5

4

3

2   National Parks

1

Projection: Conical with two standard parallels

ft   m
9000   3000
6000   2000
4500   1500
3000   1000
1200   400
600   200
0
0   200
600   2000
6000

84

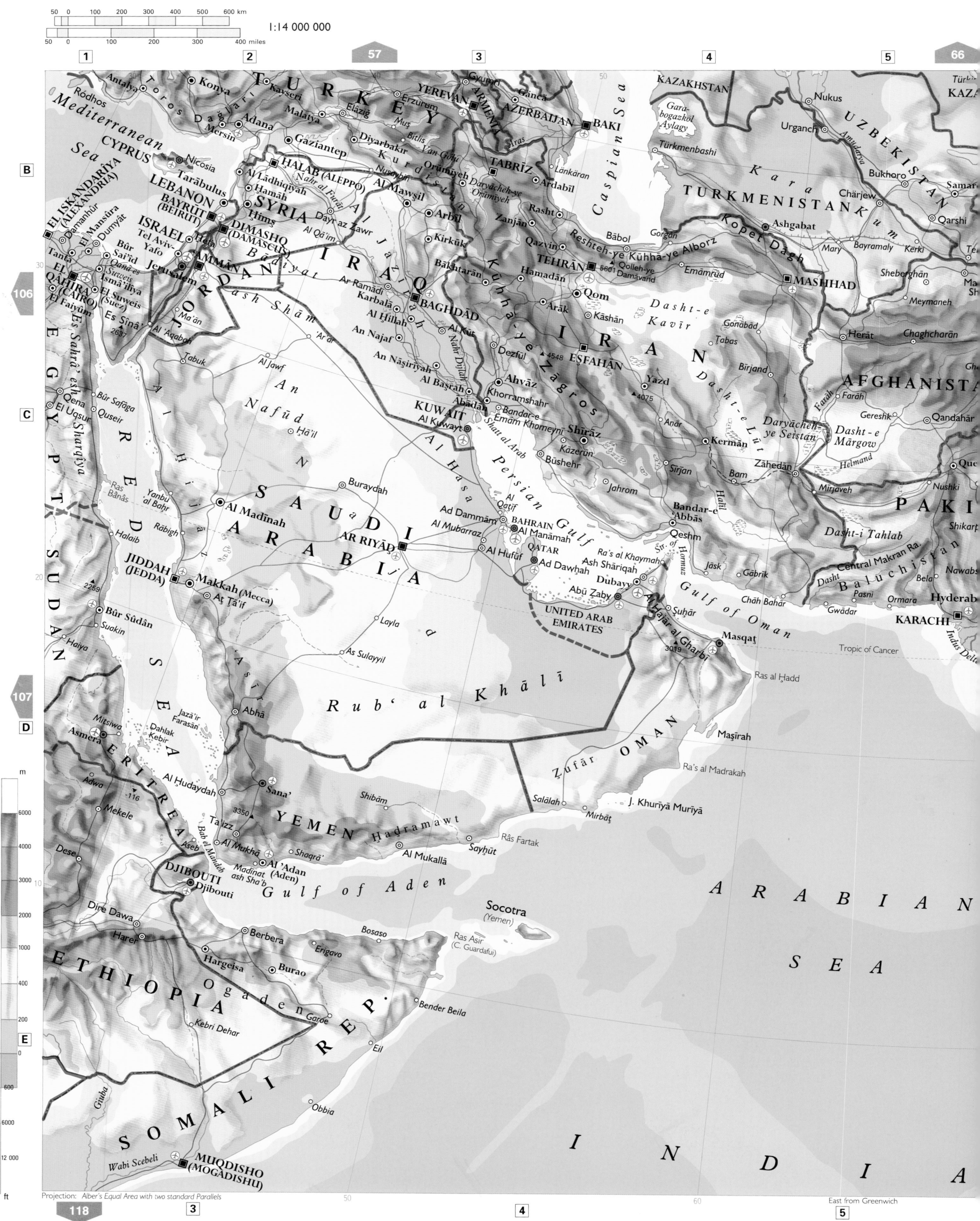

1:14 000 000

Projection: Alber's Equal Area with two standard Parallels

East from Greenwich

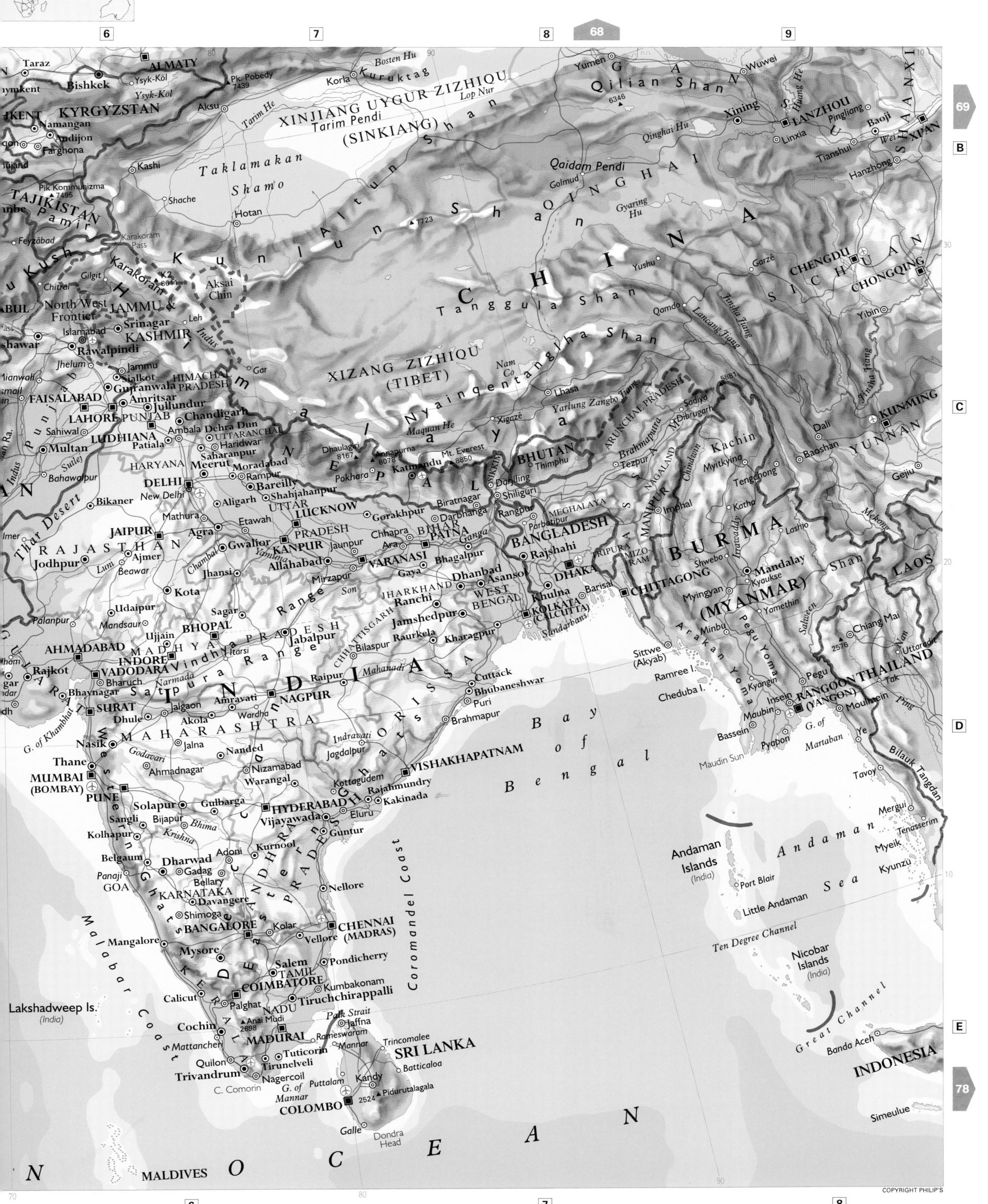

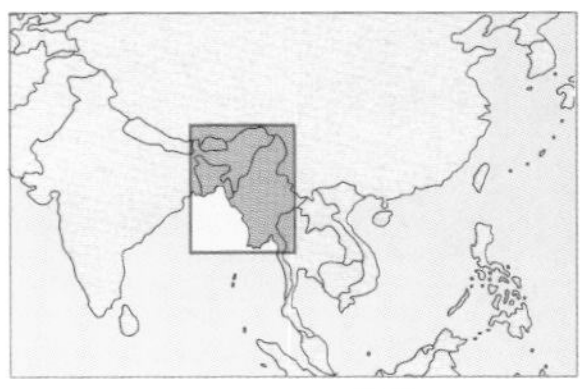

1:4 800 000

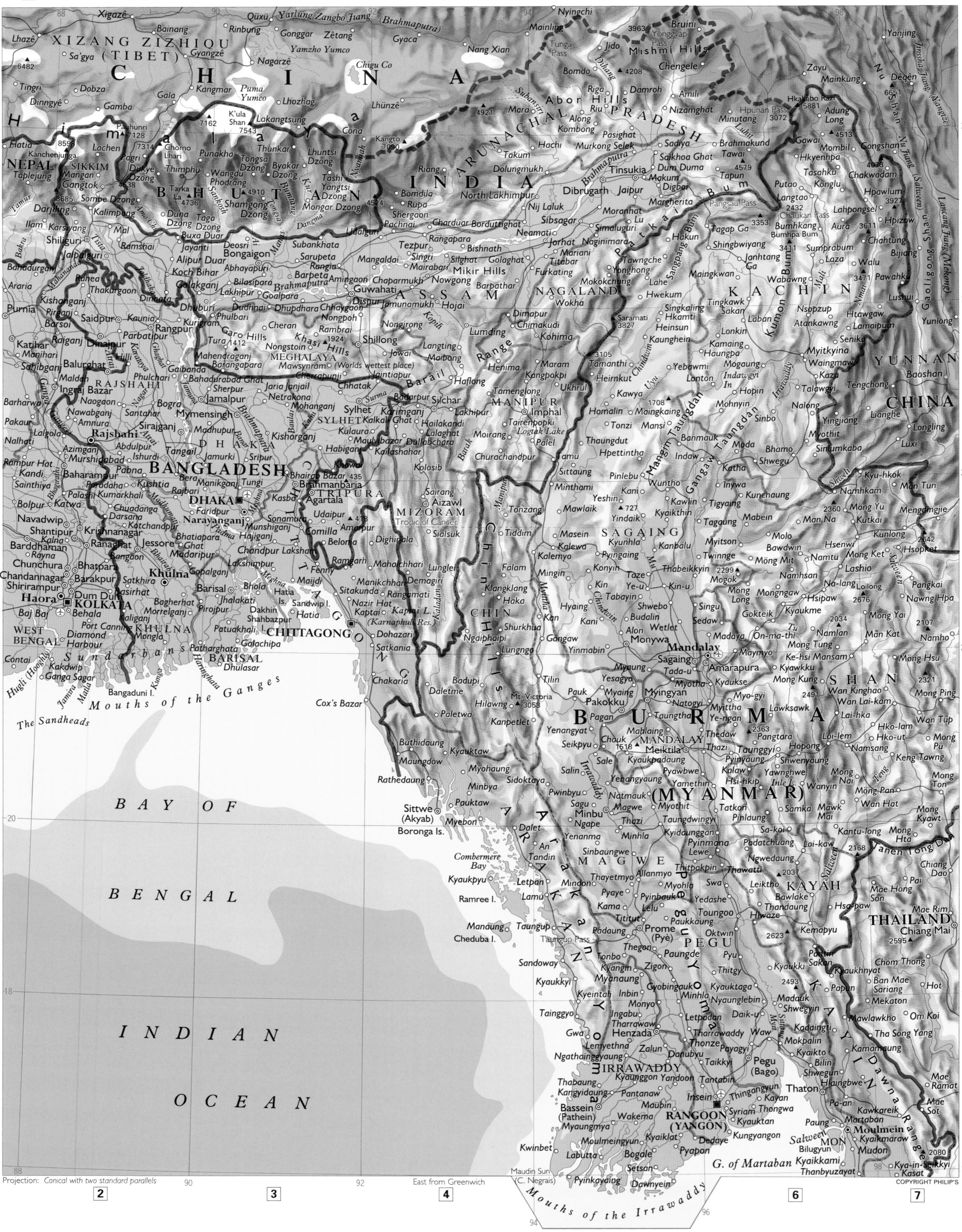

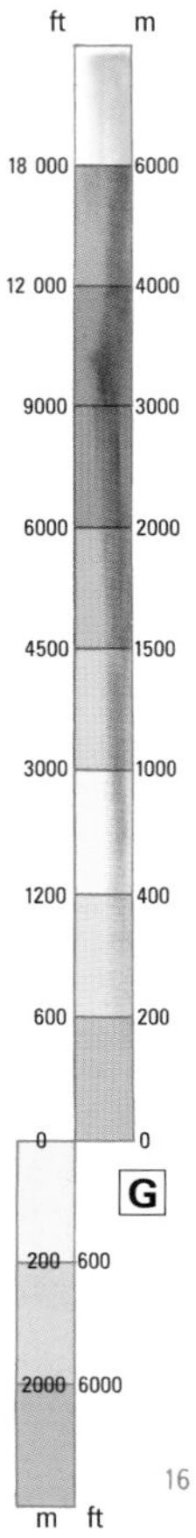

Projection: Conical with two standard parallels East from Greenwich

COPYRIGHT PHILIP'S

Major labels

CHINA

XIZANG ZIZHIQU (TIBET)

ARUNACHAL PRADESH

INDIA

NEPAL

SIKKIM

BHUTAN

ASSAM

MEGHALAYA

NAGALAND

MANIPUR

KACHIN

SAGAING

YUNNAN

CHINA

BANGLADESH

DHAKA

WEST BENGAL

RAJSHAHI

KHULNA

TRIPURA

MIZORAM

CHIN HILLS

BURMA (MYANMAR)

MANDALAY

MAGWE

PEGU

SHAN

KAYAH

THAILAND

ARAKAN

CHITTAGONG

RANGOON (YANGON)

MON

BAY OF BENGAL

INDIAN OCEAN

Mouths of the Ganges

The Sandheads

Mouths of the Irrawaddy

G. of Martaban

Tropic of Cancer

Selected cities and places

Kolkata, Haora, Dhaka, Narayanganj, Khulna, Chittagong, Cox's Bazar, Sittwe (Akyab), Mandalay, Sagaing, Amarapura, Rangoon (Yangon), Moulmein, Bassein (Pathein), Prome (Pye), Toungoo, Pegu (Bago), Shillong, Guwahati, Imphal, Kohima, Silchar, Agartala, Aizawl, Dibrugarh, Tezpur, Siliguri, Rajshahi, Thimphu, Kathmandu region

Elevation scale

ft	m
18 000	6000
12 000	4000
9000	3000
6000	2000
4500	1500
3000	1000
1200	400
600	200
0	0
200	600
2000	6000

1:5 600 000

50 0 50 100 150 200 250 300 km
50 0 50 100 150 200 miles

TURKMENISTAN · **UZBEKISTAN** · **TAJIKISTAN** · **CHINA**

AFGHANISTAN

PAKISTAN

IRAN

INDIA

ARABIAN SEA

Tropic of Cancer

Hindu Kush · *Karakoram Range*

KĀBUL · Peshawar · RAWALPINDI · Islamabad · Srinagar

Herat · Mazar-e Sharif · QONDUZ · Feyzābād · Gilgit

Qandahar · Quetta · Multan · FAISALABAD · LAHORE · Amritsar

Zāhedān · Bahawalpur · Bikaner

HYDERABAD · KARACHI · Jodhpur

Mouths of the Indus · *Rann of Kachchh* · **GUJARAT**

Thar Desert · **RAJASTHAN** · **SINDH** · **PUNJAB**

Makran Coast Range · *Central Makran Range* · *Siahan Range* · *Kirthar Range*

JAMMU AND KASHMIR

Projection: Conical with two standard parallels

East from Greenwich

COPYRIGHT PHILIP'S

ft m
18 000 6000
12 000 4000
9000 3000
6000 2000
4500 1500
3000 1000
1200 400
600 200
0 0
200 600
2000 6000
m ft

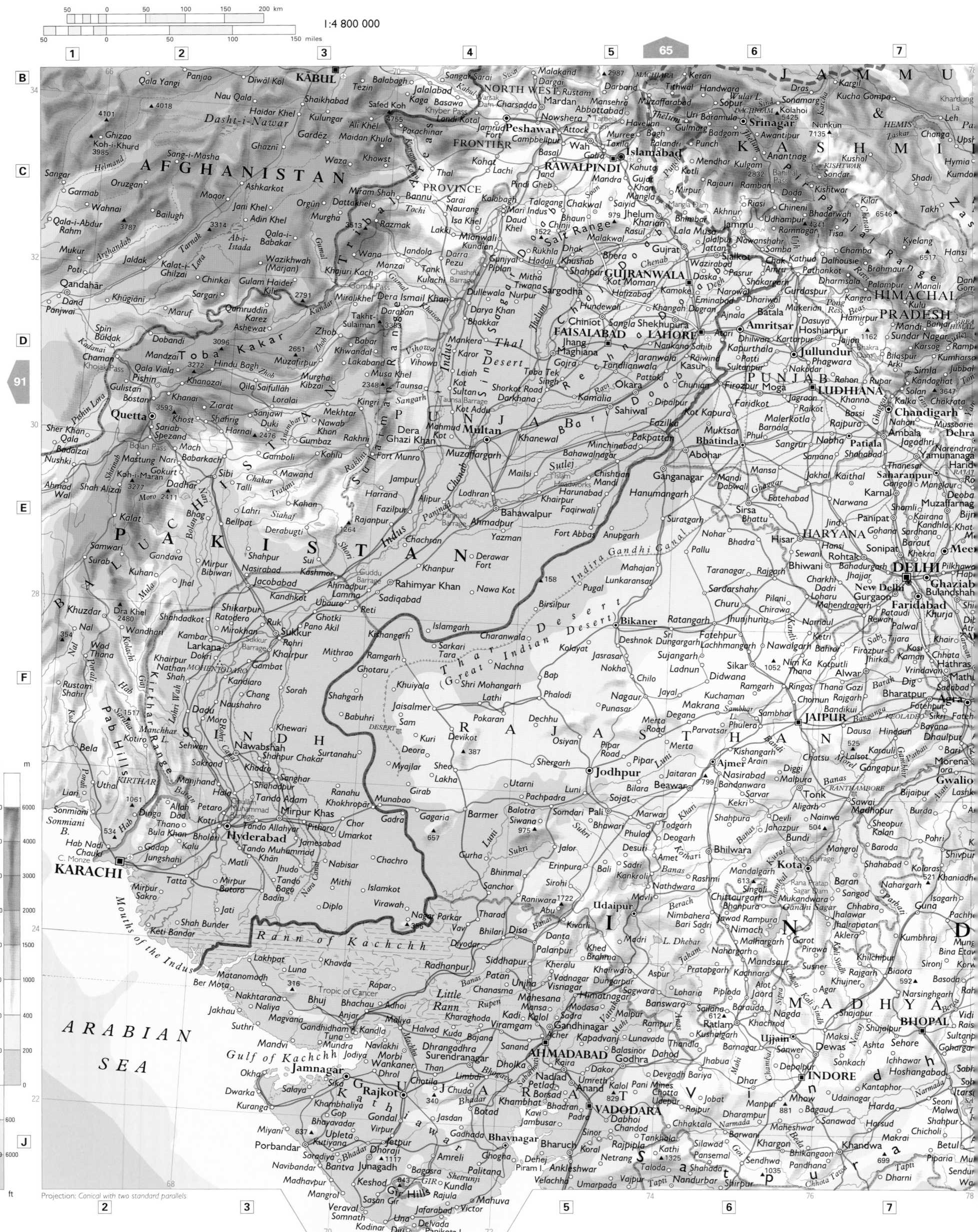

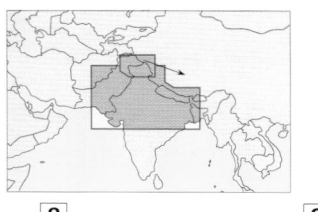

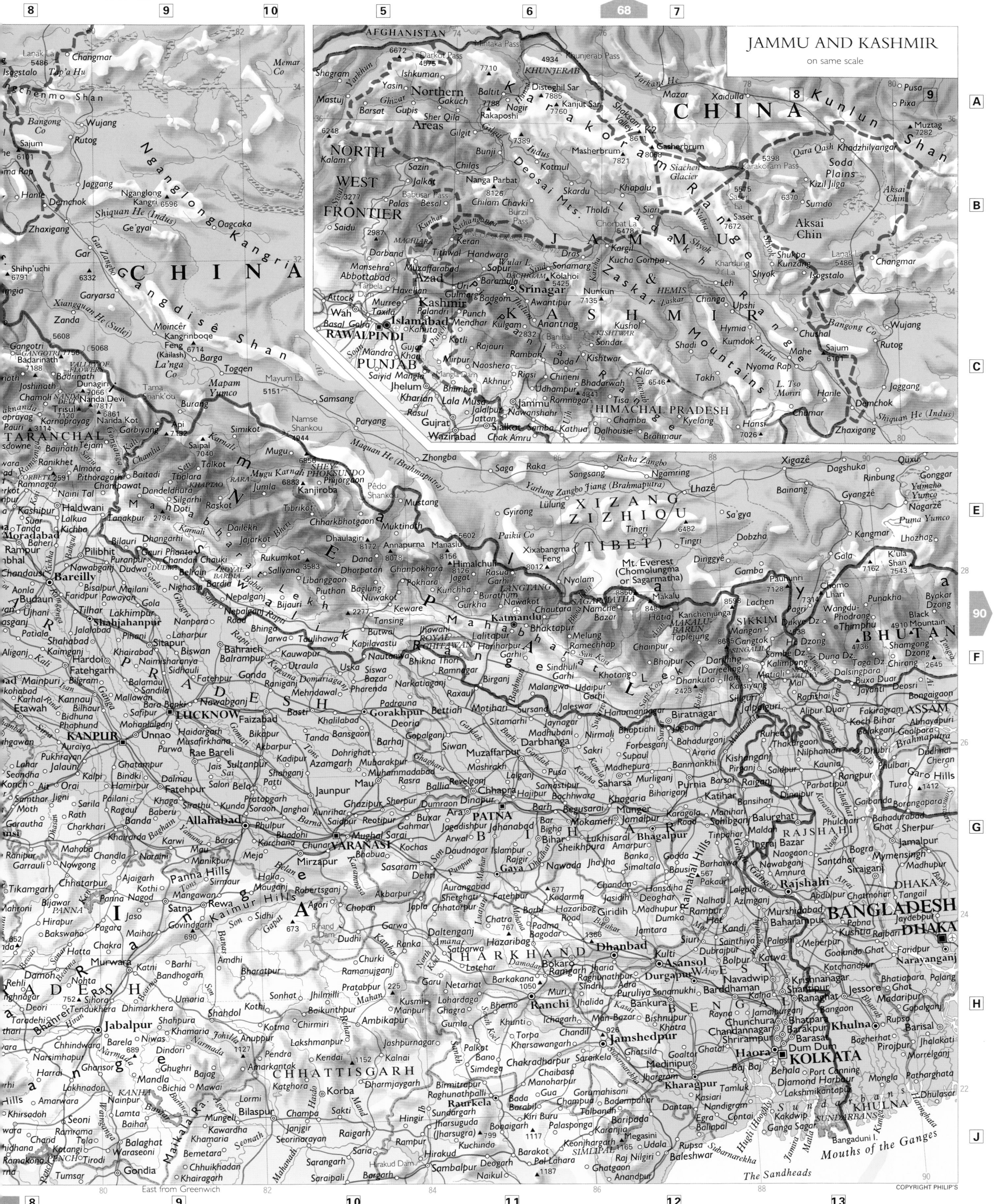

1:4 800 000

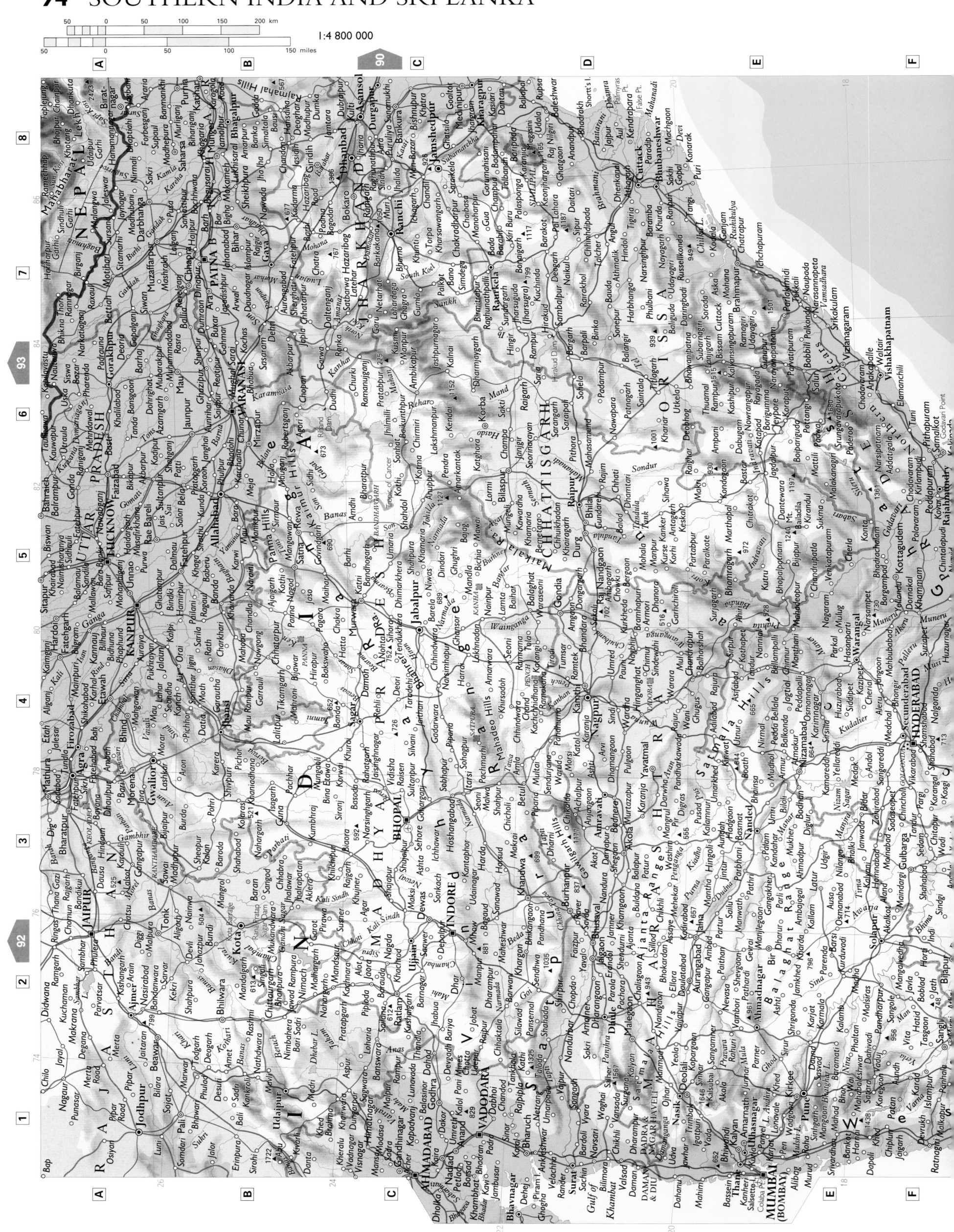

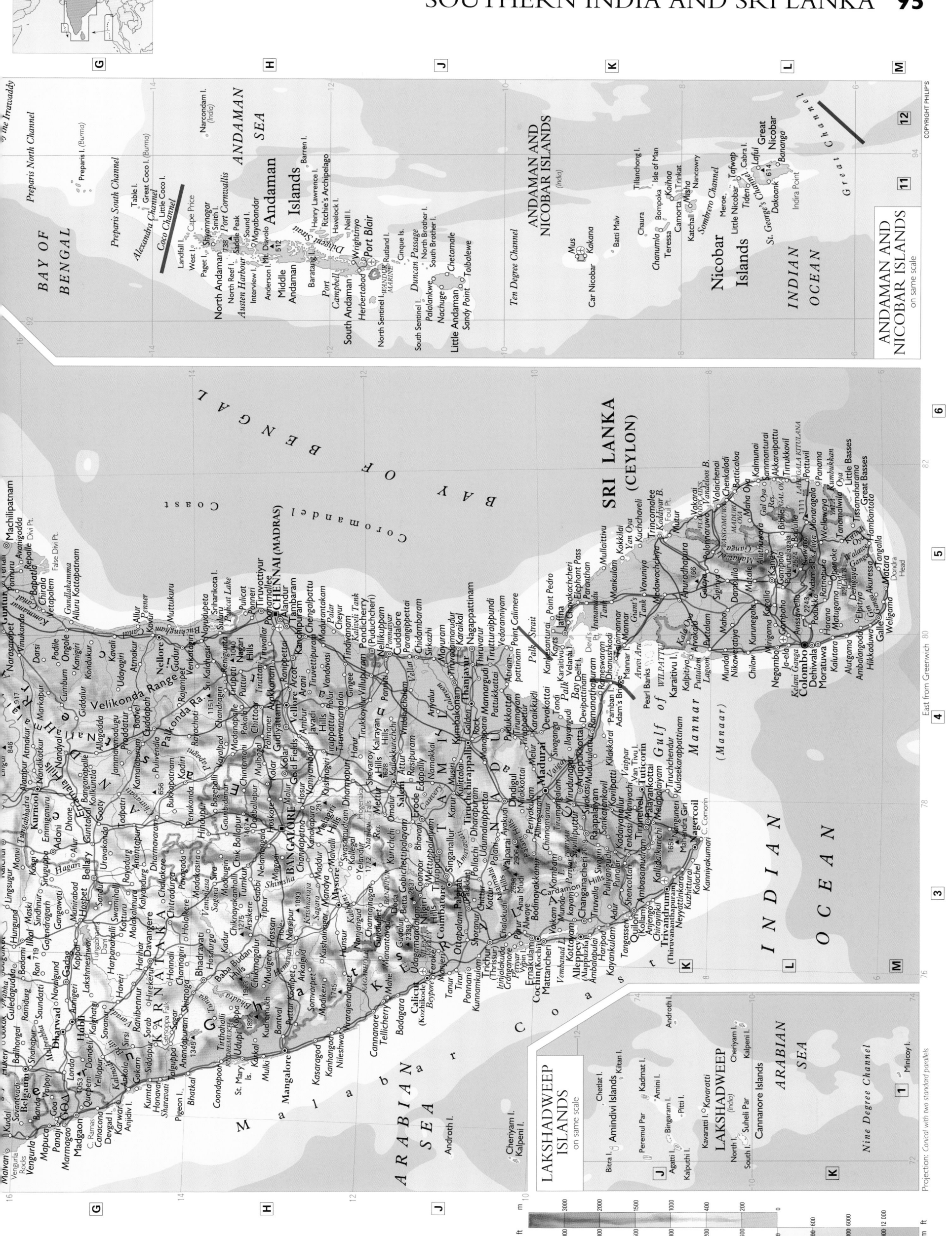

ANDAMAN AND NICOBAR ISLANDS
on same scale

LAKSHADWEEP ISLANDS
on same scale

Projection: Conical with two standard parallels

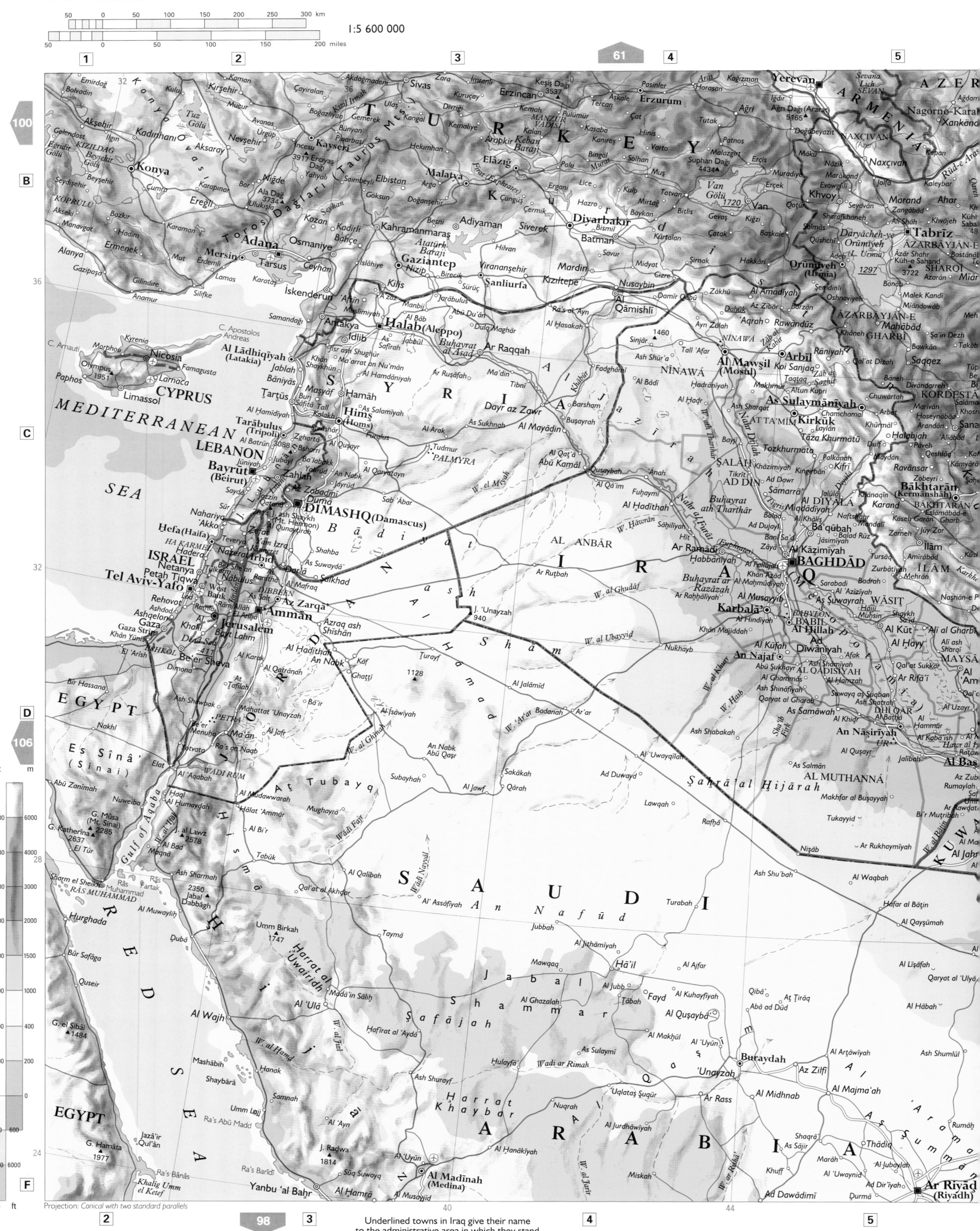

1:5 600 000

Projection: Conical with two standard parallels

Underlined towns in Iraq give their name
to the administrative area in which they stand

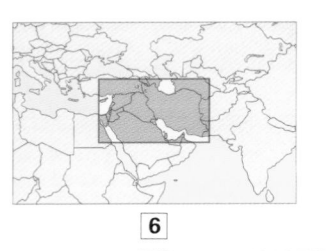

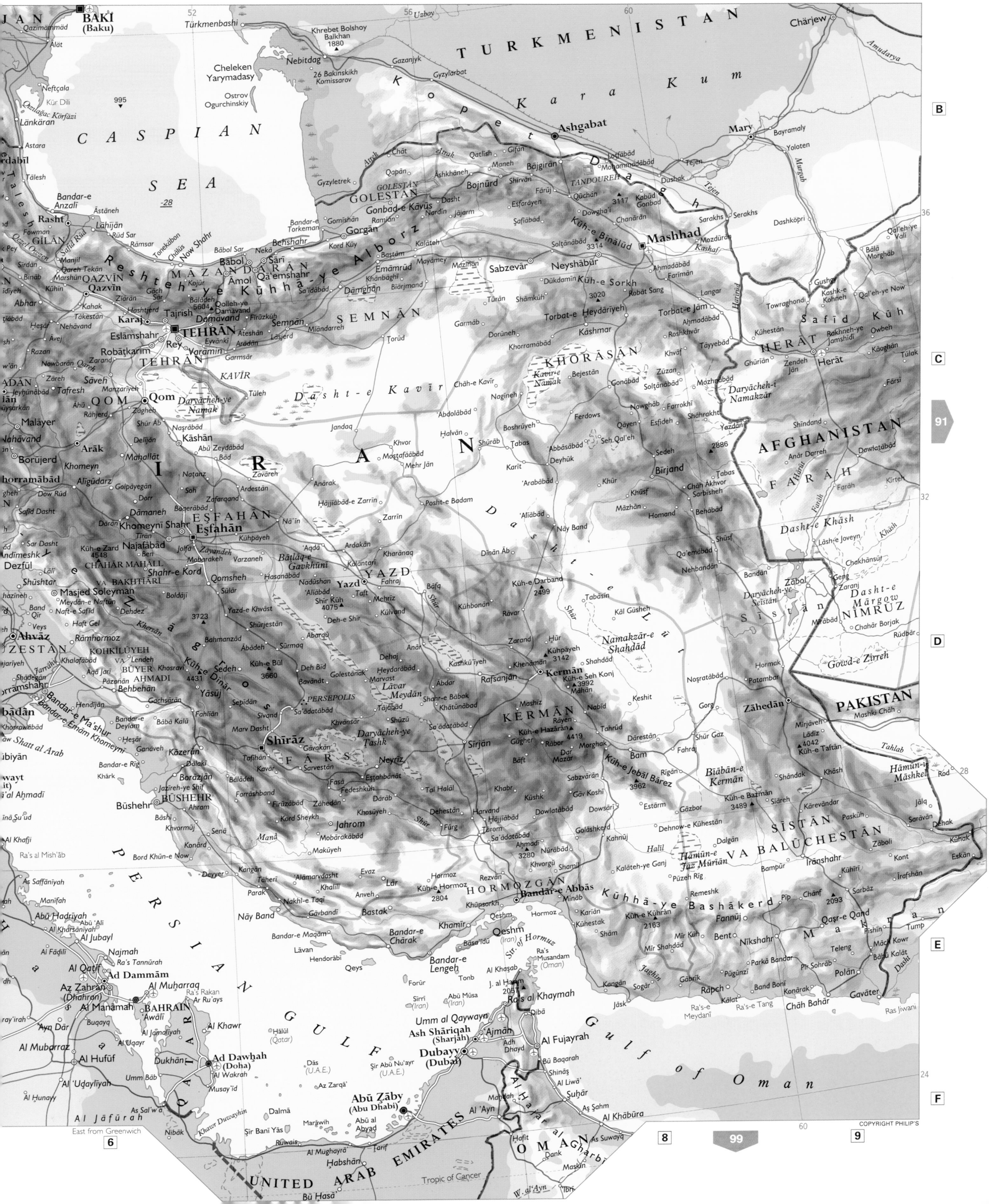

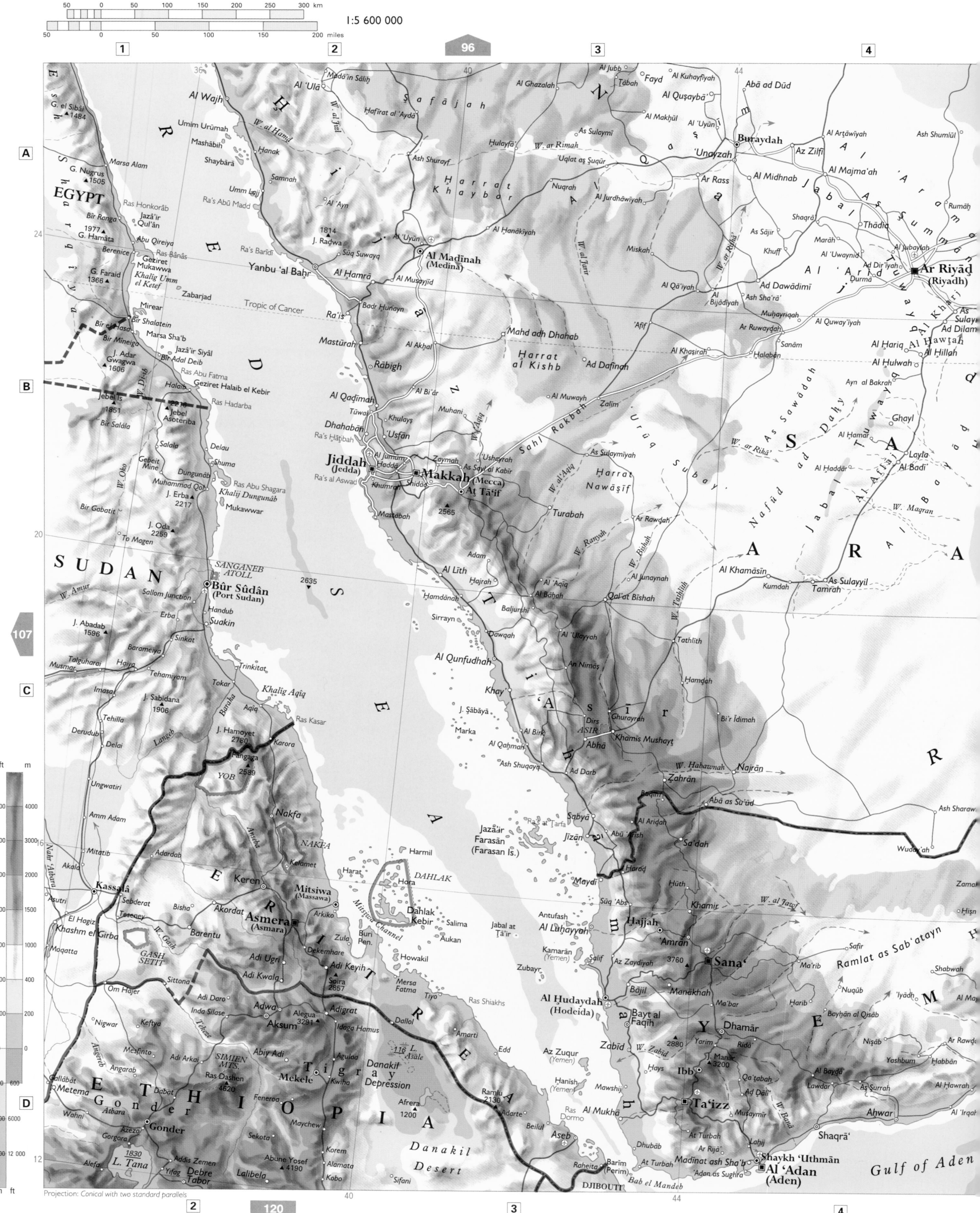

50   0   50   100   150   200   250   300 km
50   0   50   100   150   200 miles

1:5 600 000

1   2   96   3   4

ft   m
12 000   4000
9000   3000
6000   2000
4500   1500
3000   1000
1200   400
600   200
0   0
200   600
2000   6000
4000   12 000
m   ft

Projection: Conical with two standard parallels

2   120   3   4

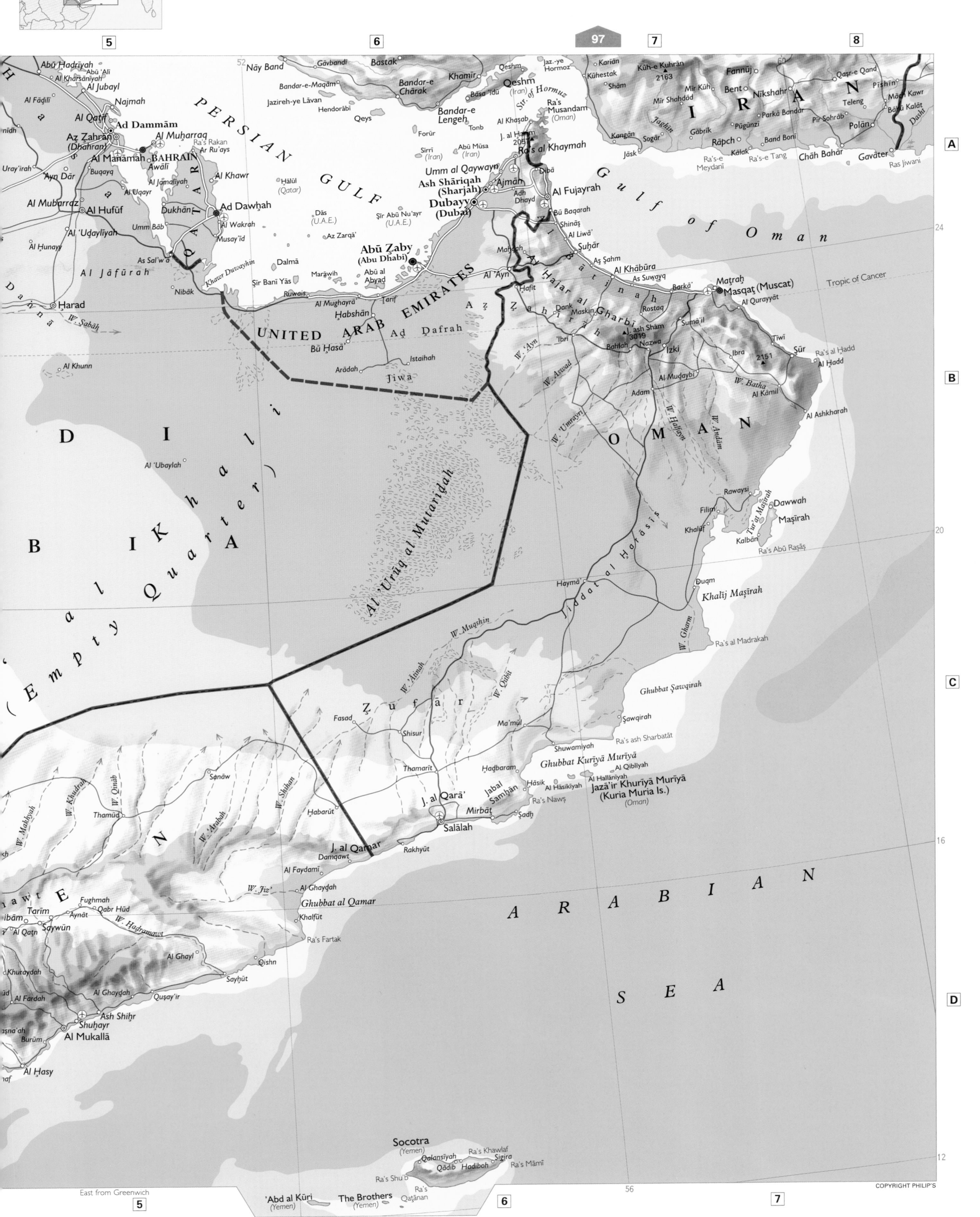

PERSIAN GULF

Abū Hadrīyah
Abū 'Alī
Al Kharsānīyah
Al Jubayl
Najmah
Al Fāḍilī
Al Qaṭīf
Az Zahrān (Dhahran)
Ad Dammām
Al Muḥarraq
Ra's Rakan
Ar Ru'ays
BAHRAIN
Al Manāmah
Awālī
Uray'irah
'Ayn Dār
Buqayq
Al Khawr
Al 'Uqayr
Al Jumaliyah
Al Mubarraz
Al Hufūf
Dukhān
Ad Dawḥah
Al Wakrah
Umm Bāb
Musay'īd
Al 'Uqaylīyah
Al Ḥunayy
As Sal'w a
Khawr Duwayhin
QATAR
Al Jāfūrah
Nibāk
Dalmā
Ṣīr Banī Yās
Marāwiḥ
Abū al Abyaḍ
Dannā
Ḥarad
W. Ṣabāḥ
Ḥabshān
Rūwais
Al Mughayrā
Ṭarīf
Al Khunn
Bū Ḥaṣā
Istaihah
Ad Ḍafrah
Arādah
Jīwā

UNITED ARAB EMIRATES

Nāy Band
Gāvbandi
Bastak
Khamir
Qeshm (Iran)
Qeshm
Str. of Hormuz
Ra's Musandam (Oman)
Bandar-e Maqām
Bandar-e Chārak
Bāsa 'Idū
Bandar-e Lengeh
Tonb
Al Khaṣab
J. al Ḥarīm 2051
Ra's al Khaymah
Dubā
Jazireh-ye Lāvan
Hendorābi
Qeys
Forūr
Umm al Qaywayn
Ash Shāriqah (Sharjah)
Ajmān
Adh Dhayd
Al Fujayrah
Sīrrī (Iran)
Abū Mūsā (Iran)
Dubayy (Dubai)
Ḥālūl (Qatar)
Dās (U.A.E.)
Ṣīr Abū Nu'ayr (U.A.E.)
Az Zarqā'
Abū Ẓaby (Abu Dhabi)
Al 'Ayn
Ḥafīt
Maḥaḍah
Al Bāṭinah
Shināṣ
Ṣuḥār
Aş Şahm
Al Khābūra
As Suwayq
Barkā
Maṭraḥ
Masqaṭ (Muscat)
Al Qurayyāt

IRAN

Jaz.-ye Hormoz
Kārian
Kūhestak
Shām
Kūh-e Kuhrān 2163
Mīr Kūh
Fannūj
Bent
Nīkshahr
Qaṣr-e Qand
Pīshīn
Māgū Kawr
Ṭaghīn
Gābrīk
Parkā Bandar
Pīr Sohrāb
Polān
Bālū Kalāt
Dashī
Kāngān
Sogār
Rāpch
Band Bonī
Jāsk
Ra's-e Meydāni
Ra's-e Tang
Chāh Bahār
Gavāter
Ras Jiwani

Gulf of Oman

24

Aẓ Ẓāhirah
Dank
Maskin
Gharbī
Ibrī
Bōtlah
Nazwa
Rostaq
Sumā'il
J. ash Shām 3019
Izki
Adam
Al Muḍaybī
Nakhl
Tiwī
Ṣūr
Ra's al Ḥadd
Al Ḥadd
Ibra 2151
Al Kāmil
Al Ashkharah

Tropic of Cancer

OMAN

RUB' AL KHALI (Empty Quarter)

Al 'Ubaylah

Al 'Urūq al Mu'tariḍah

Rawaysi
Filim
Khalūf
Kalbān
Khalīj Maṣīrah
Ra's Abū Raṣāṣ
Dawwah
Maṣīrah
T'ir al Maṣīrah

20

Haymā'
W. Muqshin
Jiddat al Ḥarāsīs
W. Gharm
Ra's al Madrakah

C

 Z u f ā r
W. Ainah
W. Qitbit
Ghubbat Ṣawqirah
Ṣawqirah
Fasad
Shisur
Ma'mūl
Ra's ash Sharbatāt
Thamarīt
Ḥaqbaram
Shuwamiyah
Sanāw
Jabal Samḥān
Ḥāsik
Ghubbat Kurīyā Murīyā
Al Qibliyah
Al Ḥāsikīyah
Al Ḥallānīyah
Jazā'ir Khurīyā Murīyā (Kuria Muria Is.) (Oman)
Thamūd
J. al Qarā'
Ra's Nawṣ
Mirbāṭ
Ṣadḥ
Ḥabarūt
Salālah
J. al Qamar
Damqawt
Rakhyūt
Al Faydāmī
W. Jiz'
Al Ghaydah
Ghubbat al Qamar
Khalfūt
Ra's Fartak

W. Masīyah
W. Qināb
W. Khudrah
W. Arabah
W. Shibam
Thamūd
HADRAMAWT
Fughmah
Tarīm
Qabr Hūd
Aynāt
Al Qaṭn
Saywūn
W. Ḥaḍramawt
Shibām
Al Ghayl
Al Ghaydah
Sayhūt
Qishn
Khuraydah
Al Fardah
Ash Shiḥr
Qusay'ir
Shuhayr
Al Mukallā
Burūm
Al Ḥasy

ARABIAN

SEA

D

16

Socotra (Yemen)
Qalansīyah
Qādib
Hadiboh
Sigira
Ra's Khawlaf
Ra's Mamī
Ra's Shu'b

'Abd al Kūri (Yemen)
The Brothers (Yemen)
Ra's Qaṭānan

12

50 25 0 25 50 75 100 125 150 175 km
1 : 4 000 000
50 25 0 25 50 75 100 125 miles

BULGARIA

B L A C K   S E A

Stara Zagora
Yambol
Aytos
Burgas
Nos Emine
Michurin
Elkhovo
Kırklareli
Demirköy
İğneada Burnu
Edirne
Orestiás
Pınarhisar
Vize
Saray
Kıyıköy
Uzunköprü
Babaeski
Lüleburgaz
Çerkezköy
Çatalca
Hayrabolu
Muratlı
Çorlu
İSTANBUL
İstanbul Boğazı (Bosporus)
Şile
Kandıra
Kerempe Burnu
İnce Burun
Sinop
İnebolu
Abana
Ayancık
Gerze
Kurucaşile
Cide
Çatalzeytin
Amasra
Kilimli
Bartın
Küre
Boyabat
Alaçam
Bafra Burnu
Zonguldak
Devrekâni
Kastamonu
Civa Burnu
Samsun
Terme
Ünye
Fatsa
İpsala
Keşan
Malkara
Tekirdağ
Büyükçekmece
Gebze
Kocaeli (İzmit)
Sakarya (Adapazarı)
Karasu
Ereğli
Kozlu
Devrek
Daday
Araç
Karabük
Tosya
Osmancık
Merzifon
Havza
Ladik
Korgan
Gürgentepe
Aybastı
Samothráki
Gökçeada
Eceabat
Gelibolu
Çanakkale Boğazı (Dardanelles)
Marmara Denizi (Sea of Marmara)
Darıca
Yalova
Orhangazi
Gemlik
İznik Gölü
Yenişehir
Geyve
Göynük
Seben
Bolu
Gerede
Çerkeş
Kurşunlu
Çankırı
İskilip
Çorum
Mecitözü
Amasya
Turhal
Erbaa
Niksar
Reşadiye
Tokat
TROY
Ezine
Bayramiç
Edremit
Balya
Susurluk
Bursa
Uludağ
İnegöl
Bilecik
Söğüt
Bozüyük
Eskişehir
Mihalıççık
Nallıhan
Beypazarı
Ayaş
Sincan
ANKARA
Kalecik
Elmadağ
Delice
Yozgat
Sorgun
Yıldızeli
Sivas
Lésvos
Ayvalık
Bergama
Soma
Akhisar
Balıkesir
Bigadiç
Dursunbey
Emet
Tavşanlı
Kütahya
Seyitgazi
Afyon (Afyonkarahisar)
Sivrihisar
Polatlı
Haymana
Bâlâ
Kırşehir
Yerköy
Kırıkkale
Keskin
Akdağmadeni
Ak Dağları
Khíos
Foça
Manisa
Menemen
Turgutlu
Salihli
Alaşehir
Uşak
Banaz
Bolvadin
Çay
Emirdağ
Yunak
Kulu
Mucur
Hacıbektaş
Ortaköy
Nevşehir
Kayseri
Bünyan
Gemerek
Şarkışla
Çeşme
Urla
İZMİR (Smyrna)
Torbalı
Ödemiş
Sarıgöl
Eşme
Uluborlu
Şuhut
Sandıklı
Dinar
Sultan Dağları
Akşehir Gölü
Akşehir
Ilgın
Sarayönü
Kadınhanı
Obruk
Şereflikoçhisar
Cihanbeyli
Tuz Gölü
Aksaray
Derinkuyu
GÖREME
Develi
Tomarza
Gürün
Darende
Sámos
Kuşadası
Aydın
Nazilli
Buldan
Çal
Çivril
Eğridir Gölü
Eğridir
Gelendost
Şarkikaraağaç
Beyşehir Gölü
Konya
Karapınar
Ereğli
Niğde
Bakırdağı
Afşin
Elbistan
Ikaría
Söke
Karacasu
Denizli
Bozdoğan
Tavas
Acıgöl
Isparta
Beyşehir
Çumra
Ulukışla
Pozantı
Kozan
Kadirli
Göksun
MILETUS
Milas
Yatağan
Muğla
Kale
Kızılhisar
Burdur
Ağlasun
Sütçüler
Seydişehir
Bozkır
Karaman
Ayrancı
Karaisalı
İmamoğlu
Kahramanmaraş
Pazarcık
Gölbaşı
Kálimnos
Bodrum
Ören
Köyceğiz
Ortaca
Dalaman
Fethiye
Korkuteli
Hadım
Toros Dağları
Mut
Silifke
Erdemli
Mersin (İçel)
Tarsus
Adana
Ceyhan
Osmaniye
İslâhiye
Gaziantep
Kilis
GREECE
Ródhos (Rhodes)
Datça
Marmaris
Kaş
Kalkan
Kemer
Antalya
Manavgat
Alanya
Gazipaşa
Anamur
Gülnar
Antalya Körfezi
Anamur Burnu
İskenderun Körfezi
İskenderun
Kırıkhan
Antakya
Reyhanlı
A'zâz
HALAB (Aleppo)
İdlib
M E D I T E R R A N E A N   S E A

CYPRUS
Rizokarpaso
C. Apostolos Andreas
Kyrenia
Morphou
Polis
Nicosia
Famagusta
Troodos
Olympus 1951
Larnaca
Paphos
Episkopi
Limassol
Al Lādhiqīyah (Latakia)
Jablah
Bāniyās
Hamāh
Maşyāf
Tartūs
Himş (Homs)
Al Hamidīyah

LEBANON
Tarābulus (Tripoli)
Zgharta
Al Batrūn
Bsharri
Jubayl
Juniyah
BAYRŪT (Beirut)
Zahlah
Saydā
DIMASHQ (Damascus)
Şūr
Qiryat Shemona
An Nabk

ISRAEL
Hefa (Haifa)
Teverya
Nazerat
'Akko
Nahariyya
Hadera
Netanya
Tel Aviv-Yafo
Nābulus
West Bank
As Salt
Irbid
AMMAN
Rehovot
Ashdod
Ashqelon
El 'Arīsh
Ramla
Jerusalem
Az Zarqā'
JORDAN

Projection: Conical with two standard parallels

Division between Greeks and Turks in Cyprus; Turks to the North.

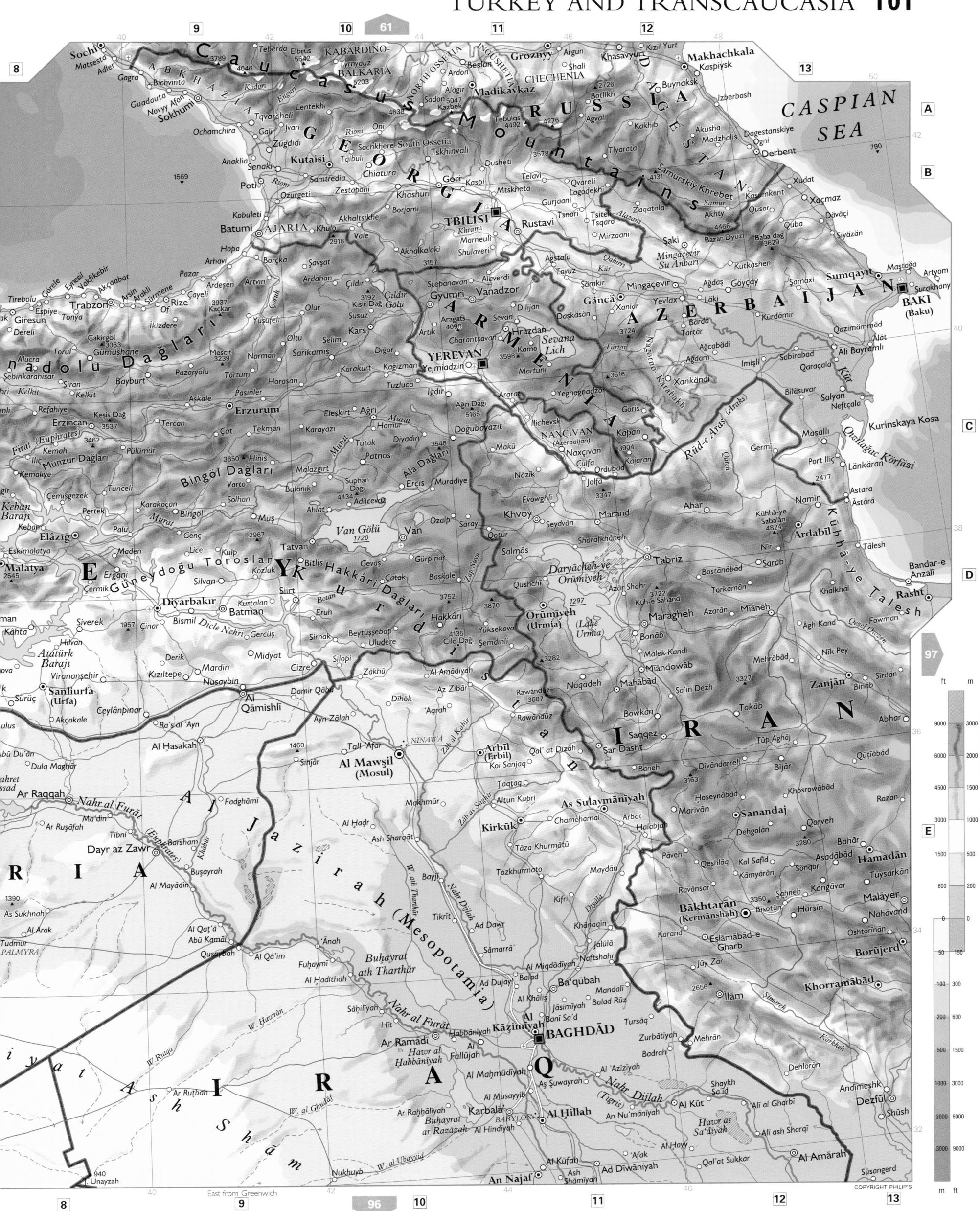

100 0 100 200 300 400 500 600 km
100 0 100 200 300 400 miles

1 : 12 000 000

101

ft m

12 000 4000

9000 3000

6000 2000

4500 1500

3000 1000

1200 400

600 200

0 0

200 600

1000 3000

2000 6000

4000 12 000

m ft

LEBANON
BAYRŪT (BEIRUT)
SYRIA
DIMASHQ (DAMASCUS)
ISRAEL
Tel Aviv-Yafo
Ashdod
Jerusalem
West Bank
'AMMĀN
Bûr Sa'îd (Port Said)
Qanâ es Suweis
Ismâ'iliya
El Suweis (Suez)
JORDAN
Ma'an
Al 'Aqabah
G. Mūsa 2637
Es Sinâ'
Khalîg el Suweis
Jabal ad Durūz 1801
Ar Rutbah
IRAQ
Karbalā
BAGHDĀD
An Najaf
Al Jawf
Rafhā
Hafar al Bāţin
An Nafūd
Tabūk
Al Muwaylih
Hā'il
Buraydah
'Unayzah
Badiyat ash Shām
Al Amarah
Ahvāz
Khorramshahr
Ābādān
Al Başrah
An Nāşirīyah
Al Kuwayt
KUWAIT
Būbiyān
J. Khārk
Al Qaţīf
Ad Dammām
Al Mubarraz
Al Hufūf
BAHRAIN
Al Manāmah
QATAR
Ad Dawħah (Doha)
Harad
AR RIYĀD (RIYADH)
Layla
As Sulayyil
UNITED ARAB EMIRATES
Abū Zaby (Abu Dhabi)
Al 'Ayn
Dubayy (Dubai)
Ash Shāriqah (Sharjah)
Ra's al-Khaymah
Ra's Musandam (Oman)
Şuħār
ESFAHĀN 4548
PERSEPOLIS
Shīrāz
Kāzerūn
Būshehr
Deyyer
Jahrom
Neyrīz
Bandar-e Abbas
Qeshm
Khamīr
Bampūr
Str. of Hormuz
Gābrik
Gulf of Oman
Khvor
Birjand
Farāh
AFGHANISTAN
Yazd
Kermān
Bam
Zābol
Daryācheh-ye Seistan
Zāhedān
Dasht-e Lut
Zagros
Persian Gulf
Kūħha-ye
Nahr Dijlah
Nahr al Furāt
Mesopotamia (Al Jazirah)
IRAN

EGYPT
Hurghada
Bûr Safâga
Qena
Quseir
El Uqsur
Idfû
Kôm Ombo
Aswân
Sadd el Aali
Buheirat en Naser
Es Sahrâ en Nûbiya
Kosha
Delgo
3rd Cataract
Dongola
4th Cataract
Kareima
Ed Debba
Wad Hamid
6th Cataract
Omdurmân
El Khartûm (Khartoum)
5th Cataract
Atbara
Berber
Abu Hamed
Nahr en Nil
El Gezira
Ed Dueim
Wad Medanî
Khashm el Girba
Kassalâ
Gedaref
Kôstî
Singa
Umm Ruwaba
Ed Damazin
SUDAN
Sûdd
Bahr-el-Jebel
Nil el Abyad
Nil el Azraq
Malakâl
Sobat
Pibor Post
Bôr
Tali Post
Juba
Mongalla
Kapoeta
Torit
Yei
Kajo Kaji 3187
Arua
Gulu
Pakwach
Lira
Moroto
UGANDA
Murchison Falls
L. Albert
L. Kyoga
Soroti
Mbale 4321
L. Masindi
Kitale
KENYA
Lokichokio
South Horn
Marsabit
Wajir
Dif
El Wak
Moyale
Mega
Lodwar
L. Turkana 375
Chew Bahir
Dolo
Lugh Ganana
Bardera
Bur Acaba
Baidoa
Belet Uen
El Dere
Lugh Ganana
MUQDISHO (MOGADISHU)
Merca
Kismayu
Giuba
Wabi Scebeli

RED SEA
Ras Bânas
Bîr Shalatein
Halaib
Ras Hadarba
Wadi Halfa
Muhammad Qol
2259
Yanbu 'al Bahr
Al Madīnah
Tropic of Cancer
Rābigh
Makkah (Mecca)
Aţ Ţā'if 2565
JIDDAH (JEDDA)
Al Līth
Turabah
Bûr Sûdân
Suakin
Sinkat
Trinkitat
Haiya
Karora 2780
Adarama
Akordat
Nakfa
Adigrat
Aksum
Adwa
Mekele
ERITREA
Asmera
Keren
Massawa
Dahlak Kebir
Zula
Adi Ugri
Al Luhayyah
Kamaran
Hanish
Farasān
Jīzān
Abhā
Najrān
Khamir
Sana'
Ta'izz
Al Hudaydah
Al Mukhā
Bab el Mandeb
Djebel Manar 3350
Nişāb
Shaqrā
Ahwar
Al' Adan (Aden)
Al Mukallā
Shibām
Sayħūt
Rās Fartak
Hadramawt
2469
YEMEN
Mirbāţ
Salālah
Zufār
Khalīf
Khalīj Maşīrah
Ras al Madrakah
J. Khurīya Murīya
Maşīrah
Ra's al Hadd
Şūr
Masqaţ
Maţraħ 3019
Nazwā
OMAN
Al 'Ubaylah
Rub' al Khālī (Empty Quarter)
Al Hasā
SAUDI ARABIA
Hijaz
'Asir
Najd

Ras Dashen 4620
Gonder
Debre Tabor
Lalibela 4190
Bahir Dar
L. Tana
1830
Bure
Debre Markos
Dese
Danakil Desert
Tendaho
L. Abbé
DJIBOUTI
Dikhil -156
Tadjoura
Djibouti
Zeila
Aseb
Berbera
Karin
Bosaso
Ras Asir
Erigavo 2406
El Gal
Dante
Ras Hafun
Bender Beila
Eil
Gardo
Garge
Las Anod
Hargeisa
Burao
Jijiga
Harer
Dire Dawa
ADDIS ABEBA
Debre Zevit
Nazret
Awash 3381
ETHIOPIA
Nekemte
Metu
Gore
Dembidolo 3202
Jima
Asela
Shashemene
Awasa
Yirga Alem 3686
Omo
Dila
Kibre Mengist
Negele
Goba
Mt. Batu 4307
Imi
Kebri Dehar
Ginir
Gando
OGADEN
SOMALI REP.
Galcaio
Obbia
Sinadogo
Ferfer
Scebeli
Arba Minch
L. Abaya
L. Shamo
Buheirat
Danakil
-116
Gulf of Aden
Abd al Kūrī
Bereda
Hadiboh
Socotra (Yemen)

INDIAN OCEAN

Projection : Sanson-Flamsteed's Sinusoidal

East from Greenwich

COPYRIGHT PHILIP'S

118

106 107

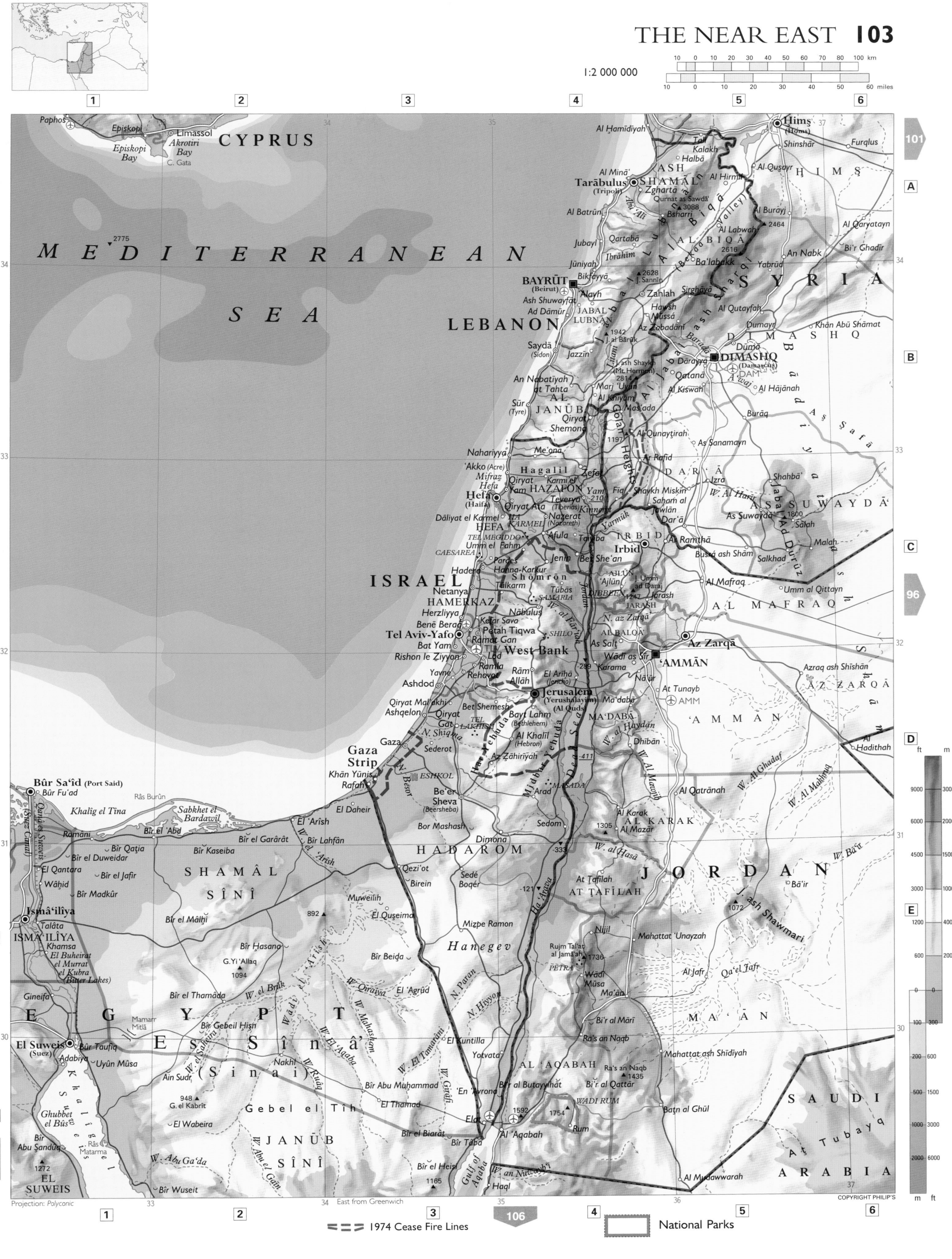

1:2 000 000

10   0   10 20 30 40 50 60 70 80   100 km

10   0   10   20   30   40   50   60 miles

1 | **2** | **3** | **4** | **5** | **6**

CYPRUS

Paphos
Episkopi
Limassol
Akrotiri
Episkopi   Bay
Bay   C. Gata

M E D I T E R R A N E A N

2775

S E A

LEBANON

BAYRŪT
(Beirut)

Al Ḥamīdīyah
Tal Kalakh
Ḥalbā
Ash SHAMĀL
Al Mīnā'
Tarābulus
(Tripoli)
Zgharta
Qurnat as Sawdā'
3088
Bsharri
Al Batrūn
Jubayl
Qartabā
Ibrāhīm
Jūniyah
Bikfayyā
J. Sannin
2628

Ḥimş
(Homs)
Shinshār
Furqlus
ḤIMŞ
Al Quşayr
Al Hirmil
Al Burayj
2464
Al Qaryatayn
An Nabk
Bi'r Ghadīr
Yabrūd

S Y R I A

Al Labwah
2616
Ba'labakk

Alayh
Ash Shuwayfāt
Ad Dāmūr
JABAL
LUBNĀN
Saydā
(Sidon)
Jazzīn
1942
Jal Bārūk
An Nabatīyah
at Taḥta
 Marj 'Uyūn
 Al Khiyām
AL
JANŪB
Şūr
(Tyre)
Qiryat
Shemona

Zaḥlah
Sirghāyā
Ḥawsh
Az Zabadānī
Ash Shaykh
(Mt. Hermon)
2814
1197
Golan
Heights
Al Qunayţirah

DIMASHQ
Dūmā
DIMASHQ
(Damascus)
DAM.
Darayyā
Qaţanā
Al Kiswah
Al Ḥājānah
Burāq
As Sanamayn
Ar Rafīd
DAR 'Ā

Khān Abū Shāmat
Dumayr
Al Quţayfah

B ā d i y a t   a s h   S h a m
Buraq

Naharīyya
'Akko (Acre)
Mifraz
Hefa
Ḥefa
(Haifa)
Qiryat Ata
Dāliyat el Karmel
HA KARMEL
Umm el Fahm
CAESAREA

Hagalil
Me'ona
Zefat
Qiryat
Yam   HAZAFON
Teverya
Yam
(Tiberias)   -210
Kinneret
Nazerat
(Nazareth)
Afula
TEL MEGIDDO
Jenin

Figl
Shaykh Miskin
Saḥam al
Juwlān
Dar'ā
Yarmūk
Ţayba
Bet She'an
IRBID

W. Al Ḥarīr
Izra
Buşrá ash Shām
Al Ramthā
Irbid
'AJLŪN
J. Umm
ad Dami
JARASH

Shahbā
AS SUWAYDĀ
As Suwaydā'
1800
Şālah
Malaḥ
Salkhad
Umm al Qiţtayn

J a b a l   a d   D u r ū z

ISRAEL

Pardes
Hanna-Karkur
Ḥadera
Netanya
HAMERKAZ
Herzliyya
Benē Beraq
Tel Aviv-Yafo
Bat Yam
Rishon le Ziyyon
Yavne
Rehovot
Ashdod
Qiryat Mal'akhi
Ashqelon
Qiryat
Gat

Shomron
Ţulkarm
Nāblus
Kefar Sava
Petaḥ Tiqwa
Ramat Gan
Lod
Ramla
West Bank
Rām
Allāh
El 'Arīḥā
(Jericho)
Jerusalem
(Yerushalayim)
(Al Quds)
Bet Shemesh
Bayt Laḥm
(Bethlehem)
Al Khalīl
(Hebron)
Az Ẓāhirīyah

Tūbās
SAMARIA
SHILO
W. al Fār'ah
AL BALQĀ'
As Salt
Wādī as Sīr
Karama
Na'ūr
Ma'daba
MA'DABA
W. al Ḥaydān
Dhībān

Az Zarqā
'AMMĀN
Azraq ash Shīshān
AZ ZARQĀ
'AMMAN
At Tunayb
AMM

Gaza
Gaza
Strip
Khān Yūnis
Rafaḥ
N. Shiqma
Sederot
ESHKOL
Be'er
Sheva
(Beersheba)
Bor Mashash
Arad
Sedom
Dimona
-333
HADAROM

Bûr Sa'îd (Port Said)
Bûr Fu'âd
Râs Burûn
Khalig el Tîna
Sabkhet el
Bardawîl
Ramâni
El 'Arîsh
El Dâheir
Bîr el 'Abd
Bîr el Garârât
Bîr Qaţia
El Qantara
Bîr el Duweidar
Bîr el Jafir
Bîr Madkûr
W. el 'Arîsh
Bîr Lahfân
Bîr Kaseiba
SHAMÂL
SÎNÎ

El Karak
AL KARAK
Al Mazar
W. al Ḥasā
1305
W. al Mūjib
Al Qaţrānah
W. Al Ghadaf
Al Ḥadithah

J O R D A N

Ismâ'ilîya
Ţalâta
ISMÂ'ILÎYA
Khamsa
El Buheirat
el Murrat
el Kubra
(Bitter Lakes)
Gineifa
Wâḥid

G. Yi 'Allaq
1094
Bîr Ḥasano
Bîr Beiḍa
Qezi'ot
Birein
Sedé
Boqér
Muweilih
El Quşeima
Mizpe Ramon
Hanegev
Nijil
-121
At Ţafilah
AT ṬAFÎLAH
1072

Bîr el Mâlḥi
892
El 'Agrûd
N. Paran
Rujm Tal'at
al Jamā'ah
1736
PETRA
Wādī
Mūsā
Ma'ān
M A 'Â N
Al Jafr
Qa'el Jafr
Mahaţtat 'Unayzah
Mahaţtat ash Shīdīyah

Bîr el Thamâda
W. el Brûk
El 'Agrûd
W. el Saleim
W. Mahashm
En 'Avrona
Bîr Abu Muḥammad
El Thamad
Bîr al Mārī
Bîr al Qaţţār
Ra's an Naqb
1435

E G Y P T

E S   S î n â '   (Sinai)

El Suweis
(Suez)
Bûr Taufiq
Adabiya
Uyûn Mûsa
948
G. el Kabrît
Ain Sudr
Nakhl
W. El Aqaba
W. El Ruaq
W. El Tamarûni
1592
Elat
Al 'Aqabah
AL 'AQABAH
1754
WADI RUM
Rum
Ra's an Naqb

Gebel el Tîh
Bîr Gebeil Ḥisn
El Kuntilla
Yotvata
'En 'Avrona
Bîr el Biarât
Bîr Ţâba
Ḥaql
Batn al Ghûl
Bā'ir
ash Shawmari

J A N Û B
S Î N Î

EL
SUWEIS
1272
Abu Sandûq
Ghubbet
el Bûs
Bîr
Ras
Matarma
W. Abu Ga'da
Bîr el Heisî
1165
W. an Nuweiba'
W. Amel Gein
SAUDI
ARABIA
At Tubayq
Al Mudawwarah

Khalig el Suweis

Gulf of
'Aqaba

m ft

COPYRIGHT PHILIP'S

1 | **2** | **3** | **4** | **5** | **6**

=== 1974 Cease Fire Lines   National Parks

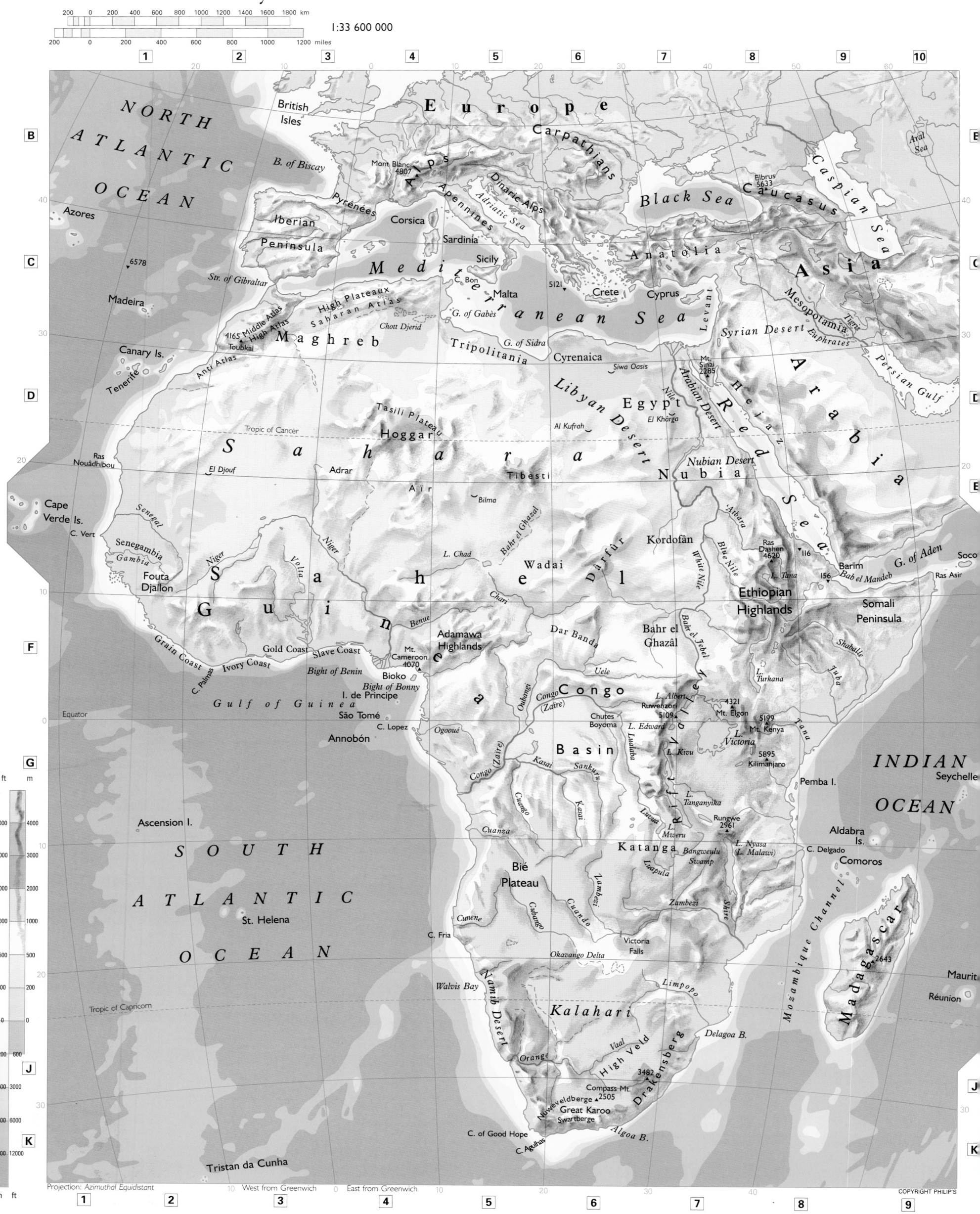

1:33 600 000

Projection: Azimuthal Equidistant

COPYRIGHT PHILIP'S

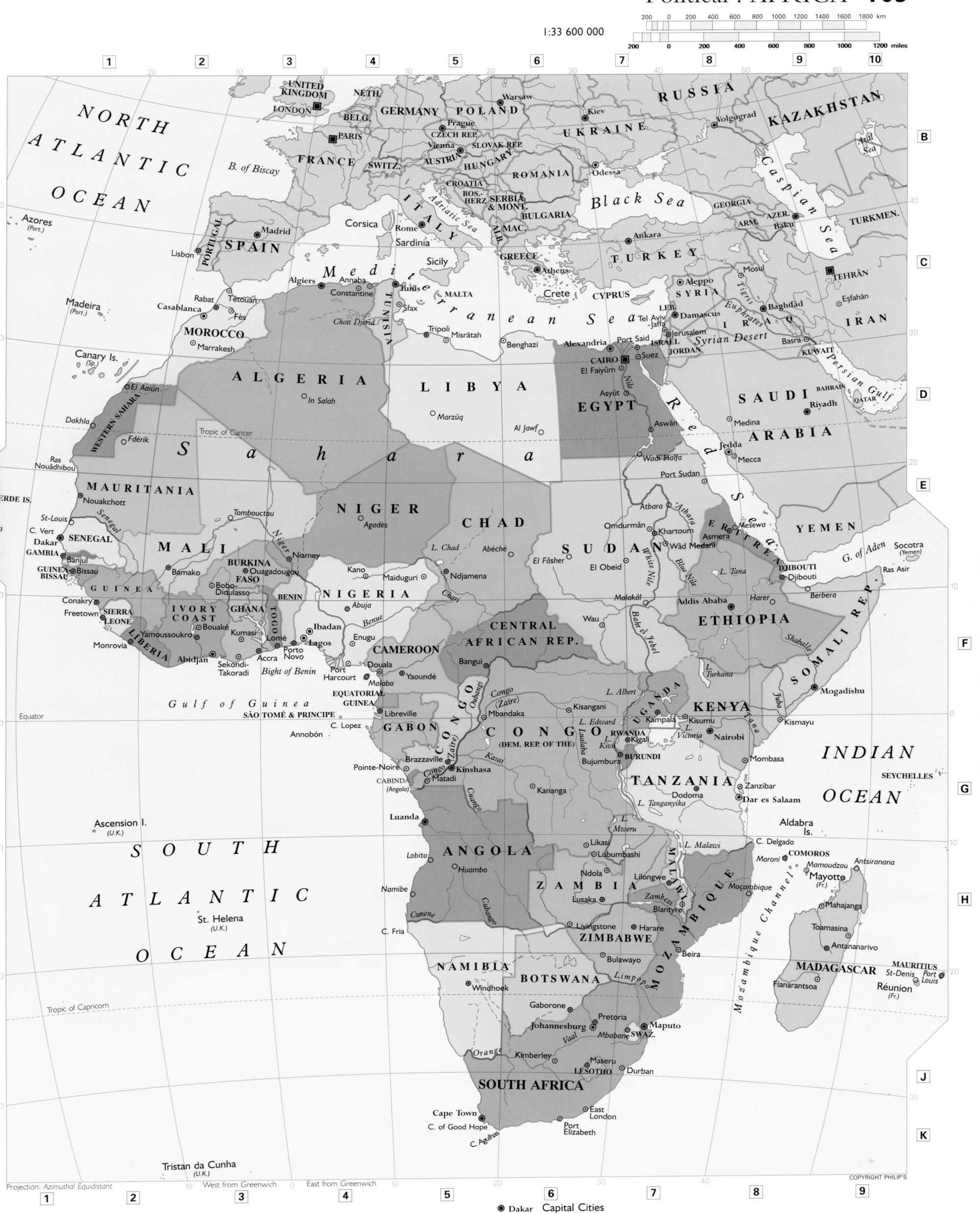

1:33 600 000

200 0 200 400 600 800 1000 1200 1400 1600 1800 km

200 0 200 400 600 800 1000 1200 miles

Projection: Azimuthal Equidistant

West from Greenwich   East from Greenwich

● Dakar Capital Cities

COPYRIGHT PHILIP'S

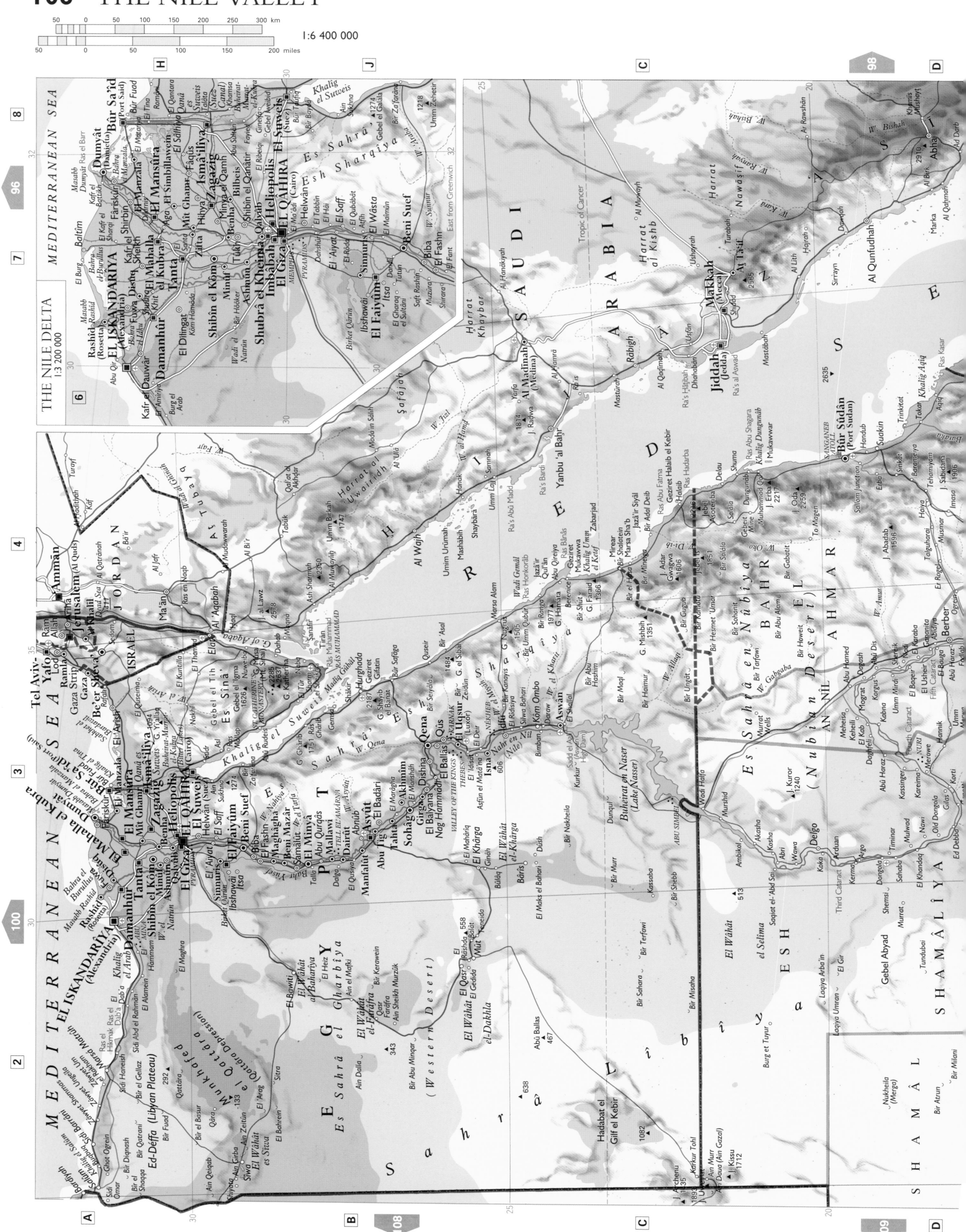

50 0   50 100 150 200 250 300 km
50 0   50 100 150 200 miles

1:6 400 000

THE NILE DELTA
1:3 200 000

MEDITERRANEAN SEA

National Parks

Nature Reserves and Game Reserves

∴ UNESCO World Heritage Sites

COPYRIGHT PHILIP'S

Projection: Lambert's Equivalent Azimuthal

East from Greenwich

1:6 400 000

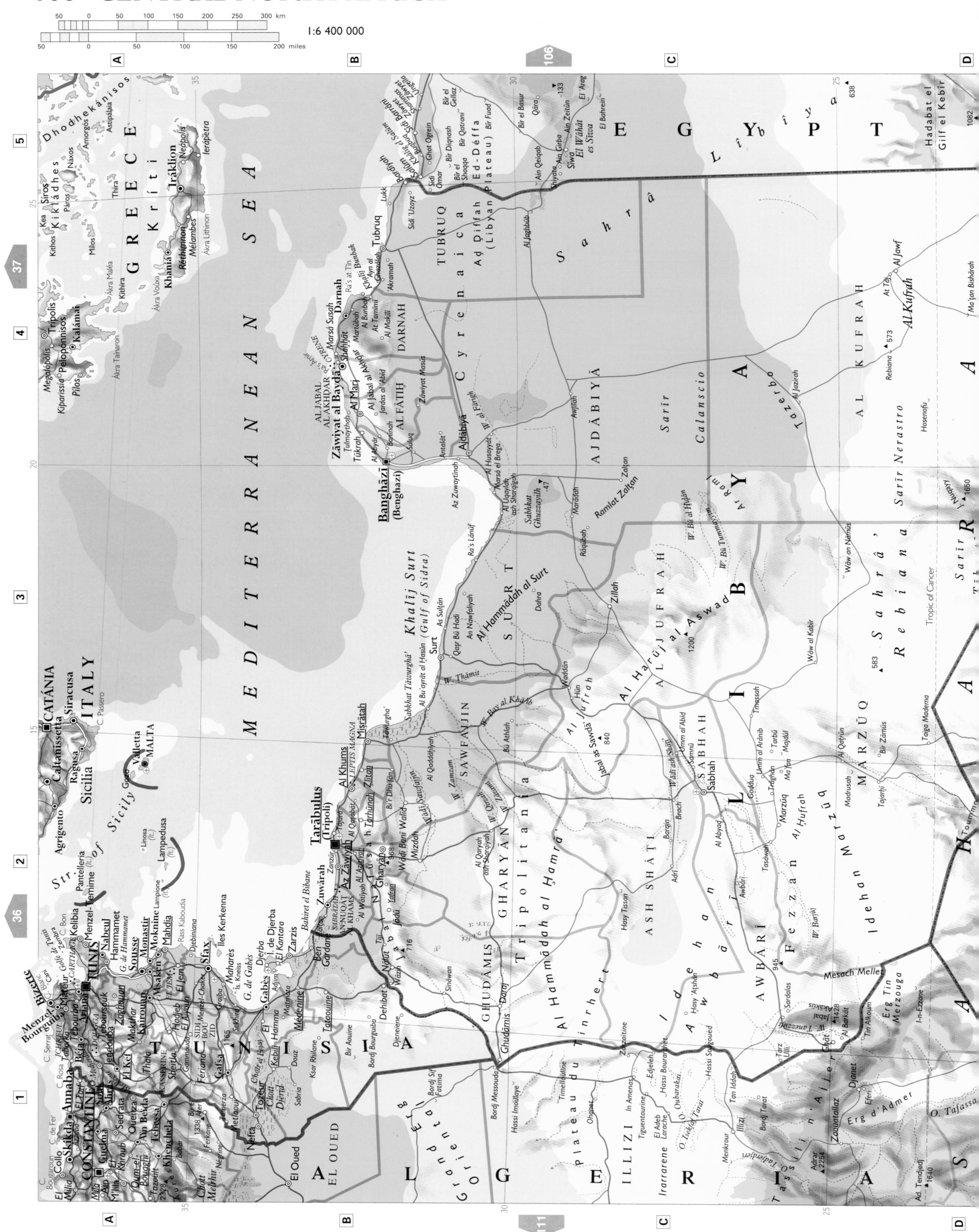

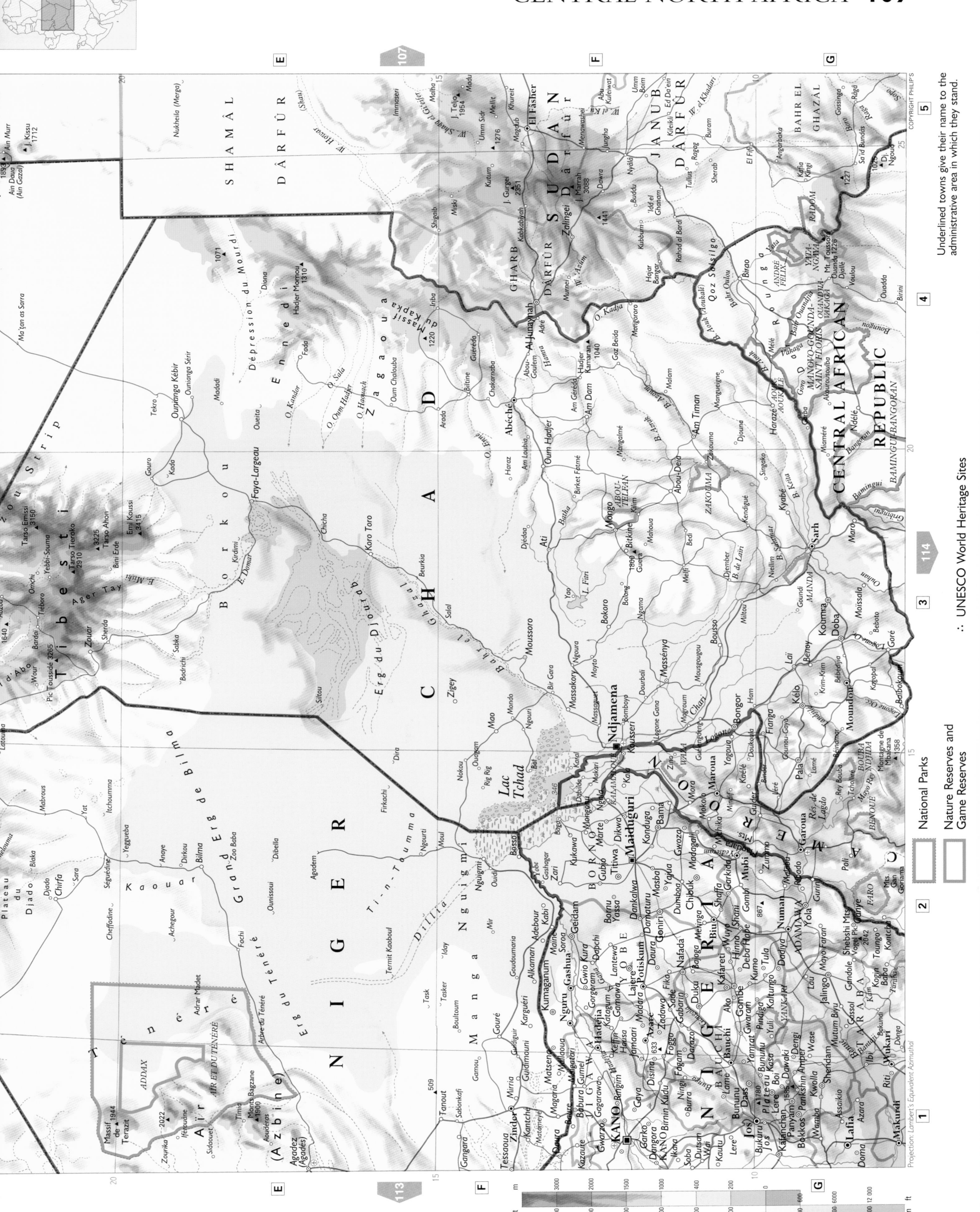

COPYRIGHT PHILIP'S

Underlined towns give their name to the administrative area in which they stand.

∴ UNESCO World Heritage Sites

National Parks

Nature Reserves and Game Reserves

Projection: Lambert's Equivalent Azimuthal

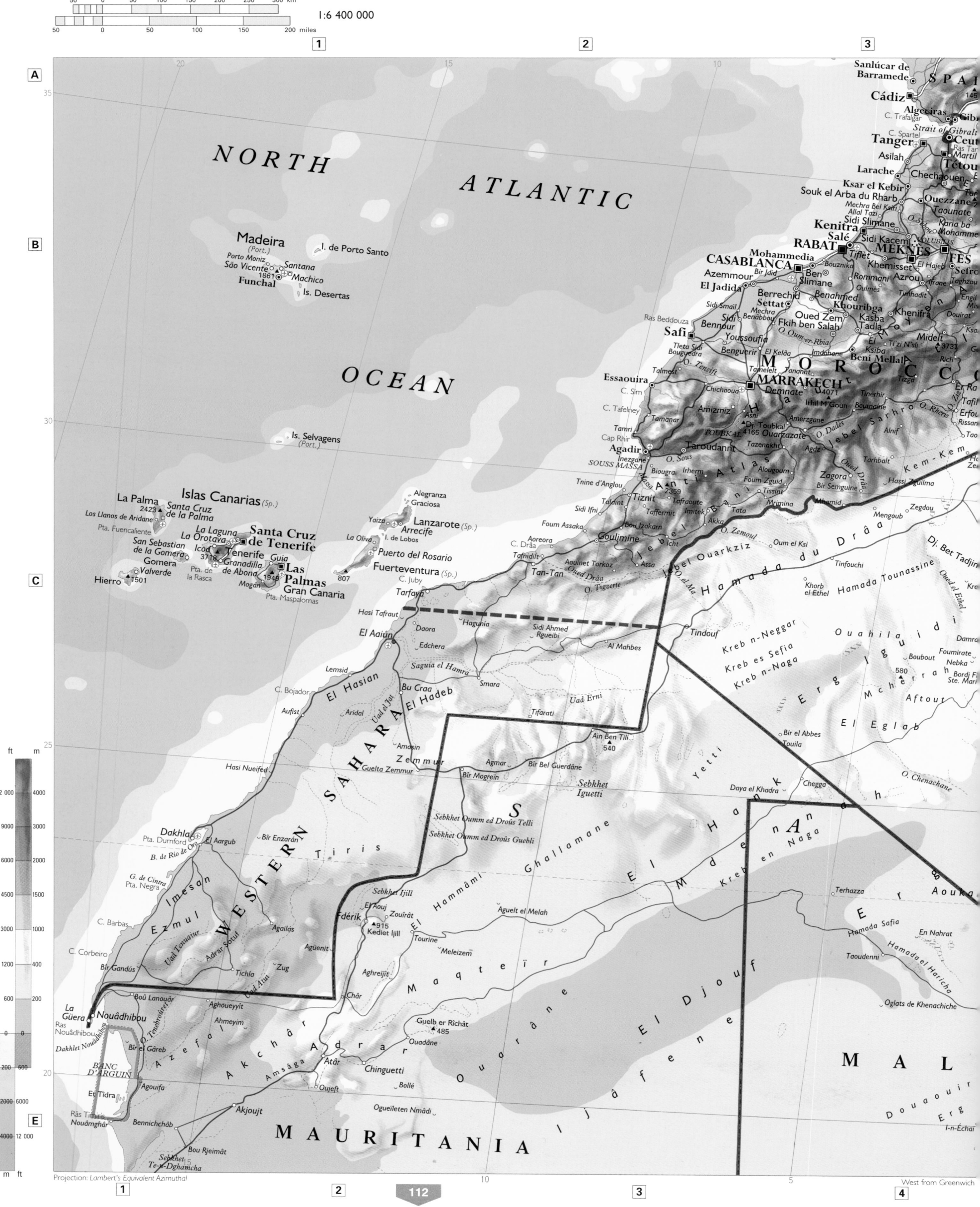

1:6 400 000

Projection: Lambert's Equivalent Azimuthal

West from Greenwich

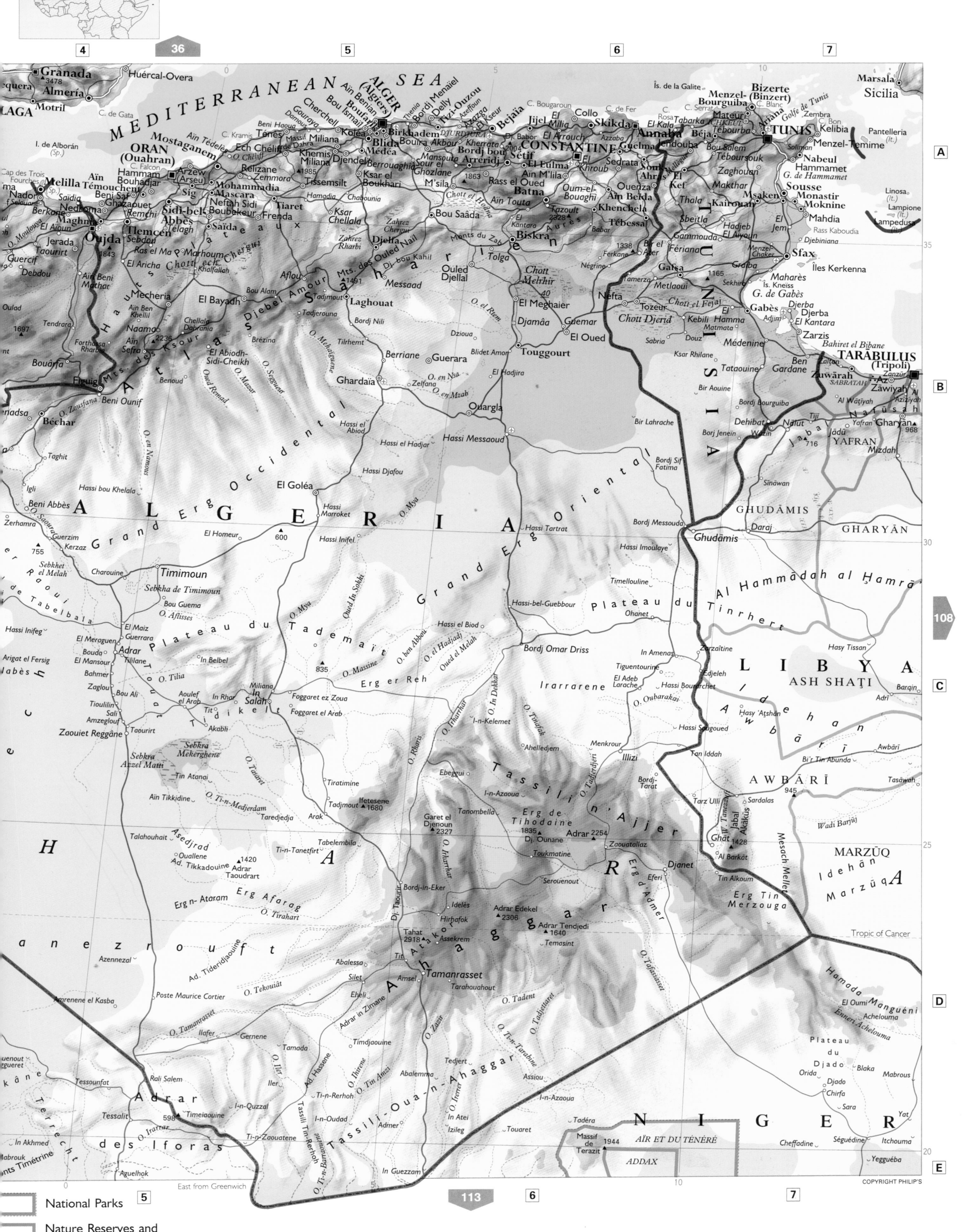

Granada
Almería
Huércal-Overa
Motril
C. de Gata
I. de Alborán (Sp.)

MEDITERRANEAN SEA

ALGER (Algiers)
Aïn Benian
Bou Ismaïl
Thenia
Bordj Menaiel
Delly
Tizi-Ouzou
Azeffoun
C. Bougaroun
Collo
C. de Fer
Skikda
Azzaba
Annaba
C. Rosa
Tabarka
Bizerte (Binzert)
Menzel-Bourguiba
Mateur
Ariana
TUNIS
Kelibia
C. Bon
Zembra
Pantelleria (It.)
Marsala
Sicilia

Mostaganem
ORAN (Ouahran)
C. Falcon
Arzew
Arseu
Mohammadia
Mascara
Neftah Sidi
Boubekeur
Sig
Ech Cheliff
Dahra
Ténès
Cherchell
Koléa
Massif Miliana
1985
Blida
Médéa
Djendel
Berrouaghia
Ksar el Boukhari
Bordj bou Arréridj
Sétif
El Eulma
El Khroub
CONSTANTINE
2004
Guelma
Sedrata
Souk Ahras
Ouenza
Aïn Beïda
El Kef
Thala
Makthar
Téboursouk
Béja
Bou Salem
Jendouba
Zaghouan
Nabeul
Hammamet
G. de Hammamet
Sousse
Monastir
Mokmine
Linosa (It.)
Lampione (It.)

Melilla
Témouchent
Aïn Bouhadjar
Beni Saf
Ghazaouet
Nedroma
Maghnia
Tlemcen
Sidi-bel-Abbès
Relizane
Tissemsilt
Ksar Chellala
M'sila
Rass el Oued
1863
Aïn Touta
Batna
Oum-el-Bouaghi
Aïn M'lila
Khenchela
Tébessa
Fériana
Gammouda
El Aiyoun
Sbeitla
Kairouan
Hadjeb
El Jem
Mahdia
Rass Kaboudia
Djebiniana

OR
Saïda
Berkane
El Aioun
Jerada
Taourirt
Oujda
1843
Sebdou
Ras el Ma
Marhoum
Saïda
Frenda
Aïn
El Aricha
Chott ech Chergui
Khalfallah
Dj ou Kahil
Aflou
1491
Bou Alam
Messaad
Ouled Djellal
Tolga
Biskra
Aurès
2328
Babar
El Kantara
Bir el Ater
1338
Fékane
Négrine
Gafsa
1165
Metlaoui
Sekhira
Maharès
Îs. Kneiss
G. de Gabès
Gabès
Adjim
Djerba
El Kantara
Zarzis
Médenine

Guercif
Debdou
Oulad
1697
Bouârfa
Figuig
Béchar
Taghit
Igli
Beni Abbès
Zemhra

Hauts Plateaux
Méchéria
El Bayadh
Brézina
El Abiodh-Sidi-Cheikh
Laghouat
Bordj Nili
Tadjerouna
Tilrhemt
Berriane
Guerara
Ghardaïa
Blidet Amor
El Hadjira
Touggourt
El Oued
Guemar
El Meghaier
Djamâa
Nefta
Tozeur
Chott el Fejaj
Kebili
Hamma
Douz
Sabria
Ksar Rhilane
Bir Aouine
Tataouine

TARĀBULUS (Tripoli)
Zuwārah
Az Zāwiyah
Zanzūr
SABRATAH
Natūsāh
Al Wāṭiyah
Gharyān
968
YAFRAN
Mizdah

GHUDĀMIS
Ghudāmis
Daraj
GHARYĀN
Al Hammādah al Hamrā

ALGERIA
Grand Erg Occidental
Timimoun
El Goléa
Hassi Messaoud
Grand Erg Oriental
Plateau du Tirhhert
LIBYA
ASH SHAŢI
Barqin
Adri

Plateau du Tademaït
Adrar
In Salah
Irarrarene
Idehan Awbārī
AWBĀRĪ
945
Ghāt
1428

Ahaggar
Tamanrasset
Tahat 2918
Tropic of Cancer

NIGER
AÏR ET DU TÉNÉRÉ
ADDAX

East from Greenwich
COPYRIGHT PHILIP'S

National Parks
Nature Reserves and Game Reserves
∴ UNESCO World Heritage Sites

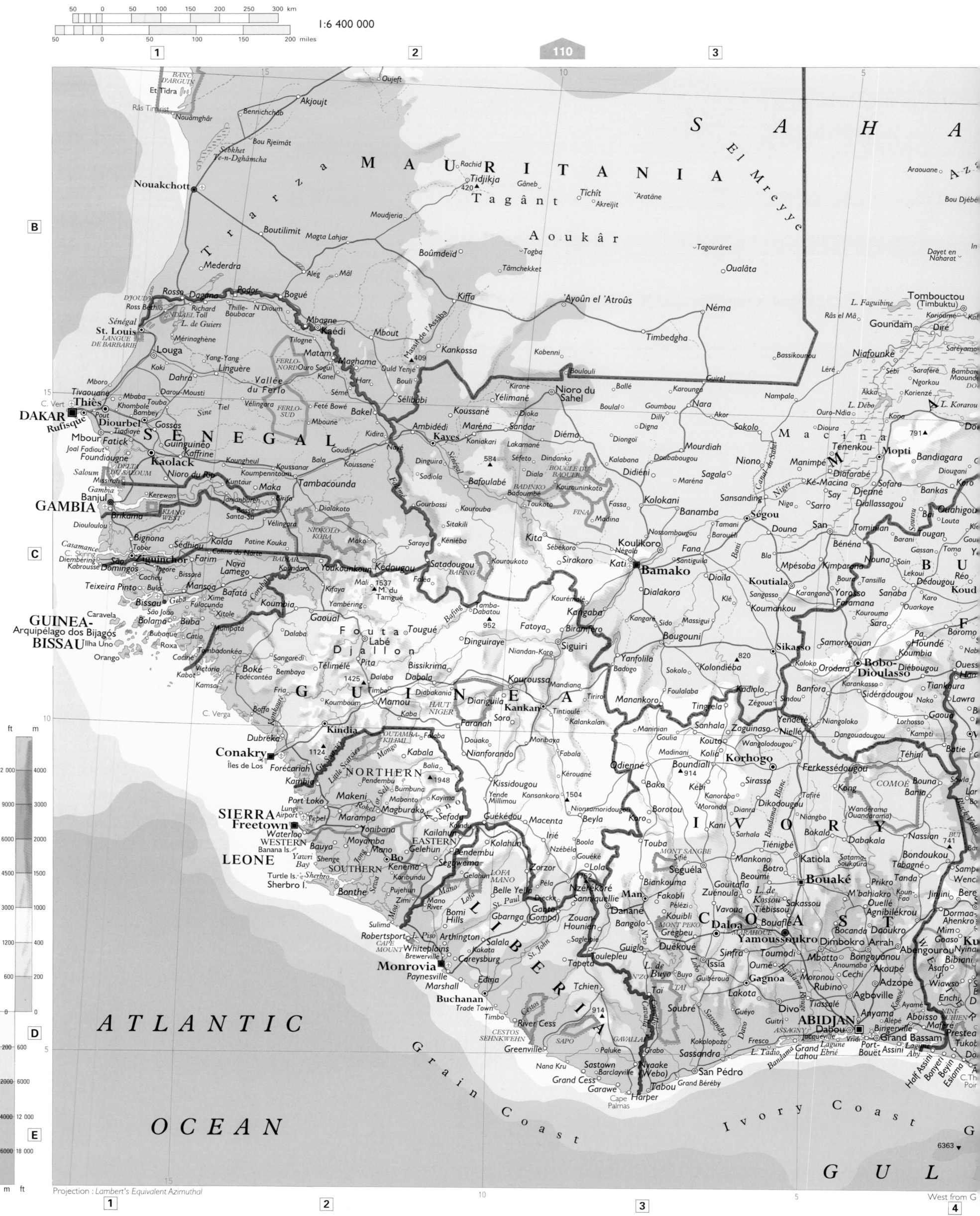

Projection : Lambert's Equivalent Azimuthal

West from G

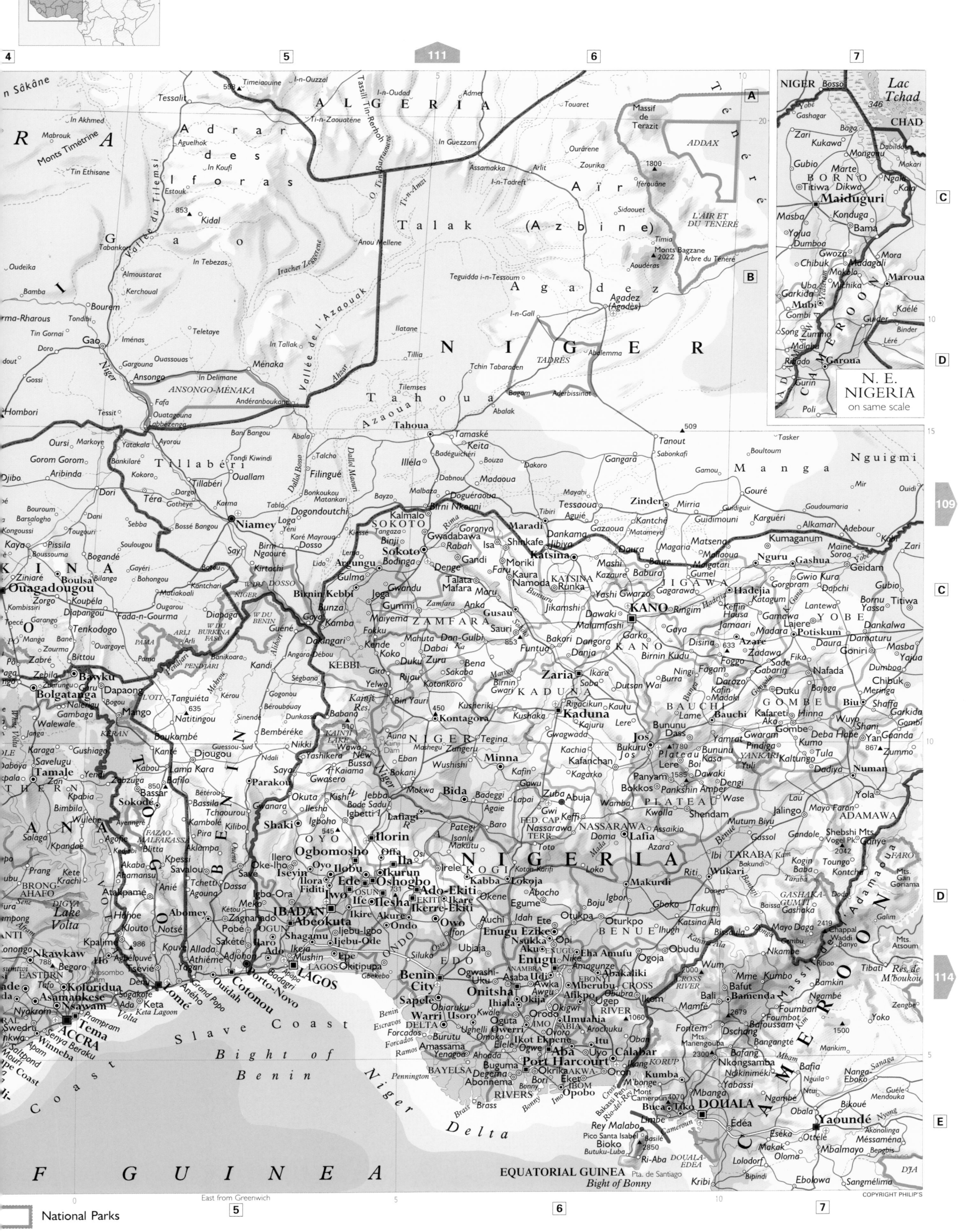

National Parks

Nature Reserves and
Game Reserves

∴ UNESCO World Heritage Sites

N. E. NIGERIA
on same scale

COPYRIGHT PHILIP'S

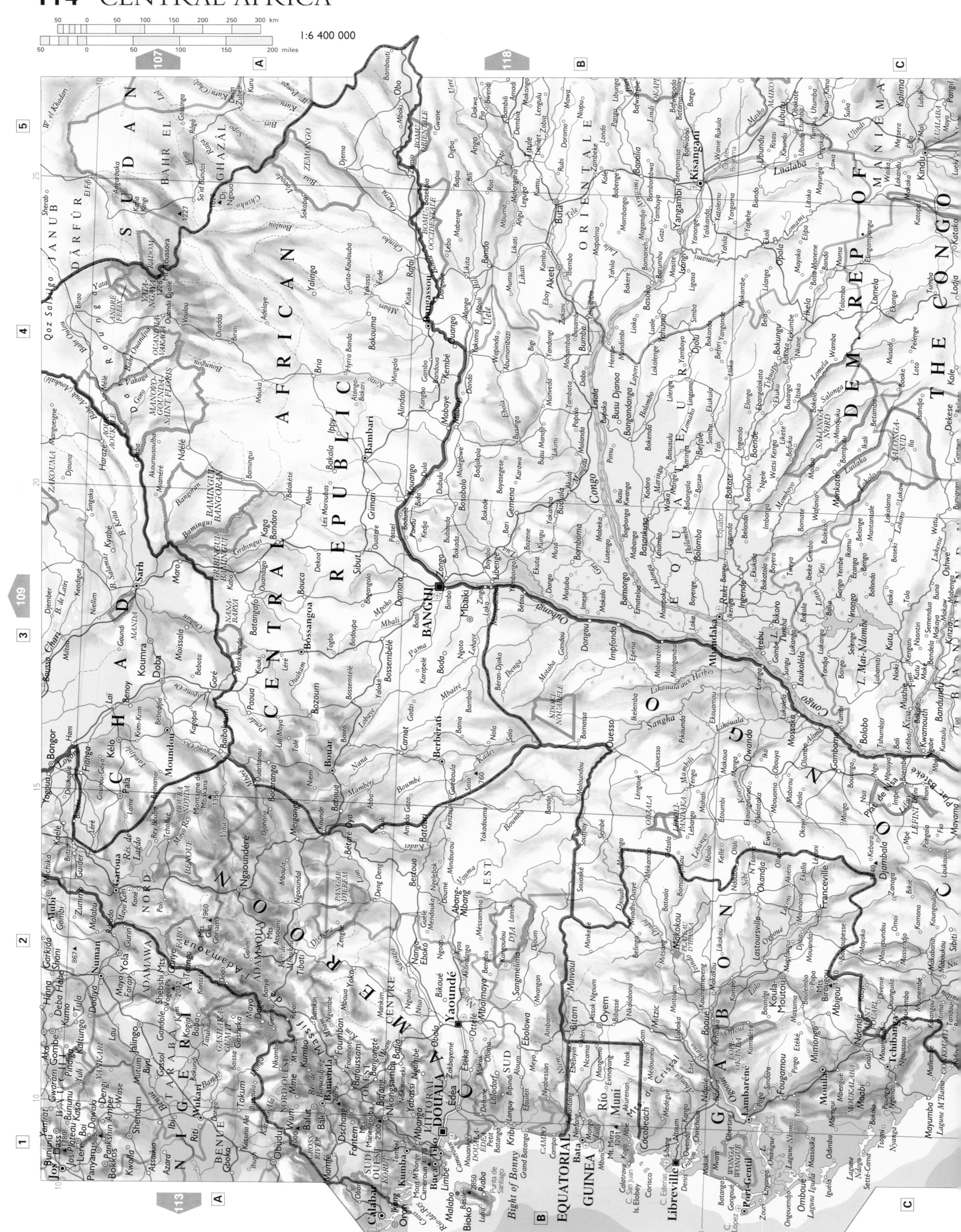

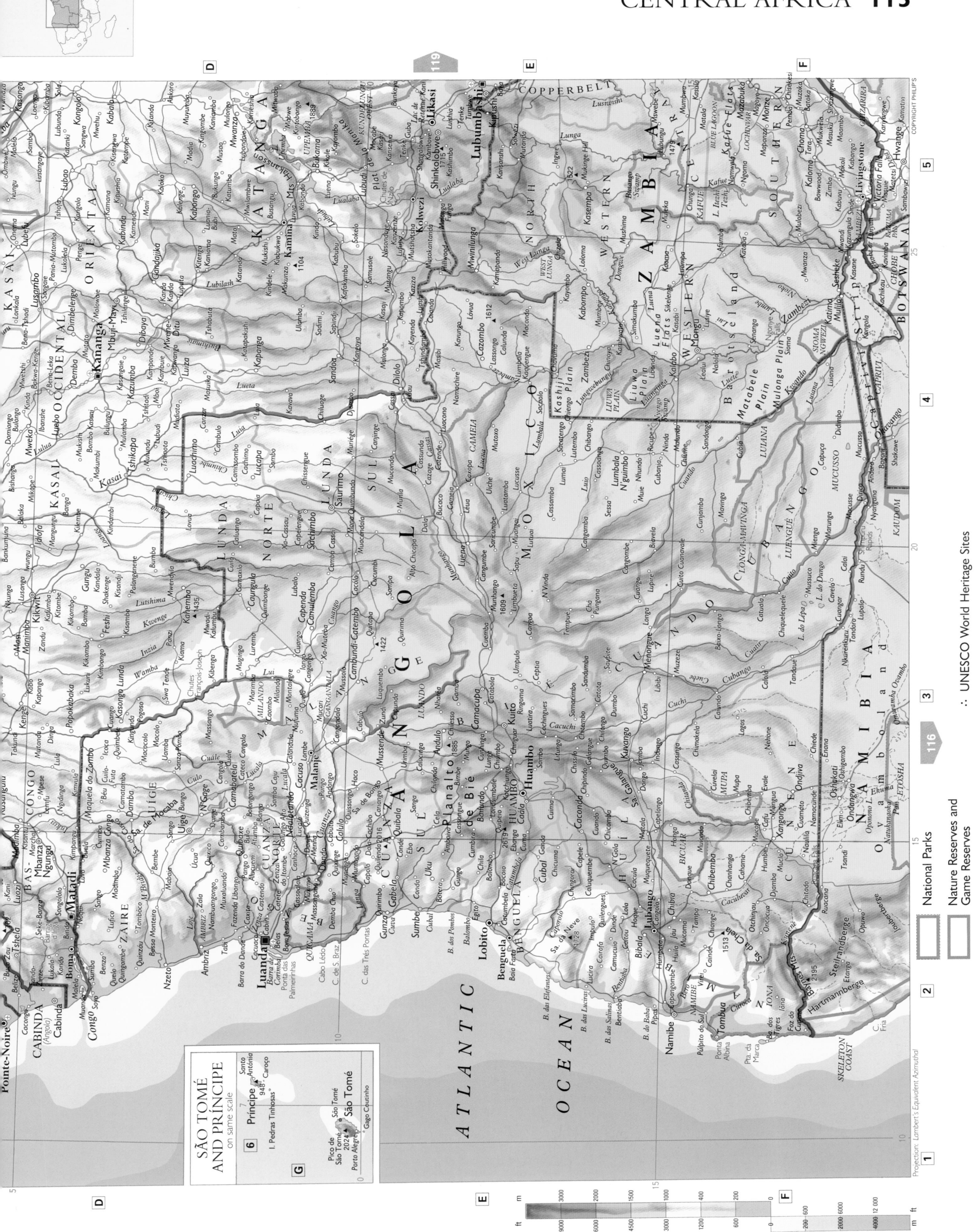

Projection: Lambert's Equivalent Azimuthal

∴ UNESCO World Heritage Sites

National Parks

Nature Reserves and
Game Reserves

**SÃO TOMÉ
AND PRÍNCIPE**
on same scale

Santo
Príncipe Antônio
948 Caroço

I. Pedras Tinhosas

São Tomé
Pico de
São Tomé
2024 São Tomé
Porto Alegre
Gago Coutinho

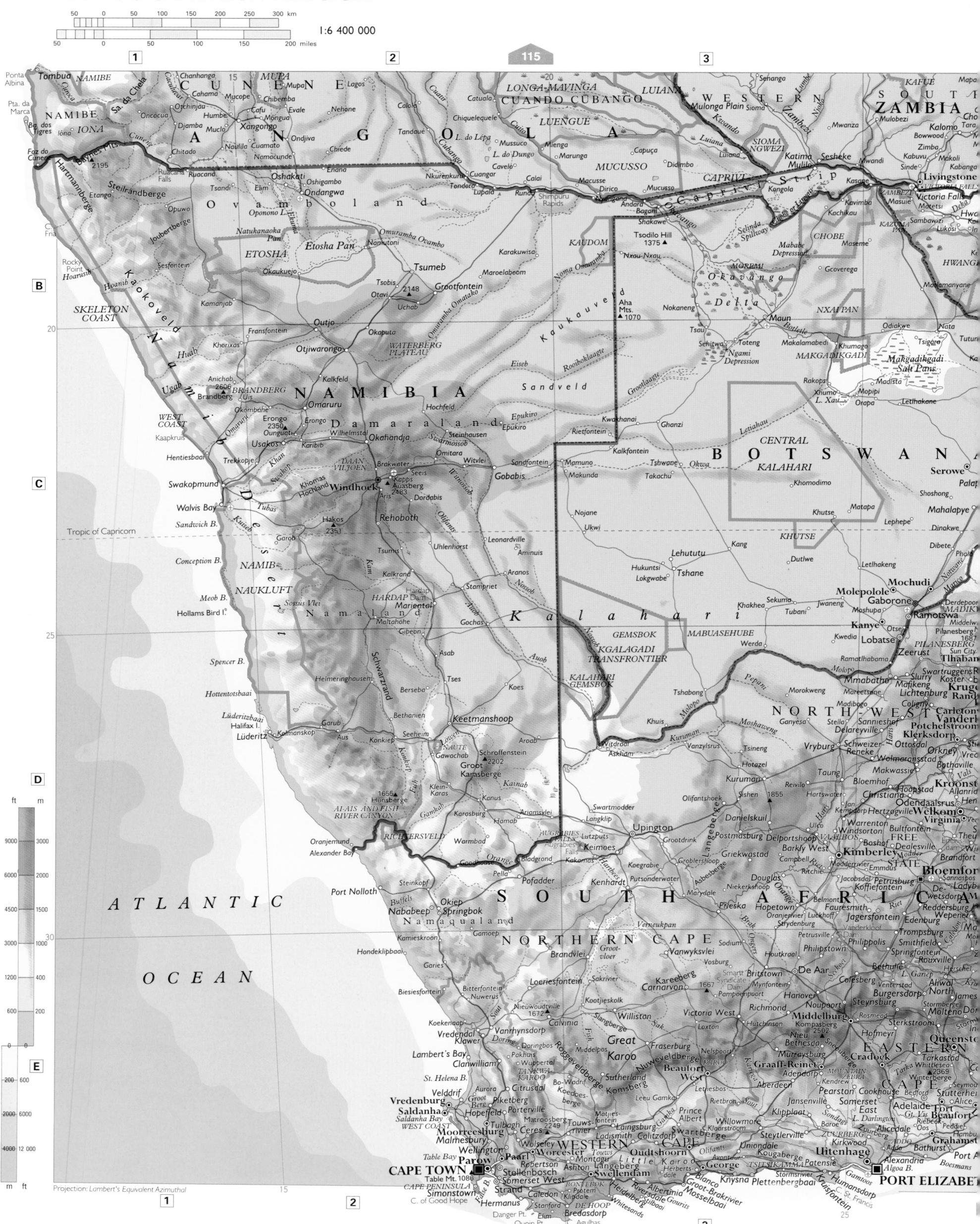

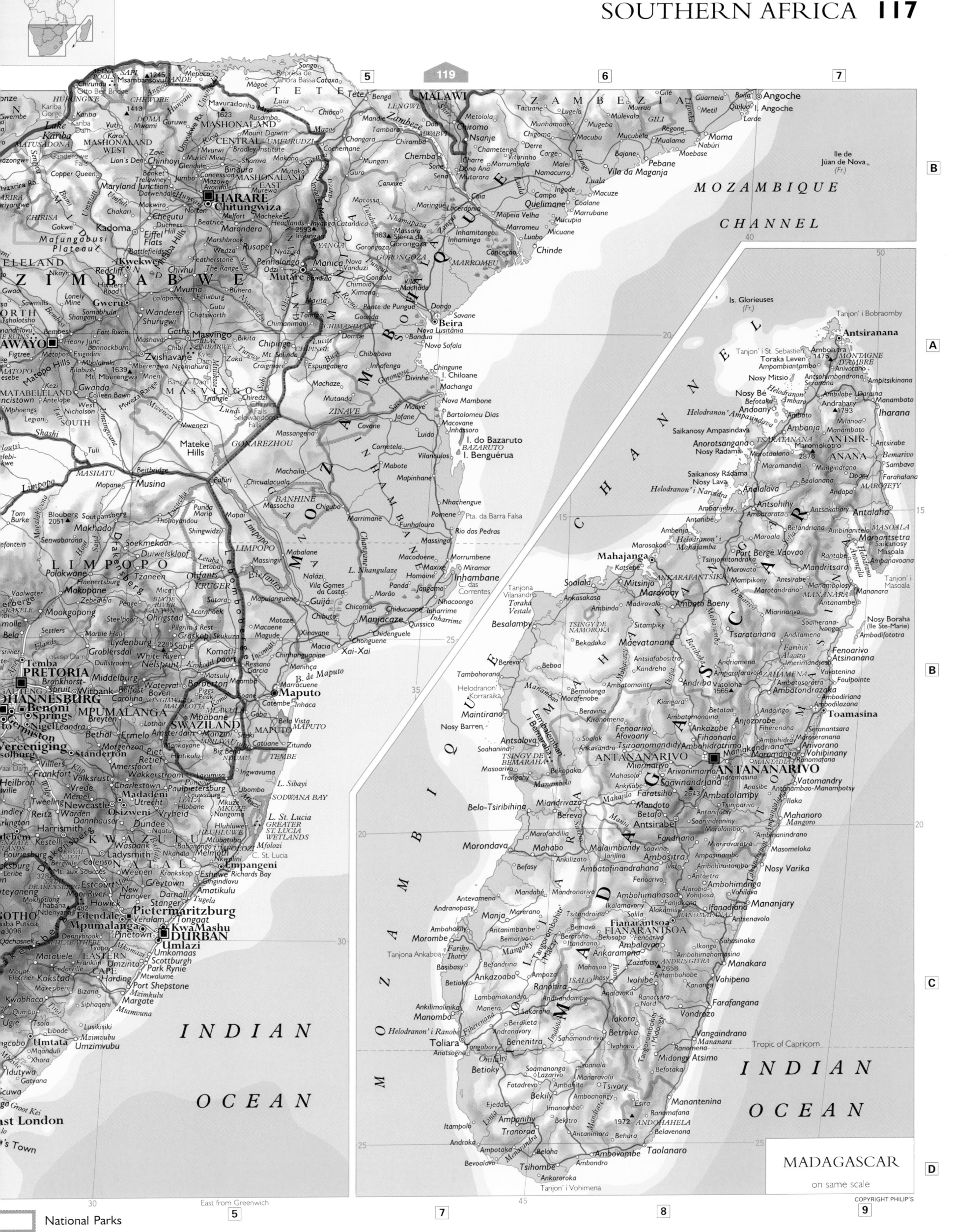

National Parks

Nature Reserves and
Game Reserves

∴ UNESCO World Heritage Sites

MADAGASCAR

on same scale

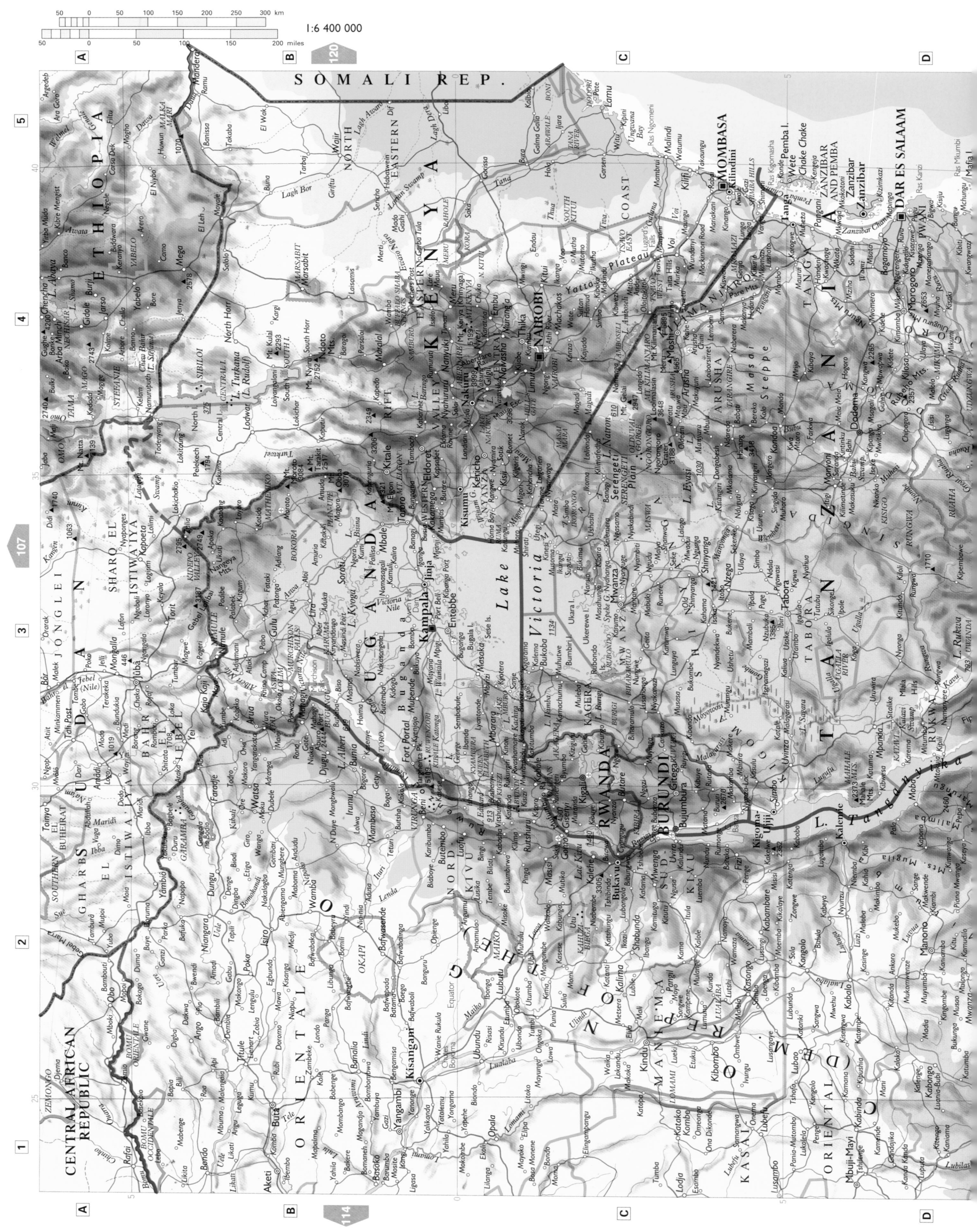

1:6 400 000

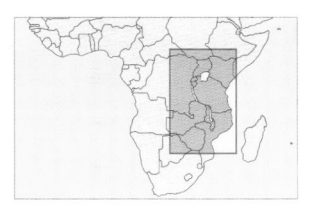

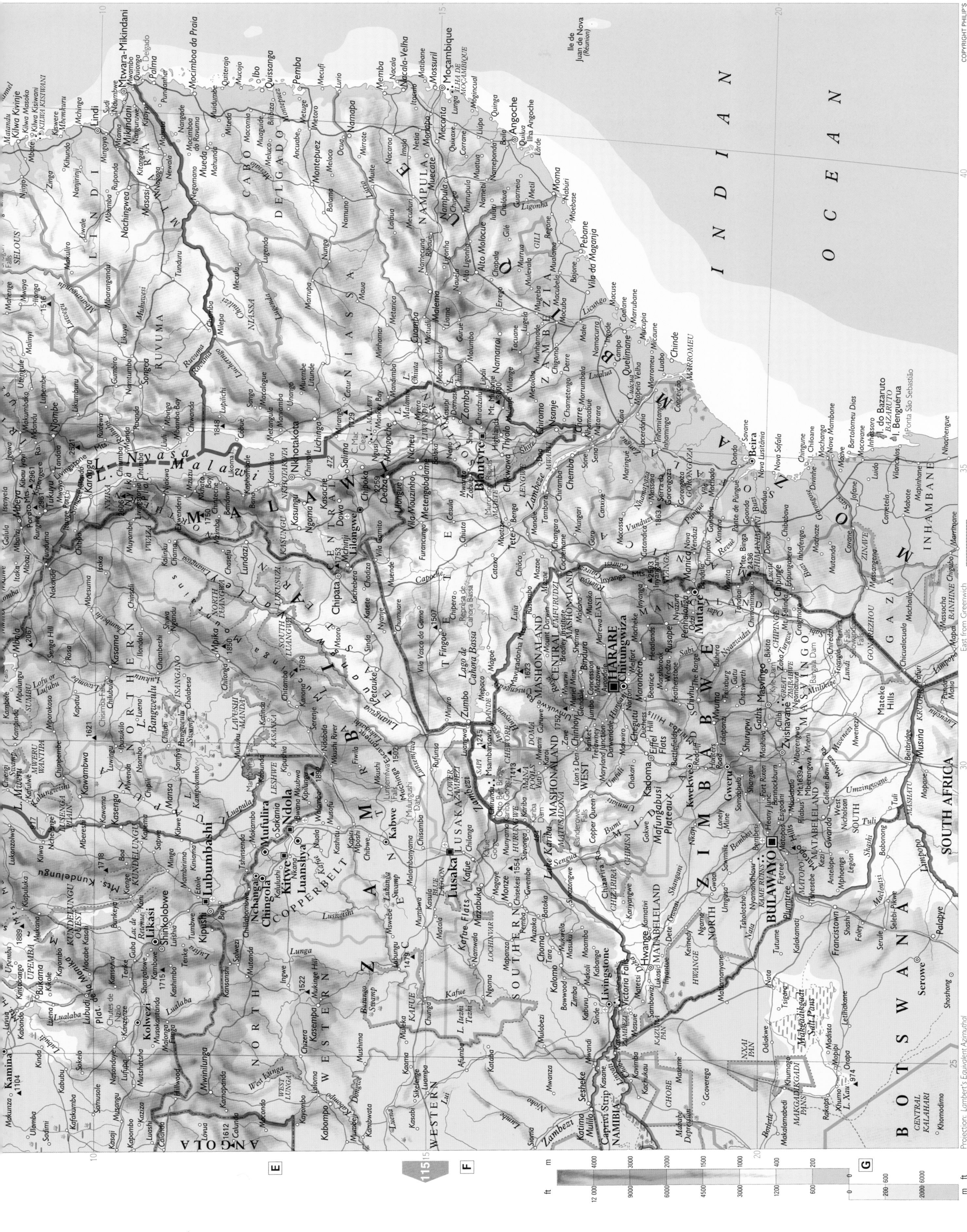

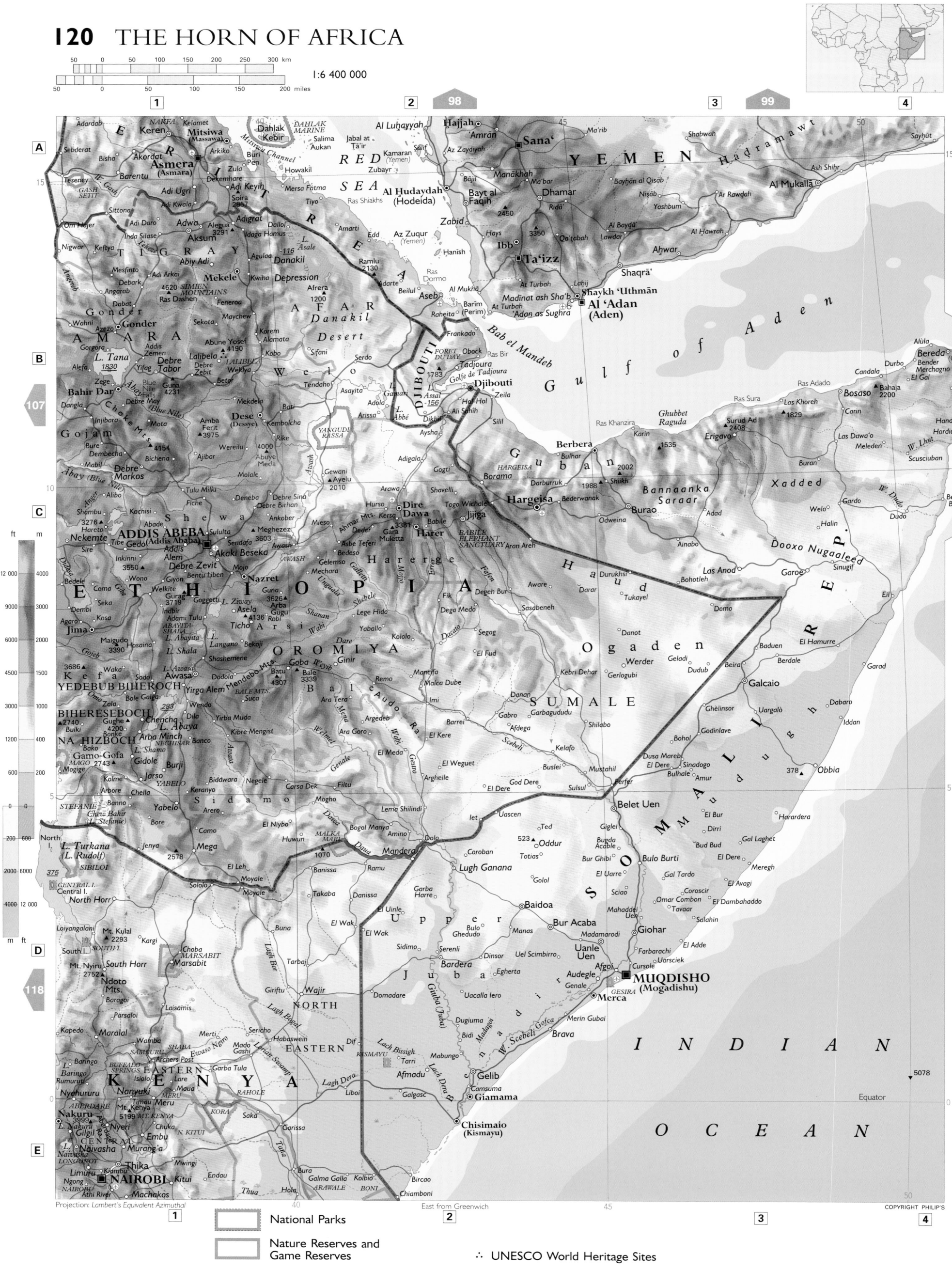

1:6 400 000

National Parks

Nature Reserves and
Game Reserves

∴ UNESCO World Heritage Sites

Projection: Lambert's Equivalent Azimuthal

East from Greenwich

COPYRIGHT PHILIP'S

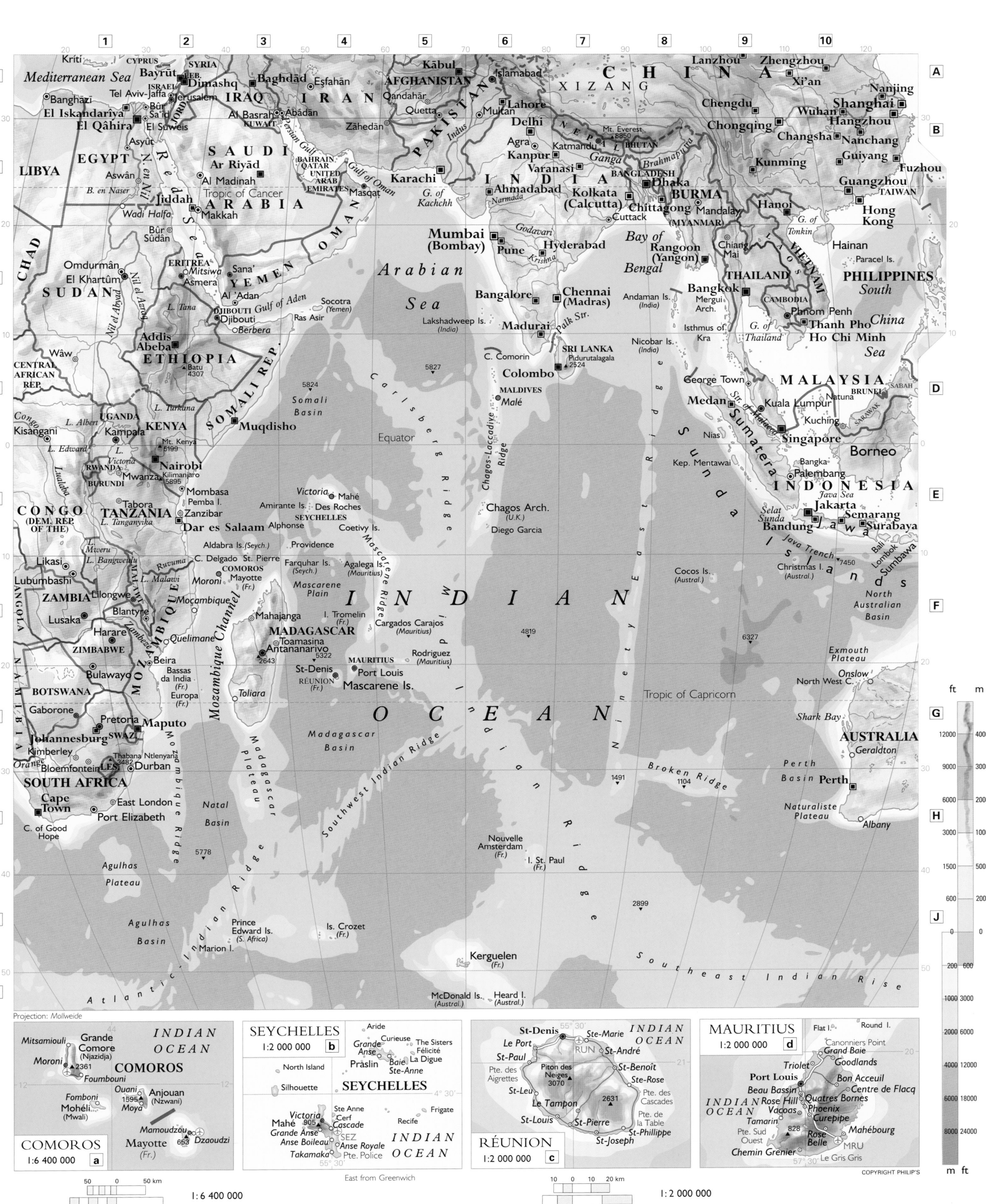

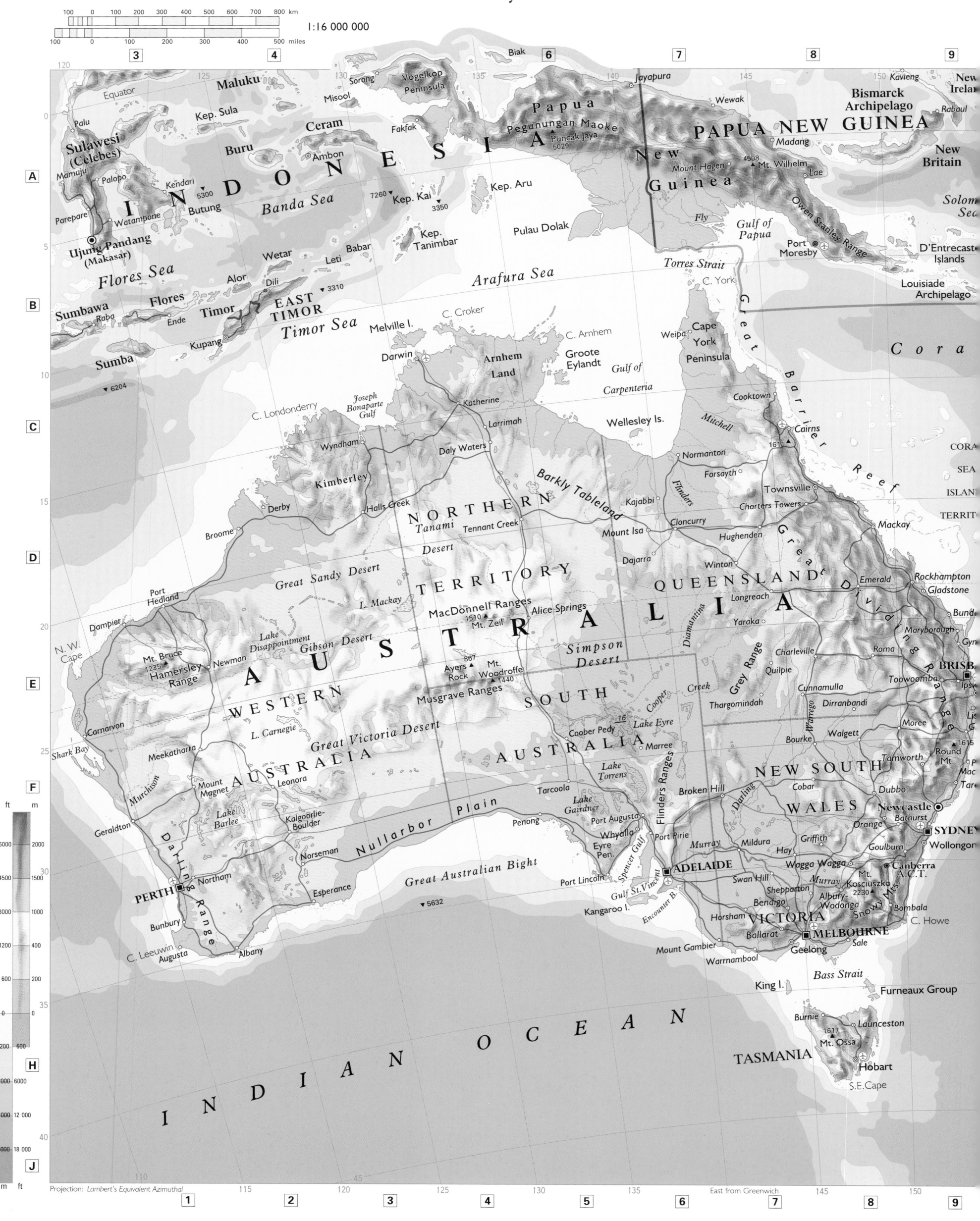

1:16 000 000

Projection: *Lambert's Equivalent Azimuthal*

East from Greenwich

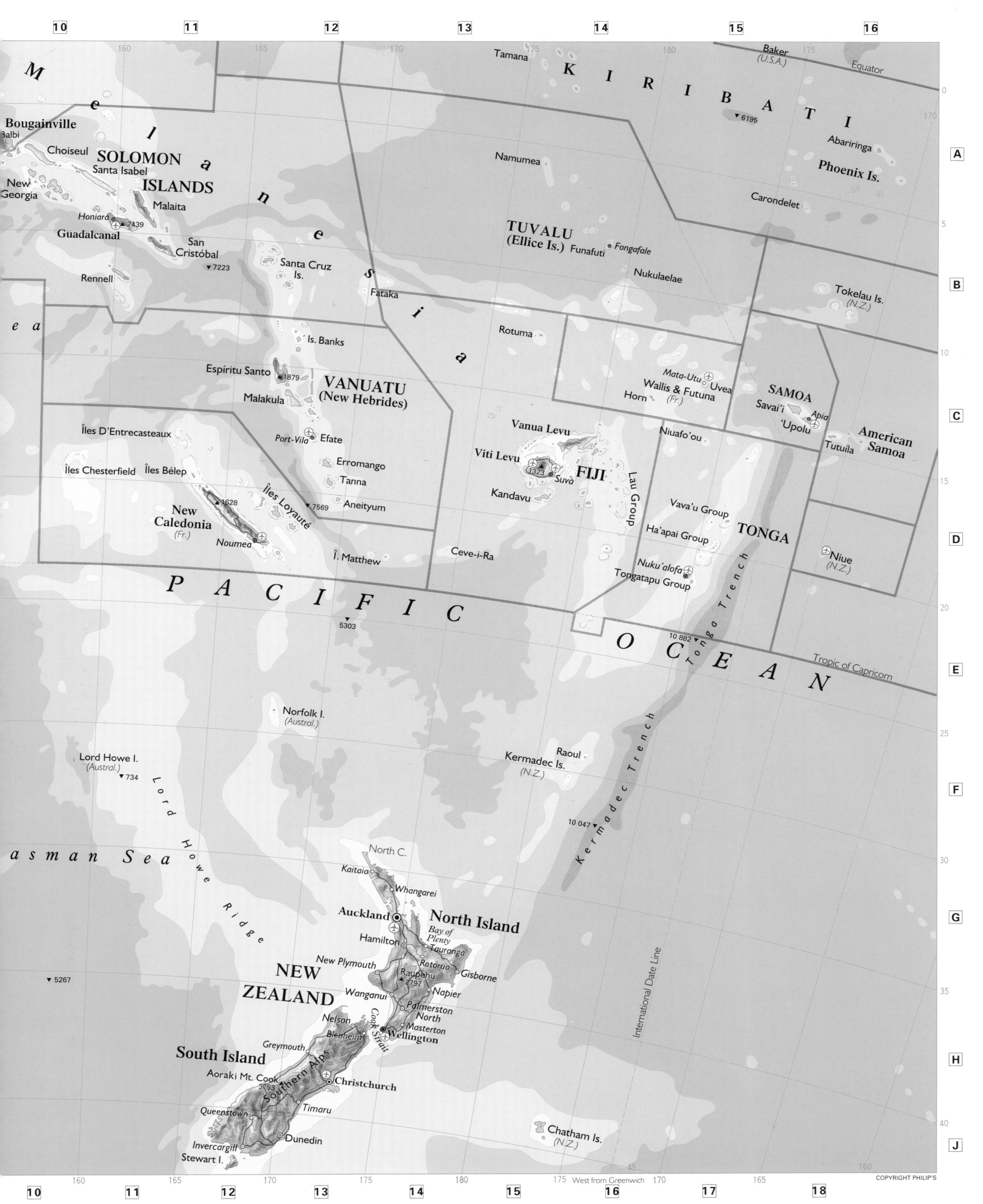

M
e
l
a
n
e
s
i
a

Bougainville
Balbi
Choiseul
Santa Isabel
New
Georgia
SOLOMON
Malaita
ISLANDS
Honiara ▲2439
Guadalcanal
San
Cristóbal
Rennell
▼7223
Santa Cruz
Is.
Fataka

Tamana
K I R I B A T I
Baker
(U.S.A.)
Equator
▼6195
Abariringa
Namumea
Phoenix Is.
Carondelet
TUVALU
(Ellice Is.) Funafuti Fongafale
Nukulaelae
Tokelau Is.
(N.Z.)
Rotuma

e
a

Is. Banks
Espíritu Santo ▲1879
VANUATU
Malakula **(New Hebrides)**
Îles D'Entrecasteaux
Port-Vila Efate
Îles Chesterfield Îles Bélep
Erromango
Tanna
Îles Loyauté
New ▲1628
Caledonia
(Fr.) Noumea
Aneityum
▼7569
Î. Matthew Ceve-i-Ra

Mata-Utu Uvea
Wallis & Futuna
Horn (Fr.)
SAMOA
Savai'i Apia
'Upolu
Tutuila
American
Samoa
Niuafo'ou
Vanua Levu
Viti Levu
▲1323 **FIJI**
Suva
Kandavu
Lau Group
Vava'u Group
Ha'apai Group **TONGA**
Niue
(N.Z.)
Nuku'alofa
Tongatapu Group
Tonga Trench

P A C I F I C
▼5303
10.882▼

O C E A N
Tropic of Capricorn

Norfolk I.
(Austral.)

Lord Howe I.
(Austral.)
▼734

Raoul
Kermadec Is.
(N.Z.)

Kermadec Trench
10 047▼

asman Sea

Lord Howe Ridge

North C.
Kaitaia
Whangarei
Auckland
North Island
Hamilton Bay of
Plenty Tauranga
New Plymouth Rotorua Gisborne
▼5267
NEW
Raupehu
Wanganui ▲2797 Napier
ZEALAND
Palmerston
Nelson North
Blenheim Masterton
Greymouth **Wellington**
Cook Strait
South Island
Aoraki Mt. Cook
3753 Christchurch
Southern Alps
Queenstown Timaru
Invercargill Dunedin
Stewart I.

International Date Line

Chatham Is.
(N.Z.)

West from Greenwich
COPYRIGHT PHILIP'S

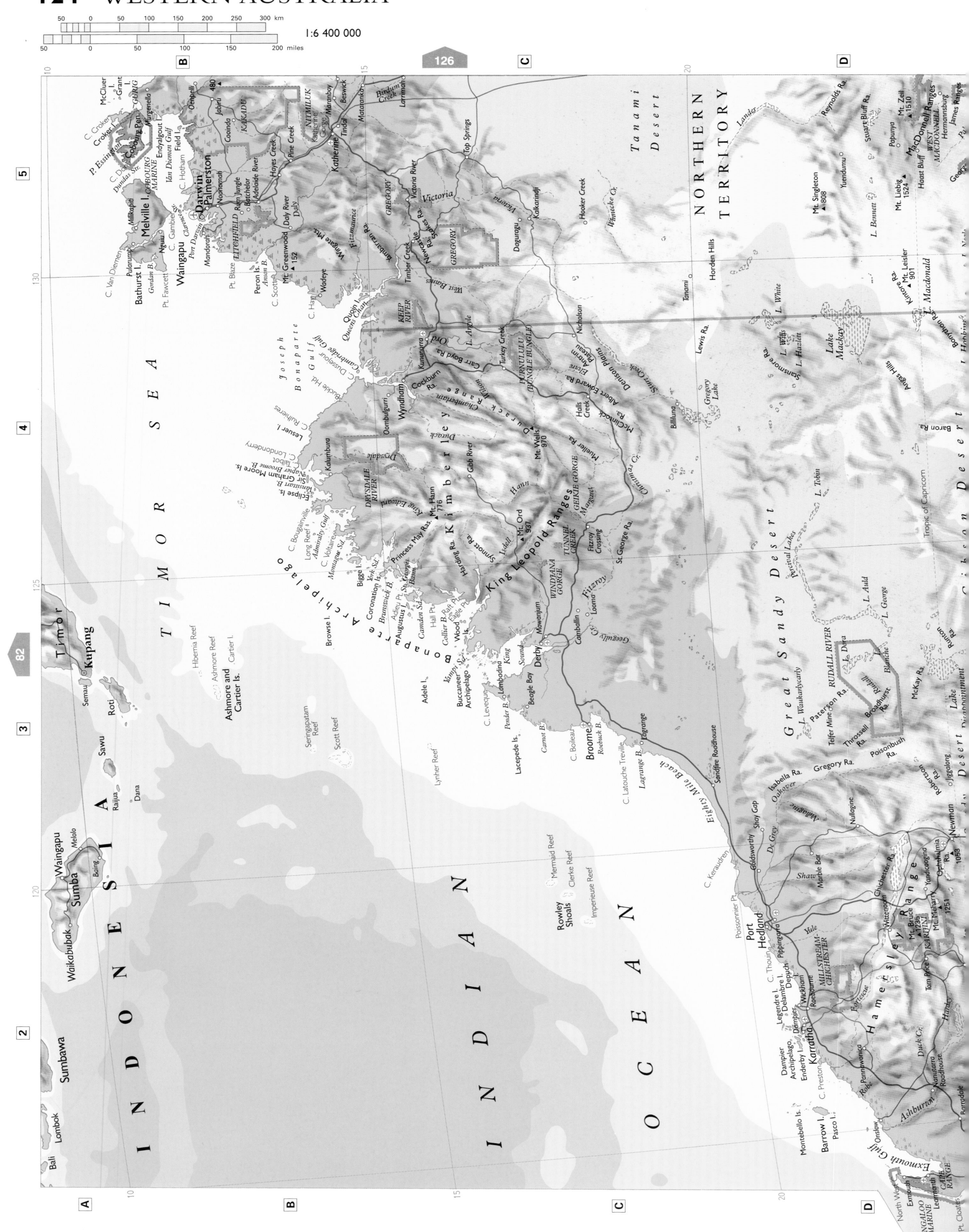

1:6 400 000

50 0 50 100 150 200 250 300 km
50 0 50 100 150 200 miles

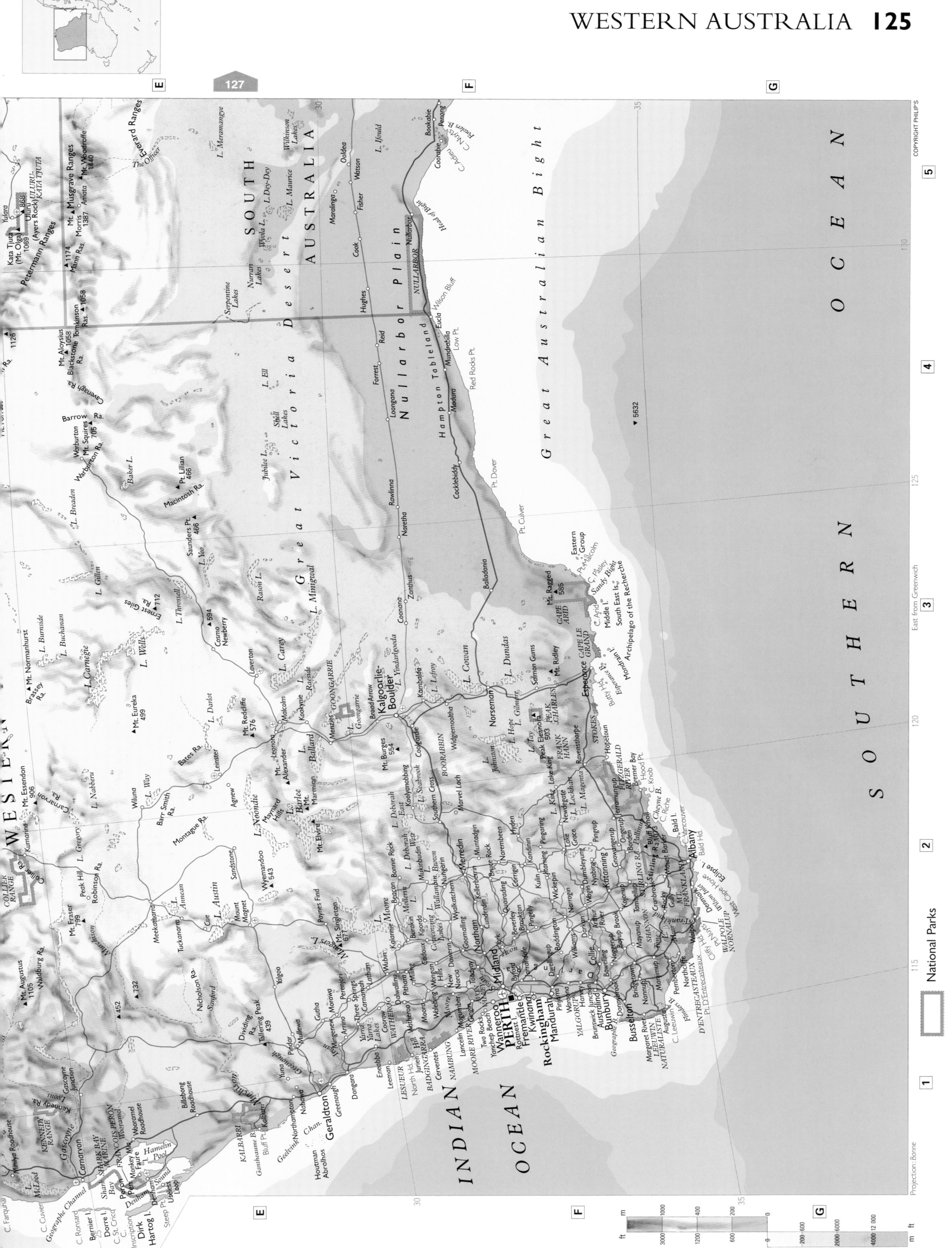

127

SOUTH

AUSTRALIA

WESTERN

Great Victoria Desert

Great Sandy Desert

Nullarbor Plain

Hampton Tableland

NULLARBOR

Great Australian Bight

SOUTHERN OCEAN

INDIAN OCEAN

PERTH
Fremantle
Mandurah
Rockingham
Kwinana
Wanneroo

Geraldton

Bunbury
Busselton

Albany

Kalgoorlie-Boulder

GOONGARRIE

Esperance

CAPE ARID

CAPE LE GRAND

FRANK HANN

STOKES

National Parks

National Parks

m
ft

3000
1200
600
200
0

9000
6000
4000
2000
1000
400
200
0

COPYRIGHT PHILIP'S

East from Greenwich

Projection: Bonne

1   2   3   4   5

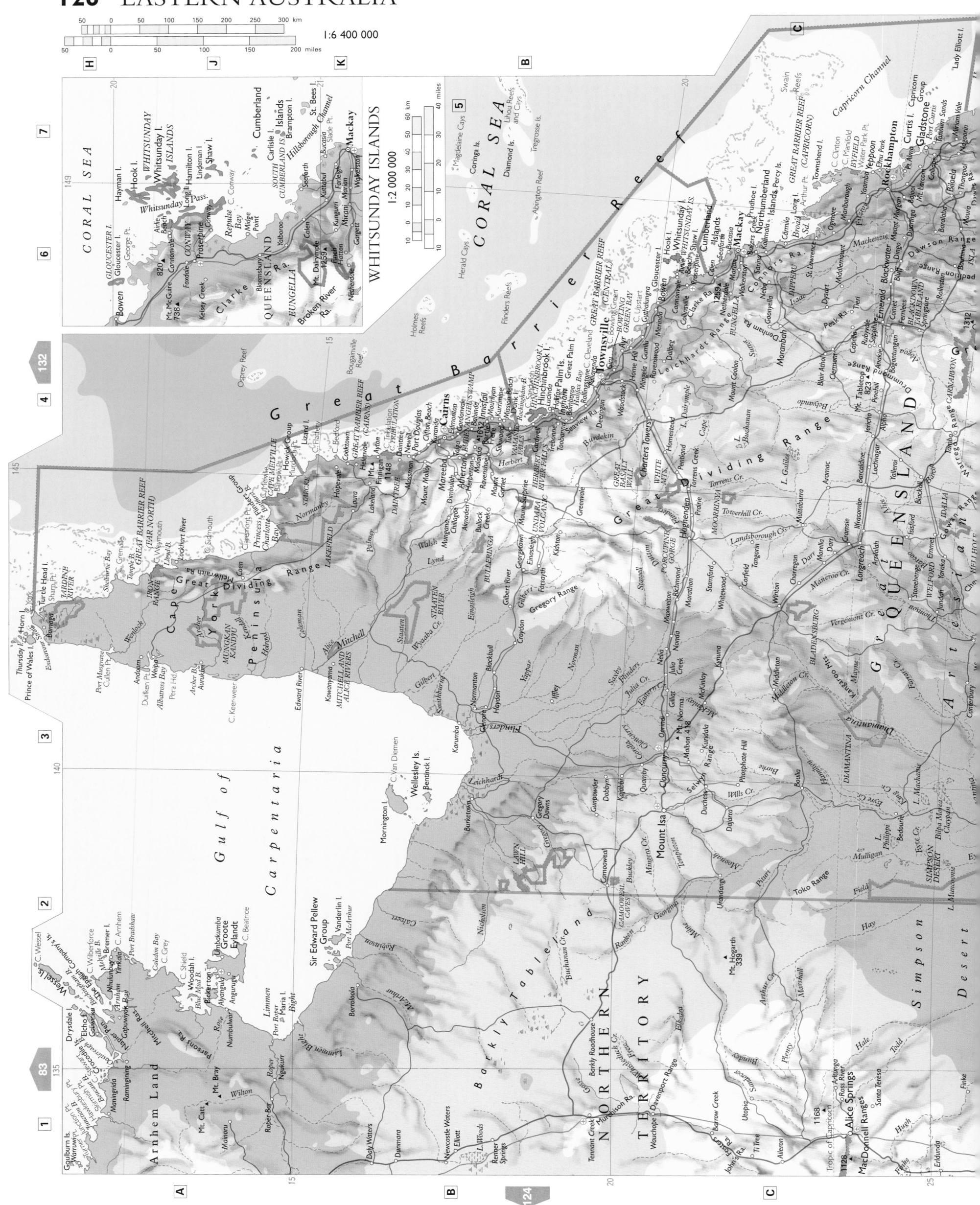

1:6 400 000

WHITSUNDAY ISLANDS

1:2 000 000

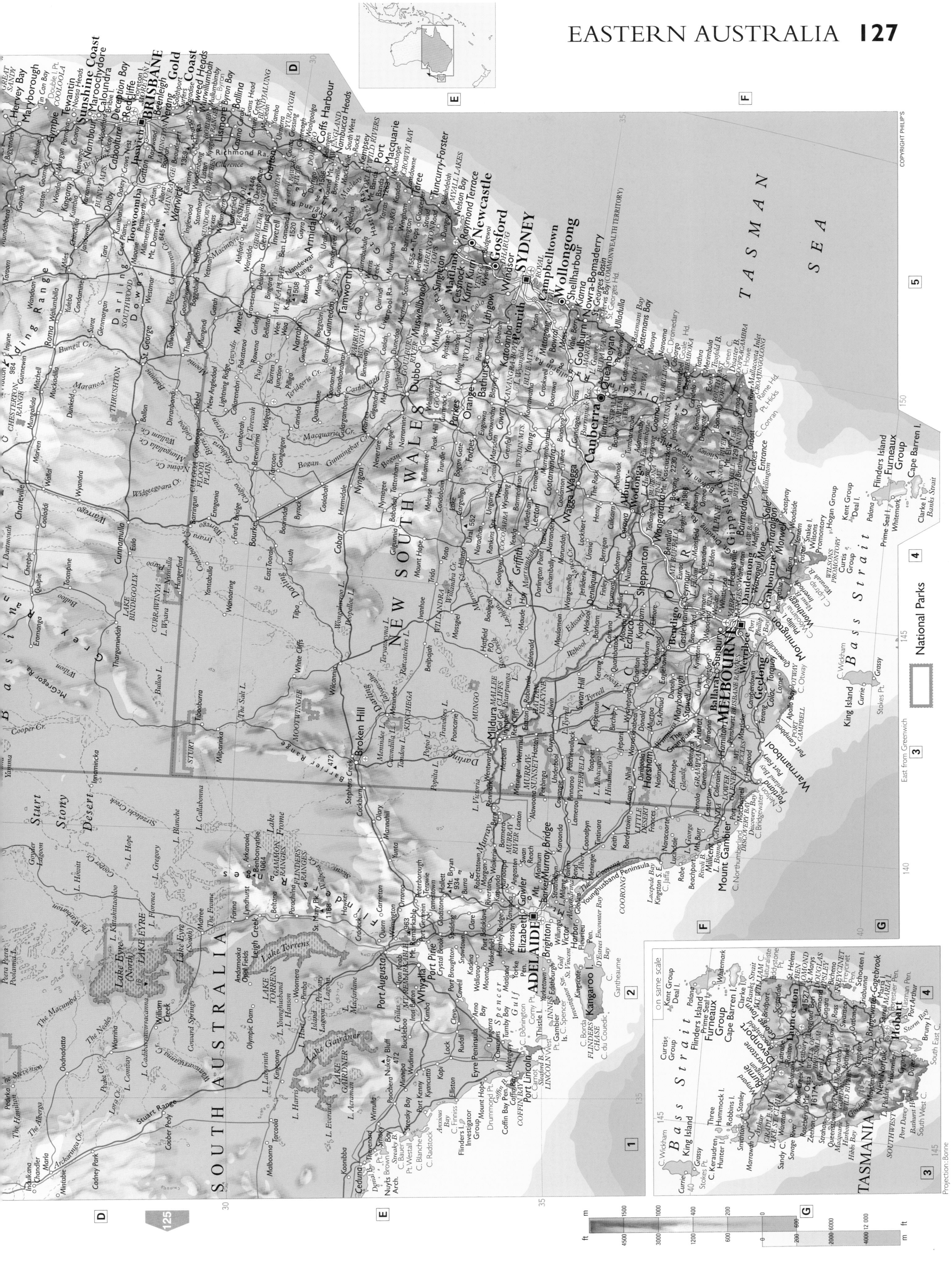

NEW SOUTH WALES

SOUTH AUSTRALIA

TASMANIA

TASMAN SEA

BRISBANE
SYDNEY
Newcastle
Gosford
Wollongong
Canberra
MELBOURNE
ADELAIDE
Hobart

Bass Strait

Gold Coast
Sunshine Coast
Coffs Harbour
Port Macquarie
Broken Hill
Furneaux Group
Flinders Island
King Island
Kangaroo I.

National Parks

on same scale

Projection: Bonne

COPYRIGHT PHILIP'S

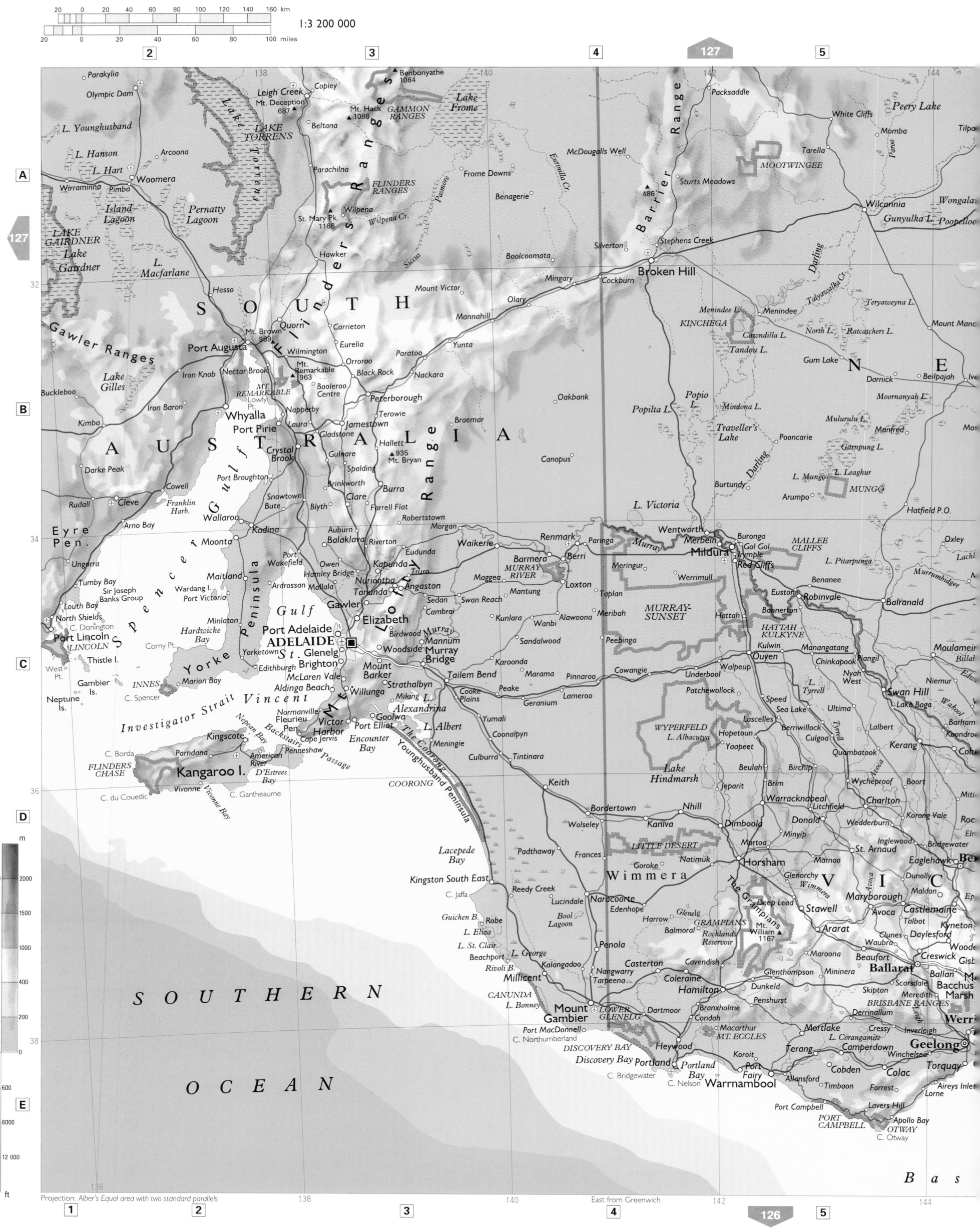

Projection: Alber's Equal area with two standard parallels

East from Greenwich

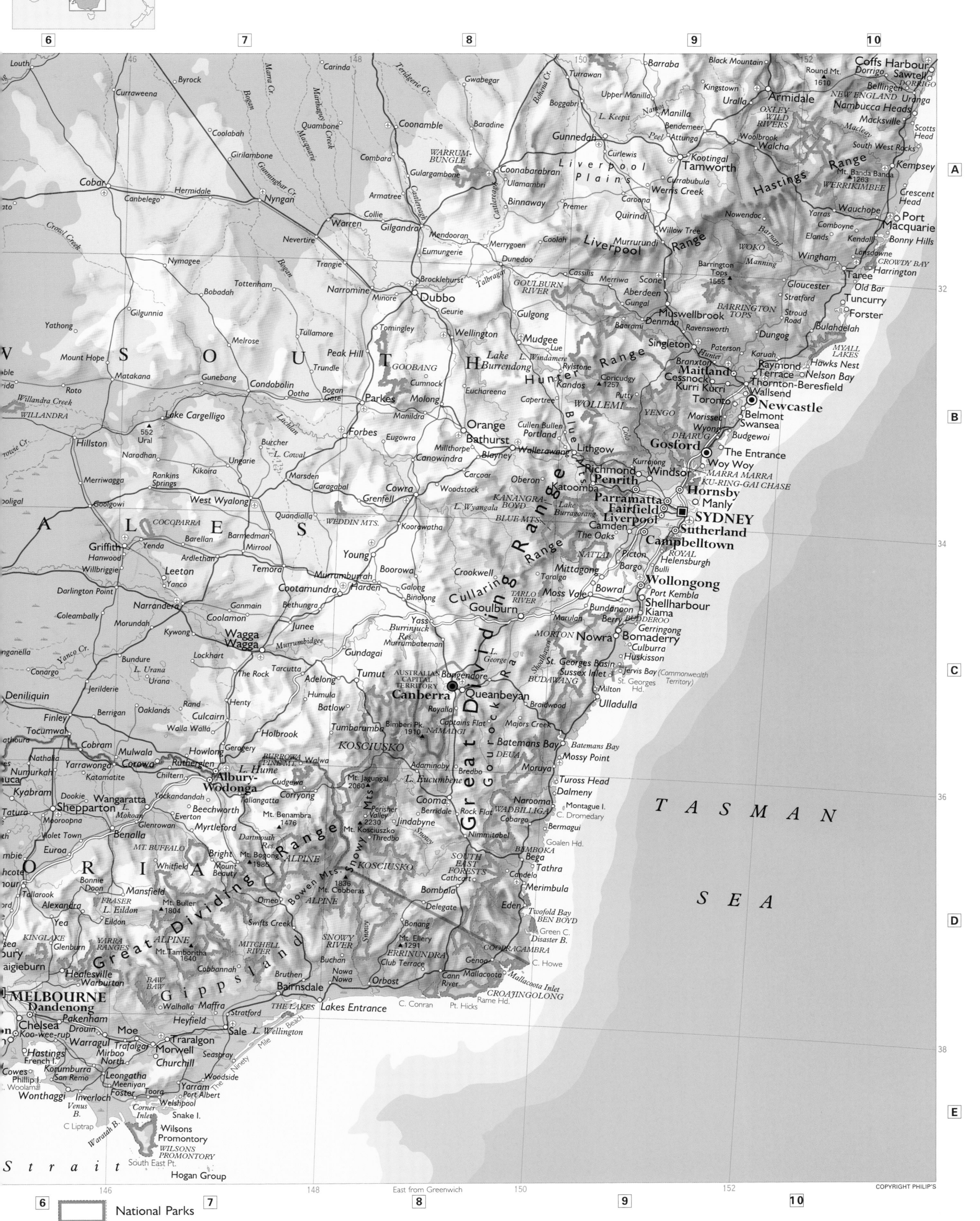

National Parks

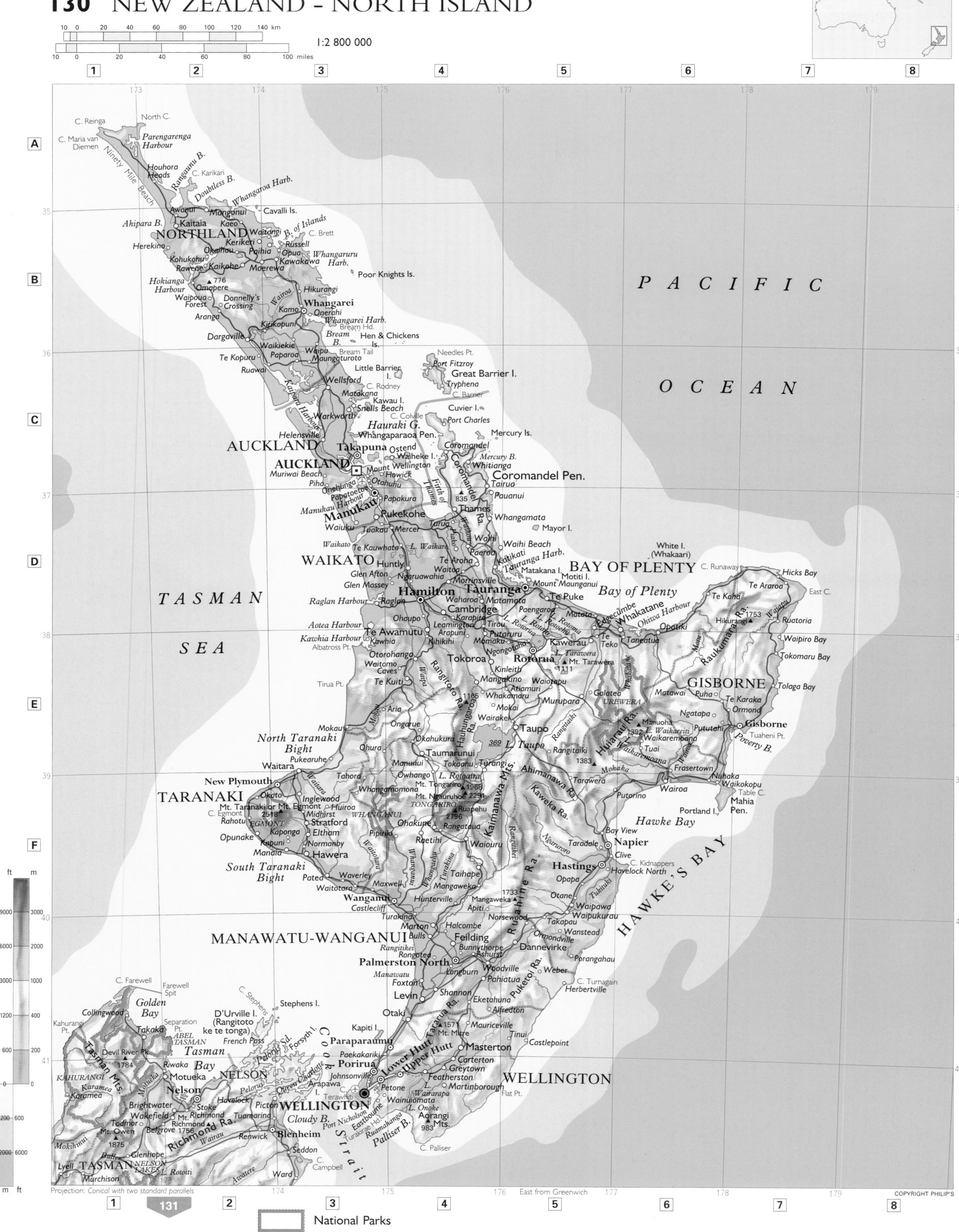

1:2 800 000

National Parks

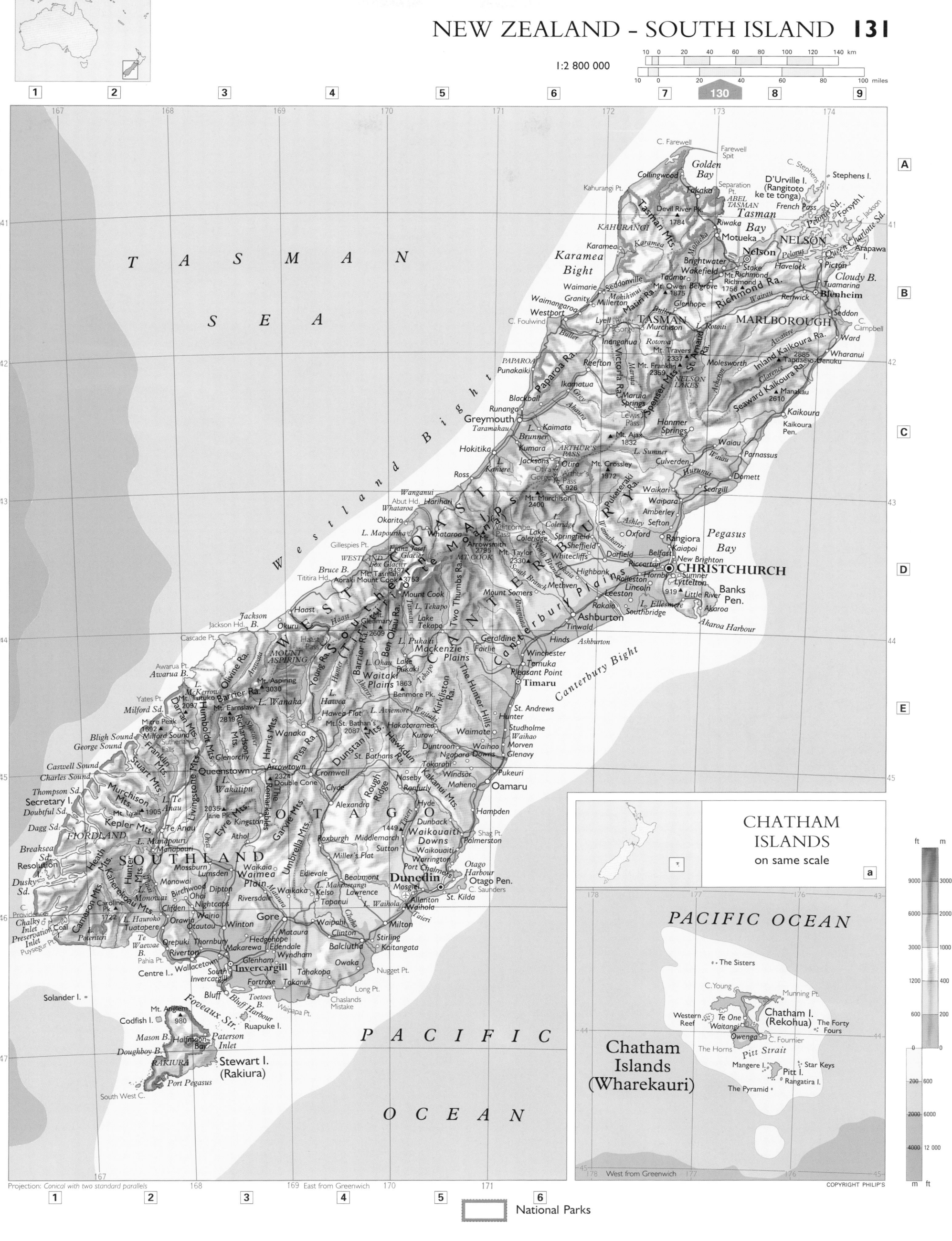

CHATHAM
ISLANDS
on same scale

PACIFIC OCEAN

Chatham
Islands
(Wharekauri)

National Parks

COPYRIGHT PHILIP'S

Projection: Conical with two standard parallels

1:5 200 000

50 0 50 100 150 200 km
50 0 50 100 150 miles

East from Greenwich

Projection: Lambert Conformal Conic

PACIFIC OCEAN

NORTH SOLOMONS

Solomon Islands

Bougainville Trench 9140

NEW IRELAND

New Ireland

St. George's Channel

Bismarck Archipelago

EAST NEW BRITAIN

New Britain

WEST NEW BRITAIN

Bismarck Sea

SOLOMON SEA

WEST SOLOMON SEA

MILNE BAY

Louisiade Archipelago

Pocklington Reef (Solomon Is.)
Rossel I.

MANUS

Admiralty Islands

St. Matthias Group

New Hanover

MADANG

MOROBE

Huon Gulf

Huon Peninsula

NORTHERN

Owen Stanley Ra.

Mt. Victoria 4035

Port Moresby

CENTRAL

Coral Sea

New Guinea

Central Range

PAPUA NEW GUINEA

WEST SEPIK

EAST SEPIK

WESTERN HIGHLANDS

SOUTHERN HIGHLANDS

ENGA

CHIMBU

EASTERN HIGHLANDS

Finisterre Ra.

Bismarck Range

WESTERN

Gulf of Papua

Torres Strait

Great Barrier Reef

AUSTRALIA

Cape York Peninsula

INDONESIA

D'Entrecasteaux Islands

Trobriand Is.

Woodlark I.

Ward Hunt Strait

Mt. Wilhelm 4508

Mt. Giluwe 4368

Mt. Kubor 3647

Mt. Michael 3647

Mt. Bangeta 4121

Mt. Balbi 2715

Mt. Takuam 2251

St. George's Channel

Schleinitz Ra.

Hans Meyer Ra.
Verron Ra.

Whiteman Ra.

Nakanai Mts.

Bowutu Mts.

Owen Stanley Range

m / ft elevation scale
4000 / 12 000
2000 / 6000
1000 / 3000
400 / 1200
200 / 600
0 / 0
200 / 600
2000 / 6000
4000 / 12 000
6000 / 18 000

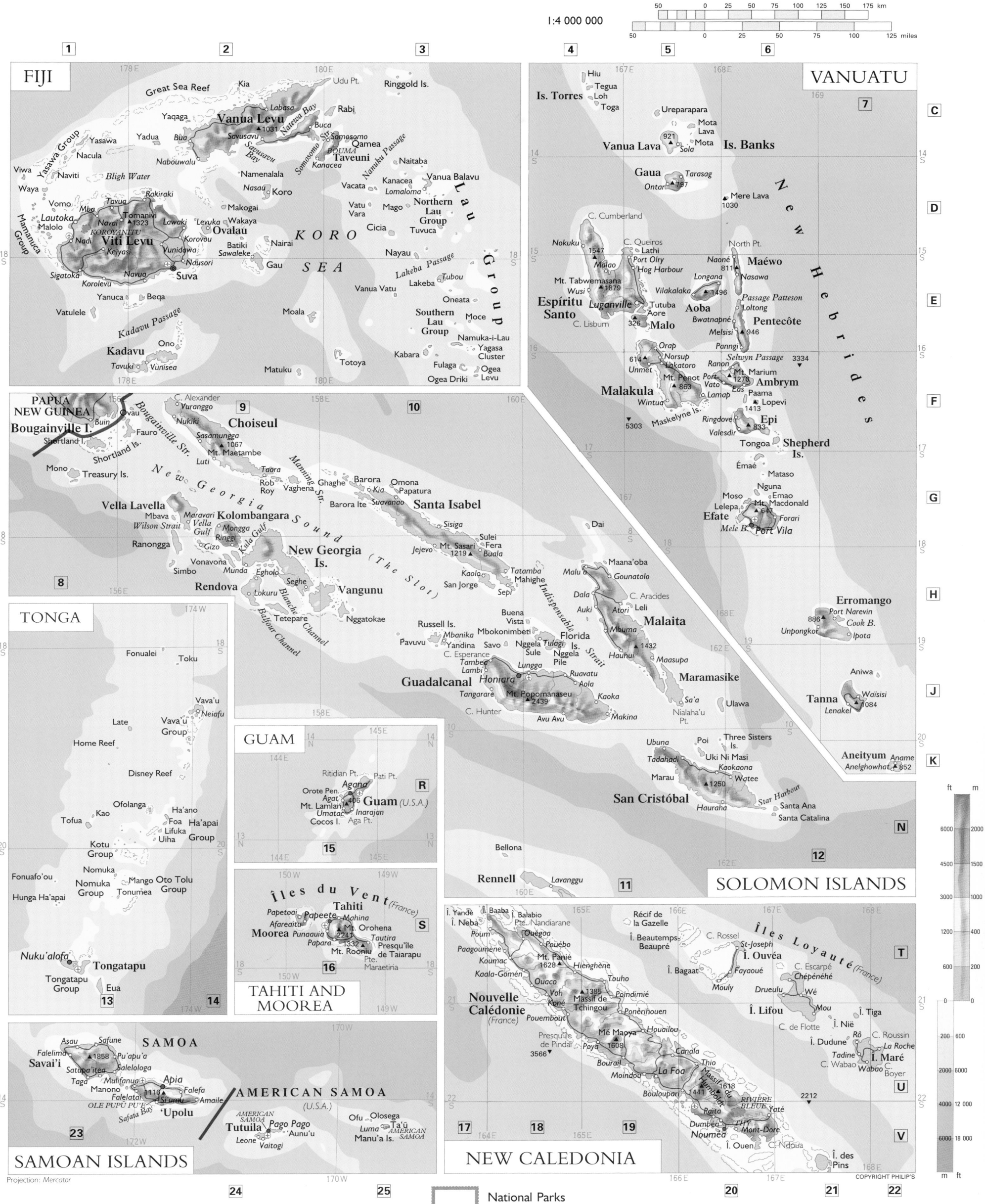

1:4 000 000

Projection: Mercator

COPYRIGHT PHILIP'S

National Parks

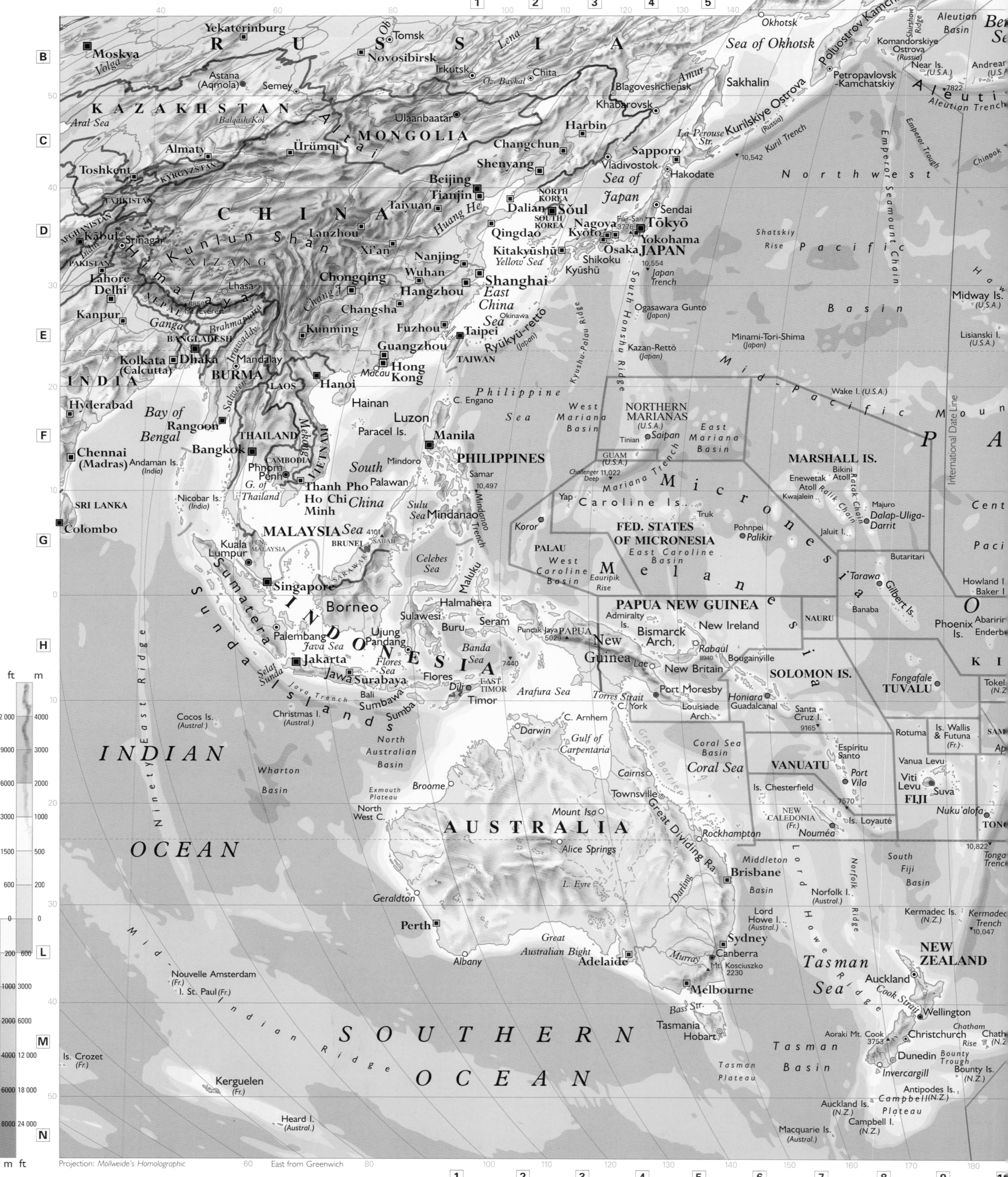

Projection: *Mollweide's Homolographic*   East from Greenwich

Arctic Circle

ALASKA
(U.S.A.)
Anchorage
5959

Juneau

Gulf of Alaska

Bristol Bay

. (U.S.A.)

Prince of Wales I.
(U.S.A.) Prince Rupert
Queen Charlotte Is.
(Canada)

CANADA

Edmonton

L. Winnipeg

NORTH

Newfoundland

Vancouver
Vancouver I. Victoria
Seattle
Portland

Calgary
Regina
Winnipeg
L. Superior

St. Lawrence
Québec
St. John's

Boise

Snake

Minneapolis
Toronto
Detroit
Chicago

Montréal
Ottawa
Buffalo
Boston
New York
Philadelphia

B

C

Northeast

Mendocino Fracture Zone C. Mendocino

Salt Lake
City
Denver
Kansas City

St. Louis
Cincinnati

Pittsburgh

Appalachian Mts.

Baltimore
Washington D.C.

ATLANTIC

D

6741

Murray Fracture Zone

4418

Sacramento
San Francisco

Colorado

UNITED STATES

Memphis

Atlanta

C. Hatteras

Bermuda
(U.K.)

Pacific

Los Angeles
San Diego

Phoenix

Oklahoma City
Dallas

Mississippi

Jacksonville

Sargasso Sea

Guadalupe
(Mex.)

Molokai Fracture Zone

Ciudad
Juárez

Houston
San Antonio

New
Orleans

Tampa

OCEAN

E

Tropic of Cancer

Basin

C. San Lucas

MEXICO

Gulf of California

Monterrey

Gulf of Mexico
Miami

BAHAMAS

West Indies

Ridge

Honolulu
Kauai Maui
Oahu HAWAIIAN IS.
4205 (U.S.A.)
Hilo
Hawaii

Guadalajara

La Habana

Canal de Yucatán

CUBA

Florida Str.

Clarion Fracture Zone Is. Revilla Gigedo
(Mex.)

Mexico
5610
Puebla

Mérida
9200

JAMAICA

7680

HAITI
DOMINICAN REP.

PUERTO
RICO
(U.S.A.)

Leeward
Is.

F

CIFIC

Acapulco

6662

GUATEMALA
Guatemala

BELIZE

HONDURAS

Kingston

Caribbean Sea

BARBADOS
Windward Is.

Middle America Trench

San Salvador
EL SALVADOR

NICARAGUA

Managua

Barranquilla

Maracaibo

I. Clipperton
(Fr.)

Guatemala
Basin

COSTA
RICA

San José
Colón Panamá

Caracas

Clipperton Fracture Zone

Cocos Ridge

PANAMA

Orinoco

VENEZUELA

G

Palmyra Is.
(U.S.A.)

Teraina
Tabuaeran
Kiritimati

I. del Coco
(Costa Rica)

I. de Malpelo
(Colombia)

Medellín

Cali
COLOMBIA

Bogotá

KIRIBATI

Jarvis I.
(U.S.A.)

Line Islands

Galápagos Fracture Zone

Galápagos
(Ecuador)

Carnegie Ridge

Quito
ECUADOR

Equator

EAN

Malden I.
Starbuck I.

Guayaquil

C. Paliñas

Iquitos

BRAZIL

H

Manihiki
Pukapuka
Plateau
Manihiki

Penrhyn
(Tongareva)

Suwarrow Is.

Vostok I.

Caroline I.
(Millennium I.)
Flint I.

Nuku Hiva

Is. Marquises
Hiva Oa

Marquesas Fracture Zone

Trujillo

East Pacific Ridge

PERU

6369

J

Australes Seamount Chain

Cook Is.
(N.Z.)

Is. de la
Société
Bora Bora
Huahine
Raiatea
Papeete

Tuamotu

Rangiroa

Tahiti

Is. Tuamotu

Lima

Cuzco
L. Titicaca
Arequipa

Nevada Ancohuma
6550

Aitutaki

FRENCH POLYNESIA

6866
Peru-Chile

Arica

La Paz
BOLIVIA

Atiu
Rarotonga
Mangaia

Is. Tubuai

Gambier Is.
Mururoa

Ridge

Oeno I.
Henderson I.

Iquique
Chile

Tropic of Capricorn

Antofagasta

PARAGUAY
Asunción

K

Pitcairn I.
(U.K.) Ducie I.

Rapa

Easter Fracture Zone

Sala-y-Gómez
(Chile)

Sala y Gómez Ridge

San Felix
(Chile)

San Ambrosio
(Chile)

8050
Trench

San Miguel
de Tucumán

I. de Pascua
(Chile)

Nazca Ridge

Porto
Alegre

Southwest

Pacific

Challenger Fracture Zone

Chile Rise

Arch. de
Juan Fernández
(Chile)

Córdoba
Aconcagua
6962
Valparaíso
Santiago

Rosario
Buenos
Aires

URUGUAY
Montevideo
Río de la Plata

L

Concepción

ARGENTINA

SOUTH

M

Basin

Pacific-Antarctic Ridge

Menard Fracture Zone

Patagonia

ATLANTIC

6212 OCEAN

Southeast
Pacific Basin

Punta Arenas
C. de Hornos

Est. de Magallanes
Tierra del Fuego

Drake Passage

Falkland Is.
(U.K.)

South Georgia
(U.K.)

N

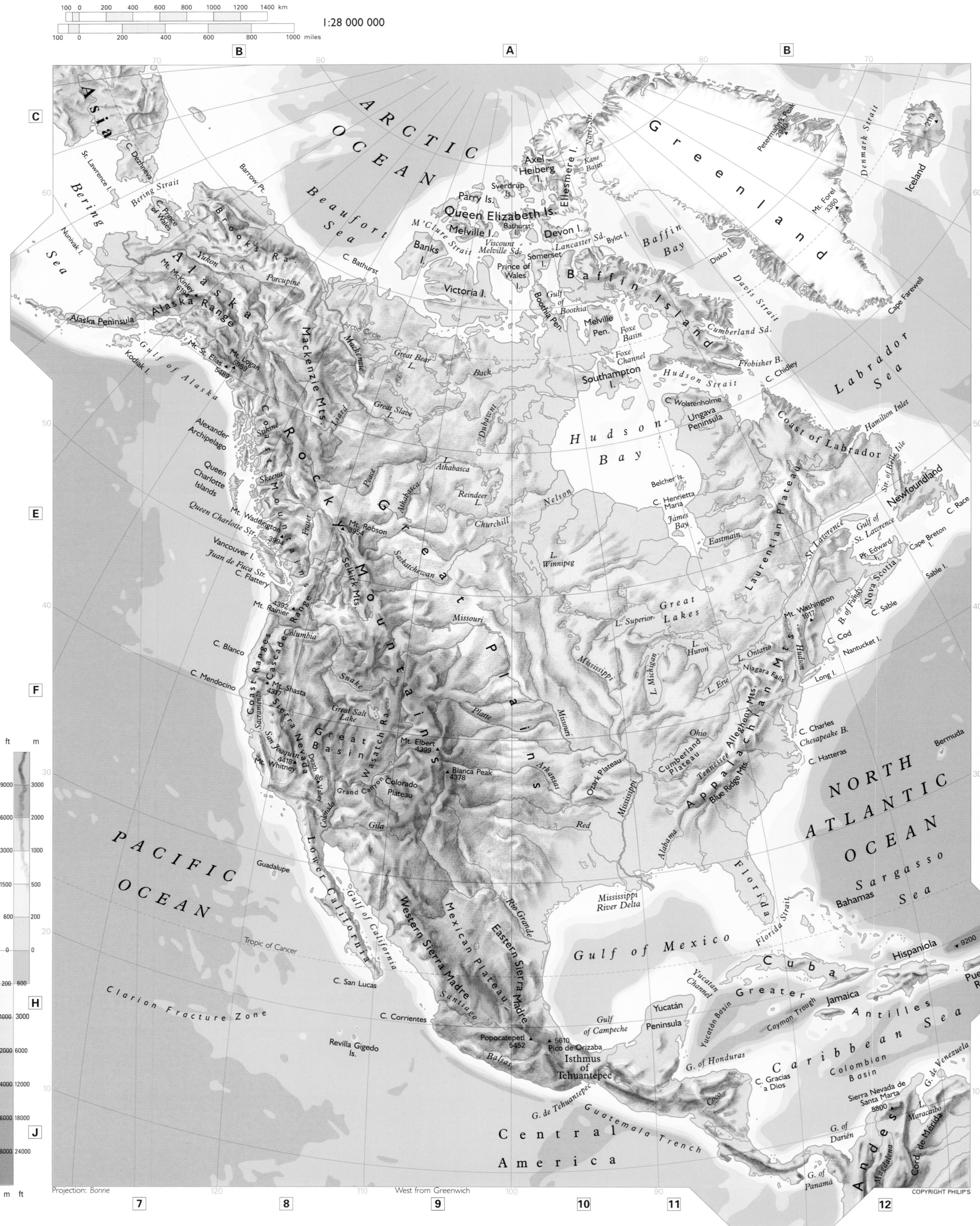

100 0   200 400 600 800 1000 1200 1400 km

1:28 000 000

100 0   200   400   600   800   1000 miles

Projection: Bonne

West from Greenwich

COPYRIGHT PHILIP'S

1:28 000 000

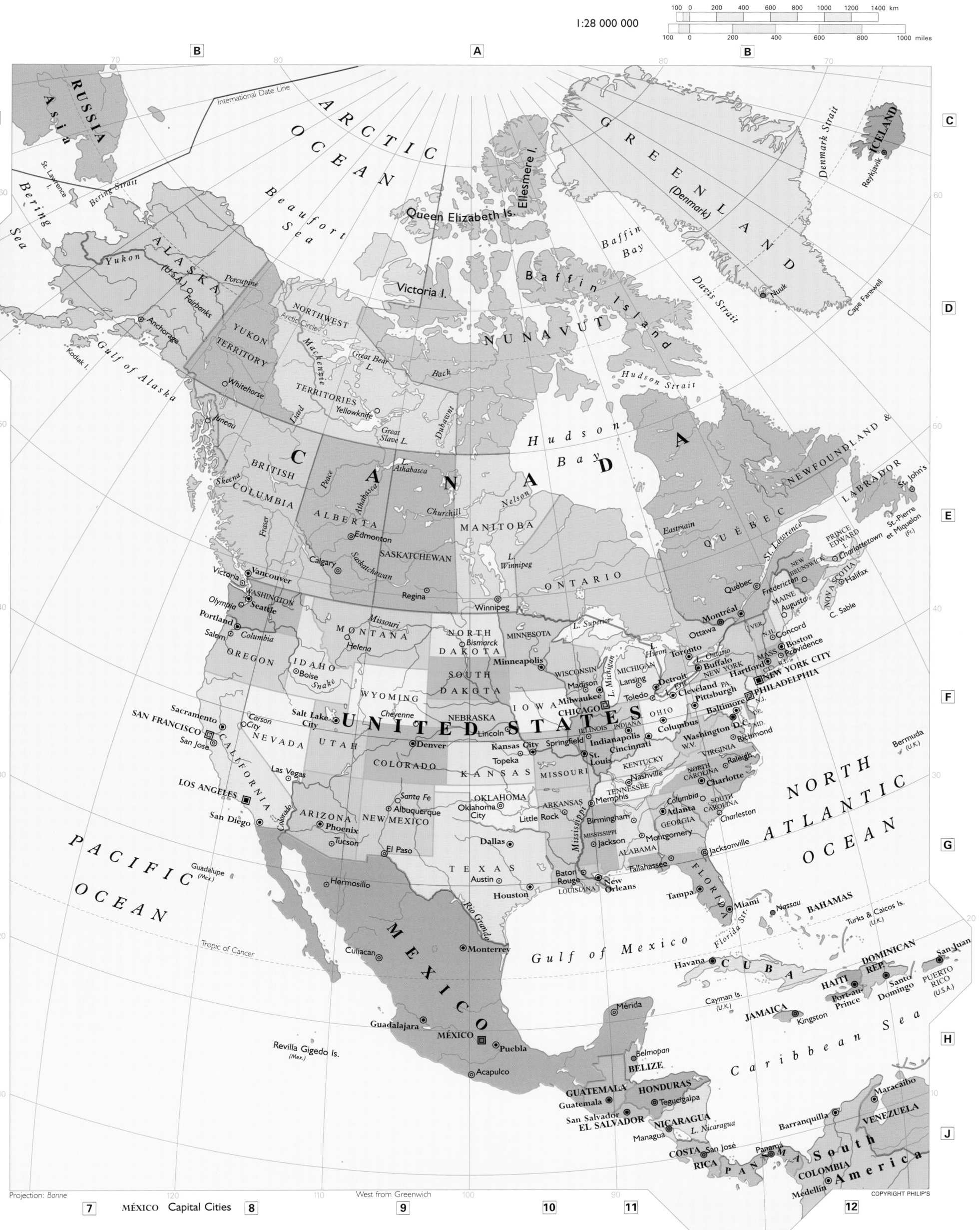

Projection: Bonne

MÉXICO Capital Cities

West from Greenwich

COPYRIGHT PHILIP'S

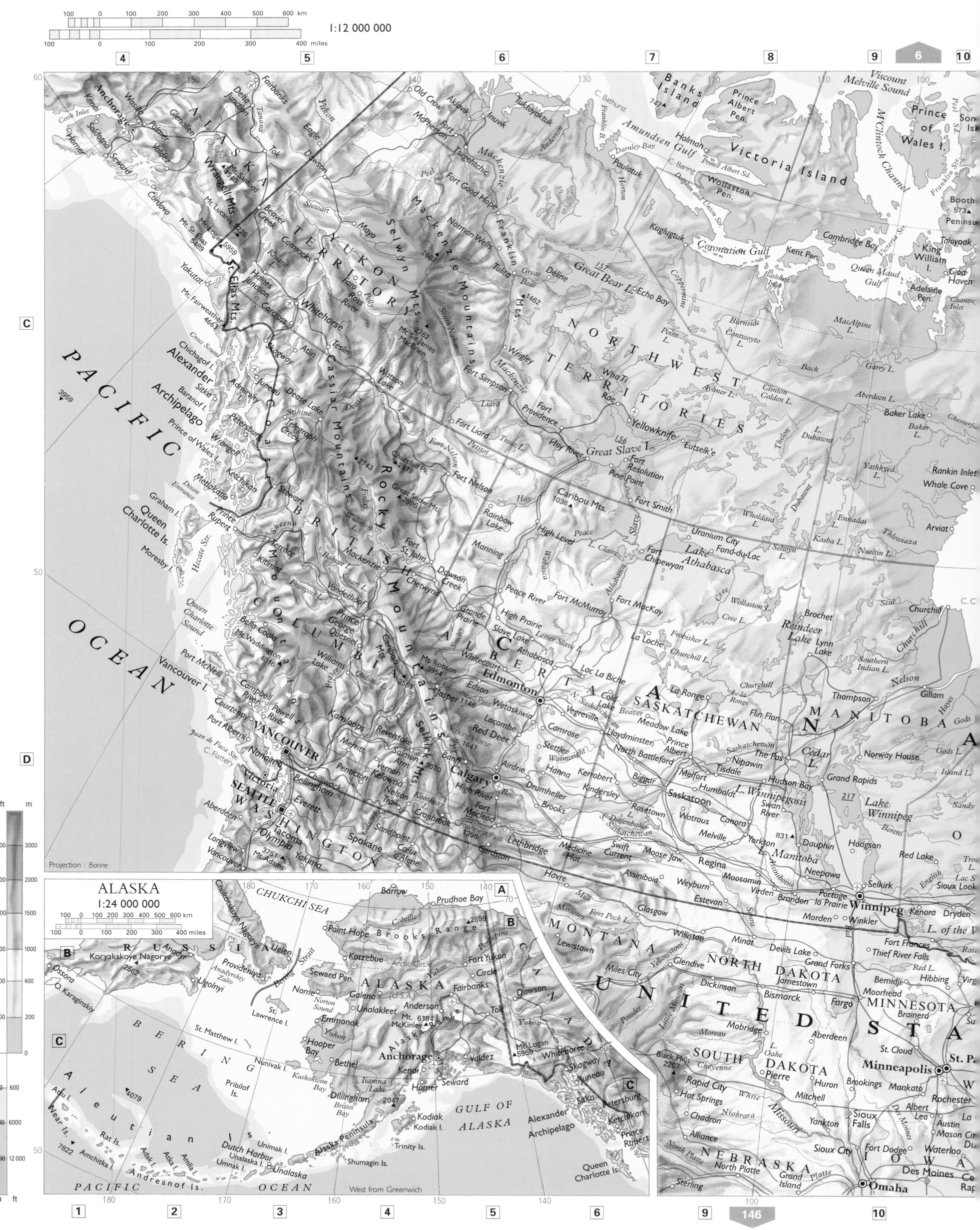

1:12 000 000

ALASKA
1:24 000 000

Projection : Bonne

West from Greenwich

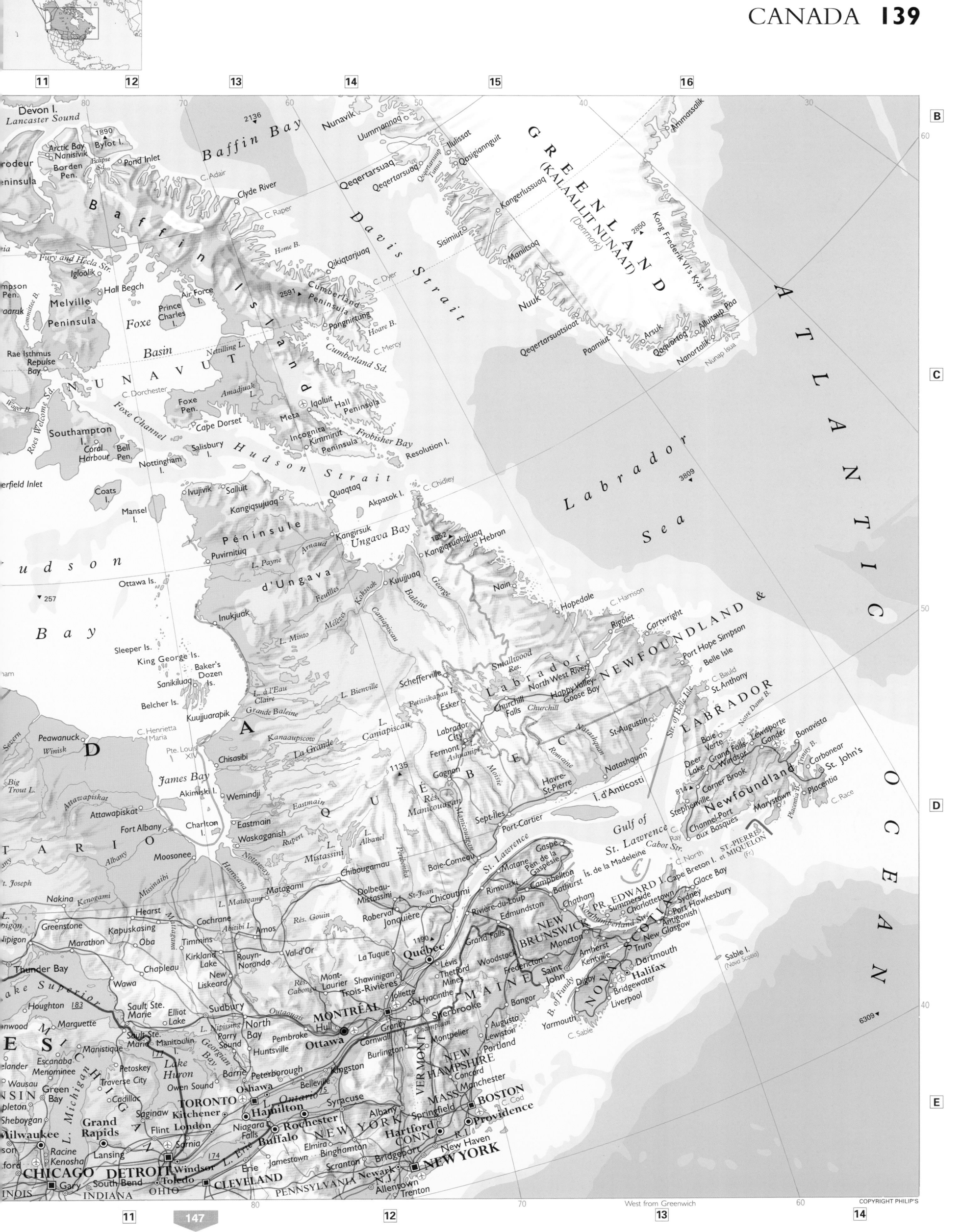

B

C

ATLANTIC

Baffin Bay

Devon I.
Lancaster Sound

Arctic Bay
Nanisivik
1890
Bylot I.
Eclipse Sd.
Pond Inlet
C. Adair

GREENLAND
(KALAALLIT NUNAAT)
(Denmark)

Uummannaq
Nunavik

Qeqertarsuaq
Qeqertarsuaq
Ilulissat
Qasigiannguit

Kangerlussuaq
2850
Kong Frederik VI's Kyst
Ammassalik

Sisimiut

Maniitsoq

Nuuk

Qeqertarsuatsiaat

Paamiut
Arsuk
Qaqortoq
Alluitsup Paa
Nanortalik
Nunap Isua

Baffin Island

Clyde River
C. Raper

Home B.
Qikiqtarjuaq

Cumberland
Peninsula
2591
Pangnirtung
Hoare B.
C. Dyer

Davis Strait

Cumberland Sd.
C. Mercy

2136

NUNAVUT

Foxe
Basin

Melville
Peninsula

Prince
Charles
I.

Air Force
I.

Hall Beach

Igloolik
Fury and Hecla Str.

Rae Isthmus
Repulse
Bay

Roes Welcome Str.

Southampton
I.
Coral
Harbour
Bell
Pen.

Nottingham
I.

Salisbury
I.

Cape Dorset

Amadjuak
L.

Meta
Incognita
Peninsula

Iqaluit
Hall
Peninsula

Kimmirut

Frobisher Bay

Resolution I.

Akpatok I.

C. Chidley

Labrador
Sea

3809

C. Dorchester
C. Henrietta
Maria

Coats
I.

Mansel
I.

Ivujivik
Salluit

Kangiqsujuaq

Quaqtaq

Hudson Strait

Hudson

257

Ottawa Is.

Inukjuak

Sleeper Is.

King George Is.

Sanikiluaq
Baker's
Dozen
Is.

Belcher Is.

Kuujjuarapik

Péninsule
d'Ungava

Puvirnituq

L. Payne
Arnaud

Kangirsuk
Ungava Bay

1852
Kangiqsualujjuaq
Hebron

Nain

Hopedale
C. Harrison

Rigolet
Cartwright

Smallwood
Res.
Port Hope Simpson
Belle Isle

NEWFOUNDLAND &
C. Bauld
St. Anthony

Bay

Pte. Louis
XIV

Big
Trout L.

Severn
Winisk

Peawanuck

C. Henrietta
Maria

Chisasibi

Kanaaupscow

La Grande

L. Bienville

Petitsikapau L.

Esker

Schefferville

Labrador

North West River
Happy Valley-
Goose Bay

Churchill
Falls
Churchill

LABRADOR

Natashquan

St-Augustin

Str. of Belle Isle
Baie
Verte
Lewisporte
Gander
Bonavista

Deer
Lake
Grand Falls
Windsor
Trinity B.
Carbonear

A

L. à l'Eau
Claire

Grande Baleine

James Bay

Akimiski I.

Wemindji

Eastmain

Waskaganish

Rupert

L.
Caniapiscau

Labrador
City
Fermont
Ashuanipi

1135

Gagnon

Rés.
Manicouagan

Mistassini

L.
Albanel

Moisie

Rés.
Gouin

Romaine

Havre-
St-Pierre

Natashquan

Natashquan

Î. d'Anticosti

814

Corner Brook

Newfoundland

Stephenville

Channel-Port
aux Basques

C. Ray

St-Pierre et
MIQUELON
(Fr)

Marystown

Placentia B.
Placentia

C. Race

St. John's

D

Big
Trout L.

Attawapiskat
Attawapiskat

Fort Albany

Charlton

Eastmain

QUÉBEC

Chibougamau

Dolbeau-
Mistassini

St-Jean

Chicoutimi

Rimouski

Matane
Pén. de
Gaspésie
Gaspé

Campbellton
Bathurst

Gulf of
St. Lawrence

Î. de la Madeleine

PR. EDWARD I.
Summerside
Charlottetown

Cape Breton I.
Sydney
Glace Bay

ATLANTIC

Sable I.
(Nova Scotia)

6309

OCEAN

ONTARIO

St. Joseph

Nakina
Kenogami

Hearst
Kapuskasing
Oba

Greenstone

Marathon

Missinaibi
Mattagami L.

Timmins

Cochrane
Abitibi L.

Kirkland
Lake

New
Liskeard

Amos

Val-d'Or

Matagami

Rouyn-
Noranda

L. Matagami

Rés.
Cabonga

Mont-
Laurier

La Tuque

Shawinigan
Trois-Rivières

1190

Québec
Lévis
Thetford
Mines

Grand Falls

Edmundston

Woodstock

NEW
BRUNSWICK

Fredericton
Saint
John

Moncton
Amherst
Chignecto
Truro

Northumberland Str.

Antigonish
Port Hawkesbury

New Glasgow

NOVA
SCOTIA

Kentville
Dartmouth
Halifax
Bridgewater
Liverpool

Digby

B. of Fundy

Yarmouth

C. Sable

Thunder Bay
Houghton
183

Wawa

Chapleau

Sudbury

Sault Ste.
Marie

Elliot
Lake

L. Nipissing

North
Bay

Pembroke

Joliette

St-Hyacinthe

MONTRÉAL
Hull
Granby
Sherbrooke

Ottawa

Cornwall

MAINE

Bangor

Augusta

Woodstock

Portland

Lake Superior

Marquette

Manistique

Sault
Ste. Marie

Manitoulin
I.

Parry
Sound

Georgian
Bay

Huntsville

Barrie

Peterborough

Belleville

Kingston

Burlington

Montpelier

VERMONT

NEW
HAMPSHIRE
Concord
Manchester

MASS.

Lewiston

MICHIGAN

Escanaba
Menominee

Petoskey

Traverse City

Cadillac

Lake
Huron

Owen Sound

Oshawa

TORONTO

Hamilton

Niagara
Falls

Buffalo

L. Erie

Rochester

Syracuse

Elmira

NEW YORK

Albany

Springfield

Hartford
CONN.

BOSTON

C. Cod

Providence

Wausau

Green
Bay

Sheboygan

L. Michigan

Milwaukee

Racine
Kenosha

Grand
Rapids

Flint

Lansing

Saginaw

London

Sarnia

Kitchener

Windsor

DETROIT

Toledo

CLEVELAND

Erie

Jamestown

Binghamton

Scranton

Newark
N.J.

NEW YORK

New Haven

Bridgeport

Allentown
Trenton

CHICAGO

Gary
South Bend

INDIANA

OHIO

PENNSYLVANIA

WISCONSIN

E

West from Greenwich

COPYRIGHT PHILIP'S

1:5 600 000

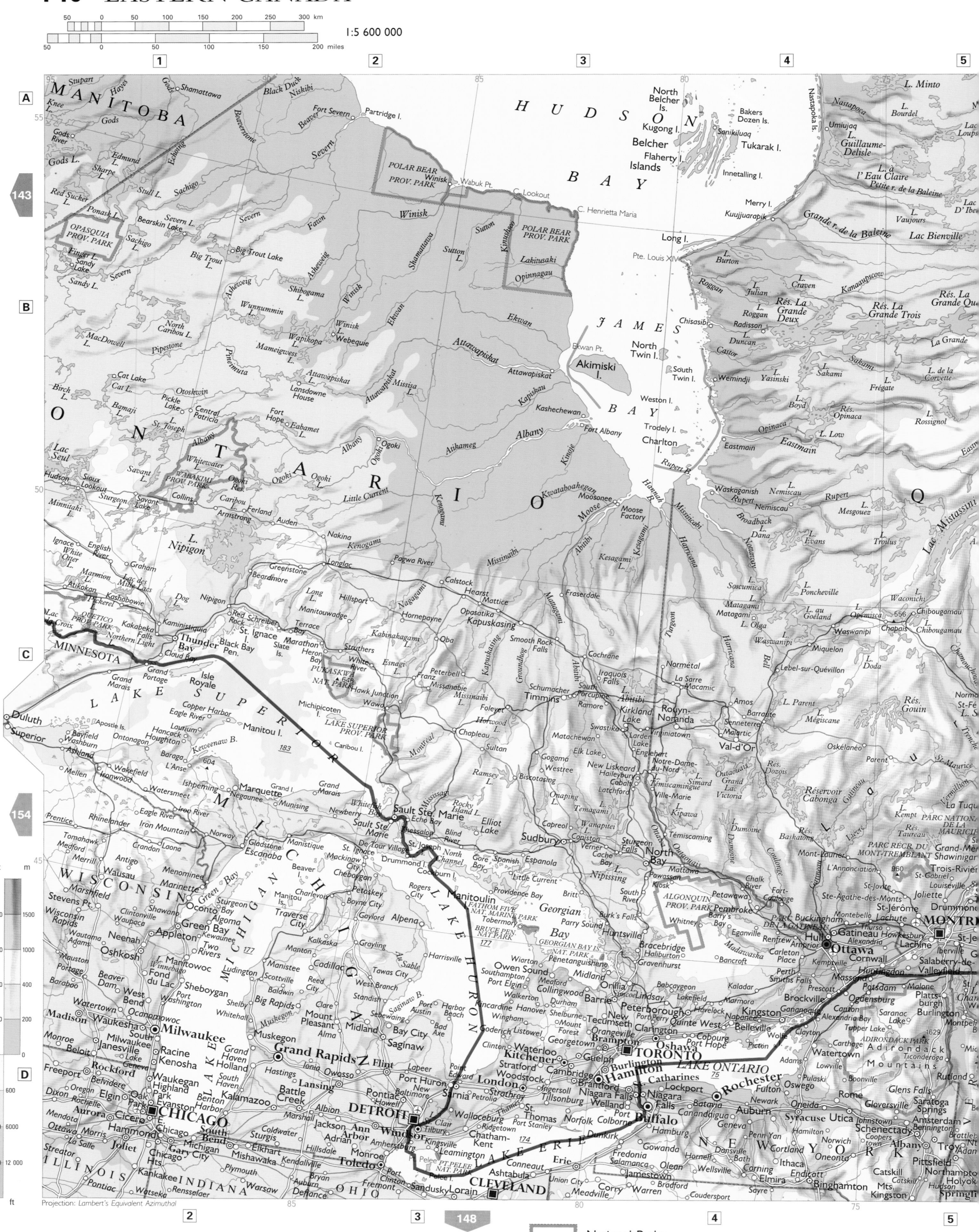

Projection: Lambert's Equivalent Azimuthal

☐ National Parks

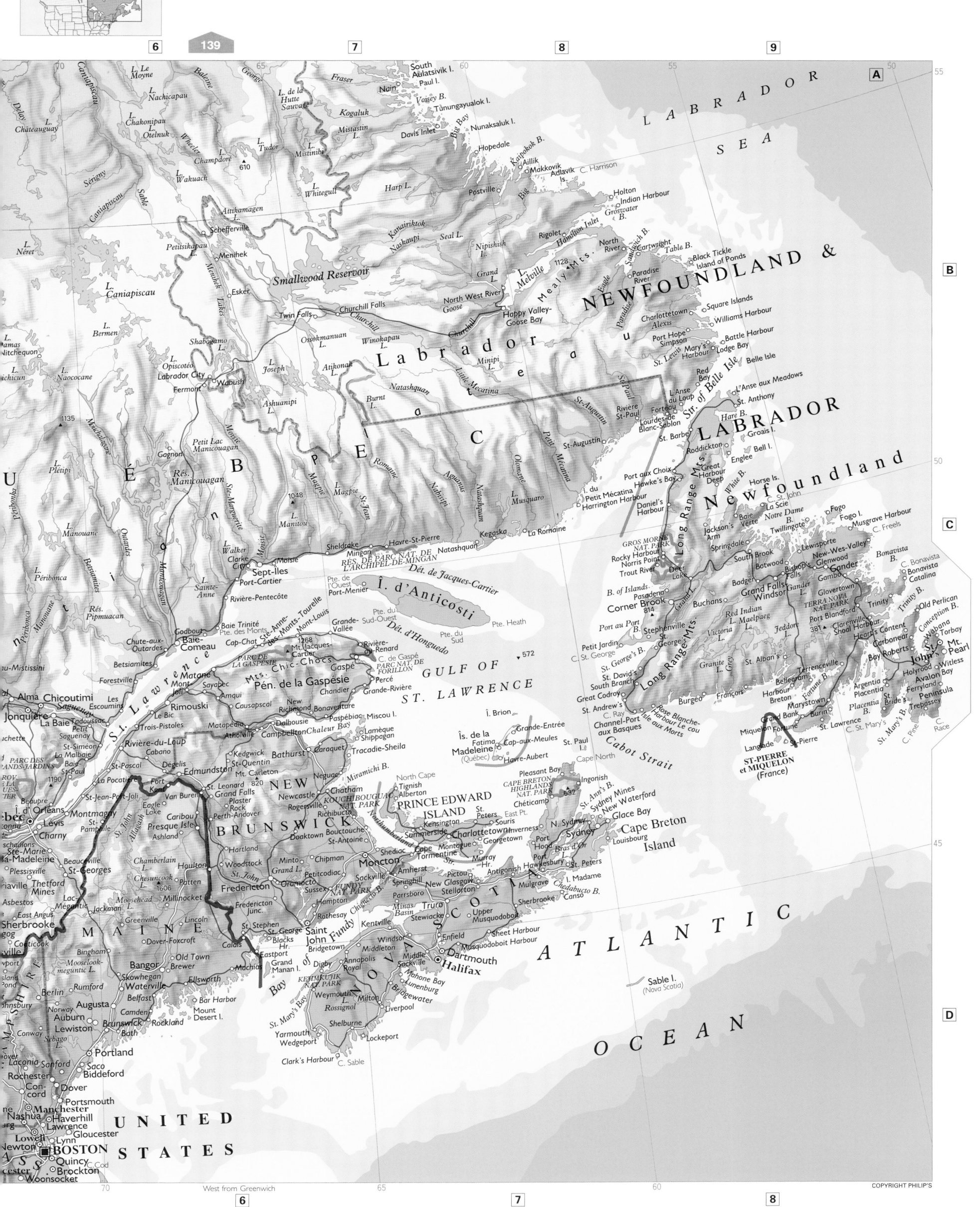

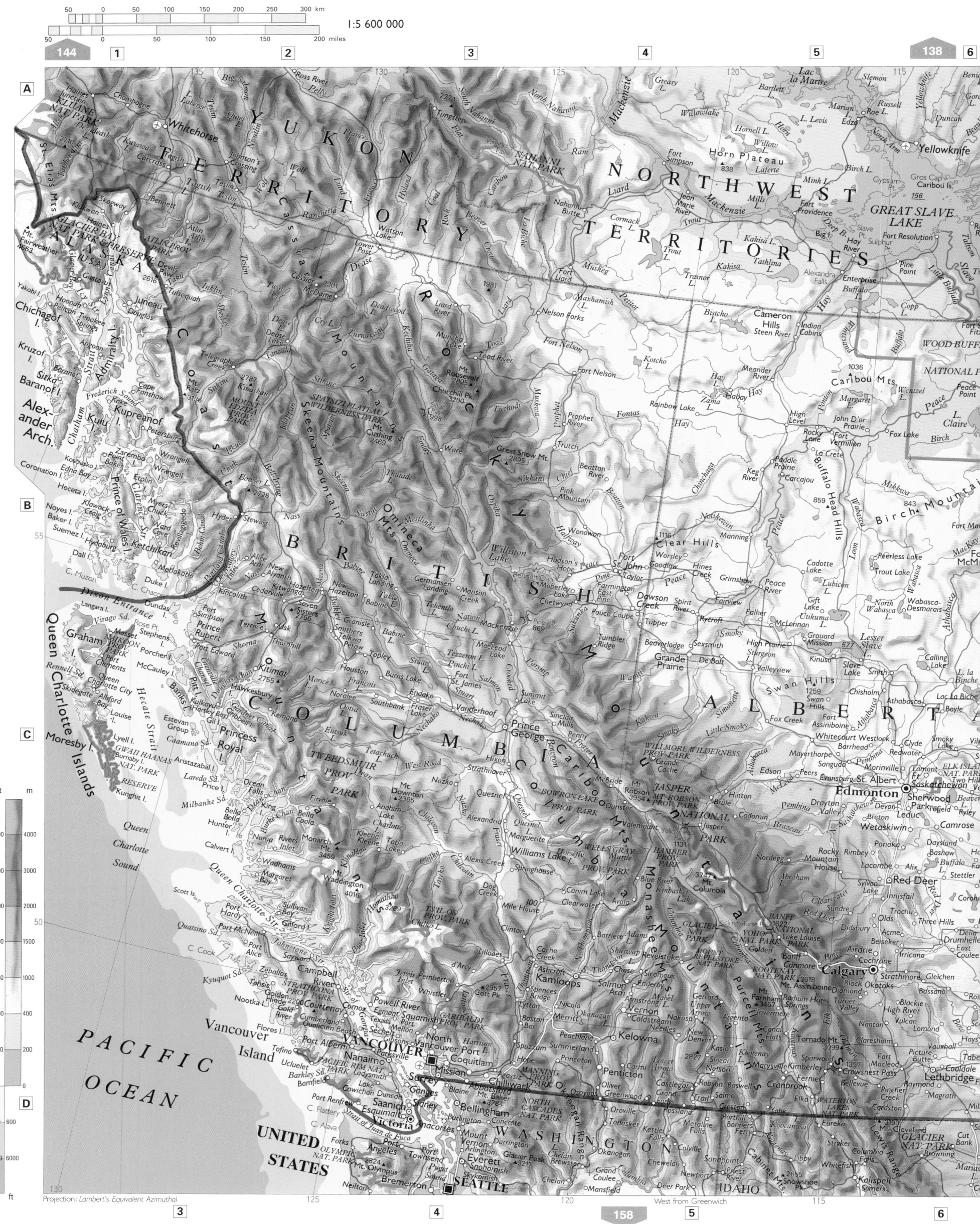

1:5 600 000

Projection: Lambert's Equivalent Azimuthal

West from Greenwich

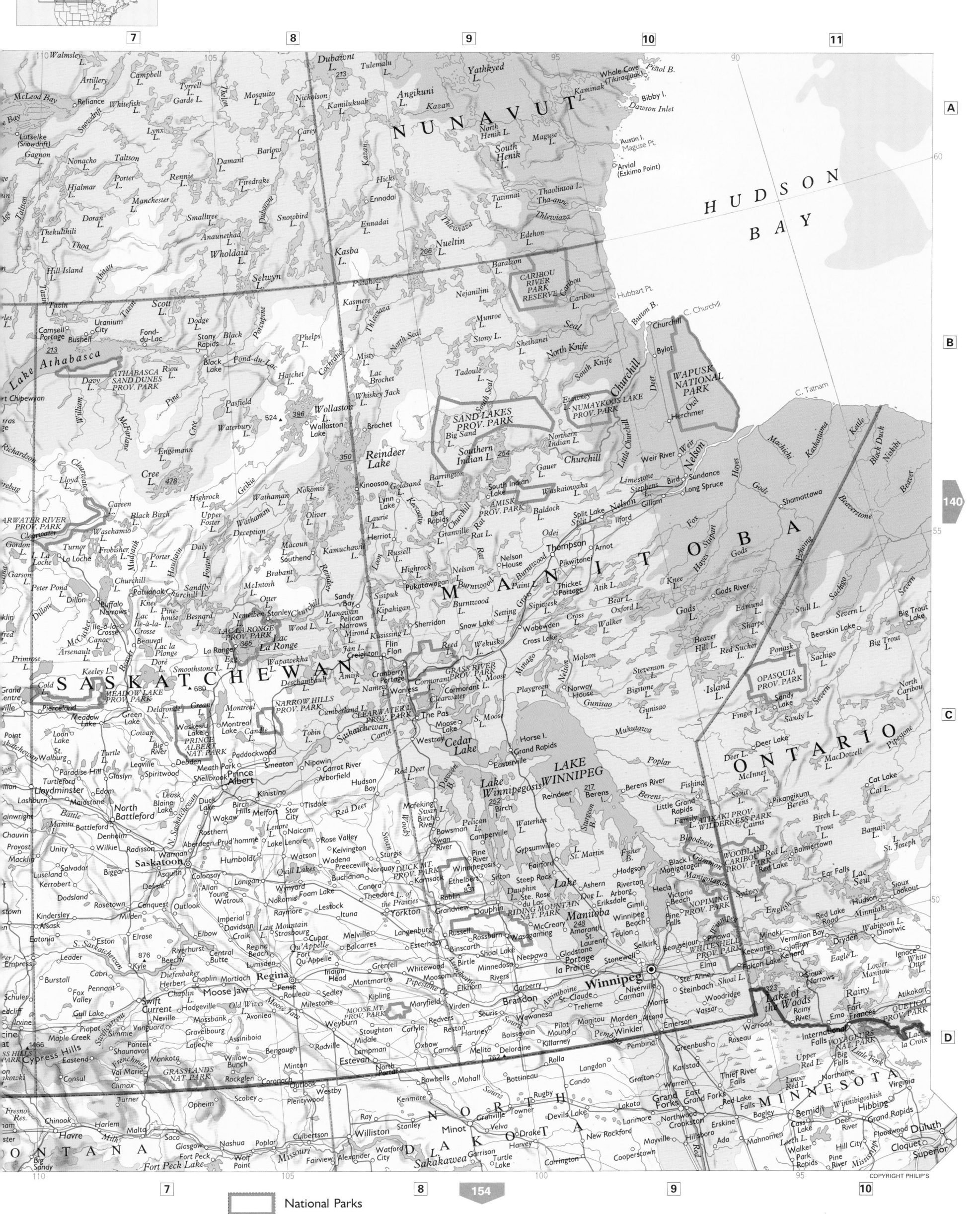

National Parks

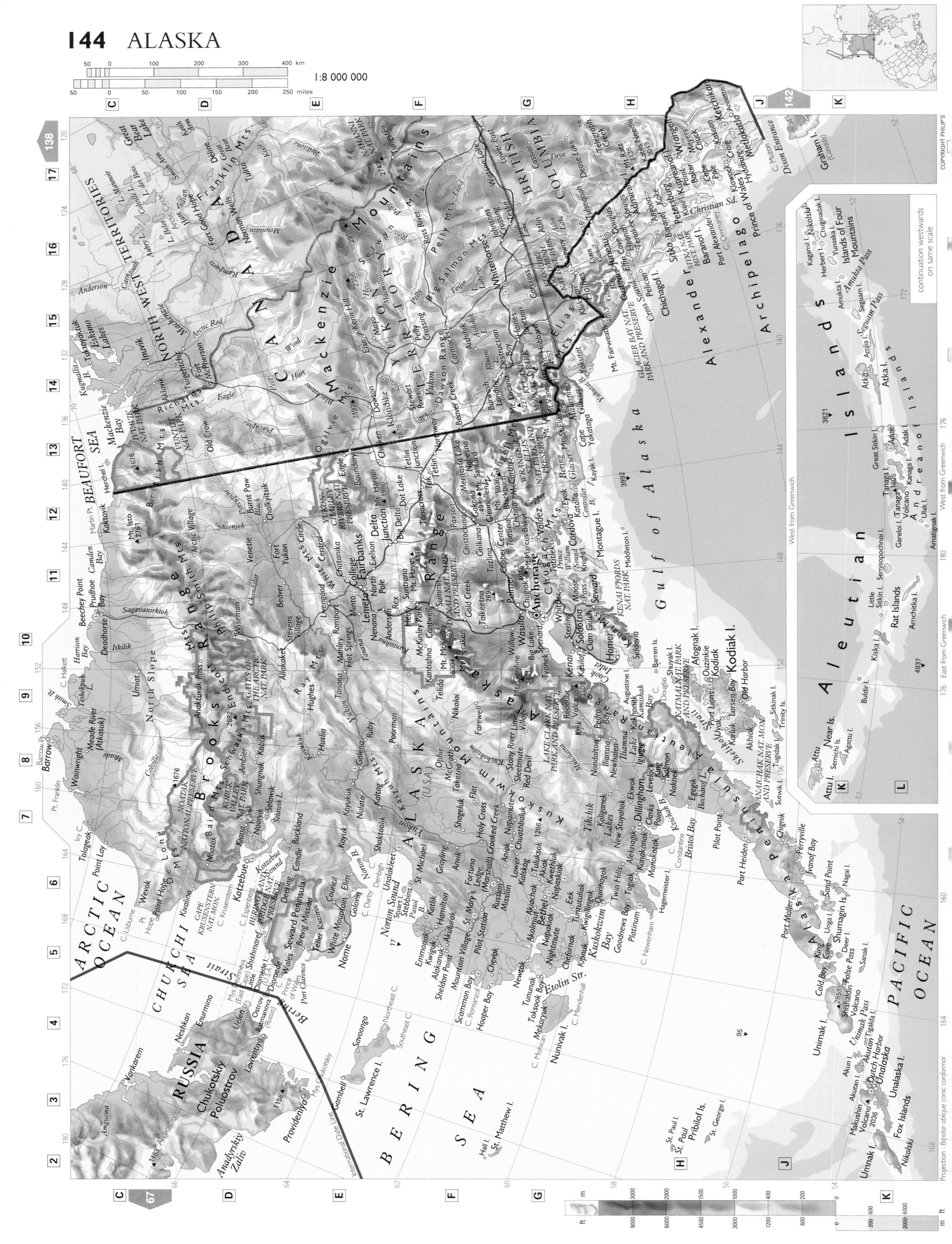

1:8 000 000

COPYRIGHT PHILIP'S

continuation westwards
on same scale

Projection: Bipolar oblique conic conformal

1:2 000 000

HAWAIIAN ISLANDS
1:20 000 000

Tropic of Cancer

PACIFIC OCEAN

H a w a i i a n   I s l a n d s

Kauai Oahu Molokai Maui
Lehua I. Niihau Lanai Kahoolawe
Kaula I. Hawaii

Kure I. Midway Is. Pearl and Hermes Reef Lisianski I. Laysan I. Maro Reef Gardner Pinnacles French Frigate Shoals Necker I. Nihoa

PACIFIC OCEAN

Projection: Albers Equal Area

National Parks

COPYRIGHT PHILIP'S

West from Greenwich

Hawaii (Big Island)

Kumukahi Cape
Keaau Kurtistown Pahoa Kalapana
Hilo Volcano Kilauea Crater
Mountain View Glenwood
Papaikou Pepeekeo Honomu Okala
Paauilo Ookala Honokaa Honokaa
Kukuihaele Kohala Mts. Waimea (Kamuela) 1678
Hawi Kapaau Nauhola Pt.
Upolu Pt. Mauna Kea ▲4205
Mauna Loa ▲4169
HAWAII VOLCANOES NATIONAL PARK
▲2096 Puu o Keokeo
Hualalai ▲2521
Holualoa Kailua Kona
Kealakekua Captain Cook Kealia
Honaunau Honuapo Bay
Keauhou Keei Papa Naalehu Kaalualu Bay
Kalae Pohue Bay Miloli Kauna Pt. Ka Lae
Malae Pt. Kiholo Bay
KALOKO-HONOKOHAU NAT. HISTORICAL PARK
PUUKOHOLA HEIAU NAT. HIST. SITE
PU'UHONUA O HONAUNAU NAT. HISTORICAL PARK
Kaiwaihae Bay

1340 ▼

PACIFIC OCEAN

Alenuihaha Channel

Maui

Hana Pauwela Paia Kahului Wailuku Waihee Waikapu
HALEAKALA NAT. PARK Haleakala Crater ▲3055
Lower Paia Puunene Pukalani Makawao
Kihei Keokea Kaupo Ulupalakua
Lahaina Olowalu Keawakapu Molokini
Puukoli Napili
Kaka Pt. Lua Makiki 450

Kealaikahiki Channel

Lanai
Lanai City 1027 Palaoa Pt.
Kaumalapau Lanaihale
Manele

Kahoolawe

Alalakeiki Channel

Pailolo Channel

Molokai
Kalaupapa Kalaupapa Kualapuu Kaunakakai
Ilio Pt. Hoolehua Maunaloa KALAUPAPA NAT. HIST. PARK
Kamakou Kamalo
Laau Pt. Kaholo Channel

Kalohi Channel

Honokohua
Nakalele Pt.
C. Halawa

Kauai Channel

Kaiwi Channel

Oahu (inset)

OAHU 1:500 000
Projection: Lambert's Conformal Conic

Kahuku Pt. Kahuku Laie Hauula Punaluu
Sunset Beach Waimea Kahana Bay Kaaawa
Kawela Waialee Kahana Kaneohe Kailua
Kaena Pt. Makaleha Pt. Waianae Kualoa Pt.
Mokapu Peninsula Kapapa I. Mokolea Rock
Mokumanu I. Kaneohe Heeia Kahaluu Ahuimanu
Puu Pauao ▲817 Kaneohe Bay
Waialua Haleiwa Wahiawa Kahana Bay
Whitmore Village Schofield Barracks
Waipio Acres Mililani Town Pearl City
Halawa Heights Honolulu
HONOLULU Waikiki Diamond Head
Kapahulu Kaimuki ▲232
Koolau Range
Koko Head Hanauma Bay
Makapuu Pt. Manana I.
Waimanalo Waimanalo Beach Maunawili
Kailua Lanikai Nuu Maunalua Bay
Waipahu Ewa Ewa Beach Honouliuli
USS ARIZONA MEMORIAL Pearl Harbor Aiea
Ford I. Sand Island HNL Keehi Lagoon
Waimanalo Kaneohe Bay
HONOLULU COUNTY Kipapa
Kunia Anahulu Helemano Kaukonahua
Waianae Mts. Kaala ▲1231 Palikea Pk. ▲944
Waianae Maili Nanakuli Makakilo City
Makaha Kaena Pt. Lualualei Pokai Bay
Kaneilio Pt. Kepuhi Pt. Lahilahi Pt.
Waialua Bay Kawailoa Beach Puaena Pt.
Waimea Bay Kaena Pt. Barbers Pt.
Mamala Bay
Waikane Waiahole Kahana
Koolaupoko
Ewa Plain

Kaiwi Channel

PACIFIC OCEAN

Oahu (main map, top)
Kahuku Pt. Kahuku Laie Hauula Kaaawa
Waialua Haleiwa Wahiawa Kaneohe Kailua Waimanalo
Oahu Waimea Aiea Ewa HONOLULU Beach
Kaena Pt. Waianae Nanakuli Barbers Pt.
Kaala 1231
446 ▼

Kauai
Mokaeae I. Kilauea Anahola
Haena Hanalei Wailua Kapaa
Mana Waimea Lihue Hanamaulu
Kawaikini 1598 Koloa
Kekaha Kapaa Nawiliwili Pt.
Nohili Pt. Ninini Pt.
Kekaha Makahuena Pt.
Waita Res.
Kaulakahi Channel

Niihau
Lehua I. Puuwai 390
Kawaihoa Pt. Pueo Pt.
Haiilii Paniau
Kawaihoa Pt.

Kauai Channel
▼3026

PACIFIC OCEAN

Projection: Albers Equal Area

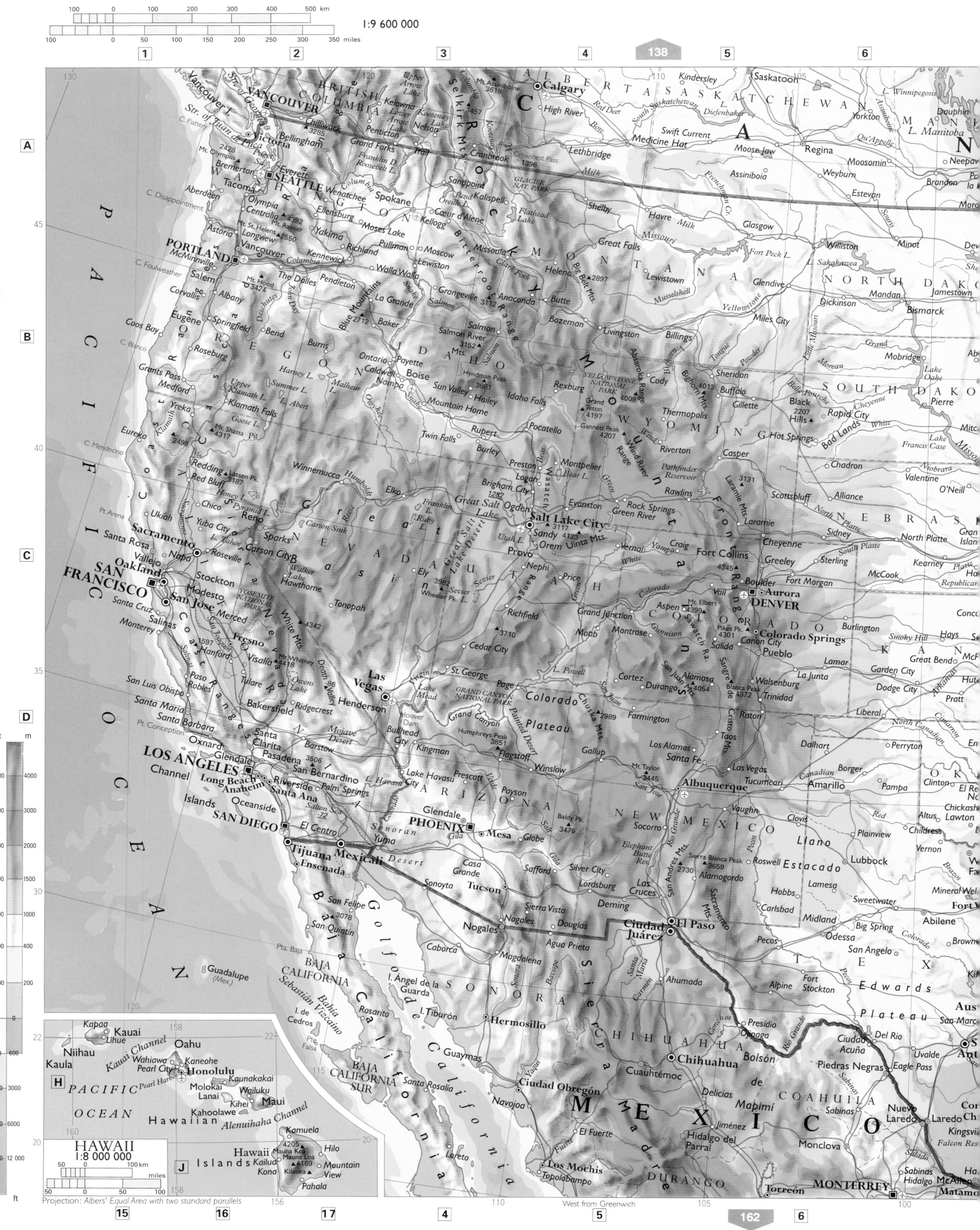

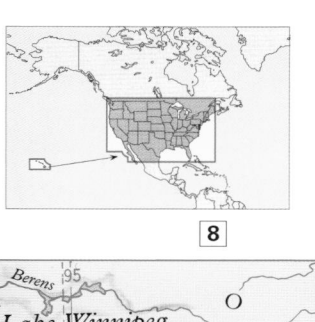

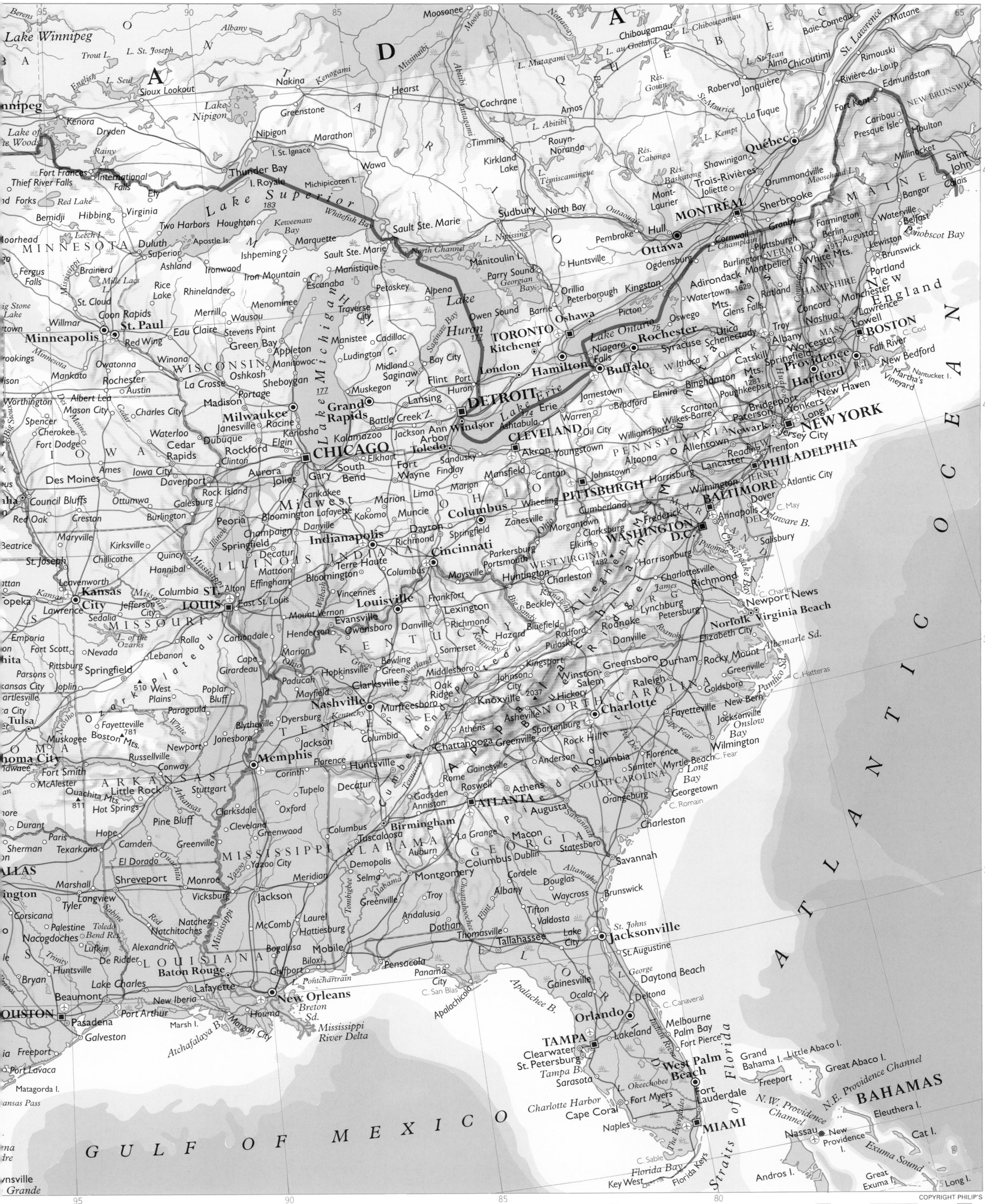

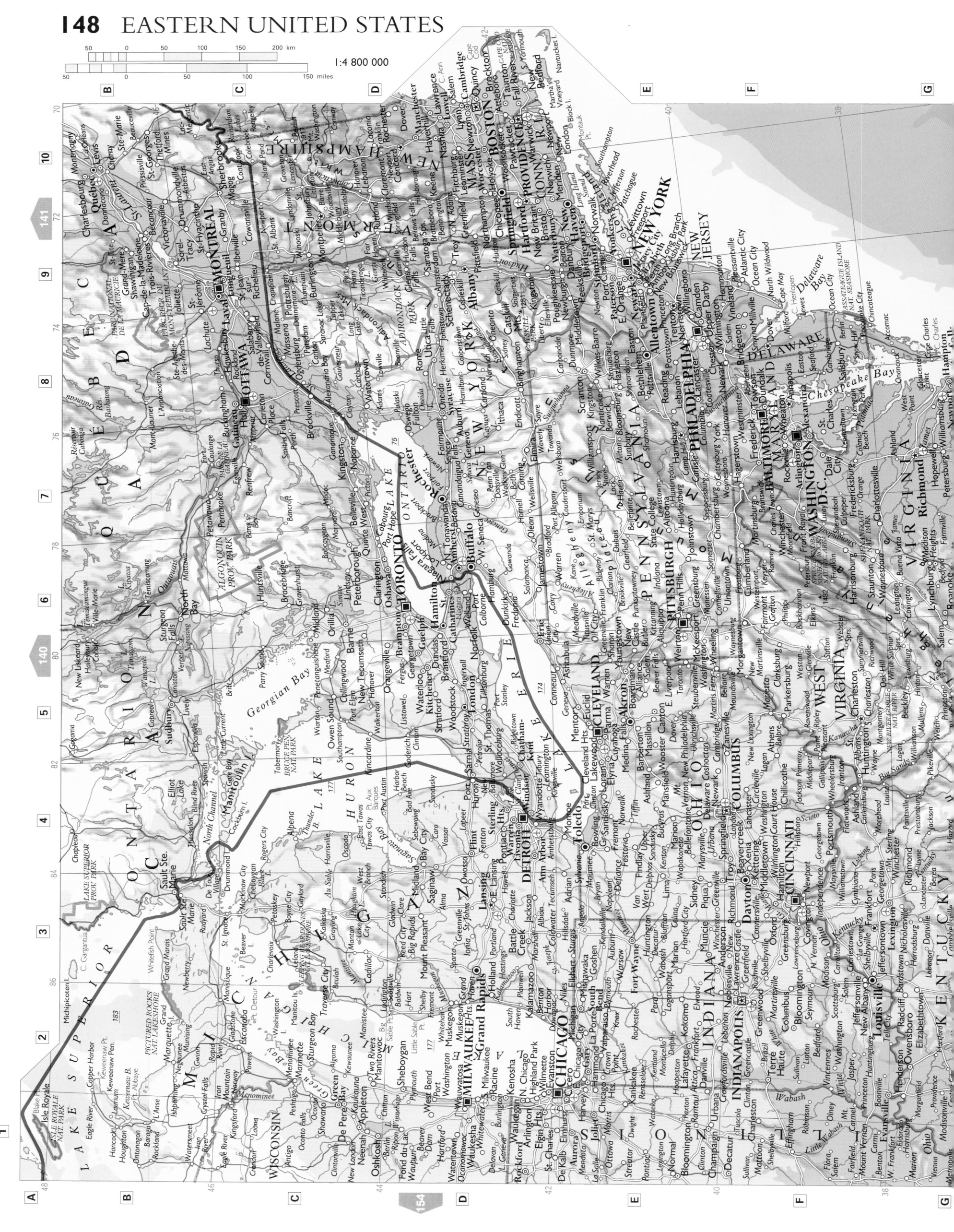

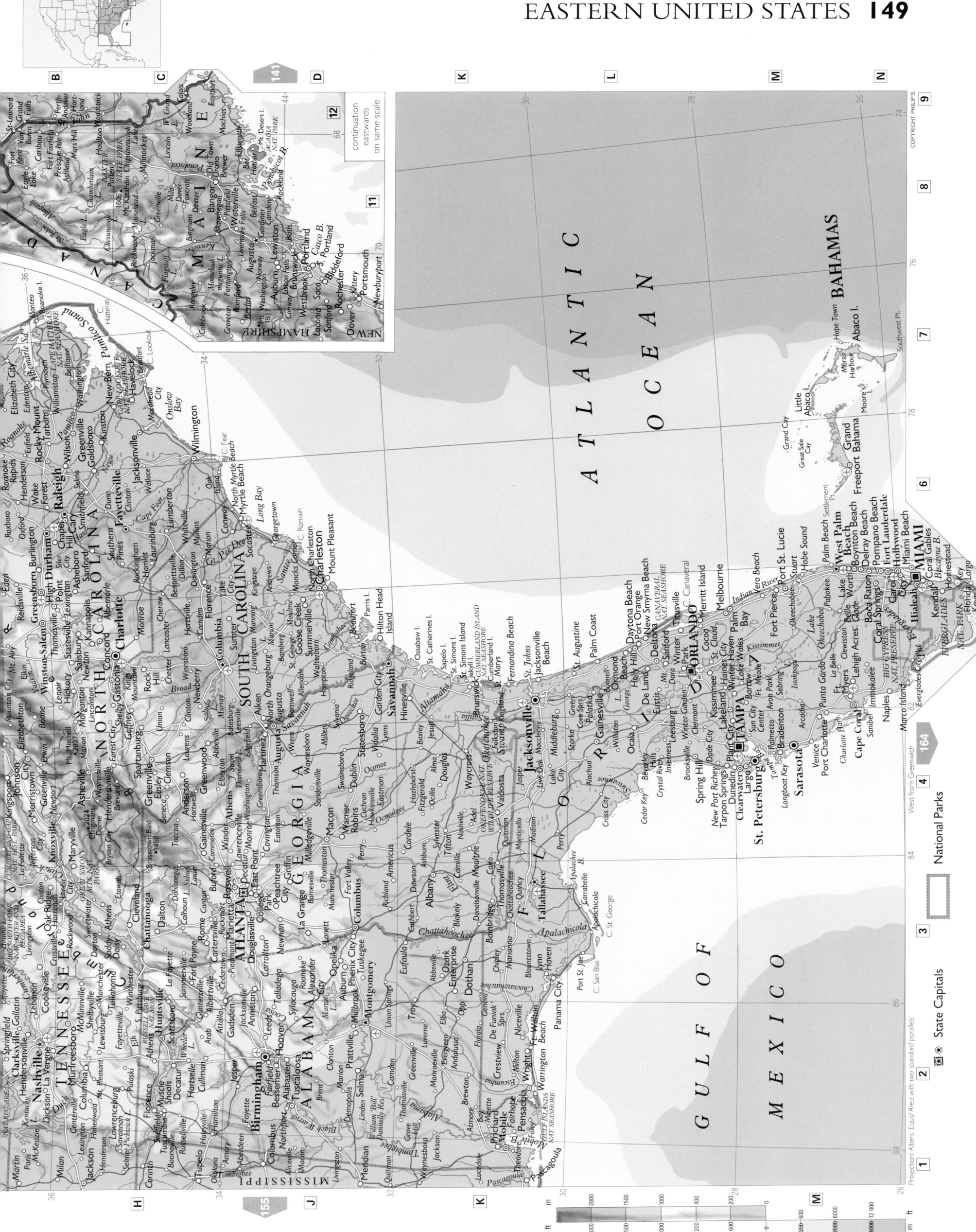

continuation eastwards on same scale

MAINE

CANADA

St-Léonard · Grand Falls · Perth Andover · Van Buren · Woodstock · Grand Lake · Eastport

Fort Kent · Caribou · Presque Isle · Ashland · Houlton · Mars Hill · Machias

Eagle Lake · Fort Fairfield · Lincoln · Old Town · Brewer · Ellsworth · Mt. Desert I. · ACADIA NAT. PARK · Schoodic Pt.

BAXTER STATE PARK · Mt. Katahdin · Chamberlain L. · Dover-Foxcroft · Bangor · Penobscot B. · Stonington · Rockland

Moosehead L. · Greenville · Dexter · Skowhegan · Waterville · Camden · Belfast

Rangeley · Kingfield · Farmington · Augusta · Gardiner · Bath · Boothbay Harbor

Mt. Washington 1917 · Norway · Lewiston · Auburn · Brunswick · Casco B. · S. Portland · Portland

Berlin · Rumford · Lisbon Falls · Saco · Biddeford

Groveton · Conway · Laconia · Sanford · Rochester · Dover · Kittery · Portsmouth · Newburyport

NEW HAMPSHIRE

ATLANTIC OCEAN

BAHAMAS

Hope Town · Abaco I. · Marsh Hbr. · Moore's I. · Little Abaco I. · Grand Cay

Great Sale Cay · Grand Bahama · Freeport · Southwest Pt.

N O R T H   C A R O L I N A

Elizabeth City · Edenton · Albemarle Sd. · Plymouth · Manteo · Roanoke I. · Kill Devil Hills

Roanoke Rapids · Enfield · Tarboro · Washington · New Bern · Pamlico Sd. · C. Hatteras · CAPE HATTERAS NAT. SEASHORE

Raleigh · Wake Forest · Goldsboro · Kinston · Havelock · Morehead City · CAPE LOOKOUT NAT. SEASHORE · C. Lookout

Durham · Smithfield · Jacksonville · Onslow Bay

Fayetteville · Clinton · Beaufort

Southern Pines · Dunn · Wilmington · C. Fear

Rockingham · Laurinburg · Lumberton · Whiteville · Long Bay

Hamlet · Whiteville

North Myrtle Beach · Myrtle Beach

S O U T H   C A R O L I N A

Cheraw · Dillon · Marion · Conway · Georgetown

Columbia · Sumter · Florence · Kingstree · C. Romani

Camden · Manning

Orangeburg · Summerville · North Charleston · Charleston · Mount Pleasant

Aiken · St. George · Goose Creek · Parris I. · Hilton Head Island

---

G E O R G I A

Augusta · Millen · Sylvania · Beaufort

Savannah · Ossabaw I. · St. Catherines I.

Statesboro · Hinesville · Sapelo I. · St. Simons Island

Vidalia · Lyons · Jesup · Brunswick · St. Simons I.

Swainsboro · Reidsville · Ludowici · CUMBERLAND ISLAND NAT. SEASHORE · Cumberland I.

Dublin · Baxley · Jesup · Kingsland · St. Marys · Fernandina Beach

Hazlehurst · Waycross · OKEFENOKEE NAT. WILDLIFE RESERVE · Folkston

---

F L O R I D A

Jacksonville · Jacksonville Beach

Lake City · Starke · St. Augustine

Gainesville · Palatka · Palm Coast

Ocala · Bunnell · Ormond · Daytona Beach

Beverly Hills · DeLand · Holly Hill · Port Orange

Inverness · Leesburg · Deltona · New Smyrna Beach

Brooksville · Eustis · Sanford · Titusville · CANAVERAL NAT. SEASHORE

Spring Hill · Clermont · Winter Garden · ORLANDO · Cocoa · Merritt Island · C. Canaveral

New Port Richey · Kissimmee · St. Cloud · Cocoa Beach

Tarpon Springs · Winter Haven · Melbourne

Dunedin · Haines City · Indian Harbour Beach

Clearwater · St. Petersburg · TAMPA · Plant City · Lakeland · Lake Wales · Vero Beach

Largo · Sun City Center · Bartow · Fort Pierce · Port St. Lucie · Stuart · Hope Sound

Bradenton · Arcadia · Sebring · Okeechobee · Palm Beach · West Palm Beach

Sarasota · Venice · Port Charlotte · Avon Park · La Belle · Belle Glade · Boynton Beach · Delray Beach

Punta Gorda · Cape Coral · Clewiston · Lehigh Acres · Lake Worth · Pompano Beach

Ft. Myers · Immokalee · BIG CYPRESS NAT. PRESERVE · Coral Springs · Fort Lauderdale

Naples · Hollywood

Marco Island · Biscayne B. · Hialeah · MIAMI · Coral Gables

EVERGLADES NAT. PARK · Kendall · Homestead · Key Largo · Florida Keys

---

A L A B A M A

Jasper · Gadsden · Anniston · Roanoke

Birmingham · Bessemer · Talladega · Alexander City · Opelika · Auburn · Phenix City

Tuscaloosa · Childersburg · Sylacauga · Tuskegee

Northport · Clanton · Prattville · Union Springs · Eufaula

Demopolis · Selma · Montgomery · Troy · Abbeville · Dothan

Linden · Camden · Greenville · Luverne · Ozark · Enterprise

Grove Hill · Evergreen · Elba · Geneva

Jackson · Brewton · Andalusia · Florala · Crestview · De Funiak Springs

Bay Minette · Atmore · Flomaton · Milton · Niceville · Fort Walton Beach

Mobile · Prichard · Pensacola · Gulf Breeze · Panama City

Mobile B. · Foley · GULF ISLANDS NAT. SEASHORE

G U L F   O F   M E X I C O

Port St. Joe · C. San Blas

Apalachicola · C. St. George

Carrabelle · Apalachee B.

Panacea · Perry

Crystal River · Cedar Key

Cross City

T E N N E S S E E

Springfield · Clarksville · Gallatin

Nashville · Hendersonville · Murfreesboro

Dickson · Columbia · Lewisburg · Winchester

Lawrenceburg · Fayetteville

National Parks

State Capitals

Projection: Albers' Equal Area with two standard parallels

COPYRIGHT PHILIP'S

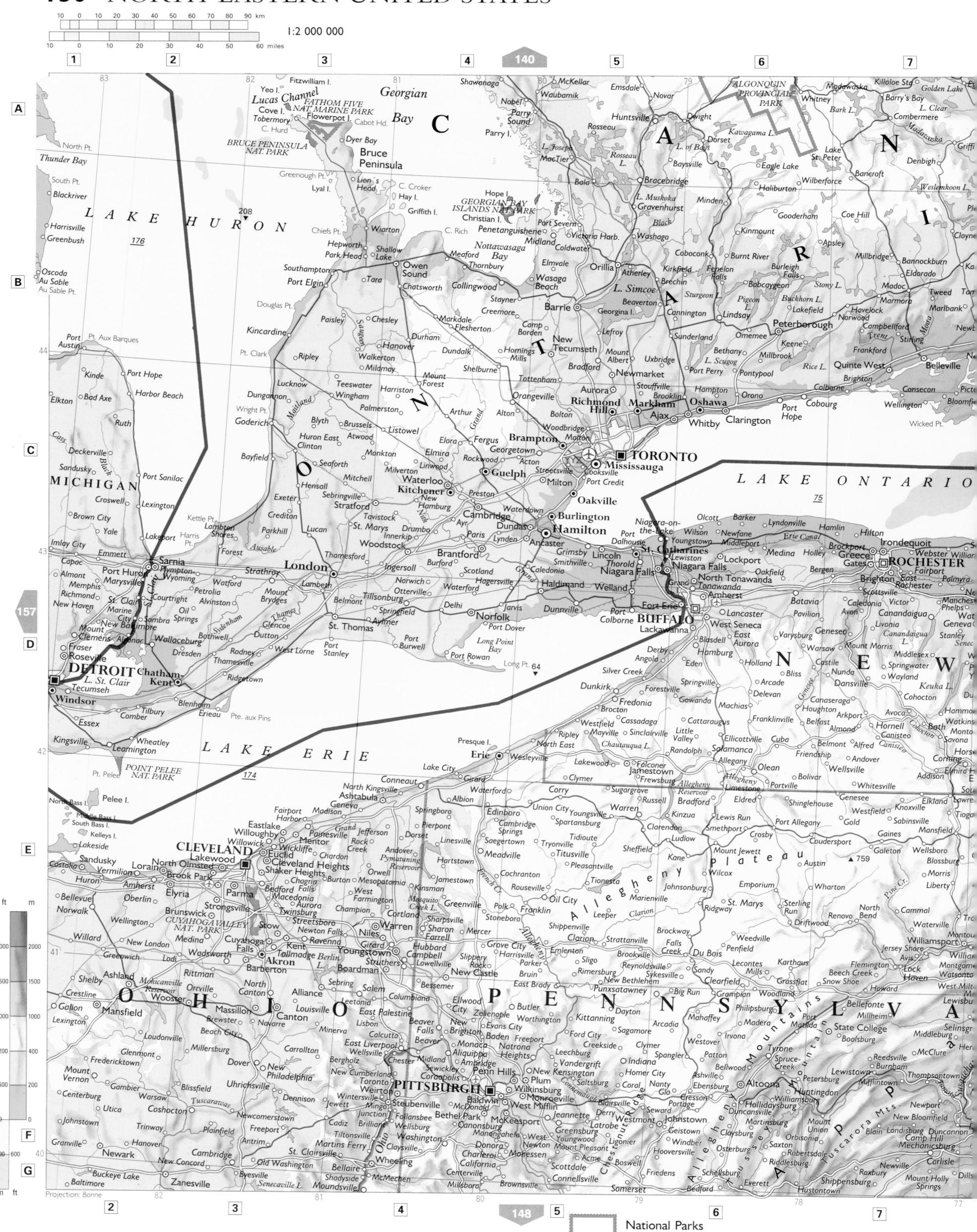

1:2 000 000

National Parks

Projection: Bonne

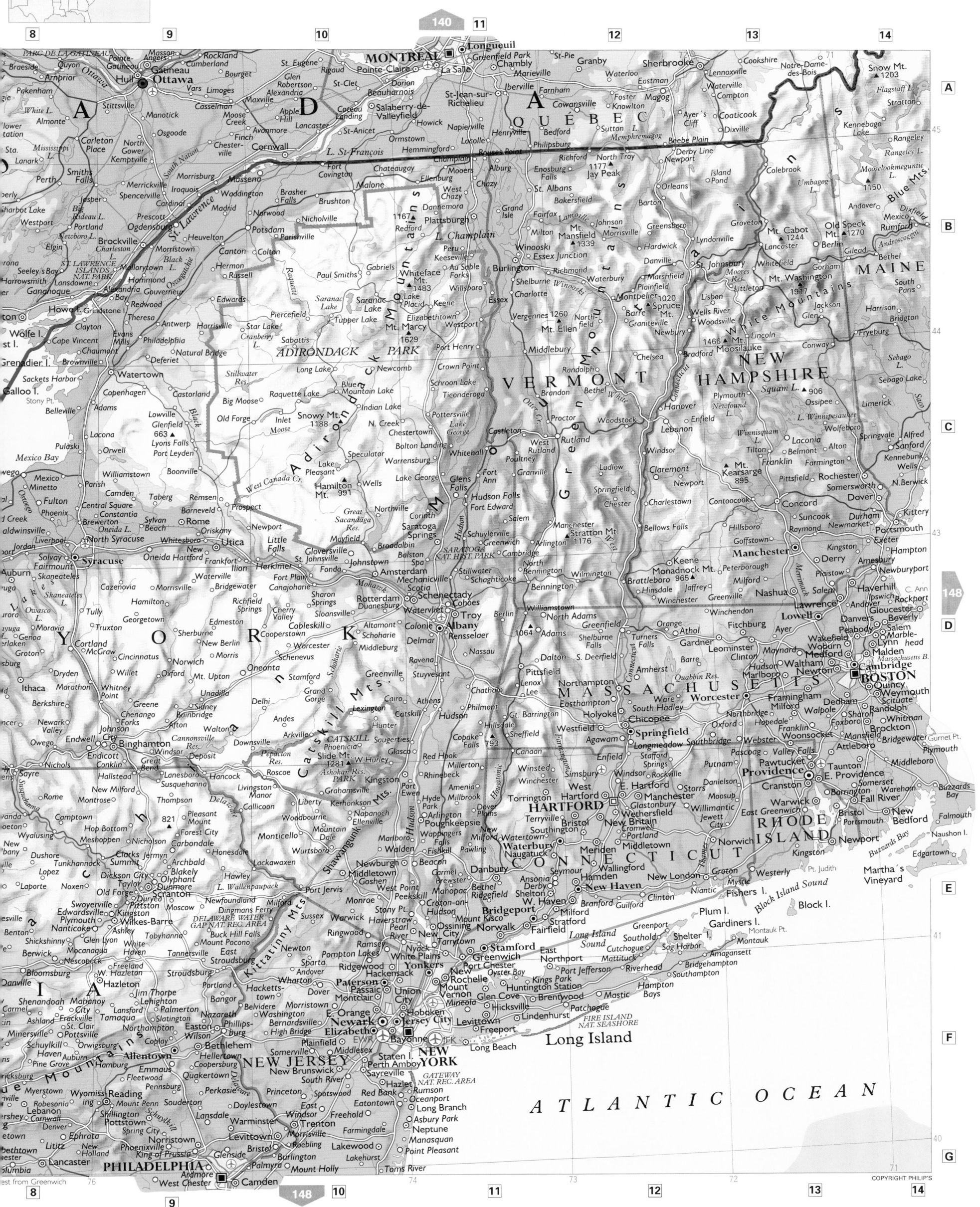

1:2 000 000

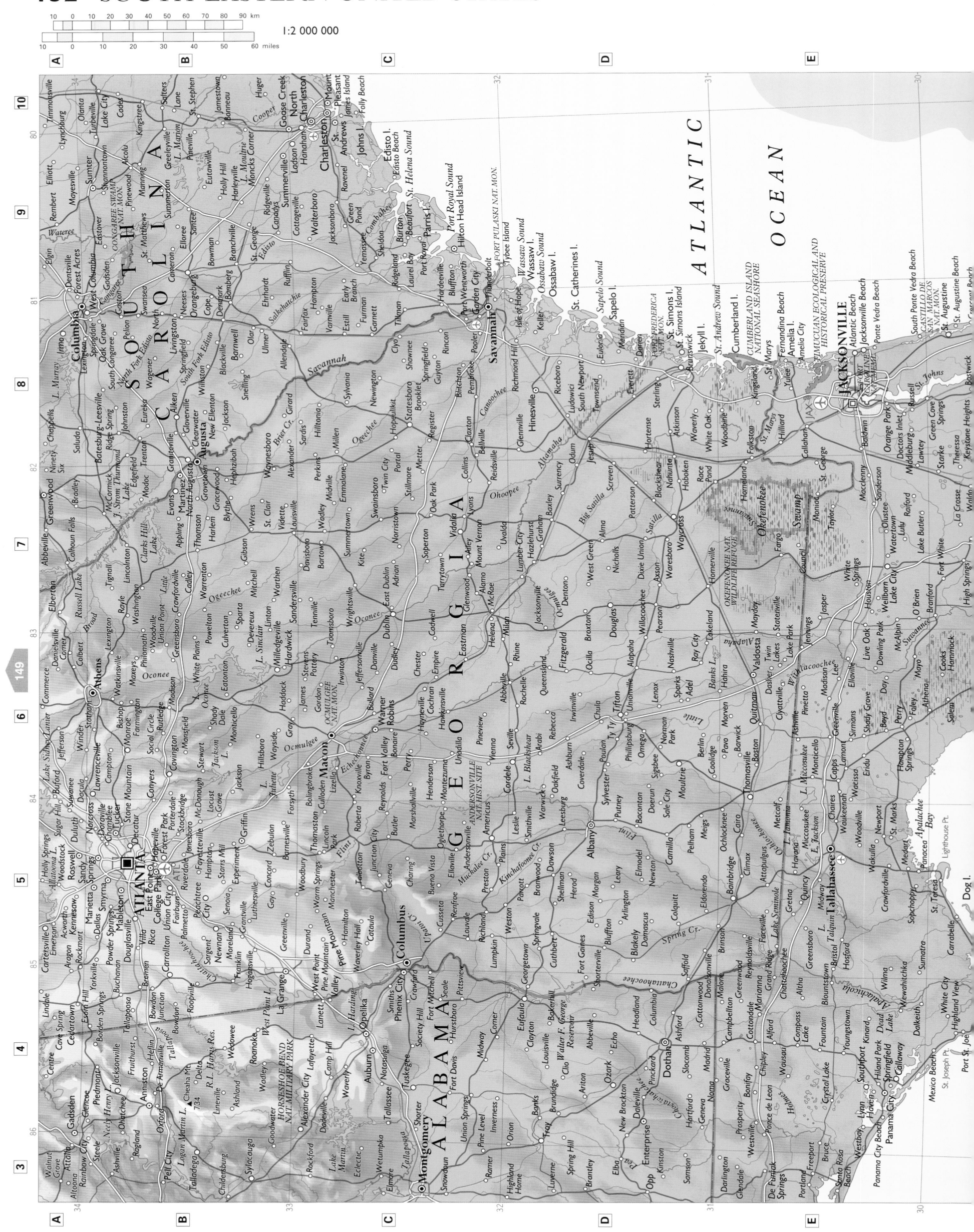

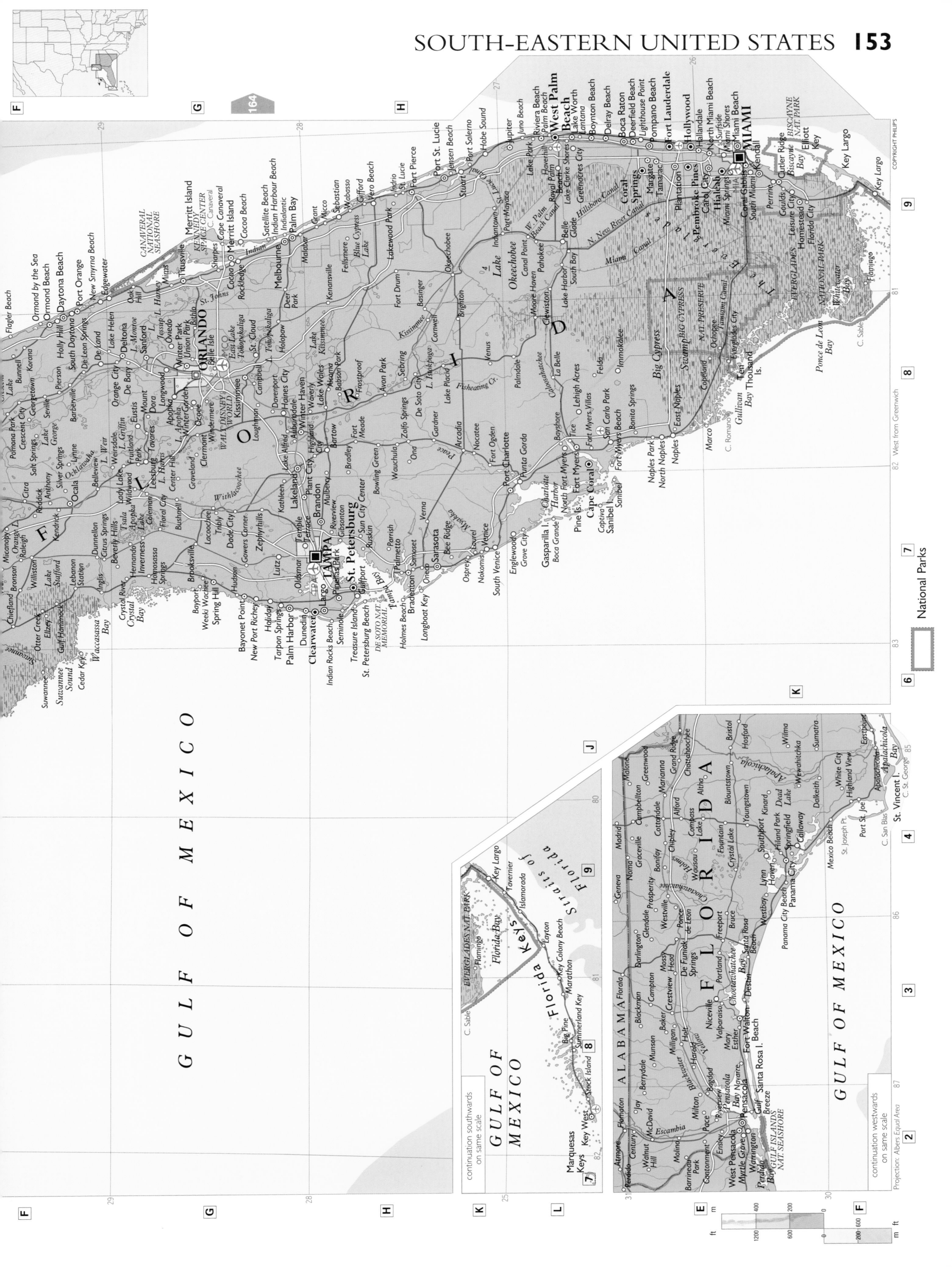

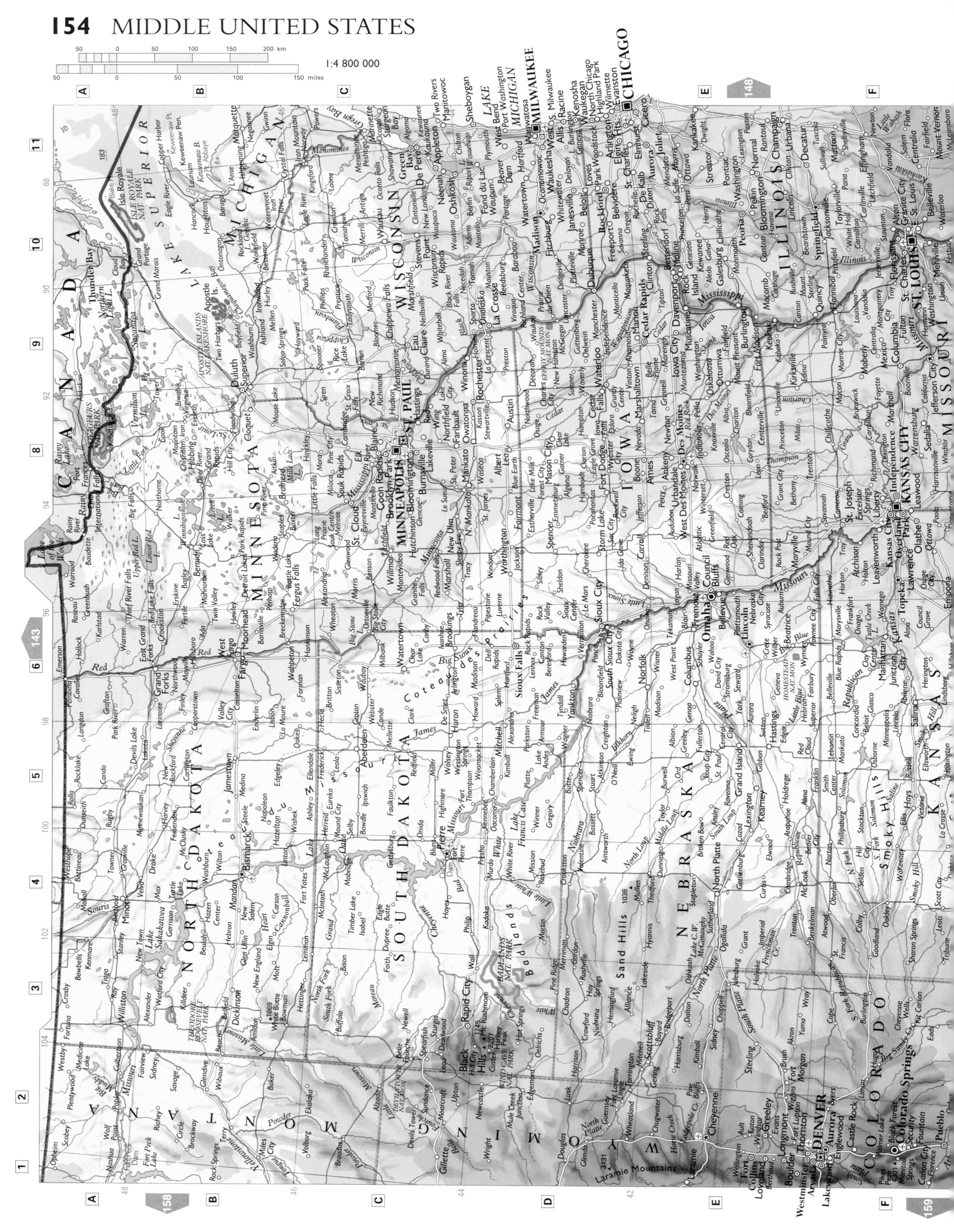

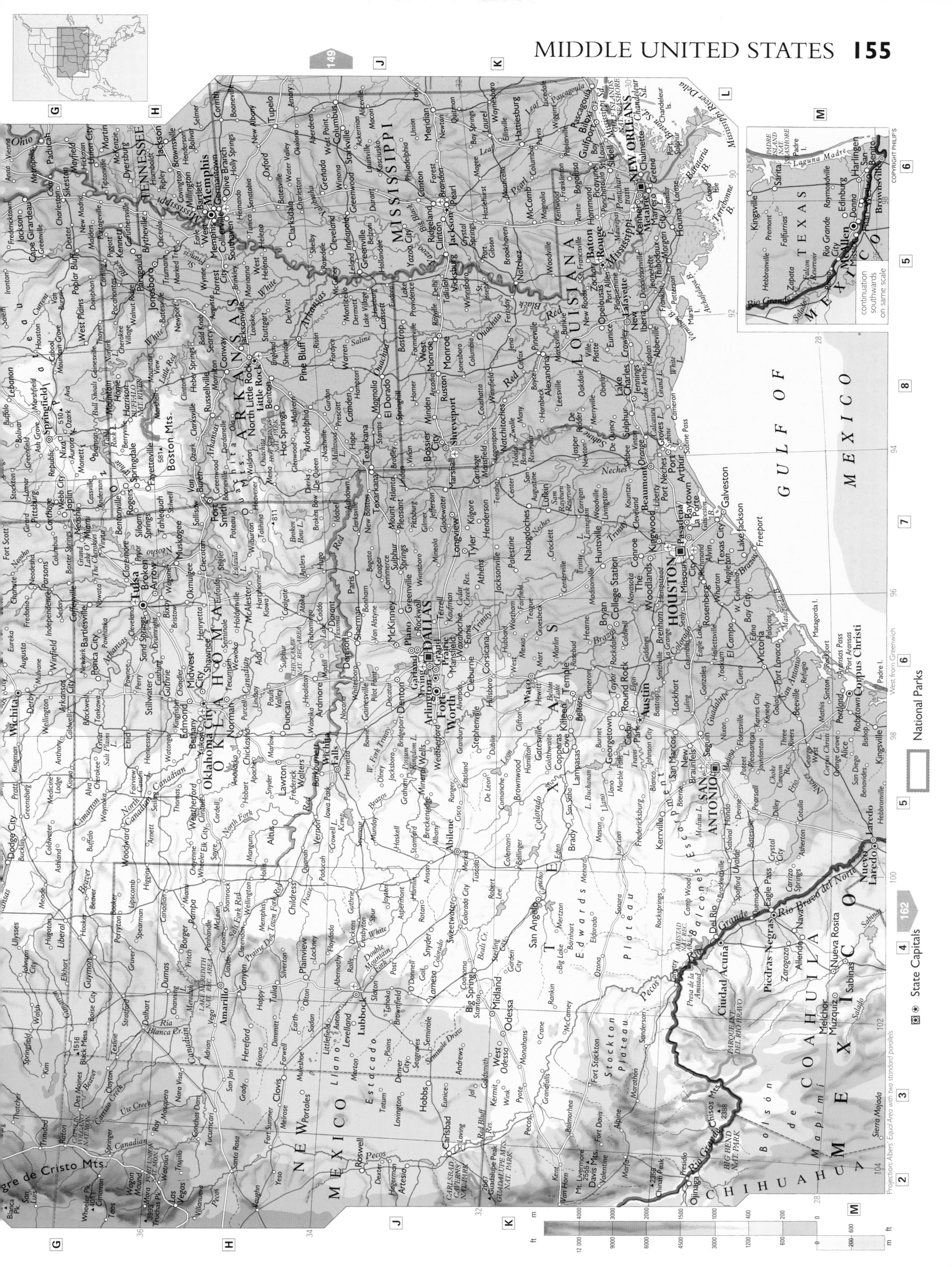

continuation southwards on same scale

West from Greenwich

National Parks

State Capitals

Projection: Albers' Equal Area with two standard parallels

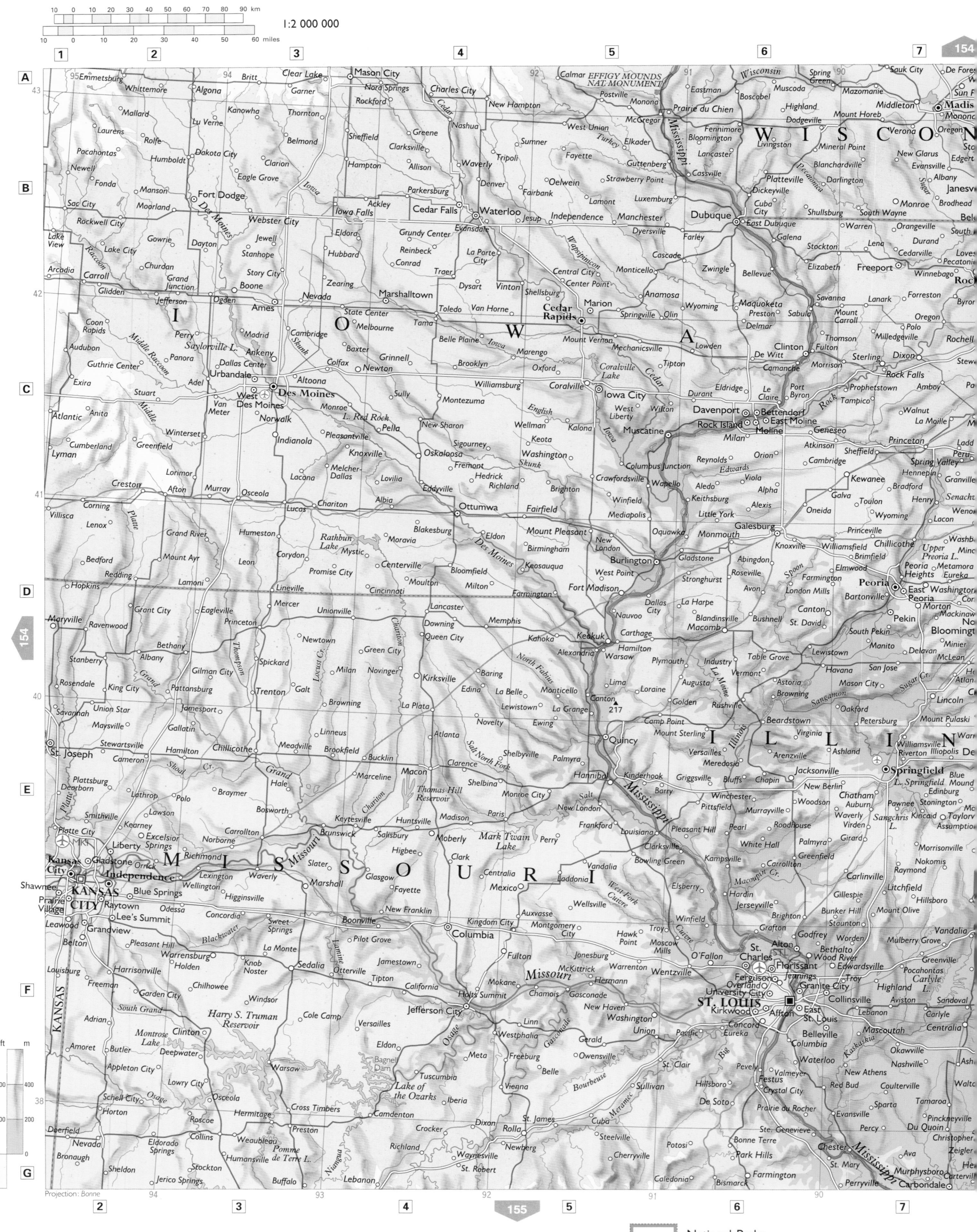

1:2 000 000

National Parks

Projection: Bonne

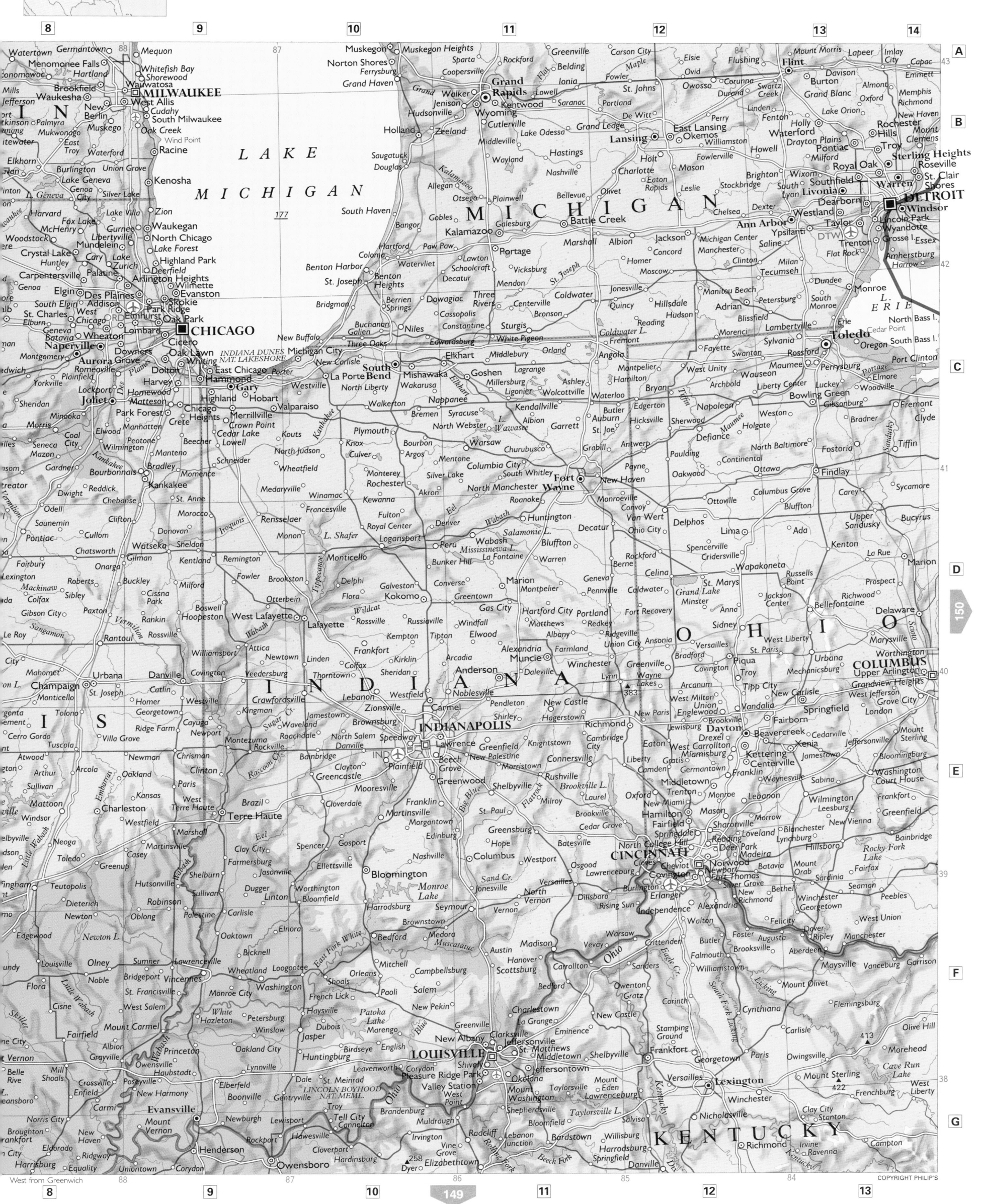

1:4 800 000

50   0   50   100   150   200 km
50   0   50   100   150 miles

A B C D E F

SASKATCHEWAN

ALBERTA

BRITISH COLUMBIA

MONTANA

WYOMING

IDAHO

WASHINGTON

OREGON

NEVADA

R O C K Y   M O U N T A I N S

Absaroka Range

Bighorn Mountains

Medicine Bow Mts.

Wind River Range

Salmon River Mountains

Bitterroot Range

Lemhi Range

Sawtooth Range

Great Salt Lake

Great Salt Lake Desert

Columbia Basin

Blue Mountains

Cascade Range

Coast Ranges

VANCOUVER

SEATTLE

PORTLAND

SACRAMENTO

Salt Lake City

Ogden

Provo

Spokane

Boise

Great Falls

Helena

Butte

Billings

Casper

Sheridan

Reno

Carson City

Eugene

Salem

Medford

Redding

Olympia

Tacoma

Bellingham

Victoria

Nanaimo

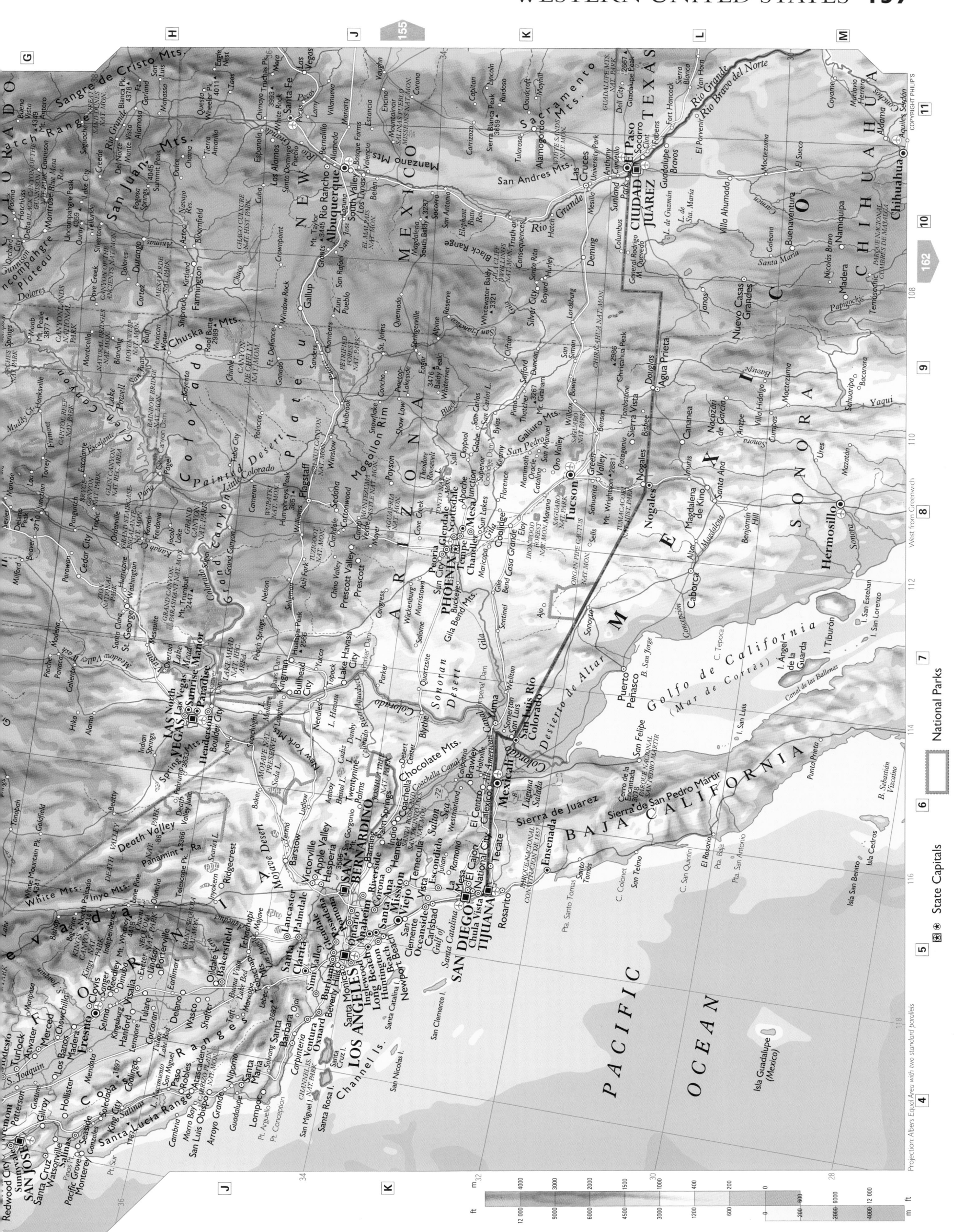

National Parks

State Capitals

Projection: Albers Equal Area with two standard parallels

West from Greenwich

COPYRIGHT PHILIP'S

1:2 000 000

10 0 10 20 30 40 50 60 70 80 90 km
10 0 10 20 30 40 50 60 miles

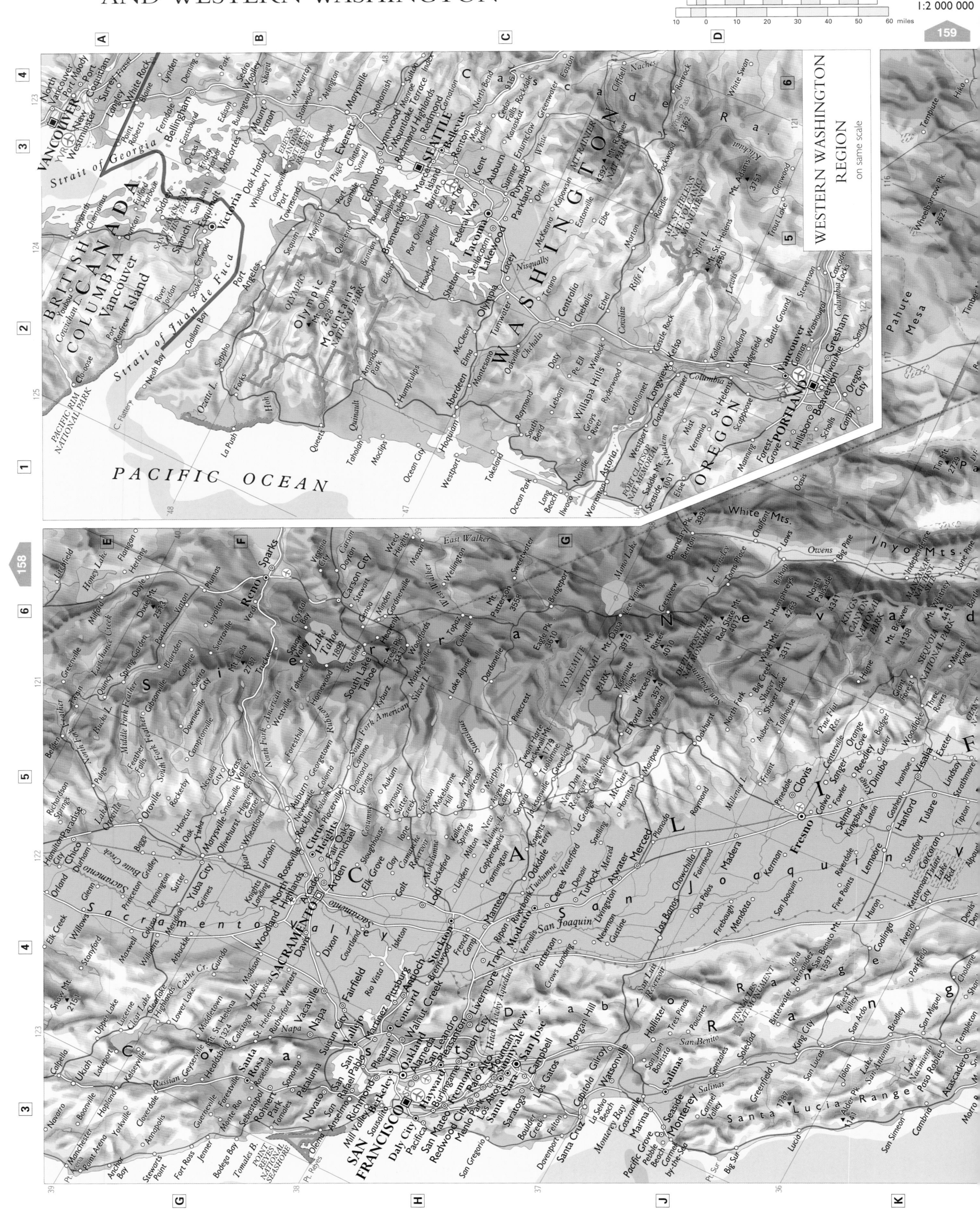

WESTERN WASHINGTON
REGION
on same scale

PACIFIC OCEAN

PACIFIC RIM NATIONAL PARK

BRITISH COLUMBIA

Vancouver Island

Strait of Georgia

Strait of Juan de Fuca

VANCOUVER

New Westminster

Victoria

SEATTLE

Tacoma

Olympic Mountains NATIONAL PARK

Mt Olympus 2428

WASHINGTON

MT RAINIER NAT PARK
Mt Rainier 4392

MT ST HELENS NAT VOLCANIC MONUMENT
Mt St Helens 2550

OREGON

PORTLAND

Vancouver

Gresham

Pahute Mesa

White Mts.

Inyo Mts.

Reno
Sparks

Lake Tahoe 1899

Carson City

SIERRA NEVADA

YOSEMITE NATIONAL PARK

KINGS CANYON NATIONAL PARK

SEQUOIA NATIONAL PARK

Mt Whitney 4418

Mt Williamson 4382

SACRAMENTO

Sacramento Valley

San Joaquin Valley

Fresno

Clovis

Visalia

Stockton

Modesto

Merced

Napa

Santa Rosa

SAN FRANCISCO

Oakland

San Jose

Salinas

Monterey

Diablo Range

Santa Lucia Range

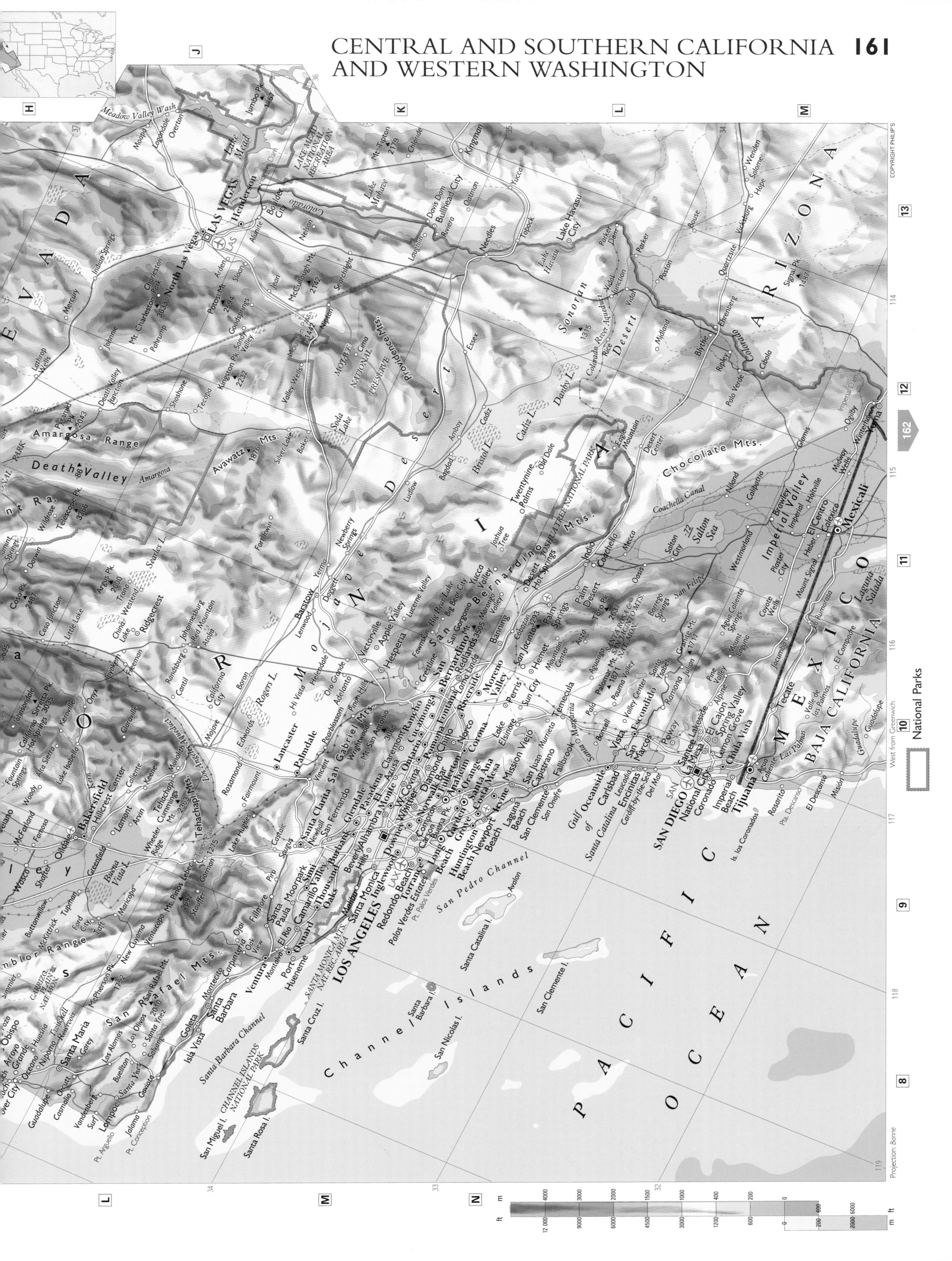

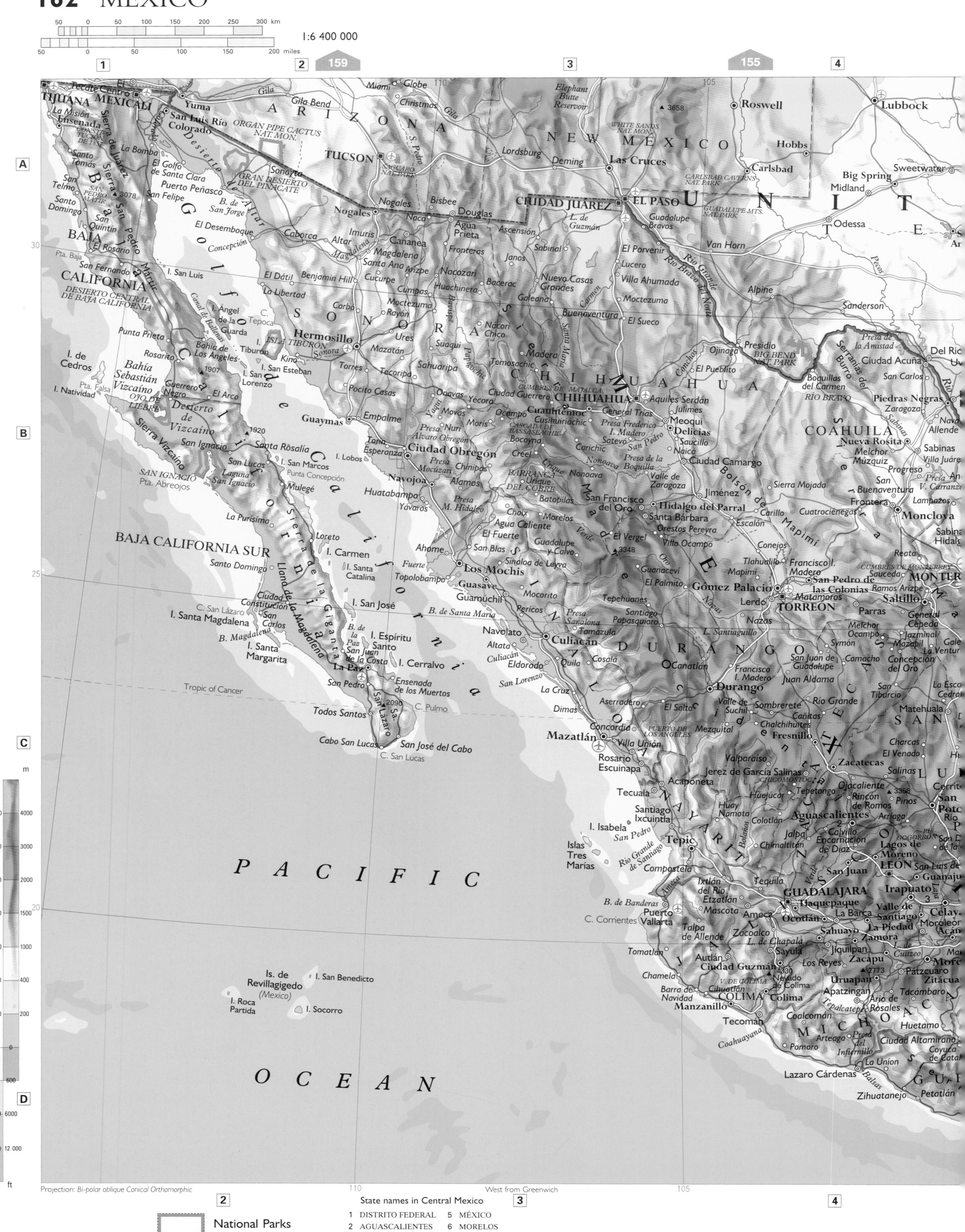

50 0 50 100 150 200 250 300 km
50 0 50 100 150 200 miles

1:6 400 000

1
2
3
4

A

B

C

D

ft   m
12 000   4000
9000   3000
6000   2000
4500   1500
3000   1000
1200   400
600   200
0   0
200   600
2000   6000
4000   12 000
m   ft

Projection: Bi-polar oblique Conical Orthomorphic

West from Greenwich

National Parks

State names in Central Mexico

1 DISTRITO FEDERAL
2 AGUASCALIENTES
3 GUANAJUATO
4 HIDALGO
5 MÉXICO
6 MORELOS
7 QUERÉTARO
8 TLAXCALA

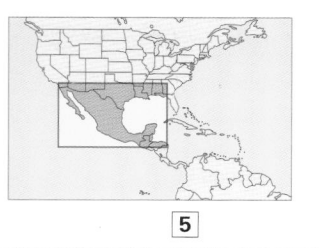

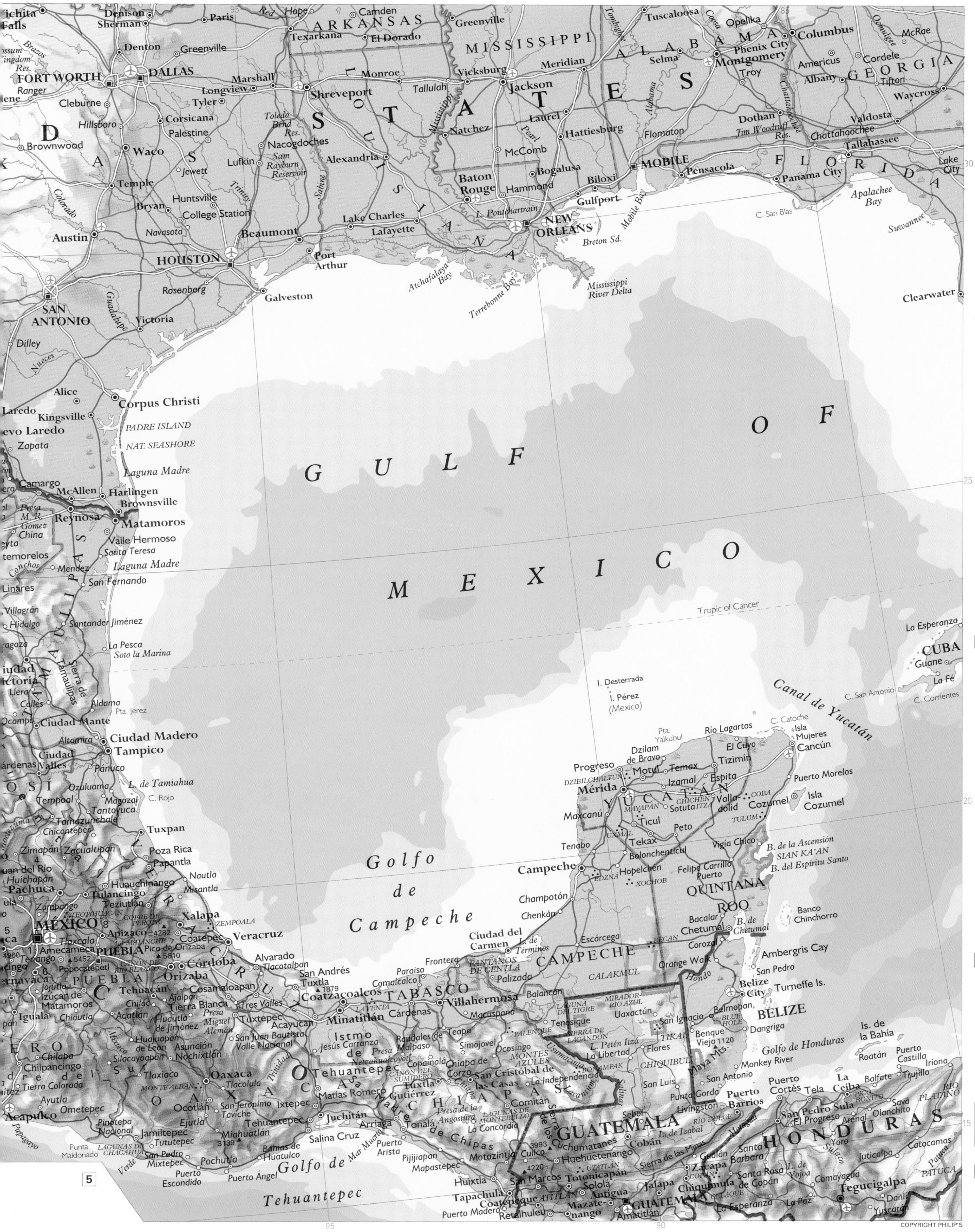

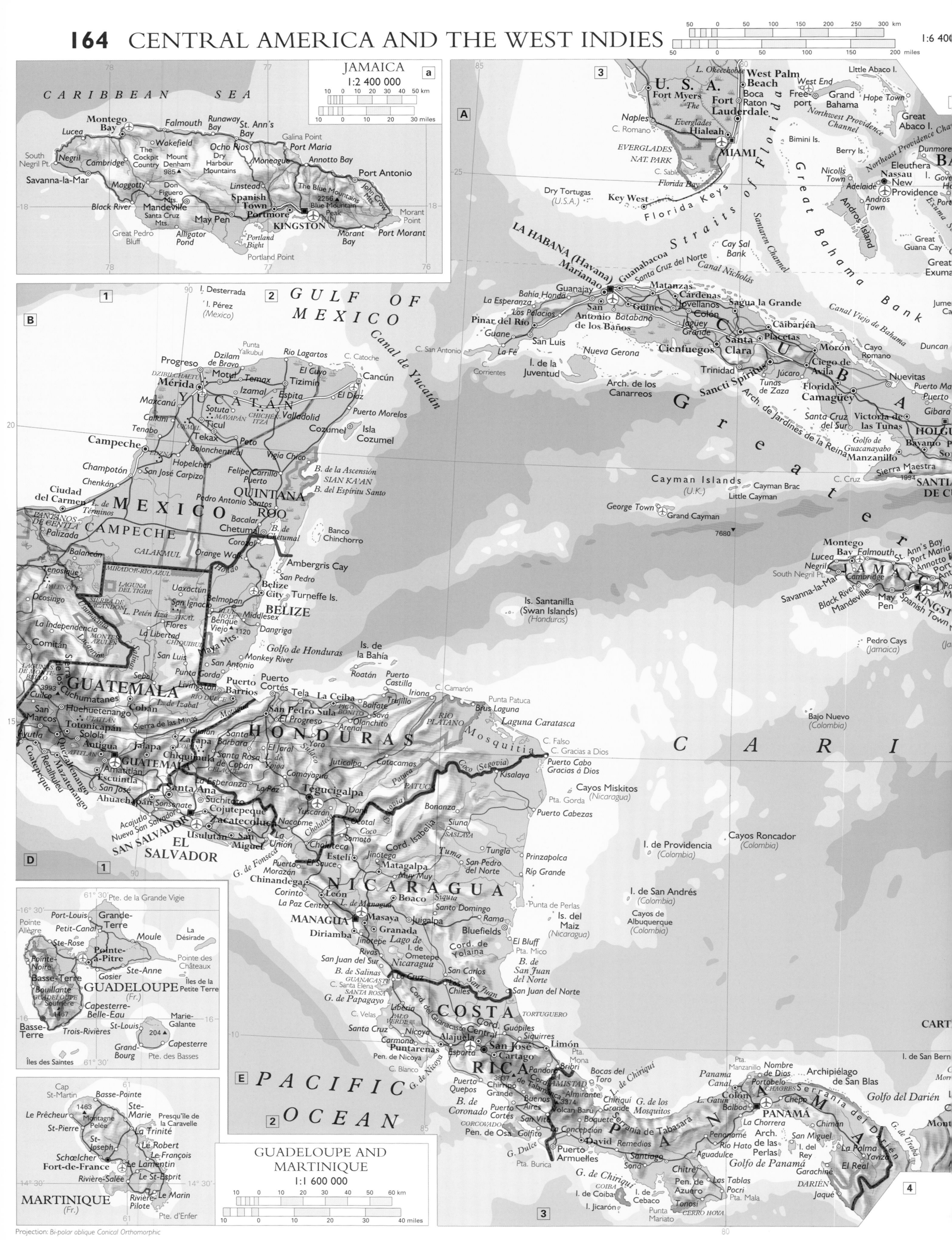

1:6 400

50 0 50 100 150 200 250 300 km
50 0 50 100 150 200 miles

JAMAICA

1:2 400 000

10 0 10 20 30 40 50 km
10 0 10 20 30 miles

CARIBBEAN SEA

South Negril Pt.
Montego Bay
Lucea
Negril
Cambridge
Falmouth
Runaway Bay
St. Ann's Bay
Wakefield
The Cockpit Country
Ocho Rios
Dry Harbour Mountains
Galina Point
Port Maria
Annotto Bay
Moneague
Port Antonio
Mount Denham 985 ▲
Don Figuero Mts.
Maggotty
Linstead
Spanish Town
The Blue Mountains
2256 ▲ Blue Mountain Peak
John Crow Mtns.
Port Morant
Black River
Mandeville
Santa Cruz Mts.
May Pen
Portmore
KINGSTON
Morant Point
Great Pedro Bluff
Savanna-la-Mar
Alligator Pond
Portland Bight
Portland Point
Morant Bay
Port Morant

GULF OF MEXICO

Canal de Yucatán

U.S.A.
West Palm Beach
Fort Myers
Naples
Fort Lauderdale
Boca Raton
West End
Freeport
Grand Bahama
Hope Town
Little Abaco I.
Great Abaco I.
EVERGLADES NAT. PARK
C. Romano
Everglades
Hialeah
MIAMI
C. Sable
Florida Bay
Dry Tortugas (U.S.A.)
Key West
Florida Keys
Straits of Florida
Bimini Is.
Berry Is.
Nicolls Town
Nassau
New Providence
Adelaide
Andros Island
Andros Town
Great Guana Cay
Eleuthera
Dunmore
Northwest Providence Channel
Northeast Providence Channel
Great Bahama Bank
Great Exuma

LA HABANA (Havana)
Mariano
Guanabacoa
Bahía Honda
La Esperanza
Guanajay
Matanzas
Santa Cruz del Norte
Cárdenas
Jovellanos
Canal Nicholás
Cay Sal Bank
Pinar del Río
Guane
Los Palacios
San Antonio de los Baños
Güines
Colón
Jagüey Grande
Sagua la Grande
Caibarién
Canal Viejo de Bahama
La Fé
San Luis
Nueva Gerona
Batabanó
Santa Clara
Placetas
Morón
Cayo Romano
Nuevitas
Corrientes
I. de la Juventud
Cienfuegos
Trinidad
Sancti Spíritus
Júcaro
Ciego de Ávila
Tunas de Zaza
Florida
Camagüey
Puerto
Gibara
HOLG
Arch. de los Canarreos
Arch. de Jardines de la Reina
Santa Cruz del Sur
Victoria de las Tunas
Bayamo
Manzanillo
G. de Guacanayabo
Sierra Maestra
1994 ▲
C. Cruz
SANTI
DE C

CUBA
GREAT
ER

Cayman Islands (U.K.)
Cayman Brac
Little Cayman
George Town
Grand Cayman
7680 ▾

Is. Santanilla (Swan Islands) (Honduras)

Montego Bay
Falmouth
St. Ann's Bay
Port Maria
Lucea
Negril
Cambridge
JAMA
Po
South Negril Pt.
Savanna-la-Mar
Black River
Mandeville
May Pen
Spanish Town
Kingst

Pedro Cays (Jamaica)

CARI

MEXICO

Progreso
Dzilam de Bravo
Río Lagartos
El Cuyo
C. Catoche
Punta Yalkubul
Mérida
Motul
Izamal
Tizimín
Cancún
Maxcanú
Temax
Espita
Calkini
YUCATÁN
Sotuta
Valladolid
Puerto Morelos
Tenabo
Tekax
Ticul
CHICHÉN ITZÁ
Cozumel
Isla Cozumel
Campeche
Hopelchén
Peto
Vigía Chico
MAYAPÁN
Champotón
Chenkán
Felipe Carrillo Puerto
B. de la Ascensión
SIAN KA'AN
Balonchenticul
Ciudad del Carmen
I. de Términos
QUINTANA ROO
Bacalar
B. del Espíritu Santo
PANTANOS DE CENTLA
Palizada
CALAKMUL
Chetumal
Corozal
Banco Chinchorro
CAMPECHE
Balancán
MIRADOR-RÍO AZUL
Orange Walk
Tenosique
LAGUNA DEL TIGRE
Uaxactún
Ambergris Cay
San Pedro
Palenque
Ocosingo
La Independencia
MONTES AZULES
Flores
L. Petén Itzá
TIKAL
BLUE HOLE ▲ 1120
Belmopan
San Ignacio
Benque Viejo
Middlesex
BELIZE
Belize City
Turneffe Is.
Comitán
LAGUNAS DE MONTE BELLO
Sebol
CHIQUIBUL
Dangriga
Sierra de los Cuchumatanes
3993 ▲
Cuilco
Huehuetenango
Cobán
L. de Izabal
Maya Mts.
Monkey River
San Luis
Golfo de Honduras
Is. de la Bahía
Roatán
Puerto Castilla
Iriona
Punta Gorda
Livingston
Puerto Barrios
Puerto Cortés
Tela
La Ceiba
Trujillo
Balfate
C. Camarón
Punta Patuca
Brus Laguna
San Marcos
UTATLÁN
Totonicapán
Sololá
Zacapa
Santa
El Progreso
San Pedro Sula
PICO BONITO
Sává
Olanchito
Arenal
Yoro
Laguna Caratasca
Ayutla
Quezaltenango
ATITLÁN
Antigua
GUATEMALA
Chiquimula
Santa Rosa de Copán
L. de Yojoa
Sulaco
RÍO PLATANO
Mosquitia
Bajo Nuevo (Colombia)
Retalhuleu
Mazatenango
Escuintla
San José
Amatitlán
Jalapa
COPÁN
Santa Bárbara
Comayagua
Juticalpa
Catacamas
C. Falso
C. Gracias a Dios
Coatepeque
Ahuachapán
Sonsonate
Santa Ana
Suchitoto
La Esperanza
La Paz
TEGUCIGALPA
Yuscarán
Danlí
Coco (Segovia)
Puerto Cabo Gracias á Dios
Kisalaya
Acajutla
Nueva San Salvador
Cojutepeque
Zacatecoluca
Nacaome
Choluteca
Yuscarán
El Paraíso
Bonanza
Siuna
SASLAYA
Cayos Miskitos (Nicaragua)
SAN SALVADOR
Usulután
San Miguel
La Unión
G. de Fonseca
Somoto
Coco
SASLAYA
Puerto Cabezas
EL SALVADOR
Puerto Morazán
El Sauce
Estelí
Jinotega
Matagalpa
Muy Muy
Cord. Isabelia
Tuma
Tungla
Prinzapolca
Cayos Roncador (Colombia)
Chinandega
León
Boaco
Siguía
San Pedro del Norte
Río Grande
Corinto
La Paz Central
L. de Managua
Juigalpa
Rama
Bluefields
I. de Providencia (Colombia)
MANAGUA
Masaya
Granada
NICARAGUA
Santo Domingo
El Bluff
I. de San Andrés (Colombia)
Diriamba
Jinotepe
Lago de Nicaragua
Cord. de Yolaina
Cord. de
Punta de Perlas
Is. del Maíz (Nicaragua)
Cayos de Albuquerque (Colombia)
Rivas
I. de Ometepe
San Juan del Sur
B. de Salinas
San Carlos
San Juan del Norte
La Cruz
C. Santa Elena
SANTA ROSA
G. de Papagayo
Los Chiles
San Juan
GUANACASTE
PALO VERDE
Liberia
Cord. de Guanacaste
Tortuguero
CART
Santa Cruz
Cañas
Cord. Central
Guápiles
Siquirres
Limón
Esparza
Puntarenas
Alajuela
SAN JOSÉ
Cartago
Pta. Manzanillo
Nombre de Dios
Archipiélago de San Blas
Carmona
Pen. de Nicoya
Quepos
Pandora
Bribri
Bocas del Toro
Panama Canal
Colón
Portobelo
Serranía de San Blas
Golfo del Darién
C. Blanco
G. de Nicoya
COSTA RICA
AMISTAD
Buenos Aires
Almirante
Chiriquí
G. de los Mosquitos
Chepo
PANAMÁ
Quepos
Palmar
Cord. de Talamanca
3374 ▲
Volcán Barú
Boquete
Concepción
David
Remedios
Río Hato
Penonomé
Aguadulce
Arch. de las Perlas
La Palma
Yaviza
CORCOVADO
Pen. de Osa
B. de Coronado
Puerto Cortés
San Vito
Golfito
Concepción
Santiago
Chitré
Las Tablas
El Real
G. Dulce
Pta. Burica
Puerto Armuelles
Sona
COIBA
I. de Coiba
I. de Cebaco
Tonosí
Pocrí
Golfo de Panamá
G. de Chiriquí
Pta. Mala
I. Jicarón
I. del Rey
San Miguel
Chiman
Garachiné
DARIÉN
G. de Urabá
Mon
I. de San Bern

PACIFIC OCEAN

GUADELOUPE

Pte. de la Grande Vigie
Port-Louis
Grande-Terre
Moule
La Désirade
Ste-Rose
Petit-Canal
Pointe-à-Pitre
Ste-Anne
Pointe des Châteaux
Pointe-Noire
Gosier
Îles de la Petite Terre
Basse-Terre
GUADELOUPE (Fr.)
Bouillante
Capesterre-Belle-Eau
Marie-Galante
Soufrière 1467 ▲
St-Louis
Basse-Terre
Trois-Rivières
Grand-Bourg
Capesterre
204 ▲
Îles des Saintes
Pte. des Basses

MARTINIQUE (Fr.)

Cap St-Martin
Basse-Pointe
Le Prêcheur
Ste-Marie
Presqu'île de la Caravelle
Montagne Pelée 1463 ▲
St-Pierre
La Trinité
Schœlcher
Le Robert
Fort-de-France
Le François
St-Joseph
Le Lamentin
Rivière-Salée
Fort-de-France
Rivière-Pilote
Le Marin
Pte. d'Enfer

GUADELOUPE AND MARTINIQUE

1:1 600 000

10 0 10 20 30 40 50 60 km
10 0 10 20 30 40 miles

Projection: Bi-polar oblique Conical Orthomorphic

PUERTO RICO
1:2 400 000 **d**

10 0 10 20 30 40 50 km
10 0 10 20 30 miles

ATLANTIC OCEAN

PUERTO RICO (U.S.A.)

Pta. Aguijereada
Isabela
Aguadilla
Arecibo
Barceloneta
Manati
Vega Baja
SAN JUAN
Bayamón
Carolina
Rio Grande
Fajardo
Dewey
Culebra
Mayagüez
San Sebastian
Adjuntas
Cordillera Central
Cerro 1338 de Punta
Utuado
Uroyan Mts.
Caguas
Cayey
Sierra de Luquillo
Naguabo
Vieques
San German
Yauco
Coamo
Humacao
Yabucoa
Esperanza
Pta. Aguila
Guanica
Ponce
Guayama
I. Caja de Muertos

VIRGIN ISLANDS
1:1 600 000 **e**

10 0 10 20 30 km
10 0 20 miles

Rufling Pt.
The Settlement
Anegada
East Pt.
Virgin Islands (U.K.)
Jost Van Dyke I.
Guana I.
Great Camanoe
Virgin Gorda
521
Beef I.
Spanish Town
Virgin Is. (U.S.A.)
Hans Lollik I.
Cruz Bay
Tortola
Road Town
Peter I.
Charlotte Amalie
St. Thomas I.
St. John I.

ST. LUCIA
1:800 000 **f**

5 0 10 km
5 0 5 10 miles

Cap Point
Pte. Hardy
Gros Islet
Esperance Bay
Castries
Marquis
Babonneau
L'Anse la Raye
Canaries
Millet
Dennery
Soufrière
Soufrière Bay
Mt. Gimie 950
Petit Piton 750
Gros Piton Pt.
796 Gros Piton
Trou Gras Pt.
Micoud
Vierge Pt.
Choiseul
Laborie
Vieux Fort
C. Moule à Chique

BARBADOS
1:800 000 **g**

5 0 10 km
5 0 5 10 miles

ATLANTIC OCEAN
Crabhill
North Point
Fustic
Spring Hall
Boscobelle
Portland
245 Belleplaine
Speightstown
Bathsheba
BARBADOS
Westmoreland
Hillcrest
Alleynes Bay
Mt. Hillaby 340
Martin's Bay
Holetown
Massiah Street
Ragged Pt.
Black Rock
Bridgefield
Jackson
Ellerton
Six Cross Roads
The Crane
Bridgetown
Ivy
Edey
Carlisle Bay
Oistins
St. Martins
Worthing
Oistins Bay
Chancery Lane
South Point

ATLANTIC OCEAN

MAS

A

Tropic of Cancer

r's Town
The Bight
Cat I.
Salvador I.
Conception I.
Rum Cay
Long I.
Clarence Town
Crooked I. Passage
Samana Cay
Crooked I.
Albert Town
Snug Corner
Plana Cays
Mira por vos Cay
Acklins I.
Hogsty Reef
y Verde
Little Inagua I.
Turks & Caicos (U.K.)
Caicos Is.
Cockburn Town
Turks Is.
Lake Rose
Great Inagua I.
Matthew Town

Baracoa
Pta. de Maisi
Maisi
Î. de la Tortue
Cap-Haïtien
Monte Cristi
LA ISABELA
Santiago de los Cabelleros
Milwaukee Deep 9200
Puerto Rico Trench
7
Jean Rabel
Port-de-Paix
Puerto Plata
San Francisco de Macorís
ANTANAMO (U.S.A.)
Cap-à-Foux
Fort Liberté
Gonaïves
La Vega
Cord. Central
Nagua
Samana
Moa
St-Marc
Hinche
Pico Duarte 3175
Sánchez
Sabana de la Mar
Hato Mayor
C. Engaño
Jérémie
Î. de la Gonâve
HAITI
PORT-AU-PRINCE
San Juan
ARMANDO BERMÚDEZ
DOMINICAN REP.
de Macorís
Higüey
Aguadilla
Bayamón
SAN JUAN
Carolina
Virgin Gorda
Anegada
Virgin Is. (U.K.)
Sombrero (U.K.)
Dame Marie
Les Cayes
Massif de la Hotte
Petit Goâve
Jacmel
2280
SIERRA DE BAHORUCO
L. Enriquillo
Azua
San Cristóbal
SANTO DOMINGO
La Romana
ESTE
Arecibo
Ponce
Tortola
Road Town
Charlotte Amalie
Fajardo
Caguas
Virgin Is. (U.S.A.)
Anguilla (U.K.)
St.-Martin (Fr.)
St.-Barthélemy (Fr.)
Pointe-à-Gravois
Aquin
Î. à Vache
Pedernales
Barahona
Bani
Compostela
I. Saona
B. de Yuma
Isla Mona (U.S.A.)
Mayagüez
PUERTO RICO (U.S.A.)
Guayama
Christiansted
Frederiksted
St. Croix (U.S.A.)
St. Maarten (Neth.)
Saba (Neth.)
St. Eustatius (Neth.)
Basseterre
ST. KITTS & NEVIS
St. John's
Antigua
Barbuda
ANTIGUA & BARBUDA
Redonda
Montserrat (U.K.)
Nevis
Guadeloupe Passage
Ste-Rose
Moule
La Désirade
GUADELOUPE (Fr.) 1467
Pointe-à-Pitre
Marie-Galante (Fr.)
Basse-Terre
Grand-Bourg
I. des Saintes (Fr.)
Dominica Passage
Portsmouth
1447
DOMINICA
Roseau
MORNE TROIS PITONS
I. de Aves (Venezuela)
Martinique Passage
Mt. Pelée 1397
Ste-Marie
Le François
Rivière-Pilote
Fort-de-France
MARTINIQUE
St. Lucia Channel (Fr.)
Castries
ST. LUCIA
Soufrière
St. Vincent Passage
Soufrière 1234
St. Vincent
Speightstown
Kingstown
Bridgetown
BARBADOS
Hillsborough
Grenadines
ST. VINCENT & THE GRENADINES
St. George's
GRENADA

Hispaniola
Antilles
Î. Beata
C. Beata

Lesser   Antilles

Leeward Islands
Lesser   Antilles
Windward Islands

B E A N   S E A

D

C

Lesser   Antilles

Aruba (Neth.)
Oranjestad
Curaçao
Bonaire
Willemstad
NETH. ANTILLES
ARC. LOS ROQUES
I. Orchila (Ven.)
I. Blanquilla (Ven.)
Is. Los Hermanos (Ven.)
Tobago
Scarborough
Pta. Gallinas
MACUIRA
C. San Román
Pen. de Paraguaná
Is. Las Aves (Ven.)
Is. Los Roques (Ven.)
Is. Los Testigos (Ven.)
NUEVA ESPARTA
I. de Margarita
Port of Spain
Galera Point
COLOMBIA
Ríohacha
Uribia
Pen. de la Guajira
Punto Fijo
I. La Tortuga (Ven.)
La Asunción
Porlamar
Pen. de Paria
Güira
TRINIDAD
Arima
Rio Claro
Santa Marta
ISLA DE SALAMANCA
GUAJIRA
Golfo de Venezuela
Punta Cardón
MEDANOS DE CORO
Puerto Cumarebo
Maiquetía
La Guaira
VARGAS
C. Codera
Cumaná
Cariaco
Carúpano
Caribe
G. de Paria San
Maturín
San Fernando
TRINIDAD & TOBAGO
Serpent's Mouth
Cienaga
San Rafael
Coro
La Vela de Coro
Tucacas
Puerto Cabello
CARACAS
Los Teques
Higuerote
Río Chico
Puerto La Cruz
Barcelona
MOCHIMA
SUCRE
Caripito
MARIUSA
DELTA
Valledupar
Villa del Rosario
Ciudad Ojeda
CUEVA DE LA QUEBRADA DEL TORO
San Felipe
Valencia
Villa de Cura
San Juan de los Morros
Aragua de Barcelona
Anaco
MONAGAS
Tucupita
Machiques
Mene Grande
FALCON
YARACUY
LARA
San Carlos
Ocumare del Tuy
Altagracia de Orituco
El Tigre
Tigre
AMACURO
Sabanalarga
Cabimas
TRUJILLO
BARQUISIMETO
Yaritagua de Barinas
El Sombrero
GUARICO
Valle de la Pascua
Santa Maria de Ipire
Ciudad Guayana
Fundación
La Concepción
MERIDA
Valera
Acarigua
El Guache
PORTUGUESA
El Baúl
Calabozo
El Tigre
Los Barrancos
Barinas
COJEDES
AGUARO-GUARIQUITO
Soledad
Plato
AGUSTIN CODAZZI
MAGDALENA
CESAR
PERIJA
ZULIA
PARAMOS DE EL TAMA
Cordi de Merida
Barinas
Libertad
San Fernando de Apure
VENEZUELA
ANZOÁTEGUI
Ciudad Bolívar
Sierra Imataca
E
Zambrano
Mompós
El Banco
SANTANDER NORTE
Ocaña
MERIDA
Santa Barbara
BARINAS
Puerto de Nutrias
Bruzual
Achaguas
Apure
Caicara
Mapire
Embalse de Guri
Upata
Caucasia
Simití
BOLÍVAR
Cúcuta
TACHIRA
CAPARA
San Carlos de Zulia
Ciudad Bolivia
Guanare
Portuguesa
San Carlos
Aragua
Orinoco
Guasipati
Tumeremo
El Callao

West from Greenwich
5
124
6
7

COPYRIGHT PHILIP'S

4000 3000 2000 1500 1000 400 200 0
12 000 9000 6000 4500 3000 1200 600 0 m
ft
600 6000 12 000 18 000 24 000 ft
200 2000 4000 6000 8000 m

□ National Parks

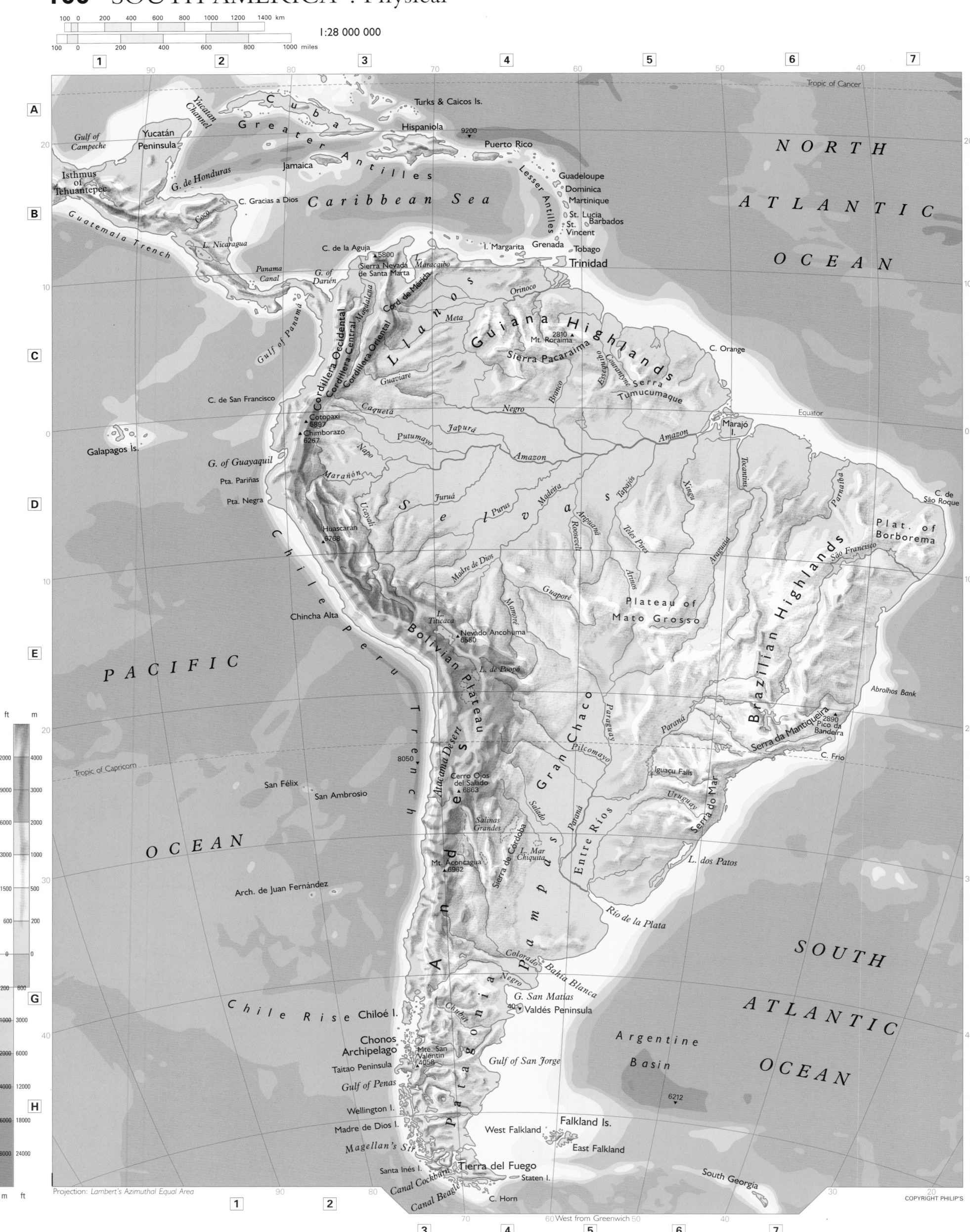

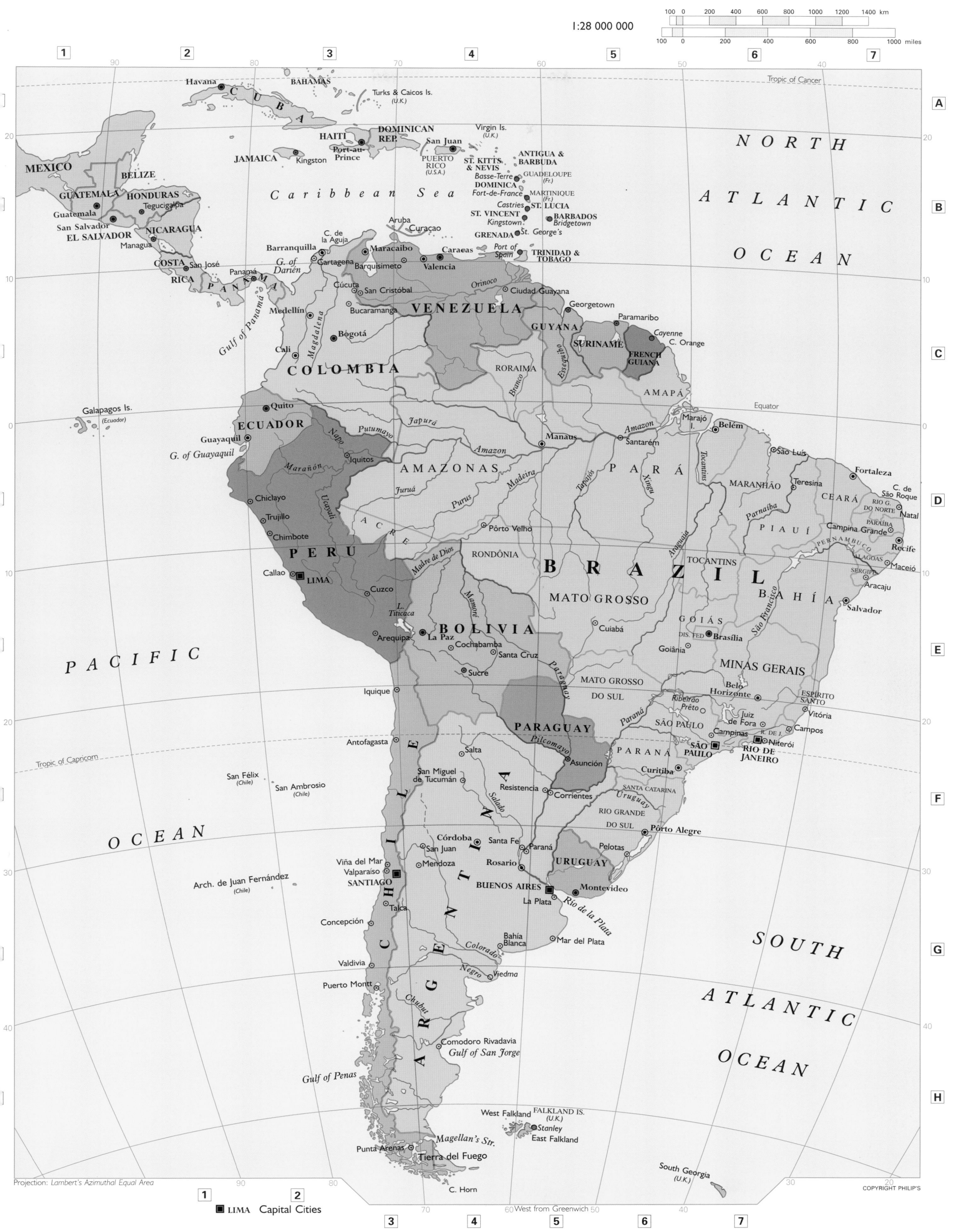

1:28 000 000

100 0 200 400 600 800 1000 1200 1400 km
100 0 200 400 600 800 1000 miles

| 1 | 2 | 3 | 4 | 5 | 6 | 7 |

Tropic of Cancer

A

NORTH

Havana
CUBA
BAHAMAS
Turks & Caicos Is.
(U.K.)

Virgin Is.
(U.K.)

HAITI **DOMINICAN REP.**
San Juan
Port-au-Prince
JAMAICA Kingston
PUERTO RICO
(U.S.A.)

ST. KITTS & NEVIS
Basse-Terre
ANTIGUA & BARBUDA
GUADELOUPE (Fr.)

ATLANTIC

MEXICO
BELIZE
GUATEMALA
HONDURAS Tegucigalpa
Guatemala
San Salvador
EL SALVADOR
NICARAGUA
Managua

Caribbean Sea

DOMINICA
Fort-de-France
Castries **ST. LUCIA**
ST. VINCENT
Kingstown
GRENADA St. George's
MARTINIQUE (Fr.)

BARBADOS
Bridgetown

B

OCEAN

COSTA RICA San José
Panamá
Barranquilla
C. de la Aguja
Aruba Curaçao
Port of Spain
TRINIDAD & TOBAGO

PANAMA
G. of Darién
Cartagena
Maracaibo
Caracas
Valencia
Barquisimeto

10

C

Medellín
San Cristóbal
Bucaramanga
VENEZUELA
Orinoco
Ciudad Guayana
Georgetown
Paramaribo
Cayenne
C. Orange

10

Cali
Bogotá
GUYANA
SURINAME
FRENCH GUIANA

COLOMBIA
RORAIMA
Branco
AMAPÁ
Essequibo

Galapagos Is.
(Ecuador)
Quito
Equator

0

ECUADOR
Guayaquil
G. of Guayaquil
Napo
Putumayo
Japurá
Amazon
Marajó I.
Belém

D

Iquitos
Marañón
AMAZONAS
Amazon
Manaus
Santarém
PARÁ
São Luís

Chiclayo
Ucayali
Juruá
Purus
Madeira
Tapajós
Xingu
Tocantins
MARANHÃO
Teresina
Fortaleza
C. de São Roque

Trujillo
ACRE
CEARÁ
RIO G. DO NORTE
Natal

Chimbote
Pôrto Velho
PIAUÍ
Parnaíba
PARAÍBA
Campina Grande

PERU
RONDÔNIA
Madre de Dios
Mamoré
BRAZIL
PERNAMBUCO
Recife

Callao
LIMA
MATO GROSSO
ALAGOAS
SERGIPE
Maceió

10

E

Cuzco
L. Titicaca
BOLIVIA
Cuiabá
Araguaia
GOIÁS
DIS. FED.
TOCANTINS
São Francisco
BAHÍA
Aracaju
Salvador

Arequipa
La Paz
Cochabamba
Santa Cruz
Brasília
Goiânia

Sucre
MINAS GERAIS

Iquique
MATO GROSSO DO SUL
Belo Horizonte
ESPÍRITO SANTO
Vitória

Antofagasta
PARAGUAY
Paraná
Ribeirão Prêto
Juiz de Fora
Campos

20

F

San Félix
(Chile)
San Ambrosio
(Chile)
Salta
Pilcomayo
Asunción
PARANÁ
SÃO PAULO
Campinas
R. DE J.
Niterói
RIO DE JANEIRO

PACIFIC
San Miguel de Tucumán
Resistencia
Corrientes
Curitiba
SANTA CATARINA
Uruguay
RIO GRANDE DO SUL

OCEAN
Arch. de Juan Fernández
(Chile)
Córdoba
San Juan
Santa Fe
Paraná
Rosario
URUGUAY
Pôrto Alegre
Pelotas

30

G

Viña del Mar
Valparaíso
SANTIAGO
Mendoza
BUENOS AIRES
Montevideo
La Plata
Río de la Plata

Talca
CHILE
ARGENTINA
Salado

Concepción
Bahía Blanca
Mar del Plata

SOUTH

Valdivia
Colorado

Puerto Montt
Negro
Viedma

40

ATLANTIC

Comodoro Rivadavia
Gulf of San Jorge

Gulf of Penas

OCEAN

H

West Falkland
FALKLAND IS. (U.K.)
Stanley
East Falkland

Punta Arenas
Magellan's Str.
Tierra del Fuego
C. Horn
South Georgia (U.K.)

West from Greenwich

COPYRIGHT PHILIP'S

Projection: Lambert's Azimuthal Equal Area

| 1 | 2 |

■ LIMA Capital Cities

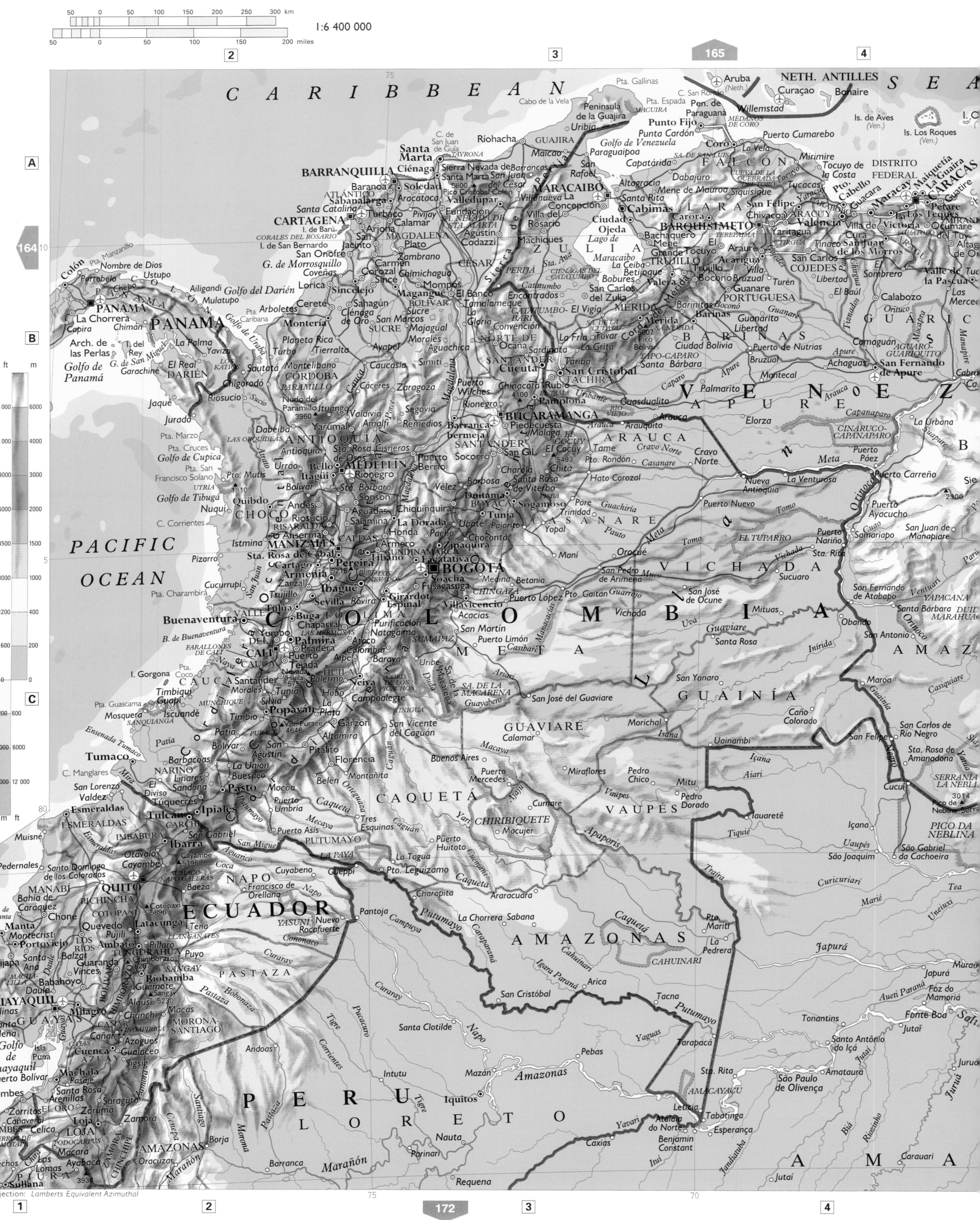

Projection: Lamberts Equivalent Azimuthal

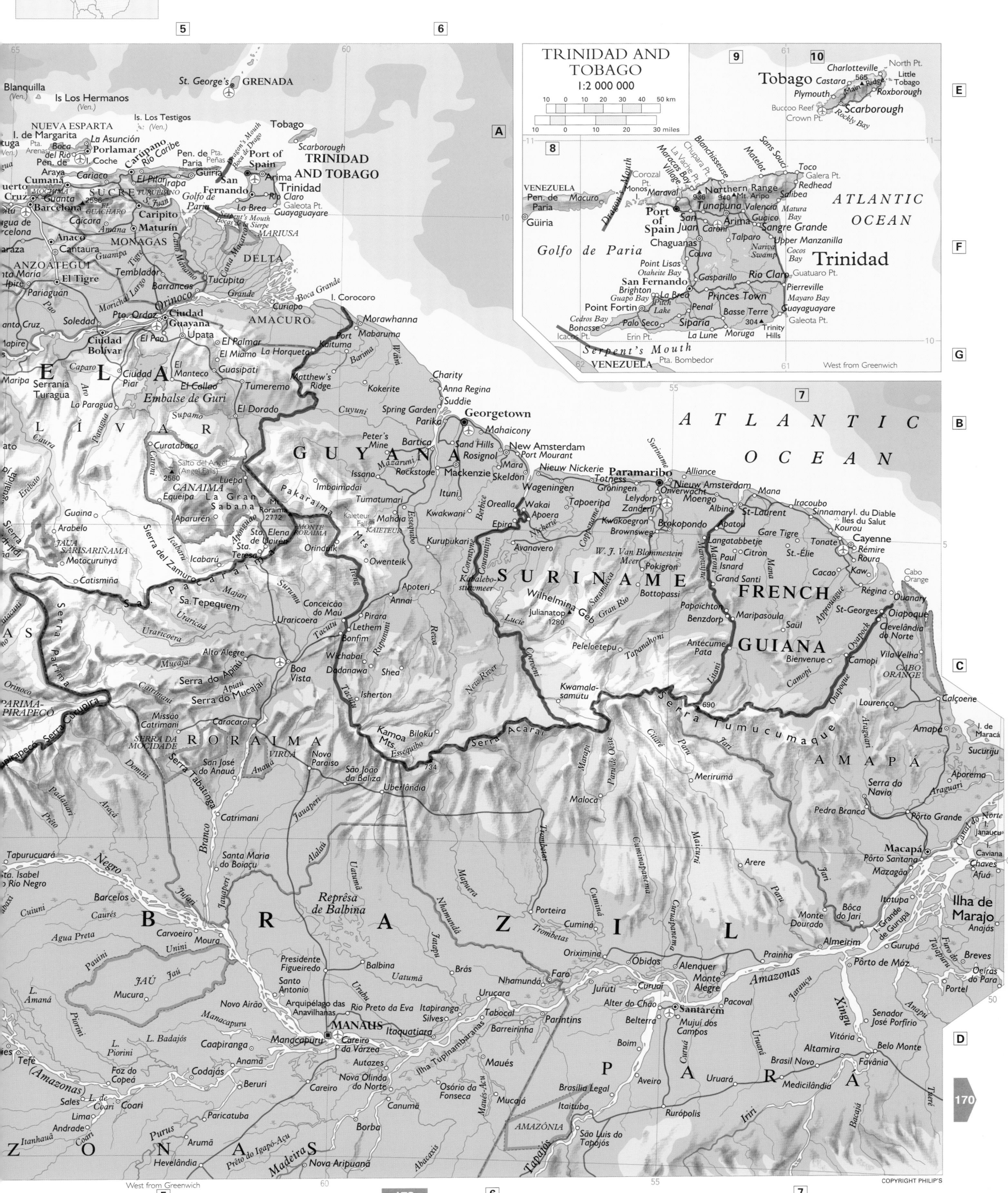

TRINIDAD AND TOBAGO
1:2 000 000

10   0   10   20   30   40   50 km
10   0   10   20   30 miles

Tobago
Charlotteville
North Pt.
Castara   565   Little
Plymouth   Man   Roxborough   Tobago
Buccoo Reef   Scarborough
Crown Pt.   Rockly Bay

ATLANTIC
OCEAN

VENEZUELA
Pen. de
Paria   Macuro
Güiria

Corozal
Pt.   La Vache   Blanchisseuse
Chupara Pt.
Maracas Bay   Sans Souci   Toco
Monos   Maraval   Maracas   Northern Range   Salibea   Galera Pt.
I.   936   940   Mt. Aripo   Redhead
Tunapuna   Valencia
Port   San   Caroni   Gugico   Sangre Grande
of Spain   Juan   Arima   Matura
Chaguanas   Talparo   Upper Manzanilla   Bay
Couva   Nariva   Cocos
Point Lisas   Gasparillo   Swamp   Bay   **Trinidad**
Otaheite Bay   Rio Claro
San Fernando   Princes Town   Pierreville
Brighton   Penal   Basse Terre   Mayaro Bay
Point Fortin   Pitch   Siparia   304   Guayaguayare
Bonasse   Lake   Palo Seco   Moruga   Trinity   Galeota Pt.
Cedros Bay   La Lune   Hills
Icacos Pt.   Erin Pt.

Golfo de Paria

Serpent's Mouth
VENEZUELA   Pta. Bombedor

West from Greenwich

ATLANTIC
OCEAN

Georgetown

GUYANA

SURINAME

Paramaribo

FRENCH
GUIANA

Cayenne

BRAZIL

MANAUS

PARÁ

AMAZONAS

RORAIMA

AMAPÁ

Macapá

Ilha de
Marajó

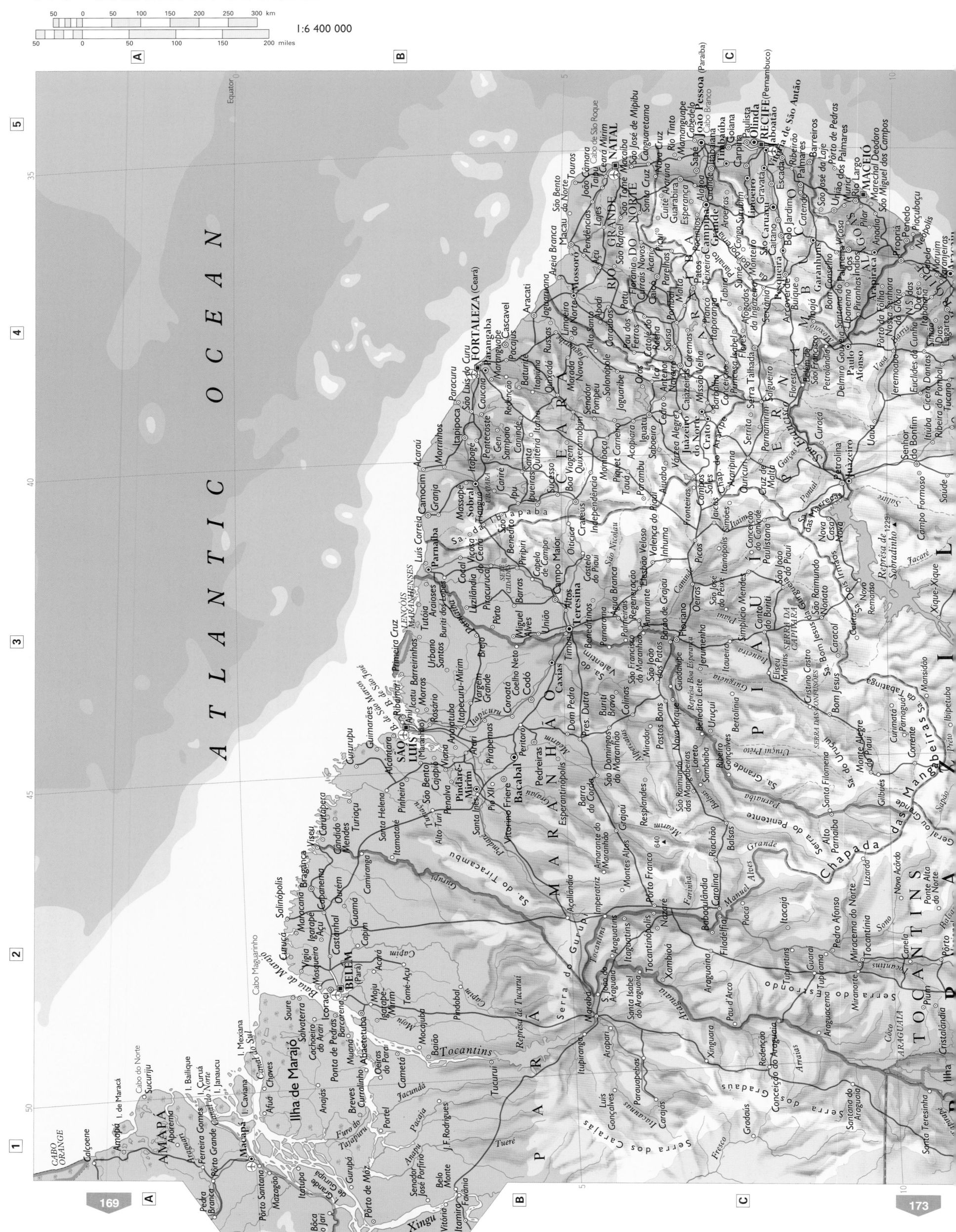

50   0   50   100   150   200   250   300 km

50   0   50   100   150   200 miles

1:6 400 000

ATLANTIC OCEAN

CABO ORANGE

AMAPÁ

Ilha de Marajó

Baía de Marajó

BELÉM (Pará)

PARÁ

MARANHÃO

SÃO LUÍS

FORTALEZA (Ceará)

CEARÁ

PIAUÍ

Teresina

RIO GRANDE DO NORTE

NATAL

JOÃO PESSOA (Paraíba)

RECIFE (Pernambuco)

MACEIÓ

ALAGOAS

TOCANTINS

Serra dos Carajás

Chapada das Mangabeiras

169   A   B   C   173

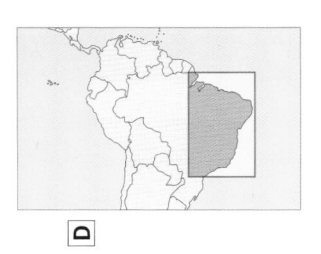

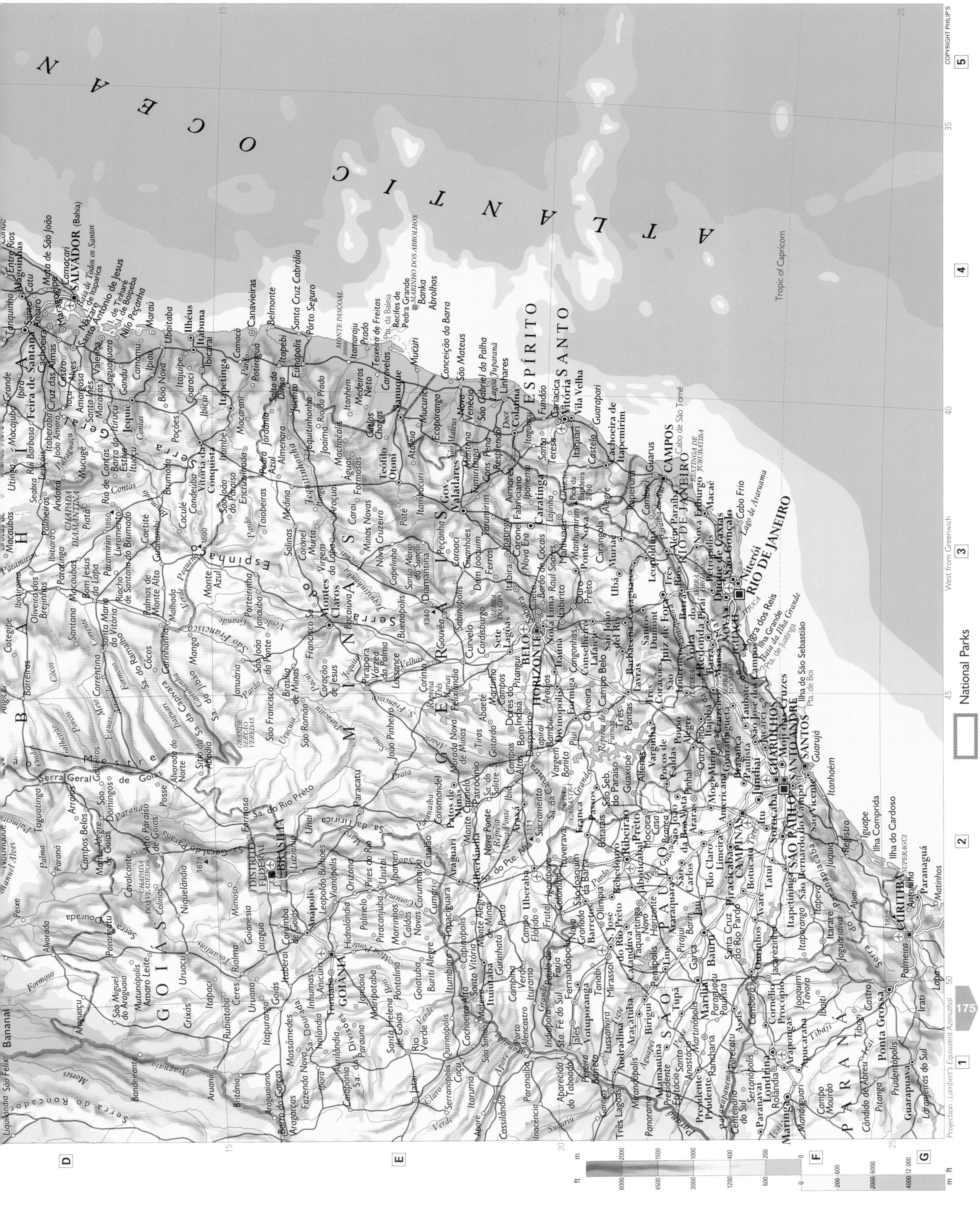
ATLANTIC OCEAN
BAHIA
MINAS GERAIS
ESPÍRITO SANTO
RIO DE JANEIRO
SÃO PAULO
PARANÁ
GOIÁS
DISTRITO FEDERAL
BRASÍLIA
SALVADOR
BELO HORIZONTE
RIO DE JANEIRO
SÃO PAULO
CURITIBA
GOIÂNIA
Vitória
CAMPOS
SANTOS
CAMPINAS
Feira de Santana
Vitória da Conquista
Montes Claros
Juiz de Fora
Niterói
Uberlândia
Ribeirão Prêto
Londrina
Tropic of Capricorn
West from Greenwich
National Parks
175
Projection: Lambert's Equivalent Azimuthal
COPYRIGHT PHILIP'S

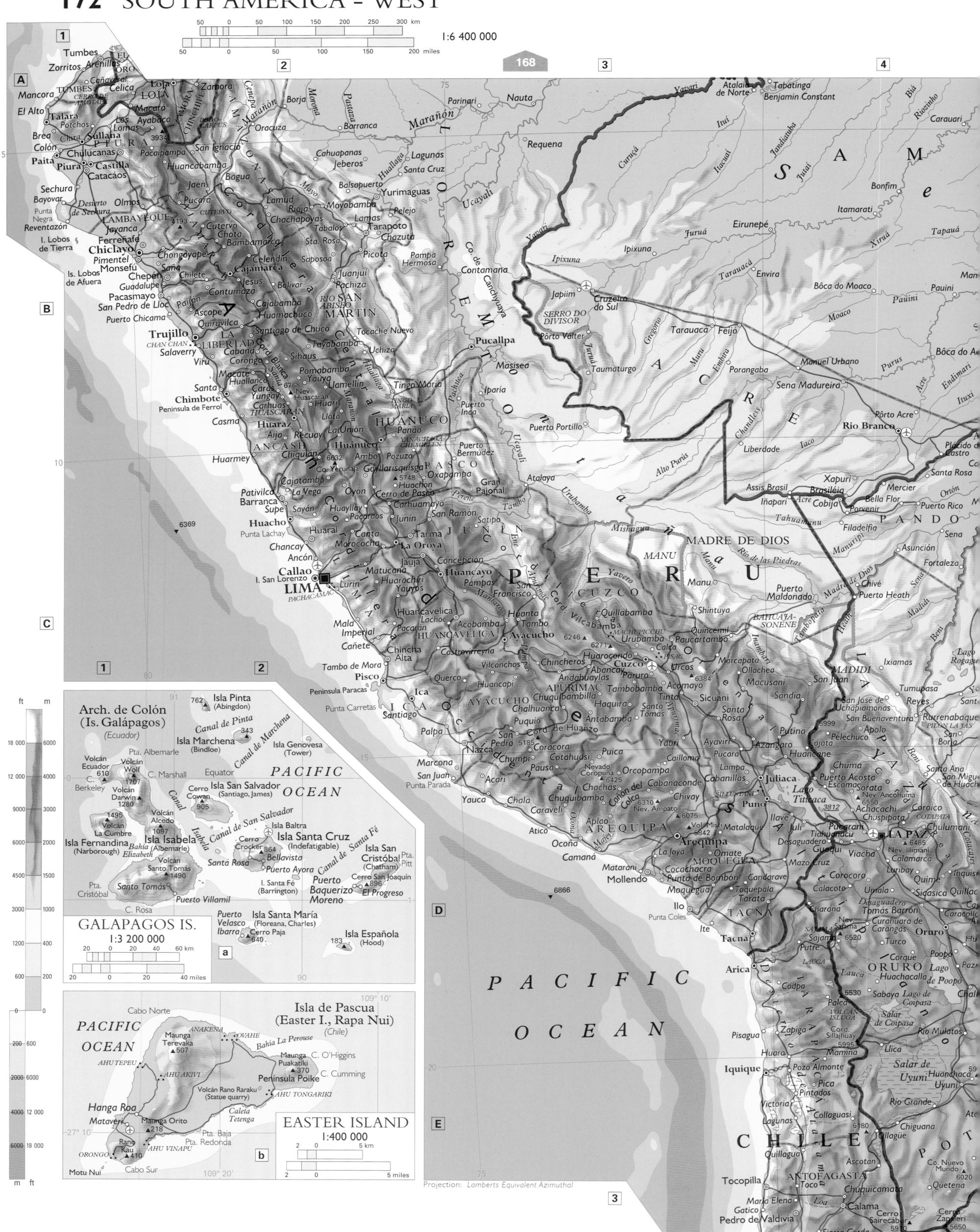

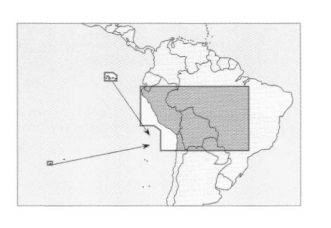

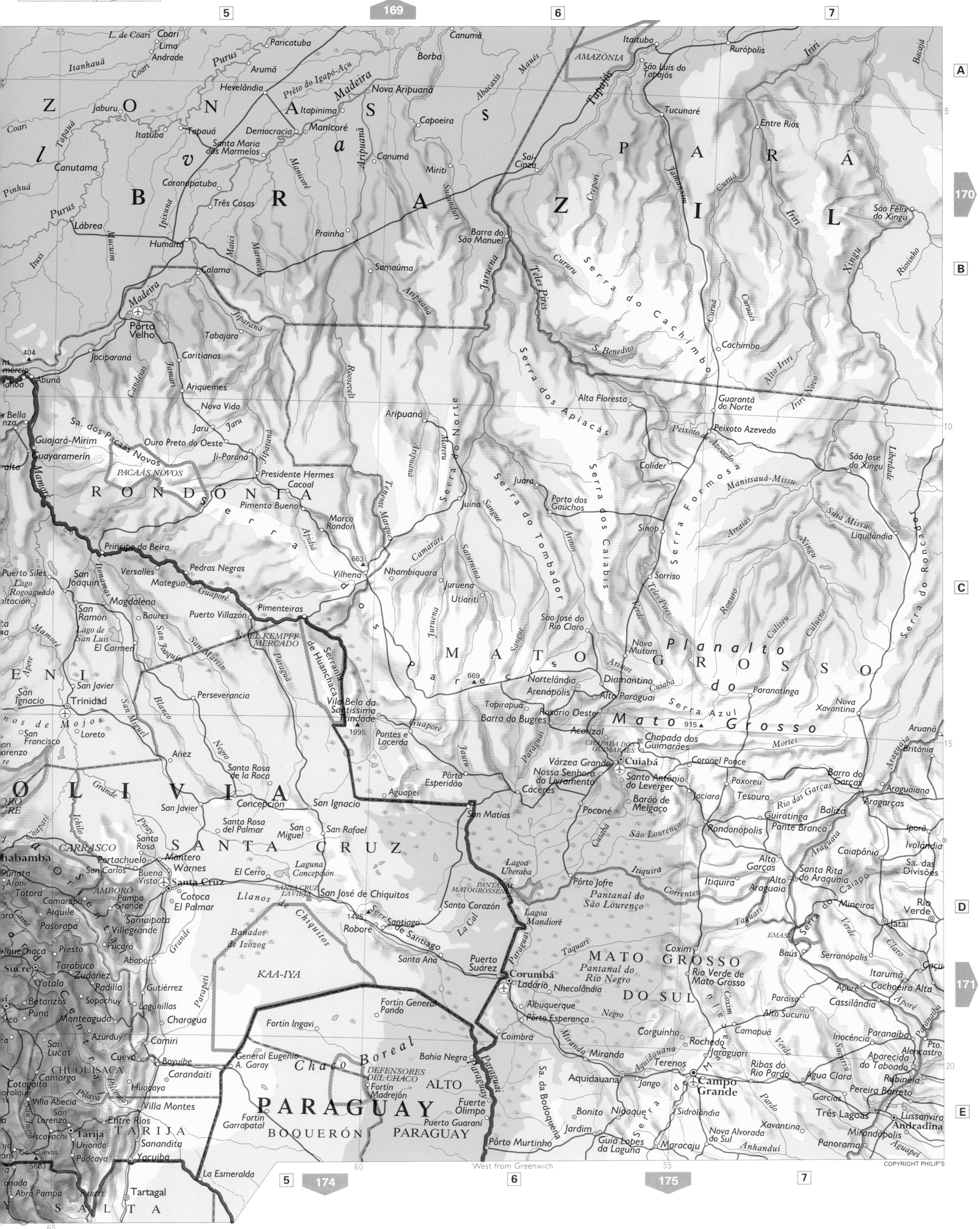

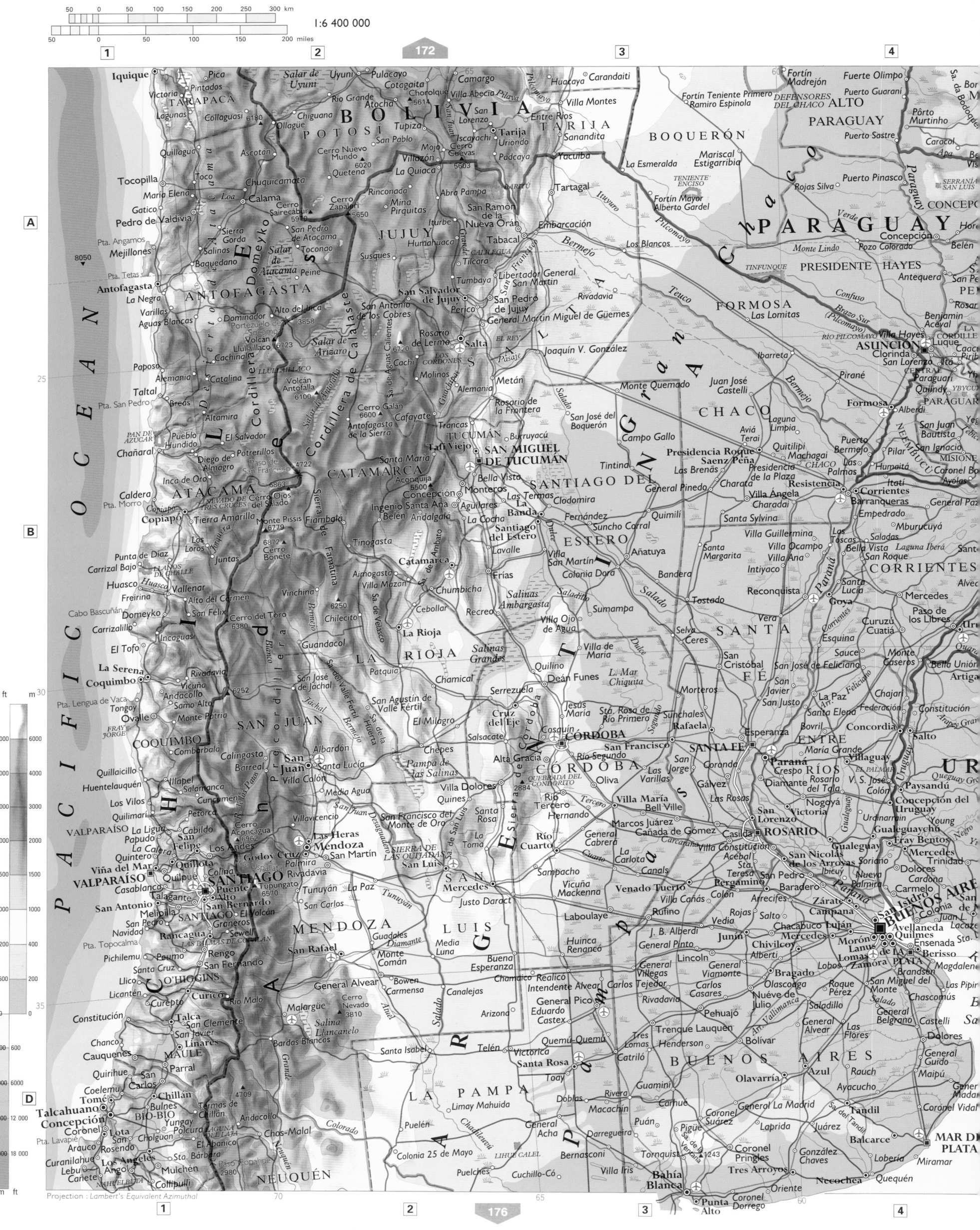

173 5 6 171 7

BELO
HORIZONTE
Nova Lima
Itabirito
Vitória
Itaquari
Vila
Velha
Guarapari
Congonhas
Conselheiro Lafaiete
Ouro Prêto
Ponte Nova
Pico da Bandeira 2890
Castelo
Cachoeiro de Itapemirim

Sidrolândia
Nioaque
Oliveira
Campo Belo
São João del Rei
Ubá
Carangola
Muriaé
Alegre

TO GROSSO
DO SUL
Laguna
Andradina
Três Lagoas
Olímpia
Mirassol
São José do Rio Prêto
Catanduva
Passos
Batatais
São Sebastião do Paraíso
Represa de Furnas
Três Pontas
Barbacena
Cataguases
Itaperuna
Cambuci

Maracaju
Nova Alvorada do Sul
Xavantina
Panorama
Araçatuba
Biguri
Penápolis
Jaboticabal
Ribeirão Prêto
Guaxupé
Alfenas
Varginha
Três Corações
Santos Dumont
Juiz de Fora
Três Rios
Leopoldina
Guarus
CAMPOS

Dourados
Rio Brilhante
Nova Andradina do Sul
Presidente Epitácio
Adamantina
Santo Anastácio
SÃO
Lins
Tupã
Bauru
PAULO
Novo Horizonte
Mococa
Casa Branca
Pouso Alegre
Pinhal
Poços de Caldas
Itajubá
Volta Redonda
Barra do Piraí
Petrópolis
RIO DE JANEIRO

Ponta Porã
Dourados
Ivinhema
Nova Andradina
Euclides da Cunha Paulista
Martinópolis
Presidente Prudente
Rancharia
Marília
Paraguaçu Paulista
Garça
Bariri
Araraquara
Rio Claro
Limeira
São Carlos
Ararás
Piracicaba
Americana
Mogi-Mirim
Cruzeiro
Guaratinguetá
Aparecida
Taubaté
Angra dos Reis
Niterói
RIO DE JANEIRO

Pedro Juan Caballero
Amambai
Mundo Novo
Salto del Guairá
Centenário do Oeste
Sertanópolis
Assis
Cambará
Ourinhos
Botucatu
Itu
Jundiaí
Sorocaba
Mogi das Cruzes
São José dos C.
Cabo Frio
L. de Araruama

CANINDÉ
Caaguazú
Curuguaty
Pôrto São José
Paranavaí
Nova Esperança
Londrina
Cornélio Procópio
Jacarèzinho
Avaré
Tatuí
Itapetininga
SÃO PAULO
Santo André
Santos
Tropic of Capricorn

Ciudad del Este
Oviedo
Iguaçú
Maringá
Mandaguari
Apucarana
Arapongas
Joaquim Távora
Itaporanga
Itararé
Itapeva
Paranapiacaba
São Bernardo do Campo
São Vicente
Itanhaém
Guarujá
Ilha de São Sebastião
Pta. de Boi

BRAZIL
Umuarama
Cianorte
Campo Mourão
Ibaiti
Tibagi
Jaguariaíva
Apiaí
Juquiá
Iguape
Ilha de São Sebastião

PARANÁ
Goio-Erê
Guaíra
Cândido de Abreu
Prudentópolis
Ponta Grossa
Palmeira
CURITIBA
Antonina
Ilha do Cardoso
Ilha Comprida
SUPERAGÜI

Cascavel
Ubiratã
Pitanga
Irati
Lapa
Paranaguá
Matinhos
Guaratuba
Joinville
São Francisco do Sul

Foz do Iguaçu
Cat. del Iguaçu
IGUAÇU
Medianeira
Francisco Beltrão
Pato Branco
Laranjeiras do Sul
União da Vitória
São Mateus do Sul
Rio Negro
Mafra

Pôrto Mendes
Toledo
Clevelândia
Palmas
Pôrto União
Espigão
Rio Negro
ATLANTIC

ALTO
Hernandárias
Itaipú
PARANÁ
Bernardo de Irigoyen
São Miguel do Oeste
Xanxerê
Caçador
Itajaí

Eldorado
Sa. da Fartura
Chapecó
Joaçaba
Santa Cecília
Blumenau
Brusque
Brusque

MISIONES
Corpus
Encarnación
Monteagudo
Frederico Westphalen
Erechim
Campos Novos
SANTA CATARINA
Curitibanos
Rio do Sul
São José
Ilha de Santa Catarina
Florianópolis

Candelaria
Leandro N. Alem
Santa Rosa
Palmeira das Missões
Passo Fundo
Lajes
São Joaquim
SÃO JOAQUIM

Santo Ângelo
Apóstoles
Ijuí
Carazinho
Lagoa Vermelha
Vacaria
Tubarão
Laguna

San Pedro
Santa Rosa
Coxilha Grande
Guaporé
São Joaquim
Criciúma
Cabo Santa Marta Grande

Santiago
São Luís Gonzaga
Cruz Alta
RIO GRANDE
Bento Gonçalves
Caxias do Sul
APARADOS DA SERRA
Araranguá
Torres

Borja
Sa. do Espinilho
Santa Maria
Santa Cruz do Sul
Montenegro
Nôvo Hamburgo
São Leopoldo
Taquara
Osorio

Ibicuy
DO SUL
Cachoeira do Sul
Canoas
Rio Pardo
Viamão
PORTO ALEGRE

Alegrete
São Gabriel
Caçapava
Sa. Encantadas
Tapes

Santana do Livramento
Dom Pedrito
Camaquã
Tapes
Mostardas
LAGOA DE PEIXE

Rivera
Santana
Bagé
Sa. do Camaquã
São Lourenço do Sul
Canguçu
Lagoa dos Patos

URUGUAY
Cuarembó
Pinheiro Machado
Pelotas
Lagoa
São José do Norte
Rio Grande

Rincón
Melo
Rio Branco
Jaguarão
Lagoa Mirim

Fraile Muerto
San Gregorio
Vergara
Lagoa Mangueira

Blanquillo
Cerro Chato
Treinta y Tres

Sarandí del Yi
José Batlle y Ordóñez
Santa Vitória do Palmar
Lascano
Chuy
SANTA TERESA

Aigua
Castillos

Tala
Minas
Piedras
Rocha

San Carlos

MONTEVIDEO
Maldonado

ATLANTIC

OCEAN

5304

National Parks

A
B
C
D

25
30
35

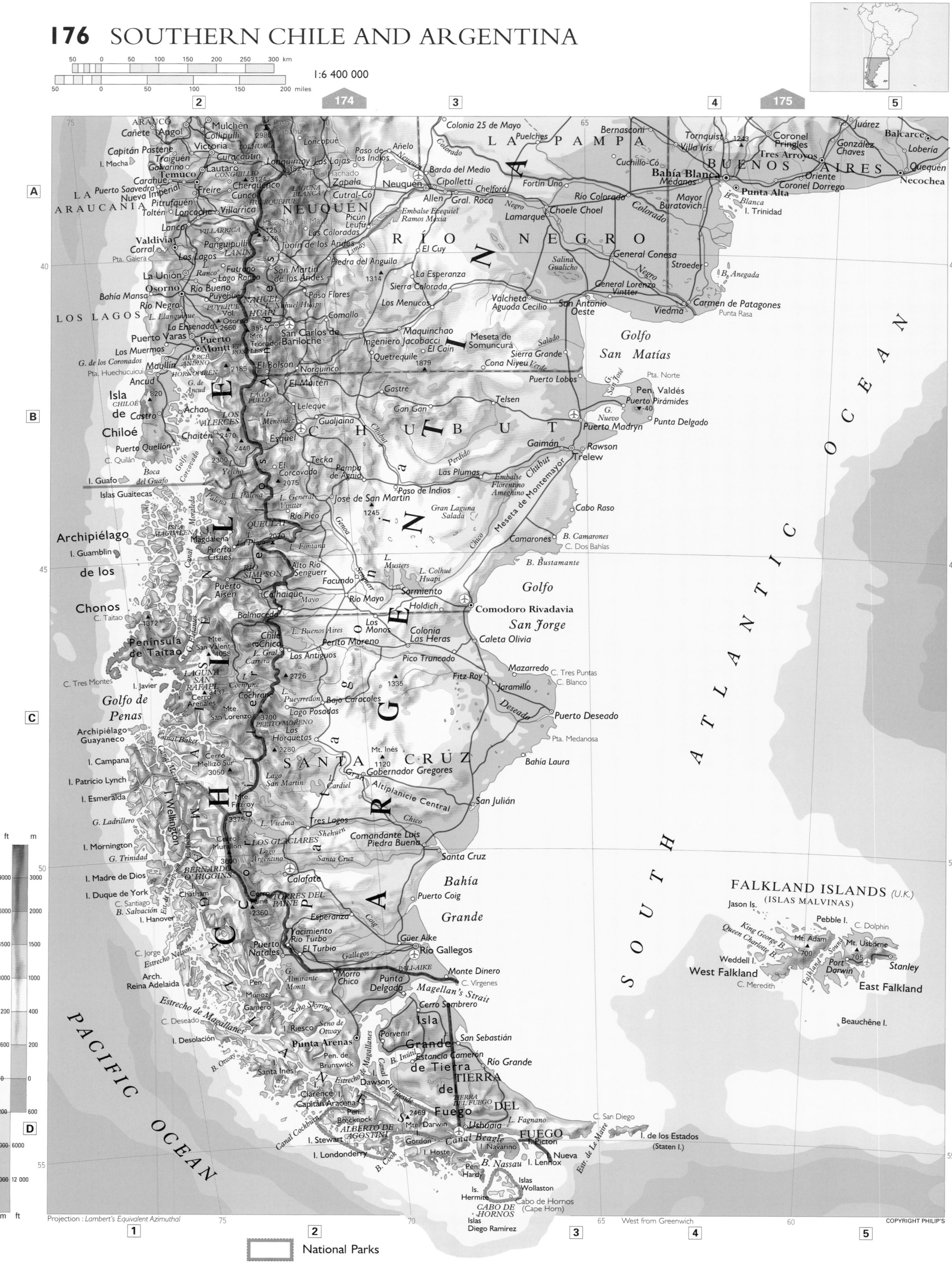

1:6 400 000

Projection : Lambert's Equivalent Azimuthal

National Parks

COPYRIGHT PHILIP'S

GEOGRAPHICAL GLOSSARY

This is a list of the geographical terms from various foreign languages that are found in the place names on the maps and in the index. Each is followed by the language and its English meaning.

Afr. Afrikaans
Alb. Albanian
Amh. Amharic
Ar. Arabic
Belo. Belorussian
Berb. Berber
Bulg. Bulgarian
Burm. Burmese
Cat. Catalan
Chin. Chinese
Czec. Czech
Dan. Danish
Dut. Dutch
Est. Estonian
Fr. French
Gae. Gaelic
Ger. German
Gr. Greek
Heb. Hebrew
Hin. Hindi
Hung. Hungarian
I.-C. Indo-Chinese
Ice. Icelandic
It. Italian
Indo. Indonesian
Jap. Japanese
Kaz. Kazakh
Kor. Korean
Kyrg. Kyrgyz
Lapp. Lapp (Sami)
Lat. Latvian
Lith. Lithuanian
Malag. Malagasy
Mong. Mongolian
Nor. Norway
Pash. Pashto
Per. Persian
Pol. Polish
Port. Portuguese
Rom. Romanian
Russ. Russian
Sin. Sinhalese
Ser.-Cr. Serbo-Croat
Slov. Slovene
Som. Somali
Sp. Spanish
Swe. Swedish
Tib. Tibetan
Turk. Turkish
Ukr. Ukrainian
Viet. Vietnamese

-á *Ice.* river
-å *Dan., Nor., Swe.* stream
-abad *Farsi, Russ.* town
Abyad *Ar.* white mountain
Ada, Adasi *Turk.* island
Addis *Amh.* new
Adrar *Ar., Ber.* mountains
Aiguille *Fr.* peak
Aïn, Aîn (A.) *Ar.* spring
Ákra *Gr.* cape, point
Akrotíri *Gr.* cape, point
Alb *Ger.* mountains
Albufera *Span.* lagoon
-ålen *Nor.* islands
Alpen *Ger.* mountain ranges
Alpes *Fr.* mountains
Alpi *It.* mountains
Alt *Ger.* old
Alta, Alto *Port.* high, upper
Altos *Span.* mountains
-älv, -älven *Swe.* stream, river
Amtskommune (Amt.) *Dan.* first-order administrative division
-ån *Swe.* river
Anse *Fr.* bay
Ao *Thai* bay
Appennino *It.* mountain range
Archipel *Fr.* archipelago
Archipiélago (Arch.) *Span.* archipelago
Arcipèlago *It.* archipelago
Arquipélago (Arq.) *Port.* archipelago
Arrecife *Span.* reef
Arroyo (Arr.) *Span.* stream
-ås, -åsen *Nor., Swe.* hill
Ayios *Gr.* island
Ayn *Ar.* well, waterhole

Baai, -baai *Afr., Dut.* bay
Bāb *Ar.* gate, strait
Bäck, -bäcken *Swe.* stream
Back, -backen, *Swe.* hill
Bad, -baden *Ger.* spa
Badia *Cat.* bay
Bādiyah, Bādiyat *Ar.* desert
Bæk *Dan.* stream
Bælt *Dan.* strait
Baharu *Malay* new
Bahia (B.) *Span.* bay
Bahiret *Ar.* lagoon
Bahr *Ar.* sea, lake, river
Bahra Bahrat *Ar.* lake
Baía (B.) *Port.* bay
Baie (B.) *Fr.* bay
Baixa, Baixo *Port.* lower
Baja, Bajo *Span.* lower
Bakke *Nor.* hill
Bala *Farsi* upper
Ballon *Fr.* dome
Baltă *Rom.* marsh, lake
Ban *Lao, Thai* village
-Bana *Jap.* cape
Banc *Fr.* bank
Banco *Span.* bank
Bandao *Chin.* peninsula
Bandar *Ar., Malay* port, harbour
Bandar *Farsi* bay
Banja *Ser.-Cr.* spa, resort
Banjaran *Malay* mountain range
Baraji *Turk.* dam
Barat *Indo., Malay* western
Barrage (Barr.) *Fr.* dam
Barragem (Barr.) *Port.* dam, reservoir
Bas, basse *Fr.* lower
Bassin *Fr.* basin
-batang *Indo.* river
Baṭlaq *Farsi* marsh
Batu *Malay* mountain
Bayt *Heb.* house, village
Bazar *Hin.* market, bazaar
-beek *Afr., Dut.* river
Be'er *Heb.* well
Bei *Chin.* north, northern
Beinn, Ben *Gae.* mountain
Beit *Heb.* village
Belaya, Belo, Beloye, Belyy *Russ.* white
Belogorye *Russ.* hills, mountain range
Bender *Som.* harbour
Berg(e), -berg(e) *Afr., Ger.* mountain(s)
-berg, -en, -et *Nor., Swe.* hill, mountain, rock
Besar *Indo., Malay* big
Bet *Heb.* house, village
Bir, Bîr, Bi'r *Ar.* well
Birkat, Birket *Ar.* lake, marsh, well
Bishti *Alb.* cape
-bjerg *Dan.* hill, point
Blaenau *Welsh* upland
-bo *Chin.* lake
Boca *Port., Span.* river mouth, inlet
Bodden *Ger.* bay, inlet
Bogaz, Boğazı *Turk.* channel, strait
Bogd *Mong.* mountain range
Bois *Fr.* woods
Boka *Ser.-Cr.* gulf, inlet
Bolshoi, Bolshaya, Bolshoye (Bol.) *Russ.* great, large
Bordj (Bj.) *Ar.* fort
-borg *Dan., Nor., Swe.* castle, fort
Bory *Pol.* woods
Bosque *Span.* woods
-botn *Nor.* valley floor
Bouche(s) *Fr.* mouth(s)
Braţul *Rom.* distributary stream, branch
-bre, -breen *Nor.* glacier
Bredning *Dan.* bay
Brücke *Ger.* bridge
-brug *Dut.* bridge
-brunn *Swe.* well, spring
Bucht *Ger.* bay
Bugt *Dan.* bay
-bugten *Dan.* bay
Buheirat *Ar.* lake, reservoir
Bukit *Malay* hill
-bukt, -a *Nor.* bay
-bukten *Swe.* bay
-bulag *Mong.* spring
Bulag *Chin.* lake
Bulu *Malay* mountain
Bum *Burm.* mountain
Bûr *Ar.* port
Burg. *Ar.* fort
Burg, -burg *Ger.* castle
Burnu, Burun *Turk.* cape
Butt *Gae.* promontory
Büyük *Turk.* big
-by *Dan., Nor., Swe.* town
-byen *Nor., Swe.* town

Cabeza *Span.* peak, hill
Cabo (C.) *Port., Span.* headland, cape
Cachoeira *Port.* waterfall
Cala Cat. *It.* bay
Camp Port. *Span.* land, field
Câmpia *Rom.* plain
Campo *It., Port., Span.* plain
Campos *Span.* upland
Canal (Can.) *Fr., Port., Span.* canal, channel
Canale (Can.) *It.* channel
Canalul (Can.) *Ser.-Cr.* canal
Cao Nguyen *Thai* plateau, tableland
Cap (C.) *Cat., Fr.* cape
Capo (C) *It.* cape
Carn *Gae.* hill
Carse *Gae.* valley
Catarata *Port., Span.* cataract
Cauce *Span.* intermittent stream
Causse *Fr.* limestone plateau
Cay, Cayi, -cay, -cayi *Turk.* river
Cayo(s) *Span.* rock(s), islet(s)
Cefn *Welsh* hill
Cerro *Span.* hill, peak
Česká, Český, České *Czec.* Czech
Chaco *Span.* jungle
Chaîne(s) *Fr.* mountain range(s)
Chang *Chin.* mountain
Chapa *Span.* hills, upland
Chapada *Port.* hills, upland
Chaung *Burm.* stream, river
Chi *Chin.* small lake
-ch'ŏn *Kor.* river
-chŏsuji *Kor.* reservoir
Chott *Ar.* salt lake, depression
Chu *Tib.* river
Chute *Fr.* waterfall
Città *It.* city
Ciudad *Span.* city
Co *Tib.* lake
Cochilla (Coch.) *Port.* hills
Col *Fr., It.* pass
Colina(s) *Span.* hill(s)
Colle *It.* pass
Colline(s) *Fr.* hill(s)
Conca *It.* plain, basin
Cordillera (Cord.) *Span.* mountain range
Costa *It., Port., Span.* coast
Côte *Fr.* coast, slope, hill
Coteaux *Fr.* hills
Cuchilla *Span.* hills
Cuenca *Span.* river basin
Cu-Lao *Viet.* island

Da *Chin.* big
Da *Viet.* river
Daban *Mong.* pass
Dağ(ı) *Turk.* mountain(s)
Dāgh *Farsi* mountain
Dağları *Turk.* mountain range
-dai, -daichi *Jap.* plateau
-Dake *Jap.* mountain
-dal, -e *Dan., Swe.* valley
-dal, -en *Swe., Nor.* valley, stream
Dalay Mong. large lake
-ðalir, -ðalur *Ice.* valley
-damm, -en *Swe.* lake
Danau *Malay* lake
Dao *Chin., Viet.* island
Dar *Ar.* region
Darya *Russ.* river
Daryācheh *Farsi* marshy lake, lake
Dasht *Farsi* desert, steppe
Daung *Burm.* mountain, hill
Dayr *Ar.* monastery
Debre *Amh.* hill
Deli *Ser.-Cr.* mountain
Deniz, -i *Turk.* sea
Département (Dépt.) *Fr.* first-order administrative division
Dere *Turk.* stream
Desierto (Des.) *Span.* desert
Détroit *Fr.* strait
Dhar *Ar.* region, mountain range
Diep *Dut.* channel
Dijk *Dut.* dyke
Ding *Chin.* mountain
Dingzi *Chin.* hill, mountain
Djebel (Dj.) *Ar.* mountain
-djúp *Ice.* fjord
-djupet *Swe.* channel, sound
-Do *Jap., Kor.* island
Dolina *Russ.* valley
Dolna, Dolni *Bulg.* lower
Dolna, Dolne, Dolny *Russ.* lower
Dolni *Czec.* lower
Dolok (D.) *Malay* mountain
-dong *Kor.* village, town
Dong *Chin.* east, eastern
Donja, Donji *Ser.-Cr.* lower
-dorf *Ger.* village
-dorp *Afr.* village
-drif *Afr.* ford
-dybet *Dan.* marine channel
Dzong *Tib.* town, settlement
Dzüün *Mong.* east, eastern

-egga *Nor.* peak
-eiland, -en (eil.) *Afr., Dut.* island(s)
Eilean *Gae.* island
-elv, -a *Nor.* river
Embalse *Span.* reservoir
'Emeq *Heb.* plain, valley
Ensenada *Span.* bay
Erg *Ar.* sand desert
Estero *Span.* estuary
Estrada *Span.* bay
Estrecho *Span.* strait
Estuaire *Fr.* estuary
Estuario *Span.* estuary
Étang *Fr.* lagoon, lake
-ey, -jar *Ice.* island(s)
-ežeras *Lith.* lake
-ezers *Lat.* lake

Falaise *Fr.* cliff
-fallet *Swe.* waterfall
Farihy *Malag.* lake
Faro *Span.* lighthouse
-feld *Ger.* field
-fell *Ice.* mountain, hill
Feng *Chin.* mountain range
Fiume (F.) *It.* river
-fjäll, -en, -et *Swe.* hill(s), mountain(s), ridge
-fjärden *Swe.* fjord
Fjeld *Dan.* mountain
-fjell, -et *Nor.* mountain range
-fjord, -en *Dan., Nor., Swe.* fjord
-fjorður *Ice.* fjord, bay, inlet
Fleuve (Fl.) *Fr.* river
-flói *Ice.* bay, marshy country
Fluss (F.) *Ger.* river
Foce, Foci *It.* mouth(s)
Folyó (F.) *Hung.* river
-fonn *Nor.* glacier
-fontein *Afr.* fountain, spring
Forêt *Fr.* forest
-fors, -en *Swe.* waterfall, rapids
-foss, -en *Ice., Nor.* waterfall
Forst *Ger.* forest
Foum *Ar.* pass
Fuente *Span.* source
-furt *Ger.* ford
Fylke *Nor.* first-order administrative division

-gang *Chin.* bay, harbour
-gang *Kor.* river
Ganga *Hin., Sin.* river
Gangri *Tib.* mountain
Gaoyuan *Chin.* plateau
-gat *Dan.* sound
-Gata *Jap.* lake
-gau *Ger.* district
-Gawa *Jap.* river
Gebel (G.) *Ar.* mountain
Gebirge (Geb.) *Ger.* hills, mountains
Gezirat, Geziret *Ar.* island
Ghat *Hin.* range of hills
Ghiol *Rom.* lake
Ghubbat *Ar.* bay, inlet
Gjiri *Alb.* bay
Gjol *Alb.* lagoon, lake
Glava (Gl.) *Ser.-Cr.* mountain, peak
Glen *Gae.* valley
Gletscher (Gl.) *Ger.* glacier
Gobi *Mong.* desert
Gol *Mong.* river
Göl *Azeri, Turk.* lake
Golfe (G.) *Fr.* gulf
Golfo (G.) *It., Span.* gulf
Gölü *Turk.* lake
Gomba *Tib.* settlement
Gora, Góra *Bulg., Russ., Ser.-Cr., Pol.* mountain
Gorje *Ser.-Cr.* hills, mountains
Gorno *Russ.* mountainous
-gorod *Russ.* small town
Gory, Góry *Pol., Russ.* mountain
-grad *Bulg. Russ., Ser.-Cr.* town, city
-grada *Russ.* ridge
Gran *It., Span.* big, great
Grand, -e *Fr.* big, great
Groot (Gt.) *Afr., Dut.* big, great
Gross, -e, -en, -er *Ger.* big, great(er)
Grupo *Span.* group
Gruppo *It.* group
Guan *Chin.* pass
Guba (G.) *Russ.* bay
-Guntō *Jap.* island group
Gunong, Gunung (G.) *Indo., Malay* mountain
Gură *Rom.* passage

Hadabat *Ar.* plateau
Hadjer *Ar.* mountain
-hafen *Ger.* harbour, port
Haff *Ger.* bay, lagoon
Hai *Chin.* lake, sea
Haixia *Chin.* channel, strait
Halbinsel *Ger.* peninsula
Halvø *Dan.* peninsula
Halvøya *Nor.* peninsula
Hāmad, Hamada, Hammādah, Hammādat *Ar.* stony desert, plateau
-hamn *Swe., Nor.* harbour, anchorage
Hāmūn *Farsi* marsh, lake
-Hantō *Jap.* peninsula
Har(e) *Heb.* hill(s), mountain(s)
Hassi (Hi.) *Ar.* well
-haug *Nor.* hill
Hav, Havet *Nor., Swe.* sea
-havn *Dan., Nor.* bay, harbour
Havre *Fr.* harbour
Hawd *Ar.* oasis
Hawr *Ar.* lake, marsh
He *Chin.* river
-hegység *Hung.* hills, forest
Heide *Ger.* heath, moor
Helodranon' *Malag.* bay
Higashi *Jap.* east, eastern
-ho *Kor.* lake
-hø *Nor.* peak
Hoch *Ger.* high
Hochland *Afr.* highland
Hoek, -hoek *Afr., Dut.* cape, point
-höfn *Ice.* harbour, port
-hög, -en, -högar, -högarna *Swe.* hill(s), peak, mountain
Höhe *Ger.* height
Hohen *Ger.* high, upper
-hoi *Chin.* bay
-høj, -e *Dan.* hills
-holm, -holme, -holmen *Dan., Nor., Swe.* island
Hon *Viet.* island
Hoog *Dut.* high
Hora *Czec., Ukr.* mountain
-horn *Ger.* peak
Hory *Czec.* mountains, hills
-hot *Mong.* town
-hoved *Dan.* point, headland, peninsula
-hrad *Czec.* town
Hráun *Ice.* lava
-hsi *Chin.* river
-hsia *Chin.* gorge, strait
-hsien *Chin.* district
Hu *Chin.* lake, reservoir
Huk *Dan., Ger.* cape
-huk *Swe.* cape
Huken *Nor.* cape

Idd *Ar.* well
Idehan *Ar., Ber.* sandy plain, dunes
-ike *Jap.* lake
Île(s) (I(s).) *Fr.* island(s)
Ilha(s) (I(s).) *Port.* island(s)
imeni *Russ.* 'in the name of'
Inish *Gae.* island
Insel(n) (I.) *Ger.* island(s)
Irmak *Turk.* river
'Irq *Ar.* dunes
Isla(s) (I(s).) *Span.* island(s)
Iso *Fin.* big, great
Isol, -a, -e (I.) *It.* island(s)
Isthme *Fr.* isthmus
Istmo *Span.* isthmus
-iwa *Jap.* island

Jabal *Ar.* mountain range
Järv *Est.* lake
järvi *Fin.* lake, bay, pond
-jaur, -javre *Lap.* lake
Jazā'ir *Ar.* islands
Jazīra, jazīrat *Ar.* island
Jazireh *Farsi* island
Jebel *Ar.* mountain
Jezero *Ser.-Cr.* lake
Jezioro *Pol.* lake
Jiang *Chin.* river
Jiao *Chin.* cape
-Jima *Jap.* island
Jøkulen *Nor.* glacier, ice cap
-joki *Fin.* river
-jökull *Ice.* glacier, ice cap
Jūras Līcis *Lat.* bay, gulf

Kaap (K.) *Afr.* cape
-kai *Jap.* bay, channel, sea
-kaikyō *Jap.* strait
-kaise *Lap.* mountain
kalnas *Lith.* hill
Kamennyy *Russ.* stony
Kampong *Cam.* village
Kampung *Malay* village
-kanaal *Dut.* canal
Kanal *Dan.* channel, gulf
Kanal *Ger., Swe.* canal
-kanal *Ser.-Cr.* channel, canal
Kanava *Fin.* canal
Kang *Kor.* river, bay
Kap (K.) *Dan., Ger.* cape, point
-kapp *Nor.* cape, point
-kaupstaður *Ice.* market town
-kaupunki *Fin.* town
Kavīr *Farsi* salt desert
Kébir *Ar.* great
Kecil *Malay* lesser, little
Kefar *Heb.* village, hamlet
-Ken *Jap.* first-order administrative division
Kep, -i (K.) *Alb.* cape
Kepulauan (Kep.) *Indo., Malay* archipelago
Keski- *Fin.* middle, central
Khalīg, Khalīj *Ar.* gulf
-khamba *Tib.* source, spring
Khawr *Ar.* bay, channel, wadi
Khlong *Thai* river
Kho Khot *Thai* isthmus
Khōr *Farsi* bay, estuary
Khrebet *Russ.* mountain range
Kita- *Jap.* north
Klein,-e, -er *Ger.* small
-klint *Dan.* cliff
Klintar *Swe.* hills
-kloof *Afr.* gorge, pass
Knude *Dan.* point
-Ko *Jap.* lake
Ko *Thai* island
-kōchi *Jap.* mountainous region
-kōgen *Jap.* plateau
Kohi *Pash.* mountains
Kol *Kaz., Kyrg.* lake
Kólpos *Gr., Turk.* gulf, bay
Kolymskoye *Russ.* mountain range
Kompong *Malay* landing place
-kop *Afr.* hill
-kopf *Ger.* hill
-köping *Swe.* market town
Körfäzi *Azer.* gulf
Körfezi *Turk.* gulf
Kosa *Russ., Ukr.* spit
-koski *Fin.* rapids
-kraal *Afr.* native village
-kraj *Czec., Pol., Ser.-Cr.* region
Krasnyy *Russ.* red
Kryazh *Russ.* ridge, hills
Kuala *Malay* bay
-kuan *Chin.* pass
Kūh(ha) *Farsi* mountain(s)
Kul *Russ.* lake
-kulle *Swe.* hill
Kum *Russ.* sandy desert
Kumpu *Fin.* hill
Kwe *Burm.* bay, gulf
-kylä *Fin.* village
Kyst, -en *Dan., Nor.* coast
Kyun(zu) *Burm.* island(s)

La *Tib.* pass
-laagte *Afr.* watercourse

Lääni Fin. first-order administrative division
Lac (L.) Fr. lake
Lacul (L.) Rom. lake, lagoon
Lago (L.) It., Port., Span. lake, lagoon
Lagoa (L.) Port. lagoon
Lagos Port., Span. lakes
Laguna (L.) It., Span. lagoon, lake
Lagune (L.) Fr. lake
-laht Est. bay
Lahti Fin. bay, gulf, cove
Lakhti Russ. bay, gulf
Lam Thai river
Lampi Fin. lake
Län Swe. first-order administrative division
Land Ger. first-order administrative division
-land Dan. region
-land Afr., Nor. land, province
Lande Fr. heath
Laut Indo. sea
Law Gae. hill, mountain
Licis Lat. gulf
Lido It. beach, shore
Liedao Chin. islands
Lilla Swe. small
Lille Dan., Nor. small
Liman Russ. bay, gulf
Límni (L.) Gr. lake
Ling Chin. mountain range
-linna Fin. fort
Llano Span. prairie, plain
Llyn Welsh lake
Loch (L.) Gae. lake, inlet
Lough (L.) Gae. lake, inlet
Lum Alb. river
Lund Dan. forest
-lund, -en Swe. wood(s)
-luoto Fin. island

-maa Est. island
Madīnat Ar. town, city
Madiq Ar. strait
Maja Alb. mountains
-mäki Fin. hill, hillside
Mal Alb. mountain
Maloye, Malyy, Malyya Russ. little, small
Mala, Mali, Malo Ser.-Cr. little, small
Malaya Belo. small
Malé Czec., Slovak small
Mali Alb. mountain
-man Kor. bay
Mar Span. lagoon, sea
Marais Fr. marsh
Mare It. sea
Mare Rom. great
Marisma Span. marsh
-mark Dan., Nor. land
Marsâ Ar. anchorage, bay, inlet
Masabb Ar. river mouth, estuary
Massif Fr. upland, mountains
Mato Port. forest
Mazar Farsi shrine, tomb
Meer, -meer Afr., Dut., Ger. lake, sea
-men Chin. bay, gorge, channel
Mesto Ser.-Cr., Czec. town
Mezzo It. middle
Midbar Heb. wilderness
Mierzeja Pol. spit
Mifraz Heb. bay
Mina Ar. port
Minami Jap. south, southern
-misaki Jap. cape, point
Mittel Ger. central, middle
-mo Nor., Swe. heath, island
-mon Swe. heath
Mong Burm. town
Mont(s) (Mt(s).) Fr. hill(s), mountain(s)
Montagna (Mt.) It. mountain
Montagne(s) (Mt(s).) Fr. hill(s), mountain(s)
Montaña(s) (Mt(s).) Span. mountain(s)
Montanyes Cat. mountains
Monte(s) (Mte(s).) It., Port., Span. mountain(s)
Monti (Mti.) It. mountains
More Russ. sea
Mörön Mong. river
Moyen Fr. central, middle
Muang Malay town
Mui Viet. cape
Mull Gae. promontory
Mund, -mund Afr. mouth
Munkhafed Ar. depression
Munte (Mte.) Rom. mount
Munţi(i) (Mti.) Rom. mountain(s)
Muong Malay village
Myit Burm. river
Myitwanya Burm. mouths of river
Mynydd Welsh mountain
-myr Nor., Swe. swamp
-mýri Ice. swamp
Mys (M.) Russ. cape

-Nada Jap. bay, gulf
-næs Dan. point, cape
Nafūd Ar. sandy desert
Nagorye Russ. hills, mountains
Nagy Hung. big
Nahal (N.) Heb. river
Nahr (N.) Ar. river, stream
Najd Ar. plateau, pass
Nakhon Thai town
Nam Kor., Viet. river
-nam Kor. south
Namakzār Per. salt flat
Nan Chin. south, southern
-nao Chin. lake
-näs Swe. cape
Neder Dut. lower
Nedre Nor. lower
Nei Chin. inner
Nek Afr. pass
-nes Ice., Nor. cape
Ness, -ness Gae. promontory, cape
Nevada, Nevado Span. snow-capped mountain
Nez Fr. cape
Nieder Ger. lower
-niemi Fin. cape, point, peninsula, island
Nieuw, -e Dut. new
Nishi Jap. west, western
Nisos, Nisoi Gr. island(s)
Nizhneye, Nizhniy Russ. lower
Nizina Belo., Pol. lowland
Nizmennost Russ. plain, lowland
Nízní Czec. lower
Noord Dut. north, northern
Nord Fr. north, northern
Norra Swe. north, northern
Nørre Dan. north, northern
Norte Port., Span. north, northern
Nos Bulg., Russ. cape, point
Nosy Malag. island
Nouveau, Nouvelle Fr. new
Nova, Novi Bulg., Port., Serb.-Cr. new
Novaya, Novo, Novoye, Novyy Russ. new
Nové, Nový Czec., Slovak new
Novo Port. new
Nowa, Nowe, Nowy Pol. new
Nudo Span. mountain
Nueva, Nuevo Span. new
Nur Chin. lake
Nur Tib. peak
Nuruu Mong. mountain range
Nusa Indo. island
Nuur Mong. lake
Ny Dan., Nor., Swe. new

-ø Dan., Nor. island
-ö Swe. island,
-öar, -na Swe. islands
Ober Ger., Ukr. upper
Oblast Russ. administrative division
Öbor Mong. inner
Occidental Fr., Span. western
-odde Dan., Nor. point, peninsula, cape
Oeste Span. west, western
Oglat Ar. well
Oji Alb. bay
Ojo Span. spring
-Oki Jap. bay
-ön Swe. island
Ondör Mong. upper
Oost(er) Dut. east(ern)
Oraşu Rom. city
Ord Gae. point
Óri Gr. mountains
Oriental, -e Fr., Span. east, eastern
Órmos Gr. bay
Óros Gr. mountain(s)
Ort Ger. point, cape
Ost Ger. east
Øst(er) Den., Nor. east(ern)
Öst(ra) Swe. east(ern)
Ostriv Ukr. island
Ostrov(a) Russ. island(s)
Otok(i) Ser.-Cr. island(s)
Ouabi, Ouadi (O.) Ar. dry watercourse, wadi
Oud, -e Dut. old
Oued, -i (O.) Ar. watercourse
Ouest Fr. west, western
Ouzan Farsi river
Ova, -si Turk. plains, lowlands
Over- (Dan.), Dut. upper
Över-, Övre Nor., Swe. upper
-øy, -a Nor. island(s)
Oya Hin. point
Oya Sin. river
Ozero, Ozera (Oz.) Russ., Ukr. lake(s)

-pää Fin. hill(s), mountain
Pahta Lapp. hill
Pampa(s) Span. plain(s)
Pantanal Port. marsh
Pantano Span. reservoir
Pantao Chin. peninsula
Parbat Urdu mountain
Pas Fr. strait
Paso (P.) Span. pass
Passage Fr. channel
Passe Fr. channel
Passo (P.) It. pass
Pasul (P.) Rom. pass
Patam Hin. small village
Patna, -patnam Hin. small village
Pegunungan Indo., Malay mountain range
Pei, -pei Chin. north
Pélagos Gr. sea
Pen Welsh hill
Peña Span. rock, peak
Pendi Chin. basin, depression
Péninsule Fr. peninsula
Penisola (Pen.) It. peninsula
Pereval (Per.) Russ. pass
Pervo-, Pervyy- Russ. first
Pertuis Fr. channel, strait
Peski Russ. sand desert
Petit, -e Fr. small
Phanom Thai mountain
Phnum Cam. mountain
Phou Lao. mountain
Phu Thai, Viet. mountain
Piano It. plain
Pic Cat., Fr. peak
Pico(s) Span. peak(s)
-piggen Dan. peak
Pik Russ. peak
Pingyuan Chin. plain
Pique Fr. peak
Piton Fr. peak
Pivostriv Ukr. peninsula
Piz, Pizzo It. peak
Plage Fr. beach
Plaine Fr. plain
Planalto Port. plateau
Planina (Pl.) Bulg., Ser.-Cr. mountain range
Plato Russ., Bulg. plateau
Playa Span. beach
-po Chin. lake, wetland
Pointe (Pte.) Fr. point, cape
Pojezierze Pol. lakes
Polder Dut. reclaimed farmland
-pólis Gr. city, town
Poluostrov (Pov.) Russ. peninsula
Połwysep Pol. peninsula
Pont Fr. bridge
Ponta (Pta.) Port. point, cape
Ponte Port. bridge
Poort Afr. passage, gate
-poort Dut. port
Porta Port. pass
Porţile Rom. gate
Portillo Span. pass
Porto It., Port., Span. port
Potámi, Potamós Gr. river
Pradesh Hin. state
Praia Port. beach, shore
Presa Span. reservoir
Presqu'île Fr. peninsula
Prokhod Bulg. pass
Proliv Russ. strait
Promontorio Span. promontory
Průsmyk (Pr.) Czec. pass
Pueblo Span. village
Puerto (Pto.) Span. port
Puig Cat. peak
Pulau (P.) Indo., Malay island
Puna Span. desert plateau
Puncak Indo. peak
Punta (Pta.) It., Span. point, peak
Puy Fr. peak

Qal'at Ar. fort
Qanat Ar. canal
Qasr Ar. fort
Qiryat Heb. town
Qiuling Chin. plateau
Qolleh Farsi mountain
-qundao Chin. islands

Rach Viet. river
Rags Lat. cape
Rambla Cat. river
Ramlat Ar. sandy desert
Rāo (R.) Port. river
Rann Hin. swampy region
Rao I.-C. river
Ras Amh., Ar., Farsi cape, point
Récif(s) Fr. reef(s)
Recife(s) Port. reef(s)
Reka Bulg. river
Repede Rom. rapids
Reprêsa Port. reservoir
Reshteh Farsi mountain range
-rettō Jap. group of islands, chain
Ria Port., Span. estuary, bay
Ribeirão (R.) Port. river
Ribera (R.) Span. river bank
Rijeka Ser.-Cr. river
Rio (R.) Port., Span. river
Rivier (R.) Afr., Dut. river
Riviera It. coastal plain, coast
Rivière (R.) Fr. river
Roca Span. rock
Rocca It. rock, peak
Roche Fr. rock
Rt Ser.-Cr. cape, point
Rubh', Rubha Gae. cape, point
-rück Ger. ridge
Rūd Farsi stream, river
Rudohorie Slovak mountains
Rzeka (R.) Pol. river

-saar Est. island
-saari Fin. island
Sabkhat, Sabkhet Ar. salt flats
Sadd Ar. dam
Sagar,-a Hin., Urdu lake
Sahrâ Ar. desert
-Saki Jap. cape, point
Salar Span. salt flat
Salina(s) Span. salt marsh(es)
-salmi Fin. strait, sound, lake, channel
Saltsjöbad Swe. resort
-Sammyaku Jap. mountain range
Samut Thai gulf
San (S.) It., Port., Span. saint
-San Jap., Kor. hill, mountain
-Sanchi Jap. mountain range
Sankt (St.) Ger., Russ. saint
-sanmaek Kor. mountain range
-sanmyaku Jap. mountain range
Santa (Sta.) It., Port., Span. saint
Santo (Sto.) It. Port., Span. saint
São (S.) Port. saint
Sarīr Ar. desert
Sasso It. mountain
Satu Rom. village
Saurums Lat. strait
Sebkha, Sebkhet Ar. salt flat
See, -see Ger. lake
-şehir Turk. town
Selat Indo., Malay strait
Selatan Indo. southern
-selkä Fin. bay, lake, ridge, hills
Selo Ser.-Cr., Russ. village
Selva Port., Span. forest, wood
Seno Span. bay, sound
Serir Ar. stony desert
Serra (Sa.) Cat., Port. range of hills
Serranía Span. mountain ridge
Severo, Severnaya, Severnoye, Severnyy (Sev.) Russ. north, northern
Sfântu Rom. saint
Shahr, -shahr Farsi city, town
Shamo Chin. desert
Shan Chin. hills, mountains
Shankou Chin. pass
Shanmo Chin. mountain range
Sharm Ar. bay
Shatt Ar. river mouth, estuary
-Shima Jap. island
Shimāli Ar. northern
-Shotō Jap. group of islands
-shui Chin. river
-shuiku Chin. reservoir
Sierra (Sa.) Span. mountain range
-sjö, -sjön, -sjø Swe., Nor. lake
-sjøen Dan. sea
-sjór Ice. lake
-sker Ice. island
-skär Swe. island, rock, cape
-skog, -skogen Nor., Swe. wood(s)
-skov Dan. forest
Slieve Gae. hill, mountain
Sø Dan., Nor. lake
Söder, Södra Swe. south, southern
Sør Nor. south, southern
Solonchak Russ. salt lake, marsh
Sønder, Søndra Dan. south, southern
Song Viet. river
Souk Ar. market
-spitze Ger. peak, mountain
-spruit Afr. stream
Sredna, Sredno Bulg. middle, central
Sredne, Sredneye Russ. middle, central
Srednja Ser.-Cr. middle, central
-stad Afr., Nor., Swe. town
-stadt Ger. town
-staður Ice. town
Stara, Stari Ser.-Cr. old
Stará, Staré, Stary Czec. old
Staraya, Staroye, Staryy Russ. old
Stare, Staro, Stary Ukr. old
Stausee Ger. reservoir
Stenón Gr. strait, pass
Step Russ. steppe
Stor, -a Swe. big
Store Dan. big
-strand Dan., Ger., Nor., Swe. beach
-strede Nor. straits
Strelka Russ. spit
-strete Nor. straits
Stretto (Str.) It. strait
Strædet (Str.) Dan. strait
-ström, -strömmen Swe. stream(s)
-stroom Afr. large river
Sud Fr. south, southern
Süd, -er Ger. south, southern
Suid Afr. south, southern
-Suidō Jap. strait, channel
Sul Port. south, southern
Sûn Burm. cape
-sund, -et Swe., Nor. sound, estuary, inlet
Sungai Indo., Malay river
Sur Span. south, southern
Sveti Bulg. saint
Syd Dan., Swe. south, southern
Sýsla Ice. first-order administrative division

-tag Uighur mountain
Tai -tai Chin. tower
-Take Jap. mountain
Tal Mong. plain, steppe
-tal Ger. valley
Tall Ar. hills
Tanjona Malag. cape, point
Tanjung, Tanjong (Tg.) Indo., Malay. cape, point
Tao Chin. island
Tasik Malay lake
Tassili Ar. rocky plateau
Tau Russ. mountain range
Taung Burm. mountain
Taungdan. Burm. mountain range
Taunggya Burm. pass
-tekojärvi Fin. reservoir
Teluk Indo., Malay bay, gulf
Ténéré Berb. desert
Tengah Indo. middle, central
-thal Ger. valley
Thok Tib. town
Tien Chin. lake, marsh
Tierra Span. land, country
Timur Indo. eastern
-tind Nor. peak
-ting Chin. mountain
Tjärn, -en, -et Swe. lake
-Tō Jap. island
Tong Kor. village, town
Tong Burm., Thai, Kor. mountain range
Tonlé Cam. lake
Top Dut. peak
-topp, -en Nor. peak
-träsk Swe. lake, swamp
Tsangpo Tib. large river
Tso Tib. lake
Tsu Jap. entrance, bay
Tsui Chin. cape, point
Tulur Ar. hill
-tunturi Fin. hill(s), mountain(s), ridge

Uad Ar. dry watercourse, wadi
Über Ger. upper
-udde, -udden Swe. point, cape
Uebi Som. river
Ujung Indo., Malay cape
Unter- Ger. lower
Us Mong. water
Ust, Ustye Russ. river mouth
Utara Indo. north, northern
Uttar Hin. north, northern
Uul Mong., Russ. mountain range

-vaara Fin. hill, mountain ridge, peak
Vaart Dut. canal
-våg Nor. bay
Val Fr., Port., Span. valley
Valea Rom. valley
-vall, -en Swe. mountain
Valle It., Span. valley
Vallée Fr. valley
Valli It. lake, lagoon
-város Hung. town
-varre Nor. mountain
Väst, Västra Swe. west, western
-vatn Ice., Nor. lake
-vatnet Nor. lake
-vatten, vattnet Swe. lake
-vecchio It. old
Vechi Rom. old
-ved, -veden Swe. hills
Veld, -veld Afr. field
Velha, Velho Port. old
Velika, Velike, Veliki, Veliko Ser.-Cr., Slov. big, large
Velikaya, Velikiy Russ. big, large
Velká, Velké, Velký Czec. big, large
Verkhne, Verkhniy Russ. upper
-vesi Fin. water, lake, bay, sound, strait
Vest, Vester, Vestre Dan., Nor. west, western
-vidda Nor. plateau
Vieille, Vieux Fr. old
Vieja, Viejo Span. old
Vig Dan. bay, inlet, cove, lagoon, lake
-vík Ice. bay
-vik, -a, -en Nor., Swe. bay, gulf, inlet, lake
Vila Port. small town
Villa Span. town
Ville Fr. town
Vinh Viet. bay
Vîrful (Vf.) Rom. peak, mountain
-viz Hung. river
-víztároló Hung. reservoir
-vlei Afr. lake, salt pan
-vliet Dut. canal
-vloer Afr. salt pan
Vodokhranilishche (Vdkhr.) Russ. reservoir
Vodoskovyshche (Vdskh.) Ukr. reservoir
Volcán (Vol.) Span. volcano, mountain
Vorota Russ. pass, channel, strait
Vostochno, Vostochnyy Russ. east, eastern
-vötn Ice. lakes
Vozvyshennost Russ. heights, uplands
Vozyera Belo. lake
Vrata Bulg. gate, pass
Vrchovina Czec. mountainous country
Vrch(y) Czec. mountain (range)
Vung Viet. bay, gulf
-vuori Fin. mountain, hill
Vychodné Slovak east, eastern
Vysochyna Ukr. upland

-waard Dut. polder
Wadi (W.) Ar. dry watercourse
Wâhât Ar. oasis
Wald Ger. forest, mountains
-Wan Chin., Jap. bay, harbour
Wāw Ar. well
Webi Amh. river
Wes Afr. west, western
Wielka, Wielki, Wielko Pol. big, large
Woestyn Afr. desert
Wysoka, Wysoki Pol. upper
Wyżyna Pol. plateau

Xi Chin. river
Xia Chin. gorge, strait
Xiao Chin. small

Yam Heb. sea
-Yama Jap. mountain
-yan Chin. gorge, island
Yang Chin. bay, sea, sound
Yangi Russ. new
Yazovir Bulg. reservoir
Yeni Turk. new
Yli Fin. upper
Ynys Welsh island
Yoma Burm. mountain range
Ytre-, Ytter- Nor., Swe. outer
-yuan Chin. stream
Yugo- Ser.-Cr. south, southern
Yunhe Chin. canal
Yuzhni, Yuzhno Russ. south, southern

-Zaki Jap. point
Zalew Pol. lagoon, swamp
Zaliv Russ. bay, gulf
-Zan Jap. mountain
Zangbo Tib. stream, river
Zapadnaya, Zapadno, Zapadnyi (Zap.) Russ. west, western
Zatoka Pol., Ukr. bay, gulf
-zee Dut. lake, sea
Zemlya Russ. land, island(s)
Zhang Chin. mountain
-zhou Chin. island
Zhong Chin. middle, central
Zhou Chin. island
Zizhiqu Chin. autonomous region
Zuid, Zuider Dut. south, southern

INDEX TO WORLD MAPS

How to use the index

The index contains the names of all the principal places and features shown on the World Maps. Each name is followed by an additional entry in italics giving the country or region within which it is located. The alphabetical order of names composed of two or more words is governed primarily by the first word and then by the second. This is an example of the rule:

Mīr Kūh, *Iran*	97 E8	26 22N 58 55 E
Mīr Shahdād, *Iran*	97 E8	26 15N 58 29 E
Mira, *Italy*	45 C9	45 26N 12 8 E
Mira por vos Cay, *Bahamas*	165 B5	22 9N 74 30W
Miraj, *India*	94 F2	16 50N 74 45 E

Physical features composed of a proper name (Erie) and a description (Lake) are positioned alphabetically by the proper name. The description is positioned after the proper name and is usually abbreviated:

Erie, L., *N. Amer.* 150 D4 42 15N 81 0W

Where a description forms part of a settlement or administrative name however, it is always written in full and put in its true alphabetic position:

Mount Olive, *U.S.A.* 156 E7 39 4N 89 44W

Names beginning with M' and Mc are indexed as if they were spelled Mac. Names beginning St. are alphabetized under Saint, but Sankt, Sint, Sant', Santa and San are all spelt in full and are alphabetized accordingly. If the same place name occurs two or more times in the index and all are in the same country, each is followed by the name of the administrative subdivision in which it is located.

The number in bold type which follows each name in the index refers to the number of the map page where that feature or place will be found. This is usually the largest scale at which the place or feature appears.

The letter and figure which are in bold type immediately after the page number give the grid square on the map page, within which the feature is situated. The letter represents the latitude and the figure the longitude. A lower case letter immediately after the page number refers to an inset map on that page.

In some cases the feature itself may fall within the specified square, while the name is outside. This is usually the case only with features which are larger than a grid square.

The geographical co-ordinates which follow the letter-figure references give the latitude and longitude of each place. The first co-ordinate indicates latitude – the distance north or south of the Equator. The second co-ordinate indicates longitude – the distance east or west of the Greenwich Meridian. Both latitude and longitude are measured in degrees and minutes (there are 60 minutes in a degree).

The latitude is followed by N(orth) or S(outh) and the longitude by E(ast) or W(est).

Rivers are indexed to their mouths or confluences, and carry the symbol ➜ after their names. The following symbols are also used in the index: ■ country, ☑ overseas territory or dependency, ☐ first order administrative area, △ national park, ◠ other park (provincial park, nature reserve or game reserve), ✈ (LHR) principal airport (and location identifier).

How to pronounce place names

English-speaking people usually have no difficulty in reading and pronouncing correctly English place names. However, foreign place name pronunciations may present many problems. Such problems can be minimised by following some simple rules. However, these rules cannot be applied to all situations, and there will be many exceptions.

1. In general, stress each syllable equally, unless your experience suggests otherwise.
2. Pronounce the letter 'a' as a broad 'a' as in 'arm'.
3. Pronounce the letter 'e' as a short 'e' as in 'elm'.
4. Pronounce the letter 'i' as a cross between a short 'i' and long 'e', as the two 'i's in 'California'.
5. Pronounce the letter 'o' as an intermediate 'o' as in 'soft'.
6. Pronounce the letter 'u' as an intermediate 'u' as in 'sure'.
7. Pronounce consonants hard, except in the Romance-language areas where 'g's are likely to be pronounced softly like 'j' in 'jam'; 'j' itself may be pronounced as 'y'; and 'x's may be pronounced as 'h'.
8. For names in mainland China, pronounce 'q' like the 'ch' in 'chin', 'x' like the 'sh' in 'she', 'zh' like the 'j' in 'jam', and 'z' as if it were spelled 'dz'. In general pronounce 'a' as in 'father', 'e' as in 'but', 'i' as in 'keep', 'o' as in 'or', and 'u' as in 'rule'.

Moreover, English has no diacritical marks (accent and pronunciation signs), although some languages do. The following is a brief and general guide to the pronunciation of those most frequently used in the principal Western European languages.

		Pronunciation as in
French	é	day and shows that the e is to be pronounced; e.g. Orléans.
	è	mare
	î	used over any vowel and does not affect pronunciation; shows contraction of the name, usually omission of 's' following a vowel.
	ç	's' before 'a', 'o' and 'u'.
	ë, ï, ü	over 'e', 'i' and 'u' when they are used with another vowel and shows that each is to be pronounced.
German	ä	fate
	ö	fur
	ü	no English equivalent; like French 'tu'
Italian	à, é	over vowels and indicates stress.
Portuguese	ã, õ	vowels pronounced nasally.
	ç	boss
	á	shows stress
	ô	shows that a vowel has an 'i' or 'u' sound combined with it.
Spanish	ñ	canyon
	ü	pronounced as w and separately from adjoining vowels.
	á	usually indicates that this is a stressed vowel.

Abbreviations

A.C.T. – Australian Capital Territory
A.R. – Autonomous Region
Afghan. – Afghanistan
Afr. – Africa
Ala. – Alabama
Alta. – Alberta
Amer. – America(n)
Arch. – Archipelago
Ariz. – Arizona
Ark. – Arkansas
Atl. Oc. – Atlantic Ocean
B. – Baie, Bahía, Bay, Bucht, Bugt
B.C. – British Columbia
Bangla. – Bangladesh
Barr. – Barrage
Bos.-H. – Bosnia-Herzegovina
C. – Cabo, Cap, Cape, Coast
C.A.R. – Central African Republic
C. Prov. – Cape Province
Calif. – California
Cat. – Catarata
Cent. – Central
Chan. – Channel
Colo. – Colorado
Conn. – Connecticut
Cord. – Cordillera
Cr. – Creek
Czech. – Czech Republic
D.C. – District of Columbia
Del. – Delaware
Dem. – Democratic
Dep. – Dependency
Des. – Desert
Dét. – Détroit
Dist. – District
Dj. – Djebel
Domin. – Dominica
Dom. Rep. – Dominican Republic
E. – East

E. Salv. – El Salvador
Eq. Guin. – Equatorial Guinea
Est. – Estrecho
Falk. Is. – Falkland Is.
Fd. – Fjord
Fla. – Florida
Fr. – French
G. – Golfe, Golfo, Gulf, Guba, Gebel
Ga. – Georgia
Gt. – Great, Greater
Guinea-Biss. – Guinea-Bissau
H.K. – Hong Kong
H.P. – Himachal Pradesh
Hants. – Hampshire
Harb. – Harbor, Harbour
Hd. – Head
Hts. – Heights
I.(s). – Île, Ilha, Insel, Isla, Island, Isle
Ill. – Illinois
Ind. – Indiana
Ind. Oc. – Indian Ocean
Ivory C. – Ivory Coast
J. – Jabal, Jebel
Jaz. – Jazīrah
Junc. – Junction
K. – Kap, Kapp
Kans. – Kansas
Kep. – Kepulauan
Ky. – Kentucky
L. – Lac, Lacul, Lago, Lagoa, Lake, Limni, Loch, Lough
La. – Louisiana
Ld. – Land
Liech. – Liechtenstein
Lux. – Luxembourg
Mad. P. – Madhya Pradesh
Madag. – Madagascar

Man. – Manitoba
Mass. – Massachusetts
Md. – Maryland
Me. – Maine
Medit. S. – Mediterranean Sea
Mich. – Michigan
Minn. – Minnesota
Miss. – Mississippi
Mo. – Missouri
Mont. – Montana
Mozam. – Mozambique
Mt.(s) – Mont, Montaña, Mountain
Mte. – Monte
Mti. – Monti
N. – Nord, Norte, North, Northern, Nouveau
N.B. – New Brunswick
N.C. – North Carolina
N. Cal. – New Caledonia
N. Dak. – North Dakota
N.H. – New Hampshire
N.I. – North Island
N.J. – New Jersey
N. Mex. – New Mexico
N.S. – Nova Scotia
N.S.W. – New South Wales
N.W.T. – North West Territory
N.Y. – New York
N.Z. – New Zealand
Nac. – Nacional
Nat. – National
Nebr. – Nebraska
Neths. – Netherlands
Nev. – Nevada
Nfld & L.. – Newfoundland and Labrador
Nic. – Nicaragua
O. – Oued, Ouadi
Occ. – Occidentale

Okla. – Oklahoma
Ont. – Ontario
Or. – Orientale
Oreg. – Oregon
Os. – Ostrov
Oz. – Ozero
P. – Pass, Passo, Pasul, Pulau
P.E.I. – Prince Edward Island
Pa. – Pennsylvania
Pac. Oc. – Pacific Ocean
Papua N.G. – Papua New Guinea
Pass. – Passage
Peg. – Pegunungan
Pen. – Peninsula, Péninsule
Phil. – Philippines
Pk. – Peak
Plat. – Plateau
Prov. – Province, Provincial
Pt. – Point
Pta. – Ponta, Punta
Pte. – Pointe
Qué. – Québec
Queens. – Queensland
R. – Rio, River
R.I. – Rhode Island
Ra. – Range
Raj. – Rajasthan
Recr. – Recreational, Récréatif
Reg. – Region
Rep. – Republic
Res. – Reserve, Reservoir
Rhld-Pfz. – Rheinland-Pfalz
S. – South, Southern, Sur
Si. Arabia – Saudi Arabia
S.C. – South Carolina
S. Dak. – South Dakota
S.I. – South Island
S. Leone – Sierra Leone
Sa. – Serra, Sierra

Sask. – Saskatchewan
Scot. – Scotland
Sd. – Sound
Serbia & M. – Serbia & Montenegro
Sev. – Severnaya
Sib. – Siberia
Sprs. – Springs
St. – Saint
Sta. – Santa
Ste. – Sainte
Sto. – Santo
Str. – Strait, Stretto
Switz. – Switzerland
Tas. – Tasmania
Tenn. – Tennessee
Terr. – Territory, Territoire
Tex. – Texas
Tg. – Tanjung
Trin. & Tob. – Trinidad & Tobago
U.A.E. – United Arab Emirates
U.K. – United Kingdom
U.S.A. – United States of America
Ut. P. – Uttar Pradesh
Va. – Virginia
Vdkhr. – Vodokhranilishche
Vdskh. – Vodoskhovyshche
Vf. – Vîrful
Vic. – Victoria
Vol. – Volcano
Vt. – Vermont
W. – Wadi, West
W. Va. – West Virginia
Wall. & F. Is. – Wallis and Futuna Is.
Wash. – Washington
Wis. – Wisconsin
Wlkp. – Wielkopolski
Wyo. – Wyoming
Yorks. – Yorkshire

A

A ’Âli an Nîl □, Sudan 107 F3 9 30N 33 0 E
A Baña, Spain 42 C2 42 58N 8 46W
A Cañiza, Spain 42 C2 42 13N 8 16W
A Coruña, Spain 42 B2 43 20N 8 25W
A Estrada, Spain 42 C2 42 43N 8 27W
A Fonsagrada, Spain 42 B3 43 8N 7 4W
A Guarda, Spain 42 C2 41 56N 8 52W
A Gudiña, Spain 42 C3 42 4N 7 8W
A Rúa, Spain 42 C3 42 24N 7 6W
Aachen, Germany 30 E2 50 45N 6 6 E
Aadorf, Switz. 33 B7 47 30N 8 55 E
Aalborg = Ålborg,
  Denmark 17 G3 57 2N 9 54 E
Aalen, Germany 31 G6 48 51N 10 6 E
Aalst, Belgium 24 D4 50 56N 4 2 E
Aalten, Neths. 24 C6 51 56N 6 35 E
Aalter, Belgium 24 C3 51 5N 3 28 E
Äänekoski, Finland 15 E21 62 36N 25 44 E
Aarau, Switz. 32 B6 47 23N 8 4 E
Aarberg, Switz. 32 B4 47 2N 7 16 E
Aarburg, Switz. 32 B5 47 19N 7 54 E
Aare →, Switz. 32 A6 47 33N 8 14 E
Aargau □, Switz. 32 B6 47 26N 8 10 E
Aarhus = Århus,
  Denmark 17 H4 56 8N 10 11 E
Aarlen = Arlon,
  Belgium 24 E5 49 42N 5 49 E
Aarschot, Belgium 24 D4 50 59N 4 49 E
Aarwangen, Switz. 32 B5 47 15N 7 46 E
Aasiaat, Greenland 10 D5 68 43N 52 56W
Ab-i-Istada, Afghan. 91 B2 32 29N 67 55 E
Ab-i-Panja =
  Pyandzh →, Asia 65 E4 37 6N 68 20 E
Aba, China 76 A3 32 59N 101 42 E
Aba, Dem. Rep. of
  the Congo 118 B3 3 58N 30 17 E
Aba, Nigeria 113 D6 5 10N 7 19 E
Âbâ, Jazîrat, Sudan 107 E3 13 30N 32 31 E
Abacaxis →, Brazil 169 D6 3 54 S 58 47W
Abaco I., Bahamas 164 A4 26 25N 77 10W
Abadab, J., Sudan 106 D4 18 53N 35 56 E
Ābādān, Iran 97 D6 30 22N 48 20 E
Abade, Ethiopia 107 F4 8 10N 38 3 E
Ābādeh, Iran 97 D7 31 8N 52 40 E
Abadin, Spain 42 B3 43 21N 7 29W
Abadla, Algeria 111 B4 31 2N 2 45W
Abaeté, Brazil 171 E2 19 9 S 45 27W
Abaeté →, Brazil 171 E2 19 9 S 45 12W
Abaetetuba, Brazil 170 B2 1 40 S 48 50W
Abagnar Qi, China 74 C9 43 52N 116 2 E
Abah, Tanjung,
  Indonesia 79 K18 8 46 S 115 38 E
Abai, Paraguay 175 B4 25 58 S 55 54W
Abak, Nigeria 113 E6 4 58N 7 50 E
Abakaliki, Nigeria 113 D6 6 22N 8 2 E
Abakan, Russia 67 D10 53 40N 91 10 E
Abala, Congo 114 C3 1 15N 15 35 E
Abala, Niger 113 C5 14 56N 3 2 E
Abalak, Niger 113 B6 15 28N 6 21 E
Abalemma, Algeria 111 D6 20 51N 5 59 E
Abalemma, Niger 113 B6 16 12N 7 50 E
Abalessa, Algeria 111 D5 22 58N 4 47 E
Abana, Turkey 100 B6 41 59N 34 1 E
Abancay, Peru 172 C3 13 35 S 72 55W
Abanga →, Gabon 114 C2 0 20 S 10 30 E
Abano Terme, Italy 45 C8 45 22N 11 46 E
Abapó, Bolivia 173 D5 18 48 S 63 25W
Abarán, Spain 41 G3 38 12N 1 23W
Abariringa, Kiribati 134 H10 2 50 S 171 40W
Abarqū, Iran 97 D7 31 10N 53 20 E
Abashiri, Japan 70 B12 44 0N 144 15 E
Abashiri-Wan, Japan 70 C12 44 0N 144 30 E
Abau, Papua N. G. 132 F5 10 11 S 148 46 E
Abaújszántó, Hungary 52 B6 48 16N 21 12 E
Abava →, Latvia 54 A8 57 6N 21 54 E
Abay = Nîl el
  Azraq →, Sudan 107 D3 15 38N 32 31 E
Abay, Kazakhstan 66 E8 49 38N 72 53 E
Abaya, L., Ethiopia 107 F4 6 30N 37 50 E
Abayita-Shala Lakes △,
  Ethiopia 107 F4 7 40N 38 37 E
Abaza, Russia 66 D9 52 39N 90 6 E
Abba, C.A.R. 114 A3 5 20N 15 11 E
Abbadia di Fiastra △,
  Italy 45 E10 43 12N 13 24 E
Abbadia San Salvatore,
  Italy 45 F8 42 53N 11 41 E
’Abbāsābād, Iran 97 C8 33 34N 58 23 E
Abbay = Nîl el
  Azraq →, Sudan 107 D3 15 38N 32 31 E
Abbaye, Pt., U.S.A. 148 B1 46 58N 88 8W
Abbazia = Opatija,
  Croatia 45 C11 45 14N 14 17 E
Abbé, L., Ethiopia 107 E5 11 8N 41 47 E
Abbeville, France 27 B8 50 6N 1 49 E
Abbeville, Ala., U.S.A. 152 D4 31 34N 85 15W
Abbeville, Ga., U.S.A. 152 D6 31 59N 83 18W
Abbeville, La., U.S.A. 155 L8 29 58N 92 8W
Abbeville, S.C., U.S.A. 152 A7 34 11N 82 23W
Abbiategrasso, Italy 44 C5 45 24N 8 54 E
Abbot Ice Shelf,
  Antarctica 7 D16 73 0 S 92 0W
Abbottabad, Pakistan 92 B5 34 10N 73 15 E
Abbou, O. ben →,
  Algeria 111 C5 28 32N 5 14 E
ABC Islands =
  Netherlands
  Antilles ⊠, W. Indies 168 A4 12 15N 69 0W
Abd al Kūrī, Yemen 99 D6 12 5N 52 20 E
Abdar, Iran 97 D7 30 16N 55 19 E
’Abdolābād, Iran 97 C8 34 12N 56 30 E
Abdulino, Russia 64 E4 53 42N 53 40 E
Abdulpur, Bangla. 90 C2 24 15N 88 59 E
Abéché, Chad 109 F4 13 50N 20 35 E
Abejar, Spain 40 D2 41 48N 2 47W
Abekr, Sudan 107 E2 12 45N 28 50 E
Abel Tasman △, N.Z. 131 A8 40 59 S 173 3 E
Abemama, Indonesia 83 C6 7 1 S 140 9 E
Abengourou, Ivory C. 112 D4 6 42N 3 27W
Abenójar, Spain 43 G6 38 53N 4 21W
Åbenrå, Denmark 17 J3 55 3N 9 25 E
Abensberg, Germany 31 G7 48 48N 11 51 E
Abeokuta, Nigeria 113 D5 7 3N 3 19 E
Aber, Uganda 118 B3 2 12N 32 25 E
Aberaeron, U.K. 21 E3 52 15N 4 15W
Aberayron =
  Aberaeron, U.K. 21 E3 52 15N 4 15W
Aberchirder, U.K. 22 D6 57 34N 2 37W
Abercorn = Mbala,
  Zambia 119 D3 8 46 S 31 24 E
Abercorn, Australia 127 G5 25 12 S 151 5 E
Aberdare, U.K. 21 F4 51 43N 3 27W
Aberdare △, Kenya 118 C4 0 22 S 36 44 E
Aberdare Ra., Kenya 118 C4 0 15 S 36 50 E
Aberdeen, Australia 129 B9 32 9 S 150 56 E
Aberdeen, China 69 G11 22 15N 114 9 E
Aberdeen, S. Africa 116 E3 32 28 S 24 2 E
Aberdeen, U.K. 22 D6 57 9N 2 5W

Aberdeen, Ala., U.S.A. 149 J1 33 49N 88 33W
Aberdeen, Idaho,
  U.S.A. 158 E7 42 57N 112 50W
Aberdeen, Md., U.S.A. 148 F7 39 31N 76 10W
Aberdeen, Ohio, U.S.A. 157 F13 38 39N 83 46W
Aberdeen, S. Dak.,
  U.S.A. 154 C5 45 28N 98 29W
Aberdeen, Wash.,
  U.S.A. 160 D3 46 59N 123 50W
Aberdeen, City of □,
  U.K. 22 D6 57 10N 2 10W
Aberdeenshire □, U.K. 22 D6 57 17N 2 36W
Aberdovey = Aberdyfi,
  U.K. 21 E3 52 33N 4 3W
Aberdyfi, U.K. 21 E3 52 33N 4 3W
Aberfeldy, U.K. 22 E5 56 37N 3 51W
Aberfoyle, U.K. 22 E4 56 11N 4 23W
Abergavenny, U.K. 21 F4 51 49N 3 1W
Abergele, U.K. 20 D4 53 17N 3 35W
Abernathy, U.S.A. 155 J4 33 50N 101 51W
Abert, L., U.S.A. 158 E3 42 38N 120 14W
Aberystwyth, U.K. 21 E3 52 25N 4 5W
Abhā, Si. Arabia 98 C3 18 0N 42 34 E
Abhar, Iran 97 B6 36 9N 49 13 E
Abhayapuri, India 90 B3 26 24N 90 38 E
Abia □, Nigeria 113 D6 5 30N 7 35 E
Abide, Turkey 49 C11 38 55N 29 20 E
Abidiya, Sudan 106 D3 18 18N 34 3 E
Abidjan, Ivory C. 112 D4 5 26N 3 58W
Abilene, Kans., U.S.A. 154 F6 38 55N 97 13W
Abilene, Tex., U.S.A. 155 J5 32 28N 99 43W
Abingdon, U.K. 21 F6 51 40N 1 17W
Abingdon, Ill., U.S.A. 156 D6 40 48N 90 24W
Abingdon, Va., U.S.A. 149 G5 36 43N 81 59W
Abingdon, I. = Pinta, I.,
  Ecuador 172 a 0 35N 90 44W
Abington Reef,
  Australia 126 B4 18 0 S 149 35 E
Abitau →, Canada 143 B7 59 53N 109 3W
Abitibi →, Canada 140 B3 51 3N 80 55W
Abitibi, L., Canada 140 C4 48 40N 79 40W
Abiy Adi, Ethiopia 107 E4 13 39N 39 3 E
Abkhaz Republic =
  Abkhazia □, Georgia 61 J5 43 12N 41 5 E
Abkhazia □, Georgia 61 J5 43 12N 41 5 E
Abminga, Australia 127 D1 26 8 S 134 51 E
Abnûb, Egypt 106 B3 27 18N 31 4 E
Åbo = Turku, Finland 15 F20 60 30N 22 19 E
Abo, Massif d', Chad 109 D3 21 41N 16 8 E
Abocho, Nigeria 113 D6 7 35N 6 56 E
Abohar, India 92 D6 30 10N 74 10 E
Aboisso, Ivory C. 112 D4 5 30N 3 5W
Abolo, Congo 114 B2 0 8N 14 16 E
Abomey, Benin 113 D5 7 10N 2 5 E
Abong-Mbang,
  Cameroon 114 B2 4 0N 13 8 E
Abongbong, Indonesia 84 B1 4 15N 96 48 E
Abonnema, Nigeria 113 E6 4 41N 6 49 E
Abony, Hungary 52 C5 47 12N 20 3 E
Abor Hills, India 94 A7 28 25N 94 45 E
Aborlan, Phil. 81 G2 9 26N 118 33 E
Aboso, Ghana 112 D4 5 23N 1 57W
Abou-Deïa, Chad 109 F3 11 20N 19 20 E
Abou-Goulem, Chad 109 F4 13 37N 21 38 E
Abou-Telfan △, Chad 109 F3 12 6N 17 38 E
Aboyne, U.K. 22 D6 57 4N 2 47W
Abra □, Phil. 80 C3 17 35N 120 45 E
Abra de Ilog, Phil. 80 E3 13 27N 120 44 E
Abra Pampa, Argentina 174 A2 22 43 S 65 42W
Abraham L., Canada 142 C5 52 15N 116 35W
Abrantes, Portugal 43 F2 39 24N 8 7W
Abreojos, Pta., Mexico 162 B2 26 50N 113 40W
Abri, Esh Shamâliya,
  Sudan 106 C3 20 50N 30 27 E
Abri, Janub Kordofân,
  Sudan 107 E3 11 40N 30 21 E
Abrolhos, Banco,
  Brazil 171 E4 18 0 S 38 0W
Abrud, Romania 53 D8 46 19N 23 5 E
Abruzzo □, Italy 45 F10 42 15N 14 0 E
Absaroka Range,
  U.S.A. 158 D9 44 45N 109 50W
Abtenau, Austria 34 D6 47 33N 13 21 E
Abu, India 92 G5 24 41N 72 50 E
Abū al Abyad, U.A.E. 97 E7 24 11N 53 50 E
Abū al Khaṣīb, Iraq 97 D6 30 25N 48 0 E
Abu ’Ali, Si. Arabia 97 E6 27 20N 49 27 E
Abu ’Ali →, Lebanon 103 A4 34 25N 35 50 E
Abu ’Arīsh, Si. Arabia 98 C3 16 53N 42 48 E
Abu Ballas, Egypt 106 C2 24 26N 27 36 E
Abu Deleiq, Sudan 107 D3 15 57N 33 48 E
Abu Dhabi = Abū
  Ẓāby, U.A.E. 97 E7 24 28N 54 22 E
Abu Dis, Sudan 106 D3 19 12N 33 38 E
Abu Dom, Sudan 107 D3 16 18N 32 25 E
Abu Du’ān, Syria 101 B1 36 25N 38 15 E
Abu el Gairi, W. →,
  Egypt 103 F2 29 35N 33 30 E
Abu Fatma, Ras, Sudan 106 C4 22 25N 36 25 E
Abu Gabra, Sudan 107 E2 11 2N 26 50 E
Abu Ga’da, W. →,
  Egypt 103 F1 29 15N 32 53 E
Abu Gelba, Sudan 107 E3 13 11N 31 52 E
Abu Gubeiha, Sudan 107 E3 11 30N 31 15 E
Abu Habl, Khawr →,
  Sudan 107 E3 12 37N 31 0 E
Abū Ḥadrīyah,
  Si. Arabia 97 E6 27 20N 48 58 E
Abu Hamed, Sudan 106 D3 19 32N 33 13 E
Abu Haraz,
  An Nîl el Azraq,
  Sudan 106 D3 18 1N 33 58 E
Abu Haraz, El Gezira,
  Sudan 107 E3 14 35N 33 30 E
Abu Haraz,
  Esh Shamâliya,
  Sudan 106 D3 19 8N 32 18 E
Abu Higar, Sudan 107 E3 12 50N 33 59 E
Abu Kamāl, Syria 101 E9 34 30N 41 0 E
Abu Kuleiwat, Sudan 107 E2 12 20N 26 0 E
Abū Madd, Ra's,
  Si. Arabia 96 E3 24 50N 37 7 E
Abu Matariq, Sudan 107 E2 10 59N 26 9 E
Abu Mendi, Ethiopia 107 E4 11 48N 35 42 E
Abū Mūsā, U.A.E. 97 E7 25 52N 55 3 E
Abū Qaṣr, Si. Arabia 96 D3 30 21N 38 34 E
Abu Qir, Egypt 106 H7 31 18N 30 0 E
Abu Qireiya, Egypt 106 C4 23 36N 35 3 E
Abū Qurqāṣ, Egypt 106 B3 28 1N 30 44 E
Abū Raṣāṣ, Ra's, Oman 99 B7 20 10N 58 38 E
Abu Shagara, Ras,
  Sudan 106 C4 21 4N 37 19 E
Abu Shanab, Sudan 107 E2 13 58N 27 49 E
Abu Simbel, Egypt 106 C3 22 18N 31 40 E
Abū Ṣukhayr, Iraq 101 G11 31 54N 44 30 E
Abu Sultan, Egypt 103 E1 30 24N 32 21 E
Abu Tabari, Sudan 106 D2 17 35N 28 20 E
Abu Tig, Egypt 106 B3 27 4N 31 15 E
Abu Tiga, Sudan 107 E3 12 47N 34 12 E
Abu Tineitin, Sudan 107 D3 15 42N 32 54 E
Abu Urruq, Sudan 107 D3 15 52N 30 25 E
Abu Zabad, Sudan 107 E2 12 25N 29 10 E
Abū Ẓāby, U.A.E. 97 E7 24 28N 54 22 E
Abū Zeydābād, Iran 97 C6 33 54N 51 45 E

Abufari, Brazil 173 B5 5 25 S 62 59W
Abuja, Nigeria 113 D6 9 5N 7 32 E
Abukuma-Gawa →,
  Japan 70 E10 38 6N 140 52 E
Abukuma-Sammyaku,
  Japan 70 F10 37 30N 140 45 E
Abulug, Phil. 80 B3 18 27N 121 27 E
Abumombazi,
  Dem. Rep. of
  the Congo 114 B4 3 42N 22 10 E
Abunã, Brazil 173 B4 9 40 S 65 20W
Abunã →, Brazil 173 B4 9 41 S 65 20W
Abune Yosef, Ethiopia 107 E4 12 5N 39 12 E
Aburatsu, Japan 72 F3 31 34N 131 24 E
Aburo, Dem. Rep. of
  the Congo 118 B3 2 4N 30 53 E
Abut Hd., N.Z. 131 D5 43 7 S 170 15 E
Abuye Meda, Ethiopia 107 E4 10 30N 39 49 E
Abuyog, Phil. 81 F5 10 45N 125 0 E
Abwong, Sudan 107 F3 9 2N 32 14 E
Aby, Sweden 17 F10 58 40N 16 10 E
Aby, Lagune, Ivory C. 112 D4 5 15 S 3 14W
Abyad, Sudan 107 E2 13 47N 26 24 E
Åbybro, Denmark 17 G3 57 10N 9 44 E
Abyei, El Salv. 164 D2 13 36N 89 50W
Açailândia, Brazil 170 C2 5 0 S 47 30W
Acámbaro, Mexico 162 D4 20 0N 100 40W
Acanthus, Greece 50 F7 40 27N 23 47 E
Acaponeta, Mexico 162 C3 22 30N 105 20W
Acapulco, Mexico 163 D5 16 51N 99 56W
Acará, Brazil 170 B2 1 57 S 48 11W
Acarai, Serra, Brazil 169 C6 1 50N 57 50W
Acaraú, Brazil 170 B3 2 53 S 40 7W
Acari, Brazil 170 C4 6 31 S 36 38W
Acarí, Peru 172 C3 15 25 S 74 36W
Acarigua, Venezuela 168 B4 9 33N 69 12W
Acatlán, Mexico 163 D5 18 10N 98 3W
Acayucan, Mexico 163 D6 17 59N 94 58W
Accéglio, Italy 44 D4 44 28N 7 0 E
Accomac, U.S.A. 148 G8 37 43N 75 40W
Accous, France 28 E3 43 0N 0 36W
Accra, Ghana 113 D4 5 35N 0 6W
Accrington, U.K. 20 D5 53 45N 2 22W
Aceh □, Indonesia 84 B1 4 15N 97 30 E
Acerra, Italy 47 B7 40 57N 14 22 E
Aceuchal, Spain 43 G4 38 39N 6 30W
Achacachi, Bolivia 172 D4 16 3 S 68 43W
Achaguas, Venezuela 168 B4 7 46N 68 14W
Achalpur, India 94 D3 21 22N 77 32 E
Achao, Chile 176 B2 42 28 S 73 30W
Acharnes = Akharnaí,
  Greece 48 C5 38 5N 23 44 E
Achegour, Niger 109 D2 19 10N 11 54 E
Acheloos →, Greece 48 C3 38 19N 21 7 E
Acheloós =
  Akheloós →, Greece 48 C3 38 19N 21 7 E
Achelouma, Niger 109 D2 18 12N 12 50 E
Achelouma, E. →,
  Niger 109 D2 15 51N 13 35 E
Achenkirch, Austria 34 D4 47 32N 11 45 E
Achensee, Austria 34 D4 47 26N 11 45 E
Acher, India 92 H5 23 10N 72 32 E
Achern, Germany 31 G4 48 37N 8 4 E
Acheron →, N.Z. 131 C8 42 16 S 173 4 E
Achill Hd., Ireland 23 C1 53 58N 10 15W
Achill I., Ireland 23 C1 53 58N 10 1W
Achim, Germany 30 B5 53 1N 9 2 E
Achinsk, Russia 67 D10 56 20N 90 20 E
Achisay = Ashchysay,
  Kazakhstan 65 B4 43 35N 68 53 E
Achit, Russia 64 C6 56 48N 57 54 E
Achouka, Gabon 114 C2 0 52 S 9 45 E
Acıgöl, Turkey 49 D11 37 50N 29 50 E
Acıpayam, Turkey 49 D11 37 26N 29 22 E
Acireale, Italy 47 E8 37 37N 15 10 E
Ackerman, U.S.A. 155 J10 33 19N 89 11W
Ackley, U.S.A. 156 B3 42 33N 93 3W
Acklins I., Bahamas 165 C5 22 30N 74 0W
Acme, Canada 142 C6 51 33N 113 30W
Acme, U.S.A. 150 F5 35 48N 101 40W
Acobamba, Peru 172 C3 12 52 S 74 35W
Acomayo, Peru 172 C3 13 55 S 71 38W
Aconcagua, Cerro,
  Argentina 174 C2 32 39 S 70 0W
Aconquija, Mt.,
  Argentina 174 B2 27 0 S 66 0W
Acopiara, Brazil 170 C4 6 6 S 39 27W
Açores, Is. dos, Atl. Oc. 8 C9 38 0N 27 0W
Acorizal, Brazil 173 D6 15 12 S 56 22W
Acornhoek, S. Africa 117 C5 24 37 S 31 2 E
Acquapendente, Italy 45 F8 42 44N 11 52 E
Acquasanta Terme,
  Italy 45 F10 42 46N 13 24 E
Acquasparta, Italy 45 F9 42 41N 12 33 E
Acquaviva delle Fonti,
  Italy 47 B9 40 54N 16 50 E
Acqui Terme, Italy 44 D5 44 41N 8 28 E
Acraman, L., Australia 127 E2 32 2 S 135 23 E
Acre = ’Akko, Israel 103 C4 32 55N 35 4 E
Acre □, Peru 172 B3 9 1 S 71 0W
Acre →, Brazil 172 B4 8 45 S 67 22W
Acri, Italy 47 C9 39 29N 16 23 E
Acs, Hungary 52 C3 47 42N 18 2 E
Actaeon Mt., St. Helena 9 h 15 58 S 5 42W
Actium, Greece 39 B2 38 57N 20 45 E
Acton, Canada 150 C4 43 38N 80 3W
Açu, Brazil 170 C4 5 34 S 36 54W
Acul = Vidin, Bulgaria 50 C6 43 59N 22 50 E
Acworth, U.S.A. 152 A5 34 4N 84 41W
Ad Dafinah, Si. Arabia 98 B3 23 18N 41 58 E
Ad Dafrah, U.A.E. 99 B6 23 30N 54 30 E
Ad Dahnā, Si. Arabia 99 A5 24 30N 48 10 E
Ad Dammām,
  Si. Arabia 97 E6 26 20N 50 5 E
Ad Dāmūr, Lebanon 103 B4 33 44N 35 27 E
Ad Dawādimī,
  Si. Arabia 98 C3 24 35N 44 15 E
Ad Dawḥah, Qatar 97 E6 25 15N 51 35 E
Ad Dawr, Iraq 101 E10 34 27N 43 47 E
Aḍ Ḍiffah, Libya 108 B4 30 30N 26 0 E
Ad Dilam, Si. Arabia 98 B4 23 55N 47 10 E
Ad Dīr’īyah, Si. Arabia 98 B4 24 44N 46 35 E
Ad Dīwānīyah, Iraq 101 F11 32 0N 45 0 E
Ad Dujayl, Iraq 101 F11 33 51N 44 14 E
Ad Duwayd, Si. Arabia 96 D4 30 15N 42 17 E
Ada, Ghana 113 D5 5 44N 0 40 E
Ada, Serbia & M. 52 E5 45 49N 20 9 E
Ada, Minn., U.S.A. 154 B6 47 18N 96 31W
Ada, Ohio, U.S.A. 157 D13 40 46N 83 49W
Ada, Okla., U.S.A. 155 H6 34 46N 96 41W
Adabiya, Egypt 103 F1 29 53N 32 28 E
Adad, Somali Rep. 120 C3 9 7N 46 20 E
Adair, C., Canada 139 A12 71 30N 71 34W
Adaja →, Spain 42 D6 41 32N 4 52W
Adak, U.S.A. 144 L3 51 45N 176 45W
Adak I., U.S.A. 144 L3 51 45N 176 45W
Ådalsbruk, Norway 18 D8 60 43N 11 19 E
Adam, Oman 99 B7 22 15N 57 28 E

Adam, Mt., Falk. Is. 9 f 51 34 S 60 4W
Adamantina, Brazil 171 F1 21 42 S 51 4W
Adamaoua, Massif de
  l', Cameroon 113 D7 7 20N 12 20 E
Adamawa □, Nigeria 113 D7 9 20N 12 30 E
Adamawa Highlands =
  Adamaoua, Massif de
  l', Cameroon 113 D7 7 20N 12 20 E
Adamello △, Italy 44 B7 46 4N 10 8 E
Adamello, Mte., Italy 44 B7 46 9N 10 30 E
Adami Tulu, Ethiopia 107 F4 7 53N 38 41 E
Adaminaby, Australia 129 C8 36 0 S 148 45 E
Adams, Mass., U.S.A. 151 D11 42 38N 73 7W
Adams, N.Y., U.S.A. 151 C8 43 49N 76 1W
Adams, Wis., U.S.A. 154 D10 43 57N 89 49W
Adams, Mt., U.S.A. 160 D5 46 12N 121 30W
Adam's Bridge,
  Sri Lanka 95 K4 9 15N 79 40 E
Adams L., Canada 142 C5 51 10N 119 40W
Adam's Peak,
  Sri Lanka 95 L5 6 48N 80 30 E
Adamuz, Spain 43 G6 38 2N 4 32W
Adana, Turkey 100 D6 37 0N 35 16 E
Adanero, Spain 42 E6 40 56N 4 36W
Adapazarı = Sakarya,
  Turkey 100 B4 40 48N 30 25 E
Adar Gwagwa, J.,
  Sudan 106 C4 22 15N 35 20 E
Adarama, Sudan 107 D3 17 10N 34 52 E
Adare, C., Antarctica 7 D11 71 0 S 171 0 E
Adarte, Eritrea 107 E5 13 18N 42 8 E
Adaut, Indonesia 83 C4 8 8 S 131 7 E
Adavale, Australia 127 D3 25 52 S 144 32 E
Adda →, Italy 44 C6 45 8N 9 53 E
Addatigala, India 94 F6 17 31N 82 3 E
Addax □, Niger 109 E1 19 17N 9 22 E
Addis Ababa = Addis
  Abeba, Ethiopia 107 F4 9 2N 38 42 E
Addis Abeba, Ethiopia 107 F4 9 2N 38 42 E
Addis Alem, Ethiopia 107 F4 9 0N 38 17 E
Addis Zemen, Ethiopia 107 E4 12 7N 37 47 E
Addison, Ill., U.S.A. 157 C8 41 55N 88 0W
Addison, N.Y., U.S.A. 150 D7 42 1N 77 14W
Addo, S. Africa 116 E4 33 32 S 25 45 E
Addo □, S. Africa 116 E4 33 30 S 25 50 E
Adebour, Niger 113 C7 13 17N 11 50 E
Adel, Ga., U.S.A. 152 D6 31 8N 83 25W
Adel, Iowa, U.S.A. 156 C2 41 37N 94 1W
Adelaide, Australia 128 C3 34 52 S 138 30 E
Adelaide, S. Africa 116 E4 32 42 S 26 20 E
Adelaide I., Antarctica 7 C17 67 15 S 68 30W
Adelaide Pen., Canada 138 B10 68 15N 97 30W
Adelaide River,
  Australia 124 B5 13 15 S 131 7 E
Adelaide Village,
  Bahamas 9 b 25 0N 77 31W
Adelanto, U.S.A. 161 L9 34 35N 117 22W
Adelaye, C.A.R. 114 A4 7 7N 22 49 E
Adelboden, Switz. 32 D5 46 29N 7 33 E
Adele I., Australia 124 C3 15 32 S 123 9 E
Adélie, Terre,
  Antarctica 7 C10 68 0 S 140 0 E
Adelie Land = Adélie,
  Terre, Antarctica 7 C10 68 0 S 140 0 E
Adelong, Australia 129 C8 35 16 S 148 4 E
Adelsk, Belarus 54 E10 53 24N 23 47 E
Ademuz, Spain 40 E3 40 5N 1 13W
Aden = Al ’Adan,
  Yemen 98 D4 12 45N 45 0 E
Aden, G. of, Asia 88 D3 12 30N 47 30 E
Adendorp, S. Africa 116 E3 32 15 S 24 30 E
Aderbissinat, Niger 113 B6 15 34N 7 54 E
Adh Dhayd, U.A.E. 97 E7 25 17N 55 53 E
Adhoi, India 92 H4 23 26N 70 32 E
Adi, Indonesia 83 B4 4 15 S 133 30 E
Adi Arkai, Ethiopia 107 E4 13 35N 37 57 E
Adi Daro, Ethiopia 107 E4 14 20N 38 14 E
Adi Keyih, Eritrea 107 E4 14 51N 39 22 E
Adi Kwala, Eritrea 107 E4 14 58N 38 48 E
Adi Ugri, Eritrea 107 E4 14 53N 38 52 E
Adieu, C., Australia 125 F5 32 0 S 132 10 E
Adieu Pt., Australia 124 C3 15 14 S 124 35 E
Adige →, Italy 45 C9 45 9N 12 20 E
Adigrat, Ethiopia 107 E4 14 20N 39 26 E
Adıgüzel Baraji, Turkey 49 C11 38 13N 29 15 E
Adilabad, India 94 E4 19 33N 78 20 E
Adilcevaz, Turkey 101 C10 38 47N 42 43 E
Adin, U.S.A. 158 F3 41 12N 120 57W
Adin Khel, Afghan. 89 C3 32 45N 68 5 E
Adirampattinam, India 95 J4 10 28N 79 20 E
Adirondack △, U.S.A. 151 C10 44 0N 74 20W
Adirondack Mts.,
  U.S.A. 151 C10 44 0N 74 0W
Adis Abeba = Addis
  Abeba, Ethiopia 107 F4 9 2N 38 42 E
Adıyaman, Turkey 101 D8 37 42N 38 16 E
Adjim, Tunisia 108 B2 33 47N 10 50 E
Adjohon, Benin 113 D5 6 41N 2 32 E
Adjud, Romania 53 D12 46 7N 27 10 E
Adjumani, Uganda 118 B3 3 20N 31 50 E
Adjuntas, Puerto Rico 165 d 18 10N 66 43W
Adlavik Is., Canada 141 B8 55 0N 58 40W
Adler, Russia 61 J4 43 28N 39 52 E
Adliswil, Switz. 33 B7 47 19N 8 32 E
Admer, Algeria 111 D6 20 21N 5 27 E
Admer, Erg d', Algeria 111 D6 24 0N 9 5 E
Admiralty G., Australia 124 B4 14 20 S 125 55 E
Admiralty I., U.S.A. 142 B2 57 30N 134 30W
Admiralty Is.,
  Papua N. G. 132 B4 2 0 S 147 0 E
Adnan Menderes,
  İzmir ✈ (ADB),
  Turkey 49 C9 38 23N 27 6 E
Ado, Nigeria 113 D5 6 36N 2 56 E
Ado-Ekiti, Nigeria 113 D6 7 38N 5 12 E
Adok, Sudan 107 F3 8 10N 30 20 E
Adola, Ethiopia 107 F5 11 14N 41 44 E
Adonara, Indonesia 82 C2 8 15 S 123 5 E
Adoni, India 95 G3 15 33N 77 18 E
Adony, Hungary 52 C3 47 6N 18 52 E
Adour →, France 28 E2 43 32N 1 32W
Adra, India 93 H12 23 30N 86 42 E
Adra, Spain 43 J7 36 43N 3 3W
Adrano, Italy 47 E7 37 40N 14 50 E
Adrar des Iforas,
  Algeria 111 C4 27 51N 0 11 E
Adrar Madet, Niger 109 E2 18 54N 10 33 E
Adrasman, Tajikistan 65 C4 40 39N 69 25 E
Adré, Chad 109 F4 13 40N 22 20 E
Adri, Libya 108 C2 27 32N 13 2 E
Ádria, Italy 45 C9 45 9N 12 3 E
Adrian, Mich., U.S.A. 157 C12 41 54N 84 2W
Adrian, Tex., U.S.A. 155 H3 35 16N 102 40W
Adrianople = Edirne,
  Turkey 51 E10 41 40N 26 34 E
Adriatic Sea, Medit. S. 12 C9 43 0N 16 0 E
Adua, Indonesia 83 B3 1 45 S 129 50 E
Adula-Gruppe, Switz. 33 D8 46 30N 9 10 E
Adung Long, Burma 90 A6 28 7N 97 42 E
Adur, India 95 K3 9 7N 76 40 E
Adwa, Ethiopia 107 E4 14 15N 38 52 E
Adygea □, Russia 61 H5 45 0N 40 0 E

Adzhar Republic =
  Ajaria □, Georgia 61 K6 41 30N 42 0 E
Adzhibakul =
  Qazimämmäd,
  Azerbaijan 61 K9 40 3N 49 0 E
Adzopé, Ivory C. 112 D4 6 7N 3 49W
Ægean Sea, Medit. S. 49 C7 38 30N 25 0 E
Aerhtai Shan, Mongolia 68 B4 46 40N 92 45 E
Ærø, Denmark 17 K4 54 52N 10 25 E
Ærøskøbing, Denmark 17 K4 54 53N 10 24 E
Aesch, Switz. 32 B5 47 28N 7 36 E
Aëtós, Greece 48 C3 38 35N 21 50 E
Afafi, Massif d', Niger 109 D3 22 11N 15 10 E
'Afak, Iraq 101 F11 32 4N 45 15 E
Afándou, Greece 38 E12 36 18N 28 12 E
Afar □, Ethiopia 107 E5 12 0N 41 0 E
Afarag, Erg, Algeria 111 D5 23 50N 2 47 E
Afareaitu, Tahiti 133 S16 17 33 S 149 47W
Åfarnes, Norway 18 E3 62 40N 7 32 E
Afdega, Ethiopia 120 C2 6 4N 43 30 E
Affoltern, Switz. 33 B6 47 17N 8 27 E
Affreville = Khemis
  Miliana, Algeria 111 A5 36 11N 2 14 E
Affton, U.S.A. 156 F6 38 33N 90 20W
Afghanistan ■, Asia 91 B2 33 0N 65 0 E
Afgoi, Somali Rep. 120 D2 2 7N 44 59 E
'Afif, Si. Arabia 98 B3 23 53N 42 56 E
Afikpo, Nigeria 113 D6 5 53N 7 54 E
Aflisses, O. →, Algeria 111 B5 34 7N 2 3 E
Aflou, Algeria 111 B5 34 7N 2 3 E
Afmadu, Somali Rep. 120 D3 0 31N 42 4 E
Afogados da Ingàzeira,
  Brazil 170 C4 7 45 S 37 39W
Afognak I., U.S.A. 144 G9 58 15N 152 30W
Afore, Papua N. G. 132 E5 9 9 S 148 23 E
Afragóla, Italy 47 B7 40 55N 14 18 E
Afram →, Ghana 113 D4 7 0N 0 52W
Afrera, Ethiopia 107 E5 13 16N 41 5 E
Africa 104 E6 10 0N 20 0 E
'Afrīn, Syria 100 D7 36 32N 36 50 E
Afşin, Turkey 100 C7 38 16N 36 54 E
Afton, Iowa, U.S.A. 156 C2 41 2N 94 12W
Afton, N.Y., U.S.A. 151 D9 42 14N 75 32W
Afton, Wyo., U.S.A. 158 E8 42 44N 110 56W
Aftout, Algeria 110 C4 26 50N 3 45W
Afuá, Brazil 169 D7 0 15 S 50 10W
'Afula, Israel 103 C4 32 37N 35 17 E
Afumba, Zambia 115 F4 15 38 S 24 56 E
Afyon, Turkey 49 C12 38 45N 30 33 E
Afyon □, Turkey 49 C12 38 30N 30 30 E
Afyonkarahisar =
  Afyon, Turkey 49 C12 38 45N 30 33 E
Aga, Egypt 106 H7 30 55N 31 10 E
Aga Pt., Guam 133 R15 13 15N 144 43 E
Agadem, Niger 109 E2 16 50N 13 11 E
Agadès = Agadez,
  Niger 113 B6 16 58N 7 59 E
Agadez, Niger 113 B6 16 58N 7 59 E
Agadir, Morocco 110 B3 30 28N 9 55W
Agaete, Canary Is. 9 e1 28 6N 15 43W
Agaie, Nigeria 113 D6 9 1N 6 18 E
Agailás, Mauritania 110 D2 23 50N 6 30W
Again, Sudan 107 E2 12 53N 29 55 E
Agana = Hagåtña, Guam 133 R15 13 28N 144 45 E
Āgapınar, Turkey 49 B12 39 48N 30 47 E
Agar, India 92 H7 23 40N 76 2 E
Agaro, Ethiopia 107 F4 7 50N 36 38 E
Agartala, India 93 H17 23 40N 91 23 E
Agaş, Romania 53 D11 46 28N 26 15 E
Agassiz, Canada 142 D4 49 14N 121 46W
Agat, Guam 133 R15 13 23N 144 40 E
Agats, Indonesia 83 C5 5 33 S 138 0 E
Agattu I., U.S.A. 144 K2 52 25N 173 35 E
Agawam, U.S.A. 151 D12 42 4N 72 37W
Agboville, Ivory C. 112 D4 5 55N 4 15W
Agbélouvé, Togo 113 D5 6 35N 1 14 E
Ağcabädi, Azerbaijan 61 K8 40 5N 47 27 E
Ağdam, Azerbaijan 61 L8 40 0N 46 58 E
Ağdaş, Azerbaijan 61 K8 40 44N 47 27 E
Agde, France 28 F7 43 19N 3 28 E
Agde, C. d', France 28 F7 43 16N 3 28 E
Agdz, Morocco 110 B3 30 47N 6 30W
Agdzhabedi =
  Ağcabädi, Azerbaijan 61 K8 40 5N 47 27 E
Agen, France 28 D4 44 12N 0 38 E
Ageo, Japan 73 B11 35 58N 139 36 E
Ager Tay, Chad 109 E3 20 0N 17 41 E
Agerbæk, Denmark 17 J2 55 36N 8 48 E
Agersø, Denmark 17 J5 55 13N 11 12 E
Ageyevo, Russia 58 E9 54 10N 36 27 E
Aggeteleki ∩, Hungary 52 B5 48 24N 20 36 E
Āgh Kand, Iran 97 B6 37 15N 48 4 E
Aghios Efstratios =
  Áyios Evstrátios,
  Greece 48 B6 39 34N 24 58 E
Aghios Oros = Áthos,
  Greece 51 F8 40 9N 24 22 E
Aghíreşu, Romania 53 D8 46 53N 23 15 E
Aghouavil, Mauritania 110 D1 21 10N 15 6W
Aghreijìt, Mauritania 110 D2 11 0N 6 1W
Aginskoye, Russia 67 D12 51 6N 114 32 E
Ağlasun, Turkey 49 D12 37 39N 30 31 E
Agly →, France 28 F7 42 46N 3 3 E
Agmar, Mauritania 110 D2 25 18N 10 50W
Agnew, Australia 125 E3 28 1 S 120 30 E
Agnibilékrou, Ivory C. 112 D4 7 10N 3 11W
Agnita, Romania 53 E9 45 59N 24 40 E
Agno, Switz. 33 E7 45 59N 8 53 E
Agnone, Italy 45 G11 41 48N 14 23 E
Agofie, Ghana 113 D5 8 27N 0 15 E
Agogna →, Italy 44 C5 45 4N 8 54 E
Agogo, Sudan 107 F2 7 50N 28 45 E
Agon Coutainville,
  France 26 C5 49 2N 1 34W
Agoo, Phil. 80 C3 16 20N 120 22 E
Ágordo, Italy 45 B9 46 18N 12 2 E
Agouna, Benin 113 D5 7 57N 1 47 E
Agout →, France 28 E5 43 47N 1 41 E
Agra, India 92 F7 27 17N 78 58 E
Agrakhanskiy
  Poluostrov, Russia 61 J8 43 42N 47 36 E
Agram = Zagreb,
  Croatia 45 C12 45 50N 15 58 E
Agramunt, Spain 40 D6 41 48N 1 6 E
Agreda, Spain 40 D3 41 51N 1 55W
Ağri, Turkey 101 C10 39 44N 43 3 E
Agri →, Italy 47 B9 40 13N 16 44 E
Ağri Daği, Turkey 101 C11 39 50N 44 15 E
Ağri Karakose = Ağri,
  Turkey 101 C10 39 44N 43 3 E
Agrigento, Italy 46 E6 37 19N 13 34 E
Agrínion, Greece 48 C3 38 37N 21 27 E
Agrónion = Agrínion,
  Greece 48 C3 38 37N 21 27 E
Agrópoli, Italy 47 B7 40 21N 14 59 E
Ağstafa, Azerbaijan 61 K7 41 7N 45 27 E

Água Branca, *Brazil* **170 C3** 5 50 S 42 40W
Agua Caliente, *Baja Calif., Mexico* **161 N10** 32 29N 116 59W
Agua Caliente, *Sinaloa, Mexico* **162 B3** 26 30N 108 20W
Agua Caliente Springs, *U.S.A.* **161 N10** 32 56N 116 19W
Água Clara, *Brazil* **173 E7** 20 25 S 52 45W
Agua Fria ⌓, *U.S.A.* **159 J8** 34 14N 112 0W
Agua Hechicero, *Mexico* **161 N10** 32 26N 116 14W
Água Preta →, *Brazil* **169 D5** 1 41 S 63 48W
Agua Prieta, *Mexico* **162 A3** 31 20N 109 32W
Aguachica, *Colombia* **168 B3** 8 19N 73 38W
Aguada Cecilio, *Argentina* **176 B3** 40 51 S 65 51W
Aguadas, *Colombia* **168 B2** 5 40N 75 38W
Aguadilla, *Puerto Rico* **165 d** 18 26N 67 10W
Aguadulce, *Panama* **164 E3** 8 15N 80 32W
Aguanga, *U.S.A.* **161 M10** 33 27N 116 51W
Aguanish, *Canada* **141 B7** 50 14N 62 2W
Aguanus →, *Canada* **141 B7** 50 13N 62 5W
Aguapeí, *Brazil* **173 D6** 16 12 S 59 43W
Aguapeí →, *Brazil* **171 F1** 21 0 S 51 0W
Aguapey →, *Argentina* **174 B4** 29 7 S 56 36W
Aguaray Guazú →, *Paraguay* **174 A4** 24 47 S 57 19W
Aguarico →, *Ecuador* **168 D2** 0 59 S 75 11W
Aguaro-Guariquito △, *Venezuela* **165 E6** 8 20N 66 35W
Aguas →, *Spain* **40 D4** 41 20N 0 30W
Aguas Blancas, *Chile* **174 A2** 24 15 S 69 55W
Aguas Calientes, Sierra de, *Argentina* **174 B2** 25 26 S 66 40W
Águas Formosas, *Brazil* **171 E3** 17 5 S 40 57W
Aguascalientes, *Mexico* **162 C4** 21 53N 102 12W
Aguascalientes □, *Mexico* **162 C4** 22 0N 102 20W
Agudo, *Spain* **43 G6** 38 59N 4 52W
Águeda, *Portugal* **42 E2** 40 34N 8 27W
Agueda →, *Spain* **42 D4** 41 2N 6 56W
Aguelhok, *Mali* **113 B5** 19 29N 0 52 E
Aguelt el Melah, *Mauritania* **110 D2** 23 3N 8 28W
Agüenit, *W. Sahara* **110 D2** 22 11N 13 8W
Aguié, *Niger* **113 C6** 13 31N 7 46 E
Aguila, Punta, *Puerto Rico* **165 d** 17 57N 67 13W
Aguilafuente, *Spain* **42 D6** 41 13N 4 7W
Aguilar, *Spain* **43 H6** 37 31N 4 40W
Aguilar de Campóo, *Spain* **42 C6** 42 47N 4 15W
Aguilares, *Argentina* **174 B2** 27 26 S 65 35W
Aguilas, *Spain* **41 H3** 37 23N 1 35W
Agüimes, *Canary Is.* **9 e1** 27 58N 15 27W
Aguja, C. de la, *Colombia* **168 A3** 11 18N 74 12W
Agujereada, Pta., *Puerto Rico* **165 d** 18 30N 67 8W
Agulaa, *Ethiopia* **107 E4** 13 40N 39 40 E
Agulhas, C., *S. Africa* **116 E3** 34 52 S 20 0 E
Agulhas Basin, *Ind. Oc.* **121 J1** 46 0 S 26 0 E
Agulhas Plateau, *Ind. Oc.* **121 H1** 40 0 S 26 0 E
Agulo, *Canary Is.* **9 e1** 28 11N 17 12W
Agung, Gunung, *Indonesia* **85 D5** 8 20 S 115 28 E
Agur, *Uganda* **118 B3** 2 28N 32 55 E
Agusan →, *Phil.* **81 G5** 9 0N 125 30 E
Agusan del Norte □, *Phil.* **81 G5** 9 20N 125 10 E
Agusan del Sur □, *Phil.* **81 G5** 8 30N 125 30 E
Agustín Codazzi, *Colombia* **168 A3** 10 2N 73 14W
Agutaya I., *Phil.* **81 F3** 11 9N 120 58 E
Ağva, *Turkey* **51 E13** 41 8N 29 51 E
Agvali, *Russia* **61 J8** 42 36N 46 8 E
Aha Mts., *Botswana* **116 B3** 19 45 S 21 0 E
Ahaggar, *Algeria* **111 D6** 23 0N 6 30 E
Ahamansu, *Ghana* **113 D5** 7 38N 0 35 E
Ahar, *Iran* **101 C12** 38 35N 47 0 E
Ahat, *Turkey* **49 C11** 38 39N 29 47 E
Ahaura →, *N.Z.* **131 C6** 42 21 S 171 34 E
Ahaus, *Germany* **30 C2** 52 4N 7 0 E
Åheim, *Norway* **18 B2** 62 2N 5 13 E
Ahelledjem, *Algeria* **111 C6** 26 37N 6 58 E
Ahimanawa Ra., *N.Z.* **130 F5** 39 3 S 176 30 E
Ahioma, *Papua N. G.* **132 F6** 10 20 S 150 33 E
Ahipara B., *N.Z.* **130 B2** 35 5 S 173 5 E
Ahir Dağı, *Turkey* **49 C12** 38 45N 30 10 E
Ahiri, *India* **94 E5** 19 30N 80 0 E
Ahlat, *Turkey* **101 C10** 38 45N 42 29 E
Ahlen, *Germany* **30 D3** 51 45N 7 53 E
Ahmad Wal, *Pakistan* **92 E1** 29 18N 65 58 E
Ahmadabad, *India* **92 H5** 23 0N 72 40 E
Aḥmadābād, *Khorāsān, Iran* **97 C9** 35 3N 60 50 E
Aḥmadābād, *Khorāsān, Iran* **97 C8** 35 49N 59 42 E
Aḥmadī, *Iran* **97 E8** 27 56N 56 42 E
Ahmadnagar, *India* **94 E2** 19 7N 74 46 E
Ahmadpur, *India* **94 E3** 18 40N 76 57 E
Ahmadpur, *Pakistan* **92 E4** 29 12N 71 10 E
Ahmadpur Lamma, *Pakistan* **92 E4** 28 19N 70 3 E
Ahmar, *Ethiopia* **107 F5** 9 20N 41 15 E
Ahmedabad = Ahmadabad, *India* **92 H5** 23 0N 72 40 E
Ahmednagar = Ahmadnagar, *India* **94 E2** 19 7N 74 46 E
Ahmetbey, *Turkey* **51 E11** 41 26N 27 34 E
Ahmetler, *Turkey* **49 C11** 38 28N 29 5 E
Ahmetli, *Turkey* **49 C9** 38 32N 27 57 E
Ahmeyim, *Mauritania* **110 D2** 20 51N 14 25W
Ahoada, *Nigeria* **113 D6** 5 8N 6 36 E
Ahome, *Mexico* **162 B3** 25 55N 109 11W
Ahon, Tarso, *Chad* **109 D3** 20 23N 18 18 E
Ahoskie, *U.S.A.* **149 G7** 36 17N 76 59W
Ahr →, *Germany* **30 E3** 50 32N 7 16 E
Ahram, *Iran* **97 D6** 28 52N 51 16 E
Ahrax Pt., *Malta* **38 F7** 36 0N 14 22 E
Ahrensbök, *Germany* **30 A6** 54 2N 10 35 E
Ahrensburg, *Germany* **30 B6** 53 40N 10 13 E
Āhū, *Iran* **97 C6** 34 33N 50 2 E
Ahu Akivi, *Chile* **172 b** 27 7 S 109 24W
Ahu Tepeu, *Chile* **172 b** 27 6 S 109 25W
Ahu Tongariki, *Chile* **172 b** 27 8 S 109 17W
Ahu Vinapu, *Chile* **172 b** 27 10 S 109 25W
Ahuachapán, *El Salv.* **164 D2** 13 54N 89 52W
Ahun, *France* **27 F9** 46 4N 2 5 E
Ahuriri →, *N.Z.* **131 E5** 44 31 S 170 12 E
Åhus, *Sweden* **17 J8** 55 56N 14 18 E
Ahvāz, *Iran* **97 D6** 31 20N 48 40 E
Ahvenanmaa, *Finland* **15 F19** 60 15N 20 0 E
Aḥwar, *Yemen* **98 D4** 13 30N 46 40 E
Ahzar →, *Mali* **113 B5** 15 30N 3 20 E
Ai →, *India* **90 B3** 26 26N 90 44 E
Ai-Ais, *Namibia* **116 D2** 27 54 S 17 59 E
Ai-Ais and Fish River Canyon △, *Namibia* **116 C2** 24 45 S 17 15 E
Aiari →, *Brazil* **168 C4** 1 22N 68 36W
Aichach, *Germany* **31 G7** 48 27N 11 8 E
Aichi □, *Japan* **73 C9** 35 0N 137 15 E
Aiduma, *Indonesia* **83 B4** 4 0 S 134 6 E
Aiduna, *Indonesia* **83 B5** 4 27 S 135 15 E
Aiea, *U.S.A.* **145 K14** 21 23N 157 56W
Aigle, *Switz.* **32 D3** 46 18N 6 58 E
Aignay-le-Duc, *France* **27 E11** 47 40N 4 43 E
Aigoual, Mt., *France* **28 D7** 44 8N 3 35 E
Aigre, *France* **28 C4** 45 54N 0 1 E
Aigrettes, Pte. des, *Réunion* **121 c** 21 3 S 55 13 E
Aigua, *Uruguay* **175 C5** 34 13 S 54 46W
Aigueperse, *France* **27 F10** 46 3N 3 13 E
Aigues →, *France* **29 D8** 44 7N 4 43 E
Aigues-Mortes, *France* **29 E8** 43 35N 4 12 E
Aigues-Mortes, G. d', *France* **29 E8** 43 31N 4 3 E
Aigües Tortes y Lago San Mauricio △, *Spain* **40 C4** 42 38N 0 31W
Aiguilles, *France* **29 D10** 44 47N 6 51 E
Aiguillon, *France* **28 D4** 44 18N 0 21 E
Aigurande, *France* **27 F8** 46 27N 1 49 E
Aihui, *China* **69 A7** 50 10N 127 30 E
Aija, *Peru* **172 B2** 9 50 S 77 45W
Aikawa, *Japan* **70 E9** 38 2N 138 15 E
Aiken, *U.S.A.* **152 B8** 33 34N 81 43W
Ailao Shan, *China* **76 F3** 24 0N 101 20 E
Aileron, *Australia* **126 C1** 22 39 S 133 20 E
Ailey, *U.S.A.* **152 C7** 32 11N 82 34W
Ailigandi, *Panama* **168 B2** 9 14N 78 1W
Aillant-sur-Tholon, *France* **27 E10** 47 52N 3 20 E
Aillik, *Canada* **141 A8** 55 11N 59 18W
Ailsa Craig, *U.K.* **22 F3** 55 15N 5 6W
Ailulual, *Papua N. G.* **132 E6** 9 38 S 150 35 E
Aim, *Russia* **67 D14** 59 0N 133 55 E
Aimere, *Indonesia* **79 F6** 8 45 S 121 3 E
Aimogasta, *Argentina* **174 B2** 28 33 S 66 50W
Aimorés, *Brazil* **171 E3** 19 30 S 41 4W
Ain □, *France* **27 F12** 46 5N 5 20 E
Ain →, *France* **29 C9** 45 45N 5 11 E
Aïn Beïda, *Algeria* **111 A6** 35 50N 7 29 E
Aïn Ben Khellil, *Algeria* **111 B4** 33 15N 0 49W
Aïn Ben Tili, *Mauritania* **110 C3** 25 59N 9 27W
Aïn Beni Mathar, *Morocco* **111 B4** 34 1N 2 0W
Aïn Benian, *Algeria* **111 A5** 36 48N 2 55 E
Ain Dalla, *Egypt* **106 B2** 27 20N 27 23 E
Ain el Mafki, *Egypt* **106 B2** 27 30N 28 15 E
Ain Girba, *Egypt* **106 B2** 29 20N 25 14 E
Aïn M'lila, *Algeria* **111 A6** 36 2N 6 35 E
Aïn Mokra = Berrahal, *Algeria* **111 A6** 36 54N 7 33 E
Ain Murr, *Sudan* **106 C2** 21 50N 25 9 E
Ain Qeiqab, *Egypt* **106 B1** 29 42N 24 55 E
Aïn Salah = In Salah, *Algeria* **111 C5** 27 10N 2 32 E
Aïn Sefra, *Algeria* **111 B4** 32 47N 0 37W
Ain Sheikh Murzûk, *Egypt* **106 B2** 26 47N 27 45 E
Ain Sudr, *Egypt* **103 F2** 29 50N 33 6 E
Ain Sukhna, *Egypt* **106 J8** 29 32N 32 20 E
Aïn Tédelès, *Algeria* **111 A5** 36 0N 0 21 E
Aïn Témouchent, *Algeria* **111 A4** 35 16N 1 8W
Aïn Tikkidine, *Algeria* **111 C5** 25 33N 1 24 E
Aïn Touta, *Algeria* **111 A6** 35 26N 5 54 E
Ain Zeitûn, *Egypt* **106 B2** 29 10N 25 48 E
Aïn Zorah, *Morocco* **111 B4** 34 37N 3 32W
Ainabo, *Somali Rep.* **120 C3** 9 0N 46 25 E
Ainaži, *Latvia* **15 H21** 57 50N 24 24 E
Aínos Óros, *Greece* **39 C2** 38 9N 20 40 E
Ainsworth, *U.S.A.* **154 D5** 42 33N 99 52W
Aintab = Gaziantep, *Turkey* **100 D7** 37 6N 37 23 E
Aioi, *Japan* **72 C6** 34 48N 134 28 E
Aiome, *Papua N. G.* **132 C3** 5 8 S 144 44 E
Aipe, *Colombia* **168 C2** 3 13N 75 15W
Aiquile, *Bolivia* **173 D4** 18 10 S 65 10W
Aïr, *Niger* **113 B6** 18 30N 8 0 E
Aïr et du Ténéré ⌓, *Niger* **109 E1** 18 12N 9 56 E
Air Force I., *Canada* **139 B12** 67 58N 74 5W
Air Hitam, *Malaysia* **87 M4** 1 55N 103 11 E
Aira, *Japan* **72 F2** 31 43N 130 43 E
Airaines, *France* **27 C8** 49 58N 1 55 E
Airão, *Brazil* **169 D5** 1 56 S 61 22W
Airdrie, *Canada* **142 C6** 51 18N 114 2W
Airdrie, *U.K.* **22 F5** 55 52N 3 57W
Aire →, *France* **27 C11** 49 18N 4 49 E
Aire →, *U.K.* **20 D7** 53 43N 0 55W
Aire, I. de l', *Spain* **38 B5** 39 48N 4 16 E
Aire-sur-la-Lys, *France* **27 B9** 50 37N 2 22 E
Aire-sur-l'Adour, *France* **28 E3** 43 42N 0 15W
Aireys Inlet, *Australia* **128 E6** 38 29 S 144 5 E
Airlie Beach, *Australia* **126 J6** 20 16 S 148 43 E
Airmadidi, *Indonesia* **82 A3** 1 25N 125 0 E
Airolo, *Switz.* **33 C7** 46 32N 8 37 E
Airvault, *France* **26 F6** 46 50N 0 8W
Aisch →, *Germany* **31 F6** 49 49N 10 58 E
Aisen □, *Chile* **176 C2** 46 30 S 73 0W
Aisne □, *France* **27 C10** 49 42N 3 40 E
Aisne →, *France* **27 C9** 49 26N 2 50 E
Ait, *India* **93 G8** 25 54N 79 14 E
Aitana, Sierra de, *Spain* **41 G4** 38 35N 0 24W
Aitape, *Papua N. G.* **132 B2** 3 11 S 142 22 E
Aitkin, *U.S.A.* **154 B8** 46 32N 93 42W
Aitolía kai Akarnanía □, *Greece* **48 C3** 38 45N 21 18 E
Aitolikón, *Greece* **48 C3** 38 26N 21 21 E
Aitutaki, *Cook Is.* **135 J12** 18 52 S 159 45 E
Aiuaba, *Brazil* **170 C3** 6 38 S 40 7W
Aiud, *Romania* **53 D8** 46 19N 23 44 E
Aix-en-Provence, *France* **29 E9** 43 32N 5 27 E
Aix-la-Chapelle = Aachen, *Germany* **30 E2** 50 45N 6 6 E
Aix-les-Bains, *France* **29 C9** 45 41N 5 53 E
Aixe-sur-Vienne, *France* **28 C5** 45 47N 1 9 E
Aiyang, Mt., *Papua N. G.* **132 C1** 5 10 S 141 20 E
Áíyina, *Greece* **48 D5** 37 45N 23 26 E
Aiyínion, *Greece* **50 F6** 40 28N 22 28 E
Aíyion, *Greece* **48 C4** 38 15N 22 5 E
Aizawl, *India* **90 D4** 23 40N 92 44 E
Aizenay, *France* **26 F5** 46 44N 1 38W
Aizkraukle, *Latvia* **15 H21** 56 36N 25 11 E
Aizpute, *Latvia* **15 H19** 56 43N 21 40 E
Aizuwakamatsu, *Japan* **70 F9** 37 30N 139 56 E
Ajaccio, *France* **29 G12** 41 55N 8 40 E
Ajaccio, G. d', *France* **29 G12** 41 52N 8 40 E
Ajai ⌓, *Uganda* **118 B3** 2 52N 31 16 E
Ajaigarh, *India* **93 G9** 24 52N 80 16 E
Ajaju →, *Colombia* **168 C3** 0 59N 72 20W
Ajalpan, *Mexico* **163 D5** 18 22N 97 15W
Ajanta, *India* **94 D2** 20 30N 75 48 E
Ajanta Ra., *India* **94 D2** 20 28N 75 50 E
Ajari Rep. = Ajaria □, *Georgia* **61 K6** 41 30N 42 0 E
Ajaria □, *Georgia* **61 K6** 41 30N 42 0 E
Ajax, *Canada* **150 C5** 43 50N 79 1W
Ajax, Mt., *N.Z.* **131 C7** 42 35 S 172 5 E
Ajdābiyā, *Libya* **108 B4** 30 54N 20 4 E
Ajdovščina, *Slovenia* **45 C10** 45 54N 13 54 E
Ajibar, *Ethiopia* **107 E4** 10 35N 38 36 E
Ajka, *Hungary* **52 C2** 47 4N 17 31 E
'Ajlūn, *Jordan* **103 C4** 32 18N 35 47 E
'Ajlūn □, *Jordan* **103 C4** 32 18N 35 47 E
'Ajmān, *U.A.E.* **97 E7** 25 25N 55 30 E
Ajmer, *India* **92 F6** 26 28N 74 37 E
Ajnala, *India* **92 D6** 31 50N 74 48 E
Ajo, *U.S.A.* **159 K7** 32 22N 112 52W
Ajo, C. de, *Spain* **42 B7** 43 31N 3 35W
Ajoie, *Switz.* **32 B4** 47 22N 7 0 E
Ajok, *Sudan* **107 F2** 9 15N 28 28 E
Ajuda, Pta. da, *Azores* **9 d3** 37 52N 25 19W
Ajuy, *Phil.* **81 F4** 11 10N 123 1 E
Ak Dağ, *Turkey* **49 E11** 36 30N 29 32 E
Ak Dağları, *Muğla, Turkey* **49 E11** 36 30N 29 30 E
Ak Dağları, *Sivas, Turkey* **100 C7** 39 32N 36 12 E
Ak-Mechet = Qyzylorda, *Kazakhstan* **65 A2** 44 48N 65 28 E
Ak-Mednet = Chornomorske, *Ukraine* **59 K7** 45 31N 32 40 E
Ak-Muz, *Kyrgyzstan* **65 C8** 41 15N 76 10 E
Ak-Sheikh = Razdolnoye, *Ukraine* **59 K7** 45 46N 33 29 E
Ak-Tüz, *Kyrgyzstan* **65 B8** 42 54N 76 7 E
Akaba, *Togo* **113 D5** 8 10N 1 2 E
Akabira, *Japan* **70 C11** 43 33N 142 5 E
Akabli, *Algeria* **111 C5** 26 49N 1 31 E
Akagera △, *Rwanda* **118 C3** 1 31 S 30 33 E
Akaishi-Dake, *Japan* **73 B10** 35 27N 138 9 E
Akaishi-Sammyaku, *Japan* **73 B10** 35 25N 138 10 E
Akaki Beseka, *Ethiopia* **107 F4** 8 55N 38 45 E
Akākūs, Jabal, *Libya* **111 C7** 25 20N 10 30 E
Akala, *Sudan* **107 D4** 15 39N 36 13 E
Akalkot, *India* **94 F3** 17 32N 76 13 E
Akamas, *Cyprus* **39 E8** 35 3N 32 18 E
Akan △, *Japan* **70 C12** 43 20N 144 20 E
Akanthou, *Cyprus* **39 E9** 35 22N 33 45 E
Akarca, *Turkey* **49 C11** 38 35N 29 35 E
Akaroa, *N.Z.* **131 D7** 43 49 S 172 59 E
Akaroa Harbour, *N.Z.* **131 D7** 43 50 S 172 55 E
Akasha, *Sudan* **106 C3** 21 10N 30 32 E
Akashi, *Japan* **72 C6** 34 45N 134 58 E
Akbarpur, *Bihar, India* **93 G10** 24 39N 83 58 E
Akbarpur, *Ut. P., India* **93 F10** 26 25N 82 32 E
Akbou, *Algeria* **111 A5** 36 31N 4 31 E
Akbulak, *Russia* **64 F5** 51 1N 55 37 E
Akçaabat, *Turkey* **101 B8** 41 1N 39 34 E
Akçadağ, *Turkey* **100 C7** 38 27N 37 43 E
Akçakale, *Turkey* **101 D8** 36 41N 38 56 E
Akçakoca, *Turkey* **100 B4** 41 5N 31 8 E
Akçaova, *Turkey* **51 E13** 41 3N 29 57 E
Akçay, *Turkey* **49 E11** 36 36N 29 45 E
Akçay →, *Turkey* **49 D10** 37 50N 28 15 E
Akchâr, *Mauritania* **110 D2** 20 20N 14 28W
Akchi-Karasu = Toktogul, *Kyrgyzstan* **65 C6** 41 50N 72 50 E
Akdağ, *Turkey* **49 C8** 38 33N 26 30 E
Akdağmadeni, *Turkey* **100 C6** 39 39N 35 53 E
Akechi, *Japan* **73 B9** 35 18N 137 23 E
Akelamo, *Indonesia* **82 A3** 1 35N 129 40 E
Åkernes, *Norway* **18 F4** 58 45N 7 30 E
Åkers styckebruk, *Sweden* **16 E11** 59 15N 17 5 E
Åkersberga, *Sweden* **16 E12** 59 29N 18 18 E
Akershus □, *Norway* **18 D8** 60 0N 11 10 E
Akeru →, *India* **94 F5** 17 25N 80 5 E
Aketi, *Dem. Rep. of the Congo* **114 B4** 2 38N 23 47 E
Akhaïa □, *Greece* **48 C3** 38 5N 21 45 E
Akhalkalaki, *Georgia* **61 K6** 41 27N 43 25 E
Akhaltsikhe, *Georgia* **61 K6** 41 40N 43 0 E
Akharnaí, *Greece* **48 C5** 38 5N 23 44 E
Akhelóös →, *Greece* **48 C3** 38 19N 21 7 E
Akhendriá, *Greece* **49 G7** 34 59N 25 13 E
Akhiok, *U.S.A.* **144 H9** 56 57N 154 10W
Akhisar, *Turkey* **49 C9** 38 56N 27 48 E
Akhladhókambos, *Greece* **48 D4** 37 31N 22 35 E
Akhmîm, *Egypt* **106 B3** 26 31N 31 47 E
Akhnur, *India* **93 C6** 32 52N 74 45 E
Akhtopol, *Bulgaria* **51 D11** 42 6N 27 56 E
Akhtuba →, *Russia* **61 G8** 47 41N 46 55 E
Akhtubinsk, *Russia* **61 F8** 48 13N 46 7 E
Akhty, *Russia* **61 K8** 41 30N 47 45 E
Akhtyrka = Okhtyrka, *Ukraine* **59 G8** 50 25N 35 0 E
Aki, *Japan* **72 D5** 33 30N 133 54 E
Aki-Nada, *Japan* **72 C4** 34 5N 132 40 E
Akiachak, *U.S.A.* **144 F7** 60 55N 161 26W
Akiak, *U.S.A.* **144 F7** 60 55N 161 13W
Akiéni, *Gabon* **114 C2** 1 11 S 13 53 E
Akimiski I., *Canada* **140 B3** 52 50N 81 30W
Akimovka, *Ukraine* **59 J8** 46 44N 35 0 E
Åkirkeby, *Denmark* **17 J8** 55 4N 14 55 E
Akita, *Japan* **70 E10** 39 45N 140 7 E
Akita □, *Japan* **70 E10** 39 40N 140 30 E
Akjoujt, *Mauritania* **112 B2** 19 45N 14 15W
Akka, *Mali* **112 B4** 15 24N 4 11W
Akka, *Morocco* **110 C3** 29 22N 8 9W
Akkaraipattu, *Sri Lanka* **95 L5** 7 13N 81 51 E
Akkaya Tepesi, *Turkey* **49 D11** 37 25N 29 38 E
Akkerman = Bilhorod-Dnistrovskyy, *Ukraine* **59 J6** 46 11N 30 23 E
Akkeshi, *Japan* **70 C12** 43 2N 144 51 E
'Akko, *Israel* **103 C4** 32 55N 35 4 E
Akkol = Aqköl, *Kazakhstan* **65 A7** 45 0N 75 39 E
Akkol = Aqköl, *Kazakhstan* **65 B5** 43 36N 70 45 E
Akköy, *Turkey* **49 D9** 37 29N 27 15 E
Aklampa, *Benin* **113 D5** 8 15N 2 10 E
Aklan □, *Phil.* **81 F4** 11 50N 122 30 E
Aklavik, *Canada* **138 B6** 68 12N 135 0W
Aklera, *India* **92 G7** 24 26N 76 32 E
Akmal-Abad = Gizhduvan, *Uzbekistan* **65 C2** 40 6N 64 41 E
Akmenė, *Lithuania* **54 B9** 56 15N 22 45 E
Akmenrags, *Latvia* **54 B8** 56 50N 21 4 E
Akmeqit, *China* **65 E8** 37 5N 76 55 E
Akmolinsk = Astana, *Kazakhstan* **66 D8** 51 10N 71 30 E
Akmonte = Almonte, *Spain* **43 H4** 37 13N 6 38W
Aknoul, *Morocco* **111 B4** 34 40N 3 55W
Akō, *Japan* **72 C6** 34 45N 134 24 E
Ako, *Nigeria* **113 C7** 10 19N 10 48 E
Akôbô, *Sudan* **107 F3** 7 47N 33 1 E
Akobo →, *Ethiopia* **107 F3** 7 48N 33 3 E
Akola, *Maharashtra, India* **94 D3** 20 42N 77 2 E
Akola, *Maharashtra, India* **94 E2** 19 32N 74 3 E
Akolmiut, *U.S.A.* **144 F7** 60 55N 162 20W
Akonolinga, *Cameroon* **113 E7** 3 50N 12 18 E
Akor, *Mali* **112 C3** 14 59N 6 58W
Akordat, *Eritrea* **107 D4** 15 30N 37 40 E
Akosombo Dam, *Ghana* **113 D5** 6 20N 0 5 E
Akot, *India* **94 D3** 21 10N 77 10 E
Akot, *Sudan* **107 F3** 6 31N 30 9 E
Akoupé, *Ivory C.* **112 D4** 6 23N 3 54W
Akourousoulba, *C.A.R.* **114 A4** 8 58N 20 46 E
Akpatok I., *Canada* **139 B13** 60 25N 68 8W
Åkrahamn, *Norway* **18 E2** 59 15N 5 10 E
'Akramah, *Libya* **108 B4** 32 2N 23 41 E
Akranes, *Iceland* **11 C4** 64 19N 22 5W
Akreïjit, *Mauritania* **112 B3** 18 19N 9 11W
Akrítas Venétiko, Ákra, *Greece* **48 E3** 36 43N 21 54 E
Akron, *Colo., U.S.A.* **154 E3** 40 10N 103 13W
Akron, *Ind., U.S.A.* **157 C10** 41 2N 86 1W
Akron, *Ohio, U.S.A.* **150 E3** 41 5N 81 31W
Akrotiri, *Cyprus* **39 F8** 34 36N 32 57 E
Akrotíri, Ákra, *Greece* **51 F9** 40 26N 25 27 E
Akrotiri Bay, *Cyprus* **39 F9** 34 35N 33 10 E
Aksai Chin, *China* **93 B8** 35 15N 79 55 E
Aksaray, *Turkey* **100 C6** 38 25N 34 2 E
Aksay, *Kazakhstan* **57 D9** 51 11N 53 0 E
Akşehir, *Turkey* **100 C4** 38 18N 31 30 E
Akşehir Gölü, *Turkey* **100 C4** 38 30N 31 25 E
Akstafa = Ağstafa, *Azerbaijan* **61 K7** 41 7N 45 27 E
Aksu, *China* **68 B3** 41 5N 80 10 E
Aksu →, *Turkey* **100 D4** 36 52N 30 57 E
Aksum, *Ethiopia* **107 E4** 14 5N 38 40 E
Aktash, *Russia* **60 C11** 55 2N 52 3 E
Aktash, *Uzbekistan* **65 D2** 39 55N 65 55 E
Aktasty, *Kazakhstan* **64 F8** 50 42N 61 42 E
Aktion, *Greece* **39 B2** 38 57N 20 46 E
Akto, *China* **65 D7** 39 5N 75 59 E
Aktogay, *Kazakhstan* **66 E8** 46 57N 79 40 E
Aktsyabrski, *Belarus* **59 F5** 52 38N 28 53 E
Aktyubinsk = Aqtöbe, *Kazakhstan* **57 D10** 50 17N 57 10 E
Aktyuz = Ak-Tüz, *Kyrgyzstan* **65 B8** 42 54N 76 7 E
Aku, *Nigeria* **113 D6** 6 40N 7 18 E
Akula, *Dem. Rep. of the Congo* **114 B4** 2 22N 20 12 E
Akulurak, *U.S.A.* **144 E6** 63 33N 164 33W
Akun I., *U.S.A.* **144 J6** 54 11N 165 32W
Akune, *Japan* **72 E2** 32 1N 130 12 E
Akure, *Nigeria* **113 D6** 7 15N 5 5 E
Akurenan, *Eq. Guin.* **114 B2** 1 2N 10 40 E
Akuressa, *Sri Lanka* **95 L5** 6 5N 80 29 E
Akureyri, *Iceland* **11 B8** 65 40N 18 6W
Akuseki-Shima, *Japan* **71 K4** 29 27N 129 37 E
Akusha, *Russia* **61 J8** 42 18N 47 30 E
Akutan, *U.S.A.* **144 J6** 54 8N 165 46W
Akutan I., *U.S.A.* **144 J6** 54 7N 165 55W
Akwa-Ibom □, *Nigeria* **113 E6** 4 30N 7 30 E
Akyab = Sittwe, *Burma* **90 E4** 20 18N 92 45 E
Akyazı, *Turkey* **100 B4** 40 40N 30 38 E
Ål, *Norway* **18 D5** 60 38N 8 33 E
Al Abyaḍ, *Libya* **108 C2** 26 49N 14 1 E
Al Abyār, *Libya* **108 B4** 32 9N 20 29 E
Al 'Adan, *Yemen* **98 D4** 12 45N 45 0 E
Al Aḥsā = Hasa □, *Si. Arabia* **97 E6** 25 50N 49 0 E
Al Ajfar, *Si. Arabia* **96 E4** 27 26N 43 0 E
Al Amādīyah, *Iraq* **101 D10** 37 5N 43 30 E
Al 'Amārah, *Iraq* **101 G12** 31 55N 47 15 E
Al 'Aqabah, *Jordan* **103 F4** 29 31N 35 0 E
Al 'Aqabah □, *Jordan* **103 F4** 29 30N 35 0 E
Al 'Aqīq, *Si. Arabia* **98 B3** 20 39N 41 25 E
Al Arak, *Syria* **101 E8** 34 38N 38 35 E
Al 'Aramah, *Si. Arabia* **96 E5** 25 30N 46 0 E
Al 'Ariḍah, *Si. Arabia* **98 C3** 17 3N 43 5 E
Al 'Arṭāwīyah, *Si. Arabia* **96 E5** 26 31N 45 20 E
Al Ashkhara, *Oman* **99 B7** 21 50N 59 30 E
Al 'Āṣimah = 'Ammān □, *Jordan* **103 D5** 31 40N 36 30 E
Al 'Assāfīyah, *Si. Arabia* **96 D3** 28 17N 38 59 E
Al 'Ayn, *Si. Arabia* **96 E3** 25 4N 38 6 E
Al 'Ayn, *U.A.E.* **97 E7** 24 15N 55 45 E
Al 'Azīzīyah, *Iraq* **101 F11** 32 54N 45 4 E
Al 'Azīzīyah, *Libya* **108 B2** 32 30N 13 1 E
Al Bāb, *Syria* **100 D7** 36 23N 37 29 E
Al Bad', *Si. Arabia* **96 D2** 28 28N 35 1 E
Al Bādī, *Iraq* **96 C4** 35 56N 41 32 E
Al Badī', *Si. Arabia* **98 B4** 22 0N 46 35 E
Al Baḥrah, *Kuwait* **96 D5** 29 40N 47 52 E
Al Baḥral Mayyit = Dead Sea, *Asia* **103 D4** 31 30N 35 30 E
Al Balqā' □, *Jordan* **103 C4** 32 5N 35 45 E
Al Barkāt, *Libya* **108 D2** 24 56N 10 14 E
Al Bārūk, J., *Lebanon* **103 B4** 33 39N 35 40 E
Al Baṣrah, *Iraq* **96 D5** 30 30N 47 50 E
Al Baṭḥā, *Iraq* **96 D5** 31 6N 45 53 E
Al Batinah, *Oman* **99 A7** 24 10N 56 50 E
Al Batrūn, *Lebanon* **103 A4** 34 15N 35 40 E
Al Bayāḍ, *Si. Arabia* **98 B4** 22 0N 47 0 E
Al Bayḍā, *Libya* **108 B4** 32 50N 21 44 E
Al Bayḍā', *Yemen* **98 D4** 14 5N 45 42 E
Al Bi'ār, *Si. Arabia* **98 B2** 22 39N 39 40 E
Al Biqā, *Lebanon* **103 A5** 34 10N 36 10 E
Al Bi'r, *Si. Arabia* **96 D3** 28 51N 36 16 E
Al Birk, *Si. Arabia* **98 C3** 18 13N 41 33 E
Al Bu'ayrāt al Ḥasūn, *Libya* **108 B3** 31 24N 15 44 E
Al Bunbah, *Libya* **108 B4** 32 24N 23 8 E
Al Burayj, *Syria* **103 A5** 34 15N 36 46 E
Al Faḍilī, *Si. Arabia* **97 E6** 26 58N 49 10 E
Al Fallūjah, *Iraq* **101 F10** 33 20N 43 55 E
Al Fātiḥ □, *Libya* **108 B4** 32 0N 21 0 E
Al Fāw, *Iraq* **97 D6** 30 0N 48 30 E
Al Faydamī, *Yemen* **99 C6** 16 25N 52 26 E
Al Fujayrah, *U.A.E.* **97 E8** 25 7N 56 18 E
Al Ghadaf, W. →, *Jordan* **103 D5** 31 26N 36 43 E
Al Ghammās, *Iraq* **96 D5** 31 45N 44 37 E
Al Gharīb, *Libya* **108 B4** 32 35N 21 11 E
Al Ghayḍah, *Yemen* **99 C6** 16 13N 52 11 E
Al Ghayḍah, *Yemen* **99 D5** 14 55N 50 0 E
Al Ghayl, *Yemen* **99 D5** 15 30N 50 54 E
Al Ghazālah, *Si. Arabia* **96 E4** 26 48N 41 19 E
Al Ḥadd, *Oman* **99 B7** 22 32N 59 48 E
Al Ḥaddār, *Si. Arabia* **98 B4** 21 58N 45 57 E
Al Ḥadīthah, *Iraq* **101 E10** 34 0N 41 13 E
Al Ḥadīthah, *Si. Arabia* **103 D6** 31 28N 37 8 E
Al Ḥaḍr, *Iraq* **101 E10** 35 35N 42 44 E
Al Hājānah, *Syria* **103 B5** 33 20N 36 33 E
Al Ḥajar al Gharbī, *Oman* **97 E8** 24 10N 56 15 E
Al Hallānīyah, *Oman* **99 C7** 17 30N 56 1 E
Al Hāmad, *Si. Arabia* **96 D3** 31 30N 39 30 E
Al Ḥamar, *Si. Arabia* **98 B4** 22 26N 46 12 E
Al Hamdāniyah, *Syria* **96 C3** 35 25N 36 50 E
Al Ḥamīdīyah, *Syria* **103 A4** 34 42N 35 57 E
Al Hammādah al Ḥamrā', *Libya* **108 C2** 29 30N 12 0 E
Al Ḥammār, *Iraq* **96 D5** 30 57N 46 51 E
Al Ḥamrā', *Si. Arabia* **96 E3** 24 2N 38 55 E
Al Ḥamzah, *Iraq* **96 D5** 31 43N 44 58 E
Al Ḥanākīyah, *Si. Arabia* **96 E4** 24 51N 40 31 E
Al Ḥarīq, *Si. Arabia* **98 B4** 23 29N 46 27 E
Al Harīr, W. →, *Syria* **103 C4** 32 44N 35 59 E
Al Harūj al Aswad, *Libya* **108 C3** 27 0N 17 10 E
Al Ḥasā, W. →, *Jordan* **103 D4** 31 4N 35 29 E
Al Ḥasakah, *Syria* **101 D9** 36 35N 40 45 E
Al Hāsikīyah, *Oman* **99 C6** 17 28N 55 36 E
Al Ḥasy, *Yemen* **99 D5** 14 3N 48 40 E
Al Ḥawrah, *Yemen* **98 D4** 13 50N 47 35 E
Al Hawtah = Laḥij, *Yemen* **98 D4** 13 4N 44 53 E
Al Ḥawṭah, *Si. Arabia* **98 B4** 23 30N 47 0 E
Al Haydān, W. →, *Jordan* **103 D4** 31 29N 35 34 E
Al Ḥayy, *Iraq* **101 F12** 32 5N 46 5 E
Al Ḥijarah, *Asia* **96 D4** 30 0N 44 0 E
Al Ḥillah, *Iraq* **101 F11** 32 30N 44 25 E
Al Ḥillah, *Si. Arabia* **98 B4** 23 35N 46 50 E
Al Hindīyah, *Iraq* **101 F11** 32 30N 44 10 E
Al Hirmil, *Lebanon* **103 A5** 34 26N 36 24 E
Al Hoceïma, *Morocco* **110 A4** 35 8N 3 58W
Al Ḥudaydah, *Yemen* **98 D3** 14 50N 43 0 E
Al Ḥufrah, *Libya* **108 C2** 25 32N 14 1 E
Al Hufūf, *Si. Arabia* **97 E6** 25 25N 49 45 E
Al Ḥulwah, *Si. Arabia* **98 B4** 23 24N 46 48 E
Al Ḥumayḍah, *Si. Arabia* **96 D2** 29 14N 34 56 E
Al Ḥunayy, *Si. Arabia* **97 E6** 25 58N 48 45 E
Al Husayyāt, *Libya* **108 B4** 30 24N 20 37 E
Al 'Irqah, *Yemen* **98 D4** 13 39N 47 22 E
Al Īsāwīyah, *Si. Arabia* **96 D3** 30 43N 37 59 E
Al Ittihad = Madīnat ash Sha'b, *Yemen* **98 D4** 12 50N 45 0 E
Al Jabal al Akhḍar, *Libya* **108 B4** 32 30N 21 30 E
Al Jabal al Akhḍar □, *Libya* **108 B4** 32 30N 21 41 E
Al Jafr, *Jordan* **103 E5** 30 18N 36 14 E
Al Jāfūrah, *Si. Arabia* **97 E7** 25 0N 50 15 E
Al Jaghbūb, *Libya* **108 C4** 29 42N 24 38 E
Al Jahrah, *Kuwait* **96 D5** 29 25N 47 40 E
Al Jalāmīd, *Si. Arabia* **96 D3** 31 20N 40 6 E
Al Jamalīyah, *Qatar* **97 E6** 25 37N 51 5 E
Al Janūb □, *Lebanon* **103 B4** 33 20N 35 20 E
Al Jawf, *Libya* **108 D4** 24 10N 23 24 E
Al Jawf, *Si. Arabia* **96 D3** 29 55N 39 40 E
Al Jazair = Algeria ■, *Africa* **111 C5** 28 30N 2 0 E
Al Jazirah, *Iraq* **101 E10** 33 30N 44 0 E
Al Jazirah, *Libya* **108 C4** 26 10N 21 20 E
Al Jithāmīyah, *Si. Arabia* **96 E4** 27 41N 41 43 E
Al Jubayl, *Si. Arabia* **97 E6** 27 0N 49 50 E
Al Jubaylah, *Si. Arabia* **96 E5** 24 55N 46 25 E
Al Jubb, *Si. Arabia* **96 E4** 27 11N 42 17 E
Al Jufrah, *Libya* **108 C3** 29 10N 16 0 E
Al Jufrah □, *Libya* **108 C3** 27 30N 17 30 E
Al Jumūm, *Si. Arabia* **98 B2** 21 37N 39 42 E
Al Junaynah, *Sudan* **109 F4** 13 27N 22 45 E
Al Kabā'ish, *Iraq* **96 D5** 30 58N 47 0 E
Al Kāmil, *Oman* **99 B7** 22 13N 59 12 E
Al Karak, *Jordan* **103 D4** 31 11N 35 42 E
Al Karak □, *Jordan* **103 E5** 31 0N 36 0 E
Al Kāẓimīyah, *Iraq* **101 F11** 33 22N 44 18 E
Al Khābūra, *Oman* **97 F8** 23 57N 57 5 E
Al Khafji, *Si. Arabia* **97 E6** 28 24N 48 29 E
Al Khalīl, *West Bank* **103 D4** 31 32N 35 6 E
Al Khāliṣ, *Iraq* **101 F11** 33 49N 44 32 E
Al Khamāsīn, *Si. Arabia* **98 B4** 20 29N 44 46 E
Al Kharj, *Si. Arabia* **98 B4** 24 0N 47 0 E
Al Kharsānīyah, *Si. Arabia* **97 E6** 27 13N 49 18 E
Al Khaṣab, *Oman* **97 E8** 26 14N 56 15 E
Al Khāṣirah, *Si. Arabia* **98 B3** 23 30N 43 47 E
Al Khawr, *Qatar* **97 E6** 25 41N 51 30 E
Al Khiḍr, *Iraq* **96 D5** 31 12N 45 33 E
Al Khiyām, *Lebanon* **103 B4** 33 20N 35 36 E
Al Khums, *Libya* **108 B2** 32 40N 14 17 E
Al Khums □, *Libya* **108 B2** 31 20N 14 10 E
Al Kiswah, *Syria* **103 B5** 33 23N 36 14 E
Al Kūfah, *Iraq* **101 F11** 32 2N 44 24 E
Al Kufrah, *Libya* **108 D4** 24 17N 23 15 E
Al Kuhayfīyah, *Si. Arabia* **96 E4** 27 12N 43 3 E
Al Kūt, *Iraq* **101 F11** 32 30N 46 0 E
Al Kuwayt, *Kuwait* **96 D5** 29 30N 48 0 E
Al Labwah, *Lebanon* **103 A5** 34 11N 36 20 E
Al Lādhiqīyah, *Syria* **100 E6** 35 30N 35 45 E
Al Līth, *Si. Arabia* **98 B3** 20 9N 40 15 E
Al Liwā', *Oman* **97 E8** 24 31N 56 36 E
Al Luḥayyah, *Yemen* **98 D3** 15 45N 42 40 E
Al Madīnah, *Iraq* **96 D5** 30 57N 47 16 E
Al Madīnah, *Si. Arabia* **96 E3** 24 35N 39 52 E
Al Mafraq, *Jordan* **103 C5** 32 17N 36 14 E
Al Mafraq □, *Jordan* **103 C5** 32 17N 36 15 E
Al Maghārīm, *Yemen* **98 D4** 15 1N 47 49 E
Al Maghreb = Morocco ■, *N. Afr.* **110 B3** 32 0N 5 50W
Al Mahbes, *W. Sahara* **110 C3** 27 10N 9 50W
Al Maḥmūdīyah, *Iraq* **101 F11** 33 3N 44 21 E
Al Majma'ah, *Si. Arabia* **96 E5** 25 57N 45 22 E
Al Makhruq, W. →, *Jordan* **103 D6** 31 28N 37 0 E
Al Makḥūl, *Si. Arabia* **96 E4** 26 37N 42 39 E
Al Makīlī, *Libya* **108 B4** 32 10N 22 17 E
Al Manāmah, *Bahrain* **97 E6** 26 10N 50 30 E
Al Maqwa', *Kuwait* **96 D5** 29 10N 47 59 E
Al Marj, *Libya* **108 B4** 32 25N 20 30 E
Al Maṭlā, *Kuwait* **96 D5** 29 24N 47 40 E
Al Mawjib, W. →, *Jordan* **103 D4** 31 28N 35 36 E
Al Mawṣil, *Iraq* **101 D10** 36 15N 43 5 E
Al Mayādin, *Syria* **101 E9** 35 1N 40 27 E
Al Mazār, *Jordan* **103 D4** 31 4N 35 41 E
Al Midhnab, *Si. Arabia* **96 E5** 25 50N 44 18 E
Al Minā', *Lebanon* **103 A4** 34 24N 35 49 E
Al Miqdādīyah, *Iraq* **101 E11** 34 0N 45 0 E
Al Mubarraz, *Si. Arabia* **97 E6** 25 30N 49 40 E
Al Mudawwarah, *Jordan* **103 F5** 29 19N 36 0 E
Al Muḍaybī, *Oman* **99 B7** 22 34N 58 7 E
Al Mughayrā', *U.A.E.* **97 E7** 24 5N 53 32 E
Al Muḥarraq, *Bahrain* **97 E6** 26 15N 50 40 E
Al Mukallā, *Yemen* **99 D5** 14 33N 49 2 E
Al Mukhā, *Yemen* **98 D3** 13 18N 43 15 E
Al Musayjīd, *Si. Arabia* **96 E3** 24 5N 39 5 E
Al Musayyib, *Iraq* **101 F11** 32 49N 44 20 E
Al Muthanná □, *Iraq* **96 D5** 30 30N 45 15 E
Al Muwayh, *Si. Arabia* **106 C5** 22 41N 41 37 E
Al Muwayliḥ, *Si. Arabia* **96 E2** 27 40N 35 30 E
Al Owuho = Otukpa, *Nigeria* **113 D6** 7 9N 7 41 E
Al Qaddāḥīyah, *Libya* **108 B3** 31 15N 15 9 E
Al Qaḍīmah, *Si. Arabia* **98 B2** 22 20N 39 13 E
Al Qādisīyah □, *Iraq* **96 D5** 32 0N 45 0 E
Al Qaḥmah, *Si. Arabia* **98 C3** 18 0N 41 41 E
Al Qā'im, *Iraq* **101 E9** 34 21N 41 7 E
Al Qalībah, *Si. Arabia* **96 D3** 28 24N 37 42 E
Al Qāmishlī, *Syria* **101 D9** 37 2N 41 14 E
Al Qaryah ash Sharqīyah, *Libya* **108 B2** 30 28N 13 40 E

Al Qaryatayn, *Syria*	**103 A6**	34 12N	37 13 E
Al Qaşabât, *Libya*	**108 B2**	32 39N	14 1 E
Al Qaşīm, *Si. Arabia*	**96 E4**	26 0N	43 0 E
Al Qaţ'ā, *Syria*	**101 E9**	34 40N	40 48 E
Al Qaţīf, *Si. Arabia*	**97 E6**	26 35N	50 0 E
Al Qaţn, *Yemen*	**99 D5**	15 51N	48 26 E
Al Qatrānah, *Jordan*	**103 D5**	31 12N	36 6 E
Al Qaţrūn, *Libya*	**108 D3**	24 56N	15 3 E
Al Qayşūmah, *Si. Arabia*	**96 D5**	28 20N	46 7 E
Al Qiblīyah, *Oman*	**99 C7**	17 30N	56 20 E
Al Quds = Jerusalem, *Israel*	**103 D4**	31 47N	35 10 E
Al Qunayţirah, *Syria*	**103 C4**	32 55N	35 45 E
Al Qunfudhah, *Si. Arabia*	**98 C3**	19 3N	41 4 E
Al Qurḩ, *Yemen*	**99 C5**	16 44N	51 29 E
Al Qurnah, *Iraq*	**96 D5**	31 1N	47 25 E
Al Quşayr, *Iraq*	**96 D5**	30 39N	45 50 E
Al Quşayr, *Syria*	**103 A5**	34 31N	36 34 E
Al Qutayfah, *Syria*	**103 B5**	33 44N	36 36 E
Al Quway'īyah, *Si. Arabia*	**98 A4**	24 3N	45 15 E
Al 'Ubaylah, *Si. Arabia*	**99 B5**	21 59N	50 57 E
Al 'Uḑaylīyah, *Si. Arabia*	**97 E6**	25 8N	49 18 E
Al 'Ulā, *Si. Arabia*	**96 E3**	26 35N	38 0 E
Al 'Ulayyah, *Si. Arabia*	**98 C3**	19 39N	41 54 E
Al Uqaylah ash Sharqīgah, *Libya*	**108 B3**	30 12N	19 10 E
Al 'Uqayr, *Si. Arabia*	**97 E6**	25 40N	50 15 E
Al 'Urūq al Mutariḑah, *Si. Arabia*	**99 B6**	21 0N	53 30 E
Al 'Uwaynid, *Si. Arabia*	**96 E5**	24 50N	46 0 E
Al 'Uwayqīlah, *Si. Arabia*	**96 D4**	30 30N	42 10 E
Al 'Uyūn, *Ḩijāz, Si. Arabia*	**96 E3**	24 33N	39 35 E
Al 'Uyūn, *Najd, Si. Arabia*	**96 E4**	26 30N	43 50 E
Al 'Uzayr, *Iraq*	**96 D5**	31 19N	47 25 E
Al Wajh, *Si. Arabia*	**96 E3**	26 10N	36 30 E
Al Wakrah, *Qatar*	**97 E6**	25 10N	51 40 E
Al Waqbah, *Si. Arabia*	**96 D5**	28 48N	45 33 E
Al Wari'āh, *Si. Arabia*	**96 E5**	27 51N	47 25 E
Al Wāţīyah, *Libya*	**108 B2**	32 28N	11 57 E
Al Yaman = Yemen ■, *Asia*	**98 D4**	15 0N	44 0 E
Ala, *Italy*	**44 C8**	45 45N	11 0 E
Ala-Buka, *Kyrgyzstan*	**65 C5**	41 23N	71 30 E
Ala Dağ, *Turkey*	**96 B2**	37 44N	35 9 E
Ala Dağları, *Turkey*	**101 C10**	39 15N	43 33 E
Ala Tau Shankou = Dzungarian Gates, *Asia*	**68 B3**	45 0N	82 0 E
Alabama □, *U.S.A.*	**149 J2**	33 0N	87 0W
Alabama →, *U.S.A.*	**149 K2**	31 8N	87 57W
Alabaster, *U.S.A.*	**149 J2**	33 15N	86 49W
Alabat I., *Phil.*	**80 D4**	14 7N	122 3 E
Alabel, *Phil.*	**81 H5**	6 4N	125 16 E
Alabule →, *Papua N. G.*	**132 E4**	8 31 S	146 56 E
Alaca, *Turkey*	**100 B6**	40 10N	34 51 E
Alacaatlı, *Turkey*	**49 B10**	39 15N	28 3 E
Alaçam, *Turkey*	**100 B6**	41 36N	35 36 E
Alaçam Dağları, *Turkey*	**49 B10**	39 18N	28 49 E
Alacant = Alicante, *Spain*	**41 G4**	38 23N	0 30W
Alaçatı, *Turkey*	**49 C8**	38 15N	26 22 E
Alachua, *U.S.A.*	**152 F7**	29 47N	82 30W
Alaejos, *Spain*	**42 D5**	41 18N	5 13W
Alaérma, *Greece*	**38 E11**	36 9N	27 57 E
Alagir, *Russia*	**61 J7**	43 3N	44 14 E
Alagna Valsésia, *Italy*	**44 C4**	45 51N	7 56 E
Alagoa de Baixo = Sertânia, *Brazil*	**170 C4**	8 5 S	37 20W
Alagoa Grande, *Brazil*	**170 C4**	7 3 S	35 35W
Alagoas = Marechal Deodoro, *Brazil*	**170 C4**	9 43 S	35 54W
Alagoas □, *Brazil*	**170 C4**	9 0 S	36 0W
Alagoinhas, *Brazil*	**171 D4**	12 7 S	38 20W
Alagón, *Spain*	**40 D3**	41 46N	1 12W
Alagón →, *Spain*	**42 F4**	39 44N	6 53W
Alagyoz = Aragats, *Armenia*	**61 K7**	40 30N	44 15 E
Alai Range, *Asia*	**65 D5**	39 45N	72 0 E
Alaior, *Spain*	**38 B5**	39 57N	4 8 E
Alajero, *Canary Is.*	**9 e1**	28 3N	17 13W
Alajuela, *Costa Rica*	**164 D3**	10 2N	84 8W
Alakamisy, *Madag.*	**117 C8**	21 19 S	47 14 E
Alakanuk, *U.S.A.*	**144 E6**	62 41N	164 37W
Alaknanda →, *India*	**93 D8**	30 8N	78 36 E
Alakurtti, *Russia*	**56 A5**	66 58N	30 25 E
Alalakeiki Channel, *U.S.A.*	**145 C5**	20 30N	156 30W
Alalapura, *Suriname*	**169 C6**	2 20N	56 25W
Alalaú →, *Brazil*	**169 D5**	0 30 S	61 9W
Alamarvdasht, *Iran*	**97 E7**	27 37N	52 59 E
Alamata, *Ethiopia*	**107 E4**	12 25N	39 33 E
Alameda, *Calif., U.S.A.*	**160 H4**	37 46N	122 15W
Alameda, *N. Mex., U.S.A.*	**159 J10**	35 11N	106 37W
Alaminos, *Phil.*	**80 C2**	16 10N	119 59 E
Alamo, *Ga., U.S.A.*	**152 C7**	32 9N	82 47W
Alamo, *Nev., U.S.A.*	**161 H11**	37 22N	115 10W
Alamo Crossing, *U.S.A.*	**161 L13**	34 16N	113 33W
Alamogordo, *U.S.A.*	**159 K11**	32 54N	105 57W
Alamos, *Mexico*	**162 B3**	27 0N	109 0W
Alamosa, *U.S.A.*	**159 H11**	37 28N	105 52W
Alampur, *India*	**95 G4**	15 55N	78 6 E
Åland = Ahvenanmaa, *Finland*	**15 F19**	60 15N	20 0 E
Aland, *India*	**94 F3**	17 36N	76 35 E
Alandroal, *Portugal*	**43 G3**	38 41N	7 24W
Ålands hav, *Europe*	**15 F18**	60 0N	19 30 E
Alandur, *India*	**95 H5**	13 0N	80 15 E
Alange, Embalse d', *Spain*	**43 G4**	38 45N	6 18W
Alania = North Ossetia □, *Russia*	**61 J7**	43 30N	44 30 E
Alanís, *Spain*	**43 G5**	38 3N	5 43W
Alanya, *Turkey*	**100 D5**	36 38N	32 0 E
Alaotra, Farihin', *Madag.*	**117 B8**	17 30 S	48 30 E
Alapaha, *U.S.A.*	**152 D6**	31 23N	83 13W
Alapayevsk, *Russia*	**64 C8**	57 52N	61 42 E
Alappuzha = Alleppey, *India*	**95 K3**	9 30N	76 28 E
Alar del Rey, *Spain*	**42 C6**	42 38N	4 20W
Alaraz, *Spain*	**42 E5**	40 45N	5 17W
Alarcón, Embalse de, *Spain*	**40 F2**	39 36N	2 10W
Alarobia-Vohiposa, *Madag.*	**117 C8**	20 59 S	47 9 E
Alaşehir, *Turkey*	**49 C10**	38 23N	28 30 E
Alaska □, *U.S.A.*	**144 E9**	64 0N	154 0W
Alaska, G. of, *Pac. Oc.*	**144 G11**	58 0N	145 0W
Alaska Peninsula, *U.S.A.*	**144 J8**	56 0N	159 0W
Alaska Range, *U.S.A.*	**144 F10**	62 50N	151 0W
Alássio, *Italy*	**44 E5**	44 0N	8 10 E
Älät, *Azerbaijan*	**61 L9**	39 58N	49 25 E
Alat, *Uzbekistan*	**65 D1**	39 24N	63 47 E
Alatri, *Italy*	**45 G10**	41 43N	13 21 E
Alatyr, *Russia*	**60 C8**	54 55N	46 35 E
Alatyr →, *Russia*	**60 C8**	54 52N	46 36 E
Alausi, *Ecuador*	**168 D2**	2 0 S	78 50W
Álava □, *Spain*	**40 C2**	42 48N	2 28W
Alava, C., *U.S.A.*	**158 B1**	48 10N	124 44W
Alaverdi, *Armenia*	**61 K7**	41 15N	44 37 E
Alavo = Alavus, *Finland*	**15 E20**	62 35N	23 36 E
Alavus, *Finland*	**15 E20**	62 35N	23 36 E
Alawoona, *Australia*	**128 C4**	34 45 S	140 30 E
'Alayh, *Lebanon*	**103 B4**	33 46N	35 33 E
Alaykuu = Kögart, *Kyrgyzstan*	**65 C7**	40 15N	74 25 E
Alazani →, *Azerbaijan*	**61 K8**	41 5N	46 40 E
Alba, *Italy*	**44 D5**	44 42N	8 2 E
Alba □, *Romania*	**53 D8**	46 10N	23 30 E
Alba Adriática, *Italy*	**45 F10**	42 50N	13 56 E
Alba de Tormes, *Spain*	**42 E5**	40 50N	5 30W
Alba-Iulia, *Romania*	**53 D8**	46 8N	23 39 E
Albac, *Romania*	**52 D7**	46 28N	22 58 E
Albacete, *Spain*	**41 F3**	39 0N	1 50W
Albacete □, *Spain*	**41 G3**	38 50N	2 0W
Albacutya, L., *Australia*	**128 C4**	35 45 S	141 58 E
Ålbæk, *Denmark*	**17 G4**	57 36N	10 25 E
Ålbæk Bugt, *Denmark*	**17 G4**	57 35N	10 40 E
Albaida, *Spain*	**41 G4**	38 51N	0 31W
Albalate de las Nogueras, *Spain*	**40 E2**	40 22N	2 18W
Albalate del Arzobispo, *Spain*	**40 D4**	41 6N	0 31W
Alban, *France*	**28 E6**	43 53N	2 28 E
Albanel, L., *Canada*	**140 B5**	50 55N	73 12W
Albania ■, *Europe*	**50 E4**	41 0N	20 0 E
Albano Laziale, *Italy*	**45 G9**	41 44N	12 39 E
Albany, *Australia*	**125 G2**	35 1 S	117 58 E
Albany, *Ga., U.S.A.*	**152 D5**	31 35N	84 10W
Albany, *Ind., U.S.A.*	**157 D11**	40 18N	85 14W
Albany, *Mo., U.S.A.*	**156 D2**	40 15N	94 20W
Albany, *N.Y., U.S.A.*	**151 D11**	42 39N	73 45W
Albany, *Oreg., U.S.A.*	**158 D2**	44 38N	123 6W
Albany, *Tex., U.S.A.*	**155 J5**	32 44N	99 18W
Albany, *Wis., U.S.A.*	**156 B7**	42 43N	89 26W
Albany →, *Canada*	**140 B3**	52 17N	81 31W
Albardón, *Argentina*	**174 C2**	31 20 S	68 30W
Albarracín, *Spain*	**40 E3**	40 25N	1 26W
Albarracín, Sierra de, *Spain*	**40 E3**	40 30N	1 30W
Albatera, *Spain*	**41 G4**	38 11N	0 52W
Albatross B., *Australia*	**126 A3**	12 45 S	141 30 E
Albatross Pt., *N.Z.*	**130 E3**	38 7 S	174 44 E
Albay □, *Phil.*	**80 E4**	13 13N	123 33 E
Albegna →, *Italy*	**45 F8**	42 30N	11 11 E
Albemarle, *U.S.A.*	**149 H5**	35 21N	80 11W
Albemarle, I. = Isabela, I., *Ecuador*	**172 a**	0 30 S	91 4W
Albemarle, Pta., *Ecuador*	**172 a**	0 11N	91 21W
Albemarle Sd., *U.S.A.*	**149 H7**	36 5N	76 0W
Albenga, *Italy*	**44 D5**	44 3N	8 13 E
Alberche →, *Spain*	**42 F6**	39 58N	4 46W
Alberdi, *Paraguay*	**174 B4**	26 14 S	58 20W
Albères, Mts., *France*	**28 F6**	42 28N	2 56 E
Ålberga, *Sweden*	**17 F10**	58 44N	16 35 E
Alberga, The →, *Australia*	**127 D2**	27 6 S	135 33 E
Albersdorf, *Germany*	**30 A5**	54 8N	9 17 E
Albert, *France*	**27 C9**	50 0N	2 38 E
Albert, L., *Africa*	**118 B3**	1 30N	31 0 E
Albert, L., *Australia*	**128 C3**	35 30 S	139 10 E
Albert Edward, Mt., *Papua N. G.*	**132 E4**	8 20 S	147 24 E
Albert Edward Ra., *Australia*	**124 C4**	18 17 S	127 57 E
Albert Lea, *U.S.A.*	**154 D8**	43 39N	93 22W
Albert National Park = Virunga △, *Dem. Rep. of the Congo*	**118 B2**	0 5N	29 38 E
Albert Nile →, *Uganda*	**118 B3**	3 36N	32 2 E
Albert Town, *Bahamas*	**165 B5**	22 37N	74 33W
Alberta □, *Canada*	**142 C6**	54 40N	115 0W
Alberti, *Argentina*	**174 D3**	35 1 S	60 16W
Albertinia, *S. Africa*	**116 E3**	34 11 S	21 34 E
Albertirsa, *Hungary*	**52 C4**	47 14N	19 37 E
Alberto de Agostini △, *Chile*	**176 D2**	54 38 S	71 37W
Alberton, *Canada*	**141 C7**	46 50N	64 0W
Albertville = Kalemie, *Dem. Rep. of the Congo*	**118 D2**	5 55 S	29 9 E
Albertville, *France*	**29 C10**	45 40N	6 22 E
Albertville, *U.S.A.*	**149 H2**	34 16N	86 13W
Albi, *France*	**28 E6**	43 56N	2 9 E
Albia, *U.S.A.*	**156 C4**	41 2N	92 48W
Albina, *Suriname*	**169 B7**	5 37N	54 15W
Albina, Ponta, *Angola*	**116 B1**	15 52 S	11 44 E
Albino, *Italy*	**44 C6**	45 46N	9 47 E
Albion, *Ill., U.S.A.*	**157 F8**	38 23N	88 4W
Albion, *Ind., U.S.A.*	**157 C11**	41 24N	85 25W
Albion, *Mich., U.S.A.*	**157 B12**	42 15N	84 45W
Albion, *Nebr., U.S.A.*	**154 E6**	41 42N	98 0W
Albion, *Pa., U.S.A.*	**150 E4**	41 53N	80 22W
Albocácer, *Spain*	**40 E5**	40 21N	0 1 E
Albolote, *Spain*	**43 H7**	37 14N	3 39W
Alborán, *Medit. S.*	**43 K7**	35 57N	3 0W
Alborea, *Spain*	**41 F3**	39 17N	1 24W
Ålborg, *Denmark*	**17 G3**	57 2N	9 54 E
Ålborg Bugt, *Denmark*	**17 H4**	56 50N	10 35 E
Alborz, Reshteh-ye Kūhhā-ye, *Iran*	**97 C7**	36 0N	52 0 E
Albosaggia, *Italy*	**33 D9**	46 8N	9 51 E
Albox, *Spain*	**41 H2**	37 23N	2 8W
Albuera, *Phil.*	**81 F5**	10 55N	124 42 E
Albufeira, *Portugal*	**43 H2**	37 5N	8 15W
Albula →, *Switz.*	**33 C8**	46 38N	9 28 E
Albuñol, *Spain*	**43 J7**	36 48N	3 11W
Albuquerque, *Brazil*	**173 D6**	19 23 S	57 26W
Albuquerque, *U.S.A.*	**159 J10**	35 5N	106 39W
Albuquerque, Cayos de, *Caribbean*	**164 D3**	12 10N	81 50W
Alburg, *U.S.A.*	**151 B11**	44 59N	73 18W
Alburno, Mte., *Italy*	**47 B8**	40 33N	15 17 E
Alburquerque, *Spain*	**43 F4**	39 15N	6 59W
Albury = Albury-Wodonga, *Australia*	**129 D7**	36 3 S	146 56 E
Albury-Wodonga, *Australia*	**129 D7**	36 3 S	146 56 E
Alcácer do Sal, *Portugal*	**43 G2**	38 22N	8 33W
Alcáçovas, *Portugal*	**43 G2**	38 23N	8 9W
Alcala, *Phil.*	**80 C3**	17 54N	121 39 E
Alcalá de Chivert, *Spain*	**40 E5**	40 19N	0 13 E
Alcalá de Guadaira, *Spain*	**43 H5**	37 20N	5 50W
Alcalá de Henares, *Spain*	**42 E7**	40 28N	3 22W
Alcalá de los Gazules, *Spain*	**43 J5**	36 29N	5 43W
Alcalá del Júcar, *Spain*	**41 F3**	39 12N	1 26W
Alcalá del Río, *Spain*	**43 H5**	37 31N	5 59W
Alcalá del Valle, *Spain*	**43 J5**	36 54N	5 10W
Alcalá la Real, *Spain*	**43 H7**	37 27N	3 57W
Álcamo, *Italy*	**46 E5**	37 59N	12 55 E
Alcanadre, *Spain*	**40 C2**	42 24N	2 7W
Alcanadre →, *Spain*	**40 D4**	41 43N	0 12W
Alcanar, *Spain*	**40 E5**	40 33N	0 28 E
Alcanede, *Portugal*	**43 F2**	39 25N	8 49W
Alcanena, *Portugal*	**43 F2**	39 27N	8 40W
Alcañices, *Spain*	**42 D4**	41 41N	6 21W
Alcaníz, *Spain*	**40 D4**	41 2N	0 8W
Alcântara, *Brazil*	**170 B3**	2 20 S	44 30W
Alcántara, *Spain*	**42 F4**	39 41N	6 57W
Alcántara, Embalse de, *Spain*	**42 F4**	39 44N	6 50W
Alcantarilla, *Spain*	**41 H3**	37 59N	1 12W
Alcaracejos, *Spain*	**43 G6**	38 24N	4 58W
Alcaraz, *Spain*	**41 G2**	38 40N	2 29W
Alcaraz, Sierra de, *Spain*	**41 G2**	38 40N	2 20W
Alcaudete, *Spain*	**43 H6**	37 35N	4 5W
Alcázar de San Juan, *Spain*	**43 F7**	39 24N	3 12W
Alcazarquivir = Ksar el Kebir, *Morocco*	**110 B3**	35 0N	6 0W
Alcedo, Volcán, *Ecuador*	**172 a**	0 24 S	91 6W
Alchevsk, *Ukraine*	**59 H10**	48 30N	38 45 E
Alcira = Alzira, *Spain*	**41 F4**	39 9N	0 30W
Alcobaça = Tucuruí, *Brazil*	**170 B2**	3 42 S	49 44W
Alcobaça, *Portugal*	**43 F2**	39 32N	8 58W
Alcobendas, *Spain*	**42 E7**	40 32N	3 38W
Alcolea del Pinar, *Spain*	**40 D2**	41 2N	2 28W
Alcoma, *U.S.A.*	**153 H8**	27 54N	81 29W
Alcora, *Spain*	**40 E4**	40 5N	0 14W
Alcorcón, *Spain*	**42 E7**	40 20N	3 50W
Alcoutim, *Portugal*	**43 H3**	37 25N	7 28W
Alcova, *U.S.A.*	**158 E10**	42 34N	106 43W
Alcoy, *Spain*	**41 G4**	38 43N	0 30W
Alcubierre, Sierra de, *Spain*	**40 D4**	41 45N	0 22W
Alcublas, *Spain*	**40 F4**	39 48N	0 43W
Alcúdia, *Spain*	**38 B4**	39 51N	3 7 E
Alcúdia, B. d', *Spain*	**38 B4**	39 47N	3 15 E
Alcudia, Sierra de la, *Spain*	**43 G6**	38 34N	4 30W
Aldabra Is., *Seychelles*	**121 E3**	9 22 S	46 28 E
Aldama, *Mexico*	**163 C5**	23 0N	98 4W
Aldan, *Russia*	**67 D13**	58 40N	125 30 E
Aldan →, *Russia*	**67 C13**	63 28N	129 35 E
Aldea, Pta. de la, *Canary Is.*	**9 e1**	28 0N	15 50W
Aldeburgh, *U.K.*	**21 E9**	52 10N	1 37 E
Alden, *Norway*	**18 C1**	61 19N	4 45 E
Alder Pk., *U.S.A.*	**160 K5**	35 53N	121 22W
Alderney, *U.K.*	**21 H5**	49 42N	2 11W
Aldershot, *U.K.*	**21 F7**	51 15N	0 44W
Aldinga Beach, *Australia*	**128 C3**	35 17 S	138 27 E
Åled, *Sweden*	**17 H6**	56 44N	12 57 E
Aledo, *U.S.A.*	**156 C6**	41 12N	90 45W
Alefa, *Ethiopia*	**107 E4**	11 55N	36 55 E
Aleg, *Mauritania*	**112 B2**	17 3N	13 55W
Alegranza, *Canary Is.*	**110 C2**	29 23N	13 32W
Alegranza, I., *Canary Is.*	**9 e2**	29 23N	13 32W
Alegre, *Brazil*	**171 F3**	20 50 S	41 30W
Alegrete, *Brazil*	**175 B4**	29 40 S	56 0W
Aleisk, *Russia*	**66 D9**	52 40N	83 0 E
Aleknagik, *U.S.A.*	**144 G8**	59 17N	158 36W
Aleksandriya = Oleksandriya, *Kirovohrad, Ukraine*	**59 H7**	48 42N	33 3 E
Aleksandriya = Oleksandriya, *Rivne, Ukraine*	**59 G4**	50 37N	26 19 E
Aleksandriyskaya, *Russia*	**61 J8**	43 58N	47 14 E
Aleksandropol = Gyumri, *Armenia*	**61 K6**	40 47N	43 50 E
Aleksandrov, *Russia*	**58 D10**	56 23N	38 44 E
Aleksandrov Gay, *Russia*	**60 E9**	50 9N	48 34 E
Aleksandrovac, *Serbia & M.*	**50 C5**	43 28N	21 3 E
Aleksandrovac, *Serbia & M.*	**50 B5**	44 28N	21 13 E
Aleksandrovka = Oleksandrovka, *Ukraine*	**59 H7**	48 55N	32 20 E
Aleksandrovka = Ordzhonikidze, *Ukraine*	**59 J8**	47 39N	34 3 E
Aleksandrovo, *Bulgaria*	**51 C8**	43 14N	24 51 E
Aleksandrovsk = Belogorsk, *Russia*	**67 D13**	51 0N	128 20 E
Aleksandrovsk = Polyarny, *Russia*	**56 A5**	69 8N	33 20 E
Aleksandrovsk = Zaporizhzhya, *Ukraine*	**59 J8**	47 50N	35 10 E
Aleksandrovsk, *Russia*	**64 B6**	59 9N	57 33 E
Aleksandrovsk-Grushevsky = Shakhty, *Russia*	**61 G5**	47 40N	40 16 E
Aleksandrovsk-Sakhalinskiy, *Russia*	**67 D15**	50 50N	142 20 E
Aleksandrów Kujawski, *Poland*	**55 F5**	52 53N	18 43 E
Aleksandrów Łódźki, *Poland*	**55 G6**	51 49N	19 17 E
Aleksandry, Z., *Russia*	**6 A10**	80 25N	48 0 E
Alekseyevka, *Samara, Russia*	**60 D10**	52 35N	51 17 E
Alekseyevka, *Voronezh, Russia*	**59 G10**	50 43N	38 40 E
Alekseyevsk = Svobodnyy, *Russia*	**67 D13**	51 20N	128 0 E
Alekseyevskoye = Qazyghurt, *Kazakhstan*	**65 C4**	41 45N	69 23 E
Aleksin, *Russia*	**58 E9**	54 31N	37 9 E
Aleksinac, *Serbia & M.*	**50 C5**	43 31N	21 42 E
Além Paraíba, *Brazil*	**171 F3**	21 52 S	42 41W
Alemania, *Argentina*	**174 B2**	25 40 S	65 30W
Alemania, *Chile*	**174 B2**	25 10 S	69 55W
Alen, *Eq. Guin.*	**114 B2**	1 58N	11 19 E
Alençon, *France*	**26 D7**	48 27N	0 4 E
Alenuihaha Channel, *U.S.A.*	**145 C6**	20 30N	156 0W
Alépé, *Ivory C.*	**112 D4**	5 29N	3 40W
Aleppo = Ḩalab, *Syria*	**100 D7**	36 10N	37 15 E
Alerce Andino △, *Chile*	**176 B2**	41 33 S	72 29W
Aléria, *France*	**29 F13**	42 5N	9 26 E
Alert, *Canada*	**6 A4**	83 2N	60 0W
Aleru, *India*	**94 F4**	17 39N	79 3 E
Alès, *France*	**29 D8**	44 9N	4 5 E
Aleşd, *Romania*	**52 C7**	47 3N	22 22 E
Alessándria, *Italy*	**44 D5**	44 54N	8 37 E
Ålestrup, *Denmark*	**17 H3**	56 42N	9 29 E
Ålesund, *Norway*	**18 B3**	62 28N	6 12 E
Alet-les-Bains, *France*	**28 F6**	42 59N	2 14 E
Aletschhorn, *Switz.*	**32 D6**	46 28N	8 0 E
Aleutian Is., *Pac. Oc.*	**138 C2**	52 0N	175 0W
Aleutian Range, *U.S.A.*	**144 G9**	60 0N	154 0W
Aleutian Trench, *Pac. Oc.*	**134 C10**	48 0N	180 0 E
Alexander, *Ga., U.S.A.*	**152 B8**	33 1N	81 53W
Alexander, *N. Dak., U.S.A.*	**154 B3**	47 51N	103 39W
Alexander, C., *Solomon Is.*	**133 L9**	6 34 S	156 32 E
Alexander, Mt., *Australia*	**125 E3**	28 58 S	120 16 E
Alexander Arch., *U.S.A.*	**144 J14**	56 0N	136 0W
Alexander Bay, *S. Africa*	**116 D2**	28 40 S	16 30 E
Alexander City, *U.S.A.*	**152 C4**	32 56N	85 58W
Alexander I., *Antarctica*	**7 C17**	69 0 S	70 0W
Alexandra, *Australia*	**129 D6**	37 8 S	145 40 E
Alexandra, *N.Z.*	**131 F4**	45 14 S	169 25 E
Alexandra Channel, *Burma*	**95 G11**	14 7N	93 13 E
Alexandra Falls, *Canada*	**142 A5**	60 29N	116 18W
Alexandretta = İskenderun, *Turkey*	**100 D7**	36 32N	36 10 E
Alexandria = El Iskandarîya, *Egypt*	**106 H7**	31 13N	29 58 E
Alexandria, *B.C., Canada*	**142 C4**	52 35N	122 27W
Alexandria, *Ont., Canada*	**140 C5**	45 19N	74 38W
Alexandria, *Romania*	**53 G10**	43 57N	25 24 E
Alexandria, *S. Africa*	**116 E4**	33 38 S	26 28 E
Alexandria, *U.K.*	**22 F4**	55 59N	4 35W
Alexandria, *Ind., U.S.A.*	**157 D11**	40 16N	85 41W
Alexandria, *Ky., U.S.A.*	**157 F12**	38 58N	84 23W
Alexandria, *La., U.S.A.*	**155 K8**	31 18N	92 27W
Alexandria, *Minn., U.S.A.*	**154 C7**	45 53N	95 22W
Alexandria, *Mo., U.S.A.*	**156 D5**	40 27N	91 28W
Alexandria, *S. Dak., U.S.A.*	**154 D6**	43 39N	97 47W
Alexandria, *Va., U.S.A.*	**148 F7**	38 48N	77 3W
Alexandria Bay, *U.S.A.*	**151 B9**	44 20N	75 55W
Alexandrina, L., *Australia*	**128 C3**	35 25 S	139 10 E
Alexandroupoli = Alexandroúpolis, *Greece*	**51 F9**	40 50N	25 54 E
Alexandroúpolis, *Greece*	**51 F9**	40 50N	25 54 E
Alexis, *U.S.A.*	**156 C6**	41 4N	90 33W
Alexis →, *Canada*	**141 B8**	52 33N	56 8W
Alexis Creek, *Canada*	**142 C4**	52 10N	123 20W
Alfabia, *Spain*	**38 B3**	39 44N	2 44 E
Alfambra, *Spain*	**40 E3**	40 33N	1 5W
Alfândega da Fé, *Portugal*	**42 D4**	41 20N	6 59W
Alfaro, *Spain*	**40 C3**	42 10N	1 50W
Alfatar, *Bulgaria*	**51 C11**	43 59N	27 13 E
Alfaz del Pi, *Spain*	**41 G4**	38 35N	0 5W
Alfeld, *Germany*	**30 D5**	51 59N	9 50 E
Alfenas, *Brazil*	**175 A6**	21 20 S	46 10W
Alfiós →, *Greece*	**48 D3**	37 40N	21 33 E
Alföld, *Hungary*	**52 D5**	46 30N	20 0 E
Alfonsine, *Italy*	**45 D9**	44 30N	12 3 E
Alford, *Aberds., U.K.*	**22 D6**	57 14N	2 41W
Alford, *Lincs., U.K.*	**20 D8**	53 15N	0 10 E
Alford, *U.S.A.*	**152 E4**	30 42N	85 24W
Ålfotbreen, *Norway*	**18 C2**	61 45N	5 39 E
Ålfoten, *Norway*	**18 C2**	61 51N	5 41 E
Alfred, *Maine, U.S.A.*	**151 C14**	43 29N	70 43W
Alfred, *N.Y., U.S.A.*	**150 D7**	42 16N	77 48W
Alfredton, *N.Z.*	**130 G4**	40 41 S	175 54 E
Alfreton, *U.K.*	**20 D6**	53 6N	1 24W
Alfta, *Sweden*	**16 C10**	61 21N	16 4 E
Alga, *Kazakhstan*	**57 E10**	49 53N	57 20 E
Algaida, *Spain*	**38 B3**	39 33N	2 53 E
Algar, *Spain*	**43 J5**	36 40N	5 39W
Ålgård, *Norway*	**18 F2**	58 46N	5 53 E
Algarinejo, *Spain*	**43 H6**	37 19N	4 9W
Algarve, *Portugal*	**43 J2**	36 58N	8 20W
Algeciras, *Spain*	**43 J5**	36 9N	5 28W
Algemesí, *Spain*	**41 F4**	39 11N	0 27W
Alger, *Algeria*	**111 A5**	36 42N	3 8 E
Alger ✈ (ALG), *Algeria*	**41 J8**	36 39N	3 13 E
Algeria ■, *Africa*	**111 C5**	28 30N	2 0 E
Alghero, *Italy*	**46 B1**	40 33N	8 19 E
Älghult, *Sweden*	**17 G9**	57 0N	15 35 E
Algiers = Alger, *Algeria*	**111 A5**	36 42N	3 8 E
Algoa B., *S. Africa*	**116 E4**	33 50 S	25 45 E
Algodonales, *Spain*	**43 J5**	36 54N	5 24W
Algodor →, *Spain*	**42 F7**	39 55N	3 53W
Algoma, *U.S.A.*	**148 C2**	44 36N	87 26W
Algona, *U.S.A.*	**156 A2**	43 4N	94 14W
Algonac, *U.S.A.*	**150 D2**	42 37N	82 32W
Algonquin ⌓, *Canada*	**140 C4**	45 50N	78 30W
Alhama de Almería, *Spain*	**43 J8**	36 57N	2 34W
Alhama de Aragón, *Spain*	**40 D3**	41 18N	1 54W
Alhama de Granada, *Spain*	**43 H7**	37 0N	3 59W
Alhama de Murcia, *Spain*	**41 H3**	37 51N	1 25W
Alhambra, *U.S.A.*	**161 L8**	34 8N	118 6W
Alhaurín el Grande, *Spain*	**43 J6**	36 39N	4 41W
Alhucemas = Al Hoceïma, *Morocco*	**110 A4**	35 8N	3 58W
'Alī al Gharbī, *Iraq*	**101 F12**	32 30N	46 45 E
'Alī ash Sharqī, *Iraq*	**101 F12**	32 7N	46 44 E
Äli Bayramlı, *Azerbaijan*	**61 L9**	39 59N	48 52 E
'Alī Khēl, *Afghan.*	**91 B3**	33 57N	69 43 E
Ali Sahîh, *Djibouti*	**107 E5**	11 10N	42 44 E
Alī Shāh, *Iran*	**96 B5**	38 9N	45 50 E
Ália, *Italy*	**46 E6**	37 47N	13 43 E
'Alīābād, *Khorāsān, Iran*	**97 C8**	32 30N	57 30 E
'Alīābād, *Kordestān, Iran*	**96 C5**	35 4N	46 58 E
'Alīābād, *Yazd, Iran*	**97 D7**	31 41N	53 49 E
Aliaga, *Spain*	**40 E4**	40 40N	0 42W
Aliağa, *Turkey*	**49 C8**	38 47N	26 59 E
Aliákmon →, *Greece*	**50 F6**	40 30N	22 36 E
Aliakmonas = Aliákmon →, *Greece*	**50 F6**	40 30N	22 36 E
Alibag, *India*	**94 E1**	18 38N	72 56 E
Alibo, *Ethiopia*	**107 F4**	9 52N	37 5 E
Alibori →, *Benin*	**113 C5**	11 56N	3 17 E
Alibunar, *Serbia & M.*	**52 E5**	45 5N	20 57 E
Alicante, *Spain*	**41 G4**	38 23N	0 30W
Alicante □, *Spain*	**41 G4**	38 30N	0 37W
Alicante ✈ (ALC), *Spain*	**41 G4**	38 14N	0 36W
Alice, *S. Africa*	**116 E4**	32 48 S	26 55 E
Alice, *U.S.A.*	**155 M5**	27 45N	98 5W
Alice →, *Queens., Australia*	**126 C3**	24 2 S	144 50 E
Alice →, *Queens., Australia*	**126 B3**	15 35 S	142 20 E
Alice →, *Papua N. G.*	**132 D1**	6 10 S	141 8 E
Alice, Punta, *Italy*	**47 C10**	39 24N	17 9 E
Alice Arm, *Canada*	**142 B3**	55 29N	129 31W
Alice Springs, *Australia*	**126 C1**	23 40 S	133 50 E
Alicedale, *S. Africa*	**116 E4**	33 15 S	26 4 E
Aliceville, *U.S.A.*	**149 J1**	33 8N	88 9W
Alichur, *Tajikistan*	**65 E6**	37 45N	73 33 E
Alicia, *Bohol, Phil.*	**81 G5**	9 54N	124 26 E
Alicia, *Isabela, Phil.*	**80 C3**	16 46N	121 42 E
Alicudi, *Italy*	**47 D7**	38 33N	14 20 E
Aliganj, *India*	**93 F8**	27 30N	79 10 E
Aligarh, *Raj., India*	**92 G7**	25 55N	76 15 E
Aligarh, *Ut. P., India*	**92 F8**	27 55N	78 10 E
Alīgūdarz, *Iran*	**97 C6**	33 25N	49 45 E
Alijó, *Portugal*	**42 D3**	41 16N	7 27W
Alikanás, *Greece*	**39 D2**	37 51N	20 47 E
Alima →, *Congo*	**114 C3**	1 35 S	16 37 E
Alimnía, *Greece*	**38 E11**	36 16N	27 43 E
Alimodian, *Phil.*	**81 F4**	10 49N	122 26 E
Alindao, *C.A.R.*	**114 A4**	5 2N	21 13 E
Alingsås, *Sweden*	**17 G6**	57 56N	12 31 E
Alipur, *Pakistan*	**92 E4**	29 25N	70 55 E
Alipur Duar, *India*	**90 B2**	26 30N	89 35 E
Aliquippa, *U.S.A.*	**150 F4**	40 37N	80 15W
Alishan, *Taiwan*	**77 F13**	23 31N	120 48 E
Aliste →, *Spain*	**42 D5**	41 34N	5 58W
Alitus = Alytus, *Lithuania*	**15 J21**	54 24N	24 3 E
Alivérion, *Greece*	**48 C6**	38 24N	24 2 E
Aliwal North, *S. Africa*	**116 E4**	30 45 S	26 45 E
Alix, *Canada*	**142 C6**	52 24N	113 11W
Aljezur, *Portugal*	**43 H2**	37 18N	8 49W
Aljustrel, *Portugal*	**43 H2**	37 55N	8 10W
Alkamari, *Niger*	**113 C7**	13 27N	11 10 E
Alkmaar, *Neths.*	**24 B4**	52 37N	4 45 E
All American Canal, *U.S.A.*	**159 K6**	32 45N	115 15W
Allacapan, *Phil.*	**80 B3**	18 15N	121 35 E
Allada, *Benin*	**113 D5**	6 41N	2 9 E
Allagadda, *India*	**95 G4**	15 8N	78 30 E
Allagash →, *U.S.A.*	**149 B11**	47 5N	69 3W
Allah Dad, *Pakistan*	**92 G2**	25 38N	67 34 E
Allahabad, *India*	**93 G9**	25 25N	81 58 E
Allakaket, *U.S.A.*	**144 C9**	66 34N	152 39W
Allal Tazi, *Morocco*	**110 B3**	34 30N	6 20W
Allan, *Canada*	**143 C7**	51 53N	106 4W
Allanche, *France*	**28 C6**	45 14N	2 57 E
Allanmyo, *Burma*	**90 F5**	19 30N	95 17 E
Allanridge, *S. Africa*	**116 D4**	27 45 S	26 40 E
Allansford, *Australia*	**128 E5**	38 26 S	142 39 E
Allanton, *N.Z.*	**131 F5**	45 55 S	170 15 E
Allaqi, Wadi →, *Egypt*	**106 C3**	23 7N	32 47 E
Allariz, *Spain*	**42 C3**	42 11N	7 50W
Allassac, *France*	**28 C5**	45 15N	1 29 E
Allatoona L., *U.S.A.*	**152 A5**	34 10N	84 44W
Ålleberg, *Sweden*	**17 F7**	58 8N	13 36 E
Allegan, *U.S.A.*	**157 B11**	42 32N	85 51W
Allegany, *U.S.A.*	**150 D6**	42 6N	78 30W
Allegheny →, *U.S.A.*	**150 F5**	40 27N	80 1W
Allegheny Mts., *U.S.A.*	**148 G6**	38 15N	80 10W
Allegheny Plateau, *U.S.A.*	**148 E6**	41 30N	78 30W
Allegheny Reservoir, *U.S.A.*	**150 E6**	41 50N	79 0W
Allègre, *France*	**28 C7**	45 12N	3 41 E
Allègre, Pte., *Guadeloupe*	**164 b**	16 22N	61 46W
Allen, *Argentina*	**176 A3**	38 58 S	67 50W
Allen, *Phil.*	**80 E5**	12 30N	124 17 E
Allen, Bog of, *Ireland*	**23 C5**	53 15N	7 0W
Allen, L., *Ireland*	**23 B3**	54 8N	8 4W
Allendale, *U.S.A.*	**152 B8**	33 1N	81 18W
Allende, *Mexico*	**162 B4**	28 20N	100 50W
Allensbach, *Germany*	**33 A8**	47 43N	9 4 E
Allenstein = Olsztyn, *Poland*	**54 E7**	53 48N	20 29 E
Allentown, *U.S.A.*	**151 F9**	40 37N	75 29W
Allentsteig, *Austria*	**34 C8**	48 41N	15 20 E
Alleppey, *India*	**95 K3**	9 30N	76 28 E
Allepuz, *Spain*	**40 E4**	40 29N	0 44W
Aller →, *Germany*	**30 C5**	52 56N	9 12 E
Alleynes B., *Barbados*	**165 g**	13 13N	59 39W
Alliance, *Suriname*	**169 B7**	5 50N	54 50W
Alliance, *Nebr., U.S.A.*	**154 D3**	42 6N	102 52W
Alliance, *Ohio, U.S.A.*	**150 F3**	40 55N	81 6W
Allier □, *France*	**27 F9**	46 25N	2 40 E
Allier →, *France*	**27 F10**	46 57N	3 4 E
Alliford Bay, *Canada*	**142 C2**	53 12N	131 58W
Alligator Pond, *Jamaica*	**164 a**	17 52N	77 34W
Allinagaram, *India*	**95 J3**	10 2N	77 30 E
Allinge, *Denmark*	**17 J8**	55 17N	14 50 E
Allison, *U.S.A.*	**156 B4**	42 45N	92 48W
Alliston = New Tecumseth, *Canada*	**140 D4**	44 9N	79 52W
Alloa, *U.K.*	**22 E5**	56 7N	3 47W
Allones, *France*	**26 D8**	48 20N	1 40 E
Allora, *Australia*	**127 D5**	28 2 S	152 0 E
Allos, *France*	**29 D10**	44 15N	6 38 E
Alluitsup Paa, *Greenland*	**10 E6**	60 30N	45 35W
Allur, *India*	**95 G5**	14 40N	80 4 E
Alluru Kottapatnam, *India*	**95 G5**	15 24N	80 7 E
Alma, *Canada*	**141 C5**	48 35N	71 40W
Alma, *Ga., U.S.A.*	**152 D7**	31 33N	82 28W
Alma, *Kans., U.S.A.*	**154 F6**	39 1N	96 17W
Alma, *Mich., U.S.A.*	**148 D3**	43 23N	84 39W
Alma, *Nebr., U.S.A.*	**154 E5**	40 6N	99 22W
Alma, *Wis., U.S.A.*	**154 C9**	44 20N	91 55W
Alma Ata = Almaty, *Kazakhstan*	**65 B8**	43 15N	76 57 E
Almacelles, *Spain*	**40 D5**	41 43N	0 27 E
Almada, *Portugal*	**43 G1**	38 40N	9 9W
Almaden, *Australia*	**126 B3**	17 22 S	144 40 E
Almadén, *Spain*	**43 G6**	38 49N	4 52W
Almalyk = Olmaliq, *Uzbekistan*	**65 C4**	40 50N	69 35 E
Almanor, L., *U.S.A.*	**158 F3**	40 14N	121 9W
Almansa, *Spain*	**41 G3**	38 51N	1 5W
Almanza, *Spain*	**42 C5**	42 39N	5 3W
Almanzor, Pico, *Spain*	**42 E5**	40 15N	5 18W
Almanzora →, *Spain*	**41 H3**	37 14N	1 46W
Almas, *Brazil*	**171 D2**	11 33 S	47 9W
Almaş, Munţii, *Romania*	**52 F7**	44 49N	22 12 E
Almassora, *Spain*	**40 F4**	39 57N	0 3W
Almaty, *Kazakhstan*	**65 B8**	43 15N	76 57 E
Almazán, *Spain*	**40 D2**	41 30N	2 30W
Almeirim, *Brazil*	**169 D7**	1 30 S	52 34W
Almeirim, *Portugal*	**43 F2**	39 12N	8 37W
Almelo, *Neths.*	**24 B6**	52 22N	6 42 E
Almenar de Soria, *Spain*	**40 D2**	41 43N	2 12W
Almenara, *Brazil*	**171 E3**	16 11 S	40 42W
Almenara, *Spain*	**40 F4**	39 46N	0 14W
Almenara, Sierra de la, *Spain*	**41 H3**	37 34N	1 32W
Almendra, Embalse de, *Spain*	**42 D4**	41 10N	6 5W
Almendralejo, *Spain*	**43 G4**	38 41N	6 26W
Almere-Stad, *Neths.*	**24 B5**	52 20N	5 15 E
Almería, *Spain*	**43 J8**	36 52N	2 27W
Almería □, *Spain*	**41 H2**	37 20N	2 20W
Almería, G. de, *Spain*	**41 J2**	36 41N	2 28W
Almetyevsk, *Russia*	**60 C11**	54 53N	52 20 E
Älmhult, *Sweden*	**17 H8**	56 33N	14 8 E
Almirante, *Panama*	**164 E3**	9 10N	82 30W
Almirante Montt, G., *Chile*	**176 D2**	51 52 S	72 50W

Almiropótamos, *Greece* **48 C6** 38 16N 24 11 E
Almirós, *Greece* **48 B4** 39 11N 22 45 E
Almiroú, Kólpos, *Greece* **39 E5** 35 23N 24 20 E
Almodôvar, *Portugal* **43 H2** 37 31N 8 2W
Almodóvar del Campo, *Spain* **43 G6** 38 43N 4 10W
Almodóvar del Río, *Spain* **43 H5** 37 48N 5 1W
Almond, *U.S.A.* **150 D7** 42 19N 77 44W
Almont, *U.S.A.* **150 D1** 42 55N 83 3W
Almonte, *Canada* **151 A8** 45 14N 76 12W
Almonte, *Spain* **43 H4** 37 13N 6 38W
Almora, *India* **93 E8** 29 38N 79 40 E
Almoradí, *Spain* **41 G4** 38 7N 0 46W
Almorox, *Spain* **42 E6** 40 14N 4 24W
Almoustarat, *Mali* **113 B5** 17 35N 0 8 E
Älmsta, *Sweden* **16 E12** 59 58N 18 50 E
Almudévar, *Spain* **40 C4** 42 3N 0 35W
Almuñécar, *Spain* **43 J7** 36 43N 3 41W
Almunge, *Sweden* **16 E12** 59 53N 18 3 E
Almuradiel, *Spain* **43 G7** 38 32N 3 28W
Alness, *U.K.* **22 D4** 57 41N 4 16W
Alnif, *Morocco* **110 B3** 31 10N 5 8W
Alnmouth, *U.K.* **20 B6** 55 24N 1 37W
Alnwick, *U.K.* **20 B6** 55 24N 1 42W
Aloi, *Uganda* **118 B3** 2 16N 33 10 E
Alon, *Burma* **90 D5** 22 12N 95 5 E
Along, *India* **90 A5** 28 10N 94 46 E
Alonissos-Voríai Sporades △, *Greece* **48 B6** 39 15N 24 5 E
Alor, *Indonesia* **82 C2** 8 15 S 124 30 E
Alor Setar, *Malaysia* **87 J3** 6 7N 100 22 E
Álora, *Spain* **43 J6** 36 49N 4 46W
Alosno, *Spain* **43 H3** 37 33N 7 7W
Alost = Aalst, *Belgium* **24 D4** 50 56N 4 2 E
Alot, *India* **92 H6** 23 56N 75 40 E
Alotau, *Papua N. G.* **132 F6** 10 16 S 150 30 E
Alougoum, *Morocco* **110 B3** 30 17N 6 56W
Aloum, *Cameroon* **114 B2** 2 16N 10 34 E
Aloysius, Mt., *Australia* **125 E4** 26 0 S 128 38 E
Alpaugh, *U.S.A.* **160 K7** 35 53N 119 29W
Alpe Apuane ⌓, *Italy* **44 D7** 44 4N 10 15 E
Alpedrinha, *Portugal* **42 E3** 40 6N 7 27W
Alpena, *U.S.A.* **148 C4** 45 4N 83 27W
Alpercatas →, *Brazil* **170 C3** 6 2 S 44 19W
Alpes-de-Haute-Provence □, *France* **29 D10** 44 8N 6 10 E
Alpes-Maritimes □, *France* **29 E11** 43 55N 7 10 E
Alpha, *Australia* **126 C4** 23 39 S 146 37 E
Alpha, *U.S.A.* **156 C6** 41 12N 90 23W
Alpha Cordillera, *Arctic* **6 A2** 84 0N 118 0W
Alphen aan den Rijn, *Neths.* **24 B4** 52 7N 4 40 E
Alphonse, *Seychelles* **121 E4** 7 0 S 52 45 E
Alpiarça, *Portugal* **43 F2** 39 15N 8 35W
Alpine, *Ariz., U.S.A.* **159 K9** 33 51N 109 9W
Alpine, *Calif., U.S.A.* **161 N10** 32 50N 116 46W
Alpine, *Tex., U.S.A.* **155 K3** 30 22N 103 40W
Alpine △, *Australia* **129 D7** 37 15 S 146 45 E
Alpnach Dorf, *Switz.* **33 C6** 46 57N 8 17 E
Alps, *Europe* **25 C8** 46 30N 9 30 E
Alpu, *Turkey* **100 C4** 39 46N 30 58 E
Alqueta, Barragem do, *Portugal* **43 G3** 38 20N 7 25W
Alrø, *Denmark* **17 J4** 55 52N 10 5 E
Als, *Denmark* **17 K3** 54 59N 9 55 E
Alsace □, *France* **27 D14** 48 15N 7 25 E
Alsask, *Canada* **143 C7** 51 21N 109 59W
Alsasua, *Spain* **40 C2** 42 54N 2 10W
Alsek →, *U.S.A.* **142 B1** 59 10N 138 12W
Alsfeld, *Germany* **30 E5** 50 44N 9 16 E
Alsten, *Norway* **14 D15** 65 58N 12 40 E
Alstermo, *Sweden* **17 H9** 56 58N 15 38 E
Alston, *U.K.* **20 C5** 54 49N 2 25W
Alta, *Norway* **14 B20** 69 57N 23 10 E
Alta, Sierra, *Spain* **40 E3** 40 31N 1 30W
Alta Floresta, *Brazil* **173 B6** 9 57 S 55 58W
Alta Gracia, *Argentina* **174 C3** 31 40 S 64 30W
Alta Sierra, *U.S.A.* **161 K8** 35 42N 118 33W
Altaelva →, *Norway* **14 B20** 69 54N 23 17 E
Altafjorden, *Norway* **14 A20** 70 5N 23 5 E
Altagracia, *Venezuela* **168 A3** 10 45N 71 30W
Altagracia de Orituco, *Venezuela* **168 B4** 9 52N 66 23W
Altai = Aerhtai Shan, *Mongolia* **68 B4** 46 40N 92 45 E
Altamachi →, *Bolivia* **172 D4** 16 8 S 66 50W
Altamaha →, *U.S.A.* **152 D8** 31 20N 81 20W
Altamira, *Brazil* **169 D7** 3 12 S 52 10W
Altamira, *Chile* **174 B2** 25 47 S 69 51W
Altamira, *Colombia* **168 C2** 2 3N 75 47W
Altamira, *Mexico* **163 C5** 22 24N 97 55W
Altamira, Cuevas de, *Spain* **42 B6** 43 20N 4 5W
Altamont, *Ill., U.S.A.* **157 E8** 39 4N 88 45W
Altamont, *N.Y., U.S.A.* **151 D10** 42 43N 74 3W
Altamont, *Oreg., U.S.A.* **158 E3** 42 12N 121 44W
Altamura, *Italy* **47 B9** 40 49N 16 33 E
Altanbulag, *Mongolia* **68 A5** 50 16N 106 30 E
Altar, *Mexico* **162 A2** 30 40N 111 50W
Altar, Desierto de, *Mexico* **162 B2** 30 10N 112 0W
Altata, *Mexico* **162 C3** 24 30N 108 0W
Altavas, *Phil.* **81 F4** 11 32N 122 29 E
Altavista, *U.S.A.* **148 G6** 37 6N 79 17W
Altay, *China* **68 B3** 47 48N 88 10 E
Altdorf, *Switz.* **33 C7** 46 52N 8 36 E
Alte Mellum, *Germany* **30 B4** 53 43N 8 10 E
Altea, *Spain* **41 G4** 38 38N 0 2W
Altenberg, *Germany* **30 E9** 50 45N 13 45 E
Altenbruch, *Germany* **30 B4** 53 49N 8 46 E
Altenburg, *Germany* **30 E8** 50 59N 12 25 E
Altenkirchen, *Mecklenburg-Vorpommern, Germany* **30 A9** 54 38N 13 22 E
Altenkirchen, *Rhld-Pfz., Germany* **30 E3** 50 41N 7 39 E
Altenmarkt, *Austria* **34 D7** 47 43N 14 39 E
Alter do Chão, *Brazil* **169 D6** 2 31 S 54 57W
Alter do Chão, *Portugal* **43 F3** 39 12N 7 40W
Altha, *U.S.A.* **152 E4** 30 34N 85 8W
Altınoluk, *Turkey* **49 B8** 39 34N 26 45 E
Altınova, *Turkey* **49 B8** 39 12N 26 47 E
Altıntaş, *Turkey* **49 B12** 39 4N 30 7 E
Altınyaka, *Turkey* **49 E12** 36 33N 30 20 E
Altınyayla, *Turkey* **49 D11** 37 0N 29 33 E
Altiplano, *Bolivia* **172 D4** 17 0 S 68 0W
Altkirch, *France* **27 E14** 47 37N 7 15 E
Altmark, *Germany* **30 C7** 52 45N 11 30 E
Altmühl →, *Germany* **31 G7** 48 54N 11 52 E
Altmühltal ⌓, *Germany* **31 G7** 48 55N 11 15 E
Altmunster, *Austria* **34 D6** 47 54N 13 45 E
Alto Adige = Trentino-Alto Adige □, *Italy* **45 B8** 46 30N 11 20 E
Alto Alegre, *Brazil* **169 C5** 2 50N 61 20W
Alto Araguaia, *Brazil* **173 D7** 17 15 S 53 20W
Alto Chicapa, *Angola* **115 E3** 10 52 S 19 17 E
Alto Cuchumatanes = Cuchumatanes, Sierra de los, *Guatemala* **164 C1** 15 35N 91 25W
Alto Cuito = Tempué, *Angola* **115 E3** 13 27 S 18 49 E
Alto del Carmen, *Chile* **174 B1** 28 46 S 70 30W
Alto del Inca, *Chile* **174 A2** 24 10 S 68 10W
Alto Garças, *Brazil* **173 D7** 16 56 S 53 32W
Alto Garda Bresciano ⌓, *Italy* **44 C7** 45 42N 10 38 E
Alto Iriri →, *Brazil* **173 B7** 8 50 S 53 25W
Alto Ligonha, *Mozam.* **119 F4** 15 30 S 38 11 E
Alto Molocue, *Mozam.* **119 F4** 15 50 S 37 35 E
Alto Paraguai, *Brazil* **173 C6** 14 30 S 56 31W
Alto Paraguay □, *Paraguay* **174 A4** 21 0 S 58 30W
Alto Paraíso de Goiás, *Brazil* **171 D2** 14 7 S 47 31W
Alto Paraná □, *Paraguay* **175 B5** 25 30 S 54 50W
Alto Parnaíba, *Brazil* **170 C2** 9 6 S 45 57W
Alto Purús →, *Peru* **172 B3** 9 12 S 70 28W
Alto Río Senguerr, *Argentina* **176 C2** 45 2 S 70 50W
Alto Santo, *Brazil* **170 C4** 5 31 S 38 15W
Alto Sucuriú, *Brazil* **173 D7** 19 19 S 52 47W
Alto Turi, *Brazil* **170 B2** 2 54 S 45 38W
Alton, *Canada* **150 C4** 43 54N 80 5W
Alton, *U.K.* **21 F7** 51 9N 0 59W
Alton, *Ill., U.S.A.* **156 F6** 38 53N 90 11W
Alton, *N.H., U.S.A.* **151 C13** 43 27N 71 13W
Altona, *Canada* **143 D9** 49 6N 97 33W
Altoona, *Ala., U.S.A.* **152 A3** 34 2N 86 20W
Altoona, *Iowa, U.S.A.* **156 C3** 41 39N 93 28W
Altoona, *Pa., U.S.A.* **150 F6** 40 31N 78 24W
Altos, *Brazil* **170 C3** 5 3 S 42 28W
Altötting, *Germany* **31 G8** 48 12N 12 39 E
Altstätten, *Switz.* **33 B9** 47 22N 9 33 E
Altun Kupri, *Iraq* **101 E11** 35 45N 44 9 E
Altun Shan, *China* **68 C3** 38 30N 88 0 E
Alturas, *U.S.A.* **158 F3** 41 29N 120 32W
Altus, *U.S.A.* **155 H5** 34 38N 99 20W
Alubijid, *Phil.* **81 G5** 8 35N 124 29 E
Alucra, *Turkey* **101 B8** 40 22N 38 47 E
Aluk, *Sudan* **107 F2** 8 25N 27 30 E
Alūksne, *Latvia* **15 H22** 57 24N 27 3 E
Alūla, *Somali Rep.* **120 B4** 11 50N 50 45 E
Alunda, *Sweden* **16 D12** 60 4N 18 5 E
Alunite, *U.S.A.* **161 K12** 35 59N 114 55W
Aluoro →, *Ethiopia* **107 F3** 8 26N 33 24 E
Alupka, *Ukraine* **59 K8** 44 23N 34 2 E
Alur, *India* **95 E3** 15 24N 77 15 E
Alur Gajah, *Malaysia* **84 B2** 2 23N 102 13 E
Alushta, *Ukraine* **59 K8** 44 40N 34 25 E
Alusi, *Indonesia* **83 C4** 7 35 S 131 40 E
Alustante, *Spain* **40 E3** 40 36N 1 40W
Alutgama, *Sri Lanka* **95 L4** 6 26N 79 59 E
Alutnuwara, *Sri Lanka* **95 L5** 7 19N 80 59 E
Alva, *U.S.A.* **155 G5** 36 48N 98 40W
Alvaiázere, *Portugal* **42 F2** 39 49N 8 23W
Älvängen, *Sweden* **17 G6** 57 58N 12 8 E
Alvão ⌓, *Portugal* **42 D3** 41 22N 7 48W
Alvarado, *Mexico* **163 D5** 18 40N 95 50W
Alvarado, *U.S.A.* **155 J6** 32 24N 97 13W
Alvarães, *Brazil* **169 D5** 3 12 S 64 50W
Alvaro Obregón, Presa, *Mexico* **162 B3** 27 55N 109 52W
Alvdal, *Norway* **18 B7** 62 6N 10 37 E
Älvdalen, *Sweden* **16 C8** 61 13N 14 4 E
Alvear, *Argentina* **174 B4** 29 5 S 56 30W
Alverca, *Portugal* **43 G1** 38 56N 9 1W
Alvesta, *Sweden* **17 H8** 56 54N 14 35 E
Ålvik, *Norway* **18 D3** 60 26N 6 26 E
Alvin, *U.S.A.* **155 L7** 29 26N 95 15W
Alvinston, *Canada* **150 D3** 42 49N 81 52W
Alvito, *Portugal* **43 G3** 38 15N 7 58W
Älvkarleby, *Sweden* **16 D11** 60 34N 17 26 E
Alvorado, *Brazil* **171 D2** 12 28 S 49 6W
Alvord Desert, *U.S.A.* **158 E4** 42 30N 118 25W
Älvros, *Sweden* **16 B8** 62 3N 14 38 E
Älvsbyn, *Sweden* **14 D19** 65 40N 21 0 E
Ålvundeid, *Norway* **18 B5** 62 45N 8 33 E
Alwar, *India* **92 F7** 27 38N 76 34 E
Alwaye, *India* **95 J3** 10 8N 76 24 E
Alxa Zuoqi, *China* **74 E3** 38 50N 105 40 E
Alyangula, *Australia* **126 A2** 13 55 S 136 30 E
Alyata = Älät, *Azerbaijan* **61 L9** 39 58N 49 25 E
Alyth, *U.K.* **22 E5** 56 38N 3 13W
Alytus, *Lithuania* **15 J21** 54 24N 24 3 E
Alzada, *U.S.A.* **154 C2** 45 2N 104 25W
Alzey, *Germany* **31 F4** 49 45N 8 7 E
Alzira, *Spain* **41 F4** 39 9N 0 30W
Am Dam, *Chad* **109 F4** 12 40N 20 35 E
Am Géréda, *Chad* **109 F4** 12 53N 21 14 E
Am Loubia, *Chad* **109 F4** 13 39N 20 8 E
Am Timan, *Chad* **109 F4** 11 0N 20 10 E
Amacayacu △, *Colombia* **168 D3** 3 21 S 70 8W
Amada Gaza, *C.A.R.* **114 B3** 4 46N 15 9 E
Amadeus, L., *Australia* **125 D5** 24 54 S 131 0 E
Amadi, *Dem. Rep. of the Congo* **118 B2** 3 40N 26 40 E
Amâdi, *Sudan* **107 F3** 5 29N 30 25 E
Amadjuak L., *Canada* **139 B12** 65 0N 71 8W
Amadora, *Portugal* **43 G1** 38 45N 9 13W
Amagansett, *U.S.A.* **151 F12** 40 59N 72 9W
Amagasaki, *Japan* **73 C7** 34 42N 135 20 E
Amager, *Denmark* **17 J6** 55 37N 12 35 E
Amagi, *Japan* **72 D2** 33 25N 130 39 E
Amagunze, *Nigeria* **113 D6** 6 20N 7 40 E
Amahai, *Indonesia* **83 C3** 3 20 S 128 55 E
Amaile, *Samoa* **133 W24** 13 59 S 171 22W
Amaimon, *Papua N. G.* **132 C3** 5 12 S 145 30 E
Amakusa-Nada, *Japan* **72 E2** 32 35N 130 5 E
Amakusa-Shotō, *Japan* **72 E2** 32 15N 130 10 E
Åmål, *Sweden* **16 E6** 59 3N 12 42 E
Amalapuram, *India* **95 F5** 16 35N 81 55 E
Amalfi, *Colombia* **168 B2** 6 55N 75 4W
Amalfi, *Italy* **47 B7** 40 38N 14 36 E
Amaliás, *Greece* **48 D3** 37 47N 21 22 E
Amalner, *India* **94 D2** 21 5N 75 5 E
Amamapare, *Indonesia* **83 B5** 4 53 S 136 38 E
Amambaí, *Brazil* **175 A4** 23 5 S 55 13W
Amambaí →, *Brazil* **175 A5** 23 22 S 53 56W
Amambay □, *Paraguay* **175 A4** 23 0 S 56 0W
Amambay, Cordillera de, *S. Amer.* **175 A4** 23 0 S 55 45W
Amami-Guntō, *Japan* **71 L4** 27 16N 129 21 E
Amami-Ō-Shima, *Japan* **71 L4** 28 0N 129 0 E
Aman, Pulau, *Malaysia* **87 c** 5 16N 100 24 E
Amana →, *Venezuela* **169 B5** 9 45N 62 39W
Amaná, L., *Brazil* **169 D5** 2 35 S 64 40W
Amanab, *Papua N. G.* **132 B1** 3 40 S 141 14 E
Amanat →, *India* **93 G11** 24 7N 84 4 E
Amanda Park, *U.S.A.* **160 C3** 47 28N 123 55W
Amangeldy, *Kazakhstan* **66 D7** 50 10N 65 10 E
Amantea, *Italy* **47 C9** 39 8N 16 4 E
Amapá, *Brazil* **169 C7** 2 5N 50 50W
Amapá □, *Brazil* **169 C7** 1 40N 52 0W
Amapari = Ferreira Gomes, *Brazil* **170 A1** 0 48N 51 8W
Amapari, *Brazil* **169 C7** 0 37N 51 39W
Amara, *Sudan* **107 E3** 10 25N 34 10 E
Amara □, *Ethiopia* **107 E4** 12 30N 37 30 E
Amaração = Luís Correia, *Brazil* **170 B3** 3 0 S 41 35W
Amarante, *Brazil* **170 C3** 6 14 S 42 50W
Amarante, *Portugal* **42 D2** 41 16N 8 5W
Amarante do Maranhão, *Brazil* **170 C2** 5 36 S 46 45W
Amaranth, *Canada* **143 C9** 50 36N 98 43W
Amarapura, *Burma* **90 E6** 21 54N 96 3 E
Amaravati →, *India* **95 J4** 11 0N 78 15 E
Amareleja, *Portugal* **43 G3** 38 12N 7 13W
Amargosa, *Brazil* **171 D4** 13 2 S 39 36W
Amargosa →, *U.S.A.* **161 J10** 36 14N 116 51W
Amargosa Range, *U.S.A.* **161 J10** 36 20N 116 45W
Amári, *Greece* **39 E5** 35 13N 24 40 E
Amarillo, *U.S.A.* **155 H4** 35 13N 101 50W
Amarkantak, *India* **93 H9** 22 40N 81 45 E
Amârna, Tell el', *Sudan* **106 B3** 27 38N 30 52 E
Amarnath, *India* **94 E1** 19 12N 73 22 E
Amaro, Mte., *Italy* **45 F11** 42 5N 14 5 E
Amaro Leite, *Brazil* **171 D2** 13 58 S 49 9W
Amarpur, *Bihar, India* **93 G12** 25 5N 87 0 E
Amarpur, *Tripura, India* **90 D3** 23 31N 91 39 E
Amarti, *Eritrea* **107 E5** 14 17N 41 6 E
Amarwara, *India* **93 H8** 22 18N 79 10 E
Amasin, *W. Sahara* **110 C2** 25 45N 13 20W
Amasra, *Turkey* **100 B5** 41 45N 32 23 E
Amassama, *Nigeria* **113 D6** 5 1N 6 2 E
Amasya, *Turkey* **100 B6** 40 40N 35 50 E
Amata, *Australia* **125 E5** 26 9 S 131 9 E
Amatauré, *Brazil* **168 D4** 3 29 S 68 6W
Amatignak I., *U.S.A.* **144 L3** 51 16N 179 6W
Amatikulu, *S. Africa* **117 D5** 29 3 S 31 33 E
Amatitlán, *Guatemala* **164 D1** 14 29N 90 38W
Amatrice, *Italy* **45 F10** 42 38N 13 17 E
Amau, *Papua N. G.* **132 F5** 10 2 S 148 34 E
Amay, *Belgium* **24 D5** 50 33N 5 19 E
Amazon = Amazonas →, *S. Amer.* **169 D7** 0 5 S 50 0W
Amazonas □, *Brazil* **173 B5** 5 0 S 65 0W
Amazonas □, *Peru* **172 B2** 5 0 S 78 0W
Amazonas □, *Venezuela* **168 C4** 3 30N 66 0W
Amazonas →, *S. Amer.* **169 D7** 0 5 S 50 0W
Amba Ferit, *Ethiopia* **107 E4** 10 55N 38 50 E
Ambad, *India* **94 E2** 19 38N 75 50 E
Ambagarh Chowki, *India* **94 D5** 20 47N 80 43 E
Ambah, *India* **92 F8** 26 43N 78 13 E
Ambahakily, *Madag.* **117 C7** 21 36 S 43 41 E
Ambahita, *Madag.* **117 C8** 24 1 S 45 16 E
Ambajogal, *India* **94 E3** 18 44N 76 23 E
Ambala, *India* **92 D7** 30 23N 76 56 E
Ambalangoda, *Sri Lanka* **95 L5** 6 15N 80 5 E
Ambalapulai, *India* **95 K3** 9 25N 76 25 E
Ambalavao, *Madag.* **117 C8** 21 50 S 46 56 E
Ambam, *Cameroon* **114 B2** 2 20N 11 15 E
Ambanja, *Madag.* **117 A8** 13 40 S 48 27 E
Ambararata, *Madag.* **117 B8** 15 3 S 48 33 E
Ambarchik, *Russia* **67 C17** 69 40N 162 20 E
Ambarijeby, *Madag.* **117 A8** 14 56 S 47 41 E
Ambaro, Helodranon', *Madag.* **117 A8** 13 23 S 48 38 E
Ambasamudram, *India* **95 K3** 8 43N 77 25 E
Ambato, *Ecuador* **168 D2** 1 5 S 78 42W
Ambato, *Madag.* **117 A8** 13 24 S 48 29 E
Ambato, Sierra de, *Argentina* **174 B2** 28 25 S 66 10W
Ambato Boeny, *Madag.* **117 B8** 16 28 S 46 43 E
Ambatofinandrahana, *Madag.* **117 C8** 20 33 S 46 48 E
Ambatolampy, *Madag.* **117 B8** 19 20 S 47 35 E
Ambatomainty, *Madag.* **117 B8** 17 41 S 45 40 E
Ambatomanoina, *Madag.* **117 B8** 18 18 S 47 37 E
Ambatondrazaka, *Madag.* **117 B8** 17 55 S 48 28 E
Ambatosoratra, *Madag.* **117 B8** 17 37 S 48 31 E
Ambelau, *Indonesia* **83 B3** 3 51 S 127 12 E
Ambelón, *Greece* **48 B4** 39 45N 22 22 E
Ambenja, *Madag.* **117 B8** 15 17 S 46 58 E
Amberg, *Germany* **31 F7** 49 26N 11 52 E
Ambergris Cay, *Belize* **163 D7** 18 0N 87 55W
Ambérieu-en-Bugey, *France* **29 C9** 45 57N 5 20 E
Amberley, *N.Z.* **131 D7** 43 9 S 172 44 E
Ambert, *France* **28 C7** 45 33N 3 44 E
Ambidédi, *Mali* **112 C2** 14 35N 11 47W
Ambikapur, *India* **93 H10** 23 15N 83 15 E
Ambikol, *Sudan* **106 C3** 21 20N 30 50 E
Ambilobé, *Madag.* **117 A8** 13 10 S 49 3 E
Ambinanindrano, *Madag.* **117 C8** 20 5 S 48 23 E
Ambinanitelo, *Madag.* **117 B8** 15 21 S 49 35 E
Ambinda, *Madag.* **117 B8** 16 25 S 45 52 E
Amble, *U.K.* **20 B6** 55 20N 1 36W
Ambler, *U.S.A.* **144 C8** 67 5N 157 52W
Ambleside, *U.K.* **20 C5** 54 26N 2 58W
Ambo, *Peru* **172 C2** 10 5 S 76 10W
Amboahangy, *Madag.* **117 C8** 24 15 S 46 22 E
Ambodifototra, *Madag.* **117 B8** 16 59 S 49 52 E
Ambodilazana, *Madag.* **117 B8** 18 6 S 49 10 E
Ambodiriana, *Madag.* **117 B8** 17 55 S 49 18 E
Ambohidratrimo, *Madag.* **117 B8** 18 50 S 47 26 E
Ambohidray, *Madag.* **117 B8** 18 36 S 48 18 E
Ambohimahamasina, *Madag.* **117 C8** 21 56 S 47 11 E
Ambohimahasoa, *Madag.* **117 C8** 21 7 S 47 13 E
Ambohimanga, *Madag.* **117 C8** 20 52 S 47 36 E
Ambohimitombo, *Madag.* **117 C8** 20 43 S 47 26 E
Ambohitra, *Madag.* **117 A8** 12 30 S 49 10 E
Amboise, *France* **26 E8** 47 24N 1 2 E
Amboiva, *Angola* **115 E2** 11 33 S 14 43 E
Ambon, *Indonesia* **82 B3** 3 43 S 128 12 E
Ambondro, *Madag.* **117 D8** 25 13 S 45 44 E
Amboró △, *Bolivia* **173 D5** 17 39 S 64 3W
Amboseli △, *Kenya* **118 C4** 2 37 S 37 13 E
Amboseli, L., *Kenya* **118 C4** 2 40 S 37 10 E
Ambositra, *Madag.* **117 C8** 20 31 S 47 25 E
Ambovombe, *Madag.* **117 D8** 25 11 S 46 5 E
Amboy, *Calif., U.S.A.* **161 L11** 34 33N 115 45W
Amboy, *Ill., U.S.A.* **156 C7** 41 44N 89 20W
Amboyna Cay, *S. China Sea* **78 C4** 7 50N 112 50 E
Ambridge, *U.S.A.* **150 F4** 40 36N 80 14W
Ambriz, *Angola* **115 D2** 7 48 S 13 8 E
Ambriz ⌓, *Angola* **115 D2** 7 56 S 10 27 E
Ambrym, *Vanuatu* **133 F6** 16 15 S 168 10 E
Ambunti, *Papua N. G.* **132 C2** 4 13 S 142 52 E
Ambur, *India* **95 H4** 12 48N 78 43 E
Amchitka I., *U.S.A.* **144 L2** 51 32N 179 0 E
Amderma, *Russia* **66 C7** 69 45N 61 30 E
Amdhi, *India* **93 H9** 23 51N 81 27 E
Ameca, *Mexico* **162 C4** 20 30N 104 0W
Ameca →, *Mexico* **162 C3** 20 40N 105 15W
Amecameca, *Mexico* **163 D5** 19 7N 98 46W
Ameland, *Neths.* **24 A5** 53 27N 5 45 E
Amélia, *Italy* **45 F9** 42 33N 12 25 E
Amelia City, *U.S.A.* **152 E8** 30 35N 81 28W
Amelia I., *U.S.A.* **152 E8** 30 40N 81 25W
Amendolara, *Italy* **47 C9** 39 57N 16 35 E
Amenia, *U.S.A.* **151 E11** 41 51N 73 33W
American Falls, *U.S.A.* **158 E7** 42 47N 112 51W
American Falls Reservoir, *U.S.A.* **158 E7** 42 47N 112 52W
American Fork, *U.S.A.* **158 F8** 40 23N 111 48W
American Highland, *Antarctica* **7 D6** 73 0 S 75 0 E
American River, *Australia* **128 C2** 35 47 S 137 46 E
American Samoa △, *Amer. Samoa* **133 X24** 14 15 S 170 28W
American Samoa ☒, *Pac. Oc.* **133 X24** 14 20 S 170 40W
Americana, *Brazil* **175 A6** 22 45 S 47 20W
Americus, *U.S.A.* **152 C5** 32 4N 84 14W
Amerigo Vespucci, Firenze ✕ (FLR), *Italy* **44 E8** 43 49N 11 13 E
Amerika = Nakhodka, *Russia* **67 E14** 42 53N 132 54 E
Amersfoort, *Neths.* **24 B5** 52 9N 5 23 E
Amersfoort, *S. Africa* **117 D4** 26 59 S 29 53 E
Amery Ice Shelf, *Antarctica* **7 C6** 69 30 S 72 0 E
Amerzgane, *Morocco* **110 B3** 31 4N 7 14W
Ames, *Spain* **42 C2** 42 54N 8 38W
Ames, *U.S.A.* **156 C3** 42 2N 93 37W
Amesbury, *U.S.A.* **151 D14** 42 51N 70 56W
Amet, *India* **92 G5** 25 18N 73 56 E
Amfíklia, *Greece* **48 C4** 38 38N 22 35 E
Amfilokhía, *Greece* **48 C3** 38 52N 21 9 E
Amfípolis, *Greece* **50 F7** 40 48N 23 52 E
Ámfissa, *Greece* **48 C4** 38 32N 22 22 E
Amga, *Russia* **67 C14** 60 50N 132 0 E
Amga →, *Russia* **67 C14** 62 38N 134 32 E
Amgaon, *India* **94 D5** 21 22N 80 22 E
Amgu, *Russia* **67 E14** 45 45N 137 15 E
Amgun →, *Russia* **67 D14** 52 56N 139 38 E
Amherst = Kyaikkami, *Burma* **90 G6** 16 4N 97 34 E
Amherst, *Canada* **141 C7** 45 48N 64 8W
Amherst, *Mass., U.S.A.* **151 D12** 42 23N 72 31W
Amherst, *N.Y., U.S.A.* **150 D6** 42 59N 78 48W
Amherst, *Ohio, U.S.A.* **150 E2** 41 24N 82 14W
Amherst I., *Canada* **151 B8** 44 8N 76 43W
Amherstburg, *Canada* **140 D3** 42 6N 83 6W
Amiata, Mte., *Italy* **45 F8** 42 53N 11 37 E
Amidon, *U.S.A.* **154 B3** 46 29N 103 19W
Amiens, *France* **27 C9** 49 54N 2 16 E
Amili, *India* **90 A5** 28 25N 95 52 E
Amindaion, *Greece* **50 F5** 40 42N 21 42 E
Amindivi Is., *India* **95 J1** 11 23N 72 23 E
Amingaon, *India* **90 B3** 26 11N 91 40 E
Amini I., *India* **95 J1** 11 6N 72 45 E
Åminne, *Sweden* **17 G7** 57 7N 14 0 E
Amino, *Ethiopia* **107 G5** 4 25N 41 52 E
Aminuis, *Namibia* **116 C2** 23 43 S 19 21 E
Āmir, Ra's, *Libya* **108 B4** 32 57N 21 43 E
Amīrābād, *Iran* **96 C5** 33 20N 46 16 E
Amirante Is., *Seychelles* **121 E4** 6 0 S 53 0 E
Amisk ⌓, *Canada* **143 B9** 56 43N 98 0W
Amisk L., *Canada* **143 C8** 54 35N 102 15W
Amistad ⌓, *U.S.A.* **155 L4** 29 32N 101 12W
Amistad, Presa de la, *Mexico* **162 B4** 29 24N 101 0W
Amite, *U.S.A.* **155 K9** 30 44N 90 30W
Amizmiz, *Morocco* **110 B3** 31 12N 8 15W
Amla, *India* **92 J8** 21 56N 78 7 E
Amlapura = Karangasem, *Indonesia* **79 J18** 8 27 S 115 37 E
Åmli, *Norway* **18 F5** 58 45N 8 32 E
Amlia I., *U.S.A.* **144 K4** 52 4N 173 30W
Amlwch, *U.K.* **20 D3** 53 24N 4 20W
Amm Adam, *Sudan* **107 D4** 16 20N 36 1 E
'Ammān, *Jordan* **103 D4** 31 57N 35 52 E
'Ammān □, *Jordan* **103 D5** 31 40N 36 30 E
'Ammān ✕ (AMM), *Jordan* **103 D5** 31 45N 36 2 E
Ammanford, *U.K.* **21 F4** 51 48N 3 59W
Ammassalik = Tasiilaq, *Greenland* **10 D7** 65 40N 37 20W
Ammerån →, *Sweden* **16 A10** 63 9N 16 13 E
Ammersee, *Germany* **31 G7** 48 0N 11 7 E
Ammochostos = Famagusta, *Cyprus* **39 E9** 35 8N 33 55 E
Ammon, *U.S.A.* **158 E8** 43 28N 111 58W
Amnat Charoen, *Thailand* **86 E5** 15 51N 104 38 E
Amnura, *Bangla.* **93 G13** 24 37N 88 25 E
Amo Jiang →, *China* **76 F3** 23 0N 101 50 E
Āmol, *Iran* **97 B7** 36 23N 52 20 E
Amoret, *U.S.A.* **156 F2** 38 15N 94 35W
Amorgós, *Greece* **49 E7** 36 50N 25 57 E
Amory, *U.S.A.* **149 J1** 33 59N 88 29W
Amos, *Canada* **140 C4** 48 35N 78 5W
Åmot, *Buskerud, Norway* **18 E6** 59 57N 9 54 E
Åmot, *Oppland, Norway* **18 D7** 61 0N 10 2 E
Åmot, *Telemark, Norway* **18 E5** 59 34N 8 0 E
Åmotfors, *Sweden* **16 E6** 59 47N 12 22 E
Åmotsdal, *Norway* **18 E5** 59 37N 8 26 E
Amour, Djebel, *Algeria* **111 B5** 33 42N 1 37 E
Amoy = Xiamen, *China* **77 E12** 24 25N 118 4 E
Ampanavoana, *Madag.* **117 B9** 15 41 S 50 22 E
Ampang, *Malaysia* **87 L3** 3 8N 101 45 E
Ampangalana, Lakandranon', *Madag.* **117 C8** 22 48 S 47 50 E
Ampani, *India* **94 E6** 19 35N 82 38 E
Ampanihy, *Madag.* **117 C7** 24 40 S 44 45 E
Amparafaravola, *Madag.* **117 B8** 17 35 S 48 13 E
Ampasinambo, *Madag.* **117 C8** 20 31 S 48 0 E
Ampasindava, Helodranon', *Madag.* **117 A8** 13 40 S 48 15 E
Ampasindava, Saikanosy, *Madag.* **117 A8** 13 42 S 47 55 E
Ampato, Nevado, *Peru* **172 D3** 15 40 S 71 56W
Ampenan, *Indonesia* **85 D5** 8 34 S 116 4 E
Amper, *Nigeria* **113 D6** 9 25N 9 40 E
Amper →, *Germany* **31 G7** 48 29N 11 55 E
Ampezzo, *Italy* **45 B9** 46 25N 12 48 E
Amphoe Kathu, *Thailand* **87 a** 7 55N 98 21 E
Amphoe Thalang, *Thailand* **87 a** 8 1N 98 20 E
Ampitsikinana, *Réunion* **117 A8** 12 57 S 49 49 E
Ampombiantambo, *Madag.* **117 A8** 12 42 S 48 57 E
Amposta, *Spain* **40 E5** 40 43N 0 34 E
Ampotaka, *Madag.* **117 D7** 25 3 S 44 41 E
Ampoza, *Madag.* **117 C7** 22 20 S 44 44 E
Amqui, *Canada* **141 C6** 48 28N 67 27W
Amrabad, *India* **95 F4** 16 23N 78 50 E
'Amrān, *Yemen* **98 D3** 15 41N 43 55 E
Amraoti = Amravati, *India* **94 D3** 20 55N 77 45 E
Amravati, *India* **94 D3** 20 55N 77 45 E
Amreli, *India* **92 J4** 21 35N 71 17 E
Amrenene el Kasba, *Algeria* **111 D5** 22 10N 0 30 E
Amriswil, *Switz.* **33 A8** 47 33N 9 18 E
Amritsar, *India* **92 D6** 31 35N 74 57 E
Amroha, *India* **93 E8** 28 53N 78 30 E
Amrum, *Germany* **30 A4** 54 38N 8 22 E
Amsâga, *Mauritania* **110 D2** 20 7N 14 10W
Amsel, *Algeria* **111 D6** 22 47N 5 29 E
Amsterdam, *Neths.* **24 B4** 52 23N 4 54 E
Amsterdam, *U.S.A.* **151 D10** 42 56N 74 11W
Amsterdam ✕ (AMS), *Neths.* **24 B4** 52 18N 4 45 E
Amsterdam, I. = Nouvelle-Amsterdam, Î., *Ind. Oc.* **121 H6** 38 30 S 77 30 E
Amstetten, *Austria* **34 C7** 48 7N 14 51 E
Amudarya, *Turkmenistan* **65 E2** 37 53N 65 15 E
Amudarya →, *Uzbekistan* **66 E6** 43 58N 59 34 E
Amukta I., *U.S.A.* **144 K5** 52 30N 171 16W
Amukta Pass, *U.S.A.* **144 L5** 52 0N 171 0W
Amulung, *Phil.* **80 C3** 17 50N 121 43 E
Amundsen Gulf, *Canada* **138 A7** 71 0N 124 0W
Amundsen-Scott, *Antarctica* **7 E** 90 0 S 166 0 E
Amundsen Sea, *Antarctica* **7 D15** 72 0 S 115 0W
Amungen, *Sweden* **16 C9** 61 10N 15 40 E
Amuntai, *Indonesia* **85 C5** 2 28 S 115 25 E
Amur, *Somali Rep.* **120 C3** 5 16N 46 30 E
Amur →, *Russia* **67 D15** 52 56N 141 10 E
Amur, W. →, *Sudan* **106 D3** 18 56N 33 34 E
Amurang, *Indonesia* **82 A2** 1 5N 124 40 E
Amurrio, *Spain* **40 B1** 43 3N 3 0W
Amursk, *Russia* **67 D14** 50 14N 136 54 E
Amusco, *Spain* **42 C6** 42 10N 4 28W
Amvrakikós Kólpos, *Greece* **48 C2** 39 0N 20 55 E
Amvrosiyivka, *Ukraine* **59 J10** 47 43N 38 30 E
Amyderya = Amudarya →, *Uzbekistan* **66 E6** 43 58N 59 34 E
Amzeglouf, *Algeria* **111 C5** 26 50N 0 1 E
An, *Burma* **90 F5** 19 48N 94 0 E
An Anbār □, *Iraq* **96 C4** 33 25N 42 0 E
An Bien, *Vietnam* **87 H5** 9 45N 105 0 E
An Hoa, *Vietnam* **86 E7** 15 40N 108 5 E
An Nabatīyah at Tahta, *Lebanon* **103 B4** 33 23N 35 27 E
An Nabk, *Si. Arabia* **96 D3** 31 20N 37 20 E
An Nabk, *Syria* **103 A5** 34 2N 36 44 E
An Nafūd, *Si. Arabia* **96 D4** 28 15N 41 0 E
An Najaf, *Iraq* **101 G11** 32 3N 44 15 E
An Nāşirīyah, *Iraq* **96 D5** 31 0N 46 15 E
An Nawfalīyah, *Libya* **108 B3** 30 54N 17 58 E
An Nhon, *Vietnam* **86 F7** 13 55N 109 7 E
An Nîl □, *Sudan* **106 D3** 19 30N 33 0 E
An Nîl el Abyad □, *Sudan* **107 E3** 14 0N 32 15 E
An Nîl el Azraq □, *Sudan* **107 E3** 11 30N 34 30 E
An Nimāş, *Si. Arabia* **98 C3** 19 7N 42 8 E
An Nu'ayrīyah, *Si. Arabia* **97 E6** 27 30N 48 30 E
An Nu'mānīyah, *Iraq* **101 F11** 32 32N 45 25 E
An Nuwayb'ī, W. →, *Si. Arabia* **103 F3** 29 18N 34 57 E
An Thoi, Dao, *Vietnam* **87 H4** 9 58N 104 0 E
An Uaimh, *Ireland* **23 C5** 53 39N 6 41W
Åna-Sira, *Norway* **18 F3** 58 17N 6 25 E
Anabanua, *Indonesia* **82 B2** 3 57 S 120 4 E
Anabar →, *Russia* **67 B12** 73 8N 113 36 E
'Anabtā, *West Bank* **103 C4** 32 19N 35 7 E
Anaco, *Venezuela* **169 B5** 9 27N 64 28W
Anaconda, *U.S.A.* **158 C7** 46 8N 112 57W
Anacortes, *U.S.A.* **160 B4** 48 30N 122 37W
Anacuao, Mt., *Phil.* **80 C3** 16 16N 121 53 E
Anadarko, *U.S.A.* **155 H5** 35 4N 98 15W
Anadia, *Brazil* **170 C4** 9 42 S 36 18W
Anadia, *Portugal* **42 E2** 40 26N 8 27W
Anadolu, *Turkey* **100 C5** 39 0N 30 0 E
Anadyr, *Russia* **67 C18** 64 35N 177 20 E
Anadyr →, *Russia* **67 C18** 64 55N 176 5 E
Anadyrskiy Zaliv, *Russia* **67 C19** 64 0N 180 0 E
Anáfi, *Greece* **49 E7** 36 22N 25 48 E
Anafonítria, *Greece* **39 D2** 37 51N 20 39 E
Anafópoulo, *Greece* **49 E7** 36 17N 25 50 E
Anaga, Pta. de, *Canary Is.* **9 e1** 28 34N 16 9W
Anagni, *Italy* **45 G10** 41 44N 13 9 E
'Ānah, *Iraq* **101 E10** 34 25N 42 0 E
Anahalu →, *U.S.A.* **145 J13** 21 37N 158 6W
Anaheim, *U.S.A.* **161 M9** 33 50N 117 55W
Anahim Lake, *Canada* **142 C3** 52 28N 125 18W
Anahola, *U.S.A.* **145 A2** 22 9N 159 19W
Anáhuac, *Mexico* **162 B4** 27 14N 100 9W
Anai Mudi, *India* **95 J3** 10 12N 77 4 E
Anaichak ⌓, *U.S.A.* **144 H8** 56 40N 157 50W
Anaimalai Hills, *India* **95 J3** 10 20N 76 40 E
Anajás, *Brazil* **170 B2** 0 59 S 49 57W
Anajatuba, *Brazil* **170 B3** 3 16 S 44 37W
Anakapalle, *India* **94 F6** 17 42N 83 6 E
Anakena, *Chile* **172 b** 27 5 S 109 20W
Anakie, *Australia* **126 C4** 23 32 S 147 45 E
Anaklia, *Georgia* **61 J5** 42 22N 41 35 E
Anaktuvuk Pass, *U.S.A.* **144 B10** 68 8N 151 45W
Analalava, *Madag.* **117 A8** 14 35 S 48 0 E
Analavoka, *Madag.* **117 C8** 22 23 S 46 30 E
Análipsis, *Greece* **38 B9** 39 36N 19 55 E
Anamã, *Brazil* **169 D5** 3 35 S 61 22W
Anambar →, *Pakistan* **92 D3** 30 15N 68 50 E
Anambas, Kepulauan, *Indonesia* **84 B3** 3 20N 106 30 E
Anambas Is. = Anambas, Kepulauan, *Indonesia* **84 B3** 3 20N 106 30 E
Anambra □, *Nigeria* **113 D6** 6 20N 7 0 E
Aname, *Vanuatu* **133 K7** 20 8 S 169 47 E
Anamosa, *U.S.A.* **156 B5** 42 7N 91 17W
Anamur, *Turkey* **100 D5** 36 8N 32 58 E
Anamur Burnu, *Turkey* **100 D5** 36 2N 32 47 E
Anan, *Japan* **72 D6** 33 54N 134 40 E
Anand, *India* **92 H5** 22 32N 72 59 E
Anandapuram, *India* **95 G2** 14 5N 75 12 E
Anandpur, *India* **94 D8** 21 16N 86 13 E
Anánes, *Greece* **48 E6** 36 33N 24 9 E
Anantapur, *India* **95 G3** 14 39N 77 42 E
Anantnag, *India* **93 C6** 33 45N 75 10 E
Ananyevo, *Kyrgyzstan* **65 B8** 42 45N 77 40 E
Ananyiv, *Ukraine* **53 C14** 47 44N 29 58 E
Anapa, *Russia* **59 K9** 44 55N 37 25 E
Anapodháris →, *Greece* **39 F6** 34 59N 25 20 E
Anápolis = Simão Dias, *Brazil* **170 D4** 10 44 S 37 49W
Anápolis, *Brazil* **171 E2** 16 15 S 48 50W
Anapu →, *Brazil* **169 D7** 1 53 S 50 53W
Anār, *Iran* **97 D7** 30 55N 55 13 E

Anār Darreh, *Afghan.* . . **91 B1** 32 46N 61 39 E
Anārak, *Iran* . . . . **97 C7** 33 25N 53 40 E
Anarisfjällen, *Sweden* . **16 A7** 63 6N 13 10 E
Anas ➤, *India* . . . . . . **92 H5** 23 26N 74 0 E
Anatolia = Anadolu,
  Turkey . . . . **100 C5** 39 0N 30 0 E
Anatsogno, *Madag.* . . . **117 C7** 23 33 S 43 46 E
Añatuya, *Argentina* . . . **174 B3** 28 20 S 62 50W
Anauá ➤, *Brazil* **169 C5** 0 58N 61 21W
Anaunethad L., *Canada* **143 A8** 60 55N 104 25W
Anavilhanas,
  Arquipélago das,
  Brazil . . . . **169 D5** 2 42 S 60 45W
Anaye, *Niger* . . . . **109 E2** 19 15N 12 50 E
Anbyŏn, *N. Korea* . . . . **75 E14** 39 1N 127 35 E
Ancares ➤, *Spain* **42 C4** 42 50N 6 40W
Ancash □, *Peru* . . . . . **172 B2** 9 30 S 77 45W
Ancaster, *Canada* **150 C5** 43 13N 79 59W
Ancenis, *France* **26 E5** 47 21N 1 10W
Anchieta = Piatã, *Brazil* **171 D3** 13 9 S 41 48W
Anch'ing = Anqing,
  China . . . . **77 B11** 30 30N 117 3 E
Ancho, Canal, *Chile* . . **176 D2** 50 0 S 74 0W
Anchor Bay, *U.S.A.* . . . **160 G3** 38 48N 123 34W
Anchorage, *U.S.A.* . . . **144 F10** 61 13N 149 54W
Anci, *China* . . . . **74 E9** 39 20N 116 40 E
Ancohuma, Nevado,
  Bolivia . . . . **172 D4** 16 0 S 68 50W
Ancón, *Peru* . . . . **172 C2** 11 50 S 77 10W
Ancona, *Italy* . . . . **45 E10** 43 38N 13 30 E
Ancud, *Chile* . . . . **176 E2** 42 0 S 73 50W
Ancud, G. de, *Chile* . . . **176 E2** 42 0 S 73 0W
Ancy-le-Franc, *France* . **27 E11** 47 46N 4 10 E
Anda, *China* . . . . **69 B7** 46 24N 125 19 E
Anda, *Phil.* . . . . **80 C2** 16 17N 119 57 E
Andacollo, *Argentina* . . **174 D1** 37 10 S 70 42W
Andacollo, *Chile* . . . . . **174 C1** 30 14 S 71 6W
Andahuaylas, *Peru* . . . **172 C3** 13 40 S 73 25W
Andaingo, *Madag.* . . . . **117 B8** 18 12 S 48 17 E
Andalgalá, *Argentina* . . **174 B2** 27 40 S 66 30W
Åndalsnes, *Norway* . . . **18 B4** 62 35N 7 43 E
Andalucía □, *Spain* . . . **43 H6** 37 35N 5 0W
Andalusia =
  Andalucía □, *Spain* . **43 H6** 37 35N 5 0W
Andalusia, *U.S.A.* **149 K2** 31 18N 86 29W
Andaman & Nicobar
  Is. □, *India* . . . . . . **95 K11** 10 0N 93 0 E
Andaman Sea, *Ind. Oc.* **95 H11** 12 30N 92 45 E
Andaman Str., *India* . . **78 B1** 13 0N 96 0 E
Andamooka Opal
  Fields, *Australia* . . . **127 E2** 30 27 S 137 9 E
Andapa, *Madag.* . . . . . **117 A8** 14 39 S 49 39 E
Andara, *Namibia* . . . . . **116 B3** 18 2 S 21 9 E
Andaraí, *Brazil* . . . . . . **171 D3** 12 48 S 41 20W
Andeer, *Switz.* . . . . . . **33 C8** 46 36N 9 26 E
Andelfingen, *Switz.* . . . **33 A7** 47 36N 8 41 E
Andelot-Blancheville,
  France . . . . **27 D12** 48 15N 5 18 E
Andenes, *Norway* . . . . **14 B17** 69 19N 16 18 E
Andenne, *Belgium* . . . . **24 D5** 50 28N 5 5 E
Andéranboukane, *Mali* **113 B5** 15 26N 3 2 E
Andermatt, *Switz.* . . . . **33 C7** 46 38N 8 35 E
Andernach, *Germany* . . **36 E4** 50 26N 7 24 E
Andernos-les-Bains,
  France **28 D2** 44 44N 1 6W
Anderslöv, *Sweden* . . . **17 J7** 55 26N 13 19 E
Anderson, *Alaska,*
  U.S.A. **144 D10** 64 25N 149 15W
Anderson, *Calif.,*
  U.S.A. **158 F2** 40 27N 122 18W
Anderson, *Ind., U.S.A.* **157 D11** 40 10N 85 41W
Anderson, *Mo., U.S.A.* **155 G7** 36 39N 94 27W
Anderson, *S.C., U.S.A.* **149 H4** 34 31N 82 39W
Anderson ➤, *Canada* . . **138 B7** 69 42N 129 0W
Andersonville, *U.S.A.* . **152 C5** 32 12N 84 9W
Andersonville △,
  U.S.A. **152 C5** 32 12N 84 8W
Anderstorp, *Sweden* . . **17 G7** 57 19N 13 39 E
Andes, *Colombia* **168 B2** 5 39N 75 54W
Andes, *U.S.A.* **151 D10** 42 12N 74 47W
Andes, Cord. de los,
  S. Amer. . . . . **172 C3** 20 0 S 68 0W
Andfjorden, *Norway* . . **14 B17** 69 10N 16 20 E
Andhra, L., *India* . . . . **94 E1** 18 54N 73 32 E
Andhra Pradesh □,
  India . . . . **94 F4** 18 0N 79 0 E
Andijon, *Uzbekistan* . . **65 C6** 41 10N 72 15 E
Andikíthira, *Greece* . . . **48 F5** 35 52N 23 15 E
Andilamena, *Madag.* . . **117 B8** 17 1 S 48 35 E
Andīmeshk, *Iran* . . . . . **97 C6** 32 27N 48 21 E
Andímilos, *Greece* . . . . **48 E6** 36 47N 24 12 E
Andíparos, *Greece* . . . . **49 D7** 37 0N 25 3 E
Andípaxos, *Greece* . . . . **48 F3** 39 9N 20 13 E
Andípsara, *Greece* . . . . **49 C7** 38 30N 25 29 E
Andírrion, *Greece* . . . . **48 C3** 38 20N 21 46 E
Andizhan = Andijon,
  Uzbekistan . . . . . . **65 C6** 41 10N 72 15 E
Andkhvoy, *Afghan.* . . . **65 E2** 36 52N 65 8 E
Andoain, *Spain* **40 B2** 43 13N 2 1W
Andoany, *Madag.* . . . . **117 A8** 13 25 S 48 16 E
Andoas, *Peru* . . . . **168 D2** 2 55 S 76 25W
Andohahela △, *Madag.* **117 C8** 24 4 S 46 44 E
Andol, *India* . . . . **94 F4** 17 51N 78 4 E
Andola, *India* . . . . **94 F3** 16 57N 76 50 E
Andongwei, *China* . . . **75 G10** 35 6N 119 20 E
Andoom, *Australia* . . . **128 A3** 12 25 S 141 53 E
Andorra, *Spain* **40 E4** 40 59N 0 28W
Andorra ■, *Europe* . . . **28 F5** 42 30N 1 30 E
Andorra La Vella,
  Andorra . . . . **28 F5** 42 31N 1 32 E
Andover, *U.K.* **21 F6** 51 12N 1 29W
Andover, *Maine, U.S.A.* **151 B14** 44 38N 70 45W
Andover, *Mass., U.S.A.* **151 D13** 42 40N 71 8W
Andover, *N.J., U.S.A.* . **151 F10** 40 59N 74 45W
Andover, *N.Y., U.S.A.* . **150 D7** 42 10N 77 48W
Andover, *Ohio, U.S.A.* . **150 E4** 41 36N 80 34W
Andøya, *Norway* . . . . . **14 B16** 69 10N 15 50 E
Andrade, *Brazil* . . . . . . **169 D5** 4 40 S 63 45W
Andradina, *Brazil* . . . . **171 F1** 20 54 S 51 23W
Andrahary, Mt.,
  Madag. . . . . **117 A8** 13 37 S 49 17 E
Andramasina, *Madag.* . **117 B8** 19 11 S 47 35 E
Andranopasy, *Madag.* . **117 C7** 21 8 S 43 44 E
Andranovory, *Madag.* . **117 C7** 23 8 S 44 10 E
Andratx, *Spain* . . . . . . **38 B9** 39 39N 2 25 E
André Félix △, *C.A.R.* . **114 A4** 9 29N 23 8 E
Andreanof Is., *U.S.A.* . **144 L4** 51 30N 176 0 W
Andrée Land,
  Greenland **10 C8** 73 40N 26 0W
Andrews, *S.C., U.S.A.* . **153 J6** 33 27N 79 34W
Andrews, *Tex., U.S.A.* . **155 J3** 32 19N 102 33W
Andria, *Italy* . . . . **47 A9** 41 13N 16 17 E
Andriamena, *Madag.* . . **117 B8** 17 26 S 47 30 E
Andriandampy, *Madag.* **117 C8** 22 45 S 45 41 E
Andriba, *Madag.* . . . . . **117 B8** 17 30 S 46 58 E
Andrijevica,
  Serbia & M. . . . . . **50 D3** 42 45N 19 48 E

Andringitra △, *Madag.* **117 C8** 22 13 S 46 5 E
Andrítsaina, *Greece* . . **48 D3** 37 29N 21 52 E
Androka, *Madag.* . . . . **117 C7** 24 58 S 44 2 E
Andropov = Rybinsk,
  Russia . . . . **58 C10** 58 5N 38 50 E
Ándros, *Greece* . . . . . . **48 D6** 37 50N 24 57 E
Andros I., *Bahamas* . . . **164 B4** 24 30N 78 0W
Andros Town,
  Bahamas **164 B4** 24 43N 77 47W
Androscoggin ➤,
  U.S.A. **151 C14** 43 58N 70 0W
Androth I., *India* . . . . . **95 J1** 10 50N 73 41 E
Andrychów, *Poland* . . . **55 J6** 49 51N 19 18 E
Andselv, *Norway* . . . . **14 B18** 69 4N 18 34 E
Andújar, *Spain* **43 G6** 38 3N 4 5W
Andulo, *Angola* . . . . . . **115 E3** 11 25 S 16 45 E
Åneby, *Norway* . . . . . . **18 D7** 60 5N 10 51 E
Åneby, *Sweden* . . . . . . **17 G8** 57 48N 14 49 E
Anegada, *Br. Virgin Is.* **165 e** 18 45N 64 20W
Anegada, B., *Argentina* **176 B4** 40 20 S 62 20W
Anegada Passage,
  W. Indies **165 C7** 18 15N 63 45W
Añeho, *Togo* . . . . **113 D5** 6 12N 1 34 E
Aneityum, *Vanuatu* . . . **133 K7** 20 12 S 169 45 E
Anelghowhat, *Vanuatu* **133 K7** 20 19 S 169 43 E
Añelo, *Argentina* . . . . . **176 A3** 38 20 S 68 45W
Anenni-Noi, *Moldova* . . **53 D14** 46 53N 29 15 E
Aneto, Pico de, *Spain* . **40 C5** 42 37N 0 40 E
Añez, *Bolivia* . . . . **173 D5** 15 40 S 63 10W
Anfu, *China* . . . . **77 D10** 27 21N 114 40 E
Ang Mo Kio, *Singapore* **87 d** 1 23N 103 50 E
Ang Thong, *Thailand* . . **86 E3** 14 35N 100 31 E
Ang Thong ➤, *Thailand* **87 H2** 9 40N 99 43 E
Ang Thong, Ko,
  Thailand . . . . **87 b** 9 37N 99 41 E
Angadanam, *Phil.* . . . . **80 C3** 16 45N 121 45 E
Angamos, Punta, *Chile* **174 A1** 23 1 S 70 32W
Angara ➤, *Russia* . . . . **67 D10** 58 5N 94 20 E
Angara-Débou, *Benin* . . **113 C5** 11 19N 3 3 E
Angarab, *Ethiopia* . . . . **107 E4** 13 11N 37 7 E
Angarbaka, *Sudan* . . . . **107 F1** 9 44N 24 44 E
Angarsk, *Russia* . . . . . **67 D11** 52 30N 104 0 E
Angas Hills, *Australia* . **124 D4** 23 0 S 127 50 E
Angaston, *Australia* . . . **128 C3** 34 30 S 139 8 E
Angat, *Phil.* . . . . **80 D3** 14 56N 121 2 E
Ånge, *Sweden* . . . . **16 B9** 62 31N 15 35 E
Ángel, Salto = Angel
  Falls, *Venezuela* . . . **169 B5** 5 57N 62 30W
Ángel de la Guarda, I.,
  Mexico **162 B2** 29 30N 113 30W
Angel Falls, *Venezuela* . **169 B5** 5 57N 62 30W
Ángeles, *Phil.* . . . . **80 D3** 15 9N 120 33 E
Ängelholm, *Sweden* . . . **17 H6** 56 15N 12 58 E
Angels Camp, *U.S.A.* . . **160 G6** 38 4N 120 32W
Ängelsberg, *Sweden* . . . **16 E10** 59 58N 16 0 E
Anger ➤, *Ethiopia* . . . . **107 F4** 9 37N 36 6 E
Angerburg =
  Węgorzewo, *Poland* . **54 D8** 54 13N 21 43 E
Angereb ➤, *Ethiopia* . . **107 E4** 13 45N 36 40 E
Ångermanälven ➤,
  Sweden . . . . **16 B11** 62 40N 18 0 E
Ångermanland, *Sweden* **14 E18** 63 36N 17 45 E
Angermünde, *Germany* **30 B9** 53 1N 14 0 E
Angers, *Canada* **151 A9** 45 31N 75 29W
Angers, *France* **26 E6** 47 30N 0 35W
Angerville, *France* . . . . **27 D9** 48 19N 2 0 E
Ångesån ➤, *Sweden* . . . **14 C20** 66 16N 22 47 E
Angical, *Brazil* . . . . . . **171 D3** 12 0 S 44 42W
Angikuni L., *Canada* . . **143 A9** 62 12N 99 59W
Angkor, *Cambodia* . . . . **86 F4** 13 22N 103 50 E
Anglem, Mt., *N.Z.* . . . . **131 G2** 46 45 S 167 53 E
Anglès, *Spain* . . . . **40 D7** 41 57N 2 38 E
Anglesey, Isle of □,
  U.K. **20 D3** 53 16N 4 18W
Anglet, *France* **28 E2** 43 29N 1 31W
Angleton, *U.S.A.* **155 L7** 29 10N 95 26W
Anglin ➤, *France* . . . . . **28 B4** 46 42N 0 52 E
Anglisidhes, *Cyprus* . . **39 E9** 34 51N 33 27 E
Anglure, *France* . . . . . **27 D10** 48 35N 3 50 E
Angmagssalik =
  Tasiilaq, *Greenland* . **10 D7** 65 40N 37 20W
Ango, *Dem. Rep. of*
  the Congo . . . . **118 B2** 4 10N 26 5 E
Angoche, *Mozam.* . . . . **119 F4** 16 8 S 39 55 E
Angoche, I., *Mozam.* . . **119 F4** 16 20 S 39 50 E
Angol, *Chile* . . . . **174 D1** 37 56 S 72 45W
Angola, *Ind., U.S.A.* . . **157 C12** 41 38N 85 0W
Angola, *N.Y., U.S.A.* . . **150 D5** 42 38N 79 2W
Angola ■, *Africa* . . . . . **115 E3** 12 0 S 18 0 E
Angoon, *U.S.A.* **144 H14** 57 30N 134 35W
Angor, *Uzbekistan* . . . . **65 E3** 37 27N 67 9 E
Angora = Ankara,
  Turkey . . . . **100 C5** 39 57N 32 54 E
Angoram, *Papua N. G.* **132 C3** 4 4 S 144 4 E
Angoulême, *France* . . . **28 C4** 45 39N 0 10 E
Angoumois, *France* . . . **28 C4** 45 50N 0 25 E
Angra do Heroísmo,
  Azores **9 d1** 38 39N 27 13W
Angra dos Reis, *Brazil* . **175 A7** 23 0 S 44 10W
Angrapa ➤, *Russia* . . . **54 D8** 54 37N 21 54 E
Angren, *Uzbekistan* . . . **65 C5** 41 1N 70 12 E
Angtassom, *Cambodia* . **87 G5** 11 1N 104 41 E
Angu, *Dem. Rep. of*
  the Congo . . . . **118 B1** 3 23N 24 30 E
Anguang, *China* . . . . . . **75 B12** 45 15N 123 45 E
Anguilla ☑, *W. Indies* . **165 C7** 18 14N 63 5W
Angul, *India* . . . . **94 D7** 20 51N 85 6 E
Anguo, *China* . . . . **74 E8** 38 28N 115 15 E
Angurugu, *Australia* . . **128 A2** 14 0 S 136 25 E
Angus □, *U.K.* **22 E6** 56 46N 2 56W
Angwa ➤, *Zimbabwe* . . **119 B5** 16 0 S 30 23 E
Anhandui ➤, *Brazil* . . . **175 A5** 21 46 S 52 9W
Anholt, *Denmark* . . . . . **17 H5** 56 42N 11 33 E
Anhui □, *China* . . . . . . **77 C8** 32 28N 111 12 E
Anhui □, *China* . . . . . . **77 C8** 32 0N 117 0 E
Anhwei = Anhui □,
  China . . . . **77 B11** 32 0N 117 0 E
Aniak, *U.S.A.* **144 F8** 61 35N 159 32W
Anichab, *Namibia* . . . . **116 C1** 21 0 S 14 46 E
Anicuns, *Brazil* . . . . . . **171 E2** 16 28 S 49 58W
Ánidhros, *Greece* . . . . . **49 E7** 36 38N 25 43 E
Anil, *Togo* . . . . **113 D5** 7 42N 1 8 E
Anil, *Brazil* . . . . **170 B3** 2 32 S 44 14W
Animas ➤, *U.S.A.* **159 H9** 36 43N 108 13W
Anina, *Romania* . . . . . . **52 E6** 45 6N 21 51 E
Anini-y, *Phil.* . . . . **81 F3** 10 25N 121 55 E
Anita, *U.S.A.* **156 E7** 41 27N 94 46W
Anivorano, *Madag.* . . . **117 B8** 18 44 S 48 58 E
Anjalankoski, *Finland* . **15 F22** 60 45N 26 51 E
Anjangaon, *India* . . . . . **94 J10** 21 10N 77 20 E
Anjar, *India* . . . . **92 H4** 23 6N 70 10 E
Anji, *China* . . . . **79 B12** 30 38N 119 40 E
Anjou, *France* **26 E6** 47 20N 0 15W
Anjouan, *Comoros Is.* . **121 a** 12 15 S 44 25 E
Anjozorobe, *Madag.* . . . **117 B8** 18 22 S 47 52 E
Anju, *N. Korea* . . . . . . **75 E13** 39 36N 125 40 E
Anka, *Nigeria* . . . . **113 C6** 12 13N 5 58 E
Ankaboa, Tanjona,
  Madag. . . . . **117 C7** 21 58 S 43 20 E

Ankang, *China* . . . . . . **74 H5** 32 40N 109 1 E
Ankara, *Turkey* . . . . . . **100 C5** 39 57N 32 54 E
Ankarafantsika △,
  Madag. . . . . **117 B8** 16 8 S 47 5 E
Ankaramena, *Madag.* . . **117 C8** 21 57 S 46 39 E
Ankarsrum, *Sweden* . . **17 G10** 57 41N 16 20 E
Ankasakasa, *Madag.* . . **117 B7** 16 21 S 44 52 E
Ankavandra, *Madag.* . . **117 B8** 18 46 S 45 18 E
Ankazoabo, *Madag.* . . . **117 C7** 22 18 S 44 31 E
Ankazobe, *Madag.* . . . . **117 B8** 18 20 S 47 10 E
Ankeny, *U.S.A.* **156 C3** 41 44N 93 36W
Ankhialo = Pomorie,
  Bulgaria . . . . **51 D11** 42 32N 27 41 E
Ankiliabo, *Madag.* . . . . **117 C7** 22 58 S 43 45 E
Ankilizato, *Madag.* . . . **117 C8** 20 25 S 45 1 E
Anking = Anqing,
  China . . . . **77 B11** 30 30N 117 3 E
Ankisabe, *Madag.* . . . . **117 B8** 19 17 S 46 29 E
Anklam, *Germany* . . . . **30 B9** 53 51N 13 41 E
Ankleshwar, *India* . . . . **94 D1** 21 38N 73 3 E
Ankober, *Ethiopia* . . . . **107 F4** 9 35N 39 40 E
Ankola, *India* . . . . **95 G2** 14 40N 74 18 E
Ankoro, *Dem. Rep. of*
  the Congo . . . . **118 D2** 6 45 S 26 55 E
Ankororoka, *Madag.* . . **117 D8** 25 30 S 45 11 E
Anlong, *China* . . . . **76 E5** 25 2N 105 27 E
Anlu, *China* . . . . **77 B9** 31 15N 113 45 E
Anmyŏn-do, *S. Korea* . **75 F14** 36 25N 126 25 E
Ånn, *Sweden* . . . . **16 A6** 63 19N 12 34 E
Ann, C., *U.S.A.* **151 D14** 42 38N 70 35W
Ann Arbor, *U.S.A.* **157 D13** 42 17N 83 45W
Anna, *Russia* . . . . **60 E5** 51 28N 40 23 E
Anna, *Ill., U.S.A.* **155 G10** 37 28N 89 15W
Anna, *Ohio, U.S.A.* . . . **157 D12** 40 24N 84 11W
Anna Regina, *Guyana* . **169 B6** 7 10N 58 30W
Annaba, *Algeria* . . . . . **111 A6** 36 50N 7 46 E
Annaberg-Buchholz,
  Germany . . . . **30 E9** 50 34N 13 0 E
Annai, *Guyana* **169 C6** 3 57N 59 8W
Annaka, *Japan* . . . . . . **73 A10** 36 19N 138 54 E
Annalee ➤, *Ireland* . . . **23 B4** 54 2N 7 24W
Annam, *Vietnam* . . . . . **86 E7** 16 0N 108 0 E
Annamitique, Chaîne,
  Asia . . . . **86 D6** 17 0N 106 0 E
Annan, *U.K.* **22 G5** 54 59N 3 16W
Annan ➤, *U.K.* **22 G5** 54 58N 3 16W
Annanberg,
  Papua N. G. . . . . . **132 C3** 4 52 S 144 42 E
Annapolis, *U.S.A.* **148 F7** 38 59N 76 30W
Annapolis Royal,
  Canada **141 D6** 44 44N 65 32W
Annapurna, *Nepal* . . . . **93 E10** 28 34N 83 50 E
Annean, L., *Australia* . **125 E2** 26 54 S 118 14 E
Anneberg, *Sweden* . . . . **17 G8** 57 44N 14 49 E
Annecy, *France* . . . . . . **29 C10** 45 55N 6 8 E
Annecy, Lac d', *France* . **29 C10** 45 52N 6 10 E
Annemasse, *France* . . . **27 F13** 46 12N 6 16 E
Annenfeld = Şämkir,
  Azerbaijan . . . . . . **61 K8** 40 50N 46 0 E
Annette I., *U.S.A.* **144 J15** 55 9N 131 28W
Annigeri, *India* . . . . . . **95 G2** 15 26N 75 26 E
Anning, *China* . . . . **76 E4** 24 55N 102 26 E
Anniston, *U.S.A.* **152 B4** 33 39N 85 50W
Annobón, *Atl. Oc.* . . . . **105 G4** 1 25 S 5 36 E
Annonay, *France* . . . . . **29 C8** 45 15N 4 40 E
Annot, *France* . . . . **29 E10** 43 58N 6 38 E
Annotto B., *Jamaica* . . **164 a** 18 17N 76 45W
Ännsjön, *Sweden* . . . . . **16 A6** 63 19N 12 34 E
Annville, *U.S.A.* **151 F8** 40 20N 76 31W
Áno Arkháňai, *Greece* . **49 F7** 35 16N 25 11 E
Áno Porróia, *Greece* . . **50 E7** 41 17N 23 2 E
Áno Síros, *Greece* . . . . **48 D6** 37 29N 24 56 E
Áno Viánnos, *Greece* . . **49 F6** 35 2N 25 21 E
Anorotsangana, *Madag.* **117 A8** 13 56 S 47 55 E
Anosibe, *Madag.* . . . . . **117 B8** 19 26 S 48 13 E
Anou Mellene, *Mali* . . . **113 B5** 17 29N 0 33 E
Anoumaba, *Ivory C.* . . **112 D4** 6 23N 4 38W
Anoyí, *Greece* . . . . **39 C2** 38 25N 20 40 E
Anóyia, *Greece* . . . . . . **39 E5** 35 16N 24 52 E
Anping, *Hebei, China* . **74 E8** 38 15N 115 30 E
Anping, *Liaoning,*
  China . . . . **75 D12** 41 5N 123 30 E
Anpu Gang, *China* . . . **76 G7** 21 25N 109 50 E
Anqing, *China* . . . . **77 B11** 30 30N 117 3 E
Anqiu, *China* . . . . **75 F10** 36 25N 119 10 E
Anren, *China* . . . . **77 D9** 26 43N 113 18 E
Ansager, *Denmark* . . . . **17 J2** 55 43N 8 45 E
Ansai, *China* . . . . **74 F5** 36 50N 109 20 E
Ansbach, *Germany* . . . **31 F6** 49 28N 10 34 E
Anse Boileau,
  Seychelles . . . . **121 b** 4 43 S 55 29 E
Anse La Raye, *St. Lucia* **165 f** 13 55N 61 3W
Anse Royale, *Seychelles* **121 b** 4 44 S 55 31 E
Anseba ➤, *Eritrea* . . . . **107 D4** 16 0N 38 30 E
Anserma, *Colombia* . . . **168 B2** 5 13N 75 48W
Ansfelden, *Austria* . . . . **34 C7** 48 12N 14 17 E
Anshan, *China* . . . . . . **75 D12** 41 5N 122 58 E
Anshun, *China* . . . . . . **76 D5** 26 18N 105 57 E
Ansião, *Portugal* **42 F2** 39 56N 8 27W
Ansley, *U.S.A.* **156 E5** 41 18N 99 23W
Ansó, *Spain* **40 C4** 42 51N 0 48W
Ansoain, *Spain* **40 C3** 42 50N 1 37W
Anson B., *Australia* . . . **124 B5** 13 20 S 130 6 E
Anson B., *Australia* . . . **124 B5** 13 20 S 130 6 E
Ansongo, *Mali* . . . . **113 B5** 15 25N 0 35 E
Ansongo-Ménaka △,
  Mali . . . . **113 B5** 15 3N 1 37 E
Ansonia, *Conn., U.S.A.* **151 E11** 41 21N 73 5W
Ansonia, *Ohio, U.S.A.* . **157 D12** 40 13N 84 38W
Ansonia, *Ohio, U.S.A.* . **157 D12** 40 13N 84 38W
Anstruther, *U.K.* **22 E6** 56 14N 2 41W
Ansudu, *Indonesia* . . . . **83 B5** 2 11 S 139 22 E
Antabamba, *Peru* . . . . **172 C3** 14 40 S 73 0W
Antagarh, *India* . . . . . . **94 D5** 20 6N 81 9 E
Antakya, *Turkey* . . . . . **100 D7** 36 14N 36 10 E
Antalaha, *Madag.* . . . . **117 A9** 14 57 S 50 20 E
Antalát, *Libya* . . . . **108 B4** 31 8N 20 42 E
Antalya, *Turkey* . . . . . **100 D4** 36 52N 30 45 E
Antalya □, *Turkey* . . . . **49 E12** 36 30N 30 0 E
Antalya Körfezi,
  Turkey . . . . **100 D4** 36 15N 31 30 E
Antambohobe, *Madag.* . **117 C8** 22 20 S 46 47 E
Antanambao-
  Manampotsy, *Madag.* **117 B8** 19 29 S 48 34 E
Antanambe, *Madag.* . . . **117 B8** 16 26 S 49 52 E
Antananarivo, *Madag.* . **117 B8** 18 55 S 47 31 E
Antananarivo □,
  Madag. . . . . **117 B8** 19 0 S 47 0 E
Antanifotsy, *Madag.* . . **117 B8** 19 39 S 47 19 E
Antanimbaribe, *Madag.* **117 C7** 21 30 S 44 48 E
Antanimora, *Madag.* . . **117 C8** 24 49 S 45 40 E
Antarctic Pen.,
  Antarctica . . . . **7 C18** 67 0 S 60 0W
Antarctica . . . . **7 E3** 90 0 S 0 0W
Antártida, Tierra de =
  Antarctica . . . . **7 E3** 90 0 S 0 0W
Antelope, *Zimbabwe* . . **119 G2** 21 2 S 28 31 E
Antenor Navarro,
  Brazil . . . . **170 C4** 6 44 S 38 27W
Antequera, *Paraguay* . . **174 A4** 24 8 S 57 7W
Antequera, *Spain* **43 H6** 37 5N 4 33W

Antero, Mt., *U.S.A.* . . . **159 G10** 38 41N 106 15W
Antevamena, *Madag.* . . **117 C7** 21 2 S 44 8 E
Anthemoús, *Greece* . . . **50 F7** 40 31N 23 15 E
Anthony, *Fla., U.S.A.* . **153 F7** 29 18N 82 7W
Anthony, *Kans., U.S.A.* **155 G5** 37 9N 98 2W
Anthony, *N. Mex.,*
  U.S.A. **159 K10** 32 0N 106 36W
Anti Atlas, *Morocco* . . . **110 C3** 30 0N 8 30W
Anti-Lebanon = Ash
  Sharqi, Al Jabal,
  Lebanon . . . . **103 B5** 33 40N 36 10 E
Antibes, *France* . . . . . . **29 E11** 43 34N 7 6 E
Antibes, C. d', *France* . **29 E11** 43 31N 7 7 E
Anticosti, Î. d', *Canada* **141 C7** 49 30N 63 0W
Antifer, C. d', *France* . . **26 C7** 49 41N 0 10 E
Antigo, *U.S.A.* **154 C10** 45 9N 89 9W
Antigonish, *Canada* . . . **141 C7** 45 38N 61 58W
Antigua, *Canary Is.* . . . **9 e2** 28 24N 14 1W
Antigua, *Guatemala* . . . **164 D1** 14 34N 90 41W
Antigua, *W. Indies* **165 C7** 17 0N 61 50W
Antigua & Barbuda ■,
  W. Indies **165 C7** 17 20N 61 48W
Antikythira =
  Andikíthira, *Greece* . **48 F5** 35 52N 23 15 E
Antilla, *Cuba* **164 B4** 20 40N 75 50W
Antilles = West Indies,
  Cent. Amer. **165 D7** 15 0N 65 0W
Antioch = Antakya,
  Turkey . . . . **100 D7** 36 14N 36 10 E
Antioch, *U.S.A.* **160 G5** 38 1N 121 48W
Antioche, Pertuis d',
  France **28 B2** 46 6N 1 20W
Antioquia, *Colombia* . . **168 B2** 6 40N 75 55W
Antioquia □, *Colombia* **168 B2** 7 0N 75 30W
Antipodes Is., *Pac. Oc.* **134 M9** 49 45 S 178 40 E
Antipolo, *Phil.* . . . . **80 D3** 14 35N 121 10 E
Antique □, *Phil.* . . . . . . **81 F4** 11 10N 122 5 E
Antiers, *U.S.A.* **155 H7** 34 14N 95 37W
Antoetra, *Madag.* . . . . **117 C8** 20 46 S 47 20 E
Antofagasta, *Chile* . . . . **174 A1** 23 50 S 70 30W
Antofagasta □, *Chile* . . **174 A2** 24 0 S 69 0W
Antofagasta de la
  Sierra, *Argentina* . . . **174 B2** 26 5 S 67 20W
Antofalla, *Argentina* . . **174 B2** 25 30 S 68 5W
Antofalla, Salar de,
  Argentina . . . . **174 B2** 25 40 S 67 45W
Anton, *U.S.A.* **155 J3** 33 49N 102 10W
Antongila, Helodrano,
  Madag. . . . . **117 B8** 15 30 S 49 50 E
Antonibé, *Madag.* . . . . **117 B8** 15 7 S 47 24 E
Antonibé, Presqu'île d',
  Madag. . . . . **117 A8** 14 55 S 47 20 E
Antonina, *Brazil* . . . . . **175 B6** 25 26 S 48 42W
António Enes =
  Angoche, *Mozam.* . . **119 F4** 16 8 S 39 55 E
Antrain, *France* **26 D5** 48 28N 1 30W
Antrim, *U.K.* **23 B5** 54 43N 6 14W
Antrim, *U.S.A.* **150 F3** 40 7N 81 21W
Antrim □, *U.K.* **23 B5** 54 56N 6 25W
Antrim, Mts. of, *U.K.* . **23 A5** 55 3N 6 14W
Antrim Plateau,
  Australia . . . . **124 C4** 18 8 S 128 20 E
Antrodoco, *Italy* . . . . . **45 F10** 42 25N 13 5 E
Antropovo, *Russia* . . . . **60 A6** 58 24N 43 6 E
Antsakabary, *Madag.* . . **117 B8** 15 3 S 48 56 E
Antsalova, *Madag.* . . . . **117 B7** 18 40 S 44 37 E
Antsenavolo, *Madag.* . . **117 C8** 21 24 S 48 3 E
Antsiafabositra, *Madag.* **117 B8** 17 18 S 46 57 E
Antsirabe,
  Antananarivo,
  Madag. . . . . **117 B8** 19 55 S 47 2 E
Antsirabe, Antsiranana,
  Madag. . . . . **117 A8** 14 0 S 49 59 E
Antsirabe, Mahajanga,
  Madag. . . . . **117 B8** 15 57 S 48 58 E
Antsiranana, *Madag.* . . **117 A8** 12 25 S 49 20 E
Antsiranana □, *Madag.* **117 A8** 12 16 S 49 17 E
Antsohihy, *Madag.* . . . **117 A8** 14 50 S 47 59 E
Antsohimbondrona
  Seranana, *Madag.* . . **117 A8** 13 7 S 48 48 E
Antu, *China* . . . . **75 C15** 42 30N 128 20 E
Antufash, *Yemen* . . . . . **98 D3** 15 42N 42 25 E
Antwerp = Antwerpen,
  Belgium . . . . **24 C4** 51 13N 4 25 E
Antwerp, *N.Y., U.S.A.* . **151 B9** 44 12N 75 37W
Antwerp, *Ohio, U.S.A.* . **157 C12** 41 11N 84 45W
Antwerpen, *Belgium* . . **24 C4** 51 13N 4 25 E
Antwerpen □, *Belgium* . **24 C4** 51 15N 4 40 E
Anukur, C.,
  Papua N. G. . . . . . **132 D5** 8 18 S 149 37 E
Anupgarh, *India* . . . . . **92 E5** 29 10N 73 10 E
Anuppur, *India* . . . . . . **93 H9** 23 6N 81 41 E
Anuradhapura,
  Sri Lanka . . . . **95 K5** 8 22N 80 28 E
Anveh, *Iran* . . . . **97 E7** 27 23N 54 11 E
Anvers = Antwerpen,
  Belgium . . . . **24 C4** 51 13N 4 25 E
Anvers I., *Antarctica* . . **7 C17** 64 30 S 63 40W
Anvik, *U.S.A.* **144 F7** 62 39N 160 13W
Anwen, *China* . . . . **77 C13** 29 4N 120 26 E
Anxi, *Fujian, China* . . . **77 E12** 25 2N 118 12 E
Anxi, *Gansu, China* . . . **68 B4** 40 30N 95 43 E
Anxian, *China* . . . . **76 B5** 31 35N 104 24 E
Anxiang, *China* . . . . . . **77 C9** 29 27N 112 11 E
Anxious B., *Australia* . . **125 E1** 33 24 S 134 45 E
Anyang, *China* . . . . . . **74 F8** 36 5N 114 21 E
Anyer-Kidul, *Indonesia* **79 G11** 6 4 S 105 53 E
Anyi, *Jiangxi, China* . . **77 C10** 28 49N 115 25 E
Anyi, *Shanxi, China* . . **74 G6** 35 2N 111 2 E
Anyuan, *China* . . . . . . **77 E10** 25 9N 115 21 E
Anyue, *China* . . . . **76 B5** 30 9N 105 50 E
Anza, *U.S.A.* **161 M10** 33 35N 116 39W
Anze, *China* . . . . **74 F7** 36 10N 112 12 E
Anzhero-Sudzhensk,
  Russia . . . . **66 D9** 56 10N 86 0 E
Anzio, *Italy* . . . . **44 A5** 41 27N 12 37 E
Anzoátegui □,
  Venezuela **169 B5** 9 0N 64 30W
Ao Makham, *Thailand* . **87 a** 7 50N 98 24 E
Ao Phangnga △,
  Thailand . . . . **87 a** 8 10N 98 32 E
Aoba, *Vanuatu* . . . . . . **133 E5** 15 25 S 167 50 E
Aoga-Shima, *Japan* . . . **73 E11** 32 28N 139 46 E
Aoiz, *Spain* **40 C3** 42 46N 1 22W
Aola, *Solomon Is.* . . . . **133 M11** 9 30 S 160 30 E
Aomen = Macau, *China* **79 G10** 22 16N 113 35 E
Aomori, *Japan* . . . . **70 D10** 40 45N 140 45 E
Aomori □, *Japan* . . . . . **70 D10** 40 45N 140 40 E
Aonla, *India* . . . . **93 E8** 28 16N 79 11 E
Aoraki Mount Cook,
  N.Z. . . . . **131 D5** 43 36 S 170 9 E
Aoral, Phnum,
  Cambodia . . . . **87 G5** 12 0N 104 15 E
Aorangi Mts., *N.Z.* . . . **130 H4** 41 28 S 175 22 E
Aore, *Vanuatu* . . . . **133 E5** 15 35 S 167 10 E
Aosta, *Italy* . . . . **44 C4** 45 45N 7 20 E
Aotearoa = New
  Zealand ■, *Oceania* **130 G5** 40 0 S 176 0 E

Aouinet Torkoz,
  Morocco **110 C3** 28 31N 9 46W
Aouk, Bahr ➤, *Africa* . **109 G3** 8 51N 18 53 E
Aouk-Aoukalé ➤,
  C.A.R. . . . . **114 A4** 9 52N 21 25 E
Aoukar, *Mali* . . . . **110 D4** 23 50 S 2 45 E
Aoukâr, *Mauritania* . . . **112 B3** 17 40N 10 0W
Aoulef el Arab, *Algeria* **111 C5** 26 55N 1 2 E
Aozou, *Chad* . . . . **109 D3** 21 45N 17 28 E
Aozou, Couloir d',
  Chad . . . . **109 D3** 22 0N 19 0 E
Apa ➤, *S. Amer.* . . . . . **174 A4** 22 6 S 58 2W
Apache, *U.S.A.* **155 H5** 34 54N 98 22W
Apache Junction,
  U.S.A. **159 K8** 33 25N 111 33W
Apalachee B., *U.S.A.* . . **152 F5** 30 0N 84 0W
Apalachicola, *U.S.A.* . . **152 F5** 29 43N 84 59W
Apalachicola ➤,
  U.S.A. **152 F5** 29 43N 84 58W
Apalachicola B., *U.S.A.* **152 F5** 29 40N 85 0W
Apam, *Ghana* **113 D4** 5 19N 0 42W
Apaporis ➤, *Colombia* . **168 D4** 1 23 S 69 25W
Aparados da Serra △,
  Brazil . . . . **175 B5** 29 10 S 50 8W
Aparecida = Bertolínia,
  Brazil . . . . **170 C3** 7 38 S 43 57W
Aparecida do Taboado,
  Brazil . . . . **171 F1** 20 5 S 51 5W
Aparri, *Phil.* . . . . **80 B3** 18 22N 121 38 E
Apărurén, *Venezuela* . . **169 B5** 5 6N 62 8W
Apateu, *Romania* . . . . . **52 D6** 46 36N 21 47 E
Apatin, *Serbia & M.* . . **52 E4** 45 40N 18 59 E
Apatity, *Russia* . . . . . . **56 A5** 67 34N 33 22 E
Apatou, *Fr. Guiana* . . . **169 B7** 5 9N 54 20W
Apatzingán, *Mexico* . . **162 D4** 19 5N 102 20W
Apawaram, *Indonesia* . **83 B5** 1 39 S 138 11 E
Apayao □, *Phil.* . . . . . . **80 B3** 18 10N 121 10 E
Apeldoorn, *Neths.* . . . . **24 C5** 52 13N 5 57 E
Apen, *Germany* . . . . . . **30 B3** 53 13N 7 48 E
Apennines =
  Appennini, *Italy* . . . **44 D7** 44 30N 10 0 E
Apenrade = Åbenrå,
  Denmark . . . . **17 J3** 55 3N 9 25 E
Apere ➤, *Bolivia* . . . . . **173 C4** 13 44 S 65 18W
Aphrodisias, *Turkey* . . **49 D10** 37 42N 28 46 E
Apia, *Samoa* . . . . **133 W24** 13 50 S 171 50W
Apiacás, Serra dos,
  Brazil . . . . **173 B6** 9 50 S 57 0W
Apiaí, *Brazil* . . . . **171 F2** 24 31 S 48 50W
Apiaú ➤, *Brazil* **169 C5** 2 39N 61 12W
Apiaú, Serra do, *Brazil* **169 C5** 2 30N 62 0W
Apidiá ➤, *Brazil* . . . . . **173 C5** 11 39 S 61 11W
Apies ➤, *S. Africa* . . . . **117 D4** 25 15 S 28 8 E
Apinajé, *Brazil* . . . . . . **171 D2** 11 31 S 48 18W
Apiti, *N.Z.* . . . . **130 H4** 39 58 S 175 54 E
Apizaco, *Mexico* **163 D5** 19 26N 98 9W
Apo, Mt., *Phil.* . . . . **81 H5** 6 53N 125 14 E
Apo East Pass, *Phil.* . . **80 E3** 12 40N 120 40 E
Apo Reef, *Phil.* . . . . . . **80 E2** 12 50N 120 50 E
Apo West Pass, *Phil.* . . **80 E2** 12 31N 120 22 E
Apodi, *Brazil* . . . . **170 C4** 5 39 S 37 48W
Apolakkiá, *Greece* . . . . **49 D9** 36 5N 27 48 E
Apolakkiá, Órmos,
  Greece . . . . **38 E11** 36 5N 27 45 E
Apolda, *Germany* . . . . . **30 D7** 51 2N 11 32 E
Apollo Bay, *Australia* . **128 F5** 38 45 S 143 40 E
Apollonia = Marsá
  Susah, *Libya* . . . . . **108 B4** 32 52N 21 59 E
Apollonia, *Greece* . . . . **48 E6** 36 58N 24 43 E
Apolo, *Bolivia* . . . . **172 C4** 14 30 S 68 30W
Apónguao ➤,
  Venezuela **169 C5** 4 48N 61 36W
Apopka, *U.S.A.* **153 G8** 28 40N 81 31W
Apopka L., *U.S.A.* **153 G8** 28 36N 81 37W
Aporé, *Brazil* . . . . **173 D7** 18 58 S 52 1W
Aporé ➤, *Brazil* . . . . . . **171 E1** 19 27 S 50 57W
Aporema, *Brazil* **170 A1** 1 14N 50 49W
Apostle Is., *U.S.A.* **154 B9** 47 0N 90 40W
Apostle Islands △,
  U.S.A. **154 B9** 46 57N 90 53W
Apóstoles, *Argentina* . . **175 B4** 28 0 S 56 0W
Apostolos Andreas, C.,
  Cyprus . . . . **39 E10** 35 42N 34 35 E
Apostolovo, *Ukraine* . . **59 J7** 47 39N 33 39 E
Apoteri, *Guyana* **169 C6** 4 2N 58 32W
Appalachian Mts.,
  U.S.A. **148 G6** 38 0N 80 0W
Äppelbo, *Sweden* . . . . . **16 D8** 60 29N 14 1 E
Appennini, *Italy* . . . . . **44 D7** 44 30N 10 0 E
Appennino Ligure,
  Italy . . . . **44 D6** 44 30N 9 0 E
Appenzell, *Switz.* . . . . . **33 B8** 47 20N 9 25 E
Appenzell-Ausser
  Rhoden □, *Switz.* . . **33 B8** 47 23N 9 23 E
Appenzell-Inner
  Rhoden □, *Switz.* . . **33 B8** 47 20N 9 25 E
Appiano, *Italy* . . . . **45 B8** 46 28N 11 15 E
Apple Hill, *Canada* . . . **151 A10** 45 13N 74 46W
Apple Valley, *U.S.A.* . . **161 L9** 34 32N 117 14W
Appleby-in-
  Westmorland, *U.K.* . **20 C5** 54 35N 2 29W
Appledore, *U.K.* **21 F3** 51 3N 4 13W
Apples, *Switz.* . . . . **32 C2** 46 33N 6 26 E
Appleton, *U.S.A.* **148 C1** 44 16N 88 25W
Appleton City, *U.S.A.* . **156 F2** 38 11N 94 2W
Appling, *U.S.A.* **152 B7** 33 33N 82 19W
Approuague,
  Fr. Guiana **169 C7** 4 20N 52 0W
Aprica, *Italy* . . . . **33 D10** 46 9N 10 6 E
Apricena, *Italy* . . . . . . **45 G12** 41 47N 15 27 E
April ➤, *Papua N. G.* . . **132 C2** 4 18 S 142 26 E
Aprília, *Italy* . . . . **46 A5** 41 36N 12 39 E
Apsheronsk, *Russia* . . **61 H4** 44 28N 39 42 E
Apsley, *Australia* **150 B6** 44 45N 78 6W
Apt, *France* . . . . **29 E9** 43 53N 5 24 E
Apuané, Alpi, *Italy* . . . **44 D7** 44 7N 10 14 E
Apuaú, *Brazil* . . . . **169 D5** 2 26 S 60 33W
Apucarana, *Brazil* . . . . **175 A5** 23 55 S 51 33W
Apulia = Púglia □, *Italy* **47 A9** 41 0N 16 30 E
Apurauan, *Phil.* . . . . . . **81 G2** 9 35N 118 20 E
Apure □, *Venezuela* . . . **168 B4** 7 10N 68 50W
Apure ➤, *Venezuela* . . . **168 B4** 7 37N 66 25W
Apurímac □, *Peru* . . . . **172 C3** 14 30 S 73 30W
Apurímac ➤, *Peru* . . . . **172 C3** 12 17 S 73 56W
Apuseni, Munții,
  Romania . . . . **52 D7** 46 30N 22 45 E
Āqā Jarī, *Iran* . . . . **97 D6** 30 42N 49 50 E
Aqaba = Al 'Aqabah,
  Jordan . . . . **103 F4** 29 31N 35 0 E
Aqaba, G. of, *Red Sea* . **96 D2** 28 15N 33 20 E
'Aqabah, Khalij al =
  Aqaba, G. of,
  Red Sea . . . . **96 D2** 28 15N 33 20 E
Aqbaqay, *Kazakhstan* . **65 A6** 45 0N 72 47 E
Aqcheh, *Afghan.* . . . . . **91 A2** 37 0N 66 5 E
'Aqdā, *Iran* . . . . **97 C7** 32 26N 53 37 E
Aqîq, *Sudan* . . . . **106 D4** 18 14N 38 12 E
Aqîq, Khalîg, *Sudan* . . **106 D4** 18 20N 38 10 E
'Aqîq, W. al =
  Sī Arabia* . . . . **98 B3** 20 16N 41 40 E

Aqköl, *Kazakhstan* ... **65 A7** 45 0N 75 39 E
Aqköl, *Kazakhstan* ... **65 B5** 43 36N 70 45 E
Aqmola = Astana,
  Kazakhstan ..... **66 D8** 51 10N 71 30 E
Aqqum, *Kazakhstan* .. **65 A2** 44 50N 65 8 E
'Aqrah, *Iraq* ..... **101 D10** 36 46N 43 45 E
Aqshī, *Kazakhstan* ... **65 B8** 43 59N 76 19 E
Aqsū, *Kazakhstan* ... **65 B4** 42 25N 69 50 E
Aqsügek, *Kazakhstan* . **65 A7** 44 37N 74 30 E
Aqtaū, *Kazakhstan* ... **65 A3** 44 26N 67 33 E
Aqtöbe, *Kazakhstan* .. **57 D10** 50 17N 57 10 E
Aquidauana, *Brazil* ... **173 E6** 20 30 S 55 50W
Aquidauana →, *Brazil* **173 D6** 19 44 S 56 50W
Aquiles Serdán, *Mexico* **162 B3** 28 37N 105 54W
Aquin, *Haiti* **165 C5** 18 16N 73 24W
Aquitain, Bassin,
  France **25 D3** 44 0N 0 30W
Aquitaine □, *France* .. **28 D3** 44 0N 0 30W
Aqyrtöbe, *Kazakhstan* . **65 B6** 42 59N 72 7 E
Aqzhar, *Kazakhstan* .. **65 B5** 43 8N 71 37 E
Ar Rachidiya = Er
  Rachidia, *Morocco* . **110 B4** 31 58N 4 20W
Ar Rafid, *Syria* ..... **103 C4** 32 57N 35 52 E
Ar Raḩḩālīyah, *Iraq* .. **101 F10** 32 44N 43 23 E
Ar Ramādī, *Iraq* .... **101 F10** 33 25N 43 20 E
Ar Raml, *Libya* ..... **103 C4** 26 45N 19 40 E
Ar Ramthā, *Jordan* .. **103 C5** 32 34N 36 0 E
Ar Raqqah, *Syria* .... **101 E8** 35 59N 39 8 E
Ar Rass, *Si. Arabia* .. **96 E4** 25 50N 43 40 E
Ar Rawḑah, *Si. Arabia* **98 B3** 21 16N 42 50 E
Ar Rawḑah, *Yemen* .. **98 D4** 14 28N 47 17 E
Ar Rawshan, *Si. Arabia* **106 C5** 20 2N 42 36 E
Ar Rifā'ī, *Iraq* ..... **96 D5** 31 50N 46 10 E
Ar Rijā', *Yemen* .... **98 D4** 13 1N 44 35 E
Ar Riyāḑ, *Si. Arabia* . **96 E5** 24 41N 46 42 E
Ar Ru'ays, *Qatar* .... **97 E6** 26 8N 51 12 E
Ar Rukhaymīyah, *Iraq* **96 D5** 29 22N 45 38 E
Ar Ruṣāfah, *Syria* ... **101 E8** 35 45N 38 49 E
Ar Ruṭbah, *Iraq* .... **101 F9** 33 0N 40 15 E
Ar Ruwayḑah,
  Si. Arabia ..... **98 B4** 23 40N 44 40 E
Ara, *India* ..... **93 G11** 25 35N 84 32 E
Ara Goro, *Ethiopia* .. **107 F5** 5 48N 41 18 E
Ara Tera, *Ethiopia* ... **107 F5** 6 38N 40 57 E
Arab, *U.S.A.* **149 H2** 34 19N 86 30W
'Arab, Bahr el →,
  Sudan ..... **107 F2** 9 0N 29 30 E
Arab, Khalīg el, *Egypt* **106 A2** 30 55N 29 0 E
Arab, Shatt al →, *Asia* **97 D6** 30 0N 48 31 E
'Araba, W. →, *Egypt* . **106 J8** 28 19N 33 31 E
'Arabābād, *Iran* .... **97 C8** 33 2N 57 41 E
'Arabah, W. →, *Yemen* **99 C5** 18 5N 51 26 E
Araban, *Turkey* ..... **100 D7** 37 25N 37 50 E
Arabatskaya Strelka,
  Ukraine ..... **59 K8** 45 40N 35 0 E
Arabba, *Italy* ..... **45 B8** 46 30N 11 52 E
Arabelo, *Venezuela* .. **169 C5** 4 55N 64 13W
Arabi, *U.S.A.* **152 D6** 31 50N 83 44W
Arabia, *Asia* ..... **62 G8** 25 0N 45 0 E
Arabian Desert = Es
  Sahrâ Esh Sharqîya,
  Egypt ..... **106 B3** 27 30N 32 30 E
Arabian Gulf = Persian
  Gulf, *Asia* ..... **97 E6** 27 0N 50 0 E
Arabian Sea, *Ind. Oc.* **88 D5** 16 0N 65 0 E
Arabistan=
  Khūzestān □, *Iran* . **97 D6** 31 0N 49 0 E
Araç, *Turkey* ..... **100 B5** 41 15N 33 21 E
Aracaju, *Brazil* ..... **170 D4** 10 55 S 37 4W
Aracataca, *Colombia* . **168 A3** 10 38N 74 9W
Aracati, *Brazil* ..... **170 B4** 4 30 S 37 44W
Araçatuba, *Brazil* ... **173 A5** 21 10 S 50 30W
Araceli, *Phil.* ..... **81 F2** 10 33N 119 59 E
Aracena, *Spain* **43 H4** 37 53N 6 38W
Aracena, Sierra de,
  Spain **43 H4** 37 50N 6 50W
Aracides, C.,
  Solomon Is. ..... **133 M11** 8 21 S 161 0 E
Aračinovo, *Macedonia* **50 D5** 42 1N 21 34 E
Araçuaí, *Brazil* ..... **171 E3** 16 52 S 42 4W
Araçuaí →, *Brazil* ... **171 E3** 16 46 S 42 2W
'Arad, *Israel* ..... **103 D4** 31 15N 35 12 E
Arad, *Romania* ..... **52 D6** 46 10N 21 20 E
Arad □, *Romania* .... **52 D6** 46 20N 22 0 E
Arada, *Chad* ..... **109 F4** 15 0N 20 20 E
Arādān, *Iran* ..... **97 C7** 35 21N 52 30 E
Aradhippou, *Cyprus* .. **39 E9** 34 57N 33 36 E
Arafura Sea, *E. Indies* **83 C5** 9 0 S 135 0 E
Aragarças, *Brazil* ... **173 D5** 15 55 S 52 15W
Aragats, *Armenia* ... **61 K7** 40 30N 44 15 E
Aragón □, *Spain* **152 A4** 34 2N 85 3W
Aragón □, *Spain* **40 D4** 41 25N 0 40W
Aragón →, *Spain* **41 C2** 42 13N 1 44W
Aragona, *Italy* ..... **46 E6** 37 24N 13 27 E
Aragua □, *Venezuela* . **168 B4** 10 0N 67 10W
Aragua de Barcelona,
  Venezuela **169 B5** 9 28N 64 49W
Araguacema, *Brazil* . **170 C2** 8 50 S 49 20W
Araguaçu = Paraguaçu
  Paulista, *Brazil* ... **175 A5** 22 22 S 50 35W
Araguaçu, *Brazil* ... **171 D2** 12 49 S 49 51W
Araguaia □, *Brazil* .. **170 D2** 10 30 S 50 0W
Araguaia →, *Brazil* .. **170 C2** 5 21 S 48 41W
Araguaiana, *Brazil* .. **173 D7** 15 43 S 51 51W
Araguaína, *Brazil* ... **170 C2** 7 12 S 48 12W
Araguari, *Brazil* .... **171 E2** 18 38 S 48 11W
Araguari →, *Brazil* .. **169 C8** 1 15N 49 55W
Araguatins, *Brazil* ... **170 C2** 5 38 S 48 7W
Arain, *India* ..... **92 F6** 26 27N 75 2 E
Araioses, *Brazil* .... **170 B3** 2 53 S 41 55W
Arak, *Algeria* ..... **111 C5** 25 20N 3 45 E
Arāk, *Iran* ..... **97 C6** 34 0N 49 40 E
Araka, *Sudan* ..... **107 G3** 4 20N 30 23 E
Arakan □, *Burma* ... **90 F5** 19 0N 94 15 E
Arakan Yoma, *Burma* **90 F5** 20 0N 94 40 E
Arákhova, *Greece* ... **48 C4** 38 28N 22 35 E
Arakkonam, *India* ... **95 H4** 13 7N 79 43 E
Arakli, *Turkey* ..... **101 B8** 41 6N 40 2 E
Araks = Aras, Rūd-
  e →, *Asia* ..... **61 K9** 40 5N 48 29 E
Aral, *Kazakhstan* ... **66 E7** 46 41N 61 45 E
Aral Sea, *Asia* ..... **66 E7** 44 30N 60 0 E
Aral Tengizi = Aral
  Sea, *Asia* ..... **66 E7** 44 30N 60 0 E
Aralsk = Aral,
  Kazakhstan ..... **66 E7** 46 41N 61 45 E
Aralskoye More = Aral
  Sea, *Asia* ..... **66 E7** 44 30N 60 0 E
Aralsor, Ozero,
  Kazakhstan ..... **61 F9** 49 5N 48 12 E
Aramac, *Australia* ... **126 C4** 22 58 S 145 14 E
Aramia →,
  Papua N. G. ..... **120 C3** 7 55 S 143 22 E
Aran →, *India* ..... **94 E4** 19 55N 78 12 E
Aran Areh, *Ethiopia* . **120 C2** 9 0N 37 0 E
Aran I., *Ireland* **23 A3** 55 0N 8 30W
Aran Is., *Ireland* **23 C2** 53 6N 9 38W
Aranda de Duero,
  Spain **42 D7** 41 39N 3 42W
Arandān, *Iran* ..... **96 C5** 35 23N 46 55 E
Arandelovac,
  Serbia & M. ..... **50 B4** 44 18N 20 34 E
Aranga, *N.Z.* ..... **130 B2** 35 44 S 173 40 E

Arani, *Bolivia* ..... **173 D4** 17 34 S 65 46W
Arani, *India* ..... **95 H4** 12 43N 79 19 E
Aranjuez, *Spain* **42 E7** 40 1N 3 40W
Aranos, *Namibia* .... **116 C2** 24 9 S 19 7 E
Aransas Pass, *U.S.A.* . **155 M6** 27 55N 97 9W
Aranyaprathet,
  Thailand ..... **86 F4** 13 41N 102 30 E
Arao, *Japan* ..... **72 E2** 32 59N 130 25 E
Araouane, *Mali* **112 B4** 18 55N 3 30W
Arapahoe, *U.S.A.* ... **154 E5** 40 18N 99 54W
Arapari, *Brazil* ..... **170 C2** 5 34 S 49 15W
Arapawa I., *N.Z.* ... **131 B9** 41 11 S 174 17 E
Arapey Grande →,
  Uruguay ..... **174 C4** 30 55 S 57 49W
Arapgir, *Turkey* .... **101 C8** 39 5N 38 30 E
Arapiraca, *Brazil* ... **170 C4** 9 45 S 36 39W
Arapongas, *Brazil* ... **173 A5** 23 29 S 51 28W
Arapuni, *N.Z.* ..... **130 E4** 38 4 S 175 39 E
Ar'ar, *Si. Arabia* ... **96 D4** 30 59N 41 2 E
Araracuara, *Colombia* **168 D3** 0 24 S 72 17W
Araranguá, *Brazil* ... **175 B6** 29 0 S 49 30W
Araraquara, *Brazil* .. **171 F2** 21 50 S 48 0W
Araras, *Brazil* ..... **171 F2** 22 22 S 47 23W
Araras, Serra das,
  Brazil ..... **175 B5** 25 0 S 53 10W
Ararat, *Armenia* .... **101 C11** 39 48N 44 50 E
Ararat, *Australia* ... **128 D5** 37 16 S 143 0 E
Ararat, Mt. = Ağrı
  Dağı, *Turkey* ..... **101 C11** 39 50N 44 15 E
Arari, *Brazil* ..... **170 B3** 3 28 S 44 47W
Araria, *India* ..... **93 F12** 26 9N 87 33 E
Araripe, Chapada do,
  Brazil ..... **170 C3** 7 20 S 40 0W
Araripina, *Brazil* ... **170 C3** 7 33 S 40 34W
Araruama, L. de, *Brazil* **171 F3** 22 53 S 42 12W
Araruna, *Brazil* .... **170 C4** 6 52 S 35 44W
Aras, Rūd-e →, *Asia* . **61 K9** 40 5N 48 29 E
Aratāne, *Mauritania* . **112 B3** 18 24N 8 32W
Araticu, *Brazil* ..... **170 B2** 1 58 S 49 51W
Arauca, *Colombia* ... **168 B3** 7 0N 70 40W
Arauca □, *Colombia* . **168 B3** 6 40N 71 0W
Arauca →, *Venezuela* **168 B4** 7 24N 66 35W
Arauco, *Chile* ..... **174 D1** 37 16 S 73 25W
Araújos, *Brazil* ..... **171 E2** 19 56 S 45 14W
Arauquita, *Colombia* . **168 B3** 7 2N 71 25W
Araure, *Venezuela* ... **168 B4** 9 34N 69 13W
Arawa, *Ethiopia* .... **107 F5** 9 57N 41 58 E
Arawale △, *Kenya* .. **118 C5** 1 24 S 40 9 E
Arawata →, *N.Z.* ... **131 E3** 44 0 S 168 40 E
Arawe Is., *Papua N. G.* **132 D5** 6 6 S 149 0 E
Araxá, *Brazil* ..... **171 E2** 19 35 S 46 55W
Araya, Pen. de,
  Venezuela **169 A5** 10 40N 64 0W
Arayat, *Phil.* ..... **80 D3** 15 10N 120 46 E
Arba Gugu, *Ethiopia* . **107 F5** 8 40N 40 15 E
Arba Minch, *Ethiopia* **107 F4** 6 0N 37 30 E
Arbat, *Iraq* ..... **101 E11** 35 25N 45 35 E
Árbatax, *Italy* ..... **46 C2** 39 56N 9 42 E
Arbedo, *Switz.* ..... **33 D8** 46 12N 9 3 E
Arbi, *Ethiopia* ..... **107 F4** 9 4N 35 7 E
Arbil, *Iraq* ..... **101 D11** 36 15N 44 5 E
Arboga, *Sweden* .... **16 E9** 59 24N 15 52 E
Arbois, *France* ..... **27 F12** 46 55N 5 46 E
Arboletes, *Colombia* . **168 B2** 8 51N 76 26W
Arbon, *Switz.* ..... **33 A8** 47 31N 9 26 E
Arbore, *Ethiopia* .... **107 F4** 5 3N 36 50 E
Arboréa, *Italy* ..... **46 C1** 39 46N 8 35 E
Arborfield, *Canada* .. **143 C8** 53 6N 103 39W
Arborg, *Canada* **143 C9** 50 54N 97 13W
Arbre du Ténéré, *Niger* **113 B7** 17 50N 10 4 E
Arbroath, *U.K.* **22 E6** 56 34N 2 35W
Arbuckle, *U.S.A.* ... **160 F4** 39 1N 122 3W
Arbus, *Italy* ..... **46 C1** 39 30N 8 33 E
Arc →, *France* ..... **29 C10** 45 34N 6 12 E
Arc-lès-Gray, *France* . **27 E12** 47 28N 5 34 E
Arcachon, *France* ... **28 D2** 44 40N 1 10W
Arcachon, Bassin d',
  France **28 D2** 44 42N 1 10W
Arcade, *Calif., U.S.A.* **161 L8** 34 2N 118 15W
Arcade, *N.Y., U.S.A.* . **150 D6** 42 32N 78 25W
Arcadia, *Fla., U.S.A.* . **153 H8** 27 13N 81 52W
Arcadia, *Ind., U.S.A.* . **157 D10** 40 11N 86 1W
Arcadia, *La., U.S.A.* .. **155 J8** 32 33N 92 55W
Arcadia, *Pa., U.S.A.* .. **150 F6** 40 47N 78 51W
Arcanum, *U.S.A.* ... **157 E12** 39 59N 84 33W
Arcata, *U.S.A.* **158 F1** 40 52N 124 5W
Arcévia, *Italy* ..... **45 E9** 43 30N 12 56 E
Archangel =
  Arkhangelsk, *Russia* **56 B7** 64 38N 40 36 E
Archar, *Bulgaria* .... **50 C6** 43 50N 22 54 E
Archbald, *U.S.A.* ... **151 E9** 41 30N 75 32W
Archbold, *U.S.A.* ... **157 C12** 41 31N 84 18W
Archena, *Spain* **41 G3** 38 9N 1 16W
Archenu, J., *Chad* .. **109 D4** 22 15N 24 45 E
Archer →, *U.S.A.* ... **153 F7** 29 32N 82 32W
Archer →, *Australia* . **126 A3** 13 28 S 141 41 E
Archer B., *Australia* . **126 A3** 13 20 S 141 30 E
Archer Bend =
  Mungkan Kandju △,
  Australia ..... **126 A3** 13 35 S 142 52 E
Archers Post, *Kenya* . **118 B4** 0 35N 37 35 E
Arches △, *U.S.A.* ... **159 G9** 38 45N 109 25W
Archidona, *Spain* ... **43 H6** 37 6N 4 22W
Archipel-de-Mingan △,
  Canada **141 B7** 50 13N 63 10W
Archipiélago Chinijo △,
  Canary Is. **9 e2** 29 20N 13 30W
Archipiélago Los
  Roques △, *Venezuela* **165 D6** 11 50N 66 44W
Arci, Mte., *Italy* .... **46 C1** 39 47N 8 45 E
Arcidosso, *Italy* .... **45 F8** 42 52N 11 33 E
Arcila = Asilah,
  Morocco **110 A3** 35 29N 6 0W
Arcipelago de la
  Maddalena △, *Italy* . **46 A2** 41 14N 9 24 E
Arcipelago Toscano △,
  Italy ..... **44 F7** 42 45N 10 15 E
Arcis-sur-Aube, *France* **27 D11** 48 32N 4 10 E
Arckaringa Cr. →,
  Australia ..... **128 D2** 28 10 S 135 22 E
Arco, *Italy* ..... **44 C7** 45 55N 10 53 E
Arco, *U.S.A.* **158 E7** 43 38N 113 18W
Arcola, *U.S.A.* **157 E8** 39 41N 88 19W
Arcoona, *Australia* .. **128 A2** 31 2 S 137 1 E
Arcos de Jalón, *Spain* **42 D2** 41 12N 2 16W
Arcos de la Frontera,
  Spain **43 J5** 36 45N 5 49W
Arcos de Valdevez,
  Portugal **42 D2** 41 55N 8 22W
Arcot, *India* ..... **95 H4** 12 53N 79 20 E
Arcoverde, *Brazil* ... **170 C4** 8 25 S 37 4W
Arcozelo, *Portugal* .. **42 E3** 40 32N 7 47W
Arctic Bay, *Canada* . **139 A11** 73 1N 85 7W
Arctic Ocean, *Arctic* . **6 B18** 78 0N 160 0W
Arctic Red River =
  Tsiigehtchic, *Canada* **138 B6** 67 15N 134 0W
Arctic Village, *U.S.A.* **144 B11** 68 8N 145 32W
Arctowski, *Antarctica* **7 C18** 62 30 S 58 0W
Arda →, *Bulgaria* ... **51 F10** 41 40N 26 30 E
Arda →, *Italy* ..... **44 C7** 45 2N 10 2 E
Ardabil, *Iran* ..... **97 B6** 38 15N 48 18 E
Ardabil □, *Iran* .... **97 B6** 38 15N 48 20 E
Ardahan, *Turkey* ... **101 B10** 41 7N 42 41 E

Ardakān = Sepīdān,
  Iran ..... **97 D7** 30 20N 52 5 E
Ardakān, *Iran* ..... **97 C7** 32 19N 53 59 E
Ardala, *Sweden* ..... **17 F7** 58 22N 13 19 E
Ardales, *Spain* **43 J6** 36 53N 4 51W
Årdalstangen, *Norway* **18 C4** 61 14N 7 43 E
Ardèche □, *France* .. **29 D8** 44 42N 4 16 E
Ardèche →, *France* .. **29 D8** 44 16N 4 39 E
Ardee, *Ireland* **23 C5** 53 52N 6 33W
Arden, *Canada* **150 B8** 44 43N 76 56W
Arden, *Denmark* .... **17 H3** 56 46N 9 52 E
Arden, *Calif., U.S.A.* . **160 G5** 38 36N 121 33W
Arden, *Nev., U.S.A.* . **163 J11** 36 1N 115 14W
Ardenne, *Belgium* ... **24 E5** 49 50N 5 5 E
Ardennes =Ardenne,
  Belgium ..... **24 E5** 49 50N 5 5 E
Ardennes □, *France* . **27 C11** 49 35N 4 40 E
Ardennes □, *France* . **27 F8** 46 45N 1 50 E
Arderin, *Ireland* **23 C4** 53 2N 7 39W
Ardeşen, *Turkey* .... **101 B9** 41 12N 41 2 E
Ardestān, *Iran* ..... **97 C7** 33 20N 52 25 E
Ardez, *Switz.* ..... **33 C10** 46 47N 10 12 E
Ardhas →, *Greece* .. **51 E10** 41 40N 26 30 E
Ardhéa, *Greece* ..... **50 F6** 40 58N 22 3 E
Ardila →, *Portugal* .. **43 G3** 38 12N 7 28W
Ardino, *Bulgaria* .... **51 E9** 41 34N 25 9 E
Ardivachar Pt., *U.K.* . **22 D1** 57 23N 7 26W
Ardlethan, *Australia* . **129 C7** 34 22 S 146 53 E
Ardmore, *Okla., U.S.A.* **155 H6** 34 10N 97 8W
Ardmore, *Pa., U.S.A.* **151 G9** 39 58N 75 18W
Ardnamurchan, Pt. of,
  U.K. **22 E2** 56 43N 6 14W
Ardnave Pt., *U.K.* ... **22 F2** 55 53N 6 20W
Ardon, *Russia* ..... **61 J7** 43 10N 44 18 E
Ardore, *Italy* ..... **47 D9** 38 11N 16 10 E
Ardrossan, *Australia* . **128 C2** 34 26 S 137 53 E
Ardrossan, *U.K.* **22 F4** 55 39N 4 49W
Ards Pen., *U.K.* **23 B6** 54 33N 5 34W
Arduan, *Sudan* ..... **106 D3** 19 54N 30 20 E
Ardud, *Romania* .... **52 C7** 47 37N 22 52 E
Åre, *Sweden* ..... **16 A7** 63 22N 13 15 E
Arecibo, *Puerto Rico* **165 d** 18 29N 66 43W
Areia Branca, *Brazil* . **170 B4** 5 0 S 37 0W
Arena, Pt., *U.S.A.* ... **160 G3** 38 57N 123 44W
Arenal, *Honduras* ... **164 C2** 15 21N 86 50W
Arenales, Cerro, *Chile* **176 C2** 47 5 S 73 40W
Arenápolis, *Brazil* ... **173 C6** 14 26 S 56 49W
Arenas = Las Arenas,
  Spain **42 B6** 43 17N 4 50W
Arenas, Pta., *Venezuela* **169 A5** 10 31N 64 14W
Arenas de San Pedro,
  Spain **42 E5** 40 12N 5 5W
Arendal, *Norway* .... **18 F5** 58 28N 8 46 E
Arendsee, *Germany* . **30 C7** 52 52N 11 27 E
Arenillas, *Ecuador* .. **168 D1** 3 33 S 80 10W
Arensburg =
  Kuressaare, *Estonia* **15 G20** 58 15N 22 30 E
Arenys de Mar, *Spain* **40 D7** 41 35N 2 33 E
Arenzano, *Italy* .... **44 D5** 44 24N 8 41 E
Arenzville, *U.S.A.* ... **156 E6** 39 53N 90 22W
Areópolis, *Greece* ... **48 E4** 36 40N 22 22 E
Arequipa, *Peru* ..... **172 D3** 16 20 S 71 30W
Arequipa □, *Peru* ... **172 D3** 16 0 S 73 0W
Arere, *Brazil* ..... **169 D7** 1 6 S 53 52W
Arès, *France* **28 D2** 44 47N 1 8W
Arévalo, *Spain* **42 D6** 41 3N 4 43W
Arezzo, *Italy* ..... **45 E8** 43 25N 11 53 E
Arga, *Turkey* ..... **96 B3** 38 21N 37 59 E
Arga →, *Spain* **40 C3** 42 18N 1 47W
Argalastí, *Greece* ... **48 B5** 39 13N 23 13 E
Argamakmur,
  Indonesia ..... **84 C2** 3 35 S 102 0 E
Argamasilla de Alba,
  Spain **43 F7** 39 8N 3 5W
Argamasilla de
  Calatrava, *Spain* .. **43 G6** 38 44N 4 4W
Arganda, *Spain* **42 E7** 40 19N 3 26W
Arganil, *Portugal* ... **42 E2** 40 13N 8 3W
Argao, *Phil.* ..... **81 G4** 9 52N 123 36 E
Argayash, *Russia* ... **64 D8** 55 29N 60 52 E
Argedeb, *Ethiopia* .. **107 F5** 6 11N 41 13 E
Argelès-Gazost, *France* **28 E3** 43 0N 0 6W
Argelès-sur-Mer,
  France ..... **28 F7** 42 34N 3 1 E
Argens →, *France* ... **29 E10** 43 24N 6 44 E
Argent-sur-Sauldre,
  France ..... **27 E9** 47 33N 2 25 E
Argenta = North Little
  Rock, *U.S.A.* **155 H8** 34 45N 92 16W
Argenta, *Canada* ... **142 C5** 50 11N 116 56W
Argenta, *Italy* ..... **45 D8** 44 37N 11 50 E
Argenta, *U.S.A.* **157 E8** 39 59N 88 49W
Argentan, *France* ... **26 D6** 48 45N 0 1 W
Argentário, Mte., *Italy* **44 F8** 42 24N 11 9 E
Argentera, *Italy* .... **28 C5** 45 6N 1 56 E
Argentera, *Italy* .... **44 D4** 44 12N 7 5 E
Argenteuil, *France* .. **27 D9** 48 57N 2 14 E
Argentia, *Canada* ... **141 C9** 47 18N 53 58W
Argentière, Aiguilles d',
  Switz. ..... **32 E4** 45 58N 7 2 E
Argentina ■, *S. Amer.* **176 B3** 35 0 S 66 0W
Argentine Basin,
  S. Amer. ..... **166 H5** 45 0 S 58 0W
Argentine Plain,
  Atl. Oc. ..... **8 L6** 45 0 S 52 0W
Argentino, L.,
  Argentina ..... **176 D2** 50 10 S 73 0W
Argenton-Château,
  France **26 F6** 46 59N 0 27W
Argenton-sur-Creuse,
  France ..... **27 F8** 46 36N 1 30 E
Arges □, *Romania* ... **53 F9** 45 0N 24 45 E
Arges →, *Romania* .. **53 F11** 44 5N 26 38 E
Arghandab →, *Afghan.* **91 C2** 31 30N 64 15 E
Argo, *Sudan* ..... **106 D3** 19 28N 30 30 E
Argolikós Kólpos,
  Greece ..... **48 D4** 37 20N 22 52 E
Argolís □, *Greece* ... **48 D4** 37 38N 22 50 E
Argonne, *France* ... **27 C12** 49 10N 5 0 E
Árgos, *Greece* ..... **48 D4** 37 40N 22 43 E
Árgos, *U.S.A.* **157 C10** 41 14N 86 15W
Árgos Orestikón,
  Greece ..... **50 F5** 40 27N 21 18 E
Argostóli =
  Argostólion, *Greece* **39 C2** 38 11N 20 29 E
Argostólion, *Greece* . **39 C2** 38 11N 20 29 E
Argostólion, Kólpos,
  Greece ..... **39 C1** 38 10N 20 27 E
Arguedas, *Spain* **40 C3** 42 11N 1 36W
Arguello, Pt., *U.S.A.* . **161 L6** 34 35N 120 39W
Arguineguín, *Canary Is.* **9 e1** 27 46N 15 41W
Argun →, *Russia* ... **61 J7** 43 18N 45 52 E
Argun →, *Russia* ... **67 D13** 53 20N 121 28 E
Argungu, *Nigeria* ... **113 C5** 12 40N 4 31 E
Arguni, *Indonesia* ... **83 B4** 3 6 S 133 42 E
Argus Pk., *U.S.A.* ... **163 K9** 35 52N 117 26W
Argyle, L., *Australia* . **124 C4** 16 20 S 128 40 E
Argyll, *U.K.* **22 E3** 56 6N 5 0W

Argyll & Bute □, *U.K.* **22 E3** 56 13N 5 28W
Arhavi, *Turkey* ..... **101 B9** 41 21N 41 18 E
Århus, *Denmark* .... **17 H4** 56 8N 10 11 E
Århus
  Amtskommune □,
  Denmark ..... **17 H4** 56 15N 10 15 E
Aria, *N.Z.* ..... **130 E4** 38 33 S 175 0 E
Ariadnoye, *Russia* .. **70 B7** 45 8N 134 25 E
Ariamsvlei, *Namibia* . **116 D2** 28 9 S 19 51 E
Ariana, *Tunisia* ..... **108 A2** 36 52N 10 12 E
Ariano Irpino, *Italy* .. **47 A8** 41 9N 15 5 E
Ariari →, *Colombia* . **168 C3** 2 35N 72 47W
Aribinda, *Burkina Faso* **113 C4** 14 17N 0 52W
Arica, *Chile* ..... **172 D3** 18 32 S 70 20W
Arica, *Colombia* .... **168 D3** 2 0 S 71 50W
Arico, *Canary Is.* ... **9 e1** 28 9N 16 29W
Arid, C., *Australia* ... **125 F3** 34 1 S 123 10 E
Arid, C., *Australia* ... **73 C7** 34 51N 135 8 E
Aridal, W. Sahara* ... **110 C2** 25 59N 13 8W
Aride, *Seychelles* .... **121 b** 4 13 S 55 40 E
Ariège □, *France* .... **28 F5** 42 56N 1 30 E
Ariège →, *France* ... **28 E5** 43 30N 1 25 E
Aries →, *Romania* .. **52 D6** 46 24N 23 20 E
Arigat el Fersig, *Algeria* **111 C4** 27 35N 2 7W
Arihā, *Israel* ..... **106 A4** 31 51N 35 27 E
Arilje, *Serbia & M.* .. **50 C4** 43 44N 20 7 E
Aríllas, Ákra, *Greece* . **38 B9** 39 43N 19 39 E
Arima, *Trin. & Tob.* . **169 F9** 10 38N 61 17W
Aringay, *Phil.* ..... **80 C3** 16 25N 120 21 E
Arinos →, *Brazil* ... **173 C6** 10 25 S 58 20W
Ario de Rosales,
  Mexico **162 D4** 19 12N 102 0W
Ariogala, *Lithuania* .. **54 C10** 55 16N 23 28 E
Aripo, Mt.,
  Trin. & Tob. **169 F9** 10 45N 61 15W
Aripuanã, *Brazil* .... **172 D5** 9 25 S 60 30W
Aripuanã □, *Brazil* .. **173 B5** 5 7 S 60 25W
Aripuanã →, *Brazil* . **173 B5** 5 5 S 63 6W
Ariquemes, *Brazil* ... **172 C5** 9 55 S 63 6W
Arisaig, *U.K.* **22 E3** 56 55N 5 51W
Arísh, W. el →, *Egypt* **106 A3** 31 9N 33 49 E
Arissa, *Ethiopia* .... **107 E5** 11 10N 41 35 E
Aristazabal I., *Canada* **142 C3** 52 40N 129 10W
Arita, *Japan* ..... **72 D1** 33 11N 129 54 E
Aritao, *Phil.* ..... **80 C3** 16 18N 121 2 E
Ariton, *U.S.A.* **152 D4** 31 36N 85 43W
Arivonimamo, *Madag.* **117 B8** 19 1 S 47 11 E
Ariyalur, *India* ..... **95 J4** 11 8N 79 8 E
Ariza, *Spain* **40 D2** 41 19N 2 3W
Arizaro, Salar de,
  Argentina ..... **174 A2** 24 40 S 67 50W
Arizona, *Argentina* .. **174 D2** 35 45 S 65 25W
Arizona □, *U.S.A.* ... **159 J8** 34 0N 112 0W
Arizpe, *Mexico* **162 A2** 30 20N 110 11W
Årjäng, *Sweden* ..... **16 E6** 59 24N 12 8 E
Arjeplog, *Sweden* ... **14 D18** 66 3N 17 54 E
Arjeplouvre =
  Arjeplog, *Sweden* .. **14 D18** 66 3N 17 54 E
Arjona, *Colombia* ... **168 A2** 10 14N 75 22W
Arjona, *Spain* **43 H6** 37 56N 4 4W
Arjuna, *Indonesia* ... **85 D4** 7 49 S 112 34 E
Arka, *Russia* ..... **67 C15** 60 15N 142 0 E
Arkadak, *Russia* .... **60 E6** 51 58N 43 30 E
Arkadelphia, *U.S.A.* . **155 H8** 34 7N 93 4W
Arkadhía □, *Greece* . **48 D4** 37 30N 22 20 E
Arkaig, L., *U.K.* **22 E3** 56 59N 5 10W
Arkalgud, *India* ..... **95 H3** 12 46N 76 3 E
Arkalyk = Arqalyk,
  Kazakhstan ..... **66 D7** 50 13N 66 50 E
Arkansas □, *U.S.A.* .. **155 H8** 35 0N 92 30W
Arkansas →, *U.S.A.* . **155 J9** 33 47N 91 4W
Arkansas City, *U.S.A.* **155 G6** 37 4N 97 2W
Arkaroola, *Australia* . **127 E2** 30 20 S 139 22 E
Arkathos →, *Greece* . **48 B3** 39 20N 21 4 E
Arkhángelo-Pashiskiy
  Zavod = Pashiya,
  Russia ..... **64 B7** 58 33N 58 26 E
Arkhángelos, Préveza,
  Greece ..... **39 A2** 39 6N 20 42 E
Arkhángelos, Ródhos,
  Greece ..... **38 E12** 36 13N 28 7 E
Arkhangelsk, *Russia* . **56 B7** 64 38N 40 36 E
Arkhangelskoye, *Russia* **60 E5** 51 32N 40 58 E
Arki, *India* ..... **92 D7** 31 9N 76 58 E
Arkiko, *Eritrea* ..... **107 D4** 15 33N 39 30 E
Arklow, *Ireland* **23 D5** 52 48N 6 10W
Árkoi, *Greece* ..... **49 D8** 37 24N 26 44 E
Arkona, Kap, *Germany* **30 A9** 54 41N 13 26 E
Arkösund, *Sweden* .. **17 F10** 58 29N 16 56 E
Arkoúdhi Nísis, *Greece* **39 B2** 38 33N 20 43 E
Arkport, *U.S.A.* **150 D7** 42 24N 77 42W
Arktícheskiy, Mys,
  Russia ..... **67 A10** 81 10N 95 0 E
Arkul, *Russia* ..... **60 B10** 57 17N 50 3 E
Arkville, *U.S.A.* **151 D10** 42 9N 74 37W
Arla, *Sweden* ..... **16 E10** 59 17N 16 40 E
Arlanda, Stockholm ✈
  (ARN), *Sweden* ... **16 E11** 59 41N 17 56 E
Arlanza →, *Spain* ... **42 C6** 42 6N 4 9W
Arlanzón →, *Spain* .. **42 C6** 42 3N 4 17W
Arlbergpass, *Austria* . **34 D3** 47 9N 10 12 E
Arles, *France* ..... **29 E8** 43 41N 4 40 E
Arlesheim, *Switz.* ... **32 B5** 47 30N 7 37 E
Arli, *Burkina Faso* ... **113 C5** 11 35N 1 28 E
Arli □, *Burkina Faso* . **113 C5** 11 35N 1 28 E
Arlington, *S. Africa* .. **117 D4** 28 1 S 27 53 E
Arlington, *Ga., U.S.A.* **152 D5** 31 26N 84 44W
Arlington, *N.Y., U.S.A.* **151 E11** 41 42N 73 54W
Arlington, *Oreg.,
  U.S.A.* **158 D3** 45 43N 120 12W
Arlington, *S. Dak.,
  U.S.A.* **154 C6** 44 22N 97 8W
Arlington, *Tex., U.S.A.* **155 J6** 32 44N 97 7W
Arlington, *Va., U.S.A.* **148 F7** 38 53N 77 7W
Arlington, *Vt., U.S.A.* **151 C11** 43 5N 73 9W
Arlington, *Wash.,
  U.S.A.* **160 B4** 48 12N 122 8W
Arlington Heights,
  U.S.A. **157 D9** 42 5N 87 59W
Arlon, *Belgium* ..... **24 E5** 49 42N 5 49 E
Arltunga, *Australia* .. **126 C1** 23 26 S 134 41 E
Armagh, *U.K.* **23 B5** 54 21N 6 39W
Armagh □, *U.K.* **23 B5** 54 18N 6 37W
Armagnac, *France* ... **28 E4** 43 44N 0 10 E
Armançon →, *France* **27 E10** 47 59N 3 30 E
Armando Bermudez △,
  Dom. Rep. **165 C5** 19 3N 71 0W
Armatree, *Australia* . **129 A8** 31 26 S 148 28 E
Armavir, *Russia* .... **61 H5** 45 2N 41 7 E
Armenia, *Colombia* .. **168 C2** 4 35N 75 45W
Armenia ■, *Asia* .... **61 K7** 40 20N 45 0 E
Armeniş, *Romania* .. **52 E7** 45 13N 22 17 E
Armenistís, Ákra,
  Greece ..... **38 E11** 36 8N 27 42 E
Armentières, *France* . **27 B9** 50 40N 2 50 E
Armero, *Colombia* .. **168 C2** 4 58N 74 54W
Armidale, *Australia* .. **129 E9** 30 30 S 151 40 E
Armilla, *Spain* **43 H7** 37 9N 3 37W
Armori, *India* ..... **94 D4** 20 20N 79 59 E
Armorique, *France* .. **26 D3** 48 23N 3 0W
Armour, *U.S.A.* **154 D5** 43 19N 98 21W
Armstrong, *B.C.,
  Canada* **142 C5** 50 25N 119 10W
Armstrong, *Ont.,
  Canada* **140 B2** 50 18N 89 4W

Armur, *India* ..... **94 E4** 18 48N 78 16 E
Armutlu, *Bursa, Turkey* **51 F12** 40 31N 28 50 E
Armutlu, *Izmir, Turkey* **49 C9** 38 24N 27 34 E
Arnaía, *Greece* ..... **50 F7** 40 30N 23 38 E
Arnarfjörður, *Iceland* . **11 B3** 65 48N 23 40W
Arnaud →, *Canada* . **139 B12** 59 59N 69 46W
Arnay-le-Duc, *France* **27 E11** 47 10N 4 27 E
Arnedillo, *Spain* **40 C2** 42 13N 2 14W
Arnedo, *Spain* **40 C2** 42 12N 2 5W
Árnes, *Iceland* **11 A5** 66 1N 21 31W
Árnes, *Norway* ..... **18 D8** 60 7N 11 28 E
Arnett, *U.S.A.* **155 G5** 36 8N 99 46W
Arnhem, *Neths.* .... **24 C5** 51 58N 5 55 E
Arnhem, C., *Australia* **126 A2** 12 20 S 137 30 E
Arnhem B., *Australia* . **126 A2** 12 20 S 136 10 E
Arnhem Land,
  Australia ..... **126 A1** 13 10 S 134 30 E
Arníssa, *Greece* .... **50 F5** 40 47N 21 49 E
Arno →, *Italy* ..... **44 E7** 43 41N 10 17 E
Arno Bay, *Australia* . **128 E2** 33 54 S 136 34 E
Arnold, *U.K.* **20 D6** 53 1N 1 7W
Arnoldstein, *Austria* . **34 E6** 46 33N 13 43 E
Arnon →, *France* ... **27 F9** 47 13N 2 1 E
Arnot, *Canada* **143 B9** 55 56N 96 41W
Arnøy, *Norway* ..... **14 A19** 70 9N 20 40 E
Arnprior, *Canada* ... **140 C4** 45 26N 76 21W
Arnsberg, *Germany* . **30 D4** 51 24N 8 5 E
Arnsberger Wald △,
  Germany ..... **30 D4** 51 25N 8 20 E
Arnstadt, *Germany* .. **30 E6** 50 50N 10 56 E
Aro →, *Venezuela* ... **169 B5** 8 1N 64 11W
Aroab, *Namibia* .... **116 D2** 26 41 S 19 39 E
Aroánia Óri, *Greece* . **48 D4** 37 56N 22 12 E
Aroche, *Spain* **43 H4** 37 56N 6 57W
Arochuku, *Nigeria* .. **113 D6** 5 21N 7 54 E
Aroeiras, *Brazil* .... **170 C4** 7 31 S 35 41W
Arolla, *Switz.* ..... **32 D4** 46 2N 7 29 E
Arolsen, *Germany* .. **30 D5** 51 23N 9 2 E
Aroma, *India* ..... **92 G5** 25 57N 77 56 E
Aron →, *France* .... **27 F10** 46 50N 3 28 E
Arona, *Canary Is.* ... **9 e1** 28 6N 16 40W
Arona, *Italy* ..... **44 C5** 45 46N 8 34 E
Aroroy, *Phil.* ..... **80 E4** 12 31N 123 24 E
Arosa, *Switz.* ..... **33 C9** 46 47N 9 41 E
Arosa, Ría de, *Spain* . **42 C2** 42 28N 8 57W
Ärøysund, *Norway* .. **18 E7** 59 10N 10 27 E
Arpajon, *France* .... **27 D9** 48 36N 2 15 E
Arpajon-sur-Cère,
  France ..... **28 D6** 44 53N 2 28 E
Arpaşu de Jos,
  Romania ..... **53 E9** 45 47N 24 37 E
Arqalyk, *Kazakhstan* **66 D7** 50 13N 66 50 E
Arque, *Bolivia* ..... **172 D4** 17 48 S 66 23W
Arrah = Ara, *India* .. **93 G11** 25 35N 84 32 E
Arrah, *Ivory C.* **112 D4** 6 40N 3 58W
Arraias, *Brazil* ..... **171 D2** 12 56 S 46 57W
Arraias, *Mato Grosso, Brazil* **173 C7** 11 10 S 53 35W
Arraias →, *Pará, Brazil* **170 C2** 7 30 S 49 20W
Arraiolos, *Portugal* .. **43 G3** 38 44N 7 59W
Arran, *U.K.* **22 F3** 55 34N 5 12W
Arras, *France* ..... **27 B9** 50 17N 2 46 E
Arrasate, *Spain* **40 B2** 43 4N 2 30W
Arrats →, *France* ... **28 D4** 44 6N 0 52 E
Arreau, *France* ..... **28 F4** 42 54N 0 22 E
Arrecife, *Canary Is.* . **9 e2** 28 57N 13 37W
Arrecifes, *Argentina* . **174 C3** 34 6 S 60 9W
Arrée, Mts. d', *France* **26 D3** 48 26N 3 55W
Arresø, *Denmark* .... **17 J6** 55 58N 12 6 E
Arriaga, *Chiapas,
  Mexico* **163 D6** 16 15N 93 52W
Arriaga,
  *San Luis Potosí,
  Mexico* **162 C4** 21 55N 101 23W
Arribes del Duero △,
  Spain **42 D4** 41 11N 6 39W
Arrilalah, *Australia* .. **126 C3** 23 43 S 143 54 E
Arrino, *Australia* .... **125 E2** 29 30 S 115 40 E
Arriondas, *Spain* **42 B5** 43 23N 5 11W
Arrojado →, *Brazil* . **171 D3** 13 24 S 43 20W
Arromanches-les-Bains,
  France **26 C6** 49 20N 0 38W
Arronches, *Portugal* . **43 F3** 39 7N 7 16W
Arros →, *France* **28 E3** 43 40N 0 2W
Arrow, L., *Ireland* ... **23 B3** 54 3N 8 19W
Arrowhead, L., *U.S.A.* **163 L9** 34 16N 117 10W
Arrowsmith, Mt., *N.Z.* **131 E3** 43 20 S 170 55 E
Arrowtown, *N.Z.* ... **131 E3** 44 57 S 168 50 E
Arroyo de la Luz, *Spain* **43 F4** 39 30N 6 38W
Arroyo del Puerco =
  Arroyo de la Luz,
  Spain **43 F4** 39 30N 6 38W
Arroyo Grande, *U.S.A.* **161 K6** 35 7N 120 35W
Års, *Denmark* ..... **17 H3** 56 48N 9 30 E
Ars, *Iran* ..... **96 B5** 37 9N 47 46 E
Ars-sur-Moselle, *France* **27 C13** 49 5N 6 4 E
Arsenault L., *Canada* . **143 B7** 55 6N 108 32W
Arsenev, *Russia* .... **70 B6** 44 10N 133 15 E
Arsi, *Ethiopia* ..... **107 F4** 7 45N 39 0 E
Arsiero, *Italy* ..... **45 C8** 45 48N 11 21 E
Arsikere, *India* ..... **95 H3** 13 15N 76 15 E
Arsin, *Turkey* ..... **101 B8** 41 3N 39 55 E
Árskógssandur, *Iceland* **11 B6** 56 N 18 27W
Ársunda, *Sweden* ... **16 D10** 60 31N 16 45 E
Árta, *Greece* ..... **38 B3** 39 8N 21 2 E
Artà, *Spain* ..... **38 B4** 39 41N 3 21 E
Arta △, *Greece* ..... **38 B3** 39 13N 21 5 E
Arteaga, *Mexico* **162 D4** 18 50N 102 20W
Arteche, *Phil.* ..... **80 E5** 12 17N 125 22 E
Arteijo = Arteixo,
  Spain **42 B2** 43 19N 8 29W
Arteixo, *Spain* **42 B2** 43 19N 8 29W
Artem = Artyom,
  Azerbaijan ..... **61 K10** 40 28N 50 20 E
Artem, *Russia* ..... **70 C6** 43 22N 132 13 E
Artemovsk, *Russia* .. **67 D10** 54 45N 93 35 E
Artemovsk, *Ukraine* . **59 H9** 48 35N 38 0 E
Artemovskiy, *Rostov,
  Russia* ..... **61 G5** 47 45N 40 16 E
Artemovskiy,
  Yekaterinburg, Russia **64 C8** 57 21N 61 54 E
Artenay, *France* .... **27 D8** 48 5N 1 50 E
Artern, *Germany* ... **30 D7** 51 22N 11 18 E
Artesa de Segre, *Spain* **40 D6** 41 54N 1 3 E
Artesia = Mosomane,
  Botswana ..... **116 C4** 24 2 S 26 19 E
Artesia, *U.S.A.* **155 J2** 32 51N 104 24W
Arth, *Switz.* ..... **33 B7** 47 4N 8 31 E
Arthez-de-Béarn, *France* **28 E3** 43 29N 0 38W
Arthington, *Liberia* .. **112 D2** 6 35N 10 45W
Arthur, *Canada* **150 C4** 43 50N 80 32W
Arthur, *U.S.A.* **157 E8** 39 43N 88 28W
Arthur →, *Australia* . **127 G3** 41 2 S 144 40 E
Arthur Cr. →,
  Australia ..... **126 C2** 22 30 S 136 25 E
Arthur Pt., *Australia* . **126 C5** 22 7 S 150 3 E
Arthur River, *Australia* **125 F2** 33 20 S 117 2 E
Arthur's Pass, *N.Z.* .. **131 C6** 42 54 S 171 35 E
Arthur's Pass △, *N.Z.* **131 C6** 42 53 S 171 42 E

Arthur's Town, *Bahamas* **165 B4** 24 38N 75 42W
Artigas = Río Branco, *Uruguay* **175 C5** 32 40 S 53 40W
Artigas, *Antarctica* **7 C18** 62 30 S 58 0W
Artigas, *Uruguay* **174 C4** 30 20 S 56 30W
Artik, *Armenia* **61 K6** 40 38N 43 58 E
Artillery L., *Canada* **143 A7** 63 9N 107 52W
Artois, *France* **27 B9** 50 20N 2 30 E
Artotína, *Greece* **48 C4** 38 42N 22 2 E
Artrutx, C. de, *Spain* **38 B4** 39 55N 3 49 E
Artsyz, *Ukraine* **53 D14** 46 4N 29 26 E
Artux, *China* **65 D8** 39 40N 76 10 E
Artvin, *Turkey* **101 B9** 41 14N 41 44 E
Artyom, *Azerbaijan* **61 K10** 40 28N 50 20 E
Aru, Kepulauan, *Indonesia* **83 C4** 6 0 S 134 30 E
Aru Is. = Aru, Kepulauan, *Indonesia* **83 C4** 6 0 S 134 30 E
Arua, *Uganda* **118 B3** 3 1N 30 58 E
Aruanã, *Brazil* **171 D1** 14 54 S 51 10W
Aruba ☒, *W. Indies* **165 D6** 12 30N 70 0W
Arudy, *France* **28 E3** 43 7N 0 28W
Arumã, *Brazil* **169 D5** 4 44 S 62 8W
Arumpo, *Australia* **128 B5** 33 48 S 142 55 E
Arun ➝, *Nepal* **93 F12** 26 55N 87 10 E
Arun ➝, *U.K.* **21 G7** 50 49N 0 33W
Arunachal Pradesh □, *India* **90 A5** 28 0N 95 0 E
Aruppukkottai, *India* **95 K4** 9 31N 78 8 E
Aruri, Selat, *Indonesia* **83 B5** 0 50 S 135 15 E
Arusha, *Tanzania* **118 C4** 3 20 S 36 40 E
Arusha □, *Tanzania* **118 C4** 4 0 S 36 30 E
Arusha △, *Tanzania* **118 C4** 3 16 S 36 47 E
Arusha Chini, *Tanzania* **118 C4** 3 32 S 37 20 E
Arut ➝, *Indonesia* **85 C4** 2 42 S 111 34 E
Aruvi ➝, *Sri Lanka* **95 K4** 8 48N 79 53 E
Aruwimi ➝, *Dem. Rep. of the Congo* **118 B1** 1 13N 23 36 E
Arvada, *Colo., U.S.A.* **154 F2** 39 48N 105 5W
Arvada, *Wyo., U.S.A.* **158 D10** 44 39N 106 8W
Arvakalu, *Sri Lanka* **95 K4** 8 20N 79 58 E
Arve ➝, *France* **27 F13** 46 11N 6 8 E
Árvi, *Greece* **39 F6** 34 59N 25 28 E
Arvi, *India* **94 D4** 20 59N 78 16 E
Arviat, *Canada* **143 A10** 61 6N 93 59W
Arvidsjaur, *Sweden* **14 D18** 65 35N 19 10 E
Arvika, *Sweden* **16 E6** 59 40N 12 36 E
Arvin, *U.S.A.* **161 K8** 35 12N 118 50W
Arwal, *India* **93 G11** 25 15N 84 41 E
Arxan, *China* **69 B6** 47 11N 119 57 E
Åryd, *Sweden* **17 H8** 56 49N 14 59 E
Aryirádhes, *Greece* **38 C9** 39 27N 19 58 E
Aryiroúpolis, *Greece* **39 E5** 35 17N 24 20 E
Arys, *Kazakhstan* **65 B4** 42 26N 68 48 E
Arys ➝, *Kazakhstan* **65 B4** 42 45N 68 15 E
Arzachena, *Italy* **46 A2** 41 5N 9 23 E
Arzamas, *Russia* **60 C6** 55 27N 43 55 E
Arzew, *Algeria* **111 A4** 35 50N 0 23W
Arzgir, *Russia* **61 H7** 45 18N 44 23 E
Arzignano, *Italy* **45 C8** 45 31N 11 20 E
Arzúa, *Spain* **42 C2** 42 56N 8 9W
Aš, *Czech Rep.* **34 A5** 50 13N 12 12 E
Ås, *Norway* **18 E7** 59 40N 10 48 E
Ås, *Sweden* **16 A8** 63 15N 14 34 E
As Pontes de García Rodríguez, *Spain* **42 B3** 43 27N 7 50W
Aş Şafā, *Syria* **103 B6** 33 10N 37 0 E
As Saffānīyah, *Si. Arabia* **97 E6** 27 55N 48 50 E
As Safīrah, *Syria* **100 D7** 36 5N 37 21 E
Aş Şahm, *Oman* **97 E8** 24 10N 56 53 E
As Sājir, *Si. Arabia* **96 E5** 25 11N 44 36 E
As Salamīyah, *Syria* **100 E7** 35 1N 37 2 E
As Salmān, *Iraq* **96 D5** 30 30N 44 32 E
As Salt, *Jordan* **103 C4** 32 2N 35 43 E
As Sal'w'a, *Qatar* **97 E6** 24 23N 50 50 E
As Samāwah, *Iraq* **96 D5** 31 15N 45 15 E
As Sanamayn, *Syria* **103 B5** 33 3N 36 10 E
As Sawādah, *Si. Arabia* **98 B4** 22 24N 44 28 E
As Sayl al Kabīr, *Si. Arabia* **98 B3** 21 38N 40 25 E
As Sohar = Şuhār, *Oman* **97 E8** 24 20N 56 40 E
As Sukhnah, *Syria* **101 E8** 34 52N 38 52 E
As Sulaymānīyah, *Iraq* **101 E11** 35 35N 45 29 E
As Sulaymānīyah, *Si. Arabia* **98 A4** 24 9N 47 18 E
As Sulaymī, *Si. Arabia* **96 E4** 26 17N 41 21 E
As Sulayyil, *Si. Arabia* **98 B4** 20 27N 45 34 E
As Sulţān, *Libya* **108 B3** 31 4N 17 8 E
As Summān, *Si. Arabia* **96 E5** 25 0N 47 0 E
Aş Şurrah, *Yemen* **98 D4** 13 57N 46 14 E
As Suwaydā', *Syria* **103 C5** 32 40N 36 30 E
As Suwaydā' □, *Syria* **103 C5** 32 45N 36 45 E
As Suwayq, *Oman* **97 F8** 23 51N 57 26 E
Aş Şuwayrah, *Iraq* **101 F11** 32 55N 45 0 E
Asa, *Kazakhstan* **65 B5** 43 2N 71 10 E
Åsa, *Sweden* **17 G6** 57 21N 12 8 E
Asab, *Namibia* **116 D2** 25 30 S 18 0 E
Asaba, *Nigeria* **113 D6** 6 12N 6 38 E
Asad, Buḩayrat al, *Syria* **101 D8** 36 0N 38 15 E
Asadābād, *Iran* **101 E13** 34 47N 48 7 E
Asafo, *Ghana* **112 D4** 6 20N 2 40W
Asahi, *Japan* **73 B12** 35 43N 140 39 E
Asahi-Gawa ➝, *Japan* **72 C5** 34 36N 133 58 E
Asahigawa, *Japan* **70 C11** 43 46N 142 22 E
Asaka, *Uzbekistan* **65 C6** 40 38N 72 15 E
Asale, L., *Ethiopia* **107 E5** 14 0N 40 20 E
Asama-Yama, *Japan* **73 A10** 36 24N 138 31 E
Asamankese, *Ghana* **113 D4** 5 50N 0 40W
Asan ➝, *India* **93 F8** 26 37N 78 24 E
Asansol, *India* **93 H12** 23 40N 87 1 E
Åsarna, *Sweden* **16 B8** 62 39N 14 22 E
Asau, *Samoa* **133 W23** 13 27 S 172 33W
Asayita, *Ethiopia* **107 E5** 11 35N 41 23 E
Asba Littoria = Asbe Teferi, *Ethiopia* **107 F5** 9 4N 40 49 E
Asbe Teferi, *Ethiopia* **107 F5** 9 4N 40 49 E
Asbesberge, *S. Africa* **116 D3** 29 0 S 23 0 E
Asbest, *Russia* **64 C8** 57 0N 61 30 E
Asbestos, *Canada* **141 C5** 45 47N 71 58W
Asbestovye Rudniki = Asbest, *Russia* **64 C8** 57 0N 61 30 E
Asbury Park, *U.S.A.* **151 F10** 40 13N 74 1W
Ascea, *Italy* **47 B8** 40 8N 15 11 E
Ascensión, *Mexico* **162 A3** 31 6N 107 59W
Ascensión, B. de la, *Mexico* **163 D7** 19 50N 87 20W
Ascension I., *Atl. Oc.* **9 g** 7 57 S 14 23W
Aschach an der Donau, *Austria* **34 C7** 48 22N 14 2 E
Aschaffenburg, *Germany* **31 F5** 49 58N 9 6 E
Aschendorf, *Germany* **30 B3** 53 3N 7 19 E
Aschersleben, *Germany* **30 D7** 51 45N 11 29 E
Asciano, *Italy* **45 E8** 43 14N 11 33 E
Áscoli Piceno, *Italy* **45 F10** 42 51N 13 34 E
Áscoli Satriano, *Italy* **47 A8** 41 11N 15 32 E
Ascona, *Switz.* **33 D7** 46 9N 8 46 E
Ascope, *Peru* **172 B2** 7 46 S 79 8W
Ascotán, *Chile* **174 A2** 21 45 S 68 17W
Ascuncion, *Phil.* **81 H5** 7 35N 125 45 E
Aseb, *Eritrea* **107 E5** 13 0N 42 40 E
Åseda, *Sweden* **17 G9** 57 10N 15 20 E
Asedjrad, *Algeria* **111 D5** 24 51N 1 29 E
Aseki, *Papua N. G.* **132 D4** 7 21 S 146 12 E
Asela, *Ethiopia* **107 F4** 8 0N 39 0 E
Åsen, *Sweden* **16 C7** 61 17N 13 50 E
Asenovgrad, *Bulgaria* **51 D8** 42 1N 24 51 E
Aserradero, *Mexico* **162 C3** 23 40N 105 43W
Asfeld, *France* **27 C11** 49 27N 4 5 E
Asfûn el Matâ'na, *Egypt* **106 B3** 25 26N 32 30 E
Åsgårdstrand, *Norway* **18 E7** 59 22N 10 27 E
Asgata, *Cyprus* **39 F9** 34 46N 33 15 E
Ash Fork, *U.S.A.* **159 J7** 35 13N 112 29W
Ash Grove, *U.S.A.* **155 G8** 37 19N 93 35W
Ash Shabakah, *Iraq* **96 D4** 30 49N 43 39 E
Ash Shamāl □, *Lebanon* **103 A5** 34 25N 36 0 E
Ash Shāmīyah, *Iraq* **101 G11** 31 55N 44 35 E
Ash Sha'rā', *Si. Arabia* **98 A4** 24 16N 44 11 E
Ash Shāriqah, *U.A.E.* **97 E7** 25 23N 55 26 E
Ash Sharmah, *Si. Arabia* **96 D2** 28 1N 35 16 E
Ash Sharqāt, *Iraq* **101 E10** 35 27N 43 16 E
Ash Sharqi, Al Jabal, *Lebanon* **103 B5** 33 40N 36 10 E
Ash Shāţi, *Libya* **108 C2** 27 30N 12 30 E
Ash Shāţi □, *Libya* **111 C7** 27 27N 13 37 E
Ash Shaţrah, *Iraq* **96 D5** 31 30N 46 10 E
Ash Shawbak, *Jordan* **96 D2** 30 32N 35 34 E
Ash Shawmari, J., *Jordan* **103 E5** 30 35N 36 35 E
Ash Shiḩr, *Yemen* **99 D5** 14 45N 49 36 E
Ash Shināfīyah, *Iraq* **96 D5** 31 35N 44 39 E
Ash Shu'bah, *Si. Arabia* **96 D5** 28 54N 44 44 E
Ash Shumlūl, *Si. Arabia* **96 E5** 26 31N 47 20 E
Ash Shuqayq, *Si. Arabia* **98 C3** 17 44N 42 1 E
Ash Shūr'a, *Iraq* **96 C4** 35 58N 43 13 E
Ash Shurayf, *Si. Arabia* **96 E3** 25 43N 39 14 E
Ash Shuwayfāt, *Lebanon* **103 B4** 33 45N 35 30 E
Asha, *Russia* **64 D6** 55 0N 57 16 E
Ashanti □, *Ghana* **113 D4** 7 30N 1 30W
Ashau, *Vietnam* **86 D6** 16 6N 107 22 E
Ashbourne, *U.K.* **20 D6** 53 2N 1 43W
Ashburn, *U.S.A.* **152 D6** 31 43N 83 39W
Ashburton, *N.Z.* **131 D6** 43 53 S 171 48 E
Ashburton ➝, *Australia* **124 D1** 21 40 S 114 56 E
Ashburton, North Branch ➝, *N.Z.* **131 D6** 43 54 S 171 44 E
Ashburton, South Branch ➝, *N.Z.* **131 D6** 43 54 S 171 44 E
Ashchysay, *Kazakhstan* **65 B4** 43 35N 68 53 E
Ashcroft, *Canada* **142 C4** 50 40N 121 20W
Ashdod, *Israel* **103 D3** 31 49N 34 35 E
Ashdown, *U.S.A.* **155 J7** 33 40N 94 8W
Asheboro, *U.S.A.* **149 H6** 35 43N 79 49W
Åsheim, *Norway* **18 C8** 61 42N 11 11 E
Ashern, *Canada* **143 C9** 51 11N 98 21W
Asherton, *U.S.A.* **155 L5** 28 27N 99 46W
Asheville, *U.S.A.* **149 H4** 35 36N 82 33W
Ashewat, *Pakistan* **92 D3** 31 22N 68 32 E
Asheweig ➝, *Canada* **140 B2** 54 17N 87 12W
Ashford, *Australia* **127 D5** 29 15 S 151 3 E
Ashford, *U.K.* **21 F8** 51 8N 0 53 E
Ashford, *U.S.A.* **152 D4** 31 11N 85 14W
Ashgabat, *Turkmenistan* **66 F6** 38 0N 57 50 E
Ashibetsu, *Japan* **70 C11** 43 31N 142 11 E
Ashikaga, *Japan* **73 A11** 36 28N 139 29 E
Ashington, *U.K.* **20 B6** 55 11N 1 33W
Ashio, *Japan* **73 A11** 36 38N 139 27 E
Ashizuri-Uwakai △, *Japan* **72 E4** 32 56N 132 32 E
Ashizuri-Zaki, *Japan* **72 E5** 32 44N 133 0 E
Ashkarkot, *Afghan.* **92 C2** 33 3N 67 58 E
Ashkhabad = Ashgabat, *Turkmenistan* **66 F6** 38 0N 57 50 E
Āshkhāneh, *Iran* **97 B8** 37 26N 56 55 E
Ashland, *Ala., U.S.A.* **152 B4** 33 16N 85 50W
Ashland, *Ill., U.S.A.* **156 E7** 39 53N 90 1W
Ashland, *Kans., U.S.A.* **155 G5** 37 11N 99 46W
Ashland, *Ky., U.S.A.* **148 F4** 38 28N 82 38W
Ashland, *Maine, U.S.A.* **149 B11** 46 38N 68 24W
Ashland, *Mont., U.S.A.* **158 D10** 45 36N 106 16W
Ashland, *Ohio, U.S.A.* **150 F2** 40 52N 82 19W
Ashland, *Oreg., U.S.A.* **158 E2** 42 12N 122 43W
Ashland, *Pa., U.S.A.* **151 F8** 40 45N 76 22W
Ashland, *Va., U.S.A.* **148 G7** 37 46N 77 29W
Ashland, *Wis., U.S.A.* **154 B9** 46 35N 90 53W
Ashley, *Ill., U.S.A.* **156 F7** 38 20N 89 11W
Ashley, *Ind., U.S.A.* **157 C11** 41 32N 85 4W
Ashley, *N. Dak., U.S.A.* **154 B5** 46 2N 99 22W
Ashley, *Pa., U.S.A.* **151 E9** 41 12N 75 55W
Ashley ➝, *N.Z.* **131 D7** 43 17 S 172 44 E
Ashmore and Cartier Is., *Ind. Oc.* **124 B3** 12 15 S 123 0 E
Ashmore Reef, *Australia* **124 B3** 12 14 S 123 5 E
Ashmûn, *Egypt* **106 H7** 30 18N 30 55 E
Ashmyany, *Belarus* **15 J21** 54 26N 25 52 E
Ashokan Reservoir, *U.S.A.* **151 E10** 41 56N 74 13W
Ashqelon, *Israel* **103 D3** 31 42N 34 35 E
Ashraf = Behshahr, *Iran* **97 B7** 36 45N 53 35 E
Ashta, *India* **92 H7** 23 1N 76 43 E
Ashtabula, *U.S.A.* **150 E4** 41 52N 80 47W
Ashti, *Maharashtra, India* **94 D4** 21 12N 78 11 E
Ashti, *Maharashtra, India* **94 E2** 18 50N 75 15 E
Ashton, *S. Africa* **116 E3** 33 50 S 20 5 E
Ashton, *U.S.A.* **158 D8** 44 4N 111 27W
Ashuanipi, L., *Canada* **141 B6** 52 45N 66 15W
Ashuapmushuan ➝, *Canada* **140 C5** 48 37N 72 20W
Ashurst, *N.Z.* **130 G4** 40 16 S 175 45 E
Ashville, *Ala., U.S.A.* **152 B3** 33 50N 86 15W
Ashville, *Fla., U.S.A.* **152 E6** 30 37N 83 39W
Ashville, *Pa., U.S.A.* **150 F6** 40 34N 78 33W
'Āşī ➝, *Asia* **100 D6** 36 1N 35 59 E
Asia **62 E11** 45 0N 75 0 E
Asia, Kepulauan, *Indonesia* **83 A4** 1 0N 131 13 E
Asiago, *Italy* **45 C8** 45 52N 11 30 E
Asidonhoppo, *Suriname* **169 C6** 3 50N 55 30W
Asifabad, *India* **94 E4** 19 20N 79 24 E
Asike, *Indonesia* **83 C6** 6 39 S 140 24 E
Asilah, *Morocco* **110 A3** 35 29N 6 0W
Asinara, *Italy* **46 A1** 41 4N 8 16 E
Asinara, G. dell', *Italy* **46 A1** 41 0N 8 30 E
Asino, *Russia* **66 D9** 57 0N 86 0 E
Asipovichy, *Belarus* **58 F5** 53 19N 28 33 E
'Asīr □, *Si. Arabia* **98 C3** 18 40N 42 30 E
Asir, Ras, *Somali Rep.* **120 B4** 11 55N 51 10 E
Aska, *India* **94 E7** 19 2N 84 42 E
Askale, *Turkey* **101 C9** 39 55N 40 41 E
Asker, *Norway* **18 E7** 59 50N 10 29 E
Askersund, *Sweden* **17 F8** 58 53N 14 55 E
Askham, *S. Africa* **116 D3** 26 59 S 20 47 E
Askim, *Norway* **18 E8** 59 35N 11 10 E
Askja, *Iceland* **11 B10** 65 3N 16 48W
Askøy, *Norway* **18 D2** 60 29N 5 10 E
Askvoll, *Norway* **18 C2** 61 21N 5 4 E
Asl, *Egypt* **106 B3** 29 33N 32 44 E
Aslan Burnu, *Turkey* **49 C8** 38 44N 26 45 E
Aslanapa, *Turkey* **49 B11** 39 13N 29 52 E
Asmār, *Afghan.* **91 B3** 35 10N 71 27 E
Asmara = Asmera, *Eritrea* **107 D4** 15 19N 38 55 E
Asmera, *Eritrea* **107 D4** 15 19N 38 55 E
Asnæs, *Denmark* **17 J4** 55 40N 11 0 E
Åsnen, *Sweden* **17 H8** 56 37N 14 45 E
Asni, *Morocco* **110 B3** 31 17N 7 58W
Aso, *Japan* **72 E3** 32 55N 131 5 E
Aso Kuju △, *Japan* **72 E3** 32 53N 131 6 E
Aso-Zan, *Japan* **72 E3** 32 53N 131 6 E
Asola, *Italy* **44 C7** 45 13N 10 24 E
Asosa, *Ethiopia* **107 E3** 10 3N 34 32 E
Asoteriba, Jebel, *Sudan* **106 C4** 21 51N 36 30 E
Aspatria, *U.K.* **20 C4** 54 47N 3 19W
Aspe, *Spain* **41 G4** 38 20N 0 40W
Aspen, *U.S.A.* **159 G10** 39 11N 106 49W
Aspendos, *Turkey* **100 D4** 36 54N 31 7 E
Aspermont, *U.S.A.* **155 J4** 33 8N 100 14W
Aspet, *France* **28 E4** 43 1N 0 48 E
Aspiring, Mt., *N.Z.* **131 E3** 44 23 S 168 46 E
Aspres-sur-Buëch, *France* **29 D9** 44 32N 5 44 E
Asprókavos, Ákra, *Greece* **38 C10** 39 21N 20 6 E
Aspromonte △, *Italy* **47 D8** 38 9N 15 58 E
Aspur, *India* **92 H6** 23 58N 74 7 E
Asquith, *Canada* **143 C7** 52 8N 107 13W
Assa, *Morocco* **110 C3** 28 35N 9 6W
Assab = Aseb, *Eritrea* **107 E5** 13 0N 42 40 E
Assâba, Massif de l', *Mauritania* **112 B2** 16 10N 11 45W
Assagny △, *Ivory C.* **112 D4** 5 10N 4 48W
Assaikio, *Nigeria* **113 D6** 8 34N 8 55 E
Assake = Asaka, *Uzbekistan* **65 C6** 40 38N 72 15 E
Assal, L., *Djibouti* **107 E5** 11 40N 42 26 E
Assam □, *India* **90 B4** 26 0N 93 0 E
Assamakka, *Niger* **113 B6** 19 21N 5 38 E
Assateague Island △, *U.S.A.* **148 F8** 38 15N 75 10W
Assaye, *India* **94 D2** 20 15N 75 53 E
Asse, *Belgium* **24 D4** 50 24N 4 10 E
Assekrem, *Algeria* **111 D6** 23 16N 5 49 E
Assémini, *Italy* **46 C1** 39 17N 9 0 E
Assen, *Neths.* **24 A6** 53 0N 6 35 E
Assens, *Denmark* **17 J3** 55 16N 9 55 E
Assini, *Ivory C.* **112 D4** 5 9N 3 17W
Assiniboia, *Canada* **143 D7** 49 40N 105 59W
Assiniboine ➝, *Canada* **143 D9** 49 53N 97 8W
Assiniboine, Mt., *Canada* **142 C5** 50 52N 115 39W
Assiou, *Algeria* **111 D6** 21 7N 7 36 E
Assis, *Brazil* **175 A5** 22 40 S 50 20W
Assis Brasil, *Brazil* **172 C4** 10 55 S 69 32W
Assisi, *Italy* **45 E9** 43 4N 12 37 E
Åsskard, *Norway* **18 A5** 63 1N 8 30 E
Assok Ngoum, *Gabon* **114 B2** 1 45N 11 39 E
Ássos, *Greece* **39 C2** 38 22N 20 33 E
Assumption, *U.S.A.* **156 E7** 39 31N 89 3W
Assynt, L., *U.K.* **22 C3** 58 10N 5 3W
Astaffort, *France* **28 D4** 44 4N 0 40 E
Astakidha, *Greece* **49 F8** 35 53N 26 50 E
Astakós, *Greece* **39 B3** 38 32N 21 5 E
Astana, *Kazakhstan* **66 D8** 51 10N 71 30 E
Āstāneh, *Iran* **97 B6** 37 17N 49 59 E
Astapovo = Lev Tolstoy, *Russia* **58 F10** 53 13N 39 29 E
Astara, *Azerbaijan* **97 B6** 38 30N 48 50 E
Āstārā, *Iran* **101 C13** 38 20N 48 52 E
Astarabad = Gorgān, *Iran* **97 B7** 36 55N 54 30 E
Asteroúsia, *Greece* **39 F6** 34 59N 25 3 E
Asti, *Italy* **44 D5** 44 54N 8 12 E
Astipálaia, *Greece* **49 E8** 36 32N 26 22 E
Astipalaia = Astipálaia, *Greece* **49 E8** 36 32N 26 22 E
Astola I., *Pakistan* **91 D1** 25 7N 63 51 E
Astorga, *Phil.* **81 H5** 6 54N 125 27 E
Astorga, *Spain* **42 C4** 42 29N 6 8W
Astoria, *Ill., U.S.A.* **156 D6** 40 14N 90 21W
Astoria, *Oreg., U.S.A.* **160 D3** 46 11N 123 50W
Åstorp, *Sweden* **17 H6** 56 6N 12 55 E
Astrakhan, *Russia* **61 G9** 46 25N 48 5 E
Astudillo, *Spain* **42 C6** 42 12N 4 22W
Asturias □, *Spain* **42 B5** 43 15N 6 0W
Asturias ✕ (OVD), *Spain* **42 B4** 43 33N 6 3W
Asunción, *Bolivia* **172 C4** 11 46 S 67 50W
Asunción, *Paraguay* **174 B4** 25 10 S 57 30W
Asunción Nochixtlán, *Mexico* **163 D5** 17 28N 97 14W
Åsunden, *Sweden* **17 F9** 58 0N 15 51 E
Asutri, *Sudan* **107 D4** 15 25N 35 45 E
Aswa ➝, *Uganda* **118 B3** 3 43N 31 55 E
Aswa-Lolim △, *Uganda* **118 B3** 2 43N 31 35 E
Aswad, Ra's al, *Si. Arabia* **98 B2** 21 20N 39 0 E
Aswân, *Egypt* **106 C3** 24 4N 32 57 E
Aswan Dam = Sadd el Aali, *Egypt* **106 C3** 23 54N 32 54 E
Asyût, *Egypt* **106 B3** 27 11N 31 4 E
Asyûti, Wadi ➝, *Egypt* **106 B3** 27 11N 31 16 E
Aszód, *Hungary* **52 C4** 47 39N 19 28 E
At-Bashy, *Kyrgyzstan* **65 C7** 41 10N 75 48 E
At-Bashy Kyrka Tooloru, *Kyrgyzstan* **65 C7** 40 50N 75 30 E
At Ţafīlah, *Jordan* **103 E4** 30 45N 35 30 E
At Ţafīlah □, *Jordan* **103 E4** 30 45N 35 30 E
Aţ Tā'if, *Si. Arabia* **98 B3** 21 5N 40 27 E
At Tāj, *Libya* **108 D4** 24 13N 23 18 E
At Ta'mīm □, *Iraq* **96 C5** 35 30N 44 20 E
At Tamīmī, *Libya* **108 B4** 32 20N 23 4 E
Aţ Ţirāq, *Si. Arabia* **96 E5** 27 19N 44 33 E
Aţ Tubayq, *Si. Arabia* **96 D3** 29 30N 37 0 E
At Turbah, *Yemen* **98 D4** 13 13N 44 7 E
At Turbah, *Yemen* **98 D3** 12 40N 43 30 E
Atabey, *Turkey* **49 D12** 37 57N 30 39 E
Atacama □, *Chile* **174 B2** 27 30 S 70 0W
Atacama, Desierto de, *Chile* **174 A2** 24 0 S 69 20W
Atacama, Salar de, *Chile* **174 A2** 23 30 S 68 20W
Ataco, *Colombia* **168 C2** 3 35N 75 23W
Atakor, *Algeria* **111 D6** 23 27N 5 31 E
Atakpamé, *Togo* **113 D5** 7 31N 1 13 E
Atalaia do Norte, *Brazil* **168 D3** 4 20 S 70 12W
Atalándi, *Greece* **48 C4** 38 39N 22 58 E
Atalaya, *Peru* **172 C3** 10 45 S 73 50W
Atalaya de Femes, *Canary Is.* **9 e2** 28 56N 13 47W
Ataléia, *Brazil* **171 E3** 18 3 S 41 6W
Atambua, *Indonesia* **82 C2** 9 7 S 124 54 E
Atami, *Japan* **73 B11** 35 5N 139 4 E
Atankawng, *Burma* **90 C6** 25 50N 97 47 E
Atapupu, *E. Timor* **82 C2** 9 0 S 124 51 E
Atâr, *Mauritania* **110 D2** 20 30N 13 5W
Ataram, Erg n-, *Algeria* **111 D5** 23 57N 2 0 E
Atarfe, *Spain* **43 H7** 37 13N 3 40W
Atari, *Pakistan* **92 D6** 30 56N 74 2 E
Atascadero, *U.S.A.* **160 K6** 35 29N 120 40W
Atasu, *Kazakhstan* **66 E8** 48 30N 71 0 E
Ataturk, Istanbul ✕ (IST), *Turkey* **51 F12** 40 59N 28 49 E
Atatürk Barajı, *Turkey* **101 D8** 37 28N 38 30 E
Atauro, *E. Timor* **82 C3** 8 10 S 125 30 E
'Atbara, *Sudan* **106 D3** 17 42N 33 59 E
'Atbara, Nahr ➝, *Sudan* **106 D3** 17 40N 33 56 E
Atbasar, *Kazakhstan* **66 D7** 51 48N 68 20 E
Atbashi = At-Bashy, *Kyrgyzstan* **65 C7** 41 10N 75 48 E
Atça, *Turkey* **49 D10** 37 53N 28 13 E
Atchafalaya B., *U.S.A.* **155 L9** 29 25N 91 25W
Atchison, *U.S.A.* **154 F7** 39 34N 95 7W
Atebubu, *Ghana* **113 D4** 7 47N 1 0W
Ateca, *Spain* **40 D3** 41 20N 1 49W
Aterno ➝, *Italy* **45 F10** 42 11N 13 51 E
Āteshān, *Iran* **97 C7** 35 35N 52 37 E
Atesine, Alpi, *Italy* **45 B8** 46 55N 11 30 E
Atessa, *Italy* **45 F11** 42 4N 14 27 E
Atfîh, *Egypt* **106 J7** 29 25N 31 15 E
Ath, *Belgium* **24 D3** 50 38N 3 47 E
Athabasca, *Canada* **142 C6** 54 45N 113 20W
Athabasca ➝, *Canada* **143 B6** 58 40N 110 50W
Athabasca, L., *Canada* **143 B7** 59 15N 109 15W
Athabasca Sand Dunes △, *Canada* **143 B7** 59 4N 108 43W
Athagarh, *India* **94 D7** 20 32N 85 37 E
Athboy, *Ireland* **23 C5** 53 37N 6 56W
Athena, *U.S.A.* **152 F6** 29 59N 83 30W
Athenry, *Ireland* **23 C3** 53 18N 8 44W
Athens = Athínai, *Greece* **48 D5** 37 58N 23 46 E
Athens, *Ala., U.S.A.* **149 H2** 34 48N 86 58W
Athens, *Ga., U.S.A.* **152 B6** 33 57N 83 23W
Athens, *N.Y., U.S.A.* **151 D11** 42 16N 73 49W
Athens, *Ohio, U.S.A.* **148 F4** 39 20N 82 6W
Athens, *Pa., U.S.A.* **151 E8** 41 57N 76 31W
Athens, *Tenn., U.S.A.* **149 H3** 35 27N 84 36W
Athens, *Tex., U.S.A.* **155 J7** 32 12N 95 51W
Athéras, *Greece* **39 C1** 38 19N 20 25 E
Atherley, *Canada* **150 B5** 44 37N 79 20W
Atherton, *Australia* **126 B4** 17 17 S 145 30 E
Athiéme, *Benin* **113 D5** 6 37N 1 40 E
Athienou, *Cyprus* **39 E9** 35 3N 33 32 E
Athina = Athínai, *Greece* **48 D5** 37 58N 23 46 E
Athínai, *Greece* **48 D5** 37 58N 23 46 E
Athínai ✕ (ATH), *Greece* **48 D5** 37 55N 23 50 E
Athlone, *Ireland* **23 C4** 53 25N 7 56W
Athmalik, *India* **94 D7** 20 43N 84 32 E
Athna, *Cyprus* **39 E9** 35 3N 33 47 E
Athni, *India* **94 F2** 16 44N 75 6 E
Athol, *N.Z.* **131 F3** 45 30 S 168 35 E
Athol, *U.S.A.* **151 D12** 42 36N 72 14W
Athol Is., *Bahamas* **9 b** 25 5N 77 16W
Atholl, Forest of, *U.K.* **22 E5** 56 51N 3 50W
Atholl, Kap, *Greenland* **10 B4** 76 25N 69 30W
Atholville, *Canada* **141 C6** 47 59N 66 43W
Áthos, *Greece* **51 F8** 40 9N 24 22 E
Athy, *Ireland* **23 C5** 53 0N 7 0W
Ati, *Chad* **109 F3** 13 13N 18 20 E
Ati, *Sudan* **107 E2** 13 5N 29 2 E
Atiak, *Uganda* **118 B3** 3 12N 32 2 E
Atiamuri, *N.Z.* **130 E5** 38 24 S 176 5 E
Atico, *Peru* **172 D3** 16 14 S 73 40W
Atienza, *Spain* **40 D2** 41 12N 2 52W
Atiit, *Sudan* **107 F3** 6 10N 30 35 E
Atik L., *Canada* **143 B9** 55 15N 96 0W
Atikaki △, *Canada* **143 C9** 51 30N 95 31W
Atikameg ➝, *Canada* **140 B3** 52 30N 82 46W
Atikokan, *Canada* **140 C1** 48 45N 91 37W
Atikonak L., *Canada* **141 B7** 52 40N 64 32W
Atimonan, *Phil.* **80 D3** 14 0N 121 55 E
'Ātinah, W. ➝, *Oman* **99 C6** 18 23N 53 28 E
Atirampattinam, *India* **95 J4** 10 28N 79 20 E
Atitlán △, *Cent. Amer.* **163 E6** 14 38N 91 10W
Atiu, *Cook Is.* **135 J12** 20 0 S 158 10W
Atka, *Russia* **67 C16** 60 50N 151 48 E
Atka, *U.S.A.* **144 K4** 52 12N 174 12W
Atka I., *U.S.A.* **144 K4** 52 7N 174 30W
Atkarsk, *Russia* **60 E7** 51 55N 45 2 E
Atkasuk = Meade River, *U.S.A.* **144 A8** 70 28N 157 24W
Atkinson, *Ga., U.S.A.* **152 D8** 31 13N 81 47W
Atkinson, *Ill., U.S.A.* **156 C6** 41 25N 90 1W
Atkinson, *Nebr., U.S.A.* **154 D5** 42 32N 98 59W
Atlanta, *Ga., U.S.A.* **152 B5** 33 45N 84 23W
Atlanta, *Ill., U.S.A.* **156 D7** 40 16N 89 14W
Atlanta, *Mo., U.S.A.* **156 E4** 39 54N 92 29W
Atlanta, *Tex., U.S.A.* **155 J7** 33 7N 94 10W
Atlanta Hartsfield International ✕ (ATL), *U.S.A.* **152 B5** 33 38N 84 26W
Atlantic, *U.S.A.* **156 C2** 41 24N 95 1W
Atlantic Beach, *U.S.A.* **152 E8** 30 20N 81 24W
Atlantic City, *U.S.A.* **148 F8** 39 21N 74 27W
Atlantic-Indian Basin, *Antarctica* **7 B4** 60 0 S 30 0 E
Atlantic-Indian Ridge, *Atl. Oc.* **8 M11** 53 0 S 5 0W
Atlantic Ocean **8 F8** 0 0 20 0W
Atlántico □, *Colombia* **168 A2** 10 45N 75 0W
Atlas Mts. = Haut Atlas, *Morocco* **110 B4** 32 30N 5 0W
Atlin, *Canada* **142 B2** 59 31N 133 41W
Atlin △, *Canada* **142 B2** 59 10N 134 30W
Atlin, L., *Canada* **142 B2** 59 26N 133 45W
Atløyna, *Norway* **18 C1** 61 21N 4 58 E
Atmakur, *Andhra Pradesh, India* **94 E4** 18 45N 78 39 E
Atmakur, *Andhra Pradesh, India* **95 G4** 14 37N 79 40 E
Atmakur, *Andhra Pradesh, India* **95 G4** 15 53N 78 35 E
Atmore, *U.S.A.* **149 K2** 31 2N 87 29W
Atna, *Norway* **18 C7** 61 44N 10 49 E
Atna ➝, *Norway* **18 C7** 61 44N 10 49 E
Atō, *Japan* **72 C3** 34 25N 131 40 E
Atocha, *Bolivia* **172 E4** 20 56 S 66 14W
Atok, *Phil.* **80 C3** 16 35N 120 41 E
Atoka, *U.S.A.* **155 H6** 34 23N 96 8W
Átokos Nisís, *Greece* **39 C2** 38 28N 20 49 E
Atolia, *U.S.A.* **161 K9** 35 19N 117 37W
Atongo-Bakari, *C.A.R.* **114 A4** 5 49N 21 35 E
Atori, *Solomon Is.* **133 M11** 8 42 S 160 59 E
Atrå, *Norway* **18 E5** 59 59N 8 45 E
Atrai ➝, *Bangla.* **90 C2** 24 7N 89 22 E
Atrak = Atrek ➝, *Turkmenistan* **97 B8** 37 35N 53 58 E
Ätran, *Sweden* **17 G6** 57 7N 12 57 E
Ätran ➝, *Sweden* **17 H6** 56 53N 12 30 E
Atrato ➝, *Colombia* **168 B2** 8 17N 76 58W
Atrauli, *India* **92 E8** 28 2N 78 20 E
Atrek ➝, *Turkmenistan* **97 B8** 37 35N 53 58 E
Atri, *Italy* **45 F10** 42 35N 13 58 E
Atsikí, *Greece* **49 B7** 39 56N 25 13 E
Atsoum, Mts., *Cameroon* **113 D7** 6 41N 12 57 E
Atsugi, *Japan* **73 B11** 35 25N 139 21 E
Atsumi, *Japan* **73 C9** 34 35N 137 4 E
Atsumi-Wan, *Japan* **73 C9** 34 44N 137 13 E
Atsuta, *Japan* **70 C10** 43 24N 141 26 E
Atsy, *Indonesia* **83 C5** 5 48 S 138 20 E
Attalla, *U.S.A.* **152 A3** 34 1N 86 6W
Attapu, *Laos* **86 E6** 14 48N 106 50 E
Attapulgus, *U.S.A.* **152 E5** 30 45N 84 29W
Attáviros, *Greece* **38 E11** 36 12N 27 50 E
Attawapiskat, *Canada* **140 B3** 52 56N 82 24W
Attawapiskat ➝, *Canada* **140 B3** 52 57N 82 18W
Attawapiskat L., *Canada* **140 B2** 52 18N 87 54W
Attersee, *Austria* **34 D6** 47 55N 13 32 E
Attica, *Ind., U.S.A.* **157 D9** 40 18N 87 15W
Attica, *Ohio, U.S.A.* **150 E2** 41 4N 82 53W
Attichy, *France* **27 C10** 49 25N 3 3 E
Attigny, *France* **27 C11** 49 28N 4 35 E
Attika = Attikí □, *Greece* **48 D5** 37 10N 23 40 E
Attikamagen L., *Canada* **141 B6** 55 0N 66 30W
Attikí □, *Greece* **48 D5** 37 10N 23 40 E
Attleboro, *U.S.A.* **151 E13** 41 57N 71 17W
Attock = Campbellpur, *Pakistan* **92 C5** 33 46N 72 26 E
Attock, *Pakistan* **92 C5** 33 52N 72 20 E
Attopeu = Attapu, *Laos* **86 E6** 14 48N 106 50 E
Attu, *U.S.A.* **144 K1** 52 56N 173 15 E
Attu I., *U.S.A.* **144 K1** 52 55N 172 55 E
Attunga, *Australia* **129 A9** 30 55 S 150 50 E
Attur, *India* **95 J4** 11 35N 78 30 E
'Atūd, *Yemen* **99 D5** 14 53N 48 10 E
Atuel ➝, *Argentina* **174 D2** 36 17 S 66 50W
Åtvidaberg, *Sweden* **17 F10** 58 12N 16 0 E
Atwater, *U.S.A.* **160 H6** 37 21N 120 37W
Atwood, *Canada* **150 C3** 43 40N 81 1W
Atwood, *Ill., U.S.A.* **157 E8** 39 48N 88 28W
Atwood, *Kans., U.S.A.* **154 F4** 39 48N 101 3W
Atyraū, *Kazakhstan* **66 E6** 47 5N 52 0 E
Au, *Austria* **33 B9** 47 19N 9 59 E
Au Sable, *U.S.A.* **150 B1** 44 25N 83 20W
Au Sable ➝, *U.S.A.* **148 C4** 44 25N 83 20W
Au Sable Forks, *U.S.A.* **151 B11** 44 27N 73 41W
Au Sable Pt., *U.S.A.* **150 B1** 44 20N 83 20W
Aubagne, *France* **29 E9** 43 17N 5 37 E
Aubarca, C. d', *Spain* **38 C1** 39 4N 1 22 E
Aube □, *France* **27 D11** 48 15N 4 10 E
Aube ➝, *France* **27 D10** 48 34N 3 43 E
Aubenas, *France* **29 D8** 44 37N 4 24 E
Aubenton, *France* **27 C11** 49 50N 4 12 E
Auberry, *U.S.A.* **160 H7** 37 7N 119 29W
Aubigny-sur-Nère, *France* **27 E9** 47 30N 2 24 E
Aubin, *France* **28 D6** 44 33N 2 15 E
Aubrac, Mts. d', *France* **28 D7** 44 40N 3 2 E
Auburn, *Australia* **128 C3** 34 1 S 138 42 E
Auburn, *Ala., U.S.A.* **152 C4** 32 36N 85 29W
Auburn, *Calif., U.S.A.* **160 G5** 38 54N 121 4W
Auburn, *Ill., U.S.A.* **156 E7** 39 36N 89 45W
Auburn, *Ind., U.S.A.* **157 C11** 41 22N 85 4W
Auburn, *Maine, U.S.A.* **149 C10** 44 6N 70 14W
Auburn, *N.Y., U.S.A.* **151 D8** 42 56N 76 34W
Auburn, *Nebr., U.S.A.* **154 E7** 40 23N 95 51W
Auburn, *Pa., U.S.A.* **151 F8** 40 36N 76 6W
Auburn, *Wash., U.S.A.* **160 C4** 47 18N 122 14W
Auburn Ra., *Australia* **127 D5** 25 15 S 150 30 E
Auburndale, *U.S.A.* **153 G8** 28 4N 81 48W
Aubusson, *France* **28 C6** 45 57N 2 11 E
Auce, *Latvia* **54 B9** 56 28N 22 53 E
Auch, *France* **28 E4** 43 39N 0 36 E
Auchi, *Nigeria* **113 D6** 7 6N 6 13 E
Auchterarder, *U.K.* **22 E5** 56 18N 3 41W
Auchtermuchty, *U.K.* **22 E5** 56 18N 3 13W
Auckland, *N.Z.* **130 C3** 36 52 S 174 46 E
Auckland □, *N.Z.* **130 E6** 36 50 S 175 0 E
Auckland Is., *Pac. Oc.* **134 N8** 50 40 S 166 5 E
Aude □, *France* **28 E6** 43 8N 2 28 E
Aude ➝, *France* **28 E7** 43 13N 3 14 E
Audegle, *Somali Rep.* **120 D2** 1 59N 44 50 E
Auden, *Canada* **140 B2** 50 14N 87 53W
Auderville, *France* **26 C5** 49 43N 1 57W
Audierne, *France* **26 D2** 48 1N 4 34W
Audincourt, *France* **27 E13** 47 30N 6 50 E
Audo Ra., *Ethiopia* **107 F5** 6 20N 41 50 E
Audubon, *U.S.A.* **156 C2** 41 43N 94 56W
Aue, *Germany* **30 E8** 50 35N 12 41 E
Auerbach, *Germany* **30 E8** 50 30N 12 24 E
Aueti Paraná ➝, *Brazil* **168 D4** 1 51 S 65 37W
Aufist, *W. Sahara* **110 C2** 25 44N 14 39W
Augathella, *Australia* **127 D4** 25 48 S 146 35 E
Aughnacloy, *U.K.* **23 B5** 54 25N 6 59W
Augrabies Falls, *S. Africa* **116 D3** 28 35 S 20 20 E
Augrabies Falls △, *S. Africa* **116 D3** 28 40 S 20 22 E
Augsburg, *Germany* **31 G6** 48 25N 10 52 E
Augsburg-Westliche Wälder △, *Germany* **31 G6** 48 22N 10 40 E
Augusta, *Australia* **125 F2** 34 19 S 115 9 E
Augusta, *Italy* **47 E8** 37 13N 15 13 E
Augusta, *Ark., U.S.A.* **155 H9** 35 17N 91 22W
Augusta, *Ga., U.S.A.* **152 B8** 33 28N 81 58W
Augusta, *Ill., U.S.A.* **156 D6** 40 14N 90 57W
Augusta, *Kans., U.S.A.* **155 G6** 37 41N 96 59W
Augusta, *Ky., U.S.A.* **157 F12** 38 47N 84 0W
Augusta, *Maine, U.S.A.* **139 D13** 44 19N 69 47W
Augusta, *Mont., U.S.A.* **158 C7** 47 30N 112 24W
Augustenborg, *Denmark* **17 K3** 54 57N 9 53 E
Augustine I., *U.S.A.* **144 G9** 59 22N 153 26W
Augusto Cardosa = Metangula, *Mozam.* **119 E3** 12 40 S 34 50 E
Augustów, *Poland* **54 E9** 53 51N 23 0 E
Augustus, Mt., *Australia* **125 D2** 24 20 S 116 50 E
Augustus I., *Australia* **124 C3** 15 20 S 124 30 E
Aukan, *Eritrea* **107 D5** 15 29N 40 50 E
Auki, *Solomon Is.* **133 M11** 8 45 S 160 42 E
Aukra, *Norway* **18 B3** 62 47N 6 55 E
Aukrug △, *Germany* **30 A5** 54 5N 9 45 E
Aukum, *U.S.A.* **160 G6** 38 34N 120 43W
Aul, *India* **94 D8** 20 41N 86 39 E
Auld, L., *Australia* **124 D3** 22 25 S 123 50 E
Auliye-Ata = Taraz, *Kazakhstan* **65 B5** 42 54N 71 22 E
Aulla, *Italy* **44 D6** 44 12N 9 58 E
Aulnay, *France* **28 B3** 46 2N 0 22W
Aulne ➝, *France* **26 D2** 48 17N 4 16W
Aulnoye-Aymeries, *France* **27 B10** 50 12N 3 50 E
Ault, *France* **26 B8** 50 8N 1 26 E
Ault, *U.S.A.* **154 E2** 40 35N 104 44W
Aulus-les-Bains, *France* **28 F5** 42 49N 1 19 E
Aumale = Sour el Ghozlane, *Algeria* **111 A5** 36 10N 3 45 E
Aumale, *France* **27 C8** 49 46N 1 46 E
Aumo, *Papua N. G.* **132 C5** 5 44 S 148 30 E

Aumont-Aubrac, *France* **28 D7** 44 43N 3 17 E
Auna, *Nigeria* **113 C5** 10 9N 4 42 E
Aundah, *India* **94 E3** 19 32N 77 3 E
Aundh, *India* **94 F2** 17 33N 74 23 E
Auning, *Denmark* **17 H4** 56 26N 10 22 E
Aunis, *France* **28 B3** 46 5N 0 50W
'Aunu'u, *Amer. Samoa* **133 X24** 14 20 S 170 31W
Auponhia, *Indonesia* **82 B3** 1 58 S 125 27 E
Aups, *France* **29 E10** 43 37N 6 15 E
Aur, Pulau, *Malaysia* **87 L5** 2 35N 104 10 E
Aura, *Burma* **90 B6** 26 59N 97 57 E
Auraiya, *India* **93 F8** 26 28N 79 33 E
Aurangabad, *Bihar, India* **93 G11** 24 45N 84 18 E
Aurangabad, *Maharashtra, India* **94 E2** 19 50N 75 23 E
Auray, *France* **26 E4** 47 40N 2 59W
Aurdal, *Norway* **18 D6** 60 55N 9 26 E
Aure, *Norway* **18 A5** 63 16N 8 33 E
Aurès, *Algeria* **111 A6** 35 8N 6 30 E
Aurich, *Germany* **30 B3** 53 28N 7 28 E
Aurilândia, *Brazil* **171 E1** 16 44 S 50 28W
Aurillac, *France* **28 D6** 44 55N 2 26 E
Aurlandsfjorden, *Norway* **18 C4** 61 3N 7 1 E
Aurlandsvangen, *Norway* **18 D4** 60 55N 7 12 E
Auronzo di Cadore, *Italy* **45 B9** 46 33N 12 26 E
Aurora = Maéwo, *Vanuatu* **133 E6** 15 10 S 168 10 E
Aurora = San Francisco, *Phil.* **80 E4** 13 21N 122 31 E
Aurora, *Canada* **150 C5** 44 0N 79 28W
Aurora, *Isabela, Phil.* **80 C3** 16 59N 121 38 E
Aurora, *Zamboanga del S., Phil.* **81 H4** 7 57N 123 36 E
Aurora, *S. Africa* **116 E2** 32 40 S 18 29 E
Aurora, *Colo., U.S.A.* **154 F2** 39 44N 104 52W
Aurora, *Ill., U.S.A.* **157 C8** 41 45N 88 19W
Aurora, *Mo., U.S.A.* **155 G8** 36 58N 93 43W
Aurora, *N.Y., U.S.A.* **151 D8** 42 45N 76 42W
Aurora, *Nebr., U.S.A.* **154 E6** 40 52N 98 0W
Aurora, *Ohio, U.S.A.* **150 E3** 41 21N 81 20W
Aurora □, *Phil.* **80 D3** 15 30N 121 30 E
Aurora △, *Phil.* **80 D3** 15 40N 121 20 E
Aursmoen, *Norway* **18 E8** 59 55N 11 26 E
Aursunden, *Norway* **18 B8** 62 40N 11 40 E
Aurukun, *Australia* **126 A3** 13 20 S 141 45 E
Aus, *Namibia* **116 D2** 26 35 S 16 12 E
Ausa, *India* **94 E3** 18 15N 76 30 E
Ausable →, *Canada* **150 C3** 43 19N 81 46W
Auschwitz = Oświęcim, *Poland* **55 H6** 50 2N 19 11 E
Auspitz = Hustopeče, *Czech Rep.* **35 C9** 48 57N 16 43 E
Aussig = Ústí nad Labem, *Czech Rep.* **34 A7** 50 41N 14 3 E
Aust-Agder □, *Norway* **18 F4** 58 45N 8 0 E
Austad, *Norway* **18 F4** 58 58N 7 37 E
Austen Harbour, *India* **95 H11** 12 55N 92 45 E
Austerlitz = Slavkov u Brna, *Czech Rep.* **35 B9** 49 10N 16 52 E
Austevoll, *Norway* **18 D2** 60 5N 5 13 E
Austin, *Ind., U.S.A.* **157 F11** 38 45N 85 49W
Austin, *Minn., U.S.A.* **154 D8** 43 40N 92 58W
Austin, *Nev., U.S.A.* **158 G5** 39 30N 117 4W
Austin, *Pa., U.S.A.* **150 E6** 41 38N 78 6W
Austin, *Tex., U.S.A.* **155 K6** 30 17N 97 45W
Austin, L., *Australia* **125 E2** 27 40 S 118 0 E
Austin I., *Canada* **143 A10** 61 10N 94 0W
Austmarka, *Norway* **18 D9** 60 6N 12 21 E
Austnes, *Norway* **18 B3** 62 38N 6 16 E
Austra, *Norway* **14 D14** 65 8N 11 55 E
Austral Is. = Tubuai Is., *French Polynesia* **135 K13** 25 0 S 150 0W
Austral Seamount Chain, *Pac. Oc.* **135 K13** 24 0 S 150 0W
Australia ■, *Oceania* **134 K5** 23 0 S 135 0 E
Australian Capital Territory □, *Australia* **129 C8** 35 30 S 149 0 E
Australind, *Australia* **125 F2** 33 17 S 115 42 E
Austria ■, *Europe* **34 E7** 47 0N 14 0 E
Austur-Skaftafellssýsla □, *Iceland* **11 C10** 64 15N 16 0W
Austvågøy, *Norway* **14 B16** 68 20N 14 40 E
Autazes, *Brazil* **169 D6** 3 35 S 59 8W
Auterive, *France* **28 E5** 43 21N 1 29 E
Authie →, *France* **27 B8** 50 22N 1 38 E
Authon-du-Perche, *France* **26 D7** 48 12N 0 54 E
Autlán, *Mexico* **162 D4** 19 40N 104 30W
Autun, *France* **27 F11** 46 58N 4 17 E
Auvergne □, *France* **28 C7** 45 20N 3 15 E
Auvergne, Mts. d', *France* **28 C6** 45 20N 2 55 E
Auvézère →, *France* **28 C4** 45 12N 0 50 E
Auxerre, *France* **27 E10** 47 48N 3 32 E
Auxi-le-Château, *France* **27 B9** 50 15N 2 8 E
Auxonne, *France* **27 E12** 47 10N 5 20 E
Auxvasse, *U.S.A.* **156 E5** 39 1N 91 54W
Auzances, *France* **27 F9** 46 2N 2 30 E
Ava, *Ill., U.S.A.* **156 G7** 37 53N 89 30W
Ava, *Mo., U.S.A.* **155 G8** 36 57N 92 40W
Avaldsnes, *Norway* **18 E2** 59 21N 5 20 E
Avallon, *France* **27 E10** 47 30N 3 53 E
Avalon, *U.S.A.* **161 M8** 33 21N 118 20W
Avalon Pen., *Canada* **141 C9** 47 30N 53 20W
Avanavero, *Suriname* **169 C6** 4 51N 57 22W
Avanigadda, *India* **95 G5** 16 0N 80 56 E
Avannaarsua □, *Greenland* **10 B5** 80 0N 55 0W
Avanos, *Turkey* **96 B2** 38 43N 34 51 E
Avaré, *Brazil* **175 A6** 23 4 S 48 58W
Ávas, *Greece* **51 F9** 40 57N 25 56 E
Avawatz Mts., *U.S.A.* **161 K10** 35 40N 116 30W
Avdan Daği, *Turkey* **51 F13** 40 23N 29 46 E
Aveiro, *Brazil* **169 D6** 3 10 S 55 5W
Aveiro, *Portugal* **42 E2** 40 37N 8 38W
Aveiro □, *Portugal* **42 E2** 40 40N 8 35W
Āvej, *Iran* **97 C6** 35 40N 49 15 E
Avellaneda, *Argentina* **174 C4** 34 50 S 58 10W
Avellino, *Italy* **47 B7** 40 54N 14 47 E
Avenal, *U.S.A.* **160 K6** 36 0N 120 8W
Avenches, *Switz.* **32 C4** 46 53N 7 2 E
Averøya, *Norway* **18 A4** 63 0N 7 35 E
Aversa, *Italy* **47 B7** 40 58N 14 12 E
Avery, *U.S.A.* **158 C6** 47 15N 115 49W
Aves, I. de, *W. Indies* **165 C7** 15 45N 63 55W
Aves, Is. las, *Venezuela* **165 D6** 12 0N 67 30W
Avesnes-sur-Helpe, *France* **27 B10** 50 8N 3 55 E
Avesnois △, *France* **27 B10** 50 10N 3 45 E
Avesta, *Sweden* **16 D10** 60 9N 16 10 E
Aveyron □, *France* **28 D6** 44 22N 2 45 E
Aveyron →, *France* **28 D5** 44 5N 1 16 E
Avezzano, *Italy* **45 F10** 42 2N 13 25 E
Avgó, *Greece* **49 F7** 35 33N 25 37 E
Aviá Terai, *Argentina* **174 B3** 26 45 S 60 50W
Aviano, *Italy* **45 B9** 46 4N 12 36 E
Aviemore, *U.K.* **22 D5** 57 12N 3 50W
Aviemore, L., *N.Z.* **131 E5** 44 37 S 170 18 E
Avigliana, *Italy* **44 C4** 45 5N 7 23 E
Avigliano, *Italy* **47 B8** 40 44N 15 43 E
Avignon, *France* **29 E8** 43 57N 4 50 E
Ávila, *Spain* **42 E6** 40 39N 4 43W
Ávila □, *Spain* **42 E6** 40 30N 5 0W
Ávila, Sierra de, *Spain* **42 E5** 40 40N 5 15W
Avila Beach, *U.S.A.* **161 K6** 35 11N 120 44W
Avilés, *Spain* **42 B5** 43 35N 5 57W
Avintes, *Portugal* **42 D2** 41 7N 8 33W
Avionárion, *Greece* **48 C6** 38 31N 24 8 E
Avis, *Portugal* **43 F3** 39 4N 7 53W
Avis, *U.S.A.* **150 E7** 41 11N 77 19W
Avísio →, *Italy* **44 B8** 46 7N 11 5 E
Avissawella, *Sri Lanka* **95 L5** 6 56N 80 11 E
Aviston, *U.S.A.* **156 F7** 38 36N 89 36W
Aviz = Avis, *Portugal* **43 F3** 39 4N 7 53W
Avize, *France* **27 D11** 48 59N 4 1 E
Avlona = Vlorë, *Albania* **50 F3** 40 32N 19 28 E
Avlum, *Denmark* **17 H2** 56 16N 8 47 E
Avoca, *Australia* **128 D5** 37 5 S 143 26 E
Avoca, *U.S.A.* **150 D7** 42 25N 77 25W
Avoca →, *Australia* **128 C5** 35 40 S 143 43 E
Avoca →, *Ireland* **23 D5** 52 48N 6 10W
Avola, *Canada* **142 C5** 51 45N 119 19W
Avola, *Italy* **47 F8** 36 56N 15 7 E
Avon, *Ill., U.S.A.* **156 D6** 40 40N 90 26W
Avon, *N.Y., U.S.A.* **150 D7** 42 55N 77 45W
Avon →, *Australia* **125 F2** 31 40 S 116 7 E
Avon →, *Bristol, U.K.* **21 F5** 51 29N 2 41W
Avon →, *Dorset, U.K.* **21 G6** 50 44N 1 46W
Avon →, *Warks., U.K.* **21 E5** 52 0N 2 8W
Avon Park, *U.S.A.* **153 H8** 27 36N 81 31W
Avondale, *Zimbabwe* **119 F3** 17 43 S 30 58 E
Avonlea, *Canada* **143 D8** 50 0N 105 0W
Avonmore, *Canada* **151 A10** 45 10N 74 58W
Avonmouth, *U.K.* **21 F5** 51 30N 2 42W
Avramov, *Bulgaria* **51 D10** 42 45N 26 38 E
Avranches, *France* **26 D5** 48 40N 1 20W
Avre →, *France* **26 D8** 48 47N 1 22 E
Avrig, *Romania* **53 E9** 45 43N 24 21 E
Avrillé, *France* **26 E6** 47 30N 0 35W
Avtovac, *Bos.-H.* **50 C2** 43 9N 18 35 E
Avu Avu, *Solomon Is.* **133 M11** 9 50 S 160 22 E
Awag el Baqar, *Sudan* **107 E3** 10 10N 33 10 E
A'waj →, *Syria* **103 B5** 33 23N 36 20 E
Awaji, *Japan* **73 C7** 34 32N 135 1 E
Awaji-Shima, *Japan* **72 C6** 34 30N 134 50 E
'Awālī, *Bahrain* **97 E6** 26 0N 50 30 E
Awantipur, *India* **93 C6** 33 55N 75 3 E
Awanui, *N.Z.* **130 B2** 35 4 S 173 17 E
Awarja →, *India* **94 F3** 17 5N 76 15 E
Awarua B., *N.Z.* **131 E3** 44 28 S 168 4 E
Awarua Pt., *N.Z.* **131 E3** 44 15 S 168 5 E
Awasa, *Ethiopia* **107 F4** 7 2N 38 28 E
Awasa, L., *Ethiopia* **107 F4** 7 0N 38 30 E
Awash, *Ethiopia* **107 F5** 9 1N 40 10 E
Awash △, *Ethiopia* **107 F5** 9 8N 40 0 E
Awash →, *Ethiopia* **107 E5** 11 45N 41 5 E
Awaso, *Ghana* **112 D4** 6 15N 2 22W
Awatere →, *N.Z.* **131 B9** 41 37 S 174 10 E
Awbārī, *Libya* **108 C2** 26 46N 12 57 E
Awbārī □, *Libya* **108 C2** 26 35N 12 46 E
Awbārī, Idehan, *Libya* **108 C2** 27 10N 11 30 E
Awe, L., *U.K.* **22 E3** 56 17N 5 16W
Aweil, *Sudan* **107 F2** 8 42N 27 20 E
Awgu, *Nigeria* **113 D6** 6 4N 7 24 E
Awjilah, *Libya* **108 C4** 29 8N 21 7 E
Awka, *Nigeria* **113 D6** 6 12N 7 5 E
Aworro, *Papua N. G.* **132 D2** 7 43 S 143 11 E
Ax-les-Thermes, *France* **28 F5** 42 44N 1 50 E
Axat, *France* **28 F6** 42 48N 2 13 E
Axe →, *U.K.* **21 F5** 50 42N 3 4W
Axel Heiberg I., *Canada* **6 B3** 80 0N 90 0W
Axim, *Ghana* **112 E4** 4 51N 2 15W
Axinim, *Brazil* **169 D6** 4 2 S 59 22W
Axintele, *Romania* **53 F11** 44 37N 26 47 E
Axioma, *Brazil* **173 B5** 6 45 S 64 31W
Axiós →, *Greece* **50 F6** 40 57N 22 35 E
Axminster, *U.K.* **21 G4** 50 46N 3 0W
Axson, *U.S.A.* **152 D7** 31 17N 82 44W
Axvall, *Sweden* **17 F7** 58 23N 13 34 E
Ay, *France* **27 C11** 49 3N 4 1 E
Ay →, *Russia* **64 C6** 56 8N 57 40 E
Ayaantang, *Eq. Guin.* **114 B2** 1 58N 10 24 E
Ayabaca, *Peru* **172 A2** 4 40 S 79 53W
Ayabe, *Japan* **73 B7** 35 20N 135 20 E
Ayacucho, *Argentina* **174 D4** 37 5 S 58 20W
Ayacucho, *Peru* **172 C3** 13 0 S 74 0W
Ayacucho □, *Peru* **172 C3** 14 0 S 74 0W
Ayaguz, *Kazakhstan* **66 E9** 48 10N 80 10 E
Ayakkuduk, *Uzbekistan* **65 C2** 41 12N 65 12 E
Ayakudi, *India* **95 J3** 10 28N 77 56 E
Ayala, *Phil.* **81 H3** 6 57N 121 57 E
Ayamé, *Ivory C.* **112 D4** 5 35N 3 9W
Ayamonte, *Spain* **43 H3** 37 12N 7 24W
Ayan, *Russia* **67 D14** 56 30N 138 16 E
Ayancık, *Turkey* **100 B6** 41 57N 34 35 E
Ayapel, *Colombia* **168 B2** 8 19N 75 9W
Ayas, *Turkey* **100 B5** 40 2N 32 21 E
Ayaviri, *Peru* **172 C3** 14 50 S 70 35W
Āybak, *Afghan.* **91 A3** 36 15N 68 5 E
Aybastı, *Turkey* **100 B7** 40 41N 37 23 E
Aydarkul Ozero, *Uzbekistan* **65 C3** 40 50N 67 10 E
Aydın, *Turkey* **100 D2** 37 51N 27 51 E
Aydın □, *Turkey* **49 D9** 37 50N 28 0 E
Aydin Dağları, *Turkey* **49 D10** 38 0N 28 0 E
Aydyrlinskiy, *Russia* **64 E7** 52 3N 59 50 E
Ayelu, *Ethiopia* **107 E5** 10 5N 40 42 E
Ayenngré, *Togo* **113 D5** 8 40N 1 1 E
Ayer, *U.S.A.* **151 D13** 42 34N 71 35W
Ayer Hitam, *Malaysia* **87 c** 5 24N 100 16 E
Ayerbe, *Spain* **40 C4** 42 17N 0 41W
Ayer's Cliff, *Canada* **151 A12** 45 10N 72 3W
Ayers Rock, *Australia* **125 E5** 25 23 S 131 5 E
Ayiá, *Greece* **48 B4** 39 43N 22 45 E
Ayia Aikateríni, Ákra, *Greece* **38 B9** 39 50N 19 50 E
Ayía Ánna, *Greece* **48 C5** 38 52N 23 24 E
Ayia Dhéka, *Greece* **39 E5** 35 3N 24 58 E
Ayia Gálini, *Greece* **39 E5** 35 6N 24 41 E
Ayía Marína, *Kásos, Greece* **49 F8** 35 27N 26 53 E
Ayía Marína, *Léros, Greece* **49 D8** 37 11N 26 48 E
Ayia Napa, *Cyprus* **39 F10** 34 59N 34 0 E
Ayía Paraskeví, *Greece* **49 B8** 39 14N 26 21 E
Ayía Phyla, *Cyprus* **39 F9** 34 43N 33 1 E
Ayía Rouméli, *Greece* **39 E4** 35 14N 23 58 E
Ayía Varvára, *Greece* **39 E6** 35 8N 25 1 E
Ayiássos, *Greece* **49 B8** 39 5N 26 23 E
Áyioi Theódhoroi, *Greece* **48 D5** 37 55N 23 9 E
Áyion Óros □, *Greece* **51 F8** 40 25N 24 6 E
Áyios Amvrósios, *Cyprus* **39 E9** 35 20N 33 35 E
Áyios Andréas, *Greece* **48 D4** 37 21N 22 45 E
Áyios Evstrátios, *Greece* **48 B6** 39 34N 24 58 E
Áyios Ioánnis, Ákra, *Greece* **39 E6** 35 20N 25 40 E
Áyios Isidhoros, *Greece* **38 E11** 36 9N 27 51 E
Áyios Kiríkos, *Greece* **49 D8** 37 34N 26 17 E
Áyios Léon, *Greece* **39 D2** 37 47N 20 43 E
Áyios Matthaíos, *Greece* **38 C9** 39 30N 19 47 E
Áyios Mírono, *Greece* **39 E6** 35 15N 25 1 E
Áyios Nikólaos, *Aitolía kai Akarnanía, Greece* **39 B2** 38 52N 20 48 E
Áyios Nikólaos, *Kríti, Greece* **39 E6** 35 11N 25 41 E
Áyios Nikólaos, *Levkás, Greece* **39 B2** 38 36N 20 34 E
Áyios Pétros, *Greece* **39 B2** 38 40N 20 36 E
Áyios Seryios, *Cyprus* **39 E9** 35 12N 33 53 E
Áyios Theodhoros, *Cyprus* **39 E10** 35 22N 34 1 E
Áyios Thomás, *Greece* **39 B2** 38 58N 20 47 E
Áyios Yeóryios, *Greece* **48 D5** 37 28N 23 57 E
Aykathonisi, *Greece* **49 D8** 37 28N 27 0 E
Aykino, *Russia* **56 B8** 62 15N 49 56 E
Aykirikçi, *Turkey* **49 B12** 39 8N 30 9 E
Aylesbury, *U.K.* **21 F7** 51 49N 0 49W
Aylmer, *Canada* **150 D4** 42 46N 80 59W
Aylmer, L., *Canada* **138 B8** 64 0N 110 8W
'Ayn, Wādī al, *Oman* **97 F7** 22 15N 55 28 E
'Ayn al Ghazālah, *Libya* **108 B4** 32 10N 23 20 E
Ayn Dār, *Si. Arabia* **97 E7** 25 55N 49 10 E
Ayn Zālah, *Iraq* **101 D10** 36 45N 42 35 E
Ayna, *Spain* **41 G2** 38 34N 2 3W
Aynabulaq, *Kazakhstan* **65 A8** 44 36N 77 56 E
Aynāt, *Yemen* **99 C5** 16 4N 49 9 E
Ayni, *Tajikistan* **65 D4** 39 23N 68 32 E
Ayod, *Sudan* **107 F3** 8 7N 31 26 E
Ayolas, *Paraguay* **174 B4** 27 10 S 56 59W
Ayom, *Sudan* **107 F2** 7 49N 28 23 E
Ayon, Ostrov, *Russia* **67 C17** 69 50N 169 0 E
Ayora, *Spain* **41 F3** 39 3N 1 3W
Ayorou, *Niger* **113 C5** 14 53N 1 0 E
Ayos, *Cameroon* **114 B2** 3 53N 12 31 E
'Ayoûn el 'Atroûs, *Mauritania* **112 B3** 16 38N 9 37W
Ayr, *Australia* **126 B4** 19 35 S 147 25 E
Ayr, *Canada* **150 C4** 43 17N 80 27W
Ayr, *U.K.* **22 F4** 55 28N 4 38W
Ayr →, *U.K.* **22 F4** 55 28N 4 38W
Ayrancı, *Turkey* **100 D5** 37 21N 33 41 E
Ayrancılar, *Turkey* **49 C9** 38 15N 27 18 E
Ayre, Pt. of, *I. of Man* **20 C3** 54 25N 4 21W
Aysha, *Ethiopia* **107 E5** 10 50N 42 23 E
Ayton, *Australia* **126 B4** 15 56 S 145 22 E
Aytos, *Bulgaria* **51 D11** 42 42N 27 16 E
Aytoska Planina, *Bulgaria* **51 D11** 42 45N 27 30 E
Ayu, Kepulauan, *Indonesia* **83 A4** 0 35N 131 5 E
Ayutla, *Guatemala* **164 D1** 14 40N 92 10W
Ayutla, *Mexico* **163 D5** 16 58N 99 17W
Ayvacık, *Turkey* **100 C2** 39 36N 26 24 E
Ayvalık, *Turkey* **49 B8** 39 20N 26 46 E
Az Zabadānī, *Syria* **103 B5** 33 43N 36 5 E
Az Ẓahirāh, *Asia* **99 B7** 23 40N 56 10 E
Az Ẓāhirīyah, *West Bank* **103 D3** 31 25N 34 58 E
Az Ẓahrān, *Si. Arabia* **97 E6** 26 10N 50 7 E
Az Zarqā, *Jordan* **103 C5** 32 5N 36 4 E
Az Zarqā', *U.A.E.* **97 E7** 24 53N 53 4 E
Az Zarqā □, *Jordan* **103 C5** 32 5N 36 4 E
Az Zāwiyah, *Libya* **108 B2** 32 52N 12 56 E
Az Zaydīyah, *Yemen* **98 D3** 15 20N 43 1 E
Az Zībār, *Iraq* **101 D11** 36 52N 44 4 E
Az Zilfī, *Si. Arabia* **96 E5** 26 12N 44 52 E
Az Zubayr, *Iraq* **96 D5** 30 26N 47 40 E
Az Zuqur, *Yemen* **98 D3** 14 0N 42 45 E
Az Zuwaytīnah, *Libya* **108 B4** 30 58N 20 7 E
Azad Kashmir □, *Pakistan* **93 C5** 33 50N 73 50 E
Azambuja, *Portugal* **43 F2** 39 4N 8 51W
Azamgarh, *India* **93 F10** 26 5N 83 13 E
Azangaro, *Peru* **172 C3** 14 55 S 70 13W
Azaoua, *Niger* **113 B5** 15 50N 4 0 E
Azaouad, *Mali* **112 B4** 19 0N 3 0W
Azaouak, Vallée de l', *Mali* **113 B5** 15 50N 3 20 E
Āzār Shahr, *Iran* **101 D11** 37 45N 45 59 E
Azara, *Nigeria* **113 D6** 8 22N 9 12 E
Azarān, *Iran* **101 D12** 37 25N 47 16 E
Azärbayjan = Azerbaijan ■, *Asia* **61 K9** 40 20N 48 0 E
Āzarbāyjān-e Gharbī □, *Iran* **96 B5** 37 0N 44 30 E
Āzarbāyjān-e Sharqī □, *Iran* **96 B5** 37 20N 47 0 E
Azare, *Nigeria* **113 C7** 11 55N 10 10 E
Azay-le-Rideau, *France* **26 E7** 47 16N 0 30 E
A'zāz, *Syria* **100 D7** 36 36N 37 4 E
Azazga, *Algeria* **111 A5** 36 48N 4 22 E
Azbine = Aïr, *Niger* **113 B6** 18 30N 8 0 E
Azefal, *Mauritania* **110 D2** 21 0N 14 45W
Azeffoun, *Algeria* **111 A5** 36 51N 4 26 E
Azemmour, *Morocco* **110 B3** 33 20N 9 20W
Azennezal, *Algeria* **111 D5** 22 58N 0 43 E
Azerbaijan ■, *Asia* **61 K9** 40 20N 48 0 E
Azerbaijchan = Azerbaijan ■, *Asia* **61 K9** 40 20N 48 0 E
Azezo, *Ethiopia* **107 E4** 12 28N 37 15 E
Azimganj, *India* **93 G13** 24 14N 88 16 E
Aznalcóllar, *Spain* **43 H4** 37 32N 6 17W
Azogues, *Ecuador* **168 D2** 2 35 S 78 0W
Azores = Açores, Is. dos, *Atl. Oc.* **8 C9** 38 0N 27 0W
Azores-Biscay Rise, *Atl. Oc.* **8 B9** 42 0N 20 0W
Azoum, B. →, *Chad* **109 F4** 10 53N 20 15 E
Azov, *Russia* **61 G4** 47 3N 39 25 E
Azov, Sea of, *Europe* **59 J9** 46 0N 36 30 E
Azovskoye More = Azov, Sea of, *Europe* **59 J9** 46 0N 36 30 E
Azpeitia, *Spain* **40 B2** 43 12N 2 19W
Azrak, B. →, *Chad* **109 F4** 10 52N 20 35 E
Azraq ash Shīshān, *Jordan* **103 D5** 31 50N 36 49 E
Azrou, *Morocco* **110 B3** 33 28N 5 19W
Aztec, *U.S.A.* **159 H10** 36 49N 107 59W
Azúa de Compostela, *Dom. Rep.* **165 C5** 18 25N 70 44W
Azuaga, *Spain* **43 G5** 38 16N 5 39W
Azuara, *Spain* **40 D4** 41 15N 0 53W
Azuay □, *Ecuador* **168 D2** 2 55 S 79 0W
Azuer →, *Spain* **43 F7** 39 8N 3 36W
Azuero, Pen. de, *Panama* **164 E3** 7 30N 80 30W
Azuga, *Romania* **53 E10** 45 27N 25 33 E
Azul, *Argentina* **174 D4** 36 42 S 59 43W
Azul, Lagoa, *Azores* **9 d3** 37 52N 25 47W
Azul, Serra, *Brazil* **173 C7** 14 50 S 54 50W
Azurduy, *Bolivia* **173 D5** 19 59 S 64 29W
Azusa, *U.S.A.* **161 L9** 34 8N 117 52W
Azzaba, *Algeria* **111 A6** 36 48N 7 6 E
Azzano Décimo, *Italy* **45 C9** 45 52N 12 56 E
Azzel Mati, Sebkra, *Algeria* **111 C5** 26 10N 0 43 E

B

Ba Be △, *Vietnam* **86 A5** 22 25N 105 37 E
Ba Don, *Vietnam* **86 D6** 17 45N 106 26 E
Ba Dong, *Vietnam* **87 H6** 9 40N 106 33 E
Ba Ngoi = Cam Lam, *Vietnam* **87 G7** 11 54N 109 10 E
Ba Tri, *Vietnam* **87 G6** 10 2N 106 36 E
Ba Vi △, *Vietnam* **86 B5** 21 1N 105 22 E
Ba Xian = Bazhou, *China* **74 E9** 39 8N 116 22 E
Baa, *Indonesia* **82 D2** 10 50 S 123 0 E
Baaba, Î., *N. Cal.* **133 T18** 20 3 S 163 59 E
Baamonde, *Spain* **42 B3** 43 7N 7 44W
Baao, *Phil.* **80 E4** 13 27N 123 22 E
Baar, *Switz.* **33 B7** 47 12N 8 32 E
Baardeere = Bardera, *Somali Rep.* **120 D2** 2 20N 42 27 E
Baarle-Nassau, *Belgium* **24 C4** 51 27N 4 56 E
Bab el Mandeb, *Red Sea* **98 D3** 12 35N 43 25 E
Baba, *Bulgaria* **50 D7** 42 44N 23 59 E
Bābā, Koh-i-, *Afghan.* **91 B2** 34 30N 67 0 E
Baba Budan Hills, *India* **95 H2** 13 30N 75 44 E
Baba Burnu, *Turkey* **49 B8** 39 29N 26 2 E
Baba dag, *Azerbaijan* **61 K9** 41 0N 48 19 E
Bābā Kalū, *Iran* **97 D6** 30 7N 50 49 E
Babaçulândia, *Brazil* **170 C2** 7 13 S 47 46W
Babadag, *Romania* **53 F13** 44 53N 28 44 E
Babadağ, *Turkey* **49 D10** 37 49N 28 52 E
Babaeski, *Turkey* **51 E11** 41 26N 27 6 E
Babahoyo, *Ecuador* **168 D2** 1 40 S 79 30W
Babai = Sarju →, *India* **93 F9** 27 21N 81 23 E
Babak, *Phil.* **81 H5** 7 8N 125 41 E
Babana, *Nigeria* **113 C5** 10 31N 3 46 E
Babanusa, *Sudan* **107 E2** 11 20N 27 48 E
Babar, *Algeria* **111 A6** 35 10N 7 6 E
Babar, *Indonesia* **83 C3** 8 0 S 129 30 E
Babar, *Pakistan* **92 D3** 31 7N 69 32 E
Babar, Kepulauan, *Indonesia* **83 C4** 8 0 S 131 30 E
Babarkach, *Pakistan* **92 E3** 29 45N 68 0 E
Babase I., *Papua N. G.* **132 B7** 4 0 S 153 42 E
Babayevo, *Russia* **58 C8** 59 24N 35 55 E
Babb, *U.S.A.* **158 B7** 48 51N 113 27W
Babenhausen, *Germany* **31 F4** 49 57N 8 57 E
Băbeni, *Romania* **53 F9** 44 59N 24 11 E
Baberu, *India* **93 G9** 25 33N 80 43 E
Babi Besar, Pulau, *Malaysia* **87 L4** 2 25N 103 59 E
Babia Gora, *Europe* **55 J6** 49 38N 19 38 E
Babian Jiang →, *China* **76 F3** 22 55N 101 47 E
Babīl □, *Iraq* **96 C5** 32 30N 44 30 E
Babile, *Ethiopia* **107 F5** 9 16N 42 11 E
Babile ⌂, *Ethiopia* **120 C2** 8 45N 42 20 E
Babimost, *Poland* **55 F2** 52 10N 15 49 E
Babinda, *Australia* **126 B4** 17 20 S 145 56 E
Babine, *Canada* **142 B3** 55 22N 126 37W
Babine →, *Canada* **142 B3** 55 45N 127 44W
Babine L., *Canada* **142 C3** 54 48N 126 0W
Babiogórski △, *Poland* **55 J6** 49 38N 19 39 E
Babo, *Indonesia* **83 B4** 2 30 S 133 30 E
Babócsa, *Hungary* **52 D2** 46 2N 17 21 E
Bābol, *Iran* **97 B7** 36 40N 52 50 E
Bābol Sar, *Iran* **97 B7** 36 45N 52 45 E
Babor, Dj., *Algeria* **111 A6** 36 31N 5 25 E
Baborów, *Poland* **55 H5** 50 7N 18 1 E
Baboua, *C.A.R.* **114 A2** 5 49N 14 58 E
Babruysk, *Belarus* **59 F5** 53 10N 29 15 E
Babson Park, *U.S.A.* **153 H8** 27 49N 81 32W
Babuhri, *India* **92 F3** 26 49N 69 43 E
Babuna, *Macedonia* **50 E5** 41 30N 21 40 E
Babura, *Nigeria* **113 C6** 12 51N 8 59 E
Babusar Pass, *Pakistan* **93 B5** 35 12N 73 59 E
Babušnica, *Serbia & M.* **50 C6** 43 7N 22 27 E
Babuyan, *Phil.* **81 F2** 10 0N 118 54 E
Babuyan Chan., *Phil.* **80 B3** 18 40N 121 30 E
Babuyan I., *Phil.* **80 B3** 19 32N 121 57 E
Babuyan Is., *Phil.* **80 B3** 19 10N 121 40 E
Babylon, *Iraq* **101 F11** 32 34N 44 22 E
Bač, *Serbia & M.* **52 E4** 45 29N 19 17 E
Bâc →, *Moldova* **53 D14** 46 55N 29 26 E
Bac Can, *Vietnam* **76 F5** 22 8N 105 49 E
Bac Giang, *Vietnam* **76 G6** 21 16N 106 11 E
Bac Lieu, *Vietnam* **87 H5** 9 17N 105 43 E
Bac Ninh, *Vietnam* **76 G6** 21 13N 106 4 E
Bac Phan, *Vietnam* **86 B5** 22 0N 105 0 E
Bac Quang, *Vietnam* **76 F5** 22 30N 104 48 E
Bacabal, *Brazil* **170 B3** 4 15 S 44 45W
Bacacay, *Phil.* **80 E4** 13 18N 123 47 E
Bacajá →, *Brazil* **169 D7** 3 25 S 51 50W
Bacalar, *Mexico* **163 D7** 18 50N 87 27W
Bacan, *Indonesia* **82 B3** 0 50 S 127 30 E
Bacan, Kepulauan, *Indonesia* **82 B3** 0 35 S 127 30 E
Bacarra, *Phil.* **80 B3** 18 15N 120 37 E
Bacău, *Romania* **53 D11** 46 35N 26 55 E
Bacău □, *Romania* **53 D11** 46 30N 26 45 E
Baccarat, *France* **27 D13** 48 28N 6 42 E
Bacchus Marsh, *Australia* **128 D6** 37 43 S 144 27 E
Bacerac, *Mexico* **162 A3** 30 18N 108 50W
Băceşti, *Romania* **53 D12** 46 50N 27 11 E
Bach, *Austria* **33 B10** 47 16N 10 25 E
Bach Long Vi, Dao, *Vietnam* **86 B6** 20 10N 107 40 E
Bach Ma △, *Vietnam* **86 D6** 16 11N 107 49 E
Bachaquero, *Venezuela* **168 B3** 9 56N 71 8W
Bacharach, *Germany* **31 E3** 50 3N 7 44 E
Bachhwara, *India* **93 G11** 25 35N 85 54 E
Bachuma, *Ethiopia* **107 F4** 6 48N 35 53 E
Bačina, *Serbia & M.* **50 C5** 43 42N 21 23 E
Back →, *Canada* **138 B9** 65 10N 104 0W
Bačka Palanka, *Serbia & M.* **52 E4** 45 17N 19 27 E
Bačka Topola, *Serbia & M.* **52 E4** 45 49N 19 39 E
Bäckebo, *Sweden* **17 H10** 56 53N 16 4 E
Bäckefors, *Sweden* **17 F6** 58 48N 12 9 E
Bäckhammar, *Sweden* **16 E8** 59 10N 14 11 E
Bački Petrovac, *Serbia & M.* **52 E4** 45 29N 19 32 E
Backnang, *Germany* **31 G5** 48 56N 9 26 E
Backstairs Passage, *Australia* **128 C3** 35 40 S 138 5 E
Baco, Mt., *Phil.* **80 E3** 12 49N 121 10 E
Bacolod, *Phil.* **81 F4** 10 40N 122 57 E
Bacon, *Phil.* **80 E5** 13 3N 124 3 E
Baconton, *U.S.A.* **152 D5** 31 23N 84 10W
Bacoor, *Phil.* **80 D3** 14 28N 120 56 E
Bacqueville-en-Caux, *France* **26 C8** 49 47N 1 0 E
Bács-Kiskun □, *Hungary* **52 D4** 46 43N 19 30 E
Bácsalmás, *Hungary* **52 D4** 46 8N 19 17 E
Bacuag = Placer, *Phil.* **81 G5** 9 36N 125 38 E
Bacuit = El Nido, *Phil.* **81 F2** 11 10N 119 25 E
Bacuk, *Malaysia* **87 J4** 6 4N 102 25 E
Bād, *Iran* **97 C7** 33 41N 52 1 E
Bad →, *U.S.A.* **154 C4** 44 21N 100 22W
Bad Aussee, *Austria* **34 D6** 47 43N 13 45 E
Bad Axe, *U.S.A.* **150 C2** 43 48N 83 0W
Bad Bergzabern, *Germany* **31 F3** 49 6N 7 59 E
Bad Berleburg, *Germany* **30 D4** 51 2N 8 26 E
Bad Bevensen, *Germany* **30 B6** 53 5N 10 35 E
Bad Bramstedt, *Germany* **30 B5** 53 55N 9 53 E
Bad Brückenau, *Germany* **31 E5** 50 18N 9 47 E
Bad Doberan, *Germany* **30 A7** 54 6N 11 53 E
Bad Driburg, *Germany* **30 D5** 51 43N 9 1 E
Bad Ems, *Germany* **31 E3** 50 20N 7 43 E
Bad Frankenhausen, *Germany* **30 D7** 51 21N 11 5 E
Bad Freienwalde, *Germany* **30 C10** 52 46N 14 1 E
Bad Goisern, *Austria* **34 D6** 47 38N 13 38 E
Bad Harzburg, *Germany* **30 D6** 51 52N 10 34 E
Bad Hersfeld, *Germany* **30 E5** 50 52N 9 42 E
Bad Hofgastein, *Austria* **34 D6** 47 17N 13 6 E
Bad Homburg, *Germany* **31 E4** 50 13N 8 38 E
Bad Honnef, *Germany* **30 E3** 50 38N 7 13 E
Bad Iburg, *Germany* **30 C4** 52 10N 8 3 E
Bad Ischl, *Austria* **34 D6** 47 44N 13 38 E
Bad Kissingen, *Germany* **31 E6** 50 11N 10 4 E
Bad Königshofen, *Germany* **31 E6** 50 17N 10 28 E
Bad Kreuznach, *Germany* **31 F3** 49 50N 7 51 E
Bad Krozingen, *Germany* **31 H3** 47 54N 7 42 E
Bad Kudowa = Kudowa-Zdrój, *Poland* **55 H3** 50 27N 16 15 E
Bad Laasphe, *Germany* **30 E4** 50 56N 8 25 E
Bad Landeck = Lądek-Zdrój, *Poland* **55 H3** 50 21N 16 53 E
Bad Langensalza, *Germany* **30 D6** 51 5N 10 38 E
Bad Lauterberg, *Germany* **30 D6** 51 38N 10 28 E
Bad Leonfelden, *Austria* **34 C7** 48 31N 14 18 E
Bad Liebenwerda, *Germany* **30 D9** 51 31N 13 24 E
Bad Mergentheim, *Germany* **31 F5** 49 28N 9 42 E
Bad Münstereifel, *Germany* **30 E2** 50 33N 6 46 E
Bad Nauheim, *Germany* **31 E4** 50 21N 8 43 E
Bad Neuenahr-Ahrweiler, *Germany* **30 E3** 50 32N 7 5 E
Bad Neustadt, *Germany* **31 E6** 50 18N 10 13 E
Bad Oeynhausen, *Germany* **30 C4** 52 12N 8 46 E
Bad Oldesloe, *Germany* **30 B6** 53 48N 10 22 E
Bad Orb, *Germany* **31 E5** 50 12N 9 22 E
Bad Polzin = Polanica-Zdrój, *Poland* **55 H3** 50 24N 16 32 E
Bad Pyrmont, *Germany* **30 D5** 51 59N 9 16 E
Bad Ragaz, *Switz.* **33 C9** 47 0N 9 30 E
Bad Reichenhall, *Germany* **31 H8** 47 43N 12 54 E
Bad Reinerz = Duszniki-Zdrój, *Poland* **55 H3** 50 24N 16 24 E
Bad Säckingen, *Germany* **31 H3** 47 33N 7 56 E
Bad Salzuflen, *Germany* **30 C4** 52 5N 8 45 E
Bad Salzungen, *Germany* **30 E6** 50 48N 10 14 E
Bad Schönfliess = Trzcińsko Zdrój, *Poland* **55 F1** 52 58N 14 35 E
Bad Schwartau, *Germany* **30 B6** 53 55N 10 41 E
Bad Segeberg, *Germany* **30 B6** 53 56N 10 17 E
Bad St. Leonhard, *Austria* **34 E7** 46 58N 14 47 E
Bad Tölz, *Germany* **31 H7** 47 45N 11 34 E
Bad Urach, *Germany* **31 G5** 48 29N 9 23 E
Bad Vöslau, *Austria* **35 D9** 47 58N 16 12 E
Bad Waldsee, *Germany* **31 H5** 47 55N 9 45 E
Bad Wildungen, *Germany* **30 D5** 51 6N 9 7 E
Bad Wimpfen, *Germany* **31 F5** 49 13N 9 11 E
Bad Windsheim, *Germany* **31 F6** 49 36N 10 25 E
Bad Zwischenahn, *Germany* **30 B4** 53 12N 8 1 E
Bada Barabil, *India* **93 H11** 22 7N 85 24 E
Badagara, *India* **95 J2** 11 35N 75 40 E
Badagri, *Nigeria* **113 D5** 6 25N 2 55 E
Badajós, L., *Brazil* **169 D5** 3 15 S 62 50W
Badajoz, *Spain* **43 G4** 38 50N 6 59W
Badajoz □, *Spain* **43 G4** 38 40N 6 30W
Badakhshān □, *Afghan.* **65 E5** 36 30N 71 0 E
Badalona, *Spain* **40 D7** 41 26N 2 15 E
Badalzai, *Afghan.* **92 E1** 29 50N 65 35 E
Badami, *India* **95 G2** 15 55N 75 41 E
Badampahar, *India* **94 C8** 22 10N 86 10 E
Badanah, *Si. Arabia* **96 D4** 30 58N 41 30 E
Badarinath, *India* **93 D8** 30 45N 79 30 E
Badarpur, *India* **90 C4** 24 54N 92 36 E
Badas, Kepulauan, *Indonesia* **84 B3** 0 45N 107 5 E
Baddo →, *Pakistan* **91 D2** 28 0N 64 20 E
Bade, *Indonesia* **83 C5** 7 10 S 139 35 E
Badeggi, *Nigeria* **113 D6** 9 1N 6 8 E
Badéguichéri, *Niger* **113 C6** 14 30N 5 22 E
Baden, *Austria* **35 C9** 48 1N 16 13 E
Baden, *Switz.* **33 B6** 47 28N 8 18 E
Baden, *U.S.A.* **150 F4** 40 38N 80 14W
Baden-Baden, *Germany* **31 G4** 48 44N 8 13 E
Baden-Württemberg □, *Germany* **31 G4** 48 20N 8 40 E
Badgastein, *Austria* **34 D6** 47 7N 13 9 E
Badger, *Canada* **141 C8** 49 0N 56 4W
Badger, *U.S.A.* **160 J7** 36 38N 119 1W
Bādghīs □, *Afghan.* **91 B1** 35 0N 63 0 E
Badgingarra △, *Australia* **125 F2** 30 23 S 115 22 E
Badgom, *India* **93 B6** 34 1N 74 45 E
Badia Polésine, *Italy* **45 C8** 45 6N 11 29 E
Badian, *Phil.* **81 G4** 9 55N 123 24 E
Badiar △, *Guinea* **112 C2** 12 30N 13 11W
Badin, *Pakistan* **91 D3** 24 38N 68 54 E
Badinka ⌂, *Mali* **112 C3** 13 31N 9 28W
Badjokola, *Dem. Rep. of the Congo* **114 B4** 3 54N 20 17 E
Badlands, *U.S.A.* **154 D3** 43 40N 102 10W
Badlands △, *U.S.A.* **154 D3** 43 38N 102 56W

Badnera, *India* **94 D3** 20 48N 77 44 E
Badoc, *Phil.* **80 C3** 17 56N 120 28 E
Badogo, *Mali* **112 C3** 11 2N 8 13W
Badoumbé, *Mali* **112 C2** 13 42N 10 15W
Badr Ḩunayn, *Si. Arabia* **98 B2** 23 44N 38 46 E
Badrah, *Iraq* **101 F11** 33 6N 45 58 E
Badrinath, *India* **93 D8** 30 44N 79 29 E
Badu I., *Papua N. G.* **132 F2** 10 5 S 142 10 E
Baduen, *Somali Rep.* **120 C3** 7 15N 47 40 E
Badulla, *Sri Lanka* **95 L5** 7 1N 81 7 E
Badung, Selat, *Indonesia* **79 K18** 8 40 S 115 22 E
Badupi, *Burma* **90 E4** 21 36N 93 27 E
Badvel, *India* **95 G4** 14 45N 79 3 E
Baena, *Spain* **43 H6** 37 37N 4 20W
Baerami, *Australia* **129 B9** 32 27 S 150 27 E
Baetov, *Kyrgyzstan* **65 C7** 41 13N 74 54 E
Baeza, *Ecuador* **168 D2** 0 25 S 77 53W
Baeza, *Spain* **43 H7** 37 57N 3 25W
Bafang, *Cameroon* **113 D7** 5 9N 10 11 E
Bafatá, *Guinea-Biss.* **112 C2** 12 8N 14 40W
Baffin B., *Canada* **139 A13** 72 0N 64 0W
Baffin I., *Canada* **139 B12** 68 0N 75 0W
Bafia, *Cameroon* **113 E7** 4 40N 11 10 E
Bafilo, *Togo* **113 D5** 9 22N 1 22 E
Bafing △, *Mali* **112 C2** 12 38N 10 28W
Bafing →, *Mali* **112 C2** 13 49N 10 50W
Bafliyūn, *Syria* **96 B3** 36 37N 36 59 E
Bafoulabé, *Mali* **112 C2** 13 50N 10 55W
Bafoussam, *Cameroon* **113 D7** 5 28N 10 25 E
Bāfq, *Iran* **97 D7** 31 40N 55 25 E
Bafra, *Turkey* **100 B6** 41 34N 35 54 E
Bafra Burnu, *Turkey* **100 B7** 41 45N 36 2 E
Bāft, *Iran* **97 D8** 29 15N 56 38 E
Bafut, *Cameroon* **113 D7** 6 6N 10 2 E
Bafwasende, *Dem. Rep. of the Congo* **118 B2** 1 3N 27 5 E
Bagaat, Î., *N. Cal.* **133 K4** 20 40 S 166 15 E
Bagabag, *Phil.* **80 C3** 16 30N 121 15 E
Bagabag I., *Papua N. G.* **132 C4** 4 48 S 146 14 E
Bagac, *Phil.* **80 D3** 14 36N 120 23 E
Bagac Bay, *Phil.* **80 D3** 14 36N 120 20 E
Bagalkot, *India* **95 F2** 16 10N 75 40 E
Bagam, *Niger* **113 B6** 15 43N 6 35 E
Bagamanoc, *Phil.* **80 E5** 13 57N 124 17 E
Bagamoyo, *Tanzania* **118 D4** 6 28 S 38 55 E
Bagan Datoh, *Malaysia* **87 L3** 3 59N 100 47 E
Bagan Serai, *Malaysia* **87 K3** 5 1N 100 32 E
Baganga, *Phil.* **81 H6** 7 34N 126 33 E
Bagani, *Namibia* **116 B3** 18 7 S 21 41 E
Bagansiapiapi, *Indonesia* **84 B2** 2 12N 100 50 E
Bagasra, *India* **92 J4** 21 30N 71 0 E
Bagata, *Dem. Rep. of the Congo* **114 C3** 3 44 S 17 57 E
Bagaud, *India* **92 H6** 22 19N 75 53 E
Bagawi, *Sudan* **107 E3** 12 20N 34 18 E
Bagbag, *Sudan* **107 D3** 15 23N 31 30 E
Bagdad, *Calif., U.S.A.* **161 L11** 34 35N 115 53W
Bagdad, *Fla., U.S.A.* **153 E2** 30 36N 87 2W
Bagdarin, *Russia* **67 D12** 54 26N 113 36 E
Bagé, *Brazil* **175 C5** 31 20 S 54 15W
Bagenalstown = Muine Bheag, *Ireland* **23 D5** 52 42N 6 58W
Bagepalli, *India* **95 H3** 13 47N 77 47 E
Bagevadi, *India* **94 F2** 16 35N 75 58 E
Baggao, *Phil.* **80 C3** 17 56N 121 46 E
Baggs, *U.S.A.* **158 F10** 41 2N 107 39W
Bagh, *Pakistan* **93 C5** 33 59N 73 45 E
Baghain →, *India* **93 G9** 25 32N 81 1 E
Baghdād, *Iraq* **101 F11** 33 20N 44 30 E
Bagherhat, *Bangla.* **90 D2** 22 40N 89 47 E
Bagheria, *Italy* **46 D6** 38 5N 13 30 E
Baghlān, *Afghan.* **91 A3** 32 12N 68 46 E
Baghlān □, *Afghan.* **91 B3** 36 0N 68 30 E
Bagley, *U.S.A.* **154 B7** 47 32N 95 24W
Bagn, *Norway* **18 D6** 60 49N 9 34 E
Bagnara Cálabra, *Italy* **47 D8** 38 17N 15 48 E
Bagnasco, *Italy* **44 D5** 44 18N 8 2 E
Bagnell Dam, *U.S.A.* **156 F4** 38 14N 92 36W
Bagnères-de-Bigorre, *France* **28 E4** 43 5N 0 9 E
Bagnères-de-Luchon, *France* **28 F4** 42 47N 0 38 E
Bagni di Lucca, *Italy* **44 D7** 44 1N 10 35 E
Bagno di Romagna, *Italy* **45 E8** 43 50N 11 57 E
Bagnoles-de-l'Orne, *France* **26 D6** 48 32N 0 25W
Bagnols-sur-Cèze, *France* **29 D8** 44 10N 4 36 E
Bagnorea = Bagnorégio, *Italy* **45 F9** 42 37N 12 5 E
Bagnorégio, *Italy* **45 F9** 42 37N 12 5 E
Bago = Pegu, *Burma* **90 G6** 17 20N 96 29 E
Bago, *Phil.* **81 F4** 10 32N 122 50 E
Bagodar, *India* **93 G11** 24 5N 85 52 E
Bagrationovsk, *Russia* **15 J19** 54 23N 20 39 E
Bagrdan, *Serbia & M.* **50 B5** 44 5N 21 11 E
Bagua, *Peru* **172 B2** 5 35 S 78 22W
Baguio, *Phil.* **80 C3** 16 26N 120 34 E
Bağyurdu, *Turkey* **49 C9** 38 25N 27 41 E
Bagzane, Monts, *Niger* **113 B6** 17 43N 8 45 E
Bah, *India* **93 F8** 26 53N 78 36 E
Bahabón de Esgueva, *Spain* **42 D7** 41 52N 3 43W
Bahadurabad Ghat, *Bangla.* **90 C2** 25 11N 89 44 E
Bahadurganj, *India* **93 F12** 26 16N 87 49 E
Bahadurgarh, *India* **92 E7** 28 40N 76 57 E
Bahama, Canal Viejo de, *W. Indies* **164 B4** 22 10N 77 30W
Bahamas ■, *N. Amer.* **165 B5** 24 0N 75 0W
Bahār, *Iran* **101 E13** 34 54N 48 26 E
Bahārak, *Afghan.* **65 E5** 37 0N 70 53 E
Baharampur, *India* **93 G13** 24 2N 88 27 E
Baharîya, El Wâhât al, *Egypt* **106 B2** 28 0N 28 50 E
Baharu Pandan = Pandan, *Malaysia* **87 d** 1 32N 103 46 E
Bahawalnagar, *Pakistan* **91 C4** 30 0N 73 15 E
Bahawalpur, *Pakistan* **91 C3** 29 24N 71 40 E
Bahçe, *Turkey* **100 D7** 37 13N 36 34 E
Bahçecik, *Turkey* **51 F13** 40 41N 29 44 E
Baheli, *Phil.* **81 F2** 10 0N 118 47 E
Baheri, *India* **93 E8** 28 45N 79 34 E
Bahgul →, *India* **93 F8** 27 45N 79 36 E
Bahi, *Tanzania* **118 D4** 5 58 S 35 21 E
Bahi Swamp, *Tanzania* **118 D4** 6 10 S 35 0 E
Bahía = Salvador, *Brazil* **171 D4** 13 0 S 38 30W
Bahía □, *Brazil* **171 D3** 12 0 S 42 0W
Bahía, Is. de la, *Honduras* **164 C2** 16 45N 86 15W
Bahía Blanca, *Argentina* **174 D3** 38 35 S 62 13W
Bahía de Caráquez, *Ecuador* **168 D1** 0 40 S 80 27W
Bahía Honda, *Cuba* **164 B3** 22 54N 83 10W
Bahía Laura, *Argentina* **176 C3** 48 10 S 66 30W
Bahía Mansa, *Chile* **176 B2** 40 33 S 73 46W
Bahía Negra, *Paraguay* **173 E6** 20 5 S 58 5W
Bahir Dar, *Ethiopia* **107 E4** 11 37N 37 10 E
Bahlah, *Oman* **99 B7** 22 58N 57 18 E
Bahmanzād, *Iran* **97 D6** 31 15N 51 47 E
Bahmer, *Algeria* **111 C4** 27 32N 0 10W
Bahr el Ahmar □, *Sudan* **106 D4** 20 0N 35 0 E
Bahr el Ghazâl □, *Sudan* **107 F2** 7 0N 28 0 E
Bahr el Jabal □, *Sudan* **107 G3** 4 0N 31 0 E
Bahraich, *India* **93 F9** 27 38N 81 37 E
Bahrain ■, *Asia* **97 E6** 26 0N 50 35 E
Bahror, *India* **92 F7** 27 51N 76 20 E
Bāhū Kalāt, *Iran* **97 E9** 25 43N 61 25 E
Bai, *Mali* **112 C4** 13 35N 3 28W
Bai Bung, Mui = Ca Mau, Mui, *Vietnam* **87 H5** 8 38N 104 44 E
Bai Duc, *Vietnam* **86 C5** 18 3N 105 49 E
Bai Thuong, *Vietnam* **86 C5** 19 54N 105 23 E
Baia de Aramă, *Romania* **52 E7** 45 0N 22 50 E
Baía dos Tigres, *Angola* **115 F2** 16 40 S 11 47 E
Baia Farta, *Angola* **115 E2** 12 40 S 13 11 E
Baia Mare, *Romania* **53 C8** 47 40N 23 35 E
Baia-Sprie, *Romania* **53 C8** 47 41N 23 43 E
Baião, *Brazil* **170 B2** 2 40 S 49 40W
Baïbokoum, *Chad* **109 G3** 7 46N 15 43 E
Baicheng, *China* **75 B12** 45 38N 122 42 E
Băicoi, *Romania* **53 E10** 45 3N 25 52 E
Baidoa, *Somali Rep.* **120 D2** 3 8N 43 30 E
Baie-Comeau, *Canada* **141 C6** 49 12N 68 10W
Baie-St-Paul, *Canada* **141 C5** 47 28N 70 32W
Baie Ste-Anne, *Seychelles* **121 b** 4 18 S 55 45 E
Baie-Trinité, *Canada* **141 C6** 49 25N 67 20W
Baie Verte, *Canada* **141 C8** 49 55N 56 12W
Baignes-Ste-Radegonde, *France* **28 C3** 45 23N 0 25W
Baigneux-les-Juifs, *France* **27 E11** 47 31N 4 39 E
Baihar, *India* **93 H9** 22 6N 80 33 E
Baihe, *China* **74 H6** 32 50N 110 5 E
Baijnath, *India* **93 E8** 29 55N 79 37 E
Baikal, L. = Baykal, Oz., *Russia* **67 D11** 53 0N 108 0 E
Baikunthpur, *India* **93 H10** 23 15N 82 33 E
Bailadila, Mt., *India* **94 E5** 18 43N 81 15 E
Baile Atha Cliath = Dublin, *Ireland* **23 C5** 53 21N 6 15W
Băile Govora, *Romania* **53 E9** 45 5N 24 11 E
Băile Herculane, *Romania* **52 F7** 44 53N 22 26 E
Băile Olăneşti, *Romania* **53 E9** 45 12N 24 14 E
Băile Tuşnad, *Romania* **53 D10** 46 9N 25 51 E
Bailén, *Spain* **43 G7** 38 8N 3 48W
Băileşti, *Romania* **53 F8** 44 1N 23 20 E
Bailhongal, *India* **95 G2** 15 55N 74 53 E
Bailique, Ilha, *Brazil* **170 A2** 1 2N 49 58W
Bailugh, *Afghan.* **91 B2** 32 40N 66 47 E
Bailundo = Luau, *Angola* **115 E4** 10 40 S 22 10 E
Bailundo, *Angola* **115 E3** 12 10 S 15 50 E
Baima, *China* **76 A3** 33 0N 100 26 E
Baimuru, *Papua N. G.* **132 D3** 7 35 S 144 51 E
Bain-de-Bretagne, *France* **26 E5** 47 50N 1 40W
Bainbridge, *Ga., U.S.A.* **152 E5** 30 55N 84 35W
Bainbridge, *Ind., U.S.A.* **157 E10** 39 46N 86 49W
Bainbridge, *N.Y., U.S.A.* **151 D9** 42 18N 75 29W
Bainbridge, *Ohio, U.S.A.* **157 E13** 39 14N 83 16W
Baing, *Indonesia* **82 D2** 10 14 S 120 34 E
Bainiu, *China* **74 H7** 32 50N 112 15 E
Bainyik, *Papua N. G.* **132 B2** 3 40 S 143 4 E
Baiona, *Spain* **42 C2** 42 6N 8 52W
Bā'ir, *Jordan* **103 E5** 30 45N 36 55 E
Baird Mts., *U.S.A.* **144 C8** 67 0N 160 0W
Bairiki = Tarawa, *Kiribati* **134 G9** 1 30N 173 0 E
Bairin Youqi, *China* **75 C10** 43 30N 118 35 E
Bairin Zuoqi, *China* **75 C10** 43 58N 119 15 E
Bairnsdale, *Australia* **129 D7** 37 48 S 147 36 E
Bais, *Phil.* **81 G4** 9 35N 123 7 E
Baisha, *China* **74 G7** 34 20N 112 32 E
Baissa, *Nigeria* **113 D7** 7 14N 10 38 E
Baitadi, *Nepal* **93 E9** 29 35N 80 25 E
Baitarani →, *India* **94 D8** 20 45N 86 48 E
Baixa Grande, *Brazil* **171 D3** 11 57 S 40 11W
Baixa Limia-Sierra do Xurés ⌓, *Spain* **42 D2** 41 59N 8 2W
Baixo-Longa, *Angola* **115 F3** 15 41 S 18 45 E
Baiyer River, *Papua N. G.* **132 C3** 5 32 S 144 9 E
Baiyin, *China* **74 F3** 36 45N 104 14 E
Baiyü, *China* **76 B2** 31 16N 98 50 E
Baiyu Shan, *China* **74 F4** 37 15N 107 30 E
Baiyuda, *Sudan* **106 D3** 17 35N 32 7 E
Baj Baj, *India* **93 H13** 22 30N 88 5 E
Baja, *Hungary* **52 D3** 46 12N 18 59 E
Baja, Pta., *Chile* **172 b** 27 10 S 109 22W
Baja, Pta., *Mexico* **162 B1** 29 50N 116 0W
Baja California, *Mexico* **162 A1** 31 10N 115 12W
Baja California □, *Mexico* **162 B2** 30 0N 115 0W
Baja California Sur □, *Mexico* **162 B2** 25 50N 111 50W
Bajag, *India* **93 H9** 22 40N 81 21 E
Bajamar, *Canary Is.* **9 e1** 28 33N 16 20W
Bajana, *India* **92 H4** 23 7N 71 49 E
Bajatrejo, *Indonesia* **79 J17** 8 29 S 114 19 E
Bajawa, *Indonesia* **82 C2** 8 47 S 120 59 E
Bajera, *Indonesia* **79 J18** 8 31 S 115 2 E
Bājgīrān, *Iran* **97 B8** 37 36N 58 24 E
Bājil, *Yemen* **98 D3** 15 4N 43 17 E
Bajimba, Mt., *Australia* **127 D5** 29 17 S 152 6 E
Bajina Bašta, *Serbia & M.* **50 C3** 43 58N 19 35 E
Bajmok, *Serbia & M.* **52 E4** 45 57N 19 24 E
Bajo Caracoles, *Argentina* **176 C2** 47 27 S 70 56W
Bajo Nuevo, *Caribbean* **164 C4** 15 40N 78 50W
Bajoga, *Nigeria* **113 C7** 10 57N 11 20 E
Bajool, *Australia* **126 C5** 23 40 S 150 35 E
Bak, *Hungary* **52 D1** 46 43N 16 51 E
Bakal, *Russia* **64 D7** 54 56N 58 48 E
Bakala, *C.A.R.* **114 A4** 6 15N 20 20 E
Bakalsky Zavod = Bakal, *Russia* **64 D7** 54 56N 58 48 E
Bakanas = Baqanas, *Kazakhstan* **65 A8** 44 50N 76 15 E
Bakar, *Croatia* **45 C11** 45 18N 14 32 E
Bakassi Pen., *Cameroon* **113 E6** 4 42N 8 20 E
Bakel, *Senegal* **112 C2** 14 56N 12 20W
Baker, *Calif., U.S.A.* **161 K10** 35 16N 116 4W
Baker, *Fla., U.S.A.* **153 E3** 30 48N 86 41W
Baker, *Mont., U.S.A.* **154 B2** 46 22N 104 17W
Baker, Canal, *Chile* **176 C2** 47 45 S 74 45W
Baker, L., *Canada* **138 B10** 64 0N 96 0W
Baker, Mt., *U.S.A.* **158 B3** 48 50N 121 49W
Baker City, *U.S.A.* **158 D5** 44 47N 117 50W
Baker I., *Pac. Oc.* **134 G10** 0 10N 176 35W
Baker I., *U.S.A.* **142 B2** 55 20N 133 40W
Baker L., *Australia* **125 E4** 26 54 S 126 5 E
Baker Lake, *Canada* **138 B10** 64 20N 96 3W
Bakere, *Dem. Rep. of the Congo* **114 B4** 1 36N 23 50 E
Bakerhill, *U.S.A.* **152 D4** 31 47N 85 18W
Bakers Creek, *Australia* **126 C4** 21 13 S 149 7 E
Bakers Dozen Is., *Canada* **140 A4** 56 45N 78 45W
Bakersfield, *Calif., U.S.A.* **161 K8** 35 23N 119 1W
Bakersfield, *Vt., U.S.A.* **151 B12** 44 45N 72 48W
Bakhchysaray, *Ukraine* **59 K7** 44 40N 33 45 E
Bakhmach, *Ukraine* **59 G7** 51 10N 32 45 E
Bakhmut = Artemovsk, *Ukraine* **59 H9** 48 35N 38 0 E
Bakht, *Uzbekistan* **65 C4** 40 43N 68 42 E
Bākhtarān, *Iran* **101 E12** 34 23N 47 0 E
Bākhtarān □, *Iran* **96 C5** 34 0N 46 30 E
Baki = Krasnyye Baki, *Russia* **60 B7** 57 8N 45 10 E
Bakı, *Azerbaijan* **61 K9** 40 29N 49 56 E
Bakır →, *Turkey* **49 C9** 38 55N 27 0 E
Bakırdaği, *Turkey* **100 C6** 38 13N 35 46 E
Bakkafjörður, *Iceland* **11 A12** 66 2N 14 48W
Bakkaflói, *Iceland* **11 A12** 66 10N 14 45W
Baklan, *Turkey* **49 C11** 38 0N 29 36 E
Bako, *Ethiopia* **107 F4** 5 51N 36 23 E
Bako, *Ivory C.* **112 D3** 9 8N 7 40W
Bakony, *Hungary* **52 C2** 47 10N 17 30 E
Bakony Forest = Bakony, *Hungary* **52 C2** 47 10N 17 30 E
Bakori, *Nigeria* **113 C6** 11 34N 7 25 E
Bakouma, *C.A.R.* **114 A4** 5 40N 22 56 E
Bakpakty = Baqbaqty, *Kazakhstan* **65 A8** 44 35N 76 40 E
Baksan, *Russia* **61 J6** 43 42N 43 32 E
Bakswaho, *India* **93 G8** 24 15N 79 18 E
Baku = Bakı, *Azerbaijan* **61 K9** 40 29N 49 56 E
Bakundi, *Nigeria* **113 D7** 8 2N 10 45 E
Bakutis Coast, *Antarctica* **7 D15** 74 0 S 120 0W
Bakwa-Kenge, *Dem. Rep. of the Congo* **115 C4** 4 51 S 22 4 E
Bakwanga = Mbuji-Mayi, *Dem. Rep. of the Congo* **118 D1** 6 9 S 23 40 E
Baky = Bakı, *Azerbaijan* **61 K9** 40 29N 49 56 E
Bala, *Canada* **150 A5** 45 1N 79 37W
Bala, *Senegal* **112 C2** 14 1N 13 8W
Bâlâ, *Turkey* **100 C5** 39 32N 33 6 E
Bala, *U.K.* **20 E4** 52 54N 3 36W
Bala, L., *U.K.* **20 E4** 52 53N 3 37W
Bālā Morghāb, *Afghan.* **91 B1** 35 35N 63 20 E
Balabac, *Phil.* **81 H1** 7 59N 117 4 E
Balabac I., *Phil.* **81 G1** 8 0N 117 0 E
Balabac Str., *E. Indies* **78 C5** 7 53N 117 5 E
Balabagh, *Afghan.* **92 B4** 34 25N 70 12 E
Ba'labakk, *Lebanon* **103 B5** 34 0N 36 10 E
Balabalangan, Kepulauan, *Indonesia* **85 C5** 2 20 S 117 30 E
Balabio, Î., *N. Cal.* **133 T18** 20 7 S 164 11 E
Bălăciţa, *Romania* **53 F8** 44 23N 23 8 E
Balad, *Iraq* **101 F11** 34 1N 44 9 E
Balad Rūz, *Iraq* **101 F11** 33 42N 45 5 E
Bālādeh, *Fārs, Iran* **97 D6** 29 17N 51 56 E
Bālādeh, *Māzandaran, Iran* **97 B6** 36 12N 51 48 E
Balaghat, *India* **94 D5** 21 49N 80 12 E
Balaghat Ra., *India* **94 E3** 18 50N 76 30 E
Balaguer, *Spain* **40 D5** 41 50N 0 50 E
Balaka, *Dem. Rep. of the Congo* **115 C3** 4 52 S 19 57 E
Balakété, *C.A.R.* **114 A3** 6 56N 19 54 E
Balakhna, *Russia* **60 B6** 56 25N 43 32 E
Balaklava, *Australia* **128 C3** 34 7 S 138 22 E
Balaklava, *Ukraine* **59 K7** 44 30N 33 30 E
Balakliya, *Ukraine* **59 H9** 49 28N 36 55 E
Balakovo, *Russia* **60 D8** 52 4N 47 55 E
Balamau, *India* **93 F9** 27 10N 80 21 E
Balamban, *Phil.* **81 F4** 10 30N 123 43 E
Balambangan, *Malaysia* **85 A5** 7 17N 116 55 E
Bălan, *Romania* **53 D10** 46 39N 25 49 E
Balancán, *Mexico* **163 D6** 17 48N 91 32W
Balanda = Kalininsk, *Russia* **60 E7** 51 30N 44 40 E
Balanga, *Phil.* **80 D3** 14 41N 120 32 E
Balangala, *Dem. Rep. of the Congo* **114 B3** 0 30N 19 56 E
Balangiga, *Phil.* **81 F5** 11 7N 125 23 E
Balangir, *India* **94 D6** 20 43N 83 35 E
Balanivka, *Ukraine* **53 B14** 48 24N 29 24 E
Balaoan, *Phil.* **80 C3** 16 49N 120 24 E
Balapur, *India* **94 D3** 20 40N 76 45 E
Balashov, *Russia* **60 E6** 51 30N 43 10 E
Balasinor, *India* **92 H5** 22 57N 73 23 E
Balasore = Baleshwar, *India* **94 D8** 21 35N 87 3 E
Balassagyarmat, *Hungary* **52 B4** 48 4N 19 15 E
Balât, *Egypt* **106 B2** 25 36N 29 19 E
Balaton, *Hungary* **52 D2** 46 50N 17 40 E
Balaton-Felvidéki △, *Hungary* **52 D2** 46 52N 17 30 E
Balatonboglár, *Hungary* **52 D2** 46 46N 17 40 E
Balatonfüred, *Hungary* **52 D2** 46 58N 17 54 E
Balatonszentgyörgy, *Hungary* **52 D2** 46 41N 17 19 E
Balayan, *Phil.* **80 E3** 13 57N 120 44 E
Balazote, *Spain* **41 G2** 38 54N 2 9W
Balbalan, *Phil.* **80 C3** 17 27N 121 12 E
Balbi, Mt., *Papua N. G.* **132 C8** 5 55 S 154 58 E
Balbieriškis, *Lithuania* **54 D10** 54 32N 23 53 E
Balbigny, *France* **29 C8** 45 49N 4 11 E
Balbina, *Brazil* **169 D6** 1 58 S 59 29W
Balbina, Reprêsa de, *Brazil* **169 D6** 2 0 S 59 30W
Balboa, *Panama* **164 E4** 8 57N 79 34W
Balbriggan, *Ireland* **23 C5** 53 37N 6 11W
Balcarce, *Argentina* **174 D4** 38 0 S 58 10W
Balcarres, *Canada* **143 C8** 50 50N 103 35W
Bălceşti, *Romania* **53 F8** 44 37N 23 57 E
Balchik, *Bulgaria* **51 C12** 43 28N 28 11 E
Balclutha, *N.Z.* **131 G4** 46 15 S 169 45 E
Balcones Escarpment, *U.S.A.* **155 L5** 29 30N 99 15W
Balçova, *Turkey* **49 C9** 38 22N 27 4 E
Bald Hd., *Australia* **125 G2** 35 6 S 118 1 E
Bald I., *Australia* **125 F2** 34 57 S 118 27 E
Bald Knob, *U.S.A.* **155 H9** 35 19N 91 34W
Baldenburg = Biały Bór, *Poland* **54 E3** 53 53N 16 51 E
Baldock L., *Canada* **143 B9** 56 33N 97 57W
Baldwin, *Fla., U.S.A.* **152 E8** 30 18N 81 59W
Baldwin, *Mich., U.S.A.* **148 D3** 43 54N 85 51W
Baldwin, *Pa., U.S.A.* **150 F5** 40 23N 79 59W
Baldwinsville, *U.S.A.* **151 C8** 43 10N 76 20W
Baldy Mt., *U.S.A.* **158 B9** 48 9N 109 39W
Baldy Peak, *U.S.A.* **159 K9** 33 54N 109 34W
Bale, *Croatia* **45 C10** 45 4N 13 46 E
Bale, *Ethiopia* **107 F5** 6 57N 40 8 E
Bale, *Ethiopia* **107 F5** 6 20N 41 30 E
Bale Mts. △, *Ethiopia* **107 F4** 6 59N 39 52 E
Baleares, Is., *Spain* **38 B4** 39 30N 3 0 E
Balearic Is. = Baleares, Is., *Spain* **38 B4** 39 30N 3 0 E
Balease, *Indonesia* **82 B2** 2 24 S 120 33 E
Baleia, Pta. da, *Brazil* **171 E4** 17 40 S 39 7W
Baleine = Whale →, *Canada* **141 A6** 58 15N 67 40W
Baleine, Petite R. de la →, *Canada* **140 A4** 56 0N 76 45W
Băleni, *Romania* **53 E12** 45 48N 27 51 E
Baler, *Phil.* **80 D3** 15 46N 121 34 E
Baler Bay, *Phil.* **80 D3** 15 50N 121 35 E
Balerna, *Switz.* **33 E8** 45 52N 9 0 E
Baleshare, *U.K.* **22 D1** 57 31N 7 22W
Baleshwar, *India* **94 D8** 21 35N 87 3 E
Balestrand, *Norway* **18 C3** 61 11N 6 31 E
Balezino, *Russia* **60 B11** 58 2N 53 6 E
Balfate, *Honduras* **164 C2** 15 48N 86 25W
Balfour Channel, *Solomon Is.* **133 M9** 8 43 S 157 27 E
Balharshah, *India* **94 E4** 19 50N 79 23 E
Bali, *Cameroon* **113 D7** 5 54N 10 0 E
Bali, *Dem. Rep. of the Congo* **114 C3** 2 50 S 16 12 E
Balí, *Greece* **39 E5** 35 25N 24 47 E
Bali, *India* **92 G5** 25 11N 73 17 E
Bali, *Indonesia* **85 D4** 8 20 S 115 0 E
Bali □, *Indonesia* **85 D4** 8 20 S 115 0 E
Bali, Selat, *Indonesia* **85 D4** 8 18 S 114 25 E
Bali Sea, *Indonesia* **85 D5** 8 0 S 115 0 E
Balia, *S. Leone* **112 D2** 9 22N 11 1W
Baliapal, *India* **93 J12** 21 40N 87 17 E
Balicuatro Is., *Phil.* **80 E5** 12 39N 124 24 E
Baliem →, *Indonesia* **83 C5** 5 44 S 138 8 E
Baligród, *Poland* **55 J9** 49 20N 22 17 E
Baliguda, *India* **94 D6** 20 12N 83 55 E
Balik Pulau, *Malaysia* **87 c** 5 21N 100 14 E
Balikeşir, *Turkey* **49 B9** 39 39N 27 53 E
Balikeşir □, *Turkey* **49 B9** 39 45N 28 0 E
Balıklıçeşme, *Turkey* **51 F11** 40 18N 27 5 E
Balikpapan, *Indonesia* **85 C5** 1 10 S 116 55 E
Balimbing, *Phil.* **81 J2** 5 5N 119 58 E
Balimo, *Papua N. G.* **132 E2** 8 6 S 142 57 E
Baling, *Malaysia* **87 K3** 5 41N 100 55 E
Balingasag, *Phil.* **81 G5** 8 45N 124 47 E
Balingen, *Germany* **31 G4** 48 16N 8 51 E
Balinţ, *Romania* **52 E6** 45 48N 21 54 E
Balintang Channel, *Phil.* **80 B3** 19 49N 121 40 E
Balintang I., *Phil.* **80 B4** 19 58N 122 9 E
Baliza, *Brazil* **173 D7** 16 0 S 52 20W
Baljurshī, *Si. Arabia* **98 C3** 19 51N 41 33 E
Balkan Mts. = Stara Planina, *Bulgaria* **50 C7** 43 15N 23 0 E
Balkh, *Afghan.* **65 E3** 36 44N 66 47 E
Balkh □, *Afghan.* **65 E3** 36 50N 67 0 E
Balkhash = Balqash, *Kazakhstan* **66 E8** 46 50N 74 50 E
Balkhash, Ozero = Balqash Köl, *Kazakhstan* **66 E8** 46 0N 74 50 E
Balkonda, *India* **94 E4** 18 52N 78 21 E
Ballachulish, *U.K.* **22 E3** 56 41N 5 8W
Balladonia, *Australia* **125 F3** 32 27 S 123 51 E
Ballaghaderreen, *Ireland* **23 C3** 53 55N 8 34W
Ballan, *Australia* **128 D6** 37 35 S 144 13 E
Ballarat, *Australia* **128 D5** 37 33 S 143 50 E
Ballard, L., *Australia* **125 E3** 29 20 S 120 40 E
Ballater, *U.K.* **22 D5** 57 3N 3 3W
Ballé, *Mali* **112 B3** 15 18N 8 33W
Ballena Gris = Ojo de Liebre ⌓, *Mexico* **162 B2** 27 50N 114 0W
Ballenas, Canal de, *Mexico* **162 B2** 29 10N 113 45W
Balleny Is., *Antarctica* **7 C11** 66 30 S 163 0 E
Balleroy, *France* **26 C6** 49 11N 0 50W
Ballerup, *Denmark* **17 J6** 55 44N 12 21 E
Ballı, *Turkey* **51 F11** 40 50N 27 3 E
Ballia, *India* **93 G11** 25 46N 84 12 E
Ballina, *Australia* **127 D5** 28 50 S 153 31 E
Ballina, *Ireland* **23 B2** 54 7N 9 9W
Ballinasloe, *Ireland* **23 C3** 53 20N 8 13W
Ballinger, *U.S.A.* **155 K5** 31 45N 99 57W
Ballinrobe, *Ireland* **23 C2** 53 38N 9 13W
Ballinskelligs B., *Ireland* **23 E1** 51 48N 10 13W
Ballon, *France* **26 D7** 48 10N 0 14 E
Ballons des Vosges ⌓, *France* **27 E14** 48 0N 7 0 E
Ballsh, *Albania* **50 F3** 40 36N 19 44 E
Ballston Spa, *U.S.A.* **151 D11** 43 0N 73 51W
Ballybunion, *Ireland* **23 D2** 52 31N 9 40W
Ballycastle, *U.K.* **23 A5** 55 12N 6 15W
Ballyclare, *U.K.* **23 B5** 54 46N 6 0W
Ballyhaunis, *Ireland* **23 C3** 53 46N 8 46W
Ballymena, *U.K.* **23 B5** 54 52N 6 17W
Ballymoney, *U.K.* **23 A5** 55 5N 6 31W
Ballymote, *Ireland* **23 B3** 54 5N 8 31W
Ballynahinch, *U.K.* **23 B6** 54 24N 5 54W
Ballyquintin Pt., *U.K.* **23 B6** 54 20N 5 30W
Ballyshannon, *Ireland* **23 B3** 54 30N 8 11W
Balmaceda, *Chile* **176 C2** 46 0 S 71 50W
Balmaseda, *Spain* **40 B1** 43 11N 3 12W
Balmazújváros, *Hungary* **52 C6** 47 37N 21 21 E
Balmertown, *Canada* **143 C10** 51 4N 93 41W
Balmhorn, *Switz.* **32 D5** 46 26N 7 42 E
Balmoral, *Australia* **128 D4** 37 15 S 141 48 E
Balmorhea, *U.S.A.* **155 K3** 30 59N 103 45W
Balochistan = Baluchistan □, *Pakistan* **91 D2** 27 30N 65 0 E
Balod, *India* **94 D5** 20 44N 81 13 E
Balombo, *Angola* **115 E2** 12 21 S 14 46 E
Balombo →, *Angola* **115 E2** 11 57 S 13 46 E
Balonne →, *Australia* **127 D4** 28 47 S 147 56 E
Balotra, *India* **92 G5** 25 50N 72 14 E
Balpyq Bī, *Kazakhstan* **65 A9** 44 52N 78 12 E
Balqash, *Kazakhstan* **66 E8** 46 50N 74 50 E
Balqash Köl, *Kazakhstan* **66 E8** 46 0N 74 50 E
Balrampur, *India* **93 F10** 27 30N 82 20 E
Balranald, *Australia* **128 C5** 34 38 S 143 33 E
Balş, *Romania* **53 F9** 44 22N 24 5 E
Balsapuerto, *Peru* **172 B2** 5 48 S 76 33W
Balsas, *Mexico* **163 D5** 18 0N 99 40W
Balsas →, *Maranhão, Brazil* **170 C3** 7 15 S 44 35W
Balsas →, *Tocantins, Brazil* **170 C2** 9 58 S 47 52W
Balsas →, *Mexico* **162 D4** 17 55N 102 10W
Bålsta, *Sweden* **16 E11** 59 35N 17 30 E
Balsthal, *Switz.* **32 B5** 47 19N 7 41 E
Balston Spa, *U.S.A.* **151 D11** 43 0N 73 52W
Balta, *Romania* **52 F7** 44 54N 22 38 E
Balta, *Ukraine* **53 B14** 48 2N 29 45 E
Baltanás, *Spain* **42 D6** 41 56N 4 15W
Bălţi, *Moldova* **53 C12** 47 48N 27 58 E
Baltic Sea, *Europe* **15 H18** 57 0N 19 0 E
Baltîm, *Egypt* **106 H7** 31 35N 31 10 E
Baltimore, *Ireland* **23 E2** 51 29N 9 22W
Baltimore, *Md., U.S.A.* **148 F7** 39 17N 76 37W
Baltimore, *Ohio, U.S.A.* **150 G2** 39 51N 82 36W
Baltit, *Pakistan* **93 A6** 36 15N 74 40 E
Baltiysk, *Russia* **15 J18** 54 41N 19 58 E
Baltiyskiy = Paldiski, *Estonia* **15 G21** 59 23N 24 9 E
Baltra, I., *Ecuador* **172 a** 0 26 S 90 16W
Baltrum, *Germany* **30 B3** 53 43N 7 24 E
Baluan I., *Papua N. G.* **132 B4** 2 33 S 147 17 E
Baluchistan □, *Pakistan* **91 D2** 27 30N 65 0 E
Balud, *Phil.* **80 E4** 12 2N 123 12 E
Balurghat, *India* **90 C2** 25 15N 88 44 E
Balvi, *Latvia* **15 H22** 57 8N 27 15 E
Balya, *Turkey* **49 B9** 39 44N 27 35 E
Balykchy, *Kyrgyzstan* **65 B8** 42 26N 76 12 E
Balzar, *Ecuador* **168 D2** 2 2 S 79 54W
Bam, *Iran* **97 D8** 29 7N 58 14 E
Bama, *China* **76 E6** 24 8N 107 12 E
Bama, *Nigeria* **113 C7** 11 33N 13 41 E
Bamaga, *Australia* **126 A3** 10 50 S 142 25 E
Bamaji L., *Canada* **140 B1** 51 9N 91 25W
Bamako, *Mali* **112 C3** 12 34N 7 55W
Bamba, *Dem. Rep. of the Congo* **115 D3** 5 45 S 18 23 E
Bamba, *Mali* **113 B4** 17 5N 1 24W
Bambamarca, *Peru* **172 B2** 6 36 S 78 32W
Bambang, *Phil.* **80 C3** 16 23N 121 6 E
Bambannan I., *Phil.* **81 J3** 5 37N 120 17 E
Bambara Maoundé, *Mali* **112 B4** 13 26N 4 3W
Bambari, *C.A.R.* **114 A4** 5 40N 20 35 E
Bambaroo, *Australia* **126 B4** 18 50 S 146 10 E
Bambaya, *Guinea* **112 D2** 10 55N 13 38W
Bamberg, *Germany* **31 F6** 49 54N 10 54 E
Bamberg, *U.S.A.* **152 B8** 33 18N 81 2W
Bambesi, *Ethiopia* **107 F3** 9 45N 34 40 E
Bambey, *Senegal* **112 C1** 14 42N 16 28W
Bambili, *Dem. Rep. of the Congo* **118 B2** 3 40N 26 0 E
Bambinga, *Dem. Rep. of the Congo* **114 C3** 3 43 S 18 53 E
Bambio, *C.A.R.* **114 B3** 3 55N 16 57 E
Bamboi, *Ghana* **112 D4** 8 13N 2 1W
Bambouti, *C.A.R.* **114 A5** 5 24N 27 12 E
Bambuí, *Brazil* **171 F2** 20 1 S 45 58W
Bamburgh, *U.K.* **20 B6** 55 37N 1 43W
Bamenda, *Cameroon* **113 D7** 5 57N 10 11 E
Bamfield, *Canada* **142 D3** 48 45N 125 10W
Bāmīān □, *Afghan.* **91 B2** 35 0N 67 0 E
Bamiancheng, *China* **75 C13** 43 15N 124 2 E
Bamingui, *C.A.R.* **114 A4** 7 34N 20 11 E
Bamingui →, *C.A.R.* **114 A3** 8 33N 19 5 E
Bamingui-Bangoran △, *C.A.R.* **114 A3** 8 30N 19 46 E
Bamkin, *Cameroon* **113 D7** 6 3N 11 27 E
Bampan, *Phil.* **80 D3** 15 40N 120 20 E
Bampūr, *Iran* **97 E9** 27 15N 60 21 E
Bamu →, *Papua N. G.* **132 E2** 8 1 S 143 33 E
Ban, *Burkina Faso* **112 C4** 14 5N 2 27W
Ban Ao Tu Khun, *Thailand* **87 a** 8 9N 98 20 E
Ban Ban, *Laos* **86 C4** 19 31N 103 30 E
Ban Bang Hin, *Thailand* **87 H2** 9 32N 98 35 E
Ban Bang Khu, *Thailand* **87 a** 7 57N 98 23 E
Ban Bang Rong, *Thailand* **87 a** 8 3N 98 25 E
Ban Bo Phut, *Thailand* **87 b** 9 33N 100 2 E
Ban Chaweng, *Thailand* **87 b** 9 32N 100 3 E
Ban Chiang Klang, *Thailand* **86 C3** 19 25N 100 55 E
Ban Chik, *Laos* **86 D4** 17 15N 102 22 E
Ban Choho, *Thailand* **86 E4** 15 2N 102 9 E
Ban Dan Lan Hoi, *Thailand* **86 D2** 17 0N 99 35 E
Ban Don = Surat Thani, *Thailand* **87 H2** 9 6N 99 20 E
Ban Don, *Vietnam* **86 F6** 12 53N 107 48 E
Ban Don, Ao →, *Thailand* **87 H2** 9 20N 99 25 E
Ban Dong, *Thailand* **86 C3** 19 30N 100 59 E
Ban Hong, *Thailand* **86 C2** 18 18N 98 50 E
Ban Hua Thanon, *Thailand* **87 b** 9 26N 100 1 E
Ban Kaeng, *Thailand* **86 D3** 17 29N 100 7 E
Ban Kantang, *Thailand* **87 J2** 7 25N 99 31 E
Ban Karon, *Thailand* **87 a** 7 51N 98 18 E
Ban Kata, *Thailand* **87 a** 7 50N 98 18 E
Ban Keun, *Laos* **86 C4** 18 22N 102 35 E
Ban Khai, *Thailand* **86 F3** 12 46N 101 18 E
Ban Kheun, *Laos* **86 B3** 20 13N 101 7 E
Ban Khlong Khian, *Thailand* **87 a** 8 10N 98 26 E
Ban Khlong Kua, *Thailand* **87 J3** 6 57N 100 8 E
Ban Khuan, *Thailand* **87 a** 8 20N 98 25 E
Ban Khuan Mao, *Thailand* **87 J2** 7 50N 99 37 E
Ban Ko Yai Chim, *Thailand* **87 G2** 11 17N 99 26 E
Ban Kok, *Thailand* **86 D4** 16 40N 103 40 E
Ban Laem, *Thailand* **86 F2** 13 13N 99 59 E
Ban Lamai, *Thailand* **87 b** 9 28N 100 3 E
Ban Lao Ngam, *Laos* **86 E6** 15 28N 106 10 E
Ban Le Kathe, *Thailand* **86 E2** 15 49N 98 53 E
Ban Lo Po Noi, *Thailand* **87 a** 8 1N 98 34 E
Ban Mae Chedi, *Thailand* **86 C2** 19 11N 99 31 E
Ban Mae Laeng, *Thailand* **86 B2** 20 1N 99 17 E
Ban Mae Nam, *Thailand* **87 b** 9 34N 100 0 E
Ban Mae Sariang, *Thailand* **86 C1** 18 10N 97 56 E
Ban Mê Thuôt = Buon Ma Thuot, *Vietnam* **86 F7** 12 40N 108 3 E
Ban Mi, *Thailand* **86 E3** 15 3N 100 32 E
Ban Muong Mo, *Laos* **86 C4** 19 4N 103 58 E
Ban Na Bo, *Thailand* **87 b** 9 19N 99 41 E
Ban Na Mo, *Laos* **86 D5** 17 7N 105 40 E
Ban Na San, *Thailand* **87 H2** 8 53N 99 52 E
Ban Na Tong, *Laos* **86 B3** 20 56N 101 47 E
Ban Nam Bac, *Laos* **86 B4** 20 38N 102 20 E
Ban Nam Ma, *Laos* **86 A3** 22 2N 101 37 E
Ban Ngang, *Laos* **86 E6** 15 59N 106 11 E
Ban Nong Bok, *Laos* **86 D5** 17 5N 104 48 E
Ban Nong Boua, *Laos* **86 E6** 15 40N 106 33 E
Ban Nong Pling, *Thailand* **86 E3** 15 40N 100 10 E
Ban Pak Chan, *Thailand* **87 G2** 10 32N 98 51 E
Ban Patong, *Thailand* **87 a** 7 54N 98 18 E
Ban Phai, *Thailand* **86 D4** 16 4N 102 44 E
Ban Phak Chit, *Thailand* **87 a** 8 0N 98 24 E
Ban Pong, *Thailand* **86 F2** 13 50N 99 55 E
Ban Rawai, *Thailand* **87 a** 7 47N 98 20 E
Ban Ron Phibun, *Thailand* **87 H2** 8 9N 99 51 E
Ban Sakhu, *Thailand* **87 a** 8 4N 98 18 E
Ban Sanam Chai, *Thailand* **87 J3** 7 33N 100 25 E

Ban Sangkha, Thailand 86 E4 14 37N 103 52 E
Ban Tak, Thailand 86 D2 17 2N 99 4 E
Ban Tako, Thailand 86 E4 14 5N 102 40 E
Ban Tha Dua, Thailand 86 D2 17 59N 98 39 E
Ban Tha Li, Thailand 86 D3 17 37N 101 25 E
Ban Tha Nun, Thailand 87 a 8 12N 98 18 E
Ban Tha Rua, Thailand 87 a 7 59N 98 22 E
Ban Tha Yu, Thailand 87 a 8 17N 98 22 E
Ban Thahine, Laos 86 E5 14 12N 105 33 E
Ban Thong Krut, Thailand 87 b 9 25N 99 57 E
Ban Xien Kok, Laos 86 B3 20 54N 100 39 E
Ban Yen Nhan, Vietnam 86 B6 20 57N 106 2 E
Banā, W. →, Yemen 98 D4 13 3N 45 24 E
Banaba, Kiribati 134 H8 0 45 S 169 50 E
Banalia, Dem. Rep. of the Congo 118 B2 1 32N 25 5 E
Banam, Cambodia 87 G5 11 20N 105 17 E
Banamba, Mali 112 C3 13 29N 7 22W
Banana Is., S. Leone 112 D2 8 7N 13 15W
Bananal, I. do, Brazil 171 D1 11 30 S 50 30W
Bananga, India 95 L11 6 57N 93 54 E
Banaras = Varanasi, India 93 G10 25 22N 83 0 E
Banas →, Gujarat, India 92 H4 23 45N 71 25 E
Banas →, Mad. P., India 93 G9 24 15N 81 30 E
Bânâs, Ras, Egypt 106 C4 23 57N 35 59 E
Banaue, Phil. 80 C3 16 55N 121 4 E
Banaz, Turkey 49 C11 38 46N 29 46 E
Banaz →, Turkey 49 C11 38 12N 29 14 E
Banbridge, U.K. 23 B5 54 22N 6 16W
Banbury, U.K. 21 E6 52 4N 1 20W
Banc d'Arguin △, Mauritania 110 D1 20 10N 16 20W
Banchory, U.K. 22 D6 57 3N 2 29W
Banco, Ethiopia 107 F4 6 12N 38 13 E
Bancroft = Chililabombwe, Zambia 119 E2 12 18 S 27 43 E
Bancroft, Canada 140 C4 45 3N 77 51W
Band, Romania 53 D9 46 30N 24 25 E
Band Bonī, Iran 97 E8 25 30N 59 33 E
Band-e Torkestan, Afghan. 91 B2 35 30N 64 0 E
Band Qīr, Iran 97 D6 31 39N 48 53 E
Banda, Cameroon 114 B2 3 58N 14 32 E
Banda, Mad. P., India 93 G8 24 3N 78 57 E
Banda, Maharashtra, India 95 G1 15 49N 73 52 E
Banda, Ut. P., India 93 G9 25 30N 80 26 E
Banda, Kepulauan, Indonesia 83 B3 4 37 S 129 50 E
Banda Aceh, Indonesia 84 A1 5 35N 95 20 E
Banda Banda, Mt., Australia 129 A10 31 10 S 152 28 E
Banda Elat, Indonesia 83 C4 5 40 S 133 5 E
Banda Is. = Banda, Kepulauan, Indonesia 83 B3 4 37 S 129 50 E
Banda Kani, Dem. Rep. of the Congo 115 C2 4 48 S 13 52 E
Banda Sea, Indonesia 82 C3 6 0 S 130 0 E
Bandai-Asahi △, Japan 70 F10 37 38N 140 5 E
Bandai-San, Japan 70 F10 37 36N 140 4 E
Bandak, Norway 18 E5 59 23N 8 29 E
Bandama →, Ivory C. 112 D3 6 32N 4 30W
Bandama Blanc →, Ivory C. 112 D3 6 55N 5 30W
Bandama Rouge →, Ivory C. 112 D4 6 55N 5 30W
Bandān, Iran 97 D9 31 23N 60 44 E
Bandanaira, Indonesia 83 B3 4 32 S 129 54 E
Bandanwara, India 92 F6 26 9N 74 38 E
Bandar = Machilipatnam, India 95 F5 16 12N 81 8 E
Bandar-e Abbās, Iran 97 E8 27 15N 56 15 E
Bandar-e Anzalī, Iran 97 B6 37 30N 49 30 E
Bandar-e Bushehr = Būshehr, Iran 97 D6 28 55N 50 55 E
Bandar-e Chārak, Iran 97 E7 26 45N 54 20 E
Bandar-e Deylam, Iran 97 D6 30 5N 50 10 E
Bandar-e Emām Khomeyni, Iran 97 D6 30 30N 49 5 E
Bandar-e Lengeh, Iran 97 E7 26 35N 54 58 E
Bandar-e Maqām, Iran 97 E7 26 56N 53 29 E
Bandar-e Ma'shur, Iran 97 D6 30 35N 49 10 E
Bandar-e Rīg, Iran 97 D6 29 29N 50 38 E
Bandar-e Torkeman, Iran 97 B7 37 0N 54 10 E
Bandar Lampung = Tanjungkarang Telukbetung, Indonesia 84 D3 5 20 S 105 10 E
Bandar Maharani = Muar, Malaysia 87 L4 2 3N 102 34 E
Bandar Penggaram = Batu Pahat, Malaysia 87 M4 1 50N 102 56 E
Bandar Seri Begawan, Brunei 85 B4 4 52N 115 0 E
Bandar Sri Aman = Sri Aman, Malaysia 85 B4 1 15N 111 32 E
Bandawe, Malawi 119 E3 11 58 S 34 5 E
Bande, Spain 42 C3 42 3N 7 58W
Bandeira, Pico da, Brazil 171 F3 20 26 S 41 47W
Bandeirante, Brazil 171 D1 13 41 S 50 48W
Bandera, Argentina 174 B3 28 55 S 62 20W
Banderas, B. de, Mexico 162 C3 20 40N 105 30W
Bandhavgarh △, India 94 C5 23 45N 81 10 E
Bandhogarh, India 93 H9 23 40N 81 2 E
Bandi →, India 92 F6 26 12N 75 47 E
Bandia →, India 94 E5 19 2N 80 28 E
Bandiagara, Mali 112 C4 14 12N 3 29W
Bandikui, India 92 F7 27 3N 76 34 E
Bandipur △, India 95 J3 11 45N 76 30 E
Bandırma, Turkey 51 F11 40 20N 28 0 E
Bandjarmasin = Banjarmasin, Indonesia 85 C4 3 20 S 114 35 E
Bandol, France 29 E9 43 8N 5 46 E
Bandon, Ireland 23 E3 51 44N 8 44W
Bandon →, Ireland 23 E3 51 43N 8 37W
Bandoua, C.A.R. 114 B4 4 39N 21 42 E
Bandula, Mozam. 119 F3 19 0 S 33 7 E
Bandundu, Dem. Rep. of the Congo 114 C3 3 15 S 17 22 E
Bandundu □, Dem. Rep. of the Congo 114 C3 3 30 S 17 30 E
Bandung, Indonesia 85 D3 6 54 S 107 36 E
Bané, Burkina Faso 113 C4 11 42N 0 15W
Băneasa, Romania 53 E12 45 56N 27 55 E
Bāneh, Iran 101 E11 35 59N 45 53 E
Bañeres, Spain 41 G4 38 44N 0 38W
Banes, Cuba 165 B4 21 0N 75 42W
Banff, Canada 142 C5 51 10N 115 34W
Banff, U.K. 22 D6 57 40N 2 33W
Banff △, Canada 142 C5 51 30N 116 15W
Banfora, Burkina Faso 112 C4 10 40N 4 40W
Bang Fai →, Laos 86 D5 16 57N 104 45 E
Bang Hieng →, Laos 86 D5 16 10N 105 10 E
Bang Krathum, Thailand 86 D3 16 34N 100 18 E
Bang Lamung, Thailand 86 F3 13 3N 100 56 E
Bang Mun Nak, Thailand 86 D3 16 2N 100 23 E
Bang Pa In, Thailand 86 E3 14 14N 100 35 E
Bang Rakam, Thailand 86 D3 16 45N 100 7 E
Bang Saphan, Thailand 87 G2 11 14N 99 28 E
Bang Thao, Thailand 87 a 7 59N 98 18 E
Banga, Angola 115 D3 8 43 S 15 13 E
Banga, Dem. Rep. of the Congo 115 D4 5 25 S 20 28 E
Banga, Aklan, Phil. 81 F4 11 38N 122 20 E
Banga, S. Cotabato, Phil. 81 H5 6 21N 124 47 E
Bangaduni I., India 90 E2 21 34N 88 52 E
Bangala Dam, Zimbabwe 119 G3 21 7 S 31 25 E
Bangalore, India 95 H3 12 59N 77 40 E
Banganapalle, India 95 G4 15 19N 78 14 E
Banganga →, India 92 F6 27 6N 77 25 E
Bangangté, Cameroon 113 D7 5 8N 10 32 E
Bangaon, India 93 H13 23 0N 88 47 E
Bangar, Phil. 80 C3 16 54N 120 25 E
Bangassou, C.A.R. 114 B4 4 55N 23 7 E
Bangeta, Mt., Papua N. G. 132 D4 6 21 S 147 3 E
Banggai, Indonesia 82 B2 1 34 S 123 30 E
Banggai, Kepulauan, Indonesia 82 B2 1 40 S 123 30 E
Banggai Arch. = Banggai, Kepulauan, Indonesia 82 B2 1 40 S 123 30 E
Banggi, Pulau, Malaysia 85 A5 7 17N 117 12 E
Banghāzī, Libya 108 B4 32 11N 20 3 E
Banghāzī □, Libya 108 B4 32 7N 20 4 E
Bangil, Indonesia 85 D4 7 36 S 112 50 E
Bangjang, Sudan 107 E3 11 23N 32 41 E
Bangka, Sulawesi, Indonesia 82 A3 1 50N 125 5 E
Bangka, Sumatera, Indonesia 84 C3 2 0 S 105 50 E
Bangka, Selat, Indonesia 84 C3 2 30 S 105 30 E
Bangka-Belitung □, Indonesia 78 E3 2 30 S 107 0 E
Bangkalan, Indonesia 85 D4 7 2 S 112 46 E
Bangkinang, Indonesia 84 B2 0 18N 101 5 E
Bangko, Indonesia 84 C2 2 5 S 102 9 E
Bangkok, Thailand 86 F3 13 45N 100 35 E
Bangladesh ■, Asia 90 C3 24 0N 90 0 E
Bangli, Indonesia 79 J18 8 27 S 115 21 E
Bangolo, Ivory C. 112 D3 7 1N 7 29W
Bangong Co, India 93 B8 35 50N 79 20 E
Bangor, Down, U.K. 23 B6 54 40N 5 40W
Bangor, Gwynedd, U.K. 20 D3 53 14N 4 8W
Bangor, Maine, U.S.A. 139 D13 44 48N 68 46W
Bangor, Mich., U.S.A. 157 B10 42 18N 86 7W
Bangor, Pa., U.S.A. 151 F9 40 52N 75 13W
Bangoran →, C.A.R. 114 A3 8 42N 19 6 E
Bangu, Dem. Rep. of the Congo 114 C3 0 3 S 19 12 E
Bangued, Phil. 80 C3 17 40N 120 37 E
Bangui, C.A.R. 114 B3 4 23N 18 35 E
Bangui, Phil. 80 B3 18 32N 120 46 E
Banguru, Dem. Rep. of the Congo 118 B2 0 30N 27 10 E
Bangweulu, L., Zambia 119 E3 11 0 S 30 0 E
Bangweulu Swamp, Zambia 119 E3 11 20 S 30 15 E
Banhine △, Mozam. 117 C5 22 49 S 32 55 E
Baní, Dom. Rep. 165 C5 18 16N 70 22W
Bani, Phil. 80 C2 16 11N 119 52 E
Bani →, Mali 112 C4 14 30N 4 12W
Bani, Jebel, Morocco 110 C3 29 16N 8 0W
Bani Bangou, Niger 113 B5 15 3N 2 42 E
Banī Sa'd, Iraq 101 F11 33 34N 44 32 E
Bania, C.A.R. 114 B3 4 1N 16 7 E
Bania, Ivory C. 112 D4 9 4N 3 6W
Baniara, Papua N. G. 132 E5 9 44 S 149 54 E
Banihal Pass, India 93 C6 33 30N 75 12 E
Banikoara, Benin 113 C5 11 18N 2 26 E
Banīnah, Libya 108 B4 32 0N 20 12 E
Bāniyās, Syria 100 E6 35 10N 36 0 E
Banja Luka, Bos.-H. 52 F2 44 49N 17 11 E
Banjar, India 92 D7 31 38N 77 21 E
Banjar, Indonesia 85 D3 7 24 S 108 30 E
Banjar →, India 93 H9 22 36N 80 22 E
Banjarmasin, Indonesia 85 C4 3 20 S 114 35 E
Banjarnegara, Indonesia 85 D3 7 24 S 109 42 E
Banjul, Gambia 112 C1 13 28N 16 40W
Banka, India 93 G12 24 53N 86 55 E
Bankas, Mali 112 C4 14 4N 3 31W
Bankeryd, Sweden 17 G8 57 53N 14 6 E
Banket, Zimbabwe 119 F3 17 27 S 30 19 E
Bankilaré, Niger 113 C5 14 35N 0 44 E
Bankot, India 94 F1 17 58N 73 2 E
Banks, U.S.A. 152 D4 31 49N 85 51W
Banks I. = Moa, I., Papua N. G. 132 F2 10 10 S 142 15 E
Banks I., B.C., Canada 142 C3 53 20N 130 0W
Banks I., N.W.T., Canada 138 A7 73 15N 121 30W
Banks Is., Vanuatu 133 C5 13 50 S 167 30 E
Banks L., U.S.A. 152 D6 31 2N 83 6W
Banks Pen., N.Z. 131 D8 43 45 S 173 15 E
Banks Str., Australia 127 G4 40 40 S 148 10 E
Bankumuna, Dem. Rep. of the Congo 115 C3 4 28 S 19 57 E
Bankura, India 93 H12 23 11N 87 18 E
Bankya, Bulgaria 50 D7 42 43N 23 8 E
Banmankhi, India 93 G12 25 53N 87 11 E
Banmauk, Burma 90 C5 24 24N 95 51 E
Bann →, Arm., U.K. 23 B5 54 30N 6 31W
Bann →, L'derry., U.K. 23 A5 55 8N 6 41W
Bannaanka Saraar, Somali Rep. 120 C3 9 25N 46 17 E
Bannalec, France 26 E3 47 57N 3 42W
Bannang Sata, Thailand 87 J3 6 16N 101 16 E
Bannerton, Australia 128 C5 34 42 S 142 47 E
Banning, U.S.A. 161 M10 33 56N 116 53W
Banningville = Bandundu, Dem. Rep. of the Congo 114 C3 3 15 S 17 22 E
Banno, Ethiopia 107 G4 4 51N 37 24 E
Bannockburn, Canada 150 B7 44 39N 77 33W
Bannockburn, U.K. 22 E5 56 5N 3 55W
Bannockburn, Zimbabwe 119 G2 20 17 S 29 48 E
Bannu, Pakistan 91 B3 33 0N 70 18 E
Bano, India 93 H11 22 40N 84 55 E
Bañolas = Banyoles, Spain 40 C7 42 16N 2 44 E
Banon, France 29 D9 44 2N 5 38 E
Baños de la Encina, Spain 43 G7 38 10N 3 46W
Baños de Molgas, Spain 42 C3 42 15N 7 40W
Bánovce nad Bebravou, Slovak Rep. 35 C11 48 44N 18 16 E
Banovići, Bos.-H. 52 F3 44 25N 18 32 E
Bansalan, Phil. 81 H5 6 55N 125 13 E
Bansgaon, India 93 F10 26 33N 83 21 E
Banská Bystrica, Slovak Rep. 35 C12 48 46N 19 14 E
Banská Štiavnica, Slovak Rep. 35 C11 48 25N 18 55 E
Bansko, Bulgaria 50 E7 41 52N 23 28 E
Banskobystrický □, Slovak Rep. 35 C12 48 20N 19 0 E
Banswara, India 92 H6 23 32N 74 24 E
Bantaeng, Indonesia 82 C1 5 32 S 119 56 E
Bantaji, Nigeria 113 D7 8 6N 10 5 E
Bantayan, Phil. 81 F4 11 10N 123 43 E
Bantayan I., Phil. 81 F4 11 13N 123 44 E
Banten, Indonesia 84 D3 6 5 S 106 8 E
Banten □, Indonesia 79 G11 6 30 S 106 0 E
Banton I., Phil. 80 E4 12 56N 122 4 E
Bantry, Ireland 23 E2 51 41N 9 27W
Bantry B., Ireland 23 E2 51 37N 9 44W
Bantul, Indonesia 85 D4 7 55 S 110 19 E
Bantva, India 92 J4 21 29N 70 12 E
Bantval, India 95 H2 12 55N 75 0 E
Banya, Bulgaria 51 D8 42 33N 24 50 E
Banyak, Kepulauan, Indonesia 84 B1 2 10N 97 10 E
Banyalbufar, Spain 38 B3 39 42N 2 31 E
Banyo, Cameroon 113 D7 6 52N 11 45 E
Banyoles, Spain 40 C7 42 16N 2 44 E
Banyuls-sur-Mer, France 28 F7 42 28N 3 8 E
Banyumas, Indonesia 85 D3 7 32 S 109 18 E
Banyuwangi, Indonesia 85 D4 8 13 S 114 21 E
Banz, Papua N. G. 132 C3 5 47 S 144 37 E
Banza, Dem. Rep. of the Congo 114 B4 0 28N 20 10 E
Banzare Coast, Antarctica 7 C9 68 0 S 125 0 E
Banzyville = Mobayi, Dem. Rep. of the Congo 114 B4 4 15N 21 8 E
Bao Ha, Vietnam 76 F5 22 11N 104 21 E
Bao Lac, Vietnam 86 A5 22 57N 105 40 E
Bao Loc, Vietnam 87 G6 11 32N 107 48 E
Bao'an = Shenzhen, China 77 F10 22 32N 114 5 E
Baocheng, China 74 H4 33 12N 106 56 E
Baode, China 74 E6 39 1N 111 5 E
Baodi, China 75 E9 39 38N 117 20 E
Baoding, China 74 E8 38 50N 115 28 E
Baoji, China 74 G4 34 20N 107 5 E
Baojing, China 76 C7 28 45N 109 41 E
Baokang, China 77 B8 31 54N 111 12 E
Baoro, C.A.R. 114 A3 5 40N 15 58 E
Baoshan, Shanghai, China 77 B13 31 27N 121 26 E
Baoshan, Yunnan, China 76 E2 25 10N 99 5 E
Baotou, China 74 D6 40 32N 110 2 E
Baotow = Baotou, China 74 D6 40 32N 110 2 E
Baoxing, China 76 B4 30 24N 102 50 E
Baoying, China 75 H10 33 17N 119 20 E
Baoyou = Ledong, China 86 C7 18 41N 109 5 E
Bap, India 92 F5 27 23N 72 18 E
Bapatla, India 95 G5 15 55N 80 30 E
Bapaume, France 27 B9 50 7N 2 50 E
Baqanas, Kazakhstan 65 A8 44 50N 76 15 E
Baqbaqty, Kazakhstan 65 A8 44 35N 76 40 E
Bāqerābād, Iran 97 C6 33 2N 51 58 E
Ba'qūbah, Iraq 101 F11 33 45N 44 50 E
Baquedano, Chile 174 A2 23 20 S 69 52W
Bar, Serbia & M. 50 D3 42 8N 19 6 E
Bar, Ukraine 59 H4 49 4N 27 40 E
Bar Bigha, India 93 G11 25 21N 85 47 E
Bar Harbor, U.S.A. 149 C11 44 23N 68 13W
Bar-le-Duc, France 27 D12 48 47N 5 10 E
Bar-sur-Aube, France 27 D11 48 14N 4 40 E
Bar-sur-Seine, France 27 D11 48 7N 4 20 E
Bara, India 93 G9 25 16N 81 43 E
Bara, Indonesia 82 B3 3 8 S 126 11 E
Bâra, Romania 53 C12 47 2N 27 3 E
Bara Banki, India 93 F9 26 55N 81 12 E
Barabai, Indonesia 85 C5 2 32 S 115 34 E
Baraboo, U.S.A. 154 D10 43 28N 89 45W
Baracoa, Cuba 165 B5 20 20N 74 30W
Baradā →, Syria 103 B5 33 33N 36 34 E
Baradero, Argentina 174 C4 33 52 S 59 29W
Baradine, Australia 129 A8 30 56 S 149 4 E
Baraga, U.S.A. 154 B10 46 47N 88 30W
Bărăganul, Romania 53 F12 44 49N 27 31 E
Barah →, India 92 F6 27 42N 77 5 E
Barahona, Dom. Rep. 165 C5 18 13N 71 7W
Barahona, Spain 40 D2 41 17N 2 39W
Barail Range, India 90 C4 25 15N 93 20 E
Barajas, Madrid ✕ (MAD), Spain 42 E7 40 26N 3 34W
Barak →, India 90 C4 24 52N 92 30 E
Baraka, Sudan 107 E2 10 59N 27 59 E
Baraka →, Sudan 106 D4 18 13N 37 35 E
Barakaldo, Spain 40 B2 43 18N 2 59W
Barakar →, India 93 G12 24 7N 86 14 E
Barakot, India 93 J11 21 33N 84 59 E
Barakpur, India 93 H13 22 44N 88 30 E
Baralaba, Australia 126 C4 24 13 S 149 50 E
Baralla, Spain 42 C3 42 53N 7 15W
Baralzon L., Canada 143 B9 60 0N 98 3W
Baram →, Malaysia 85 B4 4 35N 113 58 E
Baramati, India 94 E2 18 11N 74 33 E
Baramba, India 94 D7 20 25N 85 23 E
Barameiya, Sudan 106 D4 18 32N 36 38 E
Baramula, India 93 B6 34 15N 74 20 E
Baran, India 92 G7 25 9N 76 40 E
Baran →, Pakistan 92 G3 25 13N 68 17 E
Barañain, Spain 40 C3 42 48N 1 40W
Baranavichy, Belarus 59 F4 53 10N 26 0 E
Barani, Burkina Faso 112 C4 13 9N 3 51W
Baranoa, Colombia 168 A3 10 48N 74 55W
Baranof, U.S.A. 142 B2 57 5N 134 50W
Baranof I., U.S.A. 144 H14 57 0N 135 0W
Baranów Sandomierski, Poland 55 H8 50 29N 21 30 E
Baranowicze = Baranavichy, Belarus 59 F4 53 10N 26 0 E
Baranya □, Hungary 52 E3 46 0N 18 15 E
Barão de Cocais, Brazil 171 E3 19 56 S 43 28W
Barão de Grajaú, Brazil 170 C3 6 45 S 43 1W
Barão de Melgaço, Mato Grosso, Brazil 173 D6 16 14 S 55 52W
Barão de Melgaço, Rondônia, Brazil 173 C5 11 50 S 60 45W
Baraolt, Romania 53 D10 46 5N 25 34 E
Barapasi, Indonesia 83 B5 2 15 S 137 5 E
Barapina = Panguna, Papua N. G. 132 D8 6 21 S 155 25 E
Baras, Phil. 80 E5 13 40N 124 22 E
Barasat, India 93 H13 22 46N 88 31 E
Barat Daya, Kepulauan, Indonesia 82 C3 7 30 S 128 0 E
Baratang I., India 95 H11 12 13N 92 45 E
Barataria B., U.S.A. 155 L10 29 20N 89 55W
Barauda, India 92 H6 23 33N 75 15 E
Baraut, India 92 E7 29 13N 77 7 E
Baraya, Colombia 168 C2 3 10N 75 4W
Barbacan = Roxas, Phil. 81 F2 10 20N 119 21 E
Barbacena, Brazil 171 F3 21 15 S 43 56W
Barbacoas, Colombia 168 C2 1 45N 78 0W
Barbados ■, W. Indies 165 g 13 10N 59 30W
Barbalha, Brazil 170 C4 7 19 S 39 17W
Barban, Croatia 45 C11 45 5N 14 2 E
Barbària, C. de, Spain 38 D1 38 39N 1 24 E
Barbaros, Turkey 51 F11 40 54N 27 27 E
Barbas, C., W. Sahara 110 D1 22 20N 16 42W
Barbastro, Spain 40 C5 42 2N 0 5 E
Barbate de Franco, Spain 43 J5 36 13N 5 56W
Barbaza, Phil. 81 F4 11 12N 122 2 E
Barberino di Mugello, Italy 45 E8 44 0N 11 15 E
Barbers Pt., U.S.A. 145 K13 21 18N 158 7W
Barberton, S. Africa 117 D5 25 42 S 31 2 E
Barberton, U.S.A. 150 E3 41 0N 81 39W
Barberville, U.S.A. 153 F8 29 11N 81 26W
Barbezieux-St-Hilaire, France 28 C3 45 28N 0 9W
Barbosa, Colombia 168 B3 5 57N 73 37W
Barbourville, U.S.A. 149 G4 36 52N 83 53W
Barbuda, W. Indies 165 C7 17 30N 61 40W
Bârca, Romania 53 G8 43 59N 23 36 E
Barcaldine, Australia 126 C4 23 43 S 145 6 E
Barcarena, Brazil 170 B2 1 30 S 48 40W
Barcarrota, Spain 43 G4 38 31N 6 51W
Barce = Al Marj, Libya 108 B4 32 25N 20 30 E
Barcellona Pozzo di Gotto, Italy 47 D8 38 9N 15 13 E
Barcelona, Spain 40 D7 41 21N 2 10 E
Barcelona, Venezuela 169 A5 10 10N 64 40W
Barcelona □, Spain 40 D7 41 30N 2 0 E
Barcelona ✕ (BCN), Spain 40 D7 41 18N 2 5 E
Barceloneta, Puerto Rico 165 d 18 27N 66 32W
Barcelonette, France 29 D10 44 23N 6 40 E
Barcelos, Brazil 169 D5 1 0 S 63 0W
Barcin, Poland 55 F4 52 52N 17 55 E
Barclayville, Liberia 112 E3 4 48N 8 10W
Barcoo →, Australia 126 D3 25 30 S 142 50 E
Barcs, Hungary 52 E2 45 58N 17 28 E
Barczewo, Poland 54 E7 53 50N 20 42 E
Bärdä, Azerbaijan 61 K8 40 25N 47 10 E
Barda del Medio, Argentina 176 A3 38 45 S 68 11W
Bardaï, Chad 109 D3 21 25N 17 0 E
Bardas Blancas, Argentina 174 D2 35 49 S 69 45W
Bardawîl, Sabkhet el, Egypt 103 D2 31 10N 33 15 E
Barddhaman, India 93 H12 23 14N 87 39 E
Bardejov, Slovak Rep. 35 B14 49 18N 21 15 E
Bardera, Somali Rep. 120 D2 2 20N 42 27 E
Barð, Iceland 11 A7 66 3N 19 8W
Bárðarbunga, Iceland 11 C9 64 38N 17 32W
Barðastrandarsýsla □, Iceland 11 B3 65 40N 23 0W
Bardi, Italy 44 D6 44 38N 9 44 E
Bardīyah, Libya 108 B5 31 45N 25 5 E
Bardoli, India 94 D1 21 12N 73 5 E
Bardolino, Italy 44 C7 45 33N 10 43 E
Bardonécchia, Italy 44 C3 45 5N 6 42 E
Bardsey I., U.K. 20 E3 52 45N 4 47W
Bardstown, U.S.A. 157 G11 37 49N 85 28W
Bareilly, India 93 E8 28 22N 79 27 E
Barela, India 93 H9 23 6N 80 3 E
Barellan, Australia 129 C7 34 16 S 146 24 E
Barentin, France 26 C7 49 33N 0 58 E
Barenton, France 26 D6 48 38N 0 50W
Barents Sea, Arctic 6 B9 73 0N 39 0 E
Barentsøya, Svalbard 10 B13 78 25N 21 20 E
Barentu, Eritrea 107 D4 15 2N 37 35 E
Barfleur, France 26 C5 49 40N 1 17W
Barfleur, Pte. de, France 26 C5 49 42N 1 16W
Barfurush = Bābol, Iran 97 B7 36 40N 52 50 E
Barga, Italy 44 D7 44 4N 10 29 E
Bargal, Somali Rep. 120 B4 11 25N 51 0 E
Bargara, Australia 126 C5 24 50 S 152 25 E
Bargarh, India 94 D6 21 20N 83 37 E
Bargas, Spain 42 F6 39 56N 4 3W
Bârgăului Bistrița, Romania 53 C9 47 13N 24 46 E
Barge, Italy 44 D4 44 43N 7 20 E
Bargnop, Sudan 107 F2 9 32N 28 25 E
Bargo, Australia 129 C9 34 18 S 150 35 E
Bargteheide, Germany 30 B6 53 44N 10 14 E
Barguzin, Russia 67 D11 53 37N 109 37 E
Barh, India 93 G11 25 29N 85 46 E
Barhaj, India 93 F10 26 18N 83 44 E
Barham, Australia 128 C6 35 36 S 144 8 E
Barharwa, India 93 G12 24 52N 87 47 E
Barhi, India 93 G11 24 15N 85 25 E
Bari, Dem. Rep. of the Congo 114 B3 3 20N 19 25 E
Bari, India 92 F7 26 39N 77 39 E
Bari, Italy 47 A9 41 8N 16 51 E
Bari Doab, Pakistan 92 D5 30 20N 73 0 E
Bari Sadri, India 92 G6 24 28N 74 30 E
Bari Sardo, Italy 46 C2 39 50N 9 38 E
Barīdī, Ra's, Si. Arabia 96 E3 24 17N 37 31 E
Barīm, Yemen 98 D3 12 39N 43 25 E
Barima →, Guyana 169 B5 8 33N 60 25W
Barinas, Venezuela 168 B3 8 36N 70 15W
Barinas □, Venezuela 168 B4 8 10N 69 50W
Baring, U.S.A. 156 D4 40 15N 92 12W
Baring, C., Canada 138 B8 70 0N 117 30W
Baringa, Dem. Rep. of the Congo 114 B4 0 45N 20 52 E
Baringo, L., Kenya 118 B4 0 47N 36 16 E
Barinitas, Venezuela 168 B3 8 45N 70 25W
Baripada, India 94 D8 21 57N 86 45 E
Bariri, Brazil 171 F2 22 4 S 48 44W
Bârîs, Egypt 106 C3 24 42N 30 31 E
Barisal, Bangla. 90 D3 22 45N 90 20 E
Barisal □, Bangla. 90 D3 22 45N 90 20 E
Barisan, Bukit, Indonesia 78 E2 3 30 S 102 15 E
Barito →, Indonesia 85 C4 4 0 S 114 50 E
Baritú △, Argentina 174 A3 23 43 S 64 40W
Barjac, France 29 D8 44 20N 4 22 E
Barjols, France 29 E10 43 34N 6 2 E
Barjūj, Wadi →, Libya 108 C2 25 26N 12 12 E
Bark L., Canada 150 A7 45 27N 77 51W
Barka = Baraka →, Sudan 106 D4 18 13N 37 35 E
Barkakana, India 93 H11 23 37N 85 29 E
Barkald, Norway 16 C5 61 59N 10 53 E
Barkam, China 76 B4 31 51N 102 28 E
Barker, U.S.A. 150 C6 43 20N 78 33W
Barkley, L., U.S.A. 149 G2 37 1N 88 14W
Barkley Sound, Canada 142 D3 48 50N 125 10W
Barkly East, S. Africa 116 E4 30 58 S 27 33 E
Barkly Roadhouse, Australia 126 B2 19 52 S 135 50 E
Barkly Tableland, Australia 126 B2 17 50 S 136 40 E
Barkly West, S. Africa 116 D3 28 5 S 24 31 E
Barkol, Wadi →, Sudan 106 D3 17 40N 32 0 E
Barkol Kazak Zizhixian, China 68 B4 43 37N 93 2 E
Barla Dağı, Turkey 49 C12 38 5N 30 40 E
Bârlad, Romania 53 D12 46 15N 27 38 E
Bârlad →, Romania 53 E12 45 38N 27 32 E
Barlee, L., Australia 125 E2 29 15 S 119 30 E
Barlee, Mt., Australia 125 D4 24 38 S 128 13 E
Barletta, Italy 47 A9 41 19N 16 17 E
Barlinek, Poland 55 F2 53 0N 15 15 E
Barlovento, Canary Is. 9 e1 28 48N 17 48W
Barlovento, C. Verde Is. 9 j 17 0N 25 0W
Barlow L., Canada 143 A8 62 0N 103 0W
Barmedman, Australia 129 C7 34 9 S 147 21 E
Barmer, India 92 G4 25 45N 71 20 E
Barmera, Australia 128 C4 34 15 S 140 28 E
Barmouth, U.K. 20 E3 52 44N 4 4W
Barmstedt, Germany 30 B5 53 47N 9 46 E
Barn, The, St. Helena 9 h 15 55 S 5 40W
Barna →, India 93 G10 25 21N 83 3 E
Barnagar, India 92 H6 23 7N 75 19 E
Barnala, India 92 D6 30 23N 75 33 E
Barnard →, Australia 129 A9 31 34 S 151 25 E
Barnard Castle, U.K. 20 C6 54 33N 1 55W
Barnato, Australia 129 A6 31 38 S 145 0 E
Barnaul, Russia 66 D9 53 20N 83 40 E
Barnes, Australia 128 D6 36 2 S 144 49 E
Barnesville, U.S.A. 152 B5 33 3N 84 9W
Barnet □, U.K. 21 F7 51 38N 0 9W
Barneveld, Neths. 24 B5 52 7N 5 36 E
Barneveld, U.S.A. 151 C9 43 16N 75 14W
Barneville-Cartevert, France 26 C5 49 23N 1 46W
Barnhart, U.S.A. 155 K4 31 8N 101 10W
Barnsley, U.K. 20 D6 53 34N 1 27W
Barnstaple, U.K. 21 F3 51 5N 4 4W
Barnstaple Bay = Bideford Bay, U.K. 21 F3 51 5N 4 20W
Barnsville, U.S.A. 154 B6 46 43N 96 28W
Barnwell, U.S.A. 152 B8 33 15N 81 23W
Baro, Nigeria 113 D6 8 35N 6 18 E
Baro →, Ethiopia 107 F3 8 26N 33 13 E
Barobo, Phil. 81 G6 8 33N 126 7 E
Baroda = Vadodara, India 92 H5 22 20N 73 10 E
Baroda, India 92 G7 25 29N 76 35 E
Baroe, S. Africa 116 E3 33 13 S 24 33 E
Baron Ra., Australia 124 D4 23 30 S 127 45 E
Barong, China 76 B2 31 3N 99 20 E
Barora, Solomon Is. 133 L10 7 30 S 158 20 E
Barora Ite, Solomon Is. 133 L10 7 36 S 158 24 E
Barotse = Western □, Zambia 119 F1 15 0 S 24 4 E
Barotseland, Zambia 115 F4 15 0 S 24 0 E
Barouéli, Mali 112 C3 13 4N 6 50W
Barpali, India 94 D6 21 11N 83 35 E
Barpathar, India 90 B4 26 17N 93 53 E
Barpeta, India 90 B3 26 20N 91 10 E
Barqin, Libya 108 C2 27 33N 13 34 E
Barques, Pt. Aux, U.S.A. 150 B2 44 4N 82 58W
Barquísimeto, Venezuela 168 A4 10 4N 69 19W
Barr, Ras el, Egypt 106 H7 31 32N 31 50 E
Barr Smith Range, Australia 125 E3 27 4 S 120 20 E
Barra, Brazil 170 D3 11 5 S 43 10W
Barra, U.K. 22 E1 57 0N 7 29W
Barra, Sd. of, U.K. 22 D1 57 4N 7 25W
Barra Bonita = Ibaiti, Brazil 171 F1 23 50 S 50 10W
Barra da Estiva, Brazil 171 D3 13 38 S 41 19W
Barra de Navidad, Mexico 162 D4 19 12N 104 41W
Barra do Bugres, Brazil 173 C6 15 0 S 57 11W
Barra do Corda, Brazil 170 C2 5 30 S 45 10W
Barra do Dande, Angola 115 D2 8 28 S 13 22 E
Barra do Mendes, Brazil 171 D3 11 43 S 42 4W
Barra do Piraí, Brazil 171 F3 22 30 S 43 50W
Barra Falsa, Pta. da, Mozam. 117 C6 22 58 S 35 37 E
Barra Hd., U.K. 22 E1 56 47N 7 40W
Barra Mansa, Brazil 171 F3 22 35 S 44 12W
Barraba, Australia 129 A9 30 21 S 150 35 E
Barracão do Barreto, Brazil 173 B6 8 48 S 58 24W
Barracas al Sur = Avellaneda, Argentina 174 C4 34 50 S 58 10W
Barrackpur = Barakpur, India 93 H13 22 44N 88 30 E
Barradale Roadhouse, Australia 124 D1 22 42 S 114 58 E
Barrafranca, Italy 47 E7 37 22N 14 12 E
Barraigh = Barra, U.K. 22 E1 57 0N 7 29W
Barranca, Lima, Peru 172 C2 10 45 S 77 50W
Barranca, Loreto, Peru 168 D2 4 50 S 76 50W
Barranca del Cobre △, Mexico 162 B3 27 18N 107 40W
Barrancabermeja, Colombia 168 B3 7 0N 73 50W
Barrancas, Colombia 168 A3 10 57N 72 50W
Barrancas, Venezuela 169 B5 8 55N 62 5W
Barrancos, Portugal 43 G4 38 10N 6 58W
Barranqueras, Argentina 174 B4 27 30 S 59 0W
Barranquilla, Colombia 168 A3 11 0N 74 50W
Barras, Brazil 170 B3 4 15 S 42 18W
Barras, Colombia 168 D3 1 45 S 73 13W
Barraute, Canada 140 C4 48 26N 77 38W
Barre, Mass., U.S.A. 151 D12 42 25N 72 6W
Barre, Vt., U.S.A. 151 B12 44 12N 72 30W
Barreal, Argentina 174 C2 31 33 S 69 28W
Barrei, Ethiopia 120 C2 6 10N 42 49 E
Barreiras, Brazil 171 D3 12 8 S 45 0W
Barreirinha, Brazil 169 D6 2 47 S 57 3W
Barreirinhas, Brazil 170 B3 2 30 S 42 50W
Barreiro, Portugal 43 G1 38 40N 9 6W
Barreiros, Brazil 170 C4 8 49 S 35 12W
Barrême, France 29 E10 43 57N 6 23 E
Barren, Nosy, Madag. 117 B7 18 25 S 43 40 E
Barren I., India 95 H11 12 16N 93 51 E
Barren Is., U.S.A. 144 G9 58 55N 152 15W
Barretos, Brazil 171 F2 20 30 S 48 35W
Barrhead, Canada 142 C6 54 10N 114 24W
Barrie, Canada 140 D4 44 24N 79 40W
Barrier, C., N.Z. 130 C4 36 25 S 175 32 E
Barrier Ra., Australia 128 A4 31 0 S 141 30 E
Barrier Ra., Otago, N.Z. 131 E4 44 15 S 169 32 E
Barrier Ra., W. Coast, N.Z. 131 E3 44 30 S 168 30 E
Barrière, Canada 142 C4 51 12N 120 7W
Barrineau Park, U.S.A. 153 E2 30 42N 87 26W
Barrington, U.S.A. 151 E13 41 44N 71 18W
Barrington, I. = Santa Fé, I., Ecuador 172 a 0 49 S 90 5W
Barrington L., Canada 143 B8 56 55N 100 15W
Barrington Tops, Australia 129 B9 32 6 S 151 28 E
Barrington Tops △, Australia 129 B9 32 4 S 151 25 E
Barringun, Australia 127 D4 29 1 S 145 41 E
Barrit-Luluno = Luba, Phil. 80 C3 17 19N 120 42 E
Barro do Garças, Brazil 173 D7 15 54 S 52 16W

Barron, *U.S.A.* **154 C9** 45 24N 91 51W
Barrow, *U.S.A.* **144 A8** 71 18N 156 47W
Barrow →, *Ireland* **23 D5** 52 25N 6 58W
Barrow Creek, *Australia* **126 C1** 21 30 S 133 55 E
Barrow I., *Australia* **124 D2** 20 45 S 115 20 E
Barrow-in-Furness, *U.K.* **20 C4** 54 7N 3 14W
Barrow Pt., *Australia* **126 A3** 14 20 S 144 40 E
Barrow Pt., *U.S.A.* **144 A8** 71 10N 156 20W
Barrow Ra., *Australia* **125 E4** 26 0 S 127 40 E
Barrow Str., *Canada* **6 B3** 74 20N 95 0W
Barruecopardo, *Spain* **42 D4** 41 4N 6 40W
Barruelo de Santullán, *Spain* **42 C6** 42 54N 4 17W
Barry, *U.K.* **21 F4** 51 24N 3 16W
Barry, *U.S.A.* **156 E5** 39 42N 91 2W
Barry's Bay, *Canada* **140 C4** 45 29N 77 41W
Barsalogho, *Burkina Faso* **113 C4** 13 25N 1 3W
Barsat, *Pakistan* **93 A5** 36 10N 72 45 E
Barsham, *Syria* **101 E9** 35 21N 40 33 E
Barsi, *India* **94 E2** 18 10N 75 50 E
Barsinghausen, *Germany* **30 C5** 52 18N 9 28 E
Barskoon, *Kyrgyzstan* **65 B8** 42 10N 77 37 E
Barstow, *U.S.A.* **161 L9** 34 54N 117 1W
Bartenstein = Bartoszyce, *Poland* **54 D7** 54 15N 20 55 E
Bartfeld = Bardejov, *Slovak Rep.* **35 B14** 49 18N 21 15 E
Barth, *Germany* **30 A8** 54 22N 12 42 E
Barthélemy, Col, *Vietnam* **86 C5** 19 26N 104 6 E
Bartica, *Guyana* **169 B6** 6 25N 58 40W
Bartin, *Turkey* **100 B5** 41 38N 32 21 E
Bartle Frere, *Australia* **126 B4** 17 27 S 145 50 E
Bartlesville, *U.S.A.* **155 G7** 36 45N 95 59W
Bartlett, *Calif., U.S.A.* **160 J8** 36 29N 118 2W
Bartlett, *Tenn., U.S.A.* **155 H10** 35 12N 89 52W
Bartlett, L., *Canada* **142 A5** 63 5N 118 20W
Bartolo = Betanzos, *Bolivia* **173 D4** 19 34 S 65 27W
Bartolomeu Dias, *Mozam.* **119 G4** 21 10 S 35 8 E
Barton, *Phil.* **81 F2** 10 24N 119 8 E
Barton, *U.S.A.* **151 B12** 44 45N 72 11W
Barton upon Humber, *U.K.* **20 D7** 53 41N 0 25W
Bartonville, *U.S.A.* **156 D7** 40 39N 89 39W
Bartoszyce, *Poland* **54 D7** 54 15N 20 55 E
Bartow, *Fla., U.S.A.* **153 H8** 27 54N 81 50W
Bartow, *Ga., U.S.A.* **152 C7** 32 53N 82 29W
Barú, I. de, *Colombia* **168 A2** 10 15N 75 35W
Barú, Volcan, *Panama* **164 E3** 8 55N 82 35W
Barumba, *Dem. Rep. of the Congo* **118 B1** 1 3N 23 37 E
Barumbu, *Dem. Rep. of the Congo* **114 B4** 1 14N 23 31 E
Baruth, *Germany* **30 C9** 52 4N 13 30 E
Baruunsuu, *Mongolia* **74 C3** 43 43N 105 35 E
Barvinkove, *Ukraine* **59 H9** 48 57N 37 0 E
Bärwalde = Barwice, *Poland* **54 E3** 53 44N 16 21 E
Barwani, *India* **92 H6** 22 2N 74 57 E
Barwice, *Poland* **54 E3** 53 44N 16 21 E
Barwick, *U.S.A.* **152 E6** 30 54N 83 44W
Barycz →, *Poland* **55 G3** 51 42N 16 15 E
Barysaw, *Belarus* **58 E5** 54 17N 28 28 E
Barysh, *Russia* **60 D8** 53 39N 47 8 E
Barzān, *Iraq* **96 B5** 36 55N 44 3 E
Bârzava, *Romania* **52 D6** 46 7N 21 59 E
Bas-Congo □, *Dem. Rep. of the Congo* **115 D2** 5 0 S 15 0 E
Bas-Kouilou, *Congo* **115 C2** 4 28 S 11 42 E
Bas-Rhin □, *France* **27 D14** 48 40N 7 30 E
Bašaid, *Serbia & M.* **52 E5** 45 38N 20 25 E
Bāsa'idū, *Iran* **97 E7** 26 35N 55 20 E
Basal, *Pakistan* **92 C5** 33 33N 72 13 E
Basankusa, *Dem. Rep. of the Congo* **114 B3** 1 5N 19 50 E
Basarabeasca, *Moldova* **53 D13** 46 21N 28 58 E
Basarabi, *Romania* **53 F13** 44 10N 28 26 E
Basarabia = Bessarabiya, *Moldova* **59 J5** 47 0N 28 10 E
Basauri, *Spain* **40 B2** 43 13N 2 53W
Basawa, *Afghan.* **91 B3** 34 15N 70 50 E
Basco, *Phil.* **80 A3** 20 27N 121 58 E
Bascuñán, C., *Chile* **174 B1** 28 52 S 71 35W
Basekpio, *Dem. Rep. of the Congo* **114 B4** 4 43N 24 36 E
Basel, *Switz.* **32 A5** 47 35N 7 35 E
Basel, Euroairport ✕ (BSL), *Europe* **27 E14** 47 36N 7 33 E
Basel-Landschaft □, *Switz.* **32 B5** 47 26N 7 45 E
Basel-Stadt □, *Switz.* **32 A5** 47 35N 7 35 E
Basento →, *Italy* **47 B9** 40 20N 16 49 E
Basey, *Phil.* **81 F5** 11 17N 125 4 E
Bashākerd, Kūhhā-ye, *Iran* **97 E8** 26 42N 58 35 E
Bashanta = Gorodovikovsk, *Russia* **61 G5** 46 8N 41 58 E
Bashaw, *Canada* **142 C6** 52 35N 112 58W
Bāshī, *Iran* **97 D6** 28 41N 51 4 E
Bashkir Republic = Bashkortostan □, *Russia* **64 E6** 54 0N 57 0 E
Bashkortostan □, *Russia* **64 E6** 54 0N 57 0 E
Bashtanivka, *Ukraine* **53 E14** 45 46N 29 29 E
Basibasy, *Madag.* **117 C7** 22 10 S 43 40 E
Basilaki I., *Papua N. G.* **132 F6** 10 35 S 151 0 E
Basilan □, *Phil.* **81 H4** 6 33N 122 4 E
Basilan I., *Phil.* **81 H4** 6 35N 122 0 E
Basilan Str., *Phil.* **81 H4** 6 50N 122 0 E
Basildon, *U.K.* **21 F8** 51 34N 0 28 E
Basile, *Eq. Guin.* **113 E6** 3 42N 8 48 E
Basilicata □, *Italy* **47 B9** 40 30N 16 30 E
Basim = Washim, *India* **94 D3** 20 3N 77 0 E
Basin, *U.S.A.* **158 D9** 44 23N 108 2W
Basinger, *U.S.A.* **153 H8** 27 23N 81 2W
Basingstoke, *U.K.* **21 F6** 51 15N 1 5W
Basirhat, *Bangla.* **90 D2** 22 40N 88 54 E
Baška, *Croatia* **45 D11** 44 58N 14 45 E
Başkale, *Turkey* **101 C10** 38 2N 43 59 E
Baskatong, Rés., *Canada* **140 C4** 46 46N 75 50W
Basle = Basel, *Switz.* **32 A5** 47 35N 7 35 E
Başmakçı, *Turkey* **49 D12** 37 54N 30 1 E
Basmat, *India* **94 E3** 19 15N 77 12 E
Basoda, *India* **92 H7** 23 52N 77 54 E
Basodino, *Switz.* **33 D6** 46 25N 8 28 E
Basoko, *Dem. Rep. of the Congo* **118 B1** 1 16N 23 40 E
Basongo, *Dem. Rep. of the Congo* **115 C4** 4 15 S 20 20 E
Basque, Pays, *France* **28 E2** 43 15N 1 20W
Basque Provinces = País Vasco □, *Spain* **40 C2** 42 50N 2 45W
Basra = Al Başrah, *Iraq* **96 D5** 30 30N 47 50 E
Bass Str., *Australia* **127 F4** 39 15 S 146 30 E
Bassano, *Canada* **142 C6** 50 48N 112 20W
Bassano del Grappa, *Italy* **45 C8** 45 46N 11 44 E
Bassar, *Togo* **113 D5** 9 19N 0 57 E
Bassas da India, *Ind. Oc.* **121 G2** 22 0 S 39 0 E
Basse-Normandie □, *France* **26 D6** 48 45N 0 30W
Basse-Pointe, *Martinique* **164 c** 14 52N 61 8W
Basse Santa-Su, *Gambia* **112 C2** 13 13N 14 15W
Basse-Terre, *Guadeloupe* **164 b** 16 0N 61 44W
Basse Terre, *Trin. & Tob.* **169 F9** 10 7N 61 19W
Bassecourt, *Switz.* **32 B4** 47 20N 7 15 E
Bassein, *Burma* **90 G5** 16 45N 94 30 E
Bassein, *India* **94 E1** 19 26N 72 48 E
Basses, Pte. des, *Guadeloupe* **164 b** 15 52N 61 17W
Basses-Alpes = Alpes-de-Haute-Provence □, *France* **29 D10** 44 8N 6 10 E
Basses-Pyrénées = Pyrénées-Atlantiques □, *France* **28 E3** 43 10N 0 50W
Basseterre, *St. Kitts & Nevis* **165 C7** 17 17N 62 43W
Bassett, *U.S.A.* **154 D5** 42 35N 99 32W
Bassi, *India* **92 D7** 30 44N 76 21 E
Bassigny, *France* **27 E12** 48 0N 5 30 E
Bassikounou, *Mauritania* **112 B3** 15 55N 6 1W
Bassila, *Benin* **113 D5** 9 1N 1 46 E
Bassum, *Germany* **30 C4** 52 50N 8 40 E
Båstad, *Sweden* **17 H6** 56 25N 12 51 E
Bastak, *Iran* **97 E7** 27 15N 54 25 E
Baştām, *Iran* **97 B7** 36 29N 55 4 E
Bastar, *India* **94 E5** 19 15N 81 40 E
Bastelica, *France* **29 F13** 42 1N 9 3 E
Basti, *India* **93 F10** 26 52N 82 55 E
Bastia, *France* **29 F13** 42 40N 9 30 E
Bastogne, *Belgium* **24 D5** 50 1N 5 43 E
Bastrop, *La., U.S.A.* **155 J9** 32 47N 91 55W
Bastrop, *Tex., U.S.A.* **155 K6** 30 7N 97 19W
Basud, *Phil.* **80 D4** 14 4N 122 58 E
Basuo = Dongfang, *China* **86 C7** 18 50N 108 33 E
Basutoland = Lesotho ■, *Africa* **117 D4** 29 40 S 28 0 E
Bat Yam, *Israel* **103 C3** 32 2N 34 44 E
Bata, *Eq. Guin.* **114 B1** 1 57N 9 50 E
Bata, *Romania* **52 D7** 46 1N 22 4 E
Bataan □, *Phil.* **80 D3** 14 40N 120 25 E
Bataan △, *Phil.* **80 D3** 14 45N 120 27 E
Batabanó, *Cuba* **164 B3** 22 41N 82 18W
Batabanó, G. de, *Cuba* **164 B3** 22 30N 82 30W
Batac, *Phil.* **80 B3** 18 3N 120 34 E
Batagai, *Russia* **67 C14** 67 38N 134 38 E
Batajnica, *Serbia & M.* **50 B4** 44 54N 20 17 E
Batak, *Bulgaria* **51 E8** 41 57N 24 12 E
Batala, *India* **92 D6** 31 48N 75 12 E
Batalha, *Portugal* **42 F2** 39 40N 8 50W
Batalpashinsk = Cherkessk, *Russia* **61 H6** 44 15N 42 5 E
Batam, *Indonesia* **84 B2** 1 5N 104 3 E
Batama, *Dem. Rep. of the Congo* **118 B2** 0 58N 26 33 E
Batamay, *Russia* **67 C13** 63 30N 129 15 E
Batan I., *Albay, Phil.* **80 E4** 13 15N 124 0 E
Batan I., *Batanes, Phil.* **80 A3** 20 26N 121 58 E
Batanes □, *Phil.* **80 A3** 20 40N 121 55 E
Batanes Is., *Phil.* **80 A3** 20 30N 122 0 E
Batang, *China* **76 B2** 30 1N 99 0 E
Batang, *Indonesia* **85 D3** 6 55 S 109 45 E
Batanga, *Gabon* **114 C1** 0 21 S 9 18 E
Batangafo, *C.A.R.* **114 A3** 7 25N 18 20 E
Batangas, *Phil.* **80 E3** 13 35N 121 10 E
Batangas □, *Phil.* **80 E3** 13 40N 121 5 E
Batanghari, *Indonesia* **84 C2** 1 36 S 103 37 E
Batanta, *Indonesia* **83 B4** 0 55 S 130 40 E
Bataraza, *Phil.* **81 G1** 8 40N 117 37 E
Batas I., *Phil.* **81 F2** 11 10N 119 36 E
Batatais, *Brazil* **175 A6** 20 54 S 47 37W
Batavia = Jakarta, *Indonesia* **84 D3** 6 9 S 106 49 E
Batavia, *Ill., U.S.A.* **157 C8** 41 51N 88 19W
Batavia, *N.Y., U.S.A.* **150 D6** 43 0N 78 11W
Batavia, *Ohio, U.S.A.* **157 E12** 39 5N 84 11W
Bataysk, *Russia* **59 J10** 47 3N 39 45 E
Batbakara = Amangeldy, *Kazakhstan* **66 D7** 50 10N 65 10 E
Batchelor, *Australia* **124 B5** 13 4 S 131 1 E
Batdambang, *Cambodia* **86 F4** 13 7N 103 12 E
Batéké, Plateau, *Congo* **114 C3** 3 30 S 15 45 E
Batemans B., *Australia* **129 C9** 35 40 S 150 12 E
Batemans Bay, *Australia* **129 C9** 35 44 S 150 11 E
Bates Ra., *Australia* **125 E3** 27 27 S 121 5 E
Batesburg-Leesville, *U.S.A.* **152 B8** 33 54N 81 33W
Batesville, *Ark., U.S.A.* **155 H9** 35 46N 91 39W
Batesville, *Ind., U.S.A.* **157 E11** 39 18N 85 13W
Batesville, *Miss., U.S.A.* **155 H10** 34 19N 89 57W
Batesville, *Tex., U.S.A.* **155 L5** 28 58N 99 37W
Bath, *Canada* **151 B8** 44 11N 76 47W
Bath, *U.K.* **21 F5** 51 23N 2 22W
Bath, *Maine, U.S.A.* **149 D11** 43 55N 69 49W
Bath, *N.Y., U.S.A.* **150 D7** 42 20N 77 19W
Bath, *S.C., U.S.A.* **152 B8** 33 31N 81 51W
Bath & North East Somerset □, *U.K.* **21 F5** 51 21N 2 27W
Batha →, *Chad* **109 F3** 12 47N 17 34 E
Batheay, *Cambodia* **87 G5** 11 59N 104 57 E
Bathsheba, *Barbados* **165 g** 13 13N 59 32W
Bathurst = Banjul, *Gambia* **112 C1** 13 28N 16 40W
Bathurst, *Australia* **129 B8** 33 25 S 149 31 E
Bathurst, *Canada* **141 C6** 47 37N 65 43W
Bathurst, *S. Africa* **116 E4** 33 30 S 26 50 E
Bathurst, C., *Canada* **138 A7** 70 34N 128 0W
Bathurst B., *Australia* **126 A3** 14 16 S 144 25 E
Bathurst Harb., *Australia* **127 G4** 43 15 S 146 10 E
Bathurst I., *Australia* **124 B5** 11 30 S 130 10 E
Bathurst I., *Canada* **6 B2** 76 0N 100 30W
Bathurst Inlet, *Canada* **138 B9** 66 50N 108 1W
Bati, *Ethiopia* **107 E5** 11 10N 40 0 E
Batie, *Burkina Faso* **112 D4** 9 53N 2 53W
Batiki, *Fiji* **133 A2** 17 48 S 179 10 E
Batlow, *Australia* **129 C8** 35 31 S 148 9 E
Batman, *Turkey* **101 D9** 37 55N 41 5 E
Baţn al Ghūl, *Jordan* **103 F4** 29 36N 35 56 E
Batna, *Algeria* **111 A6** 35 34N 6 15 E
Batnfjordsøra, *Norway* **18 B4** 62 53N 7 42 E
Bato, *Catanduanes, Phil.* **80 E5** 13 36N 124 18 E
Bato, *Leyte, Phil.* **81 F5** 10 13N 124 48 E
Bato Bato, *Phil.* **81 J2** 5 6N 119 49 E
Batoala, *Gabon* **114 B2** 0 48N 13 27 E
Batobato = San Isidro, *Phil.* **81 H6** 6 50N 126 5 E
Batočina, *Serbia & M.* **50 B5** 44 7N 21 5 E
Batoka, *Zambia* **119 F2** 16 45 S 27 15 E
Baton Rouge, *U.S.A.* **155 K9** 30 27N 91 11W
Batong, Ko, *Thailand* **87 J2** 6 32N 99 12 E
Bátonyterenye, *Hungary* **52 C4** 47 59N 19 50 E
Batopilas, *Mexico* **162 B3** 27 0N 107 45W
Batouri, *Cameroon* **114 B2** 4 30N 14 25 E
Batovany = Partizánske, *Slovak Rep.* **35 C11** 48 38N 18 23 E
Båtsfjord, *Norway* **14 A23** 70 38N 29 39 E
Battambang = Batdambang, *Cambodia* **86 F4** 13 7N 103 12 E
Batti Malv, *India* **95 K11** 8 50N 92 51 E
Batticaloa, *Sri Lanka* **95 L5** 7 43N 81 45 E
Battipáglia, *Italy* **47 B7** 40 37N 14 58 E
Battle, *U.K.* **21 G8** 50 55N 0 30 E
Battle →, *Canada* **143 C7** 52 43N 108 15W
Battle Creek, *U.S.A.* **157 B11** 42 19N 85 11W
Battle Ground, *U.S.A.* **160 E4** 45 47N 122 32W
Battle Harbour, *Canada* **141 B8** 52 16N 55 35W
Battle Lake, *U.S.A.* **154 B7** 46 17N 95 43W
Battle Mountain, *U.S.A.* **158 F5** 40 38N 116 56W
Battlefields, *Zimbabwe* **119 F2** 18 37 S 29 47 E
Battleford, *Canada* **143 C7** 52 45N 108 15W
Battonya, *Hungary* **52 D6** 46 16N 21 3 E
Batu, *Ethiopia* **107 F4** 6 55N 39 45 E
Batu, Bukit, *Malaysia* **85 B4** 2 16N 113 43 E
Batu, Kepulauan, *Indonesia* **84 C1** 0 30 S 98 25 E
Batu Bora, Bukit, *Malaysia* **85 B4** 2 43N 114 43 E
Batu Caves, *Malaysia* **87 L3** 3 15N 101 40 E
Batu Ferringhi, *Malaysia* **87 c** 5 28N 100 15 E
Batu Gajah, *Malaysia* **87 K3** 4 28N 101 3 E
Batu Is. = Batu, Kepulauan, *Indonesia* **84 C1** 0 30 S 98 25 E
Batu Pahat, *Malaysia* **87 M4** 1 50N 102 56 E
Batu Puteh, Gunung, *Malaysia* **84 B2** 4 15N 101 31 E
Batuata, *Indonesia* **82 C2** 6 12 S 122 42 E
Batugondang, Tanjung, *Indonesia* **79 J17** 8 6 S 114 29 E
Batui, *Indonesia* **82 B2** 1 17 S 122 33 E
Batukau, Gunung, *Indonesia* **79 J18** 8 20 S 115 5 E
Batulaki, *Phil.* **81 J5** 5 34N 125 19 E
Batuli = San Isidro, *Phil.* **81 H6** 6 50N 126 5 E
Batumi, *Georgia* **61 K5** 41 39N 41 44 E
Batur, *Indonesia* **79 J18** 8 15 S 115 20 E
Batur, Gunung, *Indonesia* **79 J18** 8 14 S 115 23 E
Baturaja, *Indonesia* **84 C2** 4 11 S 104 15 E
Baturité, *Brazil* **170 B4** 4 28 S 38 45W
Baturiti, *Indonesia* **79 J18** 8 19 S 115 11 E
Batusangkar, *Indonesia* **84 C2** 0 27 S 100 35 E
Bau, *Malaysia* **85 B4** 1 25N 110 9 E
Bauang, *Phil.* **80 C3** 16 31N 120 20 E
Baubau, *Indonesia* **82 C2** 5 25 S 122 38 E
Baucau, *E. Timor* **82 C3** 8 27 S 126 27 E
Bauchi, *Nigeria* **113 C6** 10 22N 9 48 E
Bauchi □, *Nigeria* **113 C7** 10 30N 10 0 E
Baud, *France* **26 E3** 47 52N 3 1W
Bauda, *India* **94 D7** 20 50N 84 25 E
Baudette, *U.S.A.* **154 A7** 48 43N 94 36W
Bauen, *Switz.* **33 C7** 46 56N 8 35 E
Bauer, C., *Australia* **127 E1** 32 44 S 134 4 E
Bauerwitz = Baborów, *Poland* **55 H5** 50 7N 18 1 E
Bauguen = Salcedo, *Phil.* **81 F5** 11 9N 125 40 E
Bauhinia, *Australia* **126 C4** 24 35 S 149 18 E
Baukau = Baucau, *E. Timor* **82 C3** 8 27 S 126 27 E
Bauko, *Phil.* **80 C3** 17 0N 120 52 E
Baulai →, *Bangla.* **90 C3** 24 22N 91 1 E
Bauld, C., *Canada* **139 C14** 51 38N 55 26W
Bauma, *Switz.* **33 B7** 47 23N 8 53 E
Baumanabad = Pyandzh, *Tajikistan* **65 E4** 37 14N 69 6 E
Baume-les-Dames, *France* **27 E13** 47 22N 6 22 E
Baunatal, *Germany* **30 D5** 51 14N 9 24 E
Baunei, *Italy* **46 B2** 40 2N 9 40 E
Baure, *Nigeria* **113 C6** 12 52N 8 50 E
Baures, *Bolivia* **173 C5** 13 35 S 63 35W
Bauru, *Brazil* **175 A6** 22 10 S 49 0W
Baús, *Brazil* **173 D7** 18 22 S 52 47W
Bausi, *India* **93 G12** 24 48N 87 1 E
Bauska, *Latvia* **15 H21** 56 24N 24 15 E
Bautino, *Kazakhstan* **61 H10** 44 35N 50 14 E
Bautzen, *Germany* **30 D10** 51 10N 14 26 E
Bauya, *S. Leone* **112 D2** 8 12N 12 38W
Baūyrzhan Momyshuly, *Kazakhstan* **65 B5** 42 36N 70 47 E
Bavānāt, *Iran* **97 D7** 30 28N 53 27 E
Bavanište, *Serbia & M.* **52 F5** 44 49N 20 55 E
Bavaria = Bayern □, *Germany* **31 G7** 48 50N 12 0 E
Båven, *Sweden* **16 E10** 59 0N 16 56 E
Bavispe →, *Mexico* **162 B3** 29 30N 109 11W
Baw Baw △, *Australia* **129 D7** 37 50 S 146 17 E
Bawdwin, *Burma* **90 D6** 23 5N 97 20 E
Bawe, *Indonesia* **83 B4** 2 59 S 134 43 E
Bawean, *Indonesia* **85 D4** 5 46 S 112 35 E
Bawku, *Ghana* **113 C4** 11 3N 0 19W
Bawlake, *Burma* **90 F6** 19 11N 97 21 E
Bawolung, *China* **76 C3** 28 50N 101 16 E
Baxley, *U.S.A.* **152 D7** 31 47N 82 21W
Baxoi, *China* **76 B1** 30 1N 96 50 E
Baxter, *Iowa, U.S.A.* **156 C3** 41 49N 93 9W
Baxter, *Minn., U.S.A.* **154 B7** 46 21N 94 17W
Baxter Springs, *U.S.A.* **155 G7** 37 2N 94 44W
Baxter State △, *U.S.A.* **149 B11** 46 5N 68 57W
Bay, L. de, *Phil.* **80 D3** 14 20N 121 11 E
Bay al Khā'ib, Wādī →, *Libya* **108 B3** 30 55N 15 29 E
Bay City, *Mich., U.S.A.* **148 D4** 43 36N 83 54W
Bay City, *Tex., U.S.A.* **155 L7** 28 59N 95 58W
Bay Minette, *U.S.A.* **149 K2** 30 53N 87 46W
Bay of Plenty □, *N.Z.* **130 D5** 38 0 S 177 0 E
Bay Roberts, *Canada* **141 C9** 47 36N 53 16W
Bay St. Louis, *U.S.A.* **155 K10** 30 19N 89 20W
Bay Springs, *U.S.A.* **155 K10** 31 59N 89 17W
Bay View, *N.Z.* **130 F5** 39 25 S 176 50 E
Baya, *Dem. Rep. of the Congo* **119 E2** 11 53 S 27 25 E
Bayambang, *Phil.* **80 D3** 15 49N 120 27 E
Bayamo, *Cuba* **164 B4** 20 20N 76 40W
Bayamón, *Puerto Rico* **165 d** 18 24N 66 9W
Bayan Har Shan, *China* **68 C4** 34 0N 98 0 E
Bayan Hot = Alxa Zuoqi, *China* **74 E3** 38 50N 105 40 E
Bayan Lepas, *Malaysia* **87 c** 5 17N 100 16 E
Bayan Obo, *China* **74 D5** 41 52N 109 59 E
Bayan-Ovoo = Erdenetsogt, *Mongolia* **74 C4** 42 55N 106 5 E
Bayan-Tumen = Choybalsan, *Mongolia* **69 B6** 48 4N 114 30 E
Bayana, *India* **92 F7** 26 55N 77 18 E
Bayanaūyl, *Kazakhstan* **66 D8** 50 45N 75 45 E
Bayandalay, *Mongolia* **74 C2** 43 30N 103 29 E
Bayanhongor, *Mongolia* **68 B5** 46 8N 102 43 E
Bayard, *N. Mex., U.S.A.* **159 K9** 32 46N 108 8W
Bayard, *Nebr., U.S.A.* **154 E3** 41 45N 103 20W
Bayawan, *Phil.* **81 G4** 9 46N 122 45 E
Baybay, *Phil.* **81 F5** 10 40N 124 55 E
Bayburt, *Turkey* **101 B9** 40 15N 40 20 E
Baydhabo = Baidoa, *Somali Rep.* **120 D2** 3 8N 43 30 E
Bayelsa □, *Nigeria* **113 E6** 4 30N 6 0 E
Bayerische Alpen, *Germany* **31 H7** 47 35N 11 30 E
Bayerische Rhön △, *Germany* **31 E6** 50 15N 10 5 E
Bayerischer Spessart △, *Germany* **31 F6** 49 58N 10 15 E
Bayerischer Wald, *Germany* **31 G8** 48 56N 12 50 E
Bayern □, *Germany* **31 G7** 48 50N 12 0 E
Bayeux, *France* **26 C6** 49 17N 0 42W
Bayfield, *Canada* **150 C3** 43 34N 81 42W
Bayfield, *U.S.A.* **154 B9** 46 49N 90 49W
Baygequm, *Kazakhstan* **65 A3** 44 19N 66 27 E
Bayḩān al Qīsāb, *Yemen* **98 D4** 15 48N 45 44 E
Bayındır, *Turkey* **49 C9** 38 13N 27 39 E
Bayjī, *Iraq* **101 E10** 35 0N 43 30 E
Baykal, Oz., *Russia* **67 D11** 53 0N 108 0 E
Baykan, *Turkey* **96 B4** 38 7N 41 44 E
Baykonur = Bayqongyr, *Kazakhstan* **66 E7** 47 48N 65 50 E
Baykurt, *China* **65 D7** 39 56N 75 33 E
Baymak, *Russia* **64 E7** 52 36N 58 19 E
Baymurat, *Uzbekistan* **65 C3** 41 8N 66 25 E
Baynes Mts., *Namibia* **116 B1** 17 15 S 13 0 E
Bayombong, *Phil.* **80 C3** 16 30N 121 10 E
Bayon, *France* **27 D13** 48 30N 6 20 E
Bayona = Baiona, *Spain* **42 C2** 42 6N 8 52W
Bayonet Point, *U.S.A.* **153 G7** 28 20N 82 42W
Bayonne, *France* **28 E2** 43 30N 1 28W
Bayonne, *U.S.A.* **151 F10** 40 40N 74 7W
Bayovar, *Peru* **172 B1** 5 50 S 81 0W
Bayport, *U.S.A.* **153 G7** 28 32N 82 39W
Bayqongyr, *Kazakhstan* **66 E7** 47 48N 65 50 E
Bayram-Ali = Bayramaly, *Turkmenistan* **66 F7** 37 37N 62 10 E
Bayramaly, *Turkmenistan* **66 F7** 37 37N 62 10 E
Bayramiç, *Turkey* **49 B8** 39 48N 26 36 E
Bayreuth, *Germany* **31 F7** 49 56N 11 35 E
Bayrischzell, *Germany* **31 H8** 47 41N 12 0 E
Bayrūt, *Lebanon* **103 B4** 33 53N 35 31 E
Bays, L. of, *Canada* **150 A5** 45 15N 79 4W
Bayshore, *U.S.A.* **153 J8** 26 43N 81 50W
Baysun, *Uzbekistan* **65 D3** 38 12N 67 12 E
Baysville, *Canada* **150 A5** 45 9N 79 7W
Bayt al Faqīh, *Yemen* **98 D3** 14 31N 43 19 E
Bayt Lahm, *West Bank* **103 D4** 31 43N 35 12 E
Baytown, *U.S.A.* **155 L7** 29 43N 94 59W
Bayugan, *Phil.* **81 G5** 8 43N 125 42 E
Bayun, *Indonesia* **79 J18** 8 11 S 115 16 E
Bayville = Kirkwood, *S. Africa* **116 E4** 33 22 S 25 15 E
Bayyrqum, *Kazakhstan* **65 B4** 42 7N 68 3 E
Bayzhansay, *Kazakhstan* **65 B4** 43 14N 69 54 E
Bayzo, *Niger* **113 C5** 13 52N 4 35 E
Baza, *Spain* **43 H8** 37 30N 2 47W
Bazar Dyuzi, *Russia* **61 K8** 41 12N 47 50 E
Bazar-Korgon, *Kyrgyzstan* **65 C6** 41 0N 72 43 E
Bazardüzü = Bazar Dyuzi, *Russia* **61 K8** 41 12N 47 50 E
Bazargic = Dobrich, *Bulgaria* **51 C11** 43 37N 27 49 E
Bazarny Karabulak, *Russia* **60 D8** 52 20N 46 29 E
Bazarnyy Syzgan, *Russia* **60 D8** 53 45N 46 40 E
Bazaruto △, *Mozam.* **117 C6** 21 42 S 35 26 E
Bazaruto, I. do, *Mozam.* **117 C6** 21 40 S 35 28 E
Bazas, *France* **28 D3** 44 27N 0 13W
Bazhong, *China* **76 B6** 31 52N 106 46 E
Bazhou, *China* **74 E9** 39 8N 116 22 E
Bazmān, Kūh-e, *Iran* **97 D9** 28 4N 60 1 E
Beach, *U.S.A.* **154 B3** 46 58N 104 0W
Beach City, *U.S.A.* **150 F3** 40 39N 81 35W
Beachport, *Australia* **128 D4** 37 29 S 140 0 E
Beachy Hd., *U.K.* **21 G8** 50 44N 0 15 E
Beacon, *Australia* **125 F2** 30 26 S 117 52 E
Beacon, *U.S.A.* **151 E11** 41 30N 73 58W
Beaconsfield, *Australia* **127 G4** 41 11 S 146 48 E
Beagle, Canal, *S. Amer.* **176 E3** 55 0 S 68 30W
Beagle Bay, *Australia* **124 C3** 16 58 S 122 40 E
Bealanana, *Madag.* **117 A8** 14 33 S 48 44 E
Beals Cr. →, *U.S.A.* **155 J4** 32 10N 100 51W
Beamsville, *Canada* **150 C5** 43 12N 79 28W
Bear →, *Calif., U.S.A.* **160 G5** 38 56N 121 36W
Bear →, *Utah, U.S.A.* **146 B4** 41 30N 112 8W
Béar, C., *France* **28 F7** 42 31N 3 8 E
Bear I., *Ireland* **23 E2** 51 38N 9 50W
Bear L., *Canada* **143 B9** 55 8N 96 0W
Bear L., *U.S.A.* **158 F8** 41 59N 111 21W
Beardmore, *Canada* **140 C2** 49 36N 87 57W
Beardmore Glacier, *Antarctica* **7 E11** 84 30 S 170 0 E
Beardstown, *U.S.A.* **156 E6** 40 1N 90 26W
Bearma →, *India* **93 G8** 24 20N 79 51 E
Béarn, *France* **28 E3** 43 20N 0 30W
Bearpaw Mts., *U.S.A.* **158 B9** 48 12N 109 30W
Bearskin Lake, *Canada* **140 B1** 53 58N 91 2W
Beas →, *India* **92 D6** 31 10N 74 59 E
Beas de Segura, *Spain* **43 G8** 38 15N 2 53W
Beasain, *Spain* **40 B2** 43 3N 2 11W
Beata, C., *Dom. Rep.* **165 C5** 17 40N 71 30W
Beata, I., *Dom. Rep.* **165 C5** 17 34N 71 31W
Beatrice, *U.S.A.* **154 E6** 40 16N 96 45W
Beatrice, *Zimbabwe* **119 F3** 18 15 S 30 55 E
Beatrice, C., *Australia* **126 A2** 14 20 S 136 55 E
Beatton →, *Canada* **142 B4** 56 15N 120 45W
Beatton River, *Canada* **142 B4** 57 26N 121 20W
Beatty, *U.S.A.* **160 J10** 36 54N 116 46W
Beau Bassin, *Mauritius* **121 d** 20 13 S 57 27 E
Beauaraba = Pittsworth, *Australia* **127 D5** 27 41 S 151 37 E
Beaucaire, *France* **29 E8** 43 48N 4 39 E
Beauce, Plaine de la, *France* **27 D8** 48 10N 1 45 E
Beauceville, *Canada* **141 C5** 46 13N 70 46W
Beauchêne, I., *Falk. Is.* **9 f** 52 55 S 59 15W
Beaudesert, *Australia* **127 D5** 27 59 S 153 0 E
Beaufort, *Australia* **128 D5** 37 25 S 143 25 E
Beaufort, *France* **29 C10** 45 44N 6 34 E
Beaufort, *Malaysia* **85 A5** 5 30N 115 40 E
Beaufort, *N.C., U.S.A.* **149 H7** 34 43N 76 40W
Beaufort, *S.C., U.S.A.* **152 C9** 32 26N 80 40W
Beaufort Sea, *Arctic* **6 B1** 72 0N 140 0W
Beaufort West, *S. Africa* **116 E3** 32 18 S 22 36 E
Beaugency, *France* **27 E8** 47 47N 1 38 E
Beauharnois, *Canada* **151 A11** 45 20N 73 52W
Beaujeu, *France* **27 F11** 46 10N 4 35 E
Beaujolais, *France* **27 F11** 46 0N 4 22 E
Beaulieu →, *Canada* **142 A6** 62 3N 113 11W
Beaulieu-sur-Dordogne, *France* **28 D5** 44 58N 1 50 E
Beaulieu-sur-Mer, *France* **29 E11** 43 42N 7 20 E
Beauly, *U.K.* **22 D4** 57 30N 4 28W
Beauly →, *U.K.* **22 D4** 57 29N 4 27W
Beaumaris, *U.K.* **20 D3** 53 16N 4 6W
Beaumont, *Belgium* **24 D4** 50 15N 4 14 E
Beaumont, *France* **28 D4** 44 45N 0 46 E
Beaumont, *N.Z.* **131 F4** 45 50 S 169 33 E
Beaumont, *U.S.A.* **155 K7** 30 5N 94 6W
Beaumont-de-Lomagne, *France* **28 E5** 43 53N 1 0 E
Beaumont-le-Roger, *France* **26 C7** 49 4N 0 47 E
Beaumont-sur-Sarthe, *France* **26 D7** 48 13N 0 8 E
Beaune, *France* **27 E11** 47 2N 4 50 E
Beaune-la-Rolande, *France* **27 D9** 48 4N 2 25 E
Beaupré, *Canada* **141 C5** 47 3N 70 54W
Beaupréau, *France* **26 E6** 47 12N 1 0W
Beauraing, *Belgium* **24 D4** 50 7N 4 57 E
Beaurepaire, *France* **29 C9** 45 22N 5 1 E
Beausejour, *Canada* **143 C9** 50 5N 96 35W
Beautemps-Beaupré, Î., *N. Cal.* **133 K4** 20 24 S 166 9 E
Beauvais, *France* **27 C9** 49 25N 2 8 E
Beauval, *Canada* **143 B7** 55 9N 107 37W
Beauvoir-sur-Mer, *France* **26 F4** 46 55N 2 2W
Beauvoir-sur-Niort, *France* **28 B3** 46 12N 0 30W
Beaver, *Alaska, U.S.A.* **144 C11** 66 22N 147 24W
Beaver, *Okla., U.S.A.* **155 G4** 36 49N 100 31W
Beaver, *Pa., U.S.A.* **150 F4** 40 42N 80 19W
Beaver, *Utah, U.S.A.* **159 G7** 38 17N 112 38W
Beaver →, *B.C., Canada* **142 B4** 59 52N 124 20W
Beaver →, *Ont., Canada* **140 A2** 55 55N 87 48W
Beaver →, *Sask., Canada* **143 B7** 55 26N 107 45W
Beaver →, *U.S.A.* **155 G5** 36 35N 99 30W
Beaver City, *U.S.A.* **154 E5** 40 8N 99 50W
Beaver Creek, *Canada* **138 B5** 63 0N 141 0W
Beaver Dam, *U.S.A.* **154 D10** 43 28N 88 50W
Beaver Falls, *U.S.A.* **150 F4** 40 46N 80 20W
Beaver Hill L., *Canada* **143 C10** 54 5N 94 50W
Beaver I., *U.S.A.* **148 C3** 45 40N 85 33W
Beavercreek, *U.S.A.* **157 E12** 39 43N 84 11W
Beaverhill L., *Canada* **142 C6** 53 27N 112 32W
Beaverlodge, *Canada* **142 B5** 55 11N 119 29W
Beaverstone →, *Canada* **140 B2** 54 59N 89 25W
Beaverton, *Canada* **150 B5** 44 26N 79 9W
Beaverton, *U.S.A.* **160 E4** 45 29N 122 48W
Beawar, *India* **92 F6** 26 3N 74 18 E
Bebedouro, *Brazil* **175 A6** 21 0 S 48 25W
Bebera, Tanjung, *Indonesia* **79 K18** 8 44 S 115 51 E
Beboa, *Madag.* **117 B7** 17 22 S 44 33 E
Beboto, *Chad* **109 G3** 8 16N 16 56 E
Bebra, *Germany* **30 E5** 50 58N 9 48 E
Becan, *Mexico* **163 D7** 18 31N 89 28W
Bécancour, *Canada* **148 B9** 46 20N 72 26W
Beccles, *U.K.* **21 E9** 52 27N 1 35 E
Bečej, *Serbia & M.* **52 E5** 45 36N 20 3 E
Beceni, *Romania* **53 E11** 45 23N 26 48 E
Becerreá, *Spain* **42 C3** 42 51N 7 10W
Béchar, *Algeria* **111 B4** 31 38N 2 18W
Becharof L., *U.S.A.* **144 H8** 57 56N 156 23W
Bechuanaland = Botswana ■, *Africa* **116 C3** 22 0 S 24 0 E
Bechyně, *Czech Rep.* **34 B7** 49 17N 14 29 E
Bečkerek = Zrenjanin, *Serbia & M.* **52 E5** 45 22N 20 23 E
Beckley, *U.S.A.* **148 G5** 37 47N 81 11W
Beckum, *Germany* **30 D4** 51 45N 8 3 E
Beclean, *Romania* **53 C9** 47 11N 24 11 E
Bečov nad Teplou, *Czech Rep.* **34 A5** 50 5N 12 49 E
Bečva →, *Czech Rep.* **35 B10** 49 31N 17 20 E
Bédar, *Spain* **41 H3** 37 11N 1 59W
Bédarieux, *France* **28 E7** 43 37N 3 10 E
Beddouza, Ras, *Morocco* **110 B3** 32 33N 9 9W
Bedeau = Ras el Ma, *Algeria* **111 B4** 34 26N 0 50W
Bedele, *Ethiopia* **107 F4** 8 31N 36 23 E
Bederkesa, *Germany* **30 B4** 53 37N 8 50 E
Bederwanak, *Somali Rep.* **120 C2** 9 34N 44 23 E
Bedeso, *Ethiopia* **107 F5** 9 58N 40 52 E
Bedford, *Canada* **151 A12** 45 7N 72 59W
Bedford, *S. Africa* **116 E4** 32 40 S 26 10 E
Bedford, *U.K.* **21 E7** 52 8N 0 28W
Bedford, *Ind., U.S.A.* **157 F10** 38 52N 86 29W
Bedford, *Iowa, U.S.A.* **156 D2** 40 40N 94 44W
Bedford, *Ky., U.S.A.* **157 F11** 38 36N 85 19W
Bedford, *Ohio, U.S.A.* **150 E3** 41 23N 81 32W
Bedford, *Pa., U.S.A.* **150 F6** 40 1N 78 30W
Bedford, *Va., U.S.A.* **148 G6** 37 20N 79 31W
Bedford, C., *Australia* **126 B4** 15 14 S 145 21 E
Bedfordshire □, *U.K.* **21 E7** 52 4N 0 28W
Bedi, *Chad* **109 F3** 11 6N 18 33 E
Będków, *Poland* **55 G6** 51 36N 19 44 E
Bednja →, *Croatia* **45 B13** 46 20N 16 52 E
Bednodemyanovsk, *Russia* **60 D6** 53 55N 43 15 E
Bedok, *Singapore* **87 d** 1 19N 103 56 E
Bedónia, *Italy* **44 D6** 44 30N 9 38 E
Bedourie, *Australia* **126 C2** 24 30 S 139 30 E
Bedretto, *Switz.* **33 C7** 46 31N 8 31 E
Bedti →, *India* **95 G2** 14 50N 74 44 E
Bedum, *Neths.* **24 A6** 53 18N 6 36 E
Będzin, *Poland* **55 H6** 50 19N 19 7 E
Bee Ridge, *U.S.A.* **153 H7** 27 17N 82 29W
Beebe Plain, *Canada* **151 A12** 45 1N 72 9W
Beech Creek, *U.S.A.* **150 E7** 41 5N 77 36W
Beech Fork →, *U.S.A.* **157 G11** 37 46N 85 41W
Beech Grove, *U.S.A.* **157 E10** 39 44N 86 3W
Beecher, *U.S.A.* **157 C9** 41 21N 87 38W
Beechey Point, *U.S.A.* **144 A10** 70 29N 149 9W
Beechworth, *Australia* **129 D7** 36 22 S 146 43 E
Beef I., *Br. Virgin Is.* **165 e** 18 26N 64 30W
Beelitz, *Germany* **30 C8** 52 14N 12 58 E
Beenleigh, *Australia* **127 D5** 27 43 S 153 10 E
Be'er Menuha, *Israel* **96 D2** 30 19N 35 8 E
Be'er Sheva, *Israel* **103 D3** 31 15N 34 48 E
Beersheba = Be'er Sheva, *Israel* **103 D3** 31 15N 34 48 E
Beeskow, *Germany* **30 C10** 52 10N 14 15 E

Beestekraal, S. Africa 117 D4 25 23 S 27 38 E
Beeston, U.K. 20 E6 52 56N 1 14W
Beetzendorf, Germany 30 C7 52 42N 11 6 E
Beeville, U.S.A. 155 L6 28 24N 97 45W
Befale, Dem. Rep. of the Congo 114 B4 0 25N 20 45 E
Befandriana, Mahajanga, Madag. 117 B8 15 16 S 48 32 E
Befandriana, Toliara, Madag. 117 C7 21 55 S 44 0 E
Befasy, Madag. 117 C7 20 33 S 44 23 E
Befori, Dem. Rep. of the Congo 114 B4 0 8N 22 22 E
Befotaka, Antsiranana, Madag. 117 A8 13 15 S 48 16 E
Befotaka, Fianarantsoa, Madag. 117 C8 23 49 S 47 0 E
Bega, Australia 129 D8 36 41 S 149 51 E
Bega, Canalul, Romania 52 E5 45 37N 20 46 E
Bégard, France 26 D3 48 38N 3 18W
Beğendik, Turkey 51 F10 40 55N 26 34 E
Begndal, Norway 18 D6 60 49N 9 46 E
Begoro, Ghana 113 D4 6 23N 0 23W
Begovat = Bekabad, Uzbekistan 65 C4 40 13N 69 14 E
Begusarai, India 93 G12 25 24N 86 9 E
Behābād, Iran 97 C8 32 24N 59 47 E
Behala, India 93 H13 22 30N 88 20 E
Behara, Madag. 117 C8 24 55 S 46 20 E
Behbehān, Iran 97 D6 30 30N 50 15 E
Behm Canal, U.S.A. 142 B2 55 10N 131 0W
Behshahr, Iran 97 B7 36 45N 53 35 E
Bei Jiang →, China 77 F9 23 2N 112 58 E
Bei'an, China 69 B7 48 10N 126 20 E
Beibei, China 76 C6 29 47N 106 22 E
Beichuan, China 76 B5 31 55N 104 39 E
Beihai, China 76 G7 21 28N 109 6 E
Beijing, China 74 E9 39 55N 116 20 E
Beijing □, China 74 E9 39 55N 116 20 E
Beilau = Pilawa, Poland 55 G8 51 57N 21 32 E
Beilen, Neths. 24 B6 52 52N 6 27 E
Beiliu, China 77 F8 22 41N 110 21 E
Beilngries, Germany 31 F7 49 2N 11 28 E
Beilpajah, Australia 128 B5 32 54 S 143 52 E
Beilul, Eritrea 107 E5 13 2N 42 20 E
Béinamar, Chad 109 G3 8 40N 15 23 E
Beinn na Faoghla = Benbecula, U.K. 22 D1 57 26N 7 21W
Beipan Jiang, China 76 E5 25 7N 106 1 E
Beipiao, China 75 D11 41 52N 120 32 E
Beira, Mozam. 119 F3 19 50 S 34 52 E
Beira, Somali Rep. 120 C3 6 57N 47 19 E
Beirut = Bayrūt, Lebanon 103 B4 33 53N 35 31 E
Beiseker, Canada 142 C6 51 23N 113 32W
Beitaolaizhao, China 75 B13 44 58N 125 58 E
Beitbridge, Zimbabwe 119 G3 22 12 S 30 0 E
Beiuş, Romania 52 D7 46 40N 22 21 E
Beizhen = Binzhou, China 75 F10 37 20N 118 2 E
Beizhen, China 75 D11 41 38N 121 54 E
Beizhengzhen, China 75 B12 44 31N 123 30 E
Beja, Portugal 43 G3 38 2N 7 53W
Béja, Tunisia 108 A1 36 43N 9 12 E
Beja □, Portugal 43 H3 37 55N 7 55W
Bejaïa, Algeria 111 A6 36 42N 5 2 E
Béjar, Spain 42 E5 40 23N 5 46W
Bejestān, Iran 97 C8 34 30N 58 5 E
Bek-Budi = Qarshi, Uzbekistan 65 D2 38 53N 65 48 E
Bekaa Valley = Al Biqā, Lebanon 103 A5 34 10N 36 10 E
Bekabad, Uzbekistan 65 C4 40 13N 69 14 E
Bekasi, Indonesia 84 D3 6 14 S 106 59 E
Bekçiler, Turkey 49 E11 36 56N 29 44 E
Békés, Hungary 52 D6 46 47N 21 9 E
Békés □, Hungary 52 D6 46 45N 21 0 E
Békéscsaba, Hungary 52 D6 46 40N 21 5 E
Bekilli, Turkey 49 C11 38 17N 29 27 E
Bekily, Madag. 117 C8 24 13 S 45 19 E
Bekisopa, Madag. 117 C8 21 40 S 45 54 E
Bekitro, Madag. 117 C8 24 33 S 45 18 E
Bekodoka, Madag. 117 B8 16 58 S 45 7 E
Bekoji, Ethiopia 107 F4 7 40N 39 17 E
Bekok, Malaysia 87 L4 2 20N 103 7 E
Bekopaka, Madag. 117 B7 19 9 S 44 48 E
Bekuli, Indonesia 79 J17 8 22 S 114 13 E
Bekwai, Ghana 113 D4 6 30N 1 34W
Bela, India 93 G10 25 50N 82 0 E
Bela, Pakistan 91 D2 26 12N 66 20 E
Bela Aliança = Rio do Sul, Brazil 175 B6 27 13 S 49 37W
Bela Bela, S. Africa 117 C4 24 51 S 28 19 E
Bela Crkva, Serbia & M. 52 F6 44 55N 21 27 E
Bela Palanka, Serbia & M. 50 C6 43 13N 22 17 E
Bela Vista, Brazil 174 A4 22 12 S 56 20W
Bela Vista, Mozam. 117 D5 26 10 S 32 44 E
Bélâbre, France 28 B5 46 34N 1 8 E
Belaga, Malaysia 85 B4 2 42N 113 47 E
Belalcázar, Spain 43 G5 38 35N 5 10W
Belan →, India 93 G9 24 2N 81 45 E
Belang, Indonesia 82 A2 0 57N 124 47 E
Belanovica, Serbia & M. 50 B4 44 15N 20 23 E
Belarus ■, Europe 58 F4 53 30N 27 0 E
Belas, Angola 115 D2 8 55 S 13 9 E
Belau = Palau ■, Pac. Oc. 62 J17 7 30N 134 30 E
Belavenona, Madag. 117 C8 24 50 S 47 4 E
Belawan, Indonesia 84 B1 3 33N 98 32 E
Belaya, Ethiopia 107 E4 11 25N 36 8 E
Belaya →, Russia 66 D4 54 40N 56 0 E
Belaya Glina, Russia 61 G5 46 5N 40 48 E
Belaya Kalitva, Russia 61 F5 48 13N 40 50 E
Belaya Kholunitsa, Russia 64 B3 58 51N 50 53 E
Belaya Tserkov = Bila Tserkva, Ukraine 59 H6 49 45N 30 10 E
Belayan →, Indonesia 85 C5 0 14 S 116 36 E
Belceşti, Romania 53 C12 47 19N 27 7 E
Bełchatów, Poland 55 G6 51 21N 19 22 E
Belcher Is., Canada 140 A3 56 15N 78 45W
Belchite, Spain 40 D4 41 18N 0 43W
Belden, U.S.A. 160 E5 40 2N 121 17W
Belding, U.S.A. 157 A11 43 6N 85 14W
Belebey, Russia 64 D5 54 7N 54 7 E
Beled Weyne = Belet Uen, Somali Rep. 120 D3 4 30N 45 5 E
Belém = Palmeirais, Brazil 170 C3 6 0 S 43 0W
Belém, Brazil 170 B2 1 20 S 48 30W
Belém de São Francisco, Brazil 170 C4 8 46 S 38 58W
Belén, Argentina 174 B2 27 40 S 67 5W
Belén, Colombia 168 C2 1 26N 75 56W
Belén, Paraguay 174 A4 23 30 S 57 6W
Belen, U.S.A. 159 J10 34 40N 106 46W
Belene, Bulgaria 51 C9 43 39N 25 10 E
Beleni, Turkey 100 D7 36 31N 36 10 E
Belep, Îs., N. Cal. 123 D11 19 45 S 163 40 E
Bélesta, France 28 F5 42 55N 1 56 E
Belet Uen, Somali Rep. 120 D3 4 30N 45 5 E
Belev, Russia 58 F9 53 50N 36 5 E
Belevi, Turkey 49 C9 38 0N 27 28 E
Belfair, U.S.A. 160 C4 47 27N 122 50W
Belfast, N.Z. 131 D7 43 27 S 172 39 E
Belfast, S. Africa 117 D5 25 42 S 30 2 E
Belfast, U.K. 23 B6 54 37N 5 56W
Belfast, Maine, U.S.A. 149 C11 44 26N 69 1W
Belfast, N.Y., U.S.A. 150 D6 42 21N 78 7W
Belfast L., U.K. 23 B6 54 40N 5 50W
Belfield, U.S.A. 154 B3 46 53N 103 12W
Belfort, France 27 E13 47 38N 6 50 E
Belfort, Territoire de □, France 27 E13 47 40N 6 55 E
Belfry, U.S.A. 158 D9 45 9N 109 1W
Belgard = Białogard, Poland 54 D2 54 2N 15 58 E
Belgaum, India 95 G2 15 55N 74 35 E
Belgian Congo = Congo, Dem. Rep. of the ■, Africa 115 C4 3 0 S 23 0 E
Belgioioso, Italy 44 C6 45 10N 9 19 E
Belgium ■, Europe 24 D4 50 30N 5 0 E
Belgodère, France 29 F13 42 35N 9 1 E
Belgorod, Russia 59 G9 50 35N 36 35 E
Belgorod-Dnestrovskiy = Bilhorod-Dnistrovskyy, Ukraine 59 J6 46 11N 30 23 E
Belgrade = Beograd, Serbia & M. 50 B4 44 50N 20 37 E
Belgrade, U.S.A. 158 D8 45 47N 111 11W
Belgrove, N.Z. 131 B7 41 27 S 172 59 E
Belhaven, U.S.A. 149 H7 35 33N 76 37W
Beli Drim →, Europe 50 D4 42 6N 20 25 E
Beli Manastir, Croatia 52 E3 45 45N 18 36 E
Beli Timok →, Serbia & M. 50 C6 43 53N 22 14 E
Bélice →, Italy 46 E5 37 35N 12 55 E
Belimbing, Indonesia 79 J18 8 24 S 115 2 E
Belinga, Gabon 114 B2 1 10N 13 2 E
Belinskiy, Russia 60 D6 53 0N 43 25 E
Belinyu, Indonesia 84 C3 1 35 S 105 50 E
Beliton Is. = Belitung, Indonesia 85 C3 3 10 S 107 50 E
Belitung, Indonesia 85 C3 3 10 S 107 50 E
Beliu, Romania 52 D6 46 30N 22 0 E
Belize, Angola 115 C2 4 39 S 12 46 E
Belize ■, Cent. Amer. 163 D7 17 0N 88 30W
Belize City, Belize 163 D7 17 25N 88 10W
Beljakovci, Macedonia 50 D5 42 6N 21 59 E
Beljanica, Serbia & M. 50 B5 44 8N 21 43 E
Belkovskiy, Ostrov, Russia 67 B14 75 32N 135 44 E
Bell, U.S.A. 152 F7 29 45N 82 52W
Bell →, Canada 140 C4 49 48N 77 38W
Bell I., Canada 141 B8 50 46N 55 35W
Bell-Irving →, Canada 142 B3 56 12N 129 5W
Bell Peninsula, Canada 139 B11 63 50N 82 0W
Bell Ville, Argentina 174 C3 32 40 S 62 40W
Bella, Italy 47 B8 40 45N 15 32 E
Bella Bella, Canada 142 C3 52 10N 128 10W
Bella Coola, Canada 142 C3 52 25N 126 40W
Bella Flor, Bolivia 172 C4 11 9 S 67 49W
Bella Unión, Uruguay 174 C4 30 15 S 57 40W
Bella Vista, Corrientes, Argentina 174 B4 28 33 S 59 0W
Bella Vista, Tucuman, Argentina 174 B2 27 10 S 65 25W
Bellac, France 28 B5 46 7N 1 3 E
Bellágio, Italy 44 C6 45 59N 9 15 E
Bellaire, U.S.A. 150 F4 40 1N 80 45W
Bellária, Italy 45 D9 44 9N 12 28 E
Bellary, India 95 G3 15 10N 76 56 E
Bellata, Australia 127 D4 29 53 S 149 46 E
Bellavista, Ecuador 172 a 0 41 S 90 18W
Belle, U.S.A. 156 F5 38 17N 91 43W
Belle Fourche, U.S.A. 154 C3 44 40N 103 51W
Belle Fourche →, U.S.A. 154 C3 44 26N 102 18W
Belle Glade, U.S.A. 153 J9 26 41N 80 40W
Belle-Île, France 26 E3 47 20N 3 10W
Belle Isle, Canada 141 B8 51 57N 55 25W
Belle Isle, U.S.A. 153 G8 28 27N 81 21W
Belle Isle, Str. of, Canada 141 B8 51 30N 56 30W
Belle Plaine, U.S.A. 156 C4 41 54N 92 17W
Belle Rive, U.S.A. 157 F8 38 14N 88 45W
Belle Yella, Liberia 112 D3 7 24N 10 0W
Belledonne, France 29 C10 45 20N 6 10 E
Bellefontaine, U.S.A. 157 D13 40 22N 83 46W
Bellefonte, U.S.A. 150 F7 40 55N 77 47W
Bellegarde, France 27 E9 47 59N 2 26 E
Bellegarde-en-Marche, France 28 C6 45 59N 2 18 E
Bellegarde-sur-Valserine, France 27 F12 46 4N 5 50 E
Bellême, France 26 D7 48 22N 0 34 E
Belleoram, Canada 141 C8 47 31N 55 25W
Belleplaine, Barbados 165 g 13 15N 59 34W
Belleview, U.S.A. 153 F7 29 4N 82 3W
Belleville, Canada 140 D4 44 10N 77 23W
Belleville, France 27 F11 46 7N 4 45 E
Belleville, Ill., U.S.A. 156 F7 38 31N 89 59W
Belleville, Kans., U.S.A. 154 F6 39 50N 97 38W
Belleville, N.Y., U.S.A. 151 C8 43 46N 76 10W
Belleville-sur-Vie, France 26 F5 46 46N 1 25W
Bellevue, Canada 142 D6 49 35N 114 22W
Bellevue, Idaho, U.S.A. 158 E6 43 28N 114 16W
Bellevue, Iowa, U.S.A. 156 B6 42 16N 90 26W
Bellevue, Mich., U.S.A. 157 B11 42 27N 85 1W
Bellevue, Nebr., U.S.A. 154 E7 41 8N 95 53W
Bellevue, Ohio, U.S.A. 150 E2 41 17N 82 51W
Bellevue, Wash., U.S.A. 160 C4 47 37N 122 12W
Belley, France 29 C9 45 46N 5 41 E
Bellin = Kangirsuk, Canada 139 B13 60 0N 70 0W
Bellinge, Denmark 17 J4 55 20N 10 20 E
Bellingen, Australia 129 A10 30 25 S 152 50 E
Bellingham, U.S.A. 160 B4 48 46N 122 29W
Bellingshausen Sea, Antarctica 7 C17 66 0 S 80 0W
Bellinzona, Switz. 33 D8 46 11N 9 1 E
Bello, Colombia 168 B2 6 20N 75 33W
Bellona, Solomon Is. 133 N10 11 17 S 159 47 E
Bellows Falls, U.S.A. 151 C12 43 8N 72 27W
Bellpat, Pakistan 92 E3 29 0N 68 5 E
Bellpuig d'Urgell, Spain 40 D6 41 37N 1 1 E
Belluno, Italy 45 B9 46 9N 12 13 E
Bellville, U.S.A. 152 C8 32 9N 81 59W
Bellwood, U.S.A. 150 F6 40 36N 78 20W
Bélmez, Spain 43 G5 38 17N 5 17W
Belmond, U.S.A. 156 B3 42 51N 93 37W
Belmont, Australia 129 B9 33 4 S 151 42 E
Belmont, Canada 150 D3 42 53N 81 5W
Belmont, S. Africa 116 D3 29 28 S 24 22 E
Belmont, U.S.A. 150 D6 42 14N 78 2W
Belmonte, Brazil 171 E4 16 0 S 39 0W
Belmonte, Portugal 42 E3 40 21N 7 20W
Belmonte, Spain 41 F2 39 34N 2 43W
Belmopan, Belize 163 D7 17 18N 88 30W
Belmullet, Ireland 23 B2 54 14N 9 58W
Belo, Dem. Rep. of the Congo 114 C4 0 32 S 23 13 E
Belo Horizonte, Brazil 171 E3 19 55 S 43 56W
Belo Jardim, Brazil 170 C4 8 20 S 36 26W
Belo Monte, Brazil 169 D7 3 5 S 51 46W
Belo-sur-Mer, Madag. 117 C7 20 42 S 44 0 E
Belo-Tsiribihina, Madag. 117 B7 19 40 S 44 30 E
Belogorsk = Bilohirsk, Ukraine 59 K8 45 3N 34 35 E
Belogorsk, Russia 67 D13 51 0N 128 20 E
Belogradchik, Bulgaria 50 C6 43 53N 22 42 E
Belogradets, Bulgaria 51 C11 43 22N 27 18 E
Beloha, Madag. 117 D8 25 10 S 45 3 E
Beloit, Kans., U.S.A. 154 F5 39 28N 98 6W
Beloit, Wis., U.S.A. 156 B7 42 31N 89 2W
Belokalitvenskaya = Belaya Kalitva, Russia 61 F5 48 13N 40 50 E
Belokorovichi, Ukraine 59 G5 51 7N 28 2 E
Belomorsk, Russia 56 B5 64 35N 34 54 E
Belondo, Dem. Rep. of the Congo 114 C3 0 19 S 19 31 E
Belonge, Dem. Rep. of the Congo 114 C3 2 7 S 19 33 E
Belonia, India 90 D3 23 15N 91 30 E
Belopolye = Bilopillya, Ukraine 59 G8 51 14N 34 20 E
Belorechensk, Russia 61 H4 44 46N 39 52 E
Beloretsk, Russia 64 E7 53 58N 58 24 E
Belorussia = Belarus ■, Europe 58 F4 53 30N 27 0 E
Beloshchelye = Naryan-Mar, Russia 56 A9 67 42N 53 12 E
Beloslav, Bulgaria 51 C11 43 11N 27 42 E
Belotsarsk = Kyzyl, Russia 67 D10 51 50N 94 30 E
Belovo, Bulgaria 51 D8 42 13N 24 1 E
Belovo, Russia 66 D9 54 30N 86 0 E
Belovodsk, Ukraine 59 H10 49 13N 39 36 E
Beloyarskiy, Russia 64 C8 56 45N 61 24 E
Beloye, Ozero, Russia 58 B9 60 10N 37 35 E
Beloye More, Russia 56 A6 66 30N 38 0 E
Belozem, Bulgaria 51 D9 42 12N 25 2 E
Belozersk, Russia 58 B9 60 1N 37 45 E
Belp, Switz. 32 C5 46 53N 7 30 E
Belpasso, Italy 47 E7 37 35N 14 58 E
Belpre, U.S.A. 148 F5 39 17N 81 34W
Belrain, India 93 E9 28 23N 80 55 E
Belt, U.S.A. 158 C8 47 23N 110 55W
Beltana, Australia 128 A3 30 48 S 138 25 E
Belterra, Brazil 169 D7 2 45 S 55 0W
Beltinci, Slovenia 45 B13 46 37N 16 20 E
Belton, Mo., U.S.A. 156 F2 38 49N 94 32W
Belton, Tex., U.S.A. 155 K6 31 3N 97 28W
Belton L., U.S.A. 155 K6 31 8N 97 32W
Beltsy = Bălţi, Moldova 53 C12 47 48N 27 58 E
Belturbet, Ireland 23 B4 54 6N 7 26W
Belukha, Russia 66 E9 49 50N 86 50 E
Beluran, Malaysia 78 C5 5 48N 117 35 E
Beluša, Slovak Rep. 35 B11 49 5N 18 17 E
Belušić, Serbia & M. 50 C5 43 50N 21 10 E
Belvedere Maríttimo, Italy 47 C8 39 37N 15 52 E
Belvès, France 28 D5 44 46N 1 0 E
Belvidere, Ill., U.S.A. 154 D10 42 15N 88 50W
Belvidere, N.J., U.S.A. 151 F9 40 50N 75 5W
Belvis de la Jara, Spain 42 F6 39 45N 4 57W
Bely Bychek = Chagoda, Russia 58 C8 59 10N 35 15 E
Belyando →, Australia 126 C4 21 38 S 146 50 E
Belyy, Russia 58 E7 55 49N 33 3 E
Belyy, Ostrov, Russia 66 B8 73 30N 71 0 E
Belyy Yar, Russia 66 D9 58 26N 84 39 E
Belyye Vody = Aqsū, Kazakhstan 65 B4 42 25N 69 50 E
Belz, Ukraine 55 H11 50 23N 24 1 E
Bełżec, Poland 55 H10 50 23N 23 26 E
Belzig, Germany 30 C8 52 8N 12 35 E
Belzoni, U.S.A. 155 J9 33 11N 90 29W
Bełżyce, Poland 55 G9 51 11N 22 17 E
Bemaraha, Lembalemban' i, Madag. 117 B7 18 40 S 44 45 E
Bemarivo, Madag. 117 C7 21 45 S 44 45 E
Bemarivo →, Antsiranana, Madag. 117 A9 14 9 S 50 9 E
Bemarivo →, Mahajanga, Madag. 117 B8 15 27 S 47 40 E
Bemavo, Madag. 117 C8 21 33 S 45 25 E
Bembe, Angola 115 D2 7 3 S 14 25 E
Bembéréke, Benin 113 C5 10 11N 2 43 E
Bembesi, Zimbabwe 119 G2 20 0 S 28 58 E
Bembesi →, Zimbabwe 119 F2 18 57 S 27 47 E
Bembézar →, Spain 43 H5 37 45N 5 13W
Bembibre, Spain 42 C4 42 37N 6 25W
Bemboka △, Australia 129 D8 36 35 S 149 41 E
Bement, U.S.A. 157 E8 39 55N 88 34W
Bemetara, India 93 J9 21 42N 81 32 E
Bemidji, U.S.A. 154 B7 47 28N 94 53W
Bemolanga, Madag. 117 B8 17 44 S 45 6 E
Ben, Iran 97 C6 32 32N 50 45 E
Ben Boyd △, Australia 129 D8 37 0 S 149 55 E
Ben Cruachan, U.K. 22 E3 56 26N 5 8W
Ben Dearg, U.K. 22 D4 57 47N 4 56W
Ben En △, Vietnam 86 C5 19 37N 105 30 E
Ben Gardane, Tunisia 108 B2 33 11N 11 11 E
Ben Hope, U.K. 22 C4 58 25N 4 36W
Ben Lawers, U.K. 22 E4 56 32N 4 14W
Ben Lomond, N.S.W., Australia 127 E5 30 1 S 151 43 E
Ben Lomond, Tas., Australia 127 G4 41 38 S 147 42 E
Ben Lomond, U.K. 22 E4 56 11N 4 38W
Ben Lomond △, Australia 127 G4 41 33 S 147 39 E
Ben Luc, Vietnam 87 G6 10 39N 106 29 E
Ben Macdhui, U.K. 22 D5 57 4N 3 40W
Ben Mhor, U.K. 22 D1 57 15N 7 18W
Ben More, Arg. & Bute, U.K. 22 E2 56 26N 6 1W
Ben More, Stirl., U.K. 22 E4 56 23N 4 32W
Ben More Assynt, U.K. 22 C4 58 8N 4 52W
Ben Nevis, U.K. 22 E3 56 48N 5 1W
Ben Ohau Ra., N.Z. 131 E5 44 1 S 170 4 E
Ben Quang, Vietnam 86 D6 17 3N 106 55 E
Ben Slimane, Morocco 110 B3 33 38N 7 7W
Ben Vorlich, U.K. 22 E4 56 21N 4 14W
Ben Wyvis, U.K. 22 D4 57 40N 4 35W
Bena, Nigeria 113 C6 11 20N 5 50 E
Bena-Dibele, Dem. Rep. of the Congo 115 C4 4 4 S 22 50 E
Bena-Leka, Dem. Rep. of the Congo 115 D4 5 8 S 22 10 E
Bena-Tshadi, Dem. Rep. of the Congo 115 C4 4 40 S 22 49 E
Benadir, Somali Rep. 120 D2 1 30N 44 30 E
Benagerie, Australia 128 A4 31 25 S 140 22 E
Benahmed, Morocco 110 B3 33 4N 7 9W
Benalla, Australia 129 D7 36 30 S 146 0 E
Benalmádena, Spain 43 J6 36 36N 4 34W
Benambra, Mt., Australia 129 D7 36 31 S 147 34 E
Benanee, Australia 128 C5 34 31 S 142 52 E
Benares = Varanasi, India 93 G10 25 22N 83 0 E
Bénat, C., France 29 E10 43 5N 6 22 E
Benavente, Portugal 43 G2 38 59N 8 49W
Benavente, Spain 42 C5 42 2N 5 43W
Benavides, U.S.A. 155 M5 27 36N 98 25W
Benavides de Órbigo, Spain 42 C5 42 30N 5 54W
Benbecula, U.K. 22 D1 57 26N 7 21W
Benbonyathe, Australia 128 A3 30 25 S 139 11 E
Bend, U.S.A. 158 D3 44 4N 121 19W
Bendela, Dem. Rep. of the Congo 114 C3 3 18 S 17 36 E
Bendemeer, Australia 129 A9 30 53 S 151 8 E
Bender Beila, Somali Rep. 120 C4 9 30N 50 48 E
Bender Merchagno, Somali Rep. 120 B4 11 41N 50 34 E
Bendery = Tighina, Moldova 53 D14 46 50N 29 30 E
Bendigo, Australia 128 D6 36 40 S 144 15 E
Bendin = Będzin, Poland 55 H6 50 19N 19 7 E
Bendorf, Germany 30 E3 50 25N 7 35 E
Bendsburg = Będzin, Poland 55 H6 50 19N 19 7 E
Benē Beraq, Israel 103 C3 32 6N 34 51 E
Beneditinos, Brazil 170 C3 5 27 S 42 22W
Benedito Leite, Brazil 170 C3 7 13 S 44 34W
Bénéna, Mali 112 C4 13 9N 4 17W
Benenitra, Madag. 117 C8 23 27 S 45 5 E
Benešov, Czech Rep. 34 B7 49 46N 14 41 E
Benevento, Italy 47 A7 41 8N 14 45 E
Benfeld, France 27 D14 48 22N 7 34 E
Benga, Mozam. 119 F3 16 11 S 33 40 E
Bengal = West Bengal □, India 93 H13 23 0N 88 0 E
Bengal, Bay of, Ind. Oc. 89 D7 15 0N 90 0 E
Bengalūru = Bangalore, India 95 H3 12 59N 77 40 E
Bengbis, Cameroon 113 E7 3 27N 12 36 E
Bengbu, China 75 H9 32 58N 117 20 E
Benghazi = Banghāzī, Libya 108 B4 32 11N 20 3 E
Benghisa Point, Malta 38 F8 35 49N 14 33 E
Bengkalis, Indonesia 84 B2 1 30N 102 10 E
Bengkulu, Indonesia 84 C2 3 50 S 102 12 E
Bengkulu □, Indonesia 84 C2 3 48 S 102 16 E
Bengo, Dem. Rep. of the Congo 114 C3 2 11 S 19 5 E
Bengo □, Angola 115 D2 9 0 S 13 10 E
Bengough, Canada 143 D7 49 25N 105 10W
Bengtsfors, Sweden 16 E6 59 2N 12 14 E
Benguela, Angola 115 E2 12 37 S 13 25 E
Benguela □, Angola 115 E2 13 0 S 13 30 E
Benguerir, Morocco 110 B3 32 16N 7 56W
Benguérua, I., Mozam. 117 C6 21 58 S 35 28 E
Benguet □, Phil. 80 C3 16 30N 120 40 E
Benha, Egypt 106 H7 30 26N 31 8 E
Benham Seamount, Pac. Oc. 80 D5 15 40N 124 30 E
Beni, Dem. Rep. of the Congo 118 B2 0 30N 29 27 E
Beni □, Bolivia 173 C4 14 0 S 65 0W
Beni →, Bolivia 173 C4 10 23 S 65 24W
Beni Abbès, Algeria 111 B4 30 5N 2 5W
Beni Haoua, Algeria 111 A5 36 30N 1 30 E
Beni Mazâr, Egypt 106 B3 28 32N 30 44 E
Beni Mellal, Morocco 110 B3 32 21N 6 21W
Beni Ounif, Algeria 111 B4 32 0N 1 10W
Beni Saf, Algeria 111 A4 35 17N 1 15W
Beni Suef, Egypt 106 J7 29 5N 31 6 E
Beniah L., Canada 142 A6 63 23N 112 17W
Benicarló, Spain 40 E5 40 23N 0 23 E
Benicàssim, Spain 40 E5 40 3N 0 4 E
Benicia, U.S.A. 160 G4 38 3N 122 9W
Benidorm, Spain 41 G4 38 33N 0 9W
Benin ■, Africa 113 D5 10 0N 2 0 E
Benin →, Nigeria 113 D6 5 45N 5 4 E
Benin, Bight of, W. Afr. 113 E5 5 0N 3 0 E
Benin City, Nigeria 113 D6 6 20N 5 31 E
Benisa, Spain 41 G5 38 43N 0 3 E
Benitses, Greece 38 B9 39 32N 19 55 E
Benjamin Aceval, Paraguay 174 A4 24 58 S 57 34W
Benjamin Constant, Brazil 168 D3 4 40 S 70 15W
Benjamin Hill, Mexico 162 A2 30 10N 111 10W
Benkelman, U.S.A. 154 E4 40 3N 101 32W
Benkovac, Croatia 45 D12 44 2N 15 37 E
Benmore Pk., N.Z. 131 E5 44 25 S 170 8 E
Bennett, Canada 142 B2 59 56N 134 53W
Bennett, L., Australia 124 D5 22 50 S 131 2 E
Bennetta, Ostrov, Russia 67 B15 76 21N 148 56 E
Bennettsville, U.S.A. 149 H6 34 37N 79 41W
Bennichchãb, Mauritania 112 B1 19 32N 15 12W
Bennington, N.H., U.S.A. 151 D11 43 0N 71 55W
Bennington, Vt., U.S.A. 151 D11 42 53N 73 12W
Beno, Dem. Rep. of the Congo 114 C3 3 41 S 17 49 E
Bénodet, France 26 E2 47 53N 4 7W
Benoni, S. Africa 117 D4 26 11 S 28 18 E
Benoud, Algeria 111 B5 32 20N 0 16 E
Bénoué △, Cameroon 114 A2 8 30N 13 55 E
Benoy, Chad 109 G3 8 59N 16 19 E
Benque Viejo del Carmen, Belize 163 D7 17 5N 89 8W
Bensheim, Germany 31 F4 49 40N 8 38 E
Benson, Ariz., U.S.A. 159 L8 31 58N 110 18W
Benson, Minn., U.S.A. 154 C7 45 19N 95 36W
Bent, Iran 97 E8 26 20N 59 31 E
Benteng, Indonesia 82 C2 6 10 S 120 30 E
Bentiaba, Angola 115 E2 14 15 S 12 21 E
Bentinck I., Australia 126 B2 17 3 S 139 35 E
Bentiu, Sudan 107 F2 9 10N 29 55 E
Bento Gonçalves, Brazil 175 B5 29 10 S 51 31W
Benton, Ark., U.S.A. 155 H8 34 34N 92 35W
Benton, Calif., U.S.A. 160 H8 37 48N 118 32W
Benton, Ill., U.S.A. 156 G8 38 0N 88 55W
Benton, Pa., U.S.A. 151 E8 41 12N 76 23W
Benton Harbor, U.S.A. 157 B10 42 6N 86 27W
Benton Heights, U.S.A. 157 B10 42 7N 86 24W
Bentong, Malaysia 87 L3 3 31N 101 55 E
Bentonville, U.S.A. 155 G7 36 22N 94 13W
Bentu Liben, Ethiopia 107 F4 8 32N 38 21 E
Benue □, Nigeria 113 D6 7 20N 8 45 E
Benue →, Nigeria 113 D6 7 48N 6 46 E
Benxi, China 75 D12 41 20N 123 48 E
Benza, Dem. Rep. of the Congo 115 D2 4 49 S 13 17 E
Benzdorp, Suriname 169 C7 3 44N 54 5W
Beo, Indonesia 82 A3 4 25N 126 50 E
Beograd, Serbia & M. 50 B4 44 50N 20 37 E
Beograd ✕ (BEG), Serbia & M. 50 C4 43 49N 20 17 E
Beoumi, Ivory C. 112 D3 7 45N 5 17W
Bepan Jiang →, China 76 E6 24 55N 106 5 E
Beppu, Japan 72 D3 33 15N 131 30 E
Beppu-Wan, Japan 72 D3 33 18N 131 34 E
Beqa, Fiji 133 B2 18 23 S 178 8 E
Beqaa Valley = Al Biqā, Lebanon 103 A5 34 10N 36 10 E
Ber Mota, India 92 H3 23 27N 68 34 E
Bera, Bangla. 90 C2 24 5N 89 37 E
Berach →, India 92 G6 25 15N 75 2 E
Beraketa, Madag. 117 C7 23 7 S 44 25 E
Béran-Djoko, Congo 114 B3 3 15N 17 0 E
Berane, Serbia & M. 50 D3 42 51N 19 52 E
Berat, Albania 50 F3 40 43N 19 59 E
Berau →, Indonesia 85 B5 2 10N 117 42 E
Berau, Teluk, Indonesia 83 B4 2 30 S 132 30 E
Beravina, Madag. 117 B8 18 10 S 45 14 E
Berber, Sudan 106 D3 18 0N 34 0 E
Berbera, Somali Rep. 120 B3 10 30N 45 2 E
Berbérati, C.A.R. 114 B3 4 15N 15 40 E
Berbice →, Guyana 169 B6 6 20N 57 32W
Berceto, Italy 44 D6 44 31N 9 51 E
Berchidda, Italy 46 B2 40 47N 9 10 E
Berchtesgaden, Germany 31 H8 47 38N 13 0 E
Berchtesgaden △, Germany 31 H8 47 34N 12 55 E
Berck, France 27 B8 50 25N 1 36 E
Berdale, Somali Rep. 120 C3 7 4N 47 51 E
Berdichev = Berdychiv, Ukraine 59 H5 49 57N 28 30 E
Berdsk, Russia 66 D9 54 47N 83 2 E
Berdyansk, Ukraine 59 J9 46 45N 36 50 E
Berdyaush, Russia 64 D7 55 9N 59 9 E
Berdychiv, Ukraine 59 H5 49 57N 28 30 E
Berea, U.S.A. 148 G3 37 34N 84 17W
Berebere, Indonesia 82 A3 2 25N 128 45 E
Bereda, Somali Rep. 120 B4 11 45N 51 0 E
Berehomet, Ukraine 53 B10 48 10N 25 19 E
Berehove, Ukraine 52 B7 48 15N 22 35 E
Bereina, Papua N. G. 132 E4 8 39 S 146 30 E
Berekum, Ghana 112 D4 7 29N 2 34W
Berenice, Egypt 106 C4 24 2N 35 25 E
Berens →, Canada 143 C9 52 25N 97 2W
Berens I., Canada 143 C9 52 18N 97 18W
Berens River, Canada 143 C9 52 25N 97 0W
Beresford, U.S.A. 154 D6 43 5N 96 47W
Berestechko, Ukraine 59 G3 50 22N 25 5 E
Bereşti, Romania 53 D12 46 6N 27 50 E
Beretău →, Romania 52 C6 47 10N 21 50 E
Berettyó →, Hungary 52 D6 46 59N 21 7 E
Berettyóújfalu, Hungary 52 C6 47 13N 21 33 E
Berevo, Mahajanga, Madag. 117 B7 17 14 S 44 17 E
Berevo, Toliara, Madag. 117 B7 19 44 S 44 58 E
Bereza = Byaroza, Belarus 59 F3 52 31N 24 51 E
Berezhany, Ukraine 59 H3 49 26N 24 58 E
Berezina = Byarezina →, Belarus 59 F6 52 33N 30 14 E
Berezivka, Ukraine 59 J6 47 14N 30 55 E
Berezna, Ukraine 59 G6 51 35N 31 46 E
Bereznik, Russia 56 B7 62 51N 42 40 E
Berezniki, Russia 64 B6 59 24N 56 46 E
Berezovo, Russia 66 C7 64 0N 65 0 E
Berezyne, Ukraine 53 D14 46 14N 29 12 E
Berga, Spain 40 C6 42 6N 1 48 E
Berga, Sweden 17 G10 57 14N 16 3 E
Bergama, Turkey 49 B9 39 8N 27 11 E
Bérgamo, Italy 44 C6 45 41N 9 43 E
Bergaon, India 94 D5 20 41N 80 27 E
Bergara, Spain 40 B2 43 9N 2 28W
Bergby, Sweden 16 D11 60 57N 17 2 E
Bergedorf, Germany 30 B6 53 28N 10 6 E
Bergeforsen, Sweden 16 B11 62 32N 17 23 E
Bergen, Mecklenburg-Vorpommern, Germany 30 A9 54 25N 13 25 E
Bergen, Niedersachsen, Germany 30 C5 52 49N 9 57 E
Bergen, Neths. 24 B4 52 40N 4 43 E
Bergen, Norway 18 D2 60 20N 5 20 E
Bergen, U.S.A. 150 C7 43 5N 77 57W
Bergen ✕ (BGO), Norway 18 D2 60 17N 5 19 E
Bergen op Zoom, Neths. 24 C4 51 28N 4 18 E
Bergerac, France 28 D4 44 51N 0 30 E
Bergheim, Germany 30 E2 50 57N 6 38 E
Bergholz, U.S.A. 150 F4 40 31N 80 53W
Bergisch Gladbach, Germany 24 D7 50 59N 7 8 E
Bergisches Land △, Germany 30 E3 51 0N 7 30 E
Bergkamen, Germany 30 D3 51 37N 7 38 E
Bergkvara, Sweden 17 H10 56 23N 16 5 E
Bergshamra, Sweden 16 E12 59 38N 18 37 E
Bergsjö, Sweden 16 C11 61 59N 17 3 E
Bergstadt = Leśnica, Poland 55 H5 50 26N 18 11 E
Bergstrasse-Odenwald △, Germany 31 F1 49 45N 5 55 E
Bergues, France 27 B9 50 58N 2 24 E
Bergviken, Sweden 16 C10 61 15N 16 40 E
Bergville, S. Africa 117 D4 28 52 S 29 18 E
Berhala, Selat, Indonesia 84 C2 1 0 S 104 15 E
Berhampore = Baharampur, India 93 G13 24 2N 88 27 E
Berhampur = Brahmapur, India 94 E7 19 15N 84 54 E
Berheci →, Romania 53 E12 45 58N 27 28 E
Bering Glacier, U.S.A. 144 F12 60 20N 143 30W
Bering Land Bridge △, U.S.A. 144 C6 66 20N 165 0W
Bering Sea, Pac. Oc. 138 C1 58 0N 171 0W
Bering Strait, Pac. Oc. 144 D5 65 30N 169 0W
Beringen, Switz. 33 A7 47 38N 8 34 E
Beringovskiy, Russia 67 C18 63 3N 179 19 E
Berisso, Argentina 174 C4 34 56 S 57 50W
Berja, Spain 43 J8 36 50N 2 56W
Berkåk, Norway 18 B6 62 50N 10 0 E
Berkane, Morocco 111 B4 34 52N 2 20W
Berkeley, U.S.A. 160 H4 37 52N 122 16W
Berkeley, C., Ecuador 172 a 0 1N 91 35W
Berkner I., Antarctica 7 D18 79 30 S 50 0W
Berkovitsa, Bulgaria 50 C7 43 16N 23 8 E
Berkshire, U.S.A. 151 D8 42 19N 76 11W
Berkshire Downs, U.K. 21 F6 51 33N 1 29W
Berlanga, Spain 43 G5 38 17N 5 50W
Berlanga, I., Portugal 43 F1 39 25N 9 30W
Berlengas = Valença do Piauí, Brazil 170 C3 6 20 S 41 45W
Berlin = Kitchener, Canada 140 D3 43 27N 80 29W
Berlin, Germany 30 C9 52 30N 13 25 E
Berlin, Ga., U.S.A. 152 D6 31 4N 83 37W
Berlin, Md., U.S.A. 148 F8 38 20N 75 13W
Berlin, N.H., U.S.A. 151 B13 44 28N 71 11W
Berlin, N.Y., U.S.A. 151 D11 42 42N 73 23W
Berlin, Wis., U.S.A. 148 D1 43 58N 88 57W
Berlin □, Germany 30 C9 52 30N 13 20 E
Berlin L., U.S.A. 150 E4 41 3N 81 0W
Berlin Tegel ✕ (TXL), Germany 30 C9 52 35N 13 14 E

Berlinchen = Barlinek, Poland 55 F2 53 0N 15 15 E
Bermagui, Australia 129 D9 36 25 S 150 4 E
Bermeja, Sierra, Spain 43 J5 36 30N 5 11W
Bermejo →, Formosa, Argentina 174 B4 26 51 S 58 23W
Bermejo →, San Juan, Argentina 174 C2 32 30 S 67 30W
Bermen, L., Canada 141 B6 53 35N 68 55W
Bermeo, Spain 40 B2 43 25N 2 47W
Bermillo de Sayago, Spain 42 D4 41 22N 6 8W
Bermuda ⊠, Atl. Oc. 9 a 32 45N 65 0W
Bermuda International ✕ (BDA), Bermuda 9 a 32 22N 64 41W
Bern, Switz. 32 C4 46 57N 7 28 E
Bern □, Switz. 32 C5 46 45N 7 40 E
Bernalda, Italy 47 B9 40 24N 16 41 E
Bernalillo, U.S.A. 159 J10 35 18N 106 33W
Bernam →, Malaysia 84 B2 3 45N 101 5 E
Bernardo de Irigoyen, Argentina 175 B5 26 15 S 53 40W
Bernardo O'Higgins □, Chile 174 C1 34 15 S 70 45W
Bernardo O'Higgins △, Chile 176 C1 48 50 S 75 36W
Bernardsville, U.S.A. 151 F10 40 43N 74 34W
Bernasconi, Argentina 174 D3 37 55 S 63 44W
Bernau, Bayern, Germany 31 H8 47 47N 12 22 E
Bernau, Brandenburg, Germany 30 C9 52 40N 13 35 E
Bernay, France 26 C7 49 5N 0 35 E
Bernburg, Germany 30 D7 51 47N 11 44 E
Berndorf, Austria 34 D9 47 59N 16 1 E
Berne = Bern, Switz. 32 C4 46 57N 7 28 E
Berne = Bern □, Switz. 32 C5 46 45N 7 40 E
Berne, U.S.A. 157 D12 40 39N 84 57W
Berner Alpen, Switz. 32 D5 46 27N 7 35 E
Berneray, U.K. 22 D1 57 43N 7 11W
Bernese Oberland = Oberland, Switz. 32 C5 46 35N 7 38 E
Bernier I., Australia 125 D1 24 50 S 113 12 E
Bernina, Passo del, Switz. 33 D10 46 25N 10 2 E
Bernina, Piz, Switz. 33 D9 46 20N 9 54 E
Bernkastel-Kues, Germany 31 F3 49 55N 7 3 E
Bernstadt = Bierutów, Poland 55 G4 51 7N 17 32 E
Bernstein = Pełczyce, Poland 55 E2 53 3N 15 16 E
Bero →, Angola 115 F2 15 10 S 12 9 E
Beroroha, Madag. 117 C8 21 40 S 45 10 E
Bérouboua y, Benin 113 C5 10 34N 2 46 E
Beroun, Czech Rep. 34 B7 49 57N 14 5 E
Berounka →, Czech Rep. 34 B7 50 0N 14 22 E
Berovo, Macedonia 50 E6 41 38N 22 51 E
Berrahal, Algeria 111 A6 36 54N 7 33 E
Berre, Étang de, France 29 E9 43 27N 5 5 E
Berre-l'Étang, France 29 E9 43 27N 5 10 E
Berrechid, Morocco 110 B3 33 18N 7 36W
Berri, Australia 128 C4 34 14 S 140 35 E
Berriane, Algeria 111 B5 32 50N 3 46 E
Berridale, Australia 129 D8 36 22 S 148 48 E
Berrien Springs, U.S.A. 157 C10 41 57N 86 20W
Berrigan, Australia 129 C6 35 38 S 145 49 E
Berriwillock, Australia 128 C5 35 36 S 142 59 E
Berrouaghia, Algeria 111 A5 36 10N 2 53 E
Berry, Australia 129 C9 34 46 S 150 43 E
Berry, France 27 F8 46 50N 2 0 E
Berry Is., Bahamas 164 A4 25 40N 77 50W
Berrydale, U.S.A. 153 E2 30 53N 87 3W
Berryessa L., U.S.A. 160 G4 38 31N 122 6W
Berryville, U.S.A. 155 G8 36 22N 93 34W
Berseba, Namibia 116 D2 26 0 S 17 46 E
Bersenbrück, Germany 30 C3 52 34N 7 56 E
Bershad, Ukraine 53 B14 48 22N 29 31 E
Berthold, U.S.A. 154 A4 48 19N 101 44W
Berthoud, U.S.A. 154 E2 40 19N 105 5W
Bertincourt, France 27 B9 50 5N 2 58 E
Bertolínia, Brazil 170 C3 7 38 S 43 57W
Bertoua, Cameroon 114 B2 4 30N 13 45 E
Bertraghboy B., Ireland 23 C2 53 22N 9 54W
Bertys = Balqash, Kazakhstan 66 E8 46 50N 74 50 E
Berufjörður, Iceland 11 C12 64 48N 14 29W
Berunes, Iceland 11 C12 64 42N 14 16W
Beruri, Brazil 169 D5 3 54 S 61 22W
Berwick, U.S.A. 151 E8 41 3N 76 14W
Berwick-upon-Tweed, U.K. 20 B6 55 46N 2 0W
Berwyn Mts., U.K. 20 E4 52 54N 3 26W
Beryslav, Ukraine 59 J7 46 50N 33 30 E
Berzasca, Romania 52 F6 44 39N 21 58 E
Berzence, Hungary 52 D2 46 12N 17 11 E
Besal, Pakistan 93 B5 35 4N 73 56 E
Besalampy, Madag. 117 B7 16 43 S 44 29 E
Besançon, France 27 E13 47 15N 6 2 E
Besar, Indonesia 85 C5 2 40 S 116 0 E
Besar, Gunong, Malaysia 84 A2 5 10N 101 18 E
Besharyk, Uzbekistan 65 C5 40 26N 70 36 E
Beshenkovichi, Belarus 58 E5 55 2N 29 29 E
Beshkent, Uzbekistan 65 D2 38 49N 65 39 E
Beška, Serbia & M. 52 E5 45 8N 20 6 E
Beslan, Russia 61 J7 43 15N 44 28 E
Besna Kobila, Serbia & M. 50 D6 42 31N 22 10 E
Besnard L., Canada 143 B7 55 25N 106 0W
Besni, Turkey 100 D7 37 41N 37 52 E
Besor, N. →, Egypt 103 D3 31 28N 34 22 E
Bessa Monteiro, Angola 115 D2 7 7 S 13 44 E
Bessarabiya, Moldova 59 J5 47 0N 28 10 E
Bessarabka = Basarabeasca, Moldova 53 D13 46 21N 28 58 E
Bessèges, France 29 D8 44 18N 4 8 E
Bessemer, Ala., U.S.A. 149 J2 33 24N 86 58W
Bessemer, Mich., U.S.A. 154 B9 46 29N 90 3W
Bessemer, Pa., U.S.A. 150 F4 40 59N 80 30W
Bessin, France 26 C6 49 18N 1 0W
Bessines-sur-Gartempe, France 28 B5 46 6N 1 22 E
Beswick, Australia 124 B5 14 34 S 132 53 E
Bet She'an, Israel 103 C4 32 30N 35 30 E
Bet Shemesh, Israel 103 D4 31 44N 35 0 E
Bet Tadjine, Djebel, Algeria 110 C4 29 0N 3 30W
Betafo, Madag. 117 B8 19 50 S 46 51 E
Betamba, Dem. Rep. of the Congo 114 C4 2 17 S 21 24 E
Betancuria, Canary Is. 9 e2 28 25N 14 3W
Betancuria, Mt., Canary Is. 9 e2 28 25N 14 6W
Betania, Colombia 168 C3 4 22N 72 54W
Betanzos, Bolivia 173 D4 19 34 S 65 27W
Betanzos, Spain 42 B2 43 15N 8 12W
Bétaré Oya, Cameroon 114 A2 5 40N 14 5 E
Betatao, Madag. 117 B8 18 11 S 47 52 E
Bétera, Spain 41 F4 39 35N 0 28W
Bétérou, Benin 113 D5 9 12N 2 16 E
Bethal, S. Africa 117 D4 26 27 S 29 28 E
Bethalto, U.S.A. 156 F6 38 55N 90 2W
Bethanien, Namibia 116 D2 26 31 S 17 8 E
Bethany, Canada 150 B6 44 11N 78 34W
Bethany, Ill., U.S.A. 157 E8 39 39N 88 45W
Bethany, Mo., U.S.A. 156 D2 40 16N 94 2W
Bethany, Okla., U.S.A. 155 H6 35 31N 97 38W
Bethel, Alaska, U.S.A. 144 F7 60 48N 161 45W
Bethel, Conn., U.S.A. 151 E11 41 22N 73 25W
Bethel, Maine, U.S.A. 151 B14 44 25N 70 47W
Bethel, Ohio, U.S.A. 157 F12 38 58N 84 5W
Bethel, Vt., U.S.A. 151 C12 43 50N 72 38W
Bethel Park, U.S.A. 150 F4 40 20N 80 1W
Béthenville, France 27 C11 49 18N 4 23 E
Bethlehem = Bayt Lahm, West Bank 103 D4 31 43N 35 12 E
Bethlehem, S. Africa 117 D4 28 14 S 28 18 E
Bethlehem, U.S.A. 151 F9 40 37N 75 23W
Bethulie, S. Africa 116 E4 30 30 S 25 59 E
Béthune, France 27 B9 50 30N 2 38 E
Béthune →, France 26 C8 49 53N 1 4 E
Bethungra, Australia 129 C7 34 45 S 147 51 E
Betijoque, Venezuela 168 B3 9 23N 70 44W
Betioky, Madag. 117 C7 23 48 S 44 20 E
Betong, Malaysia 85 B4 1 24N 111 31 E
Betong, Thailand 87 K3 5 45N 101 5 E
Betoota, Australia 126 D3 25 45 S 140 42 E
Betor, Ethiopia 107 E4 11 37N 39 2 E
Bétou, Congo 114 B3 3 2N 18 32 E
Betroka, Madag. 117 C8 23 16 S 46 0 E
Betsiamites, Canada 141 C6 48 56N 68 40W
Betsiamites →, Canada 141 C6 48 56N 68 38W
Betsiboka →, Madag. 117 B8 16 3 S 46 36 E
Bettendorf, U.S.A. 156 C6 41 32N 90 30W
Bettiah, India 93 F11 26 48N 84 33 E
Bettna, Sweden 17 F10 58 55N 16 38 E
Béttola, Italy 44 D6 44 47N 9 36 E
Betul, India 94 D3 21 58N 77 59 E
Betws-y-Coed, U.K. 20 D4 53 5N 3 48W
Betxi, Spain 40 F4 39 56N 0 12W
Betzdorf, Germany 30 E3 50 46N 7 52 E
Béu, Angola 115 D3 6 15 S 15 32 E
Beuil, France 29 D10 44 6N 6 59 E
Beulah, Australia 128 C5 35 58 S 142 29 E
Beulah, Mich., U.S.A. 148 C2 44 38N 86 6W
Beulah, N. Dak., U.S.A. 154 B4 47 16N 101 47W
Beurkia, Chad 109 E3 15 20N 17 56 E
Beuthen = Bytom, Poland 55 H5 50 25N 18 54 E
Beuthen an der Oder = Bytom Odrzański, Poland 55 G2 51 44N 15 48 E
Beuvron →, France 26 E8 47 29N 1 15 E
Beveren, Belgium 24 C4 51 12N 4 16 E
Beverley, Australia 125 F2 32 9 S 116 56 E
Beverley, U.K. 20 D7 53 51N 0 26W
Beverley Hills, U.S.A. 153 G7 28 56N 82 28W
Beverly, U.S.A. 151 D14 42 33N 70 53W
Beverly Hills, U.S.A. 161 L8 34 4N 118 25W
Beverungen, Germany 30 D5 51 39N 9 22 E
Bevoalavo, Madag. 117 D7 25 13 S 45 26 E
Bewani, Papua N. G. 83 B6 3 2 S 141 10 E
Bewas →, India 93 H8 23 59N 79 21 E
Bex, Switz. 32 D4 46 15N 7 1 E
Bexhill, U.K. 21 G8 50 51N 0 29 E
Bey Dağları, Turkey 49 E12 36 38N 30 29 E
Beyānlū, Iran 96 C5 36 0N 47 51 E
Beyazköy, Turkey 51 E11 41 21N 27 42 E
Beyçayırı, Turkey 51 F10 40 15N 26 55 E
Beydağ, Turkey 49 C10 38 5N 28 13 E
Beyeğaç, Turkey 49 D10 37 14N 28 53 E
Beyin, Ghana 112 D4 5 1N 2 41W
Beykoz, Turkey 51 E13 41 8N 29 7 E
Beyla, Guinea 112 D3 8 30N 8 38W
Beynat, France 28 C5 45 8N 1 44 E
Beyneu, Kazakhstan 57 E10 45 18N 55 9 E
Beyoba, Turkey 49 C9 38 48N 27 47 E
Beyoğlu, Turkey 51 E12 41 2N 29 0 E
Beypazarı, Turkey 100 B4 40 10N 31 56 E
Beypore →, India 95 J2 11 10N 75 47 E
Beyşehir, Turkey 100 D4 37 41N 31 43 E
Beyşehir Gölü, Turkey 100 D4 37 41N 31 33 E
Beytüşşebap, Turkey 101 D10 37 35N 43 10 E
Bezau, Austria 33 B9 47 23N 9 54 E
Bezdan, Serbia & M. 52 E3 45 50N 18 57 E
Bezhetsk, Russia 58 D9 57 47N 36 39 E
Béziers, France 28 E7 43 20N 3 12 E
Bezwada = Vijayawada, India 94 F5 16 31N 80 39 E
Bhabua, India 93 G10 25 3N 83 37 E
Bhadar →, Gujarat, India 92 H5 22 17N 72 20 E
Bhadar →, Gujarat, India 92 J3 21 27N 69 47 E
Bhadarwah, India 93 C6 32 58N 75 46 E
Bhadgaon = Bhaktapur, Nepal 93 F11 27 38N 85 24 E
Bhadohi, India 93 G10 25 25N 82 34 E
Bhadra, India 92 E6 29 8N 75 14 E
Bhadra →, India 95 H2 14 0N 75 20 E
Bhadrachalam, India 94 F5 17 40N 80 53 E
Bhadrakh, India 94 D8 21 10N 86 30 E
Bhadran, India 92 H5 22 19N 72 6 E
Bhadravati, India 95 H2 13 49N 75 40 E
Bhag, Pakistan 92 E2 29 2N 67 49 E
Bhagalpur, India 93 G12 25 10N 87 0 E
Bhagirathi →, Uttaranchal, India 93 D8 30 8N 78 35 E
Bhagirathi →, W. Bengal, India 93 H13 23 25N 88 23 E
Bhainsa, India 94 E3 19 10N 77 58 E
Bhairab →, Bangla. 90 D2 22 51N 89 34 E
Bhairab Bazar, Bangla. 90 C3 24 4N 90 58 E
Bhakkar, Pakistan 91 C3 31 40N 71 5 E
Bhakra Dam, India 92 D7 31 30N 76 45 E
Bhaktapur, Nepal 93 F11 27 38N 85 24 E
Bhalki, India 94 E3 18 2N 77 13 E
Bhamo, Burma 90 C6 24 15N 97 15 E
Bhamragarh, India 94 E5 19 30N 80 40 E
Bhandara, India 94 D4 21 5N 79 42 E
Bhanpura, India 92 G6 24 31N 75 44 E
Bhanrer Ra., India 93 H8 23 40N 79 45 E
Bhaptiahi, India 93 F12 26 19N 86 44 E
Bharat = India ■, Asia 89 C6 20 0N 78 0 E
Bharatpur, Chhattisgarh, India 93 H9 23 44N 81 46 E
Bharatpur, Raj., India 92 F7 27 15N 77 30 E
Bharno, India 93 H11 23 14N 84 53 E
Bharuch, India 94 D1 21 47N 73 0 E
Bhatghar L., India 94 E1 18 10N 73 48 E
Bhatiapara Ghat, Bangla. 90 D2 23 13N 89 42 E
Bhatinda, India 92 D6 30 15N 74 57 E
Bhatkal, India 95 H2 13 58N 74 35 E
Bhatpara, India 93 H13 22 50N 88 25 E
Bhattu, India 92 E6 29 36N 75 19 E
Bhaun, Pakistan 92 C5 32 55N 72 40 E
Bhaunagar = Bhavnagar, India 94 D1 21 45N 72 10 E
Bhavani, India 95 J3 11 27N 77 43 E
Bhavnagar, India 94 D1 21 45N 72 10 E
Bhawanipatna, India 94 E5 19 55N 83 10 E
Bhawari, India 92 G5 25 42N 73 4 E
Bhayavadar, India 92 J4 21 51N 70 15 E
Bhera, Pakistan 92 C5 32 29N 72 57 E
Bhikangaon, India 92 J6 21 52N 75 57 E
Bhilai, India 94 D5 21 13N 81 26 E
Bhilainagar = Bhilai, India 94 D5 21 13N 81 26 E
Bhilsa = Vidisha, India 92 H7 23 28N 77 53 E
Bhilwara, India 92 G6 25 25N 74 38 E
Bhima →, India 94 F3 16 25N 77 17 E
Bhimavaram, India 95 F5 16 30N 81 30 E
Bhimbar, Pakistan 93 C6 32 59N 74 3 E
Bhind, India 93 F8 26 30N 78 46 E
Bhinga, India 93 F9 27 43N 81 56 E
Bhinmal, India 92 G5 25 0N 72 15 E
Bhiwandi, India 94 E1 19 20N 73 0 E
Bhiwani, India 92 E7 28 50N 76 9 E
Bhogava →, India 92 H5 22 26N 72 20 E
Bhokardan, India 94 D2 20 16N 75 46 E
Bhola, Bangla. 90 D3 22 45N 90 35 E
Bholari, Pakistan 92 G3 25 19N 68 13 E
Bhongir, India 94 F4 17 30N 78 56 E
Bhopal, India 92 H7 23 20N 77 30 E
Bhopalpatnam, India 94 E5 18 52N 80 23 E
Bhor, India 94 E1 18 12N 73 53 E
Bhubaneshwar, India 94 D7 20 15N 85 50 E
Bhuj, India 92 H3 23 15N 69 49 E
Bhumiphol Res., Thailand 86 D2 17 20N 98 40 E
Bhusawal, India 94 D2 21 3N 75 46 E
Bhutan ■, Asia 90 B3 27 25N 90 30 E
Biá →, Brazil 168 D4 3 28 S 67 23W
Biafra, B. of = Bonny, Bight of, Africa 113 E6 3 30N 9 20 E
Biak, Indonesia 83 B5 1 10 S 136 6 E
Biała, Poland 55 H4 50 24N 17 40 E
Biała →, Poland 55 H7 50 3N 20 55 E
Biała Piska, Poland 54 E9 53 37N 22 5 E
Biała Podlaska, Poland 55 F10 52 4N 23 6 E
Biała Rawska, Poland 55 G7 51 48N 20 29 E
Białobrzegi, Poland 55 G7 51 39N 20 57 E
Białogard, Poland 54 D2 54 2N 15 58 E
Białowieski △, Poland 55 F10 52 43N 23 50 E
Białowieża, Poland 55 F10 52 41N 23 49 E
Biały Bór, Poland 54 E3 53 53N 16 51 E
Białystok, Poland 55 E10 53 10N 23 10 E
Bian →, Indonesia 83 C5 8 6 S 139 58 E
Biancavilla, Italy 47 E7 37 38N 14 52 E
Bianco, Italy 47 D9 38 5N 16 9 E
Biankouma, Ivory C. 112 D3 7 50N 7 40W
Biaora, India 92 H7 23 56N 76 56 E
Bīārjmand, Iran 97 B7 36 6N 55 53 E
Biaro, Indonesia 82 A3 2 5N 125 26 E
Biarritz, France 28 E2 43 29N 1 33W
Bias, Indonesia 79 J18 8 24 S 115 36 E
Biasca, Switz. 33 D7 46 22N 8 58 E
Biavela, Angola 115 E3 14 43 S 19 47 E
Biba, Egypt 106 J7 28 55N 31 0 E
Bibai, Japan 70 C10 43 19N 141 52 E
Bibala, Angola 115 E2 14 44 S 13 24 E
Bibane, Bahiret el, Tunisia 108 B2 33 16N 11 13 E
Bibassé, Gabon 114 B2 1 27N 11 37 E
Bibbiena, Italy 45 E8 43 42N 11 49 E
Bibby I., Canada 143 A10 61 55N 93 0W
Bibel →, Spain 42 C3 42 24N 7 13W
Biberach, Germany 31 G5 48 5N 9 47 E
Biberist, Switz. 32 B5 47 11N 7 34 E
Bibi, Papua N. G. 132 C4 5 30 S 146 2 E
Bibiani, Ghana 112 D4 6 30N 2 8W
Bibile, Sri Lanka 95 L5 7 10N 81 25 E
Bibungwa, Dem. Rep. of the Congo 118 C2 2 40 S 28 15 E
Bicaj, Albania 50 E4 41 58N 20 25 E
Bicaz, Romania 53 D11 46 53N 26 5 E
Bicazu Ardelean, Romania 53 D10 46 51N 25 56 E
Biccari, Italy 47 A8 41 23N 15 12 E
Bicester, U.K. 21 F6 51 54N 1 9W
Bichena, Ethiopia 107 E4 10 28N 38 10 E
Bicheno, Australia 127 G4 41 52 S 148 18 E
Bichia, India 93 H9 22 27N 80 42 E
Bichvinta, Georgia 61 J5 43 9N 40 21 E
Bickerton I., Australia 126 A2 13 45 S 136 10 E
Bicknell, U.S.A. 157 F9 38 47N 87 19W
Bicske, Hungary 52 C3 47 29N 18 38 E
Bicuar △, Angola 115 F2 15 14 S 14 45 E
Bida, Dem. Rep. of the Congo 114 B3 4 55N 19 56 E
Bida, Nigeria 113 D6 9 3N 5 58 E
Bidar, India 94 F3 17 55N 77 35 E
Biddeford, U.S.A. 149 D10 43 30N 70 28W
Biddwara, Ethiopia 107 F4 5 11N 38 34 E
Bideford, U.K. 21 F3 51 1N 4 13W
Bideford Bay, U.K. 21 F3 51 5N 4 20W
Bidhuna, India 93 F8 26 49N 79 31 E
Bidon 5 = Poste Maurice Cortier, Algeria 111 D5 22 14N 1 2 E
Bidor, Malaysia 87 K3 4 6N 101 15 E
Bidzar, Cameroon 114 A2 9 54N 14 7 E
Bie, Sweden 16 E10 59 5N 16 12 E
Bié □, Angola 115 E3 12 30 S 17 0 E
Bié, Planalto de, Angola 115 E3 12 0 S 16 0 E
Bieber, U.S.A. 158 F3 41 7N 121 8W
Biebrza →, Poland 55 E9 53 13N 22 25 E
Biebrzański △, Poland 54 E9 53 36N 22 45 E
Biecz, Poland 55 J8 49 44N 21 15 E
Biel, Switz. 32 B4 47 8N 7 14 E
Bielawa, Poland 55 H3 50 43N 16 37 E
Bielefeld, Germany 30 C4 52 1N 8 33 E
Bielersee, Switz. 32 B4 47 6N 7 5 E
Bielitz = Bielsko-Biała, Poland 55 J6 49 50N 19 2 E
Biella, Italy 44 C5 45 34N 8 3 E
Bielsk Podlaski, Poland 55 F10 52 47N 23 12 E
Bielsko-Biała, Poland 55 J6 49 50N 19 2 E
Bien Hoa, Vietnam 87 G6 10 57N 106 49 E
Bienne = Biel, Switz. 32 B4 47 8N 7 14 E
Bienno, Italy 33 E10 45 56N 10 18 E
Bienvenida, Spain 43 G4 38 18N 6 12W
Bienvenue, Fr. Guiana 169 C7 3 0N 52 30W
Bienville, L., Canada 140 A5 55 5N 72 40W
Bière, Switz. 32 C2 46 33N 6 20 E
Bierné, France 26 E6 47 48N 0 33W
Bierun, Poland 55 H6 50 6N 19 6 E
Bierutów, Poland 55 G4 51 7N 17 32 E
Biescas, Spain 40 C4 42 37N 0 20W
Biese →, Germany 30 C7 52 53N 11 46 E
Biesiesfontein, S. Africa 116 E2 30 57 S 17 58 E
Bieszczadzki △, Poland 55 J9 49 5N 22 43 E
Bietigheim-Bissingen, Germany 31 G5 48 58N 9 8 E
Bieżuń, Poland 55 F6 52 58N 19 55 E
Biferno →, Italy 45 G12 41 59N 15 2 E
Bifoum, Gabon 114 C2 0 20 S 10 23 E
Big →, Canada 141 B8 54 50N 58 55W
Big →, U.S.A. 156 F6 38 28N 90 37W
Big B., Canada 141 A7 55 43N 60 35W
Big Bear City, U.S.A. 161 L10 34 16N 116 51W
Big Bear Lake, U.S.A. 161 L10 34 15N 116 56W
Big Belt Mts., U.S.A. 158 C8 46 30N 111 25W
Big Bend, Swaziland 117 D5 26 50 S 31 58 E
Big Bend △, U.S.A. 155 L3 29 20N 103 5W
Big Black →, U.S.A. 155 K9 32 3N 91 4W
Big Blue →, Ind., U.S.A. 157 E11 39 12N 85 56W
Big Blue →, Kans., U.S.A. 154 F6 39 35N 96 34W
Big Creek, U.S.A. 160 H7 37 11N 119 14W
Big Cypress ⌓, U.S.A. 153 J8 26 0N 81 10W
Big Cypress Swamp, U.S.A. 153 J8 26 15N 81 30W
Big Delta, U.S.A. 144 D11 64 10N 145 51W
Big Falls, U.S.A. 154 A8 48 12N 93 48W
Big Fork →, U.S.A. 154 A8 48 31N 93 43W
Big Horn Mts. = Bighorn Mts., U.S.A. 158 D10 44 30N 107 30W
Big I., Canada 142 A5 61 7N 116 45W
Big Lake, Alaska, U.S.A. 144 F10 61 20N 150 20W
Big Lake, Tex., U.S.A. 155 K4 31 12N 101 28W
Big Moose, U.S.A. 151 C10 43 49N 74 58W
Big Muddy →, U.S.A. 156 G8 38 0N 89 0W
Big Muddy Cr. →, U.S.A. 154 A2 48 8N 104 36W
Big Pine, Calif., U.S.A. 160 H8 37 10N 118 17W
Big Pine, Fla., U.S.A. 153 L8 24 40N 81 21W
Big Piney, U.S.A. 158 E8 42 32N 110 7W
Big Rapids, U.S.A. 148 D3 43 42N 85 29W
Big Rideau L., Canada 151 B8 44 40N 76 15W
Big River, Canada 143 C7 53 50N 107 0W
Big Run, U.S.A. 150 F6 40 57N 78 55W
Big Sable Pt., U.S.A. 148 C2 44 3N 86 1W
Big Salmon →, Canada 142 A2 61 52N 134 55W
Big Sand L., Canada 143 B9 57 45N 99 45W
Big Sandy, U.S.A. 158 B8 48 11N 110 7W
Big Sandy →, U.S.A. 148 F4 38 25N 82 36W
Big Sandy Cr. →, U.S.A. 154 F3 38 7N 102 29W
Big Satilla →, U.S.A. 152 D7 31 27N 82 3W
Big Sioux →, U.S.A. 154 D6 42 29N 96 27W
Big South Fork △, U.S.A. 149 G3 36 27N 84 47W
Big Spring, U.S.A. 155 J4 32 15N 101 28W
Big Stone City, U.S.A. 154 C6 45 18N 96 28W
Big Stone Gap, U.S.A. 149 G4 36 52N 82 47W
Big Stone L., U.S.A. 154 C6 45 30N 96 35W
Big Sur, U.S.A. 160 J5 36 15N 121 48W
Big Timber, U.S.A. 158 D9 45 50N 109 57W
Big Trout L., Canada 140 B2 53 40N 90 0W
Big Trout Lake, Canada 140 B2 53 45N 90 0W
Biğa, Turkey 51 F11 40 13N 27 14 E
Biga →, Turkey 51 F11 40 20N 27 14 E
Bigadiç, Turkey 49 B10 39 22N 28 7 E
Biganos, France 28 D3 44 39N 0 59W
Biggar, Canada 143 C7 52 4N 108 0W
Biggar, U.K. 22 F5 55 38N 3 32W
Bigge I., Australia 124 B4 14 35 S 125 10 E
Biggenden, Australia 127 D5 25 31 S 152 4 E
Biggleswade, U.K. 21 E7 52 5N 0 14W
Biggs, U.S.A. 160 F5 39 25N 121 43W
Bighorn, U.S.A. 158 C10 46 10N 107 27W
Bighorn →, U.S.A. 158 C10 46 10N 107 28W
Bighorn Canyon ⌓, U.S.A. 158 D9 45 10N 108 0W
Bighorn L., U.S.A. 158 D9 44 55N 108 15W
Bighorn Mts., U.S.A. 158 D10 44 30N 107 30W
Bigi, Dem. Rep. of the Congo 114 B4 3 2N 22 25 E
Bignasco, Switz. 33 D7 46 21N 8 37 E
Bignona, Senegal 112 C1 12 52N 16 14W
Bigorre, France 28 E4 43 10N 0 5 E
Bigstone L., Canada 143 C9 53 42N 95 44W
Biguglia, Étang de, France 29 F13 42 36N 9 29 E
Bigwa, Tanzania 118 D4 7 10 S 39 10 E
Bihać, Bos.-H. 45 D12 44 49N 15 57 E
Bihar, India 93 G11 25 5N 85 40 E
Bihar □, India 93 G12 25 0N 86 0 E
Biharamulo, Tanzania 118 C3 2 25 S 31 25 E
Biharamulo ⌓, Tanzania 118 C3 2 24 S 31 26 E
Bihariganj, India 93 G12 25 44N 86 59 E
Biharkeresztes, Hungary 52 C6 47 8N 21 44 E
Bihor □, Romania 52 D7 47 0N 22 10 E
Bihor, Munţii, Romania 52 D7 46 29N 22 47 E
Bijagós, Arquipélago dos, Guinea-Biss. 112 C1 11 15N 16 10W
Bijaipur, India 92 F7 26 2N 77 20 E
Bijapur, Chhattisgarh, India 94 E5 18 50N 80 50 E
Bijapur, Karnataka, India 94 F2 16 50N 75 55 E
Bījār, Iran 101 E12 35 52N 47 35 E
Bijawar, India 93 G8 24 38N 79 30 E
Bijeljina, Bos.-H. 52 F4 44 46N 19 14 E
Bijelo Polje, Serbia & M. 50 C3 43 1N 19 45 E
Bijie, China 76 D5 27 20N 105 16 E
Bijnor, India 92 E8 29 27N 78 11 E
Bikaner, India 92 E5 28 2N 73 18 E
Bikapur, India 93 F10 26 30N 82 7 E
Bikeqi, China 74 D6 40 43N 111 20 E
Bikfayyā, Lebanon 103 B4 33 55N 35 41 E
Bikié, Congo 114 C2 3 7 S 13 52 E
Bikin, Russia 67 E14 46 50N 134 20 E
Bikin →, Russia 70 A7 46 51N 134 2 E
Bikini Atoll, Marshall Is. 134 F8 12 0N 167 30 E
Bikita, Zimbabwe 117 C5 20 6 S 31 41 E
Bīkkū Bīttī, Libya 109 D3 22 0N 19 12 E
Bikoro, Dem. Rep. of the Congo 114 C3 0 48 S 18 15 E
Bikoué, Cameroon 113 E7 3 55N 11 50 E
Bila Tserkva, Ukraine 59 H6 49 45N 30 10 E
Bilanga, Burkina Faso 113 C4 12 40N 0 1W
Bilara, India 92 F5 26 14N 73 53 E
Bilasipara, India 90 B3 26 13N 90 14 E
Bilaspur, Chhattisgarh, India 93 H10 22 2N 82 15 E
Bilaspur, Punjab, India 92 D7 31 19N 76 50 E
Biläsuvar, Azerbaijan 101 C13 39 27N 48 32 E
Bilauk Taungdan, Thailand 86 F2 13 0N 99 0 E
Bilbao, Spain 40 B2 43 16N 2 56W
Bilbao ✕ (BIO), Spain 40 B2 43 18N 2 57W
Bilbeis, Egypt 106 H7 30 25N 31 34 E
Bilbo = Bilbao, Spain 40 B2 43 16N 2 56W
Bilbor, Romania 53 C10 47 6N 25 30 E
Bilche-Zolote, Ukraine 53 B10 48 47N 25 53 E
Bilciureşti, Romania 53 F10 44 44N 25 48 E
Bíldudalur, Iceland 11 B3 65 41N 23 36W
Bílé Karpaty, Europe 35 B11 49 5N 18 0 E
Bileća, Bos.-H. 50 D2 42 53N 18 27 E
Bilecik, Turkey 100 B4 40 5N 30 5 E
Biłgoraj, Poland 55 H9 50 33N 22 42 E
Bilgram, India 93 F9 27 11N 80 2 E
Bilhaur, India 93 F9 26 51N 80 5 E
Bilhorod-Dnistrovskyy, Ukraine 59 J6 46 11N 30 23 E
Bili →, Dem. Rep. of the Congo 114 B4 4 9N 22 29 E
Bilibino, Russia 67 C17 68 3N 166 20 E
Bilibiza, Mozam. 119 E5 12 30 S 40 20 E
Biliköl, Kazakhstan 65 B5 43 5N 70 45 E
Bilimora, India 94 D1 20 45N 72 57 E
Bilin, Burma 90 G6 17 14N 97 15 E
Biliran □, Phil. 81 F5 11 35N 124 28 E
Bilisht, Albania 50 F5 40 37N 21 2 E
Billabong Cr. →, Australia 128 C6 35 5 S 144 2 E
Billabong Roadhouse, Australia 125 E2 27 25 S 115 49 E
Billdal, Sweden 17 G5 57 35N 11 57 E
Billiluna, Australia 124 C4 19 37 S 127 41 E
Billings, U.S.A. 158 D9 45 47N 108 30W
Billiton Is. = Belitung, Indonesia 85 C3 3 10 S 107 50 E
Billsta, Sweden 16 A12 63 20N 18 28 E
Billund, Denmark 17 J3 55 44N 9 6 E
Bilma, Niger 109 E2 18 50N 13 30 E
Bilo Gora, Croatia 52 E2 45 53N 17 15 E
Biloela, Australia 126 C5 24 24 S 150 31 E
Bilohirsk, Ukraine 59 K8 45 3N 34 35 E
Biloku, Guyana 169 C6 1 50N 58 25W
Biloli, India 94 E3 18 46N 77 44 E
Bilopillya, Ukraine 59 G8 51 14N 34 20 E
Biloxi, U.S.A. 155 K10 30 24N 88 53W
Bilpa Morea Claypan, Australia 126 D3 25 0 S 140 0 E
Biltine, Chad 109 F4 14 40N 20 50 E
Bilugyun, Burma 90 G6 16 24N 97 32 E
Bilyarsk, Russia 60 C10 54 58N 50 22 E
Bima, Indonesia 85 D5 8 22 S 118 49 E
Bimban, Egypt 106 C3 24 24N 32 54 E
Bimbe, Angola 115 E3 11 50 S 15 50 E
Bimberi Pk., Australia 129 C8 35 44 S 148 51 E
Bimbila, Ghana 113 D5 8 54N 0 5 E
Bimbo, C.A.R. 114 B3 4 15N 18 33 E
Bimini Is., Bahamas 164 A4 25 42N 79 25W
Bin Xian, Heilongjiang, China 75 B14 45 42N 127 32 E
Bin Xian, Shaanxi, China 74 G5 35 2N 108 4 E
Bin Yauri, Nigeria 113 C5 10 46N 4 45 E
Bina-Etawah, India 92 G8 24 13N 78 14 E
Bināb, Iran 97 B6 36 35N 48 41 E
Binaiya, Indonesia 83 B3 3 11 S 129 26 E
Binalbagan, Phil. 81 F4 10 12N 122 50 E
Binalong, Australia 129 C8 34 40 S 148 39 E
Bīnālūd, Kūh-e, Iran 97 B8 36 30N 58 30 E
Binangonan de Lampon = Infanta, Phil. 80 D3 14 45N 121 39 E
Binatang = Bintangau, Malaysia 85 B4 2 10N 111 40 E
Binche, Belgium 24 D4 50 26N 4 10 E
Binchuan, China 76 E3 25 42N 100 38 E
Binda, Dem. Rep. of the Congo 115 D2 5 52 S 13 14 E
Binder, Chad 113 D7 9 56N 14 27 E
Bindki, India 93 F9 26 2N 80 36 E
Bindloe, I. = Marchena, I., Ecuador 172 a 0 19N 90 29W
Bindoy, Phil. 81 G4 9 48N 123 5 E
Bindslev, Denmark 17 G4 57 33N 10 11 E
Bindura, Zimbabwe 119 F3 17 18 S 31 18 E
Binefar, Spain 40 D5 41 51N 0 18 E
Bingara, Australia 127 D5 29 52 S 150 36 E
Bingaram I., India 95 J1 10 56N 72 17 E
Bingen, Germany 31 F3 49 57N 7 55 E
Bingerau = Węgrów, Poland 55 F9 52 24N 22 0 E
Bingerville, Ivory C. 112 D4 5 18N 3 49W
Bingham, U.S.A. 149 C11 45 3N 69 53W
Binghamton, U.S.A. 151 D9 42 6N 75 55W
Bingo-Ochiai, Japan 72 C4 34 59N 133 8 E
Bingöl, Turkey 101 C9 38 53N 40 29 E
Bingöl Dağları, Turkey 101 C9 39 16N 41 9 E
Bingsjö, Sweden 16 C9 61 1N 15 39 E
Binh Dinh = An Nhon, Vietnam 86 F7 13 55N 109 7 E
Binh Khe, Vietnam 86 F7 13 57N 108 51 E
Binh Son, Vietnam 86 E7 15 20N 108 40 E
Binhai, China 75 G10 34 2N 119 49 E
Bini Erde, Chad 109 D3 20 6N 18 1 E
Binic, France 26 D4 48 46N 2 50W
Binisatua, Spain 38 B5 39 50N 4 11 E
Binjai, Indonesia 84 B1 3 20N 98 30 E
Binji, Nigeria 113 C5 13 10N 4 55 E
Binka, India 94 D6 21 2N 83 48 E
Binnaway, Australia 129 A8 31 28 S 149 24 E
Binningen, Switz. 32 A5 47 32N 7 34 E
Binongko, Indonesia 82 C2 5 57 S 124 2 E
Binscarth, Canada 143 C8 50 37N 101 17W
Binshangul Gumuz □, Ethiopia 107 E4 11 0N 35 30 E
Bint Goda, Sudan 107 E3 13 17N 31 33 E
Bintan, Indonesia 84 B2 1 0N 104 0 E
Bintangau, Malaysia 85 B4 2 10N 111 40 E
Bintulu, Malaysia 78 D4 3 10N 113 0 E
Bintuni, Indonesia 83 B4 2 7 S 133 32 E
Bintuni, Teluk, Indonesia 83 B4 2 20 S 133 30 E
Binyang, China 76 F7 23 12N 108 47 E
Binz, Germany 30 A9 54 24N 13 35 E
Binza, Dem. Rep. of the Congo 115 C3 4 21 S 15 14 E
Binzert = Bizerte, Tunisia 108 A1 37 15N 9 50 E
Binzhou, China 75 F10 37 20N 118 2 E
Bío Bío □, Chile 174 D1 37 35 S 72 0W
Biograd na Moru, Croatia 45 E12 43 56N 15 29 E
Biogradska Gora △, Serbia & M. 50 D3 42 55N 19 40 E
Bioko, Eq. Guin. 113 E6 3 30N 8 40 E
Biokovo, Croatia 45 E14 43 23N 17 0 E
Biougra, Morocco 110 B3 30 15N 9 14W
Bipindi, Cameroon 113 E7 3 6N 10 30 E
Bir, India 94 E2 19 4N 75 46 E
Bir, Ras, Djibouti 107 E5 12 0N 43 20 E
Bîr Abu Hashim, Egypt 106 C3 23 42N 34 6 E
Bîr Abu Minqar, Egypt 106 B2 26 33N 27 33 E
Bîr Abu Muḥammad, Egypt 103 F3 29 44N 34 14 E
Bi'r ad Dabbāghāt, Jordan 103 E4 30 26N 35 32 E
Bîr Adal Deib, Sudan 106 C4 22 35N 36 10 E
Bi'r al Butayyihāt, Jordan 103 F4 29 47N 35 20 E
Bi'r al Mārī, Jordan 103 E4 30 4N 35 33 E
Bi'r al Qattār, Jordan 103 F4 29 47N 35 32 E
Bir 'Ali, Yemen 99 D5 14 1N 48 20 E
Bir Aouine, Tunisia 108 B1 32 25N 9 18 E
Bîr 'Asal, Egypt 106 B3 25 55N 34 20 E
Bir Atrun, Sudan 106 D2 18 15N 26 40 E
Bîr Beiḍa, Egypt 103 E3 30 25N 34 29 E
Bir Bel Guerdâne, Mauritania 110 C2 25 24N 10 31W
Bi'r Dhu'fān, Libya 108 B2 31 59N 14 32 E
Bîr Diqnash, Egypt 106 A2 31 3N 25 23 E
Bir el Abbes, Algeria 110 C3 26 7N 6 9W
Bîr el 'Abd, Egypt 103 D2 31 2N 33 0 E
Bir el Ater, Algeria 111 B6 34 46N 8 3 E
Bîr el Basur, Egypt 106 B2 29 51N 25 49 E
Bîr el Biarât, Egypt 103 F3 29 30N 34 43 E
Bîr el Duweidar, Egypt 103 E1 30 56N 32 32 E

Bîr el Garârât, Egypt . 103 D2 31 3N 33 34 E
Bîr el Gâreb, Mauritania . 110 D1 20 33N 16 12W
Bîr el Gellaz, Egypt . 106 A2 30 50N 26 40 E
Bîr el Heisi, Egypt . 103 F3 29 22N 34 36 E
Bîr el Jafir, Egypt . 103 E1 30 50N 32 41 E
Bîr el Mâlḥi, Egypt . 103 E2 30 38N 33 19 E
Bîr el Shaqqa, Egypt . 106 A2 30 54N 25 1 E
Bîr el Thamâda, Egypt 103 E2 30 12N 33 27 E
Bîr Enzarân, W. Sahara 110 D2 23 53N 14 32W
Bîr Fuad, Egypt . 106 A2 30 35N 26 28 E
Bîr Gandûs, W. Sahara 110 D1 21 36N 16 30W
Bîr Gara, Chad . 109 F3 13 11N 15 58 E
Bîr Gebeil Ḥiṣn, Egypt 103 E2 30 2N 33 18 E
Bi'r Ghadīr, Syria . 103 A6 34 6N 37 3 E
Bîr Haimur, Egypt . 106 C3 22 45N 33 40 E
Bîr Ḥasana, Egypt . 103 E2 30 29N 33 46 E
Bîr Hôôker, Egypt . 106 H7 30 22N 30 21 E
Bi'r Īdimah, Si. Arabia 98 C4 18 31N 44 12 E
Bîr Jdid, Morocco . 110 B3 33 26N 8 0W
Bîr Kanayis, Egypt . 106 C3 24 59N 33 15 E
Bîr Kaseiba, Egypt . 103 E2 31 0N 33 17 E
Bîr Kerawein, Egypt . 106 B2 27 10N 28 25 E
Bîr Lahfân, Egypt . 103 E2 31 0N 33 51 E
Bîr Lahrache, Algeria . 111 B6 32 1N 8 12 E
Bîr Madkûr, Egypt . 103 E1 30 44N 32 33 E
Bîr Maql, Egypt . 106 C3 23 7N 33 40 E
Bîr Mîneiga, Sudan . 106 C4 22 47N 35 12 E
Bîr Misaha, Egypt . 106 C2 22 13N 27 59 E
Bîr Mogreïn, Mauritania . 110 C2 25 10N 11 25W
Bîr Murr, Egypt . 106 C3 23 28N 30 10 E
Bi'r Muṭribah, Kuwait 96 D5 29 54N 47 17 E
Bîr Nakheila, Egypt . 106 C3 24 1N 30 50 E
Bîr Qaṭia, Egypt . 103 E1 30 58N 32 45 E
Bîr Qatrani, Egypt . 106 A2 30 55N 26 10 E
Bîr Ranga, Egypt . 106 C4 24 25N 35 15 E
Bîr Sahara, Egypt . 106 C2 22 54N 28 40 E
Bîr Seiyâla, Egypt . 106 B3 26 10N 33 50 E
Bîr Semguine, Morocco 110 B3 30 1N 5 39W
Bîr Shalatein, Egypt . 106 C4 23 5N 35 25 E
Bîr Shebb, Egypt . 106 C2 22 25N 29 40 E
Bîr Shût, Egypt . 106 C4 23 50N 35 15 E
Bîr Terfawi, Egypt . 106 C2 22 57N 28 55 E
Bi'r Tin Abunda, Libya 111 C7 26 28N 12 27 E
Bîr Umm Qubûr, Egypt 106 C3 24 35N 34 2 E
Bîr Ungât, Egypt . 106 C3 22 8N 33 48 E
Bîr Za'farâna, Egypt . 106 J8 29 10N 32 40 E
Bîr Zāmūs, Libya . 108 D3 24 16N 15 6 E
Bîr Zeidûn, Egypt . 106 B3 25 45N 33 40 E
Bira, Indonesia . 83 B4 2 3 S 132 2 E
Biramféro, Guinea . 112 C3 11 40N 9 10W
Birao, C.A.R. . 114 A4 10 20N 22 47 E
Biratnagar, Nepal . 93 F12 26 27N 87 17 E
Birawa, Dem. Rep. of the Congo . 118 C2 2 20 S 28 48 E
Birch →, Canada . 142 B6 58 28N 112 17W
Birch Hills, Canada . 143 C7 52 59N 105 25W
Birch I., Canada . 143 C9 52 26N 99 54W
Birch L., N.W.T., Canada . 142 A5 62 4N 116 33W
Birch L., Ont., Canada 140 B1 51 23N 92 18W
Birch Mts., Canada . 142 B6 57 30N 113 10W
Birch River, Canada . 143 C8 52 24N 101 6W
Birchip, Australia . 128 C5 35 56 S 142 55 E
Birchiş, Romania . 52 E7 45 58N 22 9 E
Birchwood, N.Z. . 131 F2 45 55 S 167 53 E
Bird, Canada . 143 B10 56 30N 94 13W
Bird I. = Aves, I. de, W. Indies . 165 C7 15 45N 63 55W
Bird I., Antarctica . 7 B1 54 0 S 38 0W
Birdseye, U.S.A. . 157 F10 38 19N 86 42W
Birdsville, Australia . 126 D2 25 51 S 139 20 E
Birdum Cr. →, Australia . 124 C5 15 14 S 133 0 E
Birdwood, Australia . 128 C3 34 51 S 138 58 E
Birecik, Turkey . 101 D8 37 2N 38 0 E
Birein, Israel . 103 E3 30 50N 34 28 E
Bireuen, Indonesia . 84 A1 5 14N 96 39 E
Birgu = Vittoriosa, Malta . 38 F8 35 54N 14 31 E
Biri, Norway . 18 D7 60 58N 10 35 E
Biri →, Sudan . 107 F2 7 56N 26 33 E
Birifo, Gambia . 112 C2 13 30N 14 0W
Birigui, Brazil . 175 A5 21 18 S 50 16W
Birini, C.A.R. . 114 A4 7 51N 22 24 E
Birjand, Iran . 97 C8 32 53N 59 13 E
Birkeland, Norway . 18 F4 58 24N 7 12 E
Birkenfeld, Germany . 31 F3 49 38N 7 9 E
Birkenhead, U.K. . 20 D4 53 23N 3 2W
Birkerød, Denmark . 17 J6 55 50N 12 25 E
Birket Fatmé, Chad . 109 F3 12 55N 19 7 E
Birket Qârûn, Egypt . 106 J7 29 30N 30 40 E
Birkfeld, Austria . 34 D8 47 21N 15 45 E
Birkhadem, Algeria . 111 A5 36 43N 3 3 E
Birkirkara, Malta . 38 F7 35 54N 14 28 E
Bîrlad = Bârlad, Romania . 53 D12 46 15N 27 38 E
Birlik, Kazakhstan . 65 B6 43 40N 73 49 E
Birlik, Kazakhstan . 65 A6 44 5N 73 31 E
Birmingham, U.K. . 21 E6 52 29N 1 52W
Birmingham, Ala., U.S.A. . 149 J2 33 31N 86 48W
Birmingham, Iowa, U.S.A. . 156 D5 40 53N 91 57W
Birmingham International ✕ (BHX), U.K. . 21 E6 52 26N 1 45W
Birmitrapur, India . 94 C7 22 24N 84 46 E
Birni Ngaouré, Niger . 113 C5 13 5N 2 51 E
Birni Nkonni, Niger . 113 C6 13 55N 5 15 E
Birnin Gwari, Nigeria . 113 C6 11 0N 6 45 E
Birnin Kebbi, Nigeria . 113 C5 12 32N 4 12 E
Birnin Kudu, Nigeria . 113 C6 11 30N 9 29 E
Birobidzhan, Russia . 67 E14 48 50N 132 50 E
Birougou, Mts., Gabon 114 C2 1 51 S 12 20 E
Birr, Ireland . 23 C4 53 6N 7 54W
Birrie →, Australia . 127 D4 29 43 S 146 37 E
Birs →, Switz. . 32 B5 47 24N 7 32 E
Birsilpur, India . 92 E5 28 11N 72 15 E
Birsk, Russia . 64 D5 55 25N 55 30 E
Birštonas, Lithuania . 54 D11 54 37N 24 2 E
Birtle, Canada . 143 C8 50 30N 101 5W
Biryuchiy, Ukraine . 59 J8 46 10N 35 0 E
Biržai, Lithuania . 15 H21 56 11N 24 45 E
Birzebbugga, Malta . 38 F8 35 50N 14 32 E
Birzhi = Madona, Latvia . 15 H22 56 53N 26 5 E
Birzula = Kotovsk, Ukraine . 59 J5 47 45N 29 35 E
Bisa, Indonesia . 82 B3 1 15 S 127 28 E
Bisáccia, Italy . 47 A8 41 1N 15 22 E
Bisacquino, Italy . 46 E6 37 42N 13 15 E
Bisai, Japan . 73 B8 35 16N 136 44 E
Bisalpur, India . 93 E8 28 14N 79 48 E
Bisbee, U.S.A. . 159 L9 31 27N 109 55W
Biscarrosse, France . 28 D2 44 22N 1 20W
Biscarrosse et de Parentis, Étang de, France . 28 D2 44 21N 1 10W
Biscay, B. of, Atl. Oc. . 8 B11 45 0N 2 0W
Biscay Plain, Atl. Oc. . 8 B11 45 0N 8 0W
Biscayne △, U.S.A. . 153 K9 25 25N 80 12W
Biscayne B., U.S.A. . 153 K9 25 40N 80 12W
Biscéglie, Italy . 47 A9 41 14N 16 30 E
Bischheim, France . 27 D14 48 37N 7 46 E
Bischoflack = Škofja Loka, Slovenia . 45 B11 46 9N 14 19 E
Bischofsburg = Biskupiec, Poland . 54 E7 53 53N 20 58 E
Bischofshofen, Austria 34 D6 47 26N 13 14 E
Bischofstal = Ujazd, Poland . 55 H5 50 23N 18 21 E
Bischofstein = Bisztynek, Poland . 54 D7 54 8N 20 53 E
Bischofswerda, Germany . 30 D10 51 7N 14 10 E
Bischofszell, Switz. . 33 B8 47 29N 9 15 E
Bischwiller, France . 27 D14 48 46N 7 50 E
Biscoe Is., Antarctica . 7 C17 66 0 S 67 0W
Biscoitos, Azores . 9 d1 38 47N 27 15W
Biscotasing, Canada . 140 C3 47 18N 82 9W
Biševo, Croatia . 45 F13 42 57N 16 3 E
Bisha, Eritrea . 107 D4 15 30N 37 31 E
Bishah, W. →, Si. Arabia . 98 B3 21 24N 43 26 E
Bishan, China . 76 C6 29 33N 106 12 E
Bishanga, Dem. Rep. of the Congo . 115 C4 4 31 S 21 2 E
Bishkek, Kyrgyzstan . 65 B7 42 54N 74 46 E
Bishnath, India . 90 B4 26 40N 93 10 E
Bishnupur, India . 93 H12 23 8N 87 20 E
Bisho, S. Africa . 117 E4 32 50 S 27 23 E
Bishop, Calif., U.S.A. . 160 H8 37 22N 118 24W
Bishop, Ga., U.S.A. . 152 B6 33 49N 83 26W
Bishop, Tex., U.S.A. . 155 M6 27 35N 97 48W
Bishop Auckland, U.K. 20 C6 54 39N 1 40W
Bishop's Falls, Canada 141 C8 49 2N 55 30W
Bishop's Stortford, U.K. . 21 F8 51 52N 0 10 E
Bisignano, Italy . 47 C9 39 31N 16 17 E
Bisina, L., Uganda . 118 B3 1 38N 33 56 E
Biskra, Algeria . 111 B6 34 50N 5 44 E
Biskra, Malta . 38 F7 35 58N 14 21 E
Biskupiec, Poland . 54 E7 53 53N 20 58 E
Bismarck, Mo., U.S.A. 156 G6 37 46N 90 38W
Bismarck, N. Dak., U.S.A. . 154 B4 46 48N 100 47W
Bismarck Arch., Papua N. G. . 132 B5 2 30 S 150 0 E
Bismarck Ra., Papua N. G. . 132 C3 5 35 S 145 0 E
Bismarck Sea, Papua N. G. . 132 C4 4 10 S 146 50 E
Bismarckburg = Kasanga, Tanzania . 119 D3 8 30 S 31 10 E
Bismark, Germany . 30 C7 52 40N 11 33 E
Bismil, Turkey . 101 D9 37 51N 40 40 E
Bismo, Norway . 18 C5 61 54N 8 15 E
Biso, Uganda . 118 B3 1 44N 31 26 E
Bison, U.S.A. . 154 C3 45 31N 102 28W
Bīsotūn, Iran . 101 E12 34 23N 47 26 E
Bispgården, Sweden . 16 A10 63 2N 16 40 E
Bissagos = Bijagós, Arquipélago dos, Guinea-Biss. . 112 C1 11 15N 16 10W
Bissam Cuttack, India 94 E6 19 31N 83 31 E
Bissau, Guinea-Biss. . 112 C1 11 45N 15 45W
Bissaula, Nigeria . 113 D7 7 0N 10 27 E
Bissikrima, Guinea . 112 C2 10 50N 10 58W
Bissorã, Guinea-Biss. . 112 C1 12 16N 15 35W
Bistcho L., Canada . 142 B5 59 45N 118 50W
Bistreţ, Romania . 53 G8 43 54N 23 23 E
Bistrica = Ilirska-Bistrica, Slovenia . 45 C11 45 34N 14 14 E
Bistriţa, Romania . 53 C9 47 9N 24 35 E
Bistriţa →, Romania . 53 D11 46 30N 26 57 E
Bistriţa Năsăud □, Romania . 53 C9 47 15N 24 30 E
Bistriţei, Munţii, Romania . 53 C10 47 15N 25 40 E
Biswan, India . 93 F9 27 29N 81 2 E
Bisztynek, Poland . 54 D7 54 8N 20 53 E
Bita →, C.A.R. . 114 A4 6 26N 24 43 E
Bitam, Gabon . 114 B2 2 5N 11 25 E
Bitburg, Germany . 31 F2 49 58N 6 31 E
Bitche, France . 27 C14 49 2N 7 25 E
Bithlo, U.S.A. . 153 G8 28 33N 81 6W
Bithynia, Turkey . 100 B4 40 40N 31 0 E
Bitkine, Chad . 109 F3 11 59N 18 13 E
Bitlis, Turkey . 101 C10 38 20N 42 3 E
Bitola, Macedonia . 50 E5 41 1N 21 20 E
Bitolj = Bitola, Macedonia . 50 E5 41 1N 21 20 E
Bitonto, Italy . 47 A9 41 6N 16 41 E
Bitra I., India . 95 J1 11 33N 72 9 E
Bitter Creek, U.S.A. . 158 F9 41 33N 108 33W
Bitter L. = Buheirat-Murrat-el-Kubra, Egypt . 106 H8 30 18N 32 26 E
Bitterfeld, Germany . 30 D8 51 37N 12 20 E
Bitterfontein, S. Africa 116 E2 31 1 S 18 32 E
Bitterroot →, U.S.A. . 158 C6 46 52N 114 7W
Bitterroot Range, U.S.A. . 158 D6 46 0N 114 20W
Bitterwater, U.S.A. . 160 J6 36 23N 121 0W
Bitti, Italy . 46 B2 40 29N 9 23 E
Bittou, Burkina Faso . 113 C4 11 17N 0 18W
Bitung, Indonesia . 82 A3 1 27N 125 11 E
Biu, Nigeria . 113 C7 10 40N 12 3 E
Bivolari, Romania . 53 C12 47 31N 27 27 E
Bivolu, Vf., Romania . 53 C10 47 16N 25 58 E
Biwa-Ko, Japan . 73 B8 35 15N 136 10 E
Biwabik, U.S.A. . 154 B8 47 32N 92 21W
Bixad, Romania . 53 C8 47 56N 23 28 E
Bixby, U.S.A. . 155 H7 35 57N 95 53W
Biyang, China . 74 H7 32 38N 113 21 E
Biysk, Russia . 66 D9 52 40N 85 0 E
Bizana, S. Africa . 117 E4 30 50 S 29 52 E
Bizen, Japan . 72 C6 34 43N 134 8 E
Bizerte, Tunisia . 108 A1 37 15N 9 50 E
Bjåen, Norway . 18 E4 59 37N 7 26 E
Bjargtangar, Iceland . 11 B2 65 30N 24 30W
Bjarkalundur, Iceland . 11 B4 65 33N 22 9W
Bjärnum, Sweden . 17 H7 56 17N 13 43 E
Bjästa, Sweden . 16 A12 63 12N 18 29 E
Bjelasica, Serbia & M. 50 D3 42 50N 19 40 E
Bjelašnica, Bos.-H. . 52 G3 43 43N 18 9 E
Bjelland, Norway . 18 F4 58 23N 7 32 E
Bjelovar, Croatia . 45 C13 45 56N 16 49 E
Bjerringbro, Denmark . 17 H3 56 23N 9 39 E
Bjervamoen, Norway . 18 E6 59 17N 9 5 E
Bjøberg, Norway . 18 D5 60 56N 8 13 E
Björbo, Sweden . 16 D8 60 27N 14 44 E
Bjørkelangen, Norway . 18 E8 59 53N 11 34 E
Björklinge, Sweden . 16 D11 60 2N 17 33 E
Bjørnafjorden, Norway 18 D2 60 7N 5 28 E
Björneborg = Pori, Finland . 15 F19 61 29N 21 48 E
Björneborg, Sweden . 16 E8 59 14N 14 16 E
Bjørnevatn, Norway . 14 B23 69 40N 30 0 E
Bjørnøya, Arctic . 6 B8 74 30N 19 0 E
Bjursås, Sweden . 16 D9 60 44N 15 25 E
Bjuv, Sweden . 17 H6 56 5N 12 55 E
Bla, Mali . 112 C3 12 56N 5 47W
Blace, Serbia & M. . 50 C5 43 18N 21 17 E
Blachownia, Poland . 55 H5 50 49N 18 56 E
Black = Da →, Vietnam 76 G5 21 15N 105 20 E
Black →, Canada . 150 B5 44 42N 79 19W
Black →, Alaska, U.S.A. . 144 C11 66 42N 144 42W
Black →, Ariz., U.S.A. 159 K8 33 44N 110 13W
Black →, Ark., U.S.A. 155 H9 35 38N 91 20W
Black →, La., U.S.A. . 155 K9 31 16N 91 50W
Black →, Mich., U.S.A. 150 D2 42 59N 82 27W
Black →, N.Y., U.S.A. 151 C8 43 59N 76 4W
Black →, Wis., U.S.A. 154 D9 43 57N 91 22W
Black Bay Pen., Canada 140 C2 48 38N 88 21W
Black Birch L., Canada 143 B7 56 53N 107 45W
Black Canyon of the Gunnison △, U.S.A. 159 G10 38 40N 107 35W
Black Diamond = Pittsburg, U.S.A. . 160 G5 38 2N 121 53W
Black Diamond, Canada . 142 C6 50 45N 114 14W
Black Duck →, Canada 140 A2 56 51N 89 2W
Black Forest = Schwarzwald, Germany . 31 G4 48 30N 8 20 E
Black Forest, U.S.A. . 154 F2 39 0N 104 43W
Black Hd., Ireland . 23 C2 53 9N 9 16W
Black Hills, U.S.A. . 154 D3 44 0N 103 45W
Black I., Canada . 143 C9 51 12N 96 30W
Black L., Canada . 143 B7 59 12N 105 15W
Black L., Mich., U.S.A. 148 C3 45 28N 84 16W
Black L., N.Y., U.S.A. 151 B9 44 31N 75 36W
Black Lake, Canada . 143 B7 59 11N 105 20W
Black Mesa, U.S.A. . 155 G3 36 58N 102 58W
Black Mountain, Australia . 129 A9 30 18 S 151 39 E
Black Mt. = Mynydd Du, U.K. . 21 F4 51 52N 3 50W
Black Mts., U.K. . 21 F4 51 55N 3 7W
Black Range, U.S.A. . 159 K10 33 15N 107 50W
Black River, Jamaica . 164 a 18 0N 77 50W
Black River Falls, U.S.A. . 154 C9 44 18N 90 51W
Black Rock, Australia 128 B3 32 50 S 138 44 E
Black Rock, Barbados 165 g 13 7N 59 37W
Black Sea, Eurasia . 57 F6 43 30N 35 0 E
Black Tickle, Canada . 141 B8 53 28N 55 45W
Black Volta →, Africa 112 D4 8 41N 1 33W
Black Warrior →, U.S.A. . 149 J2 32 32N 87 51W
Blackall, Australia . 126 C4 24 25 S 145 45 E
Blackball, N.Z. . 131 C6 42 22 S 171 26 E
Blackbull, Australia . 126 B3 17 55 S 141 45 E
Blackburn, U.K. . 20 D5 53 45N 2 29W
Blackburn, Mt., U.S.A. 144 F12 61 44N 143 26W
Blackburn with Darwen □, U.K. . 20 D5 53 45N 2 29W
Blackdown Tableland △, Australia . 126 C4 23 52 S 149 8 E
Blackfoot, U.S.A. . 158 E7 43 11N 112 21W
Blackfoot →, U.S.A. . 158 C7 46 52N 113 53W
Blackfoot River Reservoir, U.S.A. . 158 E8 43 0N 111 43W
Blackman, U.S.A. . 153 E3 30 56N 86 38W
Blackpool, U.K. . 20 D4 53 49N 3 3W
Blackpool □, U.K. . 20 D4 53 49N 3 3W
Blackriver, U.S.A. . 150 B1 44 46N 83 17W
Blacks Harbour, Canada . 141 C6 45 3N 66 49W
Blacksburg, U.S.A. . 148 G5 37 14N 80 25W
Blackshear, U.S.A. . 152 D7 31 18N 82 14W
Blackshear, L., U.S.A. 152 D6 31 51N 83 56W
Blacksod B., Ireland . 23 B1 54 6N 10 0W
Blackstone, U.S.A. . 148 G7 37 4N 78 0W
Blackstone Ra., Australia . 125 E4 26 0 S 128 30 E
Blackville, U.S.A. . 152 B8 33 22N 81 16W
Blackwater = West Road →, Canada . 142 C4 53 18N 122 53W
Blackwater, Australia . 126 C4 23 35 S 148 53 E
Blackwater →, Meath, Ireland . 23 C4 53 39N 6 41W
Blackwater →, Waterford, Ireland . 23 D4 52 4N 7 52W
Blackwater →, U.K. . 23 B5 54 31N 6 35W
Blackwater →, Fla., U.S.A. . 153 E2 30 36N 87 2W
Blackwater →, Mo., U.S.A. . 156 F4 38 59N 92 59W
Blackwell, U.S.A. . 155 G6 36 48N 97 17W
Blackwells Corner, U.S.A. . 161 K7 35 37N 119 47W
Blackwood, C., Papua N. G. . 132 D3 7 49 S 144 31 E
Bladensburg △, Australia . 126 C3 22 30 S 142 59 E
Blaenau Ffestiniog, U.K. . 20 E4 53 0N 3 56W
Blaenau Gwent □, U.K. 21 F4 51 48N 3 12W
Bláfell, Iceland . 11 C7 64 30N 19 51W
Bláfjall, Iceland . 11 B10 65 26N 16 50W
Blagaj, Bos.-H. . 50 C1 43 16N 17 55 E
Blagnac, France . 28 E5 43 37N 1 23 E
Blagnac, Toulouse ✕ (TLS), France . 28 E5 43 37N 1 22 E
Blagodarnoye = Blagodarnyy, Russia . 61 H6 45 7N 43 37 E
Blagodarnyy, Russia . 61 H6 45 7N 43 37 E
Blagoevgrad, Bulgaria . 50 D7 42 2N 23 5 E
Blagoveshchenka, Kazakhstan . 65 B7 43 18N 74 12 E
Blagoveshchensk, Amur, Russia . 67 D13 50 20N 127 30 E
Blagoveshchensk, Bashkortostan, Russia . 64 D5 55 1N 55 59 E
Blahkiuh, Indonesia . 79 J18 8 31 S 115 12 E
Blain, France . 26 E5 47 29N 1 45W
Blain, U.S.A. . 150 F7 40 20N 77 31W
Blaine, Minn., U.S.A. . 154 C8 45 10N 93 13W
Blaine, Wash., U.S.A. . 160 B4 48 59N 122 45W
Blaine Lake, Canada . 143 C7 52 51N 106 52W
Blair, U.S.A. . 154 E6 41 33N 96 8W
Blair Athol, Australia 126 C4 22 42 S 147 31 E
Blair Atholl, U.K. . 22 E5 56 46N 3 50W
Blairgowrie, U.K. . 22 E5 56 35N 3 21W
Blairsden, U.S.A. . 160 F6 39 47N 120 37W
Blairsville, U.S.A. . 150 F5 40 26N 79 16W
Blaj, Romania . 53 D8 46 10N 23 57 E
Blaka, Niger . 109 D2 21 21N 12 47 E
Blakang Mati, Pulau, Singapore . 87 d 1 15N 103 50 E
Blake Pt., U.S.A. . 154 A10 48 11N 88 25W
Blakely, Ga., U.S.A. . 152 D5 31 23N 84 56W
Blakely, Pa., U.S.A. . 151 E9 41 28N 75 37W
Blakeng Mati, Pulau = Sentosa, Singapore . 87 d 1 15N 103 50 E
Blakesburg, U.S.A. . 156 D4 40 58N 92 38W
Blakstad, Norway . 18 F5 58 30N 8 39 E
Blâmont, France . 27 D13 48 35N 6 50 E
Blanc, C., Spain . 38 B3 39 21N 2 51 E
Blanc, C., Tunisia . 108 A1 37 15N 9 56 E
Blanc, Mont, Europe . 29 C10 45 48N 6 50 E
Blanc-Sablon, Canada . 141 B8 51 24N 57 12W
Blanca, B., Argentina . 176 A4 39 10 S 61 30W
Blanca Peak, U.S.A. . 159 H11 37 35N 105 29W
Blanchardville, U.S.A. . 156 B7 42 49N 89 52W
Blanche, C., Australia . 127 E1 33 1 S 134 9 E
Blanche, L., S. Austral., Australia . 127 D2 29 15 S 139 40 E
Blanche, L., W. Austral., Australia 124 D3 22 25 S 123 17 E
Blanche Channel, Solomon Is. . 133 M9 8 30 S 157 30 E
Blanchester, U.S.A. . 157 E13 39 17N 83 59W
Blanchisseuse, Trin. & Tob. . 169 F9 10 48N 61 18W
Blanco, S. Africa . 116 E3 33 55 S 22 23 E
Blanco, U.S.A. . 155 K5 30 6N 98 25W
Blanco →, Argentina . 174 C2 30 20 S 68 42W
Blanco →, Bolivia . 173 C5 12 30 S 64 18W
Blanco, C., Costa Rica 164 E2 9 34N 85 8W
Blanco, C., U.S.A. . 158 E1 42 51N 124 34W
Blanda →, Iceland . 11 B6 65 37N 20 9W
Blandford Forum, U.K. 21 G5 50 51N 2 9W
Blanding, U.S.A. . 159 H9 37 37N 109 29W
Blandinsville, U.S.A. . 156 D6 40 33N 90 52W
Blanes, Spain . 40 D7 41 40N 2 48 E
Blangy-sur-Bresle, France . 27 C8 49 55N 1 37 E
Blanice →, Czech Rep. 34 B7 49 10N 14 5 E
Blankaholm, Sweden . 17 G10 57 36N 16 31 E
Blankenberge, Belgium 24 C3 51 20N 3 9 E
Blankenburg, Germany 30 D6 51 47N 10 57 E
Blanquefort, France . 28 D3 44 55N 0 38W
Blanquillo, Uruguay . 175 C4 32 53 S 55 37W
Blansko, Czech Rep. . 35 B9 49 22N 16 40 E
Blantyre, Malawi . 119 F4 15 45 S 35 0 E
Blarney, Ireland . 23 E3 51 56N 8 33W
Blasdell, U.S.A. . 150 D6 42 48N 78 50W
Blåsjø, Norway . 18 E3 59 20N 6 50 E
Błaszki, Poland . 55 G5 51 38N 18 30 E
Blatná, Czech Rep. . 34 B6 49 25N 13 52 E
Blato, Croatia . 45 F13 42 56N 16 48 E
Blatten, Switz. . 32 D5 46 20N 7 50 E
Blaubeuren, Germany . 31 G5 48 24N 9 46 E
Blaustein, Germany . 31 G5 48 25N 9 53 E
Blåvands Huk, Denmark . 17 J2 55 33N 8 4 E
Blaydon, U.K. . 20 C6 54 58N 1 42W
Blaye, France . 28 C3 45 8N 0 40W
Blaye-les-Mines, France 28 D6 44 1N 2 8 E
Blayney, Australia . 129 B8 33 32 S 149 14 E
Blaze, Pt., Australia . 124 B5 12 56 S 130 11 E
Błażowa, Poland . 55 J9 49 53N 22 7 E
Blechhammer = Blachownia, Poland . 55 H5 50 49N 18 56 E
Bleckede, Germany . 30 B6 53 17N 10 43 E
Bled, Slovenia . 45 B11 46 27N 14 7 E
Blefjell, Norway . 18 E6 59 48N 9 10 E
Bleiburg, Austria . 34 E7 46 35N 14 49 E
Blejeşti, Romania . 53 F10 44 19N 25 27 E
Blekinge, Sweden . 15 H16 56 25N 15 20 E
Blekinge län □, Sweden 17 H9 56 20N 15 20 E
Blenheim, Canada . 150 D3 42 20N 82 0W
Blenheim, N.Z. . 131 B8 41 38 S 173 57 E
Bléone →, France . 29 D10 44 5N 6 0 E
Blérancourt, France . 27 C10 49 31N 3 9 E
Bletchley, U.K. . 21 F7 51 59N 0 44W
Blida, Algeria . 111 A5 36 30N 2 49 E
Blidet Amor, Algeria . 111 B6 32 59N 5 58 E
Blidö, Sweden . 16 E12 59 37N 18 53 E
Blidsberg, Sweden . 17 G7 57 56N 13 30 E
Blieskastel, Germany . 31 F3 49 14N 7 12 E
Bligh Sound, N.Z. . 131 E2 44 47 S 167 32 E
Bligh Water, Fiji . 133 A2 17 0 S 178 0 E
Blind River, Canada . 140 C3 46 10N 82 58W
Blinisht, Albania . 50 E3 41 52N 19 59 E
Blinnenhorn, Switz. . 33 D6 46 26N 8 19 E
Bliss, Idaho, U.S.A. . 158 E6 42 56N 114 57W
Bliss, N.Y., U.S.A. . 150 D6 42 34N 78 15W
Blissfield, Mich., U.S.A. 157 C13 41 50N 83 52W
Blissfield, Ohio, U.S.A. 150 F3 40 24N 81 58W
Blitar, Indonesia . 85 D4 8 5 S 112 11 E
Blitchton, U.S.A. . 152 C8 32 12N 81 26W
Blitta, Togo . 113 D5 8 23N 1 6 E
Block I., U.S.A. . 151 E13 41 11N 71 35W
Block Island Sd., U.S.A. 151 E13 41 15N 71 40W
Bloemfontein, S. Africa 116 D4 29 6 S 26 7 E
Bloemhof, S. Africa . 116 D4 27 38 S 25 32 E
Blois, France . 26 E8 47 35N 1 20 E
Blomskog, Sweden . 16 E6 59 16N 12 2 E
Blomstermåla, Sweden 17 H10 56 59N 16 21 E
Blomvåg, Norway . 18 D1 60 32N 4 50 E
Blonay, Switz. . 32 D3 46 28N 6 54 E
Blönduós, Iceland . 11 B6 65 40N 20 12W
Blongas, Indonesia . 79 K19 8 53 S 116 2 E
Błonie, Poland . 55 F7 52 12N 20 37 E
Bloodvein →, Canada . 143 C9 51 47N 96 43W
Bloody Foreland, Ireland . 23 A3 55 10N 8 17W
Bloom = Chicago Heights, U.S.A. . 157 C9 41 30N 87 38W
Bloomer, U.S.A. . 154 C9 45 6N 91 29W
Bloomfield, Canada . 150 C7 43 59N 77 14W
Bloomfield, Ind., U.S.A. 157 E10 39 1N 86 57W
Bloomfield, Iowa, U.S.A. . 156 D4 40 45N 92 25W
Bloomfield, Ky., U.S.A. 157 G11 37 55N 85 19W
Bloomfield, N. Mex., U.S.A. . 159 H10 36 43N 107 59W
Bloomfield, Nebr., U.S.A. . 154 D6 42 36N 97 39W
Bloomingburg, U.S.A. 157 E13 39 36N 83 24W
Bloomington, Ill., U.S.A. . 156 D8 40 28N 89 0W
Bloomington, Ind., U.S.A. . 157 E10 39 10N 86 32W
Bloomington, Minn., U.S.A. . 154 C8 44 50N 93 17W
Bloomington, Wis., U.S.A. . 156 B6 42 53N 90 55W
Bloomsburg, U.S.A. . 151 F8 41 0N 76 27W
Bloomsbury, Australia 126 J6 20 48 S 148 38 E
Blora, Indonesia . 85 D4 6 57 S 111 25 E
Blossburg, U.S.A. . 150 E7 41 41N 77 4W
Blosseville Kyst, Greenland . 10 D8 68 50N 26 30W
Blotzheim, France . 32 A4 47 36N 7 29 E
Blouberg, S. Africa . 117 C4 23 8 S 28 59 E
Blountstown, U.S.A. . 152 E4 30 27N 85 3W
Bludenz, Austria . 34 D2 47 10N 9 50 E
Blue →, U.S.A. . 157 F10 38 11N 86 19W
Blue Cypress L., U.S.A. 153 H9 27 44N 80 45W
Blue Earth, U.S.A. . 154 D8 43 38N 94 6W
Blue Hole △, Belize . 164 C2 17 24N 88 30W
Blue Lagoon △, Zambia . 119 F2 15 28 S 27 26 E
Blue Mesa Reservoir, U.S.A. . 159 G10 38 28N 107 20W
Blue Mound, U.S.A. . 156 E7 39 42N 89 7W
Blue Mountain Lake, U.S.A. . 151 C10 43 52N 74 30W
Blue Mountain Pk., Jamaica . 164 a 18 3N 76 36W
Blue Mts., Australia . 129 B9 33 40 S 150 15 E
Blue Mts., Jamaica . 164 a 18 3N 76 36W
Blue Mts., Maine, U.S.A. . 151 B14 44 50N 70 35W
Blue Mts., Oreg., U.S.A. 158 D4 45 15N 119 0W
Blue Mts., Pa., U.S.A. . 151 F8 40 30N 76 30W
Blue Mts. △, Australia 129 C9 34 2 S 150 15 E
Blue Mud B., Australia 126 A2 13 30 S 136 0 E
Blue Nile = Nîl el Azraq →, Sudan . 107 D3 15 38N 32 31 E
Blue Nile Falls, Ethiopia . 107 E4 11 25N 37 45 E
Blue Rapids, U.S.A. . 154 F6 39 41N 96 39W
Blue Ridge Mts., U.S.A. 149 G5 36 30N 80 15W
Blue River, Canada . 142 C5 52 6N 119 18W
Blue Springs, U.S.A. . 156 E2 39 1N 94 17W
Bluefield, U.S.A. . 148 G5 37 15N 81 17W
Bluefields, Nic. . 164 D3 12 20N 83 50W
Bluff, Australia . 126 C4 23 35 S 149 4 E
Bluff, N.Z. . 131 G3 46 37 S 168 20 E
Bluff, U.S.A. . 159 H9 37 17N 109 33W
Bluff Harbour, N.Z. . 131 G3 46 36 S 168 21 E
Bluff Knoll, Australia . 125 F2 34 24 S 118 15 E
Bluff Pt., Australia . 125 E1 27 50 S 114 5 E
Bluffs, U.S.A. . 156 E6 39 45N 90 32W
Bluffton, Ga., U.S.A. . 152 D5 31 31N 84 52W
Bluffton, Ind., U.S.A. . 157 D11 40 44N 85 11W
Bluffton, Ohio, U.S.A. 157 D13 40 54N 83 54W
Bluffton, S.C., U.S.A. . 152 C9 32 14N 80 52W
Blumenau = Stettler, Canada . 142 C6 52 19N 112 40W
Blumenau, Brazil . 175 B6 27 0 S 49 0W
Blümisalphorn, Switz. 32 D5 46 28N 7 47 E
Blunt, U.S.A. . 154 C5 44 31N 99 59W
Bly, U.S.A. . 158 E3 42 24N 121 3W
Blyde River Canyon △, S. Africa . 117 C5 24 37 S 31 2 E
Blyth, Australia . 128 B3 33 49 S 138 28 E
Blyth, Canada . 150 C3 43 44N 81 26W
Blyth, U.K. . 20 B6 55 8N 1 31W
Blythe, Calif., U.S.A. . 161 M12 33 37N 114 36W
Blythe, Ga., U.S.A. . 152 B7 33 17N 82 12W
Blytheville, U.S.A. . 155 H10 35 56N 89 55W
Bø, Norway . 18 E6 59 25N 9 3 E
Bo, S. Leone . 112 D2 7 55N 11 50W
Bo Duc, Vietnam . 87 G6 11 58N 106 50 E
Bo Hai, China . 75 E10 39 0N 119 0 E
Bō-no-Misaki, Japan . 72 F2 31 15N 130 13 E
Bo Xian = Bozhou, China . 74 H8 33 55N 115 41 E
Boa Esperança, Brazil 169 C5 3 21N 61 23W
Boa Esperança, Represa, Brazil . 170 C3 6 50 S 43 50W
Boa Nova, Brazil . 171 D3 14 22 S 40 10W
Boa Viagem, Brazil . 170 C4 5 7 S 39 44W
Boa Vista = Tocantinópolis, Brazil . 170 C2 6 20 S 47 25W
Boa Vista, Brazil . 169 C5 2 48N 60 30W
Boa Vista, C. Verde Is. 9 j 16 0N 22 49W
Boa Vista do Erechim = Erechim, Brazil . 175 B5 27 35 S 52 15W
Boac, Phil. . 80 E3 13 27N 121 50 E
Boaco, Nic. . 164 D2 12 29N 85 35W
Bo'ai, China . 74 G7 35 10N 113 3 E
Boal, Spain . 42 B4 43 25N 6 49W
Boali, C.A.R. . 114 B3 4 48N 18 7 E
Boalsburg, U.S.A. . 150 F7 40 46N 77 47W
Boane, Mozam. . 117 D5 26 6 S 32 19 E
Boang I., Papua N. G. 132 B7 3 23 S 153 18 E
Boano, Indonesia . 82 B3 3 0 S 127 56 E
Boardman, U.S.A. . 150 E4 41 2N 80 40W
Boath, India . 94 E4 19 20N 78 20 E
Boatswain Bird I., Ascension I. . 9 g 7 56 S 14 18W
Bobadah, Australia . 129 B7 32 19 S 146 41 E
Bobai, China . 76 F7 22 17N 109 59 E
Bobbili, India . 94 E6 18 35N 83 30 E
Bòbbio, Italy . 44 D6 44 46N 9 23 E
Bobcaygeon, Canada . 140 D4 44 33N 78 33W
Boblad, India . 94 F2 17 13N 75 26 E
Böblingen, Germany . 31 G5 48 40N 9 1 E
Bobo-Dioulasso, Burkina Faso . 112 C4 11 8N 4 13W
Bobolice, Poland . 54 E3 53 58N 16 37 E
Bobon, Phil. . 80 E5 12 32N 124 34 E
Bobonaro, E. Timor . 82 C3 9 2 S 125 22 E
Bobonaza →, Ecuador 168 D2 2 36 S 76 38W
Boboshevo, Bulgaria . 50 D7 42 9N 23 0 E
Bobov Dol, Bulgaria . 50 D6 42 20N 23 0 E
Bóbr →, Poland . 55 F2 52 4N 15 4 E
Bobraomby, Tanjon' i, Madag. . 117 A8 12 40 S 49 10 E
Bobrinets, Ukraine . 59 H7 48 4N 32 5 E
Bobrov, Russia . 60 E5 51 5N 40 2 E
Bobrovitsa, Ukraine . 59 G6 50 45N 31 23 E
Bobruysk = Babruysk, Belarus . 59 F5 53 10N 29 15 E
Bobures, Venezuela . 168 B3 9 15N 71 11W
Boca de Drago, Venezuela . 169 F9 11 0N 61 50W
Bôca do Acre, Brazil . 172 B4 8 50 S 67 27W
Bôca do Jari, Brazil . 169 D7 1 7 S 51 58W
Bôca do Moaco, Brazil 172 B4 7 41 S 68 17W
Boca Grande, U.S.A. . 153 J7 26 45N 82 16W
Boca Grande, Venezuela . 169 B5 8 40N 60 40W
Boca Raton, U.S.A. . 153 J9 26 21N 80 5W
Bocaiúva, Brazil . 171 E3 17 7 S 43 49W
Bocanda, Ivory C. . 112 D4 7 5N 4 31W
Bocaranga, C.A.R. . 114 A3 7 0N 15 35 E
Bocas del Toro, Panama . 164 E3 9 15N 82 20W
Boceguillas, Spain . 42 D7 41 20N 3 39W
Bochkarevo = Belogorsk, Russia . 67 D13 51 0N 128 20 E
Bochmanivka, Ukraine 53 C14 47 40N 29 34 E
Bochnia, Poland . 55 J7 49 58N 20 27 E
Bocholt, Germany . 30 D2 51 50N 6 36 E
Bochum, Germany . 30 D3 51 28N 7 13 E
Bockenem, Germany . 30 C6 52 1N 10 8 E
Boćki, Poland . 55 F10 52 39N 23 3 E
Bocognano, France . 29 F13 42 5N 9 4 E
Bocoio, Angola . 115 E2 12 28 S 14 10 E
Boconó, Venezuela . 168 B3 9 15N 70 16W
Boconó →, Venezuela 168 B4 8 43N 69 34W
Bocoyna, Mexico . 162 B3 27 52N 107 35W
Bocşa, Romania . 52 E6 45 21N 21 47 E
Boda, C.A.R. . 114 B3 4 19N 17 26 E
Boda, Dalarna, Sweden 16 C9 61 1N 15 13 E
Böda, Kalmar, Sweden 17 G11 57 15N 17 3 E
Boda, Västernorrland, Sweden . 16 B10 62 52N 16 39 E
Bodafors, Sweden . 17 G8 57 48N 14 23 E
Bodaybo, Russia . 67 D12 57 50N 114 0 E
Boddam, U.K. . 22 B7 59 56N 1 17W
Boddington, Australia 125 F2 32 50 S 116 30 E
Bode Sadu, Nigeria . 113 D5 9 0N 4 47 E
Bodega Bay, U.S.A. . 160 G3 38 20N 123 3W
Boden, Sweden . 14 D19 65 50N 21 42 E
Bodensee, Europe . 33 A8 47 35N 9 25 E
Bodenteich, Germany . 30 C6 52 50N 10 42 E
Bodhan, India . 94 E3 18 40N 77 44 E
Bodinayakkanur, India 95 J3 10 2N 77 10 E
Bodinga, Nigeria . 113 C6 12 58N 5 10 E
Bodio, Switz. . 33 D7 46 23N 8 55 E
Bodmin, U.K. . 21 G3 50 28N 4 43W
Bodmin Moor, U.K. . 21 G3 50 33N 4 36W
Bodø, Norway . 14 C16 67 17N 14 24 E
Bodoquena, Serra da, Brazil . 173 E6 21 0 S 56 50W

Bodoupa, *C.A.R.* **114 A3** 5 43N 17 36 E
Bodrichi, *Chad* **109 E3** 19 11N 15 54 E
Bodrog →, *Hungary* **52 B6** 48 11N 21 22 E
Bodrum, *Turkey* **49 D9** 37 3N 27 30 E
Boduna, *Dem. Rep. of the Congo* **114 A3** 5 5N 19 44 E
Bódva →, *Hungary* **52 B5** 48 19N 20 45 E
Boembé, *Congo* **114 C3** 2 54 S 15 39 E
Boën, *France* **29 C8** 45 44N 4 1 E
Boende, *Dem. Rep. of the Congo* **114 C4** 0 24 S 21 12 E
Boerne, *U.S.A.* **155 L5** 29 47N 98 44W
Boesmans →, *S. Africa* **116 E4** 33 42 S 26 39 E
Boffa, *Guinea* **112 C2** 10 16N 14 3W
Bofuku, *Dem. Rep. of the Congo* **114 C4** 0 57 S 20 53 E
Bogale, *Burma* **90 G5** 16 17N 95 24 E
Bogalusa, *U.S.A.* **155 K10** 30 47N 89 52W
Bogan →, *Australia* **129 A7** 30 20 S 146 55 E
Bogan Gate, *Australia* **129 B7** 33 7 S 147 49 E
Bogandé, *Burkina Faso* **113 C4** 13 2N 0 8W
Bogangolo, *C.A.R.* **114 A3** 5 34N 18 15 E
Bogantungan, *Australia* **126 C4** 23 41 S 147 17 E
Bogata, *U.S.A.* **155 J7** 33 28N 95 13W
Bogatić, *Serbia & M.* **50 B3** 44 51N 19 30 E
Boğazkale, *Turkey* **100 B6** 40 2N 34 37 E
Boğazlıyan, *Turkey* **100 C6** 39 11N 35 14 E
Bogbonga, *Dem. Rep. of the Congo* **114 B3** 1 36N 19 24 E
Bogdanovich, *Russia* **64 C9** 56 47N 62 1 E
Bogen, *Sweden* **16 D6** 60 4N 12 33 E
Bogense, *Denmark* **17 J4** 55 34N 10 5 E
Bogetići, *Serbia & M.* **50 D2** 42 41N 18 58 E
Boggabilla, *Australia* **127 D5** 28 36 S 150 24 E
Boggabri, *Australia* **129 A9** 30 45 S 150 5 E
Boggeragh Mts., *Ireland* **23 D3** 52 2N 8 55W
Boghari = Ksar el Boukhari, *Algeria* **111 A5** 35 51N 2 52 E
Bogia, *Papua N. G.* **132 C3** 4 9 S 145 0 E
Boglan = Solhan, *Turkey* **101 C9** 38 57N 41 3 E
Bognor Regis, *U.K.* **21 G7** 50 47N 0 40W
Bogo, *Phil.* **81 F4** 11 3N 124 0 E
Bogodukhov = Bohodukhiv, *Ukraine* **59 G8** 50 9N 35 33 E
Bogol Manya, *Ethiopia* **107 G5** 4 34N 41 29 E
Bogong, Mt., *Australia* **129 D7** 36 47 S 147 17 E
Bogor, *Indonesia* **84 D3** 6 36 S 106 48 E
Bogoroditsk, *Russia* **58 F10** 53 47N 38 8 E
Bogorodsk = Noginsk, *Russia* **58 E10** 55 50N 38 25 E
Bogorodsk, *Russia* **60 B6** 56 4N 43 30 E
Bogorodskoye = Kamskoye Ustye, *Russia* **60 C9** 55 10N 49 20 E
Bogorodskoye = Leninskoye, *Russia* **60 A8** 58 23N 47 3 E
Bogoslovsky = Karpinsk, *Russia* **64 B8** 59 45N 60 1 E
Bogoso, *Ghana* **112 D4** 5 38N 2 3W
Bogotá, *Colombia* **168 C3** 4 34N 74 0W
Bogotol, *Russia* **66 D9** 56 15N 89 50 E
Bogou, *Togo* **113 C5** 10 40N 0 12 E
Bogra, *Bangla.* **90 C2** 24 51N 89 22 E
Boguchany, *Russia* **67 D10** 58 40N 97 30 E
Boguchar, *Russia* **60 F5** 49 55N 40 32 E
Bogué, *Mauritania* **112 B2** 16 45N 14 10W
Boguslav, *Ukraine* **59 H6** 49 33N 30 56 E
Boguszów-Gorce, *Poland* **55 H3** 50 45N 16 12 E
Bohain-en-Vermandois, *France* **27 C10** 49 59N 3 28 E
Bohdan, *Ukraine* **53 B9** 48 2N 24 22 E
Bohemian Forest = Böhmerwald, *Germany* **31 F9** 49 8N 13 14 E
Bohena Cr. →, *Australia* **129 A8** 30 17 S 149 42 E
Bohinjska Bistrica, *Slovenia* **45 B11** 46 17N 14 1 E
Böhmerwald, *Germany* **31 F9** 49 8N 13 14 E
Böhmisch-Brod = Český Brod, *Czech Rep.* **34 A7** 50 4N 14 52 E
Böhmisch-Leipa = Česká Lípa, *Czech Rep.* **34 A7** 50 45N 14 30 E
Böhmisch-Trübau = Česká Třebová, *Czech Rep.* **35 B9** 49 54N 16 27 E
Bohmte, *Germany* **30 C4** 52 22N 8 19 E
Bohodukhiv, *Ukraine* **59 G8** 50 9N 35 33 E
Bohol, *Somali Rep.* **120 C3** 5 45N 46 9 E
Bohol □, *Phil.* **81 G5** 9 50N 124 10 E
Bohol Sea, *Phil.* **81 G5** 9 0N 124 0 E
Bohol Str., *Phil.* **81 G4** 9 45N 123 40 E
Bohongou, *Burkina Faso* **113 C5** 12 30N 0 40 E
Böhönye, *Hungary* **52 D2** 46 25N 17 28 E
Bohorodchany, *Ukraine* **53 B9** 48 48N 24 32 E
Bohotleh, *Somali Rep.* **120 C3** 8 20N 46 25 E
Bohuslän, *Sweden* **17 F5** 58 25N 12 0 E
Boi, *Nigeria* **113 D6** 9 35N 9 27 E
Boi, Pta. de, *Brazil* **175 A6** 23 55 S 45 15W
Boiaçu, *Brazil* **169 D5** 0 27 S 61 46W
Boigu I., *Australia* **132 E2** 9 15 S 142 14 E
Boileau, C., *Australia* **124 C3** 17 40 S 122 7 E
Boim, *Brazil* **169 D6** 2 49 S 55 10W
Boing'o, *Sudan* **107 F3** 9 58N 33 44 E
Boipariguda, *India* **94 E6** 18 46N 82 26 E
Boipeba, I. de, *Brazil* **171 D4** 13 39 S 38 55W
Boiro, *Spain* **42 C2** 42 39N 8 54W
Bois →, *Brazil* **171 E1** 18 35 S 50 2W
Boise, *U.S.A.* **158 E5** 43 37N 116 13W
Boise City, *U.S.A.* **155 G3** 36 44N 102 31W
Boissevain, *Canada* **143 D8** 49 15N 100 5W
Bóite →, *Italy* **45 B9** 46 5N 12 5 E
Boitzenburg, *Germany* **30 B9** 53 16N 13 35 E
Boizenburg, *Germany* **30 B6** 53 23N 10 43 E
Bojador, C., *W. Sahara* **110 C2** 26 0N 14 30W
Bojana →, *Albania* **50 E3** 41 52N 19 22 E
Bojano, *Italy* **47 A7** 41 29N 14 29 E
Bojanowo, *Poland* **55 G3** 51 43N 16 42 E
Bøjden, *Denmark* **17 J4** 55 6N 10 7 E
Bojnūrd, *Iran* **97 B8** 37 30N 57 20 E
Bojonegoro, *Indonesia* **85 D4** 7 11 S 111 54 E
Boju, *Nigeria* **113 D6** 7 22N 7 55 E
Boka, *Serbia & M.* **52 E5** 45 22N 20 52 E
Boka Kotorska, *Serbia & M.* **50 D2** 42 23N 18 32 E
Bokada, *Dem. Rep. of the Congo* **114 B3** 4 8N 19 23 E
Bokala, *Dem. Rep. of the Congo* **114 C3** 3 8 S 17 4 E
Bokala, *Ivory C.* **112 D4** 8 31N 4 33W
Bokani, *Nigeria* **113 D6** 9 28N 5 10 E
Bokaro, *India* **93 H11** 23 46N 85 55 E
Bokatola, *Dem. Rep. of the Congo* **114 C3** 0 38 S 18 46 E
Boké, *Guinea* **112 C2** 10 56N 14 17W
Bokela, *Dem. Rep. of the Congo* **114 C4** 1 10 S 21 59 E
Bokenda, *Dem. Rep. of the Congo* **114 B4** 1 16N 21 22 E
Bokhara →, *Australia* **127 D4** 29 55 S 146 42 E
Bokkos, *Nigeria* **113 D6** 9 17N 9 1 E
Boknafjorden, *Norway* **18 E2** 59 14N 5 40 E
Bokode, *Dem. Rep. of the Congo* **114 B3** 3 55N 19 30 E
Bokolo, *Gabon* **114 C2** 2 40 S 10 10 E
Bökönbaev, *Kyrgyzstan* **65 B8** 42 10N 76 55 E
Bokondo, *Dem. Rep. of the Congo* **114 B4** 0 15N 22 32 E
Bokora ⌓, *Uganda* **118 B3** 2 12N 31 32 E
Bokoro, *Chad* **109 F3** 12 25N 17 14 E
Bokota, *Dem. Rep. of the Congo* **114 C4** 0 56 S 22 24 E
Bokote, *Dem. Rep. of the Congo* **114 C4** 0 12 S 21 8 E
Bokpyin, *Burma* **87 G2** 11 18N 98 42 E
Boksitogorsk, *Russia* **58 C7** 59 22N 33 50 E
Boku, *Papua N. G.* **132 D8** 6 34 S 155 21 E
Bokungu, *Dem. Rep. of the Congo* **114 C4** 0 35 S 22 50 E
Bol, *Chad* **109 F2** 13 30N 14 40 E
Bol, *Croatia* **45 E13** 43 18N 16 38 E
Bolama, *Guinea-Biss.* **112 C1** 11 30N 15 30W
Bolan →, *Pakistan* **92 E2** 28 38N 67 42 E
Bolan Pass, *Pakistan* **91 C2** 29 50N 67 20 E
Bolaños →, *Mexico* **162 C4** 21 14N 104 8W
Bolaños de Calatrava, *Spain* **43 G7** 38 54N 3 40W
Bolayır, *Turkey* **51 F10** 40 31N 26 45 E
Bolbec, *France* **26 C7** 49 30N 0 30 E
Boldājī, *Iran* **97 D6** 31 56N 51 3 E
Boldeşti-Scăeni, *Romania* **53 E11** 45 3N 26 2 E
Bole, *China* **68 B3** 45 11N 81 37 E
Bole, *Ethiopia* **107 F4** 6 36N 37 20 E
Bole, *Ghana* **112 D4** 9 3N 2 23W
Bolekhiv, *Ukraine* **59 H2** 49 0N 23 57 E
Boleko, *Dem. Rep. of the Congo* **114 C3** 1 35 S 19 50 E
Bolesławiec, *Poland* **55 G2** 51 17N 15 37 E
Bolgatanga, *Ghana* **113 C4** 10 44N 0 53W
Bolgrad = Bolhrad, *Ukraine* **53 E13** 45 40N 28 32 E
Bolhrad, *Ukraine* **53 E13** 45 40N 28 32 E
Bolia, *Dem. Rep. of the Congo* **114 C3** 1 36 S 18 22 E
Bolinao, *Phil.* **80 C2** 16 23N 119 54 E
Bolinao, C., *Phil.* **80 C2** 16 23N 119 55 E
Bolingbroke, *U.S.A.* **152 C6** 32 57N 83 48W
Bolingo, *Dem. Rep. of the Congo* **114 C4** 3 31 S 21 43 E
Bolintin-Vale, *Romania* **53 F10** 44 27N 25 46 E
Bolívar, *Argentina* **174 D3** 36 15 S 60 53W
Bolívar, *Antioquía, Colombia* **168 B2** 5 50N 76 1W
Bolívar, *Cauca, Colombia* **168 C2** 2 0N 77 0W
Bolívar, *Peru* **172 B2** 7 18 S 77 48W
Bolivar, *Mo., U.S.A.* **155 G8** 37 37N 93 25W
Bolivar, *N.Y., U.S.A.* **150 D6** 42 4N 78 10W
Bolivar, *Tenn., U.S.A.* **155 H10** 35 12N 89 0W
Bolívar □, *Colombia* **168 B3** 9 0N 74 40W
Bolívar □, *Ecuador* **168 D2** 1 15 S 79 5W
Bolívar □, *Venezuela* **169 B5** 6 20N 63 30W
Bolivia ■, *S. Amer.* **173 D5** 17 6 S 64 0W
Bolivian Plateau = Altiplano, *Bolivia* **172 D4** 17 0 S 68 0W
Boljevac, *Serbia & M.* **50 C5** 43 51N 21 58 E
Bolkhov, *Russia* **58 F9** 53 25N 36 0 E
Bolków, *Poland* **55 H3** 50 55N 16 6 E
Bollé, *Mauritania* **110 D2** 20 8N 11 40W
Bollebygd, *Sweden* **17 G6** 57 40N 12 35 E
Bollène, *France* **29 D8** 44 18N 4 45 E
Bollnäs, *Sweden* **16 C10** 61 21N 16 24 E
Bollon, *Australia* **127 D4** 28 2 S 147 29 E
Bollstabruk, *Sweden* **16 B11** 62 59N 17 40 E
Bolmen, *Sweden* **17 H7** 56 55N 13 40 E
Bolobo, *Dem. Rep. of the Congo* **114 C3** 2 6 S 16 20 E
Bologna, *Italy* **45 D8** 44 29N 11 20 E
Bologna ✈ (BLQ), *Italy* **45 D8** 44 34N 11 16 E
Bologoye, *Russia* **58 D8** 57 55N 34 5 E
Bolomba, *Dem. Rep. of the Congo* **114 B3** 0 35N 19 0 E
Bolombo →, *Dem. Rep. of the Congo* **114 B4** 1 32N 21 14 E
Bolonchenticul, *Mexico* **163 D7** 20 0N 89 49W
Bolondo, *Dem. Rep. of the Congo* **114 C3** 2 12 S 18 42 E
Bolong, *Chad* **109 F3** 12 3N 17 45 E
Bolong, *Phil.* **81 H4** 7 6N 122 14 E
Bolongongo, *Angola* **115 D3** 8 28 S 15 16 E
Bolótana, *Italy* **46 B1** 40 20N 8 52 E
Bolotovskoye, *Russia* **64 B9** 58 31N 62 28 E
Boloven, Cao Nguyen, *Laos* **86 E6** 15 10N 106 30 E
Bolpur, *India* **93 H12** 23 40N 87 45 E
Bolsena, *Italy* **45 F8** 42 39N 11 59 E
Bolsena, L. di, *Italy* **45 F8** 42 36N 11 56 E
Bolshakovo, *Russia* **54 D8** 54 53N 21 40 E
Bolshaya Chernigovka, *Russia* **60 D10** 52 6N 50 52 E
Bolshaya Garmanda = Evensk, *Russia* **67 C16** 62 12N 159 30 E
Bolshaya Glushitsa, *Russia* **60 D10** 52 28N 50 30 E
Bolshaya Khobda →, *Kazakhstan* **64 F5** 50 56N 54 34 E
Bolshaya Martynovka, *Russia* **61 G5** 47 19N 41 37 E
Bolshaya Tsaryovshchina = Volzhskiy, *Russia* **61 F7** 48 56N 44 46 E
Bolshaya Vradiyevka, *Ukraine* **59 J6** 47 50N 30 40 E
Bolshevik, Ostrov, *Russia* **67 B11** 78 30N 102 0 E
Bolshoy Anyuy →, *Russia* **67 C17** 68 30N 160 49 E
Bolshoy Begichev, Ostrov, *Russia* **67 B12** 74 20N 112 30 E
Bolshoy Kavkas = Caucasus Mountains, *Eurasia* **61 J7** 42 50N 44 0 E
Bolshoy Lyakhovskiy, Ostrov, *Russia* **67 B15** 73 35N 142 0 E
Bolshoy Tokmak = Tokmak, *Kyrgyzstan* **65 B7** 42 49N 75 15 E
Bolshoy Tyuters, Ostrov, *Russia* **15 G22** 59 51N 27 13 E
Bólstaðarhlíð, *Iceland* **11 B7** 65 31N 19 49W
Bolsward, *Neths.* **24 A5** 53 3N 5 32 E
Bolt Head, *U.K.* **21 G4** 50 12N 3 48W
Boltaña, *Spain* **40 C5** 42 28N 0 4 E
Boltigen, *Switz.* **32 C4** 46 38N 7 24 E
Bolton, *Canada* **150 C5** 43 54N 79 45W
Bolton, *U.K.* **20 D5** 53 35N 2 26W
Bolton Landing, *U.S.A.* **151 C11** 43 32N 73 35W
Bolu, *Turkey* **100 B4** 40 45N 31 35 E
Bolubolu, *Papua N. G.* **132 E6** 9 21 S 150 20 E
Bolungavík, *Iceland* **11 A3** 66 9N 23 15W
Boluo, *China* **77 F10** 23 3N 114 21 E
Bolvadin, *Turkey* **100 C4** 38 45N 31 4 E
Bolzano, *Italy* **45 B8** 46 31N 11 22 E
Bom Comércio, *Brazil* **173 B4** 9 45 S 65 54W
Bom Conselho, *Brazil* **170 C4** 9 10 S 36 41W
Bom Despacho, *Brazil* **171 E2** 19 43 S 45 15W
Bom Jesus, *Angola* **115 D2** 9 11 S 13 34 E
Bom Jesus, *Brazil* **170 C3** 9 4 S 44 22W
Bom Jesus da Gurguéia, Serra, *Brazil* **170 C3** 9 0 S 43 0W
Bom Jesus da Lapa, *Brazil* **171 D3** 13 15 S 43 25W
Boma, *Dem. Rep. of the Congo* **115 D2** 5 50 S 13 4 E
Bomaderry, *Australia* **129 C9** 34 52 S 150 37 E
Bomandjokou, *Congo* **114 B2** 0 34N 14 23 E
Bomaneh, *Dem. Rep. of the Congo* **114 B4** 1 18N 23 47 E
Bomassa, *Congo* **114 B3** 2 12N 16 12 E
Bomate, *Dem. Rep. of the Congo* **114 C3** 2 14N 25 15 E
Bombala, *Australia* **129 D8** 36 56 S 149 15 E
Bombarral, *Portugal* **43 F1** 39 15N 9 9W
Bombay = Mumbai, *India* **94 E1** 18 55N 72 50 E
Bombedor, Pta., *Venezuela* **169 G9** 9 53N 61 37W
Bomberai, Semenanjung, *Indonesia* **83 B4** 3 0 S 133 0 E
Bombo Kasani, *Dem. Rep. of the Congo* **115 D4** 5 51 S 21 54 E
Bomboma, *Dem. Rep. of the Congo* **114 B3** 2 25N 18 55 E
Bombombwa, *Dem. Rep. of the Congo* **118 B2** 1 40N 25 40 E
Bomboyo, *Chad* **109 F3** 12 1N 15 28 E
Bomdila, *India* **90 B4** 27 18N 92 22 E
Bomdo, *India* **90 A5** 28 44N 94 54 E
Bomi Hills, *Liberia* **112 D2** 7 1N 10 38W
Bomili, *Dem. Rep. of the Congo* **118 B2** 1 45N 27 5 E
Bømlo, *Norway* **18 E2** 59 37N 5 13 E
Bomokandi →, *Dem. Rep. of the Congo* **118 B2** 3 39N 26 8 E
Bomongo, *Dem. Rep. of the Congo* **114 B3** 1 27N 18 21 E
Bompoka, *India* **95 K11** 8 15N 93 13 E
Bomputu, *Dem. Rep. of the Congo* **114 C4** 0 23 S 20 6 E
Bomst = Babimost, *Poland* **55 F2** 52 10N 15 49 E
Bomu →, *C.A.R.* **114 B4** 4 40N 22 30 E
Bomu Occidentale ⌓, *Dem. Rep. of the Congo* **114 B4** 4 48N 24 17 E
Bomu Orientale ⌓, *Dem. Rep. of the Congo* **114 B2** 5 0N 25 50 E
Bon, C., *Tunisia* **108 A2** 37 1N 11 2 E
Bon Acceuil, *Mauritius* **121 d** 20 10 S 57 39 E
Bon Sar Pa, *Vietnam* **86 F6** 12 24N 107 35 E
Bonāb, *Iran* **101 D12** 37 20N 46 4 E
Bonaduz, *Switz.* **33 C8** 46 49N 9 25 E
Bonaigarh, *India* **93 J11** 21 50N 84 57 E
Bonaire, *Neth. Ant.* **165 D6** 12 10N 68 15W
Bonaire, *U.S.A.* **152 C6** 32 33N 83 36W
Bonampak, *Mexico* **163 D6** 16 44N 91 5W
Bonang, *Australia* **129 D8** 37 11 S 148 41 E
Bonanza, *Nic.* **164 D3** 13 54N 84 35W
Bonaparte Arch., *Australia* **124 B3** 14 0 S 124 30 E
Boñar, *Spain* **42 C5** 42 52N 5 19W
Bonar Bridge, *U.K.* **22 D4** 57 54N 4 20W
Bonasse, *Trin. & Tob.* **169 F9** 10 5N 61 54W
Bonaventure, *Canada* **141 C6** 48 5N 65 32W
Bonavista, *Canada* **141 C9** 48 40N 53 5W
Bonavista, C., *Canada* **141 C9** 48 42N 53 5W
Bonavista B., *Canada* **141 C9** 48 45N 53 25W
Bondeno, *Italy* **45 D8** 44 53N 11 25 E
Bondo, *Équateur, Dem. Rep. of the Congo* **114 C4** 1 22 S 23 54 E
Bondo, *Orientale, Dem. Rep. of the Congo* **118 B1** 3 55N 23 53 E
Bondoukou, *Ivory C.* **112 D4** 8 2N 2 47W
Bondowoso, *Indonesia* **85 D4** 7 55 S 113 49 E
Bône = Annaba, *Algeria* **111 A6** 36 50N 7 46 E
Bone, Teluk, *Indonesia* **82 B2** 4 10 S 120 50 E
Bonefish Pond, *Bahamas* **9 b** 25 59N 77 23W
Bonerate, *Indonesia* **82 C2** 7 25 S 121 5 E
Bonerate, Kepulauan, *Indonesia* **82 C2** 6 30 S 121 10 E
Bo'ness, *U.K.* **22 E5** 56 1N 3 37W
Bonete, Cerro, *Argentina* **174 B2** 27 55 S 68 40W
Bonfim = Senhor-do-Bonfim, *Brazil* **170 D3** 10 30 S 40 10W
Bonfim, *Brazil* **169 C6** 3 33N 59 25W
Bong Son = Hoai Nhon, *Vietnam* **86 E7** 14 28N 109 1 E
Bonga, *Ethiopia* **107 F4** 7 15N 36 14 E
Bongabon, *Phil.* **80 D3** 15 38N 121 8 E
Bongabong, *Phil.* **80 E3** 12 45N 121 29 E
Bongaigon, *India* **90 B3** 26 28N 90 34 E
Bongandanga, *Dem. Rep. of the Congo* **114 B4** 1 24N 21 3 E
Bongao, *Phil.* **81 J2** 5 2N 119 46 E
Bongka, *Indonesia* **82 B2** 0 58 S 121 27 E
Bongo, *Dem. Rep. of the Congo* **114 C3** 1 47 S 17 41 E
Bongo, Sa. de, *Angola* **115 E3** 10 3 S 15 15 E
Bongor, *Chad* **109 F3** 10 35N 15 20 E
Bongouanou, *Ivory C.* **112 D4** 6 42N 4 15W
Bonham, *U.S.A.* **155 J6** 33 35N 96 11W
Boni, *Mali* **112 B4** 15 3N 2 10W
Boni ⌓, *Kenya* **118 C5** 1 35 S 41 18 E
Bonifacio, *France* **29 G13** 41 24N 9 10 E
Bonifacio, Bouches de, *Medit. S.* **46 A2** 41 12N 9 15 E
Bonifay, *U.S.A.* **152 E4** 30 47N 85 41W
Bonin Is. = Ogasawara Gunto, *Pac. Oc.* **62 G18** 27 0N 142 0 E
Bonita Springs, *U.S.A.* **153 J8** 26 21N 81 47W
Bonito, *Brazil* **173** 21 8 S 56 28W
Bonke, *Ethiopia* **107 F4** 6 5N 37 16 E
Bonkoukou, *Niger* **113 C5** 14 0N 3 15 E
Bonn, *Germany* **30 E3** 50 46N 7 6 E
Bonnat, *France* **27 F8** 46 20N 1 54 E
Bonne Terre, *U.S.A.* **155 G9** 37 55N 90 33W
Bonneau, *U.S.A.* **152 B10** 33 16N 79 58W
Bonners Ferry, *U.S.A.* **158 B5** 48 42N 116 19W
Bonnétable, *France* **26 D7** 48 11N 0 25 E
Bonneval, *France* **29 C11** 45 22N 7 3 E
Bonneval-sur-Arc, *France* **26 D8** 48 11N 1 24 E
Bonneville, *France* **27 F13** 46 4N 6 24 E
Bonney, L., *Australia* **128 D4** 37 50 S 140 20 E
Bonnie Doon, *Australia* **129 D6** 37 2 S 145 53 E
Bonnie Rock, *Australia* **125 F2** 30 29 S 118 22 E
Bonny, *Nigeria* **113 E6** 4 25N 7 13 E
Bonny →, *Nigeria* **113 E6** 4 20N 7 10 E
Bonny, Bight of, *Africa* **113 E6** 3 30N 9 20 E
Bonny Hills, *Australia* **129 A10** 31 36 S 152 51 E
Bonny-sur-Loire, *France* **27 E9** 47 33N 2 50 E
Bonnyrigg, *U.K.* **22 F5** 55 53N 3 6W
Bonnyville, *Canada* **143 C6** 54 20N 110 45W
Bono, *Italy* **46 B2** 40 25N 9 2 E
Bonoi, *Indonesia* **83 B5** 1 45 S 137 41 E
Bonorva, *Italy* **46 B1** 40 25N 8 46 E
Bonsall, *U.S.A.* **161 M9** 33 16N 117 14W
Bontang, *Indonesia* **85 B5** 0 10N 117 30 E
Bontebok △, *S. Africa* **116 E3** 34 5 S 20 28 E
Bonthe, *S. Leone* **112 D2** 7 30N 12 33W
Bontoc, *Phil.* **80 C3** 17 7N 120 58 E
Bontosunggu, *Indonesia* **82 C1** 5 41 S 119 42 E
Bonyeri, *Ghana* **112 D4** 5 1N 2 46W
Bonyhád, *Hungary* **52 D3** 46 18N 18 32 E
Bonython Ra., *Australia* **124 D4** 23 40 S 128 45 E
Boo, Kepulauan, *Indonesia* **83 B3** 1 12 S 129 24 E
Bookabie, *Australia* **125 F5** 31 50 S 132 41 E
Booke, *Dem. Rep. of the Congo* **114 C4** 2 34 S 22 3 E
Booker, *U.S.A.* **155 G4** 36 27N 100 32W
Bool Lagoon, *Australia* **128 D4** 37 7 S 140 40 E
Boola, *Guinea* **112 D3** 8 22N 8 41 E
Boolcoomata, *Australia* **128 A4** 31 57 S 140 33 E
Booleroo Centre, *Australia* **128 B3** 32 53 S 138 21 E
Booligal, *Australia* **129 B6** 33 58 S 144 53 E
Boonah, *Australia* **127 D5** 27 58 S 152 41 E
Boone, *Iowa, U.S.A.* **156 B3** 42 4N 93 53W
Boone, *N.C., U.S.A.* **149 G5** 36 13N 81 41W
Booneville, *Ark., U.S.A.* **155 H8** 35 8N 93 55W
Booneville, *Miss., U.S.A.* **149 H1** 34 39N 88 34W
Boonville, *Calif., U.S.A.* **160 F3** 39 1N 123 22W
Boonville, *Ind., U.S.A.* **157 F9** 38 3N 87 16W
Boonville, *Mo., U.S.A.* **156 F4** 38 58N 92 44W
Boonville, *N.Y., U.S.A.* **151 C9** 43 29N 75 20W
Boorabbin △, *Australia* **125 F4** 31 30 S 129 57 E
Boorindal, *Australia* **127 E4** 30 22 S 146 11 E
Boorowa, *Australia* **129 C8** 34 28 S 148 44 E
Boort, *Australia* **128 D5** 36 7 S 143 46 E
Boosaaso = Bosaso, *Somali Rep.* **120 B3** 11 12N 49 18 E
Boothia, Gulf of, *Canada* **139 A11** 71 0N 90 0W
Boothia Pen., *Canada* **138 A10** 71 0N 94 0W
Bootle, *U.K.* **20 D4** 53 28N 3 1W
Booué, *Gabon* **114 C2** 0 5 S 11 55 E
Bopako, *Dem. Rep. of the Congo* **114 B4** 1 53N 21 13 E
Boppard, *Germany* **31 E3** 50 13N 7 35 E
Boquerón □, *Paraguay* **173 E5** 23 0 S 60 0W
Boquete, *Panama* **164 E3** 8 46N 82 27W
Boquilla, Presa de la, *Mexico* **162 B3** 27 40N 105 30W
Boquillas del Carmen, *Mexico* **162 B4** 29 17N 102 53W
Bor, *Czech Rep.* **34 B5** 49 41N 12 45 E
Bor, *Russia* **60 B7** 56 28N 43 59 E
Bor, *Serbia & M.* **50 B6** 44 5N 22 7 E
Bôr, *Sudan* **107 F3** 6 10N 31 40 E
Bor, *Sweden* **17 G8** 57 9N 14 10 E
Bor, *Turkey* **100 D6** 37 54N 34 32 E
Bor Döbö, *Kyrgyzstan* **65 D6** 39 31N 73 16 E
Bor Mashash, *Israel* **103 D3** 31 7N 34 50 E
Bor u Ceske Lipy = Nový Bor, *Czech Rep.* **34 A7** 50 46N 14 35 E
Bora-Bora, *French Polynesia* **135 J12** 16 30 S 151 45W
Borah Peak, *U.S.A.* **158 D7** 44 8N 113 47W
Boralday, *Kazakhstan* **65 B8** 43 20N 76 51 E
Borama, *Somali Rep.* **120 C2** 9 55N 43 7 E
Borang, *Sudan* **107 G3** 4 50N 30 59 E
Borangapara, *India* **90 C3** 25 14N 90 14 E
Borås, *Sweden* **17 G6** 57 43N 12 56 E
Borāzjān, *Iran* **97 D6** 29 22N 51 10 E
Borba, *Brazil* **169 D6** 4 12 S 59 34W
Borba, *Portugal* **43 G3** 38 50N 7 26W
Borbon, *Phil.* **81 F5** 10 50N 124 2 E
Borborema, Planalto da, *Brazil* **170 C4** 7 0 S 37 0W
Borcea, *Romania* **53 F12** 44 20N 27 45 E
Borchalo = Marneuli, *Georgia* **61 K7** 41 30N 44 48 E
Borçka, *Turkey* **101 B9** 41 25N 41 41 E
Bord Khūn-e Now, *Iran* **97 D6** 28 3N 51 28 E
Borda, C., *Australia* **128 C2** 35 45 S 136 34 E
Bordeaux, *France* **28 D3** 44 50N 0 36W
Bordeaux ✈ (BOD), *France* **28 D3** 44 50N 0 35W
Borden, *Australia* **125 F2** 34 3 S 118 12 E
Borden-Carleton, *Canada* **141 C7** 46 18N 63 47W
Borden I., *Canada* **6 B2** 78 30N 111 30W
Borden Pen., *Canada* **139 A11** 73 0N 83 0W
Borden Springs, *U.S.A.* **152 B4** 33 56N 85 28W
Border Ranges △, *Australia* **127 D5** 28 24 S 152 56 E
Borders = Scottish Borders □, *U.K.* **22 F6** 55 35N 2 50W
Bordertown, *Australia* **128 D4** 36 19 S 140 45 E
Borðeyri, *Iceland* **11 B5** 65 12N 21 6W
Bordighera, *Italy* **44 E4** 43 46N 7 39 E
Bordj bou Arreridj, *Algeria* **111 A5** 36 4N 4 45 E
Bordj Bourguiba, *Tunisia* **108 B2** 32 12N 10 2 E
Bordj Fly Ste. Marie, *Algeria* **110 C4** 27 19N 2 32W
Bordj-in-Eker, *Algeria* **111 D6** 24 9N 5 3 E
Bordj Menaïel, *Algeria* **111 A5** 36 46N 3 43 E
Bordj Messouda, *Algeria* **111 B6** 30 12N 9 25 E
Bordj Nili, *Algeria* **111 B5** 33 28N 3 2 E
Bordj Omar Driss, *Algeria* **111 C6** 28 10N 6 40 E
Bordj Sif Fatima, *Algeria* **111 B6** 31 6N 8 41 E
Bordj Tarat, *Algeria* **111 C6** 25 55N 9 3 E
Borduttighat, *India* **90 B4** 26 57N 93 58 E
Bore, *Ethiopia* **107 G4** 4 39N 37 39 E
Borehamwood, *U.K.* **21 F7** 51 40N 0 15W
Borek Wielkopolski, *Poland* **55 G4** 51 54N 17 11 E
Borensberg, *Sweden* **17 F9** 58 34N 15 17 E
Borgå = Porvoo, *Finland* **15 F21** 60 24N 25 40 E
Borgampad, *India* **94 F5** 17 39N 80 52 E
Borgarfjarðarsýsla □, *Iceland* **11 C5** 64 30N 21 30W
Borgarfjörður, *Borgarfjarðarsýsla, Iceland* **11 C4** 64 30N 22 0W
Borgarfjörður, *Norður-Múlasýsla, Iceland* **14 D7** 65 31N 13 49W
Borgarnes, *Iceland* **11 C5** 64 32N 21 55W
Børgefjellet, *Norway* **14 D15** 65 20N 13 45 E
Borger, *Neths.* **24 B6** 52 54N 6 44 E
Borger, *U.S.A.* **155 H4** 35 39N 101 24W
Borgholm, *Sweden* **17 H10** 56 52N 16 39 E
Bórgia, *Italy* **47 D9** 38 49N 16 30 E
Borgo San Dalmazzo, *Italy* **44 D4** 44 20N 7 30 E
Borgo San Donnino = Fidenza, *Italy* **44 D7** 44 52N 10 3 E
Borgo San Lorenzo, *Italy* **45 E8** 43 57N 11 23 E
Borgo Val di Taro, *Italy* **44 D6** 44 29N 9 46 E
Borgo Valsugana, *Italy* **45 B8** 46 3N 11 27 E
Borgomanero, *Italy* **44 C5** 45 42N 8 28 E
Borgorose, *Italy* **45 F10** 42 11N 13 13 E
Borgosésia, *Italy* **44 C5** 45 43N 8 16 E
Borgotaro = Borgo Val di Taro, *Italy* **44 D6** 44 29N 9 46 E
Borgund, *Norway* **18 C4** 61 3N 7 48 E
Borhoyn Tal, *Mongolia* **74 C6** 43 50N 111 58 E
Bori, *Nigeria* **113 E6** 4 42N 7 21 E
Borigumma, *India* **94 E6** 19 3N 82 33 E
Borikhane, *Laos* **86 C4** 18 33N 103 43 E
Borisoglebsk, *Russia* **60 E6** 51 27N 42 5 E
Borisov = Barysaw, *Belarus* **58 E5** 54 17N 28 28 E
Borisovgrad = Pŭrvomay, *Bulgaria* **51 D9** 42 8N 25 17 E
Borisovka, *Russia* **59 G9** 50 36N 36 1 E
Borja, *Peru* **168 D2** 4 20 S 77 40W
Borja, *Spain* **40 D3** 41 48N 1 34W
Borjas Blancas = Les Borges Blanques, *Spain* **40 D5** 41 31N 0 52 E
Borjomi, *Georgia* **61 K6** 41 48N 43 28 E
Børkop, *Denmark* **17 J3** 55 39N 9 39 E
Borkou, *Chad* **109 E3** 18 15N 18 50 E
Borkum, *Germany* **30 B2** 53 34N 6 40 E
Borlänge, *Sweden* **16 D9** 60 29N 15 26 E
Borley, C., *Antarctica* **7 C5** 66 15 S 52 30 E
Borlu, *Turkey* **49 C10** 38 44N 28 27 E
Bormida →, *Italy* **44 D5** 44 23N 8 13 E
Bórmio, *Italy* **44 B7** 46 28N 10 22 E
Borna, *Germany* **30 D8** 51 7N 12 29 E
Borne Sulinowo, *Poland* **54 E3** 53 32N 16 36 E
Borneo, *E. Indies* **85 B4** 1 0N 115 0 E
Bornholm, *Denmark* **17 J8** 55 10N 15 0 E
Bornholms Amtskommune □, *Denmark* **17 J8** 55 5N 15 0 E
Bornholmsgattet, *Europe* **17 J8** 55 15N 14 20 E
Borno, *Italy* **33 E10** 45 56N 10 12 E
Borno □, *Nigeria* **113 C7** 11 30N 13 0 E
Bornos, *Spain* **43 J5** 36 48N 5 42W
Bornova, *Turkey* **49 C9** 38 27N 27 14 E
Bornu Yassa, *Nigeria* **113 C7** 12 14N 12 25 E
Boro →, *Sudan* **107 F2** 8 52N 26 11 E
Borobudur, *Indonesia* **85 D4** 7 36 S 110 13 E
Borodino, *Russia* **58 E8** 55 31N 35 40 E
Borodino, *Ukraine* **53 D14** 46 18N 29 15 E
Borogontsy, *Russia* **67 C14** 62 42N 131 8 E
Boromo, *Burkina Faso* **112 C4** 11 45N 2 58W
Boron, *U.S.A.* **161 L9** 35 0N 117 39W
Boronga Is., *Burma* **90 F4** 19 58N 93 6 E
Borongan, *Phil.* **81 F5** 11 37N 125 26 E
Borotangba Mts., *C.A.R.* **107 F2** 6 30N 25 0 E
Borotou, *Ivory C.* **112 D3** 8 46N 7 30W
Borovan, *Bulgaria* **50 C7** 43 27N 23 45 E
Borovichi, *Russia* **58 C7** 58 25N 33 55 E
Borovsk, *Berezniki, Russia* **64 B6** 59 43N 56 40 E
Borovsk, *Moskva, Russia* **58 E9** 55 12N 36 24 E
Borrby, *Sweden* **17 J8** 55 27N 14 10 E
Borrego Springs, *U.S.A.* **161 M10** 33 15N 116 23W
Borriol, *Spain* **40 E4** 40 4N 0 4W
Borroloola, *Australia* **126 B2** 16 4 S 136 17 E
Borşa, *Cluj, Romania* **53 D8** 46 56N 23 40 E
Borşa, *Maramureş, Romania* **53 C9** 47 41N 24 50 E
Borsad, *India* **92 H5** 22 25N 72 54 E
Borsec, *Romania* **53 D10** 46 57N 25 34 E
Borshchiv, *Ukraine* **53 B11** 48 48N 26 3 E
Borsod-Abaúj-Zemplén □, *Hungary* **52 B6** 48 20N 21 0 E
Bort-les-Orgues, *France* **28 C6** 45 24N 2 29 E
Borth, *U.K.* **21 E3** 52 29N 4 2W
Börtnan, *Sweden* **16 B7** 62 45N 13 50 E
Borūjerd, *Iran* **97 C6** 33 55N 48 50 E
Borynya, *Ukraine* **55 J10** 49 4N 23 0 E
Boryslav, *Ukraine* **55 J10** 49 18N 23 28 E
Boryspil, *Ukraine* **59 G6** 50 21N 30 59 E
Borzhomi = Borjomi, *Georgia* **61 K6** 41 48N 43 28 E
Borzna, *Ukraine* **59 G7** 51 18N 32 26 E
Borzya, *Russia* **67 D12** 50 24N 116 31 E
Bosa, *Italy* **46 B1** 40 18N 8 30 E
Bosa Monene, *Dem. Rep. of the Congo* **114 C4** 1 16 S 23 40 E
Bosaga, *Turkmenistan* **65 E2** 37 33N 65 41 E
Bosambi, *Dem. Rep. of the Congo* **114 B4** 2 24N 22 39 E
Bosanska Dubica, *Bos.-H.* **45 C13** 45 10N 16 50 E
Bosanska Gradiška, *Bos.-H.* **52 E2** 45 10N 17 15 E
Bosanska Kostajnica, *Bos.-H.* **45 C13** 45 11N 16 33 E
Bosanska Krupa, *Bos.-H.* **45 D13** 44 53N 16 10 E
Bosanski Brod, *Bos.-H.* **52 E2** 45 10N 18 0 E
Bosanski Novi, *Bos.-H.* **45 C13** 45 2N 16 22 E
Bosanski Petrovac, *Bos.-H.* **45 D13** 44 35N 16 21 E
Bosanski Šamac, *Bos.-H.* **52 E3** 45 3N 18 29 E
Bosansko Grahovo, *Bos.-H.* **45 D13** 44 12N 16 26 E
Bosaso, *Somali Rep.* **120 B3** 11 12N 49 18 E
Bosavi, Mt., *Papua N. G.* **132 D2** 6 30 S 142 49 E
Boscastle, *U.K.* **21 G3** 50 41N 4 42W
Boscobel, *U.S.A.* **156 A6** 43 8N 90 42W
Boscobelle, *Barbados* **165 g** 13 17N 59 35W
Bose, *China* **76 F6** 23 53N 106 35 E
Boseki, *Dem. Rep. of the Congo* **114 C3** 2 34 S 19 38 E
Boshan, *China* **75 F9** 36 28N 117 49 E
Boshof, *S. Africa* **116 D4** 28 31 S 25 13 E
Boshrūyeh, *Iran* **97 C8** 33 50N 57 30 E
Bosilegrad, *Serbia & M.* **50 D6** 42 30N 22 27 E
Boskovice, *Czech Rep.* **35 B9** 49 29N 16 40 E
Bosna →, *Bos.-H.* **52 E3** 45 4N 18 29 E
Bosna i Hercegovina = Bosnia-Herzegovina ■, *Europe* **52 G2** 44 0N 18 0 E
Bosnia-Herzegovina ■, *Europe* **52 G2** 44 0N 18 0 E

Bosnik, Indonesia 83 B5 1 5 S 136 10 E
Bösö-Hantō, Japan 73 B12 35 20N 140 20 E
Bosobolo, Dem. Rep. of the Congo 114 B3 4 15N 19 50 E
Bosporus = Istanbul Boğazı, Turkey 51 E13 41 10N 29 10 E
Bosque Farms, U.S.A. 159 J10 34 53N 106 40W
Bossangoa, C.A.R. 114 A3 6 35N 17 30 E
Bossé Bangou, Niger 113 C5 13 20N 1 18 E
Bossembélé, C.A.R. 114 A3 5 25N 17 40 E
Bossemtélé, C.A.R. 114 A3 5 41N 16 38 E
Bossier City, U.S.A. 155 J8 32 31N 93 44W
Bosso, Niger 113 C7 13 43N 13 19 E
Bosso, Dallol →, Niger 113 C5 12 25N 2 50 E
Bostan, Pakistan 92 D2 30 26N 67 2 E
Bostānābād, Iran 101 D12 37 50N 46 50 E
Bosten Hu, China 68 B3 41 55N 87 40 E
Boston, Phil. 81 H6 7 52N 126 22 E
Boston, U.K. 20 E7 52 59N 0 2W
Boston, Ga., U.S.A. 152 E6 30 47N 83 47W
Boston, Mass., U.S.A. 151 D13 42 22N 71 4W
Boston Bar, Canada 142 D4 49 52N 121 30W
Boston Mts., U.S.A. 155 H8 35 42N 93 15W
Bostwick, U.S.A. 152 F8 29 46N 81 38W
Bosumtwi, L., Ghana 113 D4 6 30N 1 25W
Bosusulu, Dem. Rep. of the Congo 114 B4 0 50N 20 45 E
Bosut →, Croatia 52 E3 45 20N 18 45 E
Boswell, Canada 142 D5 49 28N 116 45W
Boswell, Ind., U.S.A. 157 D9 40 31N 87 23W
Boswell, Pa., U.S.A. 150 F5 40 10N 79 2W
Bosworth, U.S.A. 156 E3 39 28N 93 20W
Botad, India 92 H4 22 15N 71 40 E
Botan →, Turkey 101 D10 37 57N 42 2 E
Botene, Laos 86 D3 17 35N 101 12 E
Botera, Angola 115 E2 11 37 S 14 16 E
Botev, Bulgaria 51 D8 42 44N 24 52 E
Botevgrad, Bulgaria 50 D7 42 55N 23 47 E
Bothaville, S. Africa 116 D4 27 23 S 26 34 E
Bothnia, G. of, Europe 14 E19 62 0N 20 0 E
Bothwell, Australia 127 G4 42 20 S 147 1 E
Bothwell, Canada 150 D3 42 38N 81 52W
Boticas, Portugal 42 D3 41 41N 7 40W
Botletle →, Botswana 116 C3 20 10 S 23 15 E
Botlikh, Russia 61 J8 42 39N 46 11 E
Botna →, Moldova 53 D14 46 45N 29 34 E
Botola, Dem. Rep. of the Congo 114 C3 1 17 S 18 13 E
Botolan, Phil. 80 D3 15 17N 120 1 E
Botoroaga, Romania 53 F10 44 8N 25 32 E
Botoşani, Romania 53 C11 47 42N 26 41 E
Botoşani □, Romania 53 C11 47 50N 26 50 E
Botou, Burkina Faso 113 C5 12 42N 1 59 E
Botricello, Italy 47 D9 38 56N 16 51 E
Botro, Ivory C. 112 D3 7 51N 5 19W
Botswana ■, Africa 116 C3 22 0 S 24 0 E
Bottineau, U.S.A. 154 A4 48 50N 100 27W
Bottnaryd, Sweden 17 G7 57 47N 13 50 E
Bottopassi, Suriname 169 C6 4 14N 55 27W
Bottrop, Germany 24 C6 51 31N 6 58 E
Botucatu, Brazil 175 A6 22 55 S 48 30W
Botwood, Canada 141 C8 49 6N 55 23W
Bou Alam, Algeria 111 B5 33 50N 1 26 E
Bou Ali, Algeria 111 C4 27 11N 0 4W
Bou Djébéha, Mali 112 B4 18 25N 2 45W
Bou Guema, Algeria 111 C5 28 49N 0 19 E
Bou Ismaïl, Algeria 111 A5 36 38N 2 42 E
Bou Izakarn, Morocco 110 C3 29 12N 9 46W
Boû Lanouâr, Mauritania 110 D1 21 12N 16 34W
Boû Rjeïmât, Mauritania 112 B1 19 4N 15 3W
Bou Saâda, Algeria 111 A5 35 11N 4 9 E
Bou Salem, Tunisia 108 A1 36 45N 9 2 E
Bouaflé, Ivory C. 112 D3 7 1N 5 47W
Bouaké, Ivory C. 112 D3 7 40N 5 2W
Bouanga, Congo 114 C3 2 7 S 16 8 E
Bouar, C.A.R. 114 A3 6 0N 15 40 E
Bouârfa, Morocco 111 B4 32 32N 1 58W
Bouba Ndjida △, Cameroon 114 A2 8 50N 14 45 E
Bouboût, Algeria 110 C4 27 26N 4 30W
Bouca, C.A.R. 114 A3 6 45N 18 25 E
Boucaut B., Australia 126 A1 12 0 S 134 25 E
Bouches-du-Rhône □, France 29 E9 43 37N 5 2 E
Boucle de Baoulé △, Mali 112 C3 13 53N 9 0W
Boucles de la Seine Normande ⌂, France 26 C7 49 32N 0 35 E
Bouctouche, Canada 141 C7 46 30N 64 45W
Bouda, Algeria 111 C4 27 50N 0 27W
Boudenib, Morocco 110 B4 31 59N 3 31W
Boudry, Switz. 32 C3 46 57N 6 50 E
Boufarik, Algeria 111 A5 36 34N 2 58 E
Bougainville, C., Australia 124 B4 13 57 S 126 4 E
Bougainville I., Papua N. G. 133 L8 6 0 S 155 0 E
Bougainville Reef, Australia 126 B4 15 30 S 147 5 E
Bougainville Str., Solomon Is. 133 L9 6 40 S 156 10 E
Bougaroun, C., Algeria 111 A6 37 6N 6 30 E
Bougie = Bejaïa, Algeria 111 A6 36 42N 5 2 E
Bougouni, Mali 112 C3 11 30N 7 20W
Bouillon, Belgium 24 E5 49 44N 5 3 E
Bouïra, Algeria 111 A5 36 20N 3 59 E
Boukombé, Benin 113 C5 10 13N 1 9 E
Boulal, Mali 112 B3 15 8N 8 21W
Boulazac, France 28 C4 45 10N 0 47 E
Boulder, Colo., U.S.A. 154 E2 40 1N 105 17W
Boulder, Mont., U.S.A. 158 C7 46 14N 112 7W
Boulder City, U.S.A. 161 K12 35 59N 114 50W
Boulder Creek, U.S.A. 160 H4 37 7N 122 7W
Boulder Dam = Hoover Dam, U.S.A. 161 K12 36 1N 114 44W
Boulembo, Gabon 114 C2 1 26 S 12 0 E
Bouli, Mauritania 112 B2 15 17N 12 18W
Boulia, Australia 126 C2 22 52 S 139 51 E
Bouligny, France 27 C12 49 17N 5 45 E
Boulogne →, France 26 E5 47 12N 1 47W
Boulogne-sur-Gesse, France 28 E4 43 18N 0 38 E
Boulogne-sur-Mer, France 27 B8 50 42N 1 36 E
Bouloire, France 26 E7 47 59N 0 45 E
Boulou →, C.A.R. 114 A4 6 45N 24 16 E
Boulouli, Mali 112 B3 15 30N 9 25W
Bouloupari, N. Cal. 133 U20 21 52 S 166 4 E
Bouloupesse, Congo 114 C2 1 58 S 12 40 E
Boulsa, Burkina Faso 113 C4 12 39N 0 34W
Boultoum, Niger 113 C7 14 45N 10 25 E
Bouma △, Fiji 133 A2 16 50 S 179 52 E
Boumalne, Morocco 110 B3 31 25N 6 0W
Boumba →, Cameroon 114 B2 2 2N 15 12 E
Boumbé →, C.A.R. 114 B3 4 4N 15 23 E
Boûmdeïd, Mauritania 112 B2 17 25N 9 50W
Boun Neua, Laos 86 B3 21 38N 101 54 E
Boun Tai, Laos 86 B3 21 23N 101 58 E
Bouna, Ivory C. 112 D4 9 10N 3 0W
Boundary, U.S.A. 144 D12 64 4N 141 6W
Boundary Peak, U.S.A. 160 H8 37 51N 118 21W
Boundgi, Gabon 114 C2 1 0 S 11 51 E
Boundiali, Ivory C. 112 D3 9 30N 6 20W
Boungou →, C.A.R. 114 A4 8 21N 23 48 E
Bountiful, U.S.A. 158 F8 40 53N 111 53W
Bounty Is., Pac. Oc. 134 M9 48 0 S 178 30 E
Boura, Mali 112 C4 12 25N 4 33W
Bourail, N. Cal. 133 U19 21 34 S 165 30 E
Bourbeuse →, U.S.A. 156 F6 38 24N 90 53W
Bourbon, U.S.A. 157 C10 41 18N 86 7W
Bourbon-Lancy, France 27 F10 46 37N 3 45 E
Bourbon-l'Archambault, France 27 F10 46 36N 3 4 E
Bourbonnais, France 27 F10 46 28N 3 0 E
Bourbonnais, U.S.A. 157 C9 41 9N 87 52W
Bourbonne-les-Bains, France 27 E12 47 54N 5 45 E
Bourbourg, France 27 B9 50 56N 2 12 E
Bourdel L., Canada 140 A5 56 43N 74 10W
Bourem, Mali 113 B4 17 0N 0 24W
Bourg, France 28 C3 45 3N 0 34W
Bourg-Argental, France 29 C8 45 18N 4 32 E
Bourg-de-Péage, France 29 C9 45 2N 5 3 E
Bourg-en-Bresse, France 27 F12 46 13N 5 12 E
Bourg-Lastic, France 28 C6 45 39N 2 35 E
Bourg-Madame, France 28 F5 42 26N 1 55 E
Bourg-St-Andéol, France 29 D8 44 23N 4 39 E
Bourg-St-Maurice, France 29 C10 45 35N 6 46 E
Bourg-St. Pierre, Switz. 32 E4 45 57N 7 12 E
Bourganeuf, France 28 C5 45 57N 1 45 E
Bourgas = Burgas, Bulgaria 51 D11 42 33N 27 29 E
Bourges, France 27 E9 47 9N 2 25 E
Bourget, Canada 151 A9 45 26N 75 9W
Bourget, Lac du, France 29 C9 45 44N 5 52 E
Bourgneuf, B. de, France 26 E4 47 3N 2 10W
Bourgneuf-en-Retz, France 26 E5 47 2N 1 58W
Bourgogne □, France 27 F11 47 0N 4 50 E
Bourgoin-Jallieu, France 29 C9 45 36N 5 17 E
Bourgueil, France 26 E7 47 17N 0 10 E
Bourke, Australia 127 E4 30 8 S 145 55 E
Bourne, U.K. 20 E7 52 47N 0 22W
Bournemouth, U.K. 21 G6 50 43N 1 52W
Bournemouth □, U.K. 21 G6 50 43N 1 52W
Bouroum, Burkina Faso 113 C4 13 37N 0 39W
Bouse, U.S.A. 161 M13 33 56N 114 0W
Boussac, France 27 F9 46 22N 2 13 E
Boussé, Burkina Faso 113 C4 12 39N 1 53W
Bousso, Chad 109 F3 10 34N 16 52 E
Boussouma, Burkina Faso 113 C4 12 52N 1 13W
Boutilimit, Mauritania 112 B2 17 45N 14 40W
Boutonne →, France 28 C3 45 54N 0 50W
Bouvet I. = Bouvetøya, Antarctica 8 M12 54 26 S 3 24 E
Bouvetøya, Antarctica 8 M12 54 26 S 3 24 E
Bouxwiller, France 27 D14 48 49N 7 27 E
Bouza, Niger 113 C6 14 29N 6 2 E
Bouznika, Morocco 110 B3 33 46N 7 6W
Bouzonville, France 27 C13 49 17N 6 32 E
Bova Marina, Italy 47 E8 37 56N 15 55 E
Bovalino Marina, Italy 47 D9 38 10N 16 10 E
Bovec, Slovenia 45 B10 46 20N 13 33 E
Boven Kapuas, Pegunungan, Malaysia 85 B4 1 25N 113 15 E
Bøverdal, Norway 18 C5 61 44N 8 20 E
Bøverfjorden, Norway 18 A5 63 1N 8 32 E
Bovill, U.S.A. 158 C5 46 51N 116 24W
Bovino, Italy 47 A8 41 15N 15 20 E
Bovril, Argentina 174 C4 31 21 S 59 26W
Bow →, Canada 142 C6 49 57N 111 41W
Bow Island, Canada 158 B8 49 50N 111 23W
Bowbells, U.S.A. 154 A3 48 48N 102 15W
Bowdle, U.S.A. 154 C5 45 27N 99 39W
Bowdon, U.S.A. 152 B4 33 32N 85 15W
Bowdon Junction, U.S.A. 152 B4 33 40N 85 9W
Bowelling, Australia 125 F2 33 25 S 116 30 E
Bowen, Argentina 174 D2 35 0 S 67 31W
Bowen, Australia 126 J6 20 0 S 148 16 E
Bowen Mts., Australia 129 D7 37 0 S 147 50 E
Bowie, Ariz., U.S.A. 159 K9 32 19N 109 29W
Bowie, Tex., U.S.A. 155 J6 33 34N 97 51W
Bowkān, Iran 101 D12 36 31N 46 12 E
Bowland, Forest of, U.K. 20 D5 54 0N 2 30W
Bowling Green, Fla., U.S.A. 153 H8 27 38N 81 50W
Bowling Green, Ky., U.S.A. 148 G2 36 59N 86 27W
Bowling Green, Mo., U.S.A. 156 E5 39 21N 91 12W
Bowling Green, Ohio, U.S.A. 157 C13 41 23N 83 39W
Bowling Green, C., Australia 126 B4 19 19 S 147 25 E
Bowling Green Bay △, Australia 126 B4 19 26 S 146 57 E
Bowman, N. Dak., U.S.A. 154 B3 46 11N 103 24W
Bowman, S.C., U.S.A. 152 B9 33 21N 80 41W
Bowman I., Antarctica 7 C8 65 0 S 104 0 E
Bowmanville = Clarington, Canada 150 C6 43 55N 78 41W
Bowmore, U.K. 22 F2 55 45N 6 17W
Bowral, Australia 129 C9 34 26 S 150 27 E
Bowraville, Australia 127 E5 30 37 S 152 52 E
Bowron →, Canada 142 C4 54 3N 121 50W
Bowron Lake ⌂, Canada 142 C4 53 10N 121 5W
Bowser L., Canada 142 B3 56 30N 129 30W
Bowsman, Canada 143 C8 52 14N 101 12W
Bowutu Mts., Papua N. G. 132 D4 7 45 S 147 10 E
Bowwood, Zambia 119 F2 17 5 S 26 20 E
Box Cr. →, Australia 127 E3 34 10 S 143 50 E
Boxholm, Sweden 17 F9 58 12N 15 3 E
Boxmeer, Neths. 24 C5 51 38N 5 56 E
Boxtel, Neths. 24 C5 51 36N 5 20 E
Boyabat, Turkey 100 B6 41 28N 34 47 E
Boyabo, Dem. Rep. of the Congo 114 B3 3 43N 18 46 E
Boyaca □, Colombia 168 B3 5 30N 73 20W
Boyalıca, Turkey 51 F13 40 29N 29 33 E
Boyang, China 77 C11 29 0N 116 38 E
Boyany, Ukraine 53 B11 48 17N 26 8 E
Boyasegese, Dem. Rep. of the Congo 114 B4 3 29N 20 33 E
Boyce, U.S.A. 155 K8 31 23N 92 40W
Boyd, U.S.A. 152 E6 30 11N 83 37W
Boyd L., Canada 140 B4 52 46N 76 42W
Boyenge, Dem. Rep. of the Congo 114 B3 0 14N 18 55 E
Boyer, C., N. Cal. 133 U22 21 37 S 168 6 E
Boyera, Dem. Rep. of the Congo 114 C3 0 40 S 19 23 E
Boyle, Canada 142 C6 54 35N 112 49W
Boyle, Ireland 23 C3 53 59N 8 18W
Boyne →, Ireland 23 C5 53 43N 6 15W
Boyne City, U.S.A. 148 C3 45 13N 85 1W
Boyni Qara, Afghan. 91 A2 36 20N 67 0 E
Boynitsa, Bulgaria 50 C6 43 58N 22 32 E
Boynton Beach, U.S.A. 153 J9 26 32N 80 4W
Boyolali, Indonesia 85 D4 7 32 S 110 35 E
Boyoma, Chutes, Dem. Rep. of the Congo 118 B2 0 35N 25 23 E
Boysen Reservoir, U.S.A. 158 E9 43 25N 108 11W
Boyup Brook, Australia 125 F2 33 50 S 116 23 E
Boz Burun, Turkey 51 F12 40 32N 28 46 E
Boz Dağ, Turkey 49 D11 37 18N 29 11 E
Boz Dağları, Turkey 49 C10 38 20N 28 0 E
Bozai Gumbaz, Afghan. 65 E7 37 8N 74 0 E
Bozburun, Turkey 49 E10 36 43N 28 4 E
Bozcaada, Turkey 100 C2 39 49N 26 3 E
Bozdoğan, Turkey 49 D10 37 40N 28 17 E
Boze, Papua N. G. 132 E2 9 3 S 143 3 E
Bozeman, U.S.A. 158 D8 45 41N 111 2W
Bozen = Bolzano, Italy 45 B8 46 31N 11 22 E
Bozene, Dem. Rep. of the Congo 114 B3 2 56N 19 12 E
Boževac, Serbia & M. 50 B5 44 32N 21 24 E
Bozhou, China 74 H8 33 55N 115 41 E
Bozkır, Turkey 100 D5 37 11N 32 14 E
Bozkurt, Turkey 49 D11 37 50N 29 37 E
Bozouls, France 28 D6 44 28N 2 43 E
Bozoum, C.A.R. 114 A3 6 25N 16 35 E
Bozova, Antalya, Turkey 49 D12 37 13N 30 18 E
Bozova, Sanliurfa, Turkey 101 D8 37 21N 38 32 E
Bozovici, Romania 52 F7 44 56N 22 0 E
Bozüyük, Turkey 49 B12 39 54N 30 3 E
Bra, Italy 44 D4 44 42N 7 51 E
Braås, Sweden 17 G9 57 4N 15 3 E
Brabant □, Belgium 24 D4 50 46N 4 30 E
Brabant L., Canada 143 B8 55 58N 103 43W
Brabrand, Denmark 17 H4 56 9N 10 7 E
Brač, Croatia 45 E13 43 20N 16 40 E
Bracadale, L., U.K. 22 D2 57 20N 6 30W
Bracciano, Italy 45 F9 42 6N 12 10 E
Bracciano, L. di, Italy 45 F9 42 7N 12 14 E
Bracebridge, Canada 140 C4 45 2N 79 19W
Brach, Libya 108 C2 27 31N 14 20 E
Bracieux, France 26 E8 47 30N 1 30 E
Bräcke, Sweden 16 B9 62 45N 15 26 E
Brackettville, U.S.A. 155 L4 29 19N 100 25W
Bracki Kanal, Croatia 45 E13 43 24N 16 40 E
Bracknell, U.K. 21 F7 51 25N 0 43W
Bracknell Forest □, U.K. 21 F7 51 25N 0 44W
Brad, Romania 52 D7 46 10N 22 50 E
Brădano →, Italy 47 B9 40 23N 16 51 E
Bradenton, U.S.A. 153 H7 27 30N 82 34W
Bradford, Canada 150 B5 44 7N 79 34W
Bradford, U.K. 20 D6 53 47N 1 45W
Bradford, Ill., U.S.A. 156 C7 41 11N 89 39W
Bradford, Ohio, U.S.A. 157 D12 40 8N 84 27W
Bradford, Pa., U.S.A. 150 E6 41 58N 78 38W
Bradford, Vt., U.S.A. 151 C12 43 59N 72 9W
Bradley, Ark., U.S.A. 155 J8 33 6N 93 39W
Bradley, Calif., U.S.A. 160 K6 35 52N 120 48W
Bradley, Fla., U.S.A. 153 H8 27 48N 81 59W
Bradley, Ill., U.S.A. 157 C9 41 9N 87 52W
Bradley Institute, Zimbabwe 119 F3 17 7 S 31 25 E
Bradner, U.S.A. 157 C13 41 20N 83 26W
Brady, U.S.A. 155 K5 31 9N 99 20W
Brædstrup, Denmark 17 J3 55 58N 9 37 E
Braemar, Australia 128 B3 33 12 S 139 35 E
Braeside, Canada 151 A8 45 28N 76 24W
Braga, Portugal 42 D2 41 35N 8 25W
Braga □, Portugal 42 D2 41 30N 8 30W
Bragadiru, Romania 53 G10 43 46N 25 31 E
Bragado, Argentina 174 D3 35 2 S 60 27W
Bragança, Brazil 170 B2 1 0 S 47 2W
Bragança, Portugal 42 D4 41 48N 6 50W
Bragança □, Portugal 42 D4 41 30N 6 45W
Bragança Paulista, Brazil 175 A6 22 55 S 46 32W
Bragg's Spur = West Memphis, U.S.A. 155 H9 35 9N 90 11W
Brahestad = Raahe, Finland 14 D21 64 40N 24 28 E
Brahmakund, India 90 B6 27 52N 96 22 E
Brahmanbaria, Bangla. 90 D3 23 58N 91 15 E
Brahmani →, India 94 D8 20 39N 86 46 E
Brahmapur, India 94 E7 19 15N 84 54 E
Brahmaputra →, Asia 68 D3 23 40N 90 35 E
Braich-y-pwll, U.K. 20 E3 52 47N 4 46W
Braidwood, Australia 129 C8 35 27 S 149 49 E
Brăila, Romania 53 E12 45 19N 27 59 E
Brăila □, Romania 53 E12 45 5N 27 30 E
Brainerd, U.S.A. 154 B7 46 22N 94 12W
Braintree, U.K. 21 F8 51 53N 0 34 E
Braintree, U.S.A. 151 D14 42 13N 71 0W
Brak →, S. Africa 116 D3 29 35 S 22 55 E
Brake, Germany 30 B4 53 20N 8 28 E
Brakel, Germany 30 D5 51 42N 9 11 E
Bräkne-Hoby, Sweden 17 H9 56 14N 15 6 E
Brakwater, Namibia 116 C2 22 28 S 17 3 E
Brålanda, Sweden 17 F6 58 34N 12 21 E
Bramberg, Germany 31 E6 50 6N 10 40 E
Bramdrupdam, Denmark 17 J3 55 31N 9 28 E
Bramhapuri, India 94 D4 20 36N 79 52 E
Bramming, Denmark 17 J2 55 28N 8 42 E
Brämön, Sweden 16 B11 62 14N 17 40 E
Brampton, Canada 140 D4 43 45N 79 45W
Brampton, U.K. 20 C5 54 57N 2 44W
Bramsche, Germany 30 C3 52 24N 7 59 E
Brampton I., Australia 126 J7 20 50 S 149 17 E
Branchville, U.S.A. 152 B9 33 15N 80 49W
Branco →, Brazil 169 D5 1 20 S 61 50W
Branco, C., Brazil 170 C5 7 9 S 34 47W
Brandberg, Namibia 116 C1 21 10 S 14 33 E
Brandberg ⌂, Namibia 116 C1 21 10 S 14 30 E
Brandbu, Norway 18 D7 60 26N 10 28 E
Brande, Denmark 17 J3 55 57N 9 8 E
Brandenburg = Neubrandenburg, Germany 30 B9 53 33N 13 15 E
Brandenburg, Germany 30 C8 52 25N 12 33 E
Brandenburg, U.S.A. 157 G10 38 0N 86 10W
Brandenburg □, Germany 30 C9 52 50N 13 0 E
Brandfort, S. Africa 116 D4 28 40 S 26 30 E
Brando, France 29 F13 42 47N 9 27 E
Brandon, Canada 143 D9 49 50N 99 57W
Brandon, Fla., U.S.A. 153 H7 27 56N 82 17W
Brandon, Vt., U.S.A. 151 C11 43 48N 73 4W
Brandon B., Ireland 23 D1 52 17N 10 8W
Brandon Mt., Ireland 23 D1 52 15N 10 15W
Brandsen, Argentina 174 D4 35 10 S 58 15W
Brandvlei, S. Africa 116 E3 30 25 S 20 30 E
Brandýs nad Labem, Czech Rep. 34 A7 50 10N 14 40 E
Brăneşti, Romania 53 F11 44 27N 26 20 E
Branford, Conn., U.S.A. 151 E12 41 17N 72 49W
Branford, Fla., U.S.A. 152 F7 29 58N 82 56W
Braniewo, Poland 54 D6 54 25N 19 50 E
Bransfield Str., Antarctica 7 C18 63 0 S 59 0W
Brańsk, Poland 55 F9 52 45N 22 50 E
Branson, U.S.A. 155 G8 36 39N 93 13W
Brantford, Canada 140 D3 43 10N 80 15W
Brantley, U.S.A. 152 D3 31 35N 86 16W
Brantôme, France 28 C4 45 22N 0 39 E
Branxholme, Australia 128 D4 37 52 S 141 49 E
Branxton, Australia 129 B9 32 38 S 151 21 E
Branzi, Italy 44 B6 46 1N 9 46 E
Brás, Brazil 169 D6 2 5 S 58 10W
Bras d'Or L., Canada 141 C7 45 50N 60 50W
Brasher Falls, U.S.A. 151 B10 44 49N 74 47W
Brasil = Brazil ■, S. Amer. 171 D2 12 0 S 50 0W
Brasil, Planalto, Brazil 166 E6 18 0 S 46 30W
Brasil Novo, Brazil 169 D7 3 19 S 52 38W
Brasiléia, Brazil 172 C4 11 0 S 68 45W
Brasília, Distrito Federal, Brazil 171 E2 15 47 S 47 55W
Brasília, Minas Gerais, Brazil 171 E3 16 12 S 44 26W
Brasília △, Brazil 171 E2 15 41 S 48 8W
Brasília Legal, Brazil 169 D6 3 49 S 55 36W
Braskereidfoss, Norway 18 D8 60 44N 11 46 E
Braslaw, Belarus 15 J22 55 38N 27 0 E
Braslovče, Slovenia 45 B12 46 21N 15 3 E
Braşov, Romania 53 E10 45 38N 25 35 E
Braşov □, Romania 53 E10 45 45N 25 15 E
Brass, Nigeria 113 E6 4 35N 6 14 E
Brass →, Nigeria 113 E6 4 15N 6 13 E
Brassac-les-Mines, France 28 C7 45 24N 3 20 E
Brasschaat, Belgium 24 C4 51 19N 4 27 E
Brassey, Banjaran, Malaysia 85 B5 5 0N 117 15 E
Brassey Ra., Australia 125 E3 25 8 S 122 15 E
Brasstown Bald, U.S.A. 149 H4 34 53N 83 49W
Brastad, Sweden 17 F5 58 23N 11 30 E
Brastavăţu, Romania 53 G9 43 55N 24 24 E
Bratan = Morozov, Bulgaria 51 D9 42 30N 25 10 E
Brateş, Romania 53 E11 45 50N 26 4 E
Bratislava, Slovak Rep. 35 C10 48 10N 17 7 E
Bratislava M.R. Stefanik ✈ (BTS), Slovak Rep. 35 C10 48 11N 17 9 E
Bratislavský □, Slovak Rep. 35 C10 48 15N 17 20 E
Bratsberg = Telemark □, Norway 18 E5 59 25N 8 30 E
Bratsigovo, Bulgaria 51 D8 42 1N 24 22 E
Bratsk, Russia 67 D11 56 10N 101 30 E
Brattleboro, U.S.A. 151 D12 42 51N 72 34W
Brattvåg, Norway 18 B3 62 37N 6 25 E
Bratunac, Bos.-H. 52 F4 44 13N 19 21 E
Braunau, Austria 34 C6 48 15N 13 3 E
Braunsberg = Braniewo, Poland 54 D6 54 25N 19 50 E
Braunschweig, Germany 30 C6 52 15N 10 31 E
Braunton, U.K. 21 F3 51 7N 4 10W
Brava, C. Verde Is. 9 j 15 0N 24 40W
Brava, Somali Rep. 120 D2 1 20N 44 8 E
Bravicea, Moldova 53 C13 47 22N 28 27 E
Bråviken, Sweden 17 F10 58 38N 16 32 E
Bravo del Norte, Rio = Grande, Rio →, U.S.A. 155 N6 25 58N 97 9W
Brawley, U.S.A. 161 N11 32 59N 115 31W
Bray, Ireland 23 C5 53 13N 6 7W
Bray, Mt., Australia 126 A1 14 0 S 134 30 E
Bray, Pays de, France 25 B4 49 46N 1 26 E
Bray-sur-Seine, France 27 D10 48 25N 3 14 E
Braymer, U.S.A. 156 E3 39 35N 93 48W
Brazeau →, Canada 142 C5 52 55N 115 14W
Brazil, U.S.A. 157 E9 39 32N 87 8W
Brazil ■, S. Amer. 171 D2 12 0 S 50 0W
Brazilian Highlands = Brasil, Planalto, Brazil 166 E6 18 0 S 46 30W
Brazo Sur →, S. Amer. 174 B4 25 21 S 57 42W
Brazos →, U.S.A. 155 L7 28 53N 95 23W
Brazzaville, Congo 115 C3 4 9 S 15 12 E
Brčko, Bos.-H. 52 F3 44 54N 18 46 E
Brda →, Poland 55 E5 53 8N 18 8 E
Brdy, Czech Rep. 34 B6 49 43N 13 55 E
Brea, Peru 172 A1 4 40 S 81 7W
Breaden, L., Australia 125 E4 25 51 S 125 28 E
Breaksea Sd., N.Z. 131 F1 45 35 S 166 35 E
Bream B., N.Z. 130 B3 35 56 S 174 28 E
Bream Hd., N.Z. 130 B3 35 51 S 174 36 E
Bream Tail, N.Z. 130 C3 36 3 S 174 36 E
Breas, Chile 174 B1 25 29 S 70 24W
Breaza, Romania 53 E10 45 11N 25 40 E
Brebes, Indonesia 85 D3 6 52 S 109 3 E
Brechin, Canada 150 B5 44 32N 79 10W
Brechin, U.K. 22 E6 56 44N 2 39W
Brecht, Belgium 24 C4 51 21N 4 38 E
Breckenridge, Colo., U.S.A. 158 G10 39 29N 106 3W
Breckenridge, Minn., U.S.A. 154 B6 46 16N 96 35W
Breckenridge, Tex., U.S.A. 155 J5 32 45N 98 54W
Breckland, U.K. 21 E8 52 30N 0 40 E
Brecknock, Pen., Chile 176 D2 54 35 S 71 30W
Břeclav, Czech Rep. 35 C9 48 46N 16 53 E
Brecon, U.K. 21 F4 51 57N 3 23W
Brecon Beacons, U.K. 21 F4 51 53N 3 26W
Brecon Beacons △, U.K. 21 F4 51 50N 3 30W
Breda, Neths. 24 C4 51 35N 4 45 E
Bredaryd, Sweden 17 G7 57 10N 13 45 E
Bredasdorp, S. Africa 116 E3 34 33 S 20 2 E
Bredbo, Australia 129 C8 35 58 S 149 10 E
Brededbro, Denmark 17 J2 55 4N 8 50 E
Bredstedt, Germany 30 A4 54 37N 8 55 E
Bredy, Russia 64 E8 52 26N 60 21 E
Bree, Belgium 24 C5 51 8N 5 35 E
Bregalnica →, Macedonia 50 E6 41 43N 22 9 E
Bregenz, Austria 34 D2 47 30N 9 45 E
Bregenzer Wald, Austria 33 B9 47 20N 10 0 E
Bregovo, Bulgaria 50 B6 44 9N 22 39 E
Bréhal, France 26 D5 48 53N 1 30W
Bréhat, Î. de, France 26 D4 48 51N 3 0W
Breiðafjörður, Iceland 11 B3 65 15N 23 15W
Breiðdalsvík, Iceland 11 C13 64 44N 14 0W
Breil-sur-Roya, France 29 E11 43 56N 7 31 E
Breim, Norway 18 C3 61 44N 6 25 E
Breisach, Germany 31 G3 48 1N 7 36 E
Brejinho de Nazaré, Brazil 170 D2 11 1 S 48 34W
Brejo, Brazil 170 B3 3 41 S 42 47W
Brekke, Norway 18 C2 61 1N 5 26 E
Brekken, Norway 18 B8 62 40N 11 51 E
Brekkestø, Norway 18 F5 58 11N 8 22 E
Bremanger, Norway 18 C1 61 51N 4 58 E
Bremangerlandet, Norway 18 C1 61 51N 5 0 E
Bremen, Germany 30 B4 53 4N 8 47 E
Bremen, Ga., U.S.A. 152 B4 33 43N 85 9W
Bremen, Ind., U.S.A. 157 C10 41 27N 86 9W
Bremen □, Germany 30 B4 53 4N 8 50 E
Bremer Bay, Australia 125 F2 34 21 S 119 20 E
Bremer I., Australia 126 A2 12 5 S 136 45 E
Bremerhaven, Germany 30 B4 53 33N 8 36 E
Bremersdorp = Manzini, Swaziland 117 D5 26 30 S 31 25 E
Bremerton, U.S.A. 160 C4 47 34N 122 38W
Bremervörde, Germany 30 B5 53 29N 9 8 E
Bremgarten, Switz. 33 B6 47 22N 8 20 E
Bremnes, Norway 18 E2 59 47N 5 8 E
Bremsnes, Norway 18 A4 63 6N 7 40 E
Brenes, Spain 43 H5 37 32N 5 54W
Brenham, U.S.A. 155 K6 30 10N 96 24W
Brenne, France 28 B5 46 44N 1 14 E
Brenne ⌂, France 28 B5 46 40N 1 15 E
Brennerpass, Austria 34 D4 47 2N 11 30 E
Brennhaug, Norway 18 C6 61 54N 9 21 E
Breno, Italy 44 C7 45 57N 10 18 E
Brent, U.S.A. 149 J2 32 56N 87 10W
Brenta →, Italy 45 C9 45 11N 12 18 E
Brentwood, U.K. 21 F8 51 37N 0 19 E
Brentwood, Calif., U.S.A. 160 H5 37 56N 121 42W
Brentwood, N.Y., U.S.A. 151 F11 40 47N 73 15W
Bréscia, Italy 44 C7 45 33N 10 15 E
Breskens, Neths. 24 C3 51 23N 3 33 E
Breslau = Wrocław, Poland 55 G4 51 5N 17 5 E
Bresle →, France 26 B8 50 4N 1 22 E
Bressanone, Italy 45 B8 46 43N 11 39 E
Bressay, U.K. 22 A7 60 9N 1 6W
Bresse, France 27 F12 46 50N 5 10 E
Bressuire, France 26 F6 46 51N 0 30W
Brest, Belarus 59 F2 52 10N 23 40 E
Brest, France 26 D2 48 24N 4 31W
Brest-Litovsk = Brest, Belarus 59 F2 52 10N 23 40 E
Bretagne □, France 26 D3 48 10N 3 0W
Bretanha, Pta. da, Azores 9 d3 37 54N 25 47W
Bretçu, Romania 53 D11 46 7N 26 18 E
Bretenoux, France 28 D5 44 54N 1 51 E
Breteuil, Eure, France 26 D7 48 50N 0 57 E
Breteuil, Oise, France 27 C9 49 38N 2 18 E
Breton, Canada 142 C6 53 7N 114 28W
Breton, Pertuis, France 28 B2 46 17N 1 25W
Breton Sd., U.S.A. 155 L10 29 35N 89 15W
Brett, C., N.Z. 130 B3 35 10 S 174 20 E
Bretten, Germany 31 F4 49 2N 8 42 E
Breuil-Cervinia, Italy 44 C4 45 56N 7 38 E
Brevard, U.S.A. 149 H4 35 14N 82 44W
Breves, Brazil 170 B1 1 40 S 50 29W
Brevig Mission, U.S.A. 144 D6 65 20N 166 29W
Brevik, Norway 18 E6 59 4N 9 42 E
Brewarrina, Australia 127 E4 30 0 S 146 51 E
Brewer, U.S.A. 149 C11 44 48N 68 46W
Brewer, Mt., U.S.A. 160 J8 36 44N 118 28W
Brewerville, Liberia 112 D2 6 26N 10 47W
Brewster, N.Y., U.S.A. 151 E11 41 23N 73 37W
Brewster, Ohio, U.S.A. 150 F3 40 43N 81 36W
Brewster, Wash., U.S.A. 158 B4 48 6N 119 47W
Brewster, Kap = Kangikajik, Greenland 10 C8 70 7N 22 0W
Brewton, U.S.A. 149 K2 31 7N 87 4W
Breyten, S. Africa 117 D5 26 16 S 30 0 E
Breza, Bos.-H. 52 F3 44 2N 18 16 E
Brežice, Slovenia 45 C12 45 54N 15 35 E
Brézina, Algeria 111 B5 33 4N 1 14 E
Březnice, Czech Rep. 34 B6 49 32N 13 57 E
Breznik, Bulgaria 50 D6 42 44N 22 55 E
Brezno, Slovak Rep. 35 C12 48 50N 19 40 E
Brezoi, Romania 53 E9 45 21N 24 15 E
Brezovica, Serbia & M. 50 D5 42 15N 21 3 E
Brezovo, Bulgaria 51 D9 42 21N 25 5 E
Bria, C.A.R. 114 A4 6 30N 21 58 E
Briançon, France 29 D10 44 54N 6 39 E
Briare, France 27 E9 47 38N 2 45 E
Briático, Italy 47 D9 38 43N 16 2 E
Bribie I., Australia 127 D5 27 0 S 153 10 E
Bribri, Costa Rica 164 E3 9 38N 82 50W
Briceni, Moldova 53 B12 48 22N 27 6 E
Bricquebec, France 26 C5 49 28N 1 38W
Bridgefield, Barbados 165 g 13 9N 59 36W
Bridgehampton, U.S.A. 151 F12 40 56N 72 19W
Bridgend, U.K. 21 F4 51 30N 3 34W
Bridgend □, U.K. 21 F4 51 36N 3 36W
Bridgeport, Calif., U.S.A. 160 G7 38 15N 119 14W
Bridgeport, Conn., U.S.A. 151 E11 41 11N 73 12W
Bridgeport, Ill., U.S.A. 157 F9 38 43N 87 46W
Bridgeport, Nebr., U.S.A. 154 E3 41 40N 103 6W
Bridgeport, Tex., U.S.A. 155 J6 33 13N 97 45W
Bridger, U.S.A. 158 D9 45 18N 108 55W
Bridgeton, U.S.A. 148 F8 39 26N 75 14W
Bridgetown, Australia 125 F2 33 58 S 116 7 E
Bridgetown, Barbados 165 g 13 6N 59 37W
Bridgetown, Canada 141 D6 44 55N 65 18W
Bridgewater, Australia 128 D5 36 36 S 143 59 E
Bridgewater, Canada 141 D7 44 25N 64 31W
Bridgewater, Mass., U.S.A. 151 E14 41 59N 70 58W
Bridgewater, N.Y., U.S.A. 151 D9 42 53N 75 15W
Bridgewater, C., Australia 128 E4 38 23 S 141 23 E
Bridgewater-Gagebrook, Australia 127 G4 42 44 S 147 14 E
Bridgman, U.S.A. 157 C10 41 57N 86 33W
Bridgnorth, U.K. 21 E5 52 32N 2 25W
Bridgton, U.S.A. 151 B14 44 3N 70 42W
Bridgwater, U.K. 21 F5 51 8N 2 59W
Bridgwater B., U.K. 21 F5 51 15N 3 15W
Bridlington, U.K. 20 C7 54 5N 0 12W
Bridlington B., U.K. 20 C7 54 4N 0 10W
Bridport, Australia 127 G4 40 59 S 147 23 E
Bridport, U.K. 21 G5 50 44N 2 45W
Briec, France 26 D2 48 6N 4 0W
Brieg = Brzeg, Poland 55 H4 50 52N 17 30 E
Brienne-le-Château, France 27 D11 48 24N 4 30 E
Brienon-sur-Armançon, France 27 E10 47 59N 3 38 E
Brienz, Switz. 32 C6 46 46N 8 2 E
Brienzer Rothorn, Switz. 32 C6 46 48N 8 2 E
Brienzersee, Switz. 32 C5 46 44N 7 53 E
Brier Cr. →, U.S.A. 152 C8 33 44N 81 26W
Brière ⌂, France 26 E4 47 22N 2 13W
Brig, Switz. 32 D5 46 18N 7 59 E
Brigg, U.K. 20 D7 53 34N 0 28W
Brigham City, U.S.A. 158 F7 41 31N 112 1W
Bright, Australia 129 D7 36 42 S 146 56 E
Brighton, Australia 128 C3 35 5 S 138 30 E
Brighton, Canada 150 B7 44 2N 77 44W
Brighton, Trin. & Tob. 169 F9 10 13N 61 39W
Brighton, U.K. 21 G7 50 49N 0 7W
Brighton, Fla., U.S.A. 153 H8 27 14N 81 6W

Brighton, Ill., U.S.A. 156 E6 39 2N 90 8W
Brighton, Iowa, U.S.A. 156 C5 41 10N 91 49W
Brighton, Mich., U.S.A. 157 B13 42 32N 83 47W
Brighton, N.Y., U.S.A. 150 C7 43 8N 77 34W
Brightwater, N.Z. 131 B8 41 22 S 173 9 E
Brignogan-Plage, France 26 D2 48 40N 4 20W
Brignoles, France 29 E10 43 25N 6 5 E
Brihuega, Spain 40 E2 40 45N 2 52W
Brikama, Gambia 112 C1 13 15N 16 45W
Brilliant, U.S.A. 150 F4 40 15N 80 39W
Brilon, Germany 30 D4 51 23N 8 35 E
Brim, Australia 128 D5 36 3 S 142 27 E
Brimfield, U.S.A. 156 F4 40 50N 89 53W
Bríndisi, Italy 47 B10 40 39N 17 55 E
Brinje, Croatia 45 D12 44 59N 15 9 E
Brinkley, U.S.A. 155 H9 34 53N 91 12W
Brinkworth, Australia 128 B3 33 42 S 138 26 E
Brinnon, U.S.A. 160 C4 47 41N 122 54W
Brinson, U.S.A. 152 E5 30 59N 84 44W
Brion, I., Canada 141 C7 47 46N 61 26W
Brionne, France 26 C7 49 11N 0 43 E
Brionski, Croatia 45 D10 44 55N 13 45 E
Brioude, France 28 C7 45 18N 3 24 E
Briouze, France 26 D6 48 42N 0 23W
Brisbane, Australia 127 D5 27 25 S 153 2 E
Brisbane ➤, Australia 127 D5 27 24 S 153 9 E
Brisbane Ranges △, Australia 128 D6 37 47 S 144 16 E
Brisighella, Italy 45 D8 44 13N 11 46 E
Brissago, Switz. 33 D7 46 7N 8 43 E
Bristol, U.K. 21 F5 51 26N 2 35W
Bristol, Conn., U.S.A. 151 E12 41 40N 72 57W
Bristol, Fla., U.S.A. 152 E5 30 26N 84 59W
Bristol, Pa., U.S.A. 151 F10 40 6N 74 51W
Bristol, R.I., U.S.A. 151 E13 41 40N 71 16W
Bristol, Tenn., U.S.A. 149 G4 36 36N 82 11W
Bristol, City of □, U.K. 21 F5 51 27N 2 36W
Bristol B., U.S.A. 144 H8 58 0N 160 0W
Bristol Channel, U.K. 21 F3 51 18N 4 30W
Bristol I., Antarctica 7 B1 58 45 S 28 0W
Bristol L., U.S.A. 159 J5 34 23N 116 50W
Bristow, U.S.A. 155 H6 35 50N 96 23W
Bristow I., Papua N. G. 132 E2 8 9 S 143 14 E
Britain = Great Britain, Europe 12 E5 54 0N 2 15W
Britânia, Brazil 173 D7 15 14 S 51 9W
British Central Africa = Malawi ■, Africa 119 E3 11 55 S 34 0 E
British Columbia □, Canada 142 C3 55 0N 125 15W
British East Africa = Kenya ■, Africa 118 B4 1 0N 38 0 E
British Guiana = Guyana ■, S. Amer. 169 B6 5 0N 59 0W
British Honduras = Belize ■, Cent. Amer. 163 D7 17 0N 88 30W
British Indian Ocean Terr. = Chagos Arch. ⧫, Ind. Oc. 121 E6 6 0 S 72 0 E
British Isles, Europe 19 D5 54 0N 4 0W
British Virgin Is. ☑, W. Indies 165 e 18 30N 64 30W
Brits, S. Africa 117 D4 25 37 S 27 48 E
Britstown, S. Africa 116 E3 30 37 S 23 30 E
Britt, Canada 140 C3 45 46N 80 34W
Britt, U.S.A. 156 A3 43 6N 93 48W
Brittany = Bretagne □, France 26 D3 48 10N 3 0W
Britton, U.S.A. 154 C6 45 48N 97 45W
Brive-la-Gaillarde, France 28 C5 45 10N 1 32 E
Briviesca, Spain 42 C7 42 32N 3 19W
Brixen = Bressanone, Italy 45 B8 46 43N 11 39 E
Brixham, U.K. 21 G4 50 23N 3 31W
Brlik = Birlik, Kazakhstan 65 B6 43 40N 73 49 E
Brlik = Birlik, Kazakhstan 65 A6 44 5N 73 31 E
Brnaze, Croatia 45 E13 43 41N 16 40 E
Brnenský □, Czech Rep. 35 B9 49 10N 16 40 E
Brno, Czech Rep. 35 B9 49 10N 16 35 E
Broach = Bharuch, India 91 J4 21 47N 73 0 E
Broad ➤, Ga., U.S.A. 152 B7 33 59N 82 39W
Broad ➤, S.C., U.S.A. 149 J5 34 1N 81 4W
Broad Arrow, Australia 125 E3 30 23 S 121 15 E
Broad B., U.K. 22 C2 58 14N 6 18W
Broad Haven, Ireland 23 B2 54 20N 9 55W
Broad Law, U.K. 22 F5 55 30N 3 21W
Broad Sd., Australia 126 C4 22 0 S 149 45 E
Broadalbin, U.S.A. 151 C10 43 4N 74 12W
Broadback ➤, Canada 140 B4 51 21N 78 52W
Broadford, Australia 129 D6 37 14 S 145 4 E
Broadhurst Ra., Australia 124 D3 22 30 S 122 30 E
Broads, U.K. 21 E9 52 45N 1 30 E
Broads, The, U.K. 20 E9 52 45N 1 30 E
Broadus, U.S.A. 154 C2 45 27N 105 25W
Broager, Denmark 17 K3 54 53N 9 40 E
Broby, Sweden 17 H8 56 15N 14 4 E
Broc, Switz. 32 C4 46 37N 7 6 E
Brocēni, Latvia 54 B9 56 42N 22 32 E
Brochet, Canada 143 B8 57 53N 101 40W
Brochet, L., Canada 143 B8 58 36N 101 35W
Brocken, Germany 30 D6 51 47N 10 37 E
Brocklehurst, Australia 129 B8 32 9 S 148 38 E
Brockport, U.S.A. 150 C7 43 13N 77 56W
Brockton, U.S.A. 151 D13 42 5N 71 1W
Brockville, Canada 140 D4 44 35N 75 41W
Brockway, Mont., U.S.A. 154 B2 47 18N 105 45W
Brockway, Pa., U.S.A. 150 E6 41 15N 78 47W
Brocton, U.S.A. 150 D5 42 23N 79 26W
Brod, Macedonia 50 C3 41 32N 21 17 E
Brodarevo, Serbia & M. 50 C3 43 14N 19 44 E
Brodeur Pen., Canada 139 A11 72 30N 88 10W
Brodhead, U.S.A. 156 B7 42 37N 89 22W
Brodhead, Mt., U.S.A. 150 F7 41 39N 77 47W
Brodick, U.K. 22 F3 55 35N 5 9W
Brodnica, Poland 55 E6 53 15N 19 25 E
Brody, Ukraine 59 G3 50 5N 25 10 E
Broglie, France 26 C7 49 0N 0 30 E
Brogan, U.S.A. 158 D5 44 15N 117 31W
Broglie, France 26 C7 49 0N 0 30 E
Brok, Poland 55 F8 52 43N 21 52 E
Broken Arrow, U.S.A. 155 G7 36 3N 95 48W
Broken Bow, Nebr., U.S.A. 154 E5 41 24N 99 38W
Broken Bow, Okla., U.S.A. 155 H7 34 2N 94 44W
Broken Bow Lake, U.S.A. 155 H7 34 9N 94 40W
Broken Hill = Kabwe, Zambia 119 E2 14 30 S 28 29 E
Broken Hill, Australia 128 A4 31 58 S 141 29 E
Broken Ridge, Ind. Oc. 121 H8 30 0 S 94 0 E
Broken River Ra., Australia 126 K6 21 0 S 148 22 E
Brokind, Sweden 17 F9 58 13N 15 42 E
Brokopondo, Suriname 169 B7 5 3N 54 59W
Bromberg = Bydgoszcz, Poland 55 E5 53 10N 18 0 E

Bromley □, U.K. 21 F8 51 24N 0 2 E
Bromo, Indonesia 79 G15 7 55 S 112 55 E
Bromölla, Sweden 17 H8 56 5N 14 28 E
Bromsgrove, U.K. 21 E5 52 21N 2 2W
Brønderslev, Denmark 17 G3 57 16N 9 57 E
Brong-Ahafo □, Ghana 112 B4 7 50N 2 0W
Broni, Italy 44 C6 45 4N 9 16 E
Bronkhorstspruit, S. Africa 117 D4 25 46 S 28 45 E
Brønnøysund, Norway 14 D15 65 28N 12 14 E
Bronson, Fla., U.S.A. 153 F7 29 27N 82 39W
Bronson, Mich., U.S.A. 157 C11 41 52N 85 12W
Bronte, Italy 47 E7 37 47N 14 50 E
Bronwood, U.S.A. 152 D5 31 50N 84 22W
Brook Park, U.S.A. 150 E4 41 24N 81 51W
Brooke's Point, Phil. 81 G1 8 47N 117 50 E
Brookeland, U.S.A. 155 K8 31 6N 93 49W
Brookfield, Mo., U.S.A. 156 E8 39 47N 93 4W
Brookfield, Wis., U.S.A. 157 A8 43 4N 88 9W
Brookhaven, U.S.A. 155 K9 31 35N 90 26W
Brookings, Oreg., U.S.A. 158 E1 42 3N 124 17W
Brookings, S. Dak., U.S.A. 154 C6 44 19N 96 48W
Brookland = West Columbia, U.S.A. 152 B8 33 59N 81 4W
Brooklet, U.S.A. 152 C8 32 23N 81 40W
Brooklin, Canada 150 C6 43 55N 78 55W
Brooklyn, U.S.A. 156 C4 41 44N 92 27W
Brooklyn Park, U.S.A. 154 C8 45 6N 93 23W
Brooks, Canada 142 C6 50 35N 111 55W
Brooks Range, U.S.A. 144 C10 68 0N 152 0W
Brookston, U.S.A. 157 D10 40 36N 86 52W
Brooksville, Fla., U.S.A. 153 G7 28 33N 82 23W
Brooksville, Ky., U.S.A. 157 F12 38 41N 84 4W
Brookton, Australia 125 F2 32 22 S 117 0 E
Brookville, Ind., U.S.A. 157 E12 39 25N 85 1W
Brookville, Ohio, U.S.A. 157 E12 39 50N 84 27W
Brookville, Pa., U.S.A. 150 E5 41 10N 79 5W
Brookville L., U.S.A. 157 E11 39 28N 85 0W
Broom, L., U.K. 22 D3 57 55N 5 15W
Broome, Australia 124 C3 18 0 S 122 15 E
Broons, France 26 D4 48 20N 2 16W
Brora, U.K. 22 C5 58 0N 3 52W
Brora ➤, U.K. 22 C5 58 0N 3 51W
Brørup, Denmark 17 J2 55 29N 9 1 E
Brösarp, Sweden 17 J8 55 43N 14 6 E
Brosna ➤, Ireland 23 C4 53 14N 7 58W
Broșteni, Mehedinți, Romania 52 F7 44 45N 22 59 E
Broșteni, Suceava, Romania 53 C10 47 14N 25 43 E
Brostrud, Norway 18 D5 60 18N 8 34 E
Brotas de Macaúbas, Brazil 171 D3 12 0 S 42 38W
Brothers, U.S.A. 158 E3 43 49N 120 36W
Brothers, The, Yemen 99 D6 12 8N 53 10 E
Brøttum, Norway 18 C7 61 2N 10 34 E
Brou, France 26 D8 48 13N 1 11 E
Brouage, France 28 C2 45 52N 1 4W
Brough, U.K. 20 C5 54 32N 2 18W
Brough Hd., U.K. 22 B5 59 8N 3 20W
Broughton, U.K. 22 F5 55 37N 3 25W
Broughton Island = Qikiqtarjuaq, Canada 139 B13 67 33N 63 0W
Broumov, Czech Rep. 35 A9 50 35N 16 20 E
Brovary, Ukraine 59 G6 50 34N 30 48 E
Brovst, Denmark 17 G3 57 6N 9 31 E
Brown, L., Australia 125 F2 31 5 S 118 15 E
Brown, Mt., Australia 128 B3 32 30 S 138 0 E
Brown, Pt., Australia 127 E1 32 32 S 133 50 E
Brown City, U.S.A. 150 C2 43 13N 82 59W
Brown Willy, U.K. 21 G3 50 35N 4 37W
Brownfield, U.S.A. 155 J3 33 11N 102 17W
Browning, Ill., U.S.A. 156 D6 40 8N 90 22W
Browning, Mo., U.S.A. 156 D3 40 3N 93 12W
Browning, Mont., U.S.A. 158 B7 48 34N 113 1W
Brownsburg, U.S.A. 157 E10 39 51N 86 24W
Brownstown, U.S.A. 157 F10 38 53N 86 3W
Brownsville, Oreg., U.S.A. 158 D2 44 24N 122 59W
Brownsville, Pa., U.S.A. 150 F5 40 1N 79 53W
Brownsville, Tenn., U.S.A. 155 H10 35 36N 89 16W
Brownsville, Tex., U.S.A. 155 N6 25 54N 97 30W
Brownsweg, Suriname 169 B6 5 5N 55 15W
Brownville, U.S.A. 151 C9 44 0N 75 59W
Brownwood, U.S.A. 155 K5 31 43N 98 59W
Browse I., Australia 124 B3 14 7 S 123 33 E
Broxton, U.S.A. 152 D7 31 38N 82 53W
Broye ➤, Switz. 32 C3 46 52N 6 58 E
Bru, Norway 18 C2 61 32N 5 11 E
Bruas, Malaysia 87 K3 4 30N 100 47 E
Bruay-la-Buissière, France 27 B9 50 29N 2 33 E
Bruce, U.S.A. 152 E4 30 28N 85 58W
Bruce, Mt., Australia 124 D2 22 37 S 118 8 E
Bruce, B., N.Z. 131 D4 44 35 S 169 42 E
Bruce Pen., Canada 150 C3 45 0N 81 30W
Bruce Peninsula △, Canada 140 C3 45 14N 81 36W
Bruce Rock, Australia 125 F2 31 52 S 118 8 E
Bruche ➤, France 27 D14 48 34N 7 43 E
Bruchsal, Germany 31 F4 49 7N 8 35 E
Bruck an der Leitha, Austria 35 C9 48 1N 16 47 E
Bruck an der Mur, Austria 34 D8 47 24N 15 16 E
Brue ➤, U.K. 21 F5 51 13N 2 59W
Bruflat, Norway 18 D6 60 53N 9 37 E
Bruges = Brugge, Belgium 24 C3 51 13N 3 13 E
Brugg, Switz. 32 B6 47 29N 8 11 E
Brugge, Belgium 24 C3 51 13N 3 13 E
Bruin, U.S.A. 150 E5 41 3N 79 43W
Bruini, India 90 A6 29 10N 96 11 E
Brûlé, Canada 142 C5 53 15N 117 58W
Brûlon, France 26 D6 47 58N 0 15W
Brumado, Brazil 171 D3 14 14 S 41 40W
Brumado ➤, Brazil 171 D3 14 13 S 41 40W
Brumath, France 27 D14 48 43N 7 40 E
Brumunddal, Norway 18 D7 60 53N 10 56 E
Brundidge, U.S.A. 152 D4 31 43N 85 49W
Bruneau, U.S.A. 158 E6 42 53N 115 48W
Bruneau ➤, U.S.A. 158 E6 42 56N 115 57W
Bruneck = Brunico, Italy 45 B8 46 48N 11 56 E
Brunei = Bandar Seri Begawan, Brunei 85 B4 4 52N 115 0 E
Brunei ■, Asia 85 B4 4 50N 115 0 E
Brunflo, Sweden 16 A8 63 5N 14 50 E
Brunico, Italy 45 B8 46 48N 11 56 E
Brünig, Switz. 32 C6 46 46N 8 11 E
Brünigpass, Switz. 32 C6 46 46N 8 8 E
Brunn = Brno, Czech Rep. 35 B9 49 10N 16 35 E
Brunna, Sweden 16 E11 59 52N 17 25 E
Brunnen, Switz. 33 C7 46 59N 8 37 E
Brunner, L., N.Z. 131 C6 42 37 S 171 27 E
Brunnhöll, Iceland 11 C1 64 17N 15 26W
Brunsbüttel, Germany 30 B5 53 54N 9 6 E
Brunssum, Neths. 24 D5 50 57N 5 59 E

Brunswick = Braunschweig, Germany 30 C6 52 15N 10 31 E
Brunswick, Ga., U.S.A. 152 D8 31 10N 81 30W
Brunswick, Maine, U.S.A. 149 D11 43 55N 69 58W
Brunswick, Mo., U.S.A. 156 E3 39 26N 93 8W
Brunswick, Ohio, U.S.A. 150 E3 41 14N 81 51W
Brunswick, Pen. de, Chile 176 D2 53 30 S 71 30W
Brunswick B., Australia 124 C3 15 15 S 124 50 E
Brunswick Junction, Australia 125 F2 33 15 S 115 50 E
Bruntál, Czech Rep. 35 B10 49 59N 17 27 E
Bruny I., Australia 127 G4 43 20 S 147 15 E
Brus Laguna, Honduras 164 C3 15 47N 84 35W
Brusa = Bursa, Turkey 51 F13 40 15N 29 5 E
Brusartsi, Bulgaria 50 C7 43 40N 23 5 E
Brush, U.S.A. 154 E3 40 15N 103 37W
Brushton, U.S.A. 151 B10 44 50N 74 31W
Brusio, Switz. 33 D10 46 14N 10 8 E
Brusque, Brazil 175 B6 27 5 S 49 0W
Brussel, Belgium 24 D4 50 51N 4 21 E
Brussel ✈ (BRU), Belgium 24 D5 50 54N 4 29 E
Brussels = Brussel, Belgium 24 D4 50 51N 4 21 E
Brussels, Canada 150 C3 43 44N 81 15W
Brusy, Poland 54 E4 53 53N 17 43 E
Bruthen, Australia 129 D7 37 42 S 147 50 E
Bruvoll, Norway 18 D8 60 27N 11 29 E
Bruxelles = Brussel, Belgium 24 D4 50 51N 4 21 E
Bruyères, France 27 D13 48 10N 6 40 E
Bruz, France 26 D5 48 1N 1 46W
Brwinów, Poland 55 F7 52 9N 20 40 E
Bryagovo, Bulgaria 51 G10 41 58N 25 8 E
Bryan, Ohio, U.S.A. 157 C12 41 28N 84 33W
Bryan, Tex., U.S.A. 155 K6 30 40N 96 22W
Bryanka, Ukraine 59 H10 48 32N 38 45 E
Bryansk, Bryansk, Russia 59 F8 53 13N 34 25 E
Bryansk, Dagestan, Russia 61 H8 44 20N 47 10 E
Bryanskoye = Bryansk, Russia 61 H8 44 20N 47 10 E
Bryce Canyon △, U.S.A. 159 H7 37 30N 112 10W
Bryne, Norway 18 F2 58 44N 5 38 E
Bryson City, U.S.A. 149 H4 35 26N 83 27W
Bryukhovetskaya, Russia 59 K10 45 48N 39 0 E
Brza Palanka, Serbia & M. 50 B6 44 28N 22 27 E
Brzeg, Poland 55 H4 50 52N 17 30 E
Brzeg Dolny, Poland 55 G3 51 16N 16 41 E
Brześć Kujawski, Poland 55 F5 52 36N 18 55 E
Brześć nad Bugiem = Brest, Belarus 59 F2 52 10N 23 40 E
Brzesko, Poland 55 J7 49 59N 20 34 E
Brzeziny, Poland 55 G6 51 49N 19 42 E
Brzozów, Poland 55 J9 49 41N 22 3 E
Bsharri, Lebanon 103 A5 34 15N 36 0 E
Bū al Ḩīḑān, W. ➤, Libya 108 C3 27 25N 19 22 E
Bū Athlah, Libya 108 B3 30 15N 19 39 E
Bū Baqarah, U.A.E. 97 E8 25 35N 56 25 E
Bu Craa, W. Sahara 110 C2 26 45N 12 50W
Bū Ḩasā, U.A.E. 97 F7 23 30N 53 20 E
Bū Tummayyim, W. ➤, Libya 108 C3 26 56N 19 13 E
Bua, Fiji 133 A2 16 48 S 178 37 E
Bua ➤, Fiji 17 G6 57 14N 12 7 E
Bua Yai, Thailand 86 E4 15 33N 102 26 E
Buad I., Phil. 81 F5 11 40N 124 51 E
Buala, Solomon Is. 133 M10 8 10 S 159 35 E
Buapinang, Indonesia 82 B2 4 40 S 121 30 E
Buayan = General Santos, Phil. 81 H5 6 5N 125 14 E
Buba, Guinea-Biss. 112 C2 11 40N 14 59W
Bubanza, Burundi 114 B3 4 14N 19 38 E
Bubanza, Burundi 118 C2 3 6 S 29 23 E
Bubaque, Guinea-Biss. 112 C1 11 16N 15 51W
Bube, Ethiopia 107 F4 4 46N 35 48 E
Būbiyān, Kuwait 97 D6 29 45N 48 15 E
Buca, Turkey 49 C9 38 22N 27 11 E
Bucak, Turkey 49 D12 37 28N 30 36 E
Bucaramanga, Colombia 168 B3 7 0N 73 0W
Bucas Grande I., Phil. 81 G5 9 40N 125 57 E
Bucasia, Australia 126 K7 21 2 S 149 10 E
Bucay, Phil. 80 C3 17 32N 120 43 E
Buccaneer Arch., Australia 124 C3 16 7 S 123 20 E
Buccino, Italy 47 B8 40 38N 15 22 E
Buccoo Reef, Trin. & Tob. 169 E10 11 10N 60 51W
Bucecea, Romania 53 C11 47 47N 26 28 E
Bucegi △, Romania 53 E10 45 25N 25 25 E
Bucey-lès-Gy, France 32 B1 47 25N 5 51 E
Buchach, Ukraine 59 H3 49 5N 25 25 E
Buchan, Australia 129 D8 37 30 S 148 12 E
Buchan Ness, U.K. 22 D7 57 29N 1 46W
Buchanan, Canada 143 C8 51 40N 102 45W
Buchanan, Liberia 112 D2 5 57N 10 2W
Buchanan, Mich., U.S.A. 152 B4 33 48N 85 11W
Buchanan, Mich., U.S.A. 157 C10 41 50N 86 22W
Buchanan, L., Queens., Australia 126 C4 21 35 S 145 52 E
Buchanan, L., W. Austral., Australia 125 E3 25 33 S 123 2 E
Buchanan, L., U.S.A. 155 K5 30 45N 98 25W
Buchanan Cr. ➤, Australia 126 B2 19 13 S 136 33 E
Buchans, Canada 141 C8 48 50N 56 52W
Bucharest = București, Romania 53 F11 44 27N 26 10 E
Buchen, Germany 31 F5 49 31N 9 20 E
Bucheon = Puch'ŏn, S. Korea 57 F14 37 30N 126 50 E
Buchholz, Germany 30 B5 53 19N 9 52 E
Buchloe, Germany 31 G6 48 1N 10 44 E
Buchon, Pt., U.S.A. 160 K6 35 15N 120 54W
Buchs, Aargau, Switz. 32 B6 47 23N 8 4 E
Buchs, St. Galen, Switz. 33 B8 47 10N 9 28 E
Buciumi, Romania 53 C8 47 3N 23 1 E
Buck Hill Falls, U.S.A. 151 E9 41 11N 75 16W
Buckeye Lake, U.S.A. 150 G2 39 55N 82 29W
Buckeye, U.S.A. 159 K7 33 22N 112 35W
Buckhannon, U.S.A. 148 F5 39 0N 80 8W
Buckhaven, U.S.A. 22 E5 56 11N 3 3W
Buckie, U.K. 22 D6 57 41N 2 58W
Buckingham, Canada 140 C4 45 37N 75 24W
Buckingham, U.K. 21 F7 51 59N 0 57W
Buckingham B., Australia 126 A2 12 10 S 135 40 E

Buckingham Canal, India 95 H5 14 0N 80 5 E
Buckinghamshire □, U.K. 21 F7 51 53N 0 55W
Buckland, U.S.A. 144 D7 65 59N 161 8W
Buckle Hd., Australia 124 B4 14 26 S 127 52 E
Buckleboo, Australia 128 B2 32 54 S 136 12 E
Buckley, U.K. 20 D4 53 10N 3 5W
Buckley ➤, Australia 126 C2 20 10 S 138 49 E
Bucklin, Kans., U.S.A. 155 G5 37 33N 99 38W
Bucklin, Mo., U.S.A. 156 E4 39 47N 92 53W
Bucks L., U.S.A. 160 F5 39 54N 121 12W
Buco Zau, Angola 115 C2 4 45 S 12 33 E
Bucquoy, France 27 B9 50 9N 2 43 E
Bucureşti, Romania 53 F11 44 27N 26 10 E
București Otopeni ✈ (OTP), Romania 53 F11 44 30N 26 11 E
Bucyrus, U.S.A. 157 D14 40 48N 82 59W
Bud, Norway 18 B3 62 55N 6 55 E
Budacu, Vf., Romania 53 C10 47 7N 25 41 E
Budalin, Burma 90 D5 22 20N 95 10 E
Budaörs, Hungary 52 C3 47 27N 18 58 E
Budapest, Hungary 52 C4 47 29N 19 5 E
Budapest ✈ (BUD), Hungary 52 C4 47 29N 19 5 E
Budaun, India 93 E8 28 5N 79 10 E
Budawang △, Australia 129 C9 35 10 S 150 12 E
Budd Coast, Antarctica 7 C8 68 0 S 112 0 E
Buddenbrock = Brodnica, Poland 55 E6 53 15N 19 25 E
Budderoo △, Australia 129 C9 35 40 S 150 41 E
Buddusò, Italy 46 B2 40 35N 9 15 E
Budel, Neths. 24 C5 51 17N 5 34 E
Budennovsk, Russia 61 H7 44 50N 44 10 E
Budeşti, Romania 53 F11 44 13N 26 30 E
Budeyi, Ukraine 53 B14 48 3N 29 16 E
Budge Budge = Baj Baj, India 93 H13 22 30N 88 5 E
Budgewoi, Australia 129 B9 33 13 S 151 34 E
Bûðardalur, Iceland 11 C12 64 56N 21 46W
Bûðir, Iceland 11 C1 64 56N 14 1W
Budia, Spain 40 E2 40 38N 2 46W
Budjala, Dem. Rep. of the Congo 114 B3 2 50N 19 40 E
Budoni, Italy 46 B2 40 40N 9 45 E
Búdrio, Italy 45 D8 44 32N 11 32 E
Büdszentmihály = Tiszavasvári, Hungary 52 C6 47 58N 21 18 E
Budva, Serbia & M. 50 D2 42 17N 18 50 E
Budweis = České Budějovice, Czech Rep. 34 C7 48 55N 14 25 E
Budyonnovka = Novoazovsk, Ukraine 59 J10 47 15N 38 4 E
Budzyń, Poland 55 F3 52 54N 16 59 E
Bue, Norway 18 F2 58 40N 5 58 E
Buea, Cameroon 113 E6 4 10N 9 9 E
Buela, Angola 115 D2 5 14 S 14 33 E
Buellton, U.S.A. 161 L6 34 37N 120 12W
Buena Esperanza, Argentina 174 C2 34 45 S 65 15W
Buena Park, U.S.A. 161 M9 33 52N 117 59W
Buena Vista, Bolivia 173 D5 17 27 S 63 40W
Buena Vista, Solomon Is. 133 M11 8 52 S 160 3 E
Buena Vista, Colo., U.S.A. 159 G10 38 51N 106 8W
Buena Vista, Ga., U.S.A. 152 D5 32 19N 84 31W
Buena Vista, Va., U.S.A. 148 G6 37 44N 79 21W
Buena Vista Lake Bed, U.S.A. 161 K7 35 12N 119 18W
Buenaventura, Colombia 168 C2 3 53N 77 4W
Buenaventura, Mexico 162 B3 29 50N 107 30W
Buenaventura, B. de, Colombia 168 C2 3 48N 77 17W
Buenavista, Agusan del N., Phil. 81 G5 8 59N 125 24 E
Buenavista, Quezon, Phil. 80 E4 13 33N 122 34 E
Buendía, Embalse de, Spain 40 E2 40 25N 2 43W
Buenópolis, Brazil 171 E3 17 54 S 44 11W
Buenos Aires, Argentina 174 C4 34 30 S 58 20W
Buenos Aires, Colombia 168 C3 1 36N 73 18W
Buenos Aires, Costa Rica 164 E3 9 10N 83 20W
Buenos Aires □, Argentina 174 D4 36 30 S 60 0W
Buenos Aires, Chile 174 C2 46 35 S 72 30W
Buenos Aires, Colombia 168 C2 1 23N 77 9W
Buet, Mont, France 32 D3 46 2N 6 52 E
Buffalo, Mo., U.S.A. 155 G8 37 39N 93 6W
Buffalo, N.Y., U.S.A. 150 D6 42 53N 78 53W
Buffalo, Okla., U.S.A. 155 G5 36 50N 99 38W
Buffalo, S. Dak., U.S.A. 154 C3 45 35N 103 33W
Buffalo, Wyo., U.S.A. 158 D10 44 21N 106 42W
Buffalo ➤, Canada 155 B8 36 14N 92 36W
Buffalo ➤, S. Africa 117 D5 28 43 S 30 37 E
Buffalo Head Hills, Canada 142 B5 57 25N 115 55W
Buffalo L., Alta., Canada 142 C6 52 27N 112 54W
Buffalo L., N.W.T., Canada 142 A5 60 12N 115 25W
Buffalo Narrows, Canada 143 B7 55 51N 108 29W
Buffalo Springs △, Kenya 118 B4 0 32N 37 35 E
Buffels ➤, S. Africa 116 D2 29 36 S 17 3 E
Buford, U.S.A. 149 H4 34 10N 84 0W
Bug = Buh ➤, Ukraine 59 K7 46 59N 31 58 E
Bug ➤, Poland 55 F8 52 31N 21 5 E
Buga, Colombia 168 C2 4 0N 76 15W
Bugala I., Uganda 118 C3 0 40 S 32 0 E
Buganda, Uganda 118 C3 0 0 32 0 E
Buganga, Uganda 118 C3 0 3 S 32 0 E
Bugasong, Phil. 81 F4 11 3N 122 5 E
Bugel, Tanjung, Indonesia 85 D4 6 26 S 111 3 E
Buggenhout, Belgium 32 A5 47 51N 7 38 E
Bugibba, Malta 38 F7 35 57N 14 25 E
Buginang, Nigeria 113 C4 8 42N 6 55 E
Bugun Shara, Mongolia 68 B5 49 0N 104 0 E
Bugungu □, Uganda 118 B3 2 17N 31 50 E
Bugsuk I., Phil. 81 G1 8 12N 117 18 E
Buguey, Phil. 80 B3 18 17N 121 50 E
Bugui Pt., Phil. 81 E5 12 39N 123 30 E
Buguias, Phil. 80 C3 16 43N 120 50 E
Bugulma, Russia 64 D6 54 33N 52 48 E
Buguma, Nigeria 113 E6 4 42N 6 55 E
Bugun Shara, Mongolia 68 B5 49 0N 104 0 E
Buguruslan, Russia 64 E4 53 39N 52 26 E

Buh ➤, Ukraine 59 J6 46 59N 31 58 E
Buharkent, Turkey 49 D10 37 58N 28 44 E
Buheirat-Murrat-el-Kubra, Egypt 106 H8 30 18N 32 26 E
Buhera, Zimbabwe 117 B5 19 18 S 31 29 E
Bühl, Germany 31 G4 48 6N 8 24 E
Buhl, U.S.A. 158 E6 42 36N 114 46W
Buhuşi, Romania 53 D11 46 41N 26 45 E
Bui △, Ghana 112 D4 8 21N 2 21W
Builth Wells, U.K. 21 E4 52 9N 3 25W
Buin, Papua N. G. 133 L8 6 48 S 155 42 E
Buin, Piz, Switz. 33 C10 46 51N 10 7 E
Buíque, Brazil 170 C4 8 37 S 37 9W
Buir Nur, Mongolia 69 B6 47 50N 117 42 E
Buis-les-Baronnies, France 29 D9 44 17N 5 16 E
Buitenzorg = Bogor, Indonesia 84 D3 6 36 S 106 48 E
Buitrago del Lozoya, Spain 42 E7 40 58N 3 38W
Bujalance, Spain 43 H6 37 54N 4 23W
Bujanovac, Serbia & M. 50 D5 42 28N 21 44 E
Bujaraloz, Spain 40 D4 41 29N 0 10W
Buje, Croatia 45 C10 45 24N 13 39 E
Buji, China 69 F11 22 37N 114 5 E
Bujumbura, Burundi 118 C2 3 16 S 29 18 E
Bük, Hungary 52 C1 47 22N 16 45 E
Buk, Poland 55 F3 52 21N 16 30 E
Buka I., Papua N. G. 132 C8 5 10 S 154 35 E
Bukachacha, Russia 67 D12 52 55N 116 50 E
Bukama, Dem. Rep. of the Congo 119 D2 9 10 S 25 50 E
Bukavu, Dem. Rep. of the Congo 118 C2 2 20 S 28 52 E
Bukene, Tanzania 118 C3 4 15 S 32 48 E
Bukhara = Bukhoro, Uzbekistan 65 D2 39 48N 64 25 E
Bukhoro, Uzbekistan 65 D2 39 48N 64 25 E
Bukidnon □, Phil. 81 H5 8 0N 125 0 E
Bukima, Tanzania 118 C3 1 50 S 33 25 E
Bukit Badung, Indonesia 79 K18 8 49 S 115 10 E
Bukit Kerajaan, Malaysia 87 c 5 25N 100 15 E
Bukit Mertajam, Malaysia 87 c 5 22N 100 28 E
Bukit Ni, Malaysia 87 d 1 22N 104 12 E
Bukit Panjang, Singapore 87 d 1 23N 103 46 E
Bukit Tengah, Malaysia 87 c 5 22N 100 25 E
Bukittinggi, Indonesia 84 D2 0 20 S 100 20 E
Bükk, Hungary 52 B5 48 0N 20 30 E
Bukkapatnam, India 95 G3 14 14N 77 46 E
Bükki △, Hungary 52 B5 48 0N 20 30 E
Bukoba, Tanzania 118 C3 1 20 S 31 49 E
Bukrane, Indonesia 83 C4 7 43 S 131 9 E
Bukum, Pulau, Singapore 87 d 1 14N 103 46 E
Bukuru, Nigeria 113 D6 9 42N 8 48 E
Bukuya, Uganda 118 B3 0 40N 31 52 E
Bula, Guinea-Biss. 112 C1 12 7N 15 43W
Bula, Indonesia 83 B4 3 6 S 130 30 E
Bula, Phil. 80 E4 13 28N 123 16 E
Bula-Atumba, Angola 80 D3 15 0N 121 5 E
Bulacan □, Phil. 80 D3 15 0N 121 0 E
Bulalacao, Phil. 80 E3 12 31N 121 26 E
Bulan, Phil. 80 E4 12 40N 123 52 E
Bulanash, Russia 64 C9 57 16N 62 0 E
Bulancak, Turkey 101 B8 40 56N 38 14 E
Búland, Iceland 11 D8 63 46N 18 30W
Bulandshahr, India 93 E7 28 28N 77 51 E
Bulanık, Turkey 101 C10 39 4N 42 14 E
Bulanovo, Russia 64 E5 52 27N 55 10 E
Būlāq, Egypt 106 B3 25 10N 30 38 E
Bulawayo, Zimbabwe 119 G2 20 7 S 28 32 E
Buldan, Turkey 49 C10 38 2N 28 50 E
Buldana, India 94 D3 20 30N 76 18 E
Buldir I., U.S.A. 144 K1 52 21N 175 56 E
Buldon, Phil. 81 H5 7 33N 124 34 E
Bulgar, Russia 60 C9 54 57N 49 4 E
Bulgheria, Monte, Italy 47 B8 40 5N 15 26 E
Bulgurca, Turkey 49 C9 38 2N 27 9 E
Bulhar, Somali Rep. 120 C2 10 25N 44 30 E
Buli, Indonesia 83 B4 0 48N 128 25 E
Buli, Teluk, Indonesia 82 A3 0 48N 128 25 E
Buliluyan, C., Phil. 81 H1 8 20N 117 15 E
Bulim, Singapore 87 d 1 22N 103 43 E
Bulki, Ethiopia 107 F4 6 11N 36 31 E
Bulkley ➤, Canada 142 B3 55 15N 127 40W
Bull Shoals L., U.S.A. 155 G8 36 22N 92 35W
Bullaque ➤, Spain 43 G6 38 59N 4 17W
Bullard, U.S.A. 155 C6 32 8N 95 19W
Bullas, Spain 41 G3 38 2N 1 40W
Bulle, Switz. 32 C4 46 37N 7 3 E
Buller ➤, N.Z. 131 B6 41 44 S 171 36 E
Buller, Mt., Australia 129 D7 37 10 S 146 28 E
Buller Gorge, N.Z. 131 B7 41 40 S 172 10 E
Bullereigang ▵, Australia 126 B3 17 39 S 143 56 E
Bullhead City, U.S.A. 161 K12 35 8N 114 32W
Bulli, Australia 129 C9 34 15 S 150 57 E
Büllingen, Belgium 24 D6 50 25N 6 16 E
Bullock Creek, Australia 126 B3 17 43 S 144 31 E
Bulloo ➤, Australia 127 D3 28 43 S 142 30 E
Bulloo L., Australia 127 D3 28 43 S 142 25 E
Bulls, N.Z. 130 G4 40 10 S 175 24 E
Bully-les-Mines, France 27 B9 50 27N 2 44 E
Bulnes, Chile 174 D1 36 42 S 72 19W
Bulo Burti, Somali Rep. 120 D3 3 50N 45 33 E
Bulolo, Papua N. G. 132 D4 7 10 S 146 40 E
Bulolo ➤, Papua N. G. 132 D4 7 10 S 146 40 E
Bulolong, Dem. Rep. of the Congo 115 C4 4 45 S 21 30 E
Bulqizë, Albania 50 E4 41 30N 20 21 E
Bulsar = Valsad, India 94 D1 20 40N 72 58 E
Bultfontein, S. Africa 116 D4 28 18 S 26 10 E
Buluan, Phil. 81 H5 6 44N 124 47 E
Buluan, L., Phil. 81 H6 6 11N 124 40 E
Bulukumba, Indonesia 82 C2 5 33 S 120 11 E
Bulungkol, China 67 D13 35 36N 74 58 E
Bulungu, Dem. Rep. of the Congo 114 D4 6 4 S 21 54 E
Bulungur, Uzbekistan 65 D3 39 46N 67 16 E
Bulusan Vol., Phil. 80 E5 12 45N 124 3 E
Bumba, Bandundu, Dem. Rep. of the Congo 115 D3 6 58 S 19 19 E
Bumba, Équateur, Dem. Rep. of the Congo 114 B4 2 13N 22 30 E
Bumbești-Jiu, Romania 53 E8 45 10N 23 24 E
Bumbiri I., Tanzania 118 C3 1 40 S 31 55 E
Bumba, S. Leone 112 D2 9 2N 11 49W
Bumhkang, Burma 90 D6 26 51N 97 40 E
Bumhpa Bum, Burma 90 B6 26 51N 97 14 E

Bumi →, *Zimbabwe* .. **119 F2** 17 0 S 28 20 E
Bumtang →, *Bhutan* . **90 B3** 26 56N 90 53 E
Buna, *Dem. Rep. of the Congo* .... **114 C3** 3 14 S 18 59 E
Buna, *Kenya* .... **118 B4** 2 58N 39 30 E
Buna, *Papua N. G.* ... **132 E5** 8 42 S 148 27 E
Bunama, *Papua N. G.* **132 F6** 10 9 S 151 9 E
Bunawan, *Phil.* ...... **81 G5** 8 12N 125 57 E
Bunazi, *Tanzania* .... **118 C3** 1 3 S 31 23 E
Bunbah, Khalīj, *Libya* **108 B4** 32 20N 23 15 E
Bunbury, *Australia* ... **125 F2** 33 20 S 115 35 E
Bunclody, *Ireland* **23 D5** 52 39N 6 40W
Buncrana, *Ireland* **23 A4** 55 8N 7 27W
Bunda, *Dem. Rep. of the Congo* .... **115 C3** 4 58 S 14 29 E
Bundaberg, *Australia* . **127 C5** 24 54 S 152 22 E
Bundanoon, *Australia* **129 C9** 34 40 S 150 16 E
Bünde, *Germany* ..... **30 C4** 52 11N 8 35 E
Bundey →, *Australia* . **126 C2** 21 46 S 135 37 E
Bundi, *India* .... **92 G6** 25 30N 75 35 E
Bundjalung △, *Australia* .... **127 D5** 29 16 S 153 21 E
Bundoran, *Ireland* **23 B3** 54 28N 8 16W
Bundukia, *Sudan* .... **107 F3** 5 14N 30 55 E
Bundure, *Australia* ... **129 C7** 35 10 S 146 1 E
Bung Kan, *Thailand* .. **86 C4** 18 23N 103 37 E
Bunga →, *Nigeria* .... **113 C6** 11 23N 9 56 E
Bungay, *U.K.* .... **21 E9** 52 27N 1 28 E
Bungendore, *Australia* **129 C8** 35 14 S 149 30 E
Bungil Cr. →, *Australia* **127 D4** 27 5 S 149 5 E
Bungle Bungle = Purnululu Nat. Park △, *Australia* .. **124 C4** 17 20 S 128 20 E
Bungo, *Angola* ...... **115 D3** 7 26 S 15 33 E
Bungo, Gunung, *Malaysia* .... **85 B4** 1 16N 110 9 E
Bungo-Suidō, *Japan* .. **72 E4** 33 0N 132 15 E
Bungoma, *Kenya* ..... **118 B3** 0 34N 34 34 E
Bungotakada, *Japan* .. **72 D3** 33 35N 131 25 E
Bungu, *Tanzania* ..... **118 D4** 7 35 S 39 0 E
Bunia, *Dem. Rep. of the Congo* .... **118 B3** 1 35N 30 20 E
Bunianga, *Dem. Rep. of the Congo* .... **114 C4** 3 28 S 20 11 E
Bunji, *Pakistan* ...... **93 B6** 35 45N 74 40 E
Bunker Hill, *Ill., U.S.A.* **156 E7** 39 3N 89 57W
Bunker Hill, *Ind., U.S.A.* **157 D10** 40 40N 86 6W
Bunkie, *U.S.A.* **155 K8** 30 57N 92 11W
Bunnell, *U.S.A.* **153 F8** 29 28N 81 16W
Bunnythorpe, *N.Z.* ... **130 G4** 40 16 S 175 39 E
Buñol, *Spain* **41 F4** 39 25N 0 47W
Bunsuru, *Nigeria* .... **113 C5** 13 21N 6 23 E
Bunta, *Indonesia* .... **82 B2** 0 48 S 122 10 E
Buntok, *Indonesia* ... **85 C4** 1 40 S 114 58 E
Bununu Dass, *Nigeria* **113 C6** 10 5N 9 31 E
Bununu Kasa, *Nigeria* **113 D6** 9 51N 9 32 E
Bunya Mts. △, *Australia* .... **127 D5** 26 51 S 151 34 E
Bünyan, *Turkey* ..... **100 C6** 38 51N 35 51 E
Bunyu, *Indonesia* .... **85 B5** 3 35N 117 50 E
Bunza, *Nigeria* ...... **113 C5** 12 8N 4 0 E
Bunzlau = Bolesławiec, *Poland* .... **55 G2** 51 17N 15 37 E
Buol, *Indonesia* ..... **82 A2** 1 15N 121 32 E
Buon Brieng, *Vietnam* **86 F7** 13 9N 108 12 E
Buon Ma Thuot, *Vietnam* .... **86 F7** 12 40N 108 3 E
Buong Long, *Cambodia* **86 F6** 13 44N 106 59 E
Buorkhaya, Mys, *Russia* **67 B14** 71 50N 132 40 E
Buqayq, *Si. Arabia* ... **97 E6** 26 0N 49 45 E
Buqbuq, *Egypt* ...... **106 A2** 31 29N 25 29 E
Bur Acaba, *Somali Rep.* **120 D2** 3 12N 44 20 E
Bûr Fuad, *Egypt* .... **106 H8** 31 15N 32 20 E
Bur Ghibi, *Somali Rep.* **120 D3** 3 56N 45 7 E
Bûr Safâga, *Egypt* ... **96 E2** 26 43N 33 57 E
Bûr Sa'îd, *Egypt* .... **106 H8** 31 16N 32 18 E
Bûr Sûdân, *Sudan* ... **106 D4** 19 32N 37 9 E
Bûr Taufiq, *Egypt* ... **106 J8** 29 54N 32 32 E
Bura, *Kenya* .... **118 C4** 1 4 S 39 58 E
Burakin, *Australia* ... **125 F2** 30 31 S 117 10 E
Buram, *Sudan* .... **107 E2** 10 51N 25 9 E
Buran, *Somali Rep.* .. **120 B3** 10 14N 48 44 E
Burao, *Somali Rep.* .. **120 C3** 9 32N 45 32 E
Burāq, *Syria* .... **103 B5** 33 11N 36 29 E
Burauen, *Phil.* ...... **81 F6** 10 58N 124 53 E
Buraydah, *Si. Arabia* . **96 E4** 26 20N 43 59 E
Burbank, *U.S.A.* **161 L8** 34 11N 118 19W
Burcher, *Australia* ... **129 B7** 33 30 S 147 16 E
Burda, *India* .... **92 G6** 25 50N 77 35 E
Burdekin →, *Australia* **126 B4** 19 38 S 147 25 E
Burdeos Bay, *Phil.* ... **80 D4** 14 44N 122 6 E
Burdur, *Turkey* ...... **49 D12** 37 45N 30 17 E
Burdur □, *Turkey* .... **49 D12** 37 45N 30 0 E
Burdur Gölü, *Turkey* . **49 D12** 37 44N 30 10 E
Burdwan = Barddhaman, *India* . **93 H12** 23 14N 87 39 E
Burdwood Banks, *Atl. Oc.* .... **8 M6** 54 0 S 59 0W
Bure, *Gojam, Ethiopia* **107 E4** 10 40N 37 4 E
Bure, *Ilubabor, Ethiopia* .... **107 F4** 8 19N 35 8 E
Bure →, *U.K.* .... **20 E9** 52 38N 1 43 E
Büren, *Germany* ..... **30 D4** 51 33N 8 35 E
Bureya →, *Russia* .... **67 E13** 49 27N 129 30 E
Burford, *Canada* **150 C4** 43 7N 80 27W
Burg, *Germany* ...... **30 C7** 52 16N 11 51 E
Burg auf Fehmarn, *Germany* .... **30 A7** 54 28N 11 9 E
Burg el Arab, *Egypt* .. **106 H6** 30 54N 29 32 E
Burg et Tuyur, *Sudan* . **106 C2** 20 55N 27 56 E
Burg Stargard, *Germany* .... **30 B9** 53 29N 13 18 E
Burgas, *Bulgaria* .... **51 D11** 42 33N 27 29 E
Burgas □, *Bulgaria* .. **51 D10** 42 30N 26 50 E
Burgaski Zaliv, *Bulgaria* .... **51 D11** 42 30N 27 39 E
Burgdorf, *Germany* .. **30 C6** 52 27N 10 1 E
Burgdorf, *Switz.* ..... **32 B5** 47 3N 7 37 E
Burgenland □, *Austria* **35 D9** 47 20N 16 20 E
Burgeo, *Canada* **141 C8** 47 37N 57 38W
Burgersdorp, *S. Africa* **116 E4** 31 0 S 26 20 E
Burges, Mt., *Australia* **125 F3** 30 50 S 121 5 E
Burghausen, *Germany* **31 G8** 48 9N 12 49 E
Burghead, *U.K.* **22 D5** 57 43N 3 30W
Búrgio, *Italy* .... **46 E6** 37 36N 13 17 E
Bürglen, *Switz.* ..... **33 C7** 46 53N 8 40 E
Burglengenfeld, *Germany* .... **31 F8** 49 12N 12 2 E
Burgohondo, *Spain* .. **42 E6** 40 26N 4 47W
Burgos, *Ilocos N., Phil.* **80 B3** 18 31N 120 39 E
Burgos, *Pangasinan, Phil.* .... **80 C2** 16 4N 119 52 E
Burgos, *Spain* **42 C7** 42 21N 3 41W
Burgos □, *Spain* **42 C7** 42 21N 3 42W
Burgstädt, *Germany* .. **30 E8** 50 54N 12 49 E
Burgsvik, *Sweden* ... **17 G12** 57 3N 18 19 E
Burguillos del Cerro, *Spain* **43 G4** 38 23N 6 35W
Burgundy = Bourgogne □, *France* **27 F11** 47 0N 4 50 E
Burhaniye, *Turkey* ... **49 B8** 39 30N 26 58 E
Burhanpur, *India* .... **94 D3** 21 18N 76 14 E
Burhi Gandak →, *India* **93 G12** 25 20N 86 37 E
Burhner →, *India* .... **93 H9** 22 43N 80 31 E
Buri Pen., *Eritrea* .... **107 D4** 15 25N 39 55 E
Burias I., *Phil.* ...... **80 E4** 12 55N 123 5 E
Burias Pass, *Phil.* .... **80 E4** 13 0N 123 15 E
Burica, Pta., *Costa Rica* **164 E3** 8 3N 82 51W
Burien, *U.S.A.* **160 C4** 47 28N 122 21W
Burigi ⌓, *Tanzania* ... **118 C3** 2 20 S 31 6 E
Burigi, L., *Tanzania* .. **118 C3** 2 2 S 31 22 E
Burin, *Canada* **141 C8** 47 1N 55 14W
Buriram, *Thailand* ... **86 E4** 15 0N 103 0 E
Buriti Alegre, *Brazil* . **171 E2** 18 9 S 49 3W
Buriti Bravo, *Brazil* .. **170 C3** 5 50 S 43 50W
Buriti dos Lopes, *Brazil* **170 B3** 3 10 S 41 52W
Burj Sāfitā, *Syria* .... **100 E7** 34 48N 36 7 E
Burji, *Ethiopia* ...... **107 F4** 5 29N 37 51 E
Burkburnett, *U.S.A.* .. **155 H5** 34 6N 98 34W
Burke →, *Australia* .. **126 C2** 23 12 S 139 33 E
Burke Chan., *Canada* . **142 C3** 52 10N 127 30W
Burketown, *Australia* . **126 B2** 17 45 S 139 33 E
Burkina Faso ■, *Africa* **112 C4** 12 0N 1 0W
Burk's Falls, *Canada* . **140 C4** 45 37N 79 24W
Burlada, *Spain* **40 C3** 42 49N 1 36W
Burleigh Falls, *Canada* **150 B6** 44 33N 78 12W
Burley, *U.S.A.* **158 E7** 42 32N 113 48W
Burli, *Kazakhstan* .... **64 F4** 51 25N 52 40 E
Burlingame, *U.S.A.* .. **160 H4** 37 35N 122 21W
Burlington, *Canada* .. **140 D4** 43 18N 79 45W
Burlington, *Colo., U.S.A.* **154 F3** 39 18N 102 16W
Burlington, *Iowa, U.S.A.* **156 D5** 40 49N 91 14W
Burlington, *Kans., U.S.A.* **154 F7** 38 12N 95 45W
Burlington, *Ky., U.S.A.* **157 E12** 39 2N 84 43W
Burlington, *N.C., U.S.A.* **149 G6** 36 6N 79 26W
Burlington, *N.J., U.S.A.* **151 F10** 40 4N 74 51W
Burlington, *Vt., U.S.A.* **151 B11** 44 29N 73 12W
Burlington, *Wash., U.S.A.* **160 B4** 48 28N 122 20W
Burlington, *Wis., U.S.A.* **157 B8** 42 41N 88 17W
Burlyu-Tyube, *Kazakhstan* .... **66 E8** 46 30N 79 10 E
Burma ■, *Asia* ...... **90 E6** 21 0N 96 30 E
Burnaby I., *Canada* ... **142 C2** 52 25N 131 19W
Burnet, *U.S.A.* **155 K5** 30 45N 98 14W
Burney, *U.S.A.* **158 F3** 40 53N 121 40W
Burnham, *U.S.A.* **150 F7** 40 38N 77 34W
Burnham-on-Sea, *U.K.* **21 F5** 51 14N 3 0W
Burnie, *Australia* .... **127 G4** 41 4 S 145 56 E
Burnley, *U.K.* **20 D5** 53 47N 2 14W
Burns, *U.S.A.* **158 E4** 43 35N 119 3W
Burns Junction, *U.S.A.* **158 E5** 42 47N 117 51W
Burns Lake, *Canada* .. **142 C3** 54 20N 125 45W
Burnside →, *Canada* . **138 B9** 66 51N 108 4W
Burnside, L., *Australia* **125 E3** 25 22 S 123 0 E
Burnsville, *U.S.A.* ... **154 C8** 44 47N 93 17W
Burnt, L., *Canada* ... **141 B7** 53 35N 64 4W
Burnt Paw, *U.S.A.* ... **144 C12** 66 54N 143 44W
Burnt River, *Canada* . **150 B6** 44 41N 78 42W
Burntwood →, *Canada* **143 B9** 56 8N 96 34W
Burntwood L., *Canada* **143 B8** 55 22N 100 26W
Buronga, *Australia* ... **128 C5** 34 18 S 142 20 E
Burqān, *Kuwait* ...... **96 D5** 29 0N 47 57 E
Burra, *Australia* ..... **128 B3** 33 40 S 138 55 E
Burra, *Nigeria* ...... **113 C6** 11 0N 8 56 E
Burragorang, L., *Australia* .... **129 B9** 33 52 S 150 37 E
Burray, *U.K.* **22 C6** 58 51N 2 54W
Burrel, *Albania* ..... **50 E4** 41 36N 20 1 E
Burren △, *Ireland* **23 C3** 53 1N 8 58W
Burren Junction, *Australia* .... **127 E4** 30 7 S 148 59 E
Burrendong, L., *Australia* .... **129 B8** 32 45 S 149 10 E
Burriana, *Spain* **40 F4** 39 50N 0 4W
Burrinjuck Res., *Australia* .... **129 C8** 35 0 S 148 36 E
Burro, Serranías del, *Mexico* **162 B4** 29 0N 102 0W
Burrow Hd., *U.K.* **22 G4** 54 41N 4 24W
Burrowa Pine Mountain △, *Australia* .... **129 D7** 36 6 S 147 45 E
Burrum Coast △, *Australia* .... **127 D5** 25 13 S 152 36 E
Burruyacú, *Argentina* . **174 B3** 26 30 S 64 40W
Burry Port, *U.K.* **21 F3** 51 41N 4 15W
Bursa, *Turkey* ...... **51 F13** 40 15N 29 5 E
Burseryd, *Sweden* ... **17 G7** 57 12N 13 17 E
Burstall, *Canada* **143 C7** 50 39N 109 54W
Burton, *Mich., U.S.A.* . **157 B13** 43 0N 83 40W
Burton, *Ohio, U.S.A.* . **150 E3** 41 28N 81 8W
Burton, *S.C., U.S.A.* . **149 J5** 32 25N 80 45W
Burton, L., *Canada* ... **140 B4** 54 45N 78 20W
Burton upon Trent, *U.K.* **20 E6** 52 48N 1 38W
Burtundy, *Australia* .. **128 B5** 33 45 S 142 15 E
Buru, *Indonesia* ..... **82 B3** 3 30 S 126 30 E
Buruanga, *Phil.* ..... **81 F3** 11 51N 121 53 E
Burullus, Bahra el, *Egypt* .... **106 H7** 31 25N 31 0 E
Burûm, *Yemen* ...... **99 D5** 14 22N 48 59 E
Burûn, Râs, *Egypt* ... **103 D2** 31 14N 33 7 E
Burunday = Boralday, *Kazakhstan* .... **65 B8** 43 20N 76 51 E
Burundi ■, *Africa* .... **118 C3** 3 15 S 30 0 E
Burunny = Tsagan Aman, *Russia* ...... **61 G8** 47 34N 46 43 E
Bururi, *Burundi* ..... **118 C2** 3 57 S 29 37 E
Burutu, *Nigeria* ..... **113 D6** 5 20N 5 29 E
Burwell, *U.S.A.* **154 E5** 41 47N 99 8W
Burwick, *U.K.* **22 C5** 58 45N 2 58W
Bury, *U.K.* **20 D5** 53 35N 2 17W
Bury St. Edmunds, *U.K.* .... **21 E8** 52 15N 0 43 E
Buryatia □, *Russia* ... **67 D11** 53 0N 110 0 E
Bŭrylbaytal, *Kazakhstan* .... **65 A7** 45 5N 74 1 E
Buryn, *Ukraine* ...... **59 G7** 51 13N 33 50 E
Burzenin, *Poland* .... **55 G5** 51 28N 18 47 E
Busa, Mt., *Phil.* ..... **81 H5** 6 8N 124 39 E
Busalla, *Italy* .... **44 D5** 44 34N 8 57 E
Busan = Pusan, *S. Korea* .... **75 G15** 35 5N 129 0 E
Busanga, *Dem. Rep. of the Congo* .... **114 C4** 0 53 S 22 7 E
Busango Swamp, *Zambia* .... **119 E2** 14 15 S 25 45 E
Buşayrah, *Syria* ...... **101 E9** 35 9N 40 26 E
Busca, *Italy* .... **44 D4** 44 31N 7 29 E
Bushat, *Albania* ..... **50 E3** 41 58N 19 34 E
Būshehr, *Iran* .... **97 D6** 28 55N 50 55 E
Būshehr □, *Iran* ..... **97 D6** 28 20N 51 45 E
Bushell, *Canada* **143 B7** 59 31N 108 45W
Bushenyi, *Uganda* .... **118 C3** 0 35 S 30 10 E
Bushimaie →, *Dem. Rep. of the Congo* .... **115 D4** 6 2 S 23 45 E
Bushire = Būshehr, *Iran* **97 D6** 28 55N 50 55 E
Bushnell, *Fla., U.S.A.* . **153 G7** 28 40N 82 7W
Bushnell, *Ill., U.S.A.* .. **156 D6** 40 33N 90 31W
Bushtyna, *Ukraine* ... **53 B8** 48 3N 23 28 E
Busie, *Ghana* **112 C4** 10 29N 2 22W
Businga, *Dem. Rep. of the Congo* .... **114 B4** 3 16N 20 59 E
Buskerud □, *Norway* . **18 D5** 60 20N 9 0 E
Busko-Zdrój, *Poland* .. **55 H7** 50 28N 20 42 E
Buskul, *Kazakhstan* .. **64 E8** 53 45N 61 12 E
Buslei, *Ethiopia* ..... **120 C2** 5 28N 44 25 E
Busovača, *Bos.-H.* ... **52 F2** 44 6N 17 53 E
Buşra ash Shām, *Syria* **103 C5** 32 30N 36 25 E
Busselton, *Australia* .. **125 F2** 33 42 S 115 15 E
Busseri →, *Sudan* .... **107 F2** 7 41N 28 3 E
Busseto, *Italy* .... **44 D7** 44 59N 10 2 E
Bussière-Badil, *France* **28 C4** 45 39N 0 36 E
Bussigny, *Switz.* ..... **32 C3** 46 33N 6 33 E
Bussolengo, *Italy* .... **44 C7** 45 28N 10 51 E
Bussum, *Neths.* ..... **24 B5** 52 16N 5 10 E
Bustamante, B., *Argentina* .... **176 C3** 45 5 S 66 18W
Buşteni, *Romania* .... **53 E10** 45 24N 25 32 E
Busto, C., *Spain* **42 B4** 43 34N 6 28W
Busto Arsízio, *Italy* .. **44 C5** 45 37N 8 51 E
Busu Djanoa, *Dem. Rep. of the Congo* .... **114 B4** 1 43N 21 23 E
Busu Kwanga, *Dem. Rep. of the Congo* .... **114 B4** 1 48N 20 21 E
Busu Mandji, *Dem. Rep. of the Congo* .... **114 B4** 2 52N 21 14 E
Busuanga, *Phil.* ..... **80 E2** 12 14N 119 52 E
Busuanga I., *Phil.* ... **80 E2** 12 10N 120 0 E
Büsum, *Germany* .... **30 A4** 54 7N 8 51 E
Busungbiu, *Indonesia* . **79 J17** 8 16 S 114 58 E
Buta, *Dem. Rep. of the Congo* .... **118 B1** 2 50N 24 53 E
Butare, *Rwanda* ..... **118 C2** 2 31 S 29 52 E
Butaritari, *Kiribati* ... **134 G9** 3 30N 174 0 E
Bute, *Australia* ...... **128 B3** 33 51 S 138 2 E
Bute, *U.K.* **22 F3** 55 48N 5 2W
Bute Inlet, *Canada* ... **142 C4** 50 40N 124 53W
Butemba, *Uganda* .... **118 B3** 1 9N 31 37 E
Butembo, *Dem. Rep. of the Congo* .... **118 B2** 0 9N 29 18 E
Buteni, *Romania* ..... **52 D7** 46 19N 22 7 E
Butera, *Italy* .... **47 E7** 37 11N 14 11 E
Butha Qi, *China* ..... **69 B7** 48 0N 122 32 E
Buthidaung, *Burma* .. **90 E4** 20 52N 92 32 E
Butiaba, *Uganda* .... **118 B3** 1 50N 31 20 E
Butler, *Ga., U.S.A.* ... **152 C5** 32 33N 84 14W
Butler, *Ind., U.S.A.* .. **157 C12** 41 26N 84 52W
Butler, *Ky., U.S.A.* ... **157 F12** 38 47N 84 22W
Butler, *Mo., U.S.A.* ... **156 F2** 38 16N 94 20W
Butler, *Pa., U.S.A.* ... **150 F5** 40 52N 79 54W
Buton, *Indonesia* .... **82 C2** 5 0 S 122 45 E
Bütow = Bytów, *Poland* **54 D4** 54 10N 17 30 E
Butrint, L. e, *Albania* . **38 B10** 39 43N 20 5 E
Bütschwil, *Switz.* .... **33 B8** 47 23N 9 5 E
Butte, *Mont., U.S.A.* .. **158 C7** 46 0N 112 32W
Butte, *Nebr., U.S.A.* .. **154 D5** 42 58N 98 51W
Butte Creek →, *U.S.A.* **160 F5** 39 12N 121 56W
Butterworth = Gcuwa, *S. Africa* .... **117 E4** 32 20 S 28 11 E
Butterworth, *Malaysia* . **87 c** 5 24N 100 23 E
Buttevant, *Ireland* **23 D3** 52 14N 8 40W
Buttfield, Mt., *Australia* **125 D4** 24 45 S 128 9 E
Button B., *Canada* ... **143 B10** 58 45N 94 23W
Buttonwillow, *U.S.A.* . **161 K7** 35 24N 119 28W
Butty Hd., *Australia* .. **125 F3** 33 54 S 121 39 E
Butuan, *Phil.* .... **81 G5** 8 57N 125 33 E
Butuku-Luba, *Eq. Guin.* .... **113 E6** 3 29N 8 33 E
Butung = Buton, *Indonesia* .... **82 C2** 5 0 S 122 45 E
Buturlinovka, *Russia* . **60 E5** 50 50N 40 35 E
Butzbach, *Germany* .. **31 E4** 50 25N 8 40 E
Bützow, *Germany* ... **30 B7** 53 50N 11 58 E
Buulobarde = Bulo Burti, *Somali Rep.* ... **120 D3** 3 50N 45 33 E
Buur Hakaba = Bur Acaba, *Somali Rep.* **120 D2** 3 12N 44 20 E
Buvik, *Norway* ...... **18 A7** 63 18N 10 11 E
Buxa Duar, *India* .... **93 F13** 27 45N 89 35 E
Buxar, *India* .... **93 G10** 25 34N 83 58 E
Buxtehude, *Germany* . **30 B5** 53 28N 9 39 E
Buxton, *Guyana* **169 B6** 6 48N 58 2W
Buxton, *U.K.* **20 D6** 53 16N 1 54W
Buxy, *France* .... **27 F11** 46 44N 4 40 E
Buy, *Russia* .... **60 A5** 58 28N 41 28 E
Buynaksk, *Russia* ... **61 J8** 42 48N 47 7 E
Buyo, *Ivory C.* **112 D3** 6 21N 7 5W
Buyo, L. de, *Ivory C.* . **112 D3** 6 16N 7 10W
Büyük Menderes →, *Turkey* .... **49 D9** 37 28N 27 11 E
Büyükçekmece, *Turkey* **51 E12** 41 2N 28 35 E
Büyükkariştiran, *Turkey* .... **51 E11** 41 18N 27 33 E
Büyükkemikli Burnu, *Turkey* .... **51 F10** 40 18N 26 14 E
Büyükorhan, *Turkey* .. **49 B10** 39 46N 28 56 E
Büyükyoncalı, *Turkey* **51 E11** 41 20N 27 55 E
Buzançais, *France* .... **26 F8** 46 54N 1 25 E
Buzău, *Romania* ..... **53 E11** 45 10N 26 50 E
Buzău □, *Romania* ... **53 E11** 45 20N 26 30 E
Buzău →, *Romania* ... **53 E12** 45 26N 27 44 E
Buzău, Pasul, *Romania* **53 E11** 45 35N 26 12 E
Buzen, *Japan* .... **72 D3** 33 35N 131 5 E
Buzet, *Croatia* ...... **45 C10** 45 24N 13 58 E
Buzi →, *Mozam.* .... **119 F3** 19 50 S 34 43 E
Buziaş, *Romania* ..... **52 E6** 45 38N 21 36 E
Buzuluk, *Russia* ..... **64 E4** 52 48N 52 12 E
Buzuluk →, *Russia* ... **60 E6** 50 15N 42 7 E
Buzzards B., *U.S.A.* .. **151 E14** 41 45N 70 37W
Buzzards Bay, *U.S.A.* . **151 E14** 41 44N 70 37W
Bwagaoia, *Papua N. G.* **132 F7** 10 40 S 152 52 E
Bwana Mkubwe, *Dem. Rep. of the Congo* .... **119 E2** 13 8 S 28 38 E
Bwasa, *Dem. Rep. of the Congo* .... **114 C3** 3 55 S 18 24 E
Bwatnapné, *Vanuatu* . **133 E6** 15 41 S 168 9 E
Bwindi △, *Uganda* ... **118 C2** 1 2 S 29 42 E
Byala, *Ruse, Bulgaria* . **51 C9** 43 28N 25 44 E
Byala, *Varna, Bulgaria* **51 D11** 42 53N 27 55 E
Byala Slatina, *Bulgaria* **50 C7** 43 26N 23 58 E
Byarezina →, *Belarus* . **59 F6** 52 33N 30 14 E
Byaroza, *Belarus* .... **59 F3** 52 31N 24 51 E
Bychawa, *Poland* .... **55 G9** 51 1N 22 36 E
Byczyna, *Poland* .... **55 G5** 51 7N 18 12 E
Bydgoszcz, *Poland* ... **55 E5** 53 10N 18 0 E
Byelarus = Belarus ■, *Europe* .... **58 F4** 53 30N 27 0 E
Byelorussia = Belarus ■, *Europe* . **58 F4** 53 30N 27 0 E
Byers, *U.S.A.* **154 F2** 39 43N 104 14W
Byesville, *U.S.A.* **150 G3** 39 58N 81 32W
Byfield △, *Australia* .. **126 C5** 22 52 S 150 45 E
Byford, *Australia* .... **125 F2** 32 15 S 116 0 E
Bygdin, *Norway* ..... **18 C5** 61 21N 8 32 E
Bygland, *Norway* .... **18 F4** 58 50N 7 48 E
Byglandsfjorden, *Norway* .... **18 F4** 58 44N 7 50 E
Bygstad, *Norway* .... **18 C2** 61 23N 5 40 E
Bykhaw, *Belarus* .... **58 F6** 53 31N 30 14 E
Bykhov = Bykhaw, *Belarus* .... **58 F6** 53 31N 30 14 E
Bykle, *Norway* ...... **18 E4** 59 20N 7 22 E
Bykovo, *Russia* ..... **60 F7** 49 50N 45 25 E
Bylas, *U.S.A.* **159 K8** 33 8N 110 7W
Bylot, *Canada* **143 B10** 58 25N 94 8W
Bylot I., *Canada* **139 A12** 73 13N 78 34W
Byrd, C., *Antarctica* .. **7 C17** 69 38 S 76 7W
Byrock, *Australia* .... **129 A7** 30 40 S 146 27 E
Byron, *Ga., U.S.A.* ... **152 C6** 32 39N 83 46W
Byron, *Ill., U.S.A.* ... **156 B7** 42 8N 89 15W
Byron, C., *Australia* .. **127 D5** 28 43 S 153 38 E
Byron Bay, *Australia* . **127 D5** 28 43 S 153 37 E
Byrranga, Gory, *Russia* **67 B11** 75 0N 100 0 E
Byrranga Mts. = Byrranga, Gory, *Russia* .... **67 B11** 75 0N 100 0 E
Byrum, *Denmark* .... **17 G5** 57 16N 11 0 E
Byske, *Sweden* ..... **14 D19** 64 57N 21 11 E
Byskeälven →, *Sweden* **14 D19** 64 57N 21 13 E
Bystrovka = Kemin, *Kyrgyzstan* .... **65 B7** 42 47N 75 42 E
Bystrytsya, *Ukraine* .. **53 B9** 48 27N 24 14 E
Bystrzyca →, *Dolnośląskie, Poland* **55 G3** 51 12N 16 55 E
Bystrzyca →, *Lubelskie, Poland* .. **55 G9** 51 21N 22 46 E
Bystrzyca Kłodzka, *Poland* .... **55 H3** 50 19N 16 39 E
Bytča, *Slovak Rep.* ... **35 B11** 49 13N 18 34 E
Bytkiv, *Ukraine* ..... **53 B9** 48 38N 24 28 E
Bytom, *Poland* ..... **55 H5** 50 25N 18 54 E
Bytom Odrzański, *Poland* .... **55 G2** 51 44N 15 48 E
Bytów, *Poland* ...... **54 D4** 54 10N 17 30 E
Byumba, *Rwanda* ... **118 C3** 1 35 S 30 4 E
Bzenec, *Czech Rep.* . **35 C10** 48 58N 17 18 E
Bzura →, *Poland* .... **55 F7** 52 25N 20 15 E

C

C.W. McConaughy, L., *U.S.A.* **154 E4** 41 14N 101 40W
Ca →, *Vietnam* ..... **86 C5** 18 45N 105 45 E
Ca Mau, *Vietnam* .... **87 H5** 9 7N 105 8 E
Ca Mau, Mui, *Vietnam* **87 H5** 8 38N 104 44 E
Ca Na, *Vietnam* ..... **87 G7** 11 20N 108 54 E
Caacupé, *Paraguay* ... **174 B4** 25 23 S 57 5W
Caaguazú △, *Paraguay* **175 B4** 26 5 S 55 31W
Caála, *Angola* ...... **115 E3** 12 46 S 15 30 E
Caamaño Sd., *Canada* **142 C3** 52 55N 129 25W
Caapiranga, *Brazil* ... **169 D5** 3 18 S 61 13W
Caazapá, *Paraguay* ... **174 B4** 26 8 S 56 19W
Caazapá □, *Paraguay* **175 B4** 26 10 S 56 0W
Cabadbaran, *Phil.* .... **81 G5** 9 10N 125 38 E
Cabagan, *Phil.* ...... **80 C3** 17 26N 121 46 E
Cabalian = San Juan, *Phil.* .... **81 F5** 10 16N 125 10 E
Caballeria, C. de, *Spain* **38 A5** 40 5N 4 5 E
Cabana, *Peru* .... **172 B2** 8 25 S 78 5W
Cabana, *Spain* **42 B2** 43 13N 8 54W
Cabanaconde, *Peru* .. **172 D3** 15 38 S 71 58W
Cabañaquinta, *Spain* . **42 B5** 43 10N 5 38W
Cabanatuan, *Phil.* .... **80 D3** 15 30N 120 58 E
Cabañeros ⌓, *Spain* .. **41 F6** 39 18N 4 35W
Cabanes, *Spain* ...... **40 E5** 40 9N 0 2 E
Cabangan, *Phil.* ..... **80 D3** 15 10N 120 3 E
Cabanillas, *Peru* .... **172 D3** 15 36 S 70 28W
Cabano, *Canada* **141 C6** 47 40N 68 56W
Čabar, *Croatia* ...... **45 C11** 45 36N 14 39 E
Cabarroguis, *Phil.* ... **80 C3** 16 50N 121 30 E
Cabarruyan I., *Phil.* .. **80 C2** 16 18N 119 59 E
Cabazon, *U.S.A.* **161 M10** 33 55N 116 47W
Cabedelo, *Brazil* .... **170 C5** 7 0 S 34 50W
Cabeza del Buey, *Spain* **43 G5** 38 44N 5 13W
Cabezón de la Sal, *Spain* **42 B6** 43 18N 4 14W
Cabildo, *Chile* ...... **174 C1** 32 30 S 71 5W
Cabimas, *Venezuela* .. **168 A3** 10 23N 71 25W
Cabinda, *Angola* .... **115 D2** 5 33 S 12 11 E
Cabinda □, *Angola* ... **115 D2** 5 0 S 12 30 E
Cabinet Mts., *U.S.A.* . **158 C6** 48 0N 115 30W
Cabiri, *Angola* ...... **115 D2** 8 52 S 13 39 E
Cable Beach, *Bahamas* **9 b** 25 4N 77 24W
Cabo Blanco, *Argentina* **176 C3** 47 15 S 65 47W
Cabo de Gata-Níjar ⌓, *Spain* **41 J2** 36 51N 2 6W
Cabo de Hornos △, *Chile* .... **176 E3** 55 42 S 67 20W
Cabo Frio, *Brazil* .... **171 F3** 22 51 S 42 3W
Cabo Pantoja, *Peru* .. **168 D2** 1 0 S 75 10W
Cabo Raso, *Argentina* **176 B3** 44 20 S 65 15W
Cabo Verde = Cape Verde Is. ■, *Atl. Oc.* **8 E9** 16 0N 24 0W
Cabo Yubi = Tarfaya, *Morocco* **110 C2** 27 55N 12 55W
Cabonga, Réservoir, *Canada* **140 C4** 47 20N 76 40W
Cabool, *U.S.A.* **155 G8** 37 7N 92 6W
Caboolture, *Australia* . **127 D5** 27 5 S 152 58 E
Cabora Bassa Dam = Cahora Bassa, Represa de, *Mozam.* **119 F3** 15 20 S 32 50 E
Caborca, *Mexico* **162 A2** 30 40N 112 10W
Cabot, Mt., *U.S.A.* .. **151 B13** 44 30N 71 25W
Cabot Hd., *Canada* .. **150 A3** 45 14N 81 17W
Cabot Str., *Canada* .. **141 C8** 47 15N 59 40W
Cabra, *Spain* **43 H6** 37 30N 4 28W
Cabra del Santo Cristo, *Spain* **43 H7** 37 42N 3 16W
Cabra I., *India* ...... **95 L11** 7 18N 93 50 E
Cábras, *Italy* .... **46 C1** 39 56N 8 32 E
Cabrera, *Spain* ...... **38 B3** 39 8N 2 57 E
Cabrera △, *Spain* .... **41 F7** 39 13N 2 53 E
Cabrera, Sierra, *Spain* **42 C4** 42 12N 6 40W
Cabri, *Canada* **143 C7** 50 35N 108 25W
Cabriel →, *Spain* **41 F3** 39 14N 1 3W
Cabruta, *Venezuela* .. **168 B4** 7 50N 66 10W
Cabucgayan, *Phil.* ... **81 F5** 11 29N 124 34 E
Cabugao, *Phil.* ...... **80 C3** 17 48N 120 27 E
Cabulauan Is., *Phil.* .. **81 F3** 11 25N 120 8 E
Cabulo, *Angola* ..... **115 E3** 10 18 S 16 22 E
Caburan = Jose Abad Santos, *Phil.* ...... **81 J5** 5 55N 125 39 E
Cabuta, *Angola* ..... **115 D2** 9 48 S 14 58 E
Cabuyaro, *Colombia* .. **168 C3** 4 18N 72 49W
Cacabelos, *Spain* **42 C4** 42 36N 6 44W
Caçador, *Brazil* ..... **175 B5** 26 47 S 51 0W
Čačak, *Serbia & M.* .. **50 C4** 43 54N 20 20 E
Cacao, *Fr. Guiana* ... **169 C7** 4 33N 52 26W
Caçapava do Sul, *Brazil* **175 C5** 30 30 S 53 30W
Cáccamo, *Italy* ...... **46 E6** 37 56N 13 40 E
Cacém, *Portugal* **43 G1** 38 46N 9 18W
Cáceres, *Brazil* ..... **173 D6** 16 5 S 57 40W
Cáceres, *Colombia* .. **168 B2** 7 35N 75 20W
Cáceres, *Spain* **43 F4** 39 26N 6 23W
Cáceres □, *Spain* **42 F5** 39 45N 6 0W
Cache Bay, *Canada* .. **140 C4** 46 22N 80 0W
Cache Cr. →, *U.S.A.* . **160 G5** 38 42N 121 42W
Cache Creek, *Canada* . **142 C4** 50 48N 121 19W
Cacheu, *Guinea-Biss.* . **112 C1** 12 14N 16 8W
Cachi, *Argentina* .... **174 B2** 25 5 S 66 10W
Cachimbo, *Brazil* .... **173 B7** 8 57 S 54 54W
Cachimbo, Serra do, *Brazil* .... **173 B6** 9 30 S 55 30W
Cachimo, *Angola* .... **115 D4** 8 21 S 21 24 E
Cachinal de la Sierra, *Chile* .... **174 A2** 24 58 S 69 32W
Cachingues, *Angola* .. **115 E3** 13 5 S 16 43 E
Cachoeira = Solonópole, *Brazil* . **170 C4** 5 44 S 39 1W
Cachoeira, *Brazil* .... **171 D4** 12 30 S 39 0W
Cachoeira Alta, *Brazil* **171 E1** 18 48 S 50 58W
Cachoeira do Sul, *Brazil* .... **175 C5** 30 3 S 52 53W
Cachoeiro de Itapemirim, *Brazil* . **171 F3** 20 51 S 41 7W
Cachoeiro do Arari, *Brazil* .... **170 B2** 1 1 S 48 58W
Cachopo, *Portugal* ... **43 H3** 37 20N 7 49W
Cachuela Esperanza, *Bolivia* .... **173 C4** 10 32 S 65 38W
Cacine, *Guinea-Biss.* . **112 C1** 11 8N 14 57W
Cacoal, *Brazil* ...... **173 C5** 11 30 S 61 25W
Cacólo, *Angola* ..... **115 E3** 10 9 S 19 21 E
Caconda, *Angola* .... **115 E3** 13 48 S 15 8 E
Cacongo, *Angola* .... **115 D2** 5 11 S 12 5 E
Caçu, *Brazil* .... **171 E1** 18 37 S 51 4W
Cacuaco, *Angola* .... **115 D2** 8 47 S 13 21 E
Cacuchi →, *Angola* .. **115 E3** 14 26 S 16 46 E
Cacula, *Angola* ..... **115 E2** 14 29 S 14 10 E
Caculé, *Brazil* ...... **171 D3** 14 30 S 42 13W
Caculuvar →, *Angola* . **115 F2** 16 47 S 14 56 E
Cacuso, *Angola* ..... **115 D3** 9 25 S 15 45 E
Čadca, *Slovak Rep.* ... **35 B11** 49 26N 18 45 E
Caddo, *U.S.A.* **155 H6** 34 7N 96 16W
Cadenazzo, *Switz.* ... **33 D7** 46 9N 8 57 E
Cader Idris, *U.K.* **21 E4** 52 42N 3 53W
Cadereyta, *Mexico* ... **162 B5** 25 36N 100 0W
Cades, *U.S.A.* **152 B10** 33 47N 79 47W
Cadí, Sierra del, *Spain* **40 C6** 42 17N 1 42 E
Cadí-Moixeró ⌓, *Spain* **40 C3** 42 17N 1 44W
Cadibarrawirracanna, L., *Australia* ...... **127 D2** 28 52 S 135 27 E
Cadillac, *France* **28 D3** 44 38N 0 20W
Cadillac, *U.S.A.* **148 C3** 44 15N 85 24W
Cadiz, *Phil.* .... **81 F4** 10 57N 123 15 E
Cádiz, *Spain* **43 J4** 36 30N 6 20W
Cadiz, *Calif., U.S.A.* .. **161 L11** 34 30N 115 28W
Cadiz, *Ohio, U.S.A.* .. **150 F4** 40 22N 81 0W
Cádiz □, *Spain* **43 J5** 36 36N 5 45W
Cádiz, G. de, *Spain* .. **43 J3** 36 40N 7 0W
Cadiz L., *U.S.A.* **159 J6** 34 18N 115 24W
Cadley, *U.S.A.* **152 B7** 33 32N 82 40W
Cadney Park, *Australia* **127 D1** 27 55 S 134 3 E
Cadomin, *Canada* **142 C5** 53 2N 117 20W
Cadotte Lake, *Canada* **142 B5** 56 26N 116 23W
Cadours, *France* ..... **28 E5** 43 44N 1 2 E
Cadoux, *Australia* ... **125 F2** 30 46 S 117 7 E
Cadwell, *U.S.A.* **152 C6** 32 20N 83 3W
Caen, *France* **26 C6** 49 10N 0 22W
Caernarfon, *U.K.* **20 D3** 53 8N 4 16W
Caernarfon B., *U.K.* .. **20 D3** 53 4N 4 40W
Caernarvon = Caernarfon, *U.K.* .. **20 D3** 53 8N 4 16W
Caerphilly, *U.K.* **21 F4** 51 35N 3 13W
Caerphilly □, *U.K.* .. **21 F4** 51 37N 3 12W
Caesarea, *Israel* .... **103 C3** 32 30N 34 53 E
Caeté, *Brazil* .... **171 E3** 19 55 S 43 40W
Caetité, *Brazil* ...... **171 D3** 13 50 S 42 32W
Cafayate, *Argentina* .. **174 B2** 26 2 S 66 0W
Cafu, *Angola* .... **116 B2** 16 30 S 15 8 E
Cagayan □, *Phil.* .... **80 C3** 18 0N 121 50 E
Cagayan →, *Phil.* ... **80 B3** 18 25N 121 42 E
Cagayan de Oro, *Phil.* **81 G5** 8 30N 124 40 E
Cagayan Is., *Phil.* ... **81 G3** 9 40N 121 16 E
Cagayan Sulu I., *Phil.* **81 H2** 7 1N 118 30 E
Cagli, *Italy* .... **45 E9** 43 33N 12 39 E
Cágliari, *Italy* ...... **46 C2** 39 13N 9 7 E
Cágliari, G. di, *Italy* .. **46 C2** 39 8N 9 11 E
Cagnano Varano, *Italy* **45 G12** 41 49N 15 47 E
Cagnes-sur-Mer, *France* **29 E11** 43 40N 7 9 E
Caguán →, *Colombia* . **168 D3** 0 8 S 74 18W
Caguas, *Puerto Rico* .. **165 d** 18 14N 66 2W
Caha Mts., *Ireland* ... **23 E2** 51 45N 9 40W
Cahama, *Angola* ..... **116 B1** 16 17 S 14 19 E
Caher, *Ireland* **23 D4** 52 22N 7 56W
Cahersiveen, *Ireland* . **23 E1** 51 56N 10 14W
Cahora Bassa, L. de, *Mozam.* .... **119 F3** 15 35 S 32 0 E
Cahora Bassa, Represa de, *Mozam.* ...... **119 F3** 15 20 S 32 50 E
Cahore Pt., *Ireland* .. **23 D5** 52 33N 6 12W
Cahors, *France* ..... **28 D5** 44 27N 1 27 E
Cahuapanas, *Peru* ... **172 B2** 5 15 S 77 0W
Cahuinari △, *Colombia* **168 D3** 1 20 S 71 10W
Cahuinari →, *Colombia* .... **168 D3** 1 21 S 70 44W
Cahul, *Moldova* ..... **53 E13** 45 50N 28 15 E
Cai Bau, Dao, *Vietnam* **76 G6** 21 10N 107 27 E
Cai Nuoc, *Vietnam* ... **87 H5** 8 56N 105 1 E
Caia, *Mozam.* ...... **119 F4** 17 51 S 35 24 E
Caiabis, Serra dos, *Brazil* .... **173 C6** 11 30 S 56 30W
Caianda, *Angola* .... **119 E1** 11 2 S 23 31 E
Caiapó, Serra do, *Brazil* **173 D7** 17 0 S 52 0W
Caiapônia, *Brazil* .... **173 D7** 16 57 S 51 49W
Caibarién, *Cuba* **164 B4** 22 30N 79 30W
Caibiran, *Phil.* ...... **81 F5** 11 34N 124 35 E
Caiçara = Alvarães, *Brazil* .... **169 D5** 3 12 S 64 50W
Caicara, *Bolívar, Venezuela* **168 B4** 7 38N 66 10W
Caicara, *Monagas, Venezuela* **169 B5** 9 52N 63 38W
Caicó, *Brazil* .... **170 C4** 6 20 S 37 0W
Caicos Is., *Turks & Caicos* ... **165 B5** 21 40N 71 40W
Caicos Passage, *W. Indies* **165 B5** 22 45N 72 45W
Caidian, *China* ..... **77 B10** 30 35N 114 2 E
Cailloma, *Peru* ..... **172 D3** 15 9 S 71 45W
Căinari, *Moldova* .... **53 D14** 46 38N 29 3 E
Cainde, *Angola* ..... **115 F2** 15 29 S 13 24 E
Caine →, *Bolivia* ... **173 D4** 18 23 S 65 21W
Caird Coast, *Antarctica* **7 D1** 75 0 S 25 0W
Cairn Gorm, *U.K.* ... **22 D5** 57 7N 3 39W
Cairngorm Mts., *U.K.* . **22 D5** 57 6N 3 42W
Cairngorms △, *U.K.* .. **22 D5** 57 10N 3 50W
Cairnryan, *U.K.* **22 G3** 54 59N 5 1W
Cairns, *Australia* .... **126 B4** 16 57 S 145 45 E
Cairns L., *Canada* ... **143 C10** 51 42N 94 30W
Cairo = El Qâhira, *Egypt* .... **106 H7** 30 1N 31 14 E
Cairo, *Ga., U.S.A.* ... **152 E5** 30 52N 84 13W
Cairo, *Ill., U.S.A.* **155 G10** 37 0N 89 11W
Cairo, *N.Y., U.S.A.* .. **151 D11** 42 18N 74 0W
Cairo Montenotte, *Italy* **44 D5** 44 23N 8 16 E
Cairofa, *Angola* ..... **115 E2** 14 3 S 12 54 E
Caithness, *U.K.* **22 C5** 58 25N 3 35W
Caithness, Ord of, *U.K.* **22 C5** 58 8N 3 36W
Caitou, *Angola* ..... **115 E2** 14 28 S 13 7 E
Caiuás = Rio Brilhante, *Brazil* .... **175 A5** 21 48 S 54 33W
Caiundo, *Angola* .... **115 F3** 15 50 S 17 28 E
Caiza, *Bolivia* ...... **173 E4** 20 2 S 65 40W

Caja de Muertos, I., *Puerto Rico* . . . . **165 d** 17 54N 66 32W
Cajabamba, *Peru* . . . . . **172 B2** 7 38 S 78 4W
Cajamarca, *Peru* . . . . . **172 B2** 7 5 S 78 28W
Cajamarca ☐, *Peru* . . . **172 B2** 6 15 S 78 50W
Cajamarquilla = Bolívar, *Peru* . . . . . . **172 B2** 7 18 S 77 48W
Cajapió, *Brazil* . . . . . . **170 B3** 2 58 S 44 48W
Cajarc, *France* . . . . **28 D5** 44 29N 1 50 E
Cajas △, *Ecuador* . . . . . **168 D2** 2 48 S 79 15W
Cajatambo, *Peru* . . . . . **172 C2** 10 30 S 77 2W
Cajàzeiras, *Brazil* . . . . **170 C4** 6 52 S 38 30W
Čajetina, *Serbia & M.* . **50 C3** 43 47N 19 42 E
Cajidiocan, *Phil.* . . . . . **80 E4** 12 22N 122 41 E
Çakirgol, *Turkey* . . . . . **101 B8** 40 33N 39 40 E
Çakırlar, *Turkey* . . . . . **49 E12** 36 52N 30 33 E
Čakovec, *Croatia* . . . . . **45 B13** 46 23N 16 26 E
Çal, *Turkey* . . . . **49 C11** 38 4N 29 23 E
Cala, *Spain* **43 H4** 37 59N 6 21W
Cala →, *Spain* **43 H4** 37 38N 6 5W
Cala Cadolar, Punta de = Rotja, Pta., *Spain* . . . . **38 D2** 38 38N 1 35 E
Cala d'Or, *Spain* . . . . . **38 B4** 39 23N 3 14 E
Cala en Porter, *Spain* . **38 B5** 39 52N 4 8 E
Cala Figuera, C. de, *Spain* . . . . **38 B3** 39 27N 2 31 E
Cala Forcat, *Spain* . . . **38 B4** 40 0N 3 47 E
Cala Major, *Spain* . . . . **38 B3** 39 33N 2 37 E
Cala Mezquida = Sa Mesquida, *Spain* . . . **38 B5** 39 55N 4 16 E
Cala Millor, *Spain* . . . . **38 B4** 39 35N 3 22 E
Cala Ratjada, *Spain* . . **38 B4** 39 43N 3 27 E
Cala Santa Galdana, *Spain* . . . . **38 B4** 39 56N 3 58 E
Calabanga, *Phil.* . . . . . **80 E4** 13 42N 123 17 E
Calabar, *Nigeria* . . . . . **113 E6** 4 57N 8 20 E
Calabogie, *Canada* . . . **151 A8** 45 18N 76 43W
Calabozo, *Venezuela* . **168 B4** 9 0N 67 28W
Calábria ☐, *Italy* . . . . . **47 C9** 39 0N 16 30 E
Calábria △, *Italy* . . . . . **47 C9** 39 6N 16 35 E
Calaburras, Pta. de, *Spain* **43 J6** 36 30N 4 38W
Calaceite, *Spain* . . . . . **40 D5** 41 1N 0 11 E
Calacoto, *Bolivia* . . . . . **172 D4** 17 16 S 68 38W
Calacuccia, *France* . . . **29 F13** 42 21N 9 1 E
Calafat, *Romania* . . . . . **52 G7** 43 58N 22 59 E
Calafate, *Argentina* . . . **176 D2** 50 19 S 72 15W
Calafell, *Spain* . . . . **40 D6** 41 11N 1 34 E
Calagua Is., *Phil.* . . . . . **80 D4** 14 30N 122 55 E
Calahorra, *Spain* **40 C3** 42 18N 1 59W
Calai, *Angola* . . . . **115 F3** 17 47 S 19 41 E
Calais, *France* . . . . **27 B8** 50 57N 1 56 E
Calais, *U.S.A.* **149 C12** 45 11N 67 17W
Calakmul △, *Mexico* . . **163 D7** 18 14N 89 48W
Calalaste, Cord. de, *Argentina* . . . . **174 B2** 25 0 S 67 0W
Calama, *Brazil* . . . . **173 B5** 8 0 S 62 50W
Calama, *Chile* . . . . **174 A2** 22 30 S 68 55W
Calamar, *Bolívar, Colombia* **168 A3** 10 15N 74 55W
Calamar, *Vaupés, Colombia* **168 C3** 1 58N 72 32W
Calamarca, *Bolivia* . . . **172 D4** 16 55 S 68 9W
Calamba, *Cavite, Phil.* . **80 D3** 14 13N 121 10 E
Calamba, *Mis. Occ., Phil.* . . . . **81 G4** 8 35N 123 39 E
Calamian Group, *Phil.* . **81 F2** 11 50N 119 55 E
Calamocha, *Spain* **40 E3** 40 50N 1 17W
Calamonte, *Spain* **43 G4** 38 53N 6 23W
Călan, *Romania* . . . . . . **52 E7** 45 44N 22 59 E
Calañas, *Spain* **43 H4** 37 40N 6 53W
Calanda, *Spain* **40 E4** 40 56N 0 15W
Calandagan I., *Phil.* . . **81 F3** 10 39N 120 15 E
Calandula, *Angola* . . . **115 D3** 9 6 S 15 57 E
Calang, *Indonesia* . . . . **84 B1** 4 37N 95 37 E
Calangiánus, *Italy* . . . . **46 B2** 40 56N 9 11 E
Calanscio, Sarīr, *Libya* **108 C4** 27 30N 21 30 E
Calapan, *Phil.* . . . . **80 E3** 13 25N 121 7 E
Călăraşi, *Moldova* . . . . **53 C13** 47 16N 28 19 E
Călăraşi, *Romania* . . . . **53 F12** 44 12N 27 20 E
Călăraşi ☐, *Romania* . . **53 F12** 44 10N 27 0 E
Calasparra, *Spain* **41 G3** 38 14N 1 41W
Calatafimi, *Italy* . . . . . **46 E5** 37 55N 12 52 E
Calatagan, *Phil.* . . . . . . **80 E3** 13 50N 120 38 E
Calatayud, *Spain* **40 D3** 41 20N 1 40W
Călăţele, *Romania* . . . . **52 D8** 46 46N 23 1 E
Calato = Kálathos, *Greece* . . . . **38 E12** 36 9N 28 8 E
Calatrava, *Eq. Guin.* . . **114 B1** 1 6N 9 25 E
Calauag, *Phil.* . . . . **80 E4** 13 55N 122 15 E
Calavà, C., *Italy* . . . . . **47 D7** 38 11N 14 55 E
Calavite, C., *Phil.* . . . . **80 E3** 13 26N 120 20 E
Calavite Pass, *Phil.* . . . **80 E3** 13 36N 120 25 E
Calayan, *Phil.* . . . . **80 B3** 19 16N 121 28 E
Calayan I., *Phil.* . . . . . **80 B3** 19 20N 121 27 E
Calbayog, *Phil.* . . . . . . **80 E5** 12 4N 124 38 E
Calbiga, *Phil.* . . . . **81 F5** 11 38N 125 0 E
Calca, *Peru* . . . . **172 C3** 13 22 S 72 0W
Calcasieu L., *U.S.A.* . . **155 L8** 29 55N 93 18W
Calcutta = Kolkata, *India* . . . . **93 H13** 22 36N 88 24 E
Calcutta, *U.S.A.* **150 F4** 40 40N 80 34W
Caldaro, *Italy* . . . . **45 B8** 46 25N 11 14 E
Caldas ☐, *Colombia* . . **168 B2** 5 15N 75 30W
Caldas da Rainha, *Portugal* **43 F1** 39 24N 9 8W
Caldas de Reis, *Spain* . **42 C2** 42 36N 8 39W
Caldas Novas, *Brazil* . . **171 E2** 17 45 S 48 38W
Calder →, *U.K.* **20 D6** 53 44N 1 22W
Caldera, *Chile* . . . . **174 B1** 27 5 S 70 55W
Caldera de Taburiente △, *Canary Is.* **9 e1** 28 43N 17 52W
Caldwell, *Idaho, U.S.A.* **158 E5** 43 40N 116 41W
Caldwell, *Kans., U.S.A.* **155 G6** 37 2N 97 37W
Caldwell, *Tex., U.S.A.* . **155 K6** 30 32N 96 42W
Caledon, *S. Africa* . . . . **116 E2** 34 14 S 19 26 E
Caledon →, *S. Africa* . . **116 E4** 30 31 S 26 5 E
Caledon B., *Australia* . **126 A2** 12 45 S 137 0 E
Caledonia, *Canada* . . . **150 C5** 43 7N 79 58W
Caledonia, *Mo., U.S.A.* **156 G6** 37 45N 90 46W
Caledonia, *N.Y., U.S.A.* **150 D7** 42 58N 77 51W
Calella, *Spain* . . . . **40 D7** 41 37N 2 40 E
Calemba, *Angola* . . . . . **116 B2** 16 0 S 15 44 E
Calen, *Australia* . . . . . **126 J6** 20 56 S 148 48 E
Calenzana, *France* . . . **29 F12** 42 31N 8 51 E
Caleta Olivia, *Argentina* . . . . **176 C3** 46 25 S 67 25W
Caletones, *Chile* . . . . . **174 C1** 34 6 S 70 27W
Calexico, *U.S.A.* **161 N11** 32 40N 115 30W
Calf of Man, *I. of Man* . **20 C3** 54 3N 4 48W
Calgary, *Canada* **142 C6** 51 0N 114 10W
Calheta, *Azores* **9 d1** 38 36N 28 1W
Calheta, *Madeira* . . . . . **9 c** 32 44N 17 11W
Calheta de Nesquim, *Azores* **9 d1** 38 24N 28 5W
Calhoun, *U.S.A.* **149 H3** 34 30N 84 57W
Calhoun Falls, *U.S.A.* . **152 A7** 34 6N 82 36W
Cali, *Colombia* **168 C2** 3 25N 76 35W
Calicut, *India* . . . . **95 J2** 11 15N 75 43 E
Caliente, *U.S.A.* **159 H6** 37 37N 114 31W
California, *Mo., U.S.A.* **156 F4** 38 38N 92 34W
California, *Pa., U.S.A.* **150 F5** 40 4N 79 54W
California ☐, *U.S.A.* . . **160 H7** 37 30N 119 30W
California, Baja, *Mexico* **162 A1** 32 10N 115 12W
California, Baja, T.N. = Baja California ☐, *Mexico* **162 B2** 30 0N 115 0W
California, Baja, T.S. = Baja California Sur ☐, *Mexico* **162 B2** 25 50N 111 50W
California, G. de, *Mexico* **162 B2** 27 0N 111 0W
California City, *U.S.A.* **161 K9** 35 10N 117 55W
California Hot Springs, *U.S.A.* **161 K8** 35 51N 118 41W
Calilegua △, *Argentina* **174 B3** 25 36 S 64 50W
Călimăneşti, *Romania* . **53 E9** 45 14N 24 20 E
Călimani, Munţii, *Romania* . . . . **53 C10** 47 12N 25 0 E
Calingasta, *Argentina* . **174 C2** 31 15 S 69 30W
Calinog, *Phil.* . . . . **81 F4** 11 7N 122 32 E
Calintaan, *Phil.* . . . . . . **80 E3** 12 35N 120 57 E
Calipatria, *U.S.A.* **161 M11** 33 8N 115 31W
Calistoga, *U.S.A.* **160 G4** 38 35N 122 35W
Calitri, *Italy* . . . . **47 B8** 40 54N 15 26 E
Calitzdorp, *S. Africa* . . **116 E3** 33 33 S 21 42 E
Callabonna, L., *Australia* . . . . **127 D3** 29 40 S 140 5 E
Callac, *France* **26 D3** 48 25N 3 27W
Callahan, *U.S.A.* **152 E8** 30 34N 81 50W
Callan, *Ireland* **23 D4** 52 32N 7 24W
Callander, *U.K.* **22 E4** 56 15N 4 13W
Callang = San Manuel, *Phil.* . . . . **80 C3** 16 4N 120 40 E
Callao, *Peru* . . . . **172 C2** 12 0 S 77 0W
Callaway, *U.S.A.* **152 E4** 30 8N 85 36W
Calles, *Mexico* **163 C5** 23 2N 98 42W
Callicoon, *U.S.A.* **151 E9** 41 46N 75 3W
Calling Lake, *Canada* . **142 B6** 55 15N 113 12W
Calliope, *Australia* . . . **126 C5** 24 0 S 151 16 E
Callosa de Ensarriá, *Spain* **41 G4** 38 40N 0 8W
Callosa de Segura, *Spain* **41 G4** 38 7N 0 53W
Calmar, *U.S.A.* **156 A5** 43 11N 91 52W
Calne, *U.K.* **21 F6** 51 26N 2 0W
Calola, *Angola* . . . . **116 B2** 16 25 S 17 48 E
Calolbon = San Andres, *Phil.* . . . . **80 E5** 13 36N 124 6 E
Calonge, *Spain* . . . . . . **40 D8** 41 52N 3 5 E
Caloocan, *Phil.* . . . . . . **80 D3** 14 39N 120 58 E
Caloosahatchee →, *U.S.A.* **153 J7** 26 31N 82 1W
Calore →, *Italy* . . . . . . **47 A7** 41 11N 14 28 E
Caloundra, *Australia* . . **127 D5** 26 45 S 153 10 E
Calpe, *Spain* . . . . **41 G5** 38 39N 0 3 E
Calpella, *U.S.A.* **160 F3** 39 14N 123 12W
Calpine, *U.S.A.* **160 F6** 39 40N 120 27W
Calstock, *Canada* **140 C3** 49 47N 84 9W
Caltabellotta, *Italy* . . . **46 E6** 37 34N 13 13 E
Caltagirone, *Italy* . . . . **47 E7** 37 14N 14 31 E
Caltanissetta, *Italy* . . . **47 E7** 37 29N 14 4 E
Çaltılıbük, *Turkey* . . . . **51 G12** 39 57N 28 36 E
Caluango, *Angola* . . . . **115 D3** 8 20 S 19 39 E
Calubian, *Phil.* . . . . . . **81 F5** 11 27N 124 26 E
Calucinga, *Angola* . . . . **115 E3** 11 18 S 16 12 E
Caluire-et-Cuire, *France* . . . . **27 G11** 45 48N 4 52 E
Calulo, *Angola* . . . . . . **115 E2** 10 1 S 14 56 E
Calunda, *Angola* . . . . . **115 E4** 12 7 S 23 36 E
Caluquembe, *Angola* . . **115 E2** 13 47 S 14 44 E
Caluso, *Italy* . . . . **44 C4** 45 18N 7 53 E
Caluya I., *Phil.* . . . . . . **81 F3** 11 55N 121 34 E
Calvados ☐, *France* . . . **26 C6** 49 5N 0 15W
Calvados Chain, The, *Papua N. G.* . . . . . . **132 F7** 11 10 S 152 45 E
Calvert →, *Australia* . **126 B2** 16 17 S 137 44 E
Calvert I., *Canada* . . . **142 C3** 51 30N 128 0W
Calvert Ra., *Australia* . **124 D3** 24 0 S 122 30 E
Calvi, *France* . . . . **29 F12** 42 34N 8 45 E
Calvià, *Spain* . . . . **38 B3** 39 34N 2 31 E
Calvillo, *Mexico* **162 C4** 21 51N 102 43W
Calvinia, *S. Africa* . . . . **116 E2** 31 28 S 19 45 E
Calvo, Mte., *Italy* . . . . **45 G12** 41 44N 15 46 E
Calwa, *U.S.A.* **160 J7** 36 42N 119 46W
Calzada Almuradiel = Almuradiel, *Spain* . . **43 G7** 38 32N 3 28W
Calzada de Calatrava, *Spain* **43 G7** 38 42N 3 46W
Cam →, *U.K.* . . . . **21 E8** 52 21N 0 16 E
Cam Lam, *Vietnam* . . . . **87 G7** 11 54N 109 10 E
Cam Pha, *Vietnam* . . . . **76 G6** 21 7N 107 18 E
Cam Ranh, *Vietnam* . . **87 G7** 11 54N 109 12 E
Cam Xuyen, *Vietnam* . . **86 C6** 18 15N 106 0 E
Camabatela, *Angola* . . **115 D3** 8 20 S 15 26 E
Camacã, *Brazil* . . . . . . **171 E4** 15 24 S 39 30W
Camaçari, *Brazil* . . . . . **171 D4** 12 41 S 38 18W
Camacha, *Madeira* . . . . **9 c** 32 41N 16 49W
Camacho, *Mexico* **162 C4** 24 25N 102 18W
Camacupa, *Angola* . . . . **115 E3** 11 58 S 17 22 E
Camaguán, *Venezuela* . **168 B4** 8 6N 67 36W
Camagüey, *Cuba* **164 B4** 21 20N 77 55W
Camaiore, *Italy* . . . . . . **44 E7** 43 56N 10 18 E
Camamu, *Brazil* . . . . . . **171 D4** 13 57 S 39 7W
Camaná, *Peru* . . . . **172 D3** 16 30 S 72 50W
Camanche, *U.S.A.* **156 C6** 41 47N 90 15W
Camanche Reservoir, *U.S.A.* **160 G6** 38 14N 121 1W
Camaquã, *Brazil* . . . . . **173 D7** 19 30 S 54 5W
Camaquã, *Brazil* . . . . . **175 C5** 30 51 S 51 49W
Camaquã →, *Brazil* . . **175 C5** 31 17 S 51 47W
Câmara de Lobos, *Madeira* . . . . **9 c** 32 39N 16 59W
Camararé →, *Brazil* . . **173 C6** 12 15 S 58 55W
Camarat, C., *France* . . **29 E10** 43 12N 6 41 E
Camarès, *France* . . . . . **28 E6** 43 49N 2 53 E
Camaret-sur-Mer, *France* **26 D2** 48 16N 4 37W
Camargo, *Bolivia* . . . . . **173 E4** 20 38 S 65 15W
Camargo, *Mexico* **163 B5** 26 19N 98 50W
Camargue, *France* . . . . **29 E8** 43 34N 4 34 E
Camargue △, *France* . . **29 E8** 43 30N 4 40 E
Camarillo, *U.S.A.* **161 L7** 34 13N 119 2W
Camariñas, *Spain* **42 B1** 43 8N 9 12W
Camarines Norte ☐, *Phil.* . . . . **80 D4** 14 10N 122 45 E
Camarines Sur ☐, *Phil.* **80 E4** 13 40N 123 20 E
Camarón, C., *Honduras* **164 C2** 16 0N 85 5W
Camarones, *Argentina* **176 B3** 44 50 S 65 40W
Camarones, B., *Argentina* . . . . **176 B3** 44 45 S 65 35W
Camas, *Spain* **43 H4** 37 24N 6 2W
Camas, *U.S.A.* **160 E4** 45 35N 122 24W
Camas Valley, *U.S.A.* . **158 E2** 43 2N 123 40W
Camatambo, *Angola* . . . **115 D3** 6 31 S 15 21 E
Camataquí = Villa Abecia, *Bolivia* . . . . **174 A2** 21 0 S 68 18W
Camaxilo, *Angola* . . . . **115 D3** 8 21 S 18 56 E
Camba Cassai, *Angola* **115 D3** 9 47 S 19 9 E
Camballin, *Australia* . . **124 C3** 17 59 S 124 12 E
Cambamba, *Angola* . . . **115 D2** 8 53 S 14 44 E
Cambará, *Brazil* . . . . . **175 A5** 23 2 S 50 5W
Cambay = Khambhat, *India* . . . . **92 H5** 22 23N 72 33 E
Cambay, G. of = Khambhat, G. of, *India* . . . . **89 C6** 20 45N 72 30 E
Cambil, *Spain* **43 H7** 37 40N 3 33W
Cambo, *Angola* . . . . . . **115 D3** 10 55 S 20 6 E
Cambo-les-Bains, *France* **28 E2** 43 22N 1 23W
Cambodia ■, *Asia* . . . **86 F5** 12 15N 105 0 E
Camborne, *U.K.* **21 G2** 50 12N 5 19W
Cambrai, *Australia* . . . **128 C3** 34 40 S 139 16 E
Cambrai, *France* . . . . . **27 B10** 50 11N 3 14 E
Cambre, *Spain* **42 B2** 43 17N 8 20W
Cambria, *U.S.A.* **160 K5** 35 34N 121 5W
Cambrian Mts., *U.K.* . . **21 E4** 52 3N 3 57W
Cambridge, *Canada* . . . **140 D3** 43 23N 80 15W
Cambridge, *Jamaica* . . **164 a** 18 18N 77 54W
Cambridge, *N.Z.* . . . . . **130 D4** 37 54 S 175 29 E
Cambridge, *U.K.* . . . . . **21 E8** 52 12N 0 8 E
Cambridge, *Ill., U.S.A.* **156 C6** 41 18N 90 12W
Cambridge, *Iowa, U.S.A.* **156 C3** 41 54N 93 32W
Cambridge, *Mass., U.S.A.* **151 D13** 42 22N 71 6W
Cambridge, *Md., U.S.A.* **148 F7** 38 34N 76 5W
Cambridge, *Minn., U.S.A.* **154 C8** 45 34N 93 13W
Cambridge, *N.Y., U.S.A.* **151 C11** 43 2N 73 22W
Cambridge, *Nebr., U.S.A.* **154 E4** 40 17N 100 10W
Cambridge, *Ohio, U.S.A.* **150 F3** 40 2N 81 35W
Cambridge Bay = Ikaluktutiak, *Canada* **138 B9** 69 10N 105 0W
Cambridge City, *U.S.A.* **157 E11** 39 49N 85 10W
Cambridge G., *Australia* . . . . **124 B4** 14 55 S 128 15 E
Cambridge Springs, *U.S.A.* **150 E4** 41 48N 80 4W
Cambridgeshire ☐, *U.K.* **21 E7** 52 25N 0 7W
Cambrils, *Spain* . . . . . . **40 D6** 41 8N 1 3 E
Cambuci, *Brazil* . . . . . **171 F3** 21 35 S 41 55W
Cambulo, *Angola* . . . . . **115 D4** 7 49 S 21 15 E
Cambundi-Catembo, *Angola* . . . . **115 E3** 10 10 S 17 35 E
Camden, *Australia* . . . **129 C9** 34 1 S 150 43 E
Camden, *Ala., U.S.A.* . . **149 K2** 31 59N 87 17W
Camden, *Ark., U.S.A.* . . **155 J8** 33 35N 92 50W
Camden, *Maine, U.S.A.* **149 C11** 44 13N 69 4W
Camden, *N.J., U.S.A.* . . **151 G9** 39 56N 75 7W
Camden, *N.Y., U.S.A.* . . **151 C9** 43 20N 75 45W
Camden, *Ohio, U.S.A.* . **157 E12** 39 38N 84 39W
Camden, *S.C., U.S.A.* . . **149 H5** 34 16N 80 36W
Camden Bay, *U.S.A.* . . **144 A11** 70 10N 145 15W
Camden Sd., *Australia* **124 C3** 15 27 S 124 25 E
Camdenton, *U.S.A.* . . . **155 F8** 38 1N 92 45W
Cameia △, *Angola* . . . **115 E4** 12 5 S 21 40 E
Camelford, *U.K.* **21 G3** 50 37N 4 42W
Çameli, *Turkey* . . . . . . **49 D11** 37 5N 29 24 E
Camenca, *Moldova* . . . **53 B13** 48 3N 28 42 E
Camerino, *Italy* . . . . . . **45 E10** 43 8N 13 4 E
Cameron, *Ariz., U.S.A.* **159 J8** 35 53N 111 25W
Cameron, *La., U.S.A.* . . **155 L8** 29 48N 93 20W
Cameron, *Mo., U.S.A.* . **156 E2** 39 44N 94 14W
Cameron, *S.C., U.S.A.* . **152 B9** 33 34N 80 43W
Cameron, *Tex., U.S.A.* . **155 K6** 30 51N 96 59W
Cameron Highlands, *Malaysia* . . . . **87 K3** 4 27N 101 22 E
Cameron Hills, *Canada* **142 B5** 59 48N 118 0W
Cameron Mts., *N.Z.* . . **131 G1** 46 1 S 167 0 E
Cameroon ■, *Africa* . . **114 A2** 6 0N 12 30 E
Camerota, *Italy* . . . . . . **47 B8** 40 2N 15 22 E
Cameroun →, *Cameroon* . . . . **113 E6** 4 0N 9 35 E
Cameroun, Mt., *Cameroon* . . . . **113 E6** 4 13N 9 10 E
Cametá, *Brazil* . . . . . . **170 B2** 2 12 S 49 30W
Çamiçi Gölü, *Turkey* . . **49 D9** 37 29N 27 28 E
Camiguin ☐, *Phil.* . . . . **81 G5** 9 11N 124 42 E
Camiguin I., *Phil.* . . . . **80 B3** 18 56N 121 55 E
Camiling, *Phil.* . . . . . . **80 D3** 15 42N 120 24 E
Camilla, *U.S.A.* **152 D5** 31 14N 84 12W
Caminha, *Portugal* . . . **42 D2** 41 50N 8 50W
Camino, *U.S.A.* **160 G6** 38 44N 120 41W
Camira Creek, *Australia* . . . . **127 D5** 29 15 S 152 58 E
Camiranga, *Brazil* . . . . **170 B2** 1 48 S 46 17W
Camiri, *Bolivia* . . . . . . **173 E5** 20 3 S 63 31W
Camissombo, *Angola* . . **115 D4** 8 7 S 20 38 E
Cammal, *U.S.A.* **150 E7** 41 24N 77 28W
Cammarata, *Italy* . . . . . **46 E6** 37 38N 13 38 E
Cammin = Kamień Pomorski, *Poland* . . **54 E1** 53 57N 14 43 E
Camocim, *Brazil* . . . . . **170 B3** 2 55 S 40 50W
Camooweal, *Australia* . **126 B2** 19 56 S 138 7 E
Camooweal Caves △, *Australia* . . . . **126 C2** 20 1 S 138 11 E
Camopi, *Fr. Guiana* . . . **169 C7** 3 12N 52 17W
Camopi →, *Fr. Guiana* **169 C7** 3 10N 52 20W
Camorta, *India* . . . . . . **95 K11** 8 8N 93 30 E
Camotes Is., *Phil.* . . . . **81 F5** 10 40N 124 24 E
Camotes Sea, *Phil.* . . . **81 F5** 10 30N 124 15 E
Camp Borden, *Canada* . **150 B5** 44 18N 79 56W
Camp Coulter = Powell, *U.S.A.* **158 D9** 44 45N 108 46W
Camp Hill, *Ala., U.S.A.* **152 C4** 32 48N 85 39W
Camp Hill, *Pa., U.S.A.* **150 F8** 40 14N 76 55W
Camp Nelson, *U.S.A.* . . **161 J8** 36 8N 118 39W
Camp Pendleton, *U.S.A.* **161 M9** 33 16N 117 23W
Camp Point, *U.S.A.* . . . **156 D5** 40 3N 91 4W
Camp Verde, *U.S.A.* . . . **159 J8** 34 34N 111 51W
Camp Wood, *U.S.A.* . . . **155 L5** 29 40N 100 1W
Campagna, *Italy* . . . . . **47 B8** 40 40N 15 6 E
Campana, *Argentina* . . **174 C4** 34 10 S 58 55W
Campana, I., *Chile* . . . . **176 C1** 48 20 S 75 20W
Campanário, *Madeira* . . **9 c** 32 39N 17 2W
Campanario, *Spain* **43 G5** 38 52N 5 36W
Campánia ☐, *Italy* . . . . **47 B7** 41 0N 14 30 E
Campbell, *S. Africa* . . . **116 D3** 28 48 S 23 44 E
Campbell, *Calif., U.S.A.* **160 H5** 37 17N 121 57W
Campbell, *Fla., U.S.A.* . **153 G8** 28 16N 81 27W
Campbell, *Ohio, U.S.A.* **150 E4** 41 5N 80 37W
Campbell, C., *N.Z.* . . . **131 B9** 41 47 S 174 18 E
Campbell I., *Pac. Oc.* . . **134 N8** 52 30 S 169 0 E
Campbell L., *Canada* . . **143 A7** 63 14N 106 55W
Campbell River, *Canada* **142 C3** 50 5N 125 20W
Campbell Town, *Australia* . . . . **127 G4** 41 52 S 147 30 E
Campbellford, *Canada* **150 B7** 44 18N 77 48W
Campbellpur, *Pakistan* **92 C5** 33 46N 72 26 E
Campbellsburg, *U.S.A.* **157 F10** 38 39N 86 16W
Campbellsville, *U.S.A.* **148 G3** 37 21N 85 20W
Campbellton, *Canada* . **141 C6** 47 57N 66 43W
Campbellton, *U.S.A.* . . **152 E4** 30 57N 85 24W
Campbelltown = Bluff, *N.Z.* . . . . **131 G3** 46 37 S 168 20 E
Campbelltown, *Australia* . . . . **129 C9** 34 4 S 150 49 E
Campbeltown, *U.K.* . . . **22 F3** 55 26N 5 36W
Campeche, *Mexico* . . . **163 D6** 19 50N 90 32W
Campeche ☐, *Mexico* . . **163 D6** 19 50N 90 32W
Campeche, Golfo de, *Mexico* **163 D6** 19 30N 93 0W
Campello, *Spain* **41 G4** 38 26N 0 24W
Câmpeni, *Romania* . . . **52 D8** 46 22N 23 3 E
Camperdown, *Australia* **128 E5** 38 14 S 143 9 E
Camperville, *Canada* . . **143 C8** 51 59N 100 9W
Campi Salentina, *Italy* **47 B11** 40 24N 18 1 E
Câmpia Turzii, *Romania* . . . . **53 D8** 46 34N 23 53 E
Campidano, *Italy* . . . . . **46 C1** 39 30N 8 47 E
Campíglia Maríttima, *Italy* . . . . **44 E7** 43 4N 10 37 E
Campillo de Altobuey, *Spain* **41 F3** 39 36N 1 49W
Campillos, *Spain* **43 H6** 37 4N 4 51W
Câmpina, *Romania* . . . **53 E10** 45 10N 25 45 E
Campina Grande, *Brazil* . . . . **170 C4** 7 20 S 35 47W
Campina Verde, *Brazil* **171 E2** 19 31 S 49 28W
Campinas, *Brazil* . . . . . **175 A6** 22 50 S 47 0W
Campli, *Italy* . . . . **45 F10** 42 43N 13 41 E
Campo = Ntem →, *Cameroon* . . . . **114 B2** 2 21N 9 49 E
Campo, *Cameroon* . . . . **114 B1** 2 22N 9 50 E
Campo, *Spain* . . . . **40 C5** 42 25N 0 24 E
Campo △, *Cameroon* . . **114 B2** 2 23N 10 5 E
Campo Belo, *Brazil* . . . **171 F2** 20 52 S 45 16W
Campo de Criptana, *Spain* **43 F7** 39 24N 3 7W
Campo de Diauarum, *Brazil* . . . . **173 C7** 11 12 S 53 14W
Campo de Gibraltar, *Spain* **43 J5** 36 15N 5 25W
Campo Flórido, *Brazil* **171 E2** 19 47 S 48 35W
Campo Formoso = Campo Flórido, *Brazil* . . . . **171 E2** 19 47 S 48 35W
Campo Formoso, *Brazil* **170 D3** 10 30 S 40 20W
Campo Grande, *Brazil* **173 E7** 20 25 S 54 40W
Campo Maior, *Brazil* . . **170 B3** 4 50 S 42 12W
Campo Maior, *Portugal* **43 F3** 39 2N 7 7W
Campo Mourão, *Brazil* **175 A5** 24 3 S 52 22W
Campo Tencia, *Switz.* . . **33 D7** 46 26N 8 43 E
Campo Túres, *Italy* . . . **45 B8** 46 53N 11 55 E
Campoalegre, *Colombia* **168 C2** 2 41N 75 20W
Campobasso, *Italy* . . . . **47 A7** 41 34N 14 39 E
Campobello di Licata, *Italy* . . . . **46 E6** 37 15N 13 55 E
Campobello di Mazara, *Italy* . . . . **46 E5** 37 38N 12 45 E
Campofelice di Roccella, *Italy* . . . . . . **46 E6** 37 59N 13 53 E
Campomarino, *Italy* . . . **45 G12** 41 57N 15 2 E
Camporeale, *Italy* . . . . **46 E6** 37 54N 13 6 E
Camporrobles, *Spain* . . **40 F3** 39 39N 1 24W
Campos, *Brazil* . . . . . . **171 F3** 21 50 S 41 20W
Campos Altos, *Brazil* . . **171 E2** 19 47 S 46 10W
Campos Belos, *Brazil* . . **171 D2** 13 10 S 47 3W
Campos del Port, *Spain* **38 B4** 39 26N 3 1 E
Campos Novos, *Brazil* . **175 B5** 27 21 S 51 50W
Campos Sales, *Brazil* . . **170 C3** 7 4 S 40 23W
Camprodón, *Spain* . . . . **40 C7** 42 19N 2 23 E
Campton, *Fla., U.S.A.* . . **153 E3** 30 53N 86 31W
Campton, *Ga., U.S.A.* . . **152 B6** 33 52N 83 43W
Campton, *Ky., U.S.A.* . . **157 G13** 37 44N 83 33W
Camptonville, *U.S.A.* . . **160 F5** 39 27N 121 3W
Camptown, *U.S.A.* **151 E8** 41 44N 76 14W
Câmpulung, *Argeş, Romania* . . . . **53 E10** 45 17N 25 3 E
Câmpulung, *Suceava, Romania* . . . . **53 C10** 47 32N 25 30 E
Câmpuri, *Romania* . . . . **53 D11** 46 0N 26 50 E
Campuya →, *Peru* . . . . **168 D3** 1 40 S 73 30W
Campville, *U.S.A.* **152 F7** 29 40N 82 7W
Camrose, *Canada* **142 C6** 53 0N 112 50W
Camsell Portage, *Canada* **143 B7** 59 37N 109 15W
Camucuio, *Angola* . . . . **115 E2** 14 7 S 13 15 E
Çamyuva, *Turkey* . . . . **49 E12** 36 30N 30 30 E
Çan, *Turkey* . . . . **51 F11** 40 2N 27 3 E
Can Clavo, *Spain* . . . . . **38 D1** 38 57N 1 27 E
Can Creu, *Spain* . . . . . . **38 D1** 38 58N 1 28 E
Can Gio, *Vietnam* . . . . **87 G6** 10 25N 106 58 E
Can Tho, *Vietnam* . . . . **87 G5** 10 2N 105 46 E
Canaan, *U.S.A.* **151 D11** 42 2N 73 20W
Canacona, *India* . . . . . **95 G2** 15 1N 74 4 E
Canada ■, *N. Amer.* . . . **138 C10** 60 0N 100 0W
Canada Basin, *Arctic* . . **6 B18** 80 0N 145 0W
Cañada de Gómez, *Argentina* . . . . **174 C3** 32 40 S 61 30W
Canadian, *U.S.A.* **155 H4** 35 55N 100 23W
Canadian →, *U.S.A.* . . **155 H7** 35 28N 95 3W
Canadys, *U.S.A.* **152 B9** 33 3N 80 37W
Canajoharie, *U.S.A.* . . **151 D10** 42 54N 74 35W
Çanakkale, *Turkey* . . . . **51 F10** 40 8N 26 24 E
Çanakkale ☐, *Turkey* . . **51 F10** 40 10N 26 25 E
Çanakkale Boğazı, *Turkey* . . . . **51 F10** 40 17N 26 32 E
Canal Flats, *Canada* . . **142 C5** 50 10N 115 48W
Canal Point, *U.S.A.* . . . **153 J9** 26 52N 80 38W
Canala, *N. Cal.* . . . . . . **133 U19** 21 32 S 165 57 E
Canalejas, *Argentina* . . **174 D2** 35 15 S 66 34W
Canals, *Argentina* . . . . **174 C3** 33 35 S 62 53W
Canals, *Spain* **41 G4** 38 58N 0 35W
Canandaigua, *U.S.A.* . . **150 D7** 42 54N 77 17W
Canandaigua L., *U.S.A.* **150 D7** 42 47N 77 19W
Cananea, *Mexico* **162 A2** 31 0N 110 20W
Cañar, *Ecuador* . . . . . . **168 D2** 2 33 S 78 56W
Cañar ☐, *Ecuador* . . . . **168 D2** 2 30 S 79 0W
Canarias, Is., *Atl. Oc.* . . **9 e1** 28 30N 16 0W
Canaries, *St. Lucia* . . . **165 f** 13 55N 61 4W
Canarreos, Arch. de los, *Cuba* **164 B3** 21 35N 81 40W
Canary Is. = Canarias, Is., *Atl. Oc.* **9 e1** 28 30N 16 0W
Canaseraga, *U.S.A.* . . . **150 D7** 42 27N 77 45W
Canastra, Serra da, *Brazil* . . . . **171 F2** 20 0 S 46 20W
Canatlán, *Mexico* **162 C4** 24 31N 104 47W
Cañaveral, *Peru* . . . . . . **168 D1** 3 56 S 80 39W
Canaveral △, *U.S.A.* . . **153 G9** 28 28N 80 34W
Canaveral, C., *U.S.A.* . . **153 G9** 28 27N 80 32W
Cañaveruelas, *Spain* . . **40 E2** 40 24N 2 38W
Canavieiras, *Brazil* . . . **171 E4** 15 39 S 39 0W
Canbelego, *Australia* . . **129 A7** 31 32 S 146 18 E
Canberra, *Australia* . . . **129 C8** 35 15 S 149 8 E
Canby, *Calif., U.S.A.* . . **158 F3** 41 27N 120 52W
Canby, *Minn., U.S.A.* . . **154 C6** 44 43N 96 16W
Canby, *Oreg., U.S.A.* . . **160 E4** 45 16N 122 42W
Cancale, *France* **26 D5** 48 40N 1 50W
Canche →, *France* . . . **27 B8** 50 31N 1 39 E
Canchungo = Teixeira Pinto, *Guinea-Biss.* . **112 C1** 12 3N 16 0W
Canchyuaya, Cordillera de, *Peru* . . . . **172 B3** 7 30 S 74 0W
Cancún, *Mexico* **163 C7** 21 8N 86 44W
Candala, *Somali Rep.* . . **120 B3** 11 30N 49 58 E
Candanchu, *Spain* **40 C4** 42 47N 0 32W
Candarave, *Peru* . . . . . **172 D3** 17 15 S 70 13W
Çandarlı, *Turkey* . . . . . **49 C8** 38 56N 26 56 E
Çandarlı Körfezi, *Turkey* . . . . **49 C8** 38 52N 26 55 E
Candas, *Spain* **42 B5** 43 35N 5 45W
Candé, *France* **26 E5** 47 34N 1 2W
Candeias →, *Brazil* . . **173 B5** 8 39 S 63 31W
Candela, *Italy* . . . . **47 A8** 41 8N 15 31 E
Candelaria, *Argentina* **175 B4** 27 29 S 55 44W
Candelaria, *Canary Is.* . **9 e1** 28 22N 16 22W
Candelaria, *Phil.* . . . . . **80 E3** 13 56N 121 25 E
Candelario △, *Spain* . . **42 E5** 40 20N 5 46W
Candeleda, *Spain* **42 E5** 40 10N 5 14W
Candelo, *Australia* . . . **129 D8** 36 47 S 149 43 E
Candi Dasa, *Indonesia* **79 J18** 8 30 S 115 34 E
Candia = Iráklion, *Greece* . . . . **39 E6** 35 20N 25 12 E
Candia, Sea of = Crete, Sea of, *Greece* . . . . . **49 E7** 36 0N 25 0 E
Cândido de Abreu, *Brazil* . . . . **171 F1** 24 35 S 51 20W
Cândido Mendes, *Brazil* . . . . **170 B2** 1 27 S 45 43W
Candle, *U.S.A.* **144 D7** 65 55N 161 56W
Candle L., *Canada* **143 C7** 53 50N 105 18W
Candlemas I., *Antarctica* . . . . **7 B1** 57 3 S 26 40W
Cando, *U.S.A.* **154 A5** 48 32N 99 12W
Candon, *Phil.* . . . . **80 C3** 17 12N 120 27 E
Canea = Khaniá, *Greece* . . . . **39 E5** 35 30N 24 4 E
Canela, *Brazil* . . . . **170 D2** 10 15 S 48 25W
Canelli, *Italy* . . . . **44 D5** 44 43N 8 17 E
Canelones, *Uruguay* . . **175 C4** 34 32 S 56 17W
Canet-Plage, *France* . . **28 F7** 42 41N 3 2 E
Cañete, *Chile* . . . . **174 D1** 37 50 S 73 30W
Cañete, *Peru* . . . . **172 C2** 13 8 S 76 30W
Cañete, *Spain* **40 E3** 40 3N 1 54W
Cañete de las Torres, *Spain* **43 H6** 37 53N 4 19W
Cangamba, *Angola* . . . **115 E3** 13 40 S 19 54 E
Cangandala, *Angola* . . **115 D3** 9 45 S 16 33 E
Cangandala △, *Angola* **115 D3** 9 53 S 16 42 E
Cangas, *Spain* **42 C2** 42 16N 8 47W
Cangas de Narcea, *Spain* **42 B4** 43 10N 6 32W
Cangas de Onís, *Spain* **42 B5** 43 21N 5 8W
Cangas de Tineo = Cangas de Narcea, *Spain* **42 B4** 43 10N 6 32W
Cangnan, *China* . . . . . . **77 D13** 27 30N 120 23 E
Cangoa, *Angola* . . . . . . **115 E3** 13 8 S 18 30 E
Cangola, *Angola* . . . . . **115 D3** 7 58 S 15 53 E
Cangolo, *Angola* . . . . . **115 E2** 15 0 S 13 52 E
Cangombe, *Angola* . . . **115 E3** 14 24 S 19 59 E
Cangongo, *Angola* . . . **115 D3** 9 24 S 17 30 E
Canguaretama, *Brazil* **170 C4** 6 20 S 35 5W
Canguçu, *Brazil* . . . . . **175 C5** 31 22 S 52 43W
Canguçu, Serra do, *Brazil* . . . . **175 C5** 31 20 S 52 40W
Cangumbe, *Angola* . . . **115 E3** 11 58 S 19 12 E
Cangwu, *China* . . . . . . **77 F8** 23 25N 111 17 E
Cangxi, *China* . . . . **76 B5** 31 47N 105 59 E
Cangyuan, *China* . . . . **76 F2** 23 12N 99 14 E
Cangzhou, *China* . . . . . **74 E9** 38 19N 116 52 E
Canhoca, *Angola* . . . . . **115 D2** 9 15 S 14 41 E
Cani, I., *Tunisia* . . . . . **108 A2** 36 21N 10 5 E
Caniapiscau →, *Canada* **141 A6** 56 40N 69 30W
Caniapiscau, L. de, *Canada* **141 B6** 54 10N 69 55W
Canicattì, *Italy* . . . . . . **46 E6** 37 21N 13 51 E
Canicattini Bagni, *Italy* **47 E8** 37 2N 15 4 E
Canigao Channel, *Phil.* **81 F5** 10 15N 124 42 E
Caniles, *Spain* **43 H8** 37 26N 2 43W
Canim Lake, *Canada* . . **142 C4** 51 47N 120 54W
Canindé, *Brazil* . . . . . . **170 B4** 4 22 S 39 19W
Canindé →, *Brazil* . . . **170 C3** 6 15 S 42 52W
Canindeyu ☐, *Paraguay* **175 A5** 24 10 S 55 0W
Canino, *Italy* . . . . **45 F8** 42 28N 11 45 E
Canisteo, *U.S.A.* **150 D7** 42 16N 77 36W
Canisteo →, *U.S.A.* . . **150 D7** 42 7N 77 8W
Cañitas, *Mexico* **162 C4** 23 36N 102 43W
Cañizal, *Spain* **42 D5** 41 12N 5 22W
Canjáyar, *Spain* **43 H8** 37 1N 2 44W
Canjinge, *Angola* . . . . . **115 E4** 10 12 S 21 17 E
Çankırı, *Turkey* . . . . . . **100 B5** 40 40N 33 37 E
Cankuzo, *Burundi* . . . . **118 C3** 3 10 S 30 31 E
Canlaon, *Phil.* . . . . **81 F4** 10 22N 123 12 E
Canlaon Volcano, *Phil.* **81 F4** 10 25N 123 8 E
Canmore, *Canada* **142 C5** 51 7N 115 18W
Cann River, *Australia* . **129 D8** 37 35 S 149 7 E
Canna, *U.K.* **22 D2** 57 3N 6 33W
Cannanore, *India* . . . . **95 J2** 11 53N 75 27 E
Cannanore Is., *India* . . **95 J1** 10 30N 72 30 E
Cannelton, *U.S.A.* **157 G10** 37 55N 86 45W
Cannes, *France* . . . . . . **29 E11** 43 32N 7 1 E
Canning Town = Port Canning, *India* . . . . . **93 H13** 22 23N 88 40 E
Cannington, *Canada* . . **150 B5** 44 20N 79 2W
Cannóbio, *Italy* . . . . . . **44 B5** 46 4N 8 42 E
Cannock, *U.K.* **21 E5** 52 41N 2 1W
Cannonball →, *U.S.A.* . **154 B4** 46 20N 100 38W
Cannondale Mt., *Australia* . . . . **126 D4** 25 13 S 148 57 E
Cannonsville Reservoir, *U.S.A.* **151 D9** 42 4N 75 22W
Cannonvale, *Australia* **126 J6** 20 17 S 148 43 E
Caño Colorado, *Colombia* **168 C4** 2 18N 68 22W
Canoas, *Brazil* . . . . **175 B5** 29 56 S 51 11W
Canoe L., *Canada* **143 B7** 55 10N 108 15W
Cañon City, *U.S.A.* . . . **154 F2** 38 27N 105 14W
Cañón de Río Blanco △, *Mexico* . . **163 D5** 18 43N 97 15W
Cañón del Río Lobos △, *Spain* **42 D7** 41 46N 3 28W
Cañón del Sumidero △, *Mexico* **163 D5** 19 22N 96 24W
Canonniers Pt., *Mauritius* . . . . **121 d** 20 2 S 57 32 E
Canoochee →, *U.S.A.* . **152 D8** 31 59N 81 19W
Canopus, *Australia* . . . **128 B4** 33 29 S 140 42 E
Canora, *Canada* **143 C8** 51 40N 102 30W
Canosa di Púglia, *Italy* **47 A9** 41 13N 16 4 E
Canowindra, *Australia* **129 B8** 33 35 S 148 38 E
Canso, *Canada* **141 C7** 45 20N 61 0W
Canta, *Peru* . . . . **172 C2** 11 29 S 76 37W
Cantabria ☐, *Spain* . . . **42 B7** 43 10N 4 0W
Cantabria, Sierra de, *Spain* **40 C2** 42 40N 2 30W
Cantabrian Mts. = Cantábrica, Cordillera, *Spain* . . . **42 C5** 43 0N 5 10W
Cantábrica, Cordillera, *Spain* **42 C5** 43 0N 5 10W
Cantal ☐, *France* . . . . . **28 C6** 45 5N 2 45 E
Cantal, Plomb du, *France* . . . . **28 C6** 45 3N 2 45 E
Cantanhede, *Portugal* . **42 E2** 40 20N 8 36W
Cantaura, *Venezuela* . . **169 B5** 9 19N 64 21W
Cantavieja, *Spain* **40 E4** 40 31N 0 25W
Čantavir, *Serbia & M.* . **52 E4** 45 55N 19 46 E
Cantemir, *Moldova* . . . **53 D13** 46 17N 28 14 E
Canterbury = Invermere, *Canada* . . . **142 C5** 50 30N 116 2W
Canterbury, *Australia* . **126 D3** 25 23 S 141 53 E
Canterbury, *U.K.* . . . . . **21 F9** 51 16N 1 6 E
Canterbury ☐, *N.Z.* . . . **131 D6** 43 45 S 171 19 E
Canterbury Bight, *N.Z.* **131 E6** 44 16 S 171 55 E
Canterbury Plains, *N.Z.* **131 D6** 43 55 S 171 22 E
Cantil, *U.S.A.* **161 K9** 35 18N 117 58W

Cantilan, *Phil.* 81 G5 9 20N 125 58 E
Cantillana, *Spain* 43 H5 37 36N 5 50W
Canto do Buriti, *Brazil* 170 C3 8 7 S 42 58W
Canton = Guangzhou, *China* 77 F9 23 5N 113 10 E
Canton, *Ga., U.S.A.* 149 H3 34 14N 84 29W
Canton, *Ill., U.S.A.* 156 D6 40 33N 90 2W
Canton, *Miss., U.S.A.* 155 J9 32 37N 90 2W
Canton, *Mo., U.S.A.* 156 D5 40 8N 91 32W
Canton, *N.Y., U.S.A.* 151 B9 44 36N 75 10W
Canton, *Ohio, U.S.A.* 150 F3 40 48N 81 23W
Canton, *Pa., U.S.A.* 150 E8 41 39N 76 51W
Canton, *S. Dak., U.S.A.* 154 D6 43 18N 96 35W
Canton L., *U.S.A.* 155 G5 36 6N 98 35W
Cantonment, *U.S.A.* 153 E2 30 37N 87 20W
Cantù, *Italy* 44 C6 45 44N 9 8 E
Cantwell, *U.S.A.* 144 E10 63 24N 148 57W
Canudos, *Brazil* 173 B6 7 13 S 58 5W
Canumã, *Amazonas, Brazil* 169 D6 4 2 S 59 4W
Canumã, *Amazonas, Brazil* 173 B5 6 8 S 60 10W
Canumã →, *Brazil* 173 A6 3 55 S 59 10W
Canunda △, *Australia* 128 D4 37 42 S 140 16 E
Canutama, *Brazil* 173 B5 6 30 S 64 20W
Canutillo, *U.S.A.* 159 L10 31 55N 106 36W
Canvey, *U.K.* 21 F8 51 31N 0 37 E
Canyon, *U.S.A.* 155 H4 34 59N 101 55W
Canyon De Chelly ⌂, *U.S.A.* 159 H9 36 10N 109 20W
Canyon of the Ancients ⌂, *U.S.A.* 159 H9 37 30N 108 50W
Canyonlands △, *U.S.A.* 159 G9 38 15N 110 0W
Canyonville, *U.S.A.* 158 E2 42 56N 123 17W
Canzar, *Angola* 115 D4 7 35 S 21 34 E
Cao Bang, *Vietnam* 76 F6 22 40N 106 15 E
Cao He →, *China* 75 D13 40 10N 124 32 E
Cao Lanh, *Vietnam* 87 G5 10 27N 105 38 E
Cao Xian, *China* 74 G8 34 50N 115 35 E
Caombo, *Angola* 115 D3 8 42 S 16 33 E
Cáorle, *Italy* 45 C9 45 36N 12 53 E
Cap-aux-Meules, *Canada* 141 C7 47 23N 61 52W
Cap-Chat, *Canada* 141 C6 49 6N 66 40W
Cap-de-la-Madeleine, *Canada* 140 C5 46 22N 72 31W
Cap-Haïtien, *Haiti* 165 C5 19 40N 72 20W
Cap I., *Phil.* 81 J3 5 57N 120 6 E
Cap Pt., *St. Lucia* 165 f 14 7N 60 57W
Capac, *U.S.A.* 150 C2 43 1N 82 56W
Capáccio, *Italy* 47 B8 40 25N 15 5 E
Capaci, *Italy* 46 D6 38 10N 13 14 E
Capaia, *Angola* 115 D4 8 27 S 20 13 E
Capalonga, *Phil.* 80 D4 14 20N 122 30 E
Capanaparo →, *Venezuela* 168 B4 7 1N 67 7W
Capanema, *Brazil* 170 B2 1 12 S 47 11W
Capangombe, *Angola* 115 F2 15 6 S 13 8 E
Capánnori, *Italy* 44 E7 43 50N 10 34 E
Caparaó △, *Brazil* 171 F3 20 25 S 41 46W
Caparo →, *Barinas, Venezuela* 168 B3 7 46N 70 23W
Caparo →, *Bolívar, Venezuela* 169 B5 7 30N 64 0W
Capatárida, *Venezuela* 168 A3 11 11N 70 37W
Capayas, *Phil.* 81 F2 10 28N 119 39 E
Capbreton, *France* 28 E2 43 39N 1 26W
Capdenac, *France* 28 D6 44 34N 2 5 E
Capdepera, *Spain* 38 B4 39 42N 3 26 E
Cape →, *Australia* 126 C4 20 59 S 146 51 E
Cape Arid △, *Australia* 125 F3 33 58 S 123 13 E
Cape Barren I., *Australia* 127 G4 40 25 S 148 15 E
Cape Basin, *Atl. Oc.* 8 K12 34 0 S 7 0W
Cape Breton Highlands △, *Canada* 141 C7 46 50N 60 40W
Cape Breton I., *Canada* 141 C7 46 0N 60 30W
Cape Canaveral, *U.S.A.* 153 G9 28 24N 80 36W
Cape Charles, *U.S.A.* 148 G8 37 16N 76 1W
Cape Coast, *Ghana* 113 D4 5 5N 1 15W
Cape Cod ⌂, *U.S.A.* 148 E10 41 56N 70 6W
Cape Coral, *U.S.A.* 153 J8 26 33N 81 57W
Cape Dorset, *Canada* 139 B12 64 14N 76 32W
Cape Fear →, *U.S.A.* 149 H6 33 53N 78 1W
Cape Girardeau, *U.S.A.* 155 G10 37 19N 89 32W
Cape Hatteras ⌂, *U.S.A.* 149 H8 35 30N 75 28W
Cape Jervis, *Australia* 128 C3 35 40 S 138 5 E
Cape Krusenstern ⌂, *U.S.A.* 144 C7 67 30N 163 30W
Cape Lee △, *Australia* 125 F3 33 54 S 122 26 E
Cape Lisburne = Wevok, *U.S.A.* 144 B6 68 53N 166 13W
Cape Lookout ⌂, *U.S.A.* 149 H7 35 45N 76 25W
Cape May, *U.S.A.* 148 F8 38 56N 74 56W
Cape May Point, *U.S.A.* 147 C12 38 56N 74 58W
Cape Melville △, *Australia* 126 A3 14 26 S 144 28 E
Cape Mount △, *Liberia* 112 D2 6 44N 11 24W
Cape Peninsula △, *S. Africa* 116 E2 34 20 S 18 28 E
Cape Pole, *U.S.A.* 144 J14 55 58N 133 48W
Cape Range △, *Australia* 124 D1 22 3 S 114 0 E
Cape Tormentine, *Canada* 141 C7 46 8N 63 47W
Cape Town, *S. Africa* 116 E2 33 55 S 18 22 E
Cape Tribulation △, *Australia* 126 B4 16 5 S 145 25 E
Cape Verde Is. ■, *Atl. Oc.* 8 E9 16 0N 24 0W
Cape Vincent, *U.S.A.* 151 B8 44 8N 76 20W
Cape Yakataga, *U.S.A.* 144 F12 60 4N 142 26W
Cape York Peninsula, *Australia* 126 A3 12 0 S 142 30 E
Capela, *Brazil* 170 D4 10 30 S 37 0W
Capela de Campo, *Brazil* 170 B3 4 40 S 41 55W
Capelas, *Azores* 9 d3 37 50N 25 41W
Capele, *Angola* 115 E2 13 39 S 14 53 E
Capelengue, *Angola* 115 D3 8 53 S 19 42 E
Capelinha, *Brazil* 171 E3 17 42 S 42 31W
Capelinhos, Pta. dos, *Azores* 9 d1 38 36N 28 50W
Capella, *Australia* 126 C4 23 2 S 148 1 E
Capella, Mt., *Papua N. G.* 132 C1 5 4 S 141 8 E
Capelongo, *Angola* 115 E3 14 54 S 15 8 E
Capenda Camulemba, *Angola* 115 D3 9 24 S 18 27 E
Capendu, *France* 28 E6 43 11N 2 31 E
Capertree, *Australia* 129 B8 33 6 S 149 58 E
Capestang, *France* 28 E7 43 20N 3 2 E
Capesterre-Belle-Eau, *Guadeloupe* 164 b 16 4N 61 36W
Capesterre-de-Marie-Galante, *Guadeloupe* 164 b 15 53N 61 14W
Capim, *Brazil* 170 B2 1 41 S 47 47W
Capim →, *Brazil* 170 B2 1 40 S 47 47W
Capinópolis, *Brazil* 171 E2 18 41 S 49 35W
Capinota, *Bolivia* 172 D4 17 43 S 66 14W
Capira, *Panama* 168 B2 8 45N 79 53W
Capistrello, *Italy* 45 G10 41 57N 13 23 E
Capitan, *U.S.A.* 159 K11 33 35N 105 35W
Capitán Aracena, I., *Chile* 176 D2 54 10 S 71 20W
Capitán Arturo Prat, *Antarctica* 7 C17 63 0 S 61 0W
Capitán Pastene, *Chile* 176 A2 38 13 S 73 1W
Capitol Reef △, *U.S.A.* 159 G8 38 15N 111 10W
Capitola, *U.S.A.* 160 J5 36 59N 121 57W
Capivara, Serra da, *Brazil* 171 D3 14 35 S 45 0W
Capiz □, *Phil.* 81 F4 11 35N 122 30 E
Capizzi, *Italy* 47 E7 37 51N 14 29 E
Capoche →, *Mozam.* 119 F3 15 35 S 33 0 E
Capodichino, Nápoli ✕ (NAP), *Italy* 47 B7 40 53N 14 16 E
Capoeira, *Brazil* 173 B6 5 37 S 59 33W
Capolo, *Angola* 115 E2 10 22 S 14 7 E
Caporetto = Kobarid, *Slovenia* 45 B10 46 15N 13 30 E
Caporolo →, *Angola* 115 E2 12 56 S 12 58 E
Capoterra, *Italy* 46 C1 39 11N 8 58 E
Cappadocia, *Turkey* 100 C6 39 0N 35 0 E
Capps, *U.S.A.* 152 E6 30 24N 83 54W
Capraia, *Italy* 44 E6 43 2N 9 50 E
Caprara, Pta., *Italy* 46 A1 41 7N 8 19 E
Caprarola, *Italy* 45 F9 42 19N 12 14 E
Capreol, *Canada* 140 C3 46 43N 80 56W
Caprera, *Italy* 46 A2 41 12N 9 28 E
Capri, *Italy* 47 B7 40 33N 14 14 E
Capricorn Group, *Australia* 126 C5 23 30 S 151 55 E
Capricorn Ra., *Australia* 124 D2 23 20 S 116 50 E
Caprino Veronese, *Italy* 44 C7 45 36N 10 47 E
Caprivi Game ⌂, *Namibia* 116 B3 17 55 S 22 37 E
Caprivi Strip, *Namibia* 116 B3 18 0 S 23 0 E
Caps et Marais d'Opale ⌂, *France* 27 B9 50 40N 2 0 E
Captain Cook, *U.S.A.* 145 D6 19 30N 155 55W
Captain's Flat, *Australia* 129 C8 35 35 S 149 27 E
Captieux, *France* 28 D3 44 18N 0 16W
Captiva, *U.S.A.* 153 J7 26 31N 82 11W
Capuça, *Angola* 115 F4 17 22 S 21 18 E
Capul I., *Phil.* 80 E5 12 26N 124 10 E
Capulin Volcano ⌂, *U.S.A.* 155 G3 36 47N 103 58W
Capunda, *Angola* 115 E3 10 41 S 17 23 E
Caquetá □, *Colombia* 168 C3 1 0N 74 0W
Caquetá →, *Colombia* 168 D4 1 15 S 69 15W
Car Nicobar, *India* 95 K11 9 10N 92 47 E
Carabao I., *Phil.* 80 E3 12 4N 121 56 E
Carabobo □, *Venezuela* 168 A4 10 10N 68 5W
Caracal, *Romania* 53 F9 44 8N 24 22 E
Caracaraí, *Brazil* 169 C5 1 50N 61 8W
Caracas, *Venezuela* 168 A4 10 30N 66 55W
Caracol, *Mato Grosso do Sul, Brazil* 174 A4 22 18 S 57 1W
Caracol, *Piauí, Brazil* 170 C3 9 15 S 43 22W
Caracollo, *Bolivia* 172 D4 17 39 S 67 10W
Caraga, *Phil.* 81 H6 7 20N 126 34 E
Caragabal, *Australia* 129 B7 33 49 S 147 45 E
Caráglio, *Italy* 44 D4 44 25N 7 26 E
Carahue, *Chile* 176 A2 38 43 S 73 12W
Caraí, *Brazil* 171 E3 17 12 S 41 42W
Carajás, *Brazil* 170 C1 2 57 S 51 22W
Carajás, Serra dos, *Brazil* 170 C1 6 0 S 51 30W
Caramoan, *Phil.* 80 E4 13 46N 123 52 E
Caramoran, *Phil.* 80 D5 14 0N 124 8 E
Caranapatuba, *Brazil* 173 B5 6 38 S 62 34W
Carandaiti, *Bolivia* 173 E5 20 45 S 63 4W
Carangola, *Brazil* 171 F3 20 44 S 42 5W
Caransebeş, *Romania* 52 E7 45 28N 22 18 E
Carantec, *France* 26 D3 48 40N 3 55W
Caraparaná →, *Colombia* 168 D3 1 45 S 73 13W
Caraquet, *Canada* 141 C6 47 48N 64 57W
Caraş, *Peru* 172 B2 9 3 S 77 47W
Caraş Severin □, *Romania* 52 E7 45 10N 22 10 E
Caraşova, *Romania* 52 E6 45 11N 21 51 E
Caratasca, L., *Honduras* 164 C3 15 20N 83 40W
Caratinga, *Brazil* 171 E3 19 50 S 42 10W
Carauaí, *Brazil* 168 D4 4 52 S 66 54W
Caraúbas, *Brazil* 170 C4 5 43 S 37 33W
Caravaca de la Cruz, *Spain* 41 G3 38 8N 1 52W
Caravággio, *Italy* 44 C6 45 30N 9 38 E
Caravela, *Guinea-Biss.* 112 C1 11 30N 16 30W
Caravelas, *Brazil* 171 E4 17 45 S 39 15W
Caraveli, *Peru* 172 D3 15 45 S 73 25W
Caravelle, Presqu'île de la, *Martinique* 164 c 14 46N 60 48W
Caràzinho, *Brazil* 175 B5 28 16 S 52 46W
Carballino = O Carballiño, *Spain* 42 C2 42 26N 8 5W
Carballo, *Spain* 42 B2 43 13N 8 41W
Carberry, *Canada* 143 D9 49 50N 99 25W
Carbó, *Mexico* 162 B2 29 42N 110 58W
Carbonara, C., *Italy* 46 C2 39 6N 9 31 E
Carbondale, *Colo., U.S.A.* 158 G10 39 24N 107 13W
Carbondale, *Ill., U.S.A.* 155 G10 37 44N 89 13W
Carbondale, *Pa., U.S.A.* 151 E9 41 35N 75 30W
Carbonear, *Canada* 141 C9 47 42N 53 13W
Carboneras, *Spain* 41 J3 36 59N 1 53W
Carboneras de Guadazaón, *Spain* 40 F3 39 54N 1 50W
Carbónia, *Italy* 46 C1 39 10N 8 30 E
Carcabuey, *Spain* 43 H6 37 27N 4 17W
Carcagente = Carcaixent, *Spain* 41 F4 39 8N 0 28W
Carcaixent, *Spain* 41 F4 39 8N 0 28W
Carcajou, *Canada* 142 B5 57 47N 117 6W
Carcar, *Phil.* 81 F4 10 6N 123 38 E
Carcarana →, *Argentina* 174 C3 32 27 S 60 48W
Carcasse, C., *Haiti* 165 C5 18 30N 74 28W
Carcassonne, *France* 28 E6 43 13N 2 20 E
Carchi □, *Ecuador* 168 C2 0 45N 78 0W
Carcoar, *Australia* 129 B8 33 36 S 149 8 E
Carcross, *Canada* 142 A2 60 13N 134 45W
Çardak, *Çanakkale, Turkey* 51 F10 40 22N 26 43 E
Çardak, *Denizli, Turkey* 49 D11 37 49N 29 39 E
Cardamon Hills, *India* 95 K3 9 30N 77 15 E
Cardeña, *Spain* 43 G6 38 16N 4 20W
Cárdenas, *Cuba* 164 B3 23 0N 81 30W
Cárdenas, *San Luis Potosí, Mexico* 163 C5 22 0N 99 41W
Cárdenas, *Tabasco, Mexico* 163 D6 17 59N 93 21W
Cardenete, *Spain* 40 F3 39 46N 1 41W
Cardiel, L., *Argentina* 176 C2 48 55 S 71 10W
Cardiff, *U.K.* 21 F4 51 29N 3 10W
Cardiff □, *U.K.* 21 F4 51 31N 3 12W
Cardiff-by-the-Sea, *U.S.A.* 161 M9 33 1N 117 17W
Cardigan, *U.K.* 21 E3 52 5N 4 40W
Cardigan B., *U.K.* 21 E3 52 30N 4 30W
Cardinal, *Canada* 151 B9 44 47N 75 23W
Cardón, Punta, *Venezuela* 168 A3 11 37N 70 14W
Cardona, *Spain* 40 D6 41 56N 1 40 E
Cardona, *Uruguay* 174 C4 33 53 S 57 18W
Cardoner →, *Spain* 40 D6 41 41N 1 51 E
Cardoso, Ilha do, *Brazil* 175 B5 25 8 S 47 58W
Cardston, *Canada* 142 D6 49 15N 113 20W
Cardwell, *Australia* 126 B4 18 14 S 146 2 E
Careen L., *Canada* 143 B7 57 0N 108 11W
Carei, *Romania* 52 C7 47 40N 22 29 E
Careiro, *Brazil* 169 D6 3 12 S 59 45W
Careme = Ciremay, *Indonesia* 85 D3 6 55 S 108 27 E
Carentan, *France* 26 C5 49 19N 1 15W
Carey, *Idaho, U.S.A.* 158 E7 43 19N 113 57W
Carey, *Ohio, U.S.A.* 157 D13 40 57N 83 23W
Carey, L., *Australia* 125 E3 29 0 S 122 15 E
Carey L., *Canada* 143 A8 62 12N 102 55W
Careysburg, *Liberia* 112 D2 6 34N 10 30W
Cargados Garajos, *Ind. Oc.* 121 F4 17 0 S 59 0 E
Cargèse, *France* 29 F12 42 7N 8 35 E
Carhaix-Plouguer, *France* 26 D3 48 18N 3 36W
Carhuamayo, *Peru* 172 C2 10 51 S 76 4W
Carhuas, *Peru* 172 B2 9 15 S 77 39W
Carhué, *Argentina* 174 D3 37 10 S 62 50W
Caria, *Turkey* 49 D10 37 20N 28 10 E
Cariacica, *Brazil* 171 F3 20 16 S 40 25W
Cariaco, *Venezuela* 169 A5 10 29N 63 33W
Cariango, *Angola* 115 E3 10 37 S 15 20 E
Cariati, *Italy* 47 C9 39 30N 16 57 E
Caribbean Sea, *W. Indies* 165 D5 15 0N 75 0W
Cariboo Mts., *Canada* 142 C4 53 0N 121 0W
Caribou, *U.S.A.* 149 B12 46 52N 68 1W
Caribou →, *Man., Canada* 143 B10 59 20N 94 44W
Caribou →, *N.W.T., Canada* 142 A3 61 27N 125 45W
Caribou I., *Canada* 140 C2 47 22N 85 49W
Caribou Is., *Canada* 142 A6 61 55N 113 15W
Caribou L., *Man., Canada* 143 B9 59 21N 96 10W
Caribou L., *Ont., Canada* 140 B2 50 25N 89 5W
Caribou Mts., *Canada* 142 B5 59 12N 115 40W
Caribou River ⌂, *Canada* 143 B9 59 35N 96 35W
Caribrod = Dimitrovgrad, *Serbia & M.* 50 C6 43 2N 22 48 E
Carichic, *Mexico* 162 B3 27 56N 107 3W
Carigara, *Phil.* 81 F5 11 18N 124 41 E
Carignan, *France* 27 C12 49 38N 5 10 E
Carignano, *Italy* 44 D4 44 55N 7 40 E
Carillo, *Mexico* 162 B4 26 50N 103 55W
Carin, *Somali Rep.* 120 B3 10 59N 49 13 E
Carinda, *Australia* 129 A7 30 28 S 147 41 E
Cariñena, *Spain* 40 D3 41 20N 1 13W
Carinhanha, *Brazil* 171 D3 14 15 S 44 46W
Carinhanha →, *Brazil* 171 D3 14 20 S 43 47W
Carini, *Italy* 46 D6 38 8N 13 11 E
Cariño, *Spain* 42 B3 43 45N 7 52W
Carínola, *Italy* 46 A6 41 11N 13 58 E
Carinthia = Kärnten □, *Austria* 34 E6 46 52N 13 30 E
Caripito, *Venezuela* 169 A5 10 8N 63 6W
Cariré, *Brazil* 170 B3 3 57 S 40 27W
Caritianas, *Brazil* 173 B5 9 20 S 63 6W
Carles, *Phil.* 81 F4 11 34N 123 8 E
Carlet, *Spain* 41 F4 39 14N 0 31W
Carleton, Mt., *Canada* 141 C6 47 23N 66 53W
Carleton Place, *Canada* 140 C4 45 8N 76 9W
Carletonville, *S. Africa* 116 D4 26 23 S 27 22 E
Cârlibaba, *Romania* 53 C10 47 35N 25 8 E
Carlin, *U.S.A.* 158 F5 40 43N 116 7W
Carlingford L., *U.K.* 23 B5 54 3N 6 9W
Carlinville, *U.S.A.* 156 E7 39 17N 89 53W
Carlisle, *U.K.* 20 C5 54 54N 2 56W
Carlisle, *Ind., U.S.A.* 157 F9 38 58N 87 24W
Carlisle, *Ky., U.S.A.* 157 F12 38 19N 84 1W
Carlisle, *Pa., U.S.A.* 150 F7 40 12N 77 12W
Carlisle B., *Barbados* 165 g 13 5N 59 37W
Carlisle I., *Australia* 126 J7 20 49 S 149 18 E
Carlit, Pic, *France* 28 F5 42 35N 1 55 E
Carloforte, *Italy* 46 C1 39 8N 8 18 E
Carlos Casares, *Argentina* 174 D3 35 32 S 61 20W
Carlos Chagas, *Brazil* 171 E3 17 43 S 40 45W
Carlos Tejedor, *Argentina* 174 D3 35 25 S 62 25W
Carlow, *Ireland* 23 D5 52 50N 6 56W
Carlow □, *Ireland* 23 D5 52 43N 6 50W
Carlsbad = Karlovy Vary, *Czech Rep.* 34 A5 50 13N 12 51 E
Carlsbad, *Calif., U.S.A.* 161 M9 33 10N 117 21W
Carlsbad, *N. Mex., U.S.A.* 155 J2 32 25N 104 14W
Carlsbad Caverns △, *U.S.A.* 155 J2 32 10N 104 35W
Carlsberg Ridge, *Ind. Oc.* 121 D5 1 0N 66 0 E
Carluke, *U.K.* 22 F5 55 45N 3 50W
Carlyle, *Canada* 143 D8 49 40N 102 20W
Carlyle, *U.S.A.* 156 F7 38 37N 89 22W
Carlyle L., *U.S.A.* 156 F7 38 37N 89 21W
Carmacks, *Canada* 138 B6 62 5N 136 16W
Carmagnola, *Italy* 44 D4 44 51N 7 43 E
Carman, *Canada* 143 D9 49 30N 98 0W
Carmarthen, *U.K.* 21 F3 51 52N 4 19W
Carmarthen B., *U.K.* 21 F3 51 40N 4 30W
Carmarthenshire □, *U.K.* 21 F3 51 55N 4 13W
Carmaux, *France* 28 D6 44 3N 2 10 E
Carmel, *Ind., U.S.A.* 157 E10 39 59N 86 8W
Carmel, *N.Y., U.S.A.* 151 E11 41 26N 73 41W
Carmel-by-the-Sea, *U.S.A.* 160 J5 36 33N 121 55W
Carmel Valley, *U.S.A.* 160 J5 36 29N 121 43W
Carmelo, *Uruguay* 174 C4 34 0 S 58 20W
Carmen, *Bolivia* 172 C4 11 40 S 67 51W
Carmen, *Colombia* 168 B2 9 43N 75 8W
Carmen, *Paraguay* 175 B4 27 13 S 56 12W
Carmen, *Bohol, Phil.* 81 G5 9 50N 124 12 E
Carmen, *Cebu, Phil.* 81 F5 10 35N 124 1 E
Carmen, *Cotabato, Phil.* 81 H5 7 13N 124 45 E
Carmen, *Venezuela* 168 C4 1 16N 66 52W
Carmen →, *Mexico* 162 A3 30 42N 106 29W
Carmen, I., *Mexico* 162 B2 26 0N 111 20W
Carmen de Patagones, *Argentina* 176 B4 40 50 S 63 0W
Cármenes, *Spain* 42 C5 42 58N 5 34W
Carmensa, *Argentina* 174 D2 35 15 S 67 40W
Carmi, *Canada* 142 D5 49 36N 119 8W
Carmi, *U.S.A.* 157 F8 38 5N 88 10W
Carmichael, *U.S.A.* 160 G5 38 38N 121 19W
Carmichael Village, *Bahamas* 9 b 25 0N 77 26W
Carmila, *Australia* 126 C4 21 55 S 149 24 E
Carmona, *Costa Rica* 164 E2 10 0N 85 15W
Carmona, *Spain* 43 H5 37 28N 5 42W
Carn Ban, *U.K.* 22 D4 57 7N 4 15W
Carn Eige, *U.K.* 22 D3 57 17N 5 8W
Carnac, *France* 25 C2 47 35N 3 6W
Carnamah, *Australia* 125 E2 29 41 S 115 53 E
Carnarvon, *Australia* 125 D1 24 51 S 113 42 E
Carnarvon, *S. Africa* 116 E3 30 56 S 22 8 E
Carnarvon △, *Australia* 126 C4 24 54 S 148 2 E
Carnarvon Ra., *Queens., Australia* 126 D4 25 15 S 148 30 E
Carnarvon Ra., *W. Austral., Australia* 125 E3 25 20 S 120 45 E
Carnatic, *India* 95 K3 9 40N 77 50 E
Carnation, *U.S.A.* 160 C5 47 39N 121 55W
Carndonagh, *Ireland* 23 A4 55 16N 7 15W
Carnduff, *Canada* 143 D8 49 10N 101 50W
Carnegie, *U.S.A.* 150 F4 40 24N 80 5W
Carnegie, L., *Australia* 125 E3 26 5 S 122 30 E
Carnegie Ridge, *Pac. Oc.* 135 H19 1 0 S 87 0W
Carnic Alps = Karnische Alpen, *Europe* 34 E6 46 36N 13 0 E
Carniche Alpi = Karnische Alpen, *Europe* 34 E6 46 36N 13 0 E
Carnot, *C.A.R.* 114 B3 4 59N 15 56 E
Carnot, C., *Australia* 127 E2 34 57 S 135 38 E
Carnot B., *Australia* 124 C3 17 20 S 122 15 E
Carnoustie, *U.K.* 22 E6 56 30N 2 42W
Carnsore Pt., *Ireland* 23 D5 52 10N 6 22W
Caro, *U.S.A.* 148 D4 43 29N 83 24W
Caroço, *São Tomé & Príncipe* 115 G6 1 32N 7 27 E
Carol City, *U.S.A.* 153 K9 25 56N 80 16W
Carolina, *Brazil* 170 C2 7 10 S 47 30W
Carolina, *Puerto Rico* 165 d 18 23N 65 58W
Carolina, *S. Africa* 117 D5 26 5 S 30 6 E
Caroline I., *Kiribati* 135 H12 9 58 S 150 13W
Caroline Is., *Micronesia* 62 J17 8 0N 150 0 E
Caroline Pk., *N.Z.* 131 F2 45 57 S 167 15 E
Carondelet, *Kiribati* 123 B16 5 33 S 173 50 E
Caroni, *Trin. & Tob.* 169 F9 10 34N 61 23W
Caroní →, *Venezuela* 169 B5 8 21N 62 43W
Caroníe = Nébrodi, Monti, *Italy* 47 E7 37 54N 14 35 E
Caroona, *Australia* 129 A9 31 24 S 150 26 E
Carora, *Venezuela* 168 A3 10 11N 70 5W
Carpathians, *Europe* 37 D11 49 30N 21 0 E
Carpaţii Meridionali, *Romania* 53 E9 45 30N 25 0 E
Carpentaria, G. of, *Australia* 126 A2 14 0 S 139 0 E
Carpentersville, *U.S.A.* 157 B8 42 6N 88 17W
Carpentras, *France* 29 D9 44 3N 5 2 E
Carpi, *Italy* 44 D7 44 47N 10 53 E
Carpina, *Brazil* 170 C4 7 51 S 35 15W
Cărpineni, *Moldova* 53 D13 46 46N 28 22 E
Carpinteria, *U.S.A.* 161 L7 34 24N 119 31W
Carpio, *Spain* 42 D5 41 13N 5 7W
Carr Boyd Ra., *Australia* 124 C4 16 15 S 128 35 E
Carrabelle, *U.S.A.* 152 F5 29 51N 84 40W
Carral, *Spain* 42 B2 43 14N 8 21W
Carranglan, *Phil.* 80 D3 15 58N 121 4 E
Carranza, Presa V., *Mexico* 162 B4 27 20N 100 50W
Carrara, *Italy* 44 D7 44 5N 10 6 E
Carrascal, *Phil.* 81 G5 9 22N 125 56 E
Carrasco △, *Bolivia* 173 D5 17 23 S 64 59W
Carrascosa del Campo, *Spain* 40 E2 40 2N 2 45W
Carrauntoohill, *Ireland* 23 D2 52 0N 9 45W
Carretas, Punta, *Peru* 172 C2 14 12 S 76 17W
Carrick-on-Shannon, *Ireland* 23 C3 53 57N 8 5W
Carrick-on-Suir, *Ireland* 23 D4 52 21N 7 24W
Carrickfergus, *U.K.* 23 B6 54 43N 5 49W
Carrickmacross, *Ireland* 23 C5 53 59N 6 43W
Carrieton, *Australia* 128 B3 32 25 S 138 31 E
Carrington, *U.S.A.* 154 B5 47 27N 99 8W
Carrión →, *Spain* 42 D6 41 53N 4 32W
Carrión de los Condes, *Spain* 42 C6 42 20N 4 37W
Carrizal Bajo, *Chile* 174 B1 28 5 S 71 20W
Carrizalillo, *Chile* 174 B1 29 5 S 71 30W
Carrizo Cr. →, *U.S.A.* 155 G3 36 55N 103 55W
Carrizo Plain ⌂, *U.S.A.* 160 K7 35 12N 119 48W
Carrizo Springs, *U.S.A.* 155 L5 28 31N 99 52W
Carrizozo, *U.S.A.* 159 K11 33 38N 105 53W
Carroll, *U.S.A.* 156 B2 42 4N 94 52W
Carrollton, *Ga., U.S.A.* 152 B4 33 35N 85 5W
Carrollton, *Ill., U.S.A.* 156 E6 39 18N 90 24W
Carrollton, *Ky., U.S.A.* 157 F11 38 41N 85 11W
Carrollton, *Mo., U.S.A.* 156 E3 39 22N 93 30W
Carrollton, *Ohio, U.S.A.* 150 F3 40 34N 81 5W
Carron →, *U.K.* 22 D4 57 53N 4 22W
Carron, L., *U.K.* 22 D3 57 22N 5 35W
Carrot →, *Canada* 143 C8 53 50N 101 17W
Carrot River, *Canada* 143 C8 53 17N 103 35W
Carrouges, *France* 26 D6 48 34N 0 10W
Carrù, *Italy* 44 D4 44 29N 7 52 E
Carruthers, *Canada* 143 C7 52 52N 109 16W
Carsa Dek, *Ethiopia* 107 F4 5 13N 39 50 E
Çarşamba, *Turkey* 100 B7 41 11N 36 44 E
Carsóli, *Italy* 45 F10 42 6N 13 5 E
Carson, *Calif., U.S.A.* 161 M8 33 48N 118 17W
Carson, *N. Dak., U.S.A.* 154 B4 46 25N 101 34W
Carson →, *U.S.A.* 160 F8 39 45N 118 40W
Carson City, *Mich., U.S.A.* 157 A12 43 11N 84 51W
Carson City, *Nev., U.S.A.* 160 F7 39 10N 119 46W
Carson Sink, *U.S.A.* 158 G4 39 50N 118 25W
Carstensz Pyramid = Jaya, Puncak, *Indonesia* 83 B5 3 57 S 137 17 E
Cartagena, *Colombia* 168 A2 10 25N 75 33W
Cartagena, *Spain* 41 H4 37 38N 0 59W
Cartago, *Colombia* 168 C2 4 45N 75 55W
Cartago, *Costa Rica* 164 E3 9 50N 83 55W
Cártama, *Spain* 43 J6 36 43N 4 39W
Cartaxo, *Portugal* 43 F2 39 10N 8 47W
Cartaya, *Spain* 43 H3 37 16N 7 9W
Cartersville, *U.S.A.* 152 A5 34 10N 84 48W
Carterton, *N.Z.* 130 H4 41 2 S 175 31 E
Carterville, *U.S.A.* 156 G7 37 46N 89 5W
Carthage, *Tunisia* 46 F3 36 50N 10 21 E
Carthage, *Ill., U.S.A.* 156 D5 40 25N 91 8W
Carthage, *Mo., U.S.A.* 155 G7 37 11N 94 19W
Carthage, *N.Y., U.S.A.* 148 D8 43 59N 75 37W
Carthage, *Tex., U.S.A.* 155 J7 32 9N 94 20W
Cartier I., *Australia* 124 B3 12 31 S 123 29 E
Cartwright, *Canada* 141 B8 53 41N 56 58W
Caruaru, *Brazil* 170 C4 8 15 S 35 55W
Carúpano, *Venezuela* 169 A5 10 39N 63 15W
Caruray, *Phil.* 81 F2 10 20N 119 0 E
Carutapera, *Brazil* 170 B2 1 13 S 46 1W
Caruthersville, *U.S.A.* 155 G10 36 11N 89 39W
Carvalho, *Brazil* 169 D7 2 16 S 51 29W
Carvin, *France* 27 B9 50 30N 2 57 E
Carvoeiro, *Brazil* 169 D5 1 30 S 61 59W
Carvoeiro, C., *Portugal* 43 F1 39 21N 9 24W
Cary, *Ill., U.S.A.* 157 B8 42 13N 88 14W
Cary, *N.C., U.S.A.* 149 H6 35 47N 78 46W
Casa, Pas de la = Envalira, Port d', *Europe* 40 C6 42 33N 1 43 E
Casa Branca, *Brazil* 171 F2 21 46 S 47 4W
Casa Branca, *Portugal* 43 G2 38 29N 8 12W
Casa Grande, *U.S.A.* 159 K8 32 53N 111 45W
Casablanca, *Chile* 174 C1 33 20 S 71 25W
Casablanca, *Morocco* 110 B3 33 36N 7 36W
Casacalenda, *Italy* 45 G11 41 44N 14 51 E
Casalbordino, *Italy* 45 F11 42 9N 14 35 E
Casale Monferrato, *Italy* 44 C5 45 8N 8 27 E
Casalmaggiore, *Italy* 44 D7 44 59N 10 26 E
Casalpusterlengo, *Italy* 44 C6 45 11N 9 39 E
Casamance →, *Senegal* 112 C1 12 33N 16 46W
Casanare □, *Colombia* 168 B3 5 30N 72 0W
Casanare →, *Colombia* 168 B4 6 2N 69 51W
Casarano, *Italy* 47 B11 40 0N 18 10 E
Casares, *Spain* 43 J5 36 27N 5 16W
Casas Ibáñez, *Spain* 41 F3 39 17N 1 30W
Casasimarro, *Spain* 41 F2 39 22N 2 3W
Casatejada, *Spain* 42 F5 39 54N 5 40W
Casavieja, *Spain* 42 E6 40 17N 4 46W
Cascada de Basaseachic △, *Mexico* 162 B3 28 9N 108 15W
Cascade, *Seychelles* 121 b 4 39 S 55 29 E
Cascade, *Idaho, U.S.A.* 158 D5 44 31N 116 2W
Cascade, *Iowa, U.S.A.* 156 B6 42 18N 91 0W
Cascade, *Mont., U.S.A.* 158 C8 47 16N 111 42W
Cascade Locks, *U.S.A.* 160 E5 45 40N 121 54W
Cascade Pt., *N.Z.* 131 E3 44 1 S 168 20 E
Cascade Ra., *U.S.A.* 160 D5 47 0N 121 30W
Cascade Reservoir, *U.S.A.* 158 D5 44 32N 116 3W
Cascades, Pte. des, *Réunion* 121 c 21 9 S 55 51 E
Cascais, *Portugal* 43 G1 38 41N 9 25W
Cascavel, *Ceará, Brazil* 170 B4 4 7 S 38 14W
Cascavel, *Paraná, Brazil* 175 A5 24 57 S 53 28W
Cáscina, *Italy* 44 E7 43 41N 10 33 E
Casco B., *U.S.A.* 149 D10 43 45N 70 0W
Caselle Torinese, *Italy* 44 C4 45 10N 7 39 E
Caserta, *Italy* 47 A7 41 4N 14 20 E
Casey, *Antarctica* 7 C8 66 0 S 76 0 E
Casey, *U.S.A.* 157 E9 39 18N 87 59W
Caseyr, Raas = Asir, Ras, *Somali Rep.* 120 B4 11 55N 51 10 E
Cashel, *Ireland* 23 D4 52 30N 7 53W
Casibare →, *Colombia* 168 C3 3 48N 72 18W
Casiguran, *Phil.* 80 C4 16 22N 122 7 E
Casiguran Sound, *Phil.* 80 C3 16 6N 121 58 E
Casilda, *Argentina* 174 C3 33 10 S 61 10W
Casim = General Toshevo, *Bulgaria* 51 C12 43 42N 28 6 E
Casimcea, *Romania* 53 F13 44 45N 28 23 E
Casino, *Australia* 127 D5 28 52 S 153 3 E
Casiquiare →, *Venezuela* 168 C4 2 1N 67 7W
Casitas, *Peru* 172 A1 3 54 S 80 39W
Čáslav, *Czech Rep.* 34 B8 49 54N 15 22 E
Casma, *Peru* 172 B2 9 30 S 78 20W
Casmalia, *U.S.A.* 161 L6 34 50N 120 32W
Cásola Valsénio, *Italy* 45 D8 44 12N 11 40 E
Cásoli, *Italy* 45 F11 42 7N 14 18 E
Caspe, *Spain* 40 D4 41 14N 0 1W
Casper, *U.S.A.* 158 E10 42 51N 106 19W
Caspian Depression, *Eurasia* 61 G9 47 0N 48 0 E
Caspian Sea, *Eurasia* 57 F9 43 0N 50 0 E
Cass Lake, *U.S.A.* 154 B7 47 23N 94 37W
Cassà de la Selva, *Spain* 40 D7 41 53N 2 52 E
Cassadaga, *U.S.A.* 150 D5 42 20N 79 19W
Cassai, *Angola* 115 E4 10 33 S 21 59 E
Cassai →, *Angola* 115 E4 3 2 S 16 57 E
Cassamba, *Angola* 115 E4 13 6 S 20 18 E
Cassano allo Iónio, *Italy* 47 C9 39 47N 16 20 E
Cassel, *France* 27 B9 50 48N 2 30 E
Casselman, *Canada* 151 A9 45 19N 75 5W
Casselton, *U.S.A.* 154 B6 46 54N 97 13W
Cassiar, *Canada* 142 B3 59 16N 129 40W
Cassiar Mts., *Canada* 142 B2 59 30N 130 30W
Cassilândia, *Brazil* 173 D7 19 9 S 51 45W
Cassilis, *Australia* 129 B8 32 3 S 149 58 E
Cassinga, *Angola* 115 F3 15 5 S 16 4 E
Cassino, *Italy* 46 A6 41 30N 13 49 E
Cassis, *France* 29 E9 43 14N 5 32 E
Cassoalala, *Angola* 115 D2 9 30 S 14 22 E
Cassoango, *Angola* 115 E4 13 42 S 20 56 E
Cassongue, *Angola* 115 E3 11 53 S 15 2 E
Cassopolis, *U.S.A.* 157 C10 41 55N 86 1W
Cassunda, *Angola* 115 E4 10 57 S 21 3 E
Cassville, *Mo., U.S.A.* 155 G8 36 41N 93 52W
Cassville, *Wis., U.S.A.* 156 B6 42 43N 90 59W
Castagneto Carducci, *Italy* 44 E7 43 9N 10 36 E
Castaic, *U.S.A.* 161 L8 34 30N 118 38W
Castalia, *U.S.A.* 150 E2 41 24N 82 49W
Castanhal, *Brazil* 170 B2 1 18 S 47 55W
Castara, *Trin. & Tob.* 169 E10 11 17N 60 42W
Castasegna, *Switz.* 33 D9 46 20N 9 31 E
Castéggio, *Italy* 44 C6 45 0N 9 7 E
Castejón de Monegros, *Spain* 40 D4 41 37N 0 15W
Castèl di Sangro, *Italy* 45 G11 41 47N 14 6 E
Castèl San Giovanni, *Italy* 44 C6 45 4N 9 26 E
Castèl San Pietro Terme, *Italy* 45 D8 44 24N 11 35 E
Castelbuono, *Italy* 47 E7 37 56N 14 5 E
Castelfidardo, *Italy* 45 E10 43 28N 13 33 E
Castelfiorentino, *Italy* 44 E7 43 36N 10 58 E
Castelfranco Emília, *Italy* 44 D8 44 37N 11 3 E
Castelfranco Véneto, *Italy* 45 C8 45 40N 11 55 E
Casteljaloux, *France* 28 D4 44 19N 0 6 E
Castellabate, *Italy* 47 B7 40 17N 14 57 E
Castellammare, G. di, *Italy* 46 D5 38 8N 12 54 E
Castellammare del Golfo, *Italy* 46 D5 38 1N 12 53 E
Castellammare di Stábia, *Italy* 47 B7 40 42N 14 29 E
Castellamonte, *Italy* 44 C4 45 23N 7 42 E
Castellane, *France* 29 E10 43 50N 6 31 E
Castellaneta, *Italy* 47 B9 40 38N 16 56 E
Castelli, *Argentina* 174 D4 36 7 S 57 47W
Castelló de la Plana, *Spain* 40 F4 39 58N 0 3W
Castellón de la Plana □, *Spain* 40 E4 40 15N 0 5W
Castellote, *Spain* 40 E4 40 48N 0 15W
Castelmáuro, *Italy* 45 G11 41 50N 14 43 E
Castelnau-de-Médoc, *France* 28 C3 45 2N 0 48W
Castelnau-Magnoac, *France* 28 E4 43 17N 0 31 E
Castelnaudary, *France* 28 E5 43 20N 1 58 E
Castelnovo ne' Monti, *Italy* 44 D7 44 26N 10 24 E
Castelnuovo di Val di Cécina, *Italy* 44 E7 43 12N 10 59 E

Castelo = Manuel Urbano, *Brazil* **172 B4** 8 53 S 69 18W
Castelo, *Brazil* **171 F3** 20 33 S 41 14W
Castelo, Pta. do, *Azores* **9 d4** 36 56N 25 1W
Castelo Branco, *Azores* **9 d1** 38 31N 28 44W
Castelo Branco, *Portugal* **42 F3** 39 50N 7 31W
Castelo Branco □, *Portugal* **42 F3** 39 52N 7 45W
Castelo de Paiva, *Portugal* **42 D2** 41 2N 8 16W
Castelo de Vide, *Portugal* **43 F3** 39 25N 7 27W
Castelo do Piauí, *Brazil* **170 C3** 5 20 S 41 33W
Castelrosso = Megiste, *Greece* **49 E11** 36 8N 29 34 E
Castelsardo, *Italy* **46 B1** 40 55N 8 43 E
Castelsarrasin, *France* **28 D5** 44 2N 1 7 E
Casteltérmini, *Italy* **46 E6** 37 32N 13 39 E
Castelvetrano, *Italy* **46 E5** 37 41N 12 47 E
Castendo, *Angola* **115 D2** 8 39 S 14 10 E
Casterton, *Australia* **128 D4** 37 30 S 141 30 E
Castets, *France* **28 E2** 43 52N 1 6W
Castiglion Fiorentino, *Italy* **45 E8** 43 20N 11 55 E
Castiglione = Bou Ismaïl, *Algeria* **111 A5** 36 38N 2 42 E
Castiglione del Lago, *Italy* **45 E9** 43 7N 12 3 E
Castiglione della Pescáia, *Italy* **44 F7** 42 46N 10 53 E
Castiglione delle Stiviere, *Italy* **44 C7** 45 23N 10 29 E
Castilblanco, *Spain* **43 F5** 39 17N 5 5W
Castile, *U.S.A.* **150 D6** 42 38N 78 3W
Castilla, *Peru* **172 B1** 5 12 S 80 38W
Castilla, Playa de, *Spain* **43 J4** 37 0N 6 33W
Castilla-La Mancha □, *Spain* **12 H5** 39 30N 3 30W
Castilla y Leon □, *Spain* **42 D6** 42 0N 5 0W
Castillo de Locubín, *Spain* **43 H7** 37 32N 3 56W
Castillo de San Marcos ⌓, *U.S.A.* **152 F8** 29 54N 81 19W
Castillon-en-Couserans, *France* **28 F5** 42 56N 1 1 E
Castillonès, *France* **28 D4** 44 39N 0 37 E
Castillos, *Uruguay* **175 C5** 34 12 S 53 52W
Castle Dale, *U.S.A.* **158 G8** 39 13N 111 1W
Castle Douglas, *U.K.* **22 G5** 54 56N 3 56W
Castle Harbour, *Bermuda* **9 a** 32 21N 64 40W
Castle Rock, *Colo., U.S.A.* **154 F2** 39 22N 104 51W
Castle Rock, *Wash., U.S.A.* **160 D4** 46 17N 122 54W
Castle Rock Pt., *St. Helena* **9 h** 16 1 S 5 45W
Castlebar, *Ireland* **23 C2** 53 52N 9 18W
Castlebay, *U.K.* **22 E1** 56 57N 7 31W
Castleblaney, *Ireland* **23 B5** 54 7N 6 44W
Castlecliff, *N.Z.* **130 F4** 39 57 S 175 5 E
Castlederg, *U.K.* **23 B4** 54 42N 7 35W
Castleford, *U.K.* **20 D6** 53 43N 1 21W
Castlegar, *Canada* **142 D5** 49 20N 117 40W
Castlemaine, *Australia* **128 D6** 37 2 S 144 12 E
Castlepoint, *N.Z.* **130 G5** 40 54 S 176 15 E
Castlepollard, *Ireland* **23 C4** 53 41N 7 19W
Castlerea, *Ireland* **23 C3** 53 46N 8 29W
Castlereagh →, *Australia* **129 A7** 30 12 S 147 32 E
Castlereagh B., *Australia* **126 A2** 12 10 S 135 10 E
Castleton, *U.S.A.* **151 C11** 43 37N 73 11W
Castletown, *I. of Man* **20 C3** 54 5N 4 38W
Castletown Bearhaven, *Ireland* **23 E2** 51 39N 9 55W
Castor, *Canada* **142 C6** 52 15N 111 50W
Castor →, *Canada* **140 B4** 53 24N 78 58W
Castorland, *U.S.A.* **151 C9** 43 53N 75 31W
Castres, *France* **28 E6** 43 37N 2 13 E
Castricum, *Neths.* **24 B4** 52 33N 4 40 E
Castries, *St. Lucia* **165 f** 14 2N 60 58W
Castril, *Spain* **43 H8** 37 48N 2 46W
Castro, *Brazil* **175 A6** 24 45 S 50 0W
Castro, *Chile* **176 B2** 42 30 S 73 50W
Castro Alves, *Brazil* **171 D4** 12 46 S 39 33W
Castro del Río, *Spain* **43 H6** 37 41N 4 29W
Castro-Urdiales, *Spain* **42 B7** 43 23N 3 11W
Castro Verde, *Portugal* **43 H2** 37 41N 8 4W
Castrogiovanní = Enna, *Italy* **47 E7** 37 34N 14 16 E
Castrojeriz, *Spain* **42 C6** 42 17N 4 9W
Castropol, *Spain* **42 B4** 43 32N 7 0W
Castroreale, *Italy* **47 D8** 38 6N 15 12 E
Castrovíllari, *Italy* **47 C9** 39 49N 16 12 E
Castroville, *U.S.A.* **160 J5** 36 46N 121 45W
Castrovirreyna, *Peru* **172 C2** 13 20 S 75 18W
Castuera, *Spain* **43 G5** 38 43N 5 37W
Caswell Sound, *N.Z.* **131 E2** 44 59 S 167 8 E
Çat, *Turkey* **101 C9** 39 40N 41 3 E
Cat Ba △, *Vietnam* **86 B6** 20 47N 107 3 E
Cat Ba, Dao, *Vietnam* **86 B6** 20 50N 107 0 E
Cat I., *Bahamas* **165 B4** 24 30N 75 30W
Cat L., *Canada* **140 B1** 51 40N 91 50W
Cat Lake, *Canada* **140 B1** 51 40N 91 50W
Cat Tien △, *Vietnam* **87 G6** 11 25N 107 17 E
Čata, *Slovak Rep.* **35 D11** 47 58N 18 38 E
Catabola, *Angola* **115 E3** 12 9 S 17 16 E
Catacamas, *Honduras* **164 D2** 14 54N 85 56W
Catacáos, *Peru* **172 B1** 5 20 S 80 45W
Cataguases, *Brazil* **171 F3** 21 23 S 42 39W
Catagupan, *Phil.* **81 G1** 8 1N 116 58 E
Cataingan, *Phil.* **80 E4** 12 0N 124 0 E
Çatak, *Turkey* **101 C10** 38 1N 43 8 E
Catalão, *Brazil* **171 E2** 18 10 S 47 57W
Çatalca, *Turkey* **51 E12** 41 8N 28 27 E
Catalina, *Canada* **141 C9** 48 31N 53 4W
Catalina, *Chile* **174 B2** 25 13 S 69 43W
Catalina, *U.S.A.* **159 K8** 32 30N 110 50W
Catalonia = Cataluña □, *Spain* **40 D6** 41 40N 1 15 E
Cataluña □, *Spain* **40 D6** 41 40N 1 15 E
Çatalzeytin, *Turkey* **100 B6** 41 57N 34 12 E
Catamarca, *Argentina* **174 B2** 28 30 S 65 50W
Catamarca □, *Argentina* **174 B2** 27 0 S 65 50W
Catanauan, *Phil.* **80 E4** 13 36N 122 19 E
Catanduanes □, *Phil.* **80 E5** 13 50N 124 20 E
Catanduva, *Brazil* **175 A6** 21 5 S 48 58W
Catánia, *Italy* **47 E8** 37 30N 15 6 E
Catánia, G. di, *Italy* **47 E8** 37 24N 15 9 E
Catanzaro, *Italy* **47 D9** 38 54N 16 35 E
Catarman, *Camiguin, Phil.* **81 G5** 9 8N 124 40 E
Catarman, *N. Samar, Phil.* **80 E5** 12 28N 124 35 E
Catatumbo →, *Venezuela* **168 B3** 9 21N 71 45W
Catatumbo-Bari △, *Colombia* **165 E5** 9 3N 73 12W
Cataula, *U.S.A.* **152 C5** 32 39N 84 52W
Catbalogan, *Phil.* **81 F5** 11 46N 124 53 E
Cateco Cangola, *Angola* **115 D3** 8 28 S 15 51 E
Cateel, *Phil.* **81 H6** 7 47N 126 24 E
Cateel Bay, *Phil.* **81 H6** 7 54N 126 25 E
Catembe, *Mozam.* **117 D5** 26 0 S 32 33 E
Catende, *Angola* **115 E4** 11 14 S 21 30 E
Catende, *Brazil* **170 C4** 8 40 S 35 43W
Caterham, *U.K.* **21 F7** 51 15N 0 4W
Catete, *Angola* **115 D2** 9 6 S 13 43 E
Cathcart, *Australia* **129 D8** 36 52 S 149 24 E
Cathcart, *S. Africa* **116 E4** 32 18 S 27 10 E
Cathlamet, *U.S.A.* **160 D3** 46 12N 123 23W
Catio, *Guinea-Biss.* **112 C1** 11 17N 15 15W
Catismiña, *Venezuela* **169 C5** 4 5N 63 40W
Catita, *Brazil* **170 C3** 9 31 S 43 1W
Catlettsburg, *U.S.A.* **148 F4** 38 25N 82 36W
Catlin, *U.S.A.* **157 D9** 40 4N 87 42W
Çatma Dağı, *Turkey* **49 C11** 38 25N 29 50 E
Catmon, *Phil.* **81 F5** 10 43N 124 1 E
Catoche, C., *Mexico* **163 C7** 21 40N 87 8W
Catolé do Rocha, *Brazil* **170 C4** 6 21 S 37 45W
Catota, *Angola* **115 E3** 13 57 S 17 30 E
Cátria, Mte., *Italy* **45 E9** 43 28N 12 42 E
Catriló, *Argentina* **174 D3** 36 26 S 63 24W
Catrimani, *Brazil* **169 C5** 0 27N 61 41W
Catrimani →, *Brazil* **169 C5** 0 28N 61 44W
Catskill, *U.S.A.* **151 D11** 42 14N 73 52W
Catskill ⌓, *U.S.A.* **151 D10** 42 7N 74 39W
Catskill Mts., *U.S.A.* **151 D10** 42 10N 74 25W
Catt, Mt., *Australia* **126 A1** 13 49 S 134 23 E
Cattaraugus, *U.S.A.* **150 D6** 42 22N 78 52W
Cattaro = Kotor, *Serbia & M.* **50 D2** 42 25N 18 47 E
Catterick, *U.K.* **20 C6** 54 23N 1 37W
Cattólica, *Italy* **45 E9** 43 58N 12 44 E
Cattólica Eraclea, *Italy* **46 E6** 37 26N 13 24 E
Catu, *Brazil* **171 D4** 12 21 S 38 23W
Catuala, *Angola* **116 B2** 16 25 S 19 2 E
Catuane, *Mozam.* **117 D5** 26 48 S 32 18 E
Catubig, *Phil.* **80 E5** 12 24N 125 3 E
Catumbela, *Angola* **115 E2** 12 25 S 13 34 E
Catumbela →, *Angola* **115 E2** 12 29 S 13 28 E
Catur, *Mozam.* **119 E4** 13 45 S 35 30 E
Catwick Is., *Vietnam* **87 G7** 10 0N 109 0 E
Cauayan, *Isabela, Phil.* **80 C3** 16 56N 121 46 E
Cauayan, *Neg. Occ., Phil.* **81 G4** 9 58N 122 37 E
Cauca □, *Colombia* **168 C2** 2 30N 76 50W
Cauca →, *Colombia* **168 B3** 8 54N 74 28W
Caucaia, *Brazil* **170 B4** 3 40 S 38 35W
Caucasia, *Colombia* **168 B2** 8 0N 75 12W
Caucasus Mountains, *Eurasia* **61 J7** 42 50N 44 0 E
Caudete, *Spain* **41 G3** 38 42N 1 2W
Caudry, *France* **27 B10** 50 7N 3 22 E
Caulnes, *France* **26 D4** 48 18N 2 10W
Caulónia, *Italy* **47 D9** 38 23N 16 24 E
Caungula, *Angola* **115 D3** 8 26 S 18 38 E
Cauquenes, *Chile* **174 D1** 36 0 S 72 22W
Caura →, *Venezuela* **169 B5** 7 38N 64 53W
Caurés →, *Brazil* **169 D5** 1 21 S 62 20W
Cauresi →, *Mozam.* **119 F3** 17 8 S 33 0 E
Căuşani, *Moldova* **53 D14** 46 38N 29 25 E
Causapscal, *Canada* **141 C6** 48 19N 67 12W
Caussade, *France* **28 D5** 44 10N 1 33 E
Causse-Méjean, *France* **28 D7** 44 18N 3 42 E
Causses du Quercy ⌓, *France* **28 D5** 44 35N 1 35 E
Cauterets, *France* **28 F3** 42 52N 0 8W
Caux, Pays de, *France* **26 C7** 49 38N 0 35 E
Cava de' Tirreni, *Italy* **47 B7** 40 42N 14 42 E
Cávado →, *Portugal* **42 D2** 41 32N 8 48W
Cavagrande del Cassibile ⌓, *Italy* **47 F8** 36 58N 15 6 E
Cavaillon, *France* **29 E9** 43 50N 5 2 E
Cavalaire-sur-Mer, *France* **29 E10** 43 10N 6 33 E
Cavalcante, *Brazil* **171 D2** 13 48 S 47 30W
Cavalese, *Italy* **45 B8** 46 17N 11 27 E
Cavalier, *U.S.A.* **154 A6** 48 48N 97 37W
Cavalla = Cavally →, *Africa* **112 E3** 4 22N 7 32W
Cavalli Is., *N.Z.* **130 B2** 35 0 S 173 58 E
Cavallo, Î. de, *France* **29 G13** 41 22N 9 16 E
Cavally →, *Africa* **112 E3** 4 22N 7 32W
Cavan, *Ireland* **23 B4** 54 0N 7 22W
Cavan □, *Ireland* **23 C4** 54 1N 7 16W
Cavárzere, *Italy* **45 C9** 45 8N 12 5 E
Cavazuccherina = Iésolo, *Italy* **45 C9** 45 32N 12 38 E
Çavdarhisar, *Turkey* **49 B11** 39 12N 29 37 E
Çavdır, *Turkey* **49 D11** 37 10N 29 42 E
Cave Creek, *U.S.A.* **159 K7** 33 50N 111 57W
Cave Run L., *U.S.A.* **157 F13** 38 5N 83 25W
Cave Spring, *U.S.A.* **152 A4** 34 6N 85 20W
Cavenagh Ra., *Australia* **125 E4** 26 12 S 127 55 E
Cavendish, *Australia* **128 D5** 37 31 S 142 2 E
Caviana, I., *Brazil* **169 C7** 0 10N 50 10W
Cavite, *Phil.* **80 D3** 14 29N 120 55 E
Cavite □, *Phil.* **80 D3** 14 15N 120 50 E
Caviúna = Rolândia, *Brazil* **175 A5** 23 18 S 51 23W
Cavnic, *Romania* **53 C8** 47 40N 23 52 E
Cavour, *Italy* **44 D4** 44 47N 7 22 E
Cavtat, *Croatia* **50 D2** 42 35N 18 13 E
Cawayan, *Phil.* **81 F4** 11 56N 123 46 E
Cawayanon = Vintar, *Phil.* **80 B3** 18 14N 120 39 E
Cawndilla L., *Australia* **128 B5** 32 30 S 142 15 E
Cawnpore = Kanpur, *India* **93 F9** 26 28N 80 20 E
Caxias, *Brazil* **170 B3** 4 55 S 43 20W
Caxias do Sul, *Brazil* **175 B5** 29 10 S 51 10W
Caxito, *Angola* **115 D2** 8 30 S 13 30 E
Caxopa, *Angola* **115 E4** 11 52 S 20 52 E
Çay, *Turkey* **100 C4** 38 35N 31 1 E
Cay Pt., *Bahamas* **9 b** 25 59N 77 25W
Cay Sal Bank, *Bahamas* **164 B4** 23 45N 80 0W
Cayambe, *Napo, Ecuador* **168 C2** 0 2N 77 59W
Cayambe, *Quito, Ecuador* **168 C2** 0 3N 78 8W
Çaycuma, *Turkey* **100 B5** 41 25N 32 4 E
Çayeli, *Turkey* **101 B9** 41 5N 40 45 E
Cayenne, *Fr. Guiana* **169 B7** 5 5N 52 18W
Cayenne □, *Fr. Guiana* **169 C7** 5 0N 53 0W
Cayey, *Puerto Rico* **165 d** 18 7N 66 10W
Caygören Barajı, *Turkey* **49 B10** 39 15N 28 12 E
Cayiralan, *Turkey* **100 C6** 39 17N 35 38 E
Caylus, *France* **28 D5** 44 15N 1 47 E
Cayman Brac, *Cayman Is.* **164 C4** 19 43N 79 49W
Cayman Is. ☒, *W. Indies* **164 C3** 19 40N 80 30W
Cayman Trough, *Caribbean* **136 H11** 19 0N 81 0W
Cayres, *France* **28 D7** 44 55N 3 48 E
Cayuga, *Ind., U.S.A.* **157 E9** 39 57N 87 28W
Cayuga, *N.Y., U.S.A.* **151 D8** 42 54N 76 44W
Cayuga L., *U.S.A.* **151 D8** 42 41N 76 41W
Cazage, *Angola* **115 E4** 11 2 S 20 45 E
Cazalla de la Sierra, *Spain* **43 H5** 37 56N 5 45W
Căzăneşti, *Romania* **53 F12** 44 36N 27 3 E
Cazaubon, *France* **28 E3** 43 56N 0 3W
Cazaux et de Sanguinet, Étang de, *France* **28 D2** 44 29N 1 10W
Cazenovia, *U.S.A.* **151 D9** 42 56N 75 51W
Cazères, *France* **28 E5** 43 13N 1 5 E
Cazin, *Bos.-H.* **45 D12** 44 57N 15 57 E
Čazma, *Croatia* **45 C13** 45 45N 16 39 E
Cazombo, *Angola* **115 E4** 11 54 S 22 56 E
Cazorla, *Spain* **43 H7** 37 55N 3 2W
Cazorla, Sierra de, *Spain* **43 G8** 38 5N 2 55W
Cea →, *Spain* **42 C5** 42 0N 5 36W
Ceamurlia de Jos, *Romania* **53 F13** 44 43N 28 47 E
Ceanannus Mor, *Ireland* **23 C5** 53 44N 6 53W
Ceará = Fortaleza, *Brazil* **170 B4** 3 45 S 38 35W
Ceará □, *Brazil* **170 C4** 5 0 S 40 0W
Ceará Mirim, *Brazil* **170 C4** 5 38 S 35 25W
Ceara Plain, *Atl. Oc.* **8 F7** 2 0N 42 0W
Ceauru, L., *Romania* **53 F8** 44 58N 23 11 E
Cebaco, I. de, *Panama* **164 E3** 7 33N 81 9W
Cebollar, *Argentina* **174 B2** 29 10 S 66 35W
Cebollera, Sierra de, *Spain* **40 D2** 42 0N 2 30W
Cebreros, *Spain* **42 E6** 40 27N 4 28W
Cebu, *Phil.* **81 F4** 10 18N 123 54 E
Cebu □, *Phil.* **81 F4** 10 20N 123 40 E
Čečava, *Bos.-H.* **52 F2** 44 42N 17 44 E
Ceccano, *Italy* **46 A6** 41 34N 13 20 E
Cece, *Hungary* **52 D3** 46 46N 18 39 E
Cechi, *Ivory C.* **112 D4** 6 15N 4 25W
Cecil Plains, *Australia* **127 D5** 27 30 S 151 11 E
Cécina, *Italy* **44 E7** 43 19N 10 31 E
Cécina →, *Italy* **44 E7** 43 18N 10 29 E
Ceclavín, *Spain* **42 F4** 39 50N 6 45W
Cedar →, *U.S.A.* **156 C5** 41 17N 91 21W
Cedar City, *U.S.A.* **159 H7** 37 41N 113 4W
Cedar Creek Reservoir, *U.S.A.* **155 J6** 32 11N 96 4W
Cedar Falls, *Iowa, U.S.A.* **156 B4** 42 32N 92 27W
Cedar Falls, *Wash., U.S.A.* **160 C5** 47 25N 121 45W
Cedar Grove, *U.S.A.* **157 E12** 39 22N 84 56W
Cedar Key, *U.S.A.* **153 F6** 29 8N 83 2W
Cedar L., *Canada* **143 C9** 53 10N 100 0W
Cedar Lake, *U.S.A.* **157 C9** 41 22N 87 26W
Cedar Park, *U.S.A.* **155 K6** 30 30N 97 49W
Cedar Point, *U.S.A.* **157 C13** 41 44N 83 21W
Cedar Rapids, *U.S.A.* **156 C5** 41 59N 91 40W
Cedartown, *U.S.A.* **152 A4** 34 1N 85 15W
Cedarvale, *Canada* **142 B3** 55 1N 128 22W
Cedarville, *S. Africa* **117 E4** 30 23 S 29 3 E
Cedarville, *Ill., U.S.A.* **156 B7** 42 23N 89 38W
Cedarville, *Ohio, U.S.A.* **157 E13** 39 44N 83 49W
Cedeira, *Spain* **42 B2** 43 39N 8 2W
Cedral, *Mexico* **162 C4** 23 50N 100 42W
Cedrino →, *Italy* **46 B2** 40 11N 9 24 E
Cedro, *Brazil* **170 C4** 6 34 S 39 3W
Cedros, *Azores* **9 d1** 38 38N 28 42W
Cedros, I. de, *Mexico* **162 B1** 28 10N 115 20W
Cedros B., *Trin. & Tob.* **169 F9** 10 16N 61 54W
Ceduna, *Australia* **127 E1** 32 7 S 133 46 E
Cedynia, *Poland* **55 F1** 52 53N 14 12 E
Cée, *Spain* **42 C1** 42 57N 9 10W
Ceel Dheere = El Dere, *Somali Rep.* **120 C3** 5 22N 46 11 E
Ceerigaabo = Erigavo, *Somali Rep.* **120 B3** 10 35N 47 20 E
Cefalù, *Italy* **47 D7** 38 2N 14 1 E
Cega →, *Spain* **42 D6** 41 33N 4 46W
Cegléd, *Hungary* **52 C4** 47 11N 19 47 E
Céglie Messápico, *Italy* **47 B10** 40 39N 17 31 E
Cehegín, *Spain* **41 G3** 38 6N 1 48W
Ceheng, *China* **76 E5** 24 58N 105 48 E
Cehu-Silvaniei, *Romania* **53 C8** 47 24N 23 9 E
Ceica, *Romania* **52 D7** 46 53N 22 10 E
Ceira →, *Portugal* **42 E2** 40 13N 8 16W
Cekik, *Indonesia* **79 J17** 8 12 S 114 27 E
Cela, *Angola* **115 E3** 11 25 S 15 7 E
Čelákovice, *Czech Rep.* **34 A7** 50 10N 14 46 E
Celano, *Italy* **45 F10** 42 5N 13 33 E
Celanova, *Spain* **42 C3** 42 9N 7 58W
Celaque △, *Honduras* **164 D2** 14 30N 88 43W
Celaya, *Mexico* **162 C4** 20 31N 100 37W
Celebes = Sulawesi □, *Indonesia* **82 B2** 2 0 S 120 0 E
Celebes Sea, *Indonesia* **82 A2** 3 0N 123 0 E
Celendín, *Peru* **172 B2** 6 52 S 78 10W
Čelić, *Bos.-H.* **52 F3** 44 43N 18 49 E
Celica, *Ecuador* **168 D2** 4 7 S 79 59W
Celina, *U.S.A.* **157 D12** 40 33N 84 35W
Celinac, *Bos.-H.* **52 F2** 44 44N 17 22 E
Celje, *Slovenia* **45 B12** 46 16N 15 18 E
Celldömölk, *Hungary* **52 C2** 47 16N 17 10 E
Celle, *Germany* **30 C6** 52 37N 10 4 E
Celorico da Beira, *Portugal* **42 E3** 40 38N 7 24W
Celtic Sea, *Atl. Oc.* **8 A11** 50 9N 9 34W
Çeltikçi, *Turkey* **49 D12** 37 32N 30 29 E
Çemişgezek, *Turkey* **101 C8** 39 3N 38 56 E
Cenderwasih, Teluk, *Indonesia* **79 E9** 3 0 S 135 20 E
Cenepa →, *Peru* **168 D2** 4 40 S 78 10W
Cengong, *China* **76 D7** 27 13N 108 44 E
Ceno →, *Italy* **44 D7** 44 43N 10 5 E
Centallo, *Italy* **44 D4** 44 30N 7 35 E
Centelles, *Spain* **40 D7** 41 50N 2 14 E
Centenário do Sul, *Brazil* **171 F1** 22 48 S 51 36W
Center, *N. Dak., U.S.A.* **154 B4** 47 7N 101 18W
Center, *Tex., U.S.A.* **155 K7** 31 48N 94 11W
Center Hill, *U.S.A.* **153 G7** 28 38N 82 3W
Center Point, *U.S.A.* **156 B5** 42 12N 91 46W
Centerburg, *U.S.A.* **150 F2** 40 18N 82 42W
Centerville, *Calif., U.S.A.* **160 J7** 36 44N 119 30W
Centerville, *Iowa, U.S.A.* **156 D4** 40 44N 92 52W
Centerville, *Mich., U.S.A.* **157 C11** 41 55N 85 32W
Centerville, *Ohio, U.S.A.* **157 E12** 39 38N 84 8W
Centerville, *Pa., U.S.A.* **150 F5** 40 3N 79 59W
Centerville, *Tenn., U.S.A.* **149 H2** 35 47N 87 28W
Centerville, *Tex., U.S.A.* **155 K7** 31 16N 95 59W
Cento, *Italy* **45 D8** 44 43N 11 17 E
Central = Tsentralnyy □, *Russia* **60 D4** 52 0N 40 0 E
Central, *Brazil* **170 D3** 11 8 S 42 8W
Central, *U.S.A.* **144 D11** 65 35N 144 48W
Central □, *Ghana* **113 D4** 5 30N 1 0W
Central □, *Kenya* **118 C4** 0 30 S 37 30 E
Central □, *Malawi* **119 E3** 13 30 S 33 30 E
Central □, *Papua N. G.* **132 F5** 10 0 S 148 0 E
Central □, *Zambia* **119 E2** 14 25 S 28 50 E
Central, Cordillera, *Bolivia* **173 D5** 18 30 S 64 55W
Central, Cordillera, *Colombia* **168 C2** 5 0N 75 0W
Central, Cordillera, *Costa Rica* **164 D3** 10 10N 84 5W
Central, Cordillera, *Dom. Rep.* **165 C5** 19 15N 71 0W
Central, Cordillera, *Peru* **172 B2** 7 0 S 77 30W
Central, Cordillera, *Phil.* **80 C3** 17 20N 120 57 E
Central, Cordillera, *Puerto Rico* **165 d** 18 8N 66 35W
Central African Empire = Central African Rep. ■, *Africa* **114 A4** 7 0N 20 0 E
Central African Rep. ■, *Africa* **114 A4** 7 0N 20 0 E
Central America, *America* **136 H11** 12 0N 85 0W
Central Butte, *Canada* **143 C7** 50 48N 106 31W
Central City, *Colo., U.S.A.* **158 G11** 39 48N 105 31W
Central City, *Iowa, U.S.A.* **156 B5** 42 12N 91 32W
Central City, *Ky., U.S.A.* **148 G2** 37 18N 87 7W
Central City, *Nebr., U.S.A.* **154 E6** 41 7N 98 0W
Central I., *Kenya* **118 B4** 3 30N 36 0 E
Central Island △, *Kenya* **118 B4** 2 33N 36 1 E
Central Japan International ✈ (CJI), *Japan* **73 C8** 34 53N 136 45 E
Central Kalahari ⌓, *Botswana* **116 C3** 22 36 S 23 58 E
Central Makran Range, *Pakistan* **91 D2** 26 30N 64 15 E
Central Pacific Basin, *Pac. Oc.* **134 G10** 8 0N 175 0W
Central Patricia, *Canada* **140 B1** 51 30N 90 9W
Central Point, *U.S.A.* **158 E2** 42 23N 122 55W
Central Provinces = Madhya Pradesh □, *India* **92 J8** 22 50N 78 0 E
Central Ra., *Papua N. G.* **132 C2** 5 0 S 143 0 E
Central Russian Uplands, *Europe* **12 E13** 54 0N 36 0 E
Central Siberian Plateau, *Russia* **62 C14** 65 0N 105 0 E
Central Square, *U.S.A.* **151 C8** 43 17N 76 9W
Centralia, *Ill., U.S.A.* **156 F7** 38 32N 89 8W
Centralia, *Mo., U.S.A.* **156 E4** 39 13N 92 8W
Centralia, *Wash., U.S.A.* **160 D4** 46 43N 122 58W
Centre, *U.S.A.* **152 A4** 34 9N 85 41W
Centre de Flacq, *Mauritius* **121 d** 20 12 S 57 43 E
Century, *U.S.A.* **153 E2** 30 58N 87 16W
Cenxi, *China* **77 F8** 22 57N 110 57 E
Čeotina →, *Bos.-H.* **50 C2** 43 36N 18 50 E
Cephalonia = Kefallinía, *Greece* **39 C2** 38 15N 20 30 E
Čepin, *Croatia* **52 E3** 45 32N 18 34 E
Ceprano, *Italy* **46 A6** 41 33N 13 31 E
Ceptia, *Angola* **115 E3** 12 56 S 17 35 E
Ceptura, *Romania* **53 E11** 45 1N 26 21 E
Cepu, *Indonesia* **85 D4** 7 9 S 111 35 E
Ceram = Seram, *Indonesia* **83 B3** 3 10 S 129 0 E
Ceram Sea = Seram Sea, *Indonesia* **82 B3** 2 30 S 128 30 E
Cerbère, *France* **28 F7** 42 26N 3 10 E
Cerbicales, Îs., *France* **29 G13** 41 33N 9 22 E
Cercal, *Portugal* **43 H2** 37 48N 8 40W
Cerdaña, *Spain* **40 C6** 42 22N 1 35 E
Cère →, *France* **28 D5** 44 55N 1 49 E
Cerea, *Italy* **45 C8** 45 12N 11 13 E
Ceredigion □, *U.K.* **21 E3** 52 16N 4 15W
Ceres, *Argentina* **174 B3** 29 55 S 61 55W
Ceres, *Brazil* **171 E2** 15 17 S 49 35W
Ceres, *S. Africa* **116 E2** 33 21 S 19 18 E
Ceres, *U.S.A.* **160 H6** 37 35N 120 57W
Céret, *France* **28 F6** 42 30N 2 42 E
Cereté, *Colombia* **168 B2** 8 53N 75 48W
Cerf, *Seychelles* **121 b** 4 38 S 55 40 E
Cergy, *France* **27 C9** 49 2N 2 4 E
Cerignola, *Italy* **47 A8** 41 17N 15 53 E
Cerigo = Kíthira, *Greece* **48 E5** 36 8N 23 0 E
Cérilly, *France* **27 F9** 46 37N 2 50 E
Cerisiers, *France* **27 D10** 48 8N 3 30 E
Cerizay, *France* **26 F6** 46 50N 0 40W
Çerkeş, *Turkey* **100 B5** 40 49N 32 52 E
Çerkezköy, *Turkey* **51 E12** 41 17N 28 0 E
Cerknica, *Slovenia* **45 C11** 45 48N 14 21 E
Cerkovica, *Bulgaria* **51 C8** 43 41N 24 50 E
Cermerno, *Serbia & M.* **50 C4** 43 35N 20 25 E
Çermik, *Turkey* **101 C8** 38 8N 39 26 E
Cerna, *Romania* **53 E13** 45 4N 28 17 E
Cerna →, *Romania* **53 F8** 44 38N 23 58 E
Cernauti = Chernivtsi, *Ukraine* **53 B10** 48 15N 25 52 E
Cernavodă, *Romania* **53 F13** 44 22N 28 3 E
Cernay, *France* **27 E14** 47 44N 7 10 E
Cernik, *Croatia* **52 E2** 45 17N 17 22 E
Cerralvo, I., *Mexico* **162 C3** 24 20N 109 45W
Cërrik, *Albania* **50 E3** 41 2N 19 58 E
Cerritos, *Mexico* **162 C4** 22 27N 100 20W
Cerro Chato, *Uruguay* **175 C4** 33 6 S 55 8W
Cerro Corá △, *Paraguay* **175 A4** 22 35 S 56 2W
Cerro el Copey △, *Venezuela* **165 D7** 10 59N 63 53W
Cerro Gordo, *U.S.A.* **157 E8** 39 53N 88 44W
Cerro Hoya △, *Panama* **164 E3** 7 17N 80 45W
Cerro Saroche △, *Venezuela* **165 D6** 10 8N 69 38W
Cerro Sombrero, *Chile* **176 D3** 52 45 S 69 15W
Certaldo, *Italy* **44 E8** 43 33N 11 2 E
Cervantes, *Phil.* **80 C3** 17 0N 120 44 E
Cervaro →, *Italy* **47 A8** 41 30N 15 52 E
Cervati, Monte, *Italy* **47 B8** 40 17N 15 29 E
Cerventes, *Australia* **125 F2** 30 31 S 115 3 E
Cervera, *Spain* **40 D6** 41 40N 1 16 E
Cervera de Pisuerga, *Spain* **42 C6** 42 51N 4 30W
Cervera del Río Alhama, *Spain* **40 C3** 42 2N 1 58W
Cervéteri, *Italy* **45 F9** 42 0N 12 6 E
Cérvia, *Italy* **45 D9** 44 15N 12 22 E
Cervignano del Friuli, *Italy* **45 C10** 45 49N 13 20 E
Cervinara, *Italy* **47 A7** 41 1N 14 37 E
Cervione, *France* **29 F13** 42 20N 9 29 E
Cervo, *Spain* **42 B3** 43 40N 7 24W
César □, *Colombia* **168 B3** 9 0N 73 30W
Cesarò, *Italy* **47 E7** 37 50N 14 38 E
Cesena, *Italy* **45 D9** 44 8N 12 15 E
Cesenático, *Italy* **45 D9** 44 12N 12 24 E
Cēsis, *Latvia* **15 H21** 57 18N 25 15 E
Česká Lípa, *Czech Rep.* **34 A7** 50 45N 14 30 E
Ceská Rep. = Czech Rep. ■, *Europe* **34 B8** 50 0N 15 0 E
Česká Třebová, *Czech Rep.* **35 B9** 49 54N 16 27 E
České Budějovice, *Czech Rep.* **34 C7** 48 55N 14 25 E
České Velenice, *Czech Rep.* **34 C7** 48 45N 14 57 E
Českobudějovický □, *Czech Rep.* **34 B7** 49 10N 14 30 E
Českomoravská Vrchovina, *Czech Rep.* **34 B8** 49 30N 15 40 E
Český Brod, *Czech Rep.* **34 A7** 50 4N 14 52 E
Český Krumlov, *Czech Rep.* **34 C7** 48 43N 14 21 E
Český Těšín, *Czech Rep.* **35 B11** 49 45N 18 39 E
Česma →, *Croatia* **45 C13** 45 35N 16 29 E
Çeşme, *Turkey* **49 C8** 38 20N 26 23 E
Cessnock, *Australia* **129 B9** 32 50 S 151 21 E
Cesson-Sévigné, *France* **26 D5** 48 7N 1 36W
Cestas, *France* **28 D3** 44 44N 0 41W
Cestos →, *Liberia* **112 D3** 5 40N 9 10W
Cestos Sehnkwehn △, *Liberia* **112 D3** 5 40N 9 10W
Cetate, *Romania* **52 F8** 44 7N 23 2 E
Cetatea-Albă = Bilhorod-Dnistrovskyy, *Ukraine* **59 J6** 46 11N 30 23 E
Cetin Grad, *Croatia* **45 C12** 45 9N 15 45 E
Cetina →, *Croatia* **45 E13** 43 26N 16 42 E
Cetinje, *Serbia & M.* **50 D2** 42 23N 18 59 E
Cetraro, *Italy* **47 C8** 39 31N 15 55 E
Ceuta, *N. Afr.* **110 A3** 35 52N 5 18W
Ceva, *Italy* **44 D5** 44 23N 8 2 E
Ceve-i-Ra, *Fiji* **123 E13** 21 46 S 174 31 E
Cévennes, *France* **28 D7** 44 10N 3 50 E
Cévennes △, *France* **28 D7** 44 15N 3 45 E
Cevio, *Switz.* **33 D7** 46 19N 8 36 E
Ceyhan, *Turkey* **100 D6** 37 4N 35 47 E
Ceyhan →, *Turkey* **100 D6** 36 38N 35 40 E
Ceylânpınar, *Turkey* **101 D9** 36 50N 40 2 E
Ceylon = Sri Lanka ■, *Asia* **95 L5** 7 30N 80 50 E
Cèze →, *France* **29 D8** 44 6N 4 43 E
Cha-am, *Thailand* **86 F2** 12 48N 99 58 E
Cha Pa, *Vietnam* **86 A4** 22 20N 103 47 E
Chá Pungana, *Angola* **115 E3** 13 44 S 18 39 E
Chabanais, *France* **28 C4** 45 52N 0 48 E
Chabeuil, *France* **29 D9** 44 54N 5 3 E
Chablais, *France* **27 F13** 46 20N 6 36 E
Chablis, *France* **27 E10** 47 47N 3 48 E
Chabounia, *Algeria* **111 A5** 35 30N 2 38 E
Chacabuco, *Argentina* **174 C3** 34 40 S 60 27W
Chachapoyas, *Peru* **172 B2** 6 15 S 77 50W
Chachasp, *Peru* **172 D3** 15 30 S 72 15W
Chachoengsao, *Thailand* **86 F3** 13 42N 101 5 E
Chachro, *Pakistan* **92 G4** 25 5N 70 15 E
Chaco △, *Argentina* **174 B4** 27 0 S 59 30W
Chaco □, *Argentina* **174 B3** 26 30 S 61 0W
Chaco □, *Paraguay* **174 B4** 26 0 S 60 0W
Chaco →, *U.S.A.* **159 H9** 36 46N 108 39W
Chaco Culture △, *U.S.A.* **159 H10** 36 3N 107 58W
Chacon, C., *U.S.A.* **142 C2** 54 42N 132 0W
Chad = Oktyabrskiy, *Russia* **64 C6** 56 31N 57 12 E
Chad ■, *Africa* **109 F3** 15 0N 17 15 E
Chad, L. = Tchad, L., *Chad* **109 F2** 13 30N 14 30 E
Chadan, *Russia* **67 D10** 51 17N 91 35 E
Chadileuvú →, *Argentina* **174 D2** 37 46 S 66 0W
Chadiza, *Zambia* **119 E3** 14 45 S 32 27 E
Chadron, *U.S.A.* **154 D3** 42 50N 103 0W
Chadyr-Lunga = Ciadâr-Lunga, *Moldova* **53 D13** 46 3N 28 51 E
Chae Hom, *Thailand* **86 C2** 18 43N 99 35 E
Chae Son △, *Thailand* **86 C2** 18 42N 99 20 E
Chaek, *Kyrgyzstan* **65 C7** 41 55N 74 30 E
Chaem →, *Thailand* **86 C2** 18 11N 98 38 E
Chaeryŏng, *N. Korea* **75 E13** 38 24N 125 36 E
Chagai Hills = Chāh Gay Hills, *Afghan.* **91 C1** 29 30N 64 0 E
Chagda, *Russia* **67 D14** 58 45N 130 38 E
Chaghcharān, *Afghan.* **91 B2** 34 31N 65 15 E
Chagny, *France* **27 F11** 46 57N 4 45 E
Chagoda, *Russia* **58 C8** 59 10N 35 15 E
Chagos Arch. ☒, *Ind. Oc.* **121 E6** 6 0 S 72 0 E
Chagres △, *Panama* **164 E4** 9 33N 79 37W
Chagrin Falls, *U.S.A.* **150 E3** 41 26N 81 24W
Chaguanas, *Trin. & Tob.* **169 F9** 10 30N 61 26W
Chāh Ākhvor, *Iran* **97 C8** 32 41N 59 40 E
Chāh Bahar, *Iran* **97 E9** 25 20N 60 40 E
Chāh-e Āb, *Afghan.* **65 E4** 37 23N 69 48 E
Chāh-e Kavīr, *Iran* **97 C8** 34 29N 56 52 E
Chāh Gay Hills, *Afghan.* **91 C1** 29 30N 64 0 E
Chahār Borjak, *Afghan.* **91 C1** 30 17N 62 3 E
Chahār Mahāll va Bakhtīarī □, *Iran* **97 C6** 32 0N 49 0 E
Chahtung, *Burma* **90 B7** 26 41N 98 10 E
Chai Wan, *China* **69 G11** 22 16N 114 14 E
Chaillé-les-Marais, *France* **28 B2** 46 25N 1 2W
Chainat, *Thailand* **86 E3** 15 11N 100 8 E
Chaires, *U.S.A.* **152 E5** 30 26N 84 7W
Chaitén, *Chile* **176 B2** 42 55 S 72 43W
Chaiya, *Thailand* **87 H2** 9 23N 99 14 E
Chaiyaphum, *Thailand* **86 E4** 15 48N 102 2 E
Chaj Doab, *Pakistan* **92 C5** 32 15N 73 0 E
Chajari, *Argentina* **174 C4** 30 42 S 58 0W
Chak Amru, *Pakistan* **92 C6** 32 22N 75 11 E
Chaka, *Sudan* **107 G3** 4 49N 31 14 E
Chakar →, *Pakistan* **92 E3** 29 29N 68 2 E
Chakari, *Zimbabwe* **117 B4** 18 5 S 29 51 E
Chakaria, *Bangla.* **90 E4** 21 45N 92 5 E
Chakarnaba, *Chad* **109 F4** 14 13N 20 51 E
Chake Chake, *Tanzania* **118 D4** 5 15 S 39 45 E
Chakhānsūr, *Afghan.* **91 C1** 31 10N 62 0 E
Chakonipau, L., *Canada* **141 A6** 56 18N 68 30W
Chakradharpur, *India* **93 H11** 22 45N 85 40 E
Chakrata, *India* **92 D7** 30 42N 77 51 E
Chakwadam, *Burma* **90 B7** 27 29N 98 31 E
Chakwal, *Pakistan* **91 B4** 32 56N 72 53 E
Chala, *Peru* **172 D3** 15 48 S 74 20W
Chalais, *France* **28 C4** 45 16N 0 3 E
Chalakudi, *India* **95 J3** 10 18N 76 20 E
Chalchihuites, *Mexico* **162 C4** 23 29N 103 53W
Chalcis = Khalkís, *Greece* **48 C5** 38 27N 23 42 E
Châlette-sur-Loing, *France* **27 D9** 48 1N 2 44 E

Chaleur B., *Canada* .. 141 C6 47 55N 65 30W
Chalfant, *U.S.A.* 160 H8 37 32N 118 21W
Chalhuanca, *Peru* .. 172 C3 14 15 S 73 15W
Chalindrey, *France* .... 27 E12 47 43N 5 26 E
Chaling, *China* ...... 77 D9 26 58N 113 30 E
Chalisgaon, *India* .... 94 D2 20 30N 75 10 E
Chalk River, *Canada* . 140 C4 46 1N 77 27W
Chalkar = Shalkar,
  Kazakhstan .... 64 F3 50 40N 51 53 E
Chalkar, Ozero =
  Shalkar, Ozero,
  Kazakhstan .... 64 F3 50 35N 51 47 E
Chalky Inlet, *N.Z.* ... 131 G1 46 3 S 166 31 E
Chalkyitsik, *U.S.A.* ... 166 B5 66 39N 143 43W
Challakere, *India* .... 95 G3 14 19N 76 39 E
Challans, *France* 26 F5 46 50N 1 52W
Challapata, *Bolivia* ... 172 D4 18 53 S 66 50W
Challenger Deep,
  Pac. Oc. .... 134 F6 11 30N 142 0 E
Challenger Fracture
  Zone, *Pac. Oc.* .... 135 L17 35 0 S 105 0W
Challis, *U.S.A.* 158 D6 44 30N 114 14W
Chalmette, *U.S.A.* 155 L10 29 56N 89 58W
Chalon-sur-Saône,
  France .... 27 F11 46 48N 4 50 E
Chalonnes-sur-Loire,
  France 26 E6 47 20N 0 45W
Châlons-en-
  Champagne, *France* 27 D11 48 58N 4 20 E
Chalus, *France* ...... 28 C4 45 39N 0 58 E
Chālūs, *Iran* .... 97 B6 36 38N 51 26 E
Cham, *Germany* ...... 31 F8 49 13N 12 39 E
Cham, *Switz.* .... 33 B6 47 11N 8 28 E
Cham, Cu Lao, *Vietnam* 86 E7 15 57N 108 30 E
Chama, *U.S.A.* 159 H10 36 54N 106 35W
Chamah, Gunong,
  Malaysia .... 84 A2 5 13N 101 35 E
Chamaicó, *Argentina* . 174 D3 35 3 S 64 58W
Chaman, *Pakistan* .... 91 C2 30 58N 66 25 E
Chamba, *India* ...... 92 C7 32 35N 76 10 E
Chamba, *Tanzania* ... 119 E4 11 37 S 37 0 E
Chambal →, *India* ... 93 F8 26 29N 79 15 E
Chamberlain, *U.S.A.* . 154 D5 43 49N 99 20W
Chamberlain →,
  Australia .... 124 C4 15 30 S 127 54 E
Chamberlain L., *U.S.A.* 149 B11 46 14N 69 19W
Chambers, *U.S.A.* 159 J9 35 11N 109 26W
Chambersburg, *U.S.A.* 148 F7 39 56N 77 40W
Chambéry, *France* .... 29 C9 45 34N 5 55 E
Chamblee, *U.S.A.* 152 B5 33 53N 84 18W
Chambly, *Canada* 151 A11 45 27N 73 17W
Chambord, *Canada* ... 141 C5 48 25N 72 6W
Chamboulive, *France* . 28 C5 45 26N 1 42 E
Chambri L.,
  Papua N. G. ...... 132 C2 4 15 S 143 10 E
Chamchamal, *Iraq* ... 101 E11 35 32N 44 50 E
Chamela, *Mexico* 162 D3 19 32N 105 5W
Chamical, *Argentina* . 174 C2 30 22 S 66 27W
Chamkar Luong,
  Cambodia .... 87 G4 11 0N 103 45 E
Chamois, *U.S.A.* 156 F5 38 41N 91 46W
Chamoli, *India* ...... 93 D8 30 24N 79 21 E
Chamonix-Mont Blanc,
  France .... 29 C10 45 55N 6 51 E
Chamoson, *Switz.* .... 32 D4 46 12N 7 13 E
Champa, *India* ...... 93 H10 22 2N 82 43 E
Champagne, *Canada* . 142 A1 60 49N 136 30W
Champagne, *France* .. 27 D11 48 40N 4 20 E
Champagnole, *France* . 27 F12 46 45N 5 55 E
Champaign, *U.S.A.* .. 157 D8 40 7N 88 15W
Champassak, *Laos* ... 86 E5 14 53N 105 52 E
Champaubert, *France* . 27 D10 48 50N 3 45 E
Champawat, *India* ... 93 E9 29 20N 80 6 E
Champdeniers-St-
  Denis, *France* 28 B3 46 29N 0 25W
Champdoré, L., *Canada* 141 A6 55 55N 65 49W
Champeix, *France* .... 28 C7 45 37N 3 8 E
Champéry, *Switz.* .... 32 D3 46 11N 6 52 E
Champion, *U.S.A.* ... 150 E4 41 19N 80 51W
Champlain, *U.S.A.* ... 151 B11 44 59N 73 27W
Champlain, L., *U.S.A.* 151 B11 44 40N 73 20W
Champlitte, *France* ... 27 E12 47 32N 5 31 E
Champotón, *Mexico* . 163 D6 19 20N 90 50W
Champua, *India* ..... 93 H11 22 5N 85 40 E
Chamrajnagar, *India* . 95 J3 11 52N 76 52 E
Chamusca, *Portugal* . 43 F2 39 21N 8 29W
Chana, *Thailand* .... 87 J3 6 55N 100 44 E
Chan Chan, *Peru* .... 174 B1 26 23 S 70 40W
Chañaral, *Chile* ..... 174 B1 26 23 S 70 40W
Chanārān, *Iran* ..... 97 B8 36 39N 59 6 E
Chanasma, *India* .... 92 H5 23 44N 72 5 E
Chancay, *Peru* ...... 172 C2 11 32 S 77 25W
Chancery Lane,
  Barbados .... 165 g 13 3N 59 30W
Chanchiang =
  Zhanjiang, *China* .. 77 B8 21 15N 110 20 E
Chanco, *Chile* ...... 174 D1 35 44 S 72 32W
Chancy, *Switz.* ...... 32 D1 46 8N 5 58 E
Chand, *India* .... 93 J8 21 57N 79 7 E
Chandalar →, *U.S.A.* 144 C11 66 37N 146 0W
Chandan, *India* ..... 93 G12 24 38N 86 40 E
Chandan Chauki, *India* 93 E9 28 33N 80 47 E
Chandannagar, *India* . 93 H13 22 52N 88 24 E
Chandausi, *India* .... 93 E8 28 27N 78 49 E
Chandeleur Is., *U.S.A.* 155 L10 29 55N 88 57W
Chandeleur Sd., *U.S.A.* 155 L10 29 55N 89 0W
Chandigarh, *India* ... 92 D7 30 43N 76 47 E
Chandil, *India* ...... 93 H12 22 58N 86 3 E
Chandler, *Australia* .. 127 D1 27 0 S 133 19 E
Chandler, *Canada* ... 141 C7 48 18N 64 46W
Chandler, *Ariz., U.S.A.* 159 K8 33 18N 111 50W
Chandler, *Okla., U.S.A.* 155 H6 35 42N 96 53W
Chandless →, *Brazil* . 172 B4 9 8 S 69 51W
Chandod, *India* ..... 92 J5 21 59N 73 28 E
Chandpur, *Bangla.* .. 90 D3 23 8N 90 45 E
Chandpur, *India* .... 95 H4 13 35N 79 19 E
Chandragiri, *India* ... 95 H4 13 35N 79 19 E
Chandrapur, *India* ... 94 E5 18 33N 80 24 E
Chānf, *Iran* .... 97 E9 26 38N 60 29 E
Chang, *Pakistan* .... 92 F3 26 59N 68 30 E
Chang, Ko, *Thailand* . 87 F4 12 0N 102 23 E
Ch'ang Chiang = Chang
  Jiang →, *China* ... 77 B13 31 48N 121 10 E
Chang Jiang →, *China* 77 B13 31 48N 121 10 E
Changa, *India* ...... 93 C7 33 53N 77 35 E
Changan = Xi'an, *China* 74 G5 34 15N 109 0 E
Changanacheri, *India* . 95 K3 9 25N 76 31 E
Changane →, *Mozam.* 117 C5 24 30 S 33 30 E
Changbai, *China* .... 75 D15 41 25N 128 5 E
Changbai Shan, *China* 75 C15 42 20N 129 0 E
Changchiak'ou =
  Zhangjiakou, *China* 74 D8 40 48N 114 55 E
Changchih = Changzhi,
  China .... 74 F7 36 10N 113 6 E

Changhai = Shanghai,
  China .... 77 B13 31 15N 121 26 E
Changhua, *China* .... 77 B12 30 12N 119 12 E
Changhua, *Taiwan* ... 77 E13 24 2N 120 30 E
Changhŭng, *S. Korea* . 75 G14 34 41N 126 52 E
Changhŭngni, *N. Korea* 75 D15 40 24N 128 19 E
Changi, *Malaysia* .... 84 B2 1 23N 103 59 E
Changi, *Singapore* ... 87 d 1 23N 103 59 E
Changi, *Singapore* ✈
  (SIN), *Singapore* .. 87 M4 1 23N 103 59 E
Changjiang, *China* ... 86 C7 19 20N 108 55 E
Changjiang Shuiku,
  China .... 69 G10 22 29N 113 27 E
Changjin, *N. Korea* .. 75 D14 40 23N 127 15 E
Changjin-chōsuji,
  N. Korea .... 75 D14 40 30N 127 15 E
Changle, *China* ...... 77 E12 25 59N 119 27 E
Changli, *China* ...... 75 E10 39 40N 119 13 E
Changling, *China* .... 75 B12 44 20N 123 58 E
Changlun, *Malaysia* .. 87 J3 6 25N 100 26 E
Changning, *Hunan,*
  China .... 77 D9 26 28N 112 22 E
Changning, *Sichuan,*
  China .... 76 C5 28 40N 104 56 E
Changning, *Yunnan,*
  China .... 76 E2 24 45N 99 30 E
Changping, *China* .... 74 D9 40 14N 116 12 E
Changsha, *China* .... 77 C9 28 12N 113 0 E
Changshan, *China* ... 77 C12 28 55N 118 27 E
Changshu, *China* .... 77 B13 31 38N 120 43 E
Changshun, *China* ... 76 D6 26 3N 106 18 E
Changtai, *China* ..... 77 E11 24 35N 117 42 E
Changt'e = Chongde,
  China .... 77 B13 30 12N 120 26 E
Changting, *China* .... 77 E11 25 50N 116 22 E
Changwu, *China* ..... 74 G4 35 10N 107 45 E
Changxing, *China* .... 77 B12 31 0N 119 55 E
Changyang, *China* ... 77 B8 30 30N 111 10 E
Changyi, *China* ...... 75 F10 36 40N 119 30 E
Changyŏn, *N. Korea* . 75 E13 38 15N 125 6 E
Changyuan, *China* ... 74 G8 35 15N 114 42 E
Changzhi, *China* ..... 74 F7 36 10N 113 6 E
Changzhou, *China* ... 77 B12 31 47N 119 58 E
Chanhanga, *Angola* . 116 B1 16 0 S 14 8 E
Chania = Khaniá,
  Greece .... 39 E5 35 30N 24 4 E
Chanlar = Xanlar,
  Azerbaijan .... 61 K8 40 37N 46 12 E
Channagiri, *India* .... 95 G2 14 2N 75 56 E
Channapatna, *India* . 95 H3 12 40N 77 15 E
Channel Is., *U.K.* 21 H5 49 19N 2 24W
Channel Is., *U.S.A.* .. 161 M7 33 40N 119 15W
Channel Islands △,
  U.S.A. 161 L7 34 0N 119 24W
Channel-Port aux
  Basques, *Canada* .. 141 C8 47 30N 59 9W
Channel Tunnel,
  Europe .... 21 F9 51 0N 1 30 E
Channing, *U.S.A.* ... 155 H3 35 41N 102 20W
Chantada, *Spain* 42 C3 42 36N 7 46W
Chanthaburi, *Thailand* 86 F4 12 38N 102 12 E
Chantilly, *France* .... 27 C9 49 12N 2 29 E
Chantonnay, *France* . 26 F5 46 40N 1 3W
Chantrey Inlet, *Canada* 138 B10 67 48N 96 20W
Chanumla, *India* .... 95 K11 8 19N 93 5 E
Chanute, *U.S.A.* 155 G7 37 41N 95 27W
Chanza →, *Spain* ... 43 H3 37 32N 7 30W
Chao Hu, *China* ..... 77 B11 31 30N 117 30 E
Chao Phraya →,
  Thailand .... 86 F3 13 32N 100 36 E
Chao Phraya Lowlands,
  Thailand .... 86 E3 15 30N 100 0 E
Chaocheng, *China* ... 74 F8 36 4N 115 37 E
Chaohu, *China* ...... 77 B11 31 38N 117 50 E
Chaoyang, *Guangdong,*
  China .... 77 F11 23 17N 116 30 E
Chaoyang, *Liaoning,*
  China .... 75 D11 41 35N 120 22 E
Chaozhou, *China* .... 77 F11 23 42N 116 32 E
Chapada
  Diamantina △, *Brazil* 171 D3 12 52 S 41 30W
Chapada dos
  Guimarães, *Brazil* . 173 D6 15 26 S 55 45W
Chapada dos
  Guimarães △, *Brazil* 173 D6 15 18 S 55 54W
Chapada dos
  Veadeiros △, *Brazil* 171 D2 14 0 S 47 30W
Chapais, *Canada* 140 C5 49 47N 74 51W
Chapala, *Mozam.* ... 119 F4 15 50 S 37 35 E
Chapala, L. de, *Mexico* 162 C4 20 10N 103 20W
Chaparé →, *Bolivia* . 173 D5 15 58 S 64 42W
Chaparmukh, *India* . 90 B4 26 12N 92 31 E
Chaparral, *Colombia* . 168 C2 3 43N 75 28W
Chapayev, *Kazakhstan* 60 D9 50 25N 51 10 E
Chapayevsk, *Russia* .. 60 D9 53 0N 49 40 E
Chapecó, *Brazil* ..... 175 B5 27 14 S 52 41W
Chapel Hill, *U.S.A.* .. 149 H6 35 55N 79 4W
Chapetsk = Edinburg,
  U.S.A. 155 M5 26 18N 98 10W
Chapin, *U.S.A.* 156 E6 39 46N 90 24W
Chapleau, *Canada* ... 140 C3 47 50N 83 24W
Chaplin, *Canada* 143 C7 50 28N 106 40W
Chaplin L., *Canada* . 143 C7 50 22N 106 36W
Chaplino, *Ukraine* ... 59 H9 48 8N 36 15 E
Chaplygin, *Russia* ... 58 F11 53 15N 40 0 E
Chappell, *U.S.A.* 154 E3 41 6N 102 28W
Chappells, *U.S.A.* ... 152 A8 34 11N 81 52W
Chapra = Chhapra,
  India .... 93 G11 25 48N 84 44 E
Châr, *Mauritania* 110 D2 21 32N 12 45W
Chara, *Russia* ...... 67 D12 56 54N 118 20 E
Charadai, *Argentina* . 174 B4 27 35 S 59 55W
Charagua, *Bolivia* ... 173 D5 19 45 S 63 10W
Charalá, *Colombia* ... 168 B3 6 17N 73 10W
Charambirá, Punta,
  Colombia 168 C2 4 16N 77 32W
Charaña, *Bolivia* .... 172 D4 17 30 S 69 25W
Charantsavan, *Armenia* 61 K7 40 35N 44 41 E
Charanwala, *India* ... 92 F5 27 51N 72 10 E
Charapita, *Colombia* . 168 D3 0 37 S 74 21W
Charata, *Argentina* .. 174 B3 27 13 S 61 14W
Charcas, *Mexico* 162 C4 23 10N 101 20W
Charcoal L., *Canada* . 143 B8 58 49N 102 22W
Charcot I., *Antarctica* 7 C17 70 0 S 70 0W
Chard, *U.K.* 21 G5 50 52N 2 58W
Chardon, *U.S.A.* 150 E3 41 35N 81 12W
Charduar, *India* .... 90 B4 26 51N 92 46 E
Chardzhou = Chärjew,
  Turkmenistan .... 65 E3 39 6N 63 34 E
Charente □, *France* . 28 C4 45 50N 0 16 E
Charente →, *France* . 28 C2 45 57N 1 5W
Charente-Inférieure =
  Charente-
  Maritime □, *France* 28 C3 45 45N 0 45W
Charente-Maritime □,
  France 28 C3 45 45N 0 45W
Charenton-du-Cher,
  France .... 27 F9 46 44N 2 39 E
Chari →, *Chad* ..... 109 F2 12 58N 14 31 E
Chārīkār, *Afghan.* ... 91 B3 35 0N 69 10 E
Charing, *U.K.* ...... 21 F8 51 12N 0 49 E
Chariton, *Iowa, U.S.A.* 156 E8 41 1N 93 19W
Chariton →, *U.S.A.* . 156 E4 39 19N 92 58W

Charity, *Guyana* 169 B6 7 24N 58 36W
Chärjew, *Turkmenistan* 65 D1 39 6N 63 34 E
Charkhari, *India* .... 93 G8 25 24N 79 45 E
Charkhi Dadri, *India* . 92 E7 28 37N 76 17 E
Charleroi, *Belgium* ... 24 D4 50 24N 4 27 E
Charleroi, *U.S.A.* ... 150 F5 40 9N 79 57W
Charles, C., *U.S.A.* .. 148 G8 37 7N 75 58W
Charles, I. = Santa
  María, I., *Ecuador* . 172 a 1 17 S 90 26W
Charles City, *U.S.A.* . 156 D8 43 4N 92 41W
Charles L., *Canada* .. 143 B6 59 50N 110 33W
Charles Sound, *N.Z.* . 131 F2 45 2 S 167 4 E
Charles Town, *U.S.A.* 148 F7 39 17N 77 52W
Charlesbourg, *Canada* 141 C5 46 51N 71 16W
Charleston, *Ill., U.S.A.* 157 F8 39 30N 88 10W
Charleston, *Miss.,*
  U.S.A. 155 H9 34 1N 90 4W
Charleston, *Mo., U.S.A.* 155 G10 36 55N 89 21W
Charleston, *S.C., U.S.A.* 152 C10 32 46N 79 56W
Charleston, *W. Va.,*
  U.S.A. 148 F5 38 21N 81 38W
Charleston L., *Canada* 151 B9 44 32N 76 0W
Charleston Peak,
  U.S.A. 161 J11 36 16N 115 42W
Charlestown, *Ireland* . 23 C3 53 58N 8 48W
Charlestown, *S. Africa* 117 D4 27 26 S 29 53 E
Charlestown, *Ind.,*
  U.S.A. 157 F11 38 27N 85 40W
Charlestown, *N.H.,*
  U.S.A. 151 C12 43 14N 72 25W
Charlestown of
  Aberlour, *U.K.* 22 D5 57 28N 3 14W
Charleville = Rath
  Luirc, *Ireland* 23 D3 52 21N 8 40W
Charleville, *Australia* . 127 D4 26 24 S 146 15 E
Charleville-Mézières,
  France .... 27 C11 49 44N 4 40 E
Charlevoix, *U.S.A.* .. 148 C3 45 19N 85 16W
Charlieu, *France* .... 27 F11 46 10N 4 10 E
Charlotte, *Mich., U.S.A.* 157 B12 42 34N 84 50W
Charlotte, *N.C., U.S.A.* 149 H5 35 13N 80 51W
Charlotte, *Vt., U.S.A.* 151 B11 44 19N 73 14W
Charlotte Amalie,
  U.S. Virgin Is. .... 165 e 18 21N 64 56W
Charlotte Harbor,
  U.S.A. 153 J7 26 50N 82 10W
Charlotte L., *Canada* . 142 C3 52 12N 125 19W
Charlottenberg, *Sweden* 10 E6 59 54N 12 17 E
Charlottesville, *U.S.A.* 148 F6 38 2N 78 30W
Charlottetown,
  Nfld. & L., Canada 141 B8 52 46N 56 7W
Charlottetown, *P.E.I.,*
  Canada 141 C7 46 14N 63 8W
Charlotteville,
  Trin. & Tob. 169 E10 11 20N 60 33W
Charlton, *Australia* .. 128 D5 36 16 S 143 24 E
Charlton I., *Canada* . 140 B4 52 0N 79 20W
Charmes, *France* .... 27 D13 48 22N 6 17 E
Charmey, *Switz.* .... 32 C4 46 37N 7 10 E
Charny, *Canada* 141 C5 46 43N 71 15W
Charnyany, *Belarus* . 55 G11 51 59N 24 12 E
Charolles, *France* ... 27 F11 46 27N 4 16 E
Charost, *France* .... 27 F9 47 0N 2 7 E
Charouine, *Algeria* .. 111 C4 29 0N 0 15W
Charre, *Mozam.* .... 119 F4 17 13 S 35 10 E
Charroux, *France* ... 28 B4 46 9N 0 25 E
Charsadda, *Pakistan* . 92 B4 34 7N 71 45 E
Charshanga,
  Turkmenistan .... 65 E3 37 30N 66 1 E
Charters Towers,
  Australia .... 126 C4 20 5 S 146 13 E
Chartres, *France* .... 26 D8 48 29N 1 30 E
Chartrouse =, *France* 29 C9 45 22N 5 42 E
Charvakskoye Vdkhr.,
  Uzbekistan ...... 65 C5 41 35N 70 0 E
Chascomús, *Argentina* 174 D4 35 30 S 58 0W
Chasefu, *Zambia* ... 119 E3 11 55 S 33 8 E
Chashma Barrage,
  Pakistan .... 91 B3 32 27N 71 20 E
Chaslands Mistake,
  N.Z. .... 131 G4 46 38 S 169 22 E
Chasseneuil-sur-
  Bonnieure, *France* 28 C4 45 52N 0 29 E
Chasseron, *Switz.* ... 32 C3 46 52N 6 32 E
Chāt, *Iran* .... 97 B7 37 59N 55 16 E
Chatal Balkan = Udvoy
  Balkan, *Bulgaria* .. 51 D10 42 50N 26 50 E
Chatanika, *U.S.A.* .. 144 D11 65 7N 147 28W
Château-Arnoux-St-
  Auban, *France* ... 29 D10 44 6N 6 0 E
Château-Chinon,
  France .... 27 E10 47 4N 3 56 E
Château d'Oex, *Switz.* 32 D4 46 28N 7 8 E
Château-d'Olonne,
  France 28 B2 46 30N 1 44W
Château-du-Loir,
  France .... 26 E7 47 40N 0 25 E
Château-Gontier,
  France 26 E6 47 50N 0 48W
Château-la-Vallière,
  France .... 26 E7 47 30N 0 20 E
Château-Landon,
  France .... 27 D9 48 8N 2 40 E
Château-Renard,
  France .... 27 E9 47 56N 2 55 E
Château-Renault,
  France .... 26 E7 47 36N 0 56 E
Château-Salins, *France* 27 D13 48 50N 6 30 E
Château-Thierry,
  France .... 27 C10 49 3N 3 20 E
Châteaubourg, *France* 26 D5 48 7N 1 25W
Châteaubriant, *France* 26 E5 47 43N 1 23W
Châteaudun, *France* . 26 D8 48 3N 1 20 E
Chateaugay, *U.S.A.* . 151 B10 44 56N 74 5W
Châteaugiron, *France* 26 D5 48 3N 1 30W
Châteauguay, L.,
  Canada 141 A5 56 26N 70 3W
Châteaulin, *France* .. 26 D2 48 11N 4 8W
Châteaumeillant,
  France .... 27 F9 46 35N 2 12 E
Châteauneuf-du-Faou,
  France 26 D3 48 11N 3 50W
Châteauneuf-sur-
  Charente, *France* . 28 C3 45 36N 0 3W
Châteauneuf-sur-Cher,
  France .... 27 F9 46 52N 2 18 E
Châteauneuf-sur-Loire,
  France .... 27 E9 47 52N 2 13 E
Châteaurenard, *France* 29 E8 43 53N 4 51 E
Châteauroux, *France* . 27 F8 46 50N 1 40 E
Châteauvillain, *France* 27 D11 48 2N 4 55 E
Châteaux, Pte. des,
  Guadeloupe ...... 164 b 16 15N 61 10W
Châtel-St-Denis, *Switz.* 32 C3 46 32N 6 54 E
Châtelaillon-Plage,
  France 28 B2 46 5N 1 5W
Châtelguyon, *France* . 28 C7 45 55N 3 4 E
Châtellerault, *France* . 26 F7 46 50N 0 30 E
Châtelus-Malvaleix,
  France .... 27 F9 46 18N 2 1 E
Chatham = Chatham-
  Kent, *Canada* 140 D3 42 24N 82 11W

Chatham = Miramichi,
  Canada 141 C6 47 2N 65 28W
Chatham, *U.K.* ..... 21 F8 51 22N 0 32 E
Chatham, *Ill., U.S.A.* . 156 F7 39 40N 89 42W
Chatham, *N.Y., U.S.A.* 151 D11 42 21N 73 36W
Chatham, I. = San
  Cristóbal, I., *Ecuador* 172 a 0 50 S 89 26W
Chatham I., *Chile* .... 176 D2 50 40 S 74 25W
Chatham I., *N.Z.* .... 131 a 43 50 S 176 20W
Chatham Is., *Pac. Oc.* 130 a 44 0 S 176 40W
Chatham-Kent, *Canada* 140 D3 42 24N 82 11W
Châtillon, *Italy* ...... 44 C4 45 45N 7 37 E
Châtillon-Coligny,
  France .... 27 E9 47 50N 2 51 E
Châtillon-en-Diois,
  France .... 29 D9 44 41N 5 29 E
Châtillon-sur-Indre,
  France .... 26 F8 46 59N 1 10 E
Châtillon-sur-Loire,
  France .... 27 E9 47 35N 2 44 E
Châtillon-sur-Seine,
  France .... 27 E11 47 50N 4 33 E
Chatkal →, *Uzbekistan* 65 C5 41 38N 70 1 E
Chatkal Kyrka Tooloru,
  Kyrgyzstan .... 65 C5 41 30N 70 45 E
Chatmohar, *Bangla.* . 93 G13 24 15N 89 15 E
Chatra, *India* .... 93 G11 24 12N 84 56 E
Chatrapur, *India* .... 94 E7 19 22N 85 2 E
Chats, L. des, *Canada* 151 A8 45 30N 76 20W
Chatsu, *India* .... 92 F6 26 36N 75 57 E
Chatsworth, *Canada* . 150 B4 44 27N 80 54W
Chatsworth, *U.S.A.* . 157 D8 40 45N 88 18W
Chatsworth, *Zimbabwe* 119 F3 19 38 S 31 13 E
Chatta-Hantō, *Japan* 73 C8 34 45N 136 55 E
Chāttagām =
  Chittagong, *Bangla.* 90 D3 22 19N 91 48 E
Chattahoochee, *U.S.A.* 152 E5 30 42N 84 51W
Chattahoochee →,
  U.S.A. 152 E5 30 54N 84 57W
Chattanooga, *U.S.A.* . 149 H3 35 3N 85 19W
Chatteris, *U.K.* ..... 21 E8 52 28N 0 2 E
Chaturat, *Thailand* .. 86 E3 15 40N 101 51 E
Chatyr-Köl, *Kyrgyzstan* 65 C7 40 40N 75 18 E
Chatyr-Tash,
  Kyrgyzstan .... 65 C8 40 55N 76 25 E
Chau Doc, *Vietnam* . 87 G5 10 42N 105 7 E
Chaudes-Aigues,
  France .... 28 D7 44 51N 3 1 E
Chauffailles, *France* . 27 F11 46 13N 4 20 E
Chauk, *Burma* ...... 90 E5 20 53N 94 49 E
Chaukan Pass, *Burma* 90 B6 27 8N 97 10 E
Chaumont, *France* .. 27 D12 48 7N 5 8 E
Chaumont, *U.S.A.* .. 151 B8 44 4N 76 8W
Chaumont-en-Vexin,
  France .... 27 C8 49 16N 1 53 E
Chaumont-sur-Loire,
  France .... 26 E8 47 29N 1 11 E
Chaunay, *France* .... 28 B4 46 13N 0 9 E
Chaunskaya G., *Russia* 6 C16 69 0N 169 0 E
Chauny, *France* ..... 27 C10 49 37N 3 12 E
Chaura, *India* ...... 95 K11 8 27N 93 2 E
Chausey, Îs., *France* . 26 D5 48 52N 1 49W
Chaussin, *France* ... 27 F12 46 59N 5 22 E
Chautauqua L., *U.S.A.* 150 D5 42 10N 79 24W
Chauvay, *Kyrgyzstan* 65 C6 40 8N 72 8 E
Chauvigny, *France* .. 26 F7 46 34N 0 39 E
Chauvin, *Canada* ... 143 C6 52 45N 110 10W
Chavakachcheri,
  Sri Lanka .... 95 K5 9 39N 80 9 E
Chavanges, *France* .. 27 D11 48 30N 4 35 E
Chavantina, *Brazil* .. 173 C7 14 40 S 52 21W
Chaves, *Brazil* ...... 170 B2 0 15 S 49 55W
Chaves, *Portugal* 42 D3 41 45N 7 32W
Chavuma, *Zambia* .. 115 E4 13 4 S 22 40 E
Chawang, *Thailand* .. 87 H2 8 25N 99 30 E
Chayan = Shayan,
  Kazakhstan .... 65 B4 43 5N 69 25 E
Chaykovskiy, *Russia* . 64 C5 56 47N 54 9 E
Chazelles-sur-Lyon,
  France .... 29 C8 45 39N 4 22 E
Chazuta, *Peru* ...... 172 B2 6 30 S 76 0W
Chazy, *U.S.A.* 151 B11 44 53N 73 26W
Cheaha Mt., *U.S.A.* . 152 B3 33 29N 85 49W
Cheb, *Czech Rep.* ... 34 A5 50 9N 12 28 E
Chebanse, *U.S.A.* ... 157 D9 41 0N 87 54W
Chebarkul, *Russia* ... 64 D8 55 0N 60 25 E
Cheboksarskoye
  Vdkhr., *Russia* .... 56 B8 56 13N 46 58 E
Cheboksary, *Russia* . 60 B8 56 8N 47 12 E
Cheboygan, *U.S.A.* . 148 C3 45 39N 84 29W
Chebsara, *Russia* ... 58 C10 59 10N 38 59 E
Chech, Erg, *Africa* .. 110 D4 25 0N 2 15W
Chechaouen, *Morocco* 110 A4 35 9N 5 15W
Chechelnyk, *Ukraine* . 53 B14 48 13N 29 22 E
Chechen, Ostrov,
  Russia .... 61 H8 43 59N 47 40 E
Chechenia □, *Russia* . 61 J7 43 30N 45 29 E
Checheno-Ingush
  Republic =
  Chechenia □, *Russia* 61 J7 43 30N 45 29 E
Chechnya =
  Chechenia □, *Russia* 61 J7 43 30N 45 29 E
Chech'ŏn, *S. Korea* .. 75 F15 37 8N 128 12 E
Cȩciny, *Poland* ..... 55 H7 50 46N 20 28 E
Checotah, *U.S.A.* ... 155 H7 35 28N 95 31W
Chedabucto B., *Canada* 141 C7 45 25N 61 8W
Cheduba I., *Burma* .. 90 F4 18 45N 93 40 E
Cheepie, *Australia* ... 127 D4 26 33 S 145 1 E
Chef-Boutonne, *France* 28 B3 46 7N 0 4W
Cheffadine, *Niger* ... 109 D2 19 57N 12 11 E
Chefoo = Yantai, *China* 75 F11 37 34N 121 22 E
Chefornak, *U.S.A.* .. 144 F6 60 13N 164 12W
Chegdomyn, *Russia* . 67 D14 51 7N 133 1 E
Chegga, *Mauritania* . 110 C3 25 27N 5 40W
Chegutu, *Zimbabwe* . 119 F3 18 10 S 30 14 E
Chehalis, *U.S.A.* 160 D4 46 40N 122 58W
Chehalis →, *U.S.A.* . 160 D3 46 57N 123 50W
Cheile Nerei-
  Beuşniţa △, *Romania* 52 F6 44 56N 21 52 E
Cheiron, Mt., *France* 29 E10 43 49N 6 58 E
Cheju do, *S. Korea* .. 75 H14 33 29N 126 34 E
Chekalin, *Russia* .... 58 E9 54 10N 36 10 E
Chekhovo, *Russia* ... 54 D7 54 33N 20 43 E
Chekiang = Zhejiang □,
  China .... 77 C13 29 0N 120 0 E
Chel = Kuru, Bahr
  el →, *Sudan* ..... 107 F2 8 10N 26 50 E
Chela, Sa. da, *Angola* 116 B1 16 20 S 13 20 E
Chelan, *U.S.A.* 158 C4 47 51N 120 1W
Chelan, L., *U.S.A.* .. 158 B3 48 11N 120 30W
Chelek, *Uzbekistan* . 65 D3 39 55N 66 51 E
Cheleken,
  Turkmenistan .... 57 G9 39 34N 53 16 E
Cheleken Yarymadasy,
  Turkmenistan .... 97 B7 39 30N 53 15 E
Chelforó, *Argentina* . 176 A3 39 0 S 66 33W
Chéliff, O. →, *Algeria* 111 A5 36 0N 0 8 E
Chelkar = Shalqar,
  Kazakhstan .... 66 E6 47 48N 59 39 E
Chelkar Tengiz,
  Solonchak,
  Kazakhstan .... 66 E7 48 5N 63 7 E
Chella, *Ethiopia* .... 107 F4 6 40N 37 26 E
Chellala Dahrania,
  Algeria .... 111 B5 33 2N 0 1 E

Chelles, *France* ..... 27 D9 48 52N 2 33 E
Chełm, *Poland* ..... 55 G10 51 8N 23 30 E
Chełmno, *Poland* ... 55 E5 53 20N 18 30 E
Chelmsford, *U.K.* ... 21 F8 51 44N 0 29 E
Chełmża, *Poland* .... 55 E5 53 10N 18 39 E
Chelny = Naberezhnyye
  Chelny, *Russia* .... 60 C11 55 42N 52 19 E
Chelsea, *Australia* ... 129 E6 38 5 S 145 8 E
Chelsea, *Mich., U.S.A.* 157 B12 42 19N 84 1W
Chelsea, *Vt., U.S.A.* . 151 C12 43 59N 72 27W
Cheltenham, *U.K.* ... 21 F5 51 54N 2 4W
Chelva, *Spain* 40 F4 39 45N 1 0W
Chelyabinsk, *Russia* . 64 D8 55 10N 61 24 E
Chelyakobi = Kopeysk,
  Russia .... 64 D8 55 7N 61 37 E
Chelyuskin, C. =
  Chelyuskin, Mys,
  Russia .... 67 B11 77 30N 103 0 E
Chelyuskin, Mys,
  Russia .... 67 B11 77 30N 103 0 E
Chemainus, *Canada* . 160 B3 48 55N 123 42W
Chembar = Belinskiy,
  Russia .... 60 D6 53 0N 43 25 E
Chemillé, *France* 26 E6 47 14N 0 45W
Chemin Grenier,
  Mauritius .... 121 d 20 29 S 57 28 E
Chemnitz, *Germany* . 30 E8 50 51N 12 54 E
Chemulpho = Inch'ŏn,
  S. Korea .... 75 F14 37 27N 126 40 E
Chemult, *U.S.A.* 158 E3 43 14N 121 47W
Chen, Gora, *Russia* . 67 C15 65 16N 141 50 E
Chenab →, *Pakistan* 91 C3 30 23N 71 2 E
Chenachane, O. →,
  Algeria 110 C4 25 20N 3 20W
Chenango Forks,
  U.S.A. 151 D9 42 15N 75 51W
Chencha, *Ethiopia* ... 107 F4 6 15N 37 32 E
Chenchiang =
  Zhenjiang, *China* .. 77 A12 32 11N 119 26 E
Cheney, *U.S.A.* 158 C5 47 30N 117 35W
Chengalpattu, *India* . 95 H4 12 42N 79 58 E
Chengbu, *China* ..... 77 D8 26 18N 110 16 E
Chengcheng, *China* . 74 G5 35 8N 109 56 E
Chengchou =
  Zhengzhou, *China* . 74 G7 34 45N 113 34 E
Chengde, *China* ..... 75 D9 40 59N 117 58 E
Chengdong Hu, *China* 77 A11 32 15N 116 40 E
Chengdu, *China* .... 76 B5 30 38N 104 2 E
Chengele, *India* ..... 90 A6 28 47N 96 16 E
Chenggong, *China* .. 76 E4 24 52N 102 56 E
Chenggu, *China* .... 74 H4 33 10N 107 21 E
Chenghai, *China* .... 77 F11 23 30N 116 42 E
Chengjiang, *China* .. 76 E4 24 39N 103 0 E
Chengkou, *China* ... 76 B7 31 54N 108 31 E
Chengmai, *China* ... 86 C7 19 50N 109 58 E
Chengteh = Chengde,
  China .... 75 D9 40 59N 117 58 E
Ch'engtu = Chengdu,
  China .... 76 B5 30 38N 104 2 E
Chengwu, *China* .... 74 G8 34 58N 115 50 E
Chengxi Hu, *China* .. 77 A11 32 15N 116 10 E
Chengyang, *China* ... 75 F11 36 18N 120 21 E
Chenjiagang, *China* . 75 G10 34 23N 119 47 E
Chenkaladi, *Sri Lanka* 95 K5 7 47N 81 35 E
Chennai, *India* ...... 95 H5 13 8N 80 19 E
Chenoa, *U.S.A.* 157 D8 40 45N 88 43W
Chenôve, *France* .... 27 E12 47 16N 5 1 E
Chenxi, *China* ...... 77 C8 28 2N 110 12 E
Chenzhou, *China* ... 77 E9 25 47N 113 1 E
Cheo Reo, *Vietnam* . 78 B3 13 25N 108 28 E
Cheom Ksan,
  Cambodia .... 86 E5 14 13N 104 56 E
Chepelare, *Bulgaria* . 51 E8 41 44N 24 40 E
Chepén, *Peru* ...... 172 B2 7 15 S 79 23W
Chépénéhé, *Vanuatu* 133 K5 20 47 S 167 9 E
Chepes, *Argentina* .. 174 C2 31 20 S 66 35W
Chepo, *Panama* 164 E4 9 10N 79 6W
Chepstow, *U.K.* 21 F5 51 38N 2 41W
Cheptsa = Chaptsk →,
  Russia .... 64 B3 58 36N 50 4 E
Chequamegon B.,
  U.S.A. 154 B9 46 40N 90 30W
Cher □, *France* ..... 27 E9 47 10N 2 30 E
Cher →, *France* .... 26 E7 47 21N 0 29 E
Chéradi, *Italy* ...... 47 B10 40 27N 17 10 E
Cheran, *India* ...... 90 C3 25 45N 90 44 E
Cherasco, *Italy* ..... 44 D4 44 39N 7 51 E
Cheraw, *U.S.A.* 149 H6 34 42N 79 53W
Cherbourg, *U.K.* 26 C5 49 39N 1 40W
Cherchell, *Algeria* ... 111 A5 36 35N 2 12 E
Cherdakly, *Russia* ... 60 C9 54 25N 48 50 E
Cherdyn, *Russia* .... 64 A6 60 24N 56 29 E
Cheremkhovo, *Russia* 67 D11 53 8N 103 1 E
Cherepanovo, *Russia* 66 D9 54 15N 83 30 E
Cherepovets, *Russia* . 58 C9 59 5N 37 55 E
Chergui, Chott ech,
  Algeria .... 111 B5 34 21N 0 25 E
Chergui, Zahrez,
  Algeria .... 111 B5 35 11N 3 31 E
Cherial, *India* ...... 94 F4 17 55N 78 59 E
Cheribon = Cirebon,
  Indonesia .... 85 D3 6 45 S 108 32 E
Cherikov = Cherykaw,
  Belarus .... 58 F6 53 32N 31 20 E
Cheriyam I., *India* ... 95 J1 10 9N 73 40 E
Cherkasy, *Ukraine* .. 59 H7 49 27N 32 4 E
Cherkessk, *Russia* ... 61 H6 44 15N 42 5 E
Cherla, *India* .... 94 E5 18 5N 80 49 E
Cherlak, *Russia* ..... 66 D8 54 15N 74 55 E
Chermoz, *Russia* .... 64 B6 58 46N 56 10 E
Chernak = Shornak,
  Kazakhstan .... 65 B4 43 24N 68 2 E
Chernaya, *Russia* ... 67 B9 70 30N 89 10 E
Chernaya Kholunitsa,
  Russia .... 64 B3 58 57N 51 39 E
Chernelytsya, *Ukraine* 53 B9 48 49N 25 26 E
Cherni, *Bulgaria* .... 50 D7 42 35N 23 18 E
Chernigov = Chernihiv,
  Ukraine .... 59 G6 51 28N 31 20 E
Chernihiv, *Ukraine* .. 59 G6 51 28N 31 20 E
Chernivetska □,
  Ukraine .... 53 B10 48 30N 26 0 E
Chernivtsi, *Ukraine* .. 53 B13 48 20N 26 9 E
Chernivtsi □, *Ukraine* 53 B10 48 15N 25 52 E
Chernobyl =
  Chornobyl, *Ukraine* 59 G6 51 20N 30 15 E
Chernogorsk, *Russia* 67 D10 53 49N 91 18 E
Chernomorskoye =
  Chornomorske,
  Ukraine .... 59 K7 45 31N 32 40 E
Chernorechye =
  Dzerzhinsk, *Russia* 60 B6 56 14N 43 30 E
Chernovtsy =
  Chernivtsi, *Ukraine* 53 B10 48 15N 25 52 E
Chernushka, *Russia* . 64 C6 56 29N 56 3 E
Chernyakhovsk, *Russia* 15 J19 54 36N 21 48 E
Chernyanka, *Russia* . 59 G9 50 56N 37 49 E
Chernyayevo =
  Yangiyer, *Uzbekistan* 65 C4 40 16N 68 49 E
Chernysheyskiy, *Russia* 67 C12 63 0N 112 30 E
Chernyy Otrog, *Russia* 64 F6 51 53N 56 0 E
Chernyye Zemli, *Russia* 61 H8 46 10N 46 0 E

Cherokee, Iowa, U.S.A. 154 D7 42 45N 95 33W
Cherokee, Okla., U.S.A. 155 G5 36 45N 98 21W
Cherokee Village, U.S.A. 155 G9 36 17N 91 30W
Cherokees, Grand Lake O' The, U.S.A. 155 G7 36 28N 95 2W
Cherquenco, Chile 176 A2 38 35 S 72 0W
Cherrapunji, India 90 C3 25 17N 91 47 E
Cherry Valley, Calif., U.S.A. 161 M10 33 59N 116 57W
Cherry Valley, N.Y., U.S.A. 151 D10 42 48N 74 45W
Cherryville, U.S.A. 156 G5 37 51N 91 16W
Cherskiy, Russia 67 C17 68 45N 161 18 E
Cherskogo Khrebet, Russia 67 C15 65 0N 143 0 E
Chertkov = Chortkiv, Ukraine 59 H3 49 2N 25 46 E
Chertkovo, Russia 59 H11 49 25N 40 19 E
Cherven, Belarus 58 F5 53 45N 28 28 E
Cherven-Bryag, Bulgaria 51 C8 43 17N 24 7 E
Chervonoarmeyskoye = Volnansk, Ukraine 59 H8 48 2N 35 29 E
Chervonoarmiyske, Ukraine 53 E13 45 47N 28 44 E
Chervonohrad, Ukraine 59 G3 50 25N 24 10 E
Cherwell →, U.K. 21 F6 51 44N 1 14W
Cherykaw, Belarus 58 F6 53 32N 31 20 E
Chesapeake, U.S.A. 148 G7 36 50N 76 17W
Chesapeake B., U.S.A. 148 G7 38 0N 76 10W
Cheshire □, U.K. 20 D5 53 14N 2 30W
Cheshskaya Guba, Russia 56 A8 67 20N 47 0 E
Cheshunt, U.K. 21 F7 51 43N 0 1W
Chesil Beach, U.K. 21 G5 50 37N 2 33W
Chesley, Canada 150 B3 44 17N 81 5W
Chesnokovka = Novoaltaysk, Russia 66 D9 53 30N 84 0 E
Cheste, Spain 41 F4 39 30N 0 41W
Chester, U.K. 20 D5 53 12N 2 53W
Chester, Calif., U.S.A. 158 F3 40 19N 121 14W
Chester, Ga., U.S.A. 152 C6 32 24N 83 9W
Chester, Ill., U.S.A. 155 G10 37 55N 89 49W
Chester, Mont., U.S.A. 158 B8 48 31N 110 58W
Chester, Pa., U.S.A. 148 F8 39 51N 75 22W
Chester, S.C., U.S.A. 149 H5 34 43N 81 12W
Chester, Vt., U.S.A. 151 C12 43 16N 72 36W
Chester, W. Va., U.S.A. 150 F4 40 37N 80 34W
Chester-le-Street, U.K. 20 C6 54 51N 1 34W
Chesterfield, U.K. 20 D6 53 15N 1 25W
Chesterfield, Is., N. Cal. 134 J7 19 52 S 158 15 E
Chesterfield Inlet, Canada 138 B10 63 30N 90 45W
Chesterton Ra., Australia 127 D4 25 30 S 147 27 E
Chesterton Range △, Australia 127 D4 26 16 S 147 22 E
Chestertown, U.S.A. 151 C11 43 40N 73 48W
Chesterville, Canada 151 A9 45 6N 75 14W
Chestnut Ridge, U.S.A. 150 F5 40 20N 79 10W
Chesuncook L., U.S.A. 149 C11 46 0N 69 21W
Chetamale, India 95 J11 10 43N 92 33 E
Chéticamp, Canada 141 C7 46 37N 60 59W
Chetlat I., India 95 J1 11 42N 72 42 E
Chetrosu, Moldova 53 B12 48 5N 27 54 E
Chetumal, Mexico 163 D7 18 30N 88 20W
Chetumal, B. de, Mexico 163 D7 18 40N 88 10W
Chetwynd, Canada 142 B4 55 45N 121 36W
Chevak, U.S.A. 144 F6 61 32N 165 35W
Chevanceaux, France 28 C3 45 18N 0 14W
Cheviot, U.S.A. 157 E12 39 10N 84 37W
Cheviot, The, U.K. 20 B5 55 29N 2 9W
Cheviot Hills, U.K. 20 B5 55 20N 2 30W
Cheviot Ra., Australia 126 D3 25 20 S 143 45 E
Chew Bahir, Ethiopia 107 G4 4 40N 36 50 E
Chewelah, U.S.A. 158 B5 48 17N 117 43W
Chewore △, Zimbabwe 119 F2 16 0 S 29 52 E
Cheyenne, Okla., U.S.A. 155 H5 35 37N 99 40W
Cheyenne, Wyo., U.S.A. 154 E2 41 8N 104 49W
Cheyenne →, U.S.A. 154 C4 44 41N 101 18W
Cheyenne Wells, U.S.A. 154 F3 38 49N 102 21W
Cheyne B., Australia 125 F2 34 35 S 118 50 E
Cheyur, India 95 H5 12 21N 80 0 E
Chhabra, India 92 G7 24 40N 76 54 E
Chhaktala, India 92 H6 22 6N 74 11 E
Chhapra, India 93 G11 25 48N 84 44 E
Chhata, India 92 F7 27 42N 77 30 E
Chhatak, Bangla. 90 C3 25 5N 91 37 E
Chhatarpur, Jharkhand, India 93 G11 24 23N 84 11 E
Chhatarpur, Mad. P., India 93 G8 24 55N 79 35 E
Chhati, India 94 D5 20 47N 81 40 E
Chhattisgarh □, India 93 J10 22 0N 82 0 E
Chhaygaon, India 90 B3 26 3N 91 24 E
Chhep, Cambodia 86 F5 13 45N 105 24 E
Chhindwara, Mad. P., India 93 H8 23 3N 79 29 E
Chhindwara, Mad. P., India 93 H8 22 2N 78 59 E
Chhinhdipada, India 94 D7 21 6N 84 52 E
Chhlong, Cambodia 87 F5 12 15N 105 58 E
Chhota Tawa →, India 92 H7 22 14N 76 36 E
Chhoti Kali Sindh →, India 92 G6 24 2N 75 31 E
Chhuikhadan, India 93 J9 21 32N 80 59 E
Chhuk, Cambodia 87 G5 10 46N 104 28 E
Chi →, Thailand 86 E5 15 11N 104 43 E
Chiai, Taiwan 77 F13 23 29N 120 25 E
Chiali, Taiwan 77 F13 23 10N 120 11 E
Chiamussu = Jiamusi, China 69 B8 46 40N 130 26 E
Chianciano Terme, Italy 45 E8 43 2N 11 49 E
Chiang Dao, Thailand 86 C2 19 22N 98 58 E
Chiang Kham, Thailand 86 C3 19 32N 100 18 E
Chiang Khan, Thailand 86 D3 17 52N 101 36 E
Chiang Khong, Thailand 76 G3 20 17N 100 24 E
Chiang Mai, Thailand 86 C2 18 47N 98 59 E
Chiang Rai, Thailand 76 H2 19 52N 99 50 E
Chiang Saen, Thailand 76 G3 20 16N 100 5 E
Chiange, Angola 115 F2 15 35 S 13 40 E
Chianti, Italy 45 E8 43 32N 11 25 E
Chiapa →, Mexico 163 D6 16 42N 93 0W
Chiapa de Corzo, Mexico 163 D6 16 42N 93 0W
Chiapas □, Mexico 163 D6 17 0N 92 45W
Chiaramonte Gulfi, Italy 47 E7 37 2N 14 42 E
Chiaravalle, Italy 45 E10 43 36N 13 19 E
Chiaravalle Centrale, Italy 47 D9 38 41N 16 25 E
Chiari, Italy 44 C6 45 32N 9 56 E
Chiasso, Switz. 33 E8 45 50N 9 2 E
Chiatura, Georgia 61 J6 42 15N 43 17 E
Chiautla, Mexico 163 D5 18 18N 98 34W
Chiávari, Italy 44 D6 44 19N 9 19 E
Chiavenna, Italy 44 B6 46 19N 9 24 E
Chiba, Japan 73 B12 35 30N 140 7 E
Chiba □, Japan 73 B12 35 30N 140 20 E
Chibabava, Mozam. 117 C5 20 17 S 33 35 E
Chibango, Angola 115 E4 13 38 S 21 56 E
Chibemba, Cunene, Angola 115 F2 15 48 S 14 8 E
Chibemba, Huila, Angola 116 B2 16 20 S 15 20 E
Chibi, Zimbabwe 117 C5 20 18 S 30 25 E
Chibia, Angola 115 F2 15 10 S 13 42 E
Chibizovka = Zherdevka, Russia 60 E5 51 56N 41 29 E
Chibougamau, Canada 140 C5 49 56N 74 24W
Chibougamau, L., Canada 140 C5 49 50N 74 20W
Chibuk, Nigeria 113 C7 10 52N 12 50 E
Chibuto, Mozam. 117 C5 24 40 S 33 33 E
Chibyu = Ukhta, Russia 56 B9 63 34N 53 41 E
Chic-Chocs, Mts., Canada 141 C6 48 55N 66 0W
Chicacole = Srikakulam, India 94 E6 18 14N 83 58 E
Chicago, U.S.A. 157 E6 41 53N 87 38W
Chicago Heights, U.S.A. 157 C9 41 30N 87 38W
Chicago O'Hare International ✈ (ORD), U.S.A. 157 C9 41 59N 87 54W
Chicapa →, Dem. Rep. of the Congo 115 D4 6 25 S 20 48 E
Chicha, Chad 109 E3 16 57N 18 34 E
Chichagof I., U.S.A. 144 H14 57 30N 135 30W
Chichaoua, Morocco 110 B3 31 32N 8 44W
Chichén-Itzá, Mexico 163 C7 20 40N 88 36W
Chicheng, China 74 D8 40 55N 115 55 E
Chichester, U.K. 21 G7 50 50N 0 47W
Chichester Ra., Australia 124 D2 22 12 S 119 15 E
Chichibu, Japan 73 A11 35 59N 139 10 E
Chichibu-Tama △, Japan 73 B10 35 52N 138 42 E
Ch'ich'ihaerh = Qiqihar, China 67 E13 47 26N 124 0 E
Chicholi, India 92 H8 22 1N 77 40 E
Chickasaw △, U.S.A. 155 H6 34 26N 97 0W
Chickasha, U.S.A. 155 H6 35 3N 97 58W
Chicken, U.S.A. 144 D12 64 5N 141 56W
Chiclana de la Frontera, Spain 43 J4 36 26N 6 9W
Chiclayo, Peru 172 B2 6 42 S 79 50W
Chico, U.S.A. 160 F5 39 44N 121 50W
Chico →, Chubut, Argentina 176 B3 44 0 S 67 0W
Chico →, Santa Cruz, Argentina 176 C3 50 0 S 68 30W
Chicomba, Angola 115 E2 14 10 S 14 52 E
Chicomo, Mozam. 117 C5 24 31 S 34 6 E
Chicomostoc, Mexico 162 C4 22 28N 102 49W
Chicontepec, Mexico 163 C5 20 58N 98 10W
Chicopee, U.S.A. 151 D12 42 9N 72 37W
Chicoutimi, Canada 141 C5 48 28N 71 5W
Chicualacuala, Mozam. 117 C5 22 6 S 31 42 E
Chicuma, Angola 115 E2 13 26 S 14 50 E
Chidambaram, India 95 J4 11 20N 79 45 E
Chidenguele, Mozam. 117 C5 24 55 S 34 11 E
Chidley, C., Canada 139 B13 60 23N 64 26W
Chiducuane, Mozam. 117 C5 24 35 S 34 25 E
Chiede, Angola 116 B2 17 15 S 16 22 E
Chiefland, U.S.A. 153 F7 29 29N 82 52W
Chiefs Pt., Canada 150 B3 44 41N 81 18W
Chiem Hoa, Vietnam 86 A5 22 12N 105 17 E
Chiemsee, Germany 31 H8 47 53N 12 28 E
Chiengi, Zambia 119 D2 8 45 S 29 10 E
Chiengmai = Chiang Mai, Thailand 86 C2 18 47N 98 59 E
Chiengo, Angola 115 E4 13 20 S 21 55 E
Chienti →, Italy 45 E10 43 18N 13 45 E
Chieri, Italy 44 C4 45 1N 7 49 E
Chiers →, France 27 C11 49 39N 4 59 E
Chiesa in Valmalenco, Italy 44 B6 46 16N 9 51 E
Chiese →, Italy 44 C7 45 8N 10 25 E
Chieti, Italy 45 F11 42 21N 14 10 E
Chifeng, China 75 C10 42 18N 118 58 E
Chigasaki, Japan 73 B11 35 19N 139 24 E
Chigirin, Ukraine 59 H7 49 4N 32 38 E
Chignecto B., Canada 141 C7 45 30N 64 40W
Chignik, U.S.A. 144 H8 56 18N 158 24W
Chigorodó, Colombia 168 B2 7 41N 76 42W
Chiguana, Bolivia 174 A2 21 0 S 67 58W
Chigwell, U.K. 21 F8 51 37N 0 5 E
Chiha-ri, N. Korea 75 E14 38 40N 126 30 E
Chihli, G. of = Bo Hai, China 75 E10 39 0N 119 0 E
Chihsi = Jixi, China 75 B16 45 20N 130 50 E
Chihuahua, Mexico 162 B3 28 40N 106 3W
Chihuahua □, Mexico 162 B3 28 40N 106 3W
Chiili = Shīeli, Kazakhstan 65 A3 44 20N 66 15 E
Chik Bollapur, India 95 H3 13 25N 77 45 E
Chikalda, India 94 D3 21 24N 77 19 E
Chikhli, Ahmadabad, India 94 D1 20 45N 73 4 E
Chikhli, Maharashtra, India 94 D3 20 20N 76 18 E
Chikmagalur, India 95 H2 13 15N 75 45 E
Chiknayakanhalli, India 95 H3 13 26N 76 37 E
Chikodi, India 95 F2 16 26N 74 38 E
Chikugo, Japan 72 D2 33 14N 130 28 E
Chikuma-Gawa →, Japan 73 A10 36 59N 138 35 E
Chikushino, Japan 72 D2 33 30N 130 30 E
Chikwawa, Malawi 119 F3 16 2 S 34 50 E
Chila, Angola 115 E2 12 3 S 14 29 E
Chilac, Mexico 163 D5 18 20N 97 24W
Chilam Chavki, Pakistan 93 B6 35 5N 75 5 E
Chilanga, Zambia 119 F2 15 33 S 28 16 E
Chilapa, Mexico 163 D5 17 40N 99 11W
Chilas, Pakistan 93 B6 35 25N 74 5 E
Chilaw, Sri Lanka 95 L4 7 30N 79 50 E
Chilcotin →, Canada 142 C4 51 44N 122 23W
Childers, Australia 127 D5 25 15 S 152 17 E
Childersburg, U.S.A. 152 B3 33 16N 86 21W
Childress, U.S.A. 155 H4 34 25N 100 13W
Chile ■, S. Amer. 176 B2 35 0 S 72 0W
Chile Chico, Chile 176 C2 46 33 S 71 44W
Chile Rise, Pac. Oc. 135 L18 38 0 S 92 0W
Chilecito, Argentina 174 B2 29 10 S 67 30W
Chilesso, Angola 115 E3 11 35 S 16 34 E
Chilete, Peru 172 B2 7 10 S 78 50W
Chilhowee, U.S.A. 156 F3 38 36N 93 51W
Chilia, Braţul →, Romania 53 E14 45 14N 29 42 E
Chilik = Shelek, Kazakhstan 65 B9 43 33N 78 17 E
Chililabombwe, Zambia 119 E2 12 18 S 27 43 E
Chilin = Jilin, China 75 C14 43 44N 126 30 E
Chilka L., India 94 E7 19 40N 85 25 E
Chilko →, Canada 142 C4 52 0N 123 40W
Chilko L., Canada 142 C4 51 20N 124 10W
Chillagoe, Australia 126 B3 17 7 S 144 33 E
Chillán, Chile 174 D1 36 40 S 72 10W
Chillicothe, Ill., U.S.A. 156 D7 40 55N 89 29W
Chillicothe, Mo., U.S.A. 156 E3 39 48N 93 33W
Chillicothe, Ohio, U.S.A. 148 F4 39 20N 82 59W
Chilliwack, Canada 142 D4 49 10N 121 54W
Chilo, India 92 F5 27 25N 73 32 E
Chiloane, I., Mozam. 117 C5 20 40 S 34 55 E
Chiloé △, Chile 176 B2 42 11 S 73 59W
Chiloé, I. de, Chile 176 B2 42 30 S 73 50W
Chilonda, Angola 115 E3 11 19 S 16 12 E
Chilongo, Angola 115 E3 13 55 S 16 35 E
Chilpancingo, Mexico 163 D5 17 30N 99 30W
Chiltern, Australia 129 D7 36 10 S 146 36 E
Chiltern Hills, U.K. 21 F7 51 40N 0 53W
Chilton, U.S.A. 148 C1 44 2N 88 10W
Chiluage, Angola 115 D4 9 30 S 21 50 E
Chilubi, Zambia 119 E2 11 5 S 29 58 E
Chilubula, Zambia 119 E3 10 14 S 30 51 E
Chilumba, Malawi 119 E3 10 28 S 34 12 E
Chilung, Taiwan 77 E13 25 3N 121 45 E
Chilwa, L., Malawi 119 F4 15 15 S 35 40 E
Chimakela, Angola 115 F3 15 24 S 16 58 E
Chimakudi, India 90 C4 25 47N 93 48 E
Chimaltitán, Mexico 162 C4 21 46N 103 50W
Chimán, Panama 164 E4 8 45N 78 40W
Chimanimani, Zimbabwe 117 B5 19 48 S 32 52 E
Chimanimani △, Zimbabwe 119 F3 19 48 S 33 0 E
Chimay, Belgium 24 D4 50 3N 4 20 E
Chimayo, U.S.A. 159 H11 36 0N 105 56W
Chimbay, Uzbekistan 66 E6 42 57N 59 47 E
Chimborazo, Ecuador 168 D2 1 29 S 78 55W
Chimborazo □, Ecuador 168 D2 1 0 S 78 40W
Chimbote, Peru 172 B2 9 0 S 78 35W
Chimbu □, Papua N. G. 132 D3 6 15 S 144 50 E
Chimichagua, Colombia 168 B3 9 15N 73 49W
Chimion, Uzbekistan 65 C5 40 15N 71 32 E
Chimkent = Shymkent, Kazakhstan 65 B4 42 18N 69 36 E
Chimoio, Mozam. 119 F3 19 4 S 33 30 E
Chimpembe, Zambia 119 D2 9 31 S 29 33 E
Chimur, India 94 D4 20 30N 79 23 E
Chin □, Burma 90 D4 22 0N 93 0 E
Chin Hills, Burma 90 D4 22 30N 93 30 E
Chin Ling Shan = Qinling Shandi, China 74 H5 33 50N 108 10 E
China, Mexico 163 B5 25 40N 99 20W
China ■, Asia 69 C6 30 0N 110 0 E
China, Great Plain of, Asia 62 F15 35 0N 115 0 E
China Lake, U.S.A. 161 K9 35 44N 117 37W
Chinacota, Colombia 168 B3 7 37N 72 36W
Chinan = Jinan, China 74 F9 36 38N 117 1 E
Chinandega, Nic. 164 D2 12 35N 87 12W
Chinati Peak, U.S.A. 155 L2 29 57N 104 29W
Chinaz, Uzbekistan 65 C4 40 56N 68 46 E
Chincha Alta, Peru 172 C2 13 25 S 76 7W
Chinchaga →, Canada 142 B5 58 53N 118 20W
Chincheros, Peru 172 C3 13 30 S 73 44W
Chinchilla, Australia 127 D5 26 45 S 150 38 E
Chinchilla de Monte Aragón, Spain 41 G3 38 53N 1 40W
Chincholi, India 94 E3 17 28N 77 26 E
Chinchorro, Banco, Mexico 163 D7 18 35N 87 20W
Chinchou = Jinzhou, China 75 D11 41 5N 121 3 E
Chinchoua, Gabon 114 B1 0 1N 9 48 E
Chincoteague, U.S.A. 148 G8 37 56N 75 23W
Chinde, Mozam. 119 F4 18 35 S 36 30 E
Chindo, S. Korea 75 G14 34 28N 126 15 E
Chindwin →, Burma 90 E5 21 26N 95 15 E
Chineni, India 93 C6 33 2N 75 15 E
Chinga, Mozam. 119 F4 15 13 S 38 35 E
Chingaza △, Colombia 168 C3 4 30N 73 40W
Chingirlau, Kazakhstan 64 F5 51 7N 54 7 E
Chingola, Zambia 119 E2 12 31 S 27 53 E
Chingole, Malawi 119 E3 13 4 S 34 17 E
Chingoroi, Angola 115 E2 13 37 S 14 1 E
Ch'ingtao = Qingdao, China 75 F11 36 5N 120 20 E
Chinguar, Angola 115 E3 12 25 S 16 45 E
Chinguetti, Mauritania 110 D2 20 25N 12 24W
Chingune, Mozam. 117 C5 20 33 S 34 58 E
Chinhae, S. Korea 75 G15 35 9N 128 47 E
Chinhanguanine, Mozam. 117 D5 25 21 S 32 30 E
Chinhoyi, Zimbabwe 119 F3 17 20 S 30 8 E
Chinhsien = Jinxian, China 77 C11 28 26N 116 17 E
Chini, India 92 D8 31 32N 78 15 E
Chiniot, Pakistan 91 C4 31 45N 73 0 E
Chínipas, Mexico 162 B3 27 22N 108 32W
Chinji, Pakistan 92 C5 32 42N 72 22 E
Chinju, S. Korea 75 G15 35 12N 128 2 E
Chinkai, Afghan. 91 C2 31 57N 67 26 E
Chinkapook, Australia 128 C5 35 11 S 142 57 E
Chinkiang = Zhenjiang, China 77 A12 32 11N 119 26 E
Chinko →, C.A.R. 114 B4 4 50N 23 53 E
Chinle, U.S.A. 159 H9 36 9N 109 33W
Chinmen, Taiwan 77 E13 24 26N 118 19 E
Chinmen Tao, Taiwan 77 E12 24 27N 118 23 E
Chinnamanur, India 95 K3 9 50N 77 24 E
Chinnampo = Namp'o, N. Korea 75 E13 38 52N 125 10 E
Chinnur, India 94 E4 18 57N 79 49 E
Chino, Japan 73 B10 35 59N 138 9 E
Chino, U.S.A. 161 L9 34 1N 117 41W
Chino Valley, U.S.A. 159 J7 34 45N 112 27W
Chinon, France 26 E7 47 10N 0 15 E
Chinook, U.S.A. 158 B9 48 35N 109 14W
Chinook Trough, Pac. Oc. 134 C10 44 0N 175 0W
Chinoya, Zambia 115 E4 13 55 S 23 16 E
Chinsali, Zambia 119 E3 10 30 S 32 2 E
Chintalapudi, India 94 F5 17 4N 80 59 E
Chintamani, India 95 H4 13 26N 78 3 E
Chinwangtao = Qinhuangdao, China 75 E10 39 56N 119 30 E
Chióggia, Italy 45 C9 45 13N 12 17 E
Chíos = Khíos, Greece 49 C8 38 27N 26 9 E
Chipata, Zambia 119 E3 13 38 S 32 28 E
Chiperceni, Moldova 53 C13 47 31N 28 50 E
Chipindo, Angola 115 E3 13 49 S 15 48 E
Chipinge, Zimbabwe 119 G3 20 13 S 32 28 E
Chipinge △, Zimbabwe 119 G3 20 14 S 33 0 E
Chipiona, Spain 43 J4 36 44N 6 26W
Chipley, U.S.A. 152 E4 30 47N 85 32W
Chiplun, India 94 F1 17 31N 73 34 E
Chipman, Canada 141 C6 46 6N 65 53W
Chipoka, Malawi 119 E3 13 57 S 34 28 E
Chippenham, U.K. 21 F5 51 27N 2 6W
Chippewa →, U.S.A. 154 C8 44 25N 92 5W
Chippewa Falls, U.S.A. 154 C9 44 56N 91 24W
Chipping Norton, U.K. 21 F6 51 56N 1 32W
Chiprovtsi, Bulgaria 50 C6 43 24N 22 52 E
Chiputneticook Lakes, U.S.A. 149 C11 45 35N 67 35W
Chiputo = Vila Vasco da Gama, Mozam. 119 E3 14 54 S 32 14 E
Chiquelequele, Angola 115 F3 16 44 S 19 5 E
Chiquián, Peru 172 C2 10 10 S 77 0W
Chiquibul △, Belize 164 C2 16 49N 88 52W
Chiquimula, Guatemala 164 D2 14 51N 89 37W
Chiquinquira, Colombia 168 B3 5 37N 73 50W
Chiquitos, Llanos de, Bolivia 173 D5 18 0 S 61 30W
Chir →, Russia 61 F6 48 30N 43 0 E
Chira →, Peru 168 D1 4 54 S 81 8W
Chirala, India 95 G5 15 50N 80 26 E
Chiramba, Mozam. 119 F3 16 55 S 34 39 E
Chirawa, India 92 E6 28 14N 75 42 E
Chirayinkil, India 95 K3 8 41N 76 49 E
Chirchiq, Uzbekistan 65 C4 41 29N 69 35 E
Chiredzi, Zimbabwe 117 C5 21 0 S 31 38 E
Chirfa, Niger 109 D2 20 55N 12 22 E
Chirgua →, Venezuela 168 B4 8 54N 67 58W
Chiribiquete △, Colombia 168 C3 0 31N 72 50W
Chiricahua △, U.S.A. 159 K9 32 0N 109 20W
Chiricahua Peak, U.S.A. 159 L9 31 51N 109 18W
Chiriquí, G. de, Panama 164 E3 8 0N 82 10W
Chiriquí, L. de, Panama 164 E3 9 10N 82 0W
Chirisa △, Zimbabwe 119 F2 17 53 S 28 15 E
Chirivira Falls, Zimbabwe 119 G3 21 10 S 32 12 E
Chirnogi, Romania 53 F11 44 7N 26 32 E
Chirpan, Bulgaria 51 D9 42 10N 25 19 E
Chirripó Grande, Cerro, Costa Rica 164 E3 9 29N 83 29W
Chirundu, Zimbabwe 117 B4 16 3 S 28 50 E
Chisamba, Zambia 119 E2 14 55 S 28 20 E
Chisasibi, Canada 140 B4 53 50N 79 0W
Ch'ishan, Taiwan 77 F13 22 44N 120 31 E
Chishmy, Russia 64 D5 54 35N 55 23 E
Chisholm, Canada 142 C6 54 55N 114 10W
Chisholm, U.S.A. 154 B8 47 29N 92 53W
Chishtian Mandi, Pakistan 92 E5 29 50N 72 55 E
Chishui, China 76 C5 28 30N 105 42 E
Chishui He →, China 76 C5 28 49N 105 50 E
Chisimaio, Somali Rep. 120 E2 0 22 S 42 32 E
Chisimba Falls, Zambia 119 E3 10 12 S 30 56 E
Chişinău, Moldova 53 C13 47 2N 28 50 E
Chişinău ✈ (KIV), Moldova 53 C13 47 3N 28 46 E
Chişineu Criş, Romania 52 D6 46 32N 21 37 E
Chisone →, Italy 44 D4 44 49N 7 25 E
Chisos Mts., U.S.A. 155 L3 29 5N 103 15W
Chissenguе, Angola 115 D4 9 13 S 20 34 E
Chissilo, Angola 115 E3 13 48 S 16 31 E
Chistochina, U.S.A. 144 E11 62 34N 144 40W
Chistopol, Russia 60 C10 55 25N 50 38 E
Chita, Colombia 168 B3 6 11N 72 28W
Chita, Russia 67 D12 52 0N 113 35 E
Chitado, Angola 115 F2 17 10 S 14 8 E
Chitaldrug = Chitradurga, India 95 G3 14 14N 76 24 E
Chitanda →, Angola 115 F3 16 1 S 15 12 E
Chitapur, India 94 F3 17 10N 77 5 E
Chitembo, Angola 115 E3 13 30 S 16 50 E
Chitina, U.S.A. 144 F11 61 31N 144 26W
Chitipa, Malawi 119 D3 9 41 S 33 19 E
Chitose, Japan 70 C10 42 49N 141 39 E
Chitradurga, India 95 G3 14 14N 76 24 E
Chitrakot, India 94 E5 19 10N 81 40 E
Chitral, Pakistan 91 B3 35 50N 71 56 E
Chitravati →, India 95 G4 14 45N 78 15 E
Chitré, Panama 164 E3 7 59N 80 27W
Chittagong, Bangla. 90 D3 22 19N 91 48 E
Chittagong □, Bangla. 90 C3 24 5N 91 0 E
Chittaurgarh, India 92 G6 24 52N 74 38 E
Chittoor, India 95 H4 13 15N 79 5 E
Chittur, India 95 J3 10 40N 76 45 E
Chitungwiza, Zimbabwe 119 F3 18 0 S 31 6 E
Chiumbe →, Dem. Rep. of the Congo 115 D4 6 59 S 21 12 E
Chiumbo, Angola 115 E3 12 29 S 16 8 E
Chiume, Angola 115 F4 15 3 S 21 14 E
Chiuro, Italy 33 D9 46 10N 9 59 E
Chiusi, Italy 45 E8 43 1N 11 57 E
Chiva, Spain 41 F4 39 27N 0 41W
Chivacoa, Venezuela 168 A4 10 10N 68 54W
Chivasso, Italy 44 C4 45 11N 7 53 E
Chivay, Peru 172 D3 15 40 S 71 35W
Chivé, Bolivia 172 C4 12 23 S 68 35W
Chivhu, Zimbabwe 119 F3 19 2 S 30 52 E
Chivilcoy, Argentina 174 C4 34 55 S 60 0W
Chiwanda, Tanzania 119 E3 11 23 S 34 55 E
Chixi, China 77 G9 22 0N 112 58 E
Chizarira, Zimbabwe 119 F2 17 36 S 27 45 E
Chizarira △, Zimbabwe 119 F2 17 44 S 27 52 E
Chizela, Zambia 115 E4 13 8 S 25 0 E
Chizera, Zambia 119 E2 13 10 S 25 0 E
Chizu, Japan 72 B6 35 16N 134 14 E
Chkalov = Orenburg, Russia 64 F5 51 45N 55 6 E
Chkolovsk, Russia 60 B6 56 50N 43 10 E
Chloride, U.S.A. 161 K12 35 25N 114 12W
Chlumec nad Cidlinou, Czech Rep. 34 A8 50 9N 15 29 E
Chmielnik, Poland 55 H7 50 37N 20 43 E
Cho Bo, Vietnam 76 G5 20 46N 105 10 E
Cho-do, N. Korea 75 E13 38 30N 124 40 E
Cho Phuoc Hai, Vietnam 87 G6 10 26N 107 18 E
Choa Chu Kang, Singapore 87 d 1 22N 103 41 E
Choba, Kenya 118 B4 2 30N 38 5 E
Chobe △, Botswana 116 B4 18 37 S 24 23 E
Choch'iwŏn, S. Korea 75 F14 36 37N 127 18 E
Chocianów, Poland 55 G2 51 27N 15 55 E
Chociwel, Poland 54 E2 53 29N 15 21 E
Chocó □, Colombia 168 B2 6 0N 77 0W
Chocolate Mts., U.S.A. 161 M11 33 15N 115 15W
Choconta, Colombia 168 B3 5 9N 73 41W
Choctawhatchee →, U.S.A. 152 E3 30 25N 86 8W
Choctawhatchee B., U.S.A. 153 E3 30 20N 86 20W
Chodavaram, Andhra Pradesh, India 94 F6 17 50N 82 57 E
Chodavaram, Andhra Pradesh, India 94 F5 17 27N 81 46 E
Chodecz, Poland 55 F6 52 24N 19 2 E
Chodov, Czech Rep. 34 A5 50 15N 12 45 E
Chodziez, Poland 55 F3 52 58N 16 58 E
Choele Choel, Argentina 176 A3 39 11 S 65 40W
Chōfu, Japan 73 B11 35 39N 139 33 E
Choiseul, St. Lucia 165 f 13 47N 61 3W
Choiseul, Solomon Is. 133 L9 7 0 S 156 40 E
Choix, Mexico 162 B3 26 40N 108 23W
Chojna, Poland 55 F1 52 58N 14 25 E
Chojnice, Poland 54 E4 53 42N 17 32 E
Chojnów, Poland 55 G2 51 18N 15 58 E
Chok-Tal, Kyrgyzstan 65 B8 42 35N 76 45 E
Chōkai-San, Japan 70 E10 39 6N 140 3 E
Choke Canyon Res., U.S.A. 155 L5 28 30N 98 20W
Choke Mts., Ethiopia 107 E4 11 18N 37 15 E
Chokurdakh, Russia 67 B15 70 38N 147 55 E
Cholame, U.S.A. 160 K6 35 44N 120 18W
Cholet, France 26 E6 47 4N 0 52W
Cholguan, Chile 174 D1 37 10 S 72 3W
Cholpon-Ata, Kyrgyzstan 65 B8 42 40N 77 6 E
Choluteca, Honduras 164 D2 13 20N 87 14W
Choluteca →, Honduras 164 D2 13 0N 87 20W
Chom Bung, Thailand 86 F2 13 37N 99 36 E
Chom Thong, Thailand 86 C2 18 25N 98 41 E
Choma, Zambia 119 F2 16 48 S 26 59 E
Chomolungma = Everest, Mt., Nepal 93 E12 28 5N 86 58 E
Chomun, India 92 F6 27 15N 75 40 E
Chomutov, Czech Rep. 34 A6 50 28N 13 23 E
Chon Buri, Thailand 86 F3 13 21N 101 1 E
Chon Thanh, Vietnam 87 G6 11 24N 106 36 E
Ch'onan, S. Korea 75 F14 36 48N 127 9 E
Chone, Ecuador 168 D2 0 40 S 80 0W
Chong Kai, Cambodia 86 F4 13 57N 103 35 E
Chong Mek, Thailand 86 E5 15 10N 105 27 E
Chong Phangan, Thailand 87 b 9 39N 100 0 E
Chong Samui, Thailand 87 b 9 21N 99 50 E
Chongde, China 77 B13 30 32N 120 26 E
Chŏngdo, S. Korea 75 G15 35 38N 128 42 E
Chŏngha, S. Korea 75 F15 36 12N 129 21 E
Chŏngjin, N. Korea 75 D15 41 47N 129 50 E
Chŏngju, N. Korea 75 E13 39 40N 125 5 E
Chŏngju, S. Korea 75 F14 36 39N 127 27 E
Chongli, China 74 D8 40 58N 115 15 E
Chongming, China 77 B13 31 38N 121 23 E
Chongming Dao, China 77 B13 31 40N 121 30 E
Chongoyape, Peru 172 B2 6 35 S 79 25W
Chongqing, Chongqing, China 76 C6 29 35N 106 25 E
Chongqing, Sichuan, China 76 B4 30 38N 103 40 E
Chongqing Shi □, China 76 C6 30 0N 108 0 E
Chongren, China 77 D11 27 46N 116 3 E
Chonguene, Mozam. 117 C5 25 3 S 33 49 E
Chŏngŭp, S. Korea 75 G14 35 35N 126 50 E
Chongyi, China 77 E10 25 45N 114 29 E
Chongzuo, China 76 F6 22 23N 107 20 E
Chŏnju, S. Korea 75 G14 35 50N 127 4 E
Chonos, Arch. de los, Chile 176 C2 45 0 S 75 0W
Chop, Ukraine 52 B7 48 26N 22 12 E
Chopda, India 94 D2 21 20N 75 15 E
Chopim →, Brazil 175 B5 25 35 S 53 5W
Chor, Pakistan 92 G3 25 31N 69 46 E
Chorbat La, India 93 B7 34 42N 76 37 E
Chorley, U.K. 20 D5 53 39N 2 38W
Chorna, Ukraine 53 C14 47 36N 29 20 E
Chornobyl, Ukraine 59 G6 51 20N 30 15 E
Chornomorske, Ukraine 59 K7 45 31N 32 40 E
Chorolque, Cerro, Bolivia 174 A2 20 59 S 66 5W
Choroszcz, Poland 55 E9 53 10N 22 59 E
Chorregon, Australia 126 C3 22 40 S 143 32 E
Chorro el Indio △, Venezuela 165 E5 7 43N 72 9W
Chortkiv, Ukraine 59 H3 49 2N 25 46 E
Ch'ŏrwon, S. Korea 75 E14 38 15N 127 10 E
Chorzele, Poland 55 E7 53 15N 20 55 E
Chorzów, Poland 55 H5 50 18N 18 57 E
Chos-Malal, Argentina 174 D1 37 20 S 70 15W
Ch'osan, N. Korea 75 D13 40 50N 125 47 E
Chōshi, Japan 73 B12 35 45N 140 51 E
Choszczno, Poland 55 E2 53 7N 15 25 E
Chota, Peru 172 B2 6 33 S 78 39W
Choteau, U.S.A. 158 C7 47 49N 112 11W
Chotěboř, Czech Rep. 34 B8 49 43N 15 40 E
Chotila, India 92 H4 22 23N 71 15 E
Chotta Udepur, India 92 H6 22 19N 74 1 E
Chowchilla, U.S.A. 160 H6 37 7N 120 16W
Choybalsan, Mongolia 69 B6 48 4N 114 30 E
Chrisman, U.S.A. 157 E9 39 48N 87 41W
Christburg = Dzierzgoń, Poland 54 E6 53 58N 19 20 E
Christchurch, N.Z. 131 D7 43 33 S 172 47 E
Christchurch, U.K. 21 G6 50 44N 1 47W
Christian I., Canada 150 B4 44 50N 80 12W
Christian Sd., U.S.A. 144 J14 55 56N 134 40W
Christiana, S. Africa 116 D4 27 52 S 25 8 E
Christiansfeld, Denmark 17 J3 55 21N 9 29 E
Christianshåb = Qasigiannguit, Greenland 10 D5 68 50N 51 18W
Christiansted, U.S. Virgin Is. 165 C7 17 45N 64 42W
Christie B., Canada 143 A6 62 32N 111 10W
Christina →, Canada 143 B6 56 40N 111 3W
Christmas Cr. →, Australia 124 C4 18 29 S 125 23 E
Christmas I. = Kiritimati, Kiribati 135 G12 1 58N 157 27W
Christmas I., Ind. Oc. 121 F9 10 30 S 105 40 E
Christopher, U.S.A. 156 G7 37 59N 89 3W
Christopher L., Australia 125 D4 24 49 S 127 42 E
Christyakovo = Thorez, Ukraine 59 H10 48 4N 38 34 E
Chrudim, Czech Rep. 34 B8 49 58N 15 43 E
Chrzanów, Poland 55 H6 50 10N 19 21 E
Chtimba, Malawi 119 E3 10 35 S 34 13 E
Chū = Shū, Kazakhstan 65 B6 43 36N 73 42 E
Chū = Shū →, Kazakhstan 65 A3 45 0N 67 44 E
Chu →, Vietnam 86 C5 19 53N 105 45 E
Chu Lai, Vietnam 86 E7 15 28N 108 45 E
Chuadanga, Bangla. 90 D2 23 38N 88 51 E
Chuak, Ko, Thailand 87 b 9 28N 99 41 E
Ch'uanchou = Quanzhou, China 77 E12 24 55N 118 34 E
Chüanchow = Quanzhou, China 77 E12 24 55N 118 34 E
Chuankou, China 74 G6 34 20N 110 59 E
Chuathbaluk, U.S.A. 144 F8 61 40N 159 15W
Chubarovka = Pology, Ukraine 59 J9 47 29N 36 15 E
Chubbuck, U.S.A. 158 E7 42 55N 112 28W
Chubek = Moskovskiy, Tajikistan 65 E4 37 37N 69 42 E
Chūbu □, Japan 73 A9 36 45N 137 30 E
Chubu-Sangaku △, Japan 73 A9 36 30N 137 40 E
Chubut □, Argentina 176 B3 43 30 S 69 0W
Chubut →, Argentina 176 B3 43 20 S 65 5W
Chuchi L., Canada 142 B4 55 12N 124 30W
Chuchow = Zhuzhou, China 77 D9 27 49N 113 12 E
Chuda, India 92 H4 22 29N 71 41 E
Chudovo, Russia 58 C6 59 10N 31 41 E
Chudskoye, Ozero, Russia 15 G22 58 13N 27 30 E
Chugach Mts., U.S.A. 144 F11 60 45N 147 0W
Chugiak, U.S.A. 144 F10 61 24N 149 29W
Chuginadak I., U.S.A. 144 K5 52 50N 169 45W

Chūgoku □, *Japan* ... **72 C5** 35 0N 133 0 E
Chūgoku-Sanchi, *Japan* **72 C5** 35 0N 133 0 E
Chuguyev = Chuhuyiv,
Ukraine .... **59 H9** 49 55N 36 45 E
Chugwater, *U.S.A.* ... **154 E2** 41 46N 104 50W
Chuhuyiv, *Ukraine* ... **59 H9** 49 55N 36 45 E
Chukchi Sea, *Russia* ... **67 C19** 68 0N 175 0W
Chukotskoye Nagorye,
Russia .... **67 C18** 68 0N 175 0 E
Chula, *U.S.A.* **152 D6** 31 33N 83 32W
Chula Vista, *U.S.A.* ... **161 N9** 32 39N 117 5W
Chulakkurgan =
Sholaqqorghan,
Kazakhstan ...... **65 B4** 43 46N 69 9 E
Chulband →, *India* ... **94 D4** 20 40N 79 54 E
Chulucanas, *Peru* ... **172 B1** 5 8S 80 10W
Chulumani, *Bolivia* ... **172 D4** 16 24 S 67 31W
Chulym →, *Russia* ... **66 D9** 57 43N 83 51 E
Chum Phae, *Thailand* ... **86 D4** 16 40N 102 6 E
Chum Saeng, *Thailand* ... **86 E3** 15 55N 100 15 E
Chuma, *Bolivia* ...... **172 D4** 15 24 S 68 56W
Chumar, *India* ...... **93 C8** 32 40N 78 35 E
Chumbicha, *Argentina* ... **174 B2** 29 0 S 66 10W
Chumikan, *Russia* ... **67 D14** 54 40N 135 10 E
Chumphon, *Thailand* ... **87 G2** 10 35N 99 14 E
Chumpi, *Peru* ...... **172 D3** 15 4 S 73 46W
Chumuare, *Mozam.* ... **119 E3** 14 31 S 31 50 E
Chumunjin, *S. Korea* ... **75 F15** 37 55N 128 54 E
Chuna →, *Russia* ... **67 D10** 57 47N 94 37 E
Chun'an, *China* ...... **77 C12** 29 35N 119 3 E
Chunchura, *India* ... **93 H13** 22 53N 88 27 E
Chunga, *Zambia* ...... **119 F2** 15 0 S 26 2 E
Ch'ungch'ŏng →
Chongqing, *China* ... **76 C6** 29 35N 106 25 E
Chunggang-ŭp,
N. Korea ...... **75 D14** 41 48N 126 48 E
Chunghwa, *N. Korea* ... **75 E13** 38 52N 125 47 E
Ch'ungju, *S. Korea* ... **75 F14** 36 58N 127 58 E
Chungking =
Chongqing, *China* ... **76 C6** 29 35N 106 25 E
Chungli, *Taiwan* ... **77 E13** 24 57N 121 13 E
Ch'ungmu, *S. Korea* ... **75 G15** 34 50N 128 20 E
Chungt'iaoshan =
Zhongtiao Shan,
China .... **74 G6** 35 0N 111 10 E
Chungyang Shanmo,
Taiwan .... **77 F13** 23 10N 121 0 E
Chunian, *Pakistan* ... **89 D6** 30 57N 74 0 E
Chunya, *Tanzania* ... **119 D3** 8 30 S 33 27 E
Chunyang, *China* ... **75 C15** 43 38N 129 23 E
Chupara Pt.,
Trin. & Tob. **169 F9** 10 49N 61 22W
Chuquibamba, *Peru* ... **172 C3** 15 47 S 72 44W
Chuquibamba, *Peru* ... **172 C3** 14 7 S 72 41W
Chuquicamata, *Chile* ... **174 A2** 22 15 S 69 0W
Chuquisaca □, *Bolivia* ... **173 E5** 20 30 S 63 30W
Chur, *Switz.* ...... **33 C9** 46 52N 9 32 E
Churachandpur, *India* ... **90 C4** 24 20N 93 40 E
Church Stretton, *U.K.* ... **21 E5** 52 32N 2 48W
Churchill, *Australia* ... **129 E7** 38 19 S 146 25 E
Churchill, *Canada* ... **143 B10** 58 47N 94 11W
Churchill →, *Man.,*
Canada **143 B10** 58 47N 94 12W
Churchill →,
Nfld. & L., Canada **141 B7** 53 19N 60 10W
Churchill, C., *Canada* **143 B10** 58 46N 93 12W
Churchill Falls, *Canada* **141 B7** 53 36N 64 19W
Churchill L., *Canada* ... **143 B7** 55 55N 108 20W
Churchill Pk., *Canada* ... **142 B3** 58 10N 125 10W
Churdan, *U.S.A.* ... **156 B2** 42 9N 94 29W
Churfisten, *Switz.* ... **33 B8** 47 8N 9 17 E
Churki, *India* ...... **93 H10** 23 50N 83 12 E
Churu, *India* ...... **92 E6** 28 20N 74 50 E
Churubusco, *U.S.A.* ... **157 C11** 41 14N 85 19W
Churún Merú = Angel
Falls, *Venezuela* ... **169 B5** 5 57N 62 30W
Churwalden, *Switz.* ... **33 C9** 46 47N 9 33 E
Chushal, *India* ...... **93 C8** 33 40N 78 40 E
Chuska Mts., *U.S.A.* ... **159 H9** 36 15N 108 50W
Chusovaya →, *Russia* ... **64 B6** 58 22N 56 54 E
Chusovoy, *Russia* ... **64 B6** 58 22N 57 50 E
Chusovskoy Zavod =
Chusovoy, *Russia* ... **64 B6** 58 22N 57 50 E
Chuspita, *Bolivia* ... **172 D4** 16 18 S 67 48W
Chust = Khust, *Ukraine* **53 B8** 48 10N 23 18 E
Chust, *Uzbekistan* ... **65 E8** 41 0N 71 13 E
Chute-aux-Outardes,
Canada **141 C6** 49 7N 68 24W
Chuuronjang, *N. Korea* **75 D15** 41 35N 129 40 E
Chuvash Republic =
Chuvashia □, *Russia* **60 C8** 55 30N 47 0 E
Chuvashia □, *Russia* ... **60 C8** 55 30N 47 0 E
Chuwārtah, *Iraq* ... **96 C5** 35 43N 45 34 E
Chuxiong, *China* ... **78 D3** 25 2N 101 28 E
Chüy, *Kyrgyzstan* ... **65 B7** 42 55N 75 15 E
Chuýyen-Ko, *Japan* ... **175 C5** 33 41 S 53 27W
Chuzenji-Ko, *Japan* ... **73 A11** 36 44N 139 27 E
Chuzhou, *China* ... **77 A12** 32 19N 118 20 E
Chynadiyeve, *Ukraine* ... **52 B7** 48 29N 22 50 E
Ci Xian, *China* ...... **74 F8** 36 20N 114 25 E
Ciacova, *Romania* ... **52 E6** 45 35N 21 10 E
Ciadār-Lunga, *Moldova* **53 D13** 46 3N 28 51 E
Ciamis, *Indonesia* ... **85 D3** 7 20 S 108 21 E
Cianjur, *Indonesia* ... **84 D3** 6 49 S 107 8 E
Cianorte, *Brazil* ... **175 A5** 23 37 S 52 37W
Cibola, *U.S.A.* **161 M12** 33 17N 114 42W
Cicero, *U.S.A.* **157 C9** 41 51N 87 45W
Cícero Dantas, *Brazil* ... **170 D4** 10 36 S 38 23W
Cicia, *Fiji* .... **133 A3** 17 45 S 179 18W
Cidacos →, *Spain* ... **40 C3** 42 21N 1 38W
Cidade de Minas = Belo
Horizonte, *Brazil* ... **171 E3** 19 55 S 43 56W
Cide, *Turkey* ...... **100 B5** 41 53N 33 1 E
Ciégas del
Catatumbo □,
Venezuela **165 E5** 9 25N 71 54W
Ciechanów, *Poland* ... **55 F7** 52 52N 20 38 E
Ciechanowiec, *Poland* ... **55 F9** 52 40N 22 31 E
Ciechocinek, *Poland* ... **55 F5** 52 53N 18 45 E
Ciego de Avila, *Cuba* ... **164 B4** 21 50N 78 50W
Ciénaga, *Colombia* ... **168 A3** 11 1N 74 15W
Ciénaga de Oro,
Colombia **168 B2** 8 53N 75 37W
Ciénagas del
Catatumbo △,
Venezuela **168 B3** 9 26N 72 8W
Cienfuegos, *Cuba* ... **164 B3** 22 10N 80 30W
Cierp-Gaud, *France* ... **28 F4** 42 55N 0 40 E
Cíes, Is., *Spain* ... **42 C2** 42 12N 8 55W
Cieszanów, *Poland* ... **55 H10** 50 14N 23 16 E
Cieszyn, *Poland* ... **55 J5** 49 45N 18 35 E
Cieza, *Spain* **41 G3** 38 17N 1 23W
Çifteler, *Turkey* ... **100 C4** 39 22N 31 2 E
Cifuentes, *Spain* ... **40 E2** 40 47N 2 37 E
Cihanbeyli, *Turkey* ... **100 C5** 38 40N 32 55 E
Cihuatlán, *Mexico* ... **162 D4** 19 14N 104 35W
Cijara, Embalse de,
Spain **43 F6** 39 18N 4 35W
Cijulang, *Indonesia* ... **85 D3** 7 42 S 108 27 E
Cilacap, *Indonesia* ... **85 D3** 7 43 S 109 0 E
Çıldır, *Turkey* ...... **101 B10** 41 7N 43 8 E

Çıldır Gölü, *Turkey* ... **101 B10** 41 5N 43 15 E
Cilento e Vallo di
Diano △, *Italy* ... **47 B8** 40 15N 15 20 E
Cili, *China* ...... **77 C8** 29 30N 111 8 E
Cilibia, *Romania* ... **53 E12** 45 4N 27 4 E
Cilicia, *Turkey* ... **100 D5** 36 30N 33 40 E
Cill Chainnigh =
Kilkenny, *Ireland* ... **23 D4** 52 39N 7 15W
Cilo Dağı, *Turkey* ... **101 D10** 37 28N 43 55 E
Cima, *U.S.A.* **161 K11** 35 14N 115 30W
Cimarron, *Kans.,*
U.S.A. **155 G4** 37 48N 100 21W
Cimarron, *N. Mex.,*
U.S.A. **155 G2** 36 31N 104 55W
Cimarron →, *U.S.A.* ... **155 G6** 36 10N 96 17W
Cimişlia, *Moldova* ... **53 D13** 46 34N 28 44 E
Cimone, Mte., *Italy* ... **44 D7** 44 12N 10 42 E
Cimpu, *Indonesia* ... **82 B2** 3 25 S 120 22 E
Çınar, *Turkey* ...... **101 D9** 37 46N 40 19 E
Çınarcık, *Turkey* ... **51 F13** 40 38N 29 5 E
Cinaruco-
Capanaparo △,
Venezuela **168 B4** 6 51N 67 32W
Cinca →, *Spain* ... **40 D5** 41 26N 0 21 E
Cincar, *Bos.-H.* ... **52 G2** 43 55N 17 5 E
Cincinnati, *Iowa,*
U.S.A. **156 D4** 40 38N 92 56W
Cincinnati, *Ohio,*
U.S.A. **157 E12** 39 6N 84 31W
Cincinnati-Northern
Kentucky
International ✈
(CVG), *U.S.A.* ... **157 E12** 39 3N 84 40W
Cincinnatus, *U.S.A.* ... **151 D9** 42 33N 75 54W
Çine, *Turkey* ...... **100 D10** 37 37N 28 2 E
Ciney, *Belgium* ... **24 D5** 50 18N 5 5 E
Cíngoli, *Italy* ...... **45 E10** 43 23N 13 10 E
Cinigiano, *Italy* ... **45 F8** 42 53N 11 24 E
Cinque I., *India* ... **95 H11** 11 16N 92 42 E
Cinto, Mte., *France* ... **29 F12** 42 24N 8 54 E
Cintra, G. de,
W. Sahara **110 D1** 23 0N 16 15W
Cintruénigo, *Spain* ... **40 C3** 42 5N 1 49W
Ciocile, *Romania* ... **53 F12** 44 49N 27 14 E
Ciolăneşti din Deal,
Romania .... **53 F10** 44 19N 25 5 E
Ciorani, *Romania* ... **53 F11** 44 45N 26 25 E
Čiovo, *Croatia* ... **45 E13** 43 30N 16 17 E
Cipó, *Brazil* ...... **170 D4** 11 6 S 38 31W
Cipolletti, *Argentina* ... **176 A3** 38 56 S 67 59W
Circeo, Mte., *Italy* ... **46 A6** 41 14N 13 3 E
Çırçır, *Turkey* ...... **100 C7** 40 5N 36 49 E
Circle, *Alaska, U.S.A.* ... **144 D11** 65 50N 144 4W
Circle, *Mont., U.S.A.* ... **148 B2** 47 25N 105 35W
Circleville, *U.S.A.* ... **148 F4** 39 36N 82 57W
Circular Reef,
Papua N. G. ...... **132 B4** 3 25 S 147 47 E
Cirebon, *Indonesia* ... **85 D3** 6 45 S 108 32 E
Ciremay, *Indonesia* ... **85 D3** 6 55 S 108 27 E
Cirencester, *U.K.* ... **21 F6** 51 43N 1 57W
Cireşu, *Romania* ... **52 F7** 44 47N 22 31 E
Cirey-sur-Vezouze,
France .... **27 D13** 48 35N 6 57 E
Ciriè, *Italy* ...... **44 C4** 45 14N 7 36 E
Cirium, *Cyprus* ... **39 F8** 34 40N 32 53 E
Cirò, *Italy* ...... **47 C10** 39 23N 17 4 E
Cirò Marina, *Italy* ... **47 C10** 39 22N 17 8 E
Ciron →, *France* ... **28 D3** 44 36N 0 18W
Cisco, *U.S.A.* **155 J5** 32 23N 98 59W
Cislău, *Romania* ... **53 E11** 45 14N 26 20 E
Cisna, *Poland* ...... **55 J9** 49 12N 22 20 E
Cisnădie, *Romania* ... **53 E9** 45 42N 24 9 E
Cisne, *U.S.A.* **156 F8** 38 31N 88 26W
Cisneros, *Colombia* ... **168 B2** 6 33N 75 4W
Cissna Park, *U.S.A.* ... **157 E9** 40 34N 87 54W
Cisterna di Latina, *Italy* **46 A5** 41 35N 12 49 E
Cisternino, *Italy* ... **47 B10** 40 44N 17 25 E
Cistierna, *Spain* ... **42 C5** 42 48N 5 7W
Citaré →, *Brazil* ... **170 C7** 1 11N 54 41W
Citeli-Ckaro = Tsiteli-
Tsqaro, *Georgia* ... **61 K8** 41 33N 46 0 E
Citlaltépetl = Orizaba,
Pico de, *Mexico* ... **163 D5** 19 0N 97 20W
Citra, *U.S.A.* **153 F7** 29 25N 82 7W
Citron, *Fr. Guiana* ... **169 C7** 4 44N 53 57W
Citrus Heights, *U.S.A.* **160 G5** 38 42N 121 17W
Citrus Springs, *U.S.A.* ... **153 F7** 29 2N 82 27W
Cittrusdal, *S. Africa* ... **116 E2** 32 35 S 19 0 E
Città della Pieve, *Italy* ... **45 F9** 42 57N 12 1 E
Città di Castello, *Italy* ... **45 E9** 43 27N 12 14 E
Città Sant' Angelo,
Italy .... **45 F11** 42 32N 14 5 E
Cittadella, *Italy* ... **45 C8** 45 39N 11 47 E
Cittaducale, *Italy* ... **45 F9** 42 23N 12 57 E
Cittanova, *Italy* ... **47 D9** 38 21N 16 5 E
Ciuc, Munţii, *Romania* **53 D11** 46 25N 26 1 E
Cucaş, Vf., *Romania* ... **53 E10** 45 31N 25 56 E
Cucea, *Romania* ... **52 D7** 46 25N 22 49 E
Ciuciulea, *Moldova* ... **53 C12** 47 40N 27 29 E
Ciuciuleni, *Moldova* ... **53 C13** 47 2N 28 25 E
Ciudad Altamirano,
Mexico **162 D4** 18 20N 100 40W
Ciudad Bolívar,
Venezuela **169 B5** 8 5N 63 36W
Ciudad Camargo,
Mexico **162 B3** 27 41N 105 10W
Ciudad de Valles,
Mexico **163 C5** 22 0N 99 0W
Ciudad del Carmen,
Mexico **163 D6** 18 38N 91 50W
Ciudad del Este,
Paraguay ...... **175 B5** 25 30 S 54 50W
Ciudad Delicias =
Delicias, *Mexico* ... **162 B3** 28 10N 105 30W
Ciudad Guayana,
Venezuela **169 B5** 8 0N 62 30W
Ciudad Guerrero,
Mexico **162 B3** 28 33N 107 28W
Ciudad Guzmán,
Mexico **162 D4** 19 40N 103 30W
Ciudad Juárez, *Mexico* ... **162 A3** 31 40N 106 28W
Ciudad Madero,
Mexico **163 C5** 22 0N 98 0W
Ciudad Mante, *Mexico* ... **163 C5** 22 50N 99 0W
Ciudad Obregón,
Mexico **162 B3** 27 28N 109 59W
Ciudad Ojeda,
Venezuela **168 A3** 10 12N 71 19W
Ciudad Piar, *Venezuela* **169 B5** 7 27N 63 19W
Ciudad Porfirio Díaz =
Piedras Negras,
Mexico **162 B4** 28 42N 100 31W
Ciudad Real, *Spain* ... **43 G7** 38 59N 3 55W
Ciudad Real □, *Spain* ... **43 G7** 38 59N 4 0W
Ciudad Rodrigo, *Spain* **42 E4** 40 35N 6 32W
Ciudad Trujillo = Santo
Domingo, *Dom. Rep.* **165 C6** 18 30N 69 59W
Ciudad Victoria,
Mexico **163 C5** 23 41N 99 9W
Ciudadela, *Spain* ... **38 B4** 40 0N 3 50 E
Ciuluta, *Romania* ... **53 F12** 44 26N 27 22 E
Ciumeghiu, *Romania* ... **52 D6** 46 41N 21 35 E
Ciuperceni, *Romania* ... **52 F8** 44 54N 23 1 E
Civa Burnu, *Turkey* ... **100 B7** 41 21N 36 38 E

Cividale del Friuli, *Italy* **45 B10** 46 6N 13 25 E
Civita Castellana, *Italy* ... **45 F9** 42 18N 12 24 E
Civitanova Marche,
Italy .... **45 E10** 43 18N 13 41 E
Civitavécchia, *Italy* ... **45 F8** 42 6N 11 48 E
Civray, *France* ... **28 B4** 46 10N 0 17 E
Çivril, *Turkey* ...... **49 C11** 38 20N 29 43 E
Cixerri →, *Italy* ... **46 C1** 39 17N 8 59 E
Cixi, *China* ...... **77 B13** 30 17N 121 9 E
Cizre, *Turkey* ...... **101 D10** 37 19N 42 10 E
Cizur Mayor, *Spain* ... **40 C3** 42 47N 1 41W
Clackmannanshire □,
U.K. **22 E5** 56 10N 3 43W
Clacton-on-Sea, *U.K.* ... **21 F9** 51 47N 1 11 E
Clain →, *France* ... **26 F7** 46 47N 0 33 E
Claire, L., *Canada* ... **142 B6** 58 35N 112 5W
Clairton, *U.S.A.* ... **150 F5** 40 18N 79 53W
Clairvaux-les-Lacs,
France .... **27 F12** 46 35N 5 45 E
Claise →, *France* ... **28 B5** 46 56N 0 42 E
Clallam Bay, *U.S.A.* ... **160 B2** 48 15N 124 16W
Clam Gulch, *U.S.A.* ... **144 F10** 60 15N 151 23W
Clamecy, *France* ... **27 E10** 47 28N 3 30 E
Clanton, *U.S.A.* ... **149 J2** 32 51N 86 38W
Clanwilliam, *S. Africa* **116 E2** 32 11 S 18 52 E
Clara, *Ireland* **23 C4** 53 21N 7 37W
Claraville, *U.S.A.* ... **161 K8** 35 24N 118 20W
Clare, *Australia* ... **128 B3** 33 50 S 138 37 E
Clare, *U.S.A.* **148 D3** 43 49N 84 46W
Clare □, *Ireland* ... **23 D3** 52 45N 9 0W
Clare →, *Ireland* ... **23 C2** 53 20N 9 2W
Clare I., *Ireland* ... **23 C1** 53 49N 10 0W
Claremont, *Calif.,*
U.S.A. **161 L9** 34 6N 117 43W
Claremont, *N.H.,*
U.S.A. **151 C12** 43 23N 72 20W
Claremont Pt.,
Australia ...... **126 A3** 14 1 S 143 41 E
Claremore, *U.S.A.* ... **155 G7** 36 19N 95 36W
Claremorris, *Ireland* ... **23 C3** 53 45N 9 0W
Clarence →, *Australia* ... **156 E4** 39 45N 92 16W
Clarence →, *Australia* ... **127 D5** 29 25 S 153 22 E
Clarence →, *N.Z.* ... **131 C8** 42 10 S 173 56 E
Clarence, I., *Chile* ... **176 D2** 54 0 S 72 0W
Clarence, Port, *U.S.A.* **144 D6** 65 15N 166 40W
Clarence I.,
Ascension I. ...... **9 g** 7 55 S 14 25W
Clarence I., *Antarctica* **7 C18** 61 10 S 54 0W
Clarence Str., *Australia* **124 B5** 12 0 S 131 0 E
Clarence Town,
Bahamas **165 B5** 23 6N 74 59W
Clarendon, *Pa., U.S.A.* **150 E5** 41 47N 79 6W
Clarendon, *Tex., U.S.A.* **155 H4** 34 56N 100 53W
Clarenville-Shoal
Harbour, *Canada* ... **141 C9** 48 10N 54 1W
Clareshem, *Canada* ... **142 D6** 50 2N 113 33W
Clarie Coast, *Antarctica* **7 C9** 68 0 S 135 0 E
Clarinda, *U.S.A.* ... **154 E7** 40 44N 95 2W
Clarington, *Canada* ... **150 C6** 43 55N 78 41W
Clarion, *Iowa, U.S.A.* ... **156 B3** 42 44N 93 44W
Clarion, *Pa., U.S.A.* ... **150 E5** 41 13N 79 23W
Clarion →, *U.S.A.* ... **150 E5** 41 7N 79 41W
Clarion Fracture Zone,
Pac. Oc. **136 H7** 20 0N 120 0W
Clark, *U.S.A.* **154 C6** 44 53N 97 44W
Clark, S. Dak., *U.S.A.* ... **154 C6** 44 53N 97 44W
Clark, Pt., *Canada* ... **150 B3** 44 4N 81 45W
Clark Fork, *U.S.A.* ... **158 B5** 48 9N 116 11W
Clark Fork →, *U.S.A.* ... **158 B5** 48 9N 116 15W
Clarkdale, *U.S.A.* ... **159 J7** 34 46N 112 3W
Clarke City, *Canada* ... **141 B6** 50 12N 66 38W
Clarke I., *Australia* ... **127 G4** 40 32 S 148 10 E
Clarke Ra., *Australia* ... **126 J6** 20 40 S 148 30 E
Clark's Fork →, *U.S.A.* **158 D9** 45 39N 108 43W
Clark's Harbour,
Canada **141 D6** 43 25N 65 38W
Clarks Hill L. =
Strom Thurmond L.,
U.S.A. **152 B7** 33 40N 82 12W
Clarks Point, *U.S.A.* ... **144 G8** 58 51N 158 33W
Clarks Summit, *U.S.A.* **151 E9** 41 30N 75 42W
Clarksburg, *U.S.A.* ... **148 F5** 39 17N 80 30W
Clarksdale, *U.S.A.* ... **155 H9** 34 12N 90 35W
Clarkston, *U.S.A.* ... **158 C5** 46 25N 117 3W
Clarksville, *Ark., U.S.A.* **155 H8** 35 28N 93 28W
Clarksville, *Ind., U.S.A.* **157 F11** 38 17N 85 45W
Clarksville, *Iowa,*
U.S.A. **156 B4** 42 47N 92 40W
Clarksville, *Mo., U.S.A.* **156 E6** 39 22N 90 54W
Clarksville, *Tenn.,*
U.S.A. **149 G2** 36 32N 87 21W
Clarksville, *Tex., U.S.A.* **155 J7** 33 37N 95 3W
Claro →, *Brazil* ... **171 E1** 19 8 S 50 40W
Clatskanie, *U.S.A.* ... **160 D3** 46 6N 123 12W
Claude, *U.S.A.* ... **155 H4** 35 7N 101 22W
Claveria, *Cagayan, Phil.* **80 B3** 18 37N 121 15 E
Claveria, *Masbate, Phil.* **80 E4** 12 54N 123 15 E
Clavering Ø, *Greenland* **10 C8** 74 15N 21 0W
Claxton, *U.S.A.* ... **152 C8** 32 10N 81 55W
Clay, *U.S.A.* **160 G5** 38 17N 121 10W
Clay Center, *U.S.A.* ... **154 F6** 39 23N 97 8W
Clay City, *Ind., U.S.A.* **157 F9** 39 17N 87 7W
Clay City, *Ky., U.S.A.* ... **157 G13** 37 52N 83 55W
Claypool, *U.S.A.* ... **159 K8** 33 25N 110 51W
Claysburg, *U.S.A.* ... **150 F6** 40 17N 78 27W
Claysville, *U.S.A.* ... **150 F4** 40 7N 80 25W
Clayton, *Ala., U.S.A.* ... **152 J3** 31 53N 85 27W
Clayton, *Ind., U.S.A.* ... **157 E10** 39 41N 86 31W
Clayton, *N. Mex.,*
U.S.A. **155 G3** 36 27N 103 11W
Clayton, *N.Y., U.S.A.* ... **151 B8** 44 14N 76 5W
Clear, C., *Ireland* ... **23 E2** 51 25N 9 32W
Clear, L., *Canada* ... **150 A7** 45 26N 77 12W
Clear Hills, *Canada* ... **142 B5** 56 40N 119 30W
Clear I., *Ireland* ... **23 E2** 51 26N 9 30W
Clear L., *U.S.A.* ... **160 F4** 39 2N 122 47W
Clear Lake, *Iowa,*
U.S.A. **156 A3** 43 8N 93 23W
Clear Lake, *S. Dak.,*
U.S.A. **154 C6** 44 45N 96 41W
Clear Lake Reservoir,
U.S.A. **158 F3** 41 56N 121 5W
Clearfield, *Pa., U.S.A.* ... **150 E6** 41 2N 78 27W
Clearfield, *Utah, U.S.A.* **158 F8** 41 7N 112 2W
Clearlake, *U.S.A.* ... **158 G2** 38 57N 122 38W
Clearlake Highlands,
U.S.A. **160 G4** 38 57N 122 38W
Clearwater, *Canada* ... **142 C4** 51 38N 120 2W
Clearwater, *U.S.A.* ... **153 H7** 27 58N 82 48W
Clearwater →, *Alta.,*
Canada **142 C6** 52 22N 114 57W
Clearwater →, *Alta.,*
Canada **143 B6** 56 44N 111 23W
Clearwater L., *Canada* ... **143 C9** 53 34N 99 49W
Clearwater Lake △,
Canada **143 C8** 54 0N 101 0W
Clearwater Mts., *U.S.A.* **158 C6** 46 5N 115 20W
Clearwater River △,
Canada **143 B7** 56 55N 109 10W
Cleburne, *U.S.A.* ... **155 J6** 32 21N 97 23W
Clee Hills, *U.K.* ... **21 E5** 52 26N 2 35W
Cleethorpes, *U.K.* ... **20 D7** 53 33N 0 3W
Cleeve Cloud, *U.K.* ... **21 F6** 51 56N 2 0W

Clelles, *France* ... **29 D9** 44 50N 5 38 E
Clemson, *U.S.A.* ... **149 H4** 34 41N 82 50W
Cleopatra Needle, *Phil.* **81 F2** 10 7N 118 58 E
Clerke Reef, *Australia* ... **124 C2** 17 22 S 119 20 E
Clermont, *Australia* ... **126 C4** 22 49 S 147 39 E
Clermont, *France* ... **27 C9** 49 23N 2 24 E
Clermont, *U.S.A.* ... **153 G8** 28 33N 81 46W
Clermont-en-Argonne,
France .... **27 C12** 49 5N 5 4 E
Clermont-Ferrand,
France .... **28 C7** 45 46N 3 4 E
Clermont-l'Hérault,
France .... **28 E7** 43 38N 3 26 E
Clerval, *France* ... **27 E13** 47 25N 6 30 E
Clervaux, *Lux.* ... **24 D6** 50 4N 6 2 E
Cles, *Italy* ...... **44 B8** 46 21N 11 2 E
Cleveland, *Australia* ... **127 L5** 27 31 S 153 18 E
Clevedon, *U.K.* ... **21 F5** 51 26N 2 52W
Cleveland, *Miss., U.S.A.* **155 J9** 33 45N 90 43W
Cleveland, *Ohio, U.S.A.* **150 E3** 41 30N 81 42W
Cleveland, *Okla.,*
U.S.A. **155 G6** 36 19N 96 28W
Cleveland, *Tenn.,*
U.S.A. **149 H3** 35 10N 84 53W
Cleveland, *Tex., U.S.A.* **155 K7** 30 21N 95 5W
Cleveland, C., *Australia* **126 B4** 19 11 S 147 1 E
Cleveland, Mt., *U.S.A.* ... **158 B7** 48 56N 113 51W
Cleveland Heights,
U.S.A. **150 E3** 41 30N 81 34W
Clevelândia, *Brazil* ... **175 B5** 26 24 S 52 23W
Clevelândia do Norte,
Brazil **169 C7** 3 49N 51 52W
Cleves, *U.S.A.* ... **157 E12** 39 10N 84 45W
Clew B., *Ireland* ... **23 C2** 53 50N 9 49W
Clewiston, *U.S.A.* ... **153 J9** 26 45N 80 56W
Clifden, *Ireland* ... **23 C1** 53 29N 10 1W
Clifden, *N.Z.* ...... **131 G2** 46 1 S 167 42 E
Cliffdell, *U.S.A.* ... **160 D5** 46 56N 121 5W
Clifty Hd., *Australia* ... **125 G2** 35 1 S 116 29 E
Clifton, *Australia* ... **127 D5** 27 59 S 151 53 E
Clifton, *Ariz., U.S.A.* ... **159 K9** 33 3N 109 18W
Clifton, *Colo., U.S.A.* ... **159 G9** 39 7N 108 25W
Clifton, *Ill., U.S.A.* ... **157 D9** 40 56N 87 56W
Clifton, *Tex., U.S.A.* ... **155 K6** 31 47N 97 35W
Clifton Beach, *Australia* **126 B4** 16 46 S 145 39 E
Clifton Pt., *Bahamas* ... **164 A4** 25 1N 77 34W
Climax, *Canada* ... **143 D7** 49 10N 108 20W
Climax, *U.S.A.* ... **152 E5** 30 53N 84 26W
Clinch →, *U.S.A.* ... **149 H3** 35 53N 84 29W
Clingmans Dome,
U.S.A. **149 H4** 35 34N 83 30W
Clint, *U.S.A.* **159 L10** 31 35N 106 14W
Clinton, *B.C., Canada* ... **142 C4** 51 6N 121 35W
Clinton, *Ont., Canada* ... **140 D3** 43 37N 81 32W
Clinton, *N.Z.* ...... **131 G4** 46 12 S 169 23 E
Clinton, *Ark., U.S.A.* ... **155 H8** 35 36N 92 28W
Clinton, *Conn., U.S.A.* **151 E12** 41 17N 72 32W
Clinton, *Ill., U.S.A.* ... **156 E10** 40 9N 88 57W
Clinton, *Ind., U.S.A.* ... **157 E9** 39 40N 87 24W
Clinton, *Iowa, U.S.A.* ... **156 C6** 41 51N 90 12W
Clinton, *Mass., U.S.A.* **151 D13** 42 25N 71 41W
Clinton, *Mich., U.S.A.* **157 B13** 42 4N 83 58W
Clinton, *Miss., U.S.A.* **155 F9** 32 20N 90 20W
Clinton, *Mo., U.S.A.* ... **156 F3** 38 22N 93 46W
Clinton, *N.C., U.S.A.* ... **149 H6** 35 0N 78 22W
Clinton, *Okla., U.S.A.* ... **155 H5** 35 31N 98 58W
Clinton, *S.C., U.S.A.* ... **149 H5** 34 29N 81 53W
Clinton, *Tenn., U.S.A.* **149 G3** 36 6N 84 8W
Clinton, *Wash., U.S.A.* **160 C4** 47 59N 122 21W
Clinton, *Wis., U.S.A.* ... **157 B8** 42 34N 88 52W
Clinton C., *Australia* ... **126 C5** 22 30 S 150 45 E
Clinton Colden L.,
Canada **138 B9** 63 58N 107 27W
Clinton L., *U.S.A.* ... **157 D7** 40 15N 88 45W
Clintonville, *U.S.A.* ... **154 C10** 44 37N 88 46W
Clio, *U.S.A.* **152 D4** 31 43N 85 37W
Clipperton, I., *Pac. Oc.* **135 F17** 10 18N 109 13W
Clipperton Fracture
Zone, *Pac. Oc.* ... **135 G16** 19 0N 122 0W
Clisham, *U.K.* ... **22 D2** 57 57N 6 49W
Clisson, *France* ... **26 E5** 47 5N 1 16W
Clitheroe, *U.K.* ... **20 D5** 53 53N 2 22W
Clive, *N.Z.* ...... **130 F5** 39 36 S 176 58 E
Cliza, *Bolivia* ...... **173 D4** 17 36 S 65 56W
Clo-oose, *Canada* ... **160 B2** 48 39N 124 49W
Cloates, Pt., *Australia* **124 D1** 22 43 S 113 40 E
Clocolan, *S. Africa* ... **117 D4** 28 55 S 27 34 E
Clodomira, *Argentina* **174 B3** 27 35 S 64 14W
Clogher Hd., *Ireland* ... **23 C5** 53 48N 6 14W
Clonakilty, *Ireland* ... **23 E3** 51 37N 8 53W
Clonakilty B., *Ireland* **23 E3** 51 35N 8 51W
Cloncurry, *Australia* ... **126 C3** 20 40 S 140 28 E
Cloncurry →, *Australia* **126 B3** 18 37 S 140 40 E
Clondalkin, *Ireland* ... **23 C5** 53 19N 6 25W
Clones, *Ireland* ... **23 B4** 54 11N 7 15W
Clonmel, *Ireland* ... **23 D4** 52 21N 7 42W
Cloppenburg, *Germany* **30 C4** 52 51N 8 1 E
Cloquet, *U.S.A.* ... **154 B8** 46 43N 92 28W
Clorinda, *Argentina* ... **174 B4** 25 16 S 57 45W
Cloud Bay, *Canada* ... **140 C2** 48 5N 89 26W
Cloud Peak, *U.S.A.* ... **158 D10** 44 23N 107 11W
Cloudcroft, *U.S.A.* ... **159 K11** 32 58N 105 44W
Cloudy, *N.Z.* ...... **131 B9** 41 25 S 174 10 E
Cloverdale, *Calif.,*
U.S.A. **160 G4** 38 48N 123 1W
Cloverdale, *Ind., U.S.A.* **157 E10** 39 31N 86 48W
Cloverport, *U.S.A.* ... **157 G10** 37 50N 86 38W
Clovis, *Calif., U.S.A.* ... **160 J7** 36 49N 119 42W
Clovis, *N. Mex., U.S.A.* **155 H3** 34 24N 103 12W
Cloyes-sur-le-Loir,
France .... **26 E8** 48 0N 1 14 E
Cloyne, *Canada* ... **150 B7** 44 49N 77 11W
Club Terrace, *Australia* **129 D8** 37 35 S 148 58 E
Cluj □, *Romania* ... **53 D8** 46 45N 23 30 E
Cluj-Napoca, *Romania* **53 D8** 46 47N 23 38 E
Clunes, *Australia* ... **128 D5** 37 20 S 143 45 E
Cluny, *France* ...... **27 F11** 46 26N 4 38 E
Cluses, *France* ... **27 F13** 46 5N 6 35 E
Clusone, *Italy* ...... **44 C6** 45 53N 9 57 E
Clutha →, *N.Z.* ... **131 G4** 46 20 S 169 49 E
Clwyd →, *U.K.* ... **20 D4** 53 19N 3 31W
Clyattville, *U.S.A.* ... **152 E6** 30 43N 83 19W
Clyde, *Canada* **142 C6** 54 9N 113 39W
Clyde, *N.Z.* ...... **131 F4** 45 12 S 169 20 E
Clyde, *Ohio, U.S.A.* ... **157 C14** 41 18N 82 59W
Clyde →, *U.K.* ... **22 F4** 55 55N 4 30W
Clyde, Firth of, *U.K.* ... **22 F3** 55 22N 5 1W
Clyde Muirshiel △,
U.K. **22 F4** 55 50N 4 40W
Clyde River, *Canada* ... **139 A13** 70 30N 68 30W
Clydebank, *U.K.* ... **22 F4** 55 54N 4 23W
Clymer, *N.Y., U.S.A.* ... **150 D5** 42 1N 79 37W
Clymer, *Pa., U.S.A.* ... **150 D5** 40 40N 79 1W
Clyo, *U.S.A.* **152 C8** 32 29N 81 16W
Ćmielów, *Poland* ... **55 H8** 50 53N 21 31 E
Côa →, *Portugal* ... **42 D3** 41 5N 7 6W
Coachella, *U.S.A.* ... **161 M10** 33 41N 116 10W
Coachella Canal, *U.S.A.* **161 N12** 32 43N 114 57W
Coahoma, *U.S.A.* ... **155 J4** 32 18N 101 18W
Coahuayana →,
Mexico **162 D4** 18 41N 103 45W
Coahuila □, *Mexico* ... **162 B4** 27 0N 103 0W
Coal →, *Canada* ... **142 B3** 59 39N 126 57W

Coal City, *U.S.A.* ... **157 C8** 41 17N 88 17W
Coal, L., *N.Z.* ...... **131 G1** 46 8 S 166 40 E
Coalane, *Mozam.* ... **119 F4** 17 48 S 37 2 E
Coalcomán, *Mexico* ... **162 D4** 18 40N 103 10W
Coaldale, *Canada* ... **142 D6** 49 45N 112 35W
Coalgate, *U.S.A.* ... **155 H6** 34 32N 96 13W
Coalinga, *U.S.A.* ... **160 J6** 36 9N 120 21W
Coalisland, *U.K.* ... **23 B5** 54 33N 6 42W
Coalville, *U.K.* **21 E6** 52 44N 1 23W
Coalville, *U.S.A.* ... **158 F8** 40 55N 111 24W
Coamo, *Puerto Rico* ... **165 d** 18 5N 66 22W
Coaraci, *Brazil* ... **171 D4** 14 38 S 39 32W
Coari, *Brazil* ...... **169 D5** 4 8 S 63 7W
Coari →, *Brazil* ... **169 D5** 4 30 S 63 33W
Coari, L. de, *Brazil* ... **169 D5** 4 15 S 63 22W
Coast □, *Kenya* ... **118 C4** 2 40 S 39 45 E
Coast Mts., *Canada* ... **142 C3** 55 0N 129 20W
Coast Ranges, *U.S.A.* ... **160 G4** 39 0N 123 0W
Coatbridge, *U.K.* ... **22 F4** 55 52N 4 6W
Coatepec, *Mexico* ... **163 D5** 19 27N 96 58W
Coatepeque, *Guatemala* **164 D1** 14 46N 91 55W
Coatesville, *U.S.A.* ... **148 F8** 39 59N 75 50W
Coaticook, *Canada* ... **141 C5** 45 10N 71 46W
Coats I., *Canada* ... **139 B11** 62 30N 83 0W
Coats Land, *Antarctica* **7 D1** 77 0 S 25 0W
Coatzacoalcos, *Mexico* **163 D6** 18 7N 94 25W
Coba, *Mexico* **163 C7** 20 31N 87 39W
Cobadin, *Romania* ... **53 F13** 44 5N 28 13 E
Cobalt, *Canada* **140 C4** 47 25N 79 42W
Cobán, *Guatemala* ... **164 C1** 15 30N 90 21W
Çobanlar, *Turkey* ... **49 C12** 38 41N 30 47 E
Cobar, *Australia* ... **129 A6** 31 27 S 145 48 E
Cobargo, *Australia* ... **129 D8** 36 20 S 149 55 E
Cobbannah, *Australia* **129 D7** 37 37 S 147 13 E
Cobberas, Mt.,
Australia ...... **129 D8** 36 53 S 148 12 E
Cobden, *Australia* ... **128 E5** 38 20 S 143 3 E
Cobden, *Canada* ... **150 A8** 45 38N 76 53W
Cobh, *Ireland* **23 E3** 51 51N 8 17W
Cobija, *Bolivia* ... **172 C4** 11 0 S 68 50W
Cobleskill, *U.S.A.* ... **151 D10** 42 41N 74 29W
Coboconk, *Canada* ... **150 B6** 44 39N 78 48W
Cobourg, *Canada* ... **140 D4** 43 58N 78 10W
Cobourg, *Australia* ... **124 B5** 11 26 S 131 58 E
Cobourg Pen., *Australia* **124 B5** 11 20 S 132 15 E
Cobram, *Australia* ... **129 C6** 35 54 S 145 40 E
Cóbué, *Mozam.* ... **119 E3** 12 0 S 34 58 E
Coburg, *Germany* ... **31 E6** 50 15N 10 58 E
Coca, *Spain* **42 D6** 41 13N 4 32W
Coca →, *Ecuador* ... **168 D2** 0 29 S 76 58W
Cocachacra, *Peru* ... **172 D3** 17 5 S 71 45W
Cocal, *Brazil* ...... **170 B3** 3 28 S 41 34W
Cocanada = Kakinada,
India .... **94 F6** 16 57N 82 11 E
Cocentaina, *Spain* ... **41 G4** 38 45N 0 27W
Coche, I., *Venezuela* ... **169 A5** 10 47N 63 56W
Cochem, *Germany* ... **31 E3** 50 9N 7 9 E
Cochemane, *Mozam.* ... **119 F3** 17 0 S 32 54 E
Cochin, *India* ...... **95 K3** 9 58N 76 20 E
Cochin China = Nam-
Phan, *Vietnam* ... **87 G6** 10 30N 106 0 E
Cochran, *U.S.A.* ... **152 C6** 32 23N 83 21W
Cochrane, *Alta.,*
Canada **142 C6** 51 11N 114 30W
Cochrane, *Ont., Canada* **140 C3** 49 0N 81 0W
Cochrane, *Chile* ... **176 C2** 47 15 S 72 33W
Cochrane →, *Canada* **143 B8** 59 0N 103 40W
Cochrane, L., *Chile* ... **176 C2** 47 10 S 72 0W
Cochranton, *U.S.A.* ... **150 E4** 41 31N 80 3W
Cockburn, *Australia* ... **128 E3** 32 5 S 141 0 E
Cockburn, Canal, *Chile* **176 D2** 54 30 S 72 0W
Cockburn I., *Canada* ... **140 C3** 45 55N 83 22W
Cockburn Ra.,
Australia ...... **124 C4** 15 46 S 128 0 E
Cockermouth, *U.K.* ... **20 C4** 54 40N 3 22W
Cocklebiddy, *Australia* **125 F4** 32 0 S 126 3 E
Cockpit Country, The,
Jamaica .... **164 a** 18 15N 77 45W
Coco →, *Cent. Amer.* ... **164 D3** 15 0N 83 8W
Coco, I. del, *Pac. Oc.* ... **135 G19** 5 25N 87 55W
Coco, Pta., *Colombia* ... **168 C2** 2 58N 77 43W
Coco Channel, *Asia* ... **95 H11** 13 45N 93 10 E
Cocoa, *U.S.A.* **153 G9** 28 21N 80 44W
Cocoa Beach, *U.S.A.* ... **153 G9** 28 19N 80 37W
Cocobeach, *Gabon* ... **118 D1** 0 59N 9 34 E
Cocoparra △, *Australia* **129 C7** 34 10 S 146 12 E
Cocora, *Romania* ... **53 F12** 44 45N 27 3 E
Côcos, *Brazil* ... **171 D3** 14 10 S 44 33W
Côcos →, *Brazil* ... **171 D3** 12 44 S 44 48W
Cocos B., *Trin. & Tob.* **169 F10** 10 25N 61 2W
Cocos I., *Guam* ... **133 R15** 13 14N 144 39 E
Cocos Is., *Ind. Oc.* ... **121 D5** 12 10 S 96 55 E
Cocos Ridge, *Pac. Oc.* **135 G19** 4 0N 88 0W
Cod, C., *U.S.A.* ... **148 D10** 42 5N 70 10W
Codajás, *Brazil* ... **169 D5** 3 55 S 62 0W
Codera, C., *Venezuela* **168 A4** 10 35N 66 4W
Codfish I., *N.Z.* ... **131 G1** 46 47 S 167 38 E
Codigoro, *Italy* ... **45 D9** 44 49N 12 8 E
Codlea, *Romania* ... **53 E10** 45 42N 25 27 E
Codó, *Brazil* ...... **170 B3** 4 30 S 43 55W
Codogno, *Italy* ... **44 C6** 45 9N 9 42 E
Codpa, *Chile* ...... **172 D4** 18 50 S 69 44W
Codrói, *Italy* ... **45 C10** 45 58N 13 0 E
Codru, Munţii,
Romania .... **52 D7** 46 30N 22 15 E
Cody, *U.S.A.* **158 D9** 44 32N 109 3W
Coe Hill, *Canada* ... **150 B7** 44 52N 77 50W
Coelemu, *Chile* ... **174 D1** 36 30 S 72 48W
Coen, *Australia* ... **126 A3** 13 52 S 143 12 E
Coeroeni →, *Suriname* **169 C6** 3 21N 57 31W
Coesfeld, *Germany* ... **30 D3** 51 56N 7 10 E
Coetivy Is., *Seychelles* **121 E4** 7 8 S 56 16 E
Cœur d'Alene, *U.S.A.* ... **158 C5** 47 45N 116 51W
Cœur d'Alene L.,
U.S.A. **158 C5** 47 32N 116 48W
Coevorden, *Neths.* ... **24 B6** 52 40N 6 44 E
Cofete, *Canary Is.* ... **9 e2** 28 6N 14 23W
Coffeyville, *U.S.A.* ... **155 G7** 37 2N 95 37W
Coffin B., *Australia* ... **127 E2** 34 38 S 135 28 E
Coffin Bay, *Australia* ... **127 E2** 34 34 S 135 19 E
Coffin Bay △, *Australia* **127 E2** 34 34 S 135 14 E
Coffin Bay Peninsula,
Australia ...... **127 E2** 34 32 S 135 15 E
Coffs Harbour,
Australia ...... **129 A10** 30 16 S 153 5 E
Cofre de Perote △,
Mexico **163 D5** 19 29N 97 8W
Cofrentes, *Spain* ... **41 F3** 39 13N 1 5W
Cogalnic →, *Moldova* **53 E14** 45 49N 29 40 E
Cogealac, *Romania* ... **53 F13** 44 36N 28 36 E
Coghinas →, *Italy* ... **46 B1** 40 55N 8 48 E
Coghinas, L. del, *Italy* **46 B2** 40 46N 9 3 E
Cognac, *France* ... **28 C3** 45 41N 0 20W
Cogne, *Italy* ...... **44 C4** 45 37N 7 21 E
Cogolin, *France* ... **29 E10** 43 15N 6 32 E
Cogolludo, *Spain* ... **40 E1** 40 59N 3 10W
Cohocton, *U.S.A.* ... **150 D7** 42 30N 77 30W
Cohocton →, *U.S.A.* ... **150 D7** 42 9N 77 6W
Cohoes, *U.S.A.* ... **151 D11** 42 46N 73 42W
Cohuna, *Australia* ... **129 C6** 35 45 S 144 15 E
Coiba, I., *Panama* ... **164 E3** 7 30N 81 40W
Coig →, *Argentina* ... **176 D3** 51 0 S 69 10W

Coigeach, Rubha, U.K. 22 C3 58 6N 5 26W
Coihaique, Chile 176 C2 45 30 S 71 45W
Coimbatore, India 95 J3 11 2N 76 59 E
Coimbra, Brazil 173 D6 19 55 S 57 48W
Coimbra, Portugal 42 E2 40 15N 8 27W
Coimbra □, Portugal 42 E2 40 12N 8 25W
Coín, Spain 43 J6 36 40N 4 48W
Coipasa, L. de, Bolivia 172 D4 19 12 S 68 7W
Coipasa, Salar de, Bolivia 172 D4 19 26 S 68 9W
Cojata, Peru 172 D4 15 2 S 69 25W
Cojedes □, Venezuela 168 B4 9 20N 68 20W
Cojedes →, Venezuela 168 B4 8 34N 68 5W
Cojimies, Ecuador 168 C1 0 20N 80 0W
Cojocna, Romania 53 D8 46 45N 23 50 E
Cojutepequé, El Salv. 164 D2 13 41N 88 54W
Čoka, Serbia & M. 52 E5 45 57N 20 12 E
Cokeville, U.S.A. 158 E8 42 5N 110 57W
Colaba Pt., India 94 E1 18 54N 72 47 E
Colac, Australia 128 E5 38 21 S 143 35 E
Colachel = Kolachel, India 95 K3 8 10N 77 15 E
Colatina, Brazil 171 E3 19 32 S 40 37W
Colbeck, C., Antarctica 7 D13 77 6 S 157 48W
Colbert, U.S.A. 152 A6 34 2N 83 13W
Colborne, Canada 150 C7 44 0N 77 53W
Colby, U.S.A. 154 F4 39 24N 101 3W
Colca, Canon de, Peru 172 D3 15 50 S 72 20W
Colchester, U.K. 21 F8 51 54N 0 55 E
Cold Bay, U.S.A. 144 J7 55 12N 162 42W
Cold L., Canada 143 C7 54 33N 110 5W
Coldstream, Canada 142 C5 50 13N 119 11W
Coldstream, U.K. 22 F6 55 39N 2 15W
Coldwater, Canada 150 B5 44 42N 79 40W
Coldwater, Kans., U.S.A. 155 G5 37 16N 99 20W
Coldwater, Mich., U.S.A. 157 C11 41 57N 85 0W
Coldwater, Ohio, U.S.A. 157 D12 40 29N 84 38W
Coldwater, L., U.S.A. 157 C12 41 48N 84 59W
Cole Camp, U.S.A. 156 F3 38 28N 93 12W
Coleambally, Australia 129 C6 34 49 S 145 52 E
Colebrook, U.S.A. 151 B13 44 54N 71 30W
Coleman, Fla., U.S.A. 153 G7 28 48N 82 4W
Coleman, Tex., U.S.A. 155 K5 31 50N 99 26W
Coleman →, Australia 126 B3 15 6 S 141 38 E
Colenso, S. Africa 117 D4 28 44 S 29 50 E
Coleraine, Australia 128 D4 37 36 S 141 40 E
Coleraine, U.K. 23 A5 55 8N 6 41W
Coleridge, L., N.Z. 131 D6 43 17 S 171 30 E
Coleroon →, India 95 J4 11 25N 79 50 E
Colesberg, S. Africa 116 E4 30 45 S 25 5 E
Coleville, U.S.A. 160 G7 38 34N 119 30W
Colfax, Calif., U.S.A. 160 F6 39 6N 120 57W
Colfax, Ill., U.S.A. 157 D8 40 34N 88 37W
Colfax, Ind., U.S.A. 157 D10 40 12N 86 40W
Colfax, Iowa, U.S.A. 156 C3 41 41N 93 14W
Colfax, La., U.S.A. 155 K8 31 31N 92 42W
Colfax, Wash., U.S.A. 158 C5 46 53N 117 22W
Colhué Huapi, L., Argentina 176 C3 45 30 S 69 0W
Colibaşi, Moldova 53 E13 45 43N 28 11 E
Colibaşi, Romania 53 F9 44 56N 24 54 E
Cólico, Italy 44 B6 46 8N 9 22 E
Colíder, Brazil 173 C6 10 45 S 55 25W
Coligny, France 27 F12 46 23N 5 21 E
Coligny, S. Africa 117 D4 26 17 S 26 15 E
Colima, Mexico 162 D4 19 14N 103 43W
Colima □, Mexico 162 D4 19 10N 103 40W
Colima, Nevado de, Mexico 162 D4 19 35N 103 45W
Colina, Chile 174 C1 33 13 S 70 45W
Colina do Norte, Guinea-Biss. 112 C2 12 28N 15 0W
Colinas, Goiás, Brazil 171 D2 14 15 S 48 2W
Colinas, Maranhão, Brazil 170 C3 6 0 S 44 10W
Colindres, Spain 42 B7 43 24N 3 27W
Coll, U.K. 22 E2 56 39N 6 34W
Collaguasi, Chile 174 A2 21 5 S 68 45W
Collarada, Peña, Spain 40 C4 42 43N 0 29W
Collarenebri, Australia 127 D4 29 33 S 148 34 E
Colle di Val d'Elsa, Italy 44 E8 43 25N 11 7 E
Collécchio, Italy 44 D7 44 45N 10 13 E
Colleen Bawn, Zimbabwe 119 G2 21 0 S 29 12 E
College, U.S.A. 144 D11 64 52N 147 49W
College Park, U.S.A. 152 B5 33 40N 84 27W
College Station, U.S.A. 155 K6 30 37N 96 21W
Collesalvetti, Italy 44 E7 43 34N 10 27 E
Colli Euganei ⌂, Italy 45 C8 45 18N 11 43 E
Collie, N.S.W., Australia 129 A8 31 41 S 148 18 E
Collie, W. Austral., Australia 125 F2 33 22 S 116 8 E
Collier B., Australia 124 C3 16 10 S 124 15 E
Collier Ra., Australia 125 D2 24 45 S 119 10 E
Collier Range △, Australia 125 D2 24 39 S 119 7 E
Collierville, U.S.A. 155 H10 35 3N 89 40W
Collina, Passo di, Italy 44 D7 44 2N 10 56 E
Collingwood, Canada 140 D3 44 29N 80 13W
Collingwood, N.Z. 131 A7 40 41 S 172 40 E
Collins, Canada 140 B2 50 17N 89 27W
Collins, Ga., U.S.A. 152 C7 32 11N 82 7W
Collins, Mo., U.S.A. 156 G3 37 54N 93 37W
Collinsville, Australia 126 C4 20 30 S 147 56 E
Collinsville, U.S.A. 156 F7 38 40N 89 59W
Collipulli, Chile 174 D1 37 55 S 72 30W
Collo, Algeria 111 A6 36 58N 6 37 E
Collooney, Ireland 23 B3 54 11N 8 29W
Colmar, France 27 D14 48 5N 7 20 E
Colmars, France 29 D10 44 11N 6 39 E
Colmenar, Spain 43 J6 36 54N 4 20W
Colmenar de Oreja, Spain 42 E7 40 6N 3 25W
Colmenar Viejo, Spain 42 E7 40 39N 3 47W
Colo →, Australia 129 B9 33 25 S 150 52 E
Cologne = Köln, Germany 30 E2 50 56N 6 57 E
Colom, I. d'en, Spain 38 B5 39 58N 4 16 E
Coloma, Calif., U.S.A. 160 G6 38 48N 120 53W
Coloma, Mich., U.S.A. 157 B10 42 11N 86 19W
Colomb-Béchar = Béchar, Algeria 111 B4 31 38N 2 18W
Colombey-les-Belles, France 27 D12 48 32N 5 54 E
Colombey-les-Deux-Églises, France 27 D11 48 13N 4 50 E
Colômbia, Brazil 171 F2 20 10 S 48 40W
Colombia ■, S. Amer. 168 C3 3 45N 73 0W
Colombian Basin, S. Amer. 136 H12 14 0N 76 0W
Colombier, Switz. 32 C3 46 58N 6 53 E
Colombo, Sri Lanka 95 L4 6 56N 79 58 E
Colomiers, France 28 E5 43 36N 1 21 E
Colón, Buenos Aires, Argentina 174 C3 33 53 S 61 7W
Colón, Entre Ríos, Argentina 174 C4 32 12 S 58 10W
Colón, Cuba 164 B3 22 42N 80 54W
Colón, Panama 164 E4 9 20N 79 54W
Colón, Peru 172 A1 5 0 S 81 0W
Colón, Arch. de, Ecuador 172 a 0 0 91 0W
Colonia 25 de Mayo, Argentina 176 A3 37 48 S 67 41W
Colònia de Sant Jordi, Spain 38 B3 39 19N 2 59 E
Colonia del Sacramento, Uruguay 174 C4 34 25 S 57 50W
Colonia Dora, Argentina 174 B3 28 34 S 62 59W
Colonia Las Heras, Argentina 176 C3 46 33 S 68 57W
Colonial Beach, U.S.A. 148 F7 38 15N 76 58W
Colonie, U.S.A. 151 D11 42 43N 73 50W
Colonna, C., Italy 47 C10 39 2N 17 12 E
Colonsay, Canada 143 C7 51 59N 105 52W
Colonsay, U.K. 22 E2 56 5N 6 12W
Colorado □, U.S.A. 159 G10 39 30N 105 30W
Colorado →, Argentina 176 A4 39 50 S 62 8W
Colorado →, N. Amer. 159 L6 31 45N 114 40W
Colorado →, U.S.A. 155 L7 28 36N 95 59W
Colorado City, U.S.A. 155 J4 32 24N 100 52W
Colorado Plateau, U.S.A. 159 H8 37 0N 111 0W
Colorado River Aqueduct, U.S.A. 161 L12 34 17N 114 10W
Colorado Springs, U.S.A. 154 F2 38 50N 104 49W
Colorno, Italy 44 D7 44 56N 10 23 E
Colotlán, Mexico 162 C4 22 6N 103 16W
Colquechaca, Bolivia 173 D4 18 40 S 66 1W
Colquitt, U.S.A. 152 D5 31 10N 84 44W
Colstrip, U.S.A. 158 D10 45 53N 106 38W
Colton, U.S.A. 151 B10 44 33N 74 56W
Columbia, Ala., U.S.A. 152 D4 31 18N 85 7W
Columbia, Ill., U.S.A. 156 F6 38 27N 90 12W
Columbia, Ky., U.S.A. 148 G3 37 6N 85 18W
Columbia, La., U.S.A. 155 J8 32 6N 92 5W
Columbia, Miss., U.S.A. 155 K10 31 15N 89 50W
Columbia, Mo., U.S.A. 156 F4 38 57N 92 20W
Columbia, Pa., U.S.A. 151 F8 40 2N 76 30W
Columbia, S.C., U.S.A. 152 A8 34 0N 81 2W
Columbia, Tenn., U.S.A. 149 H2 35 37N 87 2W
Columbia →, N. Amer. 160 D2 46 15N 124 5W
Columbia, C., Canada 6 A4 83 6N 69 57W
Columbia, District of □, U.S.A. 148 F7 38 55N 77 0W
Columbia, Mt., Canada 142 C5 52 8N 117 20W
Columbia Basin, U.S.A. 158 C4 46 45N 119 5W
Columbia City, U.S.A. 157 C11 41 10N 85 29W
Columbia Falls, U.S.A. 158 B6 48 23N 114 11W
Columbia Mts., Canada 142 C5 52 0N 119 0W
Columbia Plateau, U.S.A. 158 D5 44 0N 117 30W
Columbiana, U.S.A. 150 F4 40 53N 80 42W
Columbretes, Is., Spain 40 F5 39 50N 0 50 E
Columbus, Ga., U.S.A. 152 C5 32 28N 84 59W
Columbus, Ind., U.S.A. 157 E11 39 13N 85 55W
Columbus, Kans., U.S.A. 155 G7 37 10N 94 50W
Columbus, Miss., U.S.A. 149 J1 33 30N 88 25W
Columbus, Mont., U.S.A. 158 D9 45 38N 109 15W
Columbus, N. Mex., U.S.A. 159 L10 31 50N 107 38W
Columbus, Nebr., U.S.A. 154 E6 41 26N 97 22W
Columbus, Ohio, U.S.A. 157 E13 39 58N 83 0W
Columbus, Tex., U.S.A. 155 L6 29 42N 96 33W
Columbus Grove, U.S.A. 157 D12 40 55N 84 4W
Columbus Junction, U.S.A. 156 C5 41 17N 91 22W
Colunga, Spain 42 B5 43 29N 5 16W
Colusa, U.S.A. 160 F4 39 13N 122 1W
Colville, U.S.A. 158 B5 48 33N 117 54W
Colville →, U.S.A. 144 A10 70 25N 150 30W
Colville, C., N.Z. 130 C4 36 29 S 175 21 E
Colwood, Canada 160 B3 48 26N 123 29W
Colwyn Bay, U.K. 20 D4 53 18N 3 44W
Coma, Ethiopia 107 F4 8 29N 36 53 E
Comácchio, Italy 45 D9 44 42N 12 11 E
Comalcalco, Mexico 163 D6 18 16N 93 13W
Comallo, Argentina 176 B2 41 0 S 70 5W
Comana, Romania 53 F11 44 10N 26 10 E
Comanche, U.S.A. 155 K5 31 54N 98 36W
Comandante Arbues = Mirandópolis, Brazil 175 A5 21 9 S 51 6W
Comandante Ferraz, Antarctica 7 C18 62 30 S 58 0W
Comandante Luis Piedrabuena, Argentina 176 C3 49 59 S 68 54W
Comăneşti, Romania 53 D11 46 25N 26 26 E
Comarapa, Bolivia 173 D5 17 54 S 64 29W
Comarnic, Romania 53 E10 45 15N 25 38 E
Comayagua, Honduras 164 D2 14 25N 87 37W
Combahee →, U.S.A. 149 J5 32 30N 80 31W
Combara, Australia 129 A8 31 10 S 148 22 E
Combarbalá, Chile 174 C1 31 11 S 71 2W
Combe Martin, U.K. 21 F3 51 12N 4 3W
Combeaufontaine, France 27 E12 47 38N 5 54 E
Comber, Canada 150 D2 42 14N 82 33W
Comber, U.K. 23 B6 54 33N 5 45W
Combermere, Canada 150 A7 45 22N 77 37W
Combermere Bay, Burma 90 F4 19 37N 93 34 E
Comblain-au-Pont, Belgium 24 D5 50 29N 5 35 E
Combourg, France 26 D5 48 25N 1 46W
Comboyne, Australia 129 A10 31 34 S 152 27 E
Combrailles, France 27 F9 46 8N 2 37 E
Combronde, France 28 C7 45 58N 3 5 E
Comer, Ala., U.S.A. 152 C4 32 2N 85 23W
Comer, Ga., U.S.A. 152 A6 34 4N 83 8W
Comeragh Mts., Ireland 23 D4 52 18N 7 34W
Comet, Australia 126 C4 23 36 S 148 38 E
Comilla, Bangla. 90 D3 23 28N 91 10 E
Comino, Malta 38 E7 36 1N 14 20 E
Comino, C., Italy 46 B2 40 32N 9 49 E
Cómiso, Italy 47 F7 36 56N 14 36 E
Comitán, Mexico 163 D6 16 18N 92 9W
Commentry, France 27 F9 46 20N 2 46 E
Commerce, Ga., U.S.A. 149 H4 34 12N 83 28W
Commerce, Tex., U.S.A. 155 J7 33 15N 95 54W
Commercy, France 27 D12 48 43N 5 34 E
Commissioner's Pt., Bermuda 9 a 32 19N 64 49W
Committee B., Canada 139 B11 68 30N 86 30W
Commonwealth B., Antarctica 7 C10 67 0 S 144 0 E
Commoron Cr. →, Australia 127 D5 28 22 S 150 8 E
Communism Pk. = Kommunizma, Pik, Tajikistan 65 D6 39 0N 72 2 E
Como, Italy 44 C6 45 47N 9 5 E
Como, Lago di, Italy 44 B6 46 0N 9 11 E
Comodoro Rivadavia, Argentina 176 C3 45 50 S 67 40W
Comoé △, Ivory C. 112 D4 9 0N 3 35W
Comorâşte, Romania 52 E6 45 10N 21 35 E
Comorin, C., India 95 K3 8 3N 77 40 E
Comoros ■, Ind. Oc. 121 a 12 10 S 44 15 E
Comox, Canada 142 D4 49 42N 124 55W
Compass Lake, U.S.A. 152 E4 30 36N 85 24W
Compiègne, France 27 C9 49 24N 2 50 E
Comporta, Portugal 43 G2 38 22N 8 46W
Compostela, Mexico 162 C4 21 15N 104 53W
Compostela, Phil. 81 H6 7 40N 126 2 E
Comprida, I., Brazil 175 A6 24 50 S 47 42W
Compton, Canada 151 A13 45 14N 71 49W
Compton, U.S.A. 161 M8 33 54N 118 13W
Comrat, Moldova 53 D13 46 18N 28 40 E
Con Cuong, Vietnam 86 C5 19 2N 104 54 E
Con Dao △, Vietnam 87 H6 8 42N 106 35 E
Con Son, Vietnam 87 H6 8 41N 106 37 E
Cona Niyeu, Argentina 176 B3 41 58 S 67 0W
Conakry, Guinea 112 D2 9 29N 13 49W
Conara, Australia 127 G4 41 50 S 147 26 E
Conargo, Australia 129 C6 35 16 S 145 10 E
Concarneau, France 26 E3 47 52N 3 56W
Conceição, Brazil 170 C4 7 33 S 38 31W
Conceição, Mozam. 119 F4 18 47 S 36 7 E
Conceição da Barra, Brazil 171 E4 18 35 S 39 45W
Conceição do Araguaia, Brazil 170 C2 8 0 S 49 2W
Conceição do Canindé, Brazil 170 C3 7 54 S 41 34W
Conceição do Maú, Brazil 169 C6 3 35N 59 53W
Conçeicão do Paraíba = Capela, Brazil 170 D4 10 30 S 37 0W
Concepción, Argentina 174 B2 27 20 S 65 35W
Concepción, Bolivia 173 D5 16 15 S 62 8W
Concepción, Chile 174 D1 36 50 S 73 0W
Concepción, Mexico 163 D6 18 15N 90 5W
Concepción, Paraguay 174 A4 23 22 S 57 26W
Concepción, Peru 172 C2 11 54 S 75 19W
Concepcion, Phil. 80 D3 15 27N 120 47 E
Concepción □, Chile 174 D1 37 0 S 72 30W
Concepción →, Mexico 162 A2 30 32N 113 2W
Concepción, Est. de, Chile 176 D2 50 30 S 74 55W
Concepción, L., Bolivia 173 D5 17 20 S 61 20W
Concepción, Punta, Mexico 162 B2 26 55N 111 59W
Concepción del Oro, Mexico 162 C4 24 40N 101 30W
Concepción del Uruguay, Argentina 174 C4 32 35 S 58 20W
Conception, Pt., U.S.A. 161 L6 34 27N 120 28W
Conception B., Canada 141 C9 47 45N 53 0W
Conception B., Namibia 116 C1 23 55 S 14 22 E
Conception I., Bahamas 165 B4 23 52N 75 9W
Concession, Zimbabwe 119 F3 17 27 S 30 56 E
Conchas Dam, U.S.A. 155 H2 35 22N 104 11W
Conches-en-Ouche, France 26 D7 48 58N 0 56 E
Concho, U.S.A. 159 J9 34 28N 109 36W
Concho →, U.S.A. 155 K5 31 34N 99 43W
Conchos →, Chihuahua, Mexico 162 B4 29 32N 105 0W
Conchos →, Tamaulipas, Mexico 163 B5 25 9N 98 35W
Concise, Switz. 32 C3 46 51N 6 43 E
Concord, Calif., U.S.A. 160 H4 37 59N 122 2W
Concord, Ga., U.S.A. 152 B5 33 5N 84 27W
Concord, Mich., U.S.A. 157 B12 42 11N 84 38W
Concord, Mo., U.S.A. 156 F6 38 32N 90 23W
Concord, N.C., U.S.A. 149 H5 35 25N 80 35W
Concord, N.H., U.S.A. 151 C13 43 12N 71 32W
Concordia, Argentina 174 C4 31 20 S 58 2W
Concórdia, Brazil 168 D4 4 36 S 66 36W
Concordia, Mexico 162 C3 23 18N 106 2W
Concordia, Kans., U.S.A. 154 F6 39 34N 97 40W
Concordia, Mo., U.S.A. 156 F3 38 59N 93 34W
Concrete, U.S.A. 158 B3 48 32N 121 45W
Conda, Angola 115 E2 11 9 S 14 20 E
Condah, Australia 128 D4 37 57 S 141 44 E
Condamine, Australia 127 D5 26 56 S 150 9 E
Condat, France 28 C6 45 21N 2 46 E
Condé, Angola 115 E2 10 50 S 14 37 E
Conde, Brazil 171 D4 11 49 S 37 37W
Conde, U.S.A. 154 C5 45 9N 98 6W
Condé-sur-Noireau, France 26 D6 48 51N 0 33W
Condeúba, Brazil 171 D3 14 52 S 42 0W
Condobolin, Australia 129 B7 33 4 S 147 6 E
Condom, France 28 E4 43 57N 0 22 E
Condon, U.S.A. 158 D3 45 14N 120 11W
Conegliano, Italy 45 C9 45 53N 12 18 E
Conejera, I. = Conills, I. des, Spain 38 B3 39 11N 2 58 E
Conejos, Mexico 162 B4 26 14N 103 53W
Conemaugh →, U.S.A. 150 F5 40 28N 79 19W
Conero ⌂, Italy 45 E10 43 32N 13 35 E
Conflict Group, Papua N. G. 132 F6 10 47 S 151 45 E
Confolens, France 28 B4 46 2N 0 40 E
Confuso →, Paraguay 174 B4 25 9 S 57 34W
Congaree →, U.S.A. 152 B9 33 44N 80 38W
Congaree Swamp ⌂, U.S.A. 152 B9 33 47N 80 47W
Congaz, Moldova 53 D13 46 7N 28 36 E
Congerville, U.S.A. 156 D7 40 38N 89 11W
Conghua, China 77 F9 23 36N 113 31 E
Congjiang, China 76 E7 25 43N 108 52 E
Congleton, U.K. 20 D5 53 10N 2 13W
Congo, Brazil 170 C4 7 48 S 36 40W
Congo (Brazzaville) = Congo ■, Africa 114 C3 1 0 S 16 0 E
Congo (Kinshasa) = Congo, Dem. Rep. of the ■, Africa 115 C4 3 0 S 23 0 E
Congo ■, Africa 114 C3 1 0 S 16 0 E
Congo →, Africa 115 D2 6 4 S 12 24 E
Congo, Dem. Rep. of the ■, Africa 115 C4 3 0 S 23 0 E
Congo Basin, Africa 104 G6 0 10 S 24 30 E
Congo Free State = Congo, Dem. Rep. of the ■, Africa 115 C4 3 0 S 23 0 E
Congonhas, Brazil 171 F3 20 30 S 43 52W
Congress, U.S.A. 159 J7 34 9N 112 51W
Conguillio △, Chile 176 A2 38 40 S 71 42W
Conil de la Frontera, Spain 43 J4 36 17N 6 10W
Conills, I. des, Spain 38 B3 39 11N 2 58 E
Coniston, Canada 140 C3 46 29N 80 51W
Conjeeveram = Kanchipuram, India 95 H4 12 52N 79 45 E
Conklin, Canada 143 B6 55 38N 111 5W
Conklin, U.S.A. 151 D9 42 2N 75 49W
Conkouati ⌂, Congo 114 C2 3 50 S 11 28 E
Conlendas, Pta. das, Azores 9 d1 38 38N 27 14W
Conn, L., Ireland 23 B2 54 3N 9 15W
Connacht □, Ireland 23 C2 53 43N 9 12W
Conneaut, U.S.A. 150 E4 41 57N 80 34W
Connecticut □, U.S.A. 151 E12 41 30N 72 45W
Connecticut →, U.S.A. 151 E12 41 16N 72 20W
Connell, U.S.A. 158 C4 46 40N 118 52W
Connellsville, U.S.A. 150 F5 40 1N 79 35W
Connemara, Ireland 23 C2 53 29N 9 45W
Connemara △, Ireland 23 C2 53 32N 9 52W
Conner, Phil. 80 C3 17 48N 121 19 E
Connerré, France 26 D7 48 3N 0 30 E
Connersville, U.S.A. 157 E11 39 39N 85 8W
Connors Ra., Australia 126 C4 21 40 S 149 10 E
Conoble, Australia 129 B6 32 55 S 144 33 E
Cononaco →, Ecuador 168 D2 1 32 S 75 35W
Conques, France 28 D6 44 36N 2 23 E
Conquest, Canada 143 C7 51 32N 107 14W
Conquista = Vitória da Conquista, Brazil 171 D3 14 51 S 40 51W
Conrad, Iowa, U.S.A. 156 B4 42 14N 92 52W
Conrad, Mont., U.S.A. 158 B8 48 10N 111 57W
Conran, C., Australia 129 D8 37 49 S 148 44 E
Conroe, U.S.A. 155 K7 30 19N 95 27W
Consecon, Canada 150 C7 44 0N 77 31W
Conselheiro Lafaiete, Brazil 171 F3 20 40 S 43 48W
Conselheiro Pena, Brazil 171 E3 19 10 S 41 30W
Conselve, Italy 45 C8 45 14N 11 52 E
Consett, U.K. 20 C6 54 51N 1 50W
Consort, Canada 143 C6 52 1N 110 46W
Constance = Konstanz, Germany 31 H5 47 40N 9 10 E
Constance, L. = Bodensee, Europe 33 A8 47 35N 9 25 E
Constanţa, Romania 53 F13 44 14N 28 38 E
Constanţa □, Romania 53 F13 44 15N 28 15 E
Constantia, U.S.A. 151 C8 43 15N 76 1W
Constantina, Spain 43 H5 37 51N 5 40W
Constantine, Algeria 111 A6 36 25N 6 42 E
Constantine, U.S.A. 157 C11 41 50N 85 40W
Constantine, C., U.S.A. 144 G8 58 24N 158 54W
Constitución, Chile 174 D1 35 20 S 72 30W
Constitución, Uruguay 174 C4 31 0 S 57 50W
Constitucion de 1857 △, Mexico 162 A1 32 4N 115 55W
Consuegra, Spain 43 F7 39 28N 3 36W
Consul, Canada 143 D7 49 20N 109 30W
Contact, U.S.A. 158 F6 41 46N 114 45W
Contai, India 93 J12 21 54N 87 46 E
Contamana, Peru 172 B3 7 19 S 74 55W
Contarina, Italy 45 C9 45 1N 12 13 E
Contas →, Brazil 171 D4 14 17 S 39 1W
Contes, France 29 E11 43 49N 7 19 E
Conthey, Switz. 32 D4 46 14N 7 18 E
Continental, U.S.A. 157 C12 41 6N 84 16W
Contoocook, U.S.A. 151 C13 43 13N 71 45W
Contra Costa, Mozam. 117 D5 25 9 S 33 30 E
Contres, France 26 E8 47 24N 1 26 E
Contrexéville, France 27 D12 48 10N 5 53 E
Controller B., U.S.A. 144 F11 60 7N 144 15W
Contumaza, Peru 172 B2 7 23 S 78 57W
Contwoyto L., Canada 138 B8 65 42N 110 50W
Convención, Colombia 168 B3 8 28N 73 21W
Conversano, Italy 47 B10 40 58N 17 7 E
Converse, U.S.A. 157 D11 40 35N 85 52W
Convoy, U.S.A. 157 D12 40 55N 84 43W
Conway = Conwy, U.K. 20 D4 53 17N 3 50W
Conway = Conwy →, U.K. 20 D4 53 17N 3 50W
Conway, Australia 126 J6 20 24 S 148 41 E
Conway, Ark., U.S.A. 155 H8 35 5N 92 26W
Conway, N.H., U.S.A. 151 C13 43 59N 71 7W
Conway, S.C., U.S.A. 149 J6 33 51N 79 3W
Conway, C., Australia 126 J6 20 34 S 148 46 E
Conway, L., Australia 127 D2 28 17 S 135 35 E
Conwy, U.K. 20 D4 53 17N 3 50W
Conwy □, U.K. 20 D4 53 10N 3 44W
Conwy →, U.K. 20 D4 53 17N 3 50W
Conyers, U.S.A. 152 B5 33 40N 84 1W
Coober Pedy, Australia 127 D1 29 1 S 134 43 E
Cooch Behar = Koch Bihar, India 90 B2 26 22N 89 29 E
Cooinda, Australia 124 B5 13 15 S 130 5 E
Cook, Australia 125 F5 30 37 S 130 25 E
Cook, U.S.A. 154 B8 47 49N 92 39W
Cook, B., Chile 176 E2 55 10 S 70 0W
Cook, C., Canada 142 C3 50 8N 127 55W
Cook, Mt. = Aoraki Mount Cook, N.Z. 131 D5 43 36 S 170 9 E
Cook Bay, Vanuatu 133 H7 18 46 S 169 15 E
Cook Inlet, U.S.A. 144 G10 60 0N 152 0W
Cook Is., Pac. Oc. 135 J12 17 0 S 160 0W
Cook Strait, N.Z. 130 H3 41 15 S 174 29 E
Cooke Plains, Australia 128 C3 35 23 S 139 34 E
Cookeville, U.S.A. 149 G3 36 10N 85 30W
Cookhouse, S. Africa 116 E4 32 44 S 25 47 E
Cooks Hammock, U.S.A. 152 F6 29 56N 83 17W
Cookshire, Canada 151 A13 45 25N 71 38W
Cookstown, U.K. 23 B5 54 39N 6 45W
Cooksville, Canada 150 C5 43 36N 79 35W
Cooktown, Australia 126 B4 15 30 S 145 16 E
Coolabah, Australia 129 A7 31 1 S 146 43 E
Cooladdi, Australia 127 D4 26 37 S 145 23 E
Coolah, Australia 129 A8 31 48 S 149 41 E
Coolamon, Australia 129 C7 34 46 S 147 8 E
Coolgardie, Australia 125 F3 30 55 S 121 8 E
Coolidge, Ariz., U.S.A. 159 K8 32 59N 111 31W
Coolidge, Ga., U.S.A. 152 D6 31 1N 83 52W
Coolidge Dam, U.S.A. 159 K8 33 0N 110 20W
Cooloola △, Australia 127 D5 26 13 S 153 2 E
Cooma, Australia 129 D8 36 12 S 149 8 E
Coon Rapids, Iowa, U.S.A. 156 C2 41 53N 94 41W
Coon Rapids, Minn., U.S.A. 154 C8 45 9N 93 19W
Coonabarabran, Australia 129 A8 31 14 S 149 18 E
Coonalpyn, Australia 128 C3 35 43 S 139 52 E
Coonamble, Australia 129 A8 30 56 S 148 27 E
Coonana, Australia 125 F3 31 0 S 123 0 E
Coondapoor, India 95 H2 13 42N 74 40 E
Cooninie, L., Australia 127 D2 26 4 S 139 59 E
Coonoor, India 95 J3 11 21N 76 45 E
Cooper, U.S.A. 155 J7 33 23N 95 42W
Cooper →, U.S.A. 152 C10 32 50N 79 56W
Cooper Cr. →, Australia 127 D2 28 29 S 137 46 E
Cooperstown, N. Dak., U.S.A. 154 B5 47 27N 98 8W
Cooperstown, N.Y., U.S.A. 151 D10 42 42N 74 56W
Coopersville, U.S.A. 157 A11 43 4N 85 57W
Coopracambra △, Australia 129 D8 37 20 S 149 20 E
Coorabie, Australia 125 F5 31 54 S 132 18 E
Coorong △, Australia 128 D3 36 0 S 139 29 E
Coorong, The, Australia 128 C3 35 50 S 139 20 E
Coorow, Australia 125 E2 29 53 S 116 2 E
Cooroy, Australia 127 D5 26 22 S 152 54 E
Coos Bay, U.S.A. 158 E1 43 22N 124 13W
Coosa →, U.S.A. 149 J2 32 30N 86 16W
Cootamundra, Australia 129 C8 34 36 S 148 1 E
Cootehill, Ireland 23 B4 54 4N 7 5W
Copahue Paso, Argentina 174 D1 37 49 S 71 8W
Copainalá, Mexico 163 D6 17 8N 93 11W
Copake Falls, U.S.A. 151 D11 42 7N 73 31W
Copalnic Mănăştur, Romania 53 C8 47 30N 23 41 E
Copán, Honduras 164 D2 14 50N 89 9W
Copatana, Brazil 168 D4 2 48 S 67 4W
Cope, Colo., U.S.A. 154 F3 39 40N 102 51W
Cope, S.C., U.S.A. 152 B8 33 23N 81 0W
Cope, C., Spain 41 H3 37 26N 1 28W
Copeland, U.S.A. 153 K8 25 57N 81 22W
Copenhagen = København, Denmark 17 J6 55 41N 12 34 E
Copenhagen, U.S.A. 151 C9 43 54N 75 41W
Copertino, Italy 47 B11 40 16N 18 3 E
Copiapó, Chile 174 B1 27 30 S 70 20W
Copiapó →, Chile 174 B1 27 19 S 70 56W
Coplay, U.S.A. 151 F9 40 44N 75 29W
Copley, Australia 128 A3 30 36 S 138 26 E
Copp L., Canada 142 A6 60 14N 114 40W
Copparo, Italy 45 D8 44 54N 11 49 E
Coppename →, Suriname 169 B6 5 48N 55 55W
Copper →, U.S.A. 144 F11 60 18N 145 3W
Copper Center, U.S.A. 144 F11 61 58N 145 18W
Copper City = Invermere, Canada 142 C5 50 30N 116 2W
Copper Harbor, U.S.A. 148 B2 47 28N 87 53W
Copper Queen, Zimbabwe 119 F2 17 29 S 29 18 E
Copperas Cove, U.S.A. 155 K6 31 8N 97 54W
Copperbelt □, Zambia 119 E2 13 15 S 27 30 E
Coppermine = Kugluktuk, Canada 138 B8 67 50N 115 5W
Coppermine →, Canada 138 B8 67 49N 116 4W
Copperopolis, U.S.A. 160 H6 37 58N 120 38W
Coppet, Switz. 32 D2 46 19N 6 12 E
Copşa Mică, Romania 53 D9 46 7N 24 15 E
Coquet →, U.K. 20 B6 55 20N 1 32W
Coquilhatville = Mbandaka, Dem. Rep. of the Congo 114 B3 0 1N 18 18 E
Coquille, U.S.A. 158 E1 43 11N 124 11W
Coquimbo, Chile 174 C1 30 0 S 71 20W
Coquimbo □, Chile 174 C1 31 0 S 71 0W
Corabia, Romania 53 G9 43 48N 24 30 E
Coração de Jesus, Brazil 171 E3 16 43 S 44 22W
Coracora, Peru 172 D3 15 5 S 73 45W
Coraki, Australia 127 D5 28 59 S 153 17 E
Coral, U.S.A. 150 F5 40 29N 79 10W
Coral Bay, Phil. 81 G1 8 25N 117 20 E
Coral Gables, U.S.A. 153 K9 25 45N 80 16W
Coral Harbour, Bahamas 9 b 24 58N 77 28W
Coral Harbour, Canada 139 B11 64 8N 83 10W
Coral Heights, Bahamas 9 b 25 0N 77 27W
Coral Sea, Pac. Oc. 132 F3 15 0 S 150 0 E
Coral Sea Islands Terr. □, Australia 122 D9 20 0 S 155 0 E
Coral Springs, U.S.A. 153 J9 26 16N 80 13W
Corales del Rosario △, Colombia 168 A2 10 8N 75 46W
Coralville, U.S.A. 156 C5 41 40N 91 35W
Coralville L., U.S.A. 156 C5 41 50N 91 40W
Corangamite, L., Australia 128 E5 38 5 S 143 30 E
Corantijn →, Suriname 169 B6 5 50N 57 8W
Coraopolis, U.S.A. 150 F4 40 31N 80 10W
Corato, Italy 47 A9 41 9N 16 25 E
Corbeil-Essonnes, France 27 D9 48 36N 2 26 E
Corbeiro, C., W. Sahara 110 D1 21 50N 17 0W
Corbett △, India 93 E8 29 20N 79 0 E
Corbie, France 27 C9 49 54N 2 30 E
Corbières, France 28 F6 42 55N 2 35 E
Corbigny, France 27 E10 47 16N 3 40 E
Corbin, U.S.A. 148 G3 36 57N 84 6W
Corbones →, Spain 43 H5 37 36N 5 39W
Corbu, Romania 53 F13 44 25N 28 39 E
Corby, U.K. 21 E7 52 30N 0 41W
Corcaigh = Cork, Ireland 23 E3 51 54N 8 29W
Corcoran, U.S.A. 160 J7 36 6N 119 33W
Corcovado △, Costa Rica 164 E3 8 33N 83 35W
Cordele, U.S.A. 152 D6 31 58N 83 47W
Cordell, U.S.A. 155 H5 35 17N 98 59W
Cordenòns, Italy 45 C9 45 59N 12 42 E
Cordes-sur-Ciel, France 28 D5 44 5N 1 57 E
Cordillera de los Picachos △, Colombia 168 C3 2 39N 74 30W
Cordisburgo, Brazil 171 E3 19 7 S 44 21W
Córdoba, Argentina 174 C3 31 20 S 64 10W
Córdoba, Mexico 163 D5 18 50N 97 0W
Córdoba, Spain 43 H6 37 50N 4 50W
Córdoba □, Argentina 174 C3 31 22 S 64 15W
Córdoba □, Colombia 168 B2 8 20N 75 40W
Córdoba □, Spain 43 G6 38 5N 5 0W
Córdoba, Sierra de, Argentina 174 C3 31 10 S 64 25W
Cordon, Phil. 80 C3 16 42N 121 32 E
Cordova, U.S.A. 144 F11 60 33N 145 45W
Corella, Spain 40 C3 42 7N 1 48W
Corella →, Australia 126 B3 19 34 S 140 47 E
Coremas, Brazil 170 C4 7 1 S 37 58W
Corentyne →, Guyana 169 B6 5 50N 57 8W
Corfield, Australia 126 C3 21 40 S 143 21 E
Corfu = Kérkira, Greece 38 B9 39 38N 19 50 E
Corfu ✈ (CFU), Greece 48 B1 39 35N 19 54 E
Corgo = O Corgo, Spain 42 C3 42 56N 7 25W
Corguinho, Brazil 173 D7 19 53 S 54 52W
Cori, Italy 46 A5 41 39N 12 55 E
Coria, Spain 42 F4 39 58N 6 33W
Coria del Río, Spain 43 H4 37 16N 6 3W
Coricudgy, Australia 129 B9 32 51 S 150 24 E
Corigliano Cálabro, Italy 47 C9 39 36N 16 31 E
Corimba, Barra de, Angola 115 D2 8 52 S 13 9 E
Coringa Is., Australia 126 B4 16 58 S 149 58 E
Corinth = Kórinthos, Greece 48 D4 37 56N 22 55 E
Corinth, Ky., U.S.A. 157 F12 38 30N 84 34W
Corinth, Miss., U.S.A. 149 H1 34 56N 88 31W
Corinth, N.Y., U.S.A. 151 C11 43 15N 73 49W
Corinth, G. of = Korinthiakós Kólpos, Greece 48 C4 38 16N 22 30 E
Corinth Canal, Greece 48 D4 37 58N 23 0 E
Corinto, Brazil 171 E3 18 20 S 44 30W
Corinto, Nic. 164 D2 12 30N 87 10W
Corisco, Eq. Guin. 114 B1 0 55N 9 18 E
Cork, Ireland 23 E3 51 54N 8 29W
Cork □, Ireland 23 E3 51 57N 8 40W
Cork Harbour, Ireland 23 E3 51 47N 8 16W
Corlay, France 26 D3 48 20N 3 5W
Corleone, Italy 46 E6 37 49N 13 18 E
Corleto Perticara, Italy 47 B9 40 23N 16 2 E
Çorlu, Turkey 51 E11 41 11N 27 49 E

Cormack L., *Canada* .. **142 A4** 60 56N 121 37W
Cormòns, *Italy* ..... **45 C10** 45 58N 13 28 E
Cormorant, *Canada* .. **143 C8** 54 14N 100 35W
Cormorant L., *Canada* . **143 C8** 54 15N 100 50W
Corn Is. = Maíz, Is. del,
   Nic. **164 D3** 12 15N 83 4W
Cornalvo △, *Spain* ... **43 F4** 39 1N 6 13W
Cornélio Procópio,
   Brazil .... **175 A5** 23 7 S 50 40W
Cornell, *U.S.A.* **157 D8** 41 0N 88 44W
Corner Brook, *Canada* **141 C8** 48 57N 57 58W
Corner Inlet, *Australia* **129 E7** 38 45 S 146 20 E
Corner Seamounts,
   Atl. Oc. **8 C6** 35 0N 52 0W
Cornești, *Moldova* ... **53 C13** 47 21N 28 1 E
Corneto = Tarquínia,
   Italy .... **45 F8** 42 15N 11 45 E
Corning, *Ark., U.S.A.* . **44 D7** 44 29N 10 5 E
Corning, *Ark., U.S.A.* . **155 G9** 36 25N 90 35W
Corning, *Calif., U.S.A.* **158 G2** 39 56N 122 11W
Corning, *Iowa, U.S.A.* **156 E7** 40 59N 94 44W
Corning, *N.Y., U.S.A.* **150 D7** 42 9N 77 3W
Corno Grande, *Italy* .. **45 F10** 42 28N 13 34 E
Cornwall, *Canada* ... **140 C5** 45 2N 74 44W
Cornwall, *U.S.A.* **151 F8** 40 17N 76 25W
Cornwall □, *U.K.* **21 G3** 50 26N 4 40W
Cornwell, *U.S.A.* **153 H8** 27 3N 81 35W
Corny Pt., *Australia* .. **128 C2** 34 55 S 137 0 E
Coro, *Venezuela* **168 A4** 11 25N 69 41W
Coroaci, *Brazil* ..... **171 E3** 18 35 S 42 17W
Coroatá, *Brazil* ..... **170 B3** 4 8 S 44 0W
Coroban, *Somali Rep.* **120 D2** 3 58N 42 44 E
Corocoro, *Bolivia* ... **172 D4** 17 15 S 68 28W
Corocoro, I., *Venezuela* **169 B5** 8 30N 60 10W
Coroico, *Bolivia* .... **172 D4** 16 0 S 67 50W
Coromandel, *Brazil* .. **171 E2** 18 28 S 47 13W
Coromandel, *N.Z.* ... **131 B5** 36 45 S 175 31 E
Coromandel Coast,
   India .... **95 H5** 12 30N 81 0 E
Coromandel Pen., *N.Z.* **130 C4** 37 0 S 175 45 E
Coromandel Ra., *N.Z.* **130 C4** 37 0 S 175 40 E
Coron, *Phil.* .... **80 E3** 12 1N 120 12 E
Coron Bay, *Phil.* .... **81 F3** 11 54N 120 8 E
Coron I., *Phil.* ..... **81 F3** 11 55N 120 14 E
Corona, *Calif., U.S.A.* **161 M9** 33 53N 117 34W
Corona, *N. Mex.,*
   U.S.A. **159 J11** 34 15N 105 36W
Coronach, *Canada* ... **143 D7** 49 7N 105 31W
Coronado, *U.S.A.* ... **161 N9** 32 41N 117 11W
Coronado, B. de,
   Costa Rica **164 E3** 9 0N 83 40W
Coronados, G. de los,
   Chile .... **176 B2** 41 40 S 74 0W
Coronados, Is. los,
   U.S.A. **161 N9** 32 25N 117 15W
Coronation, *Canada* .. **142 C6** 52 5N 111 27W
Coronation Gulf,
   Canada **138 B8** 68 25N 110 0W
Coronation I.,
   Antarctica .... **7 C18** 60 45 S 46 0W
Coronation Is.,
   Australia ..... **124 B3** 14 57 S 124 55 E
Coronda, *Argentina* .. **174 C3** 31 58 S 60 56W
Coronel, *Chile* ..... **174 D1** 37 0 S 73 10W
Coronel Bogado,
   Paraguay ..... **174 B4** 27 11 S 56 18W
Coronel Dorrego,
   Argentina ..... **174 D3** 38 40 S 61 10W
Coronel Fabriciano,
   Brazil .... **171 E3** 19 31 S 42 38W
Coronel Murta, *Brazil* **171 E3** 16 37 S 42 11W
Coronel Oviedo,
   Paraguay ..... **174 B4** 25 24 S 56 30W
Coronel Ponce, *Brazil* **173 D6** 15 34 S 55 1W
Coronel Pringles,
   Argentina ..... **174 D3** 38 0 S 61 30W
Coronel Suárez,
   Argentina ..... **174 D3** 37 30 S 61 52W
Coronel Vidal,
   Argentina ..... **174 D4** 37 28 S 57 45W
Corongo, *Peru* ..... **172 B2** 8 30 S 77 53W
Coropuna, Nevado,
   Peru .... **172 D3** 15 30 S 72 41W
Çorovodë, *Albania* ... **49 F4** 40 31N 20 14 E
Corowa, *Australia* ... **129 C7** 35 58 S 146 21 E
Corozal, *Colombia* ... **168 B2** 9 19N 75 18W
Corozal □, *Belize* ... **163 D7** 18 23N 88 23W
Corozal Pt.,
   Trin. & Tob. ... **169 F9** 10 45N 61 37W
Corps, *France* ...... **29 D9** 44 50N 5 56 E
Corps, *Argentina* ... **175 B4** 27 5 S 55 30W
Corpus Christi, *U.S.A.* **155 M6** 27 47N 97 24W
Corpus Christi, L.,
   U.S.A. **155 L6** 28 2N 97 52W
Corque, *Bolivia* .... **172 D4** 18 20 S 67 41W
Corral, *Chile* ...... **176 A2** 39 52 S 73 26W
Corral de Almaguer,
   Spain **42 F7** 39 45N 3 10W
Corralejo, *Canary Is.* . **9 e2** 28 43N 13 53W
Corraun Pen., *Ireland* . **23 C2** 53 54N 9 54W
Corréggio, *Italy* .... **44 D7** 44 46N 10 47 E
Corregidor, *Phil.* .... **80 D3** 14 23N 120 35 E
Corrente, *Brazil* .... **170 D2** 10 27 S 45 10W
Corrente →, *Brazil* .. **171 D3** 13 8 S 43 28W
Correntes →, *Brazil* . **173 D6** 17 38 S 55 8W
Correntes, C. das,
   Mozam. ...... **117 C6** 24 6 S 35 34 E
Correntina, *Brazil* ... **171 D3** 13 20 S 44 39W
Corrèze □, *France* ... **28 C5** 45 20N 1 45 E
Corrèze →, *France* .. **28 C5** 45 10N 1 28 E
Corrib, L., *Ireland* ... **23 C2** 53 27N 9 16W
Corridónia, *Italy* .... **45 E10** 43 15N 13 30 E
Corrientes, *Argentina* **174 B4** 27 30 S 58 45W
Corrientes □, *Argentina* **174 B4** 28 0 S 57 0W
Corrientes →,
   Argentina ..... **174 C4** 30 42 S 59 38W
Corrientes →, *Peru* .. **168 D3** 3 43 S 74 35W
Corrientes, C.,
   Colombia **168 B2** 5 30N 77 34W
Corrientes, C., *Cuba* . **164 B3** 21 43N 84 30W
Corrientes, C., *Mexico* **162 C3** 20 25N 105 42W
Corrigan, *U.S.A.* **155 K7** 31 0N 94 52W
Corrigin, *Australia* ... **125 F2** 32 20 S 117 53 E
Corry, *U.S.A.* **150 E5** 41 55N 79 39W
Corryong, *Australia* .. **129 D7** 36 12 S 147 53 E
Corse □, *France* .... **29 F13** 42 14N 9 10 E
Corse, C., *France* ... **29 E13** 43 1N 9 25 E
Corse-du-Sud □,
   France .... **29 G13** 41 45N 9 0 E
Corsica □, *France* ... **29 G13** 42 0N 9 0 E
Corsicana, *U.S.A.* ... **155 J6** 32 6N 96 28W
Corte, *France* ...... **29 F13** 42 19N 9 11 E
Corte Pinto, *Portugal* . **43 H3** 37 42N 7 29W
Cortegana, *Spain* ... **43 H4** 37 54N 6 49W
Cortes, *Phil.* ...... **81 G6** 9 17N 126 11 E
Cortés, Mar de =
   California, G. de,
   Mexico **162 B2** 27 0N 111 0W
Cortez, *U.S.A.* **159 H9** 37 21N 108 35W
Cortina d'Ampezzo,
   Italy .... **45 B9** 46 32N 12 8 E
Cortland, *N.Y., U.S.A.* **151 D8** 42 36N 76 11W

Cortland, *Ohio, U.S.A.* **150 E4** 41 20N 80 44W
Cortona, *Italy* ...... **45 E8** 43 16N 11 59 E
Corubal →,
   Guinea-Biss. ... **112 C2** 11 57N 15 5W
Coruche, *Portugal* ... **43 G2** 38 57N 8 30W
Çoruh →, *Turkey* ... **61 K5** 41 38N 41 38 E
Çorum, *Turkey* ..... **100 B6** 40 30N 34 57 E
Corumbá, *Brazil* .... **173 D6** 19 0 S 57 30W
Corumbá →, *Brazil* .. **171 E2** 18 19 S 48 55W
Corumbá de Goiás,
   Brazil .... **171 E2** 16 0 S 48 50W
Corumbaíba, *Brazil* .. **171 E2** 18 9 S 48 34W
Corund, *Romania* ... **53 D10** 46 30N 25 13 E
Corunna = A Coruña,
   Spain **42 B2** 43 20N 8 25W
Corunna, *U.S.A.* **157 B12** 42 59N 84 7W
Corvallis, *U.S.A.* **158 D2** 44 34N 123 16W
Corvette, L. de la,
   Canada **140 B5** 53 25N 74 3W
Corvo, *Azores* **9 d2** 39 42N 31 6W
Corydon, *Ind., U.S.A.* **157 F10** 38 13N 86 7W
Corydon, *Iowa, U.S.A.* **156 D3** 40 46N 93 19W
Corydon, *Ky., U.S.A.* **157 G9** 37 44N 87 43W
Cosalá, *Mexico* **162 C3** 24 28N 106 40W
Cosamaloapan, *Mexico* **163 D5** 18 23N 95 50W
Cosenza, *Italy* ...... **47 C9** 39 18N 16 15 E
Coșereni, *Romania* .. **53 F11** 44 38N 26 35 E
Coshocton, *U.S.A.* .. **150 F3** 40 16N 81 51W
Cosmo Newberry,
   Australia ..... **125 E3** 28 0 S 122 54 E
Cosne-Cours-sur-Loire,
   France .... **27 E9** 47 24N 2 54 E
Coso Junction, *U.S.A.* **161 J9** 36 3N 117 57W
Coso Pk., *U.S.A.* ... **161 J9** 36 13N 117 44W
Cospeito, *Spain* **42 B3** 43 12N 7 34W
Cosquín, *Argentina* .. **174 C3** 31 15 S 64 30W
Cossato, *Italy* ...... **44 C5** 45 34N 8 10 E
Cossé-le-Vivien, *France* **26 E6** 47 57N 0 54W
Cosson →, *France* .. **26 E8** 47 30N 1 15 E
Costa Blanca, *Spain* . **41 G4** 38 25N 0 10W
Costa Brava, *Spain* .. **40 D8** 41 30N 3 0 E
Costa del Sol, *Spain* . **43 J6** 36 30N 4 30W
Costa Dorada, *Spain* . **40 D6** 41 12N 1 15 E
Costa Mesa, *U.S.A.* . **161 M9** 33 38N 117 55W
Costa Rica ■,
   Cent. Amer. ... **164 E3** 10 0N 84 0W
Costa Smeralda, *Italy* . **46 A2** 41 5N 9 35 E
Costermansville =
   Bukavu, *Dem. Rep.*
   of the Congo ... **118 C2** 2 20 S 28 52 E
Costești, *Romania* ... **53 F9** 44 40N 24 53 E
Costigliole d'Asti, *Italy* **44 D5** 44 48N 8 11 E
Cosumnes →, *U.S.A.* **160 G5** 38 16N 121 26W
Coswig, *Sachsen,*
   Germany ...... **30 D9** 51 7N 13 34 E
Coswig,
   Sachsen-Anhalt,
   Germany ...... **30 D8** 51 53N 12 27 E
Cotabato, *Phil.* ..... **81 C2** 7 14N 124 15 E
Cotabato □, *Phil.* ... **81 H5** 7 10N 125 0 E
Cotacajes →, *Bolivia* **172 D4** 16 0 S 67 1W
Cotagaita, *Bolivia* ... **174 A2** 20 45 S 65 40W
Cotahuasi, *Peru* .... **172 D3** 15 12 S 72 50W
Côte d'Azur, *France* . **29 E11** 43 25N 7 10 E
Côte-d'Ivoire = Ivory
   Coast ■, *Africa* .. **112 D4** 7 30N 5 0W
Côte-d'Or □, *France* . **27 E11** 47 10N 4 50 E
Côte-d'Or □, *France* . **27 E11** 47 30N 4 50 E
Coteau des Prairies,
   U.S.A. **154 C6** 45 20N 97 50W
Coteau du Missouri,
   U.S.A. **154 B4** 47 0N 100 0W
Cotegipe, *Brazil* .... **171 D3** 12 2 S 44 15W
Cotentin, *France* **26 C5** 49 15N 1 30W
Côtes-d'Armor □,
   France **26 D4** 48 25N 2 40W
Côtes de Meuse, *France* **27 C12** 49 15N 5 22 E
Côtes-du-Nord = Côtes-
   d'Armor □, *France* **26 D4** 48 25N 2 40W
Cotiella, *Spain* ..... **40 C5** 42 31N 0 19 E
Cotillo, *Canary Is.* ... **9 e2** 28 41N 14 1W
Cotiujeni, *Moldova* .. **53 C13** 47 51N 28 33 E
Cotoca, *Bolivia* ..... **173 D5** 17 49 S 63 3W
Cotonou, *Benin* ..... **113 D5** 6 20N 2 25 E
Cotopaxi, *Ecuador* .. **168 D2** 0 40 S 78 30W
Cotopaxi □, *Ecuador* **168 D2** 0 39 S 78 24W
Cotopaxi □, *Ecuador* **168 D2** 0 5 S 78 55W
Cotronei, *Italy* ..... **47 C9** 39 9N 16 47 E
Cotswold Hills, *U.K.* . **21 F5** 51 42N 2 10W
Cottage Grove, *U.S.A.* **158 E2** 43 48N 123 3W
Cottageville, *U.S.A.* . **152 C9** 32 56N 80 29W
Cottbus, *Germany* ... **30 D10** 51 45N 14 20 E
Cottondale, *U.S.A.* .. **152 E4** 30 48N 85 23W
Cottonwood, *Ala.,*
   U.S.A. **152 D4** 31 3N 85 18W
Cottonwood, *Ariz.,*
   U.S.A. **159 J7** 34 45N 112 1W
Cotulla, *U.S.A.* **155 L5** 28 26N 99 14W
Coubre, Pte. de la,
   France **28 C2** 45 42N 1 15W
Couches, *France* .... **27 F11** 46 53N 4 30 E
Couço, *Portugal* **43 G2** 38 59N 8 17W
Coudersport, *U.S.A.* . **150 E6** 41 46N 78 1W
Couedic, C. du,
   Australia ..... **128 D2** 36 5 S 136 40 E
Coueron, *France* **26 E5** 47 13N 1 44W
Couesnon →, *France* . **26 D5** 48 38N 1 32W
Couhé, *France* ..... **28 B4** 46 17N 0 11 E
Coulanges-sur-Yonne,
   France .... **27 E10** 47 31N 3 33 E
Coulee City, *U.S.A.* .. **158 C4** 47 37N 119 17W
Coulman I., *Antarctica* **7 D11** 73 35 S 170 0 E
Coulommiers, *France* . **27 D10** 48 50N 3 3 E
Coulon →, *France* ... **29 E9** 43 51N 5 6 E
Coulonge →, *Canada* **140 C4** 45 52N 76 46W
Coulonges-sur-l'Autize,
   France **28 B3** 46 31N 0 36W
Coulounieix-Chamiers,
   France .... **28 C4** 45 11N 0 42 E
Coulterville, *Calif.,*
   U.S.A. **160 H6** 37 43N 120 12W
Coulterville, *Ill., U.S.A.* **156 F7** 38 11N 89 36W
Council, *Alaska, U.S.A.* **144 D7** 64 53N 163 41W
Council, *Idaho, U.S.A.* **158 D5** 44 44N 116 26W
Council Bluffs, *U.S.A.* **154 E7** 41 16N 95 52W
Council Grove, *U.S.A.* **156 F6** 38 40N 96 29W
Coupeville, *U.S.A.* ... **160 B4** 48 13N 122 41W
Courantyne →,
   S. Amer. **169 B6** 5 55N 57 5W
Courcelles, *Belgium* . **24 D4** 50 28N 4 22 E
Courchevel, *France* .. **29 C10** 45 25N 6 36 E
Courçon, *France* **28 B3** 46 15N 0 50W
Courmayeur, *Italy* ... **44 C3** 45 48N 6 58 E
Couronne, C., *France* **29 E9** 43 19N 5 3 E
Cours-la-Ville, *France* **27 F11** 46 7N 4 19 E
Coursan, *France* .... **28 E7** 43 14N 3 4 E
Courseulles-sur-Mer,
   France **26 C6** 49 20N 0 29W
Courtenay, *Canada* .. **142 D4** 49 45N 125 0W
Courtenay, *France* ... **27 D10** 48 2N 3 3 E
Courtland, *U.S.A.* ... **160 G5** 38 20N 121 34W
Courtrai = Kortrijk,
   Belgium ...... **24 D3** 50 50N 3 17 E

Courtright, *Canada* .. **150 D2** 42 49N 82 28W
Coushatta, *U.S.A.* ... **155 J8** 32 1N 93 21W
Coutances, *France* ... **26 C5** 49 3N 1 28W
Coutras, *France* **28 C3** 45 3N 0 8W
Coutts Crossing,
   Australia ..... **127 D5** 29 49 S 152 55 E
Couva, *Trin. & Tob.* . **169 F9** 10 25N 61 27W
Couvet, *Switz.* ...... **32 C3** 46 57N 6 38 E
Couvin, *Belgium* .... **24 D4** 50 3N 4 29 E
Covarrubias, *Spain* .. **42 C7** 42 4N 3 31W
Covasna, *Romania* .. **53 E11** 45 50N 26 10 E
Covasna □, *Romania* . **53 E10** 45 50N 26 0 E
Cove I., *Canada* **150 A3** 45 17N 81 44W
Coveñas, *Colombia* .. **168 B2** 9 24N 75 44W
Coventry, *U.K.* **21 E6** 52 25N 1 28W
Coverdale, *U.S.A.* ... **152 D6** 31 38N 83 58W
Covilhã, *Portugal* ... **42 E3** 40 17N 7 31W
Covington, *Ga., U.S.A.* **152 B6** 33 36N 83 51W
Covington, *Ind., U.S.A.* **157 D9** 40 9N 87 24W
Covington, *Ky., U.S.A.* **157 E12** 39 5N 84 31W
Covington, *Ohio,*
   U.S.A. **157 D12** 40 7N 84 21W
Covington, *Tenn.,*
   U.S.A. **155 H10** 35 34N 89 39W
Covington, *Va., U.S.A.* **148 G5** 37 47N 79 59W
Cowal, L., *Australia* .. **129 B7** 33 40 S 147 25 E
Cowan, Cerro, *Ecuador* **172 a** 0 2N 91 48W
Cowan, L., *Australia* . **125 F3** 31 45 S 121 45 E
Cowan L., *Canada* ... **143 C7** 54 0N 107 15W
Cowangie, *Australia* . **128 C4** 35 12 S 141 26 E
Cowansville, *Canada* . **140 C5** 45 14N 72 46W
Coward Springs,
   Australia ..... **127 D2** 29 24 S 136 49 E
Cowcowing Lakes,
   Australia ..... **125 F2** 30 55 S 117 20 E
Cowden, *U.S.A.* **157 E8** 39 15N 88 52W
Cowdenbeath, *U.K.* .. **22 E5** 56 7N 3 21W
Cowell, *Australia* .... **128 B2** 33 39 S 136 56 E
Cowes, *Australia* .... **129 E6** 38 28 S 145 14 E
Cowes, *U.K.* **21 G6** 50 45N 1 18W
Cowichan L., *Canada* **160 B2** 48 53N 124 17W
Cowlitz →, *U.S.A.* .. **160 D4** 46 6N 122 55W
Cowra, *Australia* .... **129 B8** 33 49 S 148 42 E
Cox, *Spain* **41 G4** 38 8N 0 53W
Coxilha Grande, *Brazil* **175 B5** 28 18 S 51 30W
Coxim, *Brazil* ...... **173 D7** 18 30 S 54 55W
Coxim →, *Brazil* .... **173 D7** 18 34 S 54 46W
Cox's Bazar, *Bangla.* . **90 E3** 21 26N 91 59 E
Coyote Wells, *U.S.A.* **161 N11** 32 44N 115 58W
Coyuca de Benítez,
   Mexico **163 D4** 17 1N 100 8W
Coyuca de Catalan,
   Mexico **162 D4** 18 18N 100 41W
Cozad, *U.S.A.* **154 E5** 40 52N 99 59W
Cozes, *France* **28 C3** 45 34N 0 49W
Cozumel, *Mexico* ... **163 C7** 20 31N 86 55W
Cozumel, Isla, *Mexico* **163 C7** 20 30N 86 40W
Crab Hill, *Barbados* .. **165 g** 13 19N 59 38W
Cracow = Kraków,
   Poland .... **55 H6** 50 4N 19 57 E
Cracow, *Australia* ... **127 D5** 25 17 S 150 17 E
Cradle Mt.-Lake St.
   Clair △, *Australia* . **127 G4** 41 49 S 147 56 E
Cradock, *Australia* .. **127 E2** 32 6 S 138 31 E
Cradock, *S. Africa* .. **116 E4** 32 8 S 25 36 E
Craig, *Alaska, U.S.A.* **144 J14** 55 29N 133 9W
Craig, *Colo., U.S.A.* . **158 F10** 40 31N 107 33W
Craigavon, *U.K.* **23 B5** 54 27N 6 23W
Craigieburn, *Australia* **129 D6** 37 36 S 144 56 E
Craigmore, *Zimbabwe* **119 G3** 20 28 S 32 50 E
Craik, *Canada* **143 C7** 51 3N 105 49W
Crailsheim, *Germany* . **31 F6** 49 8N 10 5 E
Craiova, *Romania* ... **53 F8** 44 21N 23 48 E
Cramsie, *Australia* ... **126 C3** 23 20 S 144 15 E
Cranberry L., *U.S.A.* . **151 B10** 44 11N 74 50W
Cranberry Portage,
   Canada **143 C8** 54 35N 101 23W
Cranbrook, *Australia* . **125 F2** 34 18 S 117 33 E
Cranbrook, *Canada* .. **142 D5** 49 30N 115 46W
Crandon, *U.S.A.* **154 C10** 45 34N 88 54W
Crane, *Oreg., U.S.A.* . **158 E4** 43 25N 118 35W
Crane, *Tex., U.S.A.* . **155 K3** 31 24N 102 21W
Cranganore, *India* ... **95 J3** 10 13N 76 13 E
Cranston, *U.S.A.* **151 E13** 41 47N 71 26W
Craon, *France* **26 E6** 47 50N 0 58W
Craonne, *France* .... **27 C10** 49 27N 3 46 E
Crapponne-sur-Arzon,
   France .... **28 C7** 45 19N 3 51 E
Crasna, *Romania* .... **53 D12** 46 32N 27 51 E
Crasna →, *Romania* . **52 C7** 47 44N 22 35 E
Crasnei, Munții,
   Romania ...... **53 C8** 47 0N 23 20 E
Crater L., *U.S.A.* **158 E2** 42 56N 122 6W
Crater Lake △, *U.S.A.* **158 E2** 42 55N 122 10W
Crater Mt., *Papua N. G.* **132 D3** 6 37 S 145 7 E
Crater Pt., *Papua N. G.* **132 C7** 5 25 S 152 9 E
Craters of the Moon △,
   U.S.A. **158 E7** 43 25N 113 30W
Crateús, *Brazil* ..... **170 C3** 5 10 S 40 39W
Crati →, *Italy* ...... **47 C9** 39 43N 16 31 E
Crato, *Brazil* .... **170 C4** 7 10 S 39 25W
Crato, *Portugal* **43 F3** 39 16N 7 39W
Craven, L., *Canada* .. **140 B4** 54 20N 76 56W
Cravo Norte, *Colombia* **168 B3** 6 18N 70 12W
Cravo Norte →,
   Colombia **168 B3** 6 18N 70 12W
Crawford, *U.S.A.* ... **154 D3** 42 41N 103 25W
Crawford, *Ala., U.S.A.* **152 C4** 32 27N 85 11W
Crawfordsville, *Ind.,*
   U.S.A. **157 D10** 40 2N 86 54W
Crawfordsville, *Iowa,*
   U.S.A. **156 C5** 41 12N 91 32W
Crawfordville, *Fla.,*
   U.S.A. **152 E5** 30 11N 84 23W
Crawfordville, *Ga.,*
   U.S.A. **152 B7** 33 33N 82 54W
Crawley, *U.K.* **21 F7** 51 7N 0 11W
Crazy Mts., *U.S.A.* .. **158 C8** 46 12N 110 20W
Crean L., *Canada* ... **143 C7** 54 5N 106 9W
Crécy-en-Ponthieu,
   France .... **27 B8** 50 15N 1 53 E
Crediton, *Canada* ... **150 C3** 43 17N 81 33W
Crediton, *U.K.* **21 G4** 50 47N 3 40W
Cree →, *Canada* **143 B7** 58 57N 105 47W
Cree →, *U.K.* **22 G4** 54 55N 4 25W
Cree L., *Canada* **143 B7** 57 30N 106 30W
Creede, *U.S.A.* **159 H10** 37 51N 106 56W
Creekside, *U.S.A.* ... **150 F5** 40 40N 79 11W
Creel, *Mexico* **162 B3** 27 45N 107 38W
Creemore, *Canada* .. **150 B4** 44 19N 80 6W
Creighton, *Canada* .. **143 C8** 54 45N 101 54W
Creighton, *U.S.A.* ... **154 D6** 42 28N 97 54W
Creil, *France* .... **27 C9** 49 15N 2 29 E
Crema, *Italy* .... **44 C7** 45 7N 9 41 E
Cremona, *Italy* ..... **44 C7** 45 7N 10 2 E
Crepaja, *Serbia & M.* **52 E5** 45 1N 20 38 E
Crepori →, *Brazil* ... **173 B6** 5 42 S 57 8W
Crépy, *France* ...... **27 C10** 49 37N 3 32 E
Crépy-en-Valois,
   France .... **27 C9** 49 14N 2 54 E
Cres, *Croatia* ...... **45 D11** 44 58N 14 25 E
Crescent Beach, *U.S.A.* **152 F8** 29 46N 81 15W
Crescent City, *Calif.,*
   U.S.A. **158 F1** 41 45N 124 12W

Crescent City, *Fla.,*
   U.S.A. **153 F8** 29 26N 81 31W
Crescent Hd., *Australia* **129 A10** 31 11 S 152 59 E
Crescent L., *U.S.A.* .. **153 F8** 29 28N 81 30W
Crescentino, *Italy* ... **44 C5** 45 11N 8 6 E
Crespo, *Argentina* ... **174 C3** 32 2 S 60 19W
Cresson, *U.S.A.* **150 F6** 40 28N 78 36W
Cressy, *Australia* .... **128 E5** 38 2 S 143 40 E
Crest, *France* .... **29 D9** 44 44N 5 2 E
Cresta, Mt., *Phil.* .... **80 C4** 17 17N 122 6 E
Crestline, *Calif., U.S.A.* **161 L9** 34 14N 117 18W
Crestline, *Ohio, U.S.A.* **150 F2** 40 47N 82 44W
Creston, *Canada* **142 D5** 49 10N 116 31W
Creston, *Calif., U.S.A.* **160 K6** 35 32N 120 33W
Creston, *Iowa, U.S.A.* **156 C2** 41 4N 94 22W
Crestview, *Calif.,*
   U.S.A. **160 H8** 37 46N 118 58W
Crestview, *Fla., U.S.A.* **153 K2** 30 46N 86 34W
Creswick, *Australia* .. **128 D5** 37 25 S 143 58 E
Crêt de la Neige,
   France .... **27 F12** 46 16N 5 58 E
Crete = Kríti, *Greece* . **39 E6** 35 15N 25 0 E
Crete, *Ill., U.S.A.* ... **157 C9** 41 27N 87 38W
Crete, *Nebr., U.S.A.* . **154 E6** 40 38N 96 58W
Crete, Sea of, *Greece* **39 E6** 36 0N 25 0 E
Créteil, *France* ..... **27 D9** 48 47N 2 28 E
Cretin, C., *Papua N. G.* **132 D4** 6 40 S 147 53 E
Creus, C. de, *Spain* . **40 C8** 42 20N 3 19 E
Creuse □, *France* ... **27 F9** 46 10N 2 0 E
Creuse →, *France* ... **28 B4** 47 0N 0 34 E
Creutzwald, *France* .. **27 C13** 49 12N 6 42 E
Creuzburg, *Germany* . **30 D6** 51 3N 10 14 E
Crèvecœur-le-Grand,
   France .... **27 C9** 49 37N 2 5 E
Crevillente, *Spain* ... **41 G4** 38 12N 0 48W
Crewe, *U.K.* **20 D5** 53 6N 2 26W
Crewkerne, *U.K.* **21 G5** 50 53N 2 48W
Crianlarich, *U.K.* **22 E4** 56 24N 4 37W
Criciúma, *Brazil* .... **175 B6** 28 40 S 49 23W
Cridersville, *U.S.A.* .. **157 D12** 40 39N 84 9W
Crieff, *U.K.* **22 E5** 56 22N 3 50W
Crikvenica, *Croatia* .. **45 C11** 45 11N 14 40 E
Crimea □, *Ukraine* .. **59 K8** 45 30N 33 10 E
Crimean Pen. =
   Krymskyy Pivostriv,
   Ukraine ...... **59 K8** 45 0N 34 0 E
Crimmitschau,
   Germany ...... **30 E8** 50 48N 12 24 E
Cristal, Mts. de, *Gabon* **114 D2** 0 30N 10 30 E
Cristalândia, *Brazil* .. **170 D2** 10 36 S 49 11W
Cristino Castro, *Brazil* **170 C3** 8 43 S 44 13W
Cristóbal, Pta., *Ecuador* **172 a** 0 54 S 91 31W
Cristuru Secuiesc,
   Romania ...... **53 D10** 46 17N 25 2 E
Crișul Alb →, *Romania* **52 D6** 46 42N 21 17 E
Crișul Negru →,
   Romania ...... **52 D6** 46 42N 21 16 E
Crișul Repede →,
   Romania ...... **52 D6** 46 55N 20 59 E
Crittenden, *U.S.A.* .. **157 F12** 38 47N 84 36W
Criuleni, *Moldova* ... **53 C14** 47 13N 29 10 E
Crivitz, *Germany* .... **30 B7** 53 34N 11 39 E
Crixás, *Brazil* ...... **171 D2** 14 27 S 49 58W
Crna →, *Macedonia* . **50 E5** 41 33N 21 59 E
Crna Gora =
   Montenegro □,
   Serbia & M. ... **50 D3** 42 40N 19 20 E
Crna Gora, *Macedonia* **50 D5** 42 10N 21 30 E
Crna Reka = Crna →,
   Macedonia .... **50 E5** 41 33N 21 59 E
Crna Trava,
   Serbia & M. ... **50 D6** 42 49N 22 19 E
Crni Drim →,
   Macedonia .... **50 E4** 41 17N 20 40 E
Crni Timok →,
   Serbia & M. ... **50 C6** 43 53N 22 15 E
Crnoljeva Planina,
   Serbia & M. ... **50 D5** 42 20N 21 0 E
Črnomelj, *Slovenia* .. **45 C12** 45 33N 15 10 E
Croagh Patrick, *Ireland* **23 C2** 53 46N 9 40W
Croajingolong △,
   Australia ..... **129 D8** 37 45 S 149 26 E
Croatia ■, *Europe* ... **45 C13** 45 20N 16 0 E
Crocker, *U.S.A.* **156 G4** 37 57N 92 16W
Crocker, Banjaran,
   Malaysia ...... **85 A5** 5 40N 116 30 E
Crocker, Cerro,
   Ecuador ...... **172 a** 0 36 S 90 21W
Crockett, *U.S.A.* **155 K7** 31 19N 95 27W
Crocodile =
   Krokodil →, *Mozam.* **117 D5** 25 14 S 32 18 E
Crocodile Is., *Australia* **126 A1** 12 3 S 134 58 E
Crocq, *France* ...... **28 C6** 45 52N 2 21 E
Crodo, *Italy* .... **44 B5** 46 13N 8 19 E
Crohy Hd., *Ireland* ... **23 B3** 54 55N 8 26W
Croisette, C., *France* . **29 E9** 43 14N 5 22 E
Croisic, Pte. du, *France* **26 E4** 47 19N 2 31W
Croix, L. La, *Canada* . **140 C1** 48 20N 92 15W
Croix-Rousse, *France* **27 D12** 49 57N 2 54W
Croker, C., *Australia* . **126 B5** 10 58 S 132 35 E
Croker, C., *Canada* .. **150 B4** 44 58N 80 59W
Croker I., *Australia* .. **124 B5** 11 12 S 132 32 E
Cromarty, *U.K.* **22 D4** 57 40N 4 2W
Cromer, *U.K.* .... **20 E9** 52 56N 1 17 E
Cromwell, *N.Z.* ..... **131 F4** 45 3 S 169 14 E
Cromwell, *U.S.A.* ... **151 E12** 41 36N 72 39W
Cronat, *France* ..... **27 F10** 46 43N 3 40 E
Crook, *U.K.* **20 C6** 54 43N 1 45W
Crooked →, *Canada* **142 C4** 54 50N 122 54W
Crooked →, *U.S.A.* . **158 D3** 44 32N 121 16W
Crooked Creek, *U.S.A.* **144 F8** 61 52N 158 7W
Crooked I., *Bahamas* . **165 B5** 22 50N 74 10W
Crooked Island
   Passage, *Bahamas* **165 B5** 22 55N 74 35W
Crookston, *Minn.,*
   U.S.A. **154 B6** 47 47N 96 37W
Crookston, *Nebr.,*
   U.S.A. **154 D4** 42 56N 100 45W
Crookwell, *Australia* . **129 C8** 34 28 S 149 24 E
Cropani-Micone △,
   Italy .... **47 D9** 38 31N 16 18 E
Crosby, *U.K.* **20 D4** 53 30N 3 3W
Crosby, *N. Dak., U.S.A.* **143 A8** 48 55N 103 18W
Crosby, *Pa., U.S.A.* . **150 E6** 41 45N 78 23W
Crosbyton, *U.S.A.* ... **155 J4** 33 40N 101 14W
Crosía, *Italy* .... **47 C9** 39 35N 16 45 E
Cross →, *Nigeria* ... **113 E6** 4 42N 8 21 E
Cross City, *U.S.A.* ... **153 G6** 29 38N 83 7W
Cross Fell, *U.K.* **20 C5** 54 43N 2 28W
Cross L., *Canada* **143 C9** 54 45N 97 30W
Cross Lake, *Canada* . **143 C9** 54 37N 97 47W
Cross River □, *Nigeria* **113 E6** 6 0N 5 50 E
Cross River △, *Nigeria* **113 D6** 5 50N 9 0 E
Cross Sound, *U.S.A.* **144 H14** 58 0N 135 0W
Cross Timbers, *U.S.A.* **156 F3** 38 1N 93 14W
Crossen = Krosno
   Odrzańskie, *Poland* **55 F2** 52 3N 15 7 E
Crossett, *U.S.A.* **155 J9** 33 8N 91 58W
Crosshaven, *Ireland* . **23 E3** 51 47N 8 17W
Crossley, Mt., *N.Z.* .. **131 C7** 42 50 S 172 5 E
Crossville, *Ill., U.S.A.* **157 F8** 38 10N 88 4W
Crossville, *Tenn.,*
   U.S.A. **149 G3** 35 57N 85 2W
Croswell, *U.S.A.* **150 C2** 43 16N 82 37W

Croton-on-Hudson,
   U.S.A. **151 E11** 41 12N 73 55W
Crotone, *Italy* ...... **47 C10** 39 5N 17 8 E
Crow →, *Canada* ... **142 B4** 59 41N 124 20W
Crow Agency, *U.S.A.* **158 D10** 45 36N 107 28W
Crow Hd., *Ireland* ... **23 E1** 51 35N 10 9W
Crowdy Bay △,
   Australia ..... **129 A10** 31 51 S 152 45 E
Crowell, *U.S.A.* **155 J5** 33 59N 99 43W
Crowl Cr. →, *Australia* **129 B6** 32 0 S 145 30 E
Crowley, *U.S.A.* **155 K8** 30 13N 92 22W
Crowley, L., *U.S.A.* .. **160 H8** 37 35N 118 42W
Crown I., *Papua N. G.* **132 C4** 5 7 S 146 58 E
Crown Point, *Ind.,*
   U.S.A. **157 C9** 41 25N 87 22W
Crown Point, *N.Y.,*
   U.S.A. **151 C11** 43 57N 73 26W
Crown Pt., *Trin. & Tob.* **169 E10** 11 18N 60 51W
Crownpoint, *U.S.A.* .. **159 J9** 35 41N 108 9W
Crows Landing, *U.S.A.* **160 H5** 37 23N 121 6W
Crows Nest, *Australia* **127 D5** 27 16 S 152 4 E
Crowsnest Pass,
   Canada **142 D6** 49 40N 114 40W
Croydon, *Australia* .. **126 B3** 18 13 S 142 14 E
Croydon □, *U.K.* **21 F7** 51 22N 0 5W
Crozet, Is., *Ind. Oc.* . **121 J4** 46 27 S 52 0 E
Crozon, *France* **26 D2** 48 15N 4 30W
Cruces, Punta,
   Colombia **168 B2** 6 39N 77 32W
Cruz, C., *Cuba* **164 C4** 19 50N 77 50W
Cruz Alta, *Brazil* .... **175 B5** 28 45 S 53 40W
Cruz Bay,
   U.S. Virgin Is. .. **165 e** 18 20N 64 48W
Cruz das Almas, *Brazil* **171 D4** 12 0 S 39 6W
Cruz de Incio, *Spain* . **42 C3** 42 39N 7 21W
Cruz de Malta, *Brazil* **170 C3** 8 15 S 40 20W
Cruz del Eje, *Argentina* **174 C3** 30 45 S 64 50W
Cruzeiro, *Brazil* ..... **171 F2** 22 33 S 45 0W
Cruzeiro do Oeste,
   Brazil .... **175 A5** 23 46 S 53 4W
Cruzeiro do Sul =
   Ioaqaba, *Brazil* .. **175 B5** 27 5 S 51 31W
Cruzeiro do Sul, *Brazil* **172 B3** 7 35 S 72 35W
Cry L., *Canada* **142 B3** 58 45N 129 0W
Crystal B., *U.S.A.* ... **153 G7** 28 50N 82 45W
Crystal Bay, *U.S.A.* .. **160 F7** 39 15N 120 0W
Crystal Brook,
   Australia ..... **128 B3** 33 21 S 138 12 E
Crystal City, *Mo.,*
   U.S.A. **156 F9** 38 13N 90 23W
Crystal City, *Tex.,*
   U.S.A. **155 L5** 28 41N 99 50W
Crystal Falls, *U.S.A.* . **148 B1** 46 5N 88 20W
Crystal Lake, *Fla.,*
   U.S.A. **152 E4** 30 26N 85 42W
Crystal Lake, *Ill.,*
   U.S.A. **157 B8** 42 14N 88 19W
Crystal River, *U.S.A.* **153 G7** 28 54N 82 35W
Crystal Springs, *U.S.A.* **155 K9** 31 59N 90 21W
Csenger, *Hungary* ... **52 C7** 47 50N 22 41 E
Csongrád, *Hungary* .. **52 D5** 46 32N 20 12 E
Csongrád □, *Hungary* **52 D5** 46 32N 20 15 E
Csorna, *Hungary* .... **52 C2** 47 38N 17 18 E
Csurgo, *Hungary* .... **52 D2** 46 16N 17 9 E
Cu Lao Hon, *Vietnam* **87 G7** 10 54N 108 18 E
Cua Rao, *Vietnam* ... **86 C5** 19 16N 104 27 E
Cuácua →, *Mozam.* . **119 F4** 17 54 S 37 0 E
Cuale, *Angola* ...... **115 G3** 7 17 S 18 9 E
Cuamato, *Angola* ... **116 B2** 17 2 S 15 7 E
Cuamba, *Mozam.* ... **117 E4** 14 45 S 36 22 E
Cuando →, *Angola* . **115 G4** 14 34 S 19 1 E
Cuando →, *Angola* . **115 H4** 17 30 S 23 15 E
Cuando Cubango □,
   Angola .... **116 B3** 16 25 S 20 0 E
Cuangar, *Angola* .... **116 B2** 17 36 S 18 39 E
Cuango = Kwango →,
   Dem. Rep. of
   the Congo ..... **114 C3** 3 14 S 17 22 E
Cuango, *Lunda Norte,*
   Angola .... **115 D3** 9 8 S 18 3 E
Cuango, *Moxico,*
   Angola .... **115 G3** 6 20 S 16 42 E
Cuango, *Uíge, Angola* **115 D3** 6 15 S 16 42 E
Cuanza →, *Angola* .. **115 D2** 9 21 S 13 9 E
Cuanza Norte □,
   Angola .... **115 D2** 8 50 S 14 30 E
Cuanza Sul □, *Angola* **115 E2** 10 50 S 14 50 E
Cuao →, *Venezuela* . **168 C4** 4 55N 67 40W
Cuarto →, *Argentina* **174 C3** 33 25 S 63 2W
Cuatir →, *Angola* ... **115 F3** 17 1 S 18 9 E
Cuatrociénegas, *Mexico* **162 B4** 26 59N 102 5W
Cuauhtémoc, *Mexico* **162 B3** 28 25N 106 52W
Cuba, *Portugal* **43 G3** 38 10N 7 54W
Cuba, *N. Mex., U.S.A.* **159 J10** 36 1N 107 4W
Cuba, *N.Y., U.S.A.* .. **150 D6** 42 13N 78 17W
Cuba ■, *W. Indies* .. **164 B4** 22 0N 79 0W
Cuba City, *U.S.A.* ... **156 D6** 42 36N 90 26W
Cubal, *Angola* ...... **115 G2** 12 26 S 14 3 E
Cubango →, *Africa* .. **116 B3** 18 50 S 22 25 E
Cubanja, *Angola* .... **115 E4** 14 49 S 21 20 E
Cubia →, *Angola* ... **115 F4** 15 58 S 21 42 E
Çubuk, *Turkey* ..... **100 B5** 40 14N 33 3 E
Cuc Phuong △, *Vietnam* **86 B5** 20 17N 105 38 E
Cuchi, *Angola* ...... **115 F3** 14 37 S 16 58 E
Cuchi →, *Angola* ... **115 F3** 15 13 S 17 20 E
Cuchillo-Có, *Argentina* **176 A4** 38 26 S 64 30W
Cuchivero →,
   Venezuela **168 B5** 7 40N 65 57W
Cuchumatanes, Sierra
   de los, *Guatemala* **164 C1** 15 35N 91 25W
Cuckfield, *U.K.* **21 F7** 51 1N 0 8W
Cucuí, *Brazil* **168 C4** 1 12N 66 50W
Cucurpe, *Mexico* ... **162 A2** 30 20N 110 43W
Cucurupí, *Colombia* . **168 C3** 4 23N 76 56W
Cúcuta, *Colombia* ... **168 B3** 7 54N 72 31W
Cudahy, *U.S.A.* **157 B9** 42 58N 87 52W
Cudalbi, *Romania* ... **53 E12** 45 46N 27 41 E
Cuddalore, *India* .... **95 J4** 11 46N 79 45 E
Cuddapan, L., *Australia* **126 D3** 25 45 S 141 26 E
Cudgewa, *Australia* .. **129 D7** 36 10 S 147 42 E
Cudillero, *Spain* **42 B4** 43 33N 6 9W
Cue, *Australia* ...... **125 E2** 27 25 S 117 54 E
Cuebe →, *Angola* ... **115 F3** 15 50 S 17 38 E
Cuéllar, *Spain* **42 D6** 41 23N 4 21W
Cuenca, *Ecuador* ... **168 D2** 2 50 S 79 9W
Cuenca, *Spain* **40 E2** 40 5N 2 10W
Cuenca □, *Spain* **40 E3** 40 0N 2 0W
Cuenca, Serranía de,
   Spain **40 F3** 39 55N 1 50W
Cuenca Alta del
   Manzanares △, *Spain* **42 E7** 40 40N 3 55W
Cuerda del Pozo,
   Embalse de la, *Spain* **42 D2** 41 51N 2 44W
Cuernavaca, *Mexico* . **163 D5** 18 55N 99 15W
Cuero, *U.S.A.* **155 L6** 29 6N 97 17W
Cuers, *France* ...... **29 E10** 43 14N 6 5 E
Cueva de la Quebrada
   del Toro △,
   Venezuela **165 D6** 10 46N 69 3W

Cueva de los Guácharos △, *Colombia* **168 C2** 1 35N 76 1W
Cuevas, Cerro, *Bolivia* **173 E4** 22 0 S 65 12W
Cuevas de Vera = Cuevas del Almanzora, *Spain* **41 H3** 37 18N 1 58W
Cuevas del Almanzora, *Spain* **41 H3** 37 18N 1 58W
Cuevo, *Bolivia* **173 E5** 20 15 S 63 30W
Cugir, *Romania* **53 E8** 45 48N 23 25 E
Cugnaux, *France* **28 E5** 43 32N 1 20 E
Cuhai-Bakony →, *Hungary* **52 C2** 47 35N 17 54 E
Cuiabá, *Brazil* **173 D6** 15 30 S 56 0W
Cuiabá →, *Brazil* **173 D6** 17 5 S 56 36W
Cuihangcun, *China* **69 G10** 22 27N 113 32 E
Cuijk, *Neths.* **24 C5** 51 44N 5 50 E
Cuilco, *Guatemala* **164 C1** 15 24N 91 58W
Cuillin Hills, *U.K.* **22 D2** 57 13N 6 15W
Cuillin Sd., *U.K.* **22 D2** 57 4N 6 20W
Cuilo = Kwilu →, *Dem. Rep. of the Congo* **115 C3** 3 22 S 17 22 E
Cuilo, *Angola* **115 D3** 8 12 S 19 28 E
Cuilo-Futa, *Angola* **115 D3** 6 28 S 15 51 E
Cuima, *Angola* **115 E3** 13 25 S 15 45 E
Cuimba, *Angola* **115 D2** 6 10 S 14 41 E
Cuiseaux, *France* **27 F12** 46 30N 5 22 E
Cuité, *Brazil* **170 C4** 6 29 S 36 9W
Cuito →, *Angola* **116 B3** 18 1 S 20 48 E
Cuito Cuanavale, *Angola* **115 F3** 15 10 S 19 10 E
Cuitzeo, L. de, *Mexico* **162 D4** 19 55N 101 5W
Cuiuni →, *Brazil* **169 D5** 0 45 S 63 7W
Cuivre →, *U.S.A.* **156 F6** 38 55N 90 44W
Cuivre, West Fork →, *U.S.A.* **156 E6** 39 2N 90 58W
Cujmir, *Romania* **52 F7** 44 13N 22 57 E
Cukai, *Malaysia* **87 K4** 4 13N 103 25 E
Culasi, *Phil.* **81 F4** 11 26N 122 3 E
Culbertson, *U.S.A.* **154 A2** 48 9N 104 31W
Culburra, *N.S.W., Australia* **129 C9** 34 56 S 150 46 E
Culburra, *S. Austral., Australia* **128 C3** 35 50 S 139 58 E
Culcairn, *Australia* **129 C7** 35 41 S 147 3 E
Culebra = Dewey, *Puerto Rico* **165 d** 18 18N 65 18W
Culebra, Isla de, *Puerto Rico* **165 d** 18 19N 65 18W
Culebra, Sierra de la, *Spain* **42 D4** 41 55N 6 20W
Culfa, *Azerbaijan* **101 C11** 38 57N 45 38 E
Culgoa, *Australia* **128 C5** 35 44 S 143 6 E
Culgoa →, *Australia* **127 D4** 29 56 S 146 20 E
Culgoa Flood Plain △, *Australia* **127 D4** 28 58 S 147 5 E
Culiacán, *Mexico* **162 C3** 24 50N 107 23W
Culiacán →, *Mexico* **162 C3** 24 30N 107 42W
Culik, *Indonesia* **79 J18** 8 21 S 115 37 E
Culion, *Phil.* **81 F3** 11 54N 119 58 E
Culion I., *Phil.* **81 F2** 11 50N 120 0 E
Culiseu →, *Brazil* **173 C7** 12 14 S 53 17W
Cúllar, *Spain* **43 H8** 37 35N 2 34W
Cullarin Ra., *Australia* **129 C8** 34 30 S 149 30 E
Cullen, *U.K.* **22 D6** 57 42N 2 49W
Cullen Bullen, *Australia* **129 B9** 33 18 S 150 2 E
Cullen Pt., *Australia* **126 A3** 11 57 S 141 54 E
Cullera, *Spain* **41 F4** 39 9N 0 17W
Cullman, *U.S.A.* **149 H2** 34 11N 86 51W
Culloden, *U.S.A.* **152 C5** 32 52N 84 6W
Cullom, *U.S.A.* **157 D8** 40 53N 88 16W
Cullompton, *U.K.* **21 G4** 50 51N 3 24W
Culo →, *Angola* **115 D3** 6 13 S 15 34 E
Culoz, *France* **29 C9** 45 47N 5 46 E
Culpeper, *U.S.A.* **148 F7** 38 30N 78 0W
Culuene →, *Brazil* **173 C7** 12 56 S 52 51W
Culver, *U.S.A.* **157 C10** 41 13N 86 25W
Culver, Pt., *Australia* **125 F3** 32 54 S 124 43 E
Culverden, *N.Z.* **131 C7** 42 47 S 172 49 E
Culverton, *U.S.A.* **152 B7** 33 19N 82 54W
Cuma, *Angola* **115 E3** 12 52 S 15 5 E
Cumaná, *Venezuela* **169 A5** 10 30N 64 5W
Cumaovası, *Turkey* **49 C9** 38 15N 27 9 E
Cumare, *Colombia* **168 C3** 0 49N 72 32W
Cumari, *Brazil* **171 E2** 18 16 S 48 11W
Cumbe = Euclides da Cunha, *Brazil* **170 D4** 10 31 S 39 1W
Cumberland, *B.C., Canada* **142 D4** 49 40N 125 0W
Cumberland, *Ont., Canada* **151 A9** 45 29N 75 24W
Cumberland, *Iowa, U.S.A.* **156 C2** 41 16N 94 52W
Cumberland, *Md., U.S.A.* **148 F6** 39 39N 78 46W
Cumberland →, *U.S.A.* **149 G2** 36 15N 87 0W
Cumberland, C., *Vanuatu* **133 D4** 14 39 S 166 37 E
Cumberland, L., *U.S.A.* **149 G3** 36 57N 84 55W
Cumberland Gap △, *U.S.A.* **149 G4** 36 36N 83 40W
Cumberland I., *U.S.A.* **152 E8** 30 50N 81 25W
Cumberland Is., *Australia* **126 J7** 20 35 S 149 10 E
Cumberland Island ⌓, *U.S.A.* **152 E8** 30 12N 81 24W
Cumberland L., *Canada* **143 C8** 54 3N 102 18W
Cumberland Pen., *Canada* **139 B13** 67 0N 64 0W
Cumberland Plateau, *U.S.A.* **149 H3** 36 0N 85 0W
Cumberland Sd., *Canada* **139 B13** 65 30N 66 0W
Cumbernauld, *U.K.* **22 F5** 55 57N 3 58W
Cumbira, *Angola* **115 E3** 12 11 S 15 8 E
Cumborah, *Australia* **127 D4** 29 40 S 147 45 E
Cumbres de Majalca △, *Mexico* **162 B3** 28 52N 106 24W
Cumbres de Monterrey △, *Mexico* **162 B4** 25 40N 100 35W
Cumbres Mayores, *Spain* **43 G4** 38 4N 6 39W
Cumbria □, *U.K.* **20 C5** 54 42N 2 52W
Cumbrian Mts., *U.K.* **20 C5** 54 30N 3 0W
Cumbum, *India* **95 G4** 15 40N 79 10 E
Cuminá, *Brazil* **169 D6** 1 57 S 56 2W
Cuminá →, *Brazil* **169 D6** 1 30 S 56 0W
Cuminapanema →, *Brazil* **169 D7** 1 9 S 54 54W
Cumming, C., *Chile* **172 b** 27 6 S 109 14W
Cummings Mt., *U.S.A.* **161 K8** 35 2N 118 34W
Cummins, *Australia* **127 E2** 34 16 S 135 43 E
Cumnock, *Australia* **129 B8** 32 59 S 148 46 E
Cumnock, *U.K.* **22 F4** 55 28N 4 17W
Cumpas, *Mexico* **162 B3** 30 0N 109 48W
Cumplida, Pta., *Canary Is.* **9 e1** 28 50N 17 48W
Çumra, *Turkey* **100 D5** 37 34N 32 45 E
Cuncumén, *Chile* **174 C1** 31 53 S 70 38W
Cunderdin, *Australia* **125 F2** 31 37 S 117 12 E
Cundinamarca □, *Colombia* **168 C3** 5 0N 74 0W
Cunene □, *Angola* **115 F3** 16 30 S 15 0 E
Cunene →, *Angola* **116 B1** 17 20 S 11 50 E
Cúneo, *Italy* **44 D4** 44 23N 7 32 E
Çüngüş, *Turkey* **96 B3** 38 13N 39 17 E
Cunhinga, *Angola* **115 E3** 12 11 S 16 47 E
Cunillera, I. = Sa Conillera, *Spain* **38 D1** 38 59N 1 13 E
Cunjamba, *Angola* **115 F4** 15 27 S 20 10 E
Cunlhat, *France* **28 C7** 45 38N 3 32 E
Cunnamulla, *Australia* **127 D4** 28 2 S 145 38 E
Cunningham, *Bahamas* **9 b** 25 5N 77 26W
Cuorgnè, *Italy* **44 C4** 45 23N 7 39 E
Cupar, *Canada* **143 C8** 50 57N 104 10W
Cupar, *U.K.* **22 E5** 56 19N 3 1W
Cupcini, *Moldova* **53 B12** 48 6N 27 23 E
Cupica, G. de, *Colombia* **168 B2** 6 25N 77 30W
Ćuprija, *Serbia & M.* **50 C5** 43 57N 21 26 E
Curaçá, *Brazil* **170 C4** 8 59 S 39 54W
Curaçao, *Neth. Ant.* **165 D6** 12 10N 69 0W
Curacautín, *Chile* **176 A2** 38 26 S 71 53W
Curador = Presidente Dutra, *Brazil* **170 C3** 5 15 S 44 30W
Curahuara de Carangas, *Bolivia* **172 D4** 17 52 S 68 26W
Curalhinho = Coelho Neto, *Brazil* **170 B3** 4 15 S 43 0W
Curanilahue, *Chile* **174 D1** 37 29 S 73 28W
Curaray →, *Peru* **168 D3** 2 20 S 74 5W
Curatabaca, *Venezuela* **169 B5** 6 19N 62 51W
Cure →, *France* **27 E10** 47 40N 3 41 E
Curepipe, *Mauritius* **121 d** 20 19 S 57 31 E
Curepto, *Chile* **174 D1** 35 8 S 72 1W
Curiapo, *Venezuela* **169 B5** 8 33N 61 5W
Curicó, *Chile* **174 C1** 34 55 S 71 20W
Curicuriari →, *Brazil* **168 D4** 0 14 S 66 48W
Curieuse, *Seychelles* **121 b** 4 15 S 55 44 E
Curimatá, *Brazil* **170 D3** 10 2 S 44 17W
Curinga, *Italy* **47 D9** 38 49N 16 19 E
Curiplaya, *Colombia* **168 C3** 0 16N 74 52W
Curitiba, *Brazil* **175 B6** 25 20 S 49 10W
Curitibanos, *Brazil* **175 B5** 27 18 S 50 36W
Curlewis, *Australia* **129 A9** 31 7 S 150 16 E
Curoca →, *Angola* **115 F2** 15 43 S 11 55 E
Currabubula, *Australia* **129 A9** 31 16 S 150 44 E
Currais Novos, *Brazil* **170 C4** 6 13 S 36 30W
Curral Velho, *C. Verde Is.* **9 j** 16 8N 22 48W
Curralinho, *Brazil* **170 B2** 1 45 S 49 46W
Currant, *U.S.A.* **158 G6** 38 51N 115 32W
Curraweena, *Australia* **129 A6** 30 47 S 145 54 E
Currawinya △, *Australia* **127 D3** 28 55 S 144 27 E
Current →, *U.S.A.* **155 G9** 36 15N 90 55W
Currie, *Australia* **127 F3** 39 56 S 143 53 E
Currie, *U.S.A.* **158 F6** 40 16N 114 45W
Cursole, *Somali Rep.* **120 D3** 2 14N 45 25 E
Curt-Bunar = Tervel, *Bulgaria* **51 C11** 43 45N 27 28 E
Curtea de Argeş, *Romania* **53 E9** 45 12N 24 42 E
Curtici, *Romania* **52 D6** 46 21N 21 18 E
Curtis, *U.S.A.* **154 E4** 40 38N 100 31W
Curtis Group, *Australia* **127 F4** 39 30 S 146 37 E
Curtis I., *Australia* **126 C5** 23 35 S 151 10 E
Curuá →, *Pará, Brazil* **169 D7** 2 24 S 54 5W
Curuá →, *Pará, Brazil* **173 B7** 5 23 S 54 22W
Curuá, I., *Brazil* **170 A1** 0 48N 50 10W
Curuaés →, *Brazil* **173 B7** 7 30 S 54 45W
Curuaí, *Brazil* **169 D6** 2 17 S 55 29W
Curuápanema →, *Brazil* **169 D6** 2 25 S 55 2W
Curuçá, *Brazil* **170 B2** 0 43 S 47 50W
Curuçá →, *Brazil* **172 B3** 4 27 S 71 23W
Curuguaty, *Paraguay* **175 A4** 24 31 S 55 42W
Curup, *Indonesia* **84 C2** 4 26 S 102 13 E
Curupira, Serra, *S. Amer.* **169 C5** 1 25N 64 30W
Cururu →, *Brazil* **173 B6** 7 12 S 58 3W
Cururupu, *Brazil* **170 B3** 1 50 S 44 50W
Curuzú Cuatiá, *Argentina* **174 B4** 29 50 S 58 5W
Curvelo, *Brazil* **171 E3** 18 45 S 44 27W
Cushing, *U.S.A.* **155 H6** 35 59N 96 46W
Cushing, Mt., *Canada* **142 B3** 57 35N 126 57W
Cusihuiriáchic, *Mexico* **162 B3** 28 10N 106 50W
Cusna, Mte., *Italy* **44 D7** 44 17N 10 23 E
Cussabat = Al Qaşabát, *Libya* **108 B2** 32 39N 14 1 E
Cusset, *France* **27 F10** 46 8N 3 28 E
Cusseta, *U.S.A.* **152 C5** 32 18N 84 47W
Cusso, Sa. do, *Angola* **115 D2** 6 30 S 14 58 E
Custer, *U.S.A.* **154 D3** 43 46N 103 36W
Cut Bank, *U.S.A.* **158 B7** 48 38N 112 20W
Cutchogue, *U.S.A.* **151 E12** 41 1N 72 30W
Cutervo, *Peru* **172 B2** 6 25 S 78 55W
Cuthbert, *U.S.A.* **152 D5** 31 46N 84 48W
Cutler, *U.S.A.* **160 J7** 36 31N 119 17W
Cutler Ridge, *U.S.A.* **153 K9** 25 35N 80 20W
Cutlerville, *U.S.A.* **157 B11** 42 50N 85 40W
Cutral-Có, *Argentina* **176 A3** 38 58 S 69 15W
Cutro, *Italy* **47 C9** 39 2N 16 59 E
Cuttaburra →, *Australia* **127 D3** 29 43 S 144 22 E
Cuttack, *India* **94 D7** 20 25N 85 57 E
Cuva →, *Angola* **115 E2** 11 42 S 14 52 E
Cuvelai, *Angola* **115 F3** 15 44 S 15 50 E
Cuvier, C., *Australia* **125 D1** 23 14 S 113 22 E
Cuvier I., *N.Z.* **130 C4** 36 27 S 175 50 E
Cuxhaven, *Germany* **30 B4** 53 51N 8 41 E
Cuyabeno, *Ecuador* **168 D2** 0 16 S 75 53W
Cuyahoga Falls, *U.S.A.* **150 E3** 41 8N 81 29W
Cuyahoga Valley △, *U.S.A.* **150 E3** 41 15N 81 33W
Cuyapo, *Phil.* **80 D3** 15 46N 120 40 E
Cuyo, *Phil.* **81 F3** 10 50N 121 5 E
Cuyo East Pass, *Phil.* **81 F3** 11 0N 121 28 E
Cuyo I., *Phil.* **81 F3** 10 51N 121 2 E
Cuyo Islands, *Phil.* **81 F3** 11 4N 120 57 E
Cuyo West Pass, *Phil.* **81 F3** 11 0N 120 30 E
Cuyuni →, *Guyana* **169 B6** 6 23N 58 41W
Cuzco, *Bolivia* **172 E4** 20 0 S 66 50W
Cuzco, *Peru* **172 C3** 13 32 S 72 0W
Cuzco □, *Peru* **172 C3** 13 31 S 71 59W
Čvrsnica, *Bos.-H.* **52 G2** 43 36N 17 35 E
Cwmbran, *U.K.* **21 F4** 51 39N 3 2W
Cyangugu, *Rwanda* **118 C2** 2 29 S 28 54 E
Cybinka, *Poland* **55 F1** 52 12N 14 46 E
Cyclades = Kikládhes, *Greece* **48 E6** 37 0N 24 30 E
Cygnet, *Australia* **127 G4** 43 8 S 147 1 E
Cynthiana, *U.S.A.* **157 F12** 38 23N 84 18W
Cypress Hills, *Canada* **143 D7** 49 40N 109 30W
Cypress Hills ⌓, *Canada* **143 D7** 49 40N 109 30W
Cyprus ■, *Asia* **39 F9** 35 0N 33 0 E
Cyrenaica, *Libya* **108 B4** 27 0N 23 0 E
Cyrene = Shaḩḩāt, *Libya* **108 B4** 32 48N 21 54 E
Cyrene, *Libya* **108 B4** 32 53N 21 52 E
Czaplinek, *Poland* **54 E3** 53 34N 16 14 E
Czar, *Canada* **143 C6** 52 27N 110 50W
Czarna →, *Łódzkie, Poland* **55 G6** 51 18N 19 55 E
Czarna →, *Świętokrzyskie, Poland* **55 H8** 50 28N 21 21 E
Czarna Białostocka, *Poland* **55 E10** 53 18N 23 17 E
Czarna Woda, *Poland* **54 E5** 53 51N 18 6 E
Czarne, *Poland* **54 E3** 53 42N 16 58 E
Czarnków, *Poland* **55 F3** 52 55N 16 38 E
Czaslau = Čáslav, *Czech Rep.* **34 B8** 49 54N 15 22 E
Czech Rep. ■, *Europe* **34 B8** 50 0N 15 0 E
Czechowice-Dziedzice, *Poland* **55 J5** 49 54N 18 59 E
Czempiń, *Poland* **55 F3** 52 9N 16 43 E
Czeremcha, *Poland* **55 F10** 52 31N 23 21 E
Czerniejewo, *Poland* **55 F4** 52 26N 17 30 E
Czernowitz = Chernivtsi, *Ukraine* **53 B10** 48 15N 25 52 E
Czersk, *Poland* **54 E4** 53 46N 17 58 E
Czerwieńsk, *Poland* **55 F2** 52 1N 15 23 E
Czerwionka-Leszczyny, *Poland* **55 H5** 50 7N 18 37 E
Częstochowa, *Poland* **55 H6** 50 49N 19 7 E
Człopa, *Poland* **55 E3** 53 6N 16 6 E
Człuchów, *Poland* **54 E4** 53 41N 17 22 E
Czortów = Chortkiv, *Ukraine* **59 H3** 49 2N 25 46 E
Czyżew-Osada, *Poland* **55 F9** 52 48N 22 19 E

D

Da →, *Vietnam* **76 G5** 21 15N 105 20 E
Da Hinggan Ling, *China* **69 B7** 48 0N 121 0 E
Da Lat, *Vietnam* **87 G7** 11 56N 108 25 E
Da Nang, *Vietnam* **86 D7** 16 4N 108 13 E
Da Qaidam, *China* **68 C4** 37 50N 95 15 E
Da Yunhe →, *China* **75 G11** 34 25N 120 5 E
Da'an, *China* **75 B13** 45 30N 124 7 E
Daan Viljoen ⌓, *Namibia* **116 C2** 22 2 S 16 45 E
Daanbantayan, *Phil.* **81 F5** 11 17N 124 2 E
Dab'a, Ras el, *Egypt* **106 H6** 31 3N 28 31 E
Daba Shan, *China* **76 B7** 32 0N 109 0 E
Dabai, *Nigeria* **113 C6** 11 25N 5 15 E
Dabajuro, *Venezuela* **168 A3** 11 2N 70 40W
Dabakala, *Ivory C.* **112 D4** 8 15N 4 20W
Dabaro, *Somali Rep.* **120 C3** 6 21N 48 43 E
Dabas, *Hungary* **52 C4** 47 11N 19 19 E
Dabat, *Ethiopia* **107 E4** 12 58N 37 41 E
Dabbagh, Jabal, *Si. Arabia* **96 E2** 27 52N 35 45 E
Dabeiba, *Colombia* **168 B2** 7 1N 76 16W
Daber = Dobra, *Poland* **54 E2** 53 34N 15 20 E
Dabhoi, *India* **92 H5** 22 10N 73 20 E
Dąbie, *Poland* **55 F5** 52 5N 18 50 E
Dabie Shan, *China* **77 B10** 31 20N 115 20 E
Dabilda, *Cameroon* **109 F2** 12 14N 14 34 E
Dabilda, *Cameroon* **113 C7** 12 45N 14 35 E
Dabnou, *Niger* **113 C6** 14 10N 5 22 E
Dabo = Pasirkuning, *Indonesia* **84 C2** 0 30 S 104 33 E
Dabola, *Guinea* **112 C2** 10 50N 11 5W
Dabou, *Ivory C.* **112 D4** 5 20N 4 23W
Daboya, *Ghana* **113 D4** 9 30N 1 20W
Dabravolya, *Belarus* **55 F10** 52 55N 23 59 E
Dąbrowa Białostocka, *Poland* **54 E10** 53 40N 23 21 E
Dąbrowa Górnicza, *Poland* **55 H6** 50 15N 19 10 E
Dąbrowa Tarnowska, *Poland* **55 H7** 50 10N 20 59 E
Dabu, *China* **77 E11** 24 22N 116 41 E
Dabugam, *India* **94 E6** 19 27N 82 26 E
Dabung, *Malaysia* **87 K4** 5 23N 102 1 E
Dabus →, *Ethiopia* **107 E4** 10 48N 35 10 E
Dacato →, *Ethiopia* **107 F5** 7 25N 42 40 E
Dacca = Dhaka, *Bangla.* **90 D3** 23 43N 90 26 E
Dacca = Dhaka □, *Bangla.* **90 C3** 24 25N 90 25 E
Dachau, *Germany* **31 G7** 48 15N 11 26 E
Dachigam △, *India* **92 B6** 34 10N 75 0 E
Dachstein, Hoher, *Austria* **34 D6** 47 28N 13 35 E
Dačice, *Czech Rep.* **34 B8** 49 5N 15 26 E
Dacula, *U.S.A.* **152 B6** 33 59N 83 54W
Dadanawa, *Guyana* **169 C6** 2 50N 59 30W
Daday, *Turkey* **100 B5** 41 28N 33 27 E
Dade City, *U.S.A.* **153 G7** 28 22N 82 11W
Dadès, Oued →, *Morocco* **110 B3** 30 58N 6 44W
Dadeville, *U.S.A.* **152 C4** 32 50N 85 46W
Dadhar, *Pakistan* **92 E2** 29 28N 67 39 E
Dadiya, *Nigeria* **113 D7** 9 35N 11 24 E
Dadra = Achalpur, *India* **94 D3** 21 22N 77 32 E
Dadra & Nagar Haveli □, *India* **94 D1** 20 5N 73 0 E
Dadri = Charkhi Dadri, *India* **92 E7** 28 37N 76 17 E
Dadu, *Pakistan* **91 D2** 26 45N 67 45 E
Dadu He →, *China* **76 C4** 29 31N 103 46 E
Daegu = Taegu, *S. Korea* **75 G15** 35 50N 128 37 E
Daejeon = Taejŏn, *S. Korea* **75 F14** 36 20N 127 28 E
Daet, *Phil.* **80 D4** 14 2N 122 55 E
Dafang, *China* **76 D5** 27 9N 105 39 E
Dağ, *Turkey* **49 D12** 37 12N 30 31 E
Dagali, *Norway* **18 D5** 60 25N 8 28 E
Dagana, *Senegal* **112 B1** 16 30N 15 35W
Dagash, *Sudan* **106 D3** 19 19N 33 25 E
Dagestan □, *Russia* **61 J8** 42 30N 47 0 E
Dagestanskiye Ogni, *Russia* **61 J9** 42 6N 48 12 E
Dagg Sd., *N.Z.* **131 F1** 45 23 S 166 45 E
Daggett, *U.S.A.* **161 L10** 34 52N 116 52W
Daghestan Republic = Dagestan □, *Russia* **61 J8** 42 30N 47 0 E
Daghfeli, *Sudan* **106 D3** 19 18N 32 40 E
Dağlıq Qarabağ = Nagorno-Karabakh □, *Azerbaijan* **101 C12** 39 55N 46 45 E
Dagmersellen, *Switz.* **32 B5** 47 13N 7 59 E
Dagö = Hiiumaa, *Estonia* **15 G20** 58 50N 22 45 E
Dagu, *China* **75 E9** 38 59N 117 40 E
Dagua, *Papua N. G.* **132 B2** 3 27 S 143 20 E
Daguan, *China* **76 D4** 27 43N 103 56 E
Dagupan, *Phil.* **80 C3** 16 3N 120 20 E
Daguragu, *Australia* **124 C5** 17 33 S 130 30 E
Dahab, *Egypt* **106 B3** 28 31N 34 31 E
Dahanu, *India* **94 E1** 19 58N 72 44 E
Dahivadi, *India* **94 F2** 17 43N 74 33 E
Dahlak △, *Eritrea* **107 D5** 15 35N 40 1 E
Dahlak Kebir, *Eritrea* **107 D5** 15 50N 40 10 E
Dahlenburg, *Germany* **30 B6** 53 11N 10 44 E
Dahlonega, *U.S.A.* **149 H4** 34 32N 83 59W
Dahme, *Germany* **30 D9** 51 52N 13 25 E
Dahod, *India* **92 H6** 22 50N 74 15 E
Dahomey = Benin ■, *Africa* **113 D5** 10 0N 2 0 E
Dahong Shan, *China* **77 B9** 31 25N 113 0 E
Dahra, *Libya* **108 C3** 29 30N 17 50 E
Dahra, *Senegal* **112 B1** 15 22N 15 30W
Dahra, Massif de, *Algeria* **111 A5** 36 7N 1 21 E
Dahshûr, *Egypt* **106 J7** 29 45N 31 14 E
Dahūk, *Iraq* **101 D10** 36 50N 43 1 E
Daḩy, Nafūd ad, *Si. Arabia* **98 B4** 22 0N 45 25 E
Dai, *Solomon Is.* **133 L11** 7 54 S 160 40 E
Dai Hao, *Vietnam* **86 C6** 18 1N 106 25 E
Dai-Sen, *Japan* **72 B5** 35 22N 133 32 E
Dai Shan, *China* **77 B14** 30 25N 122 10 E
Dai Xian, *China* **74 E7** 39 4N 112 58 E
Daicheng, *China* **74 E9** 38 42N 116 38 E
Daigo, *Japan* **73 A12** 36 46N 140 21 E
Daik-u, *Burma* **90 G6** 17 47N 96 40 E
Daimanji-San, *Japan* **72 A5** 36 14N 133 20 E
Daimiel, *Spain* **43 F7** 39 5N 3 35W
Daingean, *Ireland* **23 C4** 53 18N 7 17W
Dainkog, *China* **76 A1** 32 30N 97 58 E
Daintree, *Australia* **126 B4** 16 20 S 145 20 E
Daintree △, *Australia* **126 B4** 16 8 S 145 2 E
Daiō-Misaki, *Japan* **73 C8** 34 15N 136 45 E
Dair, J. ed, *Sudan* **107 E3** 12 27N 30 42 E
Dairen = Dalian, *China* **75 E11** 38 50N 121 40 E
Dairût, *Egypt* **106 B3** 27 34N 30 43 E
Daisen-Oki △, *Japan* **72 B5** 35 23N 133 34 E
Daisetsu-Zan, *Japan* **70 C11** 43 30N 142 57 E
Daisetsu-Zan △, *Japan* **70 C11** 43 30N 142 55 E
Daitari, *India* **94 D7** 21 10N 85 46 E
Daito, *Japan* **72 B4** 35 19N 132 58 E
Dajarra, *Australia* **126 C2** 21 42 S 139 30 E
Dajin Chuan →, *China* **76 B3** 31 16N 101 59 E
Dak Dam, *Cambodia* **86 F6** 12 20N 107 21 E
Dak Nhe, *Vietnam* **86 E6** 15 28N 107 48 E
Dak Pek, *Vietnam* **86 E6** 15 4N 107 44 E
Dak Song, *Vietnam* **87 F6** 12 19N 107 35 E
Dak Sui, *Vietnam* **86 E6** 14 55N 107 43 E
Dakar, *Senegal* **112 C1** 14 34N 17 29W
Dakhin, *Bangla.* **90 D3** 22 30N 90 45 E
Dakhla, *W. Sahara* **110 D1** 23 50N 15 53W
Dakhla, El Wâhât el-, *Egypt* **106 B2** 25 30N 28 50 E
Dakingari, *Nigeria* **113 C5** 11 37N 4 1 E
Dakoank, *India* **95 L11** 7 2N 93 43 E
Dakor, *India* **92 H5** 22 45N 73 11 E
Dakoro, *Niger* **113 C6** 14 31N 6 46 E
Dakota City, *Iowa, U.S.A.* **156 B2** 42 43N 94 12W
Dakota City, *Nebr., U.S.A.* **154 D6** 42 25N 96 25W
Đakovica, *Serbia & M.* **50 D4** 42 22N 20 26 E
Đakovo, *Croatia* **52 E3** 45 19N 18 24 E
Dal, *Norway* **18 E5** 59 53N 8 40 E
Dala, *Lunda Sul, Angola* **115 E4** 11 3 S 20 17 E
Dala, *Uíge, Angola* **115 D3** 8 5 S 15 49 E
Dala, *Solomon Is.* **133 M11** 8 30 S 160 41 E
Dala-Cachibo, *Angola* **115 E2** 10 30 S 14 41 E
Dalaas, *Austria* **33 B10** 47 7N 10 0 E
Dalaba, *Guinea* **112 C2** 10 47N 12 12W
Dalachi, *China* **74 F3** 36 48N 105 0 E
Dalagan = San Antonio, *Phil.* **80 D3** 14 57N 120 5 E
Dalaguete, *Phil.* **81 G4** 9 46N 123 32 E
Dalai Nur, *China* **74 C9** 43 20N 116 45 E
Dālakī, *Iran* **97 D6** 29 26N 51 17 E
Dalälven →, *Sweden* **16 D10** 60 12N 16 43 E
Dalaman, *Turkey* **49 E10** 36 48N 28 47 E
Dalaman →, *Turkey* **49 E10** 36 41N 28 43 E
Dalandzadgad, *Mongolia* **74 C3** 43 27N 104 30 E
Dalanganem Is., *Phil.* **81 F3** 10 40N 120 17 E
Dalap-Uliga-Darrit, *Marshall Is.* **134 G9** 7 7N 171 24 E
Dalarna, *Sweden* **16 D8** 61 0N 14 0 E
Dalarnas län □, *Sweden* **16 C8** 61 0N 14 15 E
Dalasýsla □, *Iceland* **11 B4** 65 15N 22 0W
Dalat, *Malaysia* **85 B4** 2 44N 111 56 E
Dālbandīn, *Pakistan* **91 C2** 29 0N 64 23 E
Dalbeattie, *U.K.* **22 G5** 54 56N 3 50W
Dalbeg, *Australia* **126 C4** 20 16 S 147 18 E
Dalbosjön, *Sweden* **17 F6** 58 40N 12 45 E
Dalby, *Australia* **127 D5** 27 10 S 151 17 E
Dalby, *Sweden* **17 J7** 55 40N 13 22 E
Dalby Söderskog △, *Sweden* **17 J7** 55 41N 13 21 E
Dale, *Norway* **18 C2** 61 22N 5 23 E
Dale, *U.S.A.* **157 F10** 38 10N 86 59W
Dale City, *U.S.A.* **148 F7** 38 38N 77 18W
Dale Hollow L., *U.S.A.* **149 G3** 36 32N 85 27W
Dalen, *Norway* **18 E4** 59 26N 8 0 E
Dalet, *Burma* **90 F4** 19 59N 93 51 E
Daletme, *Burma* **90 E4** 21 36N 92 46 E
Daleville, *Ala., U.S.A.* **152 D4** 31 19N 85 43W
Daleville, *Ind., U.S.A.* **157 D11** 40 7N 85 33W
Dalga, *Egypt* **106 B3** 27 39N 30 41 E
Dalgān, *Iran* **97 E8** 27 31N 59 19 E
Dalhart, *U.S.A.* **155 G3** 36 4N 102 31W
Dalhousie, *Canada* **141 C6** 48 5N 66 26W
Dalhousie, *India* **92 C6** 32 38N 75 58 E
Dali, *Shaanxi, China* **74 G5** 34 48N 109 58 E
Dali, *Yunnan, China* **76 E3** 25 40N 100 10 E
Dalian, *China* **75 E11** 38 50N 121 40 E
Daliang Shan, *China* **76 D4** 28 0N 102 45 E
Daling He →, *China* **75 D11** 40 55N 121 40 E
Dāliyat el Karmel, *Israel* **103 C4** 32 43N 35 2 E
Dalj, *Croatia* **52 E3** 45 29N 18 59 E
Dalkeith, *U.K.* **22 F5** 55 54N 3 4W
Dalkeith, *U.S.A.* **152 E4** 30 0N 85 9W
Dallas, *Ga., U.S.A.* **152 B5** 33 55N 84 51W
Dallas, *Oreg., U.S.A.* **158 D2** 44 55N 123 19W
Dallas, *Tex., U.S.A.* **155 J6** 32 47N 96 49W
Dallas Center, *U.S.A.* **156 C3** 41 41N 93 58W
Dallas City, *U.S.A.* **156 D5** 40 38N 91 10W
Dalle = Yirga Alem, *Ethiopia* **107 F4** 6 48N 38 22 E
Dallol, *Ethiopia* **107 E5** 14 14N 40 17 E
Dalmā, *U.A.E.* **97 E7** 24 30N 52 20 E
Dalmacija, *Croatia* **45 E13** 43 20N 17 0 E
Dalmas, L., *Canada* **141 B5** 53 30N 71 50W
Dalmatia = Dalmacija, *Croatia* **45 E13** 43 20N 17 0 E
Dalmatovo, *Russia* **64 C9** 56 16N 62 56 E
Dalmau, *India* **93 F9** 26 4N 81 2 E
Dalmellington, *U.K.* **22 F4** 55 19N 4 23W
Dalmeny, *Australia* **129 D9** 36 10 S 150 8 E
Dalnegorsk, *Russia* **67 E14** 44 32N 135 33 E
Dalnerechensk, *Russia* **67 E14** 45 50N 133 40 E
Dalnevostochnyy □, *Russia* **67 C14** 67 0N 140 0 E
Dalny = Dalian, *China* **75 E11** 38 50N 121 40 E
Daloa, *Ivory C.* **112 D3** 7 0N 6 30W
Dalou Shan, *China* **76 C6** 28 15N 107 0 E
Dalry, *U.K.* **22 F4** 55 42N 4 43W
Dalrymple, L., *Australia* **126 C4** 20 40 S 147 0 E
Dalrymple, Mt., *Australia* **126 K6** 21 1 S 148 39 E
Dals Långed, *Sweden* **17 F6** 58 56N 12 18 E
Dalseter, *Norway* **18 C6** 61 28N 9 26 E
Dalsjöfors, *Sweden* **17 G7** 57 46N 13 5 E
Dalsland, *Sweden* **17 F6** 58 50N 12 15 E
Dalsmynni, *Iceland* **11 C5** 64 48N 21 29W
Daltenganj, *India* **93 H11** 24 0N 84 4 E
Dalton, *Ga., U.S.A.* **149 H3** 34 46N 84 58W
Dalton, *Mass., U.S.A.* **151 D11** 42 28N 73 11W
Dalton, *Nebr., U.S.A.* **154 E3** 41 25N 102 58W
Dalton, Kap, *Greenland* **10 D8** 69 25N 24 3W
Dalton-in-Furness, *U.K.* **20 C4** 54 10N 3 11W
Dalupiri I., *Cagayan, Phil.* **80 B3** 19 5N 121 12 E
Dalupiri I., *N. Samar, Phil.* **80 E5** 12 25N 124 16 E
Dalvík, *Iceland* **11 B8** 65 58N 18 32W
Dálvvadis = Jokkmokk, *Sweden* **14 C18** 66 35N 19 50 E
Dalwallinu, *Australia* **125 F2** 30 17 S 116 40 E
Daly →, *Australia* **124 B5** 13 35 S 130 19 E
Daly City, *U.S.A.* **160 H4** 37 42N 122 28W
Daly L., *Canada* **143 B7** 56 32N 105 39W
Daly River, *Australia* **124 B5** 13 46 S 130 42 E
Daly Waters, *Australia* **126 B1** 16 15 S 133 24 E
Dalyan, *Turkey* **49 E10** 36 50N 28 39 E
Dam Doi, *Vietnam* **87 H5** 8 50N 105 12 E
Dam Ha, *Vietnam* **86 B6** 21 21N 107 36 E
Damachova, *Belarus* **55 G10** 51 45N 23 36 E
Daman, *India* **94 D1** 20 25N 72 57 E
Daman & Diu □, *India* **94 D1** 20 25N 72 58 E
Dāmaneh, *Iran* **97 C6** 33 1N 50 29 E
Damanganga →, *India* **94 D1** 20 25N 72 56 E
Damanhûr, *Egypt* **106 H7** 31 0N 30 30 E
Damant L., *Canada* **143 A7** 61 45N 105 5W
Damanzhuang, *China* **74 E9** 38 5N 116 35 E
Damar, *Indonesia* **82 C3** 7 7 S 128 40 E
Damara, *C.A.R.* **114 B3** 4 58N 18 42 E
Damaraland, *Namibia* **116 C2** 20 0 S 15 0 E
Damascus = Dimashq, *Syria* **103 B5** 33 30N 36 18 E
Damascus, *U.S.A.* **152 D5** 31 18N 84 43W
Damaturu, *Nigeria* **113 C7** 11 45N 11 55 E
Damāvand, *Iran* **97 C7** 35 47N 52 0 E
Damāvand, Qolleh-ye, *Iran* **97 C7** 35 56N 52 10 E
Damba, *Angola* **115 D3** 6 44 S 15 20 E
Dâmboviţa □, *Romania* **53 F10** 45 0N 25 30 E
Dâmboviţa →, *Romania* **53 F11** 44 12N 26 26 E
Dâmbovnic →, *Romania* **53 F10** 44 28N 25 18 E
Dambrowica = Dubrovytsya, *Ukraine* **59 G4** 51 31N 26 35 E
Dambulla, *Sri Lanka* **95 L5** 7 51N 80 39 E
Dame Marie, *Haiti* **165 C5** 18 36N 74 26W
Dāmghān, *Iran* **97 B7** 36 10N 54 17 E
Dămienesti, *Romania* **53 D11** 46 44N 26 59 E
Damietta = Dumyât, *Egypt* **106 H7** 31 24N 31 48 E
Daming, *China* **74 F8** 36 15N 115 6 E
Damīr Qābū, *Syria* **96 B4** 36 58N 41 51 E
Dammai I., *Phil.* **81 J3** 5 47N 120 25 E
Dammam = Ad Dammām, *Si. Arabia* **97 E6** 26 20N 50 5 E
Dammarie-les-Lys, *France* **27 D9** 48 31N 2 39 E
Dammartin-en-Goële, *France* **27 C9** 49 3N 2 41 E
Dammastock, *Switz.* **33 C6** 46 38N 8 24 E
Damme, *Germany* **30 C4** 52 32N 8 11 E
Damodar →, *India* **93 H12** 23 17N 87 35 E
Damoh, *India* **93 H8** 23 50N 79 28 E
Damous, *Algeria* **111 A5** 36 31N 1 42 E
Dampier, *Australia* **124 D2** 20 41 S 116 42 E
Dampier, Selat, *Indonesia* **83 B4** 0 40 S 131 0 E
Dampier Arch., *Australia* **124 D2** 20 38 S 116 32 E
Dampier Str., *Papua N. G.* **132 C5** 5 50 S 148 0 E
Dampierre-sur-Salon, *France* **32 A1** 47 33N 5 41 E
Damqawt, *Yemen* **99 C6** 16 34N 52 50 E
Damrani, *Algeria* **110 C4** 27 45N 2 56W
Damrei, Chuor Phnum, *Cambodia* **87 G4** 11 30N 103 0 E
Damroh, *India* **90 A5** 28 26N 95 14 E
Damüls, *Austria* **33 B9** 47 17N 9 53 E
Damvillers, *France* **27 C12** 49 20N 5 21 E
Dan-Gulbi, *Nigeria* **113 C6** 11 40N 6 15 E
Dana, *Indonesia* **82 D2** 11 0 S 122 52 E
Dana, L., *Canada* **140 B4** 50 53N 77 20W
Dana, Mt., *U.S.A.* **160 H7** 37 54N 119 12W
Danakil Desert, *Ethiopia* **107 E5** 12 45N 41 0 E
Danané, *Ivory C.* **112 D3** 7 16N 8 9W
Danao, *Phil.* **81 F5** 10 31N 124 1 E
Danau Poso, *Indonesia* **79 E6** 1 52 S 120 35 E
Danba, *China* **76 B3** 30 54N 101 48 E
Danbury, *U.S.A.* **151 E11** 41 24N 73 28W
Danby L., *U.S.A.* **159 J6** 34 13N 115 5W
Dand, *Afghan.* **91 C2** 31 28N 65 32 E
Dande ⌓, *Zimbabwe* **119 F3** 15 56 S 30 16 E
Dande →, *Angola* **115 D2** 6 15 S 15 34 E
Dandeldhura, *Nepal* **93 E9** 29 20N 80 35 E
Dandeli, *India* **95 G2** 15 5N 74 30 E
Dandenong, *Australia* **129 E6** 38 0 S 145 15 E
Dandîl, *Egypt* **106 J7** 29 10N 31 2 E
Dandong, *China* **75 D13** 40 10N 124 20 E
Danfeng, *China* **74 H6** 33 45N 110 25 E
Dangan Liedao, *China* **77 F10** 22 2N 114 8 E
Dangara, *Tajikistan* **65 D4** 38 6N 69 22 E
Dange, *Angola* **115 D3** 7 56 S 15 3 E
Dangé-St-Romain, *France* **28 B4** 46 56N 0 36 E
Dângeni, *Romania* **53 C11** 47 51N 26 58 E
Danger Is. = Pukapuka, *Cook Is.* **135 J11** 10 53 S 165 49W
Danger Pt., *S. Africa* **116 E2** 34 40 S 19 17 E
Danginpuri, *Indonesia* **79 K18** 8 40 S 115 13 E
Dangla, *Ethiopia* **107 E4** 11 18N 36 56 E
Dangla Shan = Tanggula Shan, *China* **68 C4** 32 40N 92 10 E
Dangora, *Nigeria* **113 C6** 11 30N 8 7 E
Dangouadougou, *Burkina Faso* **112 D4** 10 9N 4 56W
Dangrek, Phnom, *Thailand* **86 E5** 14 15N 105 0 E
Dangriga, *Belize* **163 D7** 17 0N 88 13W
Dangshan, *China* **74 G9** 34 27N 116 22 E
Dangtu, *China* **77 B12** 31 32N 118 25 E
Dangyang, *China* **77 B8** 30 52N 111 44 E
Dani, *Burkina Faso* **113 C4** 13 43N 0 10W
Daniel, *U.S.A.* **158 E8** 42 52N 110 4W
Daniel's Harbour, *Canada* **141 B8** 50 13N 57 35W
Danielskuil, *S. Africa* **116 D3** 28 11 S 23 33 E
Danielson, *U.S.A.* **151 E13** 41 48N 71 53W
Danielsville, *U.S.A.* **152 A6** 34 8N 83 13W
Danilov, *Russia* **58 C11** 58 16N 40 13 E
Danilovgrad, *Serbia & M.* **50 D3** 42 38N 19 4 E

Danilovka, Russia 60 E7 50 25N 44 12 E
Daning, China 74 F6 36 28N 110 45 E
Danish West Indies = Virgin Is. (U.S.) ☑, W. Indies 165 e 18 20N 65 0W
Danja, Nigeria 113 C6 11 21N 7 30 E
Danje-la-Menha, Angola 115 D2 9 32 S 14 39 E
Danjiangkou, China 77 A8 32 31N 111 30 E
Danjiangkou Shuiku, China 77 A8 32 37N 111 30 E
Ḑank, Oman 97 F8 23 33N 56 16 E
Dankalwa, Nigeria 113 C7 11 52N 12 12 E
Dankama, Nigeria 113 C6 13 20N 7 44 E
Dankov, Russia 58 F10 53 20N 39 5 E
Danleng, China 76 B4 30 1N 103 31 E
Danlí, Honduras 164 D2 14 4N 86 35W
Danmark = Denmark ■, Europe 17 J3 55 45N 10 0 E
Danmark Fjord, Greenland 10 A8 81 30N 22 0W
Danmarkshavn, Greenland 10 B9 76 45N 18 50W
Dannemora, U.S.A. 151 B11 44 43N 73 44W
Dannenberg, Germany 30 B7 53 6N 11 5 E
Dannevirke, N.Z. 130 G5 40 12 S 176 8 E
Dannhauser, S. Africa 117 D5 28 0 S 30 3 E
Danot, Ethiopia 120 C3 7 33N 45 17 E
Dansalan = Marawi City, Phil. 81 G5 8 0N 124 21 E
Dansville, U.S.A. 150 D7 42 34N 77 42W
Danta, India 92 G5 24 11N 72 46 E
Dantan, India 93 J12 21 57N 87 20 E
Dantewara, India 94 E5 18 54N 81 21 E
Danube = Dunărea →, Europe 53 E14 45 20N 29 40 E
Danubyu, Burma 90 G5 17 15N 95 35 E
Danvers, U.S.A. 151 D14 42 34N 70 56W
Danville, Ga., U.S.A. 152 C6 32 37N 83 15W
Danville, Ill., U.S.A. 157 D9 40 8N 87 37W
Danville, Ind., U.S.A. 157 E10 39 46N 86 32W
Danville, Ky., U.S.A. 157 G12 37 39N 84 46W
Danville, Pa., U.S.A. 151 F8 40 58N 76 37W
Danville, Va., U.S.A. 149 G6 36 36N 79 23W
Danville, Vt., U.S.A. 151 B12 44 25N 72 9W
Danyang, China 77 B12 32 0N 119 31 E
Danzhai, China 76 D6 26 11N 107 48 E
Danzhou, China 86 C7 19 31N 109 33 E
Danzig = Gdańsk, Poland 54 D5 54 22N 18 40 E
Dao = Tobias Fornier, Phil. 81 F3 10 30N 121 57 E
Dao, Phil. 81 F4 11 24N 122 41 E
Dão →, Portugal 42 E2 40 20N 8 11W
Dao Xian, China 77 E8 25 36N 111 31 E
Daocheng, China 76 C3 29 0N 100 10 E
Daora, W. Sahara 110 C2 27 5N 12 59W
Daoud = Aïn Beïda, Algeria 111 A6 35 50N 7 29 E
Daoukro, Ivory C. 112 D4 7 10N 3 58W
Dapa, Phil. 81 G6 9 46N 126 3 E
Dapaong, Togo 113 C5 10 55N 0 16 E
Dapchi, Nigeria 113 C7 12 32N 11 31 E
Dapiak, Mt., Phil. 81 G4 8 15N 123 28 E
Dapitan, Phil. 81 G4 8 39N 123 25 E
Dapoli, India 94 F1 17 46N 73 11 E
Daqing Shan, China 74 D6 40 40N 111 0 E
Daqu Shan, China 77 B14 30 25N 122 20 E
Dar Banda, Africa 104 F6 8 0N 23 0 E
Dar el Beida = Casablanca, Morocco 110 B3 33 36N 7 36W
Dar es Salaam, Tanzania 118 D4 6 50 S 39 12 E
Dar Mazār, Iran 97 D8 29 14N 57 20 E
Dar Rounga, C.A.R. 114 A4 0 45N 22 20 E
Dar'ā, Syria 103 C5 32 36N 36 7 E
Dar'ā □, Syria 103 C5 32 55N 36 10 E
Dara Dere = Zlatograd, Bulgaria 51 E9 41 22N 25 7 E
Dārāb, Iran 97 D7 28 50N 54 30 E
Daraban, Pakistan 92 D4 31 44N 70 20 E
Darabani, Romania 53 B11 48 10N 26 39 E
Darai Hills, Papua N. G. 132 D2 7 8 S 143 33 E
Daraina, Madag. 117 A8 13 12 S 49 40 E
Daraj, Libya 108 B2 30 10N 10 28 E
Daram, Phil. 81 F5 11 38N 124 48 E
Dārān, Iran 97 C6 32 59N 50 24 E
Daraut Kurgan = Daroot-Korgan, Kyrgyzstan 65 D6 39 33N 72 11 E
Daravica, Serbia & M. 50 D4 42 32N 20 8 E
Daraw, Egypt 106 C3 24 22N 32 51 E
Dārayyā, Syria 103 B5 33 28N 36 15 E
Darazo, Nigeria 113 C7 11 1N 10 24 E
Darband, Pakistan 92 B5 34 20N 72 50 E
Darband, Kūh-e, Iran 97 D8 31 34N 57 8 E
Darbhanga, India 93 F11 26 15N 85 55 E
Darburruk, Somali Rep. 120 C2 9 44N 44 31 E
Darby, C., U.S.A. 144 D7 64 19N 162 47W
D'Arcy, Canada 142 C4 50 27N 122 35W
Darda, Croatia 52 E3 45 40N 18 41 E
Dardanelle, Ark., U.S.A. 155 H8 35 13N 93 9W
Dardanelle, Calif., U.S.A. 160 G7 38 20N 119 50W
Dardanelles = Çanakkale Boğazı, Turkey 51 F10 40 17N 26 32 E
Dare →, Ethiopia 107 F5 7 20N 42 11 E
Darende, Turkey 100 C7 38 31N 37 30 E
Dārestān, Iran 97 D8 29 9N 58 42 E
Darfield, N.Z. 131 D7 43 29 S 172 7 E
Darfo, Italy 44 C7 45 53N 10 11 E
Dârfûr, Sudan 104 E6 13 40N 24 0 E
Dargai, Pakistan 92 B4 34 25N 71 55 E
Dargan Ata, Turkmenistan 66 E7 40 29N 62 10 E
Dargaville, N.Z. 130 B2 35 57 S 173 52 E
Dargol, Niger 113 C5 13 54N 1 22 E
Darhan, Mongolia 68 B5 49 37N 106 21 E
Darhan Muminggan Lianheqi, China 74 D6 41 40N 110 28 E
Dari, Sudan 107 F3 5 48N 30 26 E
Darıca, Turkey 100 B3 40 45N 29 23 E
Darien, U.S.A. 152 D8 31 23N 81 26W
Darién △, Panama 164 E4 7 36N 77 57W
Darién, G. del, Colombia 168 B2 9 0N 77 0W
Dariganga = Ovoot, Mongolia 74 B7 45 21N 113 45 E
Daringbadi, India 94 E7 19 54N 84 8 E
Darinskoye, Kazakhstan 60 E10 51 20N 51 44 E
Darjeeling = Darjiling, India 90 B2 27 3N 88 18 E
Darjiling, India 90 B2 27 3N 88 18 E
Darkan, Australia 125 F2 33 20 S 116 43 E
Darke Peak, Australia 128 B2 33 27 S 136 12 E
Darkhana, Pakistan 92 D5 30 39N 72 11 E
Darkhazīneh, Iran 97 D6 31 54N 48 39 E
Darkot Pass, Pakistan 65 E6 36 45N 73 26 E
Darling →, Australia 128 C4 34 4 S 141 54 E
Darling Downs, Australia 127 D5 27 30 S 150 30 E
Darling Ra., Australia 125 F2 32 30 S 116 0 E
Darlington, U.K. 20 C6 54 32N 1 33W
Darlington, Fla., U.S.A. 152 E3 30 57N 86 3W
Darlington, S.C., U.S.A. 149 H6 34 18N 79 52W
Darlington, Wis., U.S.A. 156 B6 42 41N 90 7W
Darlington □, U.K. 20 C6 54 32N 1 33W
Darlington, L., S. Africa 116 E4 33 10 S 25 9 E
Darlington Point, Australia 129 C7 34 37 S 146 1 E
Darlot, L., Australia 125 E3 27 48 S 121 35 E
Darłowo, Poland 54 D3 54 25N 16 25 E
Dărmăneşti, Bacău, Romania 53 D11 46 21N 26 33 E
Dărmăneşti, Suceava, Romania 53 C11 47 44N 26 9 E
Darmstadt, Germany 31 F4 49 51N 8 39 E
Darnah, Libya 108 B4 32 45N 22 45 E
Darnah □, Libya 108 B4 31 0N 23 40 E
Darnall, S. Africa 117 D5 29 23 S 31 18 E
Darney, France 27 D13 48 5N 6 2 E
Darnick, Australia 128 B5 32 48 S 143 38 E
Darnley, C., Antarctica 7 C6 68 0 S 69 0 E
Darnley B., Canada 138 B7 69 30N 123 30W
Daroca, Spain 40 D3 41 9N 1 25W
Daroot-Korgan, Kyrgyzstan 65 D6 39 33N 72 11 E
Darou-Mousti, Senegal 112 B1 15 3N 16 3W
Darr →, Australia 126 C3 23 39 S 143 50 E
Darra Pezu, Pakistan 92 C4 32 19N 70 44 E
Darran Mts., N.Z. 131 E2 44 37 S 167 59 E
Darrequeira, Argentina 174 D3 37 42 S 63 10W
Darrington, U.S.A. 158 B3 48 15N 121 36W
Darsana, Bangla. 90 D2 23 35N 88 48 E
Darsi, India 95 G4 15 46N 79 44 E
Darsser Ort, Germany 30 A8 54 28N 12 32 E
Dart →, U.K. 21 G4 50 24N 3 39W
Dart, C., Antarctica 7 D14 73 6 S 126 20W
Dartford, U.K. 21 F8 51 26N 0 13 E
Dartmoor, Australia 128 D4 37 56 S 141 19 E
Dartmoor, U.K. 21 G4 50 38N 3 57W
Dartmoor △, U.K. 21 G4 50 37N 3 59W
Dartmouth, Canada 141 D7 44 40N 63 30W
Dartmouth, U.K. 21 G4 50 21N 3 36W
Dartmouth, L., Australia 129 D7 36 34 S 147 32 E
Dartmouth Res., Australia 127 D4 26 4 S 145 18 E
Dartuch, C. = Artrutx, C. de, Spain 38 B4 39 55N 3 49 E
Daru, Papua N. G. 132 E2 9 3 S 143 13 E
Daruba, Indonesia 82 A3 2 5N 128 14 E
Daruvar, Croatia 52 E2 45 35N 17 14 E
Darvaza, Turkmenistan 66 E6 40 11N 58 24 E
Darvel, Teluk = Lahad Datu, Telok, Malaysia 85 B5 4 50N 118 20 E
Darwen, U.K. 20 D5 53 42N 2 29W
Darwendale, Zimbabwe 117 B5 17 41 S 30 33 E
Darwha, India 94 D3 20 15N 77 45 E
Darwin, Australia 124 B5 12 25 S 130 51 E
Darwin, U.S.A. 161 J9 36 15N 117 35W
Darwin, Mt., Chile 176 D3 54 47 S 69 55W
Darwin, Volcán, Ecuador 172 a 0 10 S 91 18W
Darya Khan, Pakistan 92 D4 31 48N 71 6 E
Daryapur, India 94 D3 20 55N 77 20 E
Daryoi Amu = Amudarya →, Uzbekistan 66 E6 43 58N 59 34 E
Dās, U.A.E. 97 E7 25 20N 53 30 E
Dashen, Ras, Ethiopia 107 E4 13 8N 38 26 E
Dasher, U.S.A. 152 E6 30 45N 83 13W
Dashetai, China 74 D5 41 0N 109 5 E
Dashhowuz, Turkmenistan 66 E6 41 49N 59 58 E
Dashkesan = Daşkäsän, Azerbaijan 61 K7 40 25N 46 0 E
Dashköpri, Turkmenistan 97 B9 36 16N 62 8 E
Dasht, Iran 97 B8 37 17N 56 7 E
Dasht →, Pakistan 91 D1 25 10N 61 40 E
Dasht-i-Tahlab, Pakistan 91 C1 28 40N 62 25 E
Daska, Pakistan 92 C6 32 20N 74 20 E
Daşkäsän, Azerbaijan 61 K7 40 25N 46 0 E
Dasmariñas, Phil. 80 D3 14 20N 120 56 E
Dassa, Benin 113 D5 7 46N 2 14 E
Dasuya, India 92 D6 31 49N 75 38 E
Datça, Turkey 49 E9 36 46N 27 40 E
Datia, India 93 G8 25 39N 78 27 E
Datian, China 77 E11 25 40N 117 50 E
Datong, Anhui, China 77 B11 30 48N 117 44 E
Datong, Shanxi, China 74 D7 40 6N 113 18 E
Dattakhel, Pakistan 92 C3 32 54N 69 46 E
Dattapur = Dhamangaon, India 94 D4 20 48N 78 9 E
Datteln, Germany 30 D3 51 39N 7 21 E
Datu, Tanjung, Indonesia 85 B3 2 5N 109 39 E
Datu Piang, Phil. 81 H5 7 2N 124 30 E
Datuk, Tanjong = Datu, Tanjung, Indonesia 85 B3 2 5N 109 39 E
Daua = Dawa →, Africa 107 G5 4 11N 42 6 E
Daud Khel, Pakistan 92 C4 32 53N 71 34 E
Daudnagar, India 93 G11 25 2N 84 24 E
Daugava →, Latvia 15 H21 57 4N 24 3 E
Daugavpils, Latvia 15 J22 55 53N 26 32 E
Daulatabad, India 94 E2 19 57N 75 15 E
Daule, Ecuador 168 D2 1 56 S 79 56W
Daule →, Ecuador 168 D2 2 10 S 79 52W
Daulpur, India 92 F7 26 45N 77 59 E
Daun, Germany 31 E2 50 11N 6 49 E
Daund, India 94 E2 18 26N 74 40 E
Dauphin, Canada 143 C8 51 9N 100 5W
Dauphin, U.S.A. 150 F8 40 22N 76 56W
Dauphin L., Canada 143 C9 51 20N 99 45W
Dauphiné, France 29 C9 45 15N 5 25 E
Daura, Borno, Nigeria 113 C7 11 31N 11 24 E
Daura, Katsina, Nigeria 113 C6 13 2N 8 21 E
Dausa, India 92 F7 26 52N 76 20 E
Däväçi, Azerbaijan 61 K9 41 15N 48 57 E
Davangere, India 95 G2 14 25N 75 55 E
Davao, Phil. 81 H5 7 0N 125 40 E
Davao □, Phil. 81 H5 7 0N 125 55 E
Davao del Sur □, Phil. 81 H5 6 30N 125 25 E
Davao G., Phil. 81 H5 6 30N 125 48 E
Davao Oriental □, Phil. 81 H6 7 10N 126 30 E
Dāvar Panāh = Sarāvān, Iran 97 E9 27 25N 62 15 E
Davenport, Calif., U.S.A. 160 H4 37 1N 122 12W
Davenport, Fla., U.S.A. 153 G8 28 10N 81 36W
Davenport, Iowa, U.S.A. 156 C6 41 32N 90 35W
Davenport, Wash., U.S.A. 158 C4 47 39N 118 9W
Davenport Ra., Australia 126 C1 20 28 S 134 0 E
Daventry, U.K. 21 E6 52 16N 1 10W
David, Panama 164 E3 8 30N 82 30W
David City, U.S.A. 154 E6 41 15N 97 8W
David Gorodok = Davyd Haradok, Belarus 59 F4 52 4N 27 8 E
Davidson, Canada 143 C7 51 16N 105 59W
Davis, Antarctica 7 C6 68 34 S 77 55 E
Davis, U.S.A. 160 G5 38 33N 121 44W
Davis Dam, U.S.A. 161 K12 35 11N 114 34W
Davis Inlet, Canada 141 A7 55 50N 60 59W
Davis Mts., U.S.A. 155 K2 30 50N 103 55W
Davis Sea, Antarctica 7 C7 66 0 S 92 0 E
Davis Str., N. Amer. 139 B14 65 0N 58 0W
Davisboro, U.S.A. 152 C7 32 59N 82 36W
Davison, U.S.A. 157 A13 43 2N 83 31W
Davlekanovo, Russia 64 D5 54 13N 55 3 E
Davo →, Ivory C. 112 D3 5 0N 6 10W
Davos, Switz. 33 C9 46 48N 9 49 E
Davutlar, Turkey 49 D9 37 43N 27 17 E
Davy L., Canada 143 B7 58 53N 108 18W
Davyd Haradok, Belarus 59 F4 52 4N 27 8 E
Dawa →, Africa 107 G5 4 11N 42 6 E
Dawaki, Bauchi, Nigeria 113 D6 9 25N 9 33 E
Dawaki, Kano, Nigeria 113 C6 12 5N 8 23 E
Dawei = Tavoy, Burma 86 E2 14 2N 98 12 E
Dawes Ra., Australia 126 C5 24 40 S 150 40 E
Dawley = Telford, U.K. 21 E5 52 40N 2 27W
Dawlish, U.K. 21 G4 50 35N 3 28W
Dawna Ra., Burma 86 D2 16 30N 98 30 E
Dawnyein, Burma 90 G5 15 54N 95 36 E
Dawqah, Si. Arabia 98 C3 19 36N 40 54 E
Dawros Hd., Ireland 23 B3 54 50N 8 33W
Dawson, Canada 138 B6 64 10N 139 30W
Dawson, Ga., U.S.A. 152 D5 31 46N 84 27W
Dawson, I., Chile 176 D2 53 50 S 70 50W
Dawson B., Canada 143 C8 52 53N 100 49W
Dawson Creek, Canada 142 B4 55 45N 120 15W
Dawson Inlet, Canada 143 A10 61 50N 93 25W
Dawson Ra., Australia 126 C4 24 30 S 149 48 E
Dawu, Hubei, China 77 B9 31 34N 114 7 E
Dawu, Sichuan, China 76 B3 30 55N 101 10 E
Dawwah, Oman 99 B7 20 33N 58 48 E
Dawwara, Ras id-, Malta 38 F7 35 52N 14 21 E
Dax, France 28 E2 43 44N 1 3W
Daxian, China 76 B6 31 15N 107 23 E
Daxin, China 76 F6 22 50N 107 11 E
Daxindian, China 75 F11 37 30N 120 50 E
Daxinggou, China 75 C15 43 25N 129 40 E
Daxue Shan, Sichuan, China 76 B3 30 30N 101 30 E
Daxue Shan, Yunnan, China 76 F2 23 42N 99 48 E
Day, U.S.A. 152 E6 30 12N 83 17W
Daya el Khadra, Mauritania 110 C3 25 14N 6 2W
Dayao, China 76 E3 25 43N 101 20 E
Daye, China 77 B10 30 6N 114 58 E
Dayet en Naharat, Mali 112 B4 17 39N 3 10W
Dayi, China 76 B4 30 41N 103 29 E
Daylesford, Australia 128 D6 37 21 S 144 9 E
Dayong, China 77 C8 29 11N 110 30 E
Dayr az Zawr, Syria 101 E9 35 20N 40 5 E
Daysland, Canada 142 C6 52 50N 112 20W
Dayton, Iowa, U.S.A. 156 B2 42 14N 94 6W
Dayton, Ky., U.S.A. 157 E12 39 47N 84 28W
Dayton, Nev., U.S.A. 160 F7 39 14N 119 36W
Dayton, Ohio, U.S.A. 148 F3 39 45N 84 12W
Dayton, Pa., U.S.A. 150 F5 40 53N 79 15W
Dayton, Tenn., U.S.A. 149 H3 35 30N 85 1W
Dayton, Wash., U.S.A. 158 C4 46 19N 117 59W
Dayton, Wyo., U.S.A. 158 D10 44 53N 107 16W
Daytona Beach, U.S.A. 153 F8 29 13N 81 1W
Dayu, China 77 E10 25 24N 114 22 E
Dayville, U.S.A. 158 D4 44 28N 119 32W
Dazaifu, Japan 72 D2 33 32N 130 32 E
Dazhu, China 76 B6 30 41N 107 15 E
Dazkırı, Turkey 49 D11 37 57N 29 52 E
Dazu, China 76 C5 29 40N 105 42 E
De Aar, S. Africa 116 E3 30 39 S 24 0 E
De Armanville, U.S.A. 152 B4 33 38N 85 45W
De Bary, U.S.A. 153 G8 28 54N 81 18W
De Biesbosch △, Neths. 24 C4 51 45N 4 48 E
De Forest, U.S.A. 156 A7 43 15N 89 20W
De Funiak Springs, U.S.A. 152 E3 30 43N 86 7W
De Grey →, Australia 124 D2 20 12 S 119 13 E
De Haan, Belgium 24 C3 51 16N 3 2 E
De Hoge Veluwe △, Neths. 24 B5 52 5N 5 46 E
De Hoop △, S. Africa 116 E3 34 30 S 20 28 E
De Jongs, Tg., Indonesia 83 C5 6 55 S 138 30 E
De Kalb, U.S.A. 154 E10 41 56N 88 46W
De Kennemerduinen △, Neths. 24 B4 52 27N 4 33 E
De Land, U.S.A. 153 F8 29 2N 81 18W
De Leon, U.S.A. 155 J5 32 7N 98 32W
De Leon Springs, U.S.A. 153 F8 29 7N 81 21W
De Long Mts., U.S.A. 144 B7 68 30N 163 0W
De Panne, Belgium 24 C2 51 6N 2 34 E
De Pere, U.S.A. 148 C1 44 27N 88 4W
De Queen, U.S.A. 155 H7 34 2N 94 21W
De Quincy, U.S.A. 155 K8 30 27N 93 26W
De Ridder, U.S.A. 155 K8 30 51N 93 17W
De Smet, U.S.A. 154 C6 44 23N 97 33W
De Soto, U.S.A. 156 F6 38 8N 90 34W
De Soto City, U.S.A. 153 H8 27 27N 81 24W
De Tour Village, U.S.A. 148 C4 46 0N 83 56W
De Witt, Ark., U.S.A. 155 H9 34 18N 91 20W
De Witt, Iowa, U.S.A. 156 C6 41 49N 90 33W
De Witt, Mich., U.S.A. 157 B12 42 51N 84 34W
Dead L., U.S.A. 152 E4 30 10N 85 10W
Dead Sea, Asia 103 D4 31 30N 35 30 E
Deadhorse, U.S.A. 144 A10 70 11N 148 27W
Deadman B., U.S.A. 152 F6 29 30N 83 30W
Deadwood, U.S.A. 154 C3 44 23N 103 44W
Deadwood L., Canada 142 B3 59 10N 128 30W
Deal, U.K. 21 F9 51 13N 1 25 E
Deal I., Australia 127 F4 39 30 S 147 20 E
Dealesville, S. Africa 116 D4 28 41 S 25 44 E
De'an, China 77 C10 29 21N 115 46 E
Dean →, Canada 142 C3 52 49N 126 58W
Dean, Forest of, U.K. 21 F5 51 45N 2 33W
Dean Chan., Canada 142 C3 52 30N 127 15W
Deán Funes, Argentina 174 C3 30 20 S 64 20W
Dearborn, Mich., U.S.A. 157 B13 42 19N 83 11W
Dearborn, Mo., U.S.A. 156 E2 39 32N 94 46W
Dease →, Canada 142 B3 59 56N 128 32W
Dease L., Canada 142 B2 58 40N 130 5W
Dease Lake, Canada 142 B2 58 25N 130 6W
Death Valley, U.S.A. 161 J10 36 15N 116 50W
Death Valley △, U.S.A. 161 J10 36 45N 117 15W
Death Valley Junction, U.S.A. 161 J10 36 20N 116 25W
Deauville, France 26 C7 49 23N 0 2 E
Deba, Spain 40 B2 43 18N 2 21W
Deba Habe, Nigeria 113 C7 10 14N 11 20 E
Debak, Malaysia 85 B4 1 34N 111 25 E
Debaltsevo, Ukraine 59 H10 48 22N 38 26 E
Debao, China 76 F6 23 21N 106 46 E
Debar, Macedonia 50 E4 41 31N 20 30 E
Debark, Ethiopia 107 E4 13 1N 37 48 E
Debden, Canada 143 C7 53 30N 106 50W
Debdou, Morocco 111 B4 33 59N 3 0W
Dębica, Poland 55 H8 50 2N 21 25 E
Dęblin, Poland 55 G8 51 34N 21 50 E
Dębno, Poland 55 F1 52 44N 14 41 E
Débo, L., Mali 112 B4 15 14N 4 15W
DeBolt, Canada 142 B5 55 12N 118 1W
Deborah East, L., Australia 125 F2 30 45 S 119 0 E
Deborah West, L., Australia 125 F2 30 45 S 118 50 E
Deboyne Is., Papua N. G. 132 F7 10 43 S 152 22 E
Debrc, Serbia & M. 50 B3 44 38N 19 53 E
Debre Birhan, Ethiopia 107 F4 9 41N 39 31 E
Debre Markos, Ethiopia 107 E4 10 20N 37 40 E
Debre May, Ethiopia 107 E4 11 20N 37 25 E
Debre Sina, Ethiopia 107 F4 9 51N 39 50 E
Debre Tabor, Ethiopia 107 E4 11 50N 38 26 E
Debre Zebit, Ethiopia 107 E4 11 48N 38 30 E
Debre Zevit, Ethiopia 107 F4 8 50N 39 0 E
Debrecen, Hungary 52 C6 47 33N 21 42 E
Debrzno, Poland 54 E4 53 31N 17 14 E
Dečani, Serbia & M. 50 D4 42 30N 20 18 E
Decatur, Ala., U.S.A. 149 H2 34 36N 86 59W
Decatur, Ga., U.S.A. 152 B5 33 47N 84 18W
Decatur, Ill., U.S.A. 156 E8 39 51N 88 57W
Decatur, Ind., U.S.A. 157 D12 40 50N 84 56W
Decatur, Mich., U.S.A. 157 B11 42 7N 85 58W
Decatur, Tex., U.S.A. 155 J6 33 14N 97 35W
Decazeville, France 28 D6 44 34N 2 15 E
Deccan, India 94 F4 18 0N 79 0 E
Deception, Mt., Australia 128 A3 30 42 S 138 16 E
Deception B., Papua N. G. 132 D3 7 45 S 144 40 E
Deception Bay, Australia 127 D5 27 10 S 153 5 E
Deception I., Antarctica 7 C17 63 0 S 60 15W
Deception L., Canada 143 B8 56 33N 104 13W
Dechang, China 76 D4 27 25N 102 11 E
Dechhu, India 92 F5 26 46N 72 20 E
Děčín, Czech Rep. 34 A7 50 47N 14 12 E
Decize, France 27 F10 46 50N 3 28 E
Deckerville, U.S.A. 150 C2 43 32N 82 44W
Decollatura, Italy 47 C9 39 3N 16 21 E
Decorah, U.S.A. 154 D9 43 18N 91 48W
Deda, Romania 53 D9 46 56N 24 50 E
Dedaye, Burma 90 G5 16 24N 95 53 E
Dedéagach = Alexandroúpolis, Greece 51 F9 40 50N 25 54 E
Deder, Ethiopia 107 F5 9 19N 41 27 E
Dedham, U.S.A. 151 D13 42 15N 71 10W
Dédougou, Burkina Faso 112 C4 12 30N 3 25W
Dedovichi, Russia 58 D5 57 32N 29 56 E
Dedza, Malawi 119 E3 14 20 S 34 20 E
Dee →, Aberds., U.K. 22 D6 57 9N 2 5W
Dee →, Dumf. & Gall., U.K. 22 G4 54 51N 4 3W
Dee →, Wales, U.K. 20 D4 53 22N 3 17W
Deep B., Canada 142 A5 61 15N 116 35W
Deep Bay = Chilumba, Malawi 119 E3 10 28 S 34 12 E
Deep Bay = Shenzhen Wan, China 69 G10 22 27N 113 55 E
Deep Lead, Australia 128 D5 37 0 S 142 43 E
Deepwater, Australia 127 D5 29 25 S 151 51 E
Deepwater, U.S.A. 156 F3 38 16N 93 47W
Deer →, Canada 143 B10 58 23N 94 13W
Deer I., U.S.A. 144 J7 54 55N 162 18W
Deer L., Canada 143 C10 52 40N 94 20W
Deer Lake, Nfld. & L., Canada 141 C8 49 11N 57 27W
Deer Lake, Ont., Canada 143 C10 52 36N 94 20W
Deer Lodge, U.S.A. 158 C7 46 24N 112 44W
Deer Park, Fla., U.S.A. 153 G9 28 6N 80 54W
Deer Park, Ohio, U.S.A. 157 E12 39 13N 84 23W
Deer Park, Wash., U.S.A. 158 C5 47 57N 117 28W
Deer River, U.S.A. 154 B8 47 20N 93 48W
Deeragun, Australia 126 B4 19 16 S 146 33 E
Deerdepoort, S. Africa 116 C4 24 37 S 26 27 E
Deerfield, Ill., U.S.A. 157 B9 42 10N 87 51W
Deerfield, Mo., U.S.A. 156 G2 37 50N 94 30W
Deerfield Beach, U.S.A. 153 J9 26 19N 80 6W
Deering, U.S.A. 144 C7 66 4N 162 42W
Defensores del Chaco △, Paraguay 173 E5 20 13 S 60 27W
Deferiet, U.S.A. 151 B9 44 2N 75 41W
Defiance, U.S.A. 157 C12 41 17N 84 22W
Degana, India 92 F6 26 50N 74 20 E
Dêgê, China 76 B2 31 44N 98 39 E
Degebe →, Portugal 43 G3 38 13N 7 29W
Degeberga, Sweden 17 J8 55 51N 14 5 E
Degeh Bur, Ethiopia 120 C2 8 11N 43 31 E
Dégelis, Canada 141 C6 47 30N 68 35W
Degema, Nigeria 113 E6 4 50N 6 48 E
Degerfors, Sweden 16 E8 59 15N 14 27 E
Degerhamn, Sweden 17 H10 56 20N 16 24 E
Degersheim, Switz. 33 B8 47 23N 9 12 E
Deggendorf, Germany 31 G8 48 50N 12 57 E
Degh →, Pakistan 92 D5 31 3N 73 21 E
Değirmendere, Turkey 51 F13 40 42N 29 47 E
Deh Bīd, Iran 97 D7 30 39N 53 11 E
Deh-e Shīr, Iran 97 D7 31 29N 53 45 E
Deh Nugaled = Nugaaleed, Dooxo, Somali Rep. 120 C3 8 35N 48 35 E
Dehaj, Iran 97 D7 30 42N 54 53 E
Dehak, Iran 91 D1 27 11N 62 37 E
Déhane, Cameroon 114 B2 3 30N 10 5 E
Dehdez, Iran 97 D6 31 43N 50 17 E
Dehej, India 92 J5 21 44N 72 40 E
Dehestān, Iran 97 D7 28 30N 55 35 E
Dehgolān, Iran 101 E12 35 17N 47 25 E
Dehibat, Tunisia 108 B2 32 0N 10 47 E
Dehiwala, Sri Lanka 95 L4 6 50N 79 51 E
Dehlorān, Iran 101 F12 32 41N 47 16 E
Dehnow-e Kūhestān, Iran 97 E8 27 58N 58 32 E
Dehra Dun, India 92 D8 30 20N 78 4 E
Dehri, India 93 G11 24 50N 84 15 E
Dehua, China 77 E12 25 26N 118 14 E
Dehui, China 75 B13 44 30N 125 40 E
Deim Zubeir, Sudan 107 F2 7 49N 26 16 E
Deinze, Belgium 24 D3 50 59N 3 32 E
Dej, Romania 53 C8 47 10N 23 52 E
Deje, Sweden 16 E7 59 35N 13 29 E
Dejiang, China 76 C7 28 18N 108 7 E
Deka →, Zimbabwe 116 B4 18 4 S 26 42 E
Dekemhare, Eritrea 107 D4 15 6N 39 0 E
Dekese, Dem. Rep. of the Congo 114 C4 3 24 S 21 24 E
Dekhkanabad, Uzbekistan 65 D3 38 21N 66 30 E
Dekoa, C.A.R. 114 A3 6 19N 19 4 E
Del Carmen, Phil. 81 G6 9 53N 126 2 E
Del Mar, U.S.A. 161 N9 32 58N 117 16W
Del Norte, U.S.A. 159 H10 37 41N 106 21W
Del Rio, U.S.A. 155 L4 29 22N 100 54W
Delai, Sudan 106 D4 17 21N 36 6 E
Delambre I., Australia 124 D2 20 26 S 117 5 E
Delami, Sudan 107 E3 11 38N 30 23 E
Delano, U.S.A. 161 K7 35 46N 119 15W
Delano Peak, U.S.A. 159 G7 38 22N 112 22W
Delārām, Afghan. 91 B1 32 9N 63 25 E
Delareyville, S. Africa 116 D4 26 41 S 25 26 E
Delaronde L., Canada 143 C7 54 3N 107 3W
Delavan, Ill., U.S.A. 156 D7 40 22N 89 33W
Delavan, Wis., U.S.A. 154 D10 42 38N 88 39W
Delaware, U.S.A. 157 D13 40 18N 83 4W
Delaware □, U.S.A. 148 F8 39 0N 75 20W
Delaware →, U.S.A. 151 G9 39 15N 75 20W
Delaware B., U.S.A. 148 F8 39 0N 75 10W
Delaware Water Gap ⌂, U.S.A. 151 E10 41 10N 74 55W
Delay →, Canada 141 A5 56 56N 71 28W
Delbrück, Germany 30 D4 51 46N 8 34 E
Delčevo, Macedonia 50 E6 41 58N 22 46 E
Delébio, Italy 33 D8 46 8N 9 27 E
Delegate, Australia 129 D8 37 4 S 148 56 E
Delémont, Switz. 32 B4 47 22N 7 20 E
Delevan, U.S.A. 150 D6 42 29N 78 29W
Delft, Neths. 24 B4 52 1N 4 22 E
Delft I., Sri Lanka 95 K4 9 30N 79 40 E
Delfzijl, Neths. 24 A6 53 20N 6 55 E
Delgada, Punta, Chile 176 D3 52 28 S 69 32W
Delgado, C., Mozam. 119 E5 10 45 S 40 40 E
Delgerhet, Mongolia 74 B6 45 50N 110 30 E
Delgo, Sudan 106 C3 20 6N 30 40 E
Delhi, Canada 150 D4 42 51N 80 30W
Delhi, India 92 E7 28 38N 77 17 E
Delhi, La., U.S.A. 155 J9 32 28N 91 30W
Delhi, N.Y., U.S.A. 151 D10 42 17N 74 55W
Deli Jovan, Serbia & M. 50 B6 44 13N 22 9 E
Delia, Canada 142 C6 51 38N 112 23W
Delice, Turkey 100 C6 39 54N 34 2 E
Delicias, Mexico 162 B3 28 10N 105 30W
Delījān, Iran 97 C6 33 59N 50 40 E
Delimara Point, Malta 38 F8 35 49N 14 34 E
Déline, Canada 138 B7 65 11N 123 25W
Delisle, Canada 143 C7 51 55N 107 8W
Delitzsch, Germany 30 D8 51 31N 12 20 E
Dell City, U.S.A. 159 L11 31 56N 105 12W
Dell Rapids, U.S.A. 154 D6 43 50N 96 43W
Delle, France 27 E14 47 30N 7 2 E
Dellys, Algeria 111 A5 36 57N 3 57 E
Delmar, Iowa, U.S.A. 156 C6 42 0N 90 37W
Delmar, N.Y., U.S.A. 151 D11 42 37N 73 47W
Delmenhorst, Germany 30 B4 53 3N 8 37 E
Delmiro Gouveia, Brazil 170 C4 9 24 S 38 6W
Delnice, Croatia 45 C11 45 23N 14 50 E
Delonga, Ostrova, Russia 67 B15 76 40N 149 20 E
Deloraine, Australia 127 G4 41 30 S 146 40 E
Deloraine, Canada 143 D8 49 15N 100 29W
Delphi, Greece 48 C4 38 28N 22 30 E
Delphi, U.S.A. 157 D10 40 36N 86 41W
Delphos, U.S.A. 157 D12 40 51N 84 21W
Delportshoop, S. Africa 116 D3 28 22 S 24 20 E
Delray Beach, U.S.A. 153 J9 26 28N 80 4W
Delsbo, Sweden 16 C10 61 48N 16 32 E
Delta, Ala., U.S.A. 152 B4 33 26N 85 42W
Delta, Colo., U.S.A. 159 G9 38 44N 108 4W
Delta, Utah, U.S.A. 158 G7 39 21N 112 35W
Delta □, Nigeria 113 D6 5 30N 6 0 E
Delta Amacuro □, Venezuela 169 B5 8 30N 61 30W
Delta del Ebro ⌂, Spain 40 E5 40 43N 0 43 E
Delta del Po ⌂, Italy 45 D9 44 50N 12 15 E
Delta du Saloum △, Senegal 112 C1 13 42N 16 43W
Delta Dunării ⌂, Romania 53 E14 45 15N 29 25 E
Delta Junction, U.S.A. 144 D11 64 2N 145 44W
Deltona, U.S.A. 153 G8 28 54N 81 16W
Delungra, Australia 127 D5 29 39 S 150 51 E
Delvada, India 92 J4 20 46N 71 2 E
Delvinákion, Greece 48 B2 39 57N 20 32 E
Delvinë, Albania 50 G4 39 59N 20 6 E
Delyatyn, Ukraine 53 B9 48 32N 24 38 E
Demagiri, India 90 D4 22 55N 92 48 E
Demak, Indonesia 85 D4 6 53 S 110 38 E
Demanda, Sierra de la, Spain 40 C2 42 15N 3 0W
Demavend = Damāvand, Qolleh-ye, Iran 97 C7 35 56N 52 10 E
Demba, Dem. Rep. of the Congo 115 D4 5 28 S 22 15 E
Demba Chio, Angola 115 D2 9 41 S 13 41 E
Dembecha, Ethiopia 107 E4 10 32N 37 30 E
Dembi, Ethiopia 107 F4 8 5N 36 25 E
Dembia, Dem. Rep. of the Congo 118 B2 3 33N 25 48 E
Dembica = Dębica, Poland 55 H8 50 2N 21 25 E
Dembidolo, Ethiopia 107 F3 8 34N 34 50 E
Demchok, India 93 C8 32 42N 79 29 E
Demer →, Belgium 24 D4 50 57N 4 42 E
Demetrias, Greece 48 B5 39 22N 23 1 E
Demidov, Russia 58 E6 55 16N 31 30 E
Deming, N. Mex., U.S.A. 159 K10 32 16N 107 46W
Deming, Wash., U.S.A. 160 B4 48 50N 122 13W
Demini →, Brazil 169 D5 0 46 S 62 56W
Demirci, Turkey 49 B10 39 2N 28 38 E
Demirköprü Barajı, Turkey 49 C10 38 42N 28 25 E
Demirköy, Turkey 51 E11 41 49N 27 45 E
Demmin, Germany 30 B9 53 54N 13 2 E
Demnate, Morocco 110 B3 31 44N 6 59W
Democracia, Brazil 173 B5 5 48 S 61 26W
Demonte, Italy 44 D4 44 19N 7 17 E
Demopolis, U.S.A. 149 J2 32 31N 87 50W
Dempo, Indonesia 84 C2 4 2 S 103 15 E
Demta, Indonesia 83 B6 2 20 S 140 8 E
Demyansk, Russia 58 D7 57 40N 32 27 E
Den Burg, Neths. 24 A4 53 3N 4 47 E
Den Chai, Thailand 86 D3 17 59N 100 4 E
Den Haag = 's-Gravenhage, Neths. 24 B4 52 7N 4 17 E
Den Helder, Neths. 24 B4 52 57N 4 45 E
Den Oever, Neths. 24 B5 52 56N 5 2 E
Denain, France 27 B10 50 20N 3 22 E
Denair, U.S.A. 160 H6 37 32N 120 48W
Denali △, U.S.A. 144 E10 63 30N 152 0W
Denau, Uzbekistan 65 - 38 16N 67 54 E
Denbigh, Canada 150 A7 45 8N 77 15W
Denbigh, U.K. 20 D4 53 12N 3 25W
Denbigh, C., U.S.A. 144 D7 64 23N 161 32W
Denbighshire □, U.K. 20 D4 53 8N 3 22W
Dendang, Indonesia 85 C3 3 7 S 107 56 E
Dendé = Ndindi, Gabon 114 C2 3 46 S 11 9 E
Dendermonde, Belgium 24 C4 51 2N 4 5 E
Deneba, Ethiopia 107 F4 9 47N 39 10 E
Denezhkin Kamen, Gora, Russia 64 A7 60 25N 59 32 E
Deng Deng, Cameroon 114 A2 5 12N 13 31 E
Dengchuan, China 76 E3 25 59N 100 3 E
Denge, Nigeria 113 C6 12 52N 5 21 E

Dengfeng, China . . . . . . 74 G7 34 25N 113 2 E
Dengi, Nigeria . . . . . . 113 D6 9 25N 9 55 E
Dengkou, China . . . . . . 74 D4 40 18N 106 55 E
Dengzhou, China . . . . . 77 A9 32 34N 112 4 E
Denham, Australia . . . . 125 E1 25 56 S 113 31 E
Denham, Mt., Jamaica . . 164 a 18 13N 77 32W
Denham Ra., Australia . . 126 C4 21 55 S 147 46 E
Denham Sd., Australia . . 125 E1 25 45 S 113 15 E
Denholm, Canada 143 C7 52 39N 108 1W
Denia, Spain . . . . 41 G5 38 49N 0 8 E
Denial B., Australia . . . 127 E1 32 14 S 133 32 E
Deniliquin, Australia . . 129 C6 35 30 S 144 58 E
Denis, Gabon . . . . . . 114 B1 0 19N 9 22 E
Denison, Iowa, U.S.A. . . 156 E7 42 1N 95 21W
Denison, Tex., U.S.A. . . 155 J6 33 45N 96 33W
Denison Plains,
  Australia . . . . 124 C4 18 35 S 128 0 E
Denisovka =
  Ordzhonikidze,
  Kazakhstan . . . . . 64 E8 52 27N 61 39 E
Deniyaya, Sri Lanka . . . 95 L5 6 21N 80 33 E
Denizli, Turkey . . . . . 49 D11 37 42N 29 2 E
Denizli □, Turkey . . . . 49 D11 37 45N 29 5 E
Denman, Australia . . . . 129 B9 32 24 S 150 42 E
Denman Glacier,
  Antarctica . . . . . . 7 C7 66 45 S 99 25 E
Denmark, Australia . . . 125 F2 34 59 S 117 25 E
Denmark, U.S.A. 152 B8 33 19N 81 9W
Denmark ■, Europe . . . 17 J3 55 45N 10 0 E
Denmark Str., Atl. Oc. . . 6 C6 66 0N 30 0W
Dennery, St. Lucia . . . . 165 f 13 55N 60 54W
Dennison, U.S.A. 150 F3 40 24N 81 19W
Denny, U.K. 22 E5 56 1N 3 55W
Denpasar, Indonesia . . . 85 D5 8 39 S 115 13 E
Denpasar ✈ (DPS),
  Indonesia . . . . . . 79 K18 8 44 S 115 10 E
Denton, Ga., U.S.A. . . . 153 F4 31 44N 82 42W
Denton, Mont., U.S.A. . . 158 C9 47 19N 109 57W
Denton, Tex., U.S.A. . . . 155 J6 33 13N 97 8W
D'Entrecasteaux △,
  Australia . . . . 125 F2 34 20 S 115 33 E
D'Entrecasteaux, Pt.,
  Australia . . . . 125 F2 34 50 S 115 57 E
D'Entrecasteaux Is.,
  Papua N. G. . . . . . 132 E6 9 0 S 151 0 E
Dents du Midi, Switz. . . 32 D3 46 10N 6 56 E
Dentsville, U.S.A. 152 A9 34 4N 80 58W
Denu, Ghana . . . . . . 113 D5 6 4N 1 8 E
Denver, Colo., U.S.A. . . 154 F2 39 44N 104 59W
Denver, Ind., U.S.A. . . . 150 F10 40 52N 86 5W
Denver, Iowa, U.S.A. . . 156 B4 42 40N 92 20W
Denver, Pa., U.S.A. . . . 151 F8 40 14N 76 8W
Denver City, U.S.A. . . . 155 J3 32 58N 102 50W
Denwood =
  Wainwright, Canada . 143 C6 52 50N 110 50W
Deoband, India . . . . . 93 E7 29 42N 77 43 E
Deobhog, India . . . . . 94 E6 19 53N 82 44 E
Deodrug, India . . . . . 95 F3 16 26N 76 55 E
Deogarh, Orissa, India . 94 D7 21 32N 84 45 E
Deogarh, Raj., India . . . 92 G5 25 32N 73 54 E
Deoghar, India . . . . . 93 G12 24 30N 86 42 E
Deolali, India . . . . . . 94 E1 19 58N 73 50 E
Deoli = Devli, India . . . 92 G5 25 50N 75 20 E
Déols, France . . . . . . 27 F8 46 50N 1 43 E
Deora, India . . . . 92 F4 26 22N 70 55 E
Deorha = Jubbal, India . 93 D7 31 5N 77 40 E
Deori, India . . . . 93 H8 23 24N 79 1 E
Deoria, India . . . . . . 93 F10 26 31N 83 48 E
Deosai Mts., Pakistan . . 93 B6 35 40N 75 0 E
Deosri, India . . . . . . 93 F13 26 46N 90 29 E
Depalpur, India . . . . . 92 H6 22 51N 75 33 E
Deping, China . . . . . . 75 F9 37 25N 116 58 E
Deposit, U.S.A. 151 E9 42 4N 75 25W
Depuch I., Australia . . . 124 D2 20 37 S 117 44 E
Deputatskiy, Russia . . . 67 C14 69 18N 139 54 E
Dêqên, China . . . . . . 76 C2 28 34N 98 51 E
Deqing, China . . . . . . 77 F8 23 8N 111 42 E
Dera Ghazi Khan,
  Pakistan . . . . 91 C3 30 5N 70 43 E
Dera Ismail Khan,
  Pakistan . . . . 91 C3 31 50N 70 50 E
Derabugti, Pakistan . . . 92 E3 29 2N 69 9 E
Derawar Fort, Pakistan . 92 E4 28 46N 71 20 E
Derbent, Russia . . . . . 61 J9 42 5N 48 15 E
Derbent, Turkey . . . . . 49 C10 38 11N 28 33 E
Derbent, Uzbekistan . . . 65 D3 38 13N 66 50 E
Derby, Australia . . . . . 124 C3 17 18 S 123 38 E
Derby, U.K. 20 E6 52 56N 1 28W
Derby, Conn., U.S.A. . . 151 E11 41 19N 73 5W
Derby, Kans., U.S.A. . . . 155 G6 37 33N 97 16W
Derby, N.Y., U.S.A. . . . 150 D6 42 41N 78 58W
Derby City □, U.K. . . . 20 E6 52 56N 1 28W
Derby Line, U.S.A. . . . 151 B12 45 0N 72 6W
Derbyshire □, U.K. . . . 20 E6 53 11N 1 38W
Đerdap △, Serbia & M. . 50 B6 44 40N 22 23 E
Derdepoort, S. Africa . . 116 C4 24 38 S 26 24 E
Dereceske, Hungary . . . 52 C6 47 20N 21 33 E
Dereham, U.K. . . . . . 21 E8 52 41N 0 57 E
Dereköy, Turkey . . . . . 51 B11 41 55N 27 21 E
Derg →, U.K. 23 B4 54 44N 7 26W
Derg, L., Ireland 23 D3 53 0N 8 20W
Dergachi = Derhaci,
  Ukraine . . . . 59 G9 50 9N 36 11 E
Derhaci, Ukraine . . . . 59 G9 50 9N 36 11 E
Derik, Turkey . . . . . . 101 D9 37 21N 40 18 E
Derinkuyu, Turkey . . . . 100 C6 38 22N 34 45 E
Dermantsi, Bulgaria . . . 51 C8 43 8N 24 17 E
Dermott, U.S.A. 155 J9 33 32N 91 26W
Dêrong, China . . . . . . 76 C2 28 44N 99 9 E
Derrinallum, Australia . 128 D5 37 57 S 143 15 E
Derry = Londonderry,
  U.K. 23 B4 55 0N 7 20W
Derry =
  Londonderry □, U.K. . 23 B4 55 0N 7 20W
Derry, N.H., U.S.A. . . . 151 D13 42 53N 71 19W
Derry, Pa., U.S.A. 150 F5 40 20N 79 18W
Derryveagh Mts.,
  Ireland 23 B3 54 56N 8 11W
Derudub, Sudan . . . . . 106 D4 17 31N 36 7 E
Derval, France 26 E5 47 40N 1 41W
Dervéni, Greece . . . . . 48 C4 38 8N 22 25 E
Derventa, Bos.-H. . . . . 52 F2 44 59N 17 55 E
Derwent →, Cumb.,
  U.K. 20 C4 54 39N 3 33W
Derwent →, Derby,
  U.K. 20 E6 52 57N 1 28W
Derwent →, N. Yorks.,
  U.K. 20 D7 53 45N 0 58W
Derwent Water △, U.K. . 20 C4 54 35N 3 9W
Des Moines, Iowa,
  U.S.A. 156 C3 41 35N 93 37W
Des Moines, N. Mex.,
  U.S.A. 155 G3 36 46N 103 50W
Des Moines →, U.S.A. . . 156 D5 40 23N 91 25W
Des Plaines, U.S.A. . . . 150 D2 42 2N 87 54W
Des Plaines →, U.S.A. . . 157 C8 41 23N 88 15W
Desa, Romania . . . . . 52 G8 43 54N 22 55 E
Desaguadero, Peru . . . 172 D4 16 34 S 69 3W
Desaguadero →,
  Argentina . . . . . . 174 C2 34 30 S 66 46W
Desaguadero →,
  Bolivia . . . . 172 D4 16 35 S 69 5W
Desantne, Ukraine . . . . 53 E14 45 34N 29 32 E

Desar, Malaysia . . . . . 87 d 1 31N 104 17 E
Descanso, Pta., Mexico . 161 N9 32 21N 117 3W
Descartes, France . . . . 28 B4 46 59N 0 42 E
Deschaillons-sur-St-
  Laurent, Canada . . . 141 C5 46 32N 72 7W
Deschambault L.,
  Canada 143 C8 54 50N 103 30W
Deschutes →, U.S.A. . . . 158 D3 45 38N 120 55W
Dese, Ethiopia . . . . . . 107 E4 11 5N 39 40 E
Deseado, C., Chile . . . . 176 D2 52 45 S 74 42W
Desenzano del Garda,
  Italy . . . . 44 C7 45 28N 10 32 E
Desert Center, U.S.A. . . 161 M11 33 43N 115 24W
Desert Hot Springs,
  U.S.A. 161 M10 33 58N 116 30W
Desertas, Ilhas,
  Madeira 110 B1 32 30N 16 30W
Deset, Norway . . . . . . 18 C8 61 20N 11 26 E
Deshnok, India . . . . . 92 F5 27 48N 73 21 E
Desierto Central de
  Baja California △,
  Mexico 162 B2 29 40N 114 43W
Desna →, Ukraine . . . . 59 G6 50 33N 30 32 E
Desnătui →, Romania . . 53 G8 43 53N 23 35 E
Desolación, I., Chile . . . 176 D2 53 0 S 74 0W
Despeñaperros △,
  Spain 43 G7 38 25N 3 32W
Despeñaperros, Paso,
  Spain 43 G7 38 24N 3 30W
Despotovac,
  Serbia & M. . . . . . 50 B5 44 6N 21 30 E
Dessau, Germany . . . . 30 D8 51 51N 12 14 E
Dessye = Dese,
  Ethiopia . . . . 107 E4 11 5N 39 40 E
D'Estrees B., Australia . 128 C2 35 55 S 137 45 E
Desuri, India . . . . . . 92 G5 25 18N 73 35 E
Desvres, France . . . . . 27 B8 50 40N 1 48 E
Det Udom, Thailand . . . 86 E5 14 54N 105 5 E
Deta, Romania . . . . . . 52 E6 45 24N 21 13 E
Dete, Zimbabwe . . . . . 116 B4 18 38 S 26 50 E
Đetinja →, Serbia & M. . 50 C4 43 51N 20 5 E
Detmold, Germany . . . . 30 D4 51 56N 8 52 E
Detour, Pt., U.S.A. 148 C2 45 40N 86 40W
Detroit, U.S.A. 150 D4 42 20N 83 3W
Detroit Lakes, U.S.A. . . 154 B7 46 49N 95 51W
Detroit Wayne
  County ✈ (DTW),
  U.S.A. 157 B13 42 13N 83 21W
Detskoye Selo =
  Pushkin, Russia . . . 58 C6 59 45N 30 25 E
Dettifoss, Iceland 11 B10 65 48N 16 24W
Detva, Slovak Rep. . . . 35 C12 48 34N 19 25 E
Deurne, Neths. . . . . . 24 C5 51 27N 5 49 E
Deutsch = Przemyśl,
  Poland . . . . 55 J9 49 50N 22 45 E
Deutsch Brod =
  Havlíčkův Brod,
  Czech Rep. . . . . . 34 B8 49 36N 15 33 E
Deutsch-Eylau = Iława,
  Poland . . . . 54 E6 53 36N 19 34 E
Deutsch Krone =
  Wałcz, Poland . . . . 55 E3 53 17N 16 27 E
Deutsch-
  Luxemburgischer △,
  Germany . . . . . . 31 F2 49 58N 6 12 E
Deutsche Bucht,
  Germany . . . . . . 30 A4 54 15N 8 0 E
Deutschland =
  Germany ■, Europe . 30 E6 51 0N 10 0 E
Deutschlandsberg,
  Austria . . . . 34 E8 46 49N 15 14 E
Deux-Sèvres □, France . 26 F6 46 35N 0 20W
Deva, Romania . . . . . 52 E7 45 53N 22 55 E
Deva →, Spain 42 B6 43 23N 5 36W
Devakottai, India . . . . 95 K4 9 55N 78 45 E
Devaprayag, India . . . 93 D8 30 13N 78 35 E
Devarkonda, India . . . 94 F4 16 42N 78 56 E
Devávanya, Hungary . . 52 C5 47 2N 20 59 E
Deveci Dağları, Turkey . 100 B7 40 6N 36 15 E
Devecikonağı, Turkey . . 51 G12 39 55N 28 34 E
Devecser, Hungary . . . 52 C2 47 6N 17 26 E
Develi, Turkey . . . . . 100 C6 38 23N 35 29 E
Deventer, Neths. . . . . 24 B6 52 15N 6 10 E
Devereux, U.S.A. 152 B6 33 13N 83 5W
Deveron →, U.K. 22 D6 57 41N 2 32W
Devesel, Romania . . . . 52 F7 44 28N 22 41 E
Devgad I., India . . . . . 95 G2 14 48N 74 5 E
Devgadh Bariya, India . 92 H5 22 40N 73 55 E
Devgarh, India . . . . . 95 F1 16 23N 73 23 E
Devi →, India . . . . . . 94 E8 19 59N 86 24 E
Devikot, India . . . . . . 92 F4 26 42N 71 12 E
Devil River Pk., N.Z. . . 131 A7 40 56 S 172 37 E
Devils Den, U.S.A. 160 K7 35 46N 119 58W
Devil's Island, I. =
  Diable, Île du,
  Fr. Guiana 169 B7 5 16N 52 34W
Devils Lake, U.S.A. . . . 154 A5 48 7N 98 52W
Devils Paw, Canada . . . 142 B2 58 47N 134 0W
Devils Postpile △,
  U.S.A. 160 H7 37 37N 119 5W
Devil's Pt., Sri Lanka . . 95 K5 9 26N 80 6 E
Devils Tower, U.S.A. . . 154 C2 44 31N 104 57W
Devils Tower △, U.S.A. . 154 C2 44 35N 104 43W
Devin, Bulgaria . . . . . 51 E8 41 44N 24 24 E
Devine, U.S.A. 155 L5 29 8N 98 54W
Devipattinam, India . . . 95 K4 9 23N 78 54 E
Devizes, U.K. 21 F6 51 22N 1 58W
Devli, India . . . . 92 G6 25 50N 75 20 E
Devnya, Bulgaria . . . . 51 C11 43 13N 27 33 E
Devoll →, Albania . . . . 50 F4 40 57N 20 15 E
Devon, Canada 142 C6 53 24N 113 44W
Devon □, U.K. 21 G4 50 50N 3 40W
Devon I., Canada 6 B3 75 10N 85 0W
Devonport, Australia . . 127 G4 41 10 S 146 22 E
Devonport, N.Z. . . . . . 131 B5 36 49 S 174 49 E
Devrek, Turkey . . . . . 100 B4 41 13N 31 57 E
Devrekâni, Turkey . . . . 100 B5 41 36N 33 50 E
Devrez →, Turkey . . . . 100 B6 41 5N 34 24 E
Devrukh, India . . . . . 94 F1 17 3N 73 37 E
Dewas, India . . . . . . 92 H7 22 59N 76 3 E
Dewetsdorp, S. Africa . 116 D4 29 33 S 26 39 E
Dewey, Puerto Rico . . . 165 d 18 18N 65 18W
Dexing, China . . . . . . 77 C11 28 46N 117 30 E
Dexter, Maine, U.S.A. . . 149 C11 45 1N 69 18W
Dexter, Mich., U.S.A. . . 157 B13 42 20N 83 53W
Dexter, Mo., U.S.A. . . . 155 G10 36 48N 89 57W
Dexter, N. Mex., U.S.A. . 155 J2 33 12N 104 22W
Dey-Dey, L., Australia . . 125 E5 29 12 S 131 4 E
Deyang, China . . . . . . 76 B5 31 3N 104 27 E
Deyhūk, Iran . . . . . . 101 C8 33 15N 57 30 E
Deyyer, Iran . . . . 97 E6 27 55N 51 55 E
Dezadeash L., Canada . 142 A1 60 28N 136 58W
Dezfūl, Iran . . . . 97 C6 32 20N 48 30 E
Dezhneva, Mys, Russia . 67 C19 66 5N 169 40W
Dezhou, China . . . . . . 74 F9 37 26N 116 18 E
Dhadhar →, India . . . . 93 G11 24 56N 85 24 E
Dháfni, Kríti, Greece . . 39 E6 35 13N 25 3 E
Dháfni, Pelóponnisos,
  Greece . . . . 48 D4 37 48N 22 1 E
Dhahaban, Si. Arabia . . 98 B2 21 58N 39 3 E
Dhahiriya = Aẓ
  Ẓāhirīyah, West Bank 103 D3 31 25N 34 58 E

Dhahran = Aẓ Ẓahrān,
  Si. Arabia . . . . . 97 E6 26 10N 50 7 E
Dhak, Pakistan . . . . . 92 C5 32 25N 72 33 E
Dhaka, Bangla. . . . . . 90 D3 23 43N 90 26 E
Dhaka □, Bangla. . . . 90 C4 24 25N 90 25 E
Dhali, Cyprus . . . . . . 39 E9 35 1N 33 25 E
Dhamar, Yemen . . . . . 98 D4 14 30N 44 20 E
Dhamangaon, India . . . 94 D4 20 48N 78 9 E
Dhampur, India . . . . . 93 E8 29 19N 78 33 E
Dhamra →, India . . . . 94 D8 20 47N 86 58 E
Dhamtari, India . . . . . 94 D3 20 42N 81 35 E
Dhanbad, India . . . . . 93 H12 23 50N 86 30 E
Dhankuta, Nepal . . . . 93 F12 26 55N 87 40 E
Dhanora, India . . . . . 94 D5 20 20N 80 22 E
Dhanushkodi, India . . . 95 K4 9 11N 79 24 E
Dhar, India . . . . 92 H6 22 35N 75 26 E
Dharampur, Gujarat,
  India . . . . 94 D1 20 32N 73 17 E
Dharampur, Mad. P.,
  India . . . . 92 H6 22 13N 75 18 E
Dharamsala =
  Dharmsala, India . . 92 C7 32 16N 76 23 E
Dharangaon, India . . . 94 D2 21 1N 75 16 E
Dharapuram, India . . . 95 J3 10 45N 77 34 E
Dhariwal, India . . . . . 92 D6 31 57N 75 19 E
Dharla →, Bangla. . . . 93 G13 25 46N 89 42 E
Dharmapuri, India . . . 95 H4 12 10N 78 10 E
Dharmavaram, India . . 95 G3 14 29N 77 44 E
Dharmjaygarh, India . . 93 H10 22 28N 83 13 E
Dharmsala, India . . . . 92 C7 32 16N 76 23 E
Dharni, India . . . . . . 92 J7 21 33N 76 53 E
Dharug △, Australia . . 129 B9 33 20 S 151 2 E
Dharur, India . . . . . . 94 E3 18 3N 76 8 E
Dharwad, India . . . . . 95 G2 15 30N 75 4 E
Dhasan →, India . . . . 93 G8 25 48N 79 24 E
Dhaulagiri, Nepal . . . . 93 E10 28 39N 83 28 E
Dhebar, L., India . . . . 92 G6 24 10N 74 0 E
Dheftera, Cyprus . . . . 39 E9 35 3N 33 16 E
Dhenkanal, India . . . . 94 D7 20 45N 85 35 E
Dhenoúsa, Greece . . . 49 D7 37 8N 25 48 E
Dherinia, Cyprus . . . . 39 E9 35 3N 33 57 E
Dheskáti, Greece . . . . 50 G5 39 55N 21 49 E
Dhespotikó, Greece . . . 48 E6 36 57N 24 58 E
Dhestina, Greece . . . . 48 C4 38 25N 22 31 E
Dhī Qār □, Iraq . . . . . 96 D5 31 0N 46 15 E
Dhiarrizos →, Cyprus . . 39 E8 34 41N 32 34 E
Dhílos, Greece . . . . . 49 D7 37 23N 25 15 E
Dhimitsána, Greece . . 48 D4 37 36N 22 3 E
Dhírfis Óros, Greece . . 48 C5 38 40N 23 54 E
Dhodhekánisos, Greece . 49 E8 36 35N 27 0 E
Dhodhekánisos □,
  Greece . . . . 49 E8 36 35N 27 0 E
Dhokós, Greece . . . . . 48 D5 37 20N 23 20 E
Dholiana, Greece . . . . 48 B2 39 54N 20 32 E
Dholka, India . . . . . . 92 H5 22 44N 72 29 E
Dhomokós, Greece . . . 48 B4 39 10N 22 18 E
Dhone, India . . . . . . 95 E3 15 25N 77 53 E
Dhoraji, India . . . . . . 92 J4 21 45N 70 37 E
Dhoxáton, Greece . . . 51 E8 41 9N 24 16 E
Dhubab, Yemen . . . . . 98 E3 12 56N 43 25 E
Dhuburi, India . . . . . 90 B2 26 2N 89 59 E
Dhulasar, Bangla. . . . . 90 B3 21 52N 90 14 E
Dhule, India . . . . 94 D2 20 58N 74 50 E
Dhupdhara, India . . . . 90 B3 26 10N 91 4 E
Dhuusa Mareeb =
  Dusa Mareb,
  Somali Rep. . . . . . 120 C3 5 30N 46 15 E
Di-ib, W. →, Sudan . . . 106 C4 22 38N 36 6 E
Di Linh, Vietnam . . . . 87 G7 11 35N 108 4 E
Di Linh, Cao Nguyen,
  Vietnam . . . . 87 G7 11 30N 108 0 E
Día, Greece . . . . 39 E6 35 28N 25 14 E
Diabakania, Guinea . . 112 C2 10 38N 10 58W
Diable, Île du,
  Fr. Guiana 169 B7 5 16N 52 34W
Diablo, Mt., U.S.A. . . . 160 H5 37 53N 121 56W
Diablo Range, U.S.A. . . 160 J5 37 20N 121 25W
Diafarabé, Mali 112 C4 14 9N 4 57W
Diala, Mali 112 C3 14 10N 9 58W
Dialakoto, Mali 112 C2 12 18N 7 54W
Dialakoto, Senegal . . . 112 C2 13 21N 13 19W
Diallassagou, Mali . . . 112 C4 13 47N 3 41W
Diamante, Argentina . . 174 C3 32 5 S 60 40W
Diamante →,
  Argentina . . . . . 174 C2 34 30 S 66 46W
Diamantina, Brazil . . . 171 E3 18 17 S 43 40W
Diamantina →,
  Australia . . . . . . 126 C3 23 33 S 141 23 E
Diamantina →,
  Australia . . . . . . 127 D2 26 45 S 139 10 E
Diamantina, Brazil . . . 173 C6 14 30 S 56 30W
Diamond Bar, U.S.A. . . 161 L9 34 1N 117 48W
Diamond Harbour,
  India . . . . 93 H13 22 11N 88 14 E
Diamond Head, U.S.A. . 145 K14 21 16N 157 49W
Diamond Is., Australia . 126 B5 17 25 S 151 5 E
Diamond Mts., U.S.A. . 158 G6 39 50N 115 30W
Diamond Springs,
  U.S.A. 160 G6 38 42N 120 49W
Dian Chi, China . . . . . 76 E4 24 50N 102 43 E
Dianalund, Denmark . . 17 J5 55 32N 11 30 E
Dianbai, China . . . . . 77 G8 21 33N 111 0 E
Diancheng, China . . . . 77 G8 21 33N 111 0 E
Dianjiang, China . . . . 76 B6 30 24N 107 20 E
Diano Marina, Italy . . . 46 E5 43 54N 8 5 E
Dianópolis, Brazil . . . . 171 D2 11 38 S 46 50W
Dianra, Ivory C. 112 D3 8 45N 6 14W
Diapaga, Burkina Faso . 113 C5 12 5N 1 46 E
Diapangou,
  Burkina Faso . . . . 113 C5 12 5N 0 10 E
Diariguila, Guinea . . . 112 C2 10 35N 10 2W
Diavolo, Mt., India . . . 95 H11 12 40N 92 56 E
Dībā, U.A.E. . . . . 97 E8 25 45N 56 16 E
Dibai, India . . . . 92 E8 28 13N 78 15 E
Dibaya, Dem. Rep. of
  the Congo . . . . . 115 D4 6 30 S 22 57 E
Dibaya-Lubue,
  Dem. Rep. of
  the Congo . . . . . 115 C3 4 12 S 19 54 E
Dibbeen △, Jordan . . . 103 C4 32 20N 35 45 E
Dibella, Niger . . . . . . 109 E2 17 17N 12 57 E
Dibete, Botswana . . . . 116 C4 23 45 S 26 32 E
Dibrugarh, India . . . . 90 B5 27 29N 94 55 E
Diciosânmartin =
  Târnăveni, Romania . 53 D9 46 19N 24 13 E

Dickens, U.S.A. 155 J4 33 37N 100 50W
Dickeyville, U.S.A. . . . 156 B6 42 38N 90 36W
Dickinson, U.S.A. 154 B3 46 53N 102 47W
Dick's Pt., Bahamas . . 9 b 24 N 77 18W
Dickson = Dikson,
  Russia . . . . 66 B9 73 40N 80 5 E
Dickson, U.S.A. 149 G2 36 5N 87 23W
Dickson City, U.S.A. . . 151 E9 41 29N 75 40W
Dicle Nehri →, Turkey . 101 D9 37 44N 41 0 E
Dicomano, Italy . . . . . 45 E8 43 53N 11 31 E
Didesa, W. →, Ethiopia . 107 F4 10 2N 35 32 E
Didi, Sudan . . . . 107 F3 6 18N 34 29 E
Didiéni, Mali 112 C3 13 53N 8 6W
Didsbury, Canada 142 C6 51 35N 114 10W
Didwana, India . . . . . 92 F6 27 23N 74 36 E
Die, France . . . . 29 D9 44 47N 5 22 E
Diébougou,
  Burkina Faso 112 C4 11 0N 3 15W
Diecke, Guinea 112 D3 7 27N 8 54W
Diedenhofen =
  Thionville, France . . 27 C13 49 20N 6 10 E
Diefenbaker, L.,
  Canada 143 C7 51 0N 106 55W
Diego de Almagro,
  Chile . . . . 174 B1 26 22 S 70 3W
Diego Garcia, Ind. Oc. . 121 E6 7 50 S 72 50 E
Diego Ramírez, Islas,
  Chile . . . . 176 E3 56 30 S 68 44W
Diekirch, Lux. . . . . . . 24 E6 49 52N 6 10 E
Diéma, Mali 112 C3 14 32N 9 12W
Diembéring, Senegal . . 112 C1 12 29N 16 47W
Demeisee =, Germany . 30 D4 51 20N 8 40 E
Dien Ban, Vietnam . . . 86 E7 15 53N 108 16 E
Dien Bien, Vietnam . . . 76 G4 21 20N 103 0 E
Dien Khanh, Vietnam . . 87 F7 12 15N 109 6 E
Diepholz, Germany . . . 30 C4 52 37N 8 22 E
Dieppe, France . . . . . 26 C8 49 54N 1 4 E
Dierks, U.S.A. 155 H8 34 7N 94 1W
Diest, Belgium . . . . . 24 D5 50 58N 5 4 E
Dietrich →, Canada . . . 157 E13 39 4N 88 23W
Dietikon, Switz. . . . . . 33 B6 47 24N 8 24 E
Dieulefit, France . . . . 29 D9 44 32N 5 4 E
Dieuze, France . . . . . 27 D13 48 49N 6 43 E
Dievenow = Dziwnów,
  Poland . . . . 54 E1 54 2N 14 45 E
Dif, Somali Rep. . . . . . 120 D2 0 59N 40 58 E
Differdange, Lux. . . . . 24 E5 49 31N 5 54 E
Diffun, Phil. . . . . 80 C3 16 36N 121 33 E
Dig, India . . . . 92 F7 27 28N 77 20 E
Digba, Dem. Rep. of
  the Congo . . . . . 118 B2 4 25N 25 48 E
Digboi, India . . . . . . 90 B5 27 23N 95 38 E
Digby, Canada 141 D6 44 38N 65 50W
Digges, Canada . . . . . 142 B3 62 26N 75 26 E
Dighinala, Bangla. . . . 90 D4 23 15N 92 5 E
Dighton, U.S.A. 154 F4 38 29N 100 28W
Diglur, India . . . . . . 94 E3 18 34N 77 33 E
Digna, India . . . . 92 F5 27 48N 75 1 E
Digne-les-Bains, France 29 D10 44 5N 6 12 E
Digoin, France . . . . . 27 F11 46 29N 4 1 E
Digor, Turkey . . . . . . 101 B10 40 22N 43 25 E
Digos, Phil. . . . . 81 H5 6 45N 125 20 E
Digranes, Iceland 11 A12 66 4N 14 44W
Digras, India . . . . . . 94 D3 20 7N 77 45 E
Digul →, Indonesia . . . 83 C5 7 7 S 138 42 E
Digya △, Ghana . . . . . 113 D5 7 15N 0 5 E
Dihang =
  Brahmaputra →,
  Asia . . . . 68 D3 23 40N 90 35 E
Dijlah, Nahr →, Asia . . 96 D5 31 0N 47 25 E
Dijon, France . . . . . . 27 E12 47 20N 5 3 E
Dikhil, Djibouti . . . . . 107 E5 11 8N 42 20 E
Dikili, Turkey . . . . . . 49 B8 39 4N 26 53 E
Dikirnis, Egypt . . . . . 106 H7 31 6N 31 35 E
Dikkil = Dikhil,
  Djibouti . . . . 107 E5 11 8N 42 20 E
Dikodougou, Ivory C. . . 112 D3 9 5N 5 45W
Dikomu di Kai, Botswana 116 C3 24 58 S 24 36 E
Diksmuide, Belgium . . 24 C2 51 2N 2 52 E
Dikson, Russia . . . . . 66 B9 73 40N 80 5 E
Dikwa, Nigeria . . . . . 113 C7 12 4N 13 30 E
Dila, Ethiopia . . . . . . 107 F4 6 21N 38 22 E
Dilasag, Phil. . . . . . . 80 C4 16 25N 122 11 E
Dilek Yarimadisi △,
  Turkey . . . . 49 D9 37 40N 27 10 E
Dili, E. Timor . . . . . . 82 C3 8 39 S 125 34 E
Diligent Strait, India . . 95 H11 12 11N 92 57 E
Dilijan, Armenia . . . . 65 F11 40 46N 44 57 E
Dilizhan = Dilijan,
  Armenia . . . . . . 61 K7 40 46N 44 57 E
Dilj, Croatia . . . . 52 E3 45 29N 18 1 E
Dillenburg, Germany . . 30 E4 50 43N 8 17 E
Dilley, U.S.A. 155 L5 28 40N 99 10W
Dilli = Delhi, India . . . 92 E7 28 38N 77 17 E
Dillia →, Niger . . . . . 109 F2 14 9N 12 50 E
Dilling, Sudan . . . . . . 107 E2 12 3N 29 35 E
Dillingen, Bayern,
  Germany . . . . . . 31 G6 48 36N 10 30 E
Dillingen, Saarland,
  Germany . . . . . . 31 F2 49 22N 6 43 E
Dillingham, U.S.A. . . . 144 C8 59 3N 158 28W
Dillon, Canada 143 B7 55 56N 108 35W
Dillon, Mont., U.S.A. . . 158 D7 45 13N 112 38W
Dillon, S.C., U.S.A. . . . 149 H6 34 25N 79 22W
Dillon →, Canada 143 B7 55 56N 108 56W
Dillsboro, U.S.A. 157 E11 39 1N 85 4W
Dillsburg, U.S.A. 150 F7 40 7N 77 2W
Dilly, Mali 112 C3 15 1N 7 40W
Dilolo, Dem. Rep. of
  the Congo . . . . . 115 E4 10 28 S 22 18 E
Dilove, Ukraine . . . . . 53 C9 47 56N 24 11 E
Dimapur, India . . . . . 90 C4 25 54N 93 45 E
Dimas, Mexico 162 C3 23 43N 106 47W
Dimasalang, Phil. . . . . 80 E4 12 12N 123 51 E
Dimashq, Syria . . . . . 103 B5 33 30N 36 18 E
Dimashq □, Syria . . . . 103 B5 33 30N 36 30 E
Dimbaza, S. Africa . . . 117 E4 32 50 S 27 14 E
Dimbelenge, Dem. Rep.
  of the Congo . . . . 115 D4 5 33 S 23 7 E
Dimbokro, Ivory C. . . . 112 D4 6 45N 4 46W
Dimboola, Australia . . 128 D5 36 28 S 142 7 E
Dîmboviţa →,
  Romania . . . . . . 53 F11 44 12N 26 26 E
Dimbulah, Australia . . 126 B4 17 8 S 145 4 E
Dimitrovgrad, Bulgaria . 51 C9 42 5N 25 35 E
Dimitrovgrad, Russia . . 60 C9 54 14N 49 39 E
Dimitrovo =
  Pernik, Bulgaria . . . 50 C6 43 2N 22 48 E
Dimitrovo = Pernik,
  Bulgaria . . . . . . 50 D7 42 35N 23 2 E
Dimmitt, U.S.A. 155 H3 34 33N 102 19W
Dimo, Sudan . . . . . . 107 F2 5 19N 29 10 E
Dimona, Israel . . . . . 103 D4 31 2N 35 1 E
Dimovo →, Congo . . . . 114 C2 4 13 S 12 21 E
Dinagat, Phil. . . . . . . 81 F5 10 10N 125 40 E
Dinajpur, Bangla. . . . . 91 H5 25 33N 88 43 E
Dinalupihan, Phil. . . . . 80 D3 14 53N 120 27 E
Dinan, France 26 D4 48 28N 2 2W
Dīnān Āb, Iran . . . . . 97 C8 32 4N 56 49 E

Dinant, Belgium . . . . 24 D4 50 16N 4 55 E
Dinapur, India . . . . . 93 G11 25 38N 85 5 E
Dinar, Turkey . . . . . . 49 C12 38 5N 30 10 E
Dīnār, Kūh-e, Iran . . . 97 D6 30 42N 51 46 E
Dinara Planina, Croatia . 45 D13 44 0N 16 30 E
Dinard, France 26 D4 48 38N 2 6W
Dinaric Alps = Dinara
  Planina, Croatia . . . 45 D13 44 0N 16 30 E
Dinas, Phil. . . . . 81 H4 7 38N 123 20 E
Dinde, Angola . . . . . . 115 G2 14 17 S 13 42 E
Dinder, Nahr ed →,
  Sudan . . . . 107 E3 14 6N 33 40 E
Dindi →, India . . . . . 95 F4 16 24N 78 15 E
Dindigul, India . . . . . 95 J4 10 25N 78 0 E
Dindori, India . . . . . . 93 H9 22 57N 81 5 E
Ding Xian = Dingzhou,
  China . . . . 74 E8 38 30N 114 59 E
Dinga, Dem. Rep. of
  the Congo . . . . . 115 D3 5 17 S 16 42 E
Dinga, Pakistan . . . . . 92 G2 25 26N 67 10 E
Dingalan, Phil. . . . . . 80 D3 15 18N 121 25 E
Dingalan Bay, Phil. . . . 80 D3 15 18N 121 25 E
Dingbian, China . . . . . 74 F4 37 35N 107 32 E
Dingelstädt, Germany . . 30 D6 51 18N 10 19 E
Dingle, Ireland 23 D1 52 9N 10 17W
Dingle, Sweden . . . . . 17 F5 58 32N 11 35 E
Dingle B., Ireland 23 D1 52 3N 10 20W
Dingli, Malta . . . . . . 38 f 35 52N 14 23 E
Dingmans Ferry, U.S.A. 151 E10 41 13N 74 55W
Dingnan, China . . . . . 77 E10 24 45N 115 0 E
Dingo, Australia . . . . . 126 C4 23 38 S 149 19 E
Dingolfing, Germany . . 31 G8 48 37N 12 30 E
Dingras, Phil. . . . . . . 80 B3 18 6N 120 42 E
Dingtao, China . . . . . 74 G8 35 5N 115 35 E
Dinguira, Mali 112 C2 14 11N 11 16W
Dinguiraye, Guinea . . . 112 C2 11 18N 10 49W
Dingwall, U.K. 22 D4 57 36N 4 26W
Dingxi, China . . . . . . 74 G3 35 30N 104 33 E
Dingxiang, China . . . . 74 E7 38 30N 112 58 E
Dingyuan, China . . . . 77 A11 32 32N 117 41 E
Dingzhou, China . . . . 74 E8 38 30N 114 59 E
Dinh, Mui, Vietnam . . . 87 G7 11 22N 109 1 E
Dinh Lap, Vietnam . . . 76 B6 21 33N 107 6 E
Dinhata, India . . . . . . 93 F13 26 8N 89 27 E
Dinira △, Venezuela . . 165 B6 9 57N 70 6W
Dinokwe, Botswana . . . 116 C4 23 29 S 26 37 E
Dinorwic, Canada 143 D10 49 41N 92 30W
Dinosaur △, Canada . . 142 C6 50 47N 111 30W
Dinosaur △, U.S.A. . . . 158 F9 40 30N 108 45W
Dinsor, Somali Rep. . . . 120 D2 2 24N 42 59 E
Dinuba, U.S.A. 160 J7 36 32N 119 23W
Diö, Sweden . . . . 17 H8 56 37N 14 15 E
Dioïla, Mali 112 C3 12 33N 6 50W
Dioka, Mali 112 C2 14 57N 10 4W
Diomede, U.S.A. 144 D5 65 47N 169 0W
Diona, Chad . . . . 109 E4 17 51N 22 36 E
Diongoi, Mali 112 C3 14 38N 8 34W
Diósgyőr, Hungary . . . 52 B5 48 7N 20 43 E
Diosig, Romania . . . . 52 C7 47 18N 22 2 E
Diougani, Mali 112 C4 14 19N 2 44W
Diouloulou, Senegal . . 112 C1 13 5N 16 38W
Dioura, Mali 112 C3 14 59N 5 12W
Dioura, Mali 112 C3 14 59N 5 12W
Dipaculao, Phil. . . . . . 80 D3 15 51N 121 32 E
Dipalpur, Pakistan . . . 92 D5 30 40N 73 39 E
Diplo, Pakistan . . . . . 92 G3 24 35N 69 35 E
Dipolog, Phil. . . . . . . 81 G4 8 36N 123 20 E
Dipperu △, Australia . . 126 C4 21 56 S 148 42 E
Dipton, N.Z. . . . . 131 F3 45 54 S 168 22 E
Dir, Pakistan . . . . . . 91 B3 35 8N 71 59 E
Diré, Mali 112 B4 16 20N 3 25W
Dire Dawa, Ethiopia . . 107 F5 9 35N 41 45 E
Diriamba, Nic. 164 D2 11 51N 86 19W
Dirico, Angola . . . . . . 115 F4 17 50 S 20 42 E
Dirk Hartog I.,
  Australia . . . . . . 125 E1 25 50 S 113 5 E
Dirkou, Niger . . . . . . 109 E2 19 12 53 E
Dirranbandi, Australia . 127 D4 28 33 S 148 17 E
Dirs, Si. Arabia . . . . . 98 C3 18 32N 42 5 E
Dirschau = Tczew,
  Poland . . . . 54 D5 54 8N 18 50 E
Disa, India . . . . 92 G5 24 18N 72 10 E
Disa, Sudan . . . . 107 F3 12 5N 34 15 E
Disappointment, C.,
  U.S.A. 158 C2 46 18N 124 5W
Disappointment, L.,
  Australia . . . . . . 124 D3 23 20 S 122 40 E
Disaster B., Australia . . 129 D8 37 15 S 149 58 E
Discovery B., Australia . 128 D5 38 10 S 140 40 E
Discovery B., China . . . 69 G11 22 18N 114 1 E
Disentis Muster, Switz. . 33 C7 46 42N 8 50 E
Dishna, Egypt . . . . . . 106 B3 26 9N 32 32 E
Disina, Nigeria . . . . . 113 C6 11 35N 9 50 E
Disko = Qeqertarsuaq,
  Greenland 10 D5 69 45N 53 30W
Disko Bugt, Greenland . 10 D5 69 10N 52 0W
Disna = Dzisna →,
  Belarus . . . . 58 E5 55 34N 28 12 E
Disney Reef, Tonga . . . 133 P13 19 17 S 174 7W
Dispur, India . . . . . . 90 B3 26 1N 91 52 E
Diss, U.K. . . . . 21 E9 52 23N 1 7 E
Disteghil Sar, Pakistan . 93 A6 36 20N 75 12 E
Distrito Federal □,
  Brazil . . . . 171 E2 15 45 S 47 45W
Distrito Federal □,
  Mexico 163 D5 19 15N 99 10W
Distrito Federal □,
  Venezuela 168 A4 10 30N 66 55W
Disûq, Egypt . . . . . . 106 H7 31 8N 30 35 E
Diu, India . . . . 92 J4 20 45N 70 58 E
Dīvāndarreh, Iran . . . . 101 E12 35 55N 47 2 E
Divénié, Congo . . . . . 114 C2 2 43 S 12 1 E
Dives →, France 26 C6 49 18N 0 7W
Dives-sur-Mer, France . 26 C6 49 18N 0 7W
Divi Pt., India . . . . . . 95 G5 15 59N 81 9 E
Divichi =
  Dəvəçi, Azerbaijan . 61 K9 41 15N 48 57 E
Divide, U.S.A. 158 D7 45 45N 112 45W
Dividing Ra., Australia . 125 E2 27 45 S 116 0 E
Divinópolis, Brazil . . . 171 F3 20 10 S 44 54W
Divisões, Serra dos,
  Brazil . . . . 171 E1 17 0 S 51 0W
Divjakë, Albania . . . . 50 F3 40 59N 19 32 E
Divnoye, Russia . . . . . 61 H6 45 55N 43 21 E
Divo, Ivory C. 112 D3 5 48N 5 15W
Divriği, Turkey . . . . . 101 C8 39 23N 38 7 E
Dīwāl Kol, Afghan. . . . 92 B2 34 23N 67 52 E
Dix →, U.S.A. 157 G12 37 49N 84 43W
Dixie Mts., U.S.A. . . . 159 G7 37 55N 120 16W
Dixon, Calif., U.S.A. . . 160 G5 38 27N 121 49W
Dixon, Ill., U.S.A. 156 C7 41 50N 89 29W
Dixon, Mont., U.S.A. . . 158 C6 47 19N 114 19W
Dixon Entrance, U.S.A. . 138 C6 54 30N 132 0W
Dixonville, Canada . . . 143 B5 56 32N 117 40W
Diyadin, Turkey . . . . . 101 C10 39 33N 43 40 E
Diyālā →, Iraq . . . . . 101 F11 33 14N 44 31 E
Diyarbakır, Turkey . . . 101 D9 37 55N 40 18 E

Diyodar, India ...... 92 G4 24 8N 71 50 E
Dja ◠, Cameroon .... 114 B2 3 10N 12 58 E
Djadié ➤, Gabon .... 114 B2 0 46N 12 58 E
Djado, Niger .... 109 D2 21 4N 12 14 E
Djado, Plateau du,
  Niger .... 109 D2 21 29N 12 21 E
Djakarta = Jakarta,
  Indonesia ...... 84 D3 6 9 S 106 49 E
Djalma Dutra = Miguel
  Calmon, Brazil ... 170 D3 11 26 S 40 36W
Djalma Dutra = Poções,
  Brazil .... 171 D3 14 31 S 40 21W
Djamâa, Algeria .... 111 B6 33 32N 5 59 E
Djamba, Angola .... 116 B1 16 45 S 13 58 E
Djambala, Congo ... 114 C2 2 32 S 14 30 E
Djanet, Algeria .... 111 D6 24 35N 9 32 E
Djaul I., Papua N. G. 132 B8 2 58 S 150 57 E
Djawa = Jawa,
  Indonesia ...... 85 D4 7 0 S 110 0 E
Djebiniana, Tunisia . 108 A2 35 1N 11 0 E
Djédaa, Chad ..... 109 F3 13 31N 18 34 E
Djelfa, Algeria .... 111 B5 34 40N 3 15 E
Djema, C.A.R. ..... 118 A2 6 3N 25 15 E
Djember, Chad ..... 109 F3 10 25N 17 50 E
Djembe, Dem. Rep. of
  the Congo ...... 115 D4 9 54 S 22 18 E
Djendel, Algeria ... 111 A5 36 15N 2 25 E
Djeneïene, Tunisia . 108 B3 31 45N 10 9 E
Djenné, Mali 112 C4 14 0N 4 30W
Djenoun, Garet el,
  Algeria .... 111 C6 25 4N 5 31 E
Djerba, Tunisia .... 108 B2 33 52N 10 51 E
Djerba, I. de, Tunisia 108 B2 33 50N 10 48 E
Djeréme ➤, Cameroon 114 A2 5 20N 13 24 E
Djerid, Chott, Tunisia 108 B1 33 42N 8 30 E
Djibo, Burkina Faso . 113 C4 14 9N 1 35W
Djibo, Gabon ..... 114 C2 1 20 S 13 9 E
Djibouti, Djibouti .. 107 E5 11 30N 43 5 E
Djibouti ■, Africa ... 107 E5 12 0N 43 0 E
Djohong, Cameroon . 114 A2 6 47N 14 20 E
Djolu, Dem. Rep. of
  the Congo ...... 114 B4 0 35N 22 5 E
Djouab ➤, Gabon ... 114 B2 1 13N 13 12 E
Djougou, Benin .... 113 D5 9 40N 1 45 E
Djoum, Cameroon .. 114 B2 2 41N 12 35 E
Djouna, Chad ..... 109 F4 10 27N 20 4 E
Djourab, Erg du, Chad 109 E3 16 40N 18 50 E
Djugu, Dem. Rep. of
  the Congo ...... 118 B3 1 55N 30 35 E
Djúpávík, Iceland .. 11 B5 65 55N 21 34W
Djúpivogur, Iceland . 11 C12 64 39N 14 17W
Djupvasshytta, Norway 18 B4 62 2N 7 16 E
Djurås, Sweden .... 16 D9 60 34N 15 8 E
Djurdjura ◠, Algeria 111 A5 35 20N 4 15 E
Djuró ◠, Sweden ... 17 F7 58 52S 13 28 E
Djursland, Denmark . 11 H4 56 27N 10 45 E
Dmitriya Lapteva,
  Proliv, Russia ... 67 B15 73 0N 140 0 E
Dmitriyev Lgovskiy,
  Russia .... 59 F8 52 10N 35 0 E
Dmitriyevsk =
  Makiyivka, Ukraine 59 H9 48 0N 38 0 E
Dmitriyevskoye =
  Talas, Kyrgyzstan . 65 B6 42 30N 72 13 E
Dmitrov, Russia ... 58 D9 56 25N 37 32 E
Dmitrovsk-Orlovskiy,
  Russia .... 59 F8 52 29N 35 10 E
Dnepr = Dnipro ➤,
  Ukraine .... 59 J7 46 30N 32 18 E
Dneprodzerzhinsk =
  Dniprodzerzhynsk,
  Ukraine .... 59 H8 48 32N 34 37 E
Dneprodzerzhinskoye
  Vdkhr. =
  Dniprodzerzhynske
  Vdskh., Ukraine .. 59 H8 48 49N 34 8 E
Dnepropetrovsk =
  Dnipropetrovsk,
  Ukraine .... 59 H8 48 30N 35 0 E
Dneprorudnoye =
  Dniprorudne,
  Ukraine .... 59 J8 47 21N 34 58 E
Dnestr = Dnister ➤,
  Europe .... 59 J6 46 18N 30 17 E
Dnestrovski =
  Belgorod, Russia .. 59 G9 50 35N 36 35 E
Dnieper = Dnipro ➤,
  Ukraine .... 59 J7 46 30N 32 18 E
Dniester = Dnister ➤,
  Europe .... 59 J6 46 18N 30 17 E
Dnipro ➤, Ukraine .. 59 J7 46 30N 32 18 E
Dniprodzerzhynsk,
  Ukraine .... 59 H8 48 32N 34 37 E
Dniprodzerzhynske
  Vdskh., Ukraine .. 59 H8 48 49N 34 8 E
Dnipropetrovsk,
  Ukraine .... 59 H8 48 30N 35 0 E
Dniprorudne, Ukraine 59 J8 47 21N 34 58 E
Dnister ➤, Europe .. 59 J6 46 18N 30 17 E
Dnistrovskyy Lyman,
  Ukraine .... 59 J6 46 15N 30 17 E
Dno, Russia ...... 58 D5 57 50N 29 58 E
Dnyapro = Dnipro ➤,
  Ukraine .... 59 J7 46 30N 32 18 E
Doakh, Afghan. ... 91 A3 36 31N 69 32 E
Doaktown, Canada . 141 C6 46 33N 66 8W
Doan Hung, Vietnam 76 G5 21 30N 105 10 E
Doany, Madag. .... 117 A8 14 21 S 49 30 E
Doba, Chad ...... 109 G3 8 40N 16 50 E
Dobandi, Pakistan .. 92 D2 31 13N 66 50 E
Dobbiaco, Italy .... 45 B9 46 44N 12 14 E
Dobbyn, Australia .. 126 B3 19 44 S 140 2 E
Dobczyce, Poland ... 55 J7 49 52N 20 5 E
Dobele, Latvia .... 15 H20 56 37N 23 16 E
Dobele □, Latvia ... 54 B10 56 35N 23 0 E
Döbeln, Germany .. 30 D9 51 6N 13 7 E
Doberai, Jazirah,
  Indonesia ...... 83 B4 1 25 S 133 0 E
Dobiegniew, Poland . 55 F2 52 59N 15 45 E
Doblas, Argentina .. 174 D3 37 5 S 64 0W
Dobo, Dem. Rep. of
  the Congo ...... 114 B4 2 20N 22 11 E
Dobo, Indonesia ... 83 C4 5 45 S 134 15 E
Doboj, Bos.-H. ..... 52 F3 44 46N 18 4 E
Dobra, Wielkopolskie,
  Poland .... 55 G5 51 55N 18 37 E
Dobra,
  Zachodnio-Pomorskie,
  Poland .... 54 E2 53 34N 15 20 E
Dobra, Dâmbovita,
  Romania .... 53 F10 44 52N 25 40 E
Dobra, Hunedoara,
  Romania .... 52 E7 45 54N 22 36 E
Dobre Miasto, Poland 55 E7 53 58N 20 26 E
Dobreşti, Romania .. 52 D7 46 51N 22 18 E
Dobrich, Bulgaria .. 51 C11 43 37N 27 49 E
Dobrinishta, Bulgaria 50 E7 41 49N 23 34 E
Dobříš, Czech Rep. .. 34 B7 49 46N 14 10 E
Dobrodzień, Poland . 55 H5 50 45N 18 25 E
Dobron, Ukraine ... 52 B7 48 25N 22 23 E
Dobropole, Ukraine . 59 H9 48 25N 37 2 E
Dobrovolsk, Russia . 54 D9 54 46N 22 31 E
Dobruja, Europe ... 53 F13 44 30N 28 15 E

Dobrush, Belarus .... 59 F6 52 25N 31 22 E
Dobrzany, Poland ... 54 E2 53 22N 15 25 E
Dobrzyń nad Wisłą,
  Poland .... 55 F6 52 39N 19 22 E
Doc, Mui, Vietnam .. 86 D6 17 58N 106 30 E
Doc Can I., Phil. ... 81 J2 5 55N 119 56 E
Doce ➤, Brazil .... 171 E4 19 37 S 39 49W
Docker River, Australia 125 D4 24 52 S 129 5 E
Docksta, Sweden ... 16 A12 63 3N 18 18 E
Doctor Arroyo, Mexico 162 C4 23 40N 100 11W
Doctors Inlet, U.S.A. 152 E8 30 6N 81 47W
Doda, India ...... 93 C6 33 10N 75 34 E
Doda, L., Canada .. 140 C4 49 25N 75 13W
Doda Betta, India .. 95 J3 11 24N 76 44 E
Dodaga, Indonesia . 82 A3 1 9N 128 11 E
Dodballapur, India . 95 H3 13 18N 77 32 E
Dodecanese =
  Dhodhekánisos,
  Greece .... 49 E8 36 35N 27 0 E
Dodge City, U.S.A. . 155 G5 37 45N 100 1W
Dodge L., Canada .. 143 B7 59 50N 105 36W
Dodgeville, U.S.A. . 156 B6 42 58N 90 8W
Dodo, Cameroon ... 113 D7 7 30N 12 3 E
Dodo, Sudan ...... 107 F2 5 10N 29 57 E
Dodola, Ethiopia ... 107 F4 6 59N 39 11 E
Dodoma, Tanzania . 118 D4 6 8 S 35 45 E
Dodoma □, Tanzania 118 D4 6 0 S 36 0 E
Dodona, Greece .... 48 B2 39 40N 20 46 E
Dodori ◠, Kenya ... 118 C5 1 55 S 41 7 E
Dodsland, Canada .. 143 C7 51 50N 108 45W
Dodson, U.S.A. 158 B9 48 24N 108 15W
Dodurga, Turkey ... 49 B11 39 49N 29 57 E
Doerun, U.S.A. 152 D6 31 19N 83 55W
Doesburg, Neths. ... 24 B6 52 1N 6 9 E
Dog Creek, Canada . 142 C4 51 35N 122 14W
Dog L., Man., Canada 143 C9 51 2N 98 31W
Dog L., Ont., Canada 140 C2 48 48N 89 30W
Doğanşehir, Turkey . 100 C7 38 5N 37 53 E
Dogliani, Italy ..... 44 D4 44 32 S 7 55 E
Dōgo, Japan ...... 72 A5 36 15N 133 16 E
Dōgo-San, Japan ... 72 B5 35 2N 133 13 E
Dogondoutchi, Niger 113 C5 13 38N 4 2 E
Dogran, Pakistan ... 92 D5 31 48N 73 35 E
Doğubayazıt, Turkey 101 C11 39 31N 44 5 E
Doguéraoua, Niger . 113 C6 14 0N 5 31 E
Dogura, Papua N. G. 132 F6 10 6 S 150 5 E
Doha = Ad Dawḥah,
  Qatar .... 97 E6 25 15N 51 35 E
Dohazari, Bangla. .. 90 A2 22 10N 92 5 E
Dohinog = Manukan,
  Phil. .... 81 G4 8 32N 123 12 E
Dohrighat, India ... 93 F10 26 16N 83 31 E
Dohrn Banke,
  Greenland 10 D8 65 55N 25 50W
Doi, Indonesia .... 82 A3 2 14N 127 49 E
Doi Inthanon ◠,
  Thailand .... 86 C2 18 33N 98 34 E
Doi Khuntan ◠,
  Thailand .... 86 C2 18 33N 99 14 E
Doi Luang, Thailand 86 C3 18 30N 101 0 E
Doi Luang ◠, Thailand 86 C2 19 22N 99 35 E
Doi Saket, Thailand . 86 C2 18 52N 99 9 E
Doi Suthep ◠, Thailand 86 C2 18 49N 98 53 E
Dois Irmãos, Sa., Brazil 170 C3 9 0 S 42 30W
Dojransko Jezero,
  Macedonia ..... 50 E6 41 13N 22 44 E
Dokka, Norway .... 18 D7 60 49N 10 7 E
Dokka ➤, Norway .. 18 D7 60 49N 10 7 E
Dokkum, Neths. ... 24 A5 53 20N 5 59 E
Dokri, Pakistan .... 92 F3 27 25N 68 7 E
Dokshukino =
  Nartkala, Russia .. 61 J6 43 33N 43 51 E
Dokuchayevsk, Ukraine 59 J9 47 44N 37 40 E
Dol-de-Bretagne,
  France 26 D5 48 34N 1 47W
Dolac, Serbia & M. . 50 D4 42 36N 20 36 E
Dolak, Pulau, Indonesia 83 C5 8 0 S 138 30 E
Dolbeau-Mistassini,
  Canada 141 C5 48 53N 72 14W
Dole, France ...... 27 E12 47 7N 5 31 E
Doleib, Wadi ➤, Sudan 107 E3 12 10N 33 15 E
Dolenji Logatec,
  Slovenia .... 45 C11 45 56N 14 15 E
Dolgellau, U.K. 20 E4 52 45N 3 53W
Dolgelley = Dolgellau,
  U.K. 20 E4 52 45N 3 53W
Dolhasca, Romania . 53 C11 47 26N 26 36 E
Dolianova, Italy ... 46 C2 39 22N 9 10 E
Dolinskaya = Dolynska,
  Ukraine .... 59 H7 48 6N 32 46 E
Dolj □, Romania ... 53 F8 44 10N 23 30 E
Dollard, Neths. .... 24 A7 53 20N 7 10 E
Dolna Banya, Bulgaria 50 D7 42 18N 23 44 E
Dolni Chiflik, Bulgaria 51 D11 42 59N 27 43 E
Dolní Dúbník, Bulgaria 51 C8 43 24N 24 26 E
Dolnośląskie □, Poland 55 G3 51 10N 16 30 E
Dolný Kubín,
  Slovak Rep. ..... 35 B12 49 12N 19 18 E
Dolo, Ethiopia .... 107 G5 4 11N 42 3 E
Dolo, Italy .... 45 C9 45 25N 12 5 E
Dolomites = Dolomiti,
  Italy .... 45 B8 46 23N 11 51 E
Dolomiti, Italy .... 45 B8 46 23N 11 51 E
Dolomiti Bellunesi ◠,
  Italy .... 45 B9 46 10N 12 5 E
Dolores, Argentina . 174 D4 36 20 S 57 40W
Dolores, Phil. ..... 80 E5 12 25N 125 29 E
Dolores, Uruguay .. 174 C4 33 34 S 58 15W
Dolores, U.S.A. 159 H9 37 28N 108 30W
Dolores ➤, U.S.A. .. 159 G9 38 49N 109 17W
Dolovo, Serbia & M. 52 F5 44 55N 20 52 E
Dolphin, C., Falk. Is. . 9 f
Dolphin and Union
  Str., Canada 138 B8 69 5N 114 45W
Dolsk, Poland ..... 55 G4 51 59N 17 3 E
Dolungmukh, India . 90 B5 27 30N 94 18 E
Dolyna, Ukraine ... 59 H3 48 58N 24 1 E
Dolynska, Ukraine . 59 H7 48 6N 32 46 E
Dolynske, Ukraine . 53 C14 47 32N 29 55 E
Dolynskaya, Russia . 59 J9 46 47N 37 48 E
Dom, Switz. ...... 32 E5 46 6N 7 50 E
Dom Joaquim, Brazil 171 E3 18 57 S 43 16W
Dom Pedrito, Brazil 175 C5 31 0 S 54 40W
Dom Pedro, Brazil . 170 B3 4 59 S 44 27W
Doma = Gombe,
  Nigeria .... 113 C7 10 19N 11 2 E
Doma, Nigeria .... 113 D6 8 25N 8 18 E
Doma ➤, Zimbabwe 119 F3 16 28 S 30 12 E
Domaniç, Turkey ... 49 B11 39 48N 29 36 E
Domar ◠, Chad .... 109 F3 18 11N 18 4 E
Domariaganj ➤, India 93 F10 26 17N 83 44 E
Domasi, Malawi ... 119 F4 15 15 S 35 25 E
Domat Ems, Switz. . 33 C8 46 50N 9 27 E
Domažlice, Czech Rep. 34 B5 49 28N 12 58 E
Dombarovka =
  Dombarovskiy,
  Russia .... 64 F7 50 46N 59 32 E
Dombarovskiy, Russia 64 F7 50 46N 59 32 E

Dombås, Norway ... 18 B6 62 4N 9 8 E
Dombasle-sur-Meurthe,
  France .... 27 D13 48 38N 6 21 E
Dombes, France ... 29 C9 45 58N 5 0 E
Dombóvár, Hungary 52 D3 46 21N 18 9 E
Dombrád, Hungary . 52 B6 48 13N 21 54 E
Dombrova = Dąbrowa
  Górnicza, Poland . 55 H6 50 15N 19 10 E
Dombrowitsa =
  Dubrovytsya,
  Ukraine .... 59 G4 51 31N 26 35 E
Dome Fuji, Antarctica 7 D5 77 20 S 39 45 E
Domeyko, Chile ... 174 B1 29 0 S 71 0W
Domeyko, Cordillera,
  Chile .... 174 A2 24 30 S 69 0W
Domfront, France .. 26 D6 48 37N 0 40W
Dominador, Chile .. 174 A2 24 21 S 69 20W
Dominica ■, W. Indies 165 C7 15 20N 61 20W
Dominica Passage,
  W. Indies 165 C7 15 10N 61 20W
Dominican Rep. ■,
  W. Indies 165 C5 19 0N 70 30W
Domingo, Dem. Rep.
  of the Congo .... 115 C4 4 37 S 21 15 E
Dömitz, Germany .. 30 B7 53 9N 11 16 E
Domme, France .... 28 D5 44 48N 1 12 E
Domneşti, Romania 53 E9 45 12N 24 50 E
Domo, Ethiopia ... 120 C3 7 50N 47 10 E
Domodóssola, Italy . 44 B5 46 7N 8 17 E
Domogled-Valea
  Cernei ◠, Romania 52 F7 44 52N 22 27 E
Dompaire, France .. 27 D13 48 14N 6 14 E
Dompim, Ghana ... 112 D4 5 10N 1 52W
Dompu, Indonesia . 85 D5 8 32 S 118 28 E
Domrémy-la-Pucelle,
  France .... 27 D12 48 26N 5 40 E
Domville, Mt.,
  Australia .... 127 D5 28 1 S 151 15 E
Domvraína, Greece . 48 C4 38 15N 22 59 E
Domžale, Slovenia . 45 B11 46 9N 14 35 E
Don ➤, India ..... 95 F3 16 20N 76 15 E
Don ➤, Russia .... 59 J10 47 4N 39 18 E
Don ➤, Aberds., U.K. 22 D6 57 11N 2 5W
Don ➤, S. Yorks., U.K. 20 D7 53 41N 0 52W
Don, C., Australia .. 124 B5 11 18 S 131 46 E
Don Benito, Spain . 43 G5 38 53N 5 51W
Don Figuero Mts.,
  Jamaica .... 164 a 18 5N 77 36W
Don Sak, Thailand . 87 b 9 18N 99 41 E
Dona Ana =
  Nhamaabué, Mozam. 119 F4 17 25 S 35 5 E
Doña Mencía, Spain 43 H6 37 33N 4 21W
Donaghadee, U.K. . 23 B6 54 39N 5 33W
Donald, Australia .. 128 D5 36 23 S 143 0 E
Donaldsonville, U.S.A. 155 K9 30 6N 90 59W
Donalsonville, U.S.A. 152 D5 31 3N 84 53W
Doñana ◠, Spain .. 43 J4 36 59N 6 23W
Donau = Dunărea ➤,
  Europe .... 53 E14 45 20N 29 40 E
Donau ➤, Austria .. 35 C10 48 10N 17 0 E
Donau ➤, Austria .. 35 C9 48 8N 16 44 E
Donaueschingen,
  Germany .... 31 H4 47 56N 8 29 E
Donauwörth, Germany 31 G6 48 43N 10 47 E
Doncaster, U.K. ... 20 D6 53 32N 1 6W
Dondo, Angola .... 115 D2 9 45 S 14 25 E
Dondo, Dem. Rep. of
  the Congo ...... 114 B4 4 11N 21 39 E
Dondo, Mozam. ... 119 F3 19 33 S 34 46 E
Dondo, Teluk,
  Indonesia ...... 82 A2 0 50N 120 30 E
Dondra Head,
  Sri Lanka ...... 95 M5 5 55N 80 40 E
Donduşeni, Moldova 53 B12 48 14N 27 36 E
Donegal, Ireland ... 23 B3 54 39N 8 5W
Donegal □, Ireland . 23 B4 54 53N 8 0W
Donegal B., Ireland . 23 B3 54 31N 8 49W
Donets ➤, Russia .. 61 G5 47 33N 40 55 E
Donets Basin, Ukraine 12 F13 49 0N 38 0 E
Donetsk, Ukraine .. 59 J9 48 0N 37 45 E
Dong Ba Thin, Vietnam 87 F7 12 8N 109 13 E
Dong Dang, Vietnam 76 G6 21 54N 106 42 E
Dong Giam, Vietnam 86 C5 19 25N 105 31 E
Dong Ha, Vietnam . 86 D6 16 55N 107 8 E
Dong Hoi, Vietnam . 86 D6 17 29N 106 36 E
Dong Jiang ➤, China 77 F10 23 6N 114 0 E
Dong Khe, Vietnam 86 A6 22 26N 106 27 E
Dong Ujimqin Qi,
  China .... 74 B9 45 32N 116 55 E
Dong Van, Vietnam 86 A5 23 16N 105 22 E
Dong Xoai, Vietnam 87 G6 11 32N 106 55 E
Donga, Nigeria .... 113 D7 7 45N 10 2 E
Donga ➤, Nigeria .. 113 D7 8 20N 9 58 E
Dong'an, China .... 79 D8 26 23N 111 12 E
Dongara, Australia . 125 E1 29 14 S 114 57 E
Dongargarh, India . 94 D5 21 10N 80 40 E
Dongbei, China .... 67 E13 45 0N 125 0 E
Dongchuan, China . 76 D4 26 8N 103 1 E
Dongducheon, S. Korea 75 F14 37 55N 127 7 E
Dongfang, China .. 86 C7 18 50N 108 33 E
Dongfeng, China .. 75 C13 42 40N 125 34 E
Donggala, Indonesia 82 B1 0 30 S 119 40 E
Donggan, China ... 76 F5 27 22N 105 9 E
Donggou, China ... 75 E13 39 52N 124 8 E
Dongguan, China .. 79 F9 22 58N 113 44 E
Dongguang, China . 74 F9 37 50N 116 30 E
Donghai Dao, China 77 G8 21 0N 110 15 E
Dongjingcheng, China 75 B15 44 5N 129 12 E
Dongkou, China ... 77 D8 26 1N 110 35 E
Donglan, China ... 76 E6 24 30N 107 21 E
Dongliu, China ... 77 B11 30 13N 116 55 E
Dongmen, China ... 76 F6 22 20N 107 48 E
Dongning, China .. 75 B16 44 2N 131 5 E
Dongnyi, China ... 78 D3 28 3N 100 15 E
Dongo, Angola .... 115 E3 14 36 S 15 48 E
Dongo, Dem. Rep. of
  the Congo ...... 114 B3 4 35N 18 30 E
Dongola, Sudan ... 106 D3 19 9N 30 22 E
Dongou, Congo .... 114 B3 2 0N 18 5 E
Dongping, China ... 74 G9 35 55N 116 20 E
Dongsha Dao, China 77 G11 20 45N 116 43 E
Dongsheng, China . 74 E6 39 50N 110 0 E
Dongtai, China .... 75 H11 32 51N 120 21 E
Dongting Hu, China 79 C9 29 18N 112 45 E
Dongtou, China ... 77 D13 27 51N 121 10 E
Dongwe ➤, Zambia 115 E4 15 39 S 24 15 E
Dongxiang, China .. 77 C11 28 11N 116 34 E
Dongxing, China ... 76 F7 21 34N 108 0 E
Dongyang, China .. 77 C13 29 13N 120 15 E
Dongzhi, China .... 77 B11 30 13N 117 0 E
Donington, C.,
  Australia .... 128 C2 34 45 S 136 0 E
Doniphan, U.S.A. .. 155 G9 36 37N 90 50W
Donja Stubica, Croatia 45 C12 45 59N 15 59 E
Donji Dušnik,
  Serbia & M. ..... 50 C6 43 12N 22 5 E

Donji Miholjac, Croatia 52 E3 45 45N 18 10 E
Donji Milanovac,
  Serbia & M. ..... 50 B6 44 28N 22 6 E
Donji Vakuf, Bos.-H. 52 F2 44 8N 17 24 E
Dønna, Norway .... 14 C15 66 6N 12 30 E
Donna, U.S.A. 155 M5 26 9N 98 4W
Donnaconna, Canada 141 C5 46 41N 71 41W
Donnelly's Crossing,
  N.Z. .... 130 B2 35 42 S 173 38 E
Donnybrook, Australia 125 F2 33 34 S 115 48 E
Donnybrook, S. Africa 117 D4 29 59 S 29 48 E
Donora, U.S.A. 150 F5 40 11N 79 52W
Donostia = Donostia-
  San Sebastián, Spain 40 B3 43 17N 1 58W
Donostia-San
  Sebastián, Spain . 40 B3 43 17N 1 58W
Donovan, U.S.A. ... 157 D9 40 53N 87 37W
Dongue, Angola ... 115 F2 15 28 S 14 6 E
Donskoy, Russia ... 59 F10 53 55N 38 15 E
Donsol, Phil. ..... 80 E4 12 54N 123 36 E
Donzère, France ... 29 D8 44 28N 4 43 E
Donzy, France ..... 27 E10 47 20N 3 6 E
Dookie, Australia .. 129 D6 36 33 S 145 41 E
Doon ➤, U.K. 22 F4 55 27N 4 39W
Doonbeg ➤, Ireland 23 D2 52 43N 9 31W
Doornik = Tournai,
  Belgium .... 24 D3 50 35N 3 25 E
Dora, L., Australia . 124 D3 22 0 S 123 0 E
Dora Báltea ➤, Italy 44 C5 45 11N 8 3 E
Dora Ripária ➤, Italy 44 C4 45 5N 7 44 E
Doran L., Canada .. 143 A7 61 13N 108 6W
Doraville, U.S.A. .. 152 B5 33 54N 84 17W
Dorchester, U.K. .. 21 G5 50 42N 2 27W
Dorchester, C., Canada 139 B12 65 27N 77 27W
Dordabis, Namibia . 116 C2 22 52 S 17 38 E
Dordogne □, France 28 C4 45 5N 0 40 E
Dordogne ➤, France 28 C3 45 2N 0 36W
Dordrecht, Neths. .. 24 C4 51 48N 4 39 E
Dordrecht, S. Africa 116 E4 31 20 S 27 3 E
Dore ➤, France .... 28 C7 45 50N 3 35 E
Dore, Mts., France . 28 C6 45 32N 2 50 E
Doré L., Canada ... 143 C7 54 46N 107 17W
Doré Lake, Canada . 143 C7 54 38N 107 36W
Dores da Boa
  Esperança = Boa
  Esperança, Brazil . 169 C5 3 21N 61 23W
Dores do Indaiá, Brazil 171 E2 19 27 S 45 36W
Dorfen, Germany .. 31 G8 48 16N 12 8 E
Dorgali, Italy ..... 46 B2 40 17N 9 35 E
Dori, Burkina Faso . 113 C4 14 3N 0 2W
Doring ➤, S. Africa 116 E2 31 54 S 18 39 E
Doringbos, S. Africa 116 E2 31 59 S 19 16 E
Dornie, U.K. 22 D3 57 17N 5 31W
Dornoch, U.K. 22 D4 57 53N 4 2W
Dornoch Firth, U.K. 22 D4 57 51N 4 4W
Dornogovi □, Mongolia 74 C6 44 0N 110 0 E
Doro, Mali 113 B4 16 9N 0 51W
Dorog, Hungary ... 52 C3 47 42N 18 45 E
Dorogobuzh, Russia 58 E7 54 50N 33 18 E
Dorohoi, Romania . 53 C11 47 56N 26 23 E
Döröö Nuur, Mongolia 68 B4 48 0N 93 0 E
Dorpat = Tartu, Estonia 15 G22 58 20N 26 44 E
Dorr, Iran .... 97 C6 33 17N 50 38 E
Dorre I., Australia . 125 E1 25 13 S 113 12 E
Dorrigo, Australia . 129 A10 30 20 S 152 44 E
Dorrigo □, Australia 129 A10 30 22 S 152 47 E
Dorris, U.S.A. 158 F3 41 58N 121 55W
Dorset, Canada ... 150 A6 45 14N 78 54W
Dorset, U.S.A. 150 E4 41 40N 80 40W
Dorset □, U.K. 21 G5 50 45N 2 20W
Dorsten, Germany . 24 C7 51 39N 6 58 E
Dortmund, Germany 30 D3 51 30N 7 28 E
Dortmund-Ems-
  Kanal ➤, Germany 30 D3 51 50N 7 26 E
Dörtyol, Turkey ... 100 D7 36 50N 36 13 E
Dorum, Germany .. 30 B4 53 41N 8 34 E
Doruma, Dem. Rep. of
  the Congo ...... 118 B2 4 42N 27 33 E
Dorūneh, Iran ..... 97 C8 35 10N 57 18 E
Dos Bahías, C.,
  Argentina ...... 176 E3 44 58 S 65 32W
Dos Hermanas, Spain 43 H5 37 16N 5 55W
Dos Palos, U.S.A. .. 161 J6 36 59N 120 37W
Dösemealtı, Turkey 49 D12 37 4N 30 36 E
Dosso, Niger ...... 113 C5 13 0N 3 13 E
Dosso □, Niger .... 113 C5 12 20N 3 0 E
Dothan, U.S.A. 152 D5 31 13N 85 24W
Dotnuva, Lithuania 54 C11 55 23N 23 54 E
Döttingen, Switz. .. 32 A6 47 34N 8 15 E
Doty, U.S.A. 160 D3 46 38N 123 17W
Douai, France ..... 27 B10 50 21N 3 4 E
Douako, Guinea ... 112 D2 9 45N 10 8W
Douala, Cameroon . 113 E6 4 0N 9 45 E
Douala-Édéa ◠,
  Cameroon ...... 114 B1 3 30N 9 41 E
Douaouir, Mali 110 D4 20 45N 3 0W
Douarnenez, France 26 D2 48 6N 4 21W
Doubabougou, Mali 112 C3 14 13N 7 59W
Double Cone, N.Z. . 131 F3 45 18 S 168 49 E
Double Island Pt.,
  Australia .... 127 D5 25 56 S 153 11 E
Double Mountain
  Fork ➤, U.S.A. .. 155 J4 33 16N 100 0W
Doubrava ◻,
  Czech Rep. ..... 34 A8 50 ... 15 20 E
Doubs □, France .. 27 E13 47 10N 6 20 E
Doubs ➤, France .. 27 F12 46 53N 5 1 E
Doubtful Sd., N.Z. . 131 F1 45 20 S 166 49 E
Doubtless B., N.Z. . 130 A2 34 55 S 173 26 E
Doudeville, France . 26 C7 49 43N 0 47 E
Doué-la-Fontaine,
  France 26 E6 47 11N 0 16W
Douentza, Mali .... 112 C4 14 58 S 2 48W
Douentza ◻, Mali . 112 C4 15 0N 3 0W
Dougga, Tunisia ... 108 A1 36 30N 8 55 E
Doughboy B., P.N.G. 131 H2 47 2 S 167 40 E
Douglas, I. of Man . 20 C3 54 10N 4 28W
Douglas, S. Africa . 116 D3 29 4 S 23 46 E
Douglas, Alaska, U.S.A. 144 G14 58 17N 134 24W
Douglas, Ariz., U.S.A. 159 L9 31 21N 109 33W
Douglas, Ga., U.S.A. 152 D7 31 31N 82 51W
Douglas, Mich., U.S.A. 157 B10 42 39N 86 12W
Douglas, Wyo., U.S.A. 154 D2 42 45N 105 24W
Douglas Apsley ◠,
  Australia .... 127 G4 41 45 S 148 11 E
Douglas, C.,
  Antarctica ...... 5 C11 ...
Douglas Chan., Canada 142 C3 53 40N 129 20W
Douglas Pt., Canada 150 B3 44 19N 81 37W
Douglasville, U.S.A. 152 B5 33 45N 84 45W
Douirat, Morocco .. 110 B4 33 2N 4 11W
Doukáton, Ákra,
  Greece .... 49 B2 38 34N 20 33 E
Doukoula, Cameroon 109 F2 10 10N 15 0 E
Doukoula, Cameroon 114 A2 10 0N 15 0 E

Doulevant-le-Château,
  France .... 27 D11 48 23N 4 55 E
Doullens, France ... 27 B9 50 10N 2 20 E
Doumé, Cameroon . 114 B2 4 15N 13 25 E
Doumen, China .... 77 F9 22 10N 113 18 E
Douna, Mali 112 C3 13 13N 6 0W
Dounguila, Congo . 114 C2 2 53 S 11 58 E
Dounreay, U.K. 22 C5 58 35N 3 44W
Dourada, Serra, Brazil 171 D2 13 10 S 48 45W
Dourados, Brazil .. 175 A5 22 9 S 54 50W
Dourados ➤, Brazil 175 A5 21 58 S 54 18W
Dourados, Serra dos,
  Brazil .... 175 A5 23 30 S 53 30W
Dourbali, Chad .... 109 F3 11 49N 15 52 E
Dourdan, France ... 27 D9 48 29N 2 1 E
Douro ➤, Europe .. 42 D2 41 8N 8 40W
Douvaine, France .. 27 F13 46 19N 6 16 E
Douvres-la-Délivrande,
  France 26 C6 49 17N 0 23W
Douz, Tunisia ..... 108 B1 33 25N 9 0 E
Douze ➤, France .. 28 E3 43 54N 0 30W
Dove ➤, U.K. 20 E6 52 51N 1 36W
Dove Creek, U.S.A. 159 H9 37 46N 108 54W
Dover, Australia ... 127 G4 43 18 S 147 2 E
Dover, U.K. ...... 21 F9 51 7N 1 19 E
Dover, Del., U.S.A. 148 F8 39 10N 75 32W
Dover, Ky., U.S.A. . 157 F13 38 43N 83 52W
Dover, N.H., U.S.A. 151 C14 43 12N 70 56W
Dover, N.J., U.S.A. 151 F10 40 53N 74 34W
Dover, Ohio, U.S.A. 150 F3 40 32N 81 29W
Dover, Pt., Australia 125 F4 32 32 S 125 32 E
Dover, Str. of, Europe 21 G9 51 0N 1 30 E
Dover-Foxcroft, U.S.A. 149 C11 45 11N 69 13W
Dover Plains, U.S.A. 151 E11 41 43N 73 35W
Dovey = Dyfi ➤, U.K. 21 E3 52 32N 4 3W
Dovhe, Ukraine .... 53 B8 48 22N 23 17 E
Dovlen = Devin,
  Bulgaria .... 51 E8 41 44N 24 24 E
Dovre, Norway .... 18 C6 61 58N 9 15 E
Dovrefjell, Norway . 18 B6 62 15N 9 33 E
Dovrefjell ◻, Norway 18 B6 62 15N 9 25 E
Dow Rūd, Iran .... 97 C6 33 28N 49 4 E
Dowa, Malawi ..... 119 E3 13 38 S 33 58 E
Dowagiac, U.S.A. .. 157 C10 41 59N 86 6W
Dowerin, Australia . 125 F2 31 12 S 117 2 E
Dowgha'i, Iran .... 97 B8 36 54N 58 32 E
Dowlat Yār, Afghan. 91 B2 34 30N 65 45 E
Dowlatābād, Farāh,
  Afghan. .... 91 B1 32 47N 62 40 E
Dowlatābād, Fāryāb,
  Afghan. .... 65 E2 36 26N 64 55 E
Dowlatābād, Iran .. 97 D8 28 20N 56 40 E
Dowling Park, U.S.A. 152 E6 30 15N 83 15W
Down □, U.K. 23 B5 54 23N 6 2W
Downers Grove, U.S.A. 157 C8 41 48N 88 1W
Downey, Calif., U.S.A. 161 M8 33 56N 118 7W
Downey, Idaho, U.S.A. 158 E7 42 26N 112 7W
Downham Market,
  U.K. .... 21 E8 52 37N 0 23 E
Downieville, U.S.A. 160 F6 39 34N 120 50W
Downing, U.S.A. .. 156 D4 40 29N 92 22W
Downpatrick, U.K. . 23 B6 54 20N 5 43W
Downpatrick Hd.,
  Ireland 23 B2 54 20N 9 21W
Downsville, U.S.A. 151 D10 42 5N 74 50W
Downton, Mt., Canada 142 C4 52 42N 124 52W
Dowsārī, Iran ..... 97 D8 28 25N 57 59 E
Dowshī, Afghan. .. 91 B3 35 35N 68 43 E
Doyle, U.S.A. 160 E6 40 2N 120 6W
Doylestown, U.S.A. 151 F9 40 21N 75 10W
Dōzen, Japan ..... 72 A5 36 5N 133 0 E
Dozois, Rés., Canada 140 C4 47 30N 77 5W
Dra Khel, Pakistan . 92 F2 27 58N 66 45 E
Drâa, C., Morocco . 110 C2 28 47N 11 0W
Drâa, Hamada du,
  Algeria 110 C3 28 0N 7 0W
Drâa, Oued ➤,
  Morocco 110 C2 28 40N 11 10W
Drac ➤, France .... 29 C9 45 12N 5 42 E
Dračevo, Macedonia 50 E5 41 56N 21 31 E
Drachten, Neths. .. 24 A6 53 7N 6 5 E
Drăgănești, Moldova 53 C13 47 43N 28 15 E
Drăgănești-Olt,
  Romania .... 53 F9 44 9N 24 32 E
Drăgănești-Vlașca,
  Romania .... 53 F10 44 5N 25 33 E
Dragaš, Serbia & M. 50 D4 42 5N 20 41 E
Drăgăşani, Romania 53 F9 44 39N 24 17 E
Dragichyn, Belarus . 59 F3 52 15N 25 8 E
Dragocvet, Serbia & M. 50 C5 43 58N 21 16 E
Dragon's Mouth = Boca
  de Drago, Venezuela 169 F11 11 0N 61 50W
Dragovishtitsa,
  Bulgaria .... 50 D6 42 22N 22 39 E
Draguignan, France 29 E10 43 32N 6 27 E
Drahovo, Ukraine .. 53 B8 48 14N 23 33 E
Drain, U.S.A. 158 E2 43 40N 123 19W
Drake, U.S.A. 154 B4 47 55N 100 23W
Drake Passage,
  S. Ocean .... 7 B17 58 0 S 68 0W
Drakensberg, S. Africa 117 D4 31 0 S 28 0 E
Dráma, Greece .... 51 E8 41 9N 24 10 E
Dráma □, Greece .. 51 B8 41 20N 24 0 E
Dramburg = Drawsko
  Pomorskie, Poland 54 E2 53 35N 15 50 E
Drammen, Norway . 18 E7 59 42N 10 12 E
Drangajökull, Iceland 11 A4 66 9N 22 15W
Drangedal, Norway . 18 E6 59 6N 9 3 E
Dranov, Ostrov,
  Romania .... 53 F14 44 55N 29 30 E
Dras, India .... 93 B6 34 25N 75 48 E
Drau = Drava ➤,
  Croatia .... 52 E3 45 33N 18 55 E
Drava ➤, Croatia .. 52 E3 45 33N 18 55 E
Dravinja ➤, Slovenia 45 B12 46 36N 15 5 E
Dravograd, Slovenia 45 B12 46 36N 15 5 E
Drawa ➤, Poland .. 55 F2 52 52N 15 59 E
Drawieński ◻, Poland 55 F2 53 7N 15 45 E
Drawno, Poland ... 54 E2 53 13N 15 46 E
Drawsko Pomorskie,
  Poland .... 54 E2 53 35N 15 50 E
Drayton Plains, U.S.A. 157 B13 42 42N 83 23W
Drayton Valley,
  Canada 142 C6 53 12N 114 58W
Dreieich, Germany . 31 E4 50 1N 8 41 E
Dreikikir, Papua N. G. 132 B2 3 37 S 142 46 E
Dren, Serbia & M. . 50 C4 43 8N 20 46 E
Drenthe □, Neths. . 24 B6 52 52N 6 40 E
Drepanum, C., Cyprus 49 F8 34 54N 32 19 E
Dresden, Germany . 30 D9 51 3N 13 44 E
Dreux, France ..... 26 D8 48 44N 1 23 E
Drevsjø, Norway .. 18 C9 61 53N 12 1 E
Drexel, U.S.A. 157 E12 39 45N 84 18W
Drezdenko, Poland . 55 F2 52 50N 15 49 E
Driesen = Drezdenko,
  Poland .... 55 F2 52 50N 15 49 E
Driffield, U.K. 20 C7 54 0N 0 26W
Driftwood, U.S.A. . 150 E6 41 20N 78 8W
Driggs, U.S.A. 158 E8 43 44N 111 6W
Drin ➤, Albania ... 50 D3 41 39N 19 38 E
Drin i Zi ➤, Albania 50 E3 41 37N 20 28 E
Drina ➤, Bos.-H. .. 50 B3 44 53N 19 21 E
Drincea ➤, Romania 52 F7 44 20N 22 55 E

Drinjača →, Bos.-H. . 52 F4 44 15N 19 8 E
Drissa =
  Vyerkhnyadzvinsk,
  Belarus . . . . 58 E4 55 45N 27 58 E
Driva →, Norway . . . 18 B6 62 41N 9 31 E
Drivstua, Norway . . . 18 B6 62 26N 9 47 E
Drniš, Croatia . . . . . 45 E13 43 51N 16 10 E
Drøbak, Norway . . . . 18 E7 59 39N 10 39 E
Drobeta-Turnu Severin,
  Romania . . . . 52 F7 44 39N 22 41 E
Drobin, Poland . . . . 55 F6 52 42N 19 58 E
Drochia, Moldova . . . 53 B12 48 2N 27 48 E
Drogheda, Ireland . . . 23 C5 53 43N 6 22W
Drogichin = Dragichyn,
  Belarus . . . . 59 F3 52 15N 25 8 E
Drogobych =
  Drohobych, Ukraine . 55 J10 49 20N 23 30 E
Drogobych, Poland . . 55 F9 52 42N 22 39 E
Drohobych, Ukraine . 55 J10 49 20N 23 30 E
Droichead Atha =
  Drogheda, Ireland . . 23 C5 53 43N 6 22W
Droichead Nua, Ireland 23 C5 53 11N 6 48W
Droitwich, U.K. 21 E5 52 16N 2 8W
Drôme □, France . . . 29 D9 44 38N 5 15 E
Drôme →, France . . . 29 D8 44 46N 4 46 E
Dromedary, C.,
  Australia . . . . 129 D6 36 17 S 150 10 E
Drömling △, Germany . 30 C7 52 29N 11 5 E
Dromore, U.K. 23 B4 54 31N 7 28W
Dromore West, Ireland 23 B3 54 15N 8 52W
Dronero, Italy . . . . . 44 D4 44 28N 7 22 E
Dronfield, U.K. 20 D6 53 19N 1 27W
Dronne →, France . . . 28 C3 45 2N 0 9W
Dronning Ingrid Land,
  Greenland 10 D5 66 25N 52 5W
Dronning Maud Land,
  Antarctica . . . . 7 D3 72 30 S 12 0 E
Dronninglund,
  Denmark . . . . 17 G4 57 10N 10 19 E
Dronten, Neths. . . . . 24 B5 52 32N 5 43 E
Dropt →, France . . . 28 D3 44 35N 0 6W
Drosendorf, Austria . . 34 C8 48 52N 15 37 E
Drosh, Pakistan . . . . 91 B3 35 33N 71 48 E
Droué, France . . . . . 26 D8 48 2N 1 6 E
Drouin, Australia . . . 129 E6 38 10 S 145 53 E
Drueulu, N. Cal. . . . . 133 K5 20 56 S 167 5 E
Druk Yul = Bhutan ■,
  Asia . . . . 90 B3 27 25N 90 30 E
Drumbo, Canada . . . 150 C4 43 16N 80 35W
Drumheller, Canada . . 142 C6 51 25N 112 40W
Drummond, U.S.A. . . 158 C7 46 40N 113 9W
Drummond I., U.S.A. . 148 C4 46 1N 83 39W
Drummond Pt.,
  Australia . . . . 127 E2 34 9 S 135 16 E
Drummond Ra.,
  Australia . . . . 126 C4 23 45 S 147 10 E
Drummondville,
  Canada 140 C5 45 55N 72 25W
Drumright, U.S.A. . . . 155 H6 35 59N 96 36W
Druskieniki =
  Druskininkai,
  Lithuania . . . . 15 J20 54 3N 23 58 E
Druskininkai, Lithuania 15 J20 54 3N 23 58 E
Drut →, Belarus . . . . 59 F6 53 3N 30 5 E
Druya, Belarus . . . . 58 E4 55 45N 27 28 E
Druzhba, Bulgaria . . . 51 C12 43 15N 28 1 E
Druzhina, Russia . . . 67 C15 68 14N 145 18 E
Drvar, Bos.-H. . . . . . 45 D13 44 21N 16 23 E
Drvenik, Croatia . . . . 45 E13 43 27N 16 3 E
Drwęca →, Poland . . . 55 E5 53 0N 18 42 E
Dry Harbour Mts.,
  Jamaica . . . . 164 a 18 19N 77 24W
Dry Tortugas, U.S.A. . 164 B3 24 38N 82 55W
Dryanovo, Bulgaria . . 51 D9 42 59N 25 28 E
Dryden, Canada 143 D10 49 47N 92 50W
Dryden, U.S.A. 151 D8 42 30N 76 18W
Drygalski I., Antarctica 7 C7 66 0 S 92 0 E
Drysdale →, Australia . 124 B4 13 59 S 126 51 E
Drysdale I., Australia . 126 A2 11 41 S 136 0 E
Drysdale River △,
  Australia . . . . 124 B4 14 56 S 127 2 E
Drzewica, Poland . . . 55 G7 51 27N 20 29 E
Drzewiczka →, Poland 55 G7 51 36N 20 36 E
Dschang, Cameroon . . 113 D7 5 32N 10 3 E
Du Gué →, Canada . . 140 A5 57 21N 70 45W
Du He, China . . . . . 77 A8 32 48N 110 40 E
Du Quoin, U.S.A. . . . 156 G7 38 1N 89 14W
Du'an, China . . . . . . 76 F7 23 59N 108 3 E
Duanesburg, U.S.A. . . 151 D10 42 45N 74 11W
Duaringa, Australia . . 126 C4 23 42 S 149 42 E
Duarte, Pico,
  Dom. Rep. 165 D5 19 2N 70 59W
Dubā, Si. Arabia . . . . 96 E2 27 10N 35 40 E
Dubai = Dubayy,
  U.A.E. . . . . 97 E7 25 18N 55 20 E
Dubāsari, Moldova . . 53 C14 47 15N 29 10 E
Dubāsari Vdkhr.,
  Moldova . . . . 53 C13 47 30N 29 0 E
Dubawnt →, Canada . 143 A8 64 33N 100 6W
Dubawnt L., Canada . 143 A8 63 8N 101 28W
Dubayy, U.A.E. . . . . 97 E7 25 18N 55 20 E
Dubbo, Australia . . . . 129 B8 32 11 S 148 35 E
Dubele, Dem. Rep. of
  the Congo . . . . 118 B2 2 56N 29 35 E
Dübendorf, Switz. . . . 33 B7 47 24N 8 37 E
Dubica, Croatia . . . . 45 C13 45 11N 16 48 E
Dublin, Ireland 23 C5 53 21N 6 15W
Dublin, Ga., U.S.A. . . 152 C7 32 32N 82 54W
Dublin, Tex., U.S.A. . 155 J5 32 5N 98 21W
Dublin □, Ireland . . . 23 C5 53 24N 6 20W
Dublin ✈ (DUB),
  Ireland 23 C5 53 26N 6 15W
Dubna, Russia . . . . . 58 D9 56 44N 37 10 E
Dubnica nad Váhom,
  Slovak Rep. . . . . . . 35 C11 48 58N 18 11 E
Dubno, Ukraine . . . . 59 G3 50 25N 25 45 E
Dubois, Idaho, U.S.A. . 158 D7 44 10N 112 14W
Dubois, Ind., U.S.A. . 156 F10 38 27N 86 48W
Dubois, Pa., U.S.A. . . 150 E6 41 8N 78 46W
Dubossary = Dubāsari,
  Moldova . . . . 53 C14 47 15N 29 10 E
Dubossary Vdkhr. =
  Dubāsari Vdkhr.,
  Moldova . . . . 53 C13 47 30N 29 0 E
Dubove, Ukraine . . . 53 B8 48 10N 23 53 E
Dubovka, Russia . . . . 61 F7 49 5N 44 50 E
Dubovskoye, Russia . . 61 G6 47 28N 42 46 E
Dubrajpur, India . . . 93 H12 23 48N 87 25 E
Dubréka, Guinea 112 D2 9 46N 13 31W
Dubrovitsa =
  Dubrovytsya,
  Ukraine . . . . 59 G4 51 31N 26 35 E
Dubrovnik, Croatia . . 50 D2 42 39N 18 6 E
Dubrovytsya, Ukraine . 59 G4 51 31N 26 35 E
Dubulu, Dem. Rep. of
  the Congo . . . . 114 B4 4 18N 20 16 E
Dubysa →, Lithuania . 54 C10 55 2N 23 10 E
Duchang, China . . . . 77 C11 29 18N 116 12 E
Duchesne, U.S.A. . . . 158 F8 40 10N 110 24W
Duchess, Australia . . 126 C2 21 20 S 139 50 E
Ducie I., Pac. Oc. . . . 135 K15 24 40 S 124 48W
Duck →, U.S.A. 149 G2 36 2N 87 52W
Duck Cr. →, Australia 124 D2 22 37 S 116 53 E

Duck Lake, Canada . . 143 C7 52 50N 106 16W
Duck Mountain △,
  Canada 143 C8 51 45N 101 0W
Duckwall, Mt., U.S.A. . 160 H6 37 58N 120 7W
Duda →, Colombia . . 168 C3 2 34N 74 3W
Duderstadt, Germany . 30 D6 51 31N 10 15 E
Dudhnai, India . . . . . 90 C3 25 59N 90 47 E
Düdingen, Switz. . . . . 32 C4 46 52N 7 12 E
Dudinka, Russia . . . . 67 C9 69 30N 86 13 E
Dudley, U.K. 21 E5 52 31N 2 5W
Dudley, U.S.A. 152 C6 32 32N 83 5W
Dudna →, India . . . . 94 E3 19 17N 76 54 E
Dudo, Somali Rep. . . 120 C4 9 20N 50 12 E
Dudub, Ethiopia . . . . 120 C3 6 55N 46 43 E
Dudune, İ., N. Cal. . . 133 U21 21 21 S 167 46 E
Dudwa, India . . . . . . 93 E9 28 30N 80 41 E
Dudwa △, India . . . . 93 E9 28 30N 80 40 E
Duékoué, Ivory C. . . . 112 D3 6 40N 7 15W
Dueñas, Phil. . . . . . . 81 F4 11 4N 122 37 E
Dueñas, Spain 42 D6 41 52N 4 33W
Dueré, Brazil . . . . . . 171 D2 11 20 S 49 17W
Duero = Douro →,
  Europe 42 D2 41 8N 8 40W
Dufftown, U.K. 22 D5 57 27N 3 8W
Dufourspitz, Switz. . . 32 E5 45 56N 7 52 E
Dugger, U.S.A. 157 E9 39 4N 87 18W
Dugi Otok, Croatia . . 45 D11 44 0N 15 3 E
Dugiuma, Somali Rep. 120 D2 1 15N 42 34 E
Dugo Selo, Croatia . . 45 C13 45 51N 16 18 E
Duida-Marahuaca △,
  Venezuela 168 C4 3 33N 65 33W
Duifken Pt., Australia . 126 A3 12 33 S 141 38 E
Duisburg, Germany . . 30 D2 51 26N 6 45 E
Duitama, Colombia . . 168 B3 5 50N 73 2W
Duiwelskloof, S. Africa 117 C5 23 42 S 30 10 E
Dujiangyan, China . . . 76 B4 31 2N 103 38 E
Duk Fadiat, Sudan . . 107 F3 7 45N 31 25 E
Duk Faiwil, Sudan . . 107 F3 7 30N 31 29 E
Dukat, Albania . . . . . 50 F3 40 16N 19 32 E
Dükdamīn, Iran . . . . 97 C8 35 59N 57 43 E
Dukelský Průsmyk,
  Slovak Rep. . . . . . . 35 B14 49 25N 21 42 E
Dukhān, Qatar . . . . . 97 E6 25 25N 50 50 E
Dukhovshchina, Russia 58 E7 55 15N 32 27 E
Duki, Pakistan . . . . . 91 C3 30 14N 68 25 E
Dukla, Poland . . . . . 55 J8 49 30N 21 35 E
Duku, Bauchi, Nigeria 113 C7 10 43N 10 43 E
Duku, Sokoto, Nigeria 113 C5 11 11N 4 55 E
Dula, Dem. Rep. of
  the Congo . . . . 114 B4 4 40N 20 21 E
Dulag = Datu Piang,
  Phil. . . . . 81 H5 7 2N 124 30 E
Dulce →, U.S.A. 159 H10 36 56N 107 0W
Dulce →, Argentina . . 174 C3 30 32 S 62 33W
Dulce, G., Costa Rica . 164 E3 8 40N 83 20W
Dulf, Iraq . . . . 96 C5 35 7N 45 51 E
Dülgopol, Bulgaria . . 51 C11 43 3N 27 22 E
Dulia, China . . . . . . 74 E9 39 2N 116 55 E
Dullabchara, India . . . 90 C4 24 30N 92 26 E
Dullewala, Pakistan . . 92 D4 31 50N 71 25 E
Dullstroom, S. Africa . 117 D5 25 27 S 30 7 E
Dülmen, Germany . . . 30 D3 51 49N 7 17 E
Dulovo, Bulgaria . . . . 51 C11 43 48N 27 9 E
Dulpetorpet, Norway . 18 D9 60 34N 12 19 E
Dulq Maghār, Syria . . 101 D8 36 22N 38 39 E
Duluth, Ga., U.S.A. . . 152 A5 34 0N 84 9W
Duluth, Minn., U.S.A. . 154 B8 46 47N 92 6W
Dum Dum, India . . . . 93 H13 22 39N 88 33 E
Dum Duma, India . . . 90 B5 27 40N 95 40 E
Dūmā, Syria . . . . . . 103 B5 33 34N 36 24 E
Dumaguete, Phil. . . . 81 G4 9 17N 123 15 E
Dumai, Indonesia . . . 84 B2 1 35N 101 28 E
Dumalinao, Phil. . . . 81 H4 7 49N 123 23 E
Dumanguilas Bay, Phil. 81 H4 7 34N 123 4 E
Dumanjug, Phil. . . . . 81 F4 10 4N 123 26 E
Dumaran = Araceli,
  Phil. . . . . 81 F2 10 33N 119 59 E
Dumaran, Phil. . . . . 81 F2 10 33N 119 50 E
Dumaran I., Phil. . . . 81 F2 10 33N 119 51 E
Dumarao, Phil. . . . . 81 F4 11 16N 122 41 E
Dumas, Ark., U.S.A. . 155 J9 33 53N 91 29W
Dumas, Tex., U.S.A. . 155 H4 35 52N 101 58W
Dumayr, Syria . . . . . 103 B5 33 39N 36 42 E
Dumbarton, U.K. . . . 22 F4 55 57N 4 33W
Dumbéa, N. Cal. . . . 133 V20 22 10 S 166 27 E
Dumbier, Slovak Rep. . 35 C12 48 56N 19 38 E
Dumbleyung, Australia 125 F2 33 17 S 117 42 E
Dumbo, Angola . . . . 115 E3 14 5 S 17 42 E
Dumboa, Nigeria . . . 113 C7 11 15N 12 55 E
Dumbrăveni, Romania 53 D9 46 14N 24 34 E
Dumfries, U.K. 22 F5 55 4N 3 37W
Dumfries &
  Galloway □, U.K. . . 22 F5 55 9N 3 58W
Dumingag, Phil. . . . . 81 G4 8 20N 123 20 E
Dumitrești, Romania . 53 E11 45 33N 26 55 E
Dumka, India . . . . . . 93 G12 24 12N 87 15 E
Dumlupınar, Turkey . . 49 C12 38 51N 29 54 E
Dümmer, Germany . . 30 C4 52 31N 8 20 E
Dümmer, Germany . . 30 C4 52 31N 8 21 E
Dumoine →, Canada . 140 C4 46 13N 77 51W
Dumoine, L., Canada . 140 C4 46 55N 77 55W
Dumont d'Urville,
  Antarctica . . . . 7 C10 67 0 S 110 0 E
Dumoulin Is.,
  Papua N. G. . . . . . 132 F6 10 54 S 150 46 E
Dumpu, Papua N. G. . 132 C3 5 53 S 145 44 E
Dumraon, India . . . . 93 G11 25 33N 84 8 E
Dumyât, Egypt . . . . . 106 H7 31 24N 31 48 E
Dumyât, Masabb,
  Egypt . . . . 106 H7 31 28N 31 51 E
Dún Dealgan =
  Dundalk, Ireland . . . 23 B5 54 1N 6 24W
Dún Laoghaire, Ireland 23 C5 53 17N 6 8W
Dun-le-Palestel, France 27 F8 46 18N 1 39 E
Dun-sur-Auron, France 27 F9 46 53N 2 33 E
Dun-sur-Meuse, France 27 C12 49 23N 5 11 E
Duna = Dunărea →,
  Europe . . . . 53 E14 45 20N 29 40 E
Duna →, Hungary . . . 52 E3 45 51N 18 48 E
Duna-Drava △,
  Hungary . . . . 52 D3 46 15N 18 50 E
Duna-völgyi-
  főcsatorna, Hungary . 52 D4 46 40N 19 14 E
Dunaföldvár, Hungary 52 D3 46 50N 18 57 E
Dunagiri, India . . . . 93 D8 30 31N 79 52 E
Dunaj = Dunărea →,
  Europe . . . . 53 E14 45 20N 29 40 E
Dunaj →, Slovak Rep. . 35 D11 47 50N 18 50 E
Dunajec →, Poland . . 55 H7 50 15N 20 44 E
Dunajská Streda,
  Slovak Rep. . . . . . . 35 C10 48 0N 17 37 E
Dunakeszi, Hungary . . 52 C4 47 37N 19 8 E
Dunaújváros, Hungary 52 D3 46 58N 18 57 E
Dunav = Dunărea →,
  Europe . . . . 53 E14 45 20N 29 40 E
Dunavățu de Jos,
  Romania . . . . 53 F14 44 59N 29 13 E
Dunavtsi, Bulgaria . . . 50 C6 43 57N 22 53 E

Dunay, Russia . . . . . 70 C6 42 52N 132 22 E
Dunayivtsi, Ukraine . . 53 B11 48 54N 26 50 E
Dunback, N.Z. . . . . . 131 F5 45 23 S 170 36 E
Dunbar, U.K. 22 E6 56 0N 2 31W
Dunblane, U.K. 22 E5 56 11N 3 58W
Duncan, Canada 142 D4 48 45N 123 40W
Duncan, Ariz., U.S.A. . 159 K9 32 43N 109 6W
Duncan, Okla., U.S.A. 155 H6 34 30N 97 57W
Duncan, L., Canada . . 140 B4 53 29N 77 58W
Duncan, L., Canada . . 142 A6 62 51N 113 58W
Duncan Passage, India 95 J11 11 0N 92 0 E
Duncan Town,
  Bahamas 164 B4 22 15N 75 45W
Duncannon, U.S.A. . . 150 F7 40 23N 77 2W
Duncansby Head, U.K. 23 B5 58 38N 3 1W
Duncansville, U.S.A. . 150 F6 40 25N 78 26W
Dundaga, Latvia . . . . 54 A9 57 31N 22 21 E
Dundalk, Canada . . . 150 B4 44 10N 80 24W
Dundalk, Ireland . . . 23 B5 54 1N 6 24W
Dundalk, U.S.A. 148 F7 39 16N 76 32W
Dundalk Bay, Ireland . 23 C5 53 55N 6 15W
Dundas = Uummannaq,
  Greenland 10 B4 77 0N 69 0W
Dundas = Uummannaq,
  Greenland 6 B5 70 58N 52 0W
Dundas, Canada 150 C5 43 17N 79 59W
Dundas, L., Australia . 125 F3 32 35 S 121 50 E
Dundas I., Canada . . 142 C2 54 30N 130 50W
Dundas Str., Australia 124 B5 11 15 S 131 35 E
Dundee, S. Africa . . . 117 D5 28 11 S 30 15 E
Dundee, U.K. 22 E6 56 28N 2 59W
Dundee, Mich., U.S.A. 157 C13 41 57N 83 40W
Dundee, N.Y., U.S.A. . 150 D8 42 32N 76 59W
Dundee City □, U.K. . 22 E6 56 30N 2 58W
Dundgovĭ □, Mongolia 74 B4 45 10N 106 0 E
Dundrum, U.K. 23 B6 54 16N 5 52W
Dundrum B., U.K. . . . 23 B6 54 13N 5 47W
Dunedin, N.Z. . . . . . 131 F5 45 50 S 170 33 E
Dunedin, U.S.A. 153 G7 28 1N 82 47W
Dunedoo, Australia . . 129 A8 32 0 S 149 25 E
Dunfermline, U.K. . . . 22 E5 56 5N 3 27W
Dungannon, Canada . . 150 C3 43 51N 81 36W
Dungannon, U.K. . . . 23 B5 54 31N 6 46W
Dungarpur, India . . . 92 H5 23 52N 73 45 E
Dungarvan, Ireland . . 23 D4 52 5N 7 37W
Dungarvan Harbour,
  Ireland 23 D4 52 4N 7 35W
Dungeness, U.K. . . . . 21 G8 50 54N 0 59 E
Dungo, L. do, Angola . 116 B2 17 15 S 19 0 E
Dungog, Australia . . . 129 B9 32 22 S 151 46 E
Dungu, Dem. Rep. of
  the Congo . . . . 118 B2 3 40N 28 32 E
Dungun, Malaysia . . . 87 K4 4 45N 103 25 E
Dungunāb, Sudan . . . 106 C4 21 10N 37 9 E
Dungunāb, Khalig,
  Sudan . . . . 106 C4 21 5N 37 12 E
Dunhua, China . . . . . 75 C15 43 20N 128 14 E
Dunhuang, China . . . 74 B4 40 8N 94 36 E
Dunk I., Australia . . . 126 B4 17 59 S 146 29 E
Dunkassa, Benin . . . . 113 C5 10 21N 3 10 E
Dunkeld, Queens.,
  Australia . . . . 127 E4 33 25 S 149 29 E
Dunkeld, Vic., Australia 128 E5 37 40 S 142 22 E
Dunkeld, U.K. 22 E5 56 34N 3 35W
Dunkerque, France . . 27 A9 51 2N 2 20 E
Dunkery Beacon, U.K. 21 F4 51 9N 3 36W
Dunkirk = Dunkerque,
  France . . . . 27 A9 51 2N 2 20 E
Dunkirk, U.S.A. 150 D5 42 29N 79 20W
Dunkuj, Sudan . . . . . 107 E3 12 50N 32 49 E
Dunkwa, Central,
  Ghana 112 D4 6 0N 1 47W
Dunkwa, Central,
  Ghana 113 D4 5 30N 1 0W
Dúnleary = Dún
  Laoghaire, Ireland . 23 C5 53 17N 6 8W
Dunleer, Ireland 23 C5 53 50N 6 24W
Dunmanus B., Ireland 23 E2 51 31N 9 50W
Dunmanway, Ireland . 23 E2 51 43N 9 6W
Dunmara, Australia . . 126 B1 16 42 S 133 25 E
Dunmore, U.S.A. . . . 151 E9 41 25N 75 38W
Dunmore Hd., Ireland 23 D1 52 10N 10 35W
Dunmore Town,
  Bahamas 164 A4 25 30N 76 39W
Dunn, U.S.A. 149 H6 35 19N 78 37W
Dunnellon, U.S.A. . . . 153 F7 29 3N 82 28W
Dunnet Hd., U.K. . . . 22 C5 58 40N 3 21W
Dunning, U.S.A. 154 E4 41 50N 100 6W
Dunnville, Canada . . . 150 D5 42 54N 79 36W
Dunolly, Australia . . . 128 D5 36 51 S 143 44 E
Dunoon, U.K. 22 F4 55 57N 4 56W
Dunphy, U.S.A. 158 F5 40 42N 116 31W
Dunqul, Egypt . . . . . 106 C3 23 26N 31 37 E
Duns, U.K. 22 F6 55 47N 2 20W
Dunseith, U.S.A. 154 A4 48 50N 100 3W
Dunsmuir, U.S.A. . . . 158 F2 41 13N 122 16W
Dunstable, U.K. 21 F7 51 53N 0 32W
Dunstan Mts., N.Z. . . 131 E4 44 53 S 169 35 E
Dunster, Canada 142 C5 53 8N 119 50W
Duntroon, N.Z. . . . . 131 E5 44 51 S 170 40 E
Dunvegan, Canada . . 142 B5 55 55N 118 35W
Dunvegan L., Canada . 143 A7 60 8N 107 10W
Duolun, China . . . . . 74 C9 42 12N 116 28 E
Duong Dong, Vietnam 87 G4 10 13N 103 58 E
Dupax, Phil. . . . . . . 80 C3 16 17N 121 5 E
Dupree, U.S.A. 154 C4 45 4N 101 35W
Dupuyer, U.S.A. 158 B7 48 13N 112 30W
Duqm, Oman . . . . . 99 C7 19 39N 57 42 E
Duque de Caxias,
  Brazil . . . . 171 F3 22 45 S 43 19W
Duque de York, I.,
  Chile . . . . 176 B1 50 37 S 75 25W
Durack →, Australia . . 124 C4 15 33 S 127 52 E
Durack Ra., Australia . 124 C4 16 50 S 127 40 E
Durağan, Turkey . . . . 100 B6 41 25N 35 3 E
Durak, Turkey . . . . . 49 B10 39 42N 28 17 E
Ðurakovac =
  Ðurakovac,
  Serbia & M. . . . . . 50 D4 42 43N 20 29 E
Durance →, France . . 29 E8 43 55N 4 45 E
Durand, Ga., U.S.A. . . 152 C5 32 54N 84 51W
Durand, Ill., U.S.A. . . 156 B7 42 26N 89 20W
Durand, Mich., U.S.A. 157 B13 42 55N 83 59W
Durand, Wis., U.S.A. . 154 C9 44 38N 91 58W
Durango, Mexico . . . 162 C4 24 3N 104 39W
Durango, Spain 43 B7 43 13N 2 40W
Durango, U.S.A. 159 H10 37 16N 107 53W
Durango □, Mexico . . 162 C4 25 0N 105 0W
Durankulak, Bulgaria . 51 C12 43 41N 28 32 E
Durant, Iowa, U.S.A. . 156 C6 41 36N 90 54W
Durant, Miss., U.S.A. . 155 J10 33 4N 89 51W
Durant, Okla., U.S.A. . 155 J6 33 59N 96 25W
Duratón →, Spain . . . 42 D6 41 37N 4 7W
Durazno, Uruguay . . 174 C4 33 25 S 56 31W
Durazzo = Durrës,
  Albania . . . . 50 E3 41 19N 19 28 E
Durban, France . . . . 28 F6 42 59N 2 49 E
Durban, S. Africa . . . 117 D5 29 49 S 31 1 E
Durbo, Somali Rep. . . 120 B4 11 37N 50 14 E
Durbuy, Belgium . . . . 24 D5 50 21N 5 28 E
Dúrcal, Spain 43 J7 36 59N 3 34W
Ðurđevac, Croatia . . . 45 B13 46 2N 17 3 E
Düren, Germany . . . . 30 E2 50 48N 6 29 E
Durg, India . . . . 93 J8 21 15N 81 22 E
Durgapur, India . . . . 93 H12 23 30N 87 20 E
Durham, Canada 140 D3 44 10N 80 49W

Durham, U.K. 20 C6 54 47N 1 34W
Durham, Calif., U.S.A. 160 F5 39 39N 121 48W
Durham, N.C., U.S.A. 149 H6 35 59N 78 54W
Durham, N.H., U.S.A. 151 C14 43 8N ·70 56W
Durham □, U.K. 20 C6 54 42N 1 45W
Durleşti, Moldova . . . 53 C13 47 1N 28 46 E
Durma, Si. Arabia . . . 96 E5 24 37N 46 8 E
Durmitor □,
  Serbia & M. . . . . . 50 C3 43 15N 19 5 E
Durmitor △,
  Serbia & M. . . . . . 50 C3 43 10N 19 0 E
Durness, U.K. 22 C4 58 34N 4 45W
Durnford Pta.,
  W. Sahara 110 D1 23 37N 16 0W
Durrës, Albania . . . . 50 E3 41 19N 19 28 E
Durrow, Ireland 23 D4 52 51N 7 24W
Dursey I., Ireland . . . 23 E1 51 36N 10 12W
Dursley, U.K. 21 F5 51 40N 2 21W
Dursunbey, Turkey . . 49 B10 39 35N 28 37 E
Durtal, France 26 E6 47 40N 0 18W
Duru, Dem. Rep. of
  the Congo . . . . 118 B2 4 14N 28 50 E
Duru Gölü, Turkey . . 51 E12 41 28N 28 35 E
Durusu, Turkey . . . . 51 E12 41 17N 28 41 E
Durūz, Jabal ad, Jordan 103 C5 32 35N 36 40 E
D'Urville, Tanjung,
  Indonesia . . . . 83 B5 1 28 S 137 54 E
D'Urville I., N.Z. . . . 131 A8 40 50 S 173 55 E
Duryea, U.S.A. 151 E9 41 22N 75 45W
Dusa Mareb,
  Somali Rep. . . . . . 120 C3 5 30N 46 15 E
Dūsh, Egypt . . . . . . 106 C3 24 35N 30 41 E
Dushak, Turkmenistan 66 F7 37 13N 60 1 E
Dushan, China . . . . . 76 E6 25 48N 107 30 E
Dushanbe, Tajikistan . 65 D4 38 33N 68 48 E
Dusheti, Georgia . . . . 61 J7 42 10N 44 42 E
Dushore, U.S.A. 151 E8 41 31N 76 24W
Dusky Sd., N.Z. . . . . 131 F1 45 47 S 166 30 E
Dussejour, C., Australia 124 B4 14 45 S 128 13 E
Düsseldorf, Germany . 30 D2 51 14N 6 47 E
Düsseldorf Rhein-
  Ruhr ✈ (DUS),
  Germany . . . . 30 D2 51 17N 6 46 E
Dusti, Tajikistan . . . . 65 E4 37 20N 68 40 E
Dustlik, Uzbekistan . . 65 E7 40 31N 68 2 E
Duszniki-Zdrój, Poland 55 H3 50 24N 16 24 E
Dutch East Indies =
  Indonesia ■, Asia . . 85 C4 5 0 S 115 0 E
Dutch Guiana =
  Suriname ■, S. Amer. 169 C6 4 0N 56 0W
Dutch Harbor, U.S.A. 144 K6 53 53N 166 32W
Dutlwe, Botswana . . . 116 C3 23 58 S 23 46 E
Dutsan Wai, Nigeria . 113 C6 10 50N 8 10 E
Dutton, Canada 150 D3 42 39N 81 30W
Dutton →, Australia . . 126 C3 20 44 S 143 10 E
Duved, Sweden . . . . 16 A6 63 24N 12 55 E
Düvertepe, Turkey . . 49 B10 39 14N 28 27 E
Dúvida = Roosevelt →,
  Brazil . . . . 173 B5 7 35 S 60 20W
Duwayhin, Khawr,
  U.A.E. . . . . 97 E6 24 20N 51 25 E
Duyun, China . . . . . . 76 D6 26 18N 107 29 E
Düzağaç, Turkey . . . 49 C12 38 48N 30 10 E
Düzce, Turkey . . . . . 100 B4 40 50N 31 10 E
Duzdab = Zāhedān,
  Iran . . . . 97 D9 29 30N 60 50 E
Dve Mogili, Bulgaria . 51 C9 43 35N 25 55 E
Dvigatelstroy =
  Kaspiysk, Russia . . . 61 J8 42 52N 47 40 E
Dvina, Severnaya →,
  Russia . . . . 56 B7 64 32N 40 30 E
Dvinsk = Daugavpils,
  Latvia . . . . 15 J22 55 53N 26 32 E
Dvinskaya Guba,
  Russia . . . . 56 B6 65 0N 39 0 E
Dvor, Croatia . . . . . . 45 C13 45 4N 16 22 E
Dvůr Králové nad
  Labem, Czech Rep. . 34 A8 50 27N 15 50 E
Dwarka, India . . . . . 92 H3 22 18N 69 8 E
Dwellingup, Australia . 125 F2 32 43 S 116 4 E
Dwight, U.S.A. 156 E1 41 5N 88 26W
Dyakovo, Ukraine . . . 53 B7 48 5N 23 20 E
Dyatkovo, Russia . . . 58 F8 53 40N 34 27 E
Dyatlovo = Dzyatlava,
  Belarus . . . . 58 F3 53 28N 25 28 E
Dyce, U.K. 22 D6 57 13N 2 12W
Dyer, U.S.A. 157 G10 37 49N 86 13W
Dyer, C., Canada . . . 139 B13 66 37N 61 16W
Dyer Bay, Canada . . . 150 A3 45 10N 81 20W
Dyer Plateau,
  Antarctica . . . . 7 D17 70 45 S 65 30W
Dyersburg, U.S.A. . . . 155 G10 36 3N 89 23W
Dyersville, U.S.A. . . . 156 B5 42 29N 91 8W
Dyfi →, U.K. 21 E3 52 32N 4 3W
Dyhernfurth = Brzeg
  Dolny, Poland . . . . 55 G3 51 16N 16 41 E
Dyje →, Czech Rep. . . 35 C9 48 37N 16 56 E
Dymer, Ukraine . . . . 59 G6 50 47N 30 18 E
Dynów, Poland . . . . 55 J9 49 49N 22 14 E
Dyranut, Norway . . . 18 D4 60 22N 7 31 E
Dyrhólaey, Iceland . . 19 E4 63 25N 19 6W
Dyrnes, Norway . . . . 18 A4 63 25N 7 52 E
Dysart, Australia . . . 126 C4 22 32 S 148 23 E
Dysart, U.S.A. 156 B4 42 10N 92 18W
Dyurtyuli, Russia . . . 56 D9 55 21N 54 40 E
Dyushambe =
  Dushanbe, Tajikistan . 65 D4 38 33N 68 48 E
Dyviziya, Ukraine . . . 53 E14 45 55N 29 59 E
Dzamin Üüd =
  Borhoyn Tal,
  Mongolia . . . . 74 C6 43 50N 111 58 E
Dzaoudzi, Mayotte . . 121 a 12 47 S 45 16 E
Dzaudzhikau =
  Vladikavkaz, Russia . 61 J7 43 0N 44 35 E
Dzerzhinsk, Russia . . 60 B6 56 14N 43 30 E
Dzhalal-Abad = Jalal-
  Abad, Kyrgyzstan . . 65 C6 40 56N 73 0 E
Dzhalal-Ogly =
  Stepanavan, Armenia 61 K7 41 1N 44 23 E
Dzhalinda, Russia . . . 67 D13 53 26N 124 0 E
Dzhambeyty,
  Kazakhstan . . . . . . 64 F4 50 16N 52 58 E
Dzhambul = Taraz,
  Kazakhstan . . . . . . 65 B5 42 54N 71 22 E
Dzhankoy, Ukraine . . 59 K8 45 40N 34 20 E
Dzhanybek,
  Kazakhstan . . . . . . 60 E7 49 25N 46 50 E
Dzhardzhan, Russia . . 67 C13 68 10N 124 10 E
Dzhetygara = Zhitikara,
  Kazakhstan . . . . . . 66 D7 52 30N 61 13 E
Dzhezkazgan =
  Zhezqazghan,
  Kazakhstan . . . . . . 66 E7 47 44N 67 40 E
Dzhikimde, Russia . . 67 D13 59 1N 121 47 E
Dzhizak = Jizzakh,
  Uzbekistan . . . . . . 65 E7 40 6N 67 50 E

Dzhizak = Jizzakh,
  Uzbekistan . . . . . . 65 C3 40 6N 67 50 E
Dzhugdzhur, Khrebet,
  Russia . . . . 67 D14 57 30N 138 0 E
Dzhulynk, Ukraine . . . 53 B14 48 26N 29 45 E
Dzhuma, Uzbekistan . 65 D3 39 42N 66 40 E
Dzhungarskiye
  Vorota = Dzungarian
  Gates, Asia . . . . . . 68 B3 45 0N 82 0 E
Dzhvari = Jvari,
  Georgia . . . . 61 J6 42 42N 42 4 E
Działdowo, Poland . . 55 E7 53 15N 20 15 E
Działoszyce, Poland . 55 H7 50 22N 20 20 E
Działoszyn, Poland . . 55 G5 51 6N 18 50 E
Dzibilchaltún, Mexico 163 C7 21 5N 89 36W
Dzibilchaltun, Yucatán,
  Mexico 163 C7 21 5N 89 36W
Dzierzgoń, Poland . . . 54 E6 53 58N 19 20 E
Dzierżoniów, Poland . 55 H3 50 45N 16 39 E
Dzilam de Bravo,
  Mexico 163 C7 21 24N 88 53W
Dzioua, Algeria . . . . 111 B6 33 14N 5 14 E
Dzisna, Belarus . . . . 58 E5 55 34N 28 12 E
Dzisna →, Belarus . . . 58 E5 55 34N 28 12 E
Dziwnów, Poland . . . 54 D1 54 2N 14 45 E
Dzungaria = Junggar
  Pendi, China . . . . . 68 B3 44 30N 86 0 E
Dzungarian Basin =
  Junggar Pendi, China 68 B3 44 30N 86 0 E
Dzungarian Gates, Asia 68 B3 45 0N 82 0 E
Dzuumod, Mongolia . 68 B5 47 45N 106 58 E
Dzyarzhynsk, Belarus . 58 F4 53 40N 27 1 E
Dzyatlava, Belarus . . 58 F3 53 28N 25 28 E

E

E.C. Manning △,
  Canada 142 D4 49 5N 120 45W
Eabamet L., Canada . . 140 B2 51 30N 87 46W
Eads, U.S.A. 154 F3 38 29N 102 47W
Eagar, U.S.A. 159 J9 34 6N 109 17W
Eagle, Alaska, U.S.A. . 144 D12 64 47N 141 12W
Eagle, Colo., U.S.A. . . 158 G10 39 39N 106 50W
Eagle, Idaho, U.S.A. . 158 E5 43 42N 116 21W
Eagle →, Canada . . . 141 B8 53 36N 57 26W
Eagle Butte, U.S.A. . . 154 C4 45 0N 101 10W
Eagle Cr. →, U.S.A. . 157 F11 38 36N 85 4W
Eagle Grove, U.S.A. . 156 B3 42 40N 93 54W
Eagle L., Canada . . . 143 D10 49 42N 93 13W
Eagle L., Calif., U.S.A. 158 F3 40 39N 120 45W
Eagle L., Maine, U.S.A. 149 B11 46 20N 69 22W
Eagle Lake, Canada . . 150 A6 45 8N 78 29W
Eagle Lake, Maine,
  U.S.A. 149 B11 47 3N 68 36W
Eagle Lake, Tex.,
  U.S.A. 155 L6 29 35N 96 20W
Eagle Mountain, U.S.A. 161 M11 33 49N 115 27W
Eagle Nest, U.S.A. . . 159 H11 36 33N 105 16W
Eagle Pass, U.S.A. . . . 155 L4 28 43N 100 30W
Eagle Pk., U.S.A. . . . 160 G7 38 10N 119 25W
Eagle Pt., Australia . . 124 C3 16 11 S 124 23 E
Eagle River, Mich.,
  U.S.A. 148 B1 47 24N 88 18W
Eagle River, Wis.,
  U.S.A. 154 C10 45 55N 89 15W
Eaglehawk, N.S.W.,
  Australia . . . . 127 F3 36 44 S 144 15 E
Eaglehawk, Vic.,
  Australia . . . . 128 D6 36 44 S 144 15 E
Eagles Mere, U.S.A. . 151 E8 41 25N 76 33W
Eagleville, U.S.A. . . . 156 D3 40 28N 93 59W
Ealing □, U.K. 21 F7 51 31N 0 20W
Ear Falls, Canada . . . 143 C10 50 38N 93 13W
Earle, U.S.A. 155 H9 35 16N 90 28W
Earlimart, U.S.A. . . . 161 K7 35 53N 119 16W
Earlville, U.S.A. 157 C8 41 35N 88 55W
Early Branch, U.S.A. . 152 C9 32 28N 80 55W
Earn →, U.K. 22 E5 56 21N 3 18W
Earn, L., U.K. 22 E4 56 23N 4 13W
Earnslaw, Mt., N.Z. . . 131 E3 44 32 S 168 27 E
Earth, U.S.A. 155 H3 34 14N 102 24W
Eas, Vanuatu . . . . . . 133 F6 16 20 S 168 15 E
Easley, U.S.A. 149 H4 34 50N 82 36W
East Anglia, U.K. . . . 20 E9 52 30N 1 0 E
East Angus, Canada . . 141 C5 45 30N 71 40W
East Antarctica,
  Antarctica . . . . 7 D7 80 0 S 90 0 E
East Aurora, U.S.A. . . 150 D6 42 46N 78 37W
East Ayrshire □, U.K. . 22 F4 55 26N 4 11W
East Bengal,
  Bangladesh ■, Asia . 90 C3 24 0N 90 0 E
East Beskids =
  Vychodné Beskydy,
  Europe . . . . 35 B15 49 20N 22 0 E
East Brady, U.S.A. . . 150 F5 40 59N 79 37W
East C., N.Z. . . . . . . 131 D7 37 42 S 178 35 E
East C., Papua N. G. . 132 F6 10 13 S 150 53 E
East Chicago, U.S.A. . 157 C8 41 38N 87 27W
East China Sea, Asia . 69 D7 30 0N 126 0 E
East Coulee, Canada . 142 C6 51 23N 112 27W
East Dereham =
  Dereham, U.K. . . . . 21 E8 52 41N 0 57 E
East Dublin, U.S.A. . . 152 C7 32 33N 82 52W
East Dunbartonshire □,
  U.K. 22 F4 55 57N 4 13W
East End Pt., Bahamas 9 b 25 3N 77 16W
East Falkland, Falk. Is. 9 f 51 30 S 58 30W
East Grand Forks,
  U.S.A. 154 B6 47 56N 97 1W
East Greenwich, U.S.A. 151 E13 41 40N 71 27W
East Grinstead, U.K. . 21 F8 51 7N 0 0W
East Hartford, U.S.A. . 151 E12 41 46N 72 39W
East Helena, U.S.A. . . 158 C8 46 35N 111 56W
East Indies, Asia . . . . 62 K15 0 0N 120 0 E
East Kilbride, U.K. . . 22 F4 55 46N 4 10W
East Kamma Channel,
  China . . . . 69 G11 22 14N 114 9 E
East Lansing, U.S.A. . 157 B12 42 44N 84 29W
East Liverpool, U.S.A. 150 F4 40 37N 80 35W
East London, S. Africa 117 E4 33 0 S 27 55 E
East Lothian □, U.K. . 22 F6 55 58N 2 44W
East Main = Eastmain,
  Canada 140 B4 52 10N 78 30W
East Milwaukee =
  Shorewood, U.S.A. . 157 A9 43 5N 87 54W
East Moline, U.S.A. . . 156 C6 41 30N 90 26W
East Naples, U.S.A. . . 153 J8 26 8N 81 42W
East New Britain □,
  Papua N. G. . . . . . 132 D7 6 30 S 152 30 E
East Northport, U.S.A. 151 F11 40 53N 73 20W
East Orange, U.S.A. . 151 F10 40 46N 74 13W
East Pacific Ridge,
  Pac. Oc. . . . . 135 J17 15 0 S 110 0W
East Pakistan =
  Bangladesh ■, Asia . 90 C3 24 0N 90 0 E
East Palatka, U.S.A. . 152 F8 29 39N 81 36W
East Palestine, U.S.A. 150 F4 40 50N 80 33W

East Peoria, U.S.A. 156 D7 40 40N 89 34W
East Pine, Canada 142 B4 55 48N 120 12W
East Point, U.S.A. 152 B5 33 41N 84 27W
East Providence, U.S.A. 151 E13 41 49N 71 23W
East Pt., Br. Virgin Is. 165 e 18 40N 64 18W
East Pt., Canada 141 C7 46 27N 61 58W
East Renfrewshire □, U.K. 22 F4 55 46N 4 21W
East Retford = Retford, U.K. 20 D7 53 19N 0 56W
East Riding of Yorkshire □, U.K. 20 D7 53 55N 0 30W
East Rochester, U.S.A. 150 C7 43 7N 77 29W
East St. Louis, U.S.A. 156 F6 38 37N 90 9W
East Schelde = Oosterschelde →, Neths. 24 C4 51 33N 4 0E
East Sea = Japan, Sea of, Asia 70 E7 40 0N 135 0E
East Sepik □, Papua N. G. 132 C2 4 0S 143 45E
East Siberian Sea, Russia 67 B17 73 0N 160 0E
East Stroudsburg, U.S.A. 151 E9 41 1N 75 11W
East Sussex □, U.K. 21 G8 50 56N 0 19E
East Tawas, U.S.A. 148 C4 44 17N 83 29W
East Timor ■, Asia 82 C3 8 50S 126 0E
East Tohopekaliga, Lake, U.S.A. 153 G8 28 18N 81 15W
East Toorale, Australia 127 E4 30 27S 145 28E
East Troy, U.S.A. 157 B8 42 47N 88 24W
East Walker →, U.S.A. 160 G7 38 52N 119 10W
East Windsor, U.S.A. 151 F10 40 17N 74 34W
East Youngstown = Campbell, U.S.A. 150 E4 41 5N 80 37W
Eastbourne, N.Z. 130 H3 41 19S 174 55E
Eastbourne, U.K. 21 G8 50 46N 0 18E
Eastend, Canada 143 D7 49 32N 108 50W
Easter Fracture Zone, Pac. Oc. 135 K16 25 0S 115 0W
Easter I. = Pascua, I. de, Chile 172 b 27 7S 109 23W
Eastern □, Ghana 113 D4 6 30N 0 30W
Eastern □, Kenya 118 C4 0 0 38 30E
Eastern □, S. Leone 112 D2 8 15N 11 0W
Eastern Cape □, S. Africa 116 E4 32 0S 26 0E
Eastern Cr. →, Australia 126 C3 20 40S 141 35E
Eastern Ghats, India 95 H4 14 0N 78 50E
Eastern Group = Lau Group, Fiji 133 A3 17 0S 178 30W
Eastern Group, Australia 125 F3 33 30S 124 30E
Eastern Highlands □, Papua N. G. 132 D3 6 30S 145 35E
Eastern Samar □, Phil. 81 F5 11 40N 125 40E
Eastern Transvaal = Mpumalanga □, S. Africa 117 D5 26 0S 30 0E
Easterville, Canada 143 C9 53 8N 99 49W
Easthampton, U.S.A. 151 D12 42 16N 72 40W
Eastlake, U.S.A. 150 E3 41 40N 81 26W
Eastland, U.S.A. 155 J5 32 24N 98 49W
Eastleigh, U.K. 21 G6 50 58N 1 21W
Eastmain, Canada 140 B4 52 10N 78 30W
Eastmain →, Canada 140 B4 52 27N 78 26W
Eastman, Canada 151 A12 45 18N 72 19W
Eastman, Ga., U.S.A. 152 C6 32 12N 83 11W
Eastman, Wis., U.S.A. 156 A5 43 10N 91 1W
Easton, Md., U.S.A. 148 F7 38 47N 76 5W
Easton, Pa., U.S.A. 151 F9 40 41N 75 13W
Easton, Wash., U.S.A. 160 C5 47 14N 121 11W
Eastover, U.S.A. 152 B9 33 52N 80 41W
Eastpoint, U.S.A. 152 F5 29 44N 84 53W
Eastpointe, U.S.A. 150 D2 42 27N 82 56W
Eastport, U.S.A. 149 C12 44 56N 67 0W
Eastsound, U.S.A. 160 B4 48 42N 122 55W
Eaton, Colo., U.S.A. 154 E2 40 32N 104 42W
Eaton, Ohio, U.S.A. 157 E12 39 45N 84 38W
Eaton Rapids, U.S.A. 157 B12 42 31N 84 39W
Eatonia, Canada 143 C7 51 13N 109 25W
Eatonton, U.S.A. 152 B6 33 20N 83 23W
Eatontown, U.S.A. 151 F10 40 19N 74 4W
Eatonville, U.S.A. 160 D4 46 52N 122 16W
Eau Claire, Fr. Guiana 169 C7 3 30N 53 40W
Eau Claire, U.S.A. 154 C9 44 49N 91 30W
Eau Claire, L. à l', Canada 140 A5 56 10N 74 25W
Eauze, France 28 E4 43 53N 0 7E
Eban, Nigeria 113 D5 9 40N 4 50E
Ebanga, Angola 115 E2 12 45S 14 45E
Ebangalakata, Dem. Rep. of the Congo 114 C4 0 29S 21 29E
Ebbegebirge ⌓, Germany 30 D3 51 10N 7 55E
Ebbw Vale, U.K. 21 F4 51 46N 3 12W
Ebebiyín, Eq. Guin. 114 B2 2 9N 11 20E
Ebeggui, Algeria 111 C6 26 2N 6 0E
Ebel, Gabon 114 B2 0 7N 11 5E
Ebeltoft, Denmark 17 H4 56 12N 10 41E
Ebeltoft Vig, Denmark 17 H4 56 10N 10 35E
Ebensburg, U.S.A. 150 F6 40 29N 78 44W
Ebensee, Austria 34 D6 47 48N 13 46E
Eber Gölü, Turkey 100 C4 38 38N 31 11E
Eberbach, Germany 31 F4 49 28N 8 59E
Eberswalde-Finow, Germany 30 C9 52 50N 13 49E
Ebetsu, Japan 70 C10 43 7N 141 34E
Ebey's Landing ⌓, U.S.A. 160 B4 48 13N 122 41W
Ebian, China 76 C4 29 11N 103 13E
Ebikon, Switz. 33 B6 47 5N 8 21E
Ebingen, Germany 31 G5 48 13N 9 1E
Ebino, Japan 72 E2 32 2N 130 48E
Ebnat-Kappel, Switz. 33 B8 47 16N 9 7E
Ebo, Angola 115 E2 11 40S 14 40E
Ebola →, Dem. Rep. of the Congo 114 B4 3 20N 20 57E
Eboli, Italy 47 B8 40 39N 15 2E
Ebolowa, Cameroon 113 E7 2 55N 11 10E
Ebonyi □, Nigeria 113 D6 6 20N 8 0E
Eboy, Dem. Rep. of the Congo 114 B4 2 50N 23 11E
Ebrach, Germany 31 F6 49 51N 10 29E
Ébrié, Lagune, Ivory C. 112 D4 5 12N 4 26W
Ebro →, Spain 40 E5 40 43N 0 54E
Ebro, Embalse del, Spain 42 C7 43 0N 3 58W
Ebstorf, Germany 30 B6 53 2N 10 24E
Eceabat, Turkey 51 F10 40 11N 26 21E
Ech Chéliff, Algeria 111 A5 36 10N 1 20E
Echallens, Switz. 32 C3 46 38N 6 38E
Echeconnee →, U.S.A. 152 C6 32 39N 83 36W
Echigo-Sammyaku, Japan 71 F9 36 50N 139 50E
Échirolles, France 29 C9 45 8N 5 44E
Echizen-Misaki, Japan 73 B7 35 59N 135 57E
Echmiadzin = Yejmiadzin, Armenia 61 K7 40 12N 44 19E
Echo, U.S.A. 152 D4 31 29N 85 28W
Echo Bay, N.W.T., Canada 138 B8 66 5N 117 55W
Echo Bay, Ont., Canada 140 C3 46 29N 84 4W
Echoing →, Canada 140 B1 55 51N 92 5W
Echterdingen, Stuttgart ✈ (STR), Germany 31 G5 48 42N 9 11E
Echternach, Lux. 24 E6 49 49N 6 25E
Echuca, Australia 129 D6 36 10S 144 45E
Ecija, Spain 43 H5 37 30N 5 10W
Eckental, Germany 31 F7 49 35N 11 12E
Eckernförde, Germany 30 A5 54 28N 9 50E
Eclectic, U.S.A. 152 C3 32 38N 86 2W
Eclipse I., Australia 125 G2 35 5S 117 58E
Eclipse Is., Australia 124 B4 13 54S 126 19E
Eclipse Sd., Canada 139 A11 72 38N 79 0W
Écommoy, France 26 E7 47 50N 0 17E
Economy = Ambridge, U.S.A. 150 F4 40 36N 80 14W
Ecoporanga, Brazil 171 E3 18 23S 40 50W
Écouché, France 26 D6 48 42N 0 10W
Ecrins △, France 29 D10 44 54N 6 18E
Ecuador ■, S. Amer. 168 D2 2 0S 78 0W
Ecuador, Volcán, Ecuador 172 a 1 1S 91 32W
Écueillé, France 26 E8 47 5N 1 21E
Ed, Sweden 17 F5 58 55N 11 55E
Ed Dabbura, Sudan 106 D3 17 40N 34 15E
Ed Da'ein, Sudan 107 E2 11 26N 26 9E
Ed Dâmer, Sudan 106 D3 17 27N 34 0E
Ed Dar el Beida = Casablanca, Morocco 110 B3 33 36N 7 36W
Ed Debba, Sudan 106 D3 18 0N 30 51E
Ed-Déffa, Egypt 106 A2 30 40N 26 30E
Ed Deim, Sudan 107 E2 10 10N 28 20E
Ed Dueim, Sudan 107 E3 14 0N 32 10E
Edam, Canada 143 C7 53 11N 108 46W
Edam, Neths. 24 B5 52 31N 5 3E
Edane, Sweden 16 E6 59 38N 12 49E
Edapally, India 95 J4 11 19N 78 3E
Eday, U.K. 22 B6 59 11N 2 47W
Edchera, W. Sahara 110 C2 27 2N 13 4W
Edd, Eritrea 107 E5 14 0N 41 38E
Eddrachillis B., U.K. 22 C3 58 17N 5 14W
Eddystone, U.K. 21 G3 50 11N 4 16W
Eddystone Pt., Australia 127 G4 40 59S 148 20E
Eddyville, U.S.A. 156 C4 41 9N 92 38W
Ede, Neths. 24 B5 52 4N 5 40E
Ede, Nigeria 113 D5 7 45N 4 29E
Edéa, Cameroon 113 E7 3 51N 10 9E
Edebäck, Sweden 16 D7 60 4N 13 32E
Edehon L., Canada 143 A9 60 25N 97 15W
Edekel, Adrar, Algeria 111 D6 23 56N 6 47E
Edelény, Hungary 52 B5 48 18N 20 44E
Eden = Bar Harbor, U.S.A. 149 C11 44 23N 68 13W
Eden, Australia 129 D8 37 3S 149 55E
Eden, N.C., U.S.A. 149 G6 36 29N 79 53W
Eden, N.Y., U.S.A. 150 D6 42 39N 78 55W
Eden, Tex., U.S.A. 155 K5 31 13N 99 51W
Eden →, U.K. 20 C4 54 57N 3 1W
Edenburg, S. Africa 116 D4 29 43S 25 58E
Edendale, N.Z. 131 G3 46 19S 168 48E
Edendale, S. Africa 117 D5 29 39S 30 18E
Edenderry, Ireland 23 C4 53 21N 7 4W
Edenhope, Australia 128 D4 37 4S 141 19E
Edenton, U.S.A. 149 G7 36 4N 76 39W
Edenville, S. Africa 117 D4 27 37S 27 34E
Eder →, Germany 30 D5 51 12N 9 28E
Eder-Stausee, Germany 30 D4 51 10N 8 57E
Edessa = Édhessa, Greece 50 F6 40 48N 22 5E
Edewecht, Germany 30 B3 53 8N 7 58E
Edgar, U.S.A. 154 E6 40 22N 97 58W
Edgartown, U.S.A. 151 E14 41 23N 70 31W
Edge Hill, U.K. 21 E6 52 8N 1 26W
Edgecumbe, N.Z. 130 D5 37 59S 176 47E
Edgefield, U.S.A. 152 B8 33 47N 81 56W
Edgeley, U.S.A. 154 B5 46 22N 98 43W
Edgemont, U.S.A. 154 D3 43 18N 103 50W
Edgeøya, Svalbard 6 B9 77 45N 22 30E
Edgerton, Ohio, U.S.A. 157 C12 41 27N 84 45W
Edgerton, Wis., U.S.A. 156 B7 42 50N 89 4W
Edgewater, U.S.A. 153 G9 28 59N 80 54W
Edgewood, U.S.A. 157 F8 38 55N 88 40W
Édhessa, Greece 50 F6 40 48N 22 5E
Edievale, N.Z. 131 F4 45 49S 169 22E
Edina, Liberia 112 D2 6 0N 10 10W
Edina, U.S.A. 156 D4 40 10N 92 11W
Edinboro, U.S.A. 150 E4 41 52N 80 8W
Edinburg, Ill., U.S.A. 156 E7 39 39N 89 23W
Edinburg, Ind., U.S.A. 157 E11 39 21N 85 58W
Edinburg, Tex., U.S.A. 155 M5 26 18N 98 10W
Edinburgh, U.K. 22 F5 55 57N 3 13W
Edinburgh ✈ (EDI), U.K. 22 F5 55 54N 3 22W
Edinburgh, City of □, U.K. 22 F5 55 57N 3 17W
Edineţ, Moldova 53 B12 48 9N 27 18E
Edirne, Turkey 51 E10 41 40N 26 34E
Edirne □, Turkey 51 E10 41 12N 26 30E
Edison, Ga., U.S.A. 152 D5 31 34N 84 44W
Edison, Wash., U.S.A. 160 B4 48 33N 122 27W
Edisto →, U.S.A. 152 C9 32 29N 80 21W
Edisto Beach, U.S.A. 152 C9 32 29N 80 20W
Edisto I., U.S.A. 152 C9 32 35N 80 20W
Edithburgh, Australia 128 C2 35 5S 137 43E
Edjeleh, Algeria 111 C6 28 38N 9 50E
Edmeston, U.S.A. 151 D9 42 42N 75 15W
Edmond, U.S.A. 155 H6 35 39N 97 29W
Edmonds, U.S.A. 160 C4 47 49N 122 23W
Edmonton, Australia 126 B4 17 2S 145 46E
Edmonton, Canada 142 C6 53 30N 113 30W
Edmund L., Canada 140 B1 54 45N 93 17W
Edmundston, Canada 141 C6 47 23N 68 20W
Edna, U.S.A. 155 L6 28 59N 96 39W
Edo □, Nigeria 113 D6 6 30N 6 0E
Edolo, Italy 44 B7 46 10N 10 21E
Edøy, Norway 18 A5 63 18N 8 10E
Edremit, Turkey 49 B9 39 34N 27 0E
Edremit Körfezi, Turkey 49 B8 39 30N 26 45E
Edsbro, Sweden 16 E12 59 54N 18 29E
Edsbyn, Sweden 16 C9 61 23N 15 49E
Edson, Canada 142 C5 53 35N 116 28W
Eduardo Castex, Argentina 174 D3 35 50S 64 18W
Edward →, Australia 128 C5 35 5S 143 30E
Edward, L., Africa 118 C2 0 25S 29 40E
Edward River, Australia 126 A3 14 59S 141 26E
Edward VII Land, Antarctica 7 E13 80 0S 150 0W
Edwardesabad = Bannu, Pakistan 91 B3 33 0N 70 18E
Edwards, Calif., U.S.A. 161 L9 34 55N 117 51W
Edwards, N.Y., U.S.A. 151 B9 44 20N 75 15W
Edwards →, U.S.A. 156 C6 41 9N 90 59W
Edwards Air Force Base, U.S.A. 161 L9 34 50N 117 40W
Edwards Plateau, U.S.A. 155 K4 30 45N 101 20W
Edwardsburg, U.S.A. 157 C10 41 48N 86 6W
Edwardsville, Ill., U.S.A. 156 F7 38 49N 89 58W
Edwardsville, Pa., U.S.A. 151 E9 41 15N 75 56W
Edxná, Mexico 163 D6 19 35N 90 15W
Edzo, Canada 142 A5 62 49N 116 4W
Eek, U.S.A. 144 F7 60 14N 162 2W
Eeklo, Belgium 24 C3 51 11N 3 33E
Eel →, Ind., U.S.A. 157 E10 39 7N 86 57W
Eel →, Ind., U.S.A. 157 D10 40 45N 86 22W
Eesti = Estonia ■, Europe 15 G21 58 30N 25 30E
Efate, Vanuatu 133 G6 17 40S 168 25E
Efate, I., Vanuatu 133 G6 17 40S 168 25E
Eferding, Austria 34 C7 48 18N 14 1E
Eferi, Algeria 111 D6 24 30N 9 28E
Effigy Mounds ⌓, U.S.A. 156 A5 43 5N 91 11W
Effingham, U.S.A. 157 E8 39 7N 88 33W
Effretikon, Switz. 33 B7 47 25N 8 42E
Eforie, Romania 53 F13 44 1N 28 37E
Efoulen, Cameroon 114 B2 2 46N 10 43E
Eftaløt, Norway 18 E6 59 33N 9 49E
Ega →, Spain 40 C3 42 19N 1 55W
Égadi, Ísole, Italy 46 E5 37 55N 12 16E
Egan Range, U.S.A. 158 G6 39 35N 114 55W
Eganville, Canada 140 C4 45 32N 77 5W
Egedesminde = Aasiaat, Greenland 10 D5 68 43N 52 56W
Egegik, U.S.A. 144 G8 58 13N 157 22W
Eger = Cheb, Czech Rep. 34 A5 50 9N 12 28E
Eger, Hungary 52 C5 47 53N 20 27E
Eger →, Hungary 52 C5 47 38N 20 50E
Egersund, Norway 18 F3 58 26N 6 1E
Egg, Austria 33 B9 47 26N 9 54E
Egg, Switz. 33 B7 47 18N 8 41E
Egg I., St. Helena 9 h 15 58S 5 47W
Egg L., Canada 143 B7 55 5N 105 30W
Eggedal, Norway 18 D6 60 14N 9 22E
Eggegebirge Südlicher Teutoburger Wald ⌓, Germany 30 D4 51 40N 8 59E
Eggenburg, Austria 34 C8 48 38N 15 50E
Eggenfelden, Germany 31 G8 48 23N 12 46E
Eggiwil, Switz. 32 C5 46 52N 7 47E
Egherta, Somali Rep. 120 D2 2 4N 43 11E
Éghezée, Belgium 24 D4 50 35N 4 55E
Egholo, Solomon Is. 133 M9 8 25S 157 25E
Egilsstaðir, Iceland 11 B12 65 16N 14 25W
Egio = Aíyion, Greece 48 C4 38 15N 22 5E
Egito, Angola 115 E2 12 4S 13 58E
Égletons, France 28 C6 45 24N 2 3E
Eglisau, Switz. 33 A7 47 35N 8 31E
Egmont, Canada 142 D4 49 45N 123 56W
Egmont △, N.Z. 130 F3 39 17S 174 4E
Egmont, C., N.Z. 130 F2 39 16S 173 45E
Egmont, Mt. = Taranaki, Mt., N.Z. 130 F3 39 17S 174 5E
Egra, India 93 J12 21 54N 87 32E
Eğridir, Turkey 100 D4 37 52N 30 51E
Eğridir Gölü, Turkey 100 D4 37 53N 30 50E
Egtved, Denmark 17 J3 55 38N 9 18E
Éguas →, Brazil 171 D3 13 26S 44 14W
Egum Atoll, Papua N. G. 132 E7 9 25S 152 0E
Egume, Nigeria 113 D6 7 30N 7 14E
Éguzon-Chantôme, France 27 F8 46 27N 1 33E
Egvekinot, Russia 67 C19 66 19N 179 50W
Egyek, Hungary 52 C5 47 39N 20 52E
Egypt ■, Africa 106 B3 28 0N 31 0E
Eha Amufu, Nigeria 113 D6 6 30N 7 46E
Eheli, Algeria 111 D5 22 26N 4 40E
Ehime □, Japan 72 D4 33 30N 132 40E
Ehingen, Germany 31 G5 48 16N 9 43E
Ehrenberg, U.S.A. 161 M12 33 36N 114 31W
Ehrhardt, U.S.A. 152 B8 33 6N 81 1W
Ehrwald, Austria 34 D3 47 24N 10 56E
Eibar, Spain 40 B2 43 11N 2 28W
Eibenschitz = Ivančice, Czech Rep. 35 B9 49 6N 16 23E
Eichstätt, Germany 31 G7 48 54N 11 11E
Eide, Hordaland, Norway 18 D3 60 31N 6 44E
Eide, Møre og Romsdal, Norway 18 B4 62 55N 7 27E
Eider →, Germany 30 A4 54 19N 8 57E
Eidsbugarden, Norway 18 C5 61 23N 8 16E
Eidsbygda, Norway 18 B4 62 36N 7 30E
Eidsdal, Norway 18 B4 62 16N 7 10E
Eidsvåg, Norway 18 B5 62 46N 8 2E
Eidsvold, Australia 127 D5 25 25S 151 12E
Eidsvoll, Norway 18 D8 60 19N 11 14E
Eielson, U.S.A. 144 D11 64 40N 147 4W
Eifel, Germany 31 E2 50 15N 6 50E
Eiffel Flats, Zimbabwe 119 F3 18 20S 30 0E
Eiger, Switz. 32 C6 46 34N 8 1E
Eigg, U.K. 22 E2 56 54N 6 10W
Eighty Mile Beach, Australia 124 C3 19 30S 120 40E
Eikefjord, Norway 18 C2 61 35N 5 27E
Eikelandsosen, Norway 18 D2 60 15N 5 43E
Eiken, Norway 18 F4 58 29N 7 14E
Eikeren, Norway 18 E6 59 38N 9 58E
Eiksdal, Norway 18 B5 62 28N 8 12E
Eil, Somali Rep. 120 C3 8 0N 49 50E
Eil, L., U.K. 22 E3 56 51N 5 16W
Eildon, Australia 129 D6 37 14S 145 55E
Eildon, L., Australia 129 D7 37 10S 146 0E
Eilean Sar = Western Isles □, U.K. 22 D1 57 30N 7 10W
Eilenburg, Germany 30 D8 51 27N 12 36E
Ein el Luweiqa, Sudan 107 E3 14 5N 33 50E
Eina, Norway 18 D7 60 38N 10 35E
Einarsstaðir, Iceland 11 B9 65 44N 17 24W
Einasleigh, Australia 126 B3 18 32S 144 5E
Einasleigh →, Australia 126 B3 17 30S 142 17E
Einbeck, Germany 30 D5 51 49N 9 53E
Eindhoven, Neths. 24 C5 51 26N 5 28E
Einsiedeln, Switz. 33 B7 47 7N 8 46E
Eire = Ireland ■, Europe 23 C4 53 50N 7 52W
Eiríksjökull, Iceland 11 C6 64 46N 20 24W
Eiríksstaðir, Iceland 11 B11 65 7N 15 25W
Eirunepé, Brazil 172 B4 6 35S 69 53W
Eiseb →, Namibia 116 C2 20 33S 20 59E
Eisenach, Germany 30 E6 50 58N 10 19E
Eisenberg, Germany 30 E7 50 58N 11 54E
Eisenerz, Austria 34 D7 47 32N 14 54E
Eisenhüttenstadt, Germany 30 C10 52 9N 14 38E
Eisenkappel, Austria 34 E7 46 29N 14 36E
Eisenstadt, Austria 35 D9 47 51N 16 31E
Eisenstein = Železná Ruda, Czech Rep. 34 B6 49 8N 13 15E
Eisfeld, Germany 31 E6 50 25N 10 54E
Eisleben, Germany 30 D7 51 32N 11 32E
Eislingen, Germany 31 G5 48 41N 9 42E
Eivindvik, Norway 18 D2 60 59N 5 4E
Eivissa, Spain 43 G7 38 54N 1 26E
Eixe, Serra do, Spain 42 C4 42 24N 6 54W
Ejea de los Caballeros, Spain 40 C3 42 7N 1 9W
Ejeda, Madag. 117 C7 24 20S 44 31E
Ejura, Ghana 113 D4 7 23N 1 15W
Ejutla, Mexico 163 D5 16 34N 96 44W
Ekalaka, U.S.A. 154 C2 45 53N 104 33W
Ekalla, Gabon 114 C2 1 27S 14 0E
Ekanga, Dem. Rep. of the Congo 114 C4 2 23S 23 14E
Ekenäs = Tammisaari, Finland 15 F20 60 0N 23 26E
Ekenässjön, Sweden 17 G9 57 28N 15 1E
Ekerö, Sweden 16 E11 59 16N 17 45E
Eket, Nigeria 113 E6 4 38N 7 56E
Eketahuna, N.Z. 130 G4 40 38S 175 43E
Ekhinádhes Nísoi, Greece 39 C3 38 25N 21 2E
Ekhínos, Greece 51 E9 41 16N 25 1E
Ekibastuz, Kazakhstan 66 D8 51 50N 75 10E
Ekiti □, Nigeria 113 D6 7 25N 5 20E
Ekoli, Dem. Rep. of the Congo 118 C1 0 23S 24 13E
Ekoln, Sweden 16 E11 59 45N 17 37E
Ekouamou, Congo 114 B3 0 8N 16 31E
Ekoungounou, Congo 114 C3 1 10S 15 52E
Ekshärad, Sweden 16 D7 60 10N 13 30E
Eksjö, Sweden 17 G8 57 40N 14 58E
Ekukola, Dem. Rep. of the Congo 114 C3 0 31S 18 56E
Ekuku, Dem. Rep. of the Congo 114 C4 0 41S 21 42E
Ekukula, Dem. Rep. of the Congo 114 B4 0 15N 21 30E
Ekuma →, Namibia 116 B2 18 40S 16 2E
Ekuta, Dem. Rep. of the Congo 114 B3 3 0N 18 50E
Ekwan →, Canada 140 B3 53 12N 82 15W
Ekwan Pt., Canada 140 B3 53 16N 82 7W
Ekwok, U.S.A. 144 G8 59 22N 157 30W
El Aaiún, W. Sahara 110 C2 27 9N 13 12W
El Aargub, Mauritania 110 D1 23 37N 15 52W
El Abanico, Chile 174 D1 37 20S 71 31W
El Abbasiya, Sudan 107 E3 12 10N 31 18E
El Abiodh-Sidi-Cheikh, Algeria 111 B5 32 53N 0 31E
El Adde, Somali Rep. 120 D3 2 35N 46 9E
El 'Agrûd, Egypt 103 E3 30 14N 34 24E
El Aïoun, Morocco 111 B4 34 33N 2 30W
El Ait, Sudan 107 E2 12 22N 27 27E
El 'Aiyat, Egypt 106 J7 29 36N 31 15E
El 'Alamein, Egypt 106 A2 30 48N 28 58E
El Alto, Peru 172 A1 4 15S 81 14W
El Aouj, Mauritania 110 D2 22 53N 12 49W
El 'Aqaba, W. →, Egypt 103 E2 30 7N 33 54E
El 'Arag, Egypt 106 B2 28 40N 26 20E
El Arahal, Spain 43 H5 37 15N 5 33W
El Aricha, Algeria 111 B4 34 13N 1 10W
El Arîḥâ, West Bank 103 D4 31 52N 35 27E
El 'Arîsh, Egypt 103 D2 31 8N 33 50E
El 'Arîsh, W. →, Egypt 103 D2 31 8N 33 47E
El Arrouch, Algeria 111 A6 36 37N 6 53E
El Asnam = Ech Chéliff, Algeria 111 A5 36 10N 1 20E
El Astillero, Spain 42 B7 43 24N 3 49W
El Badâri, Egypt 106 B3 27 4N 31 25E
El Bahrein, Egypt 106 B2 28 30N 26 25E
El Ballâs, Egypt 106 B3 26 2N 32 43E
El Balyana, Egypt 106 B3 26 10N 32 3E
El Banco, Colombia 168 B3 9 0N 73 58W
El Baqeir, Sudan 106 D3 18 40N 33 40E
El Barco de Ávila, Spain 42 E5 40 21N 5 31W
El Barco de Valdeorras = O Barco, Spain 42 C4 42 23N 6 58W
El Bauga, Sudan 106 D3 18 18N 33 52E
El Baúl, Venezuela 168 B4 8 57N 68 17W
El Bawiti, Egypt 106 B2 28 25N 28 45E
El Bayadh, Algeria 111 B5 33 40N 1 1E
El Bierzo, Spain 42 C4 42 45N 6 30W
El Bluff, Nic. 164 D3 11 59N 83 40W
El Bolsón, Argentina 176 B2 41 55S 71 30W
El Bonillo, Spain 41 G2 38 57N 2 35W
El Brûk, W. →, Egypt 103 E2 30 15N 33 50E
El Buheirat □, Sudan 107 F3 7 0N 30 0E
El Bur, Somali Rep. 120 D3 4 40N 46 37E
El Burgo de Osma, Spain 40 D1 41 35N 3 4W
El Caín, Argentina 176 B3 41 38S 68 19W
El Cajon, U.S.A. 161 N10 32 48N 116 58W
El Callao, Venezuela 169 B5 7 18N 61 50W
El Campo, U.S.A. 155 L6 29 12N 96 16W
El Carmen, Bolivia 173 C5 13 40S 63 55W
El Centro, U.S.A. 161 N11 32 48N 115 34W
El Cerro, Bolivia 173 D5 17 30S 61 40W
El Cerro de Andévalo, Spain 43 H4 37 45N 6 57W
El Cocuy, Colombia 168 B3 6 25N 72 27W
El Cocuy △, Colombia 168 B3 6 33N 72 5W
El Compadre, Mexico 161 N10 32 20N 116 14W
El Corcovado, Argentina 176 B2 43 25S 71 35W
El Coronil, Spain 43 H5 37 5N 5 38W
El Cuy, Argentina 176 A3 39 55S 68 25W
El Cuyo, Mexico 163 C7 21 30N 87 40W
El Dab'a, Egypt 106 H6 31 0N 28 27E
El Daheir, Egypt 103 D3 31 13N 34 10E
El Dambahaddo, Somali Rep. 120 D3 3 17N 46 40E
El Dátil, Mexico 162 B2 30 7N 112 15W
El Deir, Egypt 106 B3 25 25N 32 20E
El Dere, Ethiopia 120 C2 5 6N 43 5E
El Dere, Somali Rep. 120 D3 3 50N 47 8E
El Dere, Somali Rep. 120 C3 5 22N 46 11E
El Descanso, Mexico 161 N10 32 12N 116 58W
El Desemboque, Mexico 162 A2 30 30N 112 57W
El Dilingat, Egypt 106 H7 30 50N 30 31E
El Diviso, Colombia 168 C2 1 22N 78 14W
El Djouf, Mauritania 104 D3 20 0N 9 0W
El Dorado, Ark., U.S.A. 155 J8 33 12N 92 40W
El Dorado, Kans., U.S.A. 155 G6 37 49N 96 52W
El Dorado, Venezuela 169 B5 6 55N 61 37W
El Dorado Springs, U.S.A. 155 G8 37 52N 94 1W
El Eglab, Algeria 110 C4 26 20N 4 30W
El 'Ein, Sudan 107 D2 16 35N 29 22E
El Ejido, Spain 43 J8 36 47N 2 49W
El Escorial, Spain 42 E6 40 35N 4 7W
El Espinar, Spain 42 D6 41 43N 4 15W
El Eulma, Algeria 111 A6 36 9N 5 42E
El Faiyûm, Egypt 106 J7 29 19N 30 50E
El Fâsher, Sudan 107 E2 13 33N 25 26E
El Fashn, Egypt 106 J7 28 50N 30 54E
El Ferrol = Ferrol, Spain 42 B2 43 29N 8 15W
El Fifi, Sudan 107 E2 10 4N 25 0E
El Fud, Ethiopia 120 C2 7 15N 42 52E
El Fuerte, Mexico 162 B3 26 30N 108 40W
El Ga'a, Sudan 107 E2 14 16N 29 59E
El Gal, Somali Rep. 120 B4 10 58N 50 20E
El Garef, Sudan 107 E3 12 3N 34 19E
El Gebir, Sudan 107 E2 13 40N 29 40E
El Gedida, Egypt 106 B2 25 40N 28 30E
El Geneina = Al Junaynah, Sudan 109 F4 13 27N 22 45E
El Geteina, Sudan 107 E3 14 50N 32 27E
El Gezira □, Sudan 107 E3 15 0N 33 0E
El Gir, Sudan 106 D2 19 50N 28 18E
El Gîza, Egypt 106 J7 30 0N 31 10E
El Gogorron △, Mexico 162 C4 21 50N 100 50W
El Goléa, Algeria 111 B5 30 30N 2 50E
El Grau, Spain 41 G4 39 0N 0 7W
El Guácharo △, Venezuela 165 D7 10 8N 63 21W
El Guache △, Venezuela 165 E6 9 45N 69 30W
El Hadeb, W. Sahara 110 C2 25 51N 13 0W
El Hadjira, Algeria 111 B6 32 36N 5 30E
El Hagiz, Sudan 107 D4 15 15N 35 50E
El Hâi, Egypt 106 J7 29 39N 31 18E
El Hajeb, Morocco 110 B3 33 43N 5 13W
El Hamma, Tunisia 108 B1 33 54N 9 48E
El Hammam, Egypt 106 A2 30 52N 29 25E
El Hammâmi, Mauritania 110 D2 23 3N 11 30W
El Hamurre, Somali Rep. 120 C3 7 13N 48 54E
El Hank, Mauritania 110 D3 24 30N 7 0W
El Hasian, W. Sahara 110 C2 26 20N 14 0W
El Hawata, Sudan 107 E3 13 25N 34 42E
El Heiz, Egypt 106 B2 27 50N 28 40E
El Hideib, Sudan 107 E3 13 0N 32 50E
El Hilla, Sudan 107 E2 13 24N 27 2E
El Homeur, Algeria 111 C5 29 43N 1 45E
El 'Idisât, Egypt 106 B3 25 30N 32 35E
El Iskandarîya, Egypt 106 H7 31 13N 29 58E
El Jadida, Morocco 110 B3 33 11N 8 17W
El Jardal, Honduras 164 D2 14 54N 88 50W
El Jebelein, Sudan 107 E3 12 40N 32 55E
El Jebha, Morocco 110 A4 35 11N 4 43W
El Jem, Tunisia 108 A2 35 18N 10 42E
El Kab, Sudan 106 D3 19 27N 32 46E
El Kabrît, G., Egypt 103 F2 29 42N 33 16E
El Kafr el Sharqi, Egypt 106 H7 31 16N 31 10E
El Kala, Algeria 111 A6 36 50N 8 30E
El Kamlin, Sudan 107 D3 15 3N 33 11E
El Kantara, Algeria 111 A6 35 14N 5 45E
El Kantara, Tunisia 108 B2 33 45N 10 58E
El Karaba, Sudan 106 D3 18 32N 33 41E
El Kef, Tunisia 108 A1 36 12N 8 47E
El Kelâa, Morocco 110 B3 32 4N 7 27W
El Kere, Ethiopia 107 F5 5 50N 42 5E
El Khandaq, Sudan 106 D3 18 30N 30 30E
El Khârga, Egypt 106 B3 25 30N 30 33E
El Khartûm, Sudan 107 D3 15 31N 32 35E
El Khartûm □, Sudan 107 D3 16 0N 33 0E
El Khartûm Bahrî, Sudan 107 D3 15 40N 32 31E
El Khroub, Algeria 111 A6 36 10N 6 55E
El Kseur, Algeria 111 A5 36 46N 4 49E
El Ksiba, Morocco 110 B3 32 45N 6 1W
El Kuntilla, Egypt 103 E3 30 1N 34 45E
El Laqâwa, Sudan 107 E2 11 25N 29 1E
El Leh, Ethiopia 107 G4 3 46N 39 13E
El Leiya, Sudan 107 D4 16 15N 35 28E
El Maestrazgo, Spain 40 E4 40 30N 0 25W
El Mafâza, Sudan 107 E3 13 38N 34 30E
El Maghra, Egypt 106 A2 30 15N 28 55E
El Mahalla el Kubra, Egypt 106 H7 31 0N 31 0E
El Mahârîq, Egypt 106 B3 25 35N 30 35E
El Maîmûn, Egypt 106 J7 29 14N 31 12E
El Maitén, Argentina 176 B2 42 3S 71 10W
El Maiz, Algeria 111 C4 28 19N 0 9W
El Maks el Bahari, Egypt 106 C3 24 30N 30 40E
El Malpais ⌓, U.S.A. 159 J10 34 53N 108 0W
El Manshâh, Egypt 106 B3 26 26N 31 50E
El Mansour, Algeria 111 C4 27 47N 0 14W
El Mansûra, Egypt 106 H7 31 0N 31 19E
El Manteco, Venezuela 169 B5 7 38N 62 45W
El Manzala, Egypt 106 H7 31 10N 31 50E
El Marâgha, Egypt 106 B3 26 35N 31 10E
El Masid, Sudan 107 D3 15 15N 33 0E
El Masnou, Spain 40 D7 41 28N 2 20E
El Matariya, Egypt 106 H8 31 15N 32 0E
El Meda, Ethiopia 107 F5 5 39N 41 47E
El Medano, Canary Is. 9 e1 28 3N 16 32W
El Meghaier, Algeria 111 B6 33 55N 5 58E
El Meraguen, Algeria 111 C4 28 0N 0 7W
El Metemma, Sudan 107 D3 16 50N 33 10E
El Miamo, Venezuela 169 B5 7 39N 61 46W
El Milagro, Argentina 174 C2 30 59S 65 59W
El Milia, Algeria 111 A6 36 51N 6 13E
El Minyâ, Egypt 106 B3 28 7N 30 33E
El Monte, U.S.A. 161 L8 34 4N 118 1W
El Montseny, Spain 40 D7 41 55N 2 25E
El Mreyye, Mauritania 112 B3 18 0N 6 0W
El Nido, Phil. 81 F2 11 10N 119 25E
El Niybo, Ethiopia 107 G4 4 40N 39 55E
El Obeid, Sudan 107 E3 13 8N 30 10E
El Odaiya, Sudan 107 E2 12 8N 28 12E
El Oro, Mexico 163 D4 19 48N 100 8W
El Oro □, Ecuador 168 D2 3 30S 79 50W
El Oued, Algeria 111 B6 33 20N 6 58E
El Oumi, Niger 111 D7 20 11N 0 15E
El Palmar, Bolivia 173 D5 17 50S 63 9W
El Palmar, Venezuela 169 B5 7 58N 61 53W
El Palmar △, Argentina 174 C4 32 10S 58 31W
El Palmito, Presa, Mexico 162 B3 25 40N 105 30W
El Paso = Derby, U.S.A. 155 G6 37 33N 97 16W
El Paso, Ill., U.S.A. 156 D7 40 44N 89 1W
El Paso, Tex., U.S.A. 159 L10 31 45N 106 29W
El Paso Robles, U.S.A. 160 K6 35 38N 120 41W
El Pedernoso, Spain 41 F2 39 29N 2 45W
El Pedroso, Spain 43 H5 37 51N 5 45W
El Pilar, Venezuela 169 A5 10 32N 63 9W
El Pinacate y Gran Desierto de Altar = Gran Desierto del Pinacate △, Mexico 162 A2 31 51N 113 32W
El Pobo de Dueñas, Spain 40 E3 40 46N 1 39W
El Portal, U.S.A. 160 H7 37 41N 119 47W
El Porvenir, Mexico 162 A3 31 15N 105 51W
El Prat de Llobregat, Spain 40 D7 41 18N 2 3E
El Progreso, Ecuador 172 a 0 54S 89 33W
El Progreso, Honduras 164 C2 15 26N 87 51W
El Pueblito, Mexico 162 B3 29 3N 105 4W
El Pueblo, Canary Is. 9 e1 28 36N 17 47W
El Puente del Arzobispo, Spain 42 F5 39 48N 5 10W
El Puerto de Santa María, Spain 43 J4 36 36N 6 13W
El Qâhira, Egypt 106 H7 30 1N 31 14E
El Qantara, Egypt 103 E1 30 51N 32 20E
El Qasr, Egypt 106 B2 25 44N 28 42E
El Qubâbât, Egypt 106 J7 29 28N 31 16E
El Quseima, Egypt 103 E3 30 40N 34 15E
El Qusîya, Egypt 106 B3 27 29N 30 44E
El Râshda, Egypt 106 B2 25 36N 28 57E
El Reno, U.S.A. 146 C7 35 32N 97 57W
El Rey △, Argentina 174 A3 24 40S 64 34W
El Rîdisiya, Egypt 106 C3 24 56N 32 51E

El Rio, *U.S.A.* **161 L7** 34 14N 119 10W
El Ronquillo, *Spain* **43 H4** 37 44N 6 10W
El Roque, Pta., *Canary Is.* **9 e1** 28 10N 15 25W
El Rosarito, *Mexico* **162 B2** 28 38N 114 4W
El Rubio, *Spain* **43 H5** 37 22N 5 0W
El Saff, *Egypt* **106 J7** 29 34N 31 16 E
El Saheira, W. →, *Egypt* **103 E2** 30 5N 33 25 E
El Salto, *Mexico* **162 C3** 23 47N 105 22W
El Salvador ■, *Cent. Amer.* **164 D2** 13 50N 89 0W
El Sauce, *Nic.* **164 D2** 13 0N 86 40W
El Saucejo, *Spain* **43 H5** 37 4N 5 6W
El Shallal, *Egypt* **106 C3** 24 0N 32 53 E
El Simbillawein, *Egypt* **106 H7** 30 48N 31 13 E
El Sombrero, *Venezuela* **168 B4** 9 23N 67 3W
El Sueco, *Mexico* **162 B3** 29 54N 106 24W
El Suweis, *Egypt* **106 J8** 29 58N 32 31 E
El Tabbîn, *Egypt* **106 J7** 29 47N 31 18 E
El Tamá △, *S. Amer.* **168 B3** 7 25N 72 25W
El Tamarâni, W. →, *Egypt* **103 E3** 30 7N 34 43 E
El Thamad, *Egypt* **103 F3** 29 40N 34 28 E
El Tigre, *Venezuela* **169 B5** 8 44N 64 15W
El Tîh, Gebal, *Egypt* **103 F2** 29 40N 33 50 E
El Tîna, *Egypt* **106 H8** 31 3N 32 22 E
El Tîna, Khalîg, *Egypt* **103 D1** 31 10N 32 40 E
El Tocuyo, *Venezuela* **168 B4** 9 47N 69 48W
El Tofo, *Chile* **174 B1** 29 22 S 71 18W
El Tránsito, *Chile* **174 B1** 28 52 S 70 17W
El Tuparro △, *Colombia* **168 B4** 5 19N 68 28W
El Tûr, *Egypt* **96 D2** 28 14N 33 36 E
El Turbio, *Argentina* **176 D2** 51 45 S 72 5W
El Uinle, *Somali Rep.* **120 D2** 3 4N 41 42 E
El Uqsur, *Egypt* **106 B3** 25 41N 32 38 E
El Valle ⌓, *Spain* **41 H3** 37 56N 1 6W
El Venado, *Mexico* **162 C4** 22 56N 101 10W
El Vendrell, *Spain* **40 D6** 41 10N 1 30 E
El Vergel, *Mexico* **162 B3** 26 28N 106 22W
El Vigía, *Venezuela* **168 B3** 8 38N 71 39W
El Viso del Alcor, *Spain* **43 H5** 37 23N 5 43W
El Wabeira, *Egypt* **103 F2** 29 34N 33 6 E
El Wak, *Kenya* **118 B5** 2 49N 40 56 E
El Wak, *Somali Rep.* **120 D2** 2 44N 41 1 E
El Waqf, *Egypt* **106 B3** 25 45N 32 15 E
El Weguet, *Ethiopia* **107 F5** 5 28N 42 17 E
El Wuz, *Sudan* **107 D3** 15 5N 30 7 E
Elafónisos, *Greece* **48 E4** 36 29N 22 56 E
Elamanchili, *India* **94 F6** 17 33N 82 50 E
Élancourt, *France* **27 D8** 48 47N 1 58 E
Elands, *Australia* **129 A10** 31 37 S 152 20 E
Elandsfontein Junc. = Germiston, *S. Africa* **117 D4** 26 15 S 28 10 E
Élassa, *Greece* **49 F8** 35 18N 26 21 E
Elassón, *Greece* **48 B4** 39 53N 22 12 E
Elat, *Israel* **103 F3** 29 30N 34 56 E
Eláthia, *Greece* **48 C4** 38 37N 22 46 E
Eláti Óros, *Greece* **39 B2** 38 43N 20 39 E
Elâzığ, *Turkey* **101 C8** 38 37N 39 14 E
Elba, *Italy* **44 F7** 42 46N 10 17 E
Elba, *U.S.A.* **152 D3** 31 25N 86 4W
Elbasan, *Albania* **50 E4** 41 9N 20 9 E
Elbe, *U.S.A.* **160 D4** 46 45N 122 10W
Elbe →, *Europe* **30 B4** 53 50N 9 0 E
Elbe-Seitenkanal, *Germany* **30 C6** 52 45N 10 32 E
Elberfeld, *U.S.A.* **157 F9** 38 10N 87 27W
Elbert, Mt., *U.S.A.* **159 G10** 39 7N 106 27W
Elberton, *U.S.A.* **152 A7** 34 7N 82 52W
Elbeuf, *France* **26 C8** 49 17N 1 2 E
Elbidtan, *Turkey* **96 B3** 38 13N 37 12 E
Elbing = Elbląg, *Poland* **54 D6** 54 10N 19 25 E
Elbistan, *Turkey* **100 C7** 38 13N 37 15 E
Elbląg, *Poland* **54 D6** 54 10N 19 25 E
Elbow, *Canada* **143 C7** 51 7N 106 35W
Elbow, Pta., *W. Sahara* **110 D1** 24 5N 15 35W
Elbrus, *Asia* **61 J6** 43 21N 42 30 E
Elbufer-Drawehn ⌓, *Germany* **30 B6** 53 8N 10 58 E
Elburn, *U.S.A.* **157 C8** 41 54N 88 28W
Elburz Mts. = Alborz, Reshteh-ye Kūhhā-ye, *Iran* **97 C7** 36 0N 52 0 E
Elche, *Spain* **41 G4** 38 15N 0 42W
Elche de la Sierra, *Spain* **41 G2** 38 27N 2 3W
Elcho I., *Australia* **126 A2** 11 55 S 135 45 E
Elda, *Spain* **41 G4** 38 29N 0 47W
Elde →, *Germany* **30 B7** 53 7N 11 15 E
Eldey, *Iceland* **11 D4** 63 45N 22 55W
Eldon, *Iowa, U.S.A.* **156 D4** 40 55N 92 13W
Eldon, *Mo., U.S.A.* **156 F4** 38 21N 92 35W
Eldon, *Wash., U.S.A.* **160 C3** 47 33N 123 3W
Eldora, *U.S.A.* **156 B3** 42 22N 93 5W
Eldorado = Echo Bay, *Canada* **138 B8** 66 5N 117 55W
Eldorado, *Argentina* **175 B5** 26 28 S 54 43W
Eldorado, *Canada* **150 B7** 44 35N 77 31W
Eldorado, *Mexico* **162 C3** 24 20N 107 22W
Eldorado, *Ill., U.S.A.* **157 G8** 37 49N 88 26W
Eldorado, *Tex., U.S.A.* **155 K4** 30 52N 100 36W
Eldorendo, *U.S.A.* **152 D5** 31 3N 84 39W
Eldoret, *Kenya* **118 B4** 0 30N 35 17 E
Eldred, *U.S.A.* **150 E6** 41 58N 78 23W
Eldridge, *U.S.A.* **156 C6** 41 39N 90 35W
Elea, C., *Cyprus* **39 E10** 35 19N 34 4 E
Eleanora, Pk., *Australia* **125 F3** 32 57 S 121 9 E
Elefantes →, *Africa* **117 C5** 24 10 S 32 40 E
Elefantes, B. das, *Angola* **115 E2** 13 13 S 12 44 E
Elefantes, G., *Chile* **176 C2** 46 28 S 73 49W
Eleftherios Venizelos Airport, ✈ (ATH), *Greece* **48 D5** 37 55N 23 50 E
Elektrogorsk, *Russia* **58 E10** 55 56N 38 50 E
Elektroperedacha = Elektrogorsk, *Russia* **58 E10** 55 56N 38 50 E
Elektrostal, *Russia* **58 E10** 55 41N 38 32 E
Elektrovoz = Stupino, *Russia* **58 E10** 54 57N 38 2 E
Elele, *Nigeria* **113 D6** 5 5N 6 50 E
Elena, *Bulgaria* **51 D9** 42 55N 25 53 E
Elephant Butte Reservoir, *U.S.A.* **159 K10** 33 9N 107 11W
Elephant I., *Antarctica* **7 C18** 61 0 S 55 0W
Elephant Pass, *Sri Lanka* **95 K5** 9 35N 80 25 E
Elesbão Veloso, *Brazil* **170 C3** 6 13 S 42 8W
Eleshnitsa, *Bulgaria* **50 E7** 41 52N 23 36 E
Eleşkirt, *Turkey* **101 C10** 39 50N 42 50 E
Eleuthera, *Bahamas* **164 B4** 25 0N 76 20W
Elevsís, *Greece* **48 C5** 38 4N 23 26 E
Elevtheroúpolis, *Greece* **51 F8** 40 52N 24 20 E
Elfin Cove, *U.S.A.* **144 G13** 58 12N 136 22W
Elgå, *Norway* **18 B8** 62 10N 11 56 E
Elgepiggen, *Norway* **18 B8** 62 10N 11 21 E
Elgg, *Switz.* **33 B7** 47 29N 8 52 E
Elgin, *Canada* **151 B8** 44 36N 76 13W
Elgin, *U.K.* **22 D5** 57 39N 3 19W
Elgin, *Ill., U.S.A.* **157 B8** 42 2N 88 17W
Elgin, *N. Dak., U.S.A.* **154 B4** 46 24N 101 51W
Elgin, *Oreg., U.S.A.* **158 D5** 45 34N 117 55W
Elgin, *S.C., U.S.A.* **152 A9** 34 10N 80 48W
Elgin, *Tex., U.S.A.* **155 K6** 30 21N 97 22W
Elgoibar, *Spain* **40 B2** 43 13N 2 24W
Elgon, Mt., *Africa* **118 B3** 1 10N 34 30 E
Eliase, *Indonesia* **83 C4** 8 21 S 130 48 E
Elikón, *Greece* **48 C4** 38 18N 22 45 E
Elim, *Namibia* **116 B2** 17 48 S 15 31 E
Elim, *S. Africa* **116 E2** 34 35 S 19 45 E
Elim, *U.S.A.* **144 D7** 64 37N 162 15W
Elin Pelin, *Bulgaria* **50 D7** 42 40N 23 36 E
Elingampangu, *Dem. Rep. of the Congo* **114 C4** 2 0 S 24 4 E
Elipa, *Dem. Rep. of the Congo* **114 C4** 1 3 S 24 20 E
Eliseu Martins, *Brazil* **170 C3** 8 13 S 43 42W
Elista, *Russia* **61 G7** 46 16N 44 14 E
Eliza, L., *Australia* **128 D3** 37 15 S 139 50 E
Elizabeth, *Australia* **128 C3** 34 42 S 138 41 E
Elizabeth, *Ill., U.S.A.* **156 B6** 42 19N 90 13W
Elizabeth, *N.J., U.S.A.* **151 F10** 40 40N 74 13W
Elizabeth, B., *Ecuador* **172 a** 0 36 S 91 12W
Elizabeth City, *U.S.A.* **149 G7** 36 18N 76 14W
Elizabethton, *U.S.A.* **149 G4** 36 21N 82 13W
Elizabethtown, *Ky., U.S.A.* **157 G11** 37 42N 85 52W
Elizabethtown, *N.Y., U.S.A.* **151 B11** 44 13N 73 36W
Elizabethtown, *Pa., U.S.A.* **151 F8** 40 9N 76 36W
Elizabethville = Lubumbashi, *Dem. Rep. of the Congo* **119 E2** 11 40 S 27 28 E
Elizondo, *Spain* **40 B3** 43 12N 1 30W
Ełk, *Poland* **54 E9** 53 50N 22 21 E
Elk →, *Canada* **142 C5** 49 11N 115 14W
Ełk →, *Poland* **54 E9** 53 41N 22 28 E
Elk →, *U.S.A.* **149 H2** 34 46N 87 16W
Elk City, *U.S.A.* **155 H5** 35 25N 99 25W
Elk Creek, *U.S.A.* **160 F4** 39 36N 122 32W
Elk Grove, *U.S.A.* **160 G5** 38 25N 121 22W
Elk Island △, *Canada* **142 C6** 53 35N 112 59W
Elk Lake, *Canada* **140 C3** 47 40N 80 25W
Elk Point, *Canada* **143 C6** 53 54N 110 55W
Elk River, *Idaho, U.S.A.* **158 C5** 46 47N 116 11W
Elk River, *Minn., U.S.A.* **154 C8** 45 18N 93 35W
Elkader, *U.S.A.* **156 B5** 42 51N 91 24W
Elkedra →, *Australia* **126 C2** 21 8 S 136 22 E
Elkhart, *Ind., U.S.A.* **157 C11** 41 41N 85 58W
Elkhart, *Kans., U.S.A.* **155 G4** 37 0N 101 54W
Elkhart →, *U.S.A.* **157 C11** 41 41N 85 58W
Elkhorn, *Canada* **143 D8** 49 59N 101 14W
Elkhorn, *U.S.A.* **157 B8** 42 40N 88 33W
Elkhorn →, *U.S.A.* **154 E6** 41 8N 96 19W
Elkhovo, *Bulgaria* **51 D10** 42 10N 26 35 E
Elkin, *U.S.A.* **149 G5** 36 15N 80 51W
Elkins, *U.S.A.* **148 F6** 38 55N 79 51W
Elkland, *U.S.A.* **150 E7** 41 59N 77 19W
Elko, *Canada* **142 D5** 49 20N 115 10W
Elko, *U.S.A.* **158 F6** 40 50N 115 46W
Elkton, *U.S.A.* **150 C1** 43 49N 83 11W
Ell, L., *Australia* **125 E4** 29 13 S 127 46 E
Ellas = Greece ■, *Europe* **48 B3** 40 0N 23 0 E
Ellaville, *Fla., U.S.A.* **152 E6** 30 23N 83 10W
Ellaville, *Ga., U.S.A.* **152 C5** 32 14N 84 19W
Ellef Ringnes I., *Canada* **6 B2** 78 30N 102 2W
Ellen, Mt., *U.S.A.* **151 B12** 44 9N 72 56W
Ellenburg, *U.S.A.* **151 B11** 44 54N 73 48W
Ellendale, *U.S.A.* **154 B5** 46 0N 98 32W
Ellensburg, *U.S.A.* **158 C3** 46 59N 120 34W
Ellenville, *U.S.A.* **151 E10** 41 43N 74 24W
Ellerton, *Barbados* **165 g** 13 7N 59 33W
Ellery, Mt., *Australia* **129 D8** 37 28 S 148 47 E
Ellesmere = Scottsdale, *Australia* **127 G4** 41 9 S 147 31 E
Ellesmere, L., *N.Z.* **131 H7** 43 47 S 172 28 E
Ellesmere I., *Canada* **6 B4** 79 30N 80 0W
Ellesmere Port, *U.K.* **20 D5** 53 17N 2 54W
Ellettsville, *U.S.A.* **157 E10** 39 14N 86 38W
Ellice Is. = Tuvalu ■, *Pac. Oc.* **134 H9** 8 0 S 178 0 E
Ellicottville, *U.S.A.* **150 D6** 42 17N 78 40W
Elliot, *Australia* **126 B1** 17 33 S 133 32 E
Elliot, *S. Africa* **117 E4** 31 22 S 27 48 E
Elliot Lake, *Canada* **140 C3** 46 25N 82 35W
Elliotdale = Xhora, *S. Africa* **117 E4** 31 55 S 28 38 E
Elliott, *U.S.A.* **152 A9** 34 6N 80 10W
Elliott Key, *U.S.A.* **153 K9** 25 27N 80 12W
Ellis, *U.S.A.* **154 F5** 38 56N 99 34W
Elliston, *Australia* **127 E1** 33 39 S 134 53 E
Ellisville, *U.S.A.* **155 K10** 31 36N 89 12W
Ellon, *U.K.* **22 D6** 57 22N 2 4W
Ellora, *India* **94 D2** 20 1N 75 10 E
Ellore = Eluru, *India* **94 F5** 16 48N 81 8 E
Elloree, *U.S.A.* **152 B9** 33 32N 80 34W
Ellsworth, *Kans., U.S.A.* **154 F5** 38 44N 98 14W
Ellsworth, *Maine, U.S.A.* **149 C11** 44 33N 68 25W
Ellsworth Land, *Antarctica* **7 D16** 76 0 S 89 0W
Ellsworth Mts., *Antarctica* **7 D16** 78 30 S 85 0W
Ellwangen, *Germany* **31 G6** 48 57N 10 8 E
Ellwood City, *U.S.A.* **150 F4** 40 52N 80 17W
Ellzey, *U.S.A.* **153 F7** 29 19N 82 48W
Elm, *Switz.* **33 C8** 46 54N 9 10 E
Elm-Lappwald ⌓, *Germany* **30 C6** 52 15N 10 50 E
Elma, *Canada* **143 D9** 49 52N 95 55W
Elma, *U.S.A.* **160 D3** 47 0N 123 25W
Elmadağ, *Turkey* **100 C5** 39 55N 33 14 E
Elmalı, *Turkey* **49 E11** 36 44N 29 56 E
Elmhurst, *U.S.A.* **157 C9** 41 53N 87 56W
Elmina, *Ghana* **113 D4** 5 5N 1 21W
Elmira, *Canada* **150 C4** 43 36N 80 33W
Elmira, *U.S.A.* **150 D8** 42 6N 76 48W
Elmira Heights, *U.S.A.* **150 D8** 42 8N 76 50W
Elmodel, *U.S.A.* **152 D5** 31 21N 84 29W
Elmore, *Australia* **128 D6** 36 30 S 144 37 E
Elmore, *Ala., U.S.A.* **152 C3** 32 32N 86 19W
Elmore, *Calif., U.S.A.* **161 M11** 33 7N 115 49W
Elmore, *Minn., U.S.A.* **157 C13** 41 29N 83 18W
Elmshorn, *Germany* **30 B5** 53 43N 9 40 E
Elmvale, *Canada* **150 B5** 44 35N 79 52W
Elmwood, *U.S.A.* **156 D7** 40 47N 89 58W
Elne, *France* **28 F6** 42 36N 2 58 E
Elnesvågen, *Norway* **18 B4** 62 52N 7 10 E
Elnora, *U.S.A.* **157 F9** 38 53N 87 5W
Eloaua I., *Papua N. G.* **132 A5** 1 38 S 149 40 E
Elobey, Is., *Eq. Guin.* **114 B1** 1 1N 9 29 E
Elongo, *Dem. Rep. of the Congo* **114 C4** 0 19 S 21 39 E
Elora, *Canada* **150 C4** 43 41N 80 26W
Elorza, *Venezuela* **168 B4** 7 3N 69 31W
Elos, *Greece* **48 E4** 36 46N 22 43 E
Eloúnda, *Greece* **39 E6** 35 16N 25 42 E
Eloy, *U.S.A.* **159 K8** 32 45N 111 33W
Éloyes, *France* **27 D13** 48 6N 6 36 E
Elpitiya, *Sri Lanka* **95 L5** 6 17N 80 10 E
Elrose, *Canada* **143 C7** 51 12N 108 0W
Elsberry, *U.S.A.* **156 E6** 39 10N 90 47W
Elsdorf, *Germany* **30 E2** 50 55N 6 34 E
Elsie, *Mich., U.S.A.* **157 A12** 43 5N 84 23W
Elsie, *Oreg., U.S.A.* **160 E3** 45 52N 123 36W
Elsinore = Helsingør, *Denmark* **17 H6** 56 2N 12 35 E
Elster →, *Germany* **30 D7** 51 25N 11 57 E
Elsterwerda, *Germany* **30 D9** 51 27N 13 31 E
Eltham, *N.Z.* **130 F3** 39 26 S 174 19 E
Elton, *Russia* **61 F8** 49 5N 46 52 E
Elton, Ozero, *Russia* **61 F8** 49 5N 46 42 E
Eltville, *Germany* **31 E4** 50 2N 8 7 E
Eluru, *India* **94 F5** 16 48N 81 8 E
Elvas, *Portugal* **43 G3** 38 50N 7 10W
Elven, *France* **26 E4** 47 44N 2 36W
Elverum, *Norway* **18 D8** 60 53N 11 34 E
Elvire →, *Australia* **124 C4** 17 51 S 128 11 E
Elvire, Mt., *Australia* **125 E2** 29 22 S 119 36 E
Elvo →, *Italy* **44 C5** 45 23N 8 21 E
Elwell, L., *U.S.A.* **158 B8** 48 22N 111 17W
Elwood, *Ill., U.S.A.* **157 C8** 41 24N 88 7W
Elwood, *Ind., U.S.A.* **157 D11** 40 17N 85 50W
Elwood, *Nebr., U.S.A.* **154 E5** 40 36N 99 52W
Elx = Elche, *Spain* **41 G4** 38 15N 0 42W
Ely, *U.K.* **21 E8** 52 24N 0 16 E
Ely, *Minn., U.S.A.* **154 B9** 47 55N 91 51W
Ely, *Nev., U.S.A.* **158 G6** 39 15N 114 54W
Elyria, *U.S.A.* **150 E2** 41 22N 82 7W
Elyrus, *Greece* **48 F5** 35 15N 23 45 E
Elz →, *Germany* **31 G3** 48 18N 7 44 E
Emådalen, *Sweden* **16 C8** 61 20N 14 44 E
Émaé, *Vanuatu* **133 G6** 17 4 S 168 24 E
Emāmrūd, *Iran* **97 B7** 36 30N 55 0 E
Emån →, *Sweden* **17 G10** 57 8N 16 30 E
Emao, *Vanuatu* **133 G6** 17 29 S 168 30 E
Emas △, *Brazil* **173 D7** 18 2 S 52 50W
Emateloa, *Dem. Rep. of the Congo* **114 B3** 1 16N 18 42 E
Emba, *Kazakhstan* **66 E6** 48 50N 58 8 E
Emba →, *Kazakhstan* **57 E9** 46 55N 53 28 E
Embarcación, *Argentina* **174 A3** 23 10 S 64 0W
Embarras →, *U.S.A.* **157 F9** 38 39N 87 37W
Embarras Portage, *Canada* **143 B6** 58 27N 111 28W
Embetsu, *Japan* **70 B10** 44 44N 141 47 E
Embi = Emba, *Kazakhstan* **66 E6** 48 50N 58 8 E
Embi = Emba →, *Kazakhstan* **57 E9** 46 55N 53 28 E
Embira →, *Brazil* **172 B3** 7 19 S 70 15W
Embóna, *Greece* **38 E11** 36 13N 27 51 E
Embrach, *Switz.* **33 B7** 47 30N 8 36 E
Embrun, *France* **29 D10** 44 34N 6 30 E
Embu, *Kenya* **118 C4** 0 32 S 37 38 E
Emden, *Germany* **30 B3** 53 21N 7 12 E
Emecik, *Turkey* **49 E9** 36 46N 27 49 E
Emerald, *Queens., Australia* **126 C4** 23 32 S 148 10 E
Emerald, *Vic., Australia* **122 E8** 37 56 S 145 29 E
Emerson, *Canada* **143 D9** 49 0N 97 10W
Emerson, *U.S.A.* **152 A5** 34 8N 84 45W
Emet, *Turkey* **49 B11** 39 20N 29 15 E
Emeti, *Papua N. G.* **132 D2** 7 53 S 143 15 E
Emi Koussi, *Chad* **109 E3** 19 45N 18 55 E
Emília-Romagna □, *Italy* **44 D8** 44 45N 11 0 E
Emilius, Mte., *Italy* **44 C4** 45 45N 7 20 E
Eminabad, *Pakistan* **92 C6** 32 2N 74 8 E
Emine, Nos, *Bulgaria* **51 D11** 42 40N 27 56 E
Eminence, *U.S.A.* **157 F11** 38 22N 85 11W
Emirau I., *Papua N. G.* **132 A6** 1 40 S 150 0 E
Emirdağ, *Turkey* **100 C4** 39 2N 31 8 E
Emissi, Tarso, *Chad* **109 D3** 21 27N 18 36 E
Emlenton, *U.S.A.* **150 E5** 41 11N 79 43W
Emlichheim, *Germany* **30 C2** 52 37N 6 51 E
Emmaboda, *Sweden* **17 H9** 56 37N 15 32 E
Emmalane, *U.S.A.* **152 C7** 32 46N 82 0W
Emmaus, *S. Africa* **116 D4** 29 2 S 25 15 E
Emmaus, *U.S.A.* **151 F9** 40 32N 75 30W
Emme →, *Switz.* **32 B5** 47 14N 7 32 E
Emmeloord, *Neths.* **24 B5** 52 44N 5 46 E
Emmen, *Neths.* **24 B6** 52 48N 6 57 E
Emmen, *Switz.* **31 H4** 47 5N 8 18 E
Emmenbrücke, *Switz.* **33 B6** 47 4N 8 16 E
Emmendingen, *Germany* **31 G3** 48 6N 7 51 E
Emmental, *Switz.* **32 C4** 46 55N 7 40 E
Emmerich, *Germany* **30 D2** 51 50N 6 14 E
Emmet, *Australia* **126 C3** 24 45 S 144 30 E
Emmetsburg, *U.S.A.* **156 A2** 43 7N 94 41W
Emmett, *U.S.A.* **150 D2** 42 59N 82 46W
Emmiganuru, *India* **95 G3** 15 44N 77 29 E
Emmonak, *U.S.A.* **144 E6** 62 46N 164 30W
Emo, *Canada* **143 D10** 48 38N 93 50W
Emőd, *Hungary* **52 C5** 47 57N 20 47 E
Emona, *Bulgaria* **51 D11** 42 43N 27 53 E
Empalme, *Mexico* **162 B2** 28 1N 110 49W
Empangeni, *S. Africa* **117 D5** 28 50 S 31 52 E
Empedrado, *Argentina* **174 B4** 28 0 S 58 46W
Emperor Seamount Chain, *Pac. Oc.* **134 D9** 40 0N 170 0 E
Empingham Res. = Rutland Water, *U.K.* **21 E7** 52 39N 0 38W
Empire, *U.S.A.* **152 C6** 32 21N 83 18W
Empoli, *Italy* **44 E7** 43 43N 10 57 E
Emporia, *Kans., U.S.A.* **154 F6** 38 25N 96 11W
Emporia, *Va., U.S.A.* **149 G7** 36 42N 77 32W
Emporium, *U.S.A.* **150 E6** 41 31N 78 14W
Empress, *Canada* **143 C7** 50 57N 110 0W
Empty Quarter = Rub' al Khālī, *Si. Arabia* **99 C5** 19 0N 48 0 E
Ems →, *Germany* **30 B3** 53 20N 7 12 E
Emsdale, *Canada* **150 A5** 45 32N 79 19W
Emsdetten, *Germany* **30 C3** 52 10N 7 32 E
Emu, *China* **75 C15** 43 40N 128 6 E
Emu Park, *Australia* **126 C5** 23 13 S 150 50 E
'En 'Avrona, *Israel* **103 F4** 29 43N 35 0 E
En Gannim = Ramat Gan, *Israel* **103 C3** 32 4N 34 48 E
En Nahrat, *Mali* **110 D4** 22 55N 3 36W
En Nahud, *Sudan* **107 E2** 12 45N 28 25 E
En Nofalab, *Sudan* **107 D3** 15 52N 32 32 E
Ena, *Japan* **73 B9** 35 25N 137 25 E
Ena-San, *Japan* **73 B9** 35 26N 137 36 E
Enambú, *Colombia* **168 C3** 1 1N 70 17W
Enana, *Namibia* **116 B2** 17 30 S 16 23 E
Enånger, *Sweden* **16 C11** 61 30N 17 9 E
Enard B., *U.K.* **22 C3** 58 5N 5 20W
Enare = Inarijärvi, *Finland* **14 B22** 69 0N 28 0 E
Enarotali, *Indonesia* **83 B5** 3 55 S 136 21 E
Enbekshi, *Kazakhstan* **65 C4** 41 22N 68 3 E
Encampment, *U.S.A.* **158 F10** 41 12N 106 47W
Encantadas, Serra, *Brazil* **175 C5** 30 40 S 53 0W
Encarnación, *Paraguay* **175 B4** 27 15 S 55 50W
Encarnación de Diaz, *Mexico* **162 C4** 21 30N 102 13W
Enchi, *Ghana* **112 D4** 5 53N 2 48W
Encinitas, *U.S.A.* **161 M9** 33 3N 117 17W
Encino, *U.S.A.* **159 J11** 34 39N 105 28W
Encontrados, *Venezuela* **168 B3** 9 3N 72 14W
Encounter B., *Australia* **128 C3** 35 45 S 138 45 E
Encruzilhada, *Brazil* **171 E3** 15 31 S 40 54W
Encs, *Hungary* **52 B6** 48 20N 21 8 E
Endako, *Canada* **142 C3** 54 6N 125 2W
Ende, *Indonesia* **82 C2** 8 45 S 121 40 E
Endeavour Str., *Australia* **126 A3** 10 45 S 142 0 E
Endelave, *Denmark* **17 J4** 55 46N 10 18 E
Enden, *Norway* **18 C7** 61 47N 10 15 E
Enderbury I., *Kiribati* **134 H10** 3 8 S 171 5W
Enderby, *Canada* **142 C5** 50 35N 119 10W
Enderby I., *Australia* **124 D2** 20 35 S 116 30 E
Enderby Land, *Antarctica* **7 C5** 66 0 S 53 0 E
Enderlin, *U.S.A.* **154 B6** 46 38N 97 36W
Endicott, *U.S.A.* **151 D8** 42 6N 76 4W
Endicott Mts., *U.S.A.* **144 C10** 68 0N 152 0W
Endimari →, *Brazil* **172 B4** 8 46 S 66 7W
Endwell, *U.S.A.* **151 D8** 42 6N 76 2W
Endyalgout I., *Australia* **124 B5** 11 40 S 132 35 E
Ene →, *Peru* **172 C3** 11 10 S 74 18W
Eneabba, *Australia* **125 E2** 29 49 S 115 16 E
Energetīcheskīy, *Kazakhstan* **65 B8** 43 25N 77 1 E
Energetik, *Russia* **64 F7** 51 45N 58 45 E
Enewetak Atoll, *Marshall Is.* **134 F8** 11 30N 162 15 E
Enez, *Turkey* **51 F10** 40 45N 26 5 E
Enfer, Pte. d', *Martinique* **164 c** 14 22N 60 54W
Enfield, *Canada* **141 D7** 44 56N 63 32W
Enfield, *Conn., U.S.A.* **151 E12** 41 58N 72 36W
Enfield, *Ill., U.S.A.* **157 F8** 38 6N 88 20W
Enfield, *N.C., U.S.A.* **149 G7** 36 11N 77 41W
Enfield, *N.H., U.S.A.* **151 C12** 43 39N 72 9W
Enga □, *Papua N. G.* **132 C2** 5 30 S 143 30 E
Engadin, *Switz.* **31 J6** 46 45N 10 10 E
Engan, *Norway* **18 A5** 63 8N 8 31 E
Engaño, C., *Dom. Rep.* **165 C6** 18 30N 68 20W
Engaño, C., *Phil.* **80 B4** 18 35N 122 23 E
Engaru, *Japan* **70 B11** 44 3N 143 31 E
Engcobo, *S. Africa* **117 E4** 31 37 S 28 0 E
Engelberg, *Switz.* **33 C6** 46 48N 8 26 E
Engels, *Russia* **60 E8** 51 28N 46 6 E
Engemann L., *Canada* **143 B7** 58 0N 106 55W
Engerdal, *Norway* **18 C8** 61 45N 11 58 E
Engershatu, *Eritrea* **107 D4** 16 7N 38 34 E
Enggano, *Indonesia* **84 D2** 5 20 S 102 40 E
Engil, *Morocco* **110 B4** 33 12N 4 32W
Engineer Group, *Papua N. G.* **132 F6** 10 35 S 151 20 E
Engkilili, *Malaysia* **85 B4** 1 3N 111 42 E
England, *U.S.A.* **155 H9** 34 33N 91 58W
England □, *U.K.* **21 E5** 53 0N 2 0W
Englee, *Canada* **141 B8** 50 45N 56 5W
Englehart, *Canada* **140 C4** 47 49N 79 52W
Englewood, *Colo., U.S.A.* **154 F2** 39 39N 104 59W
Englewood, *Fla., U.S.A.* **153 J7** 26 58N 82 21W
Englewood, *Ohio, U.S.A.* **157 E12** 39 53N 84 18W
English, *U.S.A.* **157 F10** 38 20N 86 28W
English →, *Canada* **143 C10** 49 12N 91 5W
English →, *U.S.A.* **156 C5** 41 29N 91 32W
English B., *Ascension I.* **9 g** 7 54 S 14 23W
English Bazar = Ingraj Bazar, *India* **93 G13** 24 58N 88 10 E
English Channel, *Europe* **21 G6** 50 0N 2 0W
English Company's Is., The, *Australia* **126 A2** 11 50 S 136 32 E
English River, *Canada* **140 C1** 49 14N 91 0W
Engures ezers, *Latvia* **54 A10** 57 16N 23 6 E
Enguri →, *Georgia* **61 J5** 42 27N 41 38 E
Enid, *U.S.A.* **155 G6** 36 24N 97 53W
Enipévs →, *Greece* **48 B4** 39 22N 22 17 E
Enkhuizen, *Neths.* **24 B5** 52 42N 5 17 E
Enköping, *Sweden* **16 E11** 59 37N 17 4 E
Enle, *China* **76 F3** 24 0N 101 9 E
Enna, *Italy* **47 E7** 37 34N 14 16 E
Ennadai, *Canada* **143 A8** 61 8N 100 53W
Ennadai L., *Canada* **143 A8** 60 58N 101 20W
Enné, O. →, *Chad* **109 F4** 14 24N 18 45 E
Ennedi, *Chad* **109 E4** 17 15N 22 0 E
Enneri Achelouma →, *Niger* **111 D7** 21 55N 13 35 E
Enngonia, *Australia* **127 D4** 29 21 S 145 50 E
Ennigerloh, *Germany* **30 D4** 51 50N 8 2 E
Ennis, *Ireland* **23 D3** 52 51N 8 59W
Ennis, *Mont., U.S.A.* **158 D8** 45 21N 111 44W
Ennis, *Tex., U.S.A.* **155 J6** 32 20N 96 38W
Enniscorthy, *Ireland* **23 D5** 52 30N 6 34W
Enniskillen, *U.K.* **23 B4** 54 21N 7 39W
Ennistimon, *Ireland* **23 D2** 52 57N 9 17W
Enns, *Austria* **34 C7** 48 12N 14 28 E
Enns →, *Austria* **34 C7** 48 14N 14 32 E
Enontekiö, *Finland* **14 B20** 68 23N 23 37 E
Enosburg Falls, *U.S.A.* **151 B12** 44 55N 72 48W
Enping, *China* **77 F9** 22 16N 112 21 E
Enrekang, *Indonesia* **82 B1** 3 34 S 119 47 E
Enrile, *Phil.* **80 C3** 17 34N 121 42 E
Enriquillo, L., *Dom. Rep.* **165 C5** 18 20N 72 5W
Enschede, *Neths.* **24 B6** 52 13N 6 53 E
Ensenada, *Argentina* **174 C4** 34 55 S 57 55W
Ensenada, *Mexico* **162 A1** 31 50N 116 50W
Ensenada de los Muertos, *Mexico* **162 C2** 23 59N 109 50W
Enshi, *China* **76 B7** 30 18N 109 29 E
Enshū-Nada, *Japan* **73 C9** 34 27N 137 38 E
Ensiola, Pta. de n', *Spain* **38 B3** 39 7N 2 55 E
Ensisheim, *France* **27 E14** 47 50N 7 20 E
Ensley, *U.S.A.* **153 E2** 30 31N 87 16W
Entebbe, *Uganda* **118 B3** 0 4N 32 28 E
Enterprise, *Canada* **142 A5** 60 47N 115 45W
Enterprise, *Ala., U.S.A.* **152 D4** 31 19N 85 51W
Enterprise, *Oreg., U.S.A.* **158 D5** 45 25N 117 17W
Entlebuch, *Switz.* **32 C6** 46 59N 8 4 E
Entorno de Doñana ⌓, *Spain* **43 J4** 37 0N 6 26W
Entraygues-sur-Truyère, *France* **28 D6** 44 38N 2 35 E
Entre Rios = Rio Brilhante, *Brazil* **175 A5** 21 48 S 54 33W
Entre Rios = Três Rios, *Brazil* **171 F3** 22 6 S 43 15W
Entre Ríos, *Bolivia* **174 A3** 21 30 S 64 25W
Entre Rios, *Bahia, Brazil* **171 D4** 11 56 S 38 5W
Entre Rios, *Pará, Brazil* **173 B7** 5 24 S 54 21W
Entre Ríos □, *Argentina* **174 C4** 30 30 S 58 30W
Entrepeñas, Embalse de, *Spain* **40 E2** 40 34N 2 42W
Entroncamento, *Portugal* **43 F2** 39 28N 8 28W
Enugu, *Nigeria* **113 D6** 6 30N 7 30 E
Enugu □, *Nigeria* **113 D6** 6 30N 7 45 E
Enugu Ezike, *Nigeria* **113 D6** 7 0N 7 29 E
Enumclaw, *U.S.A.* **160 C5** 47 12N 121 59W
Envalira, Port d', *Europe* **40 C6** 42 33N 1 43 E
Envermeu, *France* **26 C8** 49 53N 1 15 E
Envigado, *Colombia* **168 B2** 6 10N 75 35W
Enviken, *Sweden* **16 D9** 60 49N 15 46 E
Envira, *Brazil* **172 B3** 7 18 S 70 13W
Enying, *Hungary* **52 D3** 46 56N 18 15 E
Enyonga, *Gabon* **114 C1** 0 59 S 9 22 E
Enza →, *Italy* **44 D7** 44 54N 10 31 E
Enzan, *Japan* **73 B10** 35 42N 138 44 E
Eólie, Ís., *Italy* **47 D7** 38 30N 14 57 E
Epalinges, *Switz.* **32 C3** 46 33N 6 40 E
Epanomí, *Greece* **50 F6** 40 25N 22 59 E
Epe, *Neths.* **24 B5** 52 21N 5 59 E
Epe, *Nigeria* **113 D5** 6 36N 3 59 E
Epéna, *Congo* **114 B3** 1 22N 17 29 E
Épernay, *France* **27 C10** 49 3N 3 56 E
Épernon, *France* **27 D8** 48 35N 1 40 E
Ephesus, *Turkey* **49 D9** 37 55N 27 22 E
Ephraim, *U.S.A.* **158 G8** 39 22N 111 35W
Ephrata, *Pa., U.S.A.* **151 F8** 40 11N 76 11W
Ephrata, *Wash., U.S.A.* **158 C4** 47 19N 119 33W
Epi, *Vanuatu* **133 F6** 16 43 S 168 15 E
Epidaurus Limera, *Greece* **48 E5** 36 46N 23 0 E
Épila, *Spain* **40 D3** 41 36N 1 17W
Épinac, *France* **27 F11** 46 59N 4 31 E
Épinal, *France* **27 D13** 48 10N 6 27 E
Epira, *Guyana* **169 B6** 5 5N 57 20W
Episkopi, *Cyprus* **39 F8** 34 40N 32 54 E
Episkopí, *Greece* **39 E5** 35 20N 24 20 E
Episkopi Bay, *Cyprus* **39 F8** 34 35N 32 50 E
Epitálion, *Greece* **48 D3** 37 37N 21 30 E
Eppalock, L., *Australia* **128 D6** 36 52 S 144 34 E
Eppan = Appiano, *Italy* **45 B8** 46 28N 11 15 E
Eppingen, *Germany* **31 F4** 49 8N 8 53 E
Epsom, *U.K.* **21 F7** 51 19N 0 16W
Epukiro, *Namibia* **116 C2** 21 40 S 19 9 E
Equality, *U.S.A.* **157 G8** 37 44N 88 20W
Équateur □, *Dem. Rep. of the Congo* **114 B4** 2 0N 21 0 E
Equatorial Guinea ■, *Africa* **114 B1** 2 0N 8 0 E
Equeipa, *Venezuela* **169 B5** 5 22N 62 43W
Er Hai, *China* **76 E3** 25 48N 100 11 E
Er Rachidia, *Morocco* **110 B4** 31 58N 4 20W
Er Rahad, *Sudan* **107 E3** 12 45N 30 32 E
Er Rif, *Morocco* **111 A4** 35 1N 4 1W
Er Rogel, *Sudan* **106 D4** 18 10N 35 25 E
Er Roseires, *Sudan* **107 E3** 11 55N 34 30 E
Er Rua'at, *Sudan* **107 E3** 12 21N 32 17 E
Eraclea, *Italy* **45 C9** 45 35N 12 40 E
Eran, *Phil.* **81 G1** 9 4N 117 42 E
Erandol, *India* **94 D2** 20 56N 75 20 E
Eranga, *Dem. Rep. of the Congo* **114 C3** 1 52 S 18 56 E
Erap, *Papua N. G.* **132 D4** 6 37 S 146 51 E
Erasmus = Bronkhorstspruit, *S. Africa* **117 D4** 25 46 S 28 45 E
Erave, *Papua N. G.* **132 D2** 6 39 S 144 0 E
Erave →, *Papua N. G.* **132 D3** 6 54 S 144 47 E
Erāwadī Myit = Irrawaddy →, *Burma* **90 G5** 15 50N 95 6 E
Erāwadī Myitwanya = Irrawaddy, Mouths of the, *Burma* **90 H5** 15 30N 95 0 E
Erba, *Italy* **44 C6** 45 48N 9 15 E
Erba, *Sudan* **106 D4** 19 5N 36 51 E
Erba, J., *Sudan* **106 C4** 20 48N 36 47 E
Erbaa, *Turkey* **100 B7** 40 42N 36 36 E
Erbeskopf, *Germany* **31 F3** 49 44N 7 2 E
Erbil = Arbīl, *Iraq* **101 D11** 36 15N 44 5 E
Erbu, *Ethiopia* **107 E3** 6 44N 34 53 E
Ercan, Nicosia ✈ (ECN), *Cyprus* **39 E9** 35 10N 33 30 E
Erçek, *Turkey* **96 B4** 38 39N 43 36 E
Erçis, *Turkey* **101 C10** 39 2N 43 21 E
Erciyaş Dağı, *Turkey* **96 B2** 38 30N 35 30 E
Érd, *Hungary* **52 C3** 47 22N 18 56 E
Erdao Jiang →, *China* **75 C14** 43 0N 127 0 E
Erdek, *Turkey* **51 F11** 40 23N 27 47 E
Erdély = Transilvania, *Romania* **53 D9** 46 30N 24 0 E
Erdemli, *Turkey* **100 D6** 36 36N 34 19 E
Erdene = Ulaan-Uul, *Mongolia* **74 B6** 44 13N 111 10 E
Erdenet, *Mongolia* **68 B5** 49 2N 104 5 E
Erdenetsogt, *Mongolia* **74 C4** 42 55N 106 5 E
Erding, *Germany* **31 G7** 48 18N 11 54 E
Erdre →, *France* **26 E5** 47 13N 1 32W
Erebato →, *Venezuela* **169 B5** 5 54N 64 16W
Erebus, Mt., *Antarctica* **7 D11** 77 35 S 167 0 E
Erechim, *Brazil* **175 B5** 27 35 S 52 15W
Ereğli, *Konya, Turkey* **100 D6** 37 31N 34 4 E
Ereğli, *Zonguldak, Turkey* **100 B4** 41 15N 31 24 E
Erei, Monti, *Italy* **47 E7** 37 20N 14 20 E
Erenhot, *China* **74 C7** 43 48N 112 2 E
Erenköy = Kokkina, *Cyprus* **39 E8** 35 11N 32 36 E
Eresfjord, *Norway* **18 B5** 62 40N 8 8 E
Eresma →, *Spain* **42 D6** 41 26N 4 45W
Eressós, *Greece* **49 B7** 39 11N 25 57 E
Erfenisdam, *S. Africa* **116 D4** 28 30 S 26 50 E
Erfjord, *Norway* **18 E3** 59 20N 6 14 E
Erfoud, *Morocco* **110 B4** 31 30N 4 15W
Erfstadt, *Germany* **30 E2** 50 50N 6 50 E
Erft →, *Germany* **30 D2** 51 11N 6 44 E
Erfurt, *Germany* **30 E7** 50 58N 11 2 E
Ergani, *Turkey* **101 C8** 38 17N 39 49 E
Ergel, *Mongolia* **74 C5** 43 8N 109 5 E
Ergene →, *Turkey* **51 E10** 41 1N 26 22 E
Ergeni Vozvyshennost, *Russia* **61 G7** 47 0N 44 0 E
Ērgli, *Latvia* **15 H21** 56 54N 25 38 E
Erhlin, *Taiwan* **77 F13** 23 54N 120 22 E
Eria →, *Spain* **42 C5** 42 3N 5 44W
Eriba, *Sudan* **107 D4** 16 40N 36 10 E
Eriboll, L., *U.K.* **22 C4** 58 30N 4 42W
Érice, *Italy* **46 D5** 38 2N 12 35 E
Eridu, *U.S.A.* **152 E6** 30 18N 83 45W
Erie, *Mich., U.S.A.* **157 C13** 41 47N 83 31W
Erie, *Pa., U.S.A.* **150 D4** 42 8N 80 5W
Erie, L., *N. Amer.* **150 D4** 42 15N 81 0W
Erie Canal, *U.S.A.* **150 C7** 43 5N 78 43W
Erieau, *Canada* **150 D3** 42 16N 81 57W
Erigavo, *Somali Rep.* **120 B3** 10 35N 47 20 E
Erikoúsa, *Greece* **38 B9** 39 53N 19 34 E
Eriksdale, *Canada* **143 C9** 50 52N 98 7W
Erímanthos, *Greece* **48 D3** 37 57N 21 50 E
Erimo-misaki, *Japan* **70 D11** 41 50N 143 15 E
Erin Pt., *Trin. & Tob.* **169 F9** 10 3N 61 39W
Erinpura, *India* **92 G5** 25 9N 73 3 E
Eriskay, *U.K.* **22 D1** 57 4N 7 18W
Eriswil, *Switz.* **32 B5** 47 5N 7 46 E
Erithraí, *Greece* **48 C5** 38 13N 23 20 E
Eritrea ■, *Africa* **107 E4** 14 0N 38 30 E
Erivan = Yerevan, *Armenia* **61 K7** 40 10N 44 31 E
Erjas →, *Portugal* **42 F3** 39 40N 7 1W
Erkech-Tam, *Kyrgyzstan* **65 D6** 39 41N 73 55 E

Erkech-Tam Pass, Asia 65 D7 39 46N 74 2 E
Erkelenz, Germany 30 D2 51 4N 6 19 E
Erkner, Germany 30 C9 52 25N 13 44 E
Erlangen, Germany 31 F6 49 36N 11 0 E
Erlanger, U.S.A. 157 E12 39 1N 84 36W
Erldunda, Australia 126 D1 25 14 S 133 12 E
Ermelo, Neths. 24 B5 52 18N 5 35 E
Ermelo, S. Africa 117 D4 26 31 S 29 59 E
Ermenek, Turkey 100 D5 36 38N 33 0 E
Ermil, Sudan 107 E2 13 35N 27 40 E
Ermióni, Greece 48 D5 37 23N 23 15 E
Ermones, Greece 38 B9 39 37N 19 46 E
Erne, Ireland 23 B3 54 30N 8 16W
Erne, Lower L., U.K. 23 B4 54 28N 7 47W
Erne, Upper L., U.K. 23 B4 54 14N 7 32W
Ernée, France 26 D6 48 18N 0 56W
Ernest Giles Ra., Australia 125 E3 27 0 S 123 45 E
Ernstberg, Germany 31 E2 50 13N 6 47 E
Erode, India 95 J3 11 24N 77 45 E
Eromanga, Australia 127 D3 26 40 S 143 11 E
Erongo, Namibia 116 C2 21 39 S 15 58 E
Erquy, France 26 D4 48 38N 2 29W
Err, Piz d', Switz. 33 C9 46 34N 9 43 E
Erramala Hills, India 95 G4 15 30N 78 15 E
Errer, Ethiopia 107 F5 7 32N 42 35 E
Errigal, Ireland 23 A3 55 2N 8 6W
Errinundra, Australia 129 D8 37 20 S 148 47 E
Erris Hd., Ireland 23 B1 54 19N 10 0W
Erromango, Vanuatu 133 H7 18 45 S 169 5 E
Ersekë, Albania 50 F4 40 22N 20 40 E
Érsekújvár = Nové Zámky, Slovak Rep. 35 C11 48 2N 18 8 E
Erskine, U.S.A. 154 B7 47 40N 96 0W
Erstein, France 27 D14 48 25N 7 38 E
Erstfeld, Switz. 33 C7 46 50N 8 38 E
Ertholmene, Denmark 17 J9 55 19N 15 11 E
Ertil, Russia 60 E5 51 55N 40 50 E
Ertis = Irtysh, Russia 66 C7 61 4N 68 52 E
Ertvågøy, Norway 18 A5 63 13N 8 26 E
Eruh, Turkey 101 D10 37 46N 42 13 E
Eruwa, Nigeria 113 D5 7 33N 3 26 E
Ervy-le-Châtel, France 27 D10 48 2N 3 55 E
Erwin, U.S.A. 149 G4 36 9N 82 25W
Eryuan, China 76 D2 26 7N 99 57 E
Erzgebirge, Germany 30 E8 50 27N 12 55 E
Erzin, Russia 67 D10 50 15N 95 10 E
Erzincan, Turkey 101 C8 39 46N 39 30 E
Erzurum, Turkey 101 C9 39 57N 41 15 E
Es Caló, Spain 38 D2 38 40N 1 30 E
Es Canar, Spain 38 C2 39 2N 1 36 E
Es Mercadal, Spain 38 B5 39 59N 4 5 E
Es Migjorn Gran, Spain 38 B5 39 57N 4 3 E
Es Safiya, Sudan 107 D3 15 31N 30 7 E
Es Sahrâ' Esh Sharqîya, Egypt 106 B3 27 30N 32 30 E
Es Sînâ', Egypt 106 F3 29 0N 34 0 E
Es Sûki, Sudan 107 E3 13 20N 33 58 E
Es Vedrà, Spain 38 D1 38 52N 1 12 E
Esa'ala, Papua N. G. 132 E6 9 45 S 150 49 E
Esambo, Dem. Rep. of the Congo 118 C1 3 48 S 23 30 E
Esan-Misaki, Japan 70 D10 41 40N 141 10 E
Esashi, Hokkaidō, Japan 70 B11 44 56N 142 35 E
Esashi, Hokkaidō, Japan 70 D10 41 52N 140 7 E
Esbjerg, Denmark 17 J2 55 29N 8 29 E
Esbo = Espoo, Finland 15 F21 60 12N 24 40 E
Escada, Brazil 170 C4 8 22 S 35 8W
Escalante, U.S.A. 159 H8 37 47N 111 36W
Escalante, U.S.A. 159 H8 37 24N 110 57W
Escalente, Phil. 81 F4 10 50N 123 33 E
Escalón, Mexico 162 B4 26 46N 104 20W
Escambia, U.S.A. 153 E2 30 32N 87 11W
Escanaba, U.S.A. 148 C2 45 45N 87 4W
Escarparda Pt., Phil. 80 B4 18 31N 122 13 E
Escarpé, C., Vanuatu 133 K5 20 41 S 167 13 E
Escaut = Schelde, Belgium 24 C4 51 15N 4 16 E
Esch-sur-Alzette, Lux. 24 E6 49 32N 6 0 E
Eschede, Germany 30 C6 52 44N 10 14 E
Escholzmatt, Switz. 32 C5 46 55N 7 56 E
Eschwege, Germany 30 D6 51 11N 10 2 E
Eschweiler, Germany 30 E2 50 49N 6 15 E
Escoma, Bolivia 172 D4 15 40 S 69 8W
Escondido, U.S.A. 161 M9 33 7N 117 5W
Escravos, Nigeria 113 D6 5 35N 5 10 E
Escuinapa, Mexico 162 C3 22 50N 105 50W
Escuintla, Guatemala 164 D1 14 20N 90 48W
Eséka, Cameroon 113 E7 3 41N 10 44 E
Eşen, Turkey 49 E11 36 27N 29 16 E
Esenguly, Turkmenistan 66 F6 37 37N 53 59 E
Esens, Germany 30 B3 53 38N 7 36 E
Esenyurt, Turkey 51 E12 41 3N 28 48 E
Esera, Spain 40 C5 42 6N 0 15 E
Eşfahān, Iran 97 C6 32 39N 51 43 E
Eşfahān, Iran 97 C6 32 50N 51 50 E
Esfarāyen, Iran 97 B8 37 4N 57 30 E
Esfideh, Iran 97 C8 33 39N 59 46 E
Esgueva, Spain 42 D6 41 40N 4 43W
Esh Sham = Dimashq, Syria 103 B5 33 30N 36 18 E
Esh Shamâlîya, Sudan 106 D2 19 0N 29 0 E
Esha Ness, U.K. 22 A7 60 29N 1 38W
Eshan, China 76 E4 24 11N 102 24 E
Esher, U.K. 21 F7 51 21N 0 20W
Eshkāshem = Ishkashim, Tajikistan 65 E5 36 44N 71 37 E
Eshkol, Israel 103 D3 31 20N 34 30 E
Eshowe, S. Africa 117 D5 28 50 S 31 30 E
Esiama, Ghana 112 E4 4 56N 2 25W
Esigodini, Zimbabwe 117 C4 20 18 S 28 56 E
Esik, Kazakhstan 65 B8 43 21N 77 27 E
Esil = Ishim, Russia 66 D8 57 45N 71 10 E
Esino, Italy 45 E10 43 39N 13 22 E
Esira, Madag. 117 C8 24 20 S 46 42 E
Esk, Cumb., U.K. 22 G5 54 58N 3 2W
Esk, N. Yorks., U.K. 20 C7 54 30N 0 37W
Eskān, Iran 91 D1 26 48N 63 9 E
Esker, Canada 141 B6 53 53N 66 25W
Eski-Nookat, Kyrgyzstan 65 C6 40 16N 72 36 E
Eskifjörður, Iceland 11 B13 65 3N 13 55W
Eskije = Xánthi, Greece 51 E8 41 10N 24 58 E
Eskilsäter, Sweden 17 F7 58 57N 13 10 E
Eskilstuna, Sweden 16 E10 59 22N 16 32 E
Eskimalatya, Turkey 101 C8 38 24N 38 22 E
Eskimo Point = Arviat, Canada 143 A10 61 6N 93 59W
Eskişehir, Turkey 49 B12 39 50N 30 30 E
Eskişehir, Turkey 49 B12 39 40N 31 0 E
Esla, Spain 42 D4 41 29N 6 3W
Eslāmābād-e Gharb, Iran 101 E12 34 10N 46 30 E
Eslāmshahr, Iran 97 C6 35 40N 51 10 E
Eslöv, Sweden 17 J7 55 50N 13 20 E
Eşme, Turkey 49 C10 38 23N 28 58 E
Esmeralda, I., Chile 176 C1 48 55 S 75 25W
Esmeraldas, Ecuador 168 C2 1 0N 79 40W
Esmeraldas, Ecuador 168 C2 0 40N 79 30W
Esmeraldas, Ecuador 168 C2 0 58N 79 38W
Esnagi L., Canada 140 C3 48 36N 84 33W
Esom Hill, U.S.A. 152 B4 33 57N 85 23W
Espa, Norway 18 D8 60 34N 11 16 E
Espada, Pta., Colombia 168 A3 12 5N 71 7W
Espalion, France 28 D6 44 32N 2 47 E
España = Spain, Europe 13 H5 39 0N 4 0W
Espanola, Canada 140 C3 46 15N 81 46W
Espanola, U.S.A. 159 H10 35 59N 106 5W
Española, I., Ecuador 172 a 1 23 S 89 39W
Esparreguera, Spain 40 D6 41 33N 1 52 E
Esparta, Costa Rica 164 E3 9 59N 84 40W
Espeland, Norway 18 D2 60 23N 5 28 E
Espelkamp, Germany 30 C4 52 24N 8 36 E
Espenberg, C., U.S.A. 144 C7 66 33N 163 36W
Esperança, Amazonas, Brazil 168 D4 4 24 S 69 52W
Esperança, Paraíba, Brazil 170 C4 7 1 S 35 51W
Esperance, Australia 125 F3 33 45 S 121 55 E
Esperance, C., Solomon Is. 133 M10 9 15 S 159 43 E
Esperance B., Australia 125 F3 33 48 S 121 55 E
Esperance Harbour, St. Lucia 165 f 14 4N 60 55W
Esperantinópolis, Brazil 170 B3 4 53 S 44 53W
Esperanza, Antarctica 7 C18 65 0 S 55 0W
Esperanza, Santa Cruz, Argentina 176 D2 51 1 S 70 49W
Esperanza, Santa Fe, Argentina 174 C3 31 29 S 61 3W
Esperanza, Agusan del S., Phil. 81 G5 8 43N 125 36 E
Esperanza, Masbate, Phil. 81 F5 11 45N 124 3 E
Esperanza, Puerto Rico 165 d 18 6N 65 28W
Espéraza, France 28 F6 42 56N 2 14 E
Espevær, Norway 18 E2 59 35N 5 7 E
Espichel, C., Portugal 43 G1 38 22N 9 16W
Espiel, Spain 43 G5 38 11N 5 1W
Espigão, Serra do, Brazil 175 B5 26 35 S 50 30W
Espinal, Colombia 168 C3 4 9N 74 53W
Espinar, Peru 172 C3 14 51 S 71 24W
Espinazo, Sierra del = Espinhaço, Serra do, Brazil 171 E3 17 30 S 43 30W
Espinhaço, Serra do, Brazil 171 E3 17 30 S 43 30W
Espinho, Portugal 42 D2 41 1N 8 38W
Espinilho, Serra do, Brazil 175 B5 28 30 S 55 0W
Espinosa de los Monteros, Spain 42 B7 43 5N 3 34W
Espírito Santo, Brazil 171 F3 20 0 S 40 45W
Espíritu Santo, Vanuatu 133 E4 15 15 S 166 50 E
Espíritu Santo, B. del, Mexico 163 D7 19 15N 87 0W
Espíritu Santo, I., Mexico 162 C2 24 30N 110 23W
Espita, Mexico 163 C7 21 1N 88 19W
Espiye, Turkey 101 B8 40 56N 38 43 E
Esplanada, Brazil 171 D4 11 47 S 37 57W
Espluga de Francolí, Spain 40 D6 41 24N 1 7 E
Espoo, Finland 15 F21 60 12N 24 40 E
Esprels, France 32 A2 47 32N 6 22 E
Espuña, Sierra de, Spain 41 H3 37 51N 1 35W
Espungabera, Mozam. 117 C5 20 29 S 32 45 E
Esquel, Argentina 176 B2 42 55 S 71 20W
Esquimalt, Canada 142 D4 48 26N 123 25W
Esquina, Argentina 174 C4 30 0 S 59 30W
Essandsjøen, Norway 18 A8 63 0N 12 0 E
Essaouira, Morocco 110 B3 31 32N 9 42W
Essebie, Dem. Rep. of the Congo 118 B3 2 58N 30 40 E
Essen, Belgium 24 C4 51 28N 4 28 E
Essen, Germany 30 D3 51 28N 7 2 E
Essendon, Mt., Australia 125 E3 25 0 S 120 29 E
Essequibo, Guyana 169 B6 6 50N 58 30W
Essex, Canada 150 D2 42 10N 82 49W
Essex, Calif., U.S.A. 161 L11 34 44N 115 15W
Essex, N.Y., U.S.A. 151 B11 44 19N 73 21W
Essex, U.K. 21 F8 51 54N 0 27 E
Essex Junction, U.S.A. 151 B11 44 29N 73 7W
Esslingen, Germany 31 G5 48 44N 9 18 E
Essonne, France 27 D9 48 30N 2 20 E
Estaca de Bares, C. de, Spain 42 B3 43 46N 7 42W
Estadilla, Spain 40 C5 42 4N 0 16 E
Estados, I. de Los, Argentina 176 D4 54 40 S 64 30W
Estagel, France 28 F6 42 47N 2 40 E
Eşţahbānāt, Iran 97 D7 29 8N 54 4 E
Estância, Brazil 170 D4 11 16 S 37 26W
Estancia, U.S.A. 159 J10 34 46N 106 4W
Estancia Cameron, Chile 176 D3 53 8 S 69 39W
Estārm, Iran 97 D8 28 21N 58 21 E
Estarreja, Portugal 42 E2 40 45N 8 35W
Estats, Pic d', Spain 40 C6 42 40N 1 24 E
Estavayer-le-Lac, Switz. 32 C3 46 51N 6 51 E
Estcourt, S. Africa 117 D4 29 0 S 29 53 E
Este, Italy 45 C8 45 14N 11 39 E
Este, Dom. Rep. 165 C6 18 14N 68 42W
Estelí, Nic. 164 D2 13 9N 86 22W
Estella, Spain 40 C2 42 40N 2 2W
Estellencs, Spain 38 B3 39 39N 2 29 E
Estena, Spain 43 F6 39 23N 4 44W
Estepa, Spain 43 H6 37 17N 4 52W
Estepona, Spain 43 J5 36 24N 5 7W
Esterhazy, Canada 143 C8 50 37N 102 5W
Esterias, C., Gabon 114 B1 0 40N 9 20 E
Esternay, France 27 D10 48 44N 3 33 E
Esterri d'Aneu, Spain 40 C6 42 38N 1 5 E
Estevan, Canada 143 D8 49 10N 102 59W
Estevan Group, Canada 142 C3 53 3N 129 38W
Estherville, U.S.A. 154 D7 43 24N 94 50W
Estill, U.S.A. 152 C8 32 45N 81 15W
Estissac, France 27 D10 48 16N 3 48 E
Eston, Canada 143 C7 51 8N 108 40W
Estonia, Europe 15 G21 58 30N 25 30 E
Estoril, Portugal 43 G1 38 42N 9 23W
Estouk, Mali 113 B5 18 14N 1 2 E
Estrela, Serra da, Portugal 42 E3 40 10N 7 45W
Estrella, Spain 43 G7 38 25N 3 35W
Estremoz, Portugal 43 G3 38 51N 7 39W
Estrondo, Serra do, Brazil 170 C2 7 20 S 48 0W
Esutoru = Uglegorsk, Russia 67 E15 49 5N 142 2 E
Esztergom, Hungary 52 C3 47 47N 18 44 E
Et Tîdra, Mauritania 112 B1 19 45N 16 20W
Etah, India 93 F8 27 35N 78 40 E
Étain, France 27 C12 49 13N 5 38 E
Étampes, France 27 D9 48 26N 2 10 E
Etanga, Namibia 116 B1 17 55 S 13 0 E
Étaples, France 27 B8 50 30N 1 39 E
Etawah, India 93 F8 26 48N 79 6 E
Etawney L., Canada 143 B9 57 50N 96 50W
Ete, Nigeria 113 D6 7 2N 7 28 E
Etéké, Gabon 114 C2 1 29 S 11 35 E
Ethel, U.S.A. 160 D4 46 32N 122 46W
Ethel, Oued el, Algeria 110 C4 28 31N 3 37W
Ethelbert, Canada 143 C8 51 32N 100 25W
Ethiopia, Africa 102 F3 8 0N 40 0 E
Ethiopian Highlands, Ethiopia 62 J7 10 0N 37 0 E
Etili, Turkey 51 G10 39 59N 26 54 E
Etive, L., U.K. 22 E3 56 29N 5 10W
Etna, Italy 47 E7 37 50N 14 55 E
Etna, Norway 18 C6 60 49N 10 7 E
Etne, Norway 18 E2 59 40N 5 58 E
Etoile, Dem. Rep. of the Congo 119 E2 11 33 S 27 30 E
Etolin Strait, U.S.A. 144 F6 60 20N 165 15W
Etosha, Namibia 116 B2 19 0 S 16 0 E
Etosha Pan, Namibia 116 B2 18 40 S 16 30 E
Etoumbi, Congo 114 C2 0 1 S 14 57 E
Etowah, U.S.A. 149 H3 35 20N 84 32W
Étréchy, France 27 D9 48 30N 2 12 E
Étrépagny, France 27 C8 49 18N 1 36 E
Étretat, France 26 C7 49 42N 0 12 E
Etropole, Bulgaria 51 D8 42 50N 24 0 E
Ettelbruck, Lux. 24 E6 49 51N 6 5 E
Ettlingen, Germany 31 G4 48 56N 8 25 E
Ettrick Water, U.K. 22 F6 55 31N 2 55W
Etuku, Dem. Rep. of the Congo 118 C2 3 42 S 25 45 E
Etulia, Moldova 53 E13 45 32N 28 27 E
Etzatlán, Mexico 162 C4 20 48N 104 5W
Etzná, Mexico 163 D6 19 35N 90 15W
Etzná-Tixmucuy = Edzná, Mexico 163 D6 19 35N 90 15W
Eu, France 26 B8 50 3N 1 26 E
Eua, Tonga 133 Q13 21 22 S 174 56W
Eubenangee Swamp, Australia 126 B4 16 25 S 146 1 E
Euboea = Évvoia, Greece 48 C6 38 30N 24 0 E
Eucaliptus = Tomás Barrón, Bolivia 172 D4 17 35 S 67 31W
Euchareena, Australia 129 B8 32 57 S 149 6 E
Eucla, Australia 125 F4 31 41 S 128 52 E
Euclid, U.S.A. 150 E3 41 34N 81 32W
Euclides da Cunha, Brazil 170 D4 10 31 S 39 1W
Eucumbene, L., Australia 129 D8 36 2 S 148 40 E
Eudora, U.S.A. 155 J9 33 7N 91 16W
Eudunda, Australia 128 C3 34 12 S 139 7 E
Eufaula, Ala., U.S.A. 152 D4 31 54N 85 9W
Eufaula, Okla., U.S.A. 155 H7 35 17N 95 35W
Eufaula L., U.S.A. 155 H7 35 18N 95 21W
Eugene, U.S.A. 158 E2 44 5N 123 4W
Eugowra, Australia 129 B8 33 22 S 148 24 E
Eulo, Australia 127 D4 28 10 S 145 3 E
Eulonia, U.S.A. 152 D8 31 32N 81 26W
Eumungerie, Australia 129 A8 31 56 S 148 36 E
Eungella, Australia 126 C4 20 57 S 148 40 E
Eunice, La., U.S.A. 155 K8 30 30N 92 25W
Eunice, N. Mex., U.S.A. 155 J3 32 26N 103 10W
Eupen, Belgium 24 D6 50 37N 6 3 E
Euphrates = Furāt, Nahr al, Asia 96 D5 31 0N 47 25 E
Eurapik Rise, Pac. Oc. 134 G6 2 0N 142 0 E
Eure, France 26 C8 49 10N 1 0 E
Eure, France 26 C8 49 18N 1 12 E
Eure-et-Loir, France 26 D8 48 22N 1 30 E
Eureka, Canada 6 B3 80 0N 85 56W
Eureka, Calif., U.S.A. 158 F1 40 47N 124 9W
Eureka, Ill., U.S.A. 156 D7 40 43N 89 16W
Eureka, Kans., U.S.A. 155 G6 37 49N 96 17W
Eureka, Mo., U.S.A. 156 F6 38 30N 90 38W
Eureka, Mont., U.S.A. 158 B6 48 53N 115 3W
Eureka, Nev., U.S.A. 158 G5 39 31N 115 58W
Eureka, S.C., U.S.A. 152 B8 33 42N 81 46W
Eureka, S. Dak., U.S.A. 154 C5 45 46N 99 38W
Eureka, Mt., Australia 125 E3 26 35 S 121 35 E
Eurelia, Australia 128 B3 32 33 S 138 35 E
Eurinilla Cr., Australia 128 A4 30 53 S 140 11 E
Euroa, Australia 129 D6 36 44 S 145 35 E
Europa, Île, Ind. Oc. 121 G2 22 20 S 40 22 E
Europa, Picos de, Spain 42 B6 43 10N 4 49W
Europa, Pta. de, Gib. 43 J5 36 3N 5 21W
Europe 12 E10 50 0N 20 0 E
Europoort, Neths. 24 C4 51 57N 4 10 E
Euskirchen, Germany 30 E2 50 39N 6 48 E
Eustis, U.S.A. 153 G8 28 51N 81 41W
Euston, Australia 128 C5 34 30 S 142 46 E
Eutawville, U.S.A. 152 B9 33 24N 80 21W
Eutin, Germany 30 A6 54 8N 10 36 E
Eutsuk L., Canada 142 C3 53 20N 126 45W
Eva, Brazil 169 D6 3 9 S 59 56W
Eva Perón = La Pampa, Argentina 174 D2 36 50 S 66 0W
Eva Perón = La Plata, Argentina 174 D4 35 0 S 57 55W
Evale, Angola 116 B2 16 33 S 15 44 E
Evanger, Norway 18 D3 60 39N 6 7 E
Evans, U.S.A. 154 E2 40 23N 104 41W
Evans, L., Canada 140 B4 50 50N 77 0W
Evans City, U.S.A. 150 F4 40 46N 80 4W
Evans Head, Australia 127 D5 29 7 S 153 27 E
Evans Mills, U.S.A. 151 B9 44 6N 75 48W
Evansburg, Canada 142 C5 53 36N 114 59W
Evansdale, U.S.A. 156 B4 42 30N 92 17W
Evanston, Ill., U.S.A. 157 B9 42 3N 87 41W
Evanston, Wyo., U.S.A. 158 F8 41 16N 110 58W
Evansville, Ill., U.S.A. 156 F7 38 5N 89 56W
Evansville, Ind., U.S.A. 157 G9 37 58N 87 35W
Evansville, Wis., U.S.A. 156 B7 42 47N 89 18W
Évaux-les-Bains, France 27 F9 46 12N 2 29 E
Evaz, Iran 97 E7 27 46N 53 59 E
Evciler, Afyon, Turkey 49 C11 38 3N 29 54 E
Evciler, Çanakkale, Turkey 49 B8 39 47N 26 44 E
Eveleth, U.S.A. 154 B8 47 28N 92 32W
Evensk, Russia 67 C16 62 12N 159 30 E
Evenstad, Norway 18 C8 61 25N 11 7 E
Everard, L., Australia 127 E2 31 30 S 135 0 E
Everard Ranges, Australia 125 E5 27 5 S 132 28 E
Everest, Mt., Nepal 93 E12 28 5N 86 58 E
Everett, Ga., U.S.A. 152 D8 31 24N 81 38W
Everett, Pa., U.S.A. 150 F6 40 1N 78 23W
Everett, Wash., U.S.A. 160 C4 47 59N 122 12W
Everglades, U.S.A. 153 K9 25 30N 81 0W
Everglades, The, U.S.A. 153 K9 25 50N 81 0W
Everglades City, U.S.A. 153 K8 25 52N 81 23W
Evergreen, Ala., U.S.A. 149 K2 31 26N 86 57W
Evergreen, Mont., U.S.A. 158 B6 48 9N 114 13W
Everöd, Sweden 17 J8 55 53N 14 5 E
Everton, Australia 129 D7 36 25 S 146 33 E
Evertsberg, Sweden 16 C7 61 8N 13 58 E
Evesham, U.K. 21 E6 52 6N 1 56W
Evfimía, Ayía, Greece 39 C2 38 18N 20 36 E
Evia = Évvoia, Greece 48 C6 38 30N 24 0 E
Évian-les-Bains, France 27 F13 46 24N 6 35 E
Evinayong, Eq. Guin. 114 B2 1 26N 10 35 E
Évinos, Greece 48 C3 38 27N 21 40 E
Évisa, France 29 F12 42 15N 8 48 E
Evje, Norway 18 F4 58 36N 7 51 E
Evolène, Switz. 32 D4 46 7N 7 30 E
Évora, Portugal 43 G3 38 33N 7 57W
Évora, Portugal 43 G3 38 33N 7 50W
Evowghlī, Iran 101 C11 38 43N 45 13 E
Évreux, France 26 C8 49 3N 1 8 E
Evritanía, Greece 48 B3 39 5N 21 30 E
Évron, France 26 D6 48 10N 0 24W
Évros, Greece 51 E10 41 10N 26 0 E
Évros, Greece 100 B2 41 40N 26 34 E
Evrótas, Greece 48 E4 36 50N 22 40 E
Évry, France 27 D9 48 38N 2 27 E
Évvoia, Greece 48 C6 38 30N 24 0 E
Évvoia, Greece 48 C5 38 40N 23 40 E
Evxinoúpolis, Greece 48 B4 39 12N 22 42 E
Ewa, U.S.A. 145 K13 21 20N 158 3W
Ewa Beach, U.S.A. 145 K13 21 19N 158 1W
Ewasse, Papua N. G. 132 C6 5 19 S 151 1 E
Ewe, L., U.K. 22 D3 57 49N 5 38W
Ewing, Mo., U.S.A. 156 E5 40 6N 91 43W
Ewing, Nebr., U.S.A. 154 D5 42 16N 98 21W
Ewo, Congo 114 C2 0 48 S 14 45 E
Exaltación, Bolivia 173 C4 13 10 S 65 20W
Excelsior Springs, U.S.A. 156 E2 39 20N 94 13W
Excideuil, France 28 C5 45 20N 1 4 E
Exe, U.K. 21 G4 50 41N 3 29W
Exeter, Canada 150 C3 43 21N 81 29W
Exeter, U.K. 21 G4 50 43N 3 31W
Exeter, Calif., U.S.A. 160 J7 36 18N 119 9W
Exeter, N.H., U.S.A. 151 D14 42 59N 70 57W
Exira, U.S.A. 156 C2 41 35N 94 52W
Exmoor, U.K. 21 F4 51 12N 3 45W
Exmoor, U.K. 21 F4 51 8N 3 42W
Exmouth, Australia 124 D1 21 54 S 114 10 E
Exmouth, U.K. 21 G4 50 37N 3 25W
Exmouth G., Australia 124 D1 22 15 S 114 15 E
Expedition, Australia 127 D4 25 41 S 149 7 E
Expedition Ra., Australia 126 C4 24 30 S 149 12 E
Experiment, U.S.A. 152 B5 33 17N 84 17W
Extremadura, Spain 43 F4 39 30N 6 5W
Exuma Sound, Bahamas 164 B4 24 30N 76 20W
Eyak, U.S.A. 144 F11 60 32N 145 36W
Eyasi, L., Tanzania 118 C4 3 30 S 35 0 E
Eydehamn, Norway 18 F5 58 30N 8 53 E
Eye Pen., U.K. 22 C2 58 13N 6 10W
Eyemouth, U.K. 22 F6 55 52N 2 5W
Eygues = Aigues, France 29 D8 44 7N 4 43 E
Eygurande, France 27 G9 45 40N 2 26 E
Eyjafjallajökull, Iceland 11 D7 63 38N 19 36W
Eyjafjarðarsýsla, Iceland 11 B8 65 30N 18 30W
Eyjafjörður, Iceland 11 A8 66 15N 18 30W
Eymet, France 28 D4 44 40N 0 25 E
Eymoutiers, France 28 C5 45 40N 1 45 E
Eynesil, Turkey 101 B8 41 4N 39 9 E
Eyrarbakki, Iceland 11 D5 63 52N 21 9W
Eyre (North), L., Australia 127 D2 28 30 S 137 20 E
Eyre (South), L., Australia 127 D2 29 18 S 137 25 E
Eyre, L., Australia 122 F6 29 30 S 137 26 E
Eyre Mts., N.Z. 131 F3 45 25 S 168 25 E
Eyre Pen., Australia 127 E2 33 30 S 136 17 E
Eysturoy, Færoe Is. 14 E9 62 13N 6 54W
Eyvānkī, Iran 97 C6 35 24N 51 56 E
Ez Zeidab, Sudan 106 D3 17 25N 33 55 E
Ezcaray, Spain 40 C1 42 19N 3 0W
Ežerėlis, Lithuania 54 D10 54 53N 23 37 E
Ezhou, China 77 B10 30 23N 114 50 E
Ezine, Turkey 49 B8 39 48N 26 20 E
Ezmul, Mauritania 110 D1 22 15N 15 40W
Ezouza, Cyprus 39 F8 34 44N 32 27 E

F

F.Y.R.O.M. = Macedonia, Europe 50 E5 41 53N 21 40 E
Fabala, Guinea 112 D3 9 44N 9 5W
Fabens, U.S.A. 159 L10 31 30N 106 10W
Fåberg, Norway 18 C7 61 10N 10 25 E
Fabero, Spain 42 C4 42 46N 6 37W
Fåborg, Denmark 17 J4 55 6N 10 15 E
Fabriano, Italy 45 E9 43 20N 12 54 E
Fabrichnyy, Kazakhstan 65 B8 43 9N 76 24 E
Făcăeni, Romania 53 F12 44 32N 27 53 E
Facatativá, Colombia 168 C3 4 49N 74 22W
Faceville, U.S.A. 152 E5 30 45N 84 38W
Fachi, Niger 109 E2 18 6N 11 34 E
Facundo, Argentina 176 C3 45 18 S 69 58W
Fada, Chad 109 E4 17 13N 21 34 E
Fada-n-Gourma, Burkina Faso 113 C5 12 10N 0 30 E
Fadd, Hungary 52 D3 46 28N 18 49 E
Faddeyevskiy, Ostrov, Russia 67 B15 76 0N 144 0 E
Faddor, Sudan 107 F3 8 7N 32 17 E
Fadghāmī, Syria 101 E9 35 53N 40 52 E
Fadlab, Sudan 106 D3 17 42N 34 2 E
Faenza, Italy 45 D8 44 17N 11 53 E
Færingehavn = Kangerluarsoruseq, Greenland 10 E5 63 45N 51 27W
Færoe Is. = Føroyar, Atl. Oc. 14 F9 62 0N 7 0W
Fafa, Mali 113 B5 15 22N 0 48 E
Fafe, Portugal 42 D2 41 27N 8 11W
Fagam, Nigeria 113 C7 11 1N 10 1 E
Făgăraş, Romania 53 E9 45 48N 24 58 E
Făgăras, Munţii, Romania 53 E9 45 40N 24 40 E
Fågelmara, Sweden 17 H9 56 16N 15 58 E
Fagerheim, Norway 18 D4 60 26N 7 46 E
Fagerhult, Sweden 17 G9 57 8N 15 40 E
Fagernes, Norway 18 D6 60 59N 9 14 E
Fagersta, Sweden 16 D9 60 1N 15 46 E
Făget, Romania 52 E7 45 52N 22 10 E
Făget, Munţii, Romania 53 C8 47 40N 23 10 E
Fagnano, L., Argentina 176 D3 54 30 S 68 0W
Fagnières, France 27 D11 48 58N 4 20 E
Faguibine, L., Mali 112 B4 16 45N 4 0W
Fahlīān, Iran 97 D6 30 11N 51 28 E
Fahraj, Kermān, Iran 97 D8 29 0N 59 0 E
Fahraj, Yazd, Iran 97 D7 31 46N 54 36 E
Fai Tsi Long, Vietnam 76 G6 21 0N 107 30 E
Faial, Azores 9 d1 38 34N 28 42W
Faial, Madeira 9 c 32 47N 16 53W
Faial, Canal do, Azores 9 d1 38 33N 28 35W
Faido, Switz. 33 D7 46 29N 8 48 E
Fair Haven, U.S.A. 148 D9 43 36N 73 16W
Fair Hd., U.K. 23 A5 55 14N 6 9W
Fair Isle, U.K. 19 B6 59 30N 1 40W
Fair Oaks, U.S.A. 160 G5 38 39N 121 16W
Fairbank, U.S.A. 156 B4 42 38N 92 3W
Fairbanks, Alaska, U.S.A. 144 D11 64 51N 147 43W
Fairbanks, Fla., U.S.A. 152 F7 29 44N 82 16W
Fairborn, U.S.A. 157 E12 39 49N 84 2W
Fairburn, U.S.A. 152 B5 33 34N 84 35W
Fairbury, Ill., U.S.A. 157 D8 40 45N 88 31W
Fairbury, Nebr., U.S.A. 154 E6 40 8N 97 11W
Fairfax, Ohio, U.S.A. 157 E13 39 5N 83 37W
Fairfax, S.C., U.S.A. 152 C8 32 59N 81 15W
Fairfax, Vt., U.S.A. 151 B11 44 40N 73 1W
Fairfield, Australia 129 B9 33 53 S 150 57 E
Fairfield, Ala., U.S.A. 149 J2 33 29N 86 55W
Fairfield, Calif., U.S.A. 160 G4 38 15N 122 3W
Fairfield, Conn., U.S.A. 151 E11 41 9N 73 16W
Fairfield, Idaho, U.S.A. 158 E6 43 21N 114 44W
Fairfield, Ill., U.S.A. 157 F8 38 23N 88 22W
Fairfield, Iowa, U.S.A. 156 D5 40 56N 91 57W
Fairfield, Ohio, U.S.A. 157 E12 39 21N 84 34W
Fairfield, Tex., U.S.A. 155 K7 31 44N 96 10W
Fairford, Canada 143 C9 51 37N 98 38W
Fairhope, U.S.A. 149 K2 30 31N 87 54W
Fairlie, N.Z. 131 E5 44 5 S 170 49 E
Fairmead, U.S.A. 160 H6 37 5N 120 10W
Fairmont, Minn., U.S.A. 154 D7 43 39N 94 28W
Fairmont, W. Va., U.S.A. 148 F5 39 29N 80 9W
Fairmount, Calif., U.S.A. 161 L8 34 45N 118 26W
Fairmount, N.Y., U.S.A. 151 C8 43 5N 76 12W
Fairplay, U.S.A. 159 G11 39 15N 106 2W
Fairport, U.S.A. 150 C7 43 6N 77 27W
Fairport Harbor, U.S.A. 150 E3 41 45N 81 17W
Fairview, Canada 142 B5 56 5N 118 25W
Fairview, Mont., U.S.A. 154 B2 47 51N 104 3W
Fairview, Okla., U.S.A. 155 G5 36 16N 98 29W
Fairweather, Mt., U.S.A. 142 B1 58 55N 137 32W
Faisalabad, Pakistan 91 C4 31 30N 73 5 E
Faith, U.S.A. 154 C3 45 2N 102 2W
Faizabad, India 93 F10 26 45N 82 10 E
Faizpur, India 94 D2 21 14N 75 49 E
Fajã Grande, Azores 9 d2 39 27N 31 16W
Fajardo, Puerto Rico 165 d 18 20N 65 39W
Fajr, W., Si. Arabia 96 D3 29 10N 38 10 E
Fakenham, U.K. 20 E8 52 51N 0 51 E
Fåker, Sweden 16 A8 63 0N 14 34 E
Fakfak, Indonesia 83 B4 2 55 S 132 18 E
Fakfak, Peg., Indonesia 83 B4 2 50 S 132 20 E
Fakiya, Bulgaria 51 D11 42 10N 27 6 E
Fakobli, Ivory C. 112 D3 7 23N 7 23W
Fakse, Denmark 17 J6 55 15N 12 8 E
Fakse Bugt, Denmark 17 J6 55 11N 12 15 E
Fakse Ladeplads, Denmark 17 J6 55 11N 12 9 E
Faku, China 75 C12 42 32N 123 21 E
Falaba, S. Leone 112 D2 9 54N 11 22W
Falaise, France 26 D6 48 54N 0 12W
Falaise, Mui, Vietnam 86 C5 19 6N 105 45 E
Falakrón Óros, Greece 50 E7 41 15N 23 58 E
Falam, Burma 90 D4 23 0N 93 45 E
Falces, Spain 40 C3 42 24N 1 48W
Fălciu, Romania 53 D13 46 17N 28 7 E
Falcó, C. des, Spain 38 D1 38 50N 1 23 E
Falcón, Venezuela 168 A4 11 0N 69 50W
Falcon, C., Algeria 111 A4 35 50N 0 50W
Falcón, Presa, Mexico 163 B5 26 35N 99 10W
Falcon Lake, Canada 143 D9 49 42N 95 15W
Falcon Reservoir, U.S.A. 155 M5 26 34N 99 10W
Falconara Marittima, Italy 45 E10 43 37N 13 24 E
Falcone, C. del, Italy 46 B1 40 58N 8 12 E
Falconer, U.S.A. 150 D5 42 7N 79 13W
Faléa, Mali 112 C2 12 16N 11 17W
Falefa, Samoa 133 W24 13 54 S 171 31W
Falelatai, Samoa 133 W24 13 55 S 171 59W
Falelima, Samoa 133 W23 13 32 S 172 41W
Falémé, Senegal 112 C2 14 46N 12 14W
Falenki, Russia 64 B3 58 22N 51 35 E
Falerum, Sweden 17 F10 58 8N 16 13 E
Faleshty = Făleşti, Moldova 53 C12 47 32N 27 44 E
Făleşti, Moldova 53 C12 47 32N 27 44 E
Falfurrias, U.S.A. 155 M5 27 14N 98 9W
Falher, Canada 142 B5 55 44N 117 15W
Falirakí, Greece 38 E12 36 22N 28 12 E
Falkenberg, Germany 30 D9 51 35N 13 14 E
Falkenberg, Sweden 17 H6 56 54N 12 30 E
Falkenburg = Niemodlin, Poland 55 H4 50 38N 17 38 E
Falkensee, Germany 30 C9 52 34N 13 4 E
Falkirk, U.K. 22 F5 56 0N 3 47W
Falkirk, U.K. 22 F5 55 58N 3 49W
Falkland, U.K. 22 E5 56 16N 3 12W
Falkland, East, I., Falk. Is. 176 D5 51 40 S 58 30W
Falkland, West, I., Falk. Is. 176 D4 51 40 S 60 0W
Falkland Is., Atl. Oc. 9 f 51 30 S 59 0W
Falkland Sd., Falk. Is. 9 f 52 0 S 60 0W
Falknov nad Ohří = Sokolov, Czech Rep. 34 A5 50 12N 12 40 E
Falkonéra, Greece 48 E5 36 50N 23 52 E
Falköping, Sweden 17 F7 58 12N 13 33 E
Fall River, U.S.A. 151 E13 41 43N 71 10W
Fällanden, Switz. 33 B7 47 22N 8 38 E
Fallbrook, U.S.A. 161 M9 33 23N 117 15W
Fallon, U.S.A. 158 G4 39 28N 118 47W
Falls City, U.S.A. 154 E7 40 3N 95 36W
Falls Creek, U.S.A. 150 E6 41 9N 78 48W
Falmouth, Jamaica 164 a 18 30N 77 40W
Falmouth, U.K. 21 G2 50 9N 5 5W
Falmouth, Ky., U.S.A. 157 F12 38 41N 84 20W
Falmouth, Mass., U.S.A. 151 E14 41 33N 70 37W
Falsa, Pta., Mexico 162 B1 27 51N 115 3W
False B., S. Africa 116 E2 34 15 S 18 40 E
False Divi Pt., India 95 G5 15 43N 80 50 E
False Pass, U.S.A. 144 J7 54 51N 163 25W
False Pt., India 94 D8 20 18N 86 48 E
Falso, C., Honduras 164 C3 15 12N 83 21W
Falster, Denmark 17 K5 54 45N 11 55 E
Falsterbo, Sweden 15 J15 55 23N 12 50 E
Fălticeni, Romania 53 C11 47 21N 26 20 E
Falun, Sweden 16 D9 60 37N 15 37 E
Famagusta, Cyprus 39 E9 35 8N 33 55 E
Famagusta Bay, Cyprus 39 E10 35 15N 34 0 E
Famatina, Sierra de, Argentina 174 B2 27 30 S 68 0W
Family L., Canada 143 C9 51 54N 95 27W
Famoso, U.S.A. 161 K7 35 37N 119 12W
Fan Xian, China 74 G8 35 55N 115 38 E
Fana, Mali 112 C3 13 0N 6 56W
Fanad Hd., Ireland 23 A4 55 17N 7 38W
Fanahammaren, Norway 18 D2 60 16N 5 20 E
Fanárion, Greece 48 B3 39 24N 21 47 E
Fandriana, Madag. 117 C8 20 14 S 47 21 E
Fánes-Sénnes e Braies, Italy 45 B9 46 38N 12 4 E
Fang, Thailand 76 H2 19 55N 99 13 E
Fang Xian, China 77 A8 32 3N 110 40 E
Fangaga, Sudan 106 D4 17 40N 37 50 E
Fangak, Sudan 107 F3 9 4N 30 53 E
Fangchang, China 77 B12 31 5N 118 4 E
Fangcheng, China 74 H7 33 18N 112 59 E

Fangchenggang, China . . 76 G7 21 42N 108 21 E
Fangliao, Taiwan . . . . . 77 F13 22 22N 120 38 E
Fangshan, China . . . . . 74 E6 38 3N 111 25 E
Fangzi, China . . . . 75 F10 36 33N 119 10 E
Fani i Madh →,
  Albania . . . . 50 E4 41 56N 20 16 E
Fanjakana, Madag. . . 117 C8 21 10 S 46 53 E
Fanjiatun, China . . . . 75 C13 43 40N 125 15 E
Fanling, China . . . . . . 69 F11 22 30N 114 8 E
Fannich, L., U.K. 22 D4 57 38N 4 59W
Fannūj, Iran . . . . 97 E8 26 35N 59 38 E
Fanø, Denmark . . . . . 17 J2 55 25N 8 25 E
Fano, Italy . . . . 45 E10 43 50N 13 1 E
Fanshi, China . . . . 74 E7 39 12N 113 6 E
Fao = Al Fāw, Iraq . . . 97 D6 30 0N 48 30 E
Faqirwali, Pakistan . . 92 E5 29 27N 73 0 E
Fāqūs, Egypt . . . . . . 106 H7 30 44N 31 47 E
Far East =
  Dalnevostochnyy □,
  Russia . . . . 67 C14 67 0N 140 0 E
Far East, Asia . . . . 62 E16 40 0N 130 0 E
Fara in Sabina, Italy . . 45 F9 42 12N 12 43 E
Faradje, Dem. Rep. of
  the Congo . . . . 118 B2 3 50N 29 45 E
Farafangana, Madag. . 117 C8 22 49 S 47 50 E
Farāfra, El Wâhât el-,
  Egypt . . . . 106 B2 27 15N 28 20 E
Farāh, Afghan. . . . . . 91 B1 32 20N 62 7 E
Farāh □, Afghan. . . . . 91 B1 32 25N 62 10 E
Farāh →, Afghan. . . . . 88 B5 31 27N 61 28 E
Farahalana, Madag. . . 117 A9 14 26 S 50 10 E
Faraid, Gebel, Egypt . 106 C4 23 33N 35 19 E
Farako, Ivory C. 112 D4 10 45N 6 50W
Farallones de Cali △,
  Colombia 168 C2 3 13N 76 46W
Faramana,
  Burkina Faso 112 C4 11 56N 4 45W
Faranah, Guinea 112 C2 10 3N 10 45W
Farap, Turkmenistan . . 65 D1 39 9N 63 36 E
Farasān, Jazāʾir,
  Si. Arabia . . . . 98 C3 16 45N 41 55 E
Farasan Is. = Farasān,
  Jazāʾir, Si. Arabia . . 98 C3 16 45N 41 55 E
Faratsiho, Madag. . . . 117 B8 19 24 S 46 57 E
Farbarachi, Somali Rep. 120 D3 2 30N 45 30 E
Fardes →, Spain 43 H7 37 35N 3 0W
Fareham, U.K. 21 G6 50 51N 1 11W
Farewell, U.S.A. 144 E9 62 31N 153 54W
Farewell, C., N.Z. . . . 131 A7 40 29 S 172 43 E
Farewell C. = Nunap
  Isua, Greenland 10 F6 59 48N 43 55W
Farewell Spit, N.Z. . . 131 A8 40 35 S 173 0 E
Färgelanda, Sweden . . 17 F5 58 34N 12 0 E
Farghona, Uzbekistan . 65 C5 40 23N 71 19 E
Farghonskaya Dolina,
  Uzbekistan . . . . 65 C5 40 50N 71 30 E
Fargo, Ga., U.S.A. . . . 152 E7 30 41N 82 34W
Fargo, N. Dak., U.S.A. 154 B6 46 53N 96 48W
Fàrʾiah, W. al →,
  West Bank . . . . 103 C4 32 12N 35 27 E
Faribault, U.S.A. 154 C8 44 18N 93 16W
Faridabad, India . . . . 92 E6 28 26N 77 19 E
Faridkot, India . . . . . 92 D6 30 44N 74 45 E
Faridpur, Bangla. . . . . 90 D2 23 15N 89 55 E
Faridpur, India . . . . . 93 E8 28 13N 79 33 E
Fārīgh, W. al →, Libya 108 B3 30 28N 20 44 E
Färila, Sweden . . . . . 16 C9 61 48N 15 50 E
Farim, Guinea-Biss. . . 112 C1 12 27N 15 9W
Farīmān, Iran . . . . . . 97 C8 35 40N 59 49 E
Farina, Australia . . . . 127 E2 30 3 S 138 15 E
Farinha →, Brazil . . . . 170 C2 6 51 S 47 30W
Fariones, Pta.,
  Canary Is. 9 e2 29 13N 13 28W
Fâriskûr, Egypt . . . . 106 H7 31 20N 31 43 E
Färjestaden, Sweden . . 17 H10 56 39N 16 27 E
Farkadhón, Greece . . 48 B4 39 36N 22 4 E
Farkhor = Parkhar,
  Tajikistan . . . . 65 E4 37 30N 69 34 E
Farleigh, Australia . . . 126 K7 21 4 S 149 8 E
Farley, U.S.A. 156 B6 42 27N 91 0W
Farmakonisi, Greece . . 49 D9 37 17N 27 5 E
Farmer City, U.S.A. . . 157 D8 40 15N 88 39W
Farmersburg, U.S.A. . 157 E9 39 15N 87 23W
Farmerville, U.S.A. . . 155 J8 32 47N 92 24W
Farmingdale, U.S.A. . 151 F10 40 12N 74 10W
Farmington, Canada . . 142 B4 55 54N 120 30W
Farmington, Calif.,
  U.S.A. 160 H6 37 55N 120 59W
Farmington, Ga.,
  U.S.A. 152 B6 33 47N 83 26W
Farmington, Ill., U.S.A. 156 D7 40 42N 90 0W
Farmington, Iowa,
  U.S.A. 156 D5 40 38N 91 44W
Farmington, Maine,
  U.S.A. 149 C10 44 40N 70 9W
Farmington, Mo.,
  U.S.A. 155 G9 37 47N 90 25W
Farmington, N.H.,
  U.S.A. 151 C13 43 24N 71 4W
Farmington, N. Mex.,
  U.S.A. 159 H9 36 44N 108 12W
Farmington, Utah,
  U.S.A. 158 F8 41 0N 111 12W
Farmington →, U.S.A. 151 E12 41 51N 72 38W
Farmland, U.S.A. . . . 157 D11 40 15N 85 5W
Farmville, U.S.A. . . . 148 G6 37 18N 78 24W
Färnäs, Sweden . . . . . 16 D8 61 0N 14 39 E
Farne Is., U.K. 20 B6 55 38N 1 37W
Färnebofjärden △,
  Sweden . . . . 16 D10 60 10N 16 48 E
Farnham, Canada . . . 151 A12 45 17N 72 59W
Farnham, Mt., Canada 142 C5 50 29N 116 30W
Faro, Brazil . . . . 169 D6 2 10 S 56 39W
Faro, Canada 138 B6 62 11N 133 22W
Faro, Portugal 43 H3 37 2N 7 55W
Faro, Sweden . . . . . . 15 H18 57 55N 19 5 E
Faro □, Cameroon . . . 114 A2 8 15N 12 37 E
Faro □, Portugal 43 H2 37 12N 8 10W
Faro ✈ (FAO),
  Portugal 43 H3 37 2N 7 57W
Fårösund, Sweden . . . 17 G13 57 52N 19 2 E
Farquhar, C., Australia 125 D1 23 50 S 113 36 E
Farquhar Is., Seychelles 121 F4 11 0 S 52 0 E
Farrars Cr. →,
  Australia . . . . 126 D3 25 35 S 140 43 E
Farrāshband, Iran . . . 97 D7 28 57N 52 5 E
Farrell, U.S.A. 150 E4 41 13N 80 30W
Farrell Flat, Australia . 128 B3 33 48 S 138 48 E
Farrokhī, Iran . . . . . . 97 C8 33 50N 59 31 E
Farruch, C. = Ferrutx,
  C., Spain . . . . 38 B4 39 47N 3 21 E
Fārs □, Iran . . . . 97 D7 29 30N 55 0 E
Fársala, Greece . . . . . 48 B4 39 17N 22 23 E
Fārsī, Afghan. . . . . . . 91 B1 33 47N 63 15 E
Farsø, Denmark . . . . 17 H3 56 46N 9 19 E
Farson, U.S.A. 158 E9 42 6N 109 27W
Farsund, Norway . . . . 17 J3 58 5N 6 55 E
Fartak, Râs, Si. Arabia 96 D2 28 5N 34 34 E
Fartak, Ra's, Yemen . . 99 D5 15 38N 52 15 E
Fărţăneşti, Romania . . 53 E12 45 49N 27 59 E
Fartura, Serra da,
  Brazil . . . . 175 B5 26 21 S 52 52W
Faru, Nigeria . . . . . . 113 C6 12 48N 6 12 E

Fārūj, Iran . . . . 97 B8 37 14N 58 14 E
Fårup, Denmark . . . . 17 H3 56 33N 9 51 E
Farvel, Kap = Nunap
  Isua, Greenland 10 F6 59 48N 43 55W
Farwell, U.S.A. 155 H3 34 23N 103 2W
Fāryāb □, Afghan. . . . 65 E2 36 0N 65 0 E
Fasā, Iran . . . . 97 D7 29 0N 53 39 E
Fasano, Italy . . . . 47 B10 40 50N 17 22 E
Fashoda, Sudan . . . . 107 F3 9 50N 32 2 E
Fassa, Mali . . . . 112 C3 13 26N 8 15 E
Fastiv, Ukraine . . . . . 59 G5 50 7N 29 57 E
Fastnet Rock, Ireland . 23 E2 51 22N 9 37W
Fastov = Fastiv,
  Ukraine . . . . 59 G5 50 7N 29 57 E
Fatagar, Tanjung,
  Indonesia . . . . 83 B4 2 46 S 131 57 E
Fataka, Solomon Is. . 123 C12 11 55 S 170 12 E
Fatehabad, Haryana,
  India . . . . 92 E6 29 31N 75 27 E
Fatehgarh, India . . . . 93 F8 27 25N 79 35 E
Fatehpur, Bihar, India 93 G11 24 38N 85 14 E
Fatehpur, Raj., India . 92 F6 28 0N 74 40 E
Fatehpur, Ut. P., India 93 G9 25 56N 81 13 E
Fatehpur, Ut. P., India 93 F9 27 10N 81 13 E
Fatehpur Sikri, India . 92 F6 27 6N 77 40 E
Fatesh, Russia . . . . . 59 F8 52 8N 35 57 E
Fathai, Sudan . . . . . . 107 F3 8 5N 31 48 E
Fathom Five △, Canada 140 C3 45 17N 81 40W
Fatick, Senegal 112 C1 14 19N 16 27W
Fátima, Canada 141 C7 47 24N 61 53W
Fátima, Portugal 43 F2 39 37N 8 39W
Fatoya, Guinea 112 C3 11 37N 9 10W
Fatsa, Turkey . . . . . 100 B7 41 2N 37 31 E
Fatshan = Foshan,
  China . . . . 77 F9 23 4N 113 5 E
Faucille, Col de la,
  France . . . . 27 F13 46 22N 6 2 E
Faulkton, U.S.A. 154 C5 45 2N 99 8W
Faulquemont, France . 27 C13 49 3N 6 36 E
Faure I., Australia . . . 125 E1 25 52 S 113 50 E
Fauresmith, S. Africa . 116 D4 29 44 S 25 17 E
Fauro, Solomon Is. . . 133 L9 6 55 S 156 7 E
Fauske, Norway . . . . 14 C16 67 17N 15 25 E
Fåvang, Norway . . . . 18 C7 61 27N 10 11 E
Favânia, Brazil 169 D7 3 7S 51 48W
Favara, Italy . . . . 46 E6 37 19N 13 39 E
Favárítx, C. de, Spain . 38 B5 40 0N 4 15 E
Faverges, France . . . . 29 C10 45 45N 6 17 E
Favignana, Italy . . . . 46 E5 37 56N 12 20 E
Favignana, I., Italy . . 46 E5 37 56N 12 19 E
Fawcett, Pt., Australia 124 B5 11 46 S 130 2 E
Fawn →, Canada . . . 140 A2 55 20N 87 35W
Fawnskin, U.S.A. . . . 161 L10 34 16N 116 56W
Faxaflói, Iceland 11 C3 64 29N 23 0W
Faxälven →, Sweden . 14 B10 63 13N 17 13 E
Faya-Largeau, Chad . 109 E3 17 58N 19 6 E
Fayaoué, Vanuatu . . . 133 K4 20 38 S 166 33 E
Fayd, Si. Arabia . . . . 96 E4 27 1N 42 52 E
Fayence, France . . . . 29 E10 43 38N 6 42 E
Fayette, Ala., U.S.A. . 149 J2 33 41N 87 50W
Fayette, Iowa, U.S.A. . 156 B5 42 51N 91 48W
Fayette, Mo., U.S.A. . 156 E4 39 9N 92 41W
Fayette, Ohio, U.S.A. . 157 C12 41 40N 84 20W
Fayetteville, Ark.,
  U.S.A. 155 G7 36 4N 94 10W
Fayetteville, Ga.,
  U.S.A. 152 B5 33 27N 84 27W
Fayetteville, N.C.,
  U.S.A. 149 H6 35 3N 78 53W
Fayetteville, Tenn.,
  U.S.A. 149 H2 35 9N 86 34W
Fayied, Egypt . . . . . 106 H8 30 18N 32 16 E
Fayón, Spain . . . . . . 40 D5 41 15N 0 20 E
Fazao-Malfakassa △,
  Togo . . . . 113 D5 8 45N 0 50 E
Fazenda Libongo,
  Angola . . . . 115 D2 8 24 S 13 24 E
Fazenda Nova, Brazil . 171 E1 16 11 S 50 48W
Fazilka, India . . . . . . 92 D6 30 27N 74 2 E
Fazilpur, Pakistan . . . 92 E4 29 18N 70 29 E
Fdérik, Mauritania . . . 110 D2 22 40N 12 45W
Feale →, Ireland 23 D2 52 27N 9 37W
Fear, C., U.S.A. 149 J7 33 50N 77 58W
Feather →, U.S.A. . . . 158 G3 38 47N 121 36W
Feather Falls, U.S.A. . 160 F5 39 36N 121 16W
Featherston, N.Z. . . . 130 H4 41 6 S 175 20 E
Featherstone,
  Zimbabwe . . . . 119 F3 18 42 S 30 55 E
Fécamp, France . . . . 26 C7 49 45N 0 22 E
Feda, Norway . . . . . 18 F3 58 17N 6 50 E
Fedala = Mohammedia,
  Morocco 110 B3 33 44N 7 21W
Federación, Argentina 174 C4 31 0 S 57 55W
Federal Capital
  Terr. □, Nigeria . . . 113 D6 9 0N 7 10 E
Federal Way, U.S.A. . 160 C4 47 18N 122 19W
Fedeshküh, Iran . . . . 97 D7 28 49N 53 50 E
Fedje, Norway . . . . . 18 D1 60 47N 4 43 E
Fehérgyarmat, Hungary 52 C7 47 59N 22 49 E
Fehmarn, Germany . . 30 A7 54 27N 11 7 E
Fehmarn Bælt, Europe 17 K5 54 35N 11 20 E
Fehmarn Belt =
  Fehmarn Bælt,
  Europe . . . . 17 K5 54 35N 11 20 E
Fei Xian, China . . . . . 75 G9 35 18N 117 59 E
Feijó, Brazil . . . . 172 B3 8 9 S 70 21W
Feilding, N.Z. . . . . . . 130 H5 40 13 S 175 35 E
Feira de Santana, Brazil 171 D4 12 15 S 38 57W
Feiring, Norway . . . . 18 D8 60 30N 11 0 E
Feixi, China . . . . 77 B11 31 43N 117 59 E
Feixiang, China . . . . 74 F8 36 30N 114 45 E
Fejaj, Chott el, Tunisia 108 B1 33 52N 9 14 E
Fejér □, Hungary . . . 52 C3 47 9N 18 30 E
Fejø, Denmark . . . . . 17 K5 54 55N 11 30 E
Fekete, Turkey . . . . 100 D6 37 48N 35 14 E
Fekete →, Hungary . . 52 E3 45 47N 18 15 E
Felanitx, Spain . . . . . 38 B4 39 28N 3 9 E
Felda →, Germany . . . 31 E6 50 57N 10 1 E
Feldbach, Austria . . . 34 E8 46 57N 15 52 E
Feldberg, Baden-W.,
  Germany . . . . 31 H3 47 52N 8 0 E
Feldberg,
  Mecklenburg-Vorpommern,
  Germany . . . . 30 B9 53 20N 13 25 E
Feldkirch, Austria . . . 34 D2 47 15N 9 37 E
Feldkirchen, Austria . 34 E7 46 44N 14 6 E
Felicité, Seychelles . . 121 b 4 19 S 55 52 E
Felicity, U.S.A. 157 F12 38 31N 84 6W
Felipe Carrillo Puerto,
  Mexico 163 D7 19 38N 88 3W
Felixburg, Zimbabwe . 117 B5 19 29 S 30 51 E
Felixlândia, Brazil . . . 171 E3 18 47 S 44 55W
Felixstowe, U.K. . . . . 21 F9 51 58N 1 23 E
Felletin, France . . . . 28 C6 45 53N 2 11 E
Fellingsbro, Sweden . 16 E9 59 26N 15 37 E
Fellsmere, U.S.A. . . 153 H9 27 46N 80 36W
Felsőgalla = Tatabánya,
  Hungary . . . . 52 C3 47 32N 18 25 E
Felsőszentiván,
  Hungary . . . . 52 E3 46 7N 19 2 E
Felton, U.S.A. 160 H4 37 3N 122 4W

Feltre, Italy . . . . 45 B8 46 1N 11 54 E
Femer Bælt = Fehmarn
  Bælt, Europe . . . . . 17 K5 54 35N 11 20 E
Femø, Denmark . . . . 17 K5 54 58N 11 35 E
Femunden, Norway . . 18 B8 62 10N 11 53 E
Femundsmarka △,
  Norway . . . . 18 B9 62 18N 12 6 E
Fen He →, China . . . . 74 G6 35 36N 110 42 E
Fene, Spain 42 B2 43 27N 8 9W
Fenelon Falls, Canada 150 B6 44 32N 78 45W
Fener Burnu, Turkey . 49 E9 38 58N 27 18 E
Feneroa, Ethiopia . . 107 E4 13 5N 39 3 E
Feng Xian, Jiangsu,
  China . . . . 74 G9 34 43N 116 35 E
Feng Xian, Shaanxi,
  China . . . . 74 H4 33 54N 106 40 E
Fengári, Greece . . . . 51 F9 40 25N 25 32 E
Fengcheng, Jiangxi,
  China . . . . 77 C10 28 12N 115 48 E
Fengcheng, Liaoning,
  China . . . . 75 D13 40 28N 124 5 E
Fengfeng, China . . . . 74 F8 36 28N 114 8 E
Fenggang, China . . . . 76 D6 27 57N 107 47 E
Fenghua, China . . . . 77 C13 29 40N 121 25 E
Fenghuang, China . . 76 D7 27 57N 109 29 E
Fengkai, China . . . . . 77 F8 23 24N 111 30 E
Fengkang, Taiwan . . 77 F13 22 12N 120 41 E
Fengle, China . . . . . 77 B9 31 29N 112 29 E
Fenglin, Taiwan . . . 77 F13 23 45N 121 26 E
Fengning, China . . . . 74 D9 41 10N 116 33 E
Fengqing, China . . . . 76 E2 24 38N 99 55 E
Fengqiu, China . . . . 74 G8 35 2N 114 25 E
Fengrun, China . . . . 75 E10 39 48N 118 8 E
Fengshan,
  Guangxi Zhuangzu,
  China . . . . 76 E7 24 29N 109 15 E
Fengshan,
  Guangxi Zhuangzu,
  China . . . . 76 E6 24 31N 107 3 E
Fengshan, Taiwan . . 77 F13 22 38N 120 21 E
Fengshun, China . . . 77 F11 23 46N 116 10 E
Fengtai, Anhui, China 77 A11 32 30N 116 40 E
Fengtai, Beijing, China 74 E9 39 50N 116 18 E
Fengxian, China . . . . 77 B13 30 55N 121 26 E
Fengxin, China . . . . 77 C10 28 41N 115 18 E
Fengyang, China . . . 75 H9 32 51N 117 29 E
Fengyi, China . . . . . 76 E3 25 37N 100 20 E
Fengzhen, China . . . 74 D7 40 25N 113 2 E
Feni Is., Papua N. G. 132 C7 4 0 S 153 40 E
Fennimore, U.S.A. . . 156 B6 42 59N 90 39W
Fenny, Bangla. . . . . . 90 D3 22 55N 91 32 E
Feno, C. de, France . 29 G12 41 58N 8 33 E
Fenoarivo,
  Fianarantsoa, Madag. 117 C8 21 43 S 46 24 E
Fenoarivo,
  Fianarantsoa, Madag. 117 C8 20 52 S 46 53 E
Fenoarivo Afovoany,
  Madag. . . . . 117 B8 18 26 S 46 34 E
Fenoarivo Atsinanana,
  Madag. . . . . 117 B8 17 22 S 49 25 E
Fens, The, U.K. 20 E7 52 38N 0 2W
Fensmark, Denmark . 17 J5 55 17N 11 48 E
Fenton, U.S.A. 157 B13 42 48N 83 42W
Fenxi, China . . . . . . 74 F6 36 40N 111 31 E
Fenyang, China . . . . 74 F6 37 18N 111 48 E
Fenyi, China . . . . . . 77 D10 27 45N 114 47 E
Feodosiya, Ukraine . . 59 K8 45 2N 35 16 E
Fer, C. de, Algeria . . 111 A6 37 3N 7 10 E
Fera, Solomon Is. . . 133 M10 8 6 S 159 37 E
Ferdows, Iran . . . . . 97 C8 33 58N 58 2 E
Fère-Champenoise,
  France . . . . 27 D10 48 45N 3 59 E
Fère-en-Tardenois,
  France . . . . 27 C10 49 10N 3 30 E
Ferentino, Italy . . . . 45 G10 41 42N 13 15 E
Ferfer, Somali Rep. . 120 C3 5 4N 45 9 E
Fergana = Farghona,
  Uzbekistan . . . . 65 C5 40 23N 71 19 E
Fergana Range, Asia . 65 C6 41 0N 73 50 E
Ferganskaya Dolina =
  Farghonskaya
  Dolina, Uzbekistan . 65 C5 40 50N 71 30 E
Fergus, Canada 150 C4 43 43N 80 24W
Fergus Falls, U.S.A. . 154 B6 46 17N 96 4W
Ferguson, U.S.A. . . . 156 F6 38 45N 90 18W
Fergusson I.,
  Papua N. G. . . . . . 132 E6 9 30 S 150 45 E
Fériana, Tunisia . . . 108 B1 34 59N 8 33 E
Feričanci, Croatia . . 52 E2 45 32N 18 0 E
Ferihegy, Budapest ✈
  (BUD), Hungary . . . 52 C4 47 25N 19 12 E
Ferkane, Algeria . . . 111 B6 34 37N 7 26 E
Ferkéssédougou,
  Ivory C. 112 D3 9 35N 5 6W
Ferlach, Austria . . . . 34 E7 46 32N 14 18 E
Ferland, Canada . . . 140 B2 50 19N 88 27W
Ferlo, Vallée du,
  Senegal 112 B2 15 15N 14 15W
Ferlo-Nord △, Senegal 112 B2 15 43N 14 0W
Ferlo-Sud △, Senegal 112 B2 15 43N 14 0W
Fermanagh □, U.K. . . 23 B4 54 21N 7 40W
Fermo, Italy . . . . 45 E10 43 9N 13 43 E
Fermont, Canada . . . 141 B6 52 47N 67 5W
Fermoselle, Spain . . 42 D4 41 19N 6 27W
Fermoy, Ireland 23 D3 52 9N 8 16W
Fernán Núñez, Spain . 43 H6 37 40N 4 44W
Fernández, Argentina . 174 B3 27 55 S 63 50W
Fernandina Beach,
  U.S.A. 152 E8 30 40N 81 27W
Fernando de Noronha,
  Brazil . . . . 8 G8 4 0 S 33 10W
Fernando Póo = Bioko,
  Eq. Guin. . . . . 113 E6 3 30N 8 40 E
Fernandópolis, Brazil 171 F1 20 16 S 50 14W
Ferndale, U.S.A. . . . 160 B4 48 51N 122 36W
Fernie, Canada 142 D5 49 30N 115 5W
Fernlees, Australia . . 126 C4 23 51 S 148 7 E
Fernley, U.S.A. 158 G4 39 36N 119 15W
Feroke, India . . . . . . 95 J2 11 9N 75 46 E
Ferozepore = Firozpur,
  India . . . . 92 D6 30 55N 74 40 E
Férrai, Greece . . . . . 51 F10 40 53N 26 10 E
Ferrandina, Italy . . . . 45 B9 40 29N 16 27 E
Ferrara, Italy . . . . . . 45 D8 44 50N 11 35 E
Ferrato, C., Italy . . . 46 C2 39 18N 9 38 E
Ferreira do Alentejo,
  Portugal 43 G2 38 4N 8 6W
Ferreira Gomes, Brazil 170 A1 0 48N 51 8W
Ferreñafe, Peru . . . . 172 B2 6 42 S 79 50W
Ferrerías, Spain . . . . 38 B5 39 59N 4 1 E
Ferret, C., France . . . 28 D2 44 38N 1 15W
Ferrette, France . . . . 27 E14 47 30N 7 20 E
Ferriday, U.S.A. 155 K9 31 38N 91 33W
Ferriere, Italy . . . . . . 44 D6 44 40N 9 30 E
Ferrières, France . . . 27 D9 48 5N 2 48 E
Ferrol, Spain 42 A2 43 29N 8 15W
Ferrol, Pen. de, Peru . 172 C2 9 10 S 78 35W
Ferron, U.S.A. 159 G8 39 5N 111 8W
Ferros, Brazil . . . . . . 171 E3 19 14 S 43 2W
Ferrutx, C., Spain . . . 38 B4 39 47N 3 21 E

Ferryland, Canada . . 141 C9 47 2N 52 53W
Ferrysburg, U.S.A. . . 157 A10 43 5N 86 13W
Ferryville = Menzel-
  Bourguiba, Tunisia . 108 A1 37 9N 9 49 E
Fertile, U.S.A. 154 B6 47 32N 96 17W
Fertőszentmiklós,
  Hungary . . . . 52 C1 47 35N 16 53 E
Fertőtavi △, Hungary . 52 C1 47 25N 16 50 E
Fès, Morocco 110 B4 34 0N 5 0W
Feshi, Dem. Rep. of
  the Congo . . . . 115 D3 6 8 S 18 10 E
Fessenden, U.S.A. . . 154 B5 47 39N 99 38W
Festenberg =
  Twardogóra, Poland 55 G4 51 23N 17 28 E
Festøy, Norway . . . . 18 B3 62 22N 6 19 E
Festus, U.S.A. 156 F6 38 13N 90 24W
Feté Bowé, Senegal . 112 C2 14 56N 13 30W
Feteşti, Romania . . . 53 F12 44 22N 27 51 E
Fethiye, Turkey . . . . 49 E11 36 36N 29 6 E
Fethiye Körfezi, Turkey 49 E10 36 40N 28 50 E
Fetlar, U.K. 22 A8 60 36N 0 52W
Fetsund, Norway . . . 18 E8 59 56N 11 10 E
Feuchten, Austria . . 33 B11 47 2N 10 44 E
Feuerthalen, Switz. . . 33 A7 47 37N 8 38 E
Feuilles →, Canada . . 139 C12 58 47N 70 4W
Feurs, France . . . . . 29 C8 45 45N 4 13 E
Fevik, Norway . . . . . 18 F4 58 22N 8 39 E
Feyzābād, Badākhshān,
  Afghan. . . . . 65 E5 37 7N 70 33 E
Feyzābād, Fāryāb,
  Afghan. . . . . 91 A2 36 17N 64 52 E
Fez = Fès, Morocco . 110 B4 34 0N 5 0W
Fezzan, Libya . . . . . 108 C2 27 0N 13 0 E
Fiambalá, Argentina . 174 B2 27 45 S 67 37W
Fianarantsoa, Madag. 117 C8 21 26 S 47 5 E
Fianarantsoa □, Madag. 117 B8 19 30 S 47 0 E
Fianga, Cameroon . . 109 G3 9 55N 15 9 E
Fiche, Ethiopia . . . . 107 F4 9 50N 38 46 E
Fichtelgebirge,
  Germany . . . . 31 E7 50 2N 11 55 E
Fichtelgebirge △,
  Germany . . . . 31 E8 50 8N 12 0 E
Ficksburg, S. Africa . 117 D4 28 51 S 27 53 E
Fidenza, Italy . . . . . 44 D7 44 52N 10 3 E
Fiditi, Nigeria . . . . . 113 D5 7 45N 3 53 E
Field →, Australia . . 126 C2 23 48 S 138 0 E
Field I., Australia . . 124 B5 12 5 S 132 23 E
Fieni, Romania . . . . 53 E10 45 8N 25 25 E
Fier, Albania . . . . . . 50 F3 40 43N 19 33 E
Fierzë, Albania . . . . 50 D4 42 15N 20 4 E
Fiesch, Switz. . . . . . 32 D6 46 25N 8 12 E
Fife □, U.K. 22 E5 56 15N 3 15W
Fife Ness, U.K. 22 E6 56 17N 2 35W
Fifth Cataract, Sudan 107 D3 18 22N 33 50 E
Figari, France . . . . . 29 G13 41 29N 9 7 E
Figeac, France . . . . 28 D6 44 37N 2 2 E
Figeholm, Sweden . . 17 G10 57 22N 16 33 E
Figline Valdarno, Italy 45 E8 43 37N 11 28 E
Figtree, Zimbabwe . . 119 G2 20 22 S 28 20 E
Figueira = Governador
  Valadares, Brazil . . 171 E3 18 15 S 41 57W
Figueira Castelo
  Rodrigo, Portugal . . 42 E4 40 57N 6 58W
Figueira da Foz,
  Portugal 42 E2 40 7N 8 54W
Figueiró dos Vinhos,
  Portugal 42 F2 39 55N 8 16W
Figueres, Spain . . . . 40 C7 42 18N 2 58 E
Figuig, Morocco . . . 111 B4 32 5N 1 11W
Fihaonana, Madag. . . 117 B8 18 36 S 47 12 E
Fiherenana, Madag. . 117 B8 18 29 S 48 24 E
Fiherenana →, Madag. 117 C7 23 19 S 43 37 E
Fiji ■, Pac. Oc. . . . . . 133 D9 17 20 S 179 0 E
Fika, Nigeria . . . . . . 113 C7 11 15N 11 13 E
Filabres, Sierra de los,
  Spain 43 H8 37 13N 2 20W
Filabusi, Zimbabwe . 117 C4 20 34 S 29 20 E
Filadelfia, Bolivia . . . 172 C4 11 20 S 68 46W
Filadélfia, Brazil . . . 170 C2 7 21 S 47 30W
Filadélfia, Italy . . . . 47 D9 38 47N 16 17 E
Fil'akovo, Slovak Rep. 35 C12 48 17N 19 50 E
Filey, U.K. 20 C7 54 12N 0 16W
Filey B., U.K. 20 C7 54 12N 0 15W
Filfla, Malta . . . . . . 38 F7 35 47N 14 24 E
Filiaşi, Romania . . . 53 F8 44 32N 23 31 E
Filiátes, Greece . . . . 48 B10 39 38N 20 16 E
Filiatrá, Greece . . . . 48 D3 37 9N 21 35 E
Filicudi, Italy . . . . . 47 D7 38 35N 14 33 E
Filim, Oman . . . . . . 99 B7 20 37N 58 12 E
Filingué, Niger . . . . 113 C5 14 21N 3 22 E
Filiourí →, Greece . . 51 F9 41 15N 25 40 E
Filipstad, Sweden . . 16 E8 59 43N 14 9 E
Filiput, Switz. . . . . . 33 C9 46 41N 9 40 E
Fillefjell, Norway . . 18 D5 61 8N 8 0 E
Fillmore, Calif., U.S.A. 161 L8 34 24N 118 55W
Fillmore, Utah, U.S.A. 159 G7 38 58N 112 20W
Filótion, Greece . . . 49 D8 37 8N 25 19 E
Filottrano, Italy . . . . 45 E10 43 26N 13 21 E
Filtu, Ethiopia . . . . 107 F5 5 8N 40 35 E
Fimi →, Dem. Rep. of
  the Congo . . . . 114 C3 3 1 S 16 58 E
Fîna, Mali 112 C3 13 15N 8 46W
Finale Emília, Italy . . 45 D8 44 50N 11 17 E
Finale Lígure, Italy . . 44 D5 44 10N 8 20 E
Finalmarina = Finale
  Lígure, Italy . . . . . . 44 D5 44 10N 8 20 E
Fiñana, Spain 43 H8 37 10N 2 50W
Finch, Canada 151 A9 45 11N 75 7W
Finch Hatton, Australia 126 K6 20 25 S 148 39 E
Findhorn →, U.K. . . . 22 D5 57 38N 3 38W
Findlay, U.S.A. 157 C13 41 2N 83 39W
Finger L., Canada . . 140 B1 53 33N 93 30W
Fingoè, Mozam. . . . 119 E3 14 55 S 31 50 E
Finike, Turkey . . . . 49 E12 36 21N 30 10 E
Finike Körfezi, Turkey 49 E12 36 30N 30 15 E
Finiq, Albania . . . . . 50 G4 39 54N 20 3 E
Finistère □, France . . 26 D3 48 20N 4 0W
Finisterre = Fisterra,
  Spain 42 C1 42 54N 9 16W
Finisterre, C. = Fisterra,
  C., Spain 42 C1 42 50N 9 19W
Finisterre Ra.,
  Papua N. G. . . . . . 132 D4 6 0 S 146 30 E
Finke, Australia . . . . 126 D1 25 34 S 134 35 E
Finke Gorge △,
  Australia . . . . 124 D5 24 8 S 132 49 E
Finland ■, Europe . . 14 E22 63 0N 27 0 E
Finland, G. of, Europe 15 G21 60 0N 26 0 E
Finlay →, Canada . . 142 B3 57 0N 125 10W
Finley, Australia . . . 127 F4 35 38 S 145 35 E
Finley, U.S.A. 154 B6 47 31N 97 50W
Finn →, Ireland 23 B4 54 51N 7 28W
Finnigan, Mt., Australia 126 B4 15 49 S 145 17 E
Finniss, C., Australia 127 E1 33 8 S 134 51 E
Finnmark, Norway . . 14 B20 69 37N 23 57 E
Finnsnes, Norway . . 14 B18 69 14N 18 0 E
Finnveden, Sweden . 17 H7 57 0N 14 6 E
Finschhafen,
  Papua N. G. . . . . . 132 D4 6 33 S 147 50 E

Finse, Norway . . . . . 18 D4 60 36N 7 30 E
Finspång, Sweden . . 17 F9 58 43N 15 47 E
Finsteraarhorn, Switz. 32 C6 46 31N 8 10 E
Finsterwalde, Germany 30 D9 51 37N 13 42 E
Fiora →, Italy . . . . . 45 F8 42 20N 11 34 E
Fiordland △, N.Z. . . 131 F2 45 46 S 167 0 E
Fiorenzuola d'Arda,
  Italy . . . . 44 D6 44 56N 9 55 E
Fiq, Syria . . . . 103 C4 32 46N 35 41 E
Firat = Furāt, Nahr
  al →, Asia . . . . 96 D5 31 0N 47 25 E
Fire Island △, U.S.A. 151 F11 40 38N 73 8W
Firebag →, Canada . . 143 B6 57 45 S 111 21W
Firebaugh, U.S.A. . . 160 J6 36 52N 120 27W
Firedrake L., Canada 143 A8 61 25N 104 30W
Firenze, Italy . . . . . 45 E8 43 46N 11 15 E
Firenze Amerigo
  Vespucci ✈ (FLR),
  Italy . . . . 44 E8 43 49N 11 13 E
Firenze Pisa ✈ (PSA),
  Italy . . . . 44 E7 43 40N 10 22 E
Firenzuola, Italy . . . 45 D8 44 7N 11 23 E
Firk, Sha'ib →, Iraq . 96 D5 30 59N 44 34 E
Firmi, France . . . . . 28 D6 44 33N 2 19 E
Firminy, France . . . . 29 C8 45 23N 4 18 E
Firozabad, India . . . 93 F8 27 10N 78 25 E
Firozpur, India . . . . 92 D6 30 55N 74 40 E
Firozpur-Jhirka, India 92 F7 27 48N 76 57 E
Fīrūzābād, Iran . . . . 97 D7 28 52N 52 35 E
Fīrūzkūh, Iran . . . . . 97 C7 35 50N 52 50 E
Firvale, Canada 142 C3 52 27N 126 13W
Fish →, Namibia . . . 116 D2 28 7 S 17 10 E
Fish →, Namibia . . . 116 E3 31 30 S 20 16 E
Fish River Canyon,
  Namibia . . . . 116 D2 27 40 S 17 35 E
Fisheating Cr. →,
  U.S.A. 153 J8 26 57N 81 7W
Fisher, Australia . . . 125 F5 30 30 S 131 0 E
Fisher B., Canada . . 143 C9 51 35N 97 13W
Fishers I., U.S.A. . . . 151 E13 41 15N 72 0W
Fishguard, U.K. 21 E3 52 0N 4 58W
Fishing L., Canada . . 143 C9 52 10N 95 24W
Fishkill, U.S.A. 151 E11 41 32N 73 53W
Fiskárdho, Greece . . 39 C2 38 28N 20 35 E
Fiskenæsset =
  Qeqertarsuatsiaat,
  Greenland 10 E5 63 5N 50 45W
Fismes, France . . . . 27 C10 49 20N 3 40 E
Fisterra, Spain 42 C1 42 54N 9 16W
Fisterra, C., Spain . . 42 C1 42 50N 9 19W
Fitchburg, Mass.,
  U.S.A. 151 D13 42 35N 71 48W
Fitchburg, Wis., U.S.A. 154 D10 42 58N 89 28W
Fitjar, Iceland 11 C5 64 28N 21 18W
Fitjar, Norway . . . . . 18 E2 59 55N 5 17 E
Fitri, L., Chad . . . . . 109 F3 12 50N 17 28 E
Fitz Roy, Argentina . 176 C3 47 0 S 67 0W
Fitzgerald, Canada . . 143 B6 59 51N 111 36W
Fitzgerald, U.S.A. . . 152 D6 31 43N 83 15W
Fitzgerald River △,
  Australia . . . . 125 F3 33 53 S 120 3 E
Fitzmaurice →,
  Australia . . . . 124 B5 14 45 S 130 5 E
Fitzroy →, Queens.,
  Australia . . . . 126 C5 23 32 S 150 52 E
Fitzroy →, W. Austral.,
  Australia . . . . 124 C3 17 31 S 123 35 E
Fitzroy Crossing,
  Australia . . . . 124 C4 18 9 S 125 38 E
Fitzwilliam I., Canada 150 B3 45 30N 81 45W
Fiuggi, Italy . . . . . . 45 G10 41 48N 13 13 E
Fiume = Rijeka, Croatia 45 C11 45 20N 14 21 E
Fiumicino, Roma ✈
  (FCO), Italy . . . . . . 45 G9 41 48N 12 15 E
Five Points, U.S.A. . . 160 J6 36 26N 120 6W
Fivizzano, Italy . . . . 44 D7 44 14N 10 8 E
Fizi, Dem. Rep. of
  the Congo . . . . 118 C2 4 17 S 28 55 E
Fjæra, Norway . . . . 18 E3 59 52N 6 22 E
Fjällbacka, Sweden . 17 F5 58 36N 11 17 E
Fjärdhundra, Sweden 16 E10 59 47N 16 56 E
Fjellerup, Denmark . 17 H4 56 29N 10 34 E
Fjerritslev, Denmark . 17 G3 57 5N 9 15 E
Fjugesta, Sweden . . 16 E8 59 11N 14 52 E
Fkih ben Salah,
  Morocco 110 B3 32 32N 6 45W
Flå, Norway . . . . . . 18 D6 60 25N 9 28 E
Flagler Beach, U.S.A. 153 F8 29 29N 81 8W
Flagstaff, U.S.A. . . . 159 J8 35 12N 111 39W
Flagstaff B., St. Helena 9 h 15 54 S 5 41W
Flagstaff L., U.S.A. . 149 C10 44 56N 70 18W
Flaherty I., Canada . 140 A4 56 15N 79 15W
Flåm, Norway . . . . . 18 D4 60 50N 7 7 E
Flamanville, France . 26 C5 49 32N 1 52W
Flambeau →, U.S.A. . 154 C9 45 18N 91 14W
Flamborough Hd., U.K. 20 C7 54 7N 0 5W
Flamengos, Azores . . 9 d1 38 33N 28 39W
Fläming, Germany . . 30 C8 52 6N 12 23 E
Flaming Gorge △,
  U.S.A. 158 F9 41 10N 109 25W
Flaming Gorge
  Reservoir, U.S.A. . . 158 F9 41 10N 109 25W
Flamingo, Teluk,
  Indonesia . . . . 83 C5 5 30 S 138 0 E
Flanagan, U.S.A. . . . 157 D8 40 53N 88 52W
Flanders = Flandre,
  Europe . . . . 27 B9 50 50N 2 30 E
Flandre, Europe . . . 27 B9 50 50N 2 30 E
Flandre-Occidentale =
  West-Vlaanderen □,
  Belgium . . . . 24 D2 51 0N 3 0 E
Flandre-Orientale =
  Oost-Vlaanderen □,
  Belgium . . . . 24 C3 51 5N 3 50 E
Flandreau, U.S.A. . . 154 C6 44 3N 96 36W
Flanigan, U.S.A. . . . 160 E7 40 10N 119 53W
Flannan Is., U.K. . . . 22 C1 58 9N 7 52W
Flåsjön, Sweden . . . 14 D16 64 5N 15 40 E
Flat, U.S.A. 144 D8 62 28N 158 1W
Flat →, Canada 142 A3 61 33N 125 18W
Flat I., Mauritius . . . 121 d 19 53 S 57 35 E
Flat Pt., N.Z. . . . . . 131 H5 41 14 S 175 57 E
Flat Rock, U.S.A. . . 157 B13 42 6N 83 17W
Flateyri, Iceland . . . 11 A3 66 4N 23 31W
Flathead →, U.S.A. . 158 B6 48 5N 114 5W
Flatow = Złotów,
  Poland . . . . 54 E4 53 22N 17 2 E
Flatrock →, U.S.A. . . 157 F10 39 12N 85 56W
Flattery, C., Australia 126 A4 14 58 S 145 21 E
Flattery, C., U.S.A. . 160 B2 48 23N 124 29W
Flatts Village, Bermuda 9 b 32 19N 64 44W
Flatwoods, U.S.A. . . 148 F4 38 31N 82 43W
Flèche →, Dem. Rep. of
  the Congo . . . . 118 C2 4 17 S 28 55 E
Flèche, La →, France 26 E6 47 42N 0 4W
Flecha Pt., Phil. . . . 81 H4 7 22N 123 24 E
Fleetwood, U.K. . . . 20 D4 53 55N 3 1W
Fleetwood, U.S.A. . . 151 F9 40 27N 75 49W
Flekke, U.S.A. . . . . 18 C2 61 19N 5 26 E
Flekkefjord, Norway . 18 F3 58 18N 6 39 E

Flemingsburg, U.S.A. 157 F13 38 25N 83 45W
Flemington, U.S.A. 150 E7 41 7N 77 28W
Flemish Cap, Atl. Oc. 8 B7 47 0N 45 0W
Flen, Sweden 16 E10 59 4N 16 35 E
Flensburg, Germany 30 A5 54 47N 9 27 E
Flers, France 26 D6 48 47N 0 33W
Flesberg, Norway 18 E6 59 51N 9 27 E
Flesherton, Canada 150 B4 44 16N 80 33W
Flesko, Tanjung, Indonesia 82 A2 0 29N 124 30 E
Fletcher = Aurora, U.S.A. 154 F2 39 44N 104 52W
Fleurance, France 28 E4 43 52N 0 40 E
Fleurier, Switz. 32 C3 46 54N 6 35 E
Fleurieu Pen., Australia 128 C3 35 40 S 138 5 E
Flevoland □, Neths. 24 B5 52 30N 5 30 E
Flims, Switz. 33 C8 46 50N 9 17 E
Flin Flon, Canada 143 C8 54 46N 101 53W
Flinders →, Australia 126 B3 17 36 S 140 36 E
Flinders B., Australia 125 F2 34 19 S 115 19 E
Flinders Chase △, Australia 128 C2 35 50 S 136 42 E
Flinders Group, Australia 126 A3 14 11 S 144 15 E
Flinders I., S. Austral., Australia 127 E1 33 44 S 134 41 E
Flinders I., Tas., Australia 127 G4 40 0 S 148 0 E
Flinders Ranges, Australia 128 A3 31 30 S 138 30 E
Flinders Ranges △, Australia 128 A3 31 30 S 138 40 E
Flinders Reefs, Australia 126 B4 17 37 S 148 31 E
Flint, U.K. 20 D4 53 15N 3 8W
Flint, U.S.A. 157 A13 43 1N 83 41W
Flint →, U.S.A. 152 E5 30 57N 84 34W
Flint I., Kiribati 135 J12 11 26 S 151 48W
Flintshire □, U.K. 20 D4 53 17N 3 17W
Flirsch, Austria 33 B10 47 9N 10 24 E
Flisa, Norway 18 D9 60 37N 12 0 E
Flisa →, Norway 18 D9 60 37N 12 0 E
Fliseryd, Sweden 17 G10 57 6N 16 15 E
Flix, Spain 40 D5 41 14N 0 32 E
Flixecourt, France 27 B9 50 1N 2 5 E
Floby, Sweden 17 F7 58 8N 13 20 E
Floda, Sweden 17 G6 57 49N 12 22 E
Flodden, U.K. 20 B5 55 37N 2 8W
Flogny-la-Chapelle, France 27 E10 47 57N 3 57 E
Floodplains △, Sri Lanka 95 K5 8 10N 81 10 E
Floodwood, U.S.A. 154 B8 46 55N 92 55W
Flora, Phil. 80 B3 18 14N 121 5 E
Flora, Ill., U.S.A. 156 F8 38 40N 88 29W
Flora, Ind., U.S.A. 157 D10 40 33N 86 31W
Florac, France 28 D7 44 20N 3 37 E
Florahome, U.S.A. 152 F8 29 44N 81 54W
Floral City, U.S.A. 153 G7 28 45N 82 17W
Florala, U.S.A. 149 K2 31 0N 86 20W
Florânia, Brazil 170 C4 6 8 S 36 49W
Floreana, I. = Santa María, I., Ecuador 172 a 1 17 S 90 26W
Florence = Firenze, Italy 45 E8 43 46N 11 15 E
Florence, Ala., U.S.A. 149 H2 34 48N 87 41W
Florence, Ariz., U.S.A. 159 K8 33 2N 111 23W
Florence, Colo., U.S.A. 154 F2 38 23N 105 8W
Florence, Oreg., U.S.A. 158 E1 43 58N 124 7W
Florence, S.C., U.S.A. 149 H6 34 12N 79 46W
Florence, L., Australia 127 D2 28 53 S 138 9 E
Florence Bay = Chtimba, Malawi 119 E3 10 35 S 34 13 E
Florencia, Colombia 168 C2 1 36N 75 36W
Florennes, Belgium 24 D4 50 15N 4 35 E
Florensac, France 28 E7 43 23N 3 28 E
Florenville, Belgium 24 E5 49 40N 5 19 E
Flores = Florânia, Brazil 170 C4 6 8 S 36 49W
Flores = Timon, Brazil 170 C3 5 8 S 42 52W
Flores, Azores 9 d2 39 26N 31 13W
Flores, Brazil 170 C4 7 51 S 37 59W
Flores, Guatemala 164 C2 16 59N 89 50W
Flores, Indonesia 82 C2 8 35 S 121 0 E
Flores I., Canada 142 D3 49 20N 126 10W
Flores Sea, Indonesia 82 C2 6 30 S 120 0 E
Floresta, Brazil 170 C4 8 40 S 37 26W
Floreşti, Moldova 53 C13 47 53N 28 17 E
Floresville, U.S.A. 155 L5 29 8N 98 10W
Floriano, Brazil 170 C3 6 50 S 43 0W
Florianópolis, Brazil 175 B6 27 30 S 48 30W
Florida, Cuba 164 B4 21 32N 78 14W
Florida, Uruguay 175 C4 34 7 S 56 10W
Florida □, U.S.A. 149 L5 28 0N 82 0W
Florida, Straits of, U.S.A. 164 B4 25 0N 80 0W
Florida B., U.S.A. 164 B3 25 0N 80 45W
Florida City, U.S.A. 153 K9 25 27N 80 29W
Florida Is., Solomon Is. 133 M11 9 55 S 160 15 E
Florida Keys, U.S.A. 153 L8 24 40N 81 0W
Floridablanca, Phil. 80 D3 14 59N 120 31 E
Florídia, Italy 47 E8 37 5N 15 9 E
Flórina, Greece 50 F5 40 48N 21 26 E
Flórina □, Greece 50 F5 40 45N 21 20 E
Florissant, U.S.A. 156 F6 38 48N 90 20W
Florø, Norway 18 C2 61 35N 5 1 E
Flotte, C. de, N. Cal. 133 U21 21 10 S 167 25 E
Flower Station, Canada 151 A8 45 10N 76 41W
Flowerpot I., Canada 150 A3 45 18N 81 38W
Floydada, U.S.A. 155 J4 33 59N 101 20W
Fludir, Iceland 11 C6 64 7N 20 6W
Flüelapass, Switz. 33 C9 46 46N 9 56 E
Flugmyri, Iceland 11 B7 65 34N 19 19W
Fluk, Indonesia 82 B3 1 42 S 127 44 E
Flúmen →, Spain 40 D4 41 43N 0 9W
Flumendosa →, Italy 46 C2 39 26N 9 37 E
Fluminimaggiore, Italy 46 C1 39 26N 8 30 E
Flushing = Vlissingen, Neths. 24 C3 51 26N 3 34 E
Flushing, U.S.A. 157 A13 43 4N 83 51W
Fluviá →, Spain 40 C8 42 12N 3 7 E
Fly →, Papua N. G. 132 E2 8 25 S 143 0 E
Flying Fish, C., Antarctica 7 D15 72 6 S 102 29W
Foa, Tonga 133 P13 19 45 S 174 18W
Foam Lake, Canada 143 C8 51 40N 103 32W
Foča, Bos.-H. 50 C2 43 31N 18 47 E
Foça, Turkey 49 C8 38 39N 26 46 E
Fochabers, U.K. 22 D5 57 37N 3 6W
Focşani, Romania 53 E12 45 41N 27 15 E
Fodé, C.A.R. 114 A4 5 29N 23 18 E
Fodécontéa, Guinea 112 C2 10 50N 14 22W
Fogang, China 77 F9 23 52N 113 30 E
Foggaret el Arab, Algeria 111 C5 27 13N 2 49 E
Foggaret ez Zoua, Algeria 111 C5 27 20N 2 53 E
Fóggia, Italy 47 A8 41 27N 15 34 E
Foggo, Nigeria 113 C6 11 21N 9 57 E
Foglia →, Italy 45 E9 43 55N 12 54 E
Fogo, Canada 141 C9 49 43N 54 17W
Fogo, C. Verde Is. 9 j 15 5N 24 20W
Fogo I., Canada 141 C9 49 40N 54 5W
Fohnsdorf, Austria 34 D7 47 12N 14 40 E
Föhr, Germany 30 A4 54 43N 8 30 E
Foia, Portugal 43 H2 37 19N 8 37W
Foix, France 28 E5 42 58N 1 38 E
Fojnica, Bos.-H. 52 G2 43 59N 17 51 E
Fokino, Russia 58 F8 53 30N 34 22 E
Fokís □, Greece 48 C4 38 30N 22 15 E
Fokku, Nigeria 113 C5 11 36N 4 32 E
Fokstua, Norway 18 B6 62 7N 9 17 E
Folda, Nord-Trøndelag, Norway 14 D14 64 32N 10 30 E
Folda, Nordland, Norway 14 C16 67 38N 14 50 E
Földeák, Hungary 52 D5 46 19N 20 30 E
Folégandros, Greece 48 E6 36 40N 24 55 E
Foley, Botswana 116 C4 21 34 S 27 21 E
Foley, Ala., U.S.A. 149 K2 30 24N 87 41W
Foley, Fla., U.S.A. 152 E6 30 4N 83 32W
Foleyet, Canada 140 C3 48 15N 82 25W
Folgefonni, Norway 18 D3 60 3N 6 23 E
Foligno, Italy 45 F9 42 57N 12 42 E
Folkestad, Norway 18 B3 62 7N 6 1 E
Folkestone, U.K. 21 F9 51 5N 1 12 E
Folkston, U.S.A. 152 E7 30 50N 82 0W
Folla →, Norway 18 B7 62 7N 10 37 E
Follansbee, U.S.A. 150 F4 40 19N 80 35W
Folldal, Norway 18 B6 62 8N 10 0 E
Follebu, Norway 18 C7 61 13N 10 16 E
Follónica, Italy 44 F7 42 55N 10 45 E
Follónica, G. di, Italy 44 F7 42 54N 10 43 E
Folsom L., U.S.A. 160 G5 38 42N 121 9W
Folteşti, Romania 53 E13 45 45N 28 3 E
Fomboni, Comoros Is. 121 a 12 18 S 43 46 E
Fomm ir-Rih Bay, Malta 38 F7 35 54N 14 20 E
Fond-du-Lac, Canada 143 B7 59 19N 107 12W
Fond du Lac, U.S.A. 154 D10 43 47N 88 27W
Fond-du-Lac →, Canada 143 B7 59 17N 106 0W
Fonda, Iowa, U.S.A. 156 B2 42 35N 94 51W
Fonda, N.Y., U.S.A. 151 D10 42 57N 74 22W
Fondi, Italy 46 A6 41 21N 13 25 E
Fonfría, Spain 42 D4 41 37N 6 9W
Fongafale, Tuvalu 134 H9 8 31 S 179 13 E
Fongen, Norway 18 A8 63 11N 11 38 E
Fonni, Italy 46 B2 40 7N 9 15 E
Fonsagrada = A Fonsagrada, Spain 42 B3 43 8N 7 4W
Fonseca, G. de, Cent. Amer. 164 D2 13 10N 87 40W
Font-Romeu-Odeillo-Via, France 28 F5 42 31N 2 3 E
Fontaine-Française, France 27 E12 47 32N 5 21 E
Fontainebleau, France 27 D9 48 24N 2 40 E
Fontana, U.S.A. 161 L9 34 6N 117 26W
Fontana, L., Argentina 176 B2 44 55 S 71 30W
Fontas →, Canada 142 B4 58 14N 121 48W
Fonte Boa, Brazil 168 D4 2 33 S 66 0W
Fontem, Cameroon 113 D6 5 32N 9 52 E
Fontenay-le-Comte, France 28 B3 46 28N 0 48W
Fontenelle Reservoir, U.S.A. 158 E8 42 1N 110 3W
Fontur, Iceland 14 C6 66 23N 14 32W
Fonuafo'ou, Tonga 133 Q13 20 19 S 175 25W
Fonualei, Tonga 133 P13 18 1 S 174 19W
Fonyód, Hungary 52 D2 46 44N 17 33 E
Foochow = Fuzhou, China 77 D12 26 5N 119 16 E
Foping, China 74 H5 33 41N 108 0 E
Fora →, Norway 18 B7 62 57N 10 40 E
Foraker, Mt., U.S.A. 144 E10 62 58N 151 24W
Forari, Vanuatu 133 G6 17 40 S 168 31 E
Forbach, France 27 C13 49 10N 6 52 E
Forbes, Australia 129 B8 33 22 S 148 5 E
Forbesganj, India 93 F12 26 17N 87 18 E
Forcados, Nigeria 113 D6 5 26N 5 26 E
Forcados →, Nigeria 113 D6 5 25N 5 19 E
Forcalquier, France 29 E9 43 58N 5 47 E
Forchheim, Germany 31 F7 49 43N 11 2 E
Forclaz, Col de la, Switz. 32 D4 46 3N 7 1 E
Ford City, Calif., U.S.A. 161 K7 35 9N 119 27W
Ford City, Pa., U.S.A. 150 F5 40 46N 79 32W
Ford I., U.S.A. 145 K14 21 22N 157 58W
Fordate, Indonesia 83 C4 7 0 S 131 58 E
Førde, Hordaland, Norway 18 E2 59 36N 5 27 E
Førde, Sogn og Fjordane, Norway 18 C2 61 27N 5 53 E
Førdefjorden, Norway 18 C2 61 29N 5 18 E
Førdesfjord, Norway 18 E2 59 25N 5 20 E
Ford's Bridge, Australia 127 D4 29 41 S 145 29 E
Fordyce, U.S.A. 155 J8 33 49N 92 25W
Forécariah, Guinea 112 D2 9 28N 13 10W
Forel, Mt., Greenland 10 D7 66 52N 36 55W
Foremost, Canada 142 D6 49 26N 111 34W
Forest, Canada 150 C3 43 6N 82 0W
Forest, U.S.A. 155 J10 32 22N 89 29W
Forest Acres, U.S.A. 152 A9 34 1N 80 58W
Forest City, Iowa, U.S.A. 154 D8 43 16N 93 39W
Forest City, N.C., U.S.A. 149 H5 35 20N 81 52W
Forest City, Pa., U.S.A. 151 E9 41 39N 75 28W
Forest Grove, U.S.A. 160 E3 45 31N 123 7W
Forest Park, U.S.A. 152 B5 33 37N 84 22W
Forestburg, Canada 142 C6 52 35N 112 1W
Foreste Casentinesi-Monte Falterona-Campigna △, Italy 45 E8 43 50N 11 48 E
Foresthill, U.S.A. 160 F6 39 1N 120 49W
Forestier Pen., Australia 127 G4 43 0 S 148 0 E
Forestville, Canada 141 C6 48 48N 69 2W
Forestville, Calif., U.S.A. 160 G4 38 28N 122 54W
Forestville, N.Y., U.S.A. 150 D5 42 28N 79 10W
Forêt d'Orient △, France 27 D11 48 16N 4 25 E
Forêt du Day △, Djibouti 120 B2 11 56N 42 40 E
Forez, Mts. du, France 28 C7 45 40N 3 50 E
Forfar, U.K. 22 E6 56 39N 2 53W
Forggensee, Germany 33 A11 47 35N 10 44 E
Forillon △, Canada 141 C7 48 46N 64 12W
Forks, U.S.A. 160 C2 47 57N 124 23W
Forksville, U.S.A. 151 E8 41 29N 76 35W
Forlì, Italy 45 D9 44 13N 12 3 E
Forman, U.S.A. 154 B6 46 7N 97 38W
Formazza, Italy 44 B5 46 22N 8 26 E
Formby Pt., U.K. 20 D4 53 33N 3 6W
Formentera, Spain 38 D1 38 43N 1 27 E
Formentor, C. de, Spain 38 B4 39 58N 3 13 E
Former Yugoslav Republic of Macedonia = Macedonia ■, Europe 50 E5 41 53N 21 40 E
Fórmia, Italy 46 A6 41 15N 13 37 E
Formiga, Brazil 171 F2 20 27 S 45 25W
Formigine, Italy 44 D7 44 37N 10 51 E
Formosa = Taiwan ■, Asia 77 F13 23 30N 121 0 E
Formosa, Argentina 174 B4 26 15 S 58 10W
Formosa, Brazil 171 E2 15 32 S 47 20W
Formosa □, Argentina 174 B4 25 0 S 60 0W
Formosa, Serra, Brazil 173 C6 12 0 S 55 0W
Formosa B. = Ungwana B., Kenya 118 C5 2 40 S 40 20 E
Formosa Strait = Taiwan Strait, Asia 77 E12 24 40N 120 0 E
Formoso →, Brazil 171 D2 10 34 S 49 56W
Fornells, Spain 38 A5 40 3N 4 7 E
Fornos de Algodres, Portugal 42 E3 40 38N 7 32W
Fornovo di Taro, Italy 44 D7 44 42N 10 6 E
Føroyar, Atl. Oc. 14 F9 62 0N 7 0W
Forres, U.K. 22 D5 57 37N 3 37W
Forrest, Vic., Australia 128 E5 38 33 S 143 47 E
Forrest, W. Austral., Australia 125 F4 30 51 S 128 6 E
Forrest, Mt., Australia 125 D4 24 48 S 127 45 E
Forrest City, U.S.A. 155 H9 35 1N 90 47W
Forreston, U.S.A. 156 B7 42 8N 89 35W
Fors, Sweden 16 D10 60 14N 16 20 E
Forsand, Norway 18 F3 58 54N 6 5 E
Forsayth, Australia 126 B3 18 33 S 143 34 E
Forshaga, Sweden 16 E7 59 33N 13 29 E
Förslöv, Sweden 17 H6 56 21N 12 48 E
Forsmo, Sweden 16 A11 63 16N 17 11 E
Forssa, Finland 15 F20 60 49N 23 38 E
Forst, Germany 30 D10 51 45N 14 37 E
Forster, Australia 129 B10 32 12 S 152 31 E
Forsvik, Sweden 17 F8 58 35N 14 26 E
Forsyth, Ga., U.S.A. 152 B6 33 2N 83 56W
Forsyth, Mont., U.S.A. 158 C10 46 16N 106 41W
Forsyth I., N.Z. 131 A9 40 58 S 174 5 E
Fort Abbas, Pakistan 92 E5 29 12N 72 52 E
Fort Albany, Canada 140 B3 52 15N 81 35W
Fort-Aleksandrovsky = Fort Shevchenko, Kazakhstan 61 H10 44 35N 50 23 E
Fort Ann, U.S.A. 151 C11 43 25N 73 30W
Fort Archambault = Sarh, Chad 109 G3 9 5N 18 23 E
Fort Assiniboine, Canada 142 C6 54 20N 114 45W
Fort Atkinson, U.S.A. 157 B8 42 56N 88 50W
Fort Augustus, U.K. 22 D4 57 9N 4 42W
Fort Bayard = Zhanjiang, China 77 G8 21 15N 110 20 E
Fort Beaufort, S. Africa 116 E4 32 46 S 26 40 E
Fort Benton, U.S.A. 158 C8 47 49N 110 40W
Fort Bragg, U.S.A. 158 G2 39 26N 123 48W
Fort Bridger, U.S.A. 158 F8 41 19N 110 23W
Fort Caroline ⌂, U.S.A. 152 E8 30 23N 81 30W
Fort Chipewyan, Canada 143 B6 58 42N 111 8W
Fort Clatsop ⌂, U.S.A. 160 D3 46 8N 123 53W
Fort Collins, U.S.A. 154 E2 40 35N 105 5W
Fort-Coulonge, Canada 140 C4 45 50N 76 45W
Fort Covington, U.S.A. 151 B10 44 59N 74 29W
Fort Davis, Ala., U.S.A. 152 C4 32 15N 85 43W
Fort Davis, Tex., U.S.A. 155 K3 30 35N 103 54W
Fort-de-France, Martinique 164 c 14 36N 61 2W
Fort de Kock = Bukittinggi, Indonesia 84 C2 0 20 S 100 20 E
Fort de Polignac = Illizi, Algeria 111 C6 26 31N 8 32 E
Fort de Possel = Possel, C.A.R. 114 A3 5 5N 19 10 E
Fort Defiance, U.S.A. 159 J9 35 45N 109 5W
Fort Dodge, U.S.A. 156 B2 42 30N 94 11W
Fort Drum, U.S.A. 153 H9 27 32N 80 48W
Fort Edward, U.S.A. 151 C11 43 16N 73 35W
Fort Erie, Canada 150 D6 42 54N 78 56W
Fort Fairfield, U.S.A. 149 B12 46 46N 67 50W
Fort Flatters = Bordj Omar Driss, Algeria 111 C6 28 10N 6 40 E
Fort-Foureau = Kousseri, Cameroon 109 F2 12 0N 14 55 E
Fort Frances, Canada 143 D10 48 36N 93 24W
Fort Franklin = Déline, Canada 138 B7 65 11N 123 25W
Fort Frederica ⌂, U.S.A. 152 D8 31 13N 81 23W
Fort Gaines, U.S.A. 152 D4 31 36N 85 3W
Fort Garland, U.S.A. 159 H11 37 26N 105 26W
Fort George = Chisasibi, Canada 140 B4 53 50N 79 0W
Fort George = Prince George, Canada 142 C4 53 55N 122 50W
Fort Good Hope, Canada 138 B7 66 14N 128 40W
Fort Gouraud = Fdérik, Mauritania 110 D2 22 40N 12 45W
Fort Hancock, U.S.A. 159 L11 31 18N 105 51W
Fort Hertz = Putao, Burma 90 B6 27 28N 97 30 E
Fort Hill = Chitipa, Malawi 119 D3 9 41 S 33 19 E
Fort Hope, Canada 140 B2 51 30N 88 0W
Fort Irwin, U.S.A. 161 K10 35 16N 116 34W
Fort Jameson = Chipata, Zambia 119 E3 13 38 S 32 28 E
Fort Johnston = Mangoche, Malawi 119 E4 14 25 S 35 16 E
Fort Kent, U.S.A. 149 B11 47 15N 68 36W
Fort Klamath, U.S.A. 158 E3 42 42N 122 0W
Fort Lamy = Ndjamena, Chad 109 F2 12 10N 14 59 E
Fort-Laperrine = Tamanrasset, Algeria 111 D6 22 50N 5 30 E
Fort Laramie, U.S.A. 154 D2 42 13N 104 31W
Fort Lauderdale, U.S.A. 153 J9 26 7N 80 8W
Fort Liard, Canada 142 A4 60 14N 123 30W
Fort Liberté, Haiti 165 C5 19 42N 71 51W
Fort Lupton, U.S.A. 154 E2 40 5N 104 49W
Fort MacKay, Canada 142 B6 57 12N 111 41W
Fort Macleod, Canada 142 D6 49 45N 113 30W
Fort MacMahon = El Homeur, Algeria 111 C5 29 43N 1 45 E
Fort McMurray, Canada 142 B6 56 44N 111 7W
Fort McPherson, Canada 138 B6 67 30N 134 55W
Fort Madison, U.S.A. 156 D5 40 38N 91 27W
Fort Manning = Mchinji, Malawi 119 E3 13 47 S 32 58 E
Fort Matanzas ⌂, U.S.A. 152 F8 29 43N 81 14W
Fort Meade, U.S.A. 153 H8 27 45N 81 48W
Fort Mitchell, U.S.A. 152 C4 32 20N 85 1W
Fort Morgan, U.S.A. 154 E3 40 15N 103 48W
Fort Myers, U.S.A. 153 J8 26 39N 81 52W
Fort Myers Beach, U.S.A. 153 J8 26 26N 81 52W
Fort Myers Villas, U.S.A. 153 J8 26 33N 81 52W
Fort Nelson, Canada 142 B4 58 50N 122 44W
Fort Nelson →, Canada 142 B4 59 32N 124 0W
Fort Norman = Tulita, Canada 138 B7 64 57N 125 30W
Fort Ogden, U.S.A. 153 H8 27 5N 81 57W
Fort Payne, U.S.A. 149 H3 34 26N 85 43W
Fort Peck, U.S.A. 158 B10 48 1N 106 27W
Fort Peck Dam, U.S.A. 158 C10 48 0N 106 26W
Fort Peck L., U.S.A. 158 C10 48 0N 106 26W
Fort Pierce, U.S.A. 153 H9 27 27N 80 20W
Fort Pierre, U.S.A. 154 C4 44 21N 100 22W
Fort Pierre Bordes = Ti-n-Zaouatene, Algeria 111 E5 19 55N 2 55 E
Fort Plain, U.S.A. 151 D10 42 56N 74 37W
Fort Portal, Uganda 118 B3 0 40N 30 20 E
Fort Providence, Canada 142 A5 61 3N 117 40W
Fort Pulaski ⌂, U.S.A. 152 C9 32 2N 80 56W
Fort Qu'Appelle, Canada 143 C8 50 45N 103 50W
Fort Recovery, U.S.A. 157 D12 40 25N 84 47W
Fort Resolution, Canada 142 A6 61 10N 113 40W
Fort Rixon, Zimbabwe 119 G2 20 2 S 29 17 E
Fort Rosebery = Mansa, Zambia 119 E2 11 13 S 28 55 E
Fort Ross, U.S.A. 160 G3 38 32N 123 13W
Fort-Rousset = Owando, Congo 114 C3 0 29 S 15 55 E
Fort Rupert = Waskaganish, Canada 140 B4 51 30N 78 40W
Fort St. James, Canada 142 C4 54 30N 124 10W
Fort St. John, Canada 142 B4 56 15N 120 50W
Fort Sandeman = Zhob, Pakistan 91 C3 31 20N 69 31 E
Fort Saskatchewan, Canada 142 C6 53 40N 113 15W
Fort Scott, U.S.A. 155 G7 37 50N 94 42W
Fort Severn, Canada 140 A2 56 0N 87 40W
Fort Shevchenko, Kazakhstan 61 H10 44 35N 50 23 E
Fort Simpson, Canada 142 A4 61 45N 121 15W
Fort Smith, Canada 142 B6 60 0N 111 51W
Fort Smith, U.S.A. 155 H7 35 23N 94 25W
Fort Stockton, U.S.A. 155 K3 30 53N 102 53W
Fort Sumner, U.S.A. 155 H2 34 28N 104 15W
Fort Thomas, U.S.A. 157 E12 39 5N 84 27W
Fort Thompson, U.S.A. 154 C5 44 3N 99 26W
Fort Trinquet = Bîr Mogreïn, Mauritania 110 C2 25 10N 11 25W
Fort Union ⌂, U.S.A. 155 H2 35 54N 105 1W
Fort Uritskogo = Fort Shevchenko, Kazakhstan 61 H10 44 35N 50 23 E
Fort Valley, U.S.A. 152 C6 32 33N 83 53W
Fort Vermilion, Canada 142 B5 58 24N 116 0W
Fort Walton Beach, U.S.A. 153 E3 30 25N 86 36W
Fort Wayne, U.S.A. 157 C11 41 4N 85 9W
Fort White, U.S.A. 152 F7 29 55N 82 43W
Fort William, U.K. 22 E3 56 49N 5 7W
Fort Worth, U.S.A. 155 J6 32 45N 97 18W
Fort Yates, U.S.A. 154 B4 46 5N 100 38W
Fort Yukon, U.S.A. 144 C11 66 34N 145 16W
Fortaleza = Pedra Azul, Brazil 171 E3 16 2 S 41 17W
Fortaleza, Bolivia 172 C4 12 6 S 66 49W
Fortaleza, Brazil 170 B4 3 45 S 38 35W
Forteau, Canada 141 B8 51 28N 56 58W
Fortescue →, Australia 124 D2 21 0 S 116 4 E
Forth →, U.K. 22 E5 56 9N 3 50W
Forth, Firth of, U.K. 22 E6 56 5N 2 55W
Forthassa Rharbia, Algeria 111 B4 32 52N 1 18W
Fortín Garrapatal, Paraguay 173 E5 21 27 S 61 30W
Fortín General Pando, Paraguay 173 D6 19 45 S 59 47W
Fortín Ingavi, Paraguay 173 D5 19 55 S 60 47W
Fortín Madrejón, Paraguay 173 E6 20 45 S 59 52W
Fortín Uno, Argentina 176 A3 38 50 S 65 18W
Fortore →, Italy 45 G12 41 55N 15 17 E
Fortrose, N.Z. 131 G3 46 38 S 168 45 E
Fortrose, U.K. 22 D4 57 35N 4 9W
Fortuna, Spain 41 G3 38 11N 1 7W
Fortuna, Calif., U.S.A. 158 F1 40 36N 124 9W
Fortuna, N. Dak., U.S.A. 154 A3 48 55N 103 47W
Fortuna Ledge, U.S.A. 144 F7 61 53N 162 5W
Fortune, Canada 141 C8 47 4N 55 50W
Fortune B., Canada 141 C8 47 30N 55 22W
Forūr, Iran 97 E7 26 17N 54 32 E
Fos-sur-Mer, France 29 E8 43 26N 4 56 E
Foshan, China 77 F9 23 4N 113 5 E
Fosna, Norway 14 E14 63 50N 10 20 E
Fosnavåg, Norway 18 B2 62 22N 5 38 E
Foso, Ghana 113 D4 5 43N 1 15W
Foss, Iceland 11 D9 63 51N 17 52W
Fossano, Italy 44 D4 44 33N 7 43 E
Fossil, U.S.A. 158 D3 45 0N 120 9W
Fossil Butte ⌂, U.S.A. 158 F8 41 50N 110 27W
Fossombrone, Italy 45 E9 43 41N 12 48 E
Fossvellir, Iceland 11 B12 65 27N 14 37W
Foster, Australia 129 E7 38 40 S 146 15 E
Foster, Canada 151 A12 45 17N 72 30W
Foster, U.S.A. 157 F12 38 48N 84 13W
Foster →, Canada 143 B7 55 47N 105 49W
Fosters Ra., Australia 126 C1 21 35 S 133 48 E
Fostoria, U.S.A. 157 C13 41 10N 83 25W
Fotadrevo, Madag. 117 C8 24 3 S 45 1 E
Fouesnant, France 26 E2 47 53N 4 1W
Fougamou, Gabon 114 C2 1 16 S 10 30 E
Fougères, France 26 D5 48 21N 1 14W
Foul Pt., Sri Lanka 95 K5 8 35N 81 18 E
Foula, U.K. 22 A6 60 10N 2 5W
Foulabala, Mali 112 C3 10 40N 7 20W
Foulness I., U.K. 21 F8 51 36N 0 55 E
Foulpointe, Madag. 117 B8 17 41 S 49 31 E
Foulweather, C., U.S.A. 146 B2 44 50N 124 5W
Foulwind, C., N.Z. 131 B6 41 45 S 171 28 E
Foum Assaka, Morocco 110 C2 29 8N 10 24W
Foum Zguid, Morocco 110 B3 30 2N 6 59W
Foumban, Cameroon 113 D7 5 45N 10 50 E
Foumbot, Cameroon 113 D7 5 31N 10 28 E
Foumbouni, Comoros Is. 121 a 11 52 S 43 32 E
Foumirate, Algeria 110 C4 27 30N 3 12W
Foundiougne, Senegal 112 C1 14 5N 16 32W
Fountain, Colo., U.S.A. 154 F2 38 41N 104 42W
Fountain, Fla., U.S.A. 152 E4 30 29N 85 25W
Fountain Hill, U.S.A. 159 K8 33 37N 111 43W
Fountain Springs, U.S.A. 161 K8 35 54N 118 51W
Four Mountains, Is. of, U.S.A. 144 K5 53 0N 170 0W
Fourchambault, France 27 E10 47 2N 3 3 E
Fouriesburg, S. Africa 116 D4 28 38 S 28 14 E
Fourmies, France 27 B11 50 1N 4 2 E
Fournás, Greece 48 B3 39 3N 21 52 E
Fourni = Foúrnoi, Greece 49 D8 37 36N 26 32 E
Foúrnoi, Greece 49 D8 37 36N 26 32 E
Fours, France 27 F10 46 50N 3 42 E
Fourth Cataract, Sudan 106 D3 18 47N 32 3 E
Fouschin = Fuxin, China 75 C11 42 5N 121 48 E
Fouta Djallon, Guinea 112 C2 11 20N 12 10W
Foux, Cap-à-, Haiti 165 C5 19 43N 73 27W
Foveaux Str., N.Z. 131 G3 46 42 S 168 10 E
Fowey, U.K. 21 G3 50 20N 4 39W
Fowler, Calif., U.S.A. 160 J7 36 38N 119 41W
Fowler, Colo., U.S.A. 154 F3 38 8N 104 2W
Fowler, Ind., U.S.A. 157 D9 40 37N 87 19W
Fowler, Mich., U.S.A. 157 B12 43 0N 84 45W
Fowlers B., Australia 125 F5 31 59 S 132 34 E
Fowlerville, U.S.A. 157 B12 42 40N 84 4W
Fowman, Iran 97 B6 37 13N 49 19 E
Fox →, Canada 143 B10 56 3N 93 18W
Fox Creek, Canada 142 C5 54 24N 116 48W
Fox Is., U.S.A. 144 K6 53 0N 168 0W
Fox Lake, Canada 142 B6 58 28N 114 31W
Fox Lake, U.S.A. 157 B8 42 24N 88 11W
Fox Valley, Canada 143 C7 50 30N 109 25W
Foxboro, U.S.A. 151 D13 42 4N 71 16W
Foxdale, Australia 126 J6 20 22 S 148 35 E
Foxe Basin, Canada 139 B12 66 0N 77 0W
Foxe Chan., Canada 139 B11 65 0N 80 0W
Foxe Pen., Canada 139 B12 65 0N 76 0W
Foxen, Sweden 16 E5 59 25N 11 55 E
Foxton, N.Z. 130 G4 40 29 S 175 18 E
Foyle, Lough, U.K. 23 A4 55 7N 7 4W
Foynes, Ireland 23 D2 52 37N 9 7W
Foz, Spain 42 B3 43 33N 7 20W
Foz do Copeá, Brazil 169 D5 3 52 S 63 19W
Foz do Cunene, Angola 116 B1 17 15 S 11 48 E
Foz do Gregório, Brazil 172 B3 6 47 S 70 44W
Foz do Iguaçu, Brazil 175 B5 25 30 S 54 30W
Foz do Mamoriá, Brazil 168 D4 2 27 S 66 32W
Foz do Riosinho, Brazil 172 B3 7 11 S 71 50W
Frackville, U.S.A. 151 F8 40 47N 76 14W
Fraga, Spain 40 D5 41 32N 0 21 E
Fraile Muerto, Uruguay 175 C5 32 31 S 54 32W
Fram Basin, Arctic 6 A 87 30N 80 0 E
Framingham, U.S.A. 151 D13 42 17N 71 25W
Framnes, Iceland 11 A6 66 1N 20 26W
Frampol, Poland 55 H9 50 41N 22 40 E
Franca, Brazil 171 F2 20 33 S 47 30W
Francavilla al Mare, Italy 45 F11 42 25N 14 17 E
Francavilla Fontana, Italy 47 B10 40 32N 17 35 E
France ■, Europe 25 C5 47 0N 3 0 E
Frances, Australia 128 D4 36 41 S 140 55 E
Frances →, Canada 142 A3 60 16N 129 10W
Frances L., Canada 142 A3 61 23N 129 30W
Francesville, U.S.A. 157 D10 40 59N 86 53W
Franceville, Gabon 114 C2 1 40 S 13 32 E
Franche-Comté □, France 27 F12 46 50N 5 55 E
Franches Montagnes, Switz. 32 B4 47 10N 7 0 E
Francis Case, L., U.S.A. 154 D5 43 4N 98 34W
Francisco Beltrão, Brazil 175 B5 26 5 S 53 4W
Francisco de Orellana, Ecuador 168 D2 0 28 S 76 58W
Francisco I. Madero, Coahuila, Mexico 162 B4 25 48N 103 18W
Francisco I. Madero, Durango, Mexico 162 C4 24 32N 104 22W
Francisco Sá, Brazil 171 E3 16 28 S 43 30W
Francistown, Botswana 117 C4 21 7 S 27 33 E
Francofonte, Italy 47 E7 37 14N 14 53 E
François, Canada 141 C8 47 35N 56 45W
François-Joseph, Chutes, Dem. Rep. of the Congo 115 D3 7 37 S 17 17 E
François L., Canada 142 C3 54 0N 125 30W
Francois Peron △, Australia 125 E1 25 42 S 113 33 E
Franeker, Neths. 24 A5 53 12N 5 33 E
Frank Hann △, Australia 125 F3 32 52 S 120 19 E
Frankado, Djibouti 107 E5 12 30N 43 12 E
Frankenberg, Germany 30 D4 51 3N 8 48 E
Frankenhöhe ⌂, Germany 31 F6 49 20N 10 25 E
Frankenstein = Ząbkowice Śląskie, Poland 55 H3 50 35N 16 50 E
Frankenwald, Germany 31 E7 50 20N 11 30 E
Frankenwald ⌂, Germany 31 E7 50 15N 11 30 E
Frankford, Canada 150 B7 44 12N 77 36W
Frankford, U.S.A. 156 E5 39 29N 91 19W
Frankfort, S. Africa 117 D4 27 17 S 28 30 E
Frankfort, Ind., U.S.A. 157 D10 40 17N 86 31W
Frankfort, Kans., U.S.A. 154 F6 39 42N 96 25W
Frankfort, Ky., U.S.A. 157 F12 38 12N 84 52W
Frankfort, N.Y., U.S.A. 151 C9 43 2N 75 4W
Frankfort, Ohio, U.S.A. 157 E13 39 24N 83 11W
Frankfurt, Brandenburg, Germany 30 C10 52 20N 14 32 E
Frankfurt, Hessen, Germany 31 E4 50 7N 8 41 E
Frankfurt ✕ (FRA), Germany 31 E4 50 1N 8 34 E
Fränkische Alb, Germany 31 F7 49 10N 11 23 E
Fränkische Rezat →, Germany 31 F7 49 11N 11 1 E
Fränkische Saale →, Germany 31 E5 50 3N 9 42 E
Fränkische Schweiz, Germany 31 F7 49 50N 11 16 E
Fränkische Schweiz-Veldensteiner Forst ⌂, Germany 31 F7 49 45N 11 22 E
Frankland →, Australia 125 G2 35 0 S 116 48 E
Franklin, Ga., U.S.A. 152 B4 33 17N 85 6W
Franklin, Ind., U.S.A. 157 E10 39 29N 86 3W
Franklin, Ky., U.S.A. 149 G2 36 43N 86 35W
Franklin, La., U.S.A. 155 L9 29 48N 91 30W
Franklin, Mass., U.S.A. 151 D13 42 5N 71 24W
Franklin, N.H., U.S.A. 151 C13 43 27N 71 39W
Franklin, Nebr., U.S.A. 154 E5 40 6N 98 57W
Franklin, Ohio, U.S.A. 157 E12 39 34N 84 18W
Franklin, Pa., U.S.A. 150 E5 41 24N 79 50W
Franklin, Va., U.S.A. 149 G7 36 41N 76 56W
Franklin, W. Va., U.S.A. 148 F6 38 39N 79 20W
Franklin, Pt., U.S.A. 144 A8 70 55N 158 48W
Franklin B., Canada 138 B7 69 45N 126 0W
Franklin D. Roosevelt L., U.S.A. 158 B4 48 18N 118 9W
Franklin-Gordon Wild Rivers △, Australia 127 G4 42 19 S 145 51 E
Franklin Harb., Australia 128 B2 33 43 S 136 55 E
Franklin I., Antarctica 7 D11 76 10 S 168 30 E
Franklin L., U.S.A. 158 F6 40 25N 115 22W
Franklin Mts., Canada 138 B7 65 0N 125 0W
Franklin Mts., N.Z. 131 E2 44 55 S 167 45 E
Franklin Str., Canada 138 A10 72 0N 96 0W
Franklinton, U.S.A. 155 K9 30 51N 90 9W
Franklinville, U.S.A. 150 D6 42 20N 78 27W
Franklyn Mt., N.Z. 131 C7 42 4 S 172 42 E
Franks Pk., U.S.A. 158 E9 43 58N 109 18W
Frankston, Australia 129 E6 38 8 S 145 8 E
Frånö, Sweden 16 B11 62 55N 17 50 E

Fransfontein, *Namibia* **116 C2** 20 12 S 15 1 E
Fränsta, *Sweden* **16 B10** 62 30N 16 11 E
Frantsa Iosifa, Zemlya, *Russia* **66 A6** 82 0N 55 0 E
Franz, *Canada* **140 C3** 48 25N 84 30W
Franz Josef Land = Frantsa Iosifa, Zemlya, *Russia* **66 A6** 82 0N 55 0 E
Franz Josef Strauss, München ✈ (MUC), *Germany* **31 G7** 48 20N 11 50 E
Franzburg, *Germany* **30 A8** 54 11N 12 51 E
Frascati, *Italy* **45 G9** 41 48N 12 41 E
Fraser, *U.S.A.* **150 D2** 42 32N 82 57W
Fraser △, *Australia* **129 D6** 37 9 S 145 51 E
Fraser ➝, *B.C., Canada* **142 D4** 49 7N 123 11W
Fraser ➝, *Nfld. & L., Canada* **141 A7** 56 39N 62 10W
Fraser, Mt., *Australia* **125 E2** 25 35 S 118 20 E
Fraser I., *Australia* **127 D5** 25 15 S 153 10 E
Fraser Lake, *Canada* **142 C4** 54 0N 124 50W
Fraserburg, *S. Africa* **116 E3** 31 55 S 21 30 E
Fraserburg Road = Leeu Gamka, *S. Africa* **116 E3** 32 47 S 21 59 E
Fraserburgh, *U.K.* **22 D6** 57 42N 2 1W
Fraserdale, *Canada* **140 C3** 49 55N 81 37W
Fraserpet = Kushalnagar, *India* **95 H2** 12 14N 75 57 E
Frasertown, *N.Z.* **130 E6** 38 58 S 177 28 E
Fraserville = Rivière-du-Loup, *Canada* **141 C6** 47 50N 69 30W
Frashër, *Albania* **50 F4** 40 23N 20 30 E
Frasne, *France* **27 F13** 46 50N 6 10 E
Frăteşti, *Romania* **53 G10** 43 58N 25 58 E
Frauenfeld, *Switz.* **33 A7** 47 34N 8 54 E
Frauenstadt = Wadowice, *Poland* **55 J6** 49 52N 19 30 E
Fraustadt = Wschowa, *Poland* **55 G3** 51 48N 16 20 E
Fray Bentos, *Uruguay* **174 C4** 33 10 S 58 15W
Fray Jorge △, *Chile* **174 C1** 30 42 S 71 40W
Frechilla, *Spain* **42 C6** 42 8N 4 50W
Fredericia, *Denmark* **17 J3** 55 34N 9 45 E
Frederick, *Md., U.S.A.* **148 F7** 39 25N 77 25W
Frederick, *Okla., U.S.A.* **155 H5** 34 23N 99 1W
Frederick, *S. Dak., U.S.A.* **154 C5** 45 50N 98 31W
Frederick E. Hyde Fjord, *Greenland* **10 A8** 83 25N 29 0W
Fredericksburg, *Pa., U.S.A.* **151 F8** 40 27N 76 26W
Fredericksburg, *Tex., U.S.A.* **155 K5** 30 16N 98 52W
Fredericksburg, *Va., U.S.A.* **148 F7** 38 18N 77 28W
Fredericktown, *Mo., U.S.A.* **155 G9** 37 34N 90 18W
Fredericktown, *Ohio, U.S.A.* **150 F2** 40 29N 82 33W
Frederico I. Madero, Presa, *Mexico* **162 B3** 28 7N 105 40W
Frederico Westphalen, *Brazil* **175 B5** 27 22 S 53 24W
Fredericton, *Canada* **141 C6** 45 57N 66 40W
Fredericton Junction, *Canada* **141 C6** 45 41N 66 40W
Frederiksborg Amtskommune □, *Denmark* **17 J6** 55 50N 12 10 E
Frederikshåb = Paamiut, *Greenland* **10 E6** 62 0N 49 43W
Frederikshald = Halden, *Norway* **18 E8** 59 9N 11 23 E
Frederikshamn = Hamina, *Finland* **15 F22** 60 34N 27 12 E
Frederikshavn, *Denmark* **17 G4** 57 28N 10 31 E
Frederikssund, *Denmark* **17 J6** 55 50N 12 3 E
Frederiksted, *U.S. Virgin Is.* **165 C7** 17 43N 64 53W
Frederiksværk, *Denmark* **17 J6** 55 58N 12 4 E
Fredonia, *Ariz., U.S.A.* **159 H7** 36 57N 112 32W
Fredonia, *Kans., U.S.A.* **155 G7** 37 32N 95 49W
Fredonia, *N.Y., U.S.A.* **150 D5** 42 26N 79 20W
Fredriksberg, *Sweden* **16 D8** 60 8N 14 23 E
Fredrikstad, *Norway* **18 E7** 59 13N 10 57 E
Fredriksvern = Stavern, *Norway* **18 F7** 59 0N 10 1 E
Free State □, *S. Africa* **116 D4** 28 30 S 27 0 E
Freeburg, *U.S.A.* **156 F5** 38 19N 91 56W
Freehold, *U.S.A.* **151 F10** 40 16N 74 17W
Freel Peak, *U.S.A.* **160 G7** 38 52N 119 54W
Freeland, *U.S.A.* **151 E9** 41 1N 75 54W
Freels, C., *Canada* **141 C9** 49 15N 53 30W
Freeman, *Calif., U.S.A.* **161 K9** 35 35N 117 53W
Freeman, *Mo., U.S.A.* **156 F2** 38 37N 94 30W
Freeman, *S. Dak., U.S.A.* **154 D6** 43 21N 97 26W
Freeport, *Bahamas* **164 A4** 26 30N 78 47W
Freeport, *Fla., U.S.A.* **152 E3** 30 30N 86 8W
Freeport, *Ill., U.S.A.* **156 B7** 42 17N 89 36W
Freeport, *N.Y., U.S.A.* **151 F11** 40 39N 73 35W
Freeport, *Ohio, U.S.A.* **150 F3** 40 12N 81 15W
Freeport, *Pa., U.S.A.* **150 F5** 40 41N 79 41W
Freeport, *Tex., U.S.A.* **155 L7** 28 57N 95 21W
Freetown, *S. Leone* **112 D2** 8 30N 13 17W
Frégate, L. de la, *Canada* **140 B5** 53 15N 74 45W
Fregenal de la Sierra, *Spain* **43 G4** 38 10N 6 39W
Fregene, *Italy* **45 G9** 41 51N 12 12 E
Fréhel, C., *France* **26 D4** 48 40N 2 20W
Freiberg, *Germany* **30 E9** 50 55N 13 20 E
Freibourg = Fribourg, *Switz.* **32 C4** 46 49N 7 9 E
Freiburg, *Baden-W., Germany* **31 H3** 47 59N 7 51 E
Freiburg, *Niedersachsen, Germany* **30 B5** 53 49N 9 16 E
Freiburg in Schlesien = Świebodzice, *Poland* **55 H3** 50 51N 16 20 E
Freiburger Alpen, *Switz.* **32 C4** 46 37N 7 10 E
Freienwalde = Chociwel, *Poland* **54 E2** 53 29N 15 21 E
Freilassing, *Germany* **31 H8** 47 50N 12 58 E
Freire, *Chile* **176 A2** 38 54 S 72 38W
Freirina, *Chile* **174 B1** 28 30 S 71 10W
Freising, *Germany* **31 G7** 48 24N 11 45 E
Freistadt, *Austria* **34 C7** 48 30N 14 30 E
Freital, *Germany* **30 D9** 51 1N 13 39 E
Freiwaldau = Jeseník, *Czech Rep.* **35 A10** 50 14N 17 8 E
Fréjus, *France* **29 E10** 43 25N 6 44 E
Fremantle, *Australia* **125 F2** 32 7 S 115 47 E
Fremont, *Calif., U.S.A.* **160 H4** 37 32N 121 57W
Fremont, *Ind., U.S.A.* **157 C12** 41 44N 84 56W
Fremont, *Iowa, U.S.A.* **156 C4** 41 13N 92 26W
Fremont, *Mich., U.S.A.* **148 D3** 43 28N 85 57W
Fremont, *Nebr., U.S.A.* **154 E6** 41 26N 96 30W
Fremont, *Ohio, U.S.A.* **157 C13** 41 21N 83 7W
Fremont ➝, *U.S.A.* **159 G8** 38 24N 110 42W
French Camp, *U.S.A.* **160 H5** 37 53N 121 16W
French Cays = Plana Cays, *Bahamas* **165 B5** 22 38N 73 30W
French Creek ➝, *U.S.A.* **150 E5** 41 24N 79 50W
French Frigate Shoals, *U.S.A.* **145 G10** 23 45N 166 10W
French Guiana ☒, *S. Amer.* **169 C7** 4 0N 53 0W
French Guinea = Guinea ■, *W. Afr.* **112 C2** 10 20N 11 30W
French I., *Australia* **129 E6** 38 20 S 145 22 E
French Lick, *U.S.A.* **157 F10** 38 33N 86 37W
French Pass, *N.Z.* **131 A8** 40 55 S 173 55 E
French Polynesia ☒, *Pac. Oc.* **135 K13** 20 0 S 145 0W
French Sudan = Mali ■, *Africa* **112 B4** 17 0N 3 0W
French Territory of the Afars and Issas = Djibouti ■, *Africa* **107 E5** 12 0N 43 0 E
French Togoland = Togo ■, *W. Afr.* **113 D5** 8 30N 1 35 E
Frenchburg, *U.S.A.* **157 G13** 37 57N 83 38W
Frenchman Cr. ➝, *N. Amer.* **158 B10** 48 31N 107 10W
Frenchman Cr. ➝, *U.S.A.* **154 E4** 40 14N 100 50W
Frenda, *Algeria* **111 A5** 35 2N 1 1 E
Frenštát pod Radhoštěm, *Czech Rep.* **35 B11** 49 33N 18 13 E
Fresco, *Ivory C.* **112 D3** 5 3N 5 31W
Fresco ➝, *Brazil* **173 B7** 7 15 S 51 30W
Freshfield, C., *Antarctica* **7 C10** 68 25 S 151 10 E
Fresnay-sur-Sarthe, *France* **26 D7** 48 17N 0 1 E
Fresnillo, *Mexico* **162 C4** 23 10N 103 0W
Fresno, *U.S.A.* **160 J7** 36 44N 119 47W
Fresno Alhandiga, *Spain* **42 E5** 40 42N 5 37W
Fresno Reservoir, *U.S.A.* **158 B9** 48 36N 109 57W
Fresvik, *Norway* **18 C3** 61 4N 6 55 E
Freudenstadt, *Germany* **31 G4** 48 27N 8 24 E
Freudenthal = Bruntál, *Czech Rep.* **35 B10** 49 59N 17 27 E
Frévent, *France* **27 B9** 50 15N 2 17 E
Frew ➝, *Australia* **126 C2** 20 0 S 135 38 E
Frewsburg, *U.S.A.* **150 D5** 42 3N 79 10W
Freycinet △, *Australia* **127 G4** 42 11 S 148 19 E
Freycinet Pen., *Australia* **127 G4** 42 10 S 148 25 E
Freyming-Merlebach, *France* **27 C13** 49 8N 6 48 E
Freystadt = Kisielice, *Poland* **54 E6** 53 36N 19 16 E
Freystadt = Kożuchów, *Poland* **55 G2** 51 45N 15 31 E
Freyung, *Germany* **31 G9** 48 48N 13 31 E
Fria, *Guinea* **112 C2** 10 27N 13 38W
Fria, C., *Namibia* **116 B1** 18 0 S 12 0 E
Friant, *U.S.A.* **160 J7** 36 59N 119 43W
Frías, *Argentina* **174 B2** 28 40 S 65 5W
Fribourg, *Switz.* **32 C4** 46 49N 7 9 E
Fribourg □, *Switz.* **32 C4** 46 40N 7 0 E
Frick, *Switz.* **32 A6** 47 31N 8 1 E
Fridafors, *Sweden* **17 H8** 56 25N 14 39 E
Friday Harbor, *U.S.A.* **160 B3** 48 32N 123 1W
Friedberg, *Bayern, Germany* **31 G6** 48 21N 10 59 E
Friedberg, *Hessen, Germany* **31 E4** 50 19N 8 45 E
Friedeberg = Mirsk, *Poland* **55 H2** 50 58N 15 23 E
Friedeberg in Neumark = Strzelce Krajeńskie, *Poland* **55 F2** 52 52N 15 33 E
Friedens, *U.S.A.* **150 F6** 40 3N 78 59W
Friedland = Mieroszów, *Poland* **55 H3** 50 40N 16 11 E
Friedland = Pravdinsk, *Russia* **60 B6** 56 29N 43 28 E
Friedland, *Germany* **30 B9** 53 40N 13 33 E
Friedrichshafen, *Germany* **31 H5** 47 39N 9 30 E
Friedrichskoog, *Germany* **30 A4** 54 1N 8 53 E
Friedrichstadt, *Germany* **30 A5** 54 23N 9 6 E
Friendly Is. = Tonga ■, *Pac. Oc.* **133 P13** 19 50 S 174 30W
Friendship, *U.S.A.* **150 D6** 42 12N 78 8W
Friesach, *Austria* **34 E7** 46 57N 14 24 E
Friesack, *Germany* **30 C8** 52 44N 12 34 E
Friesland □, *Neths.* **24 A5** 53 5N 5 50 E
Friesoythe, *Germany* **30 B3** 53 1N 7 51 E
Frigate, *Seychelles* **121 b** 4 35 S 55 56 E
Friggesund, *Sweden* **16 C10** 61 54N 16 33 E
Frillesås, *Sweden* **17 G6** 57 20N 12 12 E
Frinnaryd, *Sweden* **17 G8** 57 55N 14 50 E
Frio ➝, *U.S.A.* **155 L5** 28 26N 98 11W
Frio, C., *Brazil* **166 F6** 22 50 S 41 50W
Friol, *Spain* **42 B3** 43 2N 7 47W
Friona, *U.S.A.* **155 H3** 34 38N 102 43W
Frisches Haff = Zalew Wiślany, *Poland* **54 D6** 54 20N 19 50 E
Fristad, *Sweden* **17 G6** 57 50N 13 0 E
Fritch, *U.S.A.* **155 H4** 35 38N 101 36W
Fritsla, *Sweden* **17 G6** 57 33N 12 47 E
Fritzlar, *Germany* **30 D5** 51 7N 9 16 E
Friuli-Venézia Giulia □, *Italy* **45 B9** 46 0N 13 0 E
Frobisher B., *Canada* **139 B13** 62 30N 66 0W
Frobisher Bay = Iqaluit, *Canada* **139 B13** 63 44N 68 31W
Frobisher L., *Canada* **143 B7** 56 20N 108 15W
Frohavet, *Norway* **14 E13** 64 0N 9 30 E
Frohenbruck = Veselí nad Lužnicí, *Czech Rep.* **34 B7** 49 12N 14 43 E
Frohnleiten, *Austria* **34 D8** 47 16N 15 19 E
Frolovo, *Russia* **60 F6** 49 45N 43 40 E
Frombork, *Poland* **54 D6** 54 21N 19 41 E
Frome, *U.K.* **21 F5** 51 14N 2 19W
Frome ➝, *U.K.* **21 G5** 50 41N 2 6W
Frome, L., *Australia* **128 A3** 30 45 S 139 45 E
Frome, The ➝, *Australia* **127 D2** 29 8 S 137 54 E
Frome Downs, *Australia* **128 A3** 31 13 S 139 45 E
Frómista, *Spain* **42 C6** 42 16N 4 25W
Front Range, *U.S.A.* **146 C5** 40 25N 105 45W
Front Royal, *U.S.A.* **148 F6** 38 55N 78 12W
Fronteira, *Portugal* **43 F3** 39 3N 7 39W
Fronteiras, *Brazil* **170 C3** 7 5 S 40 37W
Frontera, *Canary Is.* **9 e1** 27 47N 17 59W
Frontera, *Mexico* **163 D6** 18 30N 92 40W
Fronteras, *Mexico* **162 A3** 30 56N 109 31W
Frontignan, *France* **28 E7** 43 27N 3 45 E
Frosinone, *Italy* **46 A6** 41 38N 13 19 E
Frostburg, *U.S.A.* **148 F6** 39 39N 78 56W
Frostisen, *Norway* **14 B17** 68 14N 17 10 E
Frostproof, *U.S.A.* **153 H8** 27 45N 81 32W
Frouard, *France* **27 D13** 48 47N 6 8 E
Frövi, *Sweden* **16 E9** 59 28N 15 24 E
Frøya, *Norway* **14 E13** 63 43N 8 40 E
Fruithurst, *U.S.A.* **152 B4** 33 44N 85 26W
Fruitland Park, *U.S.A.* **153 G8** 28 51N 81 54W
Frumoasa, *Romania* **53 D10** 46 28N 25 48 E
Frunze = Bishkek, *Kyrgyzstan* **65 B7** 42 54N 74 46 E
Frunze, *Kyrgyzstan* **65 C5** 40 7N 71 44 E
Frunzivka, *Ukraine* **53 C14** 47 20N 29 45 E
Fruška Gora, *Serbia & M.* **52 E4** 45 7N 19 30 E
Fruška Gora △, *Serbia & M.* **50 A3** 45 8N 19 40 E
Frutal, *Brazil* **171 F2** 20 0 S 49 0W
Frutigen, *Switz.* **32 C5** 46 35N 7 38 E
Frýdek-Místek, *Czech Rep.* **35 B11** 49 40N 18 20 E
Frýdlant, *Czech Rep.* **34 A8** 50 56N 15 9 E
Fryeburg, *U.S.A.* **151 B14** 44 1N 70 59W
Fryvaldov = Jeseník, *Czech Rep.* **35 A10** 50 14N 17 8 E
Fthiótis □, *Greece* **48 C4** 38 50N 22 25 E
Fu Jiang ➝, *China* **76 C6** 30 0N 106 16 E
Fu Xian = Wafangdian, *China* **75 E11** 39 38N 121 58 E
Fu Xian, *China* **74 G5** 36 0N 109 20 E
Fu'an, *China* **77 D12** 27 11N 119 36 E
Fubian, *China* **76 B4** 31 17N 102 22 E
Fucécchio, *Italy* **44 E7** 43 44N 10 48 E
Fucheng, *China* **74 F9** 37 50N 116 10 E
Fuchou = Fuzhou, *China* **77 D12** 26 5N 119 16 E
Fuchū, *Hiroshima, Japan* **72 C5** 34 34N 133 14 E
Fūchū, *Tōkyō, Japan* **73 B11** 35 40N 139 29 E
Fuchuan, *China* **77 E8** 24 50N 111 5 E
Fuchun Jiang ➝, *China* **77 B13** 30 5N 120 5 E
Fúcino, Piana del, *Italy* **45 F10** 42 1N 13 31 E
Fuding, *China* **77 D13** 27 20N 120 12 E
Fuencaliente, *Canary Is.* **9 e1** 28 28N 17 50W
Fuencaliente, *Spain* **43 G6** 38 25N 4 18W
Fuencaliente, Pta., *Canary Is.* **9 e1** 28 27N 17 51W
Fuengirola, *Spain* **43 J6** 36 32N 4 41W
Fuenlabrada, *Spain* **42 E7** 40 17N 3 48W
Fuensalida, *Spain* **42 E6** 40 3N 4 12W
Fuente-Álamo, *Spain* **41 G3** 38 44N 1 24W
Fuente-Álamo de Murcia, *Spain* **41 H3** 37 42N 1 6W
Fuente de Cantos, *Spain* **43 G4** 38 15N 6 18W
Fuente del Maestre, *Spain* **43 G4** 38 31N 6 28W
Fuente el Fresno, *Spain* **43 F7** 39 14N 3 46W
Fuente Obejuna, *Spain* **43 G5** 38 15N 5 25W
Fuente Palmera, *Spain* **43 H5** 37 42N 5 6W
Fuentes de Andalucía, *Spain* **43 H5** 37 28N 5 20W
Fuentes de Ebro, *Spain* **40 D4** 41 31N 0 38W
Fuentes de León, *Spain* **43 G4** 38 5N 6 32W
Fuentes de Oñoro, *Spain* **42 E4** 40 33N 6 52W
Fuentesaúco, *Spain* **42 D5** 41 15N 5 30W
Fuerte ➝, *Mexico* **162 B3** 25 50N 109 25W
Fuerte Olimpo, *Paraguay* **174 A4** 21 0 S 57 51W
Fuerteventura, *Canary Is.* **9 e2** 28 30N 14 0W
Fuerteventura ✈ (FUE), *Canary Is.* **9 e2** 28 24N 13 52W
Fufeng, *China* **74 G5** 34 22N 108 0 E
Fuga I., *Phil.* **80 B3** 18 52N 121 20 E
Fughmah, *Yemen* **99 C5** 16 9N 49 26 E
Fugong, *China* **76 D2** 27 5N 98 47 E
Fugou, *China* **74 G8** 34 3N 114 25 E
Fugu, *China* **74 E6** 39 2N 111 3 E
Fuhai, *China* **68 B3** 47 2N 87 25 E
Fuḩaymī, *Iraq* **101 E10** 34 16N 42 10 E
Fuhlsbüttel, Hamburg ✈ (HAM), *Germany* **30 B5** 53 35N 9 59 E
Fuhsien = Fu Xian, *China* **74 G5** 36 0N 109 20 E
Fuji, *Japan* **73 B10** 35 9N 138 39 E
Fuji-Hakone-Izu △, *Japan* **73 B10** 35 15N 138 45 E
Fuji-San, *Japan* **73 B10** 35 22N 138 44 E
Fuji-Yoshida, *Japan* **73 B10** 35 30N 138 46 E
Fujian □, *China* **77 E12** 26 0N 118 0 E
Fujieda, *Japan* **73 C10** 34 52N 138 16 E
Fujinomiya, *Japan* **73 B10** 35 10N 138 40 E
Fujioka, *Japan* **73 A11** 36 15N 139 5 E
Fujisawa, *Japan* **73 B11** 35 22N 139 29 E
Fujiyama, Mt. = Fuji-San, *Japan* **73 B10** 35 22N 138 44 E
Fukagawa, *Japan* **70 C11** 43 43N 142 2 E
Fukaya, *Japan* **73 A11** 36 12N 139 12 E
Fukiage, *Japan* **72 F2** 31 27N 130 17 E
Fukien = Fujian □, *China* **77 E12** 26 0N 118 0 E
Fukuchiyama, *Japan* **73 B7** 35 19N 135 9 E
Fukue-Shima, *Japan* **71 H4** 32 40N 128 45 E
Fukui, *Japan* **73 A8** 36 5N 136 10 E
Fukui □, *Japan* **73 B8** 36 0N 136 12 E
Fukuma, *Japan* **72 D2** 33 46N 130 28 E
Fukuoka, *Japan* **72 D2** 33 39N 130 21 E
Fukuoka □, *Japan* **72 D3** 33 30N 131 0 E
Fukuoka International ✈ (FUK), *Japan* **72 D2** 33 34N 130 28 E
Fukuroi, *Japan* **73 C9** 34 45N 137 55 E
Fukushima, *Japan* **70 F10** 37 44N 140 28 E
Fukushima □, *Japan* **70 F10** 37 30N 140 15 E
Fukuyama, *Japan* **72 C5** 34 35N 133 20 E
Fulacunda, *Guinea-Biss.* **112 C1** 11 44N 15 3W
Fulaga, *Fiji* **133 B3** 19 8 S 178 33W
Fulda, *Germany* **30 E5** 50 32N 9 40 E
Fulda ➝, *Germany* **30 D5** 51 25N 9 39 E
Fulford = North Miami Beach, *U.S.A.* **153 K9** 25 56N 80 10W
Fulford Harbour, *Canada* **160 B3** 48 47N 123 27W
Fuliang, *China* **77 C11** 29 23N 117 14 E
Fullerton, *Calif., U.S.A.* **161 M9** 33 53N 117 56W
Fullerton, *Nebr., U.S.A.* **154 E6** 41 22N 97 58W
Fulongquan, *China* **75 B13** 44 20N 124 42 E
Fülöpszállás, *Hungary* **52 D4** 46 49N 19 15 E
Fulton, *Ill., U.S.A.* **156 C6** 41 52N 90 11W
Fulton, *Ind., U.S.A.* **157 D10** 40 57N 86 16W
Fulton, *Mo., U.S.A.* **156 F5** 38 52N 91 57W
Fulton, *N.Y., U.S.A.* **151 C8** 43 19N 76 25W
Fuluälven ➝, *Sweden* **16 C7** 61 18N 13 4 E
Fulufjället, *Sweden* **16 C6** 61 32N 12 41 E
Fumay, *France* **27 C11** 49 58N 4 40 E
Fumel, *France* **28 D4** 44 30N 0 58 E
Fumin, *China* **76 E4** 25 10N 102 20 E
Funabashi, *Japan* **73 B12** 35 45N 140 0 E
Funafuti = Fongafale, *Tuvalu* **134 H9** 8 31 S 179 13 E
Funäsdalen, *Sweden* **16 B6** 62 33N 12 32 E
Funchal, *Madeira* **9 c** 32 38N 16 54W
Funchal ✈ (FNC), *Madeira* **9 c** 32 42N 16 45W
Fundación, *Colombia* **168 A3** 10 31N 74 11W
Fundão, *Brazil* **171 E3** 19 55 S 40 24W
Fundão, *Portugal* **42 E3** 40 8N 7 30W
Fundu Moldovei, *Romania* **53 C10** 47 32N 25 24 E
Fundulea, *Romania* **53 F11** 44 28N 26 31 E
Fundy △, *Canada* **141 C6** 45 35N 65 10W
Fundy, B. of, *Canada* **141 D6** 45 0N 66 0W
Fünfkirchen = Pécs, *Hungary* **52 D3** 46 5N 18 15 E
Funhalouro, *Mozam.* **117 C5** 23 3 S 34 25 E
Funing, *Hebei, China* **75 E10** 39 53N 119 12 E
Funing, *Jiangsu, China* **75 H10** 33 45N 119 50 E
Funing, *Yunnan, China* **76 F5** 23 35N 105 45 E
Funiu Shan, *China* **74 H7** 33 30N 112 20 E
Funsi, *Ghana* **112 C4** 10 21N 1 54W
Funtua, *Nigeria* **113 C6** 11 30N 7 18 E
Fuping, *Hebei, China* **74 E8** 38 48N 114 12 E
Fuping, *Shaanxi, China* **74 G5** 34 42N 109 10 E
Fuqing, *China* **77 E12** 25 41N 119 21 E
Fuquan, *China* **76 D6** 26 40N 107 27 E
Furano, *Japan* **70 C11** 43 21N 142 23 E
Furāt, Nahr al ➝, *Asia* **96 D5** 31 0N 47 25 E
Fūrg, *Iran* **97 D7** 28 18N 55 13 E
Furkapass, *Switz.* **33 C7** 46 34N 8 35 E
Furkating, *India* **90 B4** 26 28N 93 59 E
Furman, *U.S.A.* **152 C8** 32 41N 81 11W
Furmanov, *Russia* **60 B5** 57 10N 41 9 E
Furmanovo, *Kazakhstan* **60 F9** 49 42N 49 25 E
Furnas, *Azores* **9 d3** 37 46N 25 19W
Furnás, *Spain* **38 C2** 39 3N 1 32 E
Furnas, Reprêsa de, *Brazil* **171 F2** 20 50 S 45 30W
Furneaux Group, *Australia* **127 G4** 40 10 S 147 50 E
Furqlus, *Syria* **103 A6** 34 36N 37 8 E
Fürstenau, *Germany* **30 C3** 52 31N 7 40 E
Fürstenberg = Eisenhüttenstadt, *Germany* **30 C10** 52 9N 14 38 E
Fürstenberg, *Germany* **30 B9** 53 10N 13 8 E
Fürstenfeld, *Austria* **34 D9** 47 3N 16 3 E
Fürstenfeldbruck, *Germany* **31 G7** 48 11N 11 15 E
Fürstenwalde, *Germany* **30 C10** 52 22N 14 3 E
Fürth, *Germany* **31 F6** 49 28N 10 59 E
Furth im Wald, *Germany* **31 F8** 49 18N 12 50 E
Furtwangen, *Germany* **31 G4** 48 2N 8 12 E
Furudal, *Sweden* **16 C9** 61 10N 15 11 E
Furukawa, *Gifu, Japan* **73 A9** 36 14N 137 11 E
Furukawa, *Miyagi, Japan* **70 E10** 38 34N 140 58 E
Furulund, *Sweden* **17 J7** 55 46N 13 6 E
Fury and Hecla Str., *Canada* **139 B11** 69 56N 84 0W
Fusagasuga, *Colombia* **168 C3** 4 21N 74 22W
Fuscaldo, *Italy* **47 C9** 39 25N 16 2 E
Fushan, *Shandong, China* **75 F11** 37 30N 121 15 E
Fushan, *Shanxi, China* **74 G6** 35 58N 111 51 E
Fushë Arrëz, *Albania* **50 D4** 42 4N 20 2 E
Fushë Krujë, *Albania* **50 E3** 41 29N 19 43 E
Fushun, *Liaoning, China* **75 D12** 41 50N 123 56 E
Fushun, *Sichuan, China* **76 C5** 29 13N 104 52 E
Fusio, *Switz.* **33 D7** 46 27N 8 40 E
Fusong, *China* **75 C14** 42 20N 127 15 E
Füssen, *Germany* **31 H6** 47 34N 10 42 E
Fustic, *Barbados* **165 g** 13 16N 59 38W
Fusui, *China* **76 F6** 22 40N 107 56 E
Futago-Yama, *Japan* **72 D3** 33 35N 131 36 E
Futian, *China* **69 F11** 22 32N 114 4 E
Futog, *Serbia & M.* **52 E4** 45 15N 19 42 E
Futrono, *Chile* **176 B2** 40 8 S 72 24W
Futtsu, *Japan* **73 B10** 35 13N 139 49 E
Futuna, *Wall. & F. Is.* **134 J9** 14 25 S 178 20W
Fuwa, *Egypt* **106 H7** 31 12N 30 33 E
Fuxian Hu, *China* **76 E4** 24 30N 102 53 E
Fuxin, *China* **75 C11** 42 5N 121 48 E
Fuyang, *Anhui, China* **74 H8** 33 0N 115 48 E
Fuyang, *Zhejiang, China* **77 B12** 30 5N 119 57 E
Fuyang He ➝, *China* **74 E9** 38 12N 117 0 E
Fuying Dao, *China* **77 D13** 26 34N 120 9 E
Fuyong, *China* **69 F10** 22 40N 113 49 E
Fuyu, *Heilongjiang, China* **69 B7** 47 49N 124 27 E
Fuyu, *Jilin, China* **75 B13** 45 12N 124 43 E
Fuyuan, *China* **76 E5** 25 40N 104 16 E
Füzesgyarmat, *Hungary* **52 C6** 47 6N 21 14 E
Fuzhou, *China* **77 D12** 26 5N 119 16 E
Fylde, *U.K.* **20 D5** 53 50N 2 58W
Fyn, *Denmark* **17 J4** 55 20N 10 30 E
Fyne, L., *U.K.* **22 F3** 55 59N 5 23W
Fyns Amtskommune □, *Denmark* **17 J4** 55 15N 10 30 E
Fynshav, *Denmark* **17 K3** 54 59N 9 59 E
Fyresdal, *Norway* **18 E5** 59 11N 8 5 E
Fyresvatn, *Norway* **18 E5** 59 6N 8 10 E
Fyzabad = Faizabad, *India* **93 F10** 26 45N 82 10 E

G

Ga, *Ghana* **112 D4** 9 47N 2 30W
Gaanda, *Nigeria* **113 C7** 10 10N 12 27 E
Gabarin, *Nigeria* **113 C7** 11 8N 10 27 E
Gabas ➝, *France* **28 E3** 43 46N 0 42W
Gabela, *Angola* **115 E2** 11 0 S 14 24 E
Gaberones = Gaborone, *Botswana* **116 C4** 24 45 S 25 57 E
Gabès, *Tunisia* **108 B2** 33 53N 10 2 E
Gabès, G. de, *Tunisia* **108 B2** 34 0N 10 30 E
Gabgaba, W. ➝, *Egypt* **106 C3** 22 10N 33 5 E
Gabia, *Dem. Rep. of the Congo* **115 C3** 4 37 S 17 14 E
Gąbin, *Poland* **55 F6** 52 23N 19 41 E
Gablonz = Jablonec nad Nisou, *Czech Rep.* **34 A8** 50 43N 15 10 E
Gabon ■, *Africa* **114 C2** 0 10 S 10 0 E
Gabon ➝, *Gabon* **114 B1** 0 25N 9 20 E
Gaborone, *Botswana* **116 C4** 24 45 S 25 57 E
Gabriels, *U.S.A.* **151 B10** 44 26N 74 12W
Gābrīk, *Iran* **97 E8** 25 44N 58 28 E
Gabro, *Ethiopia* **120 C2** 6 18N 43 16 E
Gabrovo, *Bulgaria* **51 D9** 42 52N 25 19 E
Gabú = Nova Lamego, *Guinea-Biss.* **112 C2** 12 19N 14 11W
Gacé, *France* **26 D7** 48 49N 0 20 E
Gāch Sār, *Iran* **97 B6** 36 7N 51 19 E
Gachsārān, *Iran* **97 D6** 30 15N 50 45 E
Gacko, *Bos.-H.* **50 C2** 43 10N 18 33 E
Gad Hinglaj, *India* **95 F2** 16 14N 74 21 E
Gadag, *India* **95 G2** 15 30N 75 45 E
Gadaisu, *Papua N. G.* **132 F5** 10 22 S 149 46 E
Gadamai, *Sudan* **107 D4** 17 11N 36 10 E
Gadap, *Pakistan* **92 G2** 25 5N 67 28 E
Gadarwara, *India* **93 H8** 22 50N 78 50 E
Gadebusch, *Germany* **30 B7** 53 42N 11 7 E
Gadein, *Sudan* **107 F2** 8 10N 28 45 E
Gadhada, *India* **92 J4** 22 0N 71 35 E
Gadmen, *Switz.* **33 C6** 46 45N 8 16 E
Gádor, Sierra de, *Spain* **43 J8** 36 57N 2 45W
Gadra, *Pakistan* **92 G4** 25 40N 70 38 E
Gadsden, *Ala., U.S.A.* **152 A3** 34 1N 86 1W
Gadsden, *S.C., U.S.A.* **152 B9** 33 51N 80 46W
Gadwal, *India* **95 F3** 16 10N 77 50 E
Gadyach = Hadyach, *Ukraine* **59 G8** 50 21N 34 0 E
Gadzi, *C.A.R.* **114 B3** 4 47N 16 42 E
Găeşti, *Romania* **53 F10** 44 48N 25 19 E
Gaeta, *Italy* **46 A6** 41 12N 13 35 E
Gaeta, G. di, *Italy* **46 A6** 41 6N 13 30 E
Gaffney, *U.S.A.* **149 H5** 35 5N 81 39W
Gafsa, *Tunisia* **108 B1** 34 24N 8 43 E
Gag, *Indonesia* **83 B3** 0 27 S 129 52 E
Gagarawa, *Nigeria* **113 C6** 12 25N 9 32 E
Gagaria, *India* **92 G4** 25 43N 70 46 E
Gagarin, *Russia* **58 E8** 55 38N 35 0 E
Gagarin, *Uzbekistan* **65 C4** 40 39N 68 10 E
Găgăuzia □, *Moldova* **53 D13** 46 10N 28 40 E
Gaggenau, *Germany* **31 G4** 48 48N 8 18 E
Gaghamni, *Sudan* **107 E2** 11 41N 28 19 E
Gagino, *Russia* **60 C7** 55 15N 45 1 E
Gagliano del Capo, *Italy* **47 C11** 39 50N 18 22 E
Gagnef, *Sweden* **16 D9** 60 36N 15 5 E
Gagnoa, *Ivory C.* **112 D3** 6 56N 5 16W
Gagnon, *Canada* **141 B6** 51 50N 68 5W
Gagnon, L., *Canada* **143 A6** 62 3N 110 27W
Gago Coutinho, *São Tomé & Príncipe* **115 G6** 0 1 S 6 32 E
Gagra, *Georgia* **61 J5** 43 20N 40 10 E
Gahini, *Rwanda* **118 C3** 1 50 S 30 30 E
Gahmar, *India* **93 G10** 25 27N 83 49 E
Gai Xian = Gaizhou, *China* **75 D12** 40 22N 122 20 E
Gaibanda, *Bangla.* **90 C2** 25 20N 89 36 E
Gaïdhouronísi, *Greece* **39 F6** 34 53N 25 41 E
Gail, *U.S.A.* **155 J4** 32 46N 101 27W
Gail ➝, *Austria* **34 E6** 46 36N 13 53 E
Gaillac, *France* **28 E5** 43 54N 1 54 E
Gaillimh = Galway, *Ireland* **23 C2** 53 17N 9 3W
Gaillon, *France* **26 C8** 49 10N 1 20 E
Gaimán, *Argentina* **176 B3** 43 10 S 65 25W
Gaines, *U.S.A.* **150 E7** 41 46N 77 35W
Gainesville, *Fla., U.S.A.* **153 F7** 29 40N 82 20W
Gainesville, *Ga., U.S.A.* **149 H4** 34 18N 83 50W
Gainesville, *Mo., U.S.A.* **155 G8** 36 36N 92 26W
Gainesville, *Tex., U.S.A.* **155 J6** 33 38N 97 8W
Gainsborough, *U.K.* **20 D7** 53 24N 0 46W
Gairdner, L., *Australia* **128 A2** 31 30 S 136 0 E
Gairloch, *U.K.* **22 D3** 57 43N 5 41W
Gairloch, L., *U.K.* **22 D3** 57 43N 5 45W
Gais, *Switz.* **33 B8** 47 22N 9 27 E
Gaizhou, *China* **75 D12** 40 22N 122 20 E
Gaj, *Croatia* **52 E2** 45 28N 17 3 E
Gaj ➝, *Pakistan* **92 F2** 26 26N 67 21 E
Gajendragarh, *India* **95 G2** 15 44N 75 59 E
Gakona, *U.S.A.* **144 E11** 62 18N 145 18W
Gakuch, *Pakistan* **93 A5** 36 7N 73 45 E
Gal Laghet, *Somali Rep.* **120 D3** 4 9N 47 10 E
Gal Oya △, *Sri Lanka* **95 L5** 7 0N 81 20 E
Gal Oya Res., *Sri Lanka* **95 L5** 7 5N 81 30 E
Gal Tardo, *Somali Rep.* **120 D3** 3 34N 45 58 E
Galaasiya, *Uzbekistan* **65 D2** 39 51N 64 26 E
Galachipa, *Bangla.* **90 D3** 22 8N 90 26 E
Galala, Gebel el, *Egypt* **106 J8** 29 21N 32 22 E
Galán, Cerro, *Argentina* **174 B2** 25 55 S 66 52W
Galana ➝, *Kenya* **118 C5** 3 9 S 40 8 E
Galangue, *Angola* **115 E3** 13 42 S 16 9 E
Galangue, Serra, *Angola* **115 E3** 14 18 S 15 52 E
Galanta, *Slovak Rep.* **35 C10** 48 11N 17 45 E
Galapagar, *Spain* **42 E7** 40 36N 3 58W
Galápagos = Colón, Arch. de, *Ecuador* **172 a** 0 0 91 0W
Galapagos Fracture Zone, *Pac. Oc.* **135 G17** 3 0N 110 0W
Galapagos Rise, *Pac. Oc.* **135 J18** 15 0 S 95 0W
Galashiels, *U.K.* **22 F6** 55 37N 2 49W
Galatás, *Greece* **48 D5** 37 30N 23 26 E
Galatea, *N.Z.* **130 E5** 38 24 S 176 45 E
Galaţi, *Romania* **53 E13** 45 27N 28 2 E
Galaţi □, *Romania* **53 E12** 45 45N 27 30 E
Galatia, *Turkey* **100 C5** 39 30N 33 0 E
Galatina, *Italy* **47 B11** 40 10N 18 10 E
Galátone, *Italy* **47 B11** 40 9N 18 4 E
Galax, *U.S.A.* **149 G5** 36 40N 80 56W
Galaxídhion, *Greece* **48 C4** 38 22N 22 23 E
Galcaio, *Somali Rep.* **120 C3** 6 30N 47 30 E
Galdhøpiggen, *Norway* **18 C5** 61 38N 8 18 E
Galeana, *Chihuahua, Mexico* **162 A3** 30 7N 107 38W
Galeana, *Nuevo León, Mexico* **162 A3** 24 50N 100 4W
Galegu, *Sudan* **107 E4** 12 36N 35 2 E
Galela, *Indonesia* **82 A3.** 1 50N 127 49 E
Galena, *Alaska, U.S.A.* **144 D8** 64 44N 156 56W
Galena, *Ill., U.S.A.* **156 B6** 42 25N 90 26W
Galeota Pt., *Trin. & Tob.* **169 F10** 10 8N 60 59W
Galera, *Spain* **41 H2** 37 45N 2 33W
Galera, Pta., *Chile* **176 A2** 39 59 S 73 43W
Galera, Pta. da, *Azores* **9 d3** 37 42N 25 30W
Galera Pt., *Trin. & Tob.* **169 F10** 10 49N 60 54W
Galesburg, *Ill., U.S.A.* **156 D6** 40 57N 90 22W
Galesburg, *Mich., U.S.A.* **157 B11** 42 17N 85 26W
Galeton, *U.S.A.* **150 E7** 41 44N 77 39W
Galga, *Ethiopia* **107 F4** 6 39N 37 47 E
Galgasc, *Somali Rep.* **120 D2** 0 11N 41 38 E
Galheirão ➝, *Brazil* **171 D2** 12 23 S 45 5W
Galheiros, *Brazil* **171 D2** 13 18 S 46 25W
Gali, *Georgia* **61 J5** 42 37N 41 46 E
Galicea Mare, *Romania* **53 F8** 44 4N 23 19 E
Galich, *Russia* **60 A6** 58 22N 42 24 E
Galiche, *Bulgaria* **50 C7** 43 34N 23 53 E
Galicia □, *Spain* **42 C3** 42 43N 7 45W
Galičica △, *Macedonia* **50 E4** 41 2N 20 55 E
Galien, *U.S.A.* **157 C10** 41 48N 86 30W
Galilee = Hagalil, *Israel* **103 C4** 32 53N 35 18 E
Galilee, L., *Australia* **126 C4** 22 20 S 145 50 E
Galilee, Sea of = Yam Kinneret, *Israel* **103 C4** 32 45N 35 35 E
Galim, *Cameroon* **113 D7** 7 6N 12 25 E
Galina Pt., *Jamaica* **164 a** 18 24N 76 58W
Galinoporni, *Cyprus* **39 E10** 35 31N 34 18 E
Galion, *U.S.A.* **150 F2** 40 44N 82 47W
Galite, Îs. de la, *Tunisia* **111 A6** 37 30N 8 59 E
Galiuro Mts., *U.S.A.* **159 K8** 32 30N 110 20W
Galiwinku, *Australia* **126 A2** 12 2 S 135 34 E
Gallabat, *Sudan* **107 E4** 12 58N 36 11 E

Gallan Hd., *U.K.* **22 C1** 58 15N 7 2W
Gallarate, *Italy* **44 C5** 45 40N 8 48 E
Gallatin, *Mo., U.S.A.* **156 E3** 39 55N 93 58W
Gallatin, *Tenn., U.S.A.* **149 G2** 36 24N 86 27W
Galle, *Sri Lanka* **95 L5** 6 5N 80 10 E
Gállego →, *Spain* **40 D4** 41 39N 0 51W
Gallegos →, *Argentina* **176 D3** 51 35 S 69 0W
Galletti →, *Ethiopia* **107 F5** 8 46N 41 10 E
Galley Hd., *Ireland* **23 E3** 51 32N 8 55W
Galliate, *Italy* **44 C5** 45 29N 8 42 E
Gallinas, Pta., *Colombia* **168 A3** 12 28N 71 40W
Gallipoli = Gelibolu, *Turkey* **51 F10** 40 28N 26 43 E
Gallípoli, *Italy* **47 B10** 40 3N 17 58 E
Gallipolis, *U.S.A.* **148 F4** 38 49N 82 12W
Gällivare, *Sweden* **14 C19** 67 9N 20 40 E
Gallneukirchen, *Austria* **34 C7** 48 21N 14 25 E
Gällö, *Sweden* **16 B9** 62 55N 15 13 E
Gallo, C., *Italy* **46 D6** 38 13N 13 19 E
Gallocanta, L. de, *Spain* **40 E3** 40 58N 1 30W
Galloo I., *U.S.A.* **151 C8** 43 55N 76 25W
Galloway, *U.K.* **22 F4** 55 1N 4 29W
Galloway ⌓, *U.K.* **22 F4** 55 3N 4 20W
Galloway, Mull of, *U.K.* **22 G4** 54 39N 4 52W
Gallup, *U.S.A.* **159 J9** 35 32N 108 45W
Gallur, *Spain* **40 D3** 41 52N 1 19W
Gallyaaral, *Uzbekistan* **65 C3** 40 2N 67 35 E
Galong, *Australia* **129 C8** 34 37 S 148 34 E
Galoya, *Sri Lanka* **95 K5** 8 10N 80 55 E
Galt, *Calif., U.S.A.* **160 G5** 38 15N 121 18W
Galt, *Mo., U.S.A.* **156 D3** 40 8N 93 23W
Galten, *Denmark* **17 H3** 56 9N 9 54 E
Galtür, *Austria* **34 E3** 46 58N 10 11 E
Galty Mts., *Ireland* **23 D3** 52 22N 8 10W
Galtymore, *Ireland* **23 D3** 52 21N 8 11W
Galva, *U.S.A.* **156 C6** 41 10N 90 3W
Galvarino, *Chile* **176 A2** 38 24 S 72 47W
Galve de Sorbe, *Spain* **40 D1** 41 13N 3 10W
Galveston, *Ind., U.S.A.* **157 D10** 40 35N 86 11W
Galveston, *Tex., U.S.A.* **155 L7** 29 18N 94 48W
Galveston B., *U.S.A.* **155 L7** 29 36N 94 50W
Gálvez, *Argentina* **174 C3** 32 0 S 61 14W
Galway, *Ireland* **23 C2** 53 17N 9 3W
Galway □, *Ireland* **23 C2** 53 22N 9 1W
Galway B., *Ireland* **23 C2** 53 13N 9 10W
Gam, *Indonesia* **83 B4** 0 27 S 130 36 E
Gam →, *Vietnam* **86 B5** 21 55N 105 12 E
Gamagōri, *Japan* **73 C9** 34 50N 137 14 E
Gamari, L., *Ethiopia* **107 E5** 11 32N 41 40 E
Gamawa, *Nigeria* **113 C7** 12 10N 10 31 E
Gamay, *Phil.* **80 E5** 12 23N 125 18 E
Gamay Bay, *Phil.* **80 E5** 12 21N 125 21 E
Gamba, *Angola* **115 E3** 11 42 S 17 14 E
Gambaga, *Ghana* **113 C4** 10 30N 0 28W
Gambat, *Pakistan* **92 F3** 27 17N 68 26 E
Gambela, *Ethiopia* **107 F3** 8 14N 34 38 E
Gambela △, *Ethiopia* **107 F3** 8 0N 34 0 E
Gambela-Hizboch □, *Ethiopia* **107 F3** 8 0N 34 0 E
Gambell, *U.S.A.* **144 E5** 63 47N 171 45W
Gambhir →, *India* **92 F6** 26 58N 77 27 E
Gambia ■, *W. Afr.* **112 C1** 13 25N 16 0W
Gambia →, *W. Afr.* **112 C1** 13 28N 16 34W
Gambier, *U.S.A.* **150 F2** 40 22N 82 23W
Gambier, C., *Australia* **124 B5** 11 56 S 130 57 E
Gambier, Îs., *French Polynesia* **135 K14** 23 8 S 134 58W
Gambier Is., *Australia* **128 C2** 35 3 S 136 30 E
Gambier Village, *Bahamas* **9 b** 25 4N 77 30W
Gambo, *C.A.R.* **114 B4** 4 39N 22 16 E
Gambo, *Canada* **141 C9** 48 47N 54 13W
Gamboli, *Pakistan* **92 E3** 29 53N 68 24 E
Gamboma, *Congo* **114 C3** 1 55 S 15 52 E
Gamboula, *C.A.R.* **114 B3** 4 8N 15 9 E
Gambuta, *Indonesia* **82 A2** 0 30N 123 20 E
Gamka →, *S. Africa* **116 E3** 33 18 S 21 39 E
Gamkab →, *Namibia* **116 D2** 28 4 S 17 54 E
Gamla Uppsala, *Sweden* **16 E11** 59 54N 17 40 E
Gamlakarleby = Kokkola, *Finland* **14 E20** 63 50N 23 8 E
Gamleby, *Sweden* **17 G10** 57 54N 16 24 E
Gammon →, *Canada* **143 C9** 51 24N 95 44W
Gammon Ranges △, *Australia* **127 E2** 30 38 S 139 8 E
Gammouda, *Tunisia* **108 A1** 35 3N 9 39 E
Gamo-Gofa, *Ethiopia* **107 F4** 5 40N 36 40 E
Gamoda-Saki, *Japan* **72 D6** 33 50N 134 45 E
Gamou, *Niger* **113 C6** 14 20N 9 55 E
Gampaha, *Sri Lanka* **95 L4** 7 5N 79 59 E
Gampel, *Switz.* **32 D5** 46 19N 7 44 E
Gampola, *Sri Lanka* **95 L5** 7 10N 80 34 E
Gams, *Switz.* **33 B8** 47 12N 9 26 E
Gamtoos →, *S. Africa* **116 E4** 33 58 S 25 1 E
Gan, *France* **28 E3** 43 12N 0 27W
Gan Gan, *Argentina* **176 B3** 42 30 S 68 10W
Gan Goriama, Mts., *Cameroon* **113 D7** 7 44N 12 45 E
Gan Jiang →, *China* **77 C11** 29 15N 116 0 E
Ganado, *U.S.A.* **159 J9** 35 43N 109 33W
Gananita, *Sudan* **106 D3** 18 22N 33 50 E
Gananoque, *Canada* **140 D4** 44 20N 76 10W
Ganassi, *Phil.* **81 H5** 7 49N 124 6 E
Ganāveh, *Iran* **97 D6** 29 35N 50 35 E
Gäncä, *Azerbaijan* **61 K8** 40 45N 46 20 E
Gancheng, *China* **86 C7** 18 51N 108 37 E
Gand = Gent, *Belgium* **24 C3** 51 2N 3 42 E
Ganda, *Angola* **115 E2** 13 3 S 14 35 E
Gandajika, *Dem. Rep. of the Congo* **115 D4** 6 46 S 23 58 E
Gandak →, *India* **93 G11** 25 39N 85 13 E
Gandara, *Phil.* **80 E5** 12 1N 124 49 E
Gandava, *Pakistan* **91 C2** 28 32N 67 32 E
Gander, *Canada* **141 C9** 48 58N 54 35W
Gander L., *Canada* **141 C9** 48 58N 54 35W
Ganderkesee, *Germany* **30 B4** 53 2N 8 32 E
Ganderowe Falls, *Zimbabwe* **119 F2** 17 20 S 29 10 E
Gandesa, *Spain* **40 D5** 41 3N 0 26 E
Gandhi Sagar, *India* **92 G6** 24 40N 75 40 E
Gandhinagar, *India* **92 H5** 23 15N 72 45 E
Gandi, *Nigeria* **113 C6** 12 55N 5 49 E
Gandía, *Spain* **41 G4** 38 58N 0 9W
Gandino, *Italy* **44 C6** 45 49N 9 54 E
Gando, Pta., *Canary Is.* **9 e1** 27 55N 15 22W
Gandole, *Nigeria* **113 D7** 8 28N 11 35 E
Gandou, *Congo* **114 B3** 2 25N 17 25 E
Gandu, *Brazil* **171 D4** 13 45 S 39 30W
Gâneb, *Mauritania* **112 B2** 18 29N 10 8W
Ganedidalem = Gani, *Indonesia* **82 B3** 0 48 S 128 14 E
Ganetti, *Sudan* **106 D3** 18 0N 31 10 E
Ganga →, *India* **93 H14** 23 20N 90 30 E
Ganga Sagar, *India* **93 J13** 21 38N 88 5 E
Gangafani, *Mali* **112 C4** 14 20N 2 20W
Gangakher, *India* **94 E3** 18 57N 76 45 E
Gangan →, *India* **93 E8** 28 38N 78 58 E
Ganganagar, *India* **92 E5** 29 56N 73 56 E
Gangapur, *Maharashtra, India* **94 E2** 19 41N 75 1 E
Gangapur, *Raj., India* **92 F7** 26 32N 76 49 E
Gangara, *Niger* **113 C6** 14 35N 8 29 E
Gangaw, *Burma* **90 D5** 22 5N 94 5 E
Gangaw Taungdan, *Burma* **90 C6** 24 55N 96 35 E
Gangawati, *India* **95 G3** 15 30N 76 36 E
Ganges = Ganga →, *India* **93 H14** 23 20N 90 30 E
Ganges, *Canada* **142 D4** 48 51N 123 31W
Ganges, *France* **28 E7** 43 56N 3 42 E
Ganges, Mouths of the, *India* **90 E3** 21 30N 90 0 E
Gånghester, *Sweden* **17 G7** 57 42N 13 1 E
Gangi, *Italy* **47 E7** 37 48N 14 12 E
Gângiova, *Romania* **53 G8** 43 54N 23 50 E
Gangoh, *India* **92 E7** 29 46N 77 18 E
Gangotri, *India* **93 D8** 30 50N 79 10 E
Gangotri △, *India* **93 D8** 30 50N 79 10 E
Gangtok, *India* **90 B2** 27 20N 88 37 E
Gangu, *China* **74 G3** 34 40N 105 15 E
Gangwa, *Dem. Rep. of the Congo* **114 C4** 3 30 S 20 54 E
Gangyao, *China* **75 B14** 44 12N 126 37 E
Gani, *Indonesia* **82 B3** 0 48 S 128 14 E
Ganj, *India* **93 F8** 27 45N 78 57 E
Ganjam, *India* **94 E7** 19 23N 85 4 E
Ganluc, *China* **76 C4** 28 58N 102 59 E
Ganmain, *Australia* **129 C7** 34 47 S 147 1 E
Gannat, *France* **27 F10** 46 7N 3 11 E
Gannett Peak, *U.S.A.* **158 E9** 43 11N 109 39W
Ganquan, *China* **74 F5** 36 20N 109 20 E
Gänserdorf, *Austria* **35 C9** 48 20N 16 43 E
Ganshui, *China* **76 C6** 28 40N 106 40 E
Gansu □, *China* **74 G3** 36 0N 104 0 E
Ganta, *Liberia* **112 D3** 7 15N 8 59W
Gantheaume, C., *Australia* **128 D2** 36 4 S 137 32 E
Gantheaume B., *Australia* **125 E1** 27 40 S 114 10 E
Gantsevichi = Hantsavichy, *Belarus* **59 F4** 52 49N 26 30 E
Ganye, *Nigeria* **113 D7** 8 25N 12 4 E
Ganyem = Genyem, *Indonesia* **83 B6** 2 46 S 140 12 E
Ganyu, *China* **75 G10** 34 50N 119 8 E
Ganyushkino, *Kazakhstan* **61 G9** 46 35N 49 20 E
Ganzhou, *China* **77 E10** 25 51N 114 56 E
Gao, *Mali* **113 B4** 16 15N 0 5W
Gao Xian, *China* **76 C5** 28 21N 104 32 E
Gao'an, *China* **77 C10** 28 26N 115 17 E
Gaochun, *China* **77 B12** 31 20N 118 49 E
Gaohe, *China* **77 F9** 22 46N 112 57 E
Gaohebu, *China* **77 B11** 30 43N 116 49 E
Gaokeng, *China* **77 D9** 27 40N 113 58 E
Gaolan Dao, *China* **77 G9** 21 55N 113 10 E
Gaoligong Shan, *China* **76 E2** 24 45N 98 45 E
Gaomi, *China* **75 F10** 36 20N 119 42 E
Gaoping, *China* **74 G7** 35 45N 112 55 E
Gaotang, *China* **74 F9** 36 50N 116 15 E
Gaoua, *Burkina Faso* **112 C4** 10 20N 3 8W
Gaoual, *Guinea* **112 C2** 11 45N 13 25W
Gaoxiong = Kaohsiung, *Taiwan* **77 F13** 22 35N 120 16 E
Gaoyang, *China* **74 E8** 38 40N 115 45 E
Gaoyao, *China* **77 F9** 23 3N 112 27 E
Gaoyou, *China* **77 A12** 32 47N 119 26 E
Gaoyou Hu, *China* **75 H10** 32 45N 119 20 E
Gaoyuan, *China* **75 F9** 37 8N 117 58 E
Gaozhou, *China* **77 G8** 21 58N 110 50 E
Gap, *France* **29 D10** 44 33N 6 5 E
Gapan, *Phil.* **80 D3** 15 19N 120 57 E
Gapat →, *India* **93 G10** 24 30N 82 28 E
Gapuwiyak, *Australia* **126 A2** 12 25 S 135 43 E
Gar, *China* **68 C2** 32 10N 79 58 E
Garabekewül, *Turkmenistan* **65 D2** 38 30N 64 8 E
Garabogazköl Aylagy, *Turkmenistan* **57 F9** 41 0N 53 30 E
Garachico, *Canary Is.* **9 e1** 28 22N 16 46W
Garachiné, *Panama* **164 E4** 8 0N 78 12W
Garad, *Somali Rep.* **120 C3** 6 57N 49 24 E
Garafia, *Canary Is.* **9 e1** 28 48N 17 57W
Garah, *Australia* **127 D4** 29 5 S 149 38 E
Garaina, *Papua N. G.* **132 D4** 7 53 S 147 8 E
Garajonay, *Canary Is.* **9 e1** 28 7N 17 14W
Garamätnyyaz, *Turkmenistan* **65 E2** 37 45N 64 34 E
Garamba △, *Dem. Rep. of the Congo* **118 B2** 4 10N 29 40 E
Garango, *Burkina Faso* **113 C4** 11 48N 0 34W
Garanhuns, *Brazil* **170 C4** 8 50 S 36 30W
Garautha, *India* **93 G8** 25 34N 79 18 E
Garavuti, *Tajikistan* **65 E4** 37 34N 68 26 E
Garawe, *Liberia* **112 E3** 4 35N 8 0W
Garba Harre, *Somali Rep.* **120 D2** 3 19N 42 13 E
Garba Tula, *Kenya* **118 B4** 0 30N 38 32 E
Garbagududu, *Ethiopia* **120 C2** 6 12N 43 50 E
Garbahaarrey = Garba Harre, *Somali Rep.* **120 D2** 3 19N 42 13 E
Garberville, *U.S.A.* **158 F2** 40 6N 123 48W
Garbiyang, *India* **93 D9** 30 8N 80 54 E
Garbsen, *Germany* **30 C5** 52 26N 9 31 E
Garça, *Brazil* **171 F2** 22 14 S 49 37W
Garças →, *Mato Grosso, Brazil* **173 D7** 15 54 S 52 16W
Garças →, *Pernambuco, Brazil* **170 C4** 8 43 S 39 41W
Garchitorena, *Phil.* **80 E4** 13 52N 123 40 E
Garcia Hernandez, *Phil.* **81 G5** 9 37N 124 18 E
Garcias, *Brazil* **173 E7** 20 34 S 52 13W
Gard □, *France* **29 D8** 44 2N 4 10 E
Gard →, *France* **29 E8** 43 51N 4 37 E
Garda, L. di, *Italy* **44 C7** 45 40N 10 41 E
Gardanne, *France* **29 E9** 43 27N 5 27 E
Gårdby, *Sweden* **17 H10** 56 36N 16 38 E
Garde L., *Canada* **143 A7** 62 50N 106 13W
Gardelegen, *Germany* **30 C7** 52 32N 11 24 E
Garden City, *Ga., U.S.A.* **152 C8** 32 6N 81 9W
Garden City, *Idaho, U.S.A.* **158 E5** 43 38N 116 16W
Garden City, *Kans., U.S.A.* **155 G4** 37 58N 100 53W
Garden City, *Mo., U.S.A.* **156 F2** 38 34N 94 12W
Garden City, *Tex., U.S.A.* **155 K4** 31 52N 101 29W
Garden Grove, *U.S.A.* **161 M9** 33 47N 117 55W
Gardēz, *Afghan.* **91 B3** 33 37N 69 9 E
Gardhíki, *Greece* **48 C3** 38 50N 21 55 E
Garður, *Iceland* **11 A10** 66 4N 16 46W
Gardiner, *Maine, U.S.A.* **149 C11** 44 14N 69 47W
Gardiner, *Mont., U.S.A.* **158 D8** 45 2N 110 22W
Gardiners I., *U.S.A.* **151 E12** 41 6N 72 6W
Gardner, *Fla., U.S.A.* **153 H8** 27 21N 81 48W
Gardner, *Ill., U.S.A.* **157 C8** 41 12N 88 17W
Gardner, *Mass., U.S.A.* **151 D13** 42 34N 71 59W
Gardner Canal, *Canada* **142 C3** 53 27N 128 8W
Gardner Pinnacles, *U.S.A.* **145 G10** 25 0N 167 55W
Gardnerville, *U.S.A.* **160 G7** 38 56N 119 45W
Gardno, Jezioro, *Poland* **54 D4** 54 40N 17 7 E
Gardo, *Somali Rep.* **120 C3** 9 30N 49 6 E
Gardone Val Trómpia, *Italy* **44 C7** 45 41N 10 11 E
Gárdony, *Hungary* **52 C3** 47 12N 18 39 E
Gare Tigre, *Fr. Guiana* **169 C7** 4 58N 53 9W
Gareloi I., *U.S.A.* **144 L3** 51 48N 178 48W
Garešnica, *Croatia* **45 C13** 45 36N 16 56 E
Garéssio, *Italy* **44 D5** 44 12N 8 2 E
Garey, *U.S.A.* **161 L6** 34 53N 120 19W
Garfield, *U.S.A.* **158 C5** 47 1N 117 9W
Garforth, *U.K.* **20 D6** 53 47N 1 24W
Gargaliánoi, *Greece* **48 D3** 37 4N 21 38 E
Gargan, Mt., *France* **28 C5** 45 37N 1 39 E
Gargano △, *Italy* **45 G12** 41 43N 15 52 E
Gargantua, C., *Canada* **148 B3** 47 36N 85 2W
Gargett, *Australia* **126 K6** 21 9 S 148 46 E
Gargouna, *Mali* **113 B5** 15 56N 0 13 E
Gargždai, *Lithuania* **54 C8** 55 43N 21 24 E
Garhchiroli, *India* **94 D5** 20 10N 80 0 E
Gari, *Russia* **64 B9** 59 26N 62 21 E
Garibaldi ⌓, *Canada* **142 D4** 49 50N 122 40W
Gariep, L., *S. Africa* **116 E4** 30 40 S 25 40 E
Garies, *S. Africa* **116 E2** 30 32 S 17 59 E
Garigliano →, *Italy* **46 A6** 41 13N 13 45 E
Garissa, *Kenya* **118 C4** 0 25 S 39 40 E
Garkida, *Nigeria* **113 C7** 10 27N 12 36 E
Garko, *Nigeria* **113 C6** 11 45N 8 35 E
Garland, *Tex., U.S.A.* **155 J6** 32 55N 96 38W
Garland, *Utah, U.S.A.* **158 F7** 41 47N 112 10W
Garlasco, *Italy* **44 C5** 45 12N 8 55 E
Garliava, *Lithuania* **54 D10** 54 49N 23 52 E
Garlin, *France* **28 E3** 43 33N 0 16W
Garm, *Tajikistan* **65 D5** 39 0N 70 20 E
Garmāb, *Iran* **97 C8** 35 25N 56 45 E
Garmisch-Partenkirchen, *Germany* **31 H7** 47 30N 11 6 E
Garmo, Qullai = Kommunizma, Pik, *Tajikistan* **65 D6** 39 0N 72 2 E
Garmsār, *Iran* **97 C7** 35 20N 52 25 E
Garner, *U.S.A.* **156 A3** 43 6N 93 36W
Garnett, *U.S.A.* **154 F7** 38 17N 95 14W
Garnpung L., *Australia* **128 B5** 33 25 S 143 10 E
Garo Hills, *India* **90 C3** 25 30N 90 30 E
Garoe, *Somali Rep.* **120 C3** 8 25N 48 33 E
Garonne →, *France* **28 C3** 45 2N 0 36W
Garonne, Canal Latéral à la, *France* **28 D4** 44 15N 0 18 E
Garoowe = Garoe, *Somali Rep.* **120 C3** 8 25N 48 33 E
Garot, *India* **92 G6** 24 19N 75 41 E
Garoua, *Cameroon* **113 D7** 9 19N 13 21 E
Garove I., *Papua N. G.* **132 C5** 4 42 S 149 30 E
Garpenberg, *Sweden* **16 D10** 60 19N 16 12 E
Garphyttan, *Sweden* **16 E8** 59 18N 14 56 E
Garrauli, *India* **93 G8** 25 5N 79 22 E
Garrel, *Germany* **30 C4** 52 57N 8 1 E
Garrett, *U.S.A.* **157 C11** 41 21N 85 8W
Garrigues, *France* **28 E7** 43 40N 3 55 E
Garrison, *Ky., U.S.A.* **157 F13** 38 36N 83 10W
Garrison, *Mont., U.S.A.* **158 C7** 46 31N 112 49W
Garrison, *N. Dak., U.S.A.* **154 B4** 47 40N 101 25W
Garrison Res. = Sakakawea, L., *U.S.A.* **154 B4** 47 30N 101 25W
Garron Pt., *U.K.* **23 A6** 55 3N 5 59W
Garrovillas, *Spain* **43 F4** 39 40N 6 33W
Garrucha, *Spain* **41 H3** 37 11N 1 49W
Garry →, *U.K.* **22 E5** 56 44N 3 47W
Garry, L., *Canada* **138 B9** 65 58N 100 18W
Garsen, *Kenya* **118 C5** 2 20 S 40 5 E
Gärsnäs, *Sweden* **17 J8** 55 32N 14 10 E
Garson L., *Canada* **143 B6** 56 19N 110 2W
Garstang, *U.K.* **20 D5** 53 55N 2 46W
Gartempe →, *France* **28 B4** 46 47N 0 49 E
Gartz, *Germany* **30 B10** 53 13N 14 22 E
Garu, *Ghana* **113 C4** 10 55N 0 11W
Garu, *India* **93 H11** 23 40N 84 14 E
Garub, *Namibia* **116 D2** 26 37 S 16 0 E
Garut, *Indonesia* **85 D3** 7 14 S 107 53 E
Garvão, *Portugal* **43 H2** 37 42N 8 21W
Garvie Mts., *N.Z.* **131 F3** 45 30 S 168 50 E
Garwa = Garoua, *Cameroon* **113 D7** 9 19N 13 21 E
Garwa, *India* **93 G10** 24 11N 83 47 E
Garwolin, *Poland* **55 G8** 51 55N 21 38 E
Gary, *U.S.A.* **157 C9** 41 36N 87 20W
Garz, *Germany* **30 A9** 54 19N 13 20 E
Garzê, *China* **76 B3** 31 38N 100 1 E
Garzón, *Colombia* **168 C2** 2 10N 75 40W
Gas City, *U.S.A.* **157 D11** 40 29N 85 37W
Gas-San, *Japan* **70 E10** 38 32N 140 1 E
Gasan, *Phil.* **80 E3** 13 19N 121 51 E
Gasan Kuli = Esenguly, *Turkmenistan* **66 F6** 37 37N 53 59 E
Gaschurn, *Austria* **33 C10** 46 59N 10 2 E
Gascogne, *France* **28 E4** 43 45N 0 20 E
Gascogne, G. de, *Europe* **28 E2** 44 0N 2 0W
Gasconade, *U.S.A.* **156 F5** 38 40N 91 34W
Gasconade →, *U.S.A.* **156 F5** 38 41N 91 33W
Gascony = Gascogne, *France* **28 E4** 43 45N 0 20 E
Gascoyne →, *Australia* **125 D1** 24 52 S 113 37 E
Gascoyne Junction, *Australia* **125 E2** 25 2 S 115 17 E
Gascueña, *Spain* **40 E2** 40 18N 2 31W
Gash, Wadi →, *Ethiopia* **107 D4** 16 48N 35 51 E
Gash-Setit ⌓, *Eritrea* **107 D4** 15 12N 36 58 E
Gashagar, *Nigeria* **113 C7** 13 22N 12 47 E
Gashaka, *Nigeria* **113 D7** 7 20N 11 29 E
Gashaka-Gumti △, *Nigeria* **113 D7** 7 23N 11 34 E
Gasherbrum, *Pakistan* **93 B7** 35 40N 76 40 E
Gashua, *Nigeria* **113 C7** 12 54N 11 0 E
Gasmata, *Papua N. G.* **132 D6** 6 17 S 150 20 E
Gasparilla I., *U.S.A.* **153 J7** 26 46N 82 16W
Gasparillo, *Trin. & Tob.* **169 F9** 10 18N 61 26W
Gaspé, *Canada* **141 C7** 48 52N 64 30W
Gaspé, C., *Canada* **141 C7** 48 48N 64 7W
Gaspé Pen. = Gaspésie, Pén. de la, *Canada* **141 C6** 48 45N 65 40W
Gaspésie ⌓, *Canada* **141 C6** 48 55N 66 10W
Gaspésie, Pén. de la, *Canada* **141 C6** 48 45N 65 40W
Gassan, *Burkina Faso* **112 C4** 12 49N 3 12W
Gassen = Jasień, *Poland* **55 G2** 51 46N 15 0 E
Gassol, *Nigeria* **113 D7** 8 34N 10 25 E
Gasteiz = Vitoria-Gasteiz, *Spain* **40 C2** 42 50N 2 41W
Gaston, *U.S.A.* **152 B8** 33 49N 81 5W
Gastonia, *U.S.A.* **149 H5** 35 16N 81 11W
Gastoúni, *Greece* **48 D3** 37 51N 21 15 E
Gastoúri, *Greece* **38 B9** 39 34N 19 54 E
Gastre, *Argentina* **176 B3** 42 20 S 69 15W
Gästrikland, *Sweden* **16 D10** 60 45N 16 40 E
Gata, C., *Cyprus* **39 F9** 34 34N 33 2 E
Gata, C. de, *Spain* **41 J2** 36 41N 2 13W
Gata, Sierra de, *Spain* **42 E4** 40 20N 6 45W
Gataga →, *Canada* **142 B3** 58 35N 126 59W
Gătaia, *Romania* **52 E6** 45 26N 21 30 E
Gatchina, *Russia* **58 C6** 59 35N 30 9 E
Gatehouse of Fleet, *U.K.* **22 G4** 54 53N 4 12W
Gates, *U.S.A.* **150 C7** 43 9N 77 42W
Gates of the Arctic △, *U.S.A.* **144 C10** 67 20N 152 0W
Gateshead, *U.K.* **20 C6** 54 57N 1 35W
Gatesville, *U.S.A.* **155 K6** 31 26N 97 45W
Gateway ⌓, *U.S.A.* **151 F11** 40 26N 73 59W
Gaths, *Zimbabwe* **119 G3** 20 2 S 30 32 E
Gatico, *Chile* **174 A1** 22 29 S 70 20W
Gâtinais, *France* **27 D9** 48 5N 2 40 E
Gâtine, Hauteurs de, *France* **28 B3** 46 35N 0 45W
Gatineau, *Canada* **151 A9** 45 29N 75 38W
Gatineau △, *Canada* **140 C4** 45 40N 76 0W
Gatineau →, *Canada* **140 C4** 45 27N 75 42W
Gattaran, *Phil.* **80 B3** 18 4N 121 38 E
Gattinara, *Italy* **44 C5** 45 37N 8 22 E
Gatton, *Australia* **127 D5** 27 32 S 152 17 E
Gatun, L., *Panama* **164 E4** 9 7N 79 56W
Gatwick, London ✈ (LGW), *U.K.* **21 F7** 51 10N 0 11W
Gatyana, *S. Africa* **117 E4** 32 16 S 28 31 E
Gau, *Fiji* **133 B2** 18 2 S 179 18 E
Gaua, *Vanuatu* **133 D5** 14 15 S 167 30 E
Gaucín, *Spain* **43 J5** 36 31N 5 19W
Gauer L., *Canada* **143 B9** 57 0N 97 50W
Gauhati = Guwahati, *India* **90 B3** 26 10N 91 45 E
Gauja →, *Latvia* **15 H21** 57 10N 24 16 E
Gaula →, *Norway* **18 A7** 63 21N 10 14 E
Gaupne, *Norway* **18 C4** 61 25N 7 18 E
Gaurdak = Gowurdak, *Turkmenistan* **65 E3** 37 50N 66 4 E
Gauri Phanta, *India* **93 E9** 28 41N 80 36 E
Gauribidanur, *India* **95 H3** 13 37N 77 32 E
Gausta, *Norway* **18 E5** 59 48N 8 40 E
Gauteng □, *S. Africa* **117 D4** 26 0 S 28 0 E
Gāv Koshī, *Iran* **97 D8** 28 38N 57 12 E
Gāvakān, *Iran* **97 D7** 29 37N 53 10 E
Gavallai △, *Liberia* **112 D3** 5 8N 7 20W
Gavarnie, *France* **28 F3** 42 44N 0 1W
Gavāter, *Iran* **97 E9** 25 10N 61 31 E
Gāvbandī, *Iran* **97 E7** 27 12N 53 4 E
Gavdhopoúla, *Greece* **39 F5** 34 56N 24 0 E
Gávdhos, *Greece* **39 F5** 34 50N 24 5 E
Gavdos = Gávdhos, *Greece* **39 F5** 34 50N 24 5 E
Gavi, *Italy* **44 D5** 44 41N 8 49 E
Gavião, *Portugal* **43 F3** 39 28N 7 56W
Gaviota, *U.S.A.* **161 L6** 34 29N 120 13W
Gāvkhūnī, Bāţlāq-e, *Iran* **97 C7** 32 6N 52 52 E
Gävle, *Sweden* **16 D11** 60 40N 17 9 E
Gävleborgs län □, *Sweden* **16 C10** 61 30N 16 15 E
Gävlebukten, *Sweden* **16 D11** 60 40N 17 20 E
Gavorrano, *Italy* **44 F7** 42 55N 10 54 E
Gavray, *France* **26 D5** 48 55N 1 20W
Gavrilov Yam, *Russia* **58 D10** 57 18N 39 49 E
Gávrion, *Greece* **48 D6** 37 54N 24 44 E
Gawachab, *Namibia* **116 D2** 27 4 S 17 55 E
Gawai, *Burma* **90 B6** 27 56N 97 30 E
Gawilgarh Hills, *India* **94 D3** 21 15N 76 45 E
Gawler, *Australia* **128 C3** 34 30 S 138 42 E
Gawler Ranges, *Australia* **128 B2** 32 20 S 136 0 E
Gawu, *Nigeria* **113 D6** 9 14N 6 52 E
Gaxun Nur, *China* **68 B5** 42 22N 100 30 E
Gay, *Russia* **64 F7** 51 27N 58 27 E
Gay, *U.S.A.* **152 B5** 33 6N 84 35W
Gaya, *India* **93 G11** 24 47N 85 4 E
Gaya, *Niger* **113 C5** 11 52N 3 28 E
Gaya, *Nigeria* **113 C6** 11 57N 9 0 E
Gayéri, *Burkina Faso* **113 C5** 12 39N 0 29 E
Gaylord, *U.S.A.* **148 C3** 45 2N 84 41W
Gayndah, *Australia* **127 D5** 25 35 S 151 32 E
Gayny, *Russia* **64 A5** 60 18N 54 19 E
Gaysin = Haysyn, *Ukraine* **53 B14** 48 57N 29 25 E
Gayvoron = Hayvoron, *Ukraine* **53 B14** 48 22N 29 52 E
Gaza, *Gaza Strip* **103 D3** 31 30N 34 28 E
Gaza □, *Mozam.* **117 C5** 23 10 S 32 45 E
Gaza Strip ⧄, *Asia* **103 D3** 31 29N 34 25 E
Gazalkent, *Uzbekistan* **65 C4** 41 33N 69 46 E
Gazanjyk, *Turkmenistan* **97 B7** 39 16N 55 32 E
Gazaoua, *Niger* **113 C6** 13 32N 7 55 E
Gāzbor, *Iran* **97 D8** 28 5N 58 51 E
Gazelle, Récif de la, *N. Cal.* **133 T19** 20 10 S 165 30 E
Gazelle Pen., *Papua N. G.* **132 C6** 4 40 S 152 0 E
Gazi, *Dem. Rep. of the Congo* **118 B1** 1 3N 24 30 E
Gaziantep, *Turkey* **100 D7** 37 6N 37 23 E
Gazimağosa = Famagusta, *Cyprus* **39 E9** 35 8N 33 55 E
Gazipaşa, *Turkey* **100 D5** 36 16N 32 18 E
Gbarnga, *Liberia* **112 D3** 7 19N 9 13W
Gbekebo, *Nigeria* **113 D5** 6 20N 4 56 E
Gboko, *Nigeria* **113 D6** 7 17N 9 4 E
Gbongan, *Nigeria* **113 D5** 7 28N 4 20 E
Gcoverega, *Botswana* **116 B3** 19 8 S 24 18 E
Gcuwa, *S. Africa* **117 E4** 32 20 S 28 11 E
Gdańsk, *Poland* **54 D5** 54 22N 18 40 E
Gdansk ✈ (GDN), *Poland* **54 D5** 54 22N 18 30 E
Gdańska, Zatoka, *Poland* **54 D6** 54 30N 19 20 E
Gdingen = Gdynia, *Poland* **54 D5** 54 35N 18 33 E
Gdov, *Russia* **15 G22** 58 48N 27 55 E
Gdynia, *Poland* **54 D5** 54 35N 18 33 E
Geba →, *Guinea-Biss.* **112 C1** 11 46N 15 36W
Gebe, *Indonesia* **83 A3** 0 5N 129 25 E
Gebeciler, *Turkey* **49 C12** 38 46N 30 46 E
Gebeit Mine, *Sudan* **106 C4** 21 3N 36 29 E
Gebel Abyad, *Sudan* **106 D2** 19 0N 28 0 E
Gebel Iweibid, *Egypt* **106 H8** 30 8N 32 13 E
Gebze, *Turkey* **51 F13** 40 47N 29 25 E
Gecha, *Ethiopia* **107 F4** 7 30N 35 18 E
Gedaref, *Sudan* **107 E4** 14 2N 35 28 E
Gedaref □, *Sudan* **107 E4** 14 0N 35 0 E
Gede, Tanjung, *Indonesia* **84 D3** 6 46 S 105 12 E
Gediz, *Turkey* **49 B11** 39 1N 29 24 E
Gediz →, *Turkey* **49 C8** 38 35N 26 48 E
Gedo, *Ethiopia* **107 F4** 9 2N 37 25 E
Gèdre, *France* **28 F4** 42 47N 0 2 E
Gedser, *Denmark* **17 K5** 54 35N 11 55 E
Gedung, Pulau, *Malaysia* **87 c** 5 17N 100 23 E
Geegully Cr. →, *Australia* **124 C3** 18 32 S 123 41 E
Geel, *Belgium* **24 C4** 51 10N 4 59 E
Geelong, *Australia* **128 E6** 38 10 S 144 22 E
Geelvink B. = Cenderwasih, Teluk, *Indonesia* **79 E9** 3 0 S 135 20 E
Geelvink Chan., *Australia* **125 E1** 28 30 S 114 0 E
Geesthacht, *Germany* **30 B6** 53 26N 10 22 E
Geidam, *Nigeria* **113 C7** 12 57N 11 57 E
Geikie →, *Canada* **143 B8** 57 45N 103 52W
Geikie Gorge △, *Australia* **124 C4** 18 3 S 125 41 E
Geilenkirchen, *Germany* **30 E2** 50 57N 6 8 E
Geili, *Sudan* **107 D3** 16 1N 32 37 E
Geilo, *Norway* **18 D5** 60 32N 8 14 E
Geisingen, *Germany* **31 H4** 47 54N 8 38 E
Geislingen, *Germany* **31 G5** 48 37N 9 50 E
Geistown, *U.S.A.* **150 F6** 40 18N 78 52W
Geita, *Tanzania* **118 C3** 2 48 S 32 12 E
Geitastrand, *Norway* **18 A6** 63 22N 9 56 E
Geithus, *Norway* **18 E6** 59 57N 9 59 E
Gejiu, *China* **76 F4** 23 20N 103 10 E
Gel →, *Sudan* **107 F2** 7 5N 29 10 E
Gel, Meydān-e, *Iran* **97 D7** 29 4N 54 50 E
Gel River, *Sudan* **107 F2** 7 5N 29 10 E
Gela, *Italy* **47 E7** 37 4N 14 15 E
Gela, G. di, *Italy* **47 F7** 37 0N 14 20 E
Geladi, *Ethiopia* **120 C3** 6 59N 46 30 E
Gelahun, *Liberia* **112 D2** 7 55N 10 28W
Gelang Patah, *Malaysia* **87 d** 1 27N 103 35 E
Gelderland □, *Neths.* **24 B6** 52 5N 6 10 E
Geldern, *Germany* **30 D2** 51 31N 6 20 E
Geldrop, *Neths.* **24 C5** 51 25N 5 32 E
Geleen, *Neths.* **24 D5** 50 57N 5 49 E
Gelehun, *S. Leone* **112 D2** 8 20N 11 40W
Gelembe, *Turkey* **49 B9** 39 10N 27 50 E
Gelemso, *Ethiopia* **107 F5** 8 49N 40 31 E
Gelendost, *Turkey* **100 C4** 38 7N 31 1 E
Gelendzhik, *Russia* **59 K10** 44 33N 38 10 E
Gelib, *Somali Rep.* **120 D2** 0 29N 42 46 E
Gelibolu, *Turkey* **51 F10** 40 28N 26 43 E
Gelibolu Yarımadası, *Turkey* **51 F10** 40 20N 26 30 E
Gelidonya Burnu, *Turkey* **100 D4** 36 12N 30 24 E
Gelnhausen, *Germany* **31 E5** 50 11N 9 11 E
Gelnica, *Slovak Rep.* **35 C13** 48 51N 20 55 E
Gelsenkirchen, *Germany* **30 D3** 51 32N 7 6 E
Gelterkinden, *Switz.* **32 B5** 47 28N 7 51 E
Gelting, *Germany* **30 A5** 54 45N 9 53 E
Gelugur, *Malaysia* **87 c** 5 22N 100 18 E
Gemas, *Malaysia* **87 L4** 2 37N 102 36 E
Gembloux, *Belgium* **24 D4** 50 34N 4 43 E
Gembu, *Nigeria* **113 D7** 6 42N 11 10 E
Gemena, *Dem. Rep. of the Congo* **114 B3** 3 13N 19 48 E
Gemerek, *Turkey* **100 C7** 39 15N 36 10 E
Gemla, *Sweden* **17 H8** 56 52N 14 39 E
Gemlik, *Turkey* **51 F13** 40 26N 29 9 E
Gemlik Körfezi, *Turkey* **51 F12** 40 25N 28 55 E
Gemona del Friuli, *Italy* **45 B10** 46 16N 13 9 E
Gemsa, *Egypt* **106 B3** 27 39N 33 35 E
Gemsbok △, *Botswana* **116 D3** 25 5 S 21 1 E
Gemünden, *Germany* **31 E5** 50 3N 9 42 E
Genale, *Somali Rep.* **120 D2** 1 48N 44 42 E
Genale →, *Ethiopia* **107 F4** 6 2N 39 1 E
Genç, *Turkey* **101 C9** 38 44N 40 34 E
Gençay, *France* **28 B4** 46 23N 0 23 E
Geneina, Gebel, *Egypt* **106 B3** 29 2N 33 55 E
General Acha, *Argentina* **174 D3** 37 20 S 64 38W
General Alvear, *Buenos Aires, Argentina* **174 D4** 36 0 S 60 0W
General Alvear, *Mendoza, Argentina* **174 D2** 35 0 S 67 40W
General Artigas, *Paraguay* **174 B4** 26 52 S 56 16W
General Belgrano, *Argentina* **174 D4** 36 35 S 58 47W
General Bernardo O'Higgins, *Antarctica* **7 C18** 63 0 S 58 3W
General Cabrera, *Argentina* **174 C3** 32 53 S 63 52W
General Carrera, L., *Chile* **176 C2** 46 35 S 72 0W
General Cepeda, *Mexico* **162 B4** 25 23N 101 27W
General Conesa, *Argentina* **176 B4** 40 6 S 64 25W
General Eugenio A. Garay, *Paraguay* **173 E5** 20 31 S 62 8W
General Germán Busch = Villa Abecia, *Bolivia* **174 A2** 21 0 S 68 18W
General Guido, *Argentina* **174 D4** 36 40 S 57 50W
General Juan Madariaga, *Argentina* **174 D4** 37 0 S 57 0W
General La Madrid, *Argentina* **174 D3** 37 17 S 61 20W
General Lorenzo Vintter, *Argentina* **176 B4** 40 45 S 64 26W
General Luna, *Phil.* **80 E4** 13 41N 122 10 E
General MacArthur, *Phil.* **81 F5** 11 18N 125 28 E
General Martin Miguel de Güemes, *Argentina* **174 A3** 24 50 S 65 0W
General Paz, *Argentina* **174 B4** 27 45 S 57 36W
General Pico, *Argentina* **174 D3** 35 45 S 63 50W
General Pinedo, *Argentina* **174 B3** 27 15 S 61 20W
General Pinto, *Argentina* **174 C3** 34 45 S 61 50W
General Sampaio, *Brazil* **170 B4** 4 2 S 39 29W
General Santos, *Phil.* **81 H5** 6 5N 125 14 E
General Tinio, *Phil.* **80 D3** 15 39N 121 10 E
General Toshevo, *Bulgaria* **51 C12** 43 42N 28 6 E
General Trevino, *Mexico* **163 B5** 26 14N 99 29W
General Trías, *Mexico* **162 B3** 28 21N 106 22W
General Uriburu = Zárate, *Argentina* **174 C4** 34 7 S 59 0W
General Viamonte, *Argentina* **174 D3** 35 1 S 61 3W
General Villegas, *Argentina* **174 D3** 35 5 S 63 0W
General Vintter, L., *Argentina* **176 B2** 43 55 S 71 40W
Generoso, Mte., *Switz.* **33 E8** 45 56N 9 2 E
Generoso Ponce = Jaciparaná, *Brazil* **173 B5** 9 15 S 64 23W
Genesee, *Idaho, U.S.A.* **158 C5** 46 33N 116 56W
Genesee, *Pa., U.S.A.* **150 E7** 41 59N 77 54W
Genesee →, *U.S.A.* **150 C7** 43 16N 77 36W
Geneseo, *Ill., U.S.A.* **156 C6** 41 27N 90 9W
Geneseo, *N.Y., U.S.A.* **150 D7** 42 48N 77 49W
Geneva = Genève, *Switz.* **32 D2** 46 12N 6 9 E
Geneva, *Ala., U.S.A.* **152 D4** 31 2N 85 52W
Geneva, *Ga., U.S.A.* **152 C5** 32 35N 84 33W
Geneva, *Ill., U.S.A.* **157 C8** 41 53N 88 18W
Geneva, *Ind., U.S.A.* **157 D12** 40 36N 84 58W
Geneva, *N.Y., U.S.A.* **150 D8** 42 52N 76 59W

Geneva, Nebr., U.S.A. 154 E6 40 32N 97 36W
Geneva, Ohio, U.S.A. 150 E4 41 48N 80 57W
Geneva ✕ (GVA), Switz. 32 D2 46 14N 6 11 E
Geneva, L. = Léman, L., Europe 27 F13 46 26N 6 30 E
Geneva, L., U.S.A. 154 D10 42 38N 88 30W
Genève, Switz. 32 D2 46 12N 6 9 E
Genève □, Switz. 32 D2 46 10N 6 10 E
Geng, Afghan. 91 C1 31 22N 61 28 E
Gengenbach, Germany 31 G4 48 24N 8 1 E
Gengma, China 76 F2 23 32N 99 20 E
Genichesk = Henichesk, Ukraine 59 J8 46 12N 34 50 E
Genil →, Spain 43 H5 37 42N 5 19W
Genk, Belgium 24 D5 50 58N 5 32 E
Genkai-Nada, Japan 72 D2 34 0N 130 0 E
Genlis, France 27 E12 47 11N 5 12 E
Gennargentu, Mti. del, Italy 46 B2 40 1N 9 19 E
Gennes, France 26 E6 47 20N 0 17W
Genoa = Génova, Italy 44 D5 44 25N 8 57 E
Genoa, Australia 129 D8 37 29 S 149 35 E
Genoa, Ill., U.S.A. 157 B8 42 6N 88 42W
Genoa, N.Y., U.S.A. 151 D8 42 40N 76 32W
Genoa, Nebr., U.S.A. 154 E6 41 27N 97 44W
Genoa, Nev., U.S.A. 160 F7 39 2N 119 50W
Genoa →, Argentina 176 B2 44 55 S 70 5W
Genoa City, U.S.A. 157 B8 42 30N 88 20W
Génova, Italy 44 D5 44 25N 8 57 E
Genova ✕ (GOA), Italy 44 D5 44 25N 8 56 E
Génova, G. di, Italy 44 E6 44 0N 9 0 E
Genovesa, I., Ecuador 172 a 0 20N 89 58W
Genriyetty, Ostrov, Russia 67 B16 77 6N 156 30 E
Gent, Belgium 24 C3 51 2N 3 42 E
Genteng, Bali, Indonesia 79 J17 8 22 S 114 9 E
Genteng, Jawa, Indonesia 79 G12 7 22 S 106 24 E
Genthin, Germany 30 C8 52 25N 12 9 E
Gentio do Ouro, Brazil 170 D3 11 25 S 42 30W
Gentryville, U.S.A. 157 F9 38 6N 87 2W
Genyem, Indonesia 83 B6 2 46 S 140 12 E
Genzano di Lucánia, Italy 47 B9 40 51N 16 2 E
Genzano di Roma, Italy 45 G9 41 42N 12 41 E
Geoagiu, Romania 53 E8 45 55N 23 12 E
Geographe B., Australia 125 F2 33 30 S 115 15 E
Geographe Chan., Australia 125 D1 24 30 S 113 0 E
Geokchay = Göyçay, Azerbaijan 61 K8 40 42N 47 43 E
Georg Forster, Antarctica 7 D3 71 0 S 12 0 E
Georg von Neumayer, Antarctica 7 D17 71 0 S 68 30W
Georga, Zemlya, Russia 66 A5 80 30N 49 0 E
George, S. Africa 116 E3 33 58 S 22 29 E
George →, Canada 141 A6 58 49N 66 10W
George, L., N.S.W., Australia 129 C8 35 10 S 149 25 E
George, L., S. Austral., Australia 128 D4 37 25 S 140 0 E
George, L., W. Austral., Australia 124 D3 22 45 S 123 40 E
George, L., Uganda 118 B3 0 5N 30 10 E
George, L., Fla., U.S.A. 153 F8 29 17N 81 36W
George, L., N.Y., U.S.A. 151 C11 43 37N 73 33W
George Gill Ra., Australia 124 D5 24 22 S 131 45 E
George I., St. Helena 9 h 15 58 S 5 38W
George Pt., Australia 126 J6 20 6 S 148 36 E
George River = Kangiqsualujjuaq, Canada 139 C13 58 30N 65 59W
George Sound, N.Z. 131 E2 44 52 S 167 25 E
George Town, Australia 127 G4 41 6 S 146 49 E
George Town, Bahamas 164 B4 23 33N 75 47W
George Town, Cayman Is. 164 C3 19 20N 81 24W
George Town, Malaysia 87 c 5 25N 100 20 E
George V Land, Antarctica 7 C10 69 0 S 148 0 E
George VI Sound, Antarctica 7 D17 71 0 S 68 0W
George West, U.S.A. 155 L5 28 20N 98 7W
Georgetown = Janjanbureh, Gambia 112 C2 13 30N 14 47W
Georgetown, Ascension I. 9 g 7 56 S 14 25W
Georgetown, Australia 126 B3 18 17 S 143 33 E
Georgetown, Ont., Canada 140 D4 43 40N 79 56W
Georgetown, P.E.I., Canada 141 C7 46 13N 62 24W
Georgetown, Guyana 169 B6 6 50N 58 12W
Georgetown, Calif., U.S.A. 160 G6 38 54N 120 50W
Georgetown, Colo., U.S.A. 158 G11 39 42N 105 42W
Georgetown, Fla., U.S.A. 153 F8 29 23N 81 38W
Georgetown, Ga., U.S.A. 152 D4 31 53N 85 6W
Georgetown, Ill., U.S.A. 157 E9 39 59N 87 38W
Georgetown, Ky., U.S.A. 157 F12 38 13N 84 33W
Georgetown, N.Y., U.S.A. 151 D9 42 46N 75 44W
Georgetown, Ohio, U.S.A. 157 F13 38 52N 83 54W
Georgetown, S.C., U.S.A. 149 J6 33 23N 79 17W
Georgetown, Tex., U.S.A. 155 K6 30 38N 97 41W
Georgia □, U.S.A. 152 C6 32 50N 83 15W
Georgia ■, Asia 61 J6 42 0N 43 0 E
Georgia, Str. of, Canada 142 D4 49 25N 124 0W
Georgian B., Canada 140 C3 45 15N 81 0W
Georgian Bay Islands △, Canada 140 D4 44 53N 79 52W
Georgina →, Australia 126 C2 23 30 S 139 47 E
Georgina I., Canada 150 B5 44 22N 79 17W
Georgiu-Dezh = Liski, Russia 59 G10 51 3N 39 30 E
Georgiyevsk, Russia 61 H6 44 12N 43 28 E
Georgsmarienhütte, Germany 30 C4 52 13N 8 3 E
Gera, Germany 30 E8 50 53N 12 4 E
Geraardsbergen, Belgium 24 D3 50 45N 3 53 E
Geral, Serra, Bahia, Brazil 171 D3 14 0 S 41 0W
Geral, Serra, Goiás, Brazil 170 D2 11 15 S 46 30W
Geral, Serra, Sta. Catarina, Brazil 175 B6 26 25 S 50 0W
Geral de Goiás, Serra, Brazil 171 D2 12 0 S 46 0W
Geral do Paranã, Serra, Brazil 171 E2 15 0 S 47 30W
Gerald, U.S.A. 156 F5 38 24N 91 20W
Geraldine, N.Z. 131 E6 44 5 S 171 15 E
Geraldine, U.S.A. 158 C8 47 36N 110 16W
Geraldton = Innisfail, Australia 126 B4 17 33 S 146 5 E
Geraldton, Australia 125 E1 28 48 S 114 32 E
Geraldton, Canada 140 C2 49 44N 86 59W
Geranium, Australia 128 C4 35 23 S 140 11 E
Gérardmer, France 27 D13 48 3N 6 50 E
Gercüş, Turkey 101 D9 37 34N 41 23 E
Gerdine, Mt., U.S.A. 144 F9 61 35N 152 27W
Gerede, Turkey 100 B5 40 45N 32 10 E
Gerês, Sierra do, Portugal 42 D3 41 48N 8 0W
Gereshk, Afghan. 91 C2 31 47N 64 35 E
Geretsried, Germany 31 H7 47 51N 11 28 E
Gérgal, Spain 43 H2 37 7N 2 31W
Gerik, Malaysia 87 K3 5 50N 101 15 E
Gering, U.S.A. 154 E3 41 50N 103 40W
Gerlach, U.S.A. 158 F4 40 39N 119 21W
Gerlachovský štít, Slovak Rep. 35 B13 49 11N 20 7 E
Gerlogubi, Ethiopia 120 C3 6 53N 45 3 E
German East Africa = Tanzania ■, Africa 118 D3 6 0 S 34 0 E
German Planina, Macedonia 50 D6 42 20N 22 0 E
German South West Africa = Namibia ■, Africa 116 C2 22 0 S 18 9 E
Germania Land, Greenland 10 B9 77 5N 19 30W
Germansen Landing, Canada 142 B4 55 43N 124 40W
Germantown, Ohio, U.S.A. 157 E12 39 38N 84 22W
Germantown, Tenn., U.S.A. 155 M10 35 5N 89 49W
Germantown, Wis., U.S.A. 157 A8 43 14N 88 6W
Germany ■, Europe 30 E6 51 0N 10 0 E
Germencik, Turkey 49 D9 37 52N 27 37 E
Germering, Germany 31 G7 48 8N 11 22 E
Germersheim, Germany 31 F4 49 12N 8 22 E
Germī, Iran 97 B6 39 1N 48 3 E
Germiston, S. Africa 117 D4 26 15 S 28 10 E
Gernene, Algeria 111 D5 21 40N 2 24 E
Gernika-Lumo, Spain 40 B2 43 19N 2 40W
Gernsheim, Germany 31 F4 49 45N 8 30 E
Gero, Japan 73 B9 35 48N 137 14 E
Gerogery, Australia 129 C7 35 50 S 147 1 E
Gerokgak, Indonesia 79 J17 8 11 S 114 27 E
Gerolzhofen, Germany 31 F6 49 54N 10 21 E
Gerona = Girona, Spain 40 D7 41 58N 2 46 E
Gerrard, Canada 142 C5 50 30N 117 17W
Gerringong, Australia 129 C9 34 46 S 150 47 E
Gers □, France 28 E4 43 35N 0 30 E
Gers →, France 28 D4 44 9N 0 39 E
Gersfeld, Germany 30 E5 50 27N 9 56 E
Gersoppa Falls, India 95 G2 14 12N 74 46 E
Gersthofen, Germany 31 G6 48 25N 10 53 E
Gertak Sanggul, Malaysia 87 c 5 17N 100 12 E
Gertak Sanggul, Tanjung, Malaysia 87 c 5 16N 100 11 E
Gerung, Indonesia 79 K19 8 43 S 116 7 E
Géryville = El Bayadh, Algeria 111 B5 33 40N 1 1 E
Gerzat, France 28 C7 45 48N 3 8 E
Gerze, Turkey 100 B6 41 48N 35 12 E
Geseke, Germany 30 D4 51 38N 8 31 E
Geser, Indonesia 83 B4 3 50 S 130 54 E
Gesira △, Somali Rep. 120 D2 1 58N 44 59 E
Gesso →, Italy 44 D4 44 24N 7 33 E
Gestro, Wabi →, Ethiopia 107 G5 4 12N 42 2 E
Getafe, Spain 42 E7 40 18N 3 44W
Getinge, Sweden 17 H6 56 49N 12 44 E
Gettysburg, Pa., U.S.A. 148 F7 39 50N 77 14W
Gettysburg, S. Dak., U.S.A. 154 C5 45 1N 99 57W
Getxo, Spain 40 B2 43 21N 2 59W
Getz Ice Shelf, Antarctica 7 D14 75 0 S 130 0W
Geureudong, Gunong, Indonesia 84 B1 4 13N 96 42 E
Geurie, Australia 129 B8 32 22 S 148 50 E
Gevaş, Turkey 101 C10 38 15N 43 6 E
Gévaudan, France 28 D7 44 40N 3 40 E
Gevgelija, Macedonia 50 E6 41 9N 22 30 E
Gévora →, Spain 43 G4 38 53N 6 57W
Gevrai, India 94 E2 19 16N 75 45 E
Gewani, Ethiopia 107 E5 10 12N 40 40 E
Gex, France 27 F13 46 21N 6 3 E
Geyikli, Turkey 49 B8 39 48N 26 12 E
Geyser, U.S.A. 158 C8 47 16N 110 30W
Geyserville, U.S.A. 160 G4 38 42N 122 54W
Geysir, Iceland 11 C6 64 19N 20 18W
Geyve, Turkey 100 B4 40 30N 30 18 E
Ghâbat el Arab = Wang Kai, Sudan 107 F2 9 3N 29 23 E
Ghabeish, Sudan 107 E2 12 9N 27 21 E
Ghafurov, Tajikistan 65 C4 40 13N 69 43 E
Ghaggar →, India 92 E6 29 30N 74 53 E
Ghaghara →, India 93 G11 25 45N 84 40 E
Ghaghat →, Bangla. 93 G13 25 19N 89 38 E
Ghaghe, Solomon Is. 133 L10 7 24 S 158 15 E
Ghagra, India 93 H11 23 17N 84 33 E
Ghagra →, India 93 F9 27 29N 81 9 E
Ghajn Tuffieha Bay, Malta 38 F7 35 56N 14 21 E
Ghajnsielem, Malta 38 E7 36 2N 14 17 E
Ghalla, Wadi el →, Sudan 107 E2 10 25N 27 32 E
Ghana ■, W. Afr. 113 D4 8 0N 1 0W
Ghansor, India 93 H9 22 39N 80 1 E
Ghanzi, Botswana 116 C3 21 50 S 21 34 E
Gharb, Malta 38 E6 36 4N 14 13 E
Gharb el Istiwa'iya □, Sudan 107 G3 5 0N 30 0 E
Gharb Kordofân □, Sudan 107 E2 12 0N 28 0 E
Gharbîya, Es Sahrâ el, Egypt 106 B2 27 40N 26 30 E
Ghardaïa, Algeria 111 B5 32 20N 3 37 E
Ghârib, G., Egypt 106 B3 28 6N 32 54 E
Gharig, Sudan 107 E2 10 47N 27 33 E
Gharm, W. →, Oman 99 C7 19 57N 57 38 E
Gharyān, Libya 108 B2 32 10N 13 0 E
Gharyān □, Libya 108 B2 30 35N 13 0 E
Ghat, Libya 108 D2 24 59N 10 11 E
Ghatal, India 93 H12 22 40N 87 46 E
Ghatampur, India 93 F9 26 8N 80 13 E
Ghatgaon, India 94 D7 21 24N 85 53 E
Ghatprabha →, India 95 F2 16 15N 75 20 E
Ghats, Eastern, India 95 H4 14 0N 78 50 E
Ghats, Western, India 95 H2 14 0N 75 0 E
Ghatsila, India 93 H12 22 36N 86 29 E
Ghaṭṭī, Si. Arabia 96 D3 31 16N 37 31 E
Ghawdex = Gozo, Malta 38 E7 36 3N 14 15 E
Ghayl, Si. Arabia 98 B4 21 40N 46 20 E
Ghazal, Bahr el →, Chad 109 F3 13 0N 15 47 E
Ghazâl, Bahr el →, Sudan 107 F3 9 31N 30 25 E
Ghazaouet, Algeria 111 A4 35 8N 1 50W
Ghaziabad, India 92 E7 28 42N 77 26 E
Ghazipur, India 93 G10 25 38N 83 35 E
Ghaznī, Afghan. 91 B3 33 30N 68 28 E
Ghaznī □, Afghan. 91 B3 32 10N 68 20 E
Ghedi, Italy 44 C7 45 24N 10 16 E
Ghelari, Romania 52 E7 45 38N 22 45 E
Ghèlinsor, Somali Rep. 120 C3 6 28N 46 39 E
Ghent = Gent, Belgium 24 C3 51 2N 3 42 E
Gheorghe Gheorghiu-Dej = Oneşti, Romania 53 D11 46 17N 26 47 E
Gheorgheni, Romania 53 D10 46 43N 25 41 E
Gherla, Romania 53 C8 47 2N 23 57 E
Ghidigeni, Romania 53 D12 46 3N 27 30 E
Ghiffa, Italy 33 E7 45 58N 8 37 E
Ghilarza, Italy 46 B1 40 7N 8 50 E
Ghimeş-Făget, Romania 53 D11 46 35N 26 2 E
Ghīnah, Wādī al →, Si. Arabia 96 D3 30 27N 38 14 E
Ghisonaccia, France 29 F13 42 1N 9 26 E
Ghisoni, France 29 F13 42 7N 9 12 E
Ghizao, Afghan. 91 B2 33 20N 65 44 E
Ghizar →, Pakistan 93 A5 36 15N 73 43 E
Ghod →, India 94 E2 18 30N 74 35 E
Ghogha, India 94 D1 21 40N 72 20 E
Ghot Ogrein, Egypt 106 A2 31 10N 25 20 E
Ghotaru, India 92 F4 27 20N 70 1 E
Ghotki, Pakistan 92 E3 28 5N 69 21 E
Ghowr □, Afghan. 91 B2 34 0N 64 20 E
Ghudāf, W. al →, Iraq 101 F10 32 56N 43 30 E
Ghudāmis, Libya 108 B1 30 11N 9 29 E
Ghudāmis □, Libya 108 B2 30 25N 10 25 E
Ghughri, India 93 H9 22 39N 80 41 E
Ghugus, India 94 E4 19 58N 79 12 E
Ghulam Mohammad Barrage, Pakistan 92 G3 25 30N 68 20 E
Ghurayrah, Si. Arabia 98 C3 18 37N 42 41 E
Ghūrīān, Afghan. 91 B1 34 17N 61 25 E
Ghuzzayil, Sabkhat, Libya 108 C3 29 30N 19 30 E
Gia Dinh, Vietnam 87 G6 10 49N 106 42 E
Gia Lai = Plei Ku, Vietnam 86 F7 13 57N 108 0 E
Gia Nghia, Vietnam 87 G6 11 58N 107 42 E
Gia Ngoc, Vietnam 86 E7 14 50N 108 58 E
Gia Vuc, Vietnam 86 E7 14 42N 108 34 E
Giamama, Somali Rep. 120 D2 0 4N 42 44 E
Gianitsa = Yiannitsa, Greece 50 F6 40 46N 22 24 E
Giannutri, Italy 44 F8 42 15N 11 6 E
Giant Forest, U.S.A. 160 J8 36 36N 118 43W
Giant Mts. = Krkonoše, Czech Rep. 34 A8 50 50N 15 35 E
Giant Sequoia ⌂, U.S.A. 160 K8 36 0N 118 32W
Giants Causeway, U.K. 23 A5 55 16N 6 29W
Giant's Tank, Sri Lanka 95 K5 8 51N 80 2 E
Gianyar, Indonesia 79 K18 8 32 S 115 20 E
Giarabub = Al Jaghbūb, Libya 108 C4 29 42N 24 38 E
Giarre, Italy 47 E8 37 43N 15 11 E
Giaveno, Italy 44 C4 45 2N 7 21 E
Gibara, Cuba 164 B4 21 9N 76 11W
Gibb River, Australia 124 C4 16 26 S 126 26 E
Gibbon, U.S.A. 154 E5 40 45N 98 51W
Gibe →, Ethiopia 107 F4 7 20N 37 36 E
Gibellina Nuova, Italy 46 E5 37 47N 12 58 E
Gibeon, Namibia 116 D2 25 9 S 17 43 E
Gibraleón, Spain 43 H4 37 23N 6 58W
Gibraltar ☒, Europe 43 J5 36 7N 5 22W
Gibraltar, Str. of, Medit. S. 43 K5 35 55N 5 40W
Gibraltar Range △, Australia 127 D5 29 31 S 152 19 E
Gibson, U.S.A. 152 B7 33 14N 82 36W
Gibson City, U.S.A. 157 D8 40 28N 88 22W
Gibson Desert, Australia 124 D4 24 0 S 126 0 E
Gibsonburg, U.S.A. 157 C13 41 23N 83 19W
Gibsons, Canada 142 D4 49 24N 123 32W
Gibsonton, U.S.A. 153 H7 27 51N 82 23W
Gibsonville, U.S.A. 160 F6 39 46N 120 54W
Giddalur, India 95 G4 15 20N 78 57 E
Giddings, U.S.A. 155 K6 30 11N 96 56W
Gidole, Ethiopia 107 F4 5 40N 37 25 E
Giebnegáisi = Kebnekaise, Sweden 14 C18 67 53N 18 33 E
Gien, France 27 E9 47 40N 2 36 E
Giengen, Germany 31 G6 48 37N 10 14 E
Giessen, Germany 30 E4 50 34N 8 41 E
Gīfān, Iran 97 B8 37 54N 57 28 E
Gifatin, Geziret, Egypt 106 B3 27 10N 33 50 E
Gifford, U.S.A. 153 H9 27 40N 80 25W
Gifhorn, Germany 30 C6 52 30N 10 33 E
Gift Lake, Canada 142 B5 55 53N 115 49W
Gifu, Japan 73 B8 35 30N 136 45 E
Gifu □, Japan 73 B9 35 40N 137 0 E
Gigant, Russia 61 G5 46 28N 41 20 E
Giganta, Sa. de la, Mexico 162 B2 25 30N 111 30W
Gigen, Bulgaria 51 C8 43 40N 24 28 E
Gigha, U.K. 22 F3 55 42N 5 44W
Giglei, Somali Rep. 120 C3 5 25N 45 20 E
Gíglio, Italy 44 F7 42 20N 10 52 E
Gignac, France 28 E7 43 39N 3 32 E
Gignod, Italy 32 E4 45 47N 7 17 E
Gigüela →, Spain 43 F7 39 8N 3 44W
Gijón, Spain 42 B5 43 32N 5 42W
Gil I., Canada 142 C3 53 12N 129 15W
Gila →, U.S.A. 159 K6 32 43N 114 33W
Gila Bend, U.S.A. 159 K7 32 57N 112 43W
Gila Bend Mts., U.S.A. 159 K7 33 10N 113 0W
Gila Cliff Dwellings ⌂, U.S.A. 159 K9 33 2N 108 16W
Gīlān □, Iran 97 B6 37 0N 50 0 E
Gilău, Romania 53 D8 46 45N 23 23 E
Gilbert →, Australia 126 B3 16 35 S 141 15 E
Gilbert Is., Kiribati 134 G9 1 0N 172 0 E
Gilbert River, Australia 126 B3 18 9 S 142 52 E
Gilbués, Brazil 170 C2 9 50 S 45 21W
Gilead, U.S.A. 151 B14 44 24N 70 59W
Gilf el Kebîr, Hadabat el, Egypt 106 C2 23 50N 25 50 E
Gilford I., Canada 142 C3 50 40N 126 30W
Gilgandra, Australia 129 A8 31 43 S 148 39 E
Gilgil, Kenya 118 C4 0 30 S 36 20 E
Gilgit, India 93 B6 35 50N 74 15 E
Gilgit →, Pakistan 93 B6 35 44N 74 37 E
Gilgunnia, Australia 129 B7 32 26 S 146 2 E
Gili ⌂, Mozam. 119 F4 16 39 S 38 27 E
Gilimanuk, Indonesia 79 J17 8 10 S 114 26 E
Giljeva Planina, Serbia & M. 50 C3 43 9N 20 0 E
Gill Pt., St. Helena 9 h 15 58 S 5 38W
Gillam, Canada 143 B10 56 20N 94 40W
Gilleleje, Denmark 17 H6 56 8N 12 19 E
Gillen, L., Australia 125 E3 26 11 S 124 38 E
Gilles, L., Australia 128 B2 32 50 S 136 45 E
Gillespie, U.S.A. 156 E7 39 8N 89 49W
Gillespies Pt., N.Z. 131 D4 43 24 S 169 49 E
Gillette, U.S.A. 154 C2 44 18N 105 30W
Gilliat, Australia 126 C3 20 40 S 141 28 E
Gillingham, U.K. 21 F8 51 23N 0 33 E
Gilman, U.S.A. 157 D9 40 46N 88 0W
Gilman City, U.S.A. 156 D3 40 8N 93 53W
Gilmer, U.S.A. 155 J7 32 44N 94 57W
Gilmore, L., Australia 125 F3 32 29 S 121 37 E
Gilo →, Ethiopia 107 F3 8 10N 33 15 E
Gilort →, Romania 53 F8 44 38N 23 32 E
Gilroy, U.S.A. 160 H5 37 1N 121 34W
Giluwe, Mt., Papua N. G. 132 D2 6 8 S 143 52 E
Gimbi, Ethiopia 107 F4 9 3N 35 42 E
Gimie, Mt, St. Lucia 165 f 13 54N 61 0W
Gimli, Canada 143 C9 50 40N 97 0W
Gimo, Sweden 16 D12 60 11N 18 12 E
Gimone →, France 28 E5 44 0N 1 6 E
Gimont, France 28 E4 43 38N 0 52 E
Gimpu, Indonesia 82 B2 1 36 S 120 2 E
Gin →, Sri Lanka 95 L5 6 5N 80 7 E
Gin Gin, Australia 127 D5 25 0 S 151 58 E
Ginâh, Egypt 106 B3 25 21N 30 30 E
Ginatilan, Phil. 81 G4 9 34N 123 19 E
Gineifa, Egypt 106 H8 30 12N 32 25 E
Gingee, India 95 H4 12 15N 79 25 E
Gingin, Australia 125 F2 31 22 S 115 54 E
Gingindlovu, S. Africa 117 D5 29 2 S 31 30 E
Gingoog, Phil. 81 G5 8 50N 125 7 E
Ginir, Ethiopia 107 F5 7 6N 40 40 E
Gino, Pizzo di, Italy 33 D8 46 7N 9 10 E
Ginosa, Italy 47 B9 40 35N 16 45 E
Ginzo de Limia = Xinzo de Limia, Spain 42 C3 42 3N 7 47W
Giohar, Somali Rep. 120 D3 2 48N 45 30 E
Gióia, G. di, Italy 47 D8 38 30N 15 45 E
Gióia del Colle, Italy 47 B9 40 48N 16 55 E
Gióia Táuro, Italy 47 D8 38 25N 15 54 E
Gioiosa Iónica, Italy 47 D9 38 20N 16 18 E
Gioiosa Marea, Italy 47 D7 38 10N 14 54 E
Gióna, Óros, Greece 48 C4 38 38N 22 14 E
Giovi, Passo dei, Italy 44 D5 44 33N 8 57 E
Giovinazzo, Italy 47 A9 41 11N 16 40 E
Gippsland, Australia 129 D7 37 52 S 147 0 E
Gir △, India 92 J4 21 0N 71 0 E
Gir Hills, India 92 J4 21 0N 71 0 E
Girab, India 92 F4 26 2N 70 38 E
Girâfi, W. →, Egypt 103 F3 29 58N 34 39 E
Giraltovce, Slovak Rep. 35 B14 49 7N 21 32 E
Girard, Ga., U.S.A. 152 B8 33 3N 81 43W
Girard, Ill., U.S.A. 156 E7 39 27N 89 47W
Girard, Kans., U.S.A. 155 G7 37 31N 94 51W
Girard, Ohio, U.S.A. 150 E4 41 9N 80 42W
Girard, Pa., U.S.A. 150 E4 42 0N 80 19W
Girardot, Colombia 168 C3 4 18N 74 48W
Girdle Ness, U.K. 22 D6 57 9N 2 3W
Giresun, Turkey 101 B8 40 55N 38 30 E
Girga, Egypt 106 B3 26 17N 31 55 E
Girgenti = Agrigento, Italy 46 E6 37 19N 13 34 E
Girgir, C., Papua N. G. 132 B3 3 50 S 144 35 E
Giri →, Dem. Rep. of the Congo 114 B3 0 28N 17 59 E
Giri →, India 92 D7 30 28N 77 41 E
Giridih, India 93 G12 24 10N 86 21 E
Girifalco, Italy 47 D9 38 49N 16 25 E
Girilambone, Australia 129 A7 31 16 S 146 57 E
Girne = Kyrenia, Cyprus 39 E9 35 20N 33 20 E
Giro, Nigeria 113 C5 11 7N 4 42 E
Giromagny, France 27 E13 47 45N 6 50 E
Giron = Kiruna, Sweden 14 C19 67 52N 20 15 E
Girona, Spain 40 D7 41 58N 2 46 E
Girona □, Spain 40 C7 42 11N 2 30 E
Gironde □, France 28 D3 44 45N 0 30W
Gironde →, France 28 C2 45 32N 1 7W
Gironella, Spain 40 C6 42 2N 1 53 E
Girraween △, Australia 127 D5 28 46 S 151 54 E
Giru, Australia 126 B4 19 30 S 147 5 E
Girvan, U.K. 22 F4 55 14N 4 51W
Gisborne, Australia 128 D6 37 29 S 144 36 E
Gisborne, N.Z. 130 E7 38 39 S 178 5 E
Gisborne □, N.Z. 130 E6 38 30 S 178 0 E
Gisenyi, Rwanda 118 C2 1 41 S 29 15 E
Gislaved, Sweden 17 G7 57 19N 13 32 E
Gisors, France 27 C8 49 15N 1 47 E
Gissarskiy Khrebet, Tajikistan 65 D4 39 0N 69 0 E
Giswil, Switz. 32 C6 46 50N 8 11 E
Gitega, Burundi 118 C2 3 26 S 29 56 E
Githio = Yíthion, Greece 48 E4 36 46N 22 34 E
Gitschin = Jičín, Czech Rep. 34 A8 50 25N 15 28 E
Giuba →, Somali Rep. 120 D2 1 30N 42 35 E
Giubiasco, Switz. 33 D8 46 11N 9 1 E
Giugliano in Campania, Italy 47 B7 40 56N 14 12 E
Giulianova, Italy 45 F10 42 45N 13 57 E
Giurgeni, Romania 53 F12 44 45N 27 48 E
Giurgiu, Romania 53 G10 43 52N 25 57 E
Giurgiu □, Romania 53 F10 44 20N 26 0 E
Giurgiuleşti, Moldova 53 E13 45 29N 28 12 E
Give, Denmark 17 J3 55 51N 9 13 E
Givet, France 27 B11 50 8N 4 49 E
Givors, France 29 C8 45 35N 4 45 E
Givry, France 27 F11 46 41N 4 46 E
Giyon, Ethiopia 107 F4 8 33N 38 1 E
Giza = El Gîza, Egypt 106 J7 30 0N 31 10 E
Gizhduvan, Uzbekistan 65 C2 40 6N 64 41 E
Gizhiga, Russia 67 C17 62 3N 160 30 E
Gizhiginskaya Guba, Russia 67 C16 61 0N 158 0 E
Gizo, Solomon Is. 133 M9 8 7 S 156 50 E
Giżycko, Poland 54 D8 54 2N 21 48 E
Gizzeria, Italy 47 D9 38 59N 16 12 E
Gjalicë e Lumës, Mal., Albania 50 D4 42 2N 20 25 E
Gjegjan, Albania 50 E4 41 58N 20 3 E
Gjendesheim, Norway 18 C5 61 30N 8 48 E
Gjerstad, Norway 18 F6 58 54N 9 1 E
Gjevilvatnet, Norway 18 B6 62 43N 9 23 E
Gjirokastër, Albania 50 F4 40 7N 20 10 E
Gjoa Haven, Canada 138 B10 68 38N 95 53W
Gjøra, Norway 18 B6 62 33N 9 4 E
Gjøvik, Norway 18 D7 60 47N 10 43 E
Gjuhës, Kep i, Albania 50 F3 40 28N 19 15 E
Glace Bay, Canada 141 C8 46 11N 59 58W
Glacier △, Canada 142 C5 51 15N 117 30W
Glacier △, U.S.A. 158 B7 48 30N 113 18W
Glacier Bay, U.S.A. 144 G14 58 40N 136 0W
Glacier Bay △, U.S.A. 142 B1 58 45N 136 30W
Glacier Peak, U.S.A. 158 B3 48 7N 121 7W
Gladewater, U.S.A. 155 J7 32 33N 94 56W
Gladstone, Queens., Australia 126 C5 23 52 S 151 16 E
Gladstone, S. Austral., Australia 128 B3 33 15 S 138 22 E
Gladstone, Canada 143 C9 50 13N 98 57W
Gladstone, Ill., U.S.A. 156 D6 40 52N 90 57W
Gladstone, Mich., U.S.A. 148 C2 45 51N 87 1W
Gladstone, Mo., U.S.A. 156 E2 39 13N 94 35W
Gladwin, U.S.A. 148 D3 43 59N 84 29W
Glafsfjorden, Sweden 16 E6 59 30N 12 37 E
Glagah, Indonesia 79 J17 8 13 S 114 18 E
Głagów Małapolski, Poland 55 H8 50 10N 21 56 E
Glåma = Glomma →, Norway 18 E7 59 12N 10 57 E
Gláma, Iceland 11 B4 65 48N 23 0W
Glamis, U.S.A. 161 N11 32 55N 115 5W
Glamoč, Bos.-H. 45 D13 44 3N 16 51 E
Glamorgan, Vale of □, U.K. 21 F4 51 28N 3 25W
Glåmos, Norway 18 B8 62 41N 11 25 E
Glamsbjerg, Denmark 17 J4 55 17N 10 6 E
Gland, Switz. 32 D2 46 26N 6 16 E
Glarner Alpen, Switz. 33 C8 46 50N 9 0 E
Glärnisch, Switz. 33 C8 47 0N 9 0 E
Glarus, Switz. 33 B8 47 3N 9 4 E
Glarus □, Switz. 33 C8 47 0N 9 5 E
Glasco, Kans., U.S.A. 154 F6 39 22N 97 50W
Glasco, N.Y., U.S.A. 151 D11 42 3N 73 57W
Glasgow, U.K. 22 F4 55 51N 4 15W
Glasgow, Ky., U.S.A. 148 G3 37 0N 85 55W
Glasgow, Mo., U.S.A. 156 E4 39 14N 92 51W
Glasgow, Mont., U.S.A. 158 B10 48 12N 106 38W
Glasgow, City of □, U.K. 22 F4 55 51N 4 12W
Glasgow International ✕ (GLA), U.K. 22 F4 55 51N 4 21W
Glaslyn, Canada 143 C7 53 22N 108 21W
Glastonbury, U.K. 21 F5 51 9N 2 43W
Glastonbury, U.S.A. 151 E12 41 43N 72 37W
Glatt →, Switz. 33 B7 47 28N 8 32 E
Glattfelden, Switz. 33 A7 47 33N 8 30 E
Glatz = Kłodzko, Poland 55 H3 50 28N 16 38 E
Glauchau, Germany 30 E8 50 49N 12 31 E
Glava, Sweden 16 E6 59 33N 12 35 E
Glavice, Croatia 45 E13 43 43N 16 41 E
Glazov, Russia 60 A11 58 9N 52 40 E
Gleichen, Canada 142 C6 50 52N 113 3W
Gleisdorf, Austria 34 D8 47 6N 15 44 E
Gleiwitz = Gliwice, Poland 55 H5 50 22N 18 41 E
Glen, U.S.A. 151 B13 44 7N 71 11W
Glen Affric, U.K. 22 D3 57 17N 5 1W
Glen Afton, N.Z. 130 D4 37 37 S 175 4 E
Glen Canyon, U.S.A. 159 H8 37 30N 110 40W
Glen Canyon ⌂, U.S.A. 159 H8 37 15N 111 0W
Glen Canyon Dam, U.S.A. 159 H8 36 57N 111 29W
Glen Coe, U.K. 22 E3 56 40N 5 0W
Glen Cove, U.S.A. 151 F11 40 52N 73 38W
Glen Garry, U.K. 22 D3 57 3N 5 7W
Glen Innes, Australia 127 D5 29 44 S 151 44 E
Glen Lyon, U.S.A. 151 E8 41 10N 76 5W
Glen Massey, N.Z. 130 D4 37 38 S 175 2 E
Glen Mor, U.K. 22 D4 57 9N 4 37W
Glen More ⌂, U.K. 22 D5 57 8N 3 40W
Glen Moriston, U.K. 22 D4 57 11N 4 52W
Glen Robertson, Canada 151 A10 45 22N 74 30W
Glen Spean, U.K. 22 E4 56 53N 4 40W
Glen Ullin, U.S.A. 154 B4 46 49N 101 50W
Glénan, Îs. de, France 26 E3 47 42N 4 0W
Glenariff △, Ireland 23 A5 55 2N 6 10W
Glenavy, N.Z. 131 E6 44 54 S 171 7 E
Glenburn, Australia 129 D6 37 27 S 145 26 E
Glencoe, Canada 150 D3 42 45N 81 43W
Glencoe, S. Africa 117 D5 28 11 S 30 11 E
Glencoe, Ala., U.S.A. 152 B4 33 57N 85 56W
Glencoe, Minn., U.S.A. 154 C7 44 46N 94 9W
Glendale, Ariz., U.S.A. 159 K7 33 32N 112 11W
Glendale, Calif., U.S.A. 161 L8 34 9N 118 15W
Glendale, Fla., U.S.A. 152 E3 30 52N 86 7W
Glendale, Zimbabwe 119 F3 17 22 S 31 5 E
Glendive, U.S.A. 154 B2 47 7N 104 43W
Glendo, U.S.A. 154 D2 42 30N 105 2W
Glenelg, Australia 128 C3 34 58 S 138 31 E
Glenelg →, Australia 128 E4 38 4 S 140 59 E
Glenfield, U.S.A. 151 C9 43 43N 75 24W
Glengarriff, Ireland 23 E2 51 45N 9 34W
Glenham, N.Z. 131 G3 46 26 S 168 52 E
Glenhope, N.Z. 131 B7 41 40 S 172 39 E
Glenmary, Mt., N.Z. 131 D4 43 55 S 169 55 E
Glenmont, U.S.A. 150 F2 40 31N 82 6W
Glenmorgan, Australia 127 D4 27 14 S 149 42 E
Glenn, U.S.A. 160 F4 39 31N 122 1W
Glennallen, U.S.A. 144 E11 62 7N 145 33W
Glennamaddy, Ireland 23 C3 53 37N 8 33W
Glenns Ferry, U.S.A. 158 E6 42 57N 115 18W
Glennville, U.S.A. 152 D8 31 56N 81 56W
Glenorchy, Australia 128 D5 36 55 S 142 41 E
Glenorchy, N.Z. 131 E3 44 51 S 168 24 E
Glenore, Australia 126 B3 17 50 S 141 12 E
Glenreagh, Australia 127 E5 30 2 S 153 1 E
Glenrock, U.S.A. 158 E11 42 52N 105 52W
Glenrothes, U.K. 22 E5 56 12N 3 10W
Glenrowan, Australia 129 D7 36 29 S 146 13 E
Glens Falls, U.S.A. 151 C11 43 19N 73 39W
Glenside, U.S.A. 151 F9 40 6N 75 9W
Glenthompson, Australia 128 D5 37 38 S 142 38 E
Glenties, Ireland 23 B3 54 49N 8 16W
Glenveagh △, Ireland 23 A3 55 3N 8 1W
Glenville, U.S.A. 148 F5 38 56N 80 50W
Glenwood, Canada 141 C9 49 0N 54 58W
Glenwood, Ark., U.S.A. 155 H8 34 20N 93 33W
Glenwood, Ga., U.S.A. 152 C7 32 11N 82 40W
Glenwood, Hawaii, U.S.A. 145 D6 19 29N 155 9W
Glenwood, Iowa, U.S.A. 154 E7 41 3N 95 45W
Glenwood, Minn., U.S.A. 154 C7 45 39N 95 23W
Glenwood, Wash., U.S.A. 160 D5 46 1N 121 17W
Glenwood Springs, U.S.A. 158 G10 39 33N 107 19W
Gletsch, Switz. 33 C6 46 34N 8 22 E
Glettinganes, Iceland 11 B13 65 30N 13 37W
Glidden, U.S.A. 156 B2 42 4N 94 44W
Glifádha, Greece 48 D5 37 52N 23 45 E
Glimåkra, Sweden 17 H8 56 19N 14 7 E
Glina, Croatia 45 C13 45 20N 16 6 E
Glinojeck, Poland 55 F7 52 49N 20 21 E
Glittertind, Norway 18 C5 61 40N 8 32 E
Gliwice, Poland 55 H5 50 22N 18 41 E
Globe, U.S.A. 159 K8 33 24N 110 47W
Glodeanu Siliştea, Romania 53 F11 44 50N 26 48 E
Glodeni, Moldova 53 C12 47 45N 27 31 E
Glödnitz, Austria 34 E7 46 53N 14 7 E
Glogau = Głogów, Poland 55 G3 51 37N 16 5 E
Gloggnitz, Austria 34 D8 47 41N 15 56 E
Głogów, Poland 55 G3 51 37N 16 5 E
Głogówek, Poland 55 H4 50 21N 17 53 E
Glomma →, Norway 18 E7 59 12N 10 57 E
Gloria, Phil. 80 E3 12 59N 121 30 E
Glorieuses, Is., Ind. Oc. 117 A8 11 30 S 47 20 E
Glóssa, Greece 48 B5 39 10N 23 45 E

Glossop, *U.K.* **20 D6** 53 27N 1 56W
Gloucester, *Australia* . **129 B9** 32 0 S 151 59 E
Gloucester, *Papua N. G.* .... **132 C5** 5 31 S 148 31 E
Gloucester, *U.K.* **21 F5** 51 53N 2 15W
Gloucester, *U.S.A.* **151 D14** 42 37N 70 40W
Gloucester, C., *Papua N. G.* .... **132 C5** 5 26 S 148 21 E
Gloucester I., *Australia* **126 J6** 20 0 S 148 30 E
Gloucester Island △, *Australia* .... **126 J6** 20 2 S 148 30 E
Gloucester Point, *U.S.A.* **148 G7** 37 15N 76 29W
Gloucestershire □, *U.K.* **21 F5** 51 46N 2 15W
Gloversville, *U.S.A.* .. **151 C10** 43 3N 74 21W
Glovertown, *Canada* . **141 C9** 48 40N 54 3W
Gloverville, *U.S.A.* ... **152 B8** 33 32N 81 48W
Głowno, *Poland* ..... **55 G6** 51 59N 19 42 E
Głubczyce, *Poland* ... **55 H4** 50 13N 17 52 E
Glubokiy, *Russia* ..... **61 F5** 48 35N 40 25 E
Glubokoye = Hlybokaye, *Belarus* **58 E4** 55 10N 27 45 E
Głuchołazy, *Poland* .. **55 H4** 50 19N 17 24 E
Glücksburg, *Germany* **30 A5** 54 50N 9 33 E
Glückstadt, *Germany* . **30 B5** 53 45N 9 25 E
Glukhov = Hlukhiv, *Ukraine* .... **59 G7** 51 40N 33 58 E
Glusk, *Belarus* .... **59 F5** 52 53N 28 41 E
Głuszyca, *Poland* .... **55 H3** 50 41N 16 23 E
Glyngøre, *Denmark* .. **17 H2** 56 46N 8 52 E
Gmünd, *Kärnten*, *Austria* .... **34 E6** 46 54N 13 31 E
Gmünd, *Niederösterreich*, *Austria* .... **34 C8** 48 45N 15 0 E
Gmunden, *Austria* ... **34 D6** 47 55N 13 48 E
Gnali, *Gabon* .... **114 C2** 2 34 S 11 18 E
Gnarp, *Sweden* ...... **16 B11** 62 3N 17 16 E
Gnesen = Gniezno, *Poland* .... **55 F4** 52 30N 17 35 E
Gnesta, *Sweden* ...... **16 E11** 59 3N 17 17 E
Gniew, *Poland* .... **54 E5** 53 50N 18 50 E
Gniewkowo, *Poland* .. **55 F5** 52 54N 18 25 E
Gniezno, *Poland* ..... **55 F4** 52 30N 17 35 E
Gnjilane, *Serbia & M.* **50 D5** 42 28N 21 29 E
Gnoien, *Germany* .... **30 B8** 53 58N 12 41 E
Gnosjö, *Sweden* ...... **17 G7** 57 22N 13 43 E
Gnowangerup, *Australia* .... **125 F2** 33 58 S 117 59 E
Go Cong, *Vietnam* ... **87 G6** 10 22N 106 40 E
Gō-Gawa →, *Japan* .. **72 B4** 35 2N 132 13 E
Gō-no-ura, *Japan* .... **72 D1** 33 44N 129 40 E
Goa, *India* .... **95 G1** 15 33N 73 59 E
Goa, *Phil.* .... **80 E4** 13 42N 123 29 E
Goa □, *India* .... **95 G1** 15 33N 73 59 E
Goalen Hd., *Australia* **129 D9** 36 33 S 150 4 E
Goalpara, *India* ...... **90 B3** 26 10N 90 40 E
Goaltor, *India* .... **93 H12** 22 43N 87 10 E
Goalundo Ghat, *Bangla.* .... **93 H13** 23 50N 89 47 E
Goaso, *Ghana* **112 D4** 6 48N 2 30W
Goat Fell, *U.K.* **22 F3** 55 38N 5 11W
Goba, *Ethiopia* ...... **107 F4** 7 1N 39 59 E
Goba, *Mozam.* .... **117 D5** 26 15 S 32 13 E
Gobabis, *Namibia* .... **116 C2** 22 30 S 19 0 E
Gobe, *Papua N. G.* ... **132 E5** 9 4 S 149 0 E
Göbel, *Turkey* .... **51 F12** 40 0N 28 9 E
Gobernador Gregores, *Argentina* .... **176 C2** 48 46 S 70 15W
Gobi, *Asia* .... **74 C6** 44 0N 110 0 E
Gobichettipalayam, *India* .... **95 J3** 11 31N 77 21 E
Gobles, *U.S.A.* **157 B11** 42 22N 85 53W
Gobō, *Japan* .... **73 D7** 33 53N 135 10 E
Gobo, *Sudan* .... **107 F3** 5 40N 31 10 E
Göçbeyli, *Turkey* .... **49 B9** 39 13N 27 25 E
Goch, *Germany* ...... **30 D2** 51 41N 6 9 E
Gochas, *Namibia* ..... **116 C2** 24 59 S 18 55 E
Godalming, *U.K.* **21 F7** 51 11N 0 36W
Godavari →, *India* ... **94 F6** 16 25N 82 18 E
Godavari Pt., *India* .. **94 F6** 17 0N 82 20 E
Godbout, *Canada* **141 C6** 49 20N 67 38W
Godda, *India* .... **93 G12** 24 50N 87 13 E
Goddua, *Libya* .... **108 C2** 26 26N 14 19 E
Godech, *Bulgaria* .... **50 C7** 43 1N 23 4 E
Goderich, *Canada* ... **140 D3** 43 45N 81 41W
Goderville, *France* ... **26 C7** 49 38N 0 22 E
Godfrey, *U.S.A.* **156 F6** 38 58N 90 11W
Godfrey Ra., *Australia* **125 D2** 24 0 S 117 0 E
Goðafoss, *Iceland* ... **11 B9** 65 41N 17 33W
Godhavn = Qeqertarsuaq, *Greenland* **10 D5** 69 15N 53 38W
Goðdalir, *Iceland* **11 B7** 65 20N 19 6W
Godhra, *India* .... **92 H5** 22 49N 73 40 E
Godinlave, *Somali Rep.* **120 C3** 5 54N 46 38 E
Gödöllő, *Hungary* .... **52 C4** 47 38N 19 25 E
Godoy Cruz, *Argentina* **174 C2** 32 56 S 68 52W
Gods →, *Canada* **140 A1** 56 22N 92 51W
Gods L., *Canada* **140 B1** 54 40N 94 15W
Gods River, *Canada* .. **143 C10** 54 50N 94 5W
Godthåb = Nuuk, *Greenland* **10 E5** 64 10N 51 35W
Godwin Austen = K2, *Pakistan* .... **93 B7** 35 58N 76 32 E
Goeie Hoop, Kaap die = Good Hope, C. of, *S. Africa* .... **116 E2** 34 24 S 18 30 E
Goéland, L. au, *Canada* **140 C4** 49 50N 76 48W
Goélands, L. aux, *Canada* **141 A7** 55 27N 64 17W
Goeree, *Neths.* .... **24 C3** 51 50N 4 0 E
Goes, *Neths.* .... **24 C3** 51 30N 3 55 E
Goffstown, *U.S.A.* ... **151 C13** 43 1N 71 36W
Gogama, *Canada* **140 C3** 47 35N 81 43W
Gogebic, L., *U.S.A.* .. **154 B10** 46 30N 89 35W
Goggetti, *Ethiopia* ... **107 F4** 8 11N 38 35 E
Gogolin, *Poland* ..... **55 H5** 50 30N 18 0 E
Gogonou, *Benin* ..... **113 C5** 10 50N 2 50 E
Gogra = Ghaghara →, *India* .... **93 G11** 25 45N 84 40 E
Gogriâl, *Sudan* ...... **107 F2** 8 30N 28 8 E
Gogti, *Ethiopia* ...... **107 E5** 10 7N 42 51 E
Gohana, *India* .... **92 E7** 29 8N 76 42 E
Goharganj, *India* .... **92 H7** 23 1N 77 41 E
Goi →, *India* .... **92 H6** 22 4N 74 46 E
Goiana, *Brazil* .... **170 C5** 7 33 S 34 59W
Goianésia, *Brazil* .... **171 E2** 15 18 S 49 7W
Goiânia, *Brazil* ...... **171 E2** 16 43 S 49 20W
Goiás, *Brazil* .... **171 E1** 15 55 S 50 10W
Goiás □, *Brazil* ...... **170 D2** 12 10 S 48 0W
Goiatuba, *Brazil* ..... **171 E2** 18 1 S 49 23W
Goio-Erê, *Brazil* ..... **175 A5** 24 12 S 53 1W
Góis, *Portugal* **42 E2** 40 10N 8 6W
Gojam, *Ethiopia* ..... **107 E4** 10 55N 36 30 E
Gojeb, Wabi →, *Ethiopia* .... **107 F4** 7 12N 36 40 E
Gojō, *Japan* .... **73 C7** 34 21N 135 42 E
Gojra, *Pakistan* ...... **92 D5** 31 10N 72 40 E
Gokak, *India* .... **95 F2** 16 11N 74 52 E
Gokarn, *India* .... **95 G2** 14 33N 74 17 E
Gökçe = Sevana Lich, *Armenia* .... **61 K7** 40 30N 45 20 E
Gökçeada, *Turkey* ... **51 F9** 40 10N 25 50 E
Gökçedağ, *Turkey* ... **49 B10** 39 33N 28 56 E
Gökçen, *Turkey* ..... **49 C9** 38 7N 27 53 E
Gökçeören, *Turkey* ... **49 C10** 38 37N 28 35 E
Gökçeyazı, *Turkey* ... **49 B9** 39 40N 27 40 E
Gökırmak →, *Turkey* **100 B6** 41 25N 35 8 E
Gökova, *Turkey* ..... **49 D10** 37 1N 28 17 E
Gökova Körfezi, *Turkey* .... **49 E9** 36 55N 27 50 E
Göksu →, *Turkey* .... **100 D6** 36 19N 34 5 E
Göksun, *Turkey* ..... **100 C7** 38 2N 36 30 E
Gokteik, *Burma* ..... **90 D6** 22 26N 97 0 E
Göktepe, *Turkey* ..... **49 D10** 37 25N 28 34 E
Gokurt, *Pakistan* ..... **92 E2** 29 40N 67 26 E
Gokwe, *Zimbabwe* ... **117 B4** 18 7 S 28 58 E
Gol, *Norway* .... **18 D5** 60 42N 8 55 E
Gol Gol, *Australia* ... **128 C5** 34 12 S 142 14 E
Gola, *India* .... **93 E9** 28 3N 80 32 E
Golaghat, *India* ...... **90 B5** 26 30N 94 0 E
Golakganj, *India* ..... **90 B2** 26 8N 89 52 E
Golan Heights = Hagolan, *Syria* ..... **103 C4** 33 0N 35 45 E
Gołańcz, *Poland* ..... **55 F4** 52 57N 17 18 E
Golāshkerd, *Iran* ..... **97 E8** 27 59N 57 16 E
Golaya Pristen = Hola Pristan, *Ukraine* ... **59 J7** 46 29N 32 32 E
Gölbaşı, *Adiyaman*, *Turkey* .... **100 D7** 37 43N 37 25 E
Gölbaşı, *Ankara*, *Turkey* .... **100 C5** 39 47N 32 49 E
Golchikha, *Russia* .... **6 B12** 71 45N 83 30 E
Golconda, *India* ...... **94 F4** 17 24N 78 23 E
Golconda, *U.S.A.* **158 F5** 40 58N 117 30W
Gölcük, *Kocaeli*, *Turkey* .... **51 F13** 40 42N 29 48 E
Gölcük, *Niğde*, *Turkey* **100 C6** 38 14N 34 47 E
Gold, *U.S.A.* **150 E7** 41 52N 77 50W
Gold Beach, *U.S.A.* .. **158 E1** 42 25N 124 25W
Gold Coast = Ghana ■, *W. Afr.* **113 D4** 8 0N 1 0W
Gold Coast, *Australia* . **122 F9** 28 0 S 153 25 E
Gold Coast, *W. Afr.* .. **113 E4** 4 0N 1 40W
Gold Creek, *U.S.A.* .. **144 E10** 62 46N 149 41W
Gold Hill, *U.S.A.* **158 E2** 42 26N 123 3W
Gold River, *Canada* .. **142 D3** 49 46N 126 3W
Goldach, *Switz.* ...... **33 B8** 47 28N 9 28 E
Gołdap, *Poland* ...... **54 D9** 54 19N 22 18 E
Goldau, *Switz.* .... **33 B7** 47 3N 8 33 E
Goldberg = Złotoryja, *Poland* .... **55 G2** 51 8N 15 55 E
Goldberg, *Germany* .. **30 B8** 53 35N 12 4 E
Golden, *Canada* **142 C5** 51 20N 116 59W
Golden, *U.S.A.* **156 D5** 40 7N 91 1W
Golden B., *N.Z.* ...... **131 A7** 40 40 S 172 50 E
Golden Gate, *U.S.A.* . **158 H2** 37 54N 122 30W
Golden Gate Highlands △, *S. Africa* .... **117 D4** 28 40 S 28 40 E
Golden Hinde, *Canada* **142 D3** 49 40N 125 44W
Golden Lake, *Canada* **150 A7** 45 34N 77 21W
Golden Rock, *India* .. **95 J4** 10 45N 78 48 E
Golden Spike △, *U.S.A.* **158 F7** 41 37N 112 33W
Golden Vale, *Ireland* . **23 D3** 52 33N 8 17W
Goldendale, *U.S.A.* .. **158 D3** 45 49N 120 50W
Goldfield, *U.S.A.* **159 H5** 37 42N 117 14W
Goldingen = Kuldīga, *Latvia* .... **15 H19** 56 58N 21 59 E
Goldsand L., *Canada* . **143 B8** 57 2N 101 8W
Goldsboro, *U.S.A.* ... **149 H7** 35 23N 77 59W
Goldsmith, *U.S.A.* **155 K3** 31 59N 102 37W
Goldsworthy, *Australia* **124 D2** 20 21 S 119 30 E
Goldthwaite, *U.S.A.* .. **155 K5** 31 27N 98 34W
Golegã, *Portugal* **43 F2** 39 24N 8 29W
Goleniów, *Poland* .... **54 E1** 53 35N 14 50 E
Golestān □, *Iran* ..... **97 B7** 37 20N 55 25 E
Golestānak, *Iran* ..... **97 D7** 30 36N 54 14 E
Goleta, *U.S.A.* **161 L7** 34 27N 119 50W
Golfito, *Costa Rica* ... **164 E3** 8 41N 83 5W
Golfo Aranci, *Italy* ... **46 B2** 40 59N 9 38 E
Golfo di Orosei e del Gennargentu △, *Italy* **46 B2** 40 5N 9 15 E
Gölgeli Dağları, *Turkey* **49 D10** 37 10N 28 55 E
Gölhisar, *Turkey* ..... **49 D11** 37 8N 29 31 E
Goliad, *U.S.A.* **155 L6** 28 40N 97 23W
Golija, *Serbia & M.* .. **50 C2** 43 5N 18 45 E
Golija, *Serbia & M.* .. **50 C4** 43 22N 20 15 E
Golina, *Poland* .... **55 F5** 52 15N 18 4 E
Golijam Bratan = Morozov, *Bulgaria* .. **51 D9** 42 30N 25 10 E
Gölköy, *Turkey* ...... **100 B7** 40 41N 37 37 E
Gollel = Lavumisa, *Swaziland* .... **117 D5** 27 20 S 31 55 E
Göllersdorf, *Austria* .. **34 C9** 48 29N 16 7 E
Gollnow = Goleniów, *Poland* .... **54 E1** 53 35N 14 50 E
Gölmarmara, *Turkey* .. **49 C9** 38 42N 27 55 E
Golo →, *France* ..... **29 F13** 42 31N 9 32 E
Golol, *Somali Rep.* ... **120 D2** 3 38N 43 49 E
Gölova, *Turkey* ...... **49 E12** 36 48N 30 5 E
Golovin, *U.S.A.* **144 D7** 64 33N 163 2W
Golpāyegān, *Iran* ..... **97 C6** 33 27N 50 18 E
Gölpazarı, *Turkey* .... **100 B4** 40 16N 30 18 E
Golra, *Pakistan* ...... **92 C5** 33 37N 72 56 E
Golspie, *U.K.* **22 D5** 57 58N 3 59W
Golub-Dobrzyń, *Poland* .... **55 E6** 53 7N 19 2 E
Golubac, *Serbia & M.* . **50 B5** 44 38N 21 38 E
Golungo Alto, *Angola* **115 D2** 9 8 S 14 46 E
Golyam Perelik, *Bulgaria* .... **51 E8** 41 36N 24 33 E
Golyama Kamchiya →, *Bulgaria* .... **51 C11** 43 10N 27 55 E
Golyshi = Vetluzhskiy, *Russia* .... **60 A7** 58 23N 45 26 E
Goma, *Dem. Rep. of the Congo* .... **118 C2** 1 37 S 29 10 E
Gomal Pass, *Pakistan* . **92 D3** 31 56N 69 20 E
Gomati →, *India* .... **93 G10** 25 32N 83 11 E
Gombari, *Dem. Rep. of the Congo* .... **118 B2** 2 45N 29 3 E
Gombe, *Dem. Rep. of the Congo* .... **114 C3** 0 45 S 17 36 E
Gombe, *Nigeria* ...... **113 C7** 10 19N 11 2 E
Gömbe, *Turkey* ...... **49 E11** 36 33N 29 38 E
Gombe □, *Nigeria* ... **113 C7** 10 0N 11 10 E
Gombe →, *Tanzania* . **118 C3** 4 38 S 31 40 E
Gombi, *Nigeria* ...... **113 C7** 10 12N 12 30 E
Gomel = Homyel, *Belarus* .... **59 F6** 52 28N 31 0 E
Gomera, *Canary Is.* .. **9 e1** 28 7N 17 14W
Gómez Palacio, *Mexico* **162 B4** 25 40N 104 0W
Gomīshān, *Iran* .... **97 B7** 37 4N 54 6 E
Gommern, *Germany* .. **30 C7** 52 4N 11 50 E
Gomogomo, *Indonesia* **83 C4** 6 39 S 134 43 E
Gomotartsi, *Bulgaria* . **50 B6** 44 6N 22 57 E
Gompa = Ganta, *Liberia* **112 D3** 7 15N 8 59W
Gomphi, *Greece* ..... **48 B3** 39 26N 21 36 E
Goms, *Switz.* .... **32 D6** 46 27N 8 15 E
Gonābād, *Iran* .... **97 C8** 34 15N 58 45 E
Gonaïves, *Haiti* **165 C5** 19 20N 72 42W
Gonarezhou △, *Zimbabwe* .... **119 G3** 21 32 S 31 55 E
Gonâve, G. de la, *Haiti* **165 C5** 19 29N 72 42W
Gonâve, Île de la, *Haiti* **165 C5** 18 51N 73 3W
Gonbad-e Kāvūs, *Iran* **97 B7** 37 20N 55 25 E
Gönc, *Hungary* ...... **52 B6** 48 28N 21 14 E
Gonda, *India* .... **93 F9** 27 9N 81 58 E
Gondal, *India* .... **92 J4** 21 58N 70 52 E
Gonder, *Ethiopia* ..... **107 E4** 12 39N 37 30 E
Gondia, *India* .... **94 D5** 21 23N 80 10 E
Gondola, *Mozam.* .... **119 F3** 19 10 S 33 37 E
Gondomar, *Portugal* .. **42 D2** 41 10N 8 35W
Gondrecourt-le-Château, *France* ... **27 D12** 48 31N 5 30 E
Gönen, *Balıkesir*, *Turkey* .... **51 F11** 40 6N 27 39 E
Gönen, *Isparta*, *Turkey* **49 D12** 37 57N 30 31 E
Gönen →, *Turkey* .... **51 F11** 40 6N 27 39 E
Gong Xian, *China* .... **76 C5** 28 23N 104 47 E
Gong'an, *China* ...... **77 B9** 30 7N 112 12 E
Gongbei, *China* ...... **69 G10** 22 12N 113 32 E
Gongcheng, *China* ... **77 E8** 24 50N 110 49 E
Gongga Shan, *China* . **76 C3** 29 40N 101 55 E
Gongguan, *China* .... **76 G7** 21 48N 109 36 E
Gonghe, *China* ...... **68 C5** 36 18N 100 32 E
Gongming, *China* .... **69 F10** 22 47N 113 53 E
Gongo Yembe, *Dem. Rep. of the Congo* .... **114 C3** 1 58 S 18 40 E
Gongola →, *Nigeria* .. **113 D7** 9 30N 12 4 E
Gongolgon, *Australia* **127 E4** 30 21 S 146 54 E
Gongoué, *Gabon* ..... **114 C1** 0 31 S 9 13 E
Gongshan, *China* .... **76 D2** 27 43N 98 29 E
Gongtan, *China* ...... **76 C7** 28 55N 108 20 E
Gongzhuling, *China* .. **75 C13** 43 30N 124 40 E
Goniadz, *Poland* ..... **54 E9** 53 30N 22 44 E
Goniri, *Nigeria* .... **113 C7** 11 30N 12 15 E
Gonjo, *China* .... **76 B2** 30 52N 98 17 E
Gonnesa, *Italy* .... **46 C1** 39 16N 8 28 E
Gónnos, *Greece* ...... **48 B4** 39 52N 22 29 E
Gonnosfanádiga, *Italy* **46 C1** 39 29N 8 39 E
Gonzaga, *Phil.* .... **80 B4** 18 16N 122 0 E
Gonzales, *Calif.*, *U.S.A.* **160 J5** 36 30N 121 26W
Gonzales, *Tex.*, *U.S.A.* **155 L6** 29 30N 97 27W
González Chaves, *Argentina* .... **174 D3** 38 2 S 60 5W
Goobang △, *Australia* **129 B8** 33 0 S 148 32 E
Good Hope, C. of, *S. Africa* .... **116 E2** 34 24 S 18 30 E
Goodenough I., *Papua N. G.* .... **132 E6** 9 20 S 150 15 E
Gooderham, *Canada* . **150 B6** 44 54N 78 21W
Goodhouse, *S. Africa* . **116 D2** 28 57 S 18 13 E
Gooding, *U.S.A.* **158 E6** 42 56N 114 43W
Goodland, *U.S.A.* **154 F4** 39 21N 101 43W
Goodlands, *Mauritius* . **121 d** 20 2 S 57 39 E
Goodlow, *Canada* **142 B4** 56 20N 120 8W
Goodnews Bay, *U.S.A.* **144 G7** 59 7N 161 35W
Goodooga, *Australia* . **127 D4** 29 3 S 147 28 E
Goodsprings, *U.S.A.* .. **161 K11** 35 49N 115 27W
Goodwater, *U.S.A.* ... **152 B3** 33 4N 86 3W
Goole, *U.K.* **20 D7** 53 42N 0 53W
Goolgowi, *Australia* .. **129 B6** 33 58 S 145 41 E
Goolwa, *Australia* .... **128 C3** 35 30 S 138 47 E
Goomalling, *Australia* **125 F2** 31 15 S 116 49 E
Goomeri, *Australia* ... **127 D5** 26 12 S 152 6 E
Goonda, *Mozam.* ..... **119 F3** 19 48 S 33 57 E
Goondiwindi, *Australia* **127 D5** 28 30 S 150 21 E
Goongarrie △, *Australia* .... **125 F3** 30 7 S 121 30 E
Goongarrie, L., *Australia* .... **125 F3** 30 3 S 121 9 E
Goonyella, *Australia* .. **126 C4** 21 47 S 147 58 E
Goose →, *Canada* ... **141 B7** 53 20N 60 35W
Goose Creek, *U.S.A.* . **152 C9** 32 59N 80 2W
Goose L., *U.S.A.* **158 F3** 41 56N 120 26W
Gooty, *India* .... **95 G3** 15 7N 77 41 E
Gopalganj, *Bangla.* .. **90 D2** 23 1N 89 50 E
Gopalganj, *India* ..... **93 F11** 26 28N 84 30 E
Göppenstein, *Switz.* .. **32 D5** 46 23N 7 46 E
Göppingen, *Germany* . **31 G5** 48 42N 9 39 E
Gor, *Spain* **43 H8** 37 23N 2 58W
Góra, *Dolnośląskie*, *Poland* .... **55 G3** 51 40N 16 31 E
Góra, *Mazowieckie*, *Poland* .... **55 F7** 52 39N 20 6 E
Góra Kalwaria, *Poland* **55 G8** 51 59N 21 14 E
Gorakhpur, *India* .... **93 F10** 26 47N 83 23 E
Goražde, *Bos.-H.* .... **52 G3** 43 38N 18 58 E
Gorbatov, *Russia* .... **60 B6** 56 12N 43 2 E
Gorbea, Peña, *Spain* .. **40 B2** 43 1N 2 50W
Gorczański △, *Poland* **55 J7** 49 30N 20 10 E
Gorda, *U.S.A.* **160 K5** 35 53N 121 26W
Gorda, Pta., *Canary Is.* **9 e1** 28 45N 18 0W
Gorda, Pta., *Nic.* **164 D3** 14 20N 83 10W
Gordan B., *Australia* . **124 B5** 11 35 S 130 10 E
Gördes, *Turkey* ...... **49 C10** 38 54N 28 17 E
Gordon, *Ga.*, *U.S.A.* . **152 C6** 32 54N 83 20W
Gordon, *Nebr.*, *U.S.A.* **154 D3** 42 48N 102 12W
Gordon →, *Australia* . **127 G4** 42 27 S 145 30 E
Gordon, I., *Chile* .... **176 D3** 54 55 S 69 30W
Gordon L., *Alta.*, *Canada* **143 B6** 56 30N 110 25W
Gordon L., *N.W.T.*, *Canada* **142 A6** 63 5N 113 11W
Gordonvale, *Australia* **126 B4** 17 5 S 145 50 E
Goré, *Chad* .... **109 G3** 7 59N 16 31 E
Gore, *Ethiopia* .... **107 F4** 8 12N 35 32 E
Gore, *N.Z.* .... **131 G3** 46 5 S 168 58 E
Gore Bay, *Canada* ... **140 C3** 45 57N 82 28W
Görele, *Turkey* .... **101 B8** 41 2N 39 0 E
Goreme, *Turkey* ...... **100 C6** 38 35N 34 52 E
Gorey, *Ireland* **23 D5** 52 41N 6 18W
Gorg, *Iran* .... **97 D8** 29 29N 59 43 E
Gorgān, *Iran* .... **97 B7** 36 55N 54 30 E
Gorgona, *Italy* .... **44 E6** 43 26N 9 54 E
Gorgona, *Ethiopia* .... **107 E4** 12 15N 37 17 E
Gorgoram, *Nigeria* ... **113 C7** 12 40N 10 45 E
Gorham, *U.S.A.* **151 B13** 44 23N 71 10W
Gori, *Georgia* .... **61 J7** 42 0N 44 7 E
Goribidnur = Gauribidanur, *India* **95 H3** 13 37N 77 32 E
Goriganga →, *India* . **93 E9** 29 45N 80 23 E
Gorinchem, *Neths.* .. **24 C4** 51 50N 4 59 E
Gorinhatã, *Brazil* .... **171 E2** 19 15 S 49 45W
Goris, *Armenia* ...... **101 C12** 39 31N 46 22 E
Goritsy, *Russia* ...... **58 D9** 57 4N 36 43 E
Gorízia, *Italy* .... **45 C10** 45 56N 13 37 E
Gorj □, *Romania* .... **53 E8** 45 5N 23 25 E
Gorki = Horki, *Belarus* **58 E6** 54 17N 30 59 E
Gorki = Nizhniy Novgorod, *Russia* .. **60 B7** 56 20N 44 0 E
Gorkiy = Nizhniy Novgorod, *Russia* .. **60 B7** 56 20N 44 0 E
Gorkovskoye Vdkhr., *Russia* .... **60 B6** 57 2N 43 4 E
Gorleston, *U.K.* ...... **21 E9** 52 35N 1 44 E
Gorlice, *Poland* ...... **55 J8** 49 35N 21 11 E
Görlitz, *Germany* .... **30 D10** 51 9N 14 58 E
Gorlovka = Horlivka, *Ukraine* .... **59 H10** 48 19N 38 5 E
Gorman, *U.S.A.* **161 L8** 34 47N 118 51W
Gorna Djumaya = Blagoevgrad, *Bulgaria* .... **50 D7** 42 2N 23 5 E
Gorna Dzhumayo = Blagoevgrad, *Bulgaria* .... **50 D7** 42 2N 23 5 E
Gorna Oryakhovitsa, *Bulgaria* .... **51 C9** 43 7N 25 40 E
Gornja Radgona, *Slovenia* .... **45 B13** 46 40N 16 2 E
Gornja Tuzla, *Bos.-H.* **52 F3** 44 35N 18 46 E
Gornji Grad, *Slovenia* **45 B11** 46 20N 14 52 E
Gornji Milanovac, *Serbia & M.* ...... **50 B4** 44 3N 20 29 E
Gornji Vakuf, *Bos.-H.* **52 G2** 43 57N 17 34 E
Gorno Ablanovo, *Bulgaria* .... **51 C9** 43 37N 25 43 E
Gorno-Altay □, *Russia* **66 D9** 51 0N 86 0 E
Gorno-Altaysk, *Russia* **66 D9** 51 50N 86 5 E
Gorno-Badakhshan □, *Tajikistan* .... **65 D6** 38 30N 73 0 E
Gornyatski, *Russia* ... **56 A11** 67 32N 64 3 E
Gornyatskiy, *Russia* .. **61 F5** 48 18N 40 56 E
Gornyy, *Saratov*, *Russia* **60 E9** 51 50N 48 30 E
Gornyy, *Sib.*, *Russia* .. **70 B6** 44 57N 133 59 E
Goro →, *C.A.R.* ..... **114 A4** 9 14N 21 16 E
Gorodenka = Horodenka, *Ukraine* **53 B10** 48 41N 25 29 E
Gorodets, *Russia* ..... **60 B6** 56 38N 43 28 E
Gorodishche = Horodyshche, *Ukraine* .... **59 H6** 49 17N 31 27 E
Gorodishche, *Russia* .. **60 D7** 53 13N 45 40 E
Gorodnya = Horodnya, *Ukraine* .... **59 G6** 51 55N 31 33 E
Gorodok = Haradok, *Belarus* .... **58 E6** 55 30N 30 3 E
Gorodok = Horodok, *Ukraine* .... **59 H2** 49 46N 23 32 E
Gorodok = Zakamensk, *Russia* .... **67 D11** 50 23N 103 17 E
Gorodovikovsk, *Russia* **61 G5** 46 8N 41 58 E
Goroka, *Papua N. G.* . **132 D3** 6 7 S 145 25 E
Goroke, *Australia* .... **128 D4** 36 43 S 141 29 E
Gorokhov = Horokhiv, *Ukraine* .... **59 G3** 50 30N 24 45 E
Gorokhovets, *Russia* . **60 B6** 56 13N 42 39 E
Gorom Gorom, *Burkina Faso* **113 C4** 14 26N 0 14W
Goromonzi, *Zimbabwe* **119 F3** 17 52 S 31 22 E
Gorong, Kepulauan, *Indonesia* .... **83 B4** 3 59 S 131 25 E
Gorongosa △, *Mozam.* **117 B5** 18 50 S 34 29 E
Gorongose →, *Mozam.* **117 C5** 20 30 S 34 40 E
Gorongoza, *Mozam.* .. **119 F3** 18 44 S 34 2 E
Gorongoza, Sa. da, *Mozam.* .... **119 F3** 18 27 S 34 2 E
Gorontalo, *Indonesia* . **82 A2** 0 35N 123 5 E
Gorontalo □, *Indonesia* **79 D6** 0 50N 122 20 E
Goronyo, *Nigeria* .... **113 C6** 13 29N 5 39 E
Górowo Iławeckie, *Poland* .... **54 D7** 54 17N 20 30 E
Gorron, *France* **26 D6** 48 25N 0 50W
Gorshechnoye, *Russia* **59 G10** 51 31N 38 2 E
Gort, *Ireland* **23 C3** 53 3N 8 49W
Gortis, *Greece* .... **39 E5** 35 4N 24 58 E
Gorumahisani, *India* . **94 C8** 22 20N 86 24 E
Góry Bystrzyckie, *Poland* .... **55 H3** 50 16N 16 33 E
Goryachiy Klyuch, *Russia* .... **61 H4** 44 38N 39 8 E
Gorzkowice, *Poland* .. **55 G6** 51 13N 19 36 E
Górzno, *Poland* ..... **55 E6** 53 12N 19 38 E
Gorzów Śląski, *Poland* **55 G5** 51 3N 18 22 E
Gorzów Wielkopolski, *Poland* .... **55 F2** 52 43N 15 15 E
Göschenen, *Switz.* ... **33 C7** 46 40N 8 36 E
Gose, *Japan* .... **73 C7** 34 27N 135 44 E
Gosford, *Australia* ... **129 B9** 33 23 S 151 18 E
Goshen, *Calif.*, *U.S.A.* **160 J7** 36 21N 119 25W
Goshen, *Ind.*, *U.S.A.* .. **157 C11** 41 35N 85 50W
Goshen, *N.Y.*, *U.S.A.* . **151 E10** 41 24N 74 20W
Goshogawara, *Japan* . **70 D10** 40 48N 140 27 E
Goskopi = Kopeysk, *Russia* .... **64 D8** 55 7N 61 37 E
Goslar, *Germany* .... **30 D6** 51 54N 10 25 E
Gospić, *Croatia* ...... **45 D12** 44 35N 15 23 E
Gosport, *U.K.* **21 G6** 50 48N 1 9W
Gosport, *U.S.A.* **157 E10** 39 21N 86 40W
Gossa, *Norway* ...... **18 B3** 62 52N 6 50 E
Gossas, *Senegal* **112 C1** 14 28N 16 0W
Gossau, *Switz.* ...... **33 B8** 47 25N 9 15 E
Gosse →, *Australia* . **126 B1** 19 32 S 134 37 E
Gossi, *Mali* **113 B4** 15 48N 1 20W
Gossinga, *Sudan* .... **107 F2** 8 36N 25 59 E
Gostingen = Gostyń, *Poland* .... **55 G4** 51 50N 17 3 E
Gostinopolye = Volkhov, *Russia* .... **58 C7** 59 55N 32 15 E
Gostivar, *Macedonia* . **50 E4** 41 48N 20 57 E
Gostyń, *Poland* ..... **55 G4** 51 50N 17 3 E
Gostynin, *Poland* .... **55 F6** 52 26N 19 29 E
Göta älv →, *Sweden* . **17 G5** 57 42N 11 54 E
Göta kanal, *Sweden* .. **17 F9** 58 30N 15 58 E
Götaland, *Sweden* ... **17 G8** 57 30N 14 30 E
Göteborg, *Sweden* ... **17 G5** 57 43N 11 59 E
Gotemba, *Japan* ..... **73 B10** 35 18N 138 56 E
Götene, *Sweden* ..... **17 F7** 58 32N 13 30 E
Gotenhafen = Gdynia, *Poland* .... **54 D5** 54 35N 18 33 E
Goteşti, *Moldova* .... **53 D13** 46 9N 28 10 E
Gotha, *Germany* ..... **30 E6** 50 56N 10 42 E
Gothenburg = Göteborg, *Sweden* .. **17 G5** 57 43N 11 59 E
Gothenburg, *U.S.A.* .. **154 E4** 40 56N 100 10W
Gothèye, *Niger* ...... **113 C5** 13 52N 1 34 E
Gotland, *Sweden* .... **17 G12** 57 30N 18 33 E
Gotlands län □, *Sweden* **17 G12** 57 15N 18 30 E
Gotō-Rettō, *Japan* ... **71 H4** 32 55N 129 5 E
Gotse Delchev, *Bulgaria* .... **50 E7** 41 36N 23 46 E
Gotska Sandön, *Sweden* **15 G18** 58 24N 19 15 E
Gōtsu, *Japan* .... **72 C4** 35 0N 132 14 E
Gott Pk., *Canada* **142 C4** 50 18N 122 16W
Göttero, Monte, *Italy* . **44 D6** 44 22N 9 42 E
Gottesberg = Boguszów-Gorce, *Poland* .... **55 H3** 50 45N 16 12 E
Göttingen, *Germany* . **30 D5** 51 31N 9 55 E
Gottschee = Kočevje, *Slovenia* .... **45 C11** 45 39N 14 50 E
Gottwald = Zmiyev, *Ukraine* .... **59 H9** 49 39N 36 27 E
Gottwaldov = Zlín, *Czech Rep.* .... **35 B10** 49 14N 17 40 E
Götzis, *Austria* ...... **33 B9** 47 20N 9 38 E
Goubangzi, *China* .... **75 D11** 41 20N 121 52 E
Gouda, *Neths.* .... **24 B4** 52 1N 4 42 E
Goúdhoura, Ákra, *Greece* .... **39 F7** 34 59N 26 6 E
Goudiry, *Senegal* **112 C2** 14 15N 12 45W
Goudoumaria, *Niger* .. **113 C7** 13 40N 11 10 E
Gouéké, *Guinea* **112 D3** 8 2N 8 43W
Gough I., *Atl. Oc.* ... **8 L11** 40 10 S 9 45W
Gouin, Rés., *Canada* . **140 C5** 48 35N 74 40W
Gouitafla, *Ivory C.* .. **112 D3** 7 30N 5 53W
Goulburn, *Australia* .. **129 C8** 34 44 S 149 44 E
Goulburn Is., *Australia* **126 A1** 11 40 S 133 20 E
Goulburn River △, *Australia* .... **129 B9** 32 19 S 150 10 E
Goulds, *U.S.A.* **153 K9** 25 33N 80 23W
Goulia, *Ivory C.* **112 C3** 10 1N 7 11W
Goulimine, *Morocco* . **110 C3** 28 56N 10 0W
Goulmima, *Morocco* . **110 B4** 31 41N 4 57W
Goumbou, *Mali* **112 B3** 15 2N 7 25W
Gouménissa, *Greece* . **50 F6** 40 56N 22 37 E
Gounatolo, *Solomon Is.* **133 M11** 8 25 S 160 52 E
Goundam, *Mali* **112 B4** 16 27N 3 40W
Goundi, *Chad* .... **109 G3** 9 22N 17 21 E
Gounou-Gaya, *Chad* . **109 G3** 9 38N 15 31 E
Goúra, *Greece* .... **48 D4** 37 56N 22 20 E
Gouraya, *Algeria* .... **111 A5** 36 31N 1 56 E
Gourbassi, *Mali* **112 C2** 13 24N 11 38W
Gourdon, *France* ..... **28 D5** 44 44N 1 23 E
Gouré, *Niger* .... **113 C7** 14 0N 10 10 E
Gouri, *Chad* .... **109 E3** 18 50N 16 49 E
Gourin, *France* **26 D3** 48 8N 3 37W
Gourits →, *S. Africa* . **116 E3** 34 21 S 21 52 E
Gourma-Rharous, *Mali* **113 B4** 16 55N 1 50W
Goúrnais, *Greece* .... **39 E6** 35 19N 25 16 E
Gournay-en-Bray, *France* .... **27 C8** 49 29N 1 44 E
Gouro, *Chad* .... **109 E3** 19 36N 19 36 E
Gourock, *U.K.* **22 F4** 55 57N 4 49W
Gourock Ra., *Australia* **129 D8** 36 0 S 149 25 E
Goursi, *Burkina Faso* . **112 C4** 12 42N 2 37W
Gouvêa, *Brazil* ...... **171 E3** 18 27 S 43 44W
Gouverneur, *U.S.A.* .. **151 B9** 44 20N 75 28W
Gouviá, *Greece* ...... **38 B9** 39 39N 19 50 E
Gouzon, *France* ...... **27 F9** 46 12N 2 14 E
Governador Valadares, *Brazil* .... **171 E3** 18 15 S 41 57W
Governor Generoso, *Phil.* .... **81 H6** 6 39N 126 5 E
Governor's Harbour, *Bahamas* **164 A4** 25 10N 76 14W
Govindgarh, *India* .... **93 G9** 24 23N 81 18 E
Gowan Ra., *Australia* . **126 D4** 25 0 S 145 0 E
Gowanda, *U.S.A.* **150 D6** 42 28N 78 56W
Gower, *U.K.* **21 F3** 51 35N 4 10W
Gowers Corner, *U.S.A.* **153 G7** 28 20N 82 30W
Gowna, L., *Ireland* ... **23 C4** 53 51N 7 34W
Gowrie, *U.S.A.* **156 B2** 42 17N 94 17W
Gowurdak, *Turkmenistan* ...... **65 E3** 37 50N 66 4 E
Goya, *Argentina* ..... **174 B4** 29 10 S 59 10W
Göyçay, *Azerbaijan* .. **61 K8** 40 42N 47 43 E
Goyder Lagoon, *Australia* .... **127 D2** 27 3 S 138 58 E
Goyllarisquisga, *Peru* . **172 C2** 10 31 S 76 24W
Göynük, *Antalya*, *Turkey* .... **49 E12** 36 41N 30 33 E
Göynük, *Bolu*, *Turkey* **100 B4** 40 24N 30 48 E
Goz Beïda, *Chad* ..... **109 F4** 12 10N 21 20 E
Goz Regeb, *Sudan* ... **107 D4** 16 3N 35 33 E
Gozdnica, *Poland* .... **55 G2** 51 28N 15 4 E
Gozo, *Malta* .... **38 E7** 36 3N 14 15 E
Graaff-Reinet, *S. Africa* **116 E3** 32 13 S 24 32 E
Grabill, *U.S.A.* **157 C12** 41 13N 84 57W
Grabo, *Ivory C.* **112 D3** 4 57N 7 30W
Grabow, *Germany* ... **30 B7** 53 17N 11 34 E
Grabów nad Prosną, *Poland* .... **55 G5** 51 31N 18 7 E
Grabs, *Switz.* .... **33 B8** 47 11N 9 27 E
Gračac, *Croatia* ..... **45 D12** 44 18N 15 57 E
Gračanica, *Bos.-H.* .. **52 F3** 44 43N 18 18 E
Graçay, *France* ...... **27 E8** 47 10N 1 50 E
Graceville, *U.S.A.* ... **152 E4** 30 58N 85 31W
Gracewood, *U.S.A.* .. **152 B7** 33 22N 82 2W
Grachevka, *Russia* ... **64 E4** 52 55N 52 52 E
Gracias a Dios, C., *Honduras* **164 D3** 15 0N 83 10W
Graciosa, *Azores* **9 d1** 39 4N 28 0W
Graciosa, I., *Canary Is.* **9 e2** 29 15N 13 32W
Grad Sofiya □, *Bulgaria* .... **50 D7** 42 35N 23 20 E
Gradac, *Serbia & M.* .. **50 C3** 43 23N 19 9 E
Gradačac, *Bos.-H.* ... **52 F3** 44 52N 18 26 E
Gradaús, *Brazil* ...... **170 C1** 7 43 S 51 11W
Gradaús, Serra dos, *Brazil* .... **170 C1** 8 0 S 50 45W
Gradeška Planina, *Macedonia* .... **50 E6** 41 30N 22 15 E
Gradets, *Bulgaria* .... **51 D10** 42 46N 26 30 E
Gradišće, *Slovenia* ... **45 B12** 46 37N 15 50 E
Grădiştea de Munte, *Romania* .... **53 E8** 45 37N 23 13 E
Grado, *Italy* .... **45 C10** 45 40N 13 23 E
Grado, *Spain* **42 B4** 43 23N 6 4W
Grady, *U.S.A.* **155 H3** 34 49N 103 19W
Graeca, Lacul, *Romania* .... **53 F11** 44 5N 26 10 E
Grafarnes, *Iceland* ... **11 C3** 64 55N 23 16W
Grafenau, *Germany* .. **31 G9** 48 51N 13 22 E
Gräfenberg, *Germany* **31 F7** 49 39N 11 14 E
Grafham Water, *U.K.* . **21 E7** 52 19N 0 18W
Grafton, *Australia* ... **127 D5** 29 38 S 152 58 E
Grafton, *Ill.*, *U.S.A.* ... **156 F6** 38 58N 90 26W
Grafton, *N. Dak.*, *U.S.A.* **154 A6** 48 25N 97 25W
Grafton, *W. Va.*, *U.S.A.* **148 F5** 39 21N 80 2W
Graham, *Canada* **140 C1** 49 20N 90 30W
Graham, *Ga.*, *U.S.A.* . **152 D7** 31 50N 82 30W
Graham, *Tex.*, *U.S.A.* . **155 J5** 33 6N 98 35W
Graham, Mt., *U.S.A.* .. **159 K9** 32 42N 109 52W
Graham Bell, Ostrov = Greem-Bell, Ostrov, *Russia* .... **66 A7** 81 0N 62 0 E
Graham I., *Canada* ... **142 C2** 53 40N 132 30W
Graham Land, *Antarctica* .... **7 C17** 65 0 S 64 0W
Grahamstown, *S. Africa* **116 E4** 33 19 S 26 31 E
Grahamsville, *U.S.A.* . **151 E10** 41 51N 74 33W
Grahovo, *Serbia & M.* **50 D2** 42 40N 18 40 E
Graïba, *Tunisia* ...... **108 B2** 34 30N 10 13 E
Graie, Alpi, *Europe* .. **29 C11** 45 30N 7 10 E
Grain Coast, *W. Afr.* . **112 E3** 4 20N 10 0W
Grajagan, *Indonesia* .. **79 K17** 8 35 S 114 13 E
Grajagan, Teluk, *Indonesia* .... **79 K17** 8 40 S 114 18 E
Grajaú, *Brazil* .... **170 C2** 5 50 S 46 4W
Grajaú →, *Brazil* .... **170 B3** 3 41 S 44 48W
Grajewo, *Poland* ..... **54 E9** 53 39N 22 30 E
Gramada, *Bulgaria* ... **50 C6** 43 49N 22 39 E
Gramat, *France* ...... **28 D5** 44 48N 1 43 E
Grammichele, *Italy* ... **47 E7** 37 13N 14 38 E
Grámmos, Óros, *Greece* **50 F4** 40 18N 20 47 E
Grampian, *U.S.A.* **150 F6** 40 58N 78 37W
Grampian Highlands = Grampian Mts., *U.K.* **22 E5** 56 50N 4 0W
Grampian Mts., *U.K.* . **22 E5** 56 50N 4 0W
Grampians △, *Australia* **128 D5** 37 15 S 142 28 E
Grampians, The, *Australia* .... **128 D5** 37 0 S 142 20 E
Gramsh, *Albania* ..... **50 F4** 40 52N 20 12 E
Gran, *Norway* .... **18 D7** 60 23N 10 31 E
Gran →, *Suriname* .. **169 C6** 4 1N 55 30W
Gran Altiplanicie Central, *Argentina* . **176 C3** 49 0 S 69 30W
Gran Canaria, *Canary Is.* **9 e1** 27 55N 15 35W
Gran Chaco, *S. Amer.* **174 B3** 25 0 S 61 0W
Gran Desierto del Pinacate △, *Mexico* . **162 A2** 31 51N 113 32W

Gran Laguna Salada, Argentina 176 B3 44 24 S 67 23W
Gran Pajonal, Peru 172 C3 10 45 S 74 30W
Gran Paradiso, Italy 44 C4 45 33N 7 17 E
Gran Sasso d'Itália, Italy 45 F10 42 27N 13 42 E
Gran Sasso e Monti Della Laga △, Italy 45 F10 42 32N 13 22 E
Granada, Nic. 164 D2 11 58N 86 0W
Granada, Spain 43 H7 37 10N 3 35W
Granada, U.S.A. 155 F3 38 4N 102 19W
Granada □, Spain 43 H7 37 18N 3 0W
Granadilla de Abona, Canary Is. 9 e1 28 7N 16 33W
Granard, Ireland 23 C4 53 47N 7 30W
Granbury, U.S.A. 155 J6 32 27N 97 47W
Granby, Canada 140 C5 45 25N 72 45W
Granby, U.S.A. 158 F11 40 5N 105 56W
Grand →, Canada 150 D5 42 51N 79 34W
Grand →, Mich., U.S.A. 157 A10 43 4N 86 15W
Grand →, Mo., U.S.A. 156 E3 39 23N 93 7W
Grand →, S. Dak., U.S.A. 154 C4 45 40N 100 45W
Grand Anse, Seychelles 121 b 4 18 S 55 45 E
Grand Bahama I., Bahamas 164 A4 26 40N 78 30W
Grand Baie, Mauritius 121 d 20 0 S 57 35 E
Grand Bank, Canada 141 C8 47 6N 55 48W
Grand Banks, Atl. Oc. 8 B6 45 0N 52 0W
Grand Bassam, Ivory C. 112 D4 5 10N 3 49W
Grand Batanga, Cameroon 114 B1 2 50N 9 55 E
Grand Béréby, Ivory C. 112 E3 4 38N 6 55W
Grand Blanc, U.S.A. 157 B13 42 56N 83 38W
Grand-Bourg, Guadeloupe 164 b 15 53N 61 19W
Grand Canal = Yun Ho →, China 75 E9 39 10N 117 10 E
Grand Canyon, U.S.A. 159 H7 36 3N 112 9W
Grand Canyon △, U.S.A. 159 H7 36 15N 112 30W
Grand Canyon-Parashant △, U.S.A. 159 H7 36 30N 113 20W
Grand Cayman, Cayman Is. 164 C3 19 20N 81 20W
Grand Centre, Canada 143 C6 54 25N 110 13W
Grand Cess, Liberia 112 E3 4 40N 8 12W
Grand Coulee, U.S.A. 158 C4 47 57N 119 0W
Grand Coulee Dam, U.S.A. 158 C4 47 57N 118 59W
Grand Erg de Bilma, Niger 109 E2 18 30N 14 0 E
Grand Falls, Canada 141 C6 47 3N 67 44W
Grand Falls-Windsor, Canada 141 C8 48 56N 55 40W
Grand Forks, Canada 142 D5 49 0N 118 30W
Grand Forks, U.S.A. 154 B6 47 55N 97 3W
Grand Gorge, U.S.A. 151 D10 42 21N 74 29W
Grand Haven, U.S.A. 157 A10 43 4N 86 13W
Grand I., Mich., U.S.A. 148 B2 46 31N 86 40W
Grand I., N.Y., U.S.A. 150 D6 43 0N 78 58W
Grand Island, U.S.A. 154 E5 40 55N 98 21W
Grand Isle, La., U.S.A. 155 L9 29 14N 90 0W
Grand Isle, Vt., U.S.A. 151 B11 44 43N 73 18W
Grand Junction, Colo., U.S.A. 159 G9 39 4N 108 33W
Grand Junction, Iowa, U.S.A. 156 B2 42 2N 94 14W
Grand L., N.B., Canada 141 C6 45 57N 66 7W
Grand L., Nfld. & L., Canada 141 C8 49 0N 57 30W
Grand L., Nfld. & L., Canada 141 B7 53 40N 60 30W
Grand L., La., U.S.A. 155 L8 29 55N 92 47W
Grand L., Ohio, U.S.A. 157 D12 40 32N 84 25W
Grand Lahou, Ivory C. 112 D3 5 10N 5 5W
Grand Lake, U.S.A. 158 F11 40 15N 105 49W
Grand Ledge, U.S.A. 157 B12 42 45N 84 45W
Grand-Lieu, L. de, France 26 E5 47 6N 1 40W
Grand Manan I., Canada 141 D6 44 45N 66 52W
Grand Marais, Canada 154 B9 47 45N 90 25W
Grand Marais, U.S.A. 148 B3 46 40N 85 59W
Grand-Mère, Canada 140 C5 46 36N 72 40W
Grand Popo, Benin 113 D5 6 15N 1 57 E
Grand Portage, U.S.A. 154 B10 47 58N 89 41W
Grand Prairie, U.S.A. 155 J6 32 47N 97 0W
Grand Rapids = Wisconsin Rapids, U.S.A. 154 C10 44 23N 89 49W
Grand Rapids, Canada 143 C9 53 12N 99 19W
Grand Rapids, Mich., U.S.A. 157 B10 42 58N 85 40W
Grand Rapids, Minn., U.S.A. 154 B8 47 14N 93 31W
Grand Ridge, U.S.A. 152 E4 30 43N 85 1W
Grand River, U.S.A. 156 D3 40 49N 93 58W
Grand St-Bernard, Col du, Europe 32 E4 45 50N 7 10 E
Grand Santi, Fr. Guiana 169 C7 4 20N 54 24W
Grand Staircase-Escalante △, U.S.A. 159 H8 37 5N 112 0W
Grand Teton, U.S.A. 158 E8 43 54N 111 50W
Grand Teton △, U.S.A. 158 D8 43 50N 110 50W
Grand Union Canal, U.K. 21 E7 52 7N 0 53W
Grand-Vigie, Pte. de la, Guadeloupe 164 b 16 32N 61 27W
Grandas de Salime, Spain 42 B4 43 13N 6 53W
Grande →, Jujuy, Argentina 174 A2 24 20 S 65 2W
Grande →, Mendoza, Argentina 174 D2 36 52 S 69 45W
Grande →, Bolivia 173 D5 15 51 S 64 39W
Grande →, Bahia, Brazil 170 D3 11 30 S 44 30W
Grande →, Minas Gerais, Brazil 171 F1 20 6 S 51 4W
Grande →, Venezuela 169 B5 8 36N 61 39W
Grande, B., Argentina 176 D3 50 30 S 68 20W
Grande, I., Brazil 171 F3 23 9 S 44 14W
Grande, Rio →, U.S.A. 155 N6 25 58N 97 9W
Grande, Serra, Piauí, Brazil 170 C2 8 0 S 45 10W
Grande, Serra, Tocantins, Brazil 170 D2 11 15 S 46 30W
Grande Anse, Seychelles 121 b 4 40 S 55 26 E
Grande Baleine, R. de la →, Canada 140 A4 55 16N 77 47W
Grande Cache, Canada 142 C5 53 53N 119 8W
Grande Casse, Pte. de la, France 29 C10 45 24N 6 49 E
Grande Comore, Comoros Is. 121 a 11 35 S 43 20 E
Grande Dixence, Barr. de la, Switz. 32 D4 46 5N 7 23 E
Grande-Entrée, Canada 141 C7 47 30N 61 40W
Grande Prairie, Canada 142 B5 55 10N 118 50W
Grande-Rivière, Canada 141 C7 48 26N 64 30W
Grande Sertão Veredas △, Brazil 171 E2 15 10 S 45 40W
Grande-Terre, Guadeloupe 164 b 16 20N 61 25W
Grande-Vallée, Canada 141 C6 49 14N 65 8W
Grandfalls, U.S.A. 155 K3 31 20N 102 51W
Grândola, Portugal 43 G2 38 12N 8 35W
Grandpré, France 27 C11 49 20N 4 50 E
Grands Causses △, France 28 D6 44 5N 2 58 E
Grands-Jardins △, Canada 141 C5 47 41N 70 51W
Grandson, Switz. 32 C3 46 49N 6 39 E
Grandview, Canada 143 C8 51 10N 100 42W
Grandview, Mo., U.S.A. 156 F2 38 53N 94 32W
Grandview, Wash., U.S.A. 158 C4 46 15N 119 54W
Grandview Heights, U.S.A. 157 E13 39 58N 83 2W
Grandvilliers, France 27 C8 49 40N 1 57 E
Graneros, Chile 174 C1 34 5 S 70 45W
Grangemouth, U.K. 22 E5 56 1N 3 42W
Granger, U.S.A. 158 F9 41 35N 109 58W
Grängesberg, Sweden 16 D9 60 6N 15 1 E
Grangeville, U.S.A. 158 D5 45 56N 116 7W
Granisle, Canada 142 C3 54 53N 126 13W
Granite City, U.S.A. 156 F6 38 42N 90 9W
Granite Falls, U.S.A. 154 C7 44 49N 95 33W
Granite L., Canada 141 C8 48 8N 57 5W
Granite Mt., U.S.A. 161 M10 33 5N 116 28W
Granite Pk., U.S.A. 158 D9 45 10N 109 48W
Graniteville, S.C., U.S.A. 152 B8 33 34N 81 49W
Graniteville, Vt., U.S.A. 151 B12 44 8N 72 29W
Granîtogorsk, Kazakhstan 65 B6 42 44N 73 28 E
Granitola, C., Italy 46 E5 37 34N 12 39 E
Granity, N.Z. 131 B6 41 39 S 171 51 E
Granja, Brazil 170 B3 3 7 S 40 50W
Granja de Moreruela, Spain 42 D5 41 48N 5 44W
Granja de Torrehermosa, Spain 43 G5 38 19N 5 35W
Gränna, Sweden 17 F8 58 1N 14 28 E
Granollers, Spain 40 D7 41 39N 2 18 E
Gransee, Germany 30 B9 53 1N 13 8 E
Grant, Fla., U.S.A. 153 H9 27 56N 80 32W
Grant, Nebr., U.S.A. 154 E4 40 53N 101 42W
Grant, Mt., U.S.A. 158 G4 38 34N 118 48W
Grant City, U.S.A. 156 D2 40 29N 94 25W
Grant I., Australia 124 B5 11 10 S 132 52 E
Grant Range, U.S.A. 159 G6 38 30N 115 25W
Grantham, U.K. 20 E7 52 55N 0 38W
Grantown-on-Spey, U.K. 22 D5 57 20N 3 36W
Grants, U.S.A. 159 J10 35 9N 107 52W
Grants Pass, U.S.A. 158 E2 42 26N 123 19W
Grantsville, U.S.A. 158 F7 40 36N 112 28W
Grantville, U.S.A. 152 B5 33 14N 84 50W
Granville, France 26 D5 48 50N 1 35W
Granville, Ill., U.S.A. 156 C7 41 16N 89 14W
Granville, N. Dak., U.S.A. 154 A4 48 16N 100 47W
Granville, N.Y., U.S.A. 151 C11 43 24N 73 16W
Granville, Ohio, U.S.A. 150 F2 40 4N 82 31W
Granville L., Canada 143 B8 56 18N 100 30W
Granvin, Norway 18 D3 60 33N 6 45 E
Graskop, S. Africa 117 C5 24 56 S 30 49 E
Gräsö, Sweden 16 D12 60 28N 18 35 E
Grass →, Canada 143 B9 56 3N 96 33W
Grass Range, U.S.A. 158 C9 47 0N 109 0W
Grass River △, Canada 143 C8 54 40N 100 50W
Grass Valley, Calif., U.S.A. 160 F6 39 13N 121 4W
Grass Valley, Oreg., U.S.A. 158 D3 45 22N 120 47W
Grassano, Italy 47 B9 40 38N 16 17 E
Grasse, France 29 E10 43 38N 6 56 E
Grassflat, U.S.A. 150 F6 41 0N 78 6W
Grasslands △, Canada 143 D7 49 11N 107 38W
Grassy, Australia 127 G3 40 3 S 144 5 E
Gråsten, Denmark 17 K3 54 55N 9 35 E
Grästorp, Sweden 17 F6 58 20N 12 40 E
Gratis, U.S.A. 157 E12 39 38N 84 32W
Gratkorn, Austria 34 D8 47 8N 15 21 E
Gratz, U.S.A. 157 F12 38 28N 84 57W
Graubünden □, Switz. 33 C9 46 45N 9 30 E
Graudenz = Grudziądz, Poland 54 E5 53 30N 18 47 E
Graulhet, France 28 E5 43 45N 1 59 E
Graus, Spain 40 C5 42 11N 0 20 E
Gravatá, Brazil 170 C4 8 10 S 35 29W
Gravberget, Norway 18 D9 60 53N 12 14 E
Grave, Pte. de, France 28 C2 45 34N 1 4W
Gravelbourg, Canada 143 D7 49 50N 106 35W
Gravelines, France 27 A9 51 1N 2 10 E
's-Gravenhage, Neths. 24 B4 52 7N 4 17 E
Gravenhurst, Canada 140 D4 44 52N 79 20W
Gravesend, Australia 127 D5 29 35 S 150 20 E
Gravesend, U.K. 21 F8 51 26N 0 22 E
Gravina in Púglia, Italy 47 B9 40 49N 16 25 E
Gravois, Pointe-à-, Haiti 165 C5 18 15N 73 56W
Gravone →, France 29 G12 41 58N 8 45 E
Gray, France 27 E12 47 22N 5 35 E
Gray, U.S.A. 152 B6 33 1N 83 32W
Grayling, Alaska, U.S.A. 144 E7 62 57N 160 3W
Grayling, Mich., U.S.A. 148 C3 44 40N 84 43W
Grays, U.K. 21 F8 51 28N 0 21 E
Grays Harbor, U.S.A. 158 C1 46 59N 124 1W
Grays L., U.S.A. 158 E8 43 4N 111 26W
Grays River, U.S.A. 160 D3 46 21N 123 37W
Grayville, U.S.A. 157 F9 38 16N 88 0W
Grayvoron, Russia 59 G8 50 29N 35 41 E
Graz, Austria 34 D8 47 4N 15 27 E
Grdelica, Serbia & M. 50 D6 42 55N 22 3 E
Greåker, Norway 18 E8 59 16N 11 12 E
Greasy L., Canada 142 A4 62 55N 122 12W
Great Abaco I. = Abaco I., Bahamas 164 A4 26 25N 77 10W
Great Artesian Basin, Australia 126 C3 23 0 S 144 0 E
Great Australian Bight, Australia 125 F5 33 30 S 130 0 E
Great Bahama Bank, Bahamas 164 B4 23 15N 78 0W
Great Barrier I., N.Z. 130 C4 36 11 S 175 25 E
Great Barrier Reef, Australia 126 B4 18 0 S 146 50 E
Great Barrier Reef △, Australia 126 B4 20 0 S 150 0 E
Great Barrington, U.S.A. 151 D11 42 12N 73 22W
Great Basalt Wall △, Australia 126 B4 19 52 S 145 43 E
Great Basin, U.S.A. 158 G5 40 0N 117 0W
Great Basin △, U.S.A. 158 G6 38 55N 114 14W
Great Basses, Sri Lanka 95 L5 6 11N 81 29 E
Great Bear →, Canada 138 B7 65 0N 124 0W
Great Bear L., Canada 138 B7 65 30N 120 0W
Great Belt = Store Bælt, Denmark 17 J4 55 20N 11 0 E
Great Bend, Kans., U.S.A. 154 F5 38 22N 98 46W
Great Bend, Pa., U.S.A. 151 E9 41 58N 75 45W
Great Blasket I., Ireland 23 D1 52 6N 10 32W
Great Britain, Europe 12 E5 54 0N 2 15W
Great Camanoe, Br. Virgin Is. 165 e 18 30N 64 35W
Great Channel, Asia 95 L11 6 0N 94 0 E
Great Coco I., Burma 95 G11 14 7N 93 22 E
Great Codroy, Canada 141 C8 47 51N 59 16W
Great Dividing Ra., Australia 126 C4 23 0 S 146 0 E
Great Driffield = Driffield, U.K. 20 C7 54 0N 0 26W
Great Exuma I., Bahamas 164 B4 23 30N 75 50W
Great Falls, U.S.A. 158 C8 47 30N 111 17W
Great Fish = Groot Vis →, S. Africa 116 E4 33 28 S 27 5 E
Great Guana Cay, Bahamas 164 B4 24 0N 76 20W
Great Himalayan △, India 92 D7 31 30N 77 30 E
Great Inagua I., Bahamas 165 B5 21 0N 73 20W
Great Indian Desert = Thar Desert, India 92 F5 28 0N 72 0 E
Great Karoo, S. Africa 116 E3 31 55 S 21 0 E
Great Khingan Mts. = Da Hinggan Ling, China 69 B7 48 0N 121 0 E
Great Lake, Australia 127 G4 41 50 S 146 40 E
Great Lakes, N. Amer. 136 E11 46 0N 84 0W
Great Malvern, U.K. 21 E5 52 7N 2 18W
Great Miami →, U.S.A. 148 F3 39 20N 84 40W
Great Nicobar, India 95 L11 7 0N 93 50 E
Great Ormes Head, U.K. 20 D4 53 20N 3 52W
Great Ouse →, U.K. 20 E8 52 48N 0 21 E
Great Palm I., Australia 126 B4 18 45 S 146 40 E
Great Pedro Bluff, Jamaica 164 a 17 51N 77 44W
Great Plains, N. Amer. 136 E9 47 0N 105 0W
Great Ruaha →, Tanzania 118 D4 7 56 S 37 52 E
Great Sacandaga L., U.S.A. 151 C10 43 6N 74 16W
Great Saint Bernard Pass = Grand St-Bernard, Col du, Europe 32 E4 45 50N 7 10 E
Great Salt L., U.S.A. 158 F7 41 15N 112 40W
Great Salt Lake Desert, U.S.A. 158 F7 40 50N 113 30W
Great Salt Plains L., U.S.A. 155 G5 36 45N 98 8W
Great Sand Dunes △, U.S.A. 159 H11 37 48N 105 45W
Great Sandy △, Australia 127 D5 26 13 S 153 2 E
Great Sandy Desert, Australia 124 D3 21 0 S 124 0 E
Great Sangi = Sangihe, Pulau, Indonesia 82 A3 3 35N 125 30 E
Great Scarcies →, S. Leone 112 D2 9 0N 13 0W
Great Sd., Bermuda 9 a 32 17N 64 51W
Great Sea Reef, Fiji 133 A2 16 15 S 179 0 E
Great Sitkin I., U.S.A. 144 K3 52 3N 176 6W
Great Skellig, Ireland 23 E1 51 47N 10 33W
Great Slave L., Canada 142 A5 61 23N 115 38W
Great Smoky Mts. △, U.S.A. 149 H4 35 40N 83 40W
Great Snow Mt., Canada 142 B4 57 26N 124 0W
Great Stour = Stour →, U.K. 21 F9 51 18N 1 22 E
Great Victoria Desert, Australia 125 E4 29 30 S 126 30 E
Great Wall, Antarctica 7 C18 62 30 S 58 0W
Great Wall, China 74 E5 38 30N 109 30 E
Great Whale River = Kuujjuarapik, Canada 140 A4 55 20N 77 35W
Great Whernside, U.K. 20 C6 54 10N 1 58W
Great Yarmouth, U.K. 21 E9 52 37N 1 44 E
Great Zab = Zāb al Kabīr →, Iraq 101 D10 36 1N 43 24 E
Great Zimbabwe, Zimbabwe 119 G3 20 16 S 30 54 E
Greater Antilles, W. Indies 165 C5 17 40N 74 0W
Greater London □, U.K. 21 F7 51 31N 0 6W
Greater Manchester □, U.K. 20 D5 53 30N 2 15W
Greater St. Lucia Wetlands △, S. Africa 117 D5 28 6 S 32 27 E
Greater Sudbury = Sudbury, Canada 140 C3 46 30N 81 0W
Greater Sunda Is., Indonesia 78 F4 7 0 S 112 0 E
Grebbestad, Sweden 17 F5 58 42N 11 15 E
Grebenka = Hrebenka, Ukraine 59 G7 50 9N 32 22 E
Greco, C., Cyprus 39 F10 34 57N 34 5 E
Greco, Mte., Italy 45 G10 41 48N 13 58 E
Gredos, Sierra de, Spain 42 E6 40 20N 5 0W
Greece, U.S.A. 150 C7 43 13N 77 41W
Greece ■, Europe 48 B3 40 0N 23 0 E
Greeley, Colo., U.S.A. 154 E2 40 25N 104 42W
Greeley, Nebr., U.S.A. 154 E5 41 33N 98 32W
Greeleyville, U.S.A. 152 B10 33 40N 79 59W
Greem-Bell, Ostrov, Russia 66 A7 81 0N 62 0 E
Green, U.S.A. 158 E2 43 9N 123 22W
Green →, Ky., U.S.A. 148 G2 37 54N 87 30W
Green →, Utah, U.S.A. 159 G9 38 11N 109 53W
Green B., U.S.A. 148 C2 45 0N 87 30W
Green Bay, U.S.A. 148 C2 44 31N 88 0W
Green C., Australia 129 D9 37 13 S 150 1 E
Green City, U.S.A. 156 D4 40 16N 92 57W
Green Cove Springs, U.S.A. 152 F8 29 59N 81 42W
Green Is., Papua N. G. 132 C8 4 35 S 154 10 E
Green Island Bay, Phil. 81 F2 10 12N 119 22 E
Green Lake, Canada 143 C7 54 17N 107 47W
Green Mts., U.S.A. 151 C12 43 45N 72 45W
Green Pond, U.S.A. 152 C9 32 44N 80 37W
Green River, Papua N. G. 132 B1 3 54 S 141 11 E
Green River, Utah, U.S.A. 159 G8 38 59N 110 10W
Green River, Wyo., U.S.A. 158 F9 41 32N 109 28W
Green Valley, U.S.A. 159 L8 31 52N 110 56W
Greenacres City, U.S.A. 153 J9 26 38N 80 7W
Greenbank, U.S.A. 160 B4 48 6N 122 34W
Greenbush, Mich., U.S.A. 150 B1 44 35N 83 19W
Greenbush, Minn., U.S.A. 154 A6 48 42N 96 11W
Greencastle, U.S.A. 157 E10 39 38N 86 52W
Greene, Iowa, U.S.A. 156 B4 42 54N 92 48W
Greene, N.Y., U.S.A. 151 D9 42 20N 75 46W
Greenfield, Calif., U.S.A. 160 J5 36 19N 121 15W
Greenfield, Calif., U.S.A. 161 K8 35 15N 119 0W
Greenfield, Ill., U.S.A. 156 E6 39 21N 90 12W
Greenfield, Ind., U.S.A. 157 E11 39 47N 85 46W
Greenfield, Iowa, U.S.A. 156 C2 41 18N 94 28W
Greenfield, Mass., U.S.A. 151 D12 42 35N 72 36W
Greenfield, Mo., U.S.A. 155 G8 37 25N 93 51W
Greenfield, Ohio, U.S.A. 157 E13 39 21N 83 23W
Greenfield Park, Canada 151 A11 45 29N 73 29W
Greenland ☒, N. Amer. 10 D6 66 0N 45 0W
Greenland Sea, Arctic 10 B10 73 0N 10 0W
Greenock, U.K. 22 F4 55 57N 4 46W
Greenore, Ireland 23 B5 54 2N 6 8W
Greenore Pt., Ireland 23 D5 52 14N 6 19W
Greenough, Australia 125 E1 28 58 S 114 43 E
Greenough →, Australia 125 E1 28 51 S 114 38 E
Greenough Pt., Canada 150 B3 44 58N 81 26W
Greenport, U.S.A. 151 E12 41 6N 72 22W
Greensboro, Fla., U.S.A. 152 E5 30 34N 84 45W
Greensboro, Ga., U.S.A. 152 B6 33 35N 83 11W
Greensboro, N.C., U.S.A. 149 G6 36 4N 79 48W
Greensboro, Vt., U.S.A. 151 B12 44 36N 72 18W
Greensburg, Ind., U.S.A. 157 E11 39 20N 85 29W
Greensburg, Kans., U.S.A. 155 G5 37 36N 99 18W
Greensburg, Pa., U.S.A. 150 F5 40 18N 79 33W
Greenstone Pt., U.K. 22 D3 57 55N 5 37W
Greentown, U.S.A. 157 D11 40 29N 85 58W
Greenup, U.S.A. 157 E8 39 15N 88 10W
Greenvale, Australia 126 B4 18 59 S 145 7 E
Greenville, Liberia 112 D3 5 1N 9 6W
Greenville, Ala., U.S.A. 149 K2 31 50N 86 38W
Greenville, Calif., U.S.A. 160 E6 40 8N 120 57W
Greenville, Fla., U.S.A. 152 E6 30 28N 83 38W
Greenville, Ga., U.S.A. 152 B5 33 2N 84 43W
Greenville, Ill., U.S.A. 156 F7 38 53N 89 25W
Greenville, Ind., U.S.A. 157 F11 38 22N 85 59W
Greenville, Maine, U.S.A. 149 C11 45 28N 69 35W
Greenville, Mich., U.S.A. 157 A11 43 11N 85 15W
Greenville, Miss., U.S.A. 155 J9 33 24N 91 4W
Greenville, Mo., U.S.A. 155 G9 37 8N 90 27W
Greenville, N.C., U.S.A. 149 H7 35 37N 77 23W
Greenville, N.H., U.S.A. 151 D13 42 46N 71 49W
Greenville, N.Y., U.S.A. 151 D10 42 25N 74 1W
Greenville, Ohio, U.S.A. 157 D12 40 6N 84 38W
Greenville, Pa., U.S.A. 150 E4 41 24N 80 23W
Greenville, S.C., U.S.A. 149 H4 34 51N 82 24W
Greenville, Tenn., U.S.A. 149 G4 36 13N 82 51W
Greenville, Tex., U.S.A. 155 J6 33 8N 96 7W
Greenwater Lake △, Canada 143 C8 52 32N 103 30W
Greenwich, Conn., U.S.A. 151 E11 41 2N 73 38W
Greenwich, N.Y., U.S.A. 151 C11 43 5N 73 30W
Greenwich, Ohio, U.S.A. 150 E2 41 2N 82 31W
Greenwich □, U.K. 21 F8 51 29N 0 1 E
Greenwood, Canada 142 D5 49 10N 118 40W
Greenwood, Ark., U.S.A. 155 H7 35 13N 94 16W
Greenwood, Fla., U.S.A. 152 E4 30 52N 85 10W
Greenwood, Ind., U.S.A. 157 E10 39 37N 86 7W
Greenwood, Miss., U.S.A. 155 J9 33 31N 90 11W
Greenwood, S.C., U.S.A. 149 H4 34 12N 82 10W
Greenwood, Mt., Australia 124 B5 13 48 S 130 4 E
Gregbe, Ivory C. 112 D3 6 48N 6 43W
Gregório →, Brazil 172 B3 6 50 S 70 46W
Gregory, U.S.A. 154 D5 43 14N 99 20W
Gregory △, Australia 124 C5 15 38 S 131 15 E
Gregory →, Australia 126 B2 17 53 S 139 17 E
Gregory, L., S. Austral., Australia 127 D2 28 55 S 139 0 E
Gregory, L., W. Austral., Australia 125 E2 25 38 S 119 58 E
Gregory Downs, Australia 126 B2 18 35 S 138 45 E
Gregory L., Australia 124 D4 20 0 S 127 40 E
Gregory Ra., Queens., Australia 126 B3 19 30 S 143 40 E
Gregory Ra., W. Austral., Australia 124 D3 21 20 S 121 12 E
Greifenberg = Gryfice, Poland 54 E2 53 55N 15 13 E
Greifenhagen = Gryfino, Poland 55 E1 53 16N 14 29 E
Greiffenberg = Gryfów Śląski, Poland 55 G2 51 2N 15 24 E
Greiffenberg, Germany 30 B9 53 5N 13 57 E
Greifswald, Germany 30 A9 54 5N 13 23 E
Greifswalder Bodden, Germany 30 A9 54 12N 13 35 E
Grein, Austria 34 C7 48 14N 14 51 E
Greiz, Germany 30 E8 50 39N 12 10 E
Gremikha, Russia 56 A6 67 59N 39 47 E
Gremyachinsk, Russia 64 B6 58 34N 57 51 E
Grenå, Denmark 17 H4 56 25N 10 53 E
Grenada, U.S.A. 155 J10 33 47N 89 49W
Grenada ■, W. Indies 165 D7 12 10N 61 40W
Grenade, France 28 E5 43 47N 1 17 E
Grenadier I., U.S.A. 151 B8 44 3N 76 22W
Grenadines, The, St. Vincent 165 D7 12 40N 61 20W
Grenchen, Switz. 32 B4 47 12N 7 24 E
Grenen, Denmark 17 G4 57 44N 10 40 E
Grenfell, Australia 129 B8 33 52 S 148 8 E
Grenfell, Canada 143 C8 50 30N 102 56W
Grenivík, Iceland 11 B8 65 57N 18 11W
Grenjaðarstaður, Iceland 11 B9 65 49N 17 21W
Grenoble, France 29 C9 45 12N 5 42 E
Grenville, C., Australia 126 A3 12 0 S 143 13 E
Grenville Chan., Canada 142 C3 53 40N 129 46W
Gréoux-les-Bains, France 29 E9 43 45N 5 52 E
Gresham, U.S.A. 160 E4 45 30N 122 26W
Gresik, Indonesia 85 D4 7 13 S 112 38 E
Gressan, Italy 32 E4 45 43N 7 17 E
Gretna, U.K. 22 F5 55 0N 3 3W
Gretna, Fla., U.S.A. 152 E5 30 37N 84 40W
Gretna, La., U.S.A. 155 L9 29 55N 90 4W
Greven, Germany 30 C3 52 6N 7 37 E
Grevená, Greece 50 F5 40 4N 21 25 E
Grevená □, Greece 50 F5 40 2N 21 25 E
Grevenbroich, Germany 30 D2 51 5N 6 35 E
Grevenmacher, Lux. 24 E6 49 41N 6 26 E
Grevesmühlen, Germany 30 B7 53 52N 11 12 E
Grevestrand, Denmark 17 J6 55 36N 12 19 E
Grey →, Canada 141 C8 47 34N 57 6W
Grey →, N.Z. 131 C6 42 27 S 171 12 E
Grey, C., Australia 126 A2 13 0 S 136 35 E
Grey Ra., Australia 127 D3 27 0 S 143 30 E
Greybull, U.S.A. 158 D9 44 30N 108 3W
Greymouth, N.Z. 131 C6 42 29 S 171 13 E
Greystones, Ireland 23 C5 53 9N 6 5W
Greytown, N.Z. 130 H4 41 5 S 175 29 E
Greytown, S. Africa 117 D5 29 1 S 30 36 E
Gribanovskiy, Russia 60 E5 51 28N 41 50 E
Gribbell I., Canada 142 C3 53 23N 129 0W
Gribës, Mal i, Albania 50 F3 40 17N 19 45 E
Gribingui →, C.A.R. 114 A3 8 33N 19 5 E
Gribingui-Bamingui △, C.A.R. 114 A3 7 45N 19 17 E
Gridley, U.S.A. 160 F5 39 22N 121 42W
Griebeg, Ras il-, Malta 38 F7 35 58N 14 23 E
Griekwastad, S. Africa 116 D3 28 49 S 23 15 E
Griesheim, Germany 31 F4 49 51N 8 33 E
Grieskirchen, Austria 34 C6 48 16N 13 48 E
Griffin, U.S.A. 152 B5 33 15N 84 16W
Griffin, L., U.S.A. 153 G8 28 52N 81 51W
Griffith, Australia 129 C7 34 18 S 146 2 E
Griffith, Canada 150 A7 45 15N 77 10W
Griffith I., Canada 150 B4 44 50N 80 55W
Griggsville, U.S.A. 156 E6 39 43N 90 43W
Grignols, France 28 D3 44 23N 0 2W
Grigoriopol, Moldova 53 C14 47 9N 29 18 E
Grimari, C.A.R. 114 A4 5 43N 20 6 E
Grimaylov = Hrymayliv, Ukraine 59 H4 49 20N 26 5 E
Grimes, U.S.A. 160 F5 39 4N 121 54W
Grimm = Kamenskiy, Russia 60 E7 50 48N 45 25 E
Grimma, Germany 30 D8 51 14N 12 43 E
Grimmen, Germany 30 A9 54 7N 13 3 E
Grimsay, U.K. 22 D1 57 29N 7 14W
Grimsby, Canada 150 C5 43 12N 79 34W
Grimsby, U.K. 20 D7 53 34N 0 5W
Grimselpass, Switz. 33 C6 46 34N 8 23 E
Grímsey, Iceland 11 A9 66 33N 17 58W
Grimshaw, Canada 142 B5 56 10N 117 40W
Grimslöv, Sweden 17 H8 56 44N 14 34 E
Grímsstaðir, Iceland 11 B10 65 39N 16 7W
Grimstad, Norway 18 F5 58 20N 8 35 E
Grímsvötn, Iceland 11 C9 64 26N 17 22W
Grindavík, Iceland 11 D4 63 50N 22 26W
Grindelwald, Switz. 32 C6 46 38N 8 2 E
Grindsted, Denmark 17 J2 55 46N 8 55 E
Grindstone I., Canada 151 B8 44 43N 76 14W
Grindu, Romania 53 F11 44 44N 26 50 E
Grinnell, U.S.A. 156 C4 41 45N 92 43W
Grintavec, Slovenia 45 B11 46 22N 14 32 E
Gris-Nez, C., France 27 B8 50 52N 1 35 E
Grishino = Krasnoarmeisk, Ukraine 59 H9 48 18N 37 11 E
Grisolles, France 28 E5 43 49N 1 19 E
Grisons = Graubünden □, Switz. 33 C9 46 45N 9 30 E
Grisslehamn, Sweden 16 D12 60 5N 18 49 E
Grmeč Planina, Bos.-H. 45 D13 44 43N 16 16 E
Groais I., Canada 141 B8 50 55N 55 35W
Grobiņa, Latvia 54 B8 56 33N 21 10 E
Groblersdal, S. Africa 117 D4 25 15 S 29 25 E
Grobming, Austria 34 D6 47 27N 13 54 E
Grocka, Serbia & M. 50 B4 44 40N 20 42 E
Gródek, Poland 55 E10 53 6N 23 40 E
Gródek Tagiellońskí = Horodok, Ukraine 59 H2 49 46N 23 32 E
Grodekovo = Pogranichnyy, Russia 70 B5 44 25N 131 24 E
Grodków, Poland 55 H4 50 43N 17 21 E
Grodno = Hrodna, Belarus 54 E10 53 42N 23 52 E
Grodzisk Mazowiecki, Poland 55 F7 52 7N 20 37 E
Grodzisk Wielkopolski, Poland 55 F3 52 15N 16 22 E
Grodzyanka = Hrodzyanka, Belarus 58 F5 53 31N 28 42 E
Groesbeck, U.S.A. 155 K6 31 31N 96 31W
Groix, France 26 E3 47 38N 3 29W
Groix, Î. de, France 26 E3 47 38N 3 28W
Grójec, Poland 55 G7 51 50N 20 58 E
Gronau, Niedersachsen, Germany 30 C5 52 5N 9 47 E
Gronau, Nordrhein-Westfalen, Germany 30 C3 52 12N 7 2 E
Grong, Norway 14 D15 64 25N 12 8 E
Grönhögen, Sweden 17 H10 56 16N 16 24 E
Groningen, Neths. 24 A6 53 15N 6 35 E
Groningen, Suriname 169 B6 5 48N 55 28W
Groningen □, Neths. 24 A6 53 16N 6 40 E
Grønnedal = Kangilinnguit, Greenland 10 E6 61 20N 47 57W
Groom, U.S.A. 155 H4 35 12N 101 6W
Groot →, S. Africa 116 E3 33 45 S 24 36 E
Groot Berg →, S. Africa 116 E2 32 47 S 18 8 E
Groot-Brakrivier, S. Africa 116 E3 34 2 S 22 18 E
Groot Karasberge, Namibia 116 D2 27 20 S 18 40 E
Groot-Kei →, S. Africa 117 E4 32 41 S 28 22 E
Groot Vis →, S. Africa 116 E4 33 28 S 27 5 E
Grootdrink, S. Africa 116 D3 28 33 S 21 42 E
Groote Eylandt, Australia 126 A2 14 0 S 136 40 E
Grootfontein, Namibia 116 B2 19 31 S 18 6 E
Grootlaagte →, Africa 116 C3 20 55 S 21 27 E
Grootvloer →, S. Africa 116 E3 30 0 S 20 40 E
Gros C., Canada 142 A6 61 59N 113 32W
Gros Islet, St. Lucia 165 f 14 5N 60 58W
Gros Morne △, Canada 141 C8 49 40N 57 50W
Gros Piton, St. Lucia 165 f 13 49N 61 5W
Gros Piton Pt., St. Lucia 165 f 13 49N 61 5W
Grosio, Italy 44 B7 46 18N 10 16 E
Grosne →, France 27 F11 46 42N 4 56 E
Grosotto, Italy 33 D10 46 17N 10 15 E
Gross-Meseritsch = Velké Meziříčí, Czech Rep. 34 B9 49 21N 16 1 E
Gross Strehlitz = Strzelce Opolskie, Poland 55 H5 50 31N 18 18 E
Gross Wartenberg = Syców, Poland 55 G4 51 19N 17 40 E

Grossa, Pta., Spain ... **38 C2** 39 6N 1 36 E
Grosse I., U.S.A. ... **157 B13** 42 8N 83 9W
Grossenbrode,
　Germany .... **30 A7** 54 21N 11 4 E
Grossenhain, Germany **30 D9** 51 17N 13 32 E
Grosser Arber,
　Germany .... **31 F9** 49 6N 13 8 E
Grosser Plöner See,
　Germany .... **30 A6** 54 10N 10 22 E
Grosseto, Italy ...... **45 F8** 42 46N 11 8 E
Grossgerungs, Austria **34 C7** 48 34N 14 57 E
Grossglockner, Austria **34 D5** 47 5N 12 40 E
Grosswardein =
　Oradea, Romania .. **52 C6** 47 2N 21 58 E
Groswater B., Canada **141 B8** 54 20N 57 40W
Grotli, Norway ...... **18 B4** 62 2N 7 42 E
Groton, Conn., U.S.A. **151 E12** 41 21N 72 5W
Groton, N.Y., U.S.A. **151 D8** 42 36N 76 22W
Groton, S. Dak., U.S.A. **154 C5** 45 27N 98 6W
Grottáglie, Italy ...... **47 B10** 40 32N 17 26 E
Grottammare, Italy .. **47 A8** 41 4N 15 2 E
Grottammare, Italy .. **45 F10** 54 N 15 31 E
Grottkau = Grodków,
　Poland .... **55 H4** 50 43N 17 21 E
Grouard Mission,
　Canada **142 B5** 55 33N 116 9W
Grouin, Pte. du, France **26 D5** 48 43N 1 51W
Groundhog ⇸, Canada **140 C3** 48 45N 82 58W
Grouw, Neths. ...... **24 A5** 53 5N 5 51 E
Grove City, Fla., U.S.A. **153 J7** 26 56N 82 19W
Grove City, Ohio,
　U.S.A. **157 E13** 39 53N 83 6W
Grove City, Pa., U.S.A. **150 E4** 41 10N 80 5W
Grove Hill, U.S.A. .. **149 K2** 31 42N 87 47W
Groveland, Calif.,
　U.S.A. **160 H6** 37 50N 120 14W
Groveland, Fla., U.S.A. **153 G8** 28 34N 81 51W
Grover = Tiltonsville,
　U.S.A. **150 F4** 40 10N 80 41W
Grover City, U.S.A. .. **161 K6** 35 7N 120 37W
Groves, U.S.A. **155 L8** 29 57N 93 54W
Groveton, U.S.A. **151 B13** 44 36N 71 31W
Grovetown, U.S.A. .. **152 B7** 33 27N 82 12W
Grožnjan, Croatia .... **45 C10** 45 22N 13 43 E
Groznyy, Russia ..... **61 J7** 43 20N 45 45 E
Grua, Norway .... **18 D7** 60 16N 10 40 E
Grubišno Polje, Croatia **52 E2** 45 44N 17 12 E
Grudovo, Bulgaria ... **51 D11** 42 21N 27 10 E
Grudusk, Poland ..... **55 E7** 53 3N 20 38 E
Grudziądz, Poland ... **54 E5** 53 30N 18 47 E
Gruinard B., U.K. ... **22 D3** 57 56N 5 35W
Gruissan, France .... **28 E7** 43 8N 3 7 E
Grukhi = Novovyatsk,
　Russia .... **64 B2** 58 24N 49 45 E
Grumo Áppula, Italy . **47 A9** 41 1N 16 42 E
Grums, Sweden ...... **16 E7** 59 22N 13 5 E
Grünberg, Germany .. **30 E4** 50 35N 8 58 E
Grünberg in Schlesien =
　Zielona Góra,
　Poland .... **55 G2** 51 57N 15 31 E
Grund, Iceland **11 B8** 65 31N 18 9W
Gründau, Germany ... **31 E5** 50 10N 9 9 E
Grundy Center, U.S.A. **156 B4** 42 22N 92 47W
Grungedal, Norway .. **18 E4** 59 44N 7 43 E
Grünstadt, Germany .. **31 F4** 49 34N 8 9 E
Gruppo di Tessa △,
　Italy .... **44 B8** 46 47N 11 0 E
Gruvberget, Sweden .. **16 C10** 61 6N 16 10 E
Gruver, U.S.A. **155 G4** 36 16N 101 24W
Gruyères, Switz. ..... **32 C4** 46 35N 7 4 E
Gruža, Serbia & M. ... **50 C4** 43 54N 20 46 E
Gryazi, Russia .... **59 F10** 52 30N 39 58 E
Gryazovets = Borovichi,
　Russia .... **58 C7** 58 25N 33 55 E
Gryazovets, Russia ... **58 C11** 58 50N 40 10 E
Grybów, Poland ..... **55 J7** 49 36N 20 55 E
Gryckebo, Sweden ... **16 D9** 60 40N 15 29 E
Gryfice, Poland ...... **54 E2** 53 55N 15 13 E
Gryfino, Poland ..... **55 E1** 53 16N 14 29 E
Gryfów Śląski, Poland **55 G2** 51 2N 15 24 E
Grythyttan, Sweden .. **16 E8** 59 41N 14 32 E
Gstaad, Switz. ...... **32 D4** 46 28N 7 18 E
Gua Musang, Malaysia **87 K3** 4 53N 101 58 E
Guacanayabo, G. de,
　Cuba **164 B4** 20 40N 77 20W
Guacara, Venezuela .. **168 A4** 10 14N 67 53W
Guachípas ⇸,
　Argentina .... **174 B2** 25 40 S 65 30W
Guachiria ⇸,
　Colombia **168 B3** 5 27N 70 36W
Guadajoz ⇸, Spain .. **43 H6** 37 50N 4 51W
Guadalajara, Mexico .. **162 C4** 20 40N 103 20W
Guadalajara, Spain ... **40 E1** 40 37N 3 12W
Guadalajara □, Spain . **40 E2** 40 47N 2 30W
Guadalcanal,
　Solomon Is. ...... **133 M11** 9 32 S 160 12 E
Guadalcanal, Spain ... **43 G5** 38 5N 5 52W
Guadalén ⇸, Spain .. **43 G7** 38 5N 3 32W
Guadales, Argentina .. **174 C2** 34 30 S 67 55W
Guadalete ⇸, Spain .. **43 J4** 36 35N 6 13W
Guadalimar ⇸, Spain **43 G7** 38 19N 3 28W
Guadalmena ⇸, Spain **43 G8** 38 19N 2 56W
Guadalmez ⇸, Spain . **43 G5** 38 46N 5 4W
Guadalope ⇸, Spain . **40 D4** 41 15N 0 3W
Guadalquivir ⇸, Spain **43 J4** 36 47N 6 22W
Guadalupe =
　Guadeloupe ☑,
　W. Indies .... **164 b** 16 20N 61 40W
Guadalupe, Brazil .... **170 C3** 6 44 S 43 47W
Guadalupe, Mexico ... **161 N10** 32 4N 116 32W
Guadalupe, Spain **43 F5** 39 27N 5 17W
Guadalupe, U.S.A. ... **161 L6** 34 59N 120 33W
Guadalupe ⇸, Mexico **161 N10** 32 6N 116 51W
Guadalupe ⇸, U.S.A. **155 L6** 28 27N 96 47W
Guadalupe, Sierra de,
　Spain **43 F5** 39 28N 5 30W
Guadalupe Bravos,
　Mexico **162 A3** 31 20N 106 10W
Guadalupe I., Pac. Oc. **136 G8** 29 0N 118 50W
Guadalupe Mts. △,
　U.S.A. **155 K2** 31 40N 104 30W
Guadalupe Peak,
　U.S.A. **155 K2** 31 50N 104 52W
Guadalupe y Calvo,
　Mexico **162 B3** 26 6N 106 58W
Guadarrama, Sierra de,
　Spain **42 E7** 41 0N 4 0W
Guadauta, Georgia ... **61 J5** 43 7N 40 32 E
Guadeloupe △,
　Guadeloupe ...... **164 b** 16 10N 61 40W
Guadeloupe ☑,
　W. Indies .... **164 b** 16 20N 61 40W
Guadeloupe Passage,
　W. Indies **165 C7** 16 50N 62 15W
Guadelupe, Peru ..... **172 B2** 7 15 S 79 29W
Guadiana ⇸, Spain .. **43 J4** 36 55N 6 24W
Guadiana ⇸, Portugal **43 H3** 37 14N 7 22W
Guadiana Menor ⇸,
　Spain **43 H7** 37 56N 3 15W
Guadiaro ⇸, Spain .. **43 J5** 36 17N 5 17W
Guadiato ⇸, Spain ... **43 H5** 37 48N 5 9W
Guadiela ⇸, Spain ... **40 E2** 40 22N 2 49W
Guadix, Spain **43 H7** 37 18N 3 11W
Guafo, Boca del, Chile **176 B2** 43 35 S 74 0W

Guafo, I., Chile ...... **176 B2** 43 35 S 74 50W
Guaico, Trin. & Tob. . **169 F9** 10 35N 61 9W
Guainía □, Colombia . **168 C4** 2 30N 69 0W
Guainía ⇸, Colombia **168 C4** 2 1N 67 7W
Guaíra, Brazil .... **175 A5** 24 5 S 54 10W
Guaíra □, Paraguay .. **174 B4** 25 45 S 56 30W
Guaitecas, Is., Chile .. **176 B2** 44 0 S 74 30W
Guajará-Mirim, Brazil **173 C4** 10 50 S 65 20W
Guajira □, Colombia . **168 A3** 11 30N 72 30W
Guajira, Pen. de la,
　Colombia **168 A3** 12 0N 72 0W
Gualaceo, Ecuador ... **168 D2** 2 54 S 78 47W
Gualán, Guatemala ... **164 C2** 15 8N 89 22W
Gualdo Tadino, Italy . **45 E9** 43 14N 12 47 E
Gualeguay, Argentina **174 C4** 33 10 S 59 14W
Gualeguaychú,
　Argentina .... **174 C4** 33 3 S 59 31W
Gualeguay ⇸,
　Argentina .... **174 C4** 33 19 S 59 39W
Gualicho, Salina,
　Argentina .... **176 B3** 40 25 S 65 20W
Gualjaina, Argentina . **176 B2** 42 45 S 70 30W
Guam ☑, Pac. Oc. ... **133 R15** 13 27N 144 45 E
Guamá, Brazil .... **170 B2** 1 37 S 47 29W
Guamá ⇸, Brazil .... **170 B2** 1 29 S 48 30W
Guamini, Argentina .. **174 D3** 37 1 S 62 28W
Guamote, Ecuador ... **168 D2** 1 56 S 78 43W
Guampí, Sierra de,
　Venezuela **169 B4** 6 0N 65 35W
Guamúchil, Mexico .. **162 B3** 25 25N 108 3W
Guana I., Br. Virgin Is. **165 e** 18 30N 64 30W
Guanabacoa, Cuba ... **164 B3** 23 8N 82 18W
Guanacaste △,
　Costa Rica **164 D2** 10 57N 85 30W
Guanacaste, Cordillera
　del, Costa Rica ... **164 D2** 10 40N 85 4W
Guanaceví, Mexico .. **162 B3** 25 40N 106 0W
Guanahani = San
　Salvador I., Bahamas **165 B5** 24 0N 74 40W
Guanajay, Cuba **164 B3** 22 56N 82 42W
Guanajuato, Mexico .. **162 C4** 21 0N 101 20W
Guanajuato □, Mexico **162 C4** 20 40N 101 20W
Guanambi, Brazil .... **171 D3** 14 13 S 42 47W
Guanare, Venezuela .. **168 B4** 8 42N 69 12W
Guanare ⇸, Venezuela **168 B4** 8 13N 67 46W
Guanacol, Argentina . **174 B2** 29 30 S 68 40W
Guane, Cuba **164 B3** 22 10N 84 7W
Guang'an, China .... **76 B6** 30 28N 106 35 E
Guangchang, China .. **77 D11** 26 50N 116 21 E
Guangde, China ..... **77 B12** 30 54N 119 25 E
Guangdong □, China . **77 F9** 23 0N 113 0 E
Guangfeng, China ... **77 C12** 28 20N 118 15 E
Guanghan, China .... **76 B5** 30 58N 104 17 E
Guanghua, China .... **74 E8** 39 47N 114 22 E
Guangling, China .... **76 E5** 24 5N 105 4 E
Guangning, China ... **77 F9** 23 40N 112 22 E
Guangrao, China .... **75 F10** 37 5N 118 25 E
Guangshui, China .... **77 B9** 31 37N 114 0 E
Guangshun, China ... **76 D6** 26 8N 106 21 E
Guangwu, China ..... **74 F3** 37 48N 105 57 E
Guangxi Zhuangzu
　Zizhiqu □, China . **76 F7** 24 0N 109 0 E
Guangyuan, China ... **76 A5** 32 26N 105 51 E
Guangze, China ..... **77 D11** 27 30N 117 12 E
Guangzhou, China ... **77 F9** 23 5N 113 10 E
Guanhães, Brazil .... **171 E3** 18 47 S 42 57W
Guánica, Puerto Rico . **165 d** 17 58N 66 55W
Guanipa ⇸, Venezuela **169 B5** 9 56N 62 26W
Guanling, China ..... **76 E5** 25 56N 105 35 E
Guannan, China ..... **75 G10** 34 8N 119 21 E
Guanta, Venezuela ... **169 A5** 10 14N 64 36W
Guantánamo, Cuba .. **165 B4** 20 10N 75 14W
Guantánamo B., Cuba **165 C4** 19 59N 75 10W
Guantao, China ..... **74 F8** 36 42N 115 25 E
Guanyang, China .... **77 E8** 25 30N 111 8 E
Guanyun, China ..... **75 G10** 34 20N 119 18 E
Guapí, Colombia **168 C2** 2 36N 77 54W
Guápiles, Costa Rica . **164 D3** 10 10N 83 46W
Guapo B., Trin. & Tob. **169 F9** 10 12N 61 41W
Guaporé = Rondônia □,
　Brazil .... **173 C5** 10 52 S 61 57W
Guaporé, Brazil ...... **175 B5** 28 51 S 51 54W
Guaporé ⇸, Brazil ... **173 C4** 11 55 S 65 4W
Guaqui, Bolivia ...... **172 D4** 16 41 S 68 54W
Guara, Sierra de, Spain **40 C4** 42 19N 0 15W
Guarabira, Brazil .... **170 C4** 6 51 S 35 29W
Guaramacal △,
　Venezuela **165 E3** 9 13N 70 12W
Guaranda, Ecuador .. **168 D2** 1 36 S 79 0W
Guarani = Pacajus,
　Brazil .... **170 B4** 4 10 S 38 31W
Guarapari, Brazil .... **171 F3** 20 40 S 40 30W
Guarapuava, Brazil .. **171 G1** 25 20 S 51 30W
Guaratinguetá, Brazil **175 A6** 22 49 S 45 9W
Guaratuba, Brazil .... **175 B6** 25 53 S 48 38W
Guarda, Portugal **42 E3** 40 32N 7 20W
Guarda □, Portugal .. **42 E3** 40 40N 7 20W
Guardafui, C. = Asir,
　Ras, Somali Rep. .. **120 B4** 11 55N 51 10 E
Guardamar del Segura,
　Spain **41 G4** 38 5N 0 39W
Guardavalle, Italy .... **47 D9** 38 30N 16 30 E
Guárdia Sanframondi,
　Italy .... **47 A7** 41 15N 14 36 E
Guardiagrele, Italy ... **45 F11** 42 11N 14 13 E
Guardo, Spain **42 C6** 42 47N 4 50W
Guareña, Spain **43 G4** 38 51N 6 6W
Guareña ⇸, Spain ... **42 D5** 41 29N 5 23W
Guari, Papua N. G. .. **132 E4** 8 3 S 146 52 E
Guárico □, Venezuela **168 B4** 8 40N 66 35W
Guarojo ⇸, Colombia **168 C3** 4 6N 70 42W
Guarujá, Brazil ...... **175 A6** 24 2 S 46 25W
Guarulhos = Guarus,
　Brazil .... **171 F3** 21 44 S 41 20W
Guarulhos, Brazil .... **175 A6** 23 29 S 46 33W
Guarus, Brazil .... **171 F3** 21 44 S 41 20W
Guasave, Mexico **162 B3** 25 34N 108 27W
Guascama, Pta.,
　Colombia **168 C2** 2 32N 78 24W
Guasdualito, Venezuela **168 B3** 7 15N 70 44W
Guasipati, Venezuela . **169 B5** 7 28N 61 54W
Guasopa, Papua N. G. **132 E7** 9 12 S 152 58 E
Guastalla, Italy ...... **44 D7** 44 55N 10 39 E
Guatemala, Guatemala **164 D1** 14 40N 90 22W
Guatemala ■,
　Cent. Amer. **164 C1** 15 40N 90 30W
Guatemala Trench,
　Pac. Oc. **136 H10** 15 0N 95 0W
Guatire, Venezuela ... **168 A4** 10 28N 66 32W
Guatopo △, Venezuela **165 F6** 10 5N 66 38W
Guatuaro Pt.,
　Trin. & Tob. **169 F10** 10 19N 60 59W
Guaviare □, Colombia **168 C3** 2 0N 72 30W
Guaviare ⇸, Colombia **168 C4** 4 3N 67 44W
Guaxupé, Brazil ..... **175 A6** 21 10 S 47 5W
Guayabero ⇸,
　Colombia **168 C3** 2 36N 72 47W
Guayaguayare,
　Trin. & Tob. **169 F9** 10 8N 61 2W
Guayama, Puerto Rico **165 d** 17 59N 66 7W
Guayaneco, Arch.,
　Chile .... **176 C1** 47 45 S 75 10W

Guayaquil, Ecuador .. **168 D2** 2 15 S 79 52W
Guayaquil, G. de,
　Ecuador .... **168 D1** 3 10 S 81 0W
Guayaramerín, Bolivia **173 C4** 10 48 S 65 23W
Guayas ⇸, Ecuador .. **168 D2** 2 36 S 79 52W
Guaymas, Mexico **162 B2** 27 59N 110 54W
Guba, Dem. Rep. of
　the Congo .... **119 E2** 10 38 S 26 27 E
Guba, Ethiopia ...... **107 E4** 11 17N 35 20 E
Gubakha, Russia ..... **64 B6** 58 52N 57 36 E
Gūbāl, Madīq, Egypt . **106 B3** 27 30N 34 0 E
Gubam, Papua N. G. . **132 E1** 8 39 S 141 53 E
Guban, Somali Rep. .. **120 B1** 10 30N 44 0 E
Gubat, Phil. .... **80 E5** 12 55N 124 7 E
Gubbi, India .... **95 H3** 13 19N 76 56 E
Gúbbio, Italy .... **45 E9** 43 21N 12 35 E
Guben, Germany ..... **30 D10** 51 57N 14 42 E
Gubin, Poland .... **55 G1** 51 57N 14 43 E
Gubio, Nigeria ...... **113 C7** 12 30N 12 42 E
Gubkin, Russia ...... **59 G9** 51 17N 37 32 E
Gúca, Serbia & M. ... **50 C4** 43 46N 20 15 E
Gucheng, China ..... **77 A8** 32 20N 111 30 E
Gudá, Norway ...... **18 A8** 63 27N 11 36 E
Gudalur, India ...... **95 J3** 11 30N 76 29 E
Gudata = Guadauta,
　Georgia .... **61 J5** 43 7N 40 32 E
Gudbrandsdalen,
　Norway .... **15 F14** 61 33N 10 10 E
Gudená ⇸, Denmark **17 H4** 56 29N 10 13 E
Gudermes, Russia .... **61 J8** 43 24N 46 5 E
Gudhjem, Denmark .. **17 J8** 55 12N 14 58 E
Gudivada, India ..... **95 F5** 16 30N 81 3 E
Gudiyattam, India ... **95 H4** 12 57N 78 55 E
Gudur, India .... **95 G4** 14 12N 79 55 E
Gudvangen, Norway . **18 D3** 60 52N 6 49 E
Guebwiller, France ... **27 E14** 47 55N 7 12 E
Guecho = Getxo, Spain **40 B7** 43 21N 2 59W
Guékédou, Guinea ... **112 D2** 8 40N 10 5W
Guelb er Rîchât,
　Mauritania **110 D2** 21 7N 11 24W
Guélé Mendouka,
　Cameroon .... **113 E7** 4 23N 12 55 E
Guélengdeng, Chad .. **109 F3** 10 55N 15 31 E
Guelma, Algeria ..... **111 A6** 36 25N 7 29 E
Guelmine = Goulimine,
　Morocco **110 C3** 28 56N 10 0W
Guelph, Canada **140 D3** 43 35N 80 20W
Guelta Zemmur,
　W. Sahara **110 C2** 25 8N 12 22W
Guémar, Algeria ..... **111 B6** 33 30N 6 49 E
Guémené-Penfao,
　France **26 E5** 47 38N 1 50W
Guémené-sur-Scorff,
　France **26 D3** 48 4N 3 13W
Guéné, Benin .... **113 C5** 11 44N 3 16 E
Güeppí, Peru .... **168 D2** 0 7 S 75 15W
Guer Aike, Argentina . **176 D3** 51 39 S 69 35W
Guéra, Chad .... **109 F3** 11 55N 18 12 E
Guérande, France **26 E4** 47 20N 2 26W
Guerara, Algeria ..... **111 B5** 32 51N 4 22 E
Guercif, Morocco **111 B4** 34 14N 3 21W
Guéréda, Chad ...... **109 F4** 14 31N 22 5 E
Guéret, France ...... **27 F8** 46 11N 1 51 E
Guérigny, France .... **27 E10** 47 6N 3 10 E
Guernica = Gernika-
　Lumo, Spain **40 B7** 43 19N 2 40W
Guernsey, U.K. **21 H5** 49 26N 2 35W
Guernsey, U.S.A. **154 D2** 42 19N 104 45W
Guerrara, Algeria **111 C4** 28 5N 0 8W
Guerrero □, Mexico .. **163 D5** 17 30N 100 0W
Guerzim, Algeria **111 C4** 29 39N 1 40W
Guessou-Sud, Benin . **113 C5** 10 3N 2 38 E
Gueugnon, France ... **27 F11** 46 36N 4 4 E
Guéyo, Ivory C. **112 D3** 5 25N 6 5W
Gufuðalur, Iceland .. **11 B4** 65 34N 22 5W
Gughe, Ethiopia ..... **107 F4** 6 12N 37 30 E
Gūgher, Iran .... **97 D8** 29 28N 56 27 E
Guglionesi, Italy ..... **45 G11** 41 55N 14 55 E
Guhakolak, Tanjung,
　Indonesia .... **79 G11** 6 50 S 105 14 E
Guhuru = Góra, Poland **55 G3** 51 40N 16 31 E
Gui Jiang ⇸, China .. **77 F8** 23 30N 111 15 E
Guia, Canary Is. **9 e1** 28 8N 15 38W
Guia de Isora,
　Canary Is. **9 e1** 28 12N 16 46W
Guia Lopes da Laguna,
　Brazil .... **175 A4** 21 26 S 56 7W
Guiana, Venezuela ... **169 B5** 5 9N 63 36W
Guiana Highlands,
　S. Amer. **166 C4** 5 10N 60 40W
Guibéroua, Ivory C. .. **112 D3** 6 14N 6 10W
Guichen B., Australia . **128 D3** 37 0 S 139 45 E
Guichi, China .... **77 B11** 30 39N 117 19 E
Guider, Cameroon ... **113 D7** 9 56N 13 57 E
Guidiguir, Niger ..... **113 C6** 13 42N 9 31 E
Guiding, China ...... **76 D6** 26 34N 107 11 E
Guidong, China ..... **77 D9** 26 7N 113 57 E
Guidónia-Montecélio,
　Italy .... **45 F9** 42 1N 12 45 E
Guiers, L. de, Senegal . **112 B1** 16 10N 15 50W
Guigang, China ...... **76 F7** 23 8N 109 35 E
Guiglo, Ivory C. **112 D3** 6 45N 7 30W
Guihulñgan, Phil. ... **81 F4** 10 7N 123 14 E
Guijá, Mozam. ...... **117 C5** 24 27 S 33 0 E
Guijo de Coria, Spain . **42 E4** 40 6N 6 28W
Güijar, Pakistan ..... **95 C4** 32 10N 71 55 E
Guildford, U.K. **21 F7** 51 14N 0 34W
Guilford, U.S.A. **151 E12** 41 17N 72 41W
Guilin, China .... **77 E8** 25 18N 110 15 E
Guillaume-Delisle, L.,
　Canada **140 A4** 56 15N 76 17W
Guillaumes, France .. **29 D10** 44 5N 6 52 E
Guillestre, France .... **29 D10** 44 39N 6 40 E
Guilvinec, France **26 E2** 47 48N 4 17W
Güïmar, Canary Is. .. **9 e1** 28 18N 16 24W
Guimarães, Brazil .... **170 B3** 2 9 S 44 42W
Guimarães, Portugal . **42 D2** 41 28N 8 24W
Guimaras □, Phil. ... **81 F4** 10 35N 122 37 E
Guimba, Phil. .... **80 D3** 15 40N 120 46 E
Guinayangan, Phil. .. **80 E4** 13 54N 122 27 E
Guinda, U.S.A. **160 G4** 38 50N 122 12W
Guindulman, Phil. ... **81 G5** 9 46N 124 29 E
Guinea, Africa ...... **104 F4** 8 0N 8 0 E
Guinea ■, W. Afr. ... **112 C2** 10 20N 11 30W
Guinea, Gulf of,
　Atl. Oc. .... **113 E5** 3 0N 2 30 E
Guinea-Bissau ■,
　Africa **112 C2** 12 0N 15 0W
Güines, Cuba **164 B3** 22 50N 82 0W
Guingamp, France ... **26 D3** 48 34N 3 10W
Guingueiro, Senegal . **112 C1** 14 11N 15 57W
Guinguinéo, Senegal . **112 C1** 14 26N 15 57W
Guipúzcoa □, Spain .. **40 B2** 43 12N 2 15W
Guiping, China ...... **77 F8** 23 21N 110 2 E
Guipúzcoa □, Spain .. **40 B2** 43 12N 2 15W
Guir ⇸, Mali **112 B4** 14 59N 12 45W
Guir, O. ⇸, Algeria .. **111 B4** 31 29N 2 17W
Guiratinga, Brazil .... **173 D7** 16 21 S 53 45W
Guirel, Mauritania ... **112 B3** 15 30N 7 3W
Güiria, Venezuela **169 F8** 10 32N 62 18W
Guiscard, France .... **27 C10** 49 40N 3 1 E
Guise, France .... **27 C10** 49 52N 3 35 E

Guita-Koulouba,
　C.A.R. .... **114 A4** 5 58N 23 21 E
Guitiriz, Spain **42 B3** 43 11N 7 50W
Guitri, Ivory C. **112 D3** 5 30N 5 14W
Guiuan, Phil. .... **81 F5** 11 5N 125 55 E
Guixi, China .... **77 C11** 28 16N 117 15 E
Guiyang, Guizhou,
　China .... **76 D6** 26 32N 106 40 E
Guiyang, Hunan, China **77 E9** 25 46N 112 42 E
Guizhou □, China .... **76 D6** 27 0N 107 0 E
Guixi, China .... **77 D10** 27 11N 114 47 E
Gujan-Mestras, France **28 D2** 44 38N 1 4W
Gujar Khan, Pakistan **92 C5** 33 16N 73 19 E
Gujarat □, India ..... **92 H4** 23 20N 71 0 E
Gujiang, China ...... **77 D10** 27 11N 114 47 E
Gujranwala, Pakistan **91 B4** 32 10N 74 12 E
Gujrat, Pakistan ..... **91 B4** 32 40N 74 2 E
Gukovo, Russia ..... **61 F5** 48 1N 39 58 E
Gulargambone,
　Australia .... **129 A8** 31 20 S 148 30 E
Gulbarga, India ..... **94 F3** 17 20N 76 50 E
Gulbene, Latvia ..... **15 H22** 57 8N 26 52 E
Gülchö, Kyrgyzstan .. **65 C6** 40 19N 73 26 E
Guledagudda, India .. **95 F2** 16 3N 75 48 E
Gulf □, Papua N. G. . **132 D3** 8 0 S 145 0 E
Gulf, Asia .... **97 E6** 27 0N 50 0 E
Gulf, The = Persian
　Gulf, Asia .... **97 E6** 27 0N 50 0 E
Gulf Breeze, U.S.A. .. **153 E2** 30 21N 87 9W
Gulf Hammock, U.S.A. **153 F7** 29 15N 82 43W
Gulf Islands △, U.S.A. **153 D2** 30 10N 87 10W
Gulfport, Fla., U.S.A. **153 H7** 27 44N 82 43W
Gulfport, Miss., U.S.A. **155 K10** 30 22N 89 6W
Gulgong, Australia ... **129 B8** 32 20 S 149 49 E
Gulin, China .... **76 C5** 28 1N 105 50 E
Gulistan, Pakistan ... **92 D2** 30 30N 66 35 E
Guliston, Uzbekistan . **65 C6** 40 30N 68 46 E
Gulkana, U.S.A. **144 E11** 62 16N 145 23W
Gull Lake, Canada ... **143 C7** 50 10N 108 29W
Gullbrå, Norway .... **18 D3** 60 50N 6 17 E
Gullbrandstorp, Sweden **17 H6** 56 42N 12 43 E
Gullbringusýsla □,
　Iceland **11 D4** 64 0N 22 0W
Gullfoss, Iceland **11 C6** 64 20N 20 8W
Gullhaug, Norway ... **18 E7** 59 30N 10 15 E
Gullivan B., U.S.A. .. **153 K8** 25 45N 81 40W
Gullspång, Sweden .. **17 F8** 58 59N 14 6 E
Gullstein, Norway ... **18 A5** 63 13N 8 9 E
Güllük, Turkey ...... **49 D9** 37 14N 27 35 E
Güllük Dağı △, Turkey **49 E12** 37 0N 30 30 E
Güllük Körfezi, Turkey **49 D9** 37 12N 27 30 E
Gulma, Nigeria ...... **113 C5** 12 40N 4 23 E
Gulmarg, India ...... **93 B6** 34 3N 74 25 E
Gülnar, Turkey ...... **100 D5** 36 19N 33 24 E
Gulnare, Australia ... **128 B3** 33 27 S 138 27 E
Gülpınar, Turkey .... **49 B8** 39 32N 26 7 E
Gülşehir, Turkey .... **100 C6** 38 44N 34 37 E
Gulshad, Kazakhstan **66 E8** 46 45N 74 25 E
Gulsvik, Norway .... **18 D6** 60 24N 9 38 E
Gulu, Uganda .... **118 B3** 2 48N 32 17 E
Gülübovo, Bulgaria .. **51 D9** 42 8N 25 55 E
Gulud, J., Sudan ..... **107 E2** 11 41N 29 31 E
Gulwe, Tanzania ..... **118 D4** 6 30 S 36 25 E
Gulyaypole =
　Hulyaypole, Ukraine **59 J9** 47 45N 36 21 E
Gum Lake, Australia . **128 B5** 32 42 S 143 9 E
Gumaca, Phil. .... **80 E4** 13 55N 122 6 E
Gumal ⇸, Pakistan .. **92 D3** 30 4N 69 0 E
Gumbaz, Pakistan ... **92 D3** 30 2N 69 0 E
Gumbinnen = Gusev,
　Russia .... **15 J20** 54 35N 22 10 E
Gumel, Nigeria ...... **113 C6** 12 39N 9 22 E
Gumel de Hizán, Spain **40 D7** 41 46N 3 41W
Gumla, India .... **93 H11** 23 3N 84 33 E
Gumlu, Australia .... **126 B4** 19 53 S 147 41 E
Gumma □, Japan .... **73 A10** 36 30N 138 20 E
Gummersbach,
　Germany .... **30 D3** 51 1N 7 34 E
Gummi, Nigeria ..... **113 C6** 12 4N 5 9 E
Gümüldür, Turkey .. **49 C9** 38 6N 27 0 E
Gumulgina = Komotini,
　Greece .... **51 E9** 41 9N 25 26 E
Gümüşçay, Turkey .. **51 F11** 40 16N 27 17 E
Gümüşhacıköy, Turkey **100 B6** 40 50N 35 18 E
Gümüşhane, Turkey .. **101 B8** 40 30N 39 30 E
Gümüşsu, Turkey ... **49 C11** 38 14N 29 1 E
Gumzai, Indonesia ... **83 C4** 5 28 S 134 42 E
Guna, Ethiopia ...... **107 F4** 8 18N 39 52 E
Guna, India .... **92 G7** 24 40N 77 19 E
Gundagai, Australia .. **129 C8** 35 3 S 148 6 E
Gundardehi, India ... **94 D5** 20 57N 81 17 E
Gundelfingen,
　Germany .... **31 G6** 48 34N 10 22 E
Gundih, Indonesia ... **85 D4** 7 10 S 110 56 E
Gundlakamma ⇸,
　India .... **95 G5** 15 30N 80 15 E
Gundlupet, India .... **95 J3** 11 48N 76 41 E
Gunebang, Australia . **129 A8** 33 1 S 146 38 E
Gungal, Australia .... **129 B9** 32 17 S 150 32 E
Gungu, Angola ...... **115 D3** 5 43 S 19 20 E
Gunisao ⇸, Canada . **143 C9** 53 56N 97 53W
Gunisao L., Canada .. **143 C9** 53 33N 96 15W
Gunjyal, Pakistan .... **92 C4** 32 20N 71 55 E
Günlüce, Turkey ..... **49 E11** 36 50N 28 20 E
Gunnarskog, Sweden . **16 E6** 59 49N 12 34 E
Gunnbjørn Fjeld,
　Greenland **10 D8** 68 55N 29 47W
Gunnebo, Sweden ... **17 G10** 57 44N 16 32 E
Gunnedah, Australia . **129 A9** 30 59 S 150 15 E
Gunnewin, Australia . **127 D4** 25 59 S 148 33 E
Gunningbar Cr. ⇸,
　Australia .... **129 A7** 31 14 S 147 6 E
Gunnison, Colo., U.S.A. **159 G10** 38 33N 106 56W
Gunnison, Utah, U.S.A. **158 G8** 39 9N 111 49W
Gunnison ⇸, U.S.A. . **158 G9** 39 4N 108 35W
Gunpowder, Australia **126 B2** 19 42 S 139 22 E
Guntakal, India ..... **95 G3** 15 11N 77 27 E
Guntersville, U.S.A. .. **149 H2** 34 21N 86 18W
Guntong, Malaysia .. **87 K3** 4 36N 101 3 E
Guntur, India .... **95 F5** 16 23N 80 30 E
Gunungapi, Indonesia **83 C4** 6 45 S 126 30 E
Gunungsitoli, Indonesia **84 B1** 1 15N 97 30 E
Gunupur, India ..... **94 E6** 19 5N 83 50 E
Günz ⇸, Germany ... **31 G6** 48 27N 10 16 E
Gunza, Angola ...... **115 E2** 10 50 S 13 50 E
Günzburg, Germany . **31 G6** 48 26N 10 17 E
Gunzenhausen,
　Germany .... **31 F6** 49 7N 10 44 E
Guo He ⇸, China ... **75 H9** 32 59N 117 10 E
Guoyang, China ..... **75 H9** 33 32N 116 12 E
Gupis, Pakistan ..... **93 A5** 36 15N 73 20 E
Gura Humorului,
　Romania .... **53 C10** 47 35N 25 53 E
Gura-Teghii, Romania **53 E11** 45 30N 26 25 E
Gurahonţ, Romania . **52 D7** 46 16N 22 21 E
Gurdaspur, India .... **92 C6** 32 5N 75 31 E
Gurdon, U.S.A. **155 J8** 33 55N 93 9W
Gurgaon, India ...... **92 E7** 28 27N 77 1 E

Gurgaon, India ...... **92 E7** 28 27N 77 1 E
Gürgentepe, Turkey .. **100 B7** 40 51N 37 50 E
Gurghiu, Munţii,
　Romania .... **53 D10** 46 41N 25 15 E
Gurgueia ⇸, Brazil .. **170 C3** 6 50 S 43 24W
Gurha, India .... **92 G4** 25 12N 71 39 E
Guri, Embalse de,
　Venezuela **169 B5** 7 50N 62 52W
Gurig △, Australia ... **124 B5** 11 36 S 132 7 E
Gurimatu, Papua N. G. **132 D3** 6 45 S 144 45 E
Gurin, Nigeria ...... **113 D7** 9 5N 12 54 E
Gurinhatã, Brazil .... **171 E2** 19 14 S 49 48W
Gurjaani, Georgia ... **61 K7** 41 43N 45 52 E
Gurk ⇸, Austria ..... **34 E7** 46 35N 14 31 E
Gurkfeld = Krško,
　Slovenia .... **45 C12** 45 57N 15 30 E
Gurkha, Nepal ...... **93 E11** 28 5N 84 40 E
Gurley, Australia .... **129 A8** 29 45 S 149 48 E
Gurnee, U.S.A. **157 B9** 42 22N 87 55W
Gurnet Point, U.S.A. **151 D14** 42 1N 70 34W
Guro, Mozam. ...... **119 F3** 17 26 S 32 30 E
Gürpınar, Ist., Turkey **51 F12** 41 1N 28 25 E
Gürpınar, Van, Turkey **101 C10** 38 18N 43 25 E
Gürsu, Turkey ...... **51 F13** 40 13N 29 11 E
Gurué, Mozam. ...... **119 F4** 15 25 S 36 58 E
Gurun, Malaysia ..... **87 K3** 5 49N 100 27 E
Gürün, Turkey ...... **100 C7** 38 43N 37 15 E
Gurupá, Brazil ...... **169 D7** 1 25 S 51 35W
Gurupá, I. Grande de,
　Brazil .... **169 D7** 1 25 S 51 45W
Gurupi, Brazil .... **171 D2** 11 43 S 49 4W
Gurupi ⇸, Brazil .... **170 B2** 1 13 S 46 6W
Gurupi, Serra do,
　Brazil .... **170 C2** 5 0 S 47 50W
Guruwe, Zimbabwe .. **117 B5** 16 40 S 30 42 E
Guryev = Atyraū,
　Kazakhstan .... **57 E9** 47 5N 52 0 E
Guryevsk, Russia .... **54 D7** 54 47N 20 38 E
Gus-Khrustalnyy,
　Russia .... **60 C5** 55 42N 40 44 E
Gusau, Nigeria ...... **113 C6** 12 12N 6 40 E
Gusev, Russia .... **15 J20** 54 35N 22 10 E
Gushgy, Turkmenistan **66 F7** 35 20N 62 18 E
Gushi, China .... **77 A10** 32 11N 115 41 E
Gushiago, Ghana **113 D4** 9 55N 0 15W
Gusinje, Serbia & M. . **50 D3** 42 35N 19 50 E
Gusinoozersk, Russia **67 D11** 51 16N 106 27 E
Güspini, Italy .... **46 C1** 39 32N 8 37 E
Güssing, Austria .... **35 D9** 47 3N 16 20 E
Gustav Holm, Kap,
　Greenland **10 D6** 66 36N 34 15W
Gustavsberg, Sweden **16 E12** 59 19N 18 23 E
Gustavus, U.S.A. **142 B1** 58 25N 135 44W
Gustine, U.S.A. **160 H6** 37 16N 121 0W
Güstrow, Germany .. **30 B8** 53 47N 12 10 E
Gusum, Sweden ..... **17 F10** 58 16N 16 30 E
Guta = Kolárovo,
　Slovak Rep. ...... **35 D10** 47 54N 18 0 E
Gutha, Australia ..... **125 E2** 28 58 S 115 55 E
Guthalungra, Australia **126 B4** 19 52 S 147 50 E
Guthrie, Okla., U.S.A. **155 H6** 35 53N 97 25W
Guthrie, Tex., U.S.A. **155 J4** 33 37N 100 19W
Guthrie Center, U.S.A. **156 C2** 41 41N 94 30W
Gutian, China .... **77 D12** 26 32N 118 43 E
Gutiérrez, Bolivia ... **173 D5** 19 25 S 63 34W
Guttannen, Switz. ... **33 C6** 46 38N 8 18 E
Guttenberg, U.S.A. .. **156 B5** 42 47N 91 6W
Guttentag =
　Dobrodzień, Poland **55 H5** 50 45N 18 25 E
Gutu, Zimbabwe .... **117 B5** 19 41 S 31 9 E
Gutulia △, Norway .. **18 B9** 62 2N 12 11 E
Guwahati, India ..... **93 F14** 26 10N 91 45 E
Guy Fawkes River △,
　Australia .... **127 D5** 30 0 S 152 20 E
Guyana ■, S. Amer. . **169 B6** 5 0N 59 0W
Guyane française =
　French Guiana ☑,
　S. Amer. **169 C7** 4 0N 53 0W
Guyang, China ...... **74 D6** 41 0N 110 5 E
Guyenne, France .... **28 D4** 44 30N 0 40 E
Guymon, U.S.A. **155 G4** 36 41N 101 29W
Guyotville = Aïn
　Benian, Algeria ... **111 A5** 36 48N 2 55 E
Guyra, Australia ..... **127 E5** 30 15 S 151 40 E
Guyton, U.S.A. **152 C8** 32 20N 81 24W
Guyuan, Hebei, China **74 D8** 41 37N 115 40 E
Guyuan,
　Ningxia Huizu, China **74 G4** 36 0N 106 20 E
Guzar, Uzbekistan ... **65 D3** 38 36N 66 15 E
Gizelbahçe, Turkey .. **49 C8** 38 21N 26 22 E
Güzelyurt = Morphou,
　Cyprus .... **49 E8** 35 12N 32 59 E
Guzhang, China ..... **77 D8** 28 42N 109 58 E
Guzhen, China ...... **75 H9** 33 22N 117 18 E
Guzmán, L. de, Mexico **162 A3** 31 25N 107 25W
Gvardeysk, Russia ... **15 J19** 54 39N 21 5 E
Gvardeyskoye, Ukraine **59 K8** 45 7N 34 1 E
Gvarv, Norway ...... **18 E6** 59 23N 9 9 E
Gwa, Burma .... **90 G5** 17 36N 94 34 E
Gwaai, Zimbabwe ... **119 F2** 19 15 S 27 45 E
Gwaai ⇸, Zimbabwe **119 F2** 17 59 S 26 52 E
Gwabegar, Australia . **129 A8** 30 31 S 149 0 E
Gwadabawa, Nigeria **113 C6** 13 28N 5 15 E
Gwādar, Pakistan ... **91 D1** 25 10N 62 18 E
Gwagwada, Nigeria . **113 C6** 10 15N 7 15 E
Gwaii Haanas △,
　Canada **142 C2** 52 21N 131 26W
Gwalior, India ...... **93 F8** 26 12N 78 10 E
Gwanara, Nigeria ... **113 D5** 8 55N 3 9 E
Gwanda, Zimbabwe . **119 G2** 20 55 S 29 0 E
Gwandu, Nigeria .... **113 C5** 12 30N 4 41 E
Gwane, Dem. Rep. of
　the Congo .... **118 B2** 4 45N 25 48 E
Gwanju = Kwangju,
　S. Korea .... **75 G14** 35 9N 126 54 E
Gwarzo, Nigeria .... **113 C6** 11 55N 10 25 E
Gwasero, Nigeria .... **113 D5** 9 30N 7 8 E
Gwda ⇸, Poland .... **55 E3** 53 9N 16 44 E
Gweebarra B., Ireland **23 A3** 54 51N 8 23W
Gweedore, Ireland ... **23 A3** 55 3N 8 13W
Gweru, Zimbabwe ... **117 F2** 19 28 S 29 45 E
Gwi, Nigeria .... **113 C6** 9 0N 7 10 E
Gwinn, U.S.A. **156 B10** 46 19N 87 27W
Gwio Kura, Nigeria . **113 C7** 12 40N 11 2 E
Gwoza, Nigeria ...... **113 C7** 11 5N 13 40 E
Gwydir ⇸, Australia . **127 D4** 29 27 S 149 48 E
Gwynedd □, U.K. ... **20 E3** 52 52N 4 10W
Gyandzha = Gäncä,
　Azerbaijan .... **61 K8** 40 45N 46 20 E
Gyaring Hu, China .. **68 C4** 34 50N 97 40 E
Gydanskiy Poluostrov,
　Russia .... **68 C8** 70 0N 78 0 E
Gyl, Norway .... **18 B5** 62 57N 8 7 E
Gyldenløve Fjord,
　Greenland **10 E6** 64 15N 40 30W
Gympie, Australia ... **127 D5** 26 11 S 152 38 E
Gyobingauk, Burma . **90 F5** 18 13N 95 39 E
Gyōda, Japan .... **73 A11** 36 10N 139 30 E
Gyomaendrőd,
　Hungary .... **52 D5** 46 56N 20 50 E

Gyöngyös, *Hungary* . . **52 C4** 47 48N 19 56 E
Győr, *Hungary* . . . . . . **52 C2** 47 41N 17 40 E
Győr-Moson-Sopron □,
  Hungary . . . . **52 C2** 47 40N 17 20 E
Gypsum Pt., *Canada* . . **142 A6** 61 53N 114 35W
Gypsumville, *Canada* . **143 C9** 51 45N 98 40W
Gyueshevo, *Bulgaria* . . **50 D6** 42 14N 22 28 E
Gyula, *Hungary* . . . . . **52 D6** 46 38N 21 17 E
Gyumri, *Armenia* . . . . **61 K6** 40 47N 43 50 E
Gyzylarbat,
  Turkmenistan . . . . . . **66 F6** 39 4N 56 23 E
Gyzyletrek,
  Turkmenistan . . . . . . **97 B7** 37 36N 54 46 E
Gzhatsk = Gagarin,
  Russia . . . . **58 E8** 55 38N 35 0 E
Gzira, *Malta* . . . . **38 F7** 35 54N 14 29 E

H

Ha 'Arava →, *Israel* . **103 E4** 30 50N 35 20 E
Ha Coi, *Vietnam* . . . . . **76 G6** 21 26N 107 46 E
Ha Dong, *Vietnam* . . . . **76 G5** 20 58N 105 46 E
Ha Giang, *Vietnam* . . . **76 F5** 22 50N 104 59 E
Ha Karmel △, *Israel* . **103 C4** 32 45N 35 5 E
Ha Tien, *Vietnam* . . . . **87 G5** 10 23N 104 29 E
Ha Tinh, *Vietnam* . . . . **86 C5** 18 20N 105 54 E
Ha Trung, *Vietnam* . . . **86 C5** 19 58N 105 50 E
Ha Yaek Chalong,
  Thailand . . . . **87 a** 7 50N 98 22 E
Haakon VII Topp,
  Norway **10 C10** 71 0N 8 20W
Haaksbergen, *Neths.* . . **24 B6** 52 9N 6 45 E
Ha'ano, *Tonga* . . . . . **133 P13** 19 41 S 174 18W
Ha'apai Group, *Tonga* **133 P13** 19 47 S 174 27W
Haapsalu, *Estonia* . . . . **9 G20** 58 56N 23 30 E
Haarlem, *Neths.* . . . . . **24 B4** 52 23N 4 39 E
Haast, *N.Z.* . . . . **131 D4** 43 51 S 169 1 E
Haast →, *N.Z.* . . . . . **131 D4** 43 50 S 169 2 E
Haast Bluff, *Australia* . **124 D5** 23 22 S 132 0 E
Haast Pass, *N.Z.* . . . . **131 E4** 44 6 S 169 21 E
Hab →, *Pakistan* . . . . **92 G3** 24 53N 66 41 E
Hab Nadi Chauki,
  Pakistan . . . . **92 G2** 25 0N 66 50 E
Ḥabarūt, *Yemen* . . . . . **99 C6** 17 18N 52 44 E
Habaswein, *Kenya* . . . **118 B4** 1 2N 39 30 E
Ḥabawnah, W. →,
  Si. Arabia . . . . **98 C4** 17 57N 44 58 E
Habay, *Canada* **142 B5** 58 50N 118 44W
Ḥabbān, *Yemen* . . . . . **98 D4** 14 21N 47 5 E
Ḥabbānīyah, *Iraq* . . . **101 F10** 33 17N 43 29 E
Ḥabbānīyah, Hawr al,
  Iraq . . . . **101 F10** 33 17N 43 29 E
Habelschwerdt =
  Bystrzyca Kłodzka,
  Poland . . . . **55 H3** 50 19N 16 39 E
Habichtswald △,
  Germany . . . . **30 D5** 51 15N 9 15 E
Habiganj, *Bangla.* . . . . **90 C4** 24 24N 91 30 E
Habo, *Sweden* . . . . . . **17 G8** 57 55N 14 6 E
Haboro, *Japan* . . . . . . **70 B10** 44 22N 141 42 E
Ḥabshān, *U.A.E.* . . . . **97 F7** 23 50N 53 37 E
Hachenburg, *Germany* . **30 E3** 50 40N 7 49 E
Hachi, *India* . . . . **90 B5** 27 48N 94 2 E
Hachijō-Jima, *Japan* . . **73 D11** 33 5N 139 45 E
Hachiman, *Japan* . . . . **73 B8** 35 45N 136 57 E
Hachinohe, *Japan* . . . **70 D10** 40 30N 141 29 E
Hachiōji, *Japan* . . . . . **73 B11** 35 40N 139 20 E
Hachŏn, *N. Korea* . . . **75 D15** 41 29N 129 2 E
Hacıbektaş, *Turkey* . . . **100 C6** 38 56N 34 33 E
Hacılar, *Turkey* . . . . . **100 C6** 38 38N 35 26 E
Hack, Mt., *Australia* . . **128 A3** 30 45 S 138 55 E
Hackensack, *U.S.A.* . . **155 F10** 40 53N 74 3W
Hackås, *Sweden* . . . . . **16 B8** 62 56N 14 30 E
Hackettstown, *U.S.A.* . **151 F10** 40 51N 74 50W
Haco, *Angola* . . . . . . **115 E3** 10 15 S 15 44 E
Hadali, *Pakistan* . . . . . **92 C5** 32 16N 72 11 E
Hadano, *Japan* . . . . . . **73 B11** 35 22N 139 14 E
Hadarba, Ras, *Sudan* . **106 C4** 22 4N 36 51 E
Hadarom □, *Israel* . . . **103 E4** 31 0N 35 0 E
Ḥaḍbaram, *Oman* . . . . **99 C6** 17 27N 55 15 E
Ḥadd, Ra's al, *Oman* . **99 B2** 22 35N 59 50 E
Ḥaddā, *Si. Arabia* . . . . **98 B2** 21 27N 39 34 E
Haddington, *U.K.* **22 F6** 55 57N 2 47W
Haddock, *U.S.A.* **152 B6** 33 2N 83 26W
Haded Plain = Xadded,
  Somali Rep. . . . . . **120 C3** 9 46N 48 2 E
Hadejia, *Nigeria* . . . . **113 C7** 12 30N 10 5 E
Hadejia →, *Nigeria* . . **113 C7** 12 50N 10 51 E
Hadera, *Israel* . . . . . . **103 C3** 32 27N 34 55 E
Hadera, N. →, *Israel* . **103 C3** 32 28N 34 52 E
Haderslev =
  Haderslev, *Denmark* . **17 J3** 55 15N 9 30 E
Haderslev, *Denmark* . . **17 J3** 55 15N 9 30 E
Hadgaon, *India* . . . . . . **94 E3** 19 30N 77 40 E
Hadhramaut =
  Ḥaḍramawt, *Yemen* . **99 D5** 15 30N 49 30 E
Hadiboh, *Yemen* . . . . **99 D6** 12 39N 54 2 E
Hadim, *Turkey* . . . . . **100 D5** 36 59N 32 27 E
Hadjadj, O. el →,
  Algeria . . . . **111 C6** 28 18N 5 20 E
Hadjeb El Aïoun,
  Tunisia . . . . **108 A1** 35 21N 9 32 E
Hadjer Kamaran, *Chad* **109 F4** 12 41N 21 46 E
Hadjer Mornou, *Chad* **109 E4** 17 12N 23 8 E
Hadong, *S. Korea* . . . . **75 G14** 35 5N 127 44 E
Ḥaḍramawt, *Yemen* . . **99 D5** 15 30N 49 30 E
Ḥaḍramawt, W. →,
  Yemen . . . . **99 D5** 15 10N 51 8 E
Ḥaḍrānīyah, *Iraq* . . . . **96 C4** 35 38N 43 14 E
Hadrian's Wall, *U.K.* . **20 B5** 55 0N 2 30W
Hadsten, *Denmark* . . . **17 H4** 56 19N 10 3 E
Hadsund, *Denmark* . . . **17 H4** 56 44N 10 8 E
Hadyach, *Ukraine* . . . . **59 G8** 50 21N 34 0 E
Hægeland, *Norway* . . . **18 F4** 58 22N 7 45 E
Haeju, *N. Korea* . . . . . **75 E13** 38 3N 125 45 E
Haena, *U.S.A.* **145 A2** 22 14N 159 34W
Haenam, *S. Korea* . . . **75 G14** 34 34N 126 35 E
Haenertsburg, *S. Africa* **117 C4** 24 0 S 29 50 E
Haerhpin = Harbin,
  China . . . . **75 B14** 45 48N 126 40 E
Hafar al Bāṭin,
  Si. Arabia . . . . **96 D5** 28 32N 45 52 E
Hafik, *Turkey* . . . . . . **100 C7** 39 51N 37 23 E
Ḥafīrat al 'Aydā,
  Si. Arabia . . . . **96 E3** 26 26N 39 12 E
Hafit, *Oman* . . . . **97 F7** 23 59N 55 49 E
Hafizabad, *Pakistan* . . **92 C5** 32 5N 73 40 E
Haflong, *India* . . . . . . **90 C4** 25 10N 93 5 E
Hafnarfjörður, *Iceland* . **11 C5** 64 4N 21 57W
Hafnir, *Iceland* **11 D4** 63 56N 22 41W
Hafslo, *Norway* . . . . . **18 C4** 61 19N 7 10 E
Haft Gel, *Iran* . . . . . . **97 D6** 31 30N 49 32 E
Hafun, Ras,
  Somali Rep. . . . . . **102 G5** 10 29N 51 30 E
Hagalil, *Israel* . . . . . . **103 C4** 32 53N 35 18 E
Hagari →, *India* . . . . . **95 G3** 15 40N 77 0 E
Hagby, *Sweden* . . . . . **17 H10** 56 34N 16 11 E
Hagemeister I., *U.S.A.* **145 G6** 58 39N 160 54W
Hagen, *Germany* . . . . **30 D3** 51 21N 7 27 E
Hagenow, *Germany* . . . **30 B7** 53 26N 11 12 E

Hagerman, *U.S.A.* . . . **155 J2** 33 7N 104 20W
Hagerman Fossil
  Beds △, *U.S.A.* . . . **158 E6** 42 48N 114 57W
Hagerstown, *Ind.,*
  U.S.A. **157 E11** 39 55N 85 10W
Hagerstown, *Md.,*
  U.S.A. **148 F7** 39 39N 77 43W
Hagersville, *Canada* . . **150 D4** 42 58N 80 3W
Hagetmau, *France* . . . **28 E3** 43 39N 0 37W
Hagfors, *Sweden* . . . . **16 D7** 60 3N 13 45 E
Hagi, *Iceland* **11 B3** 65 28N 23 25W
Hagi, *Japan* . . . . **72 C3** 34 30N 131 22 E
Hagolan, *Syria* . . . . . **103 C4** 33 0N 35 45 E
Hagondange, *France* . . **27 C13** 49 16N 6 11 E
Hagonoy, *Phil.* . . . . . . **80 D3** 14 50N 120 44 E
Hags Hd., *Ireland* . . . **23 D2** 52 57N 9 28W
Hague, C. de la, *France* **26 C5** 49 44N 1 56W
Hague, The = 's-
  Gravenhage, *Neths.* . **24 B4** 52 7N 4 17 E
Haguenau, *France* . . . **27 D14** 48 49N 7 47 E
Hagunía, *W. Sahara* . . **110 C2** 27 26N 12 24W
Hahira, *U.S.A.* **152 E6** 30 59N 83 22W
Hai Duong, *Vietnam* . . **76 G6** 20 56N 106 19 E
Hai'an, *Guangdong,*
  China . . . . **77 G8** 20 18N 110 11 E
Hai'an, *Jiangsu, China* **77 A13** 32 37N 120 27 E
Haicheng, *Fujian,*
  China . . . . **77 E11** 24 23N 117 48 E
Haicheng, *Liaoning,*
  China . . . . **75 D12** 40 50N 122 45 E
Haidar Khel, *Afghan.* . **92 C3** 33 58N 68 38 E
Haidarâbâd =
  Hyderabad, *India* . . . **94 F4** 17 22N 78 29 E
Haidargarh, *India* . . . . **93 F9** 26 37N 81 22 E
Haifa = Ḥefa, *Israel* . . **103 C4** 32 46N 35 0 E
Haifeng, *China* . . . . . **77 F10** 22 58N 115 10 E
Haiger, *Germany* . . . . **30 E4** 50 43N 8 12 E
Haikou, *China* . . . . . . **69 D6** 20 1N 110 16 E
Ḥā'il, *Si. Arabia* . . . . . **96 E4** 27 28N 41 45 E
Hailakandi, *India* . . . . **90 C4** 24 42N 92 34 E
Hailar, *China* . . . . **69 B6** 49 10N 119 38 E
Hailey, *U.S.A.* **158 E6** 43 31N 114 19W
Haileybury, *Canada* . . **140 C4** 47 30N 79 38W
Hailin, *China* . . . . **75 B15** 44 37N 129 30 E
Hailing Dao, *China* . . **77 G8** 21 35N 111 47 E
Hailong, *China* . . . . . **75 C13** 42 32N 125 40 E
Hailuoto, *Finland* . . . . **14 D21** 65 3N 24 45 E
Haimen, *Guangdong,*
  China . . . . **77 F11** 23 15N 116 38 E
Haimen, *Jiangsu, China* **77 B13** 31 52N 121 10 E
Hainan □, *China* . . . . **69 E5** 19 0N 109 30 E
Hainan Dao, *China* . . . **86 C7** 19 0N 109 30 E
Hainan Str. =
  Qiongzhou Haixia,
  China . . . . **86 B8** 20 10N 110 15 E
Hainaut □, *Belgium* . . **24 D4** 50 30N 4 0 E
Hainburg, *Austria* . . . **35 C9** 48 9N 16 56 E
Haines, *Alaska, U.S.A.* **142 B1** 59 14N 135 26W
Haines, *Oreg., U.S.A.* **158 D5** 44 55N 117 56W
Haines City, *U.S.A.* . . **153 G8** 28 7N 81 38W
Haines Junction,
  Canada **142 A1** 60 45N 137 30W
Hainfeld, *Austria* . . . . **34 C8** 48 3N 15 48 E
Haining, *China* . . . . . **77 B13** 30 28N 120 40 E
Haiphong, *Vietnam* . . . **76 G6** 20 47N 106 41 E
Haitan Dao, *China* . . . **77 E12** 25 30N 119 45 E
Haiti ■, *W. Indies* . . . **165 C5** 19 0N 72 30W
Haiya, *Sudan* . . . . **106 D4** 18 20N 36 21 E
Haiyan, *China* . . . . . . **77 B13** 30 28N 120 58 E
Haiyang, *China* . . . . . **75 F11** 36 47N 121 9 E
Haiyuan,
  Guangxi Zhuangzu,
  China . . . . **76 F6** 22 8N 107 35 E
Haiyuan,
  Ningxia Huizu, China **74 F3** 36 35N 105 52 E
Haizhou, *China* . . . . . **75 G10** 34 37N 119 7 E
Haizhou Wan, *China* . . **75 G10** 34 50N 119 20 E
Hajar Bangar, *Sudan* . **109 F4** 10 40N 22 45 E
Hajdú-Bihar □,
  Hungary . . . . **52 C6** 47 30N 21 30 E
Hajdúböszörmény,
  Hungary . . . . **52 C6** 47 40N 21 30 E
Hajdúdorog, *Hungary* . **52 C6** 47 48N 21 30 E
Hajdúhadház, *Hungary* **52 C6** 47 40N 21 40 E
Hajdúnánás, *Hungary* . **52 C6** 47 50N 21 26 E
Hajdúsámson, *Hungary* **52 C6** 47 37N 21 42 E
Hajdúszoboszló,
  Hungary . . . . **52 C6** 47 27N 21 22 E
Hajiganj, *Bangla.* . . . . **90 D3** 23 15N 90 50 E
Hajipur, *India* . . . . . . **93 G11** 25 45N 85 13 E
Ḥajjah, *Yemen* . . . . . **98 D3** 15 42N 43 36 E
Ḥājjī Muḥsin, *Iraq* . . . **96 C5** 32 35N 45 29 E
Ḥājjīābād, *Iran* . . . . . **97 D7** 28 19N 55 55 E
Ḥājjīābād-e Zarrīn,
  Iran . . . . **97 C7** 33 9N 54 51 E
Hajnówka, *Poland* . . . **55 F10** 52 47N 23 35 E
Ḥajrah, *Si. Arabia* . . . **98 B3** 20 14N 41 3 E
Haka, *Burma* . . . . **90 D4** 22 39N 93 37 E
Hakansson, Mts.,
  Dem. Rep. of
  the Congo . . . . **119 D2** 8 40 S 25 45 E
Hakataramea, *N.Z.* . . . **131 E5** 44 43 S 170 30 E
Hakkâri, *Turkey* . . . . **101 D10** 37 34N 43 44 E
Hakkâri Dağları,
  Turkey . . . . **101 C10** 38 2N 42 58 E
Hakken-Zan, *Japan* . . **73 C7** 34 10N 135 54 E
Hakodate, *Japan* . . . . **70 D10** 41 45N 140 44 E
Hakos, *Namibia* . . . . . **116 C2** 23 13 S 16 21 E
Hakota, *Japan* . . . . . . **73 A12** 36 5N 140 30 E
Ḥaku-San, *Japan* . . . . **73 A8** 36 9N 136 46 E
Ḥaku-San □, *Japan* . . **73 A8** 36 15N 136 45 E
Hakuba, *Japan* . . . . . **73 A9** 36 42N 137 51 E
Hakui, *Japan* . . . . **71 F8** 36 53N 136 47 E
Hakun, *Burma* . . . . . . **90 B5** 26 46N 95 42 E
Hala, *Pakistan* . . . . . . **91 D3** 25 43N 68 20 E
Ḥalab, *Syria* . . . . **100 D7** 36 10N 37 15 E
Ḥalabjah, *Iraq* . . . . . **101 E11** 35 10N 45 58 E
Halach, *Turkmenistan* . **65 D2** 38 4N 64 52 E
Halaib, *Sudan* . . . . . . **106 C4** 22 12N 36 30 E
Halalii L., *U.S.A.* **145 B1** 21 52N 160 11W
Halasa, *Sudan* . . . . . . **107 E3** 14 26N 30 39 E
Hālat 'Ammār,
  Si. Arabia . . . . **96 D3** 29 10N 36 4 E
Halawa, *U.S.A.* **145 B5** 21 10N 156 43W
Halawa Heights, *U.S.A.* **145 K14** 21 23N 157 55W
Halba, *Lebanon* . . . . . **103 A5** 34 34N 36 6 E
Halberstadt, *Germany* . **30 D7** 51 54N 11 3 E
Halcombe, *N.Z.* . . . . **130 G4** 40 8 S 175 30 E
Halcon, *Phil.* . . . . **79 B6** 13 0N 121 30 E
Halcon, Mt., *Phil.* . . . **80 E3** 13 16N 121 0 E
Halde Fjäll =
  Haltiatunturi,
  Finland . . . . **14 B19** 69 17N 21 18 E
Halden, *Norway* . . . . . **18 E8** 59 9N 11 23 E
Haldensleben,
  Germany . . . . **30 C7** 52 17N 11 24 E
Haldimand, *Canada* . . **152 B4** 42 59N 79 57W
Haldwani, *India* . . . . . **93 E8** 29 31N 79 30 E
Hale, *U.S.A.* **156 E3** 39 36N 93 20W
Hale →, *Australia* . . . **126 C2** 24 56 S 135 53 E
Haleakala △, *U.S.A.* . . **145 C5** 20 40N 156 10W
Haleakala Crater,
  U.S.A. **145 C5** 20 43N 156 16W

Haleiwa, *U.S.A.* **145 J13** 21 36N 158 6W
Halesowen, *U.K.* **21 E5** 52 27N 2 3W
Halesworth, *U.K.* . . . . **21 E9** 52 20N 1 31 E
Haleyville, *U.S.A.* **149 H2** 34 14N 87 37W
Half Assini, *Ghana* . . . **112 D4** 5 1N 2 50W
Halfmoon Bay, *N.Z.* . . **131 G3** 46 50 S 168 5 E
Halfway →, *Canada* . . **142 B4** 56 12N 121 32W
Halia, *India* . . . . **93 G10** 24 50N 82 19 E
Haliburton, *Canada* . . **140 C4** 45 3N 78 30W
Halifax, *Australia* . . . . **126 B4** 18 32 S 146 22 E
Halifax, *Canada* **141 D7** 44 38N 63 35W
Halifax, *U.K.* **20 D6** 53 43N 1 52W
Halifax, *U.S.A.* **150 F8** 40 25N 76 55W
Halifax B., *Australia* . . **126 B4** 18 50 S 147 0 E
Halifax I., *Namibia* . . . **116 D2** 26 38 S 15 4 E
Ḥalīl →, *Iran* . . . . . . **97 E8** 27 40N 58 30 E
Halin, *Somali Rep.* . . . **120 C3** 9 6N 48 37 E
Halkett, C., *U.S.A.* . . . **144 A9** 70 48N 152 11W
Halkida = Khalkís,
  Greece . . . . **48 C5** 38 27N 23 42 E
Halkirk, *U.K.* **22 C5** 58 30N 3 29W
Hall Beach = Sanirajak,
  Canada **139 B11** 68 46N 81 12W
Hall I., *U.S.A.* **144 F4** 60 40N 173 6W
Hall in Tirol, *Austria* . **34 D4** 47 17N 11 30 E
Hall Pen., *Canada* . . . **139 B13** 63 30N 66 0W
Hall Pt., *Australia* . . . **124 C3** 15 40 S 124 23 E
Hallabro, *Sweden* . . . . **17 H9** 56 22N 15 5 E
Halland, *Sweden* . . . . **15 H15** 57 8N 12 47 E
Hallandale, *U.S.A.* . . . **153 K9** 25 59N 80 8W
Hallands län □, *Sweden* **17 H6** 57 0N 12 40 E
Hallands Väderö,
  Sweden . . . . **17 H6** 56 27N 12 34 E
Hallandsås, *Sweden* . . **17 H7** 56 22N 13 0 E
Hallaskar, *Norway* . . . **18 D4** 60 15N 7 9 E
Hällbybrunn, *Sweden* . **16 E10** 59 24N 16 20 E
Halle, *Belgium* . . . . . . **24 D4** 50 44N 4 13 E
Halle,
  Nordrhein-Westfalen,
  Germany . . . . **30 C4** 52 3N 8 22 E
Halle, *Sachsen-Anhalt,*
  Germany . . . . **30 D7** 51 30N 11 56 E
Hällefors, *Sweden* . . . **16 E8** 59 47N 14 31 E
Hälleforsnäs, *Sweden* . **16 E10** 59 10N 16 30 E
Hallein, *Austria* . . . . . **34 D6** 47 40N 13 5 E
Hällekis, *Sweden* . . . . **17 F7** 58 38N 13 27 E
Hallen, *Sweden* . . . . . **16 A8** 63 11N 14 4 E
Hallett, *Australia* . . . . **128 B3** 33 25 S 138 55 E
Hallettsville, *U.S.A.* . . **155 L6** 29 27N 96 57W
Hallia →, *India* . . . . . **94 F4** 16 55N 79 20 E
Hallim, *S. Korea* . . . . **75 H14** 33 24N 126 15 E
Hallingby, *Norway* . . . **18 D7** 60 7N 10 10 E
Hallingdal →, *Norway* . **18 D6** 60 40N 9 8 E
Hallingdalselvi →,
  Norway . . . . **18 D6** 60 23N 9 35 E
Hallingskarvet, *Norway* **18 D4** 60 36N 7 47 E
Hallingskeid, *Norway* . **18 D4** 60 40N 7 17 E
Hallock, *U.S.A.* **144 A6** 48 47N 96 57W
Hallormsstaður, *Iceland* **11 B12** 65 6N 14 45W
Halls Creek, *Australia* . **124 C4** 18 16 S 127 38 E
Hallsberg, *Sweden* . . . **16 E9** 59 4N 15 7 E
Hallstahammar, *Sweden* **16 E10** 59 38N 16 15 E
Hallstatt, *Austria* . . . . **34 D6** 47 33N 13 38 E
Hallstavik, *Sweden* . . . **16 D12** 60 5N 18 37 E
Hallstead, *U.S.A.* **151 E9** 41 58N 75 45W
Halmahera, *Indonesia* . **82 A3** 0 40N 128 0 E
Halmahera Sea,
  Indonesia . . . . **83 B3** 0 0N 129 0 E
Halmeu, *Romania* . . . **52 C8** 47 57N 23 2 E
Halmstad, *Sweden* . . . **17 H6** 56 41N 12 52 E
Halq el Oued, *Tunisia* . **108 A2** 36 53N 10 18 E
Hals, *Denmark* . . . . . **17 H4** 57 0N 10 18 E
Halsafjorden, *Norway* . **18 A5** 63 5N 8 10 E
Halsdanger →,
  Helsingborg = ,
  Sweden . . . . **17 H6** 56 3N 12 42 E
Hälsingland, *Sweden* . . **16 C10** 61 40N 16 5 E
Halstead, *U.K.* . . . . . **21 F8** 51 57N 0 40 E
Haltdalen, *Norway* . . . **18 B8** 62 56N 11 8 E
Haltern, *Germany* . . . . **30 D3** 51 44N 7 11 E
Haltiatunturi, *Finland* . **14 B19** 69 17N 21 18 E
Halton □, *U.K.* **20 D5** 53 22N 2 45W
Haltwhistle, *U.K.* **20 C5** 54 58N 2 26W
Ḥalūl, *Qatar* . . . . **97 E7** 25 40N 52 40 E
Halvad, *India* . . . . **92 H4** 23 1N 71 11 E
Ḥalvān, *Iran* . . . . **97 C8** 33 57N 56 15 E
Ham, *Chad* . . . . **109 F3** 10 1N 15 35 E
Ham, *France* . . . . **27 C10** 49 45N 3 4 E
Ham Tan, *Vietnam* . . . **87 G6** 10 40N 107 45 E
Ham Yen, *Vietnam* . . . **86 A5** 22 4N 105 3 E
Hamab, *Namibia* . . . . **116 D2** 28 7 S 19 16 E
Hamad, *Sudan* . . . . . **107 D3** 15 20N 33 32 E
Hamada, *Japan* . . . . . **72 C4** 34 56N 132 4 E
Hamadān, *Iran* . . . . . **97 C6** 34 52N 48 32 E
Hamadān □, *Iran* . . . . **97 C6** 35 0N 49 0 E
Hamadia, *Algeria* . . . . **111 A5** 35 28N 1 57 E
Ḥamāh, *Syria* . . . . . . **100 E7** 35 5N 36 40 E
Hamakita, *Japan* . . . . **73 C9** 34 45N 137 47 E
Hamamatsu, *Japan* . . . **73 C9** 34 45N 137 45 E
Hamar, *Norway* . . . . . **18 D8** 60 48N 11 7 E
Hamâta, Gebel, *Egypt* . **96 E2** 24 17N 35 0 E
Hambantota, *Sri Lanka* **95 L5** 6 10N 81 10 E
Hamber △, *Canada* . . **142 C5** 52 20N 118 0W
Hamburg, *Germany* . . . **30 B5** 53 33N 9 59 E
Hamburg, *Ark., U.S.A.* **155 J9** 33 14N 91 48W
Hamburg, *N.Y., U.S.A.* **150 D6** 42 43N 78 50W
Hamburg, *Pa., U.S.A.* **151 F9** 40 33N 75 59W
Hamburg □, *Germany* . **30 B5** 53 30N 10 0 E
Hamburg Fuhlsbüttel ✈
  (HAM), *Germany* . . **30 B5** 53 35N 9 59 E
Ḥamḍ, W. al →,
  Si. Arabia . . . . **96 E3** 24 55N 36 20 E
Ḥamḍah, *Si. Arabia* . . **98 C3** 19 2N 43 36 E
Ḥamḍānah, *Si. Arabia* **98 C3** 19 59N 40 34 E
Hamden, *U.S.A.* **151 E12** 41 23N 72 54W
Hamdibey, *Turkey* . . . **49 B9** 39 50N 27 15 E
Häme, *Finland* . . . . . . **15 F20** 61 38N 25 10 E
Hämeenlinna, *Finland* . **15 F21** 61 0N 24 28 E
Hamélé, *Burma* **112 C4** 10 56N 2 45W
Hamelin Pool, *Australia* **125 E1** 26 22 S 114 20 E
Hameln, *Germany* . . . **30 C5** 52 6N 9 21 E
Hamerkaz □, *Israel* . . **103 C3** 32 15N 34 55 E
Hamersley Ra.,
  Australia . . . . **124 D2** 22 0 S 117 45 E
Hamhŭng, *N. Korea* . . **75 E14** 39 54N 127 30 E
Hami, *China* . . . . **68 B4** 42 55N 93 25 E
Hamilton =
  Churchill →, *Canada* **141 B7** 53 19N 60 10W
Hamilton, *Bermuda* . . **9 a** 32 17N 64 47W
Hamilton, *Australia* . . **128 D3** 37 45 S 142 2 E
Hamilton, *Canada* . . . **150 D4** 43 15N 79 50W
Hamilton, *N.Z.* . . . . . **130 G5** 37 47 S 175 19 E
Hamilton, *U.K.* **22 F4** 55 46N 4 2W
Hamilton, *Ala., U.S.A.* **149 H1** 34 9N 87 59W
Hamilton, *Alaska,*
  U.S.A. **144 E7** 62 54N 163 53W
Hamilton, *Ill., U.S.A.* . **156 E5** 40 24N 91 21W
Hamilton, *Ind., U.S.A.* **157 C12** 41 33N 84 56W
Hamilton, *Mo., U.S.A.* **156 E2** 39 45N 94 0W
Hamilton, *Mont.,*
  U.S.A. **158 C6** 46 15N 114 10W

Hamilton, *N.Y., U.S.A.* **151 D9** 42 50N 75 33W
Hamilton, *Ohio, U.S.A.* **157 E12** 39 24N 84 34W
Hamilton, *Tex., U.S.A.* **155 K5** 31 42N 98 7W
Hamilton →, *Australia* **126 C2** 23 30 S 139 47 E
Hamilton, The =,
  Australia . . . . **127 D2** 26 40 S 135 19 E
Hamilton City, *U.S.A.* **160 F4** 39 45N 122 1W
Hamilton I., *Australia* . **126 J6** 20 21 S 148 56 E
Hamilton Inlet, *Canada* **141 B8** 54 0N 57 30W
Hamilton Mt., *U.S.A.* . **151 C10** 43 25N 74 22W
Hamina, *Finland* . . . . **15 F22** 60 34N 27 12 E
Hamipur, *H.P., India* . **92 D7** 31 41N 76 31 E
Hamirpur, *Ut. P., India* **93 G9** 25 57N 80 9 E
Hamitabat, *Turkey* . . . **51 E11** 41 24N 27 10 E
Hamlet, *U.S.A.* **149 H6** 34 53N 79 42W
Hamley Bridge,
  Australia . . . . **128 C3** 34 17 S 138 35 E
Hamlin = Hameln,
  Germany . . . . **30 C5** 52 6N 9 21 E
Hamlin, *N.Y., U.S.A.* . **150 C7** 43 17N 77 55W
Hamlin, *Tex., U.S.A.* . **155 J4** 32 53N 100 8W
Hamm, *Germany* . . . . **30 D3** 51 40N 7 50 E
Hammam Bouhadjar,
  Algeria **111 A4** 35 23N 0 58W
Hammamet, *Tunisia* . . **108 A2** 36 24N 10 38 E
Hammamet, G. de,
  Tunisia . . . . **108 A2** 36 10N 10 48 E
Hammarstrand, *Sweden* **16 A10** 63 7N 16 20 E
Hammelburg, *Germany* **31 E5** 50 6N 9 53 E
Hammeren, *Denmark* . **17 J8** 55 18N 14 47 E
Hammerfest, *Norway* . **14 A20** 70 39N 23 41 E
Hammerstein = Czarne,
  Poland . . . . **54 E3** 53 42N 16 58 E
Hammerum, *Denmark* . **17 H3** 56 9N 9 3 E
Hamminkeln, *Germany* **30 D2** 51 43N 6 35 E
Hammond, *Ind., U.S.A.* **157 E1** 41 38N 87 30W
Hammond, *La., U.S.A.* **155 K9** 30 30N 90 28W
Hammond, *N.Y.,*
  U.S.A. **151 B9** 44 27N 75 42W
Hammondsport, *U.S.A.* **150 D7** 42 25N 77 13W
Hammonton, *U.S.A.* . . **148 F8** 39 39N 74 48W
Hamneda, *Sweden* . . . **17 H7** 56 41N 13 51 E
Hamoyet, Jebel, *Sudan* **106 D4** 17 33N 38 2 E
Hampden, *N.Z.* . . . . . **131 F5** 45 18 S 170 50 E
Hampshire □, *U.K.* . . **21 F6** 51 7N 1 23W
Hampshire Downs,
  U.K. **21 F6** 51 15N 1 10W
Hampton, *N.B., Canada* **141 C6** 45 32N 65 51W
Hampton, *Ont., Canada* **150 C6** 43 58N 78 45W
Hampton, *Ark., U.S.A.* **155 J8** 33 32N 92 28W
Hampton, *Ga., U.S.A.* **152 B5** 33 23N 84 17W
Hampton, *Iowa, U.S.A.* **156 B3** 42 45N 93 13W
Hampton, *N.H., U.S.A.* **151 D14** 42 57N 70 50W
Hampton, *S.C., U.S.A.* **152 C8** 32 52N 81 7W
Hampton, *Va., U.S.A.* . **148 G7** 37 2N 76 21W
Hampton Bays, *U.S.A.* **151 F12** 40 53N 72 30W
Hampton Springs,
  U.S.A. **152 E6** 30 5N 83 40W
Hampton Tableland,
  Australia . . . . **125 F4** 32 0 S 127 0 E
Hamra, *Sweden* . . . . . **16 C8** 61 39N 14 59 E
Hamra →, *Chad* . . . . **109 F4** 12 52N 21 15 E
Hamrat esh Sheykh,
  Sudan . . . . **107 E2** 14 38N 27 55 E
Hamrun, *Malta* . . . . . **38 F8** 35 53N 14 29 E
Hamtik, *Phil.* . . . . **81 F3** 10 42N 121 59 E
Hamur, *Turkey* . . . . . **101 C10** 39 37N 43 3 E
Hamyang, *S. Korea* . . **75 G14** 35 32N 127 42 E
Han →, *China* . . . . . . **77 F11** 23 25N 116 40 E
Han Shui →, *China* . . **77 B10** 30 34N 114 17 E
Han Shui →, *Henan,*
  China . . . . **77 B10** 30 34N 114 17 E
Hana, *U.S.A.* **145 C6** 20 45N 155 59W
Hanahan, *U.S.A.* **152 C10** 32 55N 80 0W
Hanak, *Si. Arabia* . . . . **96 E3** 25 32N 37 0 E
Hanalei, *U.S.A.* **145 A2** 22 13N 159 30W
Hanamaki, *Japan* . . . . **70 E10** 39 23N 141 7 E
Hanamaulu, *U.S.A.* . . **145 B2** 21 59N 159 35W
Hanang, *Tanzania* . . . **118 C4** 4 30 S 35 25 E
Hanapepe, *U.S.A.* . . . **145 B2** 21 55N 159 35W
Hanau, *Germany* . . . . **31 E4** 50 7N 8 56 E
Hanauma B., *U.S.A.* . . **145 K14** 21 15N 157 42W
Hanbogd = Ihbulag,
  Mongolia . . . . **74 C4** 43 11N 107 10 E
Hançalar, *Turkey* . . . . **49 C11** 38 8N 29 24 E
Hăncești, *Moldova* . . . **53 D13** 46 50N 28 36 E
Hancheng, *China* . . . . **74 G6** 35 31N 110 25 E
Hanchuan, *China* . . . . **77 B9** 30 40N 113 46 E
Hanchung = Hanzhong,
  China . . . . **74 H4** 33 10N 107 1 E
Hancock, *Mich., U.S.A.* **154 B10** 47 8N 88 35W
Hancock, *N.Y., U.S.A.* **151 E9** 41 57N 75 17W
Handa, *Japan* . . . . . . **73 C8** 34 53N 136 55 E
Handa, *Somali Rep.* . . **120 B4** 10 37N 51 2 E
Handan, *China* . . . . . . **74 F8** 36 35N 114 28 E
Handeni, *Tanzania* . . . **118 C4** 5 25 S 38 2 E
Handlová, *Slovak Rep.* **35 C11** 48 45N 18 35 E
Handub, *Sudan* . . . . . **106 D4** 19 15N 37 16 E
Handwara, *India* . . . . **93 B6** 34 21N 74 20 E
Haneda, Tokyo ✈
  (HND), *Japan* . . . . **73 B11** 35 33N 139 46 E
Hanegev, *Israel* . . . . . **103 E4** 30 50N 35 0 E
Hanford, *U.S.A.* **160 J7** 36 20N 119 39W
Hanford Reach
  △, *U.S.A.* **158 C4** 46 40N 119 28W
Hang Chat, *Thailand* . . **86 C2** 18 20N 99 21 E
Hang Dong, *Thailand* . **86 C2** 18 41N 98 55 E
Hanga Roa, *Chile* . . . . **172 b** 27 8 S 109 26W
Hangang →, *S. Korea* . **75 F14** 37 50N 126 30 E
Hangayn Nuruu,
  Mongolia . . . . **68 B4** 47 30N 99 0 E
Hangchou = Hangzhou,
  China . . . . **77 B13** 30 18N 120 11 E
Hanggin Houqi, *China* . **74 D4** 40 58N 107 4 E
Hanggin Qi, *China* . . . **74 E5** 39 52N 108 50 E
Hangkong = Wuhan,
  China . . . . **77 B10** 30 31N 114 18 E
Hangku = Hangu,
  China . . . . **75 E9** 39 18N 117 53 E
Hangu, *China* . . . . . . **75 E9** 39 18N 117 53 E
Hangzhou, *China* . . . . **77 B13** 30 18N 120 11 E
Hangzhou Wan, *China* **77 B13** 30 15N 120 45 E
Hanhongor, *Mongolia* . **74 C3** 43 55N 104 28 E
Hania = Khaniá, *Greece* **49 E6** 35 30N 24 4 E
Ḥanīdh, *Si. Arabia* . . . **97 E6** 26 35N 48 38 E
Ḥanīsh, *Yemen* . . . . . **99 E3** 13 45N 42 46 E
Haniska, *Slovak Rep.* . **35 C14** 48 37N 21 15 E
Hanjiang, *China* . . . . . **77 E12** 25 26N 119 6 E
Hankinson, *U.S.A.* . . . **154 B6** 46 4N 96 54W
Hankø, *Norway* . . . . . **18 E7** 59 6N 10 50 E
Hanko, *Finland* . . . . . **15 G8** 59 50N 22 57 E
Hankou, *China* . . . . . . **77 B10** 30 35N 114 30 E
Hanksville, *U.S.A.* . . . **159 G8** 38 22N 110 43W
Hanle, *India* . . . . **89 C8** 32 42N 79 4 E
Hanmer Springs, *N.Z.* . **131 C7** 42 32 S 172 50 E
Hann →, *Australia* . . . **124 C4** 17 26 S 126 17 E
Hann, Mt., *Australia* . . **124 C4** 15 45 S 126 0 E
Hanna, *Canada* **142 C6** 51 40N 111 54W
Hanna, *U.S.A.* **158 F10** 41 52N 106 34W
Hannah B., *Canada* . . **140 B4** 51 40N 80 0W
Hannibal, *Mo., U.S.A.* **156 F9** 39 42N 91 22W
Hannibal, *N.Y., U.S.A.* **151 C8** 43 19N 76 35W
Hannik, *Sudan* . . . . . **106 D3** 18 12N 32 20 E
Hannover, *Germany* . . **30 C5** 52 22N 9 46 E

Hanö, *Sweden* . . . . . . **17 H8** 56 1N 14 50 E
Hanöbukten, *Sweden* . **17 J8** 55 35N 14 30 E
Hanoi, *Vietnam* . . . . . **76 G5** 21 5N 105 55 E
Hanover = Hannover,
  Germany . . . . **30 C5** 52 22N 9 46 E
Hanover, *Canada* **140 D3** 44 9N 81 2W
Hanover, *S. Africa* . . . **116 E3** 31 4 S 24 29 E
Hanover, *Ind., U.S.A.* . **157 F11** 38 43N 85 28W
Hanover, *N.H., U.S.A.* **151 C12** 43 42N 72 17W
Hanover, *Pa., U.S.A.* . **148 F7** 39 48N 76 59W
Hanover, I., *Chile* . . . . **176 D2** 51 0 S 74 50W
Hanpan, C.,
  Papua N. G. . . . . . **132 C8** 5 0 S 154 35 E
Hans Lollik I.,
  U.S. Virgin Is. . . . . **165 e** 18 24N 64 53W
Hans Meyer Ra.,
  Papua N. G. . . . . . **132 C7** 4 20 S 152 55 E
Hansdiha, *India* . . . . . **93 G12** 24 36N 87 5 E
Hanshou, *China* . . . . . **77 C8** 28 56N 111 50 E
Hansi, *India* . . . . **92 E6** 29 10N 75 57 E
Hanson, L., *Australia* . **128 A2** 31 0 S 136 15 E
Hanstholm, *Denmark* . **17 G2** 57 7N 8 36 E
Hantan = Handan,
  China . . . . **74 F8** 36 35N 114 28 E
Hantsavichy, *Belarus* . **59 F4** 52 49N 26 30 E
Hanumangarh, *India* . . **92 E5** 29 35N 74 19 E
Hanyin, *China* . . . . . . **76 A7** 32 54N 108 28 E
Hanyū, *Japan* . . . . . . **73 A11** 36 10N 139 32 E
Hanyuan, *China* . . . . . **76 C4** 29 21N 102 40 E
Hanzhong, *China* . . . . **74 H4** 33 10N 107 1 E
Hanzhuang, *China* . . . **75 G9** 34 33N 117 23 E
Haora, *India* . . . . **93 H13** 22 37N 88 20 E
Haouach, O. →, *Chad* **109 E4** 16 45N 19 35 E
Haoxue, *China* . . . . . . **77 B9** 30 3N 112 24 E
Haparanda, *Sweden* . . **14 D21** 65 52N 24 8 E
Hapeville, *U.S.A.* **152 B5** 33 40N 84 25W
Happy, *U.S.A.* **155 H4** 34 45N 101 52W
Happy Camp, *U.S.A.* . **158 F2** 41 48N 123 23W
Happy Valley-Goose
  Bay, *Canada* **141 B7** 53 15N 60 20W
Hapsu, *N. Korea* . . . . **75 D15** 41 13N 128 51 E
Hapur, *India* . . . . **92 E7** 28 45N 77 45 E
Ḥaql, *Si. Arabia* . . . . . **103 F3** 29 10N 34 58 E
Haquira, *Peru* . . . . . . **172 C3** 14 14 S 72 12W
Har, *Indonesia* . . . . . . **83 C4** 5 16 S 133 14 E
Har-Ayrag, *Mongolia* . **74 B5** 45 47N 109 16 E
Har Hu, *China* . . . . . . **68 C4** 38 20N 97 38 E
Har Us Nuur, *Mongolia* **68 B4** 48 0N 92 0 E
Har Yehuda, *Israel* . . . **103 D3** 31 35N 34 57 E
Ḥaraḍ, *Si. Arabia* . . . . **99 A5** 24 22N 49 0 E
Ḥaraḍ, *Yemen* . . . . . **98 D3** 16 26N 43 5 E
Haradok, *Belarus* . . . . **58 E6** 55 30N 30 3 E
Haradok, *Belarus* . . . . **59 E6** 55 30N 30 3 E
Häradsbäck, *Sweden* . . **17 H8** 56 35N 14 25 E
Haranomachi, *Japan* . . **70 F10** 37 38N 140 58 E
Harardera, *Somali Rep.* **120 D3** 4 33N 47 38 E
Harare, *Zimbabwe* . . . **119 F3** 17 43 S 31 2 E
Ḥarāsīs, Jiddat al,
  Oman . . . . **99 C7** 19 30N 56 0 E
Harat, *Eritrea* . . . . . . **107 D4** 16 5N 39 26 E
Haraz, *Chad* . . . . **109 F3** 14 20N 19 12 E
Harazé, *Chad* . . . . . . **109 G4** 9 57N 20 48 E
Harbhanga, *India* . . . . **94 J7** 20 38N 84 36 E
Harbin, *China* . . . . . . **75 B14** 45 48N 126 40 E
Harbiye, *Turkey* . . . . **100 D7** 36 10N 36 8 E
Harbo, *Sweden* . . . . . **16 D11** 60 7N 17 12 E
Harboør, *Denmark* . . . **17 H2** 56 38N 8 10 E
Harbor Beach, *U.S.A.* **150 D4** 43 51N 82 39W
Harbour Breton,
  Canada **141 C8** 47 29N 55 50W
Harbour Deep, *Canada* **141 B8** 50 25N 56 32W
Harburg, *Germany* . . . **30 B5** 53 28N 9 58 E
Harburger Berge △,
  Germany . . . . **30 B5** 53 26N 9 51 E
Hârby, *Denmark* . . . . **17 J4** 55 13N 10 7 E
Harda, *India* . . . . **92 H7** 22 27N 77 5 E
Hardangerfjorden,
  Norway . . . . **18 D3** 60 5N 6 0 E
Hardangerjøkulen,
  Norway . . . . **18 D4** 60 30N 7 27 E
Hardangervidda,
  Norway . . . . **18 D4** 60 7N 7 20 E
Hardangervidda △,
  Norway . . . . **18 D4** 60 10N 7 25 E
Hardap, *Namibia* . . . . **116 C2** 24 29 S 17 45 E
Hardap Dam, *Namibia* **116 C2** 24 32 S 17 50 E
Hardecville, *U.S.A.* . . . **152 E8** 32 17N 81 5W
Harden, *Australia* . . . . **129 C8** 34 32 S 148 24 E
Hardenberg, *Neths.* . . **24 B6** 52 34N 6 37 E
Harderwijk, *Neths.* . . . **24 B5** 52 21N 5 38 E
Hardin, *U.S.A.* **158 D10** 45 44N 107 37W
Hardin, *Ill., U.S.A.* . . . **156 K6** 39 10N 90 37W
Harding, *S. Africa* . . . **117 E4** 30 35 S 29 55 E
Harding Ra., *Australia* . **124 C3** 16 17 S 124 55 E
Hardinsburg, *U.S.A.* . . **157 G10** 37 47N 86 28W
Hardisty, *Canada* **142 C6** 52 40N 111 18W
Hardoi, *India* . . . . **93 F9** 27 26N 80 6 E
Hardwar = Haridwar,
  India . . . . **92 E8** 29 58N 78 9 E
Hardwick, *Ga., U.S.A.* **152 B6** 33 4N 83 14W
Hardwick, *Vt., U.S.A.* . **151 B12** 44 30N 72 22W
Hardwicke B., *Australia* **128 C2** 34 55 S 137 20 E
Hardy, Pen., *Chile* . . . **176 E3** 55 30 S 68 20W
Hardy, Pte., *St. Lucia* . **165 f** 14 6N 60 56W
Hare B., *Canada* **141 B8** 51 15N 55 45W
Hareid, *Norway* . . . . . **18 B3** 62 22N 6 1 E
Haren, *Germany* . . . . **30 C3** 52 47N 7 13 E
Harer, *Ethiopia* . . . . . **107 F5** 9 20N 42 8 E
Harerrge □, *Ethiopia* . **107 F5** 7 12N 42 0 E
Harestua, *Norway* . . . **18 D7** 60 11N 10 44 E
Hareto, *Ethiopia* . . . . **107 F4** 9 23N 37 6 E
Harfleur, *France* . . . . **26 C7** 49 30N 0 10 E
Hargeisa = Hargeysa,
  Somali Rep. . . . . . **120 C2** 9 30N 44 2 E
Hargeysa, *Somali Rep.* **120 B2** 9 30N 44 2 E
Harghita □, *Romania* . **53 D10** 46 30N 25 30 E
Harghita, Munții,
  Romania . . . . **53 D10** 46 25N 25 35 E
Hargshamn, *Sweden* . . **16 D12** 60 12N 18 30 E
Hari →, *Indonesia* . . . **84 C2** 1 16 S 104 5 E
Haria, *Canary Is.* **9 e2** 29 8N 13 32W
Ḥarīb, *Yemen* . . . . . . **98 D4** 14 56N 45 30 E
Haricha, Hamada el,
  Mali **110 D4** 22 40N 3 5W
Haridwar, *India* . . . . . **92 E8** 29 58N 78 9 E
Harihari, *N.Z.* . . . . . . **131 E4** 43 9 S 170 32 E
Harima-Nada, *Japan* . . **73 C7** 34 30N 134 35 E
Haringhata →, *Bangla.* **90 E2** 22 0N 89 58 E
Haripad, *India* . . . . . . **95 K3** 9 14N 76 28 E
Haripur, *Pakistan* . . . . **93 A5** 33 44N 72 55 E
Harīrūd →, *Asia* . . . . **98 B3** 37 24N 60 38 E
Härja, *Sweden* . . . . . . **16 F7** 58 1N 13 5 E
Härjedalen, *Sweden* . . **16 B7** 62 22N 13 5 E
Harlan, *Iowa, U.S.A.* . **156 E7** 41 39N 95 19W
Harlan, *Ky., U.S.A.* . . **149 G4** 36 51N 83 19W
Hârlău, *Romania* . . . . **53 C11** 47 28N 26 55 E
Harlech, *U.K.* **20 E3** 52 52N 4 6W
Harlem, *Mont., U.S.A.* **158 B9** 48 32N 108 47W
Hårlev, *Denmark* . . . . **17 J6** 55 21N 12 14 E
Harleyville, *U.S.A.* . . . **152 B9** 33 13N 80 27W
Harlingen, *Neths.* . . . . **24 A5** 53 11N 5 25 E

Harlingen, *U.S.A.* **155 M6** 26 12N 97 42W
Harlow, *U.K.* .... **21 F8** 51 46N   0 8 E
Harlowton, *U.S.A.* **158 C9** 46 26N 109 50W
Harmancık, *Turkey* .... **49 B11** 39 41N 29 9 E
Harmånger, *Sweden* ... **16 C11** 61 55N 17 20 E
Harnai, *Eritrea* .... **107 D5** 16 30N 40 10 E
Harnai, *India* .... **94 F1** 17 48N 73 6 E
Harnai, *Pakistan* ...... **92 D2** 30 6N 67 56 E
Harney, L., *U.S.A.* **153 G8** 28 45N 81 3W
Harney Basin, *U.S.A.* . **158 E4** 43 30N 119 0W
Harney L., *U.S.A.* **158 E4** 43 14N 119 8W
Harney Peak, *U.S.A.* .. **154 D3** 43 52N 103 32W
Härnön, *Sweden* ...... **16 B12** 62 36N 18 0 E
Härnösand, *Sweden* ... **16 B11** 62 38N 17 55 E
Haro, *Spain* **40 C2** 42 35N   2 55W
Harold, *U.S.A.* **153 E3** 30 40N 86 53W
Harold Pond, *Bahamas* .. **9 b** 23 7N 77 22W
Haroldswick, *U.K.* **22 A8** 60 48N   0 50W
Harp L., *Canada* **141 A7** 55 5N 61 50W
Harpanahalli, *India* ... **95 G3** 14 47N 76 2 E
Harper = Costa Mesa,
   U.S.A. **161 M9** 33 38N 117 55W
Harper, *Liberia* .... **112 E3** 4 25N   7 43 E
Harper, Mt., *U.S.A.* .. **144 D12** 64 14N 143 51W
Harplinge, *Sweden* .... **17 H6** 56 45N 12 45 E
Harr, *Mauritania* **112 B2** 25 20N 12 28W
Harrai, *India* .... **93 H8** 22 37N 79 13 E
Harrand, *Pakistan* .... **92 E4** 29 28N 70 3 E
Harrat Khaybar,
   Si. Arabia .... **106 B5** 25 30N 39 45 E
Harrat Nawāsīf,
   Si. Arabia .... **106 C5** 21 20N 42 10 E
Harricana →, *Canada* .. **140 A4** 50 56N 79 32W
Harriman, *U.S.A.* **149 H3** 35 56N 84 33W
Harrington, *Australia* .. **129 A10** 31 52 S 152 42 E
Harrington Harbour,
   Canada **141 B8** 50 31N 59 30W
Harrington Sd.,
   Bermuda .... **9 a** 32 20N 64 44W
Harris, *U.K.* **22 D2** 57 50N   6 55W
Harris, L., *Australia* ... **127 E2** 31 10 S 135 10 E
Harris, L., *U.S.A.* **153 G8** 28 47N 81 49W
Harris, Sd. of, *U.K.* .. **22 D1** 57 44N   7 6W
Harris Mts., *N.Z.* .... **131 L1** 44 49 S 168 49 E
Harrisburg, *Ill., U.S.A.* **155 G10** 37 44N 88 32W
Harrisburg, *Nebr.,*
   U.S.A. **154 E3** 41 33N 103 44W
Harrisburg, *Pa., U.S.A.* **150 F8** 40 16N 76 53W
Harrismith, *S. Africa* .. **117 D4** 28 15 S 29 8 E
Harrison, *Ark., U.S.A.* **155 G8** 36 14N 93 7W
Harrison, *Maine, U.S.A.* **151 D14** 44 7N 70 39W
Harrison, *Nebr., U.S.A.* **154 D3** 42 41N 103 53W
Harrison, C., *Canada* .. **141 B8** 54 55N 57 55W
Harrison Bay, *U.S.A.* . **144 A10** 70 40N 151 0W
Harrison L., *Canada* ... **142 D4** 49 33N 121 50W
Harrisonburg, *U.S.A.* . **148 F6** 38 27N 78 52W
Harrisonville, *U.S.A.* .. **156 F2** 38 39N 94 21W
Harriston, *Canada* **150 C4** 43 57N 80 53W
Harrisville, *Mich.,*
   U.S.A. **150 B1** 44 39N 83 17W
Harrisville, *N.Y., U.S.A.* **151 B9** 44 9N 75 19W
Harrisville, *Pa., U.S.A.* **150 E5** 41 8N 80 0W
Harrodsburg, *Ind.,*
   U.S.A. **157 E10** 39 1N 86 33W
Harrodsburg, *Ky.,*
   U.S.A. **157 G12** 37 46N 84 51W
Harrogate, *U.K.* **20 C6** 54 0N   1 33W
Harrow, *Australia* ..... **128 D4** 37 9 S 141 35 E
Harrow, *Canada* **157 B14** 42 2N 82 55W
Harrow □, *U.K.* **21 F7** 51 35N   0 21W
Harrowsmith, *Canada* . **151 B8** 44 24N 76 40W
Harry S. Truman
   Reservoir, *U.S.A.* .. **156 F3** 38 16N 93 24W
Harsefeld, *Germany* ... **30 B5** 53 27N   9 30 E
Harsewinkel, *Germany* . **30 D4** 51 56N   8 14 E
Hârşin, *Iran* .... **101 E12** 34 18N 47 33 E
Hârşova, *Romania* .... **53 F12** 44 40N 27 54 E
Harstad, *Norway* ..... **14 B17** 68 48N 16 30 E
Harsud, *India* .... **92 H7** 22 6N 76 44 E
Hart, *U.S.A.* **148 D2** 43 42N 86 22W
Hart, L., *Australia* .... **128 A2** 31 10 S 136 25 E
Hartbees →, *S. Africa* . **116 D3** 28 45 S 20 32 E
Hartberg, *Austria* ..... **34 D8** 47 17N   15 58 E
Hårteigen, *Norway* .... **18 D4** 60 11N   7 3 E
Hartford, *Ala., U.S.A.* . **153 D4** 31 6N 85 42W
Hartford, *Conn., U.S.A.* **151 E12** 41 46N 72 41W
Hartford, *Ky., U.S.A.* . **148 G2** 37 27N 86 55W
Hartford, *Mich., U.S.A.* **157 B10** 42 13N 86 10W
Hartford, *S. Dak.,*
   U.S.A. **154 D6** 43 38N 96 57W
Hartford, *Wis., U.S.A.* . **154 D10** 43 19N 88 22W
Hartford City, *U.S.A.* . **157 D11** 40 27N 85 22W
Hartland = Bela,
   Bela., S. Africa .... **117 C4** 24 51 S 28 19 E
Hartland, *Canada* **141 C6** 46 20N 67 32W
Hartland, *U.S.A.* **151 A7** 45 6N 88 21W
Hartland Pt., *U.K.* **21 F3** 51 1N   4 32W
Hartlepool, *U.K.* **20 C6** 54 42N   1 13W
Hartlepool □, *U.K.* ... **20 C6** 54 42N   1 17W
Hartley Bay, *Canada* .. **142 C3** 53 25N 129 15W
Hartmannberge,
   Namibia .... **116 B1** 17 0 S 13 0 E
Hartney, *Canada* **143 D8** 49 30N 100 35W
Hârtop, *Moldova* ...... **53 D13** 46 39N 28 44 E
Harts →, *S. Africa* .... **116 D3** 28 24 S 24 17 E
Hartselle, *U.S.A.* **149 H2** 34 27N 86 56W
Hartshorne, *U.S.A.* ... **155 H7** 34 51N 95 34W
Hartstown, *U.S.A.* **150 E4** 41 33N 80 23W
Hartsville, *U.S.A.* **149 H5** 34 23N 80 4W
Hartswater, *S. Africa* .. **116 D3** 27 34 S 24 43 E
Hartwell, *U.S.A.* **149 H4** 34 21N 82 56W
Haruku, *Indonesia* .... **82 B3** 3 34 S 128 29 E
Harunabad, *Pakistan* .. **92 E5** 29 35N 73 8 E
Harur, *India* .... **95 H4** 12 3N 78 29 E
Härür □, *Afghan.* .... **91 C1** 31 29N 61 24 E
Harvand, *Iran* .... **97 D7** 28 25N 55 43 E
Harvard, *U.S.A.* **154 B8** 42 25N 88 37W
Harvey, *Australia* ..... **125 F2** 33 5 S 115 54 E
Harvey, *Ill., U.S.A.* ... **157 C9** 41 36N 87 50W
Harvey, *N. Dak., U.S.A.* **154 B5** 47 47N 99 56W
Harwich, *U.K.* .... **21 F9** 51 56N   1 17 E
Haryana □, *India* ..... **92 E7** 29 0N 76 10 E
Haryn →, *Belarus* .... **59 F4** 52 7N 27 17 E
Harz, *Germany* .... **30 D6** 51 38N 10 44 E
Harz △, *Germany* .... **30 D7** 51 40N 10 18 E
Harzgerode, *Germany* .. **30 D7** 51 38N 11 8 E
Hasa □, *Si. Arabia* ... **97 E6** 25 50N 49 0 E
Hasaheisa, *Sudan* ..... **107 E3** 14 44N 33 20 E
Hasalbag, *China* ...... **65 E8** 37 52N 76 42 E
Hasan Kīāhfak,
   W. Sahara **110 D2** 24 54N 14 49W
Hasi Tatraut, *W. Sahara* **110 C2** 23 13N 13 15W
Hāsik, *Oman* .... **99 C6** 17 22N 55 17 E
Haskell, *U.S.A.* **155 J5** 33 10N 99 44W

Haskovo = Khaskovo,
   Bulgaria .... **51 E9** 41 56N 25 30 E
Hasköy, *Turkey* ...... **51 E10** 41 38N 26 52 E
Haslach, *Germany* .... **31 G4** 48 16N   8 5 E
Hasle, *Denmark* ...... **17 J8** 55 11N 14 44 E
Haslemere, *U.K.* **21 F7** 51 5N   0 43W
Haslev, *Denmark* ..... **17 J5** 55 18N 11 57 E
Hasparren, *France* **28 E2** 43 24N   1 18W
Hassa, *Turkey* .... **100 D7** 36 48N 36 29 E
Hassan, *India* .... **95 H3** 13 0N 76 5 E
Hassberge △, *Germany* **31 E6** 50 8N 10 45 E
Hassela, *Sweden* ..... **16 B10** 62 7N 16 42 E
Hasselt, *Belgium* ..... **24 C5** 50 56N   5 21 E
Hassene, Adrar, *Algeria* **111 D5** 21 0N   4 0 E
Hassfurt, *Germany* .... **31 E6** 50 2N 10 30 E
Hassi bou Khelala,
   Algeria **111 B4** 30 17N   0 18W
Hassi Bourarchet,
   Algeria .... **111 C6** 27 26N   9 19 E
Hassi Djafou, *Algeria* . **111 B5** 30 55N   3 35 E
Hassi el Abiod, *Algeria* **111 B5** 31 47N   3 37 E
Hassi el Biod, *Algeria* . **111 C6** 28 30N   6 0 E
Hassi el Hadjar, *Algeria* **111 B5** 31 28N   4 45 E
Hassi Imoulaye, *Algeria* **111 C6** 29 54N   9 10 E
Hassi Inifeg, *Algeria* .. **111 C4** 28 15N   1 30W
Hassi Inifel, *Algeria* ... **111 C5** 29 50N   3 41 E
Hassi Mana, *Algeria* .. **111 C4** 28 48N   2 37W
Hassi Messaoud,
   Algeria .... **111 B6** 31 51N   6 1 E
Hassi Sougoued,
   Algeria .... **111 C6** 26 50N   9 28 E
Hassi Tartrat, *Algeria* . **111 B6** 30 5N   6 28 E
Hassi Zerzour,
   Morocco **110 B4** 30 51N   3 56W
Hassi Zguilma, *Algeria* **111 B4** 30 12N   2 19W
Hässleholm, *Sweden* .. **17 H7** 56 10N 13 46 E
Hassloch, *Germany* ... **31 F4** 49 22N   8 16 E
Hästholmen, *Sweden* .. **17 F8** 58 17N 14 38 E
Hastings, *Australia* .... **129 E6** 38 18 S 145 12 E
Hastings, *N.Z.* .... **130 F5** 39 39 S 176 52 E
Hastings, *U.K.* .... **21 G8** 50 51N   0 35 E
Hastings, *Fla., U.S.A.* . **152 F8** 29 43N 81 31W
Hastings, *Mich., U.S.A.* **157 B11** 42 39N 85 17W
Hastings, *Minn., U.S.A.* **154 C8** 44 44N 92 51W
Hastings, *Nebr., U.S.A.* **154 E5** 40 35N 98 23W
Hastings Ra., *Australia* **129 A10** 31 15 S 152 14 E
Hästveda, *Sweden* .... **17 H7** 56 17N 13 55 E
Hasy 'Aţshān, *Libya* .. **108 C2** 27 20N 10 25 E
Hasy Tissan, *Libya* .... **111 C7** 28 14N 12 26 E
Hat, *Germany* .... **52 B7** 48 19N 22 38 E
Hat Yai, *Thailand* .... **87 J3** 7 1N 100 27 E
Hatanbulag = Ergel,
   Mongolia .... **74 C5** 43 8N 109 5 E
Hatay = Antalya,
   Turkey .... **100 D4** 36 52N 30 45 E
Hatch, *U.S.A.* **159 K10** 32 40N 107 9W
Hatchet L., *Canada* ... **143 B8** 58 36N 103 40W
Hațeg, *Romania* ...... **52 E7** 45 36N 22 55 E
Hateruma-Shima,
   Japan .... **71 M1** 24 3N 123 47 E
Hatfield P.O., *Australia* **128 E5** 33 54 S 143 49 E
Hatgal, *Mongolia* ..... **68 A5** 50 26N 100 9 E
Hathras, *India* .... **92 F8** 27 36N 78 6 E
Hatia, *Bangla.* .... **90 D3** 22 30N 91 5 E
Hatia Is., *Bangla.* .... **90 D3** 22 30N 91 0 E
Ḥāţibah, Ra's,
   Si. Arabia .... **106 C4** 21 55N 38 57 E
Hatid, *India* .... **94 F2** 17 17N 75 3 E
Hato Corozal,
   Colombia **168 B3** 6 11N 71 45W
Hato Mayor,
   Dom. Rep. **165 C6** 18 46N 69 15W
Hatsukaichi, *Japan* ... **72 C4** 34 22N 132 22 E
Hatta, *Japan* .... **93 G8** 24 7N 79 36 E
Hattah, *Australia* ..... **128 C5** 34 48 S 142 17 E
Hattah Kulkyne △,
   Australia .... **128 C5** 35 40 S 142 22 E
Hatteras, C., *U.S.A.* .. **149 H8** 35 14N 75 32W
Hatteras Plain, *Atl. Oc.* **8 D4** 28 0N 72 0W
Hattiesburg, *U.S.A.* ... **155 K10** 31 20N 89 17W
Hatvan, *Hungary* ..... **52 C4** 47 40N 19 45 E
Hau Bon = Cheo Reo,
   Vietnam .... **78 B3** 13 25N 108 28 E
Hau Duc, *Vietnam* .... **86 E7** 15 20N 108 13 E
Haubstadt, *U.S.A.* **157 F9** 38 12N 87 34W
Haud, *Ethiopia* ...... **120 C2** 8 0N 47 0 E
Hauganes, *Iceland* **11 B8** 65 55N 18 18W
Haugastøl, *Norway* ... **18 D4** 60 30N   7 50 E
Hauge, *Norway* ...... **18 F3** 58 20N   6 15 E
Haugesund, *Norway* .. **18 E2** 59 23N   5 13 E
Hauhui, *Solomon Is.* . **133 M11** 9 10 S 160 59 E
Hauhungaroa Ra., *N.Z.* **130 E4** 38 42 S 175 40 E
Haukeligrend, *Norway* **18 E4** 59 44N   7 33 E
Haukipudas, *Finland* .. **12 D21** 65 12N 25 20 E
Haultain →, *Canada* .. **143 B7** 55 51N 106 46W
Haungpa, *Burma* ..... **90 C6** 25 29N 96 7 E
Hauraha, *Solomon Is.* **133 N11** 10 46 S 161 59 E
Hauraki G., *N.Z.* ..... **130 C5** 36 35 S 175 5 E
Hauroko, L., *N.Z.* .... **131 F2** 45 59 S 167 21 E
Hausruck, *Austria* .... **34 C6** 48 6N 13 30 E
Hausstock, *Switz.* .... **33 C8** 46 53N   9 3 E
Haut Atlas, *Morocco* .. **110 B4** 32 30N   5 0W
Haut-Jura △, *France* .. **27 F9** 46 23N   2 23 E
Haut-Languedoc △,
   France .... **28 E6** 43 30N   2 43 E
Haut Niger △, *Guinea* **112 C2** 10 20N 10 20W
Haut-Rhin □, *France* .. **27 E14** 48 0N   7 15 E
Haut-Zaïre =
   Orientale □,
   Dem. Rep. of
   the Congo .... **118 B2** 2 20N 26 0 E
Haute-Corse □, *France* **29 F13** 42 30N   9 30 E
Haute-Garonne □,
   France .... **28 E5** 43 30N   1 30 E
Haute-Loire □, *France* **28 E7** 45 5N   3 50 E
Haute-Marne □, *France* **27 D12** 48 10N   5 20 E
Haute-Normandie □,
   France .... **26 C7** 49 20N   1 0 E
Haute-Saône □, *France* **27 E13** 47 45N   6 10 E
Haute-Savoie □, *France* **29 C10** 46 0N   6 20 E
Haute-Vienne □,
   France .... **28 C5** 45 50N   1 10 E
Hautes-Alpes □,
   France .... **29 D10** 44 42N   6 20 E
Hautes Fagnes = Hohe
   Venn, *Belgium* ..... **24 D6** 50 30N   6 5 E
Hautes Fagnes = Hohes
   Venn-Eifel △,
   Europe .... **30 E2** 50 30N   6 10 E
Hautes-Pyrénées □,
   France .... **28 F4** 43 0N   0 10 E
Hauteville-Lompnès,
   France .... **29 C9** 45 58N   5 36 E
Hautmont, *France* .... **27 B10** 50 15N   3 55 E
Hauts-de-Seine □,
   France .... **27 D9** 48 52N   2 15 E
Hauts Plateaux, *Algeria* **111 B5** 35 0N   1 0 E
Hauula, *U.S.A.* **145 K14** 21 37N 157 55W
Hauzenberg, *Germany* **31 G9** 48 40N 13 37 E
Havana = La Habana,
   Cuba **164 B3** 23 8N 82 22W
Havana, *Fla., U.S.A.* .. **152 E5** 30 37N 84 25W
Havana, *Ill., U.S.A.* ... **156 D6** 40 18N 90 4W
Havant, *U.K.* **21 G7** 50 51N   0 58W

Havârna, *Romania* .... **53 B11** 48 4N 26 43 E
Heath →, *Bolivia* ..... **172 C4** 12 31 S 68 38W
Heath, Pte., *Canada* ... **141 C7** 49 8N 61 40W
Havasor = Kızışı,
   Turkey .... **96 B4** 38 18N 43 25 E
Heathcote, *Australia* .. **129 D6** 36 56 S 144 45 E
Havasu, L., *U.S.A.* ... **161 L12** 34 18N 114 28W
Heatherwood = Edson,
   Canada **142 C5** 53 35N 116 28W
Havdhem, *Sweden* .... **17 G12** 57 10N 18 20 E
Havel →, *Germany* ... **30 C8** 52 50N 12 3 E
Heavener, *U.S.A.* **155 H7** 34 53N 94 36W
Havelian, *Pakistan* .... **92 B5** 34 2N 73 10 E
Hebbronville, *U.S.A.* .. **155 M5** 27 18N 98 41W
Havelock, *Canada* **140 D4** 44 26N 77 53W
Hebei □, *China* ...... **74 E9** 39 0N 116 0 E
Havelock, *N.Z.* ...... **131 B8** 41 17 S 173 48 E
Hebel, *Australia* ..... **127 D4** 28 58 S 147 47 E
Havelock, *U.S.A.* **149 H7** 34 53N 76 54W
Heber, *U.S.A.* **155 H9** 32 44N 115 32W
Havelock I., *India* .... **95 J11** 11 58N 93 0 E
Heber Springs, *U.S.A.* **155 H9** 35 30N 92 2W
Havelock North, *N.Z.* . **130 F5** 39 40 S 176 53 E
Hebert, *Canada* **143 C7** 50 30N 107 10W
Haverfordwest, *U.K.* .. **21 F3** 51 48N   4 58W
Hebgen L., *U.S.A.* ... **158 D8** 44 52N 111 20W
Haverhill, *U.K.* ...... **21 E8** 52 5N   0 28 E
Hebi, *China* .... **74 G8** 35 57N 114 7 E
Haverhill, *Mass., U.S.A.* **151 D13** 42 47N 71 5W
Hebrides, *U.K.* **12 D4** 57 30N   7 0W
Haveri, *India* .... **95 G2** 14 53N 75 24 E
Hebrides, Sea of the,
   U.K. **22 D2** 57 5N   7 0W
Haverstraw, *U.S.A.* ... **151 E11** 41 12N 73 58W
Hebron = Al Khalīl,
   West Bank .... **103 D4** 31 32N 35 6 E
Håverud, *Sweden* ..... **17 F6** 58 50N 12 28 E
Hebron, *Canada* **139 C13** 58 5N 62 30W
Havirga, *Mongolia* .... **74 B7** 45 41N 113 5 E
Hebron, N. Dak.,
   U.S.A. **154 B3** 46 54N 102 3W
Havířov, *Czech Rep.* . **35 B11** 49 46N 18 20 E
Hebron, Nebr., U.S.A. . **154 E6** 40 10N 97 35W
Havlíčkův Brod,
   Czech Rep. .... **34 B8** 49 36N 15 33 E
Heby, *Sweden* .... **16 E10** 59 56N 16 53 E
Havneby, *Denmark* ... **17 J2** 55 5N   8 34 E
Hecate Str., *Canada* .. **142 C2** 53 10N 130 30W
Havran, *Turkey* ...... **49 B9** 39 33N 27 6 E
Heceta I., *U.S.A.* **142 B2** 55 46N 133 40W
Havre, *U.S.A.* **158 B9** 48 33N 109 41W
Hechi, *China* .... **76 E7** 24 40N 108 2 E
Havre-Aubert, *Canada* **141 C7** 47 12N 61 56W
Hechingen, *Germany* . **31 G4** 48 21N   8 57 E
Havre-St.-Pierre,
   Canada **141 B7** 50 18N 63 33W
Hechuan, *China* ...... **76 B6** 30 2N 106 12 E
Havsa, *Turkey* .... **51 E10** 41 31N 26 48 E
Hecla, *U.S.A.* **154 C5** 45 53N 98 9W
Havza, *Turkey* .... **100 B6** 41 0N 35 35 E
Hecla I., *Canada* **143 C9** 51 10N 96 43W
Haw →, *U.S.A.* **149 H6** 35 36N 79 3W
Hedal, *Norway* ...... **18 D6** 60 37N   9 41 E
Hawaii □, *U.S.A.* **145 L8** 19 30N 156 30W
Heddal, *Norway* ..... **18 E6** 59 36N   9 9 E
Hawaii I., *Pac. Oc.* ... **145 M8** 19 30N 155 30W
Hede, *Sweden* .... **16 B7** 62 23N 13 30 E
Hawaii Volcanoes △,
   U.S.A. **145 M8** 19 23N 155 17W
Hedemora, *Sweden* ... **16 D9** 60 18N 15 58 E
Hawaiian Is., *Pac. Oc.* **135 E11** 24 0N 165 0W
Hedensted, *Denmark* . **17 J3** 55 46N   9 42 E
Hawaiian Ridge,
   Pac. Oc. **135 E11** 24 0N 165 0W
Hedeshope, N.Z. ...... **131 G3** 46 12 S 168 34 E
Hawarden, *U.S.A.* **154 D6** 43 0N 96 29W
Hedmark □, *Norway* . **18 C8** 61 17N 11 40 E
Hawea, L., *N.Z.* ..... **131 E4** 44 28 S 169 19 E
Hedrick, *U.S.A.* **156 C4** 41 11N 92 19W
Hawea Flat, *N.Z.* .... **131 E4** 44 40 S 169 19 E
Heerde, *Neths.* ...... **24 B6** 52 24N   6 2 E
Hawera, *N.Z.* .... **130 F3** 39 35 S 174 19 E
Heerenveen, *Neths.* ... **24 B5** 52 57N   5 55 E
Hawesville, *U.S.A.* ... **157 G10** 37 54N 86 45W
Heerhugowaard, *Neths.* **24 B4** 52 40N   4 51 E
Hawi, *U.S.A.* **145 C6** 20 14N 155 50W
Heerlen, *Neths.* ...... **24 D5** 50 55N   5 58 E
Hawick, *U.K.* **22 F6** 55 26N   2 47W
Heerwegen =
Hawk Junction, *Canada* **140 C3** 48 5N 84 38W
   Polkowice, *Poland* . **55 G3** 51 29N 16 3 E
Hawk Point, *U.S.A.* .. **156 F5** 38 58N 91 8W
Hefa, *Israel* .... **103 C4** 32 46N 35 0 E
Hawkdun Ra., *N.Z.* .. **131 E5** 44 53 S 170 5 E
Hefa □, *Israel* .... **103 C4** 32 40N 35 0 E
Hawke B., *N.Z.* ...... **130 F6** 39 25 S 177 20 E
Hefei, *China* .... **77 B11** 31 52N 117 18 E
Hawker, *Australia* .... **128 A3** 31 59 S 138 22 E
Hefeng, *China* .... **77 C8** 29 55N 109 52 E
Hawke's Bay □, *N.Z.* **130 F5** 39 45 S 176 35 E
Heflin, *U.S.A.* **149 H4** 33 39N 85 35W
Hawkesbury, *Canada* . **140 C5** 45 37N 74 37W
Hegalig, *Sudan* ...... **107 E3** 11 46N 30 1 E
Hawkesbury →, *Australia* **129 C5** 33 37N 129 3W
Hegang, *China* ...... **75 B8** 47 20N 130 19 E
Hawkesbury Pt.,
   Australia .... **126 A1** 11 55 S 134 5 E
Heggenes, *Norway* .... **18 C6** 61 9N   9 4 E
Hawkinsville, *U.S.A.* .. **152 C6** 32 17N 83 28W
Hegra, *Norway* ...... **16 E5** 63 31N 11 8 E
Hawks Nest, *Australia* **129 B10** 32 41 S 152 15 E
Hei Ling Chau, *China* . **69 G11** 22 15N 114 2 E
Hawley, *Minn., U.S.A.* **154 B6** 46 53N 96 19W
Heian, *Japan* .... **107 E3** 11 33N 30 31 E
Hawley, *Pa., U.S.A.* .. **151 E9** 41 28N 75 11W
Heichengzhen, *China* . **74 F4** 36 24N 106 3 E
Hawran, W. →, *Iraq* . **101 F10** 33 58N 42 34 E
Heidal, *Norway* ...... **18 C6** 61 45N   9 19 E
Hawsh Mūssā, *Lebanon* **103 B4** 33 45N 35 55 E
Heide, *Germany* ...... **30 A5** 54 11N   9 6 E
Hawthorne, *Fla., U.S.A.* **153 F7** 29 36N 82 5W
Heidelberg, *Germany* . **31 F4** 49 24N   8 42 E
Hawthorne, *Nev.,*
   U.S.A. **158 G4** 38 32N 118 38W
Heidelberg, S. Africa . **116 E3** 34 6 S 20 59 E
Hay, *Australia* .... **129 C6** 34 30 S 144 51 E
Heidenau, *Germany* .. **30 E9** 50 59N 13 52 E
Hay →, *Australia* ..... **126 C2** 24 50 S 138 0 E
Heidenheim, *Germany* **31 G6** 48 41N 10 9 E
Hay →, *Canada* **142 A5** 60 50N 116 26W
Heigun-Tō, *Japan* .... **72 D4** 33 47N 132 14 E
Hay, C., *Australia* .... **124 B4** 14 5 S 129 29 E
Heihe, *China* .... **75 B7** 50 10N 127 30 E
Hay L., *Canada* **150 B4** 44 53N 80 58W
Heijing, *China* ...... **76 E3** 25 22N 101 44 E
Hay L., *Canada* **142 B5** 58 50N 118 50W
Heijo = P'yŏngyang,
   N. Korea .... **75 E13** 39 0N 125 30 E
Hay-on-Wye, *U.K.* ... **21 E4** 52 5N   3 8W
Heilbad Heiligenstadt,
   Germany .... **30 D6** 51 22N 10 8 E
Hay River, *Canada* ... **142 A5** 60 51N 115 44W
Heilbron, S. Africa ... **117 D4** 27 16 S 27 59 E
Hay Springs, *U.S.A.* . **154 D3** 42 41N 102 41W
Heilbronn, *Germany* . **31 F5** 49 9N   9 13 E
Haya = Tehoru,
   Indonesia .... **83 B3** 3 23 S 129 30 E
Heiligenblut, *Austria* . **34 D5** 47 2N 12 51 E
Hayachine-San, *Japan* **70 E10** 39 34N 141 29 E
Heiligenhafen,
   Germany .... **30 A6** 54 22N 10 59 E
Hayange, *France* ..... **27 C13** 49 20N   6 2 E
Heilongjiang □, *China* **69 B7** 48 0N 126 0 E
Hayastan = Armenia ■,
   Asia .... **61 K7** 40 20N 45 0 E
Heilprin Land,
   Greenland **10 A7** 81 0N 33 0W
Hayato, *Japan* .... **72 J2** 31 40N 130 43 E
Heilsberg = Lidzbark
Haydarlı, *Turkey* ..... **49 C12** 38 16N 30 13 E
   Warmiński, *Poland* **54 D7** 54 7N 20 34 E
Hayden, *U.S.A.* **158 F10** 40 30N 107 16W
Heilunkiang =
Haydon, *Australia* .... **126 B3** 18 0 S 141 30 E
   Heilongjiang □,
Hayes, *U.S.A.* **154 C4** 44 23N 101 1W
   China .... **69 B7** 48 0N 126 0 E
Hayes →, *Canada* **140 A1** 57 3N 92 12W
Heim, *Norway* .... **18 A6** 63 26N   7 50 E
Hayes, Mt., *U.S.A.* ... **144 E11** 63 37N 146 43W
Heimaey, *Iceland* **11 C3** 63 26N 20 17W
Hayes Creek, *Australia* **124 B5** 13 43 S 131 22 E
Heimdal, *Norway* .... **18 A7** 63 21N 10 22 E
Hayle, *U.K.* **21 G2** 50 11N   5 26W
Heinola, *Finland* ..... **15 F22** 61 13N 26 2 E
Hayling I., *U.K.* **21 G7** 50 48N   0 59W
Heinsberg, *Germany* .. **30 D2** 51 4N   6 6 E
Haymana, *Turkey* ..... **100 C5** 39 26N 32 31 E
Heinze Kyun, *Burma* . **86 E1** 14 25N 97 45 E
Haymen I., *Australia* .. **126 J6** 20 3 S 148 52 E
Heinrikut, *Burma* .... **90 C5** 25 14N 94 44 E
Haynan, *Yemen* ...... **99 D5** 15 50N 48 18 E
Heishan, *China* ...... **75 D12** 41 40N 122 5 E
Hayrabolu, *Turkey* .... **51 E11** 41 12N 27 5 E
Heishui, Liaoning,
   China .... **75 C10** 42 8N 119 30 E
Hays, *Canada* **142 C6** 50 6N 111 48W
Heishui, Sichuan, China **76 A4** 32 4N 103 2 E
Hays, *U.S.A.* **154 F5** 38 53N 99 20W
Hejaz = Ḥijāz □,
Hays, *Yemen* .... **98 D3** 13 56N 43 29 E
   Si. Arabia .... **96 E3** 24 0N 40 0 E
Haysville, *U.S.A.* **157 F10** 38 28N 86 55W
Hejian, *China* .... **74 E9** 38 25N 116 5 E
Haysyn, *Ukraine* ..... **53 B14** 48 57N 29 25 E
Hejiang, *China* ...... **76 C5** 28 43N 105 46 E
Hayvoron, *Ukraine* ... **53 B14** 48 22N 29 52 E
Hejin, *China* .... **74 G6** 35 35N 110 42 E
Hayward, *Calif., U.S.A.* **160 H4** 37 40N 122 5W
Hekimhan, *Turkey* .... **100 C7** 38 50N 37 55 E
Hayward, *Wis., U.S.A.* **154 B9** 46 1N 91 29W
Hekinan, *Japan* ...... **73 C9** 34 52N 137 0 E
Haywards Heath, *U.K.* **21 G7** 51 0N   0 5W
Hekla, *Iceland* **11 D7** 63 56N 19 35W
Hazafon □, *Israel* .... **103 C4** 32 40N 35 20 E
Hekou, Guangdong,
Hazârân, Kûh-e, *Iran* **97 D8** 29 35N 57 20 E
   China .... **77 F9** 23 13N 112 45 E
Hazard, *U.S.A.* **148 G4** 37 15N 83 12W
Hekou, Yunnan, China **76 F4** 22 30N 103 59 E
Hazaribag, *India* ..... **93 H11** 23 58N 85 26 E
Hel, *Poland* .... **54 D5** 54 37N 18 47 E
Hazaribag Road, *India* **93 G11** 24 12N 85 57 E
Helagsfjället, *Sweden* . **16 B6** 62 54N 12 25 E
Hazebrouck, *France* .. **27 B9** 50 42N   2 31 E
Helan Shan, China .... **74 E3** 38 30N 105 55 E
Hazelton, *Canada* **142 B3** 55 20N 127 42W
Helechosa, *Spain* **37 F6** 39 22N   4 53W
Hazelton, *U.S.A.* **154 B4** 46 29N 100 17W
Helena, U.S.A. **145 J13** 21 35N 158 7W
Hazen, *U.S.A.* **154 B4** 47 18N 101 38W
Helen Atoll, Pac. Oc. .. **83 A4** 2 40N 132 0 E
Hazlehurst, Ga., *U.S.A.* **152 D7** 31 52N 82 36W
Helen Ra., *Australia* .. **128 A1** 31 20 S 134 30 E
Hazlehurst, Miss.,
   U.S.A. **155 K9** 31 52N 90 24W
Helena, *Ark., U.S.A.* . **155 H9** 34 32N 90 36W
Hazlet, *U.S.A.* **151 F10** 40 25N 74 12W
Helena, *Ga., U.S.A.* . **152 D5** 32 5N 82 55W
Hazleton, *Ind., U.S.A.* **157 F9** 38 29N 87 33W
Helena, Mont., U.S.A. **158 C7** 46 36N 112 2W
Hazleton, *Pa., U.S.A.* . **151 F9** 40 57N 75 59W
Helendale, *U.S.A.* **161 L9** 34 44N 117 19W
Hazlett, L., *Australia* . **124 D4** 21 30 S 128 48 E
Helensburgh, *Australia* **129 C9** 34 11 S 151 1 E
Hazro, *Turkey* .... **96 B4** 38 15N 40 47 E
Helensburgh, *U.K.* ... **22 E4** 56 1N   4 43W
He Xian, Anhui, China **77 B12** 31 45N 118 20 E
Helensville, *N.Z.* .... **130 C3** 36 41 S 174 29 E
He Xian,
   Guangxi Zhuangzu,
   China .... **77 E8** 24 27N 111 30 E
Helenvale, *Australia* .. **126 B3** 15 43 S 145 14 E
Head of Bight,
   Australia .... **125 F5** 31 30 S 131 25 E
Helgasjön, *Sweden* ... **17 H8** 56 55N 14 50 E
Headland, *U.S.A.* **152 D4** 31 21N 85 21W
Helgeland, *Norway* .. **14 C15** 66 7N 13 29 E
Headlands, Zimbabwe **119 F3** 18 15 S 32 2 E
Helgoland, *Germany* . **30 A3** 54 10N   7 53 E
Healdsburg, *U.S.A.* ... **160 G4** 38 37N 122 52W
Heligoland =
Healdton, *U.S.A.* **155 H6** 34 14N 97 29W
   Helgoland, *Germany* **30 A3** 54 10N   7 53 E
Healesville, *Australia* . **129 D5** 37 35 S 145 30 E
Heligoland B. =
Healy, *U.S.A.* **154 C4** 38 36N 100 37W
   Deutsche Bucht,
Heany Junction,
   Zimbabwe .... **117 C4** 20 6 S 28 54 E
   Germany .... **30 A4** 54 15N   8 0 E
Heard I., Ind. Oc. .... **121 K6** 53 0 S 74 0 E
Heliopolis, *Egypt* .... **106 H7** 30 6N 31 17 E
Heard →, *U.S.A.* **155 K6** 30 53N 96 36W
Hell, *Norway* .... **18 A7** 63 26N 10 54 E
Hearst, *Canada* **140 C3** 49 40N 83 41W
Hella, *Iceland* **11 D6** 63 50N 20 24W
Heart →, *U.S.A.* **154 B4** 46 46N 100 50W
Hellebæk, *Denmark* .. **17 H6** 56 4N 12 32 E
Heart's Content,
   Canada **141 C9** 47 54N 53 27W
Helleland, *Norway* ... **18 F3** 58 33N   6 7 E
Helleputsluis, *Neths.* . **24 C4** 51 50N   4 8 E

Hellhole Gorge △,
   Australia .... **126 D3** 25 31 S 144 12 E
Hellín, *Spain* **41 G3** 38 31N   1 40W
Hellissandur, *Iceland* . **11 C3** 64 55N 23 54W
Hells Canyon △, *U.S.A.* **158 D5** 45 30N 117 45W
Hell's Gate △, *Kenya* . **118 C4** 0 54 S 36 19 E
Hellvik, *Norway* ..... **18 F2** 58 29N   5 52 E
Helmand □, *Afghan.* . **91 C2** 31 20N 64 0 E
Helmand →, *Afghan.* **91 C1** 31 12N 61 34 E
Helme →, *Germany* .. **30 D7** 51 20N 11 21 E
Helmeringhausen,
   Namibia .... **116 D2** 25 54 S 16 57 E
Helmond, *Neths.* ..... **24 C5** 51 29N   5 41 E
Helmsdale, *U.K.* **22 C5** 58 7N   3 39W
Helmsdale →, *U.K.* .. **22 C5** 58 7N   3 40W
Helmstedt, *Germany* . **30 C7** 52 12N 11 0 E
Helper, *U.S.A.* **158 G8** 39 41N 110 51W
Helsingborg, *Sweden* . **17 H6** 56 3N 12 42 E
Helsinge, *Denmark* ... **17 H6** 56 2N 12 12 E
Helsingfors = Helsinki,
   Finland .... **15 F21** 60 15N 25 3 E
Helsingør, *Denmark* .. **17 H6** 56 2N 12 35 E
Helsinki, *Finland* .... **15 F21** 60 15N 25 3 E
Helska, Mierzeja,
   Poland .... **54 D5** 54 45N 18 40 E
Helston, *U.K.* **21 G2** 50 6N   5 17W
Helvellyn, *U.K.* **20 C4** 54 32N   3 1W
Helwân, *Egypt* .... **106 J7** 29 50N 31 20 E
Hemavati →, *India* ... **95 H3** 12 30N 76 20 E
Hemel Hempstead,
   U.K. **21 F7** 51 44N   0 28W
Hemet, *U.S.A.* **161 M10** 33 45N 116 58W
Hemingford, *U.S.A.* .. **154 D3** 42 19N 103 4W
Hemis △, *India* ..... **92 B7** 34 10N 77 15 E
Hemmingford, *Canada* **151 A11** 45 3N 73 35W
Hempstead, *U.S.A.* ... **155 K6** 30 6N 96 5W
Hemse, *Sweden* ...... **17 G12** 57 15N 18 22 E
Hemsedal, *Norway* ... **18 D5** 60 53N   8 30 E
Hemsön, *Sweden* ..... **16 B12** 62 42N 18 5 E
Hen, *Norway* .... **18 D7** 60 13N 10 14 E
Hen and Chickens Is.,
   N.Z. .... **130 B3** 35 58 S 174 45 E
Henån, *Sweden* ...... **17 F5** 58 14N 11 40 E
Henan □, *China* ..... **74 H8** 34 0N 114 0 E
Henares →, *Spain* ... **42 E7** 40 24N   3 30W
Henashi-Misaki, *Japan* **70 D9** 40 37N 139 51 E
Hendaye, *France* **28 E2** 43 23N   1 47W
Hendek, *Turkey* ..... **100 B4** 40 48N 30 44 E
Henderson, *Argentina* **174 D3** 36 18 S 61 43W
Henderson, *Ga., U.S.A.* **152 C5** 32 21N 83 47W
Henderson, *Ky., U.S.A.* **157 G9** 37 50N 87 35W
Henderson, *N.C.,*
   U.S.A. **149 G6** 36 20N 78 25W
Henderson, *Nev.,*
   U.S.A. **161 J12** 36 2N 114 59W
Henderson, *Tenn.,*
   U.S.A. **149 H1** 35 26N 88 38W
Henderson, *Tex.,*
   U.S.A. **155 J7** 32 9N 94 48W
Henderson I., Pac. Oc. **135 K15** 24 22 S 128 19W
Hendersonville, *N.C.,*
   U.S.A. **149 H4** 35 19N 82 28W
Hendersonville, *Tenn.,*
   U.S.A. **149 G2** 36 18N 86 37W
Hendijān, *Iran* .... **97 D6** 30 14N 49 43 E
Hendorābī, *Iran* ..... **97 E7** 26 40N 53 37 E
Heng Jiang, *China* .... **76 C5** 28 40N 104 25 E
Heng Xian, *China* .... **76 F7** 22 40N 109 17 E
Henganofi, Papua N. G. **132 D3** 6 15 S 145 38 E
Hengcheng, *China* .... **74 E4** 38 18N 106 28 E
Hengchun, *Taiwan* ... **77 F13** 22 0N 120 44 E
Hengdaohezi, *China* .. **75 B15** 44 52N 129 0 E
Hengelo, *Neths.* ..... **24 B6** 52 16N   6 48 E
Henggang, *China* ..... **77 C10** 28 11N 115 30 E
Hengjiang, *China* ..... **69 F11** 22 39N 114 12 E
Hengqin, *China* ...... **69 F10** 22 7N 113 34 E
Hengqin Dao, *China* . **69 G10** 22 7N 113 34 E
Hengshan, Hunan,
   China .... **77 D9** 27 16N 112 45 E
Hengshan, Shaanxi,
   China .... **74 F5** 37 58N 109 5 E
Hengshui, *China* ..... **74 F8** 37 41N 115 40 E
Hengyang, *China* ..... **77 D9** 26 59N 112 22 E
Henichesk, *Ukraine* .. **59 J8** 46 12N 34 50 E
Henin-Beaumont,
   France .... **27 B9** 50 25N   2 58 E
Hénin-Liétard = Hénin-
   Beaumont, *France* .. **27 B9** 50 25N   2 58 E
Henley-on-Thames,
   U.K. **21 F7** 51 32N   0 54W
Hennan, *Sweden* ..... **16 B9** 62 3N 15 54 E
Hennebont, *France* ... **26 E3** 47 49N   3 19W
Hennenman, S. Africa **116 D4** 27 59 S 27 1 E
Hennepin, *U.S.A.* **156 C1** 41 15N 89 21W
Hennessey, *U.S.A.* ... **155 G6** 36 6N 97 54W
Hennigsdorf, *Germany* **30 C9** 52 38N 13 12 E
Henri Pittier △,
   Venezuela .... **165 D6** 10 25 S 67 37W
Henrietta, *U.S.A.* **155 J5** 33 49N 98 12W
Henrietta, Ostrov =
   Genriyetty, Ostrov,
   Russia .... **67 B16** 77 6N 156 30 E
Henrietta Maria, C.,
   Canada **140 A3** 55 9N 82 20W
Henry, *U.S.A.* **156 C7** 41 7N 89 22W
Henry Lawrence I.,
   India .... **95 H11** 12 9N 93 5 E
Henryville, *Canada* ... **151 A11** 45 8N 73 11W
Hensall, *Canada* **150 C3** 43 26N 81 30W
Hentsted-Ulzburg,
   Germany .... **30 B6** 53 47N 10 0 E
Hentiesbaai, *Namibia* . **116 C1** 22 8 S 14 18 E
Hentiyn Nuruu,
   Mongolia .... **69 B5** 48 30N 108 30 E
Henty, *Australia* ..... **129 C7** 35 30 S 147 0 E
Henzada, *Burma* ..... **90 G5** 17 38N 95 26 E
Hephaestia, *Greece* ... **49 B7** 39 55N 25 14 E
Hephzibah, *U.S.A.* ... **152 B7** 33 14N 82 6W
Heping, *China* .... **77 E10** 24 29N 115 0 E
Heppner, *U.S.A.* **158 D4** 45 21N 119 33W
Hepu, *China* .... **76 G7** 21 40N 109 12 E
Hepworth, *Canada* ... **150 B3** 44 37N 81 9W
Heqing, *China* .... **76 D3** 26 37N 100 11 E
Hequ, *China* .... **74 E6** 39 20N 111 15 E
Héradsflói, *Iceland* ... **11 B12** 65 42N 14 12W
Héraðsvötn →, *Iceland* **11 C3** 65 45N 19 25W
Heradsbygd, *Norway* . **18 D8** 60 49N 11 39 E
Heraklion = Iráklion,
   Greece .... **39 E6** 35 20N 25 12 E
Herald Cays, *Australia* **126 B4** 16 58 S 149 9 E
Herand, *Norway* ..... **18 D3** 60 30N   6 22 E
Herāt, *Afghan.* ...... **91 B1** 34 20N 62 7 E
Herāt □, *Afghan.* .... **91 C1** 32 0N 62 0 E
Hérault □, *France* .... **28 E7** 43 34N   3 15 E
Hérault →, *France* ... **26 E8** 43 34N   3 15 E
Herbault, *France* ..... **26 E8** 47 36N   1 8 E
Herbert →, *Australia* . **126 B4** 18 31 S 146 17 E
Herbert I., *U.S.A.* ... **144 K5** 52 45N 170 7W

Herbert River Falls △, *Australia* 126 B4 18 15 S 145 32 E
Herbertabad, *India* 95 J11 11 43N 92 37 E
Herberton, *Australia* 126 B4 17 20 S 145 25 E
Herbertsdale, *S. Africa* 116 E3 34 1 S 21 46 E
Herbertville, *N.Z.* 130 G5 40 30 S 176 33 E
Herbignac, *France* 26 E4 47 27N 2 18W
Herborn, *Germany* 30 E4 50 40N 8 18 E
Herby, *Poland* 55 H5 50 45N 18 50 E
Herceg-Novi, *Serbia & M.* 50 D2 42 30N 18 33 E
Hercegfalva = Mezőfalva, *Hungary* 52 D3 46 55N 18 49 E
Herchmer, *Canada* 143 B10 57 22N 94 10W
Herculânia = Coxim, *Brazil* 173 D7 18 30 S 54 55W
Herðubreið, *Iceland* 11 B10 65 11N 16 21W
Hereford, *U.K.* 21 E5 52 4N 2 43W
Hereford, *U.S.A.* 155 H3 34 49N 102 24W
Herefordshire □, *U.K.* 21 E5 52 8N 2 40W
Herefoss, *Norway* 18 F5 58 32N 8 23 E
Herehogna, *Sweden* 18 C9 61 44N 12 8 E
Hereke, *Turkey* 51 F13 40 47N 29 38 E
Herekino, *N.Z.* 130 B2 35 18 S 173 11 E
Herencia, *Spain* 43 F7 39 21N 3 22W
Herentals, *Belgium* 24 C4 51 12N 4 51 E
Herford, *Germany* 30 C4 52 7N 8 39 E
Héricourt, *France* 27 E13 47 32N 6 45 E
Herington, *U.S.A.* 154 F6 38 40N 96 57W
Herisau, *Switz.* 33 B8 47 22N 9 17 E
Hérisson, *France* 27 F9 46 32N 2 42 E
Herkimer, *U.S.A.* 151 D10 43 0N 74 59W
Herlong, *U.S.A.* 160 E6 40 8N 120 8W
Herm, *U.K.* 21 H5 49 30N 2 28W
Hermakivka, *Ukraine* 53 B11 48 42N 26 11 E
Hermann, *U.S.A.* 156 F5 38 42N 91 27W
Hermannsbad = Ciechocinek, *Poland* 55 F5 52 53N 18 45 E
Hermannsburg, *Australia* 124 D5 23 57 S 132 45 E
Hermannsburg, *Germany* 30 C6 52 50N 10 5 E
Hermannstadt = Sibiu, *Romania* 53 E9 45 45N 24 9 E
Hermansverk, *Norway* 18 C3 61 11N 6 52 E
Hermanus, *S. Africa* 116 E2 34 27 S 19 12 E
Herment, *France* 28 C6 45 45N 2 24 E
Hermidale, *Australia* 129 A7 31 30 S 146 42 E
Hermiston, *U.S.A.* 158 D4 45 51N 119 17W
Hermit Is., *Papua N. G.* 132 A3 1 32 S 145 5 E
Hermitage, *U.S.A.* 156 G3 37 56N 93 19W
Hermite, I., *Chile* 176 E3 55 50 S 68 0W
Hermon, *U.S.A.* 151 B9 44 28N 75 14W
Hermon, Mt. = Shaykh, J. ash, *Lebanon* 103 B4 33 25N 35 50 E
Hermosillo, *Mexico* 162 B2 29 10N 111 0W
Hernád ➛, *Hungary* 52 C6 47 56N 21 8 E
Hernandarias, *Paraguay* 175 B5 25 20 S 54 40W
Hernandez, *U.S.A.* 160 J6 36 24N 120 46W
Hernando, *Argentina* 174 C3 32 28 S 63 40W
Hernando, *Fla., U.S.A.* 153 G7 28 54N 82 23W
Hernando, *Miss., U.S.A.* 155 H10 34 50N 90 0W
Hernani, *Spain* 40 B3 43 16N 1 58W
Herndon, *U.S.A.* 150 F8 40 43N 76 51W
Herne, *Germany* 24 C7 51 32N 7 14 E
Herne Bay, *U.K.* 21 F9 51 21N 1 8 E
Herning, *Denmark* 17 H2 56 8N 8 58 E
Herod, *U.S.A.* 152 D5 31 42N 84 26W
Heroica = Caborca, *Mexico* 162 A2 30 40N 112 10W
Heroica Nogales = Nogales, *Mexico* 162 A2 31 20N 110 56W
Heron Bay, *Canada* 140 C2 48 40N 86 25W
Herradura, Pta. de la, *Canary Is.* 9 e2 28 26N 14 8W
Herre, *Norway* 18 E6 59 6N 9 34 E
Herreid, *U.S.A.* 154 C4 45 50N 100 4W
Herrenberg, *Germany* 31 G4 48 35N 8 52 E
Herrera, *Spain* 43 H6 37 26N 4 55W
Herrera de Alcántara, *Spain* 43 F3 39 39N 7 25W
Herrera de Pisuerga, *Spain* 42 C6 42 35N 4 20W
Herrera del Duque, *Spain* 43 F5 39 10N 5 3W
Herrestad, *Sweden* 17 F5 58 21N 11 50 E
Herrin, *U.S.A.* 155 G10 37 48N 89 2W
Herriot, *Canada* 143 B8 56 22N 101 16W
Herrljunga, *Sweden* 17 F7 58 5N 13 1 E
Hersbruck, *Germany* 31 F7 49 30N 11 26 E
Herschel I., *Canada* 6 C1 69 35N 139 5W
Hershey, *U.S.A.* 151 F8 40 17N 76 39W
Herstal, *Belgium* 24 D5 50 40N 5 38 E
Hertford, *U.K.* 21 F7 51 48N 0 4W
Hertfordshire □, *U.K.* 21 F7 51 51N 0 5W
's-Hertogenbosch, *Neths.* 24 C5 51 42N 5 17 E
Hertsa, *Ukraine* 53 B11 48 9N 26 15 E
Hertzogville, *S. Africa* 116 D4 28 9 S 25 30 E
Hervás, *Spain* 42 E5 40 16N 5 52W
Hervey B., *Australia* 126 C5 25 0 S 152 52 E
Herzberg, *Brandenburg, Germany* 30 D9 51 41N 13 14 E
Herzberg, *Niedersachsen, Germany* 30 D6 51 38N 10 20 E
Herzliyya, *Israel* 103 C3 32 10N 34 50 E
Herzogenbuchsee, *Switz.* 32 B5 47 11N 7 42 E
Herzogenburg, *Austria* 34 C8 48 17N 15 41 E
Ḥeşār, *Fārs, Iran* 97 D6 29 52N 50 16 E
Ḥeşār, *Markazī, Iran* 97 C6 35 50N 49 12 E
Hesdin, *France* 27 B9 50 21N 2 2 E
Heshan, *China* 76 F7 23 50N 108 53 E
Heshui, *China* 74 G5 35 48N 108 0 E
Heshun, *China* 74 F7 37 22N 113 32 E
Heskestad, *Norway* 18 F3 58 28N 6 22 E
Hesperia, *U.S.A.* 161 L9 34 25N 117 18W
Hessdalen, *Norway* 18 B8 62 48N 11 10 E
Hesse = Hessen □, *Germany* 30 E4 50 30N 9 0 E
Hessen □, *Germany* 30 E4 50 30N 9 0 E
Hessenreuther und Manteler Wald ⌓, *Germany* 31 F8 49 45N 12 1 E
Hesso, *Australia* 128 B2 32 8 S 137 27 E
Hesteyri, *Iceland* 11 A4 66 20N 22 53W
Hestra, *Sweden* 17 G7 57 26N 13 35 E
Hetch Hetchy Aqueduct, *U.S.A.* 160 H5 37 29N 122 19W
Hettinger, *U.S.A.* 154 C3 46 0N 102 42W
Hettstedt, *Germany* 30 D7 51 39N 11 31 E
Heuvelton, *U.S.A.* 151 B9 44 37N 75 25W
Hevelândia, *Brazil* 169 E5 5 12 S 61 50W
Heves, *Hungary* 52 C5 47 36N 20 17 E
Heves □, *Hungary* 52 C5 47 50N 20 0 E
Hewitt, *U.S.A.* 155 K6 31 27N 97 11W
Hexham, *U.K.* 20 C5 54 58N 2 4W
Hexi, *Yunnan, China* 76 E4 24 9N 102 38 E
Hexi, *Zhejiang, China* 77 D12 27 58N 119 38 E
Hexigten Qi, *China* 75 C9 43 18N 117 30 E
Ḥeydarābād, *Iran* 97 D7 30 33N 55 38 E
Heydebreck = Kędzierzyn-Koźle, *Poland* 55 H5 50 20N 18 12 E
Heyfield, *Australia* 129 D7 37 59 S 146 47 E
Heysham, *U.K.* 20 C5 54 3N 2 53W
Heyuan, *China* 77 F10 23 39N 114 40 E
Heywood, *Australia* 128 E4 38 8 S 141 37 E
Heyworth, *U.S.A.* 156 D8 40 19N 88 59W
Heze, *China* 74 G8 35 14N 115 20 E
Hezhang, *China* 76 D5 27 8N 104 41 E
Hi, Ko, *Thailand* 87 a 7 44N 98 22 E
Hi-no-Misaki, *Japan* 72 B4 35 26N 132 38 E
Hi Vista, *U.S.A.* 161 L9 34 45N 117 46W
Hialeah, *U.S.A.* 153 K9 25 50N 80 17W
Hiawatha, *U.S.A.* 154 F7 39 51N 95 32W
Hibbing, *U.S.A.* 154 B8 47 25N 92 56W
Hibbs B., *Australia* 127 G4 42 35 S 145 15 E
Hibernia Reef, *Australia* 124 B3 12 0 S 123 23 E
Hibiki-Nada, *Japan* 72 D2 34 0N 130 0 E
Hickman, *U.S.A.* 155 G10 36 34N 89 11W
Hickory, *U.S.A.* 149 H5 35 44N 81 21W
Hicks, Pt., *Australia* 129 D8 37 49 S 149 17 E
Hicks Bay, *N.Z.* 130 D7 37 34 S 178 21 E
Hicks L., *Canada* 143 A9 61 25N 100 0W
Hicksville, *N.Y., U.S.A.* 151 F11 40 46N 73 32W
Hicksville, *Ohio, U.S.A.* 157 C12 41 18N 84 46W
Hida, *Romania* 53 C8 47 10N 23 19 E
Hida-Gawa ➛, *Japan* 73 B9 35 26N 137 3 E
Hida-Sammyaku, *Japan* 73 A9 36 30N 137 40 E
Hida-Sanchi, *Japan* 73 A9 36 10N 137 0 E
Hidaka, *Japan* 72 B6 35 30N 134 44 E
Hidaka-Sammyaku, *Japan* 70 C11 42 35N 142 45 E
Hidalgo, *Mexico* 163 C5 24 15N 99 26W
Hidalgo □, *Mexico* 163 C5 20 30N 99 10W
Hidalgo, Presa M., *Mexico* 162 B3 26 30N 108 35W
Hidalgo del Parral, *Mexico* 162 B3 26 58N 105 40W
Hiddensee, *Germany* 30 A9 54 32N 13 6 E
Hidrolândia, *Brazil* 171 E2 17 0 S 49 15W
Hieflau, *Austria* 34 D7 47 36N 14 46 E
Hiendelaencina, *Spain* 40 D2 41 5N 3 0W
Hienghène, *N. Cal.* 133 T18 20 41 S 164 56 E
Hierro, *Canary Is.* 9 e1 27 44N 18 0W
Higashi-Hiroshima, *Japan* 72 C4 34 25N 132 45 E
Higashi-Matsuyama, *Japan* 73 A11 36 2N 139 25 E
Higashiajima-San, *Japan* 70 F10 37 40N 140 10 E
Higashiōsaka, *Japan* 73 C7 34 40N 135 37 E
Higasi-Suidō, *Japan* 72 D1 34 0N 129 30 E
Higbee, *U.S.A.* 156 E4 39 19N 92 31W
Higgins, *U.S.A.* 155 G4 36 7N 100 2W
Higgins Corner, *U.S.A.* 160 F5 39 2N 121 5W
Higginsville, *U.S.A.* 156 E3 39 4N 93 43W
High Bridge, *U.S.A.* 151 F10 40 40N 74 54W
High Island Res., *China* 69 G11 22 22N 114 21 E
High Level, *Canada* 142 B5 58 31N 117 8W
High Peak, *Phil.* 80 D3 15 29N 120 7 E
High Pk., *St. Helena* 9 h 15 58 S 5 44W
High Point, *U.S.A.* 149 H6 35 57N 80 0W
High Prairie, *Canada* 142 B5 55 30N 116 30W
High River, *Canada* 142 C6 50 30N 113 50W
High Springs, *U.S.A.* 152 F7 29 50N 82 36W
High Tatra = Tatry, *Slovak Rep.* 35 B13 49 20N 20 0 E
High Veld, *Africa* 104 J6 27 0 S 27 0 E
High Wycombe, *U.K.* 21 F7 51 37N 0 45W
Highbank, *N.Z.* 131 D6 43 37 S 171 45 E
Highland, *Ill., U.S.A.* 156 F7 38 44N 89 41W
Highland, *Ind., U.S.A.* 157 C9 41 33N 87 28W
Highland, *Wis., U.S.A.* 156 A6 43 5N 90 22W
Highland □, *U.K.* 22 D4 57 17N 4 21W
Highland City, *U.S.A.* 153 H8 27 58N 81 53W
Highland Home, *U.S.A.* 152 D3 31 57N 86 19W
Highland Mills = Experiment, *U.S.A.* 152 B5 33 17N 84 17W
Highland Park, *U.S.A.* 157 B9 42 11N 87 48W
Highland View, *U.S.A.* 152 F4 29 50N 85 19W
Highlands = Fort Thomas, *U.S.A.* 157 E12 39 5N 84 27W
Highmore, *U.S.A.* 154 C5 44 31N 99 27W
Highrock L., *Man., Canada* 143 B8 55 45N 100 30W
Highrock L., *Sask., Canada* 143 B7 57 5N 105 32W
Higüey, *Dom. Rep.* 165 C6 18 37N 68 42W
Hihya, *Egypt* 106 H7 30 40N 31 36 E
Hiiumaa, *Estonia* 15 G20 58 50N 22 45 E
Híjar, *Spain* 40 D4 41 10N 0 27W
Ḥijāz □, *Si. Arabia* 96 E3 24 0N 40 0 E
Hiji, *Japan* 72 D3 33 22N 131 32 E
Hijo = Tagum, *Phil.* 81 H5 7 33N 125 53 E
Hikari, *Japan* 72 D3 33 58N 131 58 E
Hiketa, *Japan* 72 C6 34 13N 134 24 E
Hikkaduwa, *Sri Lanka* 95 L5 6 8N 80 6 E
Hikmak, Ras el, *Egypt* 106 A2 31 15N 27 51 E
Hiko, *U.S.A.* 160 H11 37 32N 115 14W
Hikone, *Japan* 73 B8 35 15N 136 10 E
Hikurangi, *Gisborne, N.Z.* 130 E5 37 55 S 178 4 E
Hikurangi, *Northland, N.Z.* 130 B3 35 36 S 174 17 E
Hiland Park, *U.S.A.* 152 E4 30 12N 85 33W
Hilawng, *Burma* 90 E4 21 23N 93 48 E
Hildburghausen, *Germany* 30 E6 50 25N 10 42 E
Hildesheim, *Germany* 30 C5 52 9N 9 56 E
Hilðarendi, *Iceland* 11 D7 63 44N 19 57W
Hill ➛, *Australia* 125 F2 30 23 S 115 3 E
Hill City, *Idaho, U.S.A.* 158 E6 43 18N 115 3W
Hill City, *Kans., U.S.A.* 154 F5 39 22N 99 51W
Hill City, *Minn., U.S.A.* 154 B8 46 59N 93 36W
Hill City, *S. Dak., U.S.A.* 154 D3 43 56N 103 35W
Hill Island L., *Canada* 143 A7 60 30N 109 50W
Hillaby, Mt., *Barbados* 165 g 13 12N 59 35W
Hillared, *Sweden* 17 G7 57 37N 13 10 E
Hillcrest, *Barbados* 165 g 13 13N 59 31W
Hillcrest Center, *U.S.A.* 161 K8 35 23N 118 57W
Hillegom, *Neths.* 24 B4 52 18N 4 35 E
Hillerød, *Denmark* 17 J6 55 56N 12 19 E
Hillerstorp, *Sweden* 17 G7 57 20N 13 52 E
Hilli, *Bangla.* 90 C2 25 17N 89 1 E
Hilliard, *U.S.A.* 152 E8 30 41N 81 55W
Hillsboro = Deerfield Beach, *U.S.A.* 153 J9 26 19N 80 6W
Hillsboro, *Ga., U.S.A.* 152 B6 33 11N 83 38W
Hillsboro, *Ill., U.S.A.* 156 E7 39 9N 89 29W
Hillsboro, *Kans., U.S.A.* 154 F6 38 21N 97 12W
Hillsboro, *Mo., U.S.A.* 156 F6 38 14N 90 34W
Hillsboro, *N. Dak., U.S.A.* 154 B6 47 26N 97 3W
Hillsboro, *Ohio, U.S.A.* 157 E13 39 12N 83 37W
Hillsboro, *Oreg., U.S.A.* 160 E4 45 31N 122 59W
Hillsboro, *Tex., U.S.A.* 155 J6 32 1N 97 8W
Hillsboro Canal, *U.S.A.* 153 J9 26 30N 80 15W
Hillsborough, *Grenada* 165 D7 12 28N 61 28W
Hillsborough, *U.S.A.* 151 C13 43 7N 71 54W
Hillsborough Channel, *Australia* 126 J7 20 56 S 149 15 E
Hillsborough Land = Belle Glade, *U.S.A.* 153 J9 26 41N 80 40W
Hillsdale, *Mich., U.S.A.* 157 C12 41 56N 84 38W
Hillsdale, *N.Y., U.S.A.* 151 D11 42 11N 73 30W
Hillsport, *Canada* 140 C2 49 27N 85 34W
Hillston, *Australia* 129 B6 33 30 S 145 31 E
Hilltonia, *U.S.A.* 152 C8 32 53N 81 40W
Hilo, *U.S.A.* 145 D6 19 44N 155 5W
Hilo B., *U.S.A.* 145 D6 19 45N 155 5W
Hilton, *U.S.A.* 150 C7 43 17N 77 48W
Hilton Head Island, *U.S.A.* 152 C9 32 13N 80 45W
Hilvan, *Turkey* 101 D8 37 34N 38 58 E
Hilversum, *Neths.* 24 B5 52 14N 5 10 E
Hilzingen, *Germany* 33 A7 47 46N 8 47 E
Himachal Pradesh □, *India* 92 D7 31 30N 77 0 E
Himalaya, *Asia* 93 E11 29 0N 84 0 E
Himamaylan, *Phil.* 81 F4 10 6N 122 52 E
Himarë, *Albania* 50 F3 40 8N 19 43 E
Hime-Jima, *Japan* 72 D3 33 43N 131 40 E
Himeji, *Japan* 72 C6 34 50N 134 40 E
Himi, *Japan* 73 A8 36 50N 136 55 E
Himmerland, *Denmark* 17 H3 56 45N 9 30 E
Ḥimş, *Syria* 103 A5 34 40N 36 45 E
Ḥimş □, *Syria* 103 A6 34 30N 37 0 E
Hinatuan, *Phil.* 81 G6 8 23N 126 20 E
Hinatuan Passage, *Phil.* 81 G5 9 45N 125 47 E
Hinche, *Haiti* 165 C5 19 9N 72 1W
Hinchinbrook I., *Australia* 126 B4 18 20 S 146 15 E
Hinchinbrook Island △, *Australia* 126 B4 18 14 S 146 6 E
Hinckley, *U.K.* 21 E6 52 33N 1 22W
Hinckley, *U.S.A.* 154 B8 46 1N 92 56W
Hindaun, *India* 92 F7 26 44N 77 5 E
Hindenburg = Zabrze, *Poland* 55 H5 50 18N 18 50 E
Hindmarsh, L., *Australia* 128 D4 36 5 S 141 55 E
Hindol, *India* 94 D7 20 40N 85 10 E
Hinds, *N.Z.* 131 D6 43 59 S 171 36 E
Hindsholm, *Denmark* 17 J4 55 30N 10 40 E
Hindu Bagh, *Pakistan* 91 C2 30 56N 67 50 E
Hindu Kush, *Asia* 65 E5 36 0N 71 0 E
Hindupur, *India* 95 H3 13 49N 77 32 E
Hines Creek, *Canada* 142 B5 56 20N 118 40W
Hinesville, *U.S.A.* 152 D8 31 51N 81 36W
Hinganghat, *India* 94 D4 20 30N 78 52 E
Hingham, *U.S.A.* 158 B8 48 33N 110 25W
Hinghwa = Xinghua, *China* 75 H10 32 58N 119 48 E
Hingir, *India* 93 J10 21 57N 83 41 E
Hingoli, *India* 94 E3 19 41N 77 15 E
Hinigaran, *Phil.* 81 F4 10 16N 122 50 E
Hinis, *Turkey* 101 C9 39 22N 41 43 E
Hinna = Imi, *Ethiopia* 107 F5 6 28N 42 10 E
Hinna, *Nigeria* 113 C7 10 25N 11 35 E
Hinnerup, *Denmark* 17 H4 56 16N 10 4 E
Hinnøya, *Norway* 14 B16 68 35N 15 50 E
Hino, *Japan* 73 C8 35 0N 136 15 E
Hinoba-an, *Phil.* 81 G4 9 35N 122 28 E
Hinojosa del Duque, *Spain* 43 G5 38 30N 5 9W
Hinokage, *Japan* 72 E3 32 39N 131 24 E
Hinsdale, *U.S.A.* 151 D12 42 47N 72 29W
Hinterrhein ➛, *Switz.* 33 C8 46 40N 9 25 E
Hinton, *Canada* 142 C5 53 26N 117 34W
Hinton, *U.S.A.* 148 G5 37 40N 80 54W
Hinuangan, *Phil.* 81 F5 10 25N 125 12 E
Hinubuan = Antipolo, *Phil.* 80 D3 14 35N 121 10 E
Hinwil, *Switz.* 33 B7 47 18N 8 51 E
Hınzır Burnu, *Turkey* 100 D6 36 19N 35 46 E
Hios = Khíos, *Greece* 49 C8 38 27N 26 9 E
Hirado, *Japan* 72 D1 33 22N 129 33 E
Hirado-Shima, *Japan* 72 D1 33 20N 129 30 E
Hirakata, *Japan* 73 C7 34 48N 135 40 E
Hirakud, *India* 94 D6 21 32N 83 51 E
Hirakud Dam, *India* 94 D6 21 32N 83 45 E
Hiran ➛, *India* 93 H8 23 6N 79 21 E
Hirapur, *India* 93 G8 24 22N 79 13 E
Hirata, *Japan* 72 B4 35 24N 132 49 E
Hiratsuka, *Japan* 73 B11 35 19N 139 21 E
Hirekerur, *India* 95 G2 14 28N 75 23 E
Hirfanlı Barajı, *Turkey* 100 C5 39 18N 33 31 E
Hirhafok, *Algeria* 111 D6 23 49N 5 45 E
Hiromi, *Japan* 72 D4 33 13N 132 36 E
Hiroo, *Japan* 70 C11 42 17N 143 19 E
Hirosaki, *Japan* 70 D10 40 34N 140 28 E
Hiroshima, *Japan* 72 C4 34 24N 132 30 E
Hiroshima □, *Japan* 72 C5 34 50N 133 0 E
Hiroshima-Wan, *Japan* 72 C4 34 5N 132 20 E
Hirschberg = Jelenia Góra, *Poland* 55 H2 50 50N 15 45 E
Hirson, *France* 27 C11 49 55N 4 4 E
Hirtshals, *Denmark* 17 G3 57 36N 9 57 E
Hisai, *Japan* 73 C8 34 40N 136 28 E
Hisar, *India* 92 E6 29 12N 75 45 E
Hisarcık, *Turkey* 49 B11 39 15N 29 14 E
Hisaria, *Bulgaria* 51 D8 42 30N 24 44 E
Hisb, Sha'ib = Ḥasb, W. ➛, *Iraq* 96 D5 31 45N 44 17 E
Ḥismá, *Si. Arabia* 96 D3 28 30N 36 0 E
Ḥişn al 'Abr, *Yemen* 98 C4 16 8N 47 14 E
Hisor, *Tajikistan* 65 D4 38 31N 68 33 E
Hispaniola, *W. Indies* 165 C5 19 0N 71 0W
Hīt, *Iraq* 101 F10 33 38N 42 49 E
Hita, *Japan* 72 D2 33 20N 130 58 E
Hitachi, *Japan* 73 A12 36 36N 140 39 E
Hitachi-Ōta, *Japan* 73 A12 36 30N 140 30 E
Hitchin, *U.K.* 21 F7 51 58N 0 16W
Hitoyoshi, *Japan* 72 E2 32 13N 130 45 E
Hitra, *Norway* 18 A5 63 30N 8 45 E
Hittisau, *Austria* 33 B9 47 28N 9 58 E
Hitzacker, *Germany* 30 B7 53 9N 11 2 E
Hiu, *Vanuatu* 133 C4 13 10 S 166 35 E
Hiuchi-Nada, *Japan* 72 C5 34 5N 133 20 E
Hiva-Oa, *French Polynesia* 135 H14 9 45 S 139 0W
Hixon, *Canada* 142 C4 53 25N 122 35W
Ḥiyyon, N. ➛, *Israel* 103 E4 30 25N 35 10 E
Hjalmar L., *Canada* 143 A7 61 33N 109 25W
Hjälmaren, *Sweden* 16 E9 59 18N 15 40 E
Hjältevad, *Sweden* 17 G9 57 38N 15 20 E
Hjartdal, *Norway* 18 E5 59 37N 8 41 E
Hjelmelandsvågen, *Norway* 18 E3 59 14N 6 10 E
Hjelset, *Norway* 18 B4 62 48N 7 30 E
Hjerkinn, *Norway* 18 B6 62 13N 9 33 E
Hjo, *Sweden* 17 F8 58 22N 14 17 E
Hjørring, *Denmark* 17 G3 57 29N 9 59 E
Hjortkvarn, *Sweden* 17 F9 58 54N 15 26 E
Hjukse, *Norway* 18 E6 59 31N 9 19 E
Hkakabo Razi, *Burma* 90 B6 28 17N 97 46 E
Hko-lam, *Burma* 90 E7 21 7N 98 5 E
Hko-ut, *Burma* 90 E7 20 58N 98 2 E
Hkyenhpa, *Burma* 90 B6 27 43N 97 25 E
Hlaingbwe, *Burma* 90 G6 17 8N 97 50 E
Hlinsko, *Czech Rep.* 34 B8 49 45N 15 54 E
Hlobane, *S. Africa* 117 D5 27 42 S 31 0 E
Hlohovec, *Slovak Rep.* 35 C10 48 26N 17 49 E
Hlučín, *Czech Rep.* 35 B11 49 54N 18 11 E
Hluhluwe, *S. Africa* 117 D5 28 1 S 32 15 E
Hluhluwe ⌓, *S. Africa* 117 C5 22 10 S 32 5 E
Hlukhiv, *Ukraine* 59 G7 51 40N 33 58 E
Hlwaze, *Burma* 90 F6 18 54N 96 37 E
Hlyboka, *Ukraine* 53 B10 48 5N 25 56 E
Hlybokaye, *Belarus* 58 E4 55 10N 27 45 E
Hnappadalssýsla □, *Iceland* 11 C4 64 50N 22 30W
Hnífsdalur, *Iceland* 11 A3 66 7N 23 8W
Hnúšt'a, *Slovak Rep.* 35 C12 48 35N 19 58 E
Ho, *Ghana* 113 D5 6 37N 0 27 E
Ho Chi Minh City = Thanh Pho Ho Chi Minh, *Vietnam* 87 G6 10 58N 106 40 E
Ho Thuong, *Vietnam* 86 C5 19 32N 105 48 E
Hoa Binh, *Vietnam* 76 G5 20 50N 105 20 E
Hoa Da, *Vietnam* 87 G7 11 16N 108 40 E
Hoa Hiep, *Vietnam* 87 G5 11 34N 105 51 E
Hoai Nhon, *Vietnam* 86 E7 14 28N 109 1 E
Hoang Lien Son, *Vietnam* 76 F4 22 0N 104 0 E
Hoanib ➛, *Namibia* 116 B2 19 27 S 12 46 E
Hoare B., *Canada* 139 B13 65 17N 62 30W
Hoarusib ➛, *Namibia* 116 B2 19 3 S 12 36 E
Hobart, *Australia* 127 G4 42 50 S 147 21 E
Hobart, *Ind., U.S.A.* 157 C9 41 32N 87 15W
Hobart, *Okla., U.S.A.* 155 H5 35 1N 99 6W
Hobbs, *U.S.A.* 155 J3 32 42N 103 8W
Hobbs Coast, *Antarctica* 7 D14 74 50 S 131 0W
Hobe Sound, *U.S.A.* 153 H9 27 4N 80 8W
Hobo, *Colombia* 168 C2 2 35N 75 30W
Hoboken, *Ga., U.S.A.* 152 D7 31 11N 82 8W
Hoboken, *N.J., U.S.A.* 151 F10 40 45N 74 4W
Hobro, *Denmark* 17 H3 56 39N 9 46 E
Hoburgen, *Sweden* 17 H12 56 55N 18 7 E
Hocalar, *Turkey* 49 C11 38 36N 30 0 E
Hochdorf, *Switz.* 33 B6 47 10N 8 17 E
Hochfeld, *Namibia* 116 C2 21 28 S 17 58 E
Hochharz △, *Germany* 30 D6 51 48N 10 38 E
Hochschwab, *Austria* 34 D8 47 35N 15 0 E
Höchstadt, *Germany* 31 F6 49 42N 10 47 E
Hochtaunus ⌓, *Germany* 31 E4 50 20N 8 30 E
Hoch'uan = Hechuan, *China* 76 B6 30 2N 106 12 E
Hochwan = Hechuan, *China* 76 B6 30 2N 106 12 E
Hockenheim, *Germany* 31 F4 49 19N 8 32 E
Hockley = Levelland, *U.S.A.* 155 J3 33 35N 102 23W
Hodaka-Dake, *Japan* 73 A9 36 17N 137 39 E
Hodeida = Al Ḥudaydah, *Yemen* 98 D3 14 50N 43 0 E
Hodgeville, *Canada* 143 C7 50 7N 106 58W
Hodgson, *Canada* 143 C9 51 13N 97 36W
Hódmezővásárhely, *Hungary* 52 D5 46 28N 20 22 E
Hodna, Chott el, *Algeria* 111 A6 35 26N 4 43 E
Hodonín, *Czech Rep.* 35 C10 48 50N 17 10 E
Hodzhambas, *Turkmenistan* 65 D2 38 7N 65 0 E
Hoeamdong, *N. Korea* 75 C16 42 30N 130 16 E
Hœdic, Î. de, *France* 26 E4 47 20N 2 53W
Hoek van Holland, *Neths.* 24 C4 52 0N 4 7 E
Hoengsŏng, *S. Korea* 75 F14 37 29N 127 59 E
Hoeryong, *N. Korea* 75 C15 42 30N 129 45 E
Hoeyang, *N. Korea* 75 E14 38 43N 127 36 E
Hof, *Germany* 31 E7 50 19N 11 55 E
Hof, *Norður-Múlasýsla, Iceland* 11 B11 65 39N 15 0W
Hof, *Suður-Múlasýsla, Iceland* 11 C12 64 33N 14 40W
Hof, *Norway* 18 E7 59 32N 10 5 E
Hofei = Hefei, *China* 77 B11 31 52N 117 18 E
Hoffell, *Iceland* 11 C11 64 23N 15 20W
Hofgeismar, *Germany* 30 D5 51 29N 9 23 E
Hofheim, *Germany* 31 E4 50 5N 8 26 E
Hofmeyr, *S. Africa* 116 E4 31 39 S 25 50 E
Höfn, *Iceland* 11 C11 64 15N 15 13W
Hofors, *Sweden* 16 D10 60 31N 16 15 E
Hofsjökull, *Iceland* 11 C8 64 49N 18 48W
Hofsós, *Iceland* 11 B7 65 53N 19 26W
Hōfu, *Japan* 72 C3 34 3N 131 34 E
Hog Harbour, *Vanuatu* 133 E5 15 8 S 167 6 E
Hog I. = Paradise I., *Bahamas* 9 b 25 6N 77 19W
Hogan Group, *Australia* 127 F4 39 13 S 147 1 E
Höganäs, *Sweden* 17 H6 56 12N 12 33 E
Hogansville, *U.S.A.* 152 B5 33 10N 84 55W
Hogarth, Mt., *Australia* 126 C2 21 48 S 136 58 E
Hogenakai Falls, *India* 95 H3 12 6N 77 50 E
Hoggar = Ahaggar, *Algeria* 111 D6 23 0N 6 30 E
Högsäter, *Sweden* 17 F6 58 38N 12 5 E
Högsby, *Sweden* 17 G10 57 10N 16 1 E
Högsjö, *Sweden* 16 E9 59 4N 15 44 E
Hogsty Reef, *Bahamas* 165 B5 21 41N 73 48W
Hoh ➛, *U.S.A.* 160 C2 47 45N 124 29W
Hohe Acht, *Germany* 31 E3 50 22N 7 0 E
Hohe Tauern, *Austria* 34 D5 47 11N 12 40 E
Hohe Tauern △, *Austria* 34 D5 47 5N 12 20 E
Hohe Venn, *Belgium* 24 D6 50 30N 6 5 E
Hohenau, *Austria* 35 C9 48 36N 16 55 E
Hohenelbe = Vrchlabí, *Czech Rep.* 34 A8 50 38N 15 37 E
Hohenems, *Austria* 34 D2 47 22N 9 42 E
Hohenloher Ebene, *Germany* 31 F5 49 14N 9 36 E
Hohenmauth = Vysoké Mýto, *Czech Rep.* 35 B9 49 58N 16 10 E
Hohensalza = Inowrocław, *Poland* 55 F5 52 50N 18 12 E
Hohensalzburg = Lunino, *Russia* 60 D7 53 38N 45 18 E
Hohenstadt = Zábřeh, *Czech Rep.* 35 B9 49 53N 16 52 E
Hohenstein = Olsztynek, *Poland* 54 E7 53 34N 20 19 E
Hohenwald, *U.S.A.* 149 H2 35 33N 87 33W
Hohenwestedt, *Germany* 30 A5 54 5N 9 40 E
Hoher Freschen, *Austria* 33 B9 47 18N 9 46 E
Hoher Rhön = Rhön, *Germany* 30 E5 50 24N 9 58 E
Hoher Vogelsberg ⌓, *Germany* 30 D5 51 45N 9 35 E
Hohes Venn-Eifel ⌓, *Europe* 30 E2 50 30N 6 10 E
Hohhot, *China* 74 D6 40 52N 111 40 E
Hóhlakas, *Greece* 38 F11 35 57N 27 53 E
Hohoe, *Ghana* 113 D5 7 8N 0 32 E
Hoi An, *Vietnam* 86 E7 15 30N 108 19 E
Hoi Xuan, *Vietnam* 76 G5 20 25N 105 9 E
Hoihow = Haikou, *China* 69 D6 20 1N 110 16 E
Hoisington, *U.S.A.* 154 F5 38 31N 98 47W
Hojai, *India* 90 B4 26 2N 92 54 E
Højer, *Denmark* 17 K2 54 58N 8 42 E
Hōjō, *Japan* 72 D4 33 58N 132 46 E
Hok, *Sweden* 17 G8 57 31N 14 16 E
Hokang = Hegang, *China* 69 B8 47 20N 130 19 E
Hökensås, *Sweden* 17 G8 58 0N 14 5 E
Hökerum, *Sweden* 17 G7 57 51N 13 16 E
Hokianga Harbour, *N.Z.* 130 B2 35 31 S 173 22 E
Hokitika, *N.Z.* 131 C5 42 42 S 171 0 E
Hokkaidō □, *Japan* 70 C11 43 30N 143 0 E
Hokksund, *Norway* 18 E6 59 48N 9 54 E
Hol-Hol, *Djibouti* 107 E5 11 20N 42 50 E
Hola Pristan, *Ukraine* 59 J7 46 29N 32 32 E
Holalkere, *India* 95 G3 14 2N 76 11 E
Hólar, *Iceland* 11 B7 65 44N 19 8W
Holbæk, *Denmark* 17 J5 55 43N 11 43 E
Holbrook, *Australia* 129 C7 35 42 S 147 18 E
Holbrook, *U.S.A.* 159 J8 34 54N 110 10W
Holden, *Mo., U.S.A.* 156 F3 38 43N 94 0W
Holden, *Utah, U.S.A.* 158 G7 39 6N 112 16W
Holdenville, *U.S.A.* 155 H6 35 5N 96 24W
Holdich, *Argentina* 176 C3 45 57 S 68 13W
Holdrege, *U.S.A.* 154 E5 40 26N 99 23W
Hole-Narsipur, *India* 95 H3 12 48N 76 16 E
Holešov, *Czech Rep.* 35 B10 49 20N 17 35 E
Holetown, *Barbados* 165 g 13 11N 59 38W
Holgate, *U.S.A.* 157 C12 41 15N 84 8W
Holguín, *Cuba* 164 B4 20 50N 76 20W
Holíč, *Slovak Rep.* 35 C10 48 49N 17 10 E
Holice, *Czech Rep.* 34 A8 50 5N 16 0 E
Holiday, *U.S.A.* 153 G7 28 13N 82 43W
Höljes, *Sweden* 16 D6 60 50N 12 35 E
Hollabrunn, *Austria* 34 C9 48 34N 16 5 E
Hollams Bird I., *Namibia* 116 C1 24 40 S 14 30 E
Holland, *Mich., U.S.A.* 157 B10 42 47N 86 7W
Holland, *N.Y., U.S.A.* 150 D6 42 38N 78 32W
Hollandale, *U.S.A.* 155 J9 33 10N 90 51W
Hollandia = Jayapura, *Indonesia* 83 B6 2 28 S 140 38 E
Holley, *U.S.A.* 150 C6 43 14N 78 2W
Hollfeld, *Germany* 31 F7 49 56N 11 18 E
Hollidaysburg, *U.S.A.* 150 F6 40 26N 78 24W
Hollis, *U.S.A.* 155 H5 34 41N 99 55W
Hollister, *Calif., U.S.A.* 160 J5 36 51N 121 24W
Hollister, *Idaho, U.S.A.* 158 E6 42 21N 114 35W
Höllviken = Höllviksnäs, *Sweden* 17 J6 55 26N 12 58 E
Höllviksnäs, *Sweden* 17 J6 55 26N 12 58 E
Holly, *U.S.A.* 157 B13 42 48N 83 38W
Holly Hill, *Fla., U.S.A.* 153 F8 29 16N 81 3W
Holly Hill, *S.C., U.S.A.* 152 B9 33 19N 80 25W
Holly Springs, *Ga., U.S.A.* 152 A5 34 10N 84 30W
Holly Springs, *Miss., U.S.A.* 155 H10 34 46N 89 27W
Hollywood, *U.S.A.* 153 J9 26 1N 80 9W
Holman, *Canada* 138 A8 70 44N 117 44W
Hólmavík, *Iceland* 11 B5 65 42N 21 40W
Holmen, *Norway* 18 D7 60 40N 10 22 E
Holmen, *U.S.A.* 154 D9 43 58N 91 15W
Holmes ➛, *U.S.A.* 152 E4 30 30N 85 50W
Holmes Beach, *U.S.A.* 153 H7 27 31N 82 43W
Holmes Reefs, *Australia* 126 B4 16 27 S 148 0 E
Holmestrand, *Norway* 18 E7 59 31N 10 14 E
Holmsjö, *Sweden* 17 H9 56 25N 15 32 E
Holmsjön, *Västernorrland, Sweden* 16 B10 62 41N 16 33 E
Holmsjön, *Västernorrland, Sweden* 16 B9 62 26N 15 20 E
Holmsland Klit, *Denmark* 17 J2 56 0N 8 5 E
Holmsund, *Sweden* 14 E19 63 41N 20 20 E
Holod, *Romania* 52 D7 46 49N 22 8 E
Holopaw, *U.S.A.* 153 G8 28 8N 81 5W
Holovne, *Ukraine* 55 G11 51 20N 24 5 E
Holøydal, *Norway* 18 B8 62 12N 11 27 E
Holozubyntsi, *Ukraine* 53 B11 48 50N 26 55 E
Holroyd ➛, *Australia* 126 A3 14 10 S 141 36 E
Holstebro, *Denmark* 17 H2 56 22N 8 37 E
Holsteinische Schweiz ⌓, *Germany* 30 A6 54 8N 10 30 E
Holsteinsborg = Sisimiut, *Greenland* 10 D5 66 40N 53 30W
Holsworthy, *U.K.* 21 G3 50 48N 4 22W
Holt, *Iceland* 11 D7 63 33N 19 48W
Holt, *Fla., U.S.A.* 153 E3 30 43N 86 45W
Holt, *Mich., U.S.A.* 157 B12 42 39N 84 31W
Holton, *Canada* 141 B8 54 31N 57 12W
Holton, *U.S.A.* 154 F7 39 28N 95 44W
Holts Summit, *U.S.A.* 156 F4 38 38N 92 7W
Holtville, *U.S.A.* 161 N11 32 49N 115 23W
Holualoa, *U.S.A.* 145 D6 19 37N 155 57W
Holum, *Norway* 18 F4 58 6N 7 32 E
Holwerd, *Neths.* 24 A5 53 22N 5 54 E
Holy Cross, *U.S.A.* 144 E8 62 12N 159 46W
Holy I., *Angl., U.K.* 20 D3 53 17N 4 37W
Holy I., *Northumberland, U.K.* 20 B6 55 40N 1 47W
Holyhead, *U.K.* 20 D3 53 18N 4 38W
Holyoke, *Colo., U.S.A.* 154 E3 40 35N 102 18W
Holyoke, *Mass., U.S.A.* 151 D12 42 12N 72 37W
Holyrood, *Canada* 141 C9 47 27N 53 8W
Holzkirchen, *Germany* 31 H7 47 52N 11 42 E
Holzminden, *Germany* 30 D5 51 50N 9 28 E
Homa Bay, *Kenya* 118 C3 0 36 S 34 30 E
Homalin, *Burma* 90 C5 24 55N 95 0 E
Homand, *Iran* 97 C8 32 28N 59 37 E
Homathko ➛, *Canada* 142 C4 51 0N 124 56W
Homberg, *Germany* 30 D5 51 2N 9 25 E
Hombori, *Mali* 113 B4 15 20N 1 38W
Homburg, *Germany* 31 F3 49 28N 7 18 E
Home B., *Canada* 139 B13 68 40N 67 10W
Home Hill, *Australia* 126 B4 19 43 S 147 25 E
Home Reef, *Tonga* 133 P13 18 59 S 174 47W
Homedale, *U.S.A.* 158 E5 43 37N 116 56W
Homeland, *U.S.A.* 152 E7 30 51N 82 1W
Homer, *Alaska, U.S.A.* 144 G10 59 39N 151 33W
Homer, *Ill., U.S.A.* 157 D9 40 4N 87 57W
Homer, *La., U.S.A.* 155 J8 32 48N 93 4W
Homer, *Mich., U.S.A.* 157 B12 42 9N 84 49W
Homer City, *U.S.A.* 150 F5 40 32N 79 10W
Homert ⌓, *Germany* 30 D4 51 15N 8 0 E
Homerville, *U.S.A.* 152 D7 31 2N 82 45W
Homestead, *Australia* 126 C4 20 20 S 145 40 E
Homestead, *U.S.A.* 153 K9 25 28N 80 29W
Homestead ⌓, *U.S.A.* 154 E6 40 17N 96 50W
Homewood, *Calif., U.S.A.* 160 F6 39 4N 120 8W
Homewood, *Ill., U.S.A.* 157 C9 41 34N 87 40W
Hommelvik, *Norway* 18 A7 63 25N 10 48 E
Hommersåk, *Norway* 18 F2 58 56N 5 50 E
Homnabad, *India* 94 F3 17 45N 77 11 E
Homoine, *Mozam.* 117 C6 23 55 S 35 8 E
Homoljske Planina, *Serbia & M.* 50 B5 44 10N 21 45 E
Homonhon I., *Phil.* 81 F5 10 44N 125 43 E
Homorod, *Romania* 53 D10 46 5N 25 15 E
Homosassa Springs, *U.S.A.* 153 G7 28 48N 82 35W
Homs = Al Khums, *Libya* 108 B2 32 40N 14 17 E

Homs = Ḥimş, Syria 103 A5 34 40N 36 45 E
Homyel, Belarus 59 F6 52 28N 31 0 E
Hon Chong, Vietnam 87 G5 10 25N 104 30 E
Hon Me, Vietnam 86 C5 19 23N 105 56 E
Honan = Henan □, China 74 H8 34 0N 114 0 E
Honaunau, U.S.A. 145 D6 19 26N 155 55W
Honavar, India 95 G2 14 17N 74 27 E
Honaz, Turkey 49 D11 37 46N 29 18 E
Honbetsu, Japan 70 C11 43 7N 143 37 E
Honcut, U.S.A. 160 F5 39 20N 121 32W
Honda, Colombia 168 B3 5 12N 74 45W
Honda Bay, Phil. 81 G2 9 53N 118 49 E
Hondarribia, Spain 40 B3 43 22N 1 47W
Hondeklipbaai, S. Africa 116 E2 30 19 S 17 17 E
Hondo, Japan 72 E2 32 27N 130 12 E
Hondo, U.S.A. 155 L5 29 21N 99 9W
Hondo, Rio →, Belize 163 D7 18 25N 88 21W
Honduras ■, Cent. Amer. 164 D2 14 40N 86 30W
Honduras, G. de, Caribbean 164 C2 16 50N 87 0W
Hønefoss, Norway 18 D7 60 10N 10 18 E
Honesdale, U.S.A. 151 E9 41 34N 75 16W
Honey L., U.S.A. 160 E6 40 15N 120 19W
Honfleur, France 26 C7 49 25N 0 13 E
Høng, Denmark 17 J5 55 31N 11 18 E
Hong →, Vietnam 76 F5 22 0N 104 0 E
Hong Gai, Vietnam 76 G6 20 57N 107 5 E
Hong He →, China 74 H8 32 25N 115 35 E
Hong Hu, China 77 C9 29 54N 113 24 E
Hong Kong □, China 77 F10 22 11N 114 14 E
Hong Kong I., China 69 G11 22 16N 114 12 E
Hong Kong International ✈ (HKG), China 69 G10 22 19N 113 57 E
Honga, Angola 115 F3 15 9 S 15 12 E
Hong'an, China 77 B10 31 20N 114 40 E
Hongch'ŏn, S. Korea 75 F14 37 44N 127 53 E
Honghai Wan, China 77 F10 22 40N 115 0 E
Honghe, China 76 F4 23 25N 102 25 E
Honghu, China 77 C9 29 50N 113 30 E
Hongjiang, China 76 D7 27 7N 109 59 E
Hongliu He →, China 74 F5 38 0N 109 50 E
Hongor, Mongolia 74 B7 45 45N 112 50 E
Hongsa, Laos 86 C3 19 43N 101 20 E
Hongshui He →, China 76 F7 23 48N 109 30 E
Hongsŏng, S. Korea 75 F14 36 37N 126 38 E
Hongtong, China 74 F6 36 16N 111 40 E
Honguedo, Détroit d', Canada 141 C7 49 15N 64 0W
Hongwon, N. Korea 75 E14 40 0N 127 56 E
Hongya, China 76 C4 29 57N 103 22 E
Hongyuan, China 76 A4 32 51N 102 40 E
Hongze Hu, China 75 H10 33 15N 118 35 E
Honiara, Solomon Is. 133 M10 9 27 S 159 57 E
Honiton, U.K. 21 G4 50 47N 3 11W
Honjō, Akita, Japan 70 E10 39 23N 140 3 E
Honjō, Gumma, Japan 73 A11 36 14N 139 11 E
Honkawane, Japan 73 B10 35 5N 138 5 E
Honkoräb, Ras, Egypt 106 C4 24 35N 35 10 E
Honnali, India 95 G2 14 15N 75 40 E
Honningsvåg, Norway 14 A21 70 59N 25 59 E
Hönö, Sweden 17 G5 57 41N 11 39 E
Honokaa, U.S.A. 145 C6 20 5N 155 28W
Honokahua, U.S.A. 145 C5 21 0N 156 40W
Honolulu, U.S.A. 145 K14 21 19N 157 52W
Honolulu International ✈ (HNL), U.S.A. 145 B4 21 19N 157 55W
Honomu, U.S.A. 145 D6 19 52N 155 7W
Honouliuli, U.S.A. 145 K13 21 22N 158 2W
Honshū, Japan 73 A8 36 0N 138 0 E
Hontoria del Pinar, Spain 40 D1 41 50N 3 10W
Honuapo B., U.S.A. 145 D6 19 5N 155 33W
Hood, I. = Española, I., Ecuador 172 a 1 23 S 89 39W
Hood, Mt., U.S.A. 158 D3 45 23N 121 42W
Hood, Pt., Australia 125 F2 34 23 S 119 34 E
Hood Pt., Papua N. G. 132 F4 10 4 S 147 45 E
Hood River, U.S.A. 158 D3 45 43N 121 31W
Hoodsport, U.S.A. 160 C3 47 24N 123 9W
Hooge, Germany 30 A4 54 34N 8 33 E
Hoogeveen, Neths. 24 B6 52 44N 6 28 E
Hoogezand-Sappemeer, Neths. 24 A6 53 9N 6 45 E
Hooghly = Hugli →, India 93 J13 21 56N 88 4 E
Hooghly-Chinsura = Chunchura, India 93 H13 22 53N 88 27 E
Hook Hd., Ireland 23 D5 52 7N 6 56W
Hook I., Australia 126 J6 20 4 S 149 0 E
Hook of Holland = Hoek van Holland, Neths. 24 C4 52 0N 4 7 E
Hooker, U.S.A. 155 G4 36 52N 101 13W
Hooker Creek, Australia 124 C5 18 23 S 130 38 E
Hoolehua, U.S.A. 145 B4 21 10N 157 5W
Hoonah, U.S.A. 142 B1 58 7N 135 27W
Hooper Bay, U.S.A. 144 F6 61 32N 166 6W
Hoopeston, U.S.A. 157 D9 40 28N 87 40W
Hoopstad, S. Africa 116 D4 27 50 S 25 55 E
Höör, Sweden 17 J7 55 56N 13 33 E
Hoorn, Neths. 24 B5 52 38N 5 4 E
Hoover, U.S.A. 149 J2 33 20N 86 11W
Hoover Dam, U.S.A. 161 K12 36 1N 114 44W
Hooversville, U.S.A. 150 F6 40 9N 78 55W
Hop Bottom, U.S.A. 151 E9 41 42N 75 46W
Hopa, Turkey 101 B9 41 28N 41 30 E
Hope, Canada 142 D4 49 25N 121 25W
Hope, Ariz., U.S.A. 161 M13 33 43N 113 42W
Hope, Ark., U.S.A. 155 J8 33 40N 93 36W
Hope, Ind., U.S.A. 157 E11 39 18N 85 46W
Hope, L., S. Austral., Australia 127 D2 28 24 S 139 18 E
Hope, L., W. Austral., Australia 125 F3 32 35 S 120 15 E
Hope, Pt., Alaska, U.S.A. 144 B6 68 21N 166 47W
Hope, Pt., Alaska, U.S.A. 6 C17 68 20N 166 50W
Hope I., Canada 150 B4 44 55N 80 11W
Hope Town, Bahamas 164 A4 26 35N 76 57W
Hopedale, Canada 141 A7 55 28N 60 13W
Hopedale, U.S.A. 151 D13 42 8N 71 33W
Hopefield, S. Africa 116 E2 33 3 S 18 22 E
Hopei = Hebei □, China 74 E9 39 0N 116 0 E
Hopelchén, Mexico 163 D7 19 46N 89 50W
Hopetoun, Vic., Australia 128 C5 35 42 S 142 22 E
Hopetoun, W. Austral., Australia 125 F3 33 57 S 120 7 E
Hopetown, S. Africa 116 D3 29 34 S 24 3 E
Hopevale, Australia 126 B4 15 16 S 145 20 E
Hopewell, U.S.A. 148 G7 37 18N 77 17W
Hopfgarten, Austria 34 D5 47 27N 12 10 E
Hopin, Burma 90 C6 24 58N 96 30 E
Hopkins, U.S.A. 156 D2 40 33N 94 49W
Hopkins, L., Australia 124 D4 24 15 S 128 35 E
Hopkinsville, U.S.A. 149 G2 36 52N 87 29W
Hopland, U.S.A. 160 G3 38 58N 123 7W
Hopong, Burma 90 E6 20 47N 97 11 E
Hopwood's Ferry = Echuca, Australia 129 D6 36 10 S 144 45 E
Hoque, Angola 115 E2 14 40 S 13 55 E
Hoquiam, U.S.A. 160 D3 46 59N 123 53W
Hora Hoverla, Ukraine 53 B9 48 7N 24 41 E
Hora Sfakion = Khóra Sfakíon, Greece 39 E5 35 15N 24 9 E
Hōrai, Japan 73 C9 34 58N 137 32 E
Horana, Sri Lanka 95 L5 6 43N 80 4 E
Horasan, Turkey 101 B10 40 3N 42 11 E
Horažďovice, Czech Rep. 34 B6 49 19N 13 42 E
Horb, Germany 31 G4 48 26N 8 47 E
Hörby, Sweden 17 J7 55 51N 13 40 E
Horcajo de Santiago, Spain 40 F1 39 50N 3 1W
Hordabø, Norway 18 D1 60 42N 4 54 E
Hordaland □, Norway 18 D3 60 25N 6 15 E
Horden Hills, Australia 124 D5 20 15 S 130 0 E
Hordio, Somali Rep. 120 B4 10 33N 51 6 E
Horezu, Romania 53 E8 45 6N 24 0 E
Horgen, Switz. 33 B7 47 15N 8 35 E
Horgoš, Serbia & M. 52 D4 46 10N 20 0 E
Hořice, Czech Rep. 34 A8 50 21N 15 39 E
Horinchove, Ukraine 53 B8 48 16N 23 26 E
Horinger, China 74 D6 40 28N 111 48 E
Horki, Belarus 58 E6 54 17N 30 59 E
Horlick Mts., Antarctica 7 E15 84 0 S 102 0W
Horlivka, Ukraine 59 H10 48 19N 38 5 E
Hormak, Iran 97 D9 29 58N 60 51 E
Hormoz, Iran 97 E7 27 35N 55 0 E
Hormoz, Jaz.-ye, Iran 97 E8 27 8N 56 28 E
Hormozgān □, Iran 97 E8 27 30N 56 0 E
Hormuz, Kūh-e, Iran 97 E7 27 27N 55 10 E
Hormuz, Str. of, The Gulf 97 E8 26 30N 56 30 E
Horn, Austria 34 C8 48 39N 15 40 E
Horn, Iceland 12 C2 66 28N 22 28W
Horn, Sweden 17 G9 57 54N 15 51 E
Horn →, Canada 142 A5 61 30N 118 1W
Horn, Cape = Hornos, C. de, Chile 176 E3 55 50 S 67 30W
Horn, Is., Wall. & F. Is. 123 C15 14 16 S 178 6W
Horn Head, Ireland 23 A3 55 14N 8 0W
Horn I., Australia 126 A3 10 37 S 142 17 E
Horn Plateau, Canada 142 A5 62 15N 119 15W
Hornachuelos, Spain 43 H5 37 50N 5 14W
Hornavan, Sweden 14 C17 66 15N 17 30 E
Hornbeck, U.S.A. 155 K8 31 20N 93 24W
Hornbjarg, Iceland 11 A4 66 28N 22 25W
Hornbrook, U.S.A. 158 F2 41 55N 122 33W
Hornburg, Germany 30 C6 52 2N 10 37 E
Hornby, N.Z. 131 D7 43 33 S 172 33 E
Horncastle, U.K. 20 D7 53 13N 0 7W
Horndal, Sweden 16 D10 60 18N 16 23 E
Hornell, U.S.A. 150 D7 42 20N 77 40W
Hornell L., Canada 142 A5 62 20N 119 25W
Hornepayne, Canada 140 C3 49 14N 84 48W
Horní Planá, Czech Rep. 34 C7 48 46N 14 2 E
Hornindal, Norway 18 C3 61 58N 6 30 E
Hornings Mills, Canada 150 B4 44 9N 80 12W
Hornitos, U.S.A. 160 H6 37 30N 120 14W
Hornopirén △, Chile 176 B2 41 58 S 72 17W
Hornos, C. de, Chile 176 E3 55 50 S 67 30W
Hornos Is., Papua N. G. 132 B4 2 12 S 147 45 E
Hornoy-le-Bourg, France 27 C8 49 50N 1 54 E
Hornsby, Australia 129 B9 33 42 S 151 2 E
Hornsea, U.K. 20 D7 53 55N 0 11W
Hornsjø, Norway 18 C7 61 19N 10 38 E
Hornslandet, Sweden 16 C11 61 35N 17 37 E
Hörnum, Germany 30 A4 54 45N 8 17 E
Horobetsu = Noboribetsu, Japan 70 C10 42 24N 141 6 E
Horodenka, Ukraine 53 B10 48 41N 25 29 E
Horodnya, Ukraine 59 G6 51 55N 31 33 E
Horodok, Khmelnytskyy, Ukraine 59 H4 49 10N 26 34 E
Horodok, Lviv, Ukraine 59 H2 49 46N 23 32 E
Horodyshche, Ukraine 59 H6 49 17N 31 27 E
Horokhiv, Ukraine 59 G3 50 30N 24 45 E
Horovice, Czech Rep. 34 B6 49 48N 13 53 E
Horqin Youyi Qianqi, China 75 A12 46 5N 122 3 E
Horqueta, Paraguay 174 A4 23 15 S 56 55W
Horred, Sweden 17 G6 57 22N 12 28 E
Horse Cr. →, U.S.A. 154 E3 41 57N 105 10W
Horse I., Canada 143 C9 53 20N 99 6W
Horse Is., Canada 141 B8 50 15N 55 50W
Horsefly L., Canada 142 C4 52 25N 121 0W
Horseheads, U.S.A. 150 D8 42 10N 76 49W
Horsens, Denmark 17 J3 55 52N 9 51 E
Horseshoe Bend ⌂, U.S.A. 152 C4 32 59N 85 44W
Horsham, Australia 128 D5 36 44 S 142 13 E
Horsham, U.K. 21 F7 51 4N 0 20W
Horšovský Týn, Czech Rep. 34 B5 49 31N 12 58 E
Horta, Azores 9 d1 38 32N 28 38W
Horten, Norway 18 E7 59 25N 10 32 E
Hortense, U.S.A. 152 B8 31 20N 81 57W
Horti, India 94 F2 17 7N 75 47 E
Hortobágy →, Hungary 52 C6 47 30N 21 6 E
Hortobágyi △, Hungary 52 C6 47 36N 21 10 E
Horton, Kans., U.S.A. 154 F7 39 40N 95 32W
Horton, Mo., U.S.A. 156 G2 37 58N 94 22W
Horton →, Canada 138 B7 69 56N 126 52W
Horw, Switz. 33 B6 47 1N 8 19 E
Horwood L., Canada 140 C3 48 5N 82 20W
Hosaina, Ethiopia 107 F4 7 30N 37 47 E
Hosdurga, India 95 H3 13 49N 76 17 E
Hosenofu, Libya 108 D4 23 41N 21 4 E
Ḥoseynābād, Khuzestān, Iran 97 C6 32 45N 48 20 E
Ḥoseynābād, Kordestān, Iran 101 E12 35 33N 47 8 E
Hosford, U.S.A. 152 E5 30 23N 84 48W
Hoshangabad, India 92 H7 22 45N 77 45 E
Hoshiarpur, India 92 D6 31 30N 75 58 E
Hoskins, Papua N. G. 132 C6 5 29 S 150 27 E
Hoskote, India 95 H3 13 4N 77 48 E
Hospental, Switz. 33 C7 46 37N 8 34 E
Hospet, India 95 G3 15 15N 76 20 E
Hoste, I., Chile 176 E3 55 0 S 69 0W
Hostens, France 28 D3 44 30N 0 40W
Hosur, India 95 H3 12 43N 77 49 E
Hot, Thailand 86 C2 18 8N 98 29 E
Hot Creek Range, U.S.A. 158 G6 38 40N 116 20W
Hot Springs = Truth or Consequences, U.S.A. 159 K10 33 8N 107 15W
Hot Springs, Ark., U.S.A. 155 H8 34 31N 93 3W
Hot Springs, S. Dak., U.S.A. 154 D3 43 26N 103 29W
Hot Springs △, U.S.A. 155 H8 34 32N 93 4W
Hotagen, Sweden 14 E16 63 59N 14 12 E
Hotan, China 68 C2 37 25N 79 55 E
Hotazel, S. Africa 116 D3 27 17 S 22 58 E
Hotchkiss, U.S.A. 159 G10 38 48N 107 43W
Hotham, C., Australia 124 B5 12 2 S 131 18 E
Hoti, Indonesia 83 B4 3 0 S 130 22 E
Hoting, Sweden 14 D17 64 8N 16 15 E
Hotolisht, Albania 50 E4 41 10N 20 25 E
Hotte, Massif de la, Haiti 165 C5 18 30N 73 45W
Hottentotsbaai, Namibia 116 D1 26 8 S 14 59 E
Hou Hai, China 69 F10 22 32N 113 56 E
Houailou, N. Cal. 133 U19 21 17 S 165 38 E
Houat, Î. de, France 26 E4 47 24N 2 58W
Houdan, France 27 D8 48 48N 1 35 E
Houei Sai, Laos 76 G3 20 18N 100 26 E
Houeillès, France 28 D4 44 12N 0 2 E
Houffalize, Belgium 24 D5 50 8N 5 48 E
Houghton, Mich., U.S.A. 154 B10 47 7N 88 34W
Houghton, N.Y., U.S.A. 150 D6 42 25N 78 10W
Houghton L., U.S.A. 148 C3 44 21N 84 44W
Houghton-le-Spring, U.K. 20 C6 54 51N 1 28W
Houhora Heads, N.Z. 130 A2 34 49 S 173 9 E
Houlton, U.S.A. 149 B12 46 8N 67 51W
Houma, U.S.A. 155 L9 29 36N 90 43W
Houmt Souk = Djerba, Tunisia 108 B2 33 52N 10 51 E
Houndé, Burkina Faso 112 C4 11 34N 3 31W
Hourtin, France 28 C2 45 11N 1 4W
Hourtin-Carcans, Étang d', France 28 C2 45 10N 1 6W
Housatonic →, U.S.A. 151 E11 41 10N 73 7W
Houston, Canada 142 C3 54 25N 126 39W
Houston, Fla., U.S.A. 152 E7 30 15N 82 54W
Houston, Mo., U.S.A. 155 G9 37 22N 91 58W
Houston, Tex., U.S.A. 155 L7 29 46N 95 22W
Hout →, S. Africa 117 C4 23 4 S 29 36 E
Houtkraal, S. Africa 116 E3 30 23 S 24 5 E
Houtman Abrolhos, Australia 125 E1 28 43 S 113 48 E
Hov, Norway 18 D7 60 42N 10 20 E
Hovd, Mongolia 68 B4 48 2N 91 37 E
Hovda, Norway 18 D6 60 53N 9 11 E
Hovden, Aust-Agder, Norway 18 E4 59 33N 7 22 E
Hovden, Sogn og Fjordane, Norway 18 C1 61 41N 4 52 E
Hove, U.K. 21 G7 50 50N 0 10W
Hovenweep ⌂, U.S.A. 159 H9 37 20N 109 0W
Hovet, Norway 18 D5 60 38N 8 8 E
Hoveyzeh, Iran 97 D6 31 27N 48 4 E
Hovgaard Ø, Greenland 10 B9 79 55N 18 50W
Hovin, Norway 18 E6 59 51N 9 0 E
Hovmantorp, Sweden 17 H9 56 47N 15 7 E
Hövsgöl, Mongolia 74 C5 43 37N 109 39 E
Hövsgöl Nuur, Mongolia 68 A5 51 0N 100 30 E
Hovsta, Sweden 16 E9 59 22N 15 15 E
Howakil, Eritrea 107 D5 15 10N 40 16 E
Howar, Wadi →, Sudan 107 D2 17 30N 27 8 E
Howard, Australia 127 D5 25 16 S 152 32 E
Howard, Pa., U.S.A. 150 F7 41 1N 77 40W
Howard, S. Dak., U.S.A. 154 C6 44 1N 97 32W
Howe, U.S.A. 158 E7 43 48N 113 0W
Howe, C., Australia 129 D9 37 30 S 150 0 E
Howe I., Canada 151 B8 44 16N 76 17W
Howell, U.S.A. 157 B13 42 36N 83 56W
Howick, Canada 151 A11 45 11N 73 51W
Howick, N.Z. 130 C3 36 54 S 174 56 E
Howick, S. Africa 117 D5 29 28 S 30 14 E
Howick Group, Australia 126 A4 14 20 S 145 30 E
Howitt, L., Australia 127 D2 27 40 S 138 40 E
Howland I., Pac. Oc. 134 G10 0 48N 176 38W
Howlong, Australia 129 C7 35 59 S 146 38 E
Howrah = Haora, India 93 H13 22 37N 88 20 E
Howth Hd., Ireland 23 C5 53 22N 6 3W
Höxter, Germany 30 D5 51 46N 9 22 E
Hoy, U.K. 22 C5 58 50N 3 15W
Hoya, Germany 30 C5 52 49N 9 8 E
Høyanger, Norway 18 C3 61 13N 6 4 E
Hoyerswerda, Germany 30 D10 51 26N 14 14 E
Hoylake, U.K. 20 D4 53 24N 3 10W
Hōyo-Kaikyō, Japan 72 D3 33 20N 131 58 E
Hoyos, Spain 42 E4 40 9N 6 45W
Hpa-an = Pa-an, Burma 90 G6 16 51N 97 40 E
Hpawlum, Burma 90 B7 27 12N 98 12 E
Hpettintha, Burma 90 C5 24 14N 95 23 E
Hpizow, Burma 90 B7 26 57N 98 24 E
Hpunan Pass, India 90 A6 28 9N 97 20 E
Hradec Králové, Czech Rep. 34 A8 50 15N 15 50 E
Hrádek, Czech Rep. 35 C9 48 46N 16 16 E
Hrafnseyri, Iceland 11 B3 65 46N 23 28W
Hranice, Czech Rep. 35 B10 49 34N 17 45 E
Hrazdan, Armenia 61 K7 40 30N 44 46 E
Hrebenka, Ukraine 59 G7 50 9N 32 22 E
Hrifunes, Iceland 11 D8 63 38N 18 30W
Hrísey, Iceland 11 B8 66 0N 18 23W
Hrodna, Belarus 54 E10 53 42N 23 52 E
Hrodzyanka, Belarus 58 F5 53 31N 28 42 E
Hron →, Slovak Rep. 35 D11 47 49N 18 45 E
Hrubieszów, Poland 55 H10 50 49N 23 51 E
Hrubý Jeseník, Czech Rep. 35 A10 50 5N 17 10 E
Hrvatska = Croatia ■, Europe 45 C13 45 20N 16 0 E
Hrymayliv, Ukraine 59 H4 49 20N 26 5 E
Hrynyava, Ukraine 53 C9 47 59N 24 53 E
Hsa-paw, Burma 90 F6 19 1N 97 30 E
Hsenwi, Burma 90 D6 23 22N 97 55 E
Hsi-hkip, Burma 90 E6 20 25N 96 42 E
Hsiamen = Xiamen, China 77 E12 24 25N 118 4 E
Hsian = Xi'an, China 74 G5 34 15N 109 0 E
Hsinchu, Taiwan 77 E13 24 48N 120 58 E
Hsinhailien = Lianyungang, China 75 G10 34 40N 119 11 E
Hsinking = Changchun, China 75 C13 43 57N 125 17 E
Hsinying, Taiwan 77 F13 23 18N 120 19 E
Hsipaw, Burma 90 D6 22 37N 97 18 E
Hsopket, Burma 76 F2 23 11N 98 26 E
Hsüchou = Xuzhou, China 75 G9 34 18N 117 10 E
Htawgaw, Burma 90 C7 25 57N 98 23 E
Hu Xian, China 74 G5 34 8N 108 42 E
Hua Hin, Thailand 86 F2 12 34N 99 58 E
Hua Xian, Henan, China 74 G8 35 30N 114 30 E
Hua Xian, Shaanxi, China 74 G5 34 30N 109 48 E
Hua'an, China 77 E11 25 1N 117 32 E
Huab →, Namibia 116 B2 20 52 S 13 25 E
Huacaya, Bolivia 173 E5 20 45 S 63 43W
Huachacalla, Bolivia 172 D4 18 45 S 68 17W
Huacheng, China 77 E10 24 4N 115 37 E
Huachinera, Mexico 162 A3 30 9N 108 55W
Huacho, Peru 172 C2 11 10 S 77 35W
Huachón, Peru 172 C2 10 35 S 76 0W
Huade, China 74 D7 41 55N 113 59 E
Huadian, China 75 C14 43 0N 126 40 E
Huadu, China 77 F9 23 22N 113 12 E
Huahiné, I., French Polynesia 135 J12 16 46 S 150 58W
Huai Had △, Thailand 86 D5 16 52N 104 17 E
Huai He →, China 77 A12 33 0N 118 30 E
Huai Nam Dang △, Thailand 86 C2 19 30N 98 30 E
Huai Yot, Thailand 87 J2 7 45N 99 37 E
Huai'an, Hebei, China 74 D8 40 30N 114 20 E
Huai'an, Jiangsu, China 75 H10 33 30N 119 10 E
Huaibei, China 74 G9 34 0N 116 48 E
Huaibin, China 77 A10 32 32N 115 27 E
Huaicho = Puerto Acosta, Bolivia 172 D4 15 32 S 69 15W
Huaide = Gongzhuling, China 75 C13 43 30N 124 40 E
Huaidezhen, China 75 C13 43 48N 124 50 E
Huaihua, China 76 D7 27 32N 109 57 E
Huaiji, China 77 F9 23 55N 112 12 E
Huainan, China 77 A11 32 38N 116 58 E
Huaining, China 77 B11 30 24N 116 40 E
Huairen, China 74 E7 39 48N 113 20 E
Huairou, China 74 D9 40 20N 116 35 E
Huaiyang, China 74 H8 33 40N 114 52 E
Huaiyin, China 75 H10 33 30N 119 2 E
Huaiyuan, Anhui, China 75 H9 32 55N 117 10 E
Huaiyuan, Guangxi Zhuangzu, China 76 E7 24 31N 108 22 E
Huajianzi, China 75 D13 41 23N 125 20 E
Huajuapan de Leon, Mexico 163 D5 17 50N 97 48W
Hualalai, U.S.A. 145 D6 19 42N 155 52W
Hualapai Peak, U.S.A. 159 J7 35 5N 113 54W
Hualien, Taiwan 77 E13 24 0N 121 30 E
Huallaga →, Peru 172 B2 5 15 S 75 30W
Huallanca, Peru 172 B2 8 50 S 77 56W
Huamachuco, Peru 172 B2 7 50 S 78 5W
Huambo, Angola 115 E3 12 42 S 15 54 E
Huambo □, Angola 115 E3 13 0 S 16 0 E
Huan Jiang →, China 74 G5 34 28N 109 0 E
Huan Xian, China 74 F4 36 33N 107 7 E
Huancabamba, Peru 172 B2 5 10 S 79 15W
Huancane, Peru 172 D4 15 10 S 69 44W
Huancapi, Peru 172 C3 13 40 S 74 0W
Huancavelica, Peru 172 C2 12 50 S 75 5W
Huancavelica □, Peru 172 C3 13 0 S 75 0W
Huancayo, Peru 172 C2 12 5 S 75 12W
Huanchaca, Bolivia 172 E4 20 15 S 66 40W
Huanchaca, Serranía de, Bolivia 173 C5 14 30 S 60 39W
Huang Hai = Yellow Sea, China 75 G12 35 0N 123 0 E
Huang He →, China 75 F10 37 55N 118 50 E
Huang Xian, China 75 F11 37 38N 120 30 E
Huangchuan, China 77 A10 32 15N 115 10 E
Huanggang, China 77 B10 30 29N 114 52 E
Huangguoshu, China 76 E5 26 0N 105 40 E
Huangling, China 74 G5 35 34N 109 15 E
Huanglong, China 74 G5 35 30N 109 59 E
Huanglongtan, China 77 A8 32 40N 110 33 E
Huangmei, China 77 B10 30 5N 115 56 E
Huangpi, China 77 B10 30 50N 114 22 E
Huangping, China 76 D6 26 52N 107 54 E
Huangshan, China 77 C12 29 42N 118 25 E
Huangshi, China 77 B10 30 10N 115 3 E
Huangsongdian, China 75 C14 43 45N 127 25 E
Huangyan, China 77 C13 28 38N 121 19 E
Huangyangsi, China 77 D8 26 33N 111 39 E
Huaning, China 76 E4 24 17N 102 56 E
Huanjiang, China 76 E7 24 50N 108 18 E
Huanta, Peru 172 C3 12 55 S 74 20W
Huantai, China 75 F9 36 58N 117 56 E
Huánuco, Peru 172 B2 9 55 S 76 15W
Huánuco □, Peru 172 B2 9 55 S 76 14W
Huanuni, Bolivia 172 D4 18 16 S 66 51W
Huanzo, Cordillera de, Peru 172 C3 14 35 S 73 20W
Huaping, China 76 D3 26 46N 101 25 E
Huara, Chile 172 D4 19 59 S 69 47W
Huaral, Peru 172 C2 11 32 S 77 13W
Huaraz, Peru 172 B2 9 30 S 77 32W
Huari, Peru 172 B2 9 14 S 77 14W
Huarmey, Peru 172 C2 10 5 S 78 5W
Huarochiri, Peru 172 C2 12 9 S 76 15W
Huarocondo, Peru 172 C3 13 26 S 72 14W
Huarong, China 77 C9 29 29N 112 30 E
Huascarán, Peru 172 B2 9 8 S 77 36W
Huascarán, Nevado, Peru 172 B2 9 7 S 77 37W
Huasco, Chile 174 B1 28 30 S 71 15W
Huasco →, Chile 174 B1 28 27 S 71 13W
Huasna, U.S.A. 161 K6 35 6N 120 24W
Huatabampo, Mexico 162 B3 26 50N 109 50W
Huauchinango, Mexico 163 C5 20 11N 98 3W
Huautla de Jiménez, Mexico 163 D5 18 8N 96 51W
Huaxi, China 76 D6 26 25N 106 40 E
Huay Namota, Mexico 162 C4 21 56N 104 30W
Huayin, China 74 G6 34 35N 110 5 E
Huayllay, Peru 172 C2 11 3 S 76 21W
Huayuan, China 76 C7 28 37N 109 29 E
Huayun, China 76 B6 30 14N 106 40 E
Huazhou, China 77 G8 21 33N 110 33 E
Hubbard, Iowa, U.S.A. 156 B3 42 18N 93 18W
Hubbard, Ohio, U.S.A. 150 E4 41 9N 80 34W
Hubbard, Tex., U.S.A. 155 K6 31 51N 96 48W
Hubbart Pt., Canada 143 B10 59 21N 94 41W
Hubei □, China 77 B9 31 0N 112 0 E
Hubli, India 95 G2 15 22N 75 15 E
Huch'ang, N. Korea 75 D14 41 25N 127 2 E
Huchow = Huzhou, China 77 B13 30 51N 120 8 E
Hucknall, U.K. 20 D6 53 3N 1 13W
Huddersfield, U.K. 20 D6 53 39N 1 47W
Hude, Germany 30 B4 53 7N 8 26 E
Hudi, Sudan 106 D3 17 43N 34 18 E
Hudiksvall, Sweden 16 C11 61 43N 17 10 E
Hudson, Canada 140 B1 50 6N 92 9W
Hudson, Fla., U.S.A. 153 G7 28 22N 82 42W
Hudson, Mass., U.S.A. 151 D13 42 23N 71 34W
Hudson, Mich., U.S.A. 157 C12 41 51N 84 21W
Hudson, N.Y., U.S.A. 151 D11 42 15N 73 46W
Hudson, Wis., U.S.A. 154 C8 44 58N 92 45W
Hudson, Wyo., U.S.A. 158 E9 42 54N 108 35W
Hudson →, U.S.A. 151 F10 40 42N 74 2W
Hudson Bay, Nunavut, Canada 139 C11 60 0N 86 0W
Hudson Bay, Sask., Canada 143 C8 52 51N 102 23W
Hudson Falls, U.S.A. 151 C11 43 18N 73 35W
Hudson Mts., Antarctica 7 D16 74 32 S 99 20W
Hudson Str., Canada 139 B13 62 0N 70 0W
Hudson's Hope, Canada 142 B4 56 0N 121 54W
Hudsonville, U.S.A. 157 B11 42 52N 85 52W
Hue, Vietnam 86 D6 16 30N 107 35 E
Huebra →, Spain 42 D4 41 2N 6 48W
Huechucuicui, Pta., Chile 176 B2 41 48 S 74 2W
Huedin, Romania 52 D8 46 52N 23 2 E
Huehuetenango, Guatemala 164 C1 15 20N 91 28W
Huejúcar, Mexico 162 C4 22 21N 103 13W
Huélamo, Spain 40 E3 40 17N 1 48W
Huelgoat, France 26 D3 48 22N 3 46W
Huelma, Spain 43 H7 37 39N 3 28W
Huelva, Spain 43 H4 37 18N 6 57W
Huelva □, Spain 43 H4 37 40N 7 0W
Huelva →, Spain 43 H5 37 27N 6 0W
Hueneme = Port Hueneme, U.S.A. 161 L7 34 7N 119 12W
Huentelauquén, Chile 174 C1 31 38 S 71 33W
Huércal-Overa, Spain 41 H3 37 23N 1 57W
Huerquehue △, Chile 176 A2 39 6 S 71 42W
Huerta, Sa. de la, Argentina 174 C2 31 10 S 67 30W
Huertas, C. de las, Spain 41 G4 38 21N 0 24W
Huerva →, Spain 40 D4 41 39N 0 52W
Huesca, Spain 40 C4 42 8N 0 25W
Huesca □, Spain 40 C5 42 20N 0 1 E
Huéscar, Spain 41 H2 37 44N 2 35W
Huetamo, Mexico 162 D4 18 36N 100 54W
Huete, Spain 40 E2 40 10N 2 43W
Huger, U.S.A. 152 B10 33 6N 79 48W
Hugh →, Australia 126 D1 25 1 S 134 1 E
Hughenden, Australia 126 C3 20 52 S 144 10 E
Hughes, Australia 125 F4 30 42 S 129 31 E
Hughes, U.S.A. 144 C9 66 3N 154 15W
Hughesville, U.S.A. 151 E8 41 14N 76 44W
Hugli →, India 93 J13 21 56N 88 4 E
Hugo, Colo., U.S.A. 154 F3 39 8N 103 28W
Hugo, Okla., U.S.A. 155 H7 34 1N 95 31W
Hugoton, U.S.A. 155 G4 37 11N 101 21W
Huhehaote = Hohhot, China 74 D6 40 52N 111 40 E
Hui Xian = Huixian, China 74 G7 35 27N 113 12 E
Hui Xian, China 74 H4 33 50N 106 4 E
Hui'an, China 77 E12 25 1N 118 43 E
Hui'anbu, China 74 F4 37 28N 106 38 E
Huiarau Ra., N.Z. 130 E5 38 45 S 176 55 E
Huichang, China 77 E10 25 32N 115 45 E
Huichapán, Mexico 163 C5 20 24N 99 40W
Huidong, Guangdong, China 77 F10 22 58N 114 43 E
Huidong, Sichuan, China 76 D4 26 34N 102 35 E
Huifa He →, China 75 C14 43 0N 127 50 E
Huíla, Angola 115 F2 15 4 S 13 32 E
Huíla □, Angola 115 E2 14 0 S 15 0 E
Huila □, Colombia 168 C2 2 30N 75 45W
Huila, Nevado del, Colombia 168 C2 3 0N 76 0W
Huilai, China 77 F11 23 0N 116 18 E
Huili, China 76 D4 26 35N 102 17 E
Huimin, China 75 F9 37 27N 117 28 E
Huinan, China 75 C14 42 40N 126 2 E
Huinca Renancó, Argentina 174 C3 34 51 S 64 22W
Huining, China 74 G3 35 38N 105 0 E
Huinong, China 74 E4 39 5N 106 35 E
Huiroa, N.Z. 130 F3 39 15 S 174 30 E
Huisache, Mexico 162 C4 22 55N 100 25W
Huishui, China 76 D6 26 7N 106 38 E
Huisne →, France 26 E7 47 59N 0 11 E
Huiting, China 74 G9 34 5N 116 5 E
Huitong, China 76 D7 26 51N 109 45 E
Huixian, China 74 G7 35 27N 113 12 E
Huixtla, Mexico 163 D6 15 9N 92 28W
Huize, China 76 D4 26 24N 103 15 E
Huizhou, China 77 F10 23 0N 114 23 E
Hukeri, India 95 F2 16 14N 74 36 E
Hukou, China 77 C11 29 45N 116 21 E
Hŭksan-chedo, S. Korea 75 G13 34 40N 125 30 E
Hukuntsi, Botswana 116 C3 23 58 S 21 45 E
Hula, Papua N. G. 132 F4 10 5 S 147 43 E
Ḩulayfā', Si. Arabia 96 E4 25 58N 40 45 E
Huld = Ulaanjirem, Mongolia 74 B3 45 5N 105 30 E
Hulin He →, China 75 B12 45 0N 122 10 E
Hull = Kingston upon Hull, U.K. 20 D7 53 45N 0 21W
Hull, Canada 140 C4 45 25N 75 44W
Hull →, U.K. 20 D7 53 44N 0 20W
Hulst, Neths. 24 C4 51 17N 4 2 E
Hultschin = Hlučín, Czech Rep. 35 B11 49 54N 18 11 E
Hultsfred, Sweden 17 G9 57 30N 15 52 E
Hulun = Hailar, China 69 B6 49 10N 119 38 E
Hulun Nur, China 69 B6 49 0N 117 30 E
Hulyaypole, Ukraine 59 J9 47 45N 36 21 E
Huma, Tanjung, Malaysia 87 c 5 29N 100 16 E
Humacao, Puerto Rico 165 d 18 9N 65 50W
Humahuaca, Argentina 174 A2 23 10 S 65 25W
Humaitá = Pôrto Válter, Brazil 172 B3 8 15 S 72 40W
Humaitá, Brazil 173 B5 7 35 S 63 1W
Humaitá, Paraguay 174 B4 27 2 S 58 31W
Humansdorp, S. Africa 116 E3 34 2 S 24 46 E
Humansville, U.S.A. 156 G3 37 48N 93 35W
Humara, J., Sudan 107 D3 16 16N 30 59 E
Humbe, Angola 116 B1 16 40 S 14 55 E
Humber →, U.K. 20 D7 53 42N 0 27W
Humboldt, Canada 143 C7 52 15N 105 9W
Humboldt, Iowa, U.S.A. 156 B2 42 44N 94 13W
Humboldt, Tenn., U.S.A. 155 H10 35 50N 88 55W
Humboldt →, U.S.A. 158 F4 39 59N 118 36W
Humboldt, Massif du, N. Cal. 133 U20 21 53 S 166 25 E
Humboldt Gletscher = Sermersuaq, Greenland 10 B4 79 30N 62 0W
Humboldt Mts., N.Z. 131 E3 44 30 S 168 15 E
Hume, U.S.A. 160 J8 36 48N 118 54W
Hume, L., Australia 129 D7 36 0 S 147 5 E
Humen, China 69 F10 22 50N 113 40 E
Humenné, Slovak Rep. 35 C14 48 55N 21 50 E
Humeston, U.S.A. 156 D3 40 52N 93 30W
Hummelsta, Sweden 16 E10 59 34N 16 58 E
Hummelvik, Norway 18 A5 63 29N 8 19 E
Hummock Hill = Whyalla, Australia 128 B2 33 2 S 137 30 E
Humpata, Angola 115 F2 15 2 S 13 24 E
Humphreys, Mt., U.S.A. 160 H8 37 17N 118 40W
Humphreys Peak, U.S.A. 159 J8 35 21N 111 41W
Humpolec, Czech Rep. 34 B8 49 31N 15 20 E
Humptulips, U.S.A. 160 C3 47 14N 123 57W
Humula, Australia 129 C7 35 30 S 147 46 E
Hūn, Libya 108 C3 29 2N 16 0 E
Hun Jiang →, China 75 D13 40 50N 125 38 E
Húnaflói, Iceland 11 B6 65 50N 20 50W
Hunan □, China 77 D9 27 30N 112 0 E
Húnavatnssýsla □, Iceland 11 B6 65 30N 20 25W
Hunchun, China 75 C16 42 52N 130 28 E
Hundested, Denmark 17 J5 55 58N 11 52 E
Hundewali, Pakistan 92 D5 31 55N 72 38 E
Hundorp, Norway 18 C7 61 33N 9 59 E
Hundred Islands △, Phil. 80 C3 16 10N 120 2 E

Hundred Mile House, *Canada* **142 C4** 51 38N 121 18W
Hundvåg, *Norway* **18 E2** 59 0N 5 43 E
Hunedoara, *Romania* **52 E7** 45 40N 22 50 E
Hunedoara □, *Romania* **52 E7** 45 50N 22 54 E
Hünfeld, *Germany* **30 E5** 50 39N 9 46 E
Hung Yen, *Vietnam* **76 G6** 20 39N 106 4 E
Hunga Ha'apai, *Tonga* **133 Q13** 20 41 S 175 7W
Hungary ■, *Europe* **35 D12** 47 20N 19 20 E
Hungary, Plain of, *Europe* **12 F10** 47 0N 20 0 E
Hungerford, *Australia* **127 D3** 28 58 S 144 24 E
Hŭngnam, *N. Korea* **75 E14** 39 49N 127 45 E
Hungt'ou Hsü, *Taiwan* **77 G13** 22 0N 121 30 E
Hungund, *India* **95 F3** 16 4N 76 3 E
Huni Valley, *Ghana* **112 D4** 5 33N 1 56W
Hunjiang, *China* **75 D14** 41 56N 126 29 E
Hunneberg, *Sweden* **17 F6** 58 18N 12 30 E
Hunnebostrand, *Sweden* **17 F5** 58 27N 11 18 E
Hunsberge, *Namibia* **116 D2** 27 45 S 17 12 E
Hunsrück, *Germany* **31 F3** 49 56N 7 27 E
Hunstanton, *U.K.* **20 E8** 52 56N 0 29 E
Hunsur, *India* **95 H3** 12 16N 76 16 E
Hunte →, *Germany* **30 B4** 53 14N 8 28 E
Hunter, *N.Z.* **131 E6** 44 36 S 171 2 E
Hunter, *U.S.A.* **151 D10** 42 13N 74 13W
Hunter →, *Australia* **129 B9** 32 52 S 151 46 E
Hunter →, *N.Z.* **131 E4** 44 21 S 169 27 E
Hunter, C., *Solomon Is.* **133 M10** 9 48 S 159 50 E
Hunter Hills, The, *N.Z.* **131 E5** 44 26 S 170 46 E
Hunter I., *Australia* **127 G3** 40 30 S 144 45 E
Hunter I., *Canada* **142 C3** 51 55N 128 0W
Hunter Mts., *N.Z.* **131 F2** 45 43 S 167 25 E
Hunter Ra., *Australia* **129 B9** 32 45 S 150 15 E
Hunters Road, *Zimbabwe* **119 F2** 19 9 S 29 49 E
Hunterville, *N.Z.* **130 F4** 39 56 S 175 35 E
Huntingburg, *U.S.A.* **157 F10** 38 18N 86 57W
Huntingdon, *Canada* **140 C5** 45 6N 74 10W
Huntingdon, *U.K.* **21 E7** 52 20N 0 11W
Huntingdon, *U.S.A.* **150 F6** 40 30N 78 1W
Huntington = Shelton, *U.S.A.* **151 E11** 41 19N 73 5W
Huntington, *Ind., U.S.A.* **157 D11** 40 53N 85 30W
Huntington, *N.Y., U.S.A.* **151 F11** 40 52N 73 26W
Huntington, *Oreg., U.S.A.* **158 D5** 44 21N 117 16W
Huntington, *Utah, U.S.A.* **158 G8** 39 20N 110 58W
Huntington, *W. Va., U.S.A.* **148 F4** 38 25N 82 27W
Huntington Beach, *U.S.A.* **161 M9** 33 40N 118 5W
Huntley, *U.S.A.* **157 B8** 42 10N 88 26W
Huntly, *N.Z.* **130 D4** 37 34 S 175 11 E
Huntly, *U.K.* **22 D6** 57 27N 2 47W
Huntsville, *Canada* **140 C4** 45 20N 79 14W
Huntsville, *Ala., U.S.A.* **149 H2** 34 44N 86 35W
Huntsville, *Mo., U.S.A.* **156 E4** 39 26N 92 33W
Huntsville, *Tex., U.S.A.* **155 K7** 30 43N 95 33W
Hunyani →, *Zimbabwe* **119 F3** 15 57 S 30 39 E
Hunyuan, *China* **74 E7** 39 42N 113 42 E
Hunza →, *India* **93 B6** 35 54N 74 20 E
Huo Xian = Huozhou, *China* **74 F6** 36 36N 111 42 E
Huon G., *Papua N. G.* **132 D4** 7 0 S 147 30 E
Huon Pen., *Papua N. G.* **132 D4** 6 20 S 147 30 E
Huong Khe, *Vietnam* **86 C5** 18 13N 105 41 E
Huonville, *Australia* **127 G4** 43 0 S 147 5 E
Huoqiu, *China* **77 A11** 32 20N 116 12 E
Huoshan, *Anhui, China* **77 A12** 32 28N 118 30 E
Huoshan, *Anhui, China* **77 B11** 31 25N 116 20 E
Huoshao Dao = Lü-Tao, *Taiwan* **77 F13** 22 40N 121 30 E
Huozhou, *China* **74 F6** 36 36N 111 42 E
Hupeh = Hubei □, *China* **77 B9** 31 0N 112 0 E
Hūr, *Iran* **97 D8** 30 50N 57 7 E
Hurbanovo, *Slovak Rep.* **35 D11** 47 51N 18 11 E
Hurd, C., *Canada* **150 A3** 45 13N 81 44W
Hure Qi, *China* **75 C11** 42 45N 121 45 E
Hurezani, *Romania* **53 F8** 44 49N 23 40 E
Hurghada, *Egypt* **106 B3** 27 15N 33 50 E
Hurley, *N. Mex., U.S.A.* **159 K9** 32 42N 108 8W
Hurley, *Wis., U.S.A.* **154 B9** 46 27N 90 11W
Huron, *Calif., U.S.A.* **160 J6** 36 12N 120 6W
Huron, *Ohio, U.S.A.* **150 E2** 41 24N 82 33W
Huron, *S. Dak., U.S.A.* **154 C5** 44 22N 98 13W
Huron, L., *U.S.A.* **150 B2** 44 30N 82 40W
Huron East, *Canada* **150 C3** 43 37N 81 18W
Hurricane, *U.S.A.* **159 H7** 37 11N 113 17W
Hurso, *Ethiopia* **107 F5** 9 35N 41 33 E
Hurstboro, *U.S.A.* **152 C4** 32 15N 85 25W
Hurungwe ⌓, *Zimbabwe* **119 F2** 16 7 S 29 5 E
Hurunui →, *N.Z.* **131 C8** 42 54 S 173 18 E
Hurup, *Denmark* **17 H2** 56 46N 8 25 E
Húsafell, *Iceland* **11 C6** 64 42N 20 53W
Húsavík, *Iceland* **11 A9** 66 3N 17 21W
Huşi, *Romania* **53 D13** 46 41N 28 7 E
Huskisson, *Australia* **129 C9** 35 2 S 150 41 E
Huskvarna, *Sweden* **17 G8** 57 47N 14 15 E
Huslia, *U.S.A.* **144 D8** 65 41N 156 24W
Husnes, *Norway* **18 E2** 59 52N 5 45 E
Hustad, *Norway* **18 B4** 62 57N 7 6 E
Hustadvika, *Norway* **18 A3** 63 0N 7 0 E
Hustontown, *U.S.A.* **150 F6** 40 3N 78 2W
Hustopeče, *Czech Rep.* **35 C9** 48 57N 16 43 E
Husum, *Germany* **30 A5** 54 28N 9 4 E
Husum, *Sweden* **16 A13** 63 21N 19 12 E
Huszt = Khust, *Ukraine* **53 B8** 48 10N 23 18 E
Hutchinson, *Kans., U.S.A.* **155 F6** 38 5N 97 56W
Hutchinson, *Minn., U.S.A.* **154 C7** 44 54N 94 22W
Ḥūth, *Yemen* **98 C3** 16 14N 43 58 E
Hutjena, *Papua N. G.* **132 C8** 5 23 S 154 42 E
Hutsonville, *U.S.A.* **157 E9** 39 7N 87 40W
Hutte Sauvage, L. de la, *Canada* **141 A7** 56 15N 64 45W
Hüttenberg, *Austria* **34 E7** 46 56N 14 33 E
Hüttener Berge ⌓, *Germany* **30 A5** 54 24N 9 40 E
Hutton, Mt., *Australia* **127 D4** 25 51 S 148 20 E
Huttwil, *Switz.* **32 B5** 47 7N 7 50 E
Huwun, *Ethiopia* **107 G5** 4 23N 40 6 E
Huy, *Belgium* **24 D5** 50 31N 5 15 E
Huzhou, *China* **77 B13** 30 51N 120 8 E
Huzurabad, *India* **94 E4** 18 12N 79 25 E
Huzurnagar, *India* **94 F4** 16 54N 79 53 E
Hvalpsund, *Denmark* **17 H3** 56 42N 9 11 E
Hvammsfjörður, *Iceland* **11 B4** 65 4N 22 5W
Hvammstangi, *Iceland* **11 B6** 65 24N 20 57W
Hvammur, *Mýrasýsla, Iceland* **11 C5** 64 50N 21 21W
Hvammur, *Skagafjarðarsýsla, Iceland* **11 B7** 65 53N 19 51W
Hvannadalshnúkur, *Iceland* **11 C10** 64 1N 16 41W
Hvanneyri, *Iceland* **11 C5** 64 34N 21 36W
Hvar, *Croatia* **45 E13** 43 11N 16 28 E
Hvarski Kanal, *Croatia* **45 E13** 43 15N 16 35 E
Hveragerði, *Iceland* **11 C5** 64 0N 21 12W
Hvítá →, *Iceland* **11 C5** 64 30N 21 58W
Hvítárvatn, *Iceland* **11 C7** 64 37N 19 50W
Hvittingfoss, *Norway* **18 E7** 59 29N 10 0 E
Hvizdets, *Ukraine* **53 B10** 48 35N 25 17 E
Hvolsvöllur, *Iceland* **11 D6** 63 45N 20 14W
Hwachŏn-chŏsuji, *S. Korea* **75 E14** 38 5N 127 50 E
Hwainan = Huainan, *China* **77 A11** 32 38N 116 58 E
Hwaiyin = Huaiyin, *China* **75 H10** 33 30N 119 2 E
Hwang Ho = Huang He →, *China* **75 F10** 37 55N 118 50 E
Hwange, *Zimbabwe* **119 F2** 18 18 S 26 30 E
Hwange △, *Zimbabwe* **116 B4** 19 0 S 26 30 E
Hwangshih = Huangshi, *China* **77 B10** 30 10N 115 3 E
Hwekum, *Burma* **90 B5** 26 7N 95 22 E
Hyaing, *Burma* **90 D5** 22 39N 94 44 E
Hyannis, *Mass., U.S.A.* **148 E10** 41 39N 70 17W
Hyannis, *Nebr., U.S.A.* **154 E4** 42 0N 101 46W
Hyargas Nuur, *Mongolia* **68 B4** 49 0N 93 0 E
Hybo, *Sweden* **16 C10** 61 49N 16 15 E
Hydaburg, *U.S.A.* **142 B2** 55 15N 132 50W
Hyde, *N.Z.* **131 F5** 45 18 S 170 16 E
Hyde Park, *Guyana* **169 B6** 6 30N 58 16W
Hyde Park, *U.S.A.* **151 E11** 41 47N 73 56W
Hyden, *Australia* **125 F2** 32 24 S 118 53 E
Hyder, *U.S.A.* **142 B2** 55 55N 130 5W
Hyderabad, *India* **94 F4** 17 22N 78 29 E
Hyderabad, *Pakistan* **91 D3** 25 23N 68 24 E
Hydra = Ídhra, *Greece* **48 D5** 37 20N 23 28 E
Hyen, *Norway* **18 C2** 61 44N 5 56 E
Hyères, *France* **29 E10** 43 8N 6 9 E
Hyères, Îs. d', *France* **29 F10** 43 0N 6 20 E
Hyesan, *N. Korea* **75 D15** 41 20N 128 10 E
Hyland →, *Canada* **142 B3** 59 52N 128 12W
Hylestad, *Norway* **18 E4** 59 6N 7 29 E
Hyllestad, *Norway* **18 C2** 61 10N 5 17 E
Hyltebruk, *Sweden* **17 H7** 56 59N 13 15 E
Hymia, *India* **93 C8** 33 40N 78 2 E
Hyndman Peak, *U.S.A.* **158 E6** 43 45N 114 8W
Hynnekleiv, *Norway* **18 F5** 58 36N 8 25 E
Hyōgo □, *Japan* **72 B6** 35 15N 134 50 E
Hyrra Banda, *C.A.R.* **114 A4** 5 58N 22 1 E
Hyrum, *U.S.A.* **158 F8** 41 38N 111 51W
Hysham, *U.S.A.* **158 C10** 46 18N 107 14W
Hythe, *U.K.* **21 F9** 51 4N 1 5 E
Hyūga, *Japan* **72 E3** 32 25N 131 35 E
Hyvinge = Hyvinkää, *Finland* **15 F21** 60 38N 24 50 E
Hyvinkää, *Finland* **15 F21** 60 38N 24 50 E

I

I-n-Azaoua, *Illizi, Algeria* **111 C6** 25 42N 6 54 E
I-n-Azaoua, *Tamanrasset, Algeria* **111 D6** 20 46N 7 32 E
I-n-Échaï, *Mali* **110 D4** 20 10N 2 5W
I-n-Gall, *Niger* **113 B6** 16 51N 7 1 E
I-n-Kelemet, *Algeria* **111 C6** 26 57N 5 47 E
I-n-Oudad, *Algeria* **111 D5** 20 17N 4 38 E
I-n-Ouzzal, *Algeria* **113 A5** 20 40N 2 35 E
I-n-Quzzal, *Algeria* **111 D5** 20 41N 2 34 E
I-n-Tadreft, *Niger* **113 B6** 19 5N 6 38 E
Iabès, Erg, *Algeria* **111 C4** 27 30N 2 2W
Iablaniţa, *Romania* **52 F7** 44 57N 22 19 E
Iaco →, *Brazil* **172 B4** 9 3 S 68 34W
Iacobeni, *Romania* **53 C10** 47 25N 25 20 E
Iaçu, *Brazil* **171 D3** 12 45 S 40 13W
Iakora, *Madag.* **117 C8** 23 6 S 46 40 E
Ialibu, *Papua N. G.* **132 D2** 6 17 S 143 59 E
Ialomiţa □, *Romania* **53 F12** 44 30N 27 30 E
Ialomiţa →, *Romania* **53 F12** 44 42N 27 51 E
Ialoveni, *Moldova* **53 D13** 46 56N 28 47 E
Ialpug →, *Moldova* **53 E13** 45 41N 28 35 E
Iamonia L., *U.S.A.* **152 E5** 30 38N 84 14W
Ianca, *Romania* **53 E12** 45 6N 27 29 E
Iara, *Romania* **53 D8** 46 31N 23 35 E
Iarda, *Ethiopia* **107 E4** 11 9N 35 53 E
Iargara, *Moldova* **53 D13** 46 24N 28 23 E
Iaşi, *Romania* **53 C12** 47 10N 27 40 E
Iaşi □, *Romania* **53 C12** 47 20N 27 0 E
Iasmos, *Greece* **51 E9** 41 8N 25 11 E
Iauaretê, *Colombia* **168 C4** 0 36N 69 12W
Ib →, *India* **93 J10** 21 34N 83 48 E
Iba, *Phil.* **80 D2** 15 22N 120 0 E
Ibadan, *Nigeria* **113 D5** 7 22N 3 58 E
Ibagué, *Colombia* **168 C2** 4 20N 75 20W
Ibaiti, *Brazil* **171 F1** 23 50 S 50 10W
Ibajay, *Phil.* **81 F4** 11 49N 122 10 E
Iballë, *Albania* **50 D4** 42 12N 20 2 E
Ibăneşti, *Botoşani, Romania* **53 B11** 48 4N 26 22 E
Ibăneşti, *Mureş, Romania* **53 D9** 46 45N 24 57 E
Ibanshe, *Dem. Rep. of the Congo* **115 C4** 4 58 S 21 30 E
Ibar →, *Serbia & M.* **50 C4** 43 43N 20 45 E
Ibara, *Japan* **72 C5** 34 36N 133 28 E
Ibaraki, *Japan* **73 C7** 34 49N 135 34 E
Ibaraki □, *Japan* **73 A12** 36 10N 140 10 E
Ibarra, *Ecuador* **168 C2** 0 21N 78 7W
Ibb, *Yemen* **98 D4** 14 2N 44 10 E
Ibba, *Sudan* **111 G11** 4 49N 29 2 E
Ibba, Bahr el →, *Sudan* **107 F2** 5 30N 28 55 E
Ibbenbüren, *Germany* **30 C3** 52 16N 7 43 E
Ibeke Gembo, *Dem. Rep. of the Congo* **114 C3** 1 24 S 18 51 E
Ibembo, *Dem. Rep. of the Congo* **118 B1** 2 35N 23 35 E
Ibenga →, *Congo* **114 B3** 2 19N 18 9 E
Ibera, L., *Argentina* **174 B4** 28 30 S 57 9W
Iberia, *U.S.A.* **156 F4** 38 5N 92 18W
Iberian Peninsula, *Europe* **12 H5** 40 0N 5 0W
Iberville, *Canada* **140 C5** 45 19N 73 17W
Iberville, Lac d', *Canada* **140 A5** 55 55N 73 15W
Ibi, *Nigeria* **113 D6** 8 15N 9 44 E
Ibi, *Spain* **41 G4** 38 38N 0 34W
Ibiá, *Brazil* **171 E2** 19 30 S 46 30W
Ibiapaba, Sa. da, *Brazil* **170 B3** 4 0 S 41 30W
Ibicaraí, *Brazil* **171 D4** 14 51 S 39 36W
Ibicuí, *Brazil* **171 D4** 14 51 S 39 59W
Ibicuí →, *Brazil* **175 B4** 29 25 S 56 47W
Ibicuy, *Argentina* **174 C4** 33 55 S 59 10W
Ibipetuba, *Brazil* **170 D3** 11 0 S 44 32W
Ibitiara, *Brazil* **171 D3** 12 39 S 42 13W
Ibiza = Eivissa, *Spain* **38 D1** 38 54N 1 26 E
Ibiza ✕ (IBZ), *Spain* **41 G6** 38 53N 1 22 E
Îblei, Monti, *Italy* **47 E7** 37 15N 14 45 E
Ibo, *Mozam.* **119 E5** 12 22 S 40 40 E
Ibonma, *Indonesia* **83 B4** 3 29 S 133 31 E
Ibotirama, *Brazil* **171 D3** 12 13 S 43 12W
Ibrāhīm →, *Lebanon* **103 A4** 34 4N 35 38 E
'Ibrī, *Oman* **97 F8** 23 14N 56 30 E
İbriktepe, *Turkey* **51 E10** 41 0N 26 30 E
Ibshawâi, *Egypt* **106 J7** 29 21N 30 40 E
Ibu, *Indonesia* **82 A3** 1 35N 127 33 E
Ibuki-Sanchi, *Japan* **73 B8** 35 25N 136 18 E
Ibusuki, *Japan* **72 F2** 31 12N 130 40 E
Ica, *Peru* **172 C2** 14 0 S 75 48W
Ica □, *Peru* **172 C2** 14 20 S 75 30W
Iça →, *Brazil* **172 A4** 2 55 S 67 58W
Icabarú, *Venezuela* **169 C5** 4 20N 61 45W
Icabarú →, *Venezuela* **169 C5** 4 45N 62 15W
Icacos Pt., *Trin. & Tob.* **169 F9** 10 3N 61 57W
Içana, *Brazil* **168 C4** 0 21N 67 19W
Içana →, *Brazil* **168 C4** 0 26N 67 19W
Icatu, *Brazil* **170 B3** 2 46 S 44 4W
Icaturama = Santa Rosa de Viterbo, *Colombia* **168 B3** 5 53N 72 59W
İçel = Mersin, *Turkey* **100 D6** 36 51N 34 36 E
Iceland ■, *Europe* **11 C8** 64 45N 19 0W
Iceland Plateau, *Arctic* **6 C7** 64 0N 10 0W
Ichalkaranji, *India* **94 F2** 16 40N 74 33 E
Ich'ang = Yichang, *China* **77 B8** 30 40N 111 20 E
Ichchapuram, *India* **94 E7** 19 10N 84 40 E
Ichhawar, *India* **92 H7** 23 1N 77 1 E
Ichihara, *Japan* **73 B12** 35 28N 140 5 E
Ichikawa, *Japan* **73 B11** 35 44N 139 55 E
Ichilo →, *Bolivia* **173 D5** 15 57 S 64 50W
Ichinohe, *Japan* **70 D10** 40 13N 141 17 E
Ichinomiya, *Gifu, Japan* **73 B8** 35 18N 136 48 E
Ichinomiya, *Kumamoto, Japan* **72 E3** 32 58N 131 5 E
Ichinoseki, *Japan* **70 E10** 38 55N 141 8 E
Ichkeul △, *Tunisia* **108 A1** 37 5N 9 37 E
Ichnya, *Ukraine* **59 G7** 50 52N 32 24 E
Icht, *Morocco* **110 C3** 29 6N 8 54W
Ichun = Yichun, *China* **69 B7** 47 44N 128 52 E
Icó, *Brazil* **170 C4** 6 24 S 38 51W
Icoca, *Angola* **115 D3** 6 12 S 16 20 E
Icod, *Canary Is.* **9 e1** 28 22N 16 43W
Icoraci, *Brazil* **170 B2** 1 18 S 48 28W
Icy C., *U.S.A.* **144 A7** 70 20N 161 52W
Ida Grove, *U.S.A.* **154 D7** 42 21N 95 28W
Idabel, *U.S.A.* **155 J7** 33 54N 94 50W
Idaga Hamus, *Ethiopia* **107 E4** 14 13N 39 48 E
Idah, *Nigeria* **113 D6** 7 5N 6 40 E
Idaho □, *U.S.A.* **158 D7** 45 0N 115 0W
Idaho City, *U.S.A.* **158 E6** 43 50N 115 50W
Idaho Falls, *U.S.A.* **158 E7** 43 30N 112 2W
Idalia △, *Australia* **126 C3** 24 49 S 144 36 E
Idanha-a-Nova, *Portugal* **42 F3** 39 50N 7 15W
Idar-Oberstein, *Germany* **31 F3** 49 43N 7 16 E
Iday, *Niger* **109 F2** 14 54N 11 33 E
'Idd el Ghanam, *Sudan* **109 F4** 11 30N 24 19 E
Iddan, *Somali Rep.* **120 C3** 6 10N 48 55 E
Idelès, *Algeria* **111 D6** 23 50N 5 53 E
Idensalmi = Iisalmi, *Finland* **14 E22** 63 32N 27 10 E
Idfû, *Egypt* **106 C3** 24 55N 32 49 E
Ídhi Óros, *Greece* **39 E5** 35 15N 24 45 E
Ídhra, *Greece* **48 D5** 37 20N 23 28 E
Idi, *Indonesia* **84 A1** 5 2N 97 37 E
Idi Amin Dada, L. = Edward, L., *Africa* **118 C2** 0 25 S 29 40 E
Idiofa, *Dem. Rep. of the Congo* **115 C3** 4 55 S 19 42 E
Idjil = Fdérik, *Mauritania* **110 D2** 22 40N 12 45W
Idkerberget, *Sweden* **16 D9** 60 22N 15 15 E
Idku, Bahra el, *Egypt* **106 H7** 31 18N 30 18 E
Idlib, *Syria* **100 E7** 35 55N 36 36 E
Idre, *Sweden* **16 C6** 61 52N 12 42 E
Idria, *U.S.A.* **160 J6** 36 25N 120 41W
Idrija, *Slovenia* **45 C11** 46 0N 14 5 E
Idritsa, *Russia* **58 D5** 56 17N 28 53 E
Idro, *Italy* **33 E10** 45 44N 10 29 E
Idutywa, *S. Africa* **117 E4** 32 8 S 28 18 E
Ieper, *Belgium* **24 D2** 50 51N 2 53 E
Ierápetra, *Greece* **39 F6** 35 1N 25 44 E
Ierissós, *Greece* **50 F7** 40 22N 23 52 E
Ierissóu Kólpos, *Greece* **50 F7** 40 27N 23 57 E
Iernut, *Romania* **53 D9** 46 27N 24 15 E
Ieshima-Shotō, *Japan* **72 C6** 34 40N 134 32 E
Iesi, *Italy* **45 E10** 43 31N 13 14 E
Iésolo, *Italy* **45 C9** 45 32N 12 38 E
Ifach, Peñón de, *Spain* **41 G5** 38 38N 0 5 E
'Ifāl, W. al →, *Si. Arabia* **96 D2** 28 7N 35 3 E
Ifanadiana, *Madag.* **117 C8** 21 19 S 47 39 E
Ife, *Nigeria* **113 D5** 7 30N 4 31 E
Iférouâne, *Niger* **113 B6** 19 5N 8 24 E
Ifetesene, *Algeria* **111 C5** 25 30N 4 33 E
Iffley, *Australia* **126 B3** 18 53 S 141 12 E
Ifon, *Nigeria* **113 D6** 6 58N 5 40 E
Iforas, Adrar des, *Africa* **111 D5** 19 40N 1 40 E
Ifould, L., *Australia* **125 F5** 30 52 S 132 6 E
Ifrane, *Morocco* **110 B3** 33 33N 5 7W
Ifugao □, *Phil.* **80 C3** 16 40N 121 10 E
Iga, *Japan* **73 C8** 34 45N 136 10 E
Iganga, *Uganda* **118 B3** 0 37N 33 28 E
Igara Paraná →, *Colombia* **168 D3** 2 9 S 71 47W
Igarapava, *Brazil* **171 F2** 20 3 S 47 47W
Igarapé Açu, *Brazil* **170 B2** 1 4 S 47 33W
Igarapé-Mirim, *Brazil* **170 B2** 1 59 S 48 58W
Igarka, *Russia* **66 C9** 67 30N 86 33 E
Igatimi, *Paraguay* **175 A4** 24 5 S 55 40W
Igatpuri, *India* **94 E1** 19 40N 73 35 E
Igbetti, *Nigeria* **113 D5** 8 44N 4 8 E
Igbo-Ora, *Nigeria* **113 D5** 7 29N 3 15 E
Igboho, *Nigeria* **113 D5** 8 53N 3 50 E
Igbor, *Nigeria* **113 D6** 7 27N 8 34 E
Iğdır, *Turkey* **101 C11** 39 55N 44 2 E
Igelfors, *Sweden* **17 F9** 58 52N 15 41 E
Iggesund, *Sweden* **16 C11** 61 39N 17 10 E
Ighil Izane = Relizane, *Algeria* **111 A5** 35 44N 0 31 E
Igiugig, *U.S.A.* **144 G9** 59 20N 155 55W
Iglau = Jihlava, *Czech Rep.* **34 B8** 49 28N 15 35 E
Iglésias, *Italy* **46 C1** 39 19N 8 32 E
Igli, *Algeria* **111 B4** 30 25N 2 19W
Iglino, *Russia* **64 D6** 54 50N 56 26 E
Igloolik, *Canada* **139 B11** 69 20N 81 49W
Igluligaarjuk = Chesterfield Inlet, *Canada* **138 B10** 63 30N 90 45W
Iglulik = Igloolik, *Canada* **139 B11** 69 20N 81 49W
'Igma, Gebel el, *Egypt* **106 B3** 28 55N 34 0 E
Ignace, *Canada* **140 C1** 49 30N 91 40W
İğneada, *Turkey* **51 E11** 41 52N 27 59 E
İğneada Burnu, *Turkey* **51 E12** 41 53N 28 2 E
Igoumenítsa, *Greece* **50 G3** 39 32N 20 18 E
Igra, *Russia* **60 B11** 57 33N 53 7 E
Iguaçu △, *Brazil* **175 B5** 25 30 S 54 0W
Iguaçu →, *Brazil* **175 B5** 25 36 S 54 36W
Iguaçu, Cat. del, *Brazil* **175 B5** 25 41 S 54 26W
Iguaçu Falls = Iguaçu, Cat. del, *Brazil* **175 B5** 25 41 S 54 26W
Iguala, *Mexico* **163 D5** 18 20N 99 40W
Igualada, *Spain* **40 D6** 41 37N 1 37 E
Iguape, *Brazil* **171 F2** 24 43 S 47 33W
Iguaratinga = São Francisco do Maranhão, *Brazil* **170 C3** 6 15 S 42 52W
Iguassu = Iguaçu →, *Brazil* **175 B5** 25 36 S 54 36W
Iguatu, *Brazil* **170 C4** 6 20 S 39 18W
Iguazú △, *Argentina* **175 B5** 25 42 S 54 22W
Iguéla, *Gabon* **114 C1** 2 0 S 9 16 E
Iguéla, Lagune, *Gabon* **114 C2** 1 48 S 9 16 E
Iguetti, Sebkhet, *Mauritania* **110 C3** 25 5N 9 50W
Iguig, *Phil.* **80 C3** 17 45N 121 44 E
Igumen = Cherven, *Belarus* **58 F5** 53 45N 28 28 E
Iharana, *Madag.* **117 A9** 13 25 S 50 0 E
Ihbulag, *Mongolia* **74 C4** 43 11N 107 10 E
Iheya-Shima, *Japan* **71 L3** 27 4N 127 58 E
Ihiala, *Nigeria* **113 D6** 5 51N 6 55 E
Ihirene →, *Algeria* **111 D5** 20 28N 4 37 E
Ihosy, *Madag.* **117 C8** 22 24 S 46 8 E
Ihotry, Farihy, *Madag.* **117 C7** 21 56 S 43 41 E
Ihu, *Papua N. G.* **132 D3** 7 55 S 145 24 E
Ihugh, *Nigeria* **113 D6** 7 2N 9 0 E
Ii, *Finland* **14 D21** 65 19N 25 22 E
Ii-Shima, *Japan* **71 L3** 26 43N 127 47 E
Iida, *Japan* **73 B9** 35 35N 137 50 E
Iijoki →, *Finland* **14 D21** 65 20N 25 20 E
Iisalmi, *Finland* **14 E22** 63 32N 27 10 E
Iiyama, *Japan* **71 F9** 36 51N 138 22 E
Iizuka, *Japan* **72 D2** 33 38N 130 42 E
Ijâfene, *Mauritania* **110 D3** 20 40N 8 0W
Ijebu-Igbo, *Nigeria* **113 D5** 6 56N 4 1 E
Ijebu-Ode, *Nigeria* **113 D5** 6 47N 3 58 E
Ijill, Sebkhet, *Mauritania* **110 D2** 22 47N 12 53W
IJmuiden, *Neths.* **24 B4** 52 28N 4 35 E
Ijo älv = Iijoki →, *Finland* **14 D21** 65 20N 25 20 E
IJssel →, *Neths.* **24 B5** 52 35N 5 50 E
IJsselmeer, *Neths.* **24 B5** 52 45N 5 20 E
Ijuí, *Brazil* **175 B5** 28 23 S 53 55W
Ijuí →, *Brazil* **175 B4** 27 58 S 55 20W
Ijūin, *Japan* **72 F2** 31 37N 130 24 E
Ik →, *Russia* **64 D4** 55 41N 53 29 E
Ikalamavony, *Madag.* **117 C8** 21 9 S 46 35 E
Ikale, *Nigeria* **113 D6** 7 40N 5 37 E
Ikali, *Dem. Rep. of the Congo* **114 C4** 2 2 S 21 4 E
Ikaluktutiak, *Canada* **138 B9** 69 10N 105 0W
Ikamatua, *N.Z.* **131 C6** 42 16 S 171 41 E
Ikang, *Nigeria* **113 E6** 4 49N 8 30 E
Ikara, *Nigeria* **113 C6** 11 12N 8 15 E
Ikare, *Nigeria* **113 D6** 7 32N 5 40 E
Ikaría, *Greece* **49 D8** 37 35N 26 10 E
Ikast, *Denmark* **17 H3** 56 8N 9 10 E
Ikeda, *Japan* **72 C5** 34 1N 133 48 E
Ikeja, *Nigeria* **113 D5** 6 36N 3 23 E
Ikela, *Dem. Rep. of the Congo* **114 C4** 1 6 S 23 6 E
Ikélemba, *Congo* **114 B3** 1 12N 16 38 E
Ikélemba →, *Dem. Rep. of the Congo* **114 B3** 0 7N 18 17 E
Ikengo, *Dem. Rep. of the Congo* **114 C3** 0 8 S 18 8 E
Ikerre-Ekiti, *Nigeria* **113 D6** 7 25N 5 19 E
Ikhtiman, *Bulgaria* **50 D7** 42 27N 23 48 E
Iki, *Japan* **72 D1** 33 45N 129 42 E
Iki-Kaikyō, *Japan* **72 D1** 33 40N 129 45 E
Ikimba L., *Tanzania* **118 C3** 1 30 S 31 20 E
Ikire, *Nigeria* **113 D5** 7 23N 4 15 E
Ikitsuki-Shima, *Japan* **72 D1** 33 23N 129 26 E
İkizdere, *Turkey* **101 B9** 40 46N 40 32 E
Iko, *Congo* **114 C3** 0 35 S 16 0 E
Ikom, *Nigeria* **113 D6** 6 0N 8 42 E
Ikomu, *Dem. Rep. of the Congo* **114 C3** 1 54 S 19 40 E
Ikongo, *Madag.* **117 C8** 21 52 S 47 27 E
Ikopa →, *Madag.* **117 B8** 16 45 S 46 40 E
Ikorongo ⌓, *Tanzania* **118 C3** 1 50 S 34 53 E
Ikot Ekpene, *Nigeria* **113 D6** 5 12N 7 40 E
Ikparjuk = Arctic Bay, *Canada* **139 A11** 73 1N 85 7W
Ikramovo = Dzhuma, *Uzbekistan* **65 D3** 39 42N 66 40 E
Ikungu, *Tanzania* **118 C3** 1 33 S 33 42 E
Ikuno, *Japan* **72 B6** 35 10N 134 48 E
Ikurun, *Nigeria* **113 D5** 7 54N 4 40 E
Il-Kullana, *Malta* **38 F7** 35 50N 14 24 E
Il-Munxar, *Malta* **38 F8** 35 51N 14 34 E
Ila, *Dem. Rep. of the Congo* **114 C4** 2 53 S 21 7 E
Ila, *Nigeria* **113 D5** 8 0N 4 39 E
Ilafer, *Algeria* **111 D5** 21 40N 1 58 E
Ilagan, *Phil.* **80 C3** 17 7N 121 53 E
Ilaka, *Madag.* **117 B8** 19 33 S 48 52 E
Īlām, *Iran* **101 F12** 33 36N 46 36 E
Ilam, *Nepal* **93 F12** 26 58N 87 58 E
Īlām □, *Iran* **96 C5** 33 0N 47 0 E
Ilan, *Taiwan* **77 E13** 24 45N 121 44 E
Ilanskiy, *Russia* **67 D10** 56 14N 96 3 E
Ilanz, *Switz.* **33 C8** 46 46N 9 12 E
Ilaro, *Nigeria* **113 D5** 6 53N 3 3 E
Ilatane, *Niger* **113 B5** 16 30N 4 45 E
Ilave, *Peru* **172 D4** 16 5 S 69 40W
Iława, *Poland* **54 E6** 53 36N 19 34 E
Ilayangudi, *India* **95 K4** 9 34N 78 37 E
Ile →, *Kazakhstan* **66 E8** 45 53N 77 10 E
Île-à-la-Crosse, *Canada* **143 B7** 55 27N 107 53W
Île-à-la-Crosse, Lac, *Canada* **143 B7** 55 40N 107 45W
Île-de-France □, *France* **27 D9** 49 0N 2 20 E
Ileanda, *Romania* **53 C8** 47 20N 23 38 E
Ilebo, *Dem. Rep. of the Congo* **115 C4** 4 17 S 20 55 E
Ilek, *Russia* **64 F4** 51 32N 53 21 E
Ilek →, *Russia* **64 F4** 51 30N 53 22 E
Iler, *Algeria* **111 D5** 20 57N 3 21 E
Iler, O. →, *Algeria* **111 D5** 20 59N 3 14 E
Ilero, *Nigeria* **113 D5** 8 0N 3 20 E
Ilesha, *Kwara, Nigeria* **113 D5** 8 57N 3 28 E
Ilesha, *Oyo, Nigeria* **113 D5** 7 37N 4 40 E
Ilet = Krasnogorskiy, *Russia* **60 B9** 56 10N 48 28 E
Iletskaya = Sol Iletsk, *Russia* **64 F5** 51 10N 55 0 E
Iletsky Gorodok = Ilek, *Russia* **64 F4** 51 32N 53 21 E
Ilford, *Canada* **143 B9** 56 4N 95 35W
Ilfracombe, *Australia* **126 C3** 23 30 S 144 30 E
Ilfracombe, *U.K.* **21 F3** 51 12N 4 8W
Ilgaz, *Turkey* **100 B5** 40 55N 33 37 E
Ilgaz Dağları, *Turkey* **100 B5** 41 10N 33 50 E
Ilgın, *Turkey* **100 C4** 38 16N 31 55 E
Ilha, Pta. da, *Azores* **9 d1** 38 25N 28 3W
Ilha de Moçambique, *Mozam.* **119 F5** 15 4 S 40 52 E
Ilha Grande, *Brazil* **169 D4** 0 27 S 65 2W
Ilha Grande, B. da, *Brazil* **171 F3** 23 9 S 44 30W
Ílhavo, *Portugal* **42 E2** 40 33N 8 43W
Ilhéus, *Brazil* **171 D4** 14 49 S 39 2W
Ili = Ile →, *Kazakhstan* **66 E8** 45 53N 77 10 E
Ilia, *Romania* **52 E7** 45 57N 22 40 E
Ilia □, *Greece* **48 D3** 37 45N 21 35 E
Iliamna, *U.S.A.* **144 G9** 59 45N 154 55W
Iliamna L., *U.S.A.* **144 G9** 59 30N 155 0W
Ilian, Mt., *Phil.* **81 F2** 10 26N 119 33 E
Iliç, *Turkey* **101 C8** 39 27N 38 33 E
Ilıca, *Turkey* **49 B9** 39 52N 27 46 E
Ilich, *Kazakhstan* **65 C4** 40 50N 68 27 E
Ilichevsk, *Azerbaijan* **101 C11** 39 22N 45 5 E
Iligan, *Phil.* **81 G5** 8 12N 124 13 E
Iligan Bay, *Phil.* **81 G5** 8 25N 124 5 E
Iligan Pt., *Phil.* **80 B4** 18 25N 122 25 E
Ilíki, L., *Greece* **48 C5** 38 24N 23 15 E
Ilin I., *Phil.* **80 E3** 12 14N 121 5 E
Ilio Pt., *U.S.A.* **145 B4** 21 13N 157 16W
Iliodhrómia, *Greece* **48 B5** 39 12N 23 50 E
Ilion, *U.S.A.* **151 D9** 43 1N 75 2W
Ilirska-Bistrica, *Slovenia* **45 C11** 45 34N 14 14 E
Iliysk = Qapshaghay, *Kazakhstan* **65 B8** 43 51N 77 14 E
Ilkal, *India* **95 G3** 15 57N 76 8 E
Ilkenau = Olkusz, *Poland* **55 H6** 50 18N 19 33 E
Ilkeston, *U.K.* **20 E6** 52 58N 1 19W
Ilkley, *U.K.* **20 D6** 53 56N 1 48W
Illampu = Ancohuma, Nevado, *Bolivia* **172 D4** 16 0 S 68 50W
Illana B., *Phil.* **81 H4** 7 35N 123 45 E
Illapel, *Chile* **174 C1** 32 0 S 71 10W
Ille-et-Vilaine □, *France* **26 D5** 48 10N 1 30W
Ille-sur-Têt, *France* **28 F6** 42 40N 2 38 E
Illéla, *Niger* **113 C6** 14 32N 5 20 E
Iller →, *Germany* **31 G5** 48 23N 9 58 E
Illertissen, *Germany* **31 G6** 48 12N 10 7 E
Illescas, *Spain* **42 E7** 40 8N 3 51W
Illetas, *Spain* **38 B3** 39 32N 2 35 E
Illichivsk, *Ukraine* **59 J6** 46 20N 30 35 E
Illiers-Combray, *France* **26 D8** 48 18N 1 15 E
Illimani, Nevado, *Bolivia* **172 D4** 16 30 S 67 50W
Illinois □, *U.S.A.* **156 D7** 40 15N 89 30W
Illinois →, *U.S.A.* **156 F6** 38 58N 90 28W
Illiopolis, *U.S.A.* **156 E7** 39 51N 89 15W
Illium = Troy, *Turkey* **49 B8** 39 57N 26 12 E
Illizi, *Algeria* **111 C6** 26 31N 8 32 E
Illkirch-Graffenstaden, *France* **27 D14** 48 34N 7 42 E
Íllora, *Spain* **43 H7** 37 17N 3 53W
Illulissat, *Greenland* **10 D5** 69 12N 51 10W
Ilm →, *Germany* **30 D7** 51 6N 11 40 E
Ilmajoki, *Finland* **15 E20** 62 44N 22 34 E
Ilmen, Ozero, *Russia* **58 C6** 58 15N 31 10 E
Ilmenau = Jordanów, *Poland* **55 J6** 49 41N 19 49 E
Ilmenau = Limanowa, *Poland* **55 J7** 49 42N 20 22 E
Ilmenau, *Germany* **30 E6** 50 41N 10 54 E
Ilnytsya, *Ukraine* **52 B8** 48 21N 23 5 E
Ilo, *Peru* **172 D3** 17 40 S 71 20W
Ilobu, *Nigeria* **113 D5** 7 45N 4 25 E
Ilocos Norte □, *Phil.* **80 B3** 18 10N 120 45 E
Ilocos Sur □, *Phil.* **80 C3** 17 20N 120 35 E
Iloilo, *Phil.* **81 F4** 10 45N 122 33 E
Iloilo □, *Phil.* **81 F4** 11 0N 122 40 E
Ilora, *Nigeria* **113 D5** 7 45N 3 50 E
Ilorin, *Nigeria* **113 D5** 8 30N 4 35 E
Ilovatka, *Russia* **60 E7** 50 30N 45 50 E
Ilovlya, *Russia* **61 F7** 49 15N 44 2 E
Ilovlya →, *Russia* **61 F7** 49 14N 44 0 E
Iłowa, *Poland* **55 G2** 51 30N 15 10 E
Ilubabor, *Ethiopia* **107 F4** 7 25N 35 0 E
Ilva Mică, *Romania* **53 C9** 47 17N 24 40 E
Ilwaco, *U.S.A.* **160 D2** 46 19N 124 3W
Ilwaki, *Indonesia* **82 C3** 7 55 S 126 30 E
Ilyichevsk = Illichivsk, *Ukraine* **59 J6** 46 20N 30 35 E
Iłża, *Poland* **55 G8** 51 10N 21 15 E
Iłżanka →, *Poland* **55 G8** 51 14N 21 48 E
Imabari, *Japan* **72 C5** 34 4N 133 0 E
Imaichi, *Japan* **73 A11** 36 43N 139 46 E
Imaloto →, *Madag.* **117 C8** 23 27 S 45 13 E
İmamoğlu, *Turkey* **100 D6** 37 15N 35 38 E
Iman = Dalnerechensk, *Russia* **67 E14** 45 50N 133 40 E
Imandra, Ozero, *Russia* **56 A5** 67 30N 33 0 E
Imanombo, *Madag.* **117 C8** 24 26 S 45 49 E
Imari, *Japan* **72 D1** 33 15N 129 52 E
Imasa, *Sudan* **106 D4** 18 0N 36 12 E
Imathía □, *Greece* **50 F6** 40 30N 22 15 E
Imatra, *Finland* **58 B5** 61 12N 28 48 E
Imazu, *Japan* **73 B8** 35 24N 136 2 E
Imbabura □, *Ecuador* **168 C2** 0 30N 78 45W
Imbaimadai, *Guyana* **169 B5** 5 44N 60 17W
Imbonga, *Dem. Rep. of the Congo* **114 C3** 0 43 S 19 44 E
Imdahane, *Morocco* **110 B3** 32 8N 7 0W
Iménas, *Mali* **113 B5** 16 20N 0 40 E
imeni 26 Bakinskikh Komissarov = Neftçala, *Azerbaijan* **97 B6** 39 19N 49 12 E
imeni 26 Bakinskikh Komissarov, *Turkmenistan* **97 B7** 39 22N 54 10 E
imeni Dvadtsati Shesti Bakinskikh Komissarov = Neftçala, *Azerbaijan* **97 B6** 39 19N 49 12 E
imeni Dzerzhinskogo = Naryan-Mar, *Russia* **56 A9** 67 42N 53 12 E
imeni Khamzy Khakimzade = Khamza, *Uzbekistan* **65 C5** 40 25N 71 29 E
imeni Mikoyana = Kara-Balta, *Kyrgyzstan* **65 B6** 42 50N 73 49 E
imeni Petrovskogo G.I. = Horodyshche, *Ukraine* **59 H6** 49 17N 31 27 E
imeni Stalina = Shakhrikhan, *Uzbekistan* **65 C6** 40 42N 72 3 E
imeni Sverdlova = Sverdlovsk, *Ukraine* **59 H10** 48 5N 39 47 E
imeni Tovarishcha Khateyevicha = Synelnykove, *Ukraine* **59 H8** 48 25N 35 30 E
imeni Tretyego Internatsionala = Novoshakhtinsk, *Russia* **59 J10** 47 46N 39 58 E
Imeri, Serra, *Brazil* **168 C4** 0 50N 65 25W
Imerimandroso, *Madag.* **117 B8** 17 26 S 48 35 E
Imesan, *Mauritania* **110 D1** 22 54N 15 30W
Imese, *Dem. Rep. of the Congo* **114 B3** 2 6N 18 9 E

Imi, *Ethiopia* **107 F5** 6 28N 42 10 E
Imishly = Imişli, *Azerbaijan* **61 L9** 39 55N 48 4 E
Imişli, *Azerbaijan* **61 L9** 39 55N 48 4 E
Imitek, *Morocco* **110 C3** 29 43N 8 10W
Imlay, *U.S.A.* **158 F4** 40 40N 118 9W
Imlay City, *U.S.A.* **150 D1** 43 2N 83 5W
Immaseri, *Sudan* **107 D2** 15 40N 25 31 E
Immenstadt, *Germany* **31 H6** 47 33N 10 13 E
Immingham, *U.K.* **20 D7** 53 37N 0 13W
Immokalee, *U.S.A.* **153 J8** 26 25N 81 25W
Imo □, *Nigeria* **113 D6** 5 30N 7 10 E
Imo →, *Nigeria* **113 E6** 4 36N 7 35 E
Ímola, *Italy* **45 D8** 44 20N 11 42 E
Imotski, *Croatia* **45 E14** 43 27N 17 12 E
Impé, *Congo* **114 C3** 2 45 S 15 16 E
Imperatorskaya Gavan = Vanino, *Russia* **67 E15** 48 50N 140 5 E
Imperatriz, *Amazonas, Brazil* **172 B4** 5 18 S 67 11W
Imperatriz, *Maranhão, Brazil* **170 C2** 5 30 S 47 29W
Impéria, *Italy* **44 E5** 43 53N 8 3 E
Imperial, *Canada* **143 C7** 51 21N 105 28W
Imperial, *Peru* **172 C2** 13 4 S 76 21W
Imperial, *Calif., U.S.A.* **161 N11** 32 51N 115 34W
Imperial, *Nebr., U.S.A.* **154 E4** 40 31N 101 39W
Imperial Beach, *U.S.A.* **161 N9** 32 35N 117 8W
Imperial Dam, *U.S.A.* **161 N12** 32 55N 114 25W
Imperial Reservoir, *U.S.A.* **161 N12** 32 53N 114 28W
Imperial Valley, *U.S.A.* **161 N11** 33 0N 115 30W
Imperieuse Reef, *Australia* **124 C2** 17 36 S 118 50 E
Impfondo, *Congo* **114 B3** 1 40N 18 0 E
Imphal, *India* **90 C4** 24 48N 93 56 E
Imphy, *France* **27 F10** 46 55N 3 16 E
Impulo, *Angola* **115 E2** 13 51 S 13 39 E
Imranlı, *Turkey* **101 C8** 39 54N 38 7 E
Imroz = Gökçeada, *Turkey* **51 F9** 40 10N 25 50 E
Imroz, *Turkey* **51 F9** 40 10N 25 55 E
Imst, *Austria* **34 D3** 47 15N 10 44 E
Imuris, *Mexico* **162 A2** 30 47N 110 52W
Imuruan B., *Phil.* **81 F2** 10 40N 119 10 E
Imus, *Phil.* **80 D3** 14 26N 120 56 E
In Akhmed, *Mali* **113 B4** 19 49N 0 56W
In Aleï, *Mali* **112 B4** 17 42N 2 30W
In Amenas, *Algeria* **111 C6** 28 5N 9 33 E
In Atei, *Algeria* **111 D6** 20 33N 6 4 E
In Belbel, *Algeria* **111 C5** 27 55N 1 12 E
In Dekkar, O. →, *Algeria* **111 C6** 27 12N 6 16 E
In Delimane, *Mali* **113 B5** 15 52N 1 31 E
In Guezzam, *Algeria* **111 E6** 19 37N 5 52 E
In Koufi, *Mali* **113 B5** 19 11N 1 25 E
In Rhar, *Algeria* **111 C5** 27 10N 1 59 E
In Salah, *Algeria* **111 C5** 27 10N 2 32 E
In Tallak, *Mali* **113 B5** 16 19N 3 15 E
In Tebezas, *Mali* **113 B5** 17 49N 1 53 E
Ina, *Japan* **73 B9** 35 50N 137 55 E
Ina, *U.S.A.* **157 F8** 38 9N 88 54W
Ina-Bonchi, *Japan* **73 B9** 35 45N 137 58 E
Inabanga, *Phil.* **81 F5** 10 2N 124 4 E
Inaguan, *Phil.* **81 G2** 9 33N 118 39 E
Inagua △, *Bahamas* **165 B5** 21 5N 73 24W
Inajá, *Brazil* **170 C4** 8 54 S 37 49W
Inambari →, *Peru* **172 C4** 12 41 S 69 44W
Inangahua, *N.Z.* **131 B6** 41 52 S 171 59 E
Inanwatan, *Indonesia* **83 B4** 2 8 S 132 10 E
Iñapari, *Peru* **172 C4** 11 0 S 69 40W
Inarajan, *Guam* **133 R15** 13 16N 144 45 E
Inari, *Finland* **14 B22** 68 54N 27 1 E
Inarijärvi, *Finland* **14 B22** 69 0N 28 0 E
Inawashiro-Ko, *Japan* **70 F10** 37 29N 140 6 E
Inazawa, *Japan* **73 B8** 35 15N 136 47 E
Inbin, *Burma* **90 F5** 18 6N 95 16 E
Inca, *Spain* **38 B3** 39 43N 2 54 E
Inca de Oro, *Chile* **174 B2** 26 45 S 69 54W
Incaguasi, *Chile* **174 B1** 29 12 S 71 5W
Ince Burun, *Turkey* **100 A6** 42 7N 34 56 E
Incekum Burnu, *Turkey* **100 D5** 36 13N 33 57 E
Incesu, *Turkey* **96 B2** 38 38N 35 11 E
Inch'ŏn, *S. Korea* **75 F14** 37 27N 126 40 E
Incio = Cruz de Incio, *Spain* **42 C3** 42 39N 7 21W
Incirliova, *Turkey* **49 D9** 37 50N 27 41 E
Incline Village, *U.S.A.* **158 G4** 39 10N 119 58W
Incomáti →, *Mozam.* **117 D5** 25 46 S 32 43 E
Incudine, Mte., *France* **29 G13** 41 50N 9 12 E
Inda Silase, *Ethiopia* **107 E4** 14 10N 38 15 E
Indal, *Sweden* **16 B11** 62 35N 17 5 E
Indalsälven →, *Sweden* **16 B11** 62 36N 17 30 E
Indaw, *Burma* **90 C6** 24 15N 96 5 E
Indawgyi In, *Burma* **90 C6** 25 8N 96 20 E
Indbir, *Ethiopia* **107 F4** 8 7N 37 52 E
Indefatigable, I. = Santa Cruz, I., *Ecuador* **172 a** 0 38 S 90 23W
Independence, *Calif., U.S.A.* **160 J8** 36 48N 118 12W
Independence, *Iowa, U.S.A.* **156 B5** 42 28N 91 54W
Independence, *Kans., U.S.A.* **155 G7** 37 14N 95 42W
Independence, *Ky., U.S.A.* **157 F12** 38 57N 84 33W
Independence, *Mo., U.S.A.* **156 E2** 39 6N 94 25W
Independence Fjord, *Greenland* **10 A8** 82 10N 29 0W
Independence Mts., *U.S.A.* **158 F5** 41 20N 116 0W
Independência, *Brazil* **170 C3** 5 23 S 40 19W
Independenţa, *Romania* **53 E12** 45 25N 27 42 E
Index, *U.S.A.* **160 C5** 47 50N 121 33W
Indi, *India* **94 F2** 17 10N 75 58 E
India ■, *Asia* **89 C6** 20 0N 78 0 E
Indialantic, *U.S.A.* **153 G9** 28 6N 80 34W
Indian →, *U.S.A.* **153 G9** 27 59N 80 34W
Indian Cabins, *Canada* **142 B5** 59 52N 117 40W
Indian Harbour, *Canada* **141 B8** 54 27N 57 13W
Indian Harbour Beach, *U.S.A.* **153 G9** 28 10N 80 35W
Indian Head, *Canada* **143 C8** 50 30N 103 41W
Indian Lake, *U.S.A.* **151 C10** 43 47N 74 16W
Indian Ocean **121 E6** 5 0 S 75 0 E
Indian Rocks Beach, *U.S.A.* **153 H7** 27 53N 82 51W
Indian Springs, *U.S.A.* **161 J11** 36 35N 115 40W
Indiana, *U.S.A.* **150 F5** 40 37N 79 9W
Indiana □, *U.S.A.* **157 E11** 40 0N 86 0W
Indiana Dunes ⌂, *U.S.A.* **157 C9** 41 40N 87 0W
Indianapolis, *U.S.A.* **157 E10** 39 46N 86 9W
Indianapolis International ✕ (IND), *U.S.A.* **157 E10** 39 43N 86 17W
Indianola, *Iowa, U.S.A.* **156 C3** 41 22N 93 34W
Indianola, *Miss., U.S.A.* **155 J9** 33 27N 90 39W
Indiantown, *U.S.A.* **153 H9** 27 1N 80 28W
Indiapora, *Brazil* **171 E1** 19 57 S 50 17W
Indiga, *Russia* **56 A8** 67 38N 49 9 E
Indigirka →, *Russia* **67 B15** 70 48N 148 54 E
Indija, *Serbia & M.* **52 E5** 45 6N 20 7 E
Indio, *U.S.A.* **161 M10** 33 43N 116 13W
Indira Gandhi Canal, *India* **92 F5** 28 0N 72 0 E
Indira Pt., *India* **95 L11** 6 44N 93 49 E
Indispensable Strait, *Solomon Is.* **133 M11** 9 0 S 160 30 E
Indo-China, *Asia* **62 H14** 15 0N 102 0 E
Indonesia ■, *Asia* **85 C4** 5 0 S 115 0 E
Indore, *India* **92 H6** 22 42N 75 53 E
Indramayu, *Indonesia* **85 D3** 6 20 S 108 19 E
Indrapura = Kerinci, *Indonesia* **84 C2** 1 40 S 101 15 E
Indravati →, *India* **94 E5** 19 20N 80 20 E
Indre □, *France* **27 F8** 46 50N 1 39 E
Indre →, *France* **26 E7** 47 16N 0 11 E
Indre Arna, *Norway* **18 D2** 60 26N 5 30 E
Indre-et-Loire □, *France* **26 E7** 47 20N 0 40 E
Indrio, *U.S.A.* **153 H9** 27 31N 80 21W
Indulkana, *Australia* **127 D1** 26 58 S 133 5 E
Indungo, *Angola* **115 E3** 14 48 S 16 17 E
Indura, *Belarus* **54 E10** 53 26N 23 53 E
Indus →, *Pakistan* **91 D2** 24 20N 67 47 E
Indus, Mouths of the, *Pakistan* **91 E3** 24 0N 68 0 E
Industry, *U.S.A.* **156 D6** 40 20N 90 36W
Inebolu, *Turkey* **100 B5** 41 55N 33 40 E
Inecik, *Turkey* **51 F11** 40 56N 27 16 E
Inegöl, *Turkey* **51 F13** 40 5N 29 31 E
Inés, Mt., *Argentina* **176 C3** 48 30 S 69 40W
Ineu, *Romania* **52 D6** 46 26N 21 51 E
Inezgane, *Morocco* **110 B3** 30 25N 9 29W
Infanta, *Phil.* **80 D3** 14 45N 121 39 E
Infantes = Villanueva de los Infantes, *Spain* **43 G7** 38 43N 3 1W
Infiernillo, Presa del, *Mexico* **162 D4** 18 9N 102 0W
Infiesto, *Spain* **42 B5** 43 21N 5 21W
Inga, Barrage d', *Dem. Rep. of the Congo* **115 D2** 5 39 S 13 39 E
Ingabu, *Burma* **90 G5** 17 37N 95 20 E
Inganda, *Dem. Rep. of the Congo* **114 C4** 0 5 S 20 57 E
Ingapirca, *Ecuador* **168 D2** 2 38 S 78 56W
Ingelstad, *Sweden* **17 H8** 56 45N 14 56 E
Ingende, *Dem. Rep. of the Congo* **114 C3** 0 12 S 18 57 E
Ingeniero Jacobacci, *Argentina* **176 B3** 41 20 S 69 36W
Ingenio, *Canary Is.* **9 e1** 27 55N 15 26W
Ingenio Santa Ana, *Argentina* **174 B2** 27 25 S 65 40W
Ingersoll, *Canada* **140 D3** 43 4N 80 55W
Ingham, *Australia* **126 B4** 18 43 S 146 10 E
Ingichka, *Uzbekistan* **65 D2** 39 47N 65 58 E
Ingleborough, *U.K.* **20 C5** 54 10N 2 22W
Inglefield Land, *Greenland* **10 B4** 78 30N 70 0W
Inglewood, *Queens., Australia* **127 D5** 28 25 S 151 2 E
Inglewood, *Vic., Australia* **128 D5** 36 29 S 143 53 E
Inglewood, *N.Z.* **130 F3** 39 9 S 174 14 E
Inglewood, *U.S.A.* **161 M8** 33 58N 118 21W
Inglis, *U.S.A.* **153 F7** 29 2N 82 40W
Ingolf Fjord, *Greenland* **10 A9** 80 35N 17 30W
Ingólfshöfði, *Iceland* **14 E5** 63 48N 16 39W
Ingolstadt, *Germany* **31 G7** 48 46N 11 26 E
Ingomar, *U.S.A.* **158 C10** 46 35N 107 23W
Ingonish, *Canada* **141 C7** 46 42N 60 18W
Ingore, *Guinea-Biss.* **112 C1** 12 24N 15 48W
Ingraj Bazar, *India* **93 G13** 24 58N 88 10 E
Ingrid Christensen Coast, *Antarctica* **7 C6** 69 30 S 76 0 E
Ingul = Inhul →, *Ukraine* **59 J7** 46 50N 32 0 E
Ingulec = Inhulec, *Ukraine* **59 J7** 47 42N 33 14 E
Ingulets = Inhulets →, *Ukraine* **59 J7** 46 46N 32 47 E
Inguri = Enguri →, *Georgia* **61 J5** 42 27N 41 38 E
Ingushetia □, *Russia* **61 J7** 43 20N 44 50 E
Ingwavuma, *S. Africa* **117 D5** 27 9 S 31 59 E
Inhaca, *Mozam.* **117 D5** 26 1 S 32 57 E
Inhafenga, *Mozam.* **117 C5** 20 36 S 33 53 E
Inhambane, *Mozam.* **117 C6** 23 54 S 35 30 E
Inhambane □, *Mozam.* **117 C5** 22 30 S 34 20 E
Inhambupe, *Brazil* **171 D4** 11 47 S 38 21W
Inhaminga, *Mozam.* **119 F4** 18 26 S 35 0 E
Inharrime, *Mozam.* **117 C6** 24 30 S 35 0 E
Inharrime →, *Mozam.* **117 C6** 24 30 S 35 0 E
Inhisar, *Turkey* **49 A12** 40 3N 30 23 E
Inhul →, *Ukraine* **59 J7** 46 50N 32 0 E
Inhulec, *Ukraine* **59 J7** 47 42N 33 14 E
Inhulets →, *Ukraine* **59 J7** 46 46N 32 47 E
Inhuma, *Brazil* **170 C3** 6 40 S 41 42W
Inhumas, *Brazil* **171 E2** 16 22 S 49 30W
Iniesta, *Spain* **41 F3** 39 27N 1 45W
Ining = Yining, *China* **66 E9** 43 58N 81 10 E
Inini □, *Fr. Guiana* **169 C7** 4 0N 53 0W
Inírida →, *Colombia* **168 C4** 3 55N 67 52W
Inishbofin, *Ireland* **23 C1** 53 37N 10 13W
Inisheer, *Ireland* **23 C2** 53 3N 9 32W
Inishfree B., *Ireland* **23 A3** 55 4N 8 23W
Inishkea North, *Ireland* **23 B1** 54 9N 10 11W
Inishkea South, *Ireland* **23 B1** 54 7N 10 12W
Inishmaan, *Ireland* **23 C2** 53 5N 9 35W
Inishmore, *Ireland* **23 C2** 53 8N 9 45W
Inishowen Pen., *Ireland* **23 A4** 55 14N 7 15W
Inishshark, *Ireland* **23 C1** 53 37N 10 16W
Inishturk, *Ireland* **23 C1** 53 42N 10 7W
Inishvickillane, *Ireland* **23 D1** 52 3N 10 37W
Injibara, *Ethiopia* **107 E4** 10 59N 37 0 E
Injune, *Australia* **127 D4** 25 53 S 148 32 E
Inkisi →, *Dem. Rep. of the Congo* **115 D3** 4 46 S 14 52 E
Inklin →, *Canada* **142 B2** 58 50N 133 10W
Inland Kaikoura Ra., *N.Z.* **131 B8** 41 59 S 173 41 E
Inland Sea = Setonaikai, *Japan* **72 C5** 34 20N 133 30 E
Inle L., *Burma* **90 E6** 20 30N 96 58 E
Inlet, *U.S.A.* **151 C10** 43 45N 74 48W
Inn →, *Austria* **34 C6** 48 35N 13 28 E
Innamincka, *Australia* **127 D3** 27 44 S 140 46 E
Innbygda, *Norway* **18 C9** 61 19N 12 17 E
Inner Hebrides, *U.K.* **22 E2** 57 0N 6 30W
Inner Mongolia = Nei Monggol Zizhiqu □, *China* **74 D7** 42 0N 112 0 E
Inner Sound, *U.K.* **22 D3** 57 30N 5 55W
Innerkip, *Canada* **150 C4** 43 13N 80 42W
Innerkirchen, *Switz.* **32 C6** 46 43N 8 14 E
Innes △, *Australia* **128 C2** 35 52 S 136 53 E
Innetalling I., *Canada* **140 A4** 56 0N 79 0W
Innisfail, *Australia* **126 B4** 17 33 S 146 5 E
Innisfail, *Canada* **142 C6** 52 2N 113 57W
In'noshima, *Japan* **72 C5** 34 19N 133 10 E
Innsbruck, *Austria* **34 D4** 47 16N 11 23 E
Innviertel, *Austria* **34 C6** 48 15N 13 15 E
Innvik, *Norway* **18 C3** 61 51N 6 37 E
Inny →, *Ireland* **23 C4** 53 30N 7 50W
Ino, *Japan* **72 D5** 33 33N 133 26 E
Inobonto, *Indonesia* **82 A2** 0 52N 123 57 E
Inocência, *Brazil* **171 E1** 19 47 S 51 48W
Inongo, *Dem. Rep. of the Congo* **114 C3** 1 55 S 18 30 E
Inoni, *Congo* **114 C3** 3 4 S 15 39 E
İnönü, *Turkey* **49 B12** 39 48N 30 9 E
Inoucdjouac = Inukjuak, *Canada* **139 C12** 58 25N 78 15W
Inowrocław, *Poland* **55 F5** 52 50N 18 12 E
Inpundong, *N. Korea* **75 D14** 41 25N 126 34 E
Inquisivi, *Bolivia* **172 D4** 16 50 S 67 10W
Ins, *Switz.* **32 B4** 47 1N 7 7 E
Inscription, C., *Australia* **125 E1** 25 29 S 112 59 E
Insein, *Burma* **90 G6** 16 50N 96 5 E
Insjön, *Sweden* **16 D9** 60 41N 15 6 E
Ińsko, *Poland* **54 E2** 53 25N 15 32 E
Insterberg = Chernyakhovsk, *Russia* **15 J19** 54 36N 21 48 E
Însurăţei, *Romania* **53 F12** 44 50N 27 40 E
Inta, *Russia* **56 A11** 66 5N 60 8 E
Intendente Alvear, *Argentina* **174 D3** 35 12 S 63 32W
Intepe, *Turkey* **49 A8** 40 1N 26 20 E
Interlachen, *U.S.A.* **153 F8** 29 37N 81 53W
Interlaken, *Switz.* **32 C5** 46 41N 7 50 E
Interlaken, *U.S.A.* **151 D8** 42 37N 76 44W
International Falls, *U.S.A.* **154 A8** 48 36N 93 25W
Interview I., *India* **95 H11** 12 55N 92 43 E
Intiyaco, *Argentina* **174 B3** 28 43 S 60 5W
Întorsura Buzăului, *Romania* **53 E11** 45 41N 26 2 E
Intragna, *Switz.* **33 D7** 46 11N 8 42 E
Intutu, *Peru* **168 D3** 3 32 S 74 48W
Inubō-Zaki, *Japan* **73 B12** 35 42N 140 52 E
Inukjuak, *Canada* **139 C12** 58 25N 78 15W
Inútil, B., *Chile* **176 D2** 53 30 S 70 15W
Inuvik, *Canada* **138 B6** 68 16N 133 40W
Inuyama, *Japan* **73 B8** 35 23N 136 56 E
Inveraray, *U.K.* **22 E3** 56 14N 5 5W
Inverbervie, *U.K.* **22 E6** 56 51N 2 17W
Invercargill, *N.Z.* **131 G3** 46 24 S 168 24 E
Inverclyde □, *U.K.* **22 F4** 55 55N 4 49W
Inverell, *Australia* **127 D5** 29 45 S 151 8 E
Invergordon, *U.K.* **22 D4** 57 41N 4 10W
Inverleigh, *Australia* **128 E6** 38 6 S 144 3 E
Inverloch, *Australia* **127 F4** 38 38 S 145 45 E
Invermere, *Canada* **142 C5** 50 30N 116 2W
Inverness, *Canada* **141 C7** 46 15N 61 19W
Inverness, *U.K.* **22 D4** 57 29N 4 13W
Inverness, *Ala., U.S.A.* **152 C4** 32 1N 85 45W
Inverness, *Fla., U.S.A.* **153 G7** 28 50N 82 20W
Inverurie, *U.K.* **22 D6** 57 17N 2 23W
Investigator Group, *Australia* **127 E1** 34 45 S 134 20 E
Investigator Str., *Australia* **128 C2** 35 30 S 137 0 E
Inya, *Russia* **66 D9** 50 28N 86 37 E
Inyanga, *Zimbabwe* **119 F3** 18 12 S 32 40 E
Inyangani, *Zimbabwe* **119 F3** 18 5 S 32 50 E
Inyantue, *Zimbabwe* **116 B4** 18 33 S 26 39 E
Inyo Mts., *U.S.A.* **160 J9** 36 40N 118 0W
Inyokern, *U.S.A.* **161 K9** 35 39N 117 49W
Inywa, *Burma* **90 D6** 23 56N 96 17 E
Inza, *Russia* **60 D8** 53 55N 46 25 E
Inzer, *Russia* **60 D10** 54 14N 57 34 E
Inzhavino, *Russia* **60 D6** 52 22N 42 30 E
Inzia →, *Dem. Rep. of the Congo* **115 C3** 3 45 S 17 57 E
Iō-Jima, *Japan* **71 J5** 30 48N 130 18 E
Ioánnina, *Greece* **48 B2** 39 42N 20 47 E
Ioánnina □, *Greece* **48 B2** 39 39N 20 57 E
Iokea, *Papua N. G.* **132 E4** 8 25 S 146 16 E
Iola, *U.S.A.* **155 G7** 37 55N 95 24W
Ioma, *Papua N. G.* **132 E4** 8 19 S 147 52 E
Ion Corvin, *Romania* **53 F12** 44 7N 27 50 E
Iôna, *Angola* **115 F2** 16 54 S 12 34 E
Iona, *U.K.* **22 E2** 56 20N 6 25W
Iona △, *Angola* **115 F2** 16 47 S 12 20 E
Ione, *U.S.A.* **160 G6** 38 21N 120 56W
Iongo, *Angola* **115 D3** 9 11 S 17 45 E
Ionia, *U.S.A.* **157 B11** 42 59N 85 4W
Ionian Is. = Iónioi Nísoi, *Greece* **39 B1** 38 40N 20 0 E
Ionian Sea, *Medit. S.* **12 H9** 37 30N 17 30 E
Iónioi Nísoi, *Greece* **39 B1** 38 40N 20 0 E
Iónioi Nísoi □, *Greece* **39 B2** 38 40N 20 0 E
Íos, *Greece* **49 E7** 36 41N 25 20 E
Iowa □, *U.S.A.* **156 C3** 42 18N 93 30W
Iowa →, *U.S.A.* **156 C5** 41 10N 91 1W
Iowa City, *U.S.A.* **156 C5** 41 40N 91 32W
Iowa Falls, *U.S.A.* **156 B3** 42 31N 93 16W
Iowa Park, *U.S.A.* **155 J5** 33 57N 98 40W
Ipala, *Tanzania* **118 C3** 4 30 S 32 52 E
Ipameri, *Brazil* **171 E2** 17 44 S 48 9W
Ipanema, *Brazil* **171 E3** 19 47 S 41 44W
Iparía, *Peru* **172 B3** 9 17 S 74 29W
Ipáti, *Greece* **48 C4** 38 52N 22 14 E
Ipatinga, *Brazil* **171 E3** 19 32 S 42 30W
Ipatovo, *Russia* **61 H6** 45 45N 42 50 E
Ipek = Peć, *Serbia & M.* **50 D4** 42 40N 20 17 E
Ipel' →, *Europe* **35 D11** 47 48N 18 53 E
Ipiales, *Colombia* **168 C2** 0 50N 77 37W
Ipiaú, *Brazil* **171 D4** 14 8 S 39 44W
Ipil, *Phil.* **81 H4** 7 47N 122 35 E
Ipin = Yibin, *China* **76 C5** 28 45N 104 32 E
Ipirá, *Brazil* **171 D4** 12 10 S 39 44W
Ipiranga, *Brazil* **168 D4** 3 13 S 65 57W
Ípiros □, *Greece* **48 B2** 39 30N 20 30 E
Ipixuna, *Brazil* **172 B3** 7 0 S 71 40W
Ipixuna →, *Amazonas, Brazil* **172 B3** 7 11 S 71 51W
Ipixuna →, *Amazonas, Brazil* **173 B5** 5 45 S 63 2W
Ipoh, *Malaysia* **87 K3** 4 35N 101 5 E
Iporá, *Brazil* **173 D7** 16 28 S 51 7W
Ipota, *Vanuatu* **133 H7** 18 52 S 169 20 E
Ippy, *C.A.R.* **114 A4** 6 5N 21 7 E
Ipsala, *Turkey* **51 F10** 40 55N 26 23 E
Ipsárion, Óros, *Greece* **51 F8** 40 40N 24 40 E
Ipsos, *Greece* **38 B9** 39 43N 19 48 E
Ipswich, *Australia* **127 D5** 27 35 S 152 40 E
Ipswich, *U.K.* **21 E9** 52 4N 1 10 E
Ipswich, *Mass., U.S.A.* **151 D14** 42 41N 70 50W
Ipswich, *S. Dak., U.S.A.* **154 C5** 45 27N 99 2W
Ipu, *Brazil* **170 B3** 4 23 S 40 44W
Ipueiras, *Brazil* **170 B3** 4 33 S 40 43W
Ipupiara, *Brazil* **171 D3** 11 49 S 42 37W
Iqaluit, *Canada* **139 B13** 63 44N 68 31W
Iquique, *Chile* **172 E3** 20 19 S 70 5W
Iquitos, *Peru* **168 D3** 3 45 S 73 10W
Ir Gannim = Bat Yam, *Israel* **103 C3** 32 2N 34 44 E
Irabu-Jima, *Japan* **71 M2** 24 50N 125 10 E
Iracoubo, *Fr. Guiana* **169 B7** 5 30N 53 10W
Īrafshān, *Iran* **97 E9** 26 42N 61 56 E
Irahuan, *Phil.* **81 G2** 9 48N 118 41 E
Iráklia, *Kikládhes, Greece* **49 E7** 36 50N 25 28 E
Iráklia, *Sérrai, Greece* **50 E7** 41 10N 23 16 E
Iraklio = Iráklion, *Greece* **39 E6** 35 20N 25 12 E
Iráklion, *Greece* **39 E6** 35 20N 25 12 E
Iráklion □, *Greece* **39 E6** 35 10N 25 10 E
Iraklion ✕ (HER), *Greece* **39 E6** 35 20N 25 15 E
Irako-Zaki, *Japan* **73 C9** 34 35N 137 1 E
Irala, *Paraguay* **175 B5** 25 55 S 54 35W
Iran ■, *Asia* **97 C7** 33 0N 53 0 E
Iran, Pegunungan, *Malaysia* **85 B4** 2 20N 114 50 E
Iran, Plateau of, *Asia* **62 F9** 32 0N 55 0 E
Iran Ra. = Iran, Pegunungan, *Malaysia* **85 B4** 2 20N 114 50 E
Iranamadu Tank, *Sri Lanka* **95 K5** 9 23N 80 29 E
Īrānshahr, *Iran* **97 E9** 27 15N 60 40 E
Irapa, *Venezuela* **169 A5** 10 34N 62 35W
Irapuato, *Mexico* **162 C4** 20 40N 101 30W
Iraq ■, *Asia* **101 F10** 33 0N 44 0 E
Irarrar, O. →, *Mali* **111 E5** 20 0N 1 30 E
Irarrarene, *Algeria* **111 C6** 27 37N 7 30 E
Irati, *Brazil* **175 B5** 25 25 S 50 38W
Irbes saurums, *Latvia* **54 A9** 57 45N 22 5 E
Irbid, *Jordan* **103 C4** 32 35N 35 48 E
Irbid □, *Jordan* **103 C5** 32 15N 36 35 E
Irbit, *Russia* **64 C9** 57 41N 63 3 E
Irebu, *Dem. Rep. of the Congo* **114 C3** 0 40 S 17 46 E
Irecê, *Brazil* **170 D3** 11 18 S 41 52W
Iregua →, *Spain* **40 C7** 42 27N 2 24 E
Ireland ■, *Europe* **23 C4** 53 50N 7 52W
Ireland I., *Bermuda* **9 a** 32 19N 64 50W
Irele, *Nigeria* **113 D6** 7 40N 5 40 E
Iremel, Gora, *Russia* **64 D7** 54 33N 58 50 E
Ireng →, *Brazil* **169 C6** 3 33N 59 51W
Irerrer, O. →, *Algeria* **111 E6** 19 25N 5 47 E
Irgiz, Bolshaya →, *Russia* **60 D9** 52 10N 49 10 E
Irharrhar, O. →, *Algeria* **111 C6** 28 3N 6 15 E
Irherm, *Morocco* **110 B3** 30 7N 8 18W
Irhil M'Goun, *Morocco* **110 B3** 31 30N 6 28W
Irhyangdong, *N. Korea* **75 D15** 41 15N 129 30 E
Iri, *S. Korea* **75 G14** 35 59N 127 0 E
Irian Barat = Papua □, *Indonesia* **83 B5** 4 0 S 137 0 E
Irian Jaya = Papua □, *Indonesia* **83 B5** 4 0 S 137 0 E
Iriba, *Chad* **109 E4** 15 7N 22 15 E
Irié, *Guinea* **112 D3** 8 15N 9 10W
Iriga, *Phil.* **80 E4** 13 25N 123 25 E
Iriklinskiy, *Russia* **64 F7** 51 39N 58 38 E
Iriklinskoye Vdkhr., *Russia* **64 F7** 52 0N 59 0 E
Iringa, *Tanzania* **118 D4** 7 48 S 35 43 E
Iringa □, *Tanzania* **118 D4** 7 48 S 35 43 E
Irinjalakuda, *India* **95 J3** 10 21N 76 14 E
Iriomote △, *Japan* **71 M1** 24 29N 123 53 E
Iriomote-Jima, *Japan* **71 M1** 24 19N 123 48 E
Iriona, *Honduras* **164 C2** 15 57N 85 11W
Iriri →, *Brazil* **169 D7** 3 52 S 52 37W
Iriri Novo →, *Brazil* **173 B7** 8 46 S 53 22W
Irish Free State = Ireland ■, *Europe* **23 C4** 53 50N 7 52W
Irish Republic ■, *Europe* **23 C4** 53 50N 7 52W
Irish Sea, *Europe* **20 D3** 53 38N 4 48W
Irkeshtam = Erkech-Tam, *Kyrgyzstan* **65 D6** 39 41N 73 55 E
Irkutsk, *Russia* **67 D11** 52 18N 104 20 E
Irlığanlı, *Turkey* **49 D11** 37 53N 29 12 E
Irma, *Canada* **143 C6** 52 55N 111 14W
Irō-Zaki, *Japan* **73 C10** 34 36N 138 51 E
Iroise, Mer d', *France* **26 D2** 48 15N 4 45W
Iron Baron, *Australia* **128 B2** 32 58 S 137 11 E
Iron Gate = Portile de Fier, *Europe* **52 F7** 44 44N 22 30 E
Iron Knob, *Australia* **128 B2** 32 46 S 137 8 E
Iron Mountain, *U.S.A.* **148 C1** 45 49N 88 4W
Iron Range △, *Australia* **126 A3** 12 34 S 143 18 E
Iron River, *U.S.A.* **154 B10** 46 6N 88 39W
Irondequoit, *U.S.A.* **150 C7** 43 13N 77 35W
Ironton, *Mo., U.S.A.* **155 G9** 37 36N 90 38W
Ironton, *Ohio, U.S.A.* **148 F4** 38 32N 82 41W
Ironwood, *U.S.A.* **154 B9** 46 27N 90 9W
Ironwood Forest ⌂, *U.S.A.* **159 K8** 32 28N 111 36W
Iroquois, *Canada* **151 B9** 44 51N 75 19W
Iroquois →, *U.S.A.* **157 C9** 41 5N 87 49W
Iroquois Falls, *Canada* **140 C3** 48 46N 80 41W
Irosin, *Phil.* **80 E5** 12 42N 124 2 E
Irpin, *Ukraine* **59 G6** 50 30N 30 15 E
Irqieqa, Ras I-, *Malta* **38 F7** 35 56N 14 29 E
Irrara Cr. →, *Australia* **127 D4** 29 35 S 145 31 E
Irrawaddy □, *Burma* **90 G5** 17 0N 95 0 E
Irrawaddy →, *Burma* **90 G5** 15 50N 95 6 E
Irrawaddy, Mouths of the, *Burma* **90 H5** 15 30N 95 0 E
Irricana, *Canada* **142 C6** 51 19N 113 37W
Irshava, *Ukraine* **52 B8** 48 19N 23 3 E
Irsina, *Italy* **47 B9** 40 45N 16 14 E
Irtysh →, *Russia* **66 C7** 61 4N 68 52 E
Irumu, *Dem. Rep. of the Congo* **118 B2** 1 32N 29 53 E
Irún, *Spain* **40 B3** 43 20N 1 52W
Iruñea = Pamplona, *Spain* **40 C3** 42 48N 1 38W
Irurzun, *Spain* **40 C3** 42 55N 1 50W
Irvine, *U.K.* **22 F4** 55 37N 4 41W
Irvine, *Calif., U.S.A.* **161 M9** 33 41N 117 46W
Irvine, *Ky., U.S.A.* **157 G13** 37 42N 83 58W
Irvinestown, *U.K.* **23 B4** 54 28N 7 39W
Irving, *U.S.A.* **155 J6** 32 49N 96 56W
Irvington, *U.S.A.* **157 G10** 37 53N 86 17W
Irvona, *U.S.A.* **150 F6** 40 46N 78 33W
Irwin →, *Australia* **125 E1** 29 15 S 114 54 E
Irwinton, *U.S.A.* **152 C6** 32 49N 83 10W
Irwinville, *U.S.A.* **152 D6** 31 39N 83 23W
Irymple, *Australia* **128 C5** 34 14 S 142 8 E
Is, Jebel, *Sudan* **106 C4** 22 3N 35 28 E
Is-sur-Tille, *France* **27 E12** 47 30N 5 8 E
Isa, *Nigeria* **113 C6** 13 14N 6 24 E
Isa Khel, *Pakistan* **92 C4** 32 41N 71 17 E
Isaac →, *Australia* **126 C4** 22 55 S 149 20 E
Isabel, *U.S.A.* **154 C4** 45 24N 101 26W
Isabela, *Basilan, Phil.* **81 H3** 6 40N 121 59 E
Isabela, *Negros, Phil.* **81 F4** 10 12N 122 59 E
Isabela, *Puerto Rico* **165 d** 18 30N 67 2W
Isabela □, *Phil.* **80 C4** 17 0N 122 0 E
Isabela, Canal, *Ecuador* **172 a** 0 20 S 90 55W
Isabela, I., *Ecuador* **172 a** 0 30 S 91 4W
Isabela, I., *Mexico* **162 C3** 21 51N 105 55W
Isabela, Cord., *Nic.* **164 D2** 13 30N 85 25W
Isabella Ra., *Australia* **124 D3** 21 0 S 121 4 E
Isaccea, *Romania* **53 E13** 45 16N 28 28 E
Ísafjarðardjúp, *Iceland* **11 A3** 66 10N 23 0W
Ísafjarðarsýsla □, *Iceland* **11 B3** 66 0N 23 0W
Ísafjörður, *Iceland* **11 A3** 66 5N 23 9W
Isagarh, *India* **92 G7** 24 48N 77 51 E
Isahaya, *Japan* **72 E2** 32 52N 130 2 E
Isaka, *Dem. Rep. of the Congo* **114 C3** 2 33 S 18 54 E
Isaka, *Tanzania* **118 C3** 3 56 S 32 59 E
Işalniţa, *Romania* **53 F8** 44 24N 23 44 E
Isalo △, *Madag.* **117 C8** 22 23 S 45 16 E
Isan →, *India* **93 F9** 26 51N 80 7 E
Isana = Içana →, *Brazil* **168 C4** 0 26N 67 19W
Isandja, *Dem. Rep. of the Congo* **114 C4** 2 59 S 21 59 E
Isangano △, *Zambia* **119 E3** 11 8 S 30 35 E
Isangi, *Dem. Rep. of the Congo* **114 B4** 0 52N 24 10 E
Isanlu Makutu, *Nigeria* **113 D6** 8 20N 5 50 E
Isar →, *Germany* **31 G8** 48 48N 12 57 E
Isarco →, *Italy* **45 B8** 46 27N 11 18 E
Ísari, *Greece* **48 D3** 37 22N 22 0 E
Isarog, Mt., *Phil.* **80 E4** 13 39N 123 23 E
Íscar, *Spain* **42 D6** 41 22N 4 32W
Iscayachi, *Bolivia* **173 E4** 21 31 S 65 3W
İscehisar, *Turkey* **49 C12** 38 51N 30 45 E
Ischgl, *Austria* **33 B10** 47 1N 10 17 E
Íschia, *Italy* **46 B6** 40 44N 13 57 E
Iscuandé, *Colombia* **168 C2** 2 28N 77 59W
Isdell →, *Australia* **124 C3** 16 27 S 124 51 E
Ise, *Japan* **73 C8** 34 25N 136 45 E
Ise-Shima △, *Japan* **73 C8** 34 25N 136 48 E
Ise-Wan, *Japan* **73 C8** 34 43N 136 43 E
Isefjord, *Denmark* **17 J5** 55 53N 11 50 E
Isel →, *Austria* **34 E5** 46 50N 12 47 E
Iseltwald, *Switz.* **32 C5** 46 43N 7 58 E
Isenthal, *Switz.* **33 C7** 46 55N 8 34 E
Iseo, *Italy* **44 C7** 45 39N 10 3 E
Iseo, L. d', *Italy* **44 C7** 45 43N 10 4 E
Iseramagazi, *Tanzania* **118 C3** 4 37 S 32 10 E
Isère □, *France* **29 C9** 45 15N 5 40 E
Isère →, *France* **29 D8** 44 59N 4 51 E
Iserlohn, *Germany* **30 D3** 51 22N 7 41 E
Isérnia, *Italy* **47 A7** 41 36N 14 14 E
Isesaki, *Japan* **73 A11** 36 19N 139 12 E
Iseyin, *Nigeria* **113 D5** 8 0N 3 36 E
Isfahan = Eşfahān, *Iran* **97 C6** 32 39N 51 43 E
Isfana, *Kyrgyzstan* **65 D4** 39 50N 69 31 E
Isfara, *Tajikistan* **65 C5** 40 7N 70 38 E
Isfjorden, *Norway* **18 B4** 62 35N 7 49 E
Ishëm, *Albania* **50 E3** 41 33N 19 34 E
Ishenga Oshwe, *Dem. Rep. of the Congo* **114 C4** 3 57 S 22 33 E
Isherton, *Guyana* **169 C6** 2 20N 59 25W
Ishigaki-Shima, *Japan* **71 M2** 24 20N 124 10 E
Ishikari-Gawa →, *Japan* **70 C10** 43 15N 141 23 E
Ishikari-Sammyaku, *Japan* **70 C11** 43 30N 143 0 E
Ishikari-Wan, *Japan* **70 C10** 43 25N 141 1 E
Ishikawa □, *Japan* **73 A8** 36 30N 136 30 E
Ishim, *Russia* **66 D7** 56 10N 69 30 E
Ishim →, *Russia* **66 D8** 57 45N 71 10 E
Ishimbay, *Russia* **64 E6** 53 28N 56 2 E
Ishinomaki, *Japan* **70 E10** 38 32N 141 20 E
Ishioka, *Japan* **73 A12** 36 11N 140 16 E
Ishizuchi-Yama, *Japan* **72 D5** 33 45N 133 6 E
Ishkashim, *Tajikistan* **65 E5** 36 44N 71 37 E
Ishkuman, *Pakistan* **93 A5** 36 30N 73 50 E
Ishpeming, *U.S.A.* **148 B2** 46 29N 87 40W
Ishtykhan, *Uzbekistan* **65 D3** 39 58N 66 29 E
Ishurdi, *Bangla.* **90 C2** 24 9N 89 3 E
Isiboro Sécure △, *Bolivia* **173 D4** 16 15 S 65 50W
Isigny-sur-Mer, *France* **26 C5** 49 19N 1 6W
Isıklar Dağı, *Turkey* **51 F11** 40 45N 27 15 E
Işıklı, *Turkey* **49 C11** 38 19N 29 51 E
Isil Kul, *Russia* **66 D8** 54 55N 71 16 E
Ísili, *Italy* **46 C2** 39 44N 9 6 E
Isiolo, *Kenya* **118 B4** 0 24N 37 33 E
Isiro, *Dem. Rep. of the Congo* **118 B2** 2 53N 27 40 E
Isisford, *Australia* **126 C3** 24 15 S 144 21 E
Iskandar, *Uzbekistan* **65 C4** 41 36N 69 41 E
İskenderun, *Turkey* **100 D7** 36 32N 36 10 E
İskenderun Körfezi, *Turkey* **100 D6** 36 40N 35 50 E
Iski-Naukat = Eski-Nookat, *Kyrgyzstan* **65 C6** 40 16N 72 36 E
Iskilip, *Turkey* **100 B6** 40 45N 34 29 E
Iskŭr →, *Bulgaria* **51 C8** 43 45N 24 25 E
Iskŭr, Yazovir, *Bulgaria* **50 D7** 42 23N 23 30 E
Iskut →, *Canada* **142 B2** 56 45N 131 49W
Isla →, *U.K.* **22 E5** 56 32N 3 20W
Isla Coiba △, *Panama* **164 E3** 7 33N 81 36W
Isla Cristina, *Spain* **43 H3** 37 13N 7 17W
Isla de Salamanca △, *Colombia* **165 D5** 10 59N 74 40W
Isla Gorge △, *Australia* **126 D4** 25 10 S 149 57 E
Isla Gorgona △, *Colombia* **168 C2** 2 59N 78 10W
Isla Guamblin △, *Chile* **176 B1** 44 50 S 75 4W
Isla Magdalena △, *Chile* **176 B2** 44 40 S 73 13W
Isla Tiburón y San Esteban ⌂, *Mexico* **162 B2** 29 0N 112 27W
Isla Vista, *U.S.A.* **161 L7** 34 25N 119 53W
Islâhiye, *Turkey* **100 D7** 37 0N 36 35 E
Islam Headworks, *Pakistan* **92 E5** 29 49N 72 33 E
Islamabad, *Pakistan* **91 B4** 33 40N 73 10 E
Islamgarh, *Pakistan* **92 F4** 27 51N 70 48 E
Islamkot, *Pakistan* **92 G4** 24 42N 70 13 E
Islamorada, *U.S.A.* **153 L9** 24 56N 80 37W
Islampur, *Bihar, India* **93 G11** 25 9N 85 12 E
Islampur, *Maharashtra, India* **94 F2** 17 2N 74 20 E
Island = Iceland ■, *Europe* **11 C8** 64 45N 19 0W
Island Bay, *Phil.* **81 G2** 9 6N 118 10 E
Island L., *Canada* **143 C10** 53 47N 94 25W
Island Lagoon, *Australia* **128 A2** 31 30 S 136 40 E
Island Pond, *U.S.A.* **151 B13** 44 49N 71 53W
Islands, B. of, *Canada* **141 C8** 49 11N 58 15W
Islands, B. of, *N.Z.* **130 B3** 35 15 S 174 6 E
Islay, *U.K.* **22 F2** 55 46N 6 10W
Isle →, *France* **28 D3** 44 55N 0 15W
Isle aux Morts, *Canada* **141 C8** 47 35N 59 0W
Isle of Hope, *U.S.A.* **152 D8** 31 58N 81 5W
Isle of Wight □, *U.K.* **21 G6** 50 41N 1 17W
Isle Royale △, *U.S.A.* **148 B1** 48 0N 88 55W
Isleton, *U.S.A.* **160 G5** 38 10N 121 37W
Ismail = Izmayil, *Ukraine* **53 E13** 45 22N 28 46 E
Ismâ'ilîya, *Egypt* **106 H8** 30 37N 32 18 E
Ismaning, *Germany* **31 G7** 48 13N 11 40 E
Isna, *Egypt* **106 B3** 25 17N 32 30 E
Isoanala, *Madag.* **117 C8** 23 50 S 45 44 E
Isogstalo, *India* **93 B8** 34 15N 78 46 E
Ísola del Liri, *Italy* **45 G10** 41 41N 13 34 E
Ísola della Scala, *Italy* **44 C7** 45 16N 11 0 E
Ísola di Capo Rizzuto, *Italy* **47 D10** 38 58N 17 6 E
Isparta, *Turkey* **49 D12** 37 47N 30 30 E
Isperikh, *Bulgaria* **51 C10** 43 43N 26 50 E
Íspica, *Italy* **47 F7** 36 47N 14 55 E
Israel ■, *Asia* **103 D3** 32 0N 34 50 E
Isratu, *Eritrea* **107 D4** 16 20N 39 53 E
Issakly, *Russia* **60 C10** 54 8N 51 32 E

Issano, *Guyana* **169 B6** 5 49N 59 26W
Issia, *Ivory C.* **112 D3** 6 33N 6 33W
Issoire, *France* **28 C7** 45 32N 3 15 E
Issoudun, *France* **27 F8** 46 57N 1 59 E
Issyk-Kul = Balykchy, *Kyrgyzstan* **65 B8** 42 26N 76 12 E
Issyk-Kul, Ozero = Ysyk-Köl, *Kyrgyzstan* **65 B8** 42 25N 77 15 E
Ist, *Croatia* **45 D11** 44 17N 14 47 E
Istaihah, *U.A.E.* **99 B6** 23 19N 54 4 E
Istállós-kő, *Hungary* **52 B5** 48 4N 20 26 E
İstanbul, *Turkey* **51 E12** 41 0N 29 0 E
İstanbul □, *Turkey* **51 E12** 41 0N 29 0 E
Istanbul ✕ (IST), *Turkey* **51 F12** 40 59N 28 49 E
İstanbul Boğazı, *Turkey* **51 E13** 41 10N 29 10 E
Isteren, *Norway* **18 B8** 61 58N 11 47 E
Istiaía, *Greece* **48 C5** 38 57N 23 9 E
Istiea = Istiaía, *Greece* **48 C5** 38 57N 23 9 E
Istmina, *Colombia* **168 B2** 5 10N 76 39W
Isto, Mt., *U.S.A.* **144 B12** 69 12N 143 48W
Istok, *Serbia & M.* **50 D4** 42 45N 20 24 E
Istokpoga, L., *U.S.A.* **153 H8** 27 23N 81 17W
Istra, *Croatia* **45 C10** 45 10N 14 0 E
Istres, *France* **29 E8** 43 31N 4 59 E
Istria = Istra, *Croatia* **45 C10** 45 10N 14 0 E
Isugod, *Phil.* **81 G2** 9 19N 118 5 E
Isulan, *Phil.* **81 H5** 6 30N 124 29 E
Itá, *Paraguay* **174 B4** 25 29 S 57 21W
Itabaiana, *Paraíba, Brazil* **170 C4** 7 18 S 35 19W
Itabaiana, *Sergipe, Brazil* **170 D4** 10 41 S 37 37W
Itabaianinha, *Brazil* **170 D4** 11 16 S 37 47W
Itaberaba, *Brazil* **171 D3** 12 32 S 40 18W
Itaberaí, *Brazil* **171 E2** 16 2 S 49 48W
Itabira, *Brazil* **171 E3** 19 37 S 43 13W
Itabirito, *Brazil* **171 F3** 20 15 S 43 48W
Itaboca, *Brazil* **169 D5** 4 50 S 62 40W
Itabuna, *Brazil* **171 D4** 14 48 S 39 16W
Itacajá, *Brazil* **170 C2** 8 19 S 47 46W
Itacaunas →, *Brazil* **170 C2** 5 21 S 49 8W
Itacuaí →, *Brazil* **172 A3** 4 20 S 70 12W
Itaguaçu, *Brazil* **171 E3** 19 48 S 40 51W
Itaguari →, *Brazil* **171 D3** 14 11 S 44 40W
Itaguatins, *Brazil* **170 C2** 5 47 S 47 29W
Itaim →, *Brazil* **170 C3** 7 2 S 42 2W
Itainópolis, *Brazil* **170 C3** 7 24 S 41 31W
Itaipú, Représa de, *Brazil* **175 B5** 25 30 S 54 30W
Itaituba, *Brazil* **169 D6** 4 10 S 55 50W
Itajaí, *Brazil* **175 B6** 27 50 S 48 39W
Itajany do Sul = Rio do Sul, *Brazil* **175 B6** 27 13 S 49 37W
Itajubá, *Brazil* **171 F2** 22 24 S 45 30W
Itajuípe, *Brazil* **171 D4** 14 41 S 39 22W
Itaka, *Tanzania* **119 D3** 8 50 S 32 49 E
Itako, *Japan* **73 B12** 35 56N 140 33 E
Itala ⌂, *S. Africa* **117 D5** 27 30 S 31 7 E
Italy ■, *Europe* **13 G8** 42 0N 13 0 E
Itamaraju, *Brazil* **171 E4** 17 4 S 39 32W
Itamarati, *Brazil* **172 B4** 6 24 S 68 15W
Itamataré, *Brazil* **170 B2** 2 16 S 46 24W
Itambacuri, *Brazil* **171 E3** 18 1 S 41 42W
Itambé, *Brazil* **171 E3** 15 15 S 40 37W
Itami, *Japan* **73 C7** 34 46N 135 25 E
Itampolo, *Madag.* **117 C7** 24 41 S 43 57 E
Itandrano, *Madag.* **117 C8** 21 47 S 45 17 E
Itanhaém, *Brazil* **171 F2** 24 11 S 46 47W
Itanhauã →, *Brazil* **169 D5** 4 45 S 63 48W
Itanhém, *Brazil* **171 E3** 17 9 S 40 20W
Itano, *Japan* **72 C6** 34 7N 134 28 E
Itapaci, *Brazil* **171 D2** 14 57 S 49 34W
Itapagé, *Brazil* **170 B4** 3 41 S 39 34W
Itaparica = Petrolândia, *Brazil* **170 C4** 9 5 S 38 20W
Itaparica, I. de, *Brazil* **171 D4** 12 54 S 38 42W
Itapebi, *Brazil* **171 E4** 15 56 S 39 32W
Itapecuru-Mirim, *Brazil* **170 B3** 3 24 S 44 20W
Itaperuna, *Brazil* **171 F3** 21 10 S 41 54W
Itapetinga, *Brazil* **171 E3** 15 15 S 40 15W
Itapetininga, *Brazil* **175 A6** 23 36 S 48 7W
Itapeva, *Brazil* **175 A6** 23 59 S 48 59W
Itapicuru →, *Bahia, Brazil* **170 D4** 11 47 S 37 32W
Itapicuru →, *Maranhão, Brazil* **170 B3** 2 52 S 44 12W
Itapinima, *Brazil* **173 B5** 5 25 S 60 44W
Itapipoca, *Brazil* **170 B4** 3 30 S 39 35W
Itapira = Ubaitaba, *Brazil* **171 D4** 14 18 S 39 20W
Itapiranga, *Brazil* **169 D6** 2 45 S 58 1W
Itapiúna, *Brazil* **170 B4** 4 33 S 38 57W
Itaporanga, *Paraíba, Brazil* **170 C4** 7 18 S 38 0W
Itaporanga, *São Paulo, Brazil* **171 F2** 23 42 S 49 29W
Itapuá □, *Paraguay* **175 B4** 26 40 S 55 40W
Itapuranga, *Brazil* **171 E2** 15 40 S 49 59W
Itaquari, *Brazil* **171 F3** 20 20 S 40 25W
Itaquatiara, *Brazil* **169 D6** 2 58 S 58 30W
Itaquí, *Brazil* **174 B4** 29 8 S 56 30W
Itararé, *Brazil* **175 A6** 24 6 S 49 23W
Itarsi, *India* **92 H7** 22 36N 77 51 E
Itarumã, *Brazil* **171 E1** 18 42 S 51 25W
Itatí, *Argentina* **174 B4** 27 16 S 58 15W
Itatiaia △, *Brazil* **175 A7** 22 22 S 44 38W
Itatira, *Brazil* **170 B4** 4 30 S 39 37W
Itatuba, *Brazil* **173 B5** 5 46 S 63 20W
Itatupa, *Brazil* **169 D7** 0 37 S 51 12W
Itaueira, *Brazil* **170 C3** 7 36 S 43 2W
Itaueira →, *Brazil* **170 C3** 6 41 S 42 55W
Itaúna, *Brazil* **171 F3** 20 4 S 44 34W
Itbayat, *Phil.* **80 A3** 20 47N 121 51 E
Itbayat I., *Phil.* **80 A3** 20 45N 121 50 E
Itchen →, *U.K.* **21 G6** 50 55N 1 22W
Itchouma, *Niger* **111 D7** 20 14N 13 32 E
Ite, *Peru* **172 D3** 17 55 S 70 57W
Itéa, *Greece* **48 C4** 38 25N 22 25 E
Itezhi Tezhi, L., *Zambia* **119 F2** 15 30 S 25 30 E
Ithaca = Itháki, *Greece* **39 C2** 38 25N 20 40 E
Ithaca, *U.S.A.* **151 D8** 42 27N 76 30W
Itháki, *Greece* **39 C2** 38 25N 20 40 E
Íti △, *Greece* **48 C4** 38 50N 22 15 E
Itinga, *Brazil* **171 E3** 16 36 S 41 47W
Itiquira, *Brazil* **173 D7** 17 12 S 54 7W
Itiquira →, *Brazil* **173 D6** 17 18 S 56 44W
Itiruçu, *Brazil* **171 D3** 13 31 S 40 9W
Itiúba, *Brazil* **170 D4** 10 43 S 39 51W
Itkilik →, *U.S.A.* **144 A10** 70 9N 150 56W
Itō, *Japan* **73 C11** 34 58N 139 5 E
Itogon, *Phil.* **80 C3** 16 22N 120 41 E
Itoigawa, *Japan* **71 F8** 37 2N 137 51 E
Itoko, *Dem. Rep. of the Congo* **114 C4** 1 0 S 21 48 E
Iton →, *France* **26 C8** 49 9N 1 12 E
Itonamas →, *Bolivia* **173 C5** 12 28 S 64 24W
Itri, *Italy* **46 A6** 41 17N 13 32 E
Itsa, *Egypt* **106 J7** 29 15N 30 47 E
Itsuki, *Japan* **72 E2** 32 24N 130 50 E
Íttiri, *Italy* **46 B1** 40 36N 8 34 E
Ittoqqortoormiit, *Greenland* **10 C8** 70 20N 23 0W
Itu, *Brazil* **175 A6** 23 17 S 47 15W
Itu, *Nigeria* **113 D6** 5 10N 7 58 E
Itu Aba I., *S. China Sea* **78 B4** 10 23N 114 21 E
Ituaçu, *Brazil* **171 D3** 13 50 S 41 18W
Ituango, *Colombia* **168 B2** 7 4N 75 45W
Ituí →, *Brazil* **168 D3** 4 38 S 70 19W
Ituiutaba, *Brazil* **171 E2** 19 0 S 49 25W
Itumbiara, *Brazil* **171 E2** 18 20 S 49 10W
Ituna, *Canada* **143 C8** 51 10N 103 24W
Itunge Port, *Tanzania* **119 D3** 9 40 S 33 55 E
Ituni, *Guyana* **169 B6** 5 28N 58 15W
Itupiranga, *Brazil* **170 C2** 5 9 S 49 20W
Iturama, *Brazil* **171 E1** 19 44 S 50 11W
Iturbe, *Argentina* **174 A2** 23 0 S 65 25W
Ituri →, *Dem. Rep. of the Congo* **118 B2** 1 40N 27 1 E
Iturup, Ostrov, *Russia* **67 E15** 45 0N 148 0 E
Ituverava, *Brazil* **171 F2** 20 20 S 47 47W
Ituxi →, *Brazil* **173 B5** 7 18 S 64 51W
Ituyuro →, *Argentina* **174 A3** 22 40 S 63 50W
Itzehoe, *Germany* **30 B5** 53 55N 9 31 E
Iuka, *U.S.A.* **157 F8** 38 37N 88 47W
Ivahona, *Madag.* **117 C8** 23 27 S 46 10 E
Ivaí →, *Brazil* **175 A5** 23 18 S 53 42W
Ivalo, *Finland* **14 B22** 68 38N 27 35 E
Ivalojoki →, *Finland* **14 B22** 68 40N 27 40 E
Ivanava, *Belarus* **59 F3** 52 7N 25 29 E
Ivančice, *Czech Rep.* **35 B9** 49 6N 16 23 E
Ivane-Puste, *Ukraine* **53 B11** 48 39N 26 10 E
Ivăneşti, *Romania* **53 D12** 46 39N 27 27 E
Ivangorod = Dęblin, *Poland* **55 G8** 51 34N 21 50 E
Ivangorod, *Russia* **58 C5** 59 27N 28 13 E
Ivanhoe, *N.S.W., Australia* **128 B6** 32 56 S 144 20 E
Ivanhoe, *Vic., Australia* **129 D6** 37 46 S 145 2 E
Ivanhoe, *Calif., U.S.A.* **160 J7** 36 23N 119 13W
Ivanhoe, *Minn., U.S.A.* **154 C6** 44 28N 96 15W
Ivanhorod, *Ukraine* **53 B14** 48 48N 29 50 E
Ivanić Grad, *Croatia* **45 C13** 45 41N 16 25 E
Ivanjica, *Serbia & M.* **50 C4** 43 35N 20 12 E
Ivanjska, *Bos.-H.* **52 F2** 44 55N 17 4 E
Ivankoyskoye Vdkhr., *Russia* **58 D9** 56 37N 36 32 E
Ivano-Frankivsk, *Ukraine* **53 B9** 48 40N 24 40 E
Ivano-Frankivska □, *Ukraine* **53 B9** 48 45N 24 30 E
Ivanof Bay, *U.S.A.* **144 J8** 55 54N 159 29W
Ivanovka, *Kyrgyzstan* **65 B7** 42 53N 75 6 E
Ivanovo = Ivanava, *Belarus* **59 F3** 52 7N 25 29 E
Ivanovo, *Russia* **58 D11** 57 5N 41 0 E
Ivanšćica, *Croatia* **45 B13** 46 12N 16 13 E
Ivashchenkovo = Chapayevsk, *Russia* **60 D9** 53 0N 49 40 E
Ivato, *Madag.* **117 C8** 20 37 S 47 10 E
Ivatsevichy, *Belarus* **59 F3** 52 43N 25 21 E
Ivaylovgrad, *Bulgaria* **51 E10** 41 32N 26 8 E
Ivdel, *Russia* **56 B11** 60 42N 60 24 E
Ivgres = Komsomolsk, *Russia* **58 D11** 57 2N 40 20 E
Ivindo →, *Gabon* **114 C2** 0 9 S 12 9 E
Ivinheima →, *Brazil* **175 A5** 23 14 S 53 42W
Ivinhema, *Brazil* **175 A5** 22 10 S 53 37W
Ivittuut, *Greenland* **10 E6** 61 14N 48 12W
Iviza = Eivissa, *Spain* **38 D1** 38 54N 1 26 E
Ivohibe, *Madag.* **117 C8** 22 31 S 46 57 E
Ivolândia, *Brazil* **171 E1** 16 34 S 50 51W
Ivory Coast, *W. Afr.* **112 E4** 4 20N 5 0W
Ivory Coast ■, *Africa* **112 D4** 7 30N 5 0W
Ivösjön, *Sweden* **17 H8** 56 8N 14 25 E
Ivrea, *Italy* **44 C4** 45 28N 7 52 E
İvrindi, *Turkey* **49 B9** 39 34N 27 30 E
Ivujivik, *Canada* **139 B12** 62 24N 77 55W
Ivvavik △, *Canada* **144 B13** 69 6N 139 30W
Ivybridge, *U.K.* **21 G4** 50 23N 3 56W
Iwai-Jima, *Japan* **72 D3** 33 47N 131 58 E
Iwaizumi, *Japan* **70 E10** 39 50N 141 45 E
Iwaki, *Japan* **71 F10** 37 3N 140 55 E
Iwakuni, *Japan* **72 C4** 34 15N 132 8 E
Iwami, *Japan* **72 B6** 35 32N 134 15 E
Iwamizawa, *Japan* **70 C10** 43 12N 141 46 E
Iwanai, *Japan* **70 C10** 42 58N 140 30 E
Iwase, *Japan* **73 A12** 36 21N 140 6 E
Iwata, *Japan* **73 C9** 34 42N 137 51 E
Iwate □, *Japan* **70 E10** 39 30N 141 30 E
Iwate-San, *Japan* **70 E10** 39 51N 141 0 E
Iwo, *Nigeria* **113 D5** 7 39N 4 9 E
Iwonicz-Zdrój, *Poland* **55 J8** 49 37N 21 47 E
Iwungu, *Dem. Rep. of the Congo* **115 D3** 5 16 S 19 17 E
Ixiamas, *Bolivia* **172 C4** 13 50 S 68 5W
Ixopo, *S. Africa* **117 E5** 30 11 S 30 5 E
Ixtepec, *Mexico* **163 D5** 16 32N 95 10W
Ixtlán del Río, *Mexico* **162 C4** 21 5N 104 21W
'Iyādh, *Yemen* **98 D4** 14 59N 46 51 E
Iyal Bakhit, *Sudan* **107 E2** 13 20N 28 39 E
Iyo, *Japan* **72 D4** 33 45N 132 45 E
Iyo-Mishima, *Japan* **72 D5** 33 58N 133 30 E
Iyo-Nada, *Japan* **72 D4** 33 40N 132 20 E
Izabal, L. de, *Guatemala* **164 C2** 15 30N 89 10W
Izamal, *Mexico* **163 C7** 20 56N 89 1W
Izberbash, *Russia* **61 J8** 42 35N 47 52 E
Izbica, *Poland* **55 H10** 50 53N 23 10 E
Izbica Kujawska, *Poland* **55 F5** 52 25N 18 40 E
Izbiceni, *Romania* **53 G9** 43 45N 24 40 E
Izena-Shima, *Japan* **71 L3** 26 56N 127 56 E
Izgrev, *Bulgaria* **51 C10** 43 36N 26 58 E
Izh →, *Russia* **64 C4** 56 9N 53 0 E
Izhevsk, *Russia* **64 C4** 56 51N 53 14 E
Izhma = Sosnogorsk, *Russia* **56 B9** 63 37N 53 51 E
Izhma →, *Russia* **56 A9** 65 19N 52 54 E
Izileg, *Algeria* **111 D6** 20 20N 6 4 E
Izkī, *Oman* **99 B7** 22 56N 57 46 E
Izmayil, *Ukraine* **53 E13** 45 22N 28 46 E
İzmir, *Turkey* **49 C9** 38 25N 27 8 E
İzmir □, *Turkey* **49 C9** 38 15N 27 40 E
İzmir Adnan Menderes ✕ (ADB), *Turkey* **49 C9** 38 23N 27 6 E
İzmir Körfezi, *Turkey* **49 C8** 38 30N 26 50 E
İzmit = Kocaeli, *Turkey* **51 F13** 40 45N 29 50 E
Iznájar, *Spain* **43 H6** 37 15N 4 19W
Iznalloz, *Spain* **43 H7** 37 24N 3 30W
İznik, *Turkey* **100 B3** 40 23N 29 46 E
İznik Gölü, *Turkey* **51 F13** 40 27N 29 30 E
Izobilno-Tishchenskoye = Izobil'nyy, *Russia* **61 H5** 45 25N 41 44 E
Izobil'nyy, *Russia* **61 H5** 45 25N 41 44 E
Izola, *Slovenia* **45 C10** 45 32N 13 39 E
Izozog, Bañados de, *Bolivia* **173 D5** 18 48 S 62 10W
Izra, *Syria* **103 C5** 32 51N 36 15 E
Iztochni Rodopi, *Bulgaria* **51 E9** 41 45N 25 30 E
Izu-Hantō, *Japan* **73 C11** 34 45N 139 0 E
Izu-Shotō, *Japan* **71 G10** 34 30N 140 0 E
Izúcar de Matamoros, *Mexico* **163 D5** 18 36N 98 28W
Izuhara, *Japan* **72 C1** 34 12N 129 17 E
Izumi, *Kagoshima, Japan* **72 E2** 32 5N 130 22 E
Izumi, *Ōsaka, Japan* **73 C7** 34 28N 135 24 E
Izumi-Sano, *Japan* **73 C7** 34 23N 135 18 E
Izumo, *Japan* **72 B4** 35 20N 132 46 E
Izyaslav, *Ukraine* **59 G4** 50 5N 26 50 E
Izyum, *Ukraine* **59 H9** 49 12N 37 19 E

J

J.F. Rodrigues, *Brazil* **170 B1** 2 55 S 50 20W
J.P. Koch Fjord, *Greenland* **10 A6** 82 45N 44 0W
J. Strom Thurmond L., *U.S.A.* **152 B7** 33 40N 82 12W
Ja-ela, *Sri Lanka* **95 L4** 7 5N 79 53 E
Jaba, *Ethiopia* **107 F4** 6 20N 35 7 E
Jabal at Tā'ir, *Red Sea* **107 D5** 15 35N 41 52 E
Jabalón →, *Spain* **43 G6** 38 53N 4 5W
Jabalpur, *India* **93 H8** 23 9N 79 58 E
Jabbūl, *Syria* **96 B3** 36 4N 37 30 E
Jabiru, *Australia* **124 B5** 12 40 S 132 53 E
Jablah, *Syria* **100 E6** 35 20N 36 0 E
Jablanac, *Croatia* **45 D11** 44 42N 14 56 E
Jablanica, *Bos.-H.* **52 G2** 43 40N 17 45 E
Jablonec nad Nisou, *Czech Rep.* **34 A8** 50 43N 15 10 E
Jablonica, *Slovak Rep.* **35 C10** 48 37N 17 26 E
Jabłonowo Pomorskie, *Poland* **54 E6** 53 23N 19 10 E
Jablunkov, *Czech Rep.* **35 B11** 49 35N 18 46 E
Jaboatão, *Brazil* **170 C4** 8 7 S 35 1W
Jabonga, *Phil.* **81 G5** 9 20N 125 32 E
Jaboticabal, *Brazil* **175 A6** 21 15 S 48 17W
Jabukovac, *Serbia & M.* **50 B6** 44 22N 22 21 E
Jaburu, *Brazil* **173 B5** 5 30 S 64 0W
Jaca, *Spain* **40 C4** 42 35N 0 33W
Jacaré →, *Brazil* **170 D3** 10 3 S 42 13W
Jacareí, *Brazil* **175 A6** 23 20 S 46 0W
Jacarèzinho, *Brazil* **175 A6** 23 5 S 49 58W
Jaciara, *Brazil* **173 D7** 15 59 S 54 57W
Jacinto, *Brazil* **171 E3** 16 10 S 40 17W
Jaciparaná, *Brazil* **173 B5** 9 15 S 64 23W
Jackman, *U.S.A.* **149 C10** 45 35N 70 17W
Jacksboro, *U.S.A.* **155 J5** 33 14N 98 15W
Jackson, *Barbados* **165 g** 13 7N 59 36W
Jackson, *Ala., U.S.A.* **149 K2** 31 31N 87 53W
Jackson, *Calif., U.S.A.* **160 G6** 38 21N 120 46W
Jackson, *Ga., U.S.A.* **152 B6** 33 20N 83 57W
Jackson, *Ky., U.S.A.* **148 G4** 37 33N 83 23W
Jackson, *Mich., U.S.A.* **157 B12** 42 15N 84 24W
Jackson, *Minn., U.S.A.* **154 D7** 43 37N 95 1W
Jackson, *Miss., U.S.A.* **155 J9** 32 18N 90 12W
Jackson, *Mo., U.S.A.* **155 G10** 37 23N 89 40W
Jackson, *N.H., U.S.A.* **151 B13** 44 10N 71 11W
Jackson, *Ohio, U.S.A.* **148 F4** 39 3N 82 39W
Jackson, *S.C., U.S.A.* **152 B8** 33 20N 81 47W
Jackson, *Tenn., U.S.A.* **149 H1** 35 37N 88 49W
Jackson, *Wyo., U.S.A.* **158 E8** 43 29N 110 46W
Jackson, C., *N.Z.* **131 A9** 40 59 S 174 20 E
Jackson B., *N.Z.* **131 D3** 43 58 S 168 42 E
Jackson Center, *U.S.A.* **157 D12** 40 27N 84 4W
Jackson Hd., *N.Z.* **131 D3** 43 58 S 168 37 E
Jackson L., *Fla., U.S.A.* **152 E5** 30 30N 84 17W
Jackson L., *Ga., U.S.A.* **152 B6** 33 19N 83 50W
Jackson L., *Wyo., U.S.A.* **158 E8** 43 52N 110 36W
Jacksons, *N.Z.* **131 C6** 42 46 S 171 32 E
Jackson's Arm, *Canada* **141 C8** 49 52N 56 47W
Jacksonville, *Ala., U.S.A.* **152 B4** 33 49N 85 46W
Jacksonville, *Ark., U.S.A.* **155 H8** 34 52N 92 7W
Jacksonville, *Calif., U.S.A.* **160 H6** 37 52N 120 24W
Jacksonville, *Fla., U.S.A.* **152 E8** 30 20N 81 39W
Jacksonville, *Ga., U.S.A.* **152 D7** 31 49N 82 59W
Jacksonville, *Ill., U.S.A.* **156 E6** 39 44N 90 14W
Jacksonville, *N.C., U.S.A.* **149 H7** 34 45N 77 26W
Jacksonville, *Tex., U.S.A.* **155 K7** 31 58N 95 17W
Jacksonville Beach, *U.S.A.* **152 E8** 30 17N 81 24W
Jacksonville International ✕ (JAX), *U.S.A.* **152 E8** 30 30N 81 41W
Jacmel, *Haiti* **165 C5** 18 14N 72 32W
Jacob Lake, *U.S.A.* **159 H7** 36 43N 112 13W
Jacobabad, *Pakistan* **91 C3** 28 20N 68 29 E
Jacobina, *Brazil* **170 D3** 11 11 S 40 30W
Jacobshagen = Dobrzany, *Poland* **54 E2** 53 22N 15 25 E
Jacques-Cartier ⌂, *Canada* **141 C5** 47 15N 71 33W
Jacques-Cartier, Dét. de, *Canada* **141 C7** 50 0N 63 30W
Jacques-Cartier, Mt., *Canada* **141 C6** 48 57N 66 0W
Jacqueville, *Ivory C.* **112 D4** 5 12N 4 25W
Jacuí →, *Brazil* **175 C5** 30 2 S 51 15W
Jacumba, *U.S.A.* **161 N10** 32 37N 116 11W
Jacundá →, *Brazil* **170 B1** 1 57 S 50 26W
Jadcherla, *India* **94 F4** 16 46N 78 9 E
Jade, *Germany* **30 B4** 53 20N 8 14 E
Jadebusen, *Germany* **30 B4** 53 29N 8 12 E
Jadotville = Likasi, *Dem. Rep. of the Congo* **119 E2** 10 55 S 26 48 E
Jadovnik, *Serbia & M.* **50 C3** 43 20N 19 45 E
Jadraque, *Spain* **40 E2** 40 55N 2 55W
Jādū, *Libya* **108 B2** 32 0N 12 0 E
Jaén, *Peru* **172 B2** 5 25 S 78 40W
Jaén, *Spain* **43 H7** 37 44N 3 43W
Jaén □, *Spain* **43 H7** 37 50N 3 30W
Jæren, *Norway* **18 F2** 58 42N 5 47 E
Jærens rev, *Norway* **18 F2** 58 45N 5 45 E
Jafarabad, *India* **92 J4** 20 52N 71 22 E
Jafène, *Africa* **110 D3** 20 35N 5 30W
Jaffa = Tel Aviv-Yafo, *Israel* **103 C3** 32 4N 34 48 E
Jaffa, C., *Australia* **128 D3** 36 58 S 139 40 E
Jaffna, *Sri Lanka* **95 K5** 9 45N 80 2 E
Jaffray, *Canada* **143 D10** 49 47N 94 26W
Jaffrey, *U.S.A.* **151 D12** 42 49N 72 2W
Jagadhri, *India* **92 D7** 30 10N 77 20 E
Jagadishpur, *India* **93 G11** 25 30N 84 21 E
Jagdalpur, *India* **94 E6** 19 3N 82 0 E
Jagersfontein, *S. Africa* **116 D4** 29 44 S 25 27 E
Jaghīn →, *Iran* **97 E8** 27 17N 57 13 E
Jagna, *Phil.* **81 G5** 9 39N 124 22 E
Jagodina, *Serbia & M.* **50 B5** 44 5N 21 15 E
Jagst →, *Germany* **31 F5** 49 14N 9 10 E
Jagtial, *India* **94 E4** 18 50N 79 0 E
Jaguaquara, *Brazil* **171 D4** 13 32 S 39 58W
Jaguariaíva, *Brazil* **175 A6** 24 10 S 49 50W
Jaguaribe, *Brazil* **170 C4** 5 53 S 38 37W
Jaguaribe →, *Brazil* **170 B4** 4 25 S 37 45W
Jaguaruana, *Brazil* **170 B4** 4 50 S 37 47W
Jagüey Grande, *Cuba* **164 B3** 22 35N 81 7W
Jagungal, Mt., *Australia* **129 D8** 36 8 S 148 22 E
Jahanabad, *India* **93 G11** 25 13N 84 59 E
Jahazpur, *India* **92 G6** 25 37N 75 17 E
Jahrom, *Iran* **97 D7** 28 30N 53 31 E
Jaicós, *Brazil* **170 C3** 7 21 S 41 8W
Jaigarh, *India* **94 F1** 17 17N 73 13 E
Jaijon, *India* **92 D7** 31 21N 76 9 E
Jailolo, *Indonesia* **82 A3** 1 5N 127 30 E
Jailolo, Selat, *Indonesia* **83 A3** 0 5N 129 5 E
Jaintiapur, *Bangla.* **90 C4** 25 8N 92 7 E
Jaipur, *Assam, India* **90 B5** 27 16N 95 24 E
Jaipur, *Raj., India* **92 F6** 27 0N 75 50 E
Jais, *India* **93 F9** 26 15N 81 32 E
Jaisalmer, *India* **92 F4** 26 55N 70 54 E
Jaisinghnagar, *India* **93 H8** 23 38N 78 34 E
Jaitaran, *India* **92 F5** 26 12N 73 56 E
Jaithari, *India* **93 H8** 23 14N 78 37 E
Jājarm, *Iran* **97 B8** 36 58N 56 27 E
Jajce, *Bos.-H.* **52 F2** 44 19N 17 17 E
Jajpur, *India* **94 D8** 20 53N 86 22 E
Jakam →, *India* **92 H6** 23 54N 74 13 E
Jakarta, *Indonesia* **84 D3** 6 9 S 106 49 E
Jakhal, *India* **92 E6** 29 48N 75 50 E
Jakhau, *India* **92 H3** 23 13N 68 43 E
Jakobshavn = Illulissat, *Greenland* **10 D5** 69 12N 51 10W
Jakobstad = Pietarsaari, *Finland* **14 E20** 63 40N 22 43 E
Jakupica, *Macedonia* **50 E5** 41 45N 21 22 E
Jal, *U.S.A.* **155 J3** 32 7N 103 12W
Jalal-Abad, *Kyrgyzstan* **65 C6** 40 56N 73 0 E
Jalālābād, *Afghan.* **91 B3** 34 30N 70 29 E
Jalalabad, *India* **93 F8** 27 41N 79 42 E
Jalalpur Jattan, *Pakistan* **92 C6** 32 38N 74 11 E
Jalama, *U.S.A.* **161 L6** 34 29N 120 29W
Jalapa, *Guatemala* **164 D2** 14 39N 89 59W
Jalapa Enríquez = Xalapa, *Mexico* **163 D5** 19 32N 96 55W
Jalasjärvi, *Finland* **15 E20** 62 29N 22 47 E
Jalaun, *India* **93 F8** 26 8N 79 25 E
Jalāzin, *Afghan.* **65 E2** 37 2N 64 49 E
Jaldak, *Afghan.* **91 C2** 31 58N 66 43 E
Jaldhaka →, *Bangla.* **90 B2** 26 16N 89 16 E
Jales, *Brazil* **171 F1** 20 10 S 50 33W
Jalesar, *India* **92 F8** 27 29N 78 19 E
Jaleswar, *Nepal* **93 F11** 26 38N 85 48 E
Jalgaon, *India* **94 D2** 21 0N 75 42 E
Jalībah, *Iraq* **96 D5** 30 35N 46 32 E
Jalingo, *Nigeria* **113 D7** 8 55N 11 25 E
Jalisco □, *Mexico* **162 D4** 20 0N 104 0W
Jalkot, *Pakistan* **93 B5** 35 14N 73 24 E
Jallas →, *Spain* **42 C1** 42 54N 9 8W
Jalna, *India* **94 E2** 19 48N 75 38 E
Jalón →, *Spain* **40 D3** 41 47N 1 4W
Jalor, *India* **92 G5** 25 21N 72 37 E
Jalpa, *Mexico* **162 C4** 21 38N 102 58W
Jalpaiguri, *India* **90 B2** 26 32N 88 46 E
Jālq, *Iran* **91 D1** 27 35N 62 46 E
Jaluit I., *Marshall Is.* **134 G8** 6 0N 169 30 E
Jalūlā, *Iraq* **101 E11** 34 16N 45 10 E
Jamaane = Giamama, *Somali Rep.* **120 D2** 0 4N 42 44 E
Jamaari, *Nigeria* **113 C6** 11 44N 9 53 E
Jamaica ■, *W. Indies* **164 a** 18 10N 77 30W
Jamalpur, *Bangla.* **90 C2** 24 52N 89 56 E
Jamalpur, *India* **93 G12** 25 18N 86 28 E
Jamalpurganj, *India* **93 H13** 23 2N 87 59 E
Jamanxim →, *Brazil* **173 A6** 4 43 S 56 18W
Jamari, *Brazil* **173 B5** 8 45 S 63 27W
Jamari →, *Brazil* **173 B5** 8 27 S 63 30W
Jamba, *Angola* **115 E3** 14 40 S 16 2 E
Jambewangi, *Indonesia* **79 J17** 8 17 S 114 7 E
Jambi, *Indonesia* **84 C2** 1 38 S 103 30 E
Jambi □, *Indonesia* **84 C2** 1 30 S 102 30 E
Jambongan, Pulau, *Malaysia* **78 C5** 6 45N 117 20 E
Jambusar, *India* **92 H5** 22 3N 72 51 E
James, *U.S.A.* **152 C6** 32 58N 83 29W
James →, *S. Dak., U.S.A.* **154 D6** 42 52N 97 18W
James →, *Va., U.S.A.* **148 G7** 36 56N 76 27W
James, I. = San Salvador, I., *Ecuador* **172 a** 0 16 S 90 42W
James B., *Canada* **140 B3** 54 0N 80 0W
James Island, *U.S.A.* **152 C10** 32 45N 79 55W
James Ranges, *Australia* **124 D5** 24 10 S 132 30 E
James Ross I., *Antarctica* **7 C18** 63 58 S 57 50W
Jamesabad, *Pakistan* **92 G3** 25 17N 69 15 E
Jameson Land, *Greenland* **10 C8** 71 0N 23 30W
Jamesport, *U.S.A.* **156 E3** 39 58N 93 48W
Jamestown = Wawa, *Canada* **140 C3** 47 59N 84 47W
Jamestown, *Australia* **128 B3** 33 10 S 138 32 E
Jamestown, *St. Helena* **9 h** 15 55 S 5 43W
Jamestown, *S. Africa* **116 E4** 31 6 S 26 45 E
Jamestown, *Ind., U.S.A.* **157 E10** 39 56N 86 38W
Jamestown, *Mo., U.S.A.* **156 F4** 38 48N 92 30W
Jamestown, *N. Dak., U.S.A.* **154 B5** 46 54N 98 42W
Jamestown, *N.Y., U.S.A.* **150 D5** 42 6N 79 14W
Jamestown, *Ohio, U.S.A.* **157 E13** 39 39N 83 33W
Jamestown, *Pa., U.S.A.* **150 E4** 41 29N 80 27W
Jamestown, *S.C., U.S.A.* **152 B10** 33 17N 79 42W
Jamīlābād, *Iran* **97 C6** 34 24N 48 28 E
Jamiltepec, *Mexico* **163 D5** 16 17N 97 49W
Jamira →, *India* **93 J13** 21 35N 88 28 E
Jämjö, *Sweden* **17 H9** 56 12N 15 49 E
Jamkhandi, *India* **94 F2** 16 30N 75 15 E
Jamkhed, *India* **94 E2** 18 43N 75 19 E
Jammalamadugu, *India* **95 G4** 14 51N 78 25 E
Jammerbugt, *Denmark* **17 G3** 57 15N 9 20 E
Jammu, *India* **92 C6** 32 43N 74 54 E
Jammu & Kashmir □, *India* **93 B7** 34 25N 77 0 E
Jamnagar, *India* **92 H4** 22 30N 70 6 E
Jamner, *India* **94 D2** 20 45N 75 52 E
Jamni →, *India* **93 G8** 25 13N 78 35 E
Jampur, *Pakistan* **91 C3** 29 39N 70 40 E
Jamrud, *Pakistan* **92 C4** 33 59N 71 24 E
Jämsä, *Finland* **15 F21** 61 53N 25 10 E
Jamshedpur, *India* **93 H12** 22 44N 86 12 E
Jamtara, *India* **93 H12** 23 59N 86 49 E
Jämtland, *Sweden* **14 E15** 63 31N 14 0 E
Jämtlands län □, *Sweden* **16 B7** 63 0N 14 40 E
Jamuna →, *Bangla.* **90 D2** 23 51N 89 45 E
Jamunamukh, *India* **90 B4** 26 6N 92 44 E
Jamurki, *Bangla.* **90 C3** 24 9N 90 2 E
Jan L., *Canada* **143 C8** 54 56N 102 55W
Jan Mayen, *Arctic* **6 B7** 71 0N 9 0W
Janakkala, *Finland* **15 F21** 60 54N 24 36 E
Janaúba, *Brazil* **171 E3** 15 48 S 43 19W
Janaucu, I., *Brazil* **170 A1** 0 30N 50 10W
Jand, *Pakistan* **92 C5** 33 30N 72 6 E
Jandaia, *Brazil* **171 E1** 17 6 S 50 7W
Jandaq, *Iran* **97 C7** 34 3N 54 22 E
Jandía, *Canary Is.* **9 e2** 28 6N 14 21W
Jandía △, *Canary Is.* **9 e2** 28 4N 14 19W
Jandía, Pta. de, *Canary Is.* **9 e2** 28 3N 14 31W
Jandiatuba →, *Brazil* **168 D4** 3 28 S 68 42W
Jandola, *Pakistan* **92 C4** 32 20N 70 9 E
Jandowae, *Australia* **127 D5** 26 45 S 151 7 E
Jándula →, *Spain* **43 G6** 38 3N 4 6W
Jane Pk., *N.Z.* **131 F3** 45 15 S 168 20 E
Janesville, *U.S.A.* **156 B7** 42 41N 89 1W
Janga, *Ghana* **113 C4** 10 5N 1 0W
Jangamo, *Mozam.* **117 C6** 24 6 S 35 21 E
Janghai, *India* **93 G10** 25 33N 82 19 E
Jango, *Brazil* **173 E6** 20 27 S 55 29W
Jangoon, *India* **94 F4** 17 44N 79 5 E
Jangy-Bazar, *Kyrgyzstan* **65 C5** 41 40N 70 53 E
Jangy-Jol, *Kyrgyzstan* **65 C6** 41 36N 72 9 E
Janhtang Ga, *Burma* **90 B6** 26 32N 96 38 E
Jani Khel, *Afghan.* **91 B3** 32 46N 68 24 E
Janikowo, *Poland* **55 F5** 52 45N 18 7 E
Janinà = Ioánnina □, *Greece* **48 B2** 39 39N 20 57 E
Janiuay, *Phil.* **81 F4** 10 58N 122 30 E
Janja, *Bos.-H.* **52 F4** 44 40N 19 14 E
Janjanbureh, *Gambia* **112 C2** 13 30N 14 47W
Janjevo, *Serbia & M.* **50 D5** 42 35N 21 19 E
Janjgir, *India* **93 J10** 22 1N 82 34 E
Janjina, *Croatia* **45 F14** 42 58N 17 25 E
Janjina, *Madag.* **117 C8** 20 30 S 45 50 E
Jankau = Janikowo, *Poland* **55 F5** 52 45N 18 7 E
Janos, *Mexico* **162 A3** 30 45N 108 10W
Jánoshalma, *Hungary* **52 D4** 46 18N 19 21 E
Jánosháza, *Hungary* **52 C2** 47 8N 17 12 E
Jánossomorja, *Hungary* **52 C2** 47 47N 17 11 E
Janów, *Poland* **55 H6** 50 44N 19 27 E
Janów Lubelski, *Poland* **55 H9** 50 48N 22 23 E
Janów Podlaski, *Poland* **55 F10** 52 11N 23 11 E
Janowiec Wielkopolski, *Poland* **55 F4** 52 45N 17 30 E
Januária, *Brazil* **171 E3** 15 25 S 44 25W
Janub △, *Sudan* **107 F2** 6 50N 28 45 E
Janub Dârfûr □, *Sudan* **107 E2** 11 0N 25 0 E
Janub Kordofân □, *Sudan* **107 E3** 12 0N 30 0 E
Janûb Sînî □, *Egypt* **103 F2** 29 30N 33 50 E
Janubio, *Canary Is.* **9 e2** 28 56N 13 50W
Janville, *France* **27 D8** 48 10N 1 50 E
Janwada, *India* **94 E3** 18 0N 77 29 E
Janzé, *France* **26 E5** 47 55N 1 28W
Jaora, *India* **92 H6** 23 40N 75 10 E
Japan ■, *Asia* **71 G8** 36 0N 136 0 E
Japan, Sea of, *Asia* **70 E7** 40 0N 135 0 E
Japan Trench, *Pac. Oc.* **62 F18** 32 0N 142 0 E
Japen = Yapen, *Indonesia* **83 B5** 1 50 S 136 0 E
Japiim, *Brazil* **172 B3** 7 37 S 72 54W
Japla, *India* **93 G11** 24 33N 84 1 E
Japurá, *Brazil* **168 D4** 1 48 S 66 34W
Japurá →, *Brazil* **168 D4** 3 8 S 65 46W
Jaquarão, *Brazil* **175 C5** 32 34 S 53 23W
Jaqué, *Panama* **164 E4** 7 27N 78 8W
Jarābulus, *Syria* **101 D8** 36 49N 38 1 E
Jaraguá, *Brazil* **171 E2** 15 45 S 49 20W
Jaraguari, *Brazil* **173 E7** 20 9 S 54 35W
Jaraicejo, *Spain* **43 F5** 39 40N 5 49W
Jaraíz de la Vera, *Spain* **42 E5** 40 4N 5 45W
Jarama →, *Spain* **42 E7** 40 24N 3 32W
Jaramānah, *Syria* **100 F7** 33 29N 36 21 E
Jaramillo, *Argentina* **176 C3** 47 10 S 67 7W
Jarandilla, *Spain* **42 E5** 40 8N 5 39W
Jaranwala, *Pakistan* **91 C4** 31 15N 73 26 E
Jarash, *Jordan* **103 C4** 32 17N 35 54 E
Jarash □, *Jordan* **103 C4** 32 17N 35 54 E
Jarauçu →, *Brazil* **169 D7** 1 48 S 52 22W
Järbo, *Sweden* **16 D10** 60 43N 16 36 E
Jarboesville = Lexington Park, *U.S.A.* **148 F7** 38 16N 76 27W
Jardas al 'Abīd, *Libya* **108 B4** 32 18N 20 59 E
Jardim, *Brazil* **174 A4** 21 28 S 56 2W
Jardín →, *Spain* **41 G2** 38 50N 2 10W
Jardine River △, *Australia* **126 A3** 11 9 S 142 21 E
Jardines de la Reina, Arch. de los, *Cuba* **164 B4** 20 50N 78 50W
Jargalang, *China* **75 C12** 43 5N 122 55 E
Jargalant = Hovd, *Mongolia* **68 B4** 48 2N 91 37 E
Jari →, *Brazil* **169 D7** 1 9 S 51 54W
Jaria Janjail, *Bangla.* **90 C3** 25 0N 90 40 E
Jarīr, W. al →, *Si. Arabia* **96 E4** 25 38N 42 30 E
Järlåsa, *Sweden* **16 E11** 59 53N 17 12 E
Jarlsberg og Larvik = Vestfold □, *Norway* **18 E7** 59 15N 10 0 E
Jarmen, *Germany* **30 B9** 53 54N 13 20 E
Järna, *Dalarna, Sweden* **16 D8** 60 33N 14 26 E
Järna, *Stockholm, Sweden* **16 E11** 59 6N 17 34 E
Jarnac, *France* **28 C3** 45 40N 0 11W
Jarny, *France* **27 C12** 49 9N 5 53 E
Jaro, *Phil.* **81 F5** 11 11N 124 47 E
Jarocin, *Poland* **55 G4** 51 59N 17 29 E
Jaroměř, *Czech Rep.* **34 A8** 50 22N 15 52 E
Jarosław, *Poland* **55 H9** 50 2N 22 42 E
Järpås, *Sweden* **17 F6** 58 23N 12 57 E
Järpen, *Sweden* **16 A7** 63 21N 13 26 E
Jarqŭrghon, *Uzbekistan* **65 E3** 37 31N 67 25 E
Jarrahdale, *Australia* **125 F2** 32 24 S 116 5 E
Jarrahi →, *Iran* **97 D6** 30 49N 48 48 E
Jarres, Plaine des, *Laos* **86 C4** 19 27N 103 10 E
Jarso, *Ethiopia* **107 F4** 5 15N 37 30 E
Jartai, *China* **74 E3** 39 45N 105 48 E
Jaru, *Brazil* **173 C5** 10 26 S 62 27W
Jaru →, *Brazil* **173 C5** 10 5 S 61 59W
Jarud Qi, *China* **75 B11** 44 28N 120 50 E
Järvenpää, *Finland* **15 F21** 60 29N 25 5 E
Jarvis, *Canada* **150 D4** 42 53N 80 6W
Jarvis I., *Pac. Oc.* **135 H12** 0 15 S 160 5W
Jarvorník, *Czech Rep.* **35 A10** 50 23N 17 2 E
Järvsö, *Sweden* **16 C10** 61 43N 16 10 E
Jarwa, *India* **93 F10** 27 38N 82 30 E
Jaša Tomić, *Serbia & M.* **52 E5** 45 26N 20 50 E
Jasaan, *Phil.* **81 G5** 8 39N 124 45 E
Jasdan, *India* **92 H4** 22 2N 71 12 E
Jashpurnagar, *India* **93 H11** 22 54N 84 9 E
Jasidih, *India* **93 G12** 24 31N 86 39 E
Jasień, *Poland* **55 G2** 51 46N 15 0 E
Jāsimīyah, *Iraq* **101 F11** 33 45N 44 41 E
Jasin, *Malaysia* **87 L4** 2 20N 102 26 E
Jāsk, *Iran* **97 E8** 25 38N 57 45 E
Jasło, *Poland* **55 J8** 49 45N 21 30 E
Jasmund, *Germany* **30 A9** 54 32N 13 35 E
Jasmund △, *Germany* **30 A9** 54 31N 13 38 E
Jaso, *India* **93 G9** 24 30N 80 29 E
Jason Is., *Falk. Is.* **9 f** 51 0 S 61 0W
Jasonville, *U.S.A.* **157 E9** 39 10N 87 12W
Jasper, *Alta., Canada* **142 C5** 52 55N 118 5W
Jasper, *Ont., Canada* **151 B9** 44 52N 75 57W
Jasper, *Ala., U.S.A.* **149 J2** 33 50N 87 17W

Jasper, *Fla., U.S.A.* . . . **152 E7** 30 31N 82 57W
Jasper, *Ind., U.S.A.* . . . **157 F10** 38 24N 86 56W
Jasper, *Tex., U.S.A.* . . . **155 K8** 30 56N 94 1W
Jasper △, *Canada* **142 C5** 52 50N 118 8W
Jasrasar, *India* . . . . . . **92 F5** 27 43N 73 49 E
Jassey = Iaşi, *Romania* **53 C12** 47 10N 27 40 E
Jastarnia, *Poland* . . . . **54 D5** 54 42N 18 40 E
Jastrebarsko, *Croatia* . **45 C12** 45 41N 15 39 E
Jastrow = Jastrowie, *Poland* . . . . **54 E3** 53 26N 16 49 E
Jastrowie, *Poland* . . . . **54 E3** 53 26N 16 49 E
Jastrzębie Zdrój, *Poland* . . . . **55 J5** 49 57N 18 35 E
Jász-Nagykun-Szolnok □, *Hungary* **52 C5** 47 15N 20 30 E
Jászapáti, *Hungary* . . . **52 C5** 47 32N 20 10 E
Jászárokszállás, *Hungary* . . . . **52 C4** 47 39N 19 58 E
Jászberény, *Hungary* . . **52 C4** 47 30N 19 55 E
Jászkisér, *Hungary* . . . **52 C5** 47 27N 20 20 E
Jászladány, *Hungary* . . **52 C5** 47 23N 20 10 E
Jataí, *Brazil* . . . . **171 E1** 17 58 S 51 48W
Jatapu ➝, *Brazil* . . . . **169 D6** 2 13 S 58 17W
Jath, *India* . . . . **94 F2** 17 3N 75 13 E
Jati, *Pakistan* . . . . **92 G3** 24 20N 68 19 E
Jatibarang, *Indonesia* . **85 D3** 6 28 S 108 18 E
Jatiluwih, *Indonesia* . . **79 J18** 8 23 S 115 8 E
Jatinegara, *Indonesia* . **84 D3** 6 13 S 106 52 E
Játiva = Xátiva, *Spain* . **41 G4** 38 59N 0 32W
Jatobá = Petrolândia, *Brazil* . . . . **170 C4** 9 5 S 38 20W
Jättendal, *Sweden* . . . . **16 C11** 61 58N 17 15 E
Jaú, *Angola* . . . . **115 F2** 15 12 S 13 31 E
Jaú, *Brazil* . . . . **175 A6** 22 10 S 48 30W
Jaú ➝, *Brazil* . . . . . . **169 D5** 1 54 S 61 26W
Jauaperí ➝, *Brazil* . . . **169 D5** 1 26 S 61 35W
Jauer = Jawor, *Poland* **55 G3** 51 4N 16 11 E
Jauja, *Peru* . . . . **172 C2** 11 45 S 75 15W
Jaunpur, *India* . . . . . . **93 G10** 25 46N 82 44 E
Jauru ➝, *Brazil* . . . . . **173 D6** 16 22 S 57 46W
Java = Jawa, *Indonesia* **85 D4** 7 0 S 110 0 E
Java Sea, *Indonesia* . . . **85 C3** 4 35 S 107 15 E
Java Trench, *Ind. Oc.* . **84 D2** 9 0 S 105 0 E
Javadi Hills, *India* . . . **95 H4** 12 40N 78 40 E
Javalambre, Sa. de, *Spain* **40 E4** 40 6N 1 0W
Jávea, *Spain* . . . . **41 G5** 38 48N 0 10 E
Javhlant = Uliastay, *Mongolia* . . . . **68 B4** 47 56N 97 28 E
Javier, I., *Chile* . . . . . . **176 C2** 47 5 S 74 25W
Javla, *India* . . . . **94 F2** 17 18N 75 9 E
Jawa, *Indonesia* . . . . . . **85 D4** 7 0 S 110 0 E
Jawa Barat □, *Indonesia* . . . . **79 G12** 7 0 S 107 0 E
Jawa Tengah □, *Indonesia* . . . . **79 G14** 7 0 S 110 0 E
Jawa Timur □, *Indonesia* . . . . **79 G15** 8 0 S 113 0 E
Jawad, *India* . . . . **92 G6** 24 36N 74 51 E
Jawf, W. al ➝, *Yemen* **98 D4** 15 50N 45 30 E
Jawhar, *India* . . . . **94 E1** 19 55N 73 14 E
Jawor, *Poland* . . . . **55 G3** 51 4N 16 11 E
Jaworzno, *Poland* . . . . **55 H6** 50 13N 19 11 E
Jaworzyna Śląska, *Poland* . . . . **55 H3** 50 55N 16 28 E
Jay, *U.S.A.* **153 E2** 30 57N 87 9W
Jay Peak, *U.S.A.* **151 B12** 44 55N 72 32W
Jaya, Puncak, *Indonesia* **83 B5** 3 57 S 137 17 E
Jayanca, *Peru* . . . . **172 B2** 6 24 S 79 50W
Jayanti, *India* . . . . **90 B2** 26 45N 89 40 E
Jayapura, *Indonesia* . . **83 B6** 2 28 S 140 38 E
Jayawijaya, Pegunungan, *Indonesia* . . . . **83 B5** 5 0 S 139 0 E
Jayrūd, *Syria* . . . . **100 F7** 33 49N 36 44 E
Jayton, *U.S.A.* **155 J4** 33 15N 100 34W
Jāz Mūrīān, Hāmūn-e, *Iran* . . . . **97 E8** 27 20N 58 55 E
Jazīreh-ye Shīf, *Iran* . . **97 D6** 29 4N 50 54 E
Jazminal, *Mexico* **162 C4** 24 56N 101 25W
Jazzīn, *Lebanon* . . . . . . **103 B4** 33 31N 35 35 E
Jean, *U.S.A.* **161 K11** 35 47N 115 20W
Jean Marie River, *Canada* **142 A4** 61 32N 120 38W
Jean-Rabel, *Haiti* **165 C5** 19 50N 73 5W
Jeanerette, *U.S.A.* **155 L9** 29 55N 91 40W
Jeanette, Ostrov = Zhannetty, Ostrov, *Russia* . . . . **67 B16** 76 43N 158 0 E
Jeannette, *U.S.A.* **150 F5** 40 20N 79 36W
Jebāl Bārez, Kūh-e, *Iran* . . . . **97 D8** 28 30N 58 20 E
Jebba, *Nigeria* . . . . **113 D5** 9 9N 4 48 E
Jebel, Bahr el ➝, *Sudan* . . . . **107 F3** 9 30N 30 25 E
Jebel Dud, *Sudan* . . . . **107 E3** 13 25N 33 9 E
Jebel Qerri, *Sudan* . . . **107 D3** 16 16N 32 50 E
Jeberos, *Peru* . . . . **172 B2** 5 15 S 76 10W
Jedburgh, *U.K.* **22 F6** 55 29N 2 33W
Jedda = Jiddah, *Si. Arabia* . . . . **98 B2** 21 29N 39 10 E
Jeddore L., *Canada* . . . **141 C8** 48 3N 55 55W
Jedlicze, *Poland* . . . . . . **55 J8** 49 43N 21 40 E
Jędrzejów, *Poland* . . . . **55 H7** 50 35N 20 15 E
Jedwabne, *Poland* . . . . **55 E9** 53 17N 22 18 E
Jeetzel ➝, *Germany* . . **30 B7** 53 9N 11 3 E
Jefferson, *Ga., U.S.A.* . **152 A6** 34 7N 83 35W
Jefferson, *Iowa, U.S.A.* **156 B2** 42 1N 94 23W
Jefferson, *Ohio, U.S.A.* **150 E4** 41 44N 80 46W
Jefferson, *Tex., U.S.A.* **155 J7** 32 46N 94 21W
Jefferson, *Wis., U.S.A.* **157 B8** 43 0N 88 48W
Jefferson, Mt., *Nev., U.S.A.* **158 G5** 38 51N 117 0W
Jefferson, Mt., *Oreg., U.S.A.* **158 D3** 44 41N 121 48W
Jefferson City, *Mo., U.S.A.* **156 F4** 38 34N 92 10W
Jefferson City, *Tenn., U.S.A.* **149 G4** 36 7N 83 30W
Jeffersontown, *U.S.A.* **157 F11** 38 12N 85 35W
Jeffersonville, *Ga., U.S.A.* **152 C6** 32 41N 83 20W
Jeffersonville, *Ind., U.S.A.* **157 F11** 38 17N 85 44W
Jeffersonville, *Ohio, U.S.A.* **157 E13** 39 39N 83 34W
Jeffrey City, *U.S.A.* . . . **158 E10** 42 30N 107 49W
Jega, *Nigeria* . . . . **113 C5** 12 15N 4 23 E
Jejevo, *Solomon Is.* . . . **133 M10** 8 6 S 159 8 E
Jeju = Cheju do, *S. Korea* . . . . **75 H14** 33 29N 126 34 E
Jēkabpils, *Latvia* . . . . . **15 H21** 56 29N 25 57 E
Jekyll I., *U.S.A.* **152 D8** 31 4N 81 25W
Jelcz-Laskowice, *Poland* . . . . **55 G4** 51 2N 17 19 E
Jelenia Góra, *Poland* . . **55 H2** 50 50N 15 45 E
Jelgava, *Latvia* . . . . . . **15 H20** 56 41N 23 49 E
Jelgava □, *Latvia* . . . . **54 B10** 56 35N 23 45 E
Jelica, *Serbia & M.* . . . **50 C4** 43 50N 20 17 E
Jelli, *Sudan* . . . . **107 F3** 5 25N 31 45 E
Jelšava, *Slovak Rep.* . . **35 C13** 48 37N 20 15 E
Jema'a Mallam = Kafanchan, *Nigeria* . **113 D6** 9 40N 8 20 E
Jemaja, *Indonesia* . . . . **87 L5** 3 5N 105 45 E
Jemaluang, *Malaysia* . . **87 L4** 2 16N 103 52 E
Jember, *Indonesia* . . . . **85 D4** 8 11 S 113 41 E
Jena, *Germany* . . . . . . **30 E7** 50 54N 11 35 E
Jena, *U.S.A.* **155 K8** 31 41N 92 8W
Jenbach, *Austria* . . . . . **34 D4** 47 24N 11 47 E
Jendouba, *Tunisia* . . . . **108 A1** 36 29N 8 47 E
Jenīn, *West Bank* . . . . **103 C4** 32 28N 35 18 E
Jenison, *U.S.A.* **157 B11** 42 54N 85 47W
Jenkins, *U.S.A.* **148 G4** 37 10N 82 38W
Jenner, *U.S.A.* **160 G3** 38 27N 123 7W
Jennings, *Fla., U.S.A.* . **152 E6** 30 36N 83 6W
Jennings, *La., U.S.A.* . . **155 K8** 30 13N 92 40W
Jennings, *Mo., U.S.A.* . **156 F6** 38 43N 90 16W
Jensen Beach, *U.S.A.* . . **153 H9** 27 15N 80 14W
Jepara, *Indonesia* . . . . **85 D3** 7 40 S 109 14 E
Jeparit, *Australia* . . . . . **128 D5** 36 8 S 142 1 E
Jequié, *Brazil* . . . . **171 D3** 13 51 S 40 5W
Jequitaí ➝, *Brazil* . . . **171 E3** 17 4 S 44 50W
Jequitinhonha, *Brazil* . **171 E3** 16 30 S 41 0W
Jequitinhonha ➝, *Brazil* . . . . **171 E4** 15 51 S 38 53W
Jerada, *Morocco* **111 B4** 34 17N 2 10W
Jerantut, *Malaysia* . . . . **87 L4** 3 56N 102 22 E
Jerejak, Pulau, *Malaysia* . . . . **87 c** 5 19N 100 19 E
Jérémie, *Haiti* **165 C5** 18 40N 74 10W
Jeremoabo, *Brazil* . . . . **170 D4** 10 4 S 38 21W
Jerez, Punta, *Mexico* . . **163 C5** 22 58N 97 40W
Jerez de García Salinas, *Mexico* **162 C4** 22 39N 103 0W
Jerez de la Frontera, *Spain* **43 J4** 36 41N 6 7W
Jerez de los Caballeros, *Spain* **43 G4** 38 20N 6 45W
Jericho = El Arīḥā, *West Bank* . . . . **103 D4** 31 52N 35 27 E
Jericho, *Australia* . . . . . **126 C4** 23 38 S 146 6 E
Jerichow, *Germany* . . . . **30 C8** 52 30N 12 1 E
Jerico Springs, *U.S.A.* . **156 G2** 37 37N 94 1W
Jerid, Chott el = Djerid, Chott, *Tunisia* . . . . . **108 B1** 33 42N 8 30 E
Jerilderie, *Australia* . . . **129 C6** 35 20 S 145 41 E
Jermyn, *U.S.A.* **151 E9** 41 31N 75 31W
Jerome, *U.S.A.* **158 E6** 42 44N 114 31W
Jerramungup, *Australia* **125 F2** 33 55 S 118 55 E
Jersey, *U.K.* **21 H5** 49 11N 2 7W
Jersey City, *U.S.A.* **151 F10** 40 44N 74 4W
Jersey Shore, *U.S.A.* . . . **150 E7** 41 12N 77 15W
Jerseyville, *U.S.A.* **156 E6** 39 7N 90 20W
Jerumenha, *Brazil* . . . . **170 C3** 7 5 S 43 30W
Jerusalem, *Israel* . . . . . **103 D4** 31 47N 35 10 E
Jervis B., *Australia* . . . **129 C9** 35 8 S 150 46 E
Jervis Inlet, *Canada* . . **142 C4** 50 0N 123 57W
Jerzu, *Italy* . . . . **46 C2** 39 47N 9 31 E
Jesenice, *Slovenia* . . . . **45 B11** 46 28N 14 3 E
Jeseník, *Czech Rep.* . . . **35 A10** 50 14N 17 8 E
Jesenké, *Slovak Rep.* . . **35 C13** 48 20N 20 10 E
Jesi = Iesi, *Italy* . . . . . **45 E10** 43 31N 13 14 E
Jessel = Jasło, *Poland* . . **55 J8** 49 45N 21 30 E
Jesselton = Kota Kinabalu, *Malaysia* . . **85 A5** 6 0N 116 4 E
Jessheim, *Norway* . . . . **18 D8** 60 9N 11 10 E
Jessnitz, *Germany* . . . . **30 D8** 51 40N 12 18 E
Jessore, *Bangla.* . . . . . . **90 D2** 23 10N 89 10 E
Jessup L., *U.S.A.* **153 G8** 28 43N 81 14W
Jesup, *Ga., U.S.A.* **152 D8** 31 36N 81 53W
Jesup, *Iowa, U.S.A.* . . . **156 B4** 42 29N 92 4W
Jesús, *Peru* . . . . **172 B2** 7 15 S 78 25W
Jesús Carranza, *Mexico* **163 D5** 17 28N 95 1W
Jesús María, *Argentina* **174 C3** 30 59 S 64 5W
Jetmore, *U.S.A.* **155 F5** 38 4N 99 54W
Jetpur, *India* . . . . **92 J4** 21 45N 70 10 E
Jeumont, *France* . . . . . . **27 B11** 50 18N 4 6 E
Jevnaker, *Norway* . . . . . **18 D7** 60 15N 10 26 E
Jewell, *U.S.A.* **156 B3** 42 20N 93 39W
Jewett, *U.S.A.* **150 F3** 40 22N 81 2W
Jewett City, *U.S.A.* **151 E13** 41 36N 71 59W
Jeyḥūnābād, *Iran* . . . . . **97 C6** 34 58N 48 59 E
Jeypore, *India* . . . . **94 E6** 18 50N 82 38 E
Jeziorak, Jezioro, *Poland* . . . . **54 E6** 53 40N 19 35 E
Jeziorany, *Poland* . . . . . **54 E7** 53 58N 20 46 E
Jeziorka ➝, *Poland* . . . **55 F8** 52 8N 21 9 E
Jha Jha, *India* . . . . **93 G12** 24 46N 86 22 E
Jhaarkand = Jharkhand □, *India* . **93 H11** 24 0N 85 50 E
Jhabua, *India* . . . . **92 H6** 22 46N 74 36 E
Jhajjar, *India* . . . . **92 E7** 28 37N 76 42 E
Jhal, *Pakistan* . . . . **92 E2** 28 17N 67 27 E
Jhal Jhao, *Pakistan* . . . . **91 D2** 26 20N 65 35 E
Jhalakati, *Bangla.* . . . . . **90 D3** 22 39N 90 12 E
Jhalawar, *India* . . . . **92 G7** 24 40N 76 10 E
Jhalida, *India* . . . . **93 H11** 23 22N 85 58 E
Jhalrapatan, *India* . . . . **92 G7** 24 33N 76 10 E
Jhang Maghiana, *Pakistan* . . . . **91 C4** 31 15N 72 22 E
Jhansi, *India* . . . . **93 G8** 25 30N 78 36 E
Jhargram, *India* . . . . . . **93 H12** 22 27N 86 59 E
Jharia, *India* . . . . **93 H12** 23 45N 86 26 E
Jharkhand □, *India* . . . **93 H11** 24 0N 85 50 E
Jharsuguda, *India* . . . . **94 D7** 21 56N 84 5 E
Jhelum, *Pakistan* . . . . . **91 B4** 33 0N 73 45 E
Jhelum ➝, *Pakistan* . . . **92 D5** 31 20N 72 10 E
Jhilmili, *India* . . . . **93 H10** 23 24N 82 51 E
Jhudo, *Pakistan* . . . . . . **92 G3** 24 58N 69 18 E
Jhunjhunu, *India* . . . . . **92 E6** 28 10N 75 30 E
Ji-Paraná, *Brazil* . . . . . **173 C5** 10 50 S 61 58W
Ji Xian, *Hebei, China* . . **75 F8** 37 35N 115 30 E
Ji Xian, *Henan, China* . **74 G8** 35 22N 114 5 E
Ji Xian, *Shanxi, China* . **74 F6** 36 7N 110 40 E
Jia Xian, *Henan, China* . **74 H7** 33 59N 113 12 E
Jia Xian, *Shaanxi, China* . . . . **74 E6** 38 12N 110 28 E
Jiading, *China* . . . . **77 B13** 31 22N 121 15 E
Jiahe, *China* . . . . **77 E9** 25 38N 112 19 E
Jiaji = Qionghai, *China* **86 C8** 19 15N 110 26 E
Jialing Jiang ➝, *China* . **76 C6** 29 30N 106 20 E
Jiamusi, *China* . . . . **69 B8** 46 40N 130 26 E
Ji'an, *Jiangxi, China* . . **77 D10** 27 6N 114 59 E
Ji'an, *Jilin, China* . . . . **75 D14** 41 5N 126 10 E
Jianchang, *China* . . . . . **75 D11** 40 55N 120 35 E
Jianchangying, *China* . . **75 D10** 40 10N 118 50 E
Jianchuan, *China* . . . . . **76 D2** 26 38N 99 55 E
Jiande, *China* . . . . **77 C12** 29 23N 119 15 E
Jiang'an, *China* . . . . . . **76 C5** 28 40N 105 3 E
Jiangbei, *China* . . . . . . **76 C6** 29 40N 106 34 E
Jiangcheng, *China* . . . . **76 F3** 22 36N 101 52 E
Jiangchuan, *China* . . . . **76 E4** 24 8N 102 39 E
Jiangdi, *China* . . . . **76 D4** 26 57N 103 37 E
Jiangdu, *China* . . . . **77 A12** 32 27N 119 36 E
Jiange, *China* . . . . **76 A5** 32 4N 105 32 E
Jianghua, *China* . . . . . . **77 E8** 25 0N 111 47 E
Jiangjin, *China* . . . . **76 C6** 29 14N 106 14 E
Jiangkou, *China* . . . . . . **76 D7** 27 40N 108 49 E
Jiangle, *China* . . . . **77 D11** 26 42N 117 23 E
Jiangling, *China* . . . . . . **77 B9** 30 25N 112 12 E
Jiangmen, *China* . . . . . . **77 F9** 22 32N 113 0 E
Jiangning, *China* . . . . . **77 B12** 31 55N 118 50 E
Jiangshan, *China* . . . . . **77 C12** 28 40N 118 37 E
Jiangsu □, *China* . . . . . **75 H11** 33 0N 120 0 E
Jiangxi □, *China* . . . . . **77 D11** 27 30N 116 0 E
Jiangyan, *China* . . . . . . **77 A13** 32 30N 120 7 E
Jiangyin, *China* . . . . . . **77 B13** 31 54N 120 17 E
Jiangyong, *China* . . . . . **77 E8** 25 20N 111 22 E
Jiangyou, *China* . . . . . . **76 B5** 31 44N 104 43 E
Jianhe, *China* . . . . **76 D7** 26 37N 108 31 E
Jianli, *China* . . . . **77 C9** 29 46N 112 56 E
Jianning, *China* . . . . . . **77 D11** 26 50N 116 50 E
Jian'ou, *China* . . . . **77 D12** 27 3N 118 17 E
Jianshi, *China* . . . . **76 B7** 30 37N 109 38 E
Jianshui, *China* . . . . . . **76 F4** 23 36N 102 43 E
Jianyang, *Fujian, China* **77 D12** 27 20N 118 5 E
Jianyang, *Sichuan, China* . . . . **76 B5** 30 24N 104 33 E
Jiao Xian = Jiaozhou, *China* . . . . **75 F11** 36 18N 120 1 E
Jiaohe, *Hebei, China* . . **74 E9** 38 2N 116 20 E
Jiaohe, *Jilin, China* . . . **75 C14** 43 40N 127 22 E
Jiaojiang, *China* . . . . . . **77 C13** 28 40N 121 24 E
Jiaoling, *China* . . . . **77 E11** 24 41N 116 12 E
Jiaozhou, *China* . . . . . . **75 F11** 36 18N 120 1 E
Jiaozhou Wan, *China* . . **75 F11** 36 5N 120 10 E
Jiaozuo, *China* . . . . **74 G7** 35 16N 113 12 E
Jiashan, *China* . . . . **77 B13** 30 55N 120 55 E
Jiashi, *China* . . . . **65 D8** 39 29N 76 39 E
Jiawang, *China* . . . . **75 G9** 34 28N 117 26 E
Jiaxiang, *China* . . . . **74 G9** 35 25N 116 20 E
Jiaxing, *China* . . . . **77 B13** 30 49N 120 45 E
Jiayi = Chiai, *Taiwan* . . **77 F13** 23 29N 120 25 E
Jiayu, *China* . . . . **77 C9** 29 55N 113 55 E
Jibão, Serra do, *Brazil* **171 D3** 14 48 S 45 0W
Jibiya, *Nigeria* . . . . **113 C6** 13 5N 7 12 E
Jibou, *Romania* . . . . . . **53 C8** 47 15N 23 17 E
Jibuti = Djibouti ■, *Africa* . . . . **107 E5** 12 0N 43 0 E
Jicarón, I., *Panama* . . . **164 E3** 7 10N 81 50W
Jičín, *Czech Rep.* . . . . . **34 A8** 50 25N 15 28 E
Jiddah, *Si. Arabia* . . . . **98 B2** 21 29N 39 10 E
Jido, *India* . . . . **90 A5** 29 2N 94 58 E
Jieshou, *China* . . . . **74 H8** 33 18N 115 22 E
Jiexiu, *China* . . . . **74 F6** 37 2N 111 55 E
Jieyang, *China* . . . . **77 F11** 23 35N 116 21 E
Jigawa □, *Nigeria* . . . . **113 C6** 12 0N 9 45 E
Jiggalong, *Australia* . . **124 D3** 23 21 S 120 47 E
Jigni, *India* . . . . **93 G8** 25 45N 79 25 E
Jihlava, *Czech Rep.* . . . **34 B8** 49 28N 15 35 E
Jihlava ➝, *Czech Rep.* . **35 C9** 48 55N 16 36 E
Jihlavský □, *Czech Rep.* **34 B8** 49 30N 15 30 E
Jihočeský □, *Czech Rep.* . . . . **34 B7** 49 8N 14 35 E
Jihomoravský □, *Czech Rep.* . . . . **35 B9** 49 5N 16 30 E
Jijel, *Algeria* . . . . **111 A6** 36 52N 5 50 E
Jijiga, *Ethiopia* . . . . . . **120 C2** 9 20N 42 50 E
Jikamshi, *Nigeria* . . . . . **113 C6** 12 12N 7 45 E
Jikau, *Sudan* . . . . **107 E3** 8 28N 33 47 E
Jilib = Gelib, *Somali Rep.* . . . . **120 D2** 0 29N 42 46 E
Jilin, *China* . . . . **75 C14** 43 44N 126 30 E
Jilin □, *China* . . . . **75 C14** 44 0N 127 0 E
Jiloca ➝, *Spain* **40 D3** 41 21N 1 39W
Jilong = Chilung, *Taiwan* . . . . **77 E13** 25 3N 121 45 E
Jim Thorpe, *U.S.A.* . . . **151 F9** 40 52N 75 44W
Jima, *Ethiopia* . . . . **107 F4** 7 40N 36 47 E
Jimbaran, Teluk, *Indonesia* . . . . **79 K18** 8 46 S 115 9 E
Jimbolia, *Romania* . . . . **52 E5** 45 47N 20 43 E
Jimena de la Frontera, *Spain* **43 J5** 36 27N 5 24W
Jiménez, *Mexico* **162 B4** 27 10N 104 54W
Jimenez, *Phil.* . . . . **81 G4** 8 20N 123 50 E
Jimo, *China* . . . . **75 F11** 36 23N 120 30 E
Jin, Kepulauan, *Indonesia* . . . . **83 C4** 6 50 S 134 40 E
Jin Jiang ➝, *China* . . . **77 C10** 28 24N 115 48 E
Jin Xian = Jinzhou, *China* . . . . **74 E8** 38 2N 115 2 E
Jin Xian, *China* . . . . . . **75 E11** 38 55N 121 42 E
Jinan, *China* . . . . **74 F9** 36 38N 117 1 E
Jinchang, *China* . . . . . . **68 C5** 38 30N 102 10 E
Jincheng, *China* . . . . . . **74 G7** 35 29N 112 50 E
Jinchuan, *China* . . . . . . **76 B4** 31 30N 102 3 E
Jind, *India* . . . . **92 E7** 29 19N 76 22 E
Jindabyne, *Australia* . . **129 D8** 36 25 S 148 35 E
Jinding, *China* . . . . **69 G10** 22 22N 113 33 E
Jindřichův Hradec, *Czech Rep.* . . . . **34 B8** 49 10N 15 2 E
Jing He ➝, *China* . . . . **74 G5** 34 27N 109 4 E
Jing Shan, *China* . . . . . **77 B8** 31 20N 111 35 E
Jing Xian, *China* . . . . . **77 B12** 30 38N 118 25 E
Jing'an, *China* . . . . **77 C10** 28 50N 115 17 E
Jingbian, *China* . . . . . . **74 F5** 37 20N 108 30 E
Jingchuan, *China* . . . . . **74 G4** 35 20N 107 20 E
Jingde, *China* . . . . **77 B12** 30 15N 118 27 E
Jingdezhen, *China* . . . . **77 C11** 29 20N 117 11 E
Jingdong, *China* . . . . . . **76 E3** 24 23N 100 47 E
Jinggangshan, *China* . . **77 D10** 26 58N 114 15 E
Jinggu, *China* . . . . **76 F3** 23 35N 100 41 E
Jinghai, *China* . . . . **74 E9** 38 55N 116 55 E
Jinghong, *China* . . . . . . **76 G3** 22 0N 100 45 E
Jingjiang, *China* . . . . . . **77 A13** 32 2N 120 16 E
Jingle, *China* . . . . **74 E6** 38 20N 111 55 E
Jingmen, *China* . . . . **77 B9** 31 0N 112 10 E
Jingning, *China* . . . . . . **74 G3** 35 30N 105 43 E
Jingpo Hu, *China* . . . . **75 C15** 43 55N 128 55 E
Jingshan, *China* . . . . . . **77 B9** 31 1N 113 7 E
Jingtai, *China* . . . . **74 F3** 37 10N 104 6 E
Jingxi, *China* . . . . **76 F6** 23 8N 106 27 E
Jingxing, *China* . . . . . . **74 E8** 38 2N 114 8 E
Jingyang, *China* . . . . . . **74 G5** 34 30N 108 50 E
Jingyu, *China* . . . . **75 C14** 42 25N 126 45 E
Jingyuan, *China* . . . . . . **74 F3** 36 30N 104 40 E
Jingzhou, *China* . . . . . . **76 D7** 26 33N 109 40 E
Jingziguan, *China* . . . . **74 H6** 33 15N 111 0 E
Jinhua, *China* . . . . **77 C12** 29 8N 119 38 E
Jining, *Nei Monggol Zizhiqu, China* . . . . **74 D7** 41 5N 113 0 E
Jining, *Shandong, China* . . . . **74 G9** 35 22N 116 34 E
Jinja, *Uganda* . . . . **118 B3** 0 25N 33 12 E
Jinjang, *Malaysia* . . . . . **87 L3** 3 13N 101 39 E
Jinji, *China* . . . . **74 F4** 37 58N 106 8 E
Jinjiang, *Fujian, China* **77 E12** 24 43N 118 33 E
Jinjiang, *Yunnan, China* **76 D3** 26 14N 100 34 E
Jinjini, *Ghana* **112 D4** 7 26N 2 42W
Jinkou, *China* . . . . **77 B10** 30 20N 114 8 E
Jinkouhe, *China* . . . . . . **76 C4** 29 18N 103 4 E
Jinmen Dao, *China* . . . . **77 E12** 24 25N 118 25 E
Jinning, *China* . . . . **76 E4** 24 38N 102 38 E
Jinotega, *Nic.* **164 D2** 13 6N 85 59W
Jinotepe, *Nic.* **164 D2** 11 50N 86 10W
Jinping, *Guizhou, China* . . . . **76 D7** 26 41N 109 10 E
Jinping, *Yunnan, China* **76 F4** 22 45N 103 18 E
Jinsha, *China* . . . . **76 D6** 27 29N 106 12 E
Jinsha Jiang ➝, *China* . **76 C5** 28 50N 104 36 E
Jinshan, *China* . . . . **77 B13** 30 54N 121 10 E
Jinshi, *China* . . . . **77 C8** 29 40N 111 50 E
Jintan, *China* . . . . **77 B12** 31 42N 119 36 E
Jintotolo Channel, *Phil.* **81 F4** 11 48N 123 5 E
Jintur, *India* . . . . **94 E3** 19 37N 76 42 E
Jinxi, *Jiangxi, China* . . **77 D11** 27 56N 116 45 E
Jinxi, *Liaoning, China* . **75 D11** 40 52N 120 50 E
Jinxian, *China* . . . . **77 C11** 28 26N 116 17 E
Jinxiang, *China* . . . . . . **74 G9** 35 5N 116 22 E
Jinyang, *China* . . . . **76 D4** 27 28N 103 5 E
Jinyun, *China* . . . . **77 C13** 28 35N 120 5 E
Jinzhai, *China* . . . . **77 B10** 31 40N 115 53 E
Jinzhou, *Hebei, China* . **74 E8** 38 2N 115 2 E
Jinzhou, *Liaoning, China* . . . . **75 D11** 41 5N 121 3 E
Jiparaná ➝, *Brazil* . . . **173 B5** 8 3 S 62 52W
Jipijapa, *Ecuador* . . . . . **168 D1** 1 0 S 80 40W
Jiquilpan, *Mexico* **162 D4** 19 57N 102 42W
Jishan, *China* . . . . **74 G6** 35 34N 110 58 E
Jishou, *China* . . . . **76 C7** 28 21N 109 43 E
Jishui, *China* . . . . **77 D10** 27 12N 115 8 E
Jisr ash Shughūr, *Syria* **100 E7** 35 49N 36 18 E
Jitarning, *Australia* . . . **125 F2** 32 48 S 117 57 E
Jitra, *Malaysia* . . . . **87 J3** 6 16N 100 25 E
Jiu ➝, *Romania* . . . . . . **53 G8** 43 47N 23 48 E
Jiudengkou, *China* . . . . **74 E4** 39 56N 106 40 E
Jiujiang, *Guangdong, China* . . . . **77 F9** 22 50N 113 0 E
Jiujiang, *Jiangxi, China* **77 C10** 29 42N 115 58 E
Jiuling Shan, *China* . . . **77 C10** 28 40N 114 40 E
Jiulong = Kowloon, *China* . . . . **77 F10** 22 19N 114 11 E
Jiulong, *China* . . . . **76 C3** 28 57N 101 31 E
Jiutai, *China* . . . . **75 B13** 44 10N 125 50 E
Jiuxincheng, *China* . . . **74 E8** 39 17N 115 59 E
Jiuyuhang, *China* . . . . . **77 B12** 30 18N 119 56 E
Jiwa, *U.A.E.* . . . . **99 B6** 23 0N 54 10 E
Jiwani, Ras, *Pakistan* . . **91 D1** 25 1N 61 44 E
Jixi, *Anhui, China* . . . . **77 B12** 30 5N 118 34 E
Jixi, *Heilongjiang, China* . . . . **75 B16** 45 20N 130 50 E
Jiyang, *China* . . . . **75 F9** 37 0N 117 12 E
Jiyuan, *China* . . . . **74 G7** 35 7N 112 57 E
Jīz', W. ➝, *Yemen* . . . . **99 C6** 16 12N 52 14 E
Jīzān, *Si. Arabia* . . . . . **98 C3** 17 0N 42 20 E
Jize, *China* . . . . **74 F8** 36 54N 114 56 E
Jizera ➝, *Czech Rep.* . . . **34 A7** 50 10N 14 43 E
Jizl, Wādī al ➝, *Si. Arabia* . . . . **96 E3** 25 39N 38 25 E
Jizō-Zaki, *Japan* . . . . . . **72 B5** 35 34N 133 20 E
Jizzakh, *Uzbekistan* . . . **65 C3** 40 6N 67 50 E
Joaçaba, *Brazil* . . . . **175 B5** 27 5 S 51 31W
Joaíma, *Brazil* . . . . **171 E3** 16 39 S 41 2W
Joal Fadiout, *Senegal* . . **112 C1** 14 9N 16 50W
João Amaro, *Brazil* . . . **171 D3** 12 46 S 40 22W
João Belo = Xai-Xai, *Mozam.* . . . . **117 D5** 25 6 S 33 31 E
João Câmara, *Brazil* . . . **170 C4** 5 32 S 35 48W
João Pessoa = Eirunepé, *Brazil* . . . **172 B4** 6 35 S 69 53W
João Pessoa = Pôrto, *Brazil* . . . . **170 B3** 3 54 S 42 42W
João Pessoa, *Brazil* . . . **170 C5** 7 10 S 34 52W
João Pinheiro, *Brazil* . . **171 E2** 17 45 S 46 10W
Joaquim Távora, *Brazil* **171 F2** 23 30 S 49 58W
Joaquín V. González, *Argentina* . . . . **174 B3** 25 10 S 64 0W
Jobat, *India* . . . . **92 H6** 22 25N 74 34 E
Jobourg, Nez de, *France* **26 C5** 49 41N 1 57W
Jódar, *Spain* **43 H7** 37 50N 3 21W
Jodhpur, *India* . . . . **92 F5** 26 23N 73 8 E
Jodiya, *India* . . . . **92 H4** 22 42N 70 18 E
Joensuu, *Finland* . . . . . **56 B4** 62 37N 29 49 E
Jōetsu, *Japan* . . . . **71 F9** 37 12N 138 10 E
Jœuf, *France* . . . . **27 C12** 49 12N 6 0 E
Jofane, *Mozam.* . . . . . . **117 C5** 21 15 S 34 18 E
Jogbani, *India* . . . . **93 F12** 26 25N 87 15 E
Jõgeva, *Estonia* . . . . . . **15 G22** 58 45N 26 24 E
Jogjakarta = Yogyakarta, *Indonesia* . . . . **85 D4** 7 49 S 110 22 E
Jōhana, *Japan* . . . . **73 A8** 36 30N 136 57 E
Johannesburg, *S. Africa* **117 D4** 26 10 S 28 2 E
Johannesburg, *U.S.A.* . . **161 K9** 35 22N 117 38W
Johannisburg = Pisz, *Poland* . . . . **54 E8** 53 38N 21 49 E
Johansfors, *Sweden* . . . **17 H9** 56 42N 15 32 E
Johilla ➝, *India* . . . . . . **93 H9** 23 37N 81 14 E
John Crow Mts., *Jamaica* . . . . **164 a** 18 5N 76 25W
John Day, *U.S.A.* **158 D4** 44 25N 118 57W
John Day ➝, *U.S.A.* . . . **158 D3** 45 44N 120 39W
John Day Fossil Beds △, *U.S.A.* **158 D4** 44 33N 119 38W
John D'Or Prairie, *Canada* **142 B5** 58 30N 115 8W
John F. Kennedy International, New York ✈ (JFK), *U.S.A.* **151 F11** 40 38N 73 47W
John F. Kennedy Space Center, *U.S.A.* **153 G9** 28 40N 80 42W
John H. Kerr Reservoir, *U.S.A.* . . . **149 G6** 36 36N 78 18W
John o' Groats, *U.K.* . . . **22 C5** 58 38N 3 4W
Johnnie, *U.S.A.* **161 J10** 36 25N 116 5W
Johns I., *U.S.A.* **152 C9** 32 40N 80 10W
John's Ra., *Australia* . . **126 C1** 21 55 S 133 23 E
Johnson, *U.S.A.* **151 B12** 44 38N 72 41W
Johnson City, *Kans., U.S.A.* **155 G4** 37 34N 101 45W
Johnson City, *N.Y., U.S.A.* **151 D9** 42 7N 75 58W
Johnson City, *Tenn., U.S.A.* **149 G4** 36 19N 82 21W
Johnson City, *Tex., U.S.A.* **155 K5** 30 17N 98 25W
Johnsonburg, *U.S.A.* . . **150 E6** 41 29N 78 41W
Johnsondale, *U.S.A.* . . . **161 K8** 35 58N 118 32W
Johnsons Crossing, *Canada* **142 A2** 60 29N 133 18W
Johnsonville, *N.Z.* . . . . **130 H3** 41 13 S 174 48 E
Johnston, *U.S.A.* **152 B8** 33 50N 81 48W
Johnston, L., *Australia* . **125 F3** 32 25 S 120 30 E
Johnston City, *U.S.A.* . . **156 G8** 37 49N 88 56W
Johnston Falls = Mambilima Falls, *Zambia* . . . . **119 E2** 10 31 S 28 45 E
Johnston I., *Pac. Oc.* . . **135 F11** 17 10N 169 8W
Johnstone Str., *Canada* **142 C3** 50 28N 126 0W
Johnstown, *N.Y., U.S.A.* **151 C10** 43 0N 74 22W
Johnstown, *Ohio, U.S.A.* **150 F2** 40 9N 82 41W
Johnstown, *Pa., U.S.A.* . **150 F6** 40 20N 78 55W
Johor □, *Malaysia* . . . . **84 B2** 2 5N 103 20 E
Johor, Selat, *Asia* . . . . **87 d** 1 28N 103 47 E
Johor Bahru, *Malaysia* . **87 d** 1 28N 103 46 E
Jõhvi, *Estonia* . . . . **15 G22** 59 22N 27 27 E
Joigny, *France* . . . . **27 E10** 47 58N 3 20 E
Joinville, *Brazil* . . . . . . **175 B6** 26 15 S 48 55W
Joinville, *France* . . . . . . **27 D12** 48 27N 5 10 E
Joinville I., *Antarctica* . **7 C18** 65 0 S 55 30W
Jojutla, *Mexico* **163 D5** 18 37N 99 11W
Jokkmokk, *Sweden* . . . . **14 C18** 66 35N 19 50 E
Jökulsá á Bru ➝, *Iceland* **11 B12** 65 40N 14 16W
Jökulsá á Fjöllum ➝, *Iceland* **11 A10** 66 10N 16 30W
Jökulsárgljúfur △, *Iceland* **11 B10** 65 56N 16 31W
Jolfā, *Āẕarbājān-e Sharqī, Iran* . . . . **101 C11** 38 57N 45 38 E
Jolfā, *Eşfahan, Iran* . . . **97 C6** 32 58N 51 37 E
Joliet, *U.S.A.* **157 C8** 41 32N 88 5W
Joliette, *Canada* **140 C5** 46 3N 73 24W
Jolo, *Phil.* . . . . **81 H3** 6 0N 121 0 E
Jolo Group, *Phil.* . . . . . **81 J3** 6 0N 121 9 E
Jolon, *U.S.A.* **160 K5** 35 58N 121 9W
Jølstravatnet, *Norway* . **18 C3** 61 32N 6 23 E
Jomalig I., *Phil.* . . . . . . **80 D4** 14 42N 122 22 E
Jombang, *Indonesia* . . . **85 D4** 7 33 S 112 14 E
Jomda, *China* . . . . **76 B2** 31 28N 98 12 E
Jona, *Switz.* . . . . **33 B7** 47 14N 8 51 E
Jonava, *Lithuania* . . . . **15 J21** 55 8N 24 12 E
Jondal, *Norway* . . . . . . **18 D3** 60 16N 6 15 E
Jones, *Phil.* . . . . **80 C3** 16 33N 121 42 E
Jones Sound, *Canada* . . **6 B3** 76 0N 85 0W
Jonesboro, *Ark., U.S.A.* **155 H9** 35 50N 90 42W
Jonesboro, *Ga., U.S.A.* . **152 B5** 33 31N 84 22W
Jonesboro, *La., U.S.A.* . **155 J8** 32 15N 92 43W
Jonesburg, *U.S.A.* **156 F5** 38 51N 91 18W
Jonesville, *Ind., U.S.A.* **157 E11** 39 5N 85 54W
Jonesville, *Mich., U.S.A.* **157 C12** 41 59N 84 40W
Jong ➝, *S. Leone* **112 D2** 7 32N 12 23W
Jonglei, *Sudan* . . . . **107 F3** 6 25N 30 50 E
Jonglei □, *Sudan* . . . . . **107 F3** 7 30N 32 30 E
Joniškis, *Lithuania* . . . **15 H20** 56 13N 23 35 E
Jönköping, *Sweden* . . . **17 G8** 57 45N 14 8 E
Jönköpings län □, *Sweden* . . . . **17 G8** 57 30N 14 30 E
Jonquière, *Canada* **141 C5** 48 27N 71 14W
Jonsered, *Sweden* . . . . . **17 G6** 57 45N 12 10 E
Jonzac, *France* **28 C3** 45 27N 0 28W
Joplin, *U.S.A.* **155 G7** 37 6N 94 31W
Jora, *India* . . . . **92 F6** 26 20N 77 49 E
Jordan, *Phil.* . . . . **81 F4** 10 40N 122 35 E
Jordan, *Mont., U.S.A.* . **158 C10** 47 19N 106 55W
Jordan, *N.Y., U.S.A.* . . **151 C8** 43 4N 76 29W
Jordan ■, *Asia* . . . . **103 E5** 31 0N 36 0 E
Jordan ➝, *Asia* . . . . . . **103 D4** 31 48N 35 32 E
Jordan Valley, *U.S.A.* . . **158 E5** 42 59N 117 3W
Jordânia, *Brazil* . . . . . . **171 E3** 15 55 S 40 11W
Jordanów, *Poland* . . . . . **55 J6** 49 41N 19 49 E
Jordet, *Norway* . . . . **18 C9** 61 25N 12 8 E
Jorge, C., *Chile* . . . . . . **176 D1** 51 40 S 75 35W
Jorgen Brønlund Fjord, *Greenland* **10 A8** 82 30N 29 0W
Jorhat, *India* . . . . **90 B5** 26 45N 94 12 E
Jorm, *Afghan.* . . . . **65 E5** 36 50N 70 52 E
Jörn, *Sweden* . . . . **14 D19** 65 4N 20 1 E
Jorong, *Indonesia* . . . . . **85 C4** 3 58 S 114 56 E
Jørpeland, *Norway* . . . . **18 E3** 59 3N 6 1 E
Jorquera ➝, *Chile* . . . . **174 B2** 28 3 S 69 58W
Jos, *Nigeria* . . . . **113 D6** 9 53N 8 51 E
Jos Plateau, *Nigeria* . . . **113 D6** 9 55N 9 0 E
Jošanička Banja, *Serbia & M.* . . . . **50 C4** 43 24N 20 47 E
Jose Abad Santos, *Phil.* **81 J5** 5 55N 125 39 E
José Batlle y Ordóñez, *Uruguay* . . . . **175 C4** 33 20 S 55 10W
José Bonifácio = Erechim, *Brazil* . . . . **175 B5** 27 35 S 52 15W
José de San Martín, *Argentina* . . . . **176 B2** 44 4 S 70 26W
Jose Panganiban, *Phil.* **80 D4** 14 17N 122 41 E
Joseni, *Romania* . . . . . . **53 D10** 46 42N 25 29 E
Joseph, L., *Nfld. & L., Canada* **141 B6** 52 45N 65 18W
Joseph, L., *Ont., Canada* **150 A5** 45 10N 79 44W
Joseph Bonaparte G., *Australia* . . . . **124 B4** 14 35 S 128 50 E
Joshinath, *India* . . . . . . **93 D8** 30 34N 79 34 E
Joshinetsu-Kōgen △, *Japan* . . . . **73 A10** 36 42N 138 32 E
Joshua Tree, *U.S.A.* . . . **161 L10** 34 8N 116 19W
Joshua Tree △, *U.S.A.* . **161 M10** 33 55N 116 0W
Josselin, *France* **26 E4** 47 57N 2 33W
Jost Van Dyke, *Br. Virgin Is.* . . . . . . **165 e** 18 29N 64 47W
Jostedal, *Norway* . . . . . **18 C4** 61 35N 7 15 E
Jostedalsbreen, *Norway* **18 C4** 61 40N 6 59 E
Jotunheimen, *Norway* . . **18 C5** 61 35N 8 25 E
Jotunheimen △, *Norway* . . . . **18 C5** 61 32N 8 25 E
Joubertberge, *Namibia* **116 B1** 18 30 S 14 0 E
Joué-lès-Tours, *France* . **26 E7** 47 21N 0 40 E
Jourdanton, *U.S.A.* . . . **155 L5** 28 55N 98 33W
Joutseno, *Finland* . . . . . **58 B5** 61 7N 28 31 E
Jovellanos, *Cuba* **164 B3** 22 40N 81 10W
Jovellar, *Phil.* . . . . **80 E4** 13 4N 123 36 E
Jowai, *India* . . . . **90 C4** 25 26N 92 12 E
Jowhar = Giohar, *Somali Rep.* . . . . **120 D3** 2 48N 45 30 E
Jowzjān □, *Afghan.* . . . **65 E3** 36 10N 66 0 E
Joyeuse, *France* . . . . . . **29 D8** 44 29N 4 16 E
Jōyō, *Japan* . . . . **73 C7** 34 50N 135 47 E
Józefów, *Lubelskie, Poland* . . . . **55 H10** 50 28N 23 2 E
Józefów, *Mazowieckie, Poland* . . . . **55 F8** 52 10N 21 11 E
Ju Xian, *China* . . . . **75 F10** 36 35N 118 20 E
Juan Aldama, *Mexico* . . **162 C4** 24 20N 103 23W
Juan Bautista Alberdi, *Argentina* . . . . **174 C3** 34 26 S 61 48W
Juan de Fuca Str., *Canada* **160 B3** 48 15N 124 0W
Juan de Nova, *Ind. Oc.* **117 B7** 17 3 S 43 45 E
Juan Fernández, Arch. de, *Pac. Oc.* . . . . . . **135 L20** 33 50 S 80 0W
Juan José Castelli, *Argentina* . . . . **174 B3** 25 27 S 60 57W
Juan L. Lacaze, *Uruguay* . . . . **174 C4** 34 26 S 57 25W
Juanjuí, *Peru* . . . . **172 B2** 7 10 S 76 45W
Juankoski, *Finland* . . . . **14 E23** 63 3N 28 19 E
Juara, *Brazil* . . . . **173 C6** 11 20 S 57 25W
Juárez, *Argentina* . . . . . **174 D4** 37 40 S 59 43W
Juárez, *Mexico* **161 N11** 32 20N 115 57W
Juárez, Sierra de, *Mexico* **162 A1** 32 0N 116 0W
Juatinga, Ponta de, *Brazil* . . . . **171 F3** 23 17 S 44 30W
Juàzeiro, *Brazil* . . . . . . **170 C3** 9 30 S 40 30W
Juàzeiro do Norte, *Brazil* . . . . **170 C4** 7 10 S 39 18W
Juba = Giuba ➝, *Somali Rep.* . . . . **120 D2** 1 30N 42 35 E
Juba, *Sudan* . . . . **107 G3** 4 50N 31 35 E
Jubany, *Antarctica* . . . . **7 C18** 62 30 S 58 0W
Jubayl, *Lebanon* . . . . . . **103 A4** 34 5N 35 39 E
Jubbah, *Si. Arabia* . . . . **96 D4** 28 2N 40 56 E
Jubbal, *India* . . . . **92 D7** 31 5N 77 40 E
Jubbulpore = Jabalpur, *India* . . . . **93 H8** 23 9N 79 58 E
Jübek, *Germany* . . . . . . **30 A5** 54 33N 9 22 E
Jubga, *Russia* . . . . **61 H4** 44 19N 38 48 E
Jubilee L., *Australia* . . **125 E4** 29 0 S 126 50 E
Juby, C., *Morocco* **110 C2** 28 0N 12 59W
Júcar = Xúquer ➝, *Spain* **41 F4** 39 5N 0 10W
Júcaro, *Cuba* **164 B4** 21 37N 78 51W
Juchitán, *Mexico* **163 D5** 16 27N 95 5W
Judaberg, *Norway* . . . . **18 E2** 59 10N 5 51 E
Judaea = Har Yehuda, *Israel* . . . . **103 D3** 31 35N 34 57 E

Judenburg, *Austria* **34 D7** 47 12N 14 38 E
Judith →, *U.S.A.* **158 C9** 47 44N 109 39W
Judith, Pt., *U.S.A.* **151 E13** 41 22N 71 29W
Judith Gap, *U.S.A.* **158 C9** 46 41N 109 45W
Juelsminde, *Denmark* **17 J4** 55 43N 10 1 E
Jufari →, *Brazil* **169 D5** 1 13 S 62 0W
Jugoslavia = Serbia & Montenegro ■, *Europe* **50 C4** 43 20N 20 0 E
Juigalpa, *Nic.* **164 D2** 12 6N 85 26W
Juillac, *France* **28 C5** 45 20N 1 19 E
Juist, *Germany* **30 B2** 53 40N 6 59 E
Juiz de Fora, *Brazil* **171 F3** 21 43 S 43 19W
Jujuy □, *Argentina* **174 A2** 23 20 S 65 40W
Jukao = Rugao, *China* **77 A13** 32 23N 120 31 E
Julesburg, *U.S.A.* **154 E3** 40 59N 102 16W
Juli, *Peru* **172 D4** 16 10 S 69 25W
Julia Cr. →, *Australia* **126 C3** 20 0 S 141 11 E
Julia Creek, *Australia* **126 C3** 20 39 S 141 44 E
Juliaca, *Peru* **172 D3** 15 25 S 70 10W
Julian, *U.S.A.* **161 M10** 33 4N 116 38W
Julian, L., *Canada* **140 B4** 54 25N 77 57W
Julian Alps = Julijske Alpe, *Slovenia* **45 B11** 46 15N 14 1 E
Juliana Top = Mandala, Puncak, *Indonesia* **83 B6** 4 44 S 140 20 E
Julianatop, *Suriname* **169 C6** 3 40N 56 30W
Julianehåb = Qaqortoq, *Greenland* **10 E6** 60 43N 46 0W
Jülich, *Germany* **30 E2** 50 55N 6 22 E
Julierpass, *Switz.* **33 D9** 46 28N 9 32 E
Juliette, L, *U.S.A.* **152 B6** 33 2N 83 50W
Julijske Alpe, *Slovenia* **45 B11** 46 15N 14 1 E
Julimes, *Mexico* **162 B3** 28 25N 105 27W
Jullundur, *India* **92 D6** 31 20N 75 40 E
Julu, *China* **74 F8** 37 15N 115 2 E
Jumbo, *Zimbabwe* **119 F3** 17 30 S 30 58 E
Jumbo Pk., *U.S.A.* **161 J12** 36 12N 114 11W
Jumentos Cays, *Bahamas* **164 B4** 23 0N 75 40W
Jumilla, *Spain* **41 G3** 38 28N 1 19W
Jumla, *Nepal* **93 E10** 29 15N 82 13 E
Jumna = Yamuna →, *India* **93 G9** 25 30N 81 53 E
Junagadh, *India* **92 J4** 21 30N 70 30 E
Junction, *Tex., U.S.A.* **155 K5** 30 29N 99 46W
Junction, *Utah, U.S.A.* **159 G7** 38 14N 112 13W
Junction B., *Australia* **126 A1** 11 52 S 133 55 E
Junction City, *Ga., U.S.A.* **152 C5** 32 36N 84 28W
Junction City, *Kans., U.S.A.* **154 F6** 39 2N 96 50W
Junction City, *Oreg., U.S.A.* **158 D2** 44 13N 123 12W
Junction Pt., *Australia* **126 A1** 11 45 S 133 50 E
Jundah, *Australia* **126 C3** 24 46 S 143 2 E
Jundiaí, *Brazil* **175 A6** 24 30 S 47 0W
Juneau, *U.S.A.* **142 B2** 58 18N 134 25W
Junee, *Australia* **129 C7** 34 53 S 147 35 E
Jungbunzlau = Mladá Boleslav, *Czech Rep.* **34 A7** 50 27N 14 53 E
Jungfrau, *Switz.* **32 C5** 46 32N 7 58 E
Junggar Pendi, *China* **68 B3** 44 30N 86 0 E
Jungsdalshytta, *Norway* **18 D4** 60 49N 7 55 E
Jungshahi, *Pakistan* **92 G2** 24 52N 67 44 E
Juniata →, *U.S.A.* **150 F7** 40 30N 77 40W
Junín, *Argentina* **174 C3** 34 33 S 60 57W
Junín, *Peru* **172 C2** 11 12 S 76 0W
Junín □, *Peru* **172 C3** 11 30 S 75 0W
Junín de los Andes, *Argentina* **176 A2** 39 45 S 71 0W
Jūniyah, *Lebanon* **103 B4** 33 59N 35 38 E
Junlian, *China* **76 C5** 28 8N 104 29 E
Junnar, *India* **94 E1** 19 12N 73 58 E
Juno Beach, *U.S.A.* **153 J9** 26 52N 80 3W
Juntas, *Chile* **174 B2** 28 24 S 69 58W
Juntura, *U.S.A.* **158 E4** 43 45N 118 5W
Juparanã, L., *Brazil* **171 E3** 19 16 S 40 8W
Jupiter, *U.S.A.* **153 J9** 26 57N 80 6W
Juquiá, *Brazil* **171 F2** 24 19 S 47 38W
Jur, Nahr el →, *Sudan* **107 F2** 8 45N 29 15 E
Jura = Jura, Mts. du, *Europe* **27 F13** 46 40N 6 5 E
Jura = Schwäbische Alb, *Germany* **31 G5** 48 20N 9 30 E
Jura, *U.K.* **22 F3** 56 0N 5 50W
Jura □, *France* **27 F12** 46 47N 5 45 E
Jura □, *Switz.* **31 H3** 47 20N 7 20 E
Jūra →, *Lithuania* **54 C9** 55 3N 22 9 E
Jura, Mts. du, *Europe* **27 F13** 46 40N 6 5 E
Jura, Sd. of, *U.K.* **22 F3** 55 57N 5 45W
Jura Suisse, *Switz.* **32 B4** 47 10N 7 0 E
Jurado, *Colombia* **168 B2** 7 7N 77 46W
Jurbarkas, *Lithuania* **15 J20** 55 4N 22 46 E
Jurien, *Australia* **125 F2** 30 18 S 115 2 E
Jurilovca, *Romania* **53 F13** 44 46N 28 52 E
Jūrmala, *Latvia* **15 H20** 56 58N 23 34 E
Jurong, *China* **77 B12** 31 57N 119 9 E
Jurong, *Singapore* **87 d** 1 19N 103 42 E
Juruá, *Brazil* **168 D4** 3 27 S 66 3W
Juruá →, *Brazil* **168 D4** 2 37 S 65 44W
Juruena, *Brazil* **173 C6** 13 0 S 58 10W
Juruena →, *Brazil* **173 B6** 7 20 S 58 3W
Juruti, *Brazil* **169 D6** 2 9 S 56 4W
Jussey, *France* **27 E12** 47 50N 5 55 E
Justo Daract, *Argentina* **174 C2** 33 52 S 65 12W
Jutaí, *Amazonas, Brazil* **168 D4** 2 44 S 66 57W
Jutaí, *Amazonas, Brazil* **172 B4** 5 11 S 68 54W
Jutaí →, *Brazil* **168 D4** 2 43 S 66 57W
Jüterbog, *Germany* **30 D9** 51 59N 13 5 E
Juticalpa, *Honduras* **164 D2** 14 40N 86 12W
Jutland = Jylland, *Denmark* **17 H3** 56 25N 9 30 E
Juventud, I. de la, *Cuba* **164 B3** 21 40N 82 40W
Juvigny-sous-Andaine, *France* **26 D6** 48 32N 0 30W
Jūy Zar, *Iran* **101 F12** 33 50N 46 18 E
Juye, *China* **74 G9** 35 22N 116 5 E
Juzennecourt, *France* **27 D11** 48 10N 4 58 E
Južni Brod = Brod, *Macedonia* **50 E5** 41 32N 21 17 E
Jvari, *Georgia* **61 J6** 42 42N 42 4 E
Jyderup, *Denmark* **17 J5** 55 40N 11 26 E
Jylland, *Denmark* **17 H3** 56 25N 9 30 E
Jyväskylä, *Finland* **15 E21** 62 14N 25 50 E

K

K2, *Pakistan* **93 B7** 35 58N 76 32 E
Ka →, *Nigeria* **113 C5** 11 40N 4 10 E
Ka Lae, *U.S.A.* **145 E6** 18 55N 155 41W
Kaa-Iya △, *Bolivia* **173 D5** 18 35 S 61 40W
Kaaawa, *U.S.A.* **145 J14** 21 33N 157 51W
Kaala, *U.S.A.* **145 J13** 21 31N 158 9W
Kaala-Gomén, *N. Cal.* **133 T18** 20 40 S 164 25 E
Kaalualu B., *U.S.A.* **145 E6** 18 58N 155 37W
Kaap Plateau, *S. Africa* **116 D3** 28 30 S 24 0 E
Kaapkruis, *Namibia* **116 C1** 21 55 S 13 57 E
Kaapstad = Cape Town, *S. Africa* **116 E2** 33 55 S 18 22 E
Kaataon, Mt., *Phil.* **81 G5** 8 10N 124 52 E
Kaba, *Guinea* **112 C2** 10 9N 11 40W
Kabacan, *Phil.* **81 H5** 7 8N 124 49 E
Kabachishche = Zelenodolsk, *Russia* **60 C9** 55 55N 48 30 E
Kabaena, *Indonesia* **82 C2** 5 15 S 122 0 E
Kabala, *S. Leone* **112 D2** 9 38N 11 37W
Kabale, *Uganda* **118 C3** 1 15 S 30 0 E
Kabalebostuwmeer, *Suriname* **169 C6** 4 45N 57 30W
Kabalo, *Dem. Rep. of the Congo* **118 D2** 6 0 S 27 0 E
Kabambare, *Dem. Rep. of the Congo* **118 C2** 4 41 S 27 39 E
Kabango, *Dem. Rep. of the Congo* **119 D2** 8 35 S 28 30 E
Kabanjahe, *Indonesia* **84 B1** 3 6N 98 30 E
Kabankalan, *Phil.* **81 G4** 9 59N 122 49 E
Kabara, *Fiji* **133 B3** 18 59 S 178 56W
Kabara, *Mali* **112 B4** 16 40N 2 50W
Kabarai, *Indonesia* **83 B4** 0 4 S 130 58 E
Kabardinka, *Russia* **59 K10** 44 40N 37 57 E
Kabardino-Balkar Republic = Kabardino-Balkaria □, *Russia* **61 J6** 43 30N 43 30 E
Kabardino-Balkaria □, *Russia* **61 J6** 43 30N 43 30 E
Kabarega Falls = Murchison Falls, *Uganda* **118 B3** 2 15N 31 30 E
Kabasalan, *Phil.* **81 H4** 7 47N 122 44 E
Kabat, *Indonesia* **79 J17** 8 16 S 114 19 E
Kabba, *Nigeria* **113 D6** 7 50N 6 3 E
Kabbani →, *India* **95 H3** 12 13N 76 54 E
Kabetogama, *U.S.A.* **154 A8** 48 28N 92 59W
Kabi, *Niger* **113 C7** 13 30N 12 35 E
Kabin Buri, *Thailand* **86 F3** 13 57N 101 43 E
Kabinakagami L., *Canada* **140 C3** 48 54N 84 25W
Kabinda, *Dem. Rep. of the Congo* **115 D4** 6 10 S 24 29 E
Kabkabīyah, *Sudan* **109 F4** 13 50N 24 0 E
Kablungu, C., *Papua N. G.* **132 D6** 6 20 S 150 1 E
Kabna, *Sudan* **106 D3** 19 6N 32 40 E
Kabo, *C.A.R.* **114 A3** 7 35N 18 38 E
Kabompo, *Zambia* **119 E1** 13 36 S 24 14 E
Kabompo →, *Zambia* **115 E4** 14 11 S 23 11 E
Kabondo, *Dem. Rep. of the Congo* **119 D2** 8 58 S 25 40 E
Kabongo, *Dem. Rep. of the Congo* **118 D2** 7 22 S 25 33 E
Kabot, *Guinea* **112 C2** 10 48N 14 57W
Kabou, *Togo* **113 D5** 9 28N 0 55 E
Kaboudia, Rass, *Tunisia* **108 A2** 35 13N 11 10 E
Kabr, *Sudan* **107 E2** 10 54N 26 50 E
Kabrousse, *Senegal* **112 C1** 12 25N 16 45W
Kabubu, *Dem. Rep. of the Congo* **115 D4** 9 42 S 24 40 E
Kabūd Gonbad, *Iran* **97 B8** 37 5N 59 45 E
Kabugao, *Phil.* **80 B3** 18 2N 121 11 E
Kābul, *Afghan.* **91 B3** 34 28N 69 11 E
Kābul □, *Afghan.* **91 B3** 34 30N 69 0 E
Kābul →, *Pakistan* **91 B4** 33 55N 72 14 E
Kabuli, *Papua N. G.* **132 B4** 2 7 S 146 40 E
Kabunga, *Dem. Rep. of the Congo* **118 C2** 1 38 S 28 3 E
Kaburuang, *Indonesia* **82 A3** 3 50N 126 30 E
Kabushiya, *Sudan* **107 D3** 16 54N 33 41 E
Kabwanga, *Dem. Rep. of the Congo* **115 D4** 7 2 S 22 36 E
Kabwe, *Zambia* **119 E2** 14 30 S 28 29 E
Kabwum, *Papua N. G.* **132 D4** 6 11 S 147 15 E
Kačanik, *Serbia & M.* **50 D5** 42 13N 21 12 E
Kačerginė, *Lithuania* **54 D10** 54 56N 23 42 E
Kachchh, Gulf of, *India* **92 H3** 22 50N 69 15 E
Kachchh, Rann of, *India* **92 H4** 24 0N 70 0 E
Kachchhidhana, *India* **93 J8** 21 44N 78 46 E
Kachebera, *Zambia* **119 E3** 13 50 S 32 50 E
Kachia, *Nigeria* **113 D6** 9 50N 7 55 E
Kachikau, *Botswana* **116 B3** 18 8 S 24 26 E
Kachin □, *Burma* **76 D1** 26 0N 97 30 E
Kachira, L., *Uganda* **118 C3** 0 40 S 31 7 E
Kachiry, *Kazakhstan* **66 D8** 53 10N 75 50 E
Kachisi, *Ethiopia* **107 F4** 9 40N 37 50 E
Kachkanar, *Russia* **64 B7** 58 42N 59 33 E
Kachnara, *India* **92 H6** 23 50N 75 6 E
Kachot, *Cambodia* **87 G4** 11 30N 103 3 E
Kaçkar, *Turkey* **101 B9** 40 45N 41 10 E
Kada, *Chad* **109 E3** 19 20N 19 39 E
Kadaingti, *Burma* **90 G6** 17 37N 97 32 E
Kadaiyanallur, *India* **95 K3** 9 3N 77 22 E
Kadan, *Czech Rep.* **34 A6** 50 23N 13 16 E
Kadan Kyun, *Burma* **86 F2** 12 30N 98 20 E
Kadanai →, *Afghan.* **92 D1** 31 22N 65 45 E
Kadarkút, *Hungary* **52 D2** 46 13N 17 39 E
Kadavu, *Fiji* **133 B2** 19 0 S 178 15 E
Kadavu Passage, *Fiji* **133 B2** 18 45 S 178 0 E
Kade, *Ghana* **113 D4** 6 7N 0 56W
Kadei →, *C.A.R.* **114 B3** 3 31N 16 3 E
Kademlija = Triglav, *Slovenia* **45 B10** 46 21N 13 50 E
Kadhimain = Al Kāẓimīyah, *Iraq* **101 F11** 33 22N 44 18 E
Kadi, *India* **92 H5** 23 18N 72 23 E
Kadiak I. = Kodiak I., *U.S.A.* **144 H9** 57 30N 152 45W
Kadina, *Australia* **128 B2** 33 55 S 137 43 E
Kadınhanı, *Turkey* **100 C5** 38 14N 32 13 E
Kadiolo, *Mali* **112 C3** 10 35N 7 41W
Kadipur, *India* **93 F10** 26 10N 82 23 E
Kadirabad, *India* **94 E2** 19 51N 75 54 E
Kadiri, *India* **95 G4** 14 12N 78 13 E
Kadirli, *Turkey* **100 D7** 37 23N 36 5 E
Kadiyevka = Stakhanov, *Ukraine* **59 H10** 48 35N 38 40 E
Kadja, O. →, *Chad* **109 F4** 12 2N 22 28 E
Kadmat I., *India* **95 J1** 11 14N 72 47 E
Kadodo, *Sudan* **107 E2** 11 4N 29 31 E
Kadoka, *U.S.A.* **154 D4** 43 50N 101 31W
Kadom, *Russia* **60 C6** 54 37N 42 30 E
Kadoma, *Zimbabwe* **119 F2** 18 20 S 29 52 E
Kâdugli, *Sudan* **107 E2** 11 0N 29 45 E
Kaduna, *Nigeria* **113 C6** 10 30N 7 21 E
Kaduna □, *Nigeria* **113 C6** 11 0N 7 30 E
Kadur, *India* **95 H3** 13 34N 76 1 E
Kaduy, *Russia* **58 C9** 59 12N 37 9 E
Kaédi, *Mauritania* **112 B2** 16 9N 13 28W
Kaélé, *Cameroon* **113 C7** 10 7N 14 27 E
Kaena Pt., *U.S.A.* **145 J13** 21 35N 158 17W
Kaeng Khoï, *Thailand* **86 E3** 14 35N 101 0 E
Kaeng Kra Chan △, *Thailand* **86 F2** 12 57N 99 23 E
Kaeng Tana △, *Thailand* **86 E5** 15 25N 105 32 E
Kaeo, *N.Z.* **130 B2** 35 6 S 173 49 E
Kaesŏng, *N. Korea* **75 F14** 37 58N 126 35 E
Kāf, *Si. Arabia* **96 D3** 31 25N 37 29 E
Kafakumba, *Dem. Rep. of the Congo* **115 D4** 9 38 S 23 46 E
Kafan = Kapan, *Armenia* **101 C12** 39 18N 46 27 E
Kafanchan, *Nigeria* **113 D6** 9 40N 8 20 E
Kafareti, *Nigeria* **113 C7** 10 25N 11 12 E
Kaffrine, *Senegal* **112 C1** 14 8N 15 36W
Kafia Kingi, *Sudan* **114 A4** 9 20N 24 25 E
Kafin, *Nigeria* **113 D6** 9 30N 7 4 E
Kafin Madaki, *Nigeria* **113 C6** 10 41N 9 46 E
Kafinda, *Zambia* **119 E3** 12 32 S 30 20 E
Kafirévs, Ákra, *Greece* **48 C6** 38 9N 24 38 E
Kafr el Battikh, *Egypt* **106 H7** 31 25N 31 44 E
Kafr el Dauwâr, *Egypt* **106 H7** 31 8N 30 8 E
Kafr el Sheikh, *Egypt* **106 H7** 31 15N 30 50 E
Kafue, *Zambia* **119 F2** 15 46 S 28 9 E
Kafue △, *Zambia* **119 F2** 15 12 S 25 38 E
Kafue Flats, *Zambia* **119 F2** 15 40 S 27 25 E
Kafulwe, *Zambia* **119 D2** 9 0 S 29 1 E
Kafumba, *Dem. Rep. of the Congo* **115 D3** 5 23 S 18 55 E
Kaga, *Afghan.* **92 B4** 34 14N 70 10 E
Kaga, *Japan* **73 A8** 36 16N 136 15 E
Kaga Bandoro, *C.A.R.* **114 A3** 7 0N 19 10 E
Kagamil I., *U.S.A.* **144 K5** 53 0N 169 43W
Kagan, *Uzbekistan* **65 D2** 39 43N 64 33 E
Kaganovich = Sokuluk, *Kyrgyzstan* **65 B7** 42 52N 74 18 E
Kaganovich = Tovarkovskiy, *Russia* **58 F10** 53 40N 38 14 E
Kaganovichabad = Kolkhozobod, *Tajikistan* **65 E4** 37 35N 68 40 E
Kaganovichevsk = Komsomolsk, *Turkmenistan* **65 D1** 39 2N 63 36 E
Kagarko, *Nigeria* **113 D6** 9 28N 7 36 E
Kagawa □, *Japan* **72 C6** 34 15N 134 0 E
Kagera □, *Tanzania* **118 C3** 2 0 S 31 30 E
Kagera →, *Uganda* **118 C3** 0 57 S 31 47 E
Kağızman, *Turkey* **101 B10** 40 5N 43 10 E
Kagmar, *Sudan* **107 E3** 14 24N 30 25 E
Kagopal, *Chad* **109 G3** 8 16N 16 23 E
Kagoshima, *Japan* **72 F2** 31 35N 130 33 E
Kagoshima □, *Japan* **72 F2** 31 30N 130 30 E
Kagoshima-Wan, *Japan* **72 F2** 31 25N 130 40 E
Kagua, *Papua N. G.* **132 D2** 6 26 S 143 48 E
Kagul = Cahul, *Moldova* **53 E13** 45 50N 28 15 E
Kahak, *Iran* **97 B6** 36 6N 49 46 E
Kahaluu, *U.S.A.* **145 K14** 21 28N 157 50W
Kahama, *Tanzania* **118 C3** 4 8 S 32 30 E
Kahan, *Pakistan* **92 E3** 29 18N 68 54 E
Kahana, *U.S.A.* **145 J14** 21 34N 157 53W
Kahana B., *U.S.A.* **145 J14** 21 35N 157 50W
Kahang, *Malaysia* **87 L4** 2 12N 103 32 E
Kahayan →, *Indonesia* **85 C4** 3 40 S 114 0 E
Kahe, *Tanzania* **118 C4** 3 30 S 37 25 E
Kahemba, *Dem. Rep. of the Congo* **115 D3** 7 18 S 18 55 E
Kaherekoau Mts., *N.Z.* **131 F2** 45 45 S 167 15 E
Kahil, Djebel bou, *Algeria* **111 B5** 34 26N 4 0 E
Kahnūj, *Iran* **97 E8** 27 55N 57 40 E
Kahoka, *U.S.A.* **156 D5** 40 25N 91 44W
Kahoolawe, *U.S.A.* **145 C5** 20 33N 156 37W
Kahramanmaraş, *Turkey* **100 D7** 37 37N 36 53 E
Kâhta, *Turkey* **101 D8** 37 46N 38 36 E
Kahuku, *U.S.A.* **145 J14** 21 41N 157 57W
Kahuku Pt., *U.S.A.* **145 J14** 21 43N 157 59W
Kahul, Ozero, *Ukraine* **53 E13** 45 24N 28 24 E
Kahului, *U.S.A.* **145 C5** 20 54N 156 28W
Kahurangi △, *N.Z.* **131 B7** 41 10 S 172 32 E
Kahurangi Pt., *N.Z.* **131 A7** 40 50 S 172 10 E
Kahuta, *Pakistan* **92 C5** 33 35N 73 24 E
Kahuzi-Biega △, *Dem. Rep. of the Congo* **118 C2** 1 50 S 27 55 E
Kai, Kepulauan, *Indonesia* **83 C4** 5 55 S 132 45 E
Kai Besar, *Indonesia* **83 C4** 5 35 S 133 0 E
Kai Is. = Kai, Kepulauan, *Indonesia* **83 C4** 5 55 S 132 45 E
Kai Kecil, *Indonesia* **83 C4** 5 45 S 132 40 E
Kai Xian, *China* **76 B7** 31 11N 108 21 E
Kaiama, *Nigeria* **113 D5** 9 36N 4 1 E
Kaiapit, *Papua N. G.* **132 D4** 6 18 S 146 18 E
Kaiapoi, *N.Z.* **131 D7** 43 24 S 172 40 E
Kaieteur Falls, *Guyana* **169 B6** 5 1N 59 10W
Kaifeng, *China* **74 G8** 34 48N 114 21 E
Kaihua, *China* **77 C12** 29 12N 118 20 E
Kaijiang, *China* **76 B6** 31 7N 107 55 E
Kaikohe, *N.Z.* **130 B2** 35 25 S 173 49 E
Kaikoura, *N.Z.* **131 C8** 42 25 S 173 43 E
Kaikoura Pen., *N.Z.* **131 C8** 42 25 S 173 43 E
Kailahun, *S. Leone* **112 D2** 8 18N 10 39W
Kailash = Kangrinboqe Feng, *China* **93 D9** 31 0N 81 25 E
Kailashahar, *India* **90 C4** 24 19N 92 0 E
Kaileuna I., *Papua N. G.* **132 E6** 8 32 S 150 57 E
Kaili, *China* **76 D6** 26 33N 107 59 E
Kailu, *China* **75 C11** 43 38N 121 18 E
Kailua, *U.S.A.* **145 K14** 21 24N 157 44W
Kailua B., *U.S.A.* **145 K14** 21 25N 157 40W
Kailua Kona, *U.S.A.* **145 D6** 19 39N 155 59W
Kaim →, *Papua N. G.* **132 D1** 6 55 S 141 33 E
Kaima, *Indonesia* **83 C5** 5 32 S 138 48 E
Kaimana, *Indonesia* **83 B4** 3 39 S 133 45 E
Kaimanawa Mts., *N.Z.* **130 F4** 39 15 S 175 56 E
Kaimata, *N.Z.* **131 C6** 42 34 S 171 28 E
Kaimganj, *India* **93 F8** 27 33N 79 24 E
Kaimon-Dake, *Japan* **72 F2** 31 11N 130 32 E
Kaimuki, *U.S.A.* **145 K14** 21 17N 157 48W
Kaimur Hills, *India* **93 G10** 24 30N 82 0 E
Kainab →, *Namibia* **116 D2** 28 32 S 19 34 E
Kainan, *Japan* **73 C7** 34 9N 135 12 E
Kainantu, *Papua N. G.* **132 D3** 6 18 S 145 52 E
Kainji Dam, *Nigeria* **113 D5** 9 55N 4 35 E
Kainji Lake △, *Nigeria* **113 C5** 10 5N 4 6 E
Kainji Res., *Nigeria* **113 C5** 10 1N 4 40 E
Kainsk = Samara, *Russia* **60 D10** 53 8N 50 6 E
Kainuu, *Finland* **14 D23** 64 30N 29 7 E
Kaipara Harbour, *N.Z.* **130 C3** 36 25 S 174 14 E
Kaiping, *China* **77 F9** 22 23N 112 42 E
Kaipokok B., *Canada* **141 B8** 54 54N 59 47W
Kaira, *India* **92 H5** 22 45N 72 50 E
Kairana, *India* **92 E7** 29 24N 77 15 E
Kairiru I., *Papua N. G.* **132 B2** 3 21 S 143 34 E
Kaironi, *Indonesia* **83 B4** 0 47 S 133 40 E
Kairouan, *Tunisia* **108 A2** 35 45N 10 5 E
Kairuku, *Papua N. G.* **132 E4** 8 51 S 146 35 E
Kaiser Wilhelm Kanal = Nord-Ostsee-Kanal, *Germany* **30 A5** 54 12N 9 32 E
Kaiser-Wilhelmsland = Papua □, *Indonesia* **83 B5** 4 0 S 137 0 E
Kaiserslautern, *Germany* **31 F3** 49 26N 7 45 E
Kaiserstuhl, *Germany* **31 G3** 48 4N 7 40 E
Kaita, *Japan* **72 C4** 34 22N 132 32 E
Kaitaia, *N.Z.* **130 B2** 35 8 S 173 17 E
Kaitangata, *N.Z.* **131 G4** 46 17 S 169 51 E
Kaithal, *India* **92 E7** 29 48N 76 26 E
Kaitu →, *Pakistan* **92 C4** 33 10N 70 30 E
Kaiwi Channel, *U.S.A.* **145 K14** 21 15N 157 30W
Kaiyang, *China* **76 D6** 27 4N 106 59 E
Kaiyuan, *Liaoning, China* **75 C13** 42 28N 124 1 E
Kaiyuan, *Yunnan, China* **76 F4** 23 40N 103 12 E
Kaiyuh Mts., *U.S.A.* **144 D8** 64 30N 158 0W
Kajaani, *Finland* **14 D22** 64 17N 27 46 E
Kajabbi, *Australia* **126 C3** 20 0 S 140 1 E
Kajana = Kajaani, *Finland* **14 D22** 64 17N 27 46 E
Kajang, *Malaysia* **87 L3** 2 59N 101 48 E
Kajaran, *Armenia* **101 C12** 39 10N 46 7 E
Kajiado, *Kenya* **118 C4** 1 53 S 36 48 E
Kajo Kaji, *Sudan* **107 G3** 3 58N 31 40 E
Kajuru, *Nigeria* **113 C6** 10 15N 7 34 E
Kajy-Say, *Kyrgyzstan* **65 B8** 42 8N 77 10 E
Kaka, *Sudan* **107 E3** 10 38N 32 10 E
Kaka Pt., *U.S.A.* **145 C5** 20 31N 156 33W
Kakabeka Falls, *Canada* **140 C2** 48 24N 89 37W
Kakadu △, *Australia* **124 B5** 12 0 S 132 3 E
Kakamas, *S. Africa* **116 D3** 28 45 S 20 33 E
Kakamega, *Kenya* **118 B3** 0 20N 34 46 E
Kakamigahara, *Japan* **73 B8** 35 28N 136 48 E
Kakana, *India* **95 K11** 9 7N 92 48 E
Kakanj, *Bos.-H.* **52 F3** 44 4N 18 4 E
Kakanui Mts., *N.Z.* **131 F5** 45 10 S 170 30 E
Kakata, *Liberia* **112 D2** 6 35N 10 20W
Kakdwip, *India* **93 J13** 21 53N 88 11 E
Kake, *Japan* **72 C4** 34 36N 132 19 E
Kake, *U.S.A.* **142 B2** 56 59N 133 57W
Kakegawa, *Japan* **73 C10** 34 45N 138 1 E
Kakeroma-Jima, *Japan* **71 K4** 28 8N 129 14 E
Kakhib, *Russia* **61 J8** 42 28N 46 34 E
Kakhonak, *U.S.A.* **144 G9** 59 26N 154 51W
Kakhovka, *Ukraine* **59 J7** 46 45N 33 30 E
Kakhovske Vdskh., *Ukraine* **59 J7** 47 5N 34 0 E
Kakinada, *India* **94 F6** 16 57N 82 11 E
Kakisa →, *Canada* **142 A5** 61 3N 118 10W
Kakisa L., *Canada* **142 A5** 60 56N 117 43W
Käkisalmi = Priozersk, *Russia* **58 B6** 61 2N 30 7 E
Kakogawa, *Japan* **72 C6** 34 46N 134 51 E
Kaktovik, *U.S.A.* **144 A12** 70 8N 143 38W
Kakum △, *Ghana* **113 D4** 5 24N 1 20W
Kakwa →, *Canada* **142 C5** 54 37N 118 28W
Kāl Gūsheh, *Iran* **97 D8** 30 59N 58 12 E
Kal Safīd, *Iran* **101 E12** 34 52N 47 23 E
Kala, *Nigeria* **113 C7** 12 2N 14 40 E
Kala Oya →, *Sri Lanka* **95 K4** 8 20N 79 45 E
Kalaa-Kebira, *Tunisia* **108 A2** 35 59N 10 32 E
Kalaallit Nunaat = Greenland ☒, *N. Amer.* **10 D6** 66 0N 45 0W
Kalabagh, *Pakistan* **92 C4** 33 0N 71 28 E
Kalabahi, *Indonesia* **82 C2** 8 13 S 124 31 E
Kalabak = Radomir, *Bulgaria* **50 D6** 42 37N 22 59 E
Kalabáka, *Greece* **48 B3** 39 42N 21 39 E
Kalabakan, *Malaysia* **85 B5** 4 25N 117 29 E
Kalabana, *Mali* **112 C3** 14 10N 8 35W
Kalabo, *Zambia* **115 E4** 14 58 S 22 40 E
Kalach, *Russia* **60 E5** 50 22N 41 0 E
Kalach na Donu, *Russia* **61 F6** 48 43N 43 32 E
Kaladan →, *Burma* **90 E4** 20 20N 93 5 E
Kaladar, *Canada* **140 D4** 44 37N 77 5W
Kalahari, *Africa* **116 C3** 24 0 S 21 30 E
Kalahari Gemsbok △, *S. Africa* **116 D3** 25 30 S 20 30 E
Kalaheo, *U.S.A.* **145 B2** 21 56N 159 32W
Kalaikhum, *Tajikistan* **65 D5** 38 28N 70 46 E
Kalajoki, *Finland* **14 D20** 64 12N 24 10 E
Kalakamati, *Botswana* **117 C4** 20 40 S 27 25 E
Kalakan, *Russia* **67 D12** 55 15N 116 45 E
K'alak'unlun Shank'ou = Karakoram Pass, *Asia* **93 B7** 35 33N 77 50 E
Kalam, *Pakistan* **93 B5** 35 34N 72 30 E
Kalama, *Dem. Rep. of the Congo* **118 C2** 2 52 S 28 35 E
Kalama, *U.S.A.* **160 E4** 46 1N 122 51W
Kalámai, *Greece* **48 D4** 37 3N 22 10 E
Kalamaloué △, *Cameroon* **109 F2** 12 9N 14 58 E
Kalamansig, *Phil.* **81 H5** 6 33N 124 3 E
Kalamariá, *Greece* **50 F6** 40 33N 22 55 E
Kalamata = Kalámai, *Greece* **48 D4** 37 3N 22 10 E
Kalamazoo, *U.S.A.* **157 B11** 42 17N 85 35W
Kalamazoo →, *U.S.A.* **157 B10** 42 40N 86 10W
Kalamb, *India* **94 E2** 18 3N 74 48 E
Kalambo Falls, *Tanzania* **119 D3** 8 37 S 31 35 E
Kalamítsi, *Greece* **39 B2** 38 45N 20 36 E
Kalamnuri, *India* **94 E3** 19 40N 77 20 E
Kálamos, *Attikí, Greece* **48 C5** 38 17N 23 52 E
Kálamos, *Levkás, Greece* **39 B2** 38 37N 20 56 E
Kálamos Nisís, *Greece* **39 B2** 38 37N 20 55 E
Kalan, *Turkey* **96 B3** 39 7N 39 32 E
Kalangadoo, *Australia* **128 D4** 37 34 S 140 41 E
Kalankalan, *Guinea* **112 C3** 10 7N 8 54W
Kalannie, *Australia* **125 F2** 30 22 S 117 5 E
Kalāntarī, *Iran* **97 C7** 32 10N 54 8 E
Kalao, *Indonesia* **82 C2** 7 21 S 121 0 E
Kalaotoa, *Indonesia* **82 C2** 7 20 S 121 50 E
Kalapana, *U.S.A.* **145 D7** 19 21N 154 59W
Kälarne, *Sweden* **16 B10** 62 59N 16 5 E
Kalasin, *Thailand* **86 D4** 16 26N 103 30 E
Kālat, *Iran* **97 E8** 25 29N 59 22 E
Kalat, *Pakistan* **91 C2** 29 8N 66 31 E
Kalāteh, *Iran* **97 B7** 36 33N 55 41 E
Kalāteh-ye Ganj, *Iran* **97 E8** 27 31N 57 55 E
Kálathos, *Greece* **38 E12** 36 9N 28 8 E
Kalatungan Mt., *Phil.* **81 H5** 7 54N 124 50 E
Kalaupapa, *U.S.A.* **145 B5** 21 12N 156 59W
Kalaupapa △, *U.S.A.* **145 B5** 21 10N 156 59W
Kalaus →, *Russia* **61 H7** 45 40N 44 7 E
Kalávrita, *Greece* **48 C4** 38 3N 22 8 E
Kalaw, *Burma* **90 E6** 20 38N 96 34 E
Kalbān, *Oman* **99 B7** 20 18N 58 38 E
Kalbarri, *Australia* **125 E1** 27 40 S 114 10 E
Kalbarri △, *Australia* **125 E1** 27 51 S 114 30 E
Kalce, *Slovenia* **36 F8** 45 54N 14 13 E
Kaldrananes, *Iceland* **11 B5** 65 45N 21 25W
Kale, *Antalya, Turkey* **49 E12** 36 14N 30 0 E
Kale, *Denizli, Turkey* **49 D10** 37 27N 28 49 E
Kalecik, *Turkey* **100 B5** 40 4N 33 26 E
Kalehe, *Dem. Rep. of the Congo* **118 C2** 2 6 S 28 50 E
Kalema, *Tanzania* **118 C3** 1 12 S 31 55 E
Kalemie, *Dem. Rep. of the Congo* **118 D2** 5 55 S 29 9 E
Kalemyo, *Burma* **90 D5** 23 11N 94 4 E
Kalety, *Poland* **55 H5** 50 35N 18 52 E
Kalewa, *Burma* **90 D5** 23 10N 94 15 E
Kaleybar, *Iran* **96 B5** 38 47N 47 2 E
Kálfafell, *Iceland* **11 D9** 63 57N 17 41W
Kalgan = Zhangjiakou, *China* **74 D8** 40 48N 114 55 E
Kalghatgi, *India* **95 G2** 15 11N 74 58 E
Kalgoorlie-Boulder, *Australia* **125 F3** 30 40 S 121 22 E
Kalhovd, *Norway* **18 D5** 60 4N 8 21 E
Kali →, *India* **93 F8** 27 6N 79 55 E
Kali Sindh →, *India* **92 G6** 25 32N 76 17 E
Kaliakra, Nos, *Bulgaria* **51 C12** 43 21N 28 30 E
Kalianda, *Indonesia* **84 D3** 5 50 S 105 45 E
Kalibo, *Phil.* **81 F4** 11 43N 122 22 E
Kaliganj, *Bangla.* **90 D2** 22 25N 89 8 E
Kalihi, *U.S.A.* **145 K14** 21 20N 157 53W
Kalima, *Dem. Rep. of the Congo* **118 C2** 2 33 S 26 32 E
Kalimantan, *Indonesia* **85 C4** 0 0 114 0 E
Kalimantan Barat □, *Indonesia* **85 C4** 0 0 110 30 E
Kalimantan Selatan □, *Indonesia* **85 C5** 2 30 S 115 30 E
Kalimantan Tengah □, *Indonesia* **85 C4** 2 0 S 113 30 E
Kalimantan Timur □, *Indonesia* **85 B5** 1 30N 116 30 E
Kálimnos, *Greece* **49 D8** 37 0N 27 0 E
Kalimpong, *India* **90 B2** 27 4N 88 35 E
Kalinadi →, *India* **95 G2** 14 50N 74 7 E
Kalinga □, *Phil.* **80 C3** 17 30N 121 20 E
Kalinin = Tver, *Russia* **58 D8** 56 55N 35 55 E
Kaliningrad, *Russia* **15 J19** 54 42N 20 32 E
Kaliningrad ✈ (KGD), *Russia* **54 D7** 54 45N 20 33 E
Kalininsk = Petrozavodsk, *Russia* **58 B8** 61 41N 34 20 E
Kalininsk, *Russia* **60 E7** 51 30N 44 40 E
Kalinkavichy, *Belarus* **59 F5** 52 12N 29 20 E
Kalinkovichi = Kalinkavichy, *Belarus* **59 F5** 52 12N 29 20 E
Kalinovik, *Bos.-H.* **50 C2** 43 31N 18 25 E
Kalipetrovo, *Bulgaria* **51 B11** 44 5N 27 14 E
Kaliro, *Uganda* **118 B3** 0 56N 33 30 E
Kalirrákhi, *Greece* **51 F8** 40 40N 24 35 E
Kalispell, *U.S.A.* **158 B6** 48 12N 114 19W
Kalisz, *Poland* **55 G5** 51 45N 18 8 E
Kalisz Pomorski, *Poland* **55 E2** 53 17N 15 55 E
Kaliua, *Tanzania* **118 D3** 5 5 S 31 48 E
Kaliveli Tank, *India* **95 H4** 12 5N 79 50 E
Kalívia Thorikoú, *Greece* **48 D5** 37 50N 23 55 E
Kalix = Kalixälven →, *Sweden* **14 D20** 65 50N 23 11 E
Kalix, *Sweden* **14 D20** 65 53N 23 12 E
Kalixälven →, *Sweden* **14 D20** 65 50N 23 11 E
Kalka, *India* **92 D7** 30 46N 76 57 E
Kalkali Ghat, *India* **90 C4** 24 36N 92 20 E
Kalkan, *Turkey* **49 E11** 36 15N 29 23 E
Kalkarindji, *Australia* **124 C5** 17 30 S 130 47 E
Kalkaska, *U.S.A.* **148 C3** 44 44N 85 11W
Kalkfeld, *Namibia* **116 C2** 20 57 S 16 14 E
Kalkfontein, *Botswana* **116 C3** 22 4 S 20 57 E
Kalkım, *Turkey* **49 B9** 39 48N 27 13 E
Kalkrand, *Namibia* **116 C2** 24 1 S 17 35 E
Kallakkurichchi, *India* **95 J4** 11 44N 79 1 E
Kallam, *India* **94 E3** 18 36N 76 2 E
Kållandsö, *Sweden* **17 F7** 58 40N 13 5 E
Kallavesi, *Finland* **14 E22** 62 58N 27 30 E
Källby, *Sweden* **17 F7** 58 30N 13 8 E
Kållered, *Sweden* **17 G6** 57 32N 12 4 E
Kallidaikurichi, *India* **95 K3** 8 38N 77 31 E
Kallies = Kalisz Pomorski, *Poland* **55 E2** 53 17N 15 55 E
Kallimasiá, *Greece* **49 C8** 38 18N 26 6 E
Kallinge, *Sweden* **17 H9** 56 15N 15 18 E
Kallithéa, *Greece* **48 D5** 37 55N 23 41 E
Kallmet, *Albania* **50 E3** 41 51N 19 41 E
Kalloní, *Greece* **49 B8** 39 14N 26 12 E
Kallonís, Kólpos, *Greece* **49 B8** 39 10N 26 10 E
Kallsjön, *Sweden* **14 E15** 63 38N 13 0 E
Kalmalo, *Nigeria* **113 C6** 13 40N 5 20 E
Kalmanstunga, *Iceland* **11 C6** 64 44N 20 48W
Kalmar, *Sweden* **17 H10** 56 40N 16 20 E
Kalmar län □, *Sweden* **17 G10** 57 25N 16 0 E
Kalmar sund, *Sweden* **17 H10** 56 40N 16 25 E
Kalmunai, *Sri Lanka* **95 L5** 7 25N 81 49 E
Kalmyk Republic = Kalmykia □, *Russia* **61 G8** 46 5N 46 1 E
Kalmykia □, *Russia* **61 G8** 46 5N 46 1 E
Kalmykovo, *Kazakhstan* **57 E9** 49 0N 51 47 E
Kalna, *India* **93 H13** 23 13N 88 25 E
Kalnai, *India* **93 H10** 22 46N 83 30 E
Kalni →, *Bangla.* **90 C3** 24 21N 91 13 E
Kalo, *Papua N. G.* **132 F4** 10 1 S 147 48 E
Kalocsa, *Hungary* **52 D4** 46 32N 19 0 E
Kalofer, *Bulgaria* **51 D8** 42 37N 24 59 E
Kalohi Channel, *U.S.A.* **145 C5** 21 0N 157 0W
Kalokhorio, *Cyprus* **39 F9** 34 51N 33 2 E
Kaloko, *Dem. Rep. of the Congo* **118 D2** 6 47 S 25 48 E
Kaloko-Honokohau △, *U.S.A.* **145 D5** 19 40N 156 1W
Kalol, *Gujarat, India* **92 H5** 22 37N 73 31 E
Kalol, *Gujarat, India* **92 H5** 23 15N 72 33 E
Kalolímnos, *Greece* **49 D9** 37 4N 27 5 E
Kalomo, *Zambia* **119 F2** 17 0 S 26 30 E
Kalona, *U.S.A.* **156 C5** 41 29N 91 43W
Kaloneróń, *Greece* **48 D3** 37 20N 21 38 E
Kalpeni I., *India* **95 J1** 10 5N 73 38 E
Kalpi, *India* **93 F8** 26 8N 79 47 E
Kalpitiya, *Sri Lanka* **95 K4** 8 14N 79 46 E
Kalputhi I., *India* **95 J1** 10 49N 72 10 E
Kalrayan Hills, *India* **95 J4** 11 45N 78 40 E
Kalsubai, *India* **94 E1** 19 35N 73 45 E
Kaltag, *U.S.A.* **144 D8** 64 20N 158 43W
Kaltbrunn, *Switz.* **33 B8** 47 13N 9 2 E
Kaltern = Caldaro, *Italy* **45 B8** 46 25N 11 14 E
Kaltungo, *Nigeria* **113 D7** 9 48N 11 19 E
Kalu, *Pakistan* **92 G2** 25 5N 67 39 E
Kaluga, *Russia* **58 E9** 54 35N 36 10 E
Kalulong, Bukit, *Malaysia* **85 B4** 3 14N 114 39 E
Kalulushi, *Zambia* **119 E2** 12 50 S 28 3 E
Kalundborg, *Denmark* **17 J5** 55 41N 11 5 E
Kalush, *Ukraine* **59 H3** 49 3N 24 23 E
Kałuszyn, *Poland* **55 F8** 52 13N 21 52 E
Kalutara, *Sri Lanka* **95 L5** 6 35N 80 0 E
Kalvåg, *Norway* **18 C1** 61 46N 4 51 E
Kalvarija, *Lithuania* **54 D10** 54 24N 23 14 E
Kalwakurti, *India* **94 F4** 16 41N 78 30 E
Kalya, *Russia* **64 A7** 60 15N 59 59 E
Kalyan, *Maharashtra, India* **94 D2** 20 30N 74 3 E
Kalyan, *Maharashtra, India* **94 E1** 19 15N 73 9 E
Kalyandurg, *India* **95 G3** 14 33N 77 6 E
Kalyani, *India* **94 F3** 17 52N 76 57 E
Kalyansingapuram, *India* **94 E6** 19 30N 83 19 E
Kalyazin, *Russia* **58 D9** 57 15N 37 55 E
Kam, *Albania* **50 D4** 42 17N 20 18 E
Kam →, *Nigeria* **113 D7** 8 15N 1 10 E
Kama, *Burma* **90 F5** 19 1N 95 4 E
Kama, *Dem. Rep. of the Congo* **118 C2** 3 30 S 27 5 E
Kama →, *Russia* **64 C5** 55 45N 52 0 E
Kamachumu, *Tanzania* **118 C3** 1 37 S 31 37 E
Kamae, *Japan* **72 E3** 32 48N 131 56 E

Kamaing, Burma 90 C6 25 26N 96 35 E
Kamaishi, Japan 70 E10 39 16N 141 53 E
Kamakou, U.S.A. 145 B5 21 7N 156 52W
Kamakura, Japan 73 B11 35 19N 139 33 E
Kamalapurum, India 95 G4 14 35N 78 39 E
Kamalété, Gabon 114 C2 0 43 S 11 49 E
Kamalia, Pakistan 92 D5 30 44N 72 42 E
Kaman, India 92 F6 27 39N 77 16 E
Kaman, Turkey 100 C5 39 22N 33 44 E
Kamana, Dem. Rep. of the Congo 115 D4 5 59 S 24 58 E
Kamananui →, U.S.A. 145 J13 21 38N 158 4W
Kamanjab, Namibia 116 B2 19 35 S 14 51 E
Kamapanda, Zambia 119 E1 12 5 S 24 0 E
Kamarān, Yemen 98 D3 15 21N 42 35 E
Kamareddi, India 94 E4 18 19N 78 21 E
Kamashi, Uzbekistan 65 D2 38 51N 65 23 E
Kamativi, Zimbabwe 116 B4 18 20 S 27 6 E
Kamba, Dem. Rep. of the Congo 115 C4 4 0 S 22 22 E
Kamba, Nigeria 113 C5 11 50N 3 45 E
Kambalda, Australia 125 F3 31 10 S 121 37 E
Kambam, India 95 K3 9 45N 77 16 E
Kambar, Pakistan 92 F3 27 37N 68 1 E
Kambarka, Russia 64 C5 56 15N 54 11 E
Kambia, S. Leone 112 D2 9 3N 12 53W
Kambolé, Togo 113 D5 8 43N 1 39 E
Kambolé, Zambia 119 D3 8 47 S 30 48 E
Kambos, Cyprus 39 E8 35 2N 32 44 E
Kambove, Dem. Rep. of the Congo 119 E2 10 51 S 26 33 E
Kambuie, Dem. Rep. of the Congo 115 D4 6 59 S 22 19 E
Kambwata, Zambia 115 E4 14 3 S 23 43 E
Kamchatka, Poluostrov, Russia 67 D16 57 0N 160 0 E
Kamchatka Pen. = Kamchatka, Poluostrov, Russia 67 D16 57 0N 160 0 E
Kamchiya →, Bulgaria 51 C11 43 4N 27 44 E
Kame Ruins, Zimbabwe 119 G2 20 7 S 28 25 E
Kamehameha Heights, U.S.A. 145 K14 21 21N 157 52W
Kamen, Russia 66 D9 53 50N 81 30 E
Kamen-Rybolov, Russia 70 B6 44 46N 132 2 E
Kamende, Dem. Rep. of the Congo 115 D4 6 26 S 24 35 E
Kamenica, Serbia & M. 50 C6 43 27N 22 27 E
Kamenica, Serbia & M. 50 B3 44 25N 19 45 E
Kamenice nad Lipou, Czech Rep. 34 B8 49 18N 15 2 E
Kamenjak, Rt, Croatia 45 D10 44 47N 13 55 E
Kamenka = Kaminka, Ukraine 59 H7 49 3N 32 6 E
Kamenka, Kazakhstan 60 E10 51 7N 50 19 E
Kamenka, Arkhangelsk, Russia 56 A7 65 58N 44 0 E
Kamenka, Penza, Russia 60 D6 53 10N 44 5 E
Kamenka, Voronezh, Russia 59 G10 50 47N 39 20 E
Kamenka Bugskaya = Kamyanka-Buzka, Ukraine 59 G3 50 8N 24 16 E
Kamenka Dneprovskaya = Kamyanka-Dniprovska, Ukraine 59 J8 47 29N 34 28 E
Kamenka-Shevchenkovskaya = Kamyanka-Buzka, Ukraine 59 G3 50 8N 24 16 E
Kamennomostskiy, Russia 61 H5 44 18N 40 13 E
Kameno, Bulgaria 51 D11 42 34N 27 18 E
Kamenolomini, Russia 61 G5 47 40N 40 14 E
Kamensk-Shakhtinskiy, Russia 61 F5 48 23N 40 20 E
Kamensk Uralskiy, Russia 64 C9 56 25N 62 2 E
Kamenskaya = Kamensk-Shakhtinskiy, Russia 61 F5 48 23N 40 20 E
Kamenskiy, Russia 60 E7 50 48N 45 25 E
Kamenskoye = Dniprodzerzhynsk, Ukraine 59 H8 48 32N 34 37 E
Kamenskoye, Russia 67 C17 62 45N 165 30 E
Kamenyak, Bulgaria 51 C10 43 24N 26 57 E
Kamenz, Germany 30 D10 51 15N 14 5 E
Kameoka, Japan 73 C7 35 0N 135 35 E
Kameyama, Japan 73 C8 34 51N 136 27 E
Kami-Jima, Japan 72 E2 32 27N 130 20 E
Kami-Koshiki-Jima, Japan 72 F1 31 50N 129 52 E
Kamiagata, Japan 72 C1 34 47N 129 24 E
Kamiah, U.S.A. 158 C5 46 14N 116 2W
Kamień Krajeński, Poland 54 E4 53 32N 17 32 E
Kamień Pomorski, Poland 54 E1 53 57N 14 43 E
Kamienna →, Poland 55 G8 51 6N 21 47 E
Kamienna Góra, Poland 55 H3 50 47N 16 2 E
Kamieńsk, Poland 55 G6 51 12N 19 29 E
Kamieskroon, S. Africa 116 E2 30 9 S 17 56 E
Kamilukuak L., Canada 143 A8 62 22N 101 40W
Kamin-Kashyrskyy, Ukraine 59 G3 51 39N 24 56 E
Kamina, Dem. Rep. of the Congo 119 D2 8 45 S 25 0 E
Kaminak L., Canada 143 A10 62 10N 95 0W
Kaministiquia, Canada 140 C1 48 32N 89 35W
Kaminka, Ukraine 59 H7 49 3N 32 6 E
Kaminoyama, Japan 70 E10 38 9N 140 17 E
Kamioka, Japan 73 A9 36 25N 137 15 E
Kamiros, Greece 38 E11 36 20N 27 56 E
Kamishak Bay, U.S.A. 144 G9 59 15N 153 45W
Kamitsushima, Japan 72 C1 34 50N 129 28 E
Kamituga, Dem. Rep. of the Congo 118 C2 3 2 S 28 10 E
Kamla →, India 93 G12 25 35N 86 36 E
Kamloops, Canada 142 C4 50 40N 120 20W
Kamnik, Slovenia 45 B11 46 14N 14 37 E
Kamo, Armenia 61 K7 40 21N 45 7 E
Kamo, Japan 70 F9 37 39N 139 3 E
Kamo, N.Z. 130 B3 35 42 S 174 20 E
Kamoa Mts., Guyana 169 C6 1 30N 59 0W
Kamogawa, Japan 73 B12 35 5N 140 5 E
Kamojima, Japan 72 C6 34 4N 134 21 E
Kamoke, Pakistan 92 C6 32 4N 74 4 E
Kamooloa, U.S.A. 145 J13 21 34N 158 7W
Kamp →, Austria 34 C8 48 23N 15 42 E
Kampala, Uganda 118 B3 0 20N 32 30 E
Kampar, Malaysia 87 K3 4 18N 101 9 E
Kampar →, Indonesia 84 B2 0 30N 103 8 E
Kampen, Neths. 24 B5 52 33N 5 53 E
Kamphaeng Phet, Thailand 86 D2 16 28N 99 30 E
Kampinoski △, Poland 55 F7 52 21N 20 40 E
Kampolombo, L., Zambia 119 E2 11 37 S 29 42 E
Kampong Chhnang, Cambodia 87 F5 12 20N 104 35 E
Kampong Pengerang, Malaysia 87 d 1 22N 104 7 E
Kampong Punggai, Malaysia 87 d 1 27N 104 18 E
Kampong Saom, Cambodia 87 G4 10 38N 103 30 E
Kampong Saom, Chaak, Cambodia 87 G4 10 50N 103 32 E
Kampong Tanjong Langsat, Malaysia 87 d 1 28N 104 1 E
Kampong Telok Ramunia, Malaysia 87 d 1 22N 104 15 E
Kampong To, Thailand 87 J3 6 3N 101 13 E
Kampot, Cambodia 87 G5 10 36N 104 10 E
Kampsville, U.S.A. 156 E6 39 18N 90 37W
Kampti, Burkina Faso 112 C4 10 7N 3 25W
Kampuchea = Cambodia ■, Asia 86 F5 12 15N 105 0 E
Kampung Air Putih, Malaysia 87 K4 4 15N 103 10 E
Kampung Jerangau, Malaysia 87 K4 4 50N 103 10 E
Kampung Raja, Malaysia 87 K4 5 45N 102 35 E
Kampungbaru = Tolitoli, Indonesia 82 A2 1 5N 120 50 E
Kamrau, Teluk, Indonesia 83 B4 3 30 S 133 36 E
Kamsack, Canada 143 C8 51 34N 101 54W
Kamsai, Guinea 112 C2 10 40N 14 36W
Kamskoye Ustye, Russia 60 C9 55 10N 49 20 E
Kamskoye Vdkhr., Russia 64 B6 58 41N 56 7 E
Kamthi, India 94 D4 21 9N 79 19 E
Kamuchawie L., Canada 143 B8 56 18N 101 59W
Kamuela, U.S.A. 145 C6 20 1N 155 41W
Kamui-Misaki, Japan 70 C10 43 20N 140 21 E
Kamundan →, Indonesia 83 B4 2 17 S 132 39 E
Kamyanets-Podilskyy, Ukraine 53 B11 48 45N 26 40 E
Kamyanka-Buzka, Ukraine 59 G3 50 8N 24 16 E
Kamyanka-Dniprovska, Ukraine 59 J8 47 29N 34 28 E
Kamyanyets, Belarus 55 F10 52 23N 23 49 E
Kamyanyuki, Belarus 55 F10 52 32N 23 49 E
Kāmyārān, Iran 101 E12 34 47N 46 56 E
Kamyshin, Russia 60 E7 50 10N 45 24 E
Kamyshlov, Russia 64 C9 56 50N 62 43 E
Kamyzyak, Russia 61 G9 46 4N 48 10 E
Kan = Gan Jiang →, China 77 C11 29 15N 116 0 E
Kan, Burma 90 D5 22 25N 94 5 E
Kan, Sudan 107 F3 9 1N 31 47 E
Kanaaupscow, Canada 139 C12 53 39N 77 9W
Kanaaupscow →, Canada 140 B4 54 2N 76 30W
Kanab, U.S.A. 159 H7 37 3N 112 32W
Kanab Cr. →, U.S.A. 159 H7 36 24N 112 38W
Kanacea, Lau Group, Fiji 133 A3 17 15 S 179 6W
Kanacea, Taveuni, Fiji 133 A2 16 59 S 179 56 E
Kanaga I., U.S.A. 144 L3 51 45N 177 22W
Kanagawa □, Japan 73 B11 35 20N 139 20 E
Kanagi, Japan 70 D10 40 54N 140 27 E
Kanairiktok →, Canada 141 A7 55 2N 60 18W
Kanakanak, U.S.A. 144 G8 59 0N 158 32W
Kanakapura, India 95 H3 12 33N 77 28 E
Kanália, Greece 48 B4 39 30N 22 53 E
Kananga, Dem. Rep. of the Congo 115 D4 5 55 S 22 18 E
Kanangra-Boyd △, Australia 129 B9 33 57 S 150 15 E
Kanash, Russia 60 C8 55 30N 47 32 E
Kanaskat, U.S.A. 160 C5 47 19N 121 54W
Kanastraíon, Ákra = Palioúrion, Ákra, Greece 50 G7 39 57N 23 45 E
Kanawha →, U.S.A. 148 F4 38 50N 82 9W
Kanazawa, Japan 73 A8 36 30N 136 38 E
Kanbalu, Burma 90 D5 23 12N 95 31 E
Kanchanaburi, Thailand 86 E2 14 2N 99 31 E
Kanchenjunga, Nepal 93 F13 27 50N 88 10 E
Kanchipuram, India 95 H4 12 52N 79 45 E
Kanchow = Ganzhou, China 77 E10 25 51N 114 56 E
Kańczuga, Poland 55 J9 49 59N 22 25 E
Kanda Kanda, Dem. Rep. of the Congo 115 D4 6 52 S 23 48 E
Kandagach = Oktyabrsk, Kazakhstan 57 E10 49 28N 57 25 E
Kandaghat, India 92 D7 30 59N 77 7 E
Kandahar = Qandahār, Afghan. 91 C2 31 32N 65 43 E
Kandahar, India 94 E3 18 52N 77 12 E
Kandala, Dem. Rep. of the Congo 115 D3 6 20 S 19 40 E
Kandalaksha, Russia 56 A5 67 9N 32 30 E
Kandalakshkiy Zaliv, Russia 56 A6 66 0N 35 0 E
Kandangan, Indonesia 85 C5 2 50 S 115 20 E
Kandanghaur, Indonesia 79 G13 6 21 S 108 6 E
Kandanos, Greece 39 E4 35 19N 23 44 E
Kandava, Latvia 53 C9 57 2N 22 46 E
Kandavu = Kadavu, Fiji 133 B2 19 0 S 178 15 E
Kandavu Passage = Kadavu Passage, Fiji 133 B2 18 45 S 178 0 E
Kandep, Papua N. G. 132 C2 5 54 S 143 32 E
Kander →, Switz. 32 C5 46 33N 7 38 E
Kandersteg, Switz. 32 D5 46 28N 7 40 E
Kandhíla, Aitolía kai Akarnanía, Greece 39 B2 38 42N 20 56 E
Kandhíla, Arkadhía, Greece 48 D4 37 46N 22 22 E
Kandhkot, Pakistan 92 E3 28 16N 69 8 E
Kandhla, India 92 E7 29 18N 77 19 E
Kandi, Benin 113 C5 11 7N 2 55 E
Kandi, India 93 H13 23 58N 88 5 E
Kandiaro, Pakistan 92 F3 27 4N 68 13 E
Kandıra, Turkey 100 B4 41 4N 30 9 E
Kandla, India 92 H4 23 0N 70 10 E
Kandor, O. →, Chad 109 E4 17 13N 20 52 E
Kandos, Australia 129 B8 32 45 S 149 58 E
Kandreho, Madag. 117 B8 17 29 S 46 6 E
Kandrian, Papua N. G. 132 D5 6 14 S 149 37 E
Kandy, Sri Lanka 95 L5 7 18N 80 43 E
Kane, U.S.A. 150 E6 41 40N 78 49W
Kane Basin, Greenland 10 B4 79 1N 70 0W
Kaneilio Pt., U.S.A. 145 K13 21 27N 158 12W
Kanel, Senegal 112 B2 15 30N 13 18W
Kaneohe, U.S.A. 145 K14 21 25N 157 48W
Kaneohe B., U.S.A. 145 K14 21 30N 157 50W
Kanevskaya, Russia 61 G4 46 3N 38 57 E
Kanfanar, Croatia 45 C10 45 7N 13 50 E
Kang, Botswana 116 C3 23 41 S 22 50 E
Kang Krung △, Thailand 87 H2 9 30N 98 50 E
Kangaamiut, Greenland 10 D5 65 50N 53 20W
Kangaba, Mali 112 C3 11 56N 8 25W
Kangal, Turkey 100 C7 39 14N 37 23 E
Kangān, Fārs, Iran 97 E7 27 50N 52 3 E
Kangān, Hormozgān, Iran 97 E8 25 48N 57 28 E
Kangar, Malaysia 87 J3 6 27N 100 12 E
Kangaré, Mali 112 C3 11 36N 8 4W
Kangaroo I., Australia 128 C2 35 45 S 137 0 E
Kangaroo Mts., Australia 126 C3 23 29 S 141 51 E
Kangasala, Finland 15 F21 61 28N 24 4 E
Kangāvar, Iran 97 C6 34 40N 48 0 E
Kangding, China 76 B3 30 2N 101 57 E
Kangdong, N. Korea 75 E14 39 9N 126 5 E
Kangean, Kepulauan, Indonesia 85 D5 6 55 S 115 23 E
Kangean Is. = Kangean, Kepulauan, Indonesia 85 D5 6 55 S 115 23 E
Kangen →, Sudan 107 F3 6 47N 33 9 E
Kangerdlugssuak, Greenland 10 D7 68 10N 32 20W
Kangerluarsoruseq, Greenland 10 E5 63 45N 51 27W
Kangerluarsoruset = Kangerluarsoruseq, Greenland 10 E5 63 45N 51 27W
Kangerlussuaq, Greenland 10 D5 66 59N 50 40W
Kanggye, N. Korea 75 D14 41 0N 126 35 E
Kanggyŏng, S. Korea 75 F14 36 10N 127 0 E
Kanghwa, S. Korea 75 F14 37 45N 126 30 E
Kangikajik, Greenland 10 C8 70 7N 22 0W
Kangilinnguit, Greenland 10 E6 61 20N 47 57W
Kangiqliniq = Rankin Inlet, Canada 138 B10 62 30N 93 0W
Kangiqsualujjuaq, Canada 139 C13 58 30N 65 59W
Kangiqsujuaq, Canada 139 B12 61 30N 72 0W
Kangiqtugaapik = Clyde River, Canada 139 A13 70 30N 68 30W
Kangirsuk, Canada 139 B13 60 0N 70 0W
Kangkar Chemaran, Malaysia 87 d 1 34N 104 12 E
Kangkar Sungai Tiram, Malaysia 87 d 1 35N 103 55 E
Kangkar Teberau, Malaysia 87 d 1 32N 103 51 E
Kangnŭng, S. Korea 75 F15 37 45N 128 54 E
Kango, Gabon 114 B2 0 11N 10 5 E
Kangoya, Dem. Rep. of the Congo 115 D4 9 55 S 22 48 E
Kangping, China 75 C12 42 43N 123 18 E
Kangpokpi, India 90 C4 25 8N 93 58 E
Kangra, India 92 C7 32 6N 76 16 E
Kangrinboqe Feng, China 93 D9 31 0N 81 25 E
Kangyidaung, Burma 90 G5 16 56N 94 54 E
Kanha △, India 93 H9 22 15N 80 40 E
Kanhan →, India 94 D4 21 4N 79 34 E
Kanhangad, India 95 H2 12 21N 74 58 E
Kanhar →, India 93 G10 24 28N 83 8 E
Kanheri, India 94 E1 19 13N 72 50 E
Kani, Sagaing, Burma 90 D5 23 52N 95 22 E
Kani, Sagaing, Burma 90 D5 22 26N 94 51 E
Kani, Ivory C. 112 D3 8 29N 6 36W
Kaniama, Dem. Rep. of the Congo 118 D1 7 30 S 24 12 E
Kaniapiskau = Caniapiscau →, Canada 141 A6 56 40N 69 30W
Kaniapiskau, L. = Caniapiscau, L. de, Canada 141 B6 54 10N 69 55W
Kanibadam, Tajikistan 65 C5 40 17N 70 25 E
Kaniere, L., N.Z. 131 C6 42 50 S 171 10 E
Kanigiri, India 95 G4 15 24N 79 31 E
Kanimekh, Uzbekistan 65 C2 40 16N 65 7 E
Kanin, Poluostrov, Russia 56 A8 68 0N 45 0 E
Kanin Nos, Mys, Russia 56 A7 68 39N 43 32 E
Kanin Pen. = Kanin, Poluostrov, Russia 56 A8 68 0N 45 0 E
Kaninë, Albania 50 F3 40 23N 19 30 E
Kaniva, Australia 128 D4 36 22 S 141 18 E
Kanjiža, Serbia & M. 52 D5 46 3N 20 4 E
Kanjut Sar, Pakistan 93 A6 36 7N 75 25 E
Kankaanpää, Finland 15 F20 61 44N 22 50 E
Kankakee, U.S.A. 157 C9 41 7N 87 52W
Kankakee →, U.S.A. 157 C8 41 23N 88 15W
Kankan, Guinea 112 C3 10 23N 9 15W
Kankendy = Xankändi, Azerbaijan 101 C12 39 52N 46 49 E
Kanker, India 94 D5 20 10N 81 40 E
Kankesanturai, Sri Lanka 95 K5 9 49N 80 2 E
Kankossa, Mauritania 112 B2 15 54N 11 31W
Kankroli, India 92 G5 25 4N 73 53 E
Kanmuri-Yama, Japan 72 C4 34 30N 132 4 E
Kannabe, Japan 72 C5 34 32N 133 23 E
Kannapolis, U.S.A. 149 H5 35 30N 80 37W
Kannauj, India 93 F8 27 3N 79 56 E
Kanniyakumari, India 95 K3 8 5N 77 34 E
Kano, Nigeria 113 C6 12 2N 8 30 E
Kano □, Nigeria 113 C6 11 30N 8 30 E
Kan'onji, Japan 72 C5 34 7N 133 39 E
Kanoroba, Ivory C. 112 D3 9 7N 6 8W
Kanowha, U.S.A. 156 B3 42 57N 93 47W
Kanowit, Malaysia 85 B4 2 14N 112 20 E
Kanoya, Japan 72 F2 31 25N 130 50 E
Kanpetlet, Burma 90 E4 21 10N 93 59 E
Kanpur, India 93 F9 26 28N 80 20 E
Kansai International ✈ (KIX), Japan 73 C7 34 27N 135 12 E
Kansas, U.S.A. 157 E9 39 33N 87 56W
Kansas □, U.S.A. 154 F6 38 30N 99 0W
Kansas →, U.S.A. 154 F7 39 7N 94 37W
Kansas City, Kans., U.S.A. 156 E2 39 7N 94 38W
Kansas City, Mo., U.S.A. 156 E2 39 6N 94 35W
Kansas City International ✈ (MCI), U.S.A. 156 E2 39 18N 94 43W
Kansenia, Dem. Rep. of the Congo 119 E2 10 20 S 26 0 E
Kansk, Russia 67 D10 56 20N 95 37 E
Kansŏng, S. Korea 75 E15 38 24N 128 30 E
Kansu = Gansu □, China 74 G3 36 0N 104 0 E
Kansu, China 65 D7 39 46N 75 2 E
Kant, Kyrgyzstan 65 B7 42 53N 74 51 E
Kantaphor, India 92 H7 22 35N 76 34 E
Kantchari, Burkina Faso 113 C5 12 37N 1 37 E
Kantché, Niger 113 C6 13 31N 8 30 E
Kanté, Togo 113 D5 9 57N 1 3 E
Kantemirovka, Russia 59 H10 49 43N 39 55 E
Kanth = Kąty Wrocławskie, Poland 55 G3 51 2N 16 45 E
Kantharalak, Thailand 86 E5 14 39N 104 39 E
Kantishna, U.S.A. 144 E10 63 31N 150 57W
Kantishna →, U.S.A. 144 D10 64 45N 149 58W
Kantli →, India 92 E6 28 20N 75 30 E
Kantō □, Japan 73 A11 36 15N 139 30 E
Kantō-Sanchi, Japan 73 B10 35 59N 138 50 E
Kantu-long, Burma 90 F6 19 57N 97 36 E
Kanturk, Ireland 23 D3 52 11N 8 54W
Kanuma, Japan 73 A11 36 34N 139 42 E
Kanus, Namibia 116 D2 27 50 S 18 39 E
Kanye, Botswana 116 C4 24 55 S 25 28 E
Kanzenze, Dem. Rep. of the Congo 119 E2 10 30 S 25 12 E
Kanzi, Ras, Tanzania 118 D4 7 1 S 39 33 E
Kao, Tonga 133 P13 19 40 S 175 1W
Kao Phara, Thailand 87 a 8 3N 98 22 E
Kaoe, Indonesia 82 A3 1 11N 127 54 E
Kaohsiung, Taiwan 77 F13 22 35N 120 16 E
Kaoka, Solomon Is. 133 M11 9 42 S 160 43 E
Kaokaona, Solomon Is. 133 N11 10 27 S 161 56 E
Kaokoveld, Namibia 116 B1 19 15 S 14 30 E
Kaolack, Senegal 112 C1 14 5N 16 8W
Kaolan = Lanzhou, China 74 F2 36 1N 103 52 E
Kaolo, Solomon Is. 133 M10 8 24 S 159 38 E
Kaoma, Zambia 115 E4 14 47 S 24 48 E
Kaoshan, China 75 B13 44 38N 124 50 E
Kaouar, Niger 109 E2 19 5N 12 52 E
Kaoyao = Zhaoqing, China 77 F9 23 0N 112 20 E
Kapaa, U.S.A. 145 A2 22 5N 159 19W
Kapadvanj, India 92 H5 23 5N 73 0 E
Kapagere, Papua N. G. 132 E4 9 46 S 147 42 E
Kapahulu, U.S.A. 145 K14 21 16N 157 49W
Kapaklı, Turkey 51 E11 41 19N 27 59 E
Kapan, Armenia 101 C12 39 18N 46 27 E
Kapanga, Bandundu, Dem. Rep. of the Congo 115 D3 5 4 S 16 58 E
Kapanga, Katanga, Dem. Rep. of the Congo 115 D4 8 30 S 22 40 E
Kapapa I., U.S.A. 145 K14 21 29N 157 48W
Kapatagan, Phil. 81 H4 7 52N 123 44 E
Kapchagai = Qapshaghay, Kazakhstan 65 B8 43 51N 77 14 E
Kapchagaiskoye Vdkhr. = Qapshaghay Bögeni, Kazakhstan 65 B8 43 45N 77 50 E
Kapela = Velika Kapela, Croatia 45 C12 45 10N 15 5 E
Kapéllo, Ákra, Greece 48 E5 36 9N 23 3 E
Kapema, Dem. Rep. of the Congo 119 E2 10 45 S 28 22 E
Kapfenberg, Austria 34 D8 47 26N 15 18 E
Kapı Dağı, Turkey 51 F11 40 28N 27 50 E
Kapia, Dem. Rep. of the Congo 115 C3 4 17 S 19 46 E
Kapiri Mposhi, Zambia 119 E2 13 59 S 28 43 E
Kāpīsā □, Afghan. 91 B3 35 0N 69 20 E
Kapiskau →, Canada 140 B3 52 47N 81 55W
Kapit, Malaysia 85 B4 2 0N 112 55 E
Kapiti I., N.Z. 130 G3 40 50 S 174 56 E
Kapka, Massif du, Chad 109 E4 15 7N 21 45 E
Kaplan, U.S.A. 155 K8 30 0N 92 17W
Kaplice, Czech Rep. 34 C7 48 42N 14 30 E
Kapoe, Thailand 87 H2 9 34N 98 32 E
Kapoeta, Sudan 107 G3 4 50N 33 35 E
Kápolnásnyék, Hungary 52 C3 47 16N 18 41 E
Kapombo, Dem. Rep. of the Congo 115 E4 10 40 S 23 30 E
Kaponga, N.Z. 130 F3 39 29 S 174 9 E
Kapos →, Hungary 52 D3 46 44N 18 30 E
Kaposvár, Hungary 52 D2 46 25N 17 47 E
Kapowsin, U.S.A. 160 D4 46 59N 122 13W
Kapp, Norway 18 D7 60 43N 10 52 E
Kappeln, Germany 30 A5 54 40N 9 55 E
Kappelshamn, Sweden 17 G12 57 52N 18 47 E
Kapps, Namibia 116 C2 22 32 S 17 18 E
Kaprije, Croatia 45 E12 43 42N 15 43 E
Kapsan, N. Korea 75 D15 41 4N 128 19 E
Kapsukas = Marijampolė, Lithuania 15 J20 54 33N 23 19 E
Kaptai, Bangla. 90 D4 22 21N 92 17 E
Kaptai L., Bangla. 90 D4 22 40N 92 20 E
Kapuas, Indonesia 85 C4 3 10 S 114 5 E
Kapuas →, Indonesia 85 C3 0 25 S 109 20 E
Kapuas Hulu, Pegunungan, Malaysia 85 B4 1 30N 113 30 E
Kapuas Hulu Ra. = Kapuas Hulu, Pegunungan, Malaysia 85 B4 1 30N 113 30 E
Kapulo, Dem. Rep. of the Congo 119 D2 8 18 S 29 15 E
Kapunda, Australia 128 C3 34 20 S 138 56 E
Kapuni, N.Z. 130 F3 39 29 S 174 8 E
Kapurthala, India 92 D6 31 23N 75 25 E
Kapuskasing, Canada 140 C3 49 25N 82 30W
Kapuskasing →, Canada 140 C3 49 49N 82 0W
Kapustin Yar, Russia 61 F7 48 37N 45 40 E
Kaputar, Australia 127 E5 30 15 S 150 10 E
Kaputir, Kenya 118 B4 2 5N 35 28 E
Kapuvár, Hungary 52 C2 47 36N 17 1 E
Kaqung, China 65 E8 38 0N 76 50 E
Kara, Russia 66 C7 69 10N 65 0 E
Karā, W. →, Si. Arabia 106 C5 20 45N 41 42 E
Kara Ada, Turkey 49 E9 36 58N 27 28 E
Kara-Balta, Kyrgyzstan 65 B6 42 50N 73 49 E
Kara Bogaz Gol, Zaliv = Garabogazköl Aylagy, Turkmenistan 57 F9 41 0N 53 30 E
Kara Burun, Turkey 49 E9 36 32N 27 58 E
Kara-Darya = Payshanba, Uzbekistan 65 C3 40 0N 66 14 E
Kara Kalpak Republic = Qoraqalpoghistan □, Uzbekistan 66 E6 43 0N 58 0 E
Kara-Köl, Kyrgyzstan 65 C6 41 40N 72 43 E
Kara-Kulja, Kyrgyzstan 65 C6 40 39N 73 26 E
Kara Kum, Turkmenistan 66 F6 39 30N 60 0 E
Kara-Saki, Japan 72 C1 34 41N 129 30 E
Kara-Say, Kyrgyzstan 65 C8 41 33N 77 54 E
Kara Sea, Russia 66 B7 75 0N 70 0 E
Kara-Suu, Kyrgyzstan 65 C6 40 44N 72 53 E
Karaadilli, Turkey 49 C12 38 18N 30 37 E
Karabash, Russia 64 D8 55 29N 60 14 E
Karabekaul = Garabekewül, Turkmenistan 65 D2 38 30N 64 8 E
Karabiğa, Turkey 51 F11 40 23N 27 17 E
Karabük, Turkey 100 B5 41 12N 32 37 E
Karabulak = Qarabulaq, Kazakhstan 65 A9 44 54N 78 30 E
Karabulak, China 65 C8 40 48N 77 32 E
Karaburun, Albania 50 F3 40 25N 19 20 E
Karaburun, Turkey 49 C8 38 41N 26 28 E
Karabutak = Qarabutaq, Kazakhstan 64 G8 49 59N 60 14 E
Karacabey, Turkey 51 F12 40 12N 28 21 E
Karacakılavuz, Turkey 51 E11 41 8N 27 21 E
Karacaköy, Turkey 51 E12 41 24N 28 22 E
Karacasu, Turkey 49 D10 37 43N 28 35 E
Karachala = Qaraçala, Azerbaijan 61 L9 39 45N 48 53 E
Karachayevsk, Russia 61 J5 43 50N 41 55 E
Karachev, Russia 59 F8 53 10N 35 5 E
Karachey-Cherkessia □, Russia 61 J5 43 40N 41 30 E
Karachi, Pakistan 91 D2 24 53N 67 0 E
Karad, India 94 F2 17 15N 74 10 E
Karadirek, Turkey 49 C12 38 34N 30 11 E
Karaga, Ghana 113 D4 9 58N 0 28W
Karaganda = Qaraghandy, Kazakhstan 66 E8 49 50N 73 10 E
Karagayly = Qaraghayly, Kazakhstan 66 E8 49 26N 76 0 E
Karaginskiy, Ostrov, Russia 67 D17 58 45N 164 0 E
Karagiye, Vpadina, Kazakhstan 57 F9 43 27N 51 45 E
Karagiye Depression = Karagiye, Vpadina, Kazakhstan 57 F9 43 27N 51 45 E
Karagola Road, India 93 G12 25 29N 87 23 E
Karagüney Dağları, Turkey 100 B6 40 30N 34 40 E
Karahallı, Turkey 49 C11 38 21N 29 33 E
Karaikal, India 95 J4 10 59N 79 50 E
Karaikkudi, India 95 J4 10 5N 78 45 E
Karaisali, Turkey 100 D6 37 16N 35 2 E
Karaiskákis, Greece 39 B3 38 35N 21 4 E
Karaitivu I., Sri Lanka 95 K4 9 45N 79 52 E
Karaj, Iran 97 C6 35 48N 51 0 E
Karak, Malaysia 87 L4 3 25N 102 2 E
Karakalpakstan = Qoraqalpoghistan □, Uzbekistan 66 E6 43 0N 58 0 E
Karakelong, Indonesia 82 A3 4 35N 126 50 E
Karakitang, Indonesia 82 A3 3 14N 125 28 E
Karaklis = Vanadzor, Armenia 61 K7 40 48N 44 30 E
Karakoçan, Turkey 101 C9 38 57N 40 2 E
Karakol, Kyrgyzstan 65 B9 42 30N 78 20 E
Karakoram Pass, Asia 93 B7 35 33N 77 50 E
Karakoram Ra., Pakistan 93 B7 35 30N 77 0 E
Karakul, Tajikistan 65 D6 39 2N 73 33 E
Karakul, Uzbekistan 65 D1 39 22N 63 50 E
Karakul, Ozero, Tajikistan 65 D6 39 5N 73 25 E
Karakurt, Turkey 101 B10 40 10N 42 37 E
Karakuwisa, Namibia 116 B2 18 56 S 19 40 E
Karal, Chad 109 F2 12 50N 14 46 E
Karalon, Russia 67 D12 57 5N 115 50 E
Karama, Jordan 103 D4 31 57N 35 35 E
Karaman, Balıkesir, Turkey 49 B9 39 39N 28 0 E
Karaman, Konya, Turkey 100 D5 37 14N 33 13 E
Karamanlı, Turkey 49 D11 37 23N 29 47 E
Karamay, China 68 B3 45 30N 84 58 E
Karambu, Indonesia 85 C5 3 53 S 116 6 E
Karamea, N.Z. 131 B7 41 14 S 172 6 E
Karamea →, N.Z. 131 B7 41 13 S 172 26 E
Karamea Bight, N.Z. 131 B6 41 22 S 171 40 E
Karamet Niyaz = Garamätnyýaz, Turkmenistan 65 E2 37 45N 64 34 E
Karamnasa →, India 93 G10 25 31N 83 52 E
Karamürsel, Turkey 51 F13 40 41N 29 36 E
Karand, Iran 101 E12 34 16N 46 15 E
Karangana, Mali 112 C3 12 15N 5 4W
Karanganyar, Indonesia 85 D3 7 38 S 109 37 E
Karangasem, Indonesia 79 J18 8 27 S 115 37 E
Karanja, Maharashtra, India 94 D4 21 11N 78 24 E
Karanja, Maharashtra, India 94 D3 20 29N 77 31 E
Karanjia, India 93 J11 21 47N 85 58 E
Karankasso, Burkina Faso 112 C4 10 50N 3 53W
Karaova, Turkey 49 D9 37 5N 27 40 E
Karapınar, Turkey 100 D5 37 41N 33 30 E
Karapiro, N.Z. 130 D4 37 53 S 175 32 E
Karas, Indonesia 83 B4 3 27 S 132 40 E
Karasburg, Namibia 116 D2 28 0 S 18 44 E
Karasino, Russia 66 C9 66 50N 86 50 E
Karasjok, Norway 14 B21 69 27N 25 30 E
Karasu, Turkey 100 B4 41 4N 30 46 E
Karasu →, Turkey 49 E12 36 18N 30 10 E
Karasubazar = Bilohirsk, Ukraine 59 K8 45 3N 34 35 E
Karasuk, Russia 66 D8 53 44N 78 2 E
Karasuyama, Japan 73 A12 36 39N 140 9 E
Karataş, Adana, Turkey 100 D6 36 36N 35 21 E
Karataş, Manisa, Turkey 49 C10 38 35N 28 16 E
Karataş Burnu, Turkey 100 D6 36 31N 35 24 E
Karatau, Khrebet = Qarataū, Kazakhstan 65 B4 43 30N 69 30 E
Karateki Shan, China 65 C8 40 40N 77 50 E
Karativu, Sri Lanka 95 K4 8 22N 79 47 E
Karatobe, Kazakhstan 64 G4 49 44N 53 30 E
Karatoprak, Turkey 49 D9 37 2N 27 15 E
Karatoya →, India 90 C2 24 7N 89 36 E
Karatsu, Japan 72 D1 33 26N 129 58 E
Karaturuk = Qaraturyq, Kazakhstan 65 B8 43 35N 77 50 E
Karaul, Russia 66 B9 70 6N 82 15 E
Karaulbazar, Uzbekistan 65 D2 39 30N 64 48 E
Karauli, India 92 F7 26 30N 77 4 E
Karavastasë, L. e, Albania 50 F3 40 55N 19 30 E
Karávi, Greece 48 E5 36 49N 23 37 E
Karavostasi, Cyprus 39 E8 35 8N 32 50 E
Karawa, Dem. Rep. of the Congo 114 B4 3 18N 20 17 E
Karawang, Indonesia 85 D3 6 30 S 107 15 E
Karawanken, Europe 34 E7 46 30N 14 40 E
Karayazı, Turkey 101 C10 39 41N 42 9 E
Karazhal, Kazakhstan 66 E8 48 2N 70 49 E
Karbalā', Iraq 101 F11 32 36N 44 3 E
Kårböle, Sweden 16 C9 61 59N 15 22 E
Karcag, Hungary 52 C5 47 19N 20 57 E
Karcha →, Pakistan 93 B7 34 45N 76 10 E
Karchana, India 93 G9 25 17N 81 56 E
Karczew, Poland 55 F8 52 5N 21 15 E
Kardam, Bulgaria 51 C12 43 45N 28 6 E
Kardeljovo = Ploče, Croatia 45 E14 43 4N 17 26 E
Kardhakata, Greece 39 C1 38 17N 20 28 E
Kardhámila, Greece 49 C8 38 35N 26 5 E
Kardhamíli, Greece 48 E4 36 53N 22 13 E

Kardhítsa, *Greece* **48 B3** 39 23N 21 54 E
Kardhítsa □, *Greece* **48 B3** 39 15N 21 50 E
Karditsa = Kardhítsa, *Greece* **48 B3** 39 23N 21 54 E
Kärdla, *Estonia* **15 G20** 59 0N 22 45 E
Kareeberge, *S. Africa* **116 E3** 30 59 S 21 50 E
Kareha →, *India* **93 G12** 25 44N 86 21 E
Kareima, *Sudan* **106 D3** 18 30N 31 49 E
Karelia □, *Russia* **56 A5** 65 30N 32 30 E
Karelian Republic = Karelia □, *Russia* **56 A5** 65 30N 32 30 E
Karelo-Finnish SSR = Karelia □, *Russia* **56 A5** 65 30N 32 30 E
Karema, *Papua N. G.* **132 E4** 9 12 S 147 18 E
Karen = Kayin □, *Burma* **90 G6** 18 0N 97 30 E
Karenni = Kayah □, *Burma* **90 F6** 19 15N 97 15 E
Karera, *India* **92 G8** 25 32N 78 9 E
Kārevāndar, *Iran* **97 E9** 27 53N 60 44 E
Kargasok, *Russia* **66 D9** 59 3N 80 53 E
Kargat, *Russia* **66 D9** 55 10N 80 15 E
Kargı, *Turkey* **100 B6** 41 11N 34 30 E
Kargil, *India* **93 B7** 34 32N 76 12 E
Kargopol, *Russia* **58 B10** 61 30N 38 58 E
Kargowa, *Poland* **55 F2** 52 5N 15 51 E
Karguéri, *Niger* **113 C7** 13 27N 10 30 E
Karhal, *India* **93 F8** 27 1N 78 57 E
Kariá, *Greece* **39 B2** 38 45N 20 39 E
Karia ba Mohammed, *Morocco* **110 B3** 34 22N 5 12W
Kariaí, *Greece* **51 F8** 40 14N 24 19 E
Karīān, *Iran* **97 E8** 26 57N 57 14 E
Karianga, *Madag.* **117 C8** 22 25 S 47 22 E
Kariba, *Zimbabwe* **119 F2** 16 28 S 28 50 E
Kariba, L., *Zimbabwe* **119 F2** 16 40 S 28 25 E
Kariba Dam, *Zimbabwe* **119 F2** 16 30 S 28 35 E
Kariba Gorge, *Zambia* **119 F2** 16 30 S 28 50 E
Karibib, *Namibia* **116 C2** 22 0 S 15 56 E
Karijini △, *Australia* **124 D2** 23 8 S 118 15 E
Karikari, C., *N.Z.* **130 A2** 34 46 S 173 24 E
Karimata, Kepulauan, *Indonesia* **85 C3** 1 25 S 109 0 E
Karimata, Selat, *Indonesia* **85 C3** 2 0 S 108 40 E
Karimata Is. = Karimata, Kepulauan, *Indonesia* **85 C3** 1 25 S 109 0 E
Karimganj, *India* **90 C4** 24 52N 92 20 E
Karimnagar, *India* **94 E4** 18 26N 79 10 E
Karimun Kecil, Pulau, *Indonesia* **87 d** 1 8N 103 22 E
Karimunjawa, Kepulauan, *Indonesia* **85 D4** 5 50 S 110 30 E
Karin, *Somali Rep.* **120 B3** 10 50N 45 52 E
Káristos, *Greece* **48 C6** 38 1N 24 29 E
Karīt, *Iran* **97 C8** 33 29N 56 55 E
Kariya, *Japan* **73 C9** 34 58N 137 1 E
Kariyangwe, *Zimbabwe* **117 B4** 18 0 S 27 38 E
Karjala, *Finland* **58 A5** 62 0N 30 25 E
Karjat, *Maharashtra, India* **94 E2** 18 33N 75 0 E
Karjat, *Maharashtra, India* **94 E1** 18 55N 73 20 E
Karkal, *India* **95 H2** 13 15N 74 56 E
Karkar, *Papua N. G.* **132 C3** 4 32 S 145 57 E
Karkar I., *Papua N. G.* **132 C4** 4 40 S 146 0 E
Karkaralinsk = Qarqaraly, *Kazakhstan* **66 E8** 49 26N 75 30 E
Karkheh →, *Iran* **96 D5** 31 2N 47 29 E
Karkinitska Zatoka, *Ukraine* **59 K7** 45 56N 33 0 E
Karkinitskiy Zaliv = Karkinitska Zatoka, *Ukraine* **59 K7** 45 56N 33 0 E
Karkuk = Kirkūk, *Iraq* **101 E11** 35 30N 44 21 E
Karkur Tohl, *Egypt* **106 C2** 22 5N 25 5 E
Karl Liebknecht, *Russia* **59 G8** 51 40N 35 35 E
Karl-Marx-Stadt = Chemnitz, *Germany* **30 E8** 50 51N 12 54 E
Karleby = Kokkola, *Finland* **14 E20** 63 50N 23 8 E
Karlholmsbruk, *Sweden* **16 D11** 60 31N 17 37 E
Karlino, *Poland* **54 D2** 54 3N 15 53 E
Karlivka, *Ukraine* **59 H8** 49 29N 35 8 E
Karlobag, *Croatia* **45 D12** 44 32N 15 5 E
Karlovac, *Croatia* **45 C12** 45 31N 15 36 E
Karlovarský □, *Czech Rep.* **34 A5** 50 10N 12 50 E
Karlovka = Karlivka, *Ukraine* **59 H8** 49 29N 35 8 E
Karlovo, *Bulgaria* **51 D8** 42 38N 24 47 E
Karlovy Vary, *Czech Rep.* **34 A5** 50 13N 12 51 E
Karlowitz = Sremski Karlovci, *Serbia & M.* **52 E4** 45 12N 19 56 E
Karlowitz = Velké Karlovice, *Czech Rep.* **35 B11** 49 20N 18 17 E
Karlsbad = Karlovy Vary, *Czech Rep.* **34 A5** 50 13N 12 51 E
Karlsborg, *Sweden* **17 F8** 58 33N 14 33 E
Karlsburg = Alba-Iulia, *Romania* **53 D8** 46 8N 23 39 E
Karlshamn, *Sweden* **17 H8** 56 10N 14 51 E
Karlshus, *Norway* **18 E7** 59 21N 10 52 E
Karlskoga, *Sweden* **16 E8** 59 28N 14 33 E
Karlskrona, *Sweden* **17 H9** 56 10N 15 35 E
Karlsruhe, *Germany* **31 F4** 49 0N 8 23 E
Karlstad = Karlovac, *Croatia* **45 C12** 45 31N 15 36 E
Karlstad, *Sweden* **16 E7** 59 23N 13 30 E
Karlstad, *U.S.A.* **154 A6** 48 35N 96 31W
Karlstadt, *Germany* **31 F5** 49 57N 9 47 E
Karluk, *U.S.A.* **144 H9** 57 34N 154 28W
Karma, *Niger* **113 C5** 13 38N 1 52 E
Karmala, *India* **94 E2** 18 25N 75 12 E
Karmana, *Uzbekistan* **65 C2** 40 8N 65 21 E
Karmėlava, *Lithuania* **54 D11** 54 58N 24 4 E
Karmi'el, *Israel* **103 C4** 32 55N 35 18 E
Karmøy, *Norway* **18 E2** 59 15N 5 15 E
Karnak, *Egypt* **106 B3** 25 43N 32 39 E
Karnal, *India* **92 E7** 29 42N 77 2 E
Karnali →, *Nepal* **93 E9** 28 45N 81 16 E
Karnaphuli Res. = Kaptai L., *Bangla.* **90 D4** 22 40N 92 20 E
Karnaprayag, *India* **93 D8** 30 16N 79 15 E
Karnataka □, *India* **95 H3** 13 15N 77 0 E
Karnes City, *U.S.A.* **155 L6** 28 53N 97 54W
Karnische Alpen, *Europe* **34 E6** 46 36N 13 0 E
Karnobat, *Bulgaria* **51 D10** 42 39N 26 59 E
Kärnten □, *Austria* **34 E6** 46 52N 13 30 E
Karo, *Mali* **112 C4** 12 16N 3 18W
Karoi, *Zimbabwe* **119 F2** 16 48 S 29 45 E
Karomatan, *Phil.* **81 H4** 7 55N 123 44 E
Karon, Ao, *Thailand* **87 a** 7 51N 98 17 E
Karonga, *Malawi* **119 D3** 9 57 S 33 55 E
Karoo △, *S. Africa* **116 E3** 32 18 S 22 27 E
Karoonda, *Australia* **128 C3** 35 1 S 139 59 E
Karor, *Pakistan* **92 D4** 31 15N 70 59 E
Karora, *Sudan* **106 D4** 17 44N 38 15 E
Káros, *Greece* **49 E7** 36 54N 25 40 E
Karosa, *Indonesia* **82 B1** 1 48 S 119 20 E
Karounga, *Mali* **112 B3** 15 20N 7 35W
Karousádhes, *Greece* **38 B9** 39 47N 19 45 E
Karpacz, *Poland* **55 H2** 50 46N 15 46 E
Karpasia, *Cyprus* **39 E10** 35 32N 34 15 E
Kárpathos, *Greece* **49 F9** 35 37N 27 10 E
Kárpathos, Stenón, *Greece* **49 F9** 36 0N 27 30 E
Karpatsky △, *Ukraine* **53 B9** 48 20N 24 35 E
Karpenísion, *Greece* **48 C3** 38 55N 21 40 E
Karpilovka = Aktsyabrski, *Belarus* **59 F5** 52 38N 28 53 E
Karpinsk, *Russia* **64 B8** 59 45N 60 1 E
Karpogory, *Russia* **56 B7** 64 0N 44 27 E
Karpuz Burnu = Apostolos Andreas, C., *Cyprus* **39 E10** 35 42N 34 35 E
Karpuzlu, *Turkey* **49 D9** 37 33N 27 51 E
Karratha, *Australia* **124 D2** 20 53 S 116 40 E
Kars, *Turkey* **101 B10** 40 40N 43 5 E
Karsakpay, *Kazakhstan* **66 E7** 47 55N 66 40 E
Karsha, *Kazakhstan* **60 F10** 49 45N 51 35 E
Karshi = Qarshi, *Uzbekistan* **65 D2** 38 53N 65 48 E
Karsiyang, *India* **90 B2** 26 56N 88 18 E
Karsog, *India* **92 D7** 31 23N 77 12 E
Karst = Kras, *Croatia* **45 C10** 45 35N 14 0 E
Kartal, *Turkey* **51 F13** 40 53N 29 11 E
Kartál Óros, *Greece* **51 E9** 41 15N 25 13 E
Kartaly, *Russia* **64 E8** 53 3N 60 40 E
Kartapur, *India* **92 D6** 31 27N 75 32 E
Karthaus, *U.S.A.* **150 E6** 41 8N 78 9W
Kartuzy, *Poland* **54 D5** 54 22N 18 10 E
Karuah, *Australia* **129 B9** 32 37 S 151 56 E
Karufa, *Indonesia* **83 B4** 3 50 S 133 20 E
Karuma ⌂, *Uganda* **118 B3** 2 5N 32 15 E
Karumba, *Australia* **126 B3** 17 31 S 140 50 E
Karumo, *Tanzania* **118 C3** 2 25 S 32 50 E
Karumwa, *Tanzania* **118 C3** 3 12 S 32 38 E
Kārūn →, *Iran* **97 D6** 30 26N 48 10 E
Karungu, *Kenya* **118 C3** 0 50 S 34 10 E
Karup, *Denmark* **17 H3** 56 19N 9 10 E
Karur, *India* **95 J4** 10 59N 78 2 E
Karviná, *Czech Rep.* **35 B11** 49 53N 18 31 E
Karwan →, *India* **92 F8** 27 26N 78 4 E
Karwendel ⌂, *Austria* **34 D4** 47 25N 11 30 E
Karwi, *India* **93 G9** 25 12N 80 57 E
Kaş, *Turkey* **49 E11** 36 11N 29 37 E
Kasaan, *U.S.A.* **144 J14** 55 32N 132 24W
Kasaba, *Turkey* **49 E11** 36 18N 29 44 E
Kasabi, *Zambia* **115 E4** 14 52 S 23 45 E
Kasache, *Malawi* **119 E3** 13 25 S 34 20 E
Kasai, *Japan* **72 C6** 34 55N 134 52 E
Kasai →, *Dem. Rep. of the Congo* **115 C3** 3 30 S 16 10 E
Kasai-Occidental □, *Dem. Rep. of the Congo* **115 D4** 6 0 S 22 0 E
Kasai-Oriental □, *Dem. Rep. of the Congo* **118 D1** 5 0 S 24 30 E
Kasaji, *Dem. Rep. of the Congo* **119 E1** 10 25 S 23 27 E
Kasama, *Japan* **73 A12** 36 23N 140 16 E
Kasama, *Zambia* **119 E3** 10 16 S 31 9 E
Kasan, *Uzbekistan* **65 D2** 39 2N 65 35 E
Kasan-dong, *N. Korea* **75 D14** 41 18N 126 55 E
Kasane, *Namibia* **116 B3** 17 34 S 24 50 E
Kasanga, *Tanzania* **119 D3** 8 30 S 31 10 E
Kasangaie, *Dem. Rep. of the Congo* **115 D4** 6 20 S 22 42 E
Kasangulu, *Dem. Rep. of the Congo* **115 C3** 4 33 S 15 15 E
Kasanka △, *Zambia* **119 E3** 11 34 S 30 15 E
Kasansay, *Uzbekistan* **65 C5** 41 15N 71 31 E
Kasaoka, *Japan* **72 C5** 34 30N 133 30 E
Kasar, Ras, *Sudan* **106 D4** 18 2N 38 36 E
Kasaragod, *India* **95 H2** 12 30N 74 58 E
Kasat, *Burma* **90 G7** 15 56N 98 13 E
Kasba, *Bangla.* **90 D3** 23 45N 91 2 E
Kasba L., *Canada* **143 A8** 60 20N 102 10W
Kasba Tadla, *Morocco* **110 B3** 32 36N 6 17W
Kaschau = Košice, *Slovak Rep.* **35 C14** 48 42N 21 15 E
Kaseda, *Japan* **72 F2** 31 25N 130 19 E
Kāseh Garān, *Iran* **96 C5** 34 5N 46 2 E
Kasempa, *Zambia* **119 E2** 13 30 S 25 44 E
Kasenga, *Dem. Rep. of the Congo* **119 E2** 10 20 S 28 45 E
Kasese, *Uganda* **118 B3** 0 13N 30 3 E
Kasevo = Neftekamsk, *Russia* **64 C5** 56 6N 54 17 E
Kasewa, *Zambia* **119 E2** 14 28 S 28 53 E
Kasganj, *India* **93 F8** 27 48N 78 42 E
Kashabowie, *Canada* **140 C1** 48 40N 90 26W
Kashaf, *Iran* **97 C9** 35 58N 61 7 E
Kāshān, *Iran* **97 C6** 34 5N 51 30 E
Kashechewan, *Canada* **140 B3** 52 18N 81 37W
Kashgar = Kashi, *China* **65 D8** 39 30N 76 2 E
Kashi, *China* **65 D8** 39 30N 76 2 E
Kashihara, *Japan* **73 C7** 34 27N 135 46 E
Kashiji Plain, *Zambia* **115 E4** 13 12 S 22 20 E
Kashima, *Ibaraki, Japan* **73 B12** 35 58N 140 38 E
Kashima, *Saga, Japan* **72 D2** 33 7N 130 6 E
Kashima-Nada, *Japan* **73 B12** 36 0N 140 45 E
Kashimbo, *Dem. Rep. of the Congo* **119 E2** 11 12 S 26 19 E
Kashin, *Russia* **58 D9** 57 20N 37 36 E
Kashing = Jiaxing, *China* **77 B13** 30 49N 120 45 E
Kashipur, *Orissa, India* **94 E6** 19 16N 83 3 E
Kashipur, *Uttaranchal, India* **93 E8** 29 15N 79 0 E
Kashira, *Russia* **58 E10** 54 45N 38 10 E
Kashiwa, *Japan* **73 B11** 35 52N 139 59 E
Kashiwabara = Severo-Kurilsk, *Russia* **67 D16** 50 40N 156 8 E
Kashiwazaki, *Japan* **71 F9** 37 22N 138 33 E
Kashk-e Kohneh, *Afghan.* **91 B1** 34 55N 62 30 E
Kashkū'īyeh, *Iran* **97 D7** 30 31N 55 40 E
Kāshmar, *Iran* **97 C8** 35 16N 58 26 E
Kashmir, *Asia* **93 C7** 34 0N 76 0 E
Kashmor, *Pakistan* **91 C3** 28 28N 69 32 E
Kashpirovka, *Russia* **60 D9** 53 0N 48 30 E
Kashun Noerh = Gaxun Nur, *China* **68 B5** 42 22N 100 30 E
Kasiari, *India* **93 H12** 22 8N 87 14 E
Kasilof, *U.S.A.* **144 F10** 60 23N 151 18W
Kasimov, *Russia* **60 C5** 54 55N 41 20 E
Kasinge, *Dem. Rep. of the Congo* **118 D2** 6 15 S 26 58 E
Kasiruta, *Indonesia* **82 B3** 0 25 S 127 12 E
Kaskaskia →, *U.S.A.* **156 G7** 37 58N 89 57W
Kaskattama →, *Canada* **143 B10** 57 3N 90 4W
Kaskelen = Qaskeleng, *Kazakhstan* **65 B8** 43 20N 76 35 E
Kaskinen, *Finland* **15 E19** 62 22N 21 15 E
Kaskö = Kaskinen, *Finland* **15 E19** 62 22N 21 15 E
Kasli, *Russia* **64 D8** 55 53N 60 46 E
Kaslo, *Canada* **142 D5** 49 55N 116 55W
Kasmere L., *Canada* **143 B8** 59 34N 101 10W
Kasongan, *Indonesia* **85 C4** 2 0 S 113 23 E
Kasongo, *Dem. Rep. of the Congo* **118 C2** 4 30 S 26 33 E
Kasongo Lunda, *Dem. Rep. of the Congo* **115 D3** 6 35 S 16 49 E
Kásos, *Greece* **49 F8** 35 20N 26 55 E
Kásos, Stenón, *Greece* **49 F8** 35 30N 26 30 E
Kaspi, *Georgia* **61 K7** 41 59N 44 26 E
Kaspichan, *Bulgaria* **51 C11** 43 18N 27 11 E
Kaspiysk, *Russia* **61 J8** 42 52N 47 40 E
Kaspiyskiy, *Russia* **61 H8** 45 22N 47 23 E
Kassab ed Doleib, *Sudan* **107 E3** 13 30N 33 35 E
Kassaba, *Egypt* **106 C2** 22 40N 29 55 E
Kassalâ, *Sudan* **107 D4** 15 30N 36 0 E
Kassalâ □, *Sudan* **107 D4** 15 20N 36 26 E
Kassándra, *Greece* **50 F7** 40 0N 23 30 E
Kassándrinon, *Greece* **50 F7** 40 1N 23 27 E
Kassel, *Germany* **30 D5** 51 18N 9 26 E
Kassinger, *Sudan* **106 D3** 18 46N 31 51 E
Kassiópi, *Greece* **38 B9** 39 48N 19 53 E
Kasson, *U.S.A.* **154 C8** 44 2N 92 45W
Kassue, *Indonesia* **83 C5** 6 58 S 139 21 E
Kastamonu, *Turkey* **100 B5** 41 25N 33 43 E
Kastav, *Croatia* **45 C11** 45 22N 14 20 E
Kastélli, *Greece* **39 E4** 35 29N 23 38 E
Kastéllion, *Greece* **39 E6** 35 12N 25 20 E
Kastellórizon = Megiste, *Greece* **49 E11** 36 8N 29 34 E
Kástellos, *Greece* **49 E9** 36 16N 27 49 E
Kastellou, Ákra, *Greece* **49 F9** 35 30N 27 15 E
Kasterlee, *Belgium* **24 C4** 51 15N 4 59 E
Kastlösa, *Sweden* **17 H10** 56 26N 16 25 E
Kastóri, *Greece* **48 D4** 37 10N 22 17 E
Kastoría, *Greece* **50 F5** 40 30N 21 19 E
Kastoría □, *Greece* **50 F5** 40 30N 21 15 E
Kastorías, Límni, *Greece* **50 F5** 40 30N 21 20 E
Kastornoye, *Russia* **59 G10** 51 55N 38 2 E
Kastós, *Greece* **39 B2** 38 34N 20 55 E
Kastós Nisís, *Greece* **39 B2** 38 35N 20 55 E
Kastrosikiá, *Greece* **39 A2** 39 6N 20 38 E
Kastrup, København ✈ (CPH), *Denmark* **17 J6** 55 37N 12 39 E
Kastsyukovichy, *Belarus* **58 F7** 53 20N 32 4 E
Kasuga, *Japan* **72 D2** 33 32N 130 26 E
Kasugai, *Japan* **73 B8** 35 12N 136 59 E
Kasukabe, *Japan* **73 B11** 35 58N 139 49 E
Kasulu, *Tanzania* **118 C3** 4 37 S 30 5 E
Kasumi, *Japan* **72 B6** 35 38N 134 38 E
Kasumiga-Ura, *Japan* **73 B12** 36 0N 140 25 E
Kasumkent, *Russia* **61 K9** 41 47N 48 15 E
Kasungu, *Malawi* **119 E3** 13 0 S 33 29 E
Kasungu △, *Malawi* **119 E3** 12 53 S 33 9 E
Kasur, *Pakistan* **91 C4** 31 5N 74 25 E
Kata Tjuta = Olga, Mt., *Australia* **125 E5** 25 20 S 130 50 E
Kataba, *Zambia* **119 F2** 16 5 S 25 10 E
Katagum, *Nigeria* **113 C7** 12 18N 10 21 E
Katahdin, Mt., *U.S.A.* **149 C11** 45 54N 68 56W
Katako Kombe, *Dem. Rep. of the Congo* **118 C1** 3 25 S 24 20 E
Katákolon, *Greece* **48 D3** 37 38N 21 19 E
Katale, *Tanzania* **118 C3** 4 52 S 31 7 E
Katalla, *U.S.A.* **144 F11** 60 12N 144 31W
Katamatite, *Australia* **129 D6** 36 6 S 145 41 E
Katanda, *Katanga, Dem. Rep. of the Congo* **118 D1** 7 52 S 24 13 E
Katanda, *Nord-Kivu, Dem. Rep. of the Congo* **118 C2** 0 55 S 29 21 E
Katanga □, *Dem. Rep. of the Congo* **118 D2** 8 0 S 25 0 E
Katangi, *India* **94 D4** 21 56N 79 50 E
Katanning, *Australia* **125 F2** 33 40 S 117 33 E
Katapakishi, *Dem. Rep. of the Congo* **115 D4** 8 15 S 22 49 E
Katastári, *Greece* **39 D2** 37 50N 20 45 E
Katav Ivanovsk, *Russia* **64 D7** 54 45N 58 12 E
Katavi △, *Tanzania* **118 D3** 6 51 S 31 3 E
Katavi Swamp, *Tanzania* **118 D3** 6 50 S 31 10 E
Kataysk, *Russia* **64 C9** 56 20N 62 30 E
Katchall, *India* **95 L11** 7 57N 93 22 E
Katchiungo, *Angola* **115 E3** 12 35 S 16 13 E
Kateríni, *Greece* **50 F6** 40 18N 22 37 E
Katghora, *India* **93 H10** 22 30N 82 33 E
Katha, *Burma* **90 C6** 24 10N 96 30 E
Katherîna, Gebel, *Egypt* **96 D2** 28 30N 33 57 E
Katherine, *Australia* **124 B5** 14 27 S 132 20 E
Katherine →, *Australia* **122 C5** 14 40 S 131 42 E
Katherine Gorge, *Australia* **124 B5** 14 18 S 132 28 E
Kathi, *India* **92 J6** 21 47N 74 3 E
Kathiawar, *India* **92 H4** 22 20N 71 0 E
Kathikas, *Cyprus* **39 F8** 34 55N 32 25 E
Kathleen, *U.S.A.* **153 G7** 28 7N 82 2W
Kathmandu = Katmandu, *Nepal* **93 F11** 27 45N 85 20 E
Kathua, *India* **92 C6** 32 23N 75 34 E
Kati, *Mali* **112 C3** 12 41N 8 4W
Katihar, *India* **93 G12** 25 34N 87 36 E
Katikati, *N.Z.* **130 D4** 37 32 S 175 57 E
Katima Mulilo, *Zambia* **116 B3** 17 28 S 24 13 E
Katimbira, *Malawi* **119 E3** 12 40 S 34 0 E
Katingan = Mendawai →, *Indonesia* **85 C4** 3 30 S 113 0 E
Katiola, *Ivory C.* **112 D3** 8 10N 5 10W
Katipunan, *Phil.* **81 G4** 8 31N 123 17 E
Katla, *Iceland* **11 D7** 63 36N 19 7W
Katlabukh, Ozero, *Ukraine* **53 E14** 45 28N 29 0 E
Katlanovo, *Macedonia* **50 E5** 41 52N 21 40 E
Katmai △, *U.S.A.* **144 G9** 58 20N 155 0W
Katmandu, *Nepal* **93 F11** 27 45N 85 20 E
Katni, *India* **93 H9** 23 51N 80 24 E
Káto Akhaïa, *Greece* **48 C3** 38 8N 21 33 E
Káto Arkhánai, *Greece* **39 E6** 35 15N 25 10 E
Káto Khorió, *Greece* **39 E6** 35 3N 25 47 E
Káto Pyrgos, *Cyprus* **39 E8** 35 11N 32 41 E
Káto Stavros, *Greece* **50 F7** 40 39N 23 43 E
Katokhí, *Greece* **48 C3** 38 26N 21 15 E
Katol, *India* **94 D4** 21 17N 78 38 E
Katompe, *Dem. Rep. of the Congo* **118 D2** 6 2 S 26 23 E
Katong, *Singapore* **87 d** 1 18N 103 53 E
Katonga →, *Uganda* **118 B3** 0 34N 31 50 E
Katoomba, *Australia* **129 B9** 33 41 S 150 19 E
Katoúna, *Greece* **48 C3** 38 47N 21 7 E
Katowice, *Poland* **55 H6** 50 17N 19 5 E
Katrancı Dağı, *Turkey* **49 D12** 37 27N 30 25 E
Katrine, L., *U.K.* **22 E4** 56 15N 4 30W
Katrineholm, *Sweden* **16 E10** 59 9N 16 12 E
Katsepe, *Madag.* **117 B8** 15 45 S 46 15 E
Katsina, *Nigeria* **113 C6** 13 0N 7 32 E
Katsina □, *Nigeria* **113 C6** 12 30N 7 30 E
Katsina Ala, *Nigeria* **113 D6** 7 10N 9 30 E
Katsina Ala →, *Nigeria* **113 D6** 7 10N 9 20 E
Katsumoto, *Japan* **72 D1** 33 51N 129 42 E
Katsuta, *Japan* **73 A12** 36 25N 140 31 E
Katsuura, *Japan* **73 B12** 35 10N 140 20 E
Katsuyama, *Fukui, Japan* **73 A8** 36 3N 136 30 E
Katsuyama, *Okayama, Japan* **72 B5** 35 5N 133 41 E
Kattakŭrgan, *Uzbekistan* **65 D3** 39 55N 66 15 E
Kattaviá, *Greece* **38 F11** 35 57N 27 46 E
Kattegat, *Denmark* **17 H5** 56 40N 11 20 E
Katthammarsvik, *Sweden* **17 G12** 57 26N 18 51 E
Kattowitz = Katowice, *Poland* **55 H6** 50 17N 19 5 E
Katul, J., *Sudan* **107 E2** 14 12N 29 25 E
Katumba, *Dem. Rep. of the Congo* **118 D2** 7 40 S 25 17 E
Katwa, *India* **93 H13** 23 30N 88 5 E
Katwijk, *Neths.* **24 B4** 52 12N 4 24 E
Kąty Wrocławskie, *Poland* **55 G3** 51 2N 16 45 E
Kauai, *U.S.A.* **145 A2** 22 3N 159 30W
Kauai Channel, *U.S.A.* **145 B3** 21 45N 158 50W
Kaub, *Germany* **31 E3** 50 5N 7 46 E
Kaudom ⌂, *Namibia* **116 B3** 18 45 S 20 51 E
Kaufbeuren, *Germany* **31 H6** 47 53N 10 37 E
Kaufman, *U.S.A.* **155 J6** 32 35N 96 19W
Kaufman Peak = Lenina, Pik, *Kyrgyzstan* **65 D6** 39 20N 72 55 E
Kauhajoki, *Finland* **15 E20** 62 25N 22 10 E
Kauhola Pt., *U.S.A.* **145 C6** 20 15N 155 47W
Kaukauna, *U.S.A.* **148 C1** 44 17N 88 17W
Kaukauveld, *Namibia* **116 C3** 20 0 S 20 15 E
Kaukonahua →, *U.S.A.* **145 J13** 21 35N 158 7W
Kaula I., *U.S.A.* **145 B1** 21 40N 160 33W
Kaulakahi Channel, *U.S.A.* **145 B2** 22 0N 159 55W
Kaumalapau, *U.S.A.* **145 C5** 20 47N 156 59W
Kauna Pt., *U.S.A.* **145 D6** 19 2N 155 53W
Kaunakakai, *U.S.A.* **145 B4** 21 6N 157 1W
Kaunas, *Lithuania* **15 J20** 54 54N 23 54 E
Kaunas ✈ (KUN), *Lithuania* **54 D11** 54 57N 24 3 E
Kaunchi = Yangiyul, *Uzbekistan* **65 C4** 41 0N 69 3 E
Kaunghein, *Burma* **90 C5** 25 41N 95 26 E
Kaunia, *Bangla.* **90 C2** 25 46N 89 26 E
Kaunos, *Turkey* **49 E10** 36 49N 28 39 E
Kaupalatmada, *Indonesia* **82 B3** 3 30 S 126 10 E
Kaupangur, *Iceland* **11 B8** 65 38N 18 2W
Kaupo, *U.S.A.* **145 C5** 20 38N 156 8W
Kaura Namoda, *Nigeria* **113 C6** 12 37N 6 33 E
Kauru, *Nigeria* **113 C6** 10 33N 8 12 E
Kautokeino, *Norway* **14 B20** 69 0N 23 4 E
Kauwapur, *India* **93 F10** 27 31N 82 18 E
Kavacha, *Russia* **67 C17** 60 16N 169 51 E
Kavadarci, *Macedonia* **50 E6** 41 26N 22 3 E
Kavajë, *Albania* **50 E3** 41 11N 19 33 E
Kavak, *Turkey* **100 B7** 41 4N 36 3 E
Kavak Dağı, *Turkey* **49 D10** 37 10N 28 2 E
Kavaklı, *Turkey* **51 E11** 41 39N 27 10 E
Kavaklıdere, *Turkey* **49 D10** 37 27N 28 21 E
Kavaklii = Topolovgrad, *Bulgaria* **51 D10** 42 5N 26 20 E
Kavala = Kaválla, *Greece* **51 F8** 40 57N 24 28 E
Kavalerovo, *Russia* **70 B7** 44 15N 135 4 E
Kavali, *India* **95 G5** 14 55N 80 1 E
Kaválla, *Greece* **51 F8** 40 57N 24 28 E
Kaválla □, *Greece* **51 E8** 41 5N 24 30 E
Kavállа Kólpos, *Greece* **51 F8** 40 50N 24 25 E
Kavār, *Iran* **97 D7** 29 11N 52 44 E
Kavaratti, *India* **95 J1** 10 34N 72 37 E
Kavaratti I., *India* **95 J1** 10 33N 72 38 E
Kavarna, *Bulgaria* **51 C12** 43 26N 28 22 E
Kavava, *Dem. Rep. of the Congo* **115 D4** 8 52 S 22 19 E
Kavi, *India* **92 H5** 22 12N 72 38 E
Kavieng, *Papua N. G.* **132 B6** 2 36 S 150 51 E
Kavimba, *Botswana* **116 B3** 18 2 S 24 38 E
Kavīr, Dasht-e, *Iran* **97 C7** 34 30N 55 0 E
Kavirondo G. = Winam G., *Kenya* **118 C3** 0 20 S 34 15 E
Kavkaz, *Russia* **59 K9** 45 20N 36 40 E
Kävlinge, *Sweden* **17 J7** 55 47N 13 9 E
Kavos, *Greece* **38 C10** 39 23N 20 3 E
Kavoúsi, *Greece* **39 E6** 35 7N 25 51 E
Kavungo, *Angola* **115 E4** 11 31 S 23 3 E
Kaw, *Fr. Guiana* **169 C7** 4 30N 52 15W
Kawa, *Sudan* **107 E3** 13 42N 32 34 E
Kawachi-Nagano, *Japan* **73 C7** 34 28N 135 31 E
Kawagama L., *Canada* **150 A6** 45 18N 78 45W
Kawagoe, *Japan* **73 B11** 35 55N 139 29 E
Kawaguchi, *Japan* **73 B11** 35 52N 139 45 E
Kawaihae B., *U.S.A.* **145 D6** 20 0N 155 50W
Kawaihoa Pt., *U.S.A.* **145 B1** 21 47N 160 12W
Kawaikimi, *U.S.A.* **145 A2** 22 5N 159 29W
Kawailoa Beach, *U.S.A.* **145 J13** 21 37N 158 5W
Kawakawa, *N.Z.* **130 B3** 35 23 S 174 6 E
Kawambwa, *Zambia* **119 D2** 9 48 S 29 3 E
Kawanabe, *Japan* **72 F2** 31 23N 130 24 E
Kawanoe, *Japan* **72 C5** 34 1N 133 34 E
Kawardha, *India* **93 J9** 22 0N 81 17 E
Kawasaki, *Japan* **73 B11** 35 31N 139 43 E
Kawasi, *Indonesia* **82 B3** 1 38 S 127 28 E
Kawau I., *N.Z.* **130 C3** 36 25 S 174 52 E
Kaweka Ra., *N.Z.* **130 F5** 39 17 S 176 19 E
Kawela, *U.S.A.* **145 J13** 21 42N 158 1W
Kawerau, *N.Z.* **130 E5** 38 7 S 176 42 E
Kawhia, *N.Z.* **130 E3** 38 4 S 174 49 E
Kawhia Harbour, *N.Z.* **130 E3** 38 5 S 174 51 E
Kawio, Kepulauan, *Indonesia* **79 D7** 4 30N 125 30 E
Kawkareik, *Burma* **90 G7** 16 33N 98 14 E
Kawlin, *Burma* **90 D5** 23 47N 95 41 E
Kawthaung, *Burma* **87 H2** 10 5N 98 36 E
Kawthoolei = Kayin □, *Burma* **90 G6** 18 0N 97 30 E
Kawthule = Kayin □, *Burma* **90 G6** 18 0N 97 30 E
Kawya, *Burma* **90 C5** 24 50N 94 58 E
Kaxholmen, *Sweden* **17 G8** 57 51N 14 19 E
Kay, *Russia* **64 B4** 59 57N 52 59 E
Kaya, *Burkina Faso* **113 C4** 13 4N 1 10W
Kayah □, *Burma* **90 F6** 19 15N 97 15 E
Kayak I., *U.S.A.* **144 G11** 59 56N 144 23W
Kayalıköy Barajı, *Turkey* **51 E11** 41 50N 27 5 E
Kayan, *Burma* **90 G6** 16 54N 96 34 E
Kayan →, *Indonesia* **85 B5** 2 55N 117 35 E
Kayankulam, *India* **95 K3** 9 10N 76 33 E
Kayasa, *Indonesia* **82 A3** 0 47N 127 38 E
Kaycee, *U.S.A.* **158 E10** 43 43N 106 38W
Kayeli, *Indonesia* **82 B3** 3 20 S 127 10 E
Kayenda, *Dem. Rep. of the Congo* **115 E4** 10 48 S 23 6 E
Kayenta, *U.S.A.* **159 H8** 36 44N 110 15W
Kayes, *Congo* **115 C2** 4 25 S 11 41 E
Kayes, *Mali* **112 C2** 14 25N 11 30W
Kayı, *Turkey* **49 B12** 39 12N 30 46 E
Kayima, *S. Leone* **112 D2** 8 54N 11 15W
Kayin □, *Burma* **90 G6** 18 0N 97 30 E
Kaymakçı, *Turkey* **49 C10** 38 10N 28 8 E
Kayoa, *Indonesia* **82 A3** 0 1N 127 28 E
Kayomba, *Zambia* **119 E1** 13 11 S 24 2 E
Kayombo, *Zambia* **115 E4** 13 3 S 23 51 E
Kayrakkumskoye Vdkhr., *Tajikistan* **65 C4** 40 20N 70 0 E
Kaysatskoye, *Russia* **60 F8** 49 47N 46 49 E
Kayseri, *Turkey* **100 C6** 38 45N 35 30 E
Kaysville, *U.S.A.* **158 F8** 41 2N 111 56W
Kayts, *Sri Lanka* **95 K4** 9 42N 79 51 E
Kayuagung, *Indonesia* **84 C2** 3 24 S 104 50 E
Kayyngdy, *Kyrgyzstan* **65 B6** 42 49N 73 41 E
Kaz Dağı, *Turkey* **49 B8** 39 42N 26 50 E
Kazachye, *Russia* **67 B14** 70 52N 135 58 E
Kazakhstan ■, *Asia* **66 E7** 50 0N 70 0 E
Kazan, *Russia* **60 C9** 55 50N 49 10 E
Kazan →, *Canada* **143 A9** 64 2N 95 29W
Kazan-Kuygan, *Kyrgyzstan* **65 C7** 41 34N 75 42 E
Kazan-Rettō, *Pac. Oc.* **134 E6** 25 0N 141 0 E
Kazanlŭk, *Bulgaria* **51 D9** 42 38N 25 20 E
Kazanskaya, *Russia* **60 F5** 49 50N 41 10 E
Kazarman, *Kyrgyzstan* **65 C6** 41 24N 73 59 E
Kazatin = Kozyatyn, *Ukraine* **59 H5** 49 45N 28 50 E
Kazaure, *Nigeria* **113 C6** 12 42N 8 28 E
Kazbek, *Russia* **61 J7** 42 42N 44 30 E
Kāzerūn, *Iran* **97 D6** 29 38N 51 40 E
Kazhim, *Russia* **64 A3** 60 21N 51 33 E
Kazi Magomed = Qazimämmäd, *Azerbaijan* **61 K9** 40 3N 49 0 E
Kazimierz Dolny, *Poland* **55 G8** 51 19N 21 57 E
Kazimierza Wielka, *Poland* **55 H7** 50 15N 20 30 E
Kazincbarcika, *Hungary* **52 B5** 48 17N 20 36 E
Kazipet, *India* **94 F4** 17 58N 79 30 E
Kaziza, *Dem. Rep. of the Congo* **115 E4** 10 42 S 23 52 E
Kazlų Rūda, *Lithuania* **54 D10** 54 46N 23 30 E
Kazo, *Japan* **73 A11** 36 7N 139 36 E
Kaztalovka, *Kazakhstan* **60 F9** 49 47N 48 43 E
Kazu, *Burma* **90 C6** 25 27N 97 46 E
Kazuma Pan △, *Zimbabwe* **119 F2** 18 20 S 25 48 E
Kazumba, *Dem. Rep. of the Congo* **115 D4** 6 25 S 22 5 E
Kazungula, *Zambia* **115 F5** 17 35 S 25 15 E
Kazuno, *Japan* **70 D10** 40 10N 140 45 E
Kazym →, *Russia* **66 C7** 63 54N 65 50 E
Kcynia, *Poland* **55 F4** 53 0N 17 30 E
Ke-hsi Mansam, *Burma* **90 E6** 21 56N 97 50 E
Ké-Macina, *Mali* **112 C3** 13 58N 5 22W
Kéa, *Greece* **48 D6** 37 35N 24 22 E
Keaau, *U.S.A.* **145 D6** 19 37N 155 2W
Keady, *U.K.* **23 B5** 54 15N 6 42W
Keahi Pt., *U.S.A.* **145 K14** 21 19N 157 59W
Keahole Pt., *U.S.A.* **145 D5** 19 44N 156 4W
Kealaikahiki Channel, *U.S.A.* **145 C5** 20 35N 156 50W
Kealaikahiki Pt., *U.S.A.* **145 C5** 20 32N 156 42W
Kealakekua, *U.S.A.* **145 D6** 19 31N 155 55W
Kealia, *U.S.A.* **145 D6** 19 24N 155 53W
Kearney, *Mo., U.S.A.* **156 E2** 39 22N 94 22W
Kearney, *Nebr., U.S.A.* **154 E5** 40 42N 99 5W
Kearny, *U.S.A.* **159 K8** 33 3N 110 55W
Kearsarge, Mt., *U.S.A.* **151 C13** 43 22N 71 50W
Keawakapu, *U.S.A.* **145 C5** 20 43N 156 27W
Keban, *Turkey* **101 C8** 38 50N 38 50 E
Keban Barajı, *Turkey* **101 C8** 38 41N 38 33 E
Kebara, *Congo* **114 C2** 2 27 S 14 25 E
Kebbi □, *Nigeria* **113 C5** 11 35N 4 0 E
Kébi, *Ivory C.* **112 D3** 9 18N 6 37W
Kebi, Mayo →, *Cameroon* **114 A2** 9 18N 13 33 E
Kebili, *Tunisia* **108 B1** 33 47N 9 0 E
Kebnekaise, *Sweden* **14 C18** 67 53N 18 33 E
Kebri Dehar, *Ethiopia* **120 C2** 6 45N 44 17 E
Kebumen, *Indonesia* **85 D3** 7 42 S 109 40 E
Kecel, *Hungary* **52 D4** 46 31N 19 16 E
Kechika →, *Canada* **142 B3** 59 41N 127 12W
Keçiborlu, *Turkey* **49 D12** 37 57N 30 18 E
Kecskemét, *Hungary* **52 D4** 46 57N 19 42 E
Kedada, *Ethiopia* **107 F4** 5 25N 35 58 E
Kedah □, *Malaysia* **84 A2** 5 50N 100 40 E
Kėdainiai, *Lithuania* **15 J21** 55 15N 24 2 E
Kedarnath, *India* **93 D8** 30 44N 79 4 E
Kedgwick, *Canada* **141 C6** 47 40N 67 20W
Kédhros Óros, *Greece* **39 E5** 35 11N 24 37 E
Kediet Ijill, *Mauritania* **110 D2** 22 38N 12 33W
Kediri, *Indonesia* **85 D4** 7 51 S 112 1 E
Kedja, *Dem. Rep. of the Congo* **114 B3** 4 50N 19 16 E
Kedjebi, *Ghana* **113 D5** 8 12N 0 25 E
Kédougou, *Senegal* **112 C2** 12 35N 12 10W
Kędzierzyn-Koźle, *Poland* **55 H5** 50 20N 18 12 E
Keehi Lagoon, *U.S.A.* **145 K14** 21 20N 157 54W
Keeler, *U.S.A.* **160 J9** 36 29N 117 52W
Keeley L., *Canada* **143 C7** 54 54N 108 8W
Keeling Is. = Cocos Is., *Ind. Oc.* **121 F8** 12 10 S 96 55 E
Keelung = Chilung, *Taiwan* **77 E13** 25 3N 121 45 E
Keene, *Canada* **150 B6** 44 15N 78 10W
Keene, *Calif., U.S.A.* **161 K8** 35 13N 118 33W
Keene, *N.H., U.S.A.* **151 D12** 42 56N 72 17W
Keene, *N.Y., U.S.A.* **151 B11** 44 16N 73 46W
Keep River △, *Australia* **124 C4** 15 49 S 129 8 E
Keeper Hill, *Ireland* **23 D3** 52 45N 8 16W
Keepit, L., *Australia* **129 A9** 30 50 S 150 30 E
Keer-Weer, C., *Australia* **126 A3** 14 0 S 141 32 E
Keeseville, *U.S.A.* **151 B11** 44 29N 73 30W
Keetmanshoop, *Namibia* **116 D2** 26 35 S 18 8 E
Keewatin, *Canada* **143 D10** 49 46N 94 34W
Keewatin →, *Canada* **143 B8** 56 29N 100 46W
Kefa, *Ethiopia* **107 F4** 6 55N 36 30 E
Kefallinía, *Greece* **39 C2** 38 15N 20 30 E
Kefallinía □, *Greece* **39 C2** 38 15N 20 30 E
Kefallinía ✈ (EFL), *Greece* **39 C1** 38 10N 20 30 E
Kefalonia = Kefallinía, *Greece* **39 C2** 38 15N 20 30 E
Kéfalos, *Greece* **49 E8** 36 45N 26 59 E
Kefamenanu, *Indonesia* **82 C2** 9 28 S 124 29 E
Kefar Sava, *Israel* **103 C3** 32 11N 34 54 E
Keffi, *Nigeria* **113 D6** 8 55N 7 43 E
Keffin Hausa, *Nigeria* **113 C6** 12 13N 9 59 E
Keflavík, *Iceland* **11 C4** 64 2N 22 35W
Keflavík ✈ (KEF), *Iceland* **11 C4** 64 0N 22 45W
Keftya, *Ethiopia* **107 E4** 13 54N 37 7 E
Keg River, *Canada* **142 B5** 57 54N 117 55W
Kegalla, *Sri Lanka* **95 L5** 7 15N 80 21 E

Kegaska, *Canada* **141 B7** 50 9N 61 18W
Keheili, *Sudan* **106 D3** 19 25N 32 50 E
Kehl, *Germany* **31 G3** 48 34N 7 50 E
Keighley, *U.K.* **20 D6** 53 52N 1 54W
Keijo = Sŏul, *S. Korea* **75 F14** 37 31N 126 58 E
Keikiwaha Pt., *U.S.A.* **145 D6** 19 31N 155 58W
Keila, *Estonia* **15 G21** 59 18N 24 25 E
Keimoes, *S. Africa* **116 D3** 28 41 S 20 59 E
Keita, *Niger* **113 C6** 14 46N 5 56 E
Keïta, B. →, *Chad* **109 G3** 9 14N 18 21 E
Keitele, *Finland* **14 E22** 63 10N 26 20 E
Keith, *Australia* **128 D4** 36 6 S 140 20 E
Keith, *U.K.* **22 D6** 57 32N 2 57W
Keithsburg, *U.S.A.* **156 C6** 41 6N 90 56W
Keiyasi, *Fiji* **133 A1** 17 53 S 177 46 E
Keizer, *U.S.A.* **158 D2** 44 57N 123 1W
Kejimkujik △, *Canada* **141 D6** 44 25N 65 25W
Kejserr Franz Joseph Fd., *Greenland* **10 C8** 73 30N 24 30W
Kekaha, *U.S.A.* **145 B2** 21 58N 159 43W
Kekri, *India* **92 G6** 26 0N 75 10 E
Keksgolm = Priozersk, *Russia* **58 B6** 61 2N 30 7 E
Kelam, *Ethiopia* **107 G4** 4 48N 35 58 E
Kelamet, *Eritrea* **107 D4** 16 0N 38 30 E
Kelan, *China* **74 E6** 38 43N 111 31 E
Kelang = Klang, *Malaysia* **87 L3** 3 2N 101 26 E
Kelang, *Indonesia* **82 B3** 3 12 S 127 44 E
Kelani Ganga →, *Sri Lanka* **95 L4** 6 58N 79 50 E
Kelantan □, *Malaysia* **84 A2** 5 10N 102 0 E
Kelantan →, *Malaysia* **87 J4** 6 13N 102 14 E
Këlcyrë, *Albania* **50 F4** 40 20N 20 12 E
Kelekçi, *Turkey* **49 D11** 37 15N 29 20 E
Keles, *Turkey* **51 G13** 39 54N 29 14 E
Keles, *Uzbekistan* **65 C4** 41 24N 69 12 E
Keles →, *Kazakhstan* **65 C4** 41 1N 68 37 E
Keleti-főcsatorna, *Hungary* **52 C6** 47 45N 21 20 E
Kelheim, *Germany* **31 G7** 48 54N 11 52 E
Kelibia, *Tunisia* **108 A2** 36 50N 11 3 E
Kelkit, *Turkey* **101 B8** 40 7N 39 16 E
Kelkit →, *Turkey* **100 B7** 40 45N 36 32 E
Kellé, *Congo* **114 C2** 0 8 S 14 38 E
Keller, *U.S.A.* **152 D8** 31 50N 81 15W
Kellerberrin, *Australia* **125 F2** 31 36 S 117 38 E
Kellett, C., *Canada* **6 B1** 72 0N 126 0W
Kelleys I., *U.S.A.* **150 E2** 41 36N 82 42W
Kellogg, *U.S.A.* **158 C5** 47 32N 116 7W
Kells = Ceanannus Mor, *Ireland* **23 C5** 53 44N 6 53W
Kelmė, *Lithuania* **54 C9** 55 38N 22 56 E
Kelmentsi, *Ukraine* **53 B11** 48 28N 26 50 E
Kélo, *Chad* **109 G3** 9 10N 15 45 E
Kelokedhara, *Cyprus* **39 F8** 34 48N 32 39 E
Kelowna, *Canada* **142 D5** 49 50N 119 25W
Kelsey Creek, *Australia* **126 J6** 20 26 S 148 31 E
Kelseyville, *U.S.A.* **160 G4** 38 59N 122 50W
Kelso, *N.Z.* **131 F4** 45 54 S 169 15 E
Kelso, *U.K.* **22 F6** 55 36N 2 26W
Kelso, *U.S.A.* **160 D4** 46 9N 122 54W
Keluang = Kluang, *Malaysia* **87 L4** 2 3N 103 18 E
Kelvington, *Canada* **143 C8** 52 10N 103 30W
Kem, *Russia* **56 B5** 65 0N 34 38 E
Kem →, *Russia* **56 B5** 64 57N 34 41 E
Kem-Kem, *Morocco* **110 B4** 30 40N 4 30W
Kema, *Indonesia* **79 D7** 1 22N 125 8 E
Kemah, *Turkey* **101 C8** 39 32N 39 5 E
Kemaliye, *Erzincan, Turkey* **101 C8** 39 16N 38 29 E
Kemaliye, *Manisa, Turkey* **49 C10** 38 27N 28 25 E
Kemalpaşa, *Turkey* **49 C9** 38 25N 27 27 E
Kemaman, *Malaysia* **78 D2** 4 12N 103 18 E
Kemano, *Canada* **142 C3** 53 35N 128 0W
Kemapyu, *Burma* **90 F6** 18 49N 97 19 E
Kemasik, *Malaysia* **87 K4** 4 25N 103 27 E
Kembani, *Indonesia* **82 B2** 1 34 S 122 54 E
Kembé, *C.A.R.* **114 B4** 4 36N 21 54 E
Kembolcha, *Ethiopia* **107 E4** 11 2N 39 42 E
Kemer, *Antalya, Turkey* **49 E12** 36 36N 30 34 E
Kemer, *Burdur, Turkey* **49 D12** 37 21N 30 4 E
Kemer, *Muğla, Turkey* **49 E11** 36 40N 29 22 E
Kemer Barajı, *Turkey* **49 D10** 37 30N 28 37 E
Kemerovo, *Russia* **66 D9** 55 20N 86 5 E
Ķemeru △, *Latvia* **54 B10** 56 58N 23 25 E
Kemi, *Finland* **14 D21** 65 44N 24 34 E
Kemi älv = Kemijoki →, *Finland* **14 D21** 65 47N 24 32 E
Kemi träsk = Kemijärvi, *Finland* **14 C22** 66 43N 27 22 E
Kemijärvi, *Finland* **14 C22** 66 43N 27 22 E
Kemijoki →, *Finland* **14 D21** 65 47N 24 32 E
Kemin, *Kyrgyzstan* **65 B7** 42 47N 75 42 E
Kemmerer, *U.S.A.* **158 F8** 41 48N 110 32W
Kemmuna = Comino, *Malta* **38 E7** 36 1N 14 20 E
Kemp, L., *U.S.A.* **155 J5** 33 46N 99 9W
Kemp Land, *Antarctica* **7 C5** 69 0 S 55 0 E
Kempas, *Malaysia* **87 d** 1 33N 103 42 E
Kempen = Kępno, *Poland* **55 G4** 51 18N 17 58 E
Kempsey, *Australia* **129 A10** 31 1 S 152 50 E
Kempt, L., *Canada* **140 C5** 47 25N 74 22W
Kempten, *Germany* **31 H6** 47 45N 10 17 E
Kempton, *Australia* **127 G4** 42 31 S 147 12 E
Kempton, *U.S.A.* **157 D10** 40 17N 86 14W
Kemptville, *Canada* **140 D4** 45 0N 75 38W
Ken →, *India* **93 G9** 25 13N 80 27 E
Kenadsa, *Algeria* **111 B4** 31 48N 2 26W
Kenai, *U.S.A.* **144 F10** 60 33N 151 16W
Kenai Fjords △, *U.S.A.* **144 E10** 59 40N 149 50W
Kenai Mts., *U.S.A.* **144 G10** 60 0N 150 0W
Kenansville, *U.S.A.* **153 H9** 27 53N 80 59W
Kendai, *India* **93 H10** 22 45N 82 37 E
Kendal, *Indonesia* **85 D4** 6 56 S 110 14 E
Kendal, *U.K.* **20 C5** 54 20N 2 44W
Kendall, *Australia* **129 A10** 31 35 S 152 44 E
Kendall, *U.S.A.* **153 K9** 25 41N 80 19W
Kendall →, *Australia* **126 A3** 14 4 S 141 35 E
Kendallville, *U.S.A.* **157 C11** 41 27N 85 16W
Kendari, *Indonesia* **82 B2** 3 50 S 122 30 E
Kendawangan, *Indonesia* **85 C4** 2 32 S 110 17 E
Kende, *Nigeria* **113 C5** 11 30N 4 12 E
Kendi, Pulau, *Malaysia* **87 c** 5 13N 100 11 E
Kendigué, *Chad* **109 F3** 10 0N 18 36 E
Kendrapara, *India* **94 D8** 20 35N 86 30 E
Këndrevicës, Maja e, *Albania* **50 F3** 40 15N 19 52 E
Kendrew, *S. Africa* **116 E3** 32 32 S 24 30 E
Kendrick, *U.S.A.* **153 F7** 29 15N 82 10W
Kene Thao, *Laos* **86 D3** 17 44N 101 10 E
Kenedy, *U.S.A.* **155 L6** 28 49N 97 51W
Kenema, *S. Leone* **112 D2** 7 50N 11 14W
Keng Kok, *Laos* **86 D5** 16 26N 105 12 E
Keng Tawng, *Burma* **90 E7** 20 45N 98 18 E
Keng Tung, *Burma* **76 G2** 21 0N 99 30 E
Kengani, *Dem. Rep. of the Congo* **114 C3** 2 59 S 17 36 E
Kenge, *Dem. Rep. of the Congo* **115 C3** 4 50 S 17 4 E
Kengeja, *Tanzania* **118 D4** 5 26 S 39 45 E
Kenhardt, *S. Africa* **116 D3** 29 19 S 21 12 E
Kéniéba, *Mali* **112 C2** 12 54N 11 17W
Kenitra, *Morocco* **110 B3** 34 15N 6 40W
Kenli, *China* **75 F10** 37 30N 118 20 E
Kenmare, *Ireland* **23 E2** 51 53N 9 36W
Kenmare, *U.S.A.* **154 A3** 48 41N 102 5W
Kenmare River, *Ireland* **23 E2** 51 48N 9 51W
Kennebago Lake, *U.S.A.* **151 A14** 45 4N 70 40W
Kennebec, *U.S.A.* **154 D5** 43 54N 99 52W
Kennebec →, *U.S.A.* **149 D11** 43 45N 69 46W
Kennebunk, *U.S.A.* **151 C14** 43 23N 70 33W
Kennedy, *Zimbabwe* **116 B4** 18 52 S 27 10 E
Kennedy, C. = Canaveral, C., *U.S.A.* **153 G9** 28 27N 80 32W
Kennedy Kanal, *Arctic* **10 A4** 80 50N 66 0W
Kennedy Ra., *Australia* **125 D2** 24 45 S 115 10 E
Kennedy Range △, *Australia* **125 D2** 24 34 S 115 2 E
Kennedy Space Center, *U.S.A.* **153 G9** 28 40N 80 42W
Kenner, *U.S.A.* **155 L9** 29 59N 90 15W
Kennesaw, *U.S.A.* **152 A5** 34 1N 84 37W
Kennet →, *U.K.* **21 F7** 51 27N 0 57W
Kenneth Ra., *Australia* **125 D2** 23 50 S 117 8 E
Kennett, *U.S.A.* **155 G9** 36 14N 90 3W
Kennewick, *U.S.A.* **158 C4** 46 12N 119 7W
Kenogami →, *Canada* **140 B3** 51 6N 84 28W
Kenora, *Canada* **143 D10** 49 47N 94 29W
Kenosha, *U.S.A.* **157 B9** 42 35N 87 49W
Kensington, *Canada* **141 C7** 46 28N 63 34W
Kent, *Ohio, U.S.A.* **150 E3** 41 9N 81 22W
Kent, *Tex., U.S.A.* **155 K2** 31 4N 104 13W
Kent, *Wash., U.S.A.* **160 C4** 47 23N 122 14W
Kent □, *U.K.* **21 F8** 51 12N 0 40 E
Kent Group, *Australia* **127 F4** 39 30 S 147 20 E
Kent Pen., *Canada* **138 B9** 68 30N 107 0W
Kentaū, *Kazakhstan* **65 B4** 43 32N 68 36 E
Kentland, *U.S.A.* **157 D9** 40 46N 87 27W
Kenton, *U.S.A.* **157 D13** 40 39N 83 37W
Kentucky □, *U.S.A.* **148 G3** 37 0N 84 0W
Kentucky →, *U.S.A.* **157 F11** 38 41N 85 11W
Kentucky L., *U.S.A.* **149 G2** 37 1N 88 16W
Kentville, *Canada* **141 C7** 45 6N 64 29W
Kentwood, *La., U.S.A.* **155 K9** 30 56N 90 31W
Kentwood, *Mich., U.S.A.* **157 B11** 42 52N 85 37W
Kenya ■, *Africa* **118 B4** 1 0N 38 0 E
Kenya, Mt., *Kenya* **118 C4** 0 10 S 37 18 E
Kenzou, *Cameroon* **114 B3** 4 10N 15 2 E
Keo Neua, Deo, *Vietnam* **86 C5** 18 23N 105 10 E
Keokea, *U.S.A.* **145 C5** 20 43N 156 22W
Keokuk, *U.S.A.* **156 D5** 40 24N 91 24W
Keoladeo △, *India* **92 F7** 27 0N 77 20 E
Keonjhargarh, *India* **93 J11** 21 28N 85 35 E
Keosauqua, *U.S.A.* **156 D5** 40 44N 91 58W
Keota, *U.S.A.* **156 C5** 41 22N 91 57W
Kep, *Cambodia* **87 G5** 10 29N 104 19 E
Kep, *Vietnam* **86 B6** 21 24N 106 16 E
Kepala Batas, *Malaysia* **87 c** 5 31N 100 26 E
Kepez, *Turkey* **51 F10** 40 5N 26 24 E
Kepi, *Indonesia* **83 C5** 6 32 S 139 19 E
Kępice, *Poland* **54 D3** 54 16N 16 51 E
Kepler Mts., *N.Z.* **131 F2** 45 25 S 167 20 E
Kępno, *Poland* **55 G4** 51 18N 17 58 E
Keppel Pt., *Papua N. G.* **132 F4** 10 10 S 147 58 E
Kepsut, *Turkey* **49 B10** 39 40N 28 9 E
Kepuhi Pt., *U.S.A.* **145 K13** 21 29N 158 14W
Kerala □, *India* **95 J3** 11 0N 76 15 E
Keram →, *Papua N. G.* **132 C3** 4 7 S 144 5 E
Kerama-Rettō, *Japan* **71 L3** 26 5N 127 15 E
Keran, *Pakistan* **93 B5** 34 35N 73 59 E
Keran △, *Togo* **113 C5** 10 9N 0 41 E
Kerang, *Australia* **128 C5** 35 40 S 143 55 E
Keranyo, *Ethiopia* **107 F4** 5 3N 38 18 E
Kerao →, *Sudan* **107 E3** 11 0N 32 41 E
Keratéa, *Greece* **48 D5** 37 48N 23 58 E
Keraudren, C., *Australia* **124 C2** 19 58 S 119 45 E
Kerava, *Finland* **15 F21** 60 25N 25 5 E
Keravat, *Papua N. G.* **132 C7** 4 17 S 152 2 E
Kerben, *Kyrgyzstan* **65 C5** 41 30N 71 45 E
Kerch, *Ukraine* **59 K9** 45 20N 36 20 E
Kerchenskiy Proliv, *Black Sea* **59 K9** 45 10N 36 30 E
Kerchoual, *Mali* **113 B5** 17 12N 0 20 E
Kerema, *Papua N. G.* **132 D3** 7 58 S 145 50 E
Kerempe Burnu, *Turkey* **100 A5** 42 2N 33 20 E
Keren, *Eritrea* **107 D4** 15 45N 38 28 E
Kerewan, *Gambia* **112 C1** 13 29N 16 10W
Kerguelen, *Ind. Oc.* **121 J5** 49 15 S 69 10 E
Keri, *Greece* **39 D2** 37 40N 20 49 E
Keri Kera, *Sudan* **107 E3** 12 21N 32 42 E
Kericho, *Kenya* **118 C4** 0 22 S 35 15 E
Kerikeri, *N.Z.* **130 B2** 35 12 S 173 59 E
Kerinci, *Indonesia* **84 C2** 1 40 S 101 15 E
Kerintji = Kerinci, *Indonesia* **84 C2** 1 40 S 101 15 E
Kerkenna, Îs., *Tunisia* **108 B2** 34 48N 11 11 E
Kerki, *Turkmenistan* **65 E2** 37 50N 65 12 E
Kerkinítis, Límni, *Greece* **50 E7** 41 12N 23 10 E
Kérkira, *Greece* **38 B9** 39 38N 19 50 E
Kérkira □, *Greece* **38 B9** 39 37N 19 50 E
Kérkira ✕ (CFU), *Greece* **48 B1** 39 35N 19 54 E
Kerkouane, *Tunisia* **46 F4** 36 58N 11 2 E
Kerkrade, *Neths.* **24 D6** 50 53N 6 4 E
Kerma, *Sudan* **106 D3** 19 33N 30 32 E
Kermadec Is., *Pac. Oc.* **134 L10** 30 0 S 178 15W
Kermadec Trench, *Pac. Oc.* **134 L10** 30 30 S 176 0W
Kermān, *Iran* **97 D8** 30 15N 57 1 E
Kerman, *U.S.A.* **160 J6** 36 43N 120 4W
Kermān □, *Iran* **97 D8** 30 0N 57 0 E
Kermān, Bīābān-e, *Iran* **97 D8** 28 45N 59 45 E
Kermānshāh = Bākhtarān, *Iran* **101 E12** 34 23N 47 0 E
Kermen, *Bulgaria* **51 D10** 42 30N 26 16 E
Kermine = Nawoiy, *Uzbekistan* **65 C2** 40 9N 65 22 E
Kermit, *U.S.A.* **155 K3** 31 52N 103 6W
Kern →, *U.S.A.* **161 K7** 35 16N 119 18W
Kernhof, *Austria* **34 D8** 47 49N 15 32 E
Kernow = Cornwall □, *U.K.* **21 G3** 50 26N 4 40W
Kerns, *Switz.* **33 C6** 46 54N 8 17 E
Kernville, *U.S.A.* **161 K8** 35 45N 118 26W
Keroh, *Malaysia* **87 K3** 5 43N 101 1 E
Kérou, *Benin* **113 C5** 10 50N 2 5 E
Kérouane, *Guinea* **112 D3** 9 15N 9 0W
Kerowagi, *Papua N. G.* **132 C3** 5 51 S 144 51 E
Kerpen, *Germany* **30 E2** 50 51N 6 41 E
Kerrera, *U.K.* **22 E3** 56 24N 5 33W
Kerrobert, *Canada* **143 C7** 51 56N 109 8W
Kerrville, *U.S.A.* **155 K5** 30 3N 99 8W
Kerry □, *Ireland* **23 D2** 52 7N 9 35W
Kerry Hd., *Ireland* **23 D2** 52 25N 9 56W
Kersa, *Ethiopia* **107 F5** 9 28N 41 48 E
Kertosono, *Indonesia* **85 D4** 7 38 S 112 9 E
Kerulen →, *Asia* **69 B6** 48 48N 117 0 E
Kervo = Kerava, *Finland* **15 F21** 60 25N 25 5 E
Kerzaz, *Algeria* **111 C4** 29 29N 1 37W
Kerzers, *Switz.* **32 C4** 46 59N 7 12 E
Kesagami →, *Canada* **140 B4** 51 40N 79 45W
Kesagami L., *Canada* **140 B3** 50 23N 80 15W
Keşan, *Turkey* **51 F10** 40 49N 26 38 E
Kesch, Piz, *Switz.* **33 C9** 46 38N 9 53 E
Kesennuma, *Japan* **70 E10** 38 54N 141 35 E
Keshit, *Iran* **97 D8** 29 43N 58 17 E
Kesigi = Kosgi, *India* **95 G3** 15 51N 77 16 E
Keşiş Dağ, *Turkey* **101 C8** 39 47N 39 46 E
Keskal, *India* **94 D5** 20 5N 81 35 E
Keskin, *Turkey* **100 C5** 39 40N 33 36 E
Kestell, *S. Africa* **117 D4** 28 17 S 28 42 E
Kestenga, *Russia* **56 A5** 65 50N 31 45 E
Keswick, *U.K.* **20 C4** 54 36N 3 8W
Keszthely, *Hungary* **52 D2** 46 50N 17 15 E
Ket →, *Russia* **66 D9** 58 55N 81 32 E
Keta, *Ghana* **113 D5** 5 49N 1 0 E
Keta Lagoon, *Ghana* **113 D5** 5 55N 1 0 E
Ketapang, *Bali, Indonesia* **79 J17** 8 9 S 114 23 E
Ketapang, *Kalimantan, Indonesia* **85 C4** 1 55 S 110 0 E
Ketchenery, *Russia* **61 G7** 47 18N 44 32 E
Ketchikan, *U.S.A.* **142 B2** 55 21N 131 39W
Ketchum, *U.S.A.* **158 E6** 43 41N 114 22W
Kete Krachi, *Ghana* **113 D4** 7 46N 0 1W
Ketef, Khalîg Umm el, *Egypt* **96 F2** 23 40N 35 35 E
Keti Bandar, *Pakistan* **92 G2** 24 8N 67 27 E
Kétou, *Benin* **113 D5** 7 25N 2 45 E
Ketri, *India* **92 E6** 28 1N 75 50 E
Kętrzyn, *Poland* **54 D8** 54 7N 21 22 E
Kettering, *U.K.* **21 E7** 52 24N 0 43W
Kettering, *U.S.A.* **157 E12** 39 41N 84 10W
Kettle →, *Canada* **143 B11** 56 40N 89 34W
Kettle Falls, *U.S.A.* **158 B4** 48 37N 118 3W
Kettle Pt., *Canada* **150 C2** 43 13N 82 1W
Kettleman City, *U.S.A.* **160 J7** 36 1N 119 58W
Kęty, *Poland* **55 J6** 49 51N 19 16 E
Keuka L., *U.S.A.* **150 D7** 42 30N 77 9W
Keuruu, *Finland* **15 E21** 62 16N 24 41 E
Kevelaer, *Germany* **30 D2** 51 36N 6 15 E
Kewanee, *U.S.A.* **156 C7** 41 14N 89 56W
Kewanna, *U.S.A.* **157 C10** 41 1N 86 25W
Kewaunee, *U.S.A.* **148 C2** 44 27N 87 31W
Keweenaw B., *U.S.A.* **148 B1** 47 0N 88 15W
Keweenaw Pen., *U.S.A.* **148 B2** 47 30N 88 0W
Keweenaw Pt., *U.S.A.* **148 B2** 47 25N 87 43W
Kexholm = Priozersk, *Russia* **58 B6** 61 2N 30 7 E
Key Colony Beach, *U.S.A.* **153 L9** 24 45N 80 57W
Key Largo, *U.S.A.* **153 K9** 25 5N 80 27W
Key West, *U.S.A.* **153 L8** 24 33N 81 48W
Keyala, *Sudan* **107 G3** 4 27N 32 52 E
Keynsham, *U.K.* **21 F5** 51 24N 2 29W
Keyser, *U.S.A.* **148 F6** 39 26N 78 59W
Keystone Heights, *U.S.A.* **152 F7** 29 47N 82 1W
Keytesville, *U.S.A.* **156 E4** 39 26N 92 56W
Kez, *Russia* **64 C4** 57 55N 53 46 E
Kezhma, *Russia* **67 D11** 58 59N 101 9 E
Kezi, *Zimbabwe* **117 C4** 20 58 S 28 32 E
Kežmarok, *Slovak Rep.* **35 B13** 49 10N 20 28 E
Kgalagadi Transfrontier ⌓, *Africa* **116 D3** 25 10 S 21 0 E
Khabarovsk, *Russia* **67 E14** 48 30N 135 5 E
Khabr, *Iran* **97 D8** 28 51N 56 22 E
Khābūr →, *Syria* **101 E9** 35 17N 40 35 E
Khachmas = Xaçmaz, *Azerbaijan* **61 K9** 41 31N 48 42 E
Khachrod, *India* **92 H6** 23 25N 75 20 E
Khadari, W. el →, *Sudan* **107 E2** 10 29N 27 15 E
Khadro, *Pakistan* **92 F3** 26 11N 68 50 E
Khadyzhensk, *Russia* **61 H4** 44 26N 39 32 E
Khadzhilyangar, *China* **93 B8** 35 45N 79 20 E
Khaga, *India* **93 G9** 25 47N 81 7 E
Khagaria, *India* **93 G12** 25 30N 86 32 E
Khaipur, *Pakistan* **92 E5** 29 34N 72 17 E
Khair, *India* **92 F7** 27 57N 77 46 E
Khairabad, *India* **93 F9** 27 33N 80 47 E
Khairagarh, *India* **93 J9** 21 27N 81 2 E
Khairpur, *Pakistan* **91 D3** 27 32N 68 49 E
Khairpur Nathan Shah, *Pakistan* **92 F2** 27 6N 67 44 E
Khairwara, *India* **92 H5** 23 58N 73 38 E
Khaisor →, *Pakistan* **92 D3** 31 17N 68 59 E
Khajuri Kach, *Pakistan* **92 C3** 32 4N 69 51 E
Khāk Dow, *Afghan.* **91 B2** 34 57N 67 16 E
Khakassia □, *Russia* **66 D9** 53 0N 90 0 E
Khakhea, *Botswana* **116 C3** 24 48 S 23 22 E
Khalafābād, *Iran* **97 D6** 30 54N 49 24 E
Khalfallah, *Algeria* **111 B5** 34 20N 0 16 E
Khalfūt, *Yemen* **99 D6** 15 52N 52 10 E
Khalilabad, *India* **93 F10** 26 48N 83 5 E
Khalīlī, *Iran* **97 E7** 27 38N 53 17 E
Khalkhāl, *Iran* **97 B6** 37 37N 48 32 E
Khálki, *Dhodhekánisos, Greece* **49 E9** 36 17N 27 35 E
Khálki, *Thessalía, Greece* **48 B4** 39 36N 22 30 E
Khalkidhikí □, *Greece* **50 F7** 40 25N 23 20 E
Khalkís, *Greece* **48 C5** 38 27N 23 42 E
Khalmer-Sede = Tazovskiy, *Russia* **66 C8** 67 30N 78 44 E
Khalmer Yu, *Russia* **66 C7** 67 58N 65 1 E
Khalturin, *Russia* **64 B2** 58 40N 48 50 E
Khalūf, *Oman* **102 C6** 20 30N 58 13 E
Kham Keut, *Laos* **86 C5** 18 15N 104 43 E
Khamaria, *India* **93 H9** 23 5N 80 48 E
Khambhaliya, *India* **92 H3** 22 14N 69 41 E
Khambhat, *India* **92 H5** 22 23N 72 33 E
Khambhat, G. of, *India* **89 C6** 20 45N 72 30 E
Khamgaon, *India* **94 D3** 20 42N 76 37 E
Khamilonísion, *Greece* **49 F8** 35 50N 26 15 E
Khamīr, *Iran* **97 E7** 26 57N 55 36 E
Khamir, *Yemen* **98 C3** 16 2N 44 0 E
Khamīs Mushayţ, *Si. Arabia* **98 C3** 18 18N 42 44 E
Khammam, *India* **94 F5** 17 11N 80 6 E
Khamsa, *Egypt* **103 E1** 30 27N 32 23 E
Khamza, *Uzbekistan* **65 C5** 40 25N 71 29 E
Khan →, *Namibia* **116 C2** 22 37 S 14 56 E
Khān Abū Shāmat, *Syria* **103 B5** 33 39N 36 53 E
Khān Azād, *Iraq* **96 C5** 33 7N 44 22 E
Khān Mujiddah, *Iraq* **96 C4** 32 21N 43 48 E
Khān Shaykhūn, *Syria* **100 E7** 35 26N 36 38 E
Khān Yūnis, *Gaza Strip* **103 D3** 31 21N 34 18 E
Khānābād, *Afghan.* **65 E4** 36 45N 69 5 E
Khanabad, *Uzbekistan* **65 C6** 40 47N 73 0 E
Khanai, *Pakistan* **92 D2** 30 30N 67 8 E
Khānaqīn, *Iraq* **101 E11** 34 23N 45 25 E
Khānbāghī, *Iran* **97 B7** 36 10N 55 25 E
Khandrá, *Greece* **49 F8** 35 3N 26 8 E
Khandūd, *Afghan.* **65 E6** 36 57N 72 19 E
Khandwa, *India* **94 D3** 21 49N 76 22 E
Khandyga, *Russia* **67 C14** 62 42N 135 35 E
Khāneh, *Iran* **96 B5** 36 41N 45 8 E
Khanewal, *Pakistan* **91 C3** 30 20N 71 55 E
Khangah Dogran, *Pakistan* **92 D5** 31 50N 73 37 E
Khanh Duong, *Vietnam* **86 F7** 12 44N 108 44 E
Khaniá, *Greece* **39 E5** 35 30N 24 4 E
Khaniá □, *Greece* **39 E5** 35 30N 24 0 E
Khanía ✕ (CHQ), *Greece* **39 E5** 35 30N 24 6 E
Khaniadhana, *India* **92 G8** 25 1N 78 8 E
Khaníon, Kólpos, *Greece* **39 E4** 35 33N 23 55 E
Khanka, L., *Asia* **67 E14** 45 0N 132 24 E
Khankendy = Xankändi, *Azerbaijan* **101 C12** 39 52N 46 49 E
Khanna, *India* **92 D7** 30 42N 76 16 E
Khanozai, *Pakistan* **92 D2** 30 37N 67 19 E
Khanpur, *Pakistan* **91 C3** 28 42N 70 35 E
Khantaū, *Kazakhstan* **65 A6** 44 13N 73 48 E
Khanty-Mansiysk, *Russia* **66 C7** 61 0N 69 0 E
Khao Laem △, *Thailand* **86 E2** 14 56N 98 31 E
Khao Laem Res., *Thailand* **86 E2** 14 50N 98 30 E
Khao Luang △, *Thailand* **87 H2** 8 34N 99 42 E
Khao Phlu, *Thailand* **87 b** 9 29N 99 59 E
Khao Pu-Khao Ya △, *Thailand* **87 J2** 7 26N 99 57 E
Khao Sam Roi Yot △, *Thailand* **87 F2** 12 13N 99 57 E
Khao Sok △, *Thailand* **87 H2** 8 55N 98 38 E
Khao Yai △, *Thailand* **86 E3** 14 21N 101 29 E
Khaoen Si Nakarin △, *Thailand* **86 E2** 14 47N 99 0 E
Khapalu, *Pakistan* **93 B7** 35 10N 76 20 E
Khapcheranga, *Russia* **67 E12** 49 42N 112 24 E
Khaptao △, *Nepal* **93 E9** 29 20N 81 10 E
Kharabali, *Russia* **61 G8** 47 25N 47 15 E
Kharaghoda, *India* **92 H4** 23 11N 71 46 E
Kharagpur, *India* **93 H12** 22 20N 87 25 E
Khárakas, *Greece* **39 E6** 35 1N 25 7 E
Kharan Kalat, *Pakistan* **91 C2** 28 34N 65 21 E
Kharānaq, *Iran* **97 C7** 32 20N 54 45 E
Kharda, *India* **94 E2** 18 40N 75 34 E
Khardung La, *India* **93 B7** 34 20N 77 43 E
Kharg = Khārk, Jazīreh-ye, *Iran* **97 D6** 29 15N 50 28 E
Khârga, El Wâhât-el, *Egypt* **106 B3** 25 10N 30 35 E
Khargon, *India* **94 D2** 21 45N 75 40 E
Khari →, *India* **92 G6** 25 54N 74 31 E
Kharian, *Pakistan* **92 C5** 32 49N 73 52 E
Khariar, *India* **94 D6** 20 17N 82 46 E
Kharit, Wadi el →, *Egypt* **106 C3** 24 26N 33 3 E
Khārk, Jazīreh-ye, *Iran* **97 D6** 29 15N 50 28 E
Kharkiv, *Ukraine* **59 H9** 49 58N 36 20 E
Kharkov = Kharkiv, *Ukraine* **59 H9** 49 58N 36 20 E
Kharmanli, *Bulgaria* **51 E9** 41 55N 25 55 E
Kharovsk, *Russia* **58 C11** 59 56N 40 13 E
Kharsawangarh, *India* **93 H11** 22 48N 85 50 E
Kharta, *Turkey* **100 B3** 40 55N 29 7 E
Khartoum = El Khartûm, *Sudan* **107 D3** 15 31N 32 35 E
Khasan, *Russia* **70 C5** 42 25N 130 40 E
Khasavyurt, *Russia* **61 J8** 43 16N 46 40 E
Khāsh, *Iran* **91 C1** 28 15N 61 15 E
Khāsh, Dasht-e, *Afghan.* **91 C1** 31 50N 62 30 E
Khashm el Girba, *Sudan* **107 E4** 14 59N 35 58 E
Khashum, *Sudan* **107 E2** 12 27N 28 2 E
Khashuri, *Georgia* **61 J6** 42 3N 43 35 E
Khasi Hills, *India* **90 C3** 25 30N 91 30 E
Khaskovo, *Bulgaria* **51 E9** 41 56N 25 30 E
Khaskovo □, *Bulgaria* **51 E9** 42 0N 25 40 E
Khatanga, *Russia* **67 B11** 72 0N 102 20 E
Khatanga →, *Russia* **67 B11** 72 55N 106 0 E
Khatauli, *India* **92 E7** 29 17N 77 43 E
Khatra, *India* **93 H12** 22 59N 86 51 E
Khātūnābād, *Iran* **97 D7** 30 1N 55 25 E
Khatyrka, *Russia* **67 C18** 62 3N 175 15 E
Khavast, *Uzbekistan* **65 C4** 40 10N 68 49 E
Khavda, *India* **92 H3** 23 51N 69 43 E
Khavdháta, *Greece* **39 D1** 38 12N 20 23 E
Khawlaf, Ra's, *Yemen* **99 D6** 12 40N 54 7 E
Khay', *Si. Arabia* **98 C3** 18 45N 41 24 E
Khaybar, Ḥarrat, *Si. Arabia* **96 E4** 25 45N 40 0 E
Khaydarken, *Kyrgyzstan* **65 D5** 39 57N 71 20 E
Khāzimiyah, *Iraq* **96 C4** 34 46N 43 37 E
Khazzān Jabal al Awliyā, *Sudan* **107 D3** 15 24N 32 20 E
Khe Bo, *Vietnam* **86 C5** 19 8N 104 41 E
Khe Long, *Vietnam* **86 B5** 21 29N 104 46 E
Khe Sanh, *Vietnam* **86 D6** 16 37N 106 45 E
Khed, *Maharashtra, India* **94 F1** 17 43N 73 27 E
Khed, *Maharashtra, India* **94 E1** 18 51N 73 56 E
Khekra, *India* **92 E7** 28 52N 77 20 E
Khem-Beldyr = Kyzyl, *Russia* **67 D10** 51 50N 94 30 E
Khemarak Phouminville, *Cambodia* **87 G4** 11 37N 102 59 E
Khemis Miliana, *Algeria* **111 A5** 36 11N 2 14 E
Khemisset, *Morocco* **110 B3** 33 50N 6 1W
Khemmarat, *Thailand* **86 D5** 16 10N 105 15 E
Khenāmān, *Iran* **97 D8** 30 27N 56 29 E
Khenchela, *Algeria* **111 A6** 35 28N 7 11 E
Khenifra, *Morocco* **110 B3** 32 58N 5 46W
Kherrata, *Algeria* **111 A6** 36 27N 5 13 E
Khersān →, *Iran* **97 D6** 31 33N 50 22 E
Khérson, *Greece* **50 E6** 41 5N 22 47 E
Kherson, *Ukraine* **59 J7** 46 35N 32 35 E
Khersónisos Akrotíri, *Greece* **39 E5** 35 30N 24 10 E
Kheta →, *Russia* **67 B11** 71 54N 102 6 E
Khewari, *Pakistan* **92 F3** 26 36N 68 52 E
Khibinogorsk = Kirovsk, *Russia* **56 A5** 67 32N 33 41 E
Khilchipur, *India* **92 G7** 24 2N 76 34 E
Khiliomódhion, *Greece* **48 D4** 37 48N 22 51 E
Khilok, *Russia* **67 D12** 51 30N 110 45 E
Khimki, *Russia* **58 E9** 55 50N 37 20 E
Khíos, *Greece* **49 C8** 38 27N 26 9 E
Khíos □, *Greece* **49 C8** 38 27N 26 9 E
Khirsadoh, *India* **93 H8** 22 11N 78 47 E
Khiuma = Hiiumaa, *Estonia* **15 G20** 58 50N 22 45 E
Khiva, *Uzbekistan* **66 E7** 41 30N 60 18 E
Khīyāv, *Iran* **96 B5** 38 30N 47 45 E
Khlebarovo, *Bulgaria* **51 C10** 43 37N 26 15 E
Khlong Khlung, *Thailand* **86 D2** 16 12N 99 43 E
Khmelnik, *Ukraine* **59 H4** 49 33N 27 58 E
Khmelnitskiy = Khmelnytskyy, *Ukraine* **59 H4** 49 23N 27 0 E
Khmelnytskyy, *Ukraine* **59 H4** 49 23N 27 0 E
Khmer Rep. = Cambodia ■, *Asia* **86 F5** 12 15N 105 0 E
Khoai, Hon, *Vietnam* **87 H5** 8 26N 104 50 E
Khodoriv, *Ukraine* **59 H3** 49 24N 24 19 E
Khodzent = Khŭjand, *Tajikistan* **65 C4** 40 17N 69 37 E
Khojak Pass, *Afghan.* **91 C2** 30 51N 66 34 E
Khok Kloi, *Thailand* **87 a** 8 17N 98 19 E
Khok Pho, *Thailand* **87 J3** 6 43N 101 6 E
Khokhropār, *Pakistan* **91 D3** 25 42N 70 12 E
Kholm, *Afghan.* **65 E3** 36 45N 67 40 E
Kholm, *Russia* **58 D6** 57 10N 31 15 E
Kholmsk, *Russia* **67 E15** 47 40N 142 5 E
Khomas Hochland, *Namibia* **116 C2** 22 40 S 16 0 E
Khombole, *Senegal* **112 C1** 14 43N 16 42W
Khomeyn, *Iran* **97 C6** 33 40N 50 7 E
Khomeynī Shahr, *Iran* **97 C6** 32 41N 51 31 E
Khomodino, *Botswana* **116 C3** 22 46 S 23 52 E
Khon Kaen, *Thailand* **86 D4** 16 30N 102 47 E
Khong →, *Cambodia* **86 F5** 13 32N 105 58 E
Khong Sedone, *Laos* **86 E5** 15 34N 105 49 E
Khonuu, *Russia* **67 C15** 66 30N 143 12 E
Khoper →, *Russia* **60 F6** 49 30N 42 20 E
Khor el 'Atash, *Sudan* **107 E3** 13 20N 34 15 E
Khóra, *Greece* **48 D3** 37 3N 21 42 E
Khóra Sfakíon, *Greece* **39 E5** 35 15N 24 9 E
Khorāsān □, *Iran* **97 C8** 34 0N 58 0 E
Khorat = Nakhon Ratchasima, *Thailand* **86 E4** 14 59N 102 12 E
Khorat, Cao Nguyen, *Thailand* **86 E4** 15 30N 102 50 E
Khorb el Ethel, *Algeria* **110 C3** 28 30N 6 17W
Khorixas, *Namibia* **116 C1** 20 16 S 14 59 E
Khorol, *Ukraine* **59 H7** 49 48N 33 15 E
Khorramābād, *Khorāsān, Iran* **97 C8** 35 6N 57 57 E
Khorramābād, *Lorestān, Iran* **97 C6** 33 30N 48 25 E
Khorrāmshahr, *Iran* **97 D6** 30 29N 48 15 E
Khorugh, *Tajikistan* **65 E5** 37 30N 71 36 E
Khosravī, *Iran* **97 D6** 30 48N 51 28 E
Khosrowābād, *Khuzestān, Iran* **97 D6** 30 10N 48 25 E
Khosrowābād, *Kordestān, Iran* **101 E12** 35 31N 47 38 E
Khost, *Pakistan* **92 D2** 30 13N 67 35 E
Khosūyeh, *Iran* **97 D7** 28 32N 54 26 E
Khotan = Hotan, *China* **68 C2** 37 25N 79 55 E
Khotyn, *Ukraine* **53 B11** 48 31N 26 27 E
Khouribga, *Morocco* **110 B3** 32 58N 6 57W
Khowai, *Bangla.* **90 C3** 24 5N 91 40 E
Khowst, *Afghan.* **91 B3** 33 22N 69 58 E
Khoyniki, *Belarus* **59 G5** 51 54N 29 55 E
Khrami →, *Georgia* **61 K7** 41 25N 45 0 E
Khrenovoye, *Russia* **60 E5** 51 4N 40 16 E
Khrisoúpolis, *Greece* **51 F8** 40 58N 24 42 E
Khristianá, *Greece* **49 E7** 36 14N 25 13 E
Khromtau, *Kazakhstan* **64 F7** 50 17N 58 27 E
Khrysokhou B., *Cyprus* **39 E8** 35 6N 32 25 E
Khtapodhiá, *Greece* **49 D7** 37 24N 25 34 E
Khu Khan, *Thailand* **86 E5** 14 42N 104 12 E
Khuan Wa, *Thailand* **87 a** 7 53N 98 17 E
Khudrah, W. →, *Yemen* **99 C5** 18 10N 50 20 E
Khudzhand = Khŭjand, *Tajikistan* **65 C4** 40 17N 69 37 E
Khuff, *Si. Arabia* **96 E5** 24 55N 44 53 E
Khūgīānī, *Afghan.* **91 C2** 31 34N 66 32 E
Khuis, *Botswana* **116 D3** 26 40 S 21 49 E
Khuiyala, *India* **92 F4** 27 9N 70 25 E
Khŭjand, *Tajikistan* **65 C4** 40 17N 69 37 E
Khujner, *India* **92 H7** 23 47N 76 36 E
Khulayş, *Si. Arabia* **98 B2** 22 9N 39 19 E
Khulna, *Bangla.* **90 D2** 22 45N 89 34 E
Khulna □, *Bangla.* **90 D2** 22 25N 89 35 E
Khulo, *Georgia* **61 K6** 41 33N 42 19 E
Khumago, *Botswana* **116 C3** 20 26 S 24 32 E
Khumrah, *Si. Arabia* **98 B2** 21 22N 39 13 E
Khunjerab △, *Pakistan* **93 A6** 36 40N 75 30 E
Khunjerab Pass = Kinjirap Daban, *Asia* **91 A4** 36 40N 75 25 E
Khūnsorkh, *Iran* **97 E8** 27 9N 56 7 E
Khunti, *India* **93 H11** 23 5N 85 17 E
Khūr, *Iran* **97 C8** 32 55N 58 18 E
Khurai, *India* **92 G8** 24 3N 78 23 E
Khuraydah, *Yemen* **99 D5** 15 33N 48 18 E
Khurayş, *Si. Arabia* **97 E6** 25 6N 48 2 E
Khurda, *India* **94 D7** 20 11N 85 37 E
Khureit, *Sudan* **107 E2** 13 59N 26 3 E
Khurīyā Murīyā, Ghubbat, *Oman* **99 C6** 17 40N 55 45 E
Khurīyā Murīyā, Jazā'ir, *Oman* **99 C6** 17 30N 55 58 E
Khurja, *India* **92 E7** 28 15N 77 58 E
Khūrmāl, *Iraq* **96 C5** 35 18N 46 2 E
Khurr, Wādī al, *Iraq* **96 C4** 32 3N 43 52 E
Khūsf, *Iran* **97 C8** 32 46N 58 53 E
Khushab, *Pakistan* **91 B4** 32 20N 72 20 E
Khust, *Ukraine* **53 B8** 48 10N 23 18 E
Khutse ⌓, *Botswana* **116 C3** 23 31 S 24 12 E
Khuzdar, *Pakistan* **91 D2** 27 52N 66 30 E
Khūzestān □, *Iran* **97 D6** 31 0N 49 0 E
Khvāf, *Iran* **97 C9** 34 33N 60 8 E
Khvājeh, *Iran* **96 B5** 38 9N 46 35 E
Khvājeh Moḩammad, Kūh-e, *Afghan.* **65 E5** 36 22N 70 17 E
Khvalynsk, *Russia* **60 D9** 52 30N 48 2 E
Khvānsār, *Iran* **97 D7** 29 56N 54 8 E
Khvatovka, *Russia* **60 D8** 52 24N 46 32 E
Khvor, *Iran* **97 C7** 33 45N 55 0 E
Khvorgū, *Iran* **97 E8** 27 34N 56 27 E
Khvormūj, *Iran* **97 D6** 28 40N 51 30 E
Khvoy, *Iran* **101 C11** 38 35N 45 0 E
Khvoynaya, *Russia* **58 C8** 58 58N 34 28 E
Khyber Pass, *Afghan.* **91 B3** 34 10N 71 8 E
Khyriv, *Ukraine* **55 J9** 49 32N 22 50 E
Kia, *Fiji* **133 A2** 16 16 S 179 8 E
Kia, *Solomon Is.* **133 L10** 7 32 S 158 26 E
Kiabukwa, *Dem. Rep. of the Congo* **119 D1** 8 40 S 24 48 E
Kiadho →, *India* **94 E3** 19 37N 77 40 E
Kiama, *Australia* **129 C9** 34 40 S 150 50 E
Kiama, *Dem. Rep. of the Congo* **115 D3** 7 19 S 17 49 E
Kiamba, *Phil.* **81 H5** 6 2N 124 46 E
Kiambi, *Dem. Rep. of the Congo* **118 D2** 7 15 S 28 0 E
Kiambu, *Kenya* **118 C4** 1 8 S 36 50 E
Kiamusze = Jiamusi, *China* **69 B8** 46 40N 130 26 E
Kian = Ji'an, *China* **75 D14** 41 5N 126 10 E
Kiana, *U.S.A.* **144 C7** 66 58N 160 26W
Kiang West △, *Gambia* **112 C1** 13 25N 15 50W
Kiangara, *Madag.* **117 B8** 17 58 S 47 2 E
Kiangsi = Jiangxi □, *China* **77 D11** 27 30N 116 0 E
Kiangsu = Jiangsu □, *China* **75 H11** 33 0N 120 0 E
Kiáton, *Greece* **48 C4** 38 1N 22 45 E
Kibæk, *Denmark* **17 H2** 56 2N 8 51 E
Kibale △, *Uganda* **118 B3** 0 16N 30 18 E
Kibanga Port, *Uganda* **118 B3** 0 10N 32 58 E

Kibangou, *Congo* **114 C2** 3 26 S 12 22 E
Kibara, *Tanzania* **118 C3** 2 8 S 33 30 E
Kibare, Mts., *Dem. Rep. of the Congo* **118 D2** 8 25 S 27 10 E
Kibawe, *Phil.* **81 H5** 7 34N 125 0 E
Kibenga, *Dem. Rep. of the Congo* **115 D3** 7 56 S 17 30 E
Kibira △, *Burundi* **118 C3** 3 6 S 30 24 E
Kibombo, *Dem. Rep. of the Congo* **118 C2** 3 57 S 25 53 E
Kibondo, *Tanzania* **118 C3** 3 35 S 30 45 E
Kibray, *Uzbekistan* **65 C4** 41 23N 69 27 E
Kibre Mengist, *Ethiopia* **107 F4** 5 54N 38 59 E
Kıbrıs = Cyprus ■, *Asia* **39 F9** 35 0N 33 0 E
Kibumbu, *Burundi* **118 C2** 3 32 S 29 45 E
Kibungo, *Rwanda* **118 C3** 2 10 S 30 32 E
Kibuye, *Burundi* **118 C2** 3 39 S 29 59 E
Kibuye, *Rwanda* **118 C2** 2 3 S 29 21 E
Kibwesa, *Tanzania* **118 D2** 6 30 S 29 58 E
Kibwezi, *Kenya* **118 C4** 2 27 S 37 57 E
Kicasalih, *Turkey* **51 E10** 41 23N 26 48 E
Kičevo, *Macedonia* **50 E4** 41 34N 20 59 E
Kichha, *India* **93 E8** 28 53N 79 30 E
Kichha →, *India* **93 E8** 28 41N 79 18 E
Kichmengskiy Gorodok, *Russia* **56 B8** 59 59N 45 48 E
Kicking Horse Pass, *Canada* **142 C5** 51 28N 116 16W
Kidal, *Mali* **113 B5** 18 26N 1 22 E
Kidapawan, *Phil.* **81 H5** 7 1N 125 3 E
Kidderminster, *U.K.* **21 E5** 52 24N 2 15W
Kidepo Valley △, *Uganda* **118 B3** 3 52N 33 50 E
Kidete, *Tanzania* **118 D4** 6 25 S 37 17 E
Kidira, *Senegal* **112 C2** 14 28N 12 13W
Kidnappers, C., *N.Z.* **130 F6** 39 38 S 177 5 E
Kidsgrove, *U.K.* **20 D5** 53 5N 2 14W
Kidston, *Australia* **126 B3** 18 52 S 144 8 E
Kidugallo, *Tanzania* **118 D4** 6 49 S 38 15 E
Kidurong, Tanjong, *Malaysia* **85 B4** 3 16N 113 3 E
Kiel, *Germany* **30 A6** 54 19N 10 8 E
Kiel Canal = Nord-Ostsee-Kanal, *Germany* **30 A5** 54 12N 9 32 E
Kiel-Kanal = Nord-Ostsee-Kanal, *Germany* **30 A5** 54 12N 9 32 E
Kielce, *Poland* **55 H7** 50 52N 20 42 E
Kielder Water, *U.K.* **20 B5** 55 11N 2 31W
Kieler Bucht, *Germany* **30 A6** 54 35N 10 25 E
Kiembara, *Burkina Faso* **112 C4** 13 15N 2 44W
Kien Binh, *Vietnam* **87 H5** 9 55N 105 19 E
Kien Tan, *Vietnam* **87 G5** 10 7N 105 17 E
Kienge, *Dem. Rep. of the Congo* **119 E2** 10 30 S 27 30 E
Kiessé, *Niger* **113 C5** 13 29N 4 1 E
Kieta, *Papua N. G.* **132 D8** 6 12 S 155 36 E
Kiev = Kyyiv, *Ukraine* **59 G6** 50 30N 30 28 E
Kifaya, *Guinea* **112 C2** 12 10N 13 4W
Kiffa, *Mauritania* **112 B2** 16 37N 11 24W
Kifisiá, *Greece* **48 C5** 38 4N 23 49 E
Kifissós →, *Greece* **48 C5** 38 35N 23 20 E
Kifrī, *Iraq* **101 E11** 34 45N 45 0 E
Kigali, *Rwanda* **118 C3** 1 59 S 30 4 E
Kigarama, *Tanzania* **118 C3** 1 1 S 31 50 E
Kigelle, *Sudan* **107 F3** 8 40N 34 2 E
Kigezi ⌓, *Uganda* **118 C2** 0 34 S 29 55 E
Kigoma □, *Tanzania* **118 D3** 5 0 S 30 0 E
Kigoma-Ujiji, *Tanzania* **118 C2** 4 55 S 29 36 E
Kigomasha, Ras, *Tanzania* **118 C4** 4 58 S 38 58 E
Kığzı, *Turkey* **96 B4** 38 18N 43 25 E
Kihei, *U.S.A.* **145 C5** 20 47N 156 28W
Kihikihi, *N.Z.* **130 E4** 38 2 S 175 22 E
Kihnu, *Estonia* **15 G21** 58 9N 24 1 E
Kiholo B., *U.S.A.* **145 D6** 19 50N 155 55W
Kii-Hantō, *Japan* **73 D7** 34 0N 135 45 E
Kii-Nagashima, *Japan* **73 C8** 34 12N 136 20 E
Kii-Sanchi, *Japan* **73 C8** 34 20N 136 0 E
Kii-Suidō, *Japan* **72 D6** 33 40N 134 45 E
Kiire, *Japan* **72 F2** 31 22N 130 33 E
Kijik, *U.S.A.* **144 F9** 60 20N 154 20W
Kikaiga-Shima, *Japan* **71 K4** 28 19N 129 59 E
Kikinda, *Serbia & M.* **52 E5** 45 50N 20 30 E
Kikládhes, *Greece* **48 E6** 37 0N 24 30 E
Kikládhes □, *Greece* **48 D6** 37 0N 25 0 E
Kikoira, *Australia* **129 B7** 33 39 S 146 40 E
Kikombo, *Bandundu, Dem. Rep. of the Congo* **115 D3** 5 37 S 18 50 E
Kikombo, *Bandundu, Dem. Rep. of the Congo* **115 D3** 5 49 S 17 45 E
Kikongo, *Dem. Rep. of the Congo* **115 C3** 4 16 S 17 17 E
Kikori, *Papua N. G.* **132 D3** 7 25 S 144 15 E
Kikori →, *Papua N. G.* **132 D3** 7 38 S 144 20 E
Kikuchi, *Japan* **72 E2** 32 59N 130 47 E
Kikwit, *Dem. Rep. of the Congo* **115 D3** 5 0 S 18 45 E
Kil, *Sweden* **16 E7** 59 30N 13 20 E
Kilafors, *Sweden* **16 C10** 61 14N 16 36 E
Kilakkarai, *India* **95 K4** 9 12N 78 47 E
Kilar, *India* **92 C7** 33 6N 76 25 E
Kilauea, *U.S.A.* **145 A2** 22 13N 159 25W
Kilauea Crater, *U.S.A.* **145 D6** 19 25N 155 17W
Kilbrannan Sd., *U.K.* **22 F3** 55 37N 5 26W
Kilchberg, *Switz.* **33 B7** 47 18N 8 33 E
Kilchu, *N. Korea* **75 D15** 40 57N 129 25 E
Kilcoy, *Australia* **127 D5** 26 59 S 152 30 E
Kildare, *Ireland* **23 C5** 53 9N 6 55W
Kildare □, *Ireland* **23 C5** 53 10N 6 50W
Kileikli, *Sudan* **107 E2** 11 25N 25 31 E
Kilembe, *Dem. Rep. of the Congo* **115 D3** 5 42 S 19 55 E
Kilen, *Norway* **18 E5** 59 20N 8 49 E
Kilfinnane, *Ireland* **23 D3** 52 21N 8 28W
Kilgore, *U.S.A.* **155 J7** 32 23N 94 53W
Kilibo, *Benin* **113 D5** 8 32N 2 38 E
Kilifi, *Kenya* **118 C4** 3 40 S 39 48 E
Kilimanjaro, *Tanzania* **118 C4** 3 7 S 37 20 E
Kilimanjaro □, *Tanzania* **118 C4** 4 0 S 38 0 E
Kilimli, *Turkey* **100 B4** 41 28N 31 50 E
Kilinailau Is., *Papua N. G.* **132 C8** 4 45 S 155 20 E
Kilindini, *Kenya* **118 C4** 4 4 S 39 40 E
Kilis, *Turkey* **100 D7** 36 42N 37 6 E
Kiliya, *Ukraine* **53 E14** 45 28N 29 16 E
Kilkee, *Ireland* **23 D2** 52 41N 9 39W
Kilkeel, *U.K.* **23 B5** 54 4N 6 0W
Kilkenny, *Ireland* **23 D4** 52 39N 7 15W
Kilkenny □, *Ireland* **23 D4** 52 35N 7 15W
Kilkieran B., *Ireland* **23 C2** 53 20N 9 41W
Kilkís, *Greece* **50 F6** 40 58N 22 57 E
Kilkís □, *Greece* **50 E6** 41 5N 22 50 E
Killala, *Ireland* **23 B2** 54 13N 9 12W
Killala B., *Ireland* **23 B2** 54 16N 9 8W
Killaloe, *Canada* **150 A7** 45 33N 77 25W
Killaloe, *Ireland* **23 D3** 52 48N 8 28W
Killarney, *Australia* **127 D5** 28 20 S 152 18 E
Killarney, *Canada* **143 D9** 49 10N 99 40W
Killarney, *Ireland* **23 D2** 52 4N 9 30W
Killarney △, *Ireland* **23 D2** 52 0N 9 33W
Killarney, L., *Bahamas* **9 b** 25 3N 77 27W
Killary Harbour, *Ireland* **23 C2** 53 38N 9 52W
Killdeer, *U.S.A.* **154 B3** 47 26N 102 48W
Killeberg, *Sweden* **17 H8** 56 29N 14 5 E
Killeen, *U.S.A.* **155 K6** 31 7N 97 44W
Killin, *U.K.* **22 E4** 56 28N 4 19W
Killíni, *Ilía, Greece* **39 D3** 37 55N 21 8 E
Killíni, *Korinthía, Greece* **48 D4** 37 54N 22 25 E
Killíni, Ákra, *Greece* **39 D3** 37 57N 21 8 E
Killorglin, *Ireland* **23 D2** 52 6N 9 47W
Killybegs, *Ireland* **23 B3** 54 38N 8 26W
Kilmarnock, *U.K.* **22 F4** 55 37N 4 29W
Kilmez, *Russia* **60 B10** 56 58N 50 55 E
Kilmez →, *Russia* **60 B10** 56 58N 50 28 E
Kilmore, *Australia* **129 D6** 37 25 S 144 53 E
Kilómetro 1082 = Joaquín V. González, *Argentina* **174 B3** 25 10 S 64 0W
Kilondo, *Tanzania* **119 D3** 9 45 S 34 20 E
Kilosa, *Tanzania* **118 D4** 6 48 S 37 0 E
Kilrush, *Ireland* **23 D2** 52 38N 9 29W
Kiltan I., *India* **95 J1** 11 29N 73 0 E
Kilwa Kisiwani, *Tanzania* **119 D4** 8 58 S 39 32 E
Kilwa Kivinje, *Tanzania* **119 D4** 8 45 S 39 25 E
Kilwa Masoko, *Tanzania* **119 D4** 8 55 S 39 30 E
Kilwinning, *U.K.* **22 F4** 55 39N 4 43W
Kim, *U.S.A.* **155 G3** 37 15N 103 21W
Kim →, *Cameroon* **113 D7** 5 28N 11 7 E
Kimaam, *Indonesia* **83 C5** 7 58 S 138 53 E
Kimamba, *Tanzania* **118 D4** 6 45 S 37 10 E
Kimba, *Australia* **128 B2** 33 8 S 136 23 E
Kimball, *Nebr., U.S.A.* **154 E3** 41 14N 103 40W
Kimball, *S. Dak., U.S.A.* **154 D5** 43 45N 98 57W
Kimbanda, *Dem. Rep. of the Congo* **115 C3** 4 16 S 18 30 E
Kimbe, *Papua N. G.* **132 C6** 5 33 S 150 11 E
Kimbe B., *Papua N. G.* **132 C6** 5 15 S 150 30 E
Kimberley, *Australia* **124 C4** 16 20 S 127 0 E
Kimberley, *Canada* **142 D5** 49 40N 115 59W
Kimberley, *S. Africa* **116 D3** 28 43 S 24 46 E
Kimberly, *U.S.A.* **158 E6** 42 32N 114 22W
Kimbongo, *Dem. Rep. of the Congo* **115 D3** 6 8 S 18 1 E
Kimch'aek, *N. Korea* **75 D15** 40 40N 129 10 E
Kimch'ŏn, *S. Korea* **75 F15** 36 11N 128 4 E
Kími, *Greece* **48 C6** 38 38N 24 6 E
Kimitsu, *Japan* **73 B10** 35 19N 139 54 E
Kimje, *S. Korea* **75 G14** 35 48N 126 45 E
Kimmirut, *Canada* **139 B13** 62 50N 69 50W
Kímolos, *Greece* **48 E6** 36 48N 24 37 E
Kimongo, *Congo* **115 C2** 4 27 S 12 53 E
Kimovsk, *Moskva, Russia* **58 E9** 55 21N 37 28 E
Kimovsk, *Tula, Russia* **58 E10** 54 0N 38 29 E
Kimpangu, *Dem. Rep. of the Congo* **115 D3** 5 52 S 15 3 E
Kimparana, *Mali* **112 C4** 12 48N 5 0W
Kimry, *Russia* **58 D9** 56 55N 37 15 E
Kimstad, *Sweden* **17 F9** 58 35N 15 58 E
Kimvula, *Dem. Rep. of the Congo* **115 D3** 5 44 S 15 58 E
Kin, *Burma* **90 D5** 22 46N 94 42 E
Kin-u, *Burma* **90 D5** 22 46N 95 37 E
Kinabalu, Gunung, *Malaysia* **85 A5** 6 3N 116 14 E
Kinard, *U.S.A.* **152 E4** 30 16N 85 15W
Kínaros, *Greece* **49 E8** 36 59N 26 15 E
Kinaskan L., *Canada* **142 B2** 57 38N 130 8W
Kinbasket L., *Canada* **142 C5** 52 0N 118 10W
Kincaid, *U.S.A.* **156 E7** 39 35N 89 25W
Kincardine, *Canada* **140 D3** 44 10N 81 40W
Kinchafoonee Cr. →, *U.S.A.* **152 D5** 31 38N 84 10W
Kinchega △, *Australia* **128 B5** 32 27 S 142 15 E
Kincolith, *Canada* **142 C3** 55 0N 129 57W
Kinda, *Kasai-Or., Dem. Rep. of the Congo* **119 D2** 9 18 S 25 4 E
Kinda, *Katanga, Dem. Rep. of the Congo* **115 C4** 4 47 S 21 48 E
Kindambi, *Dem. Rep. of the Congo* **115 D4** 5 6 S 18 14 E
Kindberg, *Austria* **34 D8** 47 30N 15 27 E
Kinde, *U.S.A.* **150 C2** 43 56N 83 0W
Kindele, *Dem. Rep. of the Congo* **115 D4** 8 39 S 24 10 E
Kinder Scout, *U.K.* **20 D6** 53 24N 1 52W
Kinderhook, *U.S.A.* **156 E5** 39 42N 91 10W
Kindersley, *Canada* **143 C7** 51 30N 109 10W
Kindia, *Guinea* **112 D2** 10 0N 12 52W
Kindley U.S.A.F. Base, *Bermuda* **9 a** 32 22N 64 42W
Kindongo, *Dem. Rep. of the Congo* **114 C3** 3 58 S 17 30 E
Kindu, *Dem. Rep. of the Congo* **118 C2** 2 55 S 25 50 E
Kinel, *Russia* **60 D10** 53 15N 50 40 E
Kineshma, *Russia* **60 B6** 57 30N 42 5 E
Kinesi, *Tanzania* **118 C3** 1 25 S 33 50 E
King, L., *Australia* **125 F2** 33 10 S 119 35 E
King, Mt., *Australia* **126 D4** 25 10 S 147 30 E
King City, *Calif., U.S.A.* **160 J5** 36 13N 121 8W
King City, *Mo., U.S.A.* **156 D2** 40 3N 94 31W
King Cove, *U.S.A.* **144 J7** 55 3N 162 19W
King Cr. →, *Australia* **126 C2** 24 35 S 139 30 E
King Edward →, *Australia* **124 B4** 14 14 S 126 35 E
King Frederick VI Land = Kong Frederik VI Kyst, *Greenland* **10 E6** 63 0N 43 0W
King George B., *Falk. Is.* **9 f** 51 30 S 60 30W
King George I., *Antarctica* **7 C18** 60 0 S 60 0W
King George Is., *Canada* **139 C11** 57 20N 80 30W
King I. = Kadan Kyun, *Burma* **86 F2** 12 30N 98 20 E
King I., *Australia* **127 F3** 39 50 S 144 0 E
King I., *Canada* **142 C3** 52 10N 127 40W
King Leopold Ranges, *Australia* **124 C4** 17 30 S 125 45 E
King of Prussia, *U.S.A.* **151 F9** 40 5N 75 23W
King Salmon, *U.S.A.* **144 G8** 58 42N 156 40W
King Sd., *Australia* **124 C3** 16 50 S 123 20 E
King Sejong, *Antarctica* **7 C18** 62 30 S 58 0W
King William I., *Canada* **138 B10** 69 10N 97 25W
King William's Town, *S. Africa* **116 E4** 32 51 S 27 22 E
Kingait = Cape Dorset, *Canada* **139 B12** 64 14N 76 32W
Kingaok = Bathurst Inlet, *Canada* **138 B9** 66 50N 108 1W
Kingaroy, *Australia* **127 D5** 26 32 S 151 51 E
Kingdom City, *U.S.A.* **156 F5** 38 56N 91 56W
Kingfisher, *U.S.A.* **155 H6** 35 52N 97 56W
Kingirbān, *Iraq* **96 C5** 34 40N 44 54 E
Kingisepp = Kuressaare, *Estonia* **15 G20** 58 15N 22 30 E
Kingisepp, *Russia* **58 C5** 59 25N 28 40 E
Kingking = Pantukan, *Phil.* **81 H5** 7 9N 125 54 E
Kinglake △, *Australia* **129 D6** 37 30 S 145 22 E
Kingman, *Ariz., U.S.A.* **161 K12** 35 12N 114 4W
Kingman, *Ind., U.S.A.* **157 E9** 39 58N 87 18W
Kingman, *Kans., U.S.A.* **155 G5** 37 39N 98 7W
Kingoonya, *Australia* **127 E2** 30 55 S 135 19 E
Kingri, *Pakistan* **92 D3** 30 27N 69 49 E
Kings →, *U.S.A.* **160 J7** 36 3N 119 50W
Kings Canyon △, *U.S.A.* **160 J8** 36 50N 118 40W
Kings County = Offaly □, *Ireland* **23 C4** 53 15N 7 30W
King's Lynn, *U.K.* **20 E8** 52 45N 0 24 E
Kings Park, *U.S.A.* **151 F11** 40 53N 73 16W
King's Peak, *U.S.A.* **158 F8** 40 46N 110 27W
Kingsbridge, *U.K.* **21 G4** 50 17N 3 47W
Kingsburg, *U.S.A.* **160 J7** 36 31N 119 33W
Kingscote, *Australia* **128 C2** 35 40 S 137 38 E
Kingscourt, *Ireland* **23 C5** 53 55N 6 48W
Kingsford, *U.S.A.* **148 C1** 45 48N 88 4W
Kingsland, *U.S.A.* **152 E8** 30 48N 81 41W
Kingsport, *U.S.A.* **149 G4** 36 33N 82 33W
Kingston, *Canada* **140 D4** 44 14N 76 30W
Kingston, *Jamaica* **164 a** 18 0N 76 50W
Kingston, *N.Z.* **131 F3** 45 20 S 168 43 E
Kingston, *N.H., U.S.A.* **151 D13** 42 56N 71 3W
Kingston, *N.Y., U.S.A.* **151 E11** 41 56N 73 59W
Kingston, *Pa., U.S.A.* **151 E9** 41 16N 75 54W
Kingston, *R.I., U.S.A.* **151 E13** 41 29N 71 30W
Kingston Pk., *U.S.A.* **161 K11** 35 45N 115 54W
Kingston South East, *Australia* **128 D3** 36 51 S 139 55 E
Kingston upon Hull, *U.K.* **20 D7** 53 45N 0 21W
Kingston upon Hull □, *U.K.* **20 D7** 53 45N 0 21W
Kingston-upon-Thames □, *U.K.* **21 F7** 51 24N 0 17W
Kingstown = Dún Laoghaire, *Ireland* **23 C5** 53 17N 6 8W
Kingstown, *Australia* **129 A9** 30 29 S 151 6 E
Kingstown, *St. Vincent* **165 D7** 13 10N 61 10W
Kingstree, *U.S.A.* **152 B10** 33 40N 79 50W
Kingsville, *Canada* **140 D3** 42 2N 82 45W
Kingsville, *U.S.A.* **155 M6** 27 31N 97 52W
Kingtechen = Jingdezhen, *China* **77 C11** 29 20N 117 11 E
Kingunda, *Dem. Rep. of the Congo* **115 D3** 6 36 S 16 58 E
Kingussie, *U.K.* **22 D4** 57 6N 4 2W
Kingwood, *U.S.A.* **155 K7** 29 54N 95 18W
Kinhwa = Jinhua, *China* **77 C12** 29 8N 119 38 E
Kınık, *Antalya, Turkey* **49 E11** 36 20N 29 20 E
Kınık, *İzmir, Turkey* **49 B9** 39 6N 27 24 E
Kinistino, *Canada* **143 C7** 52 57N 105 2W
Kinjirap Daban, *Asia* **91 A4** 36 40N 75 25 E
Kinkala, *Congo* **115 C2** 4 18 S 14 49 E
Kinki □, *Japan* **73 D8** 33 45N 136 0 E
Kinleith, *N.Z.* **130 E4** 38 20 S 175 56 E
Kinlochleven, *U.K.* **22 E4** 56 43N 5 0W
Kinmount, *Canada* **150 B6** 44 48N 78 45W
Kinmundy, *U.S.A.* **157 F8** 38 46N 88 51W
Kinn, *Norway* **18 C1** 61 34N 4 45 E
Kinna, *Sweden* **17 G6** 57 32N 12 42 E
Kinnairds Hd., *U.K.* **22 D6** 57 43N 2 1W
Kinnared, *Sweden* **17 G7** 57 2N 13 7 E
Kinnarp, *Sweden* **17 F7** 58 5N 13 32 E
Kinneviken, *Sweden* **17 F7** 58 35N 13 15 E
Kino, *Mexico* **162 B2** 28 45N 111 59W
Kinogitan, *Phil.* **81 G5** 9 0N 124 48 E
Kinoje →, *Canada* **140 B3** 52 8N 81 25W
Kinomoto, *Japan* **73 B8** 35 30N 136 13 E
Kinoni, *Uganda* **118 C3** 0 41 S 30 28 E
Kinoosao, *Canada* **143 B8** 57 5N 102 1W
Kinross, *U.K.* **22 E5** 56 13N 3 25W
Kinsale, *Ireland* **23 E3** 51 42N 8 31W
Kinsale, Old Hd. of, *Ireland* **23 E3** 51 37N 8 33W
Kinsarvik, *Norway* **18 D3** 60 22N 6 43 E
Kinsha = Chang Jiang →, *China* **77 B13** 31 48N 121 10 E
Kinshasa, *Dem. Rep. of the Congo* **115 C3** 4 20 S 15 15 E
Kinsley, *U.S.A.* **155 G5** 37 55N 99 25W
Kinsman, *U.S.A.* **150 E4** 41 26N 80 35W
Kinston, *Ala., U.S.A.* **152 D3** 31 13N 86 10W
Kinston, *N.C., U.S.A.* **149 H7** 35 16N 77 35W
Kintamani, *Indonesia* **79 J18** 8 14 S 115 19 E
Kintampo, *Ghana* **113 D4** 8 5N 1 41W
Kintap, *Indonesia* **85 C5** 3 51 S 115 13 E
Kintore, *U.K.* **22 D6** 57 14N 2 20W
Kintore Ra., *Australia* **124 D4** 23 15 S 128 47 E
Kintshua, *Dem. Rep. of the Congo* **115 C3** 4 27 S 19 38 E
Kintyre, *U.K.* **22 F3** 55 30N 5 35W
Kintyre, Mull of, *U.K.* **22 F3** 55 17N 5 47W
Kinu-Gawa →, *Japan* **73 B11** 35 36N 139 57 E
Kinushseo →, *Canada* **140 A3** 55 15N 83 45W
Kinuso, *Canada* **142 B5** 55 20N 115 25W
Kinwat, *India* **94 E4** 19 38N 78 12 E
Kinyangiri, *Tanzania* **118 C3** 4 25 S 34 37 E
Kinyeti, *Sudan* **107 G3** 3 57N 32 54 E
Kinzia, *Dem. Rep. of the Congo* **114 C3** 3 36 S 18 26 E
Kinzig →, *Germany* **31 G3** 48 36N 7 49 E
Kinzua, *U.S.A.* **150 E6** 41 52N 78 58W
Kinzua Dam, *U.S.A.* **150 E6** 41 53N 79 0W
Kióni, *Greece* **39 C2** 38 27N 20 41 E
Kiosk, *Canada* **140 C4** 46 6N 78 53W
Kiowa, *Kans., U.S.A.* **155 G5** 37 1N 98 29W
Kiowa, *Okla., U.S.A.* **155 H7** 34 43N 95 54W
Kipahigan L., *Canada* **143 B8** 55 20N 101 55W
Kipanga, *Tanzania* **118 D4** 6 15 S 35 20 E
Kipapa →, *U.S.A.* **145 K13** 21 24N 158 1W
Kiparissía, *Greece* **48 D3** 37 15N 21 40 E
Kiparissiakós Kólpos, *Greece* **48 D3** 37 25N 21 25 E
Kipawa, L., *Canada* **140 C4** 46 50N 79 0W
Kipembawe, *Tanzania* **118 D3** 7 38 S 33 27 E
Kipengere Ra., *Tanzania* **119 D3** 9 12 S 34 15 E
Kipili, *Tanzania* **118 D3** 7 28 S 30 32 E
Kipini, *Kenya* **118 C5** 2 30 S 40 32 E
Kipling, *Canada* **143 C8** 50 6N 102 38W
Kipnuk, *U.S.A.* **144 G6** 59 56N 164 3W
Kippure, *Ireland* **23 C5** 53 11N 6 21W
Kipushi, *Dem. Rep. of the Congo* **119 E2** 11 48 S 27 12 E
Kirandul, *India* **94 E5** 18 33N 81 10 E
Kirane, *Mali* **112 B2** 15 20N 10 20W
Kiranomena, *Madag.* **117 B8** 18 17 S 46 2 E
Kiraz, *Turkey* **49 C10** 38 14N 28 13 E
Kirazlı, *Turkey* **51 F10** 40 2N 26 41 E
Kirchberg, *Bern, Switz.* **32 B5** 47 5N 7 35 E
Kirchberg, *St. Galen, Switz.* **33 B8** 47 25N 9 2 E
Kirchhain, *Germany* **30 E4** 50 47N 8 56 E
Kirchheim, *Germany* **31 G5** 48 39N 9 27 E
Kirchheimbolanden, *Germany* **31 F3** 49 40N 8 0 E
Kirchschlag, *Austria* **35 D9** 47 30N 16 19 E
Kirdimi, *Chad* **109 E3** 18 11N 18 31 E
Kireç, *Turkey* **49 B10** 39 33N 28 22 E
Kirensk, *Russia* **67 D11** 57 50N 107 55 E
Kirghiz Range, *Asia* **65 B6** 42 40N 73 40 E
Kirghizia = Kyrgyzstan ■, *Asia* **65 C6** 42 0N 75 0 E
Kirghizstan = Kyrgyzstan ■, *Asia* **65 C6** 42 0N 75 0 E
Kirgiz-Kulak = Chirchiq, *Uzbekistan* **65 C4** 41 29N 69 35 E
Kirgiziya Steppe, *Eurasia* **57 E10** 50 0N 55 0 E
Kiri, *Dem. Rep. of the Congo* **114 C3** 1 29 S 19 0 E
Kiri Buru, *India* **94 D7** 22 0N 85 0 E
Kiribati ■, *Pac. Oc.* **134 H10** 5 0 S 180 0 E
Kırıkhan, *Turkey* **100 D7** 36 31N 36 21 E
Kırıkkale, *Turkey* **100 C5** 39 51N 33 32 E
Kirikopuni, *N.Z.* **130 B3** 35 50 S 174 1 E
Kirillov, *Russia* **58 C10** 59 49N 38 24 E
Kirin = Jilin, *China* **75 C14** 43 44N 126 30 E
Kirindi Oya →, *Sri Lanka* **95 L5** 6 15N 81 20 E
Kirinyaga = Kenya, Mt., *Kenya* **118 C4** 0 10 S 37 18 E
Kirishi, *Russia* **58 C7** 59 28N 31 59 E
Kirishima Yaku △, *Japan* **71 J5** 31 24N 130 50 E
Kirishima-Yama, *Japan* **72 F2** 31 58N 130 55 E
Kiritimati, *Kiribati* **135 G12** 1 58N 157 27W
Kiriwina I., *Papua N. G.* **132 E6** 8 40 S 151 6 E
Kırka, *Turkey* **49 B12** 39 17N 30 33 E
Kırkağaç, *Turkey* **49 B9** 39 8N 27 40 E
Kirkby, *U.K.* **20 D5** 53 30N 2 54W
Kirkby-in-Ashfield, *U.K.* **20 D6** 53 6N 1 14W
Kirkby Lonsdale, *U.K.* **20 C5** 54 12N 2 36W
Kirkby Stephen, *U.K.* **20 C5** 54 29N 2 21W
Kirkcaldy, *U.K.* **22 E5** 56 7N 3 9W
Kirkcudbright, *U.K.* **22 G4** 54 50N 4 2W
Kirkee, *India* **94 E1** 18 34N 73 56 E
Kirkehamn, *Norway* **18 F3** 58 14N 6 31 E
Kirkenær, *Norway* **18 D9** 60 27N 12 3 E
Kirkenes, *Norway* **14 B23** 69 40N 30 5 E
Kirkfield, *Canada* **150 B6** 44 34N 78 59W
Kirkintilloch, *U.K.* **22 F4** 55 56N 4 8W
Kirkjubæjarklaustur, *Iceland* **11 D8** 63 47N 18 4W
Kirkkonummi, *Finland* **15 F21** 60 8N 24 26 E
Kirkland, *U.S.A.* **157 B8** 42 6N 88 51W
Kirkland Lake, *Canada* **140 C3** 48 9N 80 2W
Kırklareli, *Turkey* **51 E11** 41 44N 27 15 E
Kırklareli □, *Turkey* **51 E11** 41 45N 27 15 E
Kirklin, *U.S.A.* **157 D10** 40 12N 86 22W
Kirkliston Ra., *N.Z.* **131 E5** 44 25 S 170 34 E
Kirknitz = Cerknica, *Slovenia* **45 C11** 45 48N 14 21 E
Kirksville, *U.S.A.* **156 D4** 40 12N 92 35W
Kirkūk, *Iraq* **101 E11** 35 30N 44 21 E
Kirkwall, *U.K.* **22 C6** 58 59N 2 58W
Kirkwood, *S. Africa* **116 E4** 33 22 S 25 15 E
Kirkwood, *U.S.A.* **156 F6** 38 35N 90 24W
Kirlampudi, *India* **94 F6** 17 12N 82 12 E
Kirmasti = Mustafakemalpaşa, *Turkey* **51 F12** 40 2N 28 24 E
Kirn, *Germany* **31 F3** 49 47N 7 26 E
Kirov, *Kaluga, Russia* **58 E8** 54 3N 34 20 E
Kirov, *Kirov, Russia* **64 B2** 58 35N 49 40 E
Kirovabad = Gäncä, *Azerbaijan* **61 K8** 40 45N 46 20 E
Kirovabad = Pyandzh, *Tajikistan* **65 E4** 37 14N 69 6 E
Kirovakan = Vanadzor, *Armenia* **61 K7** 40 48N 44 30 E
Kirovo = Kirovohrad, *Ukraine* **59 H7** 48 35N 32 20 E
Kirovo-Chepetsk, *Russia* **64 B3** 58 28N 50 0 E
Kirovograd = Kirovohrad, *Ukraine* **59 H7** 48 35N 32 20 E
Kirovohrad, *Ukraine* **59 H7** 48 35N 32 20 E
Kirovsk, *Russia* **56 A5** 67 32N 33 41 E
Kirovskiy = Balpyq Bī, *Kazakhstan* **65 A9** 44 52N 78 12 E
Kirovskiy, *Astrakhan, Russia* **61 H9** 45 51N 48 11 E
Kirovskiy, *Kamchatka, Russia* **67 D16** 54 27N 155 42 E
Kirovskiy, *Primorsk, Russia* **70 B6** 45 7N 133 30 E
Kirriemuir, *U.K.* **22 E5** 56 41N 3 1W
Kirs, *Russia* **64 B4** 59 21N 52 14 E
Kirsanov, *Russia* **60 D6** 52 35N 42 40 E
Kırşehir, *Turkey* **100 C6** 39 14N 34 5 E
Kirtachi, *Niger* **113 C5** 12 52N 2 30 E
Kīrteh, *Afghan.* **91 B1** 32 15N 63 0 E
Kirthar △, *Pakistan* **92 F2** 25 45N 67 30 E
Kirthar Range, *Pakistan* **91 D2** 27 0N 67 0 E
Kirtland, *U.S.A.* **159 H9** 36 44N 108 21W
Kiruna, *Sweden* **14 C19** 67 52N 20 15 E
Kirundu, *Dem. Rep. of the Congo* **118 C2** 0 50 S 25 35 E
Kirya, *Russia* **60 C8** 55 8N 46 55 E
Kiryū, *Japan* **73 A11** 36 24N 139 20 E
Kisa, *Sweden* **17 G9** 58 0N 15 39 E
Kisaga, *Tanzania* **118 C3** 4 30 S 34 23 E
Kisalaya, *Nic.* **164 D3** 14 40N 84 3W
Kisalföld, *Hungary* **52 C2** 47 30N 17 0 E
Kisambo, *Dem. Rep. of the Congo* **115 D3** 6 25 S 18 14 E
Kisámou, Kólpos, *Greece* **39 E4** 35 30N 23 38 E
Kisandji, *Dem. Rep. of the Congo* **115 D3** 6 18 S 19 16 E
Kisanga, *Dem. Rep. of the Congo* **118 B2** 2 30N 26 35 E
Kisangani, *Dem. Rep. of the Congo* **118 B2** 0 35N 25 15 E
Kisantu, *Dem. Rep. of the Congo* **115 D3** 5 7 S 15 5 E
Kisar, *Indonesia* **82 C3** 8 5 S 127 10 E
Kisaran, *Indonesia* **84 B1** 3 0N 99 37 E
Kisarawe, *Tanzania* **118 D4** 6 53 S 39 0 E
Kisarazu, *Japan* **73 B11** 35 23N 139 55 E
Kisbér, *Hungary* **52 C3** 47 30N 18 2 E
Kishanganga →, *Pakistan* **93 B5** 34 18N 73 28 E
Kishanganj, *India* **90 B2** 26 3N 88 14 E
Kishangarh, *Raj., India* **92 F6** 26 34N 74 52 E
Kishangarh, *Raj., India* **92 F4** 27 50N 70 30 E
Kishb, Ḩarrat al, *Si. Arabia* **98 B3** 22 30N 40 15 E
Kishi, *Nigeria* **113 D5** 9 1N 3 52 E
Kishinev = Chişinău, *Moldova* **53 C13** 47 2N 28 50 E
Kishiwada, *Japan* **73 C7** 34 28N 135 22 E
Kishkareny = Lazo, *Moldova* **53 C13** 47 33N 28 2 E
Kishorganj, *Bangla.* **90 C3** 24 26N 90 40 E
Kishtwar, *India* **92 C6** 33 20N 75 50 E
Kishtwar, *Jammu & Kashmir, India* **93 C6** 33 20N 75 48 E
Kishwaukee →, *U.S.A.* **156 B7** 42 12N 89 8W
Kisielice, *Poland* **54 E6** 53 36N 19 16 E
Kisigo ⌓, *Tanzania* **118 D3** 6 27 S 34 17 E
Kisii, *Kenya* **118 C3** 0 40 S 34 45 E
Kisiju, *Tanzania* **118 D4** 7 23 S 39 19 E
Kisir, *Turkey* **101 B10** 41 0N 43 5 E
Kisizi, *Uganda* **118 C2** 1 0 S 29 58 E
Kiska I., *U.S.A.* **144 L2** 51 59N 177 30 E
Kiskomárom = Zalakomár, *Hungary* **52 D2** 46 33N 17 10 E
Kiskörei-víztároló, *Hungary* **52 C5** 47 31N 20 36 E
Kiskőrös, *Hungary* **52 D4** 46 37N 19 20 E
Kiskundorozsma, *Hungary* **52 D5** 46 16N 20 5 E
Kiskunfélegyháza, *Hungary* **52 D4** 46 42N 19 53 E
Kiskunhalas, *Hungary* **52 D4** 46 28N 19 37 E
Kiskunmajsa, *Hungary* **52 D4** 46 30N 19 48 E
Kiskunsági △, *Hungary* **52 D4** 46 39N 19 30 E
Kislovodsk, *Russia* **61 J6** 43 50N 42 45 E
Kismayu = Chisimaio, *Somali Rep.* **120 E2** 0 22 S 42 32 E
Kismayu △, *Somali Rep.* **120 D2** 1 25N 41 30 E
Kiso-Gawa →, *Japan* **73 B8** 35 20N 136 45 E
Kiso-Sammyaku, *Japan* **73 B9** 35 45N 137 45 E
Kisofukushima, *Japan* **73 B9** 35 52N 137 43 E
Kisoro, *Uganda* **118 C2** 1 17 S 29 48 E
Kissidougou, *Guinea* **112 D2** 9 5N 10 5W
Kissimmee, *U.S.A.* **153 G8** 28 18N 81 24W
Kissimmee →, *U.S.A.* **153 H8** 27 9N 80 52W
Kissimmee, L., *U.S.A.* **153 H8** 27 55N 81 17W
Kississing L., *Canada* **143 B8** 55 10N 101 20W
Kissónerga, *Cyprus* **39 F8** 34 49N 32 24 E
Kissu, J., *Sudan* **106 C2** 21 37N 25 10 E
Kistanje, *Croatia* **45 E12** 43 58N 15 55 E
Kistna = Krishna →, *India* **95 G5** 15 57N 80 59 E
Kisújszállás, *Hungary* **52 C5** 47 12N 20 50 E
Kisuki, *Japan* **72 B4** 35 17N 132 54 E
Kisumu, *Kenya* **118 C3** 0 3 S 34 45 E
Kisvárda, *Hungary* **52 B7** 48 14N 22 4 E
Kiswani, *Tanzania* **118 C4** 4 5 S 37 57 E
Kiswere, *Tanzania* **119 D4** 9 27 S 39 30 E
Kit Carson, *U.S.A.* **154 F3** 38 46N 102 48W
Kita, *Mali* **112 C3** 13 5N 9 25W
Kita-Ura, *Japan* **73 B12** 36 0N 140 34 E
Kitaa □, *Greenland* **10 C6** 70 0N 47 0W
Kitab, *Uzbekistan* **65 D3** 39 7N 66 52 E
Kitaibaraki, *Japan* **71 F10** 36 50N 140 45 E
Kitakami, *Japan* **70 E10** 39 20N 141 10 E
Kitakami-Gawa →, *Japan* **70 E10** 38 25N 141 19 E
Kitakami-Sammyaku, *Japan* **70 E10** 39 30N 141 30 E
Kitakata, *Japan* **70 F9** 37 39N 139 52 E
Kitakyūshū, *Japan* **72 D2** 33 50N 130 50 E
Kitale, *Kenya* **118 B4** 1 0N 35 0 E
Kitami, *Japan* **70 C11** 43 48N 143 54 E
Kitami-Sammyaku, *Japan* **70 B11** 44 22N 142 43 E
Kitangiri, L., *Tanzania* **118 C3** 4 5 S 34 20 E
Kitano-Kaikyō, *Japan* **72 C6** 34 17N 134 58 E
Kitaotao, *Phil.* **81 H5** 7 40N 125 1 E
Kitava I., *Papua N. G.* **132 E6** 8 40 S 151 20 E
Kitaya, *Tanzania* **119 E5** 10 38 S 40 8 E
Kitcharao, *Phil.* **81 G5** 9 27N 125 36 E
Kitchener, *Canada* **140 D3** 43 27N 80 29W
Kitee, *Finland* **58 A6** 62 5N 30 8 E
Kitega = Gitega, *Burundi* **118 C2** 3 26 S 29 56 E
Kitengo, *Dem. Rep. of the Congo* **118 D1** 7 26 S 24 8 E
Kitgum, *Uganda* **118 B3** 3 17N 32 52 E
Kíthira, *Greece* **48 E5** 36 8N 23 0 E
Kíthnos, *Greece* **48 D6** 37 26N 24 27 E
Kiti, *Cyprus* **39 F9** 34 50N 33 34 E
Kiti, C., *Cyprus* **39 F9** 34 48N 33 36 E
Kitimat, *Canada* **142 C3** 54 3N 128 38W
Kitinen →, *Finland* **14 C22** 67 14N 27 27 E
Kitiyab, *Sudan* **107 D3** 17 13N 33 35 E
Kitombe, *Dem. Rep. of the Congo* **115 D3** 5 22 S 18 59 E
Kítros, *Greece* **50 F6** 40 22N 22 34 E
Kitsman, *Ukraine* **53 B10** 48 26N 25 46 E
Kitsuki, *Japan* **72 D3** 33 25N 131 37 E
Kittakittaooloo, L., *Australia* **127 D2** 28 3 S 138 14 E
Kittanning, *U.S.A.* **150 F5** 40 49N 79 31W
Kittatinny Mts., *U.S.A.* **151 F10** 41 0N 75 0W
Kittery, *U.S.A.* **149 D10** 43 5N 70 45W
Kittilä, *Finland* **14 C21** 67 40N 24 51 E
Kitui, *Kenya* **118 C4** 1 17 S 38 0 E
Kitwanga, *Canada* **142 B3** 55 6N 128 4W
Kitwe, *Zambia* **119 E2** 12 54 S 28 13 E
Kityang = Jieyang, *China* **77 F11** 23 35N 116 21 E
Kitzbühel, *Austria* **34 D5** 47 27N 12 24 E
Kitzbühler Alpen, *Austria* **34 D5** 47 20N 12 20 E
Kitzingen, *Germany* **31 F6** 49 44N 10 9 E
Kiukiang = Jiujiang, *China* **77 C10** 29 42N 115 58 E
Kiunga, *Papua N. G.* **132 D1** 6 7 S 141 18 E
Kivalina, *U.S.A.* **144 C6** 67 44N 164 33W
Kivarli, *India* **92 G5** 24 33N 72 46 E
Kivertsi, *Ukraine* **59 G3** 50 50N 25 28 E
Kividhes, *Cyprus* **39 F8** 34 46N 32 51 E
Kivik, *Sweden* **17 J8** 55 41N 14 13 E
Kivotós, *Greece* **50 F5** 40 13N 21 26 E
Kivu, L., *Dem. Rep. of the Congo* **118 C2** 1 48 S 29 0 E
Kiwai I., *Papua N. G.* **132 E2** 8 35 S 143 30 E
Kiyev = Kyyiv, *Ukraine* **59 G6** 50 30N 30 28 E
Kiyevskoye Vdkhr. = Kyyivske Vdskh., *Ukraine* **59 G6** 51 0N 30 25 E
Kıyıköy, *Turkey* **51 E12** 41 38N 28 5 E
Kizel, *Russia* **64 B6** 59 3N 57 40 E
Kiziguru, *Rwanda* **118 C3** 1 46 S 30 23 E
Kızıl Adalar, *Turkey* **51 F13** 40 52N 29 5 E
Kızıl Irmak →, *Turkey* **100 B6** 41 44N 35 58 E
Kizil Jilga, *China* **93 B8** 35 26N 78 50 E
Kizil Yurt, *Russia* **61 J8** 43 13N 46 54 E
Kızılcabölük, *Turkey* **49 D11** 37 37N 29 1 E
Kızılcadağ, *Turkey* **49 D11** 37 1N 29 58 E
Kızılcahamam, *Turkey* **100 B5** 40 30N 32 30 E
Kızılhisar, *Turkey* **100 D3** 37 32N 29 17 E
Kızılırmak, *Turkey* **100 B5** 40 21N 33 59 E
Kızılkaya, *Turkey* **49 D12** 37 18N 30 27 E
Kızılören, *Turkey* **49 C12** 38 15N 30 10 E
Kizilskoye, *Russia* **64 E7** 52 44N 58 54 E
Kızıltepe, *Turkey* **101 D9** 37 12N 40 35 E
Kizimkazi, *Tanzania* **118 D4** 6 28 S 39 30 E
Kizlyar, *Russia* **61 J8** 43 51N 46 40 E
Kizyl-Arvat = Gyzylarbat, *Turkmenistan* **66 F6** 39 4N 56 23 E

Kjellerup, *Denmark* **17 H3** 56 17N 9 25 E
Kjellmyra, *Norway* **18 D9** 60 39N 12 1 E
Kjølen, *Norway* **18 C5** 62 3N 8 45 E
Kjölur, *Iceland* **11 C7** 64 50N 19 25W
Kjósarsýsla □, *Iceland* **11 C5** 64 15N 21 30W
Kladanj, *Bos.-H.* **52 F3** 44 14N 18 42 E
Kladnica, *Serbia & M.* **50 C4** 43 23N 20 2 E
Kladno, *Czech Rep.* **34 A7** 50 10N 14 7 E
Kladovo, *Serbia & M.* **50 B6** 44 36N 22 33 E
Klæbu, *Norway* **18 A7** 63 18N 10 29 E
Klaeng, *Thailand* **86 F3** 12 47N 101 39 E
Klagan, *Malaysia* **85 A5** 5 58N 117 27 E
Klagenfurt, *Austria* **34 E7** 46 38N 14 20 E
Klaipėda, *Lithuania* **15 J19** 55 43N 21 10 E
Klaipėda □, *Lithuania* **54 C8** 55 43N 21 7 E
Klaksvík, *Færoe Is.* **14 E9** 62 14N 6 35W
Klamath →, *U.S.A.* **158 F1** 41 33N 124 5W
Klamath Falls, *U.S.A.* **158 E3** 42 13N 121 46W
Klamath Mts., *U.S.A.* **158 F2** 41 20N 123 0W
Klamono, *Indonesia* **83 B4** 1 8 S 131 30 E
Klang, *Malaysia* **87 L3** 3 2N 101 26 E
Klangklang, *Burma* **90 D4** 22 41N 93 26 E
Klanjec, *Croatia* **45 B12** 46 3N 15 45 E
Klappan →, *Canada* **142 B3** 58 0N 129 43W
Klara = Trysilelva →, *Norway* **18 C9** 61 2N 12 35 E
Klarälven →, *Sweden* **16 E7** 59 23N 13 32 E
Klässbol, *Sweden* **16 E6** 59 33N 12 45 E
Klaten, *Indonesia* **85 D4** 7 43 S 110 36 E
Klatovy, *Czech Rep.* **34 B6** 49 23N 13 18 E
Klausenburg = Cluj-Napoca, *Romania* **53 D8** 46 47N 23 38 E
Klawer, *S. Africa* **116 E2** 31 44 S 18 36 E
Klawock, *U.S.A.* **144 J14** 55 33N 133 6W
Klazienaveen, *Neths.* **24 B6** 52 44N 7 0 E
Klé, *Mali* **112 C3** 12 0N 6 28W
Kłecko, *Poland* **55 F4** 52 38N 17 25 E
Kleczew, *Poland* **55 F5** 52 22N 18 9 E
Kleena Kleene, *Canada* **142 C4** 52 0N 124 59W
Klein-Karas, *Namibia* **116 D2** 27 33 S 18 7 E
Klein-Schlatten = Zlatna, *Romania* **53 D8** 46 8N 23 11 E
Klekovača, *Bos.-H.* **45 D13** 44 25N 16 32 E
Klembivka, *Ukraine* **53 B13** 48 23N 28 25 E
Klenoec, *Macedonia* **50 E4** 41 32N 20 49 E
Klenovec, *Slovak Rep.* **35 C12** 48 36N 19 54 E
Klerksdorp, *S. Africa* **116 D4** 26 53 S 26 38 E
Kleszczele, *Poland* **55 F10** 52 35N 23 19 E
Kletnya, *Russia* **58 F7** 53 23N 33 12 E
Kletsk = Klyetsk, *Belarus* **59 F4** 53 5N 26 45 E
Kletskiy, *Russia* **61 F6** 49 16N 43 11 E
Kleve, *Germany* **30 D2** 51 47N 6 7 E
Klickitat, *U.S.A.* **158 D3** 45 49N 121 9W
Klickitat →, *U.S.A.* **160 E5** 45 42N 121 17W
Klidhes, *Cyprus* **39 E10** 35 42N 34 36 E
Klimovichi, *Belarus* **58 F6** 53 36N 32 0 E
Klin, *Russia* **58 D9** 56 20N 36 48 E
Klina, *Serbia & M.* **50 D4** 42 37N 20 35 E
Klinaklini →, *Canada* **142 C3** 51 21N 125 40W
Klintehamn, *Sweden* **17 G12** 57 24N 18 12 E
Klintsy, *Russia* **59 F7** 52 50N 32 10 E
Klip →, *S. Africa* **117 D4** 27 3 S 29 3 E
Klipdale, *S. Africa* **116 E2** 34 19 S 19 57 E
Klippan, *Sweden* **17 H7** 56 8N 13 10 E
Klipplaat, *S. Africa* **116 E3** 33 1 S 24 22 E
Klishkivtsi, *Ukraine* **53 B11** 48 26N 26 16 E
Klisura, *Bulgaria* **51 D8** 42 40N 24 28 E
Kljajićevo, *Serbia & M.* **52 E4** 45 45N 19 17 E
Ključ, *Bos.-H.* **45 D13** 44 32N 16 48 E
Kłobuck, *Poland* **55 H5** 50 55N 18 55 E
Klockestrand, *Sweden* **16 B11** 62 53N 17 55 E
Kłodawa, *Poland* **55 F5** 52 15N 18 55 E
Kłodzko, *Poland* **55 H3** 50 28N 16 38 E
Kløfta, *Norway* **18 D8** 60 4N 11 10 E
Klondike Goldrush △, *U.S.A.* **144 E14** 59 27N 135 19W
Klong Wang Chao △, *Thailand* **86 D2** 16 20N 99 9 E
Klos, *Albania* **50 E4** 41 28N 20 10 E
Klosterneuburg, *Austria* **35 C9** 48 18N 16 19 E
Klosters, *Switz.* **33 C9** 46 52N 9 52 E
Kloten, *Switz.* **33 B7** 47 27N 8 35 E
Klötze, *Germany* **30 C7** 52 37N 11 10 E
Klouto, *Togo* **113 D5** 6 57N 0 44 E
Kluane △, *Canada* **142 A1** 60 45N 139 30W
Kluane L., *Canada* **138 B6** 61 15N 138 40W
Kluang, *Malaysia* **87 L4** 2 3N 103 18 E
Kluczbork, *Poland* **55 H5** 50 58N 18 12 E
Klukhori = Karachayevsk, *Russia* **61 J5** 43 50N 41 55 E
Klukwan, *U.S.A.* **142 B1** 59 24N 135 54W
Klungkung, *Indonesia* **79 K18** 8 32 S 115 24 E
Klyetsk, *Belarus* **59 F4** 53 5N 26 45 E
Klyuchevskaya, Gora, *Russia* **67 D17** 55 50N 160 30 E
Knaben, *Norway* **18 F4** 58 40N 7 4 E
Knappavellir, *Iceland* **11 D10** 63 54N 16 36W
Knäred, *Sweden* **17 H7** 56 31N 13 19 E
Knaresborough, *U.K.* **20 C6** 54 1N 1 28W
Knarvik, *Norway* **18 D2** 60 32N 5 19 E
Knee L., *Man., Canada* **140 A1** 55 3N 94 45W
Knee L., *Sask., Canada* **143 B7** 55 51N 107 0W
Kneïss, Is., *Tunisia* **108 B2** 34 22N 10 18 E
Knezha, *Bulgaria* **51 C8** 43 30N 24 5 E
Knight I., *U.S.A.* **144 F11** 60 21N 147 45W
Knight Inlet, *Canada* **142 C3** 50 45N 125 40W
Knighton, *U.K.* **21 E4** 52 21N 3 3W
Knights Ferry, *U.S.A.* **160 H6** 37 50N 120 40W
Knights Landing, *U.S.A.* **160 G5** 38 48N 121 43W
Knightstown, *U.S.A.* **157 E11** 39 48N 85 32W
Knin, *Croatia* **45 D13** 44 3N 16 17 E
Knislinge, *Sweden* **17 H8** 56 12N 14 5 E
Knittelfeld, *Austria* **34 D7** 47 13N 14 51 E
Knivsta, *Sweden* **16 E11** 59 43N 17 48 E
Knjaževac, *Serbia & M.* **50 C6** 43 35N 22 18 E
Knob, C., *Australia* **125 F2** 34 32 S 119 16 E
Knob Lake = Schefferville, *Canada* **141 B6** 54 48N 66 50W
Knob Noster, *U.S.A.* **156 F3** 38 46N 93 33W
Knock, *Ireland* **23 C3** 53 48N 8 55W
Knockmealdown Mts., *Ireland* **23 D4** 52 14N 7 56W
Knokke-Heist, *Belgium* **24 C3** 51 21N 3 17 E
Knossós, *Greece* **39 E6** 35 16N 25 10 E
Knowlton, *Canada* **151 A12** 45 13N 72 31W
Knox, *U.S.A.* **157 C10** 41 18N 86 37W
Knox Coast, *Antarctica* **7 C8** 66 30 S 108 0 E
Knoxville, *Ga., U.S.A.* **152 C6** 32 47N 83 59W
Knoxville, *Ill., U.S.A.* **156 D6** 40 55N 90 17W
Knoxville, *Iowa, U.S.A.* **156 C4** 41 19N 93 6W
Knoxville, *Pa., U.S.A.* **150 E7** 41 57N 77 27W
Knoxville, *Tenn., U.S.A.* **149 H4** 35 58N 83 55W
Knud Rasmussen Land, *Greenland* **10 B4** 79 0N 60 0W
Knysna, *S. Africa* **116 E3** 34 2 S 23 2 E
Knyszyn, *Poland* **54 E9** 53 20N 22 56 E
Ko Kha, *Thailand* **86 C2** 18 11N 99 24 E
Kō-Saki, *Japan* **72 C1** 34 5N 129 13 E
Ko Tarutao △, *Thailand* **87 J2** 6 31N 99 26 E
Ko Yao, *Thailand* **87 a** 8 7N 98 35 E
Koartac = Quaqtaq, *Canada* **139 B13** 60 55N 69 40W
Koba, *Aru, Indonesia* **83 C4** 6 37 S 134 37 E
Koba, *Bangka, Indonesia* **84 C3** 2 26 S 106 14 E
Kobarid, *Slovenia* **45 B10** 46 15N 13 30 E
Kobayashi, *Japan* **72 F2** 31 56N 130 59 E
Kobdo = Hovd, *Mongolia* **68 B4** 48 2N 91 37 E
Kobe, *Indonesia* **82 A3** 0 26N 127 54 E
Kōbe, *Japan* **73 C7** 34 45N 135 10 E
Kobelyaky, *Ukraine* **59 H8** 49 11N 34 9 E
København, *Denmark* **17 J6** 55 41N 12 34 E
København ✖ (CPH), *Denmark* **17 J6** 55 37N 12 39 E
Københavns Amtskommune □, *Denmark* **17 J6** 55 42N 12 21 E
Kobenni, *Mauritania* **112 B3** 15 58N 9 24W
Kōbi-Sho, *Japan* **71 M1** 25 56N 123 41 E
Koblenz, *Germany* **31 E3** 50 21N 7 36 E
Koblenz, *Switz.* **32 A6** 47 37N 8 14 E
Kobo, *Dem. Rep. of the Congo* **115 C3** 4 54 S 17 9 E
Kobo, *Ethiopia* **107 E4** 12 2N 39 56 E
Kobroor, *Indonesia* **83 C4** 6 10 S 134 30 E
Kobryn, *Belarus* **59 F3** 52 15N 24 22 E
Kobuchizawa, *Japan* **73 B10** 35 52N 138 19 E
Kobuk, *U.S.A.* **144 C8** 66 55N 156 52W
Kobuk →, *U.S.A.* **144 C7** 66 54N 160 38W
Kobuk Valley △, *U.S.A.* **144 C8** 67 0N 160 0W
Kobuleti, *Georgia* **61 K5** 41 55N 41 45 E
Kobyletska Polyana, *Ukraine* **53 B9** 48 3N 24 4 E
Kobylin, *Poland* **55 G4** 51 43N 17 12 E
Kobyłka, *Poland* **55 F8** 52 21N 21 10 E
Kobylkino, *Russia* **60 C6** 54 8N 43 56 E
Koca →, *Turkey* **51 F11** 40 8N 27 57 E
Kocabaş, *Turkey* **49 D11** 37 49N 29 20 E
Kocaeli, *Turkey* **51 F13** 40 45N 29 50 E
Kocaeli □, *Turkey* **51 F13** 40 45N 29 55 E
Kočane, *Serbia & M.* **50 C5** 43 12N 21 52 E
Kočani, *Macedonia* **50 E6** 41 55N 22 25 E
Koçarlı, *Turkey* **49 D9** 37 45N 27 43 E
Koceljevo, *Serbia & M.* **50 B3** 44 28N 19 50 E
Kočevje, *Slovenia* **45 C11** 45 39N 14 50 E
Kocgiri = Zara, *Turkey* **100 C7** 39 58N 37 43 E
Koch Bihar, *India* **90 B2** 26 22N 89 29 E
Kochang, *S. Korea* **75 G14** 35 41N 127 55 E
Kochas, *India* **93 G10** 25 15N 83 56 E
Kocher →, *Germany* **31 F5** 49 13N 9 12 E
Kochi = Cochin, *India* **95 K3** 9 58N 76 20 E
Kōchi, *Japan* **72 D5** 33 30N 133 35 E
Kōchi □, *Japan* **72 D5** 33 40N 133 30 E
Kochiu = Gejiu, *China* **76 F4** 23 20N 103 10 E
Kochkor, *Kyrgyzstan* **65 B7** 42 13N 75 46 E
Kochkor-Ata, *Kyrgyzstan* **65 C6** 41 1N 72 29 E
Kock, *Poland* **55 G9** 51 38N 22 27 E
Kodaira, *Japan* **73 B11** 35 44N 139 29 E
Kodala, *India* **94 E7** 19 38N 84 57 E
Kodarma, *India* **93 G11** 24 28N 85 36 E
Koddiyar B., *Sri Lanka* **95 K5** 8 33N 81 15 E
Kode, *Sweden* **17 G5** 57 57N 11 51 E
Kodi, *Dem. Rep. of the Congo* **114 C4** 3 34 S 22 12 E
Kodi, *Indonesia* **82 C1** 9 33 S 119 0 E
Kodiak, *U.S.A.* **144 H9** 57 47N 152 24W
Kodiak I., *U.S.A.* **144 H9** 57 30N 152 45W
Kodinar, *India* **92 J4** 20 46N 70 46 E
Kodlipet, *India* **95 H2** 12 48N 75 53 E
Kodok = Fashoda, *Sudan* **107 F3** 9 50N 32 2 E
Kodok, *Sudan* **107 F3** 9 53N 32 7 E
Kodori →, *Georgia* **61 J5** 42 47N 41 10 E
Kodoro, *Dem. Rep. of the Congo* **114 B4** 1 16N 20 6 E
Kodyma, *Ukraine* **53 B14** 48 6N 29 7 E
Koedoesberge, *S. Africa* **116 E3** 32 40 S 20 11 E
Koes, *Namibia* **116 D2** 26 0 S 19 15 E
Kofarnikhon, *Tajikistan* **65 D4** 38 34N 69 1 E
Kofçaz, *Turkey* **51 E11** 41 58N 27 12 E
Koffiefontein, *S. Africa* **116 D4** 29 30 S 25 0 E
Kofiau, *Indonesia* **83 B3** 1 11 S 129 50 E
Köflach, *Austria* **34 D8** 47 4N 15 5 E
Koforidua, *Ghana* **113 D4** 6 3N 0 17W
Kōfu, *Japan* **73 B10** 35 40N 138 30 E
Koga, *Japan* **73 A11** 36 11N 139 43 E
Kogaluc →, *Canada* **141 A7** 56 12N 61 44W
Kogart, *Kyrgyzstan* **65 C7** 40 15N 74 25 E
Køge, *Denmark* **17 J6** 55 27N 12 11 E
Køge Bugt, *Denmark* **17 J6** 55 30N 12 20 E
Kogi □, *Nigeria* **113 D6** 7 45N 6 45 E
Kogin Baba, *Nigeria* **113 D7** 7 55N 11 35 E
Kogo, *Eq. Guin.* **114 B1** 1 5N 9 42 E
Koh-i-Khurd, *Afghan.* **91 B2** 33 30N 65 59 E
Koh-i-Maran, *Pakistan* **92 E2** 29 18N 66 50 E
Kohala Mts., *U.S.A.* **145 C6** 20 5N 155 45W
Kohat, *Pakistan* **92 C4** 33 40N 71 29 E
Kohima, *India* **90 C5** 25 35N 94 10 E
Kohkīlūyeh va Būyer Aḥmadi □, *Iran* **97 D6** 31 30N 50 30 E
Kohler Ra., *Antarctica* **7 D15** 77 0 S 110 0W
Kohlfurt = Węgliniec, *Poland* **55 G2** 51 18N 15 10 E
Kohlu, *Pakistan* **92 E3** 29 54N 69 15 E
Kohtla-Järve, *Estonia* **15 G22** 59 20N 27 20 E
Kohukohu, *N.Z.* **130 B2** 35 22 S 173 38 E
Kohylnyk →, *Ukraine* **53 E14** 45 49N 29 40 E
Koi Sanjaq, *Iraq* **101 D11** 36 5N 44 38 E
Koihoa, *India* **95 K11** 8 12N 93 29 E
Koilkuntla, *India* **95 G4** 15 14N 78 19 E
Koillismaa, *Finland* **14 D23** 65 44N 28 36 E
Koin-dong, *N. Korea* **75 D14** 40 28N 126 18 E
Koinare, *Bulgaria* **51 C8** 43 21N 24 8 E
Koindu, *S. Leone* **112 D2** 8 26N 10 19W
Koivisto = Primorsk, *Russia* **58 B5** 60 22N 28 37 E
Kojetín, *Czech Rep.* **35 B10** 49 21N 17 20 E
Kojŏ, *N. Korea* **75 E14** 38 58N 127 58 E
Kojonup, *Australia* **125 F2** 33 48 S 117 10 E
Kojūr, *Iran* **97 B6** 36 23N 51 43 E
Kök-Aygyr, *Kyrgyzstan* **65 C7** 40 42N 75 32 E
Kök-Janggak, *Kyrgyzstan* **65 C6** 41 2N 73 12 E
Koka, *Sudan* **106 C3** 20 5N 30 35 E
Kokand = Qŭqon, *Uzbekistan* **65 C5** 40 30N 70 57 E
Kokankishlak = Pakhtaabad, *Uzbekistan* **65 C6** 40 55N 72 29 E
Kokas, *Indonesia* **83 B4** 2 42 S 132 26 E
Kokava, *Slovak Rep.* **35 C12** 48 35N 19 50 E
Kokcha →, *Afghan.* **91 A3** 37 9N 69 24 E
Kokchetav = Kökshetaū, *Kazakhstan* **66 D7** 53 20N 69 25 E
Kokemäenjoki →, *Finland* **15 F19** 61 32N 21 44 E
Kokerite, *Guyana* **169 B6** 7 12N 59 35W
Kokhma, *Russia* **60 B5** 56 57N 41 8 E
Koki, *Senegal* **112 B1** 15 30N 15 59W
Kokiu = Gejiu, *China* **76 F4** 23 20N 103 10 E
Kokkilai, *Sri Lanka* **95 K5** 9 0N 80 57 E
Kokkina, *Cyprus* **39 E8** 35 11N 32 36 E
Kokkola, *Finland* **14 E20** 63 50N 23 8 E
Koko, *Nigeria* **113 C5** 11 28N 4 29 E
Koko Head, *U.S.A.* **145 K14** 21 16N 157 43W
Kokoda, *Papua N. G.* **132 E4** 8 54 S 147 47 E
Kokolopozo, *Ivory C.* **112 D3** 5 8N 6 5W
Kokomo, *U.S.A.* **157 D10** 40 29N 86 8W
Kokonau, *Indonesia* **83 B5** 4 43 S 136 26 E
Kokopo, *Papua N. G.* **132 C7** 4 22 S 152 19 E
Kokoro, *Niger* **113 C5** 14 12N 0 55 E
Koksan, *N. Korea* **75 E14** 38 46N 126 40 E
Köksaray, *Kazakhstan* **65 B4** 42 38N 68 9 E
Kökshetaū, *Kazakhstan* **66 D7** 53 20N 69 25 E
Koksoak →, *Canada* **139 C13** 58 30N 68 10W
Kokstad, *S. Africa* **117 E4** 30 32 S 29 29 E
Köksü, *Kazakhstan* **65 C4** 41 28N 68 1 E
Köktal, *Kazakhstan* **65 B5** 43 16N 70 18 E
Koktash = Leninskiy, *Tajikistan* **65 D4** 38 26N 68 46 E
Kokubu, *Japan* **72 F2** 31 44N 130 46 E
Kokyar, *China* **65 E8** 37 23N 77 10 E
Kola, *Indonesia* **83 C4** 5 35 S 134 30 E
Kola, *Russia* **56 A5** 68 45N 33 8 E
Kola Pen. = Kolskiy Poluostrov, *Russia* **56 A6** 67 30N 38 0 E
Kolachel, *India* **95 K3** 8 10N 77 15 E
Kolachi →, *Pakistan* **92 F2** 27 8N 67 2 E
Kolahoi, *India* **93 B6** 34 12N 75 22 E
Kolahun, *Liberia* **112 D2** 8 15N 10 4W
Kolaka, *Indonesia* **82 B2** 4 3 S 121 46 E
Kolar, *India* **95 H4** 13 12N 78 15 E
Kolar Gold Fields, *India* **95 H4** 12 58N 78 16 E
Kolaras, *India* **92 G6** 25 14N 77 36 E
Kolari, *Finland* **14 C20** 67 20N 23 48 E
Kolarovgrad = Shumen, *Bulgaria* **51 C10** 43 18N 26 55 E
Kolárovo, *Slovak Rep.* **35 D10** 47 54N 18 0 E
Kolašin, *Serbia & M.* **50 D3** 42 50N 19 31 E
Kolbäck, *Sweden* **16 E10** 59 34N 16 15 E
Kolbäcksån →, *Sweden* **16 E10** 59 36N 16 16 E
Kolbeinsstaðir, *Iceland* **11 C4** 64 59N 22 16W
Kolberg = Kołobrzeg, *Poland* **54 D2** 54 10N 15 35 E
Kolbermoor, *Germany* **31 H8** 47 51N 12 4 E
Kolbu, *Norway* **18 D7** 60 39N 10 45 E
Kolbuszowa, *Poland* **55 H8** 50 15N 21 46 E
Kolchugino = Leninsk-Kuznetskiy, *Russia* **66 D9** 54 44N 86 10 E
Kolchugino, *Russia* **58 D10** 56 17N 39 22 E
Kolda, *Senegal* **112 C2** 12 55N 14 57W
Koldegi, *Sudan* **107 E3** 12 3N 30 16 E
Kolding, *Denmark* **17 J3** 55 30N 9 29 E
Kole, *Dem. Rep. of the Congo* **114 C4** 3 16 S 22 42 E
Koléa, *Algeria* **111 A5** 36 38N 2 46 E
Kolepom = Dolak, Pulau, *Indonesia* **83 C5** 8 0 S 138 30 E
Kolguyev, Ostrov, *Russia* **56 A8** 69 20N 48 30 E
Kolhapur, *India* **94 F2** 16 43N 74 15 E
Kolia, *Ivory C.* **112 D3** 9 46N 6 28W
Koliganek, *U.S.A.* **144 G8** 59 48N 157 25W
Kolín, *Czech Rep.* **34 A8** 50 2N 15 9 E
Kolind, *Denmark* **17 H4** 56 21N 10 34 E
Kolkas rags, *Latvia* **15 H20** 57 46N 22 37 E
Kolkata, *India* **93 H13** 22 36N 88 24 E
Kolkhozobod, *Tajikistan* **65 E4** 37 35N 68 40 E
Kollam = Quilon, *India* **95 K3** 8 50N 76 38 E
Kölleda, *Germany* **30 D7** 51 11N 11 15 E
Kollegal, *India* **95 H3** 12 9N 77 9 E
Kolleru L., *India* **94 F5** 16 40N 81 10 E
Kollum, *Neths.* **24 A6** 53 17N 6 10 E
Kolmanskop, *Namibia* **116 D2** 26 45 S 15 14 E
Köln, *Germany* **30 E2** 50 56N 6 57 E
Kolno, *Poland* **54 E8** 53 25N 21 56 E
Koło, *Poland* **55 F5** 52 14N 18 40 E
Koloa, *U.S.A.* **145 B2** 21 55N 159 28W
Kołobrzeg, *Poland* **54 D2** 54 10N 15 35 E
Kolochava, *Ukraine* **53 B8** 48 26N 23 41 E
Kolokani, *Mali* **112 C3** 13 35N 7 45W
Koloko, *Burkina Faso* **112 C3** 11 5N 5 19W
Kololo, *Ethiopia* **107 F5** 7 29N 41 58 E
Kolombangara, *Solomon Is.* **133 M9** 8 0 S 157 5 E
Kolomna, *Russia* **58 E10** 55 8N 38 45 E
Kolomyya, *Ukraine* **53 B10** 48 31N 25 2 E
Kolondiéba, *Mali* **112 C3** 11 5N 6 54W
Kolonodale, *Indonesia* **82 B2** 2 0 S 121 19 E
Kolonowskie, *Poland* **55 H5** 50 39N 18 22 E
Kolosib, *India* **90 C4** 24 15N 92 45 E
Kolpashevo, *Russia* **66 D9** 58 20N 83 5 E
Kolpino, *Russia* **58 C6** 59 44N 30 39 E
Kolpny, *Russia* **59 F9** 52 17N 37 1 E
Kolskiy Poluostrov, *Russia* **56 A6** 67 30N 38 0 E
Kolskiy Zaliv, *Russia* **56 A5** 69 23N 34 0 E
Kolsva, *Sweden* **16 E9** 59 36N 15 51 E
Kolubara →, *Serbia & M.* **50 B4** 44 35N 20 15 E
Koluszki, *Poland* **55 G6** 51 45N 19 46 E
Kolwezi, *Dem. Rep. of the Congo* **119 E2** 10 40 S 25 25 E
Kolyma →, *Russia* **67 C17** 69 30N 161 0 E
Kolymskoye Nagorye, *Russia* **67 C16** 63 0N 157 0 E
Kôm Hamâda, *Egypt* **106 H7** 30 46N 30 41 E
Kôm Ombo, *Egypt* **106 C3** 24 25N 32 52 E
Komadugu Gana →, *Nigeria* **113 C7** 13 5N 12 24 E
Komagane, *Japan* **73 B9** 35 44N 137 58 E
Komaki, *Japan* **73 B8** 35 17N 136 55 E
Komandorskiye Is. = Komandorskiye Ostrova, *Russia* **67 D17** 55 0N 167 0 E
Komandorskiye Ostrova, *Russia* **67 D17** 55 0N 167 0 E
Komárno, *Slovak Rep.* **35 D11** 47 49N 18 5 E
Komarnyky, *Ukraine* **52 B8** 48 59N 23 3 E
Komárom, *Hungary* **52 C3** 47 43N 18 7 E
Komárom-Esztergom □, *Hungary* **52 C3** 47 35N 18 20 E
Komárommújváros = Komárom, *Hungary* **52 C3** 47 43N 18 7 E
Komatipoort, *S. Africa* **117 D5** 25 25 S 31 55 E
Komatou Yialou, *Cyprus* **39 E10** 35 25N 34 8 E
Komatsu, *Japan* **73 A8** 36 25N 136 30 E
Komatsushima, *Japan* **72 D6** 34 0N 134 35 E
Komavangard = Sobinka, *Russia* **58 E11** 56 0N 40 0 E
Komba, *Dem. Rep. of the Congo* **114 B4** 2 52N 24 3 E
Kombissiri, *Burkina Faso* **113 C4** 12 4N 1 20W
Kombo, *Gabon* **114 C2** 0 20 S 12 22 E
Kombong, *India* **90 A5** 28 7N 94 51 E
Kombori, *Burkina Faso* **112 C4** 13 26N 3 56W
Kombóti, *Greece* **48 B3** 39 6N 21 5 E
Komen, *Slovenia* **45 C10** 45 49N 13 45 E
Komenda, *Ghana* **113 D4** 5 4N 1 28W
Komi □, *Russia* **56 B10** 64 0N 55 0 E
Kominter = Novoshakhtinsk, *Russia* **59 J10** 47 46N 39 58 E
Komintern = Marhanets, *Ukraine* **59 J8** 47 40N 34 40 E
Komiža, *Croatia* **45 E13** 43 3N 16 11 E
Komló, *Hungary* **52 D3** 46 15N 18 16 E
Kommamur Canal, *India* **95 G5** 16 0N 80 25 E
Kommunarsk = Alchevsk, *Ukraine* **59 H10** 48 30N 38 45 E
Kommunizma, Pik, *Tajikistan* **65 D6** 39 0N 72 2 E
Komodo, *Indonesia* **82 C1** 8 37 S 119 20 E
Komoé →, *Ivory C.* **112 D4** 5 12N 3 44W
Komono, *Congo* **114 C2** 3 10 S 13 20 E
Komoran, Pulau, *Indonesia* **83 C5** 8 18 S 138 45 E
Komoro, *Japan* **73 A10** 36 19N 138 26 E
Komotau = Chomutov, *Czech Rep.* **34 A6** 50 28N 13 23 E
Komotini, *Greece* **51 E9** 41 9N 25 26 E
Komovi, *Serbia & M.* **50 D3** 42 41N 19 39 E
Kompasberg, *S. Africa* **116 E3** 31 45 S 24 32 E
Kompong Bang, *Cambodia* **87 F5** 12 24N 104 40 E
Kompong Cham, *Cambodia* **87 F5** 12 0N 105 30 E
Kompong Chhnang = Kampong Chhnang, *Cambodia* **87 F5** 12 20N 104 35 E
Kompong Chikreng, *Cambodia* **86 F5** 13 5N 104 18 E
Kompong Kleang, *Cambodia* **86 F5** 13 6N 104 8 E
Kompong Luong, *Cambodia* **87 G5** 11 49N 104 48 E
Kompong Pranak, *Cambodia* **86 F5** 13 35N 104 55 E
Kompong Som = Kampong Saom, *Cambodia* **87 G4** 10 38N 103 30 E
Kompong Som, Chhung = Kampong Saom, Chaak, *Cambodia* **87 G4** 10 50N 103 32 E
Kompong Speu, *Cambodia* **87 G5** 11 26N 104 32 E
Kompong Sralau, *Cambodia* **86 E5** 14 5N 105 46 E
Kompong Thom, *Cambodia* **86 F5** 12 35N 104 51 E
Kompong Trabeck, *Cambodia* **86 F5** 13 6N 105 14 E
Kompong Trabeck, *Cambodia* **87 G5** 11 9N 105 28 E
Kompong Trach, *Cambodia* **87 G5** 11 25N 105 48 E
Kompong Tralach, *Cambodia* **87 G5** 11 54N 104 47 E
Komrat = Comrat, *Moldova* **53 D13** 46 18N 28 40 E
Komsberg, *S. Africa* **116 E3** 32 40 S 20 45 E
Komsomolabad, *Tajikistan* **65 D4** 38 50N 69 55 E
Komsomolets, *Kazakhstan* **64 E9** 53 45N 62 2 E
Komsomolets, Ostrov, *Russia* **67 A10** 80 30N 95 0 E
Komsomolsk, *Amur, Russia* **67 D14** 50 30N 137 0 E
Komsomolsk, *Ivanovo, Russia* **58 D11** 57 2N 40 20 E
Komsomolsk, *Turkmenistan* **65 D1** 39 2N 63 36 E
Komsomolskiy, *Russia* **60 C7** 54 27N 45 33 E
Komsomolsky = Chirchiq, *Uzbekistan* **65 C4** 41 29N 69 35 E
Kömür Burnu, *Turkey* **49 C8** 38 39N 26 12 E
Kon Tum, *Vietnam* **86 E7** 14 24N 108 0 E
Kon Tum, Plateau du, *Vietnam* **86 E7** 14 30N 108 30 E
Kona, *Mali* **112 C4** 14 57N 3 53W
Konakovo, *Russia* **58 D9** 56 40N 36 51 E
Konarak, *India* **94 E8** 19 54N 86 7 E
Konarhā □, *Afghan.* **91 B3** 34 30N 71 3 E
Konārī, *Iran* **97 D6** 28 13N 51 36 E
Konch, *India* **93 G8** 26 0N 79 10 E
Konda, *Indonesia* **83 B4** 1 34 S 131 57 E
Kondagaon, *India* **94 E5** 19 35N 81 35 E
Konde, *Tanzania* **118 C4** 4 57 S 39 45 E
Kondiá, *Greece* **49 B7** 39 49N 25 10 E
Kondinin, *Australia* **125 F2** 32 34 S 118 8 E
Kondo, *Dem. Rep. of the Congo* **115 D2** 5 35 S 13 0 E
Kondoa, *Tanzania* **118 C4** 4 55 S 35 50 E
Kondókali, *Greece* **38 B9** 39 38N 19 51 E
Kondopaga, *Russia* **58 A8** 62 12N 34 17 E
Kondratyevo, *Russia* **67 D10** 57 22N 98 15 E
Kondrovo, *Russia* **58 E8** 54 48N 35 56 E
Konduga, *Nigeria* **113 C7** 11 35N 13 26 E
Kondukur, *India* **95 G4** 15 12N 79 57 E
Koné, *Cameroon* **114 A2** 8 50N 13 17 E
Koné, *N. Cal.* **133 U18** 21 4 S 164 52 E
Köneürgench, *Turkmenistan* **66 E6** 42 19N 59 10 E
Konevo, *Russia* **58 A10** 62 8N 39 20 E
Kong = Khong →, *Cambodia* **86 F5** 13 32N 105 58 E
Kong, *Ivory C.* **112 D4** 8 54N 4 36W
Kong, Koh, *Cambodia* **87 G4** 11 20N 103 0 E
Kong Christian IX Land, *Greenland* **10 D7** 68 0N 36 0W
Kong Christian X Land, *Greenland* **10 C8** 74 0N 29 0W
Kong Frederik IX Land, *Greenland* **10 D5** 67 0N 52 0W
Kong Frederik VI Kyst, *Greenland* **10 E6** 63 0N 43 0W
Kong Frederik VIII Land, *Greenland* **10 B8** 78 30N 26 0W
Kong Karls Land, *Svalbard* **10 B13** 79 0N 28 0 E
Kong Oscar Fjord, *Greenland* **10 C8** 72 20N 24 0W
Kongbo, *C.A.R.* **114 B4** 4 44N 21 23 E
Kongeå →, *Denmark* **17 J2** 55 23N 8 39 E
Kongerslev, *Denmark* **17 H4** 56 54N 10 6 E
Kongju, *S. Korea* **75 F14** 36 30N 127 0 E
Kongkemul, *Indonesia* **85 B4** 1 52N 112 11 E
Konglu, *Burma* **90 B6** 27 13N 97 57 E
Kongmoon = Jiangmen, *China* **77 F9** 22 32N 113 0 E
Kongola, *Namibia* **116 B3** 17 45 S 23 20 E
Kongolo, *Kasai-Or., Dem. Rep. of the Congo* **118 D1** 5 26 S 24 49 E
Kongolo, *Katanga, Dem. Rep. of the Congo* **118 D2** 5 22 S 27 0 E
Kongor, *Sudan* **107 F3** 7 1N 31 27 E
Kongoulou, *Cameroon* **114 B2** 2 59N 11 7 E
Kongoussi, *Burkina Faso* **113 C4** 13 19N 1 32W
Kongsberg, *Norway* **18 E6** 59 39N 9 39 E
Kongsvinger, *Norway* **18 D9** 60 12N 12 2 E
Kongwa, *Tanzania* **118 D4** 6 11 S 36 26 E
Koni, *Dem. Rep. of the Congo* **119 E2** 10 40 S 27 11 E
Koni, Mts., *Dem. Rep. of the Congo* **119 E2** 10 36 S 27 10 E
Koniakari, *Mali* **112 C2** 14 35N 10 50W
Koniecpol, *Poland* **55 H6** 50 46N 19 40 E
Königgrätz = Hradec Králové, *Czech Rep.* **34 A8** 50 15N 15 50 E
Königs Wusterhausen, *Germany* **30 C9** 52 19N 13 38 E
Königsberg = Chojna, *Poland* **55 F1** 52 58N 14 25 E
Königsberg = Kaliningrad, *Russia* **15 J19** 54 42N 20 32 E
Königsbrunn, *Germany* **31 G6** 48 16N 10 54 E
Königshütte = Chorzów, *Poland* **55 H5** 50 18N 18 57 E
Königslutter, *Germany* **30 C6** 52 15N 10 49 E
Konin, *Poland* **55 F5** 52 12N 18 15 E
Königinhof an der Elbe = Dvůr Králové nad Labem, *Czech Rep.* **34 A8** 50 27N 15 50 E
Konispol, *Albania* **38 B10** 39 42N 20 10 E
Kónitsa, *Greece* **48 A2** 40 5N 20 48 E
Köniz, *Switz.* **32 C4** 46 56N 7 25 E
Konjic, *Bos.-H.* **52 G2** 43 42N 17 58 E
Konkiep, *Namibia* **116 D2** 26 49 S 17 15 E
Konkō, *Japan* **72 C4** 34 33N 133 36 E
Konkouré →, *Guinea* **112 D2** 9 50N 13 42W
Könnern, *Germany* **30 D7** 51 41N 11 47 E
Konnur, *India* **95 F2** 16 14N 74 49 E
Kono, *S. Leone* **112 D2** 8 30N 11 5W
Konogogo, *Papua N. G.* **132 B7** 3 29 S 152 10 E
Konolfingen, *Switz.* **32 C5** 46 54N 7 38 E
Konongo, *Ghana* **113 D4** 6 40N 1 15W
Konos, *Papua N. G.* **132 B6** 3 10 S 151 44 E
Konosha, *Russia* **58 B11** 61 0N 40 5 E
Kōnosu, *Japan* **73 A11** 36 3N 139 31 E
Konotop, *Ukraine* **59 G7** 51 12N 33 7 E
Konradshof = Skawina, *Poland* **55 J6** 49 59N 19 50 E
Konsankoro, *Guinea* **112 D3** 9 2N 9 0W
Końskie, *Poland* **55 G7** 51 15N 20 23 E
Konsmo, *Norway* **18 F4** 58 16N 7 20 E
Konstadt = Wołczyn, *Poland* **55 G5** 51 1N 18 3 E
Konstancin-Jeziorna, *Poland* **55 F8** 52 5N 21 7 E
Konstantinograd = Krasnohrad, *Ukraine* **59 H8** 49 27N 35 27 E
Konstantinovka = Kostyantynivka, *Ukraine* **59 H9** 48 32N 37 39 E
Konstantinovsk, *Russia* **61 G5** 47 33N 41 10 E
Konstantynów Łódzki, *Poland* **55 G6** 51 45N 19 20 E
Konstanz, *Germany* **31 H5** 47 40N 9 10 E
Kont, *Iran* **97 E9** 26 55N 61 50 E
Konta, *India* **94 F5** 17 48N 81 23 E
Kontagora, *Nigeria* **113 C6** 10 23N 5 27 E
Kontcha, *Cameroon* **113 D7** 7 59N 12 15 E
Konya, *Turkey* **100 D5** 37 52N 32 35 E
Konya Ovası, *Turkey* **100 D5** 38 30N 33 5 E
Konyin, *Burma* **90 D5** 22 58N 94 42 E
Konz, *Germany* **31 F2** 49 42N 6 34 E
Konza, *Kenya* **118 C4** 1 45 S 37 7 E
Konzhakovskiy Kamen, Gora, *Russia* **64 B7** 59 38N 59 8 E
Koo-wee-rup, *Australia* **129 E6** 38 13 S 145 28 E
Koocanusa, L., *Canada* **158 B6** 49 20N 115 15W
Kookynie, *Australia* **125 E3** 29 17 S 121 22 E
Koolau Range, *U.S.A.* **145 J14** 21 35N 157 50W
Koolyanobbing, *Australia* **125 F2** 30 48 S 119 36 E
Koondrook, *Australia* **128 C6** 35 33 S 144 8 E
Koonibba, *Australia* **127 E1** 31 54 S 133 25 E
Koorawatha, *Australia* **129 C8** 34 2 S 148 33 E
Koorda, *Australia* **125 F2** 30 48 S 117 35 E
Kooskia, *U.S.A.* **158 C6** 46 9N 115 59W
Kootenay △, *Canada* **142 C5** 51 0N 116 0W
Kootenay →, *U.S.A.* **142 D5** 49 19N 117 39W
Kootenay L., *Canada* **158 B5** 49 45N 116 50W
Kootingal, *Australia* **129 A9** 31 3 S 151 4 E
Kootjieskolk, *S. Africa* **116 E3** 31 15 S 20 21 E
Kopa = Qopa, *Kazakhstan* **65 B7** 43 31N 75 50 E
Kopanovka, *Russia* **61 G8** 47 28N 46 50 E
Kopaonik, *Serbia & M.* **50 C4** 43 10N 20 50 E
Kopaonik △, *Serbia & M.* **50 C4** 43 20N 20 50 E
Kopargaon, *India* **94 E2** 19 51N 74 28 E
Kópasker, *Iceland* **11 A10** 66 18N 16 27W
Kópavogur, *Iceland* **11 C4** 64 6N 21 55W
Kopayhorod, *Ukraine* **53 B12** 48 52N 27 47 E
Koper, *Slovenia* **45 C10** 45 31N 13 44 E
Kopervik, *Norway* **18 E2** 59 17N 5 17 E
Kopet Dagh, *Asia* **97 B8** 38 0N 58 0 E
Kopeysk, *Russia* **64 D8** 55 7N 61 37 E
Kopi, *Australia* **127 E2** 33 24 S 135 40 E
Köping, *Sweden* **16 E10** 59 31N 16 3 E
Köpingsvik, *Sweden* **17 H10** 56 53N 16 43 E
Kopište, *Croatia* **45 F13** 42 48N 16 42 E
Koplik, *Albania* **50 D3** 42 15N 19 25 E
Köpmanholmen, *Sweden* **16 A12** 63 10N 18 35 E
Koppa, *India* **95 H2** 13 33N 75 21 E
Koppal, *India* **95 G3** 15 23N 76 5 E
Koppang, *Norway* **18 C8** 61 34N 11 3 E
Kopparberg, *Sweden* **16 E9** 59 52N 15 0 E
Koppeh Dāgh = Kopet Dagh, *Asia* **97 B8** 38 0N 58 0 E
Kopperå, *Norway* **18 A8** 63 24N 11 50 E
Koppies, *S. Africa* **117 D4** 27 20 S 27 30 E
Koppom, *Sweden* **16 E6** 59 43N 12 10 E
Koprivlen, *Bulgaria* **50 E7** 41 31N 23 53 E
Koprivnica, *Croatia* **45 B13** 46 12N 16 45 E
Kopřivnice, *Czech Rep.* **35 B11** 49 36N 18 9 E
Koprivshtitsa, *Bulgaria* **51 D8** 42 40N 24 19 E
Köprübaşı, *Turkey* **49 C10** 38 43N 28 23 E
Kopychyntsi, *Ukraine* **53 B10** 49 7N 25 58 E
Kora △, *Kenya* **118 C4** 0 14 S 38 44 E
Korab, *Macedonia* **50 E4** 41 44N 20 40 E
Korakiána, *Greece* **38 B9** 39 42N 19 45 E
Koral, *India* **92 J5** 21 50N 73 12 E
Korangal, *India* **94 E3** 17 6N 77 38 E
Koraput, *India* **94 E6** 18 50N 82 40 E
Korarou, L., *Mali* **112 B4** 15 15N 3 15W
Korba, *India* **93 H10** 22 20N 82 45 E
Korbach, *Germany* **30 D4** 51 16N 8 52 E
Korbu, G., *Malaysia* **87 K3** 4 41N 101 18 E
Korçë, *Albania* **50 F4** 40 37N 20 50 E
Korčula, *Croatia* **45 F13** 42 56N 16 57 E
Korčulanski Kanal, *Croatia* **45 E13** 43 3N 16 40 E
Kord Kūy, *Iran* **97 B7** 36 48N 54 7 E
Kord Sheykh, *Iran* **97 D7** 28 31N 52 53 E
Korday, *Kazakhstan* **65 B7** 43 3N 74 43 E
Kordestan = Kurdistan, *Asia* **101 D10** 37 20N 43 30 E

Kordestān □, *Iran* **96 C5** 36 0N 47 0 E
Koré Mayroua, *Niger* **113 C5** 13 18N 3 55 E
Korea, North ■, *Asia* **75 E14** 40 0N 127 0 E
Korea, South ■, *Asia* **75 G15** 36 0N 128 0 E
Korea Bay, *Korea* **75 E13** 39 0N 124 0 E
Korea Strait, *Asia* **75 H15** 34 0N 129 30 E
Koregaon, *India* **94 F2** 17 40N 74 10 E
Korem, *Ethiopia* **107 E4** 12 30N 39 32 E
Korenevo, *Russia* **59 G8** 51 27N 34 55 E
Korenica = Titova Korenica, *Croatia* **45 D12** 44 45N 15 41 E
Korenovsk, *Russia* **61 H4** 45 30N 39 22 E
Korets, *Ukraine* **59 G4** 50 40N 27 5 E
Korfantów, *Poland* **55 H4** 50 29N 17 36 E
Korgan, *Turkey* **100 B7** 40 44N 37 13 E
Korgus, *Sudan* **106 D3** 19 16N 33 29 E
Korhogo, *Ivory C.* **112 D3** 9 29N 5 28W
Koribundu, *S. Leone* **112 D2** 7 41N 11 46W
Korienzé, *Mali* **112 B4** 15 22N 3 50W
Korim, *Indonesia* **83 B5** 0 58 S 136 10 E
Korinthía □, *Greece* **48 D4** 37 50N 22 35 E
Korinthiakós Kólpos, *Greece* **48 C4** 38 16N 22 30 E
Kórinthos, *Greece* **48 D4** 37 56N 22 55 E
Korioumé, *Mali* **112 B4** 16 35N 3 0W
Koríssa, Límni, *Greece* **38 C9** 39 27N 19 53 E
Korithi, *Greece* **39 D2** 37 55N 20 42 E
Kōriyama, *Japan* **70 F10** 37 24N 140 23 E
Korkino, *Russia* **64 D8** 54 54N 61 23 E
Korkuteli, *Turkey* **49 D12** 37 4N 30 13 E
Korla, *China* **68 B3** 41 45N 86 4 E
Kormakiti, C., *Cyprus* **39 E8** 35 23N 32 56 E
Körmend, *Hungary* **52 C1** 47 5N 16 35 E
Kornat, *Croatia* **45 E12** 43 50N 15 20 E
Kornat △, *Croatia* **45 E12** 43 50N 15 12 E
Korneshty = Corneşti, *Moldova* **53 C13** 47 21N 28 1 E
Korneuburg, *Austria* **35 C9** 48 20N 16 20 E
Kórnik, *Poland* **55 F4** 52 15N 17 6 E
Kornsjø, *Norway* **18 F8** 58 57N 11 39 E
Koro, *Fiji* **133 A2** 17 19 S 179 23 E
Koro, *Ivory C.* **112 D3** 8 32N 7 30W
Koro, *Mali* **112 C4** 14 1N 2 58W
Koro Sea, *Fiji* **133 A3** 17 30 S 179 45W
Koro Toro, *Chad* **109 E3** 16 5N 18 30 E
Koroba, *Papua N. G.* **132 C2** 5 44 S 142 47 E
Korobkovo = Gubkin, *Russia* **59 G9** 51 17N 37 32 E
Korocha, *Russia* **59 G9** 50 54N 37 19 E
Köroğlu Dağları, *Turkey* **100 B5** 40 38N 33 0 E
Korogwe, *Tanzania* **118 D4** 5 5 S 38 25 E
Koroit, *Australia* **128 E5** 38 18 S 142 24 E
Koroleve, *Ukraine* **53 B8** 48 9N 23 8 E
Korolevu, *Fiji* **133 B1** 18 12 S 177 46 E
Korona, *U.S.A.* **153 F8** 29 25N 81 12W
Koronadal, *Phil.* **81 H5** 6 12N 125 1 E
Korong Vale, *Australia* **128 D5** 36 22 S 143 45 E
Koróni, *Greece* **48 E3** 36 48N 21 57 E
Korónia, Limni, *Greece* **50 F7** 40 47N 23 10 E
Koronís, *Greece* **49 D7** 37 12N 25 35 E
Koronowo, *Poland* **55 E4** 53 19N 17 55 E
Koropelé, *C.A.R.* **114 B3** 4 44N 17 11 E
Koropets, *Ukraine* **53 B10** 48 56N 25 10 E
Koror, *Palau* **134 G5** 7 20N 134 28 E
Körös →, *Hungary* **52 D5** 46 43N 20 12 E
Körös Maros △, *Hungary* **52 C5** 47 8N 20 52 E
Köröstarcsa, *Hungary* **52 D6** 46 53N 21 3 E
Korosten, *Ukraine* **59 G5** 50 54N 28 36 E
Korostyshev, *Ukraine* **59 G5** 50 19N 29 4 E
Korotoyak, *Russia* **59 G10** 51 1N 39 2 E
Korovou, *Fiji* **133 A2** 17 47 S 178 32 E
Koroyanitu △, *Fiji* **133 A1** 17 40 S 177 35 E
Korraraika, Helodranon' i, *Madag.* **117 B7** 17 45 S 43 57 E
Korsakov, *Russia* **67 E15** 46 36N 142 42 E
Korsberga, *Sweden* **17 G9** 57 19N 15 7 E
Korshiv, *Ukraine* **53 B10** 48 39N 25 1 E
Korshunovo, *Russia* **67 D12** 58 37N 110 10 E
Korsør, *Denmark* **17 J5** 55 20N 11 9 E
Korsun Shevchenkovskiy, *Ukraine* **59 H6** 49 26N 31 16 E
Korsze, *Poland* **54 D8** 54 11N 21 9 E
Korti, *Sudan* **106 D3** 18 6N 31 33 E
Kortrijk, *Belgium* **24 D3** 50 50N 3 17 E
Korucu, *Turkey* **49 B9** 39 28N 27 22 E
Korumburra, *Australia* **129 E6** 38 26 S 145 50 E
Korup △, *Cameroon* **114 A1** 5 15N 9 2 E
Korwai, *India* **92 G8** 24 7N 78 5 E
Koryakskoye Nagorye, *Russia* **67 C18** 61 0N 171 0 E
Koryŏng, *S. Korea* **75 G15** 35 44N 128 15 E
Koryukovka, *Ukraine* **59 G7** 51 46N 32 16 E
Kos, *Greece* **49 E9** 36 50N 27 15 E
Kos-Istek = Leninskoye, *Kazakhstan* **64 F6** 50 44N 57 53 E
Kosa, *Ethiopia* **107 F4** 7 50N 36 50 E
Kosa, *Russia* **64 B5** 59 56N 55 0 E
Kosa →, *Russia* **64 A5** 60 11N 55 10 E
Kosai, *Japan* **73 C9** 34 42N 137 32 E
Kosaya Gora, *Russia* **58 E9** 54 10N 37 30 E
Koschagyl, *Kazakhstan* **57 E9** 46 40N 54 0 E
Kościan, *Poland* **55 F3** 52 5N 16 40 E
Kościerzyna, *Poland* **54 D4** 54 8N 17 59 E
Kosciusko, *U.S.A.* **155 J10** 33 4N 89 35W
Kosciusko △, *Australia* **129 D8** 36 30 S 148 20 E
Kosciuszko, Mt., *Australia* **129 D8** 36 27 S 148 16 E
Kösély →, *Hungary* **52 C6** 47 25N 21 5 E
Kosgi, *Andhra Pradesh, India* **94 F3** 16 58N 77 43 E
Kosgi, *Andhra Pradesh, India* **95 G3** 15 51N 77 16 E
Kosh-Döbö, *Kyrgyzstan* **65 C7** 41 5N 74 15 E
Kosha, *Sudan* **106 C3** 20 50N 30 30 E
Koshava, *Bulgaria* **50 B7** 44 4N 23 2 E
Koshigaya, *Japan* **73 B11** 35 54N 139 48 E
K'oshih = Kashi, *China* **65 D8** 39 30N 76 2 E
Koshiki-Rettō, *Japan* **72 F1** 31 45N 129 49 E
Koshkonong L., *U.S.A.* **157 B8** 42 52N 88 58W
Kōshoku, *Japan* **73 A10** 36 38N 138 6 E
Koshrabad, *Uzbekistan* **65 C3** 40 18N 66 32 E
Koshu-Kavak = Krumovgrad, *Bulgaria* **51 E9** 41 29N 25 38 E
Kosi, *India* **92 F7** 27 48N 77 29 E
Kosi →, *India* **93 E8** 28 41N 78 57 E
Košice, *Slovak Rep.* **35 C14** 48 42N 21 15 E
Košický □, *Slovak Rep.* **35 C14** 48 45N 21 0 E
Kosiv, *Ukraine* **53 B10** 48 19N 25 6 E
Kosjerić, *Serbia & M.* **50 B3** 44 0N 19 55 E
Köşk, *Turkey* **49 D10** 37 50N 28 3 E
Koskinoú, *Greece* **38 E12** 36 23N 28 13 E
Koslan, *Russia* **56 B8** 63 34N 49 14 E
Köslin = Koszalin, *Poland* **54 D3** 54 11N 16 8 E
Kosmach, *Ukraine* **53 B9** 48 20N 24 50 E
Kosŏng, *N. Korea* **75 E15** 38 40N 128 22 E
Kosovo □, *Serbia & M.* **50 D4** 42 30N 21 0 E
Kosovo Polje, *Serbia & M.* **50 D5** 42 40N 21 5 E
Kosovska Kamenica, *Serbia & M.* **50 D5** 42 35N 21 35 E
Kosovska Mitrovica, *Serbia & M.* **50 D4** 42 54N 20 52 E
Kosrap, *China* **65 E8** 38 0N 76 12 E
Kossou, L. de, *Ivory C.* **112 D3** 6 59N 5 31W
Kosta, *Sweden* **17 H9** 56 50N 15 24 E
Kostajnica, *Croatia* **45 C13** 45 17N 16 30 E
Kostanjevica, *Slovenia* **45 C12** 45 51N 15 27 E
Kostenets = Pernik, *Bulgaria* **50 D7** 42 35N 23 2 E
Kostenets, *Bulgaria* **50 D7** 42 15N 23 52 E
Koster, *S. Africa* **116 D4** 25 52 S 26 54 E
Kôstî, *Sudan* **107 E3** 13 8N 32 43 E
Kostinbrod, *Bulgaria* **50 D7** 42 49N 23 13 E
Kostolac, *Serbia & M.* **50 B5** 44 37N 21 15 E
Kostopil, *Ukraine* **59 G4** 50 51N 26 22 E
Kostroma, *Russia* **58 D11** 57 50N 40 58 E
Kostromskoye Vdkhr., *Russia* **58 D11** 57 52N 40 49 E
Kostryzhivka, *Ukraine* **53 B10** 48 39N 25 43 E
Kostrzyn, *Lubuskie, Poland* **55 F1** 52 35N 14 39 E
Kostrzyn, *Wielkopolskie, Poland* **55 F4** 52 24N 17 14 E
Kostyantynivka, *Ukraine* **59 H9** 48 32N 37 39 E
Kostyukovichi = Kastsyukovichy, *Belarus* **58 F7** 53 20N 32 4 E
Koszalin, *Poland* **54 D3** 54 11N 16 8 E
Kőszeg, *Hungary* **52 C1** 47 23N 16 33 E
Kot Addu, *Pakistan* **91 C3** 30 30N 71 0 E
Kot Kapura, *India* **92 D6** 30 35N 74 50 E
Kot Moman, *Pakistan* **92 C5** 32 13N 73 0 E
Kot Sultan, *Pakistan* **92 D4** 30 46N 70 56 E
Kota, *India* **92 G6** 25 14N 75 49 E
Kota Barrage, *India* **92 G6** 25 6N 75 51 E
Kota Belud, *Malaysia* **85 A5** 6 21N 116 26 E
Kota Bharu, *Malaysia* **87 J4** 6 7N 102 14 E
Kota Kinabalu, *Malaysia* **85 A5** 6 0N 116 4 E
Kota Kubu Bharu, *Malaysia* **87 L3** 3 34N 101 39 E
Kota Tinggi, *Malaysia* **87 M4** 1 44N 103 53 E
Kotaagung, *Indonesia* **84 D2** 5 38 S 104 29 E
Kotabaru, *Indonesia* **85 C5** 3 20 S 116 20 E
Kotabumi, *Indonesia* **84 C2** 4 49 S 104 54 E
Kotagede, *Indonesia* **85 D4** 7 54 S 110 26 E
Kotamobagu, *Indonesia* **82 A2** 0 57N 124 31 E
Kotapad, *India* **94 E6** 19 9N 82 21 E
Kotawaringin, *Indonesia* **85 C4** 2 28 S 111 27 E
Kotchandpur, *Bangla.* **90 D2** 23 24N 89 1 E
Kotcho L., *Canada* **142 B4** 59 7N 121 12W
Kotdwara, *India* **93 E8** 29 45N 78 32 E
Kotel, *Bulgaria* **51 D10** 42 52N 26 26 E
Kotelnich, *Russia* **60 A9** 58 22N 48 24 E
Kotelnikovo, *Russia* **61 G6** 47 38N 43 8 E
Kotelnyy, Ostrov, *Russia* **67 B14** 75 10N 139 0 E
Kothagudam, *India* **94 F5** 17 30N 80 40 E
Kothapet, *India* **94 E4** 19 21N 79 28 E
Kothari →, *India* **92 G6** 25 20N 75 4 E
Köthen, *Germany* **30 D7** 51 45N 11 59 E
Kothi, *Chhattisgarh, India* **93 H10** 23 21N 82 3 E
Kothi, *Mad. P., India* **93 G9** 24 45N 80 40 E
Kotiro, *Pakistan* **92 F2** 26 17N 67 13 E
Kotka, *Finland* **15 F22** 60 28N 26 58 E
Kotlas, *Russia* **56 B8** 61 17N 46 43 E
Kotlenska Planina, *Bulgaria* **51 D10** 42 56N 26 30 E
Kotli, *Pakistan* **92 C5** 33 30N 73 55 E
Kotlik, *U.S.A.* **144 E7** 63 2N 163 33W
Kotma, *India* **93 H9** 23 12N 81 58 E
Kotmul, *Pakistan* **93 B6** 35 32N 75 10 E
Kotohira, *Japan* **72 C5** 34 11N 133 49 E
Koton-Karifi, *Nigeria* **113 D6** 8 0N 6 48 E
Kotonkoro, *Nigeria* **113 C6** 11 3N 5 58 E
Kotor, *Serbia & M.* **50 D2** 42 25N 18 47 E
Kotor Varoš, *Bos.-H.* **52 F2** 44 38N 17 22 E
Kotoriba, *Croatia* **45 B13** 46 23N 16 48 E
Kotovo, *Russia* **60 E7** 50 22N 44 45 E
Kotovsk, *Russia* **60 D5** 52 36N 41 32 E
Kotovsk, *Ukraine* **59 J5** 47 45N 29 35 E
Kotputli, *India* **92 F7** 27 43N 76 12 E
Kotri, *Pakistan* **91 D3** 25 22N 68 22 E
Kotri →, *India* **94 E5** 19 15N 80 35 E
Kótronas, *Greece* **48 E4** 36 38N 22 29 E
Kötschach-Mauthen, *Austria* **34 E6** 46 41N 13 1 E
Kottayam, *India* **95 K3** 9 35N 76 33 E
Kotto →, *C.A.R.* **114 B4** 4 14N 22 2 E
Kottur, *India* **95 J3** 10 34N 76 56 E
Kotu Group, *Tonga* **133 Q14** 20 0 S 173 35 E
Kotuy →, *Russia* **67 B11** 71 54N 102 6 E
Kotyuzhany, *Ukraine* **53 B12** 48 48N 27 42 E
Kotzebue, *U.S.A.* **144 C7** 66 53N 162 39W
Kotzebue Sound, *U.S.A.* **144 C7** 66 20N 163 0W
Kotzenau = Chocianów, *Poland* **55 G2** 51 27N 15 55 E
Kouango, *C.A.R.* **114 B4** 5 0N 20 10 E
Kouchibouguac △, *Canada* **141 C6** 46 50N 65 0W
Koudougou, *Burkina Faso* **112 C4** 12 10N 2 20W
Koufonísi, *Greece* **39 F7** 34 56N 26 8 E
Koufonísia, *Greece* **49 E7** 36 57N 25 35 E
Kougaberge, *S. Africa* **116 E3** 33 48 S 23 50 E
Kouibli, *Ivory C.* **112 D3** 7 15N 7 14W
Kouilou →, *Congo* **115 C2** 4 10 S 12 5 E
Kouki, *C.A.R.* **114 A3** 7 22N 17 3 E
Koula Moutou, *Gabon* **114 C2** 1 15 S 12 25 E
Koulen = Kulen, *Cambodia* **86 F5** 13 50N 104 40 E
Koulikoro, *Mali* **112 C3** 12 40N 7 50W
Kouloúra, *Greece* **38 B9** 39 42N 19 54 E
Koúm-bournoú, Ákra, *Greece* **38 E12** 36 15N 28 11 E
Koumac, *N. Cal.* **133 T18** 20 33 S 164 17 E
Koumala, *Australia* **126 C4** 21 38 S 149 15 E
Koumameyeng, *Gabon* **114 B2** 0 11N 11 51 E
Koumankou, *Mali* **112 C3** 11 58N 6 6W
Koumbia, *Burkina Faso* **112 C4** 11 10N 3 50W
Koumbia, *Guinea* **112 C2** 11 48N 13 29W
Koumboum, *Guinea* **112 C2** 10 25N 13 0W
Koumpenntoum, *Senegal* **112 C2** 13 59N 14 34W
Koumra, *Chad* **109 G3** 8 50N 17 35 E
Koun-Fao, *Ivory C.* **112 D4** 7 30N 3 15W
Koundara, *Guinea* **112 C2** 12 29N 13 18W
Koundé, *C.A.R.* **114 A2** 6 7N 14 38 E
Koundian, *Guinea* **112 C3** 13 10N 10 35W
Koungheul, *Senegal* **112 C2** 14 0N 14 50W
Koungoulou, *Congo* **114 C2** 3 31 S 13 20 E
Kounradskiy, *Kazakhstan* **66 E8** 46 59N 75 0 E
Kountze, *U.S.A.* **155 K7** 30 22N 94 19W
Koupéla, *Burkina Faso* **113 C4** 12 11N 0 21W
Kourémalé, *Mali* **112 C3** 11 59N 8 42W
Kouris →, *Cyprus* **39 F8** 34 38N 32 54 E
Kourizo, P. de, *Chad* **108 D3** 22 28N 15 27 E
Kourou, *Fr. Guiana* **169 B7** 5 9N 52 39W
Kourouba, *Mali* **112 C2** 13 22N 10 57W
Kouroukoto, *Mali* **112 C2** 12 35N 10 5W
Kourouma, *Burkina Faso* **112 C4** 11 35N 4 50W
Kourouninkoto, *Mali* **112 C3** 13 52N 9 35W
Kouroussa, *Guinea* **112 C3** 10 45N 9 45W
Koussanar, *Senegal* **112 C2** 13 52N 14 5W
Koussané, *Mali* **112 C2** 14 53N 11 14W
Koussane, *Senegal* **112 C2** 14 10N 12 22W
Kousseri, *Cameroon* **109 F2** 12 0N 14 55 E
Koutiala, *Mali* **112 C3** 12 25N 5 23W
Kouto, *Ivory C.* **112 D3** 9 53N 6 25W
Kouts, *U.S.A.* **157 C9** 41 19N 87 2W
Kouvé, *Togo* **113 D5** 6 25N 1 25 E
Kouvola, *Finland* **15 F22** 60 52N 26 43 E
Kouyi, *Congo* **114 C2** 2 29 S 12 25 E
Kouyou →, *Congo* **114 C3** 0 44 S 16 38 E
Kovačica, *Serbia & M.* **52 E5** 45 5N 20 38 E
Kovdor, *Russia* **56 A5** 67 34N 30 24 E
Kovel, *Ukraine* **59 G3** 51 11N 24 38 E
Kovilpatti, *India* **95 K3** 9 10N 77 50 E
Kovin, *Serbia & M.* **52 F5** 44 44N 20 59 E
Kovno = Kaunas, *Lithuania* **15 J20** 54 54N 23 54 E
Kovrov, *Russia* **60 B5** 56 25N 41 25 E
Kovur, *Andhra Pradesh, India* **94 F5** 17 3N 81 39 E
Kovur, *Andhra Pradesh, India* **95 G5** 14 30N 80 1 E
Kowal, *Poland* **55 F6** 52 32N 19 7 E
Kowalewo Pomorskie, *Poland* **55 E5** 53 10N 18 52 E
Kowanyama, *Australia* **126 B3** 15 29 S 141 44 E
Kowlīnī, *Afghan.* **65 E2** 37 39N 65 58 E
Kowloon, *China* **77 F10** 22 19N 114 11 E
Kowŏn, *N. Korea* **75 E14** 39 26N 127 14 E
Kōyama, *Japan* **72 F2** 31 20N 130 56 E
Koyampattur = Coimbatore, *India* **95 J3** 11 2N 76 59 E
Köyceğiz, *Turkey* **49 E10** 36 57N 28 40 E
Köyceğiz Gölü, *Turkey* **49 E10** 36 56N 28 42 E
Koytash, *Uzbekistan* **65 C3** 40 11N 67 19 E
Koyuk, *U.S.A.* **144 D7** 64 56N 161 9W
Koyukuk, *U.S.A.* **144 D8** 64 53N 157 42W
Koyukuk →, *U.S.A.* **144 D8** 64 55N 157 32W
Koyulhisar, *Turkey* **100 B7** 40 20N 37 52 E
Koyunyeri, *Turkey* **51 F10** 40 50N 26 26 E
Koza, *Japan* **71 L3** 26 19N 127 46 E
Kozak, *Turkey* **49 B9** 39 15N 27 6 E
Kozan, *Turkey* **100 D6** 37 26N 35 50 E
Kozáni, *Greece* **50 F5** 40 19N 21 47 E
Kozáni □, *Greece* **50 F5** 40 18N 21 45 E
Kozara, *Bos.-H.* **45 D14** 45 0N 17 0 E
Kozara △, *Bos.-H.* **52 F2** 45 0N 17 0 E
Kozarac, *Bos.-H.* **45 D13** 44 58N 16 48 E
Kozelets, *Ukraine* **59 G6** 50 55N 31 7 E
Kozelsk, *Russia* **58 E8** 54 2N 35 48 E
Kozhemyaki = Pervomayskiy, *Russia* **64 F5** 51 32N 55 2 E
Kozhikode = Calicut, *India* **95 J2** 11 15N 75 43 E
Kozhva, *Russia* **56 A10** 65 10N 57 0 E
Koziegłowy, *Poland* **55 H6** 50 37N 19 8 E
Kozienice, *Poland* **55 G8** 51 35N 21 34 E
Kozje, *Slovenia* **45 B12** 46 5N 15 35 E
Kozloduy, *Bulgaria* **50 C7** 43 45N 23 42 E
Kozlov = Michurinsk, *Russia* **60 D5** 52 58N 40 27 E
Kozlovets, *Bulgaria* **51 C9** 43 30N 25 20 E
Kozlovka, *Russia* **60 C9** 55 52N 48 14 E
Kozlu, *Turkey* **100 B4** 41 26N 31 45 E
Kozluk, *Turkey* **101 C9** 38 11N 41 31 E
Koźmin, *Poland* **55 G4** 51 48N 17 27 E
Kozmodemyansk, *Russia* **60 B8** 56 20N 46 36 E
Kōzu-Shima, *Japan* **73 C11** 34 13N 139 10 E
Kożuchów, *Poland* **55 G2** 51 45N 15 31 E
Kozyatyn, *Ukraine* **59 H5** 49 45N 28 50 E
Kpabia, *Ghana* **113 D4** 9 10N 0 20W
Kpalimé, *Togo* **113 D5** 6 57N 0 44 E
Kpandae, *Ghana* **113 D4** 8 30N 0 2W
Kpessi, *Togo* **113 D5** 8 4N 1 16 E
Kra, Isthmus of = Kra, Kho Khot, *Thailand* **87 G2** 10 15N 99 30 E
Kra, Kho Khot, *Thailand* **87 G2** 10 15N 99 30 E
Kra Buri, *Thailand* **87 G2** 10 22N 98 46 E
Kraai →, *S. Africa* **116 E4** 30 40 S 26 45 E
Krabi, *Thailand* **87 H2** 8 4N 98 55 E
Kracheh, *Cambodia* **86 F6** 12 32N 106 10 E
Kragan, *Indonesia* **85 D4** 6 43 S 111 38 E
Kragerø, *Norway* **18 F6** 58 52N 9 25 E
Kragujevac, *Serbia & M.* **50 B4** 44 2N 20 56 E
Krainburg = Kranj, *Slovenia* **45 B11** 46 16N 14 22 E
Krajenka, *Poland* **55 E3** 53 18N 16 59 E
Krakatau = Rakata, Pulau, *Indonesia* **84 D3** 6 10 S 105 20 E
Krakatoa = Rakata, Pulau, *Indonesia* **84 D3** 6 10 S 105 20 E
Krakau = Kraków, *Poland* **55 H6** 50 4N 19 57 E
Krakor, *Cambodia* **86 F5** 12 32N 104 12 E
Kraków, *Poland* **55 H6** 50 4N 19 57 E
Kraków ✈ (KRK), *Poland* **55 H6** 50 5N 19 52 E
Kraksaan, *Indonesia* **85 D4** 7 43 S 113 23 E
Kralanh, *Cambodia* **86 F4** 13 35N 103 25 E
Králíky, *Czech Rep.* **35 A9** 50 6N 16 45 E
Kraljevo, *Serbia & M.* **50 C4** 43 44N 20 41 E
Kralovéhradecký □, *Czech Rep.* **34 A8** 50 25N 15 50 E
Královský Chlmec, *Slovak Rep.* **35 C14** 48 27N 22 0 E
Kralupy nad Vltavou, *Czech Rep.* **34 A7** 50 13N 14 20 E
Kramatorsk, *Ukraine* **59 H9** 48 50N 37 30 E
Kramfors, *Sweden* **16 B11** 62 55N 17 48 E
Kramis, C., *Algeria* **111 A5** 36 26N 0 45 E
Kraniá, *Greece* **50 G5** 39 53N 21 18 E
Kranía Elassónas, *Greece* **48 B4** 39 57N 22 2 E
Kranídhion, *Greece* **48 D5** 37 20N 23 10 E
Kranj, *Slovenia* **45 B11** 46 16N 14 22 E
Kranjska Gora, *Slovenia* **45 B10** 46 29N 13 48 E
Krankskop, *S. Africa* **117 D5** 28 0 S 30 47 E
Kranz = Zelenogradsk, *Russia* **15 J19** 54 53N 20 29 E
Krapina, *Croatia* **45 B12** 46 10N 15 52 E
Krapina →, *Croatia* **45 C12** 45 50N 15 50 E
Krapkowice, *Poland* **55 H4** 50 29N 17 56 E
Krappitz = Krapkowice, *Poland* **55 H4** 50 29N 17 56 E
Kras, *Croatia* **45 C10** 45 35N 14 0 E
Krasavino, *Russia* **56 B8** 60 58N 46 29 E
Krashyy Klyuch, *Russia* **64 D6** 55 23N 56 39 E
Kraskino, *Russia* **67 E14** 42 44N 130 48 E
Krāslava, *Latvia* **58 E4** 55 54N 27 10 E
Kraslice, *Czech Rep.* **34 A5** 50 19N 12 31 E
Krasnaya Gorbatka, *Russia* **60 C5** 55 52N 41 45 E
Krasnaya Polyana, *Russia* **61 J5** 43 40N 40 13 E
Krasnaya Sloboda = Krasnoslobodsk, *Russia* **61 F7** 48 42N 44 33 E
Krasne, *Ukraine* **53 D14** 46 7N 29 15 E
Krasni Okny, *Ukraine* **53 C14** 47 32N 29 27 E
Kraśnik, *Poland* **55 H9** 50 55N 22 15 E
Krasnoarmeisk, *Ukraine* **59 H9** 48 18N 37 11 E
Krasnoarmeysk, *Russia* **60 E7** 51 0N 45 42 E
Krasnoarmeyskiy, *Russia* **61 G6** 47 0N 42 12 E
Krasnoarmeyskoye = Volnansk, *Ukraine* **59 H8** 48 2N 35 29 E
Krasnoarmeysky Rudnik = Dobropole, *Ukraine* **59 H9** 48 25N 37 2 E
Krasnobrod, *Poland* **55 H10** 50 33N 23 12 E
Krasnodar, *Russia* **61 H4** 45 5N 39 0 E
Krasnodon, *Ukraine* **59 H10** 48 17N 39 44 E
Krasnogorskiy, *Russia* **60 B9** 56 10N 48 28 E
Krasnograd = Krasnohrad, *Ukraine* **59 H8** 49 27N 35 27 E
Krasnogvardeysk = Bulungur, *Uzbekistan* **65 D3** 39 46N 67 16 E
Krasnogvardeysk = Gatchina, *Russia* **58 C6** 59 35N 30 9 E
Krasnogvardeysk, *Ukraine* **59 K8** 45 32N 34 16 E
Krasnogvardeyskoye, *Russia* **61 H5** 45 52N 41 33 E
Krasnohrad, *Ukraine* **59 H8** 49 27N 35 27 E
Krasnokamsk, *Russia* **64 B5** 58 4N 55 48 E
Krasnokokshaysk = Yoshkar Ola, *Russia* **60 B8** 56 38N 47 55 E
Krasnokutsk, *Ukraine* **59 G8** 50 10N 34 50 E
Krasnolesnyy, *Russia* **59 G10** 51 53N 39 35 E
Krasnoperekopsk, *Ukraine* **59 J7** 46 0N 33 54 E
Krasnorechenskiy, *Russia* **70 B7** 44 41N 135 14 E
Krasnoselkup, *Russia* **66 C9** 65 20N 82 10 E
Krasnoslobodsk, *Mordvinia, Russia* **60 C6** 54 25N 43 45 E
Krasnoslobodsk, *Volgograd, Russia* **61 F7** 48 42N 44 33 E
Krasnoturinsk, *Russia* **64 B8** 59 46N 60 12 E
Krasnoufimsk, *Russia* **64 C6** 56 36N 57 38 E
Krasnouralsk, *Russia* **64 B8** 58 21N 60 3 E
Krasnousolskiy, *Russia* **64 E6** 53 54N 56 27 E
Krasnovishersk, *Russia* **64 A6** 60 23N 57 3 E
Krasnovodsk = Türkmenbashi, *Turkmenistan* **57 G9** 40 5N 53 5 E
Krasnoyarsk, *Russia* **67 D10** 56 8N 93 0 E
Krasnoyarskiy, *Russia* **64 F7** 51 58N 59 55 E
Krasnoyarskoye, *Russia* **54 D8** 54 31N 21 56 E
Krasnoye = Krasnyy, *Russia* **58 E6** 54 25N 31 30 E
Krasnoye = Ulan Erge, *Russia* **61 G7** 46 19N 44 53 E
Krasnoye, *Russia* **64 B1** 59 15N 47 40 E
Krasnoyilsk **53 C10** 47 59N 25 38 E
Krasnozavodsk, *Russia* **58 D10** 56 27N 38 25 E
Krasnoznamensk, *Russia* **54 D9** 54 57N 22 30 E
Krasny = Kyzyl, *Russia* **67 D10** 51 50N 94 30 E
Krasny = Mozhga, *Russia* **60 B11** 56 26N 52 15 E
Krasny Boyevik = Kotovsk, *Russia* **60 D5** 52 36N 41 32 E
Krasny Sulin, *Russia* **59 J11** 47 52N 40 8 E
Krasnystaw, *Poland* **55 H10** 50 57N 23 5 E
Krasnyy, *Russia* **58 E6** 54 25N 31 30 E
Krasnyy Kholm, *Orenburg, Russia* **64 F5** 51 35N 54 9 E
Krasnyy Kholm, *Tver, Russia* **58 C9** 58 10N 37 10 E
Krasnyy Kut, *Russia* **60 E8** 50 50N 47 0 E
Krasnyy Liman, *Ukraine* **59 H9** 48 58N 37 50 E
Krasnyy Luch, *Ukraine* **59 H10** 48 13N 39 0 E
Krasnyy Profintern, *Russia* **58 D11** 57 45N 40 27 E
Krasnyy Yar, *Astrakhan, Russia* **61 G9** 46 43N 48 23 E
Krasnyy Yar, *Samara, Russia* **60 D10** 53 30N 50 22 E
Krasnyy Yar, *Volgograd, Russia* **60 E7** 50 42N 44 45 E
Krasnyye Baki, *Russia* **60 B7** 57 8N 45 10 E
Krasnyyoskolske Vdskh., *Ukraine* **59 H9** 49 27N 37 40 E
Kraszna →, *Hungary* **52 B7** 48 4N 22 20 E
Kratie = Kracheh, *Cambodia* **86 F6** 12 32N 106 10 E
Kratke Ra., *Papua N. G.* **132 D3** 6 45 S 146 0 E
Kratovo, *Macedonia* **50 D6** 42 6N 22 10 E
Krau, *Indonesia* **83 B6** 3 19 S 140 5 E
Kraulshavn = Nuussauq, *Greenland* **10 C5** 74 8N 57 3W
Kravanh, Chuor Phnum, *Cambodia* **87 G4** 12 0N 103 32 E
Kreb es Sefia, *Algeria* **110 C3** 27 12N 7 11W
Kreb n-Naga, *Algeria* **110 C3** 27 3N 7 9W
Kreb n-Neggar, *Algeria* **110 C3** 27 20N 7 15W
Krefeld, *Germany* **30 D2** 51 20N 6 33 E
Krémaston, Límni, *Greece* **48 C3** 38 52N 21 30 E
Kremen, *Croatia* **45 D12** 44 28N 15 53 E
Kremenchuk, *Ukraine* **59 H7** 49 5N 33 25 E
Kremenchuksk Vdskh., *Ukraine* **59 H7** 49 20N 32 30 E
Kremenets, *Ukraine* **59 G3** 50 8N 25 43 E
Kremennaya, *Ukraine* **59 H10** 49 1N 38 10 E
Kremges = Svitlovodsk, *Ukraine* **59 H7** 49 2N 33 13 E
Kremmen, *Germany* **30 C9** 52 45N 13 1 E
Kremmling, *U.S.A.* **158 F10** 40 4N 106 24W
Kremnica, *Slovak Rep.* **35 C11** 48 45N 18 50 E
Krems, *Austria* **34 C8** 48 25N 15 36 E
Kremsmünster, *Austria* **34 C7** 48 3N 14 8 E
Krenau = Chrzanów, *Poland* **55 H6** 50 10N 19 21 E
Kretinga, *Lithuania* **15 J19** 55 53N 21 15 E
Krettamia, *Algeria* **110 C4** 28 47N 3 27W
Krettsy, *Russia* **58 C7** 58 15N 32 30 E
Kreuzberg, *Germany* **31 E5** 50 22N 9 58 E
Kreuzburg = Kluczbork, *Poland* **55 H5** 50 58N 18 12 E
Kreuzlingen, *Switz.* **33 A8** 47 38N 9 10 E
Kreuztal, *Germany* **30 E4** 50 57N 8 0 E
Kría Vrísi, *Greece* **50 F6** 40 41N 22 18 E
Kribi, *Cameroon* **113 E6** 2 57N 9 56 E
Krichem, *Bulgaria* **51 D8** 42 8N 24 28 E
Krichev = Krychaw, *Belarus* **58 F6** 53 40N 31 41 E
Kriens, *Switz.* **33 B6** 47 2N 8 17 E
Krim, *Slovenia* **45 C11** 45 53N 14 30 E
Krim-Krim, *Chad* **109 G3** 9 0N 15 24 E
Krindachyovka = Krasnyy Luch, *Ukraine* **59 H10** 48 13N 39 0 E
Kriós, Ákra, *Greece* **39 E4** 35 13N 23 34 E
Krishna →, *India* **95 G5** 15 57N 80 59 E
Krishnagiri, *India* **95 H4** 12 32N 78 16 E
Krishnanagar, *India* **93 H13** 23 24N 88 33 E
Krishnaraja Sagara, *India* **95 H3** 12 20N 76 30 E
Kristdala, *Sweden* **17 G10** 57 24N 16 13 E
Kristians = Oppland □, *Norway* **18 C6** 61 15N 9 40 E
Kristiansand, *Norway* **18 F5** 58 8N 8 1 E
Kristianstad, *Sweden* **17 H8** 56 2N 14 9 E
Kristiansund, *Norway* **18 A4** 63 7N 7 45 E
Kristiinankaupunki, *Finland* **15 E19** 62 16N 21 21 E
Kristinehamn, *Sweden* **16 E8** 59 18N 14 7 E
Kristinestad = Kristiinankaupunki, *Finland* **15 E19** 62 16N 21 21 E
Kristinopol = Chervonohrad, *Ukraine* **59 G3** 50 25N 24 10 E
Krithotí, Ákra, *Greece* **39 B3** 38 30N 21 2 E
Kríti, *Greece* **39 E6** 35 15N 25 0 E
Kritsá, *Greece* **39 E6** 35 10N 25 41 E
Kriva →, *Macedonia* **50 D5** 42 5N 21 47 E
Kriva Palanka, *Macedonia* **50 D6** 42 11N 22 19 E
Krivaja →, *Bos.-H.* **52 F3** 44 27N 18 9 E
Krivelj, *Serbia & M.* **50 B6** 44 10N 22 5 E
Křivoklátsko ⌓, *Czech Rep.* **34 A6** 50 1N 13 51 E
Krivoy Rog = Kryvyy Rih, *Ukraine* **59 J7** 47 51N 33 20 E
Križevci, *Croatia* **45 B13** 46 3N 16 32 E
Krk, *Croatia* **45 C11** 45 8N 14 40 E
Krka △, *Croatia* **45 E12** 43 53N 15 56 E
Krka →, *Slovenia* **45 C12** 45 50N 15 30 E
Krkonoše, *Czech Rep.* **34 A8** 50 50N 15 35 E
Krkonoše △, *Czech Rep.* **34 A8** 50 43N 15 39 E
Krnjaja = Kljajićevo, *Serbia & M.* **52 E4** 45 45N 19 17 E
Krnov, *Czech Rep.* **35 A10** 50 5N 17 40 E
Krobia, *Poland* **55 G3** 51 47N 16 59 E
Krøderen, *Norway* **18 D6** 60 9N 9 49 E
Krokeaí, *Greece* **48 E4** 36 53N 22 32 E
Krokek, *Sweden* **17 F10** 58 40N 16 24 E
Krokodil →, *Mozam.* **117 D5** 25 14 S 32 18 E
Krokom, *Sweden* **16 A8** 63 20N 14 30 E
Krokowa, *Poland* **54 D5** 54 47N 18 9 E
Króksfjarðarnes, *Iceland* **11 B5** 65 27N 21 56W
Krokstadelva, *Norway* **18 E7** 59 56N 10 1 E
Krolevets, *Ukraine* **59 G7** 51 35N 33 20 E
Królewska Huta = Chorzów, *Poland* **55 H5** 50 18N 18 57 E
Kroměříž, *Czech Rep.* **35 B10** 49 18N 17 21 E
Krompachy, *Slovak Rep.* **35 C13** 48 54N 20 52 E
Kromy, *Russia* **59 F8** 52 48N 35 48 E
Kronach, *Germany* **31 E7** 50 14N 11 19 E
Kronau = Kranjska Gora, *Slovenia* **45 B10** 46 29N 13 48 E
Krong Kaoh Kong, *Cambodia* **78 B2** 11 35N 103 0 E
Kronobergs län □, *Sweden* **17 H8** 56 45N 14 30 E
Kronprins Christian Land, *Greenland* **10 A8** 80 30N 22 0W
Kronprins Frederik Land, *Greenland* **10 B5** 79 0N 55 0W
Kronprins Olav Kyst, *Antarctica* **7 C5** 69 0 S 42 0 E
Kronprinsesse Märtha Kyst, *Antarctica* **7 D2** 73 30 S 10 0W
Kronshtadt, *Russia* **58 C5** 59 57N 29 51 E
Kronstadt = Braşov, *Romania* **53 E10** 45 38N 25 35 E
Kroonstad, *S. Africa* **116 D4** 27 43 S 27 19 E
Kröpelin, *Germany* **30 A7** 54 4N 11 47 E
Kropotkin, *Russia* **61 H5** 45 28N 40 28 E
Kropp, *Germany* **30 A5** 54 24N 9 31 E
Krosna, *Lithuania* **54 D10** 54 23N 23 33 E
Krośniewice, *Poland* **55 F6** 52 15N 19 11 E
Krosno, *Poland* **55 J8** 49 42N 21 46 E
Krosno Odrzańskie, *Poland* **55 F2** 52 3N 15 7 E
Krotoszyn, *Poland* **55 G4** 51 42N 17 23 E
Krotovka, *Russia* **60 D10** 53 18N 51 10 E
Kroussón, *Greece* **39 E5** 35 13N 24 59 E
Krrabë, *Albania* **50 E3** 41 13N 20 0 E
Krško, *Slovenia* **45 C12** 45 57N 15 30 E
Krstača, *Serbia & M.* **50 D4** 42 57N 20 8 E
Kruger △, *S. Africa* **117 C5** 24 50 S 26 10 E
Krugersdorp, *S. Africa* **117 D4** 26 5 S 27 46 E
Kruisfontein, *S. Africa* **116 E3** 33 59 S 24 43 E
Krujë, *Albania* **50 E3** 41 32N 19 46 E
Krulevshchina = Krulyewshchyna, *Belarus* **58 E4** 55 5N 27 45 E
Krulyewshchyna, *Belarus* **58 E4** 55 5N 27 45 E
Krumbach, *Germany* **31 G6** 48 13N 10 22 E
Krumë, *Albania* **50 D4** 42 14N 20 28 E
Krummau = Český Krumlov, *Czech Rep.* **34 C7** 48 43N 14 21 E
Krummhübel = Karpacz, *Poland* **55 H2** 50 46N 15 46 E
Krumovgrad, *Bulgaria* **51 E9** 41 29N 25 38 E
Krung Thep = Bangkok, *Thailand* **86 F3** 13 45N 100 35 E
Krupanj, *Serbia & M.* **50 B3** 44 25N 19 22 E
Krupina, *Slovak Rep.* **35 C12** 48 22N 19 5 E
Krupinica →, *Slovak Rep.* **35 C11** 48 4N 18 55 E
Krupki, *Belarus* **58 E5** 54 19N 29 8 E
Krusenstern, C., *U.S.A.* **144 C7** 67 8N 163 45W
Kruševac, *Serbia & M.* **50 C5** 43 35N 21 28 E
Kruševo, *Macedonia* **50 E5** 41 23N 21 19 E
Krushchyov = Svitlovodsk, *Ukraine* **59 H7** 49 2N 33 13 E
Krushelnyksya, *Ukraine* **55 J10** 49 7N 23 29 E
Kruszwica, *Poland* **55 F5** 52 40N 18 20 E
Krychaw, *Belarus* **58 F6** 53 40N 31 41 E
Krymsk, *Russia* **59 K10** 44 50N 38 0 E
Krymskiy Poluostrov = Krymskyy Pivostriv, *Ukraine* **59 K8** 45 0N 34 0 E
Krymskyy Pivostriv, *Ukraine* **59 K8** 45 0N 34 0 E
Krynica, *Poland* **55 J7** 49 25N 20 57 E
Krynica Morska, *Poland* **54 D6** 54 23N 19 28 E
Krynki, *Poland* **55 E10** 53 17N 23 43 E
Krynychne, *Ukraine* **53 E13** 45 32N 28 40 E
Kryvyy Rih, *Ukraine* **59 J7** 47 51N 33 20 E
Kryzhopil, *Ukraine* **53 B13** 48 23N 28 53 E
Krzemieniec = Kremenets, *Ukraine* **59 G3** 50 8N 25 43 E
Krzepice, *Poland* **55 H5** 50 58N 18 50 E

Krzeszów, *Poland* **55 H9** 50 24N 22 21 E
Krzna →, *Poland* **55 F10** 52 8N 23 32 E
Krzywiń, *Poland* **55 G3** 51 58N 16 50 E
Krzyż Wielkopolski, *Poland* **55 F2** 52 52N 16 0 E
Ksabi, *Morocco* **110 B4** 32 51N 4 13W
Ksar Chellala, *Algeria* **111 A5** 35 13N 2 19 E
Ksar el Boukhari, *Algeria* **111 A5** 35 51N 2 52 E
Ksar el Kebir, *Morocco* **110 B3** 35 0N 6 0W
Ksar es Souk = Er Rachidia, *Morocco* **110 B4** 31 58N 4 20W
Ksar Rhilane, *Tunisia* **108 B1** 33 0N 9 39 E
Książ Wielkopolski, *Poland* **55 F4** 52 4N 17 14 E
Ksour, Mts. des, *Algeria* **111 B4** 32 45N 0 30W
Kstovo, *Russia* **60 B7** 56 12N 44 13 E
Ku, W. el →, *Sudan* **107 E2** 13 37N 25 15 E
Ku-Ring-Gai Chase △, *Australia* **129 B9** 33 39 S 151 14 E
Ku Tree Reservoir, *U.S.A.* **145 K14** 21 30N 157 59W
Kuah, *Malaysia* **87 J2** 6 19N 99 51 E
Kuala, *Indonesia* **84 B3** 2 55N 105 47 E
Kuala Belait, *Malaysia* **85 B4** 4 35N 114 11 E
Kuala Berang, *Malaysia* **87 K4** 5 5N 103 1 E
Kuala Dungun = Dungun, *Malaysia* **87 K4** 4 45N 103 25 E
Kuala Kangsar, *Malaysia* **87 K3** 4 46N 100 56 E
Kuala Kelawang, *Malaysia* **87 L4** 2 56N 102 5 E
Kuala Kerai, *Malaysia* **87 K4** 5 30N 102 12 E
Kuala Kerian, *Malaysia* **87 c** 5 10N 100 25 E
Kuala Lipis, *Malaysia* **87 K4** 4 10N 102 3 E
Kuala Lumpur, *Malaysia* **87 L3** 3 9N 101 41 E
Kuala Nerang, *Malaysia* **87 J3** 6 16N 100 37 E
Kuala Pilah, *Malaysia* **87 L4** 2 45N 102 15 E
Kuala Rompin, *Malaysia* **87 L4** 2 49N 103 29 E
Kuala Selangor, *Malaysia* **87 L3** 3 20N 101 15 E
Kuala Sepetang, *Malaysia* **87 K3** 4 49N 100 28 E
Kuala Terengganu, *Malaysia* **87 K4** 5 20N 103 8 E
Kualajelai, *Indonesia* **85 C4** 2 58 S 110 46 E
Kualakapuas, *Indonesia* **85 C4** 2 55 S 114 20 E
Kualakurun, *Indonesia* **85 C4** 1 10 S 113 50 E
Kualapembuang, *Indonesia* **85 C4** 3 14 S 112 38 E
Kualapuu, *U.S.A.* **145 B4** 21 10N 157 2W
Kualasimpang, *Indonesia* **84 B1** 4 17N 98 3 E
Kualoa Pt., *U.S.A.* **145 J14** 21 31N 157 50W
Kuamat, *Malaysia* **85 A5** 5 13N 117 30 E
Kuancheng, *China* **75 D10** 40 37N 118 30 E
Kuandang, *Indonesia* **82 A2** 0 56N 123 1 E
Kuandian, *China* **75 D13** 40 45N 124 45 E
Kuangchou = Guangzhou, *China* **77 F9** 23 5N 113 10 E
Kuanshan, *Taiwan* **77 F13** 23 3N 121 9 E
Kuantan, *Malaysia* **87 L4** 3 49N 103 20 E
Kuapa Pond, *U.S.A.* **145 K14** 21 17N 157 43W
Kuba = Quba, *Azerbaijan* **61 K9** 41 21N 48 32 E
Kuban →, *Russia* **59 K9** 45 20N 37 30 E
Kuban Depression = Prikubanskaya Nizmennost, *Russia* **61 H4** 45 39N 38 33 E
Kubenskoye, Ozero, *Russia* **58 C10** 59 40N 39 25 E
Kuberle = Krasnoarmeyskiy, *Russia* **61 G6** 47 0N 42 12 E
Küblis, *Switz.* **33 C9** 46 54N 9 45 E
Kubokawa, *Japan* **72 D5** 33 12N 133 8 E
Kubor, Mt., *Papua N. G.* **132 D3** 6 10 S 144 44 E
Kubrat, *Bulgaria* **51 C10** 43 49N 26 31 E
Kubu, *Indonesia* **79 J18** 8 16 S 115 35 E
Kubutambahan, *Indonesia* **79 J18** 8 5 S 115 10 E
Kucar, Tanjung, *Indonesia* **79 K18** 8 39 S 114 34 E
Kučevo, *Serbia & M.* **50 B5** 44 30N 21 40 E
Kucha Gompa, *India* **93 B7** 34 25N 76 56 E
Kuchaman, *India* **92 F6** 27 13N 74 47 E
Kuchchaveli, *Sri Lanka* **95 K5** 8 49N 81 6 E
Kuchenspitze, *Austria* **34 D3** 47 7N 10 12 E
Kuchinda, *India* **93 J11** 21 44N 84 21 E
Kuching, *Malaysia* **85 B4** 1 33N 110 25 E
Kuchino-eruba-Jima, *Japan* **71 J5** 30 28N 130 12 E
Kuchino-Shima, *Japan* **71 K4** 29 57N 129 55 E
Kuchinotsu, *Japan* **72 E2** 32 36N 130 11 E
Kuchl, *Austria* **34 D6** 47 37N 13 9 E
Kūchnay Darvīshān, *Afghan.* **91 C2** 30 59N 64 10 E
Kuchurhan →, *Ukraine* **53 D14** 46 33N 29 57 E
Kucing = Kuching, *Malaysia* **85 B4** 1 33N 110 25 E
Kuçovë, *Albania* **50 F3** 40 47N 19 57 E
Küçükbahçe, *Turkey* **49 C8** 38 33N 26 24 E
Küçükköy, *Turkey* **49 B8** 39 16N 26 42 E
Küçükkuyu, *Turkey* **49 B8** 39 32N 26 36 E
Küçükmenderes →, *Turkey* **49 D9** 37 57N 27 16 E
Kud →, *Pakistan* **92 F2** 26 5N 66 20 E
Kudal, *India* **95 F1** 16 2N 73 41 E
Kudalier →, *India* **94 E4** 18 35N 79 48 E
Kudamatsu, *Japan* **72 D3** 34 0N 131 52 E
Kudara, *Tajikistan* **65 D6** 38 25N 72 39 E
Kudat, *Malaysia* **85 A5** 6 55N 116 55 E
Kudelka = Asbest, *Russia* **64 C8** 57 0N 61 30 E
Kudirkos Naumiestis, *Lithuania* **54 D9** 54 46N 22 53 E
Kudowa-Zdrój, *Poland* **55 H3** 50 27N 16 15 E
Kudremukh, *India* **95 H2** 13 15N 75 20 E
Kudus, *Indonesia* **85 D4** 6 48 S 110 51 E
Kudymkar, *Russia* **64 B5** 59 1N 54 39 E
Kueiyang = Guiyang, *China* **76 D6** 26 32N 106 40 E
Kufra Oasis = Al Kufrah, *Libya* **108 D4** 24 17N 23 15 E
Kufstein, *Austria* **34 D5** 47 35N 12 11 E
Kugaaruk = Pelly Bay, *Canada* **139 B11** 68 38N 89 50W
Kugluktuk, *Canada* **138 B8** 67 50N 115 5W
Kugong I., *Canada* **140 A4** 56 18N 79 50W
Kūhak, *Iran* **91 D1** 27 12N 63 10 E
Kuhan, *Pakistan* **92 E2** 28 19N 67 14 E
Kūhbonān, *Iran* **97 D8** 31 23N 56 19 E
Kūhestak, *Iran* **97 E8** 26 47N 57 2 E
Kūhestān, *Afghan.* **91 B1** 34 39N 61 12 E
Kuhin, *Iran* **97 B6** 36 22N 49 40 E
Kūhīrī, *Iran* **97 E9** 26 55N 61 2 E
Kuhnsdorf, *Austria* **34 E7** 46 37N 14 38 E
Kūhpāyeh, *Eşfahan, Iran* **97 C7** 32 44N 52 20 E
Kūhpāyeh, *Kermān, Iran* **97 D8** 30 35N 57 15 E
Kūhrān, Kūh-e, *Iran* **97 E8** 26 46N 58 12 E
Kui Buri, *Thailand* **87 F2** 12 3N 99 52 E
Kuichong, *China* **69 F11** 22 38N 114 25 E
Kuiseb →, *Namibia* **116 C1** 22 59 S 14 31 E
Kuito, *Angola* **115 E3** 12 22 S 16 55 E
Kuiu I., *U.S.A.* **142 B2** 57 45N 134 10W
Kujang, *N. Korea* **75 E14** 39 57N 126 1 E
Kujawsko-Pomorskie □, *Poland* **54 E5** 53 20N 18 30 E
Kuji, *Japan* **70 D10** 40 11N 141 46 E
Kujū-San, *Japan* **72 D3** 33 5N 131 15 E
Kukarka = Sovetsk, *Russia* **60 B9** 57 38N 48 53 E
Kukava, *Ukraine* **53 B12** 48 37N 27 43 E
Kukavica, *Serbia & M.* **50 D5** 42 48N 21 57 E
Kukawa, *Nigeria* **113 C7** 12 58N 13 27 E
Kukës, *Albania* **50 D4** 42 5N 20 27 E
Kuki, *Japan* **73 A11** 36 4N 139 40 E
Kukipi, *Papua N. G.* **132 E4** 8 10 S 146 6 E
Kukmor, *Russia* **60 B10** 56 11N 50 54 E
Kükong = Shaoguan, *China* **77 E9** 24 48N 113 35 E
Kukuihaele, *U.S.A.* **145 C6** 20 5N 155 35W
Kukup, *Malaysia* **87 d** 1 20N 103 27 E
Kukup, Pulau, *Malaysia* **87 d** 1 18N 103 25 E
Kukvidze, *Russia* **60 E6** 50 40N 43 0 E
Kula, *Bulgaria* **50 C6** 43 52N 22 36 E
Kula, *Serbia & M.* **52 E4** 45 37N 19 32 E
Kula, *Turkey* **49 C10** 38 32N 28 40 E
Kula Gulf, *Solomon Is.* **133 M9** 8 5 S 157 18 E
Kulachi, *Pakistan* **92 D4** 31 56N 70 27 E
Kulai, *Malaysia* **87 M4** 1 44N 103 35 E
Kulaly, Ostrov, *Kazakhstan* **61 H10** 45 0N 50 0 E
Kulanak, *Kyrgyzstan* **65 C7** 41 22N 75 30 E
Kulasekarappattinam, *India* **95 K4** 8 20N 78 5 E
Kulassein I., *Phil.* **81 H3** 6 25N 120 41 E
Kulaura, *Bangla.* **90 C4** 24 32N 92 3 E
Kulautuva, *Lithuania* **54 D10** 54 56N 23 36 E
Kuldīga, *Latvia* **15 H19** 56 58N 21 59 E
Kuldīga □, *Latvia* **54 B8** 56 55N 22 0 E
Kuldja = Yining, *China* **66 E9** 43 58N 81 10 E
Kuldu, *Sudan* **107 E2** 12 50N 28 30 E
Kulebaki, *Russia* **60 C6** 55 22N 42 25 E
Kulen, *Cambodia* **86 F5** 13 50N 104 40 E
Kulen Vakuf, *Bos.-H.* **45 D13** 44 35N 16 2 E
Kulgam, *India* **93 C6** 33 36N 75 2 E
Kulgera, *Australia* **126 D1** 25 50 S 133 18 E
Kulim, *Malaysia* **87 K3** 5 22N 100 34 E
Kulin, *Australia* **125 F2** 32 40 S 118 2 E
Kulittalai, *India* **95 J4** 10 55N 78 25 E
Kulkayu = Hartley Bay, *Canada* **142 C3** 53 25N 129 15W
Kullen, *Sweden* **17 H6** 56 18N 12 26 E
Kulma Pass, *Asia* **65 D7** 38 5N 74 50 E
Kulmbach, *Germany* **31 E7** 50 6N 11 26 E
Kŭlob, *Tajikistan* **65 E4** 37 55N 69 50 E
Kulp, *Turkey* **101 C9** 38 29N 41 2 E
Kulpawn →, *Ghana* **113 D4** 10 20N 1 5W
Kulsary, *Kazakhstan* **57 E9** 46 59N 54 1 E
Kulti, *India* **93 H12** 23 43N 86 50 E
Kulu, *India* **92 D7** 31 58N 77 6 E
Kulu, *Turkey* **100 C5** 39 5N 33 4 E
Kulumadau, *Papua N. G.* **132 E7** 9 3 S 152 43 E
Kulumbura, *Australia* **124 B4** 13 55 S 126 35 E
Kulunda, *Russia* **66 D8** 52 35N 78 57 E
Kulungar, *Afghan.* **92 C3** 34 0N 69 2 E
Kūlvand, *Iran* **97 D7** 31 21N 54 35 E
Kulwin, *Australia* **128 C5** 35 0 S 142 42 E
Kulyab = Kŭlob, *Tajikistan* **65 E4** 37 55N 69 50 E
Kuma, *Japan* **72 D4** 33 39N 132 54 E
Kuma →, *Russia* **61 H8** 44 55N 47 0 E
Kumafşarı, *Turkey* **49 D11** 37 19N 29 32 E
Kumaganum, *Nigeria* **113 C7** 13 8N 10 38 E
Kumagaya, *Japan* **73 A11** 36 9N 139 22 E
Kumai, *Indonesia* **85 C4** 2 44 S 111 43 E
Kumak, *Russia* **64 F8** 51 10N 60 8 E
Kumalar Dağı, *Turkey* **49 C12** 38 15N 30 20 E
Kumamba, Kepulauan, *Indonesia* **83 B5** 1 36 S 138 45 E
Kumamoto, *Japan* **72 E2** 32 45N 130 45 E
Kumamoto □, *Japan* **72 E2** 32 55N 130 55 E
Kumano, *Japan* **73 D8** 33 54N 136 5 E
Kumano-Nada, *Japan* **73 D8** 33 47N 136 20 E
Kumanovo, *Macedonia* **50 D5** 42 9N 21 42 E
Kumar →, *Afghan.* **91 B3** 34 30N 70 28 E
Kumara, *N.Z.* **131 C6** 42 37 S 171 12 E
Kumarina, *Australia* **125 D2** 24 41 S 119 32 E
Kumarkhali, *Bangla.* **90 D2** 23 51N 89 15 E
Kumasi, *Ghana* **112 D4** 6 41N 1 38W
Kumba, *Cameroon* **113 E6** 4 36N 9 24 E
Kumbağ, *Turkey* **51 F11** 40 51N 27 27 E
Kumbakonam, *India* **95 J4** 10 58N 79 25 E
Kumbarilla, *Australia* **127 D5** 27 15 S 150 55 E
Kumbe, *Indonesia* **83 C6** 8 21 S 140 13 E
Kumbhraj, *India* **92 G7** 24 22N 77 3 E
Kumbia, *Australia* **127 D5** 26 41 S 151 39 E
Kumbo, *Cameroon* **113 D7** 6 15N 10 36 E
Kumbukkan Oya →, *Sri Lanka* **95 L5** 6 35N 81 40 E
Kŭmch'ŏn, *N. Korea* **75 E14** 38 10N 126 29 E
Kumdah, *Si. Arabia* **98 B4** 20 23N 45 5 E
Kumdok, *India* **93 C8** 33 32N 78 10 E
Kume-Shima, *Japan* **71 L3** 26 20N 126 47 E
Kumeny, *Russia* **60 A9** 58 10N 49 47 E
Kumertau, *Russia* **64 E5** 52 45N 55 57 E
Kumharsain, *India* **92 D7** 31 19N 77 27 E
Kŭmhwa, *S. Korea* **75 E14** 38 17N 127 28 E
Kumi, *Uganda* **118 B3** 1 30N 33 58 E
Kumkale, *Turkey* **51 G10** 39 59N 26 11 E
Kumkurgan = Qumqŭrghan, *Uzbekistan* **65 E3** 37 49N 67 35 E
Kumla, *Sweden* **16 E9** 59 8N 15 10 E
Kumluca, *Turkey* **49 E12** 36 22N 30 20 E
Kummerower See, *Germany* **30 B8** 53 49N 12 51 E
Kumo, *Nigeria* **113 C7** 10 1N 11 12 E
Kumo älv = Kokemäenjoki →, *Finland* **15 F19** 61 32N 21 44 E
Kumon Bum, *Burma* **90 B6** 26 30N 97 15 E
Kumotori-Yama, *Japan* **73 B10** 35 51N 138 57 E
Kumta, *India* **95 G2** 14 29N 74 25 E
Kumukahi, C., *U.S.A.* **145 D7** 19 31N 154 49W
Kumusi →, *Papua N. G.* **132 E5** 8 16 S 148 13 E
Kumylzhenskaya, *Russia* **60 F6** 49 51N 42 38 E
Kunágota, *Hungary* **52 D6** 46 26N 21 3 E
Kunak, *Malaysia* **85 B5** 4 41N 118 15 E
Kunashir, Ostrov, *Russia* **67 E15** 44 0N 146 0 E
Kunchaung, *Burma* **90 D6** 23 50N 96 35 E
Kunda, *Estonia* **15 G22** 59 30N 26 34 E
Kunda, *India* **93 G9** 25 43N 81 31 E
Kundar →, *Pakistan* **92 D3** 31 56N 69 19 E
Kundelungu △, *Dem. Rep. of the Congo* **119 E2** 10 30 S 27 40 E
Kundelungu Ouest △, *Dem. Rep. of the Congo* **119 D2** 9 55 S 27 17 E
Kundian, *Pakistan* **92 C4** 32 27N 71 28 E
Kundiawa, *Papua N. G.* **132 D3** 6 2 S 145 1 E
Kundla, *India* **92 J4** 21 21N 71 25 E
Kundur, *Indonesia* **84 C3** 3 8 S 107 48 E
Kung, Ao, *Thailand* **87 a** 8 5N 98 24 E
Kunga →, *Bangla.* **90 E2** 21 46N 89 30 E
Kungälv, *Sweden* **17 G5** 57 53N 11 59 E
Kunghit I., *Canada* **142 C2** 52 6N 131 3W
Kungrad = Qŭnghirot, *Uzbekistan* **66 E6** 43 6N 58 54 E
Kungsängen, *Sweden* **16 E11** 59 29N 17 45 E
Kungsbacka, *Sweden* **17 G6** 57 30N 12 5 E
Kungsgården, *Sweden* **16 D10** 60 37N 16 35 E
Kungshamn, *Sweden* **17 F5** 58 22N 11 15 E
Kungsör, *Sweden* **16 E10** 59 25N 16 5 E
Kungu, *Dem. Rep. of the Congo* **114 B3** 2 47N 19 12 E
Kungur, *Russia* **64 C6** 57 25N 56 57 E
Kungurri, *Australia* **126 K6** 21 4 S 148 45 E
Kungyangon, *Burma* **90 G6** 16 27N 96 20 E
Kunhar →, *Pakistan* **93 B5** 34 20N 73 30 E
Kunhegyes, *Hungary* **52 C5** 47 22N 20 36 E
Kunia, *U.S.A.* **145 K13** 21 28N 158 4W
Kunimi-Dake, *Japan* **72 E3** 32 33N 131 1 E
Kuningan, *Indonesia* **85 D3** 6 59 S 108 29 E
Kunisaki, *Japan* **72 D3** 33 33N 131 45 E
Kunjirap Daban, *Pakistan* **65 E7** 36 52N 75 27 E
Kunlara, *Australia* **128 C3** 34 54 S 139 55 E
Kunlong, *Burma* **76 F2** 23 20N 98 50 E
Kunlun Shan, *Asia* **68 C3** 36 0N 86 30 E
Kunmadaras, *Hungary* **52 C5** 47 28N 20 45 E
Kunming, *China* **76 E4** 25 1N 102 41 E
Kunnamkulam, *India* **95 J3** 10 38N 76 7 E
Kunów, *Poland* **55 H8** 50 57N 21 17 E
Kunsan, *S. Korea* **75 G14** 35 59N 126 45 E
Kunshan, *China* **77 B13** 31 22N 120 58 E
Kunszentmárton, *Hungary* **52 D5** 46 50N 20 20 E
Kunszentmiklós, *Hungary* **52 C4** 47 2N 19 8 E
Kuntaur, *Senegal* **112 C2** 13 40N 14 48W
Kunua, *Papua N. G.* **132 C8** 5 46 S 154 43 E
Kununurra, *Australia* **124 C4** 15 40 S 128 50 E
Kunwari →, *India* **93 F8** 26 26N 79 11 E
Kunya-Urgench = Köneürgench, *Turkmenistan* **66 E6** 42 19N 59 10 E
Künzelsau, *Germany* **31 F5** 49 17N 9 42 E
Kunzulu, *Dem. Rep. of the Congo* **114 C3** 3 28 S 16 12 E
Kuopio, *Finland* **14 E22** 62 53N 27 35 E
Kupa →, *Croatia* **45 C13** 45 28N 16 24 E
Kupang, *Indonesia* **82 D2** 10 19 S 123 39 E
Kupiano, *Papua N. G.* **132 F5** 10 4 S 148 14 E
Kupreanof I., *U.S.A.* **142 B2** 56 50N 133 30W
Kupres, *Bos.-H.* **52 G2** 43 56N 17 15 E
Kupyansk, *Ukraine* **59 H9** 49 52N 37 35 E
Kupyansk-Uzlovoi, *Ukraine* **59 H9** 49 40N 37 43 E
Kuqa, *China* **68 B3** 41 35N 82 30 E
Kur, *Indonesia* **83 C4** 5 20 S 132 0 E
Kür →, *Azerbaijan* **101 C13** 39 29N 49 15 E
Kur →, *Bhutan* **90 B3** 26 50N 91 0 E
Kür Dili, *Azerbaijan* **97 B6** 39 3N 49 13 E
Kura = Kür →, *Azerbaijan* **101 C13** 39 29N 49 15 E
Kurahashi-Jima, *Japan* **72 C4** 34 8N 132 31 E
Kuranda, *Australia* **126 B4** 16 48 S 145 35 E
Kuranga, *India* **92 H3** 22 4N 69 10 E
Kurashiki, *Japan* **72 C5** 34 40N 133 50 E
Kurayoshi, *Japan* **72 B5** 35 26N 133 50 E
Kürdämir, *Azerbaijan* **61 K9** 40 25N 48 3 E
Kurday = Qorday, *Kazakhstan* **65 B7** 43 21N 74 59 E
Kurdistan, *Asia* **101 D10** 37 20N 43 30 E
Kurduvadi, *India* **94 E2** 18 8N 75 29 E
Kŭrdzhali, *Bulgaria* **51 E9** 41 38N 25 21 E
Kure, *Japan* **72 C4** 34 14N 132 32 E
Küre, *Turkey* **100 B5** 41 48N 33 43 E
Küre Dağları, *Turkey* **100 B6** 41 50N 34 10 E
Kure I., *U.S.A.* **145 F8** 28 25N 178 25W
Kuressaare, *Estonia* **15 G20** 58 15N 22 30 E
Kurgan, *Russia* **66 D7** 55 26N 65 18 E
Kurgan-Tyube = Qŭrghonteppa, *Tajikistan* **65 E4** 37 50N 68 47 E
Kurganinsk, *Russia* **61 H5** 44 54N 40 34 E
Kurgannaya = Kurganinsk, *Russia* **61 H5** 44 54N 40 34 E
Kuri, *India* **92 F4** 26 37N 70 43 E
Kuria Maria Is. = Khurīyā Murīyā, Jazā'ir, *Oman* **99 C6** 17 30N 55 58 E
Kurichchi, *India* **95 J3** 11 36N 77 35 E
Kuridala, *Australia* **126 C3** 21 16 S 140 29 E
Kurigram, *Bangla.* **90 C2** 25 49N 89 39 E
Kurik, *Indonesia* **83 C5** 8 9 S 139 59 E
Kurikka, *Finland* **15 E20** 62 36N 22 24 E
Kuril Is. = Kurilskiye Ostrova, *Russia* **67 E15** 45 0N 150 0 E
Kuril Trench, *Pac. Oc.* **62 E19** 44 0N 153 0 E
Kurilsk, *Russia* **67 E15** 45 14N 147 53 E
Kurilskiye Ostrova, *Russia* **67 E15** 45 0N 150 0 E
Kurino, *Japan* **72 F2** 31 57N 130 43 E
Kurinskaya Kosa = Kür Dili, *Azerbaijan* **97 B6** 39 3N 49 13 E
Kurisches Haff = Kurshskiy Zaliv, *Russia* **15 J19** 55 9N 21 6 E
Kurkheda, *India* **94 D5** 20 37N 80 12 E
Kurkur, *Egypt* **106 C3** 23 50N 32 0 E
Kurla, *India* **94 E1** 19 5N 72 52 E
Kurlovskiy, *Russia* **60 C5** 55 25N 40 40 E
Kurmuk, *Sudan* **107 E3** 10 33N 34 21 E
Kurnool, *India* **95 G4** 15 45N 78 0 E
Kuro-Shima, *Kagoshima, Japan* **71 J4** 30 50N 129 57 E
Kuro-Shima, *Okinawa, Japan* **71 M2** 24 14N 124 1 E
Kurobe-Gawe →, *Japan* **73 A9** 36 55N 137 25 E
Kurogi, *Japan* **72 D2** 33 12N 130 40 E
Kuror, J., *Sudan* **106 C3** 20 27N 31 30 E
Kurow, *N.Z.* **131 E5** 44 44 S 170 29 E
Kurów, *Poland* **55 G9** 51 23N 22 12 E
Kurrajong, *Australia* **129 B9** 33 33 S 150 42 E
Kurram →, *Pakistan* **91 B3** 32 36N 71 20 E
Kurri Kurri, *Australia* **129 B9** 32 50 S 151 28 E
Kurrimine, *Australia* **126 B4** 17 47 S 146 6 E
Kursavka, *Russia* **61 H6** 44 29N 42 32 E
Kurse Korhi, *India* **94 D5** 20 14N 80 46 E
Kurshskaya Kosa ⌂, *Russia* **54 C7** 55 7N 20 45 E
Kurshskiy Zaliv, *Russia* **15 J19** 55 9N 21 6 E
Kuršių Nerijos △, *Lithuania* **54 C8** 55 30N 21 6 E
Kursk, *Russia* **59 G9** 51 42N 36 11 E
Kursu = Salla, *Finland* **14 C23** 66 50N 28 49 E
Kuršumlija, *Serbia & M.* **50 C5** 43 9N 21 19 E
Kuršumlijska Banja, *Serbia & M.* **50 C5** 43 3N 21 11 E
Kurşunlu, *Bursa, Turkey* **51 F13** 40 3N 29 40 E
Kurşunlu, *Çankırı, Turkey* **100 B5** 40 51N 33 15 E
Kurtalan, *Turkey* **101 D9** 37 56N 41 44 E
Kurtbey, *Turkey* **51 E10** 41 9N 26 35 E
Kürti →, *Kazakhstan* **65 A8** 44 16N 76 42 E
Kurtistown, *U.S.A.* **145 D6** 19 36N 155 4W
Kuru, *Sudan* **107 F2** 7 43N 26 31 E
Kuru, Bahr el →, *Sudan* **107 F2** 8 10N 26 50 E
Kurucaşile, *Turkey* **100 B5** 41 49N 32 42 E
Kuruçay, *Turkey* **96 B3** 39 39N 38 29 E
Kuruktag, *China* **68 B3** 41 0N 89 0 E
Kuruman, *S. Africa* **116 D3** 27 28 S 23 28 E
Kuruman →, *S. Africa* **116 D3** 26 56 S 20 39 E
Kurume, *Japan* **72 D2** 33 15N 130 30 E
Kurun →, *Sudan* **107 F3** 5 30N 34 17 E
Kurunegala, *Sri Lanka* **95 L5** 7 30N 80 23 E
Kurupukari, *Guyana* **169 C6** 4 43N 58 37W
Kurya, *Russia* **56 B10** 61 42N 57 9 E
Kus Gölü, *Turkey* **51 F11** 40 10N 27 55 E
Kusa, *Russia* **64 D7** 55 20N 59 29 E
Kuşadası, *Turkey* **100 D2** 37 52N 27 15 E
Kuşadası Körfezı, *Turkey* **49 D8** 37 56N 27 0 E
Kusamba, *Indonesia* **79 K18** 8 34 S 115 27 E
Kusatsu, *Gumma, Japan* **73 A10** 36 37N 138 36 E
Kusatsu, *Shiga, Japan* **73 C7** 34 58N 135 57 E
Kusawa L., *Canada* **142 A1** 60 20N 136 13W
Kusel, *Germany* **31 F3** 49 32N 7 24 E
Kushaka, *Nigeria* **113 C6** 10 32N 6 48 E
Kushalgarh, *India* **92 H6** 23 10N 74 27 E
Kushalnagar, *India* **95 H2** 12 14N 75 57 E
Kushchevskaya, *Russia* **61 G4** 46 33N 39 35 E
Kusheriki, *Nigeria* **113 C6** 10 33N 6 28 E
Kushikino, *Japan* **72 F2** 31 44N 130 16 E
Kushima, *Japan* **72 F3** 31 29N 131 14 E
Kushimoto, *Japan* **73 D7** 33 28N 135 47 E
Kushiro, *Japan* **70 C12** 43 0N 144 25 E
Kushiro-Gawa →, *Japan* **70 C12** 42 59N 144 23 E
Kushiro Shitsugen △, *Japan* **70 C12** 43 9N 144 26 E
Kūshk, *Iran* **97 D8** 28 46N 56 51 E
Kushka = Gushgy, *Turkmenistan* **66 F7** 35 20N 62 18 E
Kūshkī, *Iran* **96 C5** 33 31N 47 13 E
Kushnarenkovo, *Russia* **64 D5** 55 6N 55 22 E
Kushnytsya, *Ukraine* **53 B8** 48 27N 23 15 E
Kushol, *India* **93 C7** 33 40N 76 36 E
Kushrabat = Koshrabad, *Uzbekistan* **65 C3** 40 18N 66 32 E
Kushtia, *Bangla.* **90 D2** 23 55N 89 5 E
Kushum →, *Kazakhstan* **60 F10** 49 20N 50 30 E
Kushva, *Russia* **64 B7** 58 18N 59 45 E
Kuskokwim →, *U.S.A.* **144 F7** 60 5N 162 25W
Kuskokwim B., *U.S.A.* **144 G7** 59 45N 162 25W
Kuskokwim Mts., *U.S.A.* **144 E9** 62 30N 156 0W
Kusmi, *India* **93 H10** 23 17N 83 55 E
Küsnacht, *Switz.* **33 B7** 47 19N 8 35 E
Kussharo-Ko, *Japan* **70 C12** 43 38N 144 21 E
Küssnacht, *Switz.* **33 B6** 47 5N 8 26 E
Kustanay = Qostanay, *Kazakhstan* **66 D7** 53 10N 63 35 E
Küstenje = Constanţa, *Romania* **53 F13** 44 14N 28 38 E
Küstrin = Kostrzyn, *Poland* **55 F1** 52 35N 14 39 E
Kusu, *Indonesia* **82 A3** 0 53N 127 43 E
Kusu, *Japan* **72 D3** 33 16N 131 9 E
Kut, Ko, *Thailand* **87 G4** 11 40N 102 35 E
Kuta, *Indonesia* **79 K18** 8 43 S 115 11 E
Kutacane, *Indonesia* **84 B1** 3 50N 97 50 E
Kütahya, *Turkey* **49 B12** 39 30N 30 2 E
Kütahya □, *Turkey* **49 B11** 39 10N 29 30 E
Kutaisi, *Georgia* **61 J6** 42 19N 42 40 E
Kutaraja = Banda Aceh, *Indonesia* **84 A1** 5 35N 95 20 E
Kutch, Gulf of = Kachchh, Gulf of, *India* **92 H3** 22 50N 69 15 E
Kutch, Rann of = Kachchh, Rann of, *India* **92 H4** 24 0N 70 0 E
Kutina, *Croatia* **45 C13** 45 29N 16 48 E
Kutiyana, *India* **92 J4** 21 36N 70 2 E
Kutjevo, *Croatia* **52 E2** 45 23N 17 55 E
Kutkai, *Burma* **90 D6** 23 27N 97 56 E
Kutkashen, *Azerbaijan* **61 K8** 40 58N 47 47 E
Kutná Hora, *Czech Rep.* **34 B8** 49 57N 15 16 E
Kutno, *Poland* **55 F6** 52 15N 19 23 E
Kutru, *India* **94 E5** 19 5N 80 46 E
Kutse, *Botswana* **116 C3** 21 7 S 22 16 E
Kuttabul, *Australia* **126 K6** 21 1 S 148 54 E
Kutu, *Dem. Rep. of the Congo* **114 C3** 2 40 S 18 11 E
Kutu Moke, *Dem. Rep. of the Congo* **114 C3** 3 12 S 17 21 E
Kutum, *Sudan* **107 E1** 14 10N 24 40 E
Kúty, *Slovak Rep.* **35 C10** 48 40N 17 3 E
Kuty, *Ukraine* **53 B10** 48 16N 25 11 E
Kuujjuaq, *Canada* **139 C13** 58 6N 68 15W
Kuujjuarapik, *Canada* **140 A4** 55 20N 77 35W
Kuŭp-tong, *N. Korea* **75 D14** 40 45N 126 1 E
Kuusamo, *Finland* **14 D23** 65 57N 29 8 E
Kuusankoski, *Finland* **15 F22** 60 55N 26 38 E
Kuvandyk, *Russia* **64 F6** 51 28N 57 21 E
Kuvango, *Angola* **115 E3** 14 28 S 16 20 E
Kuvasay, *Uzbekistan* **65 C5** 40 18N 71 59 E
Kuvshinovo, *Russia* **58 D8** 57 2N 34 11 E
Kuwait = Al Kuwayt, *Kuwait* **96 D5** 29 30N 48 0 E
Kuwait ■, *Asia* **96 D5** 29 30N 47 30 E
Kuwana, *Japan* **73 B8** 35 5N 136 43 E
Kuwana →, *India* **93 F10** 26 25N 83 15 E
Kuybyshev = Samara, *Russia* **60 D10** 53 8N 50 6 E
Kuybyshev, *Russia* **66 D8** 55 27N 78 19 E
Kuybyshevabad = Kuybyshevskiy, *Tajikistan* **65 E4** 37 52N 68 44 E
Kuybyshevka-Vostochnaya = Belogorsk, *Russia* **67 D13** 51 0N 128 20 E
Kuybyshevo, *Ukraine* **59 J9** 47 25N 36 40 E
Kuybyshevskiy, *Tajikistan* **65 E4** 37 52N 68 44 E
Kuybyshevskoye Vdkhr., *Russia* **60 C9** 55 2N 49 30 E
Kuye He →, *China* **74 E6** 38 23N 110 46 E
Kūyeh, *Iran* **96 B5** 38 45N 47 57 E
Kuylyuk, *Uzbekistan* **65 C4** 41 14N 69 17 E
Kuyto, Ozero, *Russia* **56 B5** 65 6N 31 20 E
Kuyucak, *Turkey* **49 D10** 37 55N 28 28 E
Kuyumba, *Russia* **67 C10** 60 58N 96 59 E
Kuzey Anadolu Dağları, *Turkey* **100 B7** 41 30N 35 0 E
Kuzhitturai, *India* **95 K3** 8 18N 77 11 E
Kuzino, *Russia* **64 C7** 57 1N 59 27 E
Kuzitrin →, *U.S.A.* **144 D6** 65 10N 165 25W
Kuzmin, *Serbia & M.* **52 E4** 45 2N 19 25 E
Kuznetsk, *Russia* **60 D8** 53 12N 46 40 E
Kuznetsovo = Konakovo, *Russia* **58 D9** 56 40N 36 51 E
Kuzomen, *Russia* **56 A6** 66 22N 36 50 E
Kvænangen, *Norway* **14 A19** 70 5N 21 15 E
Kværndrup, *Denmark* **17 J4** 55 10N 10 31 E
Kvaløy, *Norway* **14 B18** 69 40N 18 30 E
Kvam, *Norway* **18 C6** 61 40N 9 42 E
Kvänum, *Sweden* **17 F7** 58 18N 13 11 E
Kvareli = Qvareli, *Georgia* **61 K7** 41 57N 45 47 E
Kvarner, *Croatia* **45 D11** 44 50N 14 10 E
Kvarnerič, *Croatia* **45 D11** 44 43N 14 37 E
Kvås, *Norway* **18 F4** 58 16N 7 14 E
Kvernaland, *Norway* **18 F2** 58 47N 5 45 E
Kvichak B., *U.S.A.* **144 G8** 58 48N 157 30W
Kvicksund, *Sweden* **16 E10** 59 27N 16 19 E
Kvikne, *Norway* **18 B7** 62 35N 10 16 E
Kvillsfors, *Sweden* **17 G9** 57 24N 15 29 E
Kvina →, *Norway* **18 F3** 58 19N 6 55 E
Kvinlog, *Norway* **18 F3** 58 31N 6 55 E
Kvirily = Zestaponi, *Georgia* **61 J6** 42 6N 43 0 E
Kvismare kanal, *Sweden* **16 E9** 59 11N 15 35 E
Kvissleby, *Sweden* **16 B11** 62 18N 17 22 E
Kviteseid, *Norway* **18 E5** 59 24N 8 29 E
Kvitøya, *Svalbard* **10 A14** 80 8N 32 35 E
Kwabhaca, *S. Africa* **117 E4** 30 51 S 29 0 E
Kwajalein, *Marshall Is.* **134 G8** 9 5N 167 20 E
Kwakhanai, *Botswana* **116 C3** 21 39 S 21 16 E
Kwakoegron, *Suriname* **169 B6** 5 12N 55 25W
Kwale, *Kenya* **118 C4** 4 15 S 39 31 E
Kwale, *Nigeria* **113 D6** 5 46N 6 26 E
Kwamalasamutu, *Suriname* **169 C6** 2 20N 56 47W
KwaMashu, *S. Africa* **117 D5** 29 45 S 30 58 E
Kwamouth, *Dem. Rep. of the Congo* **114 C3** 3 9 S 16 12 E
Kwando →, *Africa* **116 B3** 18 27 S 23 32 E
Kwangchow = Guangzhou, *China* **77 F9** 23 5N 113 10 E
Kwangdaeri, *N. Korea* **75 D14** 40 31N 127 32 E
Kwangju, *S. Korea* **75 G14** 35 9N 126 54 E
Kwango →, *Dem. Rep. of the Congo* **114 C3** 3 14 S 17 22 E
Kwangsi-Chuang = Guangxi Zhuangzu Zizhiqu □, *China* **76 F7** 24 0N 109 0 E
Kwangtung = Guangdong □, *China* **77 F9** 23 0N 113 0 E
Kwara □, *Nigeria* **113 D6** 8 45N 4 30 E
Kwataboahegan →, *Canada* **140 B3** 51 9N 80 50W
Kwatisore, *Indonesia* **83 B4** 3 18 S 134 50 E
KwaZulu Natal □, *S. Africa* **117 D5** 29 0 S 30 0 E
Kweichow = Guizhou □, *China* **76 D6** 27 0N 107 0 E
Kweilin = Guilin, *China* **77 E8** 25 18N 110 15 E
Kweisui = Hohhot, *China* **74 D6** 40 52N 111 40 E
Kweiyang = Guiyang, *China* **76 D6** 26 32N 106 40 E
Kwekwe, *Zimbabwe* **119 F2** 18 58 S 29 48 E
Kwenge →, *Dem. Rep. of the Congo* **115 C3** 4 50 S 18 44 E
Kwethluk, *U.S.A.* **144 F7** 60 49N 161 26W
Kwidzyn, *Poland* **54 E5** 53 44N 18 55 E
Kwigillingok, *U.S.A.* **144 G7** 59 51N 163 8W
Kwiguk, *U.S.A.* **144 E6** 62 46N 164 30W
Kwiha, *Ethiopia* **107 E4** 13 29N 39 32 E
Kwikila, *Papua N. G.* **132 E4** 9 49 S 147 38 E
Kwilu →, *Dem. Rep. of the Congo* **115 C3** 3 22 S 17 22 E
Kwinana New Town, *Australia* **125 F2** 32 15 S 115 47 E
Kwinbet, *Burma* **90 G5** 16 20N 94 14 E
Kwisa →, *Poland* **55 G2** 51 34N 15 24 E
Kwoka, *Indonesia* **83 B4** 0 31 S 132 27 E
Kwolla, *Nigeria* **113 D6** 9 0N 9 15 E
Kwun Tong, *China* **69 G11** 22 19N 114 13 E
Kya-in-Seikkyi, *Burma* **90 G7** 16 2N 98 8 E
Kyabé, *Chad* **109 G3** 9 30N 19 0 E
Kyabra Cr. →, *Australia* **127 D3** 25 36 S 142 55 E
Kyabram, *Australia* **129 D6** 36 19 S 145 4 E
Kyaikkami, *Burma* **90 G6** 16 4N 97 34 E
Kyaiklat, *Burma* **90 G5** 16 25N 95 40 E
Kyaikmaraw, *Burma* **90 G6** 16 23N 97 44 E
Kyaikthin, *Burma* **90 D5** 23 32N 95 40 E
Kyaikto, *Burma* **86 D1** 17 20N 97 3 E
Kyakhta, *Russia* **67 D11** 50 30N 106 25 E
Kyambura ⌂, *Uganda* **118 C3** 0 7 S 30 9 E
Kyancutta, *Australia* **127 E2** 33 8 S 135 33 E
Kyangin, *Burma* **90 F5** 18 20N 95 20 E
Kyaukhnyat, *Burma* **90 F6** 18 15N 97 31 E
Kyaukki, *Burma* **90 F6** 18 27N 96 56 E
Kyaukkyi, *Burma* **90 F5** 18 15N 94 29 E
Kyaukme, *Burma* **90 D6** 22 32N 97 2 E
Kyaukpadaung, *Burma* **90 E5** 20 52N 95 8 E
Kyaukpyu, *Burma* **90 F4** 19 28N 93 30 E
Kyaukse, *Burma* **90 E6** 21 36N 96 10 E
Kyauktaga, *Burma* **90 F6** 18 10N 96 37 E
Kyauktan, *Burma* **90 G6** 16 38N 96 19 E
Kyauktaw, *Burma* **90 E4** 20 51N 92 59 E
Kyaunggon, *Burma* **90 G5** 17 6N 95 11 E
Kyawkku, *Burma* **90 E6** 21 48N 96 56 E
Kybartai, *Lithuania* **54 D9** 54 39N 22 45 E
Kyburz, *U.S.A.* **160 G6** 38 47N 120 18W
Kyeintali, *Burma* **90 G5** 18 0N 94 29 E
Kyelang, *India* **92 C7** 32 35N 77 2 E
Kyenjojo, *Uganda* **118 B3** 0 40N 30 37 E
Kyidaunggan, *Burma* **90 F6** 19 53N 96 12 E
Kyjov, *Czech Rep.* **35 B10** 49 1N 17 7 E
Kyle, *Canada* **143 C7** 50 50N 108 2W
Kyle Dam, *Zimbabwe* **119 G3** 20 15 S 31 0 E
Kyle of Lochalsh, *U.K.* **22 D3** 57 17N 5 44W
Kyll →, *Germany* **31 F2** 49 48N 6 41 E
Kyllburg, *Germany* **31 E2** 50 2N 6 34 E
Kymijoki →, *Finland* **15 F22** 60 30N 26 55 E
Kymmene älv = Kymijoki →, *Finland* **15 F22** 60 30N 26 55 E
Kyneton, *Australia* **128 D6** 37 10 S 144 29 E
Kynuna, *Australia* **126 C3** 21 37 S 141 55 E
Kyō-ga-Saki, *Japan* **73 B7** 35 45N 135 15 E
Kyoga, L., *Uganda* **118 B3** 1 35N 33 0 E
Kyogle, *Australia* **127 D5** 28 40 S 153 0 E
Kyom →, *Sudan* **107 F2** 8 58N 28 13 E
Kyongju, *S. Korea* **75 G15** 35 51N 129 14 E
Kyŏngsŏng, *N. Korea* **75 D15** 41 35N 129 36 E
Kyōto, *Japan* **73 C7** 35 0N 135 45 E
Kyōto □, *Japan* **73 B7** 35 15N 135 45 E
Kyparissovouno, *Cyprus* **39 E9** 35 19N 33 10 E
Kyperounda, *Cyprus* **39 F8** 34 56N 32 58 E
Kypros = Cyprus ■, *Asia* **39 F9** 35 0N 33 0 E
Kyrenia, *Cyprus* **39 E9** 35 20N 33 20 E
Kyrgyzstan ■, *Asia* **65 C6** 42 0N 75 0 E
Kyritz, *Germany* **30 C8** 52 56N 12 24 E

Kyrkhult, Sweden .... 17 H8 56 22N 14 34 E
Kyrksæterøra, Norway 18 A6 63 18N 9 5 E
Kyrnasivka, Ukraine .. 53 B13 48 35N 28 58 E
Kyrnychky, Ukraine .. 53 E14 45 42N 29 4 E
Kyro älv =
Kyrönjoki ➤,
Finland .... 14 E19 63 14N 21 45 E
Kyrönjoki ➤, Finland 14 E19 63 14N 21 45 E
Kyshtym, Russia ..... 64 D8 55 42N 60 34 E
Kystatyam, Russia .... 67 C13 67 20N 123 10 E
Kysucké Nové Mesto,
Slovak Rep. .... 35 B11 49 18N 18 47 E
Kytay, Ozero, Ukraine 53 E14 45 40N 29 13 E
Kythira = Kíthira,
Greece .... 48 E5 36 8N 23 0 E
Kythréa, Cyprus ..... 39 E9 35 15N 33 29 E
Kytlym, Russia ...... 64 B7 59 30N 59 12 E
Kyu-hkok, Burma .... 90 C7 24 4N 98 4 E
Kyunhla, Burma ..... 90 D5 23 25N 95 15 E
Kyuquot Sound,
Canada 142 D3 50 2N 127 22W
Kyurdamir = Kürdämir,
Azerbaijan .... 61 K9 40 25N 48 3 E
Kyūshū, Japan ...... 72 E3 33 0N 131 0 E
Kyūshū □, Japan .... 72 E3 33 0N 131 0 E
Kyūshū-Sanchi, Japan 72 E3 32 35N 131 17 E
Kyustendil, Bulgaria .. 40 E7 42 16N 22 41 E
Kyusyur, Russia ..... 67 B13 70 19N 127 30 E
Kywong, Australia .... 129 C7 34 58 S 146 44 E
Kyyiv, Ukraine ..... 59 G6 50 30N 30 28 E
Kyyivske Vdskh.,
Ukraine .... 59 G6 51 0N 30 25 E
Kyzyl, Russia .... 67 D10 51 50N 94 30 E
Kyzyl-Adyr, Kyrgyzstan 65 B5 42 39N 71 35 E
Kyzyl-Burun = Siyäzän,
Azerbaijan .... 61 K9 41 3N 49 10 E
Kyzyl-Khoto = Kyzyl,
Russia .... 67 D10 51 50N 94 30 E
Kyzyl Kum, Uzbekistan 65 B2 42 30N 65 0 E
Kyzyl-Kyya, Kyrgyzstan 65 C6 40 16N 72 8 E
Kyzyl-Orda =
Qyzylorda,
Kazakhstan .... 65 A2 44 48N 65 28 E
Kyzyl-Suu, Kyrgyzstan 65 B9 42 20N 78 0 E
Kyzyl-Suu =
Kyrgyzstan ...... 65 D6 38 50N 70 0 E
Kyzyltepa, Uzbekistan 65 C2 40 1N 64 51 E

L

La Albuera, Spain 43 G4 38 45N 6 49W
La Alcarria, Spain 40 E2 40 31N 2 45W
La Almarcha, Spain ... 40 F2 39 41N 2 24W
La Almunia de Doña
Godina, Spain 40 D3 41 29N 1 23W
La Amistad △,
Cent. Amer. 164 E3 9 28N 83 18W
La Asunción,
Venezuela 169 A5 11 2N 63 53W
La Baie, Canada 141 C5 48 19N 70 53W
La Banda, Argentina .. 174 B3 27 45 S 64 10W
La Bañeza, Spain 42 C5 42 17N 5 54W
La Barca, Mexico 162 C4 20 20N 102 40W
La Barge, U.S.A. 158 E8 42 16N 110 12W
La Bastide-Puylaurent,
France .... 28 D7 44 35N 3 55 E
La Baule, France 26 E4 47 17N 2 24W
La Belle, Fla., U.S.A. .. 153 J8 26 46N 81 26W
La Belle, Mo., U.S.A. .. 156 D5 40 7N 91 55W
La Biche ➤, Canada .. 142 B4 59 57N 123 50W
La Biche, L., Canada .. 142 C6 54 50N 112 5W
La Bisbal d'Empordà,
Spain .... 40 D8 41 58N 3 2 E
La Blanquilla,
Venezuela 169 A5 11 51N 64 37W
La Bomba, Mexico 162 A1 31 53N 115 2W
La Brea, Trin. & Tob. .. 169 F19 10 15N 61 37W
La Brède, France 28 D3 44 41N 0 32W
La Bresse, France .... 27 D13 48 2N 6 53 E
La Bureba, Spain 42 C7 42 36N 3 24W
La Cal = Bolivia ..... 173 D6 17 27 S 58 15W
La Calera, Chile ..... 174 C1 32 50 S 71 10W
La Calle = El Kala,
Algeria .... 111 A6 36 50N 8 30 E
La Campana △, Chile . 32 58 S 71 14W
La Campiña, Spain ... 43 H6 37 45N 4 45W
La Canal = Sa Canal,
Spain .... 38 D1 38 51N 1 23 E
La Cañiza = A Cañiza,
Spain 42 C2 42 13N 8 16W
La Canourgue, France 28 D7 44 26N 3 13 E
La Capelle, France ... 27 C10 49 59N 3 50 E
La Carlota, Argentina . 174 C3 33 30 S 63 20W
La Carlota, Phil. ..... 81 F4 10 25N 122 55 E
La Carlota, Spain 43 H6 37 40N 4 56W
La Carolina, Spain ... 43 G7 38 17N 3 38W
La Castellana, Phil. .. 81 F4 10 20N 123 3 E
La Cavalerie, France . 28 D7 44 1N 3 10 E
La Ceiba, Honduras .. 164 C2 15 40N 86 50W
La Ceiba, Venezuela .. 168 C3 9 28N 71 4W
La Chaise-Dieu, France 28 C7 45 18N 3 42 E
La Chapelle d'Angillon,
France .... 27 E9 47 21N 2 25 E
La Chapelle-St-Luc,
France .... 27 D11 48 20N 4 3 E
La Chapelle-sur-Erdre,
France 26 E5 47 18N 1 34W
La Charité-sur-Loire,
France .... 27 E10 47 10N 3 1 E
La Chartre-sur-le-Loir,
France .... 26 E7 47 44N 0 34 E
La Châtaigneraie,
France 28 B3 46 39N 0 44W
La Châtre, France ... 27 F9 46 35N 2 0 E
La Chaux-de-Fonds,
Switz. .... 32 B3 47 7N 6 50 E
La Chorrera, Colombia 168 D3 0 44 S 73 1W
La Chorrera, Panama . 164 E4 8 53N 79 47W
La Ciotat, France .... 29 E9 43 10N 5 37 E
La Clayette, France .. 27 F11 46 17N 4 19 E
La Cocha, Argentina .. 174 B2 27 50 S 65 40W
La Concepción = Ri-
Aba, Eq. Guin. .... 113 E6 3 28N 8 40 E
La Concepción,
Panama 164 E3 8 31N 82 37W
La Concepción,
Venezuela 168 A3 10 30N 71 50W
La Concordia, Mexico 163 D6 16 8N 92 38W
La Coruña = A Coruña,
Spain 42 B2 43 20N 8 25W
La Coruña □, Spain .. 42 B2 43 10N 8 30W
La Côte, Switz. ...... 32 D2 46 25N 6 15 E
La Côte-St-André,
France .... 29 C9 45 24N 5 15 E
La Courtine, France .. 28 C6 45 41N 2 15 E
La Crau,
Bouches-du-Rhône,
France .... 29 E8 43 32N 4 40 E
La Crau, Var, France . 29 E10 43 9N 6 4 E
La Crescent, U.S.A. .. 154 D9 43 50N 91 18W

La Crete, Canada 142 B5 58 11N 116 24W
La Crosse, Fla., U.S.A. 152 F7 29 51N 82 24W
La Crosse, Kans.,
U.S.A. 154 F5 38 32N 99 18W
La Crosse, Wis., U.S.A. 154 D9 43 48N 91 15W
La Cruz, Costa Rica .. 164 D2 11 4N 85 39W
La Cruz, Mexico 162 C3 23 55N 106 54W
La Cumbre, Volcán,
Ecuador .... 172 a 0 21 S 91 32W
La Désirade,
Guadeloupe .... 164 b 16 18N 61 3W
La Digue, Seychelles .. 121 b 4 20 S 55 51 E
La Dorada, Colombia . 168 B3 5 30N 74 40W
La Ensenada, Chile ... 176 B2 41 12 S 72 33W
La Escondida, Mexico 162 C5 24 6N 99 55W
La Esmeralda,
Paraguay .... 174 A3 22 16 S 62 33W
La Esperanza,
Argentina .... 176 B3 40 26 S 68 32W
La Esperanza, Cuba .. 164 B3 22 46N 83 44W
La Esperanza,
Honduras 164 D2 14 15N 88 10W
La Estrada = A
Estrada, Spain 42 C2 42 43N 8 27W
La Faouët, France ... 26 D3 48 2N 3 30W
La Fayette, U.S.A. ... 149 H3 34 42N 85 17W
La Fé, Cuba 164 B3 22 2N 84 15W
La Fère, France ..... 27 C10 49 39N 3 21 E
La Ferté-Bernard,
France .... 26 D7 48 10N 0 40 E
La Ferté-Gaucher,
France .... 27 D10 48 47N 3 19 E
La Ferté-Macé, France 26 D6 48 35N 0 22W
La Ferté-St-Aubin,
France .... 27 E8 47 42N 1 57 E
La Ferté-sous-Jouarre,
France .... 27 D10 48 56N 3 8 E
La Ferté-Vidame,
France .... 26 D7 48 37N 0 53 E
La Flèche, France ... 26 E6 47 42N 0 4W
La Foa, N. Cal. ...... 133 U19 21 43 S 165 50 E
La Follette, U.S.A. ... 149 G3 36 23N 84 7W
La Fontaine, U.S.A. .. 157 D11 40 40N 85 43W
La Fregeneda, Spain .. 42 E4 40 58N 6 54W
La Fría, Venezuela ... 168 B3 8 13N 72 15W
La Fuente de San
Esteban, Spain 42 E4 40 49N 6 15W
La Gacilly, France ... 26 E4 47 45N 2 8W
La Gineta, Spain 41 F2 39 8N 2 1W
La Gloria, Colombia .. 168 B3 8 37N 73 48W
La Goulette = Halq el
Oued, Tunisia ..... 108 A2 36 53N 10 18 E
La Gran Sabana,
Venezuela 169 B5 5 30N 61 30W
La Grand'Combe,
France .... 29 D8 44 13N 4 2 E
La Grande, U.S.A. ... 158 D4 45 20N 118 5W
La Grande ➤, Canada 140 B5 53 50N 79 0W
La Grande Deux, Rés.,
Canada 140 B4 53 40N 76 55W
La Grande-Motte,
France .... 29 E8 43 23N 4 5 E
La Grande Quatre,
Rés., Canada 140 B5 54 0N 73 15W
La Grande Trois, Rés.,
Canada 140 B4 53 40N 75 10W
La Grange, Calif.,
U.S.A. 160 H6 37 42N 120 27W
La Grange, Ga., U.S.A. 152 B4 33 2N 85 2W
La Grange, Ky., U.S.A. 148 F3 38 25N 85 23W
La Grange, Ky., U.S.A. 157 F11 38 24N 85 22W
La Grange, Mo., U.S.A. 156 D5 40 3N 91 35W
La Grange, Tex., U.S.A. 155 L6 29 54N 96 52W
La Grave, France .... 29 C10 45 3N 6 18 E
La Grita, Venezuela .. 168 B3 8 8N 71 59W
La Guaira, Venezuela . 168 A4 10 36N 66 56W
La Guardia = A
Guarda, Spain 42 D2 41 56N 8 52W
La Gudiña = A Gudiña,
Spain 42 C3 42 4N 7 8W
La Güera, Mauritania . 110 D1 20 51N 17 0W
La Guerche-de-
Bretagne, France .. 26 E5 47 57N 1 16W
La Guerche-sur-
l'Aubois, France ... 27 F9 46 58N 2 56 E
La Habana, Cuba 164 B3 23 8N 82 22W
La Harpe, U.S.A. 156 D6 40 35N 90 58W
La Haute Vallée de
Chevreuse △, France 25 B3 48 35N 1 58 E
La Haye-du-Puits,
France 26 C5 49 17N 1 33W
La Horqueta,
Venezuela 169 B5 7 55N 60 20W
La Horra, Spain 42 D7 41 44N 3 53W
La Independencia,
Mexico 163 D6 16 31N 91 47W
La Isabela, Dom. Rep. 165 C5 19 58N 71 2W
La Jonquera, Spain ... 40 C7 42 25N 2 53 E
La Joya, Peru .... 172 D3 16 43 S 71 52W
La Junta, U.S.A. 155 F3 37 59N 103 33W
La Laguna, Canary Is. 9 e1 28 28N 16 18W
La Libertad, Guatemala 164 C1 16 47N 90 7W
La Libertad, Mexico .. 162 B2 29 55N 112 41W
La Libertad □, Peru .. 172 B2 8 0 S 78 30W
La Ligua, Chile ...... 174 C1 32 30 S 71 16W
La Línea de la
Concepción, Spain . 43 J5 36 15N 5 23W
La Loche, Canada 143 B7 56 29N 109 26W
La Londe-les-Maures,
France .... 29 E10 43 8N 6 14 E
La Lora, Spain 42 C7 42 45N 4 0W
La Loupe, France .... 26 D8 48 29N 1 1 E
La Louvière, Belgium . 24 D4 50 27N 4 10 E
La Lune, Trin. & Tob. . 169 F19 10 3N 61 22W
La Machine, France .. 27 F10 46 54N 3 27 E
La Maddalena, Italy .. 46 A2 41 13N 9 24 E
La Malbaie, Canada .. 141 C5 47 40N 70 10W
La Malinche △, Mexico 163 D5 19 15N 98 3W
La Mancha, Spain ... 41 F2 39 10N 2 54W
La Mariña, Spain 42 B3 43 30N 7 40W
La Martre, L., Canada 142 A5 63 15N 117 55W
La Mesa, U.S.A. 161 N9 32 46N 117 3W
La Misión, Mexico ... 162 A1 32 5N 116 50W
La Moille, U.S.A. 156 C7 41 32N 89 17W
La Moine ➤, U.S.A. .. 156 E6 39 59N 90 31W
La Monte, U.S.A. 156 F3 38 46N 93 26W
La Mothe-Achard,
France 26 F5 46 37N 1 40W
La Motte-Chalançon,
France .... 29 D9 44 30N 5 21 E
La Motte-du-Caire,
France .... 29 D10 44 21N 6 2 E
La Motte-Servolex,
France .... 29 C9 45 35N 5 53 E
La Moure, U.S.A. 154 B5 46 21N 98 18W
La Muela, Spain 40 D3 41 36N 1 7W
La Mure, France .... 29 D9 44 55N 5 48 E
La Negra, Chile ..... 174 A2 23 46 S 70 18W
La Neuveville, Switz. . 32 B4 47 4N 7 6 E
La Oliva, Canary Is. .. 9 e2 28 36N 13 57W
La Oroya, Peru ...... 172 C2 11 32 S 75 54W
La Orotava, Canary Is. 9 e1 28 22N 16 33W
La Oroya, Peru ...... 172 C2 11 32 S 75 54W
La Pacaudière, France 27 F10 46 11N 3 52 E

La Palma, Canary Is. . 9 e1 28 40N 17 50W
La Palma, Panama ... 164 E4 8 15N 78 0W
La Palma del Condado,
Spain 43 H4 37 21N 6 38W
La Paloma, Chile .... 174 C1 30 35 S 71 0W
La Pampa □, Argentina 174 D2 36 50 S 66 0W
La Paragua, Venezuela 169 B5 6 50N 63 20W
La Paya △, Colombia . 168 C2 0 0 75 5W
La Paz, Entre Ríos,
Argentina .... 174 C4 30 50 S 59 45W
La Paz, San Luis,
Argentina .... 174 C2 33 30 S 67 20W
La Paz, Bolivia ...... 172 D4 16 20 S 68 10W
La Paz, Honduras 164 D2 14 20N 87 47W
La Paz, Mexico 162 C2 24 10N 110 20W
La Paz, Abra, Phil. ... 80 C3 17 40N 120 41 E
La Paz, Tarlac, Phil. .. 80 D3 15 26N 120 45 E
La Paz □, Bolivia .... 172 D4 15 30 S 68 0W
La Paz Centro, Nic. .. 164 D2 12 20N 86 41W
La Pedrera, Colombia 168 D4 1 18 S 69 43W
La Pérade, Canada ... 141 C5 46 35N 72 12W
La Perouse, Bahía,
Chile .... 172 b 27 5 S 109 18W
La Perouse Str., Asia . 70 B11 45 40N 142 0 E
La Pesca, Mexico 163 C5 23 46N 97 47W
La Piedad, Mexico ... 162 C4 20 20N 102 1W
La Pine, U.S.A. 158 E3 43 40N 121 30W
La Plata, Argentina .. 174 C4 35 0 S 57 55W
La Plata, Colombia ... 168 C2 2 23N 75 53W
La Plata, U.S.A. 156 D4 40 2N 92 29W
La Plata ➤, Argentina 176 B2 44 55 S 71 50W
La Pobla de Lillet,
Spain .... 38 B4 39 46N 3 1 E
La Pocatière, Canada 141 C5 47 22N 70 2W
La Pola de Gordón,
Spain 42 C5 42 51N 5 41W
La Porta, France .... 29 F13 42 25N 9 21 E
La Porte, Ind., U.S.A. . 157 C10 41 36N 86 43W
La Porte, Tex., U.S.A. . 155 L7 29 39N 95 1W
La Porte City, U.S.A. . 156 D8 42 19N 92 12W
La Presanella, Italy .. 44 B7 46 13N 10 40 E
La Puebla = Sa Pobla,
Spain .... 38 B4 39 46N 3 1 E
La Puebla de Cazalla,
Spain 43 H5 37 10N 5 20W
La Puebla de los
Infantes, Spain 43 H5 37 47N 5 24W
La Puebla de
Montalbán, Spain .. 42 F6 39 52N 4 22W
La Puebla del Río,
Spain 43 H4 37 16N 6 3W
La Puerta de Segura,
Spain 43 G8 38 22N 2 45W
La Punt, Switz. ..... 33 C9 46 35N 9 56 E
La Purísima, Mexico .. 162 B2 26 10N 112 4W
La Push, U.S.A. 160 C2 47 55N 124 38W
La Quiaca, Argentina . 174 A2 22 5 S 65 35W
La Réole, France .... 28 D3 44 35N 0 1 E
La Restinga, Canary Is. 9 e1 27 38N 17 59W
La Rioja, Argentina .. 174 B2 29 20 S 67 0W
La Rioja □, Argentina 174 B2 29 30 S 67 0W
La Rioja □, Spain ... 40 C2 42 20N 2 20W
La Robla, Spain 42 C5 42 50N 5 41W
La Roche, N. Cal. .... 133 U22 21 26 S 168 2 E
La Roche, Switz. .... 32 C4 46 42N 7 7 E
La Roche-Bernard,
France 26 E4 47 31N 2 19W
La Roche-Canillac,
France .... 28 C5 45 12N 1 57 E
La Roche-en-Ardenne,
Belgium .... 24 D5 50 11N 5 35 E
La Roche-sur-Foron,
France .... 27 F13 46 4N 6 19 E
La Roche-sur-Yon,
France 26 F5 46 40N 1 25W
La Rochefoucauld,
France .... 28 C4 45 44N 0 24 E
La Rochelle, France .. 28 B2 46 10N 1 9W
La Roda, Spain 39 C3 39 13N 2 15W
La Roda de Andalucía,
Spain 43 H6 37 12N 4 46W
La Romana, Dom. Rep. 165 C6 18 27N 68 57W
La Ronge, Canada ... 143 B7 55 5N 105 20W
La Rue, U.S.A. 157 D13 40 35N 83 23W
La Rumorosa, Mexico 161 N10 32 33N 116 4W
La Sabina = Sa Savina,
Spain .... 38 D1 38 44N 1 25 E
La Sagra, Spain 41 H2 37 57N 2 35W
La Salle, U.S.A. 156 C7 41 20N 89 6W
La Sanabria, Spain ... 42 C4 42 0N 6 30W
La Santa, Canary Is. .. 9 e2 29 5N 13 40W
La Sarraz, Switz. .... 32 C3 46 38N 6 32 E
La Sarre, Canada 140 C4 48 45N 79 15W
La Scie, Canada 141 C8 49 57N 55 36W
La Selva, Spain ..... 40 C7 41 13N 1 8 E
La Selva Beach, U.S.A. 160 J5 36 56N 121 51W
La Selva del Camp,
Spain .... 40 D6 41 13N 1 8 E
La Serena, Chile .... 174 B1 29 55 S 71 10W
La Serena, Spain 43 G5 38 45N 5 40W
La Seu d'Urgell, Spain 40 C6 42 22N 1 23 E
La Seyne-sur-Mer,
France .... 29 E9 43 7N 5 52 E
La Sila, Italy .... 47 C9 39 15N 16 35 E
La Solana, Spain 43 G7 38 59N 3 14W
La Soufrière,
St. Vincent 165 D7 13 20N 61 11W
La Souterraine, France 27 F8 46 15N 1 30 E
La Spézia, Italy ..... 44 D6 44 7N 9 50 E
La Suze-sur-Sarthe,
France .... 26 E7 47 53N 0 2 E
La Tagua, Colombia .. 168 C3 0 3N 74 40W
La Teste-de-Buch,
France 28 D2 44 37N 1 8W
La Tortuga, Venezuela 169 A4 11 0N 65 22W
La Tour de Peilz, Switz. 32 D3 46 27N 6 52 E
La Tour-du-Pin, France 29 C9 45 33N 5 27 E
La Tournette, France . 32 E2 45 36N 6 15 E
La Tranche-sur-Mer,
France 26 F5 46 20N 1 27W
La Tremblade, France 28 C2 45 46N 1 8W
La Trinidad, Phil. .... 80 C3 16 28N 120 35 E
La Trinité, Martinique 164 c 14 43N 60 58W
La Tuque, Canada 140 C5 47 30N 72 50W
La Unión, Chile ..... 176 B2 40 10 S 73 0W
La Unión, Colombia .. 168 C2 1 35N 77 5W
La Unión, El Salv. ... 164 D2 13 20N 87 50W
La Unión, Mexico 162 D4 17 58N 101 49W
La Unión, Peru ...... 172 B2 9 43 S 76 45W
La Unión □, Phil. .... 80 C3 16 30N 120 25 E
La Urbana, Venezuela 168 B4 7 8N 66 56W
La Vache Pt.,
Trin. & Tob. 169 F19 10 47N 61 28W
La Vall d'Uixó, Spain . 40 F4 39 49N 0 15W
La Vecilla de Curveño,
Spain 42 C5 42 51N 5 27W
La Vega, Dom. Rep. .. 165 C5 19 20N 70 30W
La Vega, Peru .... 172 C2 10 41 S 77 44W
La Vela de Coro,
Venezuela 168 A4 11 27N 69 34W
La Veleta, Spain 43 H7 37 3N 3 22W
La Venta, Mexico 163 D6 18 8N 94 3W
La Ventura, Mexico .. 162 C4 24 38N 100 54W

La Venturosa,
Colombia 168 B4 6 8N 68 48W
La Vergne, U.S.A. 149 G2 36 1N 86 35W
La Victoria, Venezuela 168 A4 10 14N 67 20W
La Voulte-sur-Rhône,
France .... 29 D8 44 48N 4 46 E
Laa an der Thaya,
Austria .... 35 C9 48 43N 16 23 E
Laaber, Grosse ➤,
Germany .... 31 G8 48 55N 12 32 E
Laage, Germany ..... 30 B8 53 55N 12 21 E
Laas Caanood = Las
Anod, Somali Rep. . 120 C3 8 26N 47 19 E
Laatzen, Germany ... 30 C5 52 19N 9 48 E
Laau Pt., U.S.A. 145 B4 21 6N 157 19W
Laba ➤, Russia ..... 61 H4 45 11N 39 42 E
Laban, Burma ...... 90 C6 25 52N 96 40 E
Labasa, Fiji .... 133 A2 16 30 S 179 27 E
Labason, Phil. ...... 81 G4 8 4N 122 31 E
Labastide-Murat,
France .... 28 D5 44 39N 1 33 E
Labastide-Rouairoux,
France .... 28 E6 43 28N 2 39 E
Labbézenga, Mali .... 113 B5 15 2N 0 48 E
Labdah = Leptis
Magna, Libya ..... 108 B2 32 40N 14 12 E
Labe = Elbe ➤,
Europe .... 30 B4 53 50N 9 0 E
Labé, Guinea 112 C2 11 24N 12 16W
Laberge, L., Canada .. 142 A1 61 11N 135 12W
Labes = Łobez, Poland 54 E2 53 38N 15 39 E
Labian, Tanjong,
Malaysia .... 85 A5 5 9N 119 13 E
Labiau = Polessk,
Russia .... 15 J19 54 50N 21 8 E
Labig Pt., U.S.A. ..... 80 B4 18 25N 122 25 E
Labin, Croatia ...... 45 C11 45 5N 14 8 E
Labinsk, Russia ..... 61 H5 44 40N 40 48 E
Labis, Malaysia ..... 87 L4 2 22N 103 2 E
Labo, Phil. .... 80 D4 14 9N 122 51 E
Laboe, Germany ..... 30 A6 54 24N 10 13 E
Laboka, Gabon ..... 114 B2 0 19N 11 32 E
Laborec ➤,
Slovak Rep. ...... 35 C14 48 37N 21 58 E
Laborie, St. Lucia ... 165 f 13 45N 61 2W
Labouheyre, France . 28 D3 44 13N 0 55W
Laboulaye, Argentina . 174 C3 34 10 S 63 30W
Labrador, Canada ... 141 B7 53 20N 61 0W
Labrador City, Canada 141 B6 52 57N 66 55W
Labrador Sea, Atl. Oc. 137 c 57 0N 54 0W
Lábrea, Brazil ...... 173 B5 7 15 S 64 51W
Labruguière, France . 28 E6 43 33N 2 16 E
Labuan, Malaysia ... 85 A5 5 20N 115 14 E
Labuan □, Malaysia . 85 A5 5 21N 115 13 E
Labuha, Indonesia ... 83 B3 0 30 S 127 30 E
Labuhan, Indonesia .. 84 D2 6 22 S 105 50 E
Labuhanbajo, Indonesia 83 C2 8 28 S 119 54 E
Labuk, Telok, Malaysia 85 A5 6 10N 117 50 E
Labutta, Burma ..... 90 G5 16 9N 94 46 E
Labyrinth, L., Australia 127 E2 30 40 S 135 11 E
Labytnangi, Russia .. 66 C7 66 39N 66 21 E
Laç, Albania .... 50 E3 41 38N 19 43 E
Lac-Bouchette, Canada 141 C5 48 16N 72 11W
Lac Édouard, Canada 140 C5 47 40N 72 16W
Lac La Biche, Canada 142 C6 54 45N 111 58W
Lac la Martre = Wha
Ti, Canada 138 B8 63 8N 117 16W
Lac La Ronge △,
Canada 143 B7 55 9N 104 41W
Lac-Mégantic, Canada 141 C5 45 35N 70 53W
Lac Thien, Vietnam .. 86 F7 12 25N 108 11 E
Lacanau, France 28 D2 44 58N 1 7W
Lacanau, Étang de,
France 28 D2 44 58N 1 7W
Lacantún ➤, Mexico . 163 D6 16 36N 90 40W
Lacepede B., Australia 128 D3 36 40 S 139 40 E
Lacepede Is., Australia 124 C3 16 55 S 122 0 E
Lacerdónia, Mozam. . 119 F4 18 3 S 35 35 E
Lacey, U.S.A. 160 C4 47 7N 122 49W
Lachay, Pta., Peru ... 172 C2 11 17 S 77 44W
Lachen, India ...... 90 B2 27 46N 88 36 E
Lachen, Switz. ...... 33 B7 47 12N 8 51 E
Lachhmangarh, India 92 F6 27 50N 75 4 E
Lachi, Pakistan ..... 92 C4 33 25N 71 20 E
Lachine, Canada 140 C5 45 30N 73 40W
Lachlan ➤, Australia 128 C3 34 22 S 143 55 E
Lachute, Canada 140 C5 45 39N 74 21W
Lackagh Hills, Ireland 12 B3 54 59N 8 0W
Lackawanna, U.S.A. . 150 D6 42 50N 78 50W
Lackawaxen, U.S.A. . 151 E10 41 29N 74 59W
Lacolle, Canada 151 A11 45 5N 73 22W
Lacombe, Canada ... 142 C6 52 30N 113 44W
Lacon, U.S.A. 156 C7 41 2N 89 24W
Lacona, Iowa, U.S.A. 156 E8 41 12N 93 23W
Lacona, N.Y., U.S.A. . 151 C8 43 39N 76 10W
Láconi, Italy .... 46 C2 39 54N 9 4 E
Laconia, U.S.A. 151 C13 43 32N 71 28W
Lacoochee, U.S.A. ... 153 G7 28 28N 82 11W
Lacq, France 28 E3 43 25N 0 35W
Ladakh Ra., India ... 93 C8 34 0N 78 0 E
Ladário, Brazil ..... 173 D6 19 1 S 57 35W
Ladd, U.S.A. 156 C7 41 23N 89 13W
Laddonia, U.S.A. 156 F9 39 15N 91 39W
Ladik, Turkey ...... 100 B6 40 57N 35 58 E
Ladismith, S. Africa .. 116 E3 33 28 S 21 15 E
Ládispoli, Italy ..... 45 G9 41 56N 12 5 E
Ládiz, Iran .... 97 D9 28 55N 61 15 E
Ladnun, India ...... 92 F6 27 38N 74 25 E
Ladoga, L. =
Ladozhskoye Ozero,
Russia .... 58 B6 61 15N 30 30 E
Ladozhskoye Ozero,
Russia .... 58 B6 61 15N 30 30 E
Ladrillero, G., Chile .. 176 F1 49 20 S 75 35W
Ladson, U.S.A. 152 C9 32 59N 80 6W
Ladushkin, Russia ... 15 J19 54 37N 20 10 E
Lady Elliott △,
Australia .... 126 C5 24 7 S 152 42 E
Lady Grey, S. Africa . 116 E4 30 43 S 27 13 E
Lady Lake, U.S.A. ... 153 G8 28 55N 81 55W
Ladybrand, S. Africa . 116 D4 29 9 S 27 29 E
Ladybank, Canada ... 142 D4 49 0N 123 49W
Ladysmith, S. Africa . 117 D4 28 32 S 29 46 E
Ladysmith, U.S.A. ... 154 C9 45 28N 91 12W
Ladyzhyn, Ukraine .. 53 B14 48 40N 29 1 E
Lae, Papua N. G. .... 132 D4 6 40 S 147 2 E
Laem Hin Khom,
Thailand .... 87 b 9 25N 99 56 E
Laem Khat, Thailand . 87 a 8 4N 98 17 E
Laem Nga, Thailand . 87 a 7 55N 98 27 E
Laem Ngop, Thailand 87 F4 12 10N 102 26 E
Laem Phan Wa,
Thailand .... 87 a 7 47N 98 25 E

Laem Pho, Thailand . 87 J3 6 55N 101 19 E
Laem Phrom Thep,
Thailand .... 87 a 7 45N 98 19 E
Laem Riang, Thailand 87 a 8 7N 98 27 E
Laem Sam Rong,
Thailand .... 87 b 9 35N 100 4 E
Laem Son, Thailand . 87 a 7 59N 98 16 E
Laem Yamu, Thailand 87 a 7 59N 98 26 E
Lærdalsøyri, Norway . 18 C4 61 6N 7 28 E
Læsø, Denmark ..... 17 G5 57 15N 11 5 E
Læsø Rende, Denmark 17 G4 57 20N 10 45 E
Lafayette, Ala., U.S.A. 152 C4 32 54N 85 24W
Lafayette, Colo., U.S.A. 152 D7 40 0N 105 6W
Lafayette, Ind., U.S.A. 157 D10 40 25N 86 54W
Lafayette, La., U.S.A. 155 K9 30 14N 92 1W
Lafayette, Tenn., U.S.A. 149 G2 36 31N 86 2W
Laferte ➤, Canada .. 142 A5 61 53N 117 44W
Lafia, Nigeria ...... 113 D6 8 30N 8 34 E
Lafiagi, Nigeria ..... 113 D6 8 52N 5 20 E
Lafleche, Canada 143 D7 49 45N 106 40W
Lafon, Sudan .... 107 F3 5 5N 32 29 E
Laful, India .... 95 L11 7 10N 93 52 E
Lagan ➤, Russia .... 61 H8 45 22N 47 23 E
Lagan ➤, Sweden ... 17 H7 56 56N 13 58 E
Lagan ➤, Sweden ... 17 H6 56 30N 12 58 E
Lagan ➤, U.K. 12 B6 54 36N 5 55W
Laganás, Greece .... 39 D2 37 44N 20 53 E
Lagangilang, Phil. ... 80 C3 17 37N 120 44 E
Lagarfljót ➤, Iceland 11 B12 65 40N 14 18W
Lagarto, Brazil ..... 170 D4 10 54 S 37 41W
Lagawe, Phil. .... 80 C3 16 49N 121 6 E
Lagdo, Rés. de,
Cameroon .... 114 A2 8 40N 14 0 E
Lage, Germany ..... 30 D4 51 59N 8 48 E
Lågen ➤, Oppland,
Norway .... 18 C7 61 8N 10 25 E
Lågen ➤, Vestfold,
Norway .... 18 E7 59 3N 10 3 E
Lägerdorf, Germany . 30 B5 53 53N 9 34 E
Laghouat, Algeria ... 111 B5 33 50N 2 59 E
Lagmán □, Afghan. .. 91 B3 34 20N 70 0 E
Lagnieu, France .... 29 C9 45 55N 5 20 E
Lagny-sur-Marne,
France .... 27 D9 48 52N 2 44 E
Lago = Niassa □,
Mozam. .... 119 E4 13 30 S 0 E
Lago, Italy .... 47 C9 39 10N 16 9 E
Lago de Sanabria y
Entorno △, Spain .. 42 C4 42 9N 6 45W
Lago Posadas,
Argentina .... 176 C2 47 30 S 71 40W
Lago Puela △,
Argentina .... 176 B2 42 10 S 71 55W
Lago Ranco, Chile ... 176 B2 40 19 S 72 30W
Lagoa, Azores 9 d3 37 45N 25 20W
Lagoa, Portugal 43 H2 37 8N 8 27W
Lagoa do Peixe △,
Brazil .... 175 C5 31 12 S 50 55W
Lagoa Vermelha, Brazil 175 B5 28 13 S 51 32W
Lagodekhi, Georgia .. 61 K8 41 50N 46 22 E
Lagonoy = Laguna
Beach, U.S.A. 161 M9 33 33N 117 47W
Lagónegro, Italy .... 47 B8 40 8N 15 45 E
Lagonoy G., Phil. .... 80 E4 13 35N 123 50 E
Lagos, Angola ...... 115 F3 16 3 S 16 35 E
Lagos, Nigeria ...... 113 D5 6 25N 3 27 E
Lagos, Portugal 43 H2 37 5N 8 41W
Lagos □, Nigeria .... 113 D5 6 28N 3 25 E
Lagos de Moreno,
Mexico 162 C4 21 21N 101 55W
Lagrange, Australia .. 124 C3 18 45 S 121 43 E
Lagrange B., Australia 157 C11 39 85 25W
Laguardia, Spain 40 C2 42 33N 2 35W
Laguépie, France .... 28 D5 44 8N 1 57 E
Laguna = Padilla,
Bolivia .... 173 D5 19 19 S 64 20W
Laguna, Brazil ...... 175 B6 28 30 S 48 50W
Laguna □, Phil. ..... 80 D3 14 10N 121 20 E
Laguna Beach, U.S.A. 161 M9 33 33N 117 47W
Laguna Blanca □,
Argentina .... 176 A2 39 0 S 70 5W
Laguna de Duera,
Spain 42 D6 41 35N 4 43W
Laguna de la
Restinga △,
Venezuela 165 D6 10 58N 64 0W
Laguna de Tacarigua △,
Venezuela 168 A4 10 59N 64 7W
Laguna del Laja △,
Chile .... 174 D1 37 27 S 71 20W
Laguna del Tigre △,
Guatemala 164 C1 17 32N 90 56W
Laguna Limpia,
Argentina .... 174 B4 26 32 S 59 45W
Laguna San Rafael △,
Chile .... 176 C2 46 54 S 73 31W
Lagunas, Chile ..... 174 A2 21 0 S 69 45W
Lagunas de
Chacahua △, Mexico 163 D5 16 0N 97 43W
Lagunas de
Montebello △,
Mexico 163 D6 16 9N 91 41W
Lagunas de Ruidera △,
Spain 41 G2 38 57N 2 52W
Lagunillas, Bolivia ... 173 D5 19 38 S 63 43W
Lahad Datu, Malaysia 85 A5 5 0N 118 20 E
Lahad Datu, Telok,
Malaysia .... 85 D5 4 50N 118 20 E
Lahaina, U.S.A. 145 C5 20 53N 156 41W
Lahan Sai, Thailand . 87 a 14 25N 102 52 E
Lahanam, Laos ..... 86 D5 16 16N 105 16 E
Lahar, India .... 93 F8 26 12N 78 57 E
Laharpur, India ..... 93 F9 27 43N 80 56 E
Lahat, Indonesia .... 84 C2 3 45 S 103 30 E
Lahe, Burma .... 90 B5 26 20N 95 26 E
Lahewa, Indonesia .. 84 A1 1 22N 97 12 E
Lahij, Yemen .... 104 E3 13 4N 44 53 E
Lahijan, Iran .... 97 B6 37 10N 50 6 E
Lähilahi Pt., U.S.A. .. 145 K13 21 28N 158 13W
Lahn ➤, Germany ... 31 E4 50 19N 7 37 E
Laholm, Sweden .... 17 H7 56 30N 13 2 E
Laholmsbukten,
Sweden .... 17 H6 56 30N 12 45 E
Lahore, Pakistan .... 91 C4 31 32N 74 22 E
Lahpongsel, Burma .. 90 C7 27 18N 98 25 E
Lahr, Germany ...... 31 G3 48 20N 7 53 E
Lahri, Pakistan ..... 92 E3 29 11N 68 13 E
Lahti = Lahtis, Finland 15 F21 60 58N 25 40 E
Lahtis = Lahti, Finland 15 F21 60 58N 25 40 E
Lai, Chad .... 109 G3 9 25N 16 18 E
Lai Chau, Vietnam .. 76 F4 22 5N 103 3 E
Lai-hka, Burma ..... 90 E6 21 16N 97 40 E
Laiagam, Papua N. G. 132 C2 5 33 S 143 30 E

Lai'an, China 77 A12 32 28N 118 30 E
Laibach = Ljubljana, Slovenia 45 B11 46 4N 14 33 E
Laibin, China 76 F7 23 42N 109 14 E
Laie, U.S.A. 145 J14 21 39N 157 56W
Laifeng, China 76 C7 29 27N 109 20 E
L'Aigle, France 26 D7 48 46N 0 38 E
Laignes, France 27 E11 47 50N 4 20 E
L'Aiguillon-sur-Mer, France 28 B2 46 20N 1 18W
Laila = Layla, Si. Arabia 98 B4 22 10N 46 40 E
Laingsburg, S. Africa 116 E3 33 9 S 20 52 E
Lainioälven →, Sweden 14 C20 67 35N 22 40 E
Lairg, U.K. 22 C4 58 2N 4 24W
Laïri, B. de, Chad 109 F3 12 28N 16 45 E
Lais, Phil. 81 H5 6 20N 125 39 E
Laishui, China 74 E8 39 23N 115 45 E
Laissac, France 28 D6 44 23N 2 50 E
Läives, Italy 45 B8 46 26N 11 20 E
Laiwu, China 75 F9 36 15N 117 40 E
Laixi, China 75 F11 36 50N 120 31 E
Laiyang, China 75 F11 36 59N 120 45 E
Laiyuan, China 74 E8 39 20N 114 40 E
Laizhou, China 75 F10 37 8N 119 57 E
Laizhou Wan, China 75 F10 37 30N 119 30 E
Laja →, Mexico 162 C4 20 55N 100 46W
Lajeado = Guiratinga, Brazil 173 D7 16 21 S 53 45W
Lajedo, Azores 9 d2 39 23N 31 15W
Lajere, Nigeria 113 C7 12 10N 11 25 E
Lajes, Azores 9 d1 38 46N 27 6W
Lajes, Rio Grande do N., Brazil 170 C4 5 41 S 36 14W
Lajes, Sta. Catarina, Brazil 175 B5 27 48 S 50 20W
Lajes das Flores, Azores 9 d2 39 23N 31 10W
Lajes do Pico, Azores 9 d1 38 23N 28 16W
Lajinha, Brazil 171 F3 20 9 S 41 37W
Lajkovac, Serbia & M. 50 B4 44 27N 20 14 E
Lajosmizse, Hungary 52 C4 47 3N 19 32 E
Lak Sao, Laos 86 C5 18 11N 104 59 E
Láka, Greece 38 C10 39 17N 20 9 E
Lakaband, Pakistan 92 D3 31 2N 69 15 E
Lakamané, Mali 112 C3 14 35N 9 44W
Lakatoro, Vanuatu 133 F5 16 6 S 167 25 E
Lake Alfred, U.S.A. 153 G8 28 6N 81 44W
Lake Alpine, U.S.A. 160 G7 38 29N 120 0W
Lake Andes, U.S.A. 154 D5 43 9N 98 32W
Lake Arthur, U.S.A. 155 K8 30 5N 92 41W
Lake Bindegolly △, Australia 127 D3 28 0 S 144 12 E
Lake Boga, Australia 128 C5 35 26 S 143 38 E
Lake Butler, U.S.A. 152 E7 30 1N 82 21W
Lake Cargelligo, Australia 129 B7 33 15 S 146 22 E
Lake Charles, U.S.A. 155 K8 30 14N 93 13W
Lake City, Colo., U.S.A. 159 G10 38 2N 107 19W
Lake City, Fla., U.S.A. 152 E7 30 11N 82 38W
Lake City, Iowa, U.S.A. 156 B2 42 16N 94 44W
Lake City, Mich., U.S.A. 148 C3 44 20N 85 13W
Lake City, Minn., U.S.A. 154 C8 44 27N 92 16W
Lake City, Pa., U.S.A. 150 D4 42 1N 80 21W
Lake City, S.C., U.S.A. 152 B10 33 52N 79 45W
Lake Clark △, U.S.A. 144 D9 61 0N 154 0W
Lake Clarke Shores, U.S.A. 153 J9 26 39N 80 5W
Lake Coleridge, N.Z. 131 D6 43 17 S 171 30 E
Lake Cowichan, Canada 142 D4 48 49N 124 3W
Lake District △, U.K. 20 C4 54 30N 3 21W
Lake Elsinore, U.S.A. 161 M9 33 38N 117 20W
Lake Eyre △, Australia 127 D2 28 40 S 137 31 E
Lake Forest, U.S.A. 157 B9 42 15N 87 50W
Lake Gairdner △, Australia 127 E2 31 41 S 135 51 E
Lake Geneva, U.S.A. 157 B8 42 36N 88 26W
Lake George, U.S.A. 151 C11 43 26N 73 43W
Lake Grace, Australia 125 F2 33 7 S 118 28 E
Lake Harbor, U.S.A. 153 J9 26 42N 80 48W
Lake Harbour = Kimmirut, Canada 139 B13 62 50N 69 50W
Lake Havasu City, U.S.A. 161 L12 34 27N 114 22W
Lake Helen, U.S.A. 153 G8 28 59N 81 14W
Lake Hughes, U.S.A. 161 L8 34 41N 118 26W
Lake Isabella, U.S.A. 161 K8 35 38N 118 28W
Lake Jackson, U.S.A. 155 L7 29 3N 95 27W
Lake Junction, U.S.A. 158 D8 44 35N 110 28W
Lake King, Australia 125 F2 33 5 S 119 45 E
Lake Kopiago, Papua N. G. 132 C2 5 23 S 142 31 E
Lake Kutubu, Papua N. G. 132 D2 6 20 S 143 18 E
Lake Lenore, Canada 143 C8 52 24N 104 59W
Lake Louise, Canada 142 C5 51 30N 116 10W
Lake Malawi △, Malawi 119 E3 14 2 S 34 53 E
Lake Mburo △, Uganda 118 C3 0 33 S 30 56 E
Lake Mead ⌂, U.S.A. 161 K12 36 15N 114 30W
Lake Meredith ⌂, U.S.A. 155 H4 35 50N 101 50W
Lake Mills, Iowa, U.S.A. 154 D8 43 25N 93 32W
Lake Mills, Wis., U.S.A. 157 A8 43 5N 88 55W
Lake Murray, Papua N. G. 132 D1 6 48 S 141 29 E
Lake Nakura △, Kenya 118 C4 0 21 S 36 8 E
Lake Naujan △, Phil. 80 E3 13 9N 121 20 E
Lake Odessa, U.S.A. 157 B11 42 47N 85 8W
Lake Orion, U.S.A. 157 B13 42 47N 83 14W
Lake Park, Fla., U.S.A. 153 J9 26 48N 80 3W
Lake Park, Ga., U.S.A. 152 E6 30 41N 83 11W
Lake Placid, Fla., U.S.A. 153 H8 27 18N 81 22W
Lake Placid, N.Y., U.S.A. 151 B11 44 17N 73 59W
Lake Pleasant, U.S.A. 151 C10 43 28N 74 25W
Lake Providence, U.S.A. 155 J9 32 48N 91 10W
Lake Pukaki, N.Z. 131 E5 44 11 S 170 8 E
Lake Roosevelt ⌂, U.S.A. 158 C4 47 57N 118 59W
Lake St. Peter, Canada 150 A6 45 18N 78 2W
Lake Superior ⌂, Canada 140 C3 47 45N 84 45W
Lake Tekapo, N.Z. 131 D5 44 0 S 170 30 E
Lake Torrens △, Australia 127 E2 30 55 S 137 40 E
Lake View, U.S.A. 156 B1 42 18N 95 3W
Lake Villa, U.S.A. 157 B8 42 25N 88 5W
Lake Village, U.S.A. 155 J9 33 20N 91 17W
Lake Wales, U.S.A. 153 H8 27 54N 81 35W
Lake Worth, U.S.A. 153 J9 26 37N 80 3W
Lake Zurich, U.S.A. 157 B8 42 12N 88 5W
Lakeba, Fiji 133 B3 18 13 S 178 47W
Lakeba Passage, Fiji 133 B3 18 0 S 178 45W
Lakefield, Canada 140 D4 44 25N 78 16W
Lakefield △, Australia 126 B3 15 24 S 144 26 E
Lakehurst, U.S.A. 151 F10 40 1N 74 19W
Lakeland, Australia 126 B3 15 49 S 144 57 E
Lakeland, Fla., U.S.A. 153 G8 28 3N 81 57W
Lakeland, Ga., U.S.A. 152 D6 31 2N 83 4W
Lakemba = Lakeba, Fiji 133 B3 18 13 S 178 47W
Lakeport, Calif., U.S.A. 160 F4 39 3N 122 55W
Lakeport, Mich., U.S.A. 150 C2 43 7N 82 30W
Lakes Entrance, Australia 129 D8 37 50 S 148 0 E
Lakeside, Calif., U.S.A. 161 N10 32 52N 116 55W
Lakeside, Nebr., U.S.A. 154 D3 42 3N 102 26W
Lakeside, Ohio, U.S.A. 150 E2 41 32N 82 46W
Lakeview, U.S.A. 158 E3 42 11N 120 21W
Lakeville, U.S.A. 154 C8 44 39N 93 14W
Lakewood, Colo., U.S.A. 154 F2 39 44N 105 5W
Lakewood, N.J., U.S.A. 151 F10 40 6N 74 13W
Lakewood, N.Y., U.S.A. 150 D5 42 6N 79 19W
Lakewood, Ohio, U.S.A. 150 E3 41 29N 81 48W
Lakewood, Wash., U.S.A. 160 C4 47 11N 122 32W
Lakewood Park, U.S.A. 153 H9 27 30N 80 23W
Lakha, India 92 F4 26 9N 70 54 E
Lakhaniá, Greece 38 F11 35 58N 27 54 E
Lakhimpur, India 93 F9 27 57N 80 46 E
Lakhipur, Assam, India 90 C4 24 48N 93 0 E
Lakhipur, Assam, India 90 B3 26 2N 90 18 E
Lakhnadon, India 93 H8 22 36N 79 36 E
Lakhnau = Lucknow, India 93 F9 26 50N 81 0 E
Lakhonpheng, Laos 86 E5 15 54N 105 34 E
Lakhpat, India 92 H3 23 48N 68 47 E
Läki, Azerbaijan 61 K8 40 34N 47 22 E
Laki, Iceland 11 C8 64 4N 18 14W
Lakin, U.S.A. 155 G4 37 57N 101 15W
Lakitusaki →, Canada 140 B3 54 21N 82 25W
Lakki, Pakistan 92 C4 32 36N 70 55 E
Lákkoi, Greece 39 E4 35 24N 23 57 E
Lakonía □, Greece 48 E4 36 55N 22 30 E
Lakonikós Kólpos, Greece 48 E4 36 40N 22 40 E
Lakor, Indonesia 82 C3 8 15 S 128 17 E
Lakota, Ivory C. 112 D3 5 50N 5 30W
Lakota, U.S.A. 154 A5 48 2N 98 21W
Laksar, India 92 E8 29 46N 78 3 E
Laksefjorden, Norway 14 A22 70 45N 26 50 E
Lakselv, Norway 14 A21 70 2N 25 0 E
Laksettipet, India 94 E4 18 52N 79 13 E
Lakshadweep □, India 95 J1 10 0N 72 30 E
Lakshadweep Is., India 95 J1 10 0N 72 30 E
Laksham, Bangla. 90 D3 23 14N 91 8 E
Lakshimpur, Bangla. 90 D3 22 58N 90 50 E
Lakshmanpur, India 93 H10 22 58N 83 3 E
Lakshmeshwar, India 95 G2 15 9N 75 28 E
Lakshmikantapur, India 93 H13 22 5N 88 20 E
Lakuramau, Papua N. G. 132 B6 2 54 S 151 15 E
Lal-lo, Phil. 80 B3 18 12N 121 40 E
Lala, Dem. Rep. of the Congo 115 C4 4 10 S 20 30 E
Lala, Phil. 81 H4 7 59N 123 46 E
Lala Musa, Pakistan 92 C5 32 40N 73 57 E
Lalaghat, India 90 C4 24 30N 92 40 E
Lalago, Tanzania 118 C3 3 28 S 33 58 E
Lalapanzi, Zimbabwe 119 F3 19 20 S 30 15 E
Lalapaşa, Turkey 51 E10 41 49N 26 44 E
Lalbenque, France 28 D5 44 19N 1 34 E
Lalbert, Australia 128 C5 35 38 S 143 20 E
L'Albufera, Spain 41 F4 39 20N 0 27W
Lalganj, India 93 G11 25 52N 85 13 E
Lalgola, India 93 G13 24 25N 88 15 E
Lālī, Iran 97 C6 32 21N 49 6 E
Lalibela, Ethiopia 107 E4 12 3N 39 0 E
Lalin, China 75 B14 45 12N 127 0 E
Lalín, Spain 42 C2 42 40N 8 5W
Lalin He →, China 75 B13 45 32N 125 40 E
Lalinde, France 28 D4 44 50N 0 44 E
Lalitapur, Nepal 93 F11 27 40N 85 20 E
Lalitpur, India 93 G8 24 42N 78 28 E
Lalkua, India 93 E8 29 5N 79 31 E
Lalm, Norway 16 C6 61 50N 9 17 E
Lalsot, India 92 F7 26 34N 76 20 E
Lam, Vietnam 86 B6 21 21N 106 31 E
Lam Pao Res., Thailand 86 D4 16 50N 103 15 E
Lama Kara, Togo 113 D5 9 30N 1 15 E
Lamag, Malaysia 85 A5 5 29N 117 49 E
Lamaipum, Burma 90 C6 25 40N 97 57 E
Lamap, Vanuatu 133 F5 16 26 S 167 43 E
Lamar, Colo., U.S.A. 154 F3 38 5N 102 37W
Lamar, Mo., U.S.A. 155 G7 37 30N 94 16W
Lamarque, Argentina 176 A3 39 24 S 65 40W
Lamas, Peru 172 B2 6 28 S 76 31W
Lamastre, France 29 D8 44 59N 4 35 E
Lambach, Austria 34 C6 48 6N 13 51 E
Lamballe, France 26 D4 48 29N 2 31W
Lambaréné, Gabon 114 C2 0 41 S 10 12 E
Lambasa = Labasa, Fiji 133 A2 16 30 S 179 27 E
Lambay I., Ireland 23 C5 53 29N 6 1W
Lambayeque □, Peru 172 B2 6 45 S 80 0W
Lambert, C., Papua N. G. 132 C6 4 11 S 151 31 E
Lambert Glacier, Antarctica 7 D6 71 0 S 70 0 E
Lambert-St. Louis International ✕ (STL), U.S.A. 156 F6 38 45N 90 22W
Lambert's Bay, S. Africa 116 E2 32 5 S 18 17 E
Lambertville, U.S.A. 157 C13 41 46N 83 35W
Lambesc, France 29 E9 43 39N 5 16 E
Lambèse = Tazoult, Algeria 111 A6 35 29N 6 11 E
Lambeth, Canada 150 D3 42 54N 81 18W
Lambi, Solomon Is. 133 M10 9 22 S 159 39 E
Lámbia, Greece 48 D3 37 52N 21 53 E
Lambomakondro, Madag. 117 C7 22 41 S 44 44 E
Lambon, Papua N. G. 132 C7 4 45 S 152 48 E
Lambro →, Italy 44 C6 45 8N 9 32 E
Lambton Shores, Canada 150 C3 43 10N 81 56W
Lambu, Papua N. G. 132 B6 3 18 S 151 43 E
Lambunao, Phil. 81 F4 11 3N 122 29 E
Lamé, Chad 109 G2 9 15N 14 32 E
Lame, Nigeria 113 C6 10 30N 9 20 E
Lame Deer, U.S.A. 158 D10 45 37N 106 40W
Lamego, Portugal 42 D3 41 5N 7 52W
Lamèque, Canada 141 C7 47 45N 64 38W
Lameroo, Australia 128 C4 35 19 S 140 33 E
Lamesa, U.S.A. 155 J4 32 44N 101 58W
Lamía, Greece 48 C4 38 55N 22 26 E
Lamigan Pt., Phil. 81 H6 6 48N 126 21 E
Lamine →, U.S.A. 156 F4 38 59N 92 51W
Lamington △, Australia 127 D5 28 13 S 153 12 E
Lamitan, Phil. 81 H4 6 39N 122 8 E
Lamlam, Mt., Guam 133 R15 13 22N 144 41 E
Lamma I., China 69 G11 22 12N 114 8 E
Lammermuir Hills, U.K. 22 F6 55 50N 2 40W
Lammhult, Sweden 17 G8 57 10N 14 35 E
Lamoille →, U.S.A. 151 B11 44 38N 73 13W
Lamon B., Phil. 80 D4 14 30N 122 20 E
Lamongan, Indonesia 85 D4 7 7 S 112 25 E
Lamoni, U.S.A. 156 D3 40 37N 93 56W
Lamont, Canada 142 C6 53 46N 112 50W
Lamont, Calif., U.S.A. 161 K8 35 15N 118 55W
Lamont, Fla., U.S.A. 152 E6 30 23N 83 49W
Lamont, Iowa, U.S.A. 156 B5 42 35N 91 40W
Lamont, Wyo., U.S.A. 158 E10 42 13N 107 29W
Lamotte-Beuvron, France 27 E9 47 36N 2 2 E
Lampa, Peru 172 D3 15 22 S 70 22W
Lampang, Thailand 86 C2 18 16N 99 32 E
Lampasas, U.S.A. 155 K5 31 4N 98 11W
Lampazos de Naranjo, Mexico 162 B4 27 2N 100 32W
Lampedusa, Medit. S. 111 A7 35 36N 12 40 E
Lampertheim, Germany 31 F4 49 35N 8 27 E
Lampeter, U.K. 21 E3 52 7N 4 4W
Lampione, Medit. S. 108 A2 35 33N 12 20 E
Lampman, Canada 143 D8 49 25N 102 50W
Lamprechtshausen, Austria 34 D5 48 0N 12 58 E
Lampung □, Indonesia 84 D2 5 30 S 104 30 E
Lamta, India 93 H9 22 8N 80 7 E
Lamu, Burma 90 F5 19 14N 94 10 E
Lamu, Kenya 118 C5 2 16 S 40 55 E
Lamud, Peru 172 B2 6 10 S 77 57W
Lamy, U.S.A. 159 J11 35 29N 105 53W
Lan Xian, China 74 E6 38 15N 111 35 E
Lan Yu = Hungt'ou Hsü, Taiwan 77 G13 22 0N 121 30 E
Lanai, U.S.A. 145 C5 20 50N 156 55W
Lanai City, U.S.A. 145 C5 20 50N 156 55W
Lanaihale, U.S.A. 145 C5 20 49N 156 53W
Lanak La, China 93 B8 34 27N 79 32 E
Lanak'o Shank'ou = Lanak La, China 93 B8 34 27N 79 32 E
Lanao, L., Phil. 81 H5 7 52N 124 15 E
Lanao del Norte □, Phil. 81 H5 8 0N 124 10 E
Lanao del Sur □, Phil. 81 H5 7 40N 124 15 E
Lanark, Canada 151 A8 45 1N 76 22W
Lanark, U.K. 22 F5 55 40N 3 47W
Lanark, U.S.A. 156 B7 42 6N 89 50W
Lanbi Kyun, Burma 87 G2 10 50N 98 20 E
Lancang, China 76 F2 22 36N 99 58 E
Lancang Jiang →, China 76 G3 21 40N 101 10 E
Lancashire □, U.K. 20 D5 53 50N 2 48W
Lancaster, Canada 151 A10 45 10N 74 30W
Lancaster, U.K. 20 C5 54 3N 2 48W
Lancaster, Calif., U.S.A. 161 L8 34 42N 118 8W
Lancaster, Ky., U.S.A. 148 G3 37 37N 84 35W
Lancaster, Mo., U.S.A. 156 D4 40 31N 92 32W
Lancaster, N.H., U.S.A. 151 B13 44 29N 71 34W
Lancaster, N.Y., U.S.A. 150 D6 42 54N 78 40W
Lancaster, Ohio, U.S.A. 148 F4 39 43N 82 36W
Lancaster, Pa., U.S.A. 151 F8 40 2N 76 19W
Lancaster, S.C., U.S.A. 149 H5 34 43N 80 46W
Lancaster, Wis., U.S.A. 156 B6 42 51N 90 43W
Lancaster Sd., Canada 139 A11 74 13N 84 0W
Lancelin, Australia 125 F2 31 0 S 115 18 E
Lanchow = Lanzhou, China 74 F2 36 1N 103 52 E
Lanchyn, Ukraine 53 B9 48 33N 24 45 E
Lanciano, Italy 45 F11 42 14N 14 23 E
Lanco, Chile 176 A2 39 24 S 72 46W
Lancones, Peru 172 A1 4 30 S 80 30W
Lancun, China 75 F11 36 25N 120 10 E
Łańcut, Poland 55 H9 50 10N 22 13 E
Lancy, Switz. 32 D2 46 12N 6 8 E
Land Between the Lakes ⌂, U.S.A. 149 G1 36 55N 88 7W
Landau, Bayern, Germany 31 G8 48 40N 12 41 E
Landau, Rhld-Pfz., Germany 31 F4 49 12N 8 6 E
Landay, Afghan. 91 C1 30 31N 63 47 E
Landeck, Austria 34 D3 47 9N 10 34 E
Lander, U.S.A. 158 E9 42 50N 108 44W
Lander →, Australia 124 D5 22 0 S 132 0 E
Landerneau, France 26 D2 48 28N 4 17W
Landeryd, Sweden 17 G7 57 7N 13 15 E
Landes, France 28 D2 44 0N 1 0W
Landes □, France 28 E3 43 57N 0 48W
Landes de Gascogne ⌂, France 28 D3 44 23N 0 50W
Landeshut = Kamienna Góra, Poland 55 H3 50 47N 16 2 E
Landete, Spain 40 F3 39 56N 1 25W
Landfall I., India 95 H11 13 40N 93 2 E
Landi Kotal, Pakistan 92 B4 34 7N 71 6 E
Landisburg, U.S.A. 150 F7 40 21N 77 19W
Landivisiau, France 26 D2 48 31N 4 6W
Landquart, Switz. 33 C9 46 58N 9 32 E
Landquart →, Switz. 33 C9 46 50N 9 47 E
Landrecies, France 27 B10 50 7N 3 40 E
Land's End, U.K. 21 G2 50 4N 5 44W
Landsberg = Gorowo Iławeckie, Poland 54 D7 54 17N 20 30 E
Landsberg, Germany 31 G6 48 2N 10 53 E
Landsberg an der Warthe = Gorzów Wielkopolski, Poland 55 F2 52 43N 15 15 E
Landsberg in Oberschlesien = Gorzów Śląski, Poland 55 G5 51 3N 18 22 E
Landsborough Cr. →, Australia 126 C3 22 28 S 144 35 E
Landsbro, Sweden 17 G8 57 24N 14 56 E
Landshut, Germany 31 G8 48 34N 12 8 E
Landskrona, Sweden 17 J6 55 53N 12 50 E
Landstuhl, Germany 31 F3 49 24N 7 33 E
Landvetter, Sweden 17 G6 57 41N 12 17 E
Lane, U.S.A. 152 B10 33 32N 79 53W
Lanesboro, U.S.A. 151 E9 41 57N 75 34W
Lanester, France 26 E3 47 46N 3 22W
Lanett, U.S.A. 152 C4 32 52N 85 12W
Lang Qua, Vietnam 86 A5 22 16N 104 27 E
Lang Shan, China 74 D4 41 0N 106 30 E
Lang Son, Vietnam 76 G6 21 52N 106 42 E
Lang Suan, Thailand 87 H2 9 57N 99 4 E
Langå, Denmark 17 H3 56 23N 9 54 E
Langa-Langa, Dem. Rep. of the Congo 114 C3 3 50 S 15 59 E
Langadhás, Greece 50 F7 40 46N 23 6 E
Langádhia, Greece 48 D4 37 43N 22 1 E
Långan →, Sweden 16 A8 63 19N 14 44 E
Langanes, Iceland 11 A12 66 20N 14 53W
Langano, L., Ethiopia 107 F4 7 36N 38 43 E
Langar, Afghan. 65 E6 37 2N 73 47 E
Langar, Iran 97 C9 35 23N 60 25 E
Langara I., Canada 142 C2 54 14N 133 1W
Långås, Sweden 17 H6 56 58N 12 26 E
Langatabbetje, Suriname 169 C7 4 59N 54 28W
Langdai, China 76 D5 26 6N 105 21 E
Langdon, U.S.A. 154 A5 48 45N 98 22W
Långe Jan = Ölands södra udde, Sweden 17 H10 56 12N 16 23 E
Langeac, France 28 C7 45 7N 3 29 E
Langeais, France 26 E7 47 20N 0 24 E
Langeb Baraka →, Sudan 106 D4 17 28N 36 50 E
Langeberg, S. Africa 116 E3 33 55 S 21 0 E
Langeberge, S. Africa 116 D3 28 15 S 22 33 E
Langeland, Denmark 17 K4 54 56N 10 48 E
Langelands Bælt, Denmark 17 K4 54 50N 10 55 E
Langen, Austria 33 B10 47 8N 10 7 E
Langen, Hessen, Germany 31 F4 49 59N 8 40 E
Langen, Niedersachsen, Germany 30 B4 53 36N 8 36 E
Langenargen, Germany 33 A9 47 36N 9 33 E
Langenbielau = Bielawa, Poland 55 H3 50 43N 16 37 E
Langenburg, Canada 143 C8 50 51N 101 43W
Langeneß, Germany 30 A4 54 38N 8 36 E
Langenlois, Austria 34 C8 48 29N 15 40 E
Langenthal, Switz. 32 B5 47 13N 7 47 E
Langeoog, Germany 30 B3 53 45N 7 32 E
Langeskov, Denmark 17 J4 55 22N 10 35 E
Langesund, Norway 18 F6 59 0N 9 45 E
Langevåg, Norway 18 B3 62 26N 6 13 E
Länghem, Sweden 17 G7 57 36N 13 14 E
Langhirano, Italy 44 D7 44 37N 10 16 E
Langholm, U.K. 22 F5 55 9N 3 0W
Langisjór, Iceland 11 C8 64 11N 18 15W
Langjökull, Iceland 11 C6 64 39N 20 12W
Langkawi, Pulau, Malaysia 87 J2 6 25N 99 45 E
Langklip, S. Africa 116 D3 28 12 S 20 20 E
Langkon, Malaysia 85 A5 6 30N 116 40 E
Langlade, St-P. & M. 141 C8 46 50N 56 20W
Langley, Canada 160 A4 49 7N 122 39W
Langnau, Switz. 32 C5 46 56N 7 47 E
Langogne, France 28 D7 44 43N 3 50 E
Langon, France 28 D3 44 33N 0 16W
Langøya, Norway 14 B16 68 45N 14 50 E
Langreo, Spain 42 B5 43 18N 5 40W
Langres, France 27 E12 47 52N 5 20 E
Langres, Plateau de, France 27 E12 47 45N 5 3 E
Langsa, Indonesia 84 B1 4 30N 97 57 E
Långsele, Sweden 16 A11 63 12N 17 4 E
Långshyttan, Sweden 16 D10 60 27N 16 2 E
Langtang △, Nepal 93 E11 28 10N 85 30 E
Langtao, Burma 90 B6 27 15N 97 34 E
Langting, India 90 C4 25 31N 93 7 E
Langtry, U.S.A. 155 L4 29 49N 101 34W
Langu, Thailand 87 J2 6 53N 99 47 E
Langue de Barbarie △, Senegal 112 C1 14 54N 16 30W
Languedoc, France 28 E7 43 58N 3 55 E
Languedoc-Roussillon □, France 28 E6 43 25N 3 0 E
Langwang, China 69 F9 22 38N 113 27 E
Langwies, Switz. 33 C9 46 50N 9 44 E
Langxi, China 77 B12 31 10N 119 12 E
Langxiangzhen, China 74 E9 39 43N 116 8 E
Langzhong, China 76 B5 31 38N 105 58 E
Lanigan, Canada 143 C7 51 51N 105 2W
Lanín △, Argentina 176 A2 40 0 S 71 58W
Lanjigarh, India 94 E6 19 43N 83 23 E
Lankao, China 74 G8 34 48N 114 50 E
Länkäran, Azerbaijan 97 B6 38 48N 48 52 E
Lanmeur, France 26 D3 48 39N 3 43W
Lannemezan, France 28 E4 43 8N 0 23 E
Lannilis, France 26 D2 48 35N 4 32W
Lannion, France 26 D3 48 46N 3 29W
L'Annonciation, Canada 140 C5 46 25N 74 55W
Lanouaille, France 28 C5 45 24N 1 9 E
Lanping, China 76 D2 26 28N 99 15 E
Lansdale, U.S.A. 151 F9 40 14N 75 17W
Lansdowne, Australia 129 A10 31 48 S 152 30 E
Lansdowne, Canada 151 B8 44 24N 76 1W
Lansdowne, India 93 E8 29 50N 78 41 E
Lansdowne House, Canada 140 B2 52 14N 87 53W
L'Anse, U.S.A. 148 B1 46 45N 88 27W
L'Anse au Loup, Canada 141 B8 51 32N 56 50W
L'Anse aux Meadows, Canada 141 B8 51 36N 55 32W
Lansford, U.S.A. 151 F9 40 50N 75 53W
Lanshan, China 77 E9 25 24N 112 10 E
Lansing, U.S.A. 157 B12 42 44N 84 33W
Lanslebourg-Mont-Cenis, France 29 C10 45 17N 6 52 E
Lanta Yai, Ko, Thailand 87 J2 7 35N 99 3 E
Lantana, U.S.A. 153 J9 26 35N 80 3W
Lantau I., China 69 G10 22 15N 113 56 E
Lantewa, Nigeria 113 C7 12 16N 11 44 E
Lantian, China 74 G5 34 11N 109 20 E
Lanus, Argentina 174 C4 34 44 S 58 27W
Lanusei, Italy 46 C2 39 52N 9 34 E
Lanuza, Phil. 81 G6 9 14N 126 4 E
Lanxi, China 77 C12 29 13N 119 28 E
Lanzarote, Canary Is. 9 e2 29 0N 13 40W
Lanzarote ✕ (ACE), Canary Is. 9 e2 28 57N 13 40W
Lanzhou, China 74 F2 36 1N 103 52 E
Lanzo Torinese, Italy 44 C4 45 16N 7 28 E
Lao →, Italy 47 C8 39 47N 15 48 E
Lao Bao, Laos 86 D6 16 35N 106 30 E
Lao Cai, Vietnam 76 F4 22 30N 103 57 E
Laoag, Phil. 80 B3 18 7N 120 34 E
Laoang, Phil. 80 E5 12 32N 125 8 E
Laoha He →, China 75 C11 43 25N 120 35 E
Laohekou, China 77 A8 32 22N 111 38 E
Laois □, Ireland 23 D4 52 57N 7 36W
Laon, France 27 C10 49 33N 3 35 E
Laona, U.S.A. 148 C1 45 34N 88 40W
Laos ■, Asia 86 D5 17 45N 105 0 E
Lapa, Brazil 175 B6 25 46 S 49 44W
Lapac I., Phil. 81 J3 5 32N 120 47 E
Lapai, Nigeria 113 D6 9 5N 6 32 E
Lapalisse, France 27 F10 46 15N 3 38 E
Lapara I., Phil. 81 J2 5 57N 120 0 E
Lapeer, U.S.A. 157 A13 43 3N 83 19W
Lapeyrade, France 28 D3 44 4N 0 3W
Lapithos, Cyprus 39 E9 35 21N 33 11 E
Lapland = Lappland, Europe 14 B21 68 7N 24 0 E
Laporte, U.S.A. 151 E8 41 25N 76 30W
Lapovo, Serbia & M. 50 B5 44 10N 21 7 E
Lappeenranta, Finland 15 F23 61 3N 28 12 E
Lappland, Europe 14 B21 68 7N 24 0 E
Lappo = Lapua, Finland 14 E20 62 58N 23 0 E
Laprida, Argentina 174 D3 37 34 S 60 45W
Lapseki, Turkey 51 F10 40 20N 26 41 E
Laptev Sea, Russia 67 B13 76 0N 125 0 E
Lapu-Lapu, Phil. 81 F4 10 20N 123 55 E
Lapua, Finland 14 E20 62 58N 23 0 E
Lăpuş →, Romania 53 C8 47 25N 23 40 E
Lapuş, Munţii, Romania 53 C8 47 20N 23 50 E
Lăpuşna, Moldova 53 D13 46 53N 28 25 E
Łapy, Poland 55 F9 52 59N 22 52 E
Laqiya Arba'in, Sudan 106 C2 20 1N 28 1 E
Laqiya Umran, Sudan 106 D2 19 55N 28 18 E
L'Áquila, Italy 45 F10 42 22N 13 22 E
Lār, Āzarbājān-e Sharqī, Iran 96 B5 38 30N 47 52 E
Lār, Fārs, Iran 97 E7 27 40N 54 14 E
Lara, Australia 128 E6 38 2 S 144 26 E
Lara □, Venezuela 168 A4 10 10N 69 50W
Larabanga, Ghana 112 D4 9 16N 1 56W
Larache, Morocco 110 A3 35 10N 6 5W
Laragaran = Plaridel, Phil. 81 G4 8 37N 123 43 E
Laragne-Montéglin, France 29 D9 44 18N 5 49 E
Laramie, U.S.A. 154 E2 41 19N 105 35W
Laramie Mts., U.S.A. 154 E2 42 0N 105 30W
Laranjeiras, Brazil 170 D4 10 48 S 37 10W
Laranjeiras do Sul, Brazil 175 B5 25 23 S 52 23W
Larantuka, Indonesia 82 C2 8 21 S 122 55 E
Larat, Indonesia 83 C4 7 0 S 132 0 E
L'Arbresle, France 29 C8 45 50N 4 36 E
Lärbro, Sweden 17 G12 57 47N 18 50 E
Lårdal, Norway 18 E5 59 25N 8 10 E
Larde, Mozam. 119 F4 16 28 S 39 43 E
Larder Lake, Canada 140 C4 48 5N 79 40W
Lardhos, Ákra = Líndhos, Ákra, Greece 38 E12 36 4N 28 10 E
Lardhos, Órmos, Greece 38 E12 36 4N 28 2 E
Laredo, Spain 42 B7 43 26N 3 28W
Laredo, U.S.A. 155 M5 27 30N 99 30W
Laredo Sd., Canada 142 C3 52 30N 128 53W
Larena, Phil. 81 G4 9 15N 123 35 E
Largentière, France 29 D8 44 34N 4 18 E
L'Argentière-la-Bessée, France 29 D10 44 47N 6 33 E
Largo, U.S.A. 153 H7 27 55N 82 47W
Largo, Key, U.S.A. 153 K9 25 15N 80 15W
Largs, U.K. 22 F4 55 47N 4 52W
Lari, Italy 44 E7 43 34N 10 35 E
Lariang, Indonesia 82 B1 1 26 S 119 17 E
Larimore, U.S.A. 154 B6 47 54N 97 38W
Larino, Italy 45 G11 41 48N 14 54 E
Lárisa, Greece 48 B4 39 36N 22 27 E
Lárisa □, Greece 48 B4 39 39N 22 24 E
Larissa = Lárisa, Greece 48 B4 39 36N 22 27 E
Larkana, Pakistan 91 D3 27 32N 68 18 E
Larkins = South Miami, U.S.A. 153 K9 25 42N 80 18W
Larnaca, Cyprus 39 F9 34 55N 33 38 E
Larnaca ✕ (LCA), Cyprus 39 F9 34 50N 33 34 E
Larnaca Bay, Cyprus 39 F9 34 53N 33 45 E
Larne, U.K. 23 B6 54 51N 5 51W
Larned, U.S.A. 154 F5 38 11N 99 6W
Laroquebrou, France 28 D6 44 58N 2 12 E
Larose, U.S.A. 155 L9 29 34N 90 23W
Larrimah, Australia 124 C5 15 35 S 133 12 E
Larsen Bay, U.S.A. 144 H9 57 32N 153 59W
Larsen Ice Shelf, Antarctica 7 C17 67 0 S 62 0W
Laruns, France 28 F3 43 0N 0 26W
Larvik, Norway 18 E7 59 4N 10 2 E
Larzac, Causse du, France 28 E7 43 50N 3 17 E
Las Alpujarras, Spain 41 J1 36 55N 3 20W
Las Animas, U.S.A. 154 F3 38 4N 103 13W
Las Anod, Somali Rep. 120 C3 8 26N 47 19 E
Las Arenas, Spain 42 B6 43 17N 4 50W
Las Batuecas ⌂, Spain 42 E4 40 32N 6 5W
Las Bonitas, Venezuela 168 B4 7 52N 65 40W
Las Brenãs, Argentina 174 B3 27 5 S 61 7W
Las Cabezas de San Juan, Spain 43 J5 36 57N 5 58W
Las Cañadas del Teide △, Canary Is. 9 e1 28 15N 16 37W
Las Chimeneas, Mexico 161 N10 32 8N 116 5W
Las Coloradas, Argentina 176 A2 39 34 S 70 36W
Las Cruces, U.S.A. 159 K10 32 19N 106 47W
Las Flores, Argentina 174 D4 36 10 S 59 7W
Las Heras, Argentina 174 C2 32 51 S 68 49W
Las Hermosas △, Colombia 168 C2 3 48N 75 51W
Las Horquetas, Argentina 176 C2 48 14 S 71 11W
Las Khoreh, Somali Rep. 120 B3 11 10N 48 20 E
Las Lajas, Argentina 176 A2 38 30 S 70 25W
Las Lomas, Peru 172 A1 4 40 S 80 10W
Las Lomitas, Argentina 174 A3 24 43 S 60 35W
Las Marismas, Spain 43 H4 37 5N 6 20W
Las Mercedes, Venezuela 168 B4 9 7N 66 24W
Las Minas, Spain 41 G3 38 20N 1 41W
Las Navas de la Concepción, Spain 43 H5 37 56N 5 30W
Las Navas del Marqués, Spain 42 E6 40 36N 4 20W
Las Nieves, Phil. 81 G5 8 46N 125 34 E
Las Orquideas △, Colombia 168 B2 6 36N 76 16W
Las Palmas, Argentina 174 B4 27 8 S 58 45W
Las Palmas, Canary Is. 9 e1 28 7N 15 26W
Las Palmas →, Mexico 161 N10 32 26N 116 54W
Las Palmas ✕ (LPA), Canary Is. 9 e1 27 55N 15 25W
Las Palmas de Cocalán △, Chile 174 C1 34 18 S 71 4W
Las Pedroñas, Spain 41 F2 39 26N 2 40W
Las Piedras, Uruguay 175 C4 34 44 S 56 14W
Las Pipinas, Argentina 174 D4 35 30 S 57 19W
Las Plumas, Argentina 176 B3 43 40 S 67 15W
Las Rosas, Argentina 174 C3 32 30 S 61 35W
Las Rozas, Spain 42 E7 40 29N 3 52W
Las Tablas, Panama 164 E3 7 49N 80 14W
Las Termas, Argentina 174 B3 27 29 S 64 52W
Las Toscas, Argentina 174 B4 28 21 S 59 18W
Las Truchas, Mexico 162 D4 17 57N 102 13W
Las Varillas, Argentina 174 C3 31 50 S 62 50W
Las Vegas, N. Mex., U.S.A. 159 J11 35 36N 105 13W
Las Vegas, Nev., U.S.A. 161 J11 36 10N 115 9W
Las Vegas McCarran International ✕ (LAS), U.S.A. 161 J11 36 5N 115 9W
Lasa = Lhasa, China 68 D4 29 25N 90 58 E
Lasanga I., Papua N. G. 132 D4 7 25 S 147 15 E
Lasarte, Spain 40 B2 43 16N 2 1W
Lascano, Uruguay 175 C5 33 35 S 54 12W
Lascelles, Australia 128 C5 35 34 S 142 34 E
Lash-e Joveyn, Afghan. 91 C1 31 45N 61 30 E
Lashburn, Canada 143 C7 53 10N 109 40W
Lashio, Burma 90 D6 22 56N 97 45 E
Lashkar, India 92 F8 26 10N 78 10 E
Lashkar Gāh, Afghan. 91 C2 31 35N 64 21 E
Łasin, Poland 54 E6 53 30N 19 2 E
Lasíthi, Greece 39 E6 35 11N 25 31 E
Lasíthi □, Greece 39 E6 35 5N 25 50 E
Lāsjerd, Iran 97 C7 35 24N 53 4 E
Lask, Poland 55 G6 51 34N 19 8 E
Łaskarzew, Poland 55 G8 51 48N 21 36 E
Laško, Slovenia 45 B12 46 10N 15 16 E
Lassance, Brazil 171 E3 17 54 S 44 34W
Lassay-les-Châteaux, France 26 D6 48 27N 0 30W
Lassen Pk., U.S.A. 158 F3 40 29N 121 31W

Lassen Volcanic △, U.S.A. 158 F3 40 30N 121 20W
Lassongo, Angola 115 E4 12 5 S 22 46 E
Last Mountain L., Canada 143 C7 51 5N 105 14W
Lastchance Cr. →, U.S.A. 160 E5 40 2N 121 15W
Lastoursville, Gabon 114 C2 0 55 S 12 38 E
Lastovo, Croatia 45 F13 42 46N 16 55 E
Lastovski Kanal, Croatia 45 F14 42 50N 17 0 E
Lat Yao, Thailand 86 E2 15 45N 99 48 E
Latacunga, Ecuador 168 D2 0 50 S 78 35W
Latakia = Al Lādhiqīyah, Syria 100 E6 35 30N 35 45 E
Latchford, Canada 140 C4 47 20N 79 50W
Late, Tonga 133 P13 18 48 S 174 39W
Latehar, India 93 H11 23 45N 84 30 E
Laterza, Italy 47 B9 40 37N 16 48 E
Latham, Australia 125 E2 29 44 S 116 20 E
Lathen, Germany 30 C3 52 52N 7 19 E
Lathi, India 92 F4 27 43N 71 23 E
Lathi, Vanuatu 133 D5 14 57 S 167 8 E
Lathrop, U.S.A. 156 E2 39 33N 94 20W
Lathrop Wells, U.S.A. 161 J10 36 39N 116 24W
Latiano, Italy 47 B10 40 33N 17 43 E
Latina, Italy 46 A5 41 28N 12 52 E
Latisana, Italy 45 C10 45 47N 13 0 E
Latium = Lazio □, Italy 45 F9 42 10N 12 30 E
Laton, U.S.A. 160 J7 36 26N 119 41W
Latorytsya →, Slovak Rep. 35 C14 48 28N 21 50 E
Latouche Treville, C., Australia 124 C3 18 27 S 121 49 E
Latouma, Niger 109 D2 22 10N 14 50 E
Látrar, Iceland 11 A3 66 24N 23 2W
Latrobe, Australia 127 G4 41 14 S 146 30 E
Latrobe, U.S.A. 150 F5 40 19N 79 23W
Latrónico, Italy 47 B9 40 5N 16 1 E
Latur, India 94 E3 18 25N 76 40 E
Latvia ■, Europe 15 H20 56 50N 24 0 E
Lau, Nigeria 113 D7 9 11N 11 19 E
Lau Fau Shan, China 69 G10 22 28N 113 59 E
Lau Group, Fiji 133 A3 17 0 S 178 30W
Lauban = Lubań, Poland 55 G2 51 5N 15 15 E
Lauca →, Bolivia 172 D4 19 9 S 68 10W
Lauchhammer, Germany 30 D9 51 29N 13 47 E
Lauda-Königshofen, Germany 31 F5 49 33N 9 42 E
Laudal, Norway 18 F4 58 15N 7 30 E
Lauenburg = Lębork, Poland 54 D4 54 33N 17 46 E
Lauenburg, Germany 30 B6 53 22N 10 32 E
Lauenburgische Seen △, Germany 30 B6 53 38N 10 45 E
Lauf, Germany 31 F7 49 30N 11 16 E
Laufás, Iceland 11 B8 65 53N 18 4W
Läufelfingen, Switz. 32 B5 47 24N 7 52 E
Laufen, Switz. 32 B5 47 25N 7 30 E
Laugar, Iceland 11 B5 65 15N 21 48W
Laugarás, Iceland 11 C6 64 7N 20 30W
Laugarbakki, Iceland 11 B6 65 20N 20 55W
Laugarvatn, Iceland 11 C6 64 13N 20 44W
Laughlin, U.S.A. 159 J6 35 8N 114 35W
Laujar de Andarax, Spain 41 H2 37 0N 2 54W
Laukaa, Finland 15 E21 62 24N 25 56 E
Launceston, Australia 127 G4 41 24 S 147 8 E
Launceston, U.K. 21 G3 50 38N 4 22W
Laune →, Ireland 23 D2 52 7N 9 47W
Launglon Bok, Burma 86 F1 13 50N 97 54 E
Laupheim, Germany 31 G5 48 14N 9 52 E
Laura, Queens., Australia 126 B3 15 32 S 144 32 E
Laura, S. Austral., Australia 128 B3 33 10 S 138 18 E
Laureana di Borrello, Italy 47 D9 38 30N 16 5 E
Laurel, Fla., U.S.A. 153 H7 27 8N 82 27W
Laurel, Ind., U.S.A. 157 E11 39 31N 85 11W
Laurel, Miss., U.S.A. 155 K10 31 41N 89 8W
Laurel, Mont., U.S.A. 158 D9 45 40N 108 46W
Laurel Bay, U.S.A. 152 C9 32 27N 80 47W
Laurencekirk, U.K. 22 E6 56 50N 2 28W
Laurens, Iowa, U.S.A. 156 B2 42 51N 94 52W
Laurens, S.C., U.S.A. 149 H4 34 30N 82 1W
Laurentian Plateau, Canada 141 B6 52 0N 70 0W
Lauria, Italy 47 B8 40 2N 15 50 E
Laurie L., Canada 143 B8 56 35N 101 57W
Laurinburg, U.S.A. 149 H6 34 47N 79 28W
Laurium, U.S.A. 148 B1 47 14N 88 27W
Lausanne, Switz. 32 C3 46 32N 6 38 E
Laut, Indonesia 85 B3 4 45N 108 0 E
Laut, Pulau, Indonesia 85 C5 3 40 S 116 10 E
Laut Kecil, Kepulauan, Indonesia 85 C5 4 45 S 115 40 E
Lautaro, Chile 176 A2 38 31 S 72 27W
Lautem, E. Timor 82 C3 8 22 S 126 54 E
Lauterbach, Germany 30 E5 50 37N 9 24 E
Lauterbrunnen, Switz. 32 C5 46 36N 7 55 E
Lauterecken, Germany 31 F3 49 38N 7 35 E
Lautoka, Fiji 133 A1 17 37 S 177 27 E
Lauzès, France 28 D5 44 34N 1 35 E
Lava →, Russia 54 D8 54 37N 21 14 E
Lava Beds △, U.S.A. 158 F3 41 40N 121 30W
Lavagh More, Ireland 23 B3 54 46N 8 6W
Lavagna, Italy 44 D6 44 18N 9 20 E
Laval, France 26 D6 48 4N 0 48W
Lavalle, Argentina 174 B2 28 15 S 65 15W
Lavanggu, Solomon Is. 133 N11 11 36 S 160 16 E
Lavant Station, Canada 151 A8 45 3N 76 42W
Lāvar Meydān, Iran 97 D7 30 20N 54 30 E
Lávara, Greece 51 E10 41 19N 26 22 E
Lavardac, France 28 D4 44 12N 0 20 E
Lavaur, France 28 E5 43 40N 1 49 E
Lavaux, Switz. 32 D3 46 30N 6 45 E
Lavelanet, France 28 F5 42 57N 1 51 E
Lavello, Italy 47 A8 41 3N 15 48 E
L'Averdy, C., Papua N. G. 132 C8 5 33 S 155 4 E
Lavers Hill, Australia 128 E5 38 40 S 143 25 E
Laverton, Australia 125 E3 28 44 S 122 29 E
Lavik, Norway 18 C2 61 6N 5 25 E
Lavis, Italy 44 B8 46 8N 11 7 E
Lávkos, Greece 48 B5 39 9N 23 14 E
Lavos, Portugal 42 E2 40 6N 8 49W
Lavradio, Portugal 43 G1 38 40N 9 3W
Lavras, Brazil 171 F3 21 20 S 45 0W
Lavre, Portugal 43 G2 38 46N 8 22W
Lavrio = Lávrion, Greece 48 D6 37 40N 24 4 E
Lávrion, Greece 48 D6 37 40N 24 4 E
Lávris, Greece 39 E5 35 25N 24 40 E
Lavumisa, Swaziland 117 D5 27 20 S 31 55 E
Lavushi Manda △, Zambia 119 E3 12 46 S 31 0 E
Lawa, Phil. 81 H5 6 12N 125 41 E
Lawa-an, Phil. 81 F5 11 51N 125 5 E
Lawaki, Fiji 133 A2 17 40 S 178 35 E
Lawas, Malaysia 85 B5 4 55N 115 25 E
Lawdar, Yemen 98 D4 13 53N 45 52 E
Lawele, Indonesia 82 C2 5 13 S 122 57 E
Lawksawk, Burma 90 E6 21 15N 96 52 E
Lawn Hill △, Australia 126 B2 18 15 S 138 6 E
Lawowa, Indonesia 82 B2 4 26 S 122 56 E
Lawqah, Si. Arabia 96 D4 29 49N 42 45 E
Lawra, Ghana 112 C4 10 39N 2 51W
Lawrence, N.Z. 131 F4 45 55 S 169 41 E
Lawrence, Ind., U.S.A. 157 E10 39 50N 86 2W
Lawrence, Kans., U.S.A. 154 F7 38 58N 95 14W
Lawrence, Mass., U.S.A. 151 D13 42 43N 71 10W
Lawrence, Ohio, U.S.A. 148 F2 39 50N 86 2W
Lawrenceburg, Ind., U.S.A. 157 E12 39 6N 84 52W
Lawrenceburg, Ky., U.S.A. 157 F12 38 2N 84 54W
Lawrenceburg, Tenn., U.S.A. 149 H2 35 14N 87 20W
Lawrenceville, Ga., U.S.A. 152 B6 33 57N 83 59W
Lawrenceville, Ill., U.S.A. 157 F9 38 44N 87 41W
Lawrenceville, Pa., U.S.A. 150 E7 41 59N 77 8W
Laws, U.S.A. 160 H8 37 24N 118 20W
Lawson, U.S.A. 156 E2 39 26N 94 12W
Lawtey, U.S.A. 152 E7 30 3N 82 5W
Lawton, Mich., U.S.A. 157 B11 42 10N 85 50W
Lawton, Okla., U.S.A. 155 H5 34 37N 98 25W
Lawu, Indonesia 85 D4 7 40 S 111 13 E
Lawz, J. al, Si. Arabia 106 B4 28 39N 35 18 E
Laxå, Sweden 17 F8 58 59N 14 37 E
Laxamýri, Iceland 11 B9 65 58N 17 24W
Laxford, L., U.K. 22 C3 58 24N 5 6W
Laxou, France 27 D13 48 41N 6 8 E
Lay →, France 28 B2 46 18N 1 17W
Layla, Si. Arabia 98 B4 22 10N 46 40 E
Laylān, Iraq 96 C5 35 18N 44 31 E
Layon →, France 26 E6 47 20N 0 45W
Laysan I., U.S.A. 145 F9 25 50N 171 50W
Layton, Fla., U.S.A. 153 L9 24 50N 80 47W
Layton, Utah, U.S.A. 158 F7 41 4N 111 58W
Laytonville, U.S.A. 158 G2 39 41N 123 29W
Laza, Burma 90 B6 26 30N 97 38 E
Lazarāta, Greece 39 B2 38 47N 20 40 E
Lazarevac, Serbia & M. 50 B4 44 23N 20 17 E
Lazarevskoye, Russia 61 J4 43 55N 39 21 E
Lazarivo, Madag. 117 C8 23 54 S 44 59 E
Lazdijai, Lithuania 54 D10 54 14N 23 31 E
Lazi, Phil. 81 G4 9 8N 123 38 E
Lazio □, Italy 45 F9 42 10N 12 30 E
Lazo, Moldova 53 C13 47 33N 28 2 E
Lazo, Russia 70 C6 43 25N 133 55 E
Lbishchensk = Chapayev, Kazakhstan 60 E10 50 25N 51 10 E
Le Beausset, France 29 E9 43 12N 5 48 E
Le Bic, Canada 141 C6 48 20N 68 41W
Le Blanc, France 28 B5 46 37N 1 3 E
Le Bleymard, France 28 D7 44 30N 3 42 E
Le Bourgneuf-la-Fôret, France 26 D6 48 10N 0 59W
Le Brassus, Switz. 32 C2 46 35N 6 13 E
Le Bugue, France 28 D4 44 55N 0 56 E
Le Cateau Cambrésis, France 27 B10 50 7N 3 32 E
Le Caylar, France 28 E7 43 51N 3 19 E
Le Châble, Switz. 32 D4 46 5N 7 12 E
Le Chambon-Feugerolles, France 29 C8 45 24N 4 19 E
Le Châtelard, Switz. 32 D3 46 4N 6 57 E
Le Châtelet, France 28 B6 46 38N 2 16 E
Le Chesne, France 27 C11 49 30N 4 45 E
Le Cheylard, France 29 D8 44 55N 4 25 E
Le Claire, U.S.A. 156 C6 41 36N 90 21W
Le Conquet, France 26 D2 48 21N 4 46W
Le Creusot, France 27 F11 46 48N 4 24 E
Le Croisic, France 26 E4 47 18N 2 30W
Le Donjon, France 27 F10 46 22N 3 48 E
Le Dorat, France 28 B5 46 14N 1 5 E
Le François, Martinique 164 c 14 38N 60 57W
Le Gosier, Guadeloupe 164 b 16 14N 61 29W
Le Grand-Lucé, France 26 E7 47 52N 0 28 E
Le Grand-Pressigny, France 26 F7 46 55N 0 48 E
Le Grand-Quevilly, France 26 C8 49 24N 1 3 E
Le Gris Gris, Mauritius 121 d 20 31 S 57 32 E
Le Havre, France 26 C7 49 30N 0 5 E
Le Lamentin, Martinique 164 c 14 35N 61 2W
Le Lavandou, France 29 E10 43 8N 6 22 E
Le Lion-d'Angers, France 26 E6 47 37N 0 43W
Le Locle, Switz. 32 B3 47 3N 6 44 E
Le Louroux-Béconnais, France 26 E6 47 30N 0 55W
Le Luc, France 29 E10 43 23N 6 21 E
Le Lude, France 26 E7 47 39N 0 9 E
Le Maire, Estr. de, Argentina 176 D4 54 50 S 65 0W
Le Mans, France 26 E7 48 0N 0 10 E
Le Marin, Martinique 164 c 14 27N 60 55W
Le Mars, U.S.A. 154 D6 42 47N 96 10W
Le Mayet-de-Montagne, France 27 F10 46 4N 3 40 E
Le Mêle-sur-Sarthe, France 26 D7 48 31N 0 22 E
Le Moléson, Switz. 32 C4 46 33N 7 1 E
Le Monastier-sur-Gazeille, France 28 D7 44 57N 3 59 E
Le Monêtier-les-Bains, France 29 D10 44 58N 6 30 E
Le Mont-Dore, France 28 C6 45 35N 2 49 E
Le Mont-St-Michel, France 26 D5 48 40N 1 30W
Le Moule, Guadeloupe 164 b 16 20N 61 22W
Le Muy, France 29 E10 43 28N 6 34 E
Le Palais, France 26 E3 47 20N 3 10W
Le Perthus, France 28 F6 42 30N 2 53 E
Le Pont, Switz. 32 C2 46 41N 6 20 E
Le Port, Réunion 121 c 20 56 S 55 18 E
Le Prêcheur, Martinique 164 c 14 50N 61 12W
Le Puy-en-Velay, France 28 C7 45 3N 3 52 E
Le Robert, Martinique 164 c 14 40N 60 56W
Le Roy, U.S.A. 157 D8 40 21N 88 46W
Le St-Esprit, Martinique 164 c 14 34N 60 56W
Le Sentier, Switz. 32 C2 46 37N 6 15 E
Le Sueur, U.S.A. 154 C8 44 28N 93 55W
Le Tampon, Réunion 121 c 21 16 S 55 32 E
Le Teil, France 29 D8 44 33N 4 40 E
Le Teilleul, France 26 D6 48 32N 0 53W
Le Theil, France 26 D7 48 16N 0 42 E
Le Thillot, France 27 E13 47 53N 6 46 E
Le Thuy, Vietnam 86 D6 17 14N 106 49 E
Le Touquet-Paris-Plage, France 27 B8 50 30N 1 36 E
Le Tréport, France 26 B8 50 3N 1 20 E
Le Val-d'Ajol, France 27 E13 47 55N 6 30 E
Le Verdon-sur-Mer, France 28 C2 45 33N 1 4W
Le Vigan, France 28 E7 43 59N 3 36 E
Lea →, U.K. 21 F8 51 31N 0 1 E
Lea Lea, Papua N. G. 132 E4 9 17 S 146 59 E
Leach, Cambodia 87 F4 12 21N 103 46 E
Lead, U.S.A. 154 C3 44 21N 103 46W
Leader, Canada 143 C7 50 50N 109 30W
Leadville, U.S.A. 159 G10 39 15N 106 18W
Leaf →, U.S.A. 155 K10 30 59N 88 44W
Leaf Rapids, Canada 143 B9 56 30N 99 59W
Leaghur, L., Australia 128 B5 33 35 S 143 3 E
Leaksville = Eden, U.S.A. 149 G6 36 29N 79 53W
Lealui, Zambia 115 F4 15 10 S 23 2 E
Leamington, Canada 140 D3 42 3N 82 36W
Leamington, N.Z. 130 D4 37 55 S 175 30 E
Leamington, U.S.A. 158 G7 39 32N 112 17W
Leamington Spa = Royal Leamington Spa, U.K. 21 E6 52 18N 1 31W
Le'an, China 77 D10 27 22N 115 48 E
Leandro Norte Alem, Argentina 175 B4 27 34 S 55 15W
Leane, L., Ireland 23 D2 52 2N 9 32W
Learmonth, Australia 124 D1 22 13 S 114 10 E
Leary, U.S.A. 152 D5 31 29N 84 31W
Leask, Canada 143 C7 53 5N 106 45W
Leatherhead, U.K. 21 F7 51 18N 0 20W
Leavenworth, Ind., U.S.A. 157 F10 38 12N 86 21W
Leavenworth, Kans., U.S.A. 154 F7 39 19N 94 55W
Leavenworth, Wash., U.S.A. 158 C3 47 36N 120 40W
Leawood, U.S.A. 156 F2 38 57N 94 37W
Łeba, Poland 54 D4 54 45N 17 32 E
Łeba →, Poland 54 D4 54 46N 17 33 E
Lebach, Germany 31 F2 49 25N 6 54 E
Lebak, Phil. 81 H5 6 32N 124 5 E
Lebam, U.S.A. 160 D3 46 34N 123 33W
Lebane, Serbia & M. 50 D5 42 56N 21 44 E
Lebango, Congo 114 B2 0 39N 14 21 E
Lebango →, Congo 114 B2 0 2N 14 52 E
Lebanon, Ill., U.S.A. 156 F7 38 38N 89 49W
Lebanon, Ind., U.S.A. 157 D10 40 3N 86 28W
Lebanon, Kans., U.S.A. 154 F5 39 49N 98 33W
Lebanon, Ky., U.S.A. 148 G3 37 34N 85 15W
Lebanon, Mo., U.S.A. 155 G8 37 41N 92 40W
Lebanon, N.H., U.S.A. 151 C12 43 39N 72 15W
Lebanon, Ohio, U.S.A. 157 E12 39 26N 84 13W
Lebanon, Oreg., U.S.A. 158 D2 44 32N 122 55W
Lebanon, Pa., U.S.A. 151 F8 40 20N 76 26W
Lebanon, Tenn., U.S.A. 149 G2 36 12N 86 18W
Lebanon ■, Asia 103 B5 34 0N 36 0 E
Lebanon Junction, U.S.A. 157 G11 37 50N 85 44W
Lebanon Station, U.S.A. 153 F7 29 10N 82 37W
Lebec, U.S.A. 161 L8 34 50N 118 52W
Lebedyan, Russia 59 F10 53 0N 39 10 E
Lebedyn, Ukraine 59 G8 50 35N 34 30 E
Lebel-sur-Quévillon, Canada 140 C4 49 3N 76 59W
Lebo, Dem. Rep. of the Congo 114 B4 4 30N 23 58 E
Lebomboberge, S. Africa 117 C5 24 30 S 32 0 E
Lębork, Poland 54 D4 54 33N 17 46 E
Lebrija, Spain 43 J4 36 53N 6 5W
Łebsko, Jezioro, Poland 54 D4 54 40N 17 25 E
Lebu, Chile 174 D1 37 40 S 73 47W
Leca da Palmeira, Portugal 42 D2 41 12N 8 42W
Lecce, Italy 47 B11 40 23N 18 11 E
Lecco, Italy 44 C6 45 51N 9 23 E
Lecco, L. di, Italy 44 C6 45 55N 9 19 E
Lécera, Spain 40 D4 41 13N 0 43W
Lech, Austria 34 D3 47 13N 10 9 E
Lech →, Germany 31 G6 48 43N 10 56 E
Lechang, China 77 E9 25 10N 113 20 E
Lechtaler Alpen, Austria 34 D3 47 15N 10 30 E
Léconi, Gabon 114 C2 1 35 S 14 14 E
Léconi →, Gabon 114 C2 1 11 S 13 16 E
Lecontes Mills, U.S.A. 150 E6 41 5N 78 17W
Lectoure, France 28 E4 43 56N 0 38 E
Łęczna, Poland 55 G9 51 18N 22 53 E
Łęczyca, Poland 55 F6 52 5N 19 15 E
Ledang, Gunung, Malaysia 84 B2 2 22N 102 37 E
Ledesma, Spain 42 D5 41 6N 5 59W
Lediba, Dem. Rep. of the Congo 114 C3 3 1 S 16 34 E
Lédo, Cabo, Angola 115 D2 9 43 S 13 12 E
Ledong, China 86 C7 18 41N 109 5 E
Leduc, Canada 142 C6 53 15N 113 30W
Lee, Fla., U.S.A. 152 E6 30 25N 83 18W
Lee, Mass., U.S.A. 151 D11 42 19N 73 15W
Lee →, Ireland 23 E3 51 53N 8 56W
Lee Vining, U.S.A. 160 H7 37 58N 119 7W
Leech L., U.S.A. 154 B7 47 10N 94 24W
Leechburg, U.S.A. 150 F5 40 37N 79 36W
Leeds, U.K. 20 D6 53 48N 1 33W
Leeds, U.S.A. 149 J2 33 33N 86 33W
Leek, Neths. 24 A6 53 10N 6 24 E
Leek, U.K. 20 D5 53 7N 2 1W
Leeman, Australia 125 E1 29 57 S 114 58 E
Leeper, U.S.A. 150 E5 41 22N 79 18W
Leer, Germany 30 B3 53 13N 7 26 E
Lee's Summit, U.S.A. 156 F2 38 55N 94 23W
Leesburg, Fla., U.S.A. 153 G8 28 49N 81 53W
Leesburg, Ga., U.S.A. 152 D5 31 44N 84 10W
Leesburg, Ohio, U.S.A. 157 E13 39 21N 83 33W
Leeston, N.Z. 131 D7 43 45 S 172 19 E
Leesville, U.S.A. 155 K8 31 9N 93 16W
Leeton, Australia 129 C7 34 33 S 146 23 E
Leetonia, U.S.A. 150 F4 40 53N 80 45W
Leeu Gamka, S. Africa 116 E3 32 47 S 21 59 E
Leeuwarden, Neths. 24 A5 53 15N 5 48 E
Leeuwin, C., Australia 125 F2 34 20 S 115 9 E
Leeuwin Naturaliste △, Australia 125 F2 34 6 S 115 3 E
Leeward Is., Atl. Oc. 165 C7 16 30N 63 30W
Léfini, Congo 114 C3 2 55 S 15 39 E
Léfini △, Congo 114 C3 2 55 S 15 20 E
Léfini →, Congo 114 C3 2 56 S 16 9 E
Lefka, Cyprus 39 E8 35 6N 32 51 E
Lefkada = Levkás, Greece 39 B2 38 40N 20 43 E
Lefkoniko, Cyprus 39 E9 35 18N 33 44 E
Lefroy, Canada 150 B5 44 16N 79 34W
Lefroy, L., Australia 125 F3 31 21 S 121 40 E
Łeg →, Poland 55 H8 50 42N 21 50 E
Leganés, Spain 42 E7 40 19N 3 45W
Legazpi, Phil. 80 E4 13 10N 123 45 E
Lège-Cap-Ferret, France 28 D2 44 48N 1 9W
Lege Hida, Ethiopia 107 F5 7 56N 41 4 E
Legendre I., Australia 124 D2 20 22 S 116 55 E
Leghorn = Livorno, Italy 44 E7 43 33N 10 19 E
Legionowo, Poland 55 F7 52 25N 20 50 E
Legnago, Italy 45 C8 45 11N 11 18 E
Legnano, Italy 44 C5 45 36N 8 54 E
Legnica, Poland 55 G3 51 12N 16 10 E
Legrad, Croatia 45 B13 46 17N 16 51 E
Leh, India 93 B7 34 9N 77 35 E
Lehigh Acres, U.S.A. 153 J8 26 36N 81 39W
Lehighton, U.S.A. 151 F9 40 50N 75 43W
Lehliu, Romania 53 F11 44 29N 26 50 E
Leho, Sudan 107 F3 7 7N 33 52 E
Lehrte, Germany 30 C5 52 22N 9 58 E
Lehua I., U.S.A. 145 A1 22 1N 160 6W
Lehututu, Botswana 116 C3 23 54 S 21 55 E
Lei Shui →, China 77 D9 26 55N 112 35 E
Leiah, Pakistan 91 C3 30 58N 70 58 E
Leibnitz, Austria 34 E8 46 47N 15 34 E
Leibo, China 76 C4 28 11N 103 34 E
Leicester, U.K. 21 E6 52 38N 1 8W
Leicester City □, U.K. 21 E6 52 38N 1 8W
Leicestershire □, U.K. 21 E6 52 41N 1 17W
Leichhardt →, Australia 126 B2 17 35 S 139 48 E
Leichhardt Ra., Australia 126 C4 20 46 S 147 40 E
Leiden, Neths. 24 B4 52 9N 4 30 E
Leie →, Belgium 24 C3 51 2N 3 45 E
Leifers = Láives, Italy 45 B8 46 26N 11 20 E
Leigh →, Australia 128 E6 38 18 S 144 30 E
Leigh Creek, Australia 128 A3 30 38 S 138 26 E
Leikanger, Sogn og Fjordane, Norway 18 B2 62 8N 5 18 E
Leikanger, Sogn og Fjordane, Norway 18 C3 61 10N 6 51 E
Leikong, Norway 18 B2 62 15N 5 47 E
Leiktho, Burma 90 F6 19 13N 96 35 E
Leimen, Germany 31 F4 49 21N 8 41 E
Leine →, Germany 30 C5 52 43N 9 36 E
Leinefelde, Germany 30 D6 51 23N 10 19 E
Leinster, Australia 125 E3 27 51 S 120 36 E
Leinster □, Ireland 23 C4 53 3N 7 8W
Leinster, Mt., Ireland 23 D5 52 37N 6 46W
Leipalingis, Lithuania 54 D10 54 5N 23 51 E
Leipe = Lipno, Poland 55 F6 52 49N 19 15 E
Leipzig, Germany 30 D8 51 18N 12 22 E
Leira, Norway 18 D6 60 58N 9 17 E
Leiria, Portugal 42 F2 39 46N 8 53W
Leiria □, Portugal 42 F2 39 46N 8 53W
Leirvassbu, Norway 18 C5 61 33N 8 13 E
Leirvik, Norway 18 E2 59 47N 5 28 E
Leishan, China 76 D7 26 15N 108 20 E
Leisler, Mt., Australia 124 D4 23 23 S 129 20 E
Leisure City, U.S.A. 153 K9 25 31N 80 26W
Leith, U.K. 22 F5 55 59N 3 11W
Leith Hill, U.K. 21 F7 51 11N 0 22W
Leitha →, Europe 35 D10 47 50N 17 15 E
Leitrim, Ireland 23 B3 54 0N 8 5W
Leitrim □, Ireland 23 B4 54 8N 8 0W
Leitza, Spain 40 B3 43 5N 1 55W
Leiyang, China 77 D9 26 27N 112 45 E
Leizhou, China 77 G8 20 52N 110 8 E
Leizhou Bandao, China 76 G7 21 0N 110 0 E
Leizhou Wan, China 77 G8 20 50N 110 20 E
Lek →, Neths. 24 C4 51 54N 4 35 E
Leka, Norway 14 D14 65 5N 11 35 E
Lekáni, Greece 51 E8 41 10N 24 35 E
Lekbibaj, Albania 50 D3 42 17N 19 56 E
Lekeitio, Spain 40 B2 43 20N 2 32W
Lekhainá, Greece 48 D3 37 57N 21 16 E
Lekitobi, Indonesia 82 B2 1 58 S 124 33 E
Lékoli-Pandaka △, Congo 114 B2 0 41N 14 50 E
Lekoui, Burkina Faso 112 C4 12 37N 3 40W
Leksand, Sweden 16 D9 60 44N 15 1 E
Leksula, Indonesia 82 B3 3 46 S 126 31 E
Leksura = Lentekhi, Georgia 61 J6 42 47N 42 45 E
Lékva Óros, Greece 39 E5 35 18N 24 3 E
Leland, Mich., U.S.A. 148 C3 45 1N 85 45W
Leland, Miss., U.S.A. 155 J9 33 24N 90 54W
Lelång, Sweden 16 E6 59 10N 12 5 E
Leleiwi Pt., U.S.A. 145 D7 19 44N 155 0W
Lelepa, Vanuatu 133 G6 17 35 S 168 11 E
Leleque, Argentina 176 B2 42 28 S 71 0W
Lelewau, Indonesia 82 B2 3 2 S 121 5 E
Leli, Solomon Is. 133 M11 8 42 S 161 4 E
Lelu, Burma 90 F5 19 4N 95 30 E
Lelydorp, Suriname 169 B6 5 42N 55 14W
Lelystad, Neths. 24 B5 52 30N 5 25 E
Lem, Denmark 17 H2 56 1N 8 24 E
Lema, Nigeria 113 C5 12 58N 4 13 E
Lema Shilindi, Ethiopia 107 G5 4 50N 42 6 E
Léman, L., Europe 27 F13 46 26N 6 30 E
Lemankoa, Papua N. G. 132 C8 5 3 S 154 34 E
Lembar, Indonesia 79 K19 8 45 S 116 4 E
Lemberg = Lviv, Ukraine 59 H3 49 50N 24 0 E
Lembuak, Indonesia 79 K19 8 36 S 116 11 E
Lemera, Dem. Rep. of the Congo 118 C2 3 0 S 28 55 E
Lemery, Phil. 80 E3 13 51N 120 56 E
Lemeta, U.S.A. 144 D11 64 52N 147 44W
Lemfu, Dem. Rep. of the Congo 115 D3 5 18 S 15 13 E
Lemhi Ra., U.S.A. 158 D7 44 30N 113 30W
Lemmer, Neths. 24 B5 52 51N 5 43 E
Lemmon, U.S.A. 154 C3 45 57N 102 10W
Lemon Grove, U.S.A. 161 N9 32 45N 117 2W
Lemoore, U.S.A. 160 J7 36 18N 119 46W
Lempdes, France 28 C7 45 22N 3 17 E
Lemsid, W. Sahara 110 C2 26 33N 13 51W
Lemvig, Denmark 17 H2 56 33N 8 20 E
Lemyethna, Burma 90 G5 17 36N 95 9 E
Lena, U.S.A. 156 B7 42 23N 89 49W
Lena →, Russia 67 B13 72 52N 126 40 E
Lenakel, Vanuatu 133 J7 19 38 S 169 16 E
Lenart, Slovenia 45 B12 46 36N 15 48 E
Lenartovce, Slovak Rep. 35 C13 48 18N 20 19 E
Lencloître, France 26 F7 46 50N 0 20 E
Lençóis, Brazil 171 D3 12 35 S 41 24W
Lençóis Maranhenses △, Brazil 170 B3 2 30 S 43 0W
Léndas, Greece 39 F5 34 56N 24 56 E
Lendava, Slovenia 45 B13 46 35N 16 25 E
Lendeh, Iran 97 D6 30 58N 50 25 E
Lendinara, Italy 45 C8 45 5N 11 36 E
Lenger, Kazakhstan 65 B4 42 12N 69 54 E
Lengerich, Germany 30 C3 52 11N 7 52 E
Lenggong, Malaysia 87 K3 5 6N 100 58 E
Lenggries, Germany 31 H7 47 41N 11 35 E
Lengoué, Congo 114 B3 1 15N 15 38 E
Lengshuijiang, China 77 D8 27 40N 111 26 E
Lengshuitan, China 77 D8 26 27N 111 35 E
Lengua de Vaca, Pta., Chile 174 C1 30 14 S 71 38W
Lengwe △, Malawi 119 F3 16 14 S 34 45 E
Lengwethen = Lunino, Russia 60 D7 53 38N 45 18 E
Lengyeltóti, Hungary 52 D2 46 40N 17 40 E
Lengyeltótihács = Lengyeltóti, Hungary 52 D2 46 40N 17 40 E
Lenhovda, Sweden 17 G9 57 0N 15 16 E
Lenina, Kanal →, Russia 61 J7 43 44N 45 17 E
Lenina, Pik, Kyrgyzstan 65 D6 39 20N 72 55 E
Leninabad = Khŭjand, Tajikistan 65 C4 40 17N 69 37 E
Leninakan = Gyumri, Armenia 61 K6 40 47N 43 50 E
Leningrad = Sankt-Peterburg, Russia 58 C6 59 55N 30 20 E
Leningradskiy, Tajikistan 65 D5 38 6N 70 1 E
Lenino = Leninsk-Kuznetskiy, Russia 66 D9 54 44N 86 10 E
Lenino, Ukraine 59 K8 45 17N 35 46 E
Leninogorsk, Kazakhstan 66 D9 50 20N 83 30 E
Leninogorsk, Russia 64 D4 54 36N 52 30 E
Leninpol, Kyrgyzstan 65 B5 42 29N 71 55 E
Leninsk = Petrodvorets, Russia 58 C5 59 52N 29 54 E
Leninsk, Russia 61 F7 48 40N 45 15 E
Leninsk-Kuznetskiy, Russia 66 D9 54 44N 86 10 E
Leninsk-Turkmensky = Chärjew, Turkmenistan 65 D1 39 6N 63 34 E
Leninskiy, Tajikistan 65 D4 38 26N 68 46 E
Leninskoe, Kyrgyzstan 65 C6 40 40N 73 9 E
Leninskoye, Kazakhstan 64 F6 50 44N 57 53 E
Leninskoye, Russia 60 A8 58 23N 47 3 E
Lenk, Switz. 32 D4 46 27N 7 28 E
Lenkoran = Länkäran, Azerbaijan 97 B6 38 48N 48 52 E
Lenmalu, Indonesia 83 B4 1 45 S 130 15 E
Lenne →, Germany 30 D3 51 25N 7 29 E
Lennestadt, Germany 30 D4 51 8N 8 2 E
Lennox, U.S.A. 154 D6 43 21N 96 53W
Lennox, I., Chile 176 E3 55 18 S 66 50W
Lennoxville, Canada 151 A13 45 22N 71 51W
Leno, Italy 44 C7 45 22N 10 13 E
Lenoir, U.S.A. 149 H5 35 55N 81 32W
Lenoir City, U.S.A. 149 H3 35 48N 84 16W
Lenore L., Canada 143 C8 52 30N 104 59W
Lenox, Ga., U.S.A. 152 D6 31 16N 83 28W
Lenox, Iowa, U.S.A. 156 D2 40 53N 94 34W
Lenox, Mass., U.S.A. 151 D11 42 22N 73 17W
Lens, France 27 B9 50 26N 2 50 E
Lensahn, Germany 30 A6 54 13N 10 53 E
Lensk, Russia 67 C12 60 48N 114 55 E
Lensvik, Norway 18 A6 63 31N 9 48 E
Lentekhi, Georgia 61 J6 42 47N 42 45 E
Lenti, Hungary 52 D1 46 37N 16 33 E
Lentini, Italy 47 E8 37 17N 15 0 E
Lentschütz = Łęczyca, Poland 55 F6 52 5N 19 15 E
Lenwood, U.S.A. 161 L9 34 53N 117 7W
Lenya, Burma 78 B1 11 33N 98 57 E
Lenzburg, Switz. 32 B6 47 23N 8 11 E
Lenzen, Germany 30 B7 53 5N 11 29 E
Lenzerheide, Switz. 33 C9 46 44N 9 34 E
Léo, Burkina Faso 112 C4 11 3N 2 2W
Leoben, Austria 34 D8 47 22N 15 5 E
Leobschütz = Głubczyce, Poland 55 H4 50 13N 17 52 E
Leodhas = Lewis, U.K. 22 C2 58 9N 6 40W
Leola, U.S.A. 154 C5 45 43N 98 56W
Leominster, U.K. 21 E5 52 14N 2 43W
Leominster, U.S.A. 151 D13 42 32N 71 46W
León = Cotopaxi □, Ecuador 168 D2 0 5 S 78 55W
Léon, France 28 E2 43 53N 1 18W
León, Mexico 162 C4 21 7N 101 40W
León, Nic. 164 D2 12 20N 86 51W
León, Spain 42 C5 42 38N 5 34W
Leon, U.S.A. 156 D3 40 44N 93 45W
León □, Spain 42 C5 42 40N 5 55W
Leon →, U.S.A. 155 K6 31 14N 97 28W
León, Montes de, Spain 42 C4 42 30N 6 18W
Leonardo da Vinci, Roma ✕ (FCO), Italy 45 G9 41 48N 12 15 E
Leonardtown, U.S.A. 148 F7 38 17N 76 38W
Leonardville, Namibia 116 C2 23 29 S 18 49 E
Leonberg, Germany 31 G5 48 48N 9 1 E
Leonding, Austria 34 C7 48 16N 14 15 E
Leone, Amer. Samoa 133 X24 14 23 S 170 48W
Leone, Mte., Switz. 32 D6 46 15N 8 5 E
Leonessa, Italy 45 F9 42 34N 12 58 E
Leonforte, Italy 47 E7 37 38N 14 23 E
Leongatha, Australia 129 E6 38 30 S 145 58 E
Leonia, U.S.A. 152 E3 30 55N 86 1W
Leonídhion, Greece 48 D4 37 9N 22 52 E
Leonora, Australia 125 E3 28 49 S 121 19 E
Leopold II, L. = Mai-Ndombe, L., Dem. Rep. of the Congo 114 C3 2 0 S 18 20 E
Leopoldina = Aruanã, Brazil 171 D1 14 54 S 51 10W
Leopoldina = Parnamirim, Brazil 170 C4 8 5 S 39 34W
Leopoldina, Brazil 171 F3 21 28 S 42 40W
Leopoldo Bulhões, Brazil 171 E2 16 37 S 48 46W
Leopoldsburg, Belgium 24 C5 51 7N 5 13 E
Léopoldville = Kinshasa, Dem. Rep. of the Congo 115 C3 4 20 S 15 15 E
Leoti, U.S.A. 154 F4 38 29N 101 21W
Leova, Moldova 53 D13 46 28N 28 15 E
Leoville, Canada 143 C7 53 39N 107 33W
Lepe, Spain 43 H3 37 15N 7 12W
Lepel = Lyepyel, Belarus 58 E5 54 50N 28 40 E
Lepenoú, Greece 48 C3 38 42N 21 17 E
Leping, China 77 C11 28 47N 117 7 E
Lépo, L. do, Angola 116 B2 17 0 S 19 0 E
Lepontine, Alpi, Italy 33 D6 46 22N 8 27 E
Leppävirta, Finland 15 E22 62 29N 27 46 E
Lepsény, Hungary 52 D3 47 0N 18 15 E
Leptis Magna, Libya 108 B2 32 40N 14 12 E
Lequeitio = Lekeitio, Spain 40 B2 43 20N 2 32W
Lercara Friddi, Italy 46 E6 37 45N 13 36 E
Lerdo, Mexico 162 B4 25 32N 103 32W
Léré, C.A.R. 114 A3 6 46N 17 25 E
Léré, Chad 113 D7 9 39N 14 13 E
Léré, Mali 112 B4 15 45N 4 55W
Lere, Bauchi, Nigeria 113 D6 9 43N 9 18 E
Lere, Kaduna, Nigeria 113 C6 10 23N 8 35 E
Leribe, Lesotho 117 D4 28 51 S 28 3 E
Lérici, Italy 44 D6 44 4N 9 55 E
Lérida = Lleida, Spain 40 D5 41 37N 0 39 E
Lérins, Îs. de, France 29 E11 43 31N 7 3 E
Lerma, Spain 42 C7 42 0N 3 47W
Léros, Greece 49 D8 37 10N 26 50 E
Lérouville, France 27 D12 48 44N 5 30 E
Lerum, Sweden 17 G6 57 46N 12 16 E
Lerwick, U.K. 22 A7 60 9N 1 9W
Leş, Romania 52 D6 46 58N 21 50 E
Les Abrets, France 29 C9 45 32N 5 35 E
Les Andelys, France 26 C8 49 15N 1 25 E
Les Bois, Switz. 32 B3 47 11N 6 50 E

Les Borges Blanques, Spain 40 D5 41 31N 0 52 E
Les Cayes, Haiti 165 C5 18 15N 73 46W
Les Coteaux, Canada 151 A10 45 15N 74 13W
Les Diablerets, Switz. 32 D4 46 22N 7 10 E
Les Essarts, France 26 F5 46 47N 1 12W
Les Herbiers, France 26 F5 46 52N 1 1W
Les Minquiers, Plateau des, Chan. Is. 26 D4 48 58N 2 8W
Les Moroubas, C.A.R. 114 A4 6 11N 20 13 E
Les Pieux, France 26 C5 49 30N 1 48W
Les Ponts-de-Cé, France 26 E6 47 25N 0 30W
Les Riceys, France 27 E11 47 59N 4 22 E
Les Sables-d'Olonne, France 28 B2 46 30N 1 45W
Les Vans, France 29 D8 44 25N 4 7 E
Les Verrières, Switz. 32 C2 46 55N 6 28 E
Lesbos = Lésvos, Greece 49 B8 39 10N 26 20 E
L'Escala, Spain 40 C8 42 7N 3 8 E
Leschnitz = Leśnica, Poland 55 H5 50 26N 18 11 E
Leshan, China 76 C4 29 33N 103 41 E
Leshukonskoye, Russia 56 B8 64 54N 45 46 E
Leshwe ⌂, Dem. Rep. of the Congo 119 E2 12 45 S 29 30 E
Lésina, Italy 45 G12 41 52N 15 21 E
Lésina, L. di, Italy 45 G12 41 53N 15 26 E
Lesjaskog, Norway 18 B5 62 14N 8 22 E
Lesjaverk, Norway 18 B5 62 12N 8 34 E
Lesjöfors, Sweden 16 E8 59 58N 14 11 E
Leskhimstroy = Syeverodonetsk, Ukraine 59 H10 48 58N 38 35 E
Lesko, Poland 55 J9 49 30N 22 23 E
Leskov I., Antarctica 7 B1 56 0 S 28 0W
Leskovac, Serbia & M. 50 C5 43 0N 21 58 E
Leskovik, Albania 50 F4 40 10N 20 34 E
Leslau = Włocławek, Poland 55 F6 52 40N 19 3 E
Leslie, Ga., U.S.A. 152 D5 31 57N 84 5W
Leslie, Mich., U.S.A. 157 B12 42 27N 84 26W
Leśna, Poland 55 G2 51 1N 15 15 E
Lesneven, France 26 D2 48 35N 4 20W
Leśnica, Poland 55 H5 50 26N 18 11 E
Lešnica, Serbia & M. 50 B3 44 39N 19 20 E
Lesnoi = Umba, Russia 56 A5 66 42N 34 11 E
Lesnoy, Russia 64 B4 59 47N 52 9 E
Lesnoye, Russia 58 C8 58 15N 35 18 E
Lesopilnoye, Russia 70 A7 46 44N 134 20 E
Lesotho ■, Africa 117 D4 29 40 S 28 0 E
Lesozavodsk, Russia 67 E14 45 30N 133 29 E
Lesozavodsky = Novovyatsk, Russia 64 B2 58 24N 49 45 E
Lesparre-Médoc, France 28 C3 45 18N 0 57W
Lessay, France 26 C5 49 14N 1 30W
Lesse →, Belgium 24 D4 50 15N 4 54 E
Lesse et Lomme ⌂, Belgium 24 D5 50 8N 5 9 E
Lessebo, Sweden 17 H9 56 45N 15 16 E
Lesser Antilles, W. Indies 165 D7 15 0N 61 0W
Lesser Slave L., Canada 142 B5 55 30N 115 25W
Lesser Sunda Is., Indonesia 82 C1 8 0 S 120 0 E
Lessines, Belgium 24 D3 50 42N 3 50 E
Lester, U.S.A. 160 C5 47 12N 121 29W
Lester B. Pearson International, Toronto ✈ (YYZ), Canada 150 C5 43 40N 79 34W
Lestershire = Johnson City, U.S.A. 151 D9 42 7N 75 58W
Lestock, Canada 143 C8 51 19N 103 59W
Lesuer I., Australia 124 B4 13 50 S 127 17 E
Lesueur △, Australia 125 F2 30 11 S 115 10 E
Lésvos, Greece 49 B8 39 10N 26 20 E
Leszno, Poland 55 G3 51 50N 16 30 E
Letaba, S. Africa 117 C5 23 59 S 31 50 E
Letälven, Sweden 16 E8 59 5N 14 20 E
Létavértes, Hungary 52 C6 47 23N 21 55 E
Letchworth, U.K. 21 F7 51 59N 0 13W
Letea, Ostrov, Romania 53 E14 45 18N 29 20 E
Lethbridge, Canada 142 D6 49 45N 112 45W
Lethem, Guyana 169 C6 3 20N 59 50W
Leti, Kepulauan, Indonesia 82 C3 8 10 S 128 0 E
Leti Is. = Leti, Kepulauan, Indonesia 82 C3 8 10 S 128 0 E
Letiahau →, Botswana 116 C3 21 16 S 24 0 E
Leticia, Colombia 168 D4 4 9 S 70 0W
Leting, China 75 E10 39 23N 118 55 E
Letjiesbos, S. Africa 116 E3 32 34 S 22 16 E
Letlhakane, Botswana 116 C4 21 27 S 25 30 E
Letlhakeng, Botswana 116 C3 24 0 S 24 59 E
Letong, Indonesia 78 D3 2 58N 105 42 E
Letpadan, Burma 90 G5 17 45N 95 45 E
Letpan, Burma 90 F5 19 28N 94 10 E
Letsôk-aw Kyun, Burma 87 G2 11 30N 98 25 E
Letterkenny, Ireland 23 B4 54 57N 7 45W
Leu, Romania 53 F9 44 10N 24 0 E
Léua, Angola 115 E4 11 34 S 20 32 E
Leucadia, U.S.A. 161 M9 33 4N 117 18W
Leucate, France 28 F7 42 56N 3 3 E
Leucate, Étang de, France 28 F7 42 50N 3 0 E
Leuchars, U.K. 22 E6 56 24N 2 53W
Leuk, Switz. 32 D5 46 19N 7 37 E
Leukerbad, Switz. 32 D5 46 24N 7 36 E
Leuşeni, Moldova 53 D13 46 49N 28 12 E
Leuser, G., Indonesia 84 B1 3 46N 97 12 E
Leutkirch, Germany 31 H6 47 49N 10 1 E
Leutschau = Levoča, Slovak Rep. 35 B13 49 2N 20 35 E
Leuven, Belgium 24 D4 50 52N 4 42 E
Leuze-en-Hainaut, Belgium 24 D3 50 36N 3 37 E
Lev Tolstoy, Russia 58 F10 53 13N 39 29 E
Levádhia, Greece 48 C4 38 27N 22 54 E
Levan, Albania 50 F3 40 40N 19 28 E
Levanger, Norway 14 E14 63 45N 11 19 E
Levant, Î. du, France 29 E10 43 3N 6 28 E
Lévanto, Italy 44 D6 44 10N 9 38 E
Lévanzo, Italy 46 D5 38 0N 12 20 E
Leveld, Norway 18 D5 60 44N 8 13 E
Levelland, U.S.A. 155 J3 33 35N 102 23W
Levelock, U.S.A. 144 G8 59 7N 156 51W
Leven, U.K. 22 E6 56 12N 3 0W
Leven, L., U.K. 22 E5 56 12N 3 22W
Leven, Toraka, Madag. 117 A8 12 30 S 47 45 E
Leveque C., Australia 124 C3 16 20 S 123 0 E
Leverano, Italy 47 B10 40 17N 18 0 E
Leverger = Santo Antônio do Leverger, Brazil 173 D6 15 52 S 56 5W
Leverkusen, Germany 30 D3 51 1N 7 1 E
Levice, Slovak Rep. 35 C11 48 13N 18 35 E
Lévico Terme, Italy 45 C8 46 0N 11 18 E
Levie, France 29 G13 41 40N 9 7 E
Levier, France 27 F13 46 58N 6 8 E
Levin, N.Z. 130 G4 40 37 S 175 18 E
Lévis, Canada 141 C5 46 48N 71 9W
Levis, L., Canada 142 A5 62 37N 117 58W
Levítha, Greece 49 D8 37 0N 26 28 E
Levittown = Willingboro, U.S.A. 148 E8 40 3N 74 54W
Levittown, N.Y., U.S.A. 151 F11 40 44N 73 31W
Levittown, Pa., U.S.A. 151 F10 40 9N 74 51W
Levka, Bulgaria 51 E10 41 52N 26 15 E
Levkás, Greece 39 B2 38 40N 20 43 E
Levkás □, Greece 39 B2 38 45N 20 40 E
Levkímmi, Greece 38 C10 39 25N 20 3 E
Levkímmi, Ákra, Greece 38 C10 39 29N 20 4 E
Levkôsia = Nicosia, Cyprus 39 E9 35 10N 33 25 E
Levoča, Slovak Rep. 35 B13 49 2N 20 35 E
Levroux, France 27 F8 46 59N 1 38 E
Levski, Bulgaria 51 C9 43 21N 25 10 E
Levskigrad = Karlovo, Bulgaria 51 D8 42 38N 24 47 E
Levuka, Fiji 133 A2 17 34 S 179 0 E
Lewe, Burma 90 F6 19 38N 96 7 E
Lewes, U.K. 21 G8 50 52N 0 1 E
Lewes, U.S.A. 148 F8 38 46N 75 9W
Lewin Brzeski, Poland 55 H4 50 45N 17 37 E
Lewis, U.K. 22 C2 58 9N 6 40W
Lewis →, U.S.A. 160 E4 45 51N 122 48W
Lewis, Butt of, U.K. 22 C2 58 31N 6 16W
Lewis Pass, N.Z. 131 C7 42 31 S 172 11 E
Lewis Ra., Australia 124 D4 20 3 S 128 50 E
Lewis Range, U.S.A. 158 C7 48 5N 113 5W
Lewis Run, U.S.A. 150 E6 41 52N 78 40W
Lewisburg, Ohio, U.S.A. 157 E12 39 51N 84 33W
Lewisburg, Pa., U.S.A. 150 F8 40 58N 76 54W
Lewisburg, Tenn., U.S.A. 149 H2 35 27N 86 48W
Lewisburg, W. Va., U.S.A. 148 G5 37 48N 80 27W
Lewisport, U.S.A. 157 G10 37 56N 86 54W
Lewisporte, Canada 141 C8 49 15N 55 3W
Lewiston, Idaho, U.S.A. 158 C5 46 25N 117 1W
Lewiston, Maine, U.S.A. 149 C11 44 6N 70 13W
Lewiston, N.Y., U.S.A. 150 C5 43 11N 79 3W
Lewistown, Ill., U.S.A. 156 D6 40 24N 90 9W
Lewistown, Mo., U.S.A. 156 D5 40 5N 91 49W
Lewistown, Mont., U.S.A. 158 C9 47 4N 109 26W
Lewistown, Pa., U.S.A. 150 F7 40 36N 77 34W
Lexington, Ga., U.S.A. 152 B6 33 52N 83 7W
Lexington, Ill., U.S.A. 154 E10 40 39N 88 47W
Lexington, Ky., U.S.A. 157 F12 38 3N 84 30W
Lexington, Mich., U.S.A. 150 C2 43 16N 82 32W
Lexington, Mo., U.S.A. 156 E3 39 11N 93 52W
Lexington, N.C., U.S.A. 149 H5 35 49N 80 15W
Lexington, N.Y., U.S.A. 151 D10 42 15N 74 22W
Lexington, Nebr., U.S.A. 154 E5 40 47N 99 45W
Lexington, Ohio, U.S.A. 150 F2 40 41N 82 35W
Lexington, S.C., U.S.A. 152 B8 33 59N 81 11W
Lexington, Tenn., U.S.A. 149 H1 35 39N 88 24W
Lexington, Va., U.S.A. 148 G6 37 47N 79 27W
Lexington Park, U.S.A. 148 F7 38 16N 76 27W
Leyburn, U.K. 20 C6 54 19N 1 48W
Leye, China 76 E6 24 48N 106 29 E
Leyland, U.K. 20 D5 53 42N 2 43W
Leyre →, France 28 D2 44 39N 1 1W
Leysin, Switz. 32 D4 46 21N 7 1 E
Leyte, Phil. 81 F5 11 0N 125 0 E
Leyte □, Phil. 81 F5 10 30N 125 0 E
Leyte Gulf, Phil. 81 F5 10 50N 125 25 E
Leżajsk, Poland 55 H9 50 10N 22 25 E
Lezay, France 28 B3 46 15N 0 1W
Lezhë, Albania 50 E3 41 47N 19 39 E
Lezhi, China 76 B5 30 19N 104 58 E
Lézignan-Corbières, France 28 E6 43 13N 2 43 E
Lezoux, France 28 C7 45 49N 3 21 E
Lgov, Russia 59 G8 51 42N 35 16 E
Lhasa, China 68 D4 29 25N 90 58 E
Lhazê, China 68 D3 29 5N 87 38 E
Lhokkruet, Indonesia 84 B1 4 55N 95 24 E
Lhokseumawe, Indonesia 84 A1 5 10N 97 10 E
L'Hospitalet de Llobregat, Spain 40 D7 41 21N 2 6 E
Lhuntsi Dzong, Bhutan 90 B3 27 39N 91 10 E
Li, Thailand 86 D2 17 48N 98 57 E
Li Shui →, China 77 C9 29 24N 112 1 E
Li Xian, Gansu, China 74 G3 34 10N 105 5 E
Li Xian, Hebei, China 74 E8 38 30N 115 35 E
Li Xian, Hunan, China 77 C8 29 36N 111 42 E
Lia-Moya, C.A.R. 114 A3 6 54N 16 17 E
Liádhoi, Greece 49 E8 36 50N 26 11 E
Lian, Phil. 80 D3 14 3N 120 39 E
Liancheng, China 77 E11 25 42N 116 40 E
Liancourt Rocks = Tok-do, Asia 71 F5 37 15N 131 52 E
Lianga, Phil. 81 G6 8 38N 126 6 E
Lianga Bay, Phil. 81 G6 8 37N 126 12 E
Liangcheng, Nei Monggol Zizhiqu, China 74 D7 40 28N 112 25 E
Liangcheng, Shandong, China 75 G10 35 32N 119 37 E
Liangdang, China 74 H4 33 56N 106 18 E
Lianghe, China 76 E2 24 50N 98 20 E
Lianghekou, China 76 C7 29 11N 108 44 E
Liangping, China 76 B6 30 38N 107 47 E
Liangpran, Indonesia 78 D4 1 4N 114 23 E
Lianhua, China 77 D9 27 3N 113 54 E
Lianjiang, Fujian, China 77 D12 26 12N 119 27 E
Lianjiang, Guangdong, China 77 G8 21 40N 110 20 E
Lianping, China 77 E10 24 26N 114 30 E
Lianshan, China 77 E9 24 38N 112 8 E
Lianshanguan, China 75 D12 40 53N 123 43 E
Lianshui, China 75 H10 33 42N 119 20 E
Lianyuan, China 77 D8 27 40N 111 38 E
Lianyungang, China 75 G10 34 40N 119 11 E
Lianzhou, China 77 E9 24 51N 112 22 E
Liao He →, China 75 D11 41 0N 121 50 E
Liaocheng, China 74 F8 36 28N 115 58 E
Liaodong Bandao, China 75 E12 40 0N 122 30 E
Liaodong Wan, China 75 D11 40 20N 121 10 E
Liaoning □, China 75 D12 41 40N 122 30 E
Liaotung, G. of = Liaodong Wan, China 75 D11 40 20N 121 10 E
Liaoyang, China 75 D12 41 15N 122 58 E
Liaoyuan, China 75 C13 42 58N 125 2 E
Liaozhong, China 75 D12 41 23N 122 50 E
Liapádhes, Greece 38 B9 39 42N 19 40 E
Liard →, Canada 142 A4 61 51N 121 18W
Liard River, Canada 142 B3 59 25N 126 5W
Liari, Pakistan 92 G2 25 37N 66 30 E
Líbano, Colombia 168 C2 4 55N 75 4W
Libau = Liepāja, Latvia 15 H19 56 30N 21 0 E
Libby, U.S.A. 158 B6 48 23N 115 33W
Libenge, Dem. Rep. of the Congo 114 B3 3 40N 18 55 E
Liberal, U.S.A. 155 G4 37 3N 100 55W
Liberdade, Brazil 172 C3 10 5 S 70 20W
Liberdade →, Brazil 173 B7 9 40 S 52 17W
Liberec, Czech Rep. 34 A8 50 47N 15 7 E
Liberecký □, Czech Rep. 34 A8 50 45N 15 0 E
Liberia, Costa Rica 164 D2 10 40N 85 30W
Liberia ■, W. Afr. 112 D3 6 30N 9 30W
Libertad, Phil. 81 F3 11 46N 121 55 E
Libertad, Venezuela 168 B4 8 20N 69 37W
Liberty, Ind., U.S.A. 157 E12 39 38N 84 56W
Liberty, Mo., U.S.A. 156 E2 39 15N 94 25W
Liberty, N.Y., U.S.A. 151 E10 41 48N 74 45W
Liberty, Pa., U.S.A. 150 E7 41 34N 77 6W
Liberty, Tex., U.S.A. 155 K7 30 3N 94 48W
Liberty Center, U.S.A. 157 C12 41 27N 84 1W
Libertyville, U.S.A. 157 B9 42 18N 87 57W
Libiąż, Poland 55 H6 50 7N 19 21 E
Libibi, Angola 115 E3 14 42 S 17 44 E
Lîbîya, Sahrâ', Africa 108 C4 25 0N 25 0 E
Libjo, Phil. 81 F5 10 12N 125 32 E
Libmanan, Phil. 80 E4 13 42N 123 4 E
Libo, China 76 E6 25 22N 107 53 E
Libobo, Tanjung, Indonesia 82 B3 0 54 S 128 28 E
Libode, S. Africa 117 E4 31 33 S 29 2 E
Libohovë, Albania 50 F4 40 3N 20 10 E
Libona, Phil. 81 G5 8 20N 124 44 E
Libonda, Zambia 115 E4 14 28 S 23 12 E
Libourne, France 28 D3 44 55N 0 14W
Libramont, Belgium 24 E5 49 55N 5 23 E
Librazhd, Albania 50 E4 41 12N 20 22 E
Libreville, Gabon 114 B1 0 25N 9 26 E
Libya ■, N. Afr. 108 C3 27 0N 17 0 E
Libyan Desert = Lîbîya, Sahrâ', Africa 108 C4 25 0N 25 0 E
Libyan Plateau = Ed-Déffa, Egypt 106 A2 30 40N 26 30 E
Licantén, Chile 174 D1 35 55 S 72 0W
Licata, Italy 46 E6 37 6N 13 56 E
Lice, Turkey 101 C9 38 27N 40 39 E
Licheng, China 74 F7 36 28N 113 20 E
Lichfield, U.K. 21 E6 52 41N 1 49W
Lichinga, Mozam. 119 E4 13 13 S 35 11 E
Lichtenburg, S. Africa 116 D4 26 8 S 26 8 E
Lichtenfels, Germany 31 E7 50 8N 11 4 E
Lichuan, Hubei, China 76 B7 30 18N 108 57 E
Lichuan, Jiangxi, China 77 D11 27 18N 116 55 E
Licking →, U.S.A. 157 F12 39 6N 84 30W
Licosa, Punta, Italy 47 B7 40 15N 14 54 E
Licungo →, Mozam. 119 F4 17 40 S 37 15 E
Lida, Belarus 15 K21 53 53N 25 15 E
Liden, Sweden 16 B10 62 42N 16 48 E
Lidhoríkion, Greece 48 C4 38 32N 22 12 E
Lidhult, Sweden 17 H7 56 50N 13 27 E
Lidköping, Sweden 17 F7 58 31N 13 7 E
Lido, Italy 45 C9 45 25N 12 22 E
Lido, Niger 113 C5 12 54N 3 44 E
Lido di Roma = Ostia, Lido di, Italy 45 G9 41 43N 12 17 E
Lidzbark, Poland 55 E6 53 15N 19 49 E
Lidzbark Warmiński, Poland 54 D7 54 7N 20 34 E
Liebenthal = Lubomierz, Poland 55 G2 51 1N 15 31 E
Liebenwalde, Germany 30 C9 52 52N 13 24 E
Lieberose, Germany 30 D10 51 59N 14 17 E
Liebig, Mt., Australia 124 D5 23 18 S 131 22 E
Liebling, Romania 52 E6 45 36N 21 20 E
Liechtenstein ■, Europe 33 B9 47 8N 9 35 E
Liège, Belgium 24 D5 50 38N 5 35 E
Liège □, Belgium 24 D5 50 32N 5 35 E
Liegnitz = Legnica, Poland 55 G3 51 12N 16 10 E
Lienart, Dem. Rep. of the Congo 118 B2 3 3N 25 31 E
Lienyünchiangshih = Lianyungang, China 75 G10 34 40N 119 11 E
Lienz, Austria 34 E5 46 50N 12 46 E
Liepāja, Latvia 15 H19 56 30N 21 0 E
Liepāja □, Latvia 54 B8 56 30N 21 30 E
Liepājas ezers, Latvia 54 B8 56 27N 21 3 E
Lier, Belgium 24 C4 51 7N 4 34 E
Liernais, France 27 E11 47 13N 4 16 E
Liestal, Switz. 32 B5 47 29N 7 44 E
Lieşti, Romania 53 E12 45 38N 27 34 E
Lietuva = Lithuania ■, Europe 15 J20 55 30N 24 0 E
Liévin, France 27 B9 50 24N 2 47 E
Lièvre →, Canada 140 C4 45 31N 75 26W
Liezen, Austria 34 D7 47 34N 14 15 E
Liffey →, Ireland 23 C5 53 21N 6 13W
Lifford, Ireland 23 B4 54 51N 7 29W
Liffré, France 26 D5 48 12N 1 30W
Lifjell, Norway 18 E5 59 27N 8 45 E
Lifou, I., N. Cal. 133 K5 20 53 S 167 13 E
Lifudzin, Russia 70 B7 44 21N 134 58 E
Lifuka, Tonga 133 P13 19 48 S 174 21W
Ligao, Phil. 80 E4 13 14N 123 32 E
Ligasa, Dem. Rep. of the Congo 114 B4 0 44N 23 49 E
Lighthouse Point, U.S.A. 153 J9 26 15N 80 7W
Lighthouse Pt., U.S.A. 152 F5 29 54N 84 21W
Lightning Ridge, Australia 127 D4 29 22 S 148 0 E
Lignano Sabbiadoro, Italy 45 C10 45 42N 13 9 E
Ligny-en-Barrois, France 27 D12 48 36N 5 20 E
Ligonha →, Mozam. 119 F4 16 54 S 39 9 E
Ligonier, Ind., U.S.A. 157 C11 41 28N 85 35W
Ligonier, Pa., U.S.A. 150 F5 40 15N 79 14W
Ligoúrion, Greece 48 D5 37 37N 23 4 E
Ligueil, France 26 E7 47 2N 0 49 E
Liguria □, Italy 44 D5 44 30N 8 50 E
Ligurian Sea, Medit. S. 12 G7 43 20N 9 0 E
Lihir Group, Papua N. G. 132 B7 3 0 S 152 35 E
Lihir I., Papua N. G. 132 B7 3 5 S 152 35 E
Lihou Reefs and Cays, Australia 126 B5 17 25 S 151 40 E
Lihue, U.S.A. 145 B2 21 59N 159 23W
Lihué Calel △, Argentina 174 D2 38 0 S 65 10W
Lijiang, China 76 D3 26 55N 100 20 E
Likasi, Dem. Rep. of the Congo 119 E2 10 55 S 26 48 E
Likati, Dem. Rep. of the Congo 114 B4 3 20N 24 0 E
Likati →, Dem. Rep. of the Congo 114 B4 2 53N 24 3 E
Likenäs, Sweden 16 D7 60 37N 13 3 E
Likete, Dem. Rep. of the Congo 114 C4 0 48 S 21 31 E
Likhaya = Likhovskoy, Russia 59 H11 48 10N 40 10 E
Likhoslavl, Russia 58 D8 57 12N 35 30 E
Likhovskoy, Russia 59 H11 48 10N 40 10 E
Likhvin = Chekalin, Russia 58 E9 54 10N 36 10 E
Likimi, Dem. Rep. of the Congo 114 B4 2 44N 20 47 E
Likisia = Liquica, E. Timor 82 C3 8 36 S 125 19 E
Likita, Dem. Rep. of the Congo 114 B4 4 15N 23 36 E
Liknes, Norway 18 F3 58 19N 6 59 E
Likokou, Gabon 114 C2 0 12 S 12 48 E
Likoma I., Malawi 119 E3 12 3 S 34 45 E
Likouala →, Congo 114 C3 0 2N 14 53 E
Likouala aux Herbes →, Congo 114 C3 0 52 S 17 8 E
Likumburu, Tanzania 119 D4 9 43 S 35 8 E
Lilanga, Dem. Rep. of the Congo 114 C4 0 34 S 23 56 E
L'Île-Bouchard, France 26 E7 47 7N 0 26 E
L'Île-Rousse, France 29 F12 42 38N 8 57 E
Lilenga, Dem. Rep. of the Congo 114 B4 1 4N 22 2 E
Liling, China 77 D9 27 42N 113 29 E
Lilla Edet, Sweden 17 F6 58 9N 12 8 E
Lille, France 27 B10 50 38N 3 3 E
Lille Bælt, Denmark 17 J3 55 20N 9 45 E
Lillebonne, France 26 C7 49 30N 0 32 E
Lillehammer, Norway 18 C7 61 8N 10 30 E
Lillesand, Norway 18 F5 58 15N 8 23 E
Lillestrøm, Norway 18 E8 59 58N 11 5 E
Lillhärdal, Sweden 16 C8 61 51N 14 5 E
Lillian Pt., Australia 125 E4 27 40 S 126 6 E
Lillo, Spain 42 F7 39 45N 3 20W
Lillooet, Canada 142 C4 50 44N 121 57W
Lillooet →, Canada 142 D4 49 15N 121 57W
Lilongwe, Malawi 119 E3 14 0 S 33 48 E
Liloy, Phil. 81 G4 8 4N 122 39 E
Lim →, Bos.-H. 50 C3 43 45N 19 15 E
Lim Chu Kang, Singapore 87 d 1 26N 103 43 E
Lima, Brazil 169 D5 4 36 S 63 40W
Lima, Indonesia 82 B3 3 39 S 127 58 E
Lima, Peru 172 C2 12 0 S 77 0W
Lima, Ill., U.S.A. 156 D5 40 11N 91 23W
Lima, Mont., U.S.A. 158 D7 44 38N 112 36W
Lima, Ohio, U.S.A. 157 D12 40 44N 84 6W
Lima □, Peru 172 C2 12 3 S 77 3W
Lima →, Portugal 42 D2 41 41N 8 50W
Liman = Krasnyy Liman, Ukraine 59 H9 48 58N 37 50 E
Liman, Indonesia 79 G14 7 48 S 111 45 E
Liman, Russia 61 H8 45 45N 47 12 E
Limanowa, Poland 55 J7 49 42N 20 22 E
Limassol, Cyprus 39 F9 34 42N 33 1 E
Limavady, U.K. 23 A5 55 3N 6 56W
Limay →, Argentina 176 A3 39 0 S 68 0W
Limay Mahuida, Argentina 174 D2 37 10 S 66 45W
Limbach-Oberfrohna, Germany 30 E8 50 52N 12 43 E
Limbang, Brunei 85 B5 4 42N 115 6 E
Limbara, Mte., Italy 46 B2 40 51N 9 10 E
Limbaži, Latvia 15 H21 57 31N 24 42 E
Limbdi, India 92 H4 22 34N 71 51 E
Limbe, Cameroon 113 E6 4 1N 9 10 E
Limboto, Indonesia 82 A2 0 37N 122 57 E
Limbueta, Angola 115 E3 12 30 S 18 42 E
Limbuhan = Pio V. Corpuz, Phil. 81 F5 11 55N 124 2 E
Limburg, Germany 31 E4 50 22N 8 4 E
Limburg □, Belgium 24 C5 51 2N 5 25 E
Limburg □, Neths. 24 C5 51 20N 5 55 E
Lime Village, U.S.A. 144 F9 61 21N 155 28W
Limedsforsen, Sweden 16 D7 60 52N 13 25 E
Limeira = Joaçaba, Brazil 175 B5 27 5 S 51 31W
Limeira, Brazil 175 A6 22 35 S 47 28W
Limenária, Greece 51 F8 40 38N 24 32 E
Limerick, Ireland 23 D3 52 40N 8 37W
Limerick, U.S.A. 151 C14 43 41N 70 48W
Limerick □, Ireland 23 D3 52 30N 8 50W
Limestone, U.S.A. 150 D6 42 2N 78 38W
Limestone →, Canada 143 B10 56 31N 94 7W
Limestone Hill = Lackawanna, U.S.A. 150 D6 42 50N 78 50W
Limfjorden, Denmark 17 H3 56 55N 9 0 E
Limia = Lima →, Portugal 42 D2 41 41N 8 50W
Limín Khersonísou, Greece 39 E6 35 18N 25 21 E
Limingen, Norway 14 D15 64 48N 13 35 E
Limmared, Sweden 17 G7 57 34N 13 20 E
Limmat →, Switz. 33 B6 47 26N 8 20 E
Limmen Bight, Australia 126 A2 14 40 S 135 35 E
Limmen Bight →, Australia 126 B2 15 7 S 135 44 E
Límni, Greece 48 C5 38 43N 23 18 E
Límni Voulkaria, Greece 39 B2 38 52N 20 50 E
Límnos, Greece 49 B7 39 50N 25 5 E
Limoeiro, Brazil 170 C4 7 52 S 35 27W
Limoeiro do Norte, Brazil 170 C4 5 5 S 38 0W
Limoges, Canada 151 A9 45 20N 75 16W
Limoges, France 28 C5 45 50N 1 15 E
Limón, Costa Rica 164 E3 10 0N 83 2W
Limon, U.S.A. 154 F3 39 16N 103 41W
Limone Piemonte, Italy 44 D4 44 12N 7 34 E
Limousin □, France 28 C5 45 30N 1 30 E
Limousin, Plateaux du, France 28 C5 45 45N 1 15 E
Limoux, France 28 E6 43 4N 2 12 E
Limpopo □, S. Africa 117 C4 24 5 S 29 0 E
Limpopo →, Africa 117 D5 25 5 S 33 30 E
Limuru, Kenya 118 C4 1 2 S 36 35 E
Lin Xian, China 74 F6 37 57N 110 58 E
Lin'an, China 77 B12 30 15N 119 42 E
Linao Pt., Phil. 81 H4 6 46N 123 58 E
Linapacan, Phil. 81 F2 11 30N 119 52 E
Linapacan I., Phil. 81 F2 11 27N 119 49 E
Linapacan Str., Phil. 81 F2 11 37N 119 56 E
Linares, Chile 174 D1 35 50 S 71 40W
Linares, Colombia 168 C2 1 23N 77 31W
Linares, Mexico 163 C5 24 50N 99 40W
Linares, Spain 43 G7 38 10N 3 40W
Linaro, Capo, Italy 45 F8 42 2N 11 50 E
Línas Mte., Italy 46 C1 39 25N 8 38 E
Linate, Milano ✈ (LIN), Italy 44 C6 45 27N 9 16 E
Lincang, China 76 F3 23 58N 100 1 E
Lincheng, China 74 F8 37 25N 114 30 E
Linchuan, China 77 D11 27 57N 116 15 E
Lincoln = Beamsville, Canada 150 C5 43 12N 79 28W
Lincoln, Argentina 174 C3 34 55 S 61 30W
Lincoln, N.Z. 131 D7 43 38 S 172 30 E
Lincoln, U.K. 20 D7 53 14N 0 32W
Lincoln, Calif., U.S.A. 160 G5 38 54N 121 17W
Lincoln, Ill., U.S.A. 156 D7 40 9N 89 22W
Lincoln, Kans., U.S.A. 154 F5 39 3N 98 9W
Lincoln, Maine, U.S.A. 149 C11 45 22N 68 30W
Lincoln, N.H., U.S.A. 151 B13 44 3N 71 40W
Lincoln, N. Mex., U.S.A. 159 K11 33 30N 105 23W
Lincoln, Nebr., U.S.A. 154 E6 40 49N 96 41W
Lincoln Boyhood ⌂, U.S.A. 157 F10 38 7N 86 58W
Lincoln City, U.S.A. 158 D1 44 57N 124 1W
Lincoln Hav = Lincoln Sea, Arctic 10 A5 84 0N 55 0W
Lincoln Park, Ga., U.S.A. 152 C5 32 52N 84 20W
Lincoln Park, Mich., U.S.A. 157 B13 42 15N 83 11W
Lincoln Sea, Arctic 10 A5 84 0N 55 0W
Lincolnshire □, U.K. 20 D7 53 14N 0 32W
Lincolnshire Wolds, U.K. 20 D7 53 26N 0 13W
Lincolnton, Ga., U.S.A. 152 B7 33 48N 82 29W
Lincolnton, N.C., U.S.A. 149 H5 35 29N 81 16W
Lind, U.S.A. 158 C4 46 58N 118 37W
Linda, U.S.A. 160 F5 39 8N 121 34W
Lindale, U.S.A. 152 A4 34 11N 85 11W
Lindås, Norway 18 D2 60 44N 5 9 E
Lindau, Germany 31 H5 47 33N 9 42 E
Lindeman I., Australia 126 J7 20 27 S 149 3 E
Linden = Gladstone, U.S.A. 156 E2 39 13N 94 35W
Linden, Guyana 169 B6 6 0N 58 10W
Linden, Ala., U.S.A. 149 J2 32 18N 87 48W
Linden, Calif., U.S.A. 160 G5 38 1N 121 5W
Linden, Ind., U.S.A. 157 D10 40 11N 86 54W
Linden, Mich., U.S.A. 157 B13 42 49N 83 47W
Linden, Tex., U.S.A. 155 J7 33 1N 94 22W
Lindenhurst, U.S.A. 151 F11 40 41N 73 23W
Lindenow Fjord, Greenland 10 E6 60 30N 43 25W
Lindesberg, Sweden 16 E9 59 36N 15 15 E
Lindesnes, Norway 18 G4 57 58N 7 3 E
Líndhos, Greece 38 E12 36 6N 28 4 E
Líndhos, Ákra, Greece 38 E12 36 4N 28 10 E
Lindi, Tanzania 119 D4 9 58 S 39 38 E
Lindi □, Tanzania 119 D4 9 40 S 38 30 E
Lindi →, Dem. Rep. of the Congo 118 B2 0 33N 25 5 E
Lindö, Sweden 17 F10 58 37N 16 15 E
Lindome, Sweden 17 G6 57 35N 12 5 E
Lindos = Líndhos, Greece 38 E12 36 6N 28 4 E
Lindoso, Portugal 42 D2 41 52N 8 11W
Lindow, Germany 30 C8 52 58N 12 59 E
Lindsay, Canada 140 D4 44 22N 78 43W
Lindsay, Calif., U.S.A. 160 J7 36 12N 119 5W
Lindsay, Okla., U.S.A. 155 H6 34 50N 97 38W
Lindsborg, U.S.A. 154 F6 38 35N 97 40W
Lindsdal, Sweden 17 H10 56 44N 16 18 E
Line Islands, Pac. Oc. 135 H12 7 0N 160 0W
Linesville, U.S.A. 150 E4 41 39N 80 26W
Lineville, Ala., U.S.A. 152 B4 33 19N 85 45W
Lineville, Iowa, U.S.A. 156 D3 40 35N 93 32W
Linfen, China 74 F6 36 3N 111 30 E
Ling Xian, Hunan, China 77 D9 26 29N 113 48 E
Ling Xian, Shandong, China 74 F9 37 22N 116 30 E
Lingal, India 95 F4 16 17N 78 31 E
Lingao, China 86 C7 19 56N 109 42 E
Lingayen, Phil. 80 C3 16 1N 120 14 E
Lingayen G., Phil. 80 C3 16 10N 120 15 E
Lingbi, China 75 H9 33 33N 117 33 E
Lingbo, Sweden 16 C10 61 3N 16 41 E
Lingchuan, Guangxi Zhuangzu, China 77 E8 25 26N 110 21 E
Lingchuan, Shanxi, China 74 G7 35 45N 113 12 E
Lingding Yang, China 69 G10 22 25N 113 44 E
Lingen, Germany 30 C3 52 31N 7 19 E
Lingga, Indonesia 84 C2 0 12 S 104 37 E
Lingga, Kepulauan, Indonesia 84 C2 0 10 S 104 30 E
Lingga Arch. = Lingga, Kepulauan, Indonesia 84 C2 0 10 S 104 30 E
Linghem, Sweden 17 F9 58 26N 15 47 E
Lingig, Phil. 81 G6 8 2N 126 24 E
Lingle, U.S.A. 154 D2 42 8N 104 21W
Lingomo, Dem. Rep. of the Congo 114 B4 0 38N 22 3 E
Lingqiu, China 74 E8 39 28N 114 22 E
Lingshan, China 76 F7 22 25N 109 18 E
Lingshi, China 74 F6 36 48N 111 48 E
Lingshou, China 74 E8 38 20N 114 20 E
Lingshui, China 86 C8 18 27N 110 0 E
Lingsugur, India 95 F3 16 10N 76 31 E
Lingtai, China 74 G4 35 0N 107 40 E
Linguère, Senegal 112 B1 15 25N 15 5W
Lingui, China 77 E8 25 12N 110 2 E
Lingunda, Dem. Rep. of the Congo 114 C3 0 49N 21 8 E
Lingwu, China 74 E4 38 6N 106 20 E
Lingyuan, China 75 D10 41 10N 119 15 E
Lingyun, China 76 E6 25 2N 106 35 E
Linhai, China 77 C13 28 50N 121 8 E
Linhares, Brazil 171 E3 19 25 S 40 4W
Linhe, China 74 D4 40 48N 107 20 E
Linjiang, China 75 D14 41 50N 127 0 E
Linköping, Sweden 17 F9 58 28N 15 36 E
Linkou, China 75 B16 45 15N 130 18 E
Linli, China 77 C8 29 27N 111 30 E
Linlithgow = West Lothian □, U.K. 22 F5 55 54N 3 36W
Linn, U.S.A. 156 F5 38 29N 91 51W
Linneus, U.S.A. 156 E3 39 53N 93 11W
Linnhe, L., U.K. 22 E3 56 36N 5 25W
Linosa, Medit. S. 108 A2 35 51N 12 50 E
Linqi, China 74 G7 35 45N 113 52 E
Linqing, China 74 F8 36 50N 115 42 E
Linqu, China 75 F10 36 25N 118 30 E
Linru, China 74 G7 34 11N 112 52 E
Lins, Brazil 175 A6 21 40 S 49 44W
Linshui, China 76 B6 30 21N 106 57 E
Linsia = Linxia, China 68 C5 35 36N 103 10 E
Linstead, Jamaica 164 a 18 8N 77 2W
Linta →, Madag. 117 D7 25 2 S 44 5 E
Linth →, Switz. 31 H5 47 7N 9 7 E
Linthal, Switz. 33 C8 46 54N 9 0 E
Linton, Ind., U.S.A. 157 F9 39 2N 87 10W
Linton, N. Dak., U.S.A. 154 B4 46 16N 100 14W
Lintong, China 74 G5 34 20N 109 10 E
Linwood, Canada 150 C4 43 35N 80 43W
Linwu, China 77 E9 25 19N 112 31 E
Linxi, China 75 C10 43 36N 118 2 E
Linxia, China 68 C5 35 36N 103 10 E
Linxiang, China 77 C9 29 28N 113 23 E
Linyanti →, Africa 116 B4 17 50 S 25 5 E
Linyi, China 75 G10 35 5N 118 21 E
Linz, Austria 34 C7 48 18N 14 18 E
Linz, Germany 30 E3 50 34N 7 17 E
Linzhenzhen, China 74 F5 36 30N 109 59 E
Linzi, China 75 F10 36 50N 118 20 E
Lioko, Équateur, Dem. Rep. of the Congo 114 B4 0 2N 22 4 E
Lioko, Orientale, Dem. Rep. of the Congo 114 B4 1 25N 23 7 E
Liomseter, Norway 18 C6 61 15N 9 35 E
Lion, G. du, France 28 E7 43 10N 4 0 E

Lionárisso, Cyprus ... **39 E10** 35 28N 34 8 E
Lioni, Italy .... **47 B8** 40 52N 15 11 E
Lions, G. of = Lion, G.
du, France ...... **28 E7** 43 10N 4 0 E
Lion's Den, Zimbabwe **119 F3** 17 15 S 30 5 E
Lion's Head, Canada **150 B3** 44 58N 81 15W
Liouesso, Congo .... **114 B3** 1 2N 15 43 E
Liozno = Lyozna,
Belarus .... **58 E6** 55 0N 30 50 E
Lipa, Phil. .... **80 E3** 13 57N 121 10 E
Lipali, Mozam. ...... **119 F4** 15 50 S 35 50 E
Lipany, Slovak Rep. .. **53 B13** 49 9N 20 58 E
Lípari, Italy ...... **47 D7** 38 26N 14 58 E
Lípari, I., Italy .... **47 D7** 38 29N 14 58 E
Lípari, Is. = Eólie, Ís.,
Italy .... **47 D7** 38 30N 14 57 E
Lipcani, Moldova ..... **53 B11** 48 14N 26 48 E
Lipetsk, Russia ...... **59 F10** 52 37N 39 35 E
Lipiany, Poland ..... **55 E1** 53 2N 14 58 E
Liping, China ...... **76 D7** 26 15N 109 7 E
Lipkany = Lipcani,
Moldova .... **53 B11** 48 14N 26 48 E
Lipljan, Serbia & M. .. **50 D5** 42 31N 21 7 E
Lipník nad Bečvou,
Czech Rep. ...... **35 B12** 49 2N 17 36 E
Lipno, Poland ...... **55 F6** 52 49N 19 15 E
Lipova, Romania ..... **52 D6** 46 8N 21 42 E
Lipovcy Manzovka,
Russia .... **70 B5** 44 12N 132 26 E
Lipovets, Ukraine .... **59 H5** 49 12N 29 1 E
Lippe →, Germany ... **30 D2** 51 39N 6 36 E
Lippehne = Lipiany,
Poland .... **55 E1** 53 2N 14 58 E
Lippstadt, Germany ... **30 D4** 51 41N 8 22 E
Lipscomb, U.S.A. **155 G4** 36 14N 100 16W
Lipsko, Poland ..... **54 E10** 53 44N 23 24 E
Lipsko, Poland ..... **55 G8** 51 9N 21 40 E
Lipsói, Greece ..... **49 D8** 37 19N 26 50 E
Liptovský Hrádok,
Slovak Rep. ..... **35 B12** 49 2N 19 44 E
Liptovský Mikuláš,
Slovak Rep. ..... **35 B12** 49 6N 19 35 E
Liptrap, C., Australia . **129 E6** 38 50 S 145 55 E
Lipu, China .... **77 E8** 24 30N 110 22 E
Liquica, E. Timor .... **82 C3** 8 36 S 125 19 E
Liquillo, Sierra de,
Puerto Rico ..... **165 d** 18 20N 65 47W
Lira, Uganda ...... **118 B3** 2 17N 32 57 E
Liranga, Congo ..... **114 C3** 0 43 S 17 32 E
Liri →, Italy ...... **46 A6** 41 25N 13 52 E
Liria = Lliria, Spain .. **41 F4** 39 37N 0 35W
Lisakovsk, Kazakhstan **64 E9** 52 33N 62 37 E
Lisala, Dem. Rep. of
the Congo .... **116 B4** 2 12N 21 38 E
Lisboa, Portugal **43 G1** 38 42N 9 10W
Lisboa □, Portugal ... **43 F1** 39 0N 9 12W
Lisboa ✈ (LIS),
Portugal **43 G1** 38 46N 9 8W
Lisbon = Lisboa,
Portugal **43 G1** 38 42N 9 10W
Lisbon, N. Dak., U.S.A. **154 B6** 46 27N 97 41W
Lisbon, N.H., U.S.A. . **151 B13** 44 13N 71 55W
Lisbon, Ohio, U.S.A. . **150 F4** 40 46N 80 46W
Lisburn Falls, U.S.A. . **149 D10** 44 0N 70 4W
Lisburn, U.K. **23 B5** 54 31N 6 3W
Lisburne, C., U.S.A. .. **6 C17** 68 53N 166 13W
Liscannor B., Ireland . **23 D2** 52 55N 9 24W
Liscia →, Italy ..... **46 A2** 41 11N 9 9 E
Lishe Jiang →, China . **76 E3** 24 15N 101 35 E
Lishi, China .... **74 F6** 37 31N 111 8 E
Lishu, China ...... **75 C13** 43 20N 124 18 E
Lishui, Jiangsu, China **77 B12** 31 38N 119 2 E
Lishui, Zhejiang, China **77 C12** 28 28N 119 54 E
Lisianski I., Pac. Oc. . **145 F9** 26 2N 174 0W
Lisichansk =
Lysychansk, Ukraine **59 H10** 48 55N 38 30 E
Lisieux, France .... **26 C7** 49 10N 0 12 E
Liski, Russia ...... **59 G10** 51 3N 39 30 E
L'Isle-Jourdain, Gers,
France .... **28 E5** 43 36N 1 6 E
L'Isle-Jourdain, Vienne,
France .... **28 B4** 46 13N 0 31 E
L'Isle-Mont-la-Ville,
Switz. .... **32 C2** 46 37N 6 25 E
L'Isle-sur-la-Sorgue,
France .... **29 E9** 43 54N 5 2 E
Lisle-sur-Tarn, France **28 E5** 43 52N 1 49 E
Lismore, Australia ... **127 D5** 28 44 S 153 21 E
Lismore, Ireland **23 D4** 52 8N 7 55W
Lissa = Leszno, Poland **55 G3** 51 50N 16 30 E
Lista, Norway ..... **18 F3** 58 7N 6 39 E
Lister, Mt., Antarctica **7 D11** 78 0 S 162 0 E
Lister og Mandals =
Vest-Agder □,
Norway .... **18 F4** 58 30N 7 15 E
Liston, Australia .... **127 D5** 28 39 S 152 6 E
Listowel, Canada **140 D3** 43 44N 80 58W
Listowel, Ireland **23 D2** 52 27N 9 29W
Lit, Sweden .... **16 A8** 63 19N 14 51 E
Lit-et-Mixe, France .. **28 D2** 44 2N 1 15W
Litang,
Guangxi Zhuangzu,
China .... **76 F7** 23 12N 109 8 E
Litang, Sichuan, China **76 B3** 30 1N 100 17 E
Litang, Malaysia .... **85 A5** 5 27N 118 31 E
Litang Qu →, China . **76 C3** 28 4N 101 32 E
Litani →, Lebanon .. **103 B4** 33 20N 35 15 E
Litani →, Surinam .. **173 C7** 3 40N 54 0W
Litchfield, Australia .. **128 D5** 13 18 S 142 52 E
Litchfield, Calif., U.S.A. **160 E6** 40 24N 120 23W
Litchfield, Conn.,
U.S.A. **151 E11** 41 45N 73 11W
Litchfield, Ill., U.S.A. . **156 F7** 39 11N 89 39W
Litchfield, Minn.,
U.S.A. **154 C7** 45 8N 94 32W
Litchfield △, Australia **124 B5** 13 14 S 131 1 E
Liteni, Romania .... **53 C11** 47 32N 26 32 E
Lithgow, Australia ... **129 B9** 33 25 S 150 8 E
Líthinon, Ákra, Greece **39 F5** 34 55N 24 44 E
Lithuania ■, Europe . **15 J20** 55 30N 24 0 E
Litija, Slovenia .... **45 B11** 46 3N 14 50 E
Lititz, U.S.A. **151 F8** 40 9N 76 18W
Litókhoron, Greece .. **50 F6** 40 8N 22 34 E
Litoko, Dem. Rep. of
the Congo .... **114 C4** 1 13 S 24 47 E
Litoměřice, Czech Rep. **34 A7** 50 33N 14 10 E
Litomyšl, Czech Rep. . **35 B9** 49 52N 16 20 E
Litschau, Austria .... **34 C8** 48 58N 15 4 E
Little Abaco, Bahamas **164 A4** 26 50N 77 30W
Little Andaman I.,
India .... **95 J11** 10 45N 92 30 E
Little Barrier I., N.Z. . **130 C4** 36 12 S 175 8 E
Little Basses, Sri Lanka **95 L5** 6 24N 81 43 E
Little Belt Mts. =
Canada **143 B9** 57 30N 95 22W
Little Bighorn
Battlefield △, U.S.A. **158 D10** 45 34N 107 26W
Little Blue →, U.S.A. **154 F6** 39 42N 96 41W
Little Buffalo →,
Canada **142 A6** 61 0N 113 46W
Little Cayman,
Cayman Is. **164 C3** 19 41N 80 3W
Little Churchill →,
Canada **143 B9** 57 30N 95 22W

Little Coco I., Burma . **95 H11** 14 0N 93 13 E
Little Colorado →,
U.S.A. **159 H8** 36 12N 111 48W
Little Current, Canada **140 C3** 45 55N 82 0W
Little Current →,
Canada **140 B3** 50 57N 84 36W
Little Desert △,
Australia ...... **128 D4** 37 25 S 141 30 E
Little Diomede I.,
U.S.A. **144 D5** 65 45N 168 56W
Little Falls, Minn.,
U.S.A. **154 C7** 45 59N 94 22W
Little Falls, N.Y.,
U.S.A. **151 C10** 43 3N 74 51W
Little Fork →, U.S.A. **154 A8** 48 31N 93 35W
Little Grand Rapids,
Canada **143 C9** 52 0N 95 29W
Little Humboldt →,
U.S.A. **158 F5** 41 1N 117 43W
Little Inagua I.,
Bahamas **165 B5** 21 40N 73 50W
Little Karoo, S. Africa **116 E3** 33 45 S 21 0 E
Little Khingan Mts. =
Xiao Hinggan Ling,
China .... **69 B7** 49 0N 127 0 E
Little Lake, U.S.A. ... **161 K9** 35 56N 117 55W
Little Laut Is. = Laut
Kecil, Kepulauan,
Indonesia .... **85 C5** 4 45 S 115 40 E
Little Mecatina = Petit-
Mécatina →, Canada **141 B8** 50 40N 59 30W
Little Minch, U.K. ... **22 D2** 57 35N 6 45W
Little Missouri →,
U.S.A. **154 B3** 47 36N 102 25W
Little Nicobar, India .. **95 L11** 7 20N 93 40 E
Little Ouse →, U.K. . **21 E9** 52 22N 1 12 E
Little Rann, India ... **92 H4** 23 25N 71 25 E
Little Red →, U.S.A. **155 H9** 35 11N 91 27W
Little River, N.Z. ... **131 D7** 43 45 S 172 49 E
Little Ruaha →,
Tanzania ...... **118 D4** 7 57 S 37 53 E
Little Sable Pt., U.S.A. **148 D2** 43 38N 86 33W
Little Scarcies →,
S. Leone **112 D2** 8 50N 13 10W
Little Sioux →, U.S.A. **154 E6** 41 48N 96 4W
Little Sitkin I., U.S.A. **144 L2** 51 57N 178 31 E
Little Smoky →,
Canada **142 C5** 54 44N 117 11W
Little Snake →, U.S.A. **158 F9** 40 27N 108 26W
Little Sound, Bermuda **9 a** 32 15N 64 50W
Little Tobago,
Trin. & Tob. **169 E10** 11 18N 60 30W
Little Valley, U.S.A. .. **150 D6** 42 15N 78 48W
Little Wabash →,
U.S.A. **157 G8** 37 55N 88 5W
Little White →, U.S.A. **154 D4** 43 40N 100 40W
Little York, U.S.A. ... **156 C6** 41 1N 90 45W
Little Zab = Zāb aş
Şaghīr →, Iraq .. **101 E10** 35 17N 43 29 E
Littlefield, U.S.A. ... **155 J3** 33 55N 102 20W
Littlehampton, U.K. .. **21 G7** 50 49N 0 32W
Littleton, U.S.A. **151 B13** 44 18N 71 46W
Littoria = Latina, Italy **46 A5** 41 28N 12 52 E
Litunga, Angola .... **115 E3** 13 19 S 16 48 E
Litvinov, Czech Rep. . **34 A6** 50 36N 13 37 E
Liu He →, China .... **75 D11** 40 55N 121 35 E
Liu Jiang →, China .. **76 F7** 23 55N 109 30 E
Liuba, China ...... **74 H4** 33 38N 106 55 E
Liucheng, China .... **76 E7** 24 38N 109 14 E
Liugou, China ..... **75 D10** 40 57N 118 15 E
Liuhe, China ...... **75 C13** 42 17N 125 43 E
Liuheng Dao, China .. **77 C14** 29 40N 122 5 E
Liujiang, China .... **76 E7** 24 26N 109 11 E
Liukang Tenggaja =
Sabalana, Kepulauan,
Indonesia ...... **82 C1** 6 45 S 118 50 E
Liuli, Tanzania ..... **119 E3** 11 3 S 34 38 E
Liuwa Plain, Zambia . **115 E4** 14 20 S 22 30 E
Liuwa Plain △, Zambia **115 E4** 14 45 S 22 35 E
Liuyang, China ..... **77 C9** 28 10N 113 37 E
Liuzhou, China .... **76 E7** 24 22N 109 22 E
Liuzhuang, China ... **75 H11** 33 12N 120 18 E
Livada, Romania .... **52 C8** 47 52N 23 5 E
Livadherón, Greece .. **50 F5** 40 2N 21 57 E
Livadhia, Cyprus ... **39 E9** 34 57N 33 38 E
Livádhion, Greece ... **48 A4** 40 8N 22 9 E
Livadía, Albania .... **38 B10** 39 47N 20 7 E
Livadia = Levádhia,
Greece .... **48 C4** 38 27N 22 54 E
Livarot, France .... **26 D7** 48 58N 0 9 E
Live Oak, Calif., U.S.A. **160 F5** 39 17N 121 40W
Live Oak, Fla., U.S.A. **152 E7** 30 18N 82 59W
Lively, Canada **148 B5** 46 26N 81 9W
Livengood, U.S.A. ... **144 D10** 65 32N 148 33W
Liveras, Cyprus .... **39 E8** 35 23N 32 57 E
Livermore, U.S.A. ... **160 H5** 37 41N 121 47W
Livermore, Mt., U.S.A. **155 K2** 30 38N 104 11W
Livermore Falls, U.S.A. **149 C11** 44 29N 70 11W
Liverpool, Australia .. **129 B9** 33 54 S 150 58 E
Liverpool, Canada ... **141 D7** 44 5N 64 41W
Liverpool, U.K. **20 D4** 53 25N 3 0W
Liverpool, U.S.A. ... **151 C8** 43 6N 76 13W
Liverpool Bay, U.K. .. **20 D4** 53 30N 3 20W
Liverpool Plains,
Australia ...... **129 A9** 31 15 S 150 15 E
Liverpool Ra., Australia **129 A9** 31 50 S 150 30 E
Livigno, Italy ..... **44 B7** 46 35N 10 10 E
Livingston, Guatemala **164 C2** 15 50N 88 50W
Livingston, U.K. **22 F5** 55 54N 3 30W
Livingston, Ala., U.S.A. **149 J1** 32 35N 88 11W
Livingston, Calif.,
U.S.A. **160 H6** 37 23N 120 43W
Livingston, Mont.,
U.S.A. **158 D8** 45 40N 110 34W
Livingston, S.C., U.S.A. **149 J5** 33 32N 80 53W
Livingston, Tenn.,
U.S.A. **149 G3** 36 23N 85 19W
Livingston, Tex., U.S.A. **155 K7** 30 43N 94 56W
Livingston, Wis., U.S.A. **156 B6** 42 54N 90 26W
Livingston, L., U.S.A. **155 K7** 30 50N 95 10W
Livingston Manor,
U.S.A. **151 E10** 41 54N 74 50W
Livingstone, Zambia . **119 F2** 17 46 S 25 52 E
Livingstone, N.Z. ... **131 F3** 45 15 S 168 9 E
Livingstone Mts.,
Tanzania ...... **119 D3** 9 40 S 34 20 E
Livingstonia, Malawi . **119 E3** 10 38 S 34 5 E
Livno, Bos.-H. ..... **52 G2** 43 50N 17 1 E
Livny, Russia ...... **59 F9** 52 30N 37 30 E
Livonia, Mich., U.S.A. **157 B13** 42 23N 83 23W
Livonia, N.Y., U.S.A. **150 D7** 42 49N 77 40W
Livorno, Italy ..... **44 E7** 43 33N 10 19 E
Livradois-Forez △,
France .... **28 E7** 44 0N 3 0 E
Livramento = Nossa
Senhora do
Livramento, Brazil . **173 D6** 15 48 S 56 22W
Livramento, Brazil .. **175 C4** 30 55 S 55 30W
Livramento do
Brumado, Brazil .. **171 D3** 13 39 S 41 50W
Livron-sur-Drôme,
France .... **29 D8** 44 46N 4 51 E
Livyntsi, Ukraine ... **53 B11** 48 25N 24 30 E

Liwale, Tanzania ... **119 D4** 9 48 S 37 58 E
Liwiec →, Poland ... **55 F8** 52 36N 21 34 E
Liwonde, Malawi ... **119 E4** 14 48 S 35 20 E
Lixi, China .... **76 D3** 26 23N 101 59 E
Lixian, China ...... **76 B4** 31 23N 103 13 E
Lixoúrion, Greece ... **39 C2** 38 12N 20 26 E
Liyang, China ...... **77 B12** 31 26N 119 28 E
Lizard I., Australia .. **126 A4** 14 42 S 145 30 E
Lizard, Brazil ...... **170 C2** 9 36 S 46 41W
Lizella, U.S.A. **152 C6** 32 48N 83 49W
Lizzano, Italy ...... **47 B10** 40 23N 17 27 E
Ljig, Serbia & M. ... **50 B4** 44 13N 20 18 E
Ljørა →, Norway ... **18 C9** 61 23N 12 51 E
Ljørdal, Norway .... **18 C9** 61 23N 12 41 E
Ljosland, Norway ... **18 F4** 58 47N 7 22 E
Ljubija, Bos.-H. .... **45 D13** 44 55N 16 35 E
Ljubinje, Bos.-H. ... **50 D2** 42 58N 18 5 E
Ljubljana, Slovenia .. **45 B11** 46 4N 14 33 E
Ljubljana ✈ (LJU),
Slovenia .... **45 B11** 46 14N 14 33 E
Ljubno, Slovenia .... **45 B11** 46 25N 14 46 E
Ljubovija, Serbia & M. **50 B3** 44 11N 19 22 E
Ljugarn, Sweden ... **17 G12** 57 20N 18 43 E
Ljung, Sweden ..... **17 G7** 57 59N 13 3 E
Ljungan →, Sweden **16 B11** 62 18N 17 23 E
Ljungaverk, Sweden . **16 B10** 62 30N 16 5 E
Ljungby, Sweden ... **17 H7** 56 49N 13 55 E
Ljungbyholm, Sweden **17 H10** 56 39N 16 13 E
Ljungdalen, Sweden . **16 B6** 62 51N 12 47 E
Ljungsbro, Sweden .. **17 F9** 58 31N 15 30 E
Ljungskile, Sweden .. **17 F5** 58 14N 11 55 E
Ljusdal, Sweden .... **16 C10** 61 46N 16 3 E
Ljusfallshammar,
Sweden .... **17 F9** 58 48N 15 30 E
Ljusnan →, Sweden . **16 C11** 61 12N 17 8 E
Ljusne, Sweden .... **16 C11** 61 13N 17 7 E
Ljutomer, Slovenia .. **45 B13** 46 31N 16 11 E
Llagostera, Spain ... **40 D7** 41 50N 2 54 E
Llallmellín, Peru .... **172 B2** 9 0 S 76 54W
Llancanelo, Salina,
Argentina ...... **174 D2** 35 40 S 69 8W
Llandeilo, U.K. **21 F4** 51 53N 3 59W
Llandovery, U.K. ... **21 F4** 51 59N 3 48W
Llandrindod Wells,
U.K. **21 E4** 52 14N 3 22W
Llandudno, U.K. ... **20 D4** 53 19N 3 50W
Llanelli, U.K. **21 F3** 51 41N 4 10W
Llanes, Spain **42 B6** 43 25N 4 50W
Llanganates △,
Ecuador .... **168 D3** 0 51 S 78 20W
Llangollen, U.K. **20 E4** 52 58N 3 11W
Llanidloes, U.K. **21 E4** 52 27N 3 31W
Llano, U.S.A. **155 K5** 30 45N 98 41W
Llano →, U.S.A. ... **155 K5** 30 39N 98 26W
Llano Estacado, U.S.A. **155 J3** 33 30N 103 0W
Llanos, S. Amer. **166 C3** 5 0N 71 35W
Llanos de Challe △,
Chile .... **174 B1** 28 8 S 71 1W
Llanquihue, L., Chile **176 B1** 41 10 S 72 50W
Llanwrtyd Wells, U.K. **21 E4** 52 7N 3 38W
Llata, Peru .... **172 B2** 9 25 S 76 47W
Llebeig, C. des, Spain **38 B3** 39 33N 2 18 E
Lleida, Spain ...... **40 C5** 41 37N 0 39 E
Lleida □, Spain .... **40 C6** 42 6N 1 0 E
Llentrisca, C., Spain . **38 D1** 38 52N 1 15 E
Llera, Mexico **163 C5** 23 19N 99 1W
Llerena, Spain **43 G5** 38 17N 6 0W
Lleyn Peninsula, U.K. **20 E3** 52 51N 4 36W
Llica, Bolivia ...... **172 D4** 19 52 S 68 16W
Llico, Chile .... **174 C1** 34 46 S 72 5W
Lliria, Spain **41 F4** 39 37N 0 35W
Llobregat →, Spain . **40 D7** 41 19N 2 9 E
Llodio, Spain **40 B2** 43 9N 2 58W
Llorente, Phil. ..... **81 F5** 11 25N 125 33 E
Lloret de Mar, Spain . **40 D7** 41 41N 2 53 E
Lloyd B., Australia .. **126 A3** 12 45 S 143 27 E
Lloyd L., Canada ... **143 B7** 57 22N 108 57W
Lloydminster, Canada **143 C7** 53 17N 110 0W
Llucena del Cid, Spain **40 E4** 40 9N 0 17W
Llucmajor, Spain ... **38 B3** 39 29N 2 53 E
Llullaillaco △, Chile . **174 A2** 24 50 S 68 51W
Llullaillaco, Volcán,
S. Amer. .... **174 A2** 24 43 S 68 30W
Lo →, Vietnam .... **86 B5** 21 18N 105 25 E
Loa, U.S.A. **159 G8** 38 24N 111 39W
Loa →, Chile ...... **174 A1** 21 26 S 70 41W
Loaita I., S. China Sea **78 B4** 10 41N 114 25 E
Loange →, Dem. Rep.
of the Congo .... **115 C4** 4 17 S 20 2 E
Loango, Congo ..... **115 C2** 4 38 S 11 50 E
Loano, Italy .... **44 D5** 44 8N 8 15 E
Loay, Phil. .... **81 G5** 9 36N 124 1 E
Lobatse, Botswana .. **116 D4** 25 12 S 25 40 E
Löbau, Germany ... **30 D10** 51 5N 14 40 E
Lobaye →, C.A.R. .. **114 B3** 3 41N 18 35 E
Lobenstein, Germany . **30 E7** 50 25N 11 39 E
Lobería, Argentina .. **174 D4** 38 10 S 58 40W
Löberöd, Sweden ... **17 J7** 55 47N 13 31 E
Lobez, Poland ..... **54 E2** 53 38N 15 39 E
Lobito, Angola ..... **115 E2** 12 18 S 13 35 E
Lobo, Indonesia .... **83 B4** 3 45 S 134 5 E
Lobo, Phil. .... **80 E3** 13 39N 121 13 E
Lobos, Argentina ... **174 D4** 35 10 S 59 0W
Lobos, I., Mexico ... **162 B2** 27 15N 110 30W
Lobos de Afuera, Islas,
Peru .... **172 B1** 6 57 S 80 42W
Lobos de Tierra, I.,
Peru .... **172 B1** 6 27 S 80 52W
Lobva, Russia ...... **64 B8** 59 10N 60 30 E
Lobva →, Russia ... **64 B8** 59 8N 60 48 E
Łobżenica, Poland .. **55 E4** 53 18N 17 15 E
Loc Binh, Vietnam .. **86 B6** 21 46N 106 54 E
Loc Ninh, Vietnam .. **87 G6** 11 50N 106 34 E
Locarno, Switz. .... **33 D7** 46 10N 8 47 E
Loch Baghasdail =
Lochboisdale, U.K. . **22 D1** 57 9N 7 20W
Loch Garman =
Wexford, Ireland . **23 D5** 52 20N 6 28W
Loch Lomond and the
Trossachs △, U.K. . **22 E4** 56 10N 4 40W
Loch Nam Madadh =
Lochmaddy, U.K. . **22 D1** 57 36N 7 10W
Lochaber, U.K. **22 E3** 56 59N 5 1W
Locharbriggs, U.K. .. **22 F5** 55 7N 3 35W
Lochboisdale, U.K. .. **22 D1** 57 9N 7 20W
Loche, L. La, Canada **143 B7** 56 30N 109 30W
Lochem, Neths. .... **17 B6** 52 9N 6 26 E
Loches, France ..... **26 E7** 47 7N 1 0 E
Lochgilphead, U.K. .. **22 E3** 56 2N 5 26W
Lochinvar △, Zambia **119 F2** 15 55 S 27 15 E
Lochinver, U.K. **22 C3** 58 9N 5 14W
Lochmaddy, U.K. ... **22 D1** 57 36N 7 10W
Łochów, Poland ... **55 F8** 52 33N 21 42 E
Lochy, L., U.K. **22 E4** 57 0N 4 53W
Lock, Australia ..... **127 E2** 33 34 S 135 46 E
Lock Haven, U.S.A. . **150 E7** 41 8N 77 28W

Lockeford, U.S.A. ... **160 G5** 38 10N 121 9W
Lockeport, Canada .. **141 D6** 43 47N 65 4W
Lockerbie, U.K. **22 F5** 55 7N 3 21W
Lockhart, Australia .. **129 C7** 35 14 S 146 40 E
Lockhart, U.S.A. ... **155 L6** 29 53N 97 40W
Lockhart, L., Australia **126 F2** 33 15 S 119 3 E
Lockhart River,
Australia ...... **126 A3** 12 58N 143 30 E
Lockney, U.S.A. ... **155 H4** 34 7N 101 27W
Lockport, Ill., U.S.A. . **157 C8** 41 35N 88 3W
Lockport, N.Y., U.S.A. **150 C6** 43 10N 78 42W
Locminé, France ... **26 E4** 47 54N 2 51W
Locri, Italy .... **47 D9** 38 14N 16 16 E
Locronan, France ... **26 D2** 48 7N 4 15W
Locust Cr. →, U.S.A. **156 E3** 39 40N 93 17W
Locust Grove, U.S.A. **152 D5** 33 21N 84 7W
Lod, Israel .... **103 D3** 31 57N 34 54 E
Lodalskåpa, Norway . **18 C6** 61 47N 7 13 E
Lodeinoye Pole, Russia **58 B7** 60 44N 33 33 E
Lodève, France .... **28 E7** 43 44N 3 19 E
Lodge Bay, Canada . **141 B8** 52 14N 55 51W
Lodge Grass, U.S.A. . **158 D10** 45 19N 107 22W
Lodgepole Cr. →,
U.S.A. **154 E2** 41 20N 104 30W
Lodhran, Pakistan .. **92 E4** 29 32N 71 30 E
Lodi, Italy .... **44 C6** 45 19N 9 30 E
Lodi, Calif., U.S.A. .. **160 G5** 38 8N 121 16W
Lodi, Ohio, U.S.A. .. **150 E3** 41 2N 82 0W
Lodja, Dem. Rep. of
the Congo ...... **118 C1** 3 30 S 23 23 E
Lodosa, Spain **40 C2** 42 25N 2 4W
Lödöse, Sweden ... **17 F6** 58 2N 12 9 E
Lodwar, Kenya .... **118 B4** 3 10N 35 40 E
Łódź, Poland ...... **55 G6** 51 45N 19 27 E
Łódzkie □, Poland . **55 G6** 51 30N 19 10 E
Loei, Thailand .... **86 D3** 17 29N 101 35 E
Loengo, Dem. Rep. of
the Congo ...... **118 C2** 4 48 S 26 30 E
Loeriesfontein,
S. Africa .... **116 E2** 31 0 S 19 26 E
Lofa □, Liberia **112 D2** 7 35N 11 8W
Lofa Mano △, Liberia **112 D2** 7 10N 10 25W
Lofer, Austria .... **34 D5** 47 35N 12 41 E
Lofoten, Norway ... **14 B15** 68 30N 14 0 E
Lofsdalen, Sweden . **16 B7** 62 10N 13 20 E
Lofsen →, Sweden . **16 B7** 62 7N 13 57 E
Loftahammar, Sweden **17 G10** 57 54N 16 41 E
Loga, Niger .... **113 C5** 13 40N 3 15 E
Logan, Iowa, U.S.A. . **154 E7** 41 39N 95 47W
Logan, Ohio, U.S.A. . **148 F4** 39 32N 82 25W
Logan, Utah, U.S.A. . **158 F8** 41 44N 111 50W
Logan, W. Va., U.S.A. **148 G5** 37 51N 81 59W
Logan, Mt., Canada . **138 B5** 60 34N 140 23W
Logan Martin L.,
U.S.A. **152 B3** 33 26N 86 20W
Logandale, U.S.A. .. **161 J12** 36 36N 114 29W
Logansport, Ind.,
U.S.A. **157 E2** 40 45N 86 22W
Logansport, La., U.S.A. **155 K8** 31 58N 94 0W
Logirim, Sudan ... **107 G3** 4 43N 33 14 E
Logo, Sudan ...... **107 F3** 5 20N 30 18 E
Logone →, Chad ... **109 F3** 12 6N 15 2 E
Logone Gana, Chad . **109 F3** 11 36N 15 4 E
Logone Occidental →,
Chad .... **109 G3** 8 50N 16 0 E
Logone Orientale →,
Chad .... **109 G3** 9 7N 16 26 E
Logroño, Spain **40 C2** 42 28N 2 27W
Logrosán, Spain ... **43 F5** 39 20N 5 32W
Løgstør, Denmark .. **17 H3** 56 58N 9 14 E
Logtak Lake, India . **94 C4** 24 33N 93 50 E
Løgumkloster,
Denmark ...... **17 J2** 55 4N 8 57 E
Loh, Vanuatu ..... **133 C4** 13 21 S 166 38 E
Lohals, Denmark ... **17 J4** 55 8N 10 55 E
Lohardaga, India .. **93 H11** 23 27N 84 45 E
Loharia, India ..... **92 H6** 23 45N 74 14 E
Loharu, India ..... **92 E6** 28 27N 75 49 E
Lohja, Finland .... **15 F21** 60 12N 24 5 E
Löhne, Germany ... **30 C4** 52 11N 8 40 E
Lohr = Luohe, China **74 H8** 33 32N 114 2 E
Lohr, Germany .... **31 F5** 49 59N 9 35 E
Lohri Wah →, Pakistan **92 F2** 27 27N 67 37 E
Loi-kaw, Burma ... **92 F6** 19 40N 97 17 E
Loi-lem, Burma .... **90 F6** 20 56N 97 28 E
Loimaa, Finland ... **15 F20** 60 50N 23 5 E
Loir →, France **26 E6** 47 33N 0 11W
Loir-et-Cher □, France **26 E8** 47 40N 1 20 E
Loire □, France .... **29 C8** 45 40N 4 5 E
Loire →, France **26 E4** 47 16N 2 10W
Loire Anjou
Touraine △, France **26 E6** 47 14N 0 5W
Loire-Atlantique □,
France **26 E5** 47 25N 1 40W
Loiret □, France ... **27 E9** 47 55N 2 30 E
Loitz, Germany ... **30 B9** 53 58N 13 8 E
Loja, Ecuador ..... **172 A2** 3 59 S 79 16W
Loja, Spain **43 H6** 37 10N 4 10W
Loja □, Ecuador ... **168 D2** 4 0 S 79 30W
Loje →, Angola .... **115 D2** 7 49 S 13 6 E
Loji = Kawasi,
Indonesia ...... **83 B3** 1 38 S 127 28 E
Lojo = Lohja, Finland **15 F21** 60 12N 24 5 E
Løjt Kirkeby, Denmark **17 J3** 55 7N 9 26 E
Lojung, China .... **76 E7** 24 27N 109 36 E
Loka, Dem. Rep. of
the Congo ...... **114 B3** 0 20N 17 57 E
Loka, Sudan ...... **107 G3** 4 13N 31 0 E
Lokako, Dem. Rep. of
the Congo ...... **114 C4** 0 57 S 18 55 E
Lokandu, Dem. Rep. of
the Congo ...... **118 C2** 2 30 S 25 45 E
Lokaw, Dem. Rep. of
the Congo ...... **114 C4** 2 40 S 20 12 E
Løken, Norway .... **18 E8** 59 48N 11 29 E
Lokeren, Belgium .. **17 C3** 51 6N 3 59 E
Lokgwabe, Botswana **116 C3** 24 10 S 21 50 E
Lokichar, Kenya ... **118 B4** 2 23N 35 39 E
Lokichokio, Kenya .. **118 B3** 4 19N 34 13 E
Lokitaung, Kenya .. **118 B4** 4 12N 35 48 E
Lokkan tekojärvi,
Finland .... **14 C22** 67 55N 27 35 E
Løkken, Denmark .. **17 G3** 57 22N 9 41 E
Løkken, Norway ... **18 A6** 63 6N 9 43 E
Loknya, Russia .... **58 A6** 56 49N 30 4 E
Loko, Nigeria ..... **113 D6** 7 53N 7 47 E
Lokoja, Nigeria .... **113 D6** 7 47N 6 45 E
Lokolama, Dem. Rep.
of the Congo .... **114 C3** 2 35 S 19 50 E
Lokoro →, Dem. Rep.
of the Congo .... **114 C3** 1 43 S 18 23 E
Lokuru, Solomon Is. . **133 M9** 8 21 S 157 0 E
Lol →, Sudan .... **107 F2** 9 13N 26 30 E
Lola, Angola ...... **115 E2** 14 19 S 13 37 E

Lola, Guinea **112 D3** 7 52N 8 29W
Lola, Mt., U.S.A. ... **160 F6** 39 26N 120 22W
Lolibai, Gebel, Sudan **107 G3** 3 50N 33 0 E
Lolimi, Sudan ..... **107 G3** 4 35N 34 0 E
Loliondo, Tanzania . **118 C4** 2 2 S 35 39 E
Lolland, Denmark .. **17 K5** 54 45N 11 30 E
Lollar, Germany ... **30 E4** 50 37N 8 43 E
Lolo, U.S.A. **158 C6** 46 45N 114 5W
Lolodorf, Cameroon . **113 E7** 3 16N 10 49 E
Loloma, Zambia ... **115 E4** 13 24 S 24 21 E
Loltong, Vanuatu .. **133 E6** 15 32 S 168 10 E
Lom, Bulgaria ..... **50 C7** 43 48N 23 12 E
Lom, Norway ..... **18 C5** 61 50N 8 34 E
Lom →, Bulgaria .. **50 C7** 43 45N 23 9 E
Lom Kao, Thailand . **86 D3** 16 53N 101 14 E
Lom Sak, Thailand . **86 D3** 16 47N 101 15 E
Loma, U.S.A. **158 C8** 47 57N 110 30W
Loma Linda, U.S.A. **161 L9** 34 3N 117 16W
Lomako →, Dem. Rep.
of the Congo .... **114 B4** 0 50N 20 50 E
Lomalinda, Fiji .... **133 A3** 17 17 S 178 59W
Lomami →, Dem. Rep.
of the Congo .... **118 B2** 0 46N 24 16 E
Lomas de Zamóra,
Argentina ...... **174 C4** 34 45 S 58 25W
Lombadina, Australia **124 C3** 16 31 S 122 54 E
Lombard, U.S.A. ... **157 C8** 41 53N 88 1W
Lombárdia □, Italy . **44 C6** 45 40N 9 30 E
Lombardy =
Lombárdia □, Italy **44 C6** 45 40N 9 30 E
Lombe, Angola .... **115 D3** 9 27 S 16 13 E
Lombez, France ... **28 E4** 43 29N 0 55 E
Lomblen, Indonesia . **82 C3** 8 30 S 123 32 E
Lombok, Indonesia . **85 D5** 8 45 S 116 30 E
Lombok, Selat,
Indonesia ...... **79 K18** 8 30 S 115 50 E
Lomé, Togo ...... **113 D5** 6 9N 1 20 E
Lomela, Dem. Rep. of
the Congo ...... **114 C4** 2 19 S 23 15 E
Lomela →, Dem. Rep.
of the Congo .... **114 C4** 0 15 S 20 40 E
Lomianki, Poland .. **55 F7** 52 21N 20 54 E
Lomié, Cameroon .. **114 B2** 3 13N 13 38 E
Lomma, Sweden ... **17 J7** 55 43N 13 6 E
Lommel, Belgium .. **17 C5** 51 14N 5 19 E
Lomond, Canada ... **142 C6** 50 24N 112 36W
Lomond, L., U.K. .. **22 E4** 56 8N 4 38W
Lomonosov Ridge,
Arctic .... **6 A** 88 0N 140 0 E
Lomphat, Cambodia **86 F6** 13 30N 106 59 E
Lompobatang,
Indonesia ...... **82 C1** 5 24 S 119 56 E
Lompoc, U.S.A. ... **161 L6** 34 38N 120 28W
Lomsegga, Norway . **18 C5** 61 49N 8 21 E
Łomża, Poland .... **55 E9** 53 10N 22 2 E
Lon, Ko, Thailand .. **87 a** 7 47N 98 23 E
Lonavale, India .... **94 K8** 18 46N 73 29 E
Loncoche, Chile .... **176 A2** 39 20 S 72 50W
Loncopuè, Argentina **176 A2** 38 4 S 70 37W
Londa, India ...... **95 G2** 15 30N 74 30 E
Londiani, Kenya ... **118 C4** 0 10 S 35 33 E
Londinières, France **26 C8** 49 50N 1 25 E
London, Canada ... **140 D3** 42 59N 81 15W
London, U.K. **21 F7** 51 30N 0 3W
London, Ky., U.S.A. **148 G3** 37 8N 84 5W
London, Ohio, U.S.A. **157 E13** 39 53N 83 27W
London, Greater □,
U.K. **21 F7** 51 36N 0 5W
London Gatwick ✈
(LGW), U.K. **21 F7** 51 10N 0 11W
London Heathrow ✈
(LHR), U.K. **21 F7** 51 28N 0 27W
London Mills, U.S.A. **156 D6** 40 43N 90 11W
London Stansted ✈
(STN), U.K. ..... **21 F8** 51 54N 0 14 E
Londonderry, U.K. . **23 B4** 55 0N 7 20W
Londonderry □, U.K. **23 B4** 55 0N 7 20W
Londonderry, C.,
Australia ...... **124 B4** 13 45 S 126 55 E
Londonderry, I., Chile **176 E2** 55 0 S 71 0W
Londrina, Brazil ... **175 A5** 23 18 S 51 10W
Londuimbale, Angola **115 E3** 12 15 S 15 19 E
Lone Pine, U.S.A. .. **160 J8** 36 36N 118 4W
Lonely Mine,
Zimbabwe ...... **117 B4** 19 38 S 28 49 E
Long Akah, Malaysia **85 B4** 3 19N 114 47 E
Long B., U.S.A. **149 J6** 33 35N 78 45W
Long Beach, Calif.,
U.S.A. **161 M8** 33 47N 118 11W
Long Beach, N.Y.,
U.S.A. **151 F11** 40 35N 73 39W
Long Beach, Wash.,
U.S.A. **160 D2** 46 21N 124 3W
Long Branch, U.S.A. **151 F11** 40 18N 74 0W
Long Cay, Bahamas . **165 C4** 22 35N 74 20W
Long Creek, U.S.A. . **158 D4** 44 43N 119 6W
Long Eaton, U.K. .. **20 E6** 52 53N 1 15W
Long I., Australia ... **126 J6** 20 22 S 148 51 E
Long I., Bahamas ... **165 B4** 23 20N 75 10W
Long I., Canada ... **142 B4** 54 50N 79 20W
Long I., Ireland **23 E2** 51 30N 9 34W
Long I., Papua N. G. **132 C4** 5 20 S 147 5 E
Long I., U.S.A. **151 F11** 40 45N 73 30W
Long Island Sd., U.S.A. **151 E12** 41 10N 73 0W
Long L., Canada ... **140 C2** 49 30N 86 50W
Long L., U.S.A. **151 C10** 43 58N 74 25W
Long Point B., Canada **150 D4** 42 40N 80 10W
Long Prairie, U.S.A. **154 C7** 45 59N 94 52W
Long Prairie →, U.S.A. **154 C7** 46 20N 94 36W
Long Pt., Bahamas . **9 b** 21 7N 73 20W
Long Pt., Canada ... **150 D4** 42 35N 80 2W
Long Pt., U.S.A. ... **150 C3** 44 34N 80 2W
Long Point B., Canada **150 D4** 42 40N 80 10W
Long Range Mts.,
Canada **141 C8** 49 30N 57 30W
Long Reef, Australia **124 B4** 14 1 S 125 48 E
Long Spruce, Canada **143 B10** 56 24N 94 21W
Proliv = Longa,
Proliv, Russia .. **6 C16** 70 0N 175 0 E
Long Thanh, Vietnam **87 G6** 10 47N 106 57 E
Long Xian, China ... **74 G4** 34 55N 106 55 E
Long Xuyen, Vietnam **87 G5** 10 19N 105 28 E
Longá, Angola ..... **115 E3** 14 42 S 18 32 E
Longá, Greece ..... **48 E3** 36 53N 21 55 E
Longá →, Angola .. **115 E2** 10 14 S 13 29 E
Longa, Proliv, Russia **6 C16** 70 0N 175 0 E
Longa Mavinga,
Angola .... **115 F4** 16 20 S 20 15 E
Longa, Tanzania ... **114 B3** 0 50N 20 5 E
Longana, Vanuatu .. **133 E6** 15 18 S 167 55 E
Longarone, Italy ... **45 B9** 46 16N 12 18 E
Longbenton, U.K. .. **20 B6** 55 1N 1 31W
Longboat Key, U.S.A. **153 H7** 27 23N 82 39W
Longchang, China .. **76 C5** 29 18N 105 15 E
Longchi, China .... **76 C4** 29 25N 103 24 E
Longchuan,
Guangdong, China **77 E10** 24 5N 115 17 E
Longchuan, Yunnan,
China .... **76 E1** 24 23N 97 58 E

Longde, China 74 G4 35 30N 106 20 E
Longeau, France 27 E12 47 47N 5 20 E
Longford, Australia 127 G4 41 32 S 147 3 E
Longford, Ireland 23 C4 53 43N 7 49W
Longford □, Ireland 23 C4 53 42N 7 45W
Longhai, China 77 E11 24 25N 117 46 E
Longhua, Guangdong, China 69 F11 22 39N 114 0 E
Longhua, Hebei, China 75 D9 41 18N 117 45 E
Longhui, China 77 D8 27 7N 111 2 E
Longido, Tanzania 118 C4 2 43 S 36 42 E
Longiram, Indonesia 85 C5 0 5 S 115 45 E
Longkou, Jiangxi, China 77 D10 26 8N 115 10 E
Longkou, Shandong, China 75 F11 37 40N 120 18 E
Longlac, Canada 140 C2 49 45N 86 25W
Longli, China 76 D6 26 25N 106 58 E
Longlin, China 76 E5 24 47N 105 20 E
Longling, China 76 E2 24 37N 98 39 E
Longmeadow, U.S.A. 151 D12 42 3N 72 34W
Longmen, China 77 F10 23 40N 114 18 E
Longming, China 76 F6 22 59N 107 7 E
Longmont, U.S.A. 154 E2 40 10N 105 6W
Longnan, China 77 E10 24 55N 114 47 E
Longnawan, Indonesia 85 B4 1 51N 114 55 E
Longobucco, Italy 47 C9 39 27N 16 37 E
Longonot △, Kenya 120 E1 0 55 S 36 28 E
Longos, Greece 38 C10 39 16N 20 7 E
Longquan, China 77 C12 28 7N 119 10 E
Longreach, Australia 126 C3 23 28 S 144 14 E
Longshan, China 76 C7 29 29N 109 25 E
Longsheng, China 77 E8 25 48N 110 0 E
Longué-Jumelles, France 26 E6 47 22N 0 8W
Longueau, France 27 C9 49 52N 2 21 E
Longueuil, Canada 151 A11 45 32N 73 28W
Longuy, Cameroon 114 B1 3 5N 9 58 E
Longuyon, France 27 C12 49 27N 5 35 E
Longvic, France 27 E12 47 17N 5 4 E
Longview, Tex., U.S.A. 155 J7 32 30N 94 44W
Longview, Wash., U.S.A. 160 D4 46 8N 122 57W
Longwood, St. Helena 9 h 15 57 S 5 41W
Longwood, U.S.A. 153 G8 28 42N 81 21W
Longwy, France 27 C12 49 30N 5 46 E
Longxi, China 74 G3 34 53N 104 40 E
Longxue Dao, China 69 F10 22 41N 113 38 E
Longyan, China 77 E11 25 10N 117 0 E
Longyearbyen, Svalbard 6 B8 78 13N 15 40 E
Longyou, China 77 C12 29 1N 119 8 E
Longzhou, China 76 F6 22 22N 106 50 E
Lonigo, Italy 45 C8 45 23N 11 23 E
Löningen, Germany 30 C3 52 44N 7 46 E
Lonja →, Croatia 45 C13 45 22N 16 40 E
Lonkala, Dem. Rep. of the Congo 115 C4 4 37 S 23 14 E
Lonkin, Burma 90 C6 25 39N 96 22 E
Lonoke, U.S.A. 155 H9 34 47N 91 54W
Lonquimay, Chile 176 A2 38 26 S 71 14W
Lons-le-Saunier, France 27 F12 46 40N 5 31 E
Lönsboda, Sweden 17 H8 56 24N 14 20 E
Lønset, Norway 18 B4 62 46N 7 24 E
Lonton, Burma 90 C6 25 6N 96 17 E
Looe, U.K. 21 G3 50 22N 4 28W
Loogootee, U.S.A. 157 F10 38 41N 86 55W
Lookout, C., Canada 140 A3 55 18N 83 56W
Lookout, C., U.S.A. 149 H7 34 35N 76 32W
Loolmalasin, Tanzania 118 C4 3 0 S 35 53 E
Loon →, Alta., Canada 142 B5 57 8N 115 3W
Loon →, Man., Canada 143 B8 55 53N 101 59W
Loon Lake, Canada 143 C7 54 2N 109 10W
Loongana, Australia 125 F4 30 52 S 127 5 E
Loop Hd., Ireland 23 D2 52 34N 9 56W
Lop Buri, Thailand 86 E3 14 48N 100 37 E
Lop Nor = Lop Nur, China 68 B4 40 20N 90 10 E
Lop Nur, China 68 B4 40 20N 90 10 E
Lopare, Bos.-H. 52 F3 44 39N 18 46 E
Lopatin, Russia 61 J8 43 50N 47 35 E
Lopatina, Gora, Russia 67 D15 50 47N 143 10 E
Lopatino = Volzhsk, Russia 60 C9 55 57N 48 23 E
Lopaye, Sudan 107 F3 6 37N 33 40 E
Lopé-Okanda ⌂, Gabon 114 C2 0 45 S 11 34 E
Lopevi, Vanuatu 133 F6 16 30 S 168 21 E
Lopez, Phil. 80 E4 13 53N 122 15 E
Lopez, U.S.A. 151 E8 41 27N 76 20W
Lopez, C., Gabon 114 C1 0 47 S 8 40 E
López de Filippis = Mariscal Estigarribia, Paraguay 174 A3 22 3 S 60 40W
Lopori →, Dem. Rep. of the Congo 114 B3 1 14N 19 49 E
Lopphavet, Norway 14 A19 70 27N 21 15 E
Lora, Norway 18 B5 62 8N 8 45 E
Lora →, Afghan. 91 C2 31 35N 66 32 E
Lora →, Norway 18 B5 62 8N 8 42 E
Lora, Hāmūn-i-, Pakistan 91 C2 29 38N 64 58 E
Lora Cr. →, Australia 127 D2 28 10 S 135 22 E
Lora del Río, Spain 43 H5 37 39N 5 33W
Lorain, U.S.A. 150 E2 41 28N 82 11W
Loraine, U.S.A. 156 D5 40 9N 91 13W
Loralai, Pakistan 91 C3 30 20N 68 41 E
Lorca, Spain 41 H3 37 41N 1 42W
Lord Howe I., Pac. Oc. 134 L7 31 33 S 159 6 E
Lord Howe Ridge, Pac. Oc. 134 L8 30 0 S 162 30 E
Lordsburg, U.S.A. 159 K9 32 21N 108 43W
Lorengau, Papua N. G. 132 B4 2 1 S 147 15 E
Lorestan □, Iran 97 C6 33 30N 48 40 E
Loreto, Bolivia 173 D5 15 13 S 64 40W
Loreto, Brazil 170 C2 7 5 S 45 10W
Loreto, Italy 45 E10 43 26N 13 36 E
Loreto, Mexico 162 B2 26 1N 111 21W
Loreto, Phil. 81 F5 10 21N 125 34 E
Loreto □, Peru 168 D3 5 0 S 75 0W
Lorgues, France 29 E10 43 28N 6 22 E
Lorhosso, Burkina Faso 112 C4 10 17N 3 38W
Lorica, Colombia 168 B2 9 14N 75 49W
Lorient, France 26 E3 47 45N 3 23W
Lorimor, U.S.A. 156 C2 41 8N 94 3W
Lőrinci, Hungary 52 C4 47 44N 19 41 E
Lormi, India 93 H9 22 17N 81 41 E
Lorn, U.K. 22 E3 56 26N 5 10W
Lorn, Firth of, U.K. 22 E3 56 20N 5 40W
Lorne, Australia 128 E5 38 33 S 143 59 E
Loronyo, Sudan 107 G3 4 38N 32 38 E
Lorovouno, Cyprus 39 E8 35 8N 32 36 E
Lörrach, Germany 31 H3 47 36N 7 40 E
Lorraine = Baker, U.S.A. 154 B2 46 22N 104 17W
Lorraine ⌂, France 27 D12 48 55N 5 50 E
Lorraine □, France 27 D13 48 53N 6 0 E
Los, Sweden 16 C9 61 45N 15 10 E
Los, Îles de, Guinea 112 D2 9 30N 13 50W
Los Alamos, Calif., U.S.A. 161 L6 34 44N 120 17W
Los Alamos, N. Mex., U.S.A. 159 J10 35 53N 106 19W
Los Alcornocales ⌂, Spain 43 J5 36 21N 5 32W
Los Alerces △, Argentina 176 B2 42 55 S 71 55W
Los Altos, U.S.A. 160 H4 37 23N 122 7W
Los Andes, Chile 174 C1 32 50 S 70 40W
Los Angeles, Chile 174 D1 37 28 S 72 23W
Los Angeles, U.S.A. 161 M8 34 4N 118 15W
Los Angeles, Bahia de, Mexico 162 B2 28 56N 113 34W
Los Angeles Aqueduct, U.S.A. 161 K9 35 22N 118 5W
Los Angeles International ✈ (LAX), U.S.A. 161 M8 33 57N 118 25W
Los Antiguos, Argentina 176 C2 46 35 S 71 40W
Los Banos, U.S.A. 160 H6 37 4N 120 51W
Los Barrios, Spain 43 J5 36 11N 5 30W
Los Blancos, Argentina 174 A3 23 40 S 62 30W
Los Cardones △, Argentina 174 B2 25 8 S 65 55W
Los Chiles, Costa Rica 164 D3 11 2N 84 43W
Los Corrales de Buelna, Spain 42 B6 43 16N 4 4W
Los Cristianos, Canary Is. 9 e1 28 3N 16 42W
Los Gallardos, Spain 41 H3 37 10N 1 57W
Los Gatos, U.S.A. 160 H5 37 14N 121 59W
Los Glaciares △, Argentina 176 C2 50 0 S 73 55W
Los Haïtises △, Dom. Rep. 165 C6 19 4N 69 36W
Los Hermanos Is., Venezuela 169 A5 11 45N 64 25W
Los Islotes, Canary Is. 9 e2 29 4N 13 44W
Los Katios △, Colombia 168 B2 7 50N 77 10W
Los Lagos, Chile 176 A2 39 51 S 72 50W
Los Llanos de Aridane, Canary Is. 9 e1 28 38N 17 54W
Los Lomas, Peru 172 A1 4 40 S 80 10W
Los Loros, Chile 174 B1 27 50 S 70 6W
Los Lunas, U.S.A. 159 J10 34 48N 106 44W
Los Menucos, Argentina 176 B3 40 50 S 68 10W
Los Mochis, Mexico 162 B3 25 45N 108 57W
Los Monegros, Spain 40 D4 41 29N 0 13W
Los Monos, Argentina 176 C3 46 1 S 69 36W
Los Muermos, Chile 176 B2 41 24 S 73 29W
Los Nevados △, Colombia 168 C2 4 41N 75 21W
Los Nietos, Spain 41 H4 37 39N 0 47W
Los Olivos, U.S.A. 161 L6 34 40N 120 7W
Los Palacios, Cuba 164 B3 22 35N 83 15W
Los Palacios y Villafranca, Spain 43 H5 37 10N 5 55W
Los Reyes, Mexico 162 D4 19 34N 102 30W
Los Ríos □, Ecuador 168 D2 1 30 S 79 25W
Los Roques Is., Venezuela 165 D6 11 50N 66 45W
Los Santos de Maimona, Spain 43 G4 38 27N 6 22W
Los Teques, Venezuela 168 A4 10 21N 67 2W
Los Testigos, Is., Venezuela 169 A5 11 23N 63 6W
Los Vilos, Chile 174 C1 32 10 S 71 30W
Los Yébenes, Spain 43 F7 39 36N 3 55W
Loshan = Leshan, China 76 C4 29 33N 103 41 E
Łosice, Poland 55 F9 52 13N 22 43 E
Lošinj, Croatia 36 F8 44 30N 14 30 E
Loskop Dam, S. Africa 117 D4 25 23 S 29 20 E
Løsning, Denmark 17 J3 55 48N 9 42 E
Losombo, Dem. Rep. of the Congo 114 B3 1 2N 19 4 E
Losone, Switz. 33 D7 46 10N 8 45 E
Lossiemouth, U.K. 22 D5 57 42N 3 17W
Lossnen △, Sweden 16 B6 62 26N 12 45 E
Lostwithiel, U.K. 21 G3 50 24N 4 41W
Losuia, Papua N. G. 132 E6 8 30 S 151 4 E
Lot □, France 28 D5 44 39N 1 40 E
Lot →, France 28 D4 44 18N 0 20 E
Lot-et-Garonne □, France 28 D4 44 22N 0 30 E
Lota, Chile 174 D1 37 5 S 73 10W
Lotagipi Swamp, Sudan 107 G3 4 36N 34 55 E
Løten, Norway 18 D8 60 51N 11 21 E
Lotfābād, Iran 97 B8 37 32N 59 20 E
Lothair, S. Africa 117 D5 26 22 S 30 27 E
Loto, Dem. Rep. of the Congo 114 C4 2 48 S 22 3 E
Lotoi →, Dem. Rep. of the Congo 114 C3 1 35 S 18 30 E
Lotorp, Sweden 17 F9 58 44N 15 50 E
Lötschbergtunnel, Switz. 32 D5 46 26N 7 43 E
Löttorp, Sweden 17 G11 57 10N 17 0 E
Lotung, Taiwan 77 E13 24 41N 121 46 E
Lötzen = Giżycko, Poland 54 D8 54 2N 21 48 E
Lotzwil, Switz. 32 B5 47 12N 7 48 E
Lou I., Papua N. G. 132 B4 2 25 S 147 22 E
Loubomo, Congo 114 C2 4 9 S 12 47 E
Loudéac, France 26 D4 48 11N 2 47W
Loudi, China 77 D8 27 42N 111 59 E
Loudima, Congo 114 C2 4 6 S 13 5 E
Loudonville, U.S.A. 150 F2 40 38N 82 14W
Loudun, France 26 E7 47 3N 0 5 E
Loue →, France 27 E12 47 1N 5 28 E
Louga, Senegal 112 B1 15 45N 16 5W
Loughborough, U.K. 20 E6 52 47N 1 11W
Loughman, U.S.A. 153 G8 28 14N 81 34W
Loughrea, Ireland 23 C3 53 12N 8 33W
Loughros More B., Ireland 23 B3 54 48N 8 32W
Louhans, France 27 F12 46 38N 5 12 E
Louis-Gentil = Youssoufia, Morocco 110 B3 32 16N 8 31W
Louis Trichardt, S. Africa 117 C4 23 1 S 29 43 E
Louis XIV, Pte., Canada 140 B4 54 37N 79 45W
Louisa, U.S.A. 148 F4 38 7N 82 36W
Louisbourg, Canada 141 C8 45 55N 60 0W
Louisburg, U.S.A. 156 F2 38 37N 94 41W
Louise I., Canada 142 C2 52 55N 131 50W
Louiseville, Canada 140 C5 46 20N 72 56W
Louisiade Arch., Papua N. G. 132 F7 11 10 S 153 0 E
Louisiana, U.S.A. 156 E6 39 27N 91 3W
Louisiana □, U.S.A. 155 K9 30 50N 92 0W
Louisville, Ala., U.S.A. 152 D4 31 47N 85 33W
Louisville, Ga., U.S.A. 152 B7 33 0N 82 25W
Louisville, Ill., U.S.A. 157 F8 38 46N 88 30W
Louisville, Ky., U.S.A. 157 F11 38 15N 85 46W
Louisville, Miss., U.S.A. 155 J10 33 7N 89 3W
Louisville, Ohio, U.S.A. 150 F3 40 50N 81 16W
Loukoléla, Congo 114 C3 1 4 S 17 10 E
Loukouo, Congo 114 C2 3 38 S 14 39 E
Loulay, France 28 B3 46 3N 0 30W
Loulé, Portugal 43 H3 37 9N 8 0W
Louny, Czech Rep. 34 A6 50 20N 13 48 E
Loup City, U.S.A. 154 E5 41 17N 98 58W
Loups Marins, Lacs des, Canada 140 A5 56 30N 73 45W
Lourdes, France 28 E3 43 6N 0 3W
Lourenço, Brazil 169 C7 2 30N 51 40W
Lourenço Marques = Maputo, Mozam. 117 D5 25 58 S 32 32 E
Lourinhã, Portugal 43 F1 39 14N 9 17W
Loúros, Greece 39 A2 39 2N 20 47 E
Lousã, Portugal 42 E2 40 7N 8 14W
Louta, Burkina Faso 112 C4 13 30N 3 10W
Louth, Australia 129 A6 30 30 S 145 8 E
Louth, Ireland 23 C5 53 58N 6 32W
Louth, U.K. 20 D7 53 22N 0 1W
Louth □, Ireland 23 C5 53 56N 6 34W
Louth Bay, Australia 128 C1 34 33 S 135 56 E
Loutrá Aidhipsoú, Greece 48 C5 38 54N 23 2 E
Loutrá Killínis, Greece 39 D3 37 52N 21 7 E
Loutráki, Greece 48 D4 37 58N 22 57 E
Louvain = Leuven, Belgium 24 D4 50 52N 4 42 E
Louvale, U.S.A. 152 C5 32 10N 84 50W
Louviers, France 26 C8 49 12N 1 10 E
Louwsburg, S. Africa 117 D5 27 37 S 31 7 E
Lovat →, Russia 58 C6 58 14N 31 28 E
Lovćen, Serbia & M. 50 D2 42 23N 18 51 E
Lovćen △, Serbia & M. 50 D2 42 20N 18 50 E
Lovech, Bulgaria 51 C8 43 8N 24 42 E
Lovech □, Bulgaria 51 C8 43 15N 24 45 E
Loveland, Colo., U.S.A. 154 E2 40 24N 105 5W
Loveland, Ohio, U.S.A. 157 E12 39 16N 84 16W
Lovell, U.S.A. 158 D9 44 50N 108 24W
Lovelock, U.S.A. 158 F4 40 11N 118 28W
Lóvere, Italy 44 C7 45 49N 10 4 E
Loves Park, U.S.A. 156 B7 42 19N 89 3W
Lövestad, Sweden 17 J7 55 40N 13 54 E
Loviisa, Finland 15 F22 60 28N 26 12 E
Lovilia, U.S.A. 156 C4 41 8N 92 55W
Loving, U.S.A. 155 J2 32 17N 104 6W
Lovington, Ill., U.S.A. 157 E8 39 43N 88 38W
Lovington, N. Mex., U.S.A. 155 J3 32 57N 103 21W
Lovisa = Loviisa, Finland 15 F22 60 28N 26 12 E
Lovosice, Czech Rep. 34 A7 50 30N 14 2 E
Lovran, Croatia 45 C11 45 18N 14 15 E
Lovrin, Romania 52 E5 45 58N 20 48 E
Lövstabruk, Sweden 16 D11 60 25N 17 53 E
Lövstabukten, Sweden 16 D11 60 35N 17 45 E
Lóvua, Lunda Norte, Angola 115 D4 7 19 S 20 12 E
Lóvua, Moxico, Angola 115 E4 11 33 S 23 33 E
Lóvua →, Dem. Rep. of the Congo 115 D4 6 6 S 20 37 E
Low, L., Canada 140 B4 52 29N 76 17W
Low Pt., Australia 125 F4 32 25 S 127 25 E
Low Tatra = Nízké Tatry, Slovak Rep. 35 C12 48 55N 19 30 E
Lowa, Dem. Rep. of the Congo 118 C2 1 25 S 25 47 E
Lowa →, Dem. Rep. of the Congo 118 C2 1 24 S 25 51 E
Lowden, U.S.A. 156 C6 41 52N 90 56W
Lowell, Ind., U.S.A. 157 C9 41 18N 87 25W
Lowell, Mass., U.S.A. 151 D13 42 38N 71 19W
Lowell, Mich., U.S.A. 157 B11 42 56N 85 20W
Lowellville, U.S.A. 150 E4 41 2N 80 32W
Löwen = Lewin Brzeski, Poland 55 H4 50 45N 17 37 E
Löwen →, Namibia 116 D2 26 51 S 18 17 E
Löwenberg = Lwówek Śląski, Poland 55 G2 51 7N 15 38 E
Löwenstadt = Brzeziny, Poland 55 G6 51 49N 19 42 E
Lower Alkali L., U.S.A. 158 F3 41 16N 120 2W
Lower Arrow L., Canada 142 D5 49 40N 118 5W
Lower Austria = Niederösterreich □, Austria 34 C8 48 25N 15 40 E
Lower California = Baja California, Mexico 162 A1 31 10N 115 12W
Lower Glenelg △, Australia 128 E4 38 4 S 141 41 E
Lower Hutt, N.Z. 130 H3 41 10 S 174 55 E
Lower Kalskag, U.S.A. 144 F7 61 31N 160 22W
Lower Lake, U.S.A. 160 G4 38 55N 122 37W
Lower Manitou L., Canada 143 D10 49 15N 93 0W
Lower Paia, U.S.A. 145 C5 20 55N 156 23W
Lower Post, Canada 142 B3 59 58N 128 30W
Lower Red L., U.S.A. 154 B7 47 58N 95 0W
Lower Saxony = Niedersachsen □, Germany 30 C4 52 50N 9 0 E
Lower Tunguska = Tunguska, Nizhnyaya →, Russia 67 C9 65 48N 88 4 E
Lower Zambezi △, Zambia 119 F2 15 25 S 29 40 E
Lowestoft, U.K. 21 E9 52 29N 1 45 E
Lowgar □, Afghan. 91 B3 34 0N 69 0 E
Łowicz, Poland 55 F6 52 6N 19 55 E
Lowly, Pt., Australia 128 B2 33 0 S 137 46 E
Lowry City, U.S.A. 156 F3 38 8N 93 44W
Lowville, U.S.A. 151 C9 43 47N 75 29W
Loxton, Australia 128 C4 34 28 S 140 31 E
Loxton, S. Africa 116 E3 31 30 S 22 22 E
Loyalton, U.S.A. 160 F6 39 41N 120 14W
Loyalty Is. = Loyauté, Îs., N. Cal. 133 K4 20 50 S 166 30 E
Loyang = Luoyang, China 74 G7 34 40N 112 26 E
Loyauté, Îs., N. Cal. 133 K4 20 50 S 166 30 E
Loyev = Loyew, Belarus 59 G6 51 56N 30 46 E
Loyew, Belarus 59 G6 51 56N 30 46 E
Loyoro, Uganda 118 B3 3 22N 34 14 E
Lož, Slovenia 45 C11 45 43N 14 30 E
Lozère □, France 28 D7 44 35N 3 30 E
Loznica, Serbia & M. 50 B3 44 32N 19 12 E
Lozova, Ukraine 59 H9 49 0N 36 20 E
Lozva →, Russia 64 B9 59 36N 62 20 E
Lu, India 90 B5 26 58N 95 14 E
Lü Shan, China 77 C11 29 30N 115 55 E
Lü-Tao, Taiwan 77 F13 22 40N 121 30 E
Lu Verne, U.S.A. 156 B2 42 55N 94 5W
Lu Wo, China 69 F11 22 33N 114 6 E
Lua →, Dem. Rep. of the Congo 114 B3 2 46N 18 26 E
Lua Makiki, U.S.A. 145 C5 20 33N 156 37W
Luachimo, Angola 115 D4 7 23 S 20 48 E
Luacono, Angola 115 E4 11 15 S 21 37 E
Luajan →, India 93 G11 24 44N 85 1 E
Lualaba →, Dem. Rep. of the Congo 118 B2 0 26N 25 20 E
Luale, Dem. Rep. of the Congo 114 B4 1 9N 23 5 E
Luampa, Zambia 119 F1 15 4 S 24 20 E
Lu'an, China 77 B11 31 45N 116 29 E
Luan Chau, Vietnam 76 G4 21 38N 103 24 E
Luan He →, China 75 E10 39 20N 119 5 E
Luan Xian, China 75 E10 39 40N 118 40 E
Luancheng, Guangxi Zhuangzu, China 76 F7 22 48N 108 55 E
Luancheng, Hebei, China 74 F8 37 53N 114 40 E
Luanco, Spain 42 B5 43 37N 5 48W
Luanda, Angola 115 D2 8 50 S 13 15 E
Luando ⌂, Angola 115 E3 11 0 S 17 32 E
Luang, Thale, Thailand 87 J3 7 30N 100 15 E
Luang Prabang, Laos 76 H4 19 52N 102 10 E
Luanginga →, Zambia 115 F4 15 11 S 22 55 E
Luangwa, Zambia 119 F3 15 35 S 30 16 E
Luangwa →, Zambia 119 E3 14 25 S 30 25 E
Luangwa Valley, Zambia 119 E3 13 30 S 31 30 E
Luania-Bubi, Dem. Rep. of the Congo 115 D4 7 28 S 24 49 E
Luanne, China 75 D9 40 55N 117 40 E
Luanping, China 75 D9 40 53N 117 23 E
Luanshya, Zambia 119 E2 13 3 S 28 28 E
Luapula □, Zambia 119 E2 11 0 S 29 0 E
Luapula →, Africa 119 D2 9 26 S 28 33 E
Luarca, Spain 42 B4 43 32N 6 32W
Luashi, Dem. Rep. of the Congo 119 E1 10 50 S 23 36 E
Luatamba, Angola 115 E4 12 6 S 20 19 E
Luatira, Angola 115 E3 12 52 S 17 14 E
Luau, Angola 115 E4 10 40 S 22 10 E
Luba, Phil. 80 C3 17 19N 120 42 E
Lubaczów, Poland 55 H10 50 10N 23 8 E
Lubalo, Angola 115 D3 9 10 S 19 15 E
Lubamiti, Dem. Rep. of the Congo 114 C3 2 28 S 17 47 E
Lubań, Poland 55 G2 51 5N 15 15 E
Lubana, Ozero = Lubānas Ezers, Latvia 15 H22 56 45N 27 0 E
Lubānas Ezers, Latvia 15 H22 56 45N 27 0 E
Lubang, Phil. 80 E3 13 52N 120 7 E
Lubang Is., Phil. 80 E3 13 50N 120 12 E
Lubango, Angola 115 E2 14 55 S 13 30 E
Lubao, Dem. Rep. of the Congo 118 D2 5 17 S 25 42 E
Lubartów, Poland 55 G9 51 28N 22 42 E
Lubawa, Poland 54 E6 53 30N 19 48 E
Lübbecke, Germany 30 C4 52 18N 8 37 E
Lübben, Germany 30 D9 51 56N 13 54 E
Lübbenau, Germany 30 D9 51 52N 13 57 E
Lubbock, U.S.A. 155 J4 33 35N 101 51W
Lübeck, Germany 30 B6 53 52N 10 40 E
Lübecker Bucht, Germany 30 A6 54 3N 10 54 E
Lubefu, Dem. Rep. of the Congo 118 C1 4 47 S 24 27 E
Lubefu →, Dem. Rep. of the Congo 118 C1 4 10 S 23 0 E
Lubelskie □, Poland 55 G9 51 20N 22 50 E
Lüben = Lubin, Poland 55 G3 51 24N 16 11 E
Lubero = Luofu, Dem. Rep. of the Congo 118 C2 0 10 S 29 15 E
Luberon ⌂, France 29 E9 43 52N 5 25 E
Lubersac, France 28 C5 45 26N 1 23 E
Lubicon L., Canada 142 B5 56 23N 115 56W
Lubień Kujawski, Poland 55 F6 52 23N 19 9 E
Lubilash →, Dem. Rep. of the Congo 115 D4 6 2 S 23 45 E
Lubin, Poland 55 G3 51 24N 16 11 E
Lublin, Poland 55 G9 51 12N 22 38 E
Lubliniec, Poland 55 H5 50 43N 18 45 E
Lubnān = Lebanon ■, Asia 103 B5 34 0N 36 0 E
Lubnān, Jabal, Lebanon 103 B4 33 45N 35 40 E
Lubniewice, Poland 55 F2 52 31N 15 15 E
Lubny, Ukraine 59 G7 50 3N 32 58 E
Lubomierz, Poland 55 G2 51 1N 15 31 E
Luboń, Poland 55 F3 52 21N 16 51 E
Lubondaie, Dem. Rep. of the Congo 115 D4 8 1 S 26 32 E
Lubongola, Dem. Rep. of the Congo 118 C2 2 35 S 27 50 E
L'ubotín, Slovak Rep. 35 B13 49 17N 20 53 E
Lubraniec, Poland 55 F5 52 33N 18 50 E
Lubsko, Poland 55 G1 51 45N 14 57 E
Lübtheen, Germany 30 B7 53 18N 11 5 E
Lubuagan, Phil. 80 C3 17 21N 121 10 E
Lubudi, Dem. Rep. of the Congo 115 D4 6 51 S 21 18 E
Lubudi →, Kasai-Occ., Dem. Rep. of the Congo 115 C4 4 19 S 20 23 E
Lubudi →, Katanga, Dem. Rep. of the Congo 119 D2 9 0 S 25 35 E
Lubuklinggau, Indonesia 84 C2 3 15 S 102 55 E
Lubuksikaping, Indonesia 84 B2 0 10N 100 15 E
Lubumbashi, Dem. Rep. of the Congo 119 E2 11 40 S 27 28 E
Lubunda, Dem. Rep. of the Congo 118 D2 5 12 S 26 41 E
Lubungu, Zambia 119 E2 14 35 S 26 24 E
Lubuskie □, Poland 55 F2 52 10N 15 20 E
Lubutu, Dem. Rep. of the Congo 118 C2 0 45 S 26 30 E
Luc An Chau, Vietnam 86 A5 22 6N 104 43 E
Luc-en-Diois, France 29 D9 44 36N 5 28 E
Lucala, Angola 115 D3 9 7 S 15 58 E
Lucala →, Angola 115 D2 9 38 S 14 14 E
Lucan, Canada 150 C3 43 11N 81 24W
Lucania, Mt., Canada 138 B5 61 1N 140 27W
Lucapa, Angola 115 D4 8 25 S 20 45 E
Lucas, U.S.A. 156 C3 41 2N 93 29W
Lucas Channel, Canada 150 A3 45 21N 81 45W
Lucban, Phil. 80 D3 14 6N 121 33 E
Lucca, Italy 44 E7 43 50N 10 29 E
Lucé, France 26 D8 48 26N 1 27 E
Luce Bay, U.K. 22 G4 54 45N 4 48W
Lucea, Jamaica 164 a 18 27N 78 10W
Lucedale, U.S.A. 149 K1 30 56N 88 35W
Lucena, Phil. 80 E3 13 56N 121 37 E
Lucena, Spain 43 H6 37 27N 4 31W
Lučenec, Slovak Rep. 35 C12 48 18N 19 42 E
Lucens, Switz. 32 C3 46 43N 6 51 E
Lucera, Italy 47 A8 41 30N 15 20 E
Lucerne = Lake Worth, U.S.A. 153 J9 26 37N 80 3W
Lucerne = Luzern, Switz. 33 B6 47 3N 8 18 E
Lucerne, U.S.A. 160 F4 39 6N 122 48W
Lucerne Valley, U.S.A. 161 L10 34 27N 116 57W
Lucero, Mexico 162 A3 30 49N 106 30W
Luchena →, Spain 41 H3 37 44N 1 50W
Lucheng, China 74 F7 36 20N 113 11 E
Lucheringo →, Mozam. 119 E4 11 43 S 36 17 E
Luchow = Luzhou, China 76 C5 28 52N 105 20 E
Lüchow, Germany 30 C7 52 58N 11 8 E
Luchuan, China 77 F8 22 21N 110 12 E
Lucia, U.S.A. 160 J5 36 2N 121 33W
Lucie →, Suriname 169 C6 3 35N 57 38W
Lucinda, Australia 126 B4 18 32 S 146 20 E
Lucindale, Australia 128 D4 36 58 S 140 26 E
Lucira, Angola 115 E2 14 0 S 12 35 E
Luciras, B. das, Angola 115 E2 13 52 S 12 31 E
Luckau, Germany 30 D9 51 50N 13 42 E
Luckenwalde, Germany 30 C9 52 5N 13 10 E
Luckey, U.S.A. 157 C13 41 27N 83 29W
Luckhoff, S. Africa 116 D3 29 44 S 24 43 E
Lucknow, Canada 150 C3 43 57N 81 31W
Lucknow, India 93 F9 26 50N 81 0 E
Luçon, France 28 B2 46 28N 1 10W
Lucusse, Angola 115 E4 12 32 S 20 48 E
Lüda = Dalian, China 75 E11 38 50N 121 40 E
Luda Kamchiya →, Bulgaria 51 C11 43 3N 27 29 E
Ludbreg, Croatia 45 B13 46 15N 16 38 E
Lüdenscheid, Germany 30 D3 51 13N 7 37 E
Lüderitz, Namibia 116 D2 26 41 S 15 8 E
Lüderitzbaai, Namibia 116 D2 26 36 S 15 8 E
Ludhiana, India 92 D6 30 57N 75 56 E
Ludian, China 76 D4 27 10N 103 33 E
Luding Qiao, China 76 C4 29 53N 102 12 E
Lüdinghausen, Germany 30 D3 51 46N 7 27 E
Ludington, U.S.A. 148 D2 43 57N 86 27W
Ludlow, U.K. 21 E5 52 22N 2 42W
Ludlow, Calif., U.S.A. 161 L10 34 43N 116 10W
Ludlow, Pa., U.S.A. 150 E6 41 43N 78 56W
Ludlow, Vt., U.S.A. 151 C12 43 24N 72 42W
Ludowici, U.S.A. 152 D8 31 43N 81 45W
Ludus, Romania 53 D9 46 29N 24 5 E
Ludvika, Sweden 16 D9 60 8N 15 14 E
Ludwigsburg, Germany 31 G5 48 53N 9 11 E
Ludwigsfelde, Germany 30 C9 52 17N 13 17 E
Ludwigshafen, Germany 31 F4 49 29N 8 26 E
Ludwigslust, Germany 30 B7 53 19N 11 30 E
Ludza, Latvia 58 D4 56 32N 27 43 E
Lue, Australia 129 B8 32 38 S 149 50 E
Luebo, Dem. Rep. of the Congo 115 D4 5 21 S 21 23 E
Lueki, Dem. Rep. of the Congo 118 C2 3 20 S 25 48 E
Luena, Angola 115 E3 12 13 S 19 51 E
Luena, Dem. Rep. of the Congo 119 D2 9 28 S 25 43 E
Luena, Zambia 119 E3 10 40 S 30 25 E
Luena →, Angola 115 E4 12 30 S 22 34 E
Luena →, Zambia 115 E4 14 46 S 23 30 E
Luena Flats, Zambia 115 E4 14 47 S 23 17 E
Luengué ⌂, Angola 115 F3 16 55 S 19 55 E
Luenha = Ruenya →, Africa 119 F3 16 24 S 33 48 E
Luepa, Venezuela 169 B5 5 43N 61 31W
Lueta →, Dem. Rep. of the Congo 115 D4 7 4 S 21 40 E
Luete →, Zambia 115 F4 15 46 S 23 10 E
Lüeyang, China 74 H4 33 22N 106 10 E
Lufeng, Guangdong, China 77 F10 22 57N 115 38 E
Lufeng, Yunnan, China 76 E4 25 0N 102 5 E
Lufico, Angola 115 D2 6 24 S 13 23 E
Lufira →, Dem. Rep. of the Congo 119 D2 9 30 S 27 0 E
Lufkin, U.S.A. 155 K7 31 21N 94 44W
Lufupa, Dem. Rep. of the Congo 119 E1 10 37 S 24 56 E
Luga, Russia 58 C5 58 40N 29 55 E
Luga →, Russia 58 C5 59 40N 28 18 E
Lugano, Switz. 33 E7 46 1N 8 57 E
Lugano, L. di, Switz. 33 E8 46 0N 9 0 E
Lugansk = Luhansk, Ukraine 59 H10 48 38N 39 15 E
Luganville, Vanuatu 133 E5 15 27 S 167 10 E
Lugard's Falls, Kenya 118 C4 3 6 S 38 41 E
Lugela, Mozam. 119 F4 16 25 S 36 43 E
Lugenda →, Mozam. 119 E4 11 25 S 38 33 E
Lugh Ganana, Somali Rep. 120 D2 3 48N 42 34 E
Lugnaquilla, Ireland 23 D5 52 58N 6 28W
Lugo, Italy 45 D8 44 25N 11 54 E
Lugo, Spain 42 B3 43 2N 7 35W
Lugo □, Spain 42 C3 43 0N 7 30W
Lugoj, Romania 52 E6 45 42N 21 57 E
Lugovoy = Qulan, Kazakhstan 65 B6 42 55N 72 43 E
Lugus I., Phil. 81 J3 5 41N 120 50 E
Luhansk, Ukraine 59 H10 48 38N 39 15 E
Luhe, China 77 A12 32 19N 118 50 E
Luhe →, Germany 30 B6 53 23N 10 13 E
Luhit →, India 90 B5 27 48N 95 28 E
Luhuo, China 76 B3 31 21N 100 48 E
Lui →, Angola 115 D3 8 21 S 17 33 E
Lui →, Zambia 115 F4 16 18 S 23 17 E
Luia, Angola 115 D4 8 10 S 21 32 E
Luia →, Angola 115 D4 8 32 S 21 47 E
Luiana, Angola 116 B3 17 25 S 22 59 E
Luiana ⌂, Angola 115 F4 16 55 S 22 20 E
Luiana →, Angola 115 F4 17 24 S 23 3 E
Luichow = Liuzhou, China 76 E7 24 22N 109 22 E
Luichow Pen. = Leizhou Bandao, China 76 G7 21 0N 110 0 E
Luilaka →, Dem. Rep. of the Congo 114 C4 0 52 S 20 12 E
Luimneach = Limerick, Ireland 23 D3 52 40N 8 37W
Luing, U.K. 22 E3 56 14N 5 39W
Luino, Italy 44 C5 45 59N 8 44 E
Luio →, Angola 115 E4 13 17 S 21 37 E
Luís Correia, Brazil 170 B3 3 0 S 41 35W
Luís Gonçalves, Brazil 170 C1 5 37 S 50 25W
Luitpold Coast, Antarctica 7 D1 78 30 S 32 0W
Luiza, Dem. Rep. of the Congo 115 D4 7 40 S 22 30 E
Luizi, Dem. Rep. of the Congo 118 D2 6 0 S 27 25 E
Luján, Argentina 174 C4 34 45 S 59 5W
Lujiang, China 77 B11 31 20N 117 15 E
Lukala, Dem. Rep. of the Congo 115 D2 5 31 S 14 32 E
Lukang, Taiwan 77 E13 24 1N 120 22 E
Lukanga, Bandundu, Dem. Rep. of the Congo 114 C3 1 41 S 18 9 E
Lukanga, Équateur, Dem. Rep. of the Congo 114 C3 1 0 S 18 8 E
Lukanga Swamp, Zambia 119 E2 14 30 S 27 40 E
Lukavac, Bos.-H. 52 F3 44 33N 18 32 E
Lukenie →, Dem. Rep. of the Congo 114 C3 3 0 S 18 50 E
Lukhisaral, India 93 G12 25 11N 86 5 E
Lŭki, Bulgaria 51 E8 41 50N 24 43 E
Lukk, Libya 108 B4 32 1N 24 46 E
Lukolela, Équateur, Dem. Rep. of the Congo 114 C3 1 10 S 17 12 E

Lukolela, Kasai-Or., Dem. Rep. of the Congo 118 D1 5 23 S 24 32 E
Lukosi, Zimbabwe 119 F2 18 30 S 26 30 E
Lukovë, Albania 50 G3 39 59N 19 54 E
Lukovit, Bulgaria 51 C8 43 13N 24 11 E
Łuków, Poland 55 G9 51 55N 22 23 E
Lukoyanov, Russia 60 C7 55 2N 44 29 E
Luksefjell, Norway 18 E6 59 23N 9 34 E
Lukuni, Dem. Rep. of the Congo 115 D3 5 50 S 17 16 E
Lukusuzi △, Zambia 119 E3 12 43 S 32 36 E
Lula, Dem. Rep. of the Congo 115 D3 5 22 S 16 2 E
Luleå, Sweden 14 D20 65 35N 22 10 E
Luleälven →, Sweden 14 D19 65 35N 22 10 E
Lüleburgaz, Turkey 51 E11 41 23N 27 22 E
Luliang, China 76 E4 25 0N 103 40 E
Luling, U.S.A. 155 L6 29 41N 97 39W
Lulong, China 75 E10 39 53N 118 51 E
Lulonga →, Dem. Rep. of the Congo 114 B3 1 0N 18 10 E
Lulu, U.S.A. 152 E7 30 7N 82 29W
Lulu →, Dem. Rep. of the Congo 114 B4 1 18N 23 42 E
Lulua →, Dem. Rep. of the Congo 115 C4 4 30 S 20 30 E
Luluabourg = Kananga, Dem. Rep. of the Congo 115 D4 5 55 S 22 18 E
Luma, Amer. Samoa 133 X25 14 16 S 169 33W
Lumai, Angola 115 E4 13 13 S 21 25 E
Lumajang, Indonesia 85 D4 8 8 S 113 13 E
Lumaku, Gunong, Malaysia 85 B5 4 52N 115 38 E
Lumbala →, Angola 115 E4 12 39 S 22 35 E
Lumbala Kaquengue, Angola 115 E4 12 39 S 22 34 E
Lumbala N'guimbo, Angola 115 E4 14 18 S 21 18 E
Lumbe →, Zambia 115 F4 16 44 S 23 41 E
Lumber City, U.S.A. 152 D7 31 56N 82 41W
Lumberton, U.S.A. 149 H6 34 37N 79 0W
Lumding, India 90 C4 25 46N 93 10 E
Lumi, Papua N. G. 132 B2 3 30 S 142 2 E
Lumpkin, U.S.A. 152 C5 32 3N 84 48W
Lumsden, Canada 143 C8 50 39N 104 52W
Lumsden, N.Z. 131 F3 45 44 S 168 27 E
Lumut, Malaysia 87 K3 4 13N 100 37 E
Lumut, Tanjung, Indonesia 84 C3 3 50 S 105 58 E
Luna, India 92 H3 23 43N 69 16 E
Luna, Phil. 80 B3 18 18N 121 21 E
Lunan, China 76 E4 24 40N 103 18 E
Lunavada, India 92 H5 23 8N 73 37 E
Lunca, Romania 53 C10 47 22N 25 1 E
Lunca Corbului, Romania 53 F9 44 42N 24 45 E
Lund, Sweden 17 J7 55 44N 13 12 E
Lunda Norte □, Angola 115 D3 8 0 S 20 0 E
Lunda Sul □, Angola 115 D4 10 0 S 20 0 E
Lundamo, Norway 18 A7 63 9N 10 19 E
Lundazi, Zambia 119 E3 12 20 S 33 7 E
Lundenburg = Břeclav, Czech Rep. 35 C9 48 46N 16 53 E
Lunderskov, Denmark 17 J3 55 29N 9 19 E
Lundi →, Zimbabwe 119 G3 21 43 S 32 34 E
Lundu, Malaysia 85 B3 1 40N 109 50 E
Lundy, U.K. 21 F3 51 10N 4 41W
Lune →, U.K. 20 C5 54 0N 2 51W
Lüneburg, Germany 30 B6 53 15N 10 24 E
Lüneburg Heath = Lüneburger Heide, Germany 30 B6 53 10N 10 12 E
Lüneburger Heide, Germany 30 B6 53 10N 10 12 E
Lunel, France 29 E8 43 39N 4 9 E
Lünen, Germany 30 D3 51 37N 7 32 E
Lunenburg, Canada 141 D7 44 22N 64 18W
Lunéville, France 27 D13 48 36N 6 30 E
Lunga, Dem. Rep. of the Congo 115 C4 5 46 S 12 14 E
Lunga →, Zambia 119 E2 14 34 S 26 25 E
Lunge, Angola 115 E3 12 13 S 16 7 E
Lungern, Switz. 32 C6 46 48N 8 10 E
Lungga, Solomon Is. 133 M11 9 25 S 160 3 E
Lungi Airport, S. Leone 112 D2 8 40N 13 17W
Lunglei, India 90 D4 22 55N 92 45 E
Lungngo, Burma 90 E4 21 57N 93 36 E
Lungwebungu →, Zambia 115 E4 14 19 S 23 14 E
Luni, India 92 G5 26 0N 73 6 E
Luni →, India 92 G4 24 41N 71 14 E
Luninets = Luninyets, Belarus 59 F4 52 15N 26 50 E
Luning, U.S.A. 158 G4 38 30N 118 11W
Lunino, Russia 60 D7 53 38N 45 18 E
Luninyets, Belarus 59 F4 52 15N 26 50 E
Lunkaransar, India 92 E5 28 29N 73 44 E
Lunner, Norway 18 D7 60 19N 10 35 E
Lunsemfwa →, Zambia 119 E3 14 54 S 30 12 E
Lunsemfwa Falls, Zambia 119 E2 14 30 S 29 6 E
Luo He →, China 74 G6 34 35N 110 20 E
Luocheng, China 76 E7 24 48N 108 53 E
Luochuan, China 74 G5 35 45N 109 26 E
Luoci, China 76 E4 25 19N 102 18 E
Luodian, China 76 E6 25 24N 106 43 E
Luoding, China 77 F8 22 45N 111 40 E
Luofu, Dem. Rep. of the Congo 118 C2 0 10 S 29 15 E
Luohe, China 74 H8 33 32N 114 2 E
Luojiang, China 76 B5 31 18N 104 33 E
Luonan, China 74 G6 34 5N 110 10 E
Luoning, China 74 G6 34 35N 111 40 E
Luoshan, China 77 A10 32 13N 114 30 E
Luotian, China 77 B10 30 46N 115 22 E
Luoxiao Shan, China 77 D10 26 30N 114 1 E
Luoyang, China 74 G7 34 40N 112 26 E
Luoyuan, China 77 D12 26 28N 119 30 E
Luozi, Dem. Rep. of the Congo 115 C2 4 54 S 14 0 E
Luozigou, China 75 C16 43 42N 130 18 E
Lupanshui, China 76 D5 26 38N 104 48 E
Lupeni, Romania 53 E8 45 21N 23 13 E
Lupilichi, Mozam. 119 E4 11 47 S 35 13 E
Lupire, Angola 115 E3 14 36 S 19 29 E
Łupków, Poland 55 J9 49 15N 22 4 E
Lupoing, China 76 E5 24 53N 104 21 E
Lupon, Phil. 81 H6 6 54N 126 0 E
Luputa, Dem. Rep. of the Congo 115 D4 7 7 S 23 43 E
Luqa, Malta 38 F7 35 52N 14 29 E
Luquan, China 76 E4 25 35N 102 25 E
Luque, Paraguay 174 B4 25 19 S 57 25W
Luquembo, Angola 115 E3 10 44 S 17 43 E
Lūras, Italy 46 B2 40 56N 9 10 E
Luray, U.S.A. 148 F6 38 40N 78 28W
Lure, France 27 E13 47 40N 6 30 E
Luremo, Angola 115 D3 8 30 S 17 50 E
Lurgan, U.K. 23 B5 54 28N 6 19W
Luribay, Bolivia 172 D4 17 6 S 67 39W
Lurin, Peru 172 C2 12 17 S 76 52W
Lusaka, Zambia 119 F2 15 28 S 28 16 E
Lusaka □, Zambia 119 F2 15 30 S 29 0 E
Lusambo, Dem. Rep. of the Congo 118 C1 4 58 S 23 28 E
Lusancay Is. and Reefs, Papua N. G. 132 E6 8 30 S 150 30 E
Lusangaye, Dem. Rep. of the Congo 118 C2 4 54 S 26 0 E
Luseland, Canada 143 C7 52 5N 109 24W
Lusenga Plain △, Zambia 119 D2 9 22 S 29 14 E
Lusengo, Dem. Rep. of the Congo 114 B3 1 47N 19 31 E
Lushan, Henan, China 74 H7 33 45N 112 55 E
Lushan, Sichuan, China 76 B4 30 12N 102 52 E
Lushi, China 74 G6 34 3N 111 3 E
Lushnjë, Albania 50 F3 40 55N 19 41 E
Lushoto, Tanzania 118 C4 4 47 S 38 20 E
Lushui, China 76 E2 25 58N 98 44 E
Lüshun, China 75 E11 38 45N 121 15 E
Lusignan, France 28 B4 46 26N 0 8 E
Lusigny-sur-Barse, France 27 D11 48 16N 4 15 E
Lusiye, Zambia 115 F4 15 30 S 23 57 E
Lusk, U.S.A. 154 D2 42 46N 104 27W
Lussac-les-Châteaux, France 28 B4 46 24N 0 43 E
Lustenau, Austria 34 D2 47 26N 9 39 E
Lustrafjorden, Norway 18 C4 61 23N 7 25 E
Lūt, Dasht-e, Iran 97 D8 31 30N 58 0 E
Luta = Dalian, China 75 E11 38 50N 121 40 E
Lutembo, Angola 115 E4 13 26 S 21 16 E
Lutherstadt Wittenberg, Germany 30 D8 51 53N 12 39 E
Luthersville, U.S.A. 152 B5 33 13N 84 45W
Luti, Solomon Is. 133 L9 7 14 S 157 0 E
Luton, U.K. 21 F7 51 53N 0 24W
Luton □, U.K. 21 F7 51 53N 0 24W
Lutong, Malaysia 85 B4 4 28N 114 0 E
Lutry, Switz. 32 C3 46 31N 6 42 E
Łutselk'e, Canada 143 A6 62 24N 110 44W
Lutshima →, Dem. Rep. of the Congo 115 D3 5 22 S 18 59 E
Lutsk, Ukraine 59 G3 50 50N 25 15 E
Luttenberg = Ljutomer, Slovenia 45 B13 46 31N 16 11 E
Lutuai, Angola 115 E4 12 41 S 20 7 E
Lutz, U.S.A. 153 G7 28 9N 82 28W
Lützow Holmbukta, Antarctica 7 C4 69 10 S 37 30 E
Lutzputs, S. Africa 116 D3 28 3 S 20 40 E
Luuk, Phil. 81 J3 5 58N 121 18 E
Luuq = Lugh Ganana, Somali Rep. 120 D2 3 48N 42 34 E
Luverne, Ala., U.S.A. 152 D3 31 43N 86 16W
Luverne, Minn., U.S.A. 154 D6 43 39N 96 13W
Luvo, Angola 115 D2 5 51 S 14 5 E
Lúvua, Angola 115 E4 8 49 S 25 19 E
Luvua, Dem. Rep. of the Congo 119 D2 8 48 S 25 17 E
Luvua →, Dem. Rep. of the Congo 118 D2 6 50 S 27 30 E
Luvuvhu →, S. Africa 117 C5 22 25 S 31 18 E
Luwegu →, Tanzania 119 D4 8 31 S 37 23 E
Luwuk, Indonesia 82 B2 0 56 S 122 47 E
Luxembourg, Lux. 24 E6 49 37N 6 9 E
Luxembourg □, Belgium 24 E5 49 58N 5 30 E
Luxembourg ■, Europe 25 B7 49 45N 6 0 E
Luxembourg ✕ (LUX), Lux. 24 E6 49 37N 6 10 E
Luxemburg, U.S.A. 156 B5 42 36N 91 5W
Luxeuil-les-Bains, France 27 E13 47 49N 6 24 E
Luxi, Hunan, China 77 C8 28 20N 110 7 E
Luxi, Yunnan, China 76 E4 24 40N 103 55 E
Luxi, Yunnan, China 76 E2 24 27N 98 36 E
Luxor = El Uqsur, Egypt 106 B3 25 41N 32 38 E
Luy-de-Béarn →, France 28 E3 43 39N 0 48W
Luy-de-France →, France 28 E3 43 39N 0 48W
Luyi, China 74 H8 33 50N 115 35 E
Luz, Azores 9 d1 39 1N 28 0W
Luz-St-Sauveur, France 28 F4 42 53N 0 0W
Luza, Russia 56 B8 60 39N 47 10 E
Luzern, Switz. 33 B6 47 3N 8 18 E
Luzern □, Switz. 32 B5 47 2N 7 55 E
Luzhai, China 76 E7 24 29N 109 42 E
Luzhany, Ukraine 53 B10 48 22N 25 47 E
Luzhi, China 76 D5 26 21N 105 16 E
Luzhou, China 76 C5 28 52N 105 20 E
Luziânia, Brazil 171 E2 16 20 S 48 0W
Luzilândia, Brazil 170 B3 3 28 S 42 22W
Lužnice →, Czech Rep. 34 B7 49 14N 14 23 E
Luzon, Phil. 80 C3 16 0N 121 0 E
Luzon Strait, Asia 77 G13 21 0N 120 40 E
Luzy, France 27 F10 46 47N 3 58 E
Luzzi, Italy 47 C9 39 27N 16 17 E
Lviv, Ukraine 59 H3 49 50N 24 0 E
Lvov = Lviv, Ukraine 59 H3 49 50N 24 0 E
Lwówek, Poland 55 F3 52 28N 16 10 E
Lwówek Śląski, Poland 55 G2 51 7N 15 38 E
Lyakhavichy, Belarus 59 F4 53 2N 26 32 E
Lyakhovskiye, Ostrova, Russia 67 B15 73 40N 141 0 E
Lyaki = Läki, Azerbaijan 61 K8 40 34N 47 22 E
Lyal I., Canada 150 B3 44 57N 81 24W
Lyall Mt., N.Z. 131 F2 45 16 S 167 32 E
Lyallpur = Faisalabad, Pakistan 91 C4 31 30N 73 5 E
Lyalya →, Russia 64 B8 59 9N 61 29 E
Lyangar, Tajikistan 65 E6 37 3N 72 40 E
Lyaskovets, Bulgaria 51 C9 43 6N 25 44 E
Lyasnaya, Belarus 55 F10 52 9N 23 31 E
Lybster, U.K. 22 C5 58 18N 3 15W
Lycaonia, Turkey 100 D5 38 0N 33 0 E
Lychen, Germany 30 B9 53 12N 13 18 E
Lychkova, Russia 58 D7 57 55N 32 24 E
Lycia, Turkey 49 E11 36 30N 29 30 E
Lyck = Ełk, Poland 54 E9 53 50N 22 21 E
Lyckebyån →, Sweden 17 H9 56 12N 15 39 E
Lycksele, Sweden 14 D18 64 38N 18 40 E
Lycosura, Greece 48 D4 37 20N 22 3 E
Lydda = Lod, Israel 103 D3 31 57N 34 54 E
Lydenburg, S. Africa 117 D5 25 10 S 30 29 E
Lydia, Turkey 49 C10 38 48N 28 19 E
Łydynia →, Poland 55 F7 52 43N 20 26 E
Lyell, N.Z. 131 B7 41 48 S 172 4 E
Lyell I., Canada 142 C2 52 40N 131 35W
Lyepyel, Belarus 58 E5 54 50N 28 40 E
Lyford Cay, Bahamas 9 b 25 2N 77 33W
Lygnern, Sweden 17 G6 57 30N 12 15 E
Lykens, U.S.A. 151 F8 40 34N 76 42W
Lyman, Ukraine 53 E14 45 41N 29 45 E
Lyman, Iowa, U.S.A. 156 C2 30 29N 94 59W
Lyman, Wyo., U.S.A. 158 F8 41 20N 110 18W
Lymanske, Ukraine 53 D14 46 40N 29 58 E
Lyme B., U.K. 21 G4 50 42N 2 53W
Lyme Regis, U.K. 21 G5 50 43N 2 57W
Lymington, U.K. 21 G6 50 45N 1 32W
Łyna →, Poland 15 J19 54 37N 21 14 E
Lynchburg, Ohio, U.S.A. 157 E13 39 15N 83 48W
Lynchburg, S.C., U.S.A. 152 A9 34 3N 80 4W
Lynchburg, Va., U.S.A. 148 G6 37 25N 79 9W
Lynd →, Australia 126 B3 16 28 S 143 18 E
Lynd Ra., Australia 127 D4 25 30 S 149 20 E
Lynden, Canada 150 C4 43 14N 80 9W
Lynden, U.S.A. 160 B4 48 57N 122 27W
Lyndhurst, Australia 127 E2 30 15 S 138 18 E
Lyndon →, Australia 125 D1 23 29 S 114 6 E
Lyndonville, N.Y., U.S.A. 150 C6 43 20N 78 23W
Lyndonville, Vt., U.S.A. 151 B12 44 31N 72 1W
Lyngdal, Buskerud, Norway 18 E6 59 54N 9 32 E
Lyngdal, Vest-Agder, Norway 18 F4 58 8N 7 7 E
Lyngen, Norway 14 B19 69 45N 20 30 E
Lyngør, Norway 18 F6 58 38N 9 8 E
Lynher Reef, Australia 124 C3 15 27 S 121 55 E
Lynn, Ind., U.S.A. 157 D12 40 3N 84 56W
Lynn, Mass., U.S.A. 151 D14 42 28N 70 57W
Lynn Canal, U.S.A. 144 G14 58 50N 135 15W
Lynn Haven, U.S.A. 152 E4 30 15N 85 39W
Lynn Lake, Canada 143 B8 56 51N 101 3W
Lynne, U.S.A. 153 F8 29 12N 81 55W
Lynnville, U.S.A. 157 F9 38 12N 87 19W
Lynnwood, U.S.A. 160 C4 47 49N 122 19W
Lynton, U.K. 21 F4 51 13N 3 50W
Lyntupy, Belarus 15 J22 55 4N 26 23 E
Lynx L., Canada 143 A7 62 25N 106 15W
Lyon, France 29 C8 45 46N 4 50 E
Lyon St-Exupery ✕ (LYS), France 29 C9 45 44N 5 2 E
Lyonnais, France 29 C8 45 45N 4 15 E
Lyons = Lyon, France 29 C8 45 46N 4 50 E
Lyons, Ga., U.S.A. 152 C7 32 12N 82 19W
Lyons, Kans., U.S.A. 154 F5 38 21N 98 12W
Lyons, N.Y., U.S.A. 150 C8 43 5N 77 0W
Lyons →, Australia 125 E2 25 2 S 115 9 E
Lyons Falls, U.S.A. 151 C9 43 37N 75 22W
Lyozna, Belarus 58 E6 55 0N 30 50 E
Lyra Reef, Papua N. G. 132 A7 1 50 S 153 35 E
Lys = Leie →, Belgium 24 C3 51 2N 3 45 E
Lysá nad Labem, Czech Rep. 34 A7 50 11N 14 51 E
Lysebotn, Norway 18 E3 59 3N 6 37 E
Lysefjorden, Norway 18 E3 59 0N 6 23 E
Lysekil, Sweden 17 F5 58 17N 11 26 E
Lyskovo, Russia 60 B7 56 0N 45 3 E
Lyss, Switz. 32 B4 47 4N 7 19 E
Lystrup, Denmark 17 H4 56 14N 10 14 E
Lysva, Russia 64 B6 58 7N 57 49 E
Lysvik, Sweden 16 D7 60 1N 13 9 E
Lysychansk, Ukraine 59 H10 48 55N 38 30 E
Lytham St. Anne's, U.K. 20 D4 53 45N 3 0W
Lyttelton, N.Z. 131 D7 43 35 S 172 44 E
Lytton, Canada 142 C4 50 13N 121 31W
Lyuban, Russia 58 C6 59 16N 31 18 E
Lyubertsy, Russia 58 E9 55 39N 37 50 E
Lyubim, Russia 58 C11 58 20N 40 39 E
Lyubimets, Bulgaria 51 E10 41 50N 26 5 E
Lyuboml, Ukraine 55 G11 51 11N 24 4 E
Lyubotyn, Ukraine 59 H8 50 0N 36 0 E
Lyubytino, Russia 58 C7 58 50N 33 16 E
Lyudinovo, Russia 58 F8 53 52N 34 28 E

M

M.R. Gomez, Presa, Mexico 163 B5 26 10N 99 0W
M.R. Stefanik, Bratislava ✕ (BTS), Slovak Rep. 35 C10 48 11N 17 9 E
Ma →, Vietnam 76 H5 19 47N 105 56 E
Ma, O. el →, Algeria 110 C3 27 45N 7 52W
Ma'adaba, Jordan 103 E4 30 43N 35 47 E
Maamba, Zambia 116 B4 17 17 S 26 28 E
Ma'ān, Jordan 103 E4 30 12N 35 44 E
Ma'ān □, Jordan 103 F5 30 0N 36 0 E
Maana'oba, Solomon Is. 133 M11 8 17 S 160 50 E
Maanselkä, Finland 14 C23 63 52N 28 32 E
Ma'anshan, China 77 B12 31 44N 118 29 E
Maarianhamina, Finland 15 F18 60 5N 19 55 E
Maarmorilik, Greenland 10 C5 71 3N 51 0W
Ma'arrat an Nu'mān, Syria 100 E7 35 43N 36 43 E
Maas →, Neths. 24 C4 51 45N 4 32 E
Maaseik, Belgium 24 C5 51 6N 5 45 E
Maasim, Phil. 81 J5 5 52N 125 0 E
Maasin, Phil. 79 B6 10 8N 124 50 E
Maastricht, Neths. 24 D5 50 50N 5 40 E
Maasupa, Solomon Is. 133 M11 9 16 S 161 17 E
Maave, Mozam. 117 C5 21 4 S 34 47 E
Mababe Depression, Botswana 116 B3 18 50 S 24 15 E
Mabaia, Angola 115 D2 7 12 S 14 2 E
Mabalane, Mozam. 117 C5 23 37 S 32 31 E
Mabanga, Dem. Rep. of the Congo 114 B3 1 30N 19 6 E
Ma'bar, Yemen 98 D4 14 48N 44 17 E
Mabaruma, Guyana 169 B6 8 10N 59 50W
Mabein, Burma 90 D6 23 29N 96 37 E
Mabel L., Canada 142 C5 50 35N 118 43W
Mabenga, Dem. Rep. of the Congo 114 C3 3 39 S 18 40 E
Mabenge, Dem. Rep. of the Congo 118 B1 4 15N 24 12 E
Maberly, Canada 151 B8 44 50N 76 32W
Mabian, China 76 C4 28 47N 103 37 E
Mabil, Ethiopia 107 E4 10 26N 36 52 E
Mabinay, Phil. 81 G4 9 48N 122 54 E
Mabirou, Congo 114 C3 1 3 S 15 42 E
Mablethorpe, U.K. 20 D8 53 20N 0 15 E
Mableton, U.S.A. 152 B5 33 49N 84 35W
Mably, France 27 F11 46 5N 4 4 E
Maboma, Dem. Rep. of the Congo 118 B2 2 30N 28 10 E
Mabonto, S. Leone 112 D2 8 53N 11 50W
Maboukou, Congo 114 C2 3 39 S 12 31 E
Mabrouk, Mali 113 B4 19 29N 1 15W
Mabrous, Niger 109 D2 21 14N 13 35 E
Mabuasehube ⌓, Botswana 116 D3 25 5 S 21 10 E
Mabungo, Somali Rep. 120 D2 0 49N 42 35 E
Mac Bac, Vietnam 87 H6 9 46N 106 7 E
Macachín, Argentina 174 D3 37 10 S 63 43W
Macaé, Brazil 171 F3 22 20 S 41 43W
Macael, Spain 41 H2 37 20N 2 18W
Macaíba, Brazil 170 C4 5 51 S 35 21W
Macajuba, Brazil 171 D3 12 9 S 40 22W
McAlester, U.S.A. 155 H7 34 56N 95 46W
McAllen, U.S.A. 155 M5 26 12N 98 14W
McAlpin, U.S.A. 152 E7 30 8N 82 57W
MacAlpine L., Canada 138 B9 66 32N 102 45W
Macamic, Canada 140 C4 48 45N 79 0W
Macao = Macau, China 77 F9 22 12N 113 33 E
Macão, Portugal 43 F3 39 35N 7 59W
Macapá, Brazil 169 C7 0 5N 51 4W
Macará, Ecuador 168 D2 4 23 S 79 57W
Macarani, Brazil 171 E3 15 33 S 40 24W
Macarao △, Venezuela 165 D6 10 22N 67 7W
Macarena, Serranía de la, Colombia 168 C3 2 45N 73 55W
Macareo, Caño →, Venezuela 169 B5 9 47N 61 36W
Macarthur, Australia 128 E5 38 5 S 142 0 E
McArthur →, Australia 126 B2 15 54 S 136 40 E
McArthur, Port, Australia 126 B2 16 4 S 136 23 E
Macas, Ecuador 168 D2 2 19 S 78 7W
Macate, Peru 172 B2 8 48 S 78 7W
Macau, Brazil 170 C4 5 15 S 36 40W
Macau, China 77 F9 22 12N 113 33 E
Macaúbas, Brazil 171 D3 13 2 S 42 42W
Macaya →, Colombia 168 C3 0 59N 72 20W
McBride, Canada 142 C4 53 20N 120 19W
McCall, U.S.A. 158 D5 44 55N 116 6W
McCamey, U.S.A. 155 K3 31 8N 102 14W
McCammon, U.S.A. 158 E7 42 39N 112 12W
McCarthy, U.S.A. 144 F12 61 26N 142 56W
McCauley I., Canada 142 C2 53 40N 130 15W
McCleary, U.S.A. 160 C3 47 3N 123 16W
Macclenny, U.S.A. 152 E7 30 17N 82 7W
Macclesfield, U.K. 20 D5 53 15N 2 8W
M'Clintock Chan., Canada 138 A9 72 0N 102 0W
McClintock Ra., Australia 124 C4 18 44 S 127 38 E
McCloud, U.S.A. 158 F2 41 15N 122 8W
McCluer I., Australia 124 B5 11 5 S 133 0 E
McClure, U.S.A. 150 F7 40 42N 77 19W
McClure, L., U.S.A. 160 H6 37 35N 120 16W
M'Clure Str., Canada 6 B2 75 0N 119 0W
McClusky, U.S.A. 154 B4 47 29N 100 27W
McComb, U.S.A. 155 K9 31 15N 90 27W
McCook, U.S.A. 154 E4 40 12N 100 38W
McCormick, U.S.A. 152 B7 33 55N 82 17W
McCreary, Canada 143 C9 50 47N 99 29W
McCullough Mt., U.S.A. 161 K11 35 35N 115 13W
McCusker →, Canada 143 B7 55 32N 108 39W
McDame, Canada 142 B3 59 44N 128 59W
McDavid, U.S.A. 153 E2 30 52N 87 19W
McDermitt, U.S.A. 158 F5 41 59N 117 43W
McDonald, U.S.A. 150 F4 40 22N 80 14W
Macdonald, L., Australia 124 D4 23 30 S 129 0 E
Macdonald, Mt., Vanuatu 133 G6 17 36 S 168 23 E
McDonald Is., Ind. Oc. 121 K6 53 0 S 73 0 E
MacDonnell Ranges, Australia 124 D5 23 40 S 133 0 E
McDonough, U.S.A. 152 B5 33 27N 84 9W
McDougalls Well, Australia 128 A4 31 8 S 141 15 E
McDowell L., Canada 140 B1 52 15N 92 45W
Macduff, U.K. 22 D6 57 40N 2 31W
Maceda, Spain 42 C3 42 16N 7 39W
Macedonia, U.S.A. 150 E3 41 19N 81 31W
Macedonia ■, Europe 50 E5 41 53N 21 40 E
Maceió, Brazil 170 C4 9 40 S 35 41W
Maceira, Portugal 42 F2 39 41N 8 55W
Macenta, Guinea 112 D3 8 35N 9 32W
Macerata, Italy 45 E10 43 18N 13 27 E
McFarland, U.S.A. 161 K7 35 41N 119 14W
McFarlane →, Canada 143 B7 59 12N 107 58W
Macfarlane, L., Australia 128 B2 32 0 S 136 40 E
McGehee, U.S.A. 155 J9 33 38N 91 24W
McGill, U.S.A. 158 G6 39 23N 114 47W
Macgillycuddy's Reeks, Ireland 23 E2 51 58N 9 45W
McGrath, U.S.A. 144 E9 62 58N 155 36W
McGraw, U.S.A. 151 D8 42 36N 76 8W
McGregor, U.S.A. 156 A5 43 1N 91 11W
McGregor Ra., Australia 127 D3 27 0 S 142 45 E
McGuire, Mt, Australia 126 J6 20 18 S 148 23 E
Mâch Kowr, Iran 97 E9 25 48N 61 28 E
Machacalis, Brazil 171 E3 17 5 S 40 45W
Machado = Jiparaná →, Brazil 173 B5 8 3 S 62 52W
Machagai, Argentina 174 B3 26 56 S 60 2W
Machakos, Kenya 118 C4 1 30 S 37 15 E
Machala, Ecuador 168 D2 3 20 S 79 57W
Machalilla △, Ecuador 168 D1 1 24 S 80 42W
Machanga, Mozam. 117 C6 20 59 S 35 0 E
Machattie, L., Australia 126 C2 24 50 S 139 48 E
Machault, France 27 C11 49 21N 4 29 E
Machava, Mozam. 117 D5 25 54 S 32 28 E
Machece, Mozam. 119 F4 19 15 S 35 32 E
Machecoul, France 26 F5 47 0N 1 49W
Macheke, Zimbabwe 117 B5 18 5 S 31 51 E
Macheng, China 77 B10 31 12N 115 2 E
McHenry, U.S.A. 157 B8 42 21N 88 16W
Macherla, India 94 F4 16 29N 79 26 E
Machero, Spain 43 F6 39 21N 4 20W
Machgaon, India 94 D8 20 5N 86 17 E
Machhu →, India 92 H4 23 6N 70 46 E
Machiara △, Pakistan 92 B5 34 40N 73 30 E
Machias, Maine, U.S.A. 149 C12 44 43N 67 28W
Machias, N.Y., U.S.A. 150 D6 42 25N 78 30W
Machichi →, Canada 143 B10 57 3N 92 6W
Machico, Madeira 9 c 32 43N 16 44W
Machida, Japan 73 B11 35 28N 139 23 E
Machilipatnam, India 95 F5 16 12N 81 8 E
Machiques, Venezuela 168 A3 10 4N 72 34W
Machupicchu, Peru 172 C3 13 8 S 72 30W
Machynlleth, U.K. 21 E4 52 35N 3 50W
Macia, Mozam. 117 D5 25 2 S 33 8 E
Macias Nguema = Biyoga = Bioko, Eq. Guin. 113 E6 3 30N 8 40 E
Maciejowice, Poland 55 G8 51 36N 21 26 E
McIlwraith Ra., Australia 126 A3 13 50 S 143 20 E
Măcin, Romania 53 E13 45 16N 28 8 E
Macina, Mali 112 C4 14 50N 5 0W
McInnes L., Canada 143 C10 52 13N 93 45W
McIntosh, U.S.A. 154 C4 45 55N 101 21W
McIntosh L., Canada 143 B8 55 45N 105 0W
Macintosh Ra., Australia 125 E4 27 39 S 125 32 E
Macintyre →, Australia 127 D5 28 37 S 150 47 E
Macizo Galaico, Spain 42 C3 42 30N 7 30W
Mackay, Australia 126 K7 21 8 S 149 11 E
Mackay, U.S.A. 158 E7 43 55N 113 37W
MacKay →, Canada 142 B6 57 10N 111 38W
Mackay, L., Australia 124 D4 22 30 S 129 0 E
McKay Ra., Australia 124 D3 23 0 S 122 30 E
McKeesport, U.S.A. 150 F5 40 21N 79 52W
McKellar, Canada 150 A5 45 30N 79 55W
McKenna, U.S.A. 160 D4 46 56N 122 33W
Mackenzie, Canada 142 B4 55 20N 123 5W
McKenzie, U.S.A. 149 G1 36 8N 88 31W
Mackenzie →, Australia 126 C4 23 38 S 149 46 E
Mackenzie →, Canada 138 B6 69 10N 134 20W
McKenzie →, U.S.A. 158 D2 44 7N 123 6W
Mackenzie Bay, Canada 6 B1 69 0N 137 30W
Mackenzie City = Linden, Guyana 169 B6 6 0N 58 10W
Mackenzie Mts., Canada 138 B6 64 0N 130 0W
Mackenzie Plains, N.Z. 131 E5 44 10 S 170 25 E
McKerrow, L., N.Z. 131 E3 44 25 S 168 5 E
Mackheim = Maków Mazowiecki, Poland 55 F8 52 52N 21 6 E
Mackinaw, U.S.A. 156 D7 40 32N 89 21W
Mackinaw →, U.S.A. 156 D7 40 33N 89 44W
Mackinaw City, U.S.A. 148 C3 45 47N 84 44W
McKinlay, Australia 126 C3 21 16 S 141 18 E
McKinlay →, Australia 126 C3 20 50 S 141 28 E
McKinley, Mt., U.S.A. 144 E10 63 4N 151 0W
McKinley Park, U.S.A. 144 E10 63 44N 148 55W
McKinley Sea, Arctic 6 A7 82 0N 0 0W
McKinleyville, U.S.A. 158 F1 40 57N 124 6W
McKinney, U.S.A. 155 J6 33 12N 96 37W
Mackinnon Road, Kenya 118 C4 3 40 S 39 1 E
McKittrick, Calif., U.S.A. 161 K7 35 18N 119 37W
McKittrick, Mo., U.S.A. 156 F5 38 44N 91 27W
Macklin, Canada 143 C7 52 20N 109 56W
Macksville, Australia 129 A10 30 40 S 152 56 E
McLaren Vale, Australia 128 C3 35 13 S 138 31 E
McLaughlin, U.S.A. 154 C4 45 49N 100 49W
Maclean, Australia 127 D5 29 26 S 153 16 E
McLean, Ill., U.S.A. 156 D7 40 19N 89 10W
McLean, Tex., U.S.A. 155 H4 35 14N 100 36W
McLeansboro, U.S.A. 154 F10 38 6N 88 32W
Maclear, S. Africa 117 E4 31 2 S 28 23 E
Maclear, C., Malawi 119 E3 13 58 S 34 49 E
Macleay →, Australia 129 A10 30 56 S 153 0 E
McLennan, Canada 142 B5 55 42N 116 50W
MacLeod = Fort Macleod, Canada 142 D6 49 45N 113 30W
McLeod →, Canada 142 C5 54 9N 115 44W
MacLeod, B., Canada 143 A7 62 53N 110 0W
McLeod, L., Australia 125 D1 24 9 S 113 47 E
MacLeod Lake, Canada 142 C4 54 58N 123 0W
McLoughlin, Mt., U.S.A. 158 E2 42 27N 122 19W
MacMahon = Aïn Touta, Algeria 111 A6 35 26N 5 54 E
McMechen, U.S.A. 150 G4 39 57N 80 44W
McMinnville, Oreg., U.S.A. 158 D2 45 13N 123 12W
McMinnville, Tenn., U.S.A. 149 H3 35 41N 85 46W
McMurdo Sd., Antarctica 7 D11 77 0 S 170 0 E
McMurray = Fort McMurray, Canada 142 B6 56 44N 111 7W
McMurray, U.S.A. 160 B4 48 19N 122 14W
Maco, Phil. 81 H5 7 20N 125 50 E
Macocolo, Angola 115 D3 6 47 S 16 8 E
Macodoene, Mozam. 117 C6 23 32 S 35 5 E
Macolo, Angola 115 D3 7 5 S 16 42 E
Macomb, U.S.A. 156 D6 40 27N 90 40W
Macomer, Italy 46 B1 40 16N 8 47 E
Mâcon, France 27 F11 46 19N 4 50 E
Macon, Ga., U.S.A. 152 C6 32 51N 83 38W
Macon, Ill., U.S.A. 156 E8 39 43N 89 0W
Macon, Miss., U.S.A. 149 J1 33 7N 88 34W
Macon, Mo., U.S.A. 156 E4 39 44N 92 28W
Macondo, Angola 115 E4 12 37 S 23 46 E
Macossa, Mozam. 119 F3 17 55 S 33 56 E
Macoun L., Canada 143 B8 56 32N 103 40W
Macoupin Cr. →, U.S.A. 156 E6 39 11N 90 38W
Macovane, Mozam. 117 C6 21 30 S 35 2 E
McPherson = Kapuskasing, Canada 140 C3 49 25N 82 30W
McPherson, U.S.A. 154 F6 38 22N 97 40W
McPherson Pk., U.S.A. 161 L7 34 53N 119 53W
McPherson Ra., Australia 127 D5 28 15 S 153 15 E
Macquarie →, Australia 129 A7 30 7 S 147 24 E
Macquarie Harbour, Australia 127 G4 42 15 S 145 23 E
Macquarie Is., Pac. Oc. 134 N7 54 36 S 158 55 E
McRae, U.S.A. 152 C7 32 4N 82 54W
MacRobertson Land, Antarctica 7 D6 71 0 S 64 0 E
Macroom, Ireland 23 E3 51 54N 8 57W
MacTier, Canada 150 A5 45 9N 79 46W
Macubela, Mozam. 119 F4 16 53 S 37 49 E
Macugnaga, Italy 44 C4 45 58N 7 58 E
Macuira △, Colombia 165 D5 12 9N 71 21W
Macuiza, Mozam. 119 F3 18 7 S 34 29 E
Macujer, Colombia 168 C3 0 24N 73 10W
Macumba, The →, Australia 127 D2 27 52 S 137 12 E
Macuro, Venezuela 169 F9 10 42N 61 55W
Macusani, Peru 172 C3 14 4 S 70 29W
Macuse, Mozam. 119 F4 17 45 S 37 10 E
Macuspana, Mexico 163 D6 17 46N 92 36W
Macusse, Angola 116 B3 17 48 S 20 23 E
Mada →, Nigeria 113 D6 7 59N 7 55 E
Ma'dabā □, Jordan 103 D4 31 43N 35 47 E
Madadeni, S. Africa 117 D5 27 43 S 30 3 E
Madadi, Chad 109 E4 18 28N 20 45 E
Madagali, Nigeria 113 C7 10 56N 13 33 E
Madagascar ■, Africa 117 C8 20 0 S 47 0 E
Madagascar Basin, Ind. Oc. 121 G4 27 0 S 55 0 E
Madagascar Plateau, Ind. Oc. 121 G3 30 0 S 45 0 E
Madā'in Sālih, Si. Arabia 96 E3 26 46N 37 57 E
Madaipur, India 95 H3 13 56N 77 16 E
Madalena, Azores 9 d1 38 32N 28 32W
Madama, Niger 109 D2 22 0N 13 40 E
Madame, I., Canada 141 C7 45 30N 60 58W
Madan, Bulgaria 51 E8 41 30N 24 57 E
Madanapalle, India 95 H4 13 33N 78 28 E
Madang, Papua N. G. 132 C3 5 12 S 145 49 E
Madang □, Papua N. G. 132 C3 5 0 S 145 30 E
Madaoua, Niger 113 C6 14 5N 6 27 E
Madara, Nigeria 113 C7 11 45N 10 35 E
Madaripur, Bangla. 90 D3 23 19N 90 15 E
Madau I., Papua N. G. 132 E7 8 58 S 152 28 E
Madauk, Burma 90 G6 17 56N 96 52 E
Madawaska, Canada 150 A7 45 30N 78 0W
Madawaska →, Canada 140 C4 45 27N 76 21W
Madaya, Burma 90 D6 22 12N 96 10 E
Madbar, Sudan 107 F3 6 17N 30 45 E
Maddalena, Italy 46 A2 41 16N 9 23 E
Maddaloni, Italy 47 A7 41 2N 14 23 E
Maddela, Phil. 80 C3 16 21N 121 41 E
Maddur, India 95 H3 12 36N 77 4 E
Madeira, Atl. Oc. 9 c 32 50N 17 0W
Madeira, U.S.A. 157 E12 39 11N 84 22W
Madeira →, Brazil 169 D6 3 22 S 58 45W
Mädelegabel, Germany 33 B10 47 18N 10 18 E
Madeleine, Îs. de la, Canada 141 C7 47 30N 61 40W
Maden, Turkey 101 C8 38 23N 39 40 E

Madera, Mexico 162 B3 29 12N 108 7W
Madera, Calif., U.S.A. 160 J6 36 57N 120 3W
Madera, Pa., U.S.A. 150 F6 40 49N 78 26W
Madgaon, India 95 G1 15 12N 73 58 E
Madha, India 94 F2 18 0N 75 30 E
Madhavpur, India 92 J3 21 15N 69 58 E
Madhepura, India 93 F12 26 11N 86 23 E
Madhira, India 94 F5 16 55N 80 22 E
Madhubani, India 93 F12 26 21N 86 7 E
Madhugiri, India 95 H3 13 40N 77 12 E
Madhumati →, Bangla. 90 D2 22 53N 89 52 E
Madhupur, Bangla. 90 C3 24 37N 90 2 E
Madhupur, India 93 G12 24 16N 86 39 E
Madhya Pradesh □, India 92 J8 22 50N 78 0 E
Madidi →, Bolivia 172 C4 12 32 S 66 52W
Madikeri, India 95 H2 12 30N 75 45 E
Madikwe ⌓, S. Africa 117 D5 27 38 S 32 15 E
Madill, U.S.A. 155 H6 34 6N 96 46W
Madimba, Angola 115 D2 6 36 S 14 23 E
Madimba, Dem. Rep. of the Congo 115 C3 4 58 S 15 5 E
Ma'din, Syria 101 E8 35 45N 39 36 E
Madina, Mali 112 C3 13 25N 8 50W
Madinani, Ivory C. 112 D3 9 37N 6 57W
Madīnat ash Sha'b, Yemen 98 D4 12 50N 45 0 E
Madingo, Congo 114 C2 4 5 S 11 24 E
Madingou, Congo 114 C2 4 10 S 13 33 E
Madirovalo, Madag. 117 B8 16 26 S 46 32 E
Madison, Calif., U.S.A. 160 G5 38 41N 121 59W
Madison, Fla., U.S.A. 152 E6 30 28N 83 25W
Madison, Ga., U.S.A. 152 E6 33 36N 83 28W
Madison, Ind., U.S.A. 157 F11 38 44N 85 23W
Madison, Mo., U.S.A. 156 E4 39 28N 92 13W
Madison, Nebr., U.S.A. 154 E6 41 50N 97 27W
Madison, Ohio, U.S.A. 150 E3 41 46N 81 3W
Madison, S. Dak., U.S.A. 154 D6 44 0N 97 7W
Madison, Wis., U.S.A. 156 A7 43 4N 89 24W
Madison →, U.S.A. 158 D8 45 56N 111 31W
Madison Heights, U.S.A. 148 G6 37 25N 79 8W
Madisonville, Ky., U.S.A. 148 G2 37 20N 87 30W
Madisonville, Tex., U.S.A. 155 K7 30 57N 95 55W
Madista, Botswana 116 C4 21 15 S 25 6 E
Madiun, Indonesia 85 D4 7 38 S 111 32 E
Madjingo, Gabon 114 B2 1 20N 14 4 E
Madoc, Canada 150 B7 44 30N 77 28W
Madol, Sudan 107 F2 9 3N 27 45 E
Madon →, France 27 D13 48 36N 6 6 E
Madona, Latvia 15 H22 56 53N 26 5 E
Madonie, Italy 46 E6 37 50N 13 50 E
Madonna di Campíglio, Italy 33 D11 46 14N 10 49 E
Madra Dağı, Turkey 49 B9 39 23N 27 12 E
Madrakah, Ra's al, Oman 99 C7 19 0N 57 50 E
Madras = Chennai, India 95 H5 13 8N 80 19 E
Madras = Tamil Nadu □, India 95 J3 11 0N 77 0 E
Madras, U.S.A. 158 D3 44 38N 121 8W
Madre, Laguna, U.S.A. 155 M6 27 0N 97 30W
Madre, Sierra, Phil. 80 C4 17 0N 122 0 E
Madre de Dios □, Peru 172 C3 12 0 S 70 15W
Madre de Dios →, Bolivia 172 C4 10 59 S 66 8W
Madre de Dios, I., Chile 176 D1 50 20 S 75 10W
Madre del Sur, Sierra, Mexico 163 D5 17 30N 100 0W
Madre Occidental, Sierra, Mexico 162 B3 27 0N 107 0W
Madre Oriental, Sierra, Mexico 162 C5 25 0N 100 0W
Madri, India 92 G5 24 16N 73 32 E
Madrid, Spain 42 E7 40 25N 3 45W
Madrid, Ala., U.S.A. 152 D4 31 2N 85 24W
Madrid, Iowa, U.S.A. 156 C3 41 53N 93 49W
Madrid, N.Y., U.S.A. 151 B9 44 45N 75 8W
Madrid □, Spain 42 E7 40 30N 3 45W
Madrid Barajas ✕ (MAD), Spain 42 E7 40 26N 3 34W
Madridejos, Spain 43 F7 39 28N 3 33W
Madrigal de las Altas Torres, Spain 42 D6 41 5N 5 0W
Madrona, Sierra, Spain 43 G6 38 27N 4 16W
Madroñera, Spain 43 F5 39 26N 5 42W
Madrusah, Libya 108 D2 24 48N 14 32 E
Madu, Sudan 107 E2 14 37N 26 4 E
Maduo, Dem. Rep. of the Congo 114 C4 1 24 S 20 44 E
Madura, Australia 125 F4 31 55 S 127 0 E
Madura, Indonesia 79 G15 7 30 S 114 0 E
Madura, Selat, Indonesia 85 D4 7 30 S 113 20 E
Madura Oya △, Sri Lanka 95 L5 7 20N 81 10 E
Madurai, India 95 K4 9 55N 78 10 E
Madurantakam, India 95 H4 12 30N 79 50 E
Madzhalis, Russia 61 J8 42 9N 47 47 E
Mae Chan, Thailand 86 B2 20 9N 99 52 E
Mae Hong Son, Thailand 86 C2 19 16N 97 56 E
Mae Khlong →, Thailand 86 F3 13 24N 100 0 E
Mae Phrik, Thailand 86 D2 17 27N 99 7 E
Mae Ping △, Thailand 86 D2 17 37N 98 51 E
Mae Ramat, Thailand 86 D2 16 58N 98 31 E
Mae Rim, Thailand 86 C2 18 54N 98 57 E
Mae Sot, Thailand 86 D2 16 43N 98 34 E
Mae Suai, Thailand 76 H2 19 39N 99 33 E
Mae Tha, Thailand 86 C2 18 28N 99 8 E
Mae Wong △, Thailand 86 E2 15 54N 99 12 E
Mae Yom △, Thailand 86 C3 18 43N 100 15 E
Maebaru, Japan 72 D2 33 33N 130 12 E
Maebashi, Japan 73 A11 36 24N 139 4 E
Maella, Spain 40 D5 41 8N 0 7 E
Maesteg, U.K. 21 F4 51 36N 3 40W
Maestra, Sierra, Cuba 164 B4 20 15N 77 0W
Maestre de Campo I., Phil. 80 E3 12 56N 121 42 E
Maetambe, Mt., Solomon Is. 133 L9 7 3 S 157 1 E
Maevatanana, Madag. 117 B8 16 56 S 46 49 E
Maéwo, Vanuatu 133 E6 15 10 S 168 10 E
Mafa, Indonesia 82 A3 0 3N 127 53 E
Ma'fan, Libya 108 C2 25 56N 14 29 E
Mafeking = Mafikeng, S. Africa 116 D4 25 50 S 25 38 E
Mafeking, Canada 143 C8 52 40N 101 10W
Maféré, Ivory C. 112 D4 5 30N 3 2W
Mafeteng, Lesotho 116 D4 29 51 S 27 15 E
Maffra, Australia 129 D7 37 53 S 146 58 E
Mafia I., Tanzania 118 D4 7 45 S 39 50 E
Mafikeng, S. Africa 116 D4 25 50 S 25 38 E
Mafra, Brazil 175 B6 26 10 S 49 55W
Mafra, Portugal 43 G1 38 55N 9 20W
Mafungabusi Plateau, Zimbabwe 119 F2 18 30 S 29 8 E
Magadan, Russia 67 D16 59 38N 150 50 E
Magadi, India 95 H3 12 58N 77 14 E
Magadi, Kenya 118 C4 1 54 S 36 19 E
Magadi, L., Kenya 118 C4 1 54 S 36 19 E
Magaliesburg, S. Africa 117 D4 26 0 S 27 32 E
Magallanes = Punta Arenas, Chile 176 D2 53 10 S 71 0W
Magallanes, Phil. 80 E4 12 50N 123 50 E
Magallanes □, Chile 176 D2 52 0 S 72 0W
Magallanes, Estrecho de, Chile 176 D2 52 30 S 75 0W
Magaluf, Spain 38 B3 39 29N 2 32 E
Magangué, Colombia 168 B3 9 14N 74 45W
Maganoy, Phil. 81 H5 6 51N 124 31 E
Magaria, Niger 113 C6 13 4N 9 5 E
Magarida, Papua N. G. 132 F5 10 18 S 149 20 E
Magburaka, S. Leone 112 D2 8 47N 12 0W
Magdalen Is. = Madeleine, Îs. de la, Canada 141 C7 47 30N 61 40W
Magdalena, Argentina 174 D4 35 5 S 57 30W
Magdalena, Bolivia 173 C5 13 13 S 63 57W
Magdalena, Malaysia 83 B5 4 25N 117 55 E
Magdalena, Mexico 162 A2 30 50N 112 0W
Magdalena, U.S.A. 159 J10 34 7N 107 15W
Magdalena □, Colombia 168 A3 10 0N 74 0W
Magdalena →, Colombia 168 A3 11 6N 74 51W
Magdalena →, Mexico 162 A2 30 40N 112 25W
Magdalena, B., Mexico 162 C2 24 30N 112 10W
Magdalena, I., Chile 176 B2 44 40 S 73 0W
Magdalena, Llano de la, Mexico 162 C2 25 0N 111 30W
Magdeburg, Germany 30 C7 52 7N 11 38 E
Magdelaine Cays, Australia 126 B5 16 33 S 150 18 E
Magdub, Sudan 107 E2 13 42N 25 5 E
Magee, U.S.A. 155 K10 31 52N 89 44W
Magelang, Indonesia 85 D4 7 29 S 110 13 E
Magellan's Str. = Magallanes, Estrecho de, Chile 176 D2 52 30 S 75 0W
Magenta, Italy 44 C5 45 28N 8 53 E
Magenta, L., Australia 125 F2 33 30 S 119 2 E
Magerøya, Norway 14 A21 71 3N 25 40 E
Maggea, Australia 128 C4 34 28 S 140 2 E
Maggia, Switz. 33 D7 46 15N 8 42 E
Maggia →, Switz. 33 D7 46 18N 8 36 E
Maggiorasca, Mte., Italy 44 D6 44 33N 9 29 E
Maggiore, Lago, Italy 44 B5 45 57N 8 39 E
Maggotty, Jamaica 164 a 18 9N 77 46W
Maghâgha, Egypt 106 B3 28 38N 30 50 E
Maghama, Mauritania 112 B2 15 32N 12 57W
Magherafelt, U.K. 23 B5 54 45N 6 37W
Maghnia, Algeria 111 B4 34 50N 1 43W
Maghreb, N. Afr. 104 C3 32 0N 4 0W
Magione, Italy 45 E9 43 8N 12 12 E
Magistralnyy, Russia 67 D11 56 16N 107 36 E
Maglaj, Bos.-H. 52 F3 44 33N 18 7 E
Magliano in Toscana, Italy 45 F8 42 36N 11 17 E
Máglie, Italy 47 B11 40 7N 18 18 E
Magnac-Laval, France 28 B5 46 13N 1 11 E
Magnetic Pole (North), Canada 6 A2 88 30N 107 0W
Magnetic Pole (South), Antarctica 7 C9 64 8 S 138 8 E
Magnisía □, Greece 48 B5 39 15N 23 0 E
Magnitogorsk, Russia 64 E7 53 27N 59 4 E
Magnolia, Ark., U.S.A. 155 J8 33 16N 93 14W
Magnolia, Miss., U.S.A. 155 K9 31 9N 90 28W
Magnor, Norway 18 E9 59 56N 12 15 E
Magny-en-Vexin, France 27 C8 49 9N 1 47 E
Mago, Fiji 133 A3 17 26 S 179 8W
Mago △, Ethiopia 107 F4 5 40N 36 18 E
Magog, Canada 141 C5 45 18N 72 9W
Magoro, Uganda 118 B3 1 45N 34 12 E
Magoša = Famagusta, Cyprus 39 E9 35 8N 33 55 E
Magouládhes, Greece 38 B9 39 45N 19 42 E
Magoye, Zambia 119 F2 16 1 S 27 30 E
Magozal, Mexico 163 C5 21 34N 97 59W
Magpie, L., Canada 141 B7 51 0N 64 41W
Magrath, Canada 142 D6 49 25N 112 50W
Magre →, Spain 41 F4 39 11N 0 25W
Magrur, Sudan 107 E3 14 1N 30 27 E
Magrur, Wadi →, Sudan 107 D2 16 5N 26 30 E
Magsingal, Phil. 80 C3 17 41N 120 25 E
Magta Lahjar, Mauritania 112 B2 17 28N 13 17W
Maguan, China 76 F5 23 0N 104 21 E
Maguarinho, C., Brazil 170 B2 0 15 S 48 30W
Magude, Mozam. 117 D5 25 2 S 32 40 E
Maguindanao □, Phil. 81 H5 7 5N 124 0 E
Magurski △, Poland 55 J8 49 30N 21 30 E
Mağusa = Famagusta, Cyprus 39 E9 35 8N 33 55 E
Maguse L., Canada 143 A9 61 37N 95 10W
Maguse Pt., Canada 143 A10 61 20N 93 50W
Magvana, India 92 H3 23 13N 69 22 E
Magwe, Burma 90 E5 20 10N 95 0 E
Magwe, Sudan 107 G3 4 8N 32 17 E
Magwe □, Burma 90 F5 20 0N 95 0 E
Magyarorszag = Hungary ■, Europe 35 D12 47 20N 19 20 E
Maha Oya, Sri Lanka 95 L5 7 31N 81 22 E
Maha Sarakham, Thailand 86 D4 16 12N 103 16 E
Mahābād, Iran 101 D11 36 50N 45 45 E
Mahabaleshwar, India 94 F1 17 58N 73 43 E
Mahabharat Lekh, Nepal 93 E10 28 30N 82 0 E
Mahabo, Madag. 117 C7 20 23 S 44 40 E
Mahad, India 94 E1 18 6N 73 29 E
Mahadeo Uen, Somali Rep. 120 D3 2 58N 45 32 E
Mahadeo Hills, India 93 H8 22 20N 78 30 E
Mahadeopur, India 94 E5 18 48N 80 0 E
Mahaffey, U.S.A. 150 F6 40 53N 78 44W
Mahagi, Dem. Rep. of the Congo 118 B3 2 20N 31 0 E
Mahaicony, Guyana 169 B6 6 36N 57 48W
Mahajamba →, Madag. 117 B8 15 33 S 47 8 E
Mahajamba, Helodranon' i, Madag. 117 B8 15 24 S 47 5 E
Mahajan, India 92 E5 28 48N 73 56 E
Mahajanga, Madag. 117 B8 15 40 S 46 25 E
Mahajanga □, Madag. 117 B8 17 0 S 47 0 E
Mahajilo →, Madag. 117 B8 19 42 S 45 22 E
Mahakam →, Indonesia 85 C5 0 35 S 117 17 E
Mahalapye, Botswana 116 C4 23 1 S 26 51 E
Mahalchhar, Bangla. 90 D4 22 55N 92 2 E
Mahale Mts., Tanzania 118 D3 6 20 S 30 0 E
Mahale Mts. △, Tanzania 118 D2 6 10 S 29 50 E
Maḩallāt, Iran 97 C6 33 55N 50 30 E
Māhān, Iran 97 D8 30 5N 57 18 E
Mahan →, India 93 H10 23 30N 82 50 E
Mahanadi →, India 94 D8 20 20N 86 25 E
Mahananda →, India 93 G12 25 12N 87 52 E
Mahanoro, Madag. 117 B8 19 54 S 48 48 E
Mahanoy City, U.S.A. 151 F8 40 49N 76 9W
Mahaplag, Phil. 81 F5 10 35N 124 57 E
Maharashtra □, India 94 D2 20 30N 75 30 E
Maharès, Tunisia 108 B2 34 32N 10 29 E
Mahasamund, India 94 D6 21 6N 82 6 E
Mahasham, W. →, Egypt 103 E3 30 15N 34 10 E
Mahasoa, Madag. 117 C8 22 12 S 46 6 E
Mahasolo, Madag. 117 B8 19 7 S 46 22 E
Mahattat ash Shīdīyah, Jordan 103 F4 29 55N 35 55 E
Mahattat 'Unayzah, Jordan 103 E4 30 30N 35 47 E
Mahavavy →, Madag. 117 B8 15 57 S 45 54 E
Mahaweli Ganga →, Sri Lanka 95 K5 8 27N 81 13 E
Mahaxay, Laos 86 D5 17 22N 105 12 E
Mahbubabad, India 94 F5 17 42N 80 2 E
Mahbubnagar, India 94 F3 16 45N 77 59 E
Mahd adh Dhahab, Si. Arabia 98 B3 23 30N 40 52 E
Maḩḑah, Oman 97 E7 24 24N 55 59 E
Mahdia, Guyana 169 B6 5 13N 59 8W
Mahdia, Tunisia 108 A2 35 28N 11 0 E
Mahe, Jammu & Kashmir, India 93 C8 33 10N 78 32 E
Mahé, Pondicherry, India 95 J2 11 42N 75 34 E
Mahé, Seychelles 121 b 5 0 S 55 30 E
Mahé ✕ (SEZ), Seychelles 121 b 4 40 S 55 31 E
Mahebourg, Mauritius 121 d 20 24 S 57 42 E
Mahendra Giri, India 95 K3 8 20N 77 30 E
Mahendraganj, India 90 C2 25 20N 89 45 E
Mahendragarh, India 92 E7 28 17N 76 14 E
Mahenge, Tanzania 119 D4 8 45 S 36 41 E
Maheno, N.Z. 131 F5 45 10 S 170 50 E
Mahesana, India 92 H5 23 39N 72 26 E
Maheshwar, India 92 H6 22 11N 75 35 E
Mahgawan, India 93 F8 26 29N 78 37 E
Mahi →, India 92 H5 22 15N 72 55 E
Mahia Pen., N.Z. 130 F6 39 9 S 177 55 E
Mahighe, Solomon Is. 133 M10 8 30 S 159 58 E
Mahilyow, Belarus 58 F6 53 55N 30 18 E
Mahim, India 94 E1 19 39N 72 44 E
Mahina, Tahiti 133 S16 17 30 S 149 27W
Mahirija, Morocco 111 B4 34 0N 3 16W
Mahlaing, Burma 90 E5 21 6N 95 39 E
Mahmiya, Sudan 107 D3 17 12N 33 43 E
Mahmud Kot, Pakistan 92 D4 30 16N 71 0 E
Mahmudia, Romania 53 E14 45 5N 29 5 E
Mahmudiye, Turkey 49 B12 39 48N 30 15 E
Mahmutbey, Turkey 51 E12 41 3N 28 49 E
Mahnomen, U.S.A. 154 B7 47 19N 95 58W
Maho, Sri Lanka 95 L5 7 49N 80 16 E
Mahoba, India 93 G8 25 15N 79 55 E
Mahomet, U.S.A. 157 D8 40 12N 88 24W
Mahón = Maó, Spain 38 B5 39 53N 4 16 E
Mahon, Menorca ✕ (MAH), Spain 40 F9 39 50N 4 16 E
Mahone Bay, Canada 141 D7 44 30N 64 20W
Mahopac, U.S.A. 151 E11 41 22N 73 45W
Mahoua, Chad 109 F3 11 49N 18 26 E
Mährisch-Budwitz = Moravské Budějovice, Czech Rep. 34 B8 49 4N 15 49 E
Mährisch-Schönberg = Šumperk, Czech Rep. 35 B9 49 59N 16 59 E
Mährisch-Trubau = Moravská Třebová, Czech Rep. 35 B9 49 45N 16 40 E
Mahuta, Nigeria 113 C5 11 32N 4 58 E
Mahuva, India 92 J4 21 5N 71 48 E
Mahya Dağı, Turkey 51 E11 41 47N 27 36 E
Mai-Ndombe, L., Dem. Rep. of the Congo 114 C3 2 0 S 18 20 E
Mai-Sai, Thailand 76 G2 20 20N 99 55 E
Mai Thon, Ko, Thailand 87 a 7 40N 98 28 E
Maia, Azores 9 d4 36 56N 25 1W
Maia, Portugal 42 D2 41 14N 8 37W
Maia, Spain 40 B3 43 12N 1 29W
Maials, Spain 40 D5 41 22N 0 30 E
Maibong, India 90 C4 25 18N 93 10 E
Maicao, Colombia 168 A3 11 23N 72 13W
Maîche, France 27 E13 47 16N 6 48 E
Maici →, Brazil 173 B5 6 30 S 61 43W
Maicurú →, Brazil 169 D7 2 14 S 54 17W
Máida, Italy 47 D9 38 51N 16 22 E
Maidan Khula, Afghan. 91 B3 33 36N 69 50 E
Maidenhead, U.K. 21 F7 51 31N 0 42W
Maidstone, Canada 143 C7 53 5N 109 20W
Maidstone, U.K. 21 F8 51 16N 0 32 E
Maiduguri, Nigeria 113 C7 12 0N 13 20 E
Maiella △, Italy 45 F11 42 5N 14 5 E
Măieruş, Romania 53 E10 45 53N 25 31 E
Maigatari, Nigeria 113 C6 12 46N 9 27 E
Maignelay Montigny, France 27 C9 49 32N 2 30 E
Maigo, Phil. 81 G4 8 10N 123 57 E
Maigualida, Sierra, Venezuela 169 B4 5 30N 65 10W
Maigudo, Ethiopia 107 F4 7 30N 37 8 E
Maihar, India 93 G9 24 16N 80 45 E
Maihara, Japan 73 B8 35 19N 136 17 E
Maijdi, Bangla. 90 D3 22 48N 91 10 E
Maikala Ra., India 94 D5 22 0N 81 0 E
Maiko △, Dem. Rep. of the Congo 118 C2 0 30 S 27 50 E
Maikoor, Indonesia 83 C4 6 8 S 134 6 E
Mailani, India 93 E9 28 17N 80 21 E
Maili, U.S.A. 145 K13 21 25N 158 11W
Maili Pt, U.S.A. 145 K13 21 24N 158 11W
Maillezais, France 28 B3 46 22N 0 45W
Mailsi, Pakistan 92 E5 29 48N 72 15 E
Maimbung, Phil. 81 J3 5 56N 121 2 E
Main →, Germany 31 F4 50 0N 8 18 E
Main →, U.K. 23 B5 54 48N 6 18W
Main Range △, Australia 127 D5 28 11 S 152 27 E
Main Ridge, Trin. & Tob. 169 E10 11 16N 60 40W
Mainburg, Germany 31 G7 48 38N 11 47 E
Maindargi, India 94 F3 17 28N 76 18 E
Maine, France 26 D6 48 20N 0 15W
Maine □, U.S.A. 149 C11 45 20N 69 0W
Maine →, Ireland 23 D2 52 9N 9 45W
Maine-et-Loire □, France 26 E6 47 31N 0 30W
Maïne-Soroa, Niger 113 C7 13 13N 12 2 E
Maingkaing, Burma 90 C5 24 48N 95 16 E
Maingkwan, Burma 90 B6 26 15N 96 37 E
Mainit, Phil. 81 G5 9 32N 125 32 E
Mainit, L., Phil. 81 G5 9 31N 125 30 E
Mainland, Orkney, U.K. 22 C5 58 59N 3 8W
Mainland, Shet., U.K. 22 A7 60 15N 1 22W
Mainoru, Australia 126 A1 14 0 S 134 6 E
Mainpuri, India 93 F8 27 18N 79 4 E
Maintal, Germany 31 E4 50 7N 8 52 E
Maintenon, France 27 D8 48 35N 1 35 E
Maintirano, Madag. 117 B7 18 3 S 44 1 E
Mainz, Germany 31 E4 50 1N 8 14 E
Maio, C. Verde Is. 9 j 15 10N 23 10W
Maipú, Argentina 174 D4 36 52 S 57 50W
Maiquetía, Venezuela 168 A4 10 36N 66 57W
Máira →, Italy 44 D4 44 49N 7 38 E
Mairabari, India 90 B4 26 30N 92 22 E
Mairipotaba, Brazil 171 E2 17 18 S 49 28W
Maisí, Cuba 165 B5 20 17N 74 9W
Maisí, Pta. de, Cuba 165 B5 20 10N 74 10W
Maitland, N.S.W., Australia 129 B9 32 33 S 151 36 E
Maitland, S. Austral., Australia 128 C2 34 23 S 137 40 E
Maitland →, Canada 150 C3 43 45N 81 43W
Maitland, Banjaran, Malaysia 85 B5 4 55N 116 37 E
Maitri, Antarctica 7 D3 70 0 S 3 0W
Maitum, Phil. 81 H5 6 2N 124 30 E
Maiyema, Nigeria 113 C5 12 5N 4 25 E
Maiyuan, China 77 E11 25 34N 117 28 E
Maiz, Is. del, Nic. 164 D3 12 15N 83 4W
Maizuru, Japan 73 B7 35 25N 135 22 E
Majagual, Colombia 168 B3 8 33N 74 38W
Majalengka, Indonesia 85 D3 6 50 S 108 13 E
Majari →, Brazil 169 C5 3 29N 60 58W
Majdūl, Libya 108 C3 25 51N 15 7 E
Majene, Indonesia 82 B1 3 38 S 118 57 E
Majes →, Peru 172 D3 16 40 S 72 44W
Majete ⌓, Malawi 119 F3 15 54 S 34 34 E
Majevica, Bos.-H. 52 F3 44 45N 18 50 E
Maji, Ethiopia 107 F4 6 12N 35 30 E
Majiang, China 76 D6 26 28N 107 32 E
Majorca = Mallorca, Spain 38 B4 39 30N 3 0 E
Majors Creek, Australia 129 C8 35 33 S 149 45 E
Majuriã, Brazil 173 B5 7 30 S 64 55W
Majuro, Marshall Is. 134 G9 7 9N 171 12 E
Maka, Senegal 112 C2 13 40N 14 10W
Makaha, U.S.A. 145 K13 21 29N 158 13W
Makaha, Zimbabwe 117 B5 17 20 S 32 39 E
Makaha Pt., U.S.A. 145 J14 21 41N 157 56W
Makahuena Pt., U.S.A. 145 B2 21 52N 159 27W
Makak, Cameroon 113 E7 3 36N 11 0 E
Makakilo City, U.S.A. 145 K13 21 22N 158 5W
Makakou, Gabon 114 C2 0 11 S 12 12 E
Makalamabedi, Botswana 116 C3 20 19 S 23 51 E
Makale, Indonesia 82 B1 3 6 S 119 51 E
Makalu-Barun △, Nepal 93 F12 27 45N 87 10 E
Makamba, Burundi 118 C2 4 8 S 29 49 E
Makapuu Pt., U.S.A. 145 K14 21 19N 157 39W
Makarewa, N.Z. 131 G3 46 20 S 168 21 E
Makari, Cameroon 109 F2 12 35N 10 27 E
Makari, Cameroon 113 C7 12 35N 10 27 E
Makarikari = Makgadikgadi Salt Pans, Botswana 116 C4 20 40 S 25 45 E
Makarov Basin, Arctic 6 A 87 0N 150 0W
Makarovo, Russia 67 D11 57 40N 107 45 E
Makarska, Croatia 45 E14 43 20N 17 2 E
Makaryev, Russia 60 B6 57 52N 43 50 E
Makasar = Ujung Pandang, Indonesia 82 C1 5 10 S 119 20 E
Makasar, Selat, Indonesia 85 C5 1 0 S 118 20 E
Makasar, Str. of = Makasar, Selat, Indonesia 85 C5 1 0 S 118 20 E
Makat, Kazakhstan 57 E9 47 39N 53 19 E
Makaw, Dem. Rep. of the Congo 114 C3 3 29 S 18 20 E
Makawao, U.S.A. 145 C5 20 52N 156 17W
Makaya, Dem. Rep. of the Congo 114 C3 3 21 S 18 1 E
Makbon, Indonesia 83 B4 0 45 S 131 32 E
Makedonija = Macedonia ■, Europe 50 E5 41 53N 21 40 E
Makeni, S. Leone 112 D2 8 55N 12 5W
Makeyevka = Makiyivka, Ukraine 59 H9 48 0N 38 0 E
Makgadikgadi △, Botswana 116 C3 20 27 S 24 47 E
Makgadikgadi Salt Pans, Botswana 116 C4 20 40 S 25 45 E
Makhachkala, Russia 61 J8 43 0N 47 30 E
Makhado = Louis Trichardt, S. Africa 117 C4 23 1 S 29 43 E
Makhairádhon, Greece 39 D2 37 46N 20 49 E
Makharadze = Ozurgeti, Georgia 61 K5 41 55N 42 2 E
Makhfar al Buşayyah, Iraq 96 D5 30 0N 46 10 E
Makhmūr, Iraq 101 E10 35 46N 43 35 E
Makhtal, India 95 E3 16 30N 77 31 E
Makhyah, W. →, Yemen 99 C5 17 40N 49 1 E
Makian, Indonesia 82 A3 0 20N 127 20 E
Makina, Solomon Is. 133 M11 9 50 S 160 50 E
Makindu, Kenya 118 C4 2 18 S 37 50 E
Makinka = Makinsk, Kazakhstan 66 D8 52 37N 70 26 E
Makinsk, Kazakhstan 66 D8 52 37N 70 26 E
Makiv, Ukraine 53 B11 48 48N 26 43 E
Makiyivka, Ukraine 59 H9 48 0N 38 0 E
Makkah, Si. Arabia 98 B2 21 30N 39 54 E
Makkovik, Canada 141 A8 55 10N 59 10W
Makó, Hungary 52 D5 46 14N 20 33 E
Mako, Senegal 112 C2 12 52N 12 20W
Makogai, Fiji 133 A2 17 28 S 179 0 E
Makok, Gabon 114 C1 0 1 S 9 35 E
Makokou, Gabon 114 B2 0 40N 12 50 E
Makongo, Dem. Rep. of the Congo 118 B2 3 25N 26 17 E
Makoro, Dem. Rep. of the Congo 118 B2 3 10N 29 59 E
Makoua, Congo 114 C3 0 5 S 15 50 E
Maków Mazowiecki, Poland 55 F8 52 52N 21 6 E
Maków Podhalański, Poland 55 J6 49 43N 19 45 E
Makrá, Greece 49 E7 36 15N 25 54 E
Makran, Asia 91 D1 26 13N 61 30 E
Makran Coast Range, Pakistan 91 D2 25 40N 64 0 E
Makrana, India 92 F6 27 2N 74 46 E
Makrany, Belarus 55 G11 51 48N 24 17 E
Mákri, Greece 51 F9 40 52N 25 40 E
Makri, India 94 E5 19 46N 81 55 E
Makriyialos, Greece 39 E6 35 2N 25 59 E
Maktar, Tunisia 108 A1 35 48N 9 12 E
Mākū, Iran 101 C11 39 15N 44 31 E
Makum, India 90 B5 27 30N 95 23 E
Makumbi, Dem. Rep. of the Congo 115 D4 5 50 S 20 43 E
Makunda, Botswana 116 C3 22 30 S 20 7 E
Makung, Taiwan 77 F12 23 34N 119 34 E
Makunza, Dem. Rep. of the Congo 115 D4 8 52 S 24 19 E
Makurazaki, Japan 72 F2 31 15N 130 20 E
Makurdi, Nigeria 113 D6 7 43N 8 35 E
Makushin Volcano, U.S.A. 144 K6 53 53N 166 55W
Makūyeh, Iran 97 D7 28 7N 53 9 E
Makwassie, S. Africa 116 D4 27 17 S 26 0 E
Makwiro, Zimbabwe 117 B5 17 58 S 30 25 E
Mal, India 90 B2 26 51N 88 45 E
Mâl, Mauritania 112 B2 16 58N 13 23W
Mal B., Ireland 23 D2 52 50N 9 30W
Mala, Peru 172 C2 12 40 S 76 38W
Mala, Pta., Panama 164 E3 7 28N 80 2W
Mala Belozërka, Ukraine 59 J8 47 12N 34 56 E
Malá Fatra △, Slovak Rep. 35 B12 49 10N 19 0 E
Mala Kapela, Croatia 45 D12 44 45N 15 30 E
Mala Panew →, Poland 55 H4 50 43N 17 54 E
Mala Vyska, Ukraine 59 H6 48 39N 31 36 E
Malabang, Phil. 81 H5 7 36N 124 3 E
Malabar, U.S.A. 153 H9 28 0N 80 34W
Malabar Coast, India 95 J2 11 0N 75 0 E
Malabo = Rey Malabo, Eq. Guin. 113 E6 3 45N 8 50 E
Malabon, Phil. 80 D3 14 21N 121 0 E
Malabrigo = Puerto Chicama, Peru 172 B2 7 45 S 79 20W
Malabrigo Pt., Phil. 80 E3 13 36N 121 15 E
Malabu, Nigeria 113 D7 9 32N 12 28 E
Malabuñgan, Phil. 81 G1 9 3N 117 38 E
Malacca, Straits of, Indonesia 87 L3 3 0N 101 0 E
Malacky, Slovak Rep. 35 C10 48 27N 17 0 E
Malad City, U.S.A. 158 E7 42 12N 112 15W
Maladeta, Spain 40 C5 42 39N 0 39 E
Maladzyechna, Belarus 58 E4 54 20N 26 50 E
Malae Pt., U.S.A. 145 C6 20 7N 155 53W
Málaga, Colombia 168 B3 6 42N 72 44W
Málaga, Spain 43 J6 36 43N 4 23W
Málaga □, Spain 43 J6 36 38N 4 58W
Malagarasi, Tanzania 118 D3 5 5 S 30 50 E
Malagarasi →, Tanzania 118 D2 5 12 S 29 47 E
Malagasy Rep. = Madagascar ■, Africa 117 C8 20 0 S 47 0 E
Malagón, Spain 43 F7 39 11N 3 52W
Malagón →, Spain 43 H3 37 35N 7 29W
Malahide, Ireland 23 C5 53 26N 6 9W
Malaimbandy, Madag. 117 C8 20 20 S 45 36 E
Malaita, Solomon Is. 133 M11 9 0 S 161 0 E
Malakâl, Sudan 107 F3 9 33N 31 40 E
Malakanagiri, India 94 E5 18 21N 81 54 E
Malakand, Pakistan 91 B3 34 40N 71 55 E
Malakula, Vanuatu 133 F5 16 15 S 167 30 E
Malakwal, Pakistan 92 C5 32 34N 73 13 E
Malalag, Phil. 81 H5 6 36N 125 24 E
Malalaua, Papua N. G. 132 E4 8 4 S 146 10 E
Malam, Chad 109 F4 11 27N 20 59 E
Malamala, Indonesia 82 B2 3 21 S 120 55 E
Malanda, Australia 126 B4 17 22 S 145 35 E
Malang, Indonesia 85 D4 7 59 S 112 45 E
Malangas, Phil. 81 H4 7 37N 123 1 E
Malange □, Angola 115 D3 9 30 S 16 0 E
Malangen, Norway 14 B18 69 24N 18 37 E
Malanje, Angola 115 D3 9 36 S 16 17 E
Malapatan, Phil. 81 J5 5 59N 125 18 E
Mälaren, Sweden 16 E11 59 30N 17 10 E
Malargüe, Argentina 174 D2 35 32 S 69 30W
Malartic, Canada 140 C4 48 9N 78 9W
Malaryta, Belarus 55 G11 51 50N 24 3 E
Malaspina Glacier, U.S.A. 144 G12 59 50N 140 30W
Malatya, Turkey 101 C8 38 25N 38 20 E
Malawali, Malaysia 85 A5 7 3N 117 18 E
Malawi ■, Africa 119 E3 11 55 S 34 0 E
Malawi, L. = Nyasa, L., Africa 119 E3 12 30 S 34 30 E
Malay, Phil. 81 F3 11 54N 121 55 E
Malay Pen., Asia 87 J3 7 25N 100 0 E
Malaya Belozërka = Mala Belozërka, Ukraine 59 J8 47 12N 34 56 E
Malaya Vishera, Russia 58 C7 58 55N 32 25 E
Malaya Viska = Mala Vyska, Ukraine 59 H6 48 39N 31 36 E
Malaybalay, Phil. 81 G5 8 5N 125 7 E
Malāyer, Iran 97 C6 34 19N 48 51 E
Malaysia ■, Asia 85 B4 5 0N 110 0 E
Malazgirt, Turkey 101 C10 39 10N 42 33 E
Malbaza, Niger 113 C6 13 59N 5 38 E
Malbon, Australia 126 C3 21 5 S 140 17 E
Malbooma, Australia 127 E1 30 41 S 134 11 E
Malbork, Poland 54 D6 54 3N 19 1 E
Malca Dube, Ethiopia 120 C2 6 47N 42 4 E
Malcésine, Italy 44 C7 45 46N 10 48 E
Malchin, Germany 30 B8 53 44N 12 44 E
Malchow, Germany 30 B8 53 28N 12 25 E
Malcolm, Australia 125 E3 28 51 S 121 25 E
Malcolm, Pt., Australia 125 F3 33 48 S 123 45 E
Malczyce, Poland 55 G3 51 14N 16 29 E
Maldah, India 93 G13 25 2N 88 9 E
Maldegem, Belgium 24 C3 51 14N 3 26 E
Malden, Mass., U.S.A. 151 D13 42 26N 71 4W
Malden, Mo., U.S.A. 155 G10 36 34N 89 57W
Malden I., Kiribati 135 H12 4 3 S 155 1W
Maldives ■, Ind. Oc. 89 E6 5 0N 73 0 E
Maldon, Australia 128 D6 37 0 S 144 6 E
Maldon, U.K. 21 F8 51 44N 0 42 E
Maldonado, Uruguay 175 C5 34 59 S 55 0W
Maldonado, Punta, Mexico 163 D5 16 19N 98 35W
Malè, Italy 44 B7 46 21N 10 55 E
Male, Maldives 121 D6 4 0N 73 28 E
Malé Karpaty, Slovak Rep. 35 C10 48 30N 17 20 E
Maléa, Ákra, Greece 48 E5 36 28N 23 7 E
Maleas, Ákra = Maléa, Ákra, Greece 48 E5 36 28N 23 7 E
Malebo, Pool, Africa 115 C3 4 17 S 15 20 E
Malegaon, India 94 D2 20 30N 74 38 E
Malei, Mozam. 119 F4 17 12 S 36 58 E
Malek, Sudan 107 F3 6 4N 31 36 E
Malek Kandī, Iran 101 D12 37 9N 46 6 E
Malela, Bas-Congo, Dem. Rep. of the Congo 115 D2 5 59 S 12 37 E
Malela, Maniema, Dem. Rep. of the Congo 118 C2 4 22 S 26 8 E
Malema, Mozam. 119 E4 14 57 S 37 20 E
Maleme, Greece 39 E4 35 31N 23 49 E
Malendok I., Papua N. G. 132 B7 3 28 S 153 13 E
Måleräs, Sweden 17 H9 56 54N 15 34 E
Malerkotla, India 92 D6 30 32N 75 58 E
Máles, Greece 39 E6 35 6N 25 35 E
Malesherbes, France 27 D9 48 15N 2 24 E
Maleshevska Planina, Europe 50 E7 41 38N 23 7 E
Malesína, Greece 48 C5 38 37N 23 14 E
Malestroit, France 26 E4 47 49N 2 25W
Malfa, Italy 47 D7 38 35N 14 50 E
Malgobek, Russia 61 J7 43 30N 44 34 E
Malgomaj, Sweden 14 D17 64 40N 16 30 E
Malgrat de Mar, Spain 40 D7 41 39N 2 46 E
Malha, Sudan 107 D2 15 8N 25 10 E
Malhada, Brazil 171 D3 14 21 S 43 47W

Malhargarh, India ..... 92 G6   24 17N   74 59 E
Malheur →, U.S.A. ... 158 D5   44 4N 116 59W
Malheur L., U.S.A. 158 E4   43 20N 118 48W
Mali, Guinea 112 C2   12 10N 12 20W
Mali ■, Africa 112 B4   17 0N   3 0W
Mali →, Burma .... 90 C6   25 42N   97 30 E
Mali Kanal,
  Serbia & M. .... 52 E4   45 36N   19 24 E
Malibu, U.S.A. 161 L8   34 2N 118 41W
Maligaya = Gloria, Phil. 80 E3   12 59N 121 30 E
Maliku, Indonesia .... 82 B2   0 39 S 123 16 E
Malili, Indonesia ..... 82 B2   2 42 S 121 6 E
Mälilla, Sweden ...... 17 G9   57 23N   15 48 E
Malimba, Mts.,
  Dem. Rep. of
  the Congo .... 118 D2   7 30 S   29 30 E
Malin Hd., Ireland ... 23 A4   55 23N   7 23W
Malin Pen., Ireland .. 23 A4   55 20N   7 17W
Malindang, Mt., Phil. . 81 G4   8 13N 123 38 E
Malindi, Kenya ...... 118 C5   3 12 S   40 5 E
Malines = Mechelen,
  Belgium .... 24 C4   51 2N   4 29 E
Malino, Indonesia .... 82 A2   1 0N 121 0 E
Malinyi, Tanzania .... 119 D4   8 56 S   36 0 E
Malipo, China .... 76 F5   23 7N 104 42 E
Maliq, Albania ...... 50 F4   40 45N   20 48 E
Malita, Phil. .... 81 H5   6 19N 125 39 E
Maliwun, Burma ..... 78 B1   10 17N   98 40 E
Maliya, India .... 92 H4   23 5N   70 46 E
Maljenik, Serbia & M. . 50 C5   43 54N   21 43 E
Malka Mari △, Kenya . 118 B5   4 11N   40 46 E
Malkapur, India ..... 94 D1   20 53N   73 58 E
Malkara, Turkey ..... 51 F10   40 53N   26 53 E
Malkhangiri =
  Malakanagiri, India 94 E5   18 21N   81 54 E
Małkinia Górna,
  Poland .... 55 F9   52 42N   22 5 E
Malko Tŭrnovo,
  Bulgaria .... 51 E11   41 59N   27 31 E
Mallacoota, Australia . 129 D8   37 40 S 149 40 E
Mallacoota Inlet,
  Australia .... 129 D8   37 34 S 149 40 E
Mallaig, U.K. 22 D3   57 0N   5 50W
Mallala, Australia .... 128 C3   34 26 S 138 30 E
Mallaoua, Niger ..... 113 C6   13 2N   9 36 E
Mallard, U.S.A. 156 B2   42 56N   94 41W
Mallawan, India ..... 93 F9   27 4N   80 12 E
Mallawi, Egypt ...... 106 B3   27 44N   30 44 E
Mallee Cliffs △,
  Australia .... 128 C5   34 16 S 142 32 E
Mallemble, Gabon ... 114 C2   3 34 S   10 53 E
Mallemort, France ... 29 E9   43 43N   5 11 E
Málles Venosta, Italy . 44 B7   46 41N   10 32 E
Mállia, Greece ...... 39 E6   35 17N   25 32 E
Mallicolo = Malakula,
  Vanuatu .... 133 F5   16 15 S 167 30 E
Mallión, Kólpos, Greece 39 D6   35 19N   25 27 E
Mallorca, Spain ..... 38 B4   39 30N   3 0 E
Mallorytown, Canada . 151 B9   44 29N   75 53W
Mallow, Ireland 23 D3   52 8N   8 39W
Malmbäck, Sweden .. 17 H8   57 34N   14 28 E
Malmberget, Sweden . 14 C19   67 11N   20 40 E
Malmédy, Belgium ... 24 D6   50 25N   6 2 E
Malmesbury, S. Africa 116 E2   33 28 S   18 41 E
Malmivaara =
  Malmberget, Sweden 14 C19   67 11N   20 40 E
Malmköping, Sweden . 16 E10   59 8N   16 44 E
Malmö, Sweden ..... 17 J7   55 36N   12 59 E
Malmslätt, Sweden ... 17 F9   58 27N   15 33 E
Malmyzh, Russia ..... 60 B10   56 31N   50 41 E
Malnaş, Romania .... 53 D10   46 2N   25 49 E
Malo, Vanuatu ...... 133 E5   15 40 S 167 11 E
Malo Konare, Bulgaria 51 G8   42 12N   24 24 E
Maloarkhangelsk,
  Russia .... 59 F9   52 28N   36 30 E
Maloca, Brazil ...... 169 C6   1 40 S   55 57W
Maloja, Switz. ...... 33 D9   46 25N   9 35 E
Malojaross, Switz. ... 33 D9   46 25N   9 42 E
Malolo, Fiji .... 133 A1   17 45 S 177 11 E
Malolos, Phil. ...... 80 D3   14 50N 120 49 E
Malolotja △, Swaziland 117 D5   26 4 S   31 6 E
Malombe L., Malawi . 119 E4   14 40 S   35 15 E
Małomice, Poland .... 55 G2   51 34N   15 29 E
Malomir, Bulgaria ... 51 D10   42 16N   26 32 E
Malone, Fla., U.S.A. . 155 F10   30 57N   85 10W
Malone, N.Y., U.S.A. . 151 B10   44 51N   74 18W
Malong, China ...... 76 E4   25 24N 103 34 E
Malonga, Dem. Rep. of
  the Congo .... 115 E4   10 24 S   23 10 E
Malonno, Italy ...... 33 D10   46 7N   10 18 E
Małopolskie □, Poland 55 J7   49 50N   20 20 E
Malorad, Bulgaria ... 50 C7   43 28N   23 41 E
Måløy, Norway ...... 16 F11   61 57N   5 6 E
Maloyaroslavets, Russia 58 E9   55 2N   36 20 E
Malpartida, Spain 43 F4   39 26N   6 30W
Malpaso, Canary Is. . . 9 e1   27 43N   18 3W
Malpelo, I. de,
  Colombia 135 G19   4 3N   81 35W
Malpica de
  Bergantiños, Spain . 42 B2   43 19N   8 50W
Malprabha →, India .. 95 F3   16 20N   76 5 E
Malpur, India .... 92 H5   23 21N   73 27 E
Malpura, India ...... 92 F6   26 17N   75 23 E
Mals = Málles Venosta,
  Italy .... 44 B7   46 41N   10 32 E
Malsiras, India ...... 94 F2   17 52N   74 55 E
Malta, Brazil .... 170 C4   6 54 S   37 31W
Malta, Idaho, U.S.A. . 158 E7   42 18N 113 22W
Malta, Mont., U.S.A. . 158 B10   48 21N 107 52W
Malta ■, Europe ..... 38 F7   35 55N   14 26 E
Malta ✕ (MLA), Malta 38 F7   35 52N   14 29 E
Maltahöhe, Namibia .. 116 C2   24 55 S   17 0 E
Maltepe, Turkey ..... 51 F13   40 55N   29 8 E
Malters, Switz. ...... 32 B6   47 3N   8 11 E
Malton, Canada 150 C5   43 42N   79 38W
Malton, U.K. 20 C7   54 8N   0 49W
Malu'u, Solomon Is. . 133 M11   8 20 S 160 38 E
Maluku = Manolo
  Fortich, Phil. ..... 81 G5   8 28N 124 50 E
Maluku, Dem. Rep. of
  the Congo .... 114 C3   4 3 S   15 34 E
Maluku, Indonesia .... 79 E7   1 0 S 127 0 E
Maluku □, Indonesia .. 82 B3   3 0 S 128 0 E
Maluku Sea = Molucca
  Sea, Indonesia ..... 82 A3   0 0 125 0 E
Maluku Utara □,
  Indonesia .... 79 D7   1 0N 129 0 E
Malumfashi, Nigeria .. 113 C6   11 48N   7 39 E
Malunda, Indonesia ... 82 B1   3 0 S 118 50 E
Malundo, Angola .... 115 E4   14 51 S   22 0 E
Malung, Sweden ..... 16 D7   60 42N   13 44 E
Malungon, Phil. ..... 81 H5   6 16N 125 14 E
Malungsfors, Sweden . 16 D7   60 44N   13 33 E
Malur, India .... 95 H3   13 0N   77 55 E
Malvaglia, Switz. .... 33 D7   46 24N   8 59 E
Malvalli, India ...... 95 H3   12 28N   77 8 E
Malvan, India .... 95 F1   16 2N   73 30 E
Malvern, U.S.A. 155 H8   34 22N   92 49W
Malvern Hills, U.K. .. 21 E5   52 0N   2 19W
Malvik, Norway ..... 18 A7   63 25N   10 40 E

Malvinas, Is. = Falkland
  Is. ☑, Atl. Oc. .... 9 f   51 30 S   59 0W
Malý Dunaj →,
  Slovak Rep. .... 35 D11   47 45N   18 9 E
Malya, Tanzania ..... 118 C3   3 5 S   33 38 E
Malybay, Kazakhstan . 65 B9   43 30N   78 25 E
Malye Derbety, Russia 61 G7   47 57N   44 42 E
Malyn, Ukraine ...... 59 G5   50 46N   29 3 E
Malyy Lyakhovskiy,
  Ostrov, Russia ..... 67 B15   74 7N 140 36 E
Mama, Russia .... 67 D12   58 18N 112 54 E
Mamadysh, Russia ... 60 C10   55 44N   51 23 E
Mamaku, N.Z. ...... 130 E5   38 5 S 176 8 E
Mamala B., U.S.A. ... 145 K14   21 15N 157 55W
Mamanuca Group, Fiji 133 A1   17 35 S 177 5 E
Mamarr Mitlâ, Egypt . 103 E1   30 2N   32 54 E
Mamasa, Indonesia ... 82 B1   2 55 S 119 20 E
Mambajao, Phil. ..... 81 G5   9 15N 124 43 E
Mambasa, Dem. Rep. of
  the Congo .... 118 B2   1 22N   29 3 E
Mamberamo →,
  Indonesia .... 83 B5   2 0 S 137 50 E
Mambéré →, C.A.R. .. 114 B3   3 31N   16 3 E
Mambili →, Congo ... 114 B3   0 6N   16 5 E
Mambilima Falls,
  Zambia .... 119 E2   10 31 S   28 45 E
Mambirima, Dem. Rep.
  of the Congo ...... 119 E2   11 25 S   27 33 E
Mambo, Tanzania .... 118 C4   4 52 S   38 22 E
Mambrui, Kenya ..... 118 C5   3 5 S   40 5 E
Mamburao, Phil. ..... 80 E3   13 13N 120 39 E
Mameigwess L.,
  Canada 140 B2   52 35N   87 50W
Mamers, France ..... 26 D7   48 21N   0 22 E
Mamfé, Cameroon ... 113 D6   5 50N   9 15 E
Mámī, Ra's, Yemen .. 99 E6   12 32N   54 30 E
Mamiña, Chile ...... 172 E4   20 5 S   69 14W
Mammoth, U.S.A. ... 159 K8   32 43N 110 39W
Mammoth Cave △,
  U.S.A. 148 G3   37 8N   86 13W
Mamonovo, Russia ... 54 D6   54 28N   19 55 E
Mamoré →, Bolivia .. 173 C4   10 23 S   65 53W
Mamou, Guinea 112 C2   10 15N   12 0W
Mamoudzou, Mayotte 121 a   12 48 S   45 14 E
Mampatá, Guinea-Biss. 112 C2   11 54N   14 53W
Mampikony, Madag. .. 117 B8   16 6 S   47 38 E
Mampoko, Dem. Rep.
  of the Congo ...... 114 B3   0 51N   18 42 E
Mampong, Ghana 113 D4   7 6N   1 26W
Mamry, Jezioro, Poland 54 D8   54 5N   21 50 E
Mamuil Malal, Paso,
  S. Amer. .... 176 A2   39 35 S   71 28W
Mamuju, Indonesia ... 82 B1   2 41 S 118 50 E
Ma'mūl, Oman ...... 99 C6   18 8N   55 16 E
Mamuno, Botswana .. 116 C3   22 16 S   20 1 E
Mamuras, Albania ... 50 E3   41 34N   19 41 E
Man, Ivory C. 112 D3   7 30N   7 40W
Man →, India .... 94 F2   17 31N   75 32 E
Man, I. of, India .... 95 K11   8 30N   93 36 E
Man, I. of, U.K. 20 C3   54 15N   4 30W
Man-Bazar, India .... 93 H12   23 4N   86 39 E
Mān Kat, Burma ..... 90 D7   22 5N   98 1 E
Man Na, Burma ..... 90 D7   23 27N   97 19 E
Man Tun, Burma ..... 90 D7   23 52N   98 38 E
Mana, Fr. Guiana 169 B7   5 45N   53 55W
Mana, U.S.A. 145 A2   22 3N 159 47W
Mana →, Fr. Guiana . 169 B7   5 45N   53 55W
Mana Pools △,
  Zimbabwe .... 119 F2   15 56 S   29 25 E
Manaar, G. of =
  Mannar, G. of, Asia 95 K4   8 30N   79 0 E
Manabí □, Ecuador .. 168 D1   0 40 S   80 5W
Manacacías →,
  Colombia 168 C4   4 23N   72 4W
Manacapuru, Brazil .. 169 D5   3 16 S   60 37W
Manacapuru →, Brazil 169 D5   3 18 S   60 37W
Manacor, Spain ..... 38 B4   39 34N   3 13 E
Manadas, Azores 9 d1   38 38N   28 6W
Manado, Indonesia ... 82 A2   1 29N 124 51 E
Managua, Nic. 164 D2   12 6N   86 20W
Managua, L. de, Nic. . 164 D2   12 20N   86 30W
Manaia, N.Z. .... 130 F3   39 33 S 174 8 E
Manaia, N.Z. .... 130 E5   38 5 S 176 8 E
Manakara, Madag. ... 117 C8   22 8 S   48 1 E
Manakau, N.Z. ...... 131 C6   42 15 S 173 42 E
Manākhah, Yemen ... 98 D3   15 5N   43 44 E
Manali, India .... 92 C7   32 16N   77 10 E
Manam I., Papua N. G. 132 C3   4 5 S 145 0 E
Manama = Al
  Manāmah, Bahrain . 97 E6   26 10N   50 30 E
Manambao →, Madag. 117 B7   17 35 S   44 0 E
Manambato →, Madag. 117 A8   13 43 S   49 7 E
Manambolo →, Madag. 117 B7   19 18 S   44 22 E
Manambolosy, Madag. 117 B8   16 2 S   49 40 E
Mánamo, Caño →,
  Venezuela 169 B5   9 55N   62 16W
Manana I., U.S.A. ... 145 K14   21 20N 157 40W
Mananara, Madag. ... 117 B8   16 10 S   49 46 E
Mananara △, Madag. . 117 B8   16 14 S   49 45 E
Mananara →, Madag. 117 C8   23 21 S   47 42 E
Manangatang, Australia 128 C5   35 5 S 142 54 E
Mananjary, Madag. ... 117 C8   21 13 S   48 20 E
Manankoro, Mali 112 C3   10 28N   7 25W
Manantavadi, India .. 95 J3   11 49N   76 1 E
Manantenina, Madag. 117 C8   24 17 S   47 19 E
Manaos = Manaus,
  Brazil .... 169 D6   3 0 S   60 0W
Manapala, Phil. ..... 81 F4   10 58N 123 5 E
Manapire →,
  Venezuela 168 B4   7 42N   66 7W
Manapouri, N.Z. ..... 131 F2   45 34 S 167 39 E
Manapouri, L., N.Z. .. 131 F2   45 32 S 167 32 E
Manapparai, India ... 95 J4   10 36N   78 25 E
Manaqil, Sudan ..... 107 E3   14 15N   32 59 E
Manar →, India ..... 94 E3   18 50N   77 20 E
Manar, Jabal, Yemen . 98 E3   14 24N   44 17 E
Manaravolo, Madag. .. 117 C8   23 59 S   45 39 E
Manas, China .... 68 B3   44 17N   85 56 E
Manas, Somali Rep. .. 120 D2   2 57N   43 28 E
Manas →, India ..... 90 B3   26 12N   90 40 E
Manas, Gora,
  Kyrgyzstan .... 65 B5   42 22N   71 2 E
Manaslu, Nepal ..... 93 E11   28 33N   84 33 E
Manasquan, U.S.A. .. 151 F10   40 8N   74 3W
Manassa, U.S.A. 159 H11   37 11N 105 56W
Manatí, Puerto Rico . . 165 d   18 26N   66 29W
Manati B., St. Helena 9 h   16 0 S   5 46W
Manatuto, E. Timor .. 82 C3   8 30 S 126 1 E
Manau, Papua N. G. .. 132 E4   8 2 S 148 0 E
Manaung, Burma .... 90 F4   18 45N   93 40 E
Manaus, Brazil ...... 169 D6   3 0 S   60 0W
Manavgat, Turkey .... 100 D4   36 47N   31 26 E
Manawan = Rizal, Phil. 80 C3   17 51N 121 21 E
Manawan L., Canada . 143 B8   55 24N 103 14W
Manawatu →, N.Z. .. 130 G4   40 28 S 175 17 E
Manawatu-
  Wanganui □, N.Z. . 130 F4   39 50 S 175 30 E
Manay, Phil. .... 81 H6   7 17N 126 33 E
Manbij, Syria .... 100 D7   36 31N   37 57 E
Mancha Real, Spain .. 43 H7   37 48N   3 39W
Manche □, France ... 26 C5   49 10N   1 20W
Manchegorsk, Russia . 66 C4   67 54N   32 58 E
Manchester, U.K. 20 D5   53 29N   2 12W

Manchester, Calif.,
  U.S.A. 160 G3   38 58N 123 41W
Manchester, Conn.,
  U.S.A. 151 E12   41 47N   72 31W
Manchester, Ga.,
  U.S.A. 155 J3   32 51N   84 37W
Manchester, Iowa,
  U.S.A. 156 M5   42 29N   91 27W
Manchester, Ky., U.S.A. 148 G4   37 9N   83 46W
Manchester, Mich.,
  U.S.A. 157 B12   42 9N   84 2W
Manchester, N.H.,
  U.S.A. 151 D13   42 59N   71 28W
Manchester, N.Y.,
  U.S.A. 150 D7   42 56N   77 16W
Manchester, Ohio,
  U.S.A. 157 F13   38 41N   83 36W
Manchester, Pa., U.S.A. 151 F8   40 4N   76 43W
Manchester, Tenn.,
  U.S.A. 149 H2   35 29N   86 5W
Manchester, Vt., U.S.A. 151 C11   43 10N   73 5W
Manchester
  International ✕
  (MAN) U.K. 20 D5   53 21N   2 17W
Manchester L., Canada 143 A7   61 28N 107 29W
Manchhar L., Pakistan 92 F2   26 25N   67 39 E
Manchuria = Dongbei,
  China .... 67 E13   45 0N 125 0 E
Manchurian Plain,
  China .... 62 E16   47 0N 124 0 E
Manciano, Italy ..... 45 F8   42 35N   11 31 E
Mancifa, Ethiopia ... 107 F5   6 53N   41 50 E
Mancora, Peru ...... 172 A1   4 9 S   81 1W
Manhiça, Mozam. .... 117 D5   25 23 S   32 49 E
Manhuaçu, Brazil .... 171 F3   20 15 S   42 2W
Manhumirim, Brazil .. 171 F3   20 22 S   41 57W
Maní, Colombia 168 C3   4 49N   72 17W
Mania →, Madag. ... 117 B8   19 42 S   45 22 E
Maniago, Italy ...... 45 B9   46 10N   12 43 E
Manica, Mozam. ..... 117 B5   18 58 S   32 59 E
Manica □, Mozam. ... 117 B5   19 10 S   33 45 E
Manicaland □,
  Zimbabwe .... 119 F3   19 0 S   32 30 E
Manicoré, Brazil ..... 173 B5   5 48 S   61 16W
Manicoré →, Brazil .. 175 A5   23 32 S   51 42W
Manicouagan →,
  Canada 141 C6   49 30N   68 30W
Manicouagan, Rés.,
  Canada 141 B6   51 5N   68 40W
Maniema □, Dem. Rep.
  of the Congo ...... 118 C2   3 0 S   26 0 E
Manifah, Si. Arabia .. 97 E6   27 44N   49 0 E
Manifold, C., Australia 126 C5   22 41 S 150 50 E
Maniganggo, China .. 76 B3   31 56N   99 10 E
Manigotagan, Canada 143 C9   51 6N   96 18W
Manigotagan →,
  Canada 143 C9   51 7N   96 20W
Manihari, India ..... 93 G12   25 21N   87 38 E
Manihiki, Cook Is. ... 135 J11   10 24 S 161 1W
Manihiki Plateau,
  Pac. Oc. .... 135 J11   11 0 S 164 0W
Maniitsoq, Greenland . 10 D5   65 26N   52 55W
Manika, Plateau de la,
  Dem. Rep. of
  the Congo .... 119 E2   10 0 S   25 5 E
Manikchhari, Bangla. . 90 D3   22 51N   91 50 E
Manikganj, Bangla. ... 90 D3   23 52N   90 0 E
Manikpur, India ..... 93 G9   25 4N   81 7 E
Manila, Phil. .... 80 D3   14 40N 121 3 E
Manila, U.S.A. 158 F9   40 59N 109 43W
Manila B., Phil. ..... 80 D3   14 40N 120 35 E
Manildra, Australia .. 129 B8   33 11 S 148 41 E
Manilla, Australia ... 129 A9   30 45 S 150 43 E
Manimpé, Mali 112 C3   14 11N   5 28W
Maningrida, Australia 126 A1   12 3 S 134 13 E
Maninian, Ivory C. ... 112 C3   10 3N   7 52W
Manipa, Indonesia ... 82 B3   3 17 S 127 35 E
Manipur □, India .... 90 C4   25 0N   94 0 E
Manipur →, Burma .. 90 C5   23 45N   94 20 E
Manisa, Turkey ...... 49 C9   38 38N   27 30 E
Manisa □, Turkey .... 49 C9   38 38N   28 0 E
Manistee, U.S.A. 148 C2   44 15N   86 19W
Manistee →, U.S.A. .. 148 C2   44 15N   86 21W
Manistique, U.S.A. ... 148 C2   45 57N   86 15W
Manito, U.S.A. 156 D7   40 26N   89 47W
Manitoba □, Canada . 143 B9   53 30N   97 0W
Manitoba, L., Canada . 143 C9   51 0N   98 45W
Manitou, Canada 143 D9   49 15N   98 32W
Manitou, U.S.A. 141 B6   56 55N   89 17W
Manitou Beach, U.S.A. 157 C12   41 58N   84 3W
Manitou Is., U.S.A. ... 148 C3   45 8N   86 0W
Manitou L., Canada .. 143 C7   52 43N 109 43W
Manitou Springs,
  U.S.A. 154 F2   38 52N 104 55W
Manitoulin I., Canada 140 C3   45 40N   82 30W
Manitouwadge, Canada 140 C2   49 8N   85 48W
Manitowoc, U.S.A. ... 148 C2   44 5N   87 40W
Manitsauá-Missu →,
  Brazil .... 173 C7   10 58 S   53 20W
Maniyachi, India .... 95 K3   8 51N   77 55 E
Manizales, Colombia . 168 B2   5 5N   75 32W
Manja, Madag. ...... 117 C7   21 26 S   44 20 E
Manjacaze, Mozam. .. 117 C5   24 45 S   34 0 E
Manjakandriana,
  Madag. .... 117 B8   18 55 S   47 47 E
Manjeri, India ...... 95 J3   11 7N   76 11 E
Manjhand, Pakistan .. 92 G3   25 50N   68 10 E
Manjil, Iran .... 97 B6   36 46N   49 30 E
Manjimup, Australia .. 125 F2   34 15 S 116 6 E
Manjlegaon, India ... 94 E3   19 9N   76 14 E
Manjra →, India ..... 94 E3   18 49N   77 52 E
Mankato, Kans., U.S.A. 154 F5   39 47N   98 13W
Mankato, Minn., U.S.A. 154 C8   44 10N   94 0W
Mankayan, Phil. ..... 80 C3   16 52N 120 47 E
Mankayane, Swaziland 117 D5   26 40 S   31 4 E
Mankera, Pakistan ... 92 D4   31 23N   71 26 E
Mankim, Cameroon .. 113 D7   5 1N   12 0 E
Mankono, Ivory C. ... 112 D3   8 1N   6 10W
Mankota, Canada 143 D7   49 25N 107 5W
Mankulam, Sri Lanka 95 K5   9 8N   80 26 E
Manlay = Üydzin,
  Mongolia .... 74 B4   44 9N 107 0 E
Manley Hot Springs,
  U.S.A. 144 D10   65 0N 150 38W
Manlleu, Spain ...... 40 C7   42 2N   2 17 E
Manly, Australia ..... 129 B9   33 48 S 151 17 E
Manmad, India ...... 94 E2   20 18N   74 28 E
Mann Ranges, Australia 125 E5   26 6 S 130 5 E
Manna, Indonesia .... 82 E2   4 25 S 102 55 E
Mannahill, Australia . 128 B4   32 25 S 140 0 E
Mannar, Sri Lanka ... 95 K4   9 1N   79 54 E
Mannar, G. of, Asia .. 95 K4   8 30N   79 0 E
Mannar I., Sri Lanka .. 95 K4   9 5N   79 45 E
Mannargudi, India ... 95 J4   10 45N   79 51 E
Männedorf, Switz. ... 33 B8   47 15N   8 42 E
Mannheim, Germany . 31 F4   49 29N   8 29 E
Manning, Canada 142 B5   56 53N 117 39W
Manning, Oreg., U.S.A. 160 E3   45 45N 123 13W
Manning, S.C., U.S.A. . 155 J5   33 42N   80 13W
Manning →, Australia 129 A10   31 52 S 152 43 E
Mangin Taungdan,
  Burma .... 90 C5   24 15N   95 45 E
Mangindrano, Madag. 117 A8   14 17 S   48 58 E
Mangkalihat, Tanjung,
  Indonesia .... 85 B5   1 2N 118 59 E
Mangla, Pakistan .... 93 C5   33 7N   73 39 E
Mangla Dam, Pakistan 93 C5   33 9N   73 44 E

Manglares, C.,
  Colombia 168 C2   1 36N   79 2W
Manglaur, India ..... 92 E7   29 44N   77 49 E
Mangnai, China ..... 68 C4   37 52N   91 43 E
Mango, Togo .... 113 C5   10 20N   0 30 E
Mango, Tonga ...... 133 Q14   20 17 S 175 22W
Mangoche, Malawi .. 119 E4   14 25 S   35 16 E
Mangoky →, Madag. 117 C7   21 29 S   43 41 E
Mangole, Indonesia .. 82 B3   1 50 S 125 55 E
Mangombe, Dem. Rep.
  of the Congo ...... 118 C2   1 20 S   26 48 E
Mangonui, N.Z. ..... 130 B2   35 1 S 173 32 E
Mangoro →, Madag. . 117 B8   20 0 S   48 45 E
Mangrol, Mad. P., India 92 J4   21 7N   70 7 E
Mangrol, Raj., India .. 92 G6   25 20N   76 31 E
Mangrul Pir, India .. 94 D3   20 19N   77 21 E
Manguaba = Pilar,
  Brazil .... 170 C4   9 36 S   35 56W
Mangualde, Portugal . 42 E3   40 38N   7 48W
Manguéni, Chad .... 109 F4   10 30N   21 15 E
Mangueira, L. da,
  Brazil .... 175 C5   33 0 S   52 50W
Manguéni, Hamada,
  Niger .... 108 D2   22 35N   12 40 E
Mangum, U.S.A. 155 H5   34 53N   99 30W
Mangungu, Dem. Rep.
  of the Congo ...... 115 D3   5 16 S   19 36 E
Mangyshlak,
  Poluostrov,
  Kazakhstan .... 66 E6   44 30N   52 30 E
Manhattan, U.S.A. ... 154 F6   39 11N   96 35W
Manhattan, U.S.A. ... 157 C9   41 26N   87 59W
Manhiça, Mozam. .... 117 D5   25 23 S   32 49 E
Manhuaçu, Brazil .... 171 F3   20 15 S   42 2W
Manhumirim, Brazil .. 171 F3   20 22 S   41 57W
Maní, Colombia 168 C3   4 49N   72 17W
Mania →, Madag. ... 117 B8   19 42 S   45 22 E
Maniago, Italy ...... 45 B9   46 10N   12 43 E
Manica, Mozam. ..... 117 B5   18 58 S   32 59 E
Manica □, Mozam. ... 117 B5   19 10 S   33 45 E
Mano, S. Leone 112 D2   8 3N   12 2W
Mano →, Liberia 112 D2   6 56N   11 30W
Mano River, Liberia .. 112 D2   7 20N   11 6W
Manoa, Bolivia ...... 173 B4   9 40 S   65 27W
Manoharpur, India ... 93 H11   22 23N   85 12 E
Manokotak, U.S.A. ... 144 G8   58 58N 159 3W
Manokwari, Indonesia 83 B4   0 54 S 134 0 E
Manolás, Greece .... 48 C3   38 4N   21 21 E
Manolo Fortich, Phil. 81 G5   8 28N 124 50 E
Manombo, Madag. ... 117 C7   22 57 S   43 28 E
Manono, Dem. Rep. of
  the Congo .... 118 D2   7 15 S   27 25 E
Manono, Samoa ..... 133 W23   13 50 S 172 5W
Manoppello, Italy .... 45 F11   42 15N   14 3 E
Manosque, France ... 29 E9   43 49N   5 47 E
Manotick, Canada ... 151 A9   45 13N   75 41W
Manouane →, Canada 141 C5   49 30N   71 10W
Manouane, L., Canada 141 B5   50 45N   70 45W
Manovo-Gounda Saint
  Floris △, C.A.R. ... 114 A4   9 30N   21 25 E
Manp'o, N. Korea ... 75 D14   41 6N 126 24 E
Manpojin = Manp'o,
  N. Korea .... 75 D14   41 6N 126 24 E
Manpur, Chhattisgarh,
  India .... 93 H10   23 17N   83 35 E
Manpur, Chhattisgarh,
  India .... 94 D5   20 22N   80 43 E
Manpur, Mad. P., India 92 H6   22 26N   75 37 E
Manresa, Spain ..... 40 D6   41 48N   1 50 E
Mansa, Gujarat, India . 92 H5   23 27N   72 45 E
Mansa, Punjab, India . 92 E6   30 0N   75 27 E
Mansa, Zambia ...... 119 E2   11 13 S   28 55 E
Mansalay, Phil. ...... 80 E3   12 31N 121 26 E
Mânsâsen, Sweden ... 16 A8   63 5N   14 18 E
Mansehra, Pakistan .. 92 B5   34 20N   73 15 E
Mansel I., Canada ... 139 B11   62 0N   80 0W
Mansfield, Australia . 129 D7   37 4 S 146 6 E
Mansfield, U.K. 20 D6   53 9N   1 11W
Mansfield, Ga., U.S.A. 155 E3   33 31N   83 44W
Mansfield, La., U.S.A. 155 K8   32 2N   93 43W
Mansfield, Mass.,
  U.S.A. 151 D13   42 2N   71 13W
Mansfield, Ohio, U.S.A. 150 F2   40 45N   82 31W
Mansfield, Pa., U.S.A. 150 E7   41 48N   77 5W
Mansfield, Tex., U.S.A. 155 J6   32 34N   97 9W
Mansfield, Mt., U.S.A. 151 B12   44 33N   72 49W
Mansidão, Brazil .... 170 D3   10 43 S   44 2W
Mansilla de las Mulas,
  Spain 42 C5   42 30N   5 25W
Mansle, France ...... 28 C4   45 52N   0 12 E
Mansoa, Guinea-Biss. 112 C1   12 0N   15 20W
Manson Creek, Canada 142 B4   55 37N 124 32W
Mansoura, Algeria ... 111 A5   36 1N   4 31 E
Manta, Ecuador ..... 168 D1   1 0 S   80 40W
Manta, B. de, Ecuador 168 D1   0 54 S   80 44W
Mantadia △, Madag. . 117 B8   18 54 S   48 21 E
Mantalingajan, Mt.,
  Phil. .... 81 G1   8 55N 117 45 E
Mantare, Tanzania ... 118 C3   2 42 S   33 13 E
Mantaro →, Peru .... 172 C3   12 16 S   73 57W
Manteca, U.S.A. 160 H5   37 48N 121 13W
Manteca, Venezuela .. 168 B4   7 34N   69 17W
Mantena, Brazil ..... 171 E3   18 47 S   40 59W
Manteo, U.S.A. 157 C9   41 15N   87 50W
Manteo, U.S.A. 149 H8   35 55N   75 40W
Mantes-la-Jolie, France 27 D8   48 58N   1 41 E
Mantha, India ...... 94 E3   19 40N   76 23 E
Manthani, India ..... 94 E4   18 40N   79 40 E
Manti, U.S.A. 158 G8   39 16N 111 38W
Mantiqueira, Serra da,
  Brazil .... 171 F3   22 0 S   44 0W
Mantorp, Sweden .... 17 F9   58 21N   15 20 E
Mántova, Italy ...... 44 C7   45 9N   10 48 E
Mänttä, Finland ..... 15 E21   62 3N   24 40 E
Mantua = Mántova,
  Italy .... 44 C7   45 9N   10 48 E
Manturovo, Russia ... 60 A7   58 23N   44 45 E
Manu, Peru .... 172 C3   12 10 S   70 51W
Manu →, Peru ...... 172 C3   12 16 S   70 55W
Manu'a Is.,
  Amer. Samoa ..... 133 X25   14 13 S 169 35W
Manuel Alves →,
  Brazil .... 170 D2   11 19 S   48 28W
Manuel Alves
  Grande →, Brazil .. 170 C2   7 27 S   47 35W
Manuel Urbano, Brazil 172 B4   8 53 S   69 18W
Manui, Indonesia .... 82 B2   3 35 S 123 5 E
Manukan, Phil. ...... 81 G4   8 32N 123 12 E
Manukau, Phil. ...... 130 D3   37 0 S 174 52 E
Manukau Harbour,
  N.Z. .... 130 D3   37 3 S 174 45 E
Manui, India .... 95 K3   8 51N   77 55 E
Manunui, N.Z. ...... 130 E4   38 54 S 175 21 E
Manuoha, N.Z. ..... 130 E6   38 39 S 177 7 E
Manus □, Papua N. G. 132 A2   1 6 S 147 0 E
Manus □, Papua N. G. 132 B2   2 0 S 147 0 E
Manvi, India .... 95 G3   15 57N   76 59 E
Manwath, India ..... 94 E3   19 19N   76 32 E
Many, U.S.A. 155 K8   31 34N   93 29W
Manyara, L., Tanzania 118 C4   3 40 S   35 50 E
Manyas, Turkey ..... 51 F11   40 2N   27 59 E
Manyas Gölü = Kuş
  Gölü, Turkey ...... 51 F11   40 10N   27 55 E
Manyava, Ukraine ... 53 B9   48 39N   24 21 E
Manych →, Russia ... 61 G5   47 13N   40 40 E
Manych-Gudilo, Ozero,
  Russia .... 61 G6   46 24N   42 38 E
Manyonga →,
  Tanzania .... 118 C3   4 10 S   34 15 E
Manyoni, Tanzania .. 118 D3   5 45 S   34 55 E
Manzai, Pakistan .... 92 C4   32 12N   70 15 E
Manzala, Bahra el,
  Egypt .... 106 H7   31 10N   31 56 E
Manzanar △, U.S.A. . 160 J7   36 44N 119 5W
Manzanares, Spain .. 43 F7   39 2N   3 22W
Manzanillo, Cuba ... 164 B4   20 20N   77 31W
Manzanillo, Mexico .. 162 D4   19 0N 104 20W
Manzanillo, Pta.,
  Panama 164 E4   9 30N   79 40W
Manzano Mts., U.S.A. 159 J10   34 40N 106 20W
Manzarīyeh, Iran .... 97 C6   34 53N   50 50 E
Manzhouli, China ... 73 B6   49 35N 117 25 E
Manzini, Swaziland .. 117 D5   26 30 S   31 25 E
Manzou, Chad ...... 109 F3   12 26N   18 38 E
Maó, Spain .... 38 B5   39 53N   4 16 E
Maoka = Kholmsk,
  Russia .... 67 E15   47 40N 142 5 E
Maolin, China ...... 75 C12   43 42N   71 13 E
Maoming, China .... 77 G8   21 50N 110 54 E
Maopi T'ou, China .. 77 G13   21 56N 120 43 E
Maouri, Dallol →,
  Niger .... 113 C5   12 5N   3 32 E
Maoxian, China ..... 76 B4   31 41N 103 49 E
Maoxing, China ..... 75 B13   45 28N 124 40 E

Mapalma, Dem. Rep. of the Congo .... **114 B4** 2 3N 24 30 E
Mapam Yumco, China ...... **68 C3** 30 45N 81 28 E
Mapastepec, Mexico **163 D6** 15 26N 92 54W
Mapfongui, Gabon ...... **114 C2** 1 15 S 12 59 E
Maphrao, Ko, Thailand ...... **87 a** 7 56N 98 24 E
Mapi →, Indonesia ...... **83 C5** 6 55 S 139 14 E
Mapia, Kepulauan, Indonesia ...... **83 A4** 0 50N 134 20 E
Mapimí, Mexico **162 B4** 25 50N 103 50W
Mapimí, Bolsón de, Mexico **162 B4** 27 30N 104 15W
Maping, China ...... **77 B9** 31 34N 113 32 E
Mapinga, Tanzania ...... **118 D4** 6 40 S 39 12 E
Mapinhane, Mozam. ...... **117 C6** 22 20 S 35 0 E
Mapire, Venezuela **169 B5** 7 45N 64 42W
Maple →, U.S.A. **157 B12** 42 59N 84 57W
Maple Creek, Canada **143 D7** 49 55N 109 29W
Maple Valley, U.S.A. **160 C4** 47 25N 122 3W
Mapleton, U.S.A. **158 D2** 44 2N 123 52W
Mapourika, L., N.Z. ...... **131 D5** 43 16 S 170 12 E
Maprik, Papua N. G. ...... **132 B2** 3 44 S 143 3 E
Mapuca, India ...... **95 G1** 15 36N 73 46 E
Mapuera →, Brazil ...... **169 D6** 1 5 S 57 2W
Mapulanguene, Mozam. ...... **117 C5** 24 29 S 32 6 E
Maputo, Mozam. ...... **117 D5** 25 58 S 32 32 E
Maputo □, Mozam. ...... **117 D5** 26 23 S 32 48 E
Maputo →, Mozam. ...... **117 D5** 26 0 S 32 25 E
Maputo, B. de, Mozam. ...... **117 D5** 25 50 S 32 45 E
Maqiaohe, China ...... **75 B16** 44 40N 130 30 E
Maqnā, Si. Arabia ...... **96 D2** 28 25N 34 50 E
Maqran, W. →, Si. Arabia ...... **98 B4** 20 55N 47 12 E
Maqteïr, Mauritania **110 D2** 21 50N 11 40W
Maquan He = Brahmaputra →, Asia ...... **68 D3** 23 40N 90 35 E
Maqueda, Spain **42 E6** 40 4N 4 22W
Maqueda Channel, Phil. ...... **80 E5** 13 42N 124 1 E
Maquela do Zombo, Angola ...... **115 D3** 6 0 S 15 15 E
Maquinchao, Argentina ...... **176 B3** 41 15 S 68 50W
Maquoketa, U.S.A. **156 B6** 42 4N 90 40W
Mar, Serra do, Brazil ...... **175 B6** 25 30 S 49 0W
Mar Chiquita, L., Argentina ...... **174 C3** 30 40 S 62 50W
Mar del Plata, Argentina ...... **174 D4** 38 0 S 57 30W
Mar Menor, Spain **41 H4** 37 40N 0 45W
Mara, Guyana **169 B6** 6 0N 57 36W
Mara, India ...... **90 A5** 28 11N 94 14 E
Mara, Tanzania ...... **118 C3** 1 30 S 34 32 E
Mara □, Tanzania ...... **118 C3** 1 45 S 34 20 E
Maraã, Brazil ...... **168 D4** 1 52 S 65 25W
Marabá, Brazil ...... **170 C2** 5 20 S 49 5W
Maracá, I. de, Brazil **169 C7** 2 10N 50 30W
Maracaibo, Venezuela **168 A3** 10 40N 71 37W
Maracaibo, L. de, Venezuela **168 B3** 9 40N 71 30W
Maracaju, Brazil ...... **173 E6** 20 57 S 55 1W
Maracajú, Serra de, Brazil ...... **173 E6** 21 38 S 55 9W
Maracaná, Brazil ...... **170 B2** 0 46 S 47 27W
Maracás, Brazil ...... **171 D3** 13 26 S 40 18W
Maracas Bay Village, Trin. & Tob. **169 F9** 10 46N 61 28W
Maracay, Venezuela **168 A5** 10 15N 67 28W
Maracena, Spain **43 H7** 37 12N 3 38W
Marādah, Libya ...... **108 C3** 29 15N 19 15 E
Maradi, Niger ...... **113 C6** 13 29N 7 20 E
Maraetiria, Pte., Tahiti ...... **133 S16** 17 51 S 149 10W
Marāgheh, Iran ...... **101 D12** 37 30N 46 12 E
Maragogipe, Brazil ...... **171 D4** 12 46 S 38 55W
Marāh, Si. Arabia ...... **96 E5** 25 0N 45 35 E
Marahoué →, Ivory C. **112 D3** 8 0N 7 8W
Marais du Cotentin et du Bessin △, France **26 C5** 49 10N 1 30W
Marais Poitevin, Val de Sèvre et Vendée △, France **28 B3** 46 18N 0 35W
Maraisburg = Hofmeyr, S. Africa ...... **116 E4** 31 39 S 25 50 E
Marajó, B. de, Brazil ...... **170 B2** 1 0 S 49 30W
Marajó, I. de, Brazil ...... **170 B1** 1 0 S 49 30W
Marākand, Iran ...... **101 C11** 38 51N 45 16 E
Marakele △, S. Africa ...... **117 E4** 32 14 S 27 27 E
Maralal, Kenya ...... **118 B4** 1 0N 36 38 E
Maralinga, Australia ...... **125 F5** 30 13 S 131 32 E
Maram, India ...... **90 C5** 25 25N 94 6 E
Marama, Australia ...... **128 C4** 35 10 S 140 10 E
Maramag, Phil. ...... **81 H5** 7 46N 125 0 E
Maramaereğlisi, Turkey ...... **51 F11** 40 57N 27 57 E
Maramasike, Solomon Is. ...... **133 M11** 9 30 S 161 25 E
Marambio, Antarctica ...... **7 C18** 64 0 S 56 0W
Marampa, S. Leone **112 D2** 8 45N 12 28W
Maramureș □, Romania ...... **53 C9** 47 45N 24 0 E
Maran, Malaysia ...... **87 L4** 3 35N 102 45 E
Marana, U.S.A. **159 K8** 32 27N 111 13W
Maranboy, Australia ...... **124 B5** 14 40 S 132 39 E
Maranchón, Spain **40 D2** 41 6N 2 15W
Marand, Iran ...... **101 C11** 38 30N 45 45 E
Marandokhōri, Greece ...... **39 B2** 38 38N 20 39 E
Marang, Malaysia ...... **87 K4** 5 12N 103 13 E
Maranguape, Brazil ...... **170 B4** 3 55 S 38 50W
Maranhão = São Luís, Brazil ...... **170 B3** 2 39 S 44 15W
Maranhão □, Brazil ...... **170 B2** 5 0 S 46 0W
Marano, L. di, Italy ...... **45 C10** 45 44N 13 10 E
Maranoa →, Australia ...... **127 D4** 27 50 S 148 37 E
Marañón →, Peru ...... **172 A3** 4 30 S 73 35W
Marão, Mozam. ...... **117 C5** 24 18 S 34 2 E
Marapi →, Brazil **169 C6** 0 37N 55 58W
Marari, Brazil ...... **172 B4** 5 43 S 67 47W
Maraş = Kahramanmaraş, Turkey ...... **100 D7** 37 37N 36 53 E
Mărășești, Romania ...... **53 E12** 45 52N 27 14 E
Maratea, Italy ...... **47 C8** 39 59N 15 43 E
Marateca, Portugal **43 G2** 38 34N 8 40W
Marathasa, Cyprus ...... **39 F8** 34 59N 32 51 E
Marathiás, Ákra, Greece ...... **39 D2** 37 39N 20 50 E
Marathókambos, Greece ...... **49 D8** 37 43N 26 42 E
Marathon, Australia ...... **126 C3** 20 51 S 143 32 E
Marathon, Canada **140 C2** 48 44N 86 23W
Marathon, Greece ...... **38 C5** 38 11N 23 58 E
Marathon, Fla., U.S.A. **153 L8** 24 43N 81 5W
Marathon, N.Y., U.S.A. **151 D8** 42 27N 76 2W
Marathon, Tex., U.S.A. **155 K3** 30 12N 103 15W
Marathóvouno, Cyprus ...... **39 D12** 35 13N 33 37 E
Maratua, Indonesia ...... **85 B5** 2 10N 118 35 E
Maraú, Brazil ...... **171 D4** 14 6 S 39 0W
Marau, Solomon Is. ...... **133 N11** 10 31 S 161 31 E
Maraval, Trin. & Tob. **169 F9** 10 42N 61 31W
Maravari, Solomon Is. ...... **133 L9** 7 50 S 156 42 E
Maravatío, Mexico **162 D4** 19 51N 100 25W
Marawi City, Phil. ...... **81 G5** 8 0N 124 21 E
Marāwih, U.A.E. ...... **97 E7** 24 18N 53 18 E

Marazliyivka ...... **53 D15** 46 8N 30 3 E
Marbach, Switz. ...... **32 C5** 46 51N 7 53 E
Marbella, Spain **43 J6** 36 30N 4 57W
Marble Bar, Australia ...... **124 D2** 21 9 S 119 44 E
Marble Falls, U.S.A. **155 K5** 30 35N 98 16W
Marblehead, U.S.A. **151 D14** 42 30N 70 51W
Mårbu, Norway ...... **18 D5** 60 11N 8 9 E
Marburg = Maribor, Slovenia ...... **45 B12** 46 36N 15 40 E
Marburg, Germany ...... **30 E4** 50 47N 8 46 E
Marcal →, Hungary ...... **52 C2** 47 41N 17 40 E
Marcali, Hungary ...... **52 D2** 46 35N 17 25 E
Marcapata, Peru ...... **172 C3** 13 31 S 70 52W
Marcaria, Italy ...... **44 C7** 45 7N 10 32 E
Mărcăuți, Moldova ...... **53 B12** 48 20N 27 14 E
Marceline, U.S.A. **156 E4** 39 43N 92 57W
March, U.K. ...... **21 E8** 52 33N 0 5 E
Marchal, Dem. Rep. of the Congo ...... **115 D2** 5 16 S 14 58 E
Marchand = Rommani, Morocco **110 B3** 33 31N 6 40W
Marche, France ...... **28 B5** 46 5N 1 20 E
Marche □, Italy ...... **45 E10** 43 30N 13 15 E
Marche-en-Famenne, Belgium ...... **24 D5** 50 14N 5 19 E
Marchena, Spain **43 H5** 37 18N 5 23W
Marchena, Canal de, Ecuador ...... **172 a** 0 19N 90 12W
Marchena, I., Ecuador ...... **172 a** 0 19N 90 29W
Marches = Marche □, Italy ...... **45 E10** 43 30N 13 15 E
Marchesale △, Italy ...... **47 D9** 38 32N 16 13 E
Marciana Marina, Italy ...... **44 F7** 42 48N 10 12 E
Marcianise, Italy ...... **47 A7** 41 2N 14 17 E
Marcigny, France ...... **27 F11** 46 17N 4 2 E
Marcillat-en-Combraille, France ...... **27 F9** 46 12N 2 38 E
Marck, France ...... **27 B8** 50 57N 1 57 E
Marcksheim, France ...... **27 D14** 48 10N 7 30 E
Marco Island, U.S.A. **153 N5** 25 58N 81 44W
Marco Rondon, Brazil ...... **173 C5** 12 0 S 60 56W
Marcona, Peru ...... **172 D2** 15 10 S 75 0W
Marcos Juárez, Argentina ...... **174 C3** 32 42 S 62 5W
Mărculești, Moldova ...... **53 C13** 47 52N 28 14 E
Marcus Baker, Mt., U.S.A. **144 F11** 61 26N 147 45W
Marcus I. = Minami-Tori-Shima, Pac. Oc. ...... **134 E7** 24 20N 153 58 E
Marcus Necker Ridge, Pac. Oc. ...... **134 F9** 20 0N 175 0 E
Marcy, Mt., U.S.A. **151 B11** 44 7N 73 56W
Mardan, Pakistan ...... **91 B4** 34 20N 72 0 E
Mardarivka, Ukraine ...... **53 C14** 47 32N 29 44 E
Mardin, Turkey ...... **101 D9** 37 20N 40 43 E
Mårdsjö, Sweden ...... **16 A9** 63 18N 15 35 E
Maré, Î., N. Cal. ...... **13 U22** 21 30 S 168 0 E
Marécchia →, Italy ...... **45 D9** 44 4N 12 34 E
Marechal Deodoro, Brazil ...... **170 C4** 9 43 S 35 54W
Marechal Floriano = Piranhas, Brazil ...... **170 C4** 9 27 S 37 46W
Maree, L., U.K. **22 D3** 57 40N 5 26W
Mareeba, Australia ...... **126 B4** 16 59 S 145 28 E
Mareetsane, S. Africa ...... **116 D4** 26 9 S 25 25 E
Marek, Indonesia ...... **82 B2** 4 41 S 120 24 E
Maremma, Italy ...... **45 F8** 42 30N 11 30 E
Maremma →, Italy ...... **44 F8** 42 35N 11 8 E
Maréna, Kayes, Mali **112 C2** 14 36N 10 45W
Maréna, Koulikouro, Mali **112 C3** 13 55N 7 20W
Marengo, Ind., U.S.A. **157 F10** 38 22N 86 21W
Marengo, Iowa, U.S.A. **156 C4** 41 48N 92 4W
Marennes, France **28 C2** 45 49N 1 7W
Marerano, Madag. ...... **117 C7** 21 23 S 44 52 E
Maréttimo, Italy ...... **46 E5** 37 58N 12 4 E
Mareuil, France ...... **28 C4** 45 27N 0 28 E
Marfa, U.S.A. **155 K2** 30 19N 104 1W
Marganets = Marhanets, Ukraine ...... **59 J8** 47 40N 34 40 E
Margaret →, Australia ...... **124 C4** 18 9 S 125 41 E
Margaret Bay, Canada **142 C3** 51 20N 127 35W
Margaret L., Canada **142 B5** 58 56N 115 25W
Margaret River, Australia ...... **125 F2** 33 57 S 115 4 E
Margarita, I. de, Venezuela **169 A5** 11 0N 64 0W
Margarition, Greece ...... **48 B2** 39 22N 20 26 E
Margaritovo, Russia ...... **70 C7** 43 25N 134 45 E
Margate, S. Africa ...... **117 E5** 30 50 S 30 20 E
Margate, U.K. ...... **21 F9** 51 23N 1 23 E
Margate, U.S.A. **153 J9** 26 15N 80 12W
Margeride, Mts. de la, France ...... **28 D7** 44 43N 3 38 E
Marggrabowa = Olecko, Poland ...... **54 D9** 54 2N 22 31 E
Margherita, India ...... **90 B5** 27 16N 95 40 E
Margherita di Savóia, Italy ...... **47 A9** 41 22N 16 9 E
Margherita Pk., Uganda ...... **118 B3** 0 22N 29 51 E
Marghilon = Margilan, Uzbekistan ...... **65 C5** 40 27N 71 42 E
Marghita, Romania ...... **52 C7** 47 22N 22 22 E
Margilan, Uzbekistan ...... **65 C5** 40 27N 71 42 E
Margonin, Poland ...... **55 F4** 52 58N 17 5 E
Margosatubig, Phil. ...... **81 H4** 7 34N 123 10 E
Mărgow, Dasht-e, Afghan. ...... **91 C1** 30 40N 62 30 E
Marguerite, Canada **142 C4** 52 30N 122 25W
Marhanets, Ukraine ...... **59 J8** 47 40N 34 40 E
Marhoum, Algeria **111 B4** 34 27N 0 11W
Mari, Papua N. G. ...... **132 E1** 9 11 S 141 42 E
Mari El □, Russia ...... **60 B8** 56 30N 48 0 E
Mari Indus, Pakistan ...... **92 C4** 32 57N 71 34 E
Mari Republic = Mari El □, Russia ...... **60 B8** 56 30N 48 0 E
María, Sa. de, Spain **41 H2** 37 39N 2 14W
María Aurora, Phil. ...... **80 D3** 15 48N 121 28 E
María Elena, Chile ...... **174 A2** 22 18 S 69 40W
María Grande, Argentina ...... **174 C4** 31 45 S 59 55W
Maria I., N. Terr., Australia ...... **126 A2** 14 52 S 135 45 E
Maria I., Tas., Australia ...... **127 G4** 42 35 S 148 0 E
Maria Island △, Australia ...... **127 G4** 42 38 S 148 5 E
Maria Pereira, Brazil ...... **170 C4** 5 43 S 39 45W
Maria Theresiopel = Subotica, Serbia & M. ...... **52 D4** 46 6N 19 39 E
Maria van Diemen, C., N.Z. ...... **130 A1** 34 29 S 172 40 E
Mariager, Denmark ...... **17 H3** 56 40N 9 59 E
Mariager Fjord, Denmark ...... **17 H4** 56 42N 10 19 E
Mariakani, Kenya ...... **118 C4** 3 50 S 39 27 E
Mariala △, Australia ...... **127 D4** 25 57 S 145 2 E
Marian △, Australia ...... **126 K6** 21 9 S 148 57 E
Marian L., Canada **142 A5** 63 0N 116 15W
Mariana Trench, Pac. Oc. ...... **62 H18** 13 0N 145 0 E
Marianao, Cuba **164 B3** 23 8N 82 24W
Mariani, India ...... **90 B5** 26 39N 94 19 E

Marianica, Cord. = Morena, Sierra, Spain **43 G7** 38 20N 4 0W
Marianna, Ark., U.S.A. **155 H9** 34 46N 90 46W
Marianna, Fla., U.S.A. **152 E4** 30 46N 85 14W
Mariannelund, Sweden ...... **17 G9** 57 37N 15 35 E
Mariánské Lázně, Czech Rep. ...... **34 B5** 49 58N 12 41 E
Marias →, U.S.A. **158 C8** 47 56N 110 30W
Mariato, Punta, Panama **164 E3** 7 12N 80 52W
Mariazell, Austria ...... **34 D8** 47 47N 15 19 E
Ma'rib, Yemen ...... **98 D4** 15 25N 45 21 E
Maribo, Denmark ...... **17 K5** 54 48N 11 30 E
Maribor, Slovenia ...... **45 B12** 46 36N 15 40 E
Maricaban I., Phil. ...... **80 E3** 13 39N 120 53 E
Marico →, Africa ...... **116 C4** 23 35 S 26 57 E
Maricopa, Ariz., U.S.A. **159 K7** 33 4N 112 3W
Maricopa, Calif., U.S.A. **161 K7** 35 4N 119 24W
Marīdī, Sudan ...... **107 G2** 4 55N 29 25 E
Marīdī, Wadi →, Sudan ...... **107 F2** 6 5N 29 2 E
Marié →, Brazil ...... **168 D4** 0 27 S 66 26W
Marie Byrd Land, Antarctica ...... **7 D14** 79 30 S 125 0W
Marie-Galante, Guadeloupe ...... **164 b** 15 56N 61 16W
Mariecourt = Kangiqsujuaq, Canada **139 B12** 61 30N 72 0W
Mariefred, Sweden ...... **16 E11** 59 15N 17 12 E
Mariehamn = Maarianhamina, Finland ...... **15 F18** 60 5N 19 55 E
Marieholm, Sweden ...... **17 J7** 55 53N 13 10 E
Mariembourg, Belgium ...... **24 D4** 50 6N 4 31 E
Marienbad = Mariánské Lázně, Czech Rep. ...... **34 B5** 49 58N 12 41 E
Marienberg, Germany ...... **30 E9** 50 39N 13 9 E
Marienburg = Malbork, Poland ...... **54 D6** 54 3N 19 1 E
Mariental, Namibia ...... **116 C2** 24 36 S 18 0 E
Marienville, U.S.A. **150 E5** 41 28N 79 8W
Mariestad, Sweden ...... **17 F7** 58 43N 13 50 E
Marietta, Ga., U.S.A. **152 B5** 33 57N 84 33W
Marietta, Ohio, U.S.A. **148 F5** 39 25N 81 27W
Marieville, Canada **151 A11** 45 26N 73 10W
Mariga →, Nigeria ...... **113 C6** 9 40N 5 55 E
Marignac, France ...... **29 F4** 42 55N 0 38 E
Marignane, France ...... **29 E9** 43 25N 5 13 E
Marigny, France ...... **32 D3** 46 6N 6 31 E
Marihatag, Phil. ...... **81 G6** 8 48N 126 18 E
Mariinsk, Russia ...... **66 D9** 56 10N 87 20 E
Mariinsk Water = Volgo-Baltiyskiy Kanal, Russia ...... **58 B9** 60 0N 38 0 E
Mariinskiy Posad, Russia ...... **60 B8** 56 10N 47 45 E
Marijampolė, Lithuania ...... **15 J20** 54 33N 23 19 E
Marijampolė □, Lithuania ...... **54 D10** 54 34N 23 21 E
Marília, Brazil ...... **175 A6** 22 13 S 50 0W
Marimba, Angola ...... **115 D3** 8 28 S 17 8 E
Marín, Spain **42 C2** 42 23N 8 42W
Marina, U.S.A. **160 J5** 36 41N 121 48W
Marinduque, Phil. ...... **79 B6** 13 25N 122 0 E
Marinduque □, Phil. ...... **80 E4** 13 18N 122 0 E
Marine City, U.S.A. **150 D2** 42 43N 82 30W
Marineland, U.S.A. **152 F8** 29 40N 81 13W
Marineo, Italy ...... **46 E6** 37 57N 13 25 E
Marinette, U.S.A. **148 C2** 45 6N 87 38W
Maringá, Brazil ...... **175 A5** 23 26 S 52 2W
Maringa →, Dem. Rep. of the Congo ...... **114 B3** 1 14N 19 48 E
Marinha Grande, Portugal **42 F2** 39 45N 8 56W
Marinho dos Abrolhos △, Brazil ...... **171 E4** 17 50 S 39 0W
Marino, Italy ...... **45 G9** 41 46N 12 39 E
Marion, Ala., U.S.A. **149 J2** 32 38N 87 19W
Marion, Ill., U.S.A. **155 G10** 37 44N 88 56W
Marion, Ind., U.S.A. **157 D11** 40 32N 85 40W
Marion, Iowa, U.S.A. **156 B5** 42 2N 91 36W
Marion, Kans., U.S.A. **154 F6** 38 21N 97 1W
Marion, N.C., U.S.A. **149 H5** 35 41N 82 1W
Marion, Ohio, U.S.A. **157 D13** 40 35N 83 8W
Marion, S.C., U.S.A. **149 H6** 34 9N 79 24W
Marion, Va., U.S.A. **149 G5** 36 50N 81 31W
Marion, Bay, Australia ...... **128 C2** 35 12 S 136 59 E
Marion I., Ind. Oc. ...... **121 J2** 47 0 S 37 59 E
Maripa, Venezuela **169 B4** 7 26N 65 9W
Maripasoula, Fr. Guiana **169 C7** 3 40N 54 4W
Mariposa, U.S.A. **160 H7** 37 29N 119 58W
Mariscal Estigarribia, Paraguay ...... **174 A3** 22 3 S 60 40W
Marisa, Indonesia ...... **83 B6** 0 28N 121 56 E
Marismas, Spain **43 H4** 37 0N 6 20W
Marissa, U.S.A. **156 F7** 38 15N 89 45W
Maritime Alps = Maritimes, Alpes, Europe ...... **29 D11** 44 10N 7 10 E
Maritimes, Alpes, Europe ...... **29 D11** 44 10N 7 10 E
Maritsa →, Greece ...... **100 B2** 41 40N 26 34 E
Maritsá, Greece ...... **38 E12** 36 22N 28 8 E
Marium, Mt., Vanuatu ...... **133 F6** 16 15 S 168 7 E
Mariupol, Ukraine ...... **59 J9** 47 5N 37 31 E
Mariusa →, Venezuela **165 E7** 9 44N 61 27W
Marīvān, Iran ...... **101 E12** 35 30N 46 25 E
Mariveles, Phil. ...... **80 D3** 14 26N 120 29 E
Marj 'Uyūn, Lebanon ...... **103 B4** 33 20N 35 35 E
Marj = Wazikhwah, Afghan. ...... **91 B3** 32 11N 68 21 E
Mark Twain L., U.S.A. **156 E8** 39 28N 91 55W
Marka = Merca, Somali Rep. ...... **120 D2** 1 48N 44 50 E
Marka, Si. Arabia ...... **106 D5** 18 14N 41 19 E
Markam, China ...... **76 C2** 29 42N 98 38 E
Markapur, India ...... **95 G4** 15 44N 79 19 E
Markaryd, Sweden ...... **17 H7** 56 28N 13 35 E
Markat, Albania ...... **38 B10** 39 44N 20 12 E
Markdale, Canada **150 B4** 44 19N 80 39W
Marked Tree, U.S.A. **155 H9** 35 32N 90 25W
Markelsdorfer Huk, Germany ...... **30 A7** 54 33N 11 4 E
Market Drayton, U.K. **20 E5** 52 54N 2 29W
Market Harborough, U.K. **21 E7** 52 29N 0 55W
Market Rasen, U.K. **20 D7** 53 24N 0 20W
Markham, Canada **150 C5** 43 52N 79 16W
Markham →, Papua N. G. ...... **132 D4** 6 41 S 147 2 E
Markham, Mt., Antarctica ...... **7 E11** 83 0 S 164 0 E
Marki, Russia ...... **55 F8** 52 20N 21 2 E
Märkisch Friedland = Mirosławiec, Poland ...... **54 B2** 53 20N 16 5 E
Märkische Schweiz △, Germany ...... **30 C10** 52 34N 14 2 E
Markit, China ...... **65 D8** 38 53N 77 35 E
Markkleeberg, Germany ...... **30 D8** 51 16N 12 23 E
Markleeville, U.S.A. **160 G7** 38 42N 119 47W
Markounda, C.A.R. ...... **114 A3** 7 39N 16 55 E
Markoupoulo, Greece ...... **48 D5** 37 53N 23 57 E
Markovac, Serbia & M. ...... **50 B5** 44 14N 21 7 E
Markovo, Russia ...... **67 C17** 64 40N 170 24 E

Markoye, Burkina Faso ...... **113 C5** 14 39N 0 2 E
Marks, Russia ...... **60 E8** 51 45N 46 50 E
Marksshtadt = Marks, Russia ...... **60 E8** 51 45N 46 50 E
Marksville, U.S.A. **155 K8** 31 8N 92 4W
Markt Schwaben, Germany ...... **31 G7** 48 11N 11 52 E
Marktoberdorf, Germany ...... **31 H6** 47 45N 10 37 E
Marktredwitz, Germany ...... **31 E8** 50 1N 12 6 E
Marl, Germany ...... **30 D3** 51 39N 7 4 E
Marla, Australia ...... **127 D1** 27 19 S 133 33 E
Marlbank, Canada **150 B7** 44 26N 77 6W
Marlboro, Mass., U.S.A. **151 D13** 42 19N 71 33W
Marlboro, N.Y., U.S.A. **151 E11** 41 36N 73 59W
Marlborough, Australia ...... **126 C4** 22 46 S 149 52 E
Marlborough, U.K. **21 F6** 51 25N 1 43W
Marlborough □, N.Z. ...... **131 D5** 41 45 S 173 33 E
Marlborough Downs, U.K. **21 F6** 51 27N 1 53W
Marle, France ...... **27 C10** 49 43N 3 47 E
Marlin, U.S.A. **155 K6** 31 18N 96 54W
Marlow, Germany ...... **30 A8** 54 9N 12 33 E
Marlow, U.K. **21 F7** 51 34N 0 46W
Marlow, U.S.A. **155 H6** 34 39N 97 58W
Marly, Switz. ...... **32 C4** 46 47N 7 10 E
Marmagao, India ...... **95 G1** 15 25N 73 56 E
Marmande, France ...... **28 D4** 44 30N 0 10 E
Marmara, Turkey ...... **51 F11** 40 35N 27 34 E
Marmara, Sea of = Marmara Denizi, Turkey ...... **51 F12** 40 45N 28 15 E
Marmara Denizi, Turkey ...... **51 F12** 40 45N 28 15 E
Marmara Gölü, Turkey ...... **49 C10** 38 37N 28 2 E
Marmaris, Turkey ...... **49 E10** 36 50N 28 14 E
Marmaris Limanı, Turkey ...... **49 E10** 36 50N 28 19 E
Marmelos →, Brazil ...... **173 B5** 6 8 S 61 46W
Marmion, Mt., Australia ...... **125 E2** 29 16 S 119 50 E
Marmion L., Canada **140 C1** 48 55N 91 20W
Marmolada, Mte., Italy ...... **45 B8** 46 26N 11 51 E
Marmolejo, Spain **43 G6** 38 3N 4 13W
Marmora, Canada **140 D4** 44 28N 77 41W
Mármora, La, Italy ...... **46 C2** 39 59N 9 20 E
Marnay, France ...... **27 E12** 47 16N 5 48 E
Marne, Germany ...... **30 B5** 53 56N 9 2 E
Marne □, France ...... **27 D11** 48 59N 4 10 E
Marne →, France ...... **27 D9** 48 48N 2 24 E
Marneuli, Georgia ...... **61 K7** 41 30N 44 48 E
Marnia = Maghnia, Algeria **111 B4** 34 50N 1 43W
Marnoo, Australia ...... **128 D5** 36 40 S 142 52 E
Maro, Chad ...... **109 G3** 8 30N 19 0 E
Maro Reef, U.S.A. **145 F9** 25 25N 170 35W
Maroa, U.S.A. **156 D6** 40 2N 88 57W
Maroa, Venezuela **168 C4** 2 43N 67 33W
Maroala, Madag. ...... **117 B8** 15 23 S 47 59 E
Maroantsetra, Madag. ...... **117 B8** 15 26 S 49 44 E
Maroelaboom, Namibia ...... **116 B2** 19 15 S 18 53 E
Marofandilia, Madag. ...... **117 C7** 20 7 S 44 34 E
Marojejy △, Madag. ...... **117 A8** 14 26 S 49 21 E
Marolambo, Madag. ...... **117 C8** 20 2 S 48 7 E
Maromandia, Madag. ...... **117 A8** 14 13 S 48 5 E
Maromokotro, Madag. ...... **117 A8** 14 0 S 49 0 E
Marondera, Zimbabwe ...... **119 F3** 18 5 S 31 42 E
Maroni →, Fr. Guiana **169 B7** 5 30N 54 0W
Marónia, Greece ...... **51 F9** 40 53N 25 30 E
Maronne →, France ...... **28 C5** 45 5N 1 56 E
Maroochydore, Australia ...... **127 D5** 26 29 S 153 5 E
Maroona, Australia ...... **128 D5** 37 27 S 142 54 E
Maros, Indonesia ...... **82 C1** 5 0 S 119 34 E
Maros →, Hungary ...... **52 D5** 46 15N 20 13 E
Marosakoa, Madag. ...... **117 B8** 15 26 S 46 38 E
Maroseranana, Madag. ...... **117 B8** 18 32 S 48 51 E
Maróstica, Italy ...... **45 C8** 45 44N 11 40 E
Marotandrano, Madag. ...... **117 B8** 16 10 S 48 50 E
Marotaolano, Madag. ...... **117 A8** 12 47 S 49 15 E
Maroua, Cameroon ...... **113 C7** 10 40N 14 20 E
Marovato, Madag. ...... **117 B8** 15 48 S 48 5 E
Marovoay, Madag. ...... **117 B8** 16 6 S 46 39 E
Marowijne □, Suriname **169 C7** 4 0N 55 0W
Marowijne →, Suriname **169 B7** 5 45N 53 58W
Marquard, S. Africa ...... **116 D4** 28 40 S 27 28 E
Marquesas Fracture Zone, Pac. Oc. ...... **135 H15** 9 0 S 125 0W
Marquesas Is. = Marquises, Îs., French Polynesia ...... **135 H14** 9 30 S 140 0W
Marquesas Keys, U.S.A. **153 L7** 24 35N 82 10W
Marquette, U.S.A. **148 B2** 46 33N 87 24W
Marquis, St. Lucia ...... **165 f** 14 2N 60 54W
Marquise, France ...... **27 B8** 50 50N 1 40 E
Marquises, Îs., French Polynesia ...... **135 H14** 9 30 S 140 0W
Marra, Gebel, Sudan ...... **107 F2** 7 20N 27 35 E
Marra, Pta. do, Angola ...... **115 F2** 16 31 S 11 43 E
Marra Cr. →, Australia ...... **129 A7** 30 8 S 147 15 E
Marra Marra △, Australia ...... **129 B9** 33 23 S 151 4 E
Marradi, Italy ...... **45 D8** 44 4N 11 37 E
Marrakech, Morocco **110 B3** 31 9N 8 0W
Marrawah, Australia ...... **127 G3** 40 55 S 144 42 E
Marrecas, Serra das, Brazil ...... **170 C3** 9 0 S 41 0W
Marree, Australia ...... **127 D2** 29 39 S 138 1 E
Marrero, U.S.A. **155 L9** 29 54N 90 6W
Marrimane, Mozam. ...... **117 C5** 22 58 S 33 34 E
Marromeu, Mozam. ...... **117 B6** 18 15 S 36 25 E
Marroquí, Punta, Spain **43 K5** 36 0N 5 37W
Marrowie Cr. →, Australia ...... **129 B6** 33 23 S 145 40 E
Marrubane, Mozam. ...... **117 B5** 17 25 S 37 25 E
Marruás = Pôrto, Brazil ...... **170 B3** 3 54 S 42 42W
Marrubane, Mozam. ...... **119 F4** 18 0 S 37 0 E
Marrúbiu, Italy ...... **46 C1** 39 40N 8 33 E
Marrupa, Mozam. ...... **119 E4** 13 8 S 37 30 E
Mars →, France ...... **29 D8** 44 33N 3 37 E
Mars, Ascension I. ...... **9 g** 7 59 S 14 24W
Mars Hill, U.S.A. **149 B12** 46 31N 67 52W
Marsá 'Alam, Egypt ...... **106 B3** 25 5N 34 54 E
Marsá el Brega, Libya ...... **109 B9** 30 24N 19 37 E
Marsá Matrûh, Egypt ...... **106 A2** 31 19N 27 9 E
Marsá Sha'b, Sudan ...... **106 C4** 21 1N 36 46 E
Marsá Susah, Libya ...... **108 B4** 32 52N 21 59 E
Marsabit, Kenya ...... **118 B4** 2 18N 38 0 E
Marsabit △, Kenya ...... **118 B4** 2 23N 37 56 E
Marsala, Italy ...... **46 E5** 37 48N 12 26 E
Marsalforn, Malta ...... **38 E7** 36 4N 14 16 E
Marsaskala, Malta ...... **38 F8** 35 52N 14 34 E
Marsaxlokk, Malta ...... **38 F8** 35 50N 14 33 E
Marsaxlokk Bay, Malta ...... **38 F8** 35 49N 14 33 E
Marsberg, Germany ...... **30 D4** 51 27N 8 51 E
Marsciano, Italy ...... **45 F9** 42 54N 12 20 E
Marsden, Australia ...... **129 B8** 33 47 S 147 32 E
Marseillan, France ...... **28 E7** 43 23N 3 31 E
Marseille, France ...... **29 E9** 43 18N 5 23 E
Marseille ✕ (MRS), France ...... **29 E9** 43 26N 5 14 E

Marseilles = Marseille, France ...... **29 E9** 43 18N 5 23 E
Marseilles, U.S.A. **157 C8** 41 20N 88 43W
Marsh I., U.S.A. **155 L9** 29 34N 91 53W
Marshall = Fortuna Ledge, U.S.A. **144 F7** 61 53N 162 5W
Marshall, Liberia **112 D2** 6 8N 10 22W
Marshall, Ark., U.S.A. **155 H8** 35 55N 92 38W
Marshall, Ill., U.S.A. **157 E9** 39 23N 87 42W
Marshall, Mich., U.S.A. **157 B12** 42 16N 84 58W
Marshall, Minn., U.S.A. **154 C7** 44 25N 95 45W
Marshall, Mo., U.S.A. **156 F4** 39 7N 93 12W
Marshall, Tex., U.S.A. **155 J7** 32 33N 94 23W
Marshall →, Australia ...... **126 C2** 22 59 S 136 59 E
Marshall, C., Ecuador ...... **172 a** 0 1 S 91 12W
Marshall Bennett Is., Papua N. G. ...... **132 E6** 8 50 S 151 55 E
Marshall Is. ■, Pac. Oc. ...... **134 G9** 9 0N 171 0 E
Marshalltown, U.S.A. **156 B4** 42 3N 92 55W
Marshallville = Lewisporte, Canada **141 C8** 49 15N 55 3W
Marshallville, U.S.A. **152 C6** 32 27N 83 56W
Marshbrook, Zimbabwe ...... **117 B5** 18 33 S 31 9 E
Marshfield = Coos Bay, U.S.A. **158 E1** 43 22N 124 13W
Marshfield, Mo., U.S.A. **155 G8** 37 15N 92 54W
Marshfield, Vt., U.S.A. **151 B12** 44 20N 72 20W
Marshfield, Wis., U.S.A. **154 C9** 44 40N 90 10W
Marshūn, Iran ...... **97 B6** 36 19N 49 23 E
Mársico Nuovo, Italy ...... **47 B8** 40 25N 15 44 E
Märsta, Sweden ...... **16 E11** 59 37N 17 52 E
Marstal, Denmark ...... **17 K4** 54 51N 10 30 E
Marstrand, Sweden ...... **17 G5** 57 53N 11 35 E
Mart, U.S.A. **155 K6** 31 33N 96 50W
Marta →, Italy ...... **45 F8** 42 14N 11 42 E
Martaban, Burma ...... **90 G6** 16 30N 97 35 E
Martaban, G. of, Burma ...... **90 G6** 15 56N 96 30 E
Martano, Italy ...... **47 B11** 40 12N 18 18 E
Martapura, Kalimantan, Indonesia ...... **85 C4** 3 22 S 114 47 E
Martapura, Sumatera, Indonesia ...... **84 C2** 4 19 S 104 22 E
Marte, Nigeria ...... **113 C7** 12 23N 13 46 E
Martel, France ...... **28 D5** 44 57N 1 37 E
Martelange, Belgium ...... **24 E5** 49 49N 5 43 E
Martellago, Italy ...... **45 C9** 45 33N 12 9 E
Martés, Sierra, Spain **41 F4** 39 20N 1 0W
Martfű, Hungary ...... **52 C5** 47 1N 20 17 E
Marthaguy Cr. →, Australia ...... **129 A7** 30 16 S 147 35 E
Marthapal, India ...... **94 E5** 19 24N 81 37 E
Martha's Vineyard, U.S.A. **151 E14** 41 25N 70 38W
Martigné-Ferchaud, France **26 E5** 47 50N 1 20W
Martigny, Switz. ...... **32 D4** 46 6N 7 3 E
Martigues, France ...... **29 E9** 43 24N 5 4 E
Martil, Morocco **110 A3** 35 36N 5 15W
Martin, Slovak Rep. ...... **35 B11** 49 6N 18 58 E
Martin, S. Dak., U.S.A. **154 D4** 43 11N 101 44W
Martin, Tenn., U.S.A. **155 G10** 36 21N 88 51W
Martín →, Spain **40 D4** 41 18N 0 19W
Martin, L., U.S.A. **152 C4** 32 41N 85 55W
Martin Pt., U.S.A. **144 A12** 70 8N 143 16W
Martin Vaz, Atl. Oc. ...... **8 J9** 20 30 S 28 51W
Martina, Switz. ...... **33 C10** 46 53N 10 28 E
Martina Franca, Italy ...... **47 B10** 40 42N 17 20 E
Martinborough, N.Z. ...... **130 M4** 41 14 S 175 29 E
Martinez, Calif., U.S.A. **160 G4** 38 1N 122 8W
Martinez, Ga., U.S.A. **149 J4** 33 31N 82 4W
Martinho Campos, Brazil ...... **171 E2** 19 20 S 45 13W
Martinique ■, W. Indies ...... **164 c** 14 40N 61 0W
Martinique Passage, W. Indies **165 C7** 15 15N 61 0W
Martínon, Greece ...... **48 C5** 38 35N 23 12 E
Martin's Bay, Barbados ...... **165 g** 13 12N 59 29W
Martins Ferry, U.S.A. **150 F4** 40 6N 80 44W
Martinsberg, Austria ...... **34 C8** 48 22N 15 9 E
Martinsburg, Pa., U.S.A. **150 F6** 40 19N 78 20W
Martinsburg, W. Va., U.S.A. **148 F7** 39 27N 77 58W
Martinsicuro, Italy ...... **45 F10** 42 54N 13 54 E
Martinsville, Ill., U.S.A. **157 E9** 39 20N 87 53W
Martinsville, Ind., U.S.A. **157 E10** 39 26N 86 25W
Martinsville, Va., U.S.A. **149 G6** 36 41N 79 52W
Marton, N.Z. ...... **130 G4** 40 4 S 175 23 E
Martorell, Spain ...... **40 D6** 41 28N 1 56 E
Martos, Spain **43 H7** 37 44N 3 58W
Martûbah, Libya ...... **108 B4** 32 35N 22 46 E
Martuk, Kazakhstan ...... **52 N8** 50 46N 56 31 E
Martuni, Armenia ...... **61 K7** 40 9N 45 20 E
Maru, Nigeria ...... **113 C6** 12 22N 6 22 E
Marudi, Malaysia ...... **85 B4** 4 11N 114 19 E
Maruf, Afghan. ...... **91 C2** 31 30N 67 6 E
Marugame, Japan ...... **72 G6** 34 15N 133 40 E
Marui = Pagwi, Papua N. G. ...... **132 C2** 4 5 S 143 2 E
Maruia →, N.Z. ...... **131 B7** 41 47 S 172 13 E
Maruim, Brazil ...... **170 D4** 10 45 S 37 5W
Marulan, Australia ...... **129 B9** 34 43 S 150 3 E
Marunga, Angola ...... **116 B3** 17 28 S 20 2 E
Marungu, Mts., Dem. Rep. of the Congo ...... **118 D3** 7 30 S 30 0 E
Maruoka, Japan ...... **73 A8** 36 9N 136 16 E
Marv Dasht, Iran ...... **97 D7** 29 50N 52 40 E
Marvão = Castelo do Piauí, Brazil ...... **170 C3** 5 20 S 41 33W
Marvast, Iran ...... **97 D7** 30 30N 54 15 E
Marvejols, France ...... **28 D7** 44 33N 3 19 E
Marvel Loch, Australia ...... **125 F2** 31 28 S 119 29 E
Marwar, India ...... **92 G5** 25 43N 73 45 E
Mary, Turkmenistan ...... **66 F7** 37 40N 61 50 E
Mary Esther, U.S.A. **153 E3** 30 27N 86 38W
Maryborough = Port Laoise, Ireland **23 C4** 53 2N 7 18W
Maryborough, Queens., Australia ...... **127 D5** 25 31 S 152 37 E
Maryborough, Vic., Australia ...... **128 D5** 37 0 S 143 44 E
Maryfield, Canada **143 D8** 49 50N 101 35W
Maryino = Pristen, Russia ...... **59 G9** 51 15N 36 44 E
Maryland □, U.S.A. **148 F7** 39 0N 76 30W
Maryland Junction, Zimbabwe ...... **119 F3** 17 45 S 30 31 E
Maryport, U.K. **20 C4** 54 44N 3 28W
Mary's Harbour, Canada **141 B8** 52 18N 55 51W
Marystown, Canada **141 C8** 47 10N 55 10W
Marysville, Calif., U.S.A. **160 F5** 39 9N 121 35W
Marysville, Kans., U.S.A. **154 F6** 39 51N 96 39W
Marysville, Mich., U.S.A. **150 D2** 42 54N 82 29W

Marysville, *Ohio, U.S.A.* **157 D13** 40 14N 83 22W
Marysville, *Wash., U.S.A.* **160 B4** 48 3N 122 11W
Maryville, *Mo., U.S.A.* **156 D2** 40 21N 94 52W
Maryville, *Tenn., U.S.A.* **149 H4** 35 46N 83 58W
Marzo, Punta, *Colombia* **168 B2** 6 50N 77 42W
Marzūq, *Libya* **108 C2** 25 53N 13 57 E
Marzūq □, *Libya* **108 D3** 25 0N 16 0 E
Marzūq, Idehan, *Libya* **108 D2** 24 50N 13 51 E
Masada, *Israel* **103 D4** 31 15N 35 20 E
Masahunga, *Tanzania* **118 C3** 2 6 S 33 18 E
Masai, *Malaysia* **87 d** 1 29N 103 53 E
Masai Mara △, *Kenya* **118 C4** 1 25 S 35 5 E
Masai Steppe, *Tanzania* **118 C4** 4 30 S 36 30 E
Masaka, *Uganda* **118 C3** 0 21 S 31 45 E
Masalembo, Kepulauan, *Indonesia* **85 D4** 5 35 S 114 30 E
Masalima, Kepulauan, *Indonesia* **85 D5** 5 4 S 117 5 E
Masallı, *Azerbaijan* **101 C13** 39 3N 48 40 E
Masamba, *Indonesia* **82 B2** 2 30 S 120 15 E
Masan, *S. Korea* **75 G15** 35 11N 128 32 E
Masandam, Ra's, *Oman* **97 E8** 26 30N 56 30 E
Masasi, *Tanzania* **119 E4** 10 45 S 38 52 E
Masaya, *Nic.* **164 D2** 12 0N 86 7W
Masba, *Nigeria* **113 C7** 11 35N 13 1 E
Masbate, *Phil.* **80 E4** 12 21N 123 36 E
Masbate □, *Phil.* **80 E4** 12 20N 123 30 E
Masbate Pass, *Phil.* **80 E4** 12 30N 123 35 E
Máscali, *Italy* **47 E8** 37 45N 15 12 E
Mascara, *Algeria* **111 A5** 35 26N 0 6 E
Mascarene Is., *Ind. Oc.* **121 G4** 22 0 S 55 0 E
Mascarene Plain, *Ind. Oc.* **121 F4** 13 0 S 53 0 E
Mascarene Ridge, *Ind. Oc.* **121 F5** 11 0 S 61 0 E
Mascota, *Mexico* **162 C4** 20 30N 104 50W
Mascoutah, *U.S.A.* **156 F7** 38 29N 89 48W
Masein, *Burma* **90 D5** 23 22N 94 21 E
Masela, *Indonesia* **83 C3** 8 9 S 129 51 E
Maseru, *Lesotho* **116 D4** 29 18 S 27 30 E
Masfjorden, *Norway* **18 D2** 60 48N 5 18 E
Mashaba, *Zimbabwe* **119 G3** 20 2 S 30 29 E
Mashābih, *Si. Arabia* **96 E3** 25 35N 36 30 E
Mashan, *China* **76 F7** 23 40N 108 11 E
Mashar, *Sudan* **107 F2** 9 16N 26 51 E
Mashatu ⌂, *Botswana* **117 C4** 22 5 S 29 5 E
Mashegu, *Nigeria* **113 D6** 10 0N 5 35 E
Masherbrum, *Pakistan* **93 B7** 35 38N 76 18 E
Mashhad, *Iran* **97 B8** 36 20N 59 35 E
Mashi, *Nigeria* **113 C6** 13 0N 7 54 E
Mashiki, *Japan* **72 E2** 32 51N 130 53 E
Mashīz, *Iran* **97 D8** 29 56N 56 37 E
Mashkal ➝, *Pakistan* **91 D2** 26 2N 65 19 E
Māshkel, Hāmūn-i-, *Pakistan* **91 C1** 28 20N 62 56 E
Mashki Chāh, *Pakistan* **91 C1** 29 5N 62 30 E
Mashonaland Central □, *Zimbabwe* **117 B5** 17 30 S 31 0 E
Mashonaland East □, *Zimbabwe* **117 B5** 18 0 S 32 0 E
Mashonaland West □, *Zimbabwe* **117 B4** 17 30 S 29 30 E
Mashrakh, *India* **93 F11** 26 7N 84 48 E
Mashtaga = Maştağa, *Azerbaijan* **61 K10** 40 35N 49 57 E
Masi Manimba, *Dem. Rep. of the Congo* **115 C3** 4 40 S 17 54 E
Masibi, *Angola* **115 E4** 11 6 S 22 41 E
Masindi, *Uganda* **118 B3** 1 40N 31 43 E
Masindi Port, *Uganda* **118 B3** 1 43N 32 2 E
Masinloc, *Phil.* **80 D2** 15 32N 119 57 E
Maşīrah, *Oman* **99 B7** 21 0N 58 50 E
Maşīrah, Khalīj, *Oman* **99 B7** 20 10N 58 10 E
Maşīrah, Tur'at, *Oman* **99 B7** 20 30N 58 40 E
Masisea, *Peru* **172 B3** 8 35 S 74 22W
Masisi, *Dem. Rep. of the Congo* **118 C2** 1 23 S 28 49 E
Masjed Soleyman, *Iran* **97 D6** 31 55N 49 18 E
Mask, L., *Ireland* **23 C2** 53 36N 9 22W
Maskelyne Is., *Vanuatu* **133 F5** 16 32 S 167 49 E
Maski, *India* **95 G3** 15 56N 76 46 E
Maskin, *Oman* **97 F8** 23 30N 56 50 E
Maslen Nos, *Bulgaria* **51 D11** 42 18N 27 48 E
Maslinica, *Croatia* **45 E13** 43 24N 16 13 E
Maşna'ah, *Yemen* **99 D5** 14 27N 48 17 E
Masnou = El Masnou, *Spain* **40 D7** 41 28N 2 20 E
Masoala △, *Madag.* **117 B9** 15 30 S 50 12 E
Masoala, Tanjon' i, *Madag.* **117 B9** 15 59 S 50 13 E
Masoarivo, *Madag.* **117 B7** 19 3 S 44 19 E
Masohi = Amahai, *Indonesia* **83 C3** 3 20 S 128 55 E
Masomeloka, *Madag.* **117 C8** 20 17 S 48 37 E
Mason, *Mich., U.S.A.* **157 B12** 42 35N 84 27W
Mason, *Nev., U.S.A.* **160 G7** 38 56N 119 8W
Mason, *Ohio, U.S.A.* **157 E12** 39 22N 84 19W
Mason, *Tex., U.S.A.* **155 K5** 30 45N 99 14W
Mason B., *N.Z.* **131 G2** 46 55 S 167 45 E
Mason City, *Ill., U.S.A.* **156 D7** 40 12N 89 42W
Mason City, *Iowa, U.S.A.* **156 A3** 43 9N 93 12W
Maspalomas, *Canary Is.* **9 e1** 27 46N 15 35W
Maspalomas, Pta., *Canary Is.* **9 e1** 27 43N 15 36W
Masqat, *Oman* **99 B7** 23 37N 58 36 E
Massa, *Congo* **114 C3** 3 45 S 15 29 E
Massa, *Italy* **44 D7** 44 1N 10 9 E
Massa, O. ➝, *Morocco* **110 B3** 30 2N 9 40W
Massa Marittima, *Italy* **44 E7** 43 3N 10 52 E
Massachusetts □, *U.S.A.* **151 D13** 42 30N 72 0W
Massachusetts B., *U.S.A.* **151 D14** 42 20N 70 50W
Massafra, *Italy* **47 B10** 40 35N 17 7 E
Massaguet, *Chad* **109 F3** 12 28N 15 26 E
Massakory, *Chad* **109 F3** 13 0N 15 49 E
Massanella, *Spain* **38 B3** 39 48N 2 51 E
Massangano, *Angola* **115 D2** 9 40 S 14 13 E
Massangena, *Mozam.* **117 C5** 21 34 S 33 0 E
Massango, *Angola* **115 D3** 8 1 S 16 10 E
Massapê, *Brazil* **170 B3** 3 31 S 40 19W
Massat, *France* **28 F5** 42 53N 1 21 E
Massawa = Mitsiwa, *Eritrea* **107 D4** 15 35N 39 25 E
Massena, *U.S.A.* **151 B10** 44 56N 74 54W
Massénya, *Chad* **109 F3** 11 21N 16 9 E
Masset, *Canada* **142 C2** 54 2N 132 10W
Masseube, *France* **28 E4** 43 25N 0 34 E
Massiac, *France* **28 C7** 45 15N 3 11 E
Massiah Street, *Barbados* **165 g** 13 9N 59 29W
Massif Central, *France* **28 D7** 44 55N 3 0 E
Massif des Bauges ⌂, *France* **27 G13** 45 40N 6 10 E
Massigui, *Mali* **112 C3** 11 48N 6 50W
Massillon, *U.S.A.* **150 F3** 40 48N 81 32W
Massinga, *Gabon* **114 C2** 1 27 S 11 35 E
Massime, O. ➝, *Algeria* **111 C5** 36 13N 2 12 E
Massinga, *Mozam.* **117 C6** 23 15 S 35 22 E
Massingir, *Mozam.* **117 C5** 23 51 S 32 4 E
Masson-Angers, *Canada* **151 A9** 45 32N 75 25W
Masson I., *Antarctica* **7 C7** 66 10 S 93 20 E
Massouka, *Gabon* **114 C1** 1 37 S 9 56 E
Massow = Maszewo, *Poland* **54 E2** 53 29N 15 3 E
Mastābah, *Si. Arabia* **98 B2** 20 49N 39 26 E
Maştağa, *Azerbaijan* **61 K10** 40 35N 49 57 E
Mastanli = Momchilgrad, *Bulgaria* **51 E9** 41 33N 25 23 E
Masterton, *N.Z.* **130 G4** 40 56 S 175 39 E
Mastic, *U.S.A.* **151 F12** 40 47N 72 54W
Mástikho, Ákra, *Greece* **49 C8** 38 10N 26 2 E
Mastuj, *Pakistan* **93 A5** 36 20N 72 36 E
Mastung, *Pakistan* **91 C2** 29 50N 66 56 E
Mastūrah, *Si. Arabia* **98 B2** 23 7N 38 52 E
Masty, *Belarus* **58 F3** 53 27N 24 38 E
Masuda, *Japan* **72 C3** 34 40N 131 51 E
Masuika, *Dem. Rep. of the Congo* **115 D4** 7 37 S 22 32 E
Masvingo, *Zimbabwe* **119 G3** 20 8 S 30 49 E
Masvingo □, *Zimbabwe* **119 G3** 21 0 S 31 30 E
Maswa ⌂, *Tanzania* **118 C3** 2 58 S 34 19 E
Maşyāf, *Syria* **100 E7** 35 4N 36 20 E
Maszewo, *Poland* **54 E2** 53 29N 15 3 E
Mat ➝, *Albania* **50 E3** 41 40N 19 35 E
Mata de São João, *Brazil* **171 D4** 12 31 S 38 17W
Mata Utu, *Wall. & F. Is.* **123 C15** 13 17 S 176 8W
Matabele Plain, *Zambia* **115 F4** 16 20 S 23 10 E
Matabeleland North □, *Zimbabwe* **119 F2** 19 0 S 28 0 E
Matabeleland South □, *Zimbabwe* **119 G2** 21 0 S 29 0 E
Mataboor, *Indonesia* **83 B5** 1 41 S 138 3 E
Matachel ➝, *Spain* **43 G4** 38 50N 6 17W
Matachewan, *Canada* **140 C3** 47 56N 80 39W
Matacuni ➝, *Venezuela* **169 C4** 3 2N 65 16W
Matadi, *Dem. Rep. of the Congo* **115 D2** 5 52 S 13 31 E
Matagalpa, *Nic.* **164 D2** 13 0N 85 58W
Matagami, *Canada* **140 C4** 49 45N 77 34W
Matagami, L., *Canada* **140 C4** 49 50N 77 40W
Matagorda B., *U.S.A.* **155 L6** 28 40N 96 0W
Matagorda I., *U.S.A.* **155 L6** 28 15N 96 30W
Mataguinao, *Phil.* **80 E5** 12 5N 124 55 E
Matak, *Indonesia* **84 B3** 3 18N 106 16 E
Matakana, *Australia* **129 B6** 32 59 S 145 54 E
Matakana, *N.Z.* **130 C3** 36 21 S 174 43 E
Matala, *Angola* **115 E3** 14 46 S 15 4 E
Mátala, *Greece* **39 F5** 34 59N 24 45 E
Matalaque, *Peru* **172 D3** 16 26 S 70 49W
Matale, *Sri Lanka* **95 L5** 7 30N 80 37 E
Matam, *Senegal* **112 B2** 15 34N 13 17W
Matamata, *N.Z.* **130 D4** 37 48 S 175 47 E
Matameye, *Niger* **113 C6** 13 26N 8 28 E
Matamoros, *Campeche, Mexico* **163 D6** 18 50N 90 50W
Matamoros, *Coahuila, Mexico* **162 B4** 25 33N 103 15W
Matamoros, *Tamaulipas, Mexico* **163 B5** 25 50N 97 30W
Ma'ṭan as Sarra, *Libya* **109 D4** 21 45N 22 0 E
Ma'ṭan Bishārah, *Libya* **108 D4** 23 0N 22 32 E
Matana, Danau, *Indonesia* **82 B2** 2 28 S 121 20 E
Matandu ➝, *Tanzania* **119 D3** 8 45 S 34 19 E
Matane, *Canada* **141 C6** 48 50N 67 33W
Matang, *China* **76 F5** 23 30N 104 7 E
Matankari, *Niger* **113 C5** 13 46N 4 1 E
Matanomadh, *India* **92 H3** 23 33N 68 57 E
Matanzas, *Cuba* **164 B3** 23 0N 81 40W
Matapa, *Botswana* **116 C3** 23 11 S 24 39 E
Matapan, C. = Taínaron, Ákra, *Greece* **48 E4** 36 22N 22 27 E
Matapédia, *Canada* **141 C6** 48 0N 66 59W
Matapo △, *Zimbabwe* **119 G2** 20 30 S 29 40 E
Matara, *Sri Lanka* **95 M5** 5 58N 80 30 E
Mataram, *Indonesia* **85 D5** 8 35 S 116 7 E
Matarani, *Peru* **172 D3** 17 0 S 72 10W
Mataranka, *Australia* **124 B5** 14 55 S 133 4 E
Matarma, Râs, *Egypt* **103 E1** 30 27N 32 44 E
Mataró, *Spain* **40 D7** 41 32N 2 29 E
Matarraña ➝, *Spain* **40 D5** 41 14N 0 22 E
Mataruška Banja, *Serbia & M.* **50 C4** 43 40N 20 40 E
Mataso, *Vanuatu* **133 G6** 17 14 S 168 26 E
Matata, *N.Z.* **130 D5** 37 54 S 176 48 E
Matatiele, *S. Africa* **117 E4** 30 20 S 28 49 E
Mataura, *N.Z.* **131 G3** 46 11 S 168 51 E
Mataura ➝, *N.Z.* **131 G3** 46 34 S 168 44 E
Mataveri, *Chile* **172 b** 27 9 S 109 27W
Mategua, *Bolivia* **173 C5** 13 1 S 62 48W
Matehuala, *Mexico* **162 C4** 23 40N 100 40W
Mateira, *Brazil* **171 E1** 18 54 S 50 30W
Mateke, *Dem. Rep. of the Congo* **114 C3** 4 52 S 24 25 E
Mateke Hills, *Zimbabwe* **119 G3** 21 48 S 31 0 E
Matelot, *Trin. & Tob.* **169 F9** 10 50N 61 7W
Matera, *Italy* **47 B9** 40 40N 16 36 E
Matese ⌂, *Italy* **47 A7** 41 24N 14 23 E
Matese, Monti del, *Italy* **47 A7** 41 27N 14 22 E
Mátészalka, *Hungary* **52 C7** 47 58N 22 20 E
Matetsi, *Zimbabwe* **119 F2** 18 12 S 26 0 E
Mateur, *Tunisia* **108 A1** 37 0N 9 40 E
Matfors, *Sweden* **16 B11** 62 21N 17 2 E
Matha, *France* **28 C3** 45 52N 0 20W
Matheniko ⌂, *Uganda* **118 B3** 2 49N 34 27 E
Mathis, *U.S.A.* **155 L6** 28 6N 97 50W
Mathoura, *Australia* **129 C6** 35 50 S 144 55 E
Mathráki, *Greece* **38 B9** 39 48N 19 31 E
Mathura, *India* **92 F7** 27 30N 77 40 E
Mati, *Phil.* **81 H6** 6 55N 126 15 E
Matiakoali, *Burkina Faso* **113 C5** 12 28N 1 2 E
Matiali, *India* **93 F13** 26 56N 88 49 E
Matías Romero, *Mexico* **163 D5** 16 53N 95 2W
Matibane, *Mozam.* **119 E5** 14 49 S 40 45 E
Matinhos, *Brazil* **171 G2** 25 49 S 48 32W
Matiri Ra., *N.Z.* **131 B7** 41 38 S 172 20 E
Matjiesfontein, *S. Africa* **116 E3** 33 14 S 20 35 E
Matla ➝, *India* **93 J13** 21 40N 88 40 E
Matlamanyane, *Botswana* **116 B4** 19 33 S 25 57 E
Matli, *Pakistan* **92 G3** 25 2N 68 39 E
Matlock, *U.K.* **20 D6** 53 9N 1 33W
Matmata, *Tunisia* **108 B1** 33 37N 9 59 E
Matna, *Sudan* **107 E4** 13 49N 35 10 E
Matnog, *Phil.* **80 E5** 12 35N 124 5 E
Mato, *Dem. Rep. of the Congo* **115 D4** 8 1 S 24 24 E
Mato ➝, *Venezuela* **169 B4** 7 9N 65 7W
Mato, Serranía de, *Venezuela* **168 B4** 6 25N 65 25W
Mato Grosso □, *Brazil* **173 C6** 14 0 S 55 0W
Mato Grosso, Planalto do, *Brazil* **173 C7** 15 0 S 55 0W
Mato Grosso do Sul □, *Brazil* **173 D7** 18 0 S 55 0W
Mato Verde, *Brazil* **171 D1** 11 13 S 50 40W
Matobo = Matapo △, *Zimbabwe* **119 G2** 20 30 S 29 40 E
Matochkin Shar, *Russia* **66 B6** 73 10N 56 40 E
Matong, *Papua N. G.* **132 C6** 5 36 S 151 50 E
Matopo Hills, *Zimbabwe* **119 G2** 20 36 S 28 20 E
Matopos, *Zimbabwe* **119 G2** 20 20 S 28 29 E
Matosinhos, *Portugal* **42 D2** 41 11N 8 42W
Matour, *France* **27 F11** 46 19N 4 29 E
Matroosberg, *S. Africa* **116 E2** 33 23 S 19 40 E
Maṭruḥ, *Oman* **99 B7** 23 37N 58 30 E
Matsena, *Nigeria* **113 C7** 13 5N 10 5 E
Matsesta, *Russia* **61 J4** 43 34N 39 51 E
Matsu Tao, *Taiwan* **77 E13** 26 9N 119 56 E
Matsubara = Takahagi, *Japan* **71 F10** 36 43N 140 45 E
Matsudo, *Japan* **73 B11** 35 47N 139 54 E
Matsue, *Japan* **72 B5** 35 25N 133 10 E
Matsum, Ko, *Thailand* **87 b** 9 22N 99 59 E
Matsumae, *Japan* **70 D10** 41 26N 140 7 E
Matsumoto, *Japan* **73 A10** 36 15N 138 0 E
Matsusaka, *Japan* **73 C8** 34 34N 136 32 E
Matsushima, *Japan* **72 E2** 32 30N 130 25 E
Matsuura, *Japan* **72 D1** 33 20N 129 49 E
Matsuyama, *Japan* **72 D4** 33 45N 132 45 E
Matsuzaki, *Japan* **73 C10** 34 43N 138 50 E
Mattagami ➝, *Canada* **140 B3** 50 43N 81 29W
Mattancheri, *India* **95 K3** 9 50N 76 15 E
Mattawa, *Canada* **140 C4** 46 20N 78 45W
Matterhorn, *Switz.* **32 E5** 45 58N 7 39 E
Mattersburg, *Austria* **35 D9** 47 44N 16 24 E
Matteson, *U.S.A.* **157 C9** 41 30N 87 42W
Matthew, I., *N. Cal.* **123 E13** 22 29 S 171 15 E
Matthew Town, *Bahamas* **165 B5** 20 57N 73 40W
Matthews, *U.S.A.* **157 D11** 40 23N 85 30W
Matthews Ridge, *Guyana* **169 B5** 7 37N 60 10W
Mattice, *Canada* **140 C3** 49 40N 83 20W
Mattili, *India* **94 E6** 18 33N 82 12 E
Mattituck, *U.S.A.* **151 F12** 40 59N 72 32W
Mattō, *Japan* **73 A8** 36 31N 136 34 E
Mattoon, *U.S.A.* **154 F10** 39 29N 88 23W
Matuba, *Mozam.* **117 C5** 24 28 S 32 49 E
Matucana, *Peru* **172 C2** 11 55 S 76 25W
Matugama, *Sri Lanka* **95 L5** 6 31N 80 7 E
Matuku, *Papua N. G.* **132 C3** 4 54 S 145 47 E
Matuku, *Fiji* **133 B2** 19 10 S 179 44 E
Matūn = Khowst, *Afghan.* **91 B3** 33 22N 69 58 E
Matura B., *Trin. & Tob.* **169 F10** 10 39N 61 1W
Maturín, *Venezuela* **169 B5** 9 45N 63 11W
Matusadona △, *Zimbabwe* **119 F2** 16 58 S 28 42 E
Matutum, Mt., *Phil.* **81 H5** 6 22N 125 5 E
Matveyev Kurgan, *Russia* **59 J10** 47 35N 38 57 E
Matxitxako, C., *Spain* **40 B2** 43 28N 2 47W
Mau, *Mad. P., India* **93 F8** 26 17N 78 41 E
Mau, *Ut. P., India* **93 G10** 25 56N 83 33 E
Mau, *Ut. P., India* **93 G9** 25 17N 81 23 E
Mau Escarpment, *Kenya* **118 C4** 0 40 S 36 0 E
Mau Ranipur, *India* **93 G8** 25 16N 79 8 E
Mauban, *Phil.* **80 D3** 14 12N 121 44 E
Maubeuge, *France* **27 B10** 50 17N 3 57 E
Maubin, *Burma* **90 G5** 16 44N 95 39 E
Maubourguet, *France* **28 E4** 43 29N 0 1 E
Maud, Pt., *Australia* **124 D1** 23 6 S 113 45 E
Maude, *Australia* **128 C6** 34 29 S 144 18 E
Maudin Sun, *Burma* **90 G5** 16 0N 94 30 E
Maués, *Brazil* **169 D6** 3 20 S 57 45W
Maués-Acu ➝, *Brazil* **169 D6** 3 22 S 57 44W
Maughold Hd., *I. of Man* **20 C3** 54 18N 4 18W
Mauguio, *France* **28 E7** 43 37N 4 1 E
Maui, *U.S.A.* **145 C5** 20 48N 156 20W
Maulamyaing = Moulmein, *Burma* **90 G6** 16 30N 97 40 E
Maule □, *Chile* **174 D1** 36 5 S 72 30W
Mauléon-Licharre, *France* **28 E3** 43 14N 0 54W
Maullín, *Chile* **176 B2** 41 38 S 73 37W
Maulvibazar, *Bangla.* **90 C3** 24 29N 91 42 E
Maumee, *U.S.A.* **157 C13** 41 34N 83 39W
Maumee ➝, *U.S.A.* **157 C13** 41 42N 83 28W
Maumere, *Indonesia* **82 C2** 8 38 S 122 13 E
Maumusson, Pertuis de, *France* **28 C2** 45 48N 1 14W
Maun, *Botswana* **116 C3** 20 0 S 23 26 E
Mauna Kea, *U.S.A.* **145 D6** 19 50N 155 28W
Mauna Loa, *U.S.A.* **145 D6** 19 30N 155 35W
Maunaloa, *U.S.A.* **145 B4** 21 8N 157 13W
Maunalua B., *U.S.A.* **145 K14** 21 15N 157 45W
Maunawili, *U.S.A.* **145 K14** 21 23N 157 46W
Maunga Orito, *Chile* **172 b** 27 10 S 109 25W
Maunga Puakatiki, *Chile* **172 b** 27 6 S 109 15W
Maunga Terevaka, *Chile* **172 b** 27 5 S 109 23W
Maungaturoto, *N.Z.* **130 C3** 36 6 S 174 23 E
Maungdow, *Burma* **90 E4** 20 50N 92 21 E
Maungmagan Kyunzu, *Burma* **86 E1** 14 0N 97 48 E
Maupin, *U.S.A.* **158 D3** 45 11N 121 5W
Maure-de-Bretagne, *France* **26 E5** 47 59N 1 58W
Maurepas, L., *U.S.A.* **155 K9** 30 15N 90 30W
Maures, *France* **29 E10** 43 15N 6 15 E
Mauriac, *France* **28 C6** 45 13N 2 19 E
Maurice, L., *Australia* **125 E5** 29 30 S 131 0 E
Mauriceville, *N.Z.* **130 G4** 40 45 S 175 42 E
Mauricie △, *Canada* **140 C5** 46 45N 73 0W
Maurienne, *France* **29 C10** 45 13N 6 30 E
Mauritania ■, *Africa* **110 D3** 20 50N 10 0W
Mauritius ■, *Ind. Oc.* **121 d** 20 0 S 57 0 E
Mauritius ✕ (MRU), *Mauritania* **121 d** 20 25 S 57 40 E
Mauron, *France* **26 D4** 48 9N 2 18W
Maurs, *France* **28 D6** 44 43N 2 12 E
Mauston, *U.S.A.* **154 D9** 43 48N 90 5W
Mauterndorf, *Austria* **34 D6** 47 9N 13 40 E
Mauthen, *Austria* **34 E6** 46 40N 13 0 E
Mauvezin, *France* **28 E4** 43 44N 0 53 E
Mauvoisin, Barr. de, *Switz.* **32 E4** 45 58N 7 20 E
Mauzé-sur-le-Mignon, *France* **28 B3** 46 12N 0 41W
Mavaca ➝, *Venezuela* **169 C4** 2 31N 65 11W
Mavinga, *Angola* **115 F4** 15 50 S 20 21 E
Mavli, *India* **92 G5** 24 45N 73 55 E
Mavráta, *Greece* **39 C2** 38 4N 20 44 E
Mavrovë, *Albania* **50 F3** 40 26N 19 32 E
Mavrovo △, *Macedonia* **50 E4** 41 36N 20 45 E
Mavuradonha Mts., *Zimbabwe* **119 F3** 16 30 S 31 30 E
Mawa, *Dem. Rep. of the Congo* **118 B2** 2 45N 26 40 E
Mawai, *India* **93 H9** 22 30N 81 4 E
Mawana, *India* **92 E7** 29 6N 77 58 E
Mawand, *Pakistan* **92 E3** 29 33N 68 38 E
Mawasangka, *Indonesia* **82 C2** 5 17 S 122 18 E
Mawk Mai, *Burma* **90 E6** 20 14N 97 37 E
Mawlaik, *Burma* **90 D5** 23 40N 94 26 E
Mawlamyine = Moulmein, *Burma* **90 G6** 16 30N 97 40 E
Mawlawkho, *Burma* **90 G6** 17 50N 97 38 E
Mawqaq, *Si. Arabia* **96 E4** 27 25N 41 8 E
Mawshij, *Yemen* **98 D3** 13 43N 43 17 E
Mawson Base, *Antarctica* **7 C6** 67 30 S 62 53 E
Mawson Coast, *Antarctica* **7 C6** 68 30 S 63 0 E
Mawsynram, *India* **90 C3** 25 15N 91 30 E
Max, *U.S.A.* **154 B4** 47 49N 101 18W
Maxamamba = Nova Iguaçu, *Brazil* **171 F3** 22 45 S 43 28W
Maxcanú, *Mexico* **163 C6** 20 40N 92 0W
Maxesibeni, *S. Africa* **117 E4** 30 49 S 29 23 E
Maxeys, *U.S.A.* **152 B6** 33 45N 83 11W
Maxhamish L., *Canada* **142 B4** 59 50N 123 17W
Maxixe, *Mozam.* **117 C6** 23 54 S 35 17 E
Maxville, *Canada* **151 A10** 45 17N 74 51W
Maxwell, *N.Z.* **130 F3** 39 51 S 174 49 E
Maxwell, *U.S.A.* **160 F4** 39 17N 122 11W
Maxwelton, *Australia* **126 C3** 20 43 S 142 41 E
May, C., *U.S.A.* **148 F8** 38 56N 74 58W
May Jirgui, *Niger* **109 F1** 13 44N 8 8 E
May Pen, *Jamaica* **164 a** 17 58N 77 15W
May River, *Papua N. G.* **132 C1** 4 19 S 141 58 E
Maya, *Indonesia* **85 C3** 1 10 S 109 35 E
Maya ➝, *Russia* **67 D14** 60 28N 134 28 E
Maya Mts., *Belize* **163 D7** 16 30N 89 0W
Mayabandar, *India* **95 H11** 12 56N 92 56 E
Mayaguana, *Bahamas* **165 B5** 22 30N 72 44W
Mayagüez, *Puerto Rico* **165 d** 18 12N 67 9W
Mayahi, *Niger* **113 C6** 13 58N 7 40 E
Mayaky, *Ukraine* **53 C14** 47 26N 29 33 E
Mayals = Maials, *Spain* **40 D5** 41 22N 0 30 E
Mayama, *Congo* **114 C2** 3 51 S 14 54 E
Mayāmey, *Iran* **97 B7** 36 24N 55 42 E
Mayang, *China* **76 D7** 27 53N 109 49 E
Mayanup, *Australia* **125 F2** 33 57 S 116 27 E
Mayapán, *Mexico* **163 C7** 20 28N 89 11W
Mayapan, *Yucatán, Mexico* **163 C7** 20 30N 89 25W
Mayaqum, *Kazakhstan* **65 B4** 42 51N 68 3 E
Mayarí, *Cuba* **165 B4** 20 40N 75 41W
Mayaro B., *Trin. & Tob.* **169 F10** 10 14N 60 59W
Mayavaram = Mayuram, *India* **95 J4** 11 3N 79 42 E
Maybell, *U.S.A.* **158 F9** 40 31N 108 5W
Maybole, *U.K.* **22 F4** 55 21N 4 42W
Maychew, *Ethiopia* **107 E4** 12 50N 39 31 E
Maydān, *Iraq* **101 E11** 34 55N 45 37 E
Maydan, *Ukraine* **53 B8** 48 36N 23 29 E
Maydena, *Australia* **127 G4** 42 45 S 146 30 E
Maydī, *Yemen* **98 C3** 16 19N 42 48 E
Mayen, *Germany* **31 E3** 50 19N 7 13 E
Mayenne, *France* **26 D6** 48 20N 0 38W
Mayenne □, *France* **26 D6** 48 10N 0 40W
Mayenne ➝, *France* **26 E6** 47 30N 0 32W
Mayer, *U.S.A.* **159 J7** 34 24N 112 14W
Mayerthorpe, *Canada* **142 C5** 53 57N 115 8W
Mayesville, *U.S.A.* **152 A9** 34 0N 80 12W
Mayfield, *Ky., U.S.A.* **149 G1** 36 44N 88 38W
Mayfield, *N.Y., U.S.A.* **151 C10** 43 6N 74 16W
Mayhill, *U.S.A.* **159 K11** 32 53N 105 29W
Maykop, *Russia* **61 H5** 44 35N 40 10 E
Mayli-Say = Mayluu-Suu, *Kyrgyzstan* **65 C6** 41 17N 72 24 E
Mayluu-Suu, *Kyrgyzstan* **65 C6** 41 17N 72 24 E
Maymak, *Kyrgyzstan* **65 B5** 42 42N 71 13 E
Maymyo, *Burma* **86 A1** 22 2N 96 28 E
Maynard, *Mass., U.S.A.* **151 D13** 42 26N 71 27W
Maynard, *Wash., U.S.A.* **160 C4** 47 59N 122 55W
Maynard Hills, *Australia* **125 E2** 28 28 S 119 49 E
Mayne ➝, *Australia* **126 C3** 23 40 S 141 55 E
Maynooth, *Ireland* **23 C5** 53 23N 6 34W
Mayo, *Canada* **138 B6** 63 38N 135 57W
Mayo, *U.S.A.* **152 E6** 30 3N 83 10W
Mayo □, *Ireland* **23 C2** 53 53N 9 3W
Mayo ➝, *Argentina* **176 C3** 45 45 S 69 45W
Mayo ➝, *Peru* **172 B2** 6 38 S 76 15W
Mayo Bay, *Phil.* **81 H6** 6 56N 126 22 E
Mayo Daga, *Nigeria* **113 D7** 6 59N 11 25 E
Mayo Faran, *Nigeria* **113 D7** 8 57N 12 4 E
Mayoko, *Congo* **114 C2** 2 18 S 12 49 E
Mayoko, *Dem. Rep. of the Congo* **114 C4** 1 6 S 23 50 E
Mayon Volcano, *Phil.* **80 E4** 13 15N 123 41 E
Mayor Buratovich, *Argentina* **176 A4** 39 15 S 62 37W
Mayor I., *N.Z.* **130 D5** 37 16 S 176 17 E
Mayorga, *Spain* **42 C5** 42 10N 5 16W
Mayotte ☑, *Ind. Oc.* **121 a** 12 50 S 45 10 E
Mayoyao, *Phil.* **80 C3** 16 59N 121 14 E
Mayraira Pt., *Phil.* **80 B3** 18 39N 120 51 E
Maysān □, *Iraq* **96 D5** 31 55N 47 15 E
Mayskiy, *Russia* **61 J7** 43 47N 44 2 E
Maysville, *Ky., U.S.A.* **157 F13** 38 39N 83 46W
Maysville, *Mo., U.S.A.* **156 E2** 39 53N 94 22W
Mayu, *Indonesia* **82 A3** 1 30N 126 30 E
Mayumba, *Gabon* **114 C2** 3 25 S 10 39 E
Mayuram, *India* **95 J4** 11 3N 79 42 E
Mayville, *N. Dak., U.S.A.* **154 B6** 47 30N 97 20W
Mayville, *N.Y., U.S.A.* **150 D5** 42 15N 79 30W
Mayya, *Russia* **67 C14** 61 44N 130 18 E
Mazabuka, *Zambia* **119 F2** 15 52 S 27 44 E
Mazagán = El Jadida, *Morocco* **110 B3** 33 11N 8 17W
Mazagão, *Brazil* **169 D7** 0 7 S 51 16W
Mazamet, *France* **28 E6** 43 30N 2 20 E
Mazán, *Peru* **168 D3** 3 30 S 73 0W
Māzandarān □, *Iran* **97 B7** 36 30N 52 0 E
Mazapil, *Mexico* **162 C4** 24 38N 101 34W
Mazar, *China* **65 E8** 36 32N 77 1 E
Mazar, O. ➝, *Algeria* **111 B5** 31 50N 1 36 E
Mazār-e Sharīf, *Afghan.* **65 E3** 36 41N 67 0 E
Mazara del Vallo, *Italy* **46 E5** 37 39N 12 35 E
Mazarredo, *Argentina* **176 C3** 47 10 S 66 50W
Mazarrón, *Spain* **41 H3** 37 38N 1 19W
Mazarrón, G. de, *Spain* **41 H3** 37 27N 1 19W
Mazaruni ➝, *Guyana* **169 B6** 6 25N 58 35W
Mazatán, *Mexico* **162 B2** 29 0N 110 8W
Mazatenango, *Guatemala* **164 D1** 14 35N 91 30W
Mazatlán, *Mexico* **162 C3** 23 13N 106 25W
Mažeikiai, *Lithuania* **15 H20** 56 20N 22 20 E
Māzhān, *Iran* **97 C8** 32 30N 59 0 E
Mazīnān, *Iran* **97 B8** 36 19N 56 56 E
Mazo Cruz, *Peru* **172 D4** 16 45 S 69 44W
Mazoe, *Mozam.* **119 F3** 16 42 S 33 7 E
Mazoe ➝, *Mozam.* **119 F3** 16 20 S 33 30 E
Mazomanie, *U.S.A.* **156 A7** 43 11N 89 48W
Mazon, *U.S.A.* **157 C8** 41 14N 88 25W
Mazowe, *Zimbabwe* **117 B5** 17 28 S 30 58 E
Mazowieckie □, *Poland* **55 F8** 52 40N 21 0 E
Mazrūb, *Sudan* **107 E2** 14 0N 29 20 E
Mazu Dao, *China* **77 D12** 26 10N 119 55 E
Mazurian Lakes = Mazurski, Pojezierze, *Poland* **54 E7** 53 50N 21 0 E
Mazurski, Pojezierze, *Poland* **54 E7** 53 50N 21 0 E
Mazyr, *Belarus* **59 F5** 51 59N 29 15 E
Mba, *Fiji* **133 A1** 17 33 S 177 41 E
Mbaba, *Senegal* **112 C1** 14 59N 16 44W
Mbabane, *Swaziland* **117 D5** 26 18 S 31 6 E
Mbaéré ➝, *C.A.R.* **114 B3** 3 47N 17 31 E
Mbagne, *Mauritania* **112 B2** 16 6N 14 47W
M'bahiakro, *Ivory C.* **112 D4** 7 33N 4 19W
Mbaïki, *C.A.R.* **114 B3** 3 53N 18 1 E
Mbakana, Mt. de, *Cameroon* **114 A3** 7 57N 15 6 E
Mbala, *Zambia* **119 D3** 8 46 S 31 24 E
Mbalabala, *Zimbabwe* **117 C4** 20 27 S 29 3 E
Mbale, *Uganda* **118 B3** 1 8N 34 12 E
Mbali ➝, *C.A.R.* **114 B3** 4 27N 18 20 E
Mbalmayo, *Cameroon* **113 E7** 3 33N 11 33 E
Mbam ➝, *Cameroon* **113 E7** 4 24N 11 17 E
Mbamba Bay, *Tanzania* **119 E3** 11 13 S 34 49 E
Mbandaka, *Dem. Rep. of the Congo* **114 B3** 0 1N 18 18 E
Mbanga, *Cameroon* **113 E6** 4 30N 9 33 E
Mbanika, *Solomon Is.* **133 M10** 9 3 S 159 13 E
M'Banio, Lagune, *Gabon* **114 C2** 3 35 S 11 0 E
Mbanza Congo, *Angola* **115 D2** 6 18 S 14 16 E
Mbanza Ngungu, *Dem. Rep. of the Congo* **115 D2** 5 12 S 14 53 E
Mbarangandu, *Tanzania* **119 D4** 10 11 S 36 48 E
Mbarara, *Uganda* **118 C3** 0 35 S 30 40 E
Mbari ➝, *C.A.R.* **114 B4** 4 34N 22 43 E
Mbashe ➝, *S. Africa* **117 E4** 32 15 S 28 54 E
Mbatto, *Ivory C.* **112 D4** 6 28N 4 22W
Mbava, *Solomon Is.* **133 L9** 7 47 S 156 33 E
Mbé, *Cameroon* **114 C3** 3 14 S 15 50 E
Mbe, *Eq. Guin.* **114 B1** 1 47N 9 56 E
Mbengga = Beqa, *Fiji* **133 B2** 18 23 S 178 8 E
Mbengué, *Gabon* **114 C2** 2 2 S 11 7 E
Mbengui, *Gabon* **114 C2** 2 3 S 10 4 E
Mbenkuru ➝, *Tanzania* **119 D4** 9 25 S 39 50 E
Mbéré ➝, *Cameroon* **114 A3** 7 45N 15 36 E
Mberengwa, *Zimbabwe* **119 G2** 20 29 S 29 57 E
Mberengwa, Mt., *Zimbabwe* **119 G2** 20 37 S 29 55 E
Mberubu, *Nigeria* **113 D6** 6 10N 7 38 E
Mbesuma, *Zambia* **119 E3** 10 0 S 32 2 E
Mbeya, *Tanzania* **119 D3** 8 54 S 33 29 E
Mbeya □, *Tanzania* **118 D3** 8 15 S 33 30 E
Mbigou, *Gabon* **114 C2** 1 53 S 11 56 E
M'bili, *Sudan* **107 F2** 7 35N 28 15 E
Mbinga, *Tanzania* **119 E4** 10 50 S 35 0 E
Mbini = Río Muni □, *Eq. Guin.* **114 B2** 1 30N 10 0 E
Mbini, *Eq. Guin.* **114 B1** 1 35N 9 37 E
Mboi, *Dem. Rep. of the Congo* **115 D4** 6 57 S 21 54 E
Mboki, *C.A.R.* **107 F2** 5 19N 25 58 E
Mbokonimbeti, *Solomon Is.* **133 M11** 8 57 S 160 7 E
Mboli, *Dem. Rep. of the Congo* **114 B4** 4 8N 23 9 E
M'bonge, *Cameroon* **113 E6** 4 33N 9 5 E
Mboro, *Senegal* **112 B1** 15 9N 16 54W
Mboua, *Cameroon* **114 A2** 4 25N 14 16 E
M'boukou, Rés. de, *Cameroon* **113 D7** 6 23N 12 50 E
Mboune, *Senegal* **112 C2** 14 42N 13 34W
Mbouoma, *Congo* **114 C3** 0 52 S 15 4 E
Mbour, *Senegal* **112 C1** 14 22N 16 54W
Mbout, *Mauritania* **112 B2** 16 1N 12 38W
Mbrés, *C.A.R.* **114 A3** 6 40N 19 48 E
M'Bridge ➝, *Angola* **115 D2** 7 12 S 12 51 E
Mbuji-Mayi, *Dem. Rep. of the Congo* **118 D1** 6 9 S 23 40 E
Mbulu, *Tanzania* **118 C4** 3 45 S 35 30 E
Mbuma, *Dem. Rep. of the Congo* **114 B4** 3 32N 24 50 E
Mbuma, *Solomon Is.* **133 M11** 8 59 S 160 46 E
Mburucuyá, *Argentina* **174 B4** 28 1 S 58 14W
M'bwat, *Cameroon* **114 A2** 6 29N 10 45 E
McCarran International, Las Vegas ✕ (LAS), *U.S.A.* **161 J11** 36 5N 115 9W
Mcherrah, *Algeria* **110 C4** 27 0N 4 30W
Mchinja, *Tanzania* **119 D4** 9 44 S 39 45 E
Mchinji, *Malawi* **119 E3** 13 47 S 32 58 E
McMurdo, *Antarctica* **7 D11** 77 0 S 140 0 E
Mdennah, *Mauritania* **110 D3** 24 37N 6 0W
Mé Maoya, *N. Cal.* **133 U19** 21 22 S 165 22 E
Mead, L., *U.S.A.* **161 J12** 36 1N 114 44W
Meade, *U.S.A.* **155 G4** 37 17N 100 20W
Meade ➝, *U.S.A.* **144 A9** 70 52N 155 55W
Meade River, *U.S.A.* **144 A8** 70 28N 157 24W
Meadow Lake, *Canada* **143 C7** 54 10N 108 26W
Meadow Lake ⌂, *Canada* **143 C7** 54 27N 109 0W
Meadow Valley Wash ➝, *U.S.A.* **161 J12** 36 40N 114 34W
Meadville, *Mo., U.S.A.* **156 E3** 39 47N 93 18W
Meadville, *Pa., U.S.A.* **150 E4** 41 39N 80 9W
Meaford, *Canada* **140 D3** 44 36N 80 35W
Mealhada, *Portugal* **42 E2** 40 22N 8 27W
Mealy Mts., *Canada* **141 B8** 53 10N 58 0W
Meander River, *Canada* **142 B5** 59 2N 117 42W
Meares, C., *U.S.A.* **158 D2** 45 37N 124 0W
Mearim ➝, *Brazil* **170 B3** 3 4 S 44 35W
Meath □, *Ireland* **23 C5** 53 40N 6 57W
Meath Park, *Canada* **143 C7** 53 27N 105 22W
Meaulne, *France* **27 F9** 46 36N 2 36 E
Meaux, *France* **27 D9** 48 58N 2 50 E
Mebechi-Gawa ➝, *Japan* **70 D10** 40 31N 141 31 E
Mebonden, *Norway* **18 A8** 63 13N 11 2 E
Mebulu, Tanjung, *Indonesia* **79 K18** 8 50 S 115 5 E
Mecanhelas, *Mozam.* **119 F4** 15 12 S 35 54 E
Mecaya ➝, *Colombia* **168 C2** 0 29N 75 11W
Mecca = Makkah, *Si. Arabia* **98 B2** 21 30N 39 54 E
Mecca, *U.S.A.* **161 M10** 33 34N 116 5W
Mechanicsburg, *Ohio, U.S.A.* **157 D13** 40 4N 83 33W
Mechanicsburg, *Pa., U.S.A.* **150 F8** 40 13N 77 1W
Mechanicsville, *U.S.A.* **156 C5** 41 54N 91 16W
Mechanicville, *U.S.A.* **151 D11** 42 54N 73 41W
Mechara, *Ethiopia* **107 F5** 8 36N 40 20 E
Mechelen, *Belgium* **24 C4** 51 2N 4 29 E
Mecheria, *Algeria* **111 B4** 33 35N 0 18W
Mechernich, *Germany* **30 E2** 50 35N 6 39 E
Mechetinskaya, *Russia* **61 G5** 46 45N 40 32 E
Mechra Bel Ksiri, *Morocco* **110 B3** 34 34N 5 57W
Mechra Benâbbou, *Morocco* **110 B3** 32 39N 7 48W
Mecidiye, *Turkey* **51 F10** 40 38N 26 32 E
Mecitözü, *Turkey* **100 B6** 40 32N 35 17 E

Mecklenburg, Germany 36 B6 53 33N 11 40 E
Mecklenburg-Vorpommern □, Germany 30 B8 53 45N 12 15 E
Mecklenburger Bucht, Germany 30 A7 54 20N 11 40 E
Meconta, Mozam. 119 E4 14 59 S 39 50 E
Mecsek, Hungary 52 D3 46 10N 18 18 E
Meda, Portugal 42 E3 40 57N 7 18W
Medak, India 94 E4 18 1N 78 15 E
Medan, Indonesia 84 B1 3 40N 98 38 E
Médanos, Argentina 176 A4 38 50 S 62 42W
Médanos de Coro △, Venezuela 165 D6 11 35N 69 44W
Medanosa, Pta., Argentina 176 C3 48 8 S 66 0W
Medart, U.S.A. 152 E5 30 5N 84 23W
Medaryville, U.S.A. 157 C10 41 5N 86 55W
Medawachchiya, Sri Lanka 95 K5 8 30N 80 30 E
Medchal, India 94 F4 17 37N 78 29 E
Mede, Italy 44 C5 45 6N 8 44 E
Médéa, Algeria 111 A5 36 12N 2 50 E
Mededa, Bos.-H. 52 G4 43 44N 19 10 E
Médégué, Gabon 114 B2 0 37N 10 8 E
Medeiros Neto, Brazil 171 E3 17 20 S 40 14W
Medel, Pic, Switz. 33 C7 46 34N 8 55 E
Medellín, Colombia 168 B2 6 15N 75 35W
Medelpad, Sweden 16 B10 62 33N 16 30 E
Medemblik, Neths. 24 B5 52 46N 5 8 E
Médenine, Tunisia 108 B2 33 21N 10 30 E
Mederdra, Mauritania 112 B1 17 0N 15 38W
Medford, Mass., U.S.A. 151 D13 42 25N 71 7W
Medford, Oreg., U.S.A. 158 E2 42 19N 122 52W
Medford, Wis., U.S.A. 154 C9 45 9N 90 20W
Medgidia, Romania 53 F13 44 15N 28 19 E
Medi, Sudan 107 F3 5 4N 30 42 E
Media Agua, Argentina 174 C2 31 58 S 68 25W
Media Luna, Argentina 174 C2 34 45 S 66 44W
Medianeira, Brazil 175 B5 25 17 S 54 5W
Mediapolis, U.S.A. 156 D5 41 0N 91 10W
Mediaş, Romania 53 D9 46 9N 24 22 E
Medicilândia, Brazil 169 D7 3 33 S 53 8W
Medicina, Italy 45 D8 44 28N 11 38 E
Medicine Bow, U.S.A. 158 F10 41 54N 106 12W
Medicine Bow Mts., U.S.A. 158 F10 41 10N 106 25W
Medicine Bow Pk., U.S.A. 158 F10 41 21N 106 19W
Medicine Hat, Canada 143 D6 50 0N 110 45W
Medicine Lake, U.S.A. 154 A2 48 30N 104 30W
Medicine Lodge, U.S.A. 155 G5 37 17N 98 35W
Medina = Al Madīnah, Si. Arabia 96 E3 24 35N 39 52 E
Medina, Brazil 171 E3 16 15 S 41 29W
Medina, Colombia 168 C3 4 30N 73 21W
Medina, Phil. 81 G5 8 55N 125 0 E
Medina, N. Dak., U.S.A. 154 B5 46 54N 99 18W
Medina, N.Y., U.S.A. 150 C6 43 13N 78 23W
Medina, Ohio, U.S.A. 150 E3 41 8N 81 52W
Medina →, U.S.A. 155 L5 29 16N 98 29W
Medina de Pomar, Spain 42 C7 42 56N 3 29W
Medina de Ríoseco, Spain 42 D5 41 53N 5 3W
Medina del Campo, Spain 42 D6 41 18N 4 55W
Medina L., U.S.A. 155 L5 29 32N 98 56W
Medina Sidonia, Spain 43 J5 36 28N 5 57W
Medinaceli, Spain 40 D2 41 12N 2 30W
Medinipur, India 93 H12 22 25N 87 21 E
Mediterranean Sea, Europe 12 H7 35 0N 15 0 E
Medjerda, O. →, Tunisia 108 A2 37 7N 10 13 E
Mednogorsk, Russia 64 F6 51 24N 57 37 E
Medny = Mednogorsk, Russia 64 F6 51 24N 57 37 E
Médoc, France 28 C3 45 10N 0 50W
Medora, U.S.A. 157 F10 38 49N 86 10W
Médouneu, Gabon 114 B2 0 57N 10 47 E
Medulin, Croatia 45 D10 44 49N 13 55 E
Medveđa, Serbia & M. 50 D5 42 50N 21 32 E
Medvedevo, Russia 60 B8 56 37N 47 47 E
Medveditsa →, Tver, Russia 58 D9 57 5N 37 30 E
Medveditsa →, Volgograd, Russia 60 F6 49 35N 42 41 E
Medvedok, Russia 60 B10 57 20N 50 1 E
Medvezhi, Ostrava, Russia 67 B17 71 0N 161 0 E
Medvezhye = Krasnogvardeyskoye, Russia 61 H5 45 52N 41 33 E
Medvezhyegorsk, Russia 56 B5 63 0N 34 25 E
Medway □, U.K. 21 F8 51 25N 0 32 E
Medway →, U.K. 21 F8 51 27N 0 46 E
Medzev, Slovak Rep. 35 C13 48 43N 20 55 E
Medzilaborce, Slovak Rep. 35 B14 49 17N 21 52 E
Medžitlija, Macedonia 50 F5 40 56N 21 26 E
Meekatharra, Australia 125 E2 26 32 S 118 29 E
Meeker, U.S.A. 158 F10 40 2N 107 55W
Meelpaeg Res., Canada 141 C8 48 15N 56 33W
Meeniyan, Australia 129 E7 38 35 S 146 0 E
Meersburg, Germany 31 H5 47 41N 9 16 E
Meerut, India 92 E7 29 1N 77 42 E
Meeteetse, U.S.A. 158 D9 44 9N 108 52W
Mega, Ethiopia 107 G4 3 57N 38 19 E
Megálo Khorío, Greece 49 E9 36 27N 27 24 E
Megálo Petalí, Greece 48 D6 38 0N 24 15 E
Megalópolis, Greece 48 D4 37 25N 22 7 E
Meganísi Nisís, Greece 39 B2 38 38N 20 46 E
Mégara, Greece 48 D5 37 58N 23 22 E
Megasini, India 93 J12 21 38N 86 21 E
Megdhova →, Greece 48 B3 39 10N 21 45 E
Megève, France 29 C10 45 51N 6 37 E
Meghalaya □, India 90 C3 25 50N 91 0 E
Meghezez, Ethiopia 107 F4 9 18N 39 26 E
Meghna →, Bangla. 90 D3 22 50N 90 50 E
Mégiscane, L., Canada 140 C4 48 35N 75 55W
Megiste, Greece 49 E11 36 8N 29 34 E
Megra, Russia 58 B9 60 11N 37 14 E
Mehadia, Romania 52 F7 44 56N 22 23 E
Mehaïguene, O. →, Algeria 111 B5 32 15N 2 59 E
Meharry, Mt., Australia 124 D2 22 59 S 118 35 E
Mehedeby, Sweden 16 D11 60 27N 17 25 E
Mehedinţi □, Romania 52 F7 44 40N 22 45 E
Meheisa, Sudan 106 D3 19 38N 32 57 E
Mehekar, India 94 D3 20 9N 76 34 E
Mehlville, U.S.A. 154 F9 38 30N 90 19W
Mehndawal, India 93 F10 26 58N 83 5 E
Mehr Jān, Iran 97 C7 33 50N 55 6 E
Mehrābād, Iran 101 D12 36 53N 47 55 E
Mehrān, Iran 101 F12 33 7N 46 10 E
Mehrīz, Iran 97 D7 31 35N 54 28 E
Mehun-sur-Yèvre, France 27 E9 47 10N 2 13 E
Mei Jiang →, China 77 E11 24 25N 116 35 E
Mei Xian, China 74 G4 34 18N 107 55 E
Meia Ponte →, Brazil 171 E2 18 32 S 49 36W
Meicheng, China 77 C12 29 29N 119 16 E
Meichengzhen, China 77 C8 28 9N 111 40 E
Meichuan, China 77 B10 30 8N 115 31 E
Meiganga, Cameroon 114 A2 6 30N 14 25 E
Meigs, U.S.A. 152 D5 31 4N 84 6W
Meigu, China 76 C4 28 16N 103 20 E
Meiktila, Burma 90 E5 20 53N 95 54 E
Meilen, Switz. 33 B7 47 16N 8 39 E
Meinerzhagen, Germany 30 D3 51 6N 7 38 E
Meiningen, Germany 30 E6 50 34N 10 25 E
Meio →, Brazil 171 D3 13 36 S 44 7W
Meira, Serra de, Spain 42 B3 43 15N 7 15W
Meiringen, Switz. 32 C6 46 43N 8 12 E
Meishan, China 76 B4 30 3N 103 23 E
Meissen, Germany 30 D9 51 9N 13 29 E
Meissner, Germany 30 D5 51 14N 9 50 E
Meissner-Kaufunger Wald △, Germany 30 D5 51 16N 9 45 E
Meitan, China 76 D6 27 45N 107 29 E
Meizhou, China 77 E11 24 16N 116 6 E
Meja, India 93 G9 25 9N 82 7 E
Mejillones, Chile 174 A1 23 10 S 70 30W
Mékambo, Gabon 114 B2 1 2N 13 50 E
Mekdela, Ethiopia 107 E4 11 24N 39 10 E
Mekele, Ethiopia 107 E4 13 33N 39 30 E
Mekerghene, Sebkra, Algeria 111 C5 26 21N 1 30 E
Mekhomiya = Razlog, Bulgaria 50 E7 41 53N 23 28 E
Mekhtar, Pakistan 91 C3 30 30N 69 15 E
Meknès, Morocco 110 B3 33 57N 5 33W
Meko, Nigeria 113 D5 7 27N 2 52 E
Mekong →, Asia 87 H6 9 30N 106 15 E
Mekongga, Indonesia 82 E6 3 39 S 121 15 E
Mekoryuk, U.S.A. 144 F6 60 23N 166 11W
Mekrou →, Benin 113 C5 12 25N 2 50 E
Mekvari = Kür →, Azerbaijan 101 C13 39 29N 49 15 E
Mel, Italy 45 B9 46 4N 12 5 E
Melagiri Hills, India 95 H3 12 20N 77 30 E
Melah, Oued el →, Algeria 111 C6 32 20N 2 28 E
Melah, Sebkhet el, Algeria 111 C4 29 20N 1 30W
Melaka, Malaysia 87 L4 2 15N 102 15 E
Melaka □, Malaysia 84 B2 2 15N 102 15 E
Melalap, Malaysia 78 C5 5 10N 116 5 E
Mélambes, Greece 39 E5 35 8N 24 40 E
Melanesia, Pac. Oc. 134 H7 4 0 S 155 0 E
Melapalaiyam, India 95 K3 8 39N 77 44 E
Melawi →, Indonesia 85 B4 0 5N 111 29 E
Melaya, Indonesia 79 J17 8 17 S 114 30 E
Melbourne, Australia 129 D6 37 50 S 145 0 E
Melbourne, Fla., U.S.A. 153 G9 28 5N 80 37W
Melbourne, Iowa, U.S.A. 156 C3 41 57N 93 6W
Melcher-Dallas, U.S.A. 156 C3 41 14N 93 15W
Melchor Múzquiz, Mexico 162 B4 27 50N 101 30W
Melchor Ocampo, Mexico 162 C4 24 52N 101 40W
Meldal, Norway 18 A6 63 3N 9 44 E
Méldola, Italy 45 D9 44 7N 12 5 E
Meldorf, Germany 30 A5 54 5N 9 5 E
Mélé, C.A.R. 114 A4 9 46N 21 33 E
Mele B., Vanuatu 133 G6 17 44 S 168 14 E
Meleden, Somali Rep. 120 B3 10 25N 49 51 E
Melegnano, Italy 44 C6 45 21N 9 19 E
Meleizem, Mauritania 110 D2 22 19N 11 24W
Melekess = Dimitrovgrad, Russia 60 C9 54 14N 49 39 E
Melenci, Serbia & M. 52 E5 45 32N 20 20 E
Melenki, Russia 60 C5 55 20N 41 37 E
Meleuz, Russia 64 E6 52 58N 55 55 E
Mélèzes →, Canada 140 A5 57 40N 69 29W
Melfi, Chad 109 F3 11 0N 17 59 E
Melfi, Italy 47 B8 41 0N 15 39 E
Melfort, Canada 143 C8 52 50N 104 37W
Melfort, Zimbabwe 119 F3 18 0 S 31 25 E
Melgaço, Portugal 42 C2 42 7N 8 15W
Melgar de Fernamental, Spain 42 C6 42 27N 4 17W
Melgraseyri, Iceland 11 A4 66 1N 22 27W
Melhus, Norway 18 A7 63 17N 10 18 E
Melide, Spain 42 C2 42 55N 8 1W
Melide, Switz. 33 E7 45 57N 8 57 E
Meligalá, Greece 48 D3 37 15N 21 59 E
Melilla, N. Afr. 111 A4 35 21N 2 57W
Melilli, Italy 47 E8 37 11N 15 7 E
Melipilla, Chile 174 C1 33 42 S 71 15W
Mélissa, Ákra, Greece 39 E5 35 6N 24 33 E
Mélissa Óros, Greece 49 D8 37 32N 26 4 E
Melissani Cave, Greece 39 C2 38 15N 20 38 E
Melita, Canada 143 D8 49 15N 101 0W
Mélito di Porto Salvo, Italy 47 E8 37 55N 15 47 E
Melitopol, Ukraine 59 J8 46 50N 35 22 E
Melk, Austria 34 C8 48 13N 15 20 E
Mellan Fryken, Sweden 16 E7 59 45N 13 10 E
Mellansel, Sweden 14 E18 63 26N 18 19 E
Mellbystrand, Sweden 17 H6 56 30N 12 56 E
Melle, France 28 B3 46 14N 0 10W
Melle, Germany 30 C4 52 12N 8 20 E
Mellègue, O. →, Tunisia 108 A1 36 36N 9 14 E
Mellen, U.S.A. 154 B9 46 20N 90 40W
Mellerud, Sweden 17 F6 58 41N 12 28 E
Mellette, U.S.A. 154 C5 45 9N 98 30W
Mellid = Melide, Spain 42 C2 42 55N 8 1W
Mellieħa, Malta 38 F7 35 57N 14 22 E
Mellieħa Bay, Malta 38 F7 35 59N 14 22 E
Mellit, Sudan 107 E2 14 7N 25 34 E
Mellizo Sur, Cerro, Chile 176 C2 48 33 S 73 10W
Mellrichstadt, Germany 30 E6 50 25N 10 17 E
Melnik, Bulgaria 50 E7 41 30N 23 25 E
Mělník, Czech Rep. 34 A7 50 22N 14 23 E
Melnytsya Podilska, Ukraine 53 B11 48 37N 26 10 E
Melo, Uruguay 175 C5 32 20 S 54 10W
Melolo, Indonesia 82 C2 9 53 S 120 40 E
Melouprey, Cambodia 86 F5 13 48N 105 16 E
Melrhir, Chott, Algeria 111 B6 34 13N 6 30 E
Melrose, Australia 129 B7 32 42 S 146 57 E
Melrose, U.K. 22 F6 55 36N 2 43W
Melrose, Minn., U.S.A. 154 C7 45 40N 94 49W
Melrose, N. Mex., U.S.A. 155 H3 34 26N 103 38W
Mels, Switz. 33 B8 47 3N 9 25 E
Melsisi, Vanuatu 133 E6 15 46 S 168 10 E
Melstone, U.S.A. 158 C10 46 36N 107 52W
Melsungen, Germany 30 D5 51 7N 9 32 E
Melton, Australia 128 D6 37 41 S 144 35 E
Melton Mowbray, U.K. 20 E7 52 47N 0 54W
Melun, France 27 D9 48 32N 2 39 E
Melur, India 95 J4 10 2N 78 23 E
Melut, Sudan 107 E3 10 30N 32 13 E
Melville, Canada 143 C8 50 55N 102 50W
Melville, C., Australia 126 A3 14 11 S 144 30 E
Melville, C., Phil. 81 H1 7 49N 117 0 E
Melville, L., Canada 141 B8 53 30N 60 0W
Melville B., Australia 126 A2 12 0 S 136 45 E
Melville B., Greenland 10 B4 75 30N 63 0W
Melville I., Australia 124 B5 11 30 S 131 0 E
Melville I., Canada 6 B2 75 30N 112 0W
Melville Pen., Canada 139 B11 68 0N 84 0W
Mélykút, Hungary 52 D4 46 11N 19 25 E
Memaliaj, Albania 50 F3 40 25N 19 56 E
Memba, Mozam. 119 E5 14 11 S 40 30 E
Memboro, Indonesia 82 C1 9 30 S 119 30 E
Membrilla, Spain 43 G7 38 59N 3 21W
Memel = Klaipėda, Lithuania 15 J19 55 43N 21 10 E
Memel, S. Africa 117 D4 27 38 S 29 36 E
Memmingen, Germany 31 H6 47 58N 10 10 E
Mempawah, Indonesia 85 B3 0 30N 109 5 E
Memphis, Egypt 106 J7 29 52N 31 12 E
Memphis, Mich., U.S.A. 150 D2 42 54N 82 46W
Memphis, Mo., U.S.A. 156 D4 40 28N 92 10W
Memphis, Tenn., U.S.A. 155 H10 35 8N 90 3W
Memphis, Tex., U.S.A. 155 H4 34 44N 100 33W
Memphremagog, L., U.S.A. 151 B12 45 0N 72 12W
Mena, Ukraine 59 G7 51 31N 32 13 E
Mena, U.S.A. 155 H7 34 35N 94 15W
Mena →, Ethiopia 107 F5 5 40N 40 50 E
Menai Strait, U.K. 20 D3 53 11N 4 13W
Ménaka, Mali 113 B5 15 59N 2 18 E
Menan = Chao Phraya →, Thailand 86 F3 13 32N 100 36 E
Menarandra →, Madag. 117 D7 25 17 S 44 30 E
Menard, U.S.A. 155 K5 30 55N 99 47W
Menard Fracture Zone, Pac. Oc. 135 M18 43 0 S 97 0W
Menate, Indonesia 85 C4 0 12 S 113 3 E
Menawashei, Sudan 107 E1 12 41N 24 59 E
Mendawai →, Indonesia 85 C4 3 30 S 113 0 E
Mende, France 28 D7 44 31N 3 30 E
Mendebo Mts., Ethiopia 107 F4 7 0N 39 22 E
Mendeleyev Ridge, Arctic 6 B17 80 0N 178 0W
Menden, Germany 30 D3 51 26N 7 47 E
Mendenhall, C., U.S.A. 144 G6 59 45N 166 10W
Menderes, Turkey 49 C9 38 14N 27 8 E
Mendez, Mexico 163 B5 25 7N 98 34W
Mendhar, India 93 C6 33 35N 74 10 E
Mendi, Ethiopia 107 F4 9 47N 35 4 E
Mendi, Papua N. G. 132 D2 6 11 S 143 39 E
Mendip Hills, U.K. 21 F5 51 17N 2 40W
Mendocino, U.S.A. 158 G2 39 19N 123 48W
Mendocino, C., U.S.A. 158 F1 40 26N 124 25W
Mendocino Fracture Zone, Pac. Oc. 135 D13 40 0N 142 0W
Mendon, U.S.A. 157 B11 42 0N 85 27W
Mendooran, Australia 129 A8 31 50 S 149 6 E
Mendota, Calif., U.S.A. 160 J6 36 45N 120 23W
Mendota, Ill., U.S.A. 156 C7 41 33N 89 7W
Mendoyo, Indonesia 79 J17 8 23 S 114 42 E
Mendoza, Argentina 174 C2 32 50 S 68 52W
Mendoza □, Argentina 174 C2 33 0 S 69 0W
Mendrisio, Switz. 33 E7 45 52N 8 59 E
Mene Grande, Venezuela 168 B3 9 49N 70 56W
Menemen, Turkey 49 C9 38 34N 27 3 E
Menen, Belgium 24 D3 50 47N 3 7 E
Menéndez, L., Argentina 176 B2 42 40 S 71 51W
Ménerville = Thenia, Algeria 111 A5 36 44N 3 33 E
Menfi, Italy 46 E5 37 36N 12 58 E
Mengdingjie, China 76 F2 23 31N 98 58 E
Mengeš, Slovenia 45 B11 46 10N 14 35 E
Menggala, Indonesia 84 C3 4 30 S 105 15 E
Menghai, China 76 G3 21 49N 100 55 E
Mengibar, Spain 43 H7 37 58N 3 48W
Mengjin, China 74 G7 34 55N 112 45 E
Mengla, China 76 G3 21 20N 101 25 E
Menglian, China 76 F2 22 21N 99 27 E
Mengoub, Algeria 110 C3 29 49N 5 26W
Mengshan, China 77 E8 24 14N 110 55 E
Mengyin, China 75 G9 35 40N 117 58 E
Mengzhe, China 76 F3 22 2N 100 15 E
Mengzi, China 76 F4 23 20N 103 22 E
Menihek, Canada 141 B6 54 28N 56 36W
Menihek L., Canada 141 B6 54 0N 67 0W
Menin = Menen, Belgium 24 D3 50 47N 3 7 E
Menindee, Australia 128 B5 32 20 S 142 25 E
Menindee L., Australia 128 B5 32 20 S 142 25 E
Meningie, Australia 128 C3 35 50 S 139 18 E
Menjangan, Pulau, Indonesia 79 J17 8 7 S 114 31 E
Menkrour, Algeria 111 C6 26 27N 8 9 E
Menlo Park, U.S.A. 160 H4 37 27N 122 12W
Menominee, U.S.A. 148 C2 45 6N 87 37W
Menominee →, U.S.A. 148 C2 45 6N 87 36W
Menomonee Falls, U.S.A. 157 A8 43 11N 88 7W
Menomonie, U.S.A. 154 C9 44 53N 91 55W
Menongue, Angola 115 E3 14 48 S 17 52 E
Menorca, Spain 38 B5 40 0N 4 0 E
Menorca ✕ (MAH), Spain 40 F9 39 50N 4 16 E
Mentakab, Malaysia 87 L4 3 29N 102 21 E
Mentasta Lake, U.S.A. 144 E12 62 55N 143 45W
Mentawai, Kepulauan, Indonesia 84 C1 2 0 S 99 0 E
Menton, France 29 E11 43 50N 7 29 E
Mentone, U.S.A. 157 C10 41 10N 86 2W
Mentor, U.S.A. 150 E3 41 40N 81 21W
Menyamya, Papua N. G. 132 D3 7 10 S 145 59 E
Menzel-Bourguiba, Tunisia 108 A1 37 9N 9 49 E
Menzel-Chaker, Tunisia 108 B2 35 0N 10 26 E
Menzel-Temime, Tunisia 108 A2 36 46N 11 0 E
Menzelinsk, Russia 64 D4 55 47N 53 11 E
Menzies, Australia 125 E3 29 40 S 121 2 E
Meob B., Namibia 116 C1 24 25 S 14 34 E
Me'ona, Israel 103 B4 33 1N 35 15 E
Meoqui, Mexico 162 B3 28 17N 105 29W
Mepaco, Mozam. 119 F3 15 57 S 30 48 E
Meppel, Neths. 24 B6 52 42N 6 12 E
Meppen, Germany 30 C3 52 42N 7 17 E
Mequinenza, Spain 40 D5 41 22N 0 17 E
Mequinenza, Embalse de, Spain 40 D5 41 25N 0 15 E
Mequon, U.S.A. 157 A9 43 14N 87 59W
Mer, France 26 E8 47 42N 1 30 E
Merabéllou, Kólpos, Greece 39 E6 35 10N 25 50 E
Merai, Papua N. G. 132 C7 4 52 S 152 19 E
Merak, Indonesia 79 F12 6 10N 106 26 E
Meråker, Norway 18 A8 63 25N 11 46 E
Meramangye, L., Australia 125 E5 28 25 S 132 13 E
Meramec →, U.S.A. 156 F6 38 24N 90 21W
Meran = Merano, Italy 45 B8 46 40N 11 9 E
Merano, Italy 45 B8 46 40N 11 9 E
Merate, Italy 44 C6 45 42N 9 25 E
Merauke, Indonesia 83 C6 8 29 S 140 24 E
Merauke →, Indonesia 83 C6 8 30 S 140 24 E
Merbabu, Indonesia 85 D4 7 30 S 110 40 E
Merbein, Australia 128 C5 34 10 S 142 2 E
Merbuk, Gunung, Indonesia 79 J17 8 13 S 114 39 E
Merca, Somali Rep. 120 D2 1 48N 44 50 E
Mercantour △, France 29 D10 44 16N 6 43 E
Mercato Saraceno, Italy 45 E9 43 57N 12 12 E
Merced, U.S.A. 160 H6 37 18N 120 29W
Merced →, U.S.A. 160 H6 37 21N 120 59W
Merced Pk., U.S.A. 160 H7 37 36N 119 24W
Mercedes, Buenos Aires, Argentina 174 C4 34 40 S 59 30W
Mercedes, Corrientes, Argentina 174 B4 29 10 S 58 5W
Mercedes, San Luis, Argentina 174 C2 33 40 S 65 21W
Mercedes, Phil. 80 D4 14 7N 123 1 E
Mercedes, Uruguay 174 C4 33 12 S 58 0W
Merceditas, Chile 174 B1 28 20 S 70 35W
Mercer, N.Z. 130 D4 37 16 S 175 5 E
Mercer, Mo., U.S.A. 156 D3 40 31N 93 32W
Mercer, Pa., U.S.A. 150 E4 41 14N 80 15W
Mercer Island, U.S.A. 160 C4 47 35N 122 15W
Mercier, Bolivia 172 C4 10 42 S 68 5W
Mercury, U.S.A. 161 J11 36 40N 115 58W
Mercury B., N.Z. 130 C4 36 48 S 175 45 E
Mercury Is., N.Z. 130 C4 36 37 S 175 52 E
Mercy, C., Canada 139 B13 65 0N 63 30W
Merdrignac, France 26 D4 48 11N 2 27W
Mere, U.K. 21 F5 51 6N 2 16W
Mere Lava, Vanuatu 133 D6 14 25 S 168 3 E
Meredith, Australia 128 D6 37 49 S 144 5 E
Meredith, C., Falk. Is. 9 f 52 15 S 60 40W
Meredith, L., U.S.A. 155 H4 35 43N 101 33W
Meredosia, U.S.A. 156 E6 39 50N 90 34W
Merefa, Ukraine 59 H9 49 48N 36 3 E
Meregh, Somali Rep. 120 D3 3 46N 47 18 E
Merei, Romania 53 E11 45 7N 26 43 E
Merga = Nukheila, Sudan 106 D2 19 1N 26 21 E
Mergui, Burma 86 F2 12 26N 98 34 E
Mergui Arch. = Myeik Kyunzu, Burma 87 G1 11 30N 97 30 E
Meribah, Australia 128 C4 34 43 S 140 51 E
Méribel-les-Allues, France 29 C10 45 25N 6 34 E
Meriç, Turkey 51 E10 41 11N 26 25 E
Meriç →, Turkey 51 F10 40 52N 26 12 E
Mérida, Mexico 163 C7 20 58N 89 37W
Mérida, Phil. 81 F5 10 55N 124 32 E
Mérida, Spain 43 G4 38 55N 6 25W
Mérida, Venezuela 168 B3 8 24N 71 8W
Mérida □, Venezuela 168 B3 8 30N 71 10W
Mérida, Cord. de, Venezuela 168 B3 9 0N 71 0W
Meriden, U.K. 21 E6 52 26N 1 38W
Meriden, U.S.A. 151 E12 41 32N 72 48W
Meridian, Calif., U.S.A. 160 F5 39 9N 121 55W
Meridian, Ga., U.S.A. 152 D8 31 27N 81 23W
Meridian, Idaho, U.S.A. 158 E5 43 37N 116 24W
Meridian, Miss., U.S.A. 149 J1 32 22N 88 42W
Mérignac, France 28 D3 44 51N 0 39W
Merimbula, Australia 129 D8 36 53 S 149 54 E
Mérinaghène, Senegal 112 B1 15 57N 15 55W
Merinda, Australia 126 C4 20 2 S 148 11 E
Mering, Germany 31 G6 48 16N 10 59 E
Meringa, Nigeria 113 C7 10 44N 12 9 E
Meringur, Australia 128 C4 34 20 S 141 19 E
Merir, Pac. Oc. 79 D8 4 10N 132 30 E
Merirumã, Brazil 169 C7 1 15N 54 50W
Merke, Kazakhstan 65 B6 42 52N 73 11 E
Merkel, U.S.A. 155 J5 32 28N 100 1W
Mermaid Reef, Australia 124 C2 17 6 S 119 36 E
Meroe, India 95 L11 7 33N 93 33 E
Merowe, Sudan 106 D3 18 29N 31 46 E
Merredin, Australia 125 F2 31 28 S 118 18 E
Merrick, U.K. 22 F4 55 8N 4 28W
Merrickville, Canada 151 B9 44 55N 75 50W
Merrill, Oreg., U.S.A. 158 E3 42 1N 121 36W
Merrill, Wis., U.S.A. 154 C10 45 11N 89 41W
Merrillville, U.S.A. 157 C9 41 29N 87 20W
Merrimack →, U.S.A. 151 D14 42 49N 70 49W
Merriman, U.S.A. 154 D4 42 55N 101 42W
Merritt, Canada 142 C4 50 10N 120 45W
Merritt Island, U.S.A. 153 G9 28 21N 80 42W
Merriwa, Australia 129 B9 32 6 S 150 22 E
Merriwagga, Australia 129 B6 33 47 S 145 43 E
Merry I., Canada 140 A4 55 29N 77 31W
Merrygoen, Australia 129 A8 31 51 S 149 12 E
Merryville, U.S.A. 155 K8 30 45N 93 33W
Mersa Fatma, Eritrea 107 E5 14 57N 40 17 E
Mersch, Lux. 24 E6 49 44N 6 7 E
Merse →, Italy 45 E8 43 5N 11 22 E
Mersea I., U.K. 21 F8 51 47N 0 58 E
Merseburg, Germany 30 D7 51 22N 11 59 E
Mersey →, U.K. 20 D4 53 25N 3 1W
Merseyside □, U.K. 20 D4 53 31N 3 2W
Mersin, Turkey 100 D6 36 51N 34 36 E
Mersing, Malaysia 87 L4 2 25N 103 50 E
Merta, India 92 F6 26 39N 74 4 E
Merta Road, India 92 F5 26 43N 73 55 E
Merthyr Tydfil, U.K. 21 F4 51 45N 3 22W
Merthyr Tydfil □, U.K. 21 F4 51 46N 3 21W
Mértola, Portugal 43 H3 37 40N 7 40W
Mertzon, U.S.A. 155 K4 31 16N 100 49W
Méru, France 27 C9 49 13N 2 8 E
Meru, Kenya 118 B4 0 3N 37 40 E
Meru, Tanzania 118 C4 3 15 S 36 46 E
Meru △, Kenya 118 B4 0 5N 38 10 E
Merv = Mary, Turkmenistan 66 F7 37 40N 61 50 E
Merville, France 27 B9 50 38N 2 38 E
Méry-sur-Seine, France 27 D10 48 31N 3 54 E
Merzifon, Turkey 100 B6 40 53N 35 32 E
Merzig, Germany 31 F2 49 26N 6 38 E
Merzouga, Erg Tin, Algeria 111 D7 24 0N 11 4 E
Mesa, U.S.A. 159 K8 33 25N 111 50W
Mesa Verde △, U.S.A. 159 H9 37 11N 108 29W
Mesach Mellet, Libya 108 D2 24 30N 11 30 E
Mesagne, Italy 47 B10 40 34N 17 48 E
Mesanagrós, Greece 38 E11 36 1N 27 49 E
Mesaoría, Cyprus 39 E9 35 12N 33 14 E
Mesarás, Kólpos, Greece 39 E5 35 6N 24 47 E
Meschede, Germany 30 D4 51 20N 8 18 E
Mescit, Turkey 101 B9 40 21N 41 11 E
Mesemvriya = Nesebŭr, Bulgaria 51 D11 42 41N 27 46 E
Mesfinto, Ethiopia 107 E4 13 20N 37 22 E
Mesgouez, L., Canada 140 B5 51 20N 75 0W
Meshchovsk, Russia 58 E8 54 22N 35 17 E
Meshed = Mashhad, Iran 97 B8 36 20N 59 35 E
Meshkede-Ser = Bābol Sar, Iran 97 B7 36 45N 52 45 E
Meshoppen, U.S.A. 151 E8 41 36N 76 3W
Meshra er Req, Sudan 107 F2 8 25N 29 18 E
Mesilinka →, Canada 142 B4 56 6N 124 30W
Mesilla, U.S.A. 159 K10 32 16N 106 48W
Meslay-du-Maine, France 26 E6 47 58N 0 33W
Mesocco, Switz. 33 D8 46 23N 9 12 E
Mesologi = Mesolóngion, Greece 48 C3 38 21N 21 28 E
Mesolóngion, Greece 48 C3 38 21N 21 28 E
Mesopotamia = Al Jazirah, Iraq 101 E10 33 30N 44 0 E
Mesopotamia, U.S.A. 150 E4 41 27N 80 57W
Mesopótamon, Greece 48 B2 39 14N 20 32 E
Mesoraca, Italy 47 C9 39 5N 16 48 E
Mésou Volímais = Volímai, Greece 39 D2 37 52N 20 39 E
Mesquite, U.S.A. 159 H6 36 47N 114 6W
Messaad, Algeria 111 B5 34 8N 3 30 E
Messac, France 26 E5 47 49N 1 50W
Messalo →, Mozam. 119 E4 12 25 S 39 15 E
Méssaména, Cameroon 113 E7 3 48N 12 49 E
Messeue, Greece 48 D3 37 12N 21 58 E
Messier, Canal, Chile 176 C2 48 20 S 74 33W
Messina = Musina, S. Africa 117 C5 22 20 S 30 5 E
Messina, Italy 47 D8 38 11N 15 34 E
Messina, Str. di, Italy 47 D8 38 15N 15 35 E
Messíni, Greece 48 D4 37 4N 22 1 E
Messínía □, Greece 48 D3 37 10N 22 0 E
Messiniakós Kólpos, Greece 48 E4 36 45N 22 5 E
Messkirch, Germany 31 H5 47 59N 9 7 E
Messlingen, Sweden 16 B6 62 40N 12 50 E
Messonghi, Greece 38 C9 39 29N 19 56 E
Mesta →, Bulgaria 50 E7 40 54N 24 49 E
Mestá, Ákra, Greece 49 C7 38 16N 25 53 E
Mestanza, Spain 43 G6 38 35N 4 4W
Mestersvig, Greenland 10 C8 72 10N 23 40W
Mestre, Italy 45 C9 45 29N 12 15 E
Mestre, Espigão, Brazil 171 D2 12 30 S 46 10W
Mesudiye, Turkey 100 B7 40 28N 37 46 E
Meta, U.S.A. 156 F4 38 19N 92 10W
Meta □, Colombia 168 C3 3 30N 73 0W
Meta →, S. Amer. 168 B4 6 12N 67 28W
Meta Incognita Pen., Canada 139 B13 62 45N 68 30W
Metabetchouan, Canada 141 C5 48 26N 71 52W
Metairie, U.S.A. 155 L9 29 58N 90 10W
Metalici, Munţii, Romania 52 D7 46 15N 22 50 E
Metaline Falls, U.S.A. 158 B5 48 52N 117 22W
Metallifere, Colline, Italy 44 E8 43 10N 11 0 E
Metamora, U.S.A. 156 D7 40 47N 89 22W
Metán, Argentina 174 B3 25 30 S 65 0W
Metangula, Mozam. 119 E3 12 40 S 34 50 E
Metauro →, Italy 45 E10 43 50N 13 3 E
Metcalf, U.S.A. 152 E6 30 43N 83 59W
Metema, Ethiopia 107 E4 12 56N 36 13 E
Metengobalame, Mozam. 119 E3 14 49 S 34 30 E
Méthana, Greece 48 D5 37 35N 23 23 E
Methóni, Greece 48 E3 36 49N 21 42 E
Methven, N.Z. 131 D6 43 38 S 171 40 E
Metil, Mozam. 119 F4 16 24 S 39 0 E
Metkovets, Bulgaria 50 C7 43 37N 23 10 E
Metković, Croatia 45 E14 43 6N 17 39 E
Metlakatla, U.S.A. 144 J15 55 8N 131 35W
Metlaoui, Tunisia 108 B1 34 24N 8 24 E
Metlik, Papua N. G. 132 C7 4 46 S 152 55 E
Metlika, Slovenia 45 C12 45 40N 15 20 E
Metro, Indonesia 84 D3 5 5 S 105 20 E
Metropolis, U.S.A. 155 G10 37 9N 88 44W
Métsovon, Greece 48 B3 39 48N 21 12 E
Metter, U.S.A. 152 C7 32 24N 82 3W
Mettuppalaiyam, India 95 J3 11 18N 76 59 E
Mettur, India 95 J3 11 48N 77 47 E
Metu, Ethiopia 107 F4 8 18N 35 35 E
Metz, France 27 C13 49 8N 6 10 E
Metzingen, Germany 31 G5 48 31N 9 17 E
Meulaboh, Indonesia 84 B1 4 11N 96 3 E
Meung-sur-Loire, France 27 E8 47 50N 1 40 E
Meurcourt, France 32 A2 47 46N 6 14 E
Meureudu, Indonesia 84 A1 5 19N 96 10 E
Meurthe →, France 27 D13 48 47N 6 9 E
Meurthe-et-Moselle □, France 27 D13 48 52N 6 0 E
Meuse □, France 27 C12 49 8N 5 25 E
Meuse →, Europe 24 D5 50 45N 5 41 E
Meuselwitz, Germany 30 D8 51 2N 12 17 E
Meutapok, Mt., Malaysia 85 A5 5 40N 117 0 E
Mexia, U.S.A. 155 K6 31 41N 96 29W
Mexiana, I., Brazil 170 A2 0 0 49 30W
Mexicali, Mexico 161 N11 32 40N 115 30W
Mexican Plateau, Mexico 136 G9 25 0N 104 0W
Mexican Water, U.S.A. 159 H9 36 57N 109 32W
México, Mexico 163 D5 19 20N 99 10W
Mexico, Maine, U.S.A. 151 B14 44 34N 70 33W
Mexico, Mo., U.S.A. 156 E5 39 10N 91 53W
Mexico, N.Y., U.S.A. 151 C8 43 28N 76 18W
México □, Mexico 163 D5 19 20N 99 10W
Mexico ■, Cent. Amer. 162 C4 25 0N 105 0W
Mexico, G. of, Cent. Amer. 163 C7 25 0N 90 0W
Mexico B., U.S.A. 151 C8 43 35N 76 20W
Mexico Beach, U.S.A. 152 F4 29 57N 85 25W
Meydān-e Naftūn, Iran 97 D6 31 56N 49 18 E
Meydani, Ra's-e, Iran 97 E8 25 24N 59 6 E
Meyenburg, Germany 30 B8 53 18N 12 14 E
Meyers Chuck, U.S.A. 144 J14 55 45N 132 15W
Meymac, France 28 C6 45 32N 2 10 E
Meymaneh, Afghan. 91 B2 35 53N 64 38 E
Meyo, Cameroon 114 B2 2 50N 11 1 E
Meyrueis, France 28 D7 44 12N 3 27 E
Meyssac, France 28 C5 45 3N 1 40 E
Meyzieu, France 29 C8 45 46N 4 59 E
Mezdra, Bulgaria 50 C7 43 12N 23 42 E
Mèze, France 28 E7 43 27N 3 36 E
Mezen, Russia 56 A7 65 50N 44 20 E
Mezen →, Russia 56 A7 65 44N 44 22 E
Mézenc, Mt., France 29 D8 44 54N 4 11 E
Mezeş, Munţii, Romania 52 C8 47 5N 23 5 E
Mezha →, Russia 58 E6 55 44N 31 33 E
Mezhdurechenskiy, Russia 66 D7 59 36N 65 56 E
Mezhdurechye = Shali, Russia 61 J7 43 9N 45 55 E
Mezhevaya Utka = Sinegorskiy, Russia 61 G5 47 55N 40 52 E
Mézidon-Canon, France 26 C6 49 5N 0 1W
Mézières-en-Brenne, France 28 B5 46 49N 1 13 E
Mézilhac, France 29 D8 44 49N 4 21 E
Mézin, France 28 D4 44 4N 0 16 E
Mezőberény, Hungary 52 D6 46 49N 21 3 E
Mezőfalva, Hungary 52 D3 46 55N 18 49 E
Mezőhegyes, Hungary 52 D5 46 19N 20 49 E
Mezőkövácsháza, Hungary 52 D5 46 25N 20 57 E
Mezőkövesd, Hungary 52 C5 47 49N 20 35 E
Mézos, France 28 D2 44 5N 1 10W
Mezőtúr, Hungary 52 C5 47 1N 20 41 E
Mezquital, Mexico 162 C4 23 29N 104 23W
Mezzolombardo, Italy 44 B8 46 13N 11 5 E
Mfolozi →, S. Africa 117 D5 28 25 S 32 26 E

Mgarr, Malta .... 38 F7 35 55N 14 22 E
Mgarr, Gozo, Malta .... 38 2N 14 18 E
Mgeta, Tanzania .... 119 D4 8 22 S 36 6 E
Mglin, Russia .... 59 F7 53 2N 32 50 E
Mhlaba Hills, Zimbabwe ... 119 F3 18 30 S 30 30 E
Mhow, India .... 92 H6 22 33N 75 50 E
Mi-Shima, Japan .... 72 C3 34 46N 131 9 E
Miagao, Phil. .... 81 F4 10 39N 122 14 E
Miahuatlán, Mexico 163 D5 16 21N 96 36W
Miajadas, Spain 43 F5 39 9N 5 54W
Miami, Fla., U.S.A. 153 K9 25 47N 80 11W
Miami, Okla., U.S.A. .. 155 G7 36 53N 94 53W
Miami, Tex., U.S.A. ... 155 H4 35 42N 100 38W
Miami Beach, U.S.A. .. 153 K9 25 47N 80 8W
Miami Canal, U.S.A. .. 153 J9 26 30N 80 45W
Miami International ✈ (MIA), U.S.A. 153 K9 25 47N 80 17W
Miami Shores, U.S.A. . 153 K9 25 52N 80 12W
Miami Springs, U.S.A. 153 K9 25 49N 80 17W
Miamisburg, U.S.A. .. 157 E12 39 38N 84 17W
Mian Xian, China .... 74 H4 33 10N 106 32 E
Mianchi, China ...... 74 G6 34 48N 111 48 E
Mīāndarreh, Iran .... 97 C7 35 37N 53 39 E
Mīāndowāb, Iran .... 101 D12 37 0N 46 5 E
Miandrivazo, Madag. . 117 B8 19 31 S 45 29 E
Mīāneh, Iran .... 101 D12 37 30N 47 40 E
Mianning, China ..... 76 C4 28 32N 102 9 E
Mianwali, Pakistan ... 91 B3 32 38N 71 28 E
Mianyang, China ..... 76 B5 31 22N 104 47 E
Mianzhu, China ...... 76 B5 31 22N 104 7 E
Miaoli, Taiwan ...... 77 E13 24 37N 120 49 E
Miarinarivo, Antananarivo, Madag. ... 117 B8 18 57 S 46 55 E
Miarinarivo, Toamasina, Madag. 117 B8 16 38 S 48 15 E
Miarinarivo, Toamasina, Madag. 117 C8 20 13 S 47 31 E
Miass, Russia .... 64 D8 54 59N 60 6 E
Miasteczko Krajeńskie, Poland .... 55 E4 53 7N 17 1 E
Miastko, Poland ..... 54 D3 54 0N 16 58 E
Mica, S. Africa ...... 117 C5 24 10 S 30 48 E
Micanopy, U.S.A. 153 F7 29 30N 82 17W
Micăsasa, Romania ... 53 D9 46 7N 24 7 E
Micco, U.S.A. 153 H9 27 53N 80 30W
Miccosukee, U.S.A. .. 152 E5 30 36N 84 3W
Miccosukee, U.S.A. .. 152 E5 30 33N 83 53W
Michael, Mt., Papua N. G. .... 132 D3 6 27 S 145 22 E
Michalovce, Slovak Rep. ... 35 C14 48 47N 21 58 E
Michigan □, U.S.A. .. 148 C3 44 0N 85 0W
Michigan, L., U.S.A. . 148 D2 44 0N 87 0W
Michigan Center, U.S.A. ... 157 B12 42 14N 84 20W
Michigan City, U.S.A. 157 C10 41 43N 86 54W
Michika, Nigeria .... 113 C7 10 36N 13 23 E
Michipicoten I., Canada 140 C2 47 40N 85 40W
Michoacan □, Mexico 162 D4 19 0N 102 0W
Michurin, Bulgaria ... 51 D11 42 9N 27 51 E
Michurinsk, Russia ... 60 D5 52 58N 40 27 E
Mico, Pta., Nic. 164 D3 12 0N 83 30W
Miconje, Angola ..... 115 C2 4 26 S 12 48 E
Micoud, St. Lucia ... 165 f 13 49N 60 54W
Micronesia, Pac. Oc. . 134 G7 11 0N 160 0 E
Micronesia, Federated States of ■, Pac. Oc. 134 G7 9 0N 150 0 E
Mid-Indian Ridge, Ind. Oc. .... 121 H6 30 0 S 75 0 E
Mid-Oceanic Ridge, Ind. Oc. ... 134 M1 42 0 S 90 0 E
Mid-Pacific Mts., Pac. Oc. ... 134 F10 18 0N 177 0W
Midai, Indonesia .... 85 B3 3 0N 107 47 E
Midale, Canada 143 D8 49 25N 103 20W
Middelburg, Neths. ... 24 C3 51 30N 3 36 E
Middelburg, Eastern Cape, S. Africa .. 116 E4 31 30 S 25 0 E
Middelburg, Mpumalanga, S. Africa .. 117 D4 25 49 S 29 28 E
Middelfart, Denmark . 17 J3 55 30N 9 43 E
Middelpos, S. Africa . 116 E3 31 55 S 20 13 E
Middelwit, S. Africa . 116 C4 24 51 S 27 3 E
Middle →, U.S.A. 156 C3 44 25N 93 30W
Middle Alkali L., U.S.A. .. 158 F3 41 27N 120 5W
Middle America Trench, Pac. Oc. 135 F18 14 0N 95 0W
Middle Andaman I., India ... 95 H11 12 30N 92 50 E
Middle Bass I., U.S.A. 156 D2 41 41N 82 49W
Middle East, Asia ... 88 B2 38 0N 40 0 E
Middle Fork Feather →, U.S.A. 160 F5 38 33N 121 30W
Middle I., Australia .. 125 F3 34 6 S 123 11 E
Middle Loup →, U.S.A. 154 E5 41 17N 98 24W
Middle Raccoon →, U.S.A. ... 156 C3 41 35N 93 35W
Middle Sackville, Canada ... 141 D7 44 47N 63 42W
Middleboro, U.S.A. .. 151 E14 41 54N 70 55W
Middleburg, Fla., U.S.A. 152 E8 30 4N 81 52W
Middleburg, Pa., U.S.A. 150 F7 40 47N 77 3W
Middleburgh, U.S.A. . 151 D10 42 36N 74 20W
Middlebury, Ind., U.S.A. .. 157 C11 41 41N 85 42W
Middlebury, Vt., U.S.A. 151 B11 44 1N 73 10W
Middlemarch, N.Z. ... 131 F5 45 30 S 170 9 E
Middlemount, Australia 126 C4 22 50 S 148 40 E
Middleport, N.Y., U.S.A. 150 C6 43 13N 78 29W
Middleport, Ohio, U.S.A. .. 148 F4 39 0N 82 3W
Middlesboro, U.S.A. . 149 G4 36 36N 83 43W
Middlesbrough, U.K. . 20 C6 54 35N 1 13W
Middlesbrough □, U.K. 20 C6 54 28N 1 13W
Middlesex, Belize ... 164 C2 17 2N 88 31W
Middlesex, N.J., U.S.A. 151 F10 40 36N 74 30W
Middlesex, N.Y., U.S.A. 150 D7 42 42N 77 16W
Middleton, Australia . 126 C3 22 22 S 141 32 E
Middleton, Canada ... 141 D6 44 57N 65 4W
Middleton, U.S.A. ... 156 K7 43 6N 89 30W
Middleton Basin, Pac. Oc. ... 134 K7 0 0 S 156 0 E
Middleton Cr. →, Australia .. 126 C3 22 35 S 141 51 E
Middleton I., U.S.A. . 144 G11 59 26N 146 20W
Middletown, Calif., U.S.A. 160 G4 38 45N 122 37W
Middletown, Conn., U.S.A. .. 151 E12 41 34N 72 39W
Middletown, Ky., U.S.A. ... 157 F11 38 14N 85 32W
Middletown, N.Y., U.S.A. .. 151 E10 41 27N 74 25W
Middletown, Ohio, U.S.A. . 157 E12 39 31N 84 24W
Middletown, Pa., U.S.A. ... 151 F8 40 12N 76 44W

Middleville, U.S.A. ... 157 B11 42 43N 85 28W
Midelt, Morocco 110 B4 32 46N 4 44W
Midge Point, Australia 126 J6 20 39 S 148 43 E
Midhirst, N.Z. .... 130 F3 39 17 S 174 18 E
Midhurst, U.K. 21 G7 50 59N 0 44W
Midi, Yemen .... 107 D5 16 20N 42 45 E
Midi, Canal du →, France .... 28 E5 43 45N 1 21 E
Midi d'Ossau, Pic du, France 28 F3 42 50N 0 26W
Midi-Pyrénées □, France .... 28 E5 43 55N 1 45 E
Midland, Australia ... 125 F2 31 54 S 116 1 E
Midland, Canada 148 D4 44 45N 79 50W
Midland, Calif., U.S.A. 161 M12 33 52N 114 48W
Midland, Mich., U.S.A. 148 D3 43 37N 84 14W
Midland, Pa., U.S.A. . 150 F4 40 39N 80 27W
Midland, Tex., U.S.A. 155 K3 32 0N 102 3W
Midlands □, Zimbabwe 119 F2 19 40 S 29 0 E
Midleton, Ireland ... 23 E3 51 55N 8 10W
Midlothian, U.S.A. .. 155 J6 32 30N 97 0W
Midlothian □, U.K. .. 22 F5 55 51N 3 5W
Midongy, Tangorombohitr' i, Madag. .... 117 C8 23 30 S 47 0 E
Midongy Atsimo, Madag. .... 117 C8 23 35 S 47 1 E
Midou →, France 28 E3 43 54N 0 30W
Midouze →, France .. 28 E3 43 48N 0 51W
Midsayap, Phil. ..... 81 H5 7 12N 124 32 E
Midsund, Norway ... 18 B3 62 41N 6 40 E
Midtgulen, Norway .. 18 C2 61 44N 5 11 E
Midu, China .... 76 E3 25 18N 100 30 E
Midville, U.S.A. 152 C7 32 49N 82 14W
Midway, Ala., U.S.A. . 152 C4 32 5N 85 31W
Midway, Fla., U.S.A. . 152 E5 30 30N 84 27W
Midway Is., Pac. Oc. . 134 E10 28 13N 177 22W
Midway Wells, U.S.A. 161 N11 32 41N 115 7W
Midwest, U.S.A. 147 B9 42 0N 90 0W
Midwest, Wyo., U.S.A. 158 E10 43 25N 106 16W
Midwest City, U.S.A. . 155 H6 35 27N 97 14W
Midyat, Turkey ..... 101 D9 37 25N 41 23 E
Midzŏr, Bulgaria .... 50 C6 43 24N 22 40 E
Mie □, Japan .... 72 E3 34 30N 136 10 E
Mie □, Japan .... 73 C8 34 30N 136 10 E
Miechów, Poland .... 55 H7 50 21N 20 5 E
Miedwie, Jezioro, Poland .... 55 E1 53 17N 14 54 E
Międzybórz, Poland .. 55 G4 51 25N 17 34 E
Międzychód, Poland . 55 F2 52 35N 15 53 E
Międzylesie, Poland . 55 H3 50 8N 16 40 E
Międzyrzec Podlaski, Poland .... 55 G9 51 58N 22 45 E
Międzyrzecz, Poland . 55 F2 52 26N 15 35 E
Międzyzdroje, Poland 54 E1 53 56N 14 26 E
Miejska Górka, Poland 55 G3 51 39N 16 58 E
Miélan, France ...... 28 E4 43 27N 0 19 E
Mielau = Mława, Poland .... 55 E7 53 9N 20 25 E
Mielec, Poland ...... 55 H8 50 15N 21 25 E
Mienga, Angola ..... 116 B2 17 12 S 19 48 E
Miercurea-Ciuc, Romania .... 53 D10 46 21N 25 48 E
Miercurea Sibiului, Romania .... 53 D8 45 53N 23 48 E
Mieres, Spain 42 B5 43 18N 5 48W
Mieroszów, Poland .. 55 H3 50 40N 16 11 E
Mies = Stříbro, Czech Rep. .... 34 A6 49 44N 13 0 E
Mieso, Ethiopia ..... 107 F5 9 15N 40 43 E
Mieszkowice, Poland 55 F1 52 47N 14 30 E
Mifflintown, U.S.A. . 150 F7 40 34N 77 24W
Mifraz Ḥefa, Israel .. 104 C4 32 52N 35 0 E
Migennes, France ... 27 E10 47 58N 3 31 E
Migliarino, Italy .... 45 D8 44 46N 11 56 E
Migliarino-San Rossore-Massaciuccoli □, Italy .... 44 E7 43 44N 10 20 E
Miguel Alemán, Presa, Mexico 163 D5 18 15N 96 40W
Miguel Alves, Brazil . 170 B3 4 11 S 42 55W
Miguel Calmon, Brazil 170 D3 11 26 S 40 36W
Miguelturra, Spain .. 43 G7 38 58N 3 53W
Mihăileni, Romania . 53 C11 47 58N 26 9 E
Mihăileşti, Romania . 53 F10 44 20N 25 54 E
Mihailgazi, Turkey .. 49 A12 40 2N 30 34 E
Mihaliççık, Turkey .. 100 C4 39 53N 31 30 E
Mihara, Japan ...... 72 C5 34 24N 133 5 E
Mihara-Yama, Japan . 73 C11 34 43N 139 23 E
Miheşu de Cîmpie, Romania .... 53 D9 46 41N 24 9 E
Mijas, Spain 43 J6 36 36N 4 40W
Mikese, Tanzania ... 118 D4 6 48 S 37 55 E
Mikha-Tskhakaya = Senaki, Georgia .. 61 J6 42 15N 42 7 E
Mikhailovka = Mykhaylivka, Ukraine .... 59 J8 47 12N 35 15 E
Mikhaylov, Russia ... 58 E10 54 14N 39 0 E
Mikhaylovgrad = Montana, Bulgaria . 50 C7 43 27N 23 16 E
Mikhaylovka = Kimovsk, Russia ... 58 E10 54 0N 38 29 E
Mikhaylovka, Kyrgyzstan .... 65 B9 42 37N 78 20 E
Mikhaylovka, Russia . 60 E6 50 3N 43 5 E
Mikhaylovski, Russia 64 C7 56 27N 59 7 E
Mikhnevo, Russia ... 58 E9 55 4N 37 59 E
Miki, Hyōgo, Japan .. 72 C6 34 48N 134 59 E
Miki, Kagawa, Japan . 72 C6 34 12N 134 7 E
Mikinai, Greece ..... 48 D4 37 43N 22 46 E
Mikir Hills, India ... 90 B4 26 10N 93 30 E
Mikkeli, Finland .... 15 F22 61 43N 27 15 E
Mikkwa →, Canada .. 142 B6 58 25N 114 46W
Mikniya, Sudan ..... 107 D3 17 0N 33 45 E
Mikołajki, Poland ... 54 E8 53 49N 21 37 E
Míkonos, Greece .... 49 D7 37 30N 25 25 E
Mikope, Dem. Rep. of the Congo .... 115 C4 4 58 S 20 43 E
Mikoyan-Shakhar = Karachayevsk, Russia 61 J5 43 50N 41 55 E
Míkrí Préspa, Límni, Greece .... 50 F5 40 47N 21 3 E
Mikrón Dhérion, Greece .... 51 E10 41 19N 26 6 E
Mikstat, Poland ..... 55 G4 51 32N 17 59 E
Mikulov, Czech Rep. . 35 C9 48 48N 16 39 E
Mikumi, Tanzania ... 118 D4 7 26 S 37 0 E
Mikumi △, Tanzania . 118 D4 7 35 S 37 15 E
Mikun, Russia ...... 56 B9 62 20N 50 0 E
Mikuni, Japan ...... 73 A8 36 13N 136 9 E
Mikuni-Tōge, Japan . 73 A10 36 50N 138 50 E
Mikura-Jima, Japan . 73 D11 33 52N 139 36 E
Milaca, U.S.A. 154 C8 45 45N 93 39W
Milagro, Ecuador ... 168 D2 2 11 S 79 36W
Milagros, Phil. ..... 81 E5 12 13N 123 30 E
Milan = Milano, Italy 46 C6 45 28N 9 12 E
Milan, Ga., U.S.A. ... 152 C6 32 1N 83 4W
Milan, Ill., U.S.A. ... 156 E8 41 27N 90 34W
Milan, Mich., U.S.A. . 157 B13 42 5N 83 41W
Milan, Mo., U.S.A. .. 156 D3 40 12N 93 7W
Milan, Tenn., U.S.A. . 149 H1 35 55N 88 46W

Miland, Norway ..... 18 E5 59 54N 8 45 E
Milando, Angola .... 115 D3 8 45 S 17 36 E
Milando △, Angola .. 115 D3 8 45 S 17 10 E
Milang, Australia .... 128 C3 35 24 S 138 58 E
Milange, Mozam. .... 119 F4 16 3 S 35 45 E
Milano, Italy .... 46 C6 45 28N 9 12 E
Milano Linate ✈ (LIN), Italy .... 44 C6 45 27N 9 16 E
Milanoa, Madag. .... 117 A8 13 35 S 49 47 E
Milâs, Turkey .... 49 D9 37 20N 27 50 E
Milatos, Greece ..... 39 E6 35 18N 25 34 E
Milazzo, Italy .... 47 D8 38 13N 15 15 E
Milbank, U.S.A. 154 C6 45 13N 96 38W
Milbanke Sd., Canada 142 C3 52 15N 128 35W
Milden, Canada 143 C7 51 29N 107 32W
Mildenhall, U.K. .... 21 E8 52 21N 0 32 E
Mildmay, Canada 150 B3 44 3N 81 7W
Mildura, Australia ... 128 C3 34 13 S 142 9 E
Mile, China .... 76 E4 24 28N 103 20 E
Miléai, Greece ...... 48 B5 39 20N 23 9 E
Miles, Australia ..... 127 D5 26 40 S 150 9 E
Miles City, U.S.A. ... 154 B2 46 25N 105 51W
Mileşti, Moldova .... 53 C13 47 13N 28 3 E
Milestone, Canada ... 143 D8 49 59N 104 31W
Mileto, Italy .... 47 D9 38 36N 16 4 E
Miletto, Mte., Italy .. 47 A7 41 27N 14 22 E
Miletus, Turkey ..... 49 D9 37 30N 27 18 E
Milevsko, Czech Rep. 34 B7 49 27N 14 21 E
Milford, Calif., U.S.A. 160 E6 40 10N 120 22W
Milford, Conn., U.S.A. 151 E11 41 14N 73 3W
Milford, Del., U.S.A. . 148 F8 38 55N 75 26W
Milford, Ill., U.S.A. .. 157 D9 40 38N 87 42W
Milford, Mass., U.S.A. 151 D13 42 8N 71 31W
Milford, Mich., U.S.A. 157 B13 42 35N 83 36W
Milford, N.H., U.S.A. 151 D13 42 50N 71 39W
Milford, Pa., U.S.A. . 151 E10 41 19N 74 48W
Milford, Utah, U.S.A. 159 G7 38 24N 113 1W
Milford Haven, U.K. . 21 F2 51 42N 5 7W
Milford Sd., N.Z. .... 131 E2 44 41 S 167 47 E
Milh, Baḥr al = Razāzah, Buḥayrat ar, Iraq .... 101 F10 32 40N 43 35 E
Miliana, Aïn Salah, Algeria .... 106 D3 17 55N 30 20 E
Miliana, Médéa, Algeria 111 A5 36 20N 2 15 E
Milicz, Poland ...... 55 G4 51 31N 17 19 E
Milikapiti, Australia . 124 B5 11 26 S 130 40 E
Mililani Town, U.S.A. 145 K13 21 28N 158 1 W
Miling, Australia .... 125 F2 30 30 S 116 17 E
Militello in Val di Catánia, Italy .... 47 E7 37 16N 14 48 E
Militsch = Milicz, Poland .... 55 G4 51 31N 17 19 E
Milk →, U.S.A. 158 B10 48 4N 106 19W
Milk, Wadi el →, Sudan .... 106 D3 17 55N 30 20 E
Milk River, Canada .. 142 D6 49 10N 112 5W
Mill I., Antarctica ... 5 C8 66 0 S 101 30 E
Mill City, U.S.A. 158 D2 44 45N 122 29W
Mill Shoals, U.S.A. .. 157 F8 38 15N 88 21W
Mill Valley, U.S.A. ... 160 H4 37 54N 122 32W
Millárs →, Spain 40 F4 39 55N 0 1W
Millau, France ...... 28 D7 44 8N 3 4 E
Millbridge, Canada .. 150 B7 44 41N 77 36W
Millbrook, Canada ... 150 B6 44 10N 78 29W
Millbrook, Ala., U.S.A. 149 J2 32 29N 86 22W
Millbrook, N.Y., U.S.A. 151 E11 41 47N 73 42W
Mille Lacs, L. des, Canada 140 C1 48 45N 90 35W
Mille Lacs L., U.S.A. . 154 B8 46 15N 93 39W
Milledgeville, Ga., U.S.A. 152 B6 33 5N 83 14W
Milledgeville, Ill., U.S.A. .. 156 C7 41 58N 89 46W
Millen, U.S.A. 152 C8 32 48N 81 57W
Millennium I. = Caroline I., Kiribati 135 H12 9 58 S 150 13W
Miller, U.S.A. 154 C5 44 31N 98 59W
Millerovo, Russia ... 61 F5 48 57N 40 28 E
Miller's Flat, N.Z. ... 131 F4 45 39 S 169 23 E
Millersburg, Ind., U.S.A. .. 157 C11 41 32N 85 42W
Millersburg, Ohio, U.S.A. .. 150 F3 40 33N 81 55W
Millersburg, Pa., U.S.A. 150 F8 40 32N 76 58W
Millerton, N.Z. ...... 131 B6 41 39 S 171 54 E
Millerton, U.S.A. ... 151 E11 41 57N 73 31W
Millerton L., U.S.A. . 160 J7 37 1N 119 41W
Millet, St. Lucia .... 165 f 13 55N 60 59W
Millevaches, Plateau de, France .... 28 C6 45 45N 2 0 E
Millheim, U.S.A. 150 F7 40 54N 77 29W
Millicent, Australia .. 128 D4 37 34 S 140 21 E
Milligan, U.S.A. 152 E3 30 45N 86 38W
Millington, U.S.A. ... 155 H10 35 20N 89 53W
Millinocket, U.S.A. .. 149 C11 45 39N 68 43W
Millmerran, Australia 127 D5 27 53 S 151 16 E
Millom, U.K. 20 C4 54 13N 3 16W
Mills L., Canada 142 A5 61 30N 118 20W
Millsboro, U.S.A. ... 150 G5 40 0N 80 0W
Millstream-Chichester △, Australia .... 124 D2 21 35 S 117 6 E
Millthorpe, Australia 129 B8 33 26 S 149 12 E
Milltown Malbay, Ireland 23 D2 52 52N 9 24W
Millville, N.J., U.S.A. . 148 F8 39 24N 75 2W
Millville, Pa., U.S.A. . 151 E8 41 7N 76 32W
Millwood L., U.S.A. . 155 J8 33 42N 93 58W
Milna, Croatia ...... 45 E13 43 20N 16 27 E
Milne →, Australia .. 126 C2 21 10 S 137 33 E
Milne Bay □, Papua N. G. .... 132 E7 10 0 S 152 30 E
Milne Land, Greenland 10 C8 70 40N 26 30W
Milo, U.S.A. 149 C11 45 15N 68 59W
Miloliii, U.S.A. ..... 145 D6 19 11 S 155 55W
Míilos, Greece ...... 55 F4 36 44N 24 25 E
Miłosław, Poland ... 55 F4 52 12N 17 32 E
Milot, Albania ...... 50 E3 41 41N 19 43 E
Milparinka, Australia 127 D3 29 46 S 141 57 E
Milroy, U.S.A. 157 E11 39 30N 85 28W
Miltenberg, Germany 31 F5 49 41N 9 16 E
Milton, Australia .... 129 C5 35 20 S 150 27 E
Milton, N.S., Canada 141 D7 44 4N 64 45W
Milton, Ont., Canada 150 C5 43 31N 79 53W
Milton, N.Z. .... 131 G4 46 7 S 169 59 E
Milton, Calif., U.S.A. 160 G6 38 3N 120 51W
Milton, Fla., U.S.A. .. 152 E2 30 38N 87 3W
Milton, Pa., U.S.A. .. 150 F8 41 1N 76 51W
Milton, Vt., U.S.A. ... 151 B11 44 38N 73 7W
Milton, Wis., U.S.A. . 157 B8 42 47N 88 56W
Milton-Freewater, U.S.A. 158 D4 45 56N 118 23W
Milton Keynes, U.K. . 21 E7 52 1N 0 44W
Milton Keynes □, U.K. 21 E7 52 1N 0 44W
Miltou, Chad .... 109 F3 10 14N 17 26 E
Miluo, China .... 77 C9 29 0N 112 59 E
Milverton, Canada ... 150 C4 43 34N 80 55W
Milwaukee, U.S.A. .. 157 A9 43 2N 87 55W
Milwaukee Deep, Atl. Oc. 165 C6 19 50N 68 0W
Milwaukie, U.S.A. ... 160 E4 45 27N 122 38W
Mim, Ghana 112 D4 6 57N 2 33W
Mimizan, France 28 D2 44 12N 1 13W

Mimoň, Czech Rep. .. 34 A7 50 38N 14 43 E
Mimongo, Gabon ... 114 C2 1 11 S 11 36 E
Mimoso, Brazil ..... 171 E2 15 10 S 48 5W
Mims, U.S.A. 153 G9 28 40N 80 51W
Min Jiang →, Fujian, China .... 77 E12 26 0N 119 35 E
Min Jiang →, Sichuan, China .... 76 C5 28 45N 104 40 E
Min Xian, China .... 74 G3 34 25N 104 5 E
Mina Pirquitas, Argentina .... 174 A2 22 40 S 66 30W
Mīnā Su'ud, Si. Arabia 97 D6 28 45N 48 28 E
Mīnā'al Aḥmadī, Kuwait .... 97 D6 29 5N 48 10 E
Minago →, Canada .. 143 C9 54 33N 98 59W
Minaki, Canada 143 D10 49 59N 94 40W
Minakuchi, Japan ... 73 C8 34 58N 136 10 E
Minamata, Japan ... 72 E2 32 10N 130 30 E
Minami-Arapusa △, Japan .... 73 B10 35 30N 138 9 E
Minami-Tori-Shima, Pac. Oc. .... 134 E7 24 20N 153 58 E
Minas, Uruguay ..... 175 C4 34 20 S 55 10W
Minas, Sierra de las, Guatemala 164 C2 15 9N 89 31W
Minas Basin, Canada . 141 C7 45 20N 64 12W
Minas de Riotinto, Spain 43 H4 37 42N 6 35W
Minas Gerais □, Brazil 171 E2 18 50 S 46 0W
Minas Novas, Brazil . 171 E3 17 15 S 42 36W
Minatitlán, Mexico .. 163 D6 17 59N 94 31W
Minbu, Burma ...... 90 E5 20 10N 94 52 E
Minbya, Burma ..... 90 E4 20 22N 93 16 E
Minchinabad, Pakistan 92 D5 30 10N 73 34 E
Míncio →, Italy ..... 44 C7 45 4N 10 59 E
Mincol, Slovak Rep. . 35 B13 49 15N 20 58 E
Mindanao, Phil. .... 81 H5 8 0N 125 0 E
Mindanao Sea = Bohol Sea, Phil. .... 81 G5 9 0N 124 0 E
Mindanao Trench, Pac. Oc. .... 80 E5 12 0N 126 6 E
Mindel →, Germany . 31 G6 48 31N 10 23 E
Mindelheim, Germany 31 G6 48 3N 10 29 E
Mindelo, C. Verde Is. . 9 j 16 24N 25 0W
Minden, Canada 150 B6 44 55N 78 43W
Minden, Germany ... 30 C4 52 17N 8 55 E
Minden, La., U.S.A. .. 155 J8 32 37N 93 17W
Minden, Nev., U.S.A. 160 G7 38 57N 119 46W
Mindiptana, Indonesia 83 C6 5 55 S 140 22 E
Mindon, Burma ..... 90 F5 19 0N 94 44 E
Mindona L., Australia 128 B3 33 6 S 142 6 E
Mindoro, Phil. ...... 80 E3 13 0N 121 0 E
Mindoro Occidental □, Phil. .... 80 E3 13 0N 120 55 E
Mindoro Oriental □, Phil. .... 80 E3 13 0N 121 5 E
Mindoro Str., Phil. .. 80 E3 12 30N 120 30 E
Mindouli, Congo .... 115 C2 4 12 S 14 28 E
Mindourou, Cameroon 114 B2 3 29N 13 6 E
Mine, Japan .... 72 C3 34 12N 131 7 E
Minehead, U.K. 21 F4 51 12N 3 29W
Mineiros, Brazil .... 173 D7 17 34 S 52 34W
Mineola, N.Y., U.S.A. 151 F11 40 45N 73 39W
Mineola, Tex., U.S.A. 155 J7 32 40N 95 29W
Mineral King, U.S.A. . 160 J8 36 27N 118 36W
Mineral Point, U.S.A. 156 B6 42 52N 90 11W
Mineral Wells, U.S.A. 155 J5 32 48N 98 7W
Mineralnyye Vody, Russia .... 61 H6 44 15N 43 8 E
Minersville, U.S.A. .. 151 F8 40 41N 76 16W
Minerva, U.S.A. 150 F3 40 44N 81 6W
Minervino Murge, Italy 47 A9 41 5N 16 5 E
Minetto, U.S.A. 151 C8 43 24N 76 28W
Ming-Kush, Kyrgyzstan 65 C7 41 40N 74 28 E
Mingäçevir, Azerbaijan 61 K8 40 45N 47 0 E
Mingäçevir Su Anbarı, Azerbaijan .... 61 K8 40 57N 46 50 E
Mingan, Canada 141 B7 50 20N 64 0W
Mingary, Australia .. 128 B4 32 8 S 140 45 E
Mingechaur = Mingäçevir, Azerbaijan .... 61 K8 40 45N 47 0 E
Mingechaurskoye Vdkhr. = Mingäçevir Su Anbarı, Azerbaijan .... 61 K8 40 57N 46 50 E
Mingela, Australia .. 126 B4 19 52 S 146 38 E
Mingenew, Australia 125 E2 29 12 S 115 21 E
Mingera Cr. →, Australia .... 126 C2 20 38 S 137 45 E
Minggang, China ... 77 A10 32 24N 114 3 E
Mingguang, China .. 77 A11 32 47N 117 59 E
Mingin, Burma ..... 90 D5 22 50N 94 30 E
Mingir, Moldova ... 53 D13 46 40N 28 29 E
Minglanilla, Spain .. 41 F3 39 34N 1 38W
Mingo Junction, U.S.A. 150 F4 40 19N 80 37W
Mingorría, Spain ... 42 E6 40 45N 4 40W
Mingshan, China ... 76 B4 30 6N 103 10 E
Mingteke, China .... 65 E7 37 7N 75 4 E
Mingteke Daban = Mintaka Pass, Pakistan .... 65 E7 37 0N 74 58 E
Mingxi, China ...... 77 D11 26 18N 117 12 E
Mingyuegue, China . 75 C15 43 2N 128 50 E
Minhla, Magwe, Burma 90 F5 19 58N 95 3 E
Minhla, Pegu, Burma 90 G5 17 59N 95 43 E
Minho = Miño →, Spain 42 D2 41 52N 8 40W
Minho, Portugal 42 D2 41 25N 8 20W
Minho □, Portugal .. 42 D2 41 25N 8 20W
Minhou, China ...... 77 E12 26 0N 119 15 E
Miničevo, Serbia & M. 52 C7 43 42N 22 18 E
Minicoy I., India .... 95 K1 8 17N 73 2 E
Minidoka, U.S.A. ... 158 E7 42 45N 113 29W
Minier, U.S.A. 156 E9 40 26N 89 19W
Minigwal, L., Australia 125 E3 29 31 S 123 14 E
Minilya →, Australia 125 D1 23 45 S 114 0 E
Minilya Roadhouse, Australia .... 125 D1 23 55 S 114 0 E
Mininera, Australia . 128 D5 37 42 S 143 18 E
Minipi L., Canada ... 141 B7 52 25N 60 45W
Minj, Papua N. G. ... 132 C3 5 54 S 144 37 E
Mink L., Canada 142 A5 61 54N 117 40W
Minkammen, Sudan . 107 F3 6 0N 31 12 E
Minkébé, Gabon .... 114 B2 1 48N 12 48 E
Minlaton, Australia . 128 C2 34 55 S 137 35 E
Minna, Nigeria ..... 113 D6 9 37N 6 30 E
Minneapolis, Kans., U.S.A. 154 F6 39 8N 97 42W
Minneapolis, Minn., U.S.A. 154 C8 44 59N 93 16W
Minnedosa, Canada . 143 C9 50 14N 99 50W
Minnesota □, U.S.A. . 154 B8 46 0N 94 15W
Minnesund, Norway . 18 D8 60 23N 11 14 E
Minnewaukan, U.S.A. 154 A5 48 4N 99 15W
Minnipa, Australia .. 127 E2 32 51 S 135 9 E
Minnitaki L., Canada 140 C1 49 57N 92 10W
Mino, Japan .... 73 B8 35 32N 136 55 E
Miño →, Spain 42 D2 41 52N 8 40W
Mino-Kamo, Japan .. 73 B9 35 23N 137 2 E

Mino-Mikawa-Kōgen, Japan .... 73 B9 35 10N 137 23 E
Minoa, Greece ...... 49 F7 35 6N 25 45 E
Minobu, Japan ..... 73 B10 35 22N 138 26 E
Minobu-Sanchi, Japan 73 B10 35 14N 138 20 E
Minonk, U.S.A. 156 D7 40 54N 89 2W
Minooka, U.S.A. 157 C8 41 27N 88 16W
Minorca = Menorca, Spain .... 38 B5 40 0N 4 0 E
Minore, Australia ... 129 B8 32 14 S 148 27 E
Minot, U.S.A. 154 A4 48 14N 101 18W
Minqin, China ...... 74 E2 38 38N 103 20 E
Minqing, China ..... 77 D12 26 15N 118 50 E
Minsen, Germany ... 30 B3 53 41N 7 58 E
Minsk, Belarus ..... 58 F4 53 52N 27 30 E
Mińsk Mazowiecki, Poland .... 55 F8 52 10N 21 33 E
Minster, U.S.A. 157 D12 40 24N 84 23W
Mintabie, Australia . 127 D1 27 15 S 133 7 E
Mintaka Pass, Pakistan 65 E7 37 0N 74 58 E
Minthami, Burma ... 90 D5 23 5N 94 40 E
Minto, Canada 141 C6 46 5N 66 5W
Minto, U.S.A. 144 D10 64 53N 149 11W
Minto, L., Canada ... 140 A5 57 13N 75 0W
Minton, Canada 143 D8 49 10N 104 35W
Mintoum, Gabon ... 114 B2 0 27N 12 16 E
Minturn, U.S.A. 158 G10 39 35N 106 26W
Minturno, Italy ..... 46 A6 41 15N 13 45 E
Minûf, Egypt .... 106 H7 30 26N 30 52 E
Minusinsk, Russia ... 67 D10 53 43N 91 20 E
Minusio, Switz. ..... 33 D7 46 11N 8 49 E
Minutang, India .... 90 A6 28 15N 96 30 E
Minvoul, Gabon .... 114 B2 2 9N 12 8 E
Minwakh, Yemen ... 99 C5 16 48N 48 6 E
Minya el Qamh, Egypt 106 H7 30 31N 31 21 E
Minya Konka = Gongga Shan, China 76 C3 29 40N 101 55 E
Minyar, Russia ..... 64 D6 55 4N 57 33 E
Minyarskiy Zavod = Minyar, Russia ... 64 D6 55 4N 57 33 E
Miyip, Australia .... 128 D5 36 29 S 142 36 E
Minzhong, China ... 79 F10 22 37N 113 30 E
Mionica, Box-H. .... 52 F3 44 51N 18 29 E
Mionica, Serbia & M. 52 B4 44 14N 20 6 E
Miquelon, Canada .. 140 C4 49 25N 76 27W
Miquelon, St-P. & M. 141 C8 47 8N 56 22W
Mir, Niger .... 113 C7 14 5N 11 59 E
Mīr Kūh, Iran ...... 97 E8 26 22N 58 55 E
Mīr Shahdād, Iran .. 97 E8 26 15N 58 29 E
Mira, Italy .... 45 C9 45 26N 12 8 E
Mira, Portugal 42 E2 40 26N 8 44W
Mira →, Colombia .. 168 C2 1 36N 79 1W
Mira →, Portugal ... 43 H2 37 43N 8 47W
Mira por vos Cay, Bahamas 165 B5 22 9N 74 30W
Mīrābād, Afghan. ... 91 C1 30 55N 61 50 E
Miracema, Brazil ... 171 E3 21 24 S 42 10W
Miracema do Norte, Brazil .... 170 C2 9 33 S 48 24W
Mirador-Río Azul △, Guatemala 164 C2 17 45N 89 50W
Miraflores = Rovira, Colombia 168 C2 4 15N 75 20W
Miraflores, Colombia 168 C2 1 25N 72 13W
Miraj, India .... 94 F2 16 50N 74 45 E
Miram Shah, Pakistan 93 B3 33 0N 70 2 E
Miramar, Argentina . 174 D4 38 15 S 57 50W
Miramar, Mozam. ... 117 C6 23 50 S 35 35 E
Miramas, France .... 29 E8 43 33N 4 59 E
Mirambeau, France . 28 C3 45 23N 0 35W
Miramichi, Canada .. 141 C6 47 2N 65 28W
Miramichi B., Canada 141 C7 47 15N 65 0W
Miramont-de-Guyenne, France .... 28 D4 44 37N 0 21 E
Miranda, Brazil .... 173 E6 20 10 S 56 15W
Miranda □, Venezuela 168 A4 10 0N 66 25W
Miranda →, Brazil .. 173 D6 19 25 S 57 20W
Miranda de Ebro, Spain 40 C2 42 41N 2 57W
Miranda do Corvo, Portugal 42 E2 40 6N 8 20W
Miranda do Douro, Portugal 42 D4 41 30N 6 16W
Mirande, France .... 28 E4 43 31N 0 25 E
Mirandela, Portugal . 42 D3 41 32N 7 10W
Mirándola, Italy .... 44 D8 44 53N 11 4 E
Mirandópolis, Brazil 175 A5 21 9 S 51 6W
Mirango, Malawi ... 119 E3 13 32 S 34 58 E
Mirani, Australia ... 126 K6 21 9 S 148 53 E
Mirano, Italy .... 45 C9 45 30N 12 7 E
Miras, Albania ..... 50 F4 40 30N 20 56 E
Mirassol, Brazil .... 175 A6 20 46 S 49 28W
Mirbāṭ, Oman ...... 99 C6 17 0N 54 45 E
Mirboo North, Australia .... 129 E7 38 24 S 146 10 E
Mircar, Egypt ...... 106 C4 23 5N 35 41 E
Mirebeau, France ... 26 F7 46 49N 0 10 E
Mirebeau-sur-Bèze, France .... 27 E12 47 25N 5 20 E
Mirecourt, France .. 27 D13 48 20N 6 10 E
Mirgorod = Myrhorod, Ukraine .... 59 H7 49 58N 33 37 E
Miri, Malaysia ...... 85 B4 4 23N 113 59 E
Mirialguda, India ... 94 F4 16 52N 79 35 E
Miriam Vale, Australia 126 C5 24 20 S 151 33 E
Miribel, France ..... 27 G11 45 50N 4 57 E
Mirigama, Sri Lanka 95 L5 7 15N 80 8 E
Mirim, L., S. Amer. . 175 C5 32 45 S 52 50W
Mirimire, Venezuela 168 A4 11 10N 68 43W
Miriti, Brazil .... 173 B6 6 15 S 59 0W
Miriuṭ, Russia ..... 67 C12 63 33N 113 53 E
Mírobeck, Serbia & M. 52 F3 42 46N 18 6 E
Mirokhan, Pakistan . 92 F3 27 46N 68 6 E
Miromd L., Canada . 143 B8 55 6N 102 47W
Mirosławiec, Poland 54 E3 53 20N 16 5 E
Mirpur, Pakistan ... 93 C5 33 32N 73 56 E
Mirpur Batoro, Pakistan .... 92 G3 24 44N 68 16 E
Mirpur Bibiwari, Pakistan .... 92 E2 28 33N 67 44 E
Mirpur Khas, Pakistan 91 D3 25 30N 69 0 E
Mirpur Sakro, Pakistan 92 G2 24 33N 67 41 E
Mirria, Niger .... 113 C6 13 43N 9 7 E
Mirror, Canada 142 C6 52 30N 113 7W
Mirs Bay = Tai Pang Wan, China .... 69 F11 22 33N 114 24 E
Mirsk, Poland ...... 55 H2 50 58N 15 23 E
Mirtağ, Turkey ..... 96 B4 38 23N 41 56 E
Mírtou, Kólpos, Greece 39 C1 38 20N 20 27 E
Miryang, S. Korea .. 79 G15 35 31N 128 44 E
Mirzaani, Georgia .. 61 K8 41 24N 46 5 E
Mirzachul = Guliston, Uzbekistan .... 65 C4 40 29N 68 46 E
Mirzapur, India .... 93 G10 25 10N 82 34 E
Mirzapur-cum-Vindhyachal = Mirzapur, India .... 93 G10 25 10N 82 34 E
Misaki, Japan ...... 73 C7 34 18N 135 9 E
Misamis = Ozamiz, Phil. .... 81 G4 8 15N 123 50 E

Misamis Occidental □, *Phil.* **81 G4** 8 20N 123 42 E
Misamis Oriental □, *Phil.* **81 G5** 8 45N 125 0 E
Misantla, *Mexico* **163 D5** 19 56N 96 50W
Misawa, *Japan* **70 D10** 40 41N 141 24 E
Miscou I., *Canada* **141 C7** 47 57N 64 31W
Misdroy = Międzyzdroje, *Poland* **54 E1** 53 56N 14 26 E
Misericordia = Itaporanga, *Brazil* **170 C4** 7 18 S 38 0W
Misha, *India* **95 L10** 7 59N 93 20 E
Mish'āb, Ra's al, *Si. Arabia* **97 D6** 28 15N 48 43 E
Mishagua →, *Peru* **172 C3** 11 12 S 72 58W
Mishan, *China* **69 B8** 45 37N 131 48 E
Mishawaka, *U.S.A.* **157 C10** 41 40N 86 11W
Mishbih, Gebel, *Egypt* **106 C3** 22 38N 34 44 E
Mishima, *Japan* **73 B10** 35 10N 138 52 E
Mishmi Hills, *India* **90 A5** 29 0N 96 0 E
Mishō, *Japan* **72 E4** 32 57N 132 35 E
Misima I., *Papua N. G.* **132 F7** 10 40 S 152 45 E
Misión, *Mexico* **161 N10** 32 6N 116 53W
Misión Fagnano, *Argentina* **176 D3** 54 32 S 67 17W
Misiones □, *Argentina* **175 B5** 27 0 S 55 0W
Misiones □, *Paraguay* **174 B4** 27 0 S 56 0W
Miskah, *Si. Arabia* **96 E4** 24 49N 42 56 E
Miski, E. →, *Chad* **109 E3** 20 0N 17 55 E
Miskitos, Cayos, *Nic.* **164 D3** 14 26N 82 50W
Miskolc, *Hungary* **52 B5** 48 7N 20 50 E
Misoke, *Dem. Rep. of the Congo* **118 C2** 0 42 S 28 2 E
Misool, *Indonesia* **83 B4** 1 52 S 130 10 E
Mişr = Egypt ■, *Africa* **106 B3** 28 0N 31 0 E
Mişrātah, *Libya* **108 B3** 32 24N 15 3 E
Mişrātah □, *Libya* **108 C3** 33 30N 15 0 E
Missanabie, *Canada* **140 C3** 48 20N 84 6W
Missão Catrimani, *Brazil* **169 C5** 2 48N 62 18W
Missão Velha, *Brazil* **170 C4** 7 15 S 39 10W
Missinaibi →, *Canada* **140 B3** 50 43N 81 29W
Missinaibi L., *Canada* **140 C3** 48 23N 83 40W
Mission, *Canada* **142 D4** 49 10N 122 15W
Mission, *S. Dak., U.S.A.* **154 D4** 43 18N 100 39W
Mission, *Tex., U.S.A.* **155 M5** 26 13N 98 20W
Mission Beach, *Australia* **126 B4** 17 53 S 146 6 E
Mission Viejo, *U.S.A.* **161 M9** 33 36N 117 40W
Missirah, *Senegal* **112 C1** 13 40N 16 30W
Missisa L., *Canada* **140 B2** 52 20N 85 7W
Missisicabi →, *Canada* **140 B4** 51 14N 79 31W
Mississagi →, *Canada* **140 C3** 46 15N 83 9W
Mississauga, *Canada* **150 C5** 43 32N 79 35W
Mississinewa L., *U.S.A.* **157 D10** 40 46N 86 3W
Mississippi □, *U.S.A.* **155 J10** 33 0N 90 0W
Mississippi →, *U.S.A.* **155 L10** 29 9N 89 15W
Mississippi L., *Canada* **151 A8** 45 5N 76 10W
Mississippi River Delta, *U.S.A.* **155 L9** 29 10N 89 15W
Mississippi Sd., *U.S.A.* **155 K10** 30 20N 89 0W
Missoula, *U.S.A.* **158 C7** 46 52N 114 1W
Missour, *Morocco* **110 B4** 33 3N 4 0W
Missouri □, *U.S.A.* **156 E3** 38 25N 92 30W
Missouri →, *U.S.A.* **156 F6** 38 49N 90 7W
Missouri City, *U.S.A.* **155 L7** 29 37N 95 32W
Missouri Valley, *U.S.A.* **154 E7** 41 34N 95 53W
Mist, *U.S.A.* **160 E3** 45 59N 123 15W
Mistassibi →, *Canada* **141 B5** 48 53N 72 13W
Mistassini →, *Canada* **141 C5** 48 42N 72 20W
Mistassini, L., *Canada* **140 B5** 51 0N 73 30W
Mistastin L., *Canada* **141 A7** 55 57N 63 20W
Mistelbach, *Austria* **35 C9** 48 34N 16 34 E
Misterbianco, *Italy* **47 E8** 37 31N 15 1 E
Misti, Volcán, *Peru* **172 D3** 16 18 S 71 24W
Mistinibi, L., *Canada* **141 A7** 55 56N 64 17W
Mistissini, *Canada* **141 C5** 48 53N 72 12W
Mistretta, *Italy* **47 E7** 37 56N 14 22 E
Misty L., *Canada* **143 B8** 58 53N 101 40W
Misugi, *Japan* **73 C8** 34 31N 136 16 E
Misumi, *Japan* **72 E2** 32 37N 130 27 E
Misurata = Mişrātah, *Libya* **108 B3** 32 24N 15 3 E
Mît Ghamr, *Egypt* **106 H7** 30 42N 31 12 E
Mitaka, *Japan* **73 B11** 35 40N 139 33 E
Mitatib, *Sudan* **107 D4** 15 59N 36 12 E
Mitau = Jelgava, *Latvia* **15 H20** 56 41N 23 49 E
Mitava = Jelgava, *Latvia* **15 H20** 56 41N 23 49 E
Mitchell, *Australia* **127 D4** 26 29 S 147 58 E
Mitchell, *Canada* **150 C3** 43 28N 81 12W
Mitchell, *Ga., U.S.A.* **152 B7** 33 13N 82 42W
Mitchell, *Ind., U.S.A.* **157 F10** 38 44N 86 28W
Mitchell, *Nebr., U.S.A.* **154 E3** 41 57N 103 49W
Mitchell, *Oreg., U.S.A.* **158 D3** 44 34N 120 9W
Mitchell, *S. Dak., U.S.A.* **154 D6** 43 43N 98 2W
Mitchell →, *Australia* **126 B3** 15 12 S 141 35 E
Mitchell, Mt., *U.S.A.* **149 H4** 35 46N 82 16W
Mitchell and Alice Rivers △, *Australia* **126 B3** 15 28 S 142 5 E
Mitchell Ranges, *Australia* **126 A2** 12 49 S 135 36 E
Mitchell River △, *Australia* **129 D7** 37 37 S 147 22 E
Mitchelstown, *Ireland* **23 D3** 52 15N 8 16W
Mitha Tiwana, *Pakistan* **92 C5** 32 13N 72 6 E
Mithi, *Pakistan* **92 G3** 24 44N 69 48 E
Míthimna, *Greece* **49 B8** 39 20N 26 12 E
Mithrao, *Pakistan* **92 F3** 27 28N 69 40 E
Mitiamo, *Australia* **128 D6** 36 12 S 144 15 E
Mítikas, *Aitolía kai Akarnanía, Greece* **39 B2** 38 40N 20 56 E
Mítikas, *Préveza, Greece* **39 B2** 39 0N 20 42 E
Mitilíni, *Greece* **49 B8** 39 6N 26 35 E
Mitilinoí, *Greece* **49 D8** 37 42N 26 56 E
Mito, *Japan* **73 A12** 36 20N 140 30 E
Mitra, Mt., *Eq. Guin.* **114 B1** 1 23N 9 19 E
Mitre, Mt., *N.Z.* **130 G4** 40 50 S 175 30 E
Mitrofanovka, *Russia* **59 H10** 49 58N 39 42 E
Mitrovica = Kosovska Mitrovica, *Serbia & M.* **50 D4** 42 54N 20 52 E
Mitrowitz = Sremska Mitrovica, *Serbia & M.* **52 F4** 44 59N 19 38 E
Mitsamiouli, *Comoros Is.* **121 a** 11 20 S 43 16 E
Mitsang, *Gabon* **114 B2** 0 42N 12 33 E
Mitsinjo, *Madag.* **117 B8** 16 1 S 45 52 E
Mitsiwa, *Eritrea* **107 D4** 15 35N 39 25 E
Mitsiwa Channel, *Eritrea* **107 D5** 15 30N 40 0 E
Mitsukaidō, *Japan* **73 A11** 36 1N 139 59 E
Mitsushima, *Japan* **72 C1** 34 15N 129 20 E
Mittagong, *Australia* **129 C9** 34 28 S 150 29 E
Mittel Schreiberhau = Szklarska Poreba, *Poland* **55 H2** 50 50N 15 33 E
Mittelberg, *Tirol, Austria* **33 C11** 46 57N 10 53 E
Mittelberg, *Vorarlberg, Austria* **33 B10** 47 20N 10 10 E
Mittelberg, *Germany* **33 A10** 47 38N 10 26 E
Mittelfranken □, *Germany* **31 F6** 49 25N 10 40 E
Mittelland, *Switz.* **32 C4** 46 50N 7 23 E
Mittellandkanal →, *Germany* **30 C4** 52 20N 8 28 E
Mittelwalde = Międzylesie, *Poland* **55 H3** 50 8N 16 40 E
Mittenwalde, *Germany* **30 C9** 52 15N 13 31 E
Mittersill, *Austria* **34 D5** 47 16N 12 29 E
Mitterteich, *Germany* **31 F8** 49 57N 12 14 E
Mittimatalik = Pond Inlet, *Canada* **139 A12** 72 40N 77 0W
Mittweida, *Germany* **30 E8** 50 59N 12 59 E
Mitú, *Colombia* **168 C3** 1 15N 70 13W
Mituas, *Colombia* **168 C4** 3 52N 68 49W
Mitumba, *Tanzania* **118 D3** 7 8 S 31 2 E
Mitumba, Mts., *Dem. Rep. of the Congo* **118 D2** 7 0 S 27 30 E
Mitwaba, *Dem. Rep. of the Congo* **119 D2** 8 2 S 27 17 E
Mityana, *Uganda* **118 B3** 0 23N 32 2 E
Mitzic, *Gabon* **114 B2** 0 45N 11 40 E
Miura, *Japan* **73 B11** 35 12N 139 40 E
Mixteco →, *Mexico* **163 D5** 18 11N 98 30W
Miyagi □, *Japan* **70 E10** 38 15N 140 45 E
Miyāh, W. el →, *Egypt* **106 C3** 25 0N 33 23 E
Miyāh, W. el →, *Syria* **96 C3** 34 44N 39 57 E
Miyake-Jima, *Japan* **73 C11** 34 5N 139 30 E
Miyako, *Japan* **70 E10** 39 40N 141 59 E
Miyako-Jima, *Japan* **71 M2** 24 45N 125 20 E
Miyako-Rettō, *Japan* **71 M2** 24 24N 125 0 E
Miyakonojō, *Japan* **72 F3** 31 40N 131 5 E
Miyani, *India* **92 J3** 21 50N 69 26 E
Miyanojō, *Japan* **72 F2** 31 54N 130 27 E
Miyanoura-Dake, *Japan* **71 J5** 30 20N 130 31 E
Miyata, *Japan* **72 D2** 33 49N 130 42 E
Miyazaki, *Japan* **72 F3** 31 56N 131 30 E
Miyazaki □, *Japan* **72 E3** 32 30N 131 30 E
Miyazu, *Japan* **73 B7** 35 35N 135 10 E
Miyet, Bahr el = Dead Sea, *Asia* **103 D4** 31 30N 35 30 E
Miyi, *China* **76 D4** 26 47N 102 9 E
Miyoshi, *Japan* **72 C4** 34 48N 132 51 E
Miyun, *China* **74 D9** 40 28N 116 50 E
Miyun Shuiku, *China* **75 D9** 40 30N 117 0 E
Mizan Teferi, *Ethiopia* **107 F4** 6 57N 35 3 E
Mizdah, *Libya* **108 B2** 31 30N 13 0 E
Mizen Hd., *Cork, Ireland* **23 E2** 51 27N 9 50W
Mizen Hd., *Wicklow, Ireland* **23 D5** 52 51N 6 4W
Mizhhirya, *Ukraine* **53 B8** 48 32N 23 30 E
Mizhi, *China* **74 F6** 37 47N 110 12 E
Mizil, *Romania* **53 F11** 44 59N 26 29 E
Mizo Hills = Mizoram □, *India* **90 D4** 23 30N 92 40 E
Mizoram □, *India* **90 D4** 23 30N 92 40 E
Mizpe Ramon, *Israel* **103 E3** 30 34N 34 49 E
Mizuho, *Antarctica* **7 D5** 70 30 S 41 0 E
Mizuho, *Japan* **73 B7** 35 6N 135 17 E
Mizunami, *Japan* **73 B9** 35 22N 137 15 E
Mizusawa, *Japan* **70 E10** 39 8N 141 8 E
Mjällby, *Sweden* **17 H8** 56 3N 14 40 E
Mjöbäck, *Sweden* **17 G6** 57 28N 12 53 E
Mjölby, *Sweden* **17 F9** 58 20N 15 10 E
Mjølfjell, *Norway* **18 D3** 60 41N 6 55 E
Mjømna, *Norway* **18 D1** 60 55N 4 55 E
Mjörn, *Sweden* **17 G6** 57 55N 12 25 E
Mjøsa, *Norway* **18 D8** 60 40N 11 0 E
Mkata, *Tanzania* **118 D4** 5 45 S 38 20 E
Mkhaya ⌓, *Swaziland* **117 D5** 26 34 S 31 45 E
Mkokotoni, *Tanzania* **118 D4** 5 55 S 39 15 E
Mkomazi, *Tanzania* **118 C4** 4 40 S 38 7 E
Mkomazi ⌓, *Tanzania* **118 C3** 4 4 S 30 2 E
Mkomazi →, *S. Africa* **117 E5** 30 12 S 30 50 E
Mkulwe, *Tanzania* **119 D3** 8 37 S 32 20 E
Mkumbi, Ras, *Tanzania* **118 D4** 7 38 S 39 55 E
Mkushi, *Zambia* **119 E2** 14 25 S 29 15 E
Mkushi River, *Zambia* **119 E2** 13 32 S 29 45 E
Mkuze, *S. Africa* **117 D5** 27 10 S 32 0 E
Mkuze ⌓, *S. Africa* **117 D4** 29 27 S 29 30 E
Mladá Boleslav, *Czech Rep.* **34 A7** 50 27N 14 53 E
Mladenovac, *Serbia & M.* **50 B4** 44 28N 20 44 E
Mlala Hills, *Tanzania* **118 D3** 6 50 S 31 40 E
Mlange = Mulanje, *Malawi* **119 F4** 16 2 S 35 33 E
Mlava →, *Serbia & M.* **50 B5** 44 45N 21 13 E
Mława, *Poland* **55 E7** 53 9N 20 25 E
Mlawula ⌓, *Swaziland* **117 D5** 26 12 S 32 2 E
Mlinište, *Bos.-H.* **45 D13** 44 15N 16 50 E
Mljet, *Croatia* **45 F14** 42 43N 17 30 E
Mljet △, *Croatia* **45 F14** 42 45N 17 25 E
Mljetski Kanal, *Croatia* **45 F14** 42 48N 17 35 E
Młynary, *Poland* **54 D6** 54 12N 19 46 E
Mmabatho, *S. Africa* **116 D4** 25 49 S 25 30 E
Mme, *Cameroon* **113 D7** 6 18N 10 14 E
Mnichovo Hradiště, *Czech Rep.* **34 A7** 50 32N 14 59 E
Mo, *Hordaland, Norway* **18 D2** 60 49N 5 48 E
Mo, *Møre og Romsdal, Norway* **18 A5** 63 0N 8 59 E
Mo, *Telemark, Norway* **18 E4** 59 28N 7 50 E
Mo i Rana, *Norway* **14 C16** 66 20N 14 7 E
Moa, *Cuba* **165 B4** 20 40N 74 56W
Moa, *Indonesia* **82 C3** 8 0 S 128 0 E
Moa →, *S. Leone* **112 D2** 6 59N 11 36W
Moa, I., *Papua N. G.* **132 F2** 10 10 S 142 15 E
Moab, *U.S.A.* **159 G9** 38 35N 109 33W
Moabi, *Gabon* **114 C2** 2 24 S 10 59 E
Moaco →, *Brazil* **172 B4** 7 41 S 68 18W
Moala, *Fiji* **133 B2** 18 36 S 179 53 E
Moama, *Australia* **127 F3** 36 7 S 144 46 E
Moamba, *Mozam.* **117 D5** 25 36 S 32 15 E
Moapa, *U.S.A.* **161 J12** 36 40N 114 37W
Moate, *Ireland* **23 C4** 53 24N 7 44W
Moba, *Dem. Rep. of the Congo* **118 D2** 7 0 S 29 48 E
Mobara, *Japan* **73 B12** 35 25N 140 18 E
Mobārakābād, *Iran* **97 D7** 28 24N 53 20 E
Mobaye, *C.A.R.* **114 B4** 4 25N 21 5 E
Mobayi, *Dem. Rep. of the Congo* **114 B4** 4 15N 21 8 E
Mobeka, *Dem. Rep. of the Congo* **114 B3** 1 52N 19 49 E
Mobenzélé, *Congo* **114 B3** 0 56N 17 50 E
Moberley Lake, *Canada* **142 B4** 55 50N 121 44W
Moberly, *U.S.A.* **156 E4** 39 25N 92 26W
Mobile, *U.S.A.* **149 K1** 30 41N 88 3W
Mobile B., *U.S.A.* **149 K2** 30 30N 88 0W
Mobridge, *U.S.A.* **154 C4** 45 32N 100 26W
Mobutu Sese Seko, L. = Albert, L., *Africa* **118 B3** 1 30N 31 0 E
Moc Chau, *Vietnam* **86 B5** 20 50N 104 38 E
Moc Hoa, *Vietnam* **87 G5** 10 46N 105 56 E
Mocaba, Sa. de, *Angola* **115 D3** 7 12 S 15 0 E
Mocabe Kasari, *Dem. Rep. of the Congo* **119 D2** 9 58 S 26 12 E
Mocajuba, *Brazil* **170 B2** 2 35 S 49 30W
Moçambique = Mozambique ■, *Africa* **119 F4** 19 0 S 35 0 E
Moçambique, *Mozam.* **119 F5** 15 3 S 40 42 E
Moçâmedes = Namibe, *Angola* **115 F2** 15 7 S 12 11 E
Mocanaqua, *U.S.A.* **151 E8** 41 9N 76 8W
Mocapra →, *Venezuela* **168 B4** 7 56N 66 46W
Moce, *Fiji* **133 B3** 18 40 S 178 29W
Mocha = Al Mukhā, *Yemen* **98 D3** 13 18N 43 15 E
Mocha, I., *Chile* **176 A2** 38 22 S 73 56W
Mochima △, *Venezuela* **165 D7** 10 30N 64 5W
Mochudi, *Botswana* **116 C4** 24 27 S 26 7 E
Mocimboa da Praia, *Mozam.* **119 E5** 11 25 S 40 20 E
Mociu, *Romania* **53 D9** 46 46N 24 3 E
Möckeln, *Sweden* **17 H8** 56 40N 14 15 E
Mockfjärd, *Sweden* **16 D8** 60 30N 14 57 E
Moclips, *U.S.A.* **160 C2** 47 14N 124 13W
Mocoa, *Colombia* **168 C2** 1 7N 76 35W
Mococa, *Brazil* **175 A6** 21 28 S 47 0W
Mocorito, *Mexico* **162 B3** 25 30N 107 53W
Moctezuma, *Mexico* **162 B3** 29 50N 109 0W
Moctezuma →, *Mexico* **163 C5** 21 59N 98 34W
Mocuba, *Mozam.* **119 F4** 16 54 S 36 57 E
Mocúzari, Presa, *Mexico* **162 B3** 27 10N 109 10W
Moda, *Burma* **90 C6** 24 22N 96 29 E
Modane, *France* **29 C10** 45 12N 6 40 E
Modasa, *India* **92 H5** 23 30N 73 21 E
Modder →, *S. Africa* **116 D3** 29 2 S 24 37 E
Modderfontein = Niekerkshoop, *S. Africa* **116 D3** 29 19 S 22 51 E
Modderrivier, *S. Africa* **116 D3** 29 2 S 24 38 E
Módena, *Italy* **44 D7** 44 40N 10 55 E
Modena, *U.S.A.* **159 H7** 37 48N 113 56W
Modesto, *U.S.A.* **160 H6** 37 39N 121 0W
Möðrudalur, *Iceland* **11 B11** 65 22N 15 53W
Möðruvellir, *Iceland* **11 B8** 65 46N 18 15W
Módica, *Italy* **47 F7** 36 52N 14 46 E
Modimolle, *S. Africa* **117 C4** 24 42 S 28 22 E
Modjamboli, *Dem. Rep. of the Congo* **114 B4** 2 28N 22 6 E
Mödling, *Austria* **35 C9** 48 5N 16 17 E
Modo, *Sudan* **107 F3** 5 31N 30 33 E
Modoc, *U.S.A.* **152 B7** 33 44N 82 13W
Modowi, *Indonesia* **83 B4** 4 5 S 134 39 E
Modra, *Slovak Rep.* **35 C10** 48 19N 17 20 E
Modriča, *Bos.-H.* **52 F3** 44 57N 18 17 E
Moe, *Australia* **129 E7** 38 12 S 146 19 E
Moebase, *Mozam.* **119 F4** 17 3 S 38 41 E
Moëlan-sur-Mer, *France* **26 E3** 47 49N 3 38W
Moelv, *Norway* **18 D7** 60 56N 10 43 E
Moengo, *Suriname* **169 B7** 5 45N 54 20W
Moerewa, *N.Z.* **130 B3** 35 8 S 174 1 E
Moësa →, *Switz.* **33 D8** 46 12N 9 10 E
Moffat, *U.K.* **22 F5** 55 21N 3 27W
Moga, *India* **92 D6** 30 48N 75 8 E
Mogadishu = Muqdisho, *Somali Rep.* **120 D3** 2 2N 45 25 E
Mogador = Essaouira, *Morocco* **110 B3** 31 32N 9 42W
Mogadouro, *Portugal* **42 D4** 41 22N 6 47W
Mogalakwena →, *S. Africa* **117 C4** 22 38 S 28 40 E
Mogami-Gawa →, *Japan* **70 E10** 38 45N 140 0 E
Mogán, *Canary Is.* **9 e1** 27 53N 15 43W
Mogandjo, *Dem. Rep. of the Congo* **114 B4** 1 23N 24 15 E
Mogaung, *Burma* **90 C6** 25 20N 97 0 E
Mogen, *Norway* **18 D4** 60 2N 7 52 E
Mogente = Moixent, *Spain* **41 G4** 38 52N 0 45W
Mogho, *Ethiopia* **107 G5** 4 54N 40 16 E
Mogi das Cruzes, *Brazil* **175 A6** 23 31 S 46 11W
Mogi-Guaçu →, *Brazil* **175 A6** 20 53 S 48 10W
Mogi-Mirim, *Brazil* **175 A6** 22 29 S 47 0W
Mogielnica, *Poland* **55 G7** 51 42N 20 41 E
Mogige, *Ethiopia* **107 F4** 5 24N 36 14 E
Mogilev = Mahilyow, *Belarus* **58 F6** 53 55N 30 18 E
Mogilev-Podolskiy = Mohyliv-Podilskyy, *Ukraine* **53 B12** 48 26N 27 48 E
Mogilno, *Poland* **55 F4** 52 39N 17 55 E
Mogincual, *Mozam.* **119 F5** 15 35 S 40 25 E
Mogliano Véneto, *Italy* **45 C9** 45 33N 12 14 E
Mogocha, *Russia* **67 D12** 53 40N 119 50 E
Mogoi, *Indonesia* **83 B4** 1 55 S 133 10 E
Mogok, *Burma* **90 D6** 23 0N 96 40 E
Mogollon Rim, *U.S.A.* **159 J8** 34 10N 110 50W
Mógoro, *Italy* **46 C1** 39 41N 8 47 E
Mograt, *Sudan* **106 D3** 19 28N 33 16 E
Mogroum, *Chad* **109 F3** 11 6N 15 25 E
Moguer, *Spain* **43 H4** 37 15N 6 52W
Mogumber, *Australia* **125 F2** 31 2 S 116 3 E
Mohács, *Hungary* **52 E3** 45 58N 18 41 E
Mohaka →, *N.Z.* **130 F6** 39 7 S 177 12 E
Mohala, *India* **94 D5** 20 35N 80 44 E
Mohales Hoek, *Lesotho* **116 E4** 30 7 S 27 26 E
Mohali, *Congo* **114 B3** 0 15N 15 29 E
Mohall, *U.S.A.* **154 A4** 48 46N 101 31W
Moḩammadābād, *Iran* **97 B8** 37 52N 59 5 E
Mohammadia, *Algeria* **111 A5** 35 33N 0 3 E
Mohammedia, *Morocco* **110 B3** 33 44N 7 21W
Mohammerah = Khorrāmshahr, *Iran* **97 D6** 30 29N 48 15 E
Mohana, *India* **94 E7** 19 27N 84 16 E
Mohana →, *India* **93 G11** 24 43N 85 0 E
Mohanganj, *Bangla.* **90 C3** 24 54N 90 59 E
Mohanlalganj, *India* **93 F9** 26 41N 80 58 E
Mohave, L., *U.S.A.* **161 K12** 35 12N 114 34W
Mohawk →, *U.S.A.* **151 D11** 42 47N 73 41W
Moheda, *Sweden* **17 G8** 57 1N 14 35 E
Mohéli, *Comoros Is.* **121 a** 12 20 S 43 40 E
Mohenjodaro, *Pakistan* **91 D3** 27 19N 68 7 E
Moher, Cliffs of, *Ireland* **23 D2** 52 58N 9 27W
Mohican, C., *U.S.A.* **144 F6** 60 12N 167 25W
Mohicanville Reservoir, *U.S.A.* **150 F3** 40 45N 82 0W
Möhlin, *Switz.* **32 A5** 47 33N 7 51 E
Möhne →, *Germany* **30 D3** 51 29N 7 57 E
Mohnyin, *Burma* **90 C6** 24 47N 96 22 E
Mohoro, *Tanzania* **118 D4** 8 6 S 39 8 E
Mohrin = Moryń, *Poland* **55 F1** 52 51N 14 22 E
Mohyliv-Podilskyy, *Ukraine* **53 B12** 48 26N 27 48 E
Moi, *Norway* **18 F3** 58 27N 6 32 E
Moia, *Sudan* **107 F2** 5 3N 28 2 E
Moidart, L., *U.K.* **22 E3** 56 47N 5 52W
Moinabad, *India* **94 F3** 17 44N 77 16 E
Moindou, *N. Cal.* **133 U19** 21 42 S 165 41 E
Moineşti, *Romania* **53 D11** 46 28N 26 31 E
Moira →, *Canada* **150 B7** 44 21N 77 24W
Moirang, *India* **90 C4** 24 30N 93 46 E
Moirans, *France* **29 C9** 45 20N 5 33 E
Moirans-en-Montagne, *France* **27 F12** 46 26N 5 43 E
Moíres, *Greece* **39 E5** 35 4N 24 56 E
Moisaküla, *Estonia* **15 G21** 58 3N 25 12 E
Moisie, *Canada* **141 B6** 50 12N 66 1W
Moisie →, *Canada* **141 B6** 50 14N 66 5W
Moissac, *France* **28 D5** 44 7N 1 5 E
Moïssala, *Chad* **109 G3** 8 21N 17 46 E
Moita, *Portugal* **43 G2** 38 38N 8 58W
Moixent, *Spain* **41 G4** 38 52N 0 45W
Möja, *Sweden* **16 E12** 59 26N 18 55 E
Mojácar, *Spain* **41 H3** 37 6N 1 55W
Mojados, *Spain* **42 D6** 41 26N 4 40W
Mojave, *U.S.A.* **161 K8** 35 3N 118 10W
Mojave ⌓, *U.S.A.* **161 K11** 35 7N 115 30W
Mojave Desert, *U.S.A.* **161 L10** 35 0N 116 30W
Moji, *China* **65 D7** 39 0N 74 27 E
Mojiang, *China* **76 F3** 23 37N 101 35 E
Mojjo →, *Ethiopia* **107 F5** 7 55N 42 0 E
Mojkovac, *Serbia & M.* **50 D3** 42 58N 19 35 E
Mojo, *Bolivia* **174 A2** 21 48 S 65 33W
Mojo, *Ethiopia* **107 F4** 8 35N 39 5 E
Mojokerto, *Indonesia* **85 D4** 7 28 S 112 26 E
Mojos, Llanos de, *Bolivia* **173 D5** 15 10 S 65 0W
Moju, *Brazil* **170 B2** 1 53 S 48 46W
Moju →, *Brazil* **170 B2** 1 40 S 48 25W
Mokai, *N.Z.* **130 E4** 38 32 S 175 56 E
Mokambo, *Dem. Rep. of the Congo* **119 E2** 12 25 S 28 20 E
Mokameh, *India* **93 G11** 25 24N 85 55 E
Mokane, *U.S.A.* **156 F5** 38 41N 91 53W
Mokapu Peninsula, *U.S.A.* **145 K14** 21 25N 157 45W
Mokau, *N.Z.* **130 E3** 38 42 S 174 39 E
Mokau →, *N.Z.* **130 E3** 38 35 S 174 35 E
Mokelumne →, *U.S.A.* **160 G5** 38 13N 121 28W
Mokelumne Hill, *U.S.A.* **160 G6** 38 18N 120 43W
Mokhós, *Greece* **39 E6** 35 16N 25 27 E
Mokhotlong, *Lesotho* **117 D4** 29 22 S 29 2 E
Mokihinui →, *N.Z.* **131 B6** 41 33 S 171 58 E
Möklinta, *Sweden* **16 D10** 60 4N 16 33 E
Moknine, *Tunisia* **108 A2** 35 35N 10 58 E
Mokoan, L., *Australia* **129 D7** 36 27 S 146 5 E
Mokokchung, *India* **90 B5** 26 15N 94 30 E
Mokolea Rock, *U.S.A.* **145 K14** 21 27N 157 44W
Mokolo, *Cameroon* **109 F2** 10 49N 13 54 E
Mokolo, *Cameroon* **113 C7** 10 50N 13 55 E
Mokolo, *Dem. Rep. of the Congo* **114 B3** 1 55N 18 6 E
Mokolo →, *S. Africa* **117 C4** 23 14 S 27 43 E
Mokombe, *Dem. Rep. of the Congo* **114 C4** 0 14 S 23 48 E
Mokopane, *S. Africa* **117 C4** 24 10 S 28 55 E
Mokpalin, *Burma* **90 G6** 17 26N 96 53 E
Mokp'o, *S. Korea* **75 G14** 34 50N 126 25 E
Mokra Gora, *Serbia & M.* **50 D4** 42 50N 20 30 E
Mokronog, *Slovenia* **45 C12** 45 57N 15 9 E
Moksha →, *Russia* **60 C6** 54 45N 41 53 E
Mokshan, *Russia* **60 D7** 53 25N 44 35 E
Mokuaeae I., *U.S.A.* **145 A2** 22 14N 159 25W
Mokuauia I., *U.S.A.* **145 J14** 21 40N 157 56W
Mokulua Is., *U.S.A.* **145 K14** 21 24N 157 42W
Mokwa, *Nigeria* **113 D6** 9 19N 5 0 E
Mol, *Belgium* **24 C5** 51 11N 5 5 E
Mola di Bari, *Italy* **47 A10** 41 4N 17 5 E
Molakalmuru, *India* **95 G3** 14 55N 76 50 E
Molale, *Ethiopia* **107 E4** 10 10N 39 41 E
Molanda, *Dem. Rep. of the Congo* **114 B4** 2 28N 20 48 E
Moláoi, *Greece* **48 E4** 36 49N 22 56 E
Molara, *Italy* **46 B2** 40 52N 9 43 E
Molat, *Croatia* **45 D11** 44 15N 14 50 E
Molave, *Phil.* **81 G4** 8 5N 123 30 E
Molchanovo, *Russia* **66 D9** 57 40N 83 50 E
Mold, *U.K.* **20 D4** 53 9N 3 8W
Moldava nad Bodvou, *Slovak Rep.* **35 C14** 48 38N 21 0 E
Moldavia = Moldova ■, *Europe* **53 C13** 47 0N 28 0 E
Moldavia, *Romania* **53 D12** 46 30N 27 0 E
Molde, *Norway* **18 B4** 62 45N 7 9 E
Moldo Too, *Kyrgyzstan* **65 C7** 41 35N 75 0 E
Moldotau = Moldo Too, *Kyrgyzstan* **65 C7** 41 35N 75 0 E
Moldova ■, *Europe* **53 C13** 47 0N 28 0 E
Moldova Nouă, *Romania* **52 F6** 44 45N 21 41 E
Moldoveanu, Vf., *Romania* **53 E9** 45 36N 24 45 E
Moldoviţa, *Romania* **53 C10** 47 41N 25 32 E
Mole △, *Ghana* **113 D4** 9 43N 1 44W
Mole →, *U.K.* **21 F7** 51 24N 0 21W
Mole Creek, *Australia* **127 G4** 41 34 S 146 24 E
Molegbwe, *Dem. Rep. of the Congo* **114 B4** 4 12N 20 53 E
Molepolole, *Botswana* **116 C4** 24 28 S 25 28 E
Molesworth, *N.Z.* **131 C8** 42 5 S 173 16 E
Molfetta, *Italy* **47 A9** 41 12N 16 36 E
Molii Pond, *U.S.A.* **145 J14** 21 31N 157 51W
Molina de Aragón, *Spain* **40 E3** 40 46N 1 52W
Molina de Segura, *Spain* **41 G3** 38 3N 1 12W
Moline, *U.S.A.* **156 C6** 41 30N 90 31W
Molinella, *Italy* **45 D8** 44 37N 11 40 E
Molino, *U.S.A.* **153 E2** 30 43N 87 20W
Molinos, *Argentina* **174 B2** 25 28 S 66 15W
Moliro, *Dem. Rep. of the Congo* **118 D3** 8 12 S 30 30 E
Moliterno, *Italy* **47 B8** 40 14N 15 52 E
Molkom, *Sweden* **16 E7** 59 37N 13 44 E
Mölle, *Sweden* **17 H6** 56 17N 12 31 E
Molledo, *Spain* **42 B6** 43 8N 4 6W
Mollendo, *Peru* **172 D3** 17 0 S 72 0W
Mollerin, L., *Australia* **125 F2** 30 30 S 117 35 E
Mollerussa, *Spain* **40 D5** 41 37N 0 54 E
Mollina, *Spain* **43 H6** 37 8N 4 38W
Mölln, *Germany* **30 B6** 53 39N 10 32 E
Mölltorp, *Sweden* **17 F8** 58 30N 14 26 E
Mölnlycke, *Sweden* **17 G6** 57 40N 12 8 E
Molo, *Burma* **90 D6** 23 22N 96 53 E
Molochansk, *Ukraine* **59 J8** 47 15N 35 35 E
Molochnoye, Ozero, *Ukraine* **59 J8** 46 30N 35 20 E
Molodechno = Maladzyechna, *Belarus* **58 E4** 54 20N 26 50 E
Molodove, *Ukraine* **53 D14** 46 13N 29 39 E
Molokai, *U.S.A.* **145 B5** 21 8N 157 0W
Molokai Fracture Zone, *Pac. Oc.* **135 E15** 28 0N 125 0W
Molokini I., *U.S.A.* **145 C5** 20 38N 156 30W
Moloma →, *Russia* **64 B2** 58 29N 48 33 E
Molong, *Australia* **129 B8** 33 5 S 148 54 E
Molopo →, *Africa* **116 D3** 28 30 S 20 12 E
Mólos, *Greece* **48 C4** 38 47N 22 37 E
Molotov = Perm, *Russia* **64 C6** 58 0N 56 10 E
Molotov, Mys = Arkticheskiy, Mys, *Russia* **67 A10** 81 10N 95 0 E
Molotovsk = Nolinsk, *Russia* **60 B9** 57 28N 49 57 E
Molotovsk = Severodvinsk, *Russia* **56 B6** 64 27N 39 58 E
Molotovskoye = Krasnogvardeyskoye, *Russia* **61 H5** 45 52N 41 33 E
Moloundou, *Cameroon* **114 B3** 2 8N 15 15 E
Molowaie, *Dem. Rep. of the Congo* **115 D4** 5 47 S 23 18 E
Molsheim, *France* **27 D14** 48 33N 7 29 E
Molson L., *Canada* **143 C9** 54 22N 96 40W
Molteno, *S. Africa* **116 E4** 31 22 S 26 22 E
Moltrâsio, *Italy* **33 E8** 45 52N 9 6 E
Molu, *Indonesia* **83 C4** 6 45 S 131 40 E
Molucca Sea, *Indonesia* **82 A3** 0 0 125 0 E
Moluccas = Maluku, *Indonesia* **79 E7** 1 0 S 127 0 E
Molundo, *Phil.* **81 H5** 7 57N 124 23 E
Moma, *Dem. Rep. of the Congo* **118 C1** 1 35 S 23 52 E
Moma, *Mozam.* **119 F4** 16 47 S 39 4 E
Momba, *Australia* **128 A5** 30 58 S 143 30 E
Mombaça, *Brazil* **170 C4** 5 43 S 39 45W
Mombango, *Dem. Rep. of the Congo* **114 B4** 1 45N 24 26 E
Mombasa, *Kenya* **118 C4** 4 2 S 39 43 E
Mombetsu, *Japan* **70 B11** 44 21N 143 22 E
Mombil, *Burma* **90 B7** 27 46N 98 6 E
Momboyo →, *Dem. Rep. of the Congo* **114 C3** 0 16 S 19 0 E
Mombuey, *Spain* **42 C4** 42 3N 6 20W
Momchilgrad, *Bulgaria* **51 E9** 41 33N 25 23 E
Momence, *U.S.A.* **157 C9** 41 10N 87 40W
Momi, *Dem. Rep. of the Congo* **118 C2** 1 42 S 27 0 E
Momote, *Papua N. G.* **132 B4** 2 4 S 147 27 E
Mompog Pass, *Phil.* **80 E4** 13 34N 122 13 E
Mompós, *Colombia* **168 B3** 9 14N 74 26W
Møn, *Denmark* **17 K6** 54 57N 12 20 E
Mon □, *Burma* **90 G6** 16 0N 97 30 E
Mona, Canal de la = Mona Passage, *W. Indies* **165 C6** 18 30N 67 45W
Mona, Isla, *Puerto Rico* **165 C6** 18 5N 67 54W
Mona, Pta., *Costa Rica* **164 E3** 9 37N 82 36W
Mona Passage, *W. Indies* **165 C6** 18 30N 67 45W
Mona Quimbundo, *Angola* **115 D3** 9 55 S 19 58 E
Monaca, *U.S.A.* **150 F4** 40 41N 80 17W
Monaco ■, *Europe* **29 E11** 43 46N 7 23 E
Monadhliath Mts., *U.K.* **22 D4** 57 10N 4 4W
Monadnock, Mt., *U.S.A.* **151 D12** 42 52N 72 7W
Monagas □, *Venezuela* **169 B5** 9 20N 63 0W
Monaghan, *Ireland* **23 B5** 54 15N 6 57W
Monaghan □, *Ireland* **23 B5** 54 11N 6 56W
Monahans, *U.S.A.* **155 K3** 31 36N 102 54W
Monapo, *Mozam.* **119 E5** 14 56 S 40 19 E
Monar, L., *U.K.* **22 D3** 57 26N 5 8W
Monaragala, *Sri Lanka* **95 L5** 6 52N 81 22 E
Monarch Mt., *Canada* **142 C3** 51 55N 125 57W
Monashee Mts., *Canada* **142 C5** 51 0N 118 43W
Monasterevin, *Ireland* **23 C4** 53 8N 7 4W
Monastir = Bitola, *Macedonia* **50 E5** 41 1N 21 20 E
Monastir, *Tunisia* **108 A2** 35 50N 10 49 E
Moncada, *Phil.* **80 D3** 15 44N 120 34 E
Moncalieri, *Italy* **44 D4** 45 0N 7 41 E
Moncalvo, *Italy* **44 C5** 45 3N 8 16 E
Moncão, *Portugal* **42 C2** 42 4N 8 27W
Moncarapacho, *Portugal* **43 H3** 37 5N 7 46W
Moncayo, Sierra del, *Spain* **40 D3** 41 48N 1 50W
Moncha-Guba = Monchegorsk, *Russia* **56 A5** 67 54N 32 58 E
Monchegorsk, *Russia* **56 A5** 67 54N 32 58 E
Mönchengladbach, *Germany* **30 D2** 51 11N 6 27 E
Monchique, *Portugal* **43 H2** 37 19N 8 38W
Moncks Corner, *U.S.A.* **152 B9** 33 12N 80 1W
Monclova, *Mexico* **162 B4** 26 50N 101 30W
Moncontour, *France* **26 D4** 48 22N 2 38W
Moncton, *Canada* **141 C7** 46 7N 64 51W
Mondariz, *Spain* **42 C2** 42 14N 8 27W
Mondego →, *Portugal* **42 E2** 40 9N 8 52W
Mondego, C., *Portugal* **42 E2** 40 11N 8 54W
Mondeodo, *Indonesia* **82 B2** 3 34 S 122 9 E
Mondeville, *France* **26 C6** 49 10N 0 18W
Mondimbi, *Dem. Rep. of the Congo* **114 B4** 1 48N 22 46 E
Mondjuku, *Dem. Rep. of the Congo* **114 C4** 1 41 S 21 12 E
Mondo, *Chad* **109 F3** 13 47N 15 32 E
Mondolfo, *Italy* **45 E10** 43 45N 13 6 E
Mondoñedo, *Spain* **42 B3** 43 25N 7 23W
Mondovì, *Italy* **44 D4** 44 23N 7 49 E
Mondragon, *Phil.* **80 E5** 12 31N 124 45 E
Mondragone, *Italy* **46 A6** 41 7N 13 53 E
Mondrain I., *Australia* **125 F3** 34 9 S 122 14 E
Moneague, *Jamaica* **164 a** 18 16N 77 7W
Monemvasía, *Greece* **48 E5** 36 41N 23 3 E
Monessen, *U.S.A.* **150 F5** 40 9N 79 54W
Monesterio, *Spain* **43 G4** 38 6N 6 15W
Monestier-de-Clermont, *France* **29 D9** 44 55N 5 38 E
Monett, *U.S.A.* **155 G8** 36 55N 93 55W
Moneymore, *U.K.* **23 B5** 54 41N 6 40W
Monfalcone, *Italy* **45 C10** 45 49N 13 32 E
Monflanquin, *France* **28 D4** 44 32N 0 47 E
Monforte, *Portugal* **43 F3** 39 6N 7 25W
Monforte de Lemos, *Spain* **42 C3** 42 31N 7 33W
Mong Cai, *Vietnam* **86 B6** 21 27N 107 54 E
Mong Hsu, *Burma* **76 G2** 21 54N 98 30 E
Mong Hta, *Burma* **90 F7** 19 50N 98 35 E
Mong Ket, *Burma* **90 D7** 23 8N 98 22 E
Mong Kung, *Burma* **90 E6** 21 35N 97 35 E
Mong Kyawt, *Burma* **90 F7** 19 56N 98 45 E
Möng Long, *Burma* **90 D6** 22 47N 96 37 E
Möng Mit, *Burma* **90 D6** 23 7N 96 41 E
Mong Nai, *Burma* **90 E6** 20 32N 97 46 E
Möng Pan, *Burma* **90 E7** 20 19N 98 22 E
Mong Ping, *Burma* **76 G2** 21 22N 99 2 E
Mong Pu, *Burma* **90 E7** 20 55N 98 44 E
Mong Ton, *Burma* **90 E7** 20 17N 98 45 E
Mong Tung, *Burma* **90 D6** 22 2N 97 41 E
Mong Yai, *Burma* **90 D7** 22 21N 98 3 E
Möng Yu, *Burma* **90 D6** 23 30N 97 47 E
Monga, *Dem. Rep. of the Congo* **114 B4** 4 12N 22 49 E
Mongala →, *Dem. Rep. of the Congo* **114 B3** 1 53N 19 46 E
Mongalla, *Sudan* **107 F3** 5 8N 31 42 E
Mongandia, *Congo* **114 B3** 0 45N 17 11 E
Mongers, L., *Australia* **125 E2** 29 25 S 117 5 E
Mongga, *Solomon Is.* **133 L9** 7 52 S 157 0 E

Monghyr = Munger, *India* **93 G12** 25 23N 86 30 E
Mongibello = Etna, *Italy* **47 E7** 37 50N 14 55 E
Mongla, *Bangla.* **90 D2** 22 8N 89 35 E
Mongngaw, *Burma* **90 D6** 22 47N 96 59 E
Mongo, *Chad* **109 F3** 12 14N 18 43 E
Mongó, *Eq. Guin.* **114 B2** 1 52N 10 10 E
Mongo →, *S. Leone* **112 D2** 9 35N 12 10W
Mongolia ■, *Asia* **67 E10** 47 0N 103 0 E
Mongolia, Plateau of, *Asia* **62 E14** 45 0N 105 0 E
Mongomo, *Eq. Guin.* **114 B2** 1 38N 11 19 E
Mongonu, *Nigeria* **113 C7** 12 40N 13 32 E
Mongororo, *Chad* **109 F4** 12 3N 22 26 E
Mongstad, *Norway* **18 D2** 60 49N 5 2 E
Mongu, *Zambia* **115 F4** 15 16 S 23 12 E
Mônguа, *Angola* **116 B2** 16 43 S 15 20 E
Moniac, *U.S.A.* **152 E7** 30 31N 82 14W
Monifieth, *U.K.* **22 E6** 56 30N 2 48W
Monistrol-sur-Loire, *France* **29 C8** 45 17N 4 11 E
Monkayo, *Phil.* **81 H6** 7 50N 126 5 E
Monkey Bay, *Malawi* **119 E4** 14 7 S 35 1 E
Monkey Mia, *Australia* **125 E1** 25 48 S 113 43 E
Monkey River Town, *Belize* **163 D7** 16 22N 88 29W
Mońki, *Poland* **54 E9** 53 23N 22 48 E
Monkoto, *Dem. Rep. of the Congo* **114 C4** 1 38 S 20 35 E
Monkton, *Canada* **150 C3** 43 35N 81 5W
Monmouth, *U.K.* **21 F5** 51 48N 2 42W
Monmouth, *Ill., U.S.A.* **156 D6** 40 55N 90 39W
Monmouth, *Oreg., U.S.A.* **158 D2** 44 51N 123 14W
Monmouthshire □, *U.K.* **21 F5** 51 48N 2 54W
Mono, *Solomon Is.* **133 L8** 7 20 S 155 35 E
Mono L., *U.S.A.* **160 H7** 38 1N 119 1W
Monolith, *U.S.A.* **161 K8** 35 7N 118 22W
Monólithos, *Greece* **38 E11** 36 7N 27 45 E
Monon, *U.S.A.* **157 D10** 40 52N 86 53W
Monona, *Iowa, U.S.A.* **156 A5** 43 3N 91 23W
Monona, *Wis., U.S.A.* **156 A7** 43 4N 89 20W
Monongahela, *U.S.A.* **150 F5** 40 12N 79 56W
Monópoli, *Italy* **47 B10** 40 57N 17 18 E
Monor, *Hungary* **52 C4** 47 21N 19 27 E
Monos I., *Trin. & Tob.* **169 F9** 10 42N 61 44W
Monóvar, *Spain* **41 G4** 38 28N 0 53W
Monowai, *N.Z.* **131 F2** 45 53 S 167 31 E
Monowai, L., *N.Z.* **131 F2** 45 53 S 167 25 E
Monqoumba, *C.A.R.* **114 B3** 3 33N 18 40 E
Monreal del Campo, *Spain* **40 E3** 40 47N 1 20W
Monreale, *Italy* **46 D6** 38 5N 13 17 E
Monroe, *Ga., U.S.A.* **152 B6** 33 47N 83 43W
Monroe, *Iowa, U.S.A.* **156 C3** 41 31N 93 6W
Monroe, *La., U.S.A.* **155 J8** 32 30N 92 7W
Monroe, *Mich., U.S.A.* **157 C13** 41 55N 83 24W
Monroe, *N.C., U.S.A.* **149 H5** 34 59N 80 33W
Monroe, *N.Y., U.S.A.* **151 E10** 41 20N 74 11W
Monroe, *Ohio, U.S.A.* **157 E12** 39 27N 84 22W
Monroe, *Utah, U.S.A.* **159 G7** 38 38N 112 7W
Monroe, *Wash., U.S.A.* **160 C5** 47 51N 121 58W
Monroe, *Wis., U.S.A.* **156 B7** 42 36N 89 38W
Monroe, L., *U.S.A.* **153 G8** 28 50N 81 19W
Monroe City, *Ind., U.S.A.* **157 F9** 38 37N 87 20W
Monroe City, *Mo., U.S.A.* **156 E5** 39 39N 91 44W
Monroe L., *U.S.A.* **157 E10** 39 1N 86 31W
Monroeton, *U.S.A.* **151 E8** 41 43N 76 29W
Monroeville, *Ala., U.S.A.* **149 K2** 31 31N 87 20W
Monroeville, *Ind., U.S.A.* **157 D12** 40 59N 84 52W
Monroeville, *Pa., U.S.A.* **150 F5** 40 26N 79 45W
Monrovia, *Liberia* **112 D2** 6 18N 10 47W
Mons, *Belgium* **24 D3** 50 27N 3 58 E
Møns Klint, *Denmark* **17 K6** 54 57N 12 33 E
Monsaraz, *Portugal* **43 G3** 38 28N 7 22W
Monse, *Indonesia* **82 B2** 4 7 S 123 15 E
Monsefú, *Peru* **172 B2** 6 52 S 79 52W
Monségur, *France* **28 D4** 44 38N 0 4 E
Monsélice, *Italy* **45 C8** 45 14N 11 45 E
Mønshaug, *Norway* **18 D3** 60 37N 6 31 E
Mönsterås, *Sweden* **17 G10** 57 3N 16 26 E
Mont Cenis, Col du, *France* **29 C10** 45 15N 6 55 E
Mont-de-Marsan, *France* **28 E3** 43 54N 0 31W
Mont-Dore, *N. Cal.* **133 V20** 22 16 S 166 34 E
Mont Fouari ⌓, *Congo* **114 C2** 2 52 S 11 32 E
Mont-Joli, *Canada* **141 C6** 48 37N 68 10W
Mont-Laurier, *Canada* **140 C4** 46 35N 75 30W
Mont-Louis, *Canada* **141 C6** 49 15N 65 44W
Mont Peko △, *Ivory C.* **112 D3** 9 5N 7 15W
Mont-roig del Camp, *Spain* **40 D5** 41 5N 0 58 E
Mont-St-Michel, Le, *France* **26 D5** 48 40N 1 30W
Mont Sangbe △, *Ivory C.* **112 D3** 8 0N 7 10W
Mont-Tremblant ⌓, *Canada* **140 C5** 46 30N 74 30W
Montabaur, *Germany* **30 E3** 50 25N 7 50 E
Montagnac = Remchi, *Algeria* **111 A4** 35 2N 1 26W
Montagnac, *France* **28 E7** 43 29N 3 28 E
Montagnana, *Italy* **45 C8** 45 14N 11 28 E
Montagne d'Ambre △, *Madag.* **117 A8** 12 37 S 49 8 E
Montagne de Reims ⌓, *France* **27 C11** 49 8N 4 0 E
Montagu, *S. Africa* **116 E3** 33 45 S 20 8 E
Montagu I., *Antarctica* **7 B1** 58 25 S 26 20W
Montague, *Canada* **141 C7** 46 10N 62 39W
Montague, I., *Mexico* **162 A2** 31 40N 114 56W
Montague I., *Australia* **129 D9** 36 16 S 150 13 E
Montague I., *U.S.A.* **144 G11** 60 0N 147 30W
Montague Ra., *Australia* **125 E2** 27 15 S 119 30 E
Montague Sd., *Australia* **124 B4** 14 28 S 125 20 E
Montaigu, *France* **26 F5** 46 59N 1 18W
Montalbán, *Spain* **40 E4** 40 50N 0 45W
Montalbano Iónico, *Italy* **47 B9** 40 17N 16 34 E
Montalbo, *Spain* **40 F2** 39 53N 2 42W
Montalcino, *Italy* **45 E8** 43 3N 11 29 E
Montalegre, *Angola* **115 D3** 8 45 S 17 4 E
Montalegre, *Portugal* **42 D3** 41 49N 7 47W
Montalto, *Italy* **47 D8** 38 10N 15 55 E
Montalto di Castro, *Italy* **45 F8** 42 21N 11 37 E
Montalto Uffugo, *Italy* **47 C9** 39 24N 16 9 E
Montalvo, *U.S.A.* **161 L7** 34 15N 119 12W
Montamarta, *Spain* **42 D5** 41 39N 5 49W
Montana, *Bulgaria* **50 C7** 43 27N 23 16 E
Montaña, *Peru* **172 B3** 6 0 S 73 0W
Montana, *Switz.* **32 D4** 46 19N 7 29 E
Montana □, *Bulgaria* **50 C7** 43 30N 23 20 E
Montana □, *U.S.A.* **158 C9** 47 0N 110 0W
Montaña Clara, I., *Canary Is.* **9 e2** 29 17N 13 33W
Montañas de Malaga ⌓, *Spain* **43 J6** 36 48N 4 32W
Montánchez, *Spain* **43 F4** 39 15N 6 8W
Montañita, *Colombia* **168 C2** 1 22N 75 28W
Montargil, *Portugal* **43 F2** 39 5N 8 10W
Montargis, *France* **27 E9** 47 59N 2 43 E
Montauban, *France* **28 D5** 44 2N 1 21 E
Montauk, *U.S.A.* **151 E13** 41 3N 71 57W
Montauk Pt., *U.S.A.* **151 E13** 41 4N 71 52W
Montaytas, *Kazakhstan* **65 B4** 42 5N 68 59 E
Montbard, *France* **27 E11** 47 38N 4 20 E
Montbarrey, *France* **27 E12** 47 1N 5 39 E
Montbéliard, *France* **27 E13** 47 31N 6 48 E
Montblanc, *Spain* **40 D6** 41 23N 1 4 E
Montbrison, *France* **29 C8** 45 36N 4 3 E
Montcalm, Pic de, *France* **28 F5** 42 40N 1 25 E
Montceau-les-Mines, *France* **27 F11** 46 40N 4 23 E
Montcenis, *France* **29 B8** 46 47N 4 23 E
Montclair, *U.S.A.* **151 F10** 40 49N 74 13W
Montcornet, *France* **27 C11** 49 40N 4 1 E
Montcuq, *France* **28 D5** 44 21N 1 13 E
Montdidier, *France* **27 C9** 49 38N 2 35 E
Monte Albán, *Mexico* **163 D5** 17 2N 96 45W
Monte Alegre, *Brazil* **169 D7** 2 0 S 54 0W
Monte Alegre de Goiás, *Brazil* **171 D2** 13 14 S 47 10W
Monte Alegre de Minas, *Brazil* **171 E2** 18 52 S 48 52W
Monte Alegre do Piauí, *Brazil* **170 C2** 9 46 S 45 18W
Monte Azul, *Brazil* **171 E3** 15 9 S 42 53W
Monte-Carlo, *Monaco* **29 E11** 43 44N 7 25 E
Monte Carmelo, *Brazil* **171 E2** 18 43 S 47 29W
Monte Caseros, *Argentina* **174 C4** 30 10 S 57 50W
Monte Comán, *Argentina* **174 C2** 34 40 S 67 53W
Monte Cristi, *Dom. Rep.* **165 C5** 19 52N 71 39W
Monte Cucco ⌓, *Italy* **45 E9** 43 22N 12 43 E
Monte Dinero, *Argentina* **176 D3** 52 18 S 68 33W
Monte Dourado, *Brazil* **169 D7** 0 52 S 52 31W
Monte Lindo →, *Paraguay* **174 A4** 23 56 S 57 12W
Monte Pascoal △, *Brazil* **171 E4** 16 51 S 39 21W
Monte Patria, *Chile* **174 C1** 30 42 S 70 58W
Monte Quemado, *Argentina* **174 B3** 25 53 S 62 41W
Monte Redondo, *Portugal* **42 F2** 39 53N 8 50W
Monte Rio, *U.S.A.* **160 G4** 38 28N 123 0W
Monte San Giovanni Campano, *Italy* **46 A6** 41 38N 13 31 E
Monte San Giuliano = Érice, *Italy* **46 D5** 38 2N 12 35 E
Monte San Savino, *Italy* **45 E8** 43 20N 11 43 E
Monte Sant' Ángelo, *Italy* **45 G12** 41 42N 15 59 E
Monte Santu, C. di, *Italy* **46 B2** 40 5N 9 44 E
Monte Sibillini △, *Italy* **45 F10** 42 55N 13 15 E
Monte Subasio ⌓, *Italy* **45 E9** 43 5N 12 40 E
Monte Vista, *U.S.A.* **159 H10** 37 35N 106 9W
Monteagudo, *Argentina* **175 B5** 27 14 S 54 8W
Monteagudo, *Bolivia* **173 D5** 19 49 S 63 59W
Montealegre del Castillo, *Spain* **41 G3** 38 48N 1 17W
Montebello, *Canada* **140 C5** 45 40N 74 55W
Montebello Iónico, *Italy* **47 E8** 37 59N 15 45 E
Montebello Is., *Australia* **124 D2** 20 30 S 115 45 E
Montebelluna, *Italy* **45 C9** 45 47N 12 3 E
Montebourg, *France* **26 C5** 49 30N 1 20W
Montecastrilli, *Italy* **45 F9** 42 39N 12 29 E
Montecatini Terme, *Italy* **44 E7** 43 53N 10 46 E
Montecito, *U.S.A.* **161 L7** 34 26N 119 40W
Montecristi, *Ecuador* **168 D1** 1 0 S 80 40W
Montecristo, *Italy* **44 F7** 42 20N 10 19 E
Montefalco, *Italy* **45 F9** 42 54N 12 39 E
Montefiascone, *Italy* **45 F9** 42 32N 12 2 E
Montefrío, *Spain* **43 H7** 37 20N 4 0W
Montegiórgio, *Italy* **45 E10** 43 6N 13 33 E
Montego Bay, *Jamaica* **164 a** 18 28N 77 55W
Montehermoso, *Spain* **42 E4** 40 5N 6 21W
Monteiro, *Brazil* **170 C4** 7 48 S 37 2W
Montejicar, *Spain* **43 H7** 37 33N 3 30W
Monteleone di Calabria = Vibo Valéntia, *Italy* **47 D9** 38 40N 16 6 E
Montelíbano, *Colombia* **168 B2** 8 5N 75 29W
Montélimar, *France* **29 D8** 44 33N 4 45 E
Montella, *Italy* **47 B8** 40 51N 15 1 E
Montellano, *Spain* **43 J5** 36 59N 5 29W
Montello, *U.S.A.* **154 D10** 43 48N 89 20W
Montemayor, Meseta de, *Argentina* **176 B3** 44 20 S 66 10W
Montemor-o-Novo, *Portugal* **43 G2** 38 40N 8 12W
Montemor-o-Velho, *Portugal* **42 E2** 40 11N 8 40W
Montemorelos, *Mexico* **163 B5** 25 11N 99 42W
Montendre, *France* **28 C3** 45 16N 0 26W
Montenegro, *Brazil* **175 B5** 29 39 S 51 29W
Montenegro □, *Serbia & M.* **50 D3** 42 40N 19 20 E
Montenero di Bisáccia, *Italy* **45 G11** 41 57N 14 47 E
Montepuez, *Mozam.* **119 E4** 13 8 S 38 59 E
Montepuez →, *Mozam.* **119 E5** 12 32 S 40 27 E
Montepulciano, *Italy* **45 E8** 43 5N 11 47 E
Montereale, *Italy* **45 F10** 42 31N 13 15 E
Montereau-Faut-Yonne, *France* **27 D9** 48 22N 2 57 E
Monterey, *Calif., U.S.A.* **160 J5** 36 37N 121 55W
Monterey, *Ind., U.S.A.* **157 C10** 41 11N 86 30W
Monterey B., *U.S.A.* **160 J5** 36 45N 122 0W
Montería, *Colombia* **168 B2** 8 46N 75 53W
Montero, *Bolivia* **173 D5** 17 20 S 63 15W
Monteros, *Argentina* **174 B2** 27 11 S 65 30W
Monterotondo, *Italy* **45 F9** 42 3N 12 37 E
Monterrey, *Mexico* **162 B4** 25 40N 100 30W
Montes Altos, *Brazil* **170 C2** 5 50 S 47 4W
Montes Azules ⌓, *Mexico* **163 D6** 16 21N 91 3W
Montes Claros, *Brazil* **171 E3** 16 30 S 43 50W
Montesano, *U.S.A.* **160 D3** 46 59N 123 36W
Montesano sulla Marcellana, *Italy* **47 B8** 40 16N 15 42 E
Montesárchio, *Italy* **47 A7** 41 4N 14 38 E
Montescaglioso, *Italy* **47 B9** 40 33N 16 40 E
Montesilvano, *Italy* **45 F11** 42 29N 14 8 E
Montesinho ⌓, *Portugal* **42 D4** 41 54N 6 52W
Montevarchi, *Italy* **45 E8** 43 31N 11 34 E
Montevideo, *Uruguay* **175 C4** 34 50 S 56 11W
Montevideo, *U.S.A.* **154 C7** 44 57N 95 43W
Montezuma, *Ga., U.S.A.* **152 C5** 32 18N 84 2W
Montezuma, *Ind., U.S.A.* **157 E9** 39 48N 87 22W
Montezuma, *Iowa, U.S.A.* **156 C4** 41 35N 92 32W
Montezuma Castle ⌓, *U.S.A.* **159 J8** 34 34N 111 45W
Montfaucon, *France* **26 E5** 47 6N 1 7W
Montfaucon-d'Argonne, *France* **27 C12** 49 16N 5 8 E
Montfaucon-en-Velay, *France* **29 C8** 45 11N 4 20 E
Montfort-le-Gesnois, *France* **26 D7** 48 3N 0 25 E
Montfort-sur-Meu, *France* **26 D5** 48 9N 1 58W
Montfragüe ⌓, *Spain* **42 F5** 39 48N 5 52W
Montgenèvre, *France* **29 D10** 44 56N 6 43 E
Montgomery = Sahiwal, *Pakistan* **91 C4** 30 45N 73 8 E
Montgomery, *U.K.* **21 E4** 52 34N 3 8W
Montgomery, *Ala., U.S.A.* **152 C3** 32 23N 86 19W
Montgomery, *Ill., U.S.A.* **157 C8** 41 44N 88 21W
Montgomery, *Pa., U.S.A.* **150 E8** 41 10N 76 53W
Montgomery, *W. Va., U.S.A.* **148 F5** 38 11N 81 19W
Montgomery City, *U.S.A.* **156 F5** 38 59N 91 30W
Montguyon, *France* **28 C3** 45 12N 0 12W
Monthermé, *France* **27 C11** 49 52N 4 42 E
Monthey, *Switz.* **32 D3** 46 15N 6 56 E
Monthois, *France* **27 C11** 49 19N 4 43 E
Monti, *Italy* **46 B2** 40 49N 9 19 E
Monti Lucrétili ⌓, *Italy* **45 F9** 42 5N 12 50 E
Monti Picentini ⌓, *Italy* **47 B8** 40 45N 15 2 E
Monti Simbruini ⌓, *Italy* **45 G10** 41 55N 13 13 E
Monticelli d'Ongina, *Italy* **44 C6** 45 5N 9 56 E
Monticello, *Ark., U.S.A.* **155 J9** 33 38N 91 47W
Monticello, *Fla., U.S.A.* **152 E6** 30 33N 83 52W
Monticello, *Ga., U.S.A.* **152 B6** 33 18N 83 40W
Monticello, *Ill., U.S.A.* **157 D8** 40 1N 88 34W
Monticello, *Ind., U.S.A.* **157 D10** 40 45N 86 46W
Monticello, *Iowa, U.S.A.* **156 B5** 42 15N 91 12W
Monticello, *Ky., U.S.A.* **149 G3** 36 50N 84 51W
Monticello, *Minn., U.S.A.* **154 C8** 45 18N 93 48W
Monticello, *Miss., U.S.A.* **155 K9** 31 33N 90 7W
Monticello, *Mo., U.S.A.* **156 D5** 40 7N 91 43W
Monticello, *N.Y., U.S.A.* **151 E10** 41 39N 74 42W
Monticello, *Utah, U.S.A.* **159 H9** 37 52N 109 21W
Montichiari, *Italy* **44 C7** 45 25N 10 23 E
Montier-en-Der, *France* **27 D11** 48 30N 4 45 E
Montignac, *France* **28 C5** 45 4N 1 10 E
Montigny-les-Metz, *France* **27 C13** 49 7N 6 10 E
Montigny-sur-Aube, *France* **27 E11** 47 57N 4 45 E
Montijo, *Portugal* **43 G2** 38 41N 8 54W
Montijo, *Spain* **43 G4** 38 52N 6 39W
Montilla, *Spain* **43 H6** 37 36N 4 40W
Montivilliers, *France* **26 C7** 49 33N 0 12 E
Montluçon, *France* **27 F9** 46 22N 2 36 E
Montmagny, *Canada* **141 C5** 46 58N 70 34W
Montmarault, *France* **27 F9** 46 19N 2 57 E
Montmartre, *Canada* **143 C8** 50 14N 103 27W
Montmédy, *France* **27 C12** 49 30N 5 20 E
Montmélian, *France* **29 C10** 45 30N 6 4 E
Montmirail, *France* **27 D10** 48 51N 3 30 E
Montmoreau-St-Cybard, *France* **28 C4** 45 23N 0 8 E
Montmorillon, *France* **28 B4** 46 26N 0 50 E
Montmort-Lucy, *France* **27 D10** 48 55N 3 49 E
Monto, *Australia* **126 C5** 24 52 S 151 6 E
Montohora, *N.Z.* **130 E6** 38 17 S 177 32 E
Montoire-sur-le-Loir, *France* **26 E7** 47 45N 0 52 E
Montongbuwoh, *Indonesia* **79 K19** 8 33 S 116 4 E
Montório al Vomano, *Italy* **45 F10** 42 35N 13 38 E
Montoro, *Spain* **43 G6** 38 1N 4 27W
Montour Falls, *U.S.A.* **150 D8** 42 21N 76 51W
Montoursville, *U.S.A.* **150 E8** 41 15N 76 55W
Montpelier, *Idaho, U.S.A.* **158 E8** 42 19N 111 18W
Montpelier, *Ind., U.S.A.* **157 D11** 40 33N 85 17W
Montpelier, *Ohio, U.S.A.* **157 C12** 41 35N 84 37W
Montpelier, *Vt., U.S.A.* **151 B12** 44 16N 72 35W
Montpellier, *France* **28 E7** 43 37N 3 52 E
Montpezat-de-Quercy, *France* **28 D5** 44 15N 1 30 E
Montpon-Ménestérol, *France* **28 D4** 45 0N 0 11 E
Montréal, *Canada* **140 C5** 45 31N 73 34W
Montréal, *Aude, France* **28 E6** 43 13N 2 8 E
Montréal, *Gers, France* **28 E4** 43 56N 0 11 E
Montreal →, *Canada* **140 C3** 47 14N 84 39W
Montreal L., *Canada* **143 C7** 54 20N 105 45W
Montreal Lake, *Canada* **143 C7** 54 3N 105 46W
Montredon-Labessonnié, *France* **28 E6** 43 45N 2 18 E
Montrésor, *France* **26 E8** 47 10N 1 10 E
Montret, *France* **27 F12** 46 40N 5 7 E
Montreuil, *Pas-de-Calais, France* **27 B8** 50 27N 1 45 E
Montreuil, *Seine-St-Denis, France* **27 D9** 48 51N 2 27 E
Montreuil-Bellay, *France* **26 E6** 47 8N 0 9W
Montreux, *Switz.* **32 D3** 46 26N 6 55 E
Montrevel-en-Bresse, *France* **27 F12** 46 21N 5 8 E
Montrichard, *France* **26 E8** 47 20N 1 10 E
Montrose, *U.K.* **22 E6** 56 44N 2 27W
Montrose, *Colo., U.S.A.* **159 G10** 38 29N 107 53W
Montrose, *Pa., U.S.A.* **151 E9** 41 50N 75 53W
Montrose, L., *U.S.A.* **156 F3** 38 18N 93 50W
Monts, Pte. des, *Canada* **141 C6** 49 20N 67 12W
Montsalvy, *France* **28 D6** 44 41N 2 30 E
Montsant, Serra de, *Spain* **40 D6** 41 17N 1 0 E
Montsauche-les-Settons, *France* **27 E11** 47 13N 4 2 E
Montsec, Serra del, *Spain* **40 C5** 42 5N 0 45 E
Montseny ⌓, *Spain* **40 D2** 41 43N 2 22W
Montserrat, *Spain* **40 D6** 41 36N 1 49 E
Montserrat ⧄, *W. Indies* **165 C7** 16 40N 62 10W
Montuenga, *Spain* **42 D6** 41 3N 4 38W
Montuiri, *Spain* **38 B3** 39 34N 2 59 E
Monveda, *Dem. Rep. of the Congo* **114 B4** 2 52N 21 30 E
Monyo, *Burma* **90 G5** 17 59N 95 30 E
Monywa, *Burma* **90 D5** 22 7N 95 11 E
Monza, *Italy* **44 C6** 45 35N 9 16 E
Monze, *Zambia* **119 F2** 16 17 S 27 29 E
Monze, C., *Pakistan* **91 D2** 24 47N 66 37 E
Monzón, *Spain* **40 D5** 41 52N 0 10 E
Moodyville = North Vancouver, *Canada* **142 D4** 49 19N 123 4W
Mooers, *U.S.A.* **151 B11** 44 58N 73 35W
Mooi →, *S. Africa* **117 D5** 28 45 S 30 34 E
Mooi River, *S. Africa* **117 D4** 29 13 S 29 50 E
Mo'oka, *Japan* **73 A12** 36 26N 140 1 E
Moonah →, *Australia* **126 C2** 22 3 S 138 33 E
Moonda, L., *Australia* **126 D3** 25 52 S 140 25 E
Moonie, *Australia* **127 D5** 27 46 S 150 20 E
Moonie →, *Australia* **127 D4** 29 19 S 148 43 E
Moonta, *Australia* **128 C2** 34 6 S 137 32 E
Moor, Kepulauan, *Indonesia* **83 B5** 2 57 S 135 45 E
Moora, *Australia* **125 F2** 30 37 S 115 58 E
Moorcroft, *U.S.A.* **154 C2** 44 16N 104 57W
Moore →, *Australia* **125 F2** 31 22 S 115 30 E
Moore, L., *Australia* **125 E2** 29 50 S 117 35 E
Moore Haven, *U.S.A.* **153 J8** 26 50N 81 6W
Moore Park, *Australia* **126 C5** 24 43 S 152 17 E
Moore River △, *Australia* **125 F2** 31 7 S 115 39 E
Mooréa, *French Polynesia* **133 S16** 17 30 S 149 50W
Moorefield, *U.S.A.* **148 F6** 39 5N 78 59W
Moores Res., *U.S.A.* **151 B13** 44 45N 71 50W
Mooresville, *U.S.A.* **157 E10** 39 37N 86 22W
Moorfoot Hills, *U.K.* **22 F5** 55 44N 3 8W
Moorhead, *U.S.A.* **154 B6** 46 53N 96 45W
Moorland, *U.S.A.* **156 B2** 42 26N 94 18W
Moormerland, *Germany* **30 B3** 53 20N 7 20 E
Moornanyah L., *Australia* **128 B5** 33 15 S 143 42 E
Mooroopna, *Australia* **129 D6** 36 25 S 145 22 E
Moorpark, *U.S.A.* **161 L8** 34 17N 118 53W
Moorreesburg, *S. Africa* **116 E2** 33 6 S 18 38 E
Moorrinya △, *Australia* **126 C3** 21 42 S 144 58 E
Moosburg, *Germany* **31 G7** 48 27N 11 56 E
Moose →, *Canada* **140 B3** 51 20N 80 25W
Moose →, *U.S.A.* **151 C9** 43 38N 75 24W
Moose Creek, *Canada* **151 A10** 45 15N 74 58W
Moose Factory, *Canada* **140 B3** 51 16N 80 32W
Moose Jaw, *Canada* **143 C7** 50 24N 105 30W
Moose Jaw →, *Canada* **143 C7** 50 34N 105 18W
Moose Lake, *U.S.A.* **154 B8** 46 27N 92 46W
Moose Mountain ⌓, *Canada* **143 D8** 49 48N 102 25W
Moose Pass, *U.S.A.* **144 F10** 60 29N 149 22W
Moosehead L., *U.S.A.* **149 C11** 45 38N 69 40W
Mooselookmeguntic L., *U.S.A.* **149 C10** 44 55N 70 49W
Moosilauke, Mt., *U.S.A.* **151 B13** 44 3N 71 40W
Moosomin, *Canada* **143 C8** 50 9N 101 40W
Moosonee, *Canada* **140 B3** 51 17N 80 39W
Moosup, *U.S.A.* **151 E13** 41 43N 71 53W
Mootwingee △, *Australia* **128 A5** 31 10 S 142 30 E
Mopane, *S. Africa* **117 C4** 22 37 S 29 52 E
Mopeia Velha, *Mozam.* **119 F4** 17 30 S 35 40 E
Mopipi, *Botswana* **116 C3** 21 6 S 24 55 E
Mopoi, *C.A.R.* **118 A2** 5 6N 26 54 E
Mopti, *Mali* **112 C4** 14 30N 4 0W
Moqatta, *Sudan* **107 E4** 14 38N 35 50 E
Moqor, *Afghan.* **91 B2** 32 50N 67 42 E
Moquegua, *Peru* **172 D3** 17 15 S 70 46W
Moquegua □, *Peru* **172 D3** 16 50 S 70 55W
Mór, *Hungary* **52 C3** 47 25N 18 12 E
Mora, *Cameroon* **109 F2** 11 3N 14 9 E
Mora, *Cameroon* **113 C7** 11 2N 14 7 E
Móra, *Portugal* **43 G2** 38 55N 8 10W
Mora, *Spain* **43 F7** 39 41N 3 46W
Mora, *Sweden* **16 C8** 61 2N 14 38 E
Mora, *Minn., U.S.A.* **154 C8** 45 53N 93 18W
Mora, *N. Mex., U.S.A.* **159 J11** 35 58N 105 20W
Mora de Rubielos, *Spain* **40 E4** 40 15N 0 45W
Mòra d'Ebre, *Spain* **40 D5** 41 6N 0 38 E
Mòra la Nova, *Spain* **40 D5** 41 7N 0 39 E
Morača →, *Serbia & M.* **50 D3** 42 20N 19 9 E
Morada Nova, *Brazil* **170 C4** 5 7 S 38 23W
Morada Nova de Minas, *Brazil* **171 E2** 18 37 S 45 22W
Moradabad, *India* **93 E8** 28 50N 78 50 E
Morafenobe, *Madag.* **117 B7** 17 50 S 44 53 E
Morąg, *Poland* **54 E6** 53 55N 19 56 E
Moral de Calatrava, *Spain* **43 G7** 38 51N 3 33W
Moraleda, Canal, *Chile* **176 B2** 44 30 S 73 30W
Moraleja, *Spain* **42 E4** 40 6N 6 43W
Morales, *Bolívar, Colombia* **168 B3** 8 16N 73 51W
Morales, *Cauca, Colombia* **168 C2** 2 45N 76 38W
Moramanga, *Madag.* **117 B8** 18 56 S 48 12 E
Moran, *Kans., U.S.A.* **155 G7** 37 55N 95 10W
Moran, *Wyo., U.S.A.* **158 E8** 43 53N 110 37W
Moranbah, *Australia* **126 C4** 22 1 S 148 6 E
Moranhat, *India* **90 B5** 27 10N 94 50 E
Morano Cálabro, *Italy* **47 C9** 39 50N 16 8 E
Morant Bay, *Jamaica* **164 a** 17 53N 76 25W
Morant Cays, *Jamaica* **164 C4** 17 22N 76 0W
Morant Pt., *Jamaica* **164 a** 17 55N 76 12W
Morar, *India* **92 F8** 26 14N 78 14 E
Morar, L., *U.K.* **22 E3** 56 57N 5 40W
Moratalla, *Spain* **41 G3** 38 14N 1 49W
Moratuwa, *Sri Lanka* **95 L4** 6 45N 79 55 E
Morava →, *Slovak Rep.* **35 C9** 48 10N 16 59 E
Moravia, *Iowa, U.S.A.* **156 D4** 40 53N 92 49W
Moravia, *N.Y., U.S.A.* **151 D8** 42 43N 76 25W
Moravian Hts. = Českomoravská Vrchovina, *Czech Rep.* **34 B8** 49 30N 15 40 E
Moravica →, *Serbia & M.* **50 C4** 43 52N 20 8 E
Moraviţa, *Romania* **52 E6** 45 17N 21 14 E
Moravská Třebová, *Czech Rep.* **35 B9** 49 45N 16 40 E
Moravské Budějovice, *Czech Rep.* **34 B8** 49 4N 15 49 E
Morawa, *Australia* **125 E2** 29 13 S 116 0 E
Morawhanna, *Guyana* **169 B6** 8 30N 59 40W
Moray □, *U.K.* **22 D5** 57 31N 3 18W
Moray Firth, *U.K.* **22 D5** 57 40N 3 52W
Morbach, *Germany* **31 F3** 49 48N 7 6 E
Morbegno, *Italy* **44 B6** 46 8N 9 34 E
Morbi, *India* **92 H4** 22 50N 70 42 E
Morbihan □, *France* **26 E4** 47 55N 2 50W
Mörbylånga, *Sweden* **17 H10** 56 32N 16 22 E
Morcenx, *France* **28 D3** 44 3N 0 55W
Morcone, *Italy* **47 A7** 41 20N 14 40 E
Mordelles, *France* **26 D5** 48 5N 1 52W
Morden, *Canada* **143 D9** 49 15N 98 10W
Mordoğan, *Turkey* **49 C8** 38 30N 26 37 E
Mordovian Republic = Mordvinia □, *Russia* **60 C7** 54 20N 44 30 E
Mordovo, *Russia* **60 D5** 52 6N 40 50 E
Mordvinia □, *Russia* **60 C7** 54 20N 44 30 E
Mordy, *Poland* **55 F9** 52 13N 22 31 E
Møre og Romsdal □, *Norway* **18 B4** 62 30N 8 0 E
Morea, *Greece* **12 H10** 37 45N 22 10 E
Moreau →, *U.S.A.* **154 C4** 45 18N 100 43W
Morecambe, *U.K.* **20 C5** 54 5N 2 52W
Morecambe B., *U.K.* **20 C5** 54 7N 3 0W
Moree, *Australia* **127 D4** 29 28 S 149 54 E
Morehead, *Papua N. G.* **132 E1** 8 41 S 141 41 E
Morehead, *U.S.A.* **157 F13** 38 11N 83 26W
Morehead City, *U.S.A.* **149 H7** 34 43N 76 43W
Mörel, *Switz.* **32 D6** 46 22N 8 2 E
Morel →, *India* **92 F7** 26 13N 76 36 E
Moreland, *U.S.A.* **152 B5** 33 17N 84 46W
Morelia, *Mexico* **162 D4** 19 42N 101 7W
Morella, *Australia* **126 C3** 23 0 S 143 52 E
Morella, *Spain* **40 E4** 40 35N 0 5W
Morelos, *Mexico* **162 B3** 26 42N 107 40W
Morelos □, *Mexico* **163 D5** 18 40N 99 10W
Moremi ⌓, *Botswana* **116 B3** 19 18 S 23 10 E
Morena, *India* **92 F8** 26 30N 78 4 E
Morena, Sierra, *Spain* **43 G7** 38 20N 4 0W
Morenci, *U.S.A.* **157 C12** 41 43N 84 13W
Moreni, *Romania* **53 F10** 44 59N 25 36 E
Moreno Valley, *U.S.A.* **161 M10** 33 56N 117 15W
Morero, *Bolivia* **173 C4** 11 9 S 66 15W
Moreru →, *Brazil* **173 C6** 10 10 S 59 15W
Moresby I., *Canada* **142 C2** 52 30N 131 40W
Morestel, *France* **29 C9** 45 40N 5 28 E
Moreton I., *Australia* **127 D5** 27 10 S 153 25 E
Moreton Island △, *Australia* **127 D5** 27 2 S 153 24 E
Moreuil, *France* **27 C9** 49 46N 2 30 E
Morey, *Spain* **38 B4** 39 44N 3 20 E
Morez, *France* **27 F13** 46 31N 6 2 E
Morgan, *Australia* **128 C3** 34 2 S 139 35 E
Morgan, *Ga., U.S.A.* **152 D5** 31 32N 84 36W
Morgan, *Utah, U.S.A.* **158 F8** 41 2N 111 41W
Morgan City, *U.S.A.* **155 L9** 29 42N 91 12W
Morgan Hill, *U.S.A.* **160 H5** 37 8N 121 39W
Morganfield, *U.S.A.* **148 G2** 37 41N 87 55W
Morganton, *U.S.A.* **149 H5** 35 45N 81 41W
Morgantown, *Ind., U.S.A.* **157 E10** 39 22N 86 16W
Morgantown, *W. Va., U.S.A.* **148 F6** 39 38N 79 57W
Morgenzon, *S. Africa* **117 D4** 26 45 S 29 36 E
Morges, *Switz.* **32 C2** 46 31N 6 29 E
Morghak, *Iran* **97 D8** 29 7N 57 54 E
Morgongåva, *Sweden* **16 E10** 59 57N 16 58 E
Morhange, *France* **27 D13** 48 55N 6 38 E
Morhar →, *India* **93 G11** 25 29N 85 11 E
Mori, *Italy* **44 C7** 45 51N 10 59 E
Mori, *Japan* **70 C10** 42 6N 140 35 E
Moriarty, *U.S.A.* **159 J10** 34 59N 106 3W
Moribaya, *Guinea* **112 D3** 9 53N 9 32W
Morice L., *Canada* **142 C3** 53 50N 127 40W
Morichal, *Colombia* **168 C3** 2 10N 70 34W
Morichal Largo →, *Venezuela* **169 B5** 9 27N 62 25W
Moriguchi, *Japan* **73 C7** 34 44N 135 34 E
Moriki, *Nigeria* **113 C6** 12 52N 6 30 E
Morinville, *Canada* **142 C6** 53 49N 113 41W
Morioka, *Japan* **70 E10** 39 45N 141 8 E
Moris, *Mexico* **162 B3** 28 8N 108 32W
Morisset, *Australia* **129 B9** 33 6 S 151 30 E
Moriyama, *Japan* **73 B7** 35 4N 135 59 E
Morlaàs, *France* **28 E3** 43 21N 0 18W
Morlaix, *France* **26 D3** 48 36N 3 52W
Mörlunda, *Sweden* **17 G9** 57 19N 15 52 E
Mormanno, *Italy* **47 C8** 39 53N 15 59 E
Mormant, *France* **27 D9** 48 37N 2 52 E
Mornington, *Australia* **129 E6** 38 15 S 145 5 E
Mornington, I., *Chile* **176 C1** 49 50 S 75 30W
Mornington I., *Australia* **126 B2** 16 30 S 139 30 E
Mórnos →, *Greece* **48 C3** 38 25N 21 50 E
Moro, *Pakistan* **92 F2** 26 40N 68 0 E
Moro, *Sudan* **107 E3** 10 50N 30 9 E
Moro →, *Pakistan* **92 E2** 29 42N 67 22 E
Moro G., *Phil.* **81 H4** 6 30N 123 0 E
Morobe, *Papua N. G.* **132 D4** 7 49 S 147 38 E
Morobe □, *Papua N. G.* **132 D4** 7 0 S 147 0 E
Morocco, *U.S.A.* **157 D9** 40 57N 87 27W
Morocco ■, *N. Afr.* **110 B3** 32 0N 5 50W
Morococha, *Peru* **172 C2** 11 40 S 76 5W
Morogoro, *Tanzania* **118 D4** 6 50 S 37 40 E
Morogoro □, *Tanzania* **118 D4** 8 0 S 37 0 E
Moroleón, *Mexico* **162 C4** 20 8N 101 32W
Morombe, *Madag.* **117 C7** 21 45 S 43 22 E
Moron = Morong, *Phil.* **80 D3** 14 41N 120 16 E
Moron, *Argentina* **174 C4** 34 39 S 58 37W
Morón, *Cuba* **164 B4** 22 8N 78 39W
Morón de Almazán, *Spain* **40 D2** 41 29N 2 27W
Morón de la Frontera, *Spain* **43 H5** 37 6N 5 28W
Morona →, *Peru* **168 D2** 4 40 S 77 10W
Morona-Santiago □, *Ecuador* **168 D2** 2 30 S 78 0W
Morondava, *Madag.* **117 C7** 20 17 S 44 17 E
Morondo, *Ivory C.* **112 D3** 8 57N 6 47W
Morong, *Phil.* **80 D3** 14 41N 120 16 E
Morongo Valley, *U.S.A.* **161 L10** 34 3N 116 37W
Moroni, *Comoros Is.* **121 a** 11 40 S 43 16 E
Moroni, *U.S.A.* **158 G8** 39 32N 111 35W
Moronou, *Ivory C.* **112 D4** 6 16N 4 59W
Morotai, *Indonesia* **82 A3** 2 10N 128 30 E
Moroto, *Uganda* **118 B3** 2 28N 34 42 E
Moroto, Mt., *Uganda* **118 B3** 2 30N 34 43 E
Morowali, *Indonesia* **82 B2** 1 52 S 121 30 E
Morozov, *Bulgaria* **51 D9** 42 30N 25 10 E
Morozovsk, *Russia* **61 F5** 48 25N 41 50 E
Morpeth, *U.K.* **20 B6** 55 10N 1 41W
Morphou, *Cyprus* **39 E8** 35 12N 32 59 E
Morphou Bay, *Cyprus* **39 E8** 35 15N 32 50 E
Morrelganj, *Bangla.* **90 D2** 22 28N 89 51 E
Morrilton, *U.S.A.* **155 H8** 35 9N 92 44W
Morrinhos, *Ceará, Brazil* **170 B3** 3 14 S 40 7W
Morrinhos, *Minas Gerais, Brazil* **171 E2** 17 45 S 49 10W
Morrinsville, *N.Z.* **130 D4** 37 40 S 175 32 E
Morris, *Canada* **143 D9** 49 25N 97 22W
Morris, *Ill., U.S.A.* **154 E10** 41 22N 88 26W
Morris, *Minn., U.S.A.* **154 C7** 45 35N 95 55W
Morris, *N.Y., U.S.A.* **151 D9** 42 33N 75 15W
Morris, *Pa., U.S.A.* **150 E7** 41 35N 77 17W
Morris, Mt., *Australia* **125 E5** 26 9 S 131 4 E
Morris Jesup, Kap, *Greenland* **10 A7** 83 40N 34 0W
Morrisburg, *Canada* **151 B9** 44 55N 75 7W
Morrison, *U.S.A.* **156 C7** 41 49N 89 58W
Morrisonville, *U.S.A.* **156 E7** 39 25N 89 27W
Morristown, *Ariz., U.S.A.* **159 K7** 33 51N 112 37W
Morristown, *Ind., U.S.A.* **157 E11** 39 40N 85 42W
Morristown, *N.J., U.S.A.* **151 F10** 40 48N 74 29W

Morristown, N.Y., U.S.A. **151 B9** 44 35N 75 39W
Morristown, Tenn., U.S.A. **149 G4** 36 13N 83 18W
Morrisville, N.Y., U.S.A. **151 D9** 42 53N 75 35W
Morrisville, Pa., U.S.A. **151 F10** 40 13N 74 47W
Morrisville, Vt., U.S.A. **151 B12** 44 34N 72 36W
Morro, Pta., Chile **174 B1** 27 6 S 71 0W
Morro Bay, U.S.A. **160 K6** 35 22N 120 51W
Morro Chico, Chile **176 D2** 52 2 S 71 26W
Morro del Jable, Canary Is. **9 e2** 28 3N 14 23W
Morro do Chapéu, Brazil **171 D3** 11 33 S 41 9W
Morro Grande = Barão de Cocais, Brazil **171 E3** 19 56 S 43 28W
Morro Jable, Pta. de, Canary Is. **9 e2** 28 2N 14 20W
Morrocoy △, Venezuela **165 D6** 10 48N 68 13W
Morros, Brazil **170 B3** 2 52 S 44 3W
Morrosquillo, G. de, Colombia **164 E4** 9 35N 75 40W
Morrow, U.S.A. **157 E12** 39 21N 84 8W
Mörrum, Sweden **17 H8** 56 12N 14 45 E
Morrumbene, Mozam. **117 C6** 23 31 S 35 16 E
Mörrumsån →, Sweden **17 H8** 56 10N 14 45 E
Mors, Denmark **17 H2** 56 50N 8 45 E
Morshansk, Russia **60 D5** 53 28N 41 50 E
Morsi, India **94 D4** 21 21N 78 0 E
Mörsil, Sweden **16 A7** 63 19N 13 40 E
Mortagne →, France **27 D13** 48 33N 6 27 E
Mortagne-au-Perche, France **26 D7** 48 31N 0 33 E
Mortagne-sur-Gironde, France **28 C3** 45 28N 0 47W
Mortagne-sur-Sèvre, France **26 F6** 47 0N 0 59W
Mortain, France **26 D6** 48 40N 0 57W
Mortara, Italy **44 C5** 45 15N 8 44 E
Morteau, France **27 E13** 47 3N 6 35 E
Morteros, Argentina **174 C3** 30 50 S 62 0W
Mortes, R. das →, Brazil **171 D1** 11 45 S 50 44W
Mortlach, Canada **143 C7** 50 27N 106 4W
Mortlake, Australia **128 E5** 38 5 S 142 50 E
Morton, Ill., U.S.A. **156 D7** 40 37N 89 28W
Morton, Tex., U.S.A. **155 J3** 33 44N 102 46W
Morton, Wash., U.S.A. **160 D4** 46 34N 122 17W
Morton △, Australia **129 C9** 35 0 S 150 12 E
Moruga, Trin. & Tob. **169 F9** 10 4N 61 16W
Morundah, Australia **129 C7** 34 57 S 146 19 E
Moruya, Australia **129 C9** 35 58 S 150 3 E
Morvan, France **27 E11** 47 5N 4 3 E
Morvan ⌂, France **27 E11** 47 12N 4 3 E
Morven, Australia **127 D4** 26 22 S 147 5 E
Morven, N.Z. **131 E6** 44 50 S 171 6 E
Morven, U.S.A. **152 E6** 30 57N 83 30W
Morvern, U.K. **22 E3** 56 38N 5 44W
Morwell, Australia **129 E7** 38 10 S 146 22 E
Moryń, Poland **55 F1** 52 51N 14 22 E
Morzhovets, Ostrov, Russia **56 A7** 66 44N 42 35 E
Morzine, France **29 C10** 46 11N 6 42 E
Mosalsk, Russia **58 E8** 54 30N 34 55 E
Mosbach, Germany **31 F5** 49 21N 9 9 E
Mosby, Norway **18 F4** 58 12N 7 55 E
Moščenice, Croatia **45 C11** 45 17N 14 16 E
Mosciano Sant' Ángelo, Italy **45 F10** 42 42N 13 52 E
Moscos Is., Burma **86 E1** 14 0N 97 30 E
Moscow = Moskva, Russia **58 E9** 55 45N 37 35 E
Moscow, Idaho, U.S.A. **158 C5** 46 44N 117 0W
Moscow, Mich., U.S.A. **157 B12** 42 3N 84 30W
Moscow, Pa., U.S.A. **151 E9** 41 20N 75 31W
Moscow Mills, U.S.A. **156 F6** 38 57N 90 55W
Mosel →, Europe **27 B14** 50 22N 7 36 E
Moselle = Mosel →, Europe **27 B14** 50 22N 7 36 E
Moselle □, France **27 D13** 48 59N 6 33 E
Moses Lake, U.S.A. **158 C4** 47 8N 119 17W
Mosgiel, N.Z. **131 F5** 45 53 S 170 21 E
Moshaweng →, S. Africa **116 D3** 26 35 S 22 50 E
Moshi, Tanzania **118 C4** 3 22 S 37 18 E
Moshupa, Botswana **116 C4** 24 46 S 25 29 E
Mosina, Poland **55 F3** 52 15N 16 50 E
Mosite, Dem. Rep. of the Congo **114 B4** 0 53N 23 40 E
Mosjøen, Norway **14 D15** 65 51N 13 12 E
Moskenesøya, Norway **14 C15** 67 58N 13 0 E
Moskenstraumen, Norway **14 C15** 67 47N 12 45 E
Moskog, Norway **18 C2** 61 26N 6 0 E
Moskovskiy, Tajikistan **65 E4** 37 37N 69 42 E
Moskovsky = Shakhrikhan, Uzbekistan **65 C6** 40 42N 72 3 E
Moskva, Russia **58 E9** 55 45N 37 35 E
Moskva →, Russia **58 E9** 55 5N 38 51 E
Moslavačka Gora, Croatia **45 C13** 45 40N 16 37 E
Moso, Vanuatu **133 G6** 17 30 S 168 15 E
Mosomane, Botswana **116 C4** 24 2 S 26 19 E
Mosonmagyaróvár, Hungary **52 C2** 47 52N 17 18 E
Mošorin, Serbia & M. **52 E5** 45 19N 20 4 E
Mospino, Ukraine **59 J9** 47 52N 38 0 E
Mosqueiro, Brazil **170 B2** 1 10 S 48 28W
Mosquera, Colombia **168 C2** 2 35N 78 24W
Mosquero, U.S.A. **155 H3** 35 47N 103 58W
Mosqueruela, Spain **40 E4** 40 21N 0 27W
Mosquitia, Honduras **164 C3** 15 20N 84 10W
Mosquito Coast = Mosquitia, Honduras **164 C3** 15 20N 84 10W
Mosquito Creek L., U.S.A. **150 E4** 41 18N 80 46W
Mosquito L., Canada **143 A8** 62 35N 103 20W
Mosquitos, G. de los, Panama **164 E3** 9 15N 81 10W
Moss, Norway **18 E7** 59 27N 10 40 E
Moss Vale, Australia **129 C9** 34 32 S 150 25 E
Mossaka, Congo **114 C3** 1 15 S 16 45 E
Mossâmedes, Brazil **171 E1** 16 7 S 50 11W
Mossbank, Canada **143 D7** 49 56N 105 56W
Mossburn, N.Z. **131 F3** 45 41 S 168 15 E
Mosselbaai, S. Africa **116 E3** 34 11 S 22 8 E
Mossendjo, Congo **114 C2** 2 55 S 12 42 E
Mosses, Col des, Switz. **32 D4** 46 25N 7 7 E
Mossfellsbær, Iceland **11 C5** 64 11N 21 45W
Mossgiel, Australia **128 B6** 33 15 S 144 5 E
Mössingen, Germany **31 G5** 48 24N 9 4 E
Mossman, Australia **126 B4** 16 21 S 145 15 E
Mossoró, Brazil **170 C4** 5 10 S 37 15W
Mossuril, Mozam. **119 E5** 14 58 S 40 42 E
Mossy Head, U.S.A. **153 E3** 30 45N 86 19W
Mossy Point, Australia **129 C9** 35 50 S 150 11 E
Most, Czech Rep. **34 A6** 50 31N 13 38 E
Mosta, Malta **38 F7** 35 55N 14 26 E
Mostaganem, Algeria **111 A5** 35 54N 0 5 E
Mostar, Bos.-H. **52 G2** 43 22N 17 50 E
Mostardas, Brazil **175 C5** 31 2 S 50 51W
Mostefa, Rass, Tunisia **108 A2** 36 55N 11 3 E
Mosteiros, Azores **9 d3** 37 53N 25 49W
Mosterhamn, Norway **18 E2** 59 42N 5 21 E
Mostiska = Mostyska, Ukraine **55 J10** 49 48N 23 4 E
Móstoles, Spain **42 E7** 40 19N 3 53W
Mosty = Masty, Belarus **58 F3** 53 27N 24 38 E
Mostyska, Ukraine **55 J10** 49 48N 23 4 E
Mosul = Al Mawşil, Iraq **101 D10** 36 15N 43 5 E
Mosŭlpo, S. Korea **75 H14** 33 20N 126 17 E
Møsvatnet, Norway **18 E5** 59 52N 8 5 E
Mota, Ethiopia **107 E4** 11 5N 37 52 E
Mota, Vanuatu **133 C5** 13 49 S 167 42 E
Mota del Cuervo, Spain **41 F2** 39 30N 2 52W
Mota del Marqués, Spain **42 D5** 41 38N 5 11W
Mota Lava, Vanuatu **133 C5** 13 40 S 167 40 E
Motaba, Congo **114 B3** 2 6N 18 2 E
Motagua →, Guatemala **164 C2** 15 44N 88 14W
Motala, Sweden **17 F9** 58 32N 15 1 E
Motaze, Mozam. **117 C5** 24 48 S 32 52 E
Moţca, Romania **53 C11** 47 15N 26 37 E
Motegi, Japan **73 A12** 36 32N 140 11 E
Moth, India **93 G8** 25 43N 78 57 E
Motherwell, U.K. **22 F5** 55 47N 3 58W
Motihari, India **93 F11** 26 30N 84 55 E
Motilla del Palancar, Spain **41 F3** 39 34N 1 55W
Motiti I., N.Z. **130 D5** 37 38 S 176 25 E
Motnik, Slovenia **45 B11** 46 14N 14 54 E
Motocurunya, Venezuela **169 C5** 4 24N 64 5W
Motovun, Croatia **45 C10** 45 20N 13 50 E
Motozintla de Mendoza, Mexico **163 D6** 15 21N 92 14W
Motril, Spain **43 J7** 36 31N 3 37W
Motru, Romania **52 F7** 44 48N 22 59 E
Motru →, Romania **53 F8** 44 32N 23 31 E
Mott, U.S.A. **154 B3** 46 23N 102 20W
Möttling = Metlika, Slovenia **45 C12** 45 40N 15 20 E
Mòttola, Italy **47 B10** 40 38N 17 2 E
Motu →, N.Z. **130 D6** 37 51 S 177 35 E
Motu Nui, Chile **172 b** 27 12 S 109 28W
Motuba, Dem. Rep. of the Congo **114 B3** 2 20N 18 34 E
Motueka, N.Z. **131 B8** 41 7 S 173 1 E
Motueka →, N.Z. **131 B8** 41 5 S 173 1 E
Motul, Mexico **163 C7** 21 0N 89 20W
Motupena Pt., Papua N. G. **132 D8** 6 30 S 155 10 E
Mou, N. Cal. **133 U19** 21 5 S 165 26 E
Mouanda, Gabon **114 C2** 1 28 S 13 7 E
Mouchalagane →, Canada **141 B6** 50 56N 68 41W
Moúdhros, Greece **49 B7** 39 50N 25 18 E
Mouding, China **76 E3** 25 20N 101 28 E
Moudjeria, Mauritania **112 B2** 17 50N 12 28W
Moudon, Switz. **32 C3** 46 40N 6 49 E
Moudros = Moúdhros, Greece **49 B7** 39 50N 25 18 E
Mougoundou, Congo **114 C2** 2 40 S 12 41 E
Mouila, Gabon **114 C2** 1 50 S 11 0 E
Mouka, C.A.R. **114 A4** 7 16N 21 52 E
Moukalaba ⌂, Gabon **114 C2** 2 50 S 10 35 E
Moukambo, Gabon **114 C2** 3 5 S 11 38 E
Moul, Niger **109 F2** 15 5N 13 11 E
Moulamein, Australia **128 C6** 35 3 S 144 1 E
Moule à Chique, C., St. Lucia **165 f** 13 43N 60 57W
Moulianá, Greece **39 E6** 35 10N 25 59 E
Moulins, France **27 F10** 46 35N 3 19 E
Moulmein, Burma **90 G6** 16 30N 97 40 E
Moulmeingyun, Burma **90 G5** 16 23N 95 16 E
Moulouya, O. →, Morocco **111 A4** 35 5N 2 25W
Moulton, U.S.A. **156 D4** 40 41N 92 41W
Moultrie, U.S.A. **152 D6** 31 11N 83 47W
Moultrie, L., U.S.A. **152 B9** 33 20N 80 5W
Mouly, N. Cal. **133 K4** 20 47 S 166 26 E
Mounana, Gabon **114 C2** 1 18 S 13 13 E
Mound City, Mo., U.S.A. **154 E7** 40 7N 95 14W
Mound City, S. Dak., U.S.A. **154 C4** 45 44N 100 4W
Moúnda, Ákra, Greece **39 C2** 38 3N 20 47 E
Moundou, Chad **109 G3** 8 40N 16 10 E
Moundsville, U.S.A. **150 G4** 39 55N 80 44W
Mounembé, Congo **114 C2** 3 20 S 12 32 E
Moung, Cambodia **86 F4** 12 46N 103 27 E
Moungoudi, Congo **114 C2** 2 45 S 11 46 E
Mount Airy, U.S.A. **149 G5** 36 31N 80 37W
Mount Albert, Canada **150 B5** 44 8N 79 19W
Mount Apo △, Phil. **81 H5** 7 0N 125 10 E
Mount Aspiring △, N.Z. **131 E3** 44 19 S 168 47 E
Mount Ayliff = Maxesibeni, S. Africa **117 E4** 30 49 S 29 23 E
Mount Ayr, U.S.A. **156 D2** 40 43N 94 14W
Mount Barker, S. Austral., Australia **128 C3** 35 5 S 138 52 E
Mount Barker, W. Austral., Australia **125 F2** 34 38 S 117 40 E
Mount Beauty, Australia **129 D7** 36 47 S 147 10 E
Mount Brydges, Canada **150 D3** 42 54N 81 29W
Mount Buffalo △, Australia **129 D7** 36 43 S 146 46 E
Mount Burr, Australia **127 F3** 37 34 S 140 26 E
Mount Carmel = Ha Karmel △, Israel **103 C4** 32 45N 35 5 E
Mount Carmel, Ill., U.S.A. **157 F9** 38 25N 87 46W
Mount Carmel, Pa., U.S.A. **151 F8** 40 47N 76 24W
Mount Carroll, U.S.A. **156 B7** 42 6N 89 59W
Mount Charleston, U.S.A. **161 J11** 36 16N 115 37W
Mount Clemens, U.S.A. **150 D2** 42 35N 82 53W
Mount Cook, N.Z. **131 D5** 43 44 S 170 5 E
Mount Cook △, N.Z. **131 D5** 43 35 S 170 15 E
Mount Coolon, Australia **126 C4** 21 25 S 147 25 E
Mount Darwin, Zimbabwe **119 F3** 16 47 S 31 38 E
Mount Desert I., U.S.A. **149 C11** 44 21N 68 20W
Mount Dora, U.S.A. **153 G8** 28 48N 81 38W
Mount Eccles △, Australia **128 E4** 38 5 S 141 54 E
Mount Eden, U.S.A. **157 F11** 38 3N 85 9W
Mount Edgecumbe, U.S.A. **144 H14** 57 3N 135 21W
Mount Edziza ⌂, Canada **142 B2** 57 30N 130 45W
Mount Elgon △, E. Afr. **118 B3** 1 4N 34 42 E
Mount Field △, Australia **127 G4** 42 39 S 146 35 E
Mount Fletcher, S. Africa **117 E4** 30 40 S 28 30 E
Mount Forest, Canada **140 D3** 43 59N 80 43W
Mount Frere = Kwabhaca, S. Africa **117 E4** 30 51 S 29 0 E
Mount Gambier, Australia **128 D4** 37 50 S 140 46 E
Mount Garnet, Australia **126 B4** 17 37 S 145 6 E
Mount Hagen, Papua N. G. **132 C3** 5 52 S 144 16 E
Mount Holly, U.S.A. **151 G10** 39 59N 74 47W
Mount Holly Springs, U.S.A. **150 F7** 40 7N 77 12W
Mount Hope, N.S.W., Australia **129 B6** 32 51 S 145 51 E
Mount Hope, S. Austral., Australia **127 E2** 34 7 S 135 23 E
Mount Horeb, U.S.A. **156 B7** 43 1N 89 44W
Mount Isa, Australia **126 C2** 20 42 S 139 26 E
Mount Isarog △, Phil. **80 E4** 13 38N 123 24 E
Mount Jewett, U.S.A. **150 E6** 41 44N 78 39W
Mount Kaputar △, Australia **127 E5** 30 16 S 150 10 E
Mount Kenya △, Kenya **118 C4** 0 7 S 37 21 E
Mount Kilimanjaro △, Tanzania **118 C4** 3 2 S 37 19 E
Mount Kisco, U.S.A. **151 E11** 41 12N 73 44W
Mount Laguna, U.S.A. **161 N10** 32 52N 116 25W
Mount Larcom, Australia **126 C5** 23 48 S 150 59 E
Mount Lofty Ra., Australia **128 C3** 34 35 S 139 5 E
Mount McKinley = Denali △, U.S.A. **144 E10** 63 30N 152 0W
Mount Magnet, Australia **125 E2** 28 2 S 117 47 E
Mount Malindang △, Phil. **81 G4** 8 17N 123 32 E
Mount Manara, Australia **128 B5** 32 29 S 143 58 E
Mount Maunganui, N.Z. **130 D5** 37 40 S 176 14 E
Mount Molloy, Australia **126 B4** 16 42 S 145 20 E
Mount Morgan, Australia **126 C5** 23 40 S 150 25 E
Mount Morris, Mich., U.S.A. **157 A13** 43 7N 83 42W
Mount Morris, N.Y., U.S.A. **150 D7** 42 44N 77 52W
Mount Olive, U.S.A. **156 E7** 39 4N 89 44W
Mount Olivet, U.S.A. **157 F12** 38 32N 84 2W
Mount Orab, U.S.A. **157 E13** 39 2N 83 55W
Mount Pearl, Canada **141 C9** 47 31N 52 47W
Mount Penn, U.S.A. **151 F9** 40 20N 75 54W
Mount Perry, Australia **127 D5** 25 13 S 151 42 E
Mount Pleasant, Iowa, U.S.A. **156 D5** 40 58N 91 33W
Mount Pleasant, Mich., U.S.A. **148 D3** 43 36N 84 46W
Mount Pleasant, Pa., U.S.A. **150 F5** 40 9N 79 33W
Mount Pleasant, S.C., U.S.A. **152 C10** 32 47N 79 52W
Mount Pleasant, Tenn., U.S.A. **149 H2** 35 32N 87 12W
Mount Pleasant, Tex., U.S.A. **155 J7** 33 9N 94 58W
Mount Pleasant, Utah, U.S.A. **158 G8** 39 33N 111 27W
Mount Pocono, U.S.A. **151 E9** 41 7N 75 22W
Mount Pulaski, U.S.A. **156 D7** 40 1N 89 17W
Mount Pulog △, Phil. **80 C3** 16 35N 120 57 E
Mount Rainier △, U.S.A. **160 D5** 46 55N 121 50W
Mount Remarkable △, Australia **128 B3** 32 47 S 138 3 E
Mount Revelstoke △, Canada **142 C5** 51 5N 118 30W
Mount Robson ⌂, Canada **142 C5** 53 0N 119 0W
Mount St. Helens ⌂, U.S.A. **160 D4** 46 14N 122 11W
Mount Selinda, Zimbabwe **117 C5** 20 24 S 32 43 E
Mount Shasta, U.S.A. **158 F2** 41 19N 122 19W
Mount Signal, U.S.A. **161 N11** 32 39N 115 37W
Mount Somers, N.Z. **131 D6** 43 45 S 171 27 E
Mount Sterling, Ill., U.S.A. **156 E6** 39 59N 90 45W
Mount Sterling, Ky., U.S.A. **157 F13** 38 4N 83 56W
Mount Sterling, Ohio, U.S.A. **157 E13** 39 43N 83 16W
Mount Surprise, Australia **126 B3** 18 10 S 144 17 E
Mount Union, U.S.A. **150 F7** 40 23N 77 53W
Mount Upton, U.S.A. **151 D9** 42 26N 75 23W
Mount Vernon, Ga., U.S.A. **152 C7** 32 11N 82 36W
Mount Vernon, Ill., U.S.A. **148 F1** 38 19N 88 55W
Mount Vernon, Ind., U.S.A. **154 F10** 38 17N 88 57W
Mount Vernon, Ind., U.S.A. **157 G9** 37 56N 87 54W
Mount Vernon, Iowa, U.S.A. **156 C5** 41 55N 91 23W
Mount Vernon, N.Y., U.S.A. **151 F11** 40 55N 73 50W
Mount Vernon, Ohio, U.S.A. **150 F2** 40 23N 82 29W
Mount Vernon, Wash., U.S.A. **160 B4** 48 25N 122 20W
Mount Victor, Australia **128 B3** 32 11 S 139 44 E
Mount Washington, U.S.A. **157 F11** 38 3N 85 33W
Mount Wellington, N.Z. **130 C3** 36 55 S 174 52 E
Mount William △, Australia **127 G4** 40 56 S 148 14 E
Mount Zion, U.S.A. **157 E8** 39 46N 88 53W
Mountain □, Phil. **80 C3** 17 20N 121 10 E
Mountain Ash, U.K. **21 F4** 51 40N 3 23W
Mountain Center, U.S.A. **161 M10** 33 42N 116 44W
Mountain City, Nev., U.S.A. **158 F6** 41 50N 115 58W
Mountain City, Tenn., U.S.A. **149 G5** 36 29N 81 48W
Mountain Dale, U.S.A. **151 E10** 41 41N 74 32W
Mountain Grove, U.S.A. **155 G8** 37 8N 92 16W
Mountain Home, Ark., U.S.A. **155 G8** 36 20N 92 23W
Mountain Home, Idaho, U.S.A. **158 E6** 43 8N 115 41W
Mountain Iron, U.S.A. **154 B8** 47 32N 92 37W
Mountain Pass, U.S.A. **161 K11** 35 29N 115 35W
Mountain View, Ark., U.S.A. **155 H8** 35 52N 92 7W
Mountain View, Calif., U.S.A. **160 H4** 37 23N 122 5W
Mountain View, Hawaii, U.S.A. **145 D6** 19 33N 155 7W
Mountain Village, U.S.A. **144 E7** 62 5N 163 43W
Mountain Zebra △, S. Africa **116 E4** 32 14 S 25 27 E
Mountainair, U.S.A. **159 J10** 34 31N 106 15W
Mountlake Terrace, U.S.A. **160 C4** 47 47N 122 19W
Mountmellick, Ireland **23 C4** 53 7N 7 20W
Mountrath, Ireland **23 D4** 53 0N 7 28W
Moura, Australia **126 C4** 24 35 S 149 58 E
Moura, Brazil **169 D5** 1 32 S 61 38W
Moura, Portugal **43 G3** 38 7N 7 30W
Mourão, Portugal **43 G3** 38 22N 7 22W
Mourdi, Dépression du, Chad **109 E4** 18 10N 23 0 E
Mourdiah, Mali **112 C3** 14 35N 7 25W
Mourenx, France **28 E3** 43 22N 0 38W
Mouri, Ghana **113 D4** 5 6N 1 14W
Mourilyan, Australia **126 B4** 17 35 S 146 3 E
Mourmelon-le-Grand, France **27 C11** 49 8N 4 22 E
Mourne →, U.K. **23 B4** 54 52N 7 26W
Mourne Mts., U.K. **23 B5** 54 10N 6 0W
Mourniaí, Greece **39 E5** 35 29N 24 1 E
Mournies = Mourniaí, Greece **39 E5** 35 29N 24 1 E
Mouscron, Belgium **24 D3** 50 45N 3 12 E
Mousgougou, Chad **109 F3** 10 47N 16 9 E
Moussoro, Chad **109 F3** 13 41N 16 35 E
Mouthe, France **27 F13** 46 44N 6 12 E
Moutier, Switz. **32 B4** 47 16N 7 21 E
Moûtiers, France **29 C10** 45 29N 6 32 E
Moutohara, N.Z. **130 E6** 38 27 S 177 32 E
Moutong, Indonesia **82 A2** 0 28N 121 13 E
Mouy, France **27 C9** 49 18N 2 20 E
Mouyondzi, Congo **114 C2** 4 1 S 13 59 E
Mouzáki, Greece **48 B3** 39 25N 21 37 E
Mouzon, France **27 C12** 49 36N 5 5 E
Movas, Mexico **162 B3** 28 10N 109 25W
Moville, Ireland **23 A4** 55 11N 7 3W
Mowandjum, Australia **124 C3** 17 22 S 123 40 E
Moweaqua, U.S.A. **156 E7** 39 38N 89 1W
Moxico □, Angola **115 E4** 12 0 S 20 30 E
Moxotó →, Brazil **170 C4** 9 19 S 38 14W
Moy →, Ireland **23 B2** 54 8N 9 8W
Moya, Comoros Is. **121 a** 12 18 S 44 18 E
Moyale, Kenya **107 G4** 3 30N 39 0 E
Moyamba, S. Leone **112 D2** 8 4N 12 30W
Moyen Atlas, Morocco **110 B4** 33 0N 5 0W
Moyne, L. le, Canada **141 A6** 56 45N 68 47W
Moyo, Indonesia **85 D5** 8 10 S 117 40 E
Moyobamba, Peru **172 B2** 6 0 S 77 0W
Moyto, Chad **109 F3** 12 35N 16 33 E
Moyyero →, Russia **67 C11** 68 44N 103 42 E
Moyynqum, Kazakhstan **65 A6** 44 17N 72 57 E
Moyynty, Kazakhstan **66 E8** 47 10N 73 18 E
Mozambique = Moçambique, Mozam. **119 F5** 15 3 S 40 42 E
Mozambique ■, Africa **119 F4** 19 0 S 35 0 E
Mozambique Chan., Africa **117 B7** 17 30 S 42 30 E
Mozambique Ridge, Ind. Oc. **121 H2** 32 0 S 36 0 E
Mozdok, Russia **61 J7** 43 45N 44 48 E
Mozdūrān, Iran **97 B9** 36 9N 60 35 E
Mozhaysk, Russia **58 E9** 55 30N 36 2 E
Mozhga, Russia **60 B11** 56 26N 52 15 E
Mozhnābād, Iran **97 C9** 34 7N 60 6 E
Mozirje, Slovenia **45 B11** 46 22N 14 58 E
Mozyr = Mazyr, Belarus **59 F5** 51 59N 29 15 E
Mpanda, Tanzania **118 D3** 6 23 S 31 1 E
Mpé, Congo **114 C2** 2 58 S 14 38 E
Mpese, Dem. Rep. of the Congo **115 D3** 5 16 S 15 30 E
Mpésoba, Mali **112 C3** 12 31N 5 39W
Mphoengs, Zimbabwe **117 C4** 21 10 S 27 51 E
Mpika, Zambia **119 E3** 11 51 S 31 25 E
Mpoko →, C.A.R. **114 B3** 4 19N 18 33 E
Mpouya, Congo **114 C3** 2 38 S 16 13 E
Mpulungu, Zambia **119 D3** 8 51 S 31 5 E
Mpumalanga, S. Africa **117 D5** 29 50 S 30 33 E
Mpumalanga □, S. Africa **117 D5** 26 0 S 30 0 E
Mpwapwa, Tanzania **118 D4** 6 23 S 36 30 E
Mqabba, Malta **38 F7** 35 51N 14 28 E
Mqanduli, S. Africa **117 E4** 31 49 S 28 45 E
Mqinvartsveri = Kazbek, Russia **61 J7** 42 42N 44 30 E
Mrągowo, Poland **54 E8** 53 52N 21 18 E
Mramor, Serbia & M. **50 C5** 43 20N 21 45 E
Mrimina, Morocco **110 C3** 29 50N 7 9W
Mrkonjić Grad, Bos.-H. **52 F2** 44 26N 17 4 E
Mrkopalj, Croatia **45 C11** 45 21N 14 52 E
Mrocza, Poland **55 E4** 53 16N 17 35 E
Msaken, Tunisia **108 A2** 35 49N 10 33 E
Msambansovu, Zimbabwe **119 F3** 15 50 S 30 3 E
Msida, Malta **38 F7** 35 54N 14 29 E
M'sila, Algeria **111 A5** 35 46N 4 30 E
Msoro, Zambia **119 E3** 13 35 S 31 50 E
Msta →, Russia **58 C6** 58 25N 31 20 E
Mstislavl = Mstsislaw, Belarus **58 E6** 54 0N 31 50 E
Mstsislaw, Belarus **58 E6** 54 0N 31 50 E
Mszana Dolna, Poland **55 J7** 49 41N 20 5 E
Mszczonów, Poland **55 G7** 51 58N 20 33 E
Mtama, Tanzania **119 E4** 10 17 S 39 21 E
Mtamvuna →, S. Africa **117 E5** 31 6 S 30 12 E
Mtilikwe →, Zimbabwe **119 G3** 21 9 S 31 30 E
Mtima, Congo **114 C2** 3 49 S 12 7 E
Mtsensk, Russia **58 F9** 53 17N 36 36 E
Mtskheta, Georgia **61 K7** 41 52N 44 45 E
Mtubatuba, S. Africa **117 D5** 28 30 S 32 8 E
Mtwalume, S. Africa **117 E5** 30 30 S 30 38 E
Mtwara-Mikindani, Tanzania **119 E5** 10 20 S 40 20 E
Mu →, Burma **90 E5** 21 56N 95 38 E
Mu Gia, Deo, Vietnam **86 D5** 17 40N 105 47 E
Mu Ko Chang △, Thailand **87 G4** 11 59N 102 22 E
Mu Us Shamo, China **74 E5** 39 0N 109 0 E
Muacandala, Angola **115 E3** 10 2 S 19 40 E
Muaná, Brazil **170 B2** 1 25 S 49 15W
Muanda, Dem. Rep. of the Congo **115 D2** 6 0 S 12 20 E
Muang Chiang Rai = Chiang Rai, Thailand **76 H2** 19 52N 99 50 E
Muang Khong, Laos **86 E5** 14 7N 105 51 E
Muang Lamphun, Thailand **86 C2** 18 40N 99 2 E
Muang Mai, Thailand **87 a** 8 5N 98 21 E
Muang Pak Beng, Laos **76 H3** 19 54N 101 8 E
Muangai, Angola **115 E3** 12 32 S 19 55 E
Muar, Malaysia **87 L4** 2 3N 102 34 E
Muarabungo, Indonesia **84 C2** 1 28 S 102 52 E
Muaraenim, Indonesia **84 C2** 3 40 S 103 50 E
Muarajuloi, Indonesia **85 C4** 0 12 S 114 3 E
Muarakaman, Indonesia **85 C5** 0 2 S 116 45 E
Muaratebo, Indonesia **84 C2** 1 30 S 102 26 E
Muaratembesi, Indonesia **84 C2** 1 42 S 103 8 E
Muaratewe, Indonesia **85 C4** 0 58 S 114 52 E
Mubarakpur, India **93 F10** 26 6N 83 18 E
Mubarek, Uzbekistan **65 D2** 39 15N 65 9 E
Mubarraz = Al Mubarraz, Si. Arabia **97 E6** 25 30N 49 40 E
Mubende, Uganda **118 B3** 0 33N 31 22 E
Mubi, Nigeria **113 C7** 10 18N 13 16 E
Mucajá, Brazil **169 D6** 3 57 S 57 32W
Mucajaí →, Brazil **169 C5** 2 25N 60 52W
Mucajaí, Serra do, Brazil **169 C5** 2 23N 61 10W
Mucari, Angola **115 D3** 9 30 S 16 54 E
Muchachos, Roque de los, Canary Is. **9 e1** 28 44N 17 52W
Mücheln, Germany **30 D7** 51 17N 11 47 E
Muchinga Mts., Zambia **119 E3** 11 30 S 31 30 E
Muchkapskiy, Russia **60 E6** 51 52N 42 28 E
Muchuan, China **76 C5** 28 57N 103 55 E
Muck, U.K. **22 E2** 56 50N 6 15W
Muckadilla, Australia **127 D4** 26 35 S 148 23 E
Muckalee Cr. →, U.S.A. **152 D5** 31 38N 84 9W
Muckle Flugga, U.K. **22 A8** 60 51N 0 54W
Muco →, Colombia **168 C3** 4 15N 70 21W
Mucoma, Angola **115 F2** 15 18 S 13 39 E
Muconda, Angola **115 E4** 10 31 S 21 15 E
Mucope, Angola **115 F2** 16 24 S 14 52 E
Mucugê, Brazil **171 D3** 13 0 S 41 23W
Mucuim →, Brazil **173 B5** 6 33 S 64 18W
Mucur, Turkey **100 C6** 39 3N 34 22 E
Mucura, Brazil **169 D5** 2 31 S 62 43W
Mucuri, Brazil **171 E4** 18 0 S 39 36W
Mucurici, Brazil **171 E3** 18 6 S 40 31W
Mucusso, Angola **116 B3** 18 1 S 21 25 E
Mucusso ⌂, Angola **115 F4** 17 27 S 21 0 E
Muda, Canary Is. **9 e2** 28 34N 13 57W
Mudanjiang, China **75 B15** 44 38N 129 30 E
Mudanya, Turkey **51 F12** 40 25N 28 50 E
Muddebihal, India **95 F3** 16 20N 76 8 E
Muddy Cr. →, U.S.A. **159 H8** 38 24N 110 42W
Mudgee, Australia **129 B8** 32 32 S 149 31 E
Mudhol, Andhra Pradesh, India **94 E3** 18 58N 77 55 E
Mudhol, Karnataka, India **95 F2** 16 21N 75 17 E
Mudiata, Dem. Rep. of the Congo **115 D4** 7 15 S 22 1 E
Mudigere, India **95 H2** 13 8N 75 38 E
Mudjatik →, Canada **143 B7** 56 1N 107 36W
Mudon, Burma **90 G6** 16 15N 97 44 E
Mudugh, Somali Rep. **120 C3** 7 0N 47 30 E
Mudukulattur, India **95 K4** 9 21N 78 31 E
Mudurnu, Turkey **100 B4** 40 27N 31 12 E
Muecate, Mozam. **119 E4** 14 55 S 39 40 E
Mueda, Mozam. **119 E4** 11 36 S 39 28 E
Mueller Ra., Australia **124 C4** 18 18 S 126 46 E
Muende, Mozam. **119 E3** 14 28 S 33 0 E
Muerto, Mar, Mexico **163 D6** 16 10N 94 10W
Mufu Shan, China **77 C10** 29 20N 114 30 E
Mufulira, Zambia **119 E2** 12 32 S 28 15 E
Mufuma, Angola **115 D3** 9 12 S 16 29 E
Mufumbiro Range, Africa **118 C2** 1 25 S 29 30 E
Mugardos, Spain **42 B2** 43 27N 8 15W
Muge →, Portugal **43 F2** 39 8N 8 44W
Múggia, Italy **45 C10** 45 36N 13 46 E
Mughal Sarai, India **93 G10** 25 18N 83 7 E
Mughayrā', Si. Arabia **96 D3** 29 17N 37 41 E
Mugi, Japan **72 D6** 33 40N 134 25 E
Mugia = Muxía, Spain **42 B1** 43 3N 9 10W
Mugila, Mts., Dem. Rep. of the Congo **118 D2** 7 0 S 28 50 E
Muginga, Angola **115 D3** 8 21 S 17 36 E
Muğla, Turkey **49 D10** 37 15N 28 22 E
Muğla □, Turkey **49 D10** 37 15N 28 0 E
Muglad, Sudan **107 E2** 11 1N 27 50 E
Müglizh, Bulgaria **51 D9** 42 37N 25 32 E
Mugodzhary, Kazakhstan **64 G7** 49 0N 58 40 E
Mugu, Nepal **93 E10** 29 45N 82 30 E
Muhammad, Râs, Egypt **96 E2** 27 44N 34 16 E
Muhammad Qol, Sudan **106 C4** 20 53N 37 9 E
Muhammadabad, India **93 F10** 26 4N 83 25 E
Muḩayriqah, Si. Arabia **98 B4** 23 59N 45 4 E
Muhesi →, Tanzania **118 D4** 7 0 S 35 20 E
Mühlacker, Germany **31 G4** 48 57N 8 51 E
Mühldorf, Germany **31 G8** 48 14N 12 32 E
Mühlhausen = Milevsko, Czech Rep. **34 B7** 49 27N 14 21 E
Mühlhausen, Germany **30 D6** 51 12N 10 27 E
Mühlig Hofmann fjell, Antarctica **7 D3** 72 30 S 5 0 E
Mühlviertel, Austria **34 C7** 48 30N 14 10 E
Muhos, Finland **14 D22** 64 47N 25 59 E
Muhu, Estonia **15 G20** 58 36N 23 11 E
Muhutwe, Tanzania **118 C3** 1 35 S 31 45 E
Mui Wo, China **69 G10** 22 16N 113 59 E
Muie, Angola **115 E4** 14 23 S 20 25 E
Muine Bheag, Ireland **23 D5** 52 42N 6 58W
Muir, L., Australia **125 F2** 34 30 S 116 40 E
Muir of Ord, U.K. **22 D4** 57 32N 4 28W
Muisné, Ecuador **168 C1** 0 36N 80 2W
Mujnak = Muynak, Uzbekistan **66 E6** 43 44N 59 10 E
Mujuí dos Campos, Brazil **169 D7** 2 35 S 54 41W
Muka, Tanjung, Malaysia **87 c** 5 28N 100 11 E
Mukacheve, Ukraine **52 B7** 48 27N 22 45 E
Mukachevo = Mukacheve, Ukraine **52 B7** 48 27N 22 45 E
Mukah, Malaysia **85 B4** 2 55N 112 5 E
Mukandwara, India **92 G6** 24 49N 75 59 E
Mukawa, Papua N. G. **132 E5** 9 38 S 149 59 E
Mukawwa, Geziret, Egypt **106 C4** 23 55N 35 53 E
Mukawwar, Sudan **106 C4** 20 50N 37 17 E
Mukdahan, Thailand **86 D5** 16 32N 104 43 E
Mukden = Shenyang, China **75 D12** 41 48N 123 27 E
Mukerian, India **92 D6** 31 57N 75 37 E
Mukhavyets, Belarus **55 F10** 52 5N 23 39 E
Mukher, India **94 E3** 18 42N 77 22 E
Mukhtolovo, Russia **60 C6** 55 29N 43 15 E
Mukhtuya = Lensk, Russia **67 C12** 60 48N 114 55 E
Mukinbudin, Australia **125 F2** 30 55 S 118 5 E
Mukishi, Kasai-Occ., Dem. Rep. of the Congo **115 D4** 5 39 S 21 3 E
Mukishi, Katanga, Dem. Rep. of the Congo **119 D1** 8 30 S 24 44 E
Mukomuko, Indonesia **84 C2** 2 30 S 101 10 E
Mukomwenze, Dem. Rep. of the Congo **118 D2** 6 49 S 27 15 E
Mukry, Turkmenistan **65 E2** 37 54N 65 12 E
Muktsar, India **92 D6** 30 30N 74 30 E
Mukur = Moqor, Afghan. **91 B2** 32 50N 67 42 E
Mukutawa →, Canada **143 C9** 53 10N 97 24W
Mukwela, Zambia **119 F2** 17 0 S 26 40 E
Mukwonago, U.S.A. **157 B8** 42 52N 88 20W

Mul, *India* **94 D4** 20 4N 79 40 E
Mula, *Spain* **41 G3** 38 3N 1 33W
Mula →, *India* **94 E2** 18 34N 74 21 E
Mula →, *Pakistan* **92 F2** 27 57N 67 36 E
Mulamba, *Dem. Rep. of the Congo* **115 D4** 6 21 S 21 13 E
Mulanay, *Phil.* **80 E4** 13 31N 122 24 E
Mulange, *Dem. Rep. of the Congo* **118 C2** 3 40 S 27 10 E
Mulanje, *Malawi* **119 F4** 16 2 S 35 33 E
Mulanje, Mt., *Malawi* **119 F4** 16 0 S 35 30 E
Mulatupo, *Panama* **168 B2** 8 57N 77 45W
Mulbagal, *India* **95 H4** 13 10N 78 24 E
Mulberry, *U.S.A.* **153 H8** 27 54N 81 59W
Mulberry Grove, *U.S.A.* **156 F7** 38 56N 89 16W
Mulchatna →, *U.S.A.* **144 G8** 59 40N 157 7W
Mulchén, *Chile* **174 D1** 37 45 S 72 20W
Mulde →, *Germany* **30 D8** 51 53N 12 15 E
Muldraugh, *U.S.A.* **157 G11** 37 56N 85 59W
Mule Creek Junction, *U.S.A.* **154 D2** 43 19N 104 8W
Muleba, *Tanzania* **118 C3** 1 50 S 31 37 E
Mulegns, *Switz.* **33 C9** 46 32N 9 38 E
Mulejé, *Mexico* **162 B2** 26 53N 112 1W
Muleshoe, *U.S.A.* **155 H3** 34 13N 102 43W
Muletta, Gara, *Ethiopia* **107 F5** 9 15N 41 44 E
Mulgrave, *Canada* **141 C7** 45 38N 61 31W
Mulgrave I. = Badu I., *Papua N. G.* **132 F2** 10 5 S 142 10 E
Mulhacén, *Spain* **43 H7** 37 4N 3 20W
Mülheim, *Germany* **30 D2** 51 25N 6 54 E
Mulhouse, *France* **27 E14** 47 40N 7 20 E
Muli, *China* **76 D3** 27 52N 101 8 E
Muli →, *Indonesia* **83 C5** 7 16 S 138 45 E
Mulifanua, *Samoa* **133 W24** 13 50 S 171 59W
Muling, *China* **75 B16** 44 35N 130 10 E
Mulki, *India* **95 H2** 13 6N 74 48 E
Mull, *U.K.* **22 E3** 56 25N 5 56W
Mull, Sound of, *U.K.* **22 E3** 56 30N 5 50W
Mullaittivu, *Sri Lanka* **95 K5** 9 15N 80 49 E
Mullen, *U.S.A.* **154 D4** 42 3N 101 1W
Mullens, *U.S.A.* **148 G5** 37 35N 81 23W
Muller, Pegunungan, *Indonesia* **85 B4** 0 30N 113 30 E
Muller Ra., *Papua N. G.* **132 C2** 5 35 S 142 20 E
Mullet Pen., *Ireland* **23 B1** 54 13N 10 2W
Mullewa, *Australia* **125 E2** 28 29 S 115 30 E
Müllheim, *Germany* **31 H3** 47 47N 7 36 E
Mulligan →, *Australia* **126 D2** 25 0 S 139 0 E
Mullingar, *Ireland* **23 C4** 53 31N 7 21W
Mullins, *U.S.A.* **149 H6** 34 12N 79 15W
Mullsjö, *Sweden* **17 G7** 57 56N 13 55 E
Mullumbimby, *Australia* **127 D5** 28 30 S 153 30 E
Mulobezi, *Zambia* **119 F2** 16 45 S 25 7 E
Mulondo, *Angola* **115 F3** 15 41 S 15 12 E
Mulonga Plain, *Zambia* **115 F4** 16 20 S 22 40 E
Mulroy B., *Ireland* **23 A4** 55 15N 7 46W
Mulshi L., *India* **94 E1** 18 30N 73 48 E
Multai, *India* **94 D4** 21 50N 78 21 E
Multan, *Pakistan* **91 C3** 30 15N 71 36 E
Mulu, Gunung, *Malaysia* **85 B4** 4 3N 114 56 E
Mulug, *India* **94 E4** 18 11N 79 57 E
Mulumbe, Mts., *Dem. Rep. of the Congo* **119 D2** 8 40 S 27 30 E
Mulundu, *Dem. Rep. of the Congo* **115 D4** 6 40 S 20 33 E
Mulungushi Dam, *Zambia* **119 E2** 14 48 S 28 48 E
Mulurulu L., *Australia* **128 B5** 33 15 S 143 20 E
Mulvane, *U.S.A.* **155 G6** 37 29N 97 15W
Mulwad, *Sudan* **106 D3** 18 45N 30 39 E
Mulwala, *Australia* **129 C7** 35 59 S 146 0 E
Muma, *Dem. Rep. of the Congo* **114 B4** 3 25N 23 21 E
Mumbai, *India* **94 E1** 18 55N 72 50 E
Mumbeji, *Zambia* **115 E4** 13 51 S 23 39 E
Mumbondo, *Angola* **115 E2** 10 9 S 14 15 E
Mumbwa, *Zambia* **119 F2** 15 0 S 27 0 E
Mumeng, *Papua N. G.* **132 D4** 7 1 S 146 37 E
Muminabad = Leningradskiy, *Tajikistan* **65 D5** 38 6N 70 1 E
Mumra, *Russia* **61 H8** 45 45N 47 41 E
Mun →, *Thailand* **86 E5** 15 19N 105 30 E
Muna, *Indonesia* **82 B2** 5 0 S 122 30 E
Munabao, *India* **92 G4** 25 45N 70 17 E
Munakata, *Japan* **72 D2** 33 48N 130 38 E
Munamagi, *Estonia* **15 H22** 57 43N 27 4 E
Muncan, *Indonesia* **79 K18** 8 34 S 115 11 E
Muncar, *Indonesia* **79 J17** 8 26 S 114 20 E
Münchberg, *Germany* **31 E7** 50 11N 11 47 E
Müncheberg, *Germany* **30 C10** 52 30N 14 9 E
München, *Germany* **31 G7** 48 8N 11 34 E
Munchen-Gladbach = Mönchengladbach, *Germany* **30 D2** 51 11N 6 27 E
München International ✈ (MUC), *Germany* **31 G7** 48 20N 11 50 E
Münchenbuchsee, *Switz.* **32 B4** 47 1N 7 27 E
Munchique △, *Colombia* **168 C2** 2 44N 77 1W
Muncho Lake, *Canada* **142 B3** 59 0N 125 50W
Munch'ŏn, *N. Korea* **75 E14** 39 14N 127 19 E
Münchwilen, *Switz.* **33 B7** 47 28N 8 59 E
Muncie, *U.S.A.* **157 D11** 40 12N 85 23W
Muncoonie, L., *Australia* **126 D2** 25 12 S 138 40 E
Munda, *Solomon Is.* **133 M9** 8 20 S 157 16 E
Mundabbera, *Australia* **127 D5** 25 36 S 151 18 E
Mundakayam, *India* **95 K3** 9 30N 76 50 E
Mundal, *Sri Lanka* **95 L4** 7 48N 79 48 E
Munday, *U.S.A.* **155 J5** 33 27N 99 38W
Mundelein, *U.S.A.* **157 B8** 42 16N 88 0W
Münden, *Germany* **30 D5** 51 25N 9 38 E
Münden ⌓, *Germany* **30 D5** 51 28N 9 42 E
Mundiwindi, *Australia* **124 D3** 23 47 S 120 9 E
Mundo →, *Spain* **41 G2** 38 30N 2 15W
Mundo Novo, *Brazil* **171 D3** 11 50 S 40 29W
Mundra, *India* **92 H3** 22 54N 69 48 E
Mundrabilla, *Australia* **125 F4** 31 52 S 127 51 E
Munducurus, *Brazil* **169 D6** 4 47 S 58 16W
Munenga, *Angola* **115 E2** 10 2 S 14 41 E
Munera, *Spain* **41 F2** 39 2N 2 29W
Muneru →, *India* **94 F5** 16 45N 80 3 E
Mungallala, *Australia* **127 D4** 26 28 S 147 34 E
Mungallala Cr. →, *Australia* **127 D4** 28 53 S 147 5 E
Mungana, *Australia* **126 B3** 17 8 S 144 27 E
Mungaoli, *India* **92 G8** 24 24N 78 7 E
Mungari, *Mozam.* **119 F3** 17 12 S 33 30 E
Mungbere, *Dem. Rep. of the Congo* **118 B2** 2 36N 28 28 E
Mungeli, *India* **93 H9** 22 4N 81 41 E
Munger, *India* **93 G12** 25 23N 86 30 E
Mungkan Kandju △, *Australia* **126 A3** 13 35 S 142 52 E
Mungo, *Angola* **115 E3** 11 49 S 16 16 E
Mungo △, *Australia* **128 B5** 33 44 S 143 6 E
Mungo, L., *Australia* **128 B5** 33 45 S 143 0 E
Munhango, *Angola* **115 E3** 12 10 S 18 38 E
Munhango →, *Angola* **115 E4** 11 17 S 19 44 E
Munich = München, *Germany* **31 G7** 48 8N 11 34 E
Munirabad, *India* **95 F3** 15 20N 76 20 E
Munising, *U.S.A.* **148 B2** 46 25N 86 40W
Munka-Ljungby, *Sweden* **17 H6** 56 16N 12 58 E
Munkebo, *Denmark* **17 J4** 55 27N 10 34 E
Munkedal, *Sweden* **17 F5** 58 28N 11 40 E
Munkfors, *Sweden* **16 E7** 59 47N 13 30 E
Munku-Sardyk, *Russia* **67 D11** 51 45N 100 20 E
Münnerstadt, *Germany* **31 E6** 50 14N 10 12 E
Munoz, *Phil.* **80 D3** 15 43N 120 54 E
Muñoz Gamero, Pen., *Chile* **176 D2** 52 30 S 73 5W
Munroe L., *Canada* **143 B9** 59 13N 98 35W
Munsan, *S. Korea* **75 F14** 37 51N 126 48 E
Munshiganj, *Bangla.* **90 D3** 23 33N 90 32 E
Münsingen, *Switz.* **32 C5** 46 52N 7 32 E
Munson, *U.S.A.* **153 E3** 30 52N 86 52W
Munster, *France* **27 D14** 48 2N 7 8 E
Münster, *Niedersachsen, Germany* **30 C6** 52 58N 10 5 E
Münster, *Nordrhein-Westfalen, Germany* **30 D3** 51 58N 7 37 E
Münster, *Switz.* **33 D6** 46 29N 8 17 E
Munster □, *Ireland* **23 D3** 52 18N 8 44W
Münsterberg = Ziębice, *Poland* **55 H4** 50 37N 17 2 E
Muntadgin, *Australia* **125 F2** 31 45 S 118 33 E
Muntele Mare, Vf., *Romania* **53 D8** 46 30N 23 12 E
Muntok, *Indonesia* **84 C3** 2 5 S 105 10 E
Munyama, *Zambia* **119 F2** 16 5 S 28 31 E
Munzur Dağları, *Turkey* **101 C8** 39 30N 39 10 E
Muong Beng, *Laos* **76 G3** 20 23N 101 46 E
Muong Boum, *Vietnam* **76 F4** 22 24N 102 49 E
Muong Et, *Laos* **86 B5** 20 49N 104 1 E
Muong Hai, *Laos* **76 G3** 21 3N 101 49 E
Muong Hiem, *Laos* **86 B4** 20 5N 103 22 E
Muong Houn, *Laos* **76 G3** 20 8N 101 23 E
Muong Hung, *Vietnam* **76 G4** 20 56N 103 53 E
Muong Kau, *Laos* **86 E5** 15 6N 105 47 E
Muong Khao, *Laos* **86 C4** 19 38N 103 32 E
Muong Khoua, *Laos* **76 G4** 21 5N 102 31 E
Muong Liep, *Laos* **86 C3** 18 29N 101 40 E
Muong May, *Laos* **86 E6** 14 49N 106 56 E
Muong Ngeun, *Laos* **76 G3** 20 36N 101 3 E
Muong Ngoi, *Laos* **76 G4** 20 43N 102 41 E
Muong Nhie, *Vietnam* **76 F4** 22 12N 102 28 E
Muong Nong, *Laos* **86 D6** 16 22N 106 30 E
Muong Ou Tay, *Laos* **76 F3** 22 7N 101 48 E
Muong Oua, *Laos* **86 C3** 18 18N 101 20 E
Muong Peun, *Laos* **76 G4** 20 13N 103 52 E
Muong Phalane, *Laos* **86 D5** 16 39N 105 34 E
Muong Phieng, *Laos* **86 C3** 19 6N 101 32 E
Muong Phine, *Laos* **86 D6** 16 32N 106 2 E
Muong Sai, *Laos* **76 G3** 20 42N 101 59 E
Muong Saiapoun, *Laos* **86 C3** 18 24N 101 31 E
Muong Sen, *Vietnam* **86 C5** 19 24N 104 8 E
Muong Sing, *Laos* **76 G3** 21 11N 101 9 E
Muong Son, *Laos* **76 G4** 20 27N 103 19 E
Muong Soui, *Laos* **86 C4** 19 33N 102 52 E
Muong Va, *Laos* **76 G4** 21 53N 102 19 E
Muong Xia, *Vietnam* **86 B5** 20 19N 104 50 E
Muonio, *Finland* **14 C20** 67 57N 23 40 E
Muonio älv = Muonionjoki →, *Finland* **14 C20** 67 11N 23 34 E
Muonioälven = Muonionjoki →, *Finland* **14 C20** 67 11N 23 34 E
Muonionjoki →, *Finland* **14 C20** 67 11N 23 34 E
Muotathal, *Switz.* **33 C7** 46 58N 8 46 E
Mupa, *Angola* **115 F3** 16 5 S 15 50 E
Mupa △, *Angola* **115 F3** 15 55 S 15 35 E
Muping, *China* **75 F11** 37 22N 121 36 E
Mupoi, *Sudan* **107 F2** 5 28N 27 40 E
Muqaddam, Wadi →, *Sudan* **106 D3** 18 4N 31 30 E
Muqdisho, *Somali Rep.* **120 D3** 2 2N 45 25 E
Muqshin, W. →, *Oman* **99 C6** 19 44N 55 14 E
Muquequete, *Angola* **115 E2** 14 50 S 14 16 E
Mur →, *Austria* **35 E9** 46 18N 16 52 E
Mûr-de-Bretagne, *France* **26 D4** 48 12N 3 0W
Muradiye, *Manisa, Turkey* **49 C9** 38 39N 27 21 E
Muradiye, *Van, Turkey* **101 C10** 39 0N 43 44 E
Murakami, *Japan* **70 E9** 38 14N 139 29 E
Murallón, Cerro, *Chile* **176 C2** 49 48 S 73 30W
Muranda, *Rwanda* **118 C2** 1 52 S 29 20 E
Murang'a, *Kenya* **118 C4** 0 45 S 37 9 E
Murashi, *Russia* **64 B2** 59 30N 49 0 E
Murat, *France* **28 C6** 45 7N 2 53 E
Murat →, *Turkey* **101 C9** 38 46N 40 0 E
Murat Bay = Ceduna, *Australia* **127 E1** 32 7 S 133 46 E
Murat Dağı, *Turkey* **49 C11** 38 55N 29 43 E
Muratlı, *Turkey* **51 E11** 41 10N 27 29 E
Murato, *France* **29 F13** 42 35N 9 20 E
Murau, *Austria* **34 D7** 47 6N 14 10 E
Murava, *Belarus* **55 F11** 52 39N 24 15 E
Muravera, *Italy* **46 C2** 39 25N 9 34 E
Muravyevo = Mažeikiai, *Lithuania* **15 H20** 56 20N 22 20 E
Muravyovsky = Korsakov, *Russia* **67 E15** 46 36N 142 42 E
Murayama, *Japan* **70 E10** 38 30N 140 25 E
Murça, *Portugal* **42 D3** 41 24N 7 28W
Murchison, *N.Z.* **131 B7** 41 49 S 172 21 E
Murchison →, *Australia* **125 E1** 27 45 S 114 0 E
Murchison, Mt., *Antarctica* **7 D11** 73 0 S 168 0 E
Murchison, Mt., *N.Z.* **131 D6** 43 0 S 171 22 E
Murchison Falls, *Uganda* **118 B3** 2 15N 31 30 E
Murchison Falls △, *Uganda* **118 B3** 2 17N 31 48 E
Murchison Mts., *N.Z.* **131 F2** 45 13 S 167 23 E
Murchison Ra., *Australia* **126 C1** 20 0 S 134 10 E
Murchison Rapids, *Malawi* **119 F3** 15 55 S 34 35 E
Murcia, *Spain* **41 G3** 38 5N 1 10W
Murcia □, *Spain* **41 H3** 37 50N 1 30W
Murdo, *U.S.A.* **154 D4** 43 53N 100 43W
Murdoch Pt., *Australia* **126 A3** 14 37 S 144 55 E
Mürefte, *Turkey* **51 F11** 40 40N 27 14 E
Mureş □, *Romania* **53 D9** 46 45N 24 40 E
Mureş →, *Romania* **52 D5** 46 15N 20 13 E
Mureşul = Mureş →, *Romania* **52 D5** 46 15N 20 13 E
Muret, *France* **28 E5** 43 30N 1 20 E
Murewa, *Zimbabwe* **117 B5** 17 39 S 31 47 E
Murfreesboro, *N.C., U.S.A.* **149 G7** 36 27N 77 6W
Murfreesboro, *Tenn., U.S.A.* **149 H2** 35 51N 86 24W
Murg, *Switz.* **33 B8** 47 6N 9 13 E
Murgab = Murghob, *Tajikistan* **65 D7** 38 10N 74 2 E
Murgab →, *Turkmenistan* **97 B9** 38 18N 61 12 E
Murgenella, *Australia* **124 B5** 11 34 S 132 56 E
Murgeni, *Romania* **53 D13** 46 12N 28 1 E
Murgenthal, *Switz.* **32 B5** 47 16N 7 50 E
Murgha Kibzai, *Pakistan* **92 D3** 30 44N 69 25 E
Murghob, *Tajikistan* **65 D7** 38 10N 74 2 E
Murgon, *Australia* **127 D5** 26 15 S 151 54 E
Muri, *India* **93 H11** 23 22N 85 52 E
Muri, *Switz.* **33 B6** 47 17N 8 21 E
Muria, *Indonesia* **85 D4** 6 36 S 110 53 E
Muriaé, *Brazil* **171 F3** 21 8 S 42 23W
Murias de Paredes, *Spain* **42 C4** 42 52N 6 11W
Murici, *Brazil* **170 C4** 9 19 S 35 56W
Muriége, *Angola* **115 D4** 9 58 S 21 11 E
Muriel Mine, *Zimbabwe* **119 F3** 17 14 S 30 40 E
Murila, *Angola* **115 E4** 10 44 S 20 20 E
Müritz, *Germany* **30 B8** 53 25N 12 42 E
Müritz △, *Germany* **30 B8** 53 22N 12 55 E
Muriwai Beach, *N.Z.* **130 C3** 36 50 S 174 26 E
Murkong Selek, *India* **90 B5** 27 44N 95 18 E
Murliganj, *India* **93 G12** 25 54N 86 59 E
Murmansk, *Russia* **56 A5** 68 57N 33 10 E
Murnau, *Germany* **31 H7** 47 40N 11 12 E
Muro, *France* **29 F12** 42 34N 8 54 E
Muro, *Spain* **38 B4** 39 44N 3 3 E
Muro, C. de, *France* **29 G12** 41 44N 8 37 E
Muro de Alcoy, *Spain* **41 G4** 38 46N 0 26W
Muro Lucano, *Italy* **47 B8** 40 45N 15 29 E
Murom, *Russia* **60 C6** 55 35N 42 3 E
Muroran, *Japan* **70 C10** 42 25N 141 0 E
Muros, *Spain* **42 C1** 42 45N 9 5W
Muros y de Noya, Ría de, *Spain* **42 C1** 42 45N 9 0W
Muroto, *Japan* **72 D6** 33 18N 134 9 E
Muroto-Misaki, *Japan* **72 D6** 33 15N 134 10 E
Murovani Kurylivtsi, *Ukraine* **53 B12** 48 44N 27 31 E
Murowana Goślina, *Poland* **55 F3** 52 35N 17 0 E
Murphy, *U.S.A.* **158 E5** 43 13N 116 33W
Murphys, *U.S.A.* **160 G6** 38 8N 120 28W
Murphy's Station = Sunnyvale, *U.S.A.* **160 H4** 37 23N 122 2W
Murphysboro, *U.S.A.* **156 G7** 37 46N 89 20W
Murrat, *Sudan* **106 D2** 18 51N 29 33 E
Murrat Wells, *Sudan* **106 C3** 21 3N 32 55 E
Murray, *Iowa, U.S.A.* **156 C3** 41 3N 93 57W
Murray, *Ky., U.S.A.* **149 G1** 36 37N 88 19W
Murray, *Utah, U.S.A.* **158 F8** 40 40N 111 53W
Murray →, *Australia* **128 C3** 35 20 S 139 22 E
Murray, L., *Papua N. G.* **132 D1** 7 0 S 141 35 E
Murray, L., *U.S.A.* **152 A8** 34 3N 81 13W
Murray Bridge, *Australia* **128 C3** 35 6 S 139 14 E
Murray Fracture Zone, *Pac. Oc.* **135 D14** 35 0N 130 0W
Murray Harbour, *Canada* **141 C7** 46 0N 62 28W
Murray River △, *Australia* **127 E3** 34 23 S 140 32 E
Murray-Sunset △, *Australia* **128 C4** 34 45 S 141 30 E
Murraysburg, *S. Africa* **116 E3** 31 58 S 23 47 E
Murrayville, *U.S.A.* **156 E6** 39 35N 90 15W
Murree, *Pakistan* **92 C5** 33 56N 73 28 E
Murren, *Switz.* **32 C5** 46 34N 7 53 E
Murrieta, *U.S.A.* **161 M9** 33 33N 117 13W
Murro di Porco, Capo, *Italy* **47 F8** 37 0N 15 20 E
Murrumbateman, *Australia* **129 C8** 34 58 S 149 0 E
Murrumbidgee →, *Australia* **128 C5** 34 43 S 143 12 E
Murrumburrah, *Australia* **129 C8** 34 32 S 148 22 E
Murrurundi, *Australia* **129 A9** 31 42 S 150 51 E
Murshid, *Sudan* **106 C3** 21 40N 31 10 E
Murshidabad, *India* **93 G13** 24 11N 88 19 E
Murska Sobota, *Slovenia* **45 B13** 46 39N 16 12 E
Murtazapur, *India* **94 D3** 20 40N 77 25 E
Murten, *Switz.* **32 C4** 46 56N 7 4 E
Murtensee, *Switz.* **32 C4** 46 56N 7 7 E
Murtle L., *Canada* **142 C5** 52 8N 119 38W
Murtoa, *Australia* **128 D5** 36 35 S 142 28 E
Murtosa, *Portugal* **42 E2** 40 44N 8 40W
Muru →, *Brazil* **172 B3** 8 9 S 70 45W
Murud, *India* **94 E1** 18 19N 72 58 E
Murungu, *Tanzania* **118 C3** 4 12 S 31 10 E
Muruntau, *Uzbekistan* **65 C2** 41 30N 64 37 E
Murupara, *N.Z.* **130 E5** 38 28 S 176 42 E
Mururoa, *French Polynesia* **135 K14** 21 52 S 138 55W
Murwara, *India* **93 H9** 23 46N 80 28 E
Murwillumbah, *Australia* **127 D5** 28 18 S 153 27 E
Mürz →, *Austria* **34 D8** 47 30N 15 25 E
Mürzzuschlag, *Austria* **34 D8** 47 36N 15 41 E
Mus, *India* **95 K11** 9 14N 92 47 E
Muş, *Turkey* **101 C9** 38 45N 41 30 E
Musa, *Dem. Rep. of the Congo* **114 B3** 2 40N 19 18 E
Musa →, *Papua N. G.* **132 E5** 9 3 S 148 55 E
Mûsa, Gebel, *Egypt* **96 D2** 28 33N 33 59 E
Musa Khel, *Pakistan* **92 D3** 30 59N 69 52 E
Mūsa Qal'eh, *Afghan.* **91 B2** 32 20N 64 50 E
Musadi, *Dem. Rep. of the Congo* **114 C4** 2 31 S 22 50 E
Musafirkhana, *India* **93 F9** 26 22N 81 48 E
Musala, *Bulgaria* **50 D7** 42 13N 23 37 E
Musala, *Indonesia* **84 B1** 1 41N 98 28 E
Musan, *N. Korea* **75 C15** 42 12N 129 12 E
Musandam, Ra's, *Oman* **99 A7** 26 20N 56 20 E
Musangu, *Dem. Rep. of the Congo* **119 E1** 10 28 S 23 55 E
Musasa, *Tanzania* **118 C3** 3 25 S 31 30 E
Musashino, *Japan* **73 B11** 35 42N 139 34 E
Musay'īd, *Qatar* **97 E6** 25 0N 51 33 E
Musaymīr, *Yemen* **98 D4** 13 27N 44 37 E
Muscat = Masqat, *Oman* **99 B7** 23 37N 58 36 E
Muscat & Oman = Oman ■, *Asia* **99 B7** 23 0N 58 0 E
Muscatatuc →, *U.S.A.* **157 F10** 38 47N 86 9W
Muscatine, *U.S.A.* **156 C5** 41 25N 91 3W
Muschu I., *Papua N. G.* **132 B2** 3 25 S 143 35 E
Muscle Shoals, *U.S.A.* **149 H2** 34 45N 87 40W
Muscoda, *U.S.A.* **156 A6** 43 11N 90 27W
Musengezi = Unsengedsi →, *Zimbabwe* **119 F3** 15 43 S 31 14 E
Musgrave Harbour, *Canada* **141 C9** 49 27N 53 58W
Musgrave Ranges, *Australia* **125 E5** 26 0 S 132 0 E
Mushie, *Dem. Rep. of the Congo* **114 C3** 2 56 S 16 55 E
Mushima, *Zambia* **115 E4** 14 10 S 24 56 E
Mushin, *Nigeria* **113 D5** 6 32N 3 21 E
Musi →, *India* **94 F4** 16 41N 79 40 E
Musi →, *Indonesia* **84 C2** 2 20 S 104 56 E
Musina, *S. Africa* **117 C5** 22 20 S 30 5 E
Musiri, *India* **95 J4** 10 56N 78 27 E
Muskeg →, *Canada* **142 A4** 60 20N 123 20W
Muskego, *U.S.A.* **157 B8** 42 55N 88 8W
Muskegon, *U.S.A.* **157 A10** 43 14N 86 16W
Muskegon →, *U.S.A.* **148 D2** 43 14N 86 21W
Muskegon Heights, *U.S.A.* **157 A10** 43 12N 86 16W
Muskogee, *U.S.A.* **155 H7** 35 45N 95 22W
Muskoka, L., *Canada* **150 B5** 45 0N 79 25W
Muskwa →, *Canada* **142 B4** 58 47N 122 48W
Muslīmiyah, *Syria* **96 B3** 36 19N 37 12 E
Musmar, *Sudan* **106 D4** 18 13N 35 40 E
Musofu, *Zambia* **119 E2** 13 30 S 29 0 E
Musoma, *Tanzania* **118 C3** 1 30 S 33 48 E
Musquaro, L., *Canada* **141 B7** 50 38N 61 5W
Musquodoboit Harbour, *Canada* **141 D7** 44 50N 63 9W
Mussau I., *Papua N. G.* **132 A5** 1 30 S 149 40 E
Musselburgh, *U.K.* **22 F5** 55 57N 3 2W
Musselshell →, *U.S.A.* **158 C10** 47 21N 107 57W
Mussende, *Angola* **115 E3** 10 32 S 16 5 E
Mussidan, *France* **28 C4** 45 2N 0 22 E
Mussolinea di Sardegna = Arboréa, *Italy* **46 C1** 39 46N 8 35 E
Mussolo, *Angola* **115 D3** 9 59 S 17 19 E
Mussomeli, *Italy* **46 E6** 37 35N 13 45 E
Mussoorie, *India* **92 D8** 30 27N 78 6 E
Mussuco, *Angola* **116 B2** 17 2 S 19 3 E
Mustafakemalpaşa, *Turkey* **51 F12** 40 2N 28 24 E
Mustahil, *Ethiopia* **120 C2** 5 16N 44 45 E
Mustang, *Nepal* **93 E10** 29 10N 83 55 E
Musters, L., *Argentina* **176 C3** 45 20 S 69 25W
Musudan, *N. Korea* **75 D15** 40 50N 129 43 E
Muswellbrook, *Australia* **129 B9** 32 16 S 150 56 E
Muszyna, *Poland* **55 J7** 49 22N 20 55 E
Mût, *Egypt* **106 B2** 25 28N 28 58 E
Mut, *Turkey* **100 D5** 36 40N 33 28 E
Mutanda, *Dem. Rep. of the Congo* **115 D3** 5 17 S 16 34 E
Mutanda, *Mozam.* **117 C5** 21 0 S 33 34 E
Mutanda, *Zambia* **119 E2** 12 24 S 26 13 E
Mutankiang = Mudanjiang, *China* **75 B15** 44 38N 129 30 E
Mutare, *Zimbabwe* **119 F3** 18 58 S 32 38 E
Muting, *Indonesia* **83 C6** 7 23 S 140 20 E
Mutis, *Indonesia* **82 C2** 9 30 S 124 14 E
Mutki = Mirtağ, *Turkey* **96 B4** 38 23N 41 56 E
Mutoko, *Zimbabwe* **117 B5** 17 24 S 32 13 E
Mutoray, *Russia* **67 C11** 60 56N 101 0 E
Mutoto, *Dem. Rep. of the Congo* **115 D4** 5 42 S 22 42 E
Mutoxo, *Angola* **115 E4** 12 17 S 21 40 E
Mutshatsha, *Dem. Rep. of the Congo* **119 E1** 10 35 S 24 20 E
Mutsu, *Japan* **70 D10** 41 5N 140 55 E
Mutsu-Wan, *Japan* **70 D10** 41 5N 140 55 E
Muttaburra, *Australia* **126 C3** 22 38 S 144 29 E
Muttalip, *Turkey* **49 B12** 39 50N 30 32 E
Mutton I., *Ireland* **23 D2** 52 49N 9 32W
Muttra = Mathura, *India* **92 F7** 27 30N 77 40 E
Muttukuru, *India* **95 G5** 14 16N 80 6 E
Mutuáli, *Mozam.* **119 E4** 14 55 S 37 0 E
Mutum Biyu, *Nigeria* **113 D7** 8 40N 10 50 E
Mutunópolis, *Brazil* **171 D2** 13 40 S 49 15W
Mutur, *Sri Lanka* **95 K5** 8 27N 81 16 E
Muweilih, *Egypt* **103 E3** 30 42N 34 19 E
Muxaluando, *Angola* **115 D2** 8 8 S 14 18 E
Muxía, *Spain* **42 B1** 43 3N 9 10W
Muxima, *Angola* **115 D2** 9 33 S 13 58 E
Muy Muy, *Nic.* **164 D2** 12 39N 85 36W
Muyinga, *Burundi* **118 C3** 3 14 S 30 33 E
Muynak, *Uzbekistan* **66 E6** 43 44N 59 10 E
Muyunkum, Peski, *Kazakhstan* **65 A4** 44 12N 71 0 E
Muzaffarabad, *Pakistan* **93 B5** 34 25N 73 30 E
Muzaffargarh, *Pakistan* **91 C3** 30 5N 71 14 E
Muzaffarnagar, *India* **92 E7** 29 26N 77 40 E
Muzaffarpur, *India* **93 F11** 26 7N 85 23 E
Muzafirpur, *Pakistan* **92 D3** 30 58N 69 9 E
Muzeze, *Angola* **115 F3** 15 3 S 17 43 E
Muzhi, *Russia* **56 A11** 65 25N 64 40 E
Muzillac, *France* **26 E4** 47 35N 2 30W
Muzon, C., *U.S.A.* **144 J14** 54 40N 132 42W
Muztagh-Ata, *China* **65 D7** 38 17N 75 7 E
Muztor = Toktogul, *Kyrgyzstan* **65 C6** 41 50N 72 50 E
Muzūra, *Egypt* **106 J7** 28 53N 30 48 E
Mvadhi-Ousyé, *Gabon* **114 B2** 1 13N 13 12 E
Mvam, *Gabon* **114 C1** 0 13 S 9 39 E
Mvangan, *Cameroon* **114 B2** 2 17N 11 43 E
Mvôlô, *Sudan* **107 F2** 6 2N 29 53 E
Mvuma, *Zimbabwe* **119 F3** 19 16 S 30 30 E
Mvurwi, *Zimbabwe* **119 F3** 17 0 S 30 57 E
Mwabvi ⌓, *Malawi* **119 F3** 16 42 S 35 0 E
Mwadi-Kalumbu, *Dem. Rep. of the Congo* **115 D3** 7 53 S 18 43 E
Mwadui, *Tanzania* **118 C3** 3 26 S 33 32 E
Mwali = Mohéli, *Comoros Is.* **121 a** 12 20 S 43 40 E
Mwambo, *Tanzania* **119 E5** 10 30 S 40 22 E
Mwandi, *Zambia* **119 F1** 17 30 S 24 51 E
Mwanza, *Dem. Rep. of the Congo* **118 D2** 7 55 S 26 43 E
Mwanza, *Tanzania* **118 C3** 2 30 S 32 58 E
Mwanza, *Zambia* **119 F1** 16 58 S 24 28 E
Mwanza □, *Tanzania* **118 C3** 2 0 S 33 0 E
Mwaya, *Tanzania* **119 D3** 9 32 S 33 55 E
Mweelrea, *Ireland* **23 C2** 53 39N 9 49W
Mweka, *Dem. Rep. of the Congo* **115 C4** 4 50 S 21 34 E
Mwendjila, *Dem. Rep. of the Congo* **115 D3** 7 12 S 18 51 E
Mwene-Ditu, *Dem. Rep. of the Congo* **115 D4** 6 35 S 22 27 E
Mwenezi, *Zimbabwe* **119 G3** 21 15 S 30 48 E
Mwenezi →, *Mozam.* **119 G3** 22 40 S 31 50 E
Mwenga, *Dem. Rep. of the Congo* **118 C2** 3 1 S 28 28 E
Mweru, L., *Zambia* **119 D2** 9 0 S 28 40 E
Mweru Wantipa △, *Zambia* **119 D2** 8 39 S 29 25 E
Mwetshi, *Dem. Rep. of the Congo* **115 C4** 4 50 S 22 38 E
Mweza Range, *Zimbabwe* **119 G3** 21 0 S 30 0 E
Mwilambwe, *Dem. Rep. of the Congo* **118 D2** 8 7 S 25 5 E
Mwimbi, *Tanzania* **119 D3** 8 38 S 31 39 E
Mwinilunga, *Zambia* **119 E1** 11 43 S 24 25 E
My Tho, *Vietnam* **87 G6** 10 29N 106 23 E
Mya, O. →, *Algeria* **111 B5** 30 46N 4 54 E
Myajlar, *India* **92 F4** 26 15N 70 20 E
Myakka →, *U.S.A.* **153 J7** 26 56N 82 11W
Myall Lakes △, *Australia* **129 B10** 32 25 S 152 30 E
Myanaung, *Burma* **90 F5** 18 18N 95 22 E
Myanmar = Burma ■, *Asia* **90 E6** 21 0N 96 30 E
Myaung, *Burma* **90 E5** 21 50N 95 25 E
Myaungmya, *Burma* **90 G5** 16 30N 94 40 E
Myebon, *Burma* **90 E4** 20 3N 93 22 E
Myedna, *Belarus* **55 G10** 51 52N 23 42 E
Myeik Kyunzu, *Burma* **87 G1** 11 30N 97 30 E
Myers Chuck, *U.S.A.* **142 B2** 55 44N 132 11W
Myerstown, *U.S.A.* **151 F8** 40 22N 76 19W
Myingyan, *Burma* **90 E5** 21 30N 95 20 E
Myitkyina, *Burma* **90 C6** 25 24N 97 26 E
Myitson, *Burma* **90 D6** 23 16N 96 34 E
Myittha, *Burma* **90 E6** 21 25N 96 8 E
Myittha →, *Burma* **90 D5** 23 12N 94 17 E
Myjava, *Slovak Rep.* **35 C10** 48 41N 17 37 E
Mykhaylivka, *Ukraine* **59 J8** 47 12N 35 15 E
Mykines, *Færoe Is.* **14 E9** 62 7N 7 35W
Myking, *Norway* **18 D2** 60 41N 5 19 E
Mykolayiv, *Ukraine* **59 J7** 46 58N 32 0 E
Mylius Erichsen Land, *Greenland* **10 A8** 81 30N 27 0W
Mymensingh, *Bangla.* **90 C3** 24 45N 90 24 E
Mynydd Du, *U.K.* **21 F4** 51 52N 3 50W
Myo-gyi, *Burma* **90 E6** 21 27N 96 22 E
Myohaung, *Burma* **90 E4** 20 35N 93 11 E
Myohla, *Burma* **90 F5** 19 16N 95 25 E
Myotha, *Burma* **90 E5** 21 41N 95 43 E
Myothit, *Kachin, Burma* **90 C6** 24 24N 97 24 E
Myothit, *Magwe, Burma* **90 E5** 20 12N 95 27 E
Myrasýsla □, *Iceland* **11 C5** 64 45N 21 30W
Mýrdalsjökull, *Iceland* **11 D7** 63 40N 19 6W
Myrhorod, *Ukraine* **59 H7** 49 58N 33 37 E
Mýri, *Iceland* **11 B9** 65 23N 17 23W
Myrtle Beach, *U.S.A.* **149 J6** 33 42N 78 53W
Myrtle Creek, *U.S.A.* **158 E2** 43 1N 123 17W
Myrtle Grove, *U.S.A.* **153 E2** 30 23N 87 17W
Myrtle Point, *U.S.A.* **158 E1** 43 4N 124 8W
Myrtleford, *Australia* **129 D7** 36 34 S 146 44 E
Myrtou, *Cyprus* **39 E9** 35 18N 33 4 E
Myrzakent, *Kazakhstan* **65 C4** 40 40N 68 32 E
Mysen, *Norway* **18 E8** 59 33N 11 20 E
Mysia, *Turkey* **51 G11** 39 50N 27 0 E
Myślenice, *Poland* **55 J6** 49 51N 19 57 E
Myślibórz, *Poland* **55 F1** 52 55N 14 50 E
Mysłowice, *Poland* **55 H6** 50 15N 19 12 E
Myslowitz = Mysłowice, *Poland* **55 H6** 50 15N 19 12 E
Mysore = Karnataka □, *India* **95 H3** 13 15N 77 0 E
Mysore, *India* **95 H3** 12 17N 76 41 E
Mystic, *Conn., U.S.A.* **151 E13** 41 21N 71 58W
Mystic, *Iowa, U.S.A.* **156 D4** 40 47N 92 57W
Myszków, *Poland* **55 H6** 50 45N 19 22 E
Myszyniec, *Poland* **54 E8** 53 23N 21 21 E
Mythen, *Switz.* **33 B7** 47 2N 8 42 E
Mytishchi, *Russia* **58 E9** 55 50N 37 50 E
Mývatn, *Iceland* **11 B10** 65 36N 17 0W
Mzab, Oued en →, *Algeria* **111 B6** 32 15N 5 0 E
Mže →, *Czech Rep.* **34 B6** 49 46N 13 24 E
Mzimba, *Malawi* **119 E3** 11 55 S 33 39 E
Mzimkulu →, *S. Africa* **117 E5** 30 44 S 30 28 E
Mzimvubu →, *S. Africa* **117 E4** 31 38 S 29 33 E
Mzuzu, *Malawi* **119 E3** 11 30 S 33 55 E

N

Na Hearadh = Harris, *U.K.* **22 D2** 57 50N 6 55W
Na-lang, *Burma* **90 D6** 22 42N 97 33 E
Na Noi, *Thailand* **86 C3** 18 19N 100 43 E
Na Phao, *Laos* **86 D5** 17 35N 105 44 E
Na Sam, *Vietnam* **76 F6** 22 3N 106 37 E
Na San, *Vietnam* **86 B5** 21 12N 104 2 E
Na Thon, *Thailand* **87 b** 9 32N 99 56 E
Naab →, *Germany* **31 F8** 49 1N 12 2 E
Naalehu, *U.S.A.* **145 D6** 19 4N 155 35W
Na'am, *Sudan* **107 F2** 9 42N 28 27 E
Na'am →, *Sudan* **107 F2** 6 48N 29 57 E
Naantali, *Finland* **15 F19** 60 29N 22 2 E
Naas, *Ireland* **23 C5** 53 12N 6 40W
Nababeep, *S. Africa* **116 D2** 29 36 S 17 46 E
Nabadwip = Navadwip, *India* **93 H13** 23 34N 88 20 E
Nabari, *Japan* **73 C8** 34 37N 136 5 E
Nabawa, *Australia* **125 E1** 28 30 S 114 48 E
Nabberu, L., *Australia* **125 E3** 25 50 S 120 30 E
Nabburg, *Germany* **31 F8** 49 27N 12 11 E
Naberezhnyye Chelny, *Russia* **60 C11** 55 42N 52 19 E
Nabesna, *U.S.A.* **144 E12** 62 22N 143 0W
Nabeul, *Tunisia* **108 A2** 36 30N 10 44 E
Nabha, *India* **92 D7** 30 26N 76 14 E
Nabīd, *Iran* **97 D8** 29 40N 57 38 E
Nabire, *Indonesia* **83 B5** 3 15 S 135 26 E
Nabisar, *Pakistan* **92 G3** 25 8N 69 40 E
Nabisipi →, *Canada* **141 B7** 50 14N 62 13W
Nabiswera, *Uganda* **118 B3** 1 27N 32 15 E
Nāblus = Nābulus, *West Bank* **103 C4** 32 14N 35 15 E
Naboomspruit, *S. Africa* **117 C4** 24 32 S 28 40 E
Nabou, *Burkina Faso* **112 C4** 11 25N 2 50W
Nabouwalu, *Fiji* **133 A2** 17 0 S 178 45 E
Nabua, *Phil.* **80 E4** 13 24N 123 22 E
Nābulus, *West Bank* **103 C4** 32 14N 35 15 E
Nabunturan, *Phil.* **81 H5** 7 35N 125 58 E
Nacala, *Mozam.* **119 E5** 14 31 S 40 34 E
Nacala-Velha, *Mozam.* **119 E5** 14 32 S 40 34 E
Nacaome, *Honduras* **164 D2** 13 31N 87 30W
Nacaroa, *Mozam.* **119 E4** 14 22 S 39 56 E
Naches, *U.S.A.* **158 C3** 46 44N 120 42W
Naches →, *U.S.A.* **160 D6** 46 38N 120 31W
Nachicapau, L., *Canada* **141 A6** 56 40N 68 5W
Nachikatsuura, *Japan* **73 D7** 33 33N 135 58 E
Nachingwea, *Tanzania* **119 E4** 10 23 S 38 49 E
Nachna, *India* **92 F4** 27 34N 71 41 E
Náchod, *Czech Rep.* **34 A9** 50 25N 16 8 E
Nachuge, *India* **95 J11** 10 47N 92 21 E
Nacimiento L., *U.S.A.* **160 K6** 35 46N 120 53W
Nackara, *Australia* **128 B3** 32 48 S 139 12 E
Naco, *Mexico* **162 A3** 31 20N 109 56W
Nacogdoches, *U.S.A.* **155 K7** 31 36N 94 39W
Nácori Chico, *Mexico* **162 B3** 29 39N 109 1W
Nacozari, *Mexico* **162 A3** 30 24N 109 39W
Nacula, *Fiji* **133 A1** 16 54 S 177 27 E
Nådendal = Naantali, *Finland* **15 F19** 60 29N 22 2 E
Nadezhdinsky = Serov, *Russia* **64 B8** 59 29N 60 35 E
Nadi, *Fiji* **133 A1** 17 42 S 177 20 E

Nadi, *Sudan* .... **106 D3** 18 40N 33 41 E
Nadiad, *India* .... **92 H5** 22 41N 72 56 E
Nădlac, *Romania* .. **52 C5** 46 10N 20 50 E
Nador, *Morocco* **111 A4** 35 14N 2 58W
Nadur, *Malta* .... **38 F7** 35 54N 14 22 E
Nadur, *Gozo, Malta* .. **38 E2** 36 2N 14 18 E
Nadūshan, *Iran* ...... **97 C7** 32 2N 53 35 E
Nadvirna, *Ukraine* .. **53 B9** 48 37N 24 30 E
Nadvoitsy, *Russia* ... **56 B5** 63 52N 34 14 E
Nadvornaya =
  Nadvirna, *Ukraine* .. **53 B9** 48 37N 24 30 E
Nadym, *Russia* ...... **66 C8** 65 35N 72 42 E
Nadym →, *Russia* .... **66 C8** 66 12N 72 0 E
Nærbø, *Norway* ...... **18 F2** 58 40N 5 39 E
Næstved, *Denmark* .. **17 J5** 55 13N 11 44 E
Nafada, *Nigeria* ..... **113 C7** 11 8N 11 20 E
Näfels, *Switz.* .... **33 B8** 47 6N 9 4 E
Nafpaktos = Návpaktos,
  Greece .... **48 C3** 38 24N 21 50 E
Nafplio = Návplion,
  Greece .... **48 D4** 37 33N 22 50 E
Naft-e Safīd, *Iran* ... **97 D6** 31 40N 49 17 E
Naftshahr, *Iran* ..... **101 E11** 34 0N 45 30 E
Nafud Desert = An
  Nafūd, *Si. Arabia* .. **96 D4** 28 15N 41 0 E
Nafūsah, *Libya* ...... **108 B2** 32 12N 12 30 E
Nag Hammâdi, *Egypt* . **106 B3** 26 2N 32 18 E
Naga, Camarines S.,
  Phil. .... **80 E4** 13 38N 123 15 E
Naga, Cebu, *Phil.* ... **81 F4** 10 13N 123 45 E
Naga,
  Zamboanga del S.,
  Phil. .... **81 H4** 7 46N 122 45 E
Naga, Kreb en, *Africa* **110 D3** 24 12N 6 0W
Naga Hills =
  Nagaland □, *India* .. **90 B5** 26 0N 94 30 E
Naga-Shima,
  Kagoshima, Japan . . **72 E2** 32 10N 130 9 E
Naga-Shima,
  Yamaguchi, Japan . . **72 D4** 33 49N 132 5 E
Nagahama, Ehime,
  Japan .... **72 D4** 33 36N 132 29 E
Nagahama, Shiga,
  Japan .... **73 B8** 35 23N 136 16 E
Nagai, Japan .... **70 E10** 38 6N 140 2 E
Nagai I., U.S.A. **144 C8** 55 5N 160 0W
Nagaland □, India .. **90 B5** 26 0N 94 30 E
Nagambie, Australia . **129 D6** 36 47 S 145 10 E
Nagano, Japan ..... **73 A10** 36 40N 138 10 E
Nagano □, Japan ... **73 A10** 36 15N 138 0 E
Nagaoka, Japan .... **71 F9** 37 27N 138 51 E
Nagappattinam, India . **95 J4** 10 46N 79 51 E
Nagar →, Bangla. ... **90 C2** 24 27N 89 12 E
Nagar Karnul, India . **95 F4** 16 29N 78 20 E
Nagar Parkar, Pakistan **92 G4** 24 28N 70 46 E
Nagara-Gawa →,
  Japan .... **73 B8** 35 40N 136 43 E
Nagaram, India ..... **94 E5** 18 21N 80 26 E
Nagarhole △, India .. **95 J3** 12 0N 76 10 E
Nagari Hills, India .. **95 H4** 13 3N 79 45 E
Nagasaki, Japan .... **72 E1** 32 47N 129 50 E
Nagasaki □, Japan ... **72 E1** 32 50N 129 40 E
Nagato, Japan ...... **72 C3** 34 19N 131 5 E
Nagaur, India ...... **92 F5** 27 15N 73 45 E
Nagbhir, India ..... **94 D4** 20 34N 79 55 E
Nagda, India .... **92 H6** 23 27N 75 25 E
Nagercoil, India .... **95 K3** 8 12N 77 26 E
Nagina, India ...... **93 E8** 29 30N 78 30 E
Nagîneh, Iran ...... **97 C8** 34 20N 57 15 E
Naginimara, India .. **90 B5** 26 49N 94 50 E
Nagir, Pakistan .... **93 A6** 36 12N 74 42 E
Naglarby, Sweden ... **16 D9** 60 25N 15 34 E
Nagod, India .... **93 G9** 24 34N 80 36 E
Nagold, Germany ... **31 G4** 48 32N 8 43 E
Nagold →, Germany . **31 G4** 48 52N 8 42 E
Nagoorin, Australia . **126 C5** 24 17 S 151 15 E
Nagorno-Karabakh □,
  Azerbaijan .... **101 C12** 39 55N 46 45 E
Nagornyy, Russia .... **67 D13** 55 58N 124 57 E
Nagorsk, Russia ..... **64 B3** 59 18N 50 48 E
Nagoya →, Japan .... **73 B8** 35 10N 136 50 E
Nagoya ✈ (NGO),
  Japan .... **73 B8** 35 14N 136 57 E
Nagpartian = Burgos,
  Phil. .... **80 B3** 18 31N 120 39 E
Nagpur, India ...... **94 D4** 21 8N 79 10 E
Nagua, Dom. Rep. .. **165 C6** 19 23N 69 50W
Naguabo, Puerto Rico **165 d** 18 13N 65 44W
Nagyatád, Hungary .. **52 D2** 46 14N 17 22 E
Nagyecsed, Hungary . **52 C7** 47 53N 22 24 E
Nagykálló, Hungary . **52 C7** 47 53N 21 51 E
Nagykanizsa, Hungary **52 D2** 46 28N 17 0 E
Nagykáta, Hungary .. **52 C4** 47 5N 19 45 E
Nagykőrös, Hungary . **52 C4** 47 5N 19 48 E
Nagyszombat = Trnava,
  Slovak Rep. .... **35 C10** 48 23N 17 35 E
Nagyvárad = Oradea,
  Romania .... **52 B5** 47 2N 21 58 E
Naha, Japan .... **71 L3** 26 13N 127 42 E
Nahan, India .... **92 D7** 30 33N 77 18 E
Nahanni △, Canada .. **142 A4** 61 36N 125 41W
Nahanni Butte, Canada **142 A4** 61 2N 123 31W
Nahargarh, Mad. P.,
  India .... **92 G6** 24 10N 75 14 E
Nahargarh, Raj., India **92 G7** 24 55N 76 50 E
Nahariyya, Israel .... **100 F6** 33 1N 35 5 E
Nahāvand, Iran ..... **97 C6** 34 10N 48 22 E
Nahe →, Germany ... **31 F3** 49 58N 7 54 E
Nahimre, Ukraine ... **53 E13** 48 36N 28 27 E
Nahīya, W. →, Egypt . **106 B3** 28 55N 31 0 E
Nahuel Huapi △,
  Argentina .... **176 B2** 41 3 S 71 59W
Nahuel Huapi, L.,
  Argentina .... **176 B2** 41 0 S 71 32W
Nahuelbuta △, Chile . **174 D1** 37 44 S 72 57W
Nahunta, U.S.A. **152 D8** 31 12N 81 59W
Nai Yong, Thailand .. **87 a** 8 14N 98 22 E
Naic, Phil. .... **80 D3** 14 19N 120 46 E
Naicá, Mexico **162 B3** 27 53N 105 31W
Naicam, Canada **143 C8** 52 30N 104 30W
Naikliu, Indonesia .. **82 C2** 9 30 S 123 50 E
Naikoon △, Canada .. **142 C2** 53 55N 131 55W
Naikul, India .... **94 D7** 21 20N 84 58 E
Naila, Germany ..... **31 E7** 50 19N 11 42 E
Naimisharanya, India **93 F9** 27 21N 80 30 E
Nā'īn, Iran **141 A7** 56 34N 61 40W
Nā'īn, Iran .... **97 C7** 32 54N 53 0 E
Naini Tal, India .... **26 F7** 46 48N 79 30 E
Nainpur, India ...... **92 G6** 25 46N 75 51 E
Naipu, Romania ..... **55 F10** 44 12N 25 48 E
Nairai, Fiji .... **133 A2** 17 49 S 179 15 E
Nairn, U.K. **22 D5** 57 35N 3 53W
Nairobi, Kenya ..... **118 C4** 1 17 S 36 48 E
Nairobi △, Kenya ... **118 C4** 1 23 S 36 50 E
Naissaar, Estonia ... **15 G21** 59 34N 24 29 E
Naita, Mt., Ethiopia . **119 F4** 5 30N 35 18 E
Naitaba, Fiji .... **133 A3** 17 0 S 179 16W
Naivasha, Kenya .... **118 C4** 0 40 S 36 30 E
Naivasha, L., Kenya . **118 C4** 0 48 S 36 20 E
Najac, France ...... **20 D4** 44 14N 1 58 E
Najaf = An Najaf, Iraq **101 G11** 32 3N 44 15 E
Najafābād, Iran ..... **97 C6** 32 40N 51 15 E

Najd, Si. Arabia ..... **88 C3** 26 30N 42 0 E
Nájera, Spain **40 C2** 42 26N 2 48W
Najerilla →, Spain ... **40 C2** 42 32N 2 48W
Najibabad, India ... **92 E8** 29 40N 78 20 E
Najin, N. Korea ..... **75 C16** 42 12N 130 15 E
Najmah, Si. Arabia .. **97 E6** 26 42N 50 6 E
Najrān, Si. Arabia .. **98 C4** 17 34N 44 18 E
Naju, S. Korea ...... **75 G14** 35 3N 126 43 E
Naka-Gawa →, Japan **73 A12** 36 20N 140 36 E
Nakadōri-Shima, Japan **71 H4** 32 57N 129 4 E
Nakal = Nakło nad
  Notecią, Poland .... **55 E4** 53 9N 17 38 E
Nakalagba, Dem. Rep.
  of the Congo .... **118 B2** 2 50N 27 58 E
Nakalele Pt., U.S.A. .. **145 B5** 21 2N 156 35W
Nakama, Japan ..... **72 D2** 33 56N 130 43 E
Nakaminato, Japan .. **73 A12** 36 21N 140 36 E
Nakamura, Japan ... **72 E4** 32 59N 132 56 E
Nakanai Mts.,
  Papua N. G. .... **132 C6** 5 40 S 151 0 E
Nakano, Japan ...... **73 A10** 36 45N 138 22 E
Nakano-Shima, Japan **71 K4** 29 51N 129 52 E
Nakanojō, Japan .... **73 A10** 36 35N 138 51 E
Nakashibetsu, Japan . **70 C12** 43 33N 144 59 E
Nakasugawa, Japan . **73 B9** 35 29N 137 30 E
Nakfa, Eritrea ...... **107 D4** 16 40N 38 32 E
Nakfa △, Eritrea .... **107 D4** 17 28N 38 55 E
Nakha Yai, Ko,
  Thailand .... **87 a** 8 3N 98 28 E
Nakhichevan =
  Naxçıvan, Azerbaijan **101 C11** 39 12N 45 15 E
Nakhichevan Rep. =
  Naxçıvan □,
  Azerbaijan .... **101 C11** 39 25N 45 26 E
Nakhl, Egypt .... **103 F2** 29 55N 33 43 E
Nakhl-e Taqī, Iran ... **97 E7** 27 28N 52 36 E
Nakhodka, Russia ... **67 E14** 42 53N 132 54 E
Nakhon Nayok,
  Thailand .... **86 E3** 14 12N 101 13 E
Nakhon Pathom,
  Thailand .... **86 F3** 13 49N 100 3 E
Nakhon Phanom,
  Thailand .... **86 D5** 17 23N 104 43 E
Nakhon Ratchasima,
  Thailand .... **86 E4** 14 59N 102 12 E
Nakhon Sawan,
  Thailand .... **86 E3** 15 35N 100 10 E
Nakhon Si Thammarat,
  Thailand .... **87 H3** 8 29N 100 0 E
Nakhon Thai, Thailand **86 D3** 17 5N 100 44 E
Nakhtarana, India ... **92 H3** 23 20N 69 15 E
Nakina, Canada **140 B2** 50 10N 86 40W
Nakło nad Notecią,
  Poland .... **55 E4** 53 9N 17 38 E
Naknek, U.S.A. **144 G8** 58 44N 157 1W
Nako, Burkina Faso . **112 C4** 10 40N 3 4W
Nakodar, India ..... **90 D6** 31 8N 75 31 E
Nakskov, Denmark .. **17 K5** 54 50N 11 8 E
Naktong →, S. Korea . **75 G15** 35 7N 128 57 E
Nakuru, Kenya ..... **118 C4** 0 15 S 36 4 E
Nakuru, L., Kenya ... **118 C4** 0 23 S 36 5 E
Nakusp, Canada **142 C5** 50 20N 117 45W
Nal, Pakistan .... **92 F2** 27 40N 66 12 E
Nal →, Pakistan .... **91 D2** 26 20N 65 30 E
Nalázi, Mozam. ..... **117 C5** 24 3 S 33 20 E
Nalchik, Russia ..... **61 J6** 43 30N 43 33 E
Nałęczów, Poland ... **55 H12** 51 17N 22 9 E
Nalerigu, Ghana **113 C4** 10 35N 0 25W
Nalgonda, India .... **94 F4** 17 6N 79 15 E
Nalhati, India ...... **93 G12** 24 17N 87 52 E
Naliya, India .... **92 H3** 23 16N 68 50 E
Nallamalai Hills, India **95 G4** 15 30N 78 50 E
Nallhan, Turkey .... **100 B4** 40 11N 31 20 E
Nalolo, Zambia ..... **115 F4** 15 33 S 23 7 E
Nalón →, Spain **42 B4** 43 32N 6 4W
Nalong, Burma ..... **90 C6** 24 44N 97 28 E
Nālūt, Libya .... **108 B2** 31 54N 11 0 E
Nam Can, Vietnam .. **87 H5** 8 46N 104 59 E
Nam-ch'on, N. Korea **75 E14** 38 15N 126 26 E
Nam Co, China ..... **68 C4** 30 30N 90 45 E
Nam Dinh, Vietnam . **76 G6** 20 25N 106 5 E
Nam Du, Hon, Vietnam **87 H5** 9 41N 104 21 E
Nam Nao △, Thailand **86 D3** 16 44N 101 32 E
Nam Ngum Dam, Laos **86 C4** 18 35N 102 34 E
Nam-Phan, Vietnam . **87 G6** 10 30N 106 0 E
Nam Phong, Thailand **86 D4** 16 42N 102 52 E
Nam Tha, Laos ..... **76 G3** 20 58N 101 30 E
Nam Tok, Thailand . **86 E2** 14 21N 99 4 E
Namachire, Angola .. **115 E4** 11 26 S 22 43 E
Namacunde, Angola . **116 B2** 17 18 S 15 50 E
Namacurra, Mozam. . **117 B6** 17 30 S 36 50 E
Namadgi △, Australia **129 C5** 35 42 S 149 0 E
Namak, Daryācheh-ye,
  Iran .... **97 C7** 34 30N 52 0 E
Namak, Kavir-e, Iran . **97 C8** 34 30N 57 30 E
Namakkal, India .... **95 J4** 11 3N 78 13 E
Namakzār, Daryācheh-
  ye, Iran .... **91 B1** 34 0N 60 30 E
Namaland, Namibia . **116 C2** 26 0 S 17 0 E
Namangan, Uzbekistan **65 C5** 41 0N 71 40 E
Namapa, Mozam. ... **119 E4** 13 43 S 39 50 E
Namaqualand, S. Africa **116 E2** 30 0 S 17 25 E
Namasagali, Uganda . **118 B3** 1 2N 33 0 E
Namatanai,
  Papua N. G. .... **132 B7** 3 40 S 152 29 E
Namber, Indonesia .. **83 B4** 1 2 S 134 49 E
Nambour, Australia . **127 D5** 26 32 S 152 58 E
Nambouwalu =
  Nabouwalu, Fiji .... **133 A2** 17 0 S 178 45 E
Nambuangongo,
  Angola .... **116 D2** 8 1 S 14 12 E
Nambucca Heads,
  Australia .... **129 A10** 30 37 S 153 0 E
Nambung △, Australia **125 F2** 30 30 S 115 5 E
Namcha Barwa, China **68 D4** 29 40N 95 10 E
Namche Bazar, Nepal . **93 F12** 27 51N 86 47 E
Namchonjŏm = Nam-
  ch'on, N. Korea .... **75 E14** 38 15N 126 26 E
Namecunda, Mozam. . **119 E4** 14 54 S 37 37 E
Nameh, Indonesia ... **85 B5** 2 34N 116 21 E
Namen = Namur,
  Belgium .... **24 D4** 50 27N 4 52 E
Namenalala, Fiji .... **133 A2** 17 3 S 179 5 E
Nameponda, Mozam. . **119 F4** 15 50 S 39 50 E
Námest nad Oslavou,
  Czech Rep. .... **35 C9** 49 12N 16 10 E
Námestovo,
  Slovak Rep. .... **35 B12** 49 24N 19 25 E
Nametil, Mozam. .... **119 F4** 15 40 S 39 21 E
Namew L., Canada .. **143 C8** 54 14N 101 56W
Namgia, India ...... **93 D8** 31 48N 78 40 E
Namhkam, Burma ... **76 E1** 23 50N 97 41 E
Namho, Burma ..... **90 C4** 24 9N 99 1 E
Namhsan, Burma ... **90 D6** 22 48N 97 42 E
Namib Desert, Namibia **116 C2** 22 30 S 15 0 E
Namib-Naukluft △,
  Namibia .... **116 C2** 24 40 S 15 16 E
Namibe, Angola ..... **116 F2** 15 7 S 12 11 E
Namibe □, Angola ... **116 F2** 16 35 S 12 30 E
Namibe □, Angola ... **116 B1** 15 35 S 12 30 E
Namibia ■, Africa ... **116 C2** 22 0 S 18 9 E

Namibwoestyn =
  Namib Desert,
  Namibia .... **116 C2** 22 30 S 15 0 E
Namīn, Iran .... **101 C13** 38 25N 48 30 E
Namlan, Burma ..... **90 D6** 22 15N 97 24 E
Namlea, Indonesia .. **82 B3** 3 18 S 127 5 E
Namoi →, Australia . **129 A9** 30 12 S 149 30 E
Namous, O. en →,
  Algeria **111 B4** 31 0N 0 15W
Nampa, U.S.A. **158 E5** 43 34N 116 34W
Nampala, Mali **112 B3** 15 20N 5 30W
Namp'o, N. Korea ... **75 E13** 38 52N 125 10 E
Nampō-Shotō, Japan . **71 J10** 32 0N 140 0 E
Nampula, Mozam. ... **119 F4** 15 6 S 39 15 E
Namrole, Indonesia .. **82 B3** 3 46 S 126 46 E
Namsang, Burma .... **90 E6** 20 53N 97 43 E
Namsen →, Norway . **14 D14** 64 28N 11 37 E
Namslau = Namysłów,
  Poland .... **55 G4** 51 6N 17 42 E
Namsos, Norway .... **14 D14** 64 29N 11 30 E
Namtok Chat
  Trakan △, Thailand . **86 D3** 17 17N 100 40 E
Namtok Mae Surin △,
  Thailand .... **86 C2** 18 55N 98 2 E
Namtsy, Russia ..... **67 C13** 62 43N 129 37 E
Namtu, Burma ...... **90 D6** 23 5N 97 28 E
Namtumbo, Tanzania . **119 E4** 10 30 S 36 4 E
Namu, Canada **142 C3** 51 52N 127 50W
Namuka-i-Lau, Fiji .. **133 B3** 18 53 S 178 37W
Namumea, Tuvalu ... **123 B14** 5 41 S 176 9 E
Namur, Belgium .... **24 D4** 50 27N 4 52 E
Namur □, Belgium .. **24 D4** 50 17N 5 0 E
Namutoni, Namibia . **116 B2** 18 49 S 16 55 E
Namwala, Zambia ... **119 F2** 15 44 S 26 30 E
Namwŏn, S. Korea .. **75 G14** 35 23N 127 23 E
Namysłów, Poland .. **55 G4** 51 6N 17 42 E
Nan, Thailand ...... **86 C3** 18 48N 100 46 E
Nan →, Thailand ... **86 E3** 15 42N 100 9 E
Nan-ch'ang =
  Nanchang, China .. **77 C10** 28 42N 115 55 E
Nan Ling, China .... **79 E10** 25 0N 112 30 E
Nan Xian, China .... **77 C9** 29 20N 112 22 E
Nana, C.A.R. .... **114 A3** 5 0N 15 50 E
Nana, Romania ..... **53 F11** 44 17N 26 34 E
Nana-Barya →, C.A.R. **114 A3** 7 40N 17 29 E
Nana Kru, Liberia ... **112 E3** 4 55N 8 45W
Nanaimo, Canada ... **142 D4** 49 10N 124 0W
Nanakuli, U.S.A. **145 K13** 21 24N 158 9W
Nanam, N. Korea ... **75 D15** 41 44N 129 40 E
Nanan, China ...... **77 E12** 24 59N 118 21 E
Nanango, Australia .. **127 D5** 26 40 S 152 0 E
Nan'ao, China ...... **77 F11** 23 28N 117 5 E
Nanao, Japan ...... **71 F8** 37 0N 137 0 E
Nanbu, China ...... **76 B6** 31 18N 106 3 E
Nanchang, Jiangxi,
  China .... **77 C10** 28 42N 115 55 E
Nanchang, Kiangsi,
  China .... **77 C10** 28 34N 115 48 E
Nancheng, China .... **77 D11** 27 33N 116 35 E
Nanching = Nanjing,
  China .... **77 A12** 32 2N 118 47 E
Nanchong, China ... **76 B6** 30 43N 106 2 E
Nanchuan, China ... **76 C6** 29 9N 107 6 E
Nanchung = Nanchong,
  China .... **76 B6** 30 43N 106 2 E
Nancy, France ...... **19 D13** 48 42N 6 12 E
Nanda Devi, India .. **93 D8** 30 30N 79 59 E
Nanda Kot △, India . **93 D9** 30 30N 79 50 E
Nanda Kot, India ... **93 D9** 30 17N 80 5 E
Nandan, China ..... **76 E6** 24 58N 107 29 E
Nandan, Japan ..... **72 C6** 34 10N 134 42 E
Nanded, India ...... **94 E3** 19 10N 77 20 E
Nandewar Ra.,
  Australia .... **127 E5** 30 15 S 150 35 E
Nandgaon, India ... **94 D2** 20 19N 74 39 E
Nandigram, India .. **93 H12** 22 1N 87 58 E
Nandikotkur, India . **95 G4** 15 52N 78 18 E
Nandura, India ..... **94 D2** 20 52N 76 25 E
Nandurbar, India ... **94 D2** 21 20N 74 15 E
Nandyal, India ..... **95 G4** 15 30N 78 30 E
Nanfeng, Guangdong,
  China .... **77 F8** 23 45N 111 47 E
Nanfeng, Jiangxi, China **77 D11** 27 12N 116 28 E
Nanga-Eboko,
  Cameroon .... **113 E7** 4 41N 12 22 E
Nanga Parbat, Pakistan **93 B6** 35 10N 74 35 E
Nangade, Mozam. ... **119 E4** 11 5 S 39 36 E
Nangapinoh, Indonesia **85 C4** 0 20 S 111 44 E
Nangarhār □, Afghan. **91 B3** 34 20N 70 0 E
Nangatayap, Indonesia **85 C4** 1 32 S 110 34 E
Nangeya Mts., Uganda **118 B3** 3 30N 33 30 E
Nangis, France ..... **27 D10** 48 33N 3 1 E
Nangong, China .... **74 F8** 37 23N 115 22 E
Nangtud, Mt., Phil. .. **81 F4** 11 17N 122 11 E
Nanguneri, India ... **95 K3** 8 29N 77 40 E
Nangwary, Australia . **128 D4** 37 33 S 140 48 E
Nanhua, China ..... **76 E3** 25 13N 101 21 E
Nanhuang, China ... **75 F11** 36 58N 120 48 E
Nanhui, China ...... **77 B13** 31 5N 121 44 E
Nanjangud, India ... **95 H3** 12 6N 76 43 E
Nanji Shan, China .. **77 D13** 27 27N 121 4 E
Nanjian, China ..... **76 E3** 25 2N 100 25 E
Nanjiang, China .... **76 A6** 32 28N 106 51 E
Nanjing, Fujian, China **77 E11** 24 25N 117 20 E
Nanjing, Jiangsu, China **77 A12** 32 2N 118 47 E
Nanjirinji, Tanzania . **119 D4** 9 41 S 39 5 E
Nankana Sahib,
  Pakistan .... **92 D5** 31 27N 73 38 E
Nankang, China .... **77 E10** 25 40N 114 45 E
Nanking = Nanjing,
  China .... **77 A12** 32 2N 118 47 E
Nankoku, Japan .... **72 D5** 33 39N 133 44 E
Nanlang, China ..... **79 G10** 22 30N 113 32 E
Nanling, China ..... **77 B12** 30 55N 118 20 E
Nannial, India ...... **94 E4** 19 4N 79 38 E
Nanning, China ..... **76 F7** 22 48N 108 20 E
Nannup, Australia .. **125 F2** 33 59 S 115 48 E
Nanortalik, Greenland **10 E6** 60 10N 45 17W
Nanpan Jiang →,
  China .... **76 E6** 25 10N 106 5 E
Nanpara, India ..... **93 F9** 27 52N 81 33 E
Nanpi, China .... **74 E9** 38 2N 116 45 E
Nanping, Fujian, China **77 D12** 26 38N 118 10 E
Nanping, Henan, China **77 C9** 29 55N 112 3 E
Nanri Dao, China ... **77 E12** 25 15N 119 25 E
Nanripe, Mozam. ... **119 E4** 13 52 S 38 52 E
Nansei-Shotō =
  Ryūkyū-rettō, Japan **71 M3** 26 0N 126 0 E
Nansen Basin, Arctic **6 A10** 84 0N 50 0 E
Nansen Cordillera =
  Arctic .... **6 A** 87 0N 90 0 E
Nansen Land,
  Greenland **10 A6** 83 0N 43 0W
Nansen Sd., Canada . **10 A3** 81 0N 91 0W
Nansha, China ...... **69 F10** 22 45N 113 34 E
Nanshan I.,
  S. China Sea .... **78 B5** 10 45N 115 49 E
Nansio, Tanzania ... **118 C3** 2 3 S 33 4 E

Nant, France .... **28 D7** 44 1N 3 18 E
Nanterre, France ... **27 D9** 48 53N 2 13 E
Nantes, France **26 E5** 47 12N 1 33W
Nantiat, France ..... **28 B5** 46 1N 1 11 E
Nanticoke, U.S.A. .. **151 E8** 41 12N 76 0W
Nanton, Canada **142 C6** 50 21N 113 46W
Nantong, China .... **77 A13** 32 1N 120 52 E
Nantou, China ...... **69 F10** 22 32N 113 55 E
Nantou, Taiwan .... **77 F13** 23 57N 120 35 E
Nantua, France ..... **27 F12** 46 10N 5 35 E
Nantucket I., U.S.A. **148 E10** 41 16N 70 5W
Nantung = Nantong,
  China .... **77 A13** 32 1N 120 52 E
Nantwich, U.K. **20 D5** 53 4N 2 31W
Nanty Glo, U.S.A. .. **150 F6** 40 28N 78 50W
Nanuku Passage, Fiji **133 A3** 16 45 S 179 15W
Nanuque, Brazil .... **171 E3** 17 50 S 40 21W
Nanusa, Kepulauan,
  Indonesia .... **79 D7** 4 45N 127 1 E
Nanutarra Roadhouse,
  Australia .... **124 D2** 22 32 S 115 30 E
Nanxi, China .... **76 C5** 28 54N 104 59 E
Nanxiong, China ... **77 E10** 25 6N 114 15 E
Nanyang, China .... **74 H7** 33 11N 112 30 E
Nanyi Hu, China ... **77 B12** 31 5N 118 55 E
Nanyuki, Kenya .... **118 B4** 0 2N 37 4 E
Nanzhang, China ... **77 B8** 31 45N 111 50 E
Nao, C. de la, Spain . **41 G5** 38 44N 0 14 E
Naococane, L., Canada **141 B5** 52 50N 70 45W
Naogaon, Bangla. ... **90 C2** 24 52N 88 52 E
Naoné, Vanuatu .... **133 E6** 15 0 S 168 8 E
Náousa, Imathía,
  Greece .... **50 F6** 40 42N 22 9 E
Náousa, Kikládhes,
  Greece .... **49 D7** 37 7N 25 14 E
Naozhou Dao, China . **77 G8** 20 55N 110 20 E
Napa, U.S.A. **160 G4** 38 18N 122 17W
Napa →, U.S.A. **160 G4** 38 10N 122 19W
Napakiak, U.S.A. ... **144 F7** 60 42N 161 57W
Napamute, U.S.A. .. **144 F8** 61 33N 158 42W
Napanee, Canada ... **140 D4** 44 15N 77 0W
Napanoch, U.S.A. ... **151 E10** 41 44N 74 22W
Napanwainami,
  Indonesia .... **83 B3** 3 3 S 135 45 E
Napaskiak, U.S.A. ... **144 F7** 60 43N 161 55W
Nape, Laos .... **86 C5** 18 18N 105 6 E
Nape Pass = Keo Neua,
  Deo, Vietnam ...... **86 C5** 18 23N 105 10 E
Naperville, U.S.A. ... **157 C8** 41 46N 88 9W
Napf, Switz. .... **32 B5** 47 1N 7 56 E
Napier, N.Z. .... **130 F5** 39 30 S 176 56 E
Napier Broome B.,
  Australia .... **124 B4** 14 2 S 126 37 E
Napier Pen., Australia **126 A2** 12 4 S 135 43 E
Napierville, Canada . **151 A11** 45 11N 73 25W
Naples = Nápoli, Italy **47 B7** 40 50N 14 15 E
Naples, U.S.A. **153 J8** 26 8N 81 48W
Naples Park, U.S.A. . **153 J8** 26 17N 81 46W
Napo, China .... **76 F5** 23 22N 105 50 E
Napo □, Ecuador ... **168 D2** 0 30 S 77 0W
Napo →, Peru ...... **168 D3** 3 20 S 72 40W
Napoleon, N. Dak.,
  U.S.A. **154 B5** 46 30N 99 46W
Napoleon, Ohio, U.S.A. **157 C12** 41 23N 84 8W
Napoleon's Tomb,
  St. Helena .... **9 h** 15 56 S 5 42W
Nápoli, Italy .... **47 B7** 40 50N 14 15 E
Nápoli, G. di, Italy .. **47 B7** 40 43N 14 10 E
Nápoli Capodichino
  (NAP), Italy ✈ .... **47 B7** 40 53N 14 16 E
Napopo, Dem. Rep. of
  the Congo .... **118 B2** 4 15N 28 0 E
Nappanee, U.S.A. ... **157 C11** 41 27N 86 0W
Napperby, Australia . **128 B3** 33 9 S 138 7 E
Naqâda, Egypt ...... **106 B3** 25 53N 32 42 E
Naqadeh, Iran ...... **101 D11** 36 57N 45 23 E
Naqb, Ra's an, Jordan **103 F4** 30 0N 35 29 E
Naqqāsh, Iran ...... **97 C6** 35 40N 49 6 E
Nara, Japan .... **73 C7** 34 40N 135 49 E
Nara, Mali **112 B3** 15 10N 7 20W
Nara □, Japan ...... **73 C8** 34 30N 136 0 E
Nara Canal, Pakistan **92 G3** 24 30N 69 20 E
Nara Visa, U.S.A. ... **155 H3** 35 37N 103 6W
Naracoorte, Australia **128 D4** 36 58 S 140 45 E
Naradhan, Australia . **129 B7** 33 34 S 146 17 E
Naraini, India ...... **93 G9** 25 11N 80 29 E
Narasapur, India ... **94 F5** 16 26N 81 40 E
Narasaropet, India .. **95 F5** 16 14N 80 4 E
Narathiwat, Thailand **87 J3** 6 30N 101 48 E
Narayanapatnam, India **94 E5** 18 53N 83 10 E
Narayanganj, Bangla. **90 D3** 23 40N 90 33 E
Narayanpet, India .. **94 F3** 16 45N 77 30 E
Narbada =
  Narmada →, India . **92 J5** 21 38N 72 36 E
Narberth, U.K. **21 F3** 51 47N 4 44W
Narbonne, France .. **28 E7** 43 11N 3 0 E
Narborough, I. =
  Fernandina, I.,
  Ecuador .... **172 a** 0 25 S 91 30W
Narbuvollen, Norway **18 B8** 62 21N 11 27 E
Narcea →, Spain ... **42 B4** 43 33N 6 44W
Narcondam I., India . **95 H12** 13 20N 94 16 E
Nardín, Iran .... **97 B7** 37 3N 55 59 E
Nardò, Italy .... **47 B11** 40 1N 18 2 E
Narembeen, Australia **125 F2** 32 7 S 118 24 E
Narendranagar, India **92 D8** 30 10N 78 18 E
Nares Deep, Atl. Oc. **8 D6** 24 0N 57 0W
Nares Plain, Atl. Oc. . **8 D5** 22 0N 67 0W
Nares Str., Arctic ... **10 B3** 80 0N 70 0W
Naretha, Australia .. **125 F3** 31 0 S 124 45 E
Narew →, Poland ... **55 F7** 52 26N 20 41 E
Nari →, Pakistan ... **92 F2** 28 0N 67 40 E
Narin, Afghan. ..... **91 A3** 36 5N 69 0 E
Narindra, Helodranon'
  i, Madag. .... **117 A8** 14 55 S 47 30 E
Narino □, Colombia . **168 C2** 1 30N 78 0W
Narita □, Japan .... **73 B12** 35 47N 140 19 E
Narita, Tokyo ✈
  (NRT), Japan ...... **73 B12** 35 45N 140 25 E
Nariva Swamp,
  Trin. & Tob. **169 F9** 10 26N 61 4W
Närke, Sweden ..... **16 E8** 59 10N 15 0 E
Narmada →, India .. **92 J5** 21 38N 72 36 E
Narman, Turkey .... **101 B9** 40 26N 41 57 E
Narmland, Sweden .. **15 F15** 60 0N 13 30 E
Narnaul, India ..... **92 E7** 28 5N 76 11 E
Narni, Italy .... **45 F9** 42 30N 12 31 E
Naro Fominsk, Russia **58 E9** 55 23N 36 43 E
Narodnaya, Russia .. **56 A10** 65 5N 59 58 E
Narok, Kenya ...... **118 C4** 1 55 S 35 52 E
Narón, Spain **42 B2** 43 32N 8 9W
Narooma, Australia . **129 D9** 36 14 S 150 4 E
Narowal, Pakistan .. **91 B4** 32 6N 74 52 E
Narra, Phil. .... **81 G2** 9 18N 118 27 E
Narrabri, Australia .. **127 E4** 30 19 S 149 46 E
Narran →, Australia **127 D4** 28 37 S 148 12 E
Narrandera, Australia **129 C7** 34 42 S 146 31 E
Narrogin, Australia . **125 F2** 32 58 S 117 14 E
Narromine, Australia **129 B8** 32 12 S 148 12 E
Narrow Hills △,
  Canada **143 C8** 54 0N 104 37W

Narsaq, Greenland .. **10 E6** 60 57N 46 4W
Narsimhapur, India . **93 H8** 22 54N 79 14 E
Narsinghgarh, India . **92 H7** 23 45N 76 40 E
Narsinghpur, India .. **94 D7** 20 28N 85 5 E
Narsipatnam, India . **94 F6** 17 40N 82 37 E
Nartes, L., e, Albania . **50 F3** 40 32N 19 25 E
Nartkala, Russia ... **61 J6** 43 33N 43 51 E
Naruto, Kantō, Japan **73 B12** 35 36N 140 25 E
Naruto, Shikoku, Japan **72 C6** 34 11N 134 37 E
Naruto-Kaikyō, Japan **72 C6** 34 14N 134 39 E
Narva, Estonia ..... **58 C5** 59 23N 28 12 E
Narva →, Russia ... **15 G22** 59 27N 28 2 E
Narva Bay = Narva
  Laht, Estonia ...... **15 G19** 59 35N 27 35 E
Narva Laht, Estonia . **15 G19** 59 35N 27 35 E
Narvacan, Phil. ..... **80 C3** 17 25N 120 28 E
Narvik, Norway .... **14 B17** 68 28N 17 26 E
Narvskoye Vdkhr.,
  Russia .... **58 C5** 59 18N 28 14 E
Narwana, India ..... **92 E7** 29 39N 76 6 E
Narwiański △, Poland **55 E9** 52 53N 22 53 E
Naryan-Mar, Russia . **56 A9** 67 42N 53 12 E
Narym, Russia ...... **66 D9** 59 0N 81 30 E
Naryn, Kyrgyzstan .. **65 C7** 41 26N 75 58 E
Naryn →, Uzbekistan **65 C6** 40 57N 71 36 E
Nasa, Norway ...... **14 C16** 66 29N 15 23 E
Nasau, Fiji .... **133 A2** 17 9 S 179 27 E
Năsăud, Romania ... **53 C9** 47 19N 24 29 E
Nasawa, Vanuatu ... **133 E6** 15 8 S 168 8 E
Naseby, N.Z. .... **131 F5** 45 1 S 170 10 E
Naselle, U.S.A. **160 D3** 46 22N 123 49W
Naser, Buheirat en,
  Egypt .... **106 C3** 23 0N 32 30 E
Nashua, Iowa, U.S.A. **156 B4** 42 57N 92 32W
Nashua, Mont., U.S.A. **158 B10** 48 8N 106 22W
Nashua, N.H., U.S.A. **151 D13** 42 45N 71 28W
Nashville, Ark., U.S.A. **155 J8** 33 57N 93 51W
Nashville, Ga., U.S.A. **152 D6** 31 12N 83 15W
Nashville, Ill., U.S.A. **156 F7** 38 21N 89 23W
Nashville, Ind., U.S.A. **157 E10** 39 12N 86 15W
Nashville, Mich., U.S.A. **157 B11** 42 36N 85 5W
Nashville, Tenn., U.S.A. **149 G2** 36 10N 86 47W
Našice, Croatia ..... **52 E3** 45 32N 18 4 E
Nasielsk, Poland .... **55 F8** 52 35N 20 50 E
Nasik, India .... **94 E1** 19 58N 73 50 E
Nasipit, Phil. ...... **81 G5** 8 57N 125 19 E
Nasir, Sudan .... **107 F3** 8 36N 33 4 E
Nasirabad =
  Mymensingh, Bangla. **90 C3** 24 45N 90 24 E
Nasirabad, India ... **92 F6** 26 15N 74 45 E
Nasirabad, Pakistan . **92 E3** 28 23N 68 24 E
Nasiriyah = An
  Nāşiriyah, Iraq ..... **96 D5** 31 0N 46 15 E
Naskaupi →, Canada . **141 B7** 53 47N 60 51W
Naso, Italy .... **81 F3** 10 25N 121 57 E
Naso Pt., Phil. ..... **81 F3** 10 25N 121 57 E
Naşrābād, Iran ..... **97 C6** 34 8N 51 26 E
Naşrīān-e Pā'īn, Iran **96 C5** 32 52N 46 52 E
Nass →, Canada **142 C3** 55 0N 129 40W
Nassarawa, Nigeria . **113 D6** 8 32N 7 41 E
Nassarawa □, Nigeria **113 D6** 8 30N 8 20 E
Nassau, Bahamas ... **9 b** 25 5N 77 20W
Nassau, U.S.A. **151 D11** 42 31N 73 37W
Nassau, B., Chile ... **175 H3** 55 20 S 68 0W
Nassau International ✈
  (NAS), Bahamas ... **9 b** 25 3N 77 28W
Nasser, L. = Naser,
  Buheirat en, Egypt . **106 C3** 23 0N 32 30 E
Nasser City = Kôm
  Ombo, Egypt ...... **106 C3** 24 25N 32 52 E
Nassereith, Austria .. **33 B11** 47 19N 10 50 E
Nassian, Ivory C. ... **112 D4** 8 28N 3 28W
Nässjö, Sweden ..... **17 G8** 57 39N 14 42 E
Nastapoka →, Canada **140 A4** 56 55N 76 33W
Nastapoka, Is., Canada **140 A4** 56 55N 76 50W
Nasugbu, Phil. ..... **80 D3** 14 5N 120 38 E
Näsum, Sweden ..... **17 H8** 56 10N 14 29 E
Näsviken, Sweden .. **16 C10** 61 46N 16 52 E
Nata, Botswana .... **116 C4** 20 12 S 26 12 E
Nata →, Botswana .. **116 C4** 20 14 S 26 10 E
Natagaima, Colombia **168 C2** 3 37N 75 6W
Natal, Brazil .... **170 C4** 5 47 S 35 13W
Natal, Indonesia .... **84 B1** 0 35N 99 7 E
Natal Basin, Ind. Oc. **121 H2** 35 0 S 40 0 E
Natal Drakensberg △
  = S. Africa .... **117 D4** 29 27 S 29 30 E
Natalinci, Serbia & M. **52 F5** 44 15N 20 49 E
Natanz, Iran .... **97 C6** 33 30N 51 55 E
Natashquan, Canada **141 B7** 50 14N 61 46W
Natashquan →, Canada **141 B7** 50 7N 61 50W
Natchez, U.S.A. **155 K9** 31 34N 91 24W
Natchitoches, U.S.A. **155 K8** 31 46N 93 5W
Naters, Switz. ...... **32 D5** 46 19N 7 58 E
Natewa B., Fiji ..... **133 A2** 16 35 S 179 40 E
Nathalia, Australia . **129 D6** 36 1 S 145 13 E
Nathdwara, India .. **92 G5** 24 55N 73 50 E
Nati, Pta., Spain ... **38 A4** 40 3N 3 50 E
Natimuk, Australia . **128 D5** 36 42 S 142 0 E
Nation →, Canada . **142 B4** 55 30N 123 32W
National Capital
  District □,
  Papua N. G. .... **132 E4** 9 25 S 147 10 E
National City, U.S.A. **161 N9** 32 41N 117 6W
Natitingou, Benin .. **113 C5** 10 20N 1 26 E
Natividad, I., Mexico **162 B1** 27 50N 115 10W
Natividade, Brazil .. **171 D2** 11 43 S 47 47W
Natkyizin, Burma ... **86 E1** 14 57N 97 59 E
Natmauk, Burma ... **90 E5** 20 20N 95 24 E
Natogyi, Burma .... **90 E5** 21 25N 95 39 E
Natonin, Phil. ...... **80 C3** 17 8N 121 18 E
Natron, L., Tanzania **118 C4** 2 20 S 36 0 E
Natrona Heights,
  U.S.A. **150 F5** 40 37N 79 44W
Natrûn, W. el →, Egypt **106 H7** 30 25N 30 13 E
Nattai △, Australia . **129 C9** 34 12 S 150 22 E
Nättraby, Sweden .. **17 H9** 56 13N 15 31 E
Natukanaoka Pan,
  Namibia .... **116 B2** 18 40 S 15 45 E
Natuna Besar,
  Kepulauan, Indonesia **84 B3** 4 0N 108 15 E
Natuna Is. = Natuna
  Besar, Kepulauan,
  Indonesia .... **84 B3** 4 0N 108 15 E
Natuna Selatan,
  Kepulauan, Indonesia **85 B3** 2 45N 109 0 E
Natural Bridge, U.S.A. **151 B9** 44 5N 75 30W
Natural Bridges △,
  U.S.A. **159 H8** 37 36N 110 1W
Naturaliste, C.,
  Australia .... **127 G4** 40 50 S 148 15 E
Naturaliste Plateau,
  Ind. Oc. .... **121 H10** 34 0 S 112 0 E
Nau Qala, Afghan. .. **92 B3** 34 5N 68 5 E
Naucelle, France ... **28 D6** 44 11N 2 20 E
Nauders, Austria ... **34 E3** 46 54N 10 30 E
Nauen, Germany ... **30 C8** 52 36N 12 52 E
Naugard = Nowogard,
  Poland .... **54 E2** 53 41N 15 10 E
Naugatuck, U.S.A. .. **151 E11** 41 30N 73 3W
Naujaat = Repulse Bay,
  Canada **139 B11** 66 30N 86 30W
Naujan, Phil. ...... **80 E3** 13 20N 121 18 E

Naujoji Akmenė, *Lithuania* **54 B9** 56 19N 22 54 E
Naulila, *Angola* **115 F2** 17 13 S 14 39 E
Naumburg, *Germany* **30 D7** 51 9N 11 47 E
Naumburg am Queis = Nowogrodziec, *Poland* **55 G2** 51 12N 15 24 E
Naupada, *India* **94 E7** 18 34N 84 18 E
Nā'ūr at Tunayb, *Jordan* **103 D4** 31 48N 35 57 E
Nauru ■, *Pac. Oc.* **134 H8** 1 0 S 166 0 E
Naushahra = Nowshera, *Pakistan* **91 B3** 34 0N 72 0 E
Naushahro, *Pakistan* **92 F3** 26 50N 68 7 E
Naushon I., *U.S.A.* **151 E14** 41 29N 70 45W
Nausori, *Fiji* **133 B2** 18 2 S 178 32 E
Naustdal, *Norway* **18 C2** 61 31N 5 43 E
Nauta, *Peru* **168 D3** 4 31 S 73 35W
Naute ⌓, *Namibia* **116 D2** 26 55 S 17 57 E
Nautla, *Mexico* **163 C5** 20 20N 96 50W
Nauvoo, *U.S.A.* **156 D5** 40 33N 91 23W
Nava, *Mexico* **162 B4** 28 25N 100 46W
Nava, *Spain* **42 B5** 43 21N 5 31W
Nava del Rey, *Spain* **42 D5** 41 22N 5 6W
Navadwip, *India* **93 H13** 23 34N 88 20 E
Navahermosa, *Spain* **43 F6** 39 41N 4 28W
Navahrudak, *Belarus* **58 F3** 53 40N 25 50 E
Navai, *Fiji* **133 A1** 17 36 S 177 57 E
Navajo Reservoir, *U.S.A.* **159 H10** 36 48N 107 36W
Naval, *Phil.* **81 F5** 11 34N 124 23 E
Navalcarnero, *Spain* **42 E6** 40 17N 4 5W
Navalgund, *India* **95 G2** 15 34N 75 22 E
Navalmoral de la Mata, *Spain* **42 F5** 39 52N 5 33W
Navalvillar de Pela, *Spain* **43 F5** 39 9N 5 24W
Navan = An Uaimh, *Ireland* **23 C5** 53 39N 6 41W
Navanagar = Jamnagar, *India* **92 H4** 22 30N 70 6 E
Navapolatsk, *Belarus* **58 E5** 55 32N 28 37 E
Navarin, Mys, *Russia* **6 C16** 62 15N 179 5 E
Navarino, I., *Chile* **176 E3** 55 0 S 67 40W
Navarra □, *Spain* **40 C3** 42 40N 1 40W
Navarre, *Fla., U.S.A.* **153 E3** 30 24N 86 52W
Navarre, *Ohio, U.S.A.* **150 F3** 40 43N 81 31W
Navarro →, *U.S.A.* **160 F3** 39 11N 123 45W
Navas de San Juan, *Spain* **43 G7** 38 30N 3 19W
Navasota, *U.S.A.* **155 K6** 30 23N 96 5W
Navassa I., *W. Indies* **165 C5** 18 30N 75 0W
Nävekvarn, *Sweden* **17 F10** 58 38N 16 49 E
Naver →, *U.K.* **22 C4** 58 32N 4 14W
Navia, *Spain* **42 B4** 43 35N 6 42W
Navia →, *Spain* **42 B4** 43 15N 6 50W
Navia de Suarna, *Spain* **42 C3** 42 58N 7 3W
Navibandar, *India* **92 J3** 21 26N 69 48 E
Navidad, *Chile* **174 C1** 33 57 S 71 50W
Naviraí, *Brazil* **175 A5** 23 8 S 54 13W
Naviti, *Fiji* **133 A1** 17 7 S 177 15 E
Navlakhi, *India* **92 H4** 22 58N 70 28 E
Navlya, *Russia* **59 F8** 52 53N 34 30 E
Năvodari, *Romania* **53 F13** 44 19N 28 36 E
Navoi = Nawoiy, *Uzbekistan* **65 C2** 40 9N 65 22 E
Navojoa, *Mexico* **162 B3** 27 0N 109 30W
Navolato, *Mexico* **162 C3** 24 47N 107 42W
Návpaktos, *Greece* **48 C3** 38 24N 21 50 E
Návplion, *Greece* **48 D4** 37 33N 22 50 E
Navrongo, *Ghana* **113 C4** 10 51N 1 3W
Navsari, *India* **94 D1** 20 57N 72 59 E
Navua, *Fiji* **133 B2** 18 12 S 178 11 E
Nawa Kot, *Pakistan* **92 E4** 28 21N 71 24 E
Nawab Khan, *Pakistan* **92 D3** 30 17N 69 12 E
Nawabganj, *Bangla.* **90 C2** 24 35N 88 14 E
Nawabganj, *Ut. P., India* **93 F9** 26 56N 81 14 E
Nawabganj, *Ut. P., India* **93 E8** 28 32N 79 40 E
Nawabshah, *Pakistan* **91 D3** 26 15N 68 25 E
Nawada, *India* **93 G11** 24 50N 85 33 E
Nāwah, *Afghan.* **91 B2** 32 19N 67 53 E
Nawakot, *Nepal* **93 F11** 27 55N 85 10 E
Nawalgarh, *India* **92 F6** 27 50N 75 15 E
Nawanshahr, *India* **93 C6** 32 33N 74 48 E
Nawapara, *India* **94 D6** 20 46N 82 33 E
Nawar, Dasht-i-, *Afghan.* **91 B2** 33 52N 68 0 E
Nawāsīf, Ḩarrat, *Si. Arabia* **98 B3** 21 20N 42 10 E
Nawi, *Sudan* **106 D3** 18 32N 30 50 E
Nawng Hpa, *Burma* **90 D7** 22 30N 98 30 E
Nawoiy, *Uzbekistan* **65 C2** 40 9N 65 22 E
Nawş, Ra's, *Oman* **99 C6** 17 15N 55 16 E
Naxçıvan, *Azerbaijan* **101 C11** 39 12N 45 15 E
Naxçıvan □, *Azerbaijan* **101 C11** 39 25N 45 26 E
Náxos, *Greece* **49 D7** 37 8N 25 25 E
Naxxar, *Malta* **38 F7** 35 55N 14 27 E
Nay, *France* **28 E3** 43 10N 0 18W
Nay, Mui, *Vietnam* **78 B3** 12 55N 109 23 E
Nāy Band, *Būshehr, Iran* **97 E7** 27 20N 52 40 E
Nāy Band, *Khorāsān, Iran* **97 C8** 32 20N 57 34 E
Naya →, *Colombia* **168 C2** 3 13N 77 22W
Nayagarh, *India* **94 D7** 20 8N 85 6 E
Nayakhan, *Russia* **67 C16** 61 56N 159 0 E
Nayarit □, *Mexico* **162 C4** 22 0N 105 0W
Nayau, *Fiji* **133 B2** 18 6 S 178 10 E
Nayé, *Senegal* **112 C2** 14 28N 12 12W
Nayong, *China* **76 D5** 26 50N 105 20 E
Nayoro, *Japan* **70 B11** 44 21N 142 28 E
Nayudupeta, *India* **95 H4** 13 54N 79 54 E
Nayyāl, W. →, *Si. Arabia* **96 D3** 28 35N 39 4 E
Nazaré, *Bahia, Brazil* **171 D4** 13 2 S 39 0W
Nazaré, *Pará, Brazil* **173 B7** 6 25 S 52 29W
Nazaré, *Tocantins, Brazil* **170 C2** 6 23 S 47 40W
Nazaré, *Portugal* **43 F1** 39 36N 9 4W
Nazareth = Nazerat, *Israel* **103 C4** 32 42N 35 17 E
Nazareth, *U.S.A.* **151 F9** 40 44N 75 19W
Nazas, *Mexico* **162 B4** 25 10N 104 6W
Nazas →, *Mexico* **162 B4** 25 35N 103 25W
Nazca, *Peru* **172 C3** 14 50 S 74 57W
Nazca Ridge, *Pac. Oc.* **135 K19** 20 0 S 80 0W
Naze, The, *U.K.* **21 F9** 51 53N 1 18 E
Nazerat, *Israel* **103 C4** 32 42N 35 17 E
Nāzīk, *Iran* **101 C11** 39 1N 45 4 E
Nazilli, *Turkey* **49 D10** 37 55N 28 15 E
Nazir Hat, *Bangla.* **90 D3** 22 35N 91 49 E
Nazko, *Canada* **142 C4** 53 1N 123 37W
Nazko →, *Canada* **142 C4** 53 7N 123 34W
Nazret, *Ethiopia* **107 F4** 8 32N 39 22 E
Nazwa, *Oman* **99 B7** 22 56N 57 32 E
Ncama, *Eq. Guin.* **114 B2** 1 55N 10 56 E
Nchanga, *Zambia* **119 E2** 12 30 S 27 49 E
Ncheu, *Malawi* **119 E3** 14 50 S 34 47 E
Ndala, *Tanzania* **118 C3** 4 45 S 33 15 E
Ndalatando, *Angola* **115 D2** 9 12 S 14 48 E
Ndali, *Benin* **113 D5** 9 50N 2 46 E
Ndareda, *Tanzania* **118 C4** 4 12 S 35 30 E
Ndélé, *C.A.R.* **114 A4** 8 25N 20 36 E
Ndendé, *Gabon* **114 C2** 2 22 S 11 23 E
Ndiael ⌓, *Senegal* **112 B1** 16 15N 16 0W
Ndikinimeki, *Cameroon* **113 E7** 4 46N 10 50 E
Ndindi, *Gabon* **114 C2** 3 46 S 11 9 E
N'Dioum, *Senegal* **112 B2** 16 31N 14 39W
Ndjamena, *Chad* **109 F2** 12 10N 14 59 E
Ndjolé, *Gabon* **114 C2** 0 10 S 10 45 E
Ndogo, Lagune, *Gabon* **114 C2** 2 35 S 10 0 E
Ndoki-Nouabalé ⌓, *Congo* **114 B3** 2 32N 16 32 E
Ndola, *Zambia* **119 E2** 13 0 S 28 34 E
Ndoto Mts., *Kenya* **118 B4** 2 0N 37 0 E
Ndoua, C., *N. Cal.* **133 V20** 22 24 S 166 56 E
Ndouba, *Congo* **114 C2** 0 9 S 14 4 E
Nduguti, *Tanzania* **118 C3** 4 18 S 34 41 E
Ndumu ⌓, *S. Africa* **117 D5** 26 52 S 32 15 E
Nea →, *Norway* **18 A8** 63 15N 11 0 E
Néa Alikarnassós, *Greece* **49 F7** 35 18N 25 13 E
Néa Ankhíalos, *Greece* **48 B4** 39 16N 22 49 E
Néa Epídhavros, *Greece* **48 D5** 37 40N 23 7 E
Néa Flippiás, *Greece* **48 B2** 39 12N 20 53 E
Néa Ionia, *Greece* **48 B4** 39 21N 22 56 E
Néa Kallikrátia, *Greece* **50 F7** 40 21N 23 3 E
Néa Mákri, *Greece* **48 C5** 38 5N 23 59 E
Néa Moudhaniá, *Greece* **50 F7** 40 15N 23 17 E
Néa Péramos, *Attikí, Greece* **48 C5** 38 0N 23 26 E
Néa Péramos, *Kavála, Greece* **51 F8** 40 50N 24 18 E
Néa Víssi, *Greece* **51 E10** 41 34N 26 33 E
Néa Zíkhna, *Greece* **50 E7** 41 2N 23 49 E
Neagari, *Japan* **73 A8** 36 26N 136 25 E
Neagh, Lough, *U.K.* **23 B5** 54 37N 6 25W
Neah Bay, *U.S.A.* **160 B2** 48 22N 124 37W
Neale, L., *Australia* **124 D5** 24 15 S 130 0 E
Neales, The →, *Australia* **127 D2** 28 8 S 136 47 E
Neamati, *India* **90 B5** 26 50N 94 20 E
Neamţ □, *Romania* **53 C11** 47 0N 26 20 E
Neápolis, *Kozáni, Greece* **50 F5** 40 20N 21 24 E
Neápolis, *Kríti, Greece* **39 E6** 35 15N 25 37 E
Neápolis, *Lakonía, Greece* **48 E5** 36 27N 23 8 E
Near Is., *U.S.A.* **144 K1** 52 30N 174 0 E
Neath, *U.K.* **21 F4** 51 39N 3 48W
Neath Port Talbot □, *U.K.* **21 F4** 51 42N 3 45W
Neba, Î., *N. Cal.* **133 T17** 20 10 S 163 57 E
Nebbou, *Burkina Faso* **113 C4** 11 9N 1 51W
Nebelat el Hagana, *Sudan* **107 E2** 13 13N 29 2 E
Nebine Cr. →, *Australia* **127 D4** 29 27 S 146 56 E
Nebitdag, *Turkmenistan* **57 G9** 39 30N 54 22 E
Nebka, *Algeria* **110 C4** 27 28N 3 12W
Nebo, *Australia* **126 C4** 21 42 S 148 42 E
Nebolchy, *Russia* **58 C7** 59 8N 33 18 E
Nebraska □, *U.S.A.* **154 E5** 41 30N 99 30W
Nebraska City, *U.S.A.* **154 E7** 40 41N 95 52W
Nébrodi, Monti, *Italy* **47 E7** 37 54N 14 35 E
Necedah, *U.S.A.* **154 C9** 44 2N 90 4W
Nechako →, *Canada* **142 C4** 53 55N 122 42W
Neches →, *U.S.A.* **155 L8** 29 58N 93 51W
Nechisar △, *Ethiopia* **107 F4** 5 58N 37 55 E
Neckar →, *Germany* **31 F4** 49 27N 8 29 E
Neckartal-Odenwald ⌓, *Germany* **31 F5** 49 30N 9 5 E
Necker I., *U.S.A.* **145 G11** 23 35N 164 42W
Necochea, *Argentina* **174 D4** 38 30 S 58 50W
Nectar Brook, *Australia* **128 B2** 32 43 S 137 57 E
Neda, *Spain* **42 B2** 43 30N 8 9W
Nedalshytta, *Norway* **18 B9** 62 59N 12 3 E
Nedelino, *Bulgaria* **51 E9** 41 27N 25 3 E
Nedelišće, *Croatia* **45 B13** 46 23N 16 22 E
Nederland = Netherlands ■, *Europe* **24 C5** 52 0N 5 30 E
Nédha →, *Greece* **48 D3** 37 25N 21 45 E
Nedoboyivtsi, *Ukraine* **53 B11** 48 26N 26 21 E
Nedreberg, *Norway* **18 D8** 60 59N 11 41 E
Nedroma, *Algeria* **111 A4** 35 1N 1 45W
Nedstrand, *Norway* **18 E2** 59 21N 5 49 E
Needles, *Canada* **142 D5** 49 53N 118 7W
Needles, *U.S.A.* **161 L12** 34 51N 114 37W
Needles, The, *U.K.* **21 G6** 50 39N 1 35W
Needles Pt., *N.Z.* **130 C4** 36 3 S 175 25 E
Neely Henry L., *U.S.A.* **152 B3** 33 55N 86 2W
Ñeembucú □, *Paraguay* **174 B4** 27 0 S 58 0W
Neemuch = Nimach, *India* **92 G6** 24 30N 74 56 E
Neenah, *U.S.A.* **148 C1** 44 11N 88 28W
Neepawa, *Canada* **143 C9** 50 15N 99 30W
Neeses, *U.S.A.* **152 B8** 33 33N 81 7W
Nefta, *Tunisia* **108 B1** 33 53N 7 50 E
Neftah Sidi Boubekeur, *Algeria* **111 A5** 35 1N 0 4 E
Neftçala, *Azerbaijan* **97 B6** 39 19N 49 12 E
Neftechala = Neftçala, *Azerbaijan* **97 B6** 39 19N 49 12 E
Neftegorsk, *Russia* **61 H4** 44 25N 39 45 E
Neftekamsk, *Russia* **64 C5** 56 6N 54 17 E
Neftekumsk, *Russia* **61 H7** 44 46N 44 50 E
Neftenbach, *Switz.* **33 A7** 47 32N 8 41 E
Nefyn, *U.K.* **20 E3** 52 56N 4 31W
Négala, *Mali* **112 C3** 12 52N 8 30W
Negapatam = Nagappattinam, *India* **95 J4** 10 46N 79 51 E
Negara, *Indonesia* **79 J17** 8 22 S 114 37 E
Negaunee, *U.S.A.* **148 B2** 46 30N 87 36W
Negele, *Ethiopia* **107 F4** 5 20N 39 36 E
Negeri Sembilan □, *Malaysia* **84 B2** 2 45N 102 10 E
Negev Desert = Hanegev, *Israel* **103 E4** 30 50N 35 0 E
Negoiul, Vf., *Romania* **53 E9** 45 38N 24 35 E
Negombo, *Sri Lanka* **95 L4** 7 12N 79 50 E
Negotin, *Serbia & M.* **50 B6** 44 16N 22 37 E
Negotino, *Macedonia* **50 E6** 41 29N 22 7 E
Negra, Peña, *Spain* **42 C4** 42 11N 6 30W
Negra, Pta., *Mauritania* **110 D1** 22 54N 16 18W
Negra, Pta., *Peru* **172 B1** 6 6 S 81 10W
Negra Pt., *Phil.* **80 B3** 18 40N 120 50 E
Negrais, C. = Maudin Sun, *Burma* **90 G5** 16 0N 94 30 E
Negreşti, *Romania* **53 D12** 46 50N 27 30 E
Negreşti-Oaş, *Romania* **53 C8** 47 52N 23 26 E
Negril, *Jamaica* **164 a** 18 22N 78 20W
Négrine, *Algeria* **111 B6** 34 30N 7 30 E
Negro →, *Argentina* **176 B4** 41 2 S 62 47W
Negro →, *Bolivia* **173 C5** 14 11 S 63 7W
Negro →, *Brazil* **169 D6** 3 0 S 60 0W
Negro →, *Uruguay* **174 C4** 33 24 S 58 22W
Negros, *Phil.* **81 G4** 9 30N 122 40 E
Negros Occidental □, *Phil.* **81 F4** 10 0N 122 55 E
Negros Oriental □, *Phil.* **81 G4** 9 45N 123 0 E
Negru Vodă, *Romania* **53 G13** 43 47N 28 21 E
Neguac, *Canada* **141 C6** 47 15N 65 5W
Nehalem →, *U.S.A.* **160 E3** 45 40N 123 56W
Nehāvand, *Iran* **97 C6** 35 56N 49 31 E
Nehbandān, *Iran* **97 D9** 31 35N 60 5 E
Nehoiu, *Romania* **53 E11** 45 24N 26 20 E
Nei Monggol Zizhiqu □, *China* **74 D7** 42 0N 112 0 E
Neiafu, *Tonga* **133 P14** 18 39 S 173 59W
Neidenburg = Nidzica, *Poland* **55 E7** 53 25N 20 28 E
Neiges, Piton des, *Réunion* **121 c** 21 5 S 55 29 E
Neijiang, *China* **76 C5** 29 35N 104 55 E
Neikiang = Neijiang, *China* **76 C5** 29 35N 104 55 E
Neilingding Dao, *China* **69 G10** 22 25N 113 48 E
Neill I., *India* **95 J11** 11 50N 93 3 E
Neillsville, *U.S.A.* **154 C9** 44 34N 90 36W
Neilton, *U.S.A.* **158 C2** 47 25N 123 53W
Neiqiu, *China* **74 F8** 37 15N 114 30 E
Neisse = Nysa →, *Europe* **30 C10** 52 4N 14 46 E
Neiva, *Colombia* **168 C2** 2 56N 75 18W
Neixiang, *China* **74 H6** 33 10N 111 52 E
Nejanilini L., *Canada* **143 B9** 59 33N 97 48W
Nejd = Najd, *Si. Arabia* **88 C3** 26 30N 42 0 E
Nejo, *Ethiopia* **107 F4** 9 30N 35 28 E
Nekā, *Iran* **97 B7** 36 39N 53 19 E
Nekemte, *Ethiopia* **107 F4** 9 4N 36 30 E
Nêkheb, *Egypt* **106 B3** 25 10N 32 48 E
Neksø, *Denmark* **17 J9** 55 4N 15 8 E
Nelamangala, *India* **95 H3** 13 6N 77 24 E
Nelas, *Portugal* **42 E3** 40 32N 7 52W
Nelaug, *Norway* **18 F5** 58 39N 8 40 E
Nelia, *Australia* **126 C3** 20 39 S 142 12 E
Nelidovo, *Russia* **58 D7** 56 13N 32 49 E
Neligh, *U.S.A.* **154 D5** 42 8N 98 2W
Nelkan, *Russia* **67 D14** 57 40N 136 4 E
Nellikuppam, *India* **95 J4** 11 46N 79 43 E
Nellore, *India* **95 G4** 14 27N 79 59 E
Nelson, *Canada* **142 D5** 49 30N 117 20W
Nelson, *N.Z.* **131 B8** 41 18 S 173 16 E
Nelson, *U.K.* **20 D5** 53 50N 2 13W
Nelson, *Ariz., U.S.A.* **159 J7** 35 31N 113 19W
Nelson, *Nev., U.S.A.* **161 K12** 35 42N 114 50W
Nelson □, *N.Z.* **131 B8** 41 20 S 173 20 E
Nelson →, *Canada* **143 C9** 54 33N 98 2W
Nelson, C., *Australia* **128 E4** 38 26 S 141 32 E
Nelson, C., *Papua N. G.* **132 E5** 9 0 S 149 20 E
Nelson, Estrecho, *Chile* **176 D2** 51 30 S 75 0W
Nelson Bay, *Australia* **129 B10** 32 43 S 152 9 E
Nelson Forks, *Canada* **142 B4** 59 30N 124 0W
Nelson House, *Canada* **143 B9** 55 47N 98 51W
Nelson L., *Canada* **143 B8** 55 48N 100 7W
Nelson Lakes △, *N.Z.* **131 B7** 41 55 S 172 44 E
Nelspoort, *S. Africa* **116 E3** 32 7 S 23 0 E
Nelspruit, *S. Africa* **117 D5** 25 29 S 30 59 E
Néma, *Mauritania* **112 B3** 16 40N 7 15W
Neman = Nemunas →, *Lithuania* **15 J19** 55 25N 21 10 E
Neman, *Russia* **15 J20** 55 2N 22 2 E
Nembrala, *Indonesia* **82 D2** 10 53 S 122 50 E
Neméa, *Greece* **48 D4** 37 49N 22 40 E
Nemecký Brod = Havlíčkův Brod, *Czech Rep.* **34 B8** 49 36N 15 33 E
Nemeiben L., *Canada* **143 B7** 55 20N 105 20W
Nemërçkë, Mal, *Albania* **50 F4** 40 15N 20 15 E
Nemira, Vf., *Romania* **53 D11** 46 17N 26 19 E
Nemiscau, *Canada* **140 B4** 51 18N 76 54W
Nemiscau, L., *Canada* **140 B4** 51 25N 76 40W
Nemours = Ghazaouet, *Algeria* **111 A4** 35 8N 1 50W
Nemours, *France* **27 D9** 48 16N 2 40 E
Nemšová, *Slovak Rep.* **35 C11** 48 58N 18 7 E
Nemunas →, *Lithuania* **15 J19** 55 25N 21 10 E
Nemuro, *Japan* **70 C12** 43 20N 145 35 E
Nemuro-Kaikyō, *Japan* **70 C12** 43 30N 145 30 E
Nemyriv, *Ukraine* **55 H10** 50 7N 23 27 E
Nen Jiang →, *China* **75 B13** 45 28N 124 30 E
Nenagh, *Ireland* **23 D3** 52 52N 8 11W
Nenana, *U.S.A.* **144 D10** 64 34N 149 5W
Nenasi, *Malaysia* **87 L4** 3 9N 103 23 E
Nene →, *U.K.* **21 E8** 52 49N 0 11 E
Nénita, *Greece* **49 C8** 38 14N 26 6 E
Nenjiang, *China* **69 B7** 49 10N 125 10 E
Neno, *Malawi* **119 F3** 15 25 S 34 40 E
Nenzing, *Austria* **33 B9** 47 11N 9 42 E
Neodesha, *U.S.A.* **155 G7** 37 25N 95 41W
Neoga, *U.S.A.* **157 E8** 39 19N 88 27W
Neokhórion, *Aitolía kai Akarnanía, Greece* **48 C3** 38 25N 21 17 E
Neokhórion, *Árta, Greece* **48 B2** 39 4N 21 0 E
Néon Karlovásion, *Greece* **49 D8** 37 45N 26 42 E
Néon Petrítsi, *Greece* **50 E7** 41 16N 23 15 E
Neópolis, *Brazil* **170 D4** 10 18 S 36 35W
Neora Valley, *India* **93 F13** 27 0N 88 45 E
Neosho, *U.S.A.* **155 G7** 36 52N 94 22W
Neosho →, *U.S.A.* **155 H7** 36 48N 95 18W
Nepal ■, *Asia* **93 F11** 28 0N 84 30 E
Nepalganj, *Nepal* **93 E9** 28 5N 81 40 E
Nepalganj Road, *India* **93 E9** 28 1N 81 41 E
Nepean B., *Australia* **128 C2** 35 42 S 137 37 E
Nephi, *U.S.A.* **158 G8** 39 43N 111 50W
Nephin, *Ireland* **23 B2** 54 1N 9 22W
Nepi, *Italy* **45 F9** 42 14N 12 21 E
Nepomuk, *Czech Rep.* **34 B6** 49 29N 13 35 E
Neppel = Moses Lake, *U.S.A.* **158 C4** 47 8N 119 17W
Neptune, *U.S.A.* **151 F10** 40 13N 74 2W
Neptune Is., *Australia* **128 C2** 35 17 S 136 10 E
Nera →, *Italy* **45 F9** 42 26N 12 24 E
Nera →, *Romania* **52 F6** 44 48N 21 25 E
Nérac, *France* **28 D4** 44 8N 0 21 E
Nerang, *Australia* **127 D5** 27 58 S 153 20 E
Nerastro, Sarīr, *Libya* **108 D4** 24 20N 20 37 E
Neratovice, *Czech Rep.* **34 A7** 50 16N 14 31 E
Nerchinsk, *Russia* **67 D12** 52 0N 116 39 E
Nereju, *Romania* **53 E11** 45 43N 26 43 E
Nerekhta, *Russia* **58 D11** 57 26N 40 38 E
Neresnytsya, *Ukraine* **53 B8** 48 7N 23 46 E
Néret, L., *Canada* **141 B5** 54 45N 70 44W
Neretvanski Kanal, *Croatia* **45 E14** 43 7N 17 10 E
Neringa, *Lithuania* **15 J19** 55 20N 21 5 E
Neris →, *Lithuania* **15 J21** 55 8N 24 16 E
Nerja, *Spain* **43 J7** 36 43N 3 55W
Nerl →, *Russia* **58 D11** 56 11N 40 34 E
Nerpio, *Spain* **41 G2** 38 11N 2 16W
Nerva, *Spain* **43 H4** 37 42N 6 30W
Nervi, *Italy* **44 D6** 44 23N 9 2 E
Neryungri, *Russia* **67 D13** 57 38N 124 28 E
Nes, *Iceland* **11 B9** 65 53N 17 24W
Nes, *Norway* **18 D6** 60 34N 9 59 E
Nesbyen, *Norway* **18 D6** 60 34N 9 8 E
Nescopeck, *U.S.A.* **151 E8** 41 3N 76 12W
Nesebŭr, *Bulgaria* **51 D11** 42 41N 27 46 E
Neset, *Norway* **18 C7** 61 53N 10 7 E
Nesflaten, *Norway* **18 E3** 59 38N 6 48 E
Neskaupstaður, *Iceland* **11 B13** 65 9N 13 42W
Nesland, *Norway* **18 E4** 59 31N 7 59 E
Neslandsvatn, *Norway* **18 F6** 58 57N 9 10 E
Nesoddtangen, *Norway* **18 E7** 59 48N 10 40 E
Ness, L., *U.K.* **22 D4** 57 15N 4 32W
Ness City, *U.S.A.* **154 F5** 38 27N 99 54W
Nesslau, *Switz.* **33 B8** 47 14N 9 13 E
Nesterov, *Russia* **54 D9** 54 38N 22 41 E
Nesterov, *Ukraine* **59 G2** 50 4N 23 58 E
Nestórion, *Greece* **50 F5** 40 24N 21 5 E
Néstos →, *Greece* **51 E8** 41 20N 24 35 E
Nesttun, *Norway* **18 D2** 60 19N 5 20 E
Nesvady, *Slovak Rep.* **35 D11** 47 56N 18 7 E
Nesvizh = Nyasvizh, *Belarus* **59 F4** 53 14N 26 38 E
Netanya, *Israel* **103 C3** 32 20N 34 51 E
Netarhat, *India* **93 H11** 23 29N 84 16 E
Nete →, *Belgium* **24 C4** 51 7N 4 14 E
Netherdale, *Australia* **126 K6** 21 10 S 148 33 E
Netherlands ■, *Europe* **24 C5** 52 0N 5 30 E
Netherlands Antilles ⊠, *W. Indies* **168 A4** 12 15N 69 0W
Netherlands East Indies = Indonesia ■, *Asia* **85 C4** 5 0 S 115 0 E
Netherlands Guiana = Suriname ■, *S. Amer.* **169 C6** 4 0N 56 0W
Neto →, *Italy* **47 C10** 39 12N 17 9 E
Netrakona, *Bangla.* **90 C3** 24 53N 90 47 E
Netrang, *India* **92 J5** 21 39N 73 21 E
Netstal, *Switz.* **33 B8** 47 3N 9 3 E
Nettancourt, *France* **27 D11** 48 51N 4 57 E
Nettetal, *Germany* **30 D2** 51 19N 6 12 E
Nettilling L., *Canada* **139 B12** 66 30N 71 0W
Nettuno, *Italy* **46 A5** 41 27N 12 39 E
Netzahualcoyotl, Presa, *Mexico* **163 D6** 17 10N 93 30W
Neu-Bentschen = Zbąszynek, *Poland* **55 F2** 52 16N 15 51 E
Neu-Isenburg, *Germany* **31 E4** 50 3N 8 42 E
Neu-Langenburg = Tukuyu, *Tanzania* **119 D3** 9 17 S 33 35 E
Neu-Mecklenberg = New Ireland, *Papua N. G.* **132 B6** 3 20 S 151 50 E
Neu Pommern = New Britain, *Papua N. G.* **132 C6** 5 50 S 150 20 E
Neu-Sandec = Nowy Sącz, *Poland* **55 J7** 49 40N 20 41 E
Neu Sandez = Nowy Sącz, *Poland* **55 J7** 49 40N 20 41 E
Neu-Ulm, *Germany* **31 G6** 48 22N 10 0 E
Neubrandenburg, *Germany* **30 B9** 53 33N 13 15 E
Neubukow, *Germany* **30 A7** 54 2N 11 39 E
Neuburg, *Germany* **31 G7** 48 44N 11 11 E
Neuchâtel, *Switz.* **32 C3** 47 0N 6 55 E
Neuchâtel □, *Switz.* **32 C3** 47 0N 6 55 E
Neuchâtel, Lac de, *Switz.* **32 C3** 46 53N 6 50 E
Neudau, *Austria* **34 D9** 47 11N 16 6 E
Neuenberg an der Elbe = Nymburk, *Czech Rep.* **34 A8** 50 10N 15 1 E
Neuenegg, *Switz.* **32 C4** 46 54N 7 18 E
Neuenhagen, *Germany* **30 C9** 52 30N 13 38 E
Neuenhaus, *Germany* **30 C2** 52 30N 6 58 E
Neuenhof, *Switz.* **33 B6** 47 27N 8 19 E
Neuf-Brisach, *France* **27 D14** 48 1N 7 30 E
Neufahrn, *Bayern, Germany* **31 G8** 48 41N 12 11 E
Neufahrn, *Bayern, Germany* **31 G7** 48 18N 11 40 E
Neufchâteau, *Belgium* **24 E5** 49 50N 5 25 E
Neufchâteau, *France* **27 D12** 48 21N 5 40 E
Neufchâtel-en-Bray, *France* **26 C8** 49 44N 1 26 E
Neufchâtel-sur-Aisne, *France* **27 C11** 49 26N 4 1 E
Neuhaus = Jindřichův Hradec, *Czech Rep.* **34 B8** 49 10N 15 2 E
Neuhaus, *Germany* **30 B6** 53 17N 10 56 E
Neuhäusel = Nové Zámky, *Slovak Rep.* **35 C11** 48 2N 18 8 E
Neuhausen, *Switz.* **33 A7** 47 41N 8 37 E
Neuillé-Pont-Pierre, *France* **26 E7** 47 33N 0 33 E
Neuilly-St-Front, *France* **27 C10** 49 10N 3 15 E
Neukalen, *Germany* **30 B8** 53 49N 12 46 E
Neumarkt = Nowy Targ, *Poland* **55 J7** 49 29N 20 2 E
Neumarkt = Środa Śląska, *Poland* **55 G3** 51 10N 16 36 E
Neumarkt, *Germany* **31 F7** 49 26N 11 27 E
Neumarktl = Tržič, *Slovenia* **45 B11** 46 22N 14 18 E
Neumittelwalde = Międzybórz, *Poland* **55 G4** 51 25N 17 34 E
Neumünster, *Germany* **30 A5** 54 4N 9 58 E
Neung-sur-Beuvron, *France* **27 E8** 47 30N 1 50 E
Neunkirch, *Switz.* **33 A7** 47 42N 8 30 E
Neunkirchen, *Austria* **34 D9** 47 43N 16 4 E
Neunkirchen, *Germany* **31 F3** 49 20N 7 9 E
Neuquén, *Argentina* **176 A3** 38 55 S 68 0W
Neuquén □, *Argentina* **174 D2** 38 0 S 69 50W
Neuquén →, *Argentina* **176 A3** 38 59 S 68 0W
Neuruppin, *Germany* **30 C8** 52 55N 12 48 E
Neusalz an der Oder = Nowa Sól, *Poland* **55 G2** 51 48N 15 44 E
Neusäss, *Germany* **31 G6** 48 24N 10 50 E
Neusatz = Novi Sad, *Serbia & M.* **52 E4** 45 18N 19 52 E
Neuse →, *U.S.A.* **149 H7** 35 6N 76 29W
Neusiedl, *Austria* **35 D9** 47 57N 16 50 E
Neusiedler See, *Austria* **35 D9** 47 50N 16 47 E
Neusiedler See-Seewinkel △, *Austria* **35 D9** 47 50N 16 45 E
Neusohl = Banská Bystrica, *Slovak Rep.* **35 C12** 48 46N 19 14 E
Neuss, *Germany* **30 D2** 51 11N 6 42 E
Neussargues-Moissac, *France* **28 C7** 45 9N 3 0 E
Neustadt = Lwówek, *Poland* **55 F3** 52 28N 16 10 E
Neustadt = Prudnik, *Poland* **55 H4** 50 20N 17 38 E
Neustadt = Wejherowo, *Poland* **54 D5** 54 35N 18 12 E
Neustadt, *Bayern, Germany* **31 F8** 49 44N 12 10 E
Neustadt, *Bayern, Germany* **31 G7** 48 48N 11 46 E
Neustadt, *Bayern, Germany* **31 F6** 49 34N 10 37 E
Neustadt, *Bayern, Germany* **31 E7** 50 19N 11 7 E
Neustadt, *Brandenburg, Germany* **30 C8** 52 50N 12 27 E
Neustadt, *Hessen, Germany* **30 E5** 50 51N 9 9 E
Neustadt, *Niedersachsen, Germany* **30 C5** 52 30N 9 30 E
Neustadt, *Rhld-Pfz., Germany* **31 F4** 49 21N 8 10 E
Neustadt, *Sachsen, Germany* **30 D10** 51 2N 14 12 E
Neustadt, *Schleswig-Holstein, Germany* **30 A6** 54 6N 10 49 E
Neustadt, *Thüringen, Germany* **30 E7** 50 45N 11 43 E
Neustädtel = Nowe Miasteczko, *Poland* **55 G2** 51 42N 15 42 E
Neustädtl = Novo Mesto, *Slovenia* **45 C12** 45 47N 15 12 E
Neustettin = Szczecinek, *Poland* **54 E3** 53 43N 16 41 E
Neustrelitz, *Germany* **30 B9** 53 21N 13 4 E
Neutitschein = Nový Jičín, *Czech Rep.* **35 B11** 49 30N 18 2 E
Neuvic, *France* **28 C6** 45 23N 2 16 E
Neuville-sur-Saône, *France* **29 C8** 45 52N 4 51 E
Neuvy-le-Roi, *France* **26 E7** 47 36N 0 36 E
Neuvy-St-Sépulchre, *France* **27 F8** 46 35N 1 48 E
Neuvy-sur-Barangeon, *France* **27 E9** 47 20N 2 15 E
Neuwedell = Drawno, *Poland* **55 E2** 53 13N 15 46 E
Neuwerk, *Germany* **30 B4** 53 55N 8 30 E
Neuwied, *Germany* **30 E3** 50 26N 7 29 E
Neva →, *Russia* **58 C6** 59 50N 30 30 E
Nevada, *Iowa, U.S.A.* **156 B3** 42 1N 93 27W
Nevada, *Mo., U.S.A.* **155 G7** 37 51N 94 22W
Nevada □, *U.S.A.* **158 G5** 39 0N 117 0W
Nevada City, *U.S.A.* **160 F6** 39 16N 121 1W
Nevado, Cerro, *Argentina* **174 D2** 35 30 S 68 32W
Nevado de Colima = Volcán de Colima △, *Mexico* **162 D4** 19 30N 103 40W
Nevado de Tres Cruces △, *Chile* **174 B2** 27 13 S 69 5W
Nevado del Huila △, *Colombia* **168 C2** 3 5N 75 58W
Nevasa, *India* **94 E2** 19 34N 75 0 E
Neve, Sa. da, *Angola* **115 E2** 13 43 S 13 10 E
Nevel, *Russia* **58 D5** 56 0N 29 55 E
Nevers, *France* **27 F10** 47 0N 3 9 E
Nevertire, *Australia* **129 A7** 31 50 S 147 44 E
Nevesinje, *Bos.-H.* **50 C2** 43 14N 18 6 E
Neville, *Canada* **143 D7** 49 58N 107 39W
Nevinnomyssk, *Russia* **61 H6** 44 40N 42 0 E
Nevis, *St. Kitts & Nevis* **165 C7** 17 0N 62 30W
Nevlunghavn, *Norway* **18 F6** 58 58N 9 53 E
Nevoso, Mte. = Snežnik, *Slovenia* **45 C11** 45 36N 14 35 E
Nevrokop = Gotse Delchev, *Bulgaria* **50 E7** 41 36N 23 46 E
Nevşehir, *Turkey* **100 C6** 38 33N 34 40 E
Nevskoye, *Russia* **54 D9** 54 32N 22 39 E
Nevyansk, *Russia* **64 C8** 57 30N 60 13 E
New →, *Guyana* **169 C6** 3 20N 57 37W
New →, *U.S.A.* **148 F5** 38 10N 81 12W
New Aiyansh, *Canada* **142 B3** 55 12N 129 4W
New Albany, *Ind., U.S.A.* **157 F11** 38 18N 85 49W
New Albany, *Miss., U.S.A.* **155 H10** 34 29N 89 0W
New Albany, *Pa., U.S.A.* **151 E8** 41 36N 76 27W
New Amsterdam, *Guyana* **169 B6** 6 15N 57 36W
New Angledool, *Australia* **127 D4** 29 5 S 147 55 E
New Athens, *U.S.A.* **156 F7** 38 19N 89 53W
New Baltimore, *U.S.A.* **150 D2** 42 41N 82 44W
New Barbadoes = Hackensack, *U.S.A.* **151 F10** 40 53N 74 3W
New Bedford, *U.S.A.* **151 E14** 41 38N 70 56W
New Berlin = North Canton, *U.S.A.* **150 F3** 40 53N 81 24W
New Berlin, *Ill., U.S.A.* **156 E7** 39 44N 89 55W
New Berlin, *N.Y., U.S.A.* **151 D9** 42 37N 75 20W
New Berlin, *Pa., U.S.A.* **150 F8** 40 50N 76 57W
New Berlin, *Wis., U.S.A.* **157 B8** 42 59N 88 6W
New Bern, *U.S.A.* **149 H7** 35 7N 77 3W
New Bethlehem, *U.S.A.* **150 F5** 41 0N 79 20W
New Bloomfield, *U.S.A.* **150 F7** 40 25N 77 11W
New Boston, *U.S.A.* **155 J7** 33 28N 94 25W
New Braunfels, *U.S.A.* **155 L5** 29 42N 98 8W
New Brighton, *N.Z.* **131 D7** 43 29 S 172 43 E
New Brighton, *U.S.A.* **150 F4** 40 42N 80 19W
New Britain, *Papua N. G.* **132 C6** 5 50 S 150 20 E
New Britain, *U.S.A.* **151 E12** 41 40N 72 47W
New Brockton, *U.S.A.* **152 D4** 31 23N 85 56W
New Brookland = West Columbia, *U.S.A.* **152 B8** 33 59N 81 4W
New Brunswick, *U.S.A.* **151 F10** 40 30N 74 27W
New Brunswick □, *Canada* **141 C6** 46 50N 66 30W
New Buffalo, *U.S.A.* **157 C10** 41 47N 86 45W
New Bussa, *Nigeria* **113 D5** 9 53N 4 31 E
New Caledonia ⊠, *Pac. Oc.* **133 U19** 21 0 S 165 0 E
New Carlisle, *Ind., U.S.A.* **157 C10** 41 45N 86 32W
New Carlisle, *Ohio, U.S.A.* **157 E12** 39 56N 84 2W
New Castile = Castilla-La Mancha □, *Spain* **12 H5** 39 30N 3 30W
New Castle, *Ind., U.S.A.* **157 E11** 39 55N 85 22W
New Castle, *Ky., U.S.A.* **157 F11** 38 26N 85 10W
New Castle, *Pa., U.S.A.* **150 F4** 41 0N 80 21W
New City, *U.S.A.* **151 E11** 41 9N 73 59W
New Concord, *U.S.A.* **150 G3** 39 59N 81 54W
New Cumberland, *U.S.A.* **150 F4** 40 30N 80 36W
New Cuyama, *U.S.A.* **161 L7** 34 57N 119 38W
New Delhi, *India* **92 E7** 28 37N 77 13 E
New Denver, *Canada* **142 D5** 50 0N 117 25W
New Don Pedro Reservoir, *U.S.A.* **160 H6** 37 43N 120 24W
New Ellenton, *U.S.A.* **152 B8** 33 28N 81 41W
New England, *U.S.A.* **147 B12** 43 0N 71 0W
New England, *N. Dak., U.S.A.* **154 B3** 46 32N 102 52W
New England △, *Australia* **129 A10** 30 25 S 152 30 E
New England Ra., *Australia* **127 E5** 30 20 S 151 45 E
New England Seamounts, *Atl. Oc.* **8 C5** 38 0N 63 0W
New Forest, *U.K.* **21 G6** 50 53N 1 34W
New Franklin, *U.S.A.* **156 E4** 39 1N 92 44W
New Galloway, *U.K.* **22 F4** 55 5N 4 9W
New Georgia Is., *Solomon Is.* **133 M9** 8 15 S 157 30 E
New Georgia Sound, *Solomon Is.* **133 L9** 8 0 S 158 20 E
New Glarus, *U.S.A.* **156 B7** 42 49N 89 38W

New Glasgow, Canada ... **141 C7**   45 35N   62 36W
New Guinea, Oceania ... **132 C1**   4 0S 136 0 E
New Hamburg, Canada ... **150 C4**   43 23N   80 42W
New Hampshire □,
   U.S.A. **151 C13**   44 0N   71 30W
New Hampton, U.S.A. ... **156 A4**   43 3N   92 19W
New Hanover,
   Papua N. G. ...... **132 B6**   2 30 S 150 10 E
New Hanover, S. Africa **117 D5**   29 22 S   30 31 E
New Harmony, U.S.A. .. **157 F9**   38 8N   87 56W
New Hartford, U.S.A. .. **151 C9**   43 4N   75 18W
New Haven, Conn.,
   U.S.A. **151 E12**   41 18N   72 55W
New Haven, Ill., U.S.A. **157 G8**   37 55N   88   8W
New Haven, Ind.,
   U.S.A. **157 C11**   41 4N   85   1W
New Haven, Mich.,
   U.S.A. **150 D2**   42 44N   82 48W
New Haven, Mo.,
   U.S.A. **156 F5**   38 37N   91 13W
New Hazelton, Canada **150 B3**   55 20N 127 30W
New Hebrides =
   Vanuatu ■, Pac. Oc. **133 E6**   15 0S 168 0 E
New Holland, U.S.A. ... **151 F8**   40 6N   76   5W
New Iberia, U.S.A. **155 K9**   30 1N   91 49W
New Ireland,
   Papua N. G. ...... **132 B6**   3 20 S 151 50 E
New Ireland □,
   Papua N. G. ...... **132 B6**   3 0 S 151 30 E
New Jersey □, U.S.A. .. **148 E8**   40 0N   74 30W
New Kensington,
   U.S.A. **150 F5**   40 34N   79 46W
New Lexington, U.S.A. **148 F4**   39 43N   82 13W
New Liskeard, Canada **140 C4**   47 31N   79 41W
New London, Conn.,
   U.S.A. **151 E12**   41 22N   72   6W
New London, Iowa,
   U.S.A. **156 D5**   40 55N   91 24W
New London, Mo.,
   U.S.A. **156 E5**   39 35N   91 24W
New London, Ohio,
   U.S.A. **150 E2**   41 5N   82 24W
New London, Wis.,
   U.S.A. **154 C10**   44 23N   88 45W
New Madrid, U.S.A. ... **155 G10**   36 36N   89 32W
New Martinsville,
   U.S.A. **148 F5**   39 39N   80 52W
New Meadows, U.S.A. .. **158 D5**   44 58N 116 18W
New Melones L., U.S.A. **160 H6**   37 57N 120 31W
New Mexico □, U.S.A. **159 J10**   34 30N 106 0W
New Miami, U.S.A. **157 E12**   39 26N   84 32W
New Milford, Conn.,
   U.S.A. **151 E11**   41 35N   73 25W
New Milford, Pa.,
   U.S.A. **151 E9**   41 52N   75 44W
New Norcia, Australia **125 F2**   30 57 S 116 13 E
New Norfolk, Australia **127 G4**   42 46 S 147 2 E
New Orleans, U.S.A. ... **155 L9**   29 58N   90   4W
New Palestine, U.S.A. .. **157 F9**   39 45 S 85 52W
New Panamao, Phil. ... **81 J3**   5 59N 121 13 E
New Paris, U.S.A. **157 E12**   39 51N   84 48W
New Pekin, U.S.A. **157 F10**   38 31N   86   2W
New Philadelphia,
   U.S.A. **150 F3**   40 30N   81 27W
New Plymouth, N.Z. .. **130 F3**   39 4 S   174 5 E
New Plymouth, U.S.A. **158 E5**   43 58N 116 49W
New Pomerania = New
   Britain, Papua N. G. **132 C6**   5 50 S 150 20 E
New Port Richey,
   U.S.A. **153 G7**   28 16N   82 43W
New Providence,
   Bahamas .... **9 b**   25 25N   78 35W
New Quay, U.K. **21 E3**   52 13N   4 21W
New Radnor, U.K. **21 E4**   52 15N   3   9W
New Richmond,
   Canada **141 C6**   48 15N   65 45W
New Richmond, Ohio,
   U.S.A. **157 F12**   38 57N   84 17W
New Richmond, Wis.,
   U.S.A. **154 C8**   45 7N   92 32W
New River Gorge △,
   U.S.A. **148 G5**   37 53N   81   5W
New Roads, U.S.A. **155 K9**   30 42N   91 26W
New Rochelle, U.S.A. .. **151 F11**   40 55N   73 47W
New Rockford, U.S.A. **154 B5**   47 41N   99   8W
New Romney, U.K. ... **21 G8**   50 59N   0 57 E
New Ross, Ireland **23 D5**   52 23N   6 57W
New Salem, U.S.A. **154 B4**   46 51N 101 25W
New Scone = Scone,
   U.K. **22 E5**   56 25N   3 24W
New Sharon, U.S.A. ... **156 C4**   41 28N   92 39W
New Siberian I. =
   Novaya Sibir, Ostrov,
   Russia .... **67 B16**   75 10N 150 0 E
New Siberian Is. =
   Novosibirskiye
   Ostrova, Russia .... **67 B15**   75 0N 142 0 E
New Smyrna Beach,
   U.S.A. **153 F9**   29 1N   80 56W
New South Wales □,
   Australia .... **129 B7**   33 0 S 146 0 E
New Stuyahok, U.S.A. **144 G8**   59 29N 157 20W
New Tecumseth,
   Canada **140 D4**   44 9N   79 52W
New Town, U.S.A. **154 B3**   47 59N 102 30W
New Tredegar, U.K. ... **21 F4**   51 44N   3 16W
New Ulm, U.S.A. **154 C7**   44 19N   94 28W
New Vienna, U.S.A. .. **157 E13**   39 19N   83 42W
New Washington, Phil. **81 F4**   11 39N 122 26 E
New Waterford,
   Canada **141 C7**   46 13N   60   4W
New-Wes-Valley,
   Canada **141 C9**   49 8N   53 36W
New Westminster,
   Canada **160 A4**   49 13N 122 55W
New York, U.S.A. **151 F11**   40 45N   74 0W
New York □, U.S.A. .. **151 D9**   43 0N   75 0W
New York J.F.
   Kennedy
   International ✈
   (JFK), U.S.A. **151 F11**   40 38N   73 47W
New York Mts., U.S.A. **159 J6**   35 0N 115 20W
New Zealand ■,
   Oceania .... **130 G5**   40 0 S 176 0 E
Newaj →, India ...... **92 G7**   24 24N   76 49 E
Newala, Tanzania .... **119 E4**   10 58 S   39 18 E
Newark, Del., U.S.A. .. **148 F8**   39 41N   75 46W
Newark, N.J., U.S.A. .. **151 F10**   40 44N   74 10W
Newark, N.Y., U.S.A. .. **150 C7**   43 3N   77   6W
Newark, Ohio, U.S.A. **150 F2**   40 3N   82 24W
Newark International ✈
   (EWR), U.S.A. **151 F10**   40 42N   74 10W
Newark-on-Trent, U.K. **20 D7**   53 5N   0 48W
Newark Valley, U.S.A. **151 D8**   42 14N   76 11W
Newberg, Mo., U.S.A. **156 G5**   37 55N   91 54W
Newberg, Oreg., U.S.A. **158 D2**   45 18N 122 58W
Newberry, Fla., U.S.A. **153 F7**   29 39N   82 37W
Newberry, Mich.,
   U.S.A. **148 B3**   46 21N   85 30W
Newberry, S.C., U.S.A. **149 H5**   34 17N   81 37W
Newberry △, U.S.A. .. **158 E3**   43 42N 121 15W
Newberry Springs,
   U.S.A. **161 L10**   34 50N 116 41W
Newboro L., Canada ... **151 B8**   44 38N   76 20W

Newbridge = Droichead
   Nua, Ireland **23 C5**   53 11N   6 48W
Newburgh, Canada ... **150 B8**   44 19N   76 52W
Newburgh, Ind., U.S.A. **157 G9**   37 57N   87 24W
Newburgh, N.Y., U.S.A. **151 E10**   41 30N   74 1W
Newbury, U.K. **21 F6**   51 24N   1 20W
Newbury, N.H., U.S.A. **151 B12**   43 19N   72 3W
Newbury, Vt., U.S.A. **151 B12**   44 5N   72 4W
Newburyport, U.S.A. **149 D10**   42 49N   70 53W
Newcastle, Australia **129 B9**   33 0 S 151 46 E
Newcastle, N.B.,
   Canada **141 C6**   47 1N   65 38W
Newcastle, Ont.,
   Canada **140 D4**   43 55N   78 35W
Newcastle, S. Africa **117 D4**   27 45 S   29 58 E
Newcastle, U.K. **23 B6**   54 13N   5 54W
Newcastle, Calif.,
   U.S.A. **160 G5**   38 53N 121 8W
Newcastle, Wyo.,
   U.S.A. **154 D2**   43 50N 104 11W
Newcastle Emlyn, U.K. **21 E3**   52 2N   4 28W
Newcastle Ra.,
   Australia .... **124 C5**   15 45 S 130 15 E
Newcastle-under-Lyme,
   U.K. **20 D5**   53 1N   2 14W
Newcastle-upon-Tyne,
   U.K. **20 C6**   54 58N   1 36W
Newcastle Waters,
   Australia .... **126 B1**   17 30 S 133 28 E
Newcastle West,
   Ireland **23 D2**   52 27N   9 3W
Newcomb, U.S.A. **151 C10**   43 58N   74 10W
Newcomerstown,
   U.S.A. **150 F3**   40 16N   81 36W
Newdegate, Australia . **125 F2**   33 6 S 119 0 E
Newell, Australia .... **126 B4**   16 20 S 145 16 E
Newell, Iowa, U.S.A. **156 B1**   42 36N   95 0W
Newell, S. Dak., U.S.A. **154 C3**   44 43N 103 25W
Newenham, C., U.S.A. **144 G7**   58 39N 162 11W
Newfane, U.S.A. **150 C6**   43 17N   78 43W
Newfield, U.S.A. **151 D8**   42 18N   76 33W
Newfound L., U.S.A. **151 C13**   43 40N   71 47W
Newfoundland, Canada **141 C8**   49 0N   55 0W
Newfoundland, U.S.A. **151 E9**   41 18N   75 19W
Newfoundland &
   Labrador □, Canada **141 B8**   53 0N   58 0W
Newhalen, U.S.A. **144 G8**   59 43N 154 54W
Newhall, U.S.A. **161 L8**   34 23N 118 32W
Newhaven, U.K. ..... **21 G8**   50 47N   0 3 E
Newington, U.S.A. ... **152 C8**   32 35N   81 30W
Newkirk, U.S.A. **155 G6**   36 53N   97 3W
Newlyn, U.K. **21 G2**   50 6N   5 34W
Newman, Australia ... **124 D2**   23 18 S 119 45 E
Newman, Calif., U.S.A. **160 H5**   37 19N 121 1W
Newman, Ill., U.S.A. **157 F9**   39 48N   87 59W
Newmarket, Canada .. **150 B5**   44 3N   79 28W
Newmarket, Ireland .. **23 D2**   52 13N   9 0W
Newmarket, U.K. .... **21 E8**   52 15N   0 25 E
Newmarket, U.S.A. .. **151 C14**   43 4N   70 56W
Newnan, U.S.A. **152 B5**   33 23N   84 48W
Newport, Ireland **23 C2**   53 53N   9 33W
Newport, I. of W., U.K. **21 G6**   50 42N   1 17W
Newport, Newp., U.K. **21 F5**   51 35N   3 0W
Newport, Ark., U.S.A. **155 H9**   35 37N   91 16W
Newport, Fla., U.S.A. **153 F6**   30 11N   84 10W
Newport, Ind., U.S.A. **157 E9**   39 53N   87 25W
Newport, Ky., U.S.A. **157 F12**   39 5N   84 30W
Newport, N.H., U.S.A. **151 C12**   43 22N   72 10W
Newport, N.Y., U.S.A. **151 C9**   43 11N   75 1W
Newport, Oreg., U.S.A. **158 D1**   44 39N 124 3W
Newport, Pa., U.S.A. **150 F7**   40 29N   77 8W
Newport, R.I., U.S.A. **151 E13**   41 29N   71 19W
Newport, Tenn., U.S.A. **149 H4**   35 58N   83 11W
Newport, Vt., U.S.A. **151 B12**   44 56N   72 13W
Newport, Wash., U.S.A. **158 B5**   48 11N 117 3W
Newport □, U.K. **21 F5**   51 33N   3 1W
Newport Beach, U.S.A. **161 M9**   33 37N 117 56W
Newport News, U.S.A. **148 G7**   36 59N   76 25W
Newport Pagnell, U.K. **21 E7**   52 5N   0 43W
Newquay, U.K. **21 G2**   50 25N   5 6W
Newry, U.K. **23 B5**   54 11N   6 21W
Newtok, U.S.A. **144 F6**   60 56N 164 38W
Newton, Ga., U.S.A. . **152 D5**   31 19N   84 20W
Newton, Ill., U.S.A. .. **157 F8**   38 59N   88 10W
Newton, Iowa, U.S.A. **156 C3**   41 42N   93 3W
Newton, Kans., U.S.A. **156 F5**   38 3N   97 21W
Newton, Mass., U.S.A. **151 D13**   42 21N   71 12W
Newton, Miss., U.S.A. **155 J10**   32 19N   89 10W
Newton, N.C., U.S.A. **149 H5**   35 40N   81 13W
Newton, N.J., U.S.A. **151 E10**   41 3N   74 45W
Newton, Tex., U.S.A. **155 K8**   30 51N   93 46W
Newton Abbot, U.K. . **21 G4**   50 32N   3 37W
Newton Aycliffe, U.K. **20 C6**   54 37N   1 34W
Newton Falls, U.S.A. **150 E4**   41 11N   80 59W
Newton L., U.S.A. ... **157 F8**   38 55N   88 15W
Newton Stewart, U.K. **22 G4**   54 57N   4 30W
Newtonmore, U.K. ... **22 D4**   57 4N   4 8W
Newtontoppen,
   Svalbard .... **10 B12**   79 0N   17 30 E
Newtown, U.K. **21 E4**   52 31N   3 19W
Newtown, Ind., U.S.A. **157 E9**   40 13N   87 9W
Newtown, Mo., U.S.A. **156 D3**   40 22N   93 20W
Newtownabbey, U.K. . **23 B6**   54 40N   5 56W
Newtownards, U.K. .. **23 B6**   54 36N   5 42W
Newtownbarry =
   Bunclody, Ireland .. **23 D5**   52 39N   6 40W
Newtownstewart, U.K. **23 B4**   54 43N   7 23W
Newville, U.S.A. **150 F7**   40 10N   77 24W
Nexon, France ...... **28 C5**   45 41N   1 11 E
Neya, Russia .... **60 A**   58 21N   43 49 E
Neyriz, Iran .... **97 D7**   29 15N   54 19 E
Neyshābūr, Iran ..... **97 B8**   36 10N   58 50 E
Neyyattinkara, India . **95 K3**   8 26N   77 5 E
Nezametny = Aldan,
   Russia .... **67 D13**   58 40N 125 30 E
Nezhin = Nizhyn,
   Ukraine .... **59 G6**   51 5N   31 55 E
Nezperce, U.S.A. **158 C5**   46 14N 116 14W
Nezvysko, Ukraine ... **55 D10**   48 46N   25 15 E
Ngabang, Indonesia .. **85 B3**   0 23N 109 55 E
Ngabe, Congo .... **114 C3**   3 12 S   16 12 E
Ngabordamlu, Tanjung,
   Indonesia .... **83 C4**   6 56 S 134 11 E
N'Gage, Angola ..... **115 D3**   7 46 S   15 15 E
Ngaiphaipi, Burma ... **90 D4**   22 14N   93 15 E
Ngala, Nigeria ...... **113 C7**   12 20N   14 11 E
Ngama, Chad .... **109 F3**   11 45N   17 6 E
Ngambé, Centre,
   Cameroon .... **113 D7**   5 48N   11 29 E
Ngambé, Littoral,
   Cameroon .... **113 E7**   4 21N   10 40 E
Ngami Depression,
   Botswana .... **116 C3**   20 30 S   22 46 E
Ngamo, Zimbabwe ... **119 F2**   19 3 S   27 32 E
Ngangala, Sudan .... **107 G3**   4 42N   31 55 E
Nganglong Kangri,
   China .... **93 C9**   33 0N   81 0 E
Nganjuk, Indonesia ... **85 D4**   7 32 S 111 55 E
Ngao, Thailand ...... **86 C2**   18 46N   99 59 E
Ngaoundéré, Cameroon **114 A2**   7 15N   13 35 E
Ngapara, N.Z. ...... **131 E5**   44 57 S 170 46 E
Ngape, Burma ...... **90 E5**   20 2N   94 28 E
Ngara, Tanzania ..... **118 C3**   2 29 S   30 40 E

Ngaruawahia, N.Z. ... **130 D4**   37 42 S 175 11 E
Ngaruroro →, N.Z. ... **130 F5**   39 34 S 176 56 E
Ngatapa, N.Z. ...... **130 E6**   38 32 S 177 45 E
Ngathaingyaung,
   Burma .... **90 G5**   17 24N   95 5 E
Ngaruhoe, Mt., N.Z. **130 F4**   39 13 S 175 45 E
Ngawi, Indonesia .... **85 D4**   7 24 S 111 26 E
Ngele, Dem. Rep. of
   the Congo .... **114 C4**   0 30 S   20 22 E
Ngelebok, Cameroon . **114 B2**   4 16N   14 3 E
Nggatokae, Solomon Is. **133 M10**   8 45 S 158 15 E
Nggela Is., Solomon Is. **133 M11**   9 5 S 160 15 E
Nggela Pile,
   Solomon Is. ...... **133 M11**   9 5 S 160 20 E
Nggela Sule,
   Solomon Is. ...... **133 M11**   9 2 S 160 12 E
Nghia Lo, Vietnam ... **76 G5**   21 33N 104 28 E
Ngidinga, Dem. Rep. of
   the Congo .... **115 D3**   5 37 S   15 17 E
Ngo, Congo .... **114 C3**   2 29 S   15 45 E
Ngoap, Cameroon ... **114 B2**   4 9N   12 51 E
Ngoboli, Sudan ..... **107 G3**   4 57N   32 37 E
N'Gola, Angola ..... **115 E2**   14 10 S   14 30 E
Ngoma, Malawi ..... **119 E3**   13 8 S   33 45 E
Ngomahura, Zimbabwe **119 G3**   20 26 S   30 43 E
Ngomba, Tanzania ... **119 D3**   8 20 S   32 53 E
Ngongotaha, N.Z. .... **130 E5**   38 5 S 176 12 E
Ngonye Falls, Zambia **115 F4**   16 40 S   23 25 E
Ngop, Sudan .... **107 F3**   6 17N   30 9 E
Ngoring Hu, China ... **68 C4**   34 55N   97 5 E
Ngorkou, Mali **112 B4**   15 40N   3 41W
Ngorongoro, Tanzania **118 C4**   3 11 S   35 32 E
Ngorongoro △,
   Tanzania .... **118 C4**   2 40 S   35 30 E
Ngoto, C.A.R. ...... **114 B3**   3 59N   17 19 E
Ngouo, Dj., C.A.R. ... **114 A4**   7 55N   24 38 E
Ngoura, Chad .... **109 F3**   12 44N   16 21 E
Ngouri, Chad .... **109 F3**   13 38N   15 22 E
Ngourti, Niger ...... **109 E2**   15 19N   13 12 E
Ngoussou, Gabon ... **114 C2**   3 0 S   11 7 E
Ngozi, Burundi ..... **118 C2**   2 54 S   29 50 E
Ngudu, Tanzania .... **118 C3**   2 58 S   33 25 E
Nguigmi, Niger ..... **109 F2**   14 20N   13 20 E
Nguila, Cameroon ... **113 E7**   4 41N   11 43 E
Nguiu, Australia ..... **124 B5**   11 46 S 130 38 E
Ngukurr, Australia ... **126 A1**   14 44 S 134 44 E
Nguna, Vanuatu .... **133 G6**   17 26 S 168 22 E
Ngunga, Tanzania ... **118 C3**   3 37 S   33 37 E
Nguru, Nigeria ...... **113 C7**   12 56N   10 29 E
Nguru Mts., Tanzania **118 D4**   6 0 S   37 30 E
Ngusi, Malawi ...... **119 E3**   14 0 S   34 50 E
Nguyen Binh, Vietnam **76 F5**   22 39N 105 56 E
Ngwedaung, Burma . **90 F6**   19 31N   97 9 E
Nha Trang, Vietnam . **87 F7**   12 16N 109 10 E
Nhacoongo, Mozam. . **117 C6**   24 18 S   35 14 E
Nhamaabué, Mozam. **119 F4**   17 25 S   35 5 E
Nhambiquara, Brazil **173 C6**   12 50 S   59 49W
Nhamundá, Brazil ... **169 D6**   2 14 S   56 43W
Nhamundá →, Brazil **169 D6**   2 12 S   56 41W
Nhangulaze, L.,
   Mozam. .... **117 C5**   24 0 S   34 30 E
Nharêa, Angola ..... **115 E3**   11 38 S   16 58 E
Nhecolândia, Brazil .. **173 D6**   19 17 S   56 58W
Nhill, Australia ..... **128 D4**   36 18 S 141 40 E
Nho Quan, Vietnam . **76 G5**   20 18N 105 45 E
Nhulunbuy, Australia **126 A2**   12 10 S 137 20 E
Nhundo, Angola .... **115 E4**   14 25 S   21 23 E
Nia-nia, Dem. Rep. of
   the Congo .... **118 B2**   1 30N   27 40 E
Niafounké, Mali **112 B4**   16 0N   4 5W
Niagara Falls, Canada **140 D4**   43 7N   79 5W
Niagara Falls, U.S.A. **150 C6**   43 5N   79 4W
Niagara-on-the-Lake,
   Canada **150 C5**   43 15N   79 4W
Niah, Malaysia ..... **85 B4**   3 58N 113 46 E
Nialaha'u Pt.,
   Solomon Is. ...... **133 M11**   9 47 S 161 34 E
Niamey, Niger ...... **113 C5**   13 27N   2 6 E
Niandan-Koro, Guinea **112 C3**   11 5N   9 15W
Nianforando, Guinea . **112 D2**   9 37N   10 36W
Niangara, Dem. Rep. of
   the Congo .... **118 B2**   3 42N   27 50 E
Niangbo, Ivory C. ... **112 D3**   8 49N   5 10W
Niangoloko,
   Burkina Faso **112 C4**   10 15N   4 55W
Niangua →, U.S.A. .. **156 G4**   38 0N   92 48W
Niantic, U.S.A. **151 E12**   41 20N   72 11W
Niari, Congo .... **114 C2**   4 9 S   14 9 E
Niaro, Sudan .... **107 E3**   10 38N   31 31 E
Nias, Indonesia ..... **84 B1**   1 0N   97 30 E
Niassa □, Mozam. ... **119 E4**   12 4 S   36 57 E
Niassa, L., Mozam. .. **119 E4**   13 30 S   36 0 E
Nibak, Si. Arabia ... **97 E7**   24 25N   50 50 E
Nibe, Denmark ..... **17 H3**   56 59N   9 38 E
Nicaragua ■,
   Cent. Amer. **164 D2**   11 40N   85 30W
Nicaragua, L. de, Nic. **164 D2**   12 0N   85 30W
Nicastro, Italy ...... **47 D9**   38 59N   16 19 E
Nice ✈ (NCE), France **29 E11**   43 42N   7 12 E
Niceville, U.S.A. **153 F3**   30 31N   86 30W
Nichicun, L., Canada **141 B5**   53 5N   71 0W
Nichinan, Japan .... **72 F3**   31 38N 131 23 E
Nicholas Channel,
   W. Indies **164 B3**   23 30N   80 5W
Nicholasville, U.S.A. **157 G12**   37 53N   84 34W
Nicholls, U.S.A. **152 D7**   31 31N   82 38W
Nichols, U.S.A. **151 D8**   42 1N   76 22W
Nicholson, Australia **124 C4**   18 2 S 128 54 E
Nicholson, U.S.A. ... **151 E9**   41 37N   75 47W
Nicholson →, Australia **126 B2**   17 31 S 139 36 E
Nicholson L., Canada **143 A8**   62 40N 102 40W
Nicholson Ra.,
   Australia .... **125 E2**   27 15 S 116 45 E
Nicholville, U.S.A. .. **151 B10**   44 41N   74 39W
Nickerie →, Suriname **169 B6**   5 58N   57 0W
Nico Pérez = José
   Batlle y Ordóñez,
   Uruguay .... **175 C4**   33 20 S   55 10W
Nicobar Is., Ind. Oc. **95 L11**   8 0N   93 30 E
Nicola, Canada **142 C4**   50 12N 120 40W
Nicolls Town, Bahamas **164 A4**   25 8N   78 0W
Nicopolis, Greece ... **39 A2**   39 5N   20 43 E
Nicosia, Cyprus ..... **39 E9**   35 10N   33 25 E
Nicosia, Italy .... **47 E7**   37 45N   14 24 E
Nicótera, Italy ...... **47 D8**   38 33N   15 56 E
Nicoya, Costa Rica .. **164 D2**   10 9N   85 27W
Nicoya, G. de,
   Costa Rica **164 E3**   10 0N   85 0W
Nicoya, Pen. de,
   Costa Rica **164 E2**   9 45N   85 40W
Nictheroy = Niterói,
   Brazil .... **171 F3**   22 52 S   43 0W
Nida, Lithuania ..... **54 C8**   55 20N   21 4 E
Nidaros = Trondheim,
   Norway .... **18 A7**   63 36N   10 25 E
Nidau, Switz. ...... **32 B4**   47 7N   7 15 E
Nidd →, U.K. **20 D6**   53 59N   1 23W
Nidda, Germany .... **31 E5**   50 25N   9 4 E
Nidda →, Germany .. **31 E4**   50 17N   8 48 E
Nidri, Greece ...... **39 B2**   38 43N   20 42 E
Nidwalden □, Switz. **33 C6**   46 50N   8 25 E
Nidzica, Poland .... **55 E7**   53 25N   20 42 E
Nié, Ĩ., N. Cal. .... **133 U21**   21 8 S 167 35 E

Niebüll, Germany .... **30 A4**   54 46N   8 48 E
Nied →, Germany ... **27 C13**   49 23N   6 40 E
Niederaula, Germany . **30 E5**   50 47N   9 36 E
Niederbayern □,
   Germany .... **31 G8**   48 40N   12 50 E
Niederbipp, Switz. ... **32 B5**   47 16N   7 42 E
Niederbronn-les-Bains,
   France .... **27 D14**   48 57N   7 39 E
Niedere Tauern,
   Austria .... **34 D7**   47 20N   14 0 E
Niederlausitz, Germany **30 D9**   51 42N   13 59 E
Niederösterreich □,
   Austria .... **34 C8**   48 25N   15 40 E
Niedersachsen □,
   Germany .... **30 C4**   52 50N   9 0 E
Niedersächsisches
   Wattenmeer △,
   Germany .... **30 B3**   53 45N   7 30 E
Niefang, Eq. Guin. ... **114 D2**   1 50N   10 14 E
Niekerkshoop, S. Africa **116 D3**   29 19 S   22 51 E
Niellé, Ivory C. **112 C3**   10 5N   5 38W
Niellim, Chad ...... **109 G3**   9 42N   17 49 E
Niem, C.A.R. ...... **114 A3**   6 12N   15 14 E
Niemba, Dem. Rep. of
   the Congo .... **118 D2**   5 58 S   28 24 E
Niemen = Nemunas →,
   Lithuania .... **15 J19**   55 25N   21 10 E
Niemodlin, Poland ... **55 H4**   50 38N   17 38 E
Niemur, Australia ... **128 C6**   35 17 S 144 9 E
Nienburg, Germany . **30 C5**   52 39N   9 13 E
Niepolomice, Poland . **55 H7**   50 3N   20 13 E
Niers →, Germany ... **30 D1**   51 43N   5 57 E
Niesen, Switz. ...... **32 C5**   46 38N   7 39 E
Niesky, Germany .... **30 D10**   51 17N   14 49 E
Nieszawa, Poland ... **55 F5**   52 52N   18 50 E
Nieu Bethesda,
   S. Africa .... **116 E3**   31 51 S   24 34 E
Nieuw Amsterdam,
   Suriname **169 B6**   5 53N   55 5W
Nieuw Nickerie,
   Suriname **169 B6**   6 0N   56 59W
Nieuwoudtville,
   S. Africa .... **116 E2**   31 23 S   19 7 E
Nieuwpoort, Belgium **24 C2**   51 8N   2 45 E
Nieves, Pico de las,
   Canary Is. **9 e1**   27 57N   15 35W
Nièvre □, France .... **27 E10**   47 10N   3 40 E
Niğde, Mali **112 C3**   13 38N   5 27W
Niğde, Turkey ...... **100 D6**   37 58N   34 40 E
Nigel, S. Africa ..... **117 D4**   26 27 S   28 25 E
Niger □, Nigeria .... **113 D6**   10 0N   5 30 E
Niger ■, W. Afr. .... **113 B7**   17 30N   10 0 E
Niger →, W. Afr. ... **113 D6**   5 33N   6 33 E
Niger Delta, Africa .. **113 E6**   5 0N   6 0 E
Nigeria ■, W. Afr. .. **113 D6**   8 30N   8 0 E
Nighasin, India ..... **93 E9**   28 14N   80 52 E
Nightcaps, N.Z. .... **131 F3**   45 57 S 168 2 E
Nightmute, U.S.A. .. **144 F6**   60 29N 164 44W
Nigríta, Greece ..... **50 F7**   40 56N   23 29 E
Nihoa, U.S.A. **145 G11**   23 6N 161 58W
Nihon = Japan ■, Asia **71 G8**   36 0N 136 0 E
Nii-Jima, Japan .... **73 C11**   34 20N 139 15 E
Niigata, Japan ..... **70 F9**   37 58N 139 0 E
Niigata □, Japan .... **71 F9**   37 15N 138 45 E
Niihama, Japan .... **72 D5**   33 55N 133 16 E
Niihau, U.S.A. **145 B1**   21 54N 160 9W
Niimi, Japan ...... **72 C5**   34 59N 133 28 E
Niimi, Japan
Niislel Khureheh =
   Ulaanbaatar,
   Mongolia .... **67 E11**   47 55N 106 53 E
Niitsu, Japan ...... **70 F9**   37 48N 139 7 E
Nij Laluk, India .... **90 B4**   27 7N   93 56 E
Nijar, Spain **41 J2**   36 53N   2 15W
Nijil, Jordan .... **103 E4**   30 32N   35 33 E
Nijkerk, Neths. ..... **24 B5**   52 13N   5 30 E
Nijmegen, Neths. ... **24 C5**   51 50N   5 52 E
Nijverdal, Neths. ... **24 B6**   52 22N   6 28 E
Nīk Pey, Iran ...... **97 B6**   36 50N   48 10 E
Nikaweratiya,
   Sri Lanka .... **95 L5**   7 45N   80 7 E
Nike, Nigeria .... **113 D6**   6 26N   7 29 E
Nikiniki, Indonesia .. **82 C2**   9 49 S 124 30 E
Nikísiani, Greece .... **51 F8**   40 57N   24 9 E
Nikítas, Greece ..... **50 F7**   40 13N   23 43 E
Nikitinskiye promysly =
   Kirovskiy, Russia .. **61 H9**   45 51N   48 11 E
Nikki, Benin .... **113 D5**   9 58N   3 12 E
Nikkō, Japan ...... **73 A11**   36 45N 139 35 E
Nikkō △, Japan .... **71 F9**   36 56N 139 37 E
Nikolai, U.S.A. **144 F9**   63 1N 154 23W
Nikolaevskaya =
   Vaasa, Finland ... **14 E19**   63 6N   21 58 E
Nikolaistad = Vaasa,
   Finland .... **14 E19**   63 6N   21 38 E
Nikolayev = Mykolayiv,
   Ukraine .... **59 J7**   46 58N   32 0 E
Nikolayevsk, Russia . **60 E7**   50 0N   45 35 E
Nikolayevsk-na-Amur,
   Russia .... **67 D15**   53 8N 140 44 E
Nikolsburg = Mikulov,
   Czech Rep. .... **35 C9**   48 48N   16 38 E
Nikolsk, Russia ..... **60 D8**   53 49N   46 4 E
Nikolsk-Ussuriysky =
   Ussuriysk, Russia .. **67 E14**   43 48N 131 59 E
Nikolskaya Pestravka =
   Nikolsk, Russia ... **60 D8**   53 49N   46 4 E
Nikolski, U.S.A. **144 K5**   52 56N 168 52W
Nikolskoye =
   Ussuriysk, Russia .. **67 E14**   43 48N 131 59 E
Nikolskoye, Russia .. **67 D17**   55 12N 166 0 E
Nikolsky Khutor =
   Sursk, Russia .... **60 D7**   53 3N   45 40 E
Nikopol, Bulgaria ... **51 C8**   43 43N   24 54 E
Nikopol, Ukraine ... **59 J8**   47 35N   34 25 E
Niksar, Turkey ..... **100 B7**   40 31N   37 2 E
Nīkshahr, Iran ..... **97 E9**   26 15N   60 10 E
Nikšić, Serbia & M. .. **50 D2**   42 50N   18 57 E
Nîl, Nahr en →, Africa **106 H7**   30 10N   31 6 E
Nîl el Abyad →, Sudan **107 D3**   15 38N   32 31 E
Nîl el Azraq →, Sudan **107 D3**   15 38N   32 31 E
Nila, Indonesia ..... **83 C3**   6 44 S 129 31 E
Nilakkottai, India ... **95 J3**   10 10N   77 53 E
Niland, U.S.A. **161 M11**   33 14N 115 31W
Nilanga, India ...... **94 E3**   18 6N   76 46 E
Nile = Nîl, Nahr en →,
   Africa .... **106 H7**   30 10N   31 6 E
Nile Delta, Egypt ... **106 H7**   31 40N   31 0 E
Niles, Ohio, U.S.A. .. **150 E4**   41 11N   80 46W
Niles Center = Skokie,
   U.S.A. **157 B9**   42 3N   87 45W
Nileshwar, India .... **95 H2**   12 15N   75 6 E
Nilgiri Hills, India .. **95 J3**   11 30N   76 30 E
Nil Peçanha, Brazil . **171 D4**   13 37 S   39 6W
Nimach, India ...... **92 G6**   24 30N   74 56 E
Nimbahera, India ... **92 G6**   24 37N   74 45 E
Nîmes, France ...... **29 E8**   43 50N   4 23 E
Nimfaíon, Ákra =
   Pínnes, Ákra, Greece **51 F8**   40 5N   24 20 E
Nimmitabel, Australia **129 D8**   36 29 S 149 15 E
Nimneryskiy, Russia **67 D13**   57 50N 125 10 E
Nimrūz □, Afghan. .. **91 C1**   30 0N   62 0 E

Nimule, Sudan ...... **107 G3**   3 32N   32 3 E
Nimule △, Sudan .... **107 G3**   3 38N   32 2 E
Nin, Croatia .... **45 D12**   44 16N   15 12 E
Nīnawá, Iraq ...... **101 D10**   36 25N   43 10 E
Nīnawá □, Iraq ..... **96 B4**   36 15N   43 0 E
Ninda, Angola ...... **115 E4**   14 53 S   21 52 E
Nindigully, Australia **127 D4**   28 21 S 148 50 E
Nine Degree Channel,
   India .... **95 K1**   9 0N   73 0 E
Ninepin Group, China **69 G11**   22 16N 114 21 E
Ninety East Ridge,
   Ind. Oc. .... **121 E7**   1 0 S   90 0 E
Ninety Mile Beach,
   N.Z. .... **130 A1**   34 48 S 173 0 E
Ninety Mile Beach,
   The, Australia .... **129 E7**   38 15 S 147 24 E
Ninety Six, U.S.A. .. **152 A7**   34 11N   82 1W
Nineveh = Nīnawá, Iraq **101 D10**   36 25N   43 10 E
Ning Xian, China ... **74 G4**   35 30N 107 58 E
Ningaloo △, Australia **124 D1**   22 23 S 113 32 E
Ning'an, China ..... **75 B15**   44 22N 129 20 E
Ningbo, China ..... **77 C13**   29 51N 121 28 E
Ningcheng, China ... **75 D10**   41 32N 119 53 E
Ningde, China ...... **77 D12**   26 38N 119 23 E
Ningdu, China ..... **77 D10**   26 25N 115 59 E
Ningerum, Papua N. G. **132 C1**   5 41 S 141 8 E
Ninggang, China ... **77 D9**   26 42N 113 55 E
Ningguo, China .... **77 B12**   30 35N 119 0 E
Ninghai, China ..... **77 C13**   29 51N 121 45 E
Ninghua, China .... **77 D11**   26 14N 116 45 E
Ningi, Nigeria ...... **113 C6**   10 55N   9 30 E
Ningjin, China ..... **74 F8**   37 35N 114 57 E
Ningjing Shan, China **72 C2**   30 0N   98 20 E
Ningling, China .... **74 G8**   34 25N 115 22 E
Ningling, China .... **77 F6**   22 8N   109 5 E
Ningming, China ... **76 F6**   22 8N   107 4 E
Ningnan, China .... **76 D4**   27 5N   102 36 E
Ningpo = Ningbo,
   China .... **77 C13**   29 51N 121 28 E
Ningqiang, China ... **74 H4**   32 47N 106 15 E
Ningshan, China ... **74 H5**   33 21N 108 21 E
Ningsia Hui A.R. =
   Ningxia Huizu
   Zizhiqu □, China . **74 F4**   38 0N 106 0 E
Ningwu, China ..... **74 E7**   39 0N 112 18 E
Ningxia Huizu
   Zizhiqu □, China . **74 F4**   38 0N 106 0 E
Ningxiang, China ... **77 C9**   28 15N 112 30 E
Ningyang, China ... **74 G9**   35 47N 116 45 E
Ningyuan, China ... **77 E8**   25 37N 111 57 E
Ninh Binh, Vietnam **76 G5**   20 15N 105 55 E
Ninh Giang, Vietnam **86 B6**   20 44N 106 24 E
Ninh Hoa, Vietnam . **86 F7**   12 30N 109 7 E
Ninh Ma, Vietnam . **86 F7**   12 48N 109 21 E
Nini-Suhien △, Ghana **112 D4**   5 20N   2 34W
Ninigo Group,
   Papua N. G. ...... **132 A3**   1 15 S 144 17 E
Ninini Pt., U.S.A. .. **145 B2**   21 58N 159 20W
Ninove, Belgium ... **24 D4**   50 51N   4 2 E
Nioaque, Brazil .... **175 A4**   21 5 S   55 50W
Niobrara, U.S.A. ... **154 D6**   42 45N   98 2W
Niobrara →, U.S.A. . **154 D6**   42 46N   98 3W
Nioki, Dem. Rep. of
   the Congo .... **114 C3**   2 47 S   17 40 E
Niokolo-Koba △,
   Senegal **112 C2**   13 3N   13 2W
Niono, Mali **112 C3**   14 15N   6 0W
Nionsamoridougou,
   Guinea **112 D3**   8 45N   8 50W
Nioro du Rip, Senegal **112 C1**   13 40N   15 50W
Nioro du Sahel, Mali **112 B3**   15 15N   9 30W
Niort, France **28 B3**   46 19N   0 29W
Nipa, Papua N. G. .. **132 D2**   6 9 S 143 29 E
Nipani, India ...... **95 F2**   16 20N   74 25 E
Nipawin, Canada ... **143 C8**   53 20N 104 0W
Nipfjället, Sweden .. **16 C5**   61 59N   12 50 E
Nipigon, Canada ... **142 C2**   49 0N   88 17W
Nipigon, L., Canada **140 C2**   49 50N   88 30W
Nipishish L., Canada **141 B7**   54 12N   60 45W
Nipissing, L., Canada **140 C4**   46 20N   80 0W
Nipomo, U.S.A. **161 K6**   35 3N 120 29W
Nippon = Japan ■, Asia **71 G8**   36 0N 136 0 E
Nipton, U.S.A. **161 K11**   35 28N 115 16W
Niquelândia, Brazil . **171 D2**   14 33 S   48 23W
Nir, Iran .... **101 C12**   38 2N   47 59 E
Nira →, India ...... **94 F2**   17 58N   75 8 E
Nirasaki, Japan .... **73 B10**   35 42N 138 27 E
Nirmal, India ...... **94 E4**   19 3N   78 20 E
Nirmali, India ..... **93 F12**   26 20N   86 35 E
Niš, Serbia & M. ... **50 C6**   43 19N   21 58 E
Nisa, Portugal **40 F3**   39 30N   7 41W
Nişāb, Si. Arabia ... **96 D5**   29 11N   44 43 E
Nişāb, Yemen ...... **98 D4**   14 25N   46 29 E
Nišava →, Serbia & M. **50 C6**   43 3N   22 0 E
Niscemi, Italy ...... **47 E7**   37 9N   14 23 E
Nishi-Sonogi-Hantō,
   Japan .... **72 E1**   32 55N 129 45 E
Nishi-Tosa, Japan ... **72 D4**   33 13N 132 46 E
Nishinomiya, Japan . **73 C7**   34 45N 135 20 E
Nishino'omote, Japan **71 J5**   30 43N 130 59 E
Nishio, Japan ...... **73 C9**   34 52N 137 3 E
Nishiwaki, Japan ... **72 C6**   34 59N 134 58 E
Nisibin = Nusaybin,
   Turkey .... **101 D9**   37 3N   41 10 E
Nísiros, Greece ..... **49 E9**   36 35N   27 12 E
Niška Banja,
   Serbia & M. ..... **50 C6**   43 18N   22 1 E
Niskibi →, Canada .. **140 A2**   56 29N   88 9W
Nisko, Poland ...... **55 H9**   50 35N   22 7 E
Nisporeni, Moldova . **55 C13**   47 4N   28 10 E
Nisqually →, U.S.A. **160 C4**   47 6N 122 42W
Nissáki, Greece ..... **38 B9**   39 43N   19 52 E
Nissan = Sweden ■ .. **18 H5**   56 40N   12 51 E
Nissedal, Norway ... **17 G9**   59 10N   8 30 E
Nisser, Norway ..... **18 E5**   59 7N   8 28 E
Nissum Bredning,
   Denmark .... **16 H2**   56 40N   8 20 E
Nissum Fjord, Denmark **17 H2**   56 20N   8 11 E
Nistru = Dnister →,
   Europe .... **59 J6**   46 18N   30 17 E
Nisutlin →, Canada . **142 A2**   60 14N 132 34W
Nitchequon, Canada **141 B5**   53 10N   70 58W
Niterói, Brazil ..... **171 F3**   22 52 S   43 0W
Nith →, Canada **150 C4**   43 12N   80 23W
Nith →, U.K. **22 F5**   55 14N   3 33W
Nitmiluk △, Australia **124 B5**   14 6 S 132 15 E
Nitra, Slovak Rep. .. **35 C11**   48 19N   18 4 E
Nitra →, Slovak Rep. **35 D11**   47 46N   18 10 E
Nitriansky □,
   Slovak Rep. ...... **35 C11**   48 10N   18 30 E
Nittedal, Norway ... **18 F4**   49 12N   12 16 E
Nittenau, Germany . **31 F8**   49 12N   12 16 E
Niu, U.S.A. **72 G4**   31 19N 157 44W
Niuafo'ou, Tonga ... **123 D15**   15 30 S 175 58W
Niue, Cook Is. ..... **123 J11**   19 2 S 169 54W
Niulan Jiang →, China **76 D4**   27 30N 103 5 E
Niut, Indonesia ..... **85 B4**   0 55N 110 6 E
Niuzhuang, China .. **75 D12**   40 58N 122 28 E
Nivala, Finland ..... **14 E21**   63 56N   24 57 E
Nivelles, Belgium ... **24 D4**   50 35N   4 20 E
Nivernais, France ... **27 E10**   47 15N   3 30 E
Niwas, India .... **93 H9**   23 3N   80 26 E
Nixa, U.S.A. **156 G8**   37 3N   93 18W

Nixon, U.S.A. 155 L6   29 16N 97 46W
Nizam Sagar, India .... 94 E3   18 10N 77 58 E
Nizamabad, India ..... 94 E4   18 45N 78 7 E
Nizamghat, India ...... 90 A5   28 20N 95 45 E
Nizhne Kolymsk,
  Russia .... 67 C17 68 34N 160 55 E
Nizhneangarsk, Russia . 67 D11 55 47N 109 30 E
Nizhnegorskiy =
  Nyzhnohirskyy,
  Ukraine .... 59 K8   45 27N 34 38 E
Nizhnekamsk, Russia .. 60 C10 55 38N 51 49 E
Nizhnekamskoye
  Vdkhr., Russia ..... 64 D4   55 56N 52 56 E
Nizhnesaldinsky
  Zavod = Nizhnyaya
  Salda, Russia ...... 64 B8   58 8N 60 42 E
Nizhneserginsky
  Zavod = Nizhniye
  Sergi, Russia ...... 64 C7   56 40N 59 18 E
Nizhneudinsk, Russia .. 67 D10 54 54N 99 3 E
Nizhnevartovsk, Russia 66 C8   60 56N 76 38 E
Nizhniy Chir, Russia .. 61 F6   48 20N 43 5 E
Nizhniy Lomov, Russia 60 D6   53 34N 43 38 E
Nizhniy Novgorod,
  Russia .... 64 C7   56 20N 44 0 E
Nizhniy Tagil, Russia . 64 C7   57 55N 59 57 E
Nizhniye Kresty =
  Cherskiy, Russia ... 67 C17 68 45N 161 18 E
Nizhniye Sergi, Russia 64 C7   56 40N 59 18 E
Nizhnyaya Salda,
  Russia .... 64 B8   58 8N 60 42 E
Nizhyn, Ukraine ..... 59 G6   51 5N 31 55 E
Nizina Mazowiecka,
  Poland .... 55 F8   52 30N 21 0 E
Nizip, Turkey .... 100 D7   37 5N 37 50 E
Nízké Tatry,
  Slovak Rep. .... 35 C12 48 55N 19 30 E
Nízké Tatry △,
  Slovak Rep. .... 35 C12 48 55N 19 37 E
Nízký Jeseník,
  Czech Rep. .... 35 B10 49 50N 17 30 E
Nizza Monferrato, Italy 44 D5   44 46N   8 21 E
Njakwa, Malawi ...... 119 E3   11 1 S 33 56 E
Njanji, Zambia .... 119 E3   14 25 S 31 46 E
Njinjo, Tanzania ..... 119 D4   8 48 S 38 54 E
Njoko →, Zambia ..... 115 F4   17 8 S 24 4 E
Njombe, Tanzania .... 119 D3   9 20 S 34 50 E
Njombe →, Tanzania .. 118 D4   8 7 S   6 E
Njurundabommen,
  Sweden .... 16 B11 62 15N 17 25 E
Nkambe, Cameroon ... 113 D7   6 35N 10 40 E
Nkana, Zambia .... 119 E2   12 50 S 28 8 E
Nkandla, S. Africa ... 117 D5   28 37 S 31 5 E
Nkawkaw, Ghana 113 D4   6 36N   0 49W
Nkayi, Zimbabwe .... 119 F2   19 41 S 29 20 E
Nkhotakota, Malawi .. 119 E3   12 56 S 34 15 E
Nkhotakota △, Malawi 119 E3   12 50 S 34 0 E
Nkolabona, Gabon ... 114 B2   1 14N 11 43 E
Nkomi, Lagune, Gabon 114 C1   1 35 S   9 17 E
Nkone, Dem. Rep. of
  the Congo .... 114 C4   1 2 S 22 20 E
Nkongsamba,
  Cameroon .... 113 E6   4 55N   9 55 E
Nkunga, Dem. Rep. of
  the Congo .... 115 C3   4 41 S 18 34 E
Nkurenkuru, Namibia 116 B2   17 42 S 18 32 E
Nkwanta, Ghana 112 D4   6 10N   2 10W
Nmai →, Burma ..... 76 F2   25 30N 97 25 E
Noakhali = Maijdi,
  Bangla. .... 90 D3   22 48N 91 10 E
Noatak, U.S.A. 144 C7   67 34N 162 58W
Noatak △, U.S.A. 144 B8   68 10N 160 0W
Nobel, Canada 150 A4   45 25N 80 6W
Nobeoka, Japan ...... 72 E3   32 36N 131 41 E
Noble, U.S.A. 157 F8   38 42N 88 14W
Noblejas, Spain 42 F7   39 58N   3 26W
Noblesville, U.S.A. ... 157 D11 40 3N 86 1W
Noboribetsu, Japan ... 70 C10 42 24N 141 6 E
Nocatee, U.S.A. 153 H8   27 10N 81 53W
Noce →, Italy .... 44 B4   46 9N 11 4 E
Nocera Inferiore, Italy 47 B7   40 44N 14 38 E
Nocera Umbra, Italy .. 45 E9   43 5N 12 47 E
Noci, Italy .... 47 B10 40 48N 17 7 E
Nocona, U.S.A. 155 J6   33 47N 97 44W
Nocrich, Romania .... 53 E9   45 55N 24 26 E
Noda, Japan .... 73 B11 35 56N 139 52 E
Nodeland, Norway ... 18 F4   58 8N   7 51 E
Noel Kempff
  Mercado △, Bolivia 173 C5   14 9 S 60 49W
Nogal Valley =
  Nugaaleed, Dooxo,
  Somali Rep. .... 120 C3   8 35N 48 35 E
Nogales, Mexico 162 A2   31 20N 110 56W
Nogales, U.S.A. 159 L8   31 20N 110 56W
Nogaro, France 28 E3   43 45N   0 2W
Nogat →, Poland .... 54 D6   54 17N 19 17 E
Nōgata, Japan .... 72 D2   33 48N 130 44 E
Nogaysk =
  Primorskoye,
  Ukraine .... 59 J9   46 48N 36 20 E
Nogent, France ...... 27 D12 48 1N   5 0 E
Nogent-le-Rotrou,
  France .... 26 D7   48 20N   0 50 E
Nogent-sur-Seine,
  France .... 27 D10 48 30N   3 30 E
Noggerup, Australia .. 125 F2   33 32 S 116 5 E
Noginsk, Moskva,
  Russia .... 58 E10 55 50N 38 25 E
Noginsk, Tunguska,
  Russia .... 67 C10 64 30N 90 50 E
Nogoa →, Australia .. 126 C4   23 40 S 147 55 E
Nogoyá, Argentina ... 174 C4   32 24 S 59 48W
Nógrád □, Hungary .. 52 C4   48 0N 19 30 E
Noguera Pallaresa →,
  Spain .... 40 D5   41 55N   0 55 E
Noguera
  Ribagorzana →,
  Spain .... 40 D5   41 40N   0 43 E
Nohar, India .... 92 E6   29 11N 74 49 E
Nohfelden, Germany . 31 F3   49 35N   7 7 E
Nohili Pt., U.S.A. 145 A2   22 4N 159 47W
Nohta, India .... 93 H8   23 40N 79 34 E
Noia, Spain 42 C2   42 48N   8 53W
Noichi, Japan .... 72 D5   33 33N 133 42 E
Noing, Phil. .... 81 J5   5 40N 125 28 E
Noipuos, Papua N. G. 132 B6   5 35 S 141 7 E
Noire, Montagne,
  France .... 28 E6   43 28N   2 18 E
Noires, Mts., France .. 26 D3   48 11N   3 40W
Noirétable, France ... 28 C7   45 48N   3 46 E
Noirmoutier, Î. de,
  France 26 F4   46 58N   2 10W
Noirmoutier-en-l'Île,
  France 26 F4   47 0N   2 14W
Nojane, Botswana .... 116 C3   23 15 S 20 14 E
Nojima-Zaki, Japan .. 73 C11 34 54N 139 53 E
Nok Kundi, Pakistan . 91 C1   28 50N 62 45 E
Nok Ta Phao, Ko,
  Thailand .... 87 b   9 23N 99 40 E
Nokaneng, Botswana . 116 B3   19 40 S 22 17 E

Nørdstedalsseter,
  Norway .... 18 C4   61 40N   7 48 E
Nordstrand, Germany . 30 A4   54 30N   8 52 E
Nordvik, Russia ..... 67 B12 74 2N 111 32 E
Nore →, Ireland 23 D4   52 25N   6 58W
Norefjell, Norway .... 18 D6   60 16N   9 29 E
Noresund, Norway ... 18 D6   60 11N   9 37 E
Norfolk, Nebr., U.S.A. 154 D6   42 2N 97 25W
Norfolk, Va., U.S.A. . 148 G7   36 51N 76 17W
Norfolk □, U.K. ..... 21 E8   52 39N   0 54 E
Norfolk I., Pac. Oc. .. 134 K8   28 58 S 168 3 E
Norfork L., U.S.A. ... 155 G8   36 15N 92 14W
Norge = Norway ■,
  Europe .... 14 E14 63 0N 11 0 E
Norheimsund, Norway 18 D3   60 23N   6 6 E
Norilsk, Russia ...... 67 C9   69 20N 88 6 E
Norma, Mt., Australia 126 C3   20 55 S 140 42 E
Normal, U.S.A. 156 D8   40 31N 88 59W
Norman, U.S.A. 155 H6   35 13N 97 26W
Norman →, Australia . 126 B3   19 18 S 141 51 E
Norman Park, U.S.A. . 152 D6   31 16N 83 41W
Norman Wells, Canada 138 B7   65 17N 126 51W
Normanby →, Australia 126 A3   14 23 S 144 10 E
Normanby,
  Australia .... 126 A3   14 23 S 144 10 E
Normanby I.,
  Papua N. G. ...... 132 F6   10 5 S 151 5 E
Normandie, France .. 26 D6   48 30N   0 20W
Normandie-Maine △,
  France 26 D6   48 30N   0 0W
Normandy =
  Normandie, France 26 D6   48 30N   0 0W
Normandin, Canada .. 140 C5   48 49N 72 31W
Normanhurst, Mt.,
  Australia .... 125 E3   25 4 S 122 30 E
Normanton, Australia 126 B3   17 40 S 141 10 E
Normanville, Australia 128 C3   35 27 S 138 18 E
Normétal, Canada ... 140 C4   49 0N 79 22W
Norquay, Canada 143 C8   51 53N 102 5W
Norquinco, Argentina 176 E2   41 51 S 70 55W
Norra Dellen, Sweden 16 C10 61 53N 16 43 E
Norra Kvill △, Sweden 17 G9   57 46N 15 31 E
Norra Ulvön, Sweden 16 A12 63 31N 18 40 E
Norrahammar, Sweden 17 G8   57 43N 14 7 E
Norrbottens län □,
  Sweden .... 14 E14 66 50N 20 0 E
Nørre Åby, Denmark 17 J3   55 27N   9 52 E
Nørre Alslev, Denmark 17 K5   54 54N 11 52 E
Nørresundby, Denmark 17 G3   57 5N   9 52 E
Norrhult-Klavreström,
  Sweden .... 17 G9   57 7N 15 10 E
Norris City, U.S.A. .. 157 G8   37 59N 88 20W
Norris Point, Canada . 141 C8   49 31N 57 53W
Norristown, Ga., U.S.A. 152 C7   32 30N 82 30W
Norristown, Pa., U.S.A. 151 F9   40 7N 75 21W
Norrköping, Sweden .. 17 F10 58 37N 16 11 E
Norrland, Sweden ... 15 E16 62 15N 15 45 E
Norrtälje, Sweden ... 17 F11 59 46N 18 42 E
Norseman, Australia . 125 F3   32 8 S 121 43 E
Norsewood, N.Z. .... 130 G5   40 3 S 176 13 E
Norsjø, Norway ..... 18 E6   59 18N   9 20 E
Norsk, Russia .... 67 D14 52 30N 130 5 E
Norsup, Vanuatu .... 133 F5   16 3 S 167 24 E
Norte, C., Chile ..... 172 b   27 3 S 109 24W
Norte, Canal do →,
  Brazil 169 C7   0 40N 50 20W
Norte, Pta., Argentina 176 B4   42 5 S 63 46W
Norte, Pta. del,
  Canary Is. 9 e1   27 51N 17 57W
Norte, Pta. do, Azores 9 d4   37 1N 25 4W
Norte, Serra do, Brazil 173 C6   11 20 S 59 0W
Norte de Santander □,
  Colombia 168 B3   8 0N 73 0W
Norte Grande, Azores 9 d1   38 40N 28 4W
Nortelândia, Brazil .. 173 C6   14 25 S 56 48W
North, C., Canada ... 152 B8   33 37N 81 6W
North, C., Canada ... 141 C7   47 2N 60 20W
North Adams, U.S.A. 151 D11 42 42N 73 7W
North America,
  Africa 136 F10 40 0N 100 0W
North Andaman I.,
  India .... 95 H11 13 15N 92 55 E
North Arm, Canada .. 142 A5   62 0N 114 30W
North Atlantic Ocean,
  Atl. Oc. 8 C7   30 0N 50 0W
North Augusta, U.S.A. 152 B8   33 30N 81 59W
North Ayrshire □, U.K. 22 F4   55 45N   4 44W
North Baltimore,
  U.S.A. 157 C13 41 11N 83 41W
North Bass I., U.S.A. 150 E2   41 44N 82 53W
North Battleford,
  Canada 143 C7   52 50N 108 17W
North Bay, Canada .. 140 C4   46 20N 79 30W
North Belcher Is.,
  Canada 140 A4   56 50N 79 50W
North Bend, Oreg.,
  U.S.A. 158 E1   43 24N 124 14W
North Bend, Pa., U.S.A. 150 E7   41 20N 77 42W
North Bend, Wash.,
  U.S.A. 160 C5   47 30N 121 47W
North Bennington,
  U.S.A. 151 D11 42 56N 73 15W
North Berwick, U.K. . 22 E6   56 4N   2 42W
North Berwick, U.S.A. 151 D14 43 18N 70 44W
North Borneo =
  Sabah □, Malaysia . 85 A5   6 0N 117 0 E
North Brother I., India 95 J11 10 59N 92 40 E
North C., Canada 141 C7   47 5N 64 0W
North C., N.Z. ...... 130 A2   34 23 S 173 4 E
North Canadian →,
  U.S.A. 155 H7   35 16N 95 31W
North Canton, U.S.A. 150 F3   40 53N 81 24W
North Cape =
  Nordkapp, Norway . 14 A21 71 10N 25 50 E
North Cape =
  Nordkapp, Svalbard 6 A9   80 31N 20 0 E
North Caribou L.,
  Canada 140 B1   52 50N 90 40W
North Carolina □,
  U.S.A. 149 H6   35 30N 80 0W
North Cascades △,
  U.S.A. 158 B3   48 45N 121 10W
North Cay, Bahamas . 9 b   26 6N 77 26W
North Channel, Canada 150 C3   46 0N 83 0W
North Channel, U.K. . 22 F5   55 13N   5 52W
North Charleston,
  U.S.A. 152 C10 32 53N 79 58W
North Chicago, U.S.A. 157 B9   42 19N 87 51W
North College Hill,
  U.S.A. 157 E12 39 13N 84 33W
North Comino
  Channel, Malta ... 38 E7   36 1N 14 20 E
North Creek, U.S.A. . 151 C11 43 41N 73 59W
North Dakota □,
  U.S.A. 154 B5   47 30N 100 15W
North Downs, U.K. .. 21 F8   51 19N   0 1 E
North East, U.S.A. .. 150 D5   42 13N 79 50W
North East B.,
  Ascension I. ...... 9 g   7 55 S 14 21W
North East Frontier
  Agency = Arunachal
  Pradesh □, India .. 90 A5   28 0N 95 0 E

North East
  Lincolnshire □, U.K. 20 D7   53 34N   0 2W
North Eastern □,
  Kenya .... 118 B5   1 30N 40 0 E
North Esk →, U.K. .. 22 E6   56 46N   2 24W
North European Plain,
  Europe .... 12 E10 55 0N 25 0 E
North Fabius →,
  U.S.A. 156 E5   39 54N 91 30W
North Foreland, U.K. 21 F9   51 22N   1 28 E
North Fork, U.S.A. .. 160 H7   37 14N 119 21W
North Fork, Salt →,
  U.S.A. 156 E5   39 26N 91 53W
North Fork
  American →, U.S.A. 160 G5   38 57N 120 59W
North Fork Edisto →,
  U.S.A. 152 B9   33 16N 80 54W
North Fork Feather →,
  U.S.A. 160 F5   38 33N 121 30W
North Fork Grand →,
  U.S.A. 154 C3   45 47N 102 16W
North Fork Red →,
  U.S.A. 155 H5   34 24N 99 14W
North Fort Myers,
  U.S.A. 153 J8   26 41N 81 53W
North Frisian Is. =
  Nordfriesische Inseln,
  Germany .... 30 A4   54 40N   8 20 E
North Gower, Canada 151 A9   45 8N 75 43W
North Greenfield =
  West Allis, U.S.A. . 157 B8   43 1N 88 0W
North Hd., Australia . 125 F1   30 14 S 114 59 E
North Henik L.,
  Canada 143 A9   61 45N 97 40W
North Highlands,
  U.S.A. 160 G5   38 40N 121 23W
North Horr, Kenya .. 118 B4   3 20N 37 8 E
North I., India ...... 95 J1   10 8N 72 20 E
North I., Kenya ..... 118 B4   4 5N 36 5 E
North I., N.Z. ...... 130 E4   38 0 S 175 0 E
North I., Seychelles .. 121 b   4 25 S 55 13 E
North Judson, U.S.A. 157 C10 41 13N 86 46W
North Kingsville,
  U.S.A. 150 E4   41 54N 80 42W
North Kitui □, Kenya 118 C4   0 15 S 38 29 E
North Knife →,
  Canada 143 B10 58 53N 94 45W
North Koel →, India 93 G10 24 45N 83 50 E
North Korea ■, Asia . 75 E14 40 0N 127 0 E
North L., Australia .. 128 B5   32 30 S 143 5 E
North Lakhimpur,
  India .... 90 B5   27 14N 94 7 E
North Lanarkshire □,
  U.K. 22 F5   55 52N   3 56W
North Las Vegas,
  U.S.A. 161 J11 36 12N 115 7W
North Liberty, U.S.A. 157 C10 41 32N 86 26W
North Lincolnshire □,
  U.K. 20 D7   53 36N   0 30W
North Little Rock,
  U.S.A. 155 H8   34 45N 92 16W
North Loup →, U.S.A. 154 E5   41 17N 98 24W
North Luangwa △,
  Zambia .... 119 E3   11 49 S 32 9 E
North Magnetic Pole,
  Canada 6 A2   88 30N 107 0W
North Manchester,
  U.S.A. 157 D11 41 0N 85 46W
North Mankato, U.S.A. 154 C8   44 3N 94 0W
North Miami Beach,
  U.S.A. 153 K9   25 56N 80 10W
North Minch, U.K. .. 22 C3   58 5N   5 55W
North Moose L.,
  Canada 143 C8   54 11N 100 6W
North Moose L., Man.,
  Canada 143 C8   54 4N 100 12W
North Myrtle Beach,
  U.S.A. 149 J6   33 48N 78 42W
North Nahanni →,
  Canada 142 A4   62 15N 123 20W
North Naples, U.S.A. 153 J8   26 12N 81 48W
North New River
  Canal, U.S.A. 153 J9   26 30N 80 30W
North Olmsted, U.S.A. 150 E3   41 25N 81 56W
North Ossetia □, Russia 61 J7   43 30N 44 30 E
North Pagai, I. = Pagai
  Utara, Pulau,
  Indonesia .... 84 C2   2 35 S 100 0 E
North Palisade, U.S.A. 160 H8   37 6N 118 31W
North Platte, U.S.A. . 154 E4   41 8N 100 46W
North Platte →, U.S.A. 154 E4   41 7N 100 42W
North Pole, Arctic ... 6 A   90 0N   0 0 E
North Pole, U.S.A. .. 144 D11 64 45N 147 21W
North Portal, Canada 143 D8   49 0N 102 33W
North Powder, U.S.A. 158 D5   45 2N 117 55W
North Pt., Ascension I. 9 g   7 53 S 14 23W
North Pt., Barbados .. 164 C2   13 20N 59 37W
North Pt., Trin. & Tob. 169 E10 11 21N 60 31W
North Pt., U.S.A. 150 A1   45 2N 83 16W
North Pt., Vanuatu .. 133 C6   14 56 S 168 6 E
North Reef I., India . 95 H11 13 5N 92 43 E
North Rhine
  Westphalia =
  Nordrhein-
  Westfalen □,
  Germany .... 30 D3   51 45N   7 30 E
North River, Canada . 141 B8   53 49N 57 6W
North Ronaldsay, U.K. 22 B6   59 22N   2 26W
North Salem, U.S.A. 157 E10 39 52N 86 39W
North
  Saskatchewan →,
  Canada 143 C7   53 15N 105 5W
North Sea, Europe ... 19 C7   56 0N   4 0 E
North Seal →, Canada 143 B9   58 50N 98 7W
North Sentinel I., India 95 J11 11 33N 92 15 E
North Shields, Australia 128 C1   34 38 S 135 52 E
North Solomons □,
  Papua N. G. ...... 132 B8   4 0 S 155 0 E
North Somerset □,
  U.K. 21 F5   51 24N   2 45W
North Sporades =
  Vórioi Sporádhes,
  Greece .... 48 B5   39 15N 23 30 E
North Sydney, Canada 141 C7   46 12N 60 15W
North Syracuse, U.S.A. 151 C8   43 8N 76 7W
North Taranaki Bight,
  N.Z. .... 130 E3   38 50 S 174 15 E
North Thompson →,
  Canada 142 C4   50 40N 120 20W
North Tonawanda,
  U.S.A. 150 C6   43 2N 78 53W
North Troy, U.S.A. .. 151 B12 45 0N 72 24W
North Twin I., Canada 140 B4   53 20N 80 0W
North Tyne →, U.K. . 20 C5   55 0N   2 8W
North Ubian I., Phil. . 81 H3   6 9N 120 27 E
North Uist, U.K. 22 D1   57 40N   7 15W
North Union = Shaker
  Heights, U.S.A. ... 150 E3   41 29N 81 32W
North Vancouver,
  Canada 142 D4   49 19N 123 4W
North Vernon, U.S.A. 157 F11 39 0N 85 38W
North Wabasca L.,
  Canada 142 B6   56 0N 113 55W
North Walsham, U.K. 20 E9   52 50N   1 22 E

North Webster, U.S.A. 157 C11 41 25N 85 48W
North West =
  Severo-
  Zapadnyy □, Russia 66 C4   65 0N 40 0 E
North-West □,
  S. Africa .... 116 D4   27 0 S 25 0 E
North West C.,
  Australia .... 124 D1   21 45 S 114 9 E
North West Christmas
  I. Ridge, Pac. Oc. .. 135 G11   6 30N 165 0W
North West Frontier □,
  Pakistan .... 91 B3   34 0N 72 0 E
North West Highlands,
  U.K. 22 D4   57 33N   4 58W
North West River,
  Canada 141 B7   53 30N 60 10W
North Western □,
  Zambia .... 119 E2   13 30 S 25 30 E
North-Western
  Provinces and
  Oudh = Uttar
  Pradesh □, India .. 93 F9   27 0N 80 0 E
North Wildwood,
  U.S.A. 148 F8   39 0N 74 48W
North Yakima =
  Yakima, U.S.A. ... 158 C3   46 36N 120 31W
North York Moors,
  U.K. 20 C7   54 23N   0 53W
North York Moors △,
  U.K. 20 C7   54 27N   0 51W
North Yorkshire □,
  U.K. 20 C6   54 15N   1 25W
Northallerton, U.K. .. 20 C6   54 20N   1 26W
Northam, S. Africa .. 117 C4   24 56 S 27 18 E
Northam, Australia .. 125 E1   28 27 S 114 33 E
Northampton, U.K. .. 21 E7   52 15N   0 53W
Northampton, Mass.,
  U.S.A. 151 D12 42 19N 72 38W
Northampton, Pa.,
  U.S.A. 151 F9   40 41N 75 30W
Northamptonshire □,
  U.K. 21 E7   52 16N   0 55W
Northbridge, U.S.A. . 151 D13 42 9N 71 39W
Northcliffe, Australia . 125 F2   34 39 S 116 7 E
Northeast C., U.S.A. . 144 E5   63 18N 168 42W
Northeast Pacific Basin,
  Pac. Oc. 135 D13 32 0N 145 0W
Northeast Providence
  Chan., W. Indies .. 164 A4   26 0N 76 0W
Northeim, Germany . 30 D6   51 42N 10 0 E
Northern = Limpopo □,
  S. Africa .... 117 C4   24 5 S 29 0 E
Northern □, Ghana .. 113 D4   9 30N   1 0W
Northern □, Malawi . 119 E3   11 0 S 34 0 E
Northern □,
  Papua N. G. ...... 132 E5   9 0 S 148 30 E
Northern □, S. Leone 112 D2   9 15N 11 30W
Northern □, Zambia . 119 E3   10 30 S 31 0 E
Northern Areas □,
  Pakistan .... 65 E6   36 30N 73 0 E
Northern Cape □,
  S. Africa .... 116 D3   30 0 S 20 0 E
Northern Circars, India 94 F6   17 30N 82 30 E
Northern Indian L.,
  Canada 143 B9   57 20N 97 20W
Northern Ireland □,
  U.K. 23 B5   54 45N   7 0W
Northern Lau Group,
  Fiji .... 133 A3   17 30 S 178 59W
Northern Light L.,
  Canada 140 C1   48 15N 90 39W
Northern Marianas ☑,
  Pac. Oc. .... 134 F6   17 0N 145 0 E
Northern Mid-Atlantic
  Ridge, Atl. Oc. ... 8 C8   35 0N 35 0W
Northern Province □,
  S. Africa .... 117 C4   24 5 S 29 0 E
Northern Range,
  Trin. & Tob. 169 F9   10 46N 61 15W
Northern Rhodesia =
  Zambia ■, Africa .. 119 F2   15 0 S 28 0 E
Northern Samar □,
  Phil. .... 80 E5   12 30N 124 40 E
Northern Territory □,
  Australia .... 124 D5   20 0 S 133 0 E
Northfield, Minn.,
  U.S.A. 154 C8   44 27N 93 9W
Northfield, Vt., U.S.A. 151 B12 44 9N 72 40W
Northland □, N.Z. .. 130 B2   35 30 S 173 30 E
Northome, U.S.A. ... 154 B7   47 52N 94 17W
Northport, Ala., U.S.A. 149 J2   33 14N 87 35W
Northport, Wash.,
  U.S.A. 158 B5   48 55N 117 48W
Northumberland □,
  U.K. 20 B6   55 12N   2 0W
Northumberland, C.,
  Australia .... 128 E4   38 5 S 140 40 E
Northumberland Is.,
  Australia .... 126 C4   21 30 S 149 50 E
Northumberland Str.,
  Canada 141 C7   46 20N 64 0W
Northville, U.S.A. ... 151 C10 43 13N 74 11W
Northway, U.S.A. ... 144 E12 62 58N 141 56W
Northwest Pacific
  Basin, Pac. Oc. ... 134 D8   32 0N 165 0 E
Northwest Providence
  Channel, W. Indies 164 A4   26 0N 78 0W
Northwest
  Territories □,
  Canada 138 B9   63 0N 118 0W
Northwich, U.K. 20 D5   53 15N   2 31W
Northwood, Iowa,
  U.S.A. 154 D8   43 27N 93 13W
Northwood, N. Dak.,
  U.S.A. 154 B6   47 44N 97 34W
Norton, Zimbabwe .. 119 F3   17 52 S 30 40 E
Norton, U.S.A. 154 A5   39 50N 99 53W
Norton Sd., U.S.A. .. 144 E7   64 45N 161 15W
Norton Shores, U.S.A. 157 A10 43 8N 86 15W
Nortorf, Germany ... 30 A5   54 10N   9 50 E
Norwalk, Calif., U.S.A. 161 M8   33 54N 118 5W
Norwalk, Conn., U.S.A. 151 E11 41 7N 73 22W
Norwalk, Iowa, U.S.A. 156 C3   41 29N 93 41W
Norwalk, Ohio, U.S.A. 150 E2   41 15N 82 37W
Norway, Maine, U.S.A. 149 C10 44 13N 70 32W
Norway, Mich., U.S.A. 148 C2   45 47N 87 55W
Norway ■, Europe ... 14 E14 63 0N 11 0 E
Norway House, Canada 143 C9   53 59N 97 50W
Norwegian Sea, Atl. Oc. 6 C8   66 0N   1 0 E
Norwich, Canada 150 D4   42 59N 80 36W
Norwich, U.K. ...... 20 E9   52 38N   1 18 E
Norwich, Conn., U.S.A. 151 E12 41 31N 72 5W
Norwich, N.Y., U.S.A. 151 D9   42 32N 75 32W
Norwood, Canada ... 150 B7   44 23N 77 59W
Norwood, N.Y., U.S.A. 151 B10 44 45N 75 0W
Norwood, Ohio, U.S.A. 157 E12 39 10N 84 27W
Noshiro, Japan ...... 70 D10 40 12N 140 0 E
Nosovka = Nosivka,
  Ukraine .... 59 G6   50 50N 31 37 E
Nosivka, Ukraine .... 59 G6   50 50N 31 37 E
Noṣratābād, Iran .... 97 D8   29 55N 60 0 E

Noss Hd., *U.K.* **22 C5** 58 28N 3 3W
Nossa Senhora da Glória, *Brazil* **170 D4** 10 14 S 37 25W
Nossa Senhora das Dores, *Brazil* **170 D4** 10 29 S 37 13W
Nossa Senhora do Livramento, *Brazil* **173 D6** 15 48 S 56 22W
Nossebro, *Sweden* **17 F6** 58 12N 12 43 E
Nossob ➝, *S. Africa* **116 D3** 26 55 S 20 45 E
Nossombougou, *Mali* **112 C3** 13 5N 7 55W
Nosy Boraha, *Madag.* **117 B8** 16 50 S 49 55 E
Nosy Lava, *Madag.* **117 A8** 14 33 S 47 36 E
Nosy Varika, *Madag.* **117 C8** 20 35 S 48 32 E
Notasulga, *U.S.A.* **152 C4** 32 34N 85 41W
Noteć ➝, *Poland* **55 F2** 52 44N 15 26 E
Notikewin ➝, *Canada* **142 B5** 57 2N 117 38W
Notio Aigaio = Notios Aiyaíon □ **49 E7** 36 52N 25 34 E
Notios Aiyaíon □ **49 E7** 36 52N 25 34 E
Notios Evvoïkos Kólpos, *Greece* **48 C5** 38 20N 24 0 E
Noto, *Italy* **47 F8** 36 53N 15 4 E
Noto, G. di, *Italy* **47 F8** 36 50N 15 12 E
Notodden, *Norway* **18 E6** 59 35N 9 17 E
Notre Dame B., *Canada* **141 C8** 49 45N 55 30W
Notre-Dame-de-Koartac = Quaqtaq, *Qué., Canada* **139 B13** 60 55N 69 40W
Notre-Dame-de-Koartac = Quaqtaq, *Qué., Canada* **139 B13** 60 55N 69 40W
Notre-Dame-des-Bois, *Canada* **151 A13** 45 24N 71 4W
Notre-Dame-d'Ivugivic = Ivujivik, *Canada* **139 B12** 62 24N 77 55W
Notre-Dame-du-Nord, *Canada* **140 C4** 47 36N 79 30W
Notsé, *Togo* **113 D5** 7 0N 1 17 E
Nottawasaga B., *Canada* **150 B4** 44 35N 80 15W
Nottaway = Senneterre, *Canada* **140 C4** 48 25N 77 15W
Nottaway ➝, *Canada* **140 B4** 51 22N 78 55W
Nottingham, *U.K.* **20 E6** 52 58N 1 10W
Nottingham, City of □, *U.K.* **20 E6** 52 58N 1 10W
Nottingham I., *Canada* **139 B12** 63 20N 77 55W
Nottinghamshire □, *U.K.* **20 D6** 53 10N 1 3W
Nottoway ➝, *U.S.A.* **148 G7** 36 33N 76 55W
Notwane ➝, *Botswana* **116 C4** 23 35 S 26 58 E
Nouâdhibou, *Mauritania* **110 D1** 20 54N 17 0W
Nouâdhibou, Dakhlet, *Mauritania* **110 D1** 20 55N 16 52W
Nouâdhibou, Ras, *Mauritania* **110 D1** 20 50N 17 0W
Nouakchott, *Mauritania* **112 B1** 18 9N 15 58W
Nouâmghâr, *Mauritania* **112 B1** 19 20N 16 20W
Nouméa, *N. Cal.* **133 V20** 22 17 S 166 30 E
Nouna, *Burkina Faso* **112 C4** 12 45N 3 52W
Noupoort, *S. Africa* **116 E3** 31 10 S 24 57 E
Nouveau Comptoir = Wemindji, *Canada* **140 B4** 53 0N 78 49W
Nouvelle-Amsterdam, Î., *Ind. Oc.* **121 H6** 38 30 S 77 30 E
Nouvelle-Calédonie = New Caledonia ☒, *Pac. Oc.* **133 U19** 21 0 S 165 0 E
Nouzonville, *France* **27 C11** 49 48N 4 44 E
Nov = Nau, *Tajikistan* **65 C4** 40 9N 69 22 E
Nova Aripuanã, *Brazil* **169 E5** 5 8 S 60 22W
Nová Baňa, *Slovak Rep.* **35 C11** 48 28N 18 39 E
Nová Bystřice, *Czech Rep.* **34 B8** 49 2N 15 8 E
Nova Casa Nova, *Brazil* **170 C3** 9 25 S 41 5W
Nova Cruz, *Brazil* **170 C4** 6 28 S 35 25W
Nova Era, *Brazil* **171 E3** 19 45 S 43 3W
Nova Esperança, *Brazil* **175 A5** 23 8 S 52 24W
Nova Fontesvila = Vila Machado, *Mozam.* **119 F3** 19 15 S 34 14 E
Nova-Freixo = Cuamba, *Mozam.* **119 E4** 14 45 S 36 22 E
Nova Friburgo, *Brazil* **171 F3** 22 16 S 42 30W
Nova Gaia = Cambundi-Catembo, *Angola* **115 E3** 10 10 S 17 35 E
Nova Gorica, *Slovenia* **45 C10** 45 7N 13 39 E
Nova Gradiška, *Croatia* **52 E2** 45 17N 17 28 E
Nova Granada, *Brazil* **171 F2** 20 30 S 49 20W
Nova Iguaçu, *Brazil* **171 F3** 22 45 S 43 28W
Nova Iorque, *Brazil* **170 C3** 7 0 S 44 5W
Nova Kakhovka, *Ukraine* **59 J7** 46 42N 33 27 E
Nova Lamego, *Guinea-Biss.* **112 C2** 12 19N 14 11W
Nova Lima, *Brazil* **175 A7** 19 59 S 43 51W
Nova Lisboa = Huambo, *Angola* **115 E3** 12 42 S 15 54 E
Nova Lusitânia, *Mozam.* **119 F3** 19 50 S 34 34 E
Nova Mambone, *Mozam.* **117 C6** 21 0 S 35 3 E
Nova Odesa, *Ukraine* **59 J6** 47 19N 31 47 E
Nova Olinda do Norte, *Brazil* **169 D6** 3 45 S 59 3W
Nová Paka, *Czech Rep.* **34 A8** 50 29N 15 30 E
Nova Pavova, *Serbia & M.* **52 F5** 44 56N 20 14 E
Nova Ponte, *Brazil* **171 E2** 19 8 S 47 41W
Nova Scotia □, *Canada* **141 C7** 45 10N 63 0W
Nova Siri, *Italy* **47 B9** 40 10N 16 35 E
Nova Sofala, *Mozam.* **117 C5** 20 7 S 34 42 E
Nova Ushytsya, *Ukraine* **53 B12** 48 50N 27 17 E
Nova Varoš, *Serbia & M.* **50 C3** 43 29N 19 48 E
Nova Venécia, *Brazil* **171 E3** 18 45 S 40 24W
Nova Vida, *Brazil* **173 C5** 10 11 S 62 47W
Nova Zagora, *Bulgaria* **51 D10** 42 32N 26 1 E
Novaci, *Macedonia* **50 E5** 41 5N 21 29 E
Novaci, *Romania* **53 E8** 45 10N 23 42 E
Novaféltria, *Italy* **45 E9** 43 53N 12 17 E
Novannenskiy = Novoannenskiy, *Russia* **60 E6** 50 32N 42 39 E
Novar, *Canada* **150 A5** 45 27N 79 15W
Novara, *Italy* **44 C5** 45 28N 8 38 E
Novato, *U.S.A.* **160 G4** 38 6N 122 35W
Novaya Aleksandriya = Puławy, *Poland* **55 G8** 51 23N 21 59 E
Novaya Bukhara = Kagan, *Uzbekistan* **65 D2** 39 43N 64 33 E
Novaya Kakhovka = Nova Kakhovka, *Ukraine* **59 J7** 46 42N 33 27 E
Novaya Kazanka, *Kazakhstan* **61 F9** 48 56N 49 36 E
Novaya Ladoga, *Russia* **58 B7** 60 7N 32 16 E
Novaya Lyalya, *Russia* **64 B8** 59 4N 60 45 E
Novaya Pismyanka = Leninogorsk, *Kazakhstan* **66 D9** 50 20N 83 30 E
Novaya Sibir, Ostrov, *Russia* **67 B16** 75 10N 150 0 E
Novaya Zemlya, *Russia* **66 B6** 75 0N 56 0 E
Nové Město, *Slovak Rep.* **35 C10** 48 45N 17 50 E
Nové Město na Moravě, *Czech Rep.* **34 B9** 49 34N 16 5 E
Nové Město nad Metují, *Czech Rep.* **35 A9** 50 20N 16 10 E
Nové Zámky, *Slovak Rep.* **35 C11** 48 2N 18 8 E
Novelda, *Spain* **41 G4** 38 24N 0 45W
Novellara, *Italy* **44 D7** 44 51N 10 44 E
Novelty, *U.S.A.* **156 D4** 40 1N 92 12W
Noventa Vicentina, *Italy* **45 C8** 45 17N 11 32 E
Novgorod, *Russia* **58 C6** 58 30N 31 25 E
Novgorod-Severskiy = Novhorod-Siverskyy, *Ukraine* **59 G7** 52 2N 33 10 E
Novgradets = Suvorovo, *Bulgaria* **51 C11** 43 20N 27 35 E
Novhorod-Siverskyy, *Ukraine* **59 G7** 52 2N 33 10 E
Novi Bečej, *Serbia & M.* **52 E5** 45 36N 20 10 E
Novi Iskar, *Bulgaria* **50 D7** 42 48N 23 21 E
Novi Kneževac, *Serbia & M.* **52 D5** 46 4N 20 8 E
Novi Lígure, *Italy* **44 D5** 44 46N 8 47 E
Novi Pazar, *Bulgaria* **51 C11** 43 25N 27 15 E
Novi Pazar, *Serbia & M.* **50 C4** 43 12N 20 28 E
Novi Sad, *Serbia & M.* **52 E4** 45 18N 19 52 E
Novi Slankamen, *Serbia & M.* **52 E5** 45 8N 20 15 E
Novi Travnik, *Bos.-H.* **52 F2** 44 10N 17 40 E
Novi Vinodolski, *Croatia* **45 C11** 45 10N 14 48 E
Novigrad, *Istra, Croatia* **45 C10** 45 19N 13 33 E
Novigrad, *Zadar, Croatia* **45 D12** 44 10N 15 32 E
Novigradsko More, *Croatia* **45 D12** 44 12N 15 33 E
Novinger, *U.S.A.* **156 D4** 40 14N 92 43W
Novo Acôrdo, *Brazil* **170 D2** 10 10 S 46 48W
Novo Airão, *Brazil* **169 D5** 2 40 S 60 59W
Novo Aripuanã, *Brazil* **169 E5** 5 8 S 60 22W
Novo Cruzeiro, *Brazil* **171 E3** 17 29 S 41 53W
Novo Hamburgo, *Brazil* **175 B5** 29 37 S 51 7W
Novo Horizonte, *Brazil* **171 F2** 21 25 S 49 10W
Novo Ivanivka, *Ukraine* **53 E14** 45 55N 29 5 E
Novo-Mariinsk = Anadyr, *Russia* **67 C18** 64 35N 177 20 E
Novo Mesto, *Slovenia* **45 C12** 45 47N 15 12 E
Novo Miloševo, *Serbia & M.* **52 E5** 45 42N 20 20 E
Novo Nikolaevsk = Novosibirsk, *Russia* **66 D9** 55 0N 83 5 E
Novo Paraiso, *Brazil* **169 C5** 1 17N 60 28W
Novo Remanso, *Brazil* **170 C3** 9 41 S 42 4W
Novo-Sergiyevskiy, *Russia* **64 E4** 52 5N 53 38 E
Novo-Starobinsk = Salihorsk, *Belarus* **59 F4** 52 51N 27 27 E
Novo-Troitskoye = Sokuluk, *Kyrgyzstan* **65 B7** 42 52N 74 18 E
Novo Urgench = Urganch, *Uzbekistan* **66 E7** 41 40N 60 41 E
Novoaleksandrovsk = Zarasai, *Lithuania* **15 J22** 55 40N 26 20 E
Novoaleksandrovsk, *Russia* **61 H5** 45 29N 41 17 E
Novoaleksandrovskaya = Novoaleksandrovsk, *Russia* **61 H5** 45 29N 41 17 E
Novoalekseyevka, *Kazakhstan* **64 F5** 50 8N 55 39 E
Novoaltaysk, *Russia* **66 D9** 53 30N 84 0 E
Novoannenskiy, *Russia* **60 E6** 50 32N 42 39 E
Novoazovsk, *Ukraine* **59 J10** 47 15N 38 4 E
Novocheboksarsk, *Russia* **60 B8** 56 5N 47 27 E
Novocherkassk, *Russia* **61 G5** 47 27N 40 15 E
Novodevichye, *Russia* **60 D9** 53 37N 48 50 E
Novogrudok = Navahrudak, *Belarus* **58 F3** 53 40N 25 50 E
Novohrad-Volynskyy, *Ukraine* **59 G4** 50 34N 27 35 E
Novokachalinsk, *Russia* **70 B6** 45 5N 132 0 E
Novokazalinsk = Zhangaqazaly, *Kazakhstan* **66 E7** 45 48N 62 6 E
Novokhopersk, *Russia* **60 E5** 51 5N 41 39 E
Novokiyevskoye = Kraskino, *Russia* **67 E14** 42 44N 130 48 E
Novokuybyshevsk, *Russia* **60 D9** 53 7N 49 58 E
Novokuznetsk, *Russia* **66 D9** 53 45N 87 10 E
Novolyalinsky = Novaya Lyalya, *Russia* **64 B8** 59 4N 60 45 E
Novomirgorod, *Ukraine* **59 H6** 48 45N 31 33 E
Novomoskovsk, *Russia* **58 E10** 54 5N 38 15 E
Novomoskovsk, *Ukraine* **59 H8** 48 33N 35 17 E
Novonikolayevka = Novoazovsk, *Ukraine* **59 J10** 47 15N 38 4 E
Novoorsk, *Russia* **64 F7** 51 21N 59 2 E
Novopolotsk = Navapolatsk, *Belarus* **58 E5** 55 32N 28 37 E
Novorossiysk, *Russia* **59 K9** 44 43N 37 46 E
Novorossiyskoye, *Kazakhstan* **64 F7** 50 13N 58 0 E
Novorybnoye, *Russia* **67 B11** 72 50N 105 50 E
Novorzhev, *Russia* **58 D5** 57 3N 29 25 E
Novosej, *Albania* **50 E4** 41 56N 20 35 E
Novoselytsya, *Ukraine* **53 B11** 48 14N 26 15 E
Novoshakhtinsk, *Russia* **59 J10** 47 46N 39 58 E
Novosibirsk, *Russia* **66 D9** 55 0N 83 5 E
Novosibirskiye Ostrova, *Russia* **67 B15** 75 0N 142 0 E
Novosil, *Russia* **59 F9** 52 59N 37 2 E
Novosineglazovskiy, *Russia* **64 D8** 55 2N 61 21 E
Novosokolniki, *Russia* **58 D6** 56 20N 30 2 E
Novotitarovskaya, *Russia* **61 H4** 45 17N 39 2 E
Novotroitsk, *Russia* **64 F7** 51 10N 58 15 E
Novotroitskoye = Töle Bī, *Kazakhstan* **65 B6** 43 42N 73 46 E
Novoukrayinka, *Ukraine* **59 H6** 48 25N 31 30 E
Novouljanovsk, *Russia* **60 C9** 54 8N 48 24 E
Novouzensk, *Russia* **60 E9** 50 32N 48 17 E
Novovolynsk, *Ukraine* **55 H11** 50 45N 24 4 E
Novovoronezhskiy, *Russia* **59 G10** 51 19N 39 13 E
Novovoznesenovka, *Kyrgyzstan* **65 B9** 42 36N 78 44 E
Novovyatsk, *Russia* **64 B2** 58 24N 49 45 E
Novoyavoriske, *Ukraine* **55 J10** 49 53N 23 33 E
Novozybkov, *Russia* **59 F6** 52 30N 32 0 E
Novska, *Croatia* **45 C14** 45 19N 17 0 E
Novvy Urengoy, *Russia* **66 C8** 65 48N 76 52 E
Nový Bor, *Czech Rep.* **34 A7** 50 46N 14 35 E
Novy Bug = Novyy Buh, *Ukraine* **59 J7** 47 34N 32 29 E
Nový Bydžov, *Czech Rep.* **34 A8** 50 14N 15 29 E
Novy Dvor, *Belarus* **55 F11** 52 50N 24 21 E
Novy Dwór Mazowiecki, *Poland* **55 F7** 52 26N 20 44 E
Nový Jičín, *Czech Rep.* **35 B11** 49 30N 18 2 E
Novy Margelan = Farghona, *Uzbekistan* **65 C5** 40 23N 71 19 E
Novyy Afon, *Georgia* **61 J5** 43 7N 40 50 E
Novyy Bor, *Russia* **56 A9** 66 43N 52 19 E
Novyy Buh, *Ukraine* **59 J7** 47 34N 32 29 E
Novyy Oskol, *Russia* **59 G9** 50 44N 37 55 E
Novyy Port, *Russia* **66 C8** 67 40N 72 30 E
Now Shahr, *Iran* **97 B6** 36 40N 51 30 E
Nowa Deba, *Poland* **55 H8** 50 26N 21 41 E
Nowa Nowa, *Australia* **129 D8** 37 44 S 148 3 E
Nowa Ruda, *Poland* **55 H3** 50 35N 16 30 E
Nowa Sarzyna, *Poland* **55 H9** 50 21N 22 21 E
Nowa Sól, *Poland* **55 G2** 51 48N 15 44 E
Nowata, *U.S.A.* **155 G7** 36 42N 95 38W
Nowbarān, *Iran* **97 C6** 35 8N 49 42 E
Nowe, *Poland* **54 E5** 53 41N 18 44 E
Nowe Miasteczko, *Poland* **55 G2** 51 42N 15 42 E
Nowe Miasto, *Poland* **55 G7** 51 38N 20 34 E
Nowe Miasto Lubawskie, *Poland* **54 E6** 53 27N 19 33 E
Nowe Skalmierzyce, *Poland* **55 G4** 51 43N 18 0 E
Nowe Warpno, *Poland* **54 E1** 53 42N 14 18 E
Nowendoc, *Australia* **129 A9** 31 32 S 151 44 E
Nowghāb, *Iran* **97 C8** 33 53N 59 4 E
Nowgong, *Assam, India* **90 B4** 26 20N 92 50 E
Nowgong, *Mad. P., India* **93 G8** 25 4N 79 27 E
Nowogard, *Poland* **54 E2** 53 41N 15 10 E
Nowogród, *Poland* **55 E8** 53 14N 21 53 E
Nowogród Bobrzanski, *Poland* **55 G2** 51 48N 15 15 E
Nowogrodziec, *Poland* **55 G2** 51 12N 15 24 E
Noworadomsk = Radomsko, *Poland* **55 G6** 51 5N 19 28 E
Nowra, *Australia* **129 C9** 34 53 S 150 35 E
Nowrangapur, *India* **94 E6** 19 14N 82 33 E
Nowshera, *Pakistan* **91 B3** 34 0N 72 0 E
Nowy Dwór Gdański, *Poland* **54 D6** 54 13N 19 7 E
Nowy Sącz, *Poland* **55 J7** 49 40N 20 41 E
Nowy Staw, *Poland* **54 D6** 54 13N 19 2 E
Nowy Targ, *Poland* **55 J7** 49 29N 20 2 E
Nowy Tomyśl, *Poland* **55 F3** 52 19N 16 10 E
Nowy Wiśnicz, *Poland* **55 J7** 49 55N 20 28 E
Noxen, *U.S.A.* **151 E8** 41 25N 76 4W
Noxon, *U.S.A.* **158 C6** 48 0N 115 43W
Noyabr'sk, *Russia* **66 C8** 64 34N 76 21 E
Noyant, *France* **26 E7** 47 30N 0 6 E
Noyers, *France* **27 E10** 47 40N 4 0 E
Noyon, *France* **27 C9** 49 34N 2 59 E
Noyon, *Mongolia* **74 C2** 43 2N 102 4 E
Nozay, *France* **26 E5** 47 34N 1 38W
Nqutu, *S. Africa* **117 D5** 28 13 S 30 32 E
Nsa, *Congo* **114 C3** 2 22 S 15 19 E
Nsa, O. en ➝, *Algeria* **111 B6** 32 28N 5 24 E
Nsa, Plateau de, *Congo* **114 C3** 2 26 S 15 20 E
Nsanje, *Malawi* **119 F4** 16 55 S 35 12 E
Nsawam, *Ghana* **113 D4** 5 50N 0 24W
Nsok, *Eq. Guin.* **114 B2** 1 10N 11 19 E
Nsomba, *Zambia* **119 E2** 10 45 S 29 51 E
Nsontin, *Dem. Rep. of the Congo* **114 C3** 3 7 S 17 56 E
Nsopzup, *Burma* **90 C6** 25 51N 97 30 E
Nsukka, *Nigeria* **113 D6** 6 51N 7 29 E
Ntem ➝, *Cameroon* **114 B2** 2 21N 9 49 E
Ntoum, *Gabon* **114 B1** 0 22N 9 47 E
N'Tsama, *Congo* **114 C2** 0 53 S 14 44 E
Ntui, *Cameroon* **113 E7** 4 27N 11 38 E
Nu Jiang ➝, *China* **76 E2** 29 58N 97 25 E
Nu Shan, *China* **76 E2** 26 0N 99 20 E
Nuakata I., *Papua N. G.* **132 F6** 10 17 S 151 2 E
Nuba Mts. = Nubah, Jibalan, *Sudan* **107 E3** 12 0N 31 0 E
Nubah, Jibalan, *Sudan* **107 E3** 12 0N 31 0 E
Nubia, *Africa* **104 D7** 21 0N 32 0 E
Nubian Desert = Nûbîya, Es Sahrâ en, *Sudan* **106 C3** 21 30N 33 30 E
Nûbîya, Es Sahrâ en, *Sudan* **106 C3** 21 30N 33 30 E
Nubledo, *Spain* **42 B5** 43 31N 5 52W
Nuboai, *Indonesia* **83 B5** 2 10 S 136 30 E
Nubra ➝, *India* **93 B7** 34 35N 77 35 E
Nucet, *Romania* **52 D7** 46 28N 22 35 E
Nueces ➝, *U.S.A.* **155 M6** 27 51N 97 30W
Nueltin L., *Canada* **143 A9** 60 30N 99 30W
Nueva, I., *Chile* **176 E3** 55 13 S 66 30W
Nueva Antioquia, *Colombia* **168 B4** 6 5N 69 26W
Nueva Carteya, *Spain* **43 H6** 37 35N 4 28W
Nueva Ecija □, *Phil.* **80 D3** 15 35N 121 0 E
Nueva Esparta □, *Venezuela* **169 A5** 11 0N 64 0W
Nueva Gerona, *Cuba* **164 B3** 21 53N 82 49W
Nueva Imperial, *Chile* **176 A2** 38 45 S 72 58W
Nueva Palmira, *Uruguay* **174 C4** 33 52 S 58 20W
Nueva Rosita, *Mexico* **162 B4** 28 0N 101 11W
Nueva San Salvador, *El Salv.* **164 D2** 13 40N 89 18W
Nueva Tabarca, *Spain* **41 G4** 38 17N 0 30W
Nueva Vizcaya □, *Phil.* **80 C3** 16 20N 121 20 E
Nuéve de Julio, *Argentina* **174 D3** 35 30 S 61 0W
Nuevitas, *Cuba* **164 B4** 21 30N 77 20W
Nuevo, G., *Argentina* **176 B4** 43 0 S 64 30W
Nuevo Casas Grandes, *Mexico* **162 A3** 30 22N 108 0W
Nuevo Guerrero, *Mexico* **163 B5** 26 34N 99 15W
Nuevo Laredo, *Mexico* **163 B5** 27 30N 99 30W
Nuevo León □, *Mexico* **162 C5** 25 0N 100 0W
Nuevo Mundo, Cerro, *Bolivia* **172 E4** 21 55 S 66 53W
Nuevo Rocafuerte, *Ecuador* **168 D2** 0 55 S 75 27W
Nugaaleed, Dooxo, *Somali Rep.* **120 C3** 8 35N 48 35 E
Nugget Pt., *N.Z.* **131 G4** 46 27 S 169 50 E
Nugrus, Gebel, *Egypt* **106 C3** 24 47N 34 35 E
Nuguria Is., *Papua N. G.* **132 B8** 3 20 S 154 45 E
Nuhaka, *N.Z.* **130 F6** 39 3 S 177 45 E
Nuits-St-Georges, *France* **27 E11** 47 10N 4 56 E
Nukey Bluff, *Australia* **127 E2** 32 26 S 135 29 E
Nukha = Şaki, *Azerbaijan* **61 K8** 41 10N 47 5 E
Nukhayb, *Iraq* **101 F10** 32 4N 42 3 E
Nukheila, *Sudan* **106 D2** 19 1N 26 21 E
Nukiki, *Solomon Is.* **133 L9** 6 46 S 156 35 E
Nuku, *Papua N. G.* **132 B2** 3 41 S 142 28 E
Nuku-Hiva, *French Polynesia* **135 H13** 8 54 S 140 6W
Nuku'alofa, *Tonga* **133 Q14** 21 10 S 174 0W
Nukuhu, *Papua N. G.* **132 C5** 5 34 S 149 22 E
Nukulaelae, *Tuvalu* **123 B14** 9 23 S 179 52 E
Nukus, *Uzbekistan* **66 E6** 42 27N 59 41 E
Nulato, *U.S.A.* **144 D8** 64 43N 158 6W
Nules, *Spain* **40 F4** 39 51N 0 9W
Nullagine, *Australia* **124 D3** 21 53 S 120 7 E
Nullagine ➝, *Australia* **124 D3** 21 20 S 120 20 E
Nullarbor, *Australia* **125 F5** 31 28 S 130 55 E
Nullarbor △, *Australia* **125 F2** 32 39 S 115 37 E
Nullarbor Plain, *Australia* **125 F4** 31 10 S 129 0 E
Num, *Indonesia* **83 B5** 1 30 S 135 13 E
Numalla, L., *Australia* **127 D3** 28 43 S 144 20 E
Numan, *Nigeria* **113 D7** 9 29N 12 3 E
Numanuma, *Papua N. G.* **132 E6** 9 41 S 150 55 E
Numata, *Japan* **73 A11** 36 45N 139 4 E
Numatinna ➝, *Sudan* **107 F2** 7 38N 27 20 E
Numaykoos Lake ⌓, *Canada* **143 B9** 57 52N 95 58W
Numazu, *Japan* **73 B10** 35 7N 138 51 E
Numbulwar, *Australia* **126 A2** 14 15 S 135 45 E
Numedal, *Norway* **18 D6** 60 6N 9 6 E
Numfoor, *Indonesia* **83 B4** 1 0 S 134 50 E
Numurkah, *Australia* **129 D6** 36 5 S 145 26 E
Nunaksaluk I., *Canada* **141 A7** 55 49N 60 20W
Nunap Isua, *Greenland* **10 F6** 59 48N 43 55W
Nunavut □, *Canada* **139 D8** 66 0N 85 0W
Nunda, *U.S.A.* **150 D7** 42 35N 77 56W
Nuneaton, *U.K.* **21 E6** 52 32N 1 27W
Nungarin, *Australia* **125 F2** 31 12 S 118 6 E
Nungo, *Mozam.* **119 E4** 13 23 S 37 43 E
Nungwe, *Tanzania* **118 C3** 2 48 S 32 2 E
Nunivak I., *U.S.A.* **144 F6** 60 10N 166 30W
Nunkun, *India* **93 C7** 33 57N 76 2 E
Núoro, *Italy* **46 B2** 40 20N 9 20 E
Núpur, *Iceland* **11 B3** 65 56N 23 36W
Nuqayy, Jabal, *Libya* **108 D3** 23 11N 19 30 E
Nuqūb, *Yemen* **98 D4** 14 59N 45 48 E
Nuquí, *Colombia* **168 B2** 5 42N 77 17W
Nūrābād, *Iran* **97 E8** 27 47N 57 12 E
Nurabad, *Uzbekistan* **65 D3** 39 36N 66 17 E
Nurata, *Uzbekistan* **65 C2** 40 33N 65 41 E
Nurata Tizmasi, *Uzbekistan* **65 C3** 40 40N 66 30 E
Nure ➝, *Italy* **44 C6** 45 3N 9 49 E
Nurek, *Tajikistan* **65 D4** 38 23N 69 19 E
Nuremberg = Nürnberg, *Germany* **31 F7** 49 27N 11 3 E
Nuri, *Mexico* **162 B3** 28 2N 109 22W
Nuri, *Sudan* **106 D3** 18 29N 31 59 E
Nuriootpa, *Australia* **128 C3** 34 27 S 139 0 E
Nurlat, *Russia* **60 C10** 54 29N 50 45 E
Nurmes, *Finland* **14 E23** 63 33N 29 10 E
Nürnberg, *Germany* **31 F7** 49 27N 11 3 E
Nurpur, *Pakistan* **92 D4** 31 53N 71 54 E
Nurra, La, *Italy* **46 B1** 40 45N 8 15 E
Nurran, L. = Terewah, L., *Australia* **127 D4** 29 52 S 147 35 E
Nurrari Lakes, *Australia* **125 E5** 29 1 S 130 5 E
Nurri, *Italy* **46 C2** 39 43N 9 14 E
Nürtingen, *Germany* **31 G5** 48 37N 9 19 E
Nurzec ➝, *Poland* **55 F9** 52 37N 22 25 E
Nus, *Italy* **44 C4** 45 45N 7 28 E
Nusa Barung, *Indonesia* **85 D4** 8 30 S 113 30 E
Nusa Dua, *Indonesia* **79 K18** 8 48 S 115 14 E
Nusa Kambangan, *Indonesia* **85 D3** 7 40 S 108 10 E
Nusa Tenggara Barat □, *Indonesia* **85 D5** 8 50 S 117 30 E
Nusa Tenggara Timur □, *Indonesia* **82 C2** 9 30 S 122 0 E
Nusaybin, *Turkey* **101 D9** 37 3N 41 10 E
Nushki, *Pakistan* **91 C2** 29 35N 66 0 E
Nuuk, *Greenland* **10 E5** 64 10N 51 35W
Nuussauq, *Greenland* **10 C5** 74 8N 57 3W
Nuwakot, *Nepal* **93 E10** 28 10N 83 55 E
Nuwara Eliya, *Sri Lanka* **95 L5** 6 58N 80 48 E
Nuweiba', *Egypt* **96 D2** 28 59N 34 39 E
Nuwerus, *S. Africa* **116 E2** 31 8 S 18 24 E
Nuweveldberge, *S. Africa* **116 E3** 32 10 S 21 45 E
Nuyts, C., *Australia* **125 F5** 32 2 S 132 21 E
Nuyts, Pt., *Australia* **125 G2** 35 4 S 116 38 E
Nuyts Arch., *Australia* **127 E1** 32 35 S 133 20 E
Nuzvid, *India* **94 F5** 16 47N 80 53 E
N'Vinda, *Angola* **115 E3** 13 8 S 19 2 E
Nxai Pan △, *Botswana* **116 B3** 19 50 S 24 46 E
Nxau-Nxau, *Botswana* **116 B3** 18 57 S 21 4 E
Nyaake, *Liberia* **112 E3** 4 52N 7 37W
Nyabessan, *Cameroon* **114 B2** 2 28N 10 24 E
Nyabing, *Australia* **125 F2** 33 33 S 118 9 E
Nyack, *U.S.A.* **151 E11** 41 5N 73 55W
Nyagan, *Russia* **66 C7** 62 30N 65 38 E
Nyah West, *Australia* **128 C5** 35 16 S 143 21 E
Nyahanga, *Tanzania* **118 C3** 2 20 S 33 37 E
Nyahua, *Tanzania* **118 D3** 5 25 S 33 23 E
Nyahururu, *Kenya* **118 B4** 0 2N 36 27 E
Nyainqentanglha Shan, *China* **68 D4** 30 0N 90 0 E
Nyakanazi, *Tanzania* **118 C3** 3 2 S 31 10 E
Nyakrom, *Ghana* **113 D4** 5 40N 0 50W
Nyâlâ, *Sudan* **107 E1** 12 2N 24 58 E
Nyamandhlovu, *Zimbabwe* **119 F2** 19 55 S 28 16 E
Nyambiti, *Tanzania* **118 C3** 2 48 S 33 27 E
Nyamlell, *Sudan* **107 F2** 9 7N 26 59 E
Nyamwaga, *Tanzania* **118 C3** 1 27 S 34 33 E
Nyandekwa, *Tanzania* **118 C3** 3 57 S 32 32 E
Nyanding ➝, *Sudan* **107 F3** 8 40N 32 41 E
Nyandoma, *Russia* **58 B11** 61 40N 40 12 E
Nyanga △, *Zimbabwe* **119 F3** 18 17 S 32 46 E
Nyanga ➝, *Gabon* **114 C2** 2 58 S 10 15 E
Nyangana, *Namibia* **116 B3** 18 0 S 20 40 E
Nyanguge, *Tanzania* **118 C3** 2 30 S 33 12 E
Nyankpala, *Ghana* **113 D4** 9 21N 0 58W
Nyanza, *Rwanda* **118 C2** 2 20 S 29 42 E
Nyanza □, *Kenya* **118 C3** 0 10 S 34 15 E
Nyanza-Lac, *Burundi* **118 C2** 4 21 S 29 36 E
Nyaponges, *Sudan* **107 F3** 5 5N 33 45 E
Nyasa, L., *Africa* **119 E3** 12 30 S 34 30 E
Nyasaland = Malawi ■, *Africa* **119 E3** 11 55 S 34 0 E
Nyasvizh, *Belarus* **59 F4** 53 14N 26 38 E
Nyaunglebin, *Burma* **90 G6** 17 52N 96 42 E
Nyazepetrovsk, *Russia* **64 C7** 56 3N 59 36 E
Nyazura, *Zimbabwe* **119 F3** 18 40 S 32 16 E
Nyazwidzi ➝, *Zimbabwe* **119 G3** 20 0 S 31 17 E
Nybergsund, *Norway* **18 C9** 61 15N 12 19 E
Nyborg, *Denmark* **17 J4** 55 18N 10 47 E
Nybro, *Sweden* **17 H9** 56 44N 15 55 E
Nyda, *Russia* **66 C8** 66 40N 72 58 E
Nyeboe Land, *Greenland* **10 A5** 82 0N 57 0W
Nyengo Swamp, *Zambia* **115 E4** 14 51 S 22 7 E
Nyeri, *Kenya* **118 C4** 0 23 S 36 56 E
Nyerol, *Sudan* **107 F3** 8 41N 32 1 E
Nyhammar, *Sweden* **16 D8** 60 17N 14 58 E
Nyika △, *Malawi* **119 E3** 10 30 S 33 53 E
Nyinahin, *Ghana* **112 D4** 6 43N 2 3W
Nyíradony, *Hungary* **52 C6** 47 41N 21 55 E
Nyirbátor, *Hungary* **52 C7** 47 49N 22 9 E
Nyíregyháza, *Hungary* **52 C6** 47 58N 21 47 E
Nykarleby = Uusikaarlepyy, *Finland* **14 E20** 63 32N 22 31 E
Nykirke, *Norway* **18 D7** 60 54N 10 19 E
Nykøbing, *Storstrøm, Denmark* **17 K5** 54 56N 11 52 E
Nykøbing, *Vestsjælland, Denmark* **17 J5** 55 55N 11 40 E
Nykøbing, *Viborg, Denmark* **17 H2** 56 48N 8 51 E
Nyköping, *Sweden* **17 F11** 58 45N 17 1 E
Nykroppa, *Sweden* **16 E8** 59 37N 14 18 E
Nykvarn, *Sweden* **16 E11** 59 11N 17 25 E
Nyland, *Sweden* **16 A11** 63 1N 17 45 E
Nylstroom = Modimolle, *S. Africa* **117 C4** 24 42 S 28 22 E
Nymagee, *Australia* **129 B7** 32 7 S 146 20 E
Nymboida △, *Australia* **127 D5** 29 38 S 152 26 E
Nymburk, *Czech Rep.* **34 A8** 50 10N 15 1 E
Nynäshamn, *Sweden* **17 F11** 58 54N 17 57 E
Nyngan, *Australia* **129 A7** 31 30 S 147 8 E
Nyoma Rap, *India* **93 C8** 33 10N 78 40 E
Nyoman = Nemunas ➝, *Lithuania* **15 J19** 55 25N 21 10 E
Nyon, *Switz.* **32 D2** 46 23N 6 14 E
Nyong ➝, *Cameroon* **113 E6** 3 17N 9 54 E
Nyons, *France* **29 D9** 44 22N 5 10 E
Nyou, *Burkina Faso* **113 C4** 12 42N 2 1W
Nýrsko, *Czech Rep.* **34 B6** 49 18N 13 9 E
Nysa, *Poland* **55 H4** 50 30N 17 22 E
Nysa ➝, *Europe* **30 C10** 52 4N 14 46 E
Nysa Kłodzka ➝, *Poland* **55 H4** 50 49N 17 40 E
Nysäter, *Sweden* **16 E6** 59 17N 12 47 E
Nyseter, *Norway* **18 B5** 62 2N 8 20 E
Nyslott = Savonlinna, *Finland* **58 B5** 61 52N 28 53 E
Nyssa, *U.S.A.* **158 E5** 43 53N 117 0W
Nystad = Uusikaupunki, *Finland* **15 F19** 60 47N 21 25 E
Nysted, *Denmark* **17 K5** 54 40N 11 44 E
Nytva, *Russia* **64 C5** 57 56N 55 20 E
Nyunzu, *Dem. Rep. of the Congo* **118 D2** 5 57 S 27 58 E
Nyurba, *Russia* **67 C12** 63 17N 118 28 E
Nyzhankovychi, *Ukraine* **55 J9** 49 40N 22 49 E
Nyzhnohirskyy, *Ukraine* **59 K8** 45 27N 34 38 E
Nyzhny Vorota, *Ukraine* **53 B8** 48 46N 23 6 E
Nzébéla, *Guinea* **112 D3** 8 9N 9 7W
Nzega, *Tanzania* **118 C3** 4 10 S 33 12 E
Nzérékoré, *Guinea* **112 D3** 7 49N 8 48W
Nzeto, *Angola* **115 D2** 7 10 S 12 52 E
Nzilo, Chutes de, *Dem. Rep. of the Congo* **119 E2** 10 18 S 25 27 E
N'zo ⌓, *Ivory C.* **112 D3** 6 15N 7 15W
N'zo ➝, *Ivory C.* **112 D3** 6 15N 7 3W
Nzubuka, *Tanzania* **118 C3** 4 45 S 32 50 E
Nzwani = Anjouan, *Comoros Is.* **121 a** 12 15 S 44 20 E

O

O Barco, *Spain* **42 C4** 42 23N 6 58W
O Carballiño, *Spain* **42 C2** 42 26N 8 5W
O Corgo, *Spain* **42 C3** 42 56N 7 25W
O Le Pupū Pu'e △, *Samoa* **133 W24** 13 59 S 171 43W
O Pino, *Spain* **42 C2** 42 56N 8 20W
O Porriño, *Spain* **42 C2** 42 10N 8 37W
Ō-Shima, *Fukuoka, Japan* **72 D2** 30 53N 130 28 E
Ō-Shima, *Nagasaki, Japan* **72 C1** 33 29N 129 33 E
Ō-Shima, *Shizuoka, Japan* **73 C11** 34 44N 139 24 E
Oa, Mull of, *U.K.* **22 F2** 55 35N 6 20W
Oacoma, *U.S.A.* **154 D5** 43 48N 99 24W
Oahe, L., *U.S.A.* **154 C4** 44 27N 100 24W
Oahe Dam, *U.S.A.* **154 C4** 44 27N 100 24W
Oahu, *U.S.A.* **145 K14** 21 28N 157 58W
Oak Creek, *U.S.A.* **157 B9** 42 52N 87 55W
Oak Harbor, *U.S.A.* **160 B4** 48 18N 122 39W
Oak Hill, *Fla., U.S.A.* **153 G9** 28 52N 80 51W
Oak Hill, *W. Va., U.S.A.* **148 G5** 37 59N 81 9W
Oak Island, *U.S.A.* **149 J6** 33 55N 78 10W
Oak Lawn, *U.S.A.* **157 C9** 41 43N 87 44W
Oak Park, *Ga., U.S.A.* **152 C7** 32 22N 82 19W
Oak Park, *Ill., U.S.A.* **157 C9** 41 53N 87 47W
Oak Ridge, *U.S.A.* **149 G3** 36 1N 84 16W
Oak View, *U.S.A.* **161 L7** 34 24N 119 18W
Oakan-Dake, *Japan* **70 C12** 43 27N 144 10 E
Oakbank, *Australia* **128 B4** 33 4 S 140 33 E
Oakdale, *Calif., U.S.A.* **160 H6** 37 46N 120 51W
Oakdale, *La., U.S.A.* **155 K8** 30 49N 92 40W
Oakes, *U.S.A.* **154 B5** 46 8N 98 6W
Oakesdale, *U.S.A.* **158 C5** 47 8N 117 15W
Oakey, *Australia* **127 D5** 27 25 S 151 43 E
Oakfield, *Ga., U.S.A.* **152 D6** 31 47N 83 58W
Oakfield, *N.Y., U.S.A.* **150 C6** 43 4N 78 16W
Oakford, *U.S.A.* **156 D7** 40 6N 89 58W
Oakham, *U.K.* **21 E7** 52 40N 0 43W
Oakhurst, *U.S.A.* **160 H7** 37 19N 119 40W
Oakland, *Calif., U.S.A.* **160 H4** 37 49N 122 16W
Oakland, *Ill., U.S.A.* **157 E8** 39 39N 88 2W
Oakland City, *U.S.A.* **157 F9** 38 20N 87 21W
Oaklands, *Australia* **129 C7** 35 34 S 146 10 E
Oakley, *Idaho, U.S.A.* **158 E7** 42 15N 113 53W
Oakley, *Kans., U.S.A.* **154 F4** 39 8N 100 51W
Oakover ➝, *Australia* **124 D3** 21 0 S 120 40 E
Oakridge, *U.S.A.* **158 E2** 43 45N 122 28W
Oaktown, *U.S.A.* **157 F9** 38 52N 87 27W
Oakville, *Canada* **150 C5** 43 27N 79 41W
Oakville, *U.S.A.* **160 D3** 46 51N 123 14W
Oakwood, *U.S.A.* **157 C12** 41 6N 84 23W
Oamaru, *N.Z.* **131 F5** 45 5 S 170 59 E
Ōamishirasato, *Japan* **73 B12** 35 31N 140 18 E
Oancea, *Romania* **53 E12** 45 21N 27 42 E
Oarai, *Japan* **73 A12** 36 21N 140 34 E
Oasi Faunistica di Vendicari ⌓, *Italy* **47 F8** 36 49N 15 6 E
Oasis, *Calif., U.S.A.* **161 M10** 33 28N 116 6W

Oasis, *Nev., U.S.A.* **160 H9** 37 29N 117 55W
Oates Land, *Antarctica* **7 C11** 69 0 S 160 0 E
Oatlands, *Australia* **127 G4** 42 17 S 147 21 E
Oatman, *U.S.A.* **161 K12** 35 1N 114 19W
Oaxaca, *Mexico* **163 D5** 17 2N 96 40W
Oaxaca □, *Mexico* **163 D5** 17 0N 97 0W
Ob →, *Russia* **66 C7** 66 45N 69 30 E
Oba, *Canada* **140 C3** 49 4N 84 7W
Obala, *Cameroon* **113 E7** 4 9N 11 32 E
Obama, *Fukui, Japan* **73 B7** 35 30N 135 45 E
Obama, *Nagasaki, Japan* **72 E2** 32 43N 130 13 E
Oban, *Nigeria* **113 D6** 5 17N 8 33 E
Oban, *U.K.* **22 E3** 56 25N 5 29W
Obbia, *Somali Rep.* **120 C3** 5 25N 48 30 E
Obdorsk = Salekhard, *Russia* **66 C7** 66 30N 66 35 E
Ober-Aargau, *Switz.* **32 B5** 47 10N 7 45 E
Ober-engadin, *Switz.* **33 C9** 46 35N 9 55 E
Obera, *Argentina* **175 B4** 27 21 S 55 2W
Oberalppass, *Switz.* **33 C7** 46 39N 8 35 E
Oberalpstock, *Switz.* **33 C7** 46 45N 8 47 E
Oberammergau, *Germany* **31 H7** 47 36N 11 4 E
Oberasbach, *Germany* **31 F6** 49 25N 10 57 E
Oberbayern □, *Germany* **31 G7** 48 5N 11 50 E
Oberburg = Gornji Grad, *Slovenia* **45 B11** 46 20N 14 52 E
Oberdiessbach, *Switz.* **32 C5** 46 51N 7 40 E
Oberdonau = Oberösterreich □, *Austria* **34 C7** 48 10N 14 0 E
Oberdrauburg, *Austria* **34 E5** 46 44N 12 58 E
Obere Donau ⌓, *Germany* **31 G5** 48 5N 9 0 E
Oberentfelden, *Switz.* **32 B6** 47 21N 8 2 E
Oberer Bayerischer Wald ⌓, *Germany* **31 F8** 49 15N 12 40 E
Oberfranken □, *Germany* **31 E7** 50 10N 11 20 E
Oberglogau = Głogówek, *Poland* **55 H4** 50 21N 17 53 E
Oberhausen, *Germany* **30 D2** 51 28N 6 51 E
Oberkirch, *Germany* **31 G4** 48 31N 8 4 E
Oberlaibach = Vrhnika, *Slovenia* **45 C11** 45 58N 14 15 E
Oberland, *Switz.* **32 C5** 46 35N 7 38 E
Oberlausitz, *Germany* **30 D10** 51 16N 14 18 E
Oberlin, *Kans., U.S.A.* **154 F4** 39 49N 100 32W
Oberlin, *La., U.S.A.* **155 K8** 30 37N 92 46W
Oberlin, *Ohio, U.S.A.* **150 E2** 41 18N 82 13W
Obernai, *France* **27 D14** 48 28N 7 30 E
Oberndorf, *Germany* **31 G4** 48 17N 8 34 E
Obernigk = Oborniki Śląskie, *Poland* **55 G3** 51 17N 16 53 E
Oberon, *Australia* **129 B8** 33 45 S 149 52 E
Oberösterreich □, *Austria* **34 C7** 48 10N 14 0 E
Oberpfalz □, *Germany* **31 F8** 49 20N 12 10 E
Oberpfälzer Wald, *Germany* **31 F8** 49 30N 12 30 E
Oberpfälzer Wald ⌓, *Germany* **31 F8** 49 40N 12 20 E
Oberriet, *Switz.* **33 B9** 47 19N 9 34 E
Obersiggenthal, *Switz.* **33 B6** 47 29N 8 18 E
Oberstdorf, *Germany* **31 H6** 47 24N 10 15 E
Oberting, *Gabon* **114 C1** 0 22 S 9 46 E
Obertyn, *Ukraine* **53 B10** 48 42N 25 10 E
Oberursel, *Germany* **31 E4** 50 11N 8 35 E
Oberwart, *Austria* **35 D9** 47 17N 16 12 E
Oberwil, *Switz.* **32 A5** 47 32N 7 33 E
Obi, *Indonesia* **82 B3** 1 23 S 127 45 E
Obiaruku, *Nigeria* **113 D6** 5 51N 6 9 E
Óbidos, *Brazil* **169 D6** 1 50 S 55 30W
Óbidos, *Portugal* **43 F1** 39 19N 9 10W
Obigarm, *Tajikistan* **65 D4** 38 43N 69 42 E
Obihiro, *Japan* **70 C11** 42 56N 143 12 E
Obīkiik, *Tajikistan* **65 D4** 38 9N 68 39 E
Obilatu, *Indonesia* **82 B3** 1 25 S 127 20 E
Obilnoye, *Russia* **61 G7** 47 32N 44 30 E
Obing, *Germany* **31 G8** 48 0N 12 24 E
Objat, *France* **28 C5** 45 16N 1 24 E
Oblong, *U.S.A.* **157 F9** 39 0N 87 55W
Obluchye, *Russia* **67 E14** 49 1N 131 4 E
Obninsk, *Russia* **58 E9** 55 8N 36 37 E
Obo, *C.A.R.* **118 A2** 5 20N 26 32 E
Oboa, Mt., *Uganda* **118 B3** 1 45N 34 45 E
Obock, *Djibouti* **107 E5** 12 0N 43 20 E
Obodivka, *Ukraine* **53 B14** 48 24N 29 15 E
Oborniki, *Poland* **55 F3** 52 39N 16 50 E
Oborniki Śląskie, *Poland* **55 G3** 51 17N 16 53 E
Obouya, *Congo* **114 C3** 0 56 S 15 43 E
Oboyan, *Russia* **59 G9** 51 15N 36 21 E
Obozerskaya = Obozerskiy, *Russia* **56 B7** 63 34N 40 21 E
Obozerskiy, *Russia* **56 B7** 63 34N 40 21 E
Obrenovac, *Serbia & M.* **50 B4** 44 40N 20 11 E
O'Brien, *U.S.A.* **152 E7** 30 2N 82 57W
Obrovac, *Croatia* **45 D12** 44 11N 15 41 E
Obruk, *Turkey* **100 C5** 38 7N 33 12 E
Obrzycko, *Poland* **55 F3** 52 42N 16 32 E
Observatory Inlet, *Canada* **142 B3** 55 10N 129 54W
Obshchi Syrt, *Russia* **64 E4** 52 0N 53 0 E
Obskaya Guba, *Russia* **66 C8** 69 0N 73 0 E
Obuasi, *Ghana* **113 D4** 6 17N 1 40W
Obubra, *Nigeria* **113 D6** 6 8N 8 20 E
Obudu, *Nigeria* **113 D6** 6 38N 9 5 E
Obura, *Papua N. G.* **132 D3** 6 33 S 145 58 E
Obwalden □, *Switz.* **32 C6** 46 55N 8 15 E
Obzor, *Bulgaria* **51 D11** 42 50N 27 52 E
Ocala, *U.S.A.* **153 F7** 29 11N 82 8W
Ocamo →, *Venezuela* **169 C4** 2 48N 65 14W
Ocampo, *Chihuahua, Mexico* **162 B3** 28 9N 108 24W
Ocampo, *Tamaulipas, Mexico* **163 C5** 22 50N 99 20W
Ocaña, *Colombia* **168 B3** 8 15N 73 20W
Ocaña, *Spain* **42 F7** 39 55N 3 30W
Ocanomowoc, *U.S.A.* **154 D10** 43 7N 88 30W
Occidental, Cordillera, *Colombia* **168 C3** 5 0N 76 0W
Occidental, Cordillera, *Peru* **172 C3** 14 0 S 74 0W
Occidental, Grand Erg, *Algeria* **111 B5** 30 20N 1 0 E
Ocean City, *Md., U.S.A.* **148 F8** 38 20N 75 5W
Ocean City, *N.J., U.S.A.* **148 F8** 39 17N 74 35W
Ocean City, *Wash., U.S.A.* **160 C2** 47 4N 124 10W
Ocean Falls, *Canada* **142 C3** 52 18N 127 48W
Ocean I. = Banaba, *Kiribati* **134 H8** 0 45 S 169 50 E
Ocean Park, *U.S.A.* **160 D2** 46 30N 124 3W
Oceano, *U.S.A.* **161 K6** 35 6N 120 37W
Oceanport, *U.S.A.* **151 F10** 40 19N 74 3W
Oceanside, *U.S.A.* **161 M9** 33 12N 117 23W
Ochagavía, *Spain* **40 C3** 42 55N 1 5W
Ochakiv, *Ukraine* **59 J6** 46 37N 31 33 E
Ochamchira, *Georgia* **61 J5** 42 46N 41 32 E
Ocher, *Russia* **64 C5** 57 53N 54 42 E
Ochiai, *Japan* **72 B5** 35 1N 133 45 E
Ochil Hills, *U.K.* **22 E5** 56 14N 3 40W
Ochlocknee, *U.S.A.* **152 E5** 30 58N 84 3W
Ochlockonee →, *U.S.A.* **152 F5** 29 59N 84 26W
Ocho Rios, *Jamaica* **164 a** 18 24N 77 6W
Ochopee, *U.S.A.* **153 K8** 25 54N 81 18W
Ochsenfurt, *Germany* **31 F6** 49 40N 10 4 E
Ochsenhausen, *Germany* **31 G5** 48 4N 9 57 E
Ocilla, *U.S.A.* **152 D6** 31 36N 83 15W
Ockelbo, *Sweden* **16 D10** 60 54N 16 45 E
Ocmulgee ⌓, *U.S.A.* **152 C6** 32 49N 83 37W
Ocmulgee →, *U.S.A.* **152 D7** 31 58N 82 33W
Ocna Mureş, *Romania* **53 D8** 46 23N 23 55 E
Ocna Sibiului, *Romania* **53 E9** 45 52N 24 2 E
Ocnele Mari, *Romania* **53 E9** 45 8N 24 18 E
Ocniţa, *Moldova* **53 B12** 48 25N 27 30 E
Ocoee, *U.S.A.* **153 G8** 28 34N 81 33W
Ocoña, *Peru* **172 D3** 16 26 S 73 8W
Ocoña →, *Peru* **172 D3** 16 28 S 73 8W
Oconee →, *U.S.A.* **152 D7** 31 58N 82 33W
Oconee, L., *U.S.A.* **152 B6** 33 28N 83 15W
Oconomowoc, *U.S.A.* **157 A8** 43 7N 88 30W
Oconto, *U.S.A.* **148 C2** 44 53N 87 52W
Oconto Falls, *U.S.A.* **148 C1** 44 52N 88 9W
Ocosingo, *Mexico* **163 D6** 17 10N 92 15W
Ocotal, *Nic.* **164 D2** 13 41N 86 31W
Ocotlán, *Mexico* **162 C4** 20 21N 102 42W
Ocotlán de Morelos, *Mexico* **163 D5** 16 48N 96 40W
Ocreza →, *Portugal* **43 F3** 39 32N 7 50W
Ócsa, *Hungary* **52 C4** 47 17N 19 15 E
Octeville, *France* **26 C5** 49 38N 1 40W
Ocumare del Tuy, *Venezuela* **168 A4** 10 7N 66 46W
Ocuri, *Bolivia* **173 D4** 18 45 S 65 50W
Oda, *Ghana* **113 D4** 5 50N 0 51W
Ōda, *Japan* **72 B4** 35 11N 132 30 E
Oda, J., *Sudan* **106 C4** 20 21N 36 39 E
Ódáðahraun, *Iceland* **11 B9** 65 5N 17 0W
Ödåkra, *Sweden* **17 H6** 56 7N 12 45 E
Odammun →, *Indonesia* **83 C5** 6 50 S 138 45 E
Odate, *Japan* **70 D10** 40 16N 140 34 E
Odawara, *Japan* **73 B11** 35 20N 139 6 E
Odda, *Norway* **18 D3** 60 3N 6 35 E
Odder, *Denmark* **17 J4** 55 58N 10 10 E
Oddur, *Somali Rep.* **120 D2** 4 11N 43 52 E
Odei →, *Canada* **143 B9** 56 6N 96 54W
Odell, *U.S.A.* **157 C8** 41 0N 88 31W
Odemira, *Portugal* **43 H2** 37 35N 8 40W
Ödemiş, *Turkey* **49 C9** 38 15N 28 0 E
Ödenburg = Sopron, *Hungary* **52 C1** 47 45N 16 32 E
Odendaalsrus, *S. Africa* **116 D4** 27 48 S 26 45 E
Odensbacken, *Sweden* **16 E9** 59 10N 15 32 E
Odense, *Denmark* **17 J4** 55 22N 10 23 E
Odenwald = Neckartal-Odenwald ⌓, *Germany* **31 F5** 49 30N 9 5 E
Odenwald, *Germany* **31 F5** 49 35N 9 0 E
Oder →, *Europe* **30 B10** 53 33N 14 38 E
Oder-Havel Kanal, *Germany* **30 C10** 52 52N 14 2 E
Oderzo, *Italy* **45 C9** 45 47N 12 29 E
Odesa, *Ukraine* **59 J6** 46 30N 30 45 E
Ödeshög, *Sweden* **17 F8** 58 14N 14 39 E
Odessa = Odesa, *Ukraine* **59 J6** 46 30N 30 45 E
Odessa, *Canada* **151 B8** 44 17N 76 43W
Odessa, *Mo., U.S.A.* **156 F3** 39 0N 93 57W
Odessa, *Tex., U.S.A.* **155 K3** 31 52N 102 23W
Odessa, *Wash., U.S.A.* **158 C4** 47 20N 118 41W
Odiakwe, *Botswana* **116 C4** 20 12 S 25 17 E
Odiel →, *Spain* **43 H4** 37 10N 6 55W
Odienné, *Ivory C.* **112 D3** 9 30N 7 34W
Odimba, *Gabon* **114 C2** 2 2 S 9 33 E
Odintsovo, *Russia* **58 E9** 55 39N 37 15 E
Odiongan, *Phil.* **80 E3** 12 24N 121 59 E
Odobeşti, *Romania* **53 E12** 45 43N 27 4 E
Odolanów, *Poland* **55 G4** 51 34N 17 40 E
O'Donnell, *U.S.A.* **155 J4** 32 58N 101 50W
Odorheiu Secuiesc, *Romania* **53 D10** 46 21N 25 21 E
Odoyevo, *Russia* **58 F9** 53 56N 36 42 E
Odra = Oder →, *Europe* **30 B10** 53 33N 14 38 E
Odra →, *Spain* **42 C6** 42 14N 4 17W
Odum, *U.S.A.* **152 D7** 31 40N 82 2W
Odweina, *Somali Rep.* **120 C3** 9 25N 45 4 E
Odžaci, *Serbia & M.* **52 E4** 45 30N 19 17 E
Odžak, *Bos.-H.* **52 E3** 45 3N 18 18 E
Odzala, *Congo* **114 B2** 0 37N 14 37 E
Odzala △, *Congo* **114 B2** 0 55N 14 55 E
Odzi, *Zimbabwe* **117 B5** 19 0 S 32 20 E
Odzi →, *Zimbabwe* **117 B5** 19 45 S 32 23 E
Oebisfelde, *Germany* **30 C6** 52 27N 10 57 E
Oeiras = Araticu, *Brazil* **170 B2** 1 58 S 49 51W
Oeiras, *Brazil* **170 C3** 7 0 S 42 8W
Oeiras, *Portugal* **43 G1** 38 41N 9 18W
Oeiras do Para, *Brazil* **169 D8** 1 58 S 49 51W
Oelrichs, *U.S.A.* **154 D3** 43 11N 103 14W
Oels in Schlesien = Oleśnica, *Poland* **55 G4** 51 13N 17 22 E
Oelsnitz, *Germany* **31 E8** 50 24N 12 10 E
Oelwein, *U.S.A.* **156 B5** 42 41N 91 55W
Oeno I., *Pac. Oc.* **135 K14** 24 0 S 131 0W
Oenpelli, *Australia* **124 B5** 12 20 S 133 4 E
Oetz, *Austria* **34 D3** 47 13N 10 53 E
Of, *Turkey* **101 B9** 40 59N 40 23 E
O'Fallon, *U.S.A.* **156 F6** 38 49N 90 42W
Ofanto →, *Italy* **47 A9** 41 22N 16 13 E
Offa, *Nigeria* **113 D5** 8 13N 4 42 E
Offaly □, *Ireland* **23 C4** 53 15N 7 30W
Offenbach, *Germany* **31 E4** 50 6N 8 44 E
Offenburg, *Germany* **31 G3** 48 28N 7 56 E
Officer, The →, *Australia* **125 E5** 27 46 S 132 30 E
Offida, *Italy* **45 F10** 42 56N 13 41 E
Offoué →, *Gabon* **114 C2** 0 4 S 11 44 E
Ofidhousa, *Greece* **49 E8** 36 33N 26 8 E
Öflingen, *Germany* **32 A5** 47 36N 7 55 E
Ofolanga, *Tonga* **133 P14** 19 38 S 173 35W
Ofotfjorden, *Norway* **14 B17** 68 27N 17 0 E
Ofte, *Norway* **18 E5** 59 30N 8 12 E
Ofu, *Amer. Samoa* **133 X25** 14 11 S 169 41W
Ōfunato, *Japan* **70 E10** 39 4N 141 43 E
Oga, *Japan* **70 E9** 39 55N 139 50 E
Oga-Hantō, *Japan* **70 E9** 39 58N 139 47 E
Ogaden, *Ethiopia* **120 C3** 7 30N 45 30 E
Ōgaki, *Japan* **73 B8** 35 21N 136 37 E
Ogallala, *U.S.A.* **154 E4** 41 8N 101 43W
Ogan →, *Indonesia* **84 C2** 3 1 S 104 44 E
Ogasawara Gunto, *Pac. Oc.* **62 G18** 27 0N 142 0 E
Ogbomosho, *Nigeria* **113 D5** 8 1N 4 11 E
Ogden, *Iowa, U.S.A.* **156 B2** 42 2N 94 2W
Ogden, *Utah, U.S.A.* **158 F7** 41 13N 111 58W
Ogdensburg, *U.S.A.* **151 B9** 44 42N 75 30W
Ogea Driki, *Fiji* **133 B3** 19 12 S 178 27W
Ogea Levu, *Fiji* **133 B3** 19 8 S 178 24W
Ogeechee →, *U.S.A.* **152 D8** 31 50N 81 3W
Ogilby, *U.S.A.* **161 N12** 32 49N 114 50W
Oglat Beraber, *Algeria* **110 B4** 30 15N 3 34W
Oglats de Khenachiche, *Mali* **110 D4** 21 51N 3 58W
Oglesby, *U.S.A.* **156 C7** 41 18N 89 4W
Oglethorpe, *U.S.A.* **152 C5** 32 18N 84 4W
Oglio →, *Italy* **44 C7** 45 2N 10 39 E
Óglio Nord ⌓, *Italy* **44 C6** 45 22N 9 54 E
Óglio Sud ⌓, *Italy* **44 C7** 45 7N 10 24 E
Ogmore, *Australia* **126 C4** 22 37 S 149 35 E
Ognon →, *France* **27 E12** 47 16N 5 28 E
Ogoamas, *Indonesia* **82 A2** 0 50N 120 5 E
Ogoja, *Nigeria* **113 D6** 6 38N 8 39 E
Ogoki, *Canada* **140 B2** 51 38N 85 58W
Ogoki →, *Canada* **140 B2** 51 38N 85 57W
Ogoki L., *Canada* **140 B2** 50 50N 87 10W
Ogoki Res., *Canada* **140 B2** 50 45N 88 15W
Ogooué →, *Gabon* **114 C1** 1 0 S 9 0 E
Ogōri, *Japan* **72 C3** 34 6N 131 24 E
Ogosta →, *Bulgaria* **50 C7** 43 48N 23 55 E
Ogowe = Ogooué →, *Gabon* **114 C1** 1 0 S 9 0 E
Ogr = Sharafa, *Sudan* **107 E2** 11 59N 27 7 E
Ograźden, *Macedonia* **50 E6** 41 30N 22 50 E
Ogre, *Latvia* **15 H21** 56 49N 24 36 E
Ogrein, *Sudan* **106 D3** 17 55N 34 50 E
Ogulin, *Croatia* **45 C12** 45 16N 15 16 E
Ogun □, *Nigeria* **113 D5** 7 0N 3 0 E
Oguni, *Japan* **72 D3** 33 11N 131 8 E
Ögur, *Iceland* **11 A4** 66 2N 22 44W
Ogurchinskiy, Ostrov, *Turkmenistan* **97 B7** 38 55N 53 2 E
Oguta, *Nigeria* **113 D6** 5 44N 6 44 E
Ogwashi-Uku, *Nigeria* **113 D6** 6 15N 6 30 E
Ogwe, *Nigeria* **113 E6** 5 0N 7 14 E
Ohai, *N.Z.* **131 F3** 45 55 S 168 0 E
Ohakune, *N.Z.* **130 F4** 39 24 S 175 24 E
Ohanet, *Algeria* **111 C6** 28 44N 8 46 E
Ōhara, *Japan* **73 B12** 35 15N 140 23 E
O'Hare International, Chicago ✕ (ORD), *U.S.A.* **157 C9** 41 59N 87 54W
Ohata, *Japan* **70 D10** 41 24N 141 10 E
Ohatchee, *U.S.A.* **152 B4** 33 47N 86 0W
Ohau, L., *N.Z.* **131 E4** 44 15 S 169 53 E
Ohaupo, *N.Z.* **130 D4** 37 56 S 175 20 E
O'Higgins, C., *Chile* **172 b** 27 5 S 109 15W
Ohio □, *U.S.A.* **150 F2** 40 15N 82 45W
Ohio →, *U.S.A.* **157 G8** 36 59N 89 8W
Ohio City, *U.S.A.* **157 D12** 40 46N 84 37W
Ohiwa Harbour, *N.Z.* **130 D6** 37 59 S 177 10 E
Ohlau = Oława, *Poland* **55 H4** 50 57N 17 20 E
Ohře →, *Czech Rep.* **34 A7** 50 30N 14 10 E
Ohre →, *Germany* **30 C7** 52 18N 11 46 E
Ohrid, *Macedonia* **50 E4** 41 8N 20 52 E
Ohridsko Jezero, *Macedonia* **50 E4** 41 8N 20 52 E
Ohrigstad, *S. Africa* **117 C5** 24 39 S 30 36 E
Öhringen, *Germany* **31 F5** 49 12N 9 31 E
Ohura, *N.Z.* **130 E3** 38 51 S 174 59 E
Oi Qu, *China* **76 C2** 28 37N 98 16 E
Oiapoque, *Brazil* **169 C7** 3 50N 51 50W
Oiapoque →, *S. Amer.* **169 C7** 4 8N 51 40W
Oikou, *China* **75 E9** 38 35N 117 42 E
Oil City, *U.S.A.* **150 E5** 41 26N 79 42W
Oil Springs, *Canada* **150 D2** 42 47N 82 7W
Oildale, *U.S.A.* **161 K7** 35 25N 119 1W
Oinousa, *Greece* **49 C8** 38 33N 26 14 E
Oise □, *France* **27 C9** 49 28N 2 30 E
Oise →, *France* **27 C9** 49 0N 2 4 E
Oiseaux du Djoudj △, *Senegal* **112 B1** 16 24N 16 14W
Oistins, *Barbados* **165 g** 13 4N 59 33W
Oistins B., *Barbados* **165 g** 13 4N 59 33W
Ōita, *Japan* **72 D3** 33 14N 131 36 E
Ōita □, *Japan* **72 D3** 33 15N 131 30 E
Oiticica, *Brazil* **170 C3** 5 3 S 41 5W
Ojacaliente, *Mexico* **162 C4** 22 34N 102 15W
Ojai, *U.S.A.* **161 L7** 34 27N 119 15W
Ojcowski △, *Poland* **55 H6** 50 15N 19 50 E
Ojhar, *India* **94 D1** 20 6N 73 56 E
Ojinaga, *Mexico* **162 B4** 29 34N 104 25W
Ojiya, *Japan* **71 F9** 37 18N 138 48 E
Ojo de Liebre ⌓, *Mexico* **162 B2** 27 50N 114 0W
Ojos del Salado, Cerro, *Argentina* **174 B2** 27 0 S 68 40W
Oka →, *Russia* **60 B7** 56 20N 43 59 E
Okaba, *Indonesia* **83 C5** 8 6 S 139 42 E
Okahandja, *Namibia* **116 C2** 22 0 S 16 59 E
Okahukura, *N.Z.* **130 E4** 38 48 S 175 14 E
Okaihau, *N.Z.* **130 B2** 35 19 S 173 47 E
Okalataka, *Congo* **114 C2** 0 18 S 14 54 E
Okanagan L., *Canada* **142 D5** 50 0N 119 30W
Okandja, *Gabon* **114 C2** 0 35 S 13 45 E
Okano →, *Gabon* **114 C2** 0 5 S 10 57 E
Okanogan, *U.S.A.* **158 B4** 48 22N 119 35W
Okanogan →, *U.S.A.* **158 B4** 48 6N 119 44W
Okány, *Hungary* **52 D6** 46 52N 21 21 E
Okapa, *Papua N. G.* **132 D3** 6 38 S 145 39 E
Okapi △, *Dem. Rep. of the Congo* **118 B2** 2 30N 27 20 E
Okaputa, *Namibia* **116 C2** 20 5 S 17 0 E
Okara, *Pakistan* **91 C4** 30 50N 73 31 E
Okarito, *N.Z.* **131 D5** 43 15 S 170 9 E
Okato, *N.Z.* **130 F2** 39 12 S 173 53 E
Okaukuejo, *Namibia* **116 B2** 19 10 S 16 0 E
Okavango Delta, *Botswana* **116 B3** 18 45 S 22 45 E
Okavango Swamp = Okavango Delta, *Botswana* **116 B3** 18 45 S 22 45 E
Ōkawa, *Japan* **72 D2** 33 9N 130 21 E
Okawville, *U.S.A.* **156 F7** 38 26N 89 33W
Okaya, *Japan* **73 A10** 36 5N 138 10 E
Okayama, *Japan* **72 C5** 34 40N 133 54 E
Okayama □, *Japan* **72 C5** 35 0N 133 50 E
Okazaki, *Japan* **73 C9** 34 57N 137 10 E
Oke-Iho, *Nigeria* **113 D5** 8 1N 3 18 E
Okęcie, Warszawa ✕ (WAW), *Poland* **55 F7** 52 9N 20 59 E
Okeechobee, *U.S.A.* **153 H9** 27 15N 80 50W
Okeechobee, L., *U.S.A.* **153 J9** 27 0N 80 50W
Okefenokee ⌓, *U.S.A.* **152 E7** 30 44N 82 7W
Okefenokee Swamp, *U.S.A.* **152 E7** 30 40N 82 20W
Okehampton, *U.K.* **21 G4** 50 44N 4 0W
Okemos, *U.S.A.* **157 B12** 42 43N 84 26W
Okene, *Nigeria* **113 D6** 7 32N 6 11 E
Oker →, *Germany* **30 C6** 52 32N 10 22 E
Okha, *India* **92 H3** 22 27N 69 4 E
Okha, *Russia* **67 D15** 53 40N 143 0 E
Ókhi Óros, *Greece* **48 C6** 38 5N 24 25 E
Okhotsk, *Russia* **67 D15** 59 20N 143 10 E
Okhotsk, Sea of, *Asia* **67 D15** 55 0N 145 0 E
Okhotskiy Perevoz, *Russia* **67 C14** 61 52N 135 35 E
Okhtyrka, *Ukraine* **59 G8** 50 25N 35 0 E
Oki-no-Shima, *Japan* **72 E4** 32 44N 132 33 E
Oki-Shotō, *Japan* **72 A5** 36 5N 133 15 E
Okiep, *S. Africa* **116 D2** 29 39 S 17 53 E
Okigwi, *Nigeria* **113 D6** 5 52N 7 20 E
Okija, *Nigeria* **113 D6** 5 54N 6 55 E
Okinawa □, *Japan* **71 L4** 26 40N 128 0 E
Okinawa-Guntō, *Japan* **71 L4** 26 40N 128 0 E
Okinawa-Jima, *Japan* **71 L4** 26 32N 128 0 E
Okino-erabu-Shima, *Japan* **71 L4** 27 21N 128 33 E
Okitipupa, *Nigeria* **113 D5** 6 31N 4 50 E
Oklahoma □, *U.S.A.* **155 H6** 35 20N 97 30W
Oklahoma City, *U.S.A.* **155 H6** 35 30N 97 30W
Oklawaha →, *U.S.A.* **153 F8** 29 28N 81 41W
Okmulgee, *U.S.A.* **155 H7** 35 37N 95 58W
Oknitsa = Ocniţa, *Moldova* **53 B12** 48 25N 27 30 E
Oko, W. →, *Sudan* **106 C4** 21 15N 35 56 E
Okolo, *Uganda* **118 B3** 2 37N 31 8 E
Okolona, *Ky., U.S.A.* **157 F11** 38 8N 85 41W
Okolona, *Miss., U.S.A.* **155 J10** 34 0N 88 45W
Okombahe, *Namibia* **116 C2** 21 23 S 15 22 E
Okonek, *Poland* **54 E3** 53 32N 16 51 E
Okotoks, *Canada* **142 C6** 50 43N 113 58W
Okoyo, *Congo* **114 C3** 1 28 S 15 0 E
Okrika, *Nigeria* **113 E6** 4 40N 7 10 E
Oksapmin, *Papua N. G.* **132 C2** 5 17 S 142 15 E
Øksendal, *Norway* **18 B5** 62 42N 8 27 E
Oksibil, *Indonesia* **83 B6** 4 59 S 140 35 E
Øksna, *Norway* **18 D8** 60 58N 11 27 E
Oksovskiy, *Russia* **56 B6** 62 33N 39 57 E
Oktabrsk = Oktyabrsk, *Kazakhstan* **57 E10** 49 28N 57 25 E
Oktwin, *Burma* **90 F6** 18 49N 96 26 E
Oktyabr, *Kazakhstan* **65 B8** 43 41N 77 12 E
Oktyabrsk, *Kazakhstan* **57 E10** 49 28N 57 25 E
Oktyabrsk, *Russia* **60 D9** 53 11N 48 40 E
Oktyabrskiy = Aktsyabrski, *Belarus* **59 F5** 52 38N 28 53 E
Oktyabrskiy, *Bashkortostan, Russia* **64 D4** 54 28N 53 28 E
Oktyabrskiy, *Perm, Russia* **64 C6** 56 31N 57 12 E
Oktyabrskiy, *Rostov, Russia* **61 G5** 47 30N 40 4 E
Oktyabrskoy Revolyutsii, Ostrov, *Russia* **67 B10** 79 30N 97 0 E
Oktyabrskoye = Zhovtneve, *Ukraine* **59 J7** 46 54N 32 3 E
Oktyabrskoye, *Russia* **64 D9** 54 26N 62 44 E
Ōkuchi, *Japan* **72 E2** 32 4N 130 37 E
Okulovka, *Russia* **58 C7** 58 25N 33 19 E
Okuru, *N.Z.* **131 D3** 43 55 S 168 55 E
Okushiri-Tō, *Japan* **70 C9** 42 15N 139 30 E
Okuta, *Nigeria* **113 D5** 9 14N 3 12 E
Okwa →, *Botswana* **116 C3** 22 30 S 23 0 E
Ola, *U.S.A.* **155 H8** 35 2N 93 13W
Ólafsfjörður, *Iceland* **11 A8** 66 4N 18 39W
Ólafsvík, *Iceland* **11 C3** 64 53N 23 43W
Olaine, *Latvia* **54 B10** 56 48N 23 59 E
Olancha, *U.S.A.* **161 J8** 36 17N 118 1W
Olancha Pk., *U.S.A.* **161 J8** 36 15N 118 7W
Olanchito, *Honduras* **164 C2** 15 30N 86 30W
Öland, *Sweden* **17 H10** 56 45N 16 38 E
Ölands norra udde, *Sweden* **17 G11** 57 22N 17 5 E
Ölands södra udde, *Sweden* **17 H10** 56 12N 16 23 E
Olanta, *U.S.A.* **152 B10** 33 56N 79 56W
Olar, *U.S.A.* **152 B8** 33 11N 81 11W
Olargues, *France* **28 E6** 43 34N 2 53 E
Olary, *Australia* **128 B4** 32 18 S 140 19 E
Olascoaga, *Argentina* **174 D3** 35 15 S 60 39W
Olathe, *U.S.A.* **154 F7** 38 53N 94 49W
Olavarría, *Argentina* **174 D3** 36 55 S 60 20W
Oława, *Poland* **55 H4** 50 57N 17 20 E
Olbernhau, *Germany* **30 E9** 50 40N 13 19 E
Ólbia, *Italy* **46 B2** 40 55N 9 31 E
Ólbia, G. di, *Italy* **46 B2** 40 55N 9 39 E
Olching, *Germany* **31 G7** 48 12N 11 21 E
Olcott, *U.S.A.* **150 C6** 43 20N 78 42W
Old Bahama Chan. = Bahama, Canal Viejo de, *W. Indies* **164 B4** 22 10N 77 30W
Old Baldy Pk. = San Antonio, Mt., *U.S.A.* **161 L9** 34 17N 117 38W
Old Bar, *Australia* **129 A10** 31 58 S 152 35 E
Old Castile = Castilla y Leon □, *Spain* **42 D6** 42 0N 5 0W
Old Crow, *Canada* **138 B6** 67 30N 139 55W
Old Dale, *U.S.A.* **161 L11** 34 8N 115 47W
Old Forge, *N.Y., U.S.A.* **151 C10** 43 43N 74 58W
Old Forge, *Pa., U.S.A.* **151 E9** 41 22N 75 45W
Old Fort B., *Bahamas* **9 b** 25 3N 77 32W
Old Harbor, *U.S.A.* **144 H9** 57 12N 153 18W
Old Perlican, *Canada* **141 C9** 48 5N 53 1W
Old Shinyanga, *Tanzania* **118 C3** 3 33 S 33 27 E
Old Speck Mt., *U.S.A.* **151 B14** 44 34N 70 57W
Old Town, *Fla., U.S.A.* **153 F7** 29 36N 82 59W
Old Town, *Maine, U.S.A.* **149 C11** 44 56N 68 39W
Old Washington, *U.S.A.* **150 F3** 40 2N 81 27W
Old Wives L., *Canada* **143 C7** 50 5N 106 0W
Oldbury, *U.K.* **21 F5** 51 38N 2 33W
Oldcastle, *Ireland* **23 C4** 53 46N 7 10W
Oldeani, *Tanzania* **118 C4** 3 22 S 35 35 E
Olden, *Norway* **18 C3** 61 49N 6 49 E
Oldenburg, *Niedersachsen, Germany* **30 B4** 53 9N 8 13 E
Oldenburg, *Schleswig-Holstein, Germany* **30 A6** 54 17N 10 52 E
Oldenzaal, *Neths.* **24 B6** 52 19N 6 53 E
Oldham, *U.K.* **20 D5** 53 33N 2 7W
Oldman →, *Canada* **142 D6** 49 57N 111 42W
Oldmeldrum, *U.K.* **22 D6** 57 20N 2 19W
Olds, *Canada* **142 C6** 51 50N 114 10W
Oldsmar, *U.S.A.* **153 G7** 28 2N 82 40W
Olduvai Gorge, *Tanzania* **118 C4** 2 57 S 35 23 E
Oldziyt, *Mongolia* **74 B5** 44 40N 109 1 E
Ole Rømer Land, *Greenland* **10 C8** 74 10N 24 30W
Olean, *U.S.A.* **150 D6** 42 5N 78 26W
Olecko, *Poland* **54 D9** 54 2N 22 31 E
Oléggio, *Italy* **44 C5** 45 36N 8 38 E
Oleiros, *Portugal* **42 F3** 39 56N 7 56W
Oleiros, *Spain* **42 B2** 43 20N 8 19W
Olekma →, *Russia* **67 C13** 60 22N 120 42 E
Olekminsk, *Russia* **67 C13** 60 25N 120 30 E
Oleksandriya, *Kirovohrad, Ukraine* **59 H7** 48 42N 33 3 E
Oleksandriya, *Rivne, Ukraine* **59 G4** 50 37N 26 19 E
Oleksandrovka, *Ukraine* **59 H7** 48 55N 32 20 E
Olema, *U.S.A.* **160 G4** 38 3N 122 47W
Ølen, *Norway* **18 E2** 59 36N 5 48 E
Olenegorsk, *Russia* **56 A5** 68 9N 33 18 E
Olenek, *Russia* **67 C12** 68 28N 112 18 E
Olenek →, *Russia* **67 B13** 73 0N 120 10 E
Olenino, *Russia* **58 D7** 56 15N 33 30 E
Olenya = Olenegorsk, *Russia* **56 A5** 68 9N 33 18 E
Oléron, Î. d', *France* **28 C2** 45 55N 1 15W
Olesk, *Ukraine* **55 G11** 51 6N 24 11 E
Oleśnica, *Poland* **55 G4** 51 13N 17 22 E
Olesno, *Poland* **55 H5** 50 51N 18 26 E
Olevsk, *Ukraine* **59 G4** 51 12N 27 39 E
Olga, *Russia* **67 E14** 43 50N 135 14 E
Olga, L., *Canada* **140 C4** 49 47N 77 15W
Olga, Mt., *Australia* **125 E5** 25 20 S 130 50 E
Ölgiy, *Mongolia* **68 B3** 48 56N 89 57 E
Ølgod, *Denmark* **17 J2** 55 49N 8 36 E
Olhão, *Portugal* **43 H3** 37 3N 7 48W
Olhopil, *Ukraine* **53 B14** 48 12N 29 30 E
Olhovatka, *Russia* **54 D9** 54 30N 22 18 E
Olib, *Croatia* **45 D11** 44 23N 14 44 E
Oliena, *Italy* **46 B2** 40 16N 9 24 E
Oliete, *Spain* **40 D4** 41 1N 0 41W
Olifants = Elefantes →, *Africa* **117 C5** 24 10 S 32 40 E
Olifants →, *Namibia* **116 C2** 25 30 S 19 30 E
Olifantshoek, *S. Africa* **116 D3** 27 57 S 22 42 E
Ólimbos, *Greece* **49 F9** 35 44N 27 11 E
Ólimbos, Óros, *Greece* **50 F6** 40 6N 22 23 E
Olímpia, *Brazil* **175 A6** 20 44 S 48 54W
Olimpos-Beydaglari △, *Turkey* **49 E12** 36 36N 30 30 E
Olin, *U.S.A.* **156 C5** 42 0N 91 9W
Olinda, *Brazil* **170 C5** 8 1 S 34 51W
Olindiná, *Brazil* **170 D4** 11 22 S 38 21W
Olite, *Spain* **40 C3** 42 29N 1 40W
Oliva, *Argentina* **174 C3** 32 0 S 63 38W
Oliva, *Spain* **41 G4** 38 58N 0 9W
Oliva, Punta del, *Spain* **42 B5** 43 37N 5 28W
Oliva de la Frontera, *Spain* **43 G4** 38 17N 6 54W
Olivares, *Spain* **40 F2** 39 46N 2 20W
Olive Branch, *U.S.A.* **155 H10** 34 58N 89 50W
Olive Hill, *U.S.A.* **157 F13** 38 18N 83 13W
Olivehurst, *U.S.A.* **160 F5** 39 6N 121 34W
Oliveira, *Brazil* **171 F3** 20 39 S 44 50W
Oliveira de Azeméis, *Portugal* **42 E2** 40 49N 8 29W
Oliveira do Douro, *Portugal* **42 D2** 41 5N 8 2W
Oliveira dos Brejinhos, *Brazil* **171 D3** 12 19 S 42 54W
Olivenza, *Spain* **43 G3** 38 41N 7 9W
Oliver, *Canada* **142 D5** 49 13N 119 37W
Oliver L., *Canada* **143 B8** 56 56N 103 22W
Olivet, *France* **27 E8** 47 51N 1 55 E
Olivet, *U.S.A.* **157 B12** 42 27N 84 56W
Olivine Ra., *N.Z.* **131 E3** 44 15 S 168 30 E
Olivone, *Switz.* **33 C7** 46 32N 8 57 E
Olkhovka, *Russia* **60 F7** 49 48N 44 32 E
Olkusz, *Poland* **55 H6** 50 18N 19 33 E
Ollachea, *Peru* **172 C3** 13 49 S 70 29W
Ollagüe, *Chile* **174 A2** 21 15 S 68 10W
Ollon, *Switz.* **32 D3** 46 18N 7 0 E
Olloua, *Congo* **114 C2** 0 54 S 14 34 E
Olmaliq, *Uzbekistan* **65 C4** 40 50N 69 35 E
Olmedo, *Spain* **42 D6** 41 20N 4 43W
Olmeto, *France* **29 G12** 41 43N 8 55 E
Olmos, *Peru* **172 B2** 5 59 S 79 46W
Olmütz = Olomouc, *Czech Rep.* **35 B10** 49 38N 17 12 E
Olney, *Ill., U.S.A.* **157 F8** 38 44N 88 5W
Olney, *Tex., U.S.A.* **155 J5** 33 22N 98 45W
Olofström, *Sweden* **17 H8** 56 17N 14 32 E
Ololi, *Congo* **114 C2** 0 15 S 14 36 E
Oloma, *Cameroon* **113 E7** 3 29N 11 19 E
Olomane →, *Canada* **141 B7** 50 14N 60 37W
Olombo, *Congo* **114 C3** 1 18 S 15 53 E
Olomouc, *Czech Rep.* **35 B10** 49 38N 17 12 E
Olomoucký □, *Czech Rep.* **35 B10** 49 45N 17 5 E
Olonets, *Russia* **58 B7** 61 0N 32 54 E
Olongapo, *Phil.* **80 D3** 14 50N 120 18 E
Olonne-sur-Mer, *France* **28 B2** 46 32N 1 47W
Oloron, Gave d' →, *France* **28 E2** 43 33N 1 5W
Oloron-Ste-Marie, *France* **28 E3** 43 11N 0 38W
Olosega, *Amer. Samoa* **133 X25** 14 12 S 169 40W
Olosenga = Swains I., *Amer. Samoa* **135 J11** 11 11 S 171 4W
Olot, *Spain* **40 C7** 42 11N 2 30 E
Olovo, *Bos.-H.* **52 F3** 44 8N 18 35 E
Olovyannaya, *Russia* **67 D12** 50 58N 115 35 E
Olowalu, *U.S.A.* **145 C5** 20 49N 156 38W
Oloy →, *Russia* **67 C16** 66 29N 159 29 E
Olsberg, *Germany* **30 D4** 51 21N 8 31 E
Olshammar, *Sweden* **17 F8** 58 45N 14 48 E
Olshanka, *Ukraine* **59 H6** 48 16N 30 58 E
Olshany, *Ukraine* **59 G8** 50 3N 35 53 E
Olsztyn, *Poland* **54 E7** 53 48N 20 29 E
Olsztynek, *Poland* **54 E7** 53 34N 20 19 E
Olt □, *Romania* **53 F9** 44 20N 24 30 E
Olt →, *Romania* **53 G9** 43 43N 24 51 E
Oltedal, *Norway* **18 F3** 58 49N 6 2 E
Olten, *Switz.* **32 B5** 47 21N 7 53 E
Olteniţa, *Romania* **53 F11** 44 7N 26 42 E
Olton, *U.S.A.* **155 H3** 34 11N 102 8W
Oltu, *Turkey* **101 B9** 40 35N 41 58 E
Oluanpi, *Taiwan* **77 G13** 21 54N 120 51 E
Olula del Rio, *Spain* **41 H2** 37 21N 2 18W
Olur, *Turkey* **101 B10** 40 49N 42 8 E
Olustee, *U.S.A.* **152 E7** 30 12N 82 26W
Olutanga, *Phil.* **81 H4** 7 26N 122 54 E
Olutanga I., *Phil.* **81 H4** 7 22N 122 52 E
Olvega, *Spain* **40 D2** 41 47N 2 0W
Olvera, *Spain* **43 J5** 36 55N 5 18W
Olymbos, *Cyprus* **39 E9** 35 21N 33 45 E
Olympia, *Greece* **48 D3** 37 39N 21 39 E
Olympia, *U.S.A.* **160 D4** 47 3N 122 53W
Olympic △, *U.S.A.* **160 C3** 47 48N 123 30W
Olympic Dam, *Australia* **128 A2** 30 30 S 136 55 E
Olympic Mts., *U.S.A.* **160 C3** 47 55N 123 45W
Olympus, *Cyprus* **39 F8** 34 56N 32 52 E
Olympus, Mt. = Ólimbos, Óros, *Greece* **50 F6** 40 6N 22 23 E
Olympus, Mt. = Uludağ, *Turkey* **51 F13** 40 4N 29 13 E
Olympus, Mt., *U.S.A.* **160 C3** 47 48N 123 43W
Olyphant, *U.S.A.* **151 E9** 41 27N 75 36W
Om →, *Russia* **66 D8** 54 59N 73 22 E
Om Hajer, *Eritrea* **107 E4** 14 20N 36 41 E
Om Koi, *Thailand* **86 D2** 17 48N 98 22 E
Ōma, *Japan* **70 D10** 41 45N 141 5 E
Ōmachi, *Japan* **73 A9** 36 30N 137 50 E
Omae-Zaki, *Japan* **73 C10** 34 36N 138 14 E
Ōmagari, *Japan* **70 E10** 39 27N 140 29 E
Omagh, *U.K.* **23 B4** 54 36N 7 19W
Omagh □, *U.K.* **23 B4** 54 35N 7 15W
Omaha, *U.S.A.* **154 E7** 41 17N 95 58W
Omak, *U.S.A.* **158 B4** 48 25N 119 31W
Omalos, *Greece* **39 E4** 35 19N 23 55 E
Omalur, *India* **95 J4** 11 44N 78 4 E
Oman ■, *Asia* **99 B7** 23 0N 58 0 E
Oman, G. of, *Asia* **97 E8** 24 30N 58 30 E
Omapere, *N.Z.* **130 B2** 35 37 S 173 25 E
Omar Combon, *Somali Rep.* **120 D3** 3 10N 45 47 E
Omaruru, *Namibia* **116 C2** 21 26 S 16 0 E
Omaruru →, *Namibia* **116 C1** 22 7 S 14 15 E

Omate, *Peru* **172 D3** 16 45 S 71 0W
Ombai, Selat, *Indonesia* **82 C2** 8 30 S 124 50 E
Omboué, *Gabon* **114 C1** 1 35 S 9 15 E
Ombrone →, *Italy* **44 F8** 42 42N 11 5 E
Omchi, *Chad* **109 D3** 21 22N 17 53 E
Omdurmân, *Sudan* **107 D3** 15 40N 32 28 E
Ōme, *Japan* **73 B11** 35 47N 139 15 E
Omega, *U.S.A.* **152 D6** 31 21N 83 36W
Omegna, *Italy* **44 C5** 45 53N 8 24 E
Omemee, *Canada* **150 B6** 44 18N 78 33W
Omeo, *Australia* **129 D7** 37 6 S 147 36 E
Omeonga, *Dem. Rep. of the Congo* **118 C1** 3 40 S 24 22 E
Ometepe, I. de, *Nic.* **164 D2** 11 32N 85 35W
Ometepec, *Mexico* **163 D5** 16 39N 98 23W
Ōmi-Shima, *Ehime, Japan* **72 C5** 34 15N 133 0 E
Ōmi-Shima, *Yamaguchi, Japan* **72 C3** 34 25N 131 9 E
Omihachiman, *Japan* **73 B8** 35 7N 136 3 E
Ominato, *Japan* **70 D10** 41 17N 141 10 E
Omineca →, *Canada* **142 B4** 56 3N 124 16W
Omiš, *Croatia* **45 E13** 43 28N 16 40 E
Omišalj, *Croatia* **45 C11** 45 13N 14 32 E
Omitara, *Namibia* **116 C2** 22 16 S 18 2 E
Ōmiya, *Japan* **73 B11** 35 54N 139 38 E
Ommaney, C., *U.S.A.* **144 H14** 56 10N 134 40W
Omme Å →, *Denmark* **17 J2** 55 56N 8 32 E
Ommen, *Neths.* **24 B6** 52 31N 6 26 E
Ömnögovĭ □, *Mongolia* **74 C3** 43 15N 104 0 E
Omo △, *Ethiopia* **107 F4** 5 54N 35 55 E
Omo →, *Ethiopia* **107 F4** 6 25N 36 10 E
Omo Valley, *Ethiopia* **107 F4** 5 7N 36 0 E
Omodeo, L., *Italy* **46 B1** 40 8N 8 56 E
Omodhos, *Cyprus* **39 F8** 34 51N 32 48 E
Omoï, *Congo* **114 C2** 2 56 S 13 13 E
Omoko, *Nigeria* **113 D6** 5 19N 6 40 E
Omolon →, *Russia* **67 C16** 68 42N 158 36 E
Omona, *Solomon Is.* **133 L10** 7 30 S 158 43 E
Omono-Gawa →, *Japan* **70 E10** 39 46N 140 3 E
Omsk, *Russia* **66 D8** 55 0N 73 12 E
Omsukchan, *Russia* **67 C16** 62 32N 155 48 E
Ōmu, *Japan* **70 B11** 44 34N 142 58 E
Omul, Vf., *Romania* **53 E10** 45 27N 25 29 E
Omulew →, *Poland* **55 E8** 53 5N 21 33 E
Ōmura, *Japan* **72 E1** 32 56N 129 57 E
Ōmura-Wan, *Japan* **72 E1** 32 57N 129 52 E
Omuramba Omatako →, *Namibia* **116 B2** 17 45 S 20 25 E
Omuramba Ovambo →, *Namibia* **116 B2** 18 45 S 16 59 E
Omurtag, *Bulgaria* **51 C10** 43 8N 26 26 E
Ōmuta, *Japan* **72 D2** 33 5N 130 26 E
Omutninsk, *Russia* **64 B4** 58 45N 52 4 E
On-ma-thi, *Burma* **90 D6** 22 17N 96 41 E
On-Take, *Japan* **72 F2** 31 35N 130 39 E
Oña, *Spain* **42 C7** 42 43N 3 25W
Ona, *U.S.A.* **153 H8** 27 29N 81 55W
Ona Dikonde, *Dem. Rep. of the Congo* **114 C4** 3 51 S 24 11 E
Onaga, *U.S.A.* **154 F6** 39 29N 96 10W
Onalaska, *U.S.A.* **154 D9** 43 53N 91 14W
Onancock, *U.S.A.* **148 G8** 37 43N 75 45W
Onang, *Indonesia* **82 B1** 3 2 S 118 49 E
Onangue, L., *Gabon* **114 C1** 0 57 S 10 4 E
Onaping L., *Canada* **140 C3** 47 3N 81 30W
Onarga, *U.S.A.* **157 D8** 40 43N 88 1W
Oñati, *Spain* **40 B2** 43 3N 2 25W
Onavas, *Mexico* **162 B3** 28 28N 109 30W
Onawa, *U.S.A.* **154 D6** 42 2N 96 6W
Oncócua, *Angola* **116 B1** 16 30 S 13 25 E
Onda, *Spain* **40 F4** 39 55N 0 17W
Ondaejin, *N. Korea* **75 D15** 41 34N 129 40 E
Ondangwa, *Namibia* **116 B2** 17 57 S 16 4 E
Ondarroa, *Spain* **40 B2** 43 19N 2 25W
Ondas →, *Brazil* **171 D3** 12 8 S 44 55W
Ondava →, *Slovak Rep.* **35 C14** 48 27N 21 48 E
Ondjiva, *Angola* **116 B2** 16 48 S 15 50 E
Ondo, *Japan* **72 C4** 34 11N 132 32 E
Ondo, *Nigeria* **113 D5** 7 4N 4 47 E
Ondo □, *Nigeria* **113 D6** 6 45N 5 0 E
Öndörshil, *Mongolia* **74 B5** 45 13N 108 5 E
Öndverðarnes, *Iceland* **11 C2** 64 52N 24 0W
One Tree, *Australia* **127 E3** 34 11 S 144 43 E
Oneata, *Fiji* **133 B3** 18 26 S 178 25W
Oneco, *U.S.A.* **153 H7** 27 25N 82 31W
Onega, *Russia* **56 B6** 64 0N 38 10 E
Onega →, *Russia* **56 B6** 63 58N 38 2 E
Onega, G. of = Onezhskaya Guba, *Russia* **56 B6** 64 24N 36 38 E
Onega, L. = Onezhskoye Ozero, *Russia* **58 B8** 61 44N 35 22 E
Onehunga, *N.Z.* **130 C3** 36 55 S 174 48 E
Oneida, *Ill., U.S.A.* **156 C6** 41 4N 90 13W
Oneida, *N.Y., U.S.A.* **151 C9** 43 6N 75 39W
Oneida L., *U.S.A.* **151 C9** 43 12N 75 54W
O'Neill, *U.S.A.* **154 D5** 42 27N 98 39W
Onekotan, Ostrov, *Russia* **67 E16** 49 25N 154 45 E
Onema, *Dem. Rep. of the Congo* **118 C1** 4 35 S 24 30 E
Oneonta, *U.S.A.* **151 D9** 42 27N 75 4W
Onerahi, *N.Z.* **130 B3** 35 45 S 174 22 E
Oneşti, *Romania* **53 D11** 46 17N 26 47 E
Onezhskaya Guba, *Russia* **56 B6** 64 24N 36 38 E
Onezhskoye Ozero, *Russia* **58 B8** 61 44N 35 22 E
Ongarue, *N.Z.* **130 E4** 38 42 S 175 19 E
Ongea Levu = Ogea Levu, *Fiji* **133 B3** 19 8 S 178 24W
Ongers →, *S. Africa* **116 E3** 31 4 S 23 13 E
Ongerup, *Australia* **125 F2** 33 58 S 118 28 E
Ongjin, *N. Korea* **75 F13** 37 56N 125 21 E
Ongkharak, *Thailand* **86 E3** 14 8N 101 1 E
Ongniud Qi, *China* **75 C10** 43 0N 118 38 E
Ongoka, *Dem. Rep. of the Congo* **118 C2** 1 20 S 26 0 E
Ongole, *India* **95 G5** 15 33N 80 2 E
Ongon = Havirga, *Mongolia* **74 B7** 45 41N 113 5 E
Ongouendjo, *Gabon* **114 C1** 1 23 S 9 5 E
Oni, *Georgia* **61 J6** 42 33N 43 26 E
Onida, *U.S.A.* **154 C4** 44 42N 100 4W
Onilahy →, *Madag.* **117 C7** 23 34 S 43 45 E
Onitsha, *Nigeria* **113 D6** 6 6N 6 42 E
Ono, *Fiji* **133 B2** 18 55 S 178 29 E
Ono, *Fukui, Japan* **73 B8** 35 59N 136 29 E
Ono, *Hyōgo, Japan* **72 C6** 34 51N 134 56 E
Onoda, *Japan* **72 C3** 33 59N 131 11 E
Onohara, *Japan* **72 C5** 34 5N 133 40 E
Onoke, L., *N.Z.* **130 H4** 41 22 S 175 8 E
Onomichi, *Japan* **72 C5** 34 25N 133 12 E
Onpyŏng-ni, *S. Korea* **75 H14** 33 25N 126 55 E
Ons, I. de, *Spain* **42 C2** 42 23N 8 55W
Onsala, *Sweden* **17 G6** 57 26N 12 0 E
Onslow, *Australia* **124 D2** 21 40 S 115 12 E
Onslow B., *U.S.A.* **149 H7** 34 20N 77 15W
Ontake-San, *Japan* **73 B9** 35 53N 137 29 E
Ontar, *Vanuatu* **133 D5** 14 17 S 167 27 E
Ontario, *Calif., U.S.A.* **161 L9** 34 4N 117 39W
Ontario, *Oreg., U.S.A.* **158 D5** 44 2N 116 58W
Ontario □, *Canada* **140 B2** 48 0N 83 0W
Ontario, L., *N. Amer.* **150 C7** 43 20N 78 0W
Ontinyent, *Spain* **41 G4** 38 50N 0 35W
Ontonagon, *U.S.A.* **154 B10** 46 52N 89 19W
Ontur, *Spain* **41 G3** 38 38N 1 29W
Onverwacht, *Suriname* **169 B6** 5 35N 55 11W
Onyx, *U.S.A.* **161 K8** 35 41N 118 14W
Oodnadatta, *Australia* **127 D2** 27 33 S 135 30 E
Ookala, *U.S.A.* **145 C6** 20 1N 155 17W
Ooku = Ōma, *Japan* **70 D10** 41 45N 141 5 E
Ooldea, *Australia* **125 F5** 30 27 S 131 50 E
Oombulgurri, *Australia* **124 C4** 15 15 S 127 45 E
Oorindi, *Australia* **126 C3** 20 40 S 141 1 E
Oost-Vlaanderen □, *Belgium* **24 C3** 51 5N 3 50 E
Oostende, *Belgium* **24 C2** 51 15N 2 54 E
Oosterhout, *Neths.* **24 C4** 51 39N 4 47 E
Oosterschelde →, *Neths.* **24 C4** 51 33N 4 0 E
Oosterwolde, *Neths.* **24 B6** 53 0N 6 17 E
Ootacamund = Udagamandalam, *India* **95 J3** 11 30N 76 44 E
Ootha, *Australia* **129 B7** 33 6 S 147 29 E
Ootsa L., *Canada* **142 C3** 53 50N 126 2W
Op Luang △, *Thailand* **86 C2** 18 12N 98 32 E
Opaka, *Bulgaria* **51 C10** 43 28N 26 10 E
Opala, *Dem. Rep. of the Congo* **118 C1** 0 40 S 24 20 E
Opalenica, *Poland* **55 F3** 52 18N 16 24 E
Opan, *Bulgaria* **51 D9** 42 13N 25 41 E
Opanake, *Sri Lanka* **95 L5** 6 35N 80 40 E
Opapa, *N.Z.* **130 F5** 39 47 S 176 42 E
Opasatika, *Canada* **140 C3** 49 30N 82 50W
Opasquia ⌓, *Canada* **140 B1** 53 33N 93 5W
Opatija, *Croatia* **45 C11** 45 21N 14 17 E
Opatów, *Poland* **55 H8** 50 50N 21 27 E
Opava, *Czech Rep.* **35 B10** 49 57N 17 58 E
Opelika, *U.S.A.* **152 C4** 32 39N 85 23W
Opelousas, *U.S.A.* **155 K8** 30 32N 92 5W
Opémisca, L., *Canada* **140 C5** 49 56N 74 52W
Opheim, *U.S.A.* **158 B10** 48 51N 106 24W
Ophir, *U.S.A.* **144 E8** 63 10N 156 31W
Ophthalmia Ra., *Australia* **124 D2** 23 15 S 119 30 E
Opi, *Nigeria* **113 D6** 6 36N 7 28 E
Opihikao, *U.S.A.* **145 D7** 19 26N 154 53W
Opinaca →, *Canada* **140 B4** 52 15N 78 2W
Opinaca, Rés., *Canada* **140 B4** 52 39N 76 20W
Opinnagau →, *Canada* **140 B3** 54 12N 82 25W
Opiscotéo, L., *Canada* **141 B6** 53 10N 68 10W
Opobo, *Nigeria* **113 E6** 4 35N 7 34 E
Opochka, *Russia* **58 D5** 56 42N 28 45 E
Opoczno, *Poland* **55 G7** 51 22N 20 18 E
Opol, *Phil.* **81 G5** 8 31N 124 34 E
Opole, *Poland* **55 H4** 50 42N 17 58 E
Opole Lubelskie, *Poland* **55 G8** 51 9N 21 58 E
Opolskie □, *Poland* **55 H5** 50 30N 18 0 E
Opon = Lapu-Lapu, *Phil.* **81 F4** 10 20N 123 55 E
Oponono L., *Namibia* **116 B2** 18 8 S 15 45 E
Oporto = Porto, *Portugal* **42 D2** 41 8N 8 40W
Opotiki, *N.Z.* **130 E6** 38 1 S 177 19 E
Opp, *U.S.A.* **152 D3** 31 17N 86 16W
Oppdal, *Norway* **18 B6** 62 35N 9 41 E
Oppeln = Opole, *Poland* **55 H4** 50 42N 17 58 E
Óppido Mamertina, *Italy* **47 D8** 38 16N 15 59 E
Oppland □, *Norway* **18 C6** 61 15N 9 40 E
Opportunity, *U.S.A.* **158 C5** 47 39N 117 15W
Oprişor, *Romania* **52 F8** 44 17N 23 5 E
Oprtalj, *Croatia* **45 C10** 45 23N 13 50 E
Opua, *N.Z.* **130 B3** 35 19 S 174 9 E
Opunake, *N.Z.* **130 F2** 39 26 S 173 52 E
Opuwo, *Namibia* **116 B1** 18 3 S 13 45 E
Opuzen, *Croatia* **45 E14** 43 1N 17 34 E
Oquawka, *U.S.A.* **156 D6** 40 56N 90 57W
Ora, *Cyprus* **39 F9** 34 51N 33 12 E
Oracle, *U.S.A.* **159 K8** 32 37N 110 46W
Oracuzar, *Peru* **168 D2** 4 42 S 78 6W
Oradea, *Romania* **52 C6** 47 2N 21 58 E
Öræfajökull, *Iceland* **11 C10** 64 2N 16 39W
Orahovac, *Serbia & M.* **50 D4** 42 24N 20 40 E
Orahovica, *Croatia* **52 E2** 45 35N 17 52 E
Orai, *India* **93 G8** 25 58N 79 30 E
Oraison, *France* **29 E9** 43 55N 5 55 E
Oral = Zhayyq →, *Kazakhstan* **57 E9** 47 0N 51 48 E
Oral, *Kazakhstan* **60 E10** 51 20N 51 20 E
Oran, *Algeria* **111 A4** 35 45N 0 39W
Orange, *Australia* **129 B8** 33 15 S 149 7 E
Orange, *France* **29 D8** 44 8N 4 47 E
Orange, *Calif., U.S.A.* **161 M9** 33 47N 117 51W
Orange, *Mass., U.S.A.* **151 D12** 42 35N 72 19W
Orange, *Tex., U.S.A.* **155 K8** 30 6N 93 44W
Orange, *Va., U.S.A.* **148 F6** 38 15N 78 7W
Orange →, *S. Africa* **116 D2** 28 41 S 16 28 E
Orange, C., *Brazil* **169 C7** 4 20N 51 30W
Orange City, *U.S.A.* **153 G8** 28 57N 81 18W
Orange Cove, *U.S.A.* **160 J7** 36 38N 119 19W
Orange Free State = Free State □, *S. Africa* **116 D4** 28 30 S 27 0 E
Orange Grove, *U.S.A.* **155 M6** 27 58N 97 56W
Orange L., *U.S.A.* **153 F7** 29 25N 82 13W
Orange Park, *U.S.A.* **152 E8** 30 10N 81 42W
Orange River Colony = Free State □, *S. Africa* **116 D4** 28 30 S 27 0 E
Orange Walk, *Belize* **163 D7** 18 6N 88 33W
Orangeburg, *U.S.A.* **152 B9** 33 30N 80 52W
Orangeville, *Canada* **140 D3** 43 55N 80 5W
Orangeville, *U.S.A.* **156 B7** 42 28N 89 39W
Orango, *Guinea-Biss.* **112 C1** 11 5N 16 0W
Orani, *Phil.* **80 D3** 14 49N 120 32 E
Oranienburg, *Germany* **30 C9** 52 45N 13 14 E
Oranje = Orange →, *S. Africa* **116 D2** 28 41 S 16 28 E
Oranjemund, *Namibia* **116 D2** 28 38 S 16 29 E
Oranjerivier, *S. Africa* **116 D3** 29 40 S 24 12 E
Oranjestad, *Aruba* **165 D5** 12 32N 70 2W
Orap, *Vanuatu* **133 E5** 15 58 S 167 20 E
Orarak, *Sudan* **107 F3** 6 15N 32 23 E
Oras, *Phil.* **80 E5** 12 9N 125 28 E
Orašje, *Bos.-H.* **52 E3** 45 1N 18 42 E
Orăştie, *Romania* **53 E8** 45 50N 23 10 E
Orava →, *Slovak Rep.* **35 B12** 49 9N 19 8 E
Orava, Vodna nádriž, *Slovak Rep.* **35 B12** 49 25N 19 35 E
Oraviţa, *Romania* **52 E6** 45 2N 21 43 E
Orawia, *N.Z.* **131 G2** 46 1 S 167 50 E
Orb →, *France* **28 E7** 43 15N 3 18 E
Orba →, *Italy* **44 D5** 44 53N 8 37 E
Ørbæk, *Denmark* **17 J4** 55 17N 10 39 E
Orbe, *Switz.* **32 C3** 46 43N 6 32 E
Orbec, *France* **26 C7** 49 1N 0 23 E
Orbetello, *Italy* **45 F8** 42 27N 11 13 E
Órbigo →, *Spain* **42 C5** 42 5N 5 42W
Orbisonia, *U.S.A.* **150 F7** 40 15N 77 54W
Orbost, *Australia* **129 D8** 37 40 S 148 29 E
Örbyhus, *Sweden* **16 D11** 60 15N 17 43 E
Orcadas, *Antarctica* **7 C18** 60 44 S 44 37W
Orcas I., *U.S.A.* **160 B4** 48 42N 122 56W
Orce, *Spain* **41 H2** 37 44N 2 28W
Orce →, *Spain* **41 H2** 37 44N 2 28W
Orchard City, *U.S.A.* **159 G10** 38 50N 107 58W
Orchard Homes, *U.S.A.* **158 C6** 46 55N 114 4W
Orchies, *France* **27 B10** 50 28N 3 14 E
Orchila, I., *Venezuela* **165 D6** 11 48N 66 10W
Orchilla, Pta., *Canary Is.* **9 e1** 27 42N 18 10W
Órcia →, *Italy* **45 F8** 42 58N 11 21 E
Orco →, *Italy* **44 C4** 45 10N 7 52 E
Orcopampa, *Peru* **172 D3** 15 20 S 72 23W
Orcutt, *U.S.A.* **161 L6** 34 52N 120 27W
Ord, *U.S.A.* **154 E5** 41 36N 98 56W
Ord →, *Australia* **124 C4** 15 33 S 128 15 E
Ord, Mt., *Australia* **124 C4** 17 20 S 125 34 E
Ordenes = Ordes, *Spain* **42 B2** 43 5N 8 29W
Orderville, *U.S.A.* **159 H7** 37 17N 112 38W
Ordes, *Spain* **42 B2** 43 5N 8 29W
Ordesa y Monte Perido △, *Spain* **40 C4** 42 40N 0 10W
Ording = St-Peter-Ording, *Germany* **30 A4** 54 20N 8 36 E
Ordos = Mu Us Shamo, *China* **74 E5** 39 0N 109 0 E
Ordu, *Turkey* **100 B7** 40 55N 37 53 E
Ordubad, *Azerbaijan* **101 C12** 38 54N 46 1 E
Orduña, *Álava, Spain* **40 C2** 42 58N 2 58W
Orduña, *Granada, Spain* **43 H7** 37 20N 3 30W
Ordway, *U.S.A.* **154 F3** 38 13N 103 46W
Ordzhonikidze = Vladikavkaz, *Russia* **61 J7** 43 0N 44 35 E
Ordzhonikidze = Yenakiyeve, *Ukraine* **59 H10** 48 15N 38 15 E
Ordzhonikidze, *Kazakhstan* **64 E8** 52 27N 61 39 E
Ordzhonikidze, *Ukraine* **59 J8** 47 39N 34 3 E
Ordzhonikidzeabad = Kofarnikhon, *Tajikistan* **65 D4** 38 34N 69 1 E
Ore, *Dem. Rep. of the Congo* **118 B2** 3 17N 29 30 E
Ore Mts. = Erzgebirge, *Germany* **30 E8** 50 27N 12 55 E
Orealla, *Guyana* **169 B6** 5 15N 57 23W
Orebić, *Croatia* **45 F14** 43 0N 17 11 E
Örebro, *Sweden* **16 E9** 59 20N 15 18 E
Örebro län □, *Sweden* **16 E8** 59 27N 15 0 E
Orecchiella ⌓, *Italy* **44 D7** 44 16N 10 22 E
Oregon, *Ill., U.S.A.* **156 B7** 42 1N 89 20W
Oregon, *Ohio, U.S.A.* **157 C13** 41 38N 83 25W
Oregon, *Wis., U.S.A.* **156 B7** 42 56N 89 23W
Oregon □, *U.S.A.* **158 E3** 44 0N 121 0W
Oregon City, *U.S.A.* **160 E4** 45 21N 122 36W
Oregon Dunes ⌓, *U.S.A.* **158 E1** 42 3N 124 5W
Öregrund, *Sweden* **16 D12** 60 21N 18 30 E
Öregrundsgrepen, *Sweden* **16 D12** 60 25N 18 15 E
Orekhov = Orikhiv, *Ukraine* **59 J8** 47 30N 35 48 E
Orekhovo-Zuyevo, *Russia* **58 E10** 55 50N 38 55 E
Orel, *Russia* **59 F9** 52 57N 36 3 E
Orel →, *Ukraine* **59 H8** 48 40N 34 39 E
Orellana, *Spain* **43 F5** 39 1N 5 32W
Orellana, Canal de, *Spain* **43 F5** 39 2N 6 0W
Orellana, Embalse de, *Spain* **43 F5** 39 5N 5 10W
Orem, *U.S.A.* **158 F8** 40 19N 111 42W
Ören, *Turkey* **49 D9** 37 3N 27 57 E
Orenburg, *Russia* **64 F5** 51 45N 55 6 E
Örencik, *Turkey* **49 B11** 39 16N 29 33 E
Orense = Ourense, *Spain* **42 C3** 42 19N 7 55W
Orense □, *Spain* **42 C3** 42 15N 7 51W
Orepuki, *N.Z.* **131 G2** 46 19 S 167 46 E
Orestiada = Orestiás, *Greece* **51 E10** 41 30N 26 33 E
Orestiás, *Greece* **51 E10** 41 30N 26 33 E
Orestos Pereyra, *Mexico* **162 B3** 26 31N 105 40W
Øresund, *Europe* **17 J6** 55 45N 12 45 E
Oretana, Cordillera = Toledo, Montes de, *Spain* **43 F6** 39 33N 4 20W
Oreti →, *N.Z.* **131 G3** 46 28 S 168 14 E
Orford Ness, *U.K.* **21 E9** 52 5N 1 35 E
Organ Pipe Cactus ⌓, *U.S.A.* **159 K7** 32 0N 113 10W
Organos, Pta. de los, *Canary Is.* **9 e1** 28 12N 17 17W
Organyà, *Spain* **40 C6** 42 13N 1 20 E
Orgaz, *Spain* **43 F7** 39 39N 3 53W
Ørgenvika, *Norway* **18 D6** 60 17N 9 42 E
Orgeyev = Orhei, *Moldova* **53 C13** 47 24N 28 50 E
Orgūn, *Afghan.* **91 B3** 32 55N 69 12 E
Orhaneli, *Turkey* **51 G12** 39 54N 28 59 E
Orhaneli →, *Turkey* **51 G12** 39 50N 28 55 E
Orhangazi, *Turkey* **51 F13** 40 29N 29 18 E
Orhei, *Moldova* **53 C13** 47 24N 28 50 E
Orhon Gol →, *Mongolia* **68 A5** 50 21N 106 0 E
Ória, *Italy* **47 B10** 40 30N 17 38 E
Orida, *Niger* **111 D7** 21 20N 12 15 E
Oriental, Cordillera, *Bolivia* **173 D4** 17 0 S 66 0W
Oriental, Cordillera, *Colombia* **168 B3** 6 0N 73 0W
Oriental, Grand Erg, *Algeria* **111 C6** 30 0N 6 30 E
Orientale □, *Dem. Rep. of the Congo* **118 B2** 2 20N 26 0 E
Oriente, *Argentina* **174 D3** 38 44 S 60 37W
Orihuela, *Spain* **41 G4** 38 7N 0 55W
Orihuela del Tremedal, *Spain* **40 E3** 40 33N 1 39W
Orikhiv, *Ukraine* **59 J8** 47 30N 35 48 E
Orikum, *Albania* **50 F3** 40 20N 19 26 E
Orillia, *Canada* **140 D4** 44 40N 79 24W
Orinduik, *Guyana* **169 C5** 4 40N 60 3W
Orinoco →, *Venezuela* **169 B5** 9 15N 61 30W
Orion, *Canada* **143 D6** 49 27N 110 49W
Orion, *Ala., U.S.A.* **152 D4** 31 58N 86 0W
Orion, *Ill., U.S.A.* **156 C6** 41 21N 90 23W
Oriskany, *U.S.A.* **151 C9** 43 10N 75 20W
Orissa □, *India* **94 E7** 20 0N 84 0 E
Orissaare, *Estonia* **15 G20** 58 34N 23 5 E
Oristano, *Italy* **46 C1** 39 54N 8 36 E
Oristano, G. di, *Italy* **46 C1** 39 50N 8 29 E
Orituco →, *Venezuela* **168 B4** 8 45N 67 27W
Oriximina, *Brazil* **169 D6** 1 45 S 55 52W
Orizaba, *Mexico* **163 D5** 18 51N 97 6W
Orizaba, Pico de, *Mexico* **163 D5** 19 0N 97 20W
Orizare, *Bulgaria* **51 D11** 42 44N 27 39 E
Orizona, *Brazil* **171 E2** 17 3 S 48 18W
Ørje, *Norway* **18 E8** 59 29N 11 39 E
Orjen, *Bos.-H.* **50 D2** 42 35N 18 34 E
Orjiva, *Spain* **43 J7** 36 53N 3 24W
Orkanger, *Norway* **18 A6** 63 18N 9 52 E
Örkelljunga, *Sweden* **17 H7** 56 17N 13 17 E
Örken, *Sweden* **17 G9** 57 6N 15 1 E
Örkény, *Hungary* **52 C4** 47 9N 19 26 E
Orkhaniye = Botevgrad, *Bulgaria* **50 D7** 42 55N 23 47 E
Orkla →, *Norway* **18 A6** 63 18N 9 51 E
Orkney, *S. Africa* **116 D4** 26 58 S 26 40 E
Orkney □, *U.K.* **22 B5** 59 2N 3 13W
Orkney Is., *U.K.* **22 B6** 59 0N 3 0W
Orland, *Calif., U.S.A.* **160 F4** 39 45N 122 12W
Orland, *Ind., U.S.A.* **157 C11** 41 47N 85 12W
Orlando, *U.S.A.* **153 G8** 28 33N 81 23W
Orlando, C. d', *Italy* **47 D7** 38 10N 14 43 E
Orlando International ✈ (MCO), *U.S.A.* **153 G8** 28 26N 81 19W
Orléanais, *France* **27 E9** 48 0N 2 0 E
Orléans, *France* **27 E8** 47 54N 1 52 E
Orleans, *Ind., U.S.A.* **157 F10** 38 40N 86 27W
Orleans, *Vt., U.S.A.* **151 B12** 44 49N 72 12W
Orléans, Î. d', *Canada* **141 C5** 46 54N 70 58W
Orléansville = Ech Chéliff, *Algeria* **111 A5** 36 10N 1 20 E
Orlice →, *Czech Rep.* **34 A8** 50 13N 15 50 E
Orlivka, *Ukraine* **53 E13** 45 19N 28 27 E
Orlov = Khalturin, *Russia* **64 B2** 58 40N 48 50 E
Orlov, *Slovak Rep.* **35 B13** 49 17N 20 51 E
Orlov Gay, *Russia* **60 E9** 50 56N 48 19 E
Orlová, *Czech Rep.* **35 B11** 49 51N 18 26 E
Orlovat, *Serbia & M.* **52 E5** 45 14N 20 33 E
Orlovka, *Kyrgyzstan* **65 B7** 42 45N 75 36 E
Orly, Paris ✈ (ORY), *France* **27 D9** 48 44N 2 23 E
Ormara, *Pakistan* **91 D2** 25 16N 64 33 E
Ormea, *Italy* **44 D4** 44 9N 7 54 E
Ormília, *Greece* **50 F7** 40 16N 23 39 E
Ormoc, *Phil.* **81 F5** 11 0N 124 37 E
Ormond, *N.Z.* **130 E6** 38 33 S 177 56 E
Ormond Beach, *U.S.A.* **153 F8** 29 17N 81 3W
Ormond by the Sea, *U.S.A.* **153 F8** 29 21N 81 4W
Ormondville, *N.Z.* **130 G5** 40 5 S 176 19 E
Órmos Keríou, *Greece* **39 D2** 37 42N 20 53 E
Ormož, *Slovenia* **45 B13** 46 25N 16 10 E
Ormskirk, *U.K.* **20 D5** 53 35N 2 54W
Ormstown, *Canada* **151 A11** 45 8N 74 0W
Ormtjernkampen △, *Norway* **18 C6** 61 12N 9 48 E
Ornans, *France* **27 E13** 47 7N 6 10 E
Ornavasso, *Italy* **33 E6** 45 58N 8 24 E
Orne □, *France* **26 D7** 48 40N 0 5 E
Orne →, *France* **26 C6** 49 18N 0 15W
Orneta, *Poland* **54 D7** 54 8N 20 9 E
Ornö, *Sweden* **16 E12** 59 4N 18 24 E
Örnsköldsvik, *Sweden* **16 A12** 63 17N 18 40 E
Oro, *N. Korea* **75 D14** 40 1N 127 27 E
Oro →, *Mexico* **162 B3** 25 35N 105 2W
Oro Grande, *U.S.A.* **161 L9** 34 36N 117 20W
Oro Valley, *U.S.A.* **159 K8** 32 26N 110 58W
Orobie, Alpi, *Italy* **44 B6** 46 7N 10 0 E
Orobie Bergamasche ⌓, *Italy* **44 C6** 46 0N 9 45 E
Orobie Valtellinesi ⌓, *Italy* **44 B6** 46 5N 9 45 E
Orocué, *Colombia* **168 C3** 4 48N 71 20W
Orodara, *Burkina Faso* **112 C4** 11 0N 4 55W
Orodo, *Nigeria* **113 D6** 5 34N 7 4 E
Orofino, *U.S.A.* **158 C5** 46 29N 116 15W
Orohena, Mt., *Tahiti* **133 S16** 17 37 S 149 28W
Orol Dengizi = Aral Sea, *Asia* **66 E7** 44 30N 60 0 E
Oromiya □, *Ethiopia* **107 F5** 7 0N 40 0 E
Oromocto, *Canada* **141 C6** 45 54N 66 29W
Oron, *Nigeria* **113 E6** 4 48N 8 14 E
Oron, *Switz.* **32 C3** 46 34N 6 50 E
Orongo, *Chile* **172 b** 27 11 S 109 27W
Orono, *Canada* **150 C6** 43 59N 78 37W
Orono, *U.S.A.* **149 C11** 44 53N 68 40W
Oronsay, *U.K.* **22 E2** 56 1N 6 15W
Oropesa, *Spain* **42 F5** 39 57N 5 10W
Oroqen Zizhiqi, *China* **69 A7** 50 34N 123 43 E
Oroquieta, *Phil.* **81 G4** 8 32N 123 44 E
Orós, *Brazil* **170 C4** 6 15 S 38 55W
Orosei, *Italy* **46 B2** 40 23N 9 42 E
Orosei, G. di, *Italy* **46 B2** 40 15N 9 44 E
Orosháza, *Hungary* **52 D5** 46 32N 20 42 E
Oroszlány, *Hungary* **52 C3** 47 29N 18 19 E
Orote Pen., *Guam* **133 R15** 13 26N 144 38 E
Orotukan, *Russia* **67 C16** 62 16N 151 42 E
Oroville, *Calif., U.S.A.* **160 F5** 39 31N 121 33W
Oroville, *Wash., U.S.A.* **158 B4** 48 56N 119 26W
Oroville, L., *U.S.A.* **160 F5** 39 33N 121 29W
Orrefors, *Sweden* **17 H9** 56 50N 15 45 E
Orrick, *U.S.A.* **156 E2** 39 13N 94 7W
Orroroo, *Australia* **128 B3** 32 43 S 138 38 E
Orrviken, *Sweden* **16 A8** 63 6N 14 26 E
Orrville, *U.S.A.* **150 F3** 40 50N 81 46W
Orsa, *Sweden* **16 C8** 61 7N 14 37 E
Orsara di Púglia, *Italy* **47 A8** 41 17N 15 16 E
Orsasjön, *Sweden* **16 C8** 61 7N 14 37 E
Orsha, *Belarus* **58 E6** 54 30N 30 25 E
Orsières, *Switz.* **32 D4** 46 2N 7 9 E
Örsjö, *Sweden* **17 H9** 56 42N 15 45 E
Orsk, *Russia* **64 F7** 51 12N 58 34 E
Orşova, *Romania* **52 F7** 44 41N 22 25 E
Ørsta, *Norway* **18 B3** 62 13N 6 8 E
Ørsted, *Denmark* **17 H4** 56 30N 10 20 E
Örsundsbro, *Sweden* **16 E11** 59 44N 17 18 E
Orta, L. d', *Italy* **44 C5** 45 49N 8 24 E
Orta Nova, *Italy* **47 A8** 41 19N 15 42 E
Ortaca, *Turkey* **49 E10** 36 49N 28 45 E
Ortakent, *Turkey* **49 D9** 37 5N 27 21 E
Ortaklar, *Turkey* **49 D9** 37 53N 27 30 E
Ortaköy, *Çorum, Turkey* **100 B6** 40 16N 35 15 E
Ortaköy, *Niğde, Turkey* **100 C6** 38 44N 34 3 E
Orte, *Italy* **45 F9** 42 27N 12 23 E
Ortegal, C., *Spain* **42 B3** 43 43N 7 52W
Orteguaza →, *Colombia* **168 C2** 0 43N 75 16W
Ortelsburg = Szczytno, *Poland* **54 E7** 53 33N 21 0 E
Orthez, *France* **28 E3** 43 29N 0 48W
Ortigueira, *Spain* **42 B3** 43 40N 7 50W
Orting, *U.S.A.* **160 C4** 47 6N 122 12W
Ortisei, *Italy* **45 B8** 46 34N 11 40 E
Ortles, *Italy* **44 B7** 46 31N 10 33 E
Ortnevik, *Norway* **18 C3** 61 6N 6 7 E
Orto-Tokoy, *Kyrgyzstan* **65 B8** 42 20N 76 1 E
Ortón →, *Bolivia* **172 C4** 10 50 S 67 0W
Ortona, *Italy* **45 F11** 42 21N 14 24 E
Ortonville, *U.S.A.* **154 C6** 45 19N 96 27W
Orūmīyeh, *Iran* **101 D11** 37 40N 45 0 E
Orūmīyeh, Daryācheh-ye, *Iran* **101 D11** 37 50N 45 30 E
Orune, *Italy* **46 B2** 40 24N 9 22 E
Oruro, *Bolivia* **172 D4** 18 0 S 67 9W
Oruro □, *Bolivia* **172 D4** 18 40 S 67 30W
Orust, *Sweden* **17 F5** 58 10N 11 40 E
Oruzgān □, *Afghan.* **91 B2** 33 30N 66 0 E
Orvault, *France* **26 E5** 47 17N 1 38W
Orvieto, *Italy* **45 F9** 42 43N 12 7 E
Orwell, *N.Y., U.S.A.* **151 C9** 43 35N 75 50W
Orwell, *Ohio, U.S.A.* **150 E4** 41 32N 80 52W
Orwell →, *U.K.* **21 F9** 51 59N 1 18 E
Orwigsburg, *U.S.A.* **151 F8** 40 38N 76 6W
Oryakhovo, *Bulgaria* **50 C7** 43 40N 23 57 E
Orynyn, *Ukraine* **53 B11** 48 46N 26 24 E
Orzinuovi, *Italy* **44 C6** 45 24N 9 55 E
Orzyc →, *Poland* **55 F8** 52 46N 21 14 E
Orzysz, *Poland* **54 E8** 53 50N 21 58 E
Os, *Norway* **18 B8** 62 30N 11 14 E
Osa, *Russia* **64 C5** 57 17N 55 26 E
Osa →, *Norway* **18 C8** 61 18N 11 46 E
Osa →, *Poland* **54 E5** 53 33N 18 46 E
Osa, Pen. de, *Costa Rica* **164 E3** 8 0N 84 0W
Osage, *U.S.A.* **154 D8** 43 17N 92 49W
Osage →, *U.S.A.* **156 F5** 38 35N 91 57W
Osage City, *U.S.A.* **154 F7** 38 38N 95 50W
Ōsaka, *Japan* **73 C7** 34 40N 135 30 E
Ōsaka □, *Japan* **73 C7** 34 30N 135 30 E
Osaka Kansai International ✈ (KIX), *Japan* **73 C7** 34 27N 135 12 E
Ōsaka-Wan, *Japan* **73 C7** 34 30N 135 18 E
Osaki, *Japan* **72 F3** 31 25N 131 2 E
Osan, *S. Korea* **75 F14** 37 11N 127 4 E
Osawatomie, *U.S.A.* **154 F7** 38 31N 94 57W
Osborne, *U.S.A.* **154 F5** 39 26N 98 42W
Osby, *Sweden* **17 H7** 56 23N 13 59 E
Osceola, *Ark., U.S.A.* **155 H10** 35 42N 89 58W
Osceola, *Iowa, U.S.A.* **156 C3** 41 2N 93 46W
Osceola, *Mo., U.S.A.* **156 F3** 38 3N 93 42W
Oschatz, *Germany* **30 D9** 51 17N 13 6 E
Oschersleben, *Germany* **30 C7** 52 2N 11 14 E
Óschiri, *Italy* **46 B2** 40 43N 9 6 E
Oscoda, *U.S.A.* **150 B1** 44 26N 83 20W
Osečina, *Serbia & M.* **50 B3** 44 23N 19 34 E
Ösel = Saaremaa, *Estonia* **15 G20** 58 30N 22 30 E
Osensjøen, *Norway* **18 C8** 61 13N 11 50 E
Osery, *Russia* **58 E10** 54 52N 38 28 E
Osgood, *U.S.A.* **157 E11** 39 8N 85 18W
Osgoode, *Canada* **151 A9** 45 8N 75 36W
Osh, *Kyrgyzstan* **65 C6** 40 37N 72 49 E
Oshawa, *Canada* **140 D4** 43 50N 78 50W
Oshigambo, *Namibia* **116 B2** 17 45 S 16 5 E
Oshkosh, *Nebr., U.S.A.* **154 E3** 41 24N 102 21W
Oshkosh, *Wis., U.S.A.* **154 C10** 44 1N 88 33W
Oshmyany = Ashmyany, *Belarus* **15 J21** 54 26N 25 52 E
Oshnovīyeh, *Iran* **96 B5** 37 2N 45 6 E
Oshogbo, *Nigeria* **113 D5** 7 48N 4 37 E
Oshtorīnān, *Iran* **97 C6** 34 1N 48 38 E
Oshwe, *Dem. Rep. of the Congo* **114 C3** 3 25 S 19 28 E
Osi, *Nigeria* **113 D6** 8 8N 5 14 E
Osieczna, *Poland* **55 G3** 51 55N 16 40 E
Osijek, *Croatia* **52 E3** 45 34N 18 41 E
Ósilo, *Italy* **46 B1** 40 45N 8 40 E
Ósimo, *Italy* **45 E10** 43 28N 13 30 E
Osintorf, *Belarus* **58 E6** 54 40N 30 39 E
Osipenko = Berdyansk, *Ukraine* **59 J9** 46 45N 36 50 E
Osipovichi = Asipovichy, *Belarus* **58 F5** 53 19N 28 33 E
Osiyan, *India* **92 F5** 26 43N 72 55 E
Osizweni, *S. Africa* **117 D5** 27 49 S 30 7 E
Oskaloosa, *U.S.A.* **156 C4** 41 18N 92 39W
Oskarshamn, *Sweden* **17 G10** 57 15N 16 27 E
Oskarström, *Sweden* **17 H6** 56 48N 12 58 E
Oskélanéo, *Canada* **140 C4** 48 5N 75 15W
Öskemen, *Kazakhstan* **66 E9** 50 0N 82 36 E
Oskol →, *Ukraine* **59 H9** 49 6N 37 25 E
Oslo, *Norway* **18 E7** 59 55N 10 45 E
Oslo □, *Norway* **18 D7** 59 54N 10 43 E
Oslo ✈ (OSL), *Norway* **18 D8** 60 10N 11 8 E
Oslob, *Phil.* **81 G4** 9 31N 123 26 E
Oslofjorden, *Norway* **18 E7** 59 20N 10 35 E
Osmanabad, *India* **94 E3** 18 5N 76 10 E
Osmancık, *Turkey* **100 B6** 40 58N 34 47 E
Osmaniye, *Turkey* **100 D7** 37 5N 36 10 E
Osmanlı, *Turkey* **51 E10** 41 35N 26 51 E
Osmannagar, *India* **94 E4** 18 32N 79 20 E
Ösmo, *Sweden* **16 F11** 58 58N 17 55 E
Osnabrück, *Germany* **30 C4** 52 17N 8 3 E
Ośno Lubuskie, *Poland* **55 F1** 52 28N 14 51 E
Osoblaha, *Czech Rep.* **35 A10** 50 17N 17 44 E
Osogovska Planina, *Macedonia* **50 D6** 42 10N 22 30 E
Osor, *Italy* **45 D11** 44 42N 14 24 E
Osorio, *Brazil* **175 B5** 29 53 S 50 17W
Osório da Fonseca, *Brazil* **169 D6** 3 52 S 58 14W
Osorno, *Chile* **176 B2** 40 25 S 73 0W
Osorno, *Spain* **42 C6** 42 24N 4 22W
Osorno □, *Chile* **176 B2** 40 34 S 73 9W
Osorno, Vol., *Chile* **176 B2** 41 0 S 72 30W
Osoyoos, *Canada* **142 D5** 49 0N 119 30W
Osøyro, *Norway* **18 D2** 60 9N 5 30 E
Óspakseyri, *Iceland* **11 B5** 65 27N 21 26W
Ospika →, *Canada* **142 B4** 56 20N 124 0W
Osprey, *U.S.A.* **153 H7** 27 12N 82 29W
Osprey Reef, *Australia* **126 A4** 13 52 S 146 36 E
Oss, *Neths.* **24 C5** 51 46N 5 32 E
Ossa, Mt., *Australia* **127 G4** 41 52 S 146 3 E
Óssa, Óros, *Greece* **48 B4** 39 47N 22 42 E
Ossa de Montiel, *Spain* **41 G2** 38 58N 2 45W
Ossabaw I., *U.S.A.* **152 D8** 31 50N 81 5W
Ossabaw Sd., *U.S.A.* **152 D8** 31 50N 81 6W
Osse →, *France* **28 D4** 44 7N 0 17 E
Osse →, *Nigeria* **113 D6** 6 10N 5 20 E
Ossersee = Zarasai, *Lithuania* **15 J22** 55 40N 26 20 E
Ossi, *Italy* **46 B1** 40 40N 8 35 E
Ossining, *U.S.A.* **151 E11** 41 10N 73 55W
Ossipee, *U.S.A.* **151 C13** 43 41N 71 7W
Ossokmanuan L., *Canada* **141 B7** 53 25N 65 0W
Ossora, *Russia* **67 D17** 59 20N 163 13 E
Ostashkov, *Russia* **58 D7** 57 4N 33 2 E
Östavall, *Sweden* **16 B9** 62 26N 15 29 E
Østby, *Norway* **18 C9** 61 15N 12 33 E
Oste →, *Germany* **30 B5** 53 49N 9 2 E
Ostenburg = Pułtusk, *Poland* **55 F8** 52 43N 21 6 E
Ostend = Oostende, *Belgium* **24 C2** 51 15N 2 54 E
Ostend, *N.Z.* **130 C4** 36 48 S 175 2 E
Oster, *Ukraine* **59 G6** 50 57N 30 53 E
Österbotten = Pohjanmaa, *Finland* **14 E20** 62 58N 22 50 E
Osterburg, *Germany* **30 C7** 52 47N 11 45 E
Osterburg, *U.S.A.* **150 F6** 40 16N 78 31W
Osterburken, *Germany* **31 F5** 49 25N 9 26 E
Österbybruk, *Sweden* **16 D11** 60 13N 17 55 E
Österbymo, *Sweden* **17 G9** 57 49N 15 15 E
Österdalälven, *Sweden* **16 C7** 61 30N 13 45 E
Østerdalen, *Norway* **15 F14** 61 40N 10 50 E
Österfärnebo, *Sweden* **16 D10** 60 19N 16 48 E

Österforse, Sweden 16 A11 63 9N 17 3 E
Östergötlands län □, Sweden 17 F9 58 35N 15 45 E
Osterholz-Scharmbeck, Germany 30 B4 53 13N 8 47 E
Østerild, Denmark 17 G2 57 2N 8 51 E
Ostermundigen, Switz. 32 C4 46 58N 7 27 E
Östermyra = Seinäjoki, Finland 15 E20 62 40N 22 51 E
Osterode, Germany 30 D6 51 43N 10 15 E
Osterode in Ostpreussen = Ostróda, Poland 54 E6 53 42N 19 58 E
Österreich = Austria ■, Europe 34 E7 47 0N 14 0 E
Österreich ober der Ems = Oberösterreich □, Austria 34 C7 48 10N 14 0 E
Östersund, Sweden 16 A8 63 10N 14 38 E
Östervåla, Sweden 16 D11 60 11N 17 11 E
Østfold □, Norway 18 E8 59 25N 11 25 E
Ostfriesische Inseln, Germany 30 B3 53 42N 7 0 E
Ostfriesland, Germany 30 B3 53 20N 7 30 E
Östhammar, Sweden 16 D12 60 16N 18 22 E
Ostia, Lido di, Italy 45 G9 41 43N 12 17 E
Ostíglia, Italy 45 C8 45 4N 11 8 E
Östmark, Sweden 16 D6 60 17N 12 45 E
Östra Husby, Sweden 17 F10 58 35N 16 33 E
Ostrava, Czech Rep. 35 B11 49 51N 18 18 E
Ostravský □, Czech Rep. 35 B10 49 55N 17 58 E
Ostróda, Poland 54 E6 53 42N 19 58 E
Ostrogozhsk, Russia 59 G10 50 55N 39 7 E
Ostroh, Ukraine 59 G4 50 20N 26 30 E
Ostrołęka, Poland 55 E8 53 4N 21 32 E
Ostrov, Bulgaria 51 C8 43 40N 24 9 E
Ostrov, Czech Rep. 34 A5 50 18N 12 57 E
Ostrov, Romania 53 F12 44 6N 27 24 E
Ostrov, Russia 58 D5 57 25N 28 20 E
Ostrów Lubelski, Poland 55 G9 51 29N 22 51 E
Ostrów Mazowiecka, Poland 55 F8 52 50N 21 51 E
Ostrów Wielkopolski, Poland 55 G4 51 36N 17 44 E
Ostrowiec-Świętokrzyski, Poland 55 H8 50 55N 21 22 E
Ostrowo = Ostrów Wielkopolski, Poland 55 G4 51 36N 17 44 E
Ostrožac, Bos.-H. 52 G2 43 43N 17 49 E
Ostrzeszów, Poland 55 G4 51 25N 17 52 E
Ostseebad Kühlungsborn, Germany 30 A7 54 8N 11 44 E
Osttirol □, Austria 34 E5 46 50N 12 30 E
Ostuni, Italy 47 B10 40 44N 17 35 E
Ostyako-Vogulsk = Khanty-Mansiysk, Russia 66 C7 61 0N 69 0 E
Osum →, Albania 50 F4 40 40N 20 10 E
Osŭm →, Bulgaria 51 C8 43 40N 24 50 E
Ōsumi-Hantō, Japan 72 F2 31 20N 130 55 E
Ōsumi-Kaikyō, Japan 71 J5 30 55N 131 0 E
Ōsumi-Shotō, Japan 71 J5 30 30N 130 0 E
Osun □, Nigeria 113 D5 7 30N 4 30 E
Osuna, Spain 43 H5 37 14N 5 8W
Oswegatchie →, U.S.A. 151 B9 44 42N 75 30W
Oswego, U.S.A. 151 C8 43 27N 76 31W
Oswego →, U.S.A. 151 C8 43 27N 76 30W
Oswestry, U.K. 20 E4 52 52N 3 3W
Oświęcim, Poland 55 H6 50 2N 19 11 E
Ōta, Fukui, Japan 73 B8 35 57N 136 3 E
Ōta, Gumma, Japan 73 A11 36 18N 139 22 E
Ota-Gawa →, Japan 72 C4 34 21N 132 18 E
Otaci, Moldova 53 B12 48 27N 27 47 E
Otago □, N.Z. 131 E4 45 15 S 170 0 E
Otago Harbour, N.Z. 131 F5 45 47 S 170 42 E
Otago Pen., N.Z. 131 F5 45 48 S 170 39 E
Otaheite B., Trin. & Tob. 169 F9 10 15N 61 30W
Otahuhu, N.Z. 130 C3 36 56 S 174 51 E
Ōtake, Japan 72 C4 34 12N 132 13 E
Ōtaki, Japan 73 B12 35 17N 140 15 E
Otaki, N.Z. 130 G4 40 45 S 175 10 E
Otane, N.Z. 130 F5 39 54 S 176 39 E
Otar, Kazakhstan 65 B7 43 32N 75 12 E
Otaru, Japan 70 C10 43 10N 141 0 E
Otaru-Wan = Ishikari-Wan, Japan 70 C10 43 25N 141 1 E
Otautau, N.Z. 131 G3 46 9 S 168 1 E
Otava →, Czech Rep. 34 B7 49 26N 14 12 E
Otavalo, Ecuador 168 C2 0 13N 78 20W
Otavi, Namibia 116 B2 19 40 S 17 24 E
Otchinjau, Angola 116 B1 16 30 S 13 56 E
Oteiza = Marihatag, Phil. 81 G6 8 48N 126 18 E
Otelec, Romania 52 E5 45 36N 20 50 E
Otelnuk, L., Canada 141 A6 56 9N 68 12W
Oţelu Roşu, Romania 52 E7 45 32N 22 22 E
Otero de Rey = Outeiro de Rei, Spain 42 B3 43 6N 7 36W
Othello, U.S.A. 158 C4 46 50N 119 10W
Othonoí, Greece 38 B9 39 52N 19 22 E
Óthris, Óros, Greece 48 B4 39 2N 22 37 E
Oti △, Togo 113 C5 10 40N 0 35 E
Otira, N.Z. 131 C6 42 49 S 171 35 E
Otira Gorge, N.Z. 131 C6 42 53 S 171 33 E
Otjiwarongo, Namibia 116 C2 20 30 S 16 33 E
Ötmök, Kyrgyzstan 65 B6 42 20N 73 10 E
Otmuchów, Poland 55 H4 50 28N 17 10 E
Oto Tolu Group, Tonga 133 Q13 20 21 S 174 32W
Otočac, Croatia 45 D12 44 53N 15 12 E
Otoineppu, Japan 70 B11 44 44N 142 16 E
Otok, Croatia 45 E13 43 42N 16 44 E
Otomavi = Korsakov, Russia 67 E15 46 36N 142 42 E
Oton, Phil. 81 F4 10 42N 122 29 E
Otopeni, Bucureşti ✕ (OTP), Romania 53 F11 44 30N 26 11 E
Otorohanga, N.Z. 130 E4 38 12 S 175 14 E
Otoskwin →, Canada 140 B2 52 13N 88 6W
Ōtoyo, Japan 72 D5 33 43N 133 45 E
Otpor = Zabaykalsk, Russia 67 E12 49 40N 117 25 E
Otra →, Norway 18 F5 58 9N 8 1 E
Otradnyy, Russia 60 D10 53 22N 51 21 E
Otranto, Italy 47 B11 40 9N 18 28 E
Otranto, C. d', Italy 47 B11 40 7N 18 30 E
Otranto, Str. of, Italy 47 B11 40 15N 18 40 E
Otrogovo = Stepnoye, Russia 64 D8 54 4N 60 26 E
Otrokovice, Czech Rep. 35 B10 49 12N 17 32 E
Otse, S. Africa 116 D4 25 2 S 25 45 E
Otsego, U.S.A. 157 B11 42 27N 85 42W
Ōtsu, Japan 73 C7 35 0N 135 50 E
Ōtsuki, Japan 73 B10 35 36N 138 57 E
Otta, Norway 18 C6 61 46N 9 32 E
Otta →, Norway 18 C6 61 46N 9 31 E
Ottapalam, India 95 J3 10 46N 76 23 E
Ottawa = Outaouais →, Canada 140 C5 45 27N 74 8W
Ottawa, Canada 140 C4 45 27N 75 42W
Ottawa, Ill., U.S.A. 154 E10 41 21N 88 51W
Ottawa, Kans., U.S.A. 154 F7 38 37N 95 16W
Ottawa, Ohio, U.S.A. 157 C12 41 1N 84 3W
Ottawa Is., Canada 139 C11 59 35N 80 10W
Ottélé, Cameroon 113 E7 3 38N 11 19 E
Ottensheim, Austria 34 C7 48 21N 14 12 E
Otter Cr. →, U.S.A. 151 B11 44 13N 73 17W
Otter Creek, U.S.A. 153 F7 29 19N 82 46W
Otter L., Canada 143 B8 55 35N 104 39W
Otterbein, U.S.A. 157 D9 40 29N 87 6W
Otterndorf, Germany 30 B4 53 48N 8 53 E
Otterøya, Norway 18 B3 62 45N 6 50 E
Otterup, Denmark 17 J4 55 30N 10 22 E
Otterville, Canada 150 D4 42 55N 80 36W
Otterville, U.S.A. 156 F4 38 42N 93 0W
Ottery St. Mary, U.K. 21 G4 50 44N 3 17W
Ottilien Reef, Papua N. G. 132 C5 4 33 S 148 49 E
Ottmachau = Otmuchów, Poland 55 H4 50 28N 17 10 E
Otto Beit Bridge, Zimbabwe 119 F2 15 59 S 28 56 E
Ottosdal, S. Africa 116 D4 26 46 S 25 59 E
Ottoville, U.S.A. 157 D12 40 57N 84 22W
Ottumwa, U.S.A. 156 D4 41 1N 92 25W
Otu, Nigeria 113 D5 8 14N 3 22 E
Otukpa, Nigeria 113 D6 7 9N 7 41 E
Oturkpo, Nigeria 113 D6 7 16N 8 8 E
Otvazhnoye = Zhigulevsk, Russia 60 D9 53 28N 49 30 E
Otvazhny = Zhigulevsk, Russia 60 D9 53 28N 49 30 E
Otway △, Australia 128 E5 38 47 S 143 34 E
Otway, B., Chile 176 D2 53 30 S 74 0W
Otway, C., Australia 128 E5 38 52 S 143 30 E
Otway, Seno de, Chile 176 D2 53 0 S 71 30W
Otwock, Poland 55 F8 52 5N 21 20 E
Otyniya, Ukraine 53 B9 48 44N 24 51 E
Ötztaler Ache →, Austria 34 D3 47 14N 10 50 E
Ötztaler Alpen, Austria 34 E3 46 56N 11 0 E
Ou →, Laos 86 B4 20 4N 102 13 E
Ou Neua, Laos 76 F3 22 18N 101 48 E
Ou-Sammyaku, Japan 70 E10 39 20N 140 35 E
Ouachita →, U.S.A. 155 K9 31 38N 91 49W
Ouachita, L., U.S.A. 155 H8 34 34N 93 12W
Ouachita Mts., U.S.A. 155 H7 34 40N 94 25W
Ouaco, N. Cal. 133 T18 20 50 S 164 29 E
Ouadâne, Mauritania 110 D2 20 50N 11 40W
Ouadda, C.A.R. 114 A4 8 15N 22 20 E
Ouagadougou, Burkina Faso 113 C4 12 25N 1 30W
Ouagam, Chad 109 F2 14 22N 14 42 E
Ouaham →, C.A.R. 114 A3 6 35N 15 12 E
Ouahigouya, Burkina Faso 112 C4 13 31N 2 25W
Ouahila, Algeria 110 C4 27 50N 5 0W
Ouahran = Oran, Algeria 111 A4 35 45N 0 39W
Oualâta, Mauritania 112 B3 17 20N 6 55W
Ouallam, Niger 113 C5 14 23N 2 10 E
Ouallene, Algeria 111 D5 24 41N 1 11 E
Ouanary, Fr. Guiana 169 C7 4 13N 51 40W
Ouanda Djallé, C.A.R. 114 A4 8 55N 22 53 E
Ouandago, C.A.R. 114 A3 7 13N 18 50 E
Ouandjia, Bahr →, C.A.R. 114 A4 9 35N 21 43 E
Ouandjia-Vakaga △, C.A.R. 114 A4 9 2N 22 18 E
Ouango, C.A.R. 114 B4 4 19N 22 30 E
Ouani, Comoros Is. 121 a 12 9 S 44 18 E
Ouantonou, C.A.R. 114 A3 7 19N 15 18 E
Ouarâne, Mauritania 110 D2 21 0N 10 30W
Ouargaye, Burkina Faso 113 C5 11 40N 0 5 E
Ouargla, Algeria 111 B6 31 59N 5 16 E
Ouarkoye, Burkina Faso 112 C4 12 5N 3 40W
Ouarkziz, Jebel, Algeria 110 C3 28 50N 8 0W
Ouarra →, C.A.R. 114 A4 5 5N 24 26 E
Ouarzazate, Morocco 110 B3 30 55N 6 50W
Ouassouas, Mali 113 B5 16 10N 1 23 E
Ouatagouna, Mali 113 B5 15 11N 0 43 E
Ouatere, C.A.R. 114 A3 5 30N 19 8 E
Oubangi →, Dem. Rep. of the Congo 114 C3 0 30 S 17 50 E
Oubarakai, O. →, Algeria 111 C6 27 20N 9 0 E
Ouche →, France 27 E12 47 6N 5 16 E
Ouddorp, Neths. 24 C3 51 50N 3 57 E
Oude Rijn →, Neths. 24 B4 52 12N 4 24 E
Oudeïka, Mali 113 B4 17 30N 1 40W
Oudenaarde, Belgium 24 D3 50 50N 3 37 E
Oudon →, France 26 E6 47 41N 0 53W
Oudtshoorn, S. Africa 116 E3 33 35 S 22 14 E
Ouécho, N. Cal. 133 T18 20 20 S 164 26 E
Ouéga, Chad 109 E4 17 47N 20 39 E
Ouellé, Ivory C. 112 D4 7 26N 4 1W
Ouéme →, Benin 113 D5 6 30N 2 30 E
Ouen, Î., N. Cal. 133 V20 22 26 S 166 49 E
Ouenza, Algeria 111 A6 35 57N 8 4 E
Ouessa, Burkina Faso 112 C4 11 4N 2 47W
Ouessant, Î. d', France 26 D1 48 28N 5 6W
Ouesso, Congo 114 B3 1 37N 16 5 E
Ouest, Pte. de l', Canada 141 C7 49 52N 64 40W
Ouezzane, Morocco 110 B3 34 51N 5 35W
Ougarou, Burkina Faso 113 C5 12 10N 0 58 E
Oughterard, Ireland 23 C2 53 26N 9 18W
Ouhan →, Chad 109 G3 9 18N 18 14 E
Ouidah, Benin 113 D5 6 25N 2 0 E
Ouidi, Niger 113 C7 14 10N 13 0 E
Ouissongo, Angola 115 E3 7 40 S 15 41 E
Ouistreham, France 26 C6 49 17N 0 18W
Oujda, Morocco 111 B4 34 41N 1 55W
Oujeft, Mauritania 112 A2 20 2N 13 0W
Oulainen, Finland 14 D21 64 17N 24 47 E
Ould Yenjé, Mauritania 112 B2 15 38N 12 16W
Ouled Djellal, Algeria 111 B6 34 28N 5 2 E
Ouled Naïl, Mts. des, Algeria 111 B5 34 30N 3 30 E
Ouli, Cameroon 114 A2 5 12N 14 33 E
Oullins, France 29 C8 45 43N 4 49 E
Oulmès, Morocco 110 B3 33 17N 6 0W
Oulou, Bahr →, C.A.R. 114 A4 9 48N 21 32 E
Oulu, Finland 14 D21 65 1N 25 29 E
Oulujärvi, Finland 14 D22 64 25N 27 15 E
Oulujoki →, Finland 14 D21 65 1N 25 30 E
Oulx, Italy 44 C3 45 2N 6 50 E
Oum Chalouba, Chad 109 E4 15 48N 20 46 E
Oum-el-Bouaghi, Algeria 111 A6 35 55N 7 6 E
Oum-el-Ksi, Algeria 110 C3 29 4N 6 59W
Oum-er-Rbia, O. →, Morocco 110 B3 33 19N 8 21W
Oum Hadjer, Chad 109 F3 13 18N 19 41 E
Oum Hadjer, O. →, Chad 109 E4 16 38N 20 14 E
Oumé, Ivory C. 112 D3 6 21N 5 27W
Oumm ed Droûs Guebli, Sebkhet, Mauritania 110 D2 24 3N 11 45W
Oumm ed Droûs Telli, Sebkhet, Mauritania 110 D2 24 20N 11 30W
Ounane, Dj., Algeria 111 C6 25 4N 7 19 E
Ounasjoki →, Finland 14 C21 66 31N 25 40 E
Ounguati, Namibia 116 C2 22 0 S 15 46 E
Ounianga Kébir, Chad 109 E4 19 4N 20 29 E
Ounianga Sérir, Chad 109 E4 18 54N 20 51 E
Ounissoui, Niger 109 E2 17 34N 12 13 E
Our →, Lux. 24 E6 49 55N 6 5 E
Ouranópolis, Greece 50 F7 40 20N 23 59 E
Ourârene, Niger 113 B6 19 30N 7 10 E
Ourari, Tarso, Chad 109 D3 21 27N 17 27 E
Ouray, U.S.A. 159 G10 38 1N 107 40W
Ourcq →, France 27 C10 49 1N 3 1 E
Ourém, Brazil 170 B2 1 33 S 47 6W
Ourense, Spain 42 C3 42 19N 7 55W
Ouricuri, Brazil 170 C3 7 53 S 40 5W
Ourinhos, Brazil 175 A6 23 0 S 49 54W
Ourique, Portugal 43 H2 37 38N 8 16W
Ouro Fino, Brazil 175 A6 22 16 S 46 25W
Ouro-Ndia, Mali 112 B4 15 8N 4 35W
Ouro Prêto, Brazil 171 F3 20 20 S 43 30W
Ouro Prêto do Oeste, Brazil 173 C5 10 40 S 62 18W
Ouro Sogui, Senegal 112 B2 15 36N 13 19W
Oursi, Burkina Faso 113 C4 14 41N 0 27W
Ourthe →, Belgium 24 D5 50 29N 5 35 E
Ouse →, E. Susx., U.K. 21 G8 50 47N 0 4 E
Ouse →, N. Yorks., U.K. 20 D7 53 44N 0 55W
Oust, France 28 F5 42 52N 1 13 E
Oust →, France 26 E4 47 35N 2 6W
Outamba-Kilimi △, S. Leone 112 D2 9 50N 12 40W
Outaouais →, Canada 140 C5 45 27N 74 8W
Outardes →, Canada 141 C6 49 24N 69 30W
Outat Oulad el Haj, Morocco 111 B4 33 22N 3 42W
Outeiro de Rei, Spain 42 B3 43 6N 7 36W
Outer Hebrides, U.K. 22 D1 57 30N 7 40W
Outes = Serra de Outes, Spain 42 C2 42 52N 8 55W
Outjo, Namibia 116 C2 20 5 S 16 7 E
Outlook, Canada 143 C7 51 30N 107 0W
Outokumpu, Finland 14 E23 62 43N 29 1 E
Outreau, France 27 B8 50 40N 1 36 E
Ouvéa, Î., N. Cal. 133 K4 20 35 S 166 35 E
Ouvèze →, France 29 E8 43 59N 4 51 E
Ouyen, Australia 128 C5 35 1 S 142 22 E
Ouzinkie, U.S.A. 144 H9 57 56N 152 30W
Ouzouer-le-Marché, France 27 E8 47 54N 1 32 E
Ovada, Italy 44 D5 44 38N 8 38 E
Ovahe, Chile 172 b 27 5 S 109 19W
Ovalau, Fiji 133 A2 17 40 S 178 48 E
Ovalle, Chile 174 C1 30 33 S 71 18W
Ovamboland, Namibia 116 B2 18 30 S 16 0 E
Ovar, Portugal 42 E2 40 51N 8 40W
Ovau, Solomon Is. 133 L9 6 40 S 156 8 E
Overath, Germany 30 E3 50 56N 7 17 E
Overflakkee, Neths. 24 C4 51 44N 4 10 E
Overijssel □, Neths. 24 B6 52 25N 6 35 E
Overland, U.S.A. 156 F6 38 41N 90 22W
Overland Park, U.S.A. 154 F7 38 55N 94 50W
Overton, U.S.A. 161 J12 36 33N 114 27W
Övertorneå, Sweden 14 C20 66 23N 23 38 E
Överum, Sweden 17 F10 58 0N 16 20 E
Ovid, Mich., U.S.A. 157 A12 43 1N 84 22W
Ovid, N.Y., U.S.A. 151 D8 42 41N 76 49W
Ovidiopol, Ukraine 59 J6 46 15N 30 30 E
Ovidiu, Romania 53 F13 44 16N 28 34 E
Oviedo, Spain 42 B5 43 25N 5 50W
Oviedo, U.S.A. 153 G8 28 40N 81 13W
Oviksfjällen, Sweden 16 A7 63 0N 13 49 E
Oviši, Latvia 15 H19 57 33N 21 44 E
Ovoot, Mongolia 74 B7 45 21N 113 45 E
Övör Hangay □, Mongolia 74 B2 45 0N 102 30 E
Ovoro, Nigeria 113 D6 5 26N 7 16 E
Øvre Årdal, Norway 18 C4 61 19N 7 48 E
Övre Fryken, Sweden 16 E7 60 0N 13 7 E
Øvre Rendal, Norway 18 C8 61 54N 11 4 E
Øvre Rindal, Norway 18 A6 63 6N 9 10 E
Øvre Sirdal, Norway 18 F3 58 48N 6 43 E
Ovruch, Ukraine 59 G5 51 25N 28 45 E
Owaka, N.Z. 131 G4 46 27 S 169 40 E
Owambo = Ovamboland, Namibia 116 B2 18 30 S 16 0 E
Owando, Congo 114 C3 0 29 S 15 55 E
Owasco L., U.S.A. 151 D8 42 50N 76 31W
Owase, Japan 73 C8 34 7N 136 12 E
Owatonna, U.S.A. 154 C8 44 5N 93 14W
Owbeh, Afghan. 91 B1 34 28N 63 10 E
Owego, U.S.A. 151 D8 42 6N 76 16W
Owen, Australia 128 C3 34 15 S 138 32 E
Owen, Mt., N.Z. 131 B7 41 35 S 172 33 E
Owen Falls Dam, Uganda 118 B3 0 30N 33 5 E
Owen Sound, Canada 140 D3 44 35N 80 55W
Owen Stanley Ra., Papua N. G. 132 E4 8 30 S 147 0 E
Owendo, Gabon 114 B1 0 17N 9 30 E
Owens →, U.S.A. 160 J9 36 32N 117 59W
Owens L., U.S.A. 161 J9 36 26N 117 57W
Owensboro, U.S.A. 157 G9 37 46N 87 7W
Owensville, Ind., U.S.A. 157 F9 38 16N 87 41W
Owensville, Mo., U.S.A. 156 F5 38 21N 91 30W
Owenteik, Guyana 169 C6 4 27N 59 35W
Owenton, U.S.A. 157 F12 38 32N 84 50W
Owerri, Nigeria 113 D6 5 29N 7 0 E
Owhango, N.Z. 130 F4 39 0 S 175 23 E
Owingsville, U.S.A. 157 F13 38 9N 83 46W
Owl →, Canada 143 B10 57 51N 92 44W
Owo, Nigeria 113 D6 7 10N 5 39 E
Owosso, U.S.A. 157 B12 43 0N 84 10W
Owyhee, U.S.A. 158 F5 41 57N 116 6W
Owyhee →, U.S.A. 158 E5 43 49N 117 2W
Owyhee, L., U.S.A. 158 E5 43 38N 117 14W
Ox Mts. = Slieve Gamph, Ireland 23 B3 54 6N 9 0W
Oxapampa, Peru 172 C2 10 33 S 75 26W
Öxarfjörður, Iceland 11 A10 66 15N 16 45W
Oxbow, Canada 143 D8 49 14N 102 10W
Oxelösund, Sweden 17 F11 58 43N 17 5 E
Oxford, N.Z. 131 D7 43 18 S 172 11 E
Oxford, U.K. 21 F6 51 46N 1 15W
Oxford, Ala., U.S.A. 152 B4 33 36N 85 51W
Oxford, Iowa, U.S.A. 156 C5 41 43N 91 47W
Oxford, Mass., U.S.A. 151 D13 42 7N 71 52W
Oxford, Mich., U.S.A. 157 B13 42 49N 83 16W
Oxford, Miss., U.S.A. 155 H10 34 22N 89 31W
Oxford, N.C., U.S.A. 153 G6 36 19N 78 35W
Oxford, N.Y., U.S.A. 151 D9 42 27N 75 36W
Oxford, Ohio, U.S.A. 157 E12 39 31N 84 45W
Oxford L., Canada 143 C9 54 51N 95 37W
Oxfordshire □, U.K. 21 F6 51 48N 1 16W
Oxía Nisís, Greece 39 C3 38 18N 21 6 E
Oxie, Sweden 17 J7 55 33N 13 6 E
Oxílithos, Greece 48 C6 38 35N 24 7 E
Oxley, Australia 128 C6 34 11 S 144 6 E
Oxley Wild Rivers △, Australia 129 A10 30 57 S 152 12 E
Oxnard, U.S.A. 161 L7 34 12N 119 11W
Oxsjövålen, Sweden 16 B7 62 34N 13 57 E
Oxus = Amudarya →, Uzbekistan 66 E6 43 58N 59 34 E
Oy-Tal, Kyrgyzstan 65 C7 40 24N 74 6 E
Oya, Malaysia 85 B4 2 55N 111 55 E
Oyabe, Japan 73 A8 36 47N 136 56 E
Oyama, Japan 73 A11 36 18N 139 48 E
Oyambre △, Spain 42 B6 43 22N 4 21W
Oyapock →, Fr. Guiana 169 C7 4 8N 51 40W
Øye, Norway 18 F3 58 16N 6 49 E
Oyem, Gabon 114 B2 1 34N 11 31 E
Oyen, Canada 143 C6 51 22N 110 28W
Øyer, Norway 18 C7 61 16N 10 25 E
Øyeren, Norway 18 E8 59 50N 11 15 E
Oykel →, U.K. 22 D4 57 56N 4 26W
Oymyakon, Russia 67 C15 63 25N 142 44 E
Oyo, Nigeria 113 D5 7 46N 3 56 E
Oyo □, Nigeria 113 D5 8 15N 3 30 E
Oyón, Peru 172 C2 10 37 S 76 47W
Oyonnax, France 27 F12 46 16N 5 40 E
Oyrot = Gorno-Altay □, Russia 66 D9 51 0N 86 0 E
Oyrot-Tura = Gorno-Altaysk, Russia 66 D9 51 50N 86 5 E
Øyslebø, Norway 18 F4 58 9N 7 34 E
Oyster Bay, U.S.A. 151 F11 40 52N 73 32W
Oyster Harbour = Ladysmith, Canada 142 D4 49 0N 123 49W
Øystese, Norway 18 D3 60 22N 6 9 E
Oytal, Kazakhstan 65 B6 42 54N 73 17 E
Öyübari, Japan 70 C11 43 1N 142 5 E
Oyyq, Kazakhstan 65 B5 43 36N 71 16 E
Ozalp, Turkey 101 C10 38 39N 43 59 E
Ozamiz, Phil. 81 G4 8 15N 123 50 E
Ozark, Ala., U.S.A. 152 D4 31 28N 85 39W
Ozark, Ark., U.S.A. 155 H8 35 29N 93 50W
Ozark, Mo., U.S.A. 155 G8 37 1N 93 12W
Ozark Plateau, U.S.A. 155 G9 37 20N 91 40W
Ozarks, L. of the, U.S.A. 156 F4 38 12N 92 38W
Ożarów, Poland 55 H8 50 53N 21 40 E
Ózd, Hungary 52 B5 48 14N 20 15 E
Ozernoye, Russia 60 E10 51 46N 51 28 E
Ozërnyy, Russia 64 F8 51 8N 60 50 E
Ozero Svityaz, Ukraine 55 G10 51 30N 23 50 E
Ozersk, Russia 54 D8 54 25N 22 0 E
Ozette L., U.S.A. 160 B2 48 6N 124 38W
Özgön, Kyrgyzstan 65 C6 40 46N 73 18 E
Ozieri, Italy 46 B2 40 35N 9 0 E
Ozimek, Poland 55 H5 50 41N 18 11 E
Ozinki, Russia 60 E9 51 12N 49 44 E
Ozona, U.S.A. 155 K4 30 43N 101 12W
Ozorków, Poland 55 G6 51 57N 19 16 E
Ozren, Bos.-H. 52 G3 43 55N 18 29 E
Özu, Ehime, Japan 72 D4 33 30N 132 33 E
Ōzu, Kumamoto, Japan 72 E2 32 52N 130 52 E
Ozuluama, Mexico 163 C5 21 40N 97 50W
Ozun, Romania 53 E10 45 47N 25 50 E
Ozurgeti, Georgia 61 K5 41 55N 42 2 E

P

Pa, Burkina Faso 112 C4 11 33N 3 19W
Pa-an, Burma 90 G6 16 51N 97 40 E
Pa Mong Dam, Thailand 86 D4 18 0N 102 22 E
Pa Sak →, Thailand 78 B2 15 30N 101 0 E
Paagoumène, N. Cal. 133 T18 20 29 S 164 11 E
Paama, Vanuatu 133 F6 16 28 S 168 14 E
Paamiut, Greenland 10 E6 62 0N 49 43W
Paar →, Germany 31 G7 48 46N 11 36 E
Paarl, S. Africa 116 E2 33 45 S 18 56 E
Paauilo, U.S.A. 145 C6 20 2N 155 22W
Pab Hills, Pakistan 91 D2 26 30N 66 45 E
Pabbay, U.K. 22 D1 57 46N 7 14W
Pabianice, Poland 55 G6 51 40N 19 20 E
Pabna, Bangla. 90 C2 24 1N 89 18 E
Pabo, Uganda 118 B3 3 1N 32 10 E
Pacaás Novos △, Brazil 173 C5 11 0 S 63 0W
Pacaás Novos, Serra dos, Brazil 173 C5 10 45 S 64 15W
Pacaipampa, Peru 172 B2 5 35 S 79 39W
Pacaja →, Brazil 170 B1 1 56 S 50 50W
Pacajus, Brazil 170 B4 4 10 S 38 31W
Pacaraima, Sa., S. Amer. 169 C5 4 0N 62 30W
Pacarán, Peru 172 C2 12 50 S 76 3W
Pacaraos, Peru 172 C2 11 12 S 76 42W
Pacasmayo, Peru 172 B2 7 20 S 79 35W
Pace, U.S.A. 153 E2 30 36N 87 10W
Paceco, Italy 46 E5 37 59N 12 33 E
Pachacamac, Peru 172 C2 12 14 S 77 53W
Pachhar, India 92 G7 24 40N 77 42 E
Pachino, Italy 47 F8 36 43N 15 5 E
Pachitea →, Peru 172 B3 8 46 S 74 33W
Pachiza, Peru 172 B2 7 16 S 76 46W
Pachmarhi, India 93 H8 22 28N 78 26 E
Pachnai, India 90 B4 26 57N 92 19 E
Pacho, Colombia 168 B3 5 8N 74 10W
Pachora, India 94 D2 20 38N 75 29 E
Pachuca, Mexico 163 C5 20 10N 98 40W
Pacific, Canada 142 C3 54 48N 128 28W
Pacific, U.S.A. 156 F6 38 29N 90 45W
Pacific-Antarctic Ridge, Pac. Oc. 7 B13 43 0 S 115 0W
Pacific City = Huntington Beach, U.S.A. 161 M9 33 40N 118 5W
Pacific Grove, U.S.A. 160 J5 36 38N 121 56W
Pacific Ocean 135 G14 10 0N 140 0W
Pacific Palisades, U.S.A. 145 K14 21 25N 157 58W
Pacific Rim △, Canada 142 D4 48 40N 124 45W
Pacifica, U.S.A. 160 H4 37 36N 122 30W
Pacitan, Indonesia 85 D4 8 12 S 111 7 E
Packsaddle, Australia 128 A4 30 36 S 141 58 E
Packwood, U.S.A. 160 D5 46 36N 121 40W
Pacov, Czech Rep. 34 B8 49 27N 15 0 E
Pacoval, Brazil 169 D7 2 40 S 54 11W
Pacuí →, Brazil 171 E2 16 46 S 45 1W
Pacy-sur-Eure, France 26 C8 49 1N 1 23 E
Padaido, Kepulauan, Indonesia 83 B5 1 15 S 136 30 E
Padali = Amursk, Russia 67 D14 50 14N 136 54 E
Padampur, India 94 D6 20 59N 83 4 E
Padang, Indonesia 84 C2 1 0 S 100 20 E
Padang Endau, Malaysia 87 L4 2 40N 103 38 E
Padangpanjang, Indonesia 84 C2 0 40 S 100 20 E
Padangsidempuan, Indonesia 84 B1 1 30N 99 15 E
Padangtikar, Indonesia 85 C3 0 44 S 109 15 E
Padatchaung, Burma 90 F5 19 46N 94 48 E
Padauari →, Brazil 169 D5 0 15 S 64 5W
Padaung, Burma 90 F5 18 43N 95 9 E
Padborg, Denmark 17 K3 54 49N 9 21 E
Padcaya, Bolivia 173 E5 21 52 S 64 48W
Paddle Prairie, Canada 142 B5 57 57N 117 29W
Paddockwood, Canada 143 C7 53 30N 105 30W
Paderborn, Germany 30 D4 51 42N 8 45 E
Paderoo, India 94 E6 18 5N 82 40 E
Padeş, Vf., Romania 52 E7 45 40N 22 22 E
Padilla, Bolivia 173 D5 19 19 S 64 20W
Padina, Romania 53 F12 44 50N 27 8 E
Padma, India 93 G11 24 12N 85 22 E
Padma →, Bangla. 90 D3 23 22N 90 32 E
Pádova, Italy 45 C8 45 25N 11 53 E
Padra, India 92 H5 22 15N 73 7 E
Padrauna, India 93 F10 26 54N 83 59 E
Padre Burgos, Phil. 81 F5 10 1N 125 0 E
Padre I., U.S.A. 155 M6 27 10N 97 25W
Padre Island △, U.S.A. 155 M6 26 36N 97 17W
Padrón, Spain 42 C2 42 41N 8 39W
Padstow, U.K. 21 G3 50 33N 4 58W
Padthaway, Australia 128 D4 36 36 S 140 31 E
Padua = Pádova, Italy 45 C8 45 25N 11 53 E
Paducah, Ky., U.S.A. 148 G1 37 5N 88 37W
Paducah, Tex., U.S.A. 155 H4 34 1N 100 18W
Padukka, Sri Lanka 95 L5 6 50N 80 5 E
Padul, Spain 43 H7 37 1N 3 38W
Padwa, India 94 E6 18 27N 82 47 E
Paekakariki, N.Z. 130 G3 40 59 S 174 58 E
Paengaroa, N.Z. 130 D5 37 49 S 176 29 E
Paengnyŏng-do, S. Korea 75 F13 37 57N 124 40 E
Paeroa, N.Z. 130 D4 37 23 S 175 41 E
Paesana, Italy 44 D4 44 41N 7 16 E
Paete, Phil. 80 D3 14 23N 121 29 E
Pafúri, Mozam. 117 C5 22 28 S 31 17 E
Pag, Croatia 45 D12 44 25N 15 3 E
Paga, Gabon 114 C2 0 45 S 10 21 E
Paga, Ghana 113 C4 11 1N 1 8W
Pagadian, Phil. 81 H4 7 55N 123 30 E
Pagai Selatan, Pulau, Indonesia 84 C2 3 0 S 100 15 E
Pagai Utara, Pulau, Indonesia 84 C2 2 35 S 100 0 E
Pagalu = Annobón, Atl. Oc. 105 G4 1 25 S 5 36 E
Pagalungan, Phil. 81 H5 7 4N 124 41 E
Pagan, Burma 90 E5 21 10N 94 52 E
Pagara, India 93 G9 24 22N 80 1 E
Pagastikós Kólpos, Greece 48 B5 39 15N 23 0 E
Pagatan, Indonesia 85 C5 3 33 S 115 59 E
Page, U.S.A. 159 H8 36 57N 111 27W
Pagėgiai, Lithuania 54 C8 55 9N 21 54 E
Pagei, Papua N. G. 132 B1 3 2 S 141 10 E
Paget I., India 95 H11 13 26N 92 50 E
Pago Pago, Amer. Samoa 133 X24 14 16 S 170 43W
Pagosa Springs, U.S.A. 159 H10 37 16N 107 1W
Pagudpud, Phil. 80 B3 18 34N 120 47 E
Pagwa River, Canada 140 B2 50 2N 85 14W
Pagwi, Papua N. G. 132 C2 4 4 S 143 2 E
Pahala, U.S.A. 145 D6 19 12N 155 29W
Pahang □, Malaysia 84 B2 3 30N 102 45 E
Pahang →, Malaysia 87 L4 3 30N 103 9 E
Pahia Pt., N.Z. 131 G2 46 20 S 167 41 E
Pahiatua, N.Z. 130 G4 40 27 S 175 50 E
Pahoa, U.S.A. 145 D7 19 30N 154 57W
Pahokee, U.S.A. 153 J9 26 50N 80 40W
Pahrump, U.S.A. 161 J11 36 12N 115 59W
Pahute Mesa, U.S.A. 160 H10 37 20N 116 45W
Pai, Thailand 86 C2 19 19N 98 27 E
Paia, U.S.A. 145 C5 20 54N 156 22W
Paicines, U.S.A. 160 J5 36 44N 121 17W
Paide, Estonia 15 G21 58 53N 25 33 E
Paignton, U.K. 21 G4 50 26N 3 35W
Paihia, N.Z. 130 B3 35 17 S 174 6 E
Paiho, Taiwan 77 F13 23 21N 120 25 E
Paiján, Peru 172 B2 7 42 S 79 20W
Päijänne, Finland 15 F21 61 30N 25 30 E
Pailani, India 93 G9 25 45N 80 26 E
Pailin, Cambodia 86 F4 12 46N 102 36 E
Pailolo Channel, U.S.A. 145 C5 21 0N 156 40W
Paimpol, France 26 D3 48 48N 3 4W
Painan, Indonesia 84 C2 1 21 S 100 34 E
Paine, Cerro, Chile 176 D2 50 59 S 73 4W
Painesville, U.S.A. 150 E3 41 43N 81 15W
Paint Hills = Wemindji, Canada 140 B4 53 0N 78 49W
Paint L., Canada 143 B9 55 28N 97 57W
Painted Desert, U.S.A. 159 J8 36 0N 111 0W
Paintsville, U.S.A. 148 G4 37 49N 82 48W
País Vasco □, Spain 40 C2 42 50N 2 45W
Paishambe = Payshanba, Uzbekistan 65 C3 40 0N 66 14 E
Paisley, Canada 150 B3 44 18N 81 16W
Paisley, U.K. 22 F4 55 50N 4 25W
Paisley, U.S.A. 158 E3 42 42N 120 32W
Paita, N. Cal. 133 V20 22 8 S 166 22 E
Paita, Peru 172 B1 5 11 S 81 9W
Paithan, India 94 E2 19 29N 75 23 E
Paiva →, Portugal 42 D2 41 4N 8 16W
Paizhou, China 77 B9 30 12N 113 55 E
Paja, Cerro, Ecuador 172 a 1 17 S 90 26W
Pajares, Spain 42 B5 43 1N 5 46W
Pajares, Puerto de, Spain 42 C5 42 58N 5 46W
Pajarito, Colombia 168 B3 5 17N 72 43W
Pajęczno, Poland 55 G5 51 10N 19 0 E
Pak Lay, Laos 86 C3 18 15N 101 27 E
Pak Phanang, Thailand 87 H3 8 21N 100 12 E
Pak Sane, Laos 86 C4 18 22N 103 39 E
Pak Song, Laos 86 E6 15 11N 106 14 E
Pak Suong, Laos 76 H4 19 58N 102 15 E
Pak Tam Chung, China 69 G11 22 24N 114 19 E
Pakala, India 95 H4 13 29N 79 8 E
Pakaraima Mts., Guyana 169 B5 6 0N 60 0W
Pakaur, India 93 G12 24 38N 87 51 E
Pakenham, Australia 129 E6 38 6 S 145 30 E
Pakenham, Canada 151 A8 45 18N 76 18W
Pákhnes, Greece 39 E5 35 16N 24 4 E
Pakhoi = Beihai, China 76 G7 21 28N 109 6 E
Pakhtaabad, Uzbekistan 65 C6 40 55N 72 29 E
Pakhuis, S. Africa 116 E2 32 9 S 19 5 E
Pakistan ■, Asia 91 C3 30 0N 70 0 E
Pakkading, Laos 86 C4 18 19N 103 59 E
Paklay = Sayaboury, Laos 86 C3 19 15N 101 45 E
Paklenica △, Croatia 45 D12 44 20N 15 39 E
Pakokku, Burma 90 E5 21 20N 95 0 E
Pakość, Poland 55 F5 52 48N 18 6 E
Pakowki L., Canada 143 D6 49 20N 111 0W
Pakpattan, Pakistan 91 C4 30 25N 73 27 E
Pakrac, Croatia 52 E2 45 27N 17 12 E
Pakruojis, Lithuania 54 C10 55 58N 23 52 E
Paks, Hungary 52 D3 46 38N 18 55 E
Paktīā □, Afghan. 91 B3 33 30N 69 15 E
Paktīkā □, Afghan. 91 B3 32 30N 69 0 E
Pakwach, Uganda 118 B3 2 28N 31 27 E
Pakxe, Laos 86 E5 15 5N 105 52 E
Pal Lahara, India 93 J11 21 27N 85 11 E
Pala, Chad 109 G3 9 25N 15 5 E
Pala, Dem. Rep. of the Congo 118 D2 6 45 S 29 30 E
Pala, U.S.A. 161 M9 33 22N 117 5W
Palabek, Uganda 118 B3 3 22N 32 33 E
Palacios, U.S.A. 155 L6 28 42N 96 13W

Palafrugell, *Spain* 40 D8 41 55N 3 10 E
Palagiano, *Italy* 47 B10 40 35N 17 2 E
Palagonía, *Italy* 47 E7 37 19N 14 45 E
Palagruža, *Croatia* 45 F13 42 24N 16 15 E
Palaiókastron, *Greece* 39 E7 35 12N 26 15 E
Palaiokhóra, *Greece* 39 E4 35 16N 23 39 E
Pálairos, *Greece* 39 B2 38 47N 20 53 E
Palaiseau, *France* 27 D9 48 43N 2 15 E
Palakol, *India* 95 F5 16 31N 81 46 E
Palalankwe, *India* 95 J11 10 52N 92 29 E
Palam, *India* 94 E3 19 0N 77 0 E
Palamás, *Greece* 48 B4 39 26N 22 4 E
Palamòs, *Spain* 40 D8 41 50N 3 10 E
Palampur, *India* 92 C7 32 10N 76 30 E
Palamut, *Turkey* 49 C9 38 59N 27 41 E
Palana, *Australia* 127 F4 39 45 S 147 55 E
Palana, *Russia* 67 D16 59 10N 159 59 E
Palanan, *Phil.* 80 C4 17 8N 122 29 E
Palanan Bay, *Phil.* 80 C4 17 9N 122 27 E
Palanan Pt., *Phil.* 80 C4 17 17N 122 30 E
Palandri, *Pakistan* 93 C5 33 42N 73 40 E
Palanga, *Lithuania* 15 J19 55 58N 21 3 E
Palanganene, *Dem. Rep. of the Congo* 115 D3 6 32 S 18 52 E
Palangkaraya, *Indonesia* 85 C4 2 16 S 113 56 E
Palani, *India* 95 J3 10 30N 77 30 E
Palani Hills, *India* 95 J3 10 14N 77 33 E
Palanpur, *India* 92 G5 24 10N 72 25 E
Palanro, *Indonesia* 82 B1 3 21 S 119 23 E
Palaoa Pt., *U.S.A.* 145 C5 20 44N 156 58W
Palapag, *Phil.* 80 E5 12 33N 125 7 E
Palapye, *Botswana* 116 C4 22 30 S 27 7 E
Palar →, *India* 95 H5 12 27N 80 13 E
Palas, *Pakistan* 93 B5 35 4N 73 14 E
Palas de Rei, *Spain* 42 C3 42 52N 7 52W
Palashi, *India* 93 H13 23 47N 88 15 E
Palasponga, *India* 93 J11 21 47N 85 34 E
Palatine, *U.S.A.* 157 B8 42 7N 88 3W
Palatka, *Russia* 67 C16 60 6N 150 54 E
Palatka, *U.S.A.* 152 F8 29 39N 81 38W
Palau, *Italy* 46 A2 41 11N 9 23 E
Palau ■, *Pac. Oc.* 62 J17 7 30N 134 30 E
Palauk, *Burma* 86 F2 13 10N 98 40 E
Palawan, *Phil.* 81 G2 9 30N 118 30 E
Palawan □, *Phil.* 81 G2 10 0N 118 0 E
Palawan Passage, *Phil.* 81 G2 10 0N 118 0 E
Palayan, *Phil.* 80 D3 15 36N 121 8 E
Palayankottai, *India* 95 K3 8 45N 77 45 E
Palazzo, Pte., *France* 29 F12 42 28N 8 30 E
Palazzo San Gervásio, *Italy* 47 B8 40 56N 15 59 E
Palazzolo Acréide, *Italy* 47 E7 37 4N 14 54 E
Palca, *Chile* 172 D4 19 7 S 69 9W
Paldiski, *Estonia* 15 G21 59 23N 24 9 E
Pale, *Bos.-H.* 52 G3 43 50N 18 38 E
Palel, *India* 90 C5 24 27N 94 2 E
Paleleh, *Indonesia* 82 A2 1 10N 121 50 E
Palembang, *Indonesia* 84 C2 3 0 S 104 50 E
Palena →, *Chile* 176 B2 43 50 S 73 50W
Palena, L., *Chile* 176 B2 43 55 S 71 40W
Palencia, *Spain* 42 C6 42 1N 4 34W
Palencia □, *Spain* 42 C6 42 31N 4 33W
Palenque, *Mexico* 163 D6 17 31N 91 58W
Paleokastrítsa, *Greece* 38 B9 39 40N 19 41 E
Paleometokho, *Cyprus* 39 E9 35 7N 33 11 E
Palermo, *Colombia* 168 C2 2 54N 75 26W
Palermo, *Italy* 46 D6 38 7N 13 22 E
Palermo, *U.S.A.* 158 G3 39 26N 121 33W
Palermo ✕ (PMO), *Italy* 46 D6 38 11N 13 5 E
Palestina = Jordânia, *Brazil* 171 E3 15 55 S 40 11W
Palestine, *Asia* 103 D4 32 0N 35 0 E
Palestine, *Ill., U.S.A.* 157 F9 39 0N 87 37W
Palestine, *Tex., U.S.A.* 155 K7 31 46N 95 38W
Palestrina, *Italy* 45 G9 41 50N 12 53 E
Paletwa, *Burma* 90 E4 21 10N 92 50 E
Palghat, *India* 95 J3 10 46N 76 42 E
Palgrave, Mt., *Australia* 124 D2 23 22 S 115 58 E
Pali, *India* 92 G5 25 50N 73 20 E
Pali-Aike △, *Chile* 176 D3 52 6 S 69 44W
Palikea Pk., *U.S.A.* 145 K13 21 26N 158 6W
Palikir, *Micronesia* 134 G7 6 55N 158 9 E
Palimbang, *Phil.* 81 H5 6 12N 124 12 E
Palin, Mt., *Malaysia* 85 A5 6 10N 117 10 E
Palinuro, *Italy* 47 B8 40 2N 15 17 E
Palinuro, C., *Italy* 47 B8 40 2N 15 16 E
Palioúri, Ákra = Paliourion, Ákra, *Greece* 50 G7 39 57N 23 45 E
Paliourion, Ákra, *Greece* 50 G7 39 57N 23 45 E
Palisades Reservoir, *U.S.A.* 158 E8 43 20N 111 12W
Paliseul, *Belgium* 24 E5 49 54N 5 8 E
Palitana, *India* 92 J4 21 32N 71 49 E
Palizada, *Mexico* 163 D6 18 18N 92 8W
Palk Bay, *Asia* 95 K4 9 30N 79 15 E
Palk Strait, *Asia* 95 K4 10 0N 79 45 E
Palkānah, *Iraq* 96 C5 35 49N 44 26 E
Palkonda, *India* 94 E6 18 36N 83 48 E
Palkonda Ra., *India* 95 H4 13 50N 79 20 E
Palkot, *India* 93 H11 22 53N 84 39 E
Palla Road = Dinokwe, *Botswana* 116 C4 23 29 S 26 37 E
Pallanza = Verbánia, *Italy* 44 C5 45 56N 8 33 E
Pallarenda, *Australia* 126 B4 19 12 S 146 46 E
Pallasovka, *Russia* 60 E8 50 4N 47 0 E
Palleru →, *India* 94 F5 16 45N 80 2 E
Pallës, Bishti i, *Albania* 50 E3 41 24N 19 24 E
Pallinup →, *Australia* 125 F2 34 27 S 118 50 E
Pallisa, *Uganda* 118 B3 1 12N 33 43 E
Palliser, C., *N.Z.* 130 H4 41 37 S 175 14 E
Palliser B., *N.Z.* 130 H4 41 26 S 175 5 E
Pallu, *India* 92 E6 28 59N 74 14 E
Palm Bay, *U.S.A.* 153 G9 28 2N 80 35W
Palm Beach, *U.S.A.* 153 J9 26 43N 80 2W
Palm Coast, *U.S.A.* 153 F8 29 32N 81 10W
Palm Desert, *U.S.A.* 161 M10 33 43N 116 22W
Palm Harbor, *U.S.A.* 153 G7 28 5N 82 47W
Palm Is., *Australia* 126 B4 18 40 S 146 35 E
Palm Springs, *U.S.A.* 161 M10 33 50N 116 33W
Palma = Paraná, *Brazil* 171 D2 12 30 S 47 48W
Palma, *Mozam.* 119 E5 10 46 S 40 29 E
Palma →, *Brazil* 171 D2 12 33 S 47 52W
Palma, B. de, *Spain* 38 B3 39 30N 2 39 E
Palma de Mallorca, *Spain* 38 B3 39 35N 2 39 E
Palma de Mallorca ✕ (PMI), *Spain* 41 F7 39 34N 2 43 E
Palma del Río, *Spain* 43 H5 37 43N 5 17W
Palma di Montechiaro, *Italy* 46 E6 37 11N 13 46 E
Palma Nova, *Spain* 38 B3 39 32N 2 34 E
Palma Soriano, *Cuba* 164 B4 20 15N 76 0W
Palmaner, *India* 95 H4 13 12N 78 45 E
Palmares, *Brazil* 170 C4 8 41 S 35 28W
Palmarito, *Venezuela* 168 B3 7 37N 70 10W
Palmarola, *Italy* 46 B5 40 56N 12 51 E
Palmas, *Brazil* 175 B5 26 29 S 52 0W
Palmas, C., *Liberia* 112 E3 4 27N 7 46W
Pálmas, G. di, *Italy* 46 D1 39 0N 8 30 E
Palmas de Monte Alto, *Brazil* 171 D3 14 16 S 43 10W
Palmdale, *Calif., U.S.A.* 161 L8 34 35N 118 7W
Palmdale, *Fla., U.S.A.* 153 J8 26 57N 81 19W
Palmeira, *Brazil* 171 G2 25 25 S 50 0W
Palmeira das Missões, *Brazil* 175 B5 27 55 S 53 17W
Palmeira dos Índios, *Brazil* 170 C4 9 25 S 36 37W
Palmeirais, *Brazil* 170 C3 6 0 S 43 0W
Palmeiras, *Brazil* 171 D3 12 31 S 41 34W
Palmeiras →, *Brazil* 171 D2 12 22 S 47 8W
Palmeirinhas, Pta. das, *Angola* 115 D2 9 2 S 12 57 E
Palmela, *Portugal* 43 G2 38 32N 8 57W
Palmelo, *Brazil* 171 E2 17 20 S 48 27W
Palmer, *Antarctica* 7 C17 64 35 S 60 0W
Palmer, *U.S.A.* 144 F10 61 36N 149 7W
Palmer →, *Australia* 126 B3 16 0 S 142 26 E
Palmer Arch., *Antarctica* 7 C17 64 15 S 65 0W
Palmer Lake, *U.S.A.* 154 F2 39 7N 104 55W
Palmer Land, *Antarctica* 7 D18 73 0 S 63 0W
Palmerston = Darwin, *Australia* 124 B5 12 25 S 130 51 E
Palmerston, *Australia* 124 B5 12 31 S 130 59 E
Palmerston, *Canada* 150 C4 43 50N 80 51W
Palmerston, *N.Z.* 131 F5 45 29 S 170 43 E
Palmerston North, *N.Z.* 130 G4 40 21 S 175 39 E
Palmerton, *U.S.A.* 151 F9 40 48N 75 37W
Palmetto, *Fla., U.S.A.* 153 H7 27 31N 82 34W
Palmetto, *Ga., U.S.A.* 152 B5 33 31N 84 40W
Palmi, *Italy* 47 D8 38 21N 15 51 E
Palmira, *Argentina* 174 C2 32 59 S 68 34W
Palmira, *Colombia* 168 C2 3 32N 76 16W
Palmyra = Tudmur, *Syria* 101 E8 34 36N 38 15 E
Palmyra, *Ill., U.S.A.* 156 E7 39 26N 90 0W
Palmyra, *Mo., U.S.A.* 156 E5 39 48N 91 32W
Palmyra, *N.J., U.S.A.* 151 F9 40 1N 75 1W
Palmyra, *N.Y., U.S.A.* 150 C7 43 5N 77 18W
Palmyra, *Pa., U.S.A.* 151 F8 40 18N 76 36W
Palmyra, *Wis., U.S.A.* 157 B8 42 52N 88 36W
Palmyra Is., *Pac. Oc.* 135 G11 5 52N 162 5W
Palmyras = Santos Dumont, *Brazil* 171 F3 22 55 S 43 10W
Palmyras Pt., *India* 94 D8 20 46N 87 1 E
Palo, *Phil.* 81 F5 11 10N 124 59 E
Palo Alto, *U.S.A.* 160 H4 37 27N 122 10W
Palo Seco, *Trin. & Tob.* 169 F9 10 4N 61 36W
Palo Verde, *U.S.A.* 161 M12 33 26N 114 44W
Palo Verde △, *Costa Rica* 164 D2 10 21N 85 21W
Paloich, *Sudan* 107 E3 10 28N 32 32 E
Palomar Mt., *U.S.A.* 161 M10 33 22N 116 50W
Palompon, *Phil.* 81 F5 11 3N 124 23 E
Palopo, *Indonesia* 82 B2 3 0 S 120 16 E
Palos, C. de, *Spain* 41 H4 37 38N 0 40W
Palos de la Frontera, *Spain* 43 H4 37 14N 6 53W
Palos Verdes, *U.S.A.* 161 M8 33 48N 118 23W
Palos Verdes, Pt., *U.S.A.* 161 M8 33 43N 118 26W
Palpa, *Peru* 172 C2 14 30 S 75 15W
Pålsboda, *Sweden* 16 E9 59 3N 15 22 E
Palu, *Indonesia* 82 B1 1 0 S 119 52 E
Palu, *Turkey* 101 C9 38 45N 40 0 E
Paluan, *Phil.* 80 E3 13 26N 120 29 E
Paluke, *Liberia* 112 D3 5 2N 8 5W
Paluzza, *Italy* 45 B10 46 32N 13 1 E
Palwal, *India* 92 E7 28 8N 77 19 E
Pama, *Burkina Faso* 113 C5 11 19N 0 44 E
Pama ⌂, *Burkina Faso* 113 C5 11 27N 0 40 E
Pama →, *C.A.R.* 114 B3 4 23N 18 43 E
Pamanukan, *Indonesia* 85 D3 6 16 S 107 49 E
Pamban I., *India* 95 K4 9 15N 79 20 E
Pamekasan, *Indonesia* 85 D4 7 10 S 113 28 E
Pamenang, *Indonesia* 79 J19 8 24 S 116 6 E
Pamiers, *France* 28 E5 43 7N 1 39 E
Pamir, *Tajikistan* 65 E6 37 40N 73 0 E
Pamir →, *Tajikistan* 65 E6 37 1N 72 41 E
Pamirsky Post = Murghob, *Tajikistan* 65 D7 38 10N 74 2 E
Pamlico →, *U.S.A.* 149 H7 35 20N 76 28W
Pamlico Sd., *U.S.A.* 149 H8 35 20N 76 0W
Pampa, *U.S.A.* 155 H4 35 32N 100 58W
Pampa de Agma, *Argentina* 176 B3 43 45 S 69 40W
Pampa de las Salinas, *Argentina* 174 C2 32 1 S 66 58W
Pampa Grande, *Bolivia* 173 D5 18 5 S 64 6W
Pampa Hermosa, *Peru* 172 B2 7 7 S 75 4W
Pampanga □, *Phil.* 80 D3 15 4N 120 40 E
Pampanua, *Indonesia* 82 B2 4 16 S 120 8 E
Pampas, *Argentina* 174 D3 35 0 S 63 0W
Pampas, *Peru* 172 C3 12 20 S 74 50W
Pampas →, *Peru* 172 C3 13 24 S 73 12W
Pamphylia, *Turkey* 100 D4 37 0N 31 20 E
Pamplona, *Colombia* 168 B3 7 23N 72 39W
Pamplona, *Phil.* 80 B3 18 31N 121 20 E
Pamplona, *Spain* 40 C3 42 48N 1 38W
Pampoenpoort, *S. Africa* 116 E3 31 3 S 22 40 E
Pamukçu, *Turkey* 49 B9 39 30N 27 54 E
Pamukkale, *Turkey* 49 D11 37 55N 29 8 E
Pan de Azúcar △, *Chile* 174 B1 26 0 S 70 40W
Pan Xian, *China* 76 E5 25 46N 104 38 E
Pana, *U.S.A.* 156 E7 39 23N 89 5W
Panabo, *Phil.* 81 H5 7 19N 125 42 E
Panaca, *U.S.A.* 159 H6 37 47N 114 23W
Panacea, *U.S.A.* 152 E5 30 2N 84 23W
Panagyurishte, *Bulgaria* 51 D8 42 30N 24 15 E
Panaitan, *Indonesia* 84 D3 6 36 S 105 12 E
Panaji, *India* 95 G1 15 25N 73 50 E
Panamá, *Panama* 164 E4 9 0N 79 25W
Panama, *Sri Lanka* 95 L5 6 45N 81 48 E
Panama ■, *Cent. Amer.* 164 E4 8 48N 79 55W
Panamá, G. de, *Panama* 164 E4 8 4N 79 20W
Panama Canal, *Panama* 164 E4 9 10N 79 37W
Panama City, *U.S.A.* 152 E4 30 10N 85 40W
Panama City Beach, *U.S.A.* 152 E4 30 11N 85 48W
Panamint Range, *U.S.A.* 161 J9 36 20N 117 20W
Panamint Springs, *U.S.A.* 161 J9 36 20N 117 28W
Panão, *Peru* 172 B2 9 55 S 75 55W
Panaon I., *Phil.* 81 F5 10 3N 125 13 E
Panare, *Thailand* 87 J3 6 51N 101 30 E
Panarea, *Italy* 47 D8 38 38N 15 4 E
Panaro →, *Italy* 45 D8 44 55N 11 25 E
Panarukan, *Indonesia* 85 D4 7 42 S 113 56 E
Panay, *Phil.* 81 F4 11 10N 122 30 E
Panay, G., *Phil.* 79 B6 11 0N 122 30 E
Pančevo, *Serbia & M.* 52 F5 44 52N 20 41 E
Panch'iao, *Taiwan* 77 E13 25 1N 121 27 E
Panciu, *Romania* 53 E12 45 54N 27 8 E
Pancol, *Phil.* 81 F2 10 52N 119 25 E
Pancorbo, Desfiladero, *Spain* 42 C7 42 32N 3 5W
Pâncota, *Romania* 52 D6 46 20N 21 45 E
Panda, *Mozam.* 117 C5 24 2 S 34 45 E
Pandan, *Malaysia* 87 d 1 32N 103 46 E
Pandan, *Antique, Phil.* 81 F4 11 45N 122 10 E
Pandan, *Catanduanes, Phil.* 80 D5 14 3N 124 10 E
Pandan, Selat, *Singapore* 87 d 1 15N 103 44 E
Pandan Bay, *Phil.* 81 F4 11 43N 122 0 E
Pandan Tampoi = Tampoi, *Malaysia* 87 d 1 30N 103 39 E
Pandegelang, *Indonesia* 84 D3 6 25 S 106 5 E
Pandhana, *India* 92 J7 21 42N 76 13 E
Pandharkawada, *India* 94 D4 20 1N 78 32 E
Pandharpur, *India* 94 F2 17 41N 75 20 E
Pandhurna, *India* 94 D4 21 36N 78 35 E
Pando, *Uruguay* 175 C4 34 44 S 56 0W
Pando □, *Bolivia* 172 C4 11 20 S 67 40W
Pando, L. = Hope, L., *Australia* 127 D2 28 24 S 139 18 E
Pandokrátor, *Greece* 38 B9 39 45N 19 50 E
Pandora, *Costa Rica* 164 E3 9 43N 83 3W
Pandrup, *Denmark* 17 G3 57 14N 9 40 E
Pandu, *Dem. Rep. of the Congo* 114 B3 4 59N 19 16 E
Panevéggio-Pale di San Martino ⌂, *Italy* 45 B8 46 14N 11 46 E
Panevėžys, *Lithuania* 15 J21 55 42N 24 25 E
Panfilov, *Kazakhstan* 66 E8 44 10N 80 0 E
Panfilov Atyndaghy, *Kazakhstan* 65 B8 43 23N 77 7 E
Panfilovo, *Russia* 60 E6 50 25N 42 46 E
Pang Sida △, *Thailand* 86 E4 14 5N 102 17 E
Panga, *Dem. Rep. of the Congo* 118 B2 1 52N 26 18 E
Pangaíon Óros, *Greece* 51 F8 40 50N 24 0 E
Pangala, *Congo* 114 C2 3 16 S 14 34 E
Pangalanes, Canal des = Ampangalana, Lakandranon', *Madag.* 117 C8 22 48 S 47 50 E
Pangani, *Tanzania* 118 D4 5 25 S 38 58 E
Pangani →, *Tanzania* 118 D4 5 26 S 38 58 E
Pangantocan, *Phil.* 81 H5 7 50N 124 49 E
Pangar Djérem ⌂, *Cameroon* 114 A2 5 50N 13 10 E
Pangasinan □, *Phil.* 80 D3 15 55N 120 20 E
Pangfou = Bengbu, *China* 75 H9 32 58N 117 20 E
Pangil, *Dem. Rep. of the Congo* 118 C2 3 10 S 26 35 E
Pangkah, Tanjung, *Indonesia* 85 D4 6 51 S 112 33 E
Pangkai, *Burma* 90 D7 22 40N 98 40 E
Pangkajene, *Indonesia* 82 B1 4 46 S 119 34 E
Pangkalanbrandan, *Indonesia* 84 B1 4 1N 98 20 E
Pangkalanbuun, *Indonesia* 85 C4 2 41 S 111 37 E
Pangkalansusu, *Indonesia* 84 B1 4 2N 98 13 E
Pangkalpinang, *Indonesia* 84 C3 2 0 S 106 0 E
Pangkoh, *Indonesia* 85 C4 3 5 S 114 8 E
Panglao, *Phil.* 81 G4 9 35N 123 45 E
Panglao I., *Phil.* 81 G4 9 35N 123 48 E
Pangnirtung, *Canada* 139 B13 66 8N 65 43W
Pango Aluquem, *Angola* 115 D2 8 43 S 14 33 E
Pangong Tso, *India* 92 B8 34 40N 78 40 E
Pangrango, *Indonesia* 84 D3 6 46 S 107 1 E
Pangsau Pass, *Burma* 90 B6 27 15N 96 10 E
Pangtara, *Burma* 90 E6 20 57N 96 40 E
Panguipulli, *Chile* 176 A2 39 38 S 72 20W
Panguitch, *U.S.A.* 159 H7 37 50N 112 26W
Panguna, *Papua N. G.* 132 D8 6 21 S 155 25 E
Pangutaran, *Phil.* 81 H3 6 18N 120 35 E
Pangutaran Group, *Phil.* 81 H3 6 18N 120 34 E
Panhala, *India* 94 F2 16 49N 74 7 E
Panhandle, *U.S.A.* 155 H4 35 21N 101 23W
Pani Mines, *India* 92 H5 22 29N 73 50 E
Pania-Mutombo, *Dem. Rep. of the Congo* 118 D1 5 11 S 23 51 E
Paniau, *U.S.A.* 145 B1 21 56N 160 5W
Panié, Mt., *N. Cal.* 133 T18 20 36 S 164 46 E
Panikota I., *India* 92 J4 20 46N 71 21 E
Panipat, *India* 92 E7 29 25N 77 2 E
Panitan, *Phil.* 81 F4 11 28N 122 46 E
Panj = Pyandzh, *Tajikistan* 65 E4 37 14N 69 6 E
Panj = Pyandzh →, *Asia* 65 E4 37 6N 68 20 E
Panjab, *Afghan.* 91 B2 34 23N 67 1 E
Panjakent = Pendzhikent, *Tajikistan* 65 D3 39 29N 67 37 E
Panjal Range = Pir Panjal Range, *India* 92 C7 32 30N 76 50 E
Panjang, Hon, *Vietnam* 87 H4 9 20N 103 28 E
Panjgur, *Pakistan* 91 D2 27 0N 64 5 E
Panjhra →, *India* 94 D2 21 13N 74 57 E
Panji Poyon, *Tajikistan* 65 E4 37 12N 68 35 E
Panjim = Panaji, *India* 95 G1 15 25N 73 50 E
Panjin, *China* 75 D12 41 3N 122 2 E
Panjnad →, *Pakistan* 92 E4 28 57N 70 30 E
Panjwai, *Afghan.* 91 C2 31 26N 65 27 E
Pankshin, *Nigeria* 113 D6 9 16N 9 25 E
Panmunjŏm, *N. Korea* 75 F14 37 59N 126 38 E
Panna, *India* 93 G9 24 40N 80 15 E
Panna △, *India* 93 G8 24 40N 80 0 E
Panna Hills, *India* 93 G9 24 40N 81 15 E
Pannawonica, *Australia* 124 D2 21 39 S 116 19 E
Pannga, Tanjung, *Indonesia* 79 K19 8 54 S 116 2 E
Pannngi, *Vanuatu* 133 E6 15 58 S 168 12 E
Pannirtuuq = Pangnirtung, *Canada* 139 B13 66 8N 65 43W
Pano Akil, *Pakistan* 92 F3 27 51N 69 7 E
Pano Lefkara, *Cyprus* 39 F9 34 53N 33 20 E
Pano Panayia, *Cyprus* 39 F8 34 55N 32 38 E
Panora, *U.S.A.* 156 C2 41 42N 94 22W
Panorama, *Brazil* 175 A5 21 21 S 51 51W
Pánormon, *Greece* 39 E5 35 25N 24 41 E
Panruti, *India* 95 J4 11 46N 79 35 E
Pansemal, *India* 92 J6 21 39N 74 42 E
Panshan = Panjin, *China* 75 D12 41 3N 122 2 E
Panshi, *China* 75 C14 42 58N 126 5 E
Pantanal Matogrossense △, *Brazil* 173 D6 17 35 S 57 27W
Pantanaw, *Burma* 90 G5 16 59N 95 28 E
Pantanos de Centla ⌂, *Mexico* 163 D6 18 25N 92 25W
Pantar, *Indonesia* 82 C2 8 28 S 124 10 E
Pante Macassar, *E. Timor* 82 C2 9 30 S 123 58 E
Pante Makasar = Pante Macassar, *E. Timor* 82 C2 9 30 S 123 58 E
Pantelleria, *Italy* 46 F4 36 50N 11 57 E
Pantin Sakan, *Burma* 90 F6 18 38N 97 33 E
Pantoja, *Peru* 168 D2 0 58 S 75 10W
Pantón, *Spain* 42 C3 42 31N 7 37W
Pantukan, *Phil.* 81 H5 7 9N 125 54 E
Panu, *Dem. Rep. of the Congo* 114 C3 3 50 S 19 10 E
Pánuco, *Mexico* 163 C5 22 0N 98 15W
Panukulan, *Phil.* 80 D3 14 56N 121 49 E
Panvel, *India* 94 E1 18 59N 73 4 E
Panyam, *Nigeria* 113 D6 9 27N 9 8 E
Panyu = Guangzhou, *China* 77 F9 23 5N 113 10 E
Panyu, *China* 77 F9 22 51N 113 20 E
Panzhihua, *China* 76 D3 26 33N 101 44 E
Panzi, *Dem. Rep. of the Congo* 115 D3 7 17 S 18 1 E
Pao →, *Anzoátegui, Venezuela* 169 B5 8 6N 64 17W
Pao →, *Apure, Venezuela* 168 B4 8 33N 68 1W
Paochi = Baoji, *China* 74 G4 34 20N 107 5 E
Paoki = Baoji, *China* 74 G4 34 20N 107 5 E
Páola, *Italy* 47 C9 39 21N 16 2 E
Paola, *Malta* 38 F8 35 52N 14 30 E
Paola, *U.S.A.* 154 F7 38 35N 94 53W
Paoli, *U.S.A.* 157 F10 38 33N 86 28W
Paonia, *U.S.A.* 159 G10 38 52N 107 36W
Paoting = Baoding, *China* 74 E8 38 50N 115 28 E
Paot'ou = Baotou, *China* 74 D6 40 32N 110 2 E
Paoua, *C.A.R.* 114 A3 7 9N 16 20 E
Pap, *Uzbekistan* 65 C5 40 52N 71 6 E
Pápa, *Hungary* 52 C2 47 22N 17 30 E
Papa, *U.S.A.* 145 D6 19 13N 155 52W
Papa Stour, *U.K.* 22 A7 60 20N 1 42W
Papa Westray, *U.K.* 22 B6 59 20N 2 55W
Papaaloa, *U.S.A.* 145 D6 19 59N 155 13W
Papagayo →, *Mexico* 163 D5 16 36N 99 43W
Papagayo, G. de, *Costa Rica* 164 D2 10 30N 85 50W
Papagni →, *India* 95 G3 15 35N 77 45 E
Papaichton, *Fr. Guiana* 169 C7 3 48N 54 10W
Papaikou, *U.S.A.* 145 D6 19 47N 155 6W
Papakura, *N.Z.* 130 D3 37 4 S 174 59 E
Papantla, *Mexico* 163 C5 20 30N 97 30W
Papar, *Malaysia* 78 C5 5 45N 116 0 E
Papara, *Tahiti* 133 S16 17 43 S 149 22W
Paparoa, *N.Z.* 130 C3 36 6 S 174 16 E
Paparoa △, *N.Z.* 131 C6 42 7 S 171 26 E
Paparoa Ra., *N.Z.* 131 C6 42 5 S 171 35 E
Pápas, Ákra, *Greece* 48 C3 38 13N 21 20 E
Papatoetoe, *N.Z.* 130 C3 36 59 S 174 51 E
Papatura, *Solomon Is.* 133 L10 7 32 S 158 47 E
Papawai Pt., *U.S.A.* 145 C5 20 47N 156 32W
Papeete, *Tahiti* 133 S16 17 32 S 149 34W
Papenburg, *Germany* 30 B3 53 5N 7 23 E
Papetoai, *Tahiti* 133 S16 17 29 S 149 52W
Paphlagonia, *Turkey* 100 B5 41 30N 33 0 E
Paphos, *Cyprus* 39 F8 34 46N 32 25 E
Paphos ✕ (PFO), *Cyprus* 39 F8 34 43N 32 30 E
Papien Chiang = Da →, *Vietnam* 76 G5 21 15N 105 20 E
Papigochic →, *Mexico* 162 B3 29 9N 109 40W
Paposo, *Chile* 174 B1 25 0 S 70 30W
Papoutsa, *Cyprus* 39 F9 34 54N 33 4 E
Papua □, *Indonesia* 83 B5 4 0 S 137 0 E
Papua, G. of, *Papua N. G.* 132 E3 9 0 S 144 50 E
Papua New Guinea ■, *Oceania* 132 D3 8 0 S 145 0 E
Papudo, *Chile* 174 C1 32 29 S 71 27W
Papuk, *Croatia* 52 E2 45 30N 17 30 E
Papun, *Burma* 90 F6 18 2N 97 30 E
Papunya, *Australia* 124 D5 23 15 S 131 54 E
Pará = Belém, *Brazil* 170 B2 1 20 S 48 30W
Pará □, *Brazil* 173 A7 3 20 S 52 0W
Paraburdoo, *Australia* 124 D2 23 14 S 117 32 E
Paracale, *Phil.* 80 D4 14 17N 122 48 E
Paracas, Pen., *Peru* 172 C2 13 53 S 76 20W
Paracatu, *Brazil* 171 E2 17 10 S 46 50W
Paracatu →, *Brazil* 171 E2 16 30 S 45 4W
Paracel Is., *S. China Sea* 78 A4 15 50N 112 0 E
Parachilna, *Australia* 128 A3 31 10 S 138 21 E
Parachinar, *Pakistan* 91 B3 33 55N 70 5 E
Paraćin, *Serbia & M.* 50 C5 43 54N 21 27 E
Paracuru, *Brazil* 170 B4 3 24 S 39 4W
Paradas, Punta, *Peru* 172 D2 15 22 S 75 11W
Paradas, *Spain* 43 H5 37 18N 5 29W
Paradela, *Spain* 42 C3 42 44N 7 37W
Paradhísi, *Greece* 38 E12 36 18N 28 7 E
Paradip, *India* 94 D8 20 15N 86 35 E
Paradise, *Calif., U.S.A.* 160 F5 39 46N 121 37W
Paradise, *Nev., U.S.A.* 161 J11 36 9N 115 10W
Paradise →, *Canada* 141 B8 53 27N 57 19W
Paradise Hill, *Canada* 143 C7 53 32N 109 28W
Paradise I., *Bahamas* 9 b 25 6N 77 19W
Paradise River, *Canada* 141 B8 53 27N 57 17W
Paradise Valley, *U.S.A.* 158 F5 41 30N 117 32W
Parado, *Indonesia* 85 D5 8 42 S 118 30 E
Paragould, *U.S.A.* 155 G9 36 3N 90 29W
Paragua = Palawan, *Phil.* 81 G2 9 30N 118 30 E
Paraguá →, *Bolivia* 173 C5 13 34 S 61 53W
Paragua →, *Venezuela* 169 B5 6 55N 62 55W
Paraguaçu = Paraguaçu Paulista, *Brazil* 175 A5 22 22 S 50 35W
Paraguaçu →, *Brazil* 171 D4 12 45 S 38 54W
Paraguaçu Paulista, *Brazil* 175 A5 22 22 S 50 35W
Paraguaipoa, *Venezuela* 168 A3 11 21N 71 57W
Paraguaná, Pen. de, *Venezuela* 168 A3 12 0N 70 0W
Paraguarí, *Paraguay* 174 B4 25 36 S 57 0W
Paraguarí □, *Paraguay* 174 B4 26 0 S 57 10W
Paraguay ■, *S. Amer.* 174 A4 23 0 S 57 0W
Paraguay →, *Paraguay* 174 B4 27 18 S 58 38W
Paraíba = João Pessoa, *Brazil* 170 C5 7 10 S 34 52W
Paraíba □, *Brazil* 170 C4 7 0 S 36 0W
Paraíba do Sul →, *Brazil* 171 F3 21 37 S 41 3W
Parainen, *Finland* 15 F20 60 18N 22 18 E
Paraiso, *Brazil* 173 19 3 S 52 59W
Paraíso, *Mexico* 163 D6 18 24N 93 14W
Parak, *Iran* 97 E7 27 38N 52 25 E
Parakhino Paddubye, *Russia* 58 C7 58 26N 33 10 E
Parakou, *Benin* 113 D5 9 25N 2 40 E
Parakylia, *Australia* 128 A2 30 24 S 136 25 E
Paralimni, *Cyprus* 39 E9 35 2N 33 58 E
Parálion-Astrous, *Greece* 48 D4 37 25N 22 45 E
Paralkote, *India* 94 E5 19 47N 80 41 E
Parama I., *Papua N. G.* 132 E2 9 0 S 143 25 E
Paramaribo, *Suriname* 169 B6 5 50N 55 10W
Parambu, *Brazil* 170 C3 6 13 S 40 43W
Paramillo △, *Colombia* 168 B2 7 37N 76 13W
Paramillo, Nudo del, *Colombia* 168 B2 7 4N 75 55W
Paramirim, *Brazil* 171 D3 13 26 S 42 15W
Paramirim →, *Brazil* 171 D3 11 34 S 43 18W
Paramithiá, *Greece* 48 B2 39 30N 20 35 E
Páramos del Batallón y La Negra △, *Venezuela* 165 E5 8 2N 71 55W
Paramushir, Ostrov, *Russia* 67 D16 50 24N 156 0 E
Paran →, *Israel* 103 E4 30 20N 35 10 E
Paraná, *Argentina* 174 C3 31 45 S 60 30W
Paranã, *Brazil* 171 D2 12 30 S 47 48W
Paraná □, *Brazil* 175 A5 24 30 S 51 0W
Paraná →, *Argentina* 174 C4 33 43 S 59 15W
Paranã →, *Brazil* 171 D2 12 30 S 48 14W
Paranaguá, *Brazil* 175 B6 25 30 S 48 30W
Paranaíba, *Brazil* 171 E1 19 40 S 51 11W
Paranaíba →, *Brazil* 171 F1 20 6 S 51 4W
Paranapanema →, *Brazil* 175 A5 22 40 S 53 9W
Paranapiacaba, Serra do, *Brazil* 175 A6 24 31 S 48 35W
Paranas, *Phil.* 81 F5 11 42N 125 2 E
Paranavaí, *Brazil* 175 A5 23 4 S 52 56W
Parang, *Maguindanao, Phil.* 81 H5 7 23N 124 16 E
Parang, *Sulu, Phil.* 81 J3 5 55N 120 54 E
Parangaba, *Brazil* 170 B4 3 45 S 38 33W
Parangippettai, *India* 95 J4 11 30N 79 38 E
Parângul Mare, Vf., *Romania* 53 E8 45 20N 23 37 E
Paranthan, *Sri Lanka* 95 K5 9 26N 80 24 E
Paraparaumu, *N.Z.* 130 G4 40 57 S 175 3 E
Parapetí →, *Bolivia* 173 D5 18 58 S 62 21W
Parapóla, *Greece* 48 E5 36 55N 23 27 E
Paraspóri, Ákra, *Greece* 49 F9 35 55N 27 15 E
Paratinga, *Brazil* 171 D3 12 40 S 43 10W
Paratoo, *Australia* 128 B3 32 42 S 139 20 E
Paraúna, *Brazil* 171 E1 16 55 S 50 26W
Paray-le-Monial, *France* 27 F11 46 27N 4 7 E
Parbati →, *Mad. P., India* 92 G7 25 50N 76 30 E
Parbati →, *Raj., India* 92 F7 26 54N 77 53 E
Parbatipur, *Bangla.* 90 C2 25 39N 88 55 E
Parbhani, *India* 94 E3 19 8N 76 52 E
Parchim, *Germany* 30 B7 53 26N 11 52 E
Parchwitz = Prochowice, *Poland* 55 G3 51 17N 16 20 E
Parco = Sinclair, *U.S.A.* 158 F10 41 47N 107 7W
Parczew, *Poland* 55 G9 51 40N 22 52 E
Pardes Hanna-Karkur, *Israel* 103 C3 32 28N 34 57 E
Pardilla, *Spain* 42 D7 41 33N 3 43W
Pardo →, *Bahia, Brazil* 171 E4 15 40 S 39 0W
Pardo →, *Mato Grosso, Brazil* 175 A5 21 46 S 52 9W
Pardo →, *Minas Gerais, Brazil* 171 E3 15 48 S 44 48W
Pardo →, *São Paulo, Brazil* 171 F2 20 10 S 48 38W
Pardubice, *Czech Rep.* 34 A8 50 3N 15 45 E
Pardubický □, *Czech Rep.* 34 B8 49 50N 16 0 E
Pardubitz = Pardubice, *Czech Rep.* 34 A8 50 3N 15 45 E
Pare, *Indonesia* 85 D4 7 43 S 112 12 E
Pare Mts., *Tanzania* 118 C4 4 0 S 37 45 E
Parecis, Serra dos, *Brazil* 173 C6 13 0 S 60 0W
Paredes de Nava, *Spain* 42 C6 42 9N 4 42W
Parelhas, *Brazil* 170 C4 6 41 S 36 39W
Paren, *Russia* 67 C17 62 30N 163 15 E
Parenda, *India* 94 E2 18 16N 75 28 E
Parengarenga Harbour, *N.Z.* 130 A1 34 31 S 173 0 E
Parent, *Canada* 140 C5 47 55N 74 35W
Parent, L., *Canada* 140 C4 48 31N 77 1W
Parentis-en-Born, *France* 28 D2 44 21N 1 4W
Parepare, *Indonesia* 82 B1 4 0 S 119 40 E
Parfino, *Russia* 58 D6 57 59N 31 34 E
Párga, *Greece* 48 B2 39 15N 20 29 E
Pargas = Parainen, *Finland* 15 F20 60 18N 22 18 E
Pargi, *India* 94 E3 17 11N 77 53 E
Pargo, Pta. do, *Madeira* 9 c 32 49N 17 17W
Paria →, *U.S.A.* 159 H8 36 52N 111 36W
Paria, G. de, *Venezuela* 169 A5 10 20N 62 0W
Paria, Pen. de, *Venezuela* 169 A5 10 50N 62 30W
Pariaguán, *Venezuela* 169 B5 8 51N 64 34W
Pariaman, *Indonesia* 84 C2 0 47 S 100 11 E
Paricatuba, *Brazil* 169 D5 4 26 S 61 53W
Paricutín, Cerro, *Mexico* 162 D4 19 28N 102 15W
Parigi, *Java, Indonesia* 85 D3 7 42 S 108 29 E
Parigi, *Sulawesi, Indonesia* 82 B2 0 50 S 120 5 E
Parika, *Guyana* 169 B6 6 50N 58 20W
Parikkala, *Finland* 58 B5 61 33N 29 31 E
Parima, Serra, *Brazil* 169 C5 2 30N 64 0W
Parinari, *Peru* 172 A3 4 35 S 74 25W
Pariñas, Pta., *S. Amer.* 166 D2 4 30 S 82 0W
Parincea, *Romania* 53 D12 46 27N 27 9 E
Paringa, *Australia* 128 C4 34 10 S 140 46 E
Parintins, *Brazil* 169 D6 2 40 S 56 50W
Pariparit Kyun, *Burma* 90 G4 14 55N 93 45 E
Paris, *Canada* 150 C4 43 12N 80 25W
Paris, *France* 27 D9 48 50N 2 20 E
Paris, *Idaho, U.S.A.* 158 E8 42 14N 111 24W
Paris, *Ill., U.S.A.* 157 E9 39 36N 87 42W
Paris, *Ky., U.S.A.* 157 F12 38 13N 84 15W
Paris, *Mo., U.S.A.* 156 E5 39 29N 92 0W
Paris, *Tenn., U.S.A.* 149 G1 36 18N 88 19W
Paris, *Tex., U.S.A.* 155 J7 33 40N 95 33W
Paris, Ville de □, *France* 27 D9 48 50N 2 20 E
Paris Charles de Gaulle ✕ (CDG), *France* 27 D9 49 0N 2 32 E
Paris Orly ✕ (ORY), *France* 27 D9 48 44N 2 23 E
Parish, *U.S.A.* 151 C8 43 25N 76 8W
Parishville, *U.S.A.* 151 B10 44 38N 74 49W
Pariti, *Indonesia* 82 D2 10 1 S 123 45 E
Park, *U.S.A.* 160 B4 48 45N 122 18W
Park City, *U.S.A.* 155 G6 37 48N 97 20W
Park Falls, *U.S.A.* 154 C9 45 56N 90 27W
Park Forest, *U.S.A.* 157 C9 41 29N 87 40W
Park Head, *Canada* 150 B3 44 36N 81 9W
Park Hills, *Mo., U.S.A.* 155 G9 37 53N 90 28W
Park Hills, *Mo., U.S.A.* 156 G6 37 51N 90 31W
Park Range, *U.S.A.* 158 G10 40 0N 106 30W
Park Rapids, *U.S.A.* 154 B7 46 55N 95 4W
Park Ridge, *U.S.A.* 157 B9 42 2N 87 51W
Park River, *U.S.A.* 154 A6 48 24N 97 45W
Park Rynie, *S. Africa* 117 E5 30 25 S 30 45 E
Parkā Bandar, *Iran* 97 E8 25 55N 59 35 E
Parkal, *India* 94 E4 18 12N 79 43 E
Parkán = Štúrovo, *Slovak Rep.* 35 D11 47 48N 18 41 E
Parkano, *Finland* 15 E20 62 1N 23 0 E
Parkent, *Uzbekistan* 65 C4 41 18N 69 40 E
Parker, *Ariz., U.S.A.* 161 L12 34 9N 114 17W
Parker, *Pa., U.S.A.* 150 E5 41 5N 79 41W
Parker Dam, *U.S.A.* 161 L12 34 18N 114 8W
Parkersburg, *Iowa, U.S.A.* 156 B4 42 35N 92 47W
Parkersburg, *W. Va., U.S.A.* 148 F5 39 16N 81 34W
Parkes, *Australia* 129 B8 33 9 S 148 11 E
Parkfield, *U.S.A.* 160 K6 35 54N 120 26W

Parkhar, *Tajikistan* ... **65 E4** 37 30N 69 34 E
Parkhill, *Canada* **150 C3** 43 15N 81 38W
Parkland, *U.S.A.* **160 C4** 47 9N 122 26W
Parkston, *U.S.A.* **154 D6** 43 24N 97 59W
Parksville, *Canada* ... **142 D4** 49 20N 124 21W
Parla, *Spain* **42 E7** 40 14N 3 46W
Parlakimidi, *India* .... **94 E7** 18 45N 84 5 E
Parli, *India* .... **94 E3** 18 50N 76 35 E
Pârliţa, *Moldova* ..... **53 C12** 47 19N 27 52 E
Parma, *Italy* .... **44 D7** 44 48N 10 20 E
Parma, *Idaho, U.S.A.* . **158 E5** 43 47N 116 57W
Parma, *Ohio, U.S.A.* .. **150 E3** 41 23N 81 43W
Parma ➝, *Italy* ...... **44 D7** 44 56N 10 26 E
Paranaguá, *Brazil* ..... **170 D3** 10 10 S 44 38W
Parnaíba, *Brazil* ...... **170 B3** 2 54 S 41 47W
Parnaíba ➝, *Brazil* ... **170 B3** 3 0 S 41 50W
Parnamirim, *Brazil* ... **170 C4** 8 5 S 39 34W
Parnarama, *Brazil* .... **170 C3** 5 31 S 43 6W
Parnassós, *Greece* .... **48 C4** 38 35N 22 30 E
Parnassus, *N.Z.* ...... **131 C8** 42 42 S 173 23 E
Parndana, *Australia* .. **128 C2** 35 48 S 137 12 E
Parner, *India* .... **94 E2** 19 0N 74 26 E
Párnis, *Greece* .... **48 C5** 38 14N 23 45 E
Párnitha △, *Greece* .. **48 C5** 38 12N 23 44 E
Párnon Óros, *Greece* . **48 D4** 37 15N 22 45 E
Pärnu, *Estonia* .... **15 G21** 58 28N 24 33 E
Parola, *India* .... **94 D2** 20 47N 75 7 E
Paroo ➝, *Australia* .. **128 A5** 31 28 S 143 32 E
Páros, *Greece* .... **49 D7** 37 5N 25 12 E
Parowan, *U.S.A.* **159 H7** 37 51N 112 50W
Parpaillon, *France* ... **29 D10** 44 30N 6 40 E
Parral, *Chile* .... **174 D1** 36 10 S 71 52W
Parramatta, *Australia* . **129 B9** 33 48 S 151 1 E
Parras, *Mexico* **162 B4** 25 30N 102 20W
Parrett ➝, *U.K.* **21 F4** 51 12N 3 1W
Parris I., *U.S.A.* **152 C9** 32 20N 80 41W
Parrish, *U.S.A.* **153 H7** 27 35N 82 26W
Parrott, *U.S.A.* **152 D5** 31 54N 84 31W
Parrsboro, *Canada* ... **141 C7** 45 30N 64 25W
Parry I., *Canada* **150 A4** 45 18N 80 10W
Parry Is., *Canada* **6 B2** 77 0N 110 0W
Parry Sound, *Canada* . **140 C4** 45 20N 80 0W
Parsberg, *Germany* ... **31 F7** 49 10N 11 43 E
Parseier Spitze, *Austria* **33 B10** 47 10N 10 28 E
Parsęta ➝, *Poland* ... **54 D2** 54 11N 15 34 E
Parsnip ➝, *Canada* .. **142 B4** 55 10N 123 2W
Parsons, *U.S.A.* **155 G7** 37 20N 95 16W
Parsons Ra., *Australia* **126 A2** 13 30 S 135 15 E
Partabpur, *India* ..... **94 E5** 20 0N 80 42 E
Partanna, *Italy* .... **46 E5** 37 43N 12 53 E
Partenio △, *Italy* .... **47 B7** 40 56N 14 38 E
Parthenay, *France* **26 F6** 46 38N 0 16W
Partinico, *Italy* .... **46 D6** 38 3N 13 7 E
Partizánske,
Slovak Rep. .... **35 C11** 48 38N 18 23 E
Partridge I., *Canada* .. **140 A2** 55 59N 87 37W
Partur, *India* .... **94 E3** 19 40N 76 14 E
Paru ➝, *Brazil* ...... **169 D7** 1 33 S 52 38W
Parú ➝, *Venezuela* .. **168 C4** 4 20N 66 27W
Paru de Oeste ➝,
Brazil **169 C6** 1 30N 56 0W
Parucito ➝, *Venezuela* **168 B4** 5 18N 65 59W
Parur, *India* .... **95 J3** 10 13N 76 14 E
Paruro, *Peru* .... **172 C3** 13 45 S 71 50W
Parvān □, *Afghan.* ... **91 B3** 35 0N 69 0 E
Parvatipuram, *India* .. **94 E6** 18 50N 83 25 E
Parvatsar, *India* ...... **92 F6** 26 52N 74 49 E
Påryd, *Sweden* .... **17 H9** 56 34N 15 55 E
Parys, *S. Africa* ...... **116 D4** 26 52 S 27 29 E
Pas, Pta. des, *Spain* ... **38 D1** 38 46N 1 26 E
Pas-de-Calais □, *France* **27 B9** 50 30N 2 10 E
Pasada, *Spain* **42 B5** 43 23N 5 40W
Pasadena, *Canada* **141 C8** 49 1N 57 36W
Pasadena, *Calif., U.S.A.* **161 L8** 34 9N 118 9W
Pasadena, *Tex., U.S.A.* **155 L7** 29 43N 95 13W
Pasaje, *Ecuador* ...... **168 D2** 3 23 S 79 50W
Pasaje ➝, *Argentina* .. **174 B3** 25 39 S 63 56W
Paşalimanı, *Turkey* ... **51 F11** 40 29N 27 36 E
Pasar, *Indonesia* ..... **79 J17** 8 27 S 114 54 E
Pasay, *Phil.* .... **80 D3** 14 33N 121 0 E
Pascagoula, *U.S.A.* ... **155 K10** 30 21N 88 33W
Pascagoula ➝, *U.S.A.* **155 K10** 30 23N 88 37W
Paşcani, *Romania* .... **53 C11** 47 14N 26 45 E
Pasco, *U.S.A.* **158 C4** 46 14N 119 6W
Pasco □, *Peru* .... **172 C2** 10 40 S 75 0W
Pasco, Cerro de, *Peru* . **172 C2** 10 45 S 76 10W
Pasco I., *Australia* ... **124 D2** 20 57 S 115 20 E
Pascoag, *U.S.A.* **151 E13** 41 57N 71 42W
Pascua, I. de, *Chile* .. **172 b** 27 7 S 109 23W
Pasewalk, *Germany* .. **30 B9** 53 30N 13 58 E
Pasfield L., *Canada* .. **143 B7** 58 24N 105 20W
Pasha ➝, *Russia* ..... **58 B7** 60 29N 32 55 E
Pashiya, *Russia* ...... **64 B7** 58 33N 58 26 E
Pashmakli = Smolyan,
Bulgaria .... **51 E8** 41 36N 24 38 E
Pasig, *Phil.* .... **80 D3** 14 35N 121 5 E
Pasighat, *India* ...... **90 A5** 28 4N 95 21 E
Pasinler, *Turkey* ..... **101 C9** 39 59N 41 41 E
Pasir Mas, *Malaysia* .. **87 J4** 6 2N 102 8 E
Pasir Panjang,
Singapore .... **87 d** 1 18N 103 46 E
Pasir Putih, *Malaysia* . **87 K4** 5 50N 102 24 E
Pasirian, *Indonesia* ... **85 D4** 8 13 S 113 8 E
Pasirkuning, *Indonesia* **84 C2** 0 30 S 104 33 E
Påskallavik, *Sweden* .. **17 G10** 57 10N 16 26 E
Paskūh, *Iran* .... **97 E9** 27 34N 61 39 E
Pasłęk, *Poland* .... **54 D6** 54 3N 19 41 E
Pasłęka ➝, *Poland* ... **54 D6** 54 26N 19 46 E
Pasley, C., *Australia* .. **125 F3** 33 52 S 123 35 E
Pašman, *Croatia* ..... **45 E12** 43 58N 15 20 E
Pasmore ➝, *Australia* **128 A3** 31 5 S 139 49 E
Pasni, *Pakistan* ...... **91 D1** 25 15N 63 27 E
Paso Cantinela, *Mexico* **161 N11** 32 33N 115 47W
Paso de Indios,
Argentina .... **176 B3** 43 55 S 69 0W
Paso de los Indios,
Argentina .... **176 A3** 38 32 S 69 25W
Paso de los Libres,
Argentina .... **174 B4** 29 44 S 57 10W
Paso de los Toros,
Uruguay .... **174 C4** 32 45 S 56 30W
Paso Flores, *Argentina* **176 B2** 40 35 S 70 38W
Paso Robles, *U.S.A.* .. **159 J3** 35 38N 120 41W
Pasorapa, *Bolivia* .... **173 D5** 18 16 S 64 37W
Paspébiac, *Canada* ... **141 C6** 48 3N 65 17W
Pasrur, *Pakistan* ..... **92 C6** 32 16N 74 43 E
Passage West, *Ireland* . **23 E3** 51 52N 8 21W
Passaic, *U.S.A.* **151 F10** 40 51N 74 7W
Passam, *Papua N. G.* . **132 B2** 3 41 S 143 38 E
Passau, *Germany* ..... **31 G9** 48 34N 13 28 E
Passenheim = Pasym,
Poland .... **54 E7** 53 48N 20 49 E
Passero, C., *Italy* .... **47 F8** 36 41N 15 10 E
Passi, *Phil.* .... **81 F4** 11 6N 122 38 E
Passo Fundo, *Brazil* .. **175 B5** 28 10 S 52 20W
Passos, *Brazil* .... **171 F2** 20 45 S 46 37W
Passow, *Germany* .... **30 B10** 53 8N 14 6 E
Passwang, *Switz.* .... **32 B5** 47 22N 7 41 E
Passy, *France* .... **29 C10** 45 55N 6 41 E
Pastavy, *Belarus* ..... **15 J22** 55 4N 26 50 E
Pastaza □, *Ecuador* .. **168 D2** 2 0 S 77 0W
Pastaza ➝, *Peru* ..... **168 D2** 4 50 S 76 52W
Pasto, *Colombia* **168 C2** 1 13N 77 17W
Pastol B., *U.S.A.* **144 E7** 63 7N 163 15W
Pastos Bons, *Brazil* ... **170 C3** 6 36 S 44 5W
Pastrana, *Spain* **40 E2** 40 27N 2 53W
Pasuquin, *Phil.* ...... **80 B3** 18 20N 120 37 E
Pasuruan, *Indonesia* .. **85 D4** 7 40 S 112 44 E
Pasym, *Poland* .... **54 E7** 53 48N 20 49 E
Pásztó, *Hungary* ..... **52 C4** 47 52N 19 43 E
Pata, *Phil.* .... **81 J3** 5 51N 121 10 E
Pata I., *Phil.* .... **81 J3** 5 49N 121 10 E
Patagonia, *Argentina* . **176 C2** 45 0 S 69 0W
Patagonia, *U.S.A.* **159 L8** 31 33N 110 45W
Patalasang, *Indonesia* . **82 C1** 5 26 S 119 26 E
Patambar, *Iran* ...... **97 D9** 29 45N 60 17 E
Patan = Lalitapur,
Nepal .... **93 F11** 27 40N 85 20 E
Patan, *Gujarat, India* . **94 F1** 17 22N 73 57 E
Patan, *Maharashtra,*
India .... **92 H5** 23 54N 72 14 E
Patani, *Indonesia* .... **82 A3** 0 20N 128 50 E
Pătârlagele, *Romania* . **53 E11** 45 19N 26 21 E
Pataudi, *India* .... **92 E7** 28 18N 76 48 E
Patchewollock,
Australia .... **128 C5** 35 22 S 142 12 E
Patchogue, *U.S.A.* ... **151 F11** 40 46N 73 1W
Pate, *Kenya* .... **118 C5** 2 10 S 41 0 E
Patea, *N.Z.* .... **130 F3** 39 45 S 174 30 E
Pategi, *Nigeria* ...... **113 D6** 8 50N 5 45 E
Patensie, *S. Africa* ... **116 E3** 33 46 S 24 49 E
Paterna, *Spain* **41 F4** 39 30N 0 26W
Paternion, *Austria* ... **34 E6** 46 43N 13 38 E
Paternò, *Italy* .... **47 E7** 37 34N 14 54 E
Pateros, *U.S.A.* **158 B4** 48 3N 119 54W
Paterson, *Australia* .. **129 B9** 32 35 S 151 36 E
Paterson, *U.S.A.* **151 F10** 40 55N 74 11W
Paterson Inlet, *N.Z.* .. **131 G3** 46 56 S 168 12 E
Paterson Ra., *Australia* **124 D3** 21 45 S 122 10 E
Pathankot, *India* ..... **92 C6** 32 18N 75 45 E
Pathardi, *India* ...... **94 E2** 19 10N 75 11 E
Patharghata, *Bangla.* . **90 D2** 22 2N 89 58 E
Pathein = Bassein,
Burma .... **90 G5** 16 45N 94 30 E
Pathfinder Reservoir,
U.S.A. **158 E10** 42 28N 106 51W
Pathiu, *Thailand* .... **87 G2** 10 42N 99 19 E
Pathri, *India* .... **94 E3** 19 15N 76 27 E
Pathum Thani,
Thailand .... **86 E3** 14 1N 100 32 E
Pati, *Indonesia* ...... **85 D4** 6 45 S 111 1 E
Pati Pt., *Guam* ...... **133 R15** 13 40N 144 50 E
Patía, *Colombia* **168 C2** 2 4N 77 4W
Patía ➝, *Colombia* .. **168 C2** 2 13N 78 40W
Patiala, *Punjab, India* . **92 D7** 30 23N 76 26 E
Patiala, *Ut. P., India* . **93 F8** 27 43N 79 1 E
Patine Kouka, *Senegal* **112 C2** 12 45N 13 45W
Patitírion, *Greece* .... **48 B5** 39 8N 23 50 E
Pativilca, *Peru* ...... **172 C2** 10 42 S 77 48W
Patkai Bum, *India* ... **90 B5** 27 0N 95 30 E
Pátmos, *Greece* ..... **49 D8** 37 21N 26 36 E
Patna, *India* .... **93 G11** 25 35N 85 12 E
Patnagarh, *India* .... **94 D6** 20 43N 83 9 E
Patnanongan I., *Phil.* . **80 D4** 14 48N 122 11 E
Patnongon, *Phil.* .... **81 F4** 10 55N 122 0 E
Patnos, *Turkey* ...... **101 C10** 39 13N 42 51 E
Pato Branco, *Brazil* .. **175 B5** 26 13 S 52 40W
Patoka L., *U.S.A.* ... **157 F10** 38 20N 86 40W
Patong, Ao, *Thailand* . **87 a** 7 54N 98 17 E
Patonga, *Uganda* .... **118 B3** 2 45N 33 15 E
Patos, *Albania* ...... **50 F3** 40 42N 19 38 E
Patos, *Brazil* .... **170 C4** 6 55 S 37 16W
Patos, L. dos, *Brazil* . **175 C5** 31 20 S 51 0W
Patos, Río de los ➝,
Argentina .... **174 C2** 31 18 S 69 25W
Patos de Minas, *Brazil* **171 E2** 18 35 S 46 32W
Patquía, *Argentina* ... **174 C2** 30 2 S 66 55W
Patra = Pátrai, *Greece* **48 C3** 38 14N 21 47 E
Pátrai, *Greece* ...... **48 C3** 38 14N 21 47 E
Pátraikós Kólpos,
Greece .... **48 C3** 38 17N 21 30 E
Patras = Pátrai, *Greece* **48 C3** 38 14N 21 47 E
Patreksfjörður, *Iceland* **11 B2** 65 34N 24 0W
Patriarsheye =
Donskoy, *Russia* ... **58 F10** 53 55N 38 15 E
Patricio Lynch, I., *Chile* **176 C1** 48 35 S 75 30W
Patrocínio, *Brazil* .... **171 E2** 18 57 S 47 0W
Pattada, *Italy* .... **46 B2** 40 35N 9 6 E
Pattani, *Thailand* .... **87 J3** 6 48N 101 15 E
Pattaya, *Thailand* ... **78 B2** 12 52N 100 55 E
Patten, *U.S.A.* **149 C11** 46 0N 68 38W
Patterson, *Calif., U.S.A.* **160 H5** 37 28N 121 8W
Patterson, *Ga., U.S.A.* **152 D7** 31 23N 82 8W
Patterson, *La., U.S.A.* **155 L9** 29 42N 91 18W
Patterson, Mt., *U.S.A.* **160 G7** 38 29N 119 20W
Patteson, Passage,
Vanuatu .... **133 E6** 15 26 S 168 12 E
Patti, *Punjab, India* .. **92 D6** 31 17N 74 54 E
Patti, *Ut. P., India* ... **93 G10** 25 55N 82 12 E
Patti, *Italy* .... **47 D7** 38 8N 14 58 E
Pattoki, *Pakistan* .... **92 D5** 31 5N 73 52 E
Patton = Monroeville,
U.S.A. **150 F5** 40 26N 79 45W
Patton, *U.S.A.* **150 F6** 40 38N 78 39W
Pattonsburg, *U.S.A.* . **156 D2** 40 3N 94 8W
Pattukkattai, *India* ... **95 J4** 10 25N 79 20 E
Patu, *Brazil* .... **170 C4** 6 6 S 37 38W
Patuakhali, *Bangla.* .. **90 D3** 22 20N 90 25 E
Patuanak, *Canada* ... **143 B7** 55 55N 107 43W
Patuca ➝, *Honduras* . **164 D2** 15 50N 84 18W
Patuca △, *Honduras* . **164 D2** 14 30N 85 30W
Patuca, Punta,
Honduras **164 C3** 15 49N 84 14W
Pătulele, *Romania* ... **52 F7** 44 21N 22 47 E
Patur, *India* .... **94 D3** 20 27N 76 56 E
Pátzcuaro, *Mexico* ... **162 D4** 19 30N 101 40W
Pau, *France* **28 E3** 43 19N 0 25W
Pau, Gave de ➝,
France **28 E2** 43 33N 1 12W
Pau d' Arco, *Brazil* .. **170 C2** 7 30 S 49 22W
Pau dos Ferros, *Brazil* **170 C4** 6 7 S 38 10W
Pauanui, *N.Z.* ...... **130 D4** 37 1 S 175 52 E
Paucartambo, *Peru* .. **172 C3** 13 19 S 71 35W
Pauillac, *France* **28 C3** 45 11N 0 46W
Pauini, *Brazil* .... **172 B4** 7 40 S 66 58W
Pauini ➝, *Brazil* .... **169 D5** 1 42 S 62 50W
Pauk, *Burma* .... **90 E5** 21 27N 94 30 E
Paukkaung, *Burma* .. **90 F5** 18 54N 95 33 E
Pauktaw, *Burma* .... **90 E4** 20 11N 93 4 E
Paul I., *Canada* **141 A7** 56 30N 61 20W
Paul Isnard, *Fr. Guiana* **169 C7** 4 47N 54 1W
Paul Smiths, *U.S.A.* . **151 B10** 44 26N 74 15W
Paulatuk, *Canada* ... **138 B7** 69 25N 124 0W
Paulding, *U.S.A.* **157 C12** 41 8N 84 35W
Paulhan, *France* ..... **28 E7** 43 33N 3 28 E
Paulis = Isiro,
Dem. Rep. of
the Congo .... **118 B2** 2 53N 27 40 E
Paulista = Paulistana,
Brazil .... **170 C3** 8 9 S 41 9W
Paulista, *Brazil* ..... **170 C5** 7 57 S 34 53W
Paulistana, *Brazil* ... **170 C3** 8 9 S 41 9W
Paulo Afonso, *Brazil* . **170 C4** 9 21 S 38 15W
Paulo de Faria, *Brazil* . **171 F2** 20 2 S 49 24W
Paulpietersburg,
S. Africa .... **117 D5** 27 23 S 30 50 E
Pauls Valley, *U.S.A.* . **155 H6** 34 44N 97 13W
Pauma Valley, *U.S.A.* . **161 M10** 33 16N 116 58W
Paung, *Burma* ...... **90 G5** 16 37N 94 28 E
Paungde, *Burma* .... **90 F5** 18 29N 95 30 E
Pauni, *India* .... **94 D4** 20 48N 79 40 E
Pauri, *India* .... **93 D8** 30 9N 78 47 E
Pausa, *Peru* .... **172 D3** 15 16 S 73 22W
Pauto ➝, *Colombia* . **168 B3** 5 9N 70 55W
Pauwela, *U.S.A.* ... **145 C5** 20 56N 156 19W
Pavagada, *India* .... **95 G3** 14 6N 77 16 E
Pāveh, *Iran* .... **101 E12** 35 3N 46 22 E
Pavelets, *Russia* .... **58 F10** 53 49N 39 14 E
Pavia, *Italy* .... **44 C6** 45 7N 9 8 E
Pavilion, *U.S.A.* **150 D6** 42 52N 78 1W
Pavilly, *France* ..... **26 C7** 49 34N 0 57 E
Pāvilosta, *Latvia* .... **15 H19** 56 53N 21 14 E
Pavlikeni, *Bulgaria* .. **51 C9** 43 14N 25 20 E
Pavlodar, *Kazakhstan* . **66 D8** 52 33N 77 0 E
Pavlograd = Pavlohrad,
Ukraine .... **59 H8** 48 30N 35 52 E
Pavlohrad, *Ukraine* .. **59 H8** 48 30N 35 52 E
Pavlovo, *Russia* .... **60 C6** 55 58N 43 5 E
Pavlovsk, *Russia* .... **60 E5** 50 26N 40 5 E
Pavlovskaya, *Russia* . **61 G4** 46 17N 39 47 E
Pavlovskiy-Posad,
Russia .... **58 E10** 55 47N 38 42 E
Pavo, *U.S.A.* **152 E6** 30 58N 83 45W
Pavullo nel Frignano,
Italy .... **44 D7** 44 20N 10 50 E
Pavuvu, *Solomon Is.* .. **133 M10** 9 4 S 159 8 E
Paw Paw, *U.S.A.* ... **157 B11** 42 13N 85 53W
Pawahku, *Burma* .... **90 B7** 26 11N 98 40 E
Pawai, Pulau, *Singapore* **87 d** 1 11N 103 44 E
Pawan ➝, *Indonesia* . **85 C4** 1 55 S 110 0 E
Pawayan, *India* ..... **93 E9** 28 4N 80 6 E
Pawhuska, *U.S.A.* ... **155 G6** 36 40N 96 20W
Pawling, *U.S.A.* **151 E11** 41 34N 73 36W
Pawnee, *Ill., U.S.A.* .. **156 E7** 39 36N 89 35W
Pawnee, *Okla., U.S.A.* **155 G6** 36 20N 96 48W
Pawnee City, *U.S.A.* . **154 E6** 40 7N 96 9W
Pawpaw, *U.S.A.* **156 C8** 41 41N 88 59W
Pawtucket, *U.S.A.* ... **151 E13** 41 53N 71 23W
Paxi = Paxoí, *Greece* . **38 C10** 39 14N 20 12 E
Paximádhia, *Greece* .. **39 F5** 35 0N 24 35 E
Paxoí, *Greece* ...... **38 C10** 39 14N 20 12 E
Paxson, *U.S.A.* **144 E11** 63 2N 145 30W
Paxton, *U.S.A.* **157 D8** 40 27N 88 6W
Payagyi, *Burma* .... **90 G6** 17 29N 96 32 E
Payakumbuh, *Indonesia* **84 C2** 0 20 S 100 35 E
Payapa = General
Tinio, *Phil.* .... **80 D3** 15 39N 121 10 E
Payerne, *Switz.* .... **32 C3** 46 49N 6 56 E
Payette, *U.S.A.* **158 D5** 44 5N 116 56W
Paymogo, *Spain* **43 H3** 37 44N 7 21W
Payne, *U.S.A.* **157 C12** 41 5N 84 44W
Payne Bay = Kangirsuk,
Canada **139 B13** 60 0N 70 0W
Payne L., *Canada* ... **139 C12** 59 30N 74 30W
Payne Pt., *Ascension I.* **9 g** 7 57 S 14 25W
Paynes Find, *Australia* **125 E2** 29 15 S 117 42 E
Paynesville, *Liberia* .. **112 D2** 6 20N 10 45W
Paynesville, *U.S.A.* .. **154 C7** 45 23N 94 43W
Payo Obispo =
Chetumal, *Mexico* .. **163 D7** 18 30N 88 20W
Pays de la Loire □,
France **26 E6** 47 45N 0 25W
Paysandú, *Uruguay* .. **174 C4** 32 19 S 58 8W
Payshanba, *Uzbekistan* **65 C3** 40 0N 66 14 E
Payson, *Ariz., U.S.A.* . **159 J8** 34 14N 111 20W
Payson, *Utah, U.S.A.* . **158 F8** 40 3N 111 44W
Paz ➝, *Guatemala* .. **164 D1** 13 44N 90 10W
Paz, B. de la, *Mexico* . **162 C2** 24 15N 110 25W
Pāzanān, *Iran* ...... **97 D6** 30 35N 49 59 E
Pazar, *Turkey* ...... **101 B9** 41 10N 40 50 E
Pazarcık, *Turkey* ... **100 D7** 37 30N 37 17 E
Pazardzhik, *Bulgaria* . **51 D8** 42 12N 24 20 E
Pazarköy, *Turkey* ... **49 B9** 39 51N 27 24 E
Pazarlar, *Turkey* .... **49 C11** 39 0N 29 7 E
Pazaryeri, *Turkey* ... **49 B11** 40 0N 29 56 E
Pazaryolu, *Turkey* ... **101 B9** 40 21N 40 47 E
Pazin, *Croatia* ...... **45 C10** 45 14N 13 56 E
Pazña, *Bolivia* ...... **172 D4** 18 36 S 66 55W
Pčinja ➝, *Macedonia* . **50 E5** 41 50N 21 45 E
Pe Ell, *U.S.A.* **160 D3** 46 34N 123 18W
Pea ➝, *U.S.A.* **152 D4** 31 1N 85 51W
Peabody, *U.S.A.* **151 D14** 42 31N 70 56W
Peace ➝, *Canada* ... **142 B6** 59 0N 111 25W
Peace ➝, *U.S.A.* ... **153 J7** 26 56N 82 6W
Peace Point, *Canada* . **142 B6** 59 7N 112 27W
Peace River, *Canada* . **142 B5** 56 15N 117 18W
Peach Springs, *U.S.A.* **159 J7** 35 32N 113 25W
Peachland, *Canada* .. **142 D5** 49 47N 119 45W
Peachtree City, *U.S.A.* **152 B5** 33 25N 84 35W
Peak, The = Kinder
Scout, *U.K.* **20 D6** 53 24N 1 52W
Peak, The, *Ascension I.* **9 g** 7 57 S 14 20W
Peak Charles △,
Australia .... **125 F3** 32 42 S 121 10 E
Peak District △, *U.K.* . **20 D6** 53 24N 1 46W
Peak Hill, *N.S.W.,*
Australia .... **129 B8** 32 47 S 148 11 E
Peak Hill, *W. Austral.,*
Australia .... **125 E2** 25 35 S 118 43 E
Peak Ra., *Australia* .. **126 C4** 22 50 S 148 20 E
Peake, *Australia* ... **128 C3** 35 25 S 139 55 E
Peake Cr. ➝, *Australia* **127 D2** 28 2 S 136 7 E
Peal de Becerro, *Spain* **43 H7** 37 55N 3 7W
Peale, Mt., *U.S.A.* .. **159 G9** 38 26N 109 14W
Pearblossom, *U.S.A.* . **161 L9** 34 30N 117 55W
Pearl, *U.S.A.* **156 E6** 39 28N 90 38W
Pearl ➝, *U.S.A.* **155 K10** 30 11N 89 32W
Pearl and Hermes Reef,
U.S.A. **145 F8** 27 55N 175 45W
Pearl Banks, *Sri Lanka* **95 K4** 8 45N 79 45 E
Pearl City, *U.S.A.* .. **145 K14** 21 24N 157 59W
Pearl Harbor, *U.S.A.* . **145 K14** 21 21N 157 57W
Pearl River = Zhu
Jiang ➝, *China* .... **77 F9** 22 45N 113 37 E
Pearl River, *U.S.A.* .. **151 E10** 41 4N 74 2W
Pearsall, *U.S.A.* **155 L5** 28 54N 99 6W
Pearson, *U.S.A.* **152 D7** 31 18N 82 51W
Peary Land, *Greenland* **10 A7** 82 40N 33 0W
Pease ➝, *U.S.A.* ... **155 H5** 34 12N 99 2W
Peawanuck, *Canada* . **139 C11** 55 15N 85 12W
Pebane, *Mozam.* .... **119 F4** 17 10 S 38 8 E
Pebas, *Peru* .... **168 D3** 3 10 S 71 46W
Pebble, I., *Falk. Is.* .. **9 f** 51 20 S 59 40W
Pebble Beach, *U.S.A.* . **160 J5** 36 34N 121 57W
Peć, *Serbia & M.* .... **50 D4** 42 40N 20 17 E
Peçanha, *Brazil* .... **171 E3** 18 33 S 42 34W
Pecatonica, *U.S.A.* .. **156 B7** 42 19N 89 22W
Pecatonica ➝, *U.S.A.* **156 B7** 42 26N 89 12W
Péccioli, *Italy* ...... **44 E7** 43 33N 10 43 E
Pechea, *Romania* ... **53 E12** 45 36N 27 49 E
Pechenga, *Russia* ... **56 A5** 69 29N 31 4 E
Pechenizhyn, *Ukraine* . **53 B9** 48 30N 24 48 E
Pechiguera, Pta.,
Canary Is. **9 e2** 28 51N 13 53W
Pechnezhskoye Vdkhr.,
Ukraine .... **59 G9** 50 5N 36 54 E
Pechora, *Russia* .... **56 A10** 65 10N 57 11 E
Pechora ➝, *Russia* .. **56 A9** 68 13N 54 15 E
Pechorskaya Guba,
Russia .... **56 A9** 68 40N 54 0 E
Pechory, *Russia* .... **15 H22** 57 48N 27 40 E
Pecica, *Romania* .... **52 D6** 46 10N 21 3 E
Pecka, *Serbia & M.* .. **50 B3** 44 18N 19 33 E
Pécora, C., *Italy* .... **46 C1** 39 27N 8 23 E
Pecos, *N. Mex., U.S.A.* **159 J11** 35 35N 105 41W
Pecos, *Tex., U.S.A.* .. **155 K3** 31 26N 103 30W
Pecos ➝, *U.S.A.* **155 L3** 29 42N 101 22W
Pécs, *Hungary* ..... **52 D3** 46 5N 18 15 E
Pedda Bellala, *India* .. **94 E4** 19 4N 78 49 E
Peddapalli, *India* .... **94 E4** 18 40N 79 24 E
Peddapuram, *India* .. **94 F6** 17 6N 82 8 E
Pedder, L., *Australia* . **127 G4** 42 55 S 146 10 E
Peddie, *S. Africa* .... **117 E4** 33 14 S 27 7 E
Pedernales, *Dom. Rep.* **165 C5** 18 2N 71 44W
Pedernales, *Ecuador* . **168 C1** 0 5N 80 3W
Pedieos ➝, *Cyprus* .. **39 E9** 35 10N 33 54 E
Pedirka, *Australia* ... **127 D2** 26 40 S 135 14 E
Pedra Azul, *Brazil* ... **171 E3** 16 2 S 41 17W
Pedra Branca, *Brazil* . **169 C7** 0 51N 51 58W
Pedra Grande, Recifes
de, *Brazil* .... **171 E4** 17 45 S 38 58W
Pedra Lume,
C. Verde Is. .... **9 j** 16 40N 22 52W
Pedras Negras, *Brazil* . **173 C5** 12 51 S 62 54W
Pedras Tinhosas, I.,
São Tomé & Principe **115 G6** 1 22N 7 17 E
Pedreguer, *Spain* ... **41 G5** 38 48N 0 3 E
Pedreiras, *Brazil* .... **170 B3** 4 32 S 44 40W
Pedro Afonso, *Brazil* . **170 C2** 9 0 S 48 10W
Pedro Bay, *U.S.A.* ... **144 G9** 59 47N 154 7W
Pedro Cays, *Jamaica* . **164 C4** 17 5N 77 48W
Pedro Chico, *Colombia* **168 C3** 1 4N 70 25W
Pedro de Valdivia,
Chile .... **174 A2** 22 55 S 69 38W
Pedro Dorado,
Colombia **168 C3** 1 0N 70 14W
Pedro Juan Caballero,
Paraguay .... **175 A4** 22 30 S 55 40W
Pedro Muñoz, *Spain* .. **43 F8** 39 25N 2 56W
Pedrógão Grande,
Portugal **42 F2** 39 55N 8 9W
Pee Dee ➝, *U.S.A.* .. **149 J6** 33 22N 79 16W
Peebinga, *Australia* .. **128 C4** 34 52 S 140 57 E
Peebles, *U.K.* **22 F5** 55 40N 3 11W
Peebles, *U.S.A.* **157 F13** 38 57N 83 24W
Peekskill, *U.S.A.* ... **151 E11** 41 17N 73 55W
Peel, *I. of Man* **20 C3** 54 13N 4 40W
Peel ➝, *Australia* ... **129 A9** 30 50 S 150 29 E
Peel ➝, *Canada* **138 B6** 67 0N 135 0W
Peel Sd., *Canada* **138 A10** 73 0N 96 0W
Peene ➝, *Germany* .. **30 A9** 54 9N 13 46 E
Peera Peera Poolanna
L., *Australia* ...... **127 D2** 26 30 S 138 0 E
Peerless Lake, *Canada* **142 B6** 56 37N 114 40W
Peers, *Canada* **142 C5** 53 40N 116 0W
Peery L., *Australia* .. **128 A5** 30 45 S 143 35 E
Pegasus Bay, *N.Z.* ... **131 D8** 43 20 S 173 10 E
Peggau, *Austria* .... **34 D8** 47 12N 15 21 E
Pegnitz, *Germany* ... **31 F7** 49 44N 11 31 E
Pegnitz ➝, *Germany* . **31 F6** 49 30N 10 59 E
Pego, *Spain* **41 G4** 38 51N 0 8W
Pegu, *Burma* .... **90 G6** 17 20N 96 29 E
Pegu □, *Burma* ..... **90 G6** 17 30N 96 30 E
Pegu Yoma, *Burma* .. **90 F5** 19 0N 96 0 E
Pehčevo, *Macedonia* . **50 E6** 41 41N 22 55 E
Pehlivanköy, *Turkey* . **51 E10** 41 20N 26 55 E
Pehuajó, *Argentina* .. **174 D3** 35 45 S 62 0W
Pei Xian = Pizhou,
China .... **74 G9** 34 44N 116 55 E
Peian = Bei'an, *China* . **69 B7** 48 10N 126 20 E
Peihai = Beihai, *China* **76 G7** 21 28N 109 6 E
Peine, *Chile* .... **174 A2** 23 45 S 68 8W
Peine, *Germany* .... **30 C6** 52 19N 10 14 E
Peip'ing = Beijing,
China .... **74 E9** 39 55N 116 20 E
Peipus, L. =
Chudskoye, Ozero,
Russia .... **15 G22** 58 13N 27 30 E
Peissenberg, *Germany* **31 H7** 47 48N 11 4 E
Peitz, *Germany* ..... **30 D10** 51 51N 14 24 E
Peixe, *Brazil* .... **171 D2** 12 0 S 48 40W
Peixe ➝, *Brazil* ..... **171 F1** 21 31 S 51 58W
Peixoto de Azeredo ➝,
Brazil .... **173 C6** 10 6 S 55 31W
Pek ➝, *Serbia & M.* .. **50 B5** 44 45N 21 29 E
Pekalongan, *Indonesia* **85 D3** 6 53 S 109 40 E
Pekan, *Malaysia* .... **87 L4** 3 30N 103 25 E
Pekan Nenas, *Malaysia* **87 d** 1 31N 103 31 E
Pekanbaru, *Indonesia* . **84 B2** 0 30N 101 15 E
Pekang, *Taiwan* .... **77 F13** 23 34N 120 18 E
Pekin, *U.S.A.* **156 D7** 40 35N 89 40W
Peking = Beijing, *China* **74 E9** 39 55N 116 20 E
Peklevskaya =
Troitskiy, *Russia* ... **64 C9** 57 5N 63 43 E
Pekutatan, *Indonesia* . **79 J17** 8 25 S 114 49 E
Péla, *Guinea* **112 D3** 7 37N 9 7W
Pelabuhan Klang,
Malaysia .... **87 L3** 3 0N 101 23 E
Pelabuhan Ratu, Teluk,
Indonesia .... **84 D3** 7 5 S 106 30 E
Pelabuhanratu,
Indonesia .... **84 D3** 7 0 S 106 32 E
Pélagos, *Greece* .... **48 B6** 39 17N 24 4 E
Pelaihari, *Indonesia* . **85 C4** 3 55 S 114 45 E
Pelat, Mt., *France* ... **29 D10** 44 16N 6 42 E
Pełczyce, *Poland* ... **55 E2** 53 3N 15 16 E
Peleaga, Vf., *Romania* **52 E7** 45 22N 22 55 E
Pelechuco, *Bolivia* .. **172 C4** 14 48 S 69 4W
Pelée, Mt., *Martinique* **164 c** 14 48N 61 10W
Pelee, Pt., *Canada* .. **140 D3** 41 54N 82 31W
Pelee I., *Canada* **140 D3** 41 47N 82 40W
Pelejo, *Peru* .... **172 B2** 6 10 S 75 49W
Pelekech, *Kenya* .... **118 B4** 3 52N 35 8 E
Peleng, *Indonesia* ... **82 B2** 1 20 S 123 30 E
Pelenge, *Dem. Rep. of*
the Congo .... **114 C4** 2 44 S 22 39 E
Pelentong, *Malaysia* . **87 d** 1 32N 103 49 E
Pélézi, *Ivory C.* **112 D3** 7 17N 6 54W
Pelham, *U.S.A.* **152 D5** 31 8N 84 9W
Pelhřimov, *Czech Rep.* **34 B8** 49 24N 15 12 E
Pelican, *U.S.A.* **142 B1** 57 58N 136 14W
Pelican L., *Canada* .. **143 C8** 52 28N 100 20W
Pelican Narrows,
Canada **143 B8** 55 10N 102 56W
Pelion, *U.S.A.* **152 B8** 33 46N 81 15W
Pelister △, *Macedonia* **50 F5** 41 0N 21 10 E
Pelješac, *Croatia* .... **45 F14** 42 55N 17 25 E
Pelkosenniemi, *Finland* **14 C22** 67 6N 27 28 E
Pell City, *U.S.A.* **152 B3** 33 35N 86 17W
Pella, *Greece* ...... **50 F6** 40 46N 22 23 E
Pella, *S. Africa* ..... **116 D2** 29 1 S 19 6 E
Pella, *U.S.A.* **156 C4** 41 25N 92 55W
Pélla □, *Greece* .... **50 F6** 40 52N 22 0 E
Pello, *Finland* ...... **14 C21** 66 47N 23 59 E
Pellworm, *Germany* .. **30 A4** 54 31N 8 39 E
Pelly ➝, *Canada* ... **138 B6** 62 47N 137 19W
Pelly Bay, *Canada* ... **139 B11** 68 38N 89 50W
Peloponnese =
Pelopónnisos □,
Greece .... **48 D4** 37 10N 22 0 E
Pelopónnisos □, *Greece* **48 D4** 37 10N 22 0 E
Peloritani, Monti, *Italy* **47 D8** 38 3N 15 20 E
Pelorus ➝, *N.Z.* .... **131 B8** 41 16 S 173 45 E
Pelorus Sd., *N.Z.* ... **131 A8** 40 59 S 173 59 E
Pelotas, *Brazil* ..... **175 C5** 31 42 S 52 23W
Pelotas ➝, *Brazil* ... **175 B5** 27 28 S 51 55W
Pelovo, *Bulgaria* .... **51 C8** 43 26N 24 17 E
Pelplin, *Poland* ..... **54 E5** 53 55N 18 42 E
Pelvoux, Massif du,
France .... **29 D10** 44 52N 6 20 E
Pelym, *Russia* ...... **64 B9** 59 34N 63 27 E
Pelym ➝, *Russia* ... **64 B9** 59 39N 63 26 E
Pemalang, *Indonesia* . **85 D3** 6 53 S 109 23 E
Pemanggil, Pulau,
Malaysia .... **87 L5** 2 37N 104 21 E
Pematangsiantar,
Indonesia .... **84 B1** 2 57N 99 5 E
Pemba, *Mozam.* .... **119 E5** 12 58 S 40 30 E
Pemba, *Zambia* .... **119 F2** 16 30 S 27 28 E
Pemba Channel,
Tanzania .... **118 D4** 5 0 S 39 37 E
Pemba I., *Tanzania* .. **118 D4** 5 0 S 39 45 E
Pemberton, *Australia* . **125 F2** 34 30 S 116 0 E
Pemberton, *Canada* .. **142 C4** 50 25N 122 50W
Pembina, *U.S.A.* **154 A6** 48 58N 97 15W
Pembroke, *Canada* .. **140 C4** 45 50N 77 7W
Pembroke, *U.K.* **21 F3** 51 41N 4 55W
Pembroke, *U.S.A.* ... **152 C8** 32 8N 81 37W
Pembroke Pines, *U.S.A.* **153 J9** 26 5N 80 14W
Pembrokeshire □, *U.K.* **21 F3** 51 52N 4 56W
Pembrokeshire
Coast △, *U.K.* **21 F2** 51 50N 5 2W
Pembuang ➝,
Indonesia .... **85 C4** 3 24 S 112 33 E
Pen, *India* .... **94 E1** 18 45N 73 5 E
Pen-y-Ghent, *U.K.* .. **20 C5** 54 10N 2 14W
Peña, Sierra de la,
Spain **40 C4** 42 32N 0 45W
Peña de Francia, Sierra
de la, *Spain* **42 E4** 40 32N 6 10W
Penafiel, *Portugal* ... **42 D2** 41 12N 8 17W
Peñafiel, *Spain* **42 D6** 41 35N 4 7W
Peñaflor, *Spain* **43 H5** 37 43N 5 21W
Penal, *Trin. & Tob.* .. **169 F9** 10 9N 61 29W
Peñalara, *Spain* **42 E7** 40 51N 3 57W
Penalva, *Brazil* ..... **170 B2** 3 18 S 45 10W
Penamacôr, *Portugal* . **42 E3** 40 10N 7 10W
Penambulai, *Indonesia* **83 C4** 6 24 S 134 48 E
Penang = Pinang,
Malaysia .... **87 c** 5 25N 100 15 E
Penápolis, *Brazil* ... **175 A6** 21 30 S 50 0W
Peñaranda de
Bracamonte, *Spain* . **42 E5** 40 53N 5 13W
Peñarroya, *Spain* ... **40 E4** 40 25N 0 40W
Peñarroya-
Pueblonuevo, *Spain* **43 G5** 38 19N 5 16W
Penarth, *U.K.* **21 F4** 51 26N 3 11W
Peñas, C. de, *Spain* .. **42 B5** 43 42N 5 52W
Penas, G. de, *Chile* .. **176 C2** 47 0 S 75 0W
Peñas, Pta., *Venezuela* **169 A5** 11 17N 62 0W
Peñas de San Pedro,
Spain **41 G3** 38 44N 2 0W
Peñas del Chache,
Canary Is. **9 e2** 29 6N 13 33W
Peñausende, *Spain* .. **42 D5** 41 17N 5 52W
Pench △, *India* .... **93 J8** 21 45N 79 20 E
Pench ➝, *India* .... **94 D4** 21 17N 79 10 E
Pench'i = Benxi, *China* **75 D12** 41 20N 123 48 E
Pend Oreille ➝, *U.S.A.* **158 B5** 49 4N 117 37W
Pend Oreille, L., *U.S.A.* **158 C5** 48 10N 116 21W
Pendálofon, *Greece* .. **50 F5** 40 14N 21 12 E
Pendé ➝, *C.A.R.* ... **114 A3** 7 55N 16 36 E
Pendembu, *Eastern,*
S. Leone **112 D2** 8 10N 10 42W
Pendembu, *Northern,*
S. Leone **112 D2** 9 7N 11 14W
Pendências, *Brazil* ... **170 C4** 5 15 S 36 43W
Pender B., *Australia* .. **124 C3** 16 45 S 122 42 E
Pendik, *Turkey* ..... **51 F13** 40 53N 29 13 E
Pendjari △, *Benin* ... **113 C5** 11 15N 1 32 E
Pendjari ➝, *Benin* .. **113 C5** 10 55N 0 50 E
Pendleton, *Ind., U.S.A.* **157 E11** 40 0N 85 45W
Pendleton, *Oreg.,*
U.S.A. **158 D4** 45 40N 118 47W
Pendra, *India* ...... **93 H9** 22 46N 81 57 E
Pendzhikent, *Tajikistan* **65 D3** 39 29N 67 37 E
Peneda-Gerês △,
Portugal **42 D2** 41 57N 8 15W
Penedo, *Brazil* ..... **170 D4** 10 15 S 36 36W
Penelokan, *Indonesia* . **79 J18** 8 17 S 115 22 E
Penetanguishene,
Canada **140 D4** 44 50N 79 55W
Penfield, *U.S.A.* **150 E6** 41 13N 78 35W
Peng Chau, *China* ... **69 G11** 22 17N 114 2 E
Pengalengan, *Indonesia* **85 D3** 7 9 S 107 30 E
Penganga ➝, *India* .. **94 E4** 19 53N 79 9 E
Penge, *Kasai-Or.,*
Dem. Rep. of
the Congo .... **118 D1** 5 30 S 24 33 E
Penge, *Sud-Kivu,*
Dem. Rep. of
the Congo .... **118 C2** 4 27 S 28 25 E
P'enghu Ch'üntou,
Taiwan .... **77 F12** 23 34N 119 30 E
Penglai, *China* ..... **75 F11** 37 48N 120 42 E
Pengshan, *China* .... **76 B4** 30 14N 103 58 E
Pengshui, *China* .... **76 C7** 29 17N 108 12 E
Penguin, *Australia* ... **127 G4** 41 8 S 146 6 E
Pengxi, *China* ..... **76 B5** 30 44N 105 45 E
Pengze, *China* ..... **77 C11** 29 52N 116 32 E
Penhalonga, *Zimbabwe* **119 F3** 18 52 S 32 40 E
Peniche, *Portugal* ... **43 F1** 39 19N 9 22W
Penicuik, *U.K.* **22 F5** 55 50N 3 13W
Penida, Nusa, *Indonesia* **85 D5** 8 45 S 115 30 E
Penninnes, Alpes =
Pennine, Alpi, *Alps* . **31 J3** 46 4N 7 30 E
Peninsular Malaysia □,
Malaysia .... **87 L4** 4 0N 102 0 E
Peñíscola, *Spain* .... **40 E5** 40 22N 0 24 E
Penitente, Serra do,
Brazil .... **170 C2** 8 45 S 46 20W
Penki = Benxi, *China* . **75 D12** 41 20N 123 48 E
Penkridge, *U.K.* **20 E5** 52 44N 2 6W
Penmarch, *France* ... **26 E2** 47 49N 4 21W
Penmarch, Pte. de,
France **26 E2** 47 48N 4 22W
Penn = Penn Hills,
U.S.A. **150 F5** 40 28N 79 52W
Penn Hills, *U.S.A.* ... **150 F5** 40 28N 79 52W
Penn Yan, *U.S.A.* ... **150 D7** 42 40N 77 3W
Penna, Punta della,
Italy .... **45 F11** 42 10N 14 43 E
Pennant, *Canada* **143 C7** 50 32N 108 14W
Penne, *Italy* .... **45 F10** 42 27N 13 55 E
Penner ➝, *India* ... **95 G5** 14 35N 80 10 E
Penneshaw, *Australia* . **128 C2** 35 44 S 137 56 E
Pennine, Alpi, *Alps* .. **31 J3** 46 4N 7 30 E
Pennines, *U.K.* **20 C5** 54 45N 2 27W
Pennington, *U.S.A.* .. **160 F5** 39 15N 121 47W
Pennington ➝, *Nigeria* **113 E6** 4 45N 5 35 E
Pennino, Mte., *Italy* .. **45 E9** 43 6N 12 53 E
Pennsburg, *U.S.A.* .. **151 F9** 40 23N 75 29W
Pennsylvania □, *U.S.A.* **148 E7** 40 45N 77 30W
Pennville, *U.S.A.* ... **157 D11** 40 30N 85 9W
Penny, *Canada* **142 C4** 53 51N 121 20W
Peno, *Russia* ...... **58 D7** 57 2N 32 49 E
Penobscot ➝, *U.S.A.* . **149 C11** 44 30N 68 48W
Penobscot B., *U.S.A.* . **149 C11** 44 35N 68 50W
Penola, *Australia* ... **128 D4** 37 25 S 140 48 E
Penong, *Australia* ... **125 F5** 31 56 S 133 1 E

Penonomé, Panama .. 164 E3 8 31N 80 21W
Penot, Mt., Vanuatu .. 133 F5 16 20 S 167 31 E
Penrith, Australia .. 129 B9 33 43 S 150 38 E
Penrith, U.K. 20 C5 54 40N 2 45W
Penryn, U.K. 21 G2 50 9N 5 7W
Pensacola, U.S.A. ... 153 E2 30 25N 87 13W
Pensacola Bay, U.S.A. 153 E2 30 25N 87 5W
Pensacola Mts.,
 Antarctica .... 7 E1 84 0 S 40 0W
Pense, Canada 143 C8 50 25N 104 59W
Penshurst, Australia . 128 D5 37 49 S 142 20 E
Pensiangan, Malaysia . 85 B5 4 33N 116 19 E

Pentecost = Pentecôte,
 Vanuatu .... 133 E6 15 42 S 168 10 E
Pentecoste, Brazil .. 170 B4 3 48 S 39 17W
Pentecôte, Vanuatu .. 133 E6 15 42 S 168 10 E
Penticton, Canada .. 142 D5 49 30N 119 38W
Pentland, Australia .. 126 C4 20 32 S 145 25 E
Pentland Firth, U.K. . 22 C5 58 43N 3 10W
Pentland Hills, U.K. . 22 F5 55 48N 3 25W
Pentland Hills △, U.K. 22 F5 55 50N 3 20W
Penukonda, India .. 95 G3 14 5N 77 38 E
Penza, Russia ..... 60 D7 53 15N 45 5 E
Penzance, U.K. ... 21 G2 50 7N 5 33W
Penzberg, Germany .. 31 H7 47 45N 11 22 E
Penzhino, Russia ... 67 C17 63 30N 167 55 E
Penzhinskaya Guba,
 Russia .... 67 C17 61 30N 163 0 E
Penzhou, China .... 76 B4 31 4N 103 32 E
Penzlin, Germany ... 30 B9 53 30N 13 5 E
Peoria, Ariz., U.S.A. . 159 K7 33 35N 112 14W
Peoria, Ill., U.S.A. .. 156 D7 40 42N 89 36W
Peoria Heights, U.S.A. 156 D7 40 45N 89 35W
Peotone, U.S.A. ... 157 C9 41 20N 87 48W
Pepacton Reservoir,
 U.S.A. 151 D10 42 5N 74 58W
Pepani →, S. Africa .. 116 D3 25 49 S 22 47 E
Pepeekeo, U.S.A. ... 145 D6 19 51N 155 6W
Pepel, S. Leone 112 D2 8 40N 13 5W
Peqin, Albania .... 50 E3 41 3N 19 44 E
Pera Hd., Australia .. 126 A3 12 55 S 141 37 E
Perabumulih, Indonesia 84 C2 3 27 S 104 15 E
Perak □, Malaysia .. 84 A2 5 0N 101 0 E
Perak →, Malaysia .. 87 K3 4 0N 100 50 E
Perakhóra, Greece .. 48 C4 38 2N 22 56 E
Perakhórion, Greece . 39 C2 38 21N 20 43 E
Perales de Alfambra,
 Spain 40 E4 40 38N 1 0W
Perales del Puerto,
 Spain 42 E4 40 10N 6 40W
Pérama, Kérkira,
 Greece .... 38 B9 39 34N 19 54 E
Pérama, Kríti, Greece . 39 E5 35 20N 24 40 E
Perancak, Indonesia .. 79 J17 8 24 S 114 37 E
Perápohjola, Finland . 14 C22 66 16N 26 10 E
Perast, Serbia & M. .. 50 D2 42 31N 18 47 E
Peratía, Greece .... 39 B2 38 49N 20 45 E
Percé, Canada 141 C7 48 31N 64 13W
Perche, France .... 26 D8 48 31N 1 1 E
Perche →, France ... 26 D7 48 24N 0 46 E
Perche, Collines du,
 France .... 25 B4 48 30N 0 40 E
Perchtoldsdorf, Austria 35 C9 48 7N 16 16 E
Percival Lakes,
 Australia .... 124 D4 21 25 S 125 0 E
Percy, France 26 D5 48 55N 1 11W
Percy, U.S.A. 156 F7 38 5N 89 41W
Percy Is., Australia .. 126 C5 21 39 S 150 16 E
Perdido →, Argentina 176 B3 42 55 S 67 0W
Perdido, Mte., Spain .. 40 C5 42 40N 0 5 E
Perdu, Mt. = Perdido,
 Mte., Spain ...... 40 C5 42 40N 0 5 E
Perechyn, Ukraine .. 59 J19 48 44N 22 28 E
Perehinske, Ukraine . 53 B9 48 49N 24 11 E
Pereira, Colombia ... 168 C2 4 49N 75 43W
Peremul Par, India .. 95 J1 11 10N 72 4 E
Peremyshl = Przemyśl,
 Poland .... 55 J9 49 50N 22 45 E
Perené →, Peru .... 172 C3 11 9 S 74 14W
Perenjori, Australia .. 125 E2 29 26 S 116 16 E
Peresecina, Moldova . 53 C13 47 16N 28 46 E
Pereslavl-Zalesskiy,
 Russia .... 58 D10 56 45N 38 50 E
Peretu, Romania .... 53 F10 44 3N 25 5 E
Perevolotskiy, Russia . 64 F5 51 51N 54 12 E
Pereyaslav-
 Khmelnytskyy,
 Ukraine .... 59 G6 50 3N 31 28 E
Pereyma, Ukraine ... 53 B14 48 3N 29 10 E
Pérez, I., Mexico 163 C7 22 24N 89 42W
Perg, Austria ..... 34 C7 48 15N 14 38 E
Pergamino, Argentina 174 C3 33 52 S 60 30W
Pergau →, Malaysia .. 87 K3 5 23N 102 2 E
Pérgine Valsugana,
 Italy .... 45 B8 46 4N 11 14 E
Pérgola, Italy ..... 45 E9 43 34N 12 50 E
Perham, U.S.A. 154 B7 46 36N 95 34W
Perhentian, Kepulauan,
 Malaysia .... 87 K4 5 54N 102 42 E
Periam, Romania ... 52 D5 46 2N 20 52 E
Péribonka →, Canada 141 C5 48 45N 72 5W
Péribonka, L., Canada 141 B5 50 1N 71 10W
Perico, Argentina ... 174 A2 24 20 S 65 5W
Pericos, Mexico 162 C3 25 3N 107 42W
Périers, France 26 C5 49 11N 1 25W
Périgord, France ... 28 D4 45 0N 0 40 E
Périgord-Limousin □,
 France .... 28 C4 45 40N 0 50 E
Périgueux, France ... 28 C4 45 10N 0 42 E
Perijá, Venezuela ... 165 E5 9 30N 72 55W
Perijá, Sierra de,
 Colombia 168 B3 9 30N 73 3W
Perisher Valley,
 Australia .... 129 D8 36 27 S 148 25 E
Peristéra, Greece ... 48 B5 39 15N 23 58 E
Peristerona →, Cyprus 39 E9 35 8N 33 5 E
Perito Moreno,
 Argentina .... 176 C2 46 36 S 70 56W
Perito Moreno △,
 Argentina .... 176 C2 47 49 S 72 17W
Peritoró, Brazil .... 170 B3 4 20 S 44 18W
Perivol =
 Dragovishtitsa,
 Bulgaria .... 50 D6 42 22N 22 39 E
Periyakulam, India .. 95 J3 10 5N 77 32 E
Periyar △, India .... 95 K3 9 22N 77 10 E
Periyar →, India ... 95 J3 10 3N 77 10 E
Periyar, L., India ... 95 K3 9 25N 77 10 E
Perkasie, U.S.A. ... 151 F9 40 22N 75 18W
Perković, Croatia ... 45 E13 43 41N 16 10 E
Perlas, Arch. de las,
 Panama 164 E4 8 41N 79 7W
Perlas, Punta de, Nic. 164 D3 12 30N 83 30W
Perleberg, Germany .. 30 B7 53 5N 11 52 E
Perlez, Serbia & M. .. 52 E5 45 11N 20 22 E
Perlis □, Malaysia ... 84 A2 6 30N 100 15 E
Perm, Russia ...... 60 C10 58 0N 56 10 E
Përmet, Albania .... 50 F4 40 15N 20 21 E
Permskoe =
 Komsomolsk, Russia 67 D14 50 30N 137 0 E
Pernambuco = Recife,
 Brazil .... 170 C5 8 0 S 35 0W
Pernambuco □, Brazil 170 C4 8 0 S 37 0W

Pernambuco Plain,
 Atl. Oc. .... 8 G9 5 0 S 24 0W
Pernatty Lagoon,
 Australia .... 128 A2 31 30 S 137 12 E
Pernik, Bulgaria .... 50 D7 42 35N 23 2 E
Pernov = Pärnu,
 Estonia .... 15 G21 58 28N 24 33 E
Peron Is., Australia .. 124 B5 13 9 S 130 4 E
Peron Pen., Australia . 125 E1 26 0 S 113 10 E
Péronne, France .... 27 C9 49 55N 2 57 E
Perosa Argentina, Italy 44 D4 44 58N 7 10 E
Perow, Canada 142 C3 54 35N 126 10W
Perpignan, France ... 28 F6 42 42N 2 53 E
Perrégaux =
 Mohammadia,
 Algeria .... 111 A5 35 33N 0 3 E
Perrine, U.S.A. 153 K9 25 36N 80 21W
Perris, U.S.A. 161 M9 33 47N 117 14W
Perros-Guirec, France 26 D3 48 49N 3 28W
Perry, Fla., U.S.A. .. 153 F6 30 7N 83 35W
Perry, Ga., U.S.A. .. 153 C6 32 28N 83 44W
Perry, Iowa, U.S.A. .. 156 C2 41 51N 94 6W
Perry, Mich., U.S.A. . 157 B12 42 50N 84 13W
Perry, Mo., U.S.A. .. 156 E5 39 26N 91 40W
Perry, Okla., U.S.A. . 155 C6 36 17N 97 14W
Perrysburg, U.S.A. .. 157 C13 41 34N 83 38W
Perryton, U.S.A. ... 155 G4 36 24N 100 48W
Perryville, Alaska,
 U.S.A. 144 J8 55 55N 159 9W
Perryville, Mo., U.S.A. 155 G10 37 43N 89 52W
Persan, France .... 27 C9 49 9N 2 16 E
Persberg, Sweden ... 16 E8 59 47N 14 15 E
Perşembe, Turkey ... 100 B7 41 5N 37 46 E
Persepolis, Iran .... 97 D7 29 55N 52 50 E
Perseverancia, Bolivia 173 C5 14 44 S 62 48W
Pershotravensk,
 Ukraine .... 59 G4 50 13N 27 40 E
Pershotravneye =
 Pershotravensk,
 Ukraine .... 59 G4 50 13N 27 40 E
Persia = Iran ■, Asia . 97 C7 33 0N 53 0 E
Persian Gulf, Asia ... 97 E6 27 0N 50 0 E
Perstorp, Sweden ... 17 H7 56 10N 13 25 E
Pertek, Turkey .... 101 C8 38 51N 39 19 E
Perth, Australia .... 125 F2 31 57 S 115 52 E
Perth, Canada 140 D4 44 55N 76 15W
Perth, U.K. 22 E5 56 24N 3 26W
Perth & Kinross □,
 U.K. 22 E5 56 45N 3 55W
Perth Amboy, U.S.A. . 151 F10 40 31N 74 16W
Perth-Andover, Canada 141 C6 46 44N 67 42W
Perth Basin, Ind. Oc. 121 H9 30 0 S 95 0 E
Pertuis, France .... 29 E9 43 42N 5 30 E
Pertusato, C., France . 29 G13 41 21N 9 11 E
Peru, Ill., U.S.A. ... 156 C7 41 20N 89 8W
Peru, Ind., U.S.A. .. 157 D10 40 45N 86 4W
Peru, N.Y., U.S.A. .. 151 B11 44 35N 73 32W
Peru ■, S. Amer. ... 168 D2 4 0 S 75 0W
Peru Basin, Pac. Oc. . 135 J18 20 0 S 95 0W
Peru-Chile Trench,
 Pac. Oc. .... 135 K20 20 0 S 72 0W
Perúgia, Italy ..... 45 E9 43 7N 12 23 E
Perušić, Croatia .... 45 D12 44 40N 15 22 E
Pervomaysk, Russia .. 60 C6 54 56N 43 58 E
Pervomaysk, Ukraine . 59 H6 48 10N 30 46 E
Pervomayskiy, Russia 64 F5 51 32N 55 2 E
Pervouralsk, Russia .. 64 C7 56 59N 59 59 E
Pervuralsk =
 Pervouralsk, Russia 64 C7 56 59N 59 59 E
Pésaro, Italy ...... 45 E9 43 54N 12 55 E
Pescadores = P'enghu
 Ch'üntou, Taiwan .. 77 F12 23 34N 119 30 E
Péscara, Italy ..... 45 F11 42 28N 14 13 E
Péscara →, Italy ... 45 F11 42 28N 14 13 E
Peschanokopskoye,
 Russia .... 61 G5 46 14N 41 4 E
Peschanoye = Yashkul,
 Russia .... 61 G7 46 11N 45 21 E
Péscia, Italy ...... 44 E7 43 54N 10 41 E
Pescina, Italy ..... 45 F10 42 2N 13 39 E
Peseux, Switz. ..... 32 C3 46 59N 6 53 E
Peshawar, Pakistan .. 91 B3 34 2N 71 37 E
Peshkopi, Albania ... 50 E4 41 41N 20 25 E
Peshtera, Bulgaria .. 51 D8 42 2N 24 18 E
Peshtigo, U.S.A. ... 148 C2 45 4N 87 46W
Peski, Russia ..... 60 E6 51 14N 42 29 E
Peskovka, Russia ... 64 B4 59 4N 52 22 E
Pêso da Régua,
 Portugal 42 D3 41 10N 7 47W
Pesochnya = Kirov,
 Russia .... 58 E8 54 3N 34 20 E
Pesqueira, Brazil ... 170 C4 8 20 S 36 42W
Pessac, France 28 D3 44 48N 0 37W
Pessádhes, Greece ... 39 C2 38 7N 20 8 E
Pest □, Hungary .... 52 C4 47 29N 19 5 E
Pestovo = Zavolzhye,
 Russia .... 60 B6 56 37N 43 26 E
Pestovo, Russia .... 58 C8 58 33N 35 42 E
Pestravka, Russia ... 60 D9 52 28N 49 57 E
Péta, Greece ...... 48 B3 39 10N 21 2 E
Petah Tiqwa, Israel . 103 C3 32 6N 34 53 E
Petalás, Nísís, Greece 39 C3 38 37N 20 37 E
Petalídhion, Greece .. 48 E3 36 57N 21 55 E
Petaling Jaya, Malaysia 87 L3 3 4N 101 42 E
Petaloúdhes, Greece . 38 C10 36 18N 28 5 E
Petaluma, U.S.A. ... 160 G4 38 14N 122 39W
Pétange, Lux. ..... 24 E5 49 33N 5 55 E
Petaro, Pakistan ... 92 G3 25 31N 68 18 E
Petatlán, Mexico 162 D4 17 31N 101 16W
Petauke, Zambia ... 119 E3 14 14 S 31 20 E
Petawawa, Canada .. 140 C4 45 54N 77 17W
Petén Itzá, L.,
 Guatemala 164 C2 16 58N 89 50W
Peter I., Br. Virgin Is. . 165 e 18 22N 64 35W
Peter I.s Øy, Antarctica 7 C16 69 0 S 91 0W
Peter Pond L., Canada 143 B7 55 55N 108 44W
Peterbell, Canada ... 140 C3 48 36N 83 21W
Peterborough, Australia 128 B3 32 58 S 138 51 E
Peterborough, Canada 140 B6 44 20N 78 20W
Peterborough, U.K. .. 21 E7 52 35N 0 15W
Peterborough, U.S.A. . 151 D13 42 53N 71 57W
Peterborough □, U.K. 21 E7 52 35N 0 15W
Peterculter, U.K. ... 22 D6 57 6N 2 16W
Peterhead, U.K. 22 D7 57 31N 1 48W
Peterhof =
 Petrodvorets, Russia 58 C5 59 52N 29 54 E
Peterlee, U.K. 20 C6 54 47N 1 20W
Petermann Bjerg,
 Greenland 10 C8 73 7N 28 25W
Petermann Gletscher,
 Greenland 10 A4 80 30N 60 0W
Petermann Ranges,
 Australia .... 125 E5 26 0 S 130 30 E
Peter's Mine, Guyana 169 B6 6 14N 59 20W
Petersburg =
 Peterborough,
 Australia .... 128 B3 32 58 S 138 51 E
Petersburg, Alaska,
 U.S.A. 144 H14 56 48N 132 58W
Petersburg, Ill., U.S.A. 156 D7 40 1N 89 51W

Petersburg, Ind., U.S.A. 157 F9 38 30N 87 17W
Petersburg, Mich.,
 U.S.A. 157 C13 41 54N 83 43W
Petersburg, Pa., U.S.A. 150 F6 40 34N 78 3W
Petersburg, Va., U.S.A. 148 G7 37 14N 77 24W
Petersburg, W. Va.,
 U.S.A. 148 F6 39 1N 79 5W
Petersfield, U.K. ... 21 F7 51 1N 0 56W
Petershagen, Germany 30 C4 52 23N 8 58 E
Peterson, U.S.A. ... 150 D7 42 58N 77 3W
Petília Policastro, Italy 47 C9 39 7N 16 48 E
Petit Batanga,
 Cameroon .... 114 B1 3 15N 9 54 E
Petit-Canal,
 Guadeloupe ...... 164 b 16 25N 61 31W
Petit Goâve, Haiti ... 165 C5 18 27N 72 51W
Petit Jardin, Canada . 141 C8 48 28N 59 14W
Petit Lac Manicouagan,
 Canada 141 B6 51 25N 67 40W
Petit-Mécatina →,
 Canada 141 B8 50 40N 59 30W
Petit-Mécatina, Î. du,
 Canada 141 B8 50 30N 59 25W
Petit Piton, St. Lucia . 165 f 13 51N 61 5W
Petit-Saguenay, Canada 141 C5 48 15N 70 4W
Petit Saint Bernard, Col
 du, Italy .... 29 C10 45 40N 6 52 E
Petitcodiac, Canada . 141 C6 45 57N 65 11W
Petite Terre, Îles de la,
 Guadeloupe ...... 164 b 16 13N 61 9W
Petitjean = Sidi Kacem,
 Morocco 110 B3 34 11N 5 49W
Petitot →, Canada .. 142 A4 60 14N 123 29W
Petitsikapau L., Canada 141 B6 54 37N 66 25W
Petlad, India ..... 92 H5 22 30N 72 45 E
Peto, Mexico 163 C7 20 10N 88 53W
Petone, N.Z. ...... 130 H3 41 13 S 174 53 E
Petorca, Chile ..... 174 C1 32 15 S 70 56W
Petoskey, U.S.A. ... 148 C3 45 22N 84 57W
Petra, Jordan ..... 103 E4 30 20N 35 22 E
Petra, Spain ...... 38 B4 39 37N 3 6 E
Petra, Ostrova, Russia 4 B13 76 15N 118 30 E
Petra Velikogo, Zaliv,
 Russia .... 70 C6 42 40N 132 0 E
Petrel = Petrer, Spain 41 G4 38 30N 0 46W
Petrella, Monte, Italy . 46 A6 41 18N 13 40 E
Petrer, Spain 41 G4 38 30N 0 46W
Petreto-Bicchisano,
 France .... 29 G12 41 47N 8 58 E
Petrich, Bulgaria ... 50 E7 41 24N 23 13 E
Petrified Forest △,
 U.S.A. 159 J9 35 0N 109 30W
Petrijanec, Croatia .. 45 B13 46 23N 16 17 E
Petrikov = Pyetrikaw,
 Belarus .... 59 F5 52 11N 28 29 E
Petrila, Romania ... 53 E8 45 29N 23 29 E
Petrinja, Croatia ... 45 C13 45 28N 16 18 E
Petrodvorets, Russia . 58 C5 59 52N 29 54 E
Petrograd = Sankt-
 Peterburg, Russia . 58 C6 59 55N 30 20 E
Petrolândia, Brazil .. 170 C4 9 5 S 38 20W
Petrolia, Canada ... 140 D3 42 54N 82 9W
Petrolina, Brazil ... 170 C3 9 24 S 40 30W
Petromaryevka =
 Petromayevka, Ukraine 59 H6 48 10N 30 46 E
Petropavl, Kazakhstan 66 D7 54 53N 69 13 E
Petropavlovsk =
 Petropavl,
 Kazakhstan ...... 66 D7 54 53N 69 13 E
Petropavlovsk-
 Kamchatskiy, Russia 67 D16 53 3N 158 43 E
Petropavlovskiy =
 Akhtubinsk, Russia . 61 F8 48 13N 46 7 E
Petropavlovskiy =
 Severouralsk, Russia 64 A7 60 9N 59 57 E
Petrópolis, Brazil ... 171 F3 22 33 S 43 9W
Petroşani, Romania . 53 E8 45 28N 23 20 E
Petrova Gora, Croatia 45 C12 45 15N 15 45 E
Petrovac, Serbia & M. 50 D2 42 13N 18 57 E
Petrovac, Serbia & M. 50 B5 44 22N 21 26 E
Petrovaradin,
 Serbia & M. ...... 52 E4 45 16N 19 55 E
Petrovgrad = Zrenjanin,
 Serbia & M. ...... 52 E5 45 22N 20 23 E
Petrovsk, Russia ... 60 D7 52 22N 45 19 E
Petrovsk-Port =
 Makhachkala, Russia 61 J8 43 0N 47 30 E
Petrovsk-Zabaykalskiy,
 Russia .... 67 D11 51 20N 108 55 E
Petrovskaya, Russia . 59 K9 45 25N 37 58 E
Petrovskoye =
 Svetlograd, Russia . 61 H6 45 25N 42 58 E
Petrovskoye, Russia . 64 E6 53 37N 56 23 E
Petrovsky Zavod =
 Petrovsk-
 Zabaykalskiy, Russia 67 D11 51 20N 108 55 E
Petrozavodsk, Russia . 58 B8 61 41N 34 20 E
Petrus Steyn, S. Africa 117 D4 27 38 S 28 8 E
Petrusburg, S. Africa . 116 D4 29 4 S 25 26 E
Petsamo = Pechenga,
 Russia .... 56 A5 69 29N 31 4 E
Petuna = Fuyu, China 75 B13 45 12N 124 43 E
Petzeck, Austria ... 34 E5 46 57N 12 48 E
Peumo, Chile ..... 174 C1 34 21 S 71 12W
Peureulak, Indonesia . 84 B1 4 48N 97 45 E
Pevek, Russia ..... 67 C18 69 41N 171 19 E
Pevely, U.S.A. 156 F6 38 17N 90 24W
Peveragno, Italy ... 44 D4 44 20N 7 37 E
Peyrehorade, France . 28 E2 43 34N 1 7W
Peyruis, France .... 29 D9 44 1N 5 56 E
Pézenas, France .... 28 E7 43 28N 3 24 E
Pezinok, Slovak Rep. . 35 C10 48 17N 17 17 E

Phangnga, Thailand .. 87 H2 8 28N 98 30 E
Phangnga, Ao,
 Thailand .... 87 a 8 16N 98 33 E
Phanom Sarakham,
 Thailand .... 86 F3 13 45N 101 21 E
Phaphund, India ... 93 F8 26 36N 79 28 E
Pharenda, India ... 93 F10 27 5N 83 17 E
Pharr, U.S.A. 155 M5 26 12N 98 11W
Phatthalung, Thailand 87 J3 7 39N 100 6 E
Phayao, Thailand ... 86 C2 19 11N 99 55 E
Phelps, U.S.A. 150 D7 42 58N 77 3W
Phelps L., Canada .. 143 B8 59 15N 103 15W
Phenix City, U.S.A. . 149 J3 32 28N 85 0W
Phet Buri, Thailand . 86 F2 13 1N 99 55 E
Phetchabun, Thailand 86 D3 16 25N 101 8 E
Phetchabun, Thiu
 Khao, Thailand ... 86 E3 16 0N 101 20 E
Phetchaburi = Phet
 Buri, Thailand .... 86 F2 13 1N 99 55 E
Phi Phi, Ko, Thailand . 87 J2 7 45N 98 46 E
Phiafay, Laos ..... 86 E6 14 48N 106 0 E
Phibun Mangsahan,
 Thailand .... 86 E5 15 14N 105 14 E
Phichai, Thailand ... 86 D3 17 22N 100 10 E
Phichit, Thailand ... 86 D3 16 26N 100 22 E
Philadelphia, Miss.,
 U.S.A. 155 J10 32 46N 89 7W
Philadelphia, N.Y.,
 U.S.A. 151 B9 44 9N 75 43W
Philadelphia, Pa.,
 U.S.A. 151 G9 39 57N 75 10W
Philip, U.S.A. 154 C4 44 2N 101 40W
Philip Smith Mts.,
 U.S.A. 144 C11 68 0N 148 0W
Philippeville = Skikda,
 Algeria .... 111 A6 36 50N 6 58 E
Philippeville, Belgium 24 D4 50 12N 4 33 E
Philippi, U.S.A. 148 F5 39 9N 80 3W
Philippi L., Australia . 126 C2 24 20 S 138 55 E
Philippine Sea, Pac. Oc. 62 H16 18 0N 125 0 E
Philippines ■, Asia .. 80 E4 12 0N 123 0 E
Philippolis, S. Africa . 116 E4 30 15 S 25 16 E
Philippopolis = Plovdiv,
 Bulgaria .... 51 D8 42 8N 24 44 E
Philipsburg, Canada . 151 A11 45 2N 73 5W
Philipsburg, Mont.,
 U.S.A. 158 C7 46 20N 113 18W
Philipsburg, Pa., U.S.A. 150 F6 40 54N 78 13W
Philipstown =
 Daingean, Ireland . 23 C4 53 18N 7 17W
Philipstown, S. Africa 116 E3 30 28 S 24 30 E
Phillip I., Australia .. 129 E6 38 30 S 145 12 E
Phillips, U.S.A. 154 C9 45 42N 90 24W
Phillipsburg, Ga.,
 U.S.A. 152 D6 31 25N 83 30W
Phillipsburg, Kans.,
 U.S.A. 154 F5 39 45N 99 19W
Phillipsburg, N.J.,
 U.S.A. 151 F9 40 42N 75 12W
Philmont, U.S.A. ... 151 D11 42 15N 73 39W
Philomath, Ga., U.S.A. 153 H4 33 45N 82 59W
Philomath, Oreg.,
 U.S.A. 158 D2 44 32N 123 22W
Phimai, Thailand ... 86 E4 15 13N 102 30 E
Phitsanulok, Thailand 86 D3 16 50N 100 12 E
Phnom Dangrek,
 Thailand .... 78 B2 14 20N 104 0 E
Phnom Penh,
 Cambodia .... 87 G5 11 33N 104 55 E
Phnum Penh =
 Phnom Penh, Cambodia 87 G5 11 33N 104 55 E
Phoenicia, U.S.A. .. 151 D10 42 5N 74 14W
Phoenix, Mauritius .. 121 d 20 17 S 57 30 E
Phoenix, Ariz., U.S.A. 159 K7 33 27N 112 4W
Phoenix, N.Y., U.S.A. 151 C8 43 14N 76 18W
Phoenix Is., Kiribati . 132 H10 3 30 S 172 0W
Phoenixville, U.S.A. . 151 F9 40 8N 75 31W
Phon, Thailand .... 86 E4 15 49N 102 36 E
Phon Tiou, Laos ... 86 D5 17 53N 104 37 E
Phong →, Thailand . 86 A4 22 32 S 102 9 E
Phong Saly, Laos ... 76 G4 21 42N 102 9 E
Phong Tho, Vietnam . 86 A4 22 32N 103 21 E
Phonhong, Laos .... 86 C4 18 30N 102 25 E
Phonum, Thailand .. 87 H2 8 49N 98 48 E
Phosphate Hill,
 Australia .... 126 C2 21 53 S 139 58 E
Photharam, Thailand 86 F2 13 41N 99 51 E
Phra Nakhon Si
 Ayutthaya, Thailand 86 E3 14 25N 100 30 E
Phra Thong, Ko,
 Thailand .... 87 H2 9 5N 98 17 E
Phrae, Thailand .... 86 C3 18 7N 100 9 E
Phrom Phiram,
 Thailand .... 86 D3 17 2N 100 12 E
Phrygia, Turkey .... 100 C4 38 40N 30 0 E
Phu Bia, Laos ..... 86 C4 19 10N 103 0 E
Phu Chong-Na Yoi △,
 Thailand .... 86 E5 14 25N 105 30 E
Phu Dien, Vietnam .. 86 C5 18 58N 105 31 E
Phu Hin Rang Kla △,
 Thailand .... 86 D3 16 59N 101 0 E
Phu Kradung △,
 Thailand .... 86 D3 17 2N 101 44 E
Phu Loi, Laos ..... 86 B4 20 14N 103 14 E
Phu Luang △, Thailand 86 D3 17 15N 101 29 E
Phu Ly, Vietnam ... 76 G5 20 35N 105 50 E
Phu Phan △, Thailand 86 D4 17 0N 103 56 E
Phu Quoc, Dao,
 Vietnam .... 87 G4 10 20N 104 0 E
Phu Tho, Vietnam .. 76 G5 21 24N 105 13 E
Phuc Yen, Vietnam .. 76 G5 21 16N 105 45 E
Phuket, Thailand ... 87 a 7 53N 98 24 E
Phuket, Ko, Thailand . 87 a 8 0N 98 22 E
Phul, India .... 92 D6 30 19N 75 14 E
Phulad, India ..... 92 G5 25 38N 73 49 E
Phulbani, India .... 94 D7 20 28N 84 14 E
Phulbari, India .... 90 C3 25 55N 90 2 E
Phulchari, Bangla. .. 90 C2 25 11N 89 37 E
Phulera, India ..... 92 F6 26 52N 75 16 E
Phulpur, India ..... 93 G10 25 31N 82 49 E
Phun Phin, Thailand 87 H2 9 7N 99 12 E
Phuntsholing, Bhutan 93 F9 7 42 S 47 18 E
Piacá, Brazil ...... 170 C2 7 42 S 47 18 E
Piacenza, Italy ..... 44 C6 45 1N 9 40 E
Piaçabuçu, Brazil ... 170 D4 10 24 S 36 25W
Piai, Tanjung, Malaysia 87 d 1 15N 103 31 E
Piako →, N.Z. ..... 130 D4 37 12 S 175 30 E
Piana, France ..... 29 F12 42 15N 8 34 E
Piangil, Australia ... 128 C5 35 5 S 143 20 E
Pian-Upe ☐, Uganda . 118 B3 1 44N 34 20 E
Pianella, Italy ..... 45 F11 42 24N 14 2 E
Piangil, Australia ... 128 C5 35 5 S 143 20 E
Pianosa, Puglia, Italy . 45 F12 42 12N 15 44 E
Pianosa, Toscana, Italy 44 F7 42 35N 10 5 E
Pias, Portugal 43 G3 38 1N 7 29W
Piaski, Poland ..... 55 F7 52 12N 20 48 E
Piastów, Poland .... 55 F7 52 12N 20 48 E
Piatã, Brazil ...... 171 D3 13 9 S 41 48W
Piatra, Romania ... 53 G10 43 51N 25 9 E
Piatra Craiului △,
 Romania .... 53 E10 45 30N 25 12 E
Piatra Neamţ, Romania 53 D11 46 56N 26 21 E

Piatra Olt, Romania . 53 F9 44 22N 24 16 E
Piauí □, Brazil .... 170 C3 7 0 S 43 0W
Piauí →, Brazil .... 170 C3 6 38 S 42 42W
Piave →, Italy ..... 45 C9 45 32N 12 44 E
Piazza Ármerina, Italy 47 E7 37 21N 14 20 E
Pibor →, Sudan .... 107 F3 7 35N 33 0 E
Pibor Post, Sudan .. 107 F3 6 47N 33 3 E
Pica, Chile .... 172 E4 20 35 S 69 25W
Picardie □, France .. 27 C10 49 50N 3 0 E
Picardie, Plaine de,
 France .... 27 C9 50 0N 2 0 E
Picardy = Picardie □,
 France .... 27 C10 49 50N 3 0 E
Picayune, U.S.A. ... 155 K10 30 32N 89 41W
Picerno, Italy ..... 47 B8 40 38N 15 38 E
Pichhor, India ..... 93 G8 25 58N 78 20 E
Pichilemu, Chile ... 174 C1 34 22 S 72 0W
Pichincha □, Ecuador 168 D2 0 10 S 78 40W
Pichor, India ...... 92 G8 25 11N 78 11 E
Pickerel L., Canada .. 140 C1 48 40N 91 25W
Pickering, U.K. 20 C7 54 15N 0 46W
Pickering, Vale of, U.K. 20 C7 54 14N 0 45W
Pickle Lake, Canada . 138 B1 51 30N 90 12W
Pickwick L., U.S.A. . 149 H1 35 4N 88 15W
Pico, Azores 9 d1 38 28N 28 20W
Pico, Ponta do, Azores 9 d1 38 28N 28 20W
Pico Bonito △,
 Honduras 164 C2 15 34N 86 48W
Pico da Neblina △,
 Brazil 168 C4 0 19N 66 28W
Pico Truncado,
 Argentina .... 176 C3 46 40 S 68 0W
Picos, Brazil ...... 170 C3 7 5 S 41 28W
Picos de Europa △,
 Spain 42 B6 43 14N 4 59W
Picota, Peru ...... 172 B2 6 54 S 76 22W
Picton, Australia ... 129 C9 34 12 S 150 34 E
Picton, Canada 140 D4 44 1N 77 9W
Picton, N.Z. ...... 131 B9 41 18 S 174 3 E
Picton, I., Chile .... 176 E3 55 2 S 66 57W
Pictou, Canada 141 C7 45 41N 62 42W
Picture Butte, Canada 142 D6 49 55N 112 45W
Pictured Rocks △,
 U.S.A. 148 B2 46 30N 86 30W
Picuí, Brazil ...... 170 C4 6 31 S 36 21W
Picún Leufú, Argentina 176 A3 39 30 S 69 5W
Pidbuzh, Ukraine ... 55 J10 49 19N 23 14 E
Pidurutalagala,
 Sri Lanka .... 95 L5 7 10N 80 50 E
Piechowice, Poland .. 55 H2 50 51N 15 36 E
Piedecuesta, Colombia 168 B3 6 59N 73 3W
Piedimonte Matese,
 Italy .... 47 A7 41 22N 14 22 E
Piedmont =
 Piemonte □, Italy .. 44 D5 45 0N 8 0 E
Piedmont, Ala., U.S.A. 152 B4 33 55N 85 37W
Piedmont, S.C., U.S.A. 147 D10 34 0N 81 30W
Piedra →, Spain ... 40 D3 41 18N 1 47W
Piedra del Anguila,
 Argentina .... 176 B2 40 2 S 70 4W
Piedra Lais, Venezuela 168 C4 3 10N 65 50W
Piedrabuena, Spain . 43 G6 39 0N 4 10W
Piedrahita, Spain ... 42 E5 40 28N 5 23W
Piedralaves, Spain .. 42 E6 40 19N 4 42W
Piedras, R. de las →,
 Peru .... 172 C4 12 30 S 69 15W
Piedras Blancas, Spain 42 B5 43 33N 5 58W
Piedras Negras, Mexico 162 B4 28 42N 100 31W
Piedras Pt., Phil. ... 81 F2 10 11N 118 48 E
Piekar = Piekary
 Śląskie, Poland ... 55 H5 50 24N 18 57 E
Piekary Śląskie, Poland 55 H5 50 24N 18 57 E
Pieksämäki, Finland . 15 E22 62 18N 27 10 E
Piemonte □, Italy .. 44 D5 45 0N 8 0 E
Pienaarsrivier, S. Africa 117 D4 25 15 S 28 18 E
Pieniężno, Poland .. 55 G4 54 14N 20 8 E
Pieniński △, Europe . 35 B13 49 25N 20 28 E
Pieńsk, Poland .... 55 G2 51 16N 15 2 E
Piercefield, U.S.A. .. 151 B10 44 13N 74 35W
Pierceland, Canada . 143 C7 54 20N 109 46W
Pieria □, Greece ... 50 F6 40 13N 22 25 E
Pierport, U.S.A. ... 150 E4 41 45N 80 34W
Pierre, U.S.A. 154 C4 44 22N 100 21W
Pierre-Buffiere, France 28 C5 45 41N 1 22 E
Pierre-de-Bresse,
 France .... 27 F12 46 54N 5 13 E
Pierrefontaine-les-
 Varans, France .... 27 E13 47 14N 6 32 E
Pierrefort, France ... 28 D6 44 55N 2 50 E
Pierrelatte, France .. 29 D8 44 23N 4 43 E
Pierreville, Trin. & Tob. 169 F9 10 16N 61 0W
Pierson, U.S.A. 153 F8 29 14N 81 28W
Pieštany, Slovak Rep. . 35 C10 48 38N 17 55 E
Pieszyce, Poland ... 55 H3 50 43N 16 33 E
Piet Retief, S. Africa . 117 D5 27 1 S 30 50 E
Pietarsaari, Finland . 14 E20 63 40N 22 43 E
Pietermaritzburg,
 S. Africa .... 117 D5 29 35 S 30 25 E
Pietersburg =
 Polokwane, S. Africa 117 C4 23 54 S 29 25 E
Pietragalla, Italy ... 47 B8 40 45N 15 53 E
Pietrasanta, Italy ... 44 E7 43 57N 10 14 E
Pietroşia, Romania .. 53 E10 45 11N 25 26 E
Pietrosul, Vf.,
 Maramureş, Romania 53 C9 47 35N 24 43 E
Pietrosul, Vf., Suceava,
 Romania .... 53 C10 47 12N 25 18 E
Pieve di Cadore, Italy . 45 B9 46 26N 12 22 E
Pieve di Teco, Italy .. 44 D4 44 3N 7 56 E
Pievepélago, Italy ... 44 D7 44 12N 10 37 E
Pigadhítsa, Greece .. 50 G5 39 59N 21 23 E
Pigeon I., India .... 95 G2 14 2N 74 20 E
Pigeon L., Canada .. 150 B6 44 27N 78 30W
Pigna, Italy ...... 44 E4 43 56N 7 40 E
Pigüe, Argentina ... 174 D3 37 36 S 62 25W
Piha, N.Z. .... 130 C3 36 57 S 174 28 E
Pihani, India ...... 93 F9 27 36N 80 15 E
Pihlajavesi, Finland . 15 F23 61 45N 28 45 E
Pijijiapan, Mexico .. 163 D6 15 42N 93 14W
Pikalevo, Russia ... 58 C9 59 30N 34 0 E
Pikangikum Berens,
 Canada 143 C10 51 49N 94 0W
Pikes Peak, U.S.A. .. 154 F2 38 50N 105 3W
Piketberg, S. Africa .. 116 E2 32 55 S 18 40 E
Pikeville, U.S.A. ... 148 G4 37 29N 82 31W
Pikit, Phil. .... 81 H5 7 4N 124 41 E
Pikou, China ..... 75 E12 39 18N 122 22 E
Pikounda, Congo ... 114 B3 0 30N 16 44 E
Pikwitonei, Canada . 143 B9 55 35N 97 9W
Piła, Poland ...... 55 E3 53 10N 16 48 E
Pilaía, Greece ..... 50 F6 40 32N 22 59 E
Pilanesberg △, S. Africa 117 D4 25 15 S 27 4 E
Pilani, India ...... 92 E6 28 22N 75 33 E
Pilar, Brazil ...... 170 C4 9 36 S 35 56W
Pilar, Paraguay .... 174 B4 26 50 S 58 20W
Pilar, Cap d', Phil. .. 81 F5 11 29N 123 0 E
Pilar, Sorsogon, Phil. . 80 E4 12 56N 123 40 E
Pilar de la Horadada,
 Spain 41 H4 37 52N 0 47W
Pilas Group, Phil. ... 81 H5 6 45N 121 35 E

Pilat ⌂, *France* **29 C8** 45 20N 4 30 E
Pilawa, *Poland* **55 G8** 51 57N 21 32 E
Pilaya →, *Bolivia* **173 E5** 20 55 S 64 4W
Pilbara, *Australia* **124 D2** 23 35 S 117 25 E
Pilcomayo →, *Paraguay* **174 B4** 25 21 S 57 42W
Pilgrim's Rest, *S. Africa* **117 C5** 24 55 S 30 44 E
Pilgrimstad, *Sweden* **16 B9** 62 57N 15 2 E
Pílí, *Greece* **49 E9** 36 50N 27 15 E
Pili, *Phil.* **80 E4** 13 33N 123 19 E
Pilibhit, *India* **93 E8** 28 40N 79 50 E
Pilica →, *Poland* **55 G8** 51 52N 21 17 E
Pilion, *Greece* **48 B5** 39 27N 23 3 E
Pilipinas = Philippines ■, *Asia* **80 E4** 12 0N 123 0 E
Pilis, *Hungary* **52 C4** 47 17N 19 35 E
Pilisvörösvár, *Hungary* **52 C3** 47 38N 18 56 E
Pilkhawa, *India* **92 E7** 28 43N 77 42 E
Pillar B., *Ascension I.* **9 g** 7 59 S 14 21W
Pillaro, *Ecuador* **168 D2** 1 10 S 78 32W
Pillau = Baltiysk, *Russia* **15 J18** 54 41N 19 58 E
Pilliga, *Australia* **127 E4** 30 21 S 148 54 E
Pílos, *Greece* **48 E3** 36 55N 21 42 E
Pilot Grove, *U.S.A.* **156 F4** 38 53N 92 55W
Pilot Mound, *Canada* **143 D9** 49 15N 98 54W
Pilot Point, *Alaska, U.S.A.* **144 H8** 57 34N 157 35W
Pilot Point, *Tex., U.S.A.* **155 J6** 33 24N 96 58W
Pilot Rock, *U.S.A.* **158 D4** 45 29N 118 50W
Pilot Station, *U.S.A.* **144 F7** 61 56N 162 53W
Pilsen = Pilzno, *Poland* **55 J8** 49 58N 21 16 E
Pilsen = Plzeň, *Czech Rep.* **34 B6** 49 45N 13 22 E
Pilštanj, *Slovenia* **45 B12** 46 8N 15 39 E
Piltene, *Latvia* **54 A8** 57 13N 21 40 E
Pilzno, *Poland* **55 J8** 49 58N 21 16 E
Pima, *U.S.A.* **159 K9** 32 54N 109 50W
Pimba, *Australia* **128 A2** 31 18 S 136 46 E
Pimenta Bueno, *Brazil* **173 C5** 11 35 S 61 10W
Pimenteiras, *Brazil* **173 C5** 13 40 S 60 58W
Pimentel, *Peru* **172 B2** 6 45 S 79 55W
Pimu, *Dem. Rep. of the Congo* **114 B4** 1 42N 20 58 E
Pin Valley △, *India* **92 D7** 31 50N 77 50 E
Pina de Ebro, *Spain* **40 D4** 41 29N 0 33W
Pinamalayan, *Phil.* **80 E3** 13 2N 121 29 E
Pinang, *Malaysia* **87 c** 5 25N 100 15 E
Pinang □, *Malaysia* **84 A2** 5 20N 100 20 E
Pinar, C. des, *Spain* **38 B4** 39 53N 3 12 E
Pinar del Río, *Cuba* **164 B3** 22 26N 83 40W
Pınarbaşı, *Çanakkale, Turkey* **49 B8** 39 53N 26 15 E
Pınarbaşı, *Kayseri, Turkey* **100 C7** 38 43N 36 23 E
Pınarhisar, *Turkey* **51 E11** 41 37N 27 30 E
Pinatubo, Mt., *Phil.* **80 D3** 15 8N 120 21 E
Pincehely, *Hungary* **52 D3** 46 41N 18 27 E
Pinchang, *China* **76 B6** 31 36N 107 3 E
Pincher Creek, *Canada* **142 D6** 49 30N 113 57W
Pinchi L., *Canada* **142 C4** 54 38N 124 30W
Pinckard, *U.S.A.* **152 D4** 31 19N 85 33W
Pinckneyville, *U.S.A.* **156 F7** 38 5N 89 23W
Pińczów, *Poland* **55 H7** 50 32N 20 32 E
Pindaï, Presqu'île de, *N. Cal.* **133 U18** 21 20 S 164 56 E
Pindar, *Australia* **125 E2** 28 30 S 115 47 E
Pindaré →, *Brazil* **170 B3** 3 17 S 44 47W
Pindaré Mirim, *Brazil* **170 B2** 3 37 S 45 21W
Pindi Gheb, *Pakistan* **92 C5** 33 14N 72 21 E
Pindiga, *Nigeria* **113 D7** 9 58N 10 53 E
Pindobal, *Brazil* **170 B2** 3 16 S 48 25W
Pindos △, *Greece* **48 B3** 39 52N 21 11 E
Pindos Óros, *Greece* **48 B3** 40 0N 21 0 E
Pindus Mts. = Pindos Óros, *Greece* **48 B3** 40 0N 21 0 E
Pine →, *B.C., Canada* **142 B4** 56 8N 120 43W
Pine →, *Sask., Canada* **143 B7** 58 50N 105 38W
Pine, C., *Canada* **141 C9** 46 37N 53 32W
Pine Bluff, *U.S.A.* **155 H9** 34 13N 92 1W
Pine Bluffs, *U.S.A.* **154 E2** 41 11N 104 4W
Pine City, *U.S.A.* **154 C8** 45 50N 92 59W
Pine Cr. →, *U.S.A.* **150 E7** 41 10N 77 16W
Pine Creek, *Australia* **124 B5** 13 50 S 131 50 E
Pine Falls, *Canada* **143 C9** 50 34N 96 11W
Pine Flat Res., *U.S.A.* **160 J7** 36 50N 119 20W
Pine Grove, *U.S.A.* **151 F8** 40 33N 76 23W
Pine Is., *U.S.A.* **153 J7** 26 36N 82 7W
Pine Level, *U.S.A.* **152 C3** 32 4N 86 4W
Pine Mountain, *U.S.A.* **152 C5** 32 52N 84 51W
Pine Pass, *Canada* **142 B4** 55 25N 122 42W
Pine Point, *Canada* **142 A6** 60 50N 114 28W
Pine Ridge, *Australia* **129 A9** 31 30 S 150 28 E
Pine Ridge, *U.S.A.* **154 D3** 43 2N 102 33W
Pine River, *Canada* **143 C8** 51 45N 100 30W
Pine River, *U.S.A.* **154 B7** 46 43N 94 24W
Pine Valley, *U.S.A.* **161 N10** 32 50N 116 32W
Pinecrest, *U.S.A.* **160 G6** 38 12N 120 1W
Pineda de Mar, *Spain* **40 D7** 41 37N 2 42 E
Pinedale, *Calif., U.S.A.* **160 J7** 36 50N 119 48W
Pinedale, *Wyo., U.S.A.* **158 E9** 42 52N 109 52W
Pinega →, *Russia* **56 B8** 64 30N 44 19 E
Pinehill, *Australia* **126 C4** 23 38 S 146 57 E
Pinehouse L., *Canada* **143 B7** 55 32N 106 35W
Pineimuta →, *Canada* **140 B1** 52 8N 88 33W
Pinellas Park, *U.S.A.* **153 H7** 27 50N 82 43W
Pinerolo, *Italy* **44 D4** 44 53N 7 21 E
Pines, Ákra = Pínnes, Ákra, *Greece* **51 F8** 40 5N 24 20 E
Pineto, *Italy* **45 F11** 42 36N 14 4 E
Pinetop-Lakeside, *U.S.A.* **159 J9** 34 9N 109 58W
Pinetown, *S. Africa* **117 D5** 29 48 S 30 54 E
Pinetta, *U.S.A.* **152 E6** 30 36N 83 21W
Pineview, *U.S.A.* **152 C6** 32 7N 83 30W
Pineville, *La., U.S.A.* **155 K8** 31 19N 92 26W
Pineville, *S.C., U.S.A.* **152 B9** 33 26N 80 1W
Pinewood, *U.S.A.* **152 B9** 33 44N 80 27W
Piney, *France* **27 D11** 48 22N 4 21 E
Ping →, *Thailand* **86 E3** 15 42N 100 9 E
Pingaring, *Australia* **125 F2** 32 40 S 118 32 E
Pingba, *China* **76 D6** 26 23N 106 12 E
Pingbian, *China* **76 F4** 23 0N 103 45 E
Pingchuan, *China* **76 D3** 27 35N 101 55 E
Pingding, *China* **74 F7** 37 47N 113 38 E
Pingdingshan, *China* **74 H7** 33 43N 113 27 E
Pingdong, *Taiwan* **77 F13** 22 39N 120 30 E
Pingdu, *China* **75 F10** 36 42N 119 59 E
Pingelly, *Australia* **125 F2** 32 32 S 117 5 E
Pingguo, *China* **76 F6** 23 19N 107 36 E
Pinghe, *China* **77 E11** 24 17N 117 21 E
Pinghu, *China* **77 B13** 30 40N 121 2 E
Pingjiang, *China* **77 C9** 28 45N 113 36 E
Pingle, *China* **77 E8** 24 40N 110 40 E
Pingli, *China* **76 A7** 32 27N 109 22 E
Pingliang, *China* **74 G4** 35 35N 106 31 E
Pinglu, *China* **74 E7** 39 31N 112 30 E
Pingluo, *China* **74 E4** 38 52N 106 30 E
Pingnan, *Fujian, China* **77 D12** 26 55N 119 0 E
Pingnan, *Guangxi Zhuangzu, China* **77 F8** 23 33N 110 22 E
Pingo, *Gabon* **114 C2** 1 19 S 10 55 E
Pingquan, *China* **75 D10** 41 1N 118 37 E
Pingrup, *Australia* **125 F2** 33 32 S 118 29 E
Pingshan, *China* **76 C5** 28 39N 104 3 E
Pingtan, *China* **77 E12** 25 31N 119 47 E
Pingtang, *China* **76 E6** 25 49N 107 17 E
P'ingtung, *Taiwan* **77 F13** 22 38N 120 30 E
Pingwu, *China* **74 H3** 32 25N 104 30 E
Pingxiang, *Guangxi Zhuangzu, China* **76 F6** 22 6N 106 46 E
Pingxiang, *Jiangxi, China* **77 D9** 27 43N 113 48 E
Pingyao, *China* **74 F7** 37 12N 112 10 E
Pingyi, *China* **75 G9** 35 30N 117 35 E
Pingyin, *China* **74 F9** 36 20N 116 25 E
Pingyuan, *Guangdong, China* **77 E10** 24 37N 115 57 E
Pingyuan, *Shandong, China* **74 F9** 37 10N 116 22 E
Pingyuanjie, *China* **76 F4** 23 45N 103 48 E
Pinhal, *Brazil* **175 A6** 22 10 S 46 46W
Pinhal Novo, *Portugal* **43 G2** 38 38N 8 55W
Pinheiro = Icoraci, *Brazil* **170 B2** 1 18 S 48 28W
Pinheiro, *Brazil* **170 B2** 2 31 S 45 5W
Pinheiro Machado, *Brazil* **175 C5** 31 34 S 53 23W
Pinhel, *Portugal* **42 E3** 40 50N 7 1W
Pinhuá →, *Brazil* **173 B4** 6 21 S 65 0W
Pini, *Indonesia* **84 B1** 0 10N 98 40 E
Piniós →, *Ilía, Greece* **48 D3** 37 48N 21 20 E
Piniós →, *Tríkkala, Greece* **48 B4** 39 55N 22 41 E
Pinjarra, *Australia* **125 F2** 32 37 S 115 52 E
Pink Mountain, *Canada* **142 B4** 57 3N 122 52W
Pinkafeld, *Austria* **35 D9** 47 22N 16 9 E
Pinlaung, *Burma* **90 E6** 20 8N 96 47 E
Pinlebu, *Burma* **90 C5** 24 5N 95 22 E
Pinnacles, *U.S.A.* **160 J5** 36 33N 121 19W
Pinnacles ⌂, *U.S.A.* **160 J5** 36 25N 121 12W
Pinnaroo, *Australia* **128 C4** 35 17 S 140 53 E
Pinneberg, *Germany* **30 B5** 53 40N 9 48 E
Pínnes, Ákra, *Greece* **51 F8** 40 5N 24 20 E
Pino Hachado, Paso, *S. Amer.* **176 A2** 38 39 S 70 54W
Pinon Hills, *U.S.A.* **161 L9** 34 26N 117 39W
Pinos, *Mexico* **162 C4** 22 20N 101 40W
Pinos, Mt., *U.S.A.* **161 L7** 34 49N 119 8W
Pinos Pt., *U.S.A.* **159 H3** 36 38N 121 57W
Pinos Puente, *Spain* **43 H7** 37 15N 3 45W
Pinotepa Nacional, *Mexico* **163 D5** 16 19N 98 3W
Pinrang, *Indonesia* **82 B1** 3 46 S 119 41 E
Pins, Î. des, *N. Cal.* **133 V21** 22 37 S 167 30 E
Pins, Pte. aux, *Canada* **150 D3** 42 15N 81 51W
Pinsk, *Belarus* **59 F4** 52 10N 26 1 E
Pinta, Canal de, *Ecuador* **172 a** 0 27N 90 38W
Pinta, I., *Ecuador* **172 a** 0 35N 90 44W
Pintados, *Chile* **172 E4** 20 35 S 69 40W
Pintuyan, *Phil.* **81 G5** 9 57N 125 15 E
Pinukpuk, *Phil.* **80 C3** 17 35N 121 22 E
Pinyang, *China* **77 D13** 27 42N 120 31 E
Pinyug, *Russia* **64 A1** 60 5N 48 0 E
Pio Duran, *Phil.* **80 E4** 13 2N 123 25 E
Pio V. Corpuz, *Phil.* **81 F5** 11 55N 124 2 E
Pio XII, *Brazil* **170 B2** 3 53 S 45 17W
Pioche, *U.S.A.* **159 H6** 37 56N 114 27W
Piombino, *Italy* **44 F7** 42 55N 10 32 E
Piombino, Canale di, *Italy* **44 F7** 42 53N 10 30 E
Pioner, Ostrov, *Russia* **67 B10** 79 50N 92 0 E
Pionerskiy, *Russia* **54 D7** 54 56N 20 14 E
Pionki, *Poland* **55 G8** 51 29N 21 28 E
Piorini →, *Brazil* **169 D5** 3 23 S 63 30W
Piorini, L., *Brazil* **169 D5** 3 15 S 62 35W
Piotrków Trybunalski, *Poland* **55 G6** 51 23N 19 43 E
Piove di Sacco, *Italy* **45 C9** 45 18N 12 2 E
Pīp, *Iran* **97 E9** 26 45N 60 10 E
Pipar, *India* **92 F5** 26 25N 73 31 E
Pipar Road, *India* **92 F5** 26 27N 73 27 E
Piparia, *Mad. P., India* **92 H8** 22 45N 78 23 E
Piparia, *Mad. P., India* **92 J7** 21 49N 77 37 E
Pipas, *Angola* **115 E2** 14 57 S 12 11 E
Pipéri, *Greece* **48 B6** 39 20N 24 19 E
Piperno = Priverno, *Italy* **46 A6** 41 28N 13 11 E
Pipestone, *U.S.A.* **154 D6** 44 0N 96 19W
Pipestone →, *Canada* **140 B2** 52 53N 89 23W
Pipestone Cr. →, *Canada* **143 D8** 49 38N 100 15W
Pipiriki, *N.Z.* **130 F4** 39 28 S 175 5 E
Piplan, *Pakistan* **92 C4** 32 17N 71 21 E
Piploda, *India* **92 H6** 23 37N 74 56 E
Pipmuacan, Rés., *Canada* **141 C5** 49 45N 70 30W
Pippingarra, *Australia* **124 D2** 20 27 S 118 42 E
Pipriac, *France* **26 E5** 47 59N 1 58W
Piqua, *U.S.A.* **157 D12** 40 9N 84 15W
Piquet Carneiro, *Brazil* **170 C4** 5 48 S 39 25W
Piquiri →, *Brazil* **175 A5** 24 3 S 54 14W
Pir Panjal Range, *India* **92 C7** 32 30N 76 50 E
Pīr Sohrāb, *Iran* **97 E9** 25 44N 60 54 E
Pira, *Benin* **113 D5** 8 28N 1 48 E
Piracanjuba, *Brazil* **171 E2** 17 18 S 49 1W
Piracicaba, *Brazil* **175 A6** 22 45 S 47 40W
Piracuruca, *Brazil* **170 B3** 3 50 S 41 50W
Piræus = Piraiévs, *Greece* **48 D5** 37 57N 23 42 E
Piraiévs, *Greece* **48 D5** 37 57N 23 42 E
Pirajuí, *Brazil* **175 A6** 21 59 S 49 29W
Piram I., *India* **92 J5** 21 36N 72 21 E
Piran, *Slovenia* **45 C10** 45 31N 13 33 E
Pirané, *Argentina* **174 B4** 25 42 S 59 6W
Piranhas, *Brazil* **170 C4** 9 27 S 37 46W
Pirano = Piran, *Slovenia* **45 C10** 45 31N 13 33 E
Pirapemas, *Brazil* **170 B3** 3 43 S 44 14W
Pirapora, *Brazil* **171 E3** 17 20 S 44 56W
Pirara, *Guyana* **169 C6** 3 37N 59 40W
Pirawa, *India* **92 G7** 24 10N 76 2 E
Piray →, *Bolivia* **173 D5** 16 32 S 63 45W
Pirdop, *Bulgaria* **51 D8** 42 40N 24 10 E
Pireas = Piraiévs, *Greece* **48 D5** 37 57N 23 42 E
Pires do Rio, *Brazil* **171 E2** 17 18 S 48 17W
Pirganj, *Bangla.* **90 C2** 25 51N 88 24 E
Pírgos, *Ilía, Greece* **48 D3** 37 40N 21 27 E
Pírgos, *Kríti, Greece* **39 E6** 35 0N 25 9 E
Pirgovo, *Bulgaria* **51 C9** 43 44N 25 43 E
Piribebuy, *Paraguay* **174 B4** 25 26 S 57 2W
Pirimapun, *Indonesia* **83 C5** 6 20 S 138 24 E
Pirin △, *Bulgaria* **50 E7** 41 48N 23 22 E
Pirin Planina, *Bulgaria* **50 E7** 41 40N 23 30 E
Pírineos = Pyrénées, *Europe* **28 F4** 42 45N 0 18 E
Piripiri, *Brazil* **170 B3** 4 15 S 41 46W
Piritu, *Venezuela* **168 B4** 9 23N 69 12W
Pirmasens, *Germany* **31 F3** 49 12N 7 36 E
Pirna, *Germany* **30 E9** 50 57N 13 56 E
Pirojpur, *Bangla.* **90 D3** 22 35N 90 1 E
Pirot, *Serbia & M.* **50 C6** 43 9N 22 33 E
Piru, *Indonesia* **82 B3** 3 4 S 128 12 E
Piru, *U.S.A.* **161 L8** 34 25N 118 48W
Piryatin = Pyryatyn, *Ukraine* **59 G7** 50 15N 32 25 E
Piryí, *Greece* **49 C7** 38 13N 25 59 E
Pisa, *Italy* **44 E7** 43 43N 10 23 E
Pisa →, *Poland* **55 E8** 53 14N 21 52 E
Pisa, Firenze ✈ (PSA), *Italy* **44 E7** 43 40N 10 22 E
Pisa Ra., *N.Z.* **131 E4** 44 52 S 169 12 E
Pisac, *Peru* **172 C3** 13 25 S 71 50W
Pisagne, *Italy* **44 C7** 45 45N 10 10 E
Pisagua, *Chile* **172 D3** 19 40 S 70 15W
Pisarovina, *Croatia* **45 C12** 45 35N 15 50 E
Pisau, Tanjong, *Malaysia* **85 A5** 6 4N 117 59 E
Pisba △, *Colombia* **168 A3** 10 39N 74 30W
Pisco, *Peru* **172 C2** 13 50 S 76 12W
Piscu, *Romania* **53 E12** 45 30N 27 43 E
Písek, *Czech Rep.* **34 B7** 49 19N 14 10 E
Pishan, *China* **68 C2** 37 30N 78 33 E
Pishcha, *Ukraine* **55 G10** 51 35N 23 50 E
Pishchanka, *Ukraine* **53 B13** 48 12N 28 54 E
Pīshīn, *Iran* **97 E9** 26 6N 61 47 E
Pishin, *Pakistan* **92 D2** 30 35N 67 0 E
Pishin Lora →, *Pakistan* **92 E1** 29 9N 64 5 E
Pishpek = Bishkek, *Kyrgyzstan* **65 B7** 42 54N 74 46 E
Pisidia, *Turkey* **100 D4** 37 30N 31 40 E
Pising, *Indonesia* **82 C2** 5 8 S 121 53 E
Pismo Beach, *U.S.A.* **161 K6** 35 9N 120 38W
Piso, L., *Liberia* **112 D2** 6 50N 11 15W
Pissila, *Burkina Faso* **113 C4** 13 7N 0 50W
Pissis, Cerro, *Argentina* **174 B2** 27 45 S 68 48W
Pissos, *France* **28 D3** 44 19N 0 49W
Pissouri, *Cyprus* **39 F8** 34 40N 32 42 E
Pisticci, *Italy* **47 B9** 40 23N 16 33 E
Pistóia, *Italy* **44 E7** 43 55N 10 54 E
Pistol B., *Canada* **143 A10** 62 25N 92 37W
Pisuerga →, *Spain* **42 D6** 41 33N 4 52W
Pisz, *Poland* **54 E8** 53 38N 21 49 E
Pit →, *U.S.A.* **158 F2** 40 47N 122 6W
Pita, *Guinea* **112 C2** 11 5N 12 15W
Pitalito, *Colombia* **168 C2** 1 51N 76 2W
Pitanga, *Brazil* **171 F1** 24 46 S 51 44W
Pitangui, *Brazil* **171 E3** 19 40 S 44 54W
Pitarpunga, L., *Australia* **128 C5** 34 24 S 143 30 E
Pitcairn I., *Pac. Oc.* **135 K14** 25 5 S 130 5W
Pitch L., *Trin. & Tob.* **169 F9** 10 12N 61 39W
Piteå, *Sweden* **14 D19** 65 20N 21 25 E
Piteälven →, *Sweden* **14 D19** 65 20N 21 25 E
Piterka, *Russia* **60 E8** 50 41N 47 29 E
Piteşti, *Romania* **53 F9** 44 52N 24 54 E
Pithapuram, *India* **94 F6** 17 10N 82 15 E
Pithara, *Australia* **125 F2** 30 20 S 116 35 E
Píthion, *Greece* **51 E10** 41 24N 26 40 E
Pithiviers, *France* **27 D9** 48 10N 2 13 E
Pithora, *India* **94 D6** 21 16N 82 31 E
Pithoragarh, *India* **93 E9** 29 35N 80 13 E
Pithoro, *Pakistan* **92 G3** 25 31N 69 23 E
Pitigliano, *Italy* **45 F8** 42 38N 11 40 E
Pitkyaranta, *Russia* **58 B6** 61 34N 31 37 E
Pitlochry, *U.K.* **22 E5** 56 42N 3 44W
Pitogo, *Phil.* **80 E4** 13 47N 122 5 E
Pitrufquén, *Chile* **176 A2** 38 59 S 72 39W
Pitschen = Byczyna, *Poland* **55 G5** 51 7N 18 12 E
Pitsilia, *Cyprus* **39 F9** 34 55N 33 0 E
Pitt, Pta., *Ecuador* **172 a** 0 43 S 89 14W
Pitt I., *Canada* **142 C3** 53 30N 129 50W
Pitt I., *N.Z.* **131 a** 44 15 S 176 15W
Pitti I., *India* **95 J1** 10 50N 72 38 E
Pittsburg, *Calif., U.S.A.* **160 G5** 38 2N 121 53W
Pittsburg, *Kans., U.S.A.* **155 G7** 37 25N 94 42W
Pittsburg, *Tex., U.S.A.* **155 J7** 33 0N 94 59W
Pittsburgh, *U.S.A.* **150 F5** 40 26N 80 1W
Pittsfield, *Ill., U.S.A.* **156 E6** 39 36N 90 49W
Pittsfield, *Maine, U.S.A.* **149 C11** 44 47N 69 23W
Pittsfield, *Mass., U.S.A.* **151 D11** 42 27N 73 15W
Pittsfield, *N.H., U.S.A.* **151 C13** 43 18N 71 20W
Pittston, *U.S.A.* **151 E9** 41 19N 75 47W
Pittsview, *U.S.A.* **152 C4** 32 11N 85 10W
Pittsworth, *Australia* **127 D5** 27 41 S 151 37 E
Pituri →, *Australia* **126 C2** 22 35 S 138 30 E
Piuí, *Brazil* **171 F2** 20 28 S 45 58W
Pium, *Brazil* **170 D2** 10 27 S 49 11W
Piura, *Peru* **172 B1** 5 15 S 80 38W
Piura □, *Peru* **172 A2** 5 10 S 80 0W
Piva →, *Serbia & M.* **50 C2** 43 20N 18 50 E
Pivijay, *Colombia* **168 A3** 10 28N 74 37W
Piwniczna, *Poland* **55 J7** 49 27N 20 42 E
Pixley, *U.S.A.* **160 K7** 35 58N 119 18W
Piyai, *Greece* **48 B3** 39 17N 21 25 E
Pizarra, *Spain* **43 J6** 36 36N 4 42W
Pizarro, *Colombia* **168 C2** 4 58N 77 22W
Pizhou, *China* **74 G9** 34 44N 116 55 E
Pizol, *Switz.* **33 C8** 46 57N 9 23 E
Pizzo, *Italy* **47 D9** 38 44N 16 10 E
Placentia, *Canada* **141 C9** 47 20N 54 0W
Placentia B., *Canada* **141 C9** 47 0N 54 40W
Placer, *Masbate, Phil.* **81 F4** 11 52N 123 55 E
Placer, *Surigao N., Phil.* **81 G5** 9 36N 125 38 E
Placerville, *U.S.A.* **160 G6** 38 44N 120 48W
Placetas, *Cuba* **164 B4** 22 15N 79 44W
Plácido de Castro, *Brazil* **172 C4** 10 20 S 67 11W
Plačkovica, *Macedonia* **50 E6** 41 45N 22 30 E
Plaffeien, *Switz.* **32 C4** 46 45N 7 17 E
Plainfield, *Ill., U.S.A.* **157 C8** 41 37N 88 12W
Plainfield, *Ind., U.S.A.* **157 E10** 39 42N 86 24W
Plainfield, *N.J., U.S.A.* **151 F10** 40 37N 74 25W
Plainfield, *Ohio, U.S.A.* **150 F3** 40 13N 81 43W
Plainfield, *Vt., U.S.A.* **151 B12** 44 17N 72 26W
Plains, *Ga., U.S.A.* **152 C5** 32 2N 84 24W
Plains, *Mont., U.S.A.* **158 C6** 47 28N 114 53W
Plains, *Tex., U.S.A.* **155 J3** 33 11N 102 50W
Plainview, *Nebr., U.S.A.* **154 D6** 42 21N 97 47W
Plainview, *Tex., U.S.A.* **155 H4** 34 11N 101 43W
Plainwell, *U.S.A.* **157 B11** 42 27N 85 38W
Plaisance, *France* **28 E4** 43 36N 0 3 E
Plaistow, *U.S.A.* **151 D13** 42 50N 71 6W
Pláka, *Greece* **49 B7** 40 0N 25 24 E
Pláka, Ákra, *Greece* **39 E7** 35 11N 26 19 E
Plakenska Planina, *Macedonia* **50 E5** 41 14N 21 2 E
Planá, *Czech Rep.* **34 B5** 49 50N 12 44 E
Plana Cays, *Bahamas* **165 B5** 22 38N 73 30W
Planada, *U.S.A.* **160 H6** 37 16N 120 19W
Plancoët, *France* **26 D4** 48 32N 2 13W
Plandište, *Serbia & M.* **52 E6** 45 16N 21 10 E
Planeta Rica, *Colombia* **168 B2** 8 25N 75 36W
Plano, *U.S.A.* **155 J6** 33 1N 96 42W
Plant City, *U.S.A.* **153 G7** 28 1N 82 7W
Plantation, *U.S.A.* **153 J9** 26 8N 80 15W
Plaquemine, *U.S.A.* **155 K9** 30 17N 91 14W
Plaridel, *Phil.* **81 G4** 8 37N 123 43 E
Plasencia, *Spain* **42 E4** 40 3N 6 8W
Plaški, *Croatia* **45 C12** 45 4N 15 22 E
Plassen, *Norway* **18 C9** 61 9N 12 30 E
Plast, *Russia* **64 D8** 54 22N 60 50 E
Plaster City, *U.S.A.* **161 N11** 32 47N 115 51W
Plaster Rock, *Canada* **141 C6** 46 53N 67 22W
Plastun, *Russia* **70 B8** 44 45N 136 19 E
Plasy, *Czech Rep.* **34 B6** 49 56N 13 24 E
Plata, Río de la, *S. Amer.* **174 C4** 34 45 S 57 30W
Plátani →, *Italy* **46 E6** 37 23N 13 16 E
Plátanos, *Greece* **39 E4** 35 28N 23 33 E
Plataria, *Greece* **38 C10** 39 27N 20 16 E
Plateau □, *Nigeria* **113 D6** 8 30N 9 0 E
Plateau d'Ipassa ⌂, *Gabon* **114 B2** 0 26N 12 40 E
Plathe = Płoty, *Poland* **54 E2** 53 48N 15 18 E
Platí, Ákra, *Greece* **51 F8** 40 27N 24 0 E
Platinum, *U.S.A.* **144 G7** 59 1N 161 49W
Plato, *Colombia* **168 B3** 9 47N 74 47W
Platta, Piz, *Switz.* **33 D9** 46 28N 9 35 E
Platte, *U.S.A.* **154 D5** 43 23N 98 51W
Platte →, *Mo., U.S.A.* **156 E2** 39 16N 94 50W
Platte →, *Nebr., U.S.A.* **154 E7** 41 4N 95 53W
Platte City, *U.S.A.* **156 E2** 39 22N 94 47W
Platteville, *U.S.A.* **156 B6** 42 44N 90 29W
Plattling, *Germany* **31 G8** 48 46N 12 53 E
Plattsburg, *U.S.A.* **156 E2** 39 34N 94 27W
Plattsburgh, *U.S.A.* **151 B11** 44 42N 73 28W
Plattsmouth, *U.S.A.* **154 E7** 41 1N 95 53W
Plau, *Germany* **30 B8** 53 27N 12 15 E
Plauen, *Germany* **30 E8** 50 30N 12 8 E
Plauer See, *Germany* **30 B8** 53 28N 12 17 E
Plav, *Serbia & M.* **50 D3** 42 38N 19 57 E
Plavinas, *Latvia* **15 H21** 56 35N 25 46 E
Plavnica, *Serbia & M.* **50 D3** 42 20N 19 13 E
Plavno, *Croatia* **45 D13** 44 9N 16 10 E
Plavsk, *Russia* **58 F9** 53 40N 37 18 E
Playa Blanca, *Canary Is.* **9 e2** 28 55N 13 37W
Playa Blanca Sur, *Canary Is.* **9 e2** 28 51N 13 50W
Playa de las Americas, *Canary Is.* **9 e1** 28 5N 16 43W
Playa de Mogán, *Canary Is.* **9 e1** 27 48N 15 47W
Playa del Inglés, *Canary Is.* **9 e1** 27 45N 15 33W
Playa Esmerelda, *Canary Is.* **9 e2** 28 8N 14 16W
Playgreen L., *Canada* **143 C9** 54 0N 98 15W
Playiá, *Greece* **39 C2** 38 24N 20 35 E
Pleasant Bay, *Canada* **141 C7** 46 51N 60 48W
Pleasant Hill, *Calif., U.S.A.* **160 H4** 37 57N 122 4W
Pleasant Hill, *Ill., U.S.A.* **156 E6** 39 27N 90 52W
Pleasant Hill, *Mo., U.S.A.* **156 F2** 38 47N 94 16W
Pleasant Mount, *U.S.A.* **151 E9** 41 44N 75 26W
Pleasant Point, *N.Z.* **131 E6** 44 16 S 171 9 E
Pleasanton, *Calif., U.S.A.* **160 H5** 37 39N 121 52W
Pleasanton, *Tex., U.S.A.* **155 L5** 28 58N 98 29W
Pleasantville, *Iowa, U.S.A.* **156 C3** 41 23N 93 18W
Pleasantville, *N.J., U.S.A.* **148 F8** 39 24N 74 32W
Pleasantville, *Pa., U.S.A.* **150 E5** 41 35N 79 34W
Pleasure Ridge Park, *U.S.A.* **157 F11** 38 9N 85 50W
Pléaux, *France* **28 C6** 45 8N 2 13 E
Plei Ku, *Vietnam* **86 F7** 13 57N 108 0 E
Plélan-le-Grand, *France* **26 D4** 48 0N 2 7W
Pléneuf-Val-André, *France* **26 D4** 48 35N 2 32W
Plenița, *Romania* **53 F8** 44 14N 23 10 E
Plenty →, *Australia* **126 C2** 23 25 S 136 31 E
Plenty, B. of, *N.Z.* **130 D6** 37 45 S 177 0 E
Plentywood, *U.S.A.* **154 A2** 48 47N 104 34W
Plérin, *France* **26 D4** 48 32N 2 46W
Plesetsk, *Russia* **56 B7** 62 43N 40 20 E
Pleskau = Pskov, *Russia* **58 D5** 57 50N 28 25 E
Plessisville, *Canada* **141 C5** 46 14N 71 47W
Plestin-les-Grèves, *France* **26 D3** 48 40N 3 39W
Pleszew, *Poland* **55 G4** 51 53N 17 47 E
Pleternica, *Croatia* **52 E2** 45 17N 17 48 E
Plétipi, L., *Canada* **141 B5** 51 44N 70 6W
Pleven, *Bulgaria* **51 C8** 43 26N 24 37 E
Plevlja, *Serbia & M.* **50 C3** 43 21N 19 21 E
Plevna, *Canada* **150 B8** 44 58N 76 59W
Plitvička Jezera △, *Croatia* **45 D12** 44 54N 15 35 E
Plješevica, *Croatia* **45 D12** 44 45N 15 45 E
Ploaghe, *Italy* **46 B1** 40 40N 8 45 E
Ploče, *Croatia* **45 E14** 43 4N 17 26 E
Płock, *Poland* **55 F6** 52 32N 19 40 E
Plöckenpass, *Italy* **45 B9** 46 37N 12 57 E
Plöckenstein, *Germany* **31 G9** 48 46N 13 51 E
Ploemeur, *France* **26 E3** 47 44N 3 26W
Ploërmel, *France* **26 E4** 47 55N 2 26W
Plöhnen = Płońsk, *Poland* **55 F7** 52 37N 20 21 E
Ploieşti, *Romania* **53 F11** 44 57N 26 5 E
Plomárion, *Greece* **49 C8** 38 59N 26 22 E
Plombières-les-Bains, *France* **27 E13** 47 58N 6 27 E
Plomin, *Croatia* **45 C11** 45 8N 14 10 E
Plön, *Germany* **30 A6** 54 9N 10 24 E
Plonge, Lac la, *Canada* **143 B7** 55 8N 107 20W
Płońsk, *Poland* **55 F7** 52 37N 20 21 E
Plopeni, *Romania* **53 E10** 45 4N 25 59 E
Plopişului, Munţii, *Romania* **52 C7** 47 5N 22 30 E
Plotsk = Płock, *Poland* **55 F6** 52 32N 19 40 E
Płoty, *Poland* **54 E2** 53 48N 15 18 E
Plouaret, *France* **26 D3** 48 37N 3 28W
Plouay, *France* **26 E3** 47 55N 3 21W
Ploučnice →, *Czech Rep.* **34 A7** 50 46N 14 13 E
Ploudalmézeau, *France* **26 D2** 48 34N 4 41W
Plouescat, *France* **26 D2** 48 39N 4 10W
Plougasnou, *France* **26 D3** 48 42N 3 49W
Plougastel-Daoulas, *France* **26 D2** 48 22N 4 17W
Plouguerneau, *France* **26 D2** 48 36N 4 30W
Plouha, *France* **26 D4** 48 41N 2 57W
Plouhinec, *France* **26 E2** 48 0N 4 29W
Plovdiv, *Bulgaria* **51 D8** 42 8N 24 44 E
Plovdiv □, *Bulgaria* **51 D8** 42 15N 24 30 E
Plover Cove Res., *China* **69 G11** 22 28N 114 15 E
Plum, *U.S.A.* **150 F5** 40 29N 79 47W
Plum I., *U.S.A.* **151 E12** 41 11N 72 12W
Plumas, *U.S.A.* **160 F7** 39 45N 120 4W
Plummer, *U.S.A.* **158 C5** 47 20N 116 53W
Plumtree, *Zimbabwe* **119 G2** 20 27 S 27 55 E
Plungė, *Lithuania* **15 J19** 55 53N 21 59 E
Pluvigner, *France* **26 E3** 47 46N 3 1W
Plymouth, *Trin. & Tob.* **169 E10** 11 14N 60 48W
Plymouth, *U.K.* **21 G3** 50 22N 4 10W
Plymouth, *Calif., U.S.A.* **160 G6** 38 29N 120 51W
Plymouth, *Ill., U.S.A.* **156 D6** 40 18N 90 58W
Plymouth, *Ind., U.S.A.* **157 C10** 41 21N 86 19W
Plymouth, *Mass., U.S.A.* **151 E14** 41 57N 70 40W
Plymouth, *N.C., U.S.A.* **149 H7** 35 52N 76 43W
Plymouth, *N.H., U.S.A.* **151 C13** 43 46N 71 41W
Plymouth, *Pa., U.S.A.* **151 E9** 41 14N 75 57W
Plymouth, *Wis., U.S.A.* **148 D2** 43 45N 87 59W
Plympton-Wyoming, *Canada* **150 D2** 42 57N 82 7W
Plynlimon = Pumlumon Fawr, *U.K.* **21 E4** 52 28N 3 46W
Plyusa, *Russia* **58 C5** 58 28N 29 27 E
Plyusa →, *Russia* **58 C5** 59 4N 28 6 E
Plzeň, *Czech Rep.* **34 B6** 49 45N 13 22 E
Plzeňský □, *Czech Rep.* **34 B6** 49 35N 13 0 E
Pniewy, *Poland* **55 F3** 52 31N 16 16 E
Pô, *Burkina Faso* **113 C4** 11 14N 1 5W
Pô △, *Burkina Faso* **113 C4** 11 25N 1 5W
Po →, *Italy* **45 D9** 44 57N 12 4 E
Po, Foci del, *Italy* **45 D9** 44 55N 12 30 E
Po Hai = Bo Hai, *China* **75 E10** 39 0N 119 0 E
Po Toi, *China* **69 G11** 22 10N 114 16 E
Pobé, *Benin* **113 D5** 7 0N 2 56 E
Pobé, *Burkina Faso* **113 C4** 13 53N 1 42W
Pobeda, *Russia* **67 C15** 65 12N 146 12 E
Pobedy, Pik, *Kyrgyzstan* **66 E8** 42 0N 79 58 E
Pobiedziska, *Poland* **55 F4** 52 29N 17 11 E
Pobla de Segur, *Spain* **40 C5** 42 15N 0 58 E
Pobladura del Valle, *Spain* **42 C5** 42 6N 5 44W
Pobra de Trives, *Spain* **42 C3** 42 20N 7 10W
Pocahontas, *Ark., U.S.A.* **155 G9** 36 16N 90 58W
Pocahontas, *Ill., U.S.A.* **156 F7** 38 50N 89 33W
Pocahontas, *Iowa, U.S.A.* **156 B2** 42 44N 94 40W
Pocatello, *U.S.A.* **158 E7** 42 52N 112 27W
Počátky, *Czech Rep.* **34 B8** 49 15N 15 14 E
Pochep, *Russia* **59 F7** 52 58N 33 29 E
Pochinki, *Russia* **60 C7** 54 41N 44 59 E
Pochinok, *Russia* **58 E7** 54 28N 32 29 E
Pöchlarn, *Austria* **34 C8** 48 12N 15 12 E
Pochutla, *Mexico* **163 D5** 15 50N 96 31W
Poci, *Venezuela* **169 B5** 5 57N 61 29W
Pocinhos, *Brazil* **170 C4** 7 4 S 36 3W
Pocito Casas, *Mexico* **162 B2** 28 32N 111 6W
Pocking, *Germany* **31 G9** 48 23N 13 19 E
Pocklington Reef, *Papua N. G.* **132 F8** 10 51 S 155 44 E
Poções, *Brazil* **171 D3** 14 31 S 40 21W
Pocomoke City, *U.S.A.* **148 F8** 38 5N 75 34W
Poconé, *Brazil* **173 D6** 16 15 S 56 37W
Poços de Caldas, *Brazil* **175 A6** 21 50 S 46 33W
Podbořany, *Czech Rep.* **34 A6** 50 14N 13 25 E
Poddębice, *Poland* **55 G5** 51 54N 18 58 E
Poděbrady, *Czech Rep.* **34 A8** 50 9N 15 8 E
Podensac, *France* **28 D3** 44 40N 0 22W
Podenzano, *Italy* **44 D6** 44 57N 9 41 E
Podgorač, *Croatia* **52 E3** 45 27N 18 13 E
Podgorica, *Serbia & M.* **50 D3** 42 30N 19 19 E
Podgorie, *Albania* **50 F4** 40 49N 20 48 E
Podile, *India* **95 G4** 15 37N 79 37 E
Podilska Vysochyna, *Ukraine* **53 B13** 49 0N 28 0 E
Podkarpackie □, *Poland* **55 H9** 50 0N 22 10 E
Podkova, *Bulgaria* **51 E9** 41 24N 25 24 E
Podlapača, *Croatia* **45 D12** 44 37N 15 47 E
Podlaskie □, *Poland* **55 E10** 53 10N 23 0 E
Podocarpus △, *Ecuador* **168 D2** 4 13 S 79 2W
Podoleni, *Romania* **53 D11** 46 46N 26 39 E
Podolínec, *Slovak Rep.* **35 B13** 49 16N 20 31 E
Podolsk, *Russia* **58 E9** 55 25N 37 30 E
Podor, *Senegal* **112 B1** 16 40N 15 2W
Podporozhye, *Russia* **58 B8** 60 55N 34 2 E
Podu Iloaiei, *Romania* **53 C12** 47 13N 27 16 E
Podu Turcului, *Romania* **53 D12** 46 11N 27 25 E
Podujevo, *Serbia & M.* **50 D5** 42 54N 21 10 E
Podyji △, *Czech Rep.* **34 C8** 48 51N 15 57 E
Poechos, *Peru* **168 D1** 4 41 S 80 34W
Poel, *Germany* **30 B6** 54 0N 11 25 E
Pofadder, *S. Africa* **116 D2** 29 10 S 19 22 E
Poggiardo, *Italy* **47 B11** 40 3N 18 23 E
Poggibonsi, *Italy* **44 E8** 43 28N 11 9 E
Póggio Mirteto, *Italy* **45 F9** 42 16N 12 41 E
Pogoanele, *Romania* **53 F12** 44 55N 27 0 E
Pogorzela, *Poland* **55 G4** 51 50N 17 12 E
Pogoso, *Dem. Rep. of the Congo* **115 D3** 6 46 S 17 12 E
Pogradec, *Albania* **50 F4** 40 54N 20 37 E
Pogranichnyy, *Russia* **70 B5** 44 25N 131 24 E
Poh, *Indonesia* **82 B2** 0 46 S 122 51 E
P'ohang, *S. Korea* **75 F15** 36 1N 129 23 E
Pohjanmaa, *Finland* **14 E20** 62 58N 22 50 E
Pohjois-Pirkkala = Nokia, *Finland* **15 F20** 61 30N 23 30 E
Pohnpei, *Micronesia* **134 G7** 6 55N 158 10 E
Pohorelá, *Slovak Rep.* **35 C13** 48 50N 20 2 E
Pohořelice, *Czech Rep.* **35 C9** 48 59N 16 31 E
Pohorje, *Slovenia* **45 B12** 46 30N 15 20 E
Pohri, *India* **92 G6** 25 32N 77 22 E
Pohue B., *U.S.A.* **145 E6** 19 0N 155 48W
Poi, *Solomon Is.* **133 N11** 10 9 S 161 42 E
Poiana Mare, *Romania* **52 G8** 43 57N 23 5 E
Poiana Ruscăi, Munţii, *Romania* **52 E7** 45 45N 22 25 E
Poiana Stampei, *Romania* **53 C10** 47 19N 25 8 E
Poike, Península, *Chile* **172 b** 27 6 S 109 15W
Poindimié, *N. Cal.* **133 T19** 20 56 S 165 20 E
Poinsett, C., *Antarctica* **7 C8** 65 42 S 113 18 E
Point Arena, *U.S.A.* **160 G3** 38 55N 123 41W
Point Baker, *U.S.A.* **142 B2** 56 21N 133 37W
Point Calimere, *India* **95 J4** 10 17N 79 49 E
Point Edward, *Canada* **140 D3** 43 0N 82 30W
Point Fortin, *Trin. & Tob.* **169 F9** 10 10N 61 42W
Point Hope, *U.S.A.* **144 B6** 68 21N 166 47W
Point L., *Canada* **138 B8** 65 15N 113 4W
Point Lay, *U.S.A.* **144 B7** 69 46N 163 3W
Point Lisas, *Trin. & Tob.* **169 F9** 10 32N 61 30W
Point Pedro, *Sri Lanka* **95 K5** 9 50N 80 15 E
Point Pelee △, *Canada* **140 D3** 41 57N 82 31W
Point Pleasant, *N.J., U.S.A.* **151 F10** 40 5N 74 4W
Point Pleasant, *W. Va., U.S.A.* **148 F4** 38 51N 82 8W
Point Reyes ⌂, *U.S.A.* **160 G2** 38 10N 122 55W
Pointe-à-Pitre, *Guadeloupe* **164 b** 16 10N 61 32W
Pointe-au-Pic = La Malbaie, *Canada* **141 C5** 47 40N 70 10W
Pointe-Claire, *Canada* **151 A11** 45 26N 73 50W
Pointe-Gatineau, *Canada* **151 A9** 45 28N 75 42W
Pointe-Noire, *Congo* **115 C2** 4 48 S 11 53 E
Pointe Noire, *Guadeloupe* **164 b** 16 14N 61 47W
Poio, *Spain* **42 C2** 42 28N 8 41W
Poirino, *Italy* **44 D4** 44 56N 7 48 E
Poisonbush Ra., *Australia* **124 D3** 22 30 S 121 30 E
Poissonnier Pt., *Australia* **124 C2** 19 57 S 119 10 E
Poitiers, *France* **26 F7** 46 35N 0 20 E
Poitou, *France* **28 B3** 46 40N 0 10W
Poitou-Charentes □, *France* **28 B4** 46 10N 0 15 E
Poix-de-Picardie, *France* **27 C8** 49 47N 1 58 E

INDEX TO WORLD MAPS Pôrto Nacional 267

Poix-Terron, France 27 C11 49 38N 4 38 E
Pojoaque, U.S.A. 159 J11 35 54N 106 1W
Pokai B., U.S.A. 145 K13 21 27N 158 12W
Pokataroo, Australia 127 D4 29 30 S 148 36 E
Pokhara, Nepal 93 E10 28 14N 83 58 E
Pokhvistnevo, Russia 60 D11 53 36N 52 0 E
Pokigron, Suriname 169 C6 4 30N 55 22W
Poko, Dem. Rep. of the Congo 118 B2 3 7N 26 52 E
Poko, Sudan 107 F3 5 41N 31 55 E
Pokrov, Russia 58 E10 55 55N 39 7 E
Pokrovka = Kyzyl-Suu, Kyrgyzstan 65 B9 42 20N 78 0 E
Pokrovka, Kyrgyzstan 65 B5 42 45N 71 36 E
Pokrovsk = Engels, Russia 60 E8 51 28N 46 6 E
Pokrovsk, Russia 67 C13 61 29N 129 0 E
Pokrovsk-Uralskiy, Russia 64 A7 60 10N 59 49 E
Pokrovskoy = Priazovskoye, Ukraine 59 J8 46 44N 35 40 E
Pokrovskoye, Russia 59 J10 47 25N 38 54 E
Pol-e Khomri, Afghan. 91 B3 35 56N 68 42 E
Pola = Istra, Croatia 45 C10 45 10N 14 0 E
Pola = Pula, Croatia 45 D10 44 54N 13 57 E
Pola, Russia 58 D7 57 55N 32 0 E
Pola de Allande, Spain 42 B4 43 16N 6 37W
Pola de Lena, Spain 42 B5 43 10N 5 49W
Pola de Siero, Spain 42 B5 43 24N 5 39W
Pola de Somiedo, Spain 42 B4 43 5N 6 15W
Polacca, U.S.A. 159 J8 35 50N 110 23W
Polan, Iran 97 E9 25 30N 61 10 E
Pol'ana, Slovak Rep. 35 C12 48 38N 19 29 E
Poland ■, Europe 55 G3 52 0N 20 0 E
Polanica-Zdrój, Poland 55 H3 50 24N 16 32 E
Połaniec, Poland 55 H8 50 26N 21 17 E
Polanów, Poland 54 D3 54 7N 16 41 E
Polar Bear ⌂, Canada 140 A2 55 0N 83 45W
Polatlı, Turkey 100 C5 39 36N 32 9 E
Polatsk, Belarus 58 E5 55 30N 28 50 E
Polavaram, India 94 F5 17 15N 81 38 E
Polcura, Chile 174 D1 37 17 S 71 43W
Połczyn-Zdrój, Poland 54 E3 53 47N 16 5 E
Poleski △, Poland 55 G10 51 29N 23 5 E
Polessk, Russia 15 J19 54 50N 21 8 E
Polesye = Pripet Marshes, Europe 59 F5 52 10N 28 10 E
Polevskoy, Russia 64 C8 56 26N 60 11 E
Polewali, Indonesia 82 B1 3 25 S 119 20 E
Polgar, Hungary 52 C6 47 54N 21 6 E
Pŏlgyo-ri, S. Korea 75 G14 34 51N 127 21 E
Poli, Cameroon 113 C7 8 34N 13 15 E
Políaigos, Greece 48 E6 36 45N 24 38 E
Policastro, G. di, Italy 47 C8 40 0N 15 35 E
Police, Poland 54 E1 53 33N 14 33 E
Police, Pte., Seychelles 121 b 4 51 S 55 32 E
Polička, Czech Rep. 35 B9 49 43N 16 15 E
Policoro, Italy 47 B9 40 13N 16 41 E
Poligiros = Políyiros, Greece 50 F7 40 23N 23 25 E
Polignano a Mare, Italy 47 A9 41 0N 17 13 E
Poligny, France 27 F12 46 50N 5 42 E
Polikhnitas, Greece 49 B8 39 6N 26 10 E
Polillo, Phil. 80 D3 14 43N 121 56 E
Polillo Is., Phil. 80 D4 14 56N 122 0 E
Polillo Strait, Phil. 80 D3 14 44N 121 51 E
Polis, Cyprus 39 E8 35 2N 32 26 E
Polístena, Italy 47 D9 38 24N 16 4 E
Pölitz = Police, Poland 54 E1 53 33N 14 33 E
Políyiros, Greece 50 F7 40 23N 23 25 E
Polk, U.S.A. 150 E5 41 22N 79 56W
Polkowice, Poland 55 G3 51 29N 16 3 E
Polkwitz = Polkowice, Poland 55 G3 51 29N 16 3 E
Polla, Italy 47 B8 40 31N 15 29 E
Pollachi, India 95 J3 10 35N 77 0 E
Pollença, Spain 38 B4 39 54N 3 1 E
Pollença, B. de, Spain 38 B4 39 53N 3 8 E
Pollfoss, Norway 18 C4 61 58N 7 54 E
Póllica, Italy 47 B8 40 11N 15 3 E
Pollino △, Italy 47 C9 40 0N 16 12 E
Pollino, Mte., Italy 47 C9 39 55N 16 11 E
Polna, Russia 58 C5 58 31N 28 5 E
Polnovat, Russia 66 C7 63 50N 65 54 E
Polo, Ill., U.S.A. 156 C7 41 59N 89 35W
Polo, Mo., U.S.A. 156 E2 39 33N 94 3W
Pology, Ukraine 59 J9 47 29N 36 15 E
Polokwane, S. Africa 117 C4 23 54 S 29 25 E
Polonnaruwa, Sri Lanka 95 L5 7 56N 81 0 E
Polonne, Ukraine 59 G4 50 6N 27 30 E
Polonnoye = Polonne, Ukraine 59 G4 50 6N 27 30 E
Polovinka = Ugleuralskiy, Russia 64 B6 59 8N 57 35 E
Polski Trŭmbesh, Bulgaria 51 C9 43 20N 25 38 E
Polsko Kosovo, Bulgaria 51 C9 43 23N 25 38 E
Polson, U.S.A. 158 C6 47 41N 114 9W
Poltár, Slovak Rep. 35 C12 48 26N 19 48 E
Poltava, Ukraine 59 H8 49 35N 34 35 E
Poltoratsk = Ashgabat, Turkmenistan 66 F6 38 0N 57 50 E
Põltsamaa, Estonia 15 G21 58 39N 25 58 E
Polunochnoye, Russia 66 C7 60 52N 60 25 E
Polur, India 95 H4 12 32N 79 11 E
Põlva, Estonia 15 G22 58 3N 27 3 E
Polyana, Ukraine 52 B7 48 38N 22 58 E
Polyarny, Russia 56 A5 69 8N 33 20 E
Polynesia, Pac. Oc. 135 F11 10 0 S 162 0W
Polynésie française = French Polynesia ☑, Pac. Oc. 135 K13 20 0 S 145 0W
Pomabamba = Azurduy, Bolivia 173 D5 19 59 S 64 29W
Pomabamba, Peru 172 B2 8 50 S 77 28W
Pomarance, Italy 44 E7 43 18N 10 52 E
Pomaro, Mexico 162 D4 18 20N 103 18W
Pombachi = Komsomolabad, Tajikistan 65 D4 38 50N 69 55 E
Pombal, Brazil 170 C4 6 45 S 37 50W
Pombal, Portugal 42 F2 39 55N 8 40W
Pómbia, Greece 39 F5 35 0N 24 51 E
Pombos, B. dos, Angola 115 E1 11 40 S 13 47 E
Pomene, Mozam. 117 C6 22 53 S 35 33 E
Pomeroy, Ohio, U.S.A. 148 F4 39 2N 82 2W
Pomeroy, Wash., U.S.A. 158 C5 46 28N 117 36W
Pomézia, Italy 46 A5 41 40N 12 30 E
Pomichna, Ukraine 59 H6 48 13N 31 36 E
Pomio, Papua N. G. 132 C6 5 32 S 151 33 E
Pomme de Terre L., U.S.A. 156 G3 37 54N 93 19W
Pomona, Australia 127 D5 26 22 S 152 52 E
Pomona, U.S.A. 161 L9 34 4N 117 45W
Pomona Park, U.S.A. 153 F8 29 30N 81 36W
Pomorie, Bulgaria 51 D11 42 32N 27 41 E
Pomorskie ☐, Poland 54 D5 54 30N 18 0 E
Pomorskie, Pojezierze, Poland 54 E3 53 40N 16 37 E
Pomos, Cyprus 39 E8 35 9N 32 33 E
Pomos, C., Cyprus 39 E8 35 10N 32 33 E
Pompano Beach, U.S.A. 153 J9 26 14N 80 8W
Pompei, Italy 47 B7 40 45N 14 30 E
Pompey, France 27 D13 48 46N 6 6 E
Pompeys Pillar, U.S.A. 158 D10 45 59N 107 57W
Pompeys Pillar ⌂, U.S.A. 158 D10 46 0N 108 0W
Pompton Lakes, U.S.A. 151 F10 41 0N 74 17W
Ponape = Pohnpei, Micronesia 134 G7 6 55N 158 10 E
Ponask L., Canada 140 B1 54 0N 92 41W
Ponca, U.S.A. 154 D6 42 34N 96 43W
Ponca City, U.S.A. 155 G6 36 42N 97 5W
Ponce, Puerto Rico 165 d 18 1N 66 37W
Ponce de Leon, U.S.A. 152 E4 30 44N 85 56W
Ponce de Leon B., U.S.A. 153 K8 25 15N 81 10W
Ponchatoula, U.S.A. 155 K9 30 26N 90 26W
Poncheville, L., Canada 140 B4 50 10N 76 55W
Pond, U.S.A. 161 K7 35 43N 119 20W
Pond Inlet, Canada 139 A12 72 40N 77 0W
Pondicherry, India 95 J4 11 59N 79 50 E
Pondo, Papua N. G. 132 C6 4 33 S 151 38 E
Ponds, I. of, Canada 141 B8 53 27N 55 52W
Ponérihouen, N. Cal. 133 U19 21 5 S 165 24 E
Ponferrada, Spain 42 C4 42 32N 6 35W
Pongo, Wadi →, Sudan 107 F2 8 42N 27 40 E
Poniatowa, Poland 55 G9 51 11N 22 3 E
Poniec, Poland 55 G3 51 48N 16 50 E
Ponikva, Slovenia 45 B12 46 16N 15 26 E
Ponizovkino = Krasnyy Profintern, Russia 58 D11 57 45N 40 27 E
Ponnaiyar →, India 95 J4 11 50N 79 45 E
Ponnani, India 95 J2 10 45N 75 59 E
Ponneri, India 95 H5 13 20N 80 15 E
Ponnuru, India 95 F5 16 5N 80 34 E
Ponoka, Canada 142 C6 52 42N 113 40W
Ponomarevka, Russia 64 E5 53 19N 54 8 E
Ponorogo, Indonesia 85 D4 7 52 S 111 27 E
Ponot, Phil. 81 G4 8 25N 123 0 E
Ponoy, Russia 56 A7 67 0N 41 13 E
Ponoy →, Russia 56 A7 66 59N 41 17 E
Pons = Ponts, Spain 40 D6 41 55N 1 12 E
Pons, France 28 C3 45 35N 0 34W
Ponsul →, Portugal 42 F3 39 40N 7 31W
Pont-à-Mousson, France 27 D13 48 54N 6 1 E
Pont-Audemer, France 26 C7 49 21N 0 30 E
Pont-Aven, France 26 E3 47 51N 3 47W
Pont Canavese, Italy 44 C4 45 25N 7 36 E
Pont-d'Ain, France 27 F12 46 3N 5 21 E
Pont-de-Roide, France 27 E13 47 23N 6 45 E
Pont-de-Salars, France 28 D6 44 18N 2 44 E
Pont-de-Vaux, France 27 F11 46 26N 4 56 E
Pont-de-Veyle, France 27 F11 46 17N 4 53 E
Pont-du-Château, France 27 G10 45 47N 3 15 E
Pont-l'Abbé, France 26 E2 47 52N 4 15W
Pont-l'Évêque, France 26 C7 49 18N 0 11 E
Pont-St-Esprit, France 29 D8 44 16N 4 40 E
Pont-St-Martin, Italy 44 C4 45 36N 7 48 E
Pont-Ste-Maxence, France 27 C9 49 18N 2 35 E
Pont-sur-Yonne, France 27 D10 48 18N 3 10 E
Ponta de Pedras, Brazil 170 B2 1 23 S 48 52W
Ponta Delgada, Flores, Azores 9 d2 39 31N 31 13W
Ponta Delgada, São Miguel, Azores 9 d3 37 44N 25 40W
Ponta Delgada ✕ (PDL), Azores 9 d3 37 44N 25 41W
Ponta do Sol, Madeira 9 c 32 42N 17 7W
Ponta Grossa, Brazil 175 B5 25 7 S 50 10W
Ponta Pora, Brazil 175 A4 22 20 S 55 35W
Pontacq, France 28 E3 43 11N 0 8W
Pontailler-sur-Saône, France 27 E12 47 13N 5 25 E
Pontal →, Brazil 170 C3 9 8 S 40 12W
Pontalina, Brazil 171 E2 17 31 S 49 27W
Pontarlier, France 27 F13 46 54N 6 20 E
Pontassieve, Italy 45 E8 43 46N 11 26 E
Pontaumur, France 28 C6 45 52N 2 40 E
Pontcharra, France 29 C10 45 26N 6 1 E
Pontchartrain, L., U.S.A. 155 K10 30 5N 90 5W
Pontchâteau, France 26 E4 47 25N 2 5W
Ponte Alta, Serra do, Brazil 171 E2 19 42 S 47 40W
Ponte Alta do Norte, Brazil 170 D2 10 45 S 47 34W
Ponte Branca, Brazil 173 D7 16 27 S 52 40W
Ponte da Barca, Portugal 42 D2 41 48N 8 25W
Ponte de Sor, Portugal 43 F2 39 17N 8 1W
Ponte dell'Ólio, Italy 44 D6 44 52N 9 39 E
Ponte di Legno, Italy 44 B7 46 16N 10 31 E
Ponte do Lima, Portugal 42 D2 41 46N 8 35W
Ponte do Pungué, Mozam. 119 F3 19 30 S 34 33 E
Ponte-Leccia, France 29 F13 42 28N 9 13 E
Ponte nelle Alpi, Italy 45 B9 46 11N 12 16 E
Ponte Nova, Brazil 171 F3 20 25 S 42 54W
Ponte Tresa, Italy 33 E7 45 58N 8 51 E
Ponte Vedra Beach, U.S.A. 152 E8 30 15N 81 23W
Ponteareas, Spain 42 C2 42 10N 8 28W
Pontebba, Italy 45 B10 46 30N 13 18 E
Ponteceso, Spain 42 B2 43 15N 8 54W
Pontecorvo, Italy 46 A6 41 27N 13 40 E
Pontedeume, Spain 42 B2 43 24N 8 10W
Ponteix, Canada 143 D7 49 46N 107 29W
Pontes e Lacerda, Brazil 173 D6 15 12 S 59 22W
Pontevedra, Capiz, Phil. 81 F4 11 29N 122 50 E
Pontevedra, Neg. Occ., Phil. 81 F4 10 22N 122 52 E
Pontevedra, Spain 42 C2 42 26N 8 40W
Pontevedra ☐, Spain 42 C2 42 25N 8 39W
Pontevedra, R. de →, Spain 42 C2 42 22N 8 45W
Pontevico, Italy 44 C7 45 16N 10 5 E
Pontiac, Ill., U.S.A. 154 E10 40 53N 88 38W
Pontiac, Mich., U.S.A. 157 B13 42 38N 83 18W
Pontian Kechil, Malaysia 87 d 1 29N 103 23 E
Pontianak, Indonesia 85 C3 0 3 S 109 15 E
Pontine Is. = Ponziane, Ísole, Italy 46 B5 40 55N 12 57 E
Pontine Mts. = Kuzey Anadolu Dağları, Turkey 100 B7 41 30N 35 0 E
Pontínia, Italy 46 A6 41 25N 13 2 E
Pontivy, France 26 D4 48 5N 2 58W
Pontoise, France 27 C9 49 3N 2 5 E
Ponton →, Canada 142 B5 58 27N 116 11W
Pontorson, France 26 D5 48 34N 1 30W
Pontrémoli, Italy 44 D6 44 22N 9 53 E
Pontresina, Switz. 33 D9 46 29N 9 48 E
Pontrieux, France 26 D3 48 42N 3 10W
Ponts, Spain 40 D6 41 55N 1 12 E
Pontypool, Canada 150 B6 44 6N 78 38W
Pontypool, U.K. 21 F4 51 42N 3 2W
Ponza, Italy 46 B5 40 54N 12 58 E
Ponziane, Ísole, Italy 46 B5 40 55N 12 57 E
Poochera, Australia 127 E1 32 43 S 134 51 E
Poole, U.K. 21 G6 50 43N 1 59W
Poole ☐, U.K. 21 G6 50 43N 1 59W
Pooler, U.S.A. 152 C8 32 7N 81 15W
Poona = Pune, India 94 E1 18 29N 73 57 E
Poonamallee, India 95 H5 13 3N 80 10 E
Pooncarie, Australia 128 B5 33 22 S 142 31 E
Poopelloe L., Australia 128 A6 31 40 S 144 0 E
Poopó, Bolivia 172 D4 18 23 S 66 59W
Poopó, L. de, Bolivia 172 D4 18 30 S 67 35W
Poor Knights Is., N.Z. 130 B3 35 29 S 174 43 E
Poorman, U.S.A. 144 D9 64 5N 155 33W
Popa, Gabon 114 C2 1 35 S 12 32 E
Popayán, Colombia 168 C2 2 27N 76 36W
Poperinge, Belgium 24 D2 50 51N 2 42 E
Popilta L., Australia 128 B4 33 10 S 141 42 E
Popina, Bulgaria 51 B10 44 7N 26 57 E
Popio L., Australia 128 B4 33 10 S 141 52 E
Poplar, U.S.A. 154 A2 48 7N 105 12W
Poplar →, Canada 143 C9 53 0N 97 19W
Poplar Bluff, U.S.A. 155 G9 36 46N 90 24W
Poplar Head = Dothan, U.S.A. 152 D4 31 13N 85 24W
Poplarville, U.S.A. 155 K10 30 51N 89 32W
Popocatépetl, Volcán, Mexico 163 D5 19 2N 98 38W
Popokabaka, Dem. Rep. of the Congo 115 D3 5 41 S 16 40 E
Pópoli, Italy 45 F10 42 10N 13 50 E
Popolo, Dem. Rep. of the Congo 114 B4 2 22N 21 8 E
Popomanaseu, Mt., Solomon Is. 133 M11 9 40 S 160 1 E
Popondetta, Papua N. G. 132 E5 8 48 S 148 17 E
Popovača, Croatia 45 C13 45 30N 16 41 E
Popovo, Bulgaria 51 C10 43 21N 26 18 E
Poppberg, Germany 31 F7 49 26N 11 37 E
Poppi, Italy 45 E8 43 43N 11 46 E
Poprad, Slovak Rep. 35 B13 49 3N 20 18 E
Poprad →, Slovak Rep. 35 B13 49 38N 20 42 E
Poradaha, Bangla. 90 D2 23 51N 89 1 E
Porali →, Pakistan 91 D2 25 58N 66 26 E
Porangaba, Brazil 172 B3 8 48 S 70 36W
Porangahau, N.Z. 130 G5 40 17 S 176 37 E
Porangatu, Brazil 171 D2 13 26 S 49 10W
Porbandar, India 92 J3 21 44N 69 43 E
Porce →, Colombia 168 B3 7 28N 74 53W
Porcher I., Canada 142 C2 53 50N 130 30W
Porco, Bolivia 173 D4 19 50 S 65 59W
Porcos →, Brazil 171 D2 12 42 S 45 7W
Porcuna, Spain 43 H6 37 52N 4 11W
Porcupine →, Canada 143 B8 59 11N 104 46W
Porcupine →, U.S.A. 144 C11 66 34N 145 19W
Porcupine Gorge △, Australia 126 C3 20 22 S 144 26 E
Porcupine Plain, Atl. Oc. 8 B10 48 0N 8 0W
Pordenone, Italy 45 C9 45 57N 12 39 E
Pordim, Bulgaria 51 C8 43 23N 24 51 E
Pore, Colombia 168 B3 5 43N 72 0W
Poreč, Croatia 45 C10 45 14N 13 36 E
Porecatu, Brazil 171 F1 22 43 S 51 24W
Porechye = Demidov, Russia 58 E6 55 16N 31 30 E
Poretskoye, Russia 60 C8 55 9N 46 21 E
Porgera, Papua N. G. 132 C2 5 28 S 143 12 E
Pori, Finland 15 F19 61 29N 21 48 E
Porí, Greece 48 F5 35 58N 23 13 E
Porkhov, Russia 58 D5 57 45N 29 38 E
Porlamar, Venezuela 169 A5 10 57N 63 51W
Porlezza, Italy 44 B6 46 2N 9 7 E
Porma →, Spain 42 C5 42 49N 5 28W
Pornic, France 26 E4 47 7N 2 5W
Poronaysk, Russia 67 E15 49 13N 143 0 E
Póros, Attikí, Greece 48 D5 37 30N 23 30 E
Póros, Kefallinía, Greece 39 C2 38 9N 20 47 E
Póros, Levkás, Greece 39 B2 38 38N 20 43 E
Poroshiri-Dake, Japan 70 C11 42 41N 142 52 E
Poroszló, Hungary 52 C5 47 39N 20 40 E
Poroto Mts., Tanzania 119 D3 9 0 S 33 30 E
Porpoise B., Antarctica 7 C9 66 0 S 127 0 E
Porpoise Pt., Ascension I. 9 g 7 54 S 14 21W
Porquerolles, Î. de, France 29 F10 43 0N 6 13 E
Porrentruy, Switz. 32 B4 47 25N 7 6 E
Porreres, Spain 38 B4 39 31N 3 2 E
Porsangen, Norway 14 A21 70 40N 25 40 E
Porsgrunn, Norway 18 E6 59 10N 9 40 E
Port Adelaide, Australia 128 C3 34 46 S 138 30 E
Port Alberni, Canada 142 D4 49 14N 124 50W
Port Albert, Australia 129 E7 38 42 S 146 42 E
Port Alexander, U.S.A. 144 H14 56 15N 134 38W
Port Alfred, S. Africa 116 E4 33 36 S 26 55 E
Port Alice, Canada 142 C3 50 20N 127 25W
Port Allegany, U.S.A. 150 E6 41 48N 78 17W
Port Allen, U.S.A. 155 K9 30 27N 91 12W
Port Alma, Australia 126 C5 23 38 S 150 53 E
Port Angeles, U.S.A. 160 B3 48 7N 123 27W
Port Antonio, Jamaica 164 a 18 10N 76 26W
Port Aransas, U.S.A. 155 M6 27 50N 97 4W
Port Arthur, Australia 127 G4 43 7 S 147 50 E
Port Arthur, U.S.A. 155 L8 29 54N 93 56W
Port au Choix, Canada 141 B8 50 43N 57 22W
Port au Port B., Canada 141 C8 48 40N 58 50W
Port-au-Prince, Haiti 165 C5 18 40N 72 20W
Port Augusta, Australia 128 B2 32 30 S 137 50 E
Port Austin, U.S.A. 150 B2 44 3N 83 1W
Port Bell, Uganda 118 B3 0 18N 32 35 E
Port Bergé Vaovao, Madag. 117 B8 15 33 S 47 40 E
Port Blair, India 95 J11 11 40N 92 45 E
Port Blandford, Canada 141 C9 48 20N 54 10W
Port-Bouët, Ivory C. 112 D4 5 16N 3 57W
Port Bradshaw, Australia 126 A2 12 30 S 137 20 E
Port Broughton, Australia 128 B2 33 37 S 137 56 E
Port Burwell, Canada 150 D4 42 40N 80 48W
Port Byron, U.S.A. 156 C6 41 37N 90 19W
Port Campbell, Australia 128 E5 38 37 S 143 1 E
Port Campbell, India 95 J11 11 56N 92 37 E
Port Campbell △, Australia 128 E5 38 8 S 143 6 E
Port Canning, India 93 H13 22 23N 88 40 E
Port-Cartier, Canada 141 B6 50 2N 66 50W
Port Chalmers, N.Z. 131 F5 45 49 S 170 30 E
Port Charles, N.Z. 130 C4 36 33 S 175 30 E
Port Charlotte, U.S.A. 153 J7 26 59N 82 6W
Port Chester, U.S.A. 151 F11 41 0N 73 40W
Port Clements, Canada 142 C2 53 40N 132 10W
Port Clinton, U.S.A. 157 C14 41 31N 82 56W
Port Colborne, Canada 140 D4 42 50N 79 10W
Port Coquitlam, Canada 142 D4 49 15N 122 45W
Port Cornwallis, India 95 H11 13 17N 93 5 E
Port Credit, Canada 150 C5 43 33N 79 35W
Port-Cros △, France 29 F10 43 0N 6 24 E
Port Curtis, Australia 126 C5 23 57 S 151 20 E
Port d'Alcúdia, Spain 38 B4 39 50N 3 7 E
Port Dalhousie, Canada 150 C5 43 13N 79 16W
Port d'Andratx, Spain 38 B3 39 32N 2 23 E
Port Darwin, Australia 124 B5 12 24 S 130 45 E
Port Darwin, Falk. Is. 9 f 51 50 S 59 0W
Port Davey, Australia 127 G4 43 16 S 145 55 E
Port-de-Bouc, France 29 E8 43 24N 4 59 E
Port-de-Paix, Haiti 165 C5 19 50N 72 50W
Port de Pollença, Spain 38 B4 39 54N 3 4 E
Port de Sóller, Spain 38 B3 39 48N 2 42 E
Port Dickson, Malaysia 87 L3 2 30N 101 49 E
Port Douglas, Australia 126 B4 16 30 S 145 30 E
Port Dover, Canada 150 D4 42 47N 80 12W
Port Edward, Canada 142 C2 54 12N 130 10W
Port Elgin, Canada 140 D3 44 25N 81 25W
Port Elizabeth, S. Africa 116 E4 33 58 S 25 40 E
Port Ellen, U.K. 22 F2 55 38N 6 11W
Port Elliot, Australia 128 C3 35 32 S 138 41 E
Port-en-Bessin-Huppain, France 26 C6 49 21N 0 45W
Port Erin, I. of Man 20 C3 54 5N 4 45W
Port Essington, Australia 124 B5 11 15 S 132 10 E
Port Etienne = Nouâdhibou, Mauritania 110 D1 20 54N 17 0W
Port Ewen, U.S.A. 151 E11 41 54N 73 59W
Port Fairy, Australia 128 E5 38 22 S 142 12 E
Port Fitzroy, N.Z. 130 C4 36 8 S 175 20 E
Port Florence = Kisumu, Kenya 118 C3 0 3 S 34 45 E
Port Fouâd = Bûr Fuad, Egypt 106 H8 31 15N 32 20 E
Port Francqui = Ilebo, Dem. Rep. of the Congo 115 C4 4 17 S 20 55 E
Port Gamble, U.S.A. 160 C4 47 51N 122 35W
Port-Gentil, Gabon 114 C1 0 40 S 8 50 E
Port Germein, Australia 127 E2 33 1 S 138 1 E
Port Gibson, U.S.A. 155 K9 31 58N 90 59W
Port Glasgow, U.K. 22 F4 55 56N 4 41W
Port-Gueydon = Azeffoun, Algeria 111 A5 36 51N 4 26 E
Port Harcourt, Nigeria 113 E6 4 40N 7 10 E
Port Hardy, Canada 142 C3 50 41N 127 30W
Port Harrison = Inukjuak, Canada 139 C12 58 25N 78 15W
Port Hawkesbury, Canada 141 C7 45 36N 61 22W
Port Hedland, Australia 124 D2 20 25 S 118 35 E
Port Heiden, U.S.A. 144 H8 56 55N 158 41W
Port Henry, U.S.A. 151 B11 44 3N 73 28W
Port Herald = Nsanje, Malawi 119 F4 16 55 S 35 12 E
Port Hood, Canada 141 C7 46 0N 61 32W
Port Hope, Canada 140 D4 43 56N 78 20W
Port Hope, U.S.A. 150 C2 43 57N 82 43W
Port Hope Simpson, Canada 141 B8 52 33N 56 18W
Port Hueneme, U.S.A. 161 L7 34 7N 119 12W
Port Huron, U.S.A. 150 D2 42 58N 82 26W
Port Iliç, Azerbaijan 101 C13 38 53N 48 47 E
Port Jefferson, U.S.A. 151 F11 40 57N 73 3W
Port Jervis, U.S.A. 151 E10 41 22N 74 41W
Port-Joinville, France 26 F4 46 45N 2 23W
Port Katon, Russia 59 J10 46 52N 38 46 E
Port Kelang = Pelabuhan Klang, Malaysia 87 L3 3 0N 101 23 E
Port Kembla, Australia 129 C9 34 52 S 150 49 E
Port Kenny, Australia 127 E1 33 10 S 134 41 E
Port-la-Nouvelle, France 28 E7 43 1N 3 3 E
Port Lairge = Waterford, Ireland 23 D4 52 15N 7 8W
Port Laoise, Ireland 23 C4 53 2N 7 18W
Port Lavaca, U.S.A. 155 L6 28 37N 96 38W
Port Leyden, U.S.A. 151 C9 43 35N 75 21W
Port Lincoln, Australia 128 C1 34 42 S 135 52 E
Port Lions, U.S.A. 144 H9 57 52N 152 53W
Port Loko, S. Leone 112 D2 8 48N 12 46W
Port Louis, France 26 E3 47 42N 3 22W
Port-Louis, Guadeloupe 164 b 16 28N 61 32W
Port Louis, Mauritius 121 d 20 10 S 57 30 E
Port Lyautey = Kenitra, Morocco 110 B3 34 15N 6 40W
Port MacDonnell, Australia 128 E4 38 5 S 140 48 E
Port McNeill, Canada 142 C3 50 35N 127 6W
Port Macquarie, Australia 129 A10 31 25 S 152 25 E
Port Maria, Jamaica 164 a 18 22N 76 54W
Port Matilda, U.S.A. 150 F6 40 48N 78 3W
Port Mayaca, U.S.A. 153 J9 26 59N 80 36W
Port Mellon, Canada 142 D4 49 32N 123 31W
Port-Menier, Canada 141 C7 49 51N 64 15W
Port Moller, U.S.A. 144 J7 55 59N 160 34W
Port Moody, Canada 160 A4 49 17N 122 51W
Port Morant, Jamaica 164 a 17 54N 76 19W
Port Moresby, Papua N. G. 132 E4 9 24 S 147 8 E
Port Mourant, Guyana 169 B6 6 15N 57 20W
Port Musgrave, Australia 126 A3 11 55 S 141 50 E
Port Narevin, Vanuatu 133 H7 18 45 S 169 10 E
Port-Navalo, France 26 E4 47 34N 2 54W
Port Neches, U.S.A. 155 L8 30 0N 93 59W
Port Nicholson, N.Z. 130 H3 41 20 S 174 52 E
Port Nolloth, S. Africa 116 D2 29 17 S 16 52 E
Port Nouveau-Québec = Kangiqsualujjuaq, Canada 139 C13 58 30N 65 59W
Port of Spain, Trin. & Tob. 169 F9 10 40N 61 31W
Port Olry, Vanuatu 133 E5 15 1 S 167 4 E
Port Orange, U.S.A. 153 F9 29 9N 80 59W
Port Orchard, U.S.A. 160 C4 47 32N 122 38W
Port Orford, U.S.A. 158 E1 42 45N 124 30W
Port Pegasus, N.Z. 131 H2 47 12 S 167 41 E
Port Perry, Canada 140 D4 44 6N 78 56W
Port Phillip B., Australia 129 E6 38 10 S 144 50 E
Port Pirie, Australia 128 B3 33 10 S 138 1 E
Port Renfrew, Canada 142 D4 48 30N 124 20W
Port Roper, Australia 126 A2 14 45 S 135 25 E
Port Rowan, Canada 150 D4 42 40N 80 30W
Port Royal Sd., U.S.A. 152 C9 32 15N 80 40W
Port Safaga = Bûr Safâga, Egypt 96 E2 26 43N 33 57 E
Port Said = Bûr Sa'îd, Egypt 106 H8 31 16N 32 18 E
Port St. Joe, U.S.A. 152 F4 29 49N 85 18W
Port St. Johns = Umzimvubu, S. Africa 117 E4 31 38 S 29 33 E
Port-St-Louis-du-Rhône, France 29 E8 43 23N 4 49 E
Port St. Lucie, U.S.A. 153 H9 27 20N 80 20W
Port-Ste-Marie, France 28 D4 44 15N 0 25 E
Port Salerno, U.S.A. 153 H9 27 9N 80 12W
Port Sanilac, U.S.A. 150 C2 43 26N 82 33W
Port Severn, Canada 150 B5 44 48N 79 43W
Port Shepstone, S. Africa 117 E5 30 44 S 30 28 E
Port Simpson, Canada 142 C2 54 30N 130 20W
Port Stanley = Stanley, Falk. Is. 9 f 51 40 S 59 51W
Port Stanley, Canada 140 D3 42 40N 81 10W
Port Sudan = Bûr Sûdân, Sudan 106 D4 19 32N 37 9 E
Port Sulphur, U.S.A. 155 L10 29 29N 89 42W
Port-sur-Saône, France 27 E13 47 42N 6 2 E
Port Swettenham = Pelabuhan Klang, Malaysia 87 L3 3 0N 101 23 E
Port Talbot, U.K. 21 F4 51 35N 3 47W
Port Taufiq = Bûr Taufiq, Egypt 106 J8 29 54N 32 32 E
Port Townsend, U.S.A. 160 B4 48 7N 122 45W
Port-Vato, Vanuatu 133 F6 16 20 S 168 1 E
Port-Vendres, France 28 F7 42 32N 3 8 E
Port Victoria, Australia 128 C2 34 30 S 137 29 E
Port Vila, Vanuatu 133 G6 17 45 S 168 18 E
Port Vladimir, Russia 56 A5 69 25N 33 6 E
Port Wakefield, Australia 128 C3 34 12 S 138 10 E
Port Washington, U.S.A. 148 D2 43 23N 87 53W
Port Weld = Kuala Sepetang, Malaysia 87 K3 4 49N 100 28 E
Port Wentworth, U.S.A. 152 C8 32 9N 81 10W
Porta Orientalis, Romania 37 F12 45 6N 22 18 E
Portachuelo, Bolivia 173 D5 17 10 S 63 20W
Portadown, U.K. 23 B5 54 25N 6 27W
Portaferry, U.K. 23 B6 54 23N 5 33W
Portage, Mich., U.S.A. 157 B11 42 12N 85 35W
Portage, Pa., U.S.A. 150 F6 40 23N 78 41W
Portage, Wis., U.S.A. 154 D10 43 33N 89 28W
Portage →, U.S.A. 157 C14 41 31N 83 5W
Portage la Prairie, Canada 143 D9 49 58N 98 18W
Portageville, U.S.A. 155 G10 36 26N 89 42W
Portal, U.S.A. 152 C8 32 33N 81 56W
Portalegre, Portugal 43 F3 39 19N 7 25W
Portalegre ☐, Portugal 43 F3 39 20N 7 40W
Portales, U.S.A. 155 H3 34 11N 103 20W
Portarlington, Ireland 23 C4 53 9N 7 14W
Portbou, Spain 40 C8 42 25N 3 9 E
Porteira, Brazil 169 D6 1 5 S 57 4W
Porteirinha, Brazil 171 E3 15 44 S 43 2W
Portel, Brazil 170 B1 1 57 S 50 49W
Portel, Portugal 43 G3 38 19N 7 41W
Portela, Lisboa ✕ (LIS), Portugal 43 G1 38 46N 9 8W
Porter, U.S.A. 157 C9 41 36N 87 4W
Porter L., N.W.T., Canada 143 A7 61 41N 108 5W
Porter L., Sask., Canada 143 B7 56 20N 107 20W
Porterville, S. Africa 116 E2 33 0 S 19 0 E
Porterville, U.S.A. 160 J8 36 4N 119 1W
Portes-lès-Valence, France 29 D8 44 52N 4 54 E
Porthcawl, U.K. 21 F4 51 29N 3 42W
Porthill, U.S.A. 158 B5 48 59N 116 30W
Porthmadog, U.K. 20 E3 52 55N 4 8W
Portile de Fier, Europe 52 F7 44 44N 22 30 E
Portimão, Portugal 43 H2 37 8N 8 32W
Portishead, U.K. 21 F5 51 29N 2 46W
Portiţei, Gura, Romania 53 F14 44 41N 29 0 E
Portknockie, U.K. 22 D6 57 42N 2 51W
Portland, N.S.W., Australia 129 B9 33 20 S 150 0 E
Portland, Vic., Australia 128 E4 38 20 S 141 35 E
Portland, Canada 151 B8 44 42N 76 12W
Portland, Conn., U.S.A. 151 E12 41 34N 72 38W
Portland, Fla., U.S.A. 152 E3 30 31N 86 12W
Portland, Ind., U.S.A. 157 D12 40 26N 84 59W
Portland, Maine, U.S.A. 139 D12 43 39N 70 16W
Portland, Mich., U.S.A. 157 B12 42 52N 84 54W
Portland, Oreg., U.S.A. 160 E4 45 32N 122 37W
Portland, Pa., U.S.A. 151 F9 40 55N 75 6W
Portland, Tex., U.S.A. 155 M6 27 53N 97 20W
Portland ✕ (PDX), U.S.A. 160 E4 45 35N 122 36W
Portland, I. of, U.K. 21 G5 50 33N 2 26W
Portland B., Australia 128 E4 38 15 S 141 45 E
Portland Bight, Jamaica 164 a 17 52N 77 5W
Portland Bill, U.K. 21 G5 50 31N 2 28W
Portland Canal, U.S.A. 142 B2 55 56N 130 0W
Portland I., N.Z. 130 F6 39 20 S 177 51 E
Portland Pt., Ascension I. 9 g 7 59 S 14 25W
Portland Pt., Jamaica 164 a 17 42N 77 11W
Portmadoc = Porthmadog, U.K. 20 E3 52 55N 4 8W
Portmore, Jamaica 164 a 17 53N 77 53W
Porto, Brazil 170 B3 3 54 S 42 42W
Porto, France 29 F12 42 16N 8 42 E
Porto, Portugal 42 D2 41 8N 8 40W
Porto ☐, Portugal 42 D2 41 8N 8 20W
Porto, G. de, France 29 F12 42 17N 8 34 E
Pôrto Acre, Brazil 172 B4 9 34 S 67 31W
Pôrto Alegre = Luzilândia, Brazil 170 B3 3 28 S 42 22W
Pôrto Alegre, Pará, Brazil 169 D7 4 22 S 52 44W
Pôrto Alegre, Rio Grande do S., Brazil 175 C5 30 5 S 51 10W
Porto Alegre, São Tomé & Príncipe 115 G6 0 2N 6 32 E
Porto Amboim = Gunza, Angola 115 E2 10 50 S 13 50 E
Porto Amélia = Pemba, Mozam. 119 E5 12 58 S 40 30 E
Porto Azzurro, Italy 44 F7 42 46N 10 24 E
Pôrto Cajueiro, Brazil 173 C6 11 3 S 55 53W
Porto Cristo, Spain 38 B4 39 33N 3 20 E
Pôrto da Fôlha, Brazil 170 C4 9 55 S 37 17W
Pôrto de Móz, Brazil 169 D7 4 11 S 52 13W
Pôrto de Pedras, Brazil 170 C4 9 10 S 35 17W
Pôrto des Meinacos, Brazil 173 C7 12 33 S 53 7W
Pôrto dos Gaúchos, Brazil 173 C6 11 32 S 57 16W
Porto Empédocle, Italy 46 E6 37 17N 13 32 E
Pôrto Esperança, Brazil 173 D6 19 37 S 57 29W
Pôrto Esperidão, Brazil 173 D6 15 51 S 58 28W
Pôrto Formoso, Azores 9 d3 37 49N 25 25W
Pôrto Franco, Brazil 170 C2 6 20 S 47 24W
Pôrto Grande, Brazil 169 C7 0 42N 51 24W
Porto Inglês, C. Verde Is. 9 j 15 21N 23 10W
Pôrto Jofre, Brazil 173 D6 17 20 S 56 48W
Porto Lágos, Greece 51 E9 41 1N 25 6 E
Porto Lengone = Porto Azzurro, Italy 44 F7 42 46N 10 24 E
Porto Maurizio = Impéria, Italy 44 E5 43 53N 8 3 E
Pôrto Mendes, Brazil 175 A5 24 30 S 54 15W
Porto Moniz, Madeira 9 c 32 52N 17 11W
Pôrto Murtinho, Brazil 173 E6 21 45 S 57 55W
Pôrto Nacional, Brazil 170 D2 10 40 S 48 30W

Porto-Novo, Benin 113 D5 6 23N 2 42 E
Porto Petro, Spain 38 B4 39 22N 3 13 E
Porto San Giórgio, Italy 45 E10 43 11N 13 48 E
Porto Sant' Elpídio, Italy 45 E10 43 15N 13 43 E
Pôrto Santana, Brazil 169 D7 0 3 S 51 11W
Porto Santo, I. de, Madeira 110 B1 33 45N 16 25W
Porto Santo Stéfano, Italy 44 F8 42 26N 11 7 E
Pôrto São José, Brazil 175 A5 22 43 S 53 10W
Porto Seguro = Guadalupe, Brazil 170 C3 6 44 S 43 47W
Pôrto Seguro, Brazil 171 E4 16 26 S 39 5W
Porto Tolle, Italy 45 D9 44 56N 12 22 E
Porto Tórres, Italy 46 B1 40 50N 8 24 E
Pôrto União, Brazil 175 B5 26 10 S 51 10W
Pôrto Válter, Brazil 172 B3 8 15 S 72 40W
Porto-Vecchio, France 29 G13 41 35N 9 16 E
Pôrto Velho, Brazil 173 B5 8 46 S 63 54W
Portobelo, Panama 164 E4 9 35N 79 42W
Portoferráio, Italy 44 F7 42 48N 10 20 E
Portogruaro, Italy 45 C9 45 47N 12 50 E
Portola, U.S.A. 160 F6 39 49N 120 28W
Portomaggiore, Italy 45 D8 44 42N 11 48 E
Portør, Norway 18 F6 58 48N 9 28 E
Portoscuso, Italy 46 C1 39 12N 8 24 E
Portovénere, Italy 44 D6 44 3N 9 51 E
Portoviejo, Ecuador 168 D1 1 7 S 80 28W
Portpatrick, U.K. 22 G3 54 51N 5 7W
Portree, U.K. 22 D2 57 25N 6 12W
Portrush, U.K. 23 A5 55 12N 6 40W
Portsmouth, Dominica 165 C7 15 34N 61 27W
Portsmouth, U.K. 21 G6 50 48N 1 6W
Portsmouth, N.H., U.S.A. 149 D10 43 5N 70 45W
Portsmouth, Ohio, U.S.A. 148 F4 38 44N 82 57W
Portsmouth, R.I., U.S.A. 151 E13 41 36N 71 15W
Portsmouth, Va., U.S.A. 148 G7 36 50N 76 18W
Portsmouth □, U.K. 21 G6 50 48N 1 6W
Portsoy, U.K. 22 D6 57 41N 2 41W
Portstewart, U.K. 23 A5 55 11N 6 43W
Porttipahdan tekojärvi, Finland 14 B22 68 5N 26 40 E
Portugal ■, Europe 42 F3 40 0N 8 0W
Portugalete, Spain 40 B1 43 19N 3 4W
Portuguesa □, Venezuela 168 B4 9 10N 69 15W
Portuguese East Africa = Mozambique ■, Africa 119 F4 19 0 S 35 0 E
Portuguese Guinea = Guinea-Bissau ■, Africa 112 C2 12 0N 15 0W
Portuguese Timor = East Timor ■, Asia 82 C3 8 50 S 126 0 E
Portuguese West Africa = Angola ■, Africa 115 E3 12 0 S 18 0 E
Portumna, Ireland 23 C3 53 6N 8 14W
Portville, U.S.A. 150 D6 42 3N 78 20W
Porvenir, Bolivia 172 C4 11 10 S 68 50W
Porvenir, Chile 176 D2 53 10 S 70 16W
Porvoo, Finland 15 F21 60 24N 25 40 E
Porzuna, Spain 43 F6 39 9N 4 9W
Posada, Italy 46 B2 40 38N 9 43 E
Posada →, Italy 46 B2 40 39N 9 45 E
Posadas, Argentina 175 B4 27 30 S 55 50W
Posadas, Spain 43 H5 37 47N 5 11W
Poschiavo, Switz. 33 D10 46 19N 10 4 E
Posen = Poznań, Poland 55 F3 52 25N 16 55 E
Posets, Spain 40 C5 42 39N 0 25 E
Poseyville, U.S.A. 157 F9 38 10N 87 47W
Poshan = Boshan, China 75 F9 36 28N 117 49 E
Posht-e Badam, Iran 97 C7 33 2N 55 23 E
Posidhion, Ákra, Greece 50 G7 39 57N 23 30 E
Posidium, Greece 49 F9 35 30N 27 10 E
Poso, Indonesia 82 B2 1 20 S 120 55 E
Poso, Danau, Indonesia 82 B2 1 52 S 120 35 E
Posoegroenoe, Suriname 169 C6 4 23N 55 43W
Posong, S. Korea 75 G14 34 46N 127 5 E
Posse, Brazil 171 D2 14 4 S 46 18W
Possedimenti Italiani dell'Egeo = Dhodhekánisos, Greece 49 E8 36 35N 27 0 E
Possel, C.A.R. 114 A3 5 5N 19 10 E
Possession I., Antarctica 7 D11 72 4 S 172 0 E
Pössneck, Germany 30 E7 50 42N 11 35 E
Possum Kingdom L., U.S.A. 155 J5 32 52N 98 26W
Post, U.S.A. 155 J4 33 12N 101 23W
Post Falls, U.S.A. 158 C5 47 43N 116 57W
Postavy = Pastavy, Belarus 15 J22 55 4N 26 50 E
Poste-de-la-Baleine = Kuujjuarapik, Canada 140 A4 55 20N 77 35W
Poste Maurice Cortier, Algeria 111 D5 22 14N 1 2 E
Postmasburg, S. Africa 116 D3 28 18 S 23 5 E
Postojna, Slovenia 45 C11 45 46N 14 12 E
Poston, U.S.A. 161 M12 34 0N 114 24W
Postumia = Postojna, Slovenia 45 C11 45 46N 14 12 E
Postville, Canada 141 B8 54 54N 59 47W
Postville, U.S.A. 156 A5 43 5N 91 34W
Potamós, Andikíthira, Greece 48 F5 35 52N 23 15 E
Potamós, Kíthira, Greece 48 E4 36 15N 22 58 E
Potchefstroom, S. Africa 116 D4 26 41 S 27 7 E
Potcoava, Romania 53 F9 44 30N 24 39 E
Poté, Brazil 171 E3 17 49 S 41 49W
Poteau, U.S.A. 155 H7 35 3N 94 37W
Poteet, U.S.A. 155 L5 29 2N 98 35W
Potenza, Italy 47 B8 40 38N 15 48 E
Potenza →, Italy 45 E10 43 25N 13 40 E
Potenza Picena, Italy 45 E10 43 22N 13 37 E
Poteriteri, L., N.Z. 131 G2 46 5 S 167 10 E
Potgietersrus = Mokopane, S. Africa 117 C4 24 10 S 28 55 E
Poti, Georgia 61 J5 42 10N 41 38 E
Potiraguá, Brazil 171 E4 15 36 S 39 53W
Potiskum, Nigeria 113 C7 11 39N 11 2 E
Potlogi, Romania 53 F10 44 34N 25 34 E
Potomac →, U.S.A. 148 G7 38 0N 76 23W
Potosí, Bolivia 173 D4 19 38 S 65 50W
Potosi, U.S.A. 156 G6 37 56N 90 47W
Potosí □, Bolivia 172 E4 20 31 S 67 0W
Potosi Mt., U.S.A. 161 K11 35 57N 115 29W
Pototan, Phil. 81 F4 10 54N 122 38 E
Potrerillos, Chile 174 B2 26 30 S 69 30W
Potsdam, Germany 30 C9 52 25N 13 4 E
Potsdam, U.S.A. 151 B10 44 40N 74 59W
Pottangi, India 94 E6 18 34N 82 58 E
Pottenstein, Germany 31 F7 49 46N 11 24 E
Pottersville, U.S.A. 151 C11 43 43N 73 50W
Pottery Hill = Abu Ballas, Egypt 106 C2 24 26N 27 36 E
Pottstown, U.S.A. 151 F9 40 15N 75 39W
Pottsville, U.S.A. 151 F8 40 41N 76 12W
Pottuvil, Sri Lanka 95 L5 6 55N 81 50 E
P'otzu, Taiwan 77 F13 23 30N 120 25 E
Pouancé, France 26 E5 47 44N 1 10W
Pouce Coupé, Canada 142 B4 55 40N 120 10W
Pouébo, N. Cal. 133 T18 20 24 S 164 36 E
Pouembout, N. Cal. 133 U18 21 8 S 164 53 E
Poughkeepsie, U.S.A. 151 E11 41 42N 73 56W
Pouilly-sur-Loire, France 27 E9 47 17N 2 57 E
Poulan, U.S.A. 152 D6 31 31N 83 47W
Poulaphouca Res., Ireland 23 C5 53 8N 6 30W
Pouláta, Greece 39 C2 38 14N 20 36 E
Poulsbo, U.S.A. 160 C4 47 44N 122 39W
Poultney, U.S.A. 151 C11 43 31N 73 14W
Poulton-le-Fylde, U.K. 20 D5 53 51N 2 58W
Poum, N. Cal. 133 T18 20 14 S 164 2 E
Pounga-Nganda, Gabon 114 C2 2 58 S 10 51 E
Pouso Alegre, Mato Grosso, Brazil 173 C6 11 46 S 57 16W
Pouso Alegre, Minas Gerais, Brazil 175 A6 22 14 S 45 57W
Pouso Alto = Piracanjuba, Brazil 171 E2 17 18 S 49 1W
Pout, Senegal 112 C1 14 45N 17 0W
Pouthisat, Cambodia 86 F4 12 34N 103 50 E
Pouzauges, France 26 F6 46 47N 0 50W
Pova de Santa Iria, Portugal 43 G1 38 51N 9 4W
Považská Bystrica, Slovak Rep. 35 B11 49 8N 18 27 E
Povenets, Russia 56 B5 62 50N 34 50 E
Poverty B., N.Z. 130 E7 38 43 S 178 2 E
Povlen, Serbia & M. 50 B3 44 9N 19 44 E
Póvoa de Lanhosa, Portugal 42 D2 41 33N 8 15W
Póvoa de Varzim, Portugal 42 D2 41 25N 8 46W
Povoação, Azores 9 d3 37 45N 25 15W
Povorino, Russia 60 E6 51 12N 42 5 E
Povungnituk = Puvirnituq, Canada 139 B12 60 2N 77 10W
Powassan, Canada 140 C4 46 5N 79 25W
Poway, U.S.A. 161 N9 32 58N 117 2W
Powder →, U.S.A. 154 B2 46 45N 105 26W
Powder River, U.S.A. 158 E10 43 2N 106 59W
Powder Springs, U.S.A. 152 B5 33 52N 84 41W
Powell, U.S.A. 158 D9 44 45N 108 46W
Powell, L., U.S.A. 159 H8 36 57N 111 29W
Powell River, Canada 142 D4 49 50N 124 35W
Powelton, U.S.A. 152 B7 33 26N 82 52W
Power House = Drayton Valley, Canada 142 C6 53 12N 114 58W
Powers, U.S.A. 148 C2 45 41N 87 32W
Powys □, U.K. 21 E4 52 20N 3 20W
Poxoreu, Brazil 173 D7 15 50 S 54 23W
Poya, N. Cal. 133 U19 21 19 S 165 7 E
Poyang Hu, China 77 C11 29 5N 116 20 E
Poyarkovo, Russia 67 E13 49 36N 128 41 E
Poysdorf, Austria 35 C9 48 40N 16 37 E
Poza de la Sal, Spain 42 C7 42 35N 3 31W
Poza Rica, Mexico 163 C5 20 33N 97 27W
Pozanti, Turkey 100 D6 37 25N 34 50 E
Požarevac, Serbia & M. 50 B5 44 35N 21 18 E
Pozazal, Puerto, Spain 42 C6 42 56N 4 10W
Požega, Croatia 52 E2 45 20N 17 40 E
Požega, Serbia & M. 50 C4 43 53N 20 2 E
Pozhva, Russia 64 B6 59 5N 56 5 E
Poznań, Poland 55 F3 52 25N 16 55 E
Poznań ✕ (POZ), Poland 55 F3 52 26N 16 45 E
Pozo, U.S.A. 161 K6 35 20N 120 24W
Pozo Alcón, Spain 43 H8 37 42N 2 56W
Pozo Almonte, Chile 172 E4 20 10 S 69 50W
Pozo Colorado, Paraguay 174 A4 23 30 S 58 45W
Pozoblanco, Spain 43 G6 38 23N 4 51W
Pozorrubio, Phil. 80 C3 16 7N 120 33 E
Pozuzo, Peru 172 C2 10 5 S 75 35W
Pozzallo, Italy 47 F7 36 43N 14 51 E
Pozzomaggiore, Italy 46 B1 40 24N 8 39 E
Pozzuoli, Italy 47 B7 40 49N 14 7 E
Pra →, Ghana 113 D4 5 1N 1 37W
Prabuty, Poland 54 E6 53 47N 19 15 E
Prača, Bos.-H. 52 G3 43 47N 18 43 E
Prachatice, Czech Rep. 34 B6 49 1N 14 0 E
Prachin Buri, Thailand 86 E3 14 0N 101 25 E
Prachuap Khiri Khan, Thailand 87 G2 11 49N 99 48 E
Pradelles, France 28 D7 44 46N 3 52 E
Pradera, Colombia 168 C2 3 25N 76 15W
Prades, France 28 F6 42 38N 2 23 E
Prado, Brazil 171 E4 17 20 S 39 13W
Prado del Rey, Spain 43 J5 36 48N 5 33W
Præstø, Denmark 17 J6 55 8N 12 2 E
Pragersko, Slovenia 45 B12 46 27N 15 42 E
Prague = Praha, Czech Rep. 34 A7 50 5N 14 22 E
Praha, Czech Rep. 34 A7 50 5N 14 22 E
Praha ✕ (PRG), Czech Rep. 34 A7 50 7N 14 15 E
Prahecq, France 28 B3 46 19N 0 26W
Prahita →, India 94 E4 19 0N 79 55 E
Prahova □, Romania 53 E10 45 10N 26 0 E
Prahova →, Romania 53 F10 44 50N 25 50 E
Prahovo, Serbia & M. 50 B6 44 18N 22 39 E
Praia, Azores 9 d1 39 3N 27 58W
Praia, C. Verde Is. 9 j 15 2N 23 34W
Praia a Mare, Italy 47 C8 39 50N 15 45 E
Praia da Vitória, Azores 9 d1 38 44N 27 4W
Praia do Norte, Azores 9 d1 38 36N 28 46W
Praid, Romania 53 D10 46 32N 25 10 E
Prainha, Azores 9 d1 38 27N 28 12W
Prainha, Amazonas, Brazil 173 B5 7 10 S 60 30W
Prainha, Pará, Brazil 169 D7 1 45 S 53 30W
Prairie, Australia 126 C3 20 50 S 144 35 E
Prairie City, U.S.A. 158 D4 44 28N 118 43W
Prairie Dog Town Fork →, U.S.A. 155 H5 34 30N 99 23W
Prairie du Chien, U.S.A. 156 A5 43 3N 91 9W
Prairie du Rocher, U.S.A. 156 F6 38 5N 90 6W
Prairie Village, U.S.A. 156 F2 38 58N 94 38W
Prairies, L. of the, Canada 143 C8 51 16N 101 32W
Pramánda, Greece 48 B3 39 32N 21 8 E
Prampram, Ghana 113 D5 5 43N 0 8 E
Pran Buri, Thailand 86 F2 12 23N 99 55 E
Prándarjökull, Iceland 11 C12 64 40N 14 55W
Prang, Ghana 113 D4 8 1N 0 56W
Prapat, Indonesia 78 D1 2 41N 98 58 E
Praslin, Seychelles 121 b 4 18 S 55 45 E
Prasonísi, Ákra, Greece 38 F11 35 42N 27 46 E
Prassberg = Mozirje, Slovenia 45 B11 46 22N 14 58 E
Prästmon, Sweden 16 A11 63 5N 17 45 E
Praszka, Poland 55 G5 51 5N 18 31 E
Prata, Brazil 171 E2 19 25 S 48 54W
Pratabpur, India 93 H10 23 28N 83 15 E
Pratapgarh, Raj., India 92 G6 24 2N 74 40 E
Pratapgarh, Ut. P., India 93 G9 25 56N 81 59 E
Pratas Is. = Dongsha Dao, China 77 G11 20 45N 116 43 E
Prätigau, Switz. 33 C9 46 56N 9 44 E
Prato, Italy 44 E8 43 53N 11 6 E
Prato allo Stelvio, Italy 33 C11 46 37N 10 35 E
Prátola Peligna, Italy 45 F10 42 6N 13 52 E
Prats-de-Mollo-la-Preste, France 28 F6 42 25N 2 27 E
Pratt, U.S.A. 155 G5 37 39N 98 44W
Pratteln, Switz. 32 A5 47 31N 7 41 E
Prattville, U.S.A. 149 J2 32 28N 86 29W
Praust = Pruszcz Gdański, Poland 54 D5 54 17N 18 40 E
Pravara →, India 94 E2 19 35N 74 45 E
Pravdinsk, Russia 54 D8 54 27N 21 1 E
Pravdinsk, Russia 60 B6 56 29N 43 28 E
Pravets, Bulgaria 50 D7 42 53N 23 55 E
Pravia, Spain 42 B4 43 30N 6 12W
Praya, Indonesia 85 D5 8 39 S 116 17 E
Pré-en-Pail, France 26 D6 48 28N 0 12W
Precipice △, Australia 127 D5 25 18 S 150 5 E
Precordillera, Argentina 174 C2 30 0 S 69 1W
Predáppio, Italy 45 D8 44 6N 11 59 E
Predazzo, Italy 45 B8 46 19N 11 36 E
Predeal, Romania 53 E10 45 30N 25 34 E
Predejane, Serbia & M. 50 D6 42 51N 22 9 E
Preeceville, Canada 143 C8 51 57N 102 40W
Preetz, Germany 30 A6 54 14N 10 18 E
Pregolya →, Russia 54 D7 54 41N 20 22 E
Pregrada, Croatia 45 B12 46 11N 15 45 E
Preiļi, Latvia 15 H22 56 18N 26 43 E
Preko, Croatia 45 D12 44 7N 15 10 E
Prelog, Croatia 45 B13 46 18N 16 32 E
Premer, Australia 129 A8 31 29 S 149 56 E
Prémery, France 27 E10 47 10N 3 18 E
Prémia, Italy 33 D6 46 17N 8 20 E
Premià de Mar, Spain 40 D7 41 29N 2 22 E
Premont, U.S.A. 155 M5 27 22N 98 7W
Premuda, Croatia 45 D11 44 20N 14 36 E
Prentice, U.S.A. 154 C9 45 33N 90 17W
Prenzlau, Germany 30 B9 53 19N 13 50 E
Preobrazheniye, Russia 70 C6 42 54N 133 54 E
Preparis I., Burma 95 G11 14 52N 93 41 E
Preparis North Channel, Burma 95 G11 15 27N 94 5 E
Preparis South Channel, Burma 95 G11 14 33N 93 30 E
Přerov, Czech Rep. 35 B10 49 28N 17 27 E
Prescott, Canada 140 D4 44 45N 75 30W
Prescott, Ariz., U.S.A. 159 J7 34 33N 112 28W
Prescott, Ark., U.S.A. 155 J8 33 48N 93 23W
Prescott Valley, U.S.A. 159 J7 34 40N 112 18W
Preservation Inlet, N.Z. 131 G1 46 8 S 166 35 E
Preševo, Serbia & M. 50 D5 42 19N 21 39 E
Presho, U.S.A. 154 D4 43 54N 100 3W
Presicce, Italy 47 C11 39 54N 18 16 E
Presidencia de la Plaza, Argentina 174 B4 27 0 S 59 50W
Presidencia Roque Saenz Peña, Argentina 174 B3 26 45 S 60 30W
Presidente Dutra, Brazil 170 C3 5 15 S 44 30W
Presidente Epitácio, Brazil 171 F1 21 56 S 52 6W
Presidente Figueiredo, Brazil 169 D5 1 57 S 60 2W
Presidente Hayes □, Paraguay 174 A4 24 0 S 59 0W
Presidente Hermes, Brazil 173 C5 11 17 S 61 55W
Presidente Juán Perón = Chaco □, Argentina 174 B3 26 30 S 61 0W
Presidente Prudente, Brazil 175 A5 22 5 S 51 25W
Presidente Vargas = Nova Era, Brazil 171 E3 19 45 S 43 3W
Presidio, Mexico 162 B4 29 29N 104 23W
Presidio, U.S.A. 155 L2 29 34N 104 22W
Preslav, Bulgaria 51 C10 43 10N 26 52 E
Preslavska Planina, Bulgaria 51 C10 43 10N 26 45 E
Prešov, Slovak Rep. 35 B14 49 0N 21 15 E
Prešovský □, Slovak Rep. 35 B13 49 10N 21 0 E
Prespa, Bulgaria 51 E8 41 44N 24 55 E
Prespa △, Greece 50 F5 40 48N 21 4 E
Prespa, L. = Prespansko Jezero, Macedonia 50 F5 40 55N 21 0 E
Prespansko Jezero, Macedonia 50 F5 40 55N 21 0 E
Presque I., U.S.A. 150 D4 42 9N 80 6W
Presque Isle, U.S.A. 149 B12 46 41N 68 1W
Pressburg = Bratislava, Slovak Rep. 35 C10 48 10N 17 7 E
Prestatyn, U.K. 20 D4 53 20N 3 24W
Prestea, Ghana 112 D4 5 22N 2 7W
Presteigne, U.K. 21 E5 52 17N 3 0W
Přeštice, Czech Rep. 34 B6 49 34N 13 20 E
Presto, Bolivia 173 D5 18 55 S 64 56W
Preston, Canada 150 C4 43 23N 80 21W
Preston, U.K. 20 D5 53 46N 2 42W
Preston, Ga., U.S.A. 152 C5 32 4N 84 32W
Preston, Idaho, U.S.A. 158 E8 42 6N 111 53W
Preston, Iowa, U.S.A. 156 B6 42 3N 90 24W
Preston, Minn., U.S.A. 154 D8 43 40N 92 5W
Preston, Mo., U.S.A. 156 G3 37 56N 93 13W
Preston, C., Australia 124 D2 20 51 S 116 12 E
Prestonsburg, U.S.A. 148 G4 37 39N 82 46W
Prestranda, Norway 18 E6 59 6N 9 4 E
Prestwick, U.K. 22 F4 55 29N 4 37W
Prêto →, Amazonas, Brazil 169 D5 0 8 S 64 6W
Prêto →, Bahia, Brazil 170 D3 11 21 S 43 52W
Prêto do Igapó-Açu →, Brazil 169 D6 4 26 S 59 48W
Pretoria, S. Africa 117 D4 25 44 S 28 12 E
Preuilly-sur-Claise, France 26 F7 46 51N 0 56 E
Preussisch-Eylau = Bagrationovsk, Russia 15 J19 54 23N 20 39 E
Preussisch Friedland = Debrzno, Poland 54 E4 53 31N 17 14 E
Preussisch Holland = Pasłęk, Poland 54 D6 54 3N 19 41 E
Preussisch-Stargard = Starogard Gdański, Poland 54 E5 53 59N 18 30 E
Préveza, Greece 39 B2 38 57N 20 45 E
Préveza □, Greece 48 B2 39 10N 20 40 E
Préveza-Levkás ✕ (PVK), Greece 39 B2 38 57N 20 45 E
Prey Veng, Cambodia 87 G5 11 35N 105 29 E
Priazovskoye, Ukraine 59 J8 46 44N 35 40 E
Pribalkhash = Balqash, Kazakhstan 66 E8 46 50N 74 50 E
Pribilof Is., U.S.A. 144 H5 57 0N 170 0W
Priboj, Serbia & M. 50 C3 43 35N 19 32 E
Příbram, Czech Rep. 34 B7 49 41N 14 2 E
Price, U.S.A. 158 G8 39 36N 110 49W
Price, C., India 95 H11 13 34N 93 3 E
Price I., Canada 142 C3 52 23N 128 41W
Prichard, U.S.A. 149 K1 30 44N 88 5W
Priego, Spain 40 E2 40 26N 2 21W
Priego de Córdoba, Spain 43 H6 37 27N 4 12W
Priekule, Latvia 15 H19 56 26N 21 35 E
Priekulė, Lithuania 54 C8 55 33N 21 19 E
Prien, Germany 31 H8 47 51N 12 20 E
Prienai, Lithuania 15 J20 54 38N 23 57 E
Prieska, S. Africa 116 D3 29 40 S 22 42 E
Priest L., U.S.A. 158 B5 48 35N 116 52W
Priest River, U.S.A. 158 B5 48 10N 116 54W
Priest Valley, U.S.A. 160 J6 36 10N 120 39W
Prieto Diaz, Phil. 80 E5 13 2N 124 12 E
Prievidza, Slovak Rep. 35 C11 48 46N 18 36 E
Prignitz, Germany 30 B7 53 6N 11 45 E
Prijedor, Bos.-H. 45 D13 44 58N 16 41 E
Prijepolje, Serbia & M. 50 C3 43 27N 19 40 E
Prikaspiyskaya Nizmennost = Caspian Depression, Eurasia 61 G9 47 0N 48 0 E
Prikro, Ivory C. 112 D4 7 40N 3 59W
Prikubanskaya Nizmennost, Russia 61 H4 45 39N 38 33 E
Prilep, Macedonia 50 E5 41 21N 21 32 E
Priluki = Pryluky, Ukraine 59 G7 50 30N 32 24 E
Prime Seal I., Australia 127 G4 40 3 S 147 43 E
Primeira Cruz, Brazil 170 B3 2 30 S 43 26W
Primkenau = Przemków, Poland 55 G2 51 31N 15 48 E
Primorsk, Russia 54 D6 54 44N 20 0 E
Primorsk, Russia 58 B5 60 22N 28 37 E
Primorsko, Bulgaria 51 D11 42 15N 27 44 E
Primorsko-Akhtarsk, Russia 59 J10 46 2N 38 10 E
Primorskoye, Ukraine 59 J9 46 48N 36 20 E
Primrose L., Canada 143 C7 54 55N 109 45W
Prince Albert, Canada 143 C7 53 15N 105 50W
Prince Albert, S. Africa 116 E3 33 12 S 22 2 E
Prince Albert △, Canada 143 C7 54 0N 106 25W
Prince Albert Mts., Antarctica 7 D11 76 0 S 161 30 E
Prince Albert Pen., Canada 138 A8 72 30N 116 0W
Prince Albert Sd., Canada 138 A8 70 25N 115 0W
Prince Alfred, C., Canada 6 B1 74 20N 124 40W
Prince Charles I., Canada 139 B12 67 47N 76 12W
Prince Charles Mts., Antarctica 7 D6 72 0 S 67 0 E
Prince Edward I. □, Canada 141 C7 46 20N 63 20W
Prince Edward Is., Ind. Oc. 121 J2 46 35 S 38 0 E
Prince Edward Pt., Canada 150 C8 43 56N 76 52W
Prince George, Canada 142 C4 53 55N 122 50W
Prince of Wales, C., U.S.A. 144 D5 65 36N 168 5W
Prince of Wales I., Australia 126 A3 10 40 S 142 10 E
Prince of Wales I., Canada 138 A10 73 0N 99 0W
Prince of Wales I., U.S.A. 144 J14 55 47N 132 50W
Prince Patrick I., Canada 6 B2 77 0N 120 0W
Prince Regent Inlet, Canada 6 B3 73 0N 90 0W
Prince Rupert, Canada 142 C2 54 20N 130 20W
Prince William Sd., U.S.A. 144 F11 60 40N 147 0W
Princes Town, Trin. & Tob. 169 F9 10 16N 61 23W
Princesa Isabel, Brazil 170 C4 7 44 S 38 0W
Princess Charlotte B., Australia 126 A3 14 25 S 144 0 E
Princess May Ranges, Australia 124 C4 15 30 S 125 30 E
Princess Royal I., Canada 142 C3 53 0N 128 40W
Princeton, Canada 142 D4 49 27N 120 30W
Princeton, Calif., U.S.A. 160 F4 39 24N 122 1W
Princeton, Ill., U.S.A. 156 C7 41 23N 89 28W
Princeton, Ind., U.S.A. 157 F9 38 21N 87 34W
Princeton, Ky., U.S.A. 148 G2 37 7N 87 53W
Princeton, Mo., U.S.A. 156 D3 40 24N 93 35W
Princeton, N.J., U.S.A. 151 F10 40 21N 74 39W
Princeton, W. Va., U.S.A. 148 G5 37 22N 81 6W
Princeville, U.S.A. 156 D7 40 56N 89 46W
Príncipe, São Tomé & Príncipe 115 G6 1 37N 7 25 E
Príncipe, I. de, Atl. Oc. 104 F4 1 37N 7 27 E
Principe da Beira, Brazil 173 C5 12 20 S 64 30W
Prineville, U.S.A. 158 D3 44 18N 120 51W
Prins Christian Sund, Greenland 10 E6 60 4N 43 10W
Prins Harald Kyst, Antarctica 7 D4 70 0 S 35 1 E
Prins Karls Forland, Svalbard 10 B12 78 30N 11 0 E
Prinsesse Astrid Kyst, Antarctica 7 D3 70 45 S 12 30 E
Prinsesse Ragnhild Kyst, Antarctica 7 D4 70 15 S 27 30 E
Prinzapolca, Nic. 164 D3 13 20N 83 35W
Prior, C., Spain 42 B2 43 34N 8 17W
Priozersk, Russia 58 B6 61 2N 30 7 E
Pripet = Prypyat →, Europe 59 G6 51 20N 30 15 E
Pripet Marshes, Europe 59 F5 52 10N 28 10 E
Pripyat Marshes = Pripet Marshes, Europe 59 F5 52 10N 28 10 E
Pripyats = Prypyat →, Europe 59 G6 51 20N 30 15 E
Prishib = Leninsk, Russia 61 F7 48 40N 45 15 E
Prislop, Pasul, Romania 53 C9 47 37N 24 48 E
Pristen, Russia 59 G9 51 15N 36 44 E
Priština, Serbia & M. 50 D5 42 40N 21 13 E
Pritzwalk, Germany 30 B8 53 9N 12 10 E
Privas, France 29 D8 44 45N 4 37 E
Priverno, Italy 46 A6 41 28N 13 11 E
Privolzhsk, Russia 60 B5 57 23N 41 16 E
Privolzhskaya Vozvyshennost, Russia 60 E7 51 0N 46 0 E
Privolzhskiy, Russia 60 E8 51 25N 46 3 E
Privolzhskiy □, Russia 60 B10 56 0N 50 0 E
Privolzhye, Russia 60 D9 52 52N 48 33 E
Priyutnoye, Russia 61 G6 46 12N 43 40 E
Priyutovo, Russia 64 E4 53 55N 53 59 E
Prizren, Serbia & M. 50 D4 42 13N 20 45 E
Prizzi, Italy 46 E6 37 43N 13 26 E
Prnjavor, Bos.-H. 52 F2 44 52N 17 43 E
Probolinggo, Indonesia 85 D4 7 46 S 113 13 E
Prochowice, Poland 55 G3 51 17N 16 20 E
Proctor, U.S.A. 151 C11 43 40N 73 2W
Proddatur, India 95 G4 14 45N 78 30 E
Prodhromos, Cyprus 39 F8 34 57N 32 50 E
Proença-a-Nova, Portugal 42 F3 39 45N 7 54W
Profítis Ilías, Greece 38 E11 36 17N 27 56 E
Profondeville, Belgium 24 D4 50 23N 4 52 E
Progreso, Coahuila, Mexico 162 B4 27 28N 101 4W
Progreso, Yucatán, Mexico 163 C7 21 20N 89 40W
Prokhladnyy, Russia 61 J7 43 50N 44 2 E
Prokletije, Albania 50 D3 42 30N 19 45 E
Prokopyevsk, Russia 66 D9 54 0N 86 45 E
Prokuplje, Serbia & M. 50 C5 43 16N 21 36 E
Proletarsk, Russia 61 G5 46 42N 41 50 E
Proletarskaya = Proletarsk, Russia 61 G5 46 42N 41 50 E
Prome, Burma 90 F5 18 49N 95 13 E
Promise City, U.S.A. 156 D3 40 45N 93 9W
Promzino = Surskoye, Russia 60 C8 54 30N 46 44 E
Prophet →, Canada 142 B4 58 48N 122 40W
Prophet River, Canada 142 B4 58 6N 122 43W
Prophetstown, U.S.A. 156 C7 41 40N 89 56W
Propriá, Brazil 170 D4 10 13 S 36 51W
Propriano, France 29 G12 41 41N 8 52 E
Proserpine, Australia 126 J6 20 21 S 148 36 E
Proskurov = Khmelnytskyy, Ukraine 59 H4 49 23N 27 0 E
Prosna →, Poland 55 F4 52 6N 17 44 E
Prospect, N.Y., U.S.A. 151 C9 43 18N 75 9W
Prospect, Ohio, U.S.A. 157 D13 40 27N 83 11W
Prosperidad, Phil. 81 G5 8 34N 125 52 E
Prosperity, U.S.A. 152 E4 30 51N 85 56W
Prosperous B., St. Helena 9 h 15 56 S 5 39W
Prosser, U.S.A. 158 C4 46 12N 119 46W
Prossnitz = Prostějov, Czech Rep. 35 B10 49 30N 17 9 E
Prostějov, Czech Rep. 35 B10 49 30N 17 9 E
Prostki, Poland 54 E9 53 42N 22 25 E
Proston, Australia 127 D5 26 8 S 151 32 E
Proszowice, Poland 55 H7 50 13N 20 16 E
Próti, Greece 48 D3 37 5N 21 32 E
Provadiya, Bulgaria 51 C11 43 12N 27 30 E
Provence, France 29 E9 43 40N 5 46 E
Provence-Alpes-Côte d'Azur □, France 29 D10 44 0N 6 15 E
Providence, Seychelles 121 E4 9 14 S 51 2 E
Providence, Ky., U.S.A. 148 G2 37 24N 87 46W
Providence, R.I., U.S.A. 151 E13 41 49N 71 24W
Providence, C., N.Z. 131 F1 45 59 S 166 29 E
Providence Bay, Canada 140 C3 45 41N 82 15W
Providence Mts., U.S.A. 161 K11 35 10N 115 15W
Providencia, I. de, Colombia 164 D3 13 25N 81 26W
Provideniya, Russia 67 C19 64 23N 173 18W
Provins, France 27 D10 48 33N 3 15 E
Provo, U.S.A. 158 F8 40 14N 111 39W
Provost, Canada 143 C6 52 25N 110 20W
Prozor, Bos.-H. 52 G2 43 50N 17 34 E
Prrenjas, Albania 50 E4 41 4N 20 32 E
Prudentópolis, Brazil 171 G1 25 12 S 50 57W
Prudhoe Bay, U.S.A. 144 A10 70 18N 148 22W
Prudhoe I., Australia 126 C4 21 19 S 149 41 E
Prud'homme, Canada 143 C7 52 20N 105 54W
Prudnik, Poland 55 H4 50 20N 17 38 E
Prüm, Germany 31 E2 50 12N 6 25 E
Prundu, Romania 53 F11 44 6N 26 14 E
Pruszcz Gdański, Poland 54 D5 54 17N 18 40 E
Pruszków, Poland 55 F7 52 9N 20 49 E
Prut →, Romania 53 E13 45 28N 28 10 E
Prutz, Austria 33 B11 47 5N 10 40 E
Pruzhany, Belarus 59 F3 52 33N 24 28 E
Prvič, Croatia 45 D11 44 55N 14 47 E
Prydz B., Antarctica 7 C6 69 0 S 74 0 E
Pryluky, Ukraine 59 G7 50 30N 32 24 E
Pryor, U.S.A. 155 G7 36 19N 95 19W
Prypyat →, Europe 59 G6 51 20N 30 15 E
Przasnysz, Poland 55 E7 53 2N 20 54 E
Przedbórz, Poland 55 G6 51 6N 19 53 E
Przedecz, Poland 55 F5 52 20N 18 53 E
Przemków, Poland 55 G2 51 31N 15 48 E
Przemyśl, Poland 55 J9 49 50N 22 45 E
Przeworsk, Poland 55 H9 50 6N 22 32 E
Przewóz, Poland 55 G1 51 28N 14 57 E
Przhevalsk = Karakol, Kyrgyzstan 65 B9 42 30N 78 20 E
Przysucha, Poland 55 G7 51 22N 20 38 E
Psakhná, Greece 48 C5 38 34N 23 35 E
Psará, Greece 49 C7 38 37N 25 38 E
Psathoúra, Greece 48 B6 39 30N 24 12 E
Psel →, Ukraine 59 H7 49 10N 33 37 E
Pserimos, Greece 49 E9 36 56N 27 8 E
Psíra, Greece 39 E6 35 12N 25 52 E
Pskem →, Uzbekistan 65 C5 41 38N 70 1 E
Pskem Tizmasi, Uzbekistan 65 C5 42 0N 70 45 E
Pskent, Uzbekistan 65 C4 40 54N 69 20 E
Pskov, Russia 58 D5 57 50N 28 25 E
Pskovskoye, Ozero, Russia 58 D5 58 0N 27 58 E
Psunj, Croatia 52 E2 45 25N 17 19 E
Pteleón, Greece 48 B4 39 3N 22 57 E
Ptich = Ptsich →, Belarus 59 F5 52 9N 28 52 E
Ptolemaida = Ptolemaís, Greece 50 F5 40 30N 21 43 E
Ptolemaís, Greece 50 F5 40 30N 21 43 E
Ptsich →, Belarus 59 F5 52 9N 28 52 E
Ptuj, Slovenia 45 B12 46 28N 15 50 E
Ptujska Gora, Slovenia 45 B12 46 23N 15 47 E
Pu Xian, China 74 F6 36 24N 111 6 E
Pua, Thailand 86 C3 19 11N 100 55 E
Puaena Pt., U.S.A. 145 J13 21 36N 158 6W
Puán, Argentina 174 D3 37 30 S 62 45W
Pu'an, China 76 E5 25 46N 104 57 E
Puan, S. Korea 75 G14 35 44N 126 44 E
Pu'apu'a, Samoa 133 W23 13 34 S 172 9W
Pubei, China 76 F7 22 16N 109 31 E
Pucacuro →, Peru 168 D3 3 20 S 74 58W
Pucallpa, Peru 172 B3 8 25 S 74 30W
Pucará, Bolivia 173 D5 18 43 S 64 11W
Pucará, Cajamarca, Peru 172 B2 6 0 S 79 7W
Pucará, Puno, Peru 172 D3 15 5 S 70 24W
Pucarani, Bolivia 172 D4 16 23 S 68 30W
Pucheng, China 77 D12 27 59N 118 31 E
Pucheni, Romania 53 E10 45 12N 25 17 E
Puchheim, Germany 31 G7 48 9N 11 20 E
Puch'on, S. Korea 57 F14 37 30N 126 50 E
Púchov, Slovak Rep. 35 B11 49 8N 18 20 E

Pucio Pt., *Phil.* .... **81 F3** 11 46N 121 51 E
Pucioasa, *Romania* ... **53 E10** 45 5N 25 25 E
Pučišća, *Croatia* ...... **45 E13** 43 22N 16 43 E
Puck, *Poland* .... **54 D5** 54 45N 18 23 E
Pucka, Zatoka, *Poland* **54 D5** 54 30N 18 40 E
Puçol, *Spain* **41 F4** 39 37N 0 18W
Pudasjärvi, *Finland* ... **14 D22** 65 23N 26 53 E
Puding, *China* .... **76 D5** 26 18N 105 44 E
Pudozh, *Russia* ...... **58 B9** 61 48N 36 32 E
Puduchcheri = Pondicherry, *India* . **95 J4** 11 59N 79 50 E
Pudukkottai, *India* ... **95 J4** 10 28N 78 47 E
Puebla, *Mexico* **163 D5** 19 3N 98 12W
Puebla □, *Mexico* **163 D5** 18 30N 98 0W
Puebla de Alcocer, *Spain* **43 G5** 38 59N 5 14W
Puebla de Don Fadrique, *Spain* **41 H2** 37 58N 2 25W
Puebla de Don Rodrigo, *Spain* **43 F6** 39 5N 4 37W
Puebla de Guzmán, *Spain* **43 H3** 37 37N 7 15W
Puebla de la Calzada, *Spain* **43 G4** 38 54N 6 37W
Puebla de Sanabria, *Spain* **42 C4** 42 4N 6 38W
Puebla de Trives = Pobra de Trives, *Spain* **42 C3** 42 20N 7 10W
Pueblo, *U.S.A.* **154 F2** 38 16N 104 37W
Pueblo Hundido, *Chile* **174 B1** 26 20 S 70 5W
Puelches, *Argentina* .. **174 D2** 38 5 S 65 51W
Puelén, *Argentina* .... **174 D2** 37 32 S 67 38W
Puente Alto, *Chile* ... **174 C1** 33 32 S 70 35W
Puente-Genil, *Spain* .. **43 H6** 37 22N 4 47W
Puente la Reina, *Spain* **40 C3** 42 40N 1 49W
Puenteareas = Ponteareas, *Spain* .. **42 C2** 42 10N 8 28W
Puentedeume = Pontedeume, *Spain* . **42 B2** 43 24N 8 10W
Puentes de Garcia Rodriguez = As Pontes de García Rodríguez, *Spain* ... **42 B3** 43 27N 7 50W
Puerco Pt., *U.S.A.* **145 B1** 21 54N 160 4W
Pu'er, *China* .... **76 F3** 23 0N 101 15 E
Puerca, Pta., *Puerto Rico* .... **165 d** 18 13N 65 36W
Puerco →, *U.S.A.* **159 J10** 34 22N 107 50W
Puerto Acosta, *Bolivia* **172 D4** 15 32 S 69 15W
Puerto Aisén, *Chile* .. **176 C2** 45 27 S 73 0W
Puerto Ángel, *Mexico* **163 D5** 15 40N 96 29W
Puerto Arista, *Mexico* **163 D6** 15 56N 93 48W
Puerto Armuelles, *Panama* **164 E3** 8 20N 82 51W
Puerto Asis, *Colombia* **168 C2** 0 30N 76 30W
Puerto Ayacucho, *Venezuela* **168 B4** 5 40N 67 35W
Puerto Ayora, *Ecuador* **172 a** 0 45 S 90 19W
Puerto Baquerizo Moreno, *Ecuador* .. **172 a** 0 54 S 89 36W
Puerto Barrios, *Guatemala* **164 C2** 15 40N 88 32W
Puerto Bermejo, *Argentina* .... **174 B4** 26 55 S 58 34W
Puerto Bermúdez, *Peru* **172 C3** 10 20 S 74 58W
Puerto Bolívar, *Ecuador* .... **168 D2** 3 19 S 79 55W
Puerto Cabello, *Venezuela* **168 A4** 10 28N 68 1W
Puerto Cabezas, *Nic.* . **164 D3** 14 0N 83 30W
Puerto Cabo Gracias á Dios, *Nic.* **164 D3** 15 0N 83 10W
Puerto Capaz = El Jebha, *Morocco* **110 A4** 35 11N 4 43W
Puerto Carreño, *Colombia* **168 B4** 6 12N 67 22W
Puerto Castilla, *Honduras* **164 C2** 16 0N 86 0W
Puerto Chicama, *Peru* **172 B2** 7 45 S 79 20W
Puerto Cisnes, *Chile* .. **176 B2** 44 45 S 72 42W
Puerto Coig, *Argentina* **176 D3** 50 54 S 69 15W
Puerto Cortés, *Costa Rica* **164 E3** 8 55N 84 0W
Puerto Cortés, *Honduras* **164 C2** 15 51N 88 0W
Puerto Cumarebo, *Venezuela* **168 A4** 11 29N 69 30W
Puerto de Alcudia = Port d'Alcúdia, *Spain* **38 B4** 39 50N 3 7 E
Puerto de Cabras = Puerto del Rosario, *Canary Is.* **9 e2** 28 30N 13 52W
Puerto de Cabrera, *Spain* .... **38 B3** 39 8N 2 56 E
Puerto de Gran Tarajal, *Canary Is.* **9 e2** 28 13N 14 1W
Puerto de la Cruz, *Canary Is.* **9 e1** 28 24N 16 32W
Puerto de los Angeles ⌓, *Mexico* . **162 C3** 23 39N 105 45W
Puerto de Mazarrón, *Spain* **41 H3** 37 34N 1 15W
Puerto de Pozo Negro, *Canary Is.* **9 e2** 28 19N 13 55W
Puerto de Sóller = Port de Sóller, *Spain* .... **38 B3** 39 48N 2 42 E
Puerto de Somosierra, *Spain* **42 D7** 41 9N 3 35W
Puerto del Carmen, *Canary Is.* **9 e2** 28 55N 13 38W
Puerto del Rosario, *Canary Is.* **9 e2** 28 30N 13 52W
Puerto Deseado, *Argentina* .... **176 C3** 47 55 S 66 0W
Puerto Escondido, *Mexico* **163 D5** 15 50N 97 3W
Puerto Gaitán, *Colombia* **168 C3** 4 19N 72 4W
Puerto Galera, *Phil.* .. **80 E3** 13 30N 120 57 E
Puerto Guaraní, *Paraguay* .... **173 E6** 21 18 S 57 55W
Puerto Heath, *Bolivia* **172 C4** 12 34 S 68 39W
Puerto Huitoto, *Colombia* **168 C3** 0 18N 74 3W
Puerto Inca, *Peru* .... **172 B3** 9 22 S 74 54W
Puerto Inírida, *Colombia* **168 C4** 3 53N 67 52W
Puerto Juárez, *Mexico* **163 C7** 21 11N 86 49W
Puerto La Cruz, *Venezuela* **169 A5** 10 13N 64 38W
Puerto Leguízamo, *Colombia* .... **168 D3** 0 12 S 74 46W
Puerto Limón, *Colombia* **168 C3** 3 23N 73 30W
Puerto Lobos, *Argentina* .... **176 B3** 42 0 S 65 3W
Puerto López, *Colombia* **168 C3** 4 5N 72 58W
Puerto Lumbreras, *Spain* **41 H3** 37 34N 1 48W
Puerto Madryn, *Argentina* .... **176 B3** 42 48 S 65 4W
Puerto Maldonado, *Peru* .... **172 C4** 12 30 S 69 10W
Puerto Manatí, *Cuba* . **164 B4** 21 22N 76 50W
Puerto Mariti, *Colombia* .... **168 D4** 1 10 S 69 59W
Puerto Mercedes, *Colombia* **168 C3** 1 11N 72 53W
Puerto Mexico = Coatzacoalcos, *Mexico* **163 D6** 18 7N 94 25W
Puerto Miraña, *Colombia* .... **168 D3** 1 20 S 70 19W
Puerto Montt, *Chile* .. **176 B2** 41 28 S 73 0W
Puerto Morazán, *Nic.* . **164 D2** 12 51N 87 11W
Puerto Morelos, *Mexico* **163 C7** 20 49N 86 52W
Puerto Mutis, *Colombia* **168 B2** 6 14N 77 25W
Puerto Nariño, *Colombia* **168 C4** 4 56N 67 48W
Puerto Natales, *Chile* . **176 D2** 51 45 S 72 15W
Puerto Nuevo, *Colombia* **168 B4** 5 53N 69 56W
Puerto Nutrias, *Venezuela* **168 B4** 8 5N 69 18W
Puerto Ordaz, *Venezuela* **169 B5** 8 16N 62 44W
Puerto Padre, *Cuba* .. **164 B4** 21 13N 76 35W
Puerto Páez, *Venezuela* **168 B4** 6 13N 67 28W
Puerto Peñasco, *Mexico* **162 A2** 31 20N 113 33W
Puerto Pinasco, *Paraguay* .... **174 A4** 22 36 S 57 50W
Puerto Pirámides, *Argentina* .... **176 B4** 42 35 S 64 20W
Puerto Piritu, *Venezuela* **169 A4** 10 4N 65 3W
Puerto Plata, *Dom. Rep.* **165 C5** 19 48N 70 45W
Puerto Pollensa = Port de Pollença, *Spain* .. **38 B4** 39 54N 3 4 E
Puerto Portillo, *Peru* . **172 B3** 9 45 S 72 42W
Puerto Princesa, *Phil.* . **81 G2** 9 46N 118 45 E
Puerto Quellón, *Chile* **176 B2** 43 7 S 73 37W
Puerto Quepos, *Costa Rica* **164 E3** 9 29N 84 6W
Puerto Real, *Spain* ... **43 J4** 36 33N 6 12W
Puerto Rico, *Bolivia* .. **172 C4** 11 5 S 67 38W
Puerto Rico, *Canary Is.* **9 e1** 27 47N 15 42W
Puerto Rico ☒, *W. Indies* .... **165 d** 18 15N 66 45W
Puerto Rico Trench, *Atl. Oc.* **165 C6** 19 50N 66 0W
Puerto Rondón, *Colombia* **168 B3** 6 17N 71 6W
Puerto Saavedra, *Chile* **176 A2** 38 47 S 73 24W
Puerto Sastre, *Paraguay* **174 A4** 22 2 S 57 55W
Puerto Serrano, *Spain* **43 J5** 36 56N 5 33W
Puerto Siles, *Bolivia* .. **173 C4** 12 48 S 65 5W
Puerto Suárez, *Bolivia* **173 D6** 18 58 S 57 52W
Puerto Tejada, *Colombia* **168 C2** 3 14N 76 24W
Puerto Umbría, *Colombia* **168 C2** 0 52N 76 33W
Puerto Vallarta, *Mexico* **162 C3** 20 36N 105 15W
Puerto Varas, *Chile* .. **176 B2** 41 19 S 72 59W
Puerto Velasco Ibarra, *Ecuador* .... **172 a** 1 17 S 90 29W
Puerto Villamil, *Ecuador* .... **172 a** 0 56 S 91 1W
Puerto Villazón, *Bolivia* **173 C5** 13 32 S 61 57W
Puerto Wilches, *Colombia* **168 B3** 7 21N 73 54W
Puertollano, *Spain* ... **43 G6** 38 43N 4 7W
Puesto Cunambo, *Peru* **168 D2** 2 10 S 76 0W
Pueyrredón, L., *Argentina* .... **176 C2** 47 20 S 72 0W
Púez Odle ⌓, *Italy* ... **45 B8** 46 37N 11 48 E
Puffin I., *Ireland* **23 E1** 51 50N 10 24W
Pugachev, *Russia* ..... **60 D9** 52 0N 48 49 E
Pugal, *India* .... **92 E5** 28 30N 72 48 E
Puge, *China* .... **76 D4** 27 20N 102 31 E
Puge, *Tanzania* .... **118 C3** 4 45 S 33 11 E
Puget Sound, *U.S.A.* .. **158 C2** 47 50N 122 30W
Puget-Théniers, *France* **29 E10** 43 58N 6 53 E
Púglia □, *Italy* ...... **47 A9** 41 15N 16 15 E
Pugŏdong, *N. Korea* .. **75 C16** 42 5N 130 0 E
Pugu, *Tanzania* ...... **118 D4** 6 55 S 39 4 E
Pūgūnzī, *Iran* .... **97 E8** 25 49N 59 10 E
Puha, *N.Z.* .... **130 E6** 38 30 S 177 50 E
Pui, *Romania* .... **52 E8** 45 30N 23 4 E
Puica, *Peru* .... **172 C3** 15 0 S 72 53W
Puiești, *Romania* ..... **53 D12** 46 25N 27 33 E
Puig Major, *Spain* .... **38 B3** 39 48N 2 47 E
Puigcerdà, *Spain* ..... **40 C6** 42 24N 1 50 E
Puigmal, *Spain* ...... **40 C7** 42 23N 2 7 E
Puigpunyent, *Spain* ... **38 B3** 39 38N 2 32 E
Puijiang, *China* ...... **76 B4** 30 14N 103 30 E
Puisaye, Collines de la, *France* .... **27 E10** 47 37N 3 20 E
Puiseaux, *France* ..... **27 D9** 48 11N 2 30 E
Pujehun, *S. Leone* ... **112 D2** 7 23N 11 45W
Pujiang, *China* .... **77 C12** 29 29N 119 54 E
Pujili, *Ecuador* ...... **168 D2** 0 57 S 78 41W
Pujols, *France* **28 D3** 44 48N 0 2W
Pujon-chŏsuji, *N. Korea* **75 D14** 40 35N 127 35 E
Pukaki, L., *N.Z.* ...... **131 E5** 44 4 S 170 1 E
Pukalani, *U.S.A.* **145 C5** 20 51N 156 20W
Pukapuka, *Cook Is.* ... **135 J11** 10 53 S 165 49W
Pukaskwa △, *Canada* . **140 C2** 48 20N 86 0W
Pukatawagan, *Canada* **143 B8** 55 45N 101 20W
Pukchin, *N. Korea* .... **75 D13** 40 12N 125 45 E
Pukch'ŏng, *N. Korea* . **75 D15** 40 14N 128 10 E
Pukë, *Albania* .... **50 D3** 42 2N 19 53 E
Pukearuhe, *N.Z.* ..... **130 E3** 38 55 S 174 31 E
Pukekohe, *N.Z.* ...... **130 D3** 37 12 S 174 55 E
Puketeraki Ra., *N.Z.* . **131 C7** 42 58 S 172 13 E
Puketoi Ra., *N.Z.* .... **130 G5** 40 30 S 176 5 E
Pukeuri, *N.Z.* .... **131 F6** 45 4 S 171 2 E
Pukhrayan, *India* ..... **93 F8** 26 14N 79 51 E
Pukoo, *U.S.A.* **145 B5** 21 4N 156 48W
Pukou, *China* .... **77 A12** 32 7N 118 38 E
Pula, *Croatia* .... **45 D10** 44 54N 13 57 E
Pula, *Italy* .... **46 C1** 39 1N 9 0 E
Pulacayo, *Bolivia* .... **172 E4** 20 25 S 66 41W
Pulai, *Malaysia* ...... **87 d** 1 20N 103 31 E
Pulandian, *China* ..... **75 E11** 39 25N 121 58 E
Pularumpi, *Australia* . **124 B5** 11 24 S 130 26 E
Pulaski, *N.Y., U.S.A.* . **151 C8** 43 34N 76 8W
Pulaski, *Tenn., U.S.A.* . **149 H2** 35 12N 87 2W
Pulaski, *Va., U.S.A.* ... **148 G5** 37 3N 80 47W
Pulau →, *Indonesia* .. **83 C5** 5 50 S 138 15 E
Pulau Miangas, *Indonesia* .... **81 J6** 5 35N 126 34 E
Puławy, *Poland* ...... **55 G8** 51 23N 21 59 E
Pulga, *U.S.A.* **160 F5** 39 48N 121 29W
Pulgaon, *India* ...... **94 D4** 20 44N 78 21 E
Pulicat, *India* .... **95 H5** 13 25N 80 19 E
Pulicat L., *India* ..... **95 H5** 13 40N 80 15 E
Pulivendla, *India* .... **95 G4** 14 25N 78 14 E
Puliyangudi, *India* ... **95 K3** 9 11N 77 24 E
Pullman, *U.S.A.* **158 C5** 46 44N 117 10W
Pulog, Mt., *Phil.* ..... **80 C3** 16 40N 120 50 E
Púlpito do Sul, *Angola* **115 F2** 15 46 S 12 0 E
Pułtusk, *Poland* ...... **55 F8** 52 43N 21 6 E
Pülümür, *Turkey* ..... **101 C8** 39 30N 39 51 E
Pumlumon Fawr, *U.K.* **21 E4** 52 28N 3 46W
Puna, *Bolivia* .... **173 D4** 19 45 S 65 28W
Puná, I., *Ecuador* .... **168 D1** 2 55 S 80 5W
Punaauia, *Tahiti* ..... **133 S16** 17 37 S 149 34W
Punakha, *Bhutan* ..... **90 B2** 27 42N 89 52 E
Punalur, *India* .... **95 K3** 9 0N 76 56 E
Punaluu, *U.S.A.* **145 J14** 21 35N 157 53W
Punasar, *India* .... **92 F5** 27 6N 73 6 E
Punata, *Bolivia* ...... **173 D4** 17 32 S 65 50W
Punch, *India* .... **93 C6** 33 48N 74 4 E
Punch →, *Pakistan* ... **92 C5** 33 12N 73 40 E
Punda Maria, *S. Africa* **117 C5** 22 40 S 31 5 E
Pune, *India* .... **94 E1** 18 29N 73 57 E
Pungo Andongo, *Angola* .... **115 D3** 9 44 S 15 35 E
P'ungsan, *N. Korea* ... **75 D15** 40 50N 128 9 E
Pungue, Ponte de, *Mozam.* .... **119 F3** 19 0 S 34 0 E
Puning, *China* .... **77 F11** 23 20N 116 12 E
Punjab □, *India* ..... **92 D7** 31 0N 76 0 E
Punjab □, *Pakistan* .. **91 C4** 32 0N 72 30 E
Puno, *Peru* .... **172 D3** 15 55 S 70 3W
Punpun →, *India* .... **93 G11** 25 31N 85 18 E
Punta, Cerro de, *Puerto Rico* .... **165 d** 18 10N 66 37W
Punta Alta, *Argentina* **176 A4** 38 53 S 62 4W
Punta Arenas, *Chile* .. **176 D2** 53 10 S 71 0W
Punta Cardón, *Venezuela* **168 A3** 11 38N 70 14W
Punta Coles, *Peru* .... **172 D3** 17 43 S 71 23W
Punta de Bombón, *Peru* **172 D3** 17 10 S 71 48W
Punta de Díaz, *Chile* .. **174 B1** 28 0 S 70 45W
Punta del Hidalgo, *Canary Is.* **9 e1** 28 33N 16 19W
Punta Delgado, *Argentina* .... **176 B4** 42 43 S 63 38W
Punta Gorda, *Belize* .. **163 D7** 16 10N 88 45W
Punta Gorda, *U.S.A.* .. **153 J7** 26 56N 82 3W
Punta Prieta, *Mexico* . **162 B2** 28 58N 114 17W
Punta Prima, *Spain* ... **38 B5** 39 48N 4 16 E
Punta Umbría, *Spain* . **43 H4** 37 10N 6 56W
Puntarenas, *Costa Rica* **164 E3** 10 0N 84 50W
Punto Fijo, *Venezuela* **168 A3** 11 50N 70 13W
Punxsatawney, *U.S.A.* **150 F6** 40 57N 78 59W
Punyu = Guangzhou, *China* .... **77 F9** 23 5N 113 10 E
Puolo Pt., *U.S.A.* **145 B2** 21 54N 159 36W
Pupuan, *Indonesia* ... **79 J18** 8 19 S 115 0 E
Puqi, *China* .... **77 C9** 29 40N 113 50 E
Puquio, *Peru* .... **172 C3** 14 45 S 74 10W
Pur →, *Russia* .... **66 C8** 67 31N 77 55 E
Puracé △, *Colombia* .. **168 C2** 2 10N 76 21W
Puracé, Vol., *Colombia* **168 C2** 2 21N 76 23W
Puračić, *Bos.-H.* ...... **52 F3** 44 33N 18 28 E
Puralia = Puruliya, *India* .... **93 H12** 23 17N 86 24 E
Puranpur, *India* ..... **93 E9** 28 31N 80 9 E
Purari →, *Papua N. G.* **132 D3** 7 49 S 145 0 E
Purbeck, Isle of, *U.K.* . **21 G5** 50 39N 1 59W
Purcell, *U.S.A.* **155 H6** 35 1N 97 22W
Purcell Mts., *Canada* . **142 D5** 49 55N 116 15W
Puri, *India* .... **94 E7** 19 50N 85 58 E
Purificación, *Colombia* **168 C3** 3 51N 74 55W
Purmerend, *Neths.* .... **24 B4** 52 32N 4 58 E
Purna →, *India* ...... **94 E3** 19 6N 77 2 E
Purnia, *India* .... **93 G12** 25 45N 87 31 E
Purnululu Nat. Park △, *Australia* .... **124 C4** 17 20 S 128 20 E
Pursat = Pouthisat, *Cambodia* .... **86 F4** 12 34N 103 50 E
Purukcahu, *Indonesia* **85 C4** 0 35 S 114 35 E
Puruliya, *India* ...... **93 H12** 23 17N 86 24 E
Purus →, *Brazil* ..... **169 D5** 3 42 S 61 28W
Purutu I., *Papua N. G.* **132 E2** 8 24 S 143 27 E
Puruvesi, *Finland* .... **58 B5** 61 50N 29 30 E
Purvis, *U.S.A.* **155 K10** 31 9N 89 25W
Pŭrvomay, *Bulgaria* .. **51 D9** 42 8N 25 17 E
Purwa, *India* .... **93 F9** 26 28N 80 47 E
Purwakarta, *Indonesia* **85 D3** 6 35 S 107 29 E
Purwo, Tanjung, *Indonesia* .... **79 K18** 8 44 S 114 21 E
Purwodadi, *Jawa, Indonesia* .... **85 D4** 7 7 S 110 55 E
Purwodadi, *Jawa, Indonesia* .... **85 D3** 7 51 S 110 0 E
Purwokerto, *Indonesia* **85 D3** 7 25 S 109 14 E
Purworejo, *Indonesia* . **85 D4** 7 43 S 110 2 E
Puryŏng, *N. Korea* .... **75 C15** 42 5N 129 43 E
Pus →, *India* .... **94 E3** 19 55N 77 55 E
Pusa, *India* .... **93 G11** 25 59N 85 41 E
Pusad, *India* .... **94 E3** 19 56N 77 36 E
Pusan, *S. Korea* ..... **75 G15** 35 5N 129 0 E
Pushkin, *Russia* ..... **58 C6** 59 45N 30 25 E
Pushkino, *Moskva, Russia* .... **58 D9** 56 2N 37 49 E
Pushkino, *Saratov, Russia* .... **60 E8** 51 16N 47 0 E
Püspökladány, *Hungary* **52 C6** 47 19N 21 6 E
Pustoshka, *Russia* .... **58 D5** 56 20N 29 30 E
Puszczykowo, *Poland* . **55 F3** 52 18N 16 49 E
Putahow L., *Canada* .. **143 B8** 59 54N 100 40W
Putao, *Burma* .... **90 B6** 27 28N 97 30 E
Putaruru, *N.Z.* .... **130 E4** 38 2 S 175 50 E
Putbus, *Germany* ..... **30 A9** 54 22N 13 28 E
Putian, *China* .... **77 E12** 25 23N 119 0 E
Putignano, *Italy* ..... **47 B10** 40 51N 17 7 E
Putina, *Peru* .... **172 C4** 14 55 S 69 55W
Puting, Tanjung, *Indonesia* .... **85 C4** 3 31 S 111 46 E
Putlitz, *Germany* ..... **30 B8** 53 15N 12 2 E
Putna, *Romania* ..... **53 C10** 47 50N 25 33 E
Putna →, *Romania* ... **53 E12** 45 42N 27 26 E
Putnam, *U.S.A.* **151 E13** 41 55N 71 55W
Putney, *U.S.A.* **152 D5** 31 29N 84 8W
Putnok, *Hungary* ..... **52 B5** 48 18N 20 26 E
Putorana, Gory, *Russia* **67 C10** 69 0N 95 0 E
Putorino, *N.Z.* .... **130 F5** 39 4 S 176 58 E
Putrajaya, *Malaysia* .. **87 L3** 2 55N 101 40 E
Putre, *Chile* .... **172 D4** 18 12 S 69 35W
Puttalam, *Sri Lanka* .. **95 K5** 8 1N 79 55 E
Puttalam Lagoon, *Sri Lanka* .... **95 K4** 8 15N 79 45 E
Puttgarden, *Germany* . **30 A7** 54 30N 11 10 E
Püttlingen, *Germany* . **31 F2** 49 17N 6 53 E
Puttur, *Andhra Pradesh, India* .... **95 H4** 13 27N 79 33 E
Puttur, *Karnataka, India* .... **95 H2** 12 46N 75 12 E
Putty, *Australia* ..... **129 B9** 32 57 S 150 42 E
Putumayo →, *S. Amer.* **168 D4** 3 7 S 67 58W
Putuo, *China* .... **77 C14** 29 56N 122 20 E
Putussibau, *Indonesia* . **85 B4** 0 50N 112 56 E
Pututahi, *N.Z.* ...... **130 E6** 38 39 S 177 53 E
Putyla, *Ukraine* ..... **53 B10** 48 0N 25 5 E
Puu Kaaumakua, *U.S.A.* **145 K14** 21 30N 157 54W
Puu Keahiakahoe, *U.S.A.* **145 K14** 21 23N 157 49W
Puu o Keokeo, *U.S.A.* . **145 D6** 19 13N 155 44W
Puuanahulu, *U.S.A.* .. **145 D6** 19 49N 155 51W
Pu'uhonua o Hōnaunau △, *U.S.A.* **145 D6** 19 25N 155 55W
Pu'ukoholā Heiau ⌓, *U.S.A.* **145 C6** 20 1N 155 51W
Puukolii, *U.S.A.* **145 C5** 20 56N 156 41W
Puunene, *U.S.A.* **145 C5** 20 53N 156 23W
Puuwai, *U.S.A.* **145 B1** 21 54N 160 12W
Puvirnituq, *Canada* ... **139 B12** 60 2N 77 10W
Puy-de-Dôme, *France* **28 C6** 45 46N 2 57 E
Puy-de-Dôme □, *France* .... **28 C7** 45 40N 3 5 E
Puy-l'Évêque, *France* . **28 D5** 44 31N 1 9 E
Puyallup, *U.S.A.* **160 C4** 47 12N 122 18W
Puyang, *China* .... **74 G8** 35 40N 115 1 E
Puyehue, *Chile* ...... **176 B2** 40 40 S 72 37W
Puyehue △, *Chile* .... **176 B2** 40 27 S 72 6W
Puylaurens, *France* ... **28 E6** 43 35N 2 0 E
Puyo, *Ecuador* .... **168 D2** 1 28 S 77 59W
Puysegur Pt., *N.Z.* ... **131 G1** 46 9 S 166 37 E
Pūzeh Rīg, *Iran* ...... **97 E8** 27 20N 58 40 E
Puzhaykove, *Ukraine* . **53 B14** 48 7N 29 50 E
Pwani □, *Tanzania* .. **118 D4** 7 0 S 39 0 E
Pweto, *Dem. Rep. of the Congo* .... **119 D2** 8 25 S 28 51 E
Pwinbyu, *Burma* ..... **90 E5** 20 23N 94 40 E
Pwllheli, *U.K.* **20 E3** 52 53N 4 25W
Pya-ozero, *Russia* .... **56 A5** 66 5N 30 58 E
Pyana →, *Russia* .... **60 C8** 55 43N 46 1 E
Pyandzh = Dusti, *Tajikistan* .... **65 E4** 37 20N 68 40 E
Pyandzh, *Tajikistan* ... **65 E4** 37 14N 69 6 E
Pyandzh →, *Asia* .... **65 E4** 37 6N 68 20 E
Pyapon, *Burma* ...... **90 G5** 16 20N 95 40 E
Pyasina →, *Russia* ... **67 B9** 73 30N 87 0 E
Pyatigorsk, *Russia* ... **61 H6** 44 2N 43 6 E
Pyatykhatky, *Ukraine* . **59 H7** 48 28N 33 38 E
Pyawbwe, *Burma* ..... **90 E6** 20 35N 96 4 E
Pyaye, *Burma* .... **90 F5** 19 12N 95 10 E
Pydna, *Greece* .... **50 F6** 40 20N 22 34 E
Pyè = Prome, *Burma* . **90 F5** 18 49N 95 13 E
Pyetrikaw, *Belarus* ... **59 F5** 52 11N 28 29 E
Pyhäjoki, *Finland* .... **14 D21** 64 28N 24 14 E
Pyinbauk, *Burma* ..... **90 F5** 19 10N 95 12 E
Pyingaing, *Burma* .... **90 D5** 23 9N 94 50 E
Pyinkayaing, *Burma* .. **90 H5** 15 58N 94 24 E
Pyinmana, *Burma* .... **90 F6** 19 45N 96 12 E
Pyinyaung, *Burma* .... **90 E6** 20 49N 96 25 E
Pyla, C., *Cyprus* ..... **39 F9** 34 56N 33 51 E
Pymatuning Reservoir, *U.S.A.* **150 E4** 41 30N 80 28W
Pyŏktong, *N. Korea* .. **75 D13** 40 50N 125 50 E
Pyŏnggang, *N. Korea* . **75 E14** 38 24N 127 17 E
P'yŏngt'aek, *S. Korea* . **75 F14** 37 1N 127 4 E
P'yŏngyang, *N. Korea* . **75 E13** 39 0N 125 30 E
Pyote, *U.S.A.* **155 K3** 31 32N 103 8W
Pyramid L., *U.S.A.* ... **158 G4** 40 1N 119 35W
Pyramid Pk., *U.S.A.* .. **161 J10** 36 25N 116 37W
Pyramid Pt., *Ascension I.* .... **9 g** 7 55 S 14 24W
Pyramids, *Egypt* ..... **106 J7** 29 58N 31 9 E
Pyrénées, *Europe* .... **28 F4** 42 45N 0 18 E
Pyrénées △, *France* .. **28 F3** 42 52N 0 10W
Pyrénées-Atlantiques □, *France* **28 E3** 43 10N 0 50W
Pyrénées-Orientales □, *France* .... **28 F6** 42 35N 2 26 E
Pyryatyn, *Ukraine* .... **59 G7** 50 15N 32 25 E
Pyrzyce, *Poland* ..... **55 E1** 53 10N 14 55 E
Pyskowice, *Poland* ... **55 H5** 50 24N 18 38 E
Pytalovo, *Russia* .... **58 D4** 57 5N 27 55 E
Pyttegga, *Norway* .... **18 B4** 62 13N 7 42 E
Pyu, *Burma* .... **90 F6** 18 30N 96 28 E
Pyzdry, *Poland* ...... **55 F4** 52 11N 17 42 E

Q

Qaanaaq, *Greenland* .. **10 B4** 77 40N 69 0W
Qabirri →, *Azerbaijan* **61 K8** 41 3N 46 17 E
Qabr Hūd, *Yemen* ..... **99 C5** 16 9N 49 34 E
Qachasnek, *S. Africa* . **117 E4** 30 6 S 28 42 E
Qādib, *Yemen* .... **99 D6** 12 37N 53 57 E
Qa'el Jafr, *Jordan* ... **103 E5** 30 20N 36 25 E
Qa'emābād, *Iran* ..... **97 D9** 31 44N 60 2 E
Qā'emshahr, *Iran* .... **97 B7** 36 30N 52 53 E
Qagan Nur, *China* .... **74 C8** 43 30N 114 55 E
Qahar Youyi Zhongqi, *China* .... **74 D7** 41 12N 112 40 E
Qahremānshahr = Bākhtarān, *Iran* .... **101 E12** 34 23N 47 0 E
Qaidam Pendi, *China* . **68 C4** 37 0N 95 0 E
Qajarīyeh, *Iran* ...... **97 D6** 31 1N 48 22 E
Qala, *Malta* .... **38 E7** 36 2N 14 19 E
Qala, Ras il, *Malta* ... **38 E7** 36 2N 14 20 E
Qala-i-Jadid = Spīn Būldak, *Afghan.* ... **91 C2** 31 1N 66 25 E
Qala Point = Qala, Ras il, *Malta* .... **38 E7** 36 2N 14 20 E
Qala Viala, *Pakistan* .. **92 D2** 30 49N 67 17 E
Qala Yangi, *Afghan.* .. **92 B2** 34 20N 66 30 E
Qalācheh, *Afghan.* .... **91 B2** 35 30N 67 43 E
Qalaikhum = Kalaikhum, *Tajikistan* .... **65 D5** 38 28N 70 46 E
Qalansīyah, *Yemen* ... **99 D6** 12 41N 53 29 E
Qal'at al Akhḑar, *Si. Arabia* .... **96 E3** 28 0N 37 10 E
Qal'at Bīshah, *Si. Arabia* .... **98 C3** 20 0N 42 36 E
Qal'at Dīzah, *Iraq* ... **101 D11** 36 11N 45 7 E
Qalāt-i-Ghilzai, *Afghan.* .... **91 B2** 32 15N 66 58 E
Qal'at Şāliḩ, *Iraq* .... **96 D5** 31 31N 47 16 E
Qal'at Sukkar, *Iraq* .. **101 G12** 31 51N 46 5 E
Qal'eh-ye Bost, *Afghan.* **91 C2** 31 30N 64 21 E
Qal'eh-ye Now, *Afghan.* .... **91 B1** 35 0N 63 5 E
Qal'eh-ye Panjeh, *Afghan.* .... **65 E6** 37 0N 72 35 E
Qal'eh-ye Sarkari, *Afghan.* .... **91 B2** 35 54N 67 17 E
Qal'eh-ye Valī, *Afghan.* **91 B1** 35 46N 63 45 E
Qalyūb, *Egypt* .... **106 H7** 30 12N 31 11 E
Qamani'tuaq = Baker Lake, *Canada* **138 B10** 64 20N 96 3W
Qamar, Ghubbat al, *Yemen* .... **99 C6** 16 20N 52 30 E
Qamar, Jabal al, *Oman* **99 C6** 16 48N 53 15 E
Qamashi, *Uzbekistan* . **65 D3** 38 49N 66 28 E
Qamdo, *China* .... **76 B1** 31 15N 97 6 E
Qamea, *Fiji* .... **133 A3** 16 45 S 179 45W
Qammieh Point, *Malta* **38 F7** 35 58N 14 19 E
Qamruddin Karez, *Pakistan* .... **91 C3** 31 45N 68 20 E
Qandahār, *Afghan.* ... **91 C2** 31 32N 65 43 E
Qandahār □, *Afghan.* . **91 C2** 31 0N 65 0 E
Qanshenggel, *Kazakhstan* .... **65 A7** 44 53N 75 30 E
Qapān, *Iran* .... **97 B7** 37 40N 55 47 E
Qapshaghay, *Kazakhstan* .... **65 B8** 43 51N 77 14 E
Qapshaghay Bögeni, *Kazakhstan* .... **65 B8** 43 45N 77 50 E
Qaqortoq, *Greenland* . **10 E6** 60 43N 46 0W
Qâra, *Egypt* .... **106 B2** 29 38N 26 30 E
Qarā', Jabal al, *Oman* **99 C6** 17 15N 54 15 E
Qara Qash →, *China* . **93 B8** 35 0N 78 30 E
Qarabulaq, *Kazakhstan* **65 A9** 44 54N 78 30 E
Qarabulaq, *Kazakhstan* **65 B4** 42 31N 69 46 E
Qarabutaq, *Kazakhstan* **64 G8** 49 59N 60 14 E
Qaraçala, *Azerbaijan* . **61 L9** 39 45N 48 53 E
Qaradarya = Zeravshan →, *Asia* .. **65 D1** 39 22N 63 45 E
Qaradarya →, *Uzbekistan* .... **65 C2** 39 0N 63 35 E
Qaraghandy, *Kazakhstan* .... **66 E8** 49 50N 73 10 E
Qaraghayly, *Kazakhstan* .... **66 E8** 49 26N 76 0 E
Qārah, *Si. Arabia* .... **96 D4** 29 55N 40 3 E
Qarak, *China* .... **65 D8** 38 25N 77 0 E
Qarataū, *Kazakhstan* . **65 B5** 43 10N 70 28 E
Qarataū, *Kazakhstan* . **65 B4** 43 30N 69 30 E
Qaraturyq, *Kazakhstan* **65 B8** 43 35N 77 50 E
Qarāvol, *Afghan.* .... **65 E4** 37 14N 68 46 E
Qardho = Gardo, *Somali Rep.* .... **120 C3** 9 30N 49 6 E
Qardud, *Sudan* ...... **107 E2** 10 20N 29 56 E
Qareh →, *Iran* ...... **101 C12** 39 25N 47 22 E
Qareh Tekān, *Iran* ... **97 B6** 36 38N 49 29 E
Qarqan He →, *China* . **68 C3** 39 30N 88 30 E
Qarqaraly, *Kazakhstan* **66 E8** 49 26N 75 30 E
Qarqin, *Afghan.* ..... **65 E3** 37 24N 66 4 E
Qarrasa, *Sudan* ..... **107 E3** 14 38N 32 5 E
Qarshi, *Uzbekistan* ... **65 D2** 38 53N 65 48 E
Qartabā, *Lebanon* .... **103 A4** 34 4N 35 50 E
Qaryat al Gharab, *Iraq* **96 D5** 31 27N 44 48 E
Qaryat al 'Ulyā, *Si. Arabia* .... **96 E5** 27 33N 47 42 E
Qasigiannguit, *Greenland* **10 D5** 68 50N 51 18W
Qaskeleng, *Kazakhstan* **65 B8** 43 20N 76 35 E
Qasr 'Amra, *Jordan* .. **96 D3** 31 48N 36 35 E
Qaşr Bū Hadi, *Libya* . **108 B3** 31 1N 16 45 E
Qaşr-e Qand, *Iran* ... **97 E9** 26 15N 60 45 E
Qasr Farâfra, *Egypt* .. **106 B2** 27 0N 28 1 E
Qa'ṭabah, *Yemen* .... **98 D4** 13 51N 44 42 E
Qatanā, *Syria* .... **103 B5** 33 26N 36 4 E
Qaṭānan, Ra's, *Yemen* **99 D6** 12 21N 53 33 E
Qatar ■, *Asia* .... **97 E6** 25 30N 51 15 E
Qatlish, *Iran* .... **97 B8** 37 50N 57 19 E
Qattâra, *Egypt* ...... **106 A2** 30 12N 27 3 E
Qattâra, Munkhafed el, *Egypt* .... **106 B2** 29 30N 27 30 E
Qattâra Depression = Qattâra, Munkhafed el, *Egypt* .... **106 B2** 29 30N 27 30 E
Qawām al Ḩamzah = Al Ḩamzah, *Iraq* ... **96 D5** 31 43N 44 58 E
Qawra Point, *Malta* .. **38 F7** 35 58N 14 26 E
Qāyen, *Iran* .... **97 C8** 33 40N 59 10 E
Qazaqstan = Kazakhstan ■, *Asia* **66 E7** 50 0N 70 0 E
Qazimämmäd, *Azerbaijan* .... **61 K9** 40 3N 49 0 E
Qazvin, *Iran* .... **97 B6** 36 15N 50 0 E
Qazvin □, *Iran* ...... **97 B6** 36 20N 50 0 E
Qazyghurt, *Kazakhstan* **65 C4** 41 45N 69 23 E
Qeisari = Caesarea, *Israel* .... **103 C3** 32 30N 34 53 E
Qeissan, *Sudan* ..... **107 E3** 11 4N 34 40 E
Qena, *Egypt* .... **106 B3** 26 10N 32 43 E
Qena, W. →, *Egypt* .. **106 B3** 26 12N 32 44 E
Qeqertarsuaq, *Greenland* **10 D5** 69 45N 53 30W
Qeqertarsuaq, *Greenland* **10 D5** 69 15N 53 38W
Qeqertarsuatsiaat, *Greenland* **10 E5** 63 5N 50 45W
Qeshlāq, *Iran* .... **101 E12** 34 55N 46 28 E
Qeshm, *Iran* .... **97 E8** 26 55N 56 10 E
Qeys, *Iran* .... **97 E7** 26 32N 53 58 E
Qezel Owzen →, *Iran* . **97 B6** 36 45N 49 22 E
Qezi'ot, *Israel* .... **103 E3** 30 52N 34 26 E
Qi Xian, *China* ...... **74 G8** 34 40N 114 48 E
Qian Gorlos, *China* ... **75 B13** 45 5N 124 42 E
Qian Hai, *China* ..... **69 F10** 22 32N 113 54 E
Qian Xian, *China* .... **74 G5** 34 31N 108 15 E
Qiancheng, *China* .... **76 D7** 27 12N 109 50 E
Qianjiang, *Guangxi Zhuangzu, China* .... **76 F7** 23 38N 108 58 E
Qianjiang, *Hubei, China* .... **77 B9** 30 24N 112 55 E
Qianjiang, *Sichuan, China* .... **76 C7** 29 33N 108 47 E
Qianshan, *Anhui, China* **77 B11** 30 37N 116 35 E
Qianshan, *Guangdong, China* .... **69 G10** 22 15N 113 31 E
Qianwei, *China* ...... **76 C4** 29 13N 103 56 E
Qianxi, *China* .... **76 D6** 27 3N 106 3 E
Qianyang, *Hunan, China* .... **77 D8** 27 18N 110 10 E
Qianyang, *Shaanxi, China* .... **74 G4** 34 40N 107 8 E
Qianyang, *Zhejiang, China* .... **77 B12** 30 11N 119 25 E
Qi'ao, *China* .... **69 G10** 22 25N 113 39 E
Qi'ao Dao, *China* .... **69 G10** 22 25N 113 38 E
Qiaojia, *China* ...... **76 D4** 26 56N 102 58 E
Qichun, *China* ...... **77 B10** 30 18N 115 25 E
Qidong, *Hunan, China* **77 D9** 26 49N 112 7 E
Qidong, *Jiangsu, China* **77 B13** 31 48N 121 38 E
Qijiang, *China* ...... **76 C6** 28 57N 106 35 E
Qikiqtarjuaq, *Canada* . **139 B13** 67 33N 63 0W
Qila Safed, *Pakistan* .. **91 C1** 29 0N 61 30 E
Qila Saifullāh, *Pakistan* **91 C3** 30 45N 68 17 E
Qilian Shan, *China* ... **68 C4** 38 30N 96 0 E
Qimen, *China* .... **77 C11** 29 50N 117 42 E
Qin He →, *China* .... **74 G7** 35 1N 113 22 E
Qin Jiang →, *Guangxi Zhuangzu, China* .... **76 F7** 21 53N 108 35 E
Qin Jiang →, *Jiangxi, China* .... **77 D10** 26 15N 115 55 E
Qin Ling = Qinling Shandi, *China* ..... **74 H5** 33 50N 108 10 E
Qināb, W. →, *Yemen* . **99 C5** 17 55N 49 59 E
Qin'an, *China* .... **74 G3** 34 48N 105 40 E
Qing Xian, *China* .... **74 E9** 38 35N 116 45 E
Qingcheng, *China* .... **75 F9** 37 15N 117 40 E
Qingdao, *China* ...... **75 F11** 36 5N 120 20 E
Qingfeng, *China* ..... **74 G8** 35 52N 115 8 E
Qinghai □, *China* .... **68 C4** 36 0N 98 0 E
Qinghai Hu, *China* ... **68 C5** 36 40N 100 10 E
Qinghecheng, *China* .. **75 D13** 41 28N 124 15 E
Qinghemen, *China* .... **75 D11** 41 48N 121 25 E
Qingjian, *China* ..... **74 F6** 37 8N 110 8 E
Qingjiang = Huaiyin, *China* .... **75 H10** 33 30N 119 2 E
Qingliu, *China* ...... **77 D11** 26 11N 116 48 E
Qinglong, *China* ..... **76 E5** 25 49N 105 12 E
Qingping, *China* ..... **76 D6** 26 39N 107 47 E
Qingpu, *China* ...... **77 B13** 31 10N 121 6 E
Qingshui, *China* ..... **74 G4** 34 48N 106 8 E
Qingshuihe, *China* ... **74 E6** 39 55N 111 35 E
Qingtian, *China* ..... **77 C13** 28 12N 120 15 E

Qingtongxia Shuiku, China 74 F3 37 50N 105 58 E
Qingxi, China 76 D7 27 8N 108 43 E
Qingxu, China 74 F7 37 34N 112 22 E
Qingyang, Anhui, China 77 B11 30 38N 117 50 E
Qingyang, Gansu, China 74 F4 36 2N 107 55 E
Qingyi Jiang →, China 76 C4 29 32N 103 44 E
Qingyuan, Guangdong, China 77 F9 23 40N 112 59 E
Qingyuan, Liaoning, China 75 C13 42 10N 124 55 E
Qingyuan, Zhejiang, China 77 D12 27 36N 119 3 E
Qingyun, China 75 F9 37 45N 117 20 E
Qingzhen, China 76 D6 26 31N 106 25 E
Qinhuangdao, China 75 E10 39 56N 119 30 E
Qinling Shandi, China 74 H5 33 50N 108 10 E
Qinshui, China 74 G7 35 40N 112 8 E
Qinyang = Jiyuan, China 74 G7 35 7N 112 57 E
Qinyuan, China 74 F7 36 29N 112 20 E
Qinzhou, China 76 G7 21 58N 108 38 E
Qionghai, China 86 C8 19 15N 110 26 E
Qionglai, China 76 B4 30 25N 103 31 E
Qionglai Shan, China 76 B4 31 0N 102 30 E
Qiongzhou Haixia, China 86 B8 20 10N 110 15 E
Qiqihar, China 67 E13 47 26N 124 0 E
Qiraîya, W. →, Egypt 103 E3 30 27N 34 0 E
Qiryat Ata, Israel 103 C4 32 47N 35 6 E
Qiryat Gat, Israel 103 D3 31 32N 34 46 E
Qiryat Mal'akhi, Israel 103 D3 31 44N 34 44 E
Qiryat Shemona, Israel 103 B4 33 13N 35 35 E
Qiryat Yam, Israel 103 C4 32 51N 35 4 E
Qirzah, W. →, Libya 108 B2 30 56N 14 31 E
Qishan, China 74 G4 34 25N 107 38 E
Qishn, Yemen 99 D5 15 26N 51 40 E
Qitai, China 68 B3 44 2N 89 35 E
Qitbīt, W. →, Oman 99 C6 19 15N 54 23 E
Qiubei, China 76 E5 24 2N 104 12 E
Qixia, China 75 F11 37 17N 120 52 E
Qiyang, China 77 D8 26 35N 111 50 E
Qızılağac Körfäzi, Azerbaijan 97 B6 39 9N 49 0 E
Qoghaly, Kazakhstan 65 A9 44 29N 78 39 E
Qojūr, Iran 96 B5 36 12N 47 55 E
Qom, Iran 97 C6 34 40N 51 0 E
Qom □, Iran 97 C6 34 40N 51 0 E
Qomolangma Feng = Everest, Mt., Nepal 93 E12 28 5N 86 58 E
Qomsheh, Iran 97 D6 32 0N 51 55 E
Qondūz, Afghan. 65 E4 36 50N 68 50 E
Qondūz □, Afghan. 65 E4 36 50N 68 50 E
Qondūz →, Afghan. 91 A3 37 0N 68 16 E
Qopa, Kazakhstan 65 B7 43 31N 75 50 E
Qoraqalpoghistan □, Uzbekistan 66 E6 43 0N 58 0 E
Qorday, Kazakhstan 65 B7 43 21N 74 59 E
Qormi, Malta 38 F7 35 53N 14 28 E
Qorveh, Iran 101 E12 35 10N 47 48 E
Qosqudyq, Kazakhstan 65 A8 44 10N 77 18 E
Qostanay, Kazakhstan 66 D7 53 10N 63 35 E
Qotūr, Iran 101 C11 38 28N 44 25 E
Qoz Salsilgo, C.A.R. 114 A4 10 45N 22 54 E
Qrejten Point, Malta 38 F7 35 57N 14 27 E
Qu Jiang →, China 76 B6 30 1N 106 24 E
Qu Xian, China 76 B6 30 48N 106 58 E
Quabbin Reservoir, U.S.A. 151 D12 42 20N 72 20W
Quairading, Australia 125 F2 32 0 S 117 21 E
Quakenbrück, Germany 30 C3 52 41N 7 57 E
Quakertown, U.S.A. 151 F9 40 26N 75 21W
Qualicum Beach, Canada 142 D4 49 22N 124 26W
Quambatook, Australia 128 C5 35 49 S 143 34 E
Quambone, Australia 129 A7 30 57 S 147 53 E
Quamby, Australia 126 C3 20 22 S 140 17 E
Quan Long = Ca Mau, Vietnam 87 H5 9 7N 105 8 E
Quanah, U.S.A. 155 H5 34 18N 99 44W
Quandialla, Australia 129 C7 34 1 S 147 47 E
Quang Ngai, Vietnam 86 E7 15 13N 108 58 E
Quang Tri, Vietnam 86 D6 16 45N 107 13 E
Quang Yen, Vietnam 76 G6 20 56N 106 52 E
Quannan, China 77 E10 24 45N 114 33 E
Quantock Hills, U.K. 21 F4 51 8N 3 10W
Quanzhou, Fujian, China 77 E12 24 55N 118 34 E
Quanzhou, Guangxi Zhuangzu, China 77 E8 25 57N 111 5 E
Qu'Appelle, Canada 143 C8 50 33N 103 53W
Quaqtaq, Canada 139 B13 60 55N 69 40W
Quaraí, Brazil 174 C4 30 15 S 56 20W
Quarré-les-Tombes, France 27 E11 47 21N 4 0 E
Quarteira, Portugal 43 H2 37 4N 8 6W
Quartu Sant'Elena, Italy 46 C2 39 15N 9 10 E
Quartzsite, U.S.A. 161 M12 33 40N 114 13W
Quatre Bornes, Mauritius 121 d 20 15 S 57 28 E
Quatsino Sd., Canada 142 C3 50 25N 127 58W
Quba, Azerbaijan 61 K9 41 21N 48 32 E
Qūchān, Iran 97 B8 37 10N 58 27 E
Queanbeyan, Australia 129 C8 35 17 S 149 14 E
Québec, Canada 141 C5 46 52N 71 13W
Québec □, Canada 141 C6 48 0N 74 0W
Quebrada del Condorito △, Argentina 174 C3 31 49 S 64 40W
Quedlinburg, Germany 30 D7 51 47N 11 8 E
Queen Alexandra Ra., Antarctica 7 E11 85 0 S 170 0 E
Queen Charlotte B., Falk. Is. 9 f 51 50 S 60 40W
Queen Charlotte City, Canada 142 C2 53 15N 132 2W
Queen Charlotte Is., Canada 142 C2 53 20N 132 10W
Queen Charlotte Sd., Canada 142 C3 51 0N 128 0W
Queen Charlotte Sd., N.Z. 131 B9 41 10 S 174 15 E
Queen Charlotte Strait, Canada 142 C3 50 45N 127 10W
Queen City, U.S.A. 156 D4 40 25N 92 34W
Queen Elizabeth △, U.K. 22 E4 56 7N 4 30W
Queen Elizabeth △, Uganda 118 C3 0 0 30 0 E
Queen Elizabeth Is., Canada 136 B10 76 0N 95 0W
Queen Elizabeth Nat. Park = Ruwenzori △, Uganda 118 B2 0 20 S 30 0 E
Queen Mary Land, Antarctica 7 D7 70 0 S 95 0 E
Queen Maud G., Canada 138 B9 68 15N 102 30W
Queen Maud Land = Dronning Maud Land, Antarctica 7 D3 72 30 S 12 0 E
Queen Maud Mts., Antarctica 7 E13 86 0 S 160 0W
Queens Chan., Australia 124 C4 15 0 S 129 30 E
Queenscliff, Australia 128 E6 38 16 S 144 39 E
Queensland, U.S.A. 152 D6 31 46N 83 14W
Queensland □, Australia 126 C3 22 0 S 142 0 E
Queenstown = Cóbh, Ireland 23 E3 51 51N 8 17W
Queenstown, Australia 127 G4 42 4 S 145 35 E
Queenstown, N.Z. 131 F3 45 1 S 168 40 E
Queenstown, Singapore 87 d 1 18N 103 48 E
Queenstown, S. Africa 116 E4 31 52 S 26 52 E
Queets, U.S.A. 160 C2 47 32N 124 20W
Queguay Grande →, Uruguay 174 C4 32 9 S 58 9W
Queimada, Pta. da, Azores 9 d1 38 23N 28 14W
Queimadas, Brazil 170 D4 11 0 S 39 38W
Queiros, C., Vanuatu 133 D5 14 55 S 167 1 E
Quela, Angola 115 D3 9 10 S 16 56 E
Quelimane, Mozam. 119 F4 17 53 S 36 58 E
Quelo, Angola 115 D2 6 29 S 12 36 E
Quelpart = Cheju do, S. Korea 75 H14 33 29N 126 34 E
Queluz, Portugal 43 G1 38 45N 9 15W
Quemado, N. Mex., U.S.A. 159 J9 34 20N 108 30W
Quemado, Tex., U.S.A. 155 L4 28 58N 100 35W
Quemoy = Chinmen, Taiwan 77 E13 24 26N 118 19 E
Quemú-Quemú, Argentina 174 D3 36 3 S 63 36W
Quepem, India 95 G2 15 13N 74 3 E
Quequén, Argentina 174 D4 38 30 S 58 30W
Querco, Peru 172 C3 13 50 S 74 52W
Querétaro, Mexico 162 C4 20 36N 100 23W
Querétaro □, Mexico 162 C5 20 30N 100 0W
Querfurt, Germany 30 D7 51 23N 11 35 E
Quérigut, France 28 F6 42 42N 2 6 E
Querqueville, France 26 C5 49 40N 1 42W
Quesada, Spain 43 H7 37 51N 3 4W
Queshan, China 74 H8 32 55N 114 2 E
Quesnel, Canada 142 C4 53 0N 122 30W
Quesnel →, Canada 142 C4 52 58N 122 29W
Quesnel L., Canada 142 C4 52 30N 121 20W
Questa, U.S.A. 159 H11 36 42N 105 36W
Questembert, France 26 E4 47 40N 2 28W
Quetena, Bolivia 172 E4 22 10 S 67 25W
Quetico △, Canada 140 C1 48 30N 91 45W
Quetrequile, Argentina 176 B3 41 33 S 69 22W
Quetta, Pakistan 91 C2 30 15N 66 55 E
Queulat △, Chile 176 B2 44 29 S 72 24W
Quevedo, Ecuador 168 D2 1 2 S 79 29W
Queyras △, France 29 D10 44 45N 6 50 E
Quezaltenango, Guatemala 164 D1 14 50N 91 30W
Quezon, Phil. 81 G1 9 15N 117 59 E
Quezon □, Phil. 80 D3 14 40N 121 30 E
Quezon △, Phil. 80 D3 14 0N 121 55 E
Quezon City, Phil. 80 D3 14 38N 121 0 E
Qufār, Si. Arabia 96 E4 27 26N 41 37 E
Qui Nhon, Vietnam 86 F7 13 40N 109 13 E
Quibala, Angola 115 E2 10 46 S 14 59 E
Quibaxe, Angola 115 D2 8 24 S 14 27 E
Quibdo, Colombia 168 B2 5 42N 76 40W
Quiberon, France 26 E3 47 29N 3 9W
Quiberon, Presqu'île de, France 26 E3 47 30N 3 8W
Quiçama △, Angola 115 D2 9 41 S 13 35 E
Quickborn, Germany 30 B5 53 42N 9 52 E
Quiet L., Canada 142 A2 61 5N 133 5W
Quiindy, Paraguay 174 B4 25 58 S 57 14W
Quila, Mexico 162 C3 24 23N 107 13W
Quilán, C., Chile 176 B2 43 15 S 74 30W
Quilcene, U.S.A. 160 C4 47 49N 122 53W
Quilenda, Angola 115 E2 10 39 S 14 23 E
Quilengues, Angola 115 E2 14 12 S 14 12 E
Quilimarí, Chile 174 C1 32 5 S 71 30W
Quilino, Argentina 174 C3 30 14 S 64 29W
Quill Lakes, Canada 143 C8 51 55N 104 13W
Quillabamba, Peru 172 C3 12 50 S 72 50W
Quillacollo, Bolivia 172 D4 17 26 S 66 17W
Quillagua, Chile 174 A2 21 40 S 69 40W
Quillaicillo, Chile 174 C1 31 17 S 71 40W
Quillan, France 28 F6 42 53N 2 10 E
Quillota, Chile 174 C1 32 54 S 71 16W
Quilmes, Argentina 174 C4 34 43 S 58 15W
Quilon, India 95 K3 8 50N 76 38 E
Quilpie, Australia 127 D3 26 35 S 144 11 E
Quilpué, Chile 174 C1 33 5 S 71 33W
Quilua, Mozam. 119 F4 16 17 S 39 54 E
Quimbele, Angola 115 D3 6 17 S 16 41 E
Quimbo, Angola 115 E3 14 4 S 16 11 E
Quimbonge, Angola 115 D3 8 36 S 18 30 E
Quime, Bolivia 172 D4 17 2 S 67 15W
Quimili, Argentina 174 B3 27 40 S 62 30W
Quimper, France 26 E2 48 0N 4 9W
Quimperlé, France 26 E3 47 53N 3 33W
Quinault →, U.S.A. 160 C2 47 21N 124 18W
Quincemil, Peru 172 C3 13 15 S 70 40W
Quincy, Calif., U.S.A. 160 F6 39 56N 120 57W
Quincy, Fla., U.S.A. 152 E5 30 35N 84 34W
Quincy, Ill., U.S.A. 156 E5 39 56N 91 23W
Quincy, Mass., U.S.A. 151 D14 42 15N 71 0W
Quincy, Mich., U.S.A. 157 C12 41 57N 84 53W
Quincy, Wash., U.S.A. 158 C4 47 22N 119 56W
Quines, Argentina 174 C2 32 13 S 65 48W
Quinga, Mozam. 119 F5 15 49 S 40 15 E
Quingey, France 27 E12 47 7N 5 52 E
Quingombe, Angola 115 D2 6 38 S 13 1 E
Quinhagak, U.S.A. 144 G7 59 45N 161 54W
Quiniluban Group, Phil. 81 F3 11 27N 120 48 E
Quintana de la Serena, Spain 43 G5 38 45N 5 40W
Quintana Roo □, Mexico 163 D7 19 0N 88 0W
Quintanar de la Orden, Spain 43 F7 39 36N 3 5W
Quintanar de la Sierra, Spain 40 D2 41 57N 2 55W
Quintanar del Rey, Spain 41 F3 39 21N 1 56W
Quinte West, Canada 140 D4 44 10N 77 34W
Quintero, Chile 174 C1 32 45 S 71 30W
Quintin, France 26 D4 48 26N 2 56W
Quinto, Spain 40 D4 41 25N 0 32W
Quinzáu, Angola 115 D2 6 51 S 12 44 E
Quípar →, Spain 41 G3 38 15N 1 40W
Quipeio, Angola 115 E3 12 27 S 15 30 E
Quirihue, Chile 174 D1 36 15 S 72 35W
Quirima, Angola 115 E3 10 47 S 18 6 E
Quirimbo, Angola 115 E2 10 36 S 14 12 E
Quirindi, Australia 129 A9 31 28 S 150 40 E
Quirino □, Phil. 80 C3 16 15N 121 40 E
Quirinopolis, Brazil 171 E1 18 32 S 50 30W
Quiroga, Spain 42 C3 42 28N 7 18W
Quiruvilca, Peru 172 B2 8 1 S 78 19W
Quissac, France 29 E8 43 55N 4 0 E
Quissanga, Mozam. 119 E5 12 24 S 40 28 E
Quissico, Mozam. 117 C5 24 42 S 34 44 E
Quitapa, Angola 115 E3 10 20 S 18 19 E
Quitilipi, Argentina 174 B3 26 50 S 60 13W
Quitman, U.S.A. 152 E6 30 47N 83 34W
Quito, Ecuador 168 D2 0 15 S 78 35W
Quixadá, Brazil 170 B4 4 55 S 39 0W
Quixaxe, Mozam. 119 F5 15 17 S 40 4 E
Quixeramobim, Brazil 170 C4 5 12 S 39 17W
Quixico, Angola 115 D2 7 59 S 14 25 E
Quizenga, Angola 115 D3 9 21 S 15 28 E
Qujing, China 76 E4 25 32N 103 41 E
Qulan, Kazakhstan 65 B6 42 55N 72 43 E
Qul'ân, Jazâ'ir, Egypt 96 E2 24 22N 35 31 E
Qumbu, S. Africa 117 E4 31 10 S 28 48 E
Qumqŭrghan, Uzbekistan 65 E3 37 49N 67 35 E
Quneitra, Syria 103 B4 33 7N 35 48 E
Qŭnghirot, Uzbekistan 66 E6 43 6N 58 54 E
Qu'nyido, China 76 B2 31 15N 98 6 E
Quoin I., Australia 124 B4 14 54 S 129 32 E
Quoin Pt., S. Africa 116 E2 34 46 S 19 37 E
Quorn, Australia 128 B3 32 25 S 138 5 E
Qŭqon, Uzbekistan 65 C5 40 30N 70 57 E
Qurein, Sudan 107 E3 13 30N 34 50 E
Qŭrghonteppa, Tajikistan 65 E4 37 50N 68 47 E
Qurnat as Sawdā', Lebanon 103 A5 34 18N 36 6 E
Qûs, Egypt 106 B3 25 55N 32 50 E
Qusar, Azerbaijan 61 K9 41 25N 48 26 E
Quşaybā', Si. Arabia 96 E4 26 53N 43 35 E
Qusaybah, Iraq 101 E9 34 24N 40 59 E
Quşay'ir, Yemen 99 D5 14 55N 50 20 E
Quseir, Egypt 96 E2 26 7N 34 16 E
Qūshchī, Iran 101 D11 37 59N 45 3 E
Quthing, Lesotho 117 E4 30 25 S 27 36 E
Qūṭīābād, Iran 97 C6 35 47N 48 30 E
Quwo, China 74 G6 35 38N 111 25 E
Quyang, China 74 E8 38 35N 114 40 E
Quynh Nhai, Vietnam 86 B4 21 49N 103 33 E
Quyon, Canada 151 A8 45 31N 76 14W
Quzhou, China 77 C12 28 57N 118 54 E
Quzi, China 74 F4 36 20N 107 20 E
Qvareli, Georgia 61 K7 41 57N 45 47 E
Qytet Stalin = Kuçovë, Albania 50 F3 40 47N 19 57 E
Qyzylorda, Kazakhstan 65 A2 44 48N 65 28 E

R

Ra, Ko, Thailand 87 H2 9 13N 98 16 E
Raab, Austria 34 C6 48 21N 13 39 E
Raahe, Finland 14 D21 64 40N 24 28 E
Raalte, Neths. 24 B6 52 23N 6 16 E
Raasay, U.K. 22 D2 57 25N 6 4W
Raasay, Sd. of, U.K. 22 D2 57 30N 6 8W
Rab, Croatia 45 D11 44 45N 14 45 E
Raba, Indonesia 85 D5 8 36 S 118 55 E
Rába →, Hungary 52 C2 47 38N 17 38 E
Raba →, Poland 55 H7 50 8N 20 30 E
Rabaçal →, Portugal 42 D3 41 30N 7 12W
Rabah, Nigeria 113 C6 13 5N 5 30 E
Rabai, Kenya 118 C4 3 50 S 39 31 E
Rabak, Sudan 107 E3 13 9N 32 44 E
Rabaraba, Papua N. G. 132 E5 9 58 S 149 49 E
Rabastens, France 28 E5 43 50N 1 43 E
Rabastens-de-Bigorre, France 28 E4 43 23N 0 9 E
Rabat = Victoria, Malta 38 E6 36 3N 14 14 E
Rabat, Kazakhstan 65 B4 42 2N 69 31 E
Rabat, Malta 38 F7 35 53N 14 24 E
Rabat, Morocco 110 B3 34 2N 6 48W
Rabaul, Papua N. G. 132 C7 4 24 S 152 18 E
Rabi, Fiji 133 A3 16 30 S 179 59W
Rābigh, Si. Arabia 98 B2 22 50N 39 5 E
Rabka, Poland 55 J6 49 37N 19 59 E
Râbniţa, Moldova 53 C14 47 45N 29 0 E
Rābor, Iran 97 D8 29 17N 56 55 E
Rabyānah, Libya 108 D4 24 15N 22 0 E
Rača, Serbia & M. 50 B4 44 14N 21 0 E
Răcăciuni, Romania 53 D11 46 20N 26 59 E
Răcăşdia, Romania 52 F6 44 59N 21 36 E
Racconigi, Italy 44 D4 44 46N 7 46 E
Raccoon →, U.S.A. 156 C3 41 35N 93 37W
Raccoon Cr. →, U.S.A. 157 E9 39 47N 87 23W
Race, C., Canada 141 C9 46 40N 53 5W
Rach Gia, Vietnam 87 G5 10 5N 105 5 E
Rachid, Mauritania 112 B2 18 45N 11 35W
Raciąż, Poland 55 F7 52 46N 20 10 E
Racibórz, Poland 55 H5 50 7N 18 18 E
Racichy, Belarus 54 E10 53 44N 23 42 E
Racine, U.S.A. 157 B9 42 41N 87 51W
Račišdorf = Rača, Serbia & M. 50 B4 44 14N 21 0 E
Rackerby, U.S.A. 160 F5 39 26N 121 22W
Radama, Nosy, Madag. 117 A8 14 0 S 47 47 E
Radama, Saikanosy, Madag. 117 A8 14 16 S 47 53 E
Radan, Serbia & M. 50 D5 42 59N 21 29 E
Rădăuţi, Romania 53 C10 47 50N 25 59 E
Rădăuţi-Prut, Romania 53 B11 48 14N 26 48 E
Radbuza →, Czech Rep. 34 B6 49 45N 13 22 E
Radcliff, U.S.A. 157 G11 37 51N 85 57W
Radeberg, Germany 30 D9 51 7N 13 53 E
Radebeul, Germany 30 D9 51 6N 13 39 E
Radeče, Slovenia 45 B12 46 5N 15 14 E
Radekhiv, Ukraine 59 G3 50 25N 24 32 E
Radekhov = Radekhiv, Ukraine 59 G3 50 25N 24 32 E
Radenthein, Austria 34 E6 46 48N 13 43 E
Radew →, Poland 54 D2 54 2N 15 52 E
Radford, U.S.A. 148 G5 37 8N 80 34W
Radhanpur, India 92 H4 23 50N 71 38 E
Radhwa, Jabal, Si. Arabia 96 E3 24 34N 38 18 E
Radika →, Macedonia 50 E4 41 38N 20 37 E
Radisson, Qué., Canada 140 B4 53 47N 77 37W
Radisson, Sask., Canada 143 C7 52 30N 107 20W
Radium Hot Springs, Canada 142 C5 50 35N 116 2W
Radlje ob Dravi, Slovenia 45 B12 46 38N 15 13 E
Radmannsdorf = Radovljica, Slovenia 45 B11 46 22N 14 12 E
Radnevo, Bulgaria 51 D9 42 17N 25 58 E
Radnice, Czech Rep. 34 B6 49 51N 13 35 E
Radnor Forest, U.K. 21 E4 52 17N 3 10W
Radolfzell, Germany 31 H4 47 39N 8 59 E
Radom, Poland 55 G8 51 23N 21 12 E
Radom △, Sudan 114 A4 9 20N 23 50 E
Radomir, Bulgaria 50 D6 42 37N 22 59 E
Radomka →, Poland 55 G8 51 43N 21 28 E
Radomsko, Poland 55 G6 51 5N 19 28 E
Radomyshl, Ukraine 59 G5 50 30N 29 12 E
Radomyśl Wielki, Poland 55 H8 50 14N 21 15 E
Radoszyce, Poland 55 G7 51 4N 20 15 E
Radoviš, Macedonia 50 E6 41 38N 22 28 E
Radovljica, Slovenia 45 B11 46 22N 14 12 E
Radstadt, Austria 34 D6 47 24N 13 28 E
Radstock, C., Australia 127 E1 33 12 S 134 20 E
Răducăneni, Romania 53 D12 46 58N 27 54 E
Raduša, Macedonia 50 D5 42 7N 21 15 E
Radvanichy, Belarus 55 F11 52 1N 24 0 E
Radviliškis, Lithuania 15 J20 55 49N 23 33 E
Radville, Canada 143 D8 49 30N 104 15W
Radwá, J., Si. Arabia 106 C4 24 34N 38 18 E
Radymno, Poland 55 J9 49 59N 22 52 E
Radzanów, Poland 55 F7 52 56N 20 8 E
Radziejów, Poland 55 F5 52 40N 18 30 E
Radzyń Chełmiński, Poland 54 E5 53 23N 18 55 E
Radzyń Podlaski, Poland 55 G9 51 47N 22 37 E
Rae, Canada 142 A5 62 50N 116 3W
Rae Bareli, India 93 F9 26 18N 81 20 E
Rae Isthmus, Canada 139 B11 66 40N 87 30W
Raeren, Belgium 24 D6 50 41N 6 7 E
Raeside, L., Australia 125 E3 29 20 S 122 0 E
Raetihi, N.Z. 130 F4 39 25 S 175 17 E
Rafaela, Argentina 174 C3 31 10 S 61 30W
Rafah, Gaza Strip 103 D3 31 18N 34 14 E
Rafai, C.A.R. 118 B1 4 59N 23 58 E
Raffadali, Italy 46 E6 37 24N 13 32 E
Raffili, Sudan 107 F2 6 50N 28 0 E
Rafḥā, Si. Arabia 96 D4 29 35N 43 35 E
Rafsanjān, Iran 97 D8 30 30N 56 5 E
Raft Pt., Australia 124 C3 16 4 S 124 26 E
Rāgā, Sudan 107 F2 8 28N 25 41 E
Raga →, Sudan 107 F2 8 41N 25 52 E
Ragachow, Belarus 59 F6 53 8N 30 5 E
Ragag, Sudan 107 E1 10 59N 24 40 E
Ragang, Mt., Phil. 81 H5 7 43N 124 32 E
Ragay, Phil. 80 E4 13 49N 122 47 E
Ragay G., Phil. 80 E4 13 30N 122 45 E
Ragged, Mt., Australia 125 F3 33 27 S 123 25 E
Ragged Pt., Barbados 165 g 13 10N 59 26W
Rāgh, Afghan. 65 E5 37 32N 70 27 E
Raghunathpalli, India 93 H11 22 14N 84 48 E
Raghunathpur, India 93 H12 23 33N 86 40 E
Raglan, N.Z. 130 D3 37 55 S 174 55 E
Raglan Harbour, N.Z. 130 D3 37 47 S 174 50 E
Ragland, U.S.A. 152 B3 33 45N 86 9W
Ragnit = Neman, Russia 15 J20 55 2N 22 2 E
Ragusa = Dubrovnik, Croatia 50 D2 42 39N 18 6 E
Ragusa, Italy 47 F7 36 55N 14 44 E
Raha, Indonesia 82 B2 4 55 S 123 0 E
Rahad, Nahr ed →, Sudan 107 E3 14 28N 33 31 E
Rahad al Bardī, Sudan 109 F4 11 20N 23 40 E
Rahaeng = Tak, Thailand 86 D2 16 52N 99 8 E
Rahatgarh, India 93 H8 23 47N 78 22 E
Rahden, Germany 30 C4 52 26N 8 36 E
Raheb, Ras ir-, Malta 38 F7 35 54N 14 20 E
Raheita, Eritrea 107 E5 12 46N 43 4 E
Raheng = Tak, Thailand 86 D2 16 52N 99 8 E
Rahimyar Khan, Pakistan 91 C3 28 30N 70 25 E
Rāhjerd, Iran 97 C6 34 22N 50 22 E
Rahole △, Kenya 118 B4 0 5N 38 57 E
Råholt, Norway 18 D8 60 16N 11 11 E
Rahon, India 93 D7 31 3N 76 7 E
Rahotu, N.Z. 130 F2 39 20 S 173 49 E
Rahuri, India 94 E2 19 23N 74 39 E
Raiatéa, I., French Polynesia 135 J12 16 50 S 151 25W
Raichur, India 95 F3 16 10N 77 20 E
Raiford, U.S.A. 152 E7 30 4N 82 14W
Raiganj, India 93 G13 25 37N 88 10 E
Raigarh, India 94 D6 21 56N 83 25 E
Raighar, India 94 E6 19 51N 82 6 E
Raijua, Indonesia 82 D2 10 37 S 121 36 E
Raikot, India 92 D6 30 41N 75 42 E
Railton, Australia 127 G4 41 25 S 146 28 E
Rainbow Bridge △, U.S.A. 159 H8 37 5N 110 58W
Rainbow City, U.S.A. 152 B3 33 57N 86 5W
Rainbow Lake, Canada 142 B5 58 30N 119 23W
Rainier, U.S.A. 160 D4 46 53N 122 41W
Rainier, Mt., U.S.A. 160 D5 46 52N 121 46W
Rainy L., Canada 143 D10 48 42N 93 10W
Rainy River, Canada 143 D10 48 43N 94 29W
Raippaluoto, Finland 14 E19 63 13N 21 14 E
Raipur, India 94 D5 21 17N 81 45 E
Rairakhol, India 94 D7 21 4N 84 21 E
Ra'is, Si. Arabia 106 C4 23 33N 38 43 E
Raisen, India 92 H8 23 20N 77 48 E
Raisio, Finland 15 F20 60 28N 22 11 E
Raj Nandgaon, India 94 D5 21 5N 81 5 E
Raj Nilgiri, India 93 J12 21 28N 86 46 E
Raja, Ujung, Indonesia 84 B1 3 40N 96 25 E
Raja Ampat, Kepulauan, Indonesia 83 B4 0 30 S 130 0 E
Rajah Sikatuna △, Phil. 81 G5 9 40N 124 20 E
Rajahmundry, India 94 F5 17 1N 81 48 E
Rajaji △, India 92 D8 30 10N 78 20 E
Rajampet, India 95 G4 14 11N 79 10 E
Rajang →, Malaysia 85 B4 2 30N 112 0 E
Rajanpur, Pakistan 92 E4 29 6N 70 19 E
Rajapalaiyam, India 95 K3 9 25N 77 35 E
Rajapur, India 94 F1 16 40N 73 31 E
Rajasthan □, India 92 F5 26 45N 73 30 E
Rajasthan Canal = Indira Gandhi Canal, India 92 F5 28 0N 72 0 E
Rajauri, India 93 C6 33 25N 74 21 E
Rajbari, Bangla. 90 D2 23 47N 89 41 E
Rajgarh, Mad. P., India 92 G7 24 2N 76 45 E
Rajgarh, Raj., India 92 F7 27 14N 76 38 E
Rajgarh, Raj., India 92 E6 28 40N 75 25 E
Rajgir, India 93 G11 25 2N 85 25 E
Rajgród, Poland 54 E9 53 42N 22 42 E
Rajim, India 94 D5 20 58N 81 53 E
Rajkot, India 92 H4 22 15N 70 56 E
Rajmahal Hills, India 93 G12 24 30N 87 30 E
Rajpipla, India 94 D1 21 50N 73 30 E
Rajpur, India 92 H6 22 18N 74 21 E
Rajpura, India 92 D7 30 25N 76 32 E
Rajputana = Rajasthan □, India 92 F5 26 45N 73 30 E
Rajshahi, Bangla. 90 C2 24 22N 88 39 E
Rajshahi □, Bangla. 90 C2 25 0N 89 0 E
Rajula, India 92 J4 21 3N 71 26 E
Rajur, India 94 D4 20 7N 78 55 E
Rajura, India 94 E4 19 47N 79 22 E
Rakaia, N.Z. 131 D7 43 45 S 172 1 E
Rakaia →, N.Z. 131 D7 43 36 S 172 15 E
Rakan, Ra's, Qatar 97 E6 26 10N 51 20 E
Rakaposhi, Pakistan 93 A6 36 10N 74 25 E
Rakata, Pulau, Indonesia 84 D3 6 10 S 105 20 E
Rakhiv, Ukraine 53 B9 48 3N 24 12 E
Rakhni, Pakistan 92 D3 30 4N 69 56 E
Rakhni →, Pakistan 92 E3 29 31N 69 36 E
Rakhny-Lisovi, Ukraine 53 B13 48 47N 28 29 E
Rakhyūt, Oman 99 C6 16 44N 53 20 E
Rakiraki, Fiji 133 A2 17 22 S 178 11 E
Rakitnoye, Russia 70 B7 45 36N 134 17 E
Rakitovo, Bulgaria 51 E8 41 59N 24 5 E
Rakkestad, Norway 18 E8 59 25N 11 21 E
Rakoniewice, Poland 55 F3 52 10N 16 16 E
Rakops, Botswana 116 C3 21 1 S 24 28 E
Rakovica, Croatia 45 D12 44 59N 15 38 E
Rakovník, Czech Rep. 34 A6 50 6N 13 42 E
Rakovski, Bulgaria 51 D8 42 21N 24 57 E
Rakshan →, Pakistan 91 D1 27 10N 63 25 E
Rakvere, Estonia 15 G22 59 20N 26 25 E
Raleigh, Fla., U.S.A. 153 F7 29 25N 82 32W
Raleigh, N.C., U.S.A. 149 H6 35 47N 78 39W
Rali Salem, Algeria 111 D5 28 1N 1 9 E
Ralik Chain, Pac. Oc. 134 G8 8 0N 168 0 E
Ralja, Serbia & M. 50 B4 44 33N 20 34 E
Ralls, U.S.A. 155 J4 33 41N 101 24W
Ralston, U.S.A. 150 E8 41 30N 76 57W
Ram →, Canada 142 A4 62 1N 123 41W
Rām Allāh, West Bank 103 D4 31 55N 35 10 E
Rama, Nic. 164 D3 12 9N 84 15W
Ramacca, Italy 47 E7 37 23N 14 42 E
Ramachandrapuram, India 94 F6 16 50N 82 4 E
Ramagiri Udayagiri, India 94 E7 19 5N 84 18 E
Ramakona, India 93 J8 21 43N 78 50 E
Ramales de la Victoria, Spain 42 B7 43 15N 3 28W
Ramalho, Serra do, Brazil 171 D3 13 45 S 44 0W
Rāmallāh = Rām Allāh, West Bank 103 D4 31 55N 35 10 E
Raman, Thailand 87 J3 6 29N 101 18 E
Ramanathapuram, India 95 K4 9 25N 78 55 E
Ramanetaka, B. de, Madag. 117 A8 14 13 S 47 52 E
Ramanujganj, India 93 H10 23 48N 83 42 E
Ramas C., India 95 G1 15 5N 73 55 E
Ramat Gan, Israel 103 C3 32 4N 34 48 E
Ramatlhabama, S. Africa 116 D4 25 37 S 25 33 E
Ramban, India 93 C6 33 14N 75 12 E
Rambervillers, France 27 D13 48 20N 6 38 E
Rambi = Rabi, Fiji 133 A3 16 30 S 179 59W
Rambipuji, Indonesia 85 D4 8 12 S 113 37 E
Rambouillet, France 27 D8 48 39N 1 50 E
Rambrai, India 90 C3 25 40N 91 19 E
Rambutyo I., Papua N. G. 132 B4 2 18 S 147 49 E
Ramdurg, India 95 G2 15 58N 75 22 E
Rame Hd., Australia 129 D8 37 47 S 149 30 E
Ramechhap, Nepal 93 F12 27 25N 86 10 E
Ramenskoye, Russia 58 E10 55 32N 38 15 E
Ramer, U.S.A. 152 C3 32 3N 86 13W
Rameswaram, India 95 K4 9 17N 79 18 E
Ramganga →, India 93 F8 27 5N 79 58 E
Ramgarh, Bangla. 90 D3 22 59N 91 44 E
Ramgarh, Jharkhand, India 93 H11 23 40N 85 35 E
Ramgarh, Raj., India 92 F6 27 16N 75 14 E
Ramgarh, Raj., India 92 F4 27 30N 70 36 E
Rāmhormoz, Iran 97 D6 31 15N 49 35 E
Ramīān, Iran 97 B7 37 3N 55 16 E
Ramingining, Australia 126 A2 12 19 S 135 3 E
Ramla, Israel 103 D3 31 55N 34 52 E
Ramlat Zalṭan, Libya 108 C3 28 30N 19 30 E
Ramlu, Eritrea 107 E5 13 32N 41 40 E
Ramm = Rum, Jordan 103 F4 29 39N 35 26 E
Ramm, Jabal, Jordan 103 F4 29 35N 35 24 E
Râmna →, Romania 53 E12 45 36N 27 3 E
Ramnad = Ramanathapuram, India 95 K4 9 25N 78 55 E
Ramnagar, Jammu & Kashmir, India 93 C6 32 47N 75 18 E
Ramnagar, Uttaranchal, India 93 E8 29 24N 79 7 E
Ramnäs, Sweden 16 E10 59 46N 16 12 E
Râmnicu Sărat, Romania 53 E12 45 26N 27 3 E
Râmnicu Vâlcea, Romania 53 E9 45 9N 24 21 E
Ramon, Phil. 80 C3 16 50N 121 31 E
Ramon, Russia 59 G10 51 55N 39 21 E
Ramona, U.S.A. 161 M10 33 2N 116 52W
Ramonville-St-Agne, France 28 E5 43 33N 1 28 E
Ramore, Canada 140 C3 48 30N 80 25W
Ramos →, Nigeria 113 D6 5 8N 5 22 E
Ramotswa, Botswana 116 C4 24 50 S 25 52 E
Rampart, U.S.A. 144 D10 65 30N 150 10W
Rampur, H.P., India 92 D7 31 26N 77 43 E
Rampur, Mad. P., India 92 H5 23 25N 73 53 E
Rampur, Orissa, India 94 D6 21 48N 83 58 E
Rampur, Ut. P., India 93 E8 28 50N 79 5 E
Rampur Hat, India 93 G12 24 10N 87 50 E
Rampura, India 92 G6 24 30N 75 27 E
Ramrama Tola, India 93 J8 21 52N 79 55 E
Ramree I., Burma 90 F5 19 0N 93 40 E
Rāmsar, Iran 97 B6 36 53N 50 41 E
Ramsey, I. of Man 20 C3 54 20N 4 22W
Ramsey, Ill., U.S.A. 156 F7 39 8N 89 7W
Ramsey, N.J., U.S.A. 151 E10 41 4N 74 9W
Ramsey L., Canada 140 C3 47 13N 82 15W
Ramsgate, U.K. 21 F9 51 20N 1 25 E
Ramshai, India 90 B2 26 44N 88 51 E
Ramsjö, Sweden 16 B9 62 11N 15 37 E
Ramstein, Germany 31 F3 49 27N 7 32 E
Ramtek, India 94 D4 21 20N 79 15 E
Ramu →, Papua N. G. 132 C3 4 0 S 144 41 E
Ramvik, Sweden 16 B11 62 49N 17 51 E
Rana Pratap Sagar Dam, India 92 G6 24 58N 75 38 E
Ranaghat, India 93 H13 23 15N 88 35 E
Ranahu, Pakistan 92 G3 25 55N 69 45 E
Ranau, Malaysia 78 C5 6 2N 116 40 E
Rancagua, Chile 174 C1 34 10 S 70 50W
Rance →, France 26 D5 48 34N 1 59W
Rancharia, Brazil 171 F1 22 15 S 50 55W
Rancheria →, Canada 142 A3 60 13N 129 7W
Ranchester, U.S.A. 158 D10 44 54N 107 10W
Ranchi, India 93 H11 23 19N 85 27 E
Rancho Cucamonga, U.S.A. 161 L9 34 10N 117 30W
Ranco, L., Chile 176 B2 40 15 S 72 25W
Rand, Australia 129 C7 35 33 S 146 32 E
Randaberg, Norway 18 E2 59 1N 5 36 E
Randabygd, Norway 18 C3 61 51N 6 20 E
Randalstown, U.K. 23 B5 54 45N 6 19W
Randan, France 27 F10 46 2N 3 21 E
Randazzo, Italy 47 E7 37 53N 14 57 E
Rander, India 94 D1 21 14N 72 47 E
Randers, Denmark 17 H4 56 29N 10 1 E
Randers Fjord, Denmark 17 H4 56 37N 10 20 E
Randfontein, S. Africa 117 D4 26 8 S 27 45 E
Randle, U.S.A. 160 D5 46 32N 121 57W
Randolph, Mass., U.S.A. 151 D13 42 10N 71 2W
Randolph, N.Y., U.S.A. 150 D6 42 10N 78 59W
Randolph, Utah, U.S.A. 158 F8 41 40N 111 11W

Randolph, Vt., U.S.A. 151 C12 43 55N 72 40W
Randsburg, U.S.A. 161 K9 35 22N 117 39W
Randsfjorden, Norway 18 D7 60 25N 10 24 E
Randsverk, Norway 18 C6 61 44N 9 3 E
Råneälven →, Sweden 14 D20 65 50N 22 20 E
Ranenburg = Chaplygin, Russia 58 F11 53 15N 40 0 E
Ranfurly, N.Z. 131 F5 45 7 S 170 6 E
Rangae, Thailand 87 J3 6 19N 101 44 E
Rangamati, Bangla. 90 D4 22 38N 92 12 E
Rangapara, India 90 B4 26 49N 92 39 E
Rangárvallasýsla □, Iceland 11 D7 63 55N 20 0W
Rangataua, N.Z. 130 F4 39 26 S 175 28 E
Rangaunu B., N.Z. 130 A2 34 51 S 173 15 E
Rangeley, U.S.A. 149 C10 44 58N 70 39W
Rangeley L., U.S.A. 151 B14 44 55N 70 43W
Rangely, U.S.A. 158 F9 40 5N 108 48W
Ranger, U.S.A. 155 J5 32 28N 98 41W
Rangia, India 90 B3 26 28N 91 38 E
Rangiora, N.Z. 131 D7 43 19 S 172 36 E
Rangitaiki, N.Z. 130 E5 38 52 S 176 24 E
Rangitaiki →, N.Z. 130 D5 37 54 S 176 49 E
Rangitata →, N.Z. 131 D6 43 45 S 171 15 E
Rangitikei →, N.Z. 130 G4 40 17 S 175 15 E
Rangitoto ke te tonga = D'Urville I., N.Z. 131 A8 40 50 S 173 55 E
Rangitoto Ra., N.Z. 130 E4 38 25 S 175 35 E
Rangkasbitung, Indonesia 84 D3 6 21 S 106 15 E
Rangoon, Burma 90 G6 16 45N 96 20 E
Rangoon □, Burma 90 G6 17 0N 96 10 E
Rangpur, Bangla. 90 C2 25 42N 89 22 E
Rangsang, Indonesia 84 B2 1 20N 103 30 E
Rangsit, Thailand 86 F3 13 59N 100 37 E
Ranheim, Norway 18 A7 63 26N 10 32 E
Ranibennur, India 95 G2 14 35N 75 30 E
Raniganj, India 93 F9 27 3N 82 13 E
Ranikhet, India 93 E8 29 39N 79 25 E
Ranippettai, India 95 H4 12 56N 79 23 E
Rāniyah, Iraq 96 B5 36 15N 44 53 E
Ranka, India 93 H10 23 59N 83 47 E
Ranken →, Australia 126 C2 20 31 S 137 36 E
Rankin, Ill., U.S.A. 157 D9 40 28N 87 54W
Rankin, Tex., U.S.A. 155 K4 31 13N 101 56W
Rankin Inlet, Canada 138 B10 62 30N 93 0W
Rankins Springs, Australia 129 B7 33 49 S 146 14 E
Rankovicevo = Kraljevo, Serbia & M. 50 C4 43 44N 20 41 E
Rankweil, Austria 34 D2 47 17N 9 39 E
Rannoch, L., U.K. 22 E4 56 41N 4 20W
Rannoch Moor, U.K. 22 E4 56 38N 4 48W
Rano Kau, Chile 172 b 27 11 S 109 26W
Rano Raraku, Volcán, Chile 172 b 27 7 S 109 17W
Ranobe, Helodranon' i, Madag. 117 C7 23 3 S 43 33 E
Ranohira, Madag. 117 C8 22 29 S 45 24 E
Ranomafana, Toamasina, Madag. 117 B8 18 57 S 48 50 E
Ranomafana, Toliara, Madag. 117 C8 24 34 S 47 0 E
Ranomafana △, Madag. 117 C8 21 16 S 47 25 E
Ranomena, Madag. 117 C8 23 25 S 47 17 E
Ranon, Vanuatu 133 F6 16 8 S 168 7 E
Ranong, Thailand 87 H2 9 56N 98 40 E
Ranongga, Solomon Is. 133 M9 8 5 S 156 35 E
Ranotsara Nord, Madag. 117 C8 22 48 S 46 36 E
Ranpur, India 94 D7 20 5N 85 20 E
Rānsa, Iran 97 C6 33 39N 48 18 E
Ransiki, Indonesia 83 B4 1 30 S 134 10 E
Ransom, U.S.A. 157 C8 41 9N 88 39W
Rantabe, Madag. 117 B8 15 42 S 49 39 E
Rantau, Indonesia 85 C5 2 56 S 115 9 E
Rantauprapat, Indonesia 84 B1 2 15N 99 50 E
Rantemario, Indonesia 82 B1 3 15 S 119 57 E
Ranthambore △, India 92 F7 26 10N 76 30 E
Rantoul, U.S.A. 157 D8 40 19N 88 9W
Ranum, Denmark 17 H3 56 54N 9 14 E
Ranyah, W. →, Si. Arabia 98 B3 21 18N 43 20 E
Raon l'Étape, France 27 D13 48 24N 6 50 E
Raoping, China 77 F11 23 42N 117 1 E
Raoui, Erg er, Algeria 111 C4 29 0N 2 0W
Raoyang, China 74 E8 38 15N 115 45 E
Rap, Ko, Thailand 87 b 9 19N 99 58 E
Rapa, French Polynesia 135 K13 27 35 S 144 20W
Rapa Nui = Pascua, I. de, Chile 172 b 27 7 S 109 23W
Rapallo, Italy 44 D6 44 21N 9 14 E
Rapang, Indonesia 82 B1 3 50 S 119 48 E
Rapar, India 92 H4 23 34N 70 38 E
Rāpch, Iran 97 E8 25 40N 59 15 E
Raper, C., Canada 139 B13 69 44N 67 6W
Rapid City, U.S.A. 154 D3 44 5N 103 14W
Rapid River, U.S.A. 148 C2 45 55N 86 58W
Rapla, Estonia 15 G21 59 1N 24 52 E
Rapperswil, Switz. 33 B7 47 14N 8 45 E
Rapti →, India 93 F10 26 18N 83 41 E
Rapu Rapu I., Phil. 80 E5 13 12N 124 9 E
Raqaba ez Zarqa →, Sudan 107 F2 9 14N 29 44 E
Rāqūbah, Libya 108 C3 28 58N 19 2 E
Raquette →, U.S.A. 151 B10 45 0N 74 42W
Raquette Lake, U.S.A. 151 C10 43 49N 74 40W
Rara △, Nepal 93 E10 29 30N 82 10 E
Rarotonga, Cook Is. 135 K12 21 30 S 160 0W
Ra's al 'Ayn, Syria 101 D9 36 45N 40 12 E
Ra's al Khaymah, U.A.E. 97 E7 25 50N 55 59 E
Ras el Ma, Algeria 111 B4 34 26N 0 50W
Râs el Mâ, Mali 112 B4 16 35N 4 30W
Râs Ghârib, Egypt 106 B3 28 6N 33 18 E
Râs Köh, Pakistan 91 C2 28 43N 64 55 E
Ra's Lānūf, Libya 108 B3 30 46N 18 11 E
Râs Mallap, Egypt 106 B3 29 18N 32 50 E
Râs Muhammad △, Egypt 106 B3 27 45N 34 16 E
Rasa, Punta, Argentina 176 B4 40 50 S 62 15W
Rasca, Pta. de la, Canary Is. 9 e1 27 59N 16 41W
Rășcani, Moldova 53 C12 47 58N 27 33 E
Raseiniai, Lithuania 15 J20 55 25N 23 5 E
Rashad, Sudan 107 E3 11 55N 31 0 E
Rashîd, Egypt 106 H7 31 21N 30 22 E
Rashîd, Masabb, Egypt 106 H7 31 22N 30 17 E
Rashin = Najin, N. Korea 75 C16 42 12N 130 15 E
Rashmi, India 92 G6 25 4N 74 22 E
Rasht, Iran 97 B6 37 20N 49 40 E
Rasi Salai, Thailand 86 E5 15 20N 104 9 E
Rasipuram, India 95 J4 11 30N 78 15 E
Raška, Serbia & M. 50 C4 43 19N 20 39 E
Râșnov, Romania 53 E10 45 35N 25 27 E
Rason L., Australia 125 E3 28 45 S 124 25 E
Rașova, Romania 53 F12 44 15N 27 55 E
Rasovo, Bulgaria 50 C7 43 42N 23 17 E
Rasra, India 93 G10 25 50N 83 50 E
Rass el Oued, Algeria 111 A6 35 57N 5 2 E
Rasskazovo, Russia 60 D5 52 35N 41 50 E
Rast, Romania 53 G8 43 53N 23 16 E
Rastatt, Germany 31 G4 48 50N 8 11 E
Rastede, Germany 30 B4 53 15N 8 12 E
Rastenburg = Kętrzyn, Poland 54 D8 54 7N 21 22 E
Răstolița, Romania 53 D9 46 59N 24 58 E
Rastyapino = Dzerzhinsk, Russia 60 B6 56 14N 43 30 E
Rasul, Pakistan 92 C5 32 42N 73 34 E
Raszków, Poland 55 G4 51 43N 17 40 E
Rat Buri, Thailand 86 F2 13 30N 99 54 E
Rat Islands, U.S.A. 144 L2 52 0N 178 0 E
Rat L., Canada 143 B9 56 10N 99 40W
Ratak Chain, Pac. Oc. 134 G8 1 0N 170 0 E
Rätan, Sweden 16 B8 62 29N 14 33 E
Ratangarh, India 92 E6 28 5N 74 35 E
Raṭāwī, Iraq 96 D5 30 38N 47 13 E
Ratcatchers L., Australia 128 B5 32 30 S 143 12 E
Rath, India 93 G8 25 36N 79 37 E
Rath Luirc, Ireland 23 D3 52 21N 8 40W
Rathbun L., U.S.A. 156 D4 40 49N 92 53W
Rathdrum, Ireland 23 D5 52 56N 6 14W
Rathedaung, Burma 90 E4 20 29N 92 45 E
Rathenow, Germany 30 C8 52 37N 12 19 E
Rathkeale, Ireland 23 D3 52 32N 8 56W
Rathlin I., U.K. 23 A5 55 18N 6 14W
Rathmelton, Ireland 23 A4 55 2N 7 38W
Ratibor = Racibórz, Poland 55 H5 50 7N 18 18 E
Rätikon, Austria 33 B9 47 0N 9 55 E
Ratingen, Germany 30 D2 51 18N 6 52 E
Ratlam, India 92 H6 23 20N 75 0 E
Ratnagiri, India 94 F1 16 57N 73 18 E
Ratnapura, Sri Lanka 95 L5 6 40N 80 20 E
Ratodero, Pakistan 92 F3 27 48N 68 18 E
Raton, U.S.A. 155 G2 36 54N 104 24W
Ratschach = Radeče, Slovenia 45 B12 46 5N 15 14 E
Rattaphum, Thailand 87 J3 7 8N 100 16 E
Ratten, Austria 34 D8 47 28N 15 44 E
Rattray Hd., U.K. 22 D7 57 38N 1 50W
Rättvik, Sweden 16 D9 60 52N 15 7 E
Ratz, Mt., Canada 142 B2 57 23N 132 12W
Ratzebuhr = Okonek, Poland 54 E3 53 32N 16 51 E
Ratzeburg, Germany 30 B6 53 40N 10 46 E
Rau, Indonesia 82 A3 2 20N 128 10 E
Raub, Malaysia 87 L3 3 47N 101 52 E
Rauch, Argentina 174 D4 36 45 S 59 5W
Raudales de Malpaso, Mexico 163 D6 17 30N 93 30W
Raudeberg, Norway 18 C2 61 59N 5 7 E
Raufarhöfn, Iceland 11 A11 66 27N 15 57W
Raufoss, Norway 18 D7 60 44N 10 37 E
Rauhellern, Norway 18 D4 60 15N 7 50 E
Raukumara Ra., N.Z. 130 E6 38 5 S 177 55 E
Raul Soares, Brazil 171 F3 20 5 S 42 22W
Rauma, Finland 15 F19 61 10N 21 30 E
Rauma →, Norway 18 B4 62 34N 7 43 E
Raumo = Rauma, Finland 15 F19 61 10N 21 30 E
Raung, Gunung, Indonesia 79 J17 8 8 S 114 3 E
Raurkela, India 93 H11 22 14N 84 50 E
Rausu-Dake, Japan 70 B12 44 4N 145 7 E
Răut →, Moldova 53 C14 47 15N 29 9 E
Rava-Ruska, Ukraine 55 H10 50 15N 23 42 E
Rava Russkaya = Rava-Ruska, Ukraine 55 H10 50 15N 23 42 E
Ravalli, U.S.A. 158 C6 47 17N 114 11W
Ravānsar, Iran 101 E12 34 43N 46 40 E
Ravanusa, Italy 46 E6 37 16N 13 58 E
Rāvar, Iran 97 D8 31 20N 56 51 E
Ravena, U.S.A. 151 D11 42 28N 73 49W
Ravenel, U.S.A. 152 C9 32 46N 80 15W
Ravenna, Italy 45 D9 44 25N 12 12 E
Ravenna, Ky., U.S.A. 157 G13 37 42N 83 55W
Ravenna, Nebr., U.S.A. 154 E5 41 1N 98 55W
Ravenna, Ohio, U.S.A. 150 E3 41 9N 81 15W
Ravensburg, Germany 31 H5 47 46N 9 36 E
Ravenshoe, Australia 126 B4 17 37 S 145 29 E
Ravensthorpe, Australia 125 F3 33 35 S 120 2 E
Ravenswood, Australia 126 C4 20 6 S 146 54 E
Ravenswood, U.S.A. 148 F5 38 57N 81 46W
Ravensworth, Australia 129 B9 32 26 S 151 4 E
Ravenwood, U.S.A. 156 D2 40 22N 94 41W
Raver, India 94 D3 21 15N 76 2 E
Ravi →, Pakistan 92 D4 30 35N 71 49 E
Ravna Gora, Croatia 45 C11 45 24N 14 50 E
Ravna Reka, Serbia & M. 50 B5 44 1N 21 35 E
Ravne na Koroškem, Slovenia 45 B11 46 36N 14 59 E
Rawa Mazowiecka, Poland 55 G7 51 46N 20 12 E
Rawalpindi, Pakistan 91 B4 33 38N 73 8 E
Rawāndūz, Iraq 101 D11 36 40N 44 30 E
Rawang, Malaysia 87 L3 3 20N 101 35 E
Rawene, N.Z. 130 B2 35 25 S 173 32 E
Rawicz, Poland 55 G3 51 36N 16 52 E
Rawitsch = Rawicz, Poland 55 G3 51 36N 16 52 E
Rawka →, Poland 55 F7 52 9N 20 8 E
Rawlinna, Australia 125 F4 30 58 S 125 28 E
Rawlins, U.S.A. 158 F10 41 47N 107 14W
Rawlinson Ra., Australia 125 D4 24 40 S 128 30 E
Rawson, Argentina 176 B3 43 15 S 65 5W
Raxaul, India 93 F11 26 59N 84 51 E
Ray, U.S.A. 154 A3 48 21N 103 10W
Ray, C., Canada 141 C8 47 33N 59 15W
Ray City, U.S.A. 152 D6 31 5N 83 11W
Ray Mts., U.S.A. 144 D10 66 0N 152 0W
Raya Ring, Ko, Thailand 87 a 8 18N 98 29 E
Rayachoti, India 95 G4 14 4N 78 50 E
Rayadurg, India 95 G3 14 40N 76 50 E
Rayagada, India 94 E6 19 15N 83 20 E
Raychikhinsk, Russia 67 E13 49 46N 129 25 E
Rāyen, Iran 97 D8 29 34N 57 26 E
Rayevskiy, Russia 64 D5 54 4N 54 56 E
Rayle, U.S.A. 152 B7 33 48N 82 54W
Rayleigh, U.K. 21 F8 51 36N 0 37 E
Raymond, Canada 142 D6 49 30N 112 35W
Raymond, Calif., U.S.A. 160 H7 37 13N 119 54W
Raymond, Ill., U.S.A. 156 E7 39 19N 89 34W
Raymond, N.H., U.S.A. 151 C13 43 2N 71 11W
Raymond, Wash., U.S.A. 160 D3 46 41N 123 44W
Raymond Terrace, Australia 129 B9 32 45 S 151 44 E
Raymondville, U.S.A. 155 M6 26 29N 97 47W
Raymore, Canada 143 C8 51 25N 104 31W
Rayón, Mexico 162 B2 29 43N 110 35W
Rayong, Thailand 86 F3 12 40N 101 20 E
Raytown, U.S.A. 156 E2 39 1N 94 28W
Rayville, U.S.A. 155 J9 32 29N 91 46W
Raz, Pte. du, France 26 D2 48 2N 4 47W
Razan, Iran 97 C6 35 23N 49 2 E
Ražana, Serbia & M. 50 B3 44 6N 19 55 E
Ražanj, Serbia & M. 50 C5 43 40N 21 31 E
Razāzah, Buḥayrat ar, Iraq 101 F10 32 40N 43 35 E
Razazah, L. = Razāzah, Buḥayrat ar, Iraq 101 F10 32 40N 43 35 E
Razdelna, Bulgaria 51 C11 43 13N 27 41 E
Razdel'naya = Rozdilna, Ukraine 53 D15 46 50N 30 2 E
Razdolnoye, Russia 70 C5 43 30N 131 52 E
Razdolnoye, Ukraine 59 K7 45 46N 33 29 E
Razeh, Iran 97 C6 32 47N 48 9 E
Razgrad, Bulgaria 51 C10 43 33N 26 34 E
Razim, Lacul, Romania 53 F14 44 50N 29 0 E
Razlog, Bulgaria 50 E7 41 53N 23 28 E
Razmak, Pakistan 91 B3 32 45N 69 50 E
Ré, Î. de, France 28 B2 46 12N 1 30W
Reading, U.K. 21 F7 51 27N 0 58W
Reading, Mich., U.S.A. 157 C12 41 50N 84 45W
Reading, Ohio, U.S.A. 157 E12 39 13N 84 26W
Reading, Pa., U.S.A. 151 F9 40 20N 75 56W
Reading □, U.K. 21 F7 51 27N 0 58W
Real, Cordillera, Bolivia 172 D4 17 0 S 67 10W
Realicó, Argentina 174 D3 35 0 S 64 15W
Réalmont, France 28 E6 43 48N 2 10 E
Realp, Switz. 33 C6 46 36N 8 30 E
Ream, Cambodia 87 G4 10 34N 103 39 E
Reata, Mexico 162 B4 26 8N 101 5W
Reay Forest, U.K. 22 C4 58 22N 4 55W
Rebais, France 27 D10 48 50N 3 10 E
Rebi, Indonesia 83 C4 6 23 S 134 7 E
Rebiana, Libya 108 D4 24 12N 22 10 E
Rebiana, Sahrâ', Libya 108 D3 24 30N 21 0 E
Rebun-Tō, Japan 70 B10 45 23N 141 2 E
Recanati, Italy 45 E10 43 24N 13 32 E
Recaș, Romania 52 E6 45 46N 21 30 E
Recco, Italy 44 D6 44 22N 9 9 E
Recherche, Arch. of the, Australia 125 F3 34 15 S 122 50 E
Rechna Doab, Pakistan 92 D5 31 35N 73 30 E
Rechytsa, Belarus 59 F6 52 21N 30 24 E
Recife, Brazil 170 C5 8 0 S 35 0W
Recife, Seychelles 121 b 4 36 S 55 42 E
Recklinghausen, Germany 24 C7 51 37N 7 12 E
Reconquista, Argentina 174 B4 29 10 S 59 45W
Recreio, Brazil 173 B6 8 0 S 58 25W
Recreo, Argentina 174 B2 29 25 S 65 10W
Recuay, Peru 172 B2 9 43 S 77 28W
Recz, Poland 55 E2 53 16N 15 31 E
Red →, La., U.S.A. 155 K9 31 1N 91 45W
Red →, N. Dak., U.S.A. 138 C10 49 0N 97 15W
Red Bank, U.S.A. 151 F10 40 21N 74 5W
Red Bay, Canada 141 B8 51 44N 56 25W
Red Bluff, U.S.A. 158 F2 40 11N 122 15W
Red Bluff Res., U.S.A. 155 K3 31 54N 103 55W
Red Bud, U.S.A. 156 F7 38 13N 89 59W
Red Cliffs, Australia 128 C5 34 19 S 142 11 E
Red Cloud, U.S.A. 154 E5 40 5N 98 32W
Red Creek, U.S.A. 151 C8 43 14N 76 45W
Red Deer, Canada 142 C6 52 20N 113 50W
Red Deer →, Alta., Canada 143 C7 50 58N 110 0W
Red Deer →, Man., Canada 143 C8 52 53N 101 1W
Red Deer L., Canada 143 C8 52 55N 101 20W
Red Devil, U.S.A. 144 F8 61 46N 157 19W
Red Hook, U.S.A. 151 E11 41 55N 73 53W
Red Indian L., Canada 141 C8 48 35N 57 0W
Red L., Canada 143 C10 51 3N 93 49W
Red Lake, Canada 143 C10 51 3N 93 49W
Red Lake Falls, U.S.A. 154 B6 47 53N 96 16W
Red Lake Road, Canada 143 C10 49 59N 93 25W
Red Lodge, U.S.A. 158 D9 45 11N 109 15W
Red Mountain, U.S.A. 161 K9 35 37N 117 38W
Red Oak, U.S.A. 154 E7 41 1N 95 14W
Red Rock, Canada 140 C2 48 55N 88 15W
Red Rock, L., U.S.A. 156 C3 41 22N 92 59W
Red Rocks Pt., Australia 125 F4 32 13 S 127 32 E
Red Sea, Asia 88 C2 25 0N 36 0 E
Red Slate Mt., U.S.A. 160 H8 37 31N 118 52W
Red Sucker L., Canada 140 B1 54 9N 93 40W
Red Tower Pass = Turnu Roşu, P., Romania 53 E9 45 33N 24 17 E
Red Wing, U.S.A. 154 C8 44 34N 92 31W
Reda, Poland 54 D5 54 40N 18 19 E
Redang, Malaysia 87 K4 5 49N 103 2 E
Redange, Lux. 24 E5 49 46N 5 52 E
Redcar, U.K. 20 C6 54 37N 1 4W
Redcar & Cleveland □, U.K. 20 C7 54 29N 1 0W
Redcliff, Canada 158 A8 50 10N 110 50W
Redcliffe, Australia 127 D5 27 12 S 153 0 E
Redcliffe, Mt., Australia 125 E3 28 30 S 121 30 E
Reddersburg, S. Africa 116 D4 29 41 S 26 10 E
Reddick, Fla., U.S.A. 153 F7 29 22N 82 12W
Reddick, Ill., U.S.A. 157 C8 41 6N 88 15W
Redding, Calif., U.S.A. 158 F2 40 35N 122 24W
Redding, Iowa, U.S.A. 156 D2 40 36N 94 23W
Redditch, U.K. 21 E6 52 18N 1 55W
Redenção, Brazil 170 B4 4 13 S 38 43W
Redfield, U.S.A. 154 C5 44 53N 98 31W
Redford, U.S.A. 151 B11 44 38N 73 48W
Redhead, Trin. & Tob. 169 F10 10 44N 60 58W
Redkey, U.S.A. 157 D11 40 21N 85 9W
Redkino, Russia 58 D9 56 39N 36 16 E
Redlands, U.S.A. 161 M9 34 4N 117 11W
Redmond, Oreg., U.S.A. 158 D3 44 17N 121 11W
Redmond, Wash., U.S.A. 160 C4 47 41N 122 7W
Redon, France 26 E4 47 40N 2 6W
Redonda, Antigua & B. 165 C7 16 58N 62 19W
Redondela, Pta., Chile 172 b 27 10 S 109 22W
Redondela, Spain 42 C2 42 15N 8 38W
Redondo, Portugal 43 G3 38 39N 7 37W
Redondo Beach, U.S.A. 161 M8 33 50N 118 23W
Redoubt Volcano, U.S.A. 144 F9 60 29N 152 45W
Redruth, U.K. 21 G2 50 14N 5 14W
Redvers, Canada 143 D8 49 35N 101 40W
Redwater, Canada 142 C6 53 55N 113 6W
Redwood, U.S.A. 151 B9 44 18N 75 48W
Redwood △, U.S.A. 158 F1 41 40N 124 5W
Redwood City, U.S.A. 160 H4 37 30N 122 15W
Redwood Falls, U.S.A. 154 C7 44 32N 95 7W
Ree, L., Ireland 23 C3 53 35N 8 0W
Reed, L., Canada 143 C8 54 38N 100 30W
Reed City, U.S.A. 148 D3 43 53N 85 31W
Reedley, U.S.A. 160 J7 36 36N 119 27W
Reedsburg, U.S.A. 154 D9 43 32N 90 0W
Reedsport, U.S.A. 158 E1 43 42N 124 6W
Reedsville, U.S.A. 150 F7 40 39N 77 35W
Reedy Creek, Australia 128 D4 36 58 S 140 2 E
Reefton, N.Z. 131 C6 42 6 S 171 51 E
Rees, Germany 30 D2 51 46N 6 24 E
Reese →, U.S.A. 158 F5 40 48N 117 4W
Reetz = Recz, Poland 55 E2 53 16N 15 31 E
Refahiye, Turkey 101 C8 39 54N 38 47 E
Reftele, Sweden 17 G7 57 11N 13 35 E
Refugio, U.S.A. 155 L6 28 18N 97 17W
Rega →, Poland 54 D2 54 10N 15 18 E
Regalbuto, Italy 47 E7 37 39N 14 38 E
Regar = Tursunzade, Tajikistan 65 D4 38 30N 68 14 E
Regen, Germany 31 G9 48 58N 13 8 E
Regen →, Germany 31 F8 49 1N 12 6 E
Regeneração, Brazil 170 C3 6 15 S 42 41W
Regensburg, Germany 31 F8 49 1N 12 6 E
Regensdorf, Switz. 33 B6 47 26N 8 28 E
Regenstauf, Germany 31 F8 49 7N 12 8 E
Regenwalde = Resko, Poland 54 E2 53 47N 15 25 E
Reggâne = Zaouiet Reggâne, Algeria 111 C5 26 32N 0 3 E
Reggello, Italy 45 E8 43 41N 11 32 E
Réggio di Calábria, Italy 47 D8 38 6N 15 39 E
Réggio nell'Emília, Italy 44 D7 44 43N 10 36 E
Reghin, Romania 53 D9 46 46N 24 42 E
Regina, Canada 143 C8 50 27N 104 35W
Régina, Fr. Guiana 169 C7 4 19N 52 8W
Regina Beach, Canada 143 C8 50 47N 105 0W
Register, U.S.A. 152 C8 32 22N 81 53W
Registro, Brazil 175 A6 24 29 S 47 49W
Reguengos de Monsaraz, Portugal 43 G3 38 25N 7 32W
Reh, Erg er, Algeria 111 C5 27 48N 4 30 E
Rehar →, India 93 H10 23 55N 82 40 E
Rehli, India 93 H8 23 38N 79 5 E
Rehoboth, Namibia 116 C2 23 15 S 17 4 E
Rehovot, Israel 103 D3 31 54N 34 48 E
Reïbell = Ksar Chellala, Algeria 111 A5 35 13N 2 19 E
Reichenau = Rychnov nad Kněžnou, Czech Rep. 35 A9 50 10N 16 17 E
Reichenbach = Dzierżoniów, Poland 55 H3 50 45N 16 39 E
Reichenbach, Germany 30 E8 50 37N 12 17 E
Reichenbach, Switz. 32 C5 46 38N 7 42 E
Reichenberg = Liberec, Czech Rep. 34 A8 50 47N 15 7 E
Reichshof = Rzeszów, Poland 55 H8 50 5N 21 58 E
Reid, Australia 125 F4 30 49 S 128 26 E
Reiden, Switz. 32 B5 47 14N 7 59 E
Reidsville, Ga., U.S.A. 152 C7 32 6N 82 7W
Reidsville, N.C., U.S.A. 149 G6 36 21N 79 40W
Reifnig = Ribnica, Slovenia 45 C11 45 45N 14 45 E
Reigate, U.K. 21 F7 51 14N 0 12W
Reillo, Spain 40 F3 39 54N 1 53W
Reims, France 27 C11 49 15N 4 1 E
Reina Adelaida, Arch., Chile 176 D2 52 20 S 74 0W
Reina Sofia, Tenerife ✕ (TFS), Canary Is. 9 e1 28 3N 16 33W
Reinach, Aargau, Switz. 32 B6 47 14N 8 11 E
Reinach, Basel, Switz. 32 B5 47 29N 7 35 E
Reinbeck, U.S.A. 156 B4 42 19N 92 36W
Reinbek, Germany 30 B6 53 30N 10 16 E
Reindeer →, Canada 143 B8 55 36N 103 11W
Reindeer I., Canada 143 C9 52 30N 98 0W
Reindeer L., Canada 143 B8 57 15N 102 15W
Reinga, C., N.Z. 130 A1 34 25 S 172 43 E
Reinosa, Spain 42 B6 43 2N 4 15W
Reinsvoll, Norway 18 D7 60 40N 10 38 E
Reitan, Norway 18 B8 62 49N 11 22 E
Reitz, S. Africa 117 D4 27 48 S 28 29 E
Reivilo, S. Africa 116 D3 27 36 S 24 8 E
Rejaf, Sudan 107 G3 4 45N 31 35 E
Rejmyre, Sweden 17 F9 58 50N 15 55 E
Rejowiec Fabryczny, Poland 55 G10 51 5N 23 17 E
Reka →, Slovenia 45 C11 45 40N 14 0 E
Rekohua = Chatham I., N.Z. 131 a 43 50 S 176 20W
Rekovac, Serbia & M. 50 C5 43 51N 21 3 E
Reliance, Canada 143 A7 63 0N 109 20W
Relizane, Algeria 111 A5 35 44N 0 31 E
Remad, Oued →, Algeria 111 B4 33 28N 1 20W
Rémalard, France 26 D7 48 26N 0 47 E
Remarkable, Mt., Australia 128 B3 32 48 S 138 10 E
Remarkables, The, N.Z. 131 F3 45 10 S 168 50 E
Rembang, Indonesia 85 D4 6 42 S 111 21 E
Rembau, Malaysia 84 B2 2 35N 102 6 E
Rembert, U.S.A. 152 A9 34 6N 80 32W
Remchi, Algeria 111 A4 35 2N 1 26W
Remedios, Colombia 168 B3 7 2N 74 41W
Remedios, Panama 164 E3 8 15N 81 50W
Remeshk, Iran 97 E8 26 55N 58 50 E
Remetea, Romania 53 D10 46 45N 25 29 E
Remich, Lux. 24 E6 49 32N 6 22 E
Remington, U.S.A. 157 D9 40 46N 87 9W
Rémire, Fr. Guiana 169 C7 4 53N 52 17W
Remiremont, France 27 D13 48 2N 6 36 E
Remo, Ethiopia 107 F5 6 48N 41 20 E
Remontnoye, Russia 61 G6 46 34N 43 37 E
Remoulins, France 29 E8 43 55N 4 35 E
Remscheid, Germany 24 C7 51 11N 7 12 E
Ren Xian, China 74 F8 37 8N 114 40 E
Rena, Norway 18 C8 61 8N 11 20 E
Rena →, Norway 18 C8 61 8N 11 23 E
Renascença, Brazil 168 D4 3 50 S 66 21W
Rend Lake, U.S.A. 156 F8 38 2N 88 58W
Rendang, Indonesia 79 J18 8 26 S 115 25 E
Rende, Italy 47 C9 39 20N 16 11 E
Rendína, Greece 48 B3 39 4N 21 58 E
Rendova, Solomon Is. 133 M9 8 33 S 157 17 E
Rendsburg, Germany 30 A5 54 17N 9 39 E
Renens, Switz. 32 C3 46 32N 6 35 E
Renfrew, Canada 140 C4 45 30N 76 40W
Renfrewshire □, U.K. 22 F4 55 49N 4 38W
Renfroe, U.S.A. 152 C5 32 14N 84 43W
Rengat, Indonesia 84 C2 0 30 S 102 45 E
Rengo, Chile 174 C1 34 24 S 70 50W
Renhua, China 77 E9 25 5N 113 40 E
Renhuai, China 76 D6 27 48N 106 24 E
Reni, Ukraine 53 E13 45 28N 28 15 E
Renigunta, India 95 H4 13 38N 79 30 E
Renk, Sudan 107 E3 11 50N 32 50 E
Renland, Greenland 10 C8 71 10N 26 30W
Renmark, Australia 128 C4 34 11 S 140 43 E
Rennebu, Norway 18 B6 62 52N 9 49 E
Rennell, Solomon Is. 133 N11 11 40 S 160 10 E
Rennell Sd., Canada 142 C2 53 23N 132 35W
Renner Springs, Australia 126 B1 18 20 S 133 47 E
Rennes, France 26 D5 48 7N 1 41W
Rennie L., Canada 143 A7 61 32N 105 35W
Reno, U.S.A. 160 F7 39 31N 119 48W
Reno →, Italy 45 D9 44 38N 12 16 E
Renovo, U.S.A. 150 E7 41 20N 77 45W
Renqiu, China 74 E9 38 43N 116 5 E
Rens, Denmark 17 K3 54 54N 9 5 E
Renshou, China 76 C5 30 3N 104 9 E
Rensselaer, Ind., U.S.A. 157 D9 40 57N 87 9W
Rensselaer, N.Y., U.S.A. 151 D11 42 38N 73 45W
Rentería, Spain 40 B3 43 19N 1 54W
Renton, U.S.A. 160 C4 47 29N 122 12W
Renwick, N.Z. 131 B8 41 30 S 173 51 E
Réo, Burkina Faso 112 C4 12 28N 2 35W
Reo, Indonesia 82 C2 8 19 S 120 30 E
Reocín, Spain 42 B6 43 21N 4 5W
Reotipur, India 93 G10 25 33N 83 45 E
Repalle, India 95 F5 16 2N 80 45 E
Répcelak, Hungary 52 C2 47 24N 17 1 E
Reppen = Rzepin, Poland 55 F1 52 20N 14 49 E
Republic, Mo., U.S.A. 155 G8 37 7N 93 29W
Republic, Wash., U.S.A. 158 B4 48 39N 118 44W
Republican →, U.S.A. 154 F6 39 4N 96 48W
Republiek, Suriname 169 B6 5 30N 55 13W
Repulse B., Australia 126 J6 20 35 S 148 46 E
Repulse Bay, Canada 139 B11 66 30N 86 30W
Requena, Peru 172 B3 5 5 S 73 52W
Requena, Spain 41 F3 39 30N 1 4W
Réquista, France 28 D6 44 1N 2 32 E
Reşadiye = Datça, Turkey 49 E9 36 46N 27 40 E
Reşadiye, Turkey 100 B7 40 23N 37 20 E
Reşadiye Yarımadası, Turkey 49 E9 36 40N 27 45 E
Resavica, Serbia & M. 50 B5 44 4N 21 31 E
Resen, Macedonia 50 E5 41 5N 21 0 E
Reserve, U.S.A. 159 K9 33 43N 108 45W
Resht = Rasht, Iran 97 B6 37 20N 49 40 E
Résia, Italy 33 C11 46 50N 10 31 E
Resistencia, Argentina 174 B4 27 30 S 59 0W
Reşiţa, Romania 52 E6 45 18N 21 53 E
Resko, Poland 54 E2 53 47N 15 25 E
Reso = Raisio, Finland 15 F20 60 28N 22 11 E
Resolution I., Canada 139 B13 61 30N 65 0W
Resolution I., N.Z. 131 F1 45 40 S 166 40 E
Resplandes, Brazil 170 C2 6 17 S 45 13W
Resplendor, Brazil 171 E3 19 20 S 41 15W
Ressano Garcia, Mozam. 117 D5 25 25 S 32 0 E
Restinga de Jurubatiba △, Brazil 171 F3 22 5 S 41 20W
Reston, Canada 143 D8 49 33N 101 6W
Resulayn = Ceylânpınar, Turkey 101 D9 36 50N 40 2 E
Reszel, Poland 54 D8 54 4N 21 10 E
Retalhuleu, Guatemala 164 D1 14 33N 91 46W
Retenue, L. de, Dem. Rep. of the Congo 119 E2 11 0 S 27 0 E
Retezat △, Romania 52 E7 45 23N 22 56 E
Retezat, Munţii, Romania 52 E8 45 25N 23 0 E
Retford, U.K. 20 D7 53 19N 0 56W
Rethel, France 27 C11 49 30N 4 20 E
Rethem, Germany 30 C5 52 47N 9 22 E
Rethimno = Réthímnon, Greece 39 E5 35 18N 24 30 E
Réthímnon, Greece 39 E5 35 18N 24 30 E
Réthímnon □, Greece 39 E5 35 23N 24 28 E
Reti, Pakistan 92 E3 28 5N 69 48 E
Retiche, Alpi, Switz. 33 D10 46 30N 10 0 E
Retiers, France 26 E5 47 55N 1 23W
Retortillo, Spain 42 E4 40 48N 6 21W
Retournac, France 29 C8 45 12N 4 2 E
Rétság, Hungary 52 C4 47 58N 19 10 E
Rettenberg, Germany 33 A10 47 35N 10 18 E
Réunion ☑, Ind. Oc. 121 c 21 0 S 56 0 E
Reus, Spain 40 D6 41 10N 1 5 E
Reuss →, Switz. 33 B6 47 16N 8 24 E
Reuterstadt Stavenhagen, Germany 30 B8 53 42N 12 54 E
Reutlingen, Germany 31 G5 48 29N 9 12 E
Reutte, Austria 34 D3 47 29N 10 42 E
Reval = Tallinn, Estonia 15 G21 59 22N 24 48 E
Revda, Russia 64 C7 56 48N 59 57 E
Revel = Tallinn, Estonia 15 G21 59 22N 24 48 E
Revel, France 28 E6 43 28N 2 1 E
Revelganj, India 93 G11 25 50N 84 40 E
Revelstoke, Canada 142 C5 51 0N 118 10W
Reventazón, Peru 172 B1 6 10 S 80 58W
Revigny-sur-Ornain, France 27 D11 48 49N 4 59 E
Revillagigedo, Is. de, Pac. Oc. 162 D2 18 40N 112 0W
Revin, France 27 C11 49 55N 4 39 E
Revolyutsii, Pik, Tajikistan 65 D6 38 31N 72 21 E
Revolyutsiya, Qullai = Revolyutsii, Pik, Tajikistan 65 D6 38 31N 72 21 E
Revúca, Slovak Rep. 35 C13 48 41N 20 7 E
Revuè →, Mozam. 119 F3 19 50 S 34 0 E
Rewa, India 93 G9 24 33N 81 25 E
Rewa →, Guyana 169 C6 3 19N 58 42W
Rewari, India 92 E7 28 15N 76 40 E
Rex, U.S.A. 144 D10 64 13N 149 16W
Rexburg, U.S.A. 158 E8 43 49N 111 47W
Rey, Iran 97 C6 35 35N 51 25 E
Rey, I. del, Panama 164 E4 8 20N 78 30W
Rey, Mayo →, Cameroon 114 A2 8 47N 14 1 E
Rey, Rio-del-→, Cameroon 114 B1 4 31N 8 45 E
Rey Bouba, Cameroon 114 A2 8 40N 14 15 E
Rey Malabo, Eq. Guin. 113 E6 3 45N 8 50 E
Reyðarfjörður, Iceland 11 B12 65 2N 14 13W
Reyes, Bolivia 172 C4 14 19 S 67 23W
Reyes, Pt., U.S.A. 160 H3 38 0N 123 0W
Reyhanlı, Turkey 100 D7 36 16N 36 35 E
Reykholt, Árnessýsla, Iceland 11 C5 64 40N 21 18W
Reykholt, Borgarfjarðarsýsla, Iceland 11 C6 64 10N 20 25W
Reykjahlíð, Iceland 11 B10 65 40N 16 55W
Reykjanes, Iceland 11 D4 63 48N 22 40W
Reykjanes Ridge, Atl. Oc. 8 A8 59 0N 31 0W
Reykjavík, Iceland 11 C5 64 10N 21 57W
Reykjavík Keflavík ✕ (KEF), Iceland 11 C4 64 0N 22 45W
Reynolds, Ga., U.S.A. 152 C5 32 33N 84 6W
Reynolds, Ill., U.S.A. 156 C6 41 20N 90 40W
Reynolds Ra., Australia 124 D5 22 30 S 133 0 E
Reynoldsville, Ga., U.S.A. 152 E5 30 51N 84 47W
Reynoldsville, Pa., U.S.A. 150 E6 41 5N 78 58W
Reynosa, Mexico 163 B5 26 5N 98 18W
Reza'iyeh = Orūmīyeh, Iran 101 D11 37 40N 45 0 E
Rezāiyeh, L. = Orūmīyeh, Daryācheh-ye, Iran 101 D11 37 50N 45 30 E
Rēzekne, Latvia 15 H22 56 30N 27 17 E
Rezh, Russia 64 C8 57 23N 61 24 E
Rezhitsa = Rēzekne, Latvia 15 H22 56 30N 27 17 E
Rezina, Moldova 53 C14 47 45N 28 58 E
Rezovo, Bulgaria 51 D12 42 0N 28 0 E
Rezvān, Iran 97 E8 27 34N 56 6 E
Rgotina, Serbia & M. 50 B6 44 1N 22 17 E

Rhamnus, *Greece* 48 C6 38 12N 24 3 E
Rharbi, Zahrez, *Algeria* 111 B5 34 50N 2 55 E
Rharis, O. →, *Algeria* 111 C6 26 0N 5 4 E
Rhayader, *U.K.* 21 E4 52 18N 3 29W
Rheda-Wiedenbrück, *Germany* 30 D4 51 50N 8 20 E
Rhede, *Germany* 30 D2 51 50N 6 42 E
Rhein →, *Europe* 24 C6 51 52N 6 2 E
Rhein-Main-Donau-Kanal, *Germany* 31 F7 49 1N 11 27 E
Rhein-Ruhr, Düsseldorf ✈ (DUS), *Germany* 30 D2 51 17N 6 46 E
Rhein-Taunus ⌓, *Germany* 31 E4 50 10N 8 10 E
Rhein-Westerwald ⌓, *Germany* 30 E3 50 32N 7 20 E
Rheinbach, *Germany* 30 E2 50 38N 6 57 E
Rheine, *Germany* 30 C3 52 17N 7 26 E
Rheineck, *Switz.* 33 B9 47 28N 9 31 E
Rheinfall, *Switz.* 33 A7 47 40N 8 37 E
Rheinfelden, *Germany* 31 H3 47 33N 7 47 E
Rheinfelden, *Switz.* 32 A5 47 32N 7 47 E
Rheinhessen-Pfalz □, *Germany* 31 F3 49 20N 8 0 E
Rheinland-Pfalz □, *Germany* 31 E2 50 0N 7 0 E
Rheinsberg, *Germany* 30 B8 53 6N 12 54 E
Rheinwaldhorn, *Switz.* 33 D8 46 30N 9 3 E
Rheris, Oued →, *Morocco* 110 B4 30 50N 4 34W
Rhin = Rhein →, *Europe* 24 C6 51 52N 6 2 E
Rhine = Rhein →, *Europe* 24 C6 51 52N 6 2 E
Rhine, *U.S.A.* 152 D6 31 59N 83 12W
Rhinebeck, *U.S.A.* 151 E11 41 56N 73 55W
Rhineland-Palatinate = Rheinland-Pfalz □, *Germany* 31 E2 50 0N 7 0 E
Rhinelander, *U.S.A.* 154 C10 45 38N 89 25W
Rhinns Pt., *U.K.* 22 F2 55 40N 6 29W
Rhino Camp, *Uganda* 118 B3 3 0N 31 22 E
Rhir, Cap, *Morocco* 110 B3 30 38N 9 54W
Rho, *Italy* 44 C6 45 32N 9 2 E
Rhode Island □, *U.S.A.* 151 E13 41 40N 71 30W
Rhodes = Ródhos, *Greece* 38 E12 36 15N 28 10 E
Rhodesia = Zimbabwe ■, *Africa* 119 F3 19 0 S 30 0 E
Rhodope Mts. = Rhodopi Planina, *Bulgaria* 51 E8 41 40N 24 20 E
Rhodopi Planina, *Bulgaria* 51 E8 41 40N 24 20 E
Rhön, *Germany* 30 E5 50 24N 9 58 E
Rhondda, *U.K.* 21 F4 51 39N 3 31W
Rhondda Cynon Taff □, *U.K.* 21 F4 51 42N 3 27W
Rhône □, *France* 29 C8 45 54N 4 35 E
Rhône →, *France* 29 E8 43 28N 4 42 E
Rhône-Alpes □, *France* 29 C9 45 40N 6 0 E
Rhum, *U.K.* 22 E2 57 0N 6 20W
Rhyl, *U.K.* 20 D4 53 20N 3 29W
Ri-Aba, *Eq. Guin.* 113 E6 3 28N 8 40 E
Ria Formosa ⌓, *Portugal* 43 H3 37 1N 7 48W
Riachão, *Brazil* 170 C2 7 20 S 46 37W
Riacho de Santana, *Brazil* 171 D3 13 37 S 42 57W
Rialma, *Brazil* 171 E2 15 18 S 49 34W
Riang, *India* 90 B4 27 31N 92 56 E
Riangnom, *Sudan* 107 F3 9 55N 30 1 E
Riaño, *Spain* 42 C6 42 59N 4 59W
Rians, *France* 29 E9 43 37N 5 44 E
Riansáres →, *Spain* 43 F7 39 32N 3 18W
Riasi, *India* 93 C6 33 10N 74 50 E
Riau □, *Indonesia* 84 B2 0 0 102 35 E
Riau, Kepulauan, *Indonesia* 84 B2 0 30N 104 20 E
Riau Arch. = Riau, Kepulauan, *Indonesia* 84 B2 0 30N 104 20 E
Riaza, *Spain* 42 D7 41 18N 3 30W
Riaza →, *Spain* 42 D7 41 42N 3 55W
Riba de Saelices, *Spain* 40 E2 40 55N 2 17W
Riba-Roja de Turia, *Spain* 41 F4 39 33N 0 34W
Ribadavia, *Spain* 42 C2 42 17N 8 8W
Ribadeo, *Spain* 42 B3 43 35N 7 5W
Ribadesella, *Spain* 42 B5 43 30N 5 7W
Ribado, *Nigeria* 113 D7 9 16N 12 47 E
Ribamar, *Brazil* 170 B3 2 33 S 44 3W
Ribao, *Cameroon* 113 D7 6 32N 11 30 E
Ribas = Ribes de Freser, *Spain* 40 C7 42 19N 2 15 E
Ribas do Rio Pardo, *Brazil* 173 E7 20 27 S 53 46W
Ribauè, *Mozam.* 119 E4 14 57 S 38 17 E
Ribble →, *U.K.* 20 D5 53 52N 2 25W
Ribe, *Denmark* 17 J2 55 19N 8 44 E
Ribe Amtskommune □, *Denmark* 17 J2 55 35N 8 45 E
Ribeauvillé, *France* 27 D14 48 10N 7 20 E
Ribécourt-Dreslincourt, *France* 27 C9 49 30N 2 55 E
Ribeira = Santa Uxía, *Spain* 42 C2 42 36N 8 58W
Ribeira Brava, *Madeira* 9 c 32 41N 17 4W
Ribeira do Pombal, *Brazil* 170 D4 10 50 S 38 32W
Ribeira Grande, *Azores* 9 d3 37 49N 25 31W
Ribeira Grande, *C. Verde Is.* 9 j 17 0N 25 4W
Ribeirão, *Brazil* 170 C4 8 31 S 35 23W
Ribeirão Prêto, *Brazil* 175 A6 21 10 S 47 50W
Ribeiro Gonçalves, *Brazil* 170 C2 7 32 S 45 14W
Ribemont, *France* 27 C10 49 47N 3 27 E
Ribera, *Italy* 46 E6 37 30N 13 16 E
Ribérac, *France* 28 C4 45 15N 0 20 E
Riberalta, *Bolivia* 173 C4 11 0 S 66 0W
Ribes de Freser, *Spain* 40 C7 42 19N 2 15 E
Ribnica, *Slovenia* 45 C11 45 45N 14 45 E
Ribnitz-Damgarten, *Germany* 30 A8 54 15N 12 27 E
Ričany, *Czech Rep.* 34 B7 50 0N 14 40 E
Riccarton, *N.Z.* 131 D7 43 32 S 172 37 E
Ríccia, *Italy* 47 A7 41 30N 14 50 E
Riccione, *Italy* 45 E9 43 59N 12 39 E
Rice, *U.S.A.* 161 L12 34 5N 114 51W
Rice L., *Canada* 150 B6 44 12N 78 10W
Rice Lake, *U.S.A.* 154 C9 45 30N 91 44W
Riceboro, *U.S.A.* 152 D8 31 44N 81 26W
Rich, *Morocco* 110 B4 32 16N 4 30W
Rich, C., *Canada* 150 B4 44 43N 80 38W
Richard Toll, *Senegal* 112 B1 16 25N 15 42W
Richards Bay, *S. Africa* 117 D5 28 48 S 32 6 E
Richardson →, *Canada* 143 B6 58 25N 111 14W
Richardson Lakes, *U.S.A.* 148 C10 44 46N 70 58W
Richardson Mts., *N.Z.* 131 E3 44 49 S 168 34 E
Richardson Springs, *U.S.A.* 160 F5 39 51N 121 46W
Riche, C., *Australia* 125 F2 34 36 S 118 47 E
Richelieu, *France* 26 E7 47 1N 0 20 E
Richey, *U.S.A.* 154 B2 47 39N 105 4W
Richfield, *U.S.A.* 159 G8 38 46N 112 5W
Richfield Springs, *U.S.A.* 151 D10 42 51N 74 59W
Richford, *U.S.A.* 151 B12 45 0N 72 40W
Richibucto, *Canada* 141 C7 46 42N 64 54W
Richland, *Ga., U.S.A.* 152 C5 32 5N 84 40W
Richland, *Iowa, U.S.A.* 156 C5 41 13N 92 0W
Richland, *Mo., U.S.A.* 156 G4 37 51N 92 26W
Richland, *Wash., U.S.A.* 158 C4 46 17N 119 18W
Richland Center, *U.S.A.* 154 D9 43 21N 90 23W
Richlands, *U.S.A.* 148 G5 37 6N 81 48W
Richmond, *N.S.W., Australia* 129 B9 33 35 S 150 42 E
Richmond, *Queens., Australia* 126 C3 20 43 S 143 8 E
Richmond, *N.Z.* 131 B8 41 20 S 173 12 E
Richmond, *U.K.* 20 C6 54 25N 1 43W
Richmond, *Calif., U.S.A.* 160 H4 37 56N 122 21W
Richmond, *Ind., U.S.A.* 157 E12 39 50N 84 53W
Richmond, *Ky., U.S.A.* 157 G12 37 45N 84 18W
Richmond, *Mich., U.S.A.* 150 D2 42 49N 82 45W
Richmond, *Mo., U.S.A.* 156 E3 39 17N 93 58W
Richmond, *Tex., U.S.A.* 155 L7 29 35N 95 46W
Richmond, *Utah, U.S.A.* 158 F8 41 56N 111 48W
Richmond, *Va., U.S.A.* 148 G7 37 33N 77 27W
Richmond, *Vt., U.S.A.* 151 B12 44 24N 72 59W
Richmond, Mt., *N.Z.* 131 B8 41 32 S 173 22 E
Richmond Hill, *Canada* 150 C5 43 52N 79 27W
Richmond Hill, *U.S.A.* 152 D8 31 56N 81 18W
Richmond Ra., *Australia* 127 D5 29 0 S 152 45 E
Richmond Ra., *N.Z.* 131 B8 41 32 S 173 22 E
Richtersveld △, *S. Africa* 116 D2 28 15 S 17 10 E
Richterswil, *Switz.* 33 B7 47 13N 8 43 E
Richwood, *Ohio, U.S.A.* 157 D13 40 26N 83 18W
Richwood, *W. Va., U.S.A.* 148 F5 38 14N 80 32W
Ricla, *Spain* 40 D3 41 31N 1 24W
Ricupe, *Angola* 115 E4 14 37 S 21 25 E
Ridā', *Yemen* 98 D4 14 25N 44 50 E
Ridder = Leninogorsk, *Kazakhstan* 66 D9 50 20N 83 30 E
Riddes, *Switz.* 32 D4 46 11N 7 14 E
Riddlesburg, *U.S.A.* 150 F6 40 9N 78 15W
Ridge Farm, *U.S.A.* 157 E9 39 54N 87 39W
Ridge Spring, *U.S.A.* 152 B8 33 51N 81 40W
Ridgecrest, *U.S.A.* 161 K9 35 38N 117 40W
Ridgefield, *Conn., U.S.A.* 151 E11 41 17N 73 30W
Ridgefield, *Wash., U.S.A.* 160 E4 45 49N 122 45W
Ridgeland, *Miss., U.S.A.* 155 J9 32 26N 90 8W
Ridgeland, *S.C., U.S.A.* 152 C9 32 29N 80 59W
Ridgetown, *Canada* 140 D3 42 26N 81 52W
Ridgeville, *Ind., U.S.A.* 157 D11 40 18N 85 2W
Ridgeville, *S.C., U.S.A.* 152 B9 33 6N 80 19W
Ridgewood, *U.S.A.* 151 F10 40 59N 74 7W
Ridgway, *Ill., U.S.A.* 157 G8 37 48N 88 16W
Ridgway, *Pa., U.S.A.* 150 E6 41 25N 78 44W
Riding Mountain △, *Canada* 143 C9 50 50N 100 0W
Ridley, Mt., *Australia* 125 F3 33 12 S 122 7 E
Riebeek-Oos, *S. Africa* 116 E4 33 10 S 26 10 E
Ried, *Austria* 34 C6 48 14N 13 30 E
Riedlingen, *Germany* 31 G5 48 9N 9 28 E
Riedstadt, *Germany* 31 F4 49 45N 8 30 E
Riehen, *Switz.* 32 A5 47 37N 7 38 E
Rienza →, *Italy* 45 B8 46 49N 11 47 E
Riesa, *Germany* 30 D9 51 17N 13 17 E
Riesco, I., *Chile* 176 D2 52 55 S 72 40W
Riesenburg = Prabuty, *Poland* 54 E6 53 47N 19 15 E
Riesi, *Italy* 47 E7 37 17N 14 5 E
Riet →, *S. Africa* 116 D3 29 0 S 23 54 E
Rietavas, *Lithuania* 54 C8 55 44N 21 56 E
Rietbron, *S. Africa* 116 E3 32 54 S 23 10 E
Rietfontein, *Namibia* 116 C3 21 58 S 20 58 E
Rieti, *Italy* 45 F9 42 24N 12 51 E
Rieupeyroux, *France* 28 D6 44 19N 2 12 E
Riez, *France* 29 E10 43 49N 6 6 E
Rif = Er Rif, *Morocco* 111 A4 35 1N 4 1W
Riffe L., *U.S.A.* 160 D4 46 32N 122 26W
Rifle, *U.S.A.* 158 G10 39 32N 107 47W
Rift Valley, *Africa* 104 G7 7 0N 30 0 E
Rift Valley □, *Kenya* 118 B4 0 20N 36 0 E
Rig Rig, *Chad* 109 F2 14 13N 14 25 E
Riga, *India* 90 A5 28 26N 95 2 E
Rīga, *Latvia* 15 H21 56 53N 24 8 E
Rīga ✈ (RIX), *Latvia* 54 B10 56 54N 23 59 E
Riga, G. of, *Latvia* 15 H20 57 40N 23 45 E
Rigacikun, *Nigeria* 113 C6 10 40N 7 28 E
Rīgān, *Iran* 97 D8 28 37N 58 58 E
Rīgas Jūras Līcis = Riga, G. of, *Latvia* 15 H20 57 40N 23 45 E
Rigaud, *Canada* 151 A10 45 29N 74 18W
Rigby, *U.S.A.* 158 E8 43 40N 111 55W
Rīgestān, *Afghan.* 91 C2 30 15N 65 0 E
Riggins, *U.S.A.* 158 D5 45 25N 116 19W
Rignac, *France* 28 D6 44 25N 2 16 E
Rigolet, *Canada* 141 B8 54 10N 58 23W
Rihand Dam, *India* 93 G10 24 9N 83 2 E
Riihimäki, *Finland* 15 F21 60 45N 24 48 E
Riiser-Larsen-halvøya, *Antarctica* 7 C4 68 0 S 35 0 E
Rijau, *Nigeria* 113 C6 11 8N 5 17 E
Rijeka, *Croatia* 45 C11 45 20N 14 21 E
Rijeka Crnojevića, *Serbia & M.* 50 D3 42 24N 19 1 E
Rijssen, *Neths.* 24 B6 52 19N 6 31 E
Rika →, *Ukraine* 53 B8 48 11N 23 16 E
Rikā', W. ar →, *Si. Arabia* 98 B4 22 25N 44 50 E
Rike, *Ethiopia* 107 E4 10 50N 39 53 E
Rikuchū-Kaigan △, *Japan* 70 E11 39 20N 142 0 E
Rikuzentakada, *Japan* 70 E10 39 0N 141 40 E
Rila, *Bulgaria* 50 D7 42 7N 23 7 E
Rila Planina, *Bulgaria* 50 D7 42 10N 23 20 E
Riley, *U.S.A.* 158 E4 43 32N 119 28W
Rima →, *Nigeria* 113 C6 13 4N 5 10 E
Rimah, Wadi ar →, *Si. Arabia* 96 E4 26 5N 41 30 E
Rimau, Pulau, *Malaysia* 87 c 5 15N 100 16 E
Rimavská Sobota, *Slovak Rep.* 35 C13 48 22N 20 2 E
Rimbey, *Canada* 142 C6 52 35N 114 15W
Rimbo, *Sweden* 16 E12 59 44N 18 21 E
Rimersburg, *U.S.A.* 150 E5 41 3N 79 30W
Rimforsa, *Sweden* 17 F9 58 6N 15 43 E
Rimi, *Nigeria* 113 C6 12 58N 7 43 E
Rímini, *Italy* 45 D9 44 3N 12 33 E
Rimouski, *Canada* 141 C6 48 27N 68 30W
Rimrock, *U.S.A.* 160 D5 46 38N 121 10W
Rinca, *Indonesia* 82 C1 8 45 S 119 35 E
Rincon, *U.S.A.* 152 C8 32 18N 81 14W
Rincón de la Victoria, *Spain* 43 J6 36 43N 4 18W
Rincón de Romos, *Mexico* 162 C4 22 14N 102 18W
Rinconada, *Argentina* 174 A2 22 26 S 66 10W
Rind →, *India* 93 G9 25 53N 80 33 E
Rindal, *Norway* 18 A6 63 3N 9 13 E
Ringarum, *Sweden* 17 F10 58 21N 16 26 E
Ringas, *India* 92 F6 27 21N 75 34 E
Ringdove, *Vanuatu* 133 F6 16 40 S 168 10 E
Ringe, *Denmark* 17 J4 55 13N 10 28 E
Ringebu, *Norway* 18 C7 61 32N 10 7 E
Ringgi, *Solomon Is.* 133 M9 8 5 S 157 10 E
Ringgold Is., *Fiji* 133 A3 16 15 S 179 25W
Ringim, *Nigeria* 113 C6 12 13N 9 10 E
Ringkøbing, *Denmark* 17 H2 56 5N 8 15 E
Ringkøbing Amtskommune □, *Denmark* 17 H2 56 10N 8 45 E
Ringkøbing Fjord, *Denmark* 17 H2 56 0N 8 15 E
Ringoma, *Angola* 115 E3 12 25 S 17 32 E
Ringsaker, *Norway* 18 D7 60 54N 10 45 E
Ringsjön, *Sweden* 17 J7 55 55N 13 30 E
Ringsted, *Denmark* 17 J5 55 25N 11 46 E
Ringvassøy, *Norway* 14 B18 69 56N 19 15 E
Ringwood, *U.S.A.* 151 E10 41 7N 74 15W
Rinía, *Greece* 49 D7 37 23N 25 13 E
Rinjani, *Indonesia* 85 D5 8 24 S 116 28 E
Rinteln, *Germany* 30 C5 52 10N 9 8 E
Río, Punta del, *Spain* 41 J2 36 49N 2 24W
Rio Bonito = Caiapônia, *Brazil* 173 D7 16 57 S 51 49W
Rio Branco = Arcoverde, *Brazil* 170 C4 8 25 S 37 4W
Rio Branco = Paratinga, *Brazil* 171 D3 12 40 S 43 10W
Rio Branco = Roraima □, *Brazil* 169 C5 2 0N 61 30W
Rio Branco, *Brazil* 172 B4 9 58 S 67 49W
Río Branco, *Uruguay* 175 C5 32 40 S 53 40W
Río Bravo ⌓, *N. Amer.* 162 B4 29 2N 102 45W
Río Bravo del Norte →, *Mexico* 163 B5 25 57N 97 9W
Rio Brilhante, *Brazil* 175 A5 21 48 S 54 33W
Río Bueno, *Chile* 176 B2 40 19 S 72 58W
Río Caribe, *Venezuela* 169 A5 10 42N 63 7W
Río Chico, *Venezuela* 168 A4 10 19N 65 59W
Rio Claro, *Brazil* 175 A6 22 19 S 47 35W
Rio Claro, *Trin. & Tob.* 169 F9 10 20N 61 25W
Río Colorado, *Argentina* 176 A4 39 0 S 64 0W
Río Cuarto, *Argentina* 174 C3 33 10 S 64 25W
Rio das Pedras, *Mozam.* 117 C6 23 8 S 35 28 E
Rio de Contas, *Brazil* 171 D3 13 36 S 41 48W
Rio de Janeiro, *Brazil* 171 F3 23 0 S 43 12W
Rio de Janeiro □, *Brazil* 171 F3 22 50 S 43 0W
Río de Oro, B. de, *W. Sahara* 110 D1 23 45N 15 50W
Rio do Prado, *Brazil* 171 E3 16 35 S 40 34W
Rio do Sul, *Brazil* 175 B6 27 13 S 49 37W
Río Dulce △, *Guatemala* 164 C2 15 43N 88 50W
Río Gallegos, *Argentina* 176 D3 51 35 S 69 15W
Río Grande, *Argentina* 176 D3 53 50 S 67 45W
Río Grande, *Bolivia* 172 E4 20 51 S 67 17W
Rio Grande, *Brazil* 175 C5 32 0 S 52 20W
Río Grande, *Mexico* 162 C4 23 50N 103 2W
Río Grande, *Nic.* 164 D3 12 54N 83 33W
Rio Grande, *Puerto Rico* 165 d 18 23N 65 50W
Rio Grande, *U.S.A.* 155 N6 25 58N 97 9W
Rio Grande City, *U.S.A.* 155 M5 26 23N 98 49W
Río Grande de Santiago →, *Mexico* 162 C3 21 36N 105 26W
Rio Grande do Norte □, *Brazil* 170 C4 5 40 S 36 0W
Rio Grande do Sul □, *Brazil* 175 C5 30 0 S 53 0W
Rio Grande Rise, *Atl. Oc.* 8 K8 31 0 S 35 0W
Río Hato, *Panama* 164 E3 8 22N 80 10W
Río Lagartos, *Mexico* 163 C7 21 36N 88 10W
Rio Largo, *Brazil* 170 C4 9 28 S 35 50W
Rio Maior, *Portugal* 43 F2 39 19N 8 57W
Rio Marina, *Italy* 44 F7 42 49N 10 25 E
Río Mayo, *Argentina* 176 C2 45 40 S 70 15W
Río Mulatos, *Bolivia* 172 D4 19 40 S 66 50W
Río Muni □, *Eq. Guin.* 114 B2 1 30N 10 0 E
Rio Negro, *Brazil* 175 B6 26 0 S 49 55W
Río Negro, *Chile* 176 B2 40 47 S 73 14W
Rio Negro, Pantanal do, *Brazil* 173 D6 19 0 S 56 0W
Rio Novo = Ipiaú, *Brazil* 171 D4 14 8 S 39 44W
Rio Pardo = Ribas do Rio Pardo, *Brazil* 173 E7 20 27 S 53 46W
Rio Pardo, *Brazil* 175 C5 30 0 S 52 30W
Río Pico, *Argentina* 176 B2 44 0 S 70 22W
Río Pilcomayo △, *Argentina* 174 B4 25 5 S 58 5W
Río Platano ⌓, *Honduras* 164 C3 15 45N 85 0W
Rio Prêto = Ibipetuba, *Brazil* 170 D3 11 0 S 44 32W
Rio Preto da Eva, *Brazil* 169 D6 2 46 S 59 41W
Rio Rancho, *U.S.A.* 159 J10 35 14N 106 38W
Rio Real, *Brazil* 171 D4 11 28 S 37 56W
Río Seco = Villa de María, *Argentina* 174 B3 29 55 S 63 43W
Río Segundo, *Argentina* 174 C3 31 40 S 63 59W
Río Simpson △, *Chile* 176 C2 45 27 S 73 30W
Río Tercero, *Argentina* 174 C3 32 15 S 64 8W
Rio Tinto, *Brazil* 170 C4 6 48 S 35 5W
Rio Tinto, *Portugal* 42 D2 41 11N 8 34W
Río Turbio, *Argentina* 176 D2 51 32 S 72 18W
Rio Verde, *Brazil* 171 E1 17 50 S 51 0W
Río Verde, *Mexico* 163 C5 21 56N 99 59W
Rio Verde de Mato Grosso, *Brazil* 173 D7 18 56 S 54 52W
Río Viejo △, *Venezuela* 168 B3 7 15N 71 20W
Rio Vista, *U.S.A.* 160 G5 38 10N 121 42W
Ríobamba, *Ecuador* 168 D2 1 50 S 78 45W
Ríohacha, *Colombia* 168 A3 11 33N 72 55W
Rioja, *Peru* 172 B2 6 11 S 77 5W
Riom, *France* 28 C7 45 54N 3 7 E
Riom-ès-Montagnes, *France* 28 C6 45 17N 2 39 E
Rion-des-Landes, *France* 28 E3 43 55N 0 56W
Rionegro, *Antioquía, Colombia* 168 B2 6 9N 75 22W
Rionegro, *Santander, Colombia* 168 B3 7 15N 73 9W
Rionero in Vúlture, *Italy* 47 B8 40 55N 15 40 E
Rioni →, *Georgia* 61 J5 42 14N 41 44 E
Riós, *Spain* 42 D3 41 58N 7 16W
Riosinho →, *Brazil* 173 B7 7 7 S 51 39W
Ríosucio, *Caldas, Colombia* 168 B2 5 30N 75 40W
Ríosucio, *Choco, Colombia* 168 B2 7 27N 77 7W
Riou L., *Canada* 143 B7 59 7N 106 25W
Rioz, *France* 27 E13 47 26N 6 5 E
Riozinho →, *Brazil* 168 D4 2 55 S 67 7W
Ripatransone, *Italy* 45 F10 42 59N 13 46 E
Ripley, *Canada* 150 B3 44 4N 81 35W
Ripley, *Calif., U.S.A.* 161 M12 33 32N 114 39W
Ripley, *N.Y., U.S.A.* 150 D5 42 16N 79 43W
Ripley, *Ohio, U.S.A.* 157 F13 38 45N 83 51W
Ripley, *Tenn., U.S.A.* 155 H10 35 45N 89 32W
Ripley, *W. Va., U.S.A.* 148 F5 38 49N 81 43W
Ripoll, *Spain* 40 C7 42 15N 2 13 E
Ripon, *U.K.* 20 C6 54 9N 1 31W
Ripon, *Calif., U.S.A.* 160 H5 37 44N 121 7W
Ripon, *Wis., U.S.A.* 148 D1 43 51N 88 50W
Riposto, *Italy* 47 E8 37 44N 15 12 E
Rippin = Rypin, *Poland* 55 E6 53 3N 19 25 E
Risan, *Serbia & M.* 50 D2 42 32N 18 42 E
Risaralda □, *Colombia* 168 B2 5 0N 76 10W
Riscle, *France* 28 E3 43 39N 0 5W
Rishā', W. ar →, *Si. Arabia* 96 E5 25 33N 44 5 E
Rishiri-Rebun-Sarobetsu △, *Japan* 70 B10 45 26N 141 30 E
Rishiri-Tō, *Japan* 70 B10 45 11N 141 15 E
Rishon le Ẕiyyon, *Israel* 103 D3 31 58N 34 48 E
Rishtan, *Uzbekistan* 65 C5 40 20N 71 15 E
Rising Sun, *U.S.A.* 157 F12 38 57N 84 51W
Risle →, *France* 26 C7 49 26N 0 23 E
Risnjak △, *Croatia* 45 C11 45 25N 14 36 E
Rison, *U.S.A.* 155 J8 33 58N 92 11W
Risør, *Norway* 18 F6 58 43N 9 13 E
Rissani, *Morocco* 110 B4 31 18N 4 12W
Rita Blanca Cr. →, *U.S.A.* 155 H3 35 40N 102 29W
Ritchie's Arch., *India* 95 H11 12 14N 93 10 E
Riti, *Nigeria* 113 D6 7 57N 9 41 E
Ritidian Pt., *Guam* 133 R15 13 39N 144 51 E
Ritter, Mt., *U.S.A.* 160 H7 37 41N 119 12W
Rittman, *U.S.A.* 150 F3 40 58N 81 47W
Ritzville, *U.S.A.* 158 C4 47 8N 118 23W
Riu, *India* 90 A5 28 19N 95 3 E
Riva del Garda, *Italy* 44 C7 45 53N 10 50 E
Riva Lígure, *Italy* 44 E4 43 50N 7 50 E
Rivadavia, *Buenos Aires, Argentina* 174 D3 35 29 S 62 59W
Rivadavia, *Mendoza, Argentina* 174 C2 33 13 S 68 30W
Rivadavia, *Salta, Argentina* 174 A3 24 5 S 62 54W
Rivadavia, *Chile* 174 B1 29 57 S 70 35W
Rivarolo Canavese, *Italy* 44 C4 45 19N 7 43 E
Rivas, *Nic.* 164 D2 11 30N 85 50W
Rive-de-Gier, *France* 29 C8 45 32N 4 37 E
River Cess, *Liberia* 112 D3 5 30N 9 32W
River Jordan, *Canada* 160 B2 48 26N 124 3W
Rivera, *Argentina* 174 D3 37 12 S 63 14W
Rivera, *Uruguay* 175 C4 31 0 S 55 50W
Riverbank, *U.S.A.* 160 H6 37 44N 120 56W
Riverdale, *Calif., U.S.A.* 160 J7 36 26N 119 52W
Riverdale, *Ga., U.S.A.* 152 B5 33 34N 84 25W
Riverhead, *U.S.A.* 151 F12 40 55N 72 40W
Riverhurst, *Canada* 143 C7 50 55N 106 50W
Rivers, *Canada* 143 C8 50 2N 100 14W
Rivers □, *Nigeria* 113 E6 4 30N 7 10 E
Rivers Inlet, *Canada* 142 C3 51 42N 127 15W
Riversdale, *N.Z.* 131 F3 45 54 S 168 44 E
Riversdale, *S. Africa* 116 E3 34 7 S 21 15 E
Riverside, *U.S.A.* 161 M9 33 59N 117 22W
Riverton, *Australia* 128 C3 34 10 S 138 46 E
Riverton, *Canada* 143 C9 51 1N 97 0W
Riverton, *N.Z.* 131 G2 46 21 S 168 0 E
Riverton, *Ill., U.S.A.* 156 E7 39 51N 89 33W
Riverton, *Wyo., U.S.A.* 158 E9 43 2N 108 23W
Riverton Heights, *U.S.A.* 160 C4 47 28N 122 17W
Riverview, *Fla., U.S.A.* 153 H7 27 52N 82 20W
Riverview, *Fla., U.S.A.* 153 E2 30 32N 87 12W
Rives, *France* 29 C9 45 21N 5 31 E
Rivesaltes, *France* 28 F6 42 47N 2 50 E
Riviera, *U.S.A.* 161 K12 35 4N 114 35W
Riviera Beach, *U.S.A.* 153 J9 26 47N 80 3W
Riviera di Levante, *Italy* 44 D6 44 15N 9 30 E
Riviera di Ponente, *Italy* 44 D5 44 10N 8 20 E
Rivière-au-Renard, *Canada* 141 C7 48 59N 64 23W
Rivière Bleue ⌓, *N. Cal.* 133 V20 22 6 S 166 38 E
Rivière-du-Loup, *Canada* 141 C6 47 50N 69 30W
Rivière-Pentecôte, *Canada* 141 C6 49 57N 67 1W
Rivière-Pilote, *Martinique* 164 c 14 26N 60 53W
Rivière St-Paul, *Canada* 141 B8 51 28N 57 45W
Rivière-Salée, *Martinique* 164 c 14 31N 61 0W
Rivne, *Ukraine* 53 D14 46 1N 29 10 E
Rivne, *Ukraine* 59 G4 50 40N 26 10 E
Rívoli, *Italy* 44 C4 45 3N 7 31 E
Rivoli B., *Australia* 128 D4 37 32 S 140 3 E
Riwaka, *N.Z.* 131 B7 41 5 S 172 59 E
Rixheim, *France* 27 E14 47 40N 7 24 E
Riyadh = Ar Riyāḍ, *Si. Arabia* 96 E5 24 41N 46 42 E
Rizal, *Cagayan, Phil.* 80 C3 17 51N 121 21 E
Rizal, *Nueva Ecija, Phil.* 80 D3 15 43N 121 6 E
Rizal, *Zamboanga del N., Phil.* 81 G4 8 35N 123 26 E
Rize, *Turkey* 101 B9 41 0N 40 30 E
Rizhao, *China* 75 G10 35 25N 119 30 E
Rizokarpaso, *Cyprus* 39 E10 35 36N 34 23 E
Rizzuto, C., *Italy* 47 D10 38 53N 17 5 E
Rjukan, *Norway* 18 E5 59 54N 8 33 E
Rjuven, *Norway* 18 E4 59 9N 7 8 E
Ro, *Greece* 49 E11 36 9N 29 33 E
Rô, *N. Cal.* 133 U21 21 22 S 167 50 E
Roa, *Dem. Rep. of the Congo* 114 B4 3 49N 24 56 E
Roa, *Norway* 18 D7 60 17N 10 37 E
Roa, *Spain* 42 D7 41 41N 3 56W
Roachdale, *U.S.A.* 157 E10 39 51N 86 48W
Road Town, *Br. Virgin Is.* 165 e 18 27N 64 37W
Roan Plateau, *U.S.A.* 158 G9 39 20N 109 20W
Roanne, *France* 27 F11 46 3N 4 4 E
Roanoke, *Ala., U.S.A.* 152 B4 33 9N 85 22W
Roanoke, *Ind., U.S.A.* 157 D11 40 58N 85 22W
Roanoke, *Va., U.S.A.* 148 G6 37 16N 79 56W
Roanoke →, *U.S.A.* 149 H7 35 57N 76 42W
Roanoke I., *U.S.A.* 149 H8 35 55N 75 40W
Roanoke Rapids, *U.S.A.* 149 G7 36 28N 77 40W
Roatán, *Honduras* 164 C2 16 18N 86 35W
Rob Roy, *Solomon Is.* 133 L9 7 23 S 157 36 E
Robāt Sang, *Iran* 97 C8 35 35N 59 10 E
Robāṭkarīm, *Iran* 97 C6 35 25N 50 59 E
Robāṭkarīm □, *Iran* 97 B6 35 26N 50 59 E
Robbins I., *Australia* 127 G4 40 42 S 145 0 E
Róbbio, *Italy* 44 C5 45 17N 8 35 E
Robe, *Australia* 128 D3 37 11 S 139 45 E
Robe →, *Australia* 124 D2 21 42 S 116 15 E
Röbel, *Germany* 30 B8 53 22N 12 35 E
Robert Lee, *U.S.A.* 155 K4 31 54N 100 29W
Roberta, *U.S.A.* 152 C5 32 43N 84 1W
Roberts, *U.S.A.* 157 D8 40 37N 88 11W
Robertsdale, *U.S.A.* 150 F6 40 11N 78 6W
Robertsganj, *India* 93 G10 24 44N 83 4 E
Robertson, *S. Africa* 116 E2 33 46 S 19 50 E
Robertson I., *Antarctica* 7 C18 65 15 S 59 30W
Robertson Ra., *Australia* 124 D3 23 15 S 121 0 E
Robertsport, *Liberia* 112 D2 6 45N 11 26W
Robertstown, *Australia* 128 B3 33 58 S 139 5 E
Roberval, *Canada* 141 C5 48 32N 72 15W
Robeson Chan., *N. Amer.* 10 A4 82 0N 61 30W
Robesonia, *U.S.A.* 151 F8 40 21N 76 8W
Robi, *Ethiopia* 107 F4 7 52N 39 38 E
Robinson, *U.S.A.* 157 F9 39 0N 87 44W
Robinson →, *Australia* 126 B2 16 3 S 137 16 E
Robinson Ra., *Australia* 125 E2 25 40 S 119 0 E
Robinvale, *Australia* 128 C5 34 40 S 142 45 E
Robledo, *Spain* 41 G2 38 46N 2 26W
Roblin, *Canada* 143 C8 51 14N 101 21W
Roboré, *Bolivia* 173 D6 18 10 S 59 45W
Robson, *Canada* 142 D5 49 20N 117 41W
Robson, Mt., *Canada* 142 C5 53 10N 119 10W
Robstown, *U.S.A.* 155 M6 27 47N 97 40W
Roca, C. da, *Portugal* 43 G1 38 40N 9 31W
Roca Partida, I., *Mexico* 162 D2 19 1N 112 2W
Rocamadour, *France* 28 D5 44 48N 1 37 E
Rocca San Casciano, *Italy* 45 D8 44 3N 11 50 E
Roccadáspide, *Italy* 47 B8 40 27N 15 10 E
Roccastrada, *Italy* 45 F8 43 0N 11 10 E
Roccella Iónica, *Italy* 47 D9 38 19N 16 24 E
Rocha, *Uruguay* 175 C5 34 30 S 54 25W
Rochdale, *U.K.* 20 D5 53 38N 2 9W
Rochechouart, *France* 28 C4 45 50N 0 49 E
Rochedo, *Brazil* 173 D7 19 57 S 54 52W
Rochefort, *Belgium* 24 D5 50 9N 5 12 E
Rochefort, *France* 28 C3 45 56N 0 57W
Rochefort-en-Terre, *France* 26 E4 47 42N 2 22W
Rochelle, *Ga., U.S.A.* 152 D6 31 57N 83 27W
Rochelle, *Ill., U.S.A.* 156 C7 41 56N 89 4W
Rocher River, *Canada* 142 A6 61 23N 112 44W
Rocheservière, *France* 26 F5 46 57N 1 30W
Rochester, *Australia* 128 D6 36 22 S 144 41 E
Rochester, *U.K.* 21 F8 51 23N 0 31 E
Rochester, *Ind., U.S.A.* 157 C10 41 4N 86 13W
Rochester, *Minn., U.S.A.* 154 C8 44 1N 92 28W
Rochester, *N.H., U.S.A.* 151 C14 43 18N 70 59W
Rochester, *N.Y., U.S.A.* 150 C7 43 10N 77 37W
Rochester Hills, *U.S.A.* 157 B13 42 41N 83 8W
Rociu, *Romania* 53 F10 44 43N 25 2 E
Rock →, *Canada* 142 A3 60 7N 127 7W
Rock →, *U.S.A.* 156 C6 41 29N 90 37W
Rock Creek, *U.S.A.* 150 E4 41 40N 80 52W
Rock Falls, *U.S.A.* 156 C7 41 47N 89 41W
Rock Flat, *Australia* 129 D8 36 21 S 149 13 E
Rock Hill, *U.S.A.* 149 H5 34 56N 81 1W
Rock Island, *U.S.A.* 156 C6 41 30N 90 34W
Rock Port, *U.S.A.* 154 E7 40 25N 95 31W
Rock Rapids, *U.S.A.* 154 D6 43 26N 96 10W
Rock Sound, *Bahamas* 164 B4 24 54N 76 12W
Rock Springs, *Mont., U.S.A.* 158 C10 46 49N 106 15W
Rock Springs, *Wyo., U.S.A.* 158 F9 41 35N 109 14W
Rock Valley, *U.S.A.* 154 D6 43 12N 96 18W
Rockall, *Atl. Oc.* 8 A10 57 37N 13 42W
Rockdale, *Tex., U.S.A.* 155 K6 30 39N 97 0W
Rockdale, *Wash., U.S.A.* 160 C5 47 22N 121 28W
Rockeby = Mungkan Kandju △, *Australia* 126 A3 13 35 S 142 52 E
Rockefeller Plateau, *Antarctica* 7 E14 80 0 S 140 0W
Rockford, *Ala., U.S.A.* 152 C3 32 53N 86 13W
Rockford, *Ill., U.S.A.* 156 B7 42 16N 89 6W
Rockford, *Iowa, U.S.A.* 156 A4 43 3N 92 57W
Rockford, *Mich., U.S.A.* 157 A11 43 7N 85 34W
Rockford, *Ohio, U.S.A.* 157 D12 40 41N 84 39W
Rockglen, *Canada* 143 D7 49 11N 105 57W
Rockhampton, *Australia* 126 C5 23 22 S 150 32 E
Rockingham, *Australia* 125 F2 32 15 S 115 38 E
Rockingham, *U.S.A.* 149 H6 34 57N 79 46W
Rockingham B., *Australia* 126 B4 18 5 S 146 10 E
Rocklake, *U.S.A.* 154 A5 48 47N 99 15W
Rockland, *Canada* 151 A9 45 33N 75 17W
Rockland, *Idaho, U.S.A.* 158 E7 42 34N 112 53W
Rockland, *Maine, U.S.A.* 149 C11 44 6N 69 7W
Rockland, *Mich., U.S.A.* 154 B10 46 44N 89 11W
Rocklands Reservoir, *Australia* 128 D5 37 15 S 142 5 E
Rockledge, *U.S.A.* 153 G9 28 20N 80 43W
Rocklin, *U.S.A.* 160 G5 38 48N 121 14W
Rockly B., *Trin. & Tob.* 169 E10 11 9N 60 46W
Rockmart, *U.S.A.* 149 H3 34 0N 85 3W
Rockport, *Ind., U.S.A.* 157 G9 37 53N 87 3W
Rockport, *Mass., U.S.A.* 151 D14 42 39N 70 37W
Rockport, *Tex., U.S.A.* 155 L6 28 2N 97 3W
Rocksprings, *U.S.A.* 155 K4 30 1N 100 13W
Rockstone, *Guyana* 169 B6 5 59N 58 33W
Rockville, *Conn., U.S.A.* 151 E12 41 52N 72 28W
Rockville, *Ind., U.S.A.* 157 E9 39 46N 87 14W
Rockville, *Md., U.S.A.* 148 F7 39 5N 77 9W
Rockwall, *U.S.A.* 155 J6 32 56N 96 28W
Rockwell City, *U.S.A.* 156 B2 42 24N 94 38W
Rockwood, *Canada* 150 C4 43 37N 80 8W
Rockwood, *Maine, U.S.A.* 149 C11 45 41N 69 45W
Rockwood, *Tenn., U.S.A.* 149 H3 35 52N 84 41W
Rocky Ford, *U.S.A.* 154 F3 38 3N 103 43W
Rocky Fork Lake, *U.S.A.* 157 E13 39 12N 83 23W
Rocky Gully, *Australia* 125 F2 34 30 S 116 57 E
Rocky Harbour, *Canada* 141 C8 49 36N 57 55W
Rocky Island L., *Canada* 140 C3 46 55N 83 0W
Rocky Lane, *Canada* 142 B5 58 31N 116 22W
Rocky Mount, *U.S.A.* 149 H7 35 57N 77 48W
Rocky Mountain △, *U.S.A.* 158 F11 40 25N 105 45W
Rocky Mountain House, *Canada* 142 C6 52 22N 114 55W
Rocky Mts., *N. Amer.* 158 G10 49 0N 115 0W
Rocky Point, *Namibia* 116 B2 19 3 S 12 30 E

Rocroi, France .... 27 C11 49 55N 4 30 E
Rod, Pakistan .... 91 C1 28 10N 63 5 E
Roda = Stadtroda,
  Germany .... 30 E7 50 52N 11 44 E
Rødberg, Norway .... 18 D5 60 17N 8 56 E
Rødby, Denmark .... 17 K5 54 41N 11 23 E
Rødbyhavn, Denmark 17 K5 54 39N 11 22 E
Roddickton, Canada .. 141 B8 50 51N 56 8W
Rødding, Denmark .. 17 J3 55 23N 9 3 E
Rödeby, Sweden .... 17 H9 56 15N 15 37 E
Rødekro, Denmark .. 17 J3 55 4N 9 20 E
Rodenkirchen,
  Germany .... 30 B4 53 23N 8 26 E
Rodez, France ...... 28 D6 44 21N 2 33 E
Rodholívos, Greece .. 50 F7 40 55N 24 0 E
Rodhópi □, Greece .. 51 E8 41 5N 25 30 E
Rodhopoú □, Greece .. 39 E4 35 34N 23 45 E
Ródhos, Greece ...... 38 E12 36 15N 28 10 E
Ródhos ✈ (RHO),
  Greece .... 49 E10 36 23N 28 12 E
Rodi Gargánico, Italy .. 45 G12 41 55N 15 53 E
Rodna, Romania ...... 53 C9 47 35N 24 35 E
Rodnei, Munţii,
  Romania .... 53 C9 47 35N 24 35 E
Rodney, Canada 150 D3 42 34N 81 41W
Rodney, C., N.Z. .... 130 C3 36 17S 174 50 E
Rodniki, Russia .... 60 B5 57 7N 41 47 E
Rodonit, Kepi i,
  Albania .... 50 E3 41 35N 19 27 E
Rodriguez, Ind. Oc. .. 121 F5 19 45S 63 20 E
Roe ➤, Canada 23 A5 55 6N 6 59W
Roebling, U.S.A. 151 F10 40 7N 74 47W
Roebourne, Australia 124 D2 20 44S 117 9 E
Roebuck B., Australia 124 C3 18 5S 122 20 E
Roermond, Neths. .... 24 C6 51 12N 6 0 E
Roes Welcome Sd.,
  Canada 139 B11 65 0N 87 0W
Roeselare, Belgium .. 24 D3 50 57N 3 7 E
Rogachev = Ragachow,
  Belarus .... 59 F6 53 8N 30 5 E
Rogačica, Serbia & M. .. 50 B4 44 4N 19 40 E
Rogagua, L., Bolivia .. 172 C4 13 43S 66 50W
Rogaland □, Norway .. 18 E3 59 12N 6 20 E
Rogaška Slatina,
  Slovenia .... 45 B12 46 15N 15 42 E
Rogatec, Slovenia .. 45 B12 46 15N 15 46 E
Rogatica, Bos.-H. .... 52 G4 43 47N 19 0 E
Rogatyn, Ukraine .... 59 H3 49 24N 24 36 E
Rogdhia, Greece .... 39 E6 35 22N 25 1 E
Rogers, U.S.A. 155 G7 36 20N 94 7W
Rogers City, U.S.A. .. 148 C4 45 25N 83 49W
Rogersville, Canada .. 141 C6 46 44N 65 26W
Roggan ➤, Canada .. 140 B4 54 24N 79 25W
Roggan L., Canada .. 140 B4 54 8N 77 50W
Roggeveldberge,
  S. Africa .... 116 E3 32 10S 20 10 E
Roggiano Gravina, Italy 47 C9 39 37N 16 9 E
Rogliano, France .... 29 F13 42 57N 9 30 E
Rogliano, Italy ...... 47 C9 39 10N 16 19 E
Rogoaguado, L.,
  Bolivia 173 C4 13 0S 65 30W
Rogojampi, Indonesia 79 J17 8 19S 114 17 E
Rogoźno, Poland .... 55 F3 52 45N 16 59 E
Rogue ➤, U.S.A. 158 E1 42 26N 124 26W
Roha, India .... 94 E1 18 26N 73 7 E
Rohan, France 26 D4 48 4N 2 45W
Röhda, Greece ...... 38 B9 39 48N 19 46 E
Rohnert Park, U.S.A. 160 G4 38 16N 122 40W
Rohri, Pakistan .... 91 D3 27 45N 68 51 E
Rohri Canal, Pakistan 92 F3 26 15N 68 27 E
Rohtak, India ...... 92 E7 28 55N 76 43 E
Rohtisch-Sauerbrunn =
  Rogaška Slatina,
  Slovenia .... 45 B12 46 15N 15 42 E
Roi Et, Thailand .... 86 D4 16 4N 103 40 E
Roja, Latvia .... 15 H20 57 29N 22 43 E
Rojas, Argentina 174 C3 34 10S 60 45W
Rojişte, Romania .... 53 F8 44 4N 23 56 E
Rojo, C., Mexico 163 C5 21 33N 97 20W
Rokan ➤, Indonesia .. 84 B2 2 0N 100 50 E
Rokel ➤, S. Leone .. 112 D2 8 30N 12 48W
Rokiškis, Lithuania .. 15 J21 55 55N 25 35 E
Rokitno, Russia .... 34 B6 49 43N 13 35 E
Rokycany, Czech Rep. 34 B6 49 43N 13 35 E
Rolândia, Brazil 175 A5 23 5S 51 23W
Røldal, Norway .... 18 E3 59 47N 6 50 E
Rolfe, U.S.A. 156 B2 42 49N 94 31W
Rolla, Mo., U.S.A. .. 155 G9 37 57N 91 46W
Rolla, N. Dak., U.S.A. 154 A5 48 52N 99 37W
Rolle, Switz. .... 32 D2 46 28N 6 20 E
Rolleston, Australia .. 126 C4 24 28S 148 35 E
Rolleston, N.Z. .... 131 D7 43 35S 172 24 E
Rolling Fork ➤, U.S.A. 157 G11 33 55N 90 50W
Rollingstone, Australia 126 B4 19 2S 146 24 E
Rom, Norway ...... 18 F4 58 8N 7 1 E
Rom, Sudan .... 107 F3 9 54N 32 16 E
Roma, Australia .... 127 D4 26 32S 148 49 E
Roma, Italy .... 45 G9 41 54N 12 29 E
Roma, Sweden ...... 17 G12 57 32N 18 26 E
Roma ➤, Norway 155 M5 26 35N 99 1W
Roma Fiumicino ✈
  (FCO), Italy ...... 45 G9 41 48N 12 15 E
Romain C., U.S.A. .. 149 J6 33 0N 79 22W
Romaine, Canada 141 B7 50 13N 60 40W
Romaine ➤, Canada 141 B7 50 18N 63 47W
Roman, Bulgaria .... 50 C7 43 8N 23 57 E
Roman, Romania .... 53 D11 46 57N 26 55 E
Roman-Kosh, Gora,
  Ukraine .... 59 K8 44 37N 34 15 E
Romanche ➤, France 29 C9 45 5N 5 43 E
Romang, Indonesia .. 83 C3 7 30S 127 20 E
Români, Egypt ...... 103 E1 30 59N 32 38 E
Romania ■, Europe .. 53 D10 46 0N 25 0 E
Romano, Bos.-H. .... 52 G3 43 50N 18 45 E
Romano, C., U.S.A. .. 153 K8 25 51N 81 41W
Romano, Cayo, Cuba 164 B4 22 0N 77 30W
Romanov-
  Borisoglebsk =
  Tutayev, Russia .. 58 D10 57 53N 39 32 E
Romanovka =
  Basarabeasca,
  Moldova .... 53 D13 46 21N 28 58 E
Romanovo-
  Murmane =
  Murmansk, Russia .. 56 A5 68 57N 33 10 E
Romanovsk =
  Kropotkin, Russia .. 61 H5 45 28N 40 28 E
Romanovskiy Khutor =
  Kropotkin, Russia .. 61 H5 45 28N 40 28 E
Romans-sur-Isère,
  France .... 29 C9 45 3N 5 3 E
Romanshorn, Switz. .. 33 A8 47 33N 9 22 E
Romanzof C., U.S.A. 144 F6 61 49N 166 6W
Rombari, Sudan .... 107 G3 4 33N 31 2 E
Rombebai, Danau,
  Indonesia .... 83 B5 1 50S 137 53 E
Romblon, Phil. ...... 80 E4 12 33N 122 17 E
Romblon □, Phil. .... 80 E4 12 33N 122 15 E
Romblon Pass, Phil. .. 80 E4 12 27N 122 12 E
Rome = Roma, Italy .. 45 G9 41 54N 12 29 E
Rome, Ga., U.S.A. .. 149 H3 34 15N 85 10W
Rome, N.Y., U.S.A. .. 151 C9 43 13N 75 27W
Rome, Pa., U.S.A. .. 151 E8 41 51N 76 21W
Romeoville, U.S.A. .. 157 C8 41 39N 88 3W

Rometta, Italy ...... 47 D8 38 10N 15 25 E
Romilly-sur-Seine,
  France .... 27 D10 48 31N 3 44 E
Romitan, Uzbekistan .. 65 D2 39 56N 64 23 E
Rommani, Morocco .. 110 B3 33 31N 6 40W
Romney, U.S.A. 148 F6 39 21N 78 45W
Romney Marsh, U.K. 21 F8 51 2N 0 54 E
Romny, Ukraine .... 59 G7 50 48N 33 28 E
Rømø, Denmark .... 17 J2 55 10N 8 30 E
Romodan, Ukraine .. 59 G7 49 55N 33 15 E
Romodanovo, Russia 60 C7 54 26N 45 23 E
Romont, Switz. ...... 32 C3 46 42N 6 54 E
Romorantin-
  Lanthenay, France .. 27 E8 47 21N 1 45 E
Rompin ➤, Malaysia 84 B2 2 49N 103 29 E
Romsdalen, Norway .. 18 B4 62 25N 7 52 E
Romsdalsfjorden,
  Norway .... 18 B4 62 38N 7 20 E
Romsey, U.K. 21 G6 51 0N 1 29W
Ron, India .... 95 G2 15 40N 75 44 E
Ron, Vietnam ...... 86 D6 17 53N 106 27 E
Rona, U.K. 22 D3 57 34N 5 59W
Ronan, U.S.A. 158 C6 47 32N 114 6W
Roncador, Cayos,
  Colombia 164 D3 13 32N 80 4W
Roncador, Serra do,
  Brazil 171 D1 12 30S 52 30W
Ronciglione, Italy .. 45 F9 42 17N 12 13 E
Ronco ➤, Italy ...... 45 D9 44 24N 12 12 E
Ronda, Spain 43 J5 36 46N 5 12W
Ronda, Serranía de,
  Spain 43 J5 36 44N 5 3W
Rondane, Norway .. 18 C6 61 57N 9 50 E
Rondane △, Norway 18 C6 61 55N 9 44 E
Rondón, Colombia .. 168 B3 6 17N 71 6W
Rondônia, Brazil 173 C5 10 52S 61 57W
Rondônia □, Brazil .. 173 C5 11 0S 63 0W
Rondonópolis, Brazil 173 D7 16 28S 54 38W
Rondslottet, Norway 18 C6 61 55N 9 45 E
Rong, Koh, Cambodia 87 G4 10 45N 103 15 E
Rong Jiang ➤, China 76 E7 24 35N 109 20 E
Rong Xian,
  Guangxi Zhuangzu,
  China .... 77 F8 22 50N 110 31 E
Rong Xian, Sichuan,
  China .... 76 C5 29 23N 104 22 E
Rong'an, China .... 76 E7 25 14N 109 22 E
Rongchang, China .. 76 C5 29 20N 105 32 E
Ronge, L. la, Canada 143 B7 55 6N 105 17W
Rongjiang, China .. 76 E7 25 57N 108 28 E
Rongotea, N.Z. .... 130 G4 40 19S 175 25 E
Rongshui, China .... 76 E7 25 5N 109 12 E
Rønne, Denmark .... 17 J8 55 6N 14 43 E
Ronne Ice Shelf,
  Antarctica 7 D18 78 0S 60 0W
Ronneby, Sweden .. 17 H9 56 12N 15 17 E
Ronnebyån ➤, Sweden 17 H9 56 11N 15 18 E
Rönneshytta, Sweden 17 F9 58 56N 15 2 E
Ronsard, C., Australia 125 D1 24 46S 113 10 E
Ronse, Belgium .... 24 D3 50 45N 3 35 E
Ronuro ➤, Brazil .. 173 C7 11 56S 53 33W
Roodepoort, S. Africa 117 D4 26 11S 27 54 E
Roodhouse, U.S.A. .. 156 E6 39 29N 90 24W
Roof Butte, U.S.A. .. 159 H9 36 28N 109 5W
Rooiboklaagte ➤,
  Namibia .... 116 C3 20 50S 21 0 E
Roon, Indonesia .... 83 B4 2 23S 134 33 E
Rooniu, Mt., Tahiti .. 133 S16 17 49S 149 12W
Roopville, U.S.A. 152 B4 33 27N 85 8W
Roorkee, India ...... 92 E7 29 52N 77 59 E
Roosendaal, Neths. .. 24 C4 51 32N 4 29 E
Roosevelt, U.S.A. .. 158 F8 40 18N 109 59W
Roosevelt ➤, Brazil 173 B5 7 35S 60 20W
Roosevelt, Mt., Canada 142 B3 58 26N 125 20W
Roosevelt I., Antarctica 7 D12 79 30S 162 0W
Root ➤, Switz. ...... 33 B6 47 5N 8 23 E
Ropczyce, Poland .. 55 H8 50 4N 21 38 E
Roper ➤, Australia .. 126 A2 14 43S 135 27 E
Roper Bar, Australia 126 A1 14 44S 134 44 E
Roque Pérez, Argentina 174 D4 35 25S 59 24W
Roquefort, France .. 28 D3 44 2N 0 20W
Roquemaure, France 29 D8 44 3N 4 48 E
Roquetas de Mar, Spain 41 J2 36 46N 2 36W
Roquetes, Spain .... 40 E5 40 50N 0 30 E
Roquevaire, France .. 29 E9 43 20N 5 36 E
Roraima □, Brazil .. 169 C5 2 0N 61 30W
Roraima, Mt.,
  Venezuela 169 B5 5 10N 60 40W
Røros, Norway ...... 18 B8 62 35N 11 23 E
Rorschach, Switz. .. 33 B8 47 28N 9 28 E
Rosa, Zambia ...... 119 D3 9 33S 31 15 E
Rosa, C., Algeria .. 111 A6 37 0N 8 16 E
Rosa, L., Ecuador .. 172 a 1 4S 91 10W
Rosa, L., Bahamas .. 165 B5 21 0N 73 30W
Rosa, Monte, Europe .. 32 E5 45 57N 7 53 E
Rosais, Pta. dos, Azores 9 d1 38 45N 28 19W
Rosal de la Frontera,
  Spain 43 H3 37 59N 7 13W
Rosales, Phil. ...... 80 D3 15 54N 120 38 E
Rosalia, U.S.A. 158 C5 47 14N 117 22W
Rosamond, U.S.A. .. 161 L8 34 52N 118 10W
Rosans, France .... 29 D9 44 24N 5 29 E
Rosário, Argentina .. 174 C3 33 0S 60 40W
Rosário, Brazil 170 B3 3 0S 44 15W
Rosario, Baja Calif.,
  Mexico 162 B1 30 0N 115 50W
Rosario, Sinaloa,
  Mexico 162 C3 23 0N 105 52W
Rosario, Paraguay .. 174 A4 24 30S 57 35W
Rosario, Phil. ...... 81 G5 8 24N 125 59 E
Rosario, Villa del,
  Venezuela 168 A3 10 19N 72 19W
Rosario de la Frontera,
  Argentina 174 B3 25 50S 65 0W
Rosario de Lerma,
  Argentina 174 A2 24 59S 65 35W
Rosario del Tala,
  Argentina 174 C4 32 20S 59 10W
Rosário do Sul, Brazil 175 C5 30 15S 54 55W
Rosário Oeste, Brazil 173 C6 14 50S 56 25W
Rosarito, Mexico 161 N9 32 18N 117 4W
Rosarno, Italy ...... 47 D8 38 29N 15 58 E
Rosas = Roses, Spain 40 C8 42 19N 3 10 E
Roscoe, Miss., U.S.A. 156 G3 37 58N 93 48W
Roscoe, N.Y., U.S.A. 151 E10 41 56N 74 55W
Roscoff, France 26 D3 48 44N 3 58W
Roscommon, Ireland 23 C3 53 38N 8 11W
Roscommon □, Ireland 23 C3 53 49N 8 23W
Roscrea, Ireland 23 D4 52 57N 7 49W
Rose ➤, Australia .. 126 A2 14 16S 135 45 E
Rose Belle, Mauritius 121 d 20 24S 57 36 E
Rose Blanche-Harbour
  Le Cou, Canada .. 141 C8 47 38N 58 45W
Rose Hill, Mauritius .. 121 d 20 14S 57 27 E
Rose Pt., Canada 142 C2 54 11N 131 39W
Rose Valley, Canada 143 C8 52 19N 103 49W
Roseau, Dominica .. 165 C7 15 17N 61 24W
Roseau, U.S.A. 154 A7 48 51N 95 46W
Rosebery, Australia .. 127 G4 41 46S 145 33 E
Rosebud, Australia .. 128 E6 38 21S 144 54 E
Rosebud, S. Dak.,
  U.S.A. 154 D4 43 14N 100 51W
Rosebud, Tex., U.S.A. 155 K6 31 4N 96 59W
Roseburg, U.S.A. .. 158 E2 43 13N 123 20W

Rosedale, U.S.A. .. 155 J9 33 51N 91 2W
Rosehearty, U.K. .. 22 D6 57 42N 2 7W
Roseland, U.S.A. .. 160 G4 38 25N 122 43W
Rosemary, Canada .. 142 C6 50 46N 112 5W
Rosenberg = Oleśno,
  Poland .... 55 H5 50 51N 18 26 E
Rosenberg = Susz,
  Poland .... 54 E6 53 44N 19 20 E
Rosenberg, U.S.A. .. 155 L7 29 34N 95 49W
Rosendaël, France .. 27 A9 51 3N 2 24 E
Rosendal, Norway .. 18 E3 59 59N 6 0 E
Rosenheim, Germany 31 H8 47 51N 12 7 E
Roses, Spain ...... 40 C8 42 19N 3 10 E
Roses, G. de, Spain 40 C8 42 10N 3 15 E
Roseto degli Abruzzi,
  Italy .... 45 F11 42 41N 14 1 E
Rosetown, Canada .. 143 C7 51 35N 107 59W
Rosetta = Rashîd,
  Egypt .... 106 H7 31 21N 30 22 E
Roseville, Calif., U.S.A. 160 G5 38 45N 121 17W
Roseville, Ill., U.S.A. 156 D6 40 44N 90 40W
Roseville, Mich., U.S.A. 150 D2 42 30N 82 56W
Rosewood, Australia 127 D5 27 38S 152 36 E
Roshkhvâr, Iran .... 97 C8 34 58N 59 37 E
Roshtqala, Tajikistan 65 E5 37 16N 71 49 E
Rosières-en-Santerre,
  France .... 27 C9 49 49N 2 42 E
Rosignano Maríttimo,
  Italy .... 44 E7 43 24N 10 28 E
Rosignol, Guyana .. 169 B6 6 15N 57 30W
Roşiori de Vede,
  Romania .... 53 F10 44 9N 25 0 E
Rositsa, Bulgaria .... 51 C11 43 57N 27 57 E
Rositsa ➤, Bulgaria 51 C9 43 10N 25 30 E
Roskilde, Denmark .. 17 J6 55 38N 12 3 E
Roskilde
  Amtskommune □,
  Denmark .... 17 J6 55 35N 12 5 E
Roskovec, Albania .. 50 F3 40 44N 19 43 E
Roslavl, Russia .... 58 F7 53 57N 32 55 E
Rosmead, S. Africa .. 116 E4 31 29S 25 8 E
Røsnæs, Denmark .. 17 J4 55 44N 10 55 E
Rosolini, Italy ...... 47 F7 36 49N 14 57 E
Rosporden, France .. 26 E3 47 57N 3 50W
Ross, Australia ...... 127 G4 42 2S 147 30 E
Ross, N.Z. .... 131 C5 42 53S 170 49 E
Ross Béthio,
  Mauritania 112 B1 16 15N 16 8W
Ross Dependency,
  Antarctica 7 D12 76 0S 170 0W
Ross I., Antarctica .. 7 D11 77 30S 168 0 E
Ross Ice Shelf,
  Antarctica .... 7 E12 80 0S 180 0 E
Ross L., U.S.A. 158 B3 48 44N 121 4W
Ross-on-Wye, U.K. .. 21 F5 51 54N 2 34W
Ross River, Australia 126 C1 23 44S 134 30 E
Ross River, Canada .. 142 A2 62 30N 131 30W
Ross Sea, Antarctica 7 D11 74 0S 178 0 E
Rossa, Switz. .... 33 D8 46 23N 9 8 E
Rossall Pt., U.K. 20 D4 53 55N 3 3W
Rossan Pt., Ireland .. 23 B3 54 42N 8 47W
Rossburn, Canada .. 143 C8 50 40N 100 49W
Rosseau, Canada .. 150 A5 45 16N 79 39W
Rosseau, L., Canada 150 A5 45 10N 79 35W
Rössel = Reszel, Poland 54 D8 54 4N 21 10 E
Rossel, C., Vanuatu 133 K4 20 21S 166 36 E
Rossel I., Papua N. G. 132 F8 11 21S 154 9 E
Rossens, Switz. .... 32 C4 46 43N 7 7 E
Rosses, The, Ireland 23 A3 55 2N 8 20W
Rossford, U.S.A. .. 157 E4 41 36N 83 34W
Rossignol, L., Canada 140 B5 52 43N 73 40W
Rossignol L., Canada 141 D6 44 12N 65 10W
Rossiya = Russia ■,
  Eurasia .... 67 C11 62 0N 105 0 E
Rosskreppfjorden,
  Norway .... 18 E4 59 4N 7 10 E
Rossland, Canada .. 142 D5 49 6N 117 50W
Rosslare, Ireland 23 D5 52 17N 6 24W
Rosslare Harbour,
  Ireland 23 D5 52 15N 6 20W
Rosslau, Germany .. 30 D8 51 52N 12 15 E
Rosso, Mauritania .. 112 B1 16 40N 15 45W
Rosso, C., France .. 29 F12 42 13N 8 32 E
Rossosh, Russia .... 59 G10 50 15N 39 28 E
Røssvatnet, Norway 14 D16 65 45N 14 5 E
Rossville, Ill., U.S.A. 157 D9 40 23N 87 40W
Rossville, Ind., U.S.A. 157 D10 40 25N 86 36W
Røst, Norway ...... 14 C15 67 32N 12 0 E
Rostāq, Afghan. .... 65 E4 37 7N 69 49 E
Rosthern, Canada .. 143 C7 52 40N 106 20W
Rostock, Germany .. 30 A8 54 5N 12 8 E
Rostov, Don, Russia 59 J10 47 15N 39 45 E
Rostov, Yaroslavl,
  Russia .... 58 D10 57 14N 39 25 E
Rostovsevo = Bulungur,
  Uzbekistan .... 65 D3 39 46N 67 16 E
Rostrenen, France .. 26 D3 48 14N 3 21W
Roswell, Ga., U.S.A. 152 A5 34 2N 84 22W
Roswell, N. Mex.,
  U.S.A. 155 J2 33 24N 104 32W
Rot-Front =
  Dobropole, Ukraine 59 H9 48 25N 37 2 E
Rota, Spain 43 J4 36 37N 6 20W
Rotan, U.S.A. 155 J4 32 51N 100 28W
Rote Wand, Austria 33 B9 47 11N 9 59 E
Rotenburg, Hessen,
  Germany .... 30 D5 50 59N 9 44 E
Rotenburg,
  Niedersachsen,
  Germany .... 30 B5 53 6N 9 24 E
Roth, Germany ...... 31 F7 49 15N 11 5 E
Rothaargebirge,
  Germany .... 30 D4 51 2N 8 13 E
Rothaargebirge △,
  Germany .... 30 E4 51 0N 8 15 E
Rothenburg, Switz. .. 33 B6 47 6N 8 16 E
Rothenburg ob der
  Tauber, Germany .. 31 F6 49 23N 10 11 E
Rother ➤, U.K. .... 7 C17 50 59N 0 45 E
Rothera, Antarctica .. 7 C17 50 59N 0 45 E
Rotherham, U.K. 20 D6 53 26N 1 20W
Rotherham, N.Z. .... 131 C6 42 42S 172 57 E
Rothes, U.K. 22 D5 57 32N 3 13W
Rothesay, Canada .. 141 C6 45 23N 66 0W
Rothesay, U.K. 22 F3 55 50N 5 3W
Rothrist, Switz. .... 32 B5 47 18N 7 54 E
Roti, Indonesia .... 82 D2 10 50S 123 0 E
Rotja, Pta., Spain .. 38 D2 38 38N 1 35 E
Rotnes, Norway .... 18 D7 60 5N 10 51 E
Roto, Australia .... 129 B6 33 0S 145 30 E
Rotoaira, L., N.Z. .. 130 F4 39 3S 175 45 E
Rotoehu, L., N.Z. .. 130 F5 38 0S 176 26 E
Rotoma, L., N.Z. .. 130 E5 38 2S 176 35 E
Rotondo Mte., France 29 F13 42 14N 9 8 E
Rotorua, N.Z. ...... 131 B7 41 55S 172 39 E
Rotorua, N.Z. ...... 130 E5 38 9S 176 16 E
Rotorua, L., N.Z. .. 130 E5 38 5S 176 18 E
Rott ➤, Germany .. 31 G9 48 27N 13 25 E

Rotten ➤, Switz. .... 32 D5 46 18N 7 36 E
Rottenburg, Germany 31 G4 48 28N 8 55 E
Rottenmann, Austria 34 D7 47 31N 14 22 E
Rotterdam, Neths. .. 24 C4 51 55N 4 30 E
Rotterdam, U.S.A. .. 151 D10 42 48N 74 1W
Rottne, Sweden .... 17 G8 57 1N 14 54 E
Rottnest I., Australia 125 F2 32 0S 115 27 E
Rottumeroog, Neths. 24 A6 53 33N 6 34 E
Rottweil, Germany .. 31 G4 48 9N 8 37 E
Rotuma, Fiji .... 134 J9 12 25S 177 5 E
Roubaix, France .... 27 B10 50 40N 3 10 E
Roudnice nad Labem,
  Czech Rep. ...... 34 A7 50 25N 14 15 E
Rouen, France ...... 26 C8 49 27N 1 4 E
Rouergue, France .. 28 D5 44 15N 2 0 E
Rough Ridge, N.Z. .. 131 F4 45 10S 169 55 E
Rouillac, France 28 C3 45 47N 0 4W
Rouleau, Canada .. 143 C8 50 10N 104 56W
Roulers = Roeselare,
  Belgium .... 24 D3 50 57N 3 7 E
Round I., Mauritius .. 121 d 19 51S 57 45 E
Round Mountain,
  U.S.A. 158 G5 38 43N 117 4W
Round Mt., Australia 129 A10 30 26S 152 16 E
Round Rock, U.S.A. .. 155 K6 30 31N 97 41W
Roundup, U.S.A. .. 158 C9 46 27N 108 33W
Roura, Fr. Guiana .. 169 C7 4 44N 52 20W
Rousay, U.K. 22 B5 59 10N 3 2W
Rouses Point, U.S.A. 151 B11 44 59N 73 22W
Rouseville, U.S.A. .. 150 E5 41 28N 79 42W
Rousse = Ruse,
  Bulgaria .... 51 C9 43 48N 25 59 E
Roussenski Lom △,
  Bulgaria .... 51 C10 43 40N 26 10 E
Roussillon, Isère,
  France .... 29 C8 45 24N 4 49 E
Roussillon,
  Pyrénées-Or., France 28 F6 42 30N 2 35 E
Roussin, C., N. Cal. 133 U21 21 20S 167 59 E
Rouxville, S. Africa .. 116 E4 30 25S 26 50 E
Rouyn-Noranda,
  Canada 140 C4 48 20N 79 0W
Rovaniemi, Finland 14 C21 66 29N 25 41 E
Rovato, Italy ...... 44 C7 45 34N 10 0 E
Rovenki, Ukraine .. 59 H10 48 5N 39 21 E
Rovereto, Italy .... 44 C8 45 53N 11 3 E
Roverud, Norway .. 18 D9 60 15N 12 3 E
Rovigno = Rovinj,
  Croatia .... 45 C10 45 5N 13 40 E
Rovigo, Italy ...... 45 C8 45 4N 11 47 E
Rovinj, Croatia .... 45 C10 45 5N 13 40 E
Rovira, Colombia .. 168 C2 4 15N 75 20W
Rovno = Rivne,
  Ukraine .... 59 G4 50 40N 26 10 E
Rovnoye, Russia .. 60 E8 50 52N 46 3 E
Rovuma = Ruvuma ➤,
  Tanzania .... 119 E5 10 29S 40 28 E
Row'ān, Iran ...... 97 C6 35 8N 48 51 E
Rowena, Australia .. 127 D4 29 48S 148 55 E
Rowley Shoals,
  Australia .... 124 C2 17 30S 119 0 E
Roxa, Guinea-Biss. 112 C1 11 15N 15 45W
Roxas, Capiz, Phil. 81 F4 11 36N 122 49 E
Roxas, Isabela, Phil. 80 C3 17 8N 121 36 E
Roxas, Mind. Or., Phil. 80 E4 13 0N 121 8 E
Roxas, Palawan, Phil. 81 F2 10 20N 119 21 E
Roxboro, U.S.A. .. 149 G6 36 24N 78 59W
Roxborough,
  Trin. & Tob. 169 E10 11 15N 60 35W
Roxburgh, N.Z. .... 131 F4 45 33S 169 19 E
Roxbury, U.S.A. .. 150 F7 40 6N 77 39W
Roxen, Sweden .... 17 F9 58 30N 15 40 E
Roy, Mont., U.S.A. 158 C9 47 20N 108 58W
Roy, N. Mex., U.S.A. 155 H2 35 57N 104 12W
Roy, Utah, U.S.A. .. 158 F7 41 10N 112 2W
Royal △, Australia .. 129 C9 34 5S 151 5 E
Royal Bardia △, Nepal 93 E9 28 20N 81 20 E
Royal Canal, Ireland 23 C4 53 30N 7 13W
Royal Center, U.S.A. 157 D10 40 52N 86 30W
Royal Chitawan △,
  Nepal .... 93 F11 26 30N 84 30 E
Royal Leamington Spa,
  U.K. 21 E6 52 18N 1 31W
Royal Natal △,
  S. Africa .... 117 D4 28 43S 28 51 E
Royal Oak, U.S.A. .. 157 B13 42 30N 83 9W
Royal Palm Beach,
  U.S.A. 153 J9 26 41N 80 14W
Royal Tunbridge Wells,
  U.K. .... 21 F8 51 7N 0 16 E
Royale, Isle, U.S.A. 154 B10 48 0N 88 54W
Royalla, Australia .. 129 C8 35 30S 149 9 E
Royan, France 28 C2 45 37N 1 2W
Roye, France ...... 27 C9 49 42N 2 48 E
Royston, U.K. 21 E7 52 3N 0 0W
Rožaj, Serbia & M. .. 50 D4 42 50N 20 15 E
Rózan, Poland .... 55 F8 52 52N 21 25 E
Rozay-en-Brie, France 27 D9 48 41N 2 58 E
Rozdilna, Ukraine .. 53 E16 46 50N 30 2 E
Rozhnyativ, Ukraine 53 B9 48 56N 24 9 E
Rozhyshche, Ukraine 59 G3 50 54N 25 15 E
Rožmitál pod
  Třemšínem,
  Czech Rep. ...... 34 B6 49 36N 13 53 E
Rožňava, Slovak Rep. 35 C13 48 37N 20 35 E
Rozogi, Poland .... 54 E8 53 28N 21 19 E
Rozoy-sur-Serre,
  France .... 27 C11 49 40N 4 8 E
Roztocze, Poland .. 55 H10 50 37N 23 0 E
Roztoczański △,
  Poland .... 55 H10 50 35N 23 0 E
Rozzano, Italy ...... 44 C6 45 22N 9 10 E
Rrëshen, Albania .. 50 E3 41 47N 19 49 E
Rrogozhina, Albania 50 E3 41 2N 19 50 E
Rtanj, Serbia & M. .. 50 C5 43 45N 21 50 E
Rtem, O. el ➤, Algeria 111 B6 33 55N 5 37 E
Rtishchevo, Russia 60 D6 52 18N 43 46 E
Rúa = A Rúa, Spain 42 C3 42 23N 7 8W
Ruacaná, Namibia .. 116 B1 17 27S 14 21 E
Ruaha △, Tanzania 118 D3 7 41S 34 30 E
Ruahine Ra., N.Z. .. 130 H5 39 55S 176 2 E
Ruamahanga ➤, N.Z. 130 H4 41 24S 175 8 E
Ruapehu, N.Z. .... 131 G3 46 46S 168 31 E
Ruāq, W. ➤, Egypt 102 F2 30 0N 33 49 E
Ruatoria, N.Z. ...... 130 D7 37 55S 178 20 E
Ruavai, Solomon Is. 133 M11 9 26S 160 26 E
Ruawai, N.Z. ...... 130 E5 38 8S 173 59 E
Rub' al Khālī,
  Si. Arabia .... 99 C5 19 0N 48 0 E
Rubeho Mts., Tanzania 118 D4 6 50S 36 25 E
Rubezhnaya =
  Rubizhne, Ukraine 59 H10 49 6N 38 25 E
Rubezhnoye =
  Rubizhne, Ukraine 59 H10 49 6N 38 25 E
Rubh a' Mhail, U.K. 22 F2 55 56N 6 8W
Rubha Hunish, U.K. 22 D2 57 42N 6 20W
Rubha Robhanais =
  Lewis, Butt of, U.K. 22 C2 58 31N 6 16W
Rubi, Spain .... 40 D7 41 30N 2 6 E
Rubiataba, Brazil .. 171 E2 15 8S 49 48W
Rubicon ➤, U.S.A. 160 G6 38 53N 121 4W
Rubicone ➤, Italy 45 D9 44 8N 12 28 E
Rubik, Albania ...... 50 E3 41 46N 19 47 E
Rubinéia, Brazil 171 F1 20 13S 51 2W

Rubino, Ivory C. .. 112 D4 6 4N 4 18W
Rubio, Venezuela .. 168 B3 7 43N 72 22W
Rubizhne, Ukraine .. 59 H10 49 6N 38 25 E
Rubondo △, Tanzania 118 C3 2 18S 31 58 E
Ruby, U.S.A. 144 D9 64 45N 155 30W
Ruby Beach =
  Jacksonville Beach,
  U.S.A. 152 E8 30 17N 81 24W
Ruby L., U.S.A. 158 F6 40 10N 115 28W
Ruby Mts., U.S.A. .. 158 F6 40 30N 115 20W
Rubyvale, Australia 126 C4 23 25S 147 42 E
Rucheng, China .... 77 E9 25 33N 113 38 E
Ruciane-Nida, Poland 54 E8 53 40N 21 32 E
Rūd Sar, Iran ...... 97 B6 37 8N 50 18 E
Ruda, Sweden ...... 17 G10 57 6N 16 7 E
Ruda Śląska, Poland 55 H5 50 16N 18 50 E
Rudall, Australia .. 128 B2 33 43S 136 17 E
Rudall ➤, Australia 124 D3 22 34S 122 13 E
Rudall River △,
  Australia .... 124 D3 22 38S 122 30 E
Rūdbār, Afghan. .. 91 C1 30 9N 62 36 E
Rüdersdorf, Germany 30 C9 52 27N 13 47 E
Rudewa, Tanzania .. 119 E3 11 7S 34 40 E
Rudkøbing, Denmark 17 K4 54 56N 10 41 E
Rudky, Ukraine .... 55 J10 49 38N 23 29 E
Rudna, Poland .... 55 G3 51 30N 16 17 E
Rüdnichnyy,
  Kazakhstan ...... 65 A9 44 40N 78 54 E
Rudnik, Bulgaria .. 51 D11 42 36N 27 30 E
Rudnik, Serbia & M. 55 H9 50 26N 22 15 E
Rudnik, Serbia & M. 50 B4 44 7N 20 35 E
Rudnik Ingichka =
  Ingichka, Uzbekistan 65 D2 39 47N 65 58 E
Rudnya, Russia .... 58 E6 54 55N 31 7 E
Rudnytsya, Ukraine 53 B13 48 16N 28 54 E
Rudnyy, Kazakhstan 64 D7 52 57N 63 7 E
Rudo, Bos.-H. ...... 52 G4 43 41N 19 23 E
Rudolfa, Ostrov, Russia 66 A6 81 45N 58 30 E
Rudolstadt, Germany 30 E7 50 44N 11 19 E
Rudong, China .... 77 A13 32 20N 121 12 E
Rudozem, Bulgaria 51 E8 41 29N 24 51 E
Rudyard, U.S.A. .. 148 B3 46 14N 84 36W
Rue, France ...... 27 B8 50 15N 1 40 E
Ruenya ➤, Africa .. 119 F3 16 24S 33 48 E
Rufa'a, Sudan ...... 107 E3 14 44N 33 22 E
Rufflin, U.S.A. 152 B9 33 0N 80 49W
Rufiji ➤, Tanzania .. 118 D4 7 50S 39 15 E
Rufino, Argentina .. 174 C3 34 20S 62 50W
Rufisque, Senegal .. 112 C1 14 40N 17 15W
Rufling Pt.,
  Br. Virgin Is. .... 165 e 18 44N 64 27W
Rufunsa, Zambia .. 119 F2 15 4S 29 34 E
Rugao, China ...... 77 A13 32 23N 120 31 E
Rugby, U.K. 21 E6 52 23N 1 16W
Rugby, U.S.A. 154 A5 48 22N 100 0W
Rügen, Germany .. 30 A9 54 22N 13 24 E
Rügen △, Germany 30 A9 54 25N 13 25 E
Rugles, France .... 26 D7 48 50N 0 40 E
Ruhea, Bangla. .... 90 B2 26 10N 88 25 E
Ruhengeri, Rwanda 118 C2 1 30S 29 36 E
Ruhla, Germany .. 30 E6 50 54N 10 23 E
Ruhland, Germany 30 D9 51 27N 13 51 E
Ruhnu, Estonia .... 15 H20 57 48N 23 15 E
Ruhr ➤, Germany .. 30 D2 51 27N 6 43 E
Ruhuhu ➤, Tanzania 119 E3 10 31S 34 34 E
Rui Barbosa, Brazil 171 D3 12 18S 40 27W
Rui'an, China ...... 77 D13 27 47N 120 40 E
Ruichang, China .. 77 C10 29 40N 115 39 E
Ruidoso, U.S.A. .. 159 K11 33 20N 105 41W
Ruili, China ...... 76 E1 24 1N 97 43 E
Ruivo, Pico, Madeira 9 c 32 45N 16 56W
Ruj, Bulgaria ...... 50 C6 42 52N 22 34 E
Rujen, Macedonia 50 D6 42 9N 22 32 E
Rujm Tal'at al Jamā'ah,
  Jordan .... 103 E4 30 24N 35 30 E
Ruk, Pakistan ...... 92 F3 27 50N 68 42 E
Rukhla, Pakistan .. 92 C4 32 27N 71 57 E
Rukwa □, Tanzania 118 D3 7 0S 31 30 E
Rukwa, L., Tanzania 118 D3 8 0S 32 20 E
Rulhieres, C., Australia 124 B4 13 56S 127 22 E
Rum = Rhum, U.K. 22 E2 57 0N 6 20W
Rum, Jordan ...... 103 F4 29 39N 35 26 E
Rum Cay, Bahamas 165 B5 23 40N 74 58W
Rum Jungle, Australia 124 B5 13 0S 130 59 E
Ruma, Serbia & M. 52 E4 45 0N 19 50 E
Ruma △, Kenya .... 118 C3 0 39S 34 18 E
Rumāḥ, Si. Arabia 96 E5 25 29N 47 10 E
Rumania = Romania ■,
  Europe .... 53 D10 46 0N 25 0 E
Rumaylah, Iraq .... 96 D5 30 47N 47 37 E
Rumbêk, Sudan .... 107 F2 6 54N 29 37 E
Rumberpon, Indonesia 83 B4 1 35S 134 9 E
Rumford, U.S.A. .. 151 B14 44 33N 70 33W
Rumia, Poland .... 54 D10 54 37N 18 25 E
Rumilly, France .... 29 C9 45 53N 5 56 E
Rummelsburg =
  Miastko, Poland .. 54 E3 54 0N 16 58 E
Rumoi, Japan ...... 70 C10 43 56N 141 39 E
Rumonge, Burundi 118 C2 3 59S 29 26 E
Rumson, U.S.A. 151 F11 40 23N 74 0W
Rumula, Australia .. 126 B4 16 35S 145 20 E
Rumuruti, Kenya .. 118 B4 0 17N 36 32 E
Runan, China ...... 76 C8 33 0N 114 30 E
Runanga, N.Z. .... 131 C6 42 25S 171 15 E
Runaway, C., N.Z. 130 E7 37 32S 178 2 E
Runaway Bay, Jamaica 164 a 18 27N 77 20W
Runcorn, U.K. 20 D5 53 21N 2 44W
Rundu, Namibia .. 116 B2 17 52S 19 43 E
Rungwa, Tanzania .. 118 D3 6 55S 33 32 E
Rungwa ➤, Tanzania 118 D3 7 36S 31 50 E
Rungwa △, Tanzania 118 D3 6 53S 34 2 E
Rungwe, Tanzania .. 119 D3 9 11S 33 32 E
Rungwe, Mt., Tanzania 113 G6 9 8S 33 40 E
Runton Ra., Australia 124 D3 23 31S 123 6 E
Ruokolahti, Finland 15 E23 61 17N 28 50 E
Ruoqiang, China .. 68 C3 38 55N 88 10 E
Rupa, India .... 93 F18 27 15N 92 21 E
Rupar, India ...... 92 D7 31 2N 76 38 E
Rupea, Romania .. 53 D10 46 2N 25 13 E
Rupen ➤, India .... 94 H4 23 28N 71 31 E
Rupert, U.S.A. 158 E7 42 37N 113 41W
Rupert ➤, Canada 140 B4 51 29N 78 45W
Rupert B., Canada 140 B4 51 29N 78 45W
Rupert House =
  Waskaganish,
  Canada 140 B4 51 30N 78 40W
Rupsa, India ...... 93 J12 21 37N 87 1 E
Rupununi ➤, Guyana 169 C6 3 43S 58 35W
Rur ➤, Germany .. 30 D1 51 11N 5 59 E
Rurópolis, Brazil .. 170 D5 4 4S 54 59W
Rus ➤, Spain 41 F2 39 30N 3 11W
Rusambo, Zimbabwe 119 F3 16 30S 32 4 E
Ruschuk = Ruse,
  Bulgaria .... 51 C9 43 48N 25 59 E
Ruse, Bulgaria .... 51 C9 43 48N 25 59 E
Ruse □, Bulgaria .. 51 C10 43 35N 26 10 E
Ruşeţu, Romania .. 53 F12 44 57N 27 14 E
Rush, Ireland 23 C5 53 31N 6 6W

Rushan, China 75 F11 36 56N 121 30 E
Rushden, U.K. 21 E7 52 18N 0 35W
Rushikulya →, India 94 E7 19 23N 85 5 E
Rushmore, Mt., U.S.A. 154 D3 43 53N 103 28W
Rushon, Tajikistan 65 E5 37 57N 71 33 E
Rushville, Ill., U.S.A. 156 D6 40 7N 90 34W
Rushville, Ind., U.S.A. 157 E11 39 37N 85 27W
Rushville, Nebr., U.S.A. 154 D3 42 43N 102 28W
Rushworth, Australia 129 D6 36 32 S 145 1 E
Ruskin, U.S.A. 153 H7 27 43N 82 26W
Russas, Brazil 170 B4 4 55 S 37 50W
Russell, Canada 143 C8 50 50N 101 20W
Russell, N.Z. 130 B3 35 16 S 174 10 E
Russell, Fla., U.S.A. 152 E8 30 3N 81 45W
Russell, Kans., U.S.A. 154 F5 38 54N 98 52W
Russell, N.Y., U.S.A. 151 B9 44 27N 75 9W
Russell, Pa., U.S.A. 150 E5 41 56N 79 8W
Russell Cave ⌂, U.S.A. 149 H3 34 59N 85 49W
Russell Is., Solomon Is. 133 M10 9 4 S 159 12 E
Russell L., Man., Canada 143 B8 56 15N 101 30W
Russell L., N.W.T., Canada 142 A5 63 5N 115 44W
Russellkonda, India 94 E7 19 57N 84 42 E
Russells Point, U.S.A. 157 D13 40 28N 83 54W
Russellville, Ala., U.S.A. 149 H2 34 30N 87 44W
Russellville, Ark., U.S.A. 155 H8 35 17N 93 8W
Russellville, Ky., U.S.A. 149 G2 36 51N 86 53W
Rüsselsheim, Germany 31 F4 49 59N 8 23 E
Russi, Italy 45 D9 44 22N 12 2 E
Russia ■, Eurasia 67 C11 62 0N 105 0 E
Russian →, U.S.A. 160 G3 38 27N 123 8W
Russian Mission, U.S.A. 144 F7 61 47N 161 19W
Russiaville, U.S.A. 157 D10 40 25N 86 16W
Russkoye Ustie, Russia 6 B15 71 0N 149 0 E
Rust, Austria 35 D9 47 49N 16 42 E
Rustam, Pakistan 92 B5 34 25N 72 13 E
Rustam Shahr, Pakistan 92 F2 26 58N 66 6 E
Rustavi, Georgia 61 K7 41 30N 45 0 E
Rustenburg, S. Africa 116 D4 25 41 S 27 14 E
Ruston, U.S.A. 155 J8 32 32N 92 38W
Ruswil, Switz. 32 B6 47 5N 8 8 E
Rutana, Burundi 118 C3 3 55 S 30 0 E
Rute, Spain 43 H6 37 19N 4 23W
Ruteng, Indonesia 82 C2 8 35 S 120 30 E
Ruth, U.S.A. 150 C2 43 42N 82 45W
Rutherford, U.S.A. 160 G4 38 26N 122 24W
Rutherglen, Australia 129 D7 36 5 S 146 29 E
Rüti, Switz. 33 B7 47 16N 8 51 E
Rutland, U.S.A. 151 C12 43 37N 72 58W
Rutland □, U.K. 21 E7 52 38N 0 40W
Rutland I., India 95 J11 11 25N 92 10 E
Rutland Water, U.K. 21 E7 52 39N 0 38W
Rutledal, Norway 18 C2 61 4N 5 10 E
Rutledge, U.S.A. 152 B6 33 38N 83 37W
Rutledge →, Canada 143 A6 61 4N 112 0W
Rutledge L., Canada 143 A6 61 33N 110 47W
Rutqa, W. →, Syria 101 E9 34 30N 41 3 E
Rutshuru, Dem. Rep. of the Congo 118 C2 1 13 S 29 25 E
Ruvo di Púglia, Italy 47 A9 41 7N 16 29 E
Ruvu, Tanzania 118 D4 6 49 S 38 43 E
Ruvu →, Tanzania 118 D4 6 23 S 38 52 E
Ruvuba △, Burundi 118 C2 3 3 S 29 33 E
Ruvuma □, Tanzania 119 E4 10 20 S 36 0 E
Ruvuma →, Tanzania 119 E5 10 29 S 40 28 E
Ruwais, U.A.E. 97 E7 24 5N 52 50 E
Ruwenzori, Africa 118 B2 0 30N 29 55 E
Ruwenzori △, Uganda 118 B2 0 20 S 30 0 E
Ruya →, Zimbabwe 117 B5 16 27 S 32 5 E
Ruyigi, Burundi 118 C3 3 29 S 30 15 E
Ruyuan, China 77 E9 24 46N 113 16 E
Ruzayevka, Russia 60 C7 54 4N 45 0 E
Růžhevo Konare, Bulgaria 51 D8 42 23N 24 46 E
Ružomberok, Slovak Rep. 35 B12 49 3N 19 17 E
Ruzyne, Praha ✈ (PRG), Czech Rep. 34 A7 50 7N 14 15 E
Rwanda ■, Africa 118 C3 2 0 S 30 0 E
Ryakhovo, Bulgaria 51 C10 43 58N 26 18 E
Ryan, L., U.K. 22 G3 55 0N 5 2W
Ryazan, Russia 58 E10 54 40N 39 40 E
Ryazhsk, Russia 58 F11 53 45N 40 3 E
Rybache = Rybachye, Kazakhstan 66 E9 46 40N 81 20 E
Rybachiy, Russia 54 C7 55 10N 20 50 E
Rybachiy Poluostrov, Russia 56 A5 69 43N 32 0 E
Rybachye = Balykchy, Kyrgyzstan 65 B8 42 26N 76 12 E
Rybachye, Kazakhstan 66 E9 46 40N 81 20 E
Rybinsk, Russia 58 C10 58 5N 38 50 E
Rybinskoye Vdkhr., Russia 58 C10 58 30N 38 25 E
Rybnik, Poland 55 H5 50 6N 18 32 E
Rybnitsa = Râbniţa, Moldova 53 C14 47 45N 29 0 E
Rybnoye, Russia 58 E10 54 45N 39 30 E
Rychnov nad Kněžnou, Czech Rep. 35 A9 50 10N 16 17 E
Rychwał, Poland 55 F5 52 4N 18 10 E
Rycroft, Canada 142 B5 55 45N 118 40W
Ryd, Sweden 17 H8 56 27N 14 42 E
Rydaholm, Sweden 17 H8 56 59N 14 18 E
Ryde, U.K. 21 G6 50 43N 1 9W
Ryderwood, U.S.A. 160 D3 46 23N 123 3W
Rydzyna, Poland 55 G3 51 47N 16 39 E
Rye, U.K. 21 G8 50 57N 0 45 E
Rye →, U.K. 20 C7 54 11N 0 44W
Rye Bay, U.K. 21 G8 50 52N 0 49 E
Rye Patch Reservoir, U.S.A. 158 F4 40 28N 118 19W
Ryegate, U.S.A. 158 C9 46 18N 109 15W
Ryfylke, Norway 18 E3 59 25N 6 25 E
Rykene, Norway 18 F5 58 24N 8 37 E
Ryki, Poland 55 G8 51 38N 21 56 E
Rykovo = Yenakiyeve, Ukraine 59 H10 48 15N 38 15 E
Ryley, Canada 142 C6 53 17N 112 26W
Rylsk, Russia 59 G8 51 36N 34 43 E
Rylstone, Australia 129 B8 32 46 S 149 58 E
Rymanów, Poland 55 J8 49 35N 21 51 E
Ryn, Poland 54 E8 53 57N 21 34 E
Ryn Peski, Kazakhstan 61 G9 47 30N 49 0 E
Ryōhaku-Sanchi, Japan 73 A8 36 9N 136 49 E
Ryojun = Lüshun, China 75 E11 38 45N 121 15 E
Ryōtsu, Japan 70 E9 38 5N 138 26 E
Rypin, Poland 55 E6 53 3N 19 25 E
Ryssby, Sweden 17 H8 56 52N 14 10 E
Rysy, Europe 35 B13 49 10N 20 4 E
Ryūgasaki, Japan 73 B12 35 54N 140 11 E
Ryūkyū Is. = Ryūkyū-rettō, Japan 71 M3 26 0N 126 0 E
Ryūkyū-rettō, Japan 71 M3 26 0N 126 0 E
Rzepin, Poland 55 F1 52 20N 14 49 E
Rzeszów, Poland 55 J8 50 5N 21 58 E
Rzhev, Russia 58 D8 56 20N 34 20 E

S

Sa, Thailand 86 C3 18 34N 100 45 E
Sa Canal, Spain 38 D1 38 51N 1 23 E
Sa Conillera, Spain 38 D1 38 59N 1 13 E
Sa Dec, Vietnam 87 G5 10 20N 105 46 E
Sa Dragonera, Spain 38 B3 39 35N 2 19 E
Sa-koi, Burma 90 F6 19 54N 97 3 E
Sa Mesquida, Spain 38 B5 39 55N 4 16 E
Sa Pobla, Spain 38 B4 39 46N 3 1 E
Sa Savina, Spain 38 D1 38 44N 1 25 E
Sa'a, Solomon Is. 133 M11 9 43 S 161 35 E
Sa'ādatābād, Fārs, Iran 97 D7 30 10N 53 5 E
Sa'ādatābād, Hormozgān, Iran 97 D7 28 3N 55 53 E
Sa'ādatābād, Kermān, Iran 97 D7 29 40N 55 51 E
Saale →, Germany 30 D7 51 56N 11 54 E
Saaler Bodden, Germany 30 A8 54 20N 12 27 E
Saalfeld, Germany 30 E7 50 38N 11 21 E
Saalfelden, Austria 34 D5 47 25N 12 51 E
Saane →, Switz. 32 B4 47 8N 7 10 E
Saanen, Switz. 32 D4 46 29N 7 15 E
Saanich, Canada 160 B3 48 29N 123 26W
Saar →, Europe 24 E6 49 41N 6 32 E
Saar-Hunsrück ⌂, Germany 31 F2 49 30N 6 50 E
Saar in Mähren = Žďár nad Sázavou, Czech Rep. 34 B8 49 34N 15 57 E
Saarbrücken, Germany 31 F2 49 14N 6 59 E
Saarburg, Germany 31 F2 49 36N 6 32 E
Saaremaa, Estonia 15 G20 58 30N 22 30 E
Saarijärvi, Finland 15 E21 62 43N 25 16 E
Saariselkä, Finland 14 B23 68 16N 28 15 E
Saarland □, Germany 31 F2 49 20N 7 0 E
Saarlautern = Saarlouis, Germany 31 F2 49 18N 6 45 E
Saarlouis, Germany 31 F2 49 18N 6 45 E
Saas Fee, Switz. 32 D5 46 7N 7 56 E
Saaz = Žatec, Czech Rep. 34 A6 50 20N 13 32 E
Sab 'Ābar, Syria 100 F7 33 46N 37 41 E
Saba, W. Indies 165 C7 17 38N 63 14W
Šabac, Serbia & M. 50 B3 44 48N 19 42 E
Sabadell, Spain 40 D7 41 28N 2 7 E
Sabae, Japan 73 B8 35 57N 136 11 E
Sabah □, Malaysia 85 A5 6 0N 117 0 E
Sabak Bernam, Malaysia 87 L3 3 46N 100 58 E
Sabalān, Kūhhā-ye, Iran 101 C12 38 15N 47 45 E
Sabalana, Kepulauan, Indonesia 82 C1 6 45 S 118 50 E
Sábana de la Mar, Dom. Rep. 165 C6 19 7N 69 24W
Sábanalarga, Colombia 168 A3 10 38N 74 55W
Sabang, Indonesia 84 A1 5 50N 95 15 E
Săbăoani, Romania 53 C11 47 1N 26 51 E
Sabará, Brazil 171 E3 19 55 S 43 46W
Sabari →, India 94 F5 17 35N 81 16 E
Sabarmati →, India 92 H5 22 18N 72 22 E
Sab'atayn, Ramlat as, Yemen 98 D4 15 30N 46 10 E
Sabattis, U.S.A. 151 B10 44 6N 74 40W
Sabáudia, Italy 46 A6 41 18N 13 1 E
Sabaya, Bolivia 172 D4 19 1 S 68 23W
Şabāyā, Jaza'ir, Si. Arabia 98 C3 18 35N 41 3 E
Sabbio Chiese, Italy 33 E10 45 39N 10 25 E
Saberania, Indonesia 83 B5 2 5 S 138 18 E
Sabhah, Libya 108 C2 27 9N 14 29 E
Sabhah □, Libya 108 C2 26 0N 14 0 E
Sabi →, India 92 E7 28 29N 76 44 E
Sabi Game Reserve = Kruger △, S. Africa 117 C5 24 50 S 26 10 E
Sabidana, J., Sudan 106 D4 18 4N 36 50 E
Sabie, S. Africa 117 D5 25 10 S 30 48 E
Sabina, U.S.A. 157 E13 39 29N 83 38W
Sabinal, Mexico 162 A3 30 58N 107 25W
Sabinal, U.S.A. 155 L5 29 19N 99 28W
Sabiñánigo, Spain 40 C4 42 31N 0 22W
Sabinar, Punta del, Spain 41 J2 36 43N 2 44W
Sabinas, Mexico 162 B4 27 50N 101 10W
Sabinas →, Mexico 162 B4 27 37N 100 42W
Sabinas Hidalgo, Mexico 162 B4 26 33N 100 10W
Sabine →, U.S.A. 155 L8 29 59N 93 47W
Sabine L., U.S.A. 155 L8 29 53N 93 51W
Sabine Pass, U.S.A. 155 L8 29 44N 93 54W
Sabinópolis, Brazil 171 E3 18 40 S 43 6W
Sabinov, Slovak Rep. 35 B14 49 6N 21 5 E
Sabinsville, U.S.A. 150 E7 41 52N 77 31W
Sabirabad, Azerbaijan 61 K9 40 5N 48 30 E
Sabka, Chad 109 E3 19 15N 16 35 E
Sablayan, Phil. 80 E3 12 50N 120 50 E
Sable, Canada 141 A6 55 30N 68 21W
Sable, C., Canada 141 D6 43 29N 65 38W
Sable, C., U.S.A. 153 K8 25 9N 81 8W
Sable I., Canada 141 D8 44 0N 60 0W
Sable I., Papua N. G. 132 B8 3 38 S 154 42 E
Sablé-sur-Sarthe, France 26 E6 47 50N 0 20W
Saboeiro, Brazil 170 C4 6 32 S 39 54W
Sabonkafi, Niger 113 C6 14 40N 8 45 E
Sabor →, Portugal 42 D3 41 10N 7 7W
Sabou, Burkina Faso 112 C4 12 1N 2 15W
Şabrātah, Libya 108 B2 32 47N 12 29 E
Sabres, France 28 D3 44 9N 0 43W
Sabria, Tunisia 108 B1 33 22N 8 45 E
Sabrina Coast, Antarctica 7 C9 68 0 S 120 0 E
Sabtang I., Phil. 80 A3 20 19N 121 52 E
Sabugal, Portugal 42 E3 40 20N 7 5W
Sabula, U.S.A. 156 B6 42 4N 90 10W
Sabulubbek, Indonesia 84 C1 1 36 S 98 40 E
Sabuncu, Turkey 49 B12 39 33N 30 12 E
Şabyā, Si. Arabia 98 C3 17 9N 42 37 E
Sabzevār, Iran 97 B8 36 15N 57 40 E
Sabzvārān, Iran 97 D8 28 45N 57 50 E
Sac City, U.S.A. 156 B2 42 25N 95 0W
Sacaolo, Angola 115 E4 12 58 S 22 28 E
Sacatengo, Angola 115 E4 13 16 S 21 20 E
Sacedón, Spain 40 E2 40 29N 2 41W
Săcele, Romania 53 E10 45 37N 25 41 E
Sachigo →, Canada 140 A2 55 6N 88 58W
Sachigo, L., Canada 140 B1 53 50N 92 12W
Sachimbo, Angola 115 D4 9 14 S 20 16 E
Sachin, India 94 D1 21 5N 72 53 E
Sachkhere, Georgia 61 J6 42 25N 43 28 E
Sachseln, Switz. 33 C6 46 52N 8 15 E
Sachsen □, Germany 30 E9 50 55N 13 10 E
Sachsen-Anhalt □, Germany 30 D7 52 0N 12 0 E
Sächsische Schweiz △, Germany 30 E10 50 55N 14 10 E
Sacile, Italy 45 C9 45 57N 12 30 E
Sackets Harbor, U.S.A. 151 C8 43 57N 76 7W
Sackville, Canada 141 C7 45 54N 64 22W
Saco, Maine, U.S.A. 149 D10 43 30N 70 27W
Saco, Mont., U.S.A. 158 B10 48 28N 107 21W
Sacramento = Itatupa, Brazil 169 D7 0 37 S 51 12W
Sacramento, Brazil 171 E2 19 53 S 47 27W
Sacramento, U.S.A. 160 G5 38 35N 121 29W
Sacramento →, U.S.A. 160 G5 38 3N 121 56W
Sacramento Mts., U.S.A. 159 K11 32 30N 105 30W
Sacramento Valley, U.S.A. 160 G5 39 30N 122 0W
Sacratif, C., Spain 43 J7 36 42N 3 28W
Săcueni, Romania 52 C7 47 20N 22 5 E
Sada, Spain 42 B2 43 22N 8 15W
Sada-Misaki, Japan 71 H6 33 20N 132 1 E
Sada-Misaki-Hantō, Japan 72 D4 33 22N 132 1 E
Sádaba, Spain 40 C3 42 19N 1 12W
Sadabad, India 92 F8 27 27N 78 3 E
Şa'dah, Yemen 98 C3 16 15N 43 37 E
Sadani, Tanzania 118 D4 5 58 S 38 35 E
Sadao, Thailand 87 J3 6 38N 100 26 E
Sadaseopet, India 94 F3 17 38N 77 59 E
Sadd el Aali, Egypt 106 C3 23 54N 32 54 E
Saddle Mt., U.S.A. 160 E3 45 58N 123 41W
Saddle Pk., India 95 H11 13 9N 93 1 E
Saddle Pt., St. Helena 9 h 15 57 S 5 38W
Sade, Nigeria 113 C7 11 22N 10 45 E
Şadh, Oman 99 C6 17 3N 55 4 E
Sadimi, Dem. Rep. of the Congo 119 D1 9 25 S 23 32 E
Sadiola, Mali 112 C2 13 50N 11 40W
Sadiya, India 90 B5 27 50N 95 40 E
Sa'dīyah, Hawr as, Iraq 101 F12 32 15N 46 30 E
Sado, Japan 70 F9 38 0N 138 25 E
Sado →, Portugal 43 G2 38 29N 8 55W
Sadon, Russia 61 J6 42 52N 43 58 E
Sadovoye, Russia 61 G7 47 47N 44 31 E
Sadowara, Japan 72 E3 32 2N 131 26 E
Sadra, India 92 H5 23 21N 72 43 E
Sadri, India 92 G5 25 11N 73 26 E
Sæbøvik, Norway 18 E2 59 47N 5 40 E
Sæby, Denmark 17 G4 57 21N 10 30 E
Saegertown, U.S.A. 150 E4 41 43N 80 9W
Saelices, Spain 40 F2 39 55N 2 49W
Sætre, Norway 18 E7 59 41N 10 33 E
Sævareid, Norway 18 D2 60 11N 5 46 E
Safaalan, Turkey 51 E12 41 26N 28 6 E
Safaga, Egypt 106 B3 26 42N 34 0 E
Şafājah, Si. Arabia 96 E3 26 25N 39 0 E
Šafárikovo = Tornal'a, Slovak Rep. 35 C13 48 25N 20 20 E
Safata B., Samoa 133 X24 14 0 S 171 50W
Safed Koh, Afghan. 91 B3 34 0N 70 0 E
Säffle, Sweden 16 E6 59 8N 12 55 E
Safford, U.S.A. 159 K9 32 50N 109 43W
Saffron Walden, U.K. 21 E8 52 1N 0 16 E
Safi, Morocco 110 B3 32 18N 9 20W
Safia, Papua N. G. 132 E5 9 35 S 148 38 E
Safia, Hamada, Mali 110 D4 23 10N 4 15W
Şafīābād, Iran 97 B8 36 45N 57 58 E
Safīd Dasht, Iran 97 C6 33 27N 48 11 E
Safīd Kūh, Afghan. 91 B1 34 45N 63 0 E
Safīd Rūd →, Iran 97 B6 37 23N 50 11 E
Safipur, India 93 F9 26 44N 80 21 E
Safonovo, Russia 58 E7 55 4N 33 16 E
Safranbolu, Turkey 100 B5 41 15N 32 41 E
Saft Rashîn, Egypt 106 J7 28 58N 30 55 E
Safune, Samoa 133 W23 13 25 S 172 21W
Şafwān, Iraq 96 D5 30 7N 47 43 E
Sag Harbor, U.S.A. 151 F12 41 0N 72 18W
Sag Sag, Papua N. G. 132 C5 5 32 S 148 23 E
Saga, Indonesia 83 B4 2 40 S 132 55 E
Saga, Kōchi, Japan 72 D5 33 5N 133 6 E
Saga, Saga, Japan 72 D2 33 15N 130 16 E
Saga □, Japan 72 D2 33 15N 130 20 E
Sagae, Japan 70 E10 38 22N 140 17 E
Sagaing, Burma 90 E5 21 52N 95 59 E
Sagaing □, Burma 90 D5 23 55N 95 56 E
Sagala, Mali 112 C3 14 9N 6 38W
Sagami-Nada, Japan 73 C11 34 58N 139 30 E
Sagami-Wan, Japan 73 B11 35 15N 139 25 E
Sagamihara, Japan 73 B11 35 33N 139 25 E
Sagamore, U.S.A. 150 F5 40 46N 79 14W
Sagan = Żagań, Poland 55 G2 51 39N 15 22 E
Saganaga L., Canada 154 A9 48 14N 90 52W
Saganoseki, Japan 72 D3 33 15N 131 53 E
Sagar, Karnataka, India 94 F3 16 38N 76 48 E
Sagar, Karnataka, India 95 G2 14 14N 75 6 E
Sagar, Mad. P., India 93 H8 23 50N 78 44 E
Sagara, Japan 73 C10 34 41N 138 12 E
Sagara, L., Tanzania 118 D3 5 20 S 31 0 E
Sagarmatha = Everest, Mt., Nepal 93 E12 28 5N 86 58 E
Sagarmatha △, Nepal 93 F12 27 55N 86 45 E
Sagavanirktok →, U.S.A. 144 A11 70 19N 147 53W
Sagay, Phil. 81 F4 10 57N 123 25 E
Saginaw, U.S.A. 148 D4 43 26N 83 56W
Saginaw B., U.S.A. 148 D4 43 50N 83 40W
Sagleipie, Liberia 112 D3 7 0N 8 52W
Saglouc = Salluit, Canada 139 B12 62 14N 75 38W
Sagŏ-ri, S. Korea 75 G14 35 25N 126 49 E
Sagone, France 29 F12 42 7N 8 42 E
Sagone, G. de, France 29 F12 42 4N 8 40 E
Sagres, Portugal 43 J2 37 0N 8 58W
Sagu, Burma 90 E5 20 13N 94 46 E
Sagua la Grande, Cuba 164 B3 22 50N 80 10W
Saguache, U.S.A. 159 G10 38 5N 106 8W
Saguaro △, U.S.A. 159 K8 32 12N 110 38W
Saguenay →, Canada 141 C5 48 22N 71 0W
Saguia el Hamra →, W. Sahara 110 C2 27 24N 13 43W
Sagunt, Spain 40 F4 39 42N 0 18W
Sagunto = Sagunt, Spain 40 F4 39 42N 0 18W
Sagvåg, Norway 18 E2 59 46N 5 25 E
Sagwara, India 92 H6 23 41N 74 1 E
Sahaba, Sudan 106 D3 18 57N 30 25 E
Sahagún, Colombia 168 B2 8 57N 75 27W
Sahagún, Spain 42 C5 42 18N 5 2W
Saḩam al Jawlān, Syria 103 C4 32 45N 35 55 E
Sahamandrevo, Madag. 117 C8 23 15 S 45 35 E
Sahand, Kūh-e, Iran 101 D12 37 44N 46 27 E
Sahara, Africa 104 D4 23 0N 5 0 E
Saharan Atlas = Saharien, Atlas, Algeria 111 B5 33 30N 1 0 E
Saharanpur, India 92 E7 29 58N 77 33 E
Saharien, Atlas, Algeria 111 B5 33 30N 1 0 E
Saharsa, India 93 G12 25 53N 86 36 E
Sahasinaka, Madag. 117 C8 21 49 S 47 49 E
Sahaswan, India 93 E8 28 5N 78 45 E
Sahel, Africa 104 E3 12 0N 0 0 E
Sahel, Canal du, Mali 112 C3 14 20N 6 0W
Sahibganj, India 93 G12 25 12N 87 40 E
Şāḩīlīyah, Iraq 101 F10 33 43N 42 42 E
Sahiwal, Pakistan 91 C4 30 45N 73 8 E
Şaḩneh, Iran 101 E12 34 29N 47 41 E
Sahrawi = Western Sahara ■, Africa 110 D2 25 0N 13 0W
Sahrawi = Western Sahara ■, Africa 110 D2 25 0N 13 0W
Sahuaripa, Mexico 162 B3 29 0N 109 13W
Sahuarita, U.S.A. 159 L8 31 57N 110 58W
Sahuayo, Mexico 162 C4 20 4N 102 43W
Šahy, Slovak Rep. 35 C11 48 4N 18 55 E
Sai →, India 93 G10 25 39N 82 47 E
Sai Buri, Thailand 87 J3 6 43N 101 45 E
Sai-Cinza, Brazil 173 B6 6 17 S 57 42W
Sai Kung, China 69 G11 22 23N 114 16 E
Saibai I., Australia 132 E2 9 25 S 142 40 E
Sa'id Bundas, Sudan 109 G4 8 24N 24 48 E
Saïda, Algeria 111 B5 34 50N 0 11 E
Sa'īdābād = Sīrjān, Iran 97 D7 29 30N 55 45 E
Sa'īdābād, Iran 97 B7 36 8N 54 11 E
Saidaiji, Japan 72 C6 34 39N 134 2 E
Saïdia, Morocco 111 A4 35 5N 2 14W
Sa'īdīyeh, Iran 97 B6 36 20N 48 55 E
Saidor, Papua N. G. 132 C4 5 40 S 146 29 E
Saidpur, Bangla. 90 C2 25 48N 89 0 E
Saidpur, India 93 G10 25 33N 83 11 E
Saidu, Pakistan 93 B5 34 43N 72 24 E
Saignelégier, Switz. 32 B4 47 15N 7 0 E
Saignes, France 28 C6 45 20N 2 31 E
Saigō, Japan 72 A5 36 12N 133 20 E
Saigon = Thanh Pho Ho Chi Minh, Vietnam 87 G6 10 58N 106 40 E
Saijō, Japan 72 D5 33 55N 133 11 E
Saikai △, Japan 72 D1 33 12N 129 36 E
Saikanosy Masoala, Madag. 117 B9 15 45 S 50 10 E
Saikhoa Ghat, India 90 B5 27 50N 95 40 E
Saiki, Japan 72 E3 32 58N 131 51 E
Sailana, India 92 H6 23 28N 74 55 E
Saillans, France 29 D9 44 42N 5 12 E
Sailolof, Indonesia 83 B4 1 15 S 130 46 E
Sailu, India 94 E3 19 28N 76 28 E
Saimaa, Finland 15 F23 61 15N 28 15 E
Saimbeyli, Turkey 100 D7 37 59N 36 6 E
Saimen = Saimaa, Finland 15 F23 61 15N 28 15 E
Şa'in Dezh, Iran 101 D12 36 40N 46 25 E
St. Abb's Head, U.K. 22 F6 55 55N 2 8W
St-Affrique, France 28 E6 43 57N 2 53 E
St-Agrève, France 29 C8 45 0N 4 23 E
St-Aignan, France 26 E8 47 16N 1 22 E
St. Alban's, Canada 141 C8 47 51N 55 50W
St. Albans, U.K. 21 F7 51 45N 0 19W
St. Albans, Vt., U.S.A. 151 B11 44 49N 73 5W
St. Albans, W. Va., U.S.A. 148 F5 38 23N 81 50W
St. Alban's Head, U.K. 21 G5 50 34N 2 4W
St. Albert, Canada 142 C6 53 37N 113 32W
St-Amand-en-Puisaye, France 27 E10 47 32N 3 5 E
St-Amand-les-Eaux, France 27 B10 50 27N 3 25 E
St-Amand-Montrond, France 27 F9 46 43N 2 30 E
St-Amarin, France 27 E14 47 54N 7 2 E
St-Amour, France 27 F12 46 26N 5 21 E
St-André, Réunion 121 c 20 57 S 55 39 E
St-André-de-Cubzac, France 28 D3 44 59N 0 26W
St-André-les-Alpes, France 29 E10 43 58N 6 30 E
St. Andrew Sd., U.S.A. 152 E8 31 0N 81 25W
St. Andrew's, Canada 141 C8 47 45N 59 15W
St. Andrews, N.Z. 131 E6 44 33 S 171 10 E
St. Andrews, U.K. 22 E6 56 20N 2 47W
St. Andrews, U.S.A. 152 C9 32 47N 80 0W
St-Anicet, Canada 151 A10 45 8N 74 22W
St. Anne, U.S.A. 157 C9 41 1N 87 43W
St. Anns B., Canada 141 C7 46 22N 60 25W
St. Ann's Bay, Jamaica 164 a 18 26N 77 12W
St. Anthony, Canada 141 B8 51 22N 55 35W
St. Anthony, U.S.A. 158 E8 43 58N 111 41W
St-Antoine, Canada 141 C7 46 22N 64 45W
St. Anton am Arlberg, Austria 33 B10 47 8N 10 16 E
St-Antonin-Noble-Val, France 28 D5 44 10N 1 45 E
St. Arnaud = El Eulma, Algeria 111 A6 36 9N 5 42 E
St. Arnaud, Australia 128 D5 36 40 S 143 16 E
St. Arnaud Ra., N.Z. 131 C7 42 1 S 172 53 E
St-Astier, France 28 C4 45 8N 0 31 E
St-Aubin, Switz. 32 C3 46 54N 6 47 E
St-Aubin-du-Cormier, France 26 D5 48 15N 1 26W
St-Augustin, Canada 141 B8 51 13N 58 38W
St-Augustin →, Canada 141 B8 51 16N 58 40W
St. Augustine, U.S.A. 152 F8 29 54N 81 19W
St. Augustine Beach, U.S.A. 152 F8 29 51N 81 16W
St-Aulaye, France 28 C4 45 12N 0 9 E
St. Austell, U.K. 21 G3 50 20N 4 47W
St-Avold, France 27 C13 49 6N 6 43 E
St. Barbe, Canada 141 B8 51 12N 56 46W
St-Barthélemy, W. Indies 165 C7 17 50N 62 50W
St. Bathans, N.Z. 131 E4 44 53 S 169 50 E
St. Bathan's, Mt., N.Z. 131 E4 44 45 S 169 45 E
St-Béat, France 28 F4 42 55N 0 41 E
St. Bees Hd., U.K. 20 C4 54 31N 3 38W
St. Bees I., Australia 126 J7 20 56 S 149 26 E
St-Benoît, Réunion 121 c 21 2 S 55 43 E
St-Benoît-du-Sault, France 28 B5 46 26N 1 24 E
St-Bernard, Col du Grand, Europe 32 E4 45 53N 7 11 E
St-Blaise, Switz. 32 B3 47 1N 6 59 E
St-Bonnet-en-Champsaur, France 29 D10 44 40N 6 5 E
St-Brevin-les-Pins, France 26 E4 47 14N 2 10W
St-Brice-en-Coglès, France 26 D5 48 25N 1 22W
St. Bride's, Canada 141 C9 46 56N 54 10W
St. Brides B., U.K. 21 F2 51 49N 5 9W
St-Brieuc, France 26 D4 48 30N 2 46W
St-Calais, France 26 E7 47 55N 0 45 E
St-Cast-le-Guildo, France 26 D4 48 37N 2 18W
St. Catharines, Canada 140 D4 43 10N 79 15W
St. Catherine Pt., Bermuda 9 a 32 23N 64 40W
St. Catherines I., U.S.A. 152 D8 31 40N 81 10W
St. Catherine's Pt., U.K. 21 G6 50 34N 1 18W
St-Céré, France 28 D5 44 51N 1 54 E
St-Cergue, Switz. 32 D2 46 27N 6 10 E
St-Cernin, France 28 C6 45 5N 2 25 E
St-Chamond, France 29 C8 45 28N 4 31 E
St. Charles, Ill., U.S.A. 157 C8 41 54N 88 19W
St. Charles, Md., U.S.A. 148 F7 38 36N 76 56W
St. Charles, Mo., U.S.A. 156 F6 38 47N 90 29W
St-Chély-d'Apcher, France 28 D7 44 48N 3 17 E
St-Chinian, France 28 E6 43 25N 2 56 E
St. Christopher-Nevis = St. Kitts & Nevis ■, W. Indies 165 C7 17 20N 62 40W
St-Ciers-sur-Gironde, France 28 C3 45 17N 0 37W
St. Clair, Ga., U.S.A. 152 B7 33 9N 82 13W
St. Clair, Mich., U.S.A. 150 D2 42 50N 82 30W
St. Clair, Mo., U.S.A. 156 F6 38 21N 90 59W
St. Clair, Pa., U.S.A. 151 F8 40 43N 76 12W
St. Clair →, U.S.A. 150 D2 42 38N 82 31W
St. Clair, L., Australia 128 D3 37 20 S 139 55 E
St. Clair, L., Canada 140 D3 42 30N 82 45W
St. Clair, L., U.S.A. 150 D2 42 27N 82 39W
St. Clair Shores, U.S.A. 157 B14 42 30N 82 53W
St. Clairsville, U.S.A. 150 F4 40 5N 80 54W
St-Claud, France 28 C4 45 54N 0 28 E
St. Claude, Canada 143 D9 49 40N 98 20W
St-Claude, France 27 F12 46 22N 5 52 E
St. Clears, U.K. 21 F3 51 49N 4 31W
St-Clet, Canada 151 A10 45 21N 74 13W
St. Cloud, Fla., U.S.A. 153 G8 28 15N 81 17W
St. Cloud, Minn., U.S.A. 154 C7 45 34N 94 10W
St. Cricq, C., Australia 125 E1 25 17 S 113 6 E
St. Croix, U.S. Virgin Is. 165 C7 17 45N 64 45W
St. Croix →, U.S.A. 154 C8 44 45N 92 48W
St. Croix Falls, U.S.A. 154 C8 45 24N 92 38W
St-Cyprien, France 28 F7 42 37N 3 2 E
St-Cyr-sur-Mer, France 29 E9 43 11N 5 43 E
St. David, U.S.A. 156 D6 40 30N 90 3W
St. David's, Canada 141 C8 48 12N 58 52W
St. David's, U.K. 21 F2 51 53N 5 16W
St. David's Head, U.K. 21 F2 51 54N 5 19W
St. David's I., Bermuda 9 a 32 21N 64 39W
St-Denis = Sig, Algeria 111 A4 35 32N 0 12W
St-Denis, France 27 D9 48 56N 2 22 E
St-Denis, Réunion 121 c 20 52 S 55 27 E
St-Denis ✈ (RUN), Réunion 121 c 20 53 S 55 32 E
St-Dié, France 27 D13 48 17N 6 56 E
St-Dizier, France 27 D11 48 38N 4 56 E
St-Égrève, France 29 C9 45 14N 5 41 E
St. Elias, Mt., U.S.A. 144 F12 60 18N 140 56W
St. Elias Mts., N. Amer. 142 A1 60 33N 139 28W
St-Élie, Fr. Guiana 169 C7 4 49N 53 17W
St. Elmo, U.S.A. 157 E8 39 2N 88 51W
St-Eloy-les-Mines, France 27 F9 46 10N 2 51 E
St-Émilion, France 28 D3 44 53N 0 9W
St-Étienne, France 29 C8 45 27N 4 22 E
St-Étienne-de-Tinée, France 29 D10 44 16N 6 56 E
St-Étienne-du-Rouvray, France 26 C8 49 23N 1 6 E
St. Eugène, Canada 151 A10 45 30N 74 28W
St. Eustatius, W. Indies 165 C7 17 20N 63 0W
St-Exupery, Lyon ✈ (LYS), France 29 C9 45 44N 5 2 E
St-Fargeau, France 27 E10 47 39N 3 4 E
St-Félicien, Canada 140 C5 48 40N 72 25W
St. Ferdinand = Florissant, U.S.A. 156 F6 38 48N 90 20W
St-Florent, France 29 F13 42 41N 9 18 E
St-Florent, G. de, France 29 F13 42 47N 9 12 E
St-Florent-sur-Cher, France 27 F9 46 59N 2 15 E
St-Florentin, France 27 E10 48 0N 3 45 E
St-Flour, France 28 C7 45 2N 3 6 E
St. Francis, U.S.A. 154 F4 39 47N 101 48W
St. Francis →, U.S.A. 155 H9 34 38N 90 36W
St. Francis, C., S. Africa 116 E3 34 14 S 24 49 E
St. Francisville, Ill., U.S.A. 157 F9 38 36N 87 39W
St. Francisville, La., U.S.A. 155 K9 30 47N 91 23W
St-François, L., Canada 151 A10 45 10N 74 22W
St-Fulgent, France 26 F5 46 50N 1 10W
St-Gabriel, Canada 140 C5 46 17N 73 24W
St. Gallen = Sankt Gallen, Switz. 33 B8 47 26N 9 22 E
St. Gallenkirch, Austria 33 B9 47 1N 9 58 E
St-Galmier, France 27 G11 45 35N 4 19 E
St-Gaudens, France 28 E4 43 6N 0 44 E
St-Gaultier, France 26 F8 46 39N 1 26 E
St-Gengoux-le-National, France 27 F11 46 37N 4 40 E
St-Geniez-d'Olt, France 28 D6 44 27N 2 58 E
St. George, Australia 127 D4 28 1 S 148 30 E
St. George, Bermuda 9 a 32 22N 64 40W
St. George, Canada 141 C6 45 11N 66 50W
St. George, Ga., U.S.A. 152 E7 30 31N 82 2W
St. George, S.C., U.S.A. 152 B9 33 11N 80 35W
St. George, Utah, U.S.A. 159 H7 37 6N 113 35W
St. George, C., Canada 141 C8 48 30N 59 16W
St. George, C., Papua N. G. 132 C7 4 49 S 152 53 E
St. George, C., U.S.A. 152 F4 29 40N 85 5W
St. George I., Alaska, U.S.A. 144 H5 56 35N 169 35W
St. George I., Fla., U.S.A. 152 F5 29 35N 84 55W
St. George Ra., Australia 124 C4 18 40 S 125 0 E
St. George's, Canada 141 C8 48 26N 58 31W
St-Georges, Canada 141 C5 46 8N 70 40W
St-Georges, Fr. Guiana 169 C7 3 53N 51 50W
St. George's, Grenada 165 D7 12 5N 61 43W
St. George's B., Canada 141 C8 48 24N 58 53W
St. Georges Basin, N.S.W., Australia 129 C9 35 7 S 150 36 E
St. Georges Basin, W. Austral., Australia 124 C4 15 23 S 125 2 E
St. George's Channel, Europe 23 E6 52 0N 6 0W
St. George's Channel, India 95 L11 7 15N 93 43 E
St. George's Channel, Papua N. G. 132 C7 4 10 S 152 20 E
St. Georges Hd., Australia 129 C9 35 12 S 150 42 E
St. Georges I., Bermuda 9 a 32 23N 64 40W
St-Georges-lès-Baillargeaux, France 28 B4 46 41N 0 22 E
St-Germain-de-Calberte, France 28 D7 44 13N 3 48 E
St-Germain-en-Laye, France 27 D9 48 54N 2 6 E
St-Germain-Lembron, France 28 C7 45 27N 3 14 E
St-Gervais-d'Auvergne, France 27 F9 46 4N 2 50 E
St-Gervais-les-Bains, France 29 C10 45 53N 6 42 E
St-Gildas, Pte. de, France 26 E4 47 8N 2 14W
St-Gilles, France 29 E8 43 40N 4 26 E
St-Gingolph, Switz. 32 D3 46 24N 6 48 E
St-Girons, Ariège, France 28 F5 42 59N 1 8 E
St-Girons, Landes, France 28 E2 43 56N 1 18W
St. Gotthard P. = San Gottardo, P. del, Switz. 33 C7 46 33N 8 33 E
St. Helena, Atl. Oc. 9 h 15 58 S 5 42W
St. Helena, U.S.A. 158 G2 38 30N 122 28W
St. Helena, Mt., U.S.A. 160 G4 38 40N 122 36W
St. Helena B., S. Africa 116 E2 32 40 S 18 10 E
St. Helena Sd., U.S.A. 152 C9 32 15N 80 25W
St. Helens, Australia 127 G4 41 20 S 148 15 E

St. Helens, U.K. 20 D5 53 27N 2 44W
St. Helens, U.S.A. 160 E4 45 52N 122 48W
St. Helens, Mt., U.S.A. 160 D4 46 12N 122 12W
St. Helier, U.K. 21 H5 49 10N 2 7W
St-Herblain, France 26 E5 47 13N 1 40W
St-Hilaire-du-Harcouët, France 26 D5 48 35N 1 5W
St-Hippolyte, France 27 E13 47 19N 6 50 E
St-Hippolyte-du-Fort, France 28 E7 43 58N 3 52 E
St-Honoré-les-Bains, France 27 F10 46 54N 3 50 E
St-Hubert, Belgium 24 D5 50 2N 5 23 E
St-Hyacinthe, Canada 140 C5 45 40N 72 58W
St. Ignace, U.S.A. 148 C3 45 52N 84 44W
St. Ignace I., Canada 140 C2 48 45N 88 0W
St. Ignatius, U.S.A. 158 C6 47 19N 114 6W
St-Imier, Switz. 32 B3 47 9N 6 58 E
St. Ives, Cambs., U.K. 21 E7 52 20N 0 4W
St. Ives, Corn., U.K. 21 G2 50 12N 5 30W
St-James, France 26 D5 48 31N 1 20W
St. James, Minn., U.S.A. 154 D7 43 59N 94 38W
St. James, Mo., U.S.A. 156 G5 38 0N 91 37W
St-Jean →, Canada 141 B7 50 17N 64 20W
St-Jean, L., Canada 141 C5 48 40N 72 0W
St-Jean-d'Angély, France 28 C3 45 57N 0 31W
St-Jean-de-Braye, France 27 E8 47 53N 1 58 E
St-Jean-de-Luz, France 28 E2 43 23N 1 39W
St-Jean-de-Maurienne, France 29 C10 45 16N 6 21 E
St-Jean-de-Monts, France 26 F4 46 47N 2 4W
St-Jean-du-Gard, France 28 D7 44 7N 3 52 E
St-Jean-en-Royans, France 29 C9 45 1N 5 18 E
St-Jean-Pied-de-Port, France 28 E2 43 10N 1 14W
St-Jean-Port-Joli, Canada 141 C5 47 15N 70 13W
St-Jean-sur-Richelieu, Canada 140 C5 45 20N 73 20W
St-Jérôme, Canada 140 C5 45 47N 74 0W
St. Joe, U.S.A. 157 C12 41 19N 84 54W
St. John, Canada 141 C6 45 20N 66 8W
St. John, U.S.A. 155 G5 38 0N 98 46W
St. John →, Liberia 112 D2 6 40N 9 10W
St. John →, U.S.A. 149 C12 45 12N 66 5W
St. John, C., Canada 141 C8 50 0N 55 32W
St. John I., U.S. Virgin Is. 165 e 18 20N 64 42W
St. John's, Antigua & B. 165 C7 17 6N 61 51W
St. John's, Canada 141 C9 47 35N 52 40W
St. Johns, Ariz., U.S.A. 159 J9 34 30N 109 22W
St. Johns, Mich., U.S.A. 157 B12 43 0N 84 33W
St. Johns →, U.S.A. 152 E8 30 24N 81 24W
St. John's Pt., Ireland 23 B3 54 34N 8 27W
St. Johnsbury, U.S.A. 151 B12 44 25N 72 1W
St. Johnsville, U.S.A. 151 D10 43 0N 74 43W
St-Joseph, Martinique 164 c 14 39N 61 4W
St-Joseph, N. Cal. 133 K4 20 27 S 166 36 E
St-Joseph, Réunion 121 c 21 22 S 55 37 E
St. Joseph, Ill., U.S.A. 157 D8 40 7N 88 2W
St. Joseph, La., U.S.A. 155 K9 31 55N 91 14W
St. Joseph, Mich., U.S.A. 157 B10 42 6N 86 29W
St. Joseph, Mo., U.S.A. 156 E2 39 46N 94 50W
St. Joseph →, U.S.A. 157 B10 42 7N 86 29W
St. Joseph, I., Canada 140 C3 46 12N 83 58W
St. Joseph, L., Canada 140 B1 51 10N 90 35W
St. Joseph Pt., U.S.A. 152 F4 29 52N 85 24W
St-Jovite, Canada 140 C5 46 8N 74 38W
St-Juéry, France 28 E6 43 57N 2 12 E
St. Julian's, Malta 38 F7 35 55N 14 29 E
St-Julien-Chapteuil, France 29 C8 45 2N 4 4 E
St-Julien-de-Vouvantes, France 26 E5 47 38N 1 13W
St-Julien-en-Genevois, France 27 F13 46 9N 6 5 E
St-Junien, France 28 C4 45 53N 0 55 E
St-Just-en-Chaussée, France 27 C9 49 30N 2 25 E
St-Just-en-Chevalet, France 28 C7 45 55N 3 50 E
St. Kilda, N.Z. 131 F5 45 53 S 170 31 E
St. Kilda, U.K. 19 C2 57 49N 8 34W
St. Kitts & Nevis ■, W. Indies 165 C7 17 20N 62 40W
St. Laurent, Canada 143 C9 50 25N 97 58W
St-Laurent, Fr. Guiana 169 B7 5 29N 54 3W
St-Laurent-de-la-Salanque, France 28 F6 42 46N 2 59 E
St-Laurent-du-Pont, France 29 C9 45 23N 5 45 E
St-Laurent-en-Grandvaux, France 27 F12 46 35N 5 58 E
St-Laurent-Médoc, France 28 C3 45 8N 0 49W
St. Lawrence, Australia 126 C4 22 16 S 149 31 E
St. Lawrence, Canada 141 C8 46 54N 55 23W
St. Lawrence →, Canada 141 C6 49 30N 66 0W
St. Lawrence, Gulf of, Canada 141 C7 48 25N 62 0W
St. Lawrence I., U.S.A. 144 E5 63 30N 170 30W
St. Lawrence Islands △, Canada 151 B9 44 27N 75 52W
St. Leonard, Canada 141 C6 47 12N 67 58W
St-Léonard-de-Noblat, France 28 C5 45 49N 1 29 E
St. Leonhard im Pitztal, Austria 33 B11 47 4N 10 51 E
St-Leu, Réunion 121 c 21 9 S 55 18 E
St. Lewis →, Canada 141 B8 52 26N 56 11W
St-Lô, France 26 C5 49 7N 1 5W
St-Louis, France 27 E14 47 30N 7 34 E
St-Louis, Guadeloupe 164 b 15 56N 61 19W
St-Louis, Réunion 121 c 21 16 S 55 25 E
St. Louis, Senegal 112 B1 16 8N 16 27W
St. Louis, U.S.A. 156 F6 38 37N 90 12W
St. Louis →, U.S.A. 154 B8 47 15N 92 45W
St. Louis Lambert International ✕ (STL), U.S.A. 156 F6 38 45N 90 22W
St-Loup-sur-Semouse, France 27 E13 47 53N 6 16 E
St. Lucia ■, W. Indies 165 f 14 0N 60 57W
St. Lucia, L., S. Africa 117 D5 28 5 S 32 30 E
St. Lucia Channel, W. Indies 165 D7 14 15N 61 0W
St. Lucie, U.S.A. 153 H9 27 29N 80 20W
St. Lucie Canal, U.S.A. 153 H9 27 10N 80 18W
St. Maarten ⊠, W. Indies 165 C7 18 0N 63 5W
St. Magnus B., U.K. 22 A7 60 25N 1 35W
St-Maixent-l'École, France 28 B3 46 24N 0 12W
St-Malo, France 26 D4 48 39N 2 1W
St-Malo, G. de, France 26 D4 48 50N 2 30W
St-Mandrier-sur-Mer, France 29 E9 43 4N 5 57 E
St-Marc, Haiti 165 C5 19 10N 72 41W
St-Marcellin, France 29 C9 45 9N 5 20 E
St-Marcouf, Îs., France 26 C5 49 30N 1 10W
St. Maries, U.S.A. 158 C5 47 19N 116 35W
St. Marks, U.S.A. 152 E5 30 9N 84 12W
St-Martin ⊠, W. Indies 165 C7 18 0N 63 0W
St-Martin, C., Martinique 164 c 14 52N 61 14W
St. Martin, L., Canada 143 C9 51 40N 98 30W
St-Martin-de-Crau, France 29 E8 43 38N 4 48 E
St-Martin-de-Ré, France 28 B2 46 12N 1 21W
St-Martin-d'Hères, France 29 C9 45 9N 5 45 E
St-Martin-Vésubie, France 29 D11 44 4N 7 15 E
St. Martins, Barbados 165 g 13 5N 59 28W
St-Martory, France 28 E4 43 9N 0 56 E
St. Mary, U.S.A. 156 G7 37 53N 89 57W
St. Mary, Mt., Papua N. G. 132 E4 8 8 S 147 2 E
St. Mary Is., India 95 H2 13 20N 74 35 E
St. Mary Pk., Australia 128 A3 31 32 S 138 34 E
St. Marys, Australia 127 G4 41 35 S 148 11 E
St. Marys, Canada 150 C3 43 20N 81 10W
St. Mary's, Corn., U.K. 21 H1 49 55N 6 18W
St. Mary's, Orkney, U.K. 22 C6 58 54N 2 54W
St. Mary's, Alaska, U.S.A. 144 E7 62 4N 163 10W
St. Marys, Ga., U.S.A. 152 E8 30 44N 81 33W
St. Marys, Ohio, U.S.A. 157 D12 40 33N 84 24W
St. Marys, Pa., U.S.A. 150 E6 41 26N 78 34W
St. Marys →, U.S.A. 152 E8 30 43N 81 27W
St. Mary's, C., Canada 141 C9 46 50N 54 12W
St. Mary's B., Canada 141 C9 46 50N 53 50W
St. Marys Bay, Canada 141 D6 44 25N 66 10W
St-Mathieu, Pte., France 26 D2 48 20N 4 45W
St. Matthew I., U.S.A. 144 F4 60 24N 172 42W
St. Matthews, Ky., U.S.A. 157 F11 38 15N 85 39W
St. Matthews, S.C., U.S.A. 152 B9 33 40N 80 46W
St. Matthews, I. = Zadetkyi Kyun, Burma 87 G2 10 0N 98 25 E
St. Matthias Group, Papua N. G. 132 A5 1 30 S 150 0 E
St-Maurice, Switz. 32 D4 46 13N 7 0 E
St-Maurice →, Canada 140 C5 46 21N 72 31W
St. Mawes, U.K. 21 G2 50 10N 5 2W
St-Maximin-la-Ste-Baume, France 29 E9 43 27N 5 52 E
St-Médard-en-Jalles, France 28 D3 44 53N 0 43W
St-Méen-le-Grand, France 26 D4 48 11N 2 12W
St. Meinrad, U.S.A. 157 F10 38 10N 86 49W
St. Michael, U.S.A. 144 E7 63 29N 162 2W
St-Mihiel, France 27 D12 48 54N 5 32 E
St. Moritz, Switz. 31 J5 46 30N 9 51 E
St-Nazaire, France 26 E4 47 17N 2 12W
St. Neots, U.K. 21 E7 52 14N 0 15W
St-Nicolas-de-Port, France 27 D13 48 38N 6 18 E
St-Niklaas, Belgium 24 C4 51 10N 4 8 E
St. Niklaus, Switz. 32 D5 46 10N 7 49 E
St-Omer, France 27 B9 50 45N 2 15 E
St-Palais-sur-Mer, France 28 C2 45 38N 1 5W
St-Pamphile, Canada 141 C6 46 58N 69 48W
St-Pardoux-la-Rivière, France 28 C4 45 29N 0 45 E
St. Paris, U.S.A. 157 D13 40 8N 83 58W
St-Pascal, Canada 141 C6 47 32N 69 48W
St. Paul, Canada 142 C6 54 0N 111 17W
St-Paul, France 29 D10 44 31N 6 45 E
St-Paul, Réunion 121 c 20 59 S 55 17 E
St. Paul, Alaska, U.S.A. 144 H5 57 7N 170 17W
St. Paul, Ind., U.S.A. 157 E11 39 26N 85 38W
St. Paul, Minn., U.S.A. 154 C8 44 57N 93 6W
St. Paul, Nebr., U.S.A. 154 E5 41 13N 98 27W
St-Paul →, Canada 141 B8 51 27N 57 42W
St. Paul →, Liberia 112 D2 6 25N 10 48W
St. Paul, I., Ind. Oc. 121 H6 38 55 S 77 34 E
St-Paul-de-Fenouillet, France 28 F6 42 48N 2 30 E
St. Paul I., Canada 141 C7 47 12N 60 9W
St. Paul I., U.S.A. 144 H5 57 10N 170 15W
St-Paul-lès-Dax, France 28 E2 43 44N 1 3W
St. Paul Subterranean River △, Phil. 81 F2 10 10N 118 55 E
St. Paul's Bay, Malta 38 F7 35 57N 14 24 E
St-Péray, France 29 D8 44 57N 4 50 E
St. Peter, U.S.A. 154 C8 44 20N 93 57W
St-Peter-Ording, Germany 30 A4 54 20N 8 36 E
St. Peter Port, U.K. 21 H5 49 26N 2 33W
St. Peters, N.S., Canada 141 C7 45 40N 60 53W
St. Peters, P.E.I., Canada 141 C7 46 25N 62 35W
St. Petersburg = Sankt-Peterburg, Russia 58 C6 59 55N 30 20 E
St. Petersburg, U.S.A. 153 H7 27 46N 82 39W
St. Petersburg Beach, U.S.A. 153 H7 27 45N 82 45W
St-Philbert-de-Grand-Lieu, France 26 E5 47 2N 1 39W
St-Phillippe, Réunion 121 c 21 21 S 55 44 E
St-Pie, Canada 151 A12 45 30N 72 54W
St-Pierre, Martinique 164 c 14 45N 61 10W
St-Pierre, Réunion 121 c 21 19 S 55 28 E
St-Pierre, St-P. & M. 141 C8 46 46N 56 12W
St. Pierre, Seychelles 121 E3 9 20 S 46 0 E
St-Pierre, L., Canada 140 C5 46 12N 72 52W
St-Pierre-de-la-Pointe-aux-Esquimaux = Havre-St.-Pierre, Canada 141 B7 50 18N 63 33W
St-Pierre-d'Oléron, France 28 C2 45 57N 1 19W
St-Pierre-en-Port, France 26 C7 49 48N 0 30 E
St-Pierre-et-Miquelon ⊠, N. Amer. 141 C8 46 55N 56 10W
St-Pierre-le-Moûtier, France 27 F10 46 47N 3 7 E
St-Pierre-sur-Dives, France 26 C6 49 2N 0 1W
St-Pol-de-Léon, France 26 D3 48 41N 4 0W
St-Pol-sur-Mer, France 27 A9 51 1N 2 20 E
St-Pol-sur-Ternoise, France 27 B9 50 23N 2 20 E
St-Pons, France 28 E6 43 30N 2 45 E
St-Pourçain-sur-Sioule, France 27 F10 46 18N 3 18 E
St-Priest, France 29 C8 45 42N 4 57 E
St-Quay-Portrieux, France 26 D4 48 39N 2 51W
St-Quentin, Canada 141 C6 47 30N 67 23W
St-Quentin, France 27 C10 49 50N 3 16 E
St-Rambert-d'Albon, France 29 C8 45 17N 4 49 E
St-Raphaël, France 29 E10 43 25N 6 46 E
St. Regis, U.S.A. 158 C6 47 18N 115 6W
St-Renan, France 26 D2 48 26N 4 37W
St. Robert, U.S.A. 156 G4 37 48N 92 9W
St-Saëns, France 26 C8 49 41N 1 16 E
St-Savin, France 28 B4 46 34N 0 53 E
St-Savinien, France 28 C3 45 53N 0 42W
St. Sebastien, Tanjon' i, Madag. 117 A8 12 26 S 48 44 E
St-Seine-l'Abbaye, France 27 E11 47 26N 4 47 E
St-Sernin-sur-Rance, France 28 E6 43 54N 2 35 E
St-Sever, France 28 E3 43 45N 0 35W
St-Siméon, Canada 141 C6 47 51N 69 54W
St. Simons I., U.S.A. 152 D8 31 12N 81 15W
St. Simons Island, U.S.A. 149 K5 31 9N 81 22W
St. Stephen, Canada 141 C6 45 16N 67 17W
St. Stephen, U.S.A. 152 B10 33 24N 79 55W
St-Sulpice, France 28 E5 43 46N 1 41 E
St-Sulpice-Laurière, France 28 B5 46 3N 1 29 E
St-Sulpice-les-Feuilles, France 28 B5 46 19N 1 21 E
St-Syprien = St-Cyprien, France 28 F7 42 37N 3 2 E
St. Teresa, U.S.A. 152 F5 29 55N 84 27W
St-Thégonnec, France 26 D3 48 31N 3 57W
St. Thomas = Charlotte Amalie, U.S. Virgin Is. 165 e 18 21N 64 56W
St. Thomas, Canada 140 D3 42 45N 81 10W
St. Thomas Bay, Malta 38 F8 35 51N 14 34 E
St. Thomas I., U.S. Virgin Is. 165 e 18 20N 64 55W
St-Tite, Canada 140 C5 46 45N 72 34W
St-Tropez, France 29 E10 43 17N 6 38 E
St-Troud = St. Truiden, Belgium 24 D5 50 48N 5 10 E
St. Truiden, Belgium 24 D5 50 48N 5 10 E
St-Vaast-la-Hougue, France 26 C5 49 35N 1 17W
St-Valery-en-Caux, France 26 C7 49 52N 0 43 E
St-Valéry-sur-Somme, France 27 B8 50 11N 1 38 E
St-Vallier, France 27 F11 46 38N 4 22 E
St-Vallier-de-Thiey, France 29 E10 43 42N 6 51 E
St-Varent, France 26 F6 46 53N 0 13W
St-Vaury, France 28 B5 46 12N 1 46 E
St. Vincent = São Vicente, C. Verde Is. 9 j 17 0N 25 0W
St. Vincent, Italy 44 C4 45 45N 7 39 E
St. Vincent, G., Australia 128 C3 35 0 S 138 0 E
St. Vincent & the Grenadines ■, W. Indies 165 D7 13 0N 61 10W
St-Vincent-de-Tyrosse, France 28 E2 43 39N 1 19W
St. Vincent I., U.S.A. 153 F4 29 42N 85 3W
St. Vincent Passage, W. Indies 165 D7 13 30N 61 0W
St-Vith, Belgium 24 D6 50 17N 6 9 E
St-Vivien-de-Médoc, France 28 C2 45 25N 1 2W
St. Walburg, Canada 143 C7 53 39N 109 12W
St-Yrieix-la-Perche, France 28 C5 45 31N 1 12 E
Saintala, India 94 D6 20 26N 83 20 E
Ste-Adresse, France 26 C7 49 31N 0 5 E
Ste-Agathe-des-Monts, Canada 140 C5 46 3N 74 17W
Ste-Anne, Guadeloupe 164 b 16 13N 61 24W
Ste Anne, Seychelles 121 b 4 36 S 55 1 E
Ste-Anne, L., Canada 141 B6 50 0N 67 42W
Ste-Anne-des-Monts-Tourelle, Canada 141 C6 49 8N 66 30W
Ste-Croix, Switz. 32 C3 46 49N 6 34 E
Ste-Enimie, France 28 D7 44 22N 3 26 E
Ste-Foy-la-Grande, France 28 D4 44 50N 0 13 E
Ste. Genevieve, U.S.A. 156 G6 37 59N 90 2W
Ste-Hermine, France 28 B2 46 32N 1 4W
Ste-Livrade-sur-Lot, France 28 D4 44 24N 0 36 E
Ste-Marguerite →, Canada 141 B6 50 9N 66 36W
Ste-Marie, Canada 141 C5 46 26N 71 0W
Ste. Marie, Gabon 114 C2 3 48 S 11 1 E
Ste-Marie, Martinique 164 c 14 48N 61 1W
Ste-Marie, Réunion 121 c 20 53 S 55 33 E
Ste-Marie-aux-Mines, France 27 D14 48 15N 7 12 E
Ste-Maure-de-Touraine, France 26 E7 47 7N 0 37 E
Ste-Maxime, France 29 E10 43 19N 6 39 E
Ste-Menehould, France 27 C11 49 5N 4 54 E
Ste-Mère-Église, France 26 C5 49 24N 1 19W
Ste-Rose, Guadeloupe 164 b 16 20N 61 45W
Ste-Rose, Réunion 121 c 21 8 S 55 45 E
Ste. Rose du Lac, Canada 143 C9 51 4N 99 30W
Ste-Savine, France 27 D11 48 18N 4 3 E
Ste-Sigolène, France 29 C8 45 15N 4 14 E
Saintes, France 28 C3 45 45N 0 37W
Saintes, Îs. des, Guadeloupe 164 b 15 50N 61 35W
Stes-Maries-de-la-Mer, France 29 E8 43 26N 4 26 E
Saintfield, U.K. 23 B6 54 28N 5 49W
Saintonge, France 28 C3 45 40N 0 50W
Saipan, Pac. Oc. 134 F6 15 12N 145 45 E
Sairang, India 90 D4 23 50N 92 45 E
Sairecábur, Cerro, Bolivia 174 A2 22 43 S 67 54W
Saitama □, Japan 73 A11 36 25N 139 30 E
Saiteli = Kadınhanı, Turkey 100 C5 38 14N 32 13 E
Saiţi, Moldova 53 D14 46 30N 29 24 E
Saito, Japan 72 E3 32 3N 131 24 E
Saiyid, Pakistan 92 C5 33 7N 73 2 E
Saja-Besaya ⌓, Spain 42 B6 43 10N 4 9W
Sajama, Bolivia 172 D4 18 7 S 69 0W
Sajama, Nevado, Bolivia 172 D4 18 6 S 68 54W
Sajan, Serbia & M. 52 E5 45 50N 20 20 E
Sajó →, Hungary 52 C6 47 56N 21 7 E
Sajókazinc = Kazincbarcika, Hungary 52 B5 48 17N 20 36 E
Sajószentpéter, Hungary 52 B5 48 12N 20 44 E
Sajum, India 93 C8 33 20N 79 0 E
Sak →, S. Africa 116 E3 30 52 S 20 25 E
Saka Kalat, Pakistan 91 D2 27 3N 65 3 E
Sakaba, Nigeria 113 C6 11 4N 5 35 E
Sakai, Japan 73 C7 34 30N 135 30 E
Sakaide, Japan 72 C5 34 19N 133 50 E
Sakaiminato, Japan 72 B5 35 38N 133 11 E
Sakākah, Si. Arabia 96 D4 30 0N 40 8 E
Sakakawea, L., U.S.A. 154 B4 47 30N 101 25W
Sakami →, Canada 140 B4 53 40N 76 40W
Sakami, L., Canada 140 B4 53 15N 77 0W
Sâkâne, 'Erg i-n, Mali 113 A4 20 30N 1 30W
Sakania, Dem. Rep. of the Congo 119 E2 12 43 S 28 30 E
Sakar I., Papua N. G. 132 C5 5 25 S 148 6 E
Sakaraha, Madag. 117 C7 22 55 S 44 32 E
Sakartvelo = Georgia ■, Asia 61 J6 42 0N 43 0 E
Sakarya, Turkey 100 B4 40 48N 30 25 E
Sakarya →, Turkey 100 B4 41 7N 30 39 E
Sakashima-Guntō, Japan 71 M2 24 46N 124 0 E
Sakassou, Ivory C. 112 D3 7 29N 5 19W
Sakata, Japan 70 E9 38 55N 139 50 E
Sakawa, Japan 72 D5 33 28N 133 11 E
Sakchu, N. Korea 75 D13 40 23N 125 2 E
Sakeny →, Madag. 117 C8 20 0 S 45 25 E
Sakété, Benin 113 D5 6 40N 2 45 E
Sakha □, Russia 67 C13 66 0N 130 0 E
Sakhalin, Russia 67 D15 51 0N 143 0 E
Sakhalinskiy Zaliv, Russia 67 D15 54 0N 141 0 E
Sakhi Gopal, India 94 E7 19 58N 85 50 E
Şaki, Azerbaijan 61 K8 41 10N 47 5 E
Šakiai, Lithuania 15 J20 54 59N 23 2 E
Sakiz-Adasi = Khíos, Greece 49 C8 38 27N 26 9 E
Sakmara →, Russia 64 F5 51 46N 55 1 E
Sakoli, India 94 D4 21 5N 79 59 E
Sakon Nakhon, Thailand 86 D5 17 10N 104 9 E
Sakrand, Pakistan 92 F3 26 10N 68 15 E
Sakri, Maharashtra, India 93 F12 26 13N 86 5 E
Sakri, Maharashtra, India 94 D2 21 2N 74 20 E
Sakrivier, S. Africa 116 E3 30 54 S 20 28 E
Sakskøbing, Denmark 17 K5 54 49N 11 39 E
Sakti, India 93 H10 22 2N 82 58 E
Saku, Japan 73 A10 36 17N 138 31 E
Sakuma, Japan 73 B9 35 3N 137 49 E
Sakura, Japan 73 B12 35 43N 140 14 E
Sakurai, Japan 73 C7 34 30N 135 51 E
Saky, Ukraine 59 K7 45 9N 33 34 E
Sal →, Russia 61 G5 47 31N 40 45 E
Sal Rei, C. Verde Is. 9 j 16 11N 22 53W
Sala, Eritrea 107 D4 16 53N 37 36 E
Šal'a, Slovak Rep. 35 C10 48 10N 17 50 E
Sala, Sweden 16 E10 59 58N 16 35 E
Sala →, Eritrea 107 D4 16 53N 37 36 E
Sala, O. →, Chad 109 E4 17 0N 20 53 E
Sala Consilina, Italy 47 B8 40 23N 15 36 E
Sala-y-Gómez, Pac. Oc. 135 K17 26 28 S 105 28W
Salaberry-de-Valleyfield, Canada 140 C5 45 15N 74 8W
Salacgrīva, Latvia 54 A11 57 45N 24 21 E
Salada, L., Mexico 159 K6 32 20N 115 40W
Saladas, Argentina 174 B4 28 15 S 58 40W
Saladillo, Argentina 174 D4 35 40 S 59 55W
Salado →, Buenos Aires, Argentina 174 D4 35 44 S 57 22W
Salado →, La Pampa, Argentina 176 A3 37 30 S 67 0W
Salado →, Río Negro, Argentina 176 B3 41 34 S 65 3W
Salado →, Santa Fe, Argentina 174 C3 31 40 S 60 41W
Salado →, Mexico 155 M5 26 52N 99 19W
Salaga, Ghana 113 D4 8 31N 0 31W
Sālah, Syria 103 C5 32 40N 36 45 E
Şalāḩ ad Dīn □, Iraq 96 C4 34 35N 43 35 E
Sălaj □, Romania 52 C8 47 15N 23 0 E
Sálakhos, Greece 38 E11 36 17N 27 57 E
Salal, Chad 109 F3 14 48N 17 12 E
Salala, Liberia 112 D2 6 42N 10 7W
Salala, Sudan 106 C4 21 17N 36 16 E
Salālah, Oman 99 C6 16 56N 53 59 E
Salamanca, Chile 174 C1 31 46 S 70 59W
Salamanca, Spain 42 E5 40 58N 5 39W
Salamanca, U.S.A. 150 D6 42 10N 78 43W
Salamanca □, Spain 42 E5 40 57N 5 40W
Salamat, Bahr →, Chad 109 G3 9 20N 18 0 E
Salāmatābād, Iran 96 C5 35 39N 47 50 E
Salamina = Salamís, Greece 48 D5 37 56N 23 30 E
Salamina, Colombia 168 B2 5 25N 75 29W
Salamis, Cyprus 39 E9 35 11N 33 54 E
Salamís, Greece 48 D5 37 56N 23 30 E
Salamonie L., U.S.A. 157 D11 40 46N 85 37W
Salaóra, Greece 39 A2 39 2N 20 52 E
Salar de Atacama, Chile 174 A2 23 30 S 68 25W
Salar de Uyuni, Bolivia 172 E4 20 30 S 67 45W
Sălard, Romania 52 C7 47 12N 22 3 E
Salas, Spain 42 B4 43 25N 6 15W
Salas de los Infantes, Spain 42 C7 42 2N 3 17W
Salatiga, Indonesia 85 D4 7 19 S 110 30 E
Salavat, Russia 64 E5 53 21N 55 55 E
Salaverry, Peru 172 B2 8 15 S 79 0W
Salawati, Indonesia 83 B4 1 7 S 130 52 E
Salay, Phil. 81 G5 8 52N 124 47 E
Salaya, India 92 H3 22 19N 69 35 E
Salayar, Indonesia 82 C2 6 7 S 120 30 E
Salazar →, Spain 40 C3 42 40N 1 20W
Salbris, France 27 E9 47 25N 2 3 E
Salcedo, Phil. 81 F5 11 9N 125 40 E
Salcia, Romania 53 G9 43 56N 24 55 E
Sălciua, Romania 53 D8 46 24N 23 26 E
Salcombe, U.K. 21 G4 50 14N 3 47W
Saldaña, Spain 42 C6 42 32N 4 48W
Saldanha, S. Africa 116 E2 33 0 S 17 58 E
Saldanha B., S. Africa 116 E2 33 6 S 18 0 E
Saldus, Latvia 15 H20 56 38N 22 30 E
Saldus □, Latvia 54 B9 56 35N 22 30 E
Sale, Australia 129 E7 38 6 S 147 6 E
Sale, Burma 90 E5 20 50N 94 45 E
Sale, Italy 44 D5 44 59N 8 48 E
Salé, Morocco 110 B3 34 3N 6 48W
Sale, U.K. 20 D5 53 26N 2 19W
Sale City, U.S.A. 152 D5 31 16N 84 1W
Salegard = Salekhard, Russia 66 C7 66 30N 66 35 E
Salekhard, Russia 66 C7 66 30N 66 35 E
Salelologa, Samoa 133 W23 13 41 S 172 11W
Salem, India 95 J4 11 40N 78 11 E
Salem, Fla., U.S.A. 152 F6 29 53N 83 25W
Salem, Ill., U.S.A. 156 F8 38 38N 88 57W
Salem, Ind., U.S.A. 157 F10 38 36N 86 6W
Salem, Mass., U.S.A. 151 D14 42 31N 70 53W
Salem, Mo., U.S.A. 155 G9 37 39N 91 32W
Salem, N.H., U.S.A. 151 D13 42 45N 71 12W
Salem, N.J., U.S.A. 148 F8 39 34N 75 28W
Salem, N.Y., U.S.A. 151 C11 43 10N 73 20W
Salem, Ohio, U.S.A. 150 F4 40 54N 80 52W
Salem, Oreg., U.S.A. 158 D2 44 56N 123 2W
Salem, S. Dak., U.S.A. 154 D6 43 44N 97 23W
Salem, Va., U.S.A. 148 G5 37 18N 80 3W
Salemi, Italy 46 E5 37 49N 12 48 E
Sälen, Sweden 16 C7 61 15N 13 22 E
Salernes, France 29 E10 43 34N 6 15 E
Salerno, Italy 47 B7 40 41N 14 47 E
Salerno, G. di, Italy 47 B7 40 32N 14 42 E
Sales, Brazil 169 D5 4 2 S 63 40W
Salford, U.K. 20 D5 53 30N 2 18W
Salgir →, Ukraine 59 K8 45 38N 35 1 E
Salgótarján, Hungary 52 B4 48 5N 19 47 E
Salgueiro, Brazil 170 C4 8 4 S 39 6W
Salher, India 94 D1 20 40N 73 55 E
Salhus, Norway 18 D2 60 30N 5 15 E
Salibabu, Indonesia 79 D7 3 51N 126 40 E
Salibea = Salybia, Trin. & Tob. 169 F9 10 43N 61 2W
Salida, U.S.A. 146 C5 38 32N 106 0W
Salies-de-Béarn, France 28 E3 43 28N 0 56W
Şalif, Yemen 98 D3 15 18N 42 41 E
Salihli, Turkey 100 C3 38 28N 28 8 E
Salihorsk, Belarus 59 F4 52 51N 27 27 E
Salin, Burma 90 E5 20 35N 94 40 E
Salina, Italy 47 D7 38 34N 14 50 E
Salina, Kans., U.S.A. 154 F6 38 50N 97 37W
Salina, Utah, U.S.A. 159 G8 38 58N 111 51W
Salina Cruz, Mexico 163 D5 16 10N 95 10W
Salina di Margherita di Savoia ⌓, Italy 47 A9 41 23N 16 4 E
Salinas = Salinópolis, Brazil 170 B2 0 40 S 47 20W
Salinas, Brazil 171 E3 16 10 S 42 10W
Salinas, Chile 174 A2 23 31 S 69 29W
Salinas, Ecuador 168 D1 2 10 S 80 58W
Salinas, U.S.A. 160 J5 36 40N 121 39W
Salinas →, Guatemala 163 D6 16 28N 90 31W
Salinas →, U.S.A. 160 J5 36 45N 121 48W
Salinas, B. das, Angola 115 E2 14 11 S 12 21 E
Salinas, B. de, Nic. 164 D2 11 4N 85 45W
Salinas, Pampa de las, Argentina 174 C2 31 58 S 66 42W
Salinas Ambargasta, Argentina 174 B3 29 0 S 65 0W
Salinas de Hidalgo, Mexico 162 C4 22 30N 101 40W
Salinas Grandes, Argentina 174 C3 30 0 S 65 0W
Salinas Pueblo Missions ⌓, U.S.A. 159 J10 34 16N 106 5W
Saline, U.S.A. 157 B13 42 10N 83 47W
Saline →, Ark., U.S.A. 155 J8 33 10N 92 8W
Saline →, Kans., U.S.A. 154 F6 38 52N 97 30W
Saline di Trapani e Paceco ⌓, Italy 46 E5 37 59N 12 28 E
Salines, C. de ses, Spain 38 B4 39 16N 3 4 E
Salinópolis, Brazil 170 B2 0 40 S 47 20W
Salins-les-Bains, France 27 F12 46 58N 5 52 E
Salir, Portugal 43 H2 37 14N 8 2W
Salisbury = Harare, Zimbabwe 119 F3 17 43 S 31 2 E
Salisbury, U.K. 21 F6 51 4N 1 47W
Salisbury, Md., U.S.A. 148 F8 38 22N 75 36W
Salisbury, Mo., U.S.A. 156 E4 39 25N 92 48W
Salisbury, N.C., U.S.A. 149 H5 35 40N 80 29W
Salisbury I., Canada 139 B12 63 30N 77 0W
Salisbury Plain, U.K. 21 F6 51 14N 1 55W
Sălişte, Romania 53 E8 45 45N 23 56 E
Salitre →, Brazil 170 C3 9 29 S 40 39W
Salka, Nigeria 113 C5 10 20N 4 58 E
Salkehatchie →, U.S.A. 152 C9 32 37N 80 53W
Şalkhad, Syria 103 C5 32 29N 36 43 E
Salkove, Ukraine 53 B14 48 15N 29 59 E
Salla, Finland 14 C23 66 50N 28 49 E
Sallanches, France 29 C10 45 55N 6 38 E
Sallent, Spain 40 D6 41 49N 1 54 E
Salles, France 28 D3 44 33N 0 52W
Salles-Curan, France 28 D6 44 11N 2 48 E
Salling, Denmark 17 H2 56 40N 8 55 E
Salliq = Coral Harbour, Canada 139 B11 64 8N 83 10W
Sallisaw, U.S.A. 155 H7 35 28N 94 47W
Sallom Junction, Sudan 106 D4 19 17N 37 6 E
Salluit, Canada 139 B12 62 14N 75 38W
Salmās, Iran 101 C11 38 11N 44 47 E
Salmerón, Spain 40 E2 40 33N 2 29W
Salmo, Canada 142 D5 49 10N 117 20W
Salmon, U.S.A. 158 D7 45 11N 113 54W
Salmon →, Canada 142 C4 54 3N 122 40W
Salmon →, U.S.A. 158 D5 45 51N 116 47W
Salmon Arm, Canada 142 C5 50 40N 119 15W
Salmon Gums, Australia 125 F3 32 59 S 121 38 E
Salmon River Mts., U.S.A. 158 D6 45 0N 114 30W
Salo, C.A.R. 114 B3 3 10N 16 8 E
Salo, Finland 15 F20 60 22N 23 10 E
Salò, Italy 44 C7 45 36N 10 31 E
Salobreña, Spain 43 J7 36 44N 3 35W
Salome, U.S.A. 161 M13 33 47N 113 37W
Salon, India 93 F9 26 2N 81 27 E
Salon-de-Provence, France 29 E9 43 39N 5 6 E
Salonga →, Dem. Rep. of the Congo 114 C4 0 10 S 19 50 E
Salonga-Nord △, Dem. Rep. of the Congo 114 C4 1 55 S 21 45 E
Salonga-Sud △, Dem. Rep. of the Congo 114 C4 2 25 S 21 0 E
Salonica = Thessaloníki, Greece 50 F6 40 38N 22 58 E
Salonta, Romania 52 D6 46 49N 21 42 E
Salop = Shropshire □, U.K. 21 E5 52 36N 2 45W
Salor →, Spain 43 F3 39 39N 7 3W
Salou, Spain 40 D6 41 4N 1 8 E
Salou, C. de, Spain 40 D6 41 3N 1 10 E
Saloum →, Senegal 112 C1 13 50N 16 45W
Salpausselkä, Finland 15 F22 61 3N 26 15 E
Salsacate, Argentina 174 C2 31 20 S 65 5W
Salses, France 28 F6 42 50N 2 55 E
Salsette I., India 94 E1 19 5N 72 50 E
Salsk, Russia 61 G5 46 28N 41 30 E
Salso →, Italy 46 E6 37 6N 13 57 E
Salsomaggiore Terme, Italy 44 D6 44 49N 9 59 E
Salt, Spain 40 D7 41 59N 2 47 E
Salt →, Canada 142 B6 60 0N 112 25W
Salt →, Ariz., U.S.A. 159 K7 33 23N 112 19W
Salt →, Mo., U.S.A. 156 E5 39 28N 91 4W
Salt Cay, Bahamas 9 b 25 6N 77 18W
Salt Fork Red →, U.S.A. 155 H5 34 27N 99 21W
Salt L., U.S.A. 145 K14 21 21N 157 55W
Salt L., The, Australia 127 E3 30 6 S 142 8 E
Salt Lake City, U.S.A. 158 F8 40 45N 111 53W
Salt Range, Pakistan 92 C5 32 30N 72 25 E
Salt Springs, U.S.A. 153 F8 29 21N 81 44W
Salta, Argentina 174 A2 24 57 S 65 25W
Salta □, Argentina 174 A2 24 48 S 65 30W
Saltara, Italy 45 E9 43 45N 12 50 E
Saltash, U.K. 21 G3 50 24N 4 14W
Saltburn by the Sea, U.K. 20 C7 54 35N 0 58W
Saltcoats, U.K. 22 F4 55 38N 4 47W
Saltee Is., Ireland 23 D5 52 7N 6 37W
Salters, U.S.A. 152 B10 33 36N 79 51W
Saltfjellet, Norway 14 C16 66 40N 15 15 E

Saltfjorden, *Norway* **14 C16** 67 15N 14 10 E
Saltholm, *Denmark* **17 J6** 55 38N 12 43 E
Saltholmavík, *Iceland* **11 B5** 65 24N 21 57W
Saltillo, *Mexico* **162 B4** 25 25N 101 0W
Salto, *Argentina* **174 C3** 34 20 S 60 15W
Salto, *Uruguay* **174 C4** 31 27 S 57 50W
Salto da Divisa, *Brazil* **171 E4** 16 0 S 39 57W
Salto del Guaíra, *Paraguay* **175 A5** 24 3 S 54 17W
Salton City, *U.S.A.* **161 M11** 33 29N 115 51W
Salton Sea, *U.S.A.* **161 M11** 33 15N 115 45W
Saltpond, *Ghana* **113 D4** 5 15N 1 3W
Saltrød, *Norway* **18 F5** 58 30N 8 49 E
Saltsburg, *U.S.A.* **150 F5** 40 29N 79 27W
Saltsjöbaden, *Sweden* **16 E12** 59 15N 18 20 E
Saluda, *U.S.A.* **152 A8** 34 0N 81 46W
Saluda →, *U.S.A.* **149 J5** 34 1N 81 4W
Salug, *Phil.* **81 G4** 8 7N 122 47 E
Salûm, *Egypt* **106 A2** 31 31N 25 7 E
Salûm, Khâlig el, *Egypt* **106 A2** 31 35N 25 24 E
Salur, *India* **94 E6** 18 27N 83 18 E
Salut, Is. du, *Fr. Guiana* **169 B7** 5 15N 52 35W
Saluzzo, *Italy* **44 D4** 44 39N 7 29 E
Salvación, B., *Chile* **176 D1** 50 50 S 75 10W
Salvador, *Brazil* **171 D4** 13 0 S 38 30W
Salvador, *Canada* **143 C7** 52 10N 109 32W
Salvador, El ■, *Cent. Amer.* **164 D2** 13 50N 89 0W
Salvador, L., *U.S.A.* **155 L9** 29 43N 90 15W
Salvaterra, *Brazil* **170 B2** 0 46 S 48 31W
Salvaterra de Magos, *Portugal* **43 F2** 39 1N 8 47W
Salvisa, *U.S.A.* **157 G12** 37 54N 84 51W
Sálvora, I. de, *Spain* **42 C2** 42 30N 8 58W
Salween →, *Burma* **90 G6** 16 31N 97 37 E
Salyan, *Azerbaijan* **101 C13** 39 33N 48 59 E
Salybia, *Trin. & Tob.* **169 F9** 10 43N 61 2W
Salza →, *Austria* **34 D7** 47 40N 14 43 E
Salzach →, *Austria* **34 C5** 48 12N 12 56 E
Salzburg, *Austria* **34 D6** 47 48N 13 2 E
Salzburg □, *Austria* **34 D6** 47 15N 13 0 E
Salzburgen = Château-Salins, *France* **27 D13** 48 50N 6 30 E
Salzgitter, *Germany* **30 C6** 52 9N 10 19 E
Salzkotten, *Germany* **30 D4** 51 40N 8 37 E
Salzwedel, *Germany* **30 C7** 52 52N 11 10 E
Sam, *Gabon* **114 B2** 0 58N 11 16 E
Sam, *India* **92 F4** 26 50N 70 31 E
Sam Neua, *Laos* **76 G5** 20 29N 104 5 E
Sam Ngao, *Thailand* **86 D2** 17 18N 99 0 E
Sam Rayburn Reservoir, *U.S.A.* **155 K7** 31 4N 94 5W
Sam Son, *Vietnam* **86 C5** 19 44N 105 54 E
Sam Teu, *Laos* **86 C5** 19 59N 104 38 E
Sama de Langreo = Langreo, *Spain* **42 B5** 43 18N 5 40W
Samacimbo, *Angola* **115 E3** 13 33 S 16 59 E
Samagaltay, *Russia* **67 D10** 50 36N 95 3 E
Samā'il, *Oman* **99 B7** 23 40N 57 50 E
Samaipata, *Bolivia* **173 D5** 18 9 S 63 52W
Samal, *Phil.* **81 H5** 7 5N 125 42 E
Samal I., *Phil.* **81 H5** 7 3N 125 44 E
Samales Group, *Phil.* **81 J3** 6 0N 122 0 E
Samalkot, *India* **94 F6** 17 3N 82 13 E
Samâlût, *Egypt* **106 B3** 28 20N 30 42 E
Samana, *India* **92 D7** 30 10N 76 13 E
Samana Cay, *Bahamas* **165 B5** 23 3N 73 45W
Samandağı, *Turkey* **100 D6** 36 5N 35 59 E
Samandıra, *Turkey* **51 F13** 40 59N 29 13 E
Samanga, *Tanzania* **119 D4** 8 20 S 39 13 E
Samangān □, *Afghan.* **91 A3** 36 15N 68 3 E
Samangwa, *Dem. Rep. of the Congo* **118 C1** 4 23 S 24 10 E
Samani, *Japan* **70 C11** 42 7N 142 56 E
Samanli Dağları, *Turkey* **51 F13** 40 32N 29 10 E
Samar, *Phil.* **81 E5** 12 0N 125 0 E
Samar □, *Phil.* **81 F5** 11 50N 125 0 E
Samar Sea, *Phil.* **80 E5** 12 0N 124 15 E
Samara, *Russia* **60 D10** 53 8N 50 6 E
Samara →, *Russia* **60 D10** 53 10N 50 4 E
Samara →, *Ukraine* **59 H8** 48 28N 35 7 E
Samarai, *Papua N. G.* **132 F6** 10 39 S 150 41 E
Samaria = Shōmrōn, *West Bank* **103 C4** 32 15N 35 13 E
Samariá, *Greece* **39 E4** 35 17N 23 58 E
Samariá △, *Greece* **48 F5** 35 18N 23 57 E
Samariapo, *Venezuela* **168 B4** 5 15N 67 48W
Samarinda, *Indonesia* **85 C5** 0 30 S 117 9 E
Samarkand = Samarqand, *Uzbekistan* **65 D3** 39 40N 66 55 E
Samarkandsky = Temirtau, *Kazakhstan* **66 D8** 50 5N 72 56 E
Samarqand, *Uzbekistan* **65 D3** 39 40N 66 55 E
Sāmarrā', *Iraq* **101 E10** 34 12N 43 52 E
Samastipur, *India* **93 G11** 25 50N 85 50 E
Samate, *Indonesia* **83 B4** 0 58 S 131 4 E
Samaúma, *Brazil* **173 B5** 7 50 S 60 2W
Şamaxi, *Azerbaijan* **61 K9** 40 38N 48 37 E
Samba, *Équateur, Dem. Rep. of the Congo* **114 B4** 0 13N 21 25 E
Samba, *Maniema, Dem. Rep. of the Congo* **118 C2** 4 38 S 26 22 E
Samba, *India* **93 C6** 32 32N 75 10 E
Samba Caju, *Angola* **115 D3** 8 46 S 15 24 E
Sambaíba, *Brazil* **170 C2** 7 8 S 45 21W
Sambalpur, *India* **94 D7** 21 28N 84 4 E
Sambar, Tanjung, *Indonesia* **85 C4** 2 59 S 110 19 E
Sambas, *Indonesia* **85 B3** 1 20N 109 20 E
Sambava, *Madag.* **117 A9** 14 16 S 50 10 E
Sambawizi, *Zimbabwe* **119 F2** 18 24 S 26 13 E
Sambhal, *India* **93 E8** 28 35N 78 37 E
Sambhar, *India* **92 F6** 26 52N 75 6 E
Sambhar L., *India* **92 F6** 26 55N 75 12 E
Sambiase, *Italy* **47 D9** 38 58N 16 17 E
Sambir, *Ukraine* **55 J10** 49 30N 23 10 E
Sambo, *Angola* **115 E3** 13 3 S 16 8 E
Sambor, *Cambodia* **86 F6** 12 46N 106 0 E
Samborombón, B., *Argentina* **174 D4** 36 5 S 57 20W
Sambuca di Sicília, *Italy* **46 E6** 37 39N 13 7 E
Samburu ⌂, *Kenya* **118 B4** 0 37N 37 31 E
Samch'ŏk, *S. Korea* **75 F15** 37 30N 129 10 E
Samch'onp'o, *S. Korea* **75 G15** 35 0N 128 6 E
Same, *Tanzania* **118 C4** 4 2 S 37 38 E
Samedan, *Switz.* **33 C9** 46 32N 9 52 E
Samer, *France* **27 B8** 50 38N 1 44 E
Samfya, *Zambia* **119 E2** 11 22 S 29 31 E
Samḩān, Jabal, *Oman* **99 C6** 17 12N 54 55 E
Sámi, *Greece* **39 C2** 38 15N 20 39 E
Samka, *Burma* **90 E6** 20 9N 96 57 E
Şämkir, *Azerbaijan* **61 K8** 40 50N 46 0 E
Şamlı, *Turkey* **49 B9** 39 48N 27 51 E
Sammanturai, *Sri Lanka* **95 L5** 7 36N 81 39 E
Samnah, *Si. Arabia* **96 E3** 25 10N 37 15 E
Samnaun, *Switz.* **33 C10** 46 57N 10 22 E
Samnū, *Libya* **108 C2** 27 15N 14 55 E
Samo Alto, *Chile* **174 C1** 30 22 S 71 0W
Samoa ■, *Pac. Oc.* **133 X24** 14 0 S 172 0W
Samoan Is., *Pac. Oc.* **133 X24** 14 0 S 171 0W
Samobor, *Croatia* **45 C12** 45 47N 15 44 E
Samoëns, *France* **27 F13** 46 5N 6 45 E
Samokov, *Bulgaria* **50 D7** 42 18N 23 35 E
Šamorín, *Slovak Rep.* **35 C10** 48 2N 17 19 E
Samorogouan, *Burkina Faso* **112 C4** 11 21N 4 57W
Sámos, *Greece* **49 D8** 37 45N 26 50 E
Samoš, *Serbia & M.* **52 E5** 45 13N 20 46 E
Samos, *Spain* **42 C3** 42 44N 7 20W
Sámos □, *Greece* **49 D8** 37 45N 26 50 E
Samoset, *U.S.A.* **153 H7** 27 28N 82 33W
Samosir, *Indonesia* **84 B1** 2 55N 98 50 E
Samothráki = Mathráki, *Greece* **38 B9** 39 48N 19 31 E
Samothráki, *Greece* **51 F9** 40 28N 25 28 E
Samoylovka, *Russia* **60 E6** 51 12N 43 43 E
Sampa, *Angola* **115 E3** 10 38 S 18 56 E
Sampa, *Ghana* **112 D4** 8 0N 2 36W
Sampacho, *Argentina* **174 C3** 33 20 S 64 50W
Sampalan, *Indonesia* **79 K18** 8 41 S 115 34 E
Sampang, *Indonesia* **85 D4** 7 11 S 113 13 E
Samper de Calanda, *Spain* **40 D4** 41 11N 0 28W
Sampéyre, *Italy* **44 D4** 44 34N 7 11 E
Sampit, *Indonesia* **85 C4** 2 34 S 113 0 E
Sampit →, *Indonesia* **85 C4** 2 44 S 112 54 E
Sampit, Teluk, *Indonesia* **85 C4** 3 5 S 113 3 E
Sampsoús, *Greece* **39 A2** 39 5N 20 45 E
Sampun, *Papua N. G.* **132 C7** 5 21 S 152 8 E
Samrong, *Cambodia* **86 E4** 14 15N 103 30 E
Samrong, *Thailand* **86 E3** 15 10N 100 40 E
Samsø, *Denmark* **17 J4** 55 50N 10 35 E
Samsø Bælt, *Denmark* **17 J4** 55 45N 10 45 E
Samson, *U.S.A.* **152 D3** 31 7N 86 3W
Samsun, *Turkey* **100 B7** 41 15N 36 22 E
Samtredia, *Georgia* **61 J6** 42 7N 42 24 E
Samui, Ko, *Thailand* **87 b** 9 30N 100 0 E
Samur →, *Russia* **61 K9** 41 53N 48 32 E
Samurskiy Khrebet, *Russia* **61 K8** 41 55N 47 11 E
Samusole, *Dem. Rep. of the Congo* **119 E1** 10 2 S 24 0 E
Samut Prakan, *Thailand* **86 F3** 13 32N 100 40 E
Samut Songkhram →, *Thailand* **78 B1** 13 24N 100 1 E
Samwari, *Pakistan* **92 E2** 28 30N 66 46 E
San, *Mali* **112 C4** 13 15N 4 57W
San →, *Cambodia* **86 F5** 13 32N 105 57 E
San →, *Poland* **55 H8** 50 45N 21 51 E
San Adrián, *Spain* **40 C3** 42 20N 1 56W
San Adrián, C. de, *Spain* **42 B2** 43 21N 8 50W
San Agustín, *Colombia* **168 C2** 1 53N 76 16W
San Agustin, *Phil.* **80 E4** 12 34N 122 6 E
San Agustin, C., *Phil.* **81 H6** 6 20N 126 13 E
San Agustín de Valle Fértil, *Argentina* **174 C2** 30 35 S 67 30W
San Ambrosio, *Pac. Oc.* **135 K20** 26 28 S 79 53W
San Andreas, *U.S.A.* **160 G6** 38 12N 120 41W
San Andres, *Catanduanes, Phil.* **80 E5** 13 36N 124 6 E
San Andres, *Romblon, Phil.* **80 E4** 13 19N 122 41 E
San Andres, *Romblon, Phil.* **80 E4** 12 31N 122 2 E
San Andrés, I. de, *Caribbean* **164 D3** 12 42N 81 46W
San Andrês del Rabanedo, *Spain* **42 C5** 42 37N 5 36W
San Andres Mts., *U.S.A.* **159 K10** 33 0N 106 30W
San Andrés Tuxtla, *Mexico* **163 D5** 18 30N 95 20W
San Angelo, *U.S.A.* **155 K4** 31 28N 100 26W
San Anselmo, *U.S.A.* **160 H4** 37 59N 122 34W
San Antonio, *Belize* **163 D7** 16 15N 89 2W
San Antonio, *Chile* **174 C1** 33 40 S 71 40W
San Antonio, *Phil.* **80 D3** 14 57N 120 5 E
San Antonio, *N. Mex., U.S.A.* **159 K10** 33 55N 106 52W
San Antonio, *Tex., U.S.A.* **155 L5** 29 25N 98 30W
San Antonio, *Venezuela* **168 C4** 3 30N 66 44W
San Antonio →, *U.S.A.* **155 L6** 28 30N 96 54W
San Antonio, C., *Argentina* **174 D4** 36 15 S 56 40W
San Antonio, C. de, *Cuba* **164 B3** 21 50N 84 57W
San Antonio, C. de, *Spain* **41 G5** 38 48N 0 12 E
San Antonio, Mt., *U.S.A.* **161 L9** 34 17N 117 38W
San Antonio Bay, *Phil.* **81 G1** 8 38N 117 35 E
San Antonio de los Baños, *Cuba* **164 B3** 22 54N 82 31W
San Antonio de los Cobres, *Argentina* **174 A2** 24 10 S 66 17W
San Antonio Oeste, *Argentina* **176 B4** 40 40 S 65 0W
San Arcángelo, *Italy* **47 B9** 40 14N 16 14 E
San Ardo, *U.S.A.* **160 J6** 36 1N 120 54W
San Augustín, *Canary Is.* **9 e1** 27 47N 15 32W
San Augustine, *U.S.A.* **155 K7** 31 30N 94 7W
San Bartolomé, *Canary Is.* **9 e2** 28 59N 13 37W
San Bartolomé de Tirajana, *Canary Is.* **9 e1** 27 54N 15 34W
San Bartolomeo in Galdo, *Italy* **47 A8** 41 24N 15 1 E
San Benedetto del Tronto, *Italy* **45 F10** 42 57N 13 53 E
San Benedetto Po, *Italy* **44 C7** 45 2N 10 55 E
San Benedicto, I., *Mexico* **162 D2** 19 18N 110 49W
San Benito, *U.S.A.* **155 M6** 26 8N 97 38W
San Benito →, *U.S.A.* **160 J5** 36 53N 121 34W
San Benito Mt., *U.S.A.* **160 J6** 36 22N 120 37W
San Bernadino, *Switz.* **33 D8** 46 27N 9 12 E
San Bernardino, *U.S.A.* **161 L9** 34 7N 117 19W
San Bernardino, Paso del, *Switz.* **33 D8** 46 28N 9 11 E
San Bernardino Mts., *U.S.A.* **161 L10** 34 10N 116 45W
San Bernardino Str., *Phil.* **80 E5** 13 0N 125 0 E
San Bernardo, *Chile* **174 C1** 33 40 S 70 50W
San Bernardo, I. de, *Colombia* **168 B2** 9 45N 75 50W
San-Beyse = Choybalsan, *Mongolia* **69 B6** 48 4N 114 30 E
San Blas, *Mexico* **162 B3** 26 4N 108 46W
San Blas, Arch. de, *Panama* **164 E4** 9 50N 78 31W
San Blas, C., *U.S.A.* **152 F4** 29 40N 85 21W
San Bonifacio, *Italy* **45 C8** 45 24N 11 16 E
San Borja, *Bolivia* **172 C4** 14 50 S 66 52W
San Buenaventura = Ventura, *U.S.A.* **161 L7** 34 17N 119 18W
San Buenaventura, *Bolivia* **172 C4** 14 28 S 67 35W
San Buenaventura, *Mexico* **162 B4** 27 5N 101 32W
San Carlo Park, *U.S.A.* **153 J8** 26 28N 81 49W
San Carlos = Butuku-Luba, *Eq. Guin.* **113 E6** 3 29N 8 33 E
San Carlos = Sant Carles, *Spain* **38 C2** 39 3N 1 34 E
San Carlos, *Argentina* **174 C2** 33 50 S 69 0W
San Carlos, *Bolivia* **173 D5** 17 24 S 63 45W
San Carlos, *Chile* **174 D1** 36 10 S 72 0W
San Carlos, *Baja Calif. S., Mexico* **162 C2** 24 47N 112 6W
San Carlos, *Coahuila, Mexico* **162 B4** 29 0N 100 54W
San Carlos, *Nic.* **164 D3** 11 12N 84 50W
San Carlos, *Neg. Occ., Phil.* **81 F4** 10 29N 123 25 E
San Carlos, *Pangasinan, Phil.* **80 D3** 15 55N 120 20 E
San Carlos, *Uruguay* **175 C5** 34 46 S 54 58W
San Carlos, *U.S.A.* **159 K8** 33 21N 110 27W
San Carlos, *Amazonas, Venezuela* **168 C4** 1 55N 67 4W
San Carlos, *Cojedes, Venezuela* **168 B4** 9 40N 68 36W
San Carlos de Bariloche, *Argentina* **176 B2** 41 10 S 71 25W
San Carlos de la Rápita = Sant Carles de la Ràpita, *Spain* **40 E5** 40 37N 0 35 E
San Carlos de Río Negro, *Venezuela* **168 C4** 1 55N 67 4W
San Carlos del Zulia, *Venezuela* **168 B3** 9 1N 71 55W
San Carlos L., *U.S.A.* **159 K8** 33 11N 110 32W
San Cataldo, *Italy* **46 E6** 37 29N 13 59 E
San Celoni = Sant Celoni, *Spain* **40 D7** 41 42N 2 30 E
San Clemente, *Chile* **174 D1** 35 30 S 71 29W
San Clemente, *Spain* **41 F2** 39 24N 2 25W
San Clemente, *U.S.A.* **161 M9** 33 26N 117 37W
San Clemente I., *U.S.A.* **161 N8** 32 53N 118 29W
San Cristóbal = Es Migjorn Gran, *Spain* **38 B5** 39 57N 4 3 E
San Cristóbal, *Argentina* **174 C3** 30 20 S 61 10W
San Cristóbal, *Colombia* **168 D3** 2 18 S 73 2W
San Cristóbal, *Dom. Rep.* **165 C5** 18 25N 70 6W
San Cristóbal, *Solomon Is.* **133 N11** 10 30 S 161 0 E
San Cristóbal, *Venezuela* **168 B3** 7 46N 72 14W
San Cristóbal, I., *Ecuador* **172 a** 0 50 S 89 26W
San Cristóbal de la Casas, *Mexico* **163 D6** 16 50N 92 33W
San Damiano d'Asti, *Italy* **44 D5** 44 50N 8 4 E
San Daniele del Friuli, *Italy* **45 B10** 46 9N 13 1 E
San Diego, *Calif., U.S.A.* **161 N9** 32 43N 117 9W
San Diego, *Tex., U.S.A.* **155 M5** 27 46N 98 14W
San Diego, C., *Argentina* **176 D3** 54 40 S 65 10W
San Diego de la Unión, *Mexico* **162 C4** 21 28N 100 52W
San Diego International ✕ (SAN), *U.S.A.* **161 N9** 32 44N 117 11W
San Dimitri, Ras, *Malta* **38 E6** 36 4N 14 11 E
San Dimitri Point = San Dimitri, Ras, *Malta* **38 E6** 36 4N 14 11 E
San Donà di Piave, *Italy* **45 C9** 45 38N 12 34 E
San Estanislao, *Paraguay* **174 A4** 24 39 S 56 26W
San Esteban △, *Venezuela* **168 A4** 10 24N 67 58W
San Esteban de Gormaz, *Spain* **40 D1** 41 34N 3 13W
San Eugenio = Artigas, *Uruguay* **174 C4** 30 20 S 56 30W
San Felice Circeo, *Italy* **46 A6** 41 14N 13 5 E
San Felice sul Panaro, *Italy* **45 D8** 44 50N 11 8 E
San Felipe, *Chile* **174 C1** 32 43 S 70 42W
San Felipe, *Colombia* **168 C4** 1 55N 67 6W
San Felipe, *Mexico* **162 A2** 31 0N 114 52W
San Felipe, *Phil.* **80 D3** 15 4N 120 4 E
San Felipe, *Venezuela* **168 A4** 10 20N 68 44W
San Felipe →, *U.S.A.* **161 M11** 33 12N 115 49W
San Félix, *Chile* **174 B1** 28 56 S 70 28W
San Félix, *Pac. Oc.* **135 K20** 26 23 S 80 0W
San Fernando = Sant Ferran, *Spain* **38 D1** 38 42N 1 28 E
San Fernando, *Chile* **174 C1** 34 30 S 71 0W
San Fernando, *Baja Calif., Mexico* **162 B1** 29 55N 115 10W
San Fernando, *Tamaulipas, Mexico* **163 C5** 24 51N 98 10W
San Fernando, *Cebu, Phil.* **81 F4** 10 10N 123 42 E
San Fernando, *La Union, Phil.* **80 C3** 16 40N 120 23 E
San Fernando, *Pampanga, Phil.* **80 D3** 15 5N 120 37 E
San Fernando, *Romblon, Phil.* **80 E4** 12 18N 122 36 E
San Fernando, *Spain* **43 J4** 36 28N 6 17W
San Fernando, *Trin. & Tob.* **169 F9** 10 16N 61 28W
San Fernando, *U.S.A.* **161 L8** 34 17N 118 26W
San Fernando de Apure, *Venezuela* **168 B4** 7 54N 67 15W
San Fernando de Atabapo, *Venezuela* **168 C4** 4 3N 67 42W
San Fernando di Púglia, *Italy* **47 A9** 41 18N 16 5 E
San Francisco, *Argentina* **174 C3** 31 30 S 62 5W
San Francisco, *Bolivia* **173 D4** 15 16 S 65 31W
San Francisco, *Peru* **172 C3** 12 36 S 73 49W
San Francisco, *Agusan del S., Phil.* **81 G5** 8 30N 125 56 E
San Francisco, *Cebu, Phil.* **81 F5** 10 39N 124 23 E
San Francisco, *Quezon, Phil.* **80 E4** 13 21N 122 31 E
San Francisco, *S. Leyte, Phil.* **81 F5** 10 4N 125 9 E
San Francisco, *U.S.A.* **160 H4** 37 47N 122 25W
San Francisco →, *U.S.A.* **159 K9** 32 59N 109 22W
San Francisco, C. de, *Colombia* **168 B2** 6 18N 77 29W
San Francisco, Paso de, *S. Amer.* **174 B2** 27 0 S 68 0W
San Francisco de Macorís, *Dom. Rep.* **165 C5** 19 19N 70 15W
San Francisco del Monte de Oro, *Argentina* **174 C2** 32 36 S 66 8W
San Francisco del Oro, *Mexico* **162 B3** 26 52N 105 50W
San Francisco International ✕ (SFO), *U.S.A.* **160 H4** 37 37N 122 22W
San Francisco Javier = Sant Francesc de Formentera, *Spain* **38 D1** 38 42N 1 26 E
San Fratello, *Italy* **47 D7** 38 1N 14 36 E
San Gabriel, *Chile* **174 C1** 33 47 S 70 15W
San Gabriel, *Ecuador* **168 C2** 0 36N 77 49W
San Gabriel Mts., *U.S.A.* **161 L9** 34 20N 118 0W
San Gavino Monreale, *Italy* **46 C1** 39 33N 8 47 E
San German, *Puerto Rico* **165 d** 18 4N 67 4W
San Gil, *Colombia* **168 B3** 6 33N 73 8W
San Giljan = St. Julian's, *Malta* **38 F7** 35 55N 14 29 E
San Gimignano, *Italy* **44 E8** 43 28N 11 2 E
San Giórgio di Nogaro, *Italy* **45 C10** 45 50N 13 13 E
San Giórgio Iónico, *Italy* **47 B10** 40 27N 17 23 E
San Giovanni Bianco, *Italy* **44 C6** 45 52N 9 39 E
San Giovanni in Fiore, *Italy* **47 C9** 39 15N 16 42 E
San Giovanni in Persiceto, *Italy* **45 D8** 44 38N 11 11 E
San Giovanni Rotondo, *Italy* **45 G12** 41 42N 15 44 E
San Giovanni Valdarno, *Italy* **45 E8** 43 34N 11 32 E
San Giuliano Terme, *Italy* **44 E7** 43 46N 10 26 E
San Gorgonio Mt., *U.S.A.* **161 L10** 34 7N 116 51W
San Gottardo, P. del, *Switz.* **33 C7** 46 33N 8 33 E
San Gregorio, *Uruguay* **175 C4** 32 37 S 55 40W
San Gregorio, *U.S.A.* **160 H4** 37 20N 122 23W
San Guiseppe Jato, *Italy* **46 E6** 37 57N 13 11 E
San Ignacio, *Belize* **163 D7** 17 10N 89 5W
San Ignacio, *Beni, Bolivia* **173 C4** 14 53 S 65 36W
San Ignacio, *Santa Cruz, Bolivia* **173 D5** 16 20 S 60 55W
San Ignacio, *Mexico* **162 B2** 27 27N 113 0W
San Ignacio, *Paraguay* **174 B4** 26 52 S 57 3W
San Ignacio, *Peru* **172 B2** 5 8 S 78 59W
San Ignacio ⌓, *Mexico* **162 B2** 27 0N 113 10W
San Ignacio, L., *Mexico* **162 B2** 26 50N 113 11W
San Ildefonso, C., *Phil.* **80 C4** 16 0N 122 1 E
San Isidro, *Argentina* **174 C4** 34 29 S 58 31W
San Isidro, *Phil.* **81 H6** 6 50N 126 5 E
San Isidro de Potot = Burgos, *Phil.* **80 C2** 16 4N 119 52 E
San Jacinto, *Colombia* **168 B2** 9 50N 75 8W
San Jacinto, *Phil.* **80 E4** 12 34N 123 44 E
San Jacinto, *U.S.A.* **161 M10** 33 47N 116 57W
San Jaime = Sant Jaume, *Spain* **38 B5** 39 54N 4 4 E
San Javier, *Misiones, Argentina* **175 B4** 27 55 S 55 5W
San Javier, *Santa Fe, Argentina* **174 C4** 30 40 S 59 55W
San Javier, *Beni, Bolivia* **173 C5** 14 34 S 64 42W
San Javier, *Santa Cruz, Bolivia* **173 D5** 16 18 S 62 30W
San Javier, *Chile* **174 D1** 35 40 S 71 45W
San Javier, *Spain* **41 H4** 37 49N 0 50W
San Jeronimo Taviche, *Mexico* **163 D5** 16 38N 96 32W
San Joaquín, *Bolivia* **173 C5** 13 4 S 64 49W
San Joaquin, *Phil.* **81 F4** 10 35N 122 8 E
San Joaquin, *U.S.A.* **160 J6** 36 36N 120 11W
San Joaquín →, *Bolivia* **173 C5** 13 8 S 63 41W
San Joaquin →, *U.S.A.* **160 G5** 38 4N 121 51W
San Joaquin, Cerro, *Ecuador* **172 a** 0 53 S 89 30W
San Joaquin Valley, *U.S.A.* **160 J6** 37 20N 121 0W
San Jon, *U.S.A.* **155 H3** 35 6N 103 20W
San Jordi = Sant Jordi, *Spain* **38 B3** 39 33N 2 46 E
San Jorge, *Argentina* **174 C3** 31 54 S 61 50W
San Jorge, *Solomon Is.* **133 M10** 8 28 S 159 38 E
San Jorge, B. de, *Mexico* **162 A2** 31 20N 113 20W
San Jorge, G., *Argentina* **176 C3** 46 0 S 66 0W
San José = San Josep, *Spain* **38 D1** 38 55N 1 18 E
San José, *Costa Rica* **164 E3** 9 55N 84 2W
San José, *Guatemala* **164 D1** 14 0N 90 50W
San José, *Mexico* **162 C2** 25 0N 110 50W
San Jose, *Mind. Occ., Phil.* **80 E3** 12 27N 121 4 E
San Jose, *Nueva Ecija, Phil.* **80 D3** 15 45N 120 55 E
San Jose, *Calif., U.S.A.* **160 H5** 37 20N 121 53W
San Jose, *Ill., U.S.A.* **156 D7** 40 18N 89 36W
San Jose →, *U.S.A.* **159 J10** 34 25N 106 45W
San José, Golfo, *Argentina* **176 B4** 42 20 S 64 18W
San Jose de Buenavista, *Phil.* **79 B6** 10 45N 121 56 E
San José de Chiquitos, *Bolivia* **173 D5** 17 53 S 60 50W
San José de Feliciano, *Argentina* **174 C4** 30 26 S 58 46W
San José de Jáchal, *Argentina* **174 C2** 30 15 S 68 46W
San José de Mayo, *Uruguay* **174 C4** 34 27 S 56 40W
San José de Ocune, *Colombia* **168 C3** 4 15N 70 20W
San José de Uchapiamonas, *Bolivia* **172 C4** 14 13 S 68 5W
San José del Cabo, *Mexico* **162 C3** 23 0N 109 40W
San José del Guaviare, *Colombia* **168 C3** 2 35N 72 38W
San Jose del Monte, *Phil.* **80 D3** 14 49N 121 3 E
San José do Anauá, *Brazil* **169 C5** 0 58N 61 22W
San Josep, *Spain* **38 D1** 38 55N 1 18 E
San Juan, *Argentina* **174 C2** 31 30 S 68 30W
San Juan, *Colombia* **168 B2** 8 46N 76 32W
San Juan, *Mexico* **162 C4** 21 20N 102 50W
San Juan, *Ica, Peru* **172 D2** 15 22 S 75 7W
San Juan, *Puno, Peru* **172 C4** 14 2 S 69 19W
San Juan, *Batangas, Phil.* **80 E3** 13 50N 121 24 E
San Juan, *S. Leyte, Phil.* **81 F5** 10 16N 125 10 E
San Juan, *Puerto Rico* **165 d** 18 28N 66 7W
San Juan, *Trin. & Tob.* **169 F9** 10 39N 61 29W
San Juan □, *Argentina* **174 C2** 31 9 S 69 0W
San Juan →, *Argentina* **174 C2** 32 20 S 67 25W
San Juan →, *Bolivia* **173 E4** 21 2 S 65 19W
San Juan →, *Colombia* **168 C2** 4 3N 77 27W
San Juan →, *Nic.* **164 D3** 10 56N 83 42W
San Juan →, *U.S.A.* **159 H8** 37 16N 110 26W
San Juan →, *Venezuela* **169 A5** 10 14N 62 38W
San Juan, C., *Eq. Guin.* **114 B1** 1 5N 9 20 E
San Juan Bautista = Sant Joan Baptista, *Spain* **38 C2** 39 5N 1 31 E
San Juan Bautista = Villahermosa, *Mexico* **163 D6** 17 59N 92 55W
San Juan Bautista, *Paraguay* **174 B4** 26 37 S 57 6W
San Juan Bautista, *U.S.A.* **160 J5** 36 51N 121 32W
San Juan Bautista Valle Nacional, *Mexico* **163 D5** 17 47N 96 19W
San Juan Capistrano, *U.S.A.* **161 M9** 33 30N 117 40W
San Juan Cr. →, *U.S.A.* **160 J5** 35 40N 120 22W
San Juan de Alicante, *Spain* **41 G4** 38 24N 0 26W
San Juan de Guadalupe, *Mexico* **162 C4** 24 38N 102 44W
San Juan de Guía, Cabo de, *Colombia* **168 A3** 11 21N 73 59W
San Juan de la Costa, *Mexico* **162 C2** 24 23N 110 45W
San Juan de los Morros, *Venezuela* **168 B4** 9 55N 67 21W
San Juan de Manapiare, *Venezuela* **168 B4** 5 15N 66 5W
San Juan de Villa Hermosa = Villahermosa, *Mexico* **163 D6** 17 59N 92 55W
San Juan del César, *Colombia* **168 A3** 10 46N 73 1W
San Juan del Norte, *Nic.* **164 D3** 10 58N 83 40W
San Juan del Norte, B. de, *Nic.* **164 D3** 11 0N 83 40W
San Juan del Río, *Mexico* **163 C5** 20 25N 100 0W
San Juan del Sur, *Nic.* **164 D2** 11 20N 85 51W
San Juan I., *U.S.A.* **160 B3** 48 32N 123 5W
San Juan Island △, *U.S.A.* **160 B4** 48 27N 123 0W
San Juan Mts., *U.S.A.* **159 H10** 37 30N 107 0W
San Julián, *Argentina* **176 C3** 49 15 S 67 45W
San Julian, *Phil.* **81 F5** 11 45N 125 27 E
San Just, Sierra de, *Spain* **40 E4** 40 45N 0 49W
San Justo, *Argentina* **174 C3** 30 47 S 60 30W
San Kamphaeng, *Thailand* **86 C2** 18 45N 99 8 E
San Lázaro, C., *Mexico* **162 C2** 24 50N 112 18W
San Lázaro, Sa., *Mexico* **162 C3** 23 25N 110 0W
San Leandro, *U.S.A.* **160 H4** 37 44N 122 9W
San Leonardo de Yagüe, *Spain* **40 D1** 41 51N 3 5W
San Lorenzo = Sant Llorenç des Cardassar, *Spain* **38 B4** 39 37N 3 17 E
San Lorenzo, *Argentina* **174 C3** 32 45 S 60 45W
San Lorenzo, *Beni, Bolivia* **173 D4** 15 22 S 65 48W
San Lorenzo, *Tarija, Bolivia* **173 E5** 21 26 S 64 47W
San Lorenzo, *Ecuador* **168 C2** 1 15N 78 50W
San Lorenzo, *Paraguay* **174 B4** 25 20 S 57 32W
San Lorenzo →, *Mexico* **162 C3** 24 15N 107 24W
San Lorenzo, I., *Mexico* **162 B2** 28 35N 112 50W
San Lorenzo, I., *Peru* **172 C2** 12 7 S 77 15W
San Lorenzo, Mte., *Argentina* **176 C2** 47 40 S 72 20W
San Lorenzo de la Parrilla, *Spain* **40 F2** 39 51N 2 22W
San Lorenzo de Morunys = Sant Llorenç de Morunys, *Spain* **40 C6** 42 8N 1 35 E
San Lucas, *Bolivia* **173 E4** 20 5 S 65 7W
San Lucas, *Baja Calif. S., Mexico* **162 C3** 22 53N 109 54W
San Lucas, *Baja Calif. S., Mexico* **162 B2** 27 10N 112 14W
San Lucas, *U.S.A.* **160 J5** 36 8N 121 1W
San Lucas, C., *Mexico* **162 C3** 22 50N 110 0W
San Lúcido, *Italy* **47 C9** 39 18N 16 3 E
San Luis = Entre Ríos, *Bolivia* **174 A3** 21 30 S 64 25W
San Luis = Sevilla, *Colombia* **168 C2** 4 16N 75 57W
San Luis, *Argentina* **174 C2** 33 20 S 66 20W
San Luis, *Cuba* **164 B3** 22 17N 83 46W
San Luis, *Guatemala* **164 C2** 16 14N 89 27W
San Luis, *Ariz., U.S.A.* **159 K6** 32 29N 114 47W
San Luis, *Colo., U.S.A.* **159 H11** 37 12N 105 25W
San Luis □, *Argentina* **174 C2** 34 0 S 66 0W
San Luis, I., *Mexico* **162 B2** 29 58N 114 26W
San Luis, L. de, *Bolivia* **173 C5** 13 45 S 64 0W
San Luis, Sierra de, *Argentina* **174 C2** 32 30 S 66 10W
San Luis de la Paz, *Mexico* **162 C4** 21 19N 100 32W
San Luis Obispo, *U.S.A.* **161 K6** 35 17N 120 40W
San Luis Potosí, *Mexico* **162 C4** 22 9N 100 59W
San Luis Potosí □, *Mexico* **162 C4** 22 10N 101 0W
San Luis Reservoir, *U.S.A.* **160 H5** 37 4N 121 5W
San Luis Río Colorado, *Mexico* **162 A2** 32 29N 114 58W
San Manuel, *Phil.* **80 C3** 16 4N 120 40 E
San Manuel, *U.S.A.* **159 K8** 32 36N 110 38W
San Marco, C., *Italy* **46 C1** 39 51N 8 26 E
San Marco Argentano, *Italy* **47 C9** 39 33N 16 7 E
San Marco in Lámis, *Italy* **45 G12** 41 43N 15 38 E
San Marcos, *Colombia* **168 B2** 8 39N 75 8W
San Marcos, *Guatemala* **164 D1** 14 59N 91 52W
San Marcos, *Mexico* **162 B2** 27 13N 112 6W
San Marcos, *Calif., U.S.A.* **161 M9** 33 9N 117 10W
San Marcos, *Tex., U.S.A.* **155 L6** 29 53N 97 56W
San Mariano, *Phil.* **80 C4** 17 0N 122 2 E
San Marino, *San Marino* **45 E9** 43 55N 12 30 E
San Marino ■, *Europe* **45 E9** 43 56N 12 25 E
San Martín = Tarapoto, *Peru* **172 B2** 6 30 S 76 20W
San Martin, *Antarctica* **7 C17** 68 11 S 67 0W
San Martín, *Argentina* **174 C2** 33 5 S 68 28W
San Martín, *Colombia* **168 C3** 3 42N 73 42W
San Martín □, *Peru* **172 B2** 7 0 S 76 50W
San Martín →, *Bolivia* **173 C5** 13 8 S 63 43W

San Martín, L.,
  Argentina .... **176 C2** 48 50 S 72 50W
San Martín de la Vega,
  Spain **42 E7** 40 13N 3 34W
San Martín de los
  Andes, Argentina **176 B2** 40 10 S 71 20W
San Martín de
  Valdeiglesias, Spain **42 E6** 40 21N 4 24W
San Mateo = Sant
  Mateu, Baleares,
  Spain .... **38 C1** 39 3N 1 23 E
San Mateo = Sant
  Mateu, Valencia,
  Spain .... **40 E5** 40 28N 0 10 E
San Mateo, Phil. .... **80 C3** 16 54N 121 33 E
San Mateo, U.S.A. ... **160 H4** 37 34N 122 19W
San Matías, Bolivia .. **173 D6** 16 25 S 58 20W
San Matías, G.,
  Argentina .... **176 B4** 41 30 S 64 0W
San Miguel =
  Linapacan, Phil. .. **81 F2** 11 30N 119 52 E
San Miguel = Sant
  Miguel, Spain .... **38 C1** 39 3N 1 26 E
San Miguel = Sarrat,
  Phil. .... **80 B3** 18 9N 120 39 E
San Miguel, Bolivia .. **173 C5** 16 42 S 61 1W
San Miguel, El Salv. . **164 D2** 13 30N 88 12W
San Miguel, Panama .. **164 E4** 8 27N 78 55W
San Miguel, Bulacan,
  Phil. .... **80 D3** 15 9N 120 59 E
San Miguel, Palawan,
  Phil. .... **81 F2** 11 30N 119 51 E
San Miguel, Surigao S.,
  Phil. .... **81 G5** 9 3N 125 59 E
San Miguel, U.S.A. ... **160 K6** 35 45N 120 42W
San Miguel →, Bolivia **173 C5** 13 52 S 63 56W
San Miguel →,
  S. Amer. **168 C2** 0 25N 76 30W
San Miguel, Golfo de,
  Panama **168 B2** 8 22N 78 17W
San Miguel de Huachi,
  Bolivia .... **172 D4** 15 40 S 67 15W
San Miguel de
  Tucumán, Argentina **174 B2** 26 50 S 65 20W
San Miguel del Monte,
  Argentina .... **174 D4** 35 23 S 58 50W
San Miguel I., U.S.A. **161 L6** 34 2N 120 23W
San Miguel Is., Phil. . **80 E2** 7 45N 118 28 E
San Miniato, Italy .... **44 E7** 43 41N 10 51 E
San Narciso, Phil. ... **80 E4** 13 34N 122 34 E
San Nicolás, Canary Is. **9 e1** 27 58N 15 47W
San Nicolas, Phil. .... **80 B3** 18 10N 120 36 E
San Nicolás de los
  Arroyas, Argentina **174 C3** 33 25 S 60 10W
San Nicolas I., U.S.A. **161 M7** 33 15N 119 30W
San Onofre, Colombia **168 B2** 9 44N 75 32W
San Onofre, U.S.A. ... **161 M9** 33 22N 117 34W
San Pablo, Bolivia ... **174 A2** 21 43 S 66 38W
San Pablo, Isabela, Phil. **80 C3** 17 27N 121 48 E
San Pablo, Laguna,
  Phil. .... **80 D3** 14 11N 121 31 E
San Pablo, U.S.A. **160 H4** 37 58N 122 21W
San Pablo de Manta =
  Manta, Ecuador .. **168 D1** 1 0 S 80 40W
San Páolo di Civitate,
  Italy .... **45 G12** 41 44N 15 15 E
San Pascual, Phil. ... **80 E4** 13 8N 122 59 E
San Pedro,
  Buenos Aires,
  Argentina .... **174 C4** 33 40 S 59 40W
San Pedro, Misiones,
  Argentina .... **175 B5** 26 30 S 54 10W
San Pedro, Chile .... **174 C1** 33 54 S 71 28W
San Pedro, Colombia . **168 C3** 4 56N 71 53W
San Pédro, Ivory C. .. **112 E3** 4 50N 6 33W
San Pedro, Mexico ... **163 C2** 23 55N 110 17W
San Pedro, Peru ..... **172 C4** 14 49 S 74 5W
San Pedro □, Paraguay **174 A4** 24 0 S 57 0W
San Pedro →,
  Chihuahua, Mexico **162 B3** 28 20N 106 10W
San Pedro →, Nayarit,
  Mexico **162 C3** 21 45N 105 30W
San Pedro →, U.S.A. **159 K8** 32 59N 110 47W
San Pedro, Pta., Chile **174 B1** 25 30 S 70 38W
San Pedro, Sierra de,
  Spain **43 F4** 39 18N 6 40W
San Pedro Channel,
  U.S.A. **161 M8** 33 30N 118 25W
San Pedro de Arimena,
  Colombia **168 C3** 4 37N 71 42W
San Pedro de Atacama,
  Chile .... **174 A2** 22 55 S 68 15W
San Pedro de Jujuy,
  Argentina .... **174 A3** 24 12 S 64 55W
San Pedro de las
  Colonias, Mexico . **162 B4** 25 50N 102 59W
San Pedro de Lloc,
  Peru .... **172 B2** 7 15 S 79 28W
San Pedro de Macorís,
  Dom. Rep. **165 C6** 18 30N 69 18W
San Pedro del Norte,
  Nic. **164 D3** 13 4N 84 33W
San Pedro del Paraná,
  Paraguay .... **174 B4** 26 43 S 56 13W
San Pedro del Pinatar,
  Spain **41 H4** 37 50N 0 50W
San Pedro Mártir △,
  Mexico **162 A1** 31 0N 115 21W
San Pedro Mártir,
  Sierra, Mexico ... **162 A1** 31 0N 115 30W
San Pedro Mixtepec,
  Mexico **163 D5** 16 2N 97 7W
San Pedro Ocampo =
  Melchor Ocampo,
  Mexico **162 C4** 24 52N 101 40W
San Pedro Sula,
  Honduras **164 C2** 15 30N 88 0W
San Pietro, Italy ..... **46 C1** 39 8N 8 17 E
San Pietro Vernótico,
  Italy .... **47 B11** 40 29N 18 0 E
San Quintín, Mexico . **162 A1** 30 29N 115 57W
San Rafael, Argentina **174 C2** 34 40 S 68 21W
San Rafael, Bolivia .. **173 D5** 16 45 S 60 34W
San Rafael, Calif.,
  U.S.A. **160 H4** 37 58N 122 32W
San Rafael, N. Mex.,
  U.S.A. **159 J10** 35 7N 107 53W
San Rafael, Venezuela **168 A3** 10 42N 71 46W
San Rafael Mt., U.S.A. **161 L7** 34 41N 119 52W
San Rafael Mts., U.S.A. **161 L7** 34 40N 119 50W
San Ramón, Bolivia .. **173 C5** 13 17 S 64 43W
San Ramón, Peru .... **172 C2** 11 8 S 75 20W
San Ramón de la Nueva
  Orán, Argentina .. **174 A3** 23 10 S 64 20W
San Remo, Australia . **129 E6** 38 33 S 145 22 E
San Remo, Italy ..... **44 E4** 43 49N 7 46 E
San Román, C.,
  Venezuela **168 A3** 12 12N 70 0W
San Roque, Argentina **174 B4** 28 25 S 58 45W
San Roque, Phil. .... **80 E5** 12 37N 124 52 E
San Roque, Spain **43 J5** 36 17N 5 21W
San Rosendo, Chile .. **174 D1** 37 16 S 72 43W
San Saba, U.S.A. **155 K5** 31 12N 98 43W
San Salvador, El Salv. **164 D2** 13 40N 89 10W

San Salvador, Spain . **38 B4** 39 27N 3 11 E
San Salvador, Canal de,
  Ecuador .... **172 a** 0 25 S 90 30W
San Salvador, I.,
  Ecuador .... **172 a** 0 16 S 90 42W
San Salvador de Jujuy,
  Argentina .... **174 A3** 24 10 S 64 48W
San Salvador I.,
  Bahamas **165 B5** 24 0N 74 40W
San Salvo, Italy ..... **45 F11** 42 3N 14 44 E
San Sebastián =
  Donostia-San
  Sebastián, Spain .. **40 B3** 43 17N 1 58W
San Sebastián,
  Argentina .... **176 D3** 53 10 S 68 30W
San Sebastian,
  Puerto Rico ...... **165 d** 18 20N 66 59W
San Sebastián de la
  Gomera, Canary Is. **9 e1** 28 5N 17 7W
San Serra = Son Serra,
  Spain .... **38 B4** 39 43N 3 13 E
San Servatore Marche,
  Italy .... **45 E10** 43 13N 13 10 E
San Severo, Italy .... **45 G12** 41 41N 15 23 E
San Simeon, U.S.A. . **160 K5** 35 39N 121 11W
San Simon, U.S.A. ... **159 K9** 32 16N 109 14W
San Stéfano di Cadore,
  Italy .... **45 B9** 46 34N 12 33 E
San Stino di Livenza,
  Italy .... **45 C9** 45 44N 12 41 E
San Telmo = Sant Telm,
  Spain .... **38 B3** 39 35N 2 21 E
San Telmo, Mexico .. **162 A1** 30 58N 116 6W
San Teodoro, Phil. .. **80 E3** 13 26N 121 1 E
San Tiburcio, Mexico **162 C4** 24 8N 101 32W
San Valentin, Mte.,
  Chile .... **176 C2** 46 30 S 73 30W
San Vicente de
  Alcántara, Spain .. **43 F3** 39 22N 7 8W
San Vicente de la
  Barquera, Spain ... **42 B6** 43 23N 4 29W
San Vicente del
  Caguán, Colombia . **168 C3** 2 7N 74 46W
San Vicente del
  Raspeig, Spain **41 G4** 38 24N 0 31W
San Vincenzo, Italy .. **44 E7** 43 6N 10 32 E
San Vito, Costa Rica . **164 E3** 8 50N 82 58W
San Vito, Italy ...... **46 C2** 39 26N 9 32 E
San Vito, C., Italy ... **46 D5** 38 11N 12 41 E
San Vito al
  Tagliamento, Italy . **45 C9** 45 54N 12 52 E
San Vito Chietino, Italy **45 F11** 42 18N 14 27 E
San Vito dei Normanni,
  Italy .... **47 B10** 40 39N 17 42 E
San Yanaro, Colombia **168 C4** 2 47N 69 42W
Saña, Peru .... **172 B2** 6 54 S 79 36W
Sana', Yemen .... **98 D4** 15 27N 44 12 E
Sana →, Bos.-H. .... **45 C13** 45 3N 16 23 E
Sanaba, Burkina Faso **112 C4** 12 25N 3 47W
Şanäfir, Si. Arabia ... **106 B3** 27 56N 34 42 E
Sanaga →, Cameroon **113 E6** 3 35N 9 38 E
Sanak I., U.S.A. **144 J7** 54 25N 162 40W
Sanalona, Presa, Mexico **162 C3** 24 50N 107 20W
Sanám, Si. Arabia ... **98 B4** 2 4 S 125 58 E
Sanana, Indonesia ... **83 B3** 2 4 S 125 58 E
Sanand, India .... **92 H5** 22 59N 72 25 E
Sanandaj, Iran ...... **101 E12** 35 18N 47 1 E
Sanandita, Bolivia ... **174 A3** 21 40 S 63 45W
Sanaroa I., Papua N. G. **132 E6** 9 37 S 151 0 E
Sanary-sur-Mer, France **29 E9** 43 7N 5 49 E
Sanäw, Yemen ...... **99 C5** 17 50N 51 5 E
Sanawad, India ...... **92 H7** 22 11N 76 5 E
Sanbe-San, Japan ... **72 B4** 35 6N 132 38 E
Sancellas = Sencelles,
  Spain .... **38 B3** 39 39N 2 54 E
Sancergues, France .. **27 E9** 47 10N 2 54 E
Sancerre, France .... **27 E9** 47 20N 2 50 E
Sancerrois, Collines du,
  France .... **27 E9** 47 20N 2 40 E
Sancha He →, China **76 D6** 26 48N 106 7 E
Sanchahe, China .... **75 B14** 44 50N 126 2 E
Sanchakou, China ... **65 D9** 39 47N 78 20 E
Sánchez, Dom. Rep. . **165 C6** 19 15N 69 36W
Sanchez-Mira, Phil. . **80 B3** 18 34N 121 14 E
Sanchor, India ...... **92 G4** 24 45N 71 55 E
Sanco Pt., Phil. ..... **81 G6** 8 15N 126 27 E
Sancoins, France .... **27 F9** 46 47N 2 55 E
Sancti Spíritus, Cuba **164 B4** 21 52N 79 33W
Sancy, Puy de, France **28 C6** 45 32N 2 50 E
Sand, Norway .... **18 E3** 59 29N 6 16 E
Sand →, S. Africa ... **117 C5** 22 25 S 30 5 E
Sand Cr. →, U.S.A. . **157 K11** 39 30N 85 51W
Sand Hills, Guyana .. **169 B6** 6 27N 58 19W
Sand Hills, U.S.A. ... **154 D4** 42 10N 101 30W
Sand I., U.S.A. **145 K14** 21 19N 157 53W
Sand Lakes △, Canada **143 B9** 57 51N 98 32W
Sand Point, U.S.A. .. **144 J7** 55 20N 160 30W
Sand Springs, U.S.A. . **155 G6** 36 9N 96 7W
Sanda, Japan .... **73 C7** 34 53N 135 14 E
Sandakan, Malaysia .. **85 A5** 5 53N 118 4 E
Sandalwood, Australia **128 C4** 34 55 S 140 9 E
Sandan = Sambor,
  Cambodia .... **86 F6** 12 46N 106 0 E
Sandane, Norway .... **18 C3** 61 46N 6 13 E
Sandanski, Bulgaria .. **50 E7** 41 35N 23 16 E
Sandaré, Mali **112 C2** 14 40N 10 15W
Sandared, Sweden ... **17 G6** 57 43N 12 47 E
Sandarne, Sweden ... **16 C11** 61 16N 17 9 E
Sanday, U.K. **22 B6** 59 16N 2 31W
Sande,
  Møre og Romsdal,
  Norway .... **18 B2** 62 15N 5 27 E
Sande,
  Sogn og Fjordane,
  Norway .... **18 C2** 61 20N 5 47 E
Sande, Vestfold,
  Norway .... **18 E7** 59 36N 10 12 E
Sandefjord, Norway .. **18 E7** 59 10N 10 15 E
Sandeid, Norway .... **18 E2** 59 33N 5 52 E
Sanders, Ariz., U.S.A. **159 J9** 35 13N 109 20W
Sanders, Ky., U.S.A. . **157 F12** 38 40N 84 56W
Sanderson, Fla., U.S.A. **152 E7** 30 15N 82 16W
Sanderson, Tex., U.S.A. **155 K3** 30 9N 102 24W
Sandersville, U.S.A. . **152 C7** 32 59N 82 48W
Sandfire Roadhouse,
  Australia .... **124 C3** 19 45 S 121 15 E
Sandfloegga, Norway **18 E4** 59 58N 7 10 E
Sandfly L., Canada .. **143 B7** 55 43N 106 6W
Sandfontein, Namibia **116 C2** 23 48 S 19 1 E
Sandhammaren, C.,
  Sweden .... **17 J8** 55 23N 14 14 E
Sandheads, The, India **90 E2** 21 10N 88 30 E
Sandía, Peru .... **172 C4** 14 10 S 69 30W
Sandikli, Turkey .... **49 C12** 38 30N 30 17 E
Sandila, India .... **93 F9** 27 5N 80 31 E
Sandilands, Bahamas **9 b** 25 3N 77 19W
Sandnes, Aust-Agder,
  Norway .... **18 F4** 58 53N 7 45 E
Sandnes, Rogaland,
  Norway .... **18 F2** 58 50N 5 45 E
Sandnessjøen, Norway **14 C15** 66 2N 12 38 E
Sandoa, Dem. Rep. of
  the Congo .... **115 D4** 9 41 S 23 0 E
Sandomierz, Poland . **55 H8** 50 40N 21 43 E

Sândominic, Romania **53 D10** 46 35N 25 47 E
Sandona, Colombia .. **168 C2** 1 17N 77 28W
Sandongo, Angola ... **115 F4** 15 30 S 21 28 E
Sandoval, U.S.A. **156 F7** 38 37N 89 7W
Sandover →, Australia **126 C2** 21 43 S 136 32 E
Sandoway, Burma ... **90 F5** 18 20N 94 30 E
Sandoy, Faeroe Is. .. **14 F9** 61 52N 6 46W
Sandpoint, U.S.A. ... **158 B5** 48 17N 116 33W
Sandray, U.K. **20 E1** 56 53N 7 31W
Sandringham, U.K. .. **20 E8** 52 51N 0 31 E
Sandstone, Australia **125 E2** 27 59 S 119 16 E
Sandu, China .... **76 E6** 26 0N 107 52 E
Sandumba, Angola .. **115 E3** 13 45 S 17 34 E
Sandur, India .... **95 F3** 15 6N 76 33 E
Sandusky, Mich., U.S.A. **150 C2** 43 25N 82 50W
Sandusky, Ohio, U.S.A. **156 E2** 41 27N 82 42W
Sandusky →, U.S.A. . **157 C14** 41 27N 83 0W
Sandvig, Sweden .... **17 J8** 55 18N 14 47 E
Sandvika, Norway ... **18 E7** 59 54N 10 31 E
Sandviken, Sweden .. **16 D10** 60 38N 16 46 E
Sandwich, C., Australia **126 B4** 18 14 S 146 18 E
Sandwich B., Canada **141 B8** 53 40N 57 15W
Sandwich B., Namibia **116 C1** 23 25 S 14 20 E
Sandwip I., Bangla. . **90 D3** 22 30N 91 25 E
Sandy, Oreg., U.S.A. **160 E4** 45 24N 122 16W
Sandy, Pa., U.S.A. .. **150 E6** 41 6N 78 46W
Sandy, Utah, U.S.A. . **158 F8** 40 35N 111 50W
Sandy B., St. Helena **9 h** 16 0 S 5 43W
Sandy Bay, Canada .. **143 B8** 55 31N 102 19W
Sandy Bight, Australia **125 F3** 33 50 S 123 20 E
Sandy C., Queens.,
  Australia .... **126 C5** 24 42 S 153 15 E
Sandy C., Tas.,
  Australia .... **127 G3** 41 25 S 144 45 E
Sandy Cay, Bahamas **165 B4** 23 13N 75 18W
Sandy Cr. →, U.S.A. **158 F9** 41 51N 109 47W
Sandy L., Canada **140 B1** 53 2N 93 0W
Sandy Lake, Canada . **140 B1** 53 0N 93 15W
Sandy Point, India .. **95 J11** 10 32N 92 22 E
Sandy Springs, U.S.A. **152 B5** 33 56N 84 23W
Sandy Valley, U.S.A. **161 K11** 35 49N 115 36W
Sânfälless △, Sweden **16 B7** 62 17N 13 35 E
Sanford, Fla., U.S.A. **153 G8** 28 48N 81 16W
Sanford, Maine, U.S.A. **149 D10** 43 27N 70 47W
Sanford, N.C., U.S.A. **149 H6** 35 29N 79 1W
Sanford →, Australia **125 E2** 27 22 S 115 53 E
Sanford, Mt., U.S.A. **144 E11** 62 13N 144 9W
Sang-i-Masha, Afghan. **92 C2** 33 8N 67 27 E
Sanga, Angola .... **115 E3** 11 9 S 15 21 E
Sanga, Mozam. ...... **119 E4** 12 22 S 35 21 E
Sanga →, Congo .... **114 C3** 1 5 S 17 0 E
Sangaie, Dem. Rep. of
  the Congo .... **115 D4** 6 48 S 22 46 E
Sangamner, India ... **94 E2** 19 37N 74 15 E
Sangamon →, U.S.A. **154 E9** 38 12N 117 15 E
Sanganeb Atoll △,
  Sudan .... **106 D4** 19 33N 37 11 E
Sangar, Afghan. .... **92 C1** 32 56N 65 30 E
Sangar, Russia ...... **67 C13** 64 2N 127 31 E
Sangar Sarai, Afghan. **92 B4** 34 27N 70 35 E
Sangareddi, India ... **94 F4** 17 38N 78 7 E
Sangaredi, Guinea .. **112 C2** 11 7N 13 52W
Sangarh →, Pakistan **92 D4** 30 43N 70 44 E
Sangasangadalam,
  Indonesia .... **85 C5** 0 36 S 117 13 E
Sangasso, Mali **112 C3** 12 5N 5 35W
Sangatte, France .... **27 B8** 50 56N 1 44 E
Sangay, Ecuador .... **168 D2** 2 0 S 78 20W
Sangay △, Ecuador .. **168 D2** 2 15 S 78 26W
Sangchris L., U.S.A. **156 F7** 39 35N 89 30W
Sange, Dem. Rep. of
  the Congo .... **118 D2** 6 58 S 28 21 E
Sangeang, Indonesia **85 D5** 8 12 S 119 6 E
Sângeorz-Băi, Romania **53 C9** 47 22N 24 41 E
Sanger, U.S.A. **160 J7** 36 42N 119 33W
Sangerhausen,
  Germany .... **30 D7** 51 28N 11 18 E
Sanggan He →, China **74 E9** 38 12N 117 15 E
Sanggau, Indonesia .. **85 B4** 0 5N 110 30 E
Sanghar, Pakistan ... **92 F3** 26 2N 68 57 E
Sanghe, Kepulauan,
  Indonesia .... **82 A3** 3 0N 125 30 E
Sanghe, Pulau,
  Indonesia .... **82 A3** 3 35N 125 30 E
Sangju, S. Korea .... **75 F15** 36 25N 128 10 E
Sangkapura, Indonesia **85 D4** 5 52 S 112 40 E
Sangkhla, Thailand .. **86 E2** 14 57N 98 28 E
Sangkulirang, Indonesia **85 B5** 0 59N 117 58 E
Sangla, Pakistan .... **92 D5** 31 43N 73 23 E
Sangli, India .... **94 F2** 16 55N 74 33 E
Sangmélima, Cameroon **113 E7** 2 57N 12 1 E
Sango, Angola .... **115 D2** 9 51 S 15 44 E
Sangod, India .... **92 G7** 24 55N 76 17 E
Sangole, India .... **94 F2** 17 26N 75 12 E
Sangorodok = Ust-
  Vorkuta, Russia .. **56 A11** 67 24N 64 0 E
Sangpang Bum, Burma **90 B5** 26 30N 95 50 E
Sangre de Cristo Mts.,
  U.S.A. **155 G2** 37 30N 105 20W
Sangre Grande,
  Trin. & Tob. **169 F9** 10 35N 61 8W
Sangro →, Italy ..... **45 F11** 42 14N 14 32 E
Sangrur, India ...... **92 D6** 30 59N 75 25 E
Sangudo, Canada ... **142 C6** 53 50N 114 54W
Sangue →, Brazil ... **173 C6** 11 1 S 58 39W
Sangüesa, Spain **40 C3** 42 37N 1 17W
Sanguinaires, Îs.,
  France .... **29 G12** 41 51N 8 36 E
Sangzhi, China ...... **77 C8** 29 25N 110 12 E
Sanhala, Ivory C. ... **112 C3** 10 3N 6 51W
Sanibel, U.S.A. **153 J7** 26 26N 82 1W
Sanibel I., U.S.A. ... **153 J7** 26 26N 82 6W
Sanikiluaq, Canada . **139 C12** 56 32N 79 14W
Sanin-Kaigan △, Japan **72 B6** 35 39N 134 37 E
Sanirajak, Canada .. **139 B11** 68 46N 81 2W
Sanjawi, Pakistan ... **92 D3** 30 17N 68 21 E
Sanje, Uganda ...... **118 C3** 0 49 S 31 30 E
Sanjiang, China ..... **76 E7** 25 48N 109 37 E
Sanjo, Japan .... **70 F9** 37 37N 138 57 E
Sankarankovil, India **95 K3** 9 10N 77 35 E
Sankh →, India ..... **93 H11** 22 15N 84 48 E
Sankosh →, India ... **90 B2** 26 24N 89 47 E
Sankt Andrä, Austria **34 E7** 46 46N 14 50 E
Sankt Antönien, Switz. **33 C9** 46 58N 9 48 E
Sankt Augustin,
  Germany .... **30 E3** 50 45N 7 10 E
Sankt Blasien,
  Germany .... **31 H4** 47 47N 8 7 E
Sankt Gallen, Switz. . **33 B8** 47 26N 9 22 E
Sankt Gallen □, Switz. **33 B8** 47 25N 9 22 E
Sankt Goar, Germany **31 E3** 50 12N 7 43 E
Sankt Ingbert,
  Germany .... **31 F3** 49 16N 7 6 E
Sankt Johann im
  Pongau, Austria .. **34 D6** 47 22N 13 12 E
Sankt Johann in Tirol,
  Austria .... **34 D5** 47 30N 12 25 E
Sankt Marein = Smarje,
  Slovenia .... **45 B12** 46 15N 15 34 E
Sankt Margrethen,
  Switz. .... **33 B9** 47 28N 9 37 E

Sankt Michel = Mikkeli,
  Finland .... **15 F22** 61 43N 27 15 E
Sankt Moritz, Switz. . **33 D9** 46 30N 9 50 E
Sankt-Peterburg, Russia **58 C6** 59 55N 30 20 E
Sankt Pölten, Austria **34 C8** 48 12N 15 38 E
Sankt Ulrich = Ortisei,
  Italy .... **45 B8** 46 34N 11 40 E
Sankt Valentin, Austria **34 C7** 48 11N 14 33 E
Sankt Veit an der Glan,
  Austria .... **34 E7** 46 47N 14 22 E
Sankt Wendel,
  Germany .... **31 F3** 49 27N 7 9 E
Sankt Wolfgang,
  Austria .... **34 D6** 47 43N 13 27 E
Sankuru →, Dem. Rep.
  of the Congo ..... **115 C4** 4 17 S 20 25 E
Sanliurfa, Turkey .... **101 D8** 37 12N 38 50 E
Sanlúcar de Barrameda,
  Spain **43 J4** 36 46N 6 21W
Sanlúcar la Mayor,
  Spain **43 H4** 37 26N 6 18W
Sanluri, Italy .... **46 C1** 39 34N 8 54 E
Sânmartin, Romania **53 D10** 46 19N 25 58 E
Sanmen, China ...... **77 C13** 29 5N 121 35 E
Sanmenxia, China ... **74 G6** 34 47N 111 12 E
Sanming, China ..... **77 D11** 26 15N 117 40 E
Sannan, Japan ...... **73 B7** 35 2N 135 1 E
Sannaspos, S. Africa **116 D4** 29 6 S 26 34 E
Sannat, Malta .... **38 E6** 36 1N 14 15 E
Sannicandro Gargánico,
  Italy .... **45 G12** 41 50N 15 34 E
Sännicolau Mare,
  Romania .... **52 D5** 46 5N 20 39 E
Sannieshof, S. Africa **116 D4** 26 30 S 25 47 E
Sannin, J., Lebanon . **103 B4** 33 57N 35 52 E
Sanniquellie, Liberia . **112 D3** 7 19N 8 38W
Sannûr, W. →, Egypt **106 B3** 28 35N 31 3 E
Sano, Japan .... **73 A11** 36 19N 139 35 E
Sanoe, Antarctica ... **7 D2** 70 20 S 9 0W
Sanok, Poland ...... **55 J9** 49 35N 22 10 E
Sanquhar, U.K. **22 F5** 55 22N 3 54W
Sanquianga △,
  Colombia **168 C2** 2 33N 78 14W
Sans Souci,
  Trin. & Tob. **169 F9** 10 50N 61 0W
Sansanding, Mali ... **112 C3** 13 48N 6 0W
Sansepolcro, Italy ... **45 E9** 43 34N 12 8 E
Sansha, China .... **77 D13** 26 58N 120 12 E
Sanshui, China ...... **77 F9** 23 10N 112 56 E
Sanski Most, Bos.-H. **45 D13** 44 46N 16 40 E
Sansui, China .... **76 D7** 26 58N 108 39 E
Sant Antoni Abat,
  Spain .... **38 D1** 38 59N 1 19 E
Sant Boi de Llobregat,
  Spain .... **40 D7** 41 21N 2 2 E
Sant Carles, Spain .. **38 C2** 39 3N 1 34 E
Sant Carles de la
  Ràpita, Spain ..... **40 E5** 40 37N 0 35 E
Sant Celoni, Spain .. **40 D7** 41 42N 2 30 E
Sant Feliu de Guíxols,
  Spain .... **40 D8** 41 45N 3 1 E
Sant Feliu de Llobregat,
  Spain .... **40 D7** 41 23N 2 2 E
Sant Ferran, Spain .. **38 D1** 38 42N 1 28 E
Sant Francesc de
  Formentera, Spain **38 D1** 38 42N 1 26 E
Sant Jaume, Spain .. **38 B5** 39 54N 4 4 E
Sant Joan Baptista,
  Spain .... **38 C2** 39 5N 1 31 E
Sant Jordi, Ibiza, Spain **38 D1** 38 53N 1 24 E
Sant Jordi, Mallorca,
  Spain .... **38 B3** 39 33N 2 46 E
Sant Jordi, G. de, Spain **40 E6** 40 53N 1 2 E
Sant Llorenç de
  Morunys, Spain .. **40 C6** 42 8N 1 35 E
Sant Llorenç del Munt
  y l'Obac △, Spain **40 D3** 41 39N 1 55W
Sant Llorenç des
  Cardassar, Spain . **38 B4** 39 37N 3 17 E
Sant Mateu, Baleares,
  Spain .... **38 C1** 39 3N 1 23 E
Sant Mateu, Valencia,
  Spain .... **40 E5** 40 28N 0 10 E
Sant Miguel, Spain .. **38 C1** 39 3N 1 26 E
Sant Telm, Spain ... **38 B3** 39 35N 2 21 E
Santa, Peru .... **172 B2** 8 59 S 78 40W
Sant' Ágata Militello,
  Italy .... **47 D7** 38 2N 14 8 E
Santa Agnés, Spain . **38 C1** 39 3N 1 21 E
Santa Ana, Beni,
  Bolivia .... **173 C4** 13 50 S 65 40W
Santa Ana, La Paz,
  Bolivia .... **172 D4** 15 31 S 67 30W
Santa Ana, Santa Cruz,
  Bolivia .... **173 D6** 18 43 S 58 44W
Santa Ana, Santa Cruz,
  Bolivia .... **173 D5** 16 37 S 60 43W
Santa Ana, Ecuador . **168 D1** 1 16 S 80 20W
Santa Ana, El Salv. . **164 D2** 14 0N 89 31W
Santa Ana, Mexico .. **162 A2** 30 31N 111 8W
Santa Ana, Phil. .... **80 B4** 18 28N 122 20 E
Santa Ana, Solomon Is. **133 N12** 10 50 S 162 30 E
Santa Ana, U.S.A. .. **161 M9** 33 46N 117 52W
Santa Ana →,
  Venezuela **168 B3** 9 30N 71 57W
Sant' Ángelo
  Lodigiano, Italy .. **44 C6** 45 14N 9 25 E
Sant' Antíoco, Italy . **46 C1** 39 4N 8 27 E
Santa Bárbara,
  Santa Maria, Azores **9 d4** 36 59N 25 4W
Santa Bárbara,
  Terceira, Azores . **9 d1** 38 41N 27 20W
Santa Bárbara, Chile **174 D1** 37 40 S 72 1W
Santa Bárbara,
  Colombia **168 B2** 5 53N 75 35W
Santa Barbara,
  Honduras **164 D2** 14 53N 88 14W
Santa Bárbara, Mexico **162 B3** 26 48N 105 50W
Santa Bárbara, Spain **40 E5** 40 42N 0 29 E
Santa Bárbara, U.S.A. **161 L7** 34 25N 119 42W
Santa Bárbara,
  Amazonas,
  Venezuela **168 C4** 3 57N 67 6W
Santa Bárbara, Barinas,
  Venezuela **168 B3** 7 47N 71 10W
Santa Bárbara, Mt.,
  Spain **41 H2** 37 23N 2 50W
Santa Bárbara, Serra
  de, Azores **9 d1** 38 41N 27 22W
Santa Barbara Channel,
  U.S.A. **161 L7** 34 15N 120 0W
Santa Barbara I., U.S.A. **161 M7** 33 29N 119 2W
Santa Catalina,
  Colombia **168 A2** 10 36N 75 17W
Santa Catalina, Phil. **81 G4** 9 22N 122 59 E
Santa Catalina,
  Solomon Is. ...... **133 N12** 10 53 S 162 29 E
Santa Catalina, Gulf of,
  U.S.A. **161 N9** 33 10N 117 50W
Santa Catalina, I.,
  Mexico **162 B2** 25 40N 110 50W
Santa Catalina I.,
  U.S.A. **161 M8** 33 23N 118 25W
Santa Catarina □,
  Brazil .... **175 B6** 27 25 S 48 30W

Santa Catarina, I. de,
  Brazil .... **175 B6** 27 30 S 48 40W
Santa Caterina di
  Pittinuri, Italy ... **46 B1** 40 6N 8 27 E
Santa Caterina
  Villarmosa, Italy . **47 E7** 37 35N 14 2 E
Santa Cecília, Brazil **175 B5** 26 56 S 50 18W
Santa Clara, Cuba .. **164 B4** 22 20N 80 0W
Santa Clara, Calif.,
  U.S.A. **160 H5** 37 21N 121 57W
Santa Clara, Utah,
  U.S.A. **159 H7** 37 8N 113 39W
Santa Clara, El Golfo
  de, Mexico **162 A2** 31 42N 114 30W
Santa Clara de Olimar,
  Uruguay .... **175 C5** 32 50 S 54 54W
Santa Clarita, U.S.A. **161 L8** 34 24N 118 30W
Santa Clotilde, Peru **168 D3** 2 33 S 73 45W
Santa Coloma de
  Farners, Spain ... **40 D7** 41 50N 2 39 E
Santa Coloma de
  Gramenet, Spain . **40 D7** 41 27N 2 13 E
Santa Comba, Spain **42 B2** 43 2N 8 49W
Santa Croce Camerina,
  Italy .... **47 F7** 36 50N 14 31 E
Santa Croce di
  Magliano, Italy ... **45 G11** 41 42N 14 59 E
Santa Cruz, Argentina **176 D3** 50 0 S 68 32W
Santa Cruz, Bolivia . **173 D5** 17 43 S 63 10W
Santa Cruz, Brazil .. **170 C4** 6 13 S 36 1W
Santa Cruz, Chile ... **174 C1** 34 38 S 71 27W
Santa Cruz, Costa Rica **164 D2** 10 15N 85 35W
Santa Cruz, Madeira **9 c** 32 42N 16 46W
Santa Cruz, Peru ... **172 B2** 5 40 S 75 56W
Santa Cruz,
  Davao del S., Phil. **81 H5** 6 50N 125 25 E
Santa Cruz, Laguna,
  Phil. .... **80 D3** 14 20N 121 24 E
Santa Cruz,
  Marinduque, Phil. **80 E4** 13 28N 122 2 E
Santa Cruz, Mind. Occ.,
  Phil. .... **80 E3** 13 4N 120 43 E
Santa Cruz, Zambales,
  Phil. .... **80 D2** 14 53N 119 55 E
Santa Cruz, U.S.A. .. **160 J4** 36 58N 122 1W
Santa Cruz, Venezuela **168 B5** 8 3N 64 27W
Santa Cruz □,
  Argentina .... **176 C3** 49 0 S 70 0W
Santa Cruz □, Bolivia **173 D5** 17 43 S 63 10W
Santa Cruz →,
  Argentina .... **176 D3** 50 10 S 68 20W
Santa Cruz, I., Ecuador **172 a** 0 38 S 90 23W
Santa Cruz Cabrália,
  Brazil .... **171 E4** 16 17 S 39 2W
Santa Cruz da Graciosa,
  Azores **9 d1** 39 5N 28 1W
Santa Cruz das Flores,
  Azores **9 d2** 39 27N 31 7W
Santa Cruz de Bravo =
  Felipe Carrillo
  Puerto, Mexico ... **163 D7** 19 38N 88 3W
Santa Cruz de la Palma,
  Canary Is. **9 e1** 28 41N 17 46W
Santa Cruz de la
  Palma ✈ (SPC),
  Canary Is. **9 e1** 28 40N 17 45W
Santa Cruz de Mudela,
  Spain **43 G7** 38 39N 3 28W
Santa Cruz de Tenerife,
  Canary Is. **9 e1** 28 28N 16 15W
Santa Cruz del Norte,
  Cuba **164 B3** 23 9N 81 55W
Santa Cruz del
  Retamar, Spain .. **42 E6** 40 8N 4 14W
Santa Cruz del Sur,
  Cuba **164 B4** 20 44N 78 0W
Santa Cruz do Rio
  Pardo, Brazil ..... **175 A6** 22 54 S 49 37W
Santa Cruz do Sul,
  Brazil .... **175 B5** 29 42 S 52 25W
Santa Cruz I.,
  Solomon Is. **161 M7** 34 1N 119 43W
Santa Cruz Is.,
  Solomon Is. ...... **134 J8** 10 30 S 166 0 E
Santa Cruz la Vieja △,
  Bolivia .... **173 D5** 17 55 S 60 50W
Santa Cruz Mts.,
  Jamaica .... **164 a** 17 58N 77 43W
Santa Domingo, Cay,
  Bahamas **164 B4** 21 25N 75 15W
Sant' Egídio alla
  Vibrata, Italy .... **45 F10** 42 49N 13 42 E
Santa Elena, Argentina **174 C4** 30 58 S 59 47W
Santa Elena, Ecuador **168 D1** 2 16 S 80 52W
Santa Elena, Phil. .. **80 D4** 14 12N 122 24 E
Santa Elena, C.,
  Costa Rica **164 D2** 10 54N 85 56W
Sant' Eufémia, G. di,
  Italy .... **47 D9** 38 51N 16 4 E
Santa Eulàlia des Riu,
  Spain .... **38 D2** 38 59N 1 32 E
Santa Fe, Argentina . **174 C3** 31 35 S 60 41W
Santa Fe,
  Nueva Viscaya, Phil. **80 C3** 16 10N 120 57 E
Santa Fe, Romblon,
  Phil. .... **80 E4** 12 10N 122 2 E
Santa Fe, Spain **43 H7** 37 11N 3 43W
Santa Fe, U.S.A. **159 J11** 35 41N 105 57W
Santa Fé □, Argentina **174 C3** 31 50 S 60 55W
Santa Fe, Canal de,
  Ecuador .... **172 a** 0 48 S 89 55W
Santa Fé, I., Ecuador **172 a** 0 49 S 90 3W
Santa Fé do Sul, Brazil **175 F11** 20 13 S 50 56W
Santa Filomena, Brazil **170 C2** 9 6 S 45 50W
Santa Fiora, Italy ... **45 F8** 42 50N 11 35 E
Santa Gertrudis, Spain **38 C1** 39 0N 1 26 E
Santa Giustina, Italy **45 B9** 46 10N 12 5 E
Santa Helena, Brazil **170 B2** 2 14 S 45 18W
Santa Helena de Goiás,
  Brazil .... **171 E1** 17 53 S 50 35W
Santa Inês, Bahia,
  Brazil .... **171 D4** 13 17 S 39 48W
Santa Inês, Maranhão,
  Brazil .... **170 B2** 3 39 S 45 20W
Santa Inés, Spain ... **43 G5** 38 32N 5 37W
Santa Inés, I., Chile **176 D2** 54 0 S 73 0W
Santa Isabel = Rey
  Malabo, Eq. Guin. **113 E6** 3 45N 8 50 E
Santa Isabel, Argentina **174 D2** 36 10 S 66 54W
Santa Isabel,
  Solomon Is. ...... **133 M10** 8 0 S 159 0 E
Santa Isabel, Pico,
  Eq. Guin. .... **113 E6** 3 36N 8 49 E
Santa Isabel do
  Araguaia, Brazil . **170 C2** 6 7 S 48 19W
Santa Isabel do Morro,
  Brazil .... **171 D1** 11 34 S 50 40W
Santa Isabel do Río
  Negro, Brazil .... **169 D4** 0 24 S 65 2W
Santa Lucía, Corrientes,
  Argentina .... **174 B4** 28 58 S 59 5W
Santa Lucía, San Juan,
  Argentina .... **174 C2** 31 30 S 68 30W
Santa Lucia, Phil. .. **80 C3** 17 7N 120 27 E
Santa Lucía, Spain .. **41 H4** 37 35N 0 58W

Santa Lucia, Uruguay 174 C4 34 27 S 56 24W
Santa Lucia Range, U.S.A. 160 K5 36 0N 121 20W
Santa Luzia = Luziânia, Brazil 171 E2 16 20 S 48 0W
Santa Luzia, C. Verde Is. 9 j 16 50N 24 35W
Santa Magdalena, I., Mexico 162 C2 24 40N 112 15W
Santa Margarita, Argentina 174 D3 38 28 S 61 35W
Santa Margarita, Spain 38 B4 39 42N 3 6 E
Santa Margarita, U.S.A. 160 K6 35 23N 120 37W
Santa Margarita →, U.S.A. 161 M9 33 13N 117 23W
Santa Margarita, I., Mexico 162 C2 24 30N 111 50W
Santa Margherita, Italy 46 D1 38 58N 8 58 E
Santa Margherita Ligure, Italy 44 D6 44 20N 9 11 E
Santa María, Argentina 174 B2 26 40 S 66 0W
Santa Maria, Azores 9 d4 36 58N 25 6W
Santa Maria, Brazil 175 B5 29 40 S 53 48W
Santa Maria, C. Verde Is. 9 j 16 31N 22 53W
Santa Maria, Ilocos S., Phil. 80 C3 17 22N 120 29 E
Santa Maria, Isabela, Phil. 80 C3 17 28N 121 45 E
Santa Maria, Switz. 33 C10 46 36N 10 25 E
Santa Maria, U.S.A. 161 L6 34 57N 120 26W
Santa María →, Mexico 162 A3 31 0N 107 14W
Santa María, B. de, Mexico 162 B3 25 10N 108 40W
Santa Maria, C. de, Portugal 43 J3 36 58N 7 53W
Santa María, I., Ecuador 172 a 1 17 S 90 26W
Santa Maria Cápua Vétere, Italy 47 A7 41 5N 14 15 E
Santa Maria da Feira, Portugal 42 E2 40 55N 8 35W
Santa Maria da Vitória, Brazil 171 D3 13 24 S 44 12W
Santa María de Ipire, Venezuela 169 B4 8 49N 65 19W
Santa Maria del Camí, Spain 38 B3 39 38N 2 47 E
Santa Maria di Léuca, C., Italy 47 C11 39 47N 18 22 E
Santa Maria do Boiaçu, Brazil 169 D5 0 25 S 61 48W
Santa Maria do Suaçuí, Brazil 171 E3 18 12 S 42 25W
Santa Maria dos Marmelos, Brazil 173 B5 6 7 S 61 51W
Santa María la Real de Nieva, Spain 42 D6 41 4N 4 24W
Santa Marinella, Italy 45 F8 42 2N 11 52 E
Santa Marta, Colombia 168 A3 11 15N 74 13W
Santa Marta, Sierra Nevada de, Colombia 168 A3 10 55N 73 50W
Santa Marta de Tormes, Spain 42 E5 40 57N 5 38W
Santa Marta Grande, C., Brazil 175 B6 28 43 S 48 50W
Santa Marta Ortigueira, Ría de, Spain 42 B3 43 44N 7 45W
Santa Maura = Levkás, Greece 39 B2 38 40N 20 43 E
Santa Monica, U.S.A. 161 M8 34 1N 118 29W
Santa Monica Mts. ⌂, U.S.A. 161 L8 34 4N 118 44W
Santa Olalla, Huelva, Spain 43 H4 37 54N 6 14W
Santa Olalla, Toledo, Spain 42 E6 40 2N 4 25W
Santa Paula, U.S.A. 161 L7 34 21N 119 4W
Santa Pola, Spain 41 G4 38 13N 0 35W
Santa Ponça, Spain 38 B3 39 30N 2 28 E
Santa Quitéria, Brazil 170 B3 4 20 S 40 10W
Santa Rita = Itumbiara, Brazil 171 E2 18 20 S 49 10W
Santa Rita, Brazil 168 D4 3 29 S 69 19W
Santa Rita, Colombia 168 C4 4 53N 68 24W
Santa Rita, Phil. 81 F5 11 27N 124 56 E
Santa Rita, U.S.A. 159 K10 32 48N 108 4W
Santa Rita, Venezuela 168 A3 10 32N 71 32W
Santa Rita do Araguaia = Guiratinga, Brazil 173 D7 16 21 S 53 45W
Santa Rita do Araquaia, Brazil 173 D7 17 20 S 53 12W
Santa Rosa = Bella Unión, Uruguay 174 C4 30 15 S 57 40W
Santa Rosa, La Pampa, Argentina 174 D3 36 40 S 64 17W
Santa Rosa, San Luis, Argentina 174 C2 32 21 S 65 10W
Santa Rosa, Beni, Bolivia 172 C4 14 10 S 66 53W
Santa Rosa, Pando, Bolivia 172 C4 10 36 S 67 20W
Santa Rosa, Santa Cruz, Bolivia 173 D5 17 7 S 63 35W
Santa Rosa, Brazil 175 B5 27 52 S 54 29W
Santa Rosa, Colombia 168 C4 3 32N 69 48W
Santa Rosa, El Oro, Ecuador 168 D2 3 27 S 79 58W
Santa Rosa, Galápagos Is., Ecuador 172 a 0 40 S 90 25W
Santa Rosa, Puno, Peru 172 C3 14 30 S 70 50W
Santa Rosa, San Martin, Peru 172 B2 6 41 S 76 37W
Santa Rosa, Phil. 80 D3 15 25N 120 57 E
Santa Rosa, Calif., U.S.A. 160 G4 38 26N 122 43W
Santa Rosa, N. Mex., U.S.A. 155 H2 34 57N 104 41W
Santa Rosa, Venezuela 168 C4 1 29N 66 55W
Santa Rosa and San Jacinto Mts. ⌂, U.S.A. 161 M10 33 28N 116 20W
Santa Rosa Beach, U.S.A. 152 E3 30 22N 86 14W
Santa Rosa de Amanadona, Venezuela 168 C4 1 29N 66 55W
Santa Rosa de Cabal, Colombia 168 C2 4 52N 75 38W
Santa Rosa de Copán, Honduras 164 D2 14 47N 88 46W
Santa Rosa de la Roca, Bolivia 173 D5 16 3 S 61 34W
Santa Rosa de Osos, Colombia 168 B2 6 39N 75 28W
Santa Rosa de Río Primero, Argentina 174 C3 31 8 S 63 20W
Santa Rosa de Viterbo, Colombia 168 B3 5 53N 72 59W
Santa Rosa del Palmar, Bolivia 173 D5 16 54 S 62 24W
Santa Rosa I., Calif., U.S.A. 161 M6 33 58N 120 6W
Santa Rosa I., Fla., U.S.A. 153 E3 30 20N 86 50W
Santa Rosa Range, U.S.A. 158 F5 41 45N 117 40W
Santa Rosalía, Mexico 162 B2 27 20N 112 20W
Santa Sylvina, Argentina 174 B3 27 50 S 61 10W
Santa Tecla = Nueva San Salvador, El Salv. 164 D2 13 40N 89 18W
Santa Teresa, Argentina 174 C3 33 25 S 60 47W
Santa Teresa, Australia 126 C1 24 8 S 134 22 E
Santa Teresa, Brazil 171 E3 19 55 S 40 36W
Santa Teresa, Mexico 163 B5 25 17N 97 51W
Santa Teresa, Venezuela 169 C5 4 43N 61 4W
Santa Teresa △, Uruguay 175 C5 33 57 S 53 31W
Santa Teresa di Riva, Italy 47 E8 37 57N 15 22 E
Santa Teresa Gallura, Italy 46 A2 41 14N 9 11 E
Santa Teresinha, Brazil 170 D1 10 28 S 50 31W
Santa Uxía, Spain 42 C2 42 36N 8 58W
Santa Vitória, Brazil 171 E1 18 50 S 50 8W
Santa Vitória do Palmar, Brazil 175 C5 33 32 S 53 25W
Santa Ynez →, U.S.A. 161 L6 35 41N 120 36W
Santa Ynez Mts., U.S.A. 161 L6 34 30N 120 0W
Santa Ysabel, U.S.A. 161 M10 33 7N 116 40W
Santadi, Italy 46 C1 39 5N 8 43 E
Santaella, Spain 43 H6 37 34N 4 51W
Santahar, Bangla. 90 C2 24 48N 88 59 E
Santai, China 76 B5 31 5N 104 58 E
Santaluz, Brazil 170 D4 11 15 S 39 22W
Santana = Uruaçu, Brazil 171 D2 14 30 S 49 10W
Santana, Brazil 171 D3 13 2 S 44 5W
Santana, Madeira 9 c 32 48N 16 52W
Sântana, Romania 52 D6 46 20N 21 30 E
Santana, Coxilha de, Brazil 175 C4 30 50 S 55 35W
Santana do Ipanema, Brazil 170 C4 9 22 S 37 14W
Santana do Livramento, Brazil 175 C4 30 55 S 55 30W
Santana do Paranaíba = Paranaíba, Brazil 173 D7 19 40 S 51 11W
Santander, Colombia 168 C2 3 1N 76 28W
Santander, Phil. 81 G4 9 25N 123 20 E
Santander, Spain 42 B7 43 27N 3 51W
Santander □, Colombia 168 B3 7 0N 73 15W
Santander Jiménez, Mexico 163 C5 24 11N 98 29W
Santanilla, Is., Honduras 164 C3 17 22N 83 57W
Santanyí, Spain 38 B4 39 20N 3 5 E
Santaquin, U.S.A. 158 G8 39 59N 111 47W
Santarcángelo di Romagna, Italy 45 D9 44 4N 12 26 E
Santarém, Brazil 169 D7 2 25 S 54 42W
Santarém, Portugal 43 F2 39 12N 8 42W
Santarém □, Portugal 43 F2 39 10N 8 40W
Santaren Channel, W. Indies 164 B4 24 0N 79 30W
Santee, U.S.A. 161 N10 32 50N 116 58W
Santee →, U.S.A. 149 J6 33 7N 79 17W
Santéramo in Colle, Italy 47 B9 40 49N 16 45 E
Santerno →, Italy 45 D8 44 34N 11 58 E
Santhià, Italy 44 C5 45 22N 8 10 E
Santi-Quaranta = Sarandë, Albania 38 B9 39 52N 19 55 E
Santiago = São Tiago, C. Verde Is. 9 j 15 0N 23 40W
Santiago, Bolivia 173 D6 18 19 S 59 34W
Santiago, Brazil 175 B5 29 11 S 54 52W
Santiago, Canary Is. 9 e1 28 2N 17 12W
Santiago, Chile 174 C1 33 24 S 70 40W
Santiago, Panama 164 E3 8 0N 81 0W
Santiago, Peru 172 C2 14 11 S 75 43W
Santiago, Ilocos S., Phil. 80 C3 17 18N 120 27 E
Santiago, Isabela, Phil. 80 C3 16 41N 121 33 E
Santiago □, Chile 174 C1 33 30 S 70 50W
Santiago →, Mexico 136 G9 25 11N 105 26W
Santiago →, Peru 168 D2 4 27 S 77 38W
Santiago, C., Chile 176 D1 50 46 S 75 27W
Santiago, I. = San Salvador, I., Ecuador 172 a 0 16 S 90 42W
Santiago, Punta de, Eq. Guin. 113 E6 3 12N 8 40 E
Santiago, Serranía de, Bolivia 173 D6 18 25 S 59 25W
Santiago de Chuco, Peru 172 B2 8 9 S 78 11W
Santiago de Compostela, Spain 42 C2 42 52N 8 37W
Santiago de Cuba, Cuba 164 C4 20 0N 75 49W
Santiago de los Cabelleros, Dom. Rep. 165 C5 19 30N 70 40W
Santiago del Estero, Argentina 174 B3 27 50 S 64 15W
Santiago del Estero □, Argentina 174 B3 27 40 S 63 15W
Santiago del Teide, Canary Is. 9 e1 28 17N 16 48W
Santiago do Boqueirão = Santiago, Brazil 175 B5 29 11 S 54 52W
Santiago do Cacém, Portugal 43 G2 38 1N 8 42W
Santiago Ixcuintla, Mexico 162 C3 21 50N 105 11W
Santiago Papasquiaro, Mexico 162 C3 25 0N 105 20W
Santiaguillo, L. de, Mexico 162 C4 24 50N 104 50W
Santiguila, Mali 112 C3 12 42N 7 25W
Santillana, Spain 42 B6 43 24N 4 6W
Säntis, Switz. 33 B8 47 15N 9 22 E
Santisteban del Puerto, Spain 43 G7 38 17N 3 15W
Santo →, Peru 172 B2 8 56 S 78 37W
Santo Amaro, Brazil 171 D4 12 30 S 38 43W
Santo Anastácio, Brazil 175 A5 21 58 S 51 39W
Santo André, Brazil 175 A6 23 39 S 46 29W
Santo Ângelo, Brazil 175 B5 28 15 S 54 15W
Santo Antão, C. Verde Is. 9 j 16 52N 25 10W
Santo Antônia, São Tomé & Príncipe 115 G6 1 37N 7 27 E
Santo Antonio, Brazil 169 D5 2 24 S 60 58W
Santo Antônio da Cachoeira = Itaguatins, Brazil 170 C2 5 47 S 47 29W
Santo Antônio de Jesus, Brazil 171 D4 12 58 S 39 16W
Santo Antônio do Abaixo = Santo Antônio do Leverger, Brazil 173 D6 15 52 S 56 5W
Santo Antônio do Içá, Brazil 168 D4 3 5 S 67 57W
Santo Antônio do Leverger, Brazil 173 D6 15 52 S 56 5W
Santo Corazón, Bolivia 173 D6 18 0 S 58 45W
Santo Domingo, Dom. Rep. 165 C6 18 30N 69 59W
Santo Domingo, Baja Calif., Mexico 162 A1 30 43N 116 2W
Santo Domingo, Baja Calif. S., Mexico 162 B2 25 32N 112 2W
Santo Domingo, Nic. 164 D3 12 14N 84 59W
Santo Domingo de la Calzada, Spain 40 C2 42 26N 2 57W
Santo Domingo de los Colorados, Ecuador 168 D2 0 15 S 79 9W
Santo Domingo Pueblo, U.S.A. 159 J10 35 31N 106 22W
Santo Stéfano di Camastro, Italy 47 D7 38 1N 14 22 E
Santo Tirso, Portugal 42 D2 41 21N 8 28W
Santo Tomás, Ecuador 172 a 0 51 S 91 2W
Santo Tomás, Mexico 162 A1 31 33N 116 24W
Santo Tomás, Peru 172 C3 14 26 S 72 8W
Santo Tomás, Volcán, Ecuador 172 a 0 48 S 91 7W
Santo Tomé, Argentina 175 B4 28 40 S 56 5W
Santo Tomé de Guayana = Ciudad Guayana, Venezuela 169 B5 8 0N 62 30W
Santomera, Spain 41 G3 38 4N 1 3W
Santoña, Spain 42 B7 43 29N 3 27W
Santoríni = Thíra, Greece 49 E7 36 23N 25 27 E
Santos, Brazil 175 A6 24 0 S 46 20W
Santos, Sierra de los, Spain 43 G5 38 7N 5 12W
Santos Dumont, Brazil 171 F3 22 55 S 43 10W
Santos Plateau, India 8 J7 26 0 S 42 0W
Sanur, Indonesia 79 K18 8 41 S 115 15 E
Sanwer, India 92 H6 22 59N 75 50 E
Sanxenxo, Spain 42 C2 42 24N 8 49W
Sanxiang, China 69 G9 22 21N 113 25 E
Sanya, China 86 C7 18 14N 109 29 E
San'yō, Japan 72 C3 34 2N 131 5 E
Sanyuan, China 74 G5 34 35N 108 58 E
Sanyuki-Sammyaku, Japan 72 C6 34 5N 134 0 E
Sanza Pombo, Angola 115 D3 7 18 S 15 56 E
São Bartolomeu de Messines, Portugal 43 H2 37 15N 8 17W
São Benedito = Beneditinos, Brazil 170 C3 5 27 S 42 22W
São Benedito, Brazil 170 B3 4 3 S 40 53W
São Benedito →, Brazil 173 B6 9 11 S 57 2W
São Bento, Brazil 170 B3 2 42 S 44 50W
São Bento do Norte, Brazil 170 C4 5 4 S 36 2W
São Bernardo do Campo, Brazil 171 F2 23 45 S 46 34W
São Borja, Brazil 175 B4 28 39 S 56 0W
São Brás de Alportel, Portugal 43 H3 37 8N 7 37W
São Braz, C. de, Angola 115 D2 9 58 S 13 19 E
São Caitano, Brazil 170 C4 8 21 S 36 6W
São Carlos, Brazil 175 A6 22 0 S 47 50W
São Cristóvão, Brazil 170 D4 11 1 S 37 15W
São Domingos, Brazil 171 D2 13 25 S 46 19W
São Domingos, Guinea-Biss. 112 C1 12 19N 16 13W
São Domingos da Boa Vista = Capim, Brazil 170 B2 1 41 S 47 47W
São Domingos do Capim = Capim, Brazil 170 B2 1 41 S 47 47W
São Domingos do Maranhão, Brazil 170 C3 5 42 S 44 22W
São Felipe = Içana, Brazil 168 C4 0 21N 67 19W
São Felippe = Eirunepé, Brazil 172 B4 6 35 S 69 53W
São Félix, Brazil 171 D1 11 36 S 50 39W
São Felix do Xingu, Brazil 173 B7 6 38 S 51 59W
São Filipe, C. Verde Is. 9 j 15 2N 24 30W
São Francisco = Itapagé, Brazil 170 B4 3 41 S 39 34W
São Francisco, Brazil 171 E3 16 0 S 44 50W
São Francisco →, Brazil 170 D4 10 30 S 36 24W
São Francisco do Maranhão, Brazil 170 C3 6 15 S 42 52W
São Francisco do Sul, Brazil 175 B6 26 15 S 48 36W
São Gabriel, Brazil 175 C5 30 20 S 54 20W
São Gabriel da Cachoeira, Brazil 168 D4 0 8 S 67 5W
São Gabriel da Palha, Brazil 171 E3 18 47 S 40 39W
São Gonçalo = Araripina, Brazil 170 C3 7 33 S 40 34W
São Gonçalo, Brazil 171 F3 22 48 S 43 5W
São Gotardo, Brazil 171 E2 19 19 S 46 3W
Sao Hill, Tanzania 119 D4 8 20 S 35 12 E
São João, Guinea-Biss. 112 C1 11 32N 15 25W
São João da Baliza, Brazil 169 C6 0 52N 59 52W
São João da Boa Vista, Brazil 175 A6 22 0 S 46 52W
São João da Madeira, Portugal 42 E2 40 54N 8 30W
São João da Pesqueira, Portugal 42 D3 41 8N 7 24W
São João da Ponte, Brazil 171 E3 15 56 S 44 1W
São João do Montenegro = Montenegro, Brazil 175 B5 29 39 S 51 29W
São João del Rei, Brazil 171 F3 21 8 S 44 15W
São João do Araguaia, Brazil 170 C2 5 23 S 48 46W
São João do Paraíso, Brazil 171 E3 15 19 S 42 1W
São João do Piauí, Brazil 170 C3 8 21 S 42 15W
São João dos Patos, Brazil 170 C3 6 30 S 43 42W
São Joaquim, Amazonas, Brazil 168 D4 0 1 S 67 16W
São Joaquim, Sta. Catarina, Brazil 175 B6 28 18 S 49 56W
São Joaquim △, Brazil 175 B6 28 12 S 49 37W
São Joaquim da Barra, Brazil 171 F2 20 35 S 47 53W
São Jorge, Azores 9 d1 38 38N 28 3W
São Jorge, Canal de, Azores 9 d1 38 30N 28 0W
São Jorge, Pta. de, Azores 9 d1 38 42N 27 3W
São Jorge, Pta. de, Madeira 9 c 32 50N 16 53W
São José, Brazil 175 B5 27 38 S 48 39W
São José, B. de, Brazil 170 B3 2 38 S 44 4W
São José da Lagoa = Nova Era, Brazil 171 E3 19 45 S 43 3W
São José da Laje, Brazil 170 C4 9 1 S 36 3W
São José de Mipibu, Brazil 170 C4 6 5 S 35 15W
São José de Tocantins = Niquelândia, Brazil 171 D2 14 33 S 48 23W
São José do Norte, Brazil 175 C5 32 1 S 52 3W
São José do Peixe, Brazil 170 C3 7 24 S 42 34W
São José do Rio Prêto, Brazil 175 A6 20 50 S 49 20W
São José dos Campos, Brazil 175 A6 23 7 S 45 52W
São José dos Cocais = Nossa Senhora do Livramento, Brazil 173 D6 15 48 S 56 22W
São José dos Matões = Parnarama, Brazil 170 C3 5 31 S 43 6W
São Leopoldo, Brazil 175 B5 29 50 S 51 10W
São Lourenço, Brazil 171 F2 22 7 S 45 3W
São Lourenço →, Brazil 173 D6 17 53 S 57 27W
São Lourenço, Pantanal do, Brazil 173 D6 17 30 S 56 20W
São Lourenço, Pta. de, Madeira 9 c 32 44N 16 39W
São Lourenço do Sul, Brazil 175 C5 31 22 S 51 58W
São Luís, Brazil 170 B3 2 39 S 44 15W
São Luís do Curu, Brazil 170 B4 3 40 S 39 14W
São Luís do Tapojós, Brazil 169 D6 4 25 S 56 12W
São Luís Gonzaga = Ipixuna, Brazil 172 B3 7 0 S 71 40W
São Luís Gonzaga, Brazil 175 B5 28 25 S 55 0W
São Marcos →, Brazil 171 E2 18 15 S 47 37W
São Marcos, B. de, Brazil 170 B3 2 0 S 44 0W
São Martinho da Cortiça, Portugal 42 E2 40 18N 8 8W
São Mateus, Azores 9 d1 38 26N 28 27W
São Mateus, Brazil 171 E4 18 44 S 39 50W
São Mateus →, Brazil 171 E4 18 35 S 39 44W
São Mateus do Sul, Brazil 175 B5 25 52 S 50 23W
São Miguel, Azores 9 d3 37 47N 25 30W
São Miguel do Araguaia, Brazil 171 D1 13 19 S 50 13W
São Miguel do Guamá = Guamá, Brazil 170 B2 1 37 S 47 29W
São Miguel do Oeste, Brazil 175 B5 26 45 S 53 34W
São Miguel dos Campos, Brazil 170 C4 9 47 S 36 5W
São Nicolau, C. Verde Is. 9 j 16 20N 24 20W
São Nicolau →, Angola 115 E2 14 16 S 12 22 E
São Nicolau →, Brazil 170 C3 5 45 S 42 2W
São Paulo, Brazil 175 A6 23 32 S 46 37W
São Paulo □, Brazil 175 A6 22 0 S 49 0W
São Paulo, I., Atl. Oc. 8 F9 0 56N 29 22W
São Paulo de Olivença, Brazil 168 D4 3 27 S 68 48W
São Pedro, Atl. Oc. 8 F9 0 56N 29 22W
São Pedro do Sul, Portugal 42 E2 40 46N 8 4W
São Rafael, Brazil 170 C4 5 47 S 36 55W
São Raimundo das Mangabeiras, Brazil 170 C2 7 1 S 45 29W
São Raimundo Nonato, Brazil 170 C3 9 1 S 42 42W
São Romão, Brazil 171 E2 16 22 S 45 4W
São Roque, Madeira 9 c 32 46N 16 48W
São Roque, C. de, Brazil 170 C4 5 30 S 35 16W
São Roque do Pico, Azores 9 d1 38 31N 28 19W
São Salvador do Congo = Mbanza Congo, Angola 115 D2 6 18 S 14 16 E
São Sebastião, Azores 9 d1 38 39N 27 6W
São Sebastião, I. de, Brazil 175 A6 23 50 S 45 18W
São Sebastião do Paraíso, Brazil 175 A6 20 54 S 46 59W
São Simão, Brazil 171 E1 18 56 S 50 30W
São Teotónio, Portugal 43 H2 37 30N 8 42W
São Tiago, C. Verde Is. 9 j 15 0N 23 40W
São Tomé, Brazil 170 C4 5 58 S 36 4W
São Tomé, São Tomé & Príncipe 115 G6 0 10N 6 39 E
São Tomé, C. de, Brazil 171 F3 22 0 S 40 59W
São Tomé, Pico de, São Tomé & Príncipe 115 G6 0 16N 6 33 E
São Tomé & Príncipe ■, Africa 115 G6 0 12N 6 39 E
São Vicente = Araguatins, Brazil 170 C2 5 38 S 48 7W
São Vicente, Brazil 175 A6 23 57 S 46 23W
São Vicente, C. Verde Is. 9 j 17 0N 25 0W
São Vicente, Madeira 9 c 32 48N 17 3W
São Vicente, C. de, Portugal 43 H1 37 0N 9 0W
Saona, I., Dom. Rep. 165 C6 18 10N 68 40W
Saône →, France 27 G11 45 44N 4 50 E
Saône-et-Loire □, France 27 F11 46 30N 4 50 E
Saonek, Indonesia 83 B4 0 22 S 130 55 E
Saoura, O. →, Algeria 111 C4 29 0N 0 55W
Sápai, Greece 51 E9 41 2N 25 43 E
Sapam, Ao, Thailand 87 a 8 0N 98 26 E
Sapanca, Turkey 100 B4 40 41N 30 16 E
Sapão →, Brazil 170 D2 11 1 S 45 32W
Saparua, Indonesia 82 B3 3 33 S 128 40 E
Sapé, Brazil 170 C4 7 6 S 35 13W
Sape, Indonesia 85 D5 8 34 S 118 59 E
Sapele, Nigeria 113 D6 5 50N 5 40 E
Sapelo I., U.S.A. 152 D8 31 25N 81 12W
Sapelo Sound, U.S.A. 152 D8 31 30N 81 10W
Saphane, Turkey 49 B11 39 1N 29 13 E
Sapi ⌂, Zimbabwe 119 F2 15 48 S 29 42 E
Sapiéntza, Greece 48 E3 36 45N 21 43 E
Sapindji, Dem. Rep. of the Congo 115 D4 9 39 S 23 12 E
Sapo △, Liberia 112 D3 5 15N 8 30W
Sapone, Burkina Faso 113 C4 12 3N 1 35W
Saposoa, Peru 172 B2 6 55 S 76 45W
Sapotskina, Belarus 54 E10 53 49N 23 40 E
Sapouy, Burkina Faso 113 C4 11 34N 1 44W
Sapozhok, Russia 60 D5 53 59N 40 41 E
Sapphire, Australia 126 C4 23 28 S 147 43 E
Sappho, U.S.A. 160 B2 48 4N 124 16W
Sapporo, Japan 70 C10 43 0N 141 21 E
Sapri, Italy 47 B8 40 4N 15 38 E
Sapu, Angola 115 E3 12 28 S 19 26 E
Sapudi, Indonesia 85 D4 7 6 S 114 20 E
Sapulpa, U.S.A. 155 H6 35 59N 96 5W
Saqqez, Iran 101 D12 36 15N 46 20 E
Sar Dasht, Āzarbāyjān-e Gharbī, Iran 101 D11 36 9N 45 28 E
Sar Dasht, Khuzestān, Iran 97 C6 32 32N 48 52 E
Sar-e Pol, Afghan. 91 A2 36 10N 66 0 E
Sar-e Pol □, Afghan. 91 A2 36 20N 65 50 E
Sar Gachīneh = Yāsūj, Iran 97 D6 30 31N 51 31 E
Sar Planina, Macedonia 50 E4 42 0N 21 0 E
Sara, Burkina Faso 112 C4 11 40N 3 53W
Sara, Niger 109 D2 20 46N 12 35 E
Sara, Phil. 81 F4 11 16N 123 1 E
Šara △, Serbia & M. 50 D5 42 12N 21 0 E
Sara Buri = Saraburi, Thailand 86 E3 14 30N 100 55 E
Sarāb, Iran 101 D12 37 55N 47 40 E
Sarabadi, Iraq 96 C5 33 1N 44 48 E
Saraburi, Thailand 86 E3 14 30N 100 55 E
Saradiya, India 92 J4 21 34N 70 2 E
Saraféré, Mali 112 B4 15 50N 3 40W
Saragossa = Zaragoza, Spain 40 D4 41 39N 0 53W
Saraguro, Ecuador 168 D2 3 35 S 79 16W
Sarai Naurang, Pakistan 92 C4 32 50N 70 47 E
Saraikela, India 93 H11 22 42N 85 56 E
Saraipali, India 94 D6 21 20N 82 59 E
Saraiu, Romania 53 F13 44 43N 28 10 E
Sarajevo, Bos.-H. 52 G3 43 52N 18 26 E
Sarakhs, Turkmenistan 97 B9 36 32N 61 13 E
Saraktash, Russia 64 F7 51 47N 56 22 E
Saramacca →, Suriname 169 B6 5 50N 55 55W
Saramati, Burma 90 C5 25 44N 95 2 E
Saran, Gunung, Indonesia 85 C4 0 30 S 111 25 E
Saranac, U.S.A. 157 B11 42 56N 85 13W
Saranac L., U.S.A. 151 B10 44 20N 74 10W
Saranac Lake, U.S.A. 151 B10 44 20N 74 8W
Saranda, Tanzania 118 D3 5 45 S 34 59 E
Sarandë, Albania 38 B9 39 52N 19 55 E
Sarandí del Yí, Uruguay 175 C4 33 18 S 55 38W
Sarandí Grande, Uruguay 174 C4 33 44 S 56 20W
Sarangani □, Phil. 81 J5 5 45N 125 20 E
Sarangani B., Phil. 81 J5 6 0N 125 13 E
Sarangani Is., Phil. 81 J5 5 25N 125 25 E
Sarangarh, India 94 D6 21 30N 83 5 E
Saranovo = Septemvri, Bulgaria 51 D8 42 13N 24 6 E
Saransk, Russia 60 C7 54 10N 45 10 E
Sarapul, Russia 64 C4 56 28N 53 48 E
Sarar Plain = Bannaanka Saraar, Somali Rep. 120 C3 9 25N 46 17 E
Sarasota, U.S.A. 153 H7 27 20N 82 32W
Sarata, Ukraine 53 D14 46 1N 29 40 E
Sarata →, Ukraine 53 E14 45 51N 29 41 E
Saratoga, Calif., U.S.A. 160 H4 37 16N 122 2W
Saratoga, Wyo., U.S.A. 158 F10 41 27N 106 49W
Saratoga △, U.S.A. 151 D11 43 0N 73 37W
Saratoga Springs, U.S.A. 151 C11 43 5N 73 47W
Saratok, Malaysia 78 D4 1 55N 111 17 E
Saratov, Russia 60 E7 51 30N 46 2 E
Sarāvān, Iran 97 E9 27 25N 62 15 E
Saravane, Laos 86 E6 15 43N 106 25 E
Sarawak □, Malaysia 85 B4 2 0N 113 0 E
Saray, Tekirdağ, Turkey 51 E11 41 26N 27 55 E
Saray, Van, Turkey 101 C11 38 38N 44 9 E
Saray Komar = Pyandzh, Tajikistan 65 E4 37 14N 69 6 E
Saraya, Guinea 112 C2 12 50N 11 45W
Saraya, Senegal 112 C2 12 50N 11 45W
Sarayçık, Turkey 49 B11 39 1N 29 49 E
Sarayköy, Turkey 49 D10 37 55N 28 54 E
Saraylar, Turkey 51 F11 40 39N 27 40 E
Sarayönü, Turkey 100 C5 38 16N 32 24 E
Sarbāz, Iran 97 E9 26 38N 61 19 E
Sarbīsheh, Iran 97 C8 32 30N 59 40 E
Sárbogárd, Hungary 52 D3 46 50N 18 40 E
Sarca →, Italy 44 C7 45 52N 10 52 E
Sarcelles, France 27 D9 49 1N 2 23 E
Sardalas, Libya 108 C2 25 50N 10 34 E
Sardarova Karakhana = Leninskiy, Tajikistan 65 D4 38 26N 68 46 E
Sardarshahr, India 92 E6 28 30N 74 29 E
Sardegna □, Italy 46 B1 40 0N 9 0 E
Sardhana, India 92 E7 29 9N 77 39 E
Sardina, Pta., Canary Is. 9 e1 28 9N 15 44W
Sardinata, Colombia 168 B3 8 5N 72 48W
Sardinia = Sardegna □, Italy 46 B1 40 0N 9 0 E
Sardinia, U.S.A. 157 F13 39 0N 83 49W
Sardis, Turkey 49 C10 38 28N 28 2 E
Sardis, U.S.A. 152 C8 32 58N 81 46W
Sārdūīyeh = Dar Mazār, Iran 97 D8 29 14N 57 20 E
Saren, Indonesia 79 J18 8 26 S 115 34 E
S'Arenal, Spain 38 B3 39 30N 2 45 E
Sarentino, Italy 45 B8 46 38N 11 21 E
Saréyamou, Mali 112 B4 16 7N 3 10W
Sargans, Switz. 33 B8 47 3N 9 15 E
Sargasso Sea, Atl. Oc. 8 D4 27 0N 72 0W
Sargent, U.S.A. 152 B5 33 26N 84 52W
Sargodha, Pakistan 91 B4 32 10N 72 40 E
Sarh, Chad 109 G3 9 5N 18 23 E
Sarhala, Ivory C. 112 D3 8 22N 6 8W
Sarhro, Jebel, Morocco 110 B4 31 6N 5 0W
Sārī, Iran 97 B7 36 30N 53 4 E
Sari d'Orcino, France 29 F12 42 3N 8 49 E
Sária, Greece 49 F9 35 54N 27 17 E
Saria, India 93 J10 21 38N 83 22 E
Sariab, Pakistan 92 D2 30 6N 66 59 E
Sarıbeyler, Turkey 49 B9 39 24N 27 35 E
Saricumbe, Angola 115 E3 12 12 S 19 46 E
Sarıgöl, Turkey 100 C3 38 14N 28 41 E
Sarıkamiş, Turkey 101 B10 40 22N 42 35 E
Sarıkaya, Turkey 100 C6 39 29N 35 22 E
Sarikei, Malaysia 85 B4 2 8N 111 30 E
Sarıköy, Turkey 51 F11 40 12N 27 37 E
Sarila, India 93 G8 25 46N 79 41 E
Sarina, Australia 126 C4 21 22 S 149 13 E
Sariñena, Spain 40 D4 41 47N 0 10W
Sariri, Papua N. G. 132 E5 9 11 S 148 35 E
Sarita, U.S.A. 155 M6 27 13N 97 47W
Sariwŏn, N. Korea 75 E13 38 31N 125 46 E
Sariyer Barajı, Turkey 100 B4 40 2N 31 33 E
Sarıyer, Turkey 51 E13 41 10N 29 3 E
Sarju →, India 93 F9 27 21N 81 23 E
Sark, U.K. 21 H5 49 25N 2 22W
Sarkad, Hungary 52 D6 46 47N 21 23 E
Sarkari Tala, India 92 F4 27 39N 70 52 E
Şarkışla, Turkey 100 C7 39 21N 36 25 E
Şarköy, Turkey 51 F11 40 36N 27 6 E
Sarlat-la-Canéda, France 28 D5 44 54N 1 13 E
Sărmăşag, Romania 52 C7 47 21N 22 50 E
Sărmaşu, Romania 53 D9 46 45N 24 13 E
Sarmi, Indonesia 83 B5 1 49 S 138 44 E
Sarmiento, Argentina 176 C3 45 35 S 69 5W
Sarmizegetusa, Romania 52 E7 45 31N 22 47 E
Särna, Sweden 16 C7 61 41N 13 8 E

Sarnano, *Italy* **45 E10** 43 2N 13 18 E
Sarnen, *Switz.* **32 C6** 46 53N 8 13 E
Sarnia, *Canada* **140 D3** 42 58N 82 23W
Sarno, *Italy* **47 B7** 40 49N 14 37 E
Sarnthein = Sarentino, *Italy* **45 B8** 46 38N 11 21 E
Särö, *Sweden* **17 G5** 57 31N 11 57 E
Saroako, *Indonesia* **82 B2** 2 31 S 121 22 E
Sarolangun, *Indonesia* **84 C2** 2 19 S 102 42 E
Saronikós Kólpos, *Greece* **48 D5** 37 45N 23 45 E
Saronno, *Italy* **44 C6** 45 38N 9 2 E
Saros Körfezi, *Turkey* **51 F10** 40 30N 26 15 E
Sárospatak, *Hungary* **52 B6** 48 18N 21 33 E
Sarowbī, *Afghan.* **91 B3** 34 36N 69 44 E
Sarpsborg, *Norway* **18 E8** 59 16N 11 7 E
Sarracín, *Spain* **42 C7** 42 15N 3 45W
Sarralbe, *France* **27 D14** 49 0N 7 1 E
Sarrat, *Phil.* **80 B3** 18 9N 120 39 E
Sarre = Saar →, *Europe* **24 E6** 49 41N 6 32 E
Sarre, *Italy* **44 C4** 45 40N 7 15 E
Sarre-Union, *France* **27 D14** 48 57N 7 4 E
Sarrebourg, *France* **27 D14** 48 43N 7 3 E
Sarreguemines, *France* **27 C14** 49 5N 7 4 E
Sarria, *Spain* **42 C3** 42 49N 7 29W
Sarrión, *Spain* **40 E4** 40 9N 0 49W
Sarro, *Mali* **112 C3** 13 40N 5 15W
Sarstedt, *Germany* **30 C5** 52 14N 9 52 E
Sartène, *France* **29 G12** 41 38N 8 58 E
Sarthe □, *France* **26 D7** 48 10N 0 10 E
Sarthe →, *France* **26 E6** 47 33N 0 31W
Sartilly, *France* **26 D5** 48 45N 1 28W
Saruhanlı, *Turkey* **49 C9** 38 44N 27 36 E
Săruleşti, *Romania* **53 F11** 44 25N 26 39 E
Saruna →, *Pakistan* **92 F2** 26 31N 67 7 E
Sarupeta, *India* **90 B3** 26 30N 91 5 E
Saruwaged Ra., *Papua N. G.* **132 D4** 6 13 S 146 45 E
Sárvár, *Hungary* **52 C1** 47 15N 16 56 E
Sarvar, *India* **92 F6** 26 4N 75 0 E
Sarvestān, *Iran* **97 D7** 29 20N 53 10 E
Särvfjället, *Sweden* **16 B7** 62 42N 13 30 E
Sárviz →, *Hungary* **52 D3** 46 24N 18 41 E
Sary-Tash, *Kyrgyzstan* **65 D6** 39 44N 73 15 E
Saryaghash, *Kazakhstan* **65 C4** 41 27N 69 9 E
Sarybulaq, *Kazakhstan* **65 B5** 43 23N 71 29 E
Sarych, Mys, *Ukraine* **59 K7** 44 25N 33 45 E
Sarykemer, *Kazakhstan* **65 B5** 43 0N 71 30 E
Sarykolskiy Khrebet, *Tajikistan* **65 D7** 38 30N 74 30 E
Saryözek, *Kazakhstan* **65 A8** 44 22N 77 59 E
Saryshagan, *Kazakhstan* **66 E8** 46 12N 73 38 E
Sarzana, *Italy* **44 D6** 44 7N 9 58 E
Sarzeau, *France* **26 E4** 47 31N 2 48W
Sasabeneh, *Ethiopia* **120 C2** 7 59N 44 43 E
Sasamungga, *Solomon Is.* **133 L9** 7 0 S 156 50 E
Sasan Gir, *India* **92 J4** 21 10N 70 36 E
Sasaram, *India* **93 G11** 24 57N 84 5 E
Sasari, Mt., *Solomon Is.* **133 M10** 8 10 S 159 30 E
Sasayama, *Japan* **73 B7** 35 4N 135 13 E
Sasebo, *Japan* **72 D1** 33 10N 129 43 E
Saser, *India* **93 B7** 34 50N 77 50 E
Saskatchewan □, *Canada* **143 C7** 54 40N 106 0W
Saskatchewan →, *Canada* **143 C8** 53 37N 100 40W
Saskatoon, *Canada* **143 C7** 52 10N 106 38W
Saskylakh, *Russia* **67 B12** 71 55N 114 1 E
Saslaya △, *Nic.* **164 D2** 13 45N 85 4W
Sasolburg, *S. Africa* **117 D4** 26 46 S 27 49 E
Sasovo, *Russia* **60 C5** 54 25N 41 55 E
Sassandra, *Ivory C.* **112 E3** 4 55N 6 8W
Sassandra →, *Ivory C.* **112 E3** 4 58N 6 5W
Sássari, *Italy* **46 B1** 40 43N 8 34 E
Sassnitz, *Germany* **30 A9** 54 29N 13 39 E
Sasso Marconi, *Italy* **45 D8** 44 24N 11 15 E
Sassocorvaro, *Italy* **45 E9** 43 47N 12 30 E
Sassoferrato, *Italy* **45 E9** 43 26N 12 51 E
Sasstown, *Liberia* **112 E3** 4 45N 8 27W
Sassuolo, *Italy* **44 D7** 44 33N 10 47 E
Sástago, *Spain* **40 D4** 41 19N 0 21W
Sastöbe, *Kazakhstan* **65 B4** 42 33N 70 0 E
Sasvad, *India* **94 E2** 18 20N 74 2 E
Sasyk, Ozero, *Ukraine* **53 E14** 45 45N 29 20 E
Sata-Misaki, *Japan* **72 F2** 31 0N 130 40 E
Satadougou, *Mali* **112 C2** 12 25N 11 25W
Satakunda = Satakunta, *Finland* **15 F20** 61 45N 23 0 E
Satakunta, *Finland* **15 F20** 61 45N 23 0 E
Satama-Soukoura, *Ivory C.* **112 D4** 7 55N 4 27W
Satara, *India* **94 F1** 17 44N 73 58 E
Satara, *S. Africa* **117 C5** 24 29 S 31 47 E
Satbarwa, *India* **93 H11** 23 55N 84 16 E
Satellite Beach, *U.S.A.* **153 G9** 28 10N 80 36W
Såtenäs, *Sweden* **17 F6** 58 27N 12 41 E
Säter, *Sweden* **16 D9** 60 21N 15 45 E
Satevó, *Mexico* **162 B3** 27 57N 106 7W
Satilla →, *U.S.A.* **152 E8** 30 59N 81 29W
Satipo, *Peru* **172 C3** 11 15 S 74 25W
Satka, *Russia* **64 D7** 55 3N 59 1 E
Satkania, *Bangla.* **90 D4** 22 4N 92 3 E
Satkhira, *Bangla.* **90 D2** 22 43N 89 8 E
Satmala Hills, *Andhra Pradesh, India* **94 E4** 19 45N 78 45 E
Satmala Hills, *Maharashtra, India* **94 D2** 20 15N 74 40 E
Satna, *India* **93 G9** 24 35N 80 50 E
Šator, *Bos.-H.* **45 D13** 44 11N 16 37 E
Sátoraljaújhely, *Hungary* **52 B6** 48 25N 21 41 E
Satpura △, *India* **92 H8** 22 40N 78 15 E
Satpura Ra., *India* **94 D3** 21 25N 76 10 E
Satrup, *Germany* **30 A5** 54 41N 9 36 E
Satsuma-Hantō, *Japan* **72 F2** 31 25N 130 25 E
Satsuna-Shotō, *Japan* **71 K5** 30 0N 130 0 E
Sattahip, *Thailand* **86 F3** 12 41N 100 54 E
Sattenapalle, *India* **95 F5** 16 25N 80 6 E
Satu Mare, *Romania* **52 C7** 47 46N 22 55 E
Satu Mare □, *Romania* **52 C8** 47 45N 23 0 E
Satui, *Indonesia* **85 C5** 3 50 S 115 27 E
Satun, *Thailand* **87 J3** 6 43N 100 2 E
Satupa'itea, *Samoa* **133 W23** 13 45 S 172 18W
Saturnina →, *Brazil* **173 C6** 12 15 S 58 10W
Sauce = Juan L. Lacaze, *Uruguay* **174 C4** 34 26 S 57 25W
Sauce, *Argentina* **174 C4** 30 5 S 58 46W
Sauceda, *Mexico* **162 B4** 25 55N 101 18W
Saucillo, *Mexico* **162 B3** 28 1N 105 17W
Sauda, *Norway* **18 E3** 59 40N 6 20 E
Saūdakent, *Kazakhstan* **65 B4** 43 48N 69 58 E
Saudasjøen, *Norway* **18 E3** 59 38N 6 17 E
Saúde, *Brazil* **170 D3** 10 56 S 40 24W
Sauðarkrókur, *Iceland* **11 B7** 65 45N 19 40W
Saudi Arabia ■, *Asia* **96 B3** 26 0N 44 0 E
Sauerland, *Germany* **36 C4** 51 12N 7 59 E
Saugatuck, *U.S.A.* **157 B10** 42 40N 86 12W
Saugeen →, *Canada* **150 B3** 44 30N 81 22W
Saugerties, *U.S.A.* **151 D11** 42 5N 73 57W
Saugues, *France* **28 D7** 44 58N 3 32 E
Saugus, *U.S.A.* **161 L8** 34 25N 118 32W
Saujbulagh = Mahābād, *Iran* **101 D11** 36 50N 45 45 E
Saujon, *France* **28 C3** 45 41N 0 55W
Sauk Centre, *U.S.A.* **154 C7** 45 44N 94 57W
Sauk City, *U.S.A.* **156 A7** 43 17N 89 43W
Sauk Rapids, *U.S.A.* **154 C7** 45 35N 94 10W
Saül, *Fr. Guiana* **169 C7** 3 37N 53 12W
Sauland, *Norway* **18 E5** 59 37N 8 56 E
Saulgau, *Germany* **31 G5** 48 1N 9 29 E
Saulieu, *France* **27 E11** 47 17N 4 14 E
Sault, *France* **29 D9** 44 6N 5 24 E
Sault Ste. Marie, *Canada* **140 C3** 46 30N 84 20W
Sault Ste. Marie, *U.S.A.* **139 D11** 46 30N 84 21W
Saumlaki, *Indonesia* **83 C4** 7 55 S 131 20 E
Saumur, *France* **26 E6** 47 15N 0 5W
Saundatti, *India* **95 G2** 15 47N 75 7 E
Saunders, C., *N.Z.* **131 F5** 45 53 S 170 45 E
Saunders I., *Antarctica* **7 B1** 57 48 S 26 28W
Saunders Point, *Australia* **125 E4** 27 52 S 125 38 E
Saunemin, *U.S.A.* **157 D8** 40 54N 88 24W
Saupite, *Angola* **115 E3** 13 54 S 17 43 E
Saurbær, *Borgarfjarðarsýsla, Iceland* **11 C5** 64 24N 21 35W
Saurbær, *Eyjafjarðarsýsla, Iceland* **11 B8** 65 27N 18 13W
Sauri, *Nigeria* **113 C6** 11 42N 6 44 E
Saurimo, *Angola* **115 D4** 9 40 S 20 12 E
Sausalito, *U.S.A.* **160 H4** 37 51N 122 29W
Sausapor, *Indonesia* **83 B4** 0 31 S 132 4 E
Sautatá, *Colombia* **168 B2** 7 50N 77 4W
Sauveterre-de-Béarn, *France* **28 E3** 43 24N 0 57W
Sauzé-Vaussais, *France* **28 B4** 46 8N 0 8 E
Savá, *Honduras* **164 C2** 15 32N 86 15W
Sava, *Italy* **47 B10** 40 24N 17 33 E
Sava →, *Serbia & M.* **52 F5** 44 50N 20 26 E
Savage, *U.S.A.* **154 B2** 47 27N 104 21W
Savage I. = Niue, *Cook Is.* **135 J11** 19 2 S 169 54W
Savage River, *Australia* **127 G4** 41 31 S 145 14 E
Savai'i, *Samoa* **133 W23** 13 28 S 172 24W
Savalou, *Benin* **113 D5** 7 57N 1 58 E
Savane, *Mozam.* **119 F4** 19 37 S 35 8 E
Savanna, *U.S.A.* **156 B6** 42 5N 90 8W
Savanna-la-Mar, *Jamaica* **164 a** 18 10N 78 10W
Savannah, *Ga., U.S.A.* **152 C8** 32 5N 81 6W
Savannah, *Mo., U.S.A.* **156 E2** 39 56N 94 50W
Savannah, *Tenn., U.S.A.* **149 H1** 35 14N 88 15W
Savannah →, *U.S.A.* **152 C9** 32 2N 80 53W
Savannah Beach = Tybee Island , *U.S.A.* **152 C9** 32 1N 80 51W
Savannakhet, *Laos* **86 D5** 16 30N 104 49 E
Savant L., *Canada* **140 B1** 50 16N 90 44W
Savant Lake, *Canada* **140 B1** 50 14N 90 40W
Savantvadi, *India* **95 G1** 15 55N 73 54 E
Savanur, *India* **95 G2** 14 59N 75 21 E
Săvârşin, *Romania* **52 D7** 46 1N 22 14 E
Savaştepe, *Turkey* **49 B9** 39 22N 27 42 E
Savda, *India* **94 D2** 21 9N 75 56 E
Savé, *Benin* **113 D5** 8 2N 2 29 E
Save →, *France* **28 E5** 43 47N 1 17 E
Save →, *Mozam.* **117 C5** 21 16 S 34 0 E
Sāveh, *Iran* **97 C6** 35 2N 50 20 E
Savelugu, *Ghana* **113 D4** 9 38N 0 54W
Savenay, *France* **26 E5** 47 20N 1 55W
Săveni, *Romania* **53 C11** 47 57N 26 52 E
Saverdun, *France* **28 E5** 43 14N 1 34 E
Saverne, *France* **27 D14** 48 43N 7 20 E
Savièse, *Switz.* **32 D4** 46 17N 7 22 E
Savigliano, *Italy* **44 D4** 44 38N 7 40 E
Savigny-sur-Braye, *France* **26 E7** 47 53N 0 49 E
Sávio →, *Italy* **45 D9** 44 19N 12 20 E
Šavnik, *Serbia & M.* **50 D3** 42 59N 19 10 E
Savo, *Finland* **14 E22** 62 45N 27 30 E
Savo, *Solomon Is.* **133 M10** 9 8 S 159 48 E
Savognin, *Switz.* **33 C9** 46 36N 9 37 E
Savoie □, *France* **29 C10** 45 26N 6 25 E
Savolax = Savo, *Finland* **14 E22** 62 45N 27 30 E
Savona, *Italy* **44 D5** 44 17N 8 30 E
Savona, *U.S.A.* **150 D7** 42 17N 77 13W
Savonlinna, *Finland* **58 B5** 61 52N 28 53 E
Savoonga, *U.S.A.* **144 E5** 63 42N 170 29W
Savoy = Savoie □, *France* **29 C10** 45 26N 6 25 E
Şavşat, *Turkey* **101 B10** 41 15N 42 20 E
Sävsjö, *Sweden* **17 G8** 57 20N 14 40 E
Savur, *Turkey* **96 B4** 37 34N 40 53 E
Savusavu, *Fiji* **133 A2** 16 34 S 179 15 E
Savusavu B., *Fiji* **133 A2** 16 45 S 179 15 E
Sawahlunto, *Indonesia* **84 C2** 0 40 S 100 52 E
Sawai, *Indonesia* **83 B3** 3 0 S 129 5 E
Sawai Madhopur, *India* **92 G7** 26 0N 76 25 E
Sawaleke, *Fiji* **133 A2** 17 59 S 179 18 E
Sawang Daen Din, *Thailand* **86 D4** 17 28N 103 28 E
Sawankhalok, *Thailand* **86 D2** 17 19N 99 50 E
Sawara, *Japan* **73 B12** 35 55N 140 30 E
Sawatch Range, *U.S.A.* **159 G10** 38 30N 106 30W
Sawdā', Jabal as, *Libya* **108 C3** 28 51N 15 12 E
Sawel Mt., *U.K.* **23 B4** 54 50N 7 2W
Sawfajjin □, *Libya* **108 B3** 31 0N 15 0 E
Sawfajjin, W. →, *Libya* **108 B2** 31 41N 14 44 E
Sawi, *Thailand* **87 G2** 10 14N 99 5 E
Sawla, *Ghana* **112 D4** 9 17N 2 25W
Sawmills, *Zimbabwe* **119 F2** 19 30 S 28 2 E
Şawqirah, *Oman* **99 C7** 18 7N 56 32 E
Şawqirah, Ghubbat, *Oman* **99 C7** 18 35N 57 0 E
Sawtell, *Australia* **129 A10** 30 19 S 153 6 E
Sawtooth ⌓, *U.S.A.* **158 D6** 44 0N 114 50W
Sawtooth Range, *U.S.A.* **158 E6** 44 3N 114 58W
Sawu, *Indonesia* **82 C2** 10 35 S 121 50 E
Sawu Sea, *Indonesia* **82 C2** 9 30 S 121 50 E
Saxby →, *Australia* **126 B3** 18 25 S 140 53 E
Saxmundham, *U.K.* **21 E9** 52 13N 1 30 E
Saxon, *Switz.* **32 D4** 46 9N 7 11 E
Saxony = Sachsen □, *Germany* **30 E9** 50 55N 13 10 E
Saxony, Lower = Niedersachsen □, *Germany* **30 C4** 52 50N 9 0 E
Saxton, *U.S.A.* **150 F6** 40 13N 78 15W
Say, *Mali* **112 C4** 13 50N 4 57W
Say, *Niger* **113 C5** 13 8N 2 22 E
Saya, *Nigeria* **113 D5** 9 30N 3 18 E
Sayabec, *Canada* **141 C6** 48 35N 67 41W
Sayaboury, *Laos* **86 C3** 19 15N 101 45 E
Sayán, *Peru* **172 C2** 11 8 S 77 12W
Sayan, Vostochnyy, *Russia* **67 D10** 54 0N 96 0 E
Sayan, Zapadnyy, *Russia* **67 D10** 52 30N 94 0 E
Saydā, *Lebanon* **103 B4** 33 35N 35 25 E
Sayghān, *Afghan.* **91 B2** 35 10N 67 55 E
Sayhandulaan = Oldziyt, *Mongolia* **74 B5** 44 40N 109 1 E
Sayḩūt, *Yemen* **99 D5** 15 12N 51 10 E
Sayiádha, *Greece* **38 B10** 39 38N 20 12 E
Saykhin, *Kazakhstan* **61 F8** 48 50N 46 47 E
Saylac = Zeila, *Somali Rep.* **120 B2** 11 21N 43 30 E
Saylorville L., *U.S.A.* **156 C3** 41 48N 93 46W
Saynshand, *Mongolia* **69 B6** 44 55N 110 11 E
Sayō, *Japan* **72 C6** 34 59N 134 22 E
Sayre, *Okla., U.S.A.* **155 H5** 35 18N 99 38W
Sayre, *Pa., U.S.A.* **151 E8** 41 59N 76 32W
Sayreville, *U.S.A.* **151 F10** 40 28N 74 22W
Sayula, *Mexico* **162 D4** 19 50N 103 40W
Sayward, *Canada* **142 C3** 50 21N 125 55W
Saywūn, *Yemen* **99 D5** 15 56N 48 47 E
Saza, *Japan* **72 D1** 33 14N 129 39 E
Sazanit, *Albania* **50 F3** 40 30N 19 20 E
Sázava →, *Czech Rep.* **34 B7** 49 53N 14 24 E
Sazin, *Pakistan* **93 B5** 35 35N 73 30 E
Sazlika →, *Bulgaria* **51 E9** 41 59N 25 50 E
Sbeïtla, *Tunisia* **108 A1** 35 12N 9 7 E
Scaër, *France* **26 D3** 48 2N 3 42W
Scafell Pike, *U.K.* **20 C4** 54 27N 3 14W
Scalea, *Italy* **47 C8** 39 49N 15 47 E
Scalloway, *U.K.* **22 A7** 60 9N 1 17W
Scalpay, *U.K.* **22 D3** 57 18N 6 0W
Scammon Bay, *U.S.A.* **144 F6** 61 51N 165 35W
Scandia, *Canada* **142 C6** 50 20N 112 2W
Scandiano, *Italy* **44 D7** 44 36N 10 43 E
Scandicci, *Italy* **45 E8** 43 45N 11 11 E
Scandinavia, *Europe* **14 E16** 64 0N 12 0 E
Scansano, *Italy* **45 F8** 42 41N 11 20 E
Scapa Flow, *U.K.* **22 C5** 58 53N 3 3W
Scappoose, *U.S.A.* **160 E4** 45 45N 122 53W
Scarámia, Capo, *Italy* **47 F7** 36 47N 14 29 E
Scarba, *U.K.* **22 E3** 56 11N 5 43W
Scarborough, *Trin. & Tob.* **169 E10** 11 11N 60 42W
Scarborough, *U.K.* **20 C7** 54 17N 0 24W
Scarborough Shoal, *S. China Sea* **80 D1** 15 0N 117 50 E
Scargill, *N.Z.* **131 C7** 42 56 S 172 58 E
Scariff I., *Ireland* **23 E1** 51 44N 10 15W
Scarp, *U.K.* **22 C1** 58 1N 7 8W
Scarpanto = Kárpathos, *Greece* **49 F9** 35 37N 27 10 E
Scarpe-Escaut ⌓, *France* **27 B10** 50 26N 3 23 E
Scarsdale, *Australia* **128 D5** 37 41 S 143 39 E
Scebeli, Wabi →, *Somali Rep.* **120 D2** 2 0N 44 0 E
Šćedro, *Croatia* **45 E13** 43 6N 16 43 E
Schaal See, *Germany* **30 B6** 53 36N 10 55 E
Schaalsee ⌓, *Germany* **30 B6** 53 40N 10 59 E
Schaan, *Liech.* **33 B9** 47 10N 9 31 E
Schaffhausen, *Switz.* **33 A7** 47 42N 8 39 E
Schaffhausen □, *Switz.* **33 A7** 47 42N 8 36 E
Schagen, *Neths.* **24 B4** 52 49N 4 48 E
Schaghticoke, *U.S.A.* **151 D11** 42 54N 73 35W
Schangnau, *Switz.* **32 C5** 46 50N 7 47 E
Schänis, *Switz.* **33 B8** 47 10N 9 3 E
Schärding, *Austria* **34 C6** 48 27N 13 27 E
Scharfenwiese = Ostrołęka, *Poland* **55 E8** 53 4N 21 32 E
Scharhörn, *Germany* **30 B4** 53 57N 8 24 E
Schässburg = Sighişoara, *Romania* **53 D9** 46 12N 24 50 E
Scheessel, *Germany* **30 B5** 53 10N 9 29 E
Schefferville, *Canada* **141 B6** 54 48N 66 50W
Scheibbs, *Austria* **34 C8** 48 1N 15 9 E
Scheidt = Schelde →, *Belgium* **24 C4** 51 15N 4 16 E
Schelde →, *Belgium* **24 C4** 51 15N 4 16 E
Schell City, *U.S.A.* **156 F2** 38 1N 94 7W
Schell Creek Ra., *U.S.A.* **158 G6** 39 15N 114 30W
Schellsburg, *U.S.A.* **150 F6** 40 3N 78 39W
Schemnitz = Banská Štiavnica, *Slovak Rep.* **35 C11** 48 25N 18 55 E
Schenectady, *U.S.A.* **151 D11** 42 49N 73 57W
Schenevus, *U.S.A.* **151 D10** 42 33N 74 50W
Scherfede, *Germany* **30 D5** 51 32N 9 2 E
Schesaplana, *Switz.* **33 B9** 47 5N 9 43 E
Schesslitz, *Germany* **31 F7** 49 58N 11 1 E
Schiedam, *Neths.* **24 C4** 51 55N 4 25 E
Schieratz = Sieradz, *Poland* **55 G5** 51 37N 18 41 E
Schiermonnikoog, *Neths.* **24 A6** 53 30N 6 15 E
Schiers, *Switz.* **33 C9** 46 58N 9 41 E
Schiltigheim, *France* **27 D14** 48 35N 7 45 E
Schio, *Italy* **45 C8** 45 43N 11 21 E
Schiphol, Amsterdam ✈ (AMS), *Neths.* **24 B4** 52 18N 4 45 E
Schippenbeil = Sępopol, *Poland* **54 D8** 54 16N 21 2 E
Schivelbein = Świdwin, *Poland* **54 E2** 53 47N 15 49 E
Schladming, *Austria* **34 D6** 47 23N 13 41 E
Schlanders = Silandro, *Italy* **44 B7** 46 38N 10 46 E
Schlawa = Sława, *Poland* **55 G3** 51 52N 16 2 E
Schlei →, *Germany* **30 A5** 54 40N 10 0 E
Schleiden, *Germany* **30 E2** 50 31N 6 28 E
Schleinitz Ra., *Papua N. G.* **132 B6** 3 0 S 151 30 E
Schleiz, *Germany* **30 E7** 50 35N 11 49 E
Schlesiersee = Sława, *Poland* **55 G3** 51 52N 16 2 E
Schleswig, *Germany* **30 A5** 54 31N 9 34 E
Schleswig-Holstein □, *Germany* **30 A5** 54 30N 9 30 E
Schlettstadt = Sélestat, *France* **27 D14** 48 16N 7 26 E
Schlichtingsheim = Szlichtyngowa, *Poland* **55 G3** 51 42N 16 15 E
Schlieren, *Switz.* **33 B6** 47 26N 8 27 E
Schlochau = Człuchów, *Poland* **54 E4** 53 41N 17 22 E
Schloppe = Człopa, *Poland* **55 E3** 53 6N 16 6 E
Schlüchtern, *Germany* **31 E5** 50 20N 9 32 E
Schmalkalden, *Germany* **30 E6** 50 44N 10 26 E
Schmölln, *Germany* **30 E8** 50 54N 12 19 E
Schneeberg, *Austria* **34 D8** 47 47N 15 48 E
Schneeberg, *Germany* **30 E8** 50 35N 12 38 E
Schneidemühl = Piła, *Poland* **55 E3** 53 10N 16 48 E
Schneider, *U.S.A.* **157 C9** 41 13N 87 28W
Schneverdingen, *Germany* **30 B5** 53 7N 9 48 E
Schœlcher, *Martinique* **164 c** 14 36N 61 7W
Schoharie, *U.S.A.* **151 D10** 42 40N 74 19W
Schoharie Cr. →, *U.S.A.* **151 D10** 42 57N 74 18W
Scholls, *U.S.A.* **160 E4** 45 24N 122 56W
Schönau = Swierzawa, *Poland* **55 G2** 51 1N 15 54 E
Schönberg, *Mecklenburg-Vorpommern, Germany* **30 B6** 53 52N 10 56 E
Schönberg, *Schleswig-Holstein, Germany* **30 A6** 54 23N 10 21 E
Schönbuch ⌓, *Germany* **31 G5** 48 35N 9 2 E
Schönebeck, *Germany* **30 C7** 52 2N 11 44 E
Schönenwerd, *Switz.* **32 B6** 47 23N 8 0 E
Schongau, *Germany* **31 H6** 47 47N 10 53 E
Schöningen, *Germany* **30 C6** 52 8N 10 56 E
Schönlanke = Trzcianka, *Poland* **55 E3** 53 3N 16 25 E
Schönstein = Šoštanj, *Slovenia* **45 B12** 46 23N 15 4 E
Schoolcraft, *U.S.A.* **157 B11** 42 7N 85 38W
Schopfheim, *Germany* **31 H3** 47 38N 7 50 E
Schorndorf, *Germany* **31 G5** 48 47N 9 32 E
Schortens, *Germany* **30 B3** 53 31N 7 56 E
Schouten I., *Australia* **127 G4** 42 20 S 148 20 E
Schouten Is. = Supiori, *Indonesia* **83 B5** 1 0 S 136 0 E
Schouten Is., *Papua N. G.* **132 B3** 3 30 S 144 30 E
Schouwen, *Neths.* **24 C3** 51 43N 3 45 E
Schramberg, *Germany* **31 G4** 48 13N 8 22 E
Schrankogel, *Austria* **34 D4** 47 3N 11 7 E
Schreckhorn, *Switz.* **32 C6** 46 36N 8 7 E
Schreiber, *Canada* **140 C2** 48 45N 87 20W
Schrems, *Austria* **34 C8** 48 47N 15 4 E
Schrobenhausen, *Germany* **31 G7** 48 34N 11 16 E
Schröcken, *Austria* **33 B10** 47 17N 10 5 E
Schroffenstein, *Namibia* **116 D2** 27 11 S 18 42 E
Schroon Lake, *U.S.A.* **151 C11** 43 50N 73 46W
Schröttersberg = Płock, *Poland* **55 F6** 52 32N 19 40 E
Schruns, *Austria* **34 D2** 47 5N 9 56 E
Schuchye = Shchuchinsk, *Kazakhstan* **66 D8** 52 56N 70 12 E
Schuler, *Canada* **143 C6** 50 20N 110 6W
Schuls, *Switz.* **33 C10** 46 48N 10 18 E
Schumacher, *Canada* **140 C3** 48 30N 81 16W
Schüpfen, *Switz.* **32 B4** 47 2N 7 24 E
Schüpfheim, *Switz.* **32 C6** 46 57N 8 2 E
Schurz, *U.S.A.* **158 G4** 38 57N 118 49W
Schuyler, *U.S.A.* **154 E6** 41 27N 97 4W
Schuylerville, *U.S.A.* **151 C11** 43 6N 73 35W
Schuylkill →, *U.S.A.* **151 G9** 39 53N 75 12W
Schuylkill Haven, *U.S.A.* **151 F8** 40 37N 76 11W
Schwabach, *Germany* **31 F7** 49 19N 11 2 E
Schwaben □, *Germany* **31 G6** 48 15N 10 30 E
Schwäbisch-Fränkischer Wald ⌓, *Germany* **31 G5** 49 0N 9 30 E
Schwäbisch Gmünd, *Germany* **31 G5** 48 48N 9 47 E
Schwäbisch Hall, *Germany* **31 F5** 49 6N 9 44 E
Schwäbische Alb, *Germany* **31 G5** 48 20N 9 30 E
Schwabmünchen, *Germany* **31 G6** 48 10N 10 46 E
Schwalmstadt, *Germany* **30 E5** 50 55N 9 10 E
Schwanden, *Switz.* **33 C8** 46 58N 9 5 E
Schwandorf, *Germany* **31 F8** 49 20N 12 7 E
Schwaner, Pegunungan, *Indonesia* **85 C4** 1 0 S 112 30 E
Schwanewede, *Germany* **30 B4** 53 14N 8 35 E
Schwarmstedt, *Germany* **30 C5** 52 39N 9 38 E
Schwarze Elster →, *Germany* **30 D8** 51 48N 12 50 E
Schwarzenberg, *Germany* **30 E8** 50 32N 12 47 E
Schwarzenburg, *Switz.* **32 C4** 46 49N 7 20 E
Schwarzrand, *Namibia* **116 D2** 25 37 S 16 50 E
Schwarzwald, *Germany* **31 G4** 48 30N 8 20 E
Schwatka Mts., *U.S.A.* **144 C8** 67 20N 156 30W
Schwaz, *Austria* **34 D4** 47 20N 11 44 E
Schwechat, *Austria* **35 C9** 48 8N 16 28 E
Schwechat, Wien ✈ (VIA), *Austria* **35 C9** 48 7N 16 35 E
Schwedt, *Germany* **30 B10** 53 3N 14 16 E
Schweidnitz = Świdnica, *Poland* **55 H3** 50 50N 16 30 E
Schweinfurt, *Germany* **31 E6** 50 3N 10 14 E
Schweiz = Svizzer △, *Switz.* **33 C10** 46 40N 10 10 E
Schweiz = Switzerland ■, *Europe* **32 D6** 46 30N 8 0 E
Schweizer Mittelland, *Switz.* **32 C4** 47 0N 7 15 E
Schweizer-Reneke, *S. Africa* **116 D4** 27 11 S 25 18 E
Schwenningen = Villingen-Schwenningen, *Germany* **31 G4** 48 3N 8 26 E
Schwerin = Skwierzyna, *Poland* **55 F2** 52 33N 15 30 E
Schwerin, *Germany* **30 B7** 53 36N 11 22 E
Schweriner See, *Germany* **30 B7** 53 43N 11 28 E
Schwetzingen, *Germany* **31 F4** 49 23N 8 35 E
Schwiebus = Świebodzin, *Poland* **55 F2** 52 15N 15 31 E
Schwyz, *Switz.* **33 B7** 47 2N 8 39 E
Schwyz □, *Switz.* **33 B7** 47 2N 8 39 E
Sciacca, *Italy* **46 E6** 37 31N 13 3 E
Sciao, *Somali Rep.* **120 D3** 3 26N 45 21 E
Scicli, *Italy* **47 F7** 36 47N 14 42 E
Sciliar ⌓, *Italy* **45 B8** 46 28N 11 35 E
Scilla, *Italy* **47 D8** 38 15N 15 43 E
Scilly, Isles of, *U.K.* **21 H1** 49 56N 6 22W
Ścinawa, *Poland* **55 G3** 51 25N 16 26 E
Scione, *Greece* **50 G7** 39 57N 23 36 E
Scioto →, *U.S.A.* **157 D13** 38 44N 83 1W
Scituate, *U.S.A.* **151 D14** 42 12N 70 44W
Scobey, *U.S.A.* **154 A2** 48 47N 105 25W
Scone, *Australia* **129 B9** 32 5 S 150 52 E
Scone, *U.K.* **22 E5** 56 25N 3 24W
Scordia, *Italy* **47 E7** 37 18N 14 51 E
Scoresby Sund, *Greenland* **10 C8** 70 28N 21 46W
Scoresbysund = Ittoqqortoormiit, *Greenland* **10 C8** 70 20N 23 0W
Scorniceşti, *Romania* **53 F9** 44 34N 24 33 E
Scotia, *Calif., U.S.A.* **158 F1** 40 29N 124 6W
Scotia, *N.Y., U.S.A.* **151 D11** 42 50N 73 58W
Scotia Sea, *Antarctica* **7 B18** 56 5 S 56 0W
Scotland, *Canada* **150 C4** 43 1N 80 22W
Scotland □, *U.K.* **22 E5** 57 0N 4 0W
Scott, *Antarctica* **7 D11** 77 0 S 165 0 E
Scott, C., *Australia* **124 B4** 13 30 S 129 49 E
Scott City, *U.S.A.* **154 F4** 38 29N 100 54W
Scott Glacier, *Antarctica* **7 C8** 66 15 S 100 5 E
Scott I., *Antarctica* **7 C11** 67 0 S 179 0 E
Scott Is., *Canada* **142 C3** 50 48N 128 40W
Scott L., *Canada* **143 B7** 59 55N 106 18W
Scott Reef, *Australia* **124 B3** 14 0 S 121 50 E
Scottburgh, *S. Africa* **117 E5** 30 15 S 30 47 E
Scottdale, *U.S.A.* **150 F5** 40 6N 79 35W
Scottish Borders □, *U.K.* **22 F6** 55 35N 2 50W
Scotts Head, *Australia* **129 A10** 30 45 S 153 0 E
Scottsbluff, *U.S.A.* **154 E3** 41 52N 103 40W
Scottsboro, *U.S.A.* **149 H3** 34 40N 86 2W
Scottsburg, *U.S.A.* **157 F11** 38 41N 85 47W
Scottsdale, *Australia* **127 G4** 41 9 S 147 31 E
Scottsdale, *U.S.A.* **159 K7** 33 29N 111 56W
Scottsville, *Ky., U.S.A.* **149 G2** 36 45N 86 11W
Scottsville, *N.Y., U.S.A.* **150 C7** 43 2N 77 47W
Scottville, *U.S.A.* **148 D2** 43 58N 86 17W
Scranton, *U.S.A.* **151 E9** 41 25N 75 40W
Screven, *U.S.A.* **152 D7** 31 29N 82 1W
Scugog, L., *Canada* **150 B6** 44 10N 78 55W
Sculeni, *Moldova* **53 C12** 47 20N 27 37 E
Scunthorpe, *U.K.* **20 D7** 53 36N 0 39W
Scuol Schuls, *Switz.* **33 C10** 46 48N 10 17 E
Scusciuban, *Somali Rep.* **120 B4** 10 18N 50 12 E
Scutari = Shkodër, *Albania* **50 D3** 42 4N 19 32 E
Scutari = Üsküdar, *Turkey* **51 F13** 41 0N 29 5 E
Sea Lake, *Australia* **128 C5** 35 28 S 142 55 E
Seabra = Tarauacá, *Brazil* **172 B3** 8 6 S 70 48W
Seabra, *Brazil* **171 D3** 12 25 S 41 46W
Seabrook, L., *Australia* **125 F2** 30 55 S 119 40 E
Seaford, *U.K.* **21 G8** 50 47N 0 7 E
Seaford, *U.S.A.* **148 F8** 38 39N 75 37W
Seaforth, *Australia* **126 J6** 20 55 S 148 57 E
Seaforth, *Canada* **150 C3** 43 35N 81 25W
Seaforth, L., *U.K.* **22 D2** 57 52N 6 36W
Seagraves, *U.S.A.* **155 J3** 32 57N 102 34W
Seaham, *U.K.* **20 C6** 54 50N 1 20W
Seal →, *Canada* **143 B10** 59 4N 94 48W
Seal L., *Canada* **141 B7** 54 20N 61 30W
Seale, *U.S.A.* **152 C4** 32 18N 85 10W
Sealy, *U.S.A.* **155 L6** 29 47N 96 9W
Seaman, *U.S.A.* **157 F13** 38 57N 83 34W
Searchlight, *U.S.A.* **161 K12** 35 28N 114 55W
Searcy, *U.S.A.* **155 H9** 35 15N 91 44W
Searles L., *U.S.A.* **161 K9** 35 44N 117 21W
Seascale, *U.K.* **20 C4** 54 24N 3 29W
Seaside, *Calif., U.S.A.* **160 J5** 36 37N 121 50W
Seaside, *Oreg., U.S.A.* **160 E3** 46 0N 123 56W
Seaspray, *Australia* **129 E7** 38 25 S 147 15 E
Seattle, *U.S.A.* **160 C4** 47 36N 122 20W
Seattle-Tacoma International ✈ (SEA), *U.S.A.* **160 C4** 47 27N 122 18W
Seaview Ra., *Australia* **126 B4** 18 40 S 145 45 E
Seaward Kaikoura Ra., *N.Z.* **131 C8** 42 10 S 173 44 E
Seba, *Indonesia* **82 D2** 10 29 S 121 50 E
Sebago L., *U.S.A.* **151 C14** 43 52N 70 34W
Sebago Lake, *U.S.A.* **151 C14** 43 51N 70 34W
Sebangka, *Indonesia* **84 B2** 0 7N 104 36 E
Sebastian, *U.S.A.* **153 H9** 27 49N 80 28W
Sebastián Vizcaíno, B., *Mexico* **162 B2** 28 0N 114 30W
Sebastopol = Sevastopol, *Ukraine* **59 K7** 44 35N 33 30 E
Sebastopol, *U.S.A.* **160 G4** 38 24N 122 49W
Sebba, *Burkina Faso* **113 C5** 13 35N 0 32 E
Sebderat, *Eritrea* **107 D4** 15 26N 36 42 E
Sebdou, *Algeria* **111 B4** 34 38N 1 19W
Sébé →, *Gabon* **114 C2** 1 2 S 13 6 E
Sébékoro, *Mali* **112 C3** 12 58N 9 0W
Seben, *Turkey* **100 B4** 40 24N 31 34 E
Sebeş, *Romania* **53 E8** 45 58N 23 34 E
Sebeşului, Munţii, *Romania* **53 E8** 45 36N 23 40 E
Sebewaing, *U.S.A.* **148 D4** 43 44N 83 27W
Sebezh, *Russia* **58 D5** 56 14N 28 22 E
Sebha = Sabhah, *Libya* **108 C2** 27 9N 14 29 E
Sébi, *Mali* **112 B4** 15 50N 4 12W
Şebinkarahisar, *Turkey* **101 B8** 40 22N 38 28 E
Sebiş, *Romania* **52 D7** 46 23N 22 13 E
Seblat, *Indonesia* **84 C2** 3 14 S 101 38 E
Sebnitz, *Germany* **30 E10** 50 58N 14 15 E
Sebou, Oued →, *Morocco* **110 B3** 34 16N 6 40W
Sebring, *Fla., U.S.A.* **153 H8** 27 30N 81 27W
Sebring, *Ohio, U.S.A.* **150 F3** 40 55N 81 2W
Sebringville, *Canada* **150 C3** 43 24N 81 4W
Sebta = Ceuta, *N. Afr.* **110 A3** 35 52N 5 18W
Sebuku, *Indonesia* **85 C5** 3 30 S 116 25 E
Sebuku, Teluk, *Malaysia* **85 B5** 4 0N 118 10 E
Sečanj, *Serbia & M.* **52 E5** 45 25N 20 47 E
Secchia →, *Italy* **44 C8** 45 4N 11 0 E
Sechelt, *Canada* **142 D4** 49 25N 123 42W
Sechura, *Peru* **172 B1** 5 39 S 80 50W
Sechura, Desierto de, *Peru* **172 B1** 6 0 S 80 30W
Seclin, *France* **27 B10** 50 33N 3 2 E
Secondigny, *France* **26 F6** 46 37N 0 26W
Sečovce, *Slovak Rep.* **35 C14** 48 42N 21 40 E
Secretary I., *N.Z.* **131 F1** 45 15 S 166 56 E
Secunderabad, *India* **94 F4** 17 28N 78 30 E
Sécure →, *Bolivia* **173 D5** 15 10 S 64 52W
Security, *U.S.A.* **154 F2** 38 45N 104 45W
Sedalia, *U.S.A.* **156 F3** 38 42N 93 14W
Sedam, *India* **94 E3** 17 11N 77 17 E
Sedan, *Australia* **128 C3** 34 34 S 139 19 E
Sedan, *France* **27 C11** 49 43N 4 57 E
Sedan, *U.S.A.* **155 G6** 37 8N 96 11W
Sedano, *Spain* **42 C7** 42 43N 3 49W
Sedaw, *Burma* **90 D6** 22 19N 96 19 E
Sedbergh, *U.K.* **20 C5** 54 20N 2 31W
Seddon, *N.Z.* **131 B9** 41 40 S 174 7 E
Seddonville, *N.Z.* **131 B7** 41 33 S 172 1 E
Sedé Boqér, *Israel* **103 E3** 30 52N 34 47 E
Sedeh, *Fārs, Iran* **97 D7** 30 45N 52 11 E
Sedeh, *Khorāsān, Iran* **97 C8** 33 20N 59 14 E
Séderon, *France* **29 D9** 44 12N 5 32 E
Sederot, *Israel* **103 D3** 31 32N 34 37 E
Sédhiou, *Senegal* **112 C1** 12 44N 15 30W
Sedico, *Italy* **45 B9** 46 8N 12 6 E
Sedlčany, *Czech Rep.* **34 B7** 49 40N 14 25 E
Sedley, *Canada* **143 C8** 50 10N 104 0W
Sedona, *U.S.A.* **159 J8** 34 52N 111 46W
Sedova, Pik, *Russia* **66 B6** 73 29N 54 58 E
Sedrata, *Algeria* **111 A6** 36 7N 7 31 E
Sedro Woolley, *U.S.A.* **160 B4** 48 30N 122 14W
Sedrun, *Switz.* **33 C7** 46 36N 8 47 E
Šeduva, *Lithuania* **54 C10** 55 45N 23 45 E
Sędziszów, *Poland* **55 H7** 50 35N 20 4 E
Sędziszów Małapolski, *Poland* **55 H8** 50 5N 21 45 E
Seebad Ahlbeck, *Germany* **30 B10** 53 56N 14 10 E
Seeburg = Jeziorany, *Poland* **54 E7** 53 58N 20 46 E
Seefeld in Tirol, *Austria* **34 D4** 47 19N 11 13 E
Seehausen, *Germany* **30 C7** 52 54N 11 45 E
Seeheim, *Namibia* **116 D2** 26 50 S 17 45 E

Seeheim-Jugenheim, Germany **31 F4** 49 49N 8 40 E
Seeis, Namibia **116 C2** 22 29 S 17 39 E
Seekoei →, S. Africa **116 E4** 30 18 S 25 1 E
Seeley's Bay, Canada **151 B8** 44 29N 76 14W
Seelow, Germany **30 C10** 52 32N 14 23 E
Sées, France **26 D7** 48 38N 0 10 E
Seesen, Germany **30 D6** 51 54N 10 10 E
Seevetal, Germany **30 B6** 53 26N 10 1 E
Seewinkel = Neusiedler See-Seewinkel △, Austria **35 D9** 47 50N 16 45 E
Sefadu, S. Leone **112 D2** 8 35N 10 58W
Seferihisar, Turkey **49 C8** 38 10N 26 50 E
Séfeto, Mali **112 C3** 14 8N 9 49W
Sefrou, Morocco **110 B4** 33 52N 4 52W
Sefton, N.Z. **131 D7** 43 15 S 172 41 E
Sefuri-San, Japan **72 D2** 33 28N 130 18 E
Sefwi Bekwai, Ghana **112 D4** 6 10N 2 25W
Seg-ozero, Russia **56 B5** 63 20N 33 46 E
Segaf, Kepulauan, Indonesia **83 B4** 2 10 S 130 28 E
Segag, Ethiopia **120 C2** 7 39N 42 50 E
Segamat, Malaysia **87 L4** 2 30N 102 50 E
Şegarcea, Romania **53 F8** 44 6N 23 43 E
Ségbana, Benin **113 C5** 10 55N 3 42 E
Segbwema, S. Leone **112 D2** 8 0N 11 0W
Seget, Indonesia **83 B4** 1 24 S 130 58 E
Segewold = Sigulda, Latvia **15 H21** 57 10N 24 55 E
Segezha, Russia **56 B5** 63 44N 34 19 E
Seggueur, O. →, Algeria **111 B5** 32 14N 1 48 E
Seghe, Solomon Is. **133 M9** 8 32 S 157 54 E
Segonzac, France **28 C3** 45 36N 0 14W
Segorbe, Spain **40 F4** 39 50N 0 30W
Ségou, Mali **112 C3** 13 30N 6 16W
Segovia = Coco →, Cent. Amer. **164 D3** 15 0N 83 8W
Segovia, Colombia **168 B3** 7 7N 74 42W
Segovia, Spain **42 E6** 40 57N 4 10W
Segovia □, Spain **42 E6** 40 55N 4 10W
Segré, France **26 E6** 47 40N 0 52W
Segre →, Spain **40 D5** 41 40N 0 43 E
Seguam I., U.S.A. **144 K4** 52 19N 172 30W
Seguam Pass, U.S.A. **144 L4** 52 0N 172 30W
Séguédine, Niger **109 D2** 20 9N 12 55 E
Séguéla, Ivory C. **112 D3** 7 55N 6 40W
Séguénéga, Burkina Faso **113 C4** 13 25N 1 58W
Seguin, U.S.A. **155 L6** 29 34N 97 58W
Segundo →, Argentina **174 C3** 30 53 S 62 44W
Segura →, Spain **41 G4** 38 3N 0 44W
Segura, Sierra de, Spain **41 G2** 38 5N 2 45W
Seh Konj, Kūh-e, Iran **97 D8** 30 6N 57 30 E
Seh Qal'eh, Iran **97 C8** 33 40N 58 24 E
Sehitwa, Botswana **116 C3** 20 30 S 22 30 E
Sehlabathebe △, Lesotho **117 D4** 29 53 S 29 7 E
Sehore, India **92 H7** 23 10N 77 5 E
Sehulea, Papua N. G. **132 E6** 9 58 S 151 10 E
Sehwan, Pakistan **91 D2** 26 28N 67 53 E
Şeica Mare, Romania **53 D9** 46 1N 24 7 E
Seikpyu, Burma **90 E5** 20 54N 94 48 E
Seil, U.K. **22 E3** 56 18N 5 38W
Seiland, Norway **14 A20** 70 25N 23 15 E
Seilhac, France **28 C5** 45 22N 1 43 E
Seiling, U.S.A. **155 G5** 36 9N 98 56W
Seille →, Moselle, France **27 C13** 49 7N 6 11 E
Seille →, Saône-et-Loire, France **27 F11** 46 31N 4 57 E
Sein, Î. de, France **26 D2** 48 2N 4 52W
Seinäjoki, Finland **15 E20** 62 40N 22 51 E
Seine →, France **26 C7** 49 26N 0 26 E
Seine, B. de la, France **26 C6** 49 40N 0 40W
Seine-et-Marne □, France **27 D10** 48 45N 3 0 E
Seine-Inférieure = Seine-Maritime □, France **26 C7** 49 40N 1 0 E
Seine-Maritime □, France **26 C7** 49 40N 1 0 E
Seine-St-Denis □, France **27 D9** 48 58N 2 24 E
Seini, Romania **53 C8** 47 44N 23 21 E
Seirijai, Lithuania **54 D10** 54 14N 23 49 E
Seis de Septiembre = Moron, Argentina **174 C4** 34 39 S 58 37W
Seistan = Sīstān, Asia **97 D9** 30 50N 61 0 E
Seistan, Daryācheh-ye = Sīstān, Daryācheh-ye, Iran **97 D9** 31 0N 61 0 E
Seitler = Nyzhnohirskyy, Ukraine **59 K8** 45 27N 34 38 E
Sejerø, Denmark **17 J5** 55 54N 11 9 E
Sejerø Bugt, Denmark **17 J5** 55 53N 11 15 E
Sejny, Poland **54 D10** 54 6N 23 21 E
Seka, Ethiopia **107 F4** 8 10N 36 52 E
Sekayu, Indonesia **84 C2** 2 51 S 103 51 E
Seke, Tanzania **118 C3** 3 20 S 33 31 E
Seke-Banza, Dem. Rep. of the Congo **115 D2** 5 20 S 13 16 E
Sekenke, Tanzania **118 C3** 4 18 S 34 11 E
Sekhira, Tunisia **108 B2** 34 20N 10 5 E
Seki, Japan **73 B8** 35 29N 136 55 E
Seki, Turkey **49 E11** 36 48N 29 33 E
Sekigahara, Japan **73 B8** 35 22N 136 28 E
Sekondi-Takoradi, Ghana **112 E4** 4 58N 1 45W
Sekota, Ethiopia **107 E4** 12 40N 39 2 E
Seksna, Russia **58 C10** 59 13N 38 30 E
Sekudai, Malaysia **87 d** 1 32N 103 39 E
Sekuma, Botswana **116 C3** 24 36 S 23 50 E
Selah, U.S.A. **158 C3** 46 39N 120 32W
Selama, Malaysia **87 K3** 5 12N 100 42 E
Selangor □, Malaysia **84 B2** 3 10N 101 30 E
Selárgius, Italy **46 C2** 39 16N 9 10 E
Selaru, Indonesia **83 C4** 8 9 S 131 0 E
Selatan, Selat, Malaysia **87 c** 5 15N 100 20 E
Selawik, U.S.A. **144 C8** 66 36N 160 0W
Selawik L., U.S.A. **144 C7** 66 30N 160 45W
Selb, Germany **31 E8** 50 10N 12 7 E
Selbusjøen, Norway **18 A7** 63 15N 10 50 E
Selby, U.K. **20 D6** 53 47N 1 5W
Selby, U.S.A. **154 C4** 45 31N 100 2W
Selca, Croatia **45 E13** 43 20N 16 50 E
Selçuk, Turkey **49 D9** 37 56N 27 22 E
Selden, U.S.A. **154 F4** 39 33N 100 34W
Seldovia, U.S.A. **144 G10** 59 26N 151 43W
Sele →, Italy **47 B7** 40 29N 14 56 E
Selebi-Pikwe, Botswana **117 C4** 21 58 S 27 48 E
Selemdzha →, Russia **67 D13** 51 42N 128 53 E
Selendi, Manisa, Turkey **49 C10** 38 43N 28 50 E
Selendi, Manisa, Turkey **49 C9** 38 46N 27 53 E
Selenga = Selenge Mörön →, Asia **68 A5** 52 16N 106 16 E
Selenge, Dem. Rep. of the Congo **114 C3** 1 58 S 18 11 E
Selenge Mörön →, Asia **68 A5** 52 16N 106 16 E
Selenicë, Albania **50 F3** 40 33N 19 39 E
Selenter See, Germany **30 A6** 54 18N 10 26 E
Sélestat, France **27 D14** 48 16N 7 26 E
Seletan, Tanjung, Indonesia **85 C4** 4 10 S 114 40 E
Selevac, Serbia & M. **50 B4** 44 28N 20 52 E
Selfoss, Iceland **11 D6** 63 56N 21 0W
Sélibabi, Mauritania **112 B2** 15 10N 12 15W
Seliger, Ozero, Russia **58 D7** 57 15N 33 0 E
Seligman, U.S.A. **159 J7** 35 20N 112 53W
Şelim, Turkey **101 B10** 40 30N 42 46 E
Selîma, El Wâhât el, Sudan **106 C2** 21 22N 29 19 E
Selimiye, Turkey **49 D9** 37 24N 27 40 E
Selinda Spillway →, Botswana **116 B3** 18 35 S 23 10 E
Selinoús, Greece **48 D3** 37 35N 21 37 E
Selinsgrove, U.S.A. **150 F8** 40 48N 76 52W
Selizharovo, Russia **58 D7** 56 51N 33 27 E
Selje, Norway **18 B2** 62 3N 5 22 E
Seljord, Norway **18 E5** 59 30N 8 40 E
Selkirk, Canada **143 C9** 50 10N 96 55W
Selkirk, U.K. **22 F6** 55 33N 2 50W
Selkirk I. = Horse I., Canada **143 C9** 53 20N 99 6W
Selkirk Mts., Canada **138 C8** 51 15N 117 40W
Sellafield, U.K. **20 C4** 54 25N 3 29W
Sellama, Sudan **107 E2** 12 51N 29 46 E
Selliá, Greece **39 E5** 35 12N 24 23 E
Sellières, France **27 F12** 46 50N 5 32 E
Sells, U.S.A. **159 L8** 31 55N 111 53W
Sellye, Hungary **52 E2** 45 52N 17 51 E
Selma, Ala., U.S.A. **149 J2** 32 25N 87 1W
Selma, Calif., U.S.A. **160 J7** 36 34N 119 37W
Selma, N.C., U.S.A. **149 H6** 35 32N 78 17W
Selmer, U.S.A. **149 H1** 35 10N 88 36W
Selong, Indonesia **85 D5** 8 39 S 116 32 E
Selongey, France **27 E12** 47 36N 5 11 E
Selouane, Morocco **111 A4** 35 7N 2 57W
Selous ⌓, Tanzania **119 D4** 8 37 S 37 42 E
Selowandoma Falls, Zimbabwe **119 G3** 21 15 S 31 50 E
Selpele, Indonesia **83 B4** 0 1 S 130 5 E
Selsey Bill, U.K. **21 G7** 50 43N 0 47W
Seltso, Russia **58 F8** 53 22N 34 4 E
Seltz, France **27 D15** 48 54N 8 4 E
Selu, Indonesia **83 C4** 7 32 S 130 55 E
Sélune →, France **26 D5** 48 38N 1 22W
Selva = La Selva del Camp, Spain **40 D6** 41 13N 1 8 E
Selva, Argentina **174 B3** 29 50 S 62 0W
Selva Lancandona = Montes Azules ⌓, Mexico **163 D6** 16 21N 91 3W
Selvagens, Ilhas, Madeira **110 B1** 30 5N 15 55W
Selvas, Brazil **172 B4** 6 30 S 67 0W
Selwyn L., Canada **143 B8** 60 0N 104 30W
Selwyn Mts., Canada **138 B6** 63 0N 130 0W
Selwyn Passage, Vanuatu **133 F6** 16 3 S 168 12 E
Selwyn Ra., Australia **126 C3** 21 10 S 140 0 E
Selyatyn, Ukraine **53 C10** 47 50N 25 12 E
Sem, Norway **18 E7** 59 14N 10 17 E
Sem Kolodezey = Lenino, Ukraine **59 K8** 45 17N 35 46 E
Semadrek = Samothráki, Greece **51 F9** 40 28N 25 28 E
Seman →, Albania **50 F3** 40 47N 19 30 E
Semara, W. Sahara **110 C2** 26 48N 11 41W
Semarang, Indonesia **85 D4** 7 0 S 110 26 E
Sematan, Malaysia **85 B3** 1 48N 109 46 E
Semau, Indonesia **82 D2** 10 13 S 123 22 E
Sembabule, Uganda **118 C3** 0 4 S 31 25 E
Sembawang, Singapore **87 d** 1 27N 103 50 E
Sembé, Congo **114 B2** 1 39N 14 36 E
Sembung, Indonesia **79 J18** 8 28 S 115 11 E
Şemdinli, Turkey **101 D11** 37 18N 44 35 E
Sémé, Senegal **112 B2** 15 4N 13 41W
Semeih, Sudan **107 E3** 12 43N 30 53 E
Semenanjung Blambangan, Indonesia **79 K17** 8 42 S 114 29 E
Semendua, Dem. Rep. of the Congo **114 C3** 3 10 S 18 6 E
Semenov, Russia **60 B7** 56 43N 44 30 E
Semenovka, Chernihiv, Ukraine **59 F7** 52 8N 32 36 E
Semenovka, Kremenchuk, Ukraine **59 H7** 49 37N 33 10 E
Semeru, Indonesia **85 D4** 8 4 S 112 55 E
Semey, Kazakhstan **66 D9** 50 30N 80 10 E
Semichi Is., U.S.A. **144 K1** 52 42N 174 0 E
Semikarakorskiy, Russia **61 G5** 47 31N 40 48 E
Semiluki, Russia **59 G10** 51 41N 39 2 E
Seminoe Reservoir, U.S.A. **158 F10** 42 9N 106 55W
Seminole, Fla., U.S.A. **153 H7** 27 50N 82 47W
Seminole, Okla., U.S.A. **155 H6** 35 14N 96 41W
Seminole, Tex., U.S.A. **155 J3** 32 43N 102 39W
Seminole, L., U.S.A. **152 E5** 30 43N 84 52W
Seminole Draw →, U.S.A. **155 J3** 32 27N 102 20W
Semipalatinsk = Semey, Kazakhstan **66 D9** 50 30N 80 10 E
Semirara I., Phil. **80 E3** 12 4N 121 23 E
Semirara Is., Phil. **81 F3** 12 0N 121 20 E
Semisopochnoi I., U.S.A. **144 L2** 51 55N 179 36 E
Semitau, Indonesia **85 B4** 0 29N 111 57 E
Semiyarka, Kazakhstan **66 D8** 50 55N 78 23 E
Semiyarskoye = Semiyarka, Kazakhstan **66 D8** 50 55N 78 23 E
Semlin = Zemun, Serbia & M. **50 B4** 44 51N 20 25 E
Semmering P., Austria **34 D8** 47 41N 15 45 E
Semnān, Iran **97 C7** 35 40N 53 23 E
Semnān □, Iran **97 C7** 36 0N 54 0 E
Sempang Mengayou, Tanjong, Malaysia **85 A5** 7 0N 116 40 E
Semporna, Malaysia **85 B5** 4 30N 118 33 E
Semuda, Indonesia **85 C4** 2 51 S 112 58 E
Semur-en-Auxois, France **27 E11** 47 30N 4 20 E
Semyonovka = Arsenev, Russia **70 B6** 44 10N 133 15 E
Semyonovskoye = Bereznik, Russia **56 B7** 62 51N 42 40 E
Sen →, Cambodia **78 B3** 13 45N 105 12 E
Sena, Bolivia **172 C4** 11 32 S 67 11W
Senā, Iran **97 D6** 28 27N 51 36 E
Sena, Mozam. **119 F4** 17 25 S 35 0 E
Sena →, Bolivia **172 C4** 11 31 S 67 11W
Sena Madureira, Brazil **172 B4** 9 5 S 68 45W
Senachwine L., U.S.A. **156 C7** 41 10N 89 18W
Senador José Porfírio, Brazil **169 D7** 2 35 S 51 55W
Senador Pompeu, Brazil **170 C4** 5 40 S 39 20W
Senaja, Malaysia **85 A5** 6 45N 117 3 E
Senaki, Georgia **61 J6** 42 15N 42 7 E
Senang, Pulau, Singapore **87 d** 1 10N 103 44 E
Senanga, Zambia **115 F4** 16 7 S 23 16 E
Senatobia, U.S.A. **155 H10** 34 37N 89 58W
Sencelles, Spain **38 B3** 39 39N 2 54 E
Sendafa, Ethiopia **107 F4** 9 11N 39 3 E
Sendai, Kagoshima, Japan **72 F2** 31 50N 130 20 E
Sendai, Miyagi, Japan **70 E10** 38 15N 140 53 E
Sendai-Wan, Japan **70 E10** 38 15N 141 0 E
Senden, Bayern, Germany **31 G6** 48 19N 10 4 E
Senden, Nordrhein-Westfalen, Germany **30 D3** 51 52N 7 22 E
Sendhwa, India **92 J6** 21 41N 75 6 E
Sendurjana, India **94 D4** 21 32N 78 17 E
Sene →, Ghana **113 D4** 7 30N 0 33W
Senec, Slovak Rep. **35 C10** 48 12N 17 23 E
Seneca, Ill., U.S.A. **157 C8** 41 19N 88 37W
Seneca, S.C., U.S.A. **149 H4** 34 41N 82 57W
Seneca Falls, U.S.A. **151 D8** 42 55N 76 48W
Seneca L., U.S.A. **150 D8** 42 40N 76 54W
Senecaville L., U.S.A. **150 G3** 39 55N 81 25W
Senegal ■, W. Afr. **112 C2** 14 30N 14 30W
Sénégal →, W. Afr. **112 B1** 15 48N 16 32W
Senegambia, Africa **104 E2** 12 45N 12 0W
Senegambia & Niger = Mali ■, Africa **112 B4** 17 0N 3 0W
Senekal, S. Africa **117 D4** 28 20 S 27 36 E
Senftenberg, Germany **30 D10** 51 32N 14 0 E
Senga Hill, Zambia **119 D3** 9 19 S 31 11 E
Senge Khambab = Indus →, Pakistan **91 D2** 24 20N 67 47 E
Sengiley, Russia **60 D9** 53 58N 48 46 E
Sengua →, Zimbabwe **119 F2** 17 7 S 28 5 E
Senguerr →, Argentina **176 C3** 45 35 S 68 50W
Senhor-do-Bonfim, Brazil **170 D3** 10 30 S 40 10W
Senica, Slovak Rep. **35 C10** 48 41N 17 25 E
Senigállia, Italy **45 E10** 43 43N 13 13 E
Seniku, Burma **90 C6** 25 32N 97 48 E
Senio →, Italy **45 D9** 44 35N 12 15 E
Senirkent, Turkey **49 C12** 38 6N 30 33 E
Senise, Italy **47 B9** 40 9N 16 17 E
Senj, Croatia **45 D11** 45 0N 14 58 E
Senja, Norway **14 B17** 69 25N 17 30 E
Senkaku-Shotō, Japan **71 L1** 25 45N 124 0 E
Senkuang, Indonesia **87 d** 1 11N 104 2 E
Senlis, France **27 C9** 49 13N 2 35 E
Senmonorom, Cambodia **86 F6** 12 27N 107 12 E
Sennâr, Sudan **107 E3** 13 30N 33 35 E
Sennar □, Sudan **107 E3** 13 0N 34 0 E
Senneterre, Canada **140 C4** 48 25N 77 15W
Senno, Belarus **58 E5** 54 45N 29 43 E
Sénnori, Italy **46 B1** 40 47N 8 35 E
Seno, Laos **86 D5** 16 35N 104 50 E
Senoia, U.S.A. **152 B5** 33 18N 84 33W
Senonches, France **26 D8** 48 34N 1 2 E
Senorbì, Italy **46 C2** 39 32N 9 8 E
Senožeče, Slovenia **45 C11** 45 43N 14 3 E
Sens, France **27 D10** 48 11N 3 15 E
Senta, Serbia & M. **52 E5** 45 55N 20 3 E
Sentani, Indonesia **83 B6** 2 36 S 140 37 E
Sentani, Danau, Indonesia **83 B6** 2 36 S 140 34 E
Sentery = Lubao, Dem. Rep. of the Congo **118 D2** 5 17 S 25 42 E
Sentinel, U.S.A. **159 K7** 32 52N 113 13W
Šentjur, Slovenia **45 B12** 46 14N 15 24 E
Sentolo, Indonesia **85 D4** 7 55 S 110 13 E
Sentosa, Singapore **87 d** 1 15N 103 50 E
Senya Beraku, Ghana **113 D4** 5 28N 0 31W
Seo de Urgel = La Seu d'Urgell, Spain **40 C6** 42 22N 1 23 E
Seohara, India **93 E8** 29 15N 78 33 E
Seonath →, India **93 J10** 21 44N 82 28 E
Seondha, India **93 F8** 26 9N 78 48 E
Seoni, India **93 H8** 22 5N 79 30 E
Seoni Malwa, India **92 H8** 22 27N 77 28 E
Seoriuarayan, India **94 D6** 21 45N 82 34 E
Seoul = Sŏul, S. Korea **75 F14** 37 31N 126 58 E
Separation Pt., N.Z. **131 A7** 40 47 S 172 59 E
Sepatini →, Brazil **172 B4** 7 36 S 65 24W
Sepi, Solomon Is. **133 M10** 8 31 S 159 52 E
Sepīdān, Iran **97 D7** 30 20N 52 5 E
Sepik →, Papua N. G. **132 B3** 3 49 S 144 30 E
Sepo-ri, N. Korea **75 E14** 38 57N 127 25 E
Sępólno Krajeńskie, Poland **54 E4** 53 26N 17 30 E
Sepone, Laos **86 D6** 16 45N 106 13 E
Sępopol, Poland **54 D8** 54 16N 21 2 E
Sept-Îles, Canada **141 B6** 50 13N 66 22W
Septemvri, Bulgaria **51 D8** 42 13N 24 6 E
Sepúlveda, Spain **42 D7** 41 18N 3 45W
Sequeros, Spain **42 E4** 40 31N 6 2W
Sequim, U.S.A. **160 B3** 48 5N 123 6W
Sequoia △, U.S.A. **160 J8** 36 30N 118 30W
Sera, Indonesia **83 C4** 7 40 S 131 5 E
Serafimovich, Russia **60 F6** 49 36N 42 43 E
Seraing, Belgium **24 D5** 50 35N 5 32 E
Serakhis →, Cyprus **39 E8** 35 13N 32 55 E
Seram, Indonesia **83 B3** 3 10 S 129 0 E
Seram Sea, Indonesia **82 B3** 2 30 S 128 30 E
Seranantsara, Madag. **117 B8** 18 30 S 49 5 E
Serang, Indonesia **84 D3** 6 8 S 106 10 E
Serangoon, Singapore **87 d** 1 23N 103 54 E
Serasan, Indonesia **85 B3** 2 29N 109 4 E
Seravezza, Italy **44 E7** 43 59N 10 13 E
Şerbettar, Turkey **51 E10** 41 27N 26 46 E
Serbia □, Serbia & M. **50 C5** 43 30N 21 0 E
Serbia & Montenegro ■, Europe **50 C4** 43 20N 20 0 E
Şercaia, Romania **53 E10** 45 49N 25 9 E
Serdo, Ethiopia **107 E5** 11 56N 41 14 E
Serdobol = Sortavala, Russia **58 B6** 61 42N 30 41 E
Serdobsk, Russia **60 D7** 52 28N 44 10 E
Sered', Slovak Rep. **35 C10** 48 17N 17 44 E
Sereda = Furmanov, Russia **60 B5** 57 10N 41 9 E
Seredka, Russia **58 C5** 58 12N 28 10 E
Serednye, Ukraine **52 B7** 48 32N 22 30 E
Şereflikoçhisar, Turkey **100 C5** 38 56N 33 32 E
Seregno, Italy **44 C6** 45 39N 9 12 E
Seremban, Malaysia **87 L3** 2 43N 101 53 E
Serengeti △, Tanzania **118 C3** 2 11 S 35 0 E
Serengeti Plain, Tanzania **118 C4** 2 40 S 35 0 E
Serenje, Zambia **119 E3** 13 14 S 30 15 E
Seret →, Ukraine **53 B10** 48 37N 25 52 E
Sereth = Siret →, Romania **53 E12** 45 24N 28 1 E
Sergach, Russia **60 C7** 55 30N 45 30 E
Sergen, Turkey **51 E11** 41 41N 27 42 E
Sergino, Russia **66 C7** 62 25N 65 12 E
Sergiopol = Ayaguz, Kazakhstan **66 E9** 48 10N 80 10 E
Sergipe □, Brazil **170 D4** 10 30 S 37 30W
Sergiyev Posad, Russia **58 D10** 56 20N 38 10 E
Sergo = Stakhanov, Ukraine **59 H10** 48 35N 38 40 E
Seria, Brunei **85 B4** 4 37N 114 23 E
Serian, Malaysia **85 B4** 1 10N 110 31 E
Seriate, Italy **44 C6** 45 41N 9 43 E
Seribu, Kepulauan, Indonesia **84 D3** 5 36 S 106 33 E
Sérifontaine, France **27 C8** 49 20N 1 45 E
Sérifos, Greece **48 D6** 37 9N 24 30 E
Sérignan, France **28 E7** 43 17N 3 17 E
Sérigny →, Canada **141 A6** 56 47N 66 0W
Serik, Turkey **100 D4** 36 55N 31 7 E
Serikbuya, China **65 D8** 39 21N 77 50 E
Seringapatam Reef, Australia **124 B3** 13 38 S 122 5 E
Serinhisar, Turkey **49 D11** 37 36N 29 18 E
Seririt, Indonesia **79 J17** 8 12 S 114 56 E
Sermaize-les-Bains, France **27 D11** 48 47N 4 54 E
Sermata, Indonesia **83 C3** 8 15 S 128 50 E
Sermersuaq, Greenland **10 B4** 79 30N 62 0W
Sérmide, Italy **45 D8** 45 0N 11 18 E
Sernovodsk, Russia **60 D10** 53 54N 51 16 E
Sernur, Russia **60 B9** 56 52N 49 2 E
Serock, Poland **55 F8** 52 31N 21 4 E
Serón, Spain **41 H2** 37 20N 2 29W
Seròs, Spain **40 D5** 41 27N 0 24 E
Serouenout, Algeria **111 D6** 24 18N 7 25 E
Serov, Russia **64 B8** 59 29N 60 35 E
Serowe, Botswana **116 C4** 22 25 S 26 43 E
Serpa, Portugal **43 H3** 37 57N 7 38W
Serpeddí, Punta, Italy **46 C2** 39 22N 9 18 E
Serpentara, Italy **46 C2** 39 8N 9 36 E
Serpentine Lakes, Australia **125 E4** 28 30 S 129 10 E
Serpent's Mouth = Sierpe, Bocas de la, Venezuela **169 G9** 10 0N 61 30W
Serpis →, Spain **41 G4** 38 59N 0 9W
Serpneve, Ukraine **53 D14** 46 18N 29 1 E
Serpukhov, Russia **58 E9** 54 55N 37 28 E
Serra da Bocaina △, Brazil **171 F3** 23 0 S 44 40W
Serra da Canastra △, Brazil **171 F2** 20 3 S 46 50W
Serra da Capivara △, Brazil **170 C3** 8 42 S 42 15W
Serra da Estrela ⌓, Portugal **42 E3** 40 27N 7 33W
Serra das Confusões △, Brazil **170 C3** 8 50 S 43 50W
Serra de Outes, Spain **42 C2** 42 52N 8 55W
Serra do Cipó △, Brazil **171 E3** 19 14 S 43 23W
Serra do Navio, Brazil **169 C7** 0 59N 52 3W
Serra do Salitre, Brazil **171 E2** 19 6 S 46 41W
Serra dos Orgãos △, Brazil **171 F3** 22 25 S 43 8W
Serra San Bruno, Italy **47 D9** 38 35N 16 20 E
Serra Talhada, Brazil **170 C4** 7 59 S 38 18W
Serradilla, Spain **42 F4** 39 50N 6 9W
Sérrai, Greece **50 E7** 41 5N 23 31 E
Sérrai □, Greece **50 E7** 41 5N 23 37 E
Serramanna, Italy **46 C1** 39 25N 8 55 E
Serranía de la Neblina △, Venezuela **168 C4** 1 5N 65 51W
Serranía San Luís △, Paraguay **174 A4** 22 35 S 57 22W
Serranópolis, Brazil **173** 18 16 S 52 0W
Serras d'Aire e Candeeiros ⌓, Portugal **43 F2** 39 31N 8 48W
Serrat, C., Tunisia **108 A1** 37 14N 9 10 E
Serravalle, Italy **33 E6** 45 41N 8 18 E
Serravalle Scrívia, Italy **44 D5** 44 43N 8 51 E
Serre-Ponçon, L. de, France **29 D10** 44 22N 6 20 E
Serres = Sérrai, Greece **50 E7** 41 5N 23 31 E
Serres, France **29 D9** 44 26N 5 43 E
Serrezuela, Argentina **174 C2** 30 40 S 65 20W
Serrinha, Brazil **171 D4** 11 39 S 39 0W
Serrita, Brazil **170 C4** 7 56 S 39 19W
Sersale, Italy **47 C9** 39 1N 16 43 E
Sertã, Portugal **42 F2** 39 48N 8 6W
Sertânia, Brazil **170 C4** 8 5 S 37 20W
Sertanópolis, Brazil **175 A5** 23 4 S 51 2W
Sêrtar, China **76 A3** 32 20N 100 41 E
Sertig, Switz. **33 C9** 46 44N 9 52 E
Serua, Indonesia **83 C4** 6 18 S 130 1 E
Serui, Indonesia **83 B5** 1 53 S 136 10 E
Serule, Botswana **116 C4** 21 57 S 27 20 E
Sérvia, Greece **50 F6** 40 11N 22 0 E
Serzedelo, Portugal **42 D2** 41 24N 8 14W
Ses Salines, Spain **38 B4** 39 21N 3 3 E
Sesayap →, Indonesia **85 B5** 3 36N 117 15 E
Sese Is., Uganda **118 C3** 0 20 S 32 20 E
Sesepe, Indonesia **82 B3** 1 30 S 127 59 E
Sesfontein, Namibia **116 B1** 19 7 S 13 39 E
Sesheke, Zambia **116 B3** 17 29 S 24 13 E
Sésia →, Italy **44 C5** 45 5N 8 37 E
Sesimbra, Portugal **43 G1** 38 28N 9 6W
S'Espalmador, Spain **38 D1** 38 47N 1 26 E
S'Espardell, Spain **38 D1** 38 48N 1 29 E
Sessa, Angola **115 E4** 13 56 S 20 38 E
Sessa Aurunca, Italy **46 A6** 41 14N 13 56 E
Sesser, U.S.A. **156 F7** 38 5N 89 1W
S'Estanyol, Spain **38 B3** 39 22N 2 54 E
Sestao, Spain **40 B2** 43 18N 3 0W
Sesto Calende, Italy **44 C5** 45 44N 8 37 E
Sesto San Giovanni, Italy **44 C6** 45 32N 9 14 E
Sestri Levante, Italy **44 D6** 44 16N 9 24 E
Sestriere, Italy **44 D3** 44 57N 6 53 E
Sestroretsk, Russia **58 B6** 60 5N 29 58 E
Sestrunj, Croatia **45 D11** 44 10N 15 0 E
Sestu, Italy **46 C2** 39 18N 9 5 E
Sesvenna, Switz. **33 C10** 46 42N 10 25 E
Setaka, Japan **72 D2** 33 9N 130 28 E
Setana, Japan **70 C9** 42 26N 139 51 E
Sète, France **28 E7** 43 25N 3 42 E
Sete Cidades △, Brazil **170 B3** 4 0 S 41 37W
Sete Lagôas, Brazil **171 E3** 19 27 S 44 16W
Setesdalsheiene, Norway **18 E3** 59 28N 7 10 E
Sétif, Algeria **111 A6** 36 9N 5 26 E
Seto, Japan **73 B9** 35 14N 137 6 E
Setonaikai, Japan **72 C5** 34 20N 133 30 E
Setonaikai △, Japan **72 C5** 34 15N 133 15 E
Setsan, Burma **90 G5** 16 3N 95 23 E
Settat, Morocco **110 B3** 33 0N 7 40W
Setté-Cama, Gabon **114 C1** 2 32 S 9 45 E
Séttimo Torinese, Italy **44 C4** 45 9N 7 46 E
Setting L., Canada **143 C9** 55 0N 98 38W
Settle, U.K. **20 C5** 54 5N 2 16W
Settlement Pt., Bahamas **149 M6** 26 40N 79 0W
Settlers, S. Africa **117 C4** 25 2 S 28 30 E
Setúbal, Portugal **43 G2** 38 30N 8 58W
Setúbal □, Portugal **43 G2** 38 25N 8 35W
Setúbal, B. de, Portugal **43 G2** 38 40N 8 56W
Seugne →, France **28 C3** 45 42N 0 32W
Seul, Lac, Canada **140 B1** 50 20N 92 30W
Seulimeum, Indonesia **84 A1** 5 27N 95 15 E
Seurre, France **27 F12** 47 0N 5 8 E
Seuzach, Switz. **33 A7** 47 32N 8 49 E
Sevan, Armenia **61 K7** 40 33N 44 56 E
Sevan, Ozero = Sevana Lich, Armenia **61 K7** 40 30N 45 20 E
Sevana Lich, Armenia **61 K7** 40 30N 45 20 E
Sevastopol, Ukraine **59 K7** 44 35N 33 30 E
Sevelen, Switz. **33 B8** 47 7N 9 28 E
Seven Islands = Sept-Îles, Canada **141 B6** 50 13N 66 22W
Seven Sisters, Canada **142 C3** 54 56N 128 10W
Sever →, Spain **43 F3** 39 40N 7 32W
Sévérac-le-Château, France **28 D7** 44 20N 3 5 E
Severn →, Canada **140 A2** 56 2N 87 36W
Severn →, U.K. **21 F5** 51 35N 2 40W
Severn L., Canada **140 B1** 53 54N 90 48W
Severnaya Zemlya, Russia **67 B10** 79 0N 100 0 E
Severnyye Uvaly, Russia **64 B2** 60 0N 50 0 E
Severo-Kurilsk, Russia **67 D16** 50 40N 156 8 E
Severo-Yeniseyskiy, Russia **67 C10** 60 22N 93 1 E
Severo-Zapadnyy □, Russia **66 C4** 65 0N 40 0 E
Severočeský □, Czech Rep. **34 A7** 50 30N 14 0 E
Severodonetsk = Syeverodonetsk, Ukraine **59 H10** 48 58N 38 35 E
Severodvinsk, Russia **56 B6** 64 27N 39 58 E
Severomoravský □, Czech Rep. **35 B10** 49 38N 17 40 E
Severomorsk, Russia **56 A5** 69 5N 33 27 E
Severouralsk, Russia **64 A7** 60 9N 59 57 E
Sevier, U.S.A. **159 G7** 38 39N 112 11W
Sevier →, U.S.A. **159 G7** 39 4N 113 6W
Sevier Desert, U.S.A. **158 G7** 39 40N 112 45W
Sevier L., U.S.A. **158 G7** 38 54N 113 9W
Sevilla, Colombia **168 C2** 4 16N 75 57W
Sevilla, Spain **43 H5** 37 23N 5 58W
Sevilla □, Spain **43 H5** 37 25N 5 30W
Seville = Sevilla, Spain **43 H5** 37 23N 5 58W
Seville, Fla., U.S.A. **153 F8** 29 19N 81 30W
Seville, Ga., U.S.A. **152 D6** 31 58N 83 36W
Sevlievo, Bulgaria **51 C9** 43 2N 25 6 E
Sevnica, Slovenia **45 B12** 46 2N 15 19 E
Sèvre-Nantaise →, France **26 E5** 47 12N 1 33W
Sèvre-Niortaise →, France **28 B3** 46 28N 0 50W
Sevsk, Russia **59 F8** 52 10N 34 30 E
Sewa →, S. Leone **112 D2** 7 20N 12 10W
Sewani, India **92 E6** 28 58N 75 39 E
Seward, Alaska, U.S.A. **144 F10** 60 7N 149 27W
Seward, Nebr., U.S.A. **154 E6** 40 55N 97 6W
Seward, Pa., U.S.A. **150 F5** 40 25N 79 1W
Seward Peninsula, U.S.A. **144 D6** 65 30N 166 0W
Sewell, Chile **174 C1** 34 10 S 70 23W
Sewer, Indonesia **83 C4** 5 53 S 134 40 E
Sewickley, U.S.A. **150 F4** 40 32N 80 12W
Sexsmith, Canada **142 B5** 55 21N 118 47W
Seychelles ■, Ind. Oc. **121 b** 5 0 S 56 0 E
Seyðisfjörður, Iceland **11 B13** 65 16N 13 57W
Seydişehir, Turkey **100 D4** 37 25N 31 51 E
Seydvān, Iran **101 C11** 38 34N 45 2 E
Seyhan →, Turkey **100 D6** 36 43N 34 53 E
Seyhan Barajı, Turkey **100 D6** 37 2N 35 18 E
Seyitgazi, Turkey **49 B12** 39 27N 30 43 E
Seyitömer, Turkey **49 B11** 39 34N 29 52 E
Seym →, Ukraine **59 G7** 51 27N 32 34 E
Seymen, Turkey **51 E11** 41 6N 27 57 E
Seymour, Australia **129 D6** 37 0 S 145 10 E
Seymour, S. Africa **117 E4** 32 33 S 26 46 E
Seymour, Conn., U.S.A. **151 E11** 41 24N 73 4W
Seymour, Ind., U.S.A. **157 F11** 38 58N 85 53W
Seymour, Tex., U.S.A. **155 J5** 33 35N 99 16W
Seyne, France **29 D10** 44 21N 6 22 E
Seyssel, France **29 C9** 45 57N 5 50 E
Sežana, Slovenia **45 C10** 45 43N 13 41 E
Sézanne, France **27 D10** 48 40N 3 40 E
Sezze, Italy **46 A6** 41 30N 13 3 E
Sfântu Gheorghe, Covasna, Romania **53 E10** 45 52N 25 48 E
Sfântu Gheorghe, Tulcea, Romania **53 F14** 44 53N 29 36 E
Sfântu Gheorghe, Braţul →, Romania **53 F14** 44 51N 29 36 E
Sfax, Tunisia **108 B2** 34 49N 10 48 E
Sha Tau Kok, China **69 F11** 22 33N 114 13 E
Sha Tin, China **69 G11** 22 23N 114 12 E
Sha Xi →, China **77 D12** 26 35N 118 0 E
Sha Xian, China **77 D11** 26 23N 117 45 E
Shaanxi □, China **74 G5** 35 0N 109 0 E
Shaarikhan = Shakhrikhan, Uzbekistan **65 C6** 40 42N 72 3 E
Shaartuz, Tajikistan **65 E4** 37 16N 68 8 E
Shaba = Katanga □, Dem. Rep. of the Congo **118 D2** 8 0 S 25 0 E
Shaba ⌓, Kenya **118 B4** 0 38N 37 48 E
Shaballe = Scebeli, Wabi →, Somali Rep. **120 D2** 2 0N 44 0 E
Shabla, Bulgaria **51 C12** 43 31N 28 32 E
Shabogamo L., Canada **141 B6** 53 15N 66 30W
Shabunda, Dem. Rep. of the Congo **118 C2** 2 40 S 27 16 E
Shabwah, Yemen **98 D4** 15 22N 47 1 E
Shache, China **65 D8** 38 20N 77 10 E
Shackleton Ice Shelf, Antarctica **7 C8** 66 0 S 100 0 E
Shackleton Inlet, Antarctica **7 E11** 83 0 S 160 0 E
Shādegān, Iran **97 D6** 30 40N 48 38 E
Shadi, China **77 D10** 26 7N 114 47 E
Shadi, India **93 C7** 33 24N 77 14 E
Shadrinsk, Russia **64 C9** 56 5N 63 32 E
Shady Dale, U.S.A. **152 B6** 33 24N 83 36W
Shady Grove, U.S.A. **152 E6** 30 17N 83 38W
Shadyside, U.S.A. **150 G4** 39 58N 80 45W
Shafer, L., U.S.A. **157 D10** 40 46N 86 46W
Shaffa, Nigeria **113 C7** 10 30N 12 6 E
Shafter, U.S.A. **161 K7** 35 30N 119 16W
Shaftesbury, U.K. **21 F5** 51 0N 2 11W
Shag Pt., N.Z. **131 F5** 45 29 S 170 52 E
Shag Rocks, Atl. Oc. **8 M7** 53 0 S 41 0W
Shagamu, Nigeria **113 D5** 6 51N 3 39 E
Shageluk, U.S.A. **144 E8** 62 41N 159 34W
Shaghan, Kazakhstan **65 A2** 44 53N 64 57 E
Shagram, Pakistan **93 A5** 36 24N 72 20 E
Shah Alam, Malaysia **84 B2** 3 5N 101 30 E
Shah Alizai, Pakistan **92 E2** 29 25N 66 33 E
Shah Bunder, Pakistan **92 G2** 24 13N 67 56 E
Shāh Jūy, Afghan. **91 B2** 32 31N 67 25 E
Shahabad, Andhra Pradesh, India **94 F4** 17 10N 78 7 E
Shahabad, Karnataka, India **94 F3** 17 10N 76 54 E
Shahabad, Punjab, India **92 D7** 30 10N 76 55 E
Shahabad, Raj., India **92 G7** 25 15N 77 11 E
Shahabad, Ut. P., India **93 F8** 27 36N 79 56 E

Shahada, *India* **94 D2** 21 33N 74 30 E
Shahadpur, *Pakistan* **92 G3** 25 55N 68 35 E
Shahapur, *India* **95 G2** 15 50N 74 34 E
Shahba, *Syria* **103 C5** 32 52N 36 38 E
Shahbazpur I., *Bangla.* **90 D3** 22 30N 90 45 E
Shahdād, *Iran* **97 D8** 30 30N 57 40 E
Shahdād, Namakzār-e, *Iran* **97 D8** 30 20N 58 20 E
Shahdadkot, *Pakistan* **91 D2** 27 50N 67 55 E
Shahdol, *India* **93 H9** 23 19N 81 26 E
Shahe, *China* **74 F8** 37 0N 114 32 E
Shahganj, *India* **93 F10** 26 3N 82 44 E
Shaḩḩāt, *Libya* **108 B4** 32 48N 21 54 E
Shahīdān, *Afghan.* **91 A2** 36 42N 67 49 E
Shahjahanpur, *India* **93 F8** 27 54N 79 57 E
Shahpur, *Karnataka, India* **94 F3** 16 40N 76 48 E
Shahpur, *Mad. P., India* **92 H7** 22 12N 77 58 E
Shahpur, *Baluchistan, Pakistan* **92 E3** 28 46N 68 27 E
Shahpur, *Punjab, Pakistan* **92 C5** 32 17N 72 26 E
Shahpur Chakar, *Pakistan* **92 F3** 26 9N 68 39 E
Shahpura, *Mad. P., India* **93 H9** 23 10N 80 45 E
Shahpura, *Raj., India* **92 G6** 25 38N 74 56 E
Shahr-e Bābak, *Iran* **97 D7** 30 7N 55 9 E
Shahr-e Kord, *Iran* **97 C6** 32 15N 50 55 E
Shāhrakht, *Iran* **97 C9** 33 38N 60 16 E
Shahrig, *Pakistan* **91 C2** 30 15N 67 40 E
Shahukou, *China* **74 D7** 40 20N 112 18 E
Shaikhabad, *Afghan.* **91 B3** 34 2N 68 45 E
Shajapur, *India* **92 H7** 23 27N 76 21 E
Shajing, *China* **69 F10** 22 44N 113 48 E
Shakargarh, *Pakistan* **92 C6** 32 17N 75 10 E
Shakawe, *Botswana* **116 B3** 18 28 S 21 49 E
Shakenge, *Dem. Rep. of the Congo* **115 D3** 6 14 S 18 41 E
Shaker Heights, *U.S.A.* **150 E3** 41 29N 81 32W
Shakhimardan = Khamza, *Uzbekistan* **65 C5** 40 25N 71 29 E
Shakhrikhan, *Uzbekistan* **65 C6** 40 42N 72 3 E
Shakhrisabz, *Uzbekistan* **65 D3** 39 3N 66 50 E
Shakhristan, *Tajikistan* **65 D4** 39 47N 68 49 E
Shakhty, *Russia* **61 G5** 47 40N 40 16 E
Shakhtyorskoye = Pershotravensk, *Ukraine* **59 G4** 50 13N 27 40 E
Shakhunya, *Russia* **60 B8** 57 40N 46 46 E
Shaki, *Nigeria* **113 D5** 8 41N 3 21 E
Shākir, *Egypt* **106 B3** 27 30N 33 59 E
Shakpak, *Kazakhstan* **65 B4** 43 15N 69 20 E
Shaksam Valley, *Asia* **93 A7** 36 0N 76 20 E
Shaktoolik, *U.S.A.* **144 D7** 64 20N 161 9W
Shala, L., *Ethiopia* **107 F4** 7 30N 38 30 E
Shali, *Russia* **61 J7** 43 9N 45 55 E
Shalkar, *Kazakhstan* **64 F3** 50 40N 51 53 E
Shalkar, Ozero, *Kazakhstan* **64 F3** 50 35N 51 47 E
Shallow Lake, *Canada* **150 B3** 44 36N 81 5W
Shalqar, *Kazakhstan* **66 E6** 47 48N 59 39 E
Shalskiy, *Russia* **58 B8** 61 48N 35 58 E
Shaluli Shan, *China* **76 B2** 30 40N 99 55 E
Shām, *Iran* **97 E8** 26 39N 57 21 E
Shām, Bādiyat ash, *Asia* **96 C3** 32 0N 40 0 E
Shām, J. ash, *Oman* **99 B7** 23 10N 57 5 E
Shamâl Bahr el Ghazal □, *Sudan* **107 F2** 8 0N 27 30 E
Shamâl Dârfûr □, *Sudan* **107 E2** 15 0N 25 0 E
Shamâl Kordofân □, *Sudan* **107 E3** 15 0N 30 0 E
Shamâl Sînî □, *Egypt* **103 E2** 30 30N 33 30 E
Shamaldy-Say, *Kyrgyzstan* **65 C6** 41 12N 72 11 E
Shamattawa, *Canada* **140 A1** 55 51N 92 5W
Shamattawa →, *Canada* **140 A2** 55 1N 85 23W
Shambe, *Sudan* **107 F3** 7 8N 30 46 E
Shambe △, *Sudan* **107 F3** 6 57N 30 50 E
Shambu, *Ethiopia* **107 F4** 9 32N 37 3 E
Shamgong Dzong, *Bhutan* **90 B3** 27 13N 90 35 E
Shamīl, *Iran* **97 E8** 27 30N 56 55 E
Shamkhor = Şämkir, *Azerbaijan* **61 K8** 40 50N 46 0 E
Shāmkūh, *Iran* **97 C8** 35 47N 57 50 E
Shamli, *India* **92 E7** 29 32N 77 18 E
Shammar, Jabal, *Si. Arabia* **96 E4** 27 40N 41 0 E
Shamo = Gobi, *Asia* **74 C6** 44 0N 110 0 E
Shamo, L., *Ethiopia* **107 F4** 5 45N 37 30 E
Shamokin, *U.S.A.* **151 F8** 40 47N 76 34W
Shamrock, *U.S.A.* **155 H4** 35 13N 100 15W
Shamshabad, *India* **94 F4** 17 15N 78 25 E
Shamva, *Zimbabwe* **119 F3** 17 20 S 31 32 E
Shan □, *Burma* **90 E7** 21 30N 98 30 E
Shan Xian, *China* **74 G9** 34 50N 116 5 E
Shana = Kurilsk, *Russia* **67 E15** 45 14N 147 53 E
Shanan →, *Ethiopia* **107 F5** 8 0N 40 20 E
Shanchengzhen, *China* **75 C13** 42 20N 125 20 E
Shāndak, *Iran* **97 D9** 28 28N 60 27 E
Shandon, *U.S.A.* **160 K6** 35 39N 120 23W
Shandong □, *China* **75 G10** 36 0N 118 0 E
Shandong Bandao, *China* **75 F11** 37 0N 121 0 E
Shang Xian = Shangzhou, *China* **74 H5** 33 50N 109 58 E
Shangalowe, *Dem. Rep. of the Congo* **119 E2** 10 50 S 26 30 E
Shangani, *Zimbabwe* **117 B4** 19 41 S 29 20 E
Shangani →, *Zimbabwe* **119 F2** 18 41 S 27 10 E
Shangbancheng, *China* **75 D10** 40 50N 118 1 E
Shangcheng, *China* **77 B10** 31 47N 115 26 E
Shangchuan Dao, *China* **77 G9** 21 40N 112 50 E
Shangdu, *China* **74 D7** 41 30N 113 30 E
Shanggao, *China* **77 C10** 28 17N 114 55 E
Shanghai, *China* **77 B13** 31 15N 121 26 E
Shanghai Shi □, *China* **77 B13** 31 0N 121 30 E
Shanghang, *China* **77 E11** 25 2N 116 23 E
Shanghe, *China* **75 F9** 37 20N 117 10 E
Shangjao = Shangrao, *China* **77 C11** 28 25N 117 59 E
Shanglin, *China* **76 F7** 23 27N 108 33 E
Shangnan, *China* **74 H6** 33 32N 110 50 E
Shangqiu, *China* **74 G8** 34 26N 115 36 E
Shangrao, *China* **77 C11** 28 25N 117 59 E
Shangshui, *China* **69 C6** 33 42N 114 35 E
Shangsi, *China* **76 F6** 22 8N 107 58 E
Shangyou, *China* **77 E10** 25 48N 114 32 E
Shangyu, *China* **77 B13** 30 3N 120 52 E
Shangzhi, *China* **75 B14** 45 22N 127 56 E
Shangzhou, *China* **74 H5** 33 50N 109 58 E
Shanhetun, *China* **75 B14** 44 33N 127 15 E
Shani, *Nigeria* **113 C7** 10 14N 12 2 E
Shanklin, *U.K.* **21 G6** 50 38N 1 11W
Shannon, *Greenland* **10 B9** 75 10N 18 30W
Shannon, *N.Z.* **130 G4** 40 33 S 175 25 E
Shannon △, *Australia* **125 F2** 31 55 S 117 51 E
Shannon →, *Ireland* **23 D2** 52 35N 9 30W
Shannon, Mouth of the, *Ireland* **23 D2** 52 30N 9 55W
Shannon Airport, *Ireland* **23 D3** 52 42N 8 57W
Shannontown, *U.S.A.* **152 B9** 33 53N 80 21W
Shansi = Shanxi □, *China* **74 F7** 37 0N 112 0 E
Shantar, Ostrov Bolshoy, *Russia* **67 D14** 55 9N 137 40 E
Shantipur, *India* **93 H13** 23 17N 88 25 E
Shantou, *China* **77 F11** 23 18N 116 40 E
Shantung = Shandong □, *China* **75 G10** 36 0N 118 0 E
Shanwei, *China* **77 F10** 22 48N 115 22 E
Shanxi □, *China* **74 F7** 37 0N 112 0 E
Shanyang, *China* **74 H5** 33 31N 109 55 E
Shanyin, *China* **74 E7** 39 25N 112 56 E
Shaodong, *China* **77 D8** 27 15N 111 43 E
Shaoguan, *China* **77 E9** 24 48N 113 35 E
Shaohing = Shaoxing, *China* **77 C13** 30 0N 120 35 E
Shaoshan, *China* **77 D9** 27 55N 112 33 E
Shaowu, *China* **77 D11** 27 22N 117 28 E
Shaoxing, *China* **77 C13** 30 0N 120 35 E
Shaoyang, *Hunan, China* **77 D8** 26 59N 111 20 E
Shaoyang, *Hunan, China* **77 D8** 27 14N 111 25 E
Shap, *U.K.* **20 C5** 54 32N 2 40W
Shapinsay, *U.K.* **22 B6** 59 3N 2 51W
Shaqq el Gi'eifer →, *Sudan* **107 D2** 15 16N 26 0 E
Shaqra', *Si. Arabia* **96 E5** 25 15N 45 16 E
Shaqrā', *Yemen* **98 D4** 13 22N 45 44 E
Sharafa, *Sudan* **107 E2** 11 59N 27 7 E
Sharafkhāneh, *Iran* **101 C11** 38 11N 45 29 E
Sharashova, *Belarus* **55 F11** 52 34N 24 12 E
Sharavati →, *India* **95 G2** 14 20N 74 25 E
Sharbatāt, Ra's ash, *Oman* **99 C7** 17 56N 56 21 E
Sharbot Lake, *Canada* **151 B8** 44 46N 76 41W
Shardara, *Kazakhstan* **65 C3** 41 15N 67 0 E
Shardara, Step, *Kazakhstan* **65 C3** 42 20N 68 0 E
Shardara Bögeni, *Kazakhstan* **65 C4** 41 10N 68 15 E
Shargun, *Uzbekistan* **65 D3** 38 35N 67 58 E
Sharhorod, *Ukraine* **53 B13** 48 45N 28 5 E
Shari, *Japan* **70 C12** 43 55N 144 40 E
Sharjah = Ash Shāriqah, *U.A.E.* **97 E7** 25 23N 55 26 E
Shark B., *Australia* **125 E1** 25 30 S 113 32 E
Shark Bay ⌓, *Australia* **125 F2** 32 49 S 118 49 E
Sharm el Sheikh, *Egypt* **106 B3** 27 53N 34 18 E
Sharon, *Mass., U.S.A.* **151 D13** 42 7N 71 11W
Sharon, *Pa., U.S.A.* **150 E4** 41 14N 80 31W
Sharon, *Wis., U.S.A.* **157 B8** 42 30N 88 44W
Sharon Springs, *Kans., U.S.A.* **154 F4** 38 54N 101 45W
Sharon Springs, *N.Y., U.S.A.* **151 D10** 42 48N 74 37W
Sharonville, *U.S.A.* **157 E12** 39 16N 84 25W
Sharp Pk., *Phil.* **81 J5** 5 58N 125 31 E
Sharp Pt., *Australia* **126 A3** 10 58 S 142 43 E
Sharpe L., *Canada* **140 B1** 54 24N 93 40W
Sharpes, *U.S.A.* **153 G9** 28 26N 80 46W
Sharpsville, *U.S.A.* **150 E4** 41 15N 80 29W
Sharq el Istiwa'iya □, *Sudan* **107 G3** 5 0N 33 0 E
Sharya, *Russia* **60 A7** 58 22N 45 20 E
Shasha, *Ethiopia* **107 F4** 6 29N 35 59 E
Shashemene, *Ethiopia* **107 F4** 7 13N 38 33 E
Shashi, *Botswana* **117 C4** 21 15 S 27 27 E
Shashi, *China* **77 B9** 30 25N 112 14 E
Shashi →, *Africa* **119 G2** 21 14 S 29 20 E
Shasta, Mt., *U.S.A.* **158 F2** 41 25N 122 12W
Shasta L., *U.S.A.* **158 F2** 40 43N 122 25W
Shatawi, *Sudan* **107 E3** 14 39N 32 6 E
Shāţi', Wādī ash →, *Libya* **108 C3** 27 30N 15 0 E
Shatilki = Svyetlahorsk, *Belarus* **59 F5** 52 38N 29 46 E
Shatsk, *Russia* **60 C5** 54 5N 41 45 E
Shatsk, *Ukraine* **55 G10** 51 29N 23 55 E
Shatskiy Rise, *Pac. Oc.* **134 D7** 34 0N 157 0 E
Shatskyi ⌓, *Ukraine* **55 G10** 51 30N 23 52 E
Shatt al Arab, *Asia* **97 D6** 30 0N 48 31 E
Shatt al'Arab →, *Iraq* **88 C3** 29 57N 48 34 E
Shatura, *Russia* **58 E10** 55 33N 39 21 E
Shaturtof = Shatura, *Russia* **58 E10** 55 33N 39 21 E
Shäüildir, *Kazakhstan* **65 B4** 42 47N 68 3 E
Shaumyani = Shulaveri, *Georgia* **61 K7** 41 22N 44 45 E
Shaunavon, *Canada* **143 D7** 49 35N 108 25W
Shaver L., *U.S.A.* **160 H7** 37 9N 119 18W
Shavli = Šiauliai, *Lithuania* **15 J20** 55 56N 23 15 E
Shaw →, *Australia* **124 D2** 20 21 S 119 17 E
Shaw I., *Australia* **126 J7** 20 30 S 149 2 E
Shawanaga, *Canada* **150 A4** 45 31N 80 17W
Shawangunk Mts., *U.S.A.* **151 E10** 41 35N 74 30W
Shawano, *U.S.A.* **148 C1** 44 47N 88 36W
Shawinigan, *Canada* **140 C5** 46 35N 72 50W
Shawnee, *Ga., U.S.A.* **152 C8** 32 29N 81 25W
Shawnee, *Kans., U.S.A.* **156 E2** 39 1N 94 43W
Shawnee, *Okla., U.S.A.* **155 H6** 35 20N 96 55W
Shay Gap, *Australia* **124 D3** 20 30 S 120 10 E
Shayan, *Kazakhstan* **65 B4** 43 5N 69 25 E
Shayang, *China* **77 B9** 30 42N 112 29 E
Shaybārā, *Si. Arabia* **96 E3** 25 26N 36 47 E
Shayib el Banat, Gebel, *Egypt* **106 B3** 26 59N 33 29 E
Shaykh, J. ash, *Lebanon* **103 B4** 33 25N 35 50 E
Shaykh Miskīn, *Syria* **103 C5** 32 49N 36 9 E
Shaykh Sa'īd, *Iraq* **101 F12** 32 34N 46 17 E
Shaykh 'Uthmān, *Yemen* **98 D4** 12 52N 44 59 E
Shaymak, *Tajikistan* **65 E7** 37 33N 74 50 E
Shaytansky Zavod = Pervouralsk, *Russia* **64 C7** 56 59N 59 59 E
Shazud, *Tajikistan* **65 E6** 37 45N 72 25 E
Shcheglovo = Kemerovo, *Russia* **66 D9** 55 20N 86 5 E
Shchekino, *Russia* **58 E9** 54 1N 37 34 E
Shcherbakov = Rybinsk, *Russia* **58 C10** 58 5N 38 50 E
Shchigry, *Russia* **59 G9** 51 55N 36 58 E
Shchors, *Ukraine* **59 G6** 51 48N 31 56 E
Shchuchinsk, *Kazakhstan* **66 D8** 52 56N 70 12 E
Shchuchye, *Russia* **64 D9** 55 12N 62 46 E
She Xian, *Anhui, China* **77 C12** 29 50N 118 25 E
She Xian, *Hebei, China* **74 F7** 36 30N 113 40 E
Shea, *Guyana* **169 C6** 2 48N 59 4W
Shebekino, *Russia* **59 G9** 50 28N 36 54 E
Shebele = Scebeli, Wabi →, *Somali Rep.* **120 D2** 2 0N 44 0 E
Sheberghān, *Afghan.* **65 E2** 36 40N 65 45 E
Sheboygan, *U.S.A.* **148 D2** 43 46N 87 45W
Shebshi Mts., *Nigeria* **113 D7** 8 30N 12 0 E
Shediac, *Canada* **141 C7** 46 14N 64 32W
Sheelin, L., *Ireland* **23 C4** 53 48N 7 20W
Sheenjek →, *U.S.A.* **144 C11** 66 45N 144 33W
Sheep Haven, *Ireland* **23 A4** 55 11N 7 52W
Sheerness, *U.K.* **21 F8** 51 26N 0 47 E
Sheet Harbour, *Canada* **141 D7** 44 56N 62 31W
Sheffield, *N.Z.* **131 D7** 43 23 S 172 1 E
Sheffield, *U.K.* **20 D6** 53 23N 1 28W
Sheffield, *Ala., U.S.A.* **149 H2** 34 46N 87 41W
Sheffield, *Ill., U.S.A.* **156 C7** 41 21N 89 44W
Sheffield, *Iowa, U.S.A.* **156 B3** 42 54N 93 13W
Sheffield, *Mass., U.S.A.* **151 D11** 42 5N 73 21W
Sheffield, *Pa., U.S.A.* **150 E5** 41 42N 79 3W
Shegaon, *India* **94 D3** 20 48N 76 47 E
Sheghnān, *Afghan.* **65 E5** 37 37N 71 36 E
Shehojele, *Ethiopia* **107 E4** 10 40N 35 9 E
Shehong, *China* **76 B5** 30 54N 105 18 E
Shehuen →, *Argentina* **176 C3** 49 35 S 69 34W
Sheikh Idris, *Sudan* **107 E3** 11 43N 33 30 E
Sheikhpura, *India* **93 G11** 25 9N 85 53 E
Shek Hasan, *Ethiopia* **107 E4** 12 5N 35 58 E
Shekhupura, *Pakistan* **91 C4** 31 42N 73 58 E
Sheki = Şaki, *Azerbaijan* **61 K8** 41 10N 47 5 E
Shekki = Zhongshan, *China* **77 F9** 22 26N 113 20 E
Shekou, *China* **69 G10** 22 30N 113 55 E
Shelbina, *U.S.A.* **156 E4** 39 47N 92 2W
Shelburn, *U.S.A.* **157 E9** 39 11N 87 24W
Shelburne, *N.S., Canada* **141 D6** 43 47N 65 20W
Shelburne, *Ont., Canada* **140 D3** 44 4N 80 15W
Shelburne, *U.S.A.* **151 B11** 44 23N 73 14W
Shelburne B., *Australia* **126 A3** 11 50 S 142 50 E
Shelburne Falls, *U.S.A.* **151 D12** 42 36N 72 45W
Shelby, *Mich., U.S.A.* **148 D2** 43 37N 86 22W
Shelby, *Miss., U.S.A.* **155 J9** 33 57N 90 46W
Shelby, *Mont., U.S.A.* **158 B8** 48 30N 111 51W
Shelby, *N.C., U.S.A.* **149 H5** 35 17N 81 32W
Shelby, *Ohio, U.S.A.* **150 F2** 40 53N 82 40W
Shelbyville, *Ill., U.S.A.* **154 F10** 39 24N 88 48W
Shelbyville, *Ind., U.S.A.* **157 E11** 39 31N 85 47W
Shelbyville, *Ky., U.S.A.* **157 F11** 38 13N 85 14W
Shelbyville, *Mo., U.S.A.* **156 E4** 39 48N 92 2W
Shelbyville, *Tenn., U.S.A.* **149 H2** 35 29N 86 28W
Shelbyville, L., *U.S.A.* **157 E8** 39 26N 88 46W
Sheldon, *Ill., U.S.A.* **157 D9** 40 46N 87 34W
Sheldon, *Iowa, U.S.A.* **154 D7** 43 11N 95 51W
Sheldon, *Mo., U.S.A.* **156 G2** 37 40N 94 18W
Sheldon, *S.C., U.S.A.* **152 C9** 32 36N 80 48W
Sheldon Point, *U.S.A.* **144 E6** 62 32N 164 52W
Sheldrake, *Canada* **141 B7** 50 20N 64 51W
Shelek, *Kazakhstan* **65 B9** 43 33N 78 17 E
Shelengo, Khawr →, *Sudan* **107 E2** 10 33N 28 40 E
Shelikhova, Zaliv, *Russia* **67 D16** 59 30N 157 0 E
Shelikof Strait, *U.S.A.* **144 H9** 57 30N 155 0W
Shell Beach = Huntington Beach, *U.S.A.* **161 M9** 33 40N 118 5W
Shell Lakes, *Australia* **125 E4** 29 20 S 127 30 E
Shellbrook, *Canada* **143 C7** 53 13N 106 24W
Shellharbour, *Australia* **129 C9** 34 31 S 150 51 E
Shellman, *U.S.A.* **152 D5** 31 46N 84 37W
Shellsburg, *U.S.A.* **156 B5** 42 6N 91 52W
Shelon →, *Russia* **58 C6** 58 13N 30 47 E
Shelter Bay = Port-Cartier, *Canada* **141 B6** 50 2N 66 50W
Shelter I, *U.S.A.* **151 E12** 41 5N 72 21W
Shelton, *Conn., U.S.A.* **151 E11** 41 19N 73 5W
Shelton, *Wash., U.S.A.* **160 C3** 47 13N 123 6W
Shemakha = Şamaxi, *Azerbaijan* **61 K9** 40 38N 48 37 E
Shëmri, *Albania* **50 D4** 42 7N 20 13 E
Shemsi, *Sudan* **106 D2** 19 2N 29 57 E
Shen Xian, *China* **74 F8** 36 15N 115 40 E
Shenandoah, *Iowa, U.S.A.* **154 E7** 40 46N 95 22W
Shenandoah, *Pa., U.S.A.* **151 F8** 40 49N 76 12W
Shenandoah, *Va., U.S.A.* **148 F6** 38 29N 78 37W
Shenandoah △, *U.S.A.* **148 F6** 38 35N 78 22W
Shenandoah →, *U.S.A.* **148 F7** 39 19N 77 44W
Shenchi, *China* **74 E7** 39 8N 112 10 E
Shencottah, *India* **95 K3** 8 59N 77 18 E
Shendam, *Nigeria* **113 D6** 8 49N 9 30 E
Shendî, *Sudan* **107 D3** 16 46N 33 22 E
Shendurni, *India* **94 D2** 20 39N 75 36 E
Shenge, *S. Leone* **112 D2** 7 54N 12 55W
Shengfang, *China* **74 E9** 39 3N 116 42 E
Shenggeldi, *Kazakhstan* **65 B8** 43 59N 77 27 E
Shëngjergj, *Albania* **50 E4** 41 17N 20 10 E
Shëngjin, *Albania* **50 E3** 41 50N 19 35 E
Shengzhou, *China* **77 C13** 29 35N 120 50 E
Shenjingzi, *China* **75 B13** 44 40N 124 30 E
Shenmu, *China* **74 E6** 38 50N 110 29 E
Shennongjia, *China* **77 B8** 31 43N 110 44 E
Shenqiu, *China* **74 H8** 33 25N 115 5 E
Shensi = Shaanxi □, *China* **74 G5** 35 0N 109 0 E
Shenyang, *China* **75 D12** 41 48N 123 27 E
Shenzhen, *China* **77 F10** 22 32N 114 5 E
Shenzhen ✈ (SZX), *China* **69 F10** 22 41N 113 49 E
Shenzhen Shuiku, *China* **69 F11** 22 34N 114 8 E
Shenzhen Wan, *China* **69 G10** 22 27N 113 55 E
Sheo, *India* **92 F4** 26 11N 71 15 E
Shepetivka, *Ukraine* **59 G4** 50 10N 27 10 E
Shepetovka = Shepetivka, *Ukraine* **59 G4** 50 10N 27 10 E
Shepherd Is., *Vanuatu* **133 F6** 16 55 S 168 36 E
Shepherdsville, *U.S.A.* **157 G11** 37 59N 85 43W
Shepparton, *Australia* **129 D6** 36 23 S 145 26 E
Sheppey, I. of, *U.K.* **21 F8** 51 25N 0 48 E
Shepton Mallet, *U.K.* **21 F5** 51 11N 2 33W
Sheqi, *China* **74 H7** 33 12N 112 57 E
Sher Khan Qala, *Afghan.* **91 C2** 29 53N 66 13 E
Sher Qila, *Pakistan* **93 A6** 36 7N 74 2 E
Sherab, *Sudan* **107 E1** 10 44N 24 41 E
Sherabad, *Uzbekistan* **65 E3** 37 40N 67 1 E
Sherborne, *U.K.* **21 G5** 50 57N 2 31W
Sherbro →, *S. Leone* **112 D2** 7 45N 12 55W
Sherbro I., *S. Leone* **112 D2** 7 30N 12 40W
Sherbrooke, *N.S., Canada* **141 C7** 45 8N 61 59W
Sherbrooke, *Qué., Canada* **141 C5** 45 28N 71 57W
Sherburne, *U.S.A.* **151 D9** 42 41N 75 30W
Sherburne Reef, *Papua N. G.* **132 B5** 3 20 S 148 0 E
Sherda, *Chad* **109 D3** 20 7N 16 46 E
Shereik, *Sudan* **106 D3** 18 44N 33 47 E
Shergaon, *India* **90 B4** 27 7N 92 16 E
Shergarh, *India* **92 F5** 26 20N 72 18 E
Sherghati, *India* **93 G11** 24 34N 84 47 E
Sheridan, *Ark., U.S.A.* **155 H8** 34 19N 92 24W
Sheridan, *Ill., U.S.A.* **157 C8** 41 32N 88 41W
Sheridan, *Ind., U.S.A.* **157 D10** 40 8N 86 13W
Sheridan, *Wyo., U.S.A.* **158 D10** 44 48N 106 58W
Sheringham, *U.K.* **20 E9** 52 56N 1 13 E
Sherkin I., *Ireland* **23 E2** 51 28N 9 26W
Sherkot, *India* **93 E8** 29 22N 78 35 E
Sherman, *U.S.A.* **155 J6** 33 40N 96 35W
Sherpur, *Bangla.* **90 C3** 25 0N 90 0 E
Sherpur, *India* **93 G10** 25 34N 83 47 E
Sherridon, *Canada* **143 B8** 55 8N 101 5W
Sherwood, *U.S.A.* **157 C12** 41 17N 84 33W
Sherwood Forest, *U.K.* **20 D6** 53 6N 1 7W
Sherwood Park, *Canada* **142 C6** 53 31N 113 19W
Sheslay →, *Canada* **142 B2** 58 48N 132 5W
Shethanei L., *Canada* **143 B9** 58 48N 97 50W
Shetland □, *U.K.* **22 A7** 60 30N 1 30W
Shetland Is., *U.K.* **22 A7** 60 30N 1 30W
Shetrunji →, *India* **92 J5** 21 19N 72 7 E
Sheung Shui, *China* **69 F11** 22 31N 114 7 E
Shevaroy Hills, *India* **95 J4** 11 58N 78 12 E
Shevchenkovo = Dolynska, *Ukraine* **59 H7** 48 6N 32 46 E
Shevchenkovo, *Ukraine* **53 E14** 45 33N 29 20 E
Shevgaon, *India* **94 E2** 19 21N 75 14 E
Shewa, *Ethiopia* **107 F4** 9 33N 38 10 E
Shewa Gimira, *Ethiopia* **107 F4** 7 4N 35 51 E
Shey-Phoksundo △, *Nepal* **93 E10** 29 30N 82 45 E
Sheyenne →, *U.S.A.* **154 B6** 47 2N 96 50W
Shibām, *Yemen* **99 D5** 15 59N 48 36 E
Shibata, *Japan* **70 F9** 37 57N 139 20 E
Shibecha, *Japan* **70 C12** 43 17N 144 36 E
Shibetsu, *Japan* **70 B11** 44 10N 142 23 E
Shibîn el Kôm, *Egypt* **106 H7** 30 31N 30 55 E
Shibîn el Qanâtir, *Egypt* **106 H7** 30 19N 31 19 E
Shibing, *China* **76 D7** 27 2N 108 7 E
Shibogama L., *Canada* **140 B2** 53 35N 88 15W
Shibukawa, *Japan* **73 A11** 36 29N 139 0 E
Shibushi, *Japan* **72 F3** 31 25N 131 8 E
Shibushi-Wan, *Japan* **72 F3** 31 24N 131 8 E
Shicheng, *China* **77 D11** 26 22N 116 20 E
Shickshinny, *U.S.A.* **151 E8** 41 9N 76 9W
Shickshock Mts. = Chic-Chocs, Mts., *Canada* **141 C6** 48 55N 66 0W
Shidād, *Si. Arabia* **98 B3** 21 19N 40 3 E
Shidao, *China* **75 F12** 36 50N 122 25 E
Shidian, *China* **76 E2** 24 40N 99 5 E
Shido, *Japan* **72 C6** 34 19N 134 10 E
Shiel, L., *U.K.* **22 E3** 56 48N 5 34W
Shield, C., *Australia* **126 A2** 13 20 S 136 20 E
Shīeli, *Kazakhstan* **65 A3** 44 20N 66 15 E
Shifang, *China* **76 B5** 31 8N 104 10 E
Shiga □, *Japan* **73 B8** 35 20N 136 0 E
Shigaib, *Sudan* **109 E4** 15 5N 23 35 E
Shigu, *China* **76 D2** 26 51N 99 56 E
Shiguaigou, *China* **74 D6** 40 52N 110 15 E
Shihan, W. →, *Yemen* **99 C5** 17 24N 51 26 E
Shihchiachuangi = Shijiazhuang, *China* **74 E8** 38 2N 114 28 E
Shihezi, *China* **68 B3** 44 15N 86 2 E
Shiiba, *Japan* **72 E3** 32 29N 131 4 E
Shijak, *Albania* **50 E3** 41 21N 19 33 E
Shijiazhuang, *China* **74 E8** 38 2N 114 28 E
Shijiu Hu, *China* **77 B12** 31 25N 118 50 E
Shikarpur, *India* **92 E8** 28 17N 78 7 E
Shikarpur, *Pakistan* **91 D3** 27 57N 68 39 E
Shikhrany = Kanash, *Russia* **60 C8** 55 30N 47 32 E
Shikine-Jima, *Japan* **73 C11** 34 19N 139 13 E
Shikohabad, *India* **93 F8** 27 6N 78 36 E
Shikoku, *Japan* **72 D5** 33 30N 133 30 E
Shikoku □, *Japan* **72 D5** 33 30N 133 30 E
Shikoku-Sanchi, *Japan* **72 D5** 33 30N 133 30 E
Shikotsu-Ko, *Japan* **70 C10** 42 45N 141 25 E
Shikotsu-Tōya △, *Japan* **70 C10** 44 4N 145 8 E
Shikuka = Poronaysk, *Russia* **67 E15** 49 13N 143 0 E
Shiliguri, *India* **90 B2** 26 45N 88 25 E
Shiliu = Changjiang, *China* **86 C7** 19 20N 108 55 E
Shilka, *Russia* **67 D12** 52 0N 115 55 E
Shilka →, *Russia* **67 D13** 53 20N 121 26 E
Shillelagh, *Ireland* **23 D5** 52 45N 6 32W
Shillington, *U.S.A.* **151 F9** 40 18N 75 58W
Shillong, *India* **90 C3** 25 35N 91 53 E
Shilo, *West Bank* **103 C4** 32 4N 35 18 E
Shilong, *China* **77 F9** 23 5N 113 52 E
Shilou, *China* **74 F6** 37 0N 110 48 E
Shilovo, *Russia* **60 C5** 54 25N 40 57 E
Shima-Hantō, *Japan* **73 C8** 34 22N 136 45 E
Shimabara, *Japan* **72 E2** 32 48N 130 20 E
Shimada, *Japan* **73 C10** 34 49N 138 10 E
Shimane □, *Japan* **72 C4** 35 0N 132 30 E
Shimane-Hantō, *Japan* **72 B5** 35 30N 133 0 E
Shimanovsk, *Russia* **67 D13** 52 15N 127 30 E
Shimba Hills ⌓, *Kenya* **118 C4** 4 14 S 39 25 E
Shimen, *China* **77 C8** 29 35N 111 20 E
Shimenjie, *China* **77 C11** 29 29N 116 48 E
Shimian, *China* **76 C4** 29 17N 102 23 E
Shimizu, *Japan* **73 C10** 35 0N 138 30 E
Shimo-Jima, *Japan* **72 E2** 32 15N 130 7 E
Shimo-Koshiki-Jima, *Japan* **72 F1** 31 40N 129 43 E
Shimoda, *Japan* **73 C10** 34 40N 138 57 E
Shimodate, *Japan* **73 A11** 36 20N 139 55 E
Shimoga, *India* **95 H2** 13 57N 75 32 E
Shimoni, *Kenya* **118 C4** 4 38 S 39 20 E
Shimonita, *Japan* **73 A10** 36 13N 138 47 E
Shimonoseki, *Japan* **72 D2** 33 58N 130 55 E
Shimotsuma, *Japan* **73 A11** 36 11N 139 58 E
Shimpuru Rapids, *Namibia* **116 B2** 17 45 S 19 55 E
Shimsha →, *India* **95 H3** 13 15N 77 10 E
Shimsk, *Russia* **58 C6** 58 15N 30 50 E
Shin, L., *U.K.* **22 C4** 58 5N 4 30W
Shin-Nan'yō, *Japan* **72 C3** 34 3N 131 49 E
Shin-Tone-Gawa →, *Japan* **73 B12** 35 44N 140 51 E
Shinan, *China* **76 F7** 22 44N 109 53 E
Shinano-Gawa →, *Japan* **71 F9** 36 50N 138 30 E
Shināş, *Oman* **97 E8** 24 46N 56 28 E
Shīndand, *Afghan.* **91 B1** 33 12N 62 8 E
Shingbwiyang, *Burma* **90 B6** 26 41N 96 13 E
Shinglehouse, *U.S.A.* **150 E6** 41 58N 78 12W
Shingū, *Japan* **73 D7** 33 40N 135 55 E
Shingwidzi, *S. Africa* **117 C5** 23 5 S 31 25 E
Shinji, *Japan* **72 B4** 35 24N 132 54 E
Shinji-Ko, *Japan* **72 B4** 35 26N 132 57 E
Shinjō, *Japan* **70 E10** 38 46N 140 18 E
Shinkafe, *Nigeria* **113 C6** 13 8N 6 29 E
Shinminato, *Japan* **73 A9** 36 47N 137 4 E
Shinshār, *Syria* **103 A5** 34 36N 36 43 E
Shinshiro, *Japan* **73 C9** 34 54N 137 30 E
Shintuya, *Peru* **172 C3** 12 41 S 71 15W
Shinyanga, *Tanzania* **118 C3** 3 45 S 33 27 E
Shinyanga □, *Tanzania* **118 C3** 3 50 S 34 0 E
Shio-no-Misaki, *Japan* **73 D7** 33 25N 135 45 E
Shiogama, *Japan* **70 E10** 38 19N 141 1 E
Shiojiri, *Japan* **73 A9** 36 6N 137 58 E
Shipchenski Prokhod, *Bulgaria* **51 D9** 42 45N 25 15 E
Shiping, *China* **76 F4** 23 45N 102 23 E
Shippagan, *Canada* **141 C7** 47 45N 64 45W
Shippensburg, *U.S.A.* **150 F7** 40 3N 77 31W
Shippenville, *U.S.A.* **150 E5** 41 15N 79 28W
Shiprock, *U.S.A.* **159 H9** 36 47N 108 41W
Shiqian, *China* **76 D7** 27 32N 108 13 E
Shiqma, N. →, *Israel* **103 D3** 31 37N 34 30 E
Shiquan, *China* **74 H5** 33 5N 108 15 E
Shiquan He = Indus →, *Pakistan* **91 D2** 24 20N 67 47 E
Shīr Khān, *Afghan.* **65 E4** 37 11N 68 36 E
Shīr Kūh, *Iran* **97 D7** 31 39N 54 3 E
Shirabad = Sherabad, *Uzbekistan* **65 E3** 37 40N 67 1 E
Shiragami-Misaki, *Japan* **70 D10** 41 24N 140 12 E
Shirahama, *Japan* **73 D7** 33 41N 135 20 E
Shirakawa, *Fukushima, Japan* **71 F10** 37 7N 140 13 E
Shirakawa, *Gifu, Japan* **73 A8** 36 17N 136 56 E
Shirane-San, *Gumma, Japan* **73 A11** 36 48N 139 22 E
Shirane-San, *Yamanashi, Japan* **73 B10** 35 42N 138 9 E
Shiraoi, *Japan* **70 C10** 42 33N 141 21 E
Shīrāz, *Iran* **97 D7** 29 42N 52 30 E
Shirbīn, *Egypt* **106 H7** 31 11N 31 32 E
Shire →, *Africa* **119 F4** 17 42 S 35 19 E
Shiretoko-Misaki, *Japan* **70 B12** 44 21N 145 20 E
Shirin, *Uzbekistan* **65 C4** 40 14N 69 7 E
Shirinab →, *Pakistan* **92 D2** 30 15N 66 28 E
Shiriya-Zaki, *Japan* **70 D10** 41 25N 141 30 E
Shirley, *U.S.A.* **157 E11** 39 53N 85 35W
Shiroishi, *Japan* **70 F10** 38 0N 140 37 E
Shirol, *India* **94 F2** 16 47N 74 41 E
Shirpur, *India* **94 D2** 21 21N 74 57 E
Shirshow Ridge, *Pac. Oc.* **134 B8** 58 0N 170 0 E
Shīrvān, *Iran* **97 B8** 37 30N 57 50 E
Shirwa, L. = Chilwa, L., *Malawi* **119 F4** 15 15 S 35 40 E
Shishaldin Volcano, *U.S.A.* **144 J7** 54 45N 163 58W
Shishi, *China* **77 E12** 24 44N 118 37 E
Shishmaref, *U.S.A.* **144 C6** 66 15N 166 4W
Shishou, *China* **77 C9** 29 38N 112 22 E
Shitai, *China* **77 B11** 30 12N 117 25 E
Shively, *U.S.A.* **157 F11** 38 12N 85 49W
Shivpuri, *India* **92 G7** 25 26N 77 42 E
Shixian, *China* **75 C15** 43 5N 129 50 E
Shixing, *China* **77 E10** 24 46N 114 5 E
Shiyan, *Guangdong, China* **69 F10** 22 42N 113 56 E
Shiyan, *Hubei, China* **77 A8** 32 35N 110 45 E
Shiyan Shuiku, *China* **69 F10** 22 42N 113 54 E
Shiyata, *Egypt* **106 B2** 29 25N 25 7 E
Shizhu, *China* **76 C7** 29 58N 108 7 E
Shizong, *China* **76 E5** 24 50N 104 0 E
Shizuishan, *China* **74 E4** 39 15N 106 50 E
Shizuoka, *Japan* **73 C10** 34 57N 138 24 E
Shizuoka □, *Japan* **73 B10** 35 15N 138 40 E
Shklov = Shklow, *Belarus* **58 E6** 54 16N 30 15 E
Shklow, *Belarus* **58 E6** 54 16N 30 15 E
Shkodër, *Albania* **50 D3** 42 4N 19 32 E
Shkodra = Shkodër, *Albania* **50 D3** 42 4N 19 32 E
Shkumbini →, *Albania* **50 E3** 41 2N 19 31 E
Shmidta, Ostrov, *Russia* **67 A10** 81 0N 91 0 E
Shō-Gawa →, *Japan* **73 A9** 36 47N 137 4 E
Shoal Cr. →, *U.S.A.* **156 E3** 39 44N 93 32W
Shoal L., *Canada* **143 D9** 49 33N 95 1W
Shoal Lake, *Canada* **143 C8** 50 30N 100 35W
Shoalhaven →, *Australia* **129 C9** 34 54 S 150 42 E
Shoals, *U.S.A.* **157 F10** 38 40N 86 47W
Shōbara, *Japan* **72 C5** 34 51N 133 1 E
Shōdo-Shima, *Japan* **72 C6** 34 30N 134 15 E
Shokpar = Shoqpar, *Kazakhstan* **65 B7** 43 49N 74 21 E
Sholapur = Solapur, *India* **94 F2** 17 43N 75 56 E
Sholaqqŭrghan, *Kazakhstan* **65 B4** 43 46N 69 9 E
Shōmrōn, *West Bank* **103 C4** 32 15N 35 13 E
Shoqpar, *Kazakhstan* **65 B7** 43 49N 74 21 E
Shoranur, *India* **95 J3** 10 46N 76 19 E
Shorapur, *India* **95 F3** 16 31N 76 48 E
Shoreham by Sea, *U.K.* **21 G7** 50 50N 0 16W
Shorewood, *U.S.A.* **157 A9** 43 5N 87 54W
Shori →, *Pakistan* **92 E3** 28 29N 69 44 E
Shorkot Road, *Pakistan* **92 D5** 30 47N 72 15 E
Shornak, *Kazakhstan* **65 B4** 43 24N 68 2 E
Shorter, *U.S.A.* **152 C4** 32 24N 85 57W
Shorterville, *U.S.A.* **152 D4** 31 34N 85 6W
Shortland I., *Solomon Is.* **133 L8** 7 0 S 155 45 E
Shortland Is., *Solomon Is.* **133 L8** 7 0 S 156 0 E
Shortt's I., *India* **94 D8** 20 47N 87 4 E
Shoshone, *Calif., U.S.A.* **161 K10** 35 58N 116 16W
Shoshone, *Idaho, U.S.A.* **158 E6** 42 56N 114 25W
Shoshone L., *U.S.A.* **158 D8** 44 22N 110 43W
Shoshone Mts., *U.S.A.* **158 G5** 39 20N 117 25W
Shoshong, *Botswana* **116 C4** 22 56 S 26 31 E
Shoshoni, *U.S.A.* **158 E9** 43 14N 108 7W
Shostka, *Ukraine* **59 G7** 51 57N 33 32 E
Shotor Khūn, *Afghan.* **91 B2** 34 19N 64 56 E
Shotover →, *N.Z.* **131 E3** 44 59 S 168 41 E
Shou Xian, *China* **77 A11** 32 37N 116 42 E
Shouchang, *China* **77 C12** 29 18N 119 12 E
Shouguang, *China* **75 F10** 37 52N 118 45 E
Shouning, *China* **77 D12** 27 27N 119 31 E
Shouyang, *China* **74 F7** 37 54N 113 8 E
Show Low, *U.S.A.* **159 J9** 34 15N 110 2W
Showa, *Japan* **73 B10** 35 36N 138 29 E
Shpola, *Ukraine* **59 H6** 49 1N 31 30 E
Shpykiv, *Ukraine* **53 B13** 48 47N 28 34 E
Shqipëria = Albania ■, *Europe* **50 E4** 41 0N 20 0 E
Shreveport, *U.S.A.* **155 J8** 32 31N 93 45W
Shrewsbury, *U.K.* **21 E5** 52 43N 2 45W
Shri Mohangarh, *India* **92 F4** 27 17N 71 18 E
Shrigonda, *India* **94 E2** 18 37N 74 41 E
Shrirampur, *India* **93 H13** 22 44N 88 21 E
Shropshire □, *U.K.* **21 E5** 52 36N 2 45W
Shū, *Kazakhstan* **65 B6** 43 36N 73 42 E
Shū →, *Kazakhstan* **65 A3** 45 0N 67 44 E
Shuangbai, *China* **76 E3** 24 42N 101 38 E
Shuangcheng, *China* **75 B14** 45 20N 126 15 E
Shuangfeng, *China* **77 D9** 27 29N 112 11 E
Shuanggou, *China* **75 G9** 34 2N 117 30 E
Shuangjiang, *China* **76 F2** 23 26N 99 58 E
Shuangliao, *China* **75 C12** 43 29N 123 30 E
Shuangshanzi, *China* **75 D10** 40 20N 119 8 E
Shuangyang, *China* **75 C13** 43 28N 125 40 E
Shuangyashan, *China* **69 B8** 46 28N 131 5 E
Shu'b, Ra's, *Yemen* **99 D6** 12 30N 53 25 E
Shubra el Kheima, *Egypt* **106 H7** 30 6N 31 15 E
Shubra Khit, *Egypt* **106 H7** 31 2N 30 42 E
Shucheng, *China* **77 B11** 31 28N 116 57 E
Shufu, *China* **65 D7** 39 27N 75 52 E
Shugozero, *Russia* **58 C8** 59 54N 34 10 E
Shuguri Falls, *Tanzania* **119 D4** 8 33 S 37 22 E
Shuḩayr, *Yemen* **99 D5** 14 41N 49 23 E

Shuiji, China 77 D12 27 13N 118 20 E
Shuiye, China 74 F8 36 7N 114 8 E
Shujalpur, India 92 H7 23 18N 76 46 E
Shukpa Kunzang, India 93 B8 34 22N 78 22 E
Shulan, China 75 B14 44 28N 127 0 E
Shulaveri, Georgia 61 K7 41 22N 44 45 E
Shule, China 65 D8 39 25N 76 3 E
Shullsburg, U.S.A. 156 B6 42 35N 90 13W
Shumagin Is., U.S.A. 144 J8 55 7N 160 30W
Shumen, Bulgaria 51 C10 43 18N 26 55 E
Shumerlya, Russia 60 C8 55 30N 46 25 E
Shumikha, Russia 64 D9 55 10N 63 15 E
Shunchang, China 77 D11 26 54N 117 48 E
Shunde, China 77 F9 22 42N 113 14 E
Shungay, Kazakhstan 61 F8 48 30N 46 45 E
Shungnak, U.S.A. 144 C8 66 52N 157 9W
Shuo Xian = Shuozhou, China 74 E7 39 20N 112 33 E
Shuozhou, China 74 E7 39 20N 112 33 E
Shūr →, Fārs, Iran 97 D7 28 30N 55 0 E
Shūr →, Kermān, Iran 97 D8 30 52N 57 37 E
Shūr →, Yazd, Iran 97 D7 31 45N 55 15 E
Shūr Āb, Iran 97 C6 34 23N 51 11 E
Shūr Gaz, Iran 97 D8 29 10N 59 20 E
Shūrāb, Iran 97 C8 33 43N 56 29 E
Shurab, Tajikistan 65 C5 40 3N 70 33 E
Shurchi, Uzbekistan 65 E3 37 59N 67 47 E
Shūrjestān, Iran 97 D7 31 24N 52 25 E
Shurkhua, Burma 90 D4 22 15N 93 38 E
Shurugwi, Zimbabwe 119 F3 19 40 S 30 0 E
Shūsf, Iran 97 D9 31 50N 60 5 E
Shūsh, Iran 101 F13 32 11N 48 15 E
Shūshtar, Iran 97 D6 32 0N 48 50 E
Shuswap L., Canada 142 C5 50 55N 119 3W
Shuya, Russia 60 B5 56 50N 41 28 E
Shuyak I., U.S.A. 144 G9 58 31N 152 30W
Shuyang, China 75 G10 34 10N 118 42 E
Shuzenji, Japan 73 C10 34 58N 138 56 E
Shūzū, Iran 97 D7 29 52N 54 30 E
Shwangliao = Liaoyuan, China 75 C13 42 58N 125 2 E
Shwebo, Burma 90 D5 22 30N 95 45 E
Shwegu, Burma 90 C6 24 15N 96 26 E
Shwegun, Burma 90 G6 17 9N 97 39 E
Shwegyin, Burma 90 G6 17 55N 96 53 E
Shweli →, Burma 90 D6 23 45N 96 45 E
Shwenyaung, Burma 90 E6 20 46N 96 57 E
Shyamnagar, India 95 H11 13 21N 92 57 E
Shyghanaq, Kazakhstan 65 A6 45 6N 73 59 E
Shyghanaq, Kazakhstan 65 A5 44 49N 70 0 E
Shymkent, Kazakhstan 65 B4 42 18N 69 36 E
Shyok, India 93 B8 34 13N 78 12 E
Shyok →, Pakistan 93 B6 35 13N 75 53 E
Shyroke, Ukraine 52 B8 48 13N 23 6 E
Shyroke, Ukraine 53 E15 45 59N 30 5 E
Si Chon, Thailand 87 H2 9 0N 99 54 E
Si Kiang = Xi Jiang →, China 77 F9 22 5N 113 20 E
Si Lanna △, Thailand 86 C2 19 17N 99 12 E
Si-ngan = Xi'an, China 74 G5 34 15N 109 0 E
Si Prachan, Thailand 86 E3 14 37N 100 9 E
Si Racha, Thailand 86 F3 13 10N 100 48 E
Si Xian, China 75 H9 33 30N 117 50 E
Siachen Glacier, Asia 93 B7 35 20N 77 30 E
Siahaf →, Pakistan 92 E3 29 3N 68 57 E
Siahan Range, Pakistan 91 D2 27 30N 64 40 E
Siak →, Indonesia 84 B2 1 13N 102 9 E
Siaksriindrapura, Indonesia 84 B2 0 51N 102 0 E
Sialkot, Pakistan 91 B4 32 32N 74 30 E
Sialsuk, India 90 D4 23 24N 92 45 E
Sialum, Papua N. G. 132 D4 6 5 S 147 36 E
Siam = Thailand ■, Asia 86 E4 16 0N 102 0 E
Sian = Xi'an, China 74 G5 34 15N 109 0 E
Sian Ka'an ⌂, Mexico 163 D7 19 35N 87 40W
Siangtan = Xiangtan, China 77 D9 27 51N 112 54 E
Sianów, Poland 54 D3 54 13N 16 18 E
Siantan, Indonesia 84 B3 3 10N 106 15 E
Siàpo →, Venezuela 168 C4 2 7N 66 28W
Siāreh, Iran 97 D9 28 5N 60 14 E
Siargao I., Phil. 81 G6 9 52N 126 3 E
Siari, Pakistan 93 B7 34 55N 76 40 E
Siasi, Phil. 79 C6 5 34N 120 50 E
Siasi I., Phil. 81 J3 5 33N 120 51 E
Siassi, Papua N. G. 132 C4 5 40 S 147 51 E
Siátista, Greece 50 F5 40 15N 21 33 E
Siaton, Phil. 81 G4 9 4N 123 2 E
Siau, Indonesia 82 A3 2 50N 125 25 E
Šiauliai, Lithuania 15 J20 55 56N 23 15 E
Šiauliai □, Lithuania 54 C10 55 56N 23 19 E
Siazan = Siyäzän, Azerbaijan 61 K9 41 3N 49 10 E
Sibâi, Gebel el, Egypt 96 E2 25 45N 34 10 E
Sibang, Gabon 114 B1 0 25N 9 31 E
Sibang, Indonesia 79 K18 8 34 S 115 13 E
Sibay, Russia 64 E7 52 42N 58 39 E
Sibay I., Phil. 81 F3 11 51N 121 29 E
Sibayi, L., S. Africa 117 D5 27 20 S 32 45 E
Sibdu, Sudan 107 E2 10 57N 26 17 E
Šibenik, Croatia 45 E12 43 48N 15 54 E
Siberia = Sibirskiy □, Russia 67 D10 58 0N 90 0 E
Siberia, Russia 6 D13 60 0N 100 0 E
Siberut, Indonesia 84 C1 1 30 S 99 0 E
Sibi, Pakistan 91 C2 29 30N 67 54 E
Sibil = Oksibil, Indonesia 83 B6 4 59 S 140 35 E
Sibiloi △, Kenya 118 B4 4 0N 36 20 E
Sibirskiy □, Russia 67 D10 58 0N 90 0 E
Sibiti, Congo 114 C2 3 38 S 13 19 E
Sibiu, Romania 53 E9 45 45N 24 9 E
Sibiu □, Romania 53 E9 45 50N 24 15 E
Sibium Mts., Papua N. G. 132 E5 9 19 S 148 25 E
Sibley, Ill., U.S.A. 157 D8 40 35N 88 23W
Sibley, Iowa, U.S.A. 154 D7 43 24N 95 45W
Sibolga, Indonesia 84 B1 1 42N 98 45 E
Sibsagar, India 90 B5 27 0N 94 36 E
Sibu, Malaysia 85 B4 2 18N 111 49 E
Sibuco, Phil. 81 H4 7 20N 122 10 E
Sibuguey B., Phil. 81 H4 7 50N 122 45 E
Sibut, C.A.R. 114 A3 5 46N 19 10 E
Sibutu, Phil. 85 B5 4 45N 119 30 E
Sibutu Group, Phil. 81 J2 4 45N 119 20 E
Sibutu Passage, E. Indies 81 J3 4 50N 120 0 E
Sibuyan I., Phil. 80 E4 12 25N 122 40 E
Sibuyan Sea, Phil. 80 E4 12 30N 122 20 E
Sic, Romania 53 D8 46 56N 23 53 E
Sicamous, Canada 142 C5 50 49N 119 0W
Sicapoo, Mt., Phil. 80 B3 18 1N 120 56 E
Sicasica, Bolivia 172 D4 17 22 S 67 45W
Siccus →, Australia 128 A3 31 55 S 139 17 E
Sichelberg = Sierpc, Poland 55 F6 52 55N 19 43 E
Sichuan □, China 76 B5 30 30N 103 0 E
Sichuan Pendi, China 76 B5 31 0N 105 0 E
Sicilia, Italy 47 E7 37 30N 14 30 E
Sicily = Sicilia, Italy 47 E7 37 30N 14 30 E
Sicily, Str. of 46 E4 37 35N 11 56 E
Sicuani, Peru 172 C3 14 21 S 71 10W
Šid, Serbia & M. 52 E4 45 8N 19 14 E
Sidamo, Ethiopia 107 G4 5 0N 37 50 E
Sidaouet, Niger 113 B6 18 34N 8 3 E
Sidári, Greece 38 B9 39 47N 19 41 E
Siddapur, India 95 G2 14 20N 74 53 E
Siddhapur, India 92 H5 23 56N 72 25 E
Siddipet, India 94 E4 18 5N 78 51 E
Sidensjö, Sweden 16 A12 63 18N 18 17 E
Sidéradougou, Burkina Faso 112 C4 10 42N 4 12W
Siderno, Italy 47 D9 38 16N 16 18 E
Sidhauli, India 93 F9 27 17N 80 50 E
Sídheros, Ákra, Greece 39 E7 35 19N 26 19 E
Sidhi, India 93 G9 24 25N 81 53 E
Sidhirókastron, Greece 50 E7 41 13N 23 24 E
Sîdi Abd el Rahmân, Egypt 106 A2 30 55N 29 44 E
Sidi Ahmed Rgueibi, W. Sahara 110 C2 27 32N 11 16W
Sîdi Barrâni, Egypt 106 A2 31 38N 25 58 E
Sidi-bel-Abbès, Algeria 111 A4 35 13N 0 39W
Sidi Bennour, Morocco 110 B3 32 40N 8 25W
Sidi Haneish, Egypt 106 A2 31 10N 27 35 E
Sidi Ifni, Morocco 110 C2 29 29N 10 12W
Sidi Kacem, Morocco 110 B3 34 11N 5 49W
Sîdi Omar, Egypt 106 A1 31 24N 24 57 E
Sidi Slimane, Morocco 110 B3 34 16N 5 56W
Sidi Smaïl, Morocco 110 B3 32 50N 8 31W
Sîdî 'Uzayz, Libya 108 B4 31 41N 24 55 E
Siding No 14 = Ponoka, Canada 142 C6 52 42N 113 40W
Sidlaw Hills, U.K. 22 E5 56 32N 3 2W
Sidley, Mt., Antarctica 7 D14 77 2 S 126 2W
Sidmouth, U.K. 21 G4 50 40N 3 15W
Sidmouth, C., Australia 126 A3 13 25 S 143 36 E
Sidney, Canada 142 D4 48 39N 123 24W
Sidney, Mont., U.S.A. 154 B2 47 43N 104 9W
Sidney, N.Y., U.S.A. 151 D9 42 19N 75 24W
Sidney, Nebr., U.S.A. 154 E3 41 8N 102 59W
Sidney, Ohio, U.S.A. 157 D12 40 17N 84 9W
Sidney Lanier, L., U.S.A. 153 B4 34 10N 84 4W
Sido, Mali 112 C3 11 37N 7 29W
Sidoarjo, Indonesia 85 D4 7 27 S 112 43 E
Sidoktaya, Burma 90 E5 20 27N 94 15 E
Sidon = Saydā, Lebanon 103 B4 33 35N 35 25 E
Sidra, G. of = Surt, Khalīj, Libya 108 B3 31 40N 18 30 E
Sidrolândia, Brazil 173 20 55 S 54 58W
Siedlce, Poland 55 F9 52 10N 22 20 E
Sieg →, Germany 30 E3 50 46N 7 6 E
Siegburg, Germany 30 E3 50 47N 7 12 E
Siegen, Germany 30 E4 50 51N 8 0 E
Siem Pang, Cambodia 86 E6 14 7N 106 23 E
Siem Reap = Siemreab, Cambodia 86 F4 13 20N 103 52 E
Siemiatycze, Poland 55 F9 52 27N 22 53 E
Siemreab, Cambodia 86 F4 13 20N 103 52 E
Siena, Italy 45 E8 43 19N 11 21 E
Sieniawa, Poland 55 H9 50 11N 22 38 E
Sienyang = Xianyang, China 74 G5 34 20N 108 40 E
Sieradz, Poland 55 G5 51 37N 18 41 E
Sieraków, Poland 55 F3 52 39N 16 2 E
Sierck-les-Bains, France 27 C13 49 26N 6 20 E
Sierning, Austria 34 C7 48 2N 14 18 E
Sierpc, Poland 55 F6 52 55N 19 43 E
Sierpe, Bocas de la, Venezuela 169 G9 10 0N 61 30W
Sierra Blanca, U.S.A. 159 L11 31 11N 105 22W
Sierra Blanca Peak, U.S.A. 159 K11 33 23N 105 49W
Sierra City, U.S.A. 160 F6 39 34N 120 38W
Sierra Colorada, Argentina 176 B3 40 35 S 67 50W
Sierra de Aracena y Picos de Aroche ⌂, Spain 43 H4 37 53N 6 41W
Sierra de Bahoruco △, Dom. Rep. 165 C5 18 10N 71 25W
Sierra de Baza ⌂, Spain 41 H2 37 20N 2 48W
Sierra de Castril ⌂, Spain 41 H2 37 54N 2 50W
Sierra de Espuña ⌂, Spain 41 H3 37 50N 1 31W
Sierra de Grazalema ⌂, Spain 43 J5 36 31N 5 28W
Sierra de Gredos ⌂, Spain 42 E5 40 17N 5 17W
Sierra de Hornachuelos ⌂, Spain 43 H5 37 56N 5 14W
Sierra de Huétor ⌂, Spain 43 H7 37 14N 3 30W
Sierra de La Culata △, Venezuela 165 E5 8 45N 71 10W
Sierra de la Culata △, Venezuela 168 B3 8 48N 70 56W
Sierra de la Macarena △, Colombia 168 A3 11 19N 74 1W
Sierra de Lancandón △, Guatemala 164 C1 16 59N 90 23W
Sierra de las Nieves ⌂, Spain 43 J6 36 42N 5 0W
Sierra de las Quijadas △, Argentina 174 C2 32 29 S 67 5W
Sierra de María-Los Vélez ⌂, Spain 41 H2 37 41N 2 10W
Sierra de San Luis △, Venezuela 165 D6 11 20N 69 43W
Sierra de San Luis △, Venezuela 168 A4 11 11N 69 33W
Sierra de Yeguas, Spain 43 H6 37 7N 4 52W
Sierra del São Mamede ⌂, Portugal 43 F3 39 17N 7 18W
Sierra Gorda, Chile 174 A2 22 50 S 69 15W
Sierra Grande, Argentina 176 B3 41 36 S 65 22W
Sierra Leone ■, W. Afr. 112 D2 9 0N 12 0W
Sierra Leone Rise, Atl. Oc. 8 F9 7 0N 22 0W
Sierra Madre, Mexico 163 D6 16 0N 93 0W
Sierra Mágina ⌂, Spain 43 H7 37 44N 3 28W
Sierra Mojada, Mexico 162 B4 27 19N 103 42W
Sierra Nevada, Spain 43 H7 37 3N 3 15W
Sierra Nevada, U.S.A. 160 H8 39 0N 120 30W
Sierra Nevada ⌂, Spain 43 H7 37 4N 3 7W
Sierra Nevada △, Venezuela 165 E5 8 35N 70 45W
Sierra Nevada de Santa Marta △, Colombia 165 D5 10 56N 73 36W
Sierra Norte de Seville ⌂, Spain 43 H5 37 55N 5 46W
Sierra Subbéticas ⌂, Spain 43 H6 37 26N 4 18W
Sierra Vista, U.S.A. 159 L8 31 33N 110 18W
Sierras de Cardeña y Montoro ⌂, Spain 43 G6 38 13N 4 15W
Sierras de Cazorla, Segura y las Villas ⌂, Spain 41 J2 37 0N 2 45W
Sierraville, U.S.A. 160 F6 39 36N 120 22W
Sierre, Switz. 32 D5 46 17N 7 31 E
Sifani, Ethiopia 107 E5 12 18N 40 19 E
Sifié, Ivory C. 112 D3 8 0N 7 5W
Sífnos, Greece 48 E6 37 0N 24 45 E
Sifton, Canada 143 C8 51 21N 100 8W
Sifton Pass, Canada 142 B3 57 52N 126 15W
Sig, Algeria 111 A4 35 32N 0 12W
Sigaboy = Governor Generoso, Phil. 81 H6 6 39N 126 5 E
Sigatoka, Fiji 133 B1 18 8 S 177 32 E
Sigdal, Norway 18 D6 60 3N 9 38 E
Sigean, France 28 E6 43 2N 2 58 E
Siggiewi, Malta 38 F7 35 51N 14 26 E
Sighetu-Marmaţiei, Romania 53 C8 47 57N 23 52 E
Sighişoara, Romania 53 D9 46 12N 24 50 E
Sigira, Yemen 99 D6 12 37N 54 20 E
Sigiriya, Sri Lanka 95 L5 7 57N 80 45 E
Sigli, Indonesia 84 A1 5 25N 96 0 E
Siglufjörður, Iceland 11 A8 66 12N 18 55W
Siglunes, Iceland 11 A8 66 12N 18 50W
Sigmaringen, Germany 31 G5 48 5N 9 12 E
Signa, Italy 44 E8 43 45N 11 10 E
Signakhi = Tsnori, Georgia 61 K7 41 40N 45 57 E
Signal, U.S.A. 161 L13 34 30N 113 38W
Signal de Botrang, Belgium 24 D6 50 29N 6 4 E
Signal Pk., U.S.A. 161 M12 33 20N 114 2W
Signau, Switz. 32 C5 46 56N 7 45 E
Signy I., Antarctica 7 C18 60 45 S 45 56W
Signy-l'Abbaye, France 27 C11 49 40N 4 25 E
Sigourney, U.S.A. 156 C4 41 20N 92 12W
Sigsbee, U.S.A. 152 D6 31 16N 83 52W
Sigsig, Ecuador 168 D2 3 0 S 78 50W
Sigüenza, Spain 40 D2 41 3N 2 40W
Siguiri, Guinea 112 C3 11 31N 9 10W
Sigulda, Latvia 15 H21 57 10N 24 55 E
Sihanoukville = Kampong Saom, Cambodia 87 G4 10 38N 103 30 E
Sihaus, Peru 172 B2 8 40 S 77 40W
Sihawa, India 94 D5 20 19N 81 55 E
Sihora, India 93 H9 23 29N 80 6 E
Sihui, China 77 F9 23 20N 112 40 E
Siikajoki →, Finland 14 D21 64 50N 24 43 E
Siilinjärvi, Finland 14 E22 63 4N 27 39 E
Siirt, Turkey 101 D9 37 57N 41 55 E
Sijarira Ra. = Chizarira, Zimbabwe 119 F2 17 36 S 27 45 E
Sijungjung, Indonesia 84 C2 0 42 S 100 58 E
Sika, India 92 H3 22 26N 69 47 E
Sikani Chief →, Canada 142 B4 57 47N 122 15W
Sikao, Thailand 87 J2 7 34N 99 21 E
Sikar, India 92 F6 27 33N 75 10 E
Sikasso, Mali 112 C3 11 18N 5 35W
Sikelenge, Zambia 115 E4 14 53 S 24 14 E
Sikeston, U.S.A. 155 G10 36 53N 89 35W
Sikhote Alin, Khrebet, Russia 67 E14 45 0N 136 0 E
Sikhote Alin Ra. = Sikhote Alin, Khrebet, Russia 67 E14 45 0N 136 0 E
Sikiá, Greece 50 F7 40 2N 23 56 E
Síkinos, Greece 49 E7 36 40N 25 8 E
Sikkim □, India 90 B2 27 50N 88 30 E
Siklós, Hungary 52 E3 45 50N 18 19 E
Sil →, Spain 42 C3 42 27N 7 43W
Silacayoapan, Mexico 163 D5 17 30N 98 9W
Šilalė, Lithuania 54 C9 55 28N 22 12 E
Silam, Malaysia 81 J2 4 59N 118 12 E
Silandro, Italy 44 B7 46 38N 10 46 E
Silang, Phil. 80 D3 14 14N 120 58 E
Silawad, India 92 J6 21 54N 74 54 E
Silay, Phil. 81 F4 10 47N 122 58 E
Silba, Croatia 45 D11 44 24N 14 41 E
Silchar, India 90 C4 24 49N 92 48 E
Sildegapet, Norway 18 B2 62 5N 5 0 E
Şile, Turkey 51 E13 41 10N 29 37 E
Silent Valley △, India 95 J3 11 10N 76 20 E
Siler City, U.S.A. 149 H6 35 44N 79 28W
Sileru →, India 94 F5 17 49N 81 24 E
Silesia = Śląsk, Poland 36 C9 51 0N 16 30 E
Silet, Algeria 111 D5 22 44N 4 37 E
Silgarhi Doti, Nepal 93 E9 29 15N 81 0 E
Silghat, India 90 B4 26 35N 93 0 E
Silhouette, Seychelles 121 b 4 29 S 55 12 E
Silí, Burkina Faso 112 C4 11 37N 2 30W
Silifke, Turkey 100 D5 36 22N 33 58 E
Siliguri = Shiliguri, India 90 B2 26 45N 88 25 E
Siling Co, China 68 C3 31 50N 89 20 E
Silistea Nouă, Romania 53 F10 44 23N 25 1 E
Silistra, Bulgaria 51 B11 44 6N 27 19 E
Silivri, Turkey 51 E12 41 4N 28 14 E
Siljan, Norway 18 E6 59 18N 9 42 E
Siljan, Sweden 16 D8 60 55N 14 45 E
Siljansnäs, Sweden 16 D8 60 47N 14 52 E
Silkeborg, Denmark 17 H3 56 10N 9 32 E
Silkwood, Australia 126 B4 17 45 S 146 2 E
Silla, Spain 41 F4 39 22N 0 25W
Sillajhuay, Cordillera, Chile 172 D4 19 46 S 68 40W
Sillamäe, Estonia 15 G22 59 24N 27 45 E
Sillé-le-Guillaume, France 26 D6 48 10N 0 8W
Silleda, Spain 42 C2 42 42N 8 14W
Sillein = Žilina, Slovak Rep. 35 B11 49 12N 18 42 E
Sillod, India 94 D2 20 18N 75 39 E
Silloth, U.K. 20 C4 54 52N 3 23W
Sillustani, Peru 172 D3 15 50 S 70 7W
Sĩlo, Greece 51 E9 41 10N 25 53 E
Siloam Springs, U.S.A. 155 G7 36 11N 94 32W
Silopi, Turkey 101 D10 37 15N 42 27 E
Silsbee, U.S.A. 155 K7 30 21N 94 11W
Siltou, Chad 109 E3 16 46N 15 33 E
Siluko, Nigeria 113 D6 6 35N 5 10 E
Šilutė, Lithuania 15 J19 55 21N 21 33 E
Silva Porto = Kuito, Angola 115 E3 12 22 S 16 55 E
Silvan, Turkey 101 C9 38 7N 41 2 E
Silvani, India 93 H8 23 18N 78 25 E
Silvaplana, Switz. 33 D9 46 28N 9 48 E
Silver City, U.S.A. 159 K9 32 46N 108 17W
Silver Cr. →, U.S.A. 158 E4 43 16N 119 13W
Silver Creek, U.S.A. 150 D5 42 33N 79 10W
Silver Grove, U.S.A. 157 E12 39 2N 84 24W
Silver L., U.S.A. 160 G6 38 39N 120 6W
Silver Lake, Calif., U.S.A. 161 K10 35 21N 116 7W
Silver Lake, Ind., U.S.A. 157 C11 41 4N 85 53W
Silver Lake, Oreg., U.S.A. 158 E3 43 8N 121 3W
Silver Lake, Wis., U.S.A. 157 B8 42 33N 88 13W
Silver Springs, U.S.A. 153 F7 29 13N 82 3W
Silverdalen, Sweden 17 G9 57 32N 15 45 E
Silverton, Australia 128 A4 31 52 S 141 10 E
Silverton, Colo., U.S.A. 159 H10 37 49N 107 40W
Silverton, Tex., U.S.A. 155 H4 34 28N 101 19W
Silves, Brazil 169 D6 2 54 S 58 27W
Silves, Portugal 43 H2 37 11N 8 26W
Silvi Marina, Italy 45 F11 42 34N 14 5 E
Silvia, Colombia 168 C2 2 37N 76 21W
Silvies →, U.S.A. 158 E4 43 34N 119 2W
Silvrettahorn, Switz. 33 C10 46 50N 10 6 E
Silwa Bahari, Egypt 106 C3 24 45N 32 55 E
Silz, Austria 34 D3 47 16N 10 56 E
Sim, C., Morocco 110 B3 31 26N 9 51W
Simakumba, Zambia 115 E4 14 12 S 23 16 E
Simaltala, India 93 G12 24 43N 86 33 E
Simaluguri, India 90 B5 26 55N 94 46 E
Simanggang = Sri Aman, Malaysia 85 B4 1 15N 111 32 E
Simão, China 76 F3 22 47N 101 5 E
Simão Dias, Brazil 170 D4 10 44 S 37 49W
Simara I., Phil. 80 E4 12 48N 122 3 E
Simard, L., Canada 140 C4 47 40N 78 40W
Şimareh →, Iran 101 F12 33 9N 47 41 E
Simav, Turkey 49 B10 39 4N 28 58 E
Simav →, Turkey 51 F12 40 23N 28 31 E
Simav Dağları, Turkey 49 B10 39 10N 28 30 E
Simba, Dem. Rep. of the Congo 114 B4 0 38N 22 59 E
Simba, Tanzania 118 C4 2 10 S 37 36 E
Simbach, Germany 31 G9 48 16N 13 2 E
Simberi I., Papua N. G. 132 B7 2 38 S 152 0 E
Simbirsk, Russia 60 C9 54 20N 48 25 E
Simbo, Solomon Is. 133 M9 8 16 S 156 33 E
Simbo, Tanzania 118 C2 4 51 S 29 41 E
Simcoe, Canada 140 D3 42 50N 80 20W
Simcoe, L., Canada 140 D4 44 25N 79 20W
Simdega, India 93 H11 22 37N 84 31 E
Simeonovgrad, Bulgaria 51 D9 42 1N 25 50 E
Simeria, Romania 52 E8 45 51N 23 1 E
Simeto →, Italy 47 E8 37 24N 15 6 E
Simeulue, Indonesia 84 B1 2 45N 95 45 E
Simferopol, Ukraine 59 K8 44 55N 34 3 E
Sími, Greece 49 E9 36 35N 27 50 E
Simi Valley, U.S.A. 161 L8 34 16N 118 47W
Simien Mts. △, Ethiopia 107 E4 13 19N 38 0 E
Simikot, Nepal 93 E9 30 0N 81 50 E
Simití, Colombia 168 B3 7 58N 73 57W
Simitli, Bulgaria 50 E7 41 52N 23 7 E
Simla, India 92 D7 31 2N 77 9 E
Simlångsdalen, Sweden 17 H7 56 43N 13 6 E
Şimleu-Silvaniei, Romania 52 C7 47 17N 22 50 E
Simlipal △, India 93 J12 21 45N 86 30 E
Simme →, Switz. 32 C4 46 38N 7 25 E
Simmern, Germany 31 F3 49 58N 7 30 E
Simmie, Canada 143 D7 49 56N 108 6W
Simmler, U.S.A. 161 K7 35 21N 119 59W
Simnas, Lithuania 54 D10 54 24N 23 39 E
Simo älv = Simojoki →, Finland 14 D21 65 35N 25 1 E
Simões, Brazil 170 C3 7 36 S 40 49W
Simojoki →, Finland 14 D21 65 35N 25 1 E
Simojovel, Mexico 163 D6 17 12N 92 38W
Simonette →, Canada 142 B5 55 9N 118 15W
Šimonovany = Partizánske, Slovak Rep. 35 C11 48 38N 18 23 E
Simonstown, S. Africa 116 E2 34 14 S 18 26 E
Simontornya, Hungary 52 D3 46 45N 18 33 E
Simpang Empat, Malaysia 87 c 5 27N 100 29 E
Simpangkiri →, Indonesia 84 B1 2 50N 97 40 E
Simplício Mendes, Brazil 170 C3 7 51 S 41 54W
Simplon, Switz. 32 D6 46 12N 8 4 E
Simplonpass, Switz. 32 D6 46 15N 8 3 E
Simplontunnel, Switz. 32 D6 46 15N 8 7 E
Simpson, Mt., Papua N. G. 132 F5 10 2 S 149 34 E
Simpson Desert, Australia 126 D2 25 0 S 137 0 E
Simpson Desert △, Australia 126 C2 24 59 S 138 21 E
Simpson Pen., Canada 139 B11 68 34N 88 45W
Simpungdong, N. Korea 75 D15 40 56N 129 29 E
Simrishamn, Sweden 17 J8 55 33N 14 22 E
Simsbury, U.S.A. 151 E12 41 53N 72 48W
Simunjan, Malaysia 85 B4 1 25N 110 45 E
Simunul, Phil. 81 J2 4 54N 119 51 E
Simushir, Ostrov, Russia 67 E16 46 50N 152 30 E
Sin Cowe I., S. China Sea 78 C4 9 53N 114 19 E
Sina →, India 94 F2 17 30N 75 55 E
Sinabang, Indonesia 84 B1 2 30N 96 24 E
Sinadogo, Somali Rep. 120 C3 5 50N 47 0 E
Sinai = Es Sînâ', Egypt 103 F3 29 0N 34 0 E
Sinai, Mt. = Mûsa, Gebel, Egypt 96 D2 28 33N 33 59 E
Sinai Peninsula, Egypt 62 G7 29 30N 34 0 E
Sinaia, Romania 53 E10 45 21N 25 38 E
Sinait, Phil. 80 C3 17 52N 120 27 E
Sinako, Mt., Phil. 81 H5 7 30N 125 17 E
Sinaloa □, Mexico 162 C3 25 0N 107 30W
Sinaloa de Leyva, Mexico 162 B3 25 50N 108 20W
Sinalunga, Italy 45 E8 43 12N 11 44 E
Sinan, China 76 D7 27 56N 108 13 E
Sinandrei, Romania 52 E6 45 52N 21 13 E
Sinarádhes, Greece 38 B9 39 34N 19 51 E
Sināwan, Libya 108 B2 31 0N 10 37 E
Sinbaungwe, Burma 90 F5 19 43N 95 10 E
Sinbo, Burma 90 C6 24 46N 97 3 E
Sincan, Turkey 100 B5 39 58N 32 36 E
Sincanli, Turkey 49 C12 38 45N 30 15 E
Sincé, Colombia 168 B2 9 15N 75 9W
Sincelejo, Colombia 168 B2 9 18N 75 24W
Sinch'ang, N. Korea 75 D15 40 7N 128 28 E
Sinchang-ni, N. Korea 75 E14 39 24N 126 8 E
Sinclair, U.S.A. 158 F10 41 47N 107 7W
Sinclair, L., U.S.A. 152 B6 33 8N 83 12W
Sinclair Mills, Canada 142 C4 54 5N 121 40W
Sinclair's B., U.K. 22 C5 58 31N 3 5W
Sinclairville, U.S.A. 150 D5 42 16N 79 16W
Sind = Sindh □, Pakistan 91 D3 26 0N 69 0 E
Sind, Pakistan 92 G3 26 0N 68 30 E
Sind →, Jammu & Kashmir, India 93 B6 34 18N 74 45 E
Sind →, Mad. P., India 93 F8 26 26N 79 13 E
Sind Sagar Doab, Pakistan 92 D4 32 0N 71 30 E
Sindal, Denmark 17 G4 57 28N 10 10 E
Sindangan, Phil. 81 G4 8 10N 123 5 E
Sindangan Bay, Phil. 81 G4 8 11N 122 50 E
Sindangbarang, Indonesia 85 D3 7 27 S 107 1 E
Sindara, Gabon 114 C2 1 7 S 10 41 E
Sinde, Zambia 119 F2 17 28 S 25 51 E
Sindelfingen, Germany 31 G4 48 42N 9 0 E
Sindewahi, India 94 D4 20 17N 79 39 E
Sindgi, India 94 F3 16 55N 76 14 E
Sindh □, Pakistan 91 D3 26 0N 69 0 E
Sindhnur, India 95 F3 15 47N 76 46 E
Sindi, India 94 D4 20 48N 78 52 E
Sındırgı, Turkey 49 B10 39 13N 28 10 E
Sindou, Burkina Faso 112 C3 10 35N 5 4W
Sindri, India 93 H12 23 45N 86 42 E
Sine →, Senegal 112 C1 14 10N 16 28W
Sineglazovo = Novosineglazovskiy, Russia 64 D8 55 2N 61 21 E
Sinegorskiy, Russia 61 G5 47 55N 40 52 E
Sinekli, Turkey 51 E12 41 14N 28 12 E
Sinelnikove = Synelnykove, Ukraine 59 H8 48 25N 35 30 E
Sinendé, Benin 113 C5 10 20N 2 22 E
Sines, Portugal 43 H2 37 56N 8 51W
Sines, C. de, Portugal 43 H2 37 58N 8 53W
Sineu, Spain 38 B4 39 38N 3 1 E
Sinewit, Mt., Papua N. G. 132 C7 4 44 S 152 2 E
Sinfra, Ivory C. 112 D3 6 35N 5 56W
Sing Buri, Thailand 86 E3 14 53N 100 25 E
Sing Sing = Ossining, U.S.A. 151 E11 41 10N 73 55W
Singa, Sudan 107 E3 13 10N 33 57 E
Singako, Chad 109 G3 9 50N 19 24 E
Singalila △, India 93 F13 27 10N 88 5 E
Singanallur, India 95 J3 11 2N 77 1 E
Singapore ■, Asia 87 d 1 17N 103 51 E
Singapore, Straits of, Asia 87 d 1 15N 104 0 E
Singapore Changi ✕ (SIN), Singapore 87 M4 1 23N 103 59 E
Singaraja, Indonesia 85 D5 8 7 S 115 6 E
Singatoka = Sigatoka, Fiji 133 B1 18 8 S 177 32 E
Singen, Germany 31 H4 47 45N 8 50 E
Singida, Tanzania 118 C3 4 49 S 34 48 E
Singida □, Tanzania 118 D3 6 0 S 34 30 E
Singitikós Kólpos, Greece 50 F7 40 6N 24 0 E
Singkaling Hkamti, Burma 90 C5 26 0N 95 39 E
Singkang, Indonesia 82 B2 4 8 S 120 1 E
Singkawang, Indonesia 85 B3 1 0N 108 57 E
Singkep, Indonesia 78 E2 0 30 S 104 25 E
Singleton, Australia 129 B9 32 33 S 151 0 E
Singleton, Mt., N. Terr., Australia 124 D5 22 0 S 130 46 E
Singleton, Mt., W. Austral., Australia 125 E2 29 27 S 117 15 E
Singö, Sweden 16 D12 60 12N 18 45 E
Singoli, India 92 G6 25 0N 75 22 E
Singora = Songkhla, Thailand 87 J3 7 13N 100 37 E
Singosan, N. Korea 75 E14 38 52N 127 25 E
Singri, India 90 B4 26 36N 92 29 E
Singsås, Norway 18 B7 62 56N 10 37 E
Singu, Burma 90 D6 22 33N 96 0 E
Sinhgarh, India 94 E1 18 22N 73 45 E
Sinhung, N. Korea 75 D14 40 11N 127 34 E
Siniátsikon, Óros, Greece 50 F5 40 25N 21 35 E
Siniloan, Phil. 80 D3 14 25N 121 27 E
Sining = Xining, China 68 C5 36 34N 101 40 E
Siniscóla, Italy 46 B2 40 34N 9 41 E
Sinj, Croatia 45 E13 43 42N 16 39 E
Sinjai, Indonesia 82 C2 5 7 S 120 20 E
Sinjajevina, Serbia & M. 50 D3 42 57N 19 22 E
Sinjār, Iraq 101 D9 36 19N 41 52 E
Sinkat, Sudan 106 D4 18 55N 36 49 E
Sinkiang Uighur = Xinjiang Uygur Zizhiqu □, China 68 C3 42 0N 86 0 E
Sinlumkaba, Burma 90 C6 24 16N 97 31 E
Sinmak, N. Korea 75 E14 38 25N 126 14 E
Sinnai, Italy 46 C2 39 18N 9 13 E
Sinnar, India 94 E2 19 48N 74 0 E
Sinni →, Italy 47 B9 40 8N 16 41 E
Sinnuris, Egypt 106 J7 29 26N 30 31 E
Sinoie, Lacul, Romania 53 F13 44 35N 28 50 E
Sinop, Turkey 100 A6 42 1N 35 11 E
Sinor, India 92 J5 21 55N 73 20 E
Sinp'o, N. Korea 75 E15 40 0N 128 13 E
Sins, Switz. 33 B6 47 12N 8 24 E
Sinsheim, Germany 31 F4 49 15N 8 52 E
Sinsiang = Xinxiang, China 74 G7 35 18N 113 50 E
Sinsk, Russia 67 C13 61 8N 126 48 E
Sintang, Indonesia 85 B4 0 5N 111 35 E
Sinton, U.S.A. 155 L6 28 2N 97 31W
Sintra, Portugal 43 G1 38 47N 9 25W
Sintra-Cascais ⌂, Portugal 43 G1 38 50N 9 25W
Sinugif, Somali Rep. 120 C3 8 33N 48 59 E
Sinŭiju, N. Korea 75 D13 40 5N 124 24 E
Sinyukha →, Ukraine 59 H6 48 3N 30 51 E
Sinzig, Germany 30 E3 50 32N 7 14 E
Sio →, Hungary 52 D3 46 20N 18 53 E
Siocon, Phil. 81 H4 7 40N 122 10 E
Siófok, Hungary 52 D3 46 54N 18 3 E
Sioma, Zambia 115 F4 16 40 S 23 32 E
Sioma Ngwezi △, Zambia 115 F4 17 14 S 23 26 E
Sion, Switz. 32 D4 46 14N 7 20 E
Sion Mills, U.K. 23 B4 54 48N 7 29W
Sioux Center, U.S.A. 154 D6 43 5N 96 11W
Sioux City, U.S.A. 154 D6 42 30N 96 24W
Sioux Falls, U.S.A. 154 D6 43 33N 96 44W
Sioux Lookout, Canada 140 B1 50 10N 91 50W
Sioux Narrows, Canada 143 D10 49 25N 94 10W
Sipalay, Phil. 81 G4 9 45N 122 24 E
Šipan, Croatia 50 D1 42 45N 17 52 E
Sipang, Tanjong, Malaysia 85 B4 1 48N 110 20 E
Siparia, Trin. & Tob. 169 F9 10 8N 61 31W
Sipil Dağı △, Turkey 49 C9 38 35N 27 30 E
Siping, China 75 C13 43 8N 124 21 E
Sipiwesk L., Canada 143 B9 55 5N 97 35W
Siple, Antarctica 7 D7 75 0 S 84 0W
Sipocot, Phil. 80 E4 13 46N 122 58 E
Šipovo, Bos.-H. 52 F2 44 16N 17 6 E
Sipra →, India 92 H6 23 55N 75 28 E
Sipur, India 94 D7 21 11N 85 9 E
Sipura, Indonesia 84 C1 2 18 S 99 40 E
Siquia →, Nic. 164 D3 12 10N 84 20W
Siquijor, Phil. 81 G4 9 12N 123 35 E
Siquijor □, Phil. 81 G4 9 11N 123 35 E
Siquirres, Costa Rica 164 D3 10 6N 83 30W
Siquisique, Venezuela 168 A4 10 34N 69 42W
Şīr Abu Nu'ayr, U.A.E. 97 E7 25 20N 54 20 E
Şīr Banī Yās, U.A.E. 97 E7 24 19N 52 37 E
Sir Edward Pellew Group, Australia 126 B2 15 40 S 137 10 E
Sir Graham Moore Is., Australia 124 B4 13 53 S 126 34 E
Sir James MacBrien, Mt., Canada 138 B7 62 7N 127 41W
Sir Joseph Banks Group, Australia 128 C2 34 36 S 136 16 E
Sira, India 95 H3 13 41N 76 49 E
Sira, Norway 18 F3 58 24N 6 40 E
Sira →, Norway 18 F3 58 23N 6 34 E
Siracusa, Italy 47 E8 37 4N 15 17 E
Sirajganj, Bangla. 90 C2 24 25N 89 47 E
Sirakoro, Mali 112 C3 12 41N 9 14W
Şiran, Turkey 101 B8 40 11N 39 7 E

Sirasso, *Ivory C.* **112 D3** 9 16N 6 6W
Sīrathu, *India* ...... **93 G9** 25 39N 81 19 E
Sirawai, *Phil.* ...... **81 H4** 7 34N 122 8 E
Sirdalsvatnet, *Norway* .. **18 F3** 58 34N 6 43 E
Sïrdän, *Iran* ...... **97 B6** 36 39N 49 12 E
Sirdaryo = Syrdarya ➔,
  Uzbekistan ...... **65 C4** 40 50N 68 40 E
Sirdaryo = Syrdarya ➔,
  Kazakhstan ...... **66 E7** 46 3N 61 0 E
Sire, *Ethiopia* ..... **107 F4** 6 55N 35 36 E
Siren, *U.S.A.* **154 C8** 45 47N 92 24W
Sirente-Velino △, *Italy* .. **41 F10** 42 10N 13 32 E
Sirer, *Spain* ...... **38 D1** 38 56N 1 22 E
Siret, *Romania* ..... **53 C11** 47 55N 26 5 E
Siret ➔, *Romania* .... **53 E12** 45 24N 28 1 E
Sireväg, *Norway* .... **18 F2** 58 30N 5 48 E
Sirghāyā, *Syria* ..... **103 B5** 33 51N 36 8 E
Şiria, *Romania* ..... **52 D6** 46 16N 21 38 E
Sirik, Tanjong,
  Malaysia ...... **85 B4** 2 47N 111 15 E
Sirinath △, *Thailand* ... **87 a** 8 6N 98 17 E
Sirino, *Mte., Italy* ... **47 B8** 40 7N 15 50 E
Sïrjän, *Iran* ...... **97 D7** 29 30N 55 45 E
Sirkali = Sirkazhi, *India* . **95 J4** 11 15N 79 41 E
Sirkazhi, *India* ..... **95 J4** 11 15N 79 41 E
Sirmans, *U.S.A.* **152 E6** 30 21N 83 39W
Sirmaur, *India* ..... **93 G9** 24 51N 81 23 E
Sírna, *Greece* ..... **49 E8** 36 22N 26 42 E
Sirnach, *Switz.* ..... **29 B7** 47 28N 8 59 E
Şırnak, *Turkey* ..... **101 D10** 37 32N 42 28 E
Sirohi, *India* ...... **92 G5** 24 52N 72 53 E
Sironj, *India* ...... **92 G7** 24 5N 77 39 E
Síros, *Greece* ..... **48 D6** 37 28N 24 57 E
Siroz = Sérrai, *Greece* .. **50 E7** 41 5N 23 31 E
Sirpur, *India* ...... **94 E4** 19 29N 79 36 E
Sirrayn, *Si. Arabia* ... **98 C3** 19 38N 40 36 E
Sirretta Pk., *U.S.A.* ... **161 K8** 35 56N 118 19W
Sïrrï, *Iran* ...... **97 E7** 25 55N 54 32 E
Sirsa, *India* ...... **92 E6** 29 33N 75 4 E
Sirsa ➔, *India* ..... **93 F8** 26 51N 79 4 E
Sirsi, *India* ...... **95 G2** 14 40N 74 49 E
Sirsilla, *India* ..... **94 E4** 18 23N 78 50 E
Siruela, *Spain* **43 G5** 38 58N 5 3W
Siruguppa, *India* .... **95 F3** 15 38N 76 54 E
Sirur, *India* ...... **94 E2** 18 50N 74 23 E
Sisak, *Croatia* ..... **45 C13** 45 30N 16 21 E
Sisaket, *Thailand* ... **86 E5** 15 8N 104 23 E
Sisante, *Spain* **41 F2** 39 25N 2 12W
Sisargas, Is., *Spain* ... **42 B2** 43 21N 8 50W
Sishen, *S. Africa* ... **116 D3** 27 47 S 22 59 E
Sishui, *Henan, China* .. **74 G7** 34 48N 113 15 E
Sishui, *Shandong,*
  China .... **75 G9** 35 42N 117 18 E
Sisiga, *Solomon Is.* .. **133 L10** 7 54 S 159 10 E
Sisimiut, *Greenland* .. **10 D5** 66 40N 53 30W
Sisipuk L., *Canada* .. **143 B8** 55 45N 101 50W
Sisophon, *Cambodia* .. **86 F4** 13 38N 102 59 E
Sissach, *Switz.* .... **32 B5** 47 27N 7 48 E
Sissano, *Papua N. G.* . **132 B2** 3 0 S 142 3 E
Sisseton, *U.S.A.* ... **154 C6** 45 40N 97 3W
Sisson = Mount Shasta,
  U.S.A. **158 F2** 41 19N 122 19W
Sissonne, *France* .... **27 C10** 49 34N 3 51 E
Sïstän, *Asia* ...... **97 D9** 30 50N 61 0 E
Sïstän, Daryâcheh-ye,
  Iran .... **97 D9** 31 0N 61 0 E
Sïstän va
  Balüchestän □, *Iran* . **97 E9** 27 0N 62 0 E
Sisteron, *France* .... **29 D9** 44 12N 5 57 E
Sisters, *U.S.A.* **158 D3** 44 18N 121 33W
Sisters, The, *Seychelles* **121 b** 4 16 S 55 52 E
Sisters Pk., *Ascension I.* **9 g** 7 56 S 14 22W
Siswa Bazar, *India* .. **93 F10** 27 9N 83 46 E
Sitakili, *Mali* **112 C2** 13 7N 11 14W
Sitakunda, *Bangla.* .. **90 D3** 22 37N 91 39 E
Sitamarhi, *India* .... **93 F11** 26 37N 85 30 E
Sitampiky, *Madag.* .. **117 B8** 16 41 S 46 6 E
Sitangkai, *Phil.* .... **81 J2** 4 40N 119 24 E
Sitapur, *India* ..... **93 F9** 27 38N 80 45 E
Siteki, *Swaziland* ... **117 D5** 26 32 S 31 58 E
Sitges, *Spain* ..... **40 D6** 41 17N 1 47 E
Sithoniá, *Greece* ... **50 F7** 40 0N 23 45 E
Sitía, *Greece* ..... **49 E7** 35 13N 26 6 E
Sítia △ (JSH), *Greece* . **49 E7** 35 13N 26 5 E
Sitio da Abadia, *Brazil* . **171 D2** 14 48 S 46 16W
Sitka, *U.S.A.* **142 B1** 57 3N 135 20W
Sitka △, *U.S.A.* **144 E14** 57 3N 135 19W
Sitkinak I., *U.S.A.* .. **144 H9** 56 33N 154 10W
Sitoti, *Botswana* ... **116 C3** 23 15 S 23 40 E
Sitra, *Egypt* ...... **106 B2** 28 40N 26 53 E
Sittang Myit ➔, *Burma* . **90 G6** 17 20N 96 45 E
Sittard, *Neths.* .... **24 C5** 51 0N 5 52 E
Sittaung, *Burma* .... **90 C5** 24 10N 94 29 E
Sittensen, *Germany* .. **30 B5** 53 17N 9 32 E
Sittingbourne, *U.K.* .. **21 F8** 51 21N 0 45 E
Sittona, *Eritrea* .... **107 E4** 14 25N 37 23 E
Sittoung = Sittang
  Myit ➔, *Burma* .... **90 G6** 17 20N 96 45 E
Sittwe, *Burma* ..... **90 C4** 20 18N 92 45 E
Situbondo, *Indonesia* . **79 G16** 7 42 S 114 0 E
Si'umu, *Samoa* .... **133 X24** 14 1 S 171 48W
Siuna, *Nic.* **164 D3** 13 37N 84 45W
Siuri, *India* ...... **93 H12** 23 50N 87 34 E
Siutghiol, Lacul,
  Romania .... **53 F13** 44 15N 28 35 E
Sivaganga, *India* ... **95 K4** 9 50N 78 28 E
Sivagiri, *India* ..... **95 K3** 9 16N 77 26 E
Sivakasi, *India* .... **95 K3** 9 24N 77 47 E
Sïvand, *Iran* ...... **97 D7** 30 5N 52 55 E
Sivas, *Turkey* ..... **100 C7** 39 43N 36 58 E
Sivasamudram, *India* . **95 H3** 12 16N 77 10 E
Sivaslı, *Turkey* .... **49 C11** 38 31N 29 42 E
Siverek, *Turkey* .... **101 D8** 37 50N 39 19 E
Sivomaskinskiy, *Russia* **54 A11** 66 40N 62 35 E
Sívota, *Greece* ..... **38 C10** 39 24N 20 13 E
Sivrihisar, *Turkey* .. **100 C4** 39 30N 31 35 E
Sívros, *Greece* ..... **39 B2** 38 40N 20 39 E
Sîwa, *Egypt* ...... **106 B2** 29 11N 25 31 E
Siwa, El Wâhât es,
  Egypt .... **106 B2** 29 10N 25 30 E
Siwa Oasis = Sîwa, El
  Wâhât es, *Egypt* ... **106 B2** 29 10N 25 30 E
Siwalik Range, *Nepal* . **93 F10** 28 0N 83 0 E
Siwan, *India* ...... **93 F11** 26 13N 84 21 E
Siwana, *India* ..... **92 G5** 25 38N 72 25 E
Six Cross Roads,
  Barbados .... **165 g** 13 7N 59 28W
Sixmilebridge, *Ireland* . **23 D3** 52 44N 8 46W
Sixth Cataract, *Sudan* . **107 D3** 16 20N 32 42 E
Siyâh Koh, *Afghan.* .. **91 B2** 34 50N 67 40 E
Siyâl, Jazâ'ir, *Egypt* . **106 C4** 22 49N 36 12 E
Siyäzän, *Azerbaijan* .. **61 K9** 41 3N 49 10 E
Siziwang Qi, *China* .. **74 D6** 41 25N 111 40 E
Sjælland, *Denmark* .. **17 J5** 55 30N 11 30 E
Sjællands Odde,
  Denmark .... **17 J5** 55 58N 11 24 E
Sjenica, *Serbia & M.* . **50 C8** 43 19N 20 0 E
Sjoa, *Norway* ..... **18 C6** 61 41N 9 33 E
Sjöbo, *Sweden* ..... **17 J7** 55 37N 13 45 E
Sjøholt, *Norway* .... **18 B3** 62 27N 6 52 E
Sjøli, *Norway* ..... **18 C6** 61 29N 11 18 E
Sjötofta, *Sweden* ... **17 G7** 57 22N 13 17 E
Sjötorp, *Sweden* ... **17 F8** 58 50N 14 0 E

Sjumen = Shumen,
  Bulgaria .... **51 C10** 43 18N 26 55 E
Sjuntorp, *Sweden* ... **17 F6** 58 12N 12 13 E
Skåbu, *Norway* ..... **18 C6** 61 32N 9 24 E
Skadarsko Jezero,
  Serbia & M. ...... **50 D3** 42 10N 19 20 E
Skadovsk, *Ukraine* .. **59 J7** 46 17N 32 52 E
Skælskør, *Denmark* .. **17 J5** 55 15N 11 18 E
Skærbæk, *Denmark* .. **17 J2** 55 9N 8 45 E
Skaftafell, *Iceland* .. **11 C9** 64 1N 17 0W
Skaftafell △, *Iceland* . **11 C9** 64 1N 16 50W
Skagafjarðarsýsla □,
  Iceland **11 B7** 65 30N 19 0W
Skagafjörður, *Iceland* . **11 B7** 65 54N 19 35W
Skagastølstindane,
  Norway .... **18 C4** 61 28N 7 52 E
Skagaströnd, *Iceland* . **11 B6** 65 50N 20 19W
Skagatá, *Iceland* ... **11 A6** 66 7N 20 8W
Skagen, *Denmark* ... **16 E8** 57 43N 10 35 E
Skagen, *Sweden* .... **16 E8** 59 0N 14 20 E
Skagerrak, *Denmark* . **17 G2** 57 30N 9 0 E
Skagit ➔, *U.S.A.* ... **160 B4** 48 23N 122 22W
Skagway, *U.S.A.* ... **144 G14** 59 28N 135 19W
Skála, *Greece* ..... **39 C2** 38 5N 20 47 E
Skala nad Zbruczem =
  Skala-Podilska,
  Ukraine .... **53 B11** 48 50N 26 15 E
Skala-Podilska, *Ukraine* **53 B11** 48 50N 26 15 E
Skala Podolskaya =
  Skala-Podilska,
  Ukraine .... **53 B11** 48 50N 26 15 E
Skalat, *Ukraine* .... **59 H3** 49 23N 25 55 E
Skálavík, *Iceland* ... **11 A3** 66 11N 23 29W
Skalbmierz, *Poland* .. **55 H7** 50 20N 20 25 E
Skälderviken, *Sweden* . **17 H6** 56 22N 12 30 E
Skålevik, *Norway* ... **18 F5** 58 5N 8 1 E
Skalica, *Slovak Rep.* . **35 C10** 48 50N 17 15 E
Skallingen, *Denmark* . **17 J2** 55 32N 8 13 E
Skalni Dol =
  Kamenyak, *Bulgaria* . **51 C10** 43 24N 26 57 E
Skanderborg, *Denmark* **17 H3** 56 2N 9 55 E
Skåne, *Sweden* .... **17 J7** 55 59N 13 30 E
Skåne län □, *Sweden* . **17 J7** 55 59N 13 30 E
Skaneateles, *U.S.A.* . **151 D8** 42 57N 76 26W
Skaneateles L., *U.S.A.* **151 D8** 42 51N 76 22W
Skånevik, *Norway* ... **18 E2** 59 43N 5 53 E
Skänninge, *Sweden* .. **17 F9** 58 24N 15 5 E
Skanör med Falsterbo,
  Sweden .... **17 J6** 55 24N 12 50 E
Skántzoúra, *Greece* .. **48 B6** 39 5N 24 6 E
Skara, *Sweden* ..... **17 F7** 58 25N 13 30 E
Skärblacka, *Sweden* . **17 F9** 58 35N 15 54 E
Skarð, *Iceland* **11 B4** 65 17N 22 19W
Skardu, *Pakistan* ... **93 B6** 35 20N 75 44 E
Skåre, *Norway* ..... **18 E3** 59 55N 6 36 E
Skåre, *Sweden* ..... **16 E7** 59 26N 13 26 E
Skärhamn, *Sweden* .. **17 G5** 57 59N 11 34 E
Skarnes, *Norway* ... **18 D6** 60 15N 11 41 E
Skarszewy, *Poland* .. **54 D5** 54 4N 18 25 E
Skaryszew, *Poland* .. **55 G8** 51 19N 21 15 E
Skarżysko-Kamienna,
  Poland .... **55 G7** 51 7N 20 52 E
Skattkärr, *Sweden* .. **16 E7** 59 25N 13 40 E
Skattungbyn, *Sweden* . **16 C8** 61 10N 14 56 E
Skawina, *Poland* ... **55 J6** 49 59N 19 50 E
Skebobruk, *Sweden* .. **16 E12** 59 58N 18 36 E
Skeena ➔, *Canada* .. **142 C2** 54 9N 130 5W
Skeena Mts., *Canada* . **142 B3** 56 40N 128 30W
Skegness, *U.K.* ..... **20 D8** 53 9N 0 20 E
Skei, *Norway* ...... **18 C3** 61 34N 6 5 E
Skeiðarársandur,
  Iceland **11 D9** 63 54N 17 14W
Skeiðisfoss, *Iceland* .. **11 D7** 63 26N 19 11W
Skeldon, *Guyana* ... **169 B6** 5 55N 57 20W
Skeleton Coast △,
  Namibia .... **116 C1** 20 0 S 13 20 E
Skellefteå, *Sweden* .. **14 D19** 64 45N 20 50 E
Skellefteälven ➔,
  Sweden .... **14 D19** 64 45N 21 10 E
Skellefteahamn, *Sweden* **14 D19** 64 40N 21 9 E
Skender Vakuf, *Bos.-H.* **44 C7** 44 29N 17 22 E
Skerries, The, *U.K.* .. **20 D3** 53 25N 4 36W
Skhidnytsya, *Ukraine* . **59 H7** 49 20N 23 20 E
Skhíza, *Greece* ..... **48 E3** 36 41N 21 40 E
Skhoinoúsa, *Greece* . **49 E7** 36 53N 25 31 E
Ski, *Norway* ...... **18 E7** 59 43N 10 52 E
Skíathos, *Greece* ... **48 B5** 39 12N 23 30 E
Skibbereen, *Ireland* .. **23 E2** 51 33N 9 16W
Skiddaw, *U.K.* **20 C4** 54 39N 3 9W
Skidegate, *Canada* .. **142 C2** 53 15N 132 1W
Skídhra, *Greece* .... **50 F6** 40 46N 22 10 E
Skien, *Norway* ..... **18 E6** 59 12N 9 35 E
Skierniewice, *Poland* . **55 G7** 51 58N 20 10 E
Skikda, *Algeria* .... **114 A6** 36 50N 6 58 E
Skillet ➔, *U.S.A.* ... **157 F8** 38 5N 88 5W
Skillingaryd, *Sweden* . **17 G8** 57 27N 14 5 E
Skillinge, *Sweden* ... **17 J8** 55 30N 14 16 E
Skilloura, *Cyprus* ... **39 D2** 35 14N 33 10 E
Skinári, Ákra, *Greece* . **39 D2** 37 56N 20 42 E
Skinnastaður, *Iceland* . **11 A10** 66 1N 16 27W
Skinnskatteberg,
  Sweden .... **16 E9** 59 50N 15 42 E
Skipton, *Australia* .. **128 D5** 37 39 S 143 40 E
Skipton, *U.K.* **20 D5** 53 58N 2 3W
Skiptvet, *Norway* ... **18 E8** 59 28N 11 11 E
Skíring, C., *Senegal* .. **112 C1** 12 26N 16 46W
Skirmish Pt., *Australia* . **126 A11** 11 59 S 134 17 E
Skiropoúla, *Greece* .. **48 C6** 38 50N 24 21 E
Skíros, *Greece* ..... **48 C6** 38 55N 24 34 E
Skivarp, *Sweden* ... **17 J7** 55 26N 13 34 E
Skive, *Denmark* .... **17 H3** 56 33N 9 2 E
Skjærhalden, *Norway* . **18 E8** 59 2N 11 2 E
Skjálfandafljót ➔,
  Iceland **11 B9** 65 59N 17 25W
Skjálfandi, *Iceland* .. **11 A9** 66 5N 17 30W
Skjeberg, *Norway* ... **18 E8** 59 12N 11 12 E
Skjern, *Denmark* ... **17 J2** 55 57N 8 30 E
Skjold, *Norway* .... **18 E2** 59 31N 5 34 E
Skjolden, *Norway* ... **18 C4** 61 29N 7 40 E
Skjöldólfsstaðir, *Iceland* **11 B11** 65 19N 15 7W
Skjønhaug, *Norway* . **18 E8** 59 39N 11 18 E
Skobelev = Farghona,
  Uzbekistan ...... **65 C5** 40 23N 71 19 E
Skobeleva, Pik,
  Kyrgyzstan ...... **65 D6** 39 48N 72 36 E
Skoczów, *Poland* ... **55 J5** 49 49N 18 45 E
Škofja Loka, *Slovenia* . **45 B11** 46 9N 14 19 E
Skógar, *Iceland* **11 D7** 63 23N 19 27W
Skógarnes, *Iceland* .. **11 C4** 64 46N 22 34W
Skoghall, *Sweden* ... **16 E7** 59 19N 16 29 E
Skogstorp, *Sweden* .. **16 E10** 59 19N 16 29 E
Skoki, *Poland* ..... **55 F4** 52 40N 17 11 E
Skokie, *U.S.A.* **157 B9** 42 3N 87 45W
Skollenborg, *Norway* . **18 E6** 59 39N 9 39 E
Skópelos, *Greece* ... **48 B5** 39 9N 23 47 E
Skopí, *Greece* ..... **49 E7** 35 11N 26 2 E
Skopin, *Russia* ..... **58 F10** 53 55N 39 32 E
Skopje, *Macedonia* .. **50 D5** 42 1N 21 26 E
Skopje ✕ (SKP),
  Macedonia ...... **50 E5** 41 59N 21 29 E
Skoppum, *Norway* .. **18 E7** 59 25N 10 26 E
Skórcz, *Poland* .... **54 E5** 53 47N 18 30 E

Skørping, *Denmark* .. **17 H3** 56 50N 9 53 E
Skotfoss, *Norway* ... **18 E6** 59 12N 9 30 E
Skotterud, *Norway* .. **18 D9** 60 0N 12 7 E
Skövde, *Sweden* .... **17 F7** 58 24N 13 50 E
Skovorodino, *Russia* . **67 D13** 54 0N 124 0 E
Skowhegan, *U.S.A.* . **149 C11** 44 46N 69 43W
Skradin, *Croatia* .... **45 E12** 43 52N 15 53 E
Skrea, *Sweden* ..... **17 H6** 56 53N 12 34 E
Skreia, *Norway* .... **18 D7** 60 40N 10 56 E
Skrim, *Norway* ..... **18 E6** 59 31N 9 38 E
Skrunda, *Latvia* .... **54 B9** 56 41N 22 1 E
Skrwa ➔, *Poland* ... **55 F6** 52 35N 19 32 E
Skudeneshavn, *Norway* **18 E2** 59 10N 5 10 E
Skuleskogen △, *Sweden* **16 A12** 63 6N 18 30 E
Skull, *Ireland* **23 E2** 51 32N 9 34W
Skultorp, *Sweden* ... **17 F7** 58 24N 13 51 E
Skultuna, *Sweden* .. **16 E10** 59 43N 16 25 E
Skunk ➔, *U.S.A.* ... **156 D5** 40 42N 91 7W
Skuodas, *Lithuania* .. **15 H19** 56 16N 21 33 E
Skurup, *Sweden* .... **17 J7** 55 28N 13 30 E
Skutskär, *Sweden* .. **16 D11** 60 37N 17 25 E
Skútustaðir, *Iceland* . **11 B9** 65 34N 17 2W
Skvyra, *Ukraine* .... **59 H5** 49 44N 29 40 E
Skwierzyna, *Poland* .. **55 F2** 52 33N 15 30 E
Skye, *U.K.* **22 D2** 57 15N 6 10W
Skykomish, *U.S.A.* .. **158 C3** 47 42N 121 22W
Skyring, Seno, *Chile* .. **176 D3** 52 35 S 72 0W
Skyros = Skíros, *Greece* **48 C6** 38 55N 24 34 E
Skyttorp, *Sweden* ... **16 D11** 60 5N 17 44 E
Slade Pt., *Australia* .. **126 K7** 21 5 S 149 13 E
Slættaratindur,
  Færoe Is. **14 E9** 62 18N 7 1W
Slagelse, *Denmark* .. **17 J5** 55 23N 11 19 E
Slamet, *Indonesia* ... **85 D3** 7 16 S 109 8 E
Slaney ➔, *Ireland* ... **23 D5** 52 26N 6 33W
Slangberge, *S. Africa* . **116 E3** 31 32 S 20 48 E
Slânic, *Romania* .... **53 E10** 45 14N 25 58 E
Slano, *Croatia* ..... **50 D1** 42 48N 17 53 E
Slantsy, *Russia* .... **58 C5** 59 7N 28 5 E
Slaný, *Czech Rep.* ... **34 A7** 50 13N 14 6 E
Śląsk, *Poland* ..... **36 C9** 51 0N 16 30 E
Śląskie □, *Poland* ... **55 H6** 50 30N 19 0 E
Slätbaken, *Sweden* .. **17 F10** 58 25N 16 45 E
Slate Is., *Canada* ... **140 C2** 48 40N 87 0W
Slater, *U.S.A.* **156 E3** 39 13N 93 4W
Slatina, *Croatia* .... **52 E2** 45 42N 17 45 E
Slatina, *Romania* ... **53 F9** 44 28N 24 22 E
Slatina Timiş, *Romania* **52 F7** 45 15N 22 17 E
Slatington, *U.S.A.* .. **151 F9** 40 45N 75 37W
Slaton, *U.S.A.* **155 J4** 33 26N 101 39W
Slave ➔, *Canada* ... **142 A6** 61 18N 113 39W
Slave Coast, *W. Afr.* . **113 D5** 6 0 S 2 30 E
Slave Lake, *Canada* .. **142 B6** 55 17N 114 43W
Slave Pt., *Canada* ... **142 A5** 61 11N 115 56W
Slavgorod, *Russia* .. **68 D8** 53 1N 78 37 E
Slavinja, *Serbia & M.* . **50 C6** 43 9N 22 50 E
Slavkov u Brna,
  Czech Rep. ...... **35 B9** 49 10N 16 52 E
Slavkovský Les △,
  Czech Rep. ...... **34 A5** 50 5N 12 44 E
Slavonija, *Europe* ... **52 E2** 45 20N 17 40 E
Slavonski Brod, *Croatia* **52 E3** 45 11N 18 1 E
Slavsk, *Russia* ..... **54 C8** 55 3N 21 41 E
Slavska, *Ukraine* ... **53 B8** 48 51N 23 27 E
Slavskoye, *Russia* .. **54 D7** 54 30N 20 27 E
Slavuta, *Ukraine* ... **59 G4** 50 15N 27 2 E
Slavyanka, *Russia* .. **70 C5** 42 53N 131 21 E
Slavyanovo, *Bulgaria* . **51 C8** 43 28N 24 52 E
Slavyansk = Slovyansk,
  Ukraine .... **59 H9** 48 55N 37 36 E
Slavyansk-na-Kubani,
  Russia .... **59 K10** 45 15N 38 11 E
Sława, *Poland* ..... **55 G3** 51 52N 16 2 E
Slawharad, *Belarus* .. **58 F6** 53 27N 31 0 E
Sławno, *Poland* .... **54 D3** 54 20N 16 41 E
Sławoborze, *Poland* . **54 E2** 53 55N 15 42 E
Sleaford, *U.K.* **20 D7** 53 0N 0 24W
Sleaford B., *Australia* . **127 E2** 34 55 S 135 45 E
Sleat, Sd. of, *U.K.* ... **22 D3** 57 5N 5 47W
Sleðbrjótur, *Iceland* .. **11 B12** 65 34N 14 30W
Sleeper Is., *Canada* .. **139 C11** 58 30N 81 0W
Sleeping Bear Dunes △,
  U.S.A. **148 C2** 44 50N 86 5W
Sleepy Eye, *U.S.A.* .. **154 C7** 44 18N 94 43W
Sleetmute, *U.S.A.* .. **144 F8** 61 42N 157 10W
Sleman, *Indonesia* .. **85 D4** 7 40 S 110 20 E
Slemon L., *Canada* .. **142 A5** 63 13N 116 4W
Slesin, *Poland* ..... **55 F5** 52 22N 18 14 E
Slide Mt., *U.S.A.* ... **151 E10** 42 0N 74 25W
Slidell, *U.S.A.* **155 K10** 30 17N 89 47W
Sliema, *Malta* ..... **38 F8** 35 55N 14 30 E
Slieve Aughty, *Ireland* . **23 C3** 53 4N 8 30W
Slieve Bloom, *Ireland* . **23 C4** 53 4N 7 40W
Slieve Donard, *Ireland* . **23 B6** 54 11N 5 55W
Slieve Gamph, *Ireland* . **23 B3** 54 6N 8 42W
Slieve Gullion, *Ireland* . **23 B5** 54 7N 6 26W
Slieve League, *Ireland* . **23 B3** 54 40N 8 42W
Slieve Mish, *Ireland* .. **23 D2** 52 12N 9 50W
Slievenamon, *Ireland* . **23 D4** 52 25N 7 34W
Sligeach = Sligo, *Ireland* **23 B3** 54 16N 8 28W
Sligo, *Ireland* **23 B3** 54 16N 8 28W
Sligo, *U.S.A.* **150 E5** 41 6N 79 29W
Sligo □, *Ireland* **23 B4** 54 8N 8 42W
Sligo B., *Ireland* **23 B3** 54 18N 8 40W
Slippery Rock, *U.S.A.* . **150 E4** 41 3N 80 3W
Slite, *Sweden* ..... **17 G12** 57 42N 18 48 E
Sliven, *Bulgaria* .... **51 D10** 42 42N 26 19 E
Slivnitsa, *Bulgaria* .. **50 D7** 42 50N 23 0 E
Sljeme, *Croatia* .... **45 C12** 45 57N 15 58 E
Sloan, *U.S.A.* **161 K11** 35 57N 115 13W
Sloansville, *U.S.A.* .. **151 D10** 42 45N 74 22W
Slobidka, *Ukraine* ... **53 C14** 47 54N 29 15 E
Slobodskoy, *Russia* . **64 B3** 58 40N 50 6 E
Slobozia, *Moldova* .. **53 D14** 46 45N 29 42 E
Slobozia, *Argeş,*
  Romania .... **53 F10** 44 30N 25 14 E
Slobozia, *Ialomiţa,*
  Romania .... **53 F12** 44 34N 27 23 E
Slocan, *Canada* **142 D5** 49 48N 117 28W
Slocomb, *U.S.A.* ... **152 D4** 31 7N 85 36W
Slomikino =
  Furmanovo,
  Kazakhstan ...... **60 F9** 49 42N 49 25 E
Słomniki, *Poland* ... **55 H7** 50 16N 20 4 E
Slonim, *Belarus* .... **59 F3** 53 4N 25 19 E
Slot, The = New
  Georgia Sound,
  Solomon Is. ...... **133 L9** 8 0 S 158 0 E
Slough, *U.K.* **21 F7** 51 30N 0 36W
Slough □, *U.K.* **21 F7** 51 30N 0 36W
Sloughhouse, *U.S.A.* . **160 G5** 38 26N 121 12W
Slovak Rep. ■, *Europe* **35 C13** 48 30N 20 0 E
Slovakia = Slovak
  Rep. ■, *Europe* ... **35 C13** 48 30N 20 0 E
Slovakian Ore Mts. =
  Slovenské
  Rudohorie,
  Slovak Rep. ...... **35 C12** 48 45N 20 0 E
Slovenia = Slovenija ■,
  Europe .... **45 C11** 45 58N 14 30 E
Slovenija ■, *Europe* .. **45 C11** 45 58N 14 30 E
Slovenj Gradec,
  Slovenia .... **45 B12** 46 31N 15 5 E

Slovenska = Slovak
  Rep. ■, *Europe* ... **35 C13** 48 30N 20 0 E
Slovenska Bistrica,
  Slovenia .... **45 B12** 46 24N 15 35 E
Slovenské Konjice,
  Slovenia .... **45 B12** 46 20N 15 28 E
Slovenské Rudohorie,
  Slovak Rep. ...... **35 C12** 48 45N 20 0 E
Slovenský Raj △,
  Slovak Rep. ...... **35 C13** 48 55N 20 25 E
Slovyansk, *Ukraine* .. **59 H9** 48 55N 37 36 E
Słowiński ➔, *Poland* . **54 D4** 54 43N 17 26 E
Słubice, *Poland* .... **55 F1** 52 22N 14 35 E
Sluch ➔, *Ukraine* ... **59 G4** 51 37N 26 38 E
Sluis, *Neths.* ...... **24 C3** 51 18N 3 23 E
Slünchev Bryag,
  Bulgaria .... **51 D11** 42 40N 27 41 E
Slunj, *Croatia* ..... **45 C12** 45 6N 15 33 E
Słupca, *Poland* .... **55 F4** 52 15N 17 52 E
Słupia ➔, *Poland* ... **54 D3** 54 35N 16 51 E
Słupsk, *Poland* ..... **54 D4** 54 30N 17 3 E
Slurry, *S. Africa* .... **116 D4** 25 49 S 25 42 E
Slutsk = Pavlovsk,
  Russia .... **60 E5** 50 26N 40 5 E
Slutsk, *Belarus* ..... **59 F4** 53 2N 27 31 E
Slyne Hd., *Ireland* ... **23 C1** 53 25N 10 10W
Slyudyanka, *Russia* .. **67 D11** 51 40N 103 40 E
Smaalenene =
  Østfold □, *Norway* .. **18 E8** 59 25N 11 30 E
Småland, *Sweden* ... **17 G9** 57 15N 15 25 E
Smålandsfarvandet,
  Denmark .... **17 J5** 55 10N 11 20 E
Smålandsstenar,
  Sweden .... **17 G7** 57 10N 13 25 E
Smaldeel = Theunissen,
  S. Africa .... **116 D4** 28 26 S 26 43 E
Smalltree L., *Canada* . **143 A8** 61 0N 105 0W
Smallwood Res.,
  Canada **141 B7** 54 5N 64 30W
Smarhon, *Belarus* ... **58 E4** 54 20N 26 24 E
Smarje, *Slovenia* ... **45 B12** 46 15N 15 34 E
Smartt Syndicate Dam,
  S. Africa .... **116 E3** 30 45 S 23 10 E
Smartville, *U.S.A.* .. **160 F5** 39 13N 121 18W
Smeaton, *Canada* ... **143 C8** 53 30N 104 49W
Smedby, *Sweden* ... **17 H10** 56 41N 16 13 E
Smederevo,
  Serbia & M. ...... **50 B4** 44 40N 20 57 E
Smederevska Palanka,
  Serbia & M. ...... **50 B4** 44 22N 20 58 E
Smedjebacken, *Sweden* **16 D9** 60 8N 15 25 E
Smela = Smila, *Ukraine* **59 H6** 49 15N 31 58 E
Smerwick Harbour,
  Ireland **23 D1** 52 12N 10 23W
Smethport, *U.S.A.* .. **150 E6** 41 49N 78 27W
Smidovich, *Russia* .. **67 E14** 48 36N 133 49 E
Śmigiel, *Poland* .... **55 F3** 52 1N 16 32 E
Smila, *Ukraine* .... **59 H6** 49 15N 31 58 E
Smilyan, *Bulgaria* .. **51 E8** 41 29N 24 46 E
Smith, *Canada* **142 B6** 55 10N 114 0W
Smith B., *U.S.A.* ... **144 A9** 70 30N 154 20W
Smith Center, *U.S.A.* . **154 F5** 39 47N 98 47W
Smith I., *India* ..... **95 H11** 13 20N 93 4 E
Smith River ➔, *U.S.A.* **158 F2** 41 55N 124 4W
Smith Sd., *N. Amer.* . **10 B3** 78 25N 74 0W
Smithburne ➔,
  Australia .... **126 B3** 17 3 S 140 57 E
Smithers, *Canada* ... **142 C3** 54 45N 127 10W
Smithfield, *S. Africa* . **117 E4** 30 9 S 26 30 E
Smithfield, *N.C., U.S.A.* **149 H6** 35 31N 78 21W
Smithfield, *Utah, U.S.A.* **158 F8** 41 50N 111 50W
Smiths, *U.S.A.* **152 C4** 32 32N 85 6W
Smiths Falls, *Canada* . **140 D4** 44 55N 76 0W
Smithton, *Australia* .. **127 G4** 40 53 S 145 6 E
Smithville, *Canada* .. **150 C5** 43 6N 79 33W
Smithville, *Ga., U.S.A.* **152 D5** 31 54N 84 15W
Smithville, *Mo., U.S.A.* **156 E2** 39 23N 94 35W
Smithville, *Tex., U.S.A.* **155 K6** 30 1N 97 10W
Smoky ➔, *Canada* .. **142 B5** 56 10N 117 21W
Smoky Bay, *Australia* . **127 E1** 32 22 S 134 13 E
Smoky Hill ➔, *U.S.A.* **154 F6** 39 4N 96 48W
Smoky Hills, *U.S.A.* . **154 F5** 39 15N 99 30W
Smoky Lake, *Canada* . **142 C6** 54 10N 112 30W
Smøla, *Norway* .... **18 A5** 63 23N 8 3 E
Smolensk, *Russia* ... **58 E7** 54 45N 32 5 E
Smolikas, Óros, *Greece* **50 F4** 40 9N 20 58 E
Smolník, *Slovak Rep.* . **35 C13** 48 43N 20 44 E
Smolyan, *Bulgaria* .. **51 E8** 41 36N 24 38 E
Smooth Rock Falls,
  Canada **140 C3** 49 17N 81 37W
Smoothstone L.,
  Canada **143 C7** 54 40N 106 50W
Smorgon = Smarhon,
  Belarus .... **58 E4** 54 20N 26 24 E
Smotrych, *Ukraine* .. **53 B11** 48 57N 26 33 E
Smotrych ➔, *Ukraine* **53 B11** 48 34N 26 53 E
Smulţi, *Romania* ... **53 E12** 45 57N 27 44 E
Smyadovo, *Bulgaria* . **51 C11** 43 2N 27 1 E
Smygehamn, *Sweden* . **17 J7** 55 21N 13 22 E
Smyrna = İzmir, *Turkey* **49 C9** 38 25N 27 8 E
Smyrna, *Del., U.S.A.* . **148 F8** 39 18N 75 36W
Smyrna, *Ga., U.S.A.* . **152 B5** 33 53N 84 31W
Snæfell, *Iceland* **11 C11** 64 48N 15 34W
Snaefell, *I. of Man* .. **20 C3** 54 16N 4 27W
Snæfellsjökull, *Iceland* **11 C3** 64 49N 23 46W
Snæfellsnessýsla □,
  Iceland **11 C3** 65 0N 22 0W
Snake ➔, *U.S.A.* ... **158 C4** 46 12N 119 2W
Snake I., *Australia* .. **129 F7** 38 47 S 146 33 E
Snake Range, *U.S.A.* . **158 G6** 39 0N 114 20W
Snake River Plain,
  U.S.A. **158 E7** 42 50N 113 0W
Snasahögarna, *Sweden* **16 A8** 63 13N 12 21 E
Snåsavatnet, *Norway* . **14 D14** 64 12N 12 0 E
Snedsted, *Denmark* .. **17 H2** 56 55N 8 32 E
Sneek, *Neths.* ..... **24 A5** 53 2N 5 40 E
Sneeuberge, *S. Africa* . **116 E3** 31 46 S 24 20 E
Snejbjerg, *Denmark* . **17 H2** 56 9N 8 54 E
Snelling, *U.S.A.* **160 H6** 37 31N 120 26W
Snelling, S.C., *U.S.A.* . **152 B8** 33 15N 81 27W
Snells Beach, *N.Z.* .. **130 C3** 36 25 S 174 44 E
Snezhnoye, *Ukraine* .. **59 J10** 48 0N 38 58 E
Snežka, *Europe* .... **36 C5** 50 41N 15 50 E
Snežnik, *Slovenia* ... **45 C11** 45 36N 14 35 E
Śniadowo, *Poland* .. **55 E8** 53 1N 22 6 E
Sniardwy, Jezioro,
  Poland .... **54 E8** 53 48N 21 50 E
Śniežka, *Europe* .... **34 A8** 50 44N 15 44 E
Snigirevka =
  Snihurivka, *Ukraine* . **59 J7** 47 2N 32 49 E
Snihurivka, *Ukraine* . **59 J7** 47 2N 32 49 E
Snillfjord, *Norway* ... **18 A4** 63 26N 9 16 E
Snina, *Slovak Rep.* ... **35 C15** 48 58N 22 9 E
Snizort, L., *U.K.* **22 D2** 57 33N 6 28W
Snøhetta, *Norway* ... **18 B6** 62 19N 9 16 E
Snohomish, *U.S.A.* .. **160 C4** 47 55N 122 6W
Snønuten, *Norway* .. **18 E3** 59 31N 6 52 E
Snøtinden, *Norway* .. **14 C16** 66 39N 13 50 E
Snøul, *Cambodia* ... **87 F6** 12 4N 106 26 E
Snovsk = Shchors,
  Ukraine .... **59 G6** 51 48N 31 56 E
Snow Hill, *U.S.A.* ... **148 F8** 38 11N 75 24W
Snow Lake, *Canada* . **143 C8** 54 52N 100 3W

Snow Mt., *Calif., U.S.A.* **160 F4** 39 23N 122 45W
Snow Mt., *Maine,*
  U.S.A. **151 A14** 45 18N 70 48W
Snow Shoe, *U.S.A.* .. **150 E7** 41 2N 77 57W
Snowbird L., *Canada* . **143 A8** 60 45N 103 0W
Snowdon, *U.K.* **20 D3** 53 4N 4 5W
Snowdonia △, *U.K.* .. **20 D4** 53 7N 3 59W
Snowdoun, *U.S.A.* .. **152 C3** 32 15N 86 18W
Snowdrift = Łutselk'e,
  Canada **143 A6** 62 24N 110 44W
Snowdrift ➔, *Canada* . **143 A6** 62 24N 110 44W
Snowflake, *U.S.A.* .. **159 J8** 34 30N 110 5W
Snowshoe Pk., *U.S.A.* **158 B6** 48 13N 115 41W
Snowtown, *Australia* . **128 B3** 33 46 S 138 14 E
Snowville, *U.S.A.* ... **158 F7** 41 58N 112 43W
Snowy ➔, *Australia* . **129 D8** 37 46 S 148 30 E
Snowy Mt., *U.S.A.* .. **151 C10** 43 42N 74 23W
Snowy Mts., *Australia* **129 D8** 36 30 S 148 20 E
Snowy River △,
  Australia .... **129 D7** 37 15 S 147 29 E
Snug Corner, *Bahamas* **53 B10** 48 27N 25 38 E
Snyatyn, *Ukraine* ... **53 B10** 48 27N 25 38 E
Snyder, *Okla., U.S.A.* . **155 H5** 34 40N 98 57W
Snyder, *Tex., U.S.A.* . **155 J4** 32 44N 100 55W
Soacha, *Colombia* .. **168 C3** 4 35N 74 13W
Soahanina, *Madag.* .. **117 B7** 18 42 S 44 13 E
Soalala, *Madag.* .... **117 B8** 16 6 S 45 20 E
Soaloka, *Madag.* ... **117 B8** 18 32 S 45 15 E
Soamanonga, *Madag.* **117 C7** 23 52 S 44 47 E
Soan ➔, *Pakistan* .. **92 C4** 33 1N 71 44 E
Soanierana-Ivongo,
  Madag. .... **117 B8** 16 55 S 49 35 E
Soanindraniny, *Madag.* **117 B8** 19 54 S 47 14 E
Şoarş, *Romania* .... **53 E9** 45 56N 24 55 E
Soasiu, *Indonesia* ... **82 A3** 0 40N 127 26 E
Soavina, *Indonesia* .. **117 C8** 20 23 S 46 56 E
Soavinandriana,
  Madag. .... **117 B8** 19 9 S 46 45 E
Sob ➔, *Ukraine* .... **53 B14** 48 40N 29 15 E
Soba, *Nigeria* ..... **113 C6** 10 58N 8 4 E
Sobat, Nahr ➔, *Sudan* **107 F3** 9 22N 31 33 E
Sobėšlav, *Czech Rep.* . **34 B7** 49 16N 14 45 E
Sobger ➔, *Indonesia* . **83 B6** 3 42 S 140 16 E
Sobhapur, *India* .... **92 H8** 22 47N 78 17 E
Sobinka, *Russia* .... **58 E11** 56 0N 40 0 E
Sobo-Yama, *Japan* .. **72 E3** 32 51N 131 22 E
Sobol, *Russia* ..... **55 H3** 50 54N 16 44 E
Sobra, *Croatia* ..... **45 F14** 42 44N 17 34 E
Sobradinho, Reprêsa
  de, *Brazil* ...... **170 C3** 9 30 S 42 0W
Sobral, *Brazil* ..... **170 B3** 3 50 S 40 20W
Sobrance, *Slovak Rep.* **35 C15** 48 45N 22 11 E
Sobreira Formosa,
  Portugal **42 F3** 39 46N 7 51W
Soc Giang, *Vietnam* . **76 F6** 22 54N 106 1 E
Soc Trang, *Vietnam* . **87 H5** 9 37N 105 50 E
Soča ➔, *Europe* .... **34 E6** 46 20N 13 40 E
Socastee, *U.S.A.* **149 J6** 33 41N 79 1W
Sochaczew, *Poland* .. **55 F7** 52 15N 20 13 E
Soch'e = Shache, *China* **61 J4** 43 35N 39 40 E
Sochi, *Russia* ..... **61 J4** 43 35N 39 40 E
Social Circle, *U.S.A.* . **152 B6** 33 39N 83 43W
Société, Îs. de la,
  French Polynesia ... **135 J12** 17 0 S 151 0W
Society Hill, *U.S.A.* .. **152 C4** 32 26N 85 27W
Society Is. = Société, Îs.
  de la,
  French Polynesia ... **135 J12** 17 0 S 151 0W
Socompa, Portezuelo
  de, *Chile* .... **174 A2** 24 27 S 68 18W
Socorro = Fronteiras,
  Brazil .... **170 C3** 7 5 S 40 37W
Socorro, *Colombia* .. **168 B3** 6 29N 73 16W
Socorro, *Phil.* ..... **81 G5** 9 37N 125 58 E
Socorro, N. Mex.,
  U.S.A. **159 J10** 34 4N 106 54W
Socorro, *Tex., U.S.A.* . **159 L10** 31 39N 106 18W
Socorro, I., *Mexico* .. **162 D2** 18 45N 110 58W
Socotra, *Yemen* ... **99 D6** 12 30N 54 0 E
Socovos, *Spain* **41 G3** 38 20N 1 58W
Socuéllamos, *Spain* . **41 F2** 39 16N 2 47W
Soda Plains, *India* .. **93 B8** 35 30N 79 0 E
Soda Springs, *U.S.A.* . **158 E8** 42 39N 111 36W
Sodankylä, *Finland* .. **14 C22** 67 29N 26 40 E
Soddy-Daisy, *U.S.A.* . **149 H3** 35 17N 85 10W
Söderala, *Sweden* ... **16 C10** 61 17N 16 55 E
Södersen ➔, *Sweden* . **17 H7** 56 13N 13 3 E
Söderbärke, *Sweden* . **16 D9** 60 16N 15 20 E
Söderfors, *Sweden* .. **16 D11** 60 23N 17 25 E
Söderhamn, *Sweden* . **16 C11** 61 18N 17 10 E
Söderköping, *Sweden* . **17 F10** 58 31N 16 35 E
Södermanland, *Sweden* **16 F11** 58 56N 16 55 E
Södermanlands län □,
  Sweden .... **15 G17** 58 56N 16 55 E
Södertälje, *Sweden* .. **16 E11** 59 12N 17 39 E
Sodiri, *Sudan* ..... **107 E2** 14 27N 29 0 E
Sodo, *Ethiopia* ..... **107 F4** 7 0N 37 41 E
Södra Dellen, *Sweden* **16 C10** 61 48N 16 43 E
Södra Finnskoga,
  Sweden .... **16 D6** 60 42N 12 34 E
Södra Sandby, *Sweden* **17 J7** 55 43N 13 21 E
Södra Ulvön, *Sweden* **16 B12** 62 59N 18 38 E
Södra Vi, *Sweden* ... **17 G9** 57 45N 15 45 E
Sodražica, *Slovenia* .. **45 C11** 45 45N 14 39 E
Sodus, *U.S.A.* **150 C7** 43 14N 77 4W
Sodwana Bay △,
  S. Africa .... **117 D5** 27 35 S 32 43 E
Soekmekaar, *S. Africa* **117 C4** 23 30 S 29 55 E
Soest, *Germany* .... **30 D4** 51 34N 8 7 E
Soest, *Neths.* ...... **24 B5** 52 9N 5 19 E
Sofádhes, *Greece* ... **38 B4** 39 20N 22 4 E
Sofala □, *Mozam.* ... **117 B5** 19 30 S 34 30 E
Sofara, *Mali* **112 C4** 13 59N 4 9W
Sofia = Sofiya, *Bulgaria* **50 D7** 42 45N 23 20 E
Sofia ➔, *Madag.* .... **117 B8** 15 27 S 47 23 E
Sofievka, *Ukraine* ... **59 H7** 48 1N 33 9 E
Sofikón, *Greece* .... **50 D7** 37 47N 23 3 E
Sofiya, *Bulgaria* .... **50 D7** 42 45N 23 20 E
Sofiya ✕ (SOF),
  Bulgaria .... **50 D7** 42 46N 23 28 E
Sofievka = Volnansk,
  Ukraine .... **59 H8** 48 25N 35 29 E
Sōfu-Gan, *Japan* ... **71 K10** 29 49N 140 21 E
Sogakofe, *Ghana* ... **113 D5** 6 2N 0 39 E
Sogamoso, *Colombia* **168 B3** 5 43N 72 56W
Sogār, *Iran* .... **97 E8** 25 53N 58 6 E
Sögel, *Germany* .... **30 C3** 52 51N 7 31 E
Sogeri, *Papua N. G.* . **132 E4** 9 26 S 147 35 E
Sogndalsfjøra,
  Norway .... **18 C3** 61 40N 6 45 E
Søgne, *Norway* ..... **18 F4** 58 5N 7 48 E
Sognefjorden, *Norway* **18 C2** 61 10N 5 50 E
Sogod, *Phil.* ...... **81 F5** 10 28N 124 59 E
Söğüt, Bilecik, *Turkey* **49 D11** 37 2N 29 12 E
Söğüt, Burdur, *Turkey* **49 D11** 37 2N 29 12 E
Söğüt Dağı, *Turkey* .. **49 E10** 36 40N 28 3 E
Söğütköy, *Turkey* ... **75 H14** 33 5N 130 3 E
Sögwipo, *S. Korea* .. **59 J7** 47 2N 32 49 E
Soh, *Iran* .... **97 C6** 33 26N 51 27 E
Sohâg, *Egypt* ..... **106 B3** 26 33N 31 43 E

Sohagpur, *India* **92 H8** 22 42N 78 12 E
Sohano, *Papua N. G.* **132 C8** 5 22 S 154 37 E
Sohela, *India* **94 D6** 21 18N 83 24 E
Sŏhori, *N. Korea* **75 D15** 40 7N 128 23 E
Soignies, *Belgium* **24 D4** 50 35N 4 5 E
Soin, *Burkina Faso* **112 C4** 12 47N 3 50W
Soira, *Eritrea* **107 E4** 14 45N 39 30 E
Soissons, *France* **27 C10** 49 25N 3 19 E
Sōja, *Japan* **72 C5** 34 40N 133 45 E
Sojat, *India* **92 G5** 25 55N 73 45 E
Sok →, *Russia* **60 D10** 53 24N 50 8 E
Sokal, *Ukraine* **59 G3** 50 31N 24 15 E
Söke, *Turkey* **49 D9** 37 48N 27 28 E
Sokelo, *Dem. Rep. of the Congo* **119 D1** 9 55 S 24 36 E
Sokh, *Uzbekistan* **65 D5** 39 56N 71 9 E
Sokhós, *Greece* **50 F7** 40 48N 23 22 E
Sokhumi, *Georgia* **61 J5** 43 0N 41 0 E
Sokki, Oued In →, *Algeria* **111 C5** 29 30N 3 42 E
Sokna, *Norway* **18 D6** 60 16N 9 58 E
Soknedal, *Norway* **18 B7** 62 57N 10 13 E
Soko Banja, *Serbia & M.* **50 C5** 43 40N 21 51 E
Soko Islands, *China* **69 G10** 22 10N 113 54 E
Sokodé, *Togo* **113 D5** 9 0N 1 11 E
Sokol, *Russia* **58 C11** 59 30N 40 5 E
Sokolac, *Bos.-H.* **52 G3** 43 56N 18 48 E
Sokółka, *Poland* **54 E10** 53 25N 23 30 E
Sokolo, *Ségou, Mali* **112 C3** 14 53N 6 8W
Sokolo, *Sikasso, Mali* **112 C3** 10 52N 6 59W
Sokolov, *Czech Rep.* **34 A5** 50 12N 12 40 E
Sokołów Małpolski, *Poland* **55 H9** 50 12N 22 7 E
Sokołów Podlaski, *Poland* **55 F9** 52 25N 22 15 E
Sokoły, *Poland* **55 F9** 52 59N 22 42 E
Sokoto, *Nigeria* **113 C6** 13 2N 5 16 E
Sokoto □, *Nigeria* **113 C6** 12 30N 6 0 E
Sokoto →, *Nigeria* **113 C5** 11 20N 4 10 E
Sokuluk, *Kyrgyzstan* **65 B7** 42 52N 74 18 E
Sokyrnytsya, *Ukraine* **53 B8** 48 7N 23 23 E
Sokyryany, *Ukraine* **53 B12** 48 27N 27 25 E
Sol Iletsk, *Russia* **64 F5** 51 10N 55 0 E
Sola, *Norway* **18 F2** 58 53N 5 36 E
Sola, *Vanuatu* **133 C5** 13 51 S 167 33 E
Sola →, *Poland* **55 H6** 50 4N 19 15 E
Solai, *Kenya* **118 B4** 0 2N 36 12 E
Solan, *India* **92 D7** 30 55N 77 7 E
Solana, *Phil.* **80 C3** 17 39N 121 41 E
Solander I., *N.Z.* **131 G1** 46 34 S 166 54 E
Solano, *Phil.* **80 C3** 16 31N 121 15 E
Solapur, *India* **94 F2** 17 43N 75 56 E
Solca, *Romania* **53 C10** 47 40N 25 50 E
Solda Gölü, *Turkey* **49 D11** 37 33N 29 42 E
Soldănești, *Moldova* **53 C13** 47 49N 28 48 E
Soldeu, *Andorra* **40 C6** 42 35N 1 40 E
Soldin = Myślibórz, *Poland* **55 F1** 52 55N 14 50 E
Soldotna, *U.S.A.* **144 F10** 60 29N 151 3W
Soléa, *Cyprus* **39 E9** 35 5N 33 4 E
Solec Kujawski, *Poland* **55 E5** 53 5N 18 14 E
Soledad, *Colombia* **168 A3** 10 55N 74 46W
Soledad, *U.S.A.* **160 J5** 36 26N 121 20W
Soledad, *Venezuela* **169 B5** 8 10N 63 34W
Søllen, *Norway* **18 C8** 61 53N 11 31 E
Solent, The, *U.K.* **21 G6** 50 45N 1 25W
Solenzara, *France* **29 G13** 41 53N 9 23 E
Solesmes, *France* **27 B10** 50 10N 3 30 E
Solfonn, *Norway* **18 D3** 60 2N 6 57 E
Solhan, *Turkey* **101 C9** 38 57N 41 3 E
Sølheim, *Norway* **18 D2** 60 53N 5 27 E
Soligalich, *Russia* **56 C7** 59 5N 42 10 E
Soligorsk = Salihorsk, *Belarus* **59 F4** 52 51N 27 27 E
Solihull, *U.K.* **21 E6** 52 26N 1 47W
Solikamsk, *Russia* **64 B6** 59 38N 56 50 E
Solila, *Madag.* **117 C8** 21 25 S 46 37 E
Solimões = Amazonas →, *S. Amer.* **169 D7** 0 5 S 50 0W
Solin, *Croatia* **45 E13** 43 33N 16 30 E
Solingen, *Germany* **30 D3** 51 10N 7 5 E
Sollebrunn, *Sweden* **17 F6** 58 8N 12 32 E
Sollefteå, *Sweden* **16 A11** 63 12N 17 20 E
Sollentuna, *Sweden* **16 E11** 59 26N 17 56 E
Sóller, *Spain* **38 B3** 39 46N 2 43 E
Sollerön, *Sweden* **16 D8** 60 55N 14 37 E
Solling, *Germany* **30 D5** 51 42N 9 38 E
Solling-Vogler ⌓, *Germany* **30 D5** 51 45N 9 32 E
Solnechnogorsk, *Russia* **58 D9** 56 10N 36 57 E
Solo →, *Indonesia* **79 G15** 6 47 S 112 22 E
Solofra, *Italy* **47 B7** 40 50N 14 51 E
Sologne, *France* **27 E8** 47 40N 1 45 E
Solok, *Indonesia* **84 C2** 0 45 S 100 40 E
Sololá, *Guatemala* **164 D1** 14 49N 91 10W
Solomon, N. Fork →, *U.S.A.* **154 F5** 39 29N 98 26W
Solomon, S. Fork →, *U.S.A.* **154 F5** 39 25N 99 12W
Solomon Is., *Papua N. G.* **132 D8** 6 0 S 155 0 E
Solomon Is. ■, *Pac. Oc.* **133 L8** 6 0 S 155 0 E
Solomon Sea, *Papua N. G.* **132 D6** 7 0 S 150 0 E
Solon, *China* **69 B7** 46 32N 121 10 E
Solon Springs, *U.S.A.* **154 B9** 46 22N 91 49W
Solonópole, *Brazil* **170 C4** 5 44 S 39 1W
Solor, *Indonesia* **82 C2** 8 27 S 123 0 E
Solotcha, *Russia* **58 E10** 54 48N 39 53 E
Solothurn, *Switz.* **32 B5** 47 13N 7 32 E
Solothurn □, *Switz.* **32 B5** 47 18N 7 40 E
Solotvyn, *Ukraine* **53 B9** 48 42N 24 25 E
Solsona, *Spain* **40 C6** 42 0N 1 31 E
Solsvik, *Norway* **18 D1** 60 26N 4 58 E
Solt, *Hungary* **52 D4** 46 45N 19 1 E
Šolta, *Croatia* **45 E13** 43 24N 16 15 E
Solṭānābād, *Khorāsān, Iran* **97 C8** 34 13N 59 58 E
Solṭānābād, *Khorāsān, Iran* **97 B8** 36 29N 58 5 E
Soltau, *Germany* **30 C5** 52 59N 9 50 E
Soltsy, *Russia* **58 C6** 58 10N 30 30 E
Solund, *Norway* **18 C1** 61 5N 4 50 E
Solunska Glava, *Macedonia* **50 E5** 41 44N 21 31 E
Solvang, *U.S.A.* **161 L6** 34 36N 120 8W
Solvay, *U.S.A.* **151 C8** 43 3N 76 13W
Sölvesborg, *Sweden* **17 H8** 56 5N 14 35 E
Solvychegodsk, *Russia* **56 B8** 61 21N 46 56 E
Solway Firth, *U.K.* **22 D4** 54 49N 3 35W
Solwezi, *Zambia* **119 E2** 12 11 S 26 21 E
Sōma, *Japan* **70 F10** 37 40N 140 50 E
Soma, *Turkey* **49 B9** 39 10N 27 35 E
Somabhula, *Zimbabwe* **117 B4** 19 42 S 29 40 E
Somali = Sumale □, *Ethiopia* **120 C2** 7 0N 45 0 E
Somali Basin, *Ind. Oc.* **121 D4** 3 0N 53 0 E
Somali Pen., *Africa* **104 F8** 7 0N 46 0 E
Somali Rep. ■, *Africa* **120 C3** 7 0N 47 0 E
Somalia = Somali Rep. ■, *Africa* **120 C3** 7 0N 47 0 E
Sombe Dzong, *Bhutan* **90 B2** 27 13N 89 8 E
Sombernon, *France* **27 E11** 47 20N 4 40 E
Sombo, *Angola* **115 D4** 8 42 S 20 59 E
Sombor, *Serbia & M.* **52 E4** 45 46N 19 9 E
Sombra, *Canada* **150 D2** 42 43N 82 29W
Sombrerete, *Mexico* **162 C4** 23 40N 103 40W
Sombrero, *Anguilla* **165 C7** 18 37N 63 30W
Sombrero Channel, *India* **95 L11** 7 41N 93 35 E
Şomcuta Mare, *Romania* **53 C8** 47 31N 23 28 E
Somdari, *India* **92 G5** 25 47N 72 38 E
Someido ⌓, *Spain* **42 B4** 43 5N 6 11W
Somers, *U.S.A.* **158 B6** 48 5N 114 13W
Somerset, *Bermuda* **9 a** 32 17N 64 52W
Somerset, *Ky., U.S.A.* **148 G3** 37 5N 84 36W
Somerset, *Mass., U.S.A.* **151 E13** 41 47N 71 8W
Somerset, *Pa., U.S.A.* **150 F5** 40 1N 79 5W
Somerset □, *U.K.* **21 F5** 51 9N 3 0W
Somerset East, *S. Africa* **116 E4** 32 42 S 25 35 E
Somerset I., *Bermuda* **9 a** 32 17N 64 52W
Somerset I., *Canada* **138 A10** 73 30N 93 0W
Somerset West, *S. Africa* **116 E2** 34 8 S 18 50 E
Somersworth, *U.S.A.* **151 C14** 43 16N 70 52W
Somerton, *U.S.A.* **159 K6** 32 36N 114 43W
Somerville, *U.S.A.* **151 F10** 40 35N 74 38W
Someş →, *Romania* **52 C7** 47 49N 22 43 E
Someşul Mare →, *Romania* **53 C8** 47 9N 23 55 E
Somme □, *France* **27 C9** 49 57N 2 20 E
Somme →, *France* **27 B8** 50 11N 1 38 E
Somme, B. de la, *France* **26 B8** 50 14N 1 33 E
Sommen, *Jönköping, Sweden* **17 F8** 58 12N 14 58 E
Sommen, *Östergötland, Sweden* **17 F9** 58 0N 15 15 E
Sommepy-Tahure, *France* **27 C11** 49 15N 4 31 E
Sömmerda, *Germany* **30 D7** 51 9N 11 7 E
Sommerfeld = Lubsko, *Poland* **55 G1** 51 45N 14 57 E
Sommesous, *France* **27 D11** 48 44N 4 12 E
Sommières, *France* **29 E8** 43 47N 4 6 E
Somnath, *India* **92 J4** 20 53N 70 22 E
Somogy □, *Hungary* **52 D2** 46 19N 17 30 E
Somogyszob, *Hungary* **52 D2** 46 18N 17 20 E
Somosomo, *Fiji* **133 A3** 16 47 S 179 58W
Somosomo Str., *Fiji* **133 A3** 16 0 S 180 0 E
Somoto, *Nic.* **164 D2** 13 28N 86 37W
Sompolno, *Poland* **55 F5** 52 26N 18 30 E
Somport, Puerto de, *Spain* **40 C4** 42 48N 0 31W
Somuncurá, Meseta de, *Argentina* **176 B3** 41 30 S 67 0W
Somvarpet, *India* **95 H2** 12 36N 75 52 E
Son, *Norway* **18 E7** 59 32N 10 42 E
Son →, *India* **93 G11** 25 42N 84 52 E
Son Ha, *Vietnam* **86 E7** 15 3N 108 34 E
Son Hoa, *Vietnam* **86 F7** 13 2N 108 58 E
Son La, *Vietnam* **76 G4** 21 20N 103 50 E
Son Serra, *Spain* **38 B4** 39 43N 3 13 E
Son Servera, *Spain* **38 B4** 39 37N 3 21 E
Son Tay, *Vietnam* **76 G5** 21 8N 105 30 E
Soná, *Panama* **164 E3** 8 0N 81 20W
Sonamarg, *India* **93 B6** 34 18N 75 21 E
Sonamukhi, *India* **93 H12** 23 18N 87 27 E
Sonamura, *India* **93 H12** 23 18N 87 27 E
Sonar →, *India* **93 G8** 24 24N 79 56 E
Sŏnch'ŏn, *N. Korea* **75 E13** 39 48N 124 55 E
Sondags →, *S. Africa* **116 E4** 33 44 S 25 51 E
Sóndalo, *Italy* **44 B7** 46 20N 10 19 E
Sondar, *India* **93 C6** 33 28N 75 56 E
Søndeled, *Norway* **18 F6** 58 46N 9 3 E
Sønder Felding, *Denmark* **17 J2** 55 57N 8 47 E
Sønder Omme, *Denmark* **17 J2** 55 50N 8 54 E
Sønderborg, *Denmark* **17 K3** 54 55N 9 49 E
Sønderjyllands Amtskommune □, *Denmark* **17 J3** 55 10N 9 10 E
Sondershausen, *Germany* **30 D6** 51 22N 10 51 E
Sondre Bergenhaus = Hordaland □, *Norway* **18 D3** 60 25N 6 15 E
Søndre Strømfjord = Kangerlussuaq, *Greenland* **10 D5** 66 59N 50 40W
Søndre Trøndhjem = Sør-Trøndelag □, *Norway* **18 A7** 63 0N 11 0 E
Sóndrio, *Italy* **44 B6** 46 10N 9 52 E
Sondur →, *India* **94 D6** 20 40N 82 1 E
Sone, *Mozam.* **119 F3** 17 23 S 34 55 E
Sonepur, *India* **94 D6** 20 55N 83 50 E
Sonfim, *Brazil* **172 B4** 6 0 S 67 52W
Song, *Nigeria* **113 D7** 9 49N 12 39 E
Song, *Thailand* **86 C3** 18 28N 100 11 E
Song Cau, *Vietnam* **86 F7** 13 27N 109 18 E
Song-Köl, *Kyrgyzstan* **65 C7** 41 50N 75 12 E
Song Xian, *China* **74 G7** 34 12N 112 8 E
Songadh, *India* **94 D1** 21 9N 73 33 E
Songan, *Indonesia* **79 J18** 8 13 S 115 24 E
Songavatnet, *Norway* **18 E4** 59 52N 7 32 E
Songch'ŏn, *N. Korea* **75 E14** 39 12N 126 15 E
Songea, *Tanzania* **119 E4** 10 40 S 35 40 E
Songeons, *France* **27 C8** 49 32N 1 50 E
Songgang, *China* **69 F10** 22 46N 113 50 E
Songhua Hu, *China* **75 C14** 43 35N 126 50 E
Songhua Jiang →, *China* **69 B8** 47 45N 132 30 E
Songimvelo ⌓, *S. Africa* **117 D5** 25 50 S 31 2 E
Songjiang, *China* **77 B13** 31 1N 121 12 E
Sŏngjin = Kimch'aek, *N. Korea* **75 D15** 40 40N 129 10 E
Songjin, *N. Korea* **75 D15** 40 40N 129 10 E
Songjŏng-ni, *S. Korea* **75 G14** 35 8N 126 47 E
Songkan, *China* **76 C6** 28 35N 106 52 E
Songkhla, *Thailand* **87 J3** 7 13N 100 37 E
Songming, *China* **76 E4** 25 12N 103 2 E
Songnam, *S. Korea* **57 F14** 37 25N 127 10 E
Songnim, *N. Korea* **75 E13** 38 45N 125 39 E
Songo, *Angola* **115 D2** 7 22 S 14 51 E
Songololo = Mbanza Ngungu, *Dem. Rep. of the Congo* **115 D2** 5 12 S 14 53 E
Songololo, *Dem. Rep. of the Congo* **115 D2** 5 42 S 14 2 E
Songpan, *China* **76 A4** 32 40N 103 30 E
Songtao, *China* **76 C7** 28 11N 109 10 E
Songwe, *Dem. Rep. of the Congo* **118 C2** 3 20 S 26 16 E
Songwe →, *Africa* **119 D3** 9 44 S 33 58 E
Songxi, *China* **77 D12** 27 31N 118 44 E
Songzi, *China* **77 B8** 30 12N 111 45 E
Sonhat, *India* **93 H10** 23 29N 82 31 E
Sonid Youqi, *China* **74 C7** 42 45N 112 48 E
Sonipat, *India* **92 E7** 29 0N 77 5 E
Sonkach, *India* **92 H7** 22 59N 76 21 E
Sonkovo, *Russia* **58 D9** 57 50N 37 5 E
Sonmiani, *Pakistan* **91 D2** 25 25N 66 40 E
Sonmiani B., *Pakistan* **92 G2** 25 15N 66 30 E
Sonnino, *Italy* **46 A6** 41 25N 13 14 E
Sono →, *Minas Gerais, Brazil* **171 E2** 17 2 S 45 32W
Sono →, *Tocantins, Brazil* **170 C2** 9 58 S 48 11W
Sonobe, *Japan* **73 B7** 35 6N 135 28 E
Sonogno, *Switz.* **33 D7** 46 22N 8 47 E
Sonoma, *U.S.A.* **160 G4** 38 18N 122 28W
Sonora, *Calif., U.S.A.* **160 H6** 37 59N 120 23W
Sonora, *Tex., U.S.A.* **155 K4** 30 34N 100 39W
Sonora □, *Mexico* **162 B2** 29 0N 111 0W
Sonora →, *Mexico* **162 B2** 28 50N 111 33W
Sonoran Desert, *U.S.A.* **161 L12** 33 40N 114 15W
Sonoyta, *Mexico* **162 A2** 31 51N 112 50W
Sonqor, *Iran* **101 E12** 34 47N 47 36 E
Sŏnsan, *S. Korea* **75 F15** 36 14N 128 17 E
Sonseca, *Spain* **43 F7** 39 42N 3 57W
Sonsón, *Colombia* **168 B2** 5 43N 75 18W
Sonsonate, *El Salv.* **164 D2** 13 43N 89 44W
Sonstorp, *Sweden* **17 F9** 58 44N 15 38 E
Sonthofen, *Germany* **31 H6** 47 30N 10 16 E
Soochow = Suzhou, *China* **77 B13** 31 19N 120 38 E
Sooke, *Canada* **160 B3** 48 13N 123 43W
Soomaaliya = Somali Rep. ■, *Africa* **120 C3** 7 0N 47 0 E
Sop Hao, *Laos* **76 G5** 20 33N 104 27 E
Sop Prap, *Thailand* **86 D2** 17 53N 99 20 E
Sopachuy, *Bolivia* **173 D5** 19 29 S 64 31W
Sopchoppy, *U.S.A.* **152 E5** 30 4N 84 29W
Sopelana, *Spain* **40 B2** 43 23N 2 58W
Soperton, *U.S.A.* **152 C7** 32 23N 82 35W
Sopi, *Indonesia* **82 A3** 2 34N 128 28 E
Sopo, Nahr →, *Sudan* **107 F2** 8 40N 26 30 E
Sopot, *Bulgaria* **51 D8** 42 39N 24 45 E
Sopot, *Poland* **54 D5** 54 27N 18 31 E
Sopot, *Serbia & M.* **50 B4** 44 29N 20 36 E
Sopotnica, *Macedonia* **50 E5** 41 18N 21 13 E
Sopron, *Hungary* **52 C1** 47 45N 16 32 E
Sopur, *India* **93 B6** 34 18N 74 27 E
Sør-Rondane, *Antarctica* **7 D4** 72 0 S 25 0 E
Sør-Trøndelag □, *Norway* **18 A7** 63 0N 11 0 E
Sora, *Italy* **45 G10** 41 43N 13 37 E
Sorab, *India* **95 G2** 14 23N 75 6 E
Sorada, *India* **94 E7** 19 45N 84 26 E
Sorah, *Pakistan* **92 F3** 27 13N 68 56 E
Soråker, *Sweden* **16 B11** 62 30N 17 32 E
Sorano, *Italy* **45 F8** 42 41N 11 43 E
Soraon, *India* **93 G9** 25 37N 81 51 E
Sorata, *Bolivia* **172 D4** 15 50 S 68 40W
Sorbas, *Spain* **41 H2** 37 6N 2 7W
Sörbygden, *Sweden* **16 B10** 62 48N 16 12 E
Sore, *France* **28 D3** 44 18N 0 35W
Sorel-Tracy, *Canada* **140 C5** 46 0N 73 10W
Sörenberg, *Switz.* **32 C6** 46 50N 8 2 E
Soresina, *Italy* **44 C6** 45 17N 9 51 E
Sørfjorden, *Norway* **18 D3** 60 20N 6 37 E
Sörforsa, *Sweden* **16 C10** 61 43N 16 58 E
Sórgono, *Italy* **46 B2** 40 1N 9 6 E
Sorgues, *France* **29 D8** 44 1N 4 53 E
Sorgun, *Turkey* **100 C6** 39 46N 35 11 E
Sori, *Papua N. G.* **132 A4** 1 58 S 146 42 E
Soria, *Spain* **40 D2** 41 43N 2 32W
Soria □, *Spain* **40 D2** 41 46N 2 28W
Soriano, *Uruguay* **174 C4** 33 24 S 58 19W
Soriano nel Cimino, *Italy* **45 F9** 42 25N 12 14 E
Sorkh, Kuh-e, *Iran* **97 C8** 35 40N 58 30 E
Sorø, *Denmark* **17 J5** 55 26N 11 32 E
Soro, *Guinea* **112 C3** 10 9N 9 48W
Soroca, *Moldova* **53 B13** 48 8N 28 12 E
Sorocaba, *Brazil* **175 A6** 23 31 S 47 27W
Sorochinsk, *Russia* **64 E4** 52 26N 53 10 E
Soroka = Belomorsk, *Russia* **56 B5** 64 35N 34 54 E
Soroki = Soroca, *Moldova* **53 B13** 48 8N 28 12 E
Sorokino = Krasnodon, *Ukraine* **59 H10** 48 17N 39 44 E
Sorong, *Indonesia* **83 B4** 0 55 S 131 15 E
Soroní, *Greece* **38 E12** 36 21N 28 1 E
Soroti, *Uganda* **118 B3** 1 43N 33 35 E
Sørøya, *Norway* **14 A20** 70 40N 22 30 E
Sørøyane, *Norway* **18 B2** 62 25N 5 32 E
Sørøysundet, *Norway* **14 A20** 70 25N 23 0 E
Sorraia →, *Portugal* **43 G2** 38 55N 8 53W
Sorrell, *Australia* **127 G4** 42 47 S 147 34 E
Sorrento, *Italy* **47 B7** 40 37N 14 22 E
Sorsele, *Sweden* **14 D17** 65 31N 17 30 E
Sörsjön, *Sweden* **16 C7** 61 24N 13 5 E
Sorso, *Italy* **46 B1** 40 48N 8 34 E
Sorsogon, *Phil.* **80 E5** 13 0N 124 0 E
Sorsogon □, *Phil.* **80 E4** 12 50N 123 55 E
Sortavala, *Russia* **58 B6** 61 42N 30 41 E
Sortino, *Italy* **47 E8** 37 9N 15 2 E
Sortland, *Norway* **14 B16** 68 42N 15 25 E
Sørum, *Norway* **18 D7** 60 30N 10 17 E
Sørvika, *Norway* **18 B8** 62 25N 11 54 E
Sorvizhi, *Russia* **60 B9** 57 52N 48 32 E
Sos del Rey Católico, *Spain* **40 C3** 42 30N 1 13W
Sŏsan, *S. Korea* **75 F14** 36 47N 126 27 E
Sosaq, *Kazakhstan* **65 A4** 44 9N 68 27 E
Soscumica, L., *Canada* **140 B4** 50 15N 77 27W
Sösdala, *Sweden* **17 H7** 56 2N 13 41 E
Sosna →, *Russia* **59 F10** 52 42N 38 55 E
Sosnogorsk, *Russia* **56 B9** 63 37N 53 51 E
Sosnovka, *Kyrgyzstan* **65 B6** 42 40N 73 50 E
Sosnovka, *Kirov, Russia* **60 B10** 56 17N 51 17 E
Sosnovka, *Tambov, Russia* **60 D5** 53 13N 41 24 E
Sosnovy Bor, *Russia* **58 C5** 59 55N 29 6 E
Sosnowiec, *Poland* **55 H6** 50 20N 19 10 E
Sosnowitz = Sosnowiec, *Poland* **55 H6** 50 20N 19 10 E
Soso, *C.A.R.* **114 B3** 3 55N 15 30 E
Sospel, *France* **29 E11** 43 52N 7 27 E
Sossus Vlei, *Namibia* **116 C2** 24 40 S 15 23 E
Šoštanj, *Slovenia* **45 B12** 46 23N 15 4 E
Sŏsura, *N. Korea* **75 C16** 42 16N 130 36 E
Sosva, *Russia* **64 B8** 59 10N 61 50 E
Sosva →, *Russia* **64 B9** 59 21N 62 23 E
Sosvinsky Zavod = Sosva, *Russia* **64 B8** 59 10N 61 50 E
Sot →, *India* **93 F8** 27 27N 79 37 E
Sotaseter, *Norway* **18 C4** 61 49N 7 43 E
Sotavento, *C. Verde Is.* **9 j** 15 0N 25 0W
Sotkamo, *Finland* **14 D23** 64 8N 28 23 E
Soto del Barco, *Spain* **42 B4** 43 32N 6 4W
Soto la Marina →, *Mexico* **163 C5** 23 40N 97 40W
Soto y Amío, *Spain* **42 C5** 42 46N 5 53W
Sotrondio, *Spain* **42 B5** 43 17N 5 36W
Sotuf, Adrar, *W. Sahara* **110 D1** 21 42N 15 36W
Sotuta, *Mexico* **163 C7** 20 29N 89 43W
Souanké, *Congo* **114 B2** 2 10N 14 3 E
Soubré, *Ivory C.* **112 D3** 5 50N 6 35W
Souderton, *U.S.A.* **151 F9** 40 19N 75 19W
Soúdha, *Greece* **39 E5** 35 29N 24 4 E
Soúdhas, Kólpos, *Greece* **39 E5** 35 25N 24 10 E
Soufflay, *Congo* **114 B2** 2 1N 14 54 E
Souflíon, *Greece* **51 E10** 41 12N 26 18 E
Soufrière, *Guadeloupe* **164 b** 16 5N 61 40W
Soufrière, *St. Lucia* **165 f** 13 51N 61 3W
Soufrière Bay, *Dominica* **165 f** 13 53N 61 6W
Souillac, *France* **28 D5** 44 53N 1 29 E
Souilly, *France* **27 C12** 49 3N 5 17 E
Souk-Ahras, *Algeria* **111 A6** 36 23N 7 57 E
Souk el Arba du Rharb, *Morocco* **110 B3** 34 43N 5 59W
Soukhouma, *Laos* **86 E5** 14 38N 105 48 E
Sŏul, *S. Korea* **75 F14** 37 31N 126 58 E
Soulac-sur-Mer, *France* **28 C2** 45 30N 1 7W
Soulári, *Greece* **39 C1** 38 10N 20 25 E
Soulougou, *Burkina Faso* **113 C5** 13 1N 0 25 E
Soultz-sous-Forêts, *France* **27 D14** 48 57N 7 52 E
Sound, The = Øresund, *Europe* **17 J6** 55 45N 12 45 E
Sound, The, *U.K.* **21 G3** 50 20N 4 10W
Sound I., *India* **95 H11** 12 58N 92 59 E
Soúnion, Ákra, *Greece* **48 D6** 37 37N 24 1 E
Sour el Ghozlane, *Algeria* **111 A5** 36 10N 3 45 E
Sources, Mt. aux, *Lesotho* **117 D4** 28 45 S 28 50 E
Soure, *Brazil* **170 B2** 0 35 S 48 30W
Soure, *Portugal* **42 E2** 40 4N 8 38W
Souris, *Man., Canada* **143 D8** 49 40N 100 20W
Souris, *P.E.I., Canada* **141 C7** 46 21N 62 15W
Souris →, *Canada* **154 A4** 49 40N 99 34W
Sourou →, *Africa* **112 C4** 12 45N 3 25W
Soúrpi, *Greece* **48 B4** 39 6N 22 54 E
Sous, O. →, *Morocco* **110 B3** 30 27N 9 31W
Sousa, *Brazil* **170 C4** 6 45 S 38 10W
Sousel, *Brazil* **170 B1** 2 38 S 52 29W
Sousel, *Portugal* **43 G3** 38 57N 7 40W
Souss-Massa △, *Morocco* **110 B3** 31 26N 9 35W
Sousse, *Tunisia* **108 A2** 35 50N 10 38 E
Soustons, *France* **28 E2** 43 45N 1 19W
Sout →, *S. Africa* **116 E2** 31 35 S 18 24 E
South Africa ■, *Africa* **116 E3** 32 0 S 23 0 E
South America **166 E5** 10 0 S 60 0W
South Andaman, *India* **95 J11** 11 45N 92 10 E
South Atlantic Ocean **8 J10** 20 0 S 10 0W
South Aulatsivik I., *Canada* **141 A7** 56 45N 61 30W
South Australia □, *Australia* **128 B3** 32 0 S 139 0 E
South Ayrshire □, *U.K.* **22 F4** 55 18N 4 41W
South Baldy, *U.S.A.* **159 J10** 34 6N 107 11W
South Bass I., *U.S.A.* **150 E2** 41 38N 82 53W
South Bay, *U.S.A.* **153 J9** 26 40N 80 43W
South Beach, *Bahamas* **9 b** 25 1N 77 20W
South Beloit, *U.S.A.* **156 B7** 42 29N 89 2W
South Bend, *Ind., U.S.A.* **157 C10** 41 41N 86 15W
South Bend, *Wash., U.S.A.* **160 D3** 46 40N 123 48W
South Boston, *U.S.A.* **149 G6** 36 42N 78 54W
South Branch, *Canada* **141 C8** 47 55N 59 2W
South Brook, *Canada* **141 C8** 49 26N 56 5W
South Brother I., *India* **95 J11** 10 56N 92 37 E
South C. = Ka Lae, *U.S.A.* **145 E6** 18 55N 155 41W
South Carolina □, *U.S.A.* **149 J5** 34 0N 81 0W
South Charleston, *U.S.A.* **148 F5** 38 22N 81 44W
South China Sea, *Asia* **80 D2** 10 0N 113 0 E
South Comino Channel, *Malta* **38 F7** 36 0N 14 20 E
South Congaree, *U.S.A.* **152 B8** 33 53N 81 9W
South Cotabato □, *Phil.* **81 J5** 6 0N 125 0 E
South Cumberland Is. △, *Australia* **126 J7** 20 42 S 149 11 E
South Dakota □, *U.S.A.* **154 C5** 44 15N 100 0W
South Daytona, *U.S.A.* **153 F8** 29 10N 81 0W
South Deerfield, *U.S.A.* **151 D12** 42 29N 72 37W
South Downs, *U.K.* **21 G7** 50 52N 0 25W
South East B., *Ascension I.* **9 g** 7 57 S 14 18W
South East C., *Australia* **127 G4** 43 40 S 146 50 E
South East Forests △, *Australia* **129 D8** 37 0 S 149 30 E
South-East Indian Rise, *Ind. Oc.* **7 B10** 43 0 S 80 0 E
South East Is., *Australia* **125 F3** 34 17 S 123 30 E
South Elgin, *U.S.A.* **157 C8** 42 0N 88 18W
South Esk →, *U.K.* **22 E6** 56 43N 2 31W
South Foreland, *U.K.* **21 F9** 51 8N 1 24 E
South Fork American →, *U.S.A.* **160 G5** 38 45N 121 5W
South Fork Edisto →, *U.S.A.* **152 B9** 33 16N 80 54W
South Fork Feather →, *U.S.A.* **160 F5** 39 17N 121 36W
South Fork Grand →, *U.S.A.* **154 C3** 45 43N 102 17W
South Fork Licking →, *U.S.A.* **157 F12** 38 40N 84 18W
South Fork Republican →, *U.S.A.* **154 E4** 40 3N 101 31W
South Georgia, *Antarctica* **7 B1** 54 30 S 37 0W
South Gloucestershire □, *U.K.* **21 F5** 51 32N 2 28W
South Grand →, *U.S.A.* **156 F3** 38 17N 93 25W
South Hadley, *U.S.A.* **151 D12** 42 16N 72 35W
South Haven, *U.S.A.* **157 B10** 42 24N 86 16W
South Henik L., *Canada* **143 A9** 61 30N 97 20W
South Honshu Ridge, *Pac. Oc.* **134 E6** 23 0N 143 0 E
South Horr, *Kenya* **118 B4** 2 12N 36 56 E
South I., *India* **95 J1** 10 3N 72 17 E
South I., *Kenya* **118 B4** 2 35N 36 35 E
South I., *N.Z.* **131 E5** 44 0 S 170 0 E
South Indian Lake, *Canada* **143 B9** 56 47N 98 56W
South Invercargill, *N.Z.* **131 G3** 46 26 S 168 23 E
South Island △, *Kenya* **118 B4** 2 39N 36 35 E
South Kitui ⌓, *Kenya* **118 C4** 1 48 S 38 46 E
South Knife →, *Canada* **143 B10** 58 55N 94 37W
South Koel →, *India* **93 H11** 22 32N 85 14 E
South Korea ■, *Asia* **75 G15** 36 0N 128 0 E
South Lake Tahoe, *U.S.A.* **160 G6** 38 57N 119 59W
South Lanarkshire □, *U.K.* **22 F5** 55 37N 3 53W
South Loup →, *U.S.A.* **154 E5** 41 4N 98 39W
South Luangwa △, *Zambia* **119 E3** 13 0 S 31 20 E
South Lyon, *U.S.A.* **157 B13** 42 28N 83 39W
South Magnetic Pole, *Antarctica* **7 C9** 64 8 S 138 8 E
South Miami, *U.S.A.* **153 K9** 25 42N 80 18W
South Milwaukee, *U.S.A.* **157 B9** 42 55N 87 52W
South Molton, *U.K.* **21 F4** 51 1N 3 51W
South Monroe, *U.S.A.* **157 C13** 41 54N 83 26W
South Moose L., *Canada* **143 C8** 53 46N 100 8W
South Nahanni →, *Canada* **142 A4** 61 3N 123 21W
South Nation →, *Canada* **151 A9** 45 34N 75 6W
South Natuna Is. = Natuna Selatan, Kepulauan, *Indonesia* **85 B3** 2 45N 109 0 E
South Negril Pt., *Jamaica* **164 a** 18 16N 78 22W
South Newport, *U.S.A.* **152 D8** 31 38N 81 24W
South Orkney Is., *Antarctica* **7 C18** 63 0 S 45 0W
South Ossetia □, *Georgia* **61 J7** 42 21N 44 2 E
South Pagai, I. = Pagai Selatan, Pulau, *Indonesia* **84 C2** 3 0 S 100 15 E
South Paris, *U.S.A.* **151 B14** 44 14N 70 31W
South Pekin, *U.S.A.* **156 D7** 40 30N 89 39W
South Pittsburg, *U.S.A.* **149 H3** 35 1N 85 42W
South Platte →, *U.S.A.* **154 E4** 41 7N 100 42W
South Pole, *Antarctica* **7 E** 90 0 S 0 0W
South Ponte Vedra Beach, *U.S.A.* **152 E8** 30 3N 81 20W
South Porcupine, *Canada* **140 C3** 48 30N 81 12W
South Portland, *U.S.A.* **149 D10** 43 38N 70 15W
South Pt., *Ascension I.* **9 g** 8 0 S 14 24W
South Pt., *Barbados* **165 g** 13 2N 59 32W
South Pt., *U.S.A.* **150 B1** 44 52N 83 19W
South River, *Canada* **140 C4** 45 52N 79 23W
South River, *U.S.A.* **151 F10** 40 27N 74 23W
South Ronaldsay, *U.K.* **22 C6** 58 48N 2 58W
South Sandwich Is., *Antarctica* **7 B1** 57 0 S 27 0W
South Sandwich Trench, *Atl. Oc.* **8 M9** 56 0 S 24 0W
South Saskatchewan →, *Canada* **143 C7** 53 15N 105 5W
South Seal →, *Canada* **143 B9** 58 48N 98 8W
South Sentinel I., *India* **95 J11** 10 59N 92 14 E
South Shetland Is., *Antarctica* **7 C18** 62 0 S 59 0W
South Shields, *U.K.* **20 C6** 55 0N 1 25W
South Sioux City, *U.S.A.* **154 D6** 42 28N 96 24W
South Taranaki Bight, *N.Z.* **130 F3** 39 40 S 174 5 E
South Thompson →, *Canada* **142 C4** 50 40N 120 20W
South Twin I., *Canada* **140 B4** 53 7N 79 52W
South Tyne →, *U.K.* **20 C5** 54 59N 2 8W
South Ubian, *Phil.* **81 J3** 5 11N 120 30 E
South Uist, *U.K.* **22 D1** 57 20N 7 15W
South Valley, *U.S.A.* **159 J10** 35 1N 106 41W
South Venice, *U.S.A.* **153 H7** 27 3N 82 25W
South Wayne, *U.S.A.* **156 B7** 42 34N 89 53W
South West Africa = Namibia ■, *Africa* **116 C2** 22 0 S 18 9 E
South West B., *Ascension I.* **9 g** 7 58 S 14 25W
South West B., *Bahamas* **9 b** 25 0N 77 32W
South West C., *Australia* **127 G4** 43 34 S 146 3 E
South West C., *N.Z.* **131 H2** 47 17 S 167 28 E
South West Pt., *Papua N. G.* **132 B4** 2 14 S 146 34 E
South West Pt., *St. Helena* **9 h** 15 59 S 5 48W
South West Rocks, *Australia* **129 A10** 30 52 S 153 3 E
South Whitley, *U.S.A.* **157 C11** 41 5N 85 38W
South Williamsport, *U.S.A.* **150 E8** 41 13N 77 0W
South Yarmouth, *U.S.A.* **148 E10** 41 40N 70 10W
South Yemen = Yemen ■, *Asia* **98 D4** 15 0N 44 0 E
South Yorkshire □, *U.K.* **20 D6** 53 27N 1 36W
Southampton, *Canada* **140 D3** 44 30N 81 25W
Southampton, *U.K.* **21 G6** 50 54N 1 23W
Southampton, *U.S.A.* **151 F12** 40 53N 72 23W
Southampton □, *U.K.* **21 G6** 50 54N 1 23W
Southampton I., *Canada* **139 B11** 64 30N 84 0W
Southaven, *U.S.A.* **155 H9** 34 59N 90 2W
Southbank, *Canada* **142 C3** 54 2N 125 46W
Southbridge, *N.Z.* **131 D7** 43 48 S 172 16 E
Southbridge, *U.S.A.* **151 D12** 42 5N 72 2W
Southeast C., *U.S.A.* **144 E5** 62 56N 169 39W
Southeast Pacific Basin, *Pac. Oc.* **7 C15** 16 30 S 92 0W
Southend, *Canada* **143 B8** 56 19N 103 22W
Southend-on-Sea, *U.K.* **21 F8** 51 32N 0 44 E
Southend-on-Sea □, *U.K.* **21 F8** 51 32N 0 44 E
Southern = Janub △, *Sudan* **107 F2** 6 50N 28 45 E
Southern = Yedebub Biheroch Bihereseboch na Hizboch □, *Ethiopia* **107 F4** 12 0N 36 0 E
Southern = Yuzhnyy □, *Russia* **61 H5** 44 0N 40 0 E
Southern □, *Malawi* **119 F4** 15 0 S 35 0 E
Southern □, *S. Leone* **112 D2** 8 0N 12 30W
Southern □, *Zambia* **119 F2** 16 20 S 26 20 E
Southern Alps, *N.Z.* **131 D5** 43 41 S 170 11 E
Southern Cross, *Australia* **125 F2** 31 12 S 119 15 E
Southern Highlands □, *Papua N. G.* **132 D2** 6 15 S 143 25 E
Southern Indian L., *Canada* **143 B9** 57 10N 98 30W
Southern Lau Group, *Fiji* **133 B3** 18 40 S 178 40W
Southern Leyte □, *Phil.* **81 F5** 10 30N 125 10 E
Southern Mid-Atlantic Ridge, *Atl. Oc.* **8 J10** 21 0 S 13 0W
Southern Ocean, *Antarctica* **7 C6** 62 0 S 60 0 E
Southern Pines, *U.S.A.* **149 H6** 35 11N 79 24W
Southern Rhodesia = Zimbabwe ■, *Africa* **119 F3** 19 0 S 30 0 E
Southern Uplands, *U.K.* **22 F5** 55 28N 3 52W
Southfield, *U.S.A.* **157 B13** 42 29N 83 17W
Southington, *U.S.A.* **151 E12** 41 36N 72 53W
Southland □, *N.Z.* **131 F3** 45 30 S 168 0 E
Southold, *U.S.A.* **151 E12** 41 4N 72 26W
Southport, *Australia* **127 D5** 27 58 S 153 25 E
Southport, *U.K.* **20 D4** 53 39N 3 0W
Southport, *Fla., U.S.A.* **152 E4** 30 17N 85 38W
Southport, *N.Y., U.S.A.* **150 D8** 42 3N 76 49W
Southwest △, *Australia* **127 G4** 43 8 S 146 5 E

Southwest Indian Ridge, *Ind. Oc.* **121 H4** 30 0 S 59 0 E
Southwest Pacific Basin, *Pac. Oc.* **135 L13** 40 0 S 140 0W
Southwestern Pacific Basin, *Pac. Oc.* **7 A12** 42 0 S 170 0W
Southwold, *U.K.* **21 E9** 52 20N 1 41 E
Southwood △, *Australia* **127 D5** 27 48 S 150 8 E
Soutpansberg, *S. Africa* **117 C4** 23 0 S 29 30 E
Souvigny, *France* **27 F10** 46 33N 3 10 E
Sovata, *Romania* **53 D10** 46 35N 25 3 E
Soverato, *Italy* **47 D9** 38 41N 16 33 E
Sovet, *Kyrgyzstan* **65 C5** 40 11N 71 20 E
Sovetsk, *Kaliningrad, Russia* **15 J19** 55 6N 21 50 E
Sovetsk, *Kirov, Russia* **60 B9** 57 38N 48 53 E
Sovetskaya Gavan = Vanino, *Russia* **67 E15** 48 50N 140 5 E
Sovetskoye = Zelenokumsk, *Russia* **61 H6** 44 24N 44 0 E
Sovicille, *Italy* **45 E8** 43 17N 11 13 E
Søvik, *Norway* **18 B3** 62 33N 6 17 E
Soweto, *S. Africa* **117 D4** 26 14 S 27 54 E
Sōya-Kaikyō = La Perouse Str., *Asia* **70 B11** 45 40N 142 0 E
Sōya-Misaki, *Japan* **70 B10** 45 30N 141 55 E
Soyaux, *France* **28 C4** 45 39N 0 12 E
Soyo, *Angola* **115 D2** 6 13 S 12 20 E
Sozh →, *Belarus* **59 F6** 51 57N 30 48 E
Sozopol, *Bulgaria* **51 D11** 42 23N 27 42 E
Spa, *Belgium* **24 D5** 50 29N 5 53 E
Spaccaforno = Íspica, *Italy* **47 F7** 36 47N 14 55 E
Spain ■, *Europe* **13 H5** 39 0N 4 0W
Spalato = Split, *Croatia* **45 E13** 43 31N 16 26 E
Spalding, *Australia* **128 B3** 33 30 S 138 37 E
Spalding, *U.K.* **20 E7** 52 48N 0 9W
Spangler, *U.S.A.* **150 F6** 40 39N 78 48W
Spanish, *Canada* **140 C3** 46 12N 82 20W
Spanish Fork, *U.S.A.* **158 F8** 40 7N 111 39W
Spanish Pt., *Bermuda* **9 a** 32 18N 64 49W
Spanish Town, *Br. Virgin Is.* **165 e** 17 43N 64 26W
Spanish Town, *Jamaica* **164 a** 18 0N 76 57W
Sparks, *Ga., U.S.A.* **152 D6** 31 11N 83 26W
Sparks, *Nev., U.S.A.* **160 F7** 39 32N 119 45W
Sparreholm, *Sweden* **16 E10** 59 4N 16 49 E
Sparta = Spárti, *Greece* **48 D4** 37 5N 22 25 E
Sparta, *Ga., U.S.A.* **152 B7** 33 17N 82 58W
Sparta, *Ill., U.S.A.* **156 F7** 38 8N 89 42W
Sparta, *Mich., U.S.A.* **157 A11** 43 10N 85 42W
Sparta, *N.J., U.S.A.* **151 E10** 41 2N 74 38W
Sparta, *Wis., U.S.A.* **154 D9** 43 56N 90 49W
Spartanburg, *U.S.A.* **149 H5** 34 56N 81 57W
Spartansburg, *U.S.A.* **150 E5** 41 49N 79 41W
Spartel, C., *Morocco* **110 A3** 35 47N 5 56W
Spárti, *Greece* **48 D4** 37 5N 22 25 E
Spartivento, C., *Calabria, Italy* **47 E9** 37 55N 16 4 E
Spartivento, C., *Sard., Italy* **46 D1** 38 53N 8 50 E
Spartokhóri, *Greece* **39 B2** 38 40N 20 46 E
Sparwood, *Canada* **142 D6** 49 44N 114 53W
Spas-Demensk, *Russia* **58 E7** 54 20N 34 0 E
Spas-Klepiki, *Russia* **58 E11** 55 10N 40 10 E
Spassk = Bednodemyanovsk, *Russia* **60 D6** 53 55N 43 15 E
Spassk Dalniy, *Russia* **67 E14** 44 40N 132 48 E
Spassk-Ryazanskiy, *Russia* **58 E11** 54 24N 40 25 E
Spátha, Ákra, *Greece* **39 E4** 35 42N 23 43 E
Spatsizi →, *Canada* **142 B3** 57 42N 128 7W
Spatsizi Plateau Wilderness △, *Canada* **142 B3** 57 40N 128 0W
Spean →, *U.K.* **22 E4** 56 55N 4 59W
Spearfish, *U.S.A.* **154 C3** 44 30N 103 52W
Spearman, *U.S.A.* **155 G4** 36 12N 101 12W
Speculator, *U.S.A.* **151 C10** 43 30N 74 25W
Speed, *Australia* **128 C5** 35 21 S 142 27 E
Speedway, *U.S.A.* **157 E10** 39 47N 86 15W
Speer, *Switz.* **33 B8** 47 12N 9 8 E
Speery I., *St. Helena* **9 h** 16 1 S 5 46W
Speia, *Moldova* **53 D14** 46 59N 29 19 E
Speightstown, *Barbados* **165 g** 13 15N 59 39W
Speke Gulf, *Tanzania* **118 C3** 2 20 S 32 50 E
Spello, *Italy* **45 F9** 42 59N 12 40 E
Spenard, *U.S.A.* **144 F10** 61 11N 149 55W
Spence Bay = Taloyoak, *Canada* **138 B10** 69 32N 93 32W
Spencer, *Idaho, U.S.A.* **158 D7** 44 22N 112 11W
Spencer, *Ind., U.S.A.* **157 E10** 39 17N 86 46W
Spencer, *Iowa, U.S.A.* **154 D7** 43 9N 95 9W
Spencer, *N.Y., U.S.A.* **151 D8** 42 13N 76 30W
Spencer, *Nebr., U.S.A.* **154 D5** 42 53N 98 42W
Spencer, C., *Australia* **128 C2** 35 20 S 136 53 E
Spencer B., *Namibia* **116 D1** 25 30 S 14 47 E
Spencer G., *Australia* **128 C2** 34 0 S 137 20 E
Spencerville, *Canada* **151 B9** 44 51N 75 33W
Spencerville, *U.S.A.* **157 D12** 40 43N 84 21W
Spences Bridge, *Canada* **142 C4** 50 25N 121 20W
Spennymoor, *U.K.* **20 C6** 54 42N 1 36W
Spenser Mts., *N.Z.* **131 C7** 42 15 S 172 45 E
Spentrup, *Denmark* **17 H4** 56 33N 10 2 E
Sperillen, *Norway* **18 D7** 60 28N 10 3 E
Sperkhiós →, *Greece* **48 C4** 38 57N 22 3 E
Sperrin Mts., *U.K.* **23 B5** 54 50N 7 0W
Spessart, *Germany* **31 F5** 49 56N 9 18 E
Spetalen, *Norway* **18 E7** 59 18N 10 45 E
Spétsai, *Greece* **48 D5** 37 15N 23 10 E
Spey →, *U.K.* **22 D5** 57 40N 3 6W
Speyer, *Germany* **31 F4** 49 29N 8 25 E
Spezand, *Pakistan* **92 E2** 29 59N 67 0 E
Spezzano Albanese, *Italy* **47 C9** 39 40N 16 19 E
Spickard, *U.S.A.* **156 D3** 40 14N 93 36W
Spiekeroog, *Germany* **30 B3** 53 46N 7 42 E
Spiez, *Switz.* **32 C5** 46 40N 7 40 E
Spili, *Greece* **39 E5** 35 13N 24 31 E
Spilimbergo, *Italy* **45 B9** 46 7N 12 54 E
Spīn Būldak, *Afghan.* **91 D5** 31 1N 66 25 E
Spinalónga, *Greece* **39 E6** 35 18N 25 44 E
Spinazzola, *Italy* **47 B9** 40 58N 16 5 E
Spineni, *Romania* **53 F9** 44 43N 24 37 E
Spirding = Śniardwy, Jezioro, *Poland* **54 E8** 53 48N 21 50 E
Spirit Lake, *U.S.A.* **160 D4** 46 15N 122 9W
Spirit River, *Canada* **142 B5** 55 45N 118 50W
Spiritwood, *Canada* **143 C7** 53 24N 107 33W
Spišská Nová Ves, *Slovak Rep.* **35 C13** 48 58N 20 34 E
Spišské Podhradie, *Slovak Rep.* **35 B13** 49 0N 20 48 E
Spital, *Austria* **34 D7** 47 42N 14 18 E
Spithead, *U.K.* **21 G6** 50 45N 1 10W
Spittal an der Drau, *Austria* **34 E6** 46 48N 13 31 E
Spitzbergen = Svalbard, *Arctic* **6 B8** 78 0N 17 0 E
Spjelkavik, *Norway* **18 B3** 62 28N 6 22 E
Split, *Croatia* **45 E13** 43 31N 16 26 E
Split ✕ (SPU), *Croatia* **45 E13** 43 33N 16 15 E
Split L., *Canada* **143 B9** 56 8N 96 15W
Split Lake, *Canada* **143 B9** 56 8N 96 15W
Splitski Kanal, *Croatia* **45 E13** 43 31N 16 20 E
Splügen, *Switz.* **33 C8** 46 34N 9 21 E
Splügenpass, *Switz.* **33 D8** 46 30N 9 20 E
Spofford, *U.S.A.* **155 L4** 29 10N 100 25W
Spokane, *U.S.A.* **158 C5** 47 40N 117 24W
Spoleto, *Italy* **45 F9** 42 44N 12 44 E
Sponvika, *Norway* **18 E8** 59 7N 11 15 E
Spoon →, *U.S.A.* **156 D6** 40 19N 90 4W
Spooner, *U.S.A.* **154 C9** 45 50N 91 53W
Sporyy Navolok, Mys, *Russia* **66 B7** 75 50N 68 40 E
Sprague, *U.S.A.* **158 C5** 47 18N 117 59W
Spratly I., *S. China Sea* **78 C4** 8 38N 111 55 E
Spratly Is., *S. China Sea* **78 C4** 8 20N 112 0 E
Spray, *U.S.A.* **158 D4** 44 50N 119 48W
Spreča →, *Bos.-H.* **52 F3** 44 44N 18 6 E
Spree →, *Germany* **30 C9** 52 32N 13 13 E
Spreewald, *Germany* **30 D9** 51 58N 13 51 E
Spremberg, *Germany* **30 D10** 51 34N 14 22 E
Sprengisandur, *Iceland* **11 B4** 64 52N 18 7W
Spring City, *U.S.A.* **151 F9** 40 11N 75 33W
Spring Cr. →, *U.S.A.* **152 E5** 30 54N 84 45W
Spring Creek, *U.S.A.* **158 F6** 40 45N 115 38W
Spring Garden, *Guyana* **169 B6** 6 59N 58 31W
Spring Garden, *U.S.A.* **160 F6** 39 52N 120 47W
Spring Green, *U.S.A.* **156 A6** 43 11N 90 4W
Spring Hall, *Barbados* **165 g** 13 18N 59 36W
Spring Hill, *Ala., U.S.A.* **152 D4** 31 42N 85 58W
Spring Hill, *Fla., U.S.A.* **153 G7** 28 27N 82 41W
Spring Mts., *U.S.A.* **159 H6** 36 0N 115 45W
Spring Valley, *Calif., U.S.A.* **161 N10** 32 45N 117 5W
Spring Valley, *Ill., U.S.A.* **156 C7** 41 20N 89 12W
Springbok, *S. Africa* **116 D2** 29 42 S 17 54 E
Springboro, *U.S.A.* **150 E4** 41 48N 80 22W
Springdale, *Canada* **141 C8** 49 30N 56 6W
Springdale, *Ark., U.S.A.* **155 G7** 36 11N 94 8W
Springdale, *Ohio, U.S.A.* **157 E12** 39 17N 84 29W
Springe, *Germany* **30 C5** 52 13N 9 33 E
Springer, *U.S.A.* **155 G2** 36 22N 104 36W
Springerville, *U.S.A.* **159 J9** 34 8N 109 17W
Springfield, *Canada* **150 D4** 42 50N 80 56W
Springfield, *N.Z.* **131 D6** 43 19 S 171 56 E
Springfield, *Colo., U.S.A.* **155 G3** 37 24N 102 37W
Springfield, *Fla., U.S.A.* **152 E4** 30 10N 85 37W
Springfield, *Ga., U.S.A.* **152 C8** 32 22N 81 18W
Springfield, *Ill., U.S.A.* **156 E7** 39 48N 89 39W
Springfield, *Ky., U.S.A.* **157 G11** 37 41N 85 13W
Springfield, *Mass., U.S.A.* **151 D12** 42 6N 72 35W
Springfield, *Mo., U.S.A.* **155 G8** 37 13N 93 17W
Springfield, *Ohio, U.S.A.* **157 E13** 39 55N 83 49W
Springfield, *Oreg., U.S.A.* **158 D2** 44 3N 123 1W
Springfield, *S.C., U.S.A.* **152 B8** 33 30N 81 17W
Springfield, *Tenn., U.S.A.* **149 G2** 36 31N 86 53W
Springfield, *Vt., U.S.A.* **151 C12** 43 18N 72 29W
Springfield, L., *U.S.A.* **156 E7** 39 46N 89 36W
Springfontein, *S. Africa* **116 E4** 30 15 S 25 40 E
Springhill, *Canada* **141 C7** 45 40N 64 4W
Springhill, *U.S.A.* **155 J8** 33 0N 93 28W
Springhouse, *Canada* **142 C4** 51 56N 122 7W
Springs, *S. Africa* **117 D4** 26 13 S 28 25 E
Springsure, *Australia* **126 C4** 24 8 S 148 6 E
Springvale, *Ga., U.S.A.* **152 D5** 31 50N 84 53W
Springvale, *Maine, U.S.A.* **151 C14** 43 28N 70 48W
Springville, *Calif., U.S.A.* **160 J8** 36 8N 118 49W
Springville, *Iowa, U.S.A.* **156 B5** 42 3N 91 27W
Springville, *N.Y., U.S.A.* **150 D6** 42 31N 78 40W
Springville, *Utah, U.S.A.* **158 F8** 40 10N 111 37W
Springwater, *U.S.A.* **150 D7** 42 38N 77 35W
Sprottau = Szprotawa, *Poland* **55 G2** 51 33N 15 35 E
Spruce-Creek, *U.S.A.* **150 F6** 40 36N 78 9W
Spruce Knob-Seneca Rocks △, *U.S.A.* **148 F6** 38 50N 79 30W
Spruce Mt., *U.S.A.* **151 B12** 44 12N 72 19W
Spur, *U.S.A.* **155 J4** 33 28N 100 52W
Spurn Hd., *U.K.* **20 D8** 53 35N 0 8 E
Spuž, *Serbia & M.* **50 D3** 42 32N 19 10 E
Spuzzum, *Canada* **142 D4** 49 37N 121 23W
Spydeberg, *Norway* **18 E8** 59 36N 11 5 E
Squam L., *U.S.A.* **151 C13** 43 45N 71 32W
Squamish, *Canada* **142 D4** 49 45N 123 10W
Square Islands, *Canada* **141 B8** 52 47N 55 47W
Squillace, G. di, *Italy* **47 D9** 38 45N 16 50 E
Squinzano, *Italy* **47 B11** 40 26N 18 2 E
Squires, Mt., *Australia* **125 E4** 26 14 S 127 28 E
Sragen, *Indonesia* **85 D4** 7 26 S 111 2 E
Srbac, *Bos.-H.* **52 E2** 45 7N 17 30 E
Srbica, *Serbia & M.* **50 D4** 42 45N 20 47 E
Srbija = Serbia □, *Serbia & M.* **50 C5** 43 30N 21 0 E
Srbobran, *Serbia & M.* **52 E4** 45 32N 19 48 E
Sre Ambel, *Cambodia* **87 G4** 11 8N 103 46 E
Sre Khtum, *Cambodia* **87 F6** 12 10N 106 52 E
Sre Umbell = Sre Ambel, *Cambodia* **87 G4** 11 8N 103 46 E
Srebrenica, *Bos.-H.* **52 F4** 44 6N 19 18 E
Sredinny Ra. = Sredinnyy Khrebet, *Russia* **67 D16** 57 0N 160 0 E
Sredinnyy Khrebet, *Russia* **67 D16** 57 0N 160 0 E
Središće, *Slovenia* **45 B13** 46 24N 16 17 E
Sredna Gora, *Bulgaria* **51 D8** 42 40N 24 20 E
Srednekolymsk, *Russia* **67 C16** 67 27N 153 40 E
Sredni Rodopi, *Bulgaria* **51 E8** 41 40N 24 45 E
Srednogorie, *Bulgaria* **51 D8** 42 43N 24 10 E
Śrem, *Poland* **55 F4** 52 6N 17 2 E
Sremska Mitrovica, *Serbia & M.* **52 F4** 44 59N 19 38 E
Sremski Karlovci, *Serbia & M.* **52 E4** 45 12N 19 56 E
Srepok →, *Cambodia* **86 F6** 13 33N 106 16 E
Sretensk, *Russia* **67 D12** 52 10N 117 40 E
Sri Aman, *Malaysia* **85 B4** 1 15N 111 32 E
Sri Kalahasti, *India* **95 H4** 13 45N 79 44 E
Sri Lanka ■, *Asia* **95 L5** 7 30N 80 50 E
Sriharikota I., *India* **95 H5** 13 40N 80 20 E
Srikakulam, *India* **94 E6** 18 14N 83 58 E
Srinagar, *India* **93 B6** 34 5N 74 50 E
Srinagarind Res., *Thailand* **86 E2** 14 35N 99 0 E
Sripur, *Bangla.* **90 C3** 24 14N 90 30 E
Srivardhan, *India* **94 E1** 18 4N 73 3 E
Srivilliputtur, *India* **95 K3** 9 31N 77 40 E
Środa Śląska, *Poland* **55 G3** 51 10N 16 36 E
Środa Wielkopolski, *Poland* **55 F4** 52 15N 17 19 E
Srono, *Indonesia* **79 J17** 8 24 S 114 16 E
Srpska Crnja, *Serbia & M.* **52 E5** 45 38N 20 44 E
Srpski Itebej, *Serbia & M.* **52 E5** 45 35N 20 44 E
Srungavarapukota, *India* **94 E6** 18 7N 83 10 E
Staaten →, *Australia* **126 B3** 16 24 S 141 17 E
Staaten River △, *Australia* **126 B3** 16 15 S 142 40 E
Staberhuk, *Germany* **30 A7** 54 23N 11 18 E
Stade, *Germany* **30 B5** 53 35N 9 29 E
Staðarfell, *Iceland* **11 B4** 65 7N 22 12W
Staðarhólskirkja, *Iceland* **11 B5** 65 23N 21 58W
Staðastaður, *Iceland* **11 C3** 64 49N 23 1W
Stadhavet, *Norway* **18 B3** 62 13N 5 0 E
Staður, *Húnavatnssýsla, Iceland* **11 B5** 65 9N 21 3W
Staður, *Ísafjarðarsýsla, Iceland* **11 A4** 66 15N 22 50W
Stadlandet, *Norway* **18 B2** 62 10N 5 10 E
Stadskanaal, *Neths.* **24 A6** 53 4N 6 55 E
Stadtallendorf, *Germany* **30 E5** 50 48N 9 1 E
Stadthagen, *Germany* **30 C5** 52 19N 9 13 E
Stadtlohn, *Germany* **30 D2** 51 59N 6 55 E
Stadtroda, *Germany* **30 E7** 50 52N 11 44 E
Stäfa, *Switz.* **33 B7** 47 14N 8 45 E
Stafafell, *Iceland* **11 C12** 64 25N 14 52W
Staffa, *U.K.* **22 E2** 56 27N 6 21W
Staffanstorp, *Sweden* **17 J7** 55 39N 13 13 E
Stafford, *U.K.* **20 E5** 52 49N 2 7W
Stafford, *U.S.A.* **155 G5** 37 58N 98 36W
Stafford, L., *U.S.A.* **153 F7** 29 20N 82 29W
Stafford Springs, *U.S.A.* **151 E12** 41 57N 72 18W
Staffordshire □, *U.K.* **20 E5** 52 53N 2 10W
Stagnone, *Italy* **46 E5** 37 53N 12 26 E
Stagnone di Marsala △, *Italy* **46 E5** 37 52N 12 26 E
Staines, *U.K.* **21 F7** 51 26N 0 29W
Stainz, *Austria* **34 E8** 46 53N 15 17 E
Stakhanov, *Ukraine* **59 H10** 48 35N 38 40 E
Stalać, *Serbia & M.* **50 C5** 43 43N 21 28 E
Stalden, *Switz.* **32 D5** 46 14N 7 52 E
Stalin = Kuçovë, *Albania* **50 F3** 40 47N 19 57 E
Stalin = Varna, *Bulgaria* **51 C11** 43 13N 27 56 E
Stalin, Pk. = Musala, *Bulgaria* **50 D7** 42 13N 23 37 E
Stalin Pk. = Gerlachovský štit, *Slovak Rep.* **35 B13** 49 11N 20 7 E
Stalin Pk. = Kommunizma, Pik, *Tajikistan* **65 D6** 39 0N 72 2 E
Stalinabad = Dushanbe, *Tajikistan* **65 D4** 38 33N 68 48 E
Stalingrad = Volgograd, *Russia* **61 F7** 48 40N 44 25 E
Staliniri = Tskhinvali, *Georgia* **61 J7** 42 14N 44 1 E
Stalino = Shakhrikhan, *Uzbekistan* **65 C6** 40 42N 72 3 E
Stalinogorsk = Novomoskovsk, *Russia* **58 E10** 54 5N 38 15 E
Stalinogrod = Katowice, *Poland* **55 H6** 50 17N 19 5 E
Stalinsk = Novokuznetsk, *Russia* **66 D9** 53 45N 87 10 E
Stalinstadt = Eisenhüttenstadt, *Germany* **30 C10** 52 9N 14 38 E
Stallarholmen, *Sweden* **16 E11** 59 22N 17 12 E
Ställdalen, *Sweden* **16 E8** 59 56N 14 56 E
Stalowa Wola, *Poland* **55 H9** 50 34N 22 3 E
Stalybridge, *U.K.* **20 D5** 53 28N 2 3W
Stamford, *Australia* **126 C3** 21 15 S 143 46 E
Stamford, *U.K.* **21 E7** 52 39N 0 29W
Stamford, *Conn., U.S.A.* **151 E11** 41 3N 73 32W
Stamford, *N.Y., U.S.A.* **151 D10** 42 25N 74 38W
Stamford, *Tex., U.S.A.* **155 J5** 32 57N 99 48W
Stamnes, *Norway* **18 D2** 60 40N 5 45 E
Stamping Ground, *U.S.A.* **157 F12** 38 16N 84 41W
Stampriet, *Namibia* **116 C2** 24 20 S 18 28 E
Stamps, *U.S.A.* **155 J8** 33 22N 93 30W
Stanberry, *U.S.A.* **156 D2** 40 13N 94 35W
Stančevo = Kalipetrovo, *Bulgaria* **51 B11** 44 5N 27 14 E
Standerton, *S. Africa* **117 D4** 26 55 S 29 7 E
Standish, *U.S.A.* **148 D4** 43 59N 83 57W
Stanford, *S. Africa* **116 E2** 34 26 S 19 29 E
Stanford, *U.S.A.* **158 C8** 47 9N 110 13W
Stånga, *Sweden* **17 G12** 57 17N 18 29 E
Stange, *Norway* **18 D8** 60 43N 11 5 E
Stanger, *S. Africa* **117 D5** 29 27 S 31 14 E
Stängselåsen = Salpausselkä, *Finland* **15 F22** 61 3N 26 15 E
Stangvik, *Norway* **18 B5** 62 55N 8 28 E
Stanhope, *Australia* **129 D6** 36 27 S 144 59 E
Stanhope, *U.S.A.* **156 B3** 42 17N 93 48W
Stanimaka = Asenovgrad, *Bulgaria* **51 D8** 42 1N 24 51 E
Stanišić, *Serbia & M.* **52 E4** 45 56N 19 10 E
Stanislaus →, *U.S.A.* **160 H5** 37 40N 121 14W
Stanislav = Ivano-Frankivsk, *Ukraine* **53 B9** 48 40N 24 40 E
Stanisławów = Ivano-Frankivsk, *Ukraine* **53 B9** 48 40N 24 40 E
Stanisławów, *Poland* **55 F8** 52 18N 21 33 E
Stanley, *Australia* **127 G4** 40 46 S 145 19 E
Stanley, *China* **69 G11** 22 13N 114 12 E
Stanley, *Falk. Is.* **9 f** 51 40 S 59 51W
Stanley, *U.K.* **20 C6** 54 53N 1 41W
Stanley, *Idaho, U.S.A.* **158 D6** 44 13N 114 56W
Stanley, *N. Dak., U.S.A.* **154 A3** 48 19N 102 23W
Stanley, *N.Y., U.S.A.* **150 D7** 42 48N 77 6W
Stanley Falls = Boyoma, Chutes, *Dem. Rep. of the Congo* **118 B2** 0 35N 25 23 E
Stanley Mission, *Canada* **143 B8** 55 25N 104 33W
Stanley Pool = Malebo, Pool, *Africa* **115 C3** 4 17 S 15 20 E
Stanley Res., *India* **95 J3** 11 50N 77 40 E
Stanleyville = Kisangani, *Dem. Rep. of the Congo* **118 B2** 0 35N 25 15 E
Stanovoy Khrebet, *Russia* **67 D13** 55 0N 130 0 E
Stanovoy Ra. = Stanovoy Khrebet, *Russia* **67 D13** 55 0N 130 0 E
Stans, *Switz.* **33 C6** 46 58N 8 21 E
Stansmore Ra., *Australia* **124 D4** 21 23 S 128 33 E
Stansted, London ✕ (STN), *U.K.* **21 F8** 51 54N 0 14 E
Stanthorpe, *Australia* **127 D5** 28 36 S 151 59 E
Stanton, *Ky., U.S.A.* **157 G13** 37 54N 83 52W
Stanton, *Tex., U.S.A.* **155 J4** 32 8N 101 48W
Stantsiya Regar = Tursunzade, *Tajikistan* **65 D4** 38 30N 68 14 E
Stanwood, *U.S.A.* **160 B4** 48 15N 122 23W
Staples, *U.S.A.* **154 B7** 46 21N 94 48W
Stapleton, *U.S.A.* **154 E4** 41 29N 100 31W
Stąporków, *Poland* **55 G7** 51 9N 20 31 E
Star City, *Canada* **143 C8** 52 50N 104 20W
Star Harbour, *Solomon Is.* **133 N12** 10 47 S 162 19 E
Star Lake, *U.S.A.* **151 B9** 44 10N 75 2W
Stará Ďala = Hurbanovo, *Slovak Rep.* **35 D11** 47 51N 18 11 E
Stará L'ubovňa, *Slovak Rep.* **35 B13** 49 18N 20 42 E
Stara Moravica, *Serbia & M.* **52 E4** 45 50N 19 30 E
Stara Pazova, *Serbia & M.* **52 F5** 44 58N 20 10 E
Stara Planina, *Bulgaria* **50 C7** 43 15N 23 0 E
Stara Sil, *Ukraine* **55 J9** 49 29N 22 58 E
Stará Turá, *Slovak Rep.* **35 C10** 48 47N 17 42 E
Stara Ushytsya, *Ukraine* **53 B12** 48 35N 27 8 E
Stara Zagora, *Bulgaria* **51 D9** 42 26N 25 39 E
Starachowice, *Poland* **55 G8** 51 3N 21 2 E
Staraya Russa, *Russia* **58 D6** 57 58N 31 23 E
Starbuck I., *Kiribati* **135 H12** 5 37 S 155 55W
Starchiojd, *Romania* **53 E11** 45 19N 26 11 E
Starcke △, *Australia* **126 A4** 14 56 S 145 2 E
Stargard in Pommern = Stargard Szczeciński, *Poland* **54 E2** 53 20N 15 0 E
Stargard Szczeciński, *Poland* **54 E2** 53 20N 15 0 E
Stårheim, *Norway* **18 C2** 61 56N 5 40 E
Stari Bar, *Serbia & M.* **50 D3** 42 7N 19 10 E
Stari Bečej = Bečej, *Serbia & M.* **52 E5** 45 36N 20 3 E
Stari Trg, *Slovenia* **45 C12** 45 29N 15 7 E
Staritsa, *Russia* **58 D8** 56 33N 34 55 E
Starke, *U.S.A.* **152 F7** 29 57N 82 7W
Starkville, *U.S.A.* **155 J10** 33 28N 88 49W
Starnberg, *Germany* **31 H7** 48 0N 11 21 E
Starnberger See, *Germany* **31 H7** 47 54N 11 19 E
Starobilsk, *Ukraine* **59 H10** 49 16N 39 0 E
Starodub, *Russia* **59 F7** 52 30N 32 50 E
Starogard Gdański, *Poland* **54 E5** 53 59N 18 30 E
Starokonstantinov = Starokonstyantyniv, *Ukraine* **59 H4** 49 48N 27 10 E
Starokonstyantyniv, *Ukraine* **59 H4** 49 48N 27 10 E
Starokozache, *Ukraine* **53 D14** 46 20N 29 59 E
Starominskaya, *Russia* **59 J10** 46 33N 39 0 E
Staroshcherbinovskaya, *Russia* **59 J10** 46 40N 38 53 E
Starrs Mill, *U.S.A.* **152 B5** 33 19N 84 31W
Start Pt., *U.K.* **21 G4** 50 13N 3 39W
Stary Chardzhuy = Komsomolsk, *Turkmenistan* **65 D1** 39 2N 63 36 E
Stary Sącz, *Poland* **55 J7** 49 33N 20 35 E
Staryy Biryuzyak, *Russia* **61 H8** 44 46N 46 50 E
Staryy Chartoriysk, *Ukraine* **59 G3** 51 15N 25 54 E
Staryy Krym, *Ukraine* **59 K8** 45 3N 35 8 E
Staryy Margilan = Margilan, *Uzbekistan* **65 C5** 40 27N 71 42 E
Staryy Oskol, *Russia* **59 G9** 51 19N 37 55 E
Staryy Sambir, *Ukraine* **55 J9** 49 27N 22 59 E
Stassfurt, *Germany* **30 D7** 51 51N 11 35 E
Staszów, *Poland* **55 H8** 50 33N 21 10 E
State Center, *U.S.A.* **156 B3** 42 1N 93 10W
State College, *U.S.A.* **150 F7** 40 48N 77 52W
Stateline, *U.S.A.* **160 G7** 38 57N 119 56W
Staten, I. = Estados, I. de Los, *Argentina* **176 D4** 54 40 S 64 30W
Staten I., *U.S.A.* **151 F10** 40 35N 74 9W
Statenville, *U.S.A.* **152 E6** 30 42N 83 2W
Statesboro, *U.S.A.* **152 C8** 32 27N 81 47W
Statesville, *U.S.A.* **149 H5** 35 47N 80 53W
Statham, *U.S.A.* **152 B6** 33 58N 83 35W
Stathelle, *Norway* **18 E6** 59 3N 9 41 E
Statia = St. Eustatius, *W. Indies* **165 C7** 17 20N 63 0W
Stauffer, *U.S.A.* **161 L7** 34 45N 119 3W
Staunton, *Ill., U.S.A.* **156 F7** 39 1N 89 47W
Staunton, *Va., U.S.A.* **148 F6** 38 9N 79 4W
Stavanger = Rogaland □, *Norway* **18 E3** 59 12N 6 20 E
Stavanger, *Norway* **18 F2** 58 57N 5 40 E
Stavelot, *Belgium* **24 D5** 50 23N 5 55 E
Stavern, *Norway* **18 F7** 59 0N 10 1 E
Stavoren, *Neths.* **24 B5** 52 53N 5 22 E
Stavropol, *Russia* **61 H6** 45 5N 42 0 E
Stavros, *Cyprus* **39 E8** 35 1N 32 38 E
Stavrós, *Ithaki, Greece* **39 C2** 38 27N 20 39 E
Stavrós, *Kriti, Greece* **39 E5** 35 12N 24 45 E
Stavrós, Ákra, *Greece* **39 E5** 35 26N 24 58 E
Stavroúpolis, *Greece* **51 E8** 41 12N 24 45 E
Stawell, *Australia* **128 D5** 37 5 S 142 47 E
Stawell →, *Australia* **126 C3** 20 20 S 142 55 E
Stawiski, *Poland* **54 E9** 53 22N 22 9 E
Stawiszyn, *Poland* **55 G5** 51 56N 18 4 E
Stayner, *Canada* **150 B4** 44 25N 80 5W
Stayton, *U.S.A.* **158 D2** 44 48N 122 48W
Steamboat Springs, *U.S.A.* **158 F10** 40 29N 106 50W
Steane, *Norway* **18 E5** 59 16N 8 33 E
Stebbins, *U.S.A.* **144 E7** 63 31N 162 17W
Steblevë, *Albania* **50 E4** 41 23N 20 33 E
Steckborn, *Switz.* **33 A7** 47 44N 8 59 E
Steele, *Ala., U.S.A.* **152 B3** 33 56N 86 12W
Steele, *N. Dak., U.S.A.* **154 B5** 46 51N 99 55W
Steelton, *U.S.A.* **150 F8** 40 14N 76 50W
Steelville, *U.S.A.* **156 G5** 37 58N 91 22W
Steen River, *Canada* **142 B5** 59 40N 117 12W
Steenkool = Bintuni, *Indonesia* **83 B4** 2 7 S 133 32 E
Steens Mt., *U.S.A.* **158 E4** 42 35N 118 40W
Steenstrup Gletscher, *Greenland* **10 B5** 75 15N 57 0W
Steenwijk, *Neths.* **24 B6** 52 47N 6 7 E
Steep Pt., *Australia* **125 E1** 26 8 S 113 8 E
Steep Rock, *Canada* **143 C9** 51 30N 98 48W
Ştefan Vodă, *Moldova* **53 D14** 46 27N 29 42 E
Ştefăneşti, *Romania* **53 C12** 47 44N 27 15 E
Stefanie L. = Chew Bahir, *Ethiopia* **107 G4** 4 40N 36 50 E
Stefanie L. △, *Ethiopia* **107 G4** 4 55N 36 55 E
Stefansson Bay, *Antarctica* **7 C5** 67 20 S 59 8 E
Steffisburg, *Switz.* **32 C5** 46 47N 7 38 E
Stege, *Denmark* **17 K6** 54 59N 12 18 E
Stegi = Siteki, *Swaziland* **117 D5** 26 32 S 31 58 E
Stegman = Artesia, *U.S.A.* **155 J2** 32 51N 104 24W
Ştei, *Romania* **52 D7** 46 32N 22 27 E
Steiermark □, *Austria* **34 D8** 47 26N 15 10 E
Steigerwald, *Germany* **31 F6** 49 44N 10 26 E
Steigerwald △, *Germany* **31 F6** 49 50N 10 30 E
Steilacoom, *U.S.A.* **160 C4** 47 10N 122 36W
Steilrandberge, *Namibia* **116 B1** 17 45 S 13 20 E
Stein = Kamnik, *Slovenia* **45 B11** 46 14N 14 37 E
Stein am Rhein, *Switz.* **33 A7** 47 39N 8 51 E
Steinbach, *Canada* **143 D9** 49 32N 96 40W
Steinfurt, *Germany* **30 C3** 52 9N 7 20 E
Steinhatchee, *U.S.A.* **152 F6** 29 40N 83 23W
Steinhausen, *Namibia* **116 C2** 21 49 S 18 20 E
Steinheim, *Germany* **30 D5** 51 51N 9 5 E
Steinhuder Meer, *Germany* **30 C5** 52 29N 9 21 E
Steinhuder Meer △, *Germany* **30 C5** 52 30N 9 16 E
Steinkjer, *Norway* **14 D14** 64 1N 11 31 E
Steinkopf, *S. Africa* **116 D2** 29 18 S 17 43 E
Steinshamn, *Norway* **18 B3** 62 47N 6 28 E
Steinwald △, *Germany* **31 F8** 49 55N 12 8 E
Stellarton, *Canada* **141 C7** 45 32N 62 30W
Stellenbosch, *S. Africa* **116 E2** 33 58 S 18 50 E
Stelvio, Paso dello, *Italy* **33 C10** 46 32N 10 27 E
Stenay, *France* **27 C12** 49 29N 5 12 E
Stendal, *Germany* **30 C7** 52 36N 11 53 E
Stende, *Latvia* **54 A9** 57 11N 22 33 E
Stenhamra, *Sweden* **16 E11** 59 20N 17 41 E
Stenón Ithákis, *Greece* **39 C2** 38 22N 20 39 E
Stenón Kerkiras, *Greece* **38 B10** 39 36N 20 5 E
Stenshuvud △, *Sweden* **17 J8** 55 39N 14 15 E
Stenstorp, *Sweden* **17 F7** 58 17N 13 45 E
Stenungsund, *Sweden* **17 F5** 58 6N 11 50 E
Steornabhaigh = Stornoway, *U.K.* **22 C2** 58 13N 6 23W
Stepanakert = Xankändi, *Azerbaijan* **101 C12** 39 52N 46 49 E
Stepanavan, *Armenia* **61 K7** 41 1N 44 23 E
Stephens, C., *N.Z.* **131 A8** 40 42 S 173 58 E
Stephens Creek, *Australia* **128 A4** 31 50 S 141 30 E
Stephens I., *Canada* **142 C2** 54 10N 130 45W
Stephens I., *N.Z.* **131 A9** 40 40 S 174 1 E
Stephens L., *Canada* **143 B9** 56 32N 95 0W
Stephenville, *Canada* **141 C8** 48 31N 58 35W
Stephenville, *U.S.A.* **155 J5** 32 13N 98 12W
Stepnica, *Poland* **54 E1** 53 38N 14 36 E
Stepnoi = Elista, *Russia* **61 G7** 46 16N 44 14 E
Stepnoye, *Russia* **64 D8** 54 4N 60 26 E
Steppe, *Asia* **62 D9** 50 0N 50 0 E
Stereá Ellas □, *Greece* **48 C4** 38 50N 23 0 E
Sterkstroom, *S. Africa* **116 E4** 31 32 S 26 32 E
Sterling, *Alaska, U.S.A.* **144 F10** 60 32N 150 46W
Sterling, *Colo., U.S.A.* **154 E3** 40 37N 103 13W
Sterling, *Ga., U.S.A.* **152 D8** 31 16N 81 34W
Sterling, *Ill., U.S.A.* **156 C7** 41 48N 89 42W
Sterling, *Kans., U.S.A.* **154 F5** 38 13N 98 12W
Sterling City, *U.S.A.* **155 K4** 31 51N 101 0W
Sterling Heights, *U.S.A.* **157 B13** 42 35N 83 0W
Sterling Run, *U.S.A.* **150 E6** 41 25N 78 12W
Sterlitamak, *Russia* **64 E6** 53 40N 56 0 E
Sternberg, *Germany* **30 B7** 53 42N 11 50 E
Šternberk, *Czech Rep.* **35 B10** 49 45N 17 15 E
Stérnes, *Greece* **39 E5** 35 30N 24 9 E
Sterzing = Vipiteno, *Italy* **45 B8** 46 54N 11 26 E
Stettin = Szczecin, *Poland* **54 E1** 53 27N 14 27 E
Stettiner Haff, *Germany* **30 B10** 53 47N 14 15 E
Stettler, *Canada* **142 C6** 52 19N 112 40W
Steubenville, *U.S.A.* **150 F4** 40 22N 80 37W
Stevenage, *U.K.* **21 F7** 51 55N 0 13W
Stevens Point, *U.S.A.* **154 C10** 44 31N 89 34W
Stevens Pottery, *U.S.A.* **152 C6** 32 57N 83 17W
Stevens Village, *U.S.A.* **144 C10** 66 1N 149 6W
Stevenson, *U.S.A.* **160 E5** 45 42N 121 53W
Stevenson, The →, *Australia* **127 D2** 27 6 S 135 33 E
Stevenson L., *Canada* **143 C9** 53 55N 96 0W
Stevensville, *U.S.A.* **158 C6** 46 30N 114 5W
Stevns Klint, *Denmark* **17 J6** 55 17N 12 28 E
Steward, *U.S.A.* **156 C7** 41 51N 89 1W
Stewardson, *U.S.A.* **157 F8** 39 16N 88 38W
Stewart, *Canada* **142 B3** 55 56N 129 57W
Stewart, *Ga., U.S.A.* **152 B6** 33 25N 83 52W
Stewart, *Nev., U.S.A.* **160 F7** 39 5N 119 46W
Stewart →, *Canada* **138 B6** 63 19N 139 26W
Stewart, C., *Australia* **126 A1** 11 57 S 134 56 E
Stewart, I., *Chile* **176 D2** 54 50 S 71 15W
Stewart I., *N.Z.* **131 G2** 46 58 S 167 54 E
Stewarts Point, *U.S.A.* **160 G3** 38 39N 123 24W
Stewartsville, *U.S.A.* **156 E2** 39 45N 94 30W
Stewartville, *U.S.A.* **154 D8** 43 51N 92 29W
Stewiacke, *Canada* **141 C7** 45 9N 63 22W
Steynsburg, *S. Africa* **116 E4** 31 15 S 25 49 E
Steyr, *Austria* **34 C7** 48 3N 14 25 E
Steyr →, *Austria* **34 C7** 48 3N 14 25 E
Steytlerville, *S. Africa* **116 E3** 33 17 S 24 19 E
Stia, *Italy* **45 E8** 43 48N 11 42 E
Stigler, *U.S.A.* **155 H7** 35 15N 95 8W
Stigliano, *Italy* **47 B9** 40 24N 16 14 E
Stigtomta, *Sweden* **17 F10** 58 47N 16 48 E
Stikine →, *Canada* **142 B2** 56 40N 132 30W
Stilfontein, *S. Africa* **116 D4** 26 51 S 26 50 E
Stilís, *Greece* **48 C4** 38 55N 22 47 E
Stillmore, *U.S.A.* **152 C7** 32 27N 82 13W
Stillwater, *Minn., U.S.A.* **147 A8** 45 3N 92 49W
Stillwater, *N.Y., U.S.A.* **151 D11** 42 55N 73 41W
Stillwater, *Okla., U.S.A.* **155 G6** 36 7N 97 4W
Stillwater Range, *U.S.A.* **158 G4** 39 50N 118 5W
Stillwater Reservoir, *U.S.A.* **151 C9** 43 54N 75 3W
Stilo, Pta., *Italy* **47 D9** 38 25N 16 35 E
Stilwell, *U.S.A.* **155 H7** 35 49N 94 38W
Stînga Nistrului □, *Moldova* **53 C14** 47 20N 29 15 E
Štip, *Macedonia* **50 E6** 41 42N 22 10 E
Stira, *Greece* **48 C6** 38 9N 24 14 E
Stirling, *Canada* **150 B7** 44 18N 77 33W
Stirling, *N.Z.* **131 G4** 46 14 S 169 49 E
Stirling, *U.K.* **22 E5** 56 8N 3 57W
Stirling □, *U.K.* **22 E4** 56 12N 4 18W
Stirling Ra., *Australia* **125 F2** 34 23 S 118 0 E
Stirling Range △, *Australia* **125 F2** 34 26 S 118 20 E
Stittsville, *Canada* **151 A9** 45 15N 75 55W
Stjernøya, *Norway* **14 A20** 70 20N 22 40 E
Stjørdalshalsen, *Norway* **18 A7** 63 29N 10 51 E
Stock Island, *U.S.A.* **153 L8** 24 32N 81 34W
Stockach, *Germany* **31 H5** 47 50N 9 1 E
Stockaryd, *Sweden* **17 G8** 57 19N 14 36 E
Stockbridge, *Ga., U.S.A.* **152 B5** 33 33N 84 14W

Stockbridge, *Mich., U.S.A.* **157 B12** 42 27N 84 11W
Stockerau, *Austria* **35 C9** 48 24N 16 12 E
Stockholm, *Sweden* **16 E12** 59 20N 18 3 E
Stockholm Arlanda ✈ (ARN), *Sweden* **16 E11** 59 41N 17 56 E
Stockholms län □, *Sweden* **16 E12** 59 30N 18 20 E
Stockhorn, *Switz.* **32 C5** 46 42N 7 33 E
Stockport, *U.K.* **20 D5** 53 25N 2 9W
Stocksbridge, *U.K.* **20 D6** 53 29N 1 35W
Stockton, *Calif., U.S.A.* **160 H5** 37 58N 121 17W
Stockton, *Ill., U.S.A.* **156 B6** 42 21N 90 1W
Stockton, *Kans., U.S.A.* **154 F5** 39 26N 99 16W
Stockton, *Mo., U.S.A.* **155 G8** 37 42N 93 48W
Stockton-on-Tees, *U.K.* **20 C6** 54 35N 1 19W
Stockton-on-Tees □, *U.K.* **20 C6** 54 35N 1 19W
Stockton Plateau, *U.S.A.* **155 K3** 30 30N 102 30W
Stoczek Łukowski, *Poland* **55 G8** 51 58N 21 58 E
Stöde, *Sweden* **16 B10** 62 28N 16 35 E
Stoeng Treng, *Cambodia* **86 F5** 13 31N 105 58 E
Stoer, Pt. of, *U.K.* **22 C3** 58 16N 5 23W
Stogovo, *Macedonia* **50 E4** 41 31N 20 38 E
Stoholm, *Denmark* **17 H3** 56 30N 9 8 E
Stoke, *N.Z.* **131 B8** 41 19 S 173 14 E
Stoke-on-Trent, *U.K.* **20 D5** 53 1N 2 11W
Stoke-on-Trent □, *U.K.* **20 D5** 53 1N 2 11W
Stokes △, *Australia* **125 E2** 29 55 S 115 6 E
Stokes Pt., *Australia* **127 G3** 40 10 S 143 56 E
Stokes Ra., *Australia* **124 C5** 15 50 S 130 50 E
Stokkseyri, *Iceland* **11 D5** 63 50N 21 2W
Stokksnes, *Iceland* **11 C12** 64 14N 14 58W
Stokmarknes, *Norway* **14 B16** 68 34N 14 54 E
Stolac, *Bos.-H.* **50 C1** 43 5N 17 59 E
Stolberg, *Germany* **30 E2** 50 47N 6 13 E
Stolbovoy, Ostrov, *Russia* **67 B14** 74 44N 135 14 E
Stolbtsy = Stowbtsy, *Belarus* **58 F4** 53 30N 26 43 E
Stolin, *Belarus* **59 G4** 51 53N 26 50 E
Stöllet, *Sweden* **16 D7** 60 26N 13 15 E
Stolnici, *Romania* **53 F9** 44 31N 24 48 E
Stolp = Słupsk, *Poland* **54 D4** 54 30N 17 3 E
Stolpmünde = Ustka, *Poland* **54 D3** 54 35N 16 55 E
Stomíon, *Greece* **39 E4** 35 21N 23 32 E
Ston, *Croatia* **45 F14** 42 51N 17 43 E
Stone, *U.K.* **20 E5** 52 55N 2 9W
Stone Mountain, *U.S.A.* **152 B5** 33 49N 84 10W
Stoneboro, *U.S.A.* **150 E4** 41 20N 80 7W
Stonehaven, *U.K.* **22 E6** 56 59N 2 12W
Stonehenge, *Australia* **126 C3** 24 22 S 143 17 E
Stonehenge, *U.K.* **21 F6** 51 9N 1 45W
Stonewall, *Canada* **143 C9** 50 10N 97 19W
Stongfjorden, *Norway* **18 C2** 61 26N 5 10 E
Stonington, *U.S.A.* **156 E7** 39 44N 89 12W
Stony L., *Man., Canada* **143 B9** 58 51N 98 40W
Stony L., *Ont., Canada* **150 B6** 44 30N 78 5W
Stony Point, *U.S.A.* **151 E11** 41 14N 73 59W
Stony Pt., *U.S.A.* **151 C8** 43 50N 76 18W
Stony Rapids, *Canada* **143 B7** 59 16N 105 50W
Stony River, *U.S.A.* **144 F8** 61 47N 156 35W
Stony Tunguska = Tunguska, Podkamennaya →, *Russia* **67 C10** 61 50N 90 13 E
Stonyford, *U.S.A.* **160 F4** 39 23N 122 33W
Stopnica, *Poland* **55 H7** 50 27N 20 57 E
Storå, *Sweden* **16 E9** 59 42N 15 6 E
Storå →, *Denmark* **17 H2** 56 20N 8 19 E
Stora Gla, *Sweden* **16 E6** 59 30N 12 30 E
Stora Le, *Sweden* **16 E5** 59 5N 11 55 E
Stora Lulevatten, *Sweden* **14 C18** 67 10N 19 30 E
Stóra-Vatnshorn, *Iceland* **11 B5** 65 4N 21 33W
Storavan, *Sweden* **14 D18** 65 45N 18 10 E
Stord, *Norway* **18 E2** 59 52N 5 23 E
Stordal, *Norway* **18 B4** 62 23N 7 0 E
Store Bælt, *Denmark* **17 J4** 55 20N 11 0 E
Store Heddinge, *Denmark* **17 J6** 55 18N 12 23 E
Store Jukleggi, *Norway* **18 C5** 61 3N 8 12 E
Store Koldewey, *Greenland* **10 B9** 76 30N 19 0W
Store Mosse △, *Sweden* **17 G7** 57 18N 13 55 E
Store Sølnkletten, *Norway* **18 C7** 61 59N 10 16 E
Store Sotra, *Norway* **18 D1** 60 18N 5 4 E
Storebro, *Sweden* **17 G9** 57 35N 15 52 E
Støren, *Norway* **18 A7** 63 3N 10 18 E
Storerikvollen, *Norway* **18 A8** 63 7N 11 58 E
Storfjellseter, *Norway* **18 C7** 61 40N 10 30 E
Storfjorden, *Norway* **18 B3** 62 28N 6 35 E
Storfors, *Sweden* **16 E8** 59 32N 14 17 E
Stóridalur, *Iceland* **11 D7** 63 38N 19 57W
Stórinúpur, *Iceland* **11 C6** 64 3N 20 10W
Storli, *Norway* **18 B6** 62 42N 9 5 E
Storlien, *Sweden* **16 A6** 63 19N 12 6 E
Storm B., *Australia* **127 G4** 43 10 S 147 30 E
Storm Lake, *U.S.A.* **154 D7** 42 39N 95 13W
Stormberge, *S. Africa* **116 E4** 31 16 S 26 17 E
Stormsrivier, *S. Africa* **116 E3** 33 59 S 23 52 E
Stornoway, *U.K.* **22 C2** 58 13N 6 23W
Storo, *Italy* **44 C7** 45 51N 10 35 E
Storozhinets = Storozhynets, *Ukraine* **53 B10** 48 14N 25 45 E
Storozhynets, *Ukraine* **53 B10** 48 14N 25 45 E
Storrs, *U.S.A.* **151 E12** 41 49N 72 15W
Storsjøen, *Hedmark, Norway* **18 D8** 60 20N 11 40 E
Storsjøen, *Hedmark, Norway* **18 C8** 61 30N 11 14 E
Storsjön, *Gävleborg, Sweden* **16 D10** 60 35N 16 45 E
Storsjön, *Jämtland, Sweden* **16 B7** 62 48N 13 7 E
Storsjön, *Jämtland, Sweden* **16 A8** 63 9N 14 30 E
Storstrøms Amtskommune □, *Denmark* **17 J5** 54 50N 11 45 E
Storuman, *Sweden* **14 D17** 65 5N 17 10 E
Storuman, *Sweden* **14 D17** 65 13N 16 50 E
Stóruvellir, *Iceland* **11 B9** 65 30N 17 29W
Storvätteshågna, *Sweden* **16 B6** 62 6N 12 30 E
Storvigelen, *Norway* **18 B9** 62 32N 12 2 E
Storvik, *Sweden* **16 D10** 60 35N 16 33 E
Storvreta, *Sweden* **16 E11** 59 58N 17 44 E
Story City, *U.S.A.* **156 B3** 42 11N 93 36W
Stouffville, *Canada* **150 C5** 43 58N 79 15W
Stoughton, *Canada* **143 D8** 49 40N 103 0W
Stoughton, *U.S.A.* **156 B8** 42 55N 89 13W
Stour →, *Dorset, U.K.* **21 G6** 50 43N 1 47W
Stour →, *Kent, U.K.* **21 F9** 51 18N 1 22 E
Stour →, *Suffolk, U.K.* **21 F9** 51 57N 1 4 E
Stourbridge, *U.K.* **21 E5** 52 28N 2 8W
Stout L., *Canada* **143 C10** 52 0N 94 40W
Stove Pipe Wells Village, *U.S.A.* **161 J9** 36 35N 117 11W
Støvring, *Denmark* **17 H3** 56 54N 9 50 E
Stow, *U.S.A.* **150 E3** 41 10N 81 27W
Stowbtsy, *Belarus* **58 F4** 53 30N 26 43 E
Stowmarket, *U.K.* **21 E9** 52 12N 1 0 E
Strabane, *U.K.* **23 B4** 54 50N 7 27W
Stracin, *Macedonia* **50 D6** 42 13N 22 2 E
Stradella, *Italy* **44 C6** 45 5N 9 18 E
Strahan, *Australia* **127 G4** 42 9 S 145 20 E
Strajitsa, *Bulgaria* **51 C9** 43 14N 25 58 E
Strakonice, *Czech Rep.* **34 B6** 49 15N 13 53 E
Straldzha, *Bulgaria* **51 D10** 42 35N 26 40 E
Stralsund, *Germany* **30 A9** 54 18N 13 4 E
Strand, *Norway* **18 C8** 61 17N 11 17 E
Strand, *S. Africa* **116 E2** 34 9 S 18 48 E
Stranda, *Møre og Romsdal, Norway* **18 B3** 62 19N 6 58 E
Stranda, *Nord-Trøndelag, Norway* **14 E14** 63 33N 10 14 E
Strandasýsla □, *Iceland* **11 B5** 65 45N 21 45W
Strandby, *Denmark* **17 G4** 57 30N 10 29 E
Strangford L., *U.K.* **23 B6** 54 30N 5 37W
Strängnäs, *Sweden* **16 E11** 59 23N 17 2 E
Stranraer, *U.K.* **22 G3** 54 54N 5 1W
Strasbourg, *Canada* **143 C8** 51 4N 104 55W
Strasbourg, *France* **27 D14** 48 35N 7 42 E
Strasburg, *Germany* **30 B9** 53 30N 13 43 E
Strășeni, *Moldova* **53 C13** 47 8N 28 36 E
Stråssa, *Sweden* **16 E9** 59 44N 15 12 E
Strassburg = Aiud, *Romania* **53 D8** 46 19N 23 44 E
Stratford, *N.S.W., Australia* **129 B9** 32 7 S 151 55 E
Stratford, *Vic., Australia* **129 D7** 37 59 S 147 7 E
Stratford, *Canada* **140 D3** 43 23N 81 0W
Stratford, *N.Z.* **130 F3** 39 20 S 174 19 E
Stratford, *Calif., U.S.A.* **160 J7** 36 11N 119 49W
Stratford, *Conn., U.S.A.* **151 E11** 41 12N 73 8W
Stratford, *Tex., U.S.A.* **155 G3** 36 20N 102 4W
Stratford-upon-Avon, *U.K.* **21 E6** 52 12N 1 42W
Strath Spey, *U.K.* **22 D5** 57 9N 3 49W
Strathalbyn, *Australia* **128 C3** 35 13 S 138 53 E
Strathaven, *U.K.* **22 F4** 55 40N 4 5W
Strathcona ⌓, *Canada* **142 D3** 49 38N 125 40W
Strathmore, *Canada* **142 C6** 51 5N 113 18W
Strathmore, *U.K.* **22 E5** 56 37N 3 7W
Strathmore, *U.S.A.* **160 J7** 36 9N 119 4W
Strathnaver, *Canada* **142 C4** 53 20N 122 33W
Strathpeffer, *U.K.* **22 D4** 57 35N 4 32W
Strathroy, *Canada* **140 D3** 42 58N 81 38W
Strathy Pt., *U.K.* **22 C4** 58 36N 4 1W
Strattanville, *U.S.A.* **150 E5** 41 12N 79 19W
Stratton, *U.S.A.* **151 A14** 45 8N 70 26W
Stratton Mt., *U.S.A.* **151 C12** 43 4N 72 55W
Straubing, *Germany* **31 G8** 48 52N 12 34 E
Straumnes, *Iceland* **11 A3** 66 26N 23 8W
Strausberg, *Germany* **30 C9** 52 35N 13 54 E
Strawberry →, *U.S.A.* **158 F8** 40 10N 110 24W
Strawberry Point, *U.S.A.* **156 B5** 42 41N 91 32W
Strážnice, *Czech Rep.* **35 C10** 48 54N 17 19 E
Streaky B., *Australia* **127 E1** 32 48 S 134 13 E
Streaky Bay, *Australia* **127 E1** 32 51 S 134 18 E
Streator, *U.S.A.* **154 E10** 41 8N 88 50W
Středočeský □, *Czech Rep.* **34 B7** 49 55N 14 30 E
Streetsboro, *U.S.A.* **150 E3** 41 14N 81 21W
Streetsville, *Canada* **150 C5** 43 35N 79 42W
Strehaia, *Romania* **53 F8** 44 37N 23 10 E
Strehlen = Strzelin, *Poland* **55 H4** 50 46N 17 2 E
Strelcha, *Bulgaria* **51 D8** 42 25N 24 19 E
Strelka, *Russia* **67 D10** 58 5N 93 3 E
Streng →, *Cambodia* **86 F4** 13 12N 103 37 E
Stresa, *Italy* **44 C5** 45 52N 8 28 E
Streymoy, *Færoe Is.* **14 E9** 62 8N 7 5W
Strezhevoy, *Russia* **66 C8** 60 42N 77 34 E
Stříbro, *Czech Rep.* **34 A6** 49 44N 13 0 E
Strickland →, *Papua N. G.* **132 D1** 7 35 S 141 36 E
Striegau = Strzegom, *Poland* **55 H3** 50 58N 16 20 E
Strilky, *Ukraine* **55 J9** 49 20N 22 59 E
Strimón →, *Greece* **50 F7** 40 46N 23 51 E
Strimonas = Strimón →, *Greece* **50 F7** 40 46N 23 51 E
Strimonikós Kólpos, *Greece* **50 F7** 40 33N 24 0 E
Stroeder, *Argentina* **176 B4** 40 12 S 62 37W
Strofádhes, *Greece* **48 D3** 37 15N 21 0 E
Stroma, *U.K.* **22 C5** 58 41N 3 7W
Stromberg-Heuchelberg ⌓, *Germany* **31 F4** 49 2N 8 50 E
Strómboli, *Italy* **47 D8** 38 47N 15 13 E
Stromeferry, *U.K.* **22 D3** 57 21N 5 33W
Strømmen, *Norway* **18 E7** 59 58N 10 59 E
Stromness, *U.K.* **22 C5** 58 58N 3 17W
Strömsbruk, *Sweden* **16 C11** 61 52N 17 18 E
Stromsburg, *U.S.A.* **154 E6** 41 7N 97 36W
Strömsnäsbruk, *Sweden* **17 H7** 56 35N 13 45 E
Strömstad, *Sweden* **17 F5** 58 56N 11 10 E
Strömsund, *Sweden* **14 E16** 63 51N 15 33 E
Stronghurst, *U.S.A.* **156 D6** 40 45N 90 55W
Strongilí, *Greece* **49 E11** 36 6N 29 42 E
Stróngoli, *Italy* **47 C10** 39 16N 17 3 E
Strongsville, *U.S.A.* **150 E3** 41 19N 81 50W
Stronie Śląskie, *Poland* **55 H3** 50 18N 16 53 E
Stronsay, *U.K.* **22 B6** 59 7N 2 35W
Stropkov, *Slovak Rep.* **35 B14** 49 13N 21 39 E
Stroud, *U.K.* **21 F5** 51 45N 2 13W
Stroud Road, *Australia* **129 B9** 32 18 S 151 57 E
Stroudsburg, *U.S.A.* **151 F9** 40 59N 75 12W
Stroumbi, *Cyprus* **39 F8** 34 53N 32 29 E
Struer, *Denmark* **17 H2** 56 30N 8 35 E
Struga, *Macedonia* **50 E4** 41 11N 20 44 E
Strugi Krasnyye, *Russia* **58 C5** 58 21N 29 1 E
Strumica, *Macedonia* **50 E6** 41 28N 22 41 E
Strumica →, *Europe* **50 E7** 41 20N 23 22 E
Strumok, *Ukraine* **53 E14** 45 43N 29 27 E
Struthers, *Canada* **140 C2** 48 41N 85 51W
Struthers, *U.S.A.* **150 E4** 41 4N 80 39W
Stryama, *Bulgaria* **51 D8** 42 16N 24 54 E
Stryker, *U.S.A.* **158 B6** 48 41N 114 46W
Stryków, *Poland* **55 G6** 51 55N 19 33 E
Stryn, *Norway* **18 C3** 61 54N 6 43 E
Stryy, *Ukraine* **59 H2** 49 16N 23 48 E
Strzegom, *Poland* **55 H3** 50 58N 16 20 E
Strzelce Krajeńskie, *Poland* **55 F2** 52 52N 15 33 E
Strzelce Opolskie, *Poland* **55 H5** 50 31N 18 18 E
Strzelecki Cr. →, *Australia* **127 D2** 29 37 S 139 59 E
Strzelin, *Poland* **55 H4** 50 46N 17 2 E
Strzelno, *Poland* **55 F5** 52 35N 18 9 E
Strzybnica, *Poland* **55 H5** 50 28N 18 48 E
Strzyżów, *Poland* **55 J8** 49 52N 21 47 E
Stuart, *Fla., U.S.A.* **153 H9** 27 12N 80 15W
Stuart, *Iowa, U.S.A.* **156 C2** 41 30N 94 19W
Stuart, *Nebr., U.S.A.* **154 D5** 42 36N 99 8W
Stuart →, *Canada* **142 C4** 54 0N 123 35W
Stuart Bluff Ra., *Australia* **124 D5** 22 50 S 131 52 E
Stuart I., *U.S.A.* **144 E7** 63 35N 162 30W
Stuart L., *Canada* **142 C4** 54 30N 124 30W
Stuart Mts., *N.Z.* **131 F2** 45 2 S 167 39 E
Stuart Ra., *Australia* **127 D1** 29 10 S 134 56 E
Stubbekøbing, *Denmark* **17 K6** 54 53N 12 9 E
Stuben, *Austria* **34 D3** 47 10N 10 8 E
Štubnianske Teplice = Turčianske Teplice, *Slovak Rep.* **35 C11** 48 52N 18 52 E
Studen Kladenets, Yazovir, *Bulgaria* **51 E9** 41 37N 25 30 E
Studenka, *Czech Rep.* **35 B11** 49 44N 18 5 E
Studholme, *N.Z.* **131 E6** 44 42 S 171 9 E
Stugudal, *Norway* **18 B8** 62 53N 11 53 E
Stugun, *Sweden* **16 A9** 63 10N 15 40 E
Stühlingen, *Germany* **33 A6** 47 44N 8 26 E
Stuhlweissenburg = Székesfehérvár, *Hungary* **52 C3** 47 15N 18 25 E
Stuhm = Sztum, *Poland* **54 E6** 53 55N 19 1 E
Stuhr, *Germany* **30 B4** 53 5N 8 44 E
Stull L., *Canada* **140 B1** 54 24N 92 34W
Stung Treng = Stoeng Treng, *Cambodia* **86 F5** 13 31N 105 58 E
Stupart →, *Canada* **140 A1** 56 0N 93 25W
Stupava, *Slovak Rep.* **35 C10** 48 17N 17 2 E
Stupino, *Russia* **58 E10** 54 57N 38 2 E
Sturgeon B., *Canada* **143 C9** 52 0N 97 50W
Sturgeon Bay, *U.S.A.* **148 C2** 44 50N 87 23W
Sturgeon Falls, *Canada* **140 C4** 46 25N 79 57W
Sturgeon L., *Alta., Canada* **142 B5** 55 6N 117 32W
Sturgeon L., *Ont., Canada* **140 C1** 50 0N 90 45W
Sturgeon L., *Ont., Canada* **150 B6** 44 28N 78 43W
Sturgis, *Canada* **143 C8** 51 56N 102 36W
Sturgis, *Mich., U.S.A.* **157 C11** 41 48N 85 25W
Sturgis, *S. Dak., U.S.A.* **154 C3** 44 25N 103 31W
Sturkö, *Sweden* **17 H9** 56 5N 15 42 E
Štúrovo, *Slovak Rep.* **35 D11** 47 48N 18 41 E
Sturt △, *Australia* **127 D3** 27 17 S 141 37 E
Sturt Cr. →, *Australia* **124 C4** 19 8 S 127 50 E
Sturt Stony Desert, *Australia* **127 D2** 28 30 S 141 0 E
Sturts Meadows, *Australia* **128 A4** 31 18 S 141 42 E
Stutterheim, *S. Africa* **116 E4** 32 33 S 27 28 E
Stuttgart, *Germany* **31 G5** 48 48N 9 11 E
Stuttgart, *U.S.A.* **155 H9** 34 30N 91 33W
Stuttgart Echterdingen ✈ (STR), *Germany* **31 G5** 48 42N 9 11 E
Stutthof = Sztutowo, *Poland* **54 D6** 54 20N 19 15 E
Stuyvesant, *U.S.A.* **151 D11** 42 23N 73 45W
Stykkishólmur, *Iceland* **11 B4** 65 2N 22 40W
Styria = Steiermark □, *Austria* **34 D8** 47 26N 15 0 E
Styrsö, *Sweden* **17 G5** 57 37N 11 46 E
Su-no-Saki, *Japan* **73 C11** 34 58N 139 45 E
Su Xian = Suzhou, *China* **74 H9** 33 41N 116 59 E
Suakin, *Sudan* **106 D4** 19 8N 37 20 E
Suan, *N. Korea* **75 E14** 38 42N 126 22 E
Süanhwa = Xuanhua, *China* **74 D8** 40 40N 115 2 E
Suapure →, *Venezuela* **168 B4** 6 48N 67 1W
Suaqui, *Mexico* **162 B3** 29 12N 109 41W
Suar, *India* **93 E8** 29 2N 79 3 E
Suatá →, *Venezuela* **169 B4** 7 52N 65 22W
Suau, *Papua N. G.* **132 F6** 10 37 S 150 2 E
Suavanao, *Solomon Is.* **133 L10** 7 35 S 158 47 E
Suba Talan, *Malaysia* **81 H1** 6 22N 117 38 E
Subang, *Indonesia* **85 D3** 6 34 S 107 45 E
Subankhata, *India* **90 B3** 26 48N 91 25 E
Subansiri →, *India* **90 B4** 26 48N 93 50 E
Subarnagiri, *India* **94 E6** 19 50N 83 51 E
Subarnarekha →, *India* **93 H12** 22 34N 87 24 E
Subayhah, *Si. Arabia* **96 D3** 30 2N 38 50 E
Subcetate, *Romania* **52 E8** 45 36N 23 0 E
Subi, *Indonesia* **85 B3** 2 58N 108 50 E
Subiaco, *Italy* **45 G10** 41 56N 13 5 E
Subotica, *Serbia & M.* **52 D4** 46 6N 19 39 E
Suca, *Ethiopia* **107 F4** 6 31N 39 14 E
Suceava, *Romania* **53 C11** 47 38N 26 16 E
Suceava □, *Romania* **53 C10** 47 37N 25 40 E
Suceava →, *Romania* **53 C11** 47 32N 26 32 E
Sucesso, *Brazil* **170 B3** 4 56 S 40 32W
Sucha-Beskidzka, *Poland* **55 J6** 49 44N 19 35 E
Suchań, *Poland* **55 E2** 53 18N 15 18 E
Suchan, *Russia* **70 C6** 43 8N 133 9 E
Suchedniów, *Poland* **55 G7** 51 3N 20 49 E
Suchitoto, *El Salv.* **164 D2** 13 56N 89 0W
Suchou = Suzhou, *China* **77 B13** 31 19N 120 38 E
Süchow = Xuzhou, *China* **75 G9** 34 18N 117 10 E
Suchowola, *Poland* **54 E10** 53 33N 23 3 E
Sucio →, *Colombia* **168 B2** 7 27N 77 7W
Suck →, *Ireland* **23 C3** 53 17N 8 3W
Suckling, Mt., *Papua N. G.* **132 E5** 9 49 S 148 53 E
Sucre, *Bolivia* **173 D4** 19 0 S 65 15W
Sucre, *Colombia* **168 B3** 8 49N 74 44W
Sucre □, *Colombia* **168 B2** 8 50N 75 40W
Sucre □, *Venezuela* **169 A5** 10 25N 63 30W
Sucuaro, *Colombia* **168 C4** 4 34N 68 50W
Sućuraj, *Croatia* **45 E14** 43 10N 17 8 E
Sucuriju, *Brazil* **170 A2** 1 39N 49 57W
Sucuriú →, *Brazil* **173 E7** 20 47 S 51 38W
Sud, Pte. du, *Canada* **141 C7** 49 3N 62 14W
Sud-Kivu □, *Dem. Rep. of the Congo* **118 C2** 3 0 S 28 30 E
Sud-Ouest, Pte., *Canada* **141 C7** 49 23N 63 36W
Sud-Ouest, Pte., *Mauritius* **121 d** 20 28 S 57 18 E
Suda →, *Russia* **58 C9** 59 0N 37 40 E
Sudak, *Ukraine* **59 K8** 44 51N 34 57 E
Sudan, *U.S.A.* **155 H3** 34 4N 102 32W
Sudan ■, *Africa* **107 E3** 15 0N 30 0 E
Sudauen = Suwałki, *Poland* **54 D9** 54 8N 22 59 E
Sudbury, *Canada* **140 C3** 46 30N 81 0W
Sudbury, *U.K.* **21 E8** 52 2N 0 45 E
Sûdd, *Sudan* **107 F3** 8 20N 30 0 E
Suddie, *Guyana* **169 B6** 7 8N 58 29W
Sudeifel = Deutsch-Luxemburgischer ⌓, *Germany* **31 F2** 49 58N 6 12 E
Süderbrarup, *Germany* **30 A5** 54 38N 9 45 E
Süderlügum, *Germany* **30 A4** 54 52N 8 54 E
Süderoogsand, *Germany* **30 A4** 54 27N 8 28 E
Sudeten Mts. = Sudety, *Europe* **35 A9** 50 20N 16 45 E
Sudety, *Europe* **35 A9** 50 20N 16 45 E
Súðavík, *Iceland* **11 A3** 66 2N 23 0W
Südheide ⌓, *Germany* **30 C6** 52 46N 10 10 E
Suður-múlasýsla □, *Iceland* **11 C12** 65 0N 14 30W
Suður-þingeyjarsýsla □, *Iceland* **11 B9** 65 30N 17 0W
Suðureyri, *Iceland* **11 A3** 66 7N 23 32W
Suðuroy, *Færoe Is.* **14 F9** 61 32N 6 50W
Sudi, *Tanzania* **119 E4** 10 11 S 39 57 E
Sudirman, Pegunungan, *Indonesia* **83 B5** 4 30 S 137 0 E
Sudiți, *Romania* **53 F12** 44 35N 27 38 E
Sudogda, *Russia* **60 C5** 55 55N 40 50 E
Sudong, Pulau, *Singapore* **87 d** 1 12N 103 43 E
Sudostroy = Severodvinsk, *Russia* **56 B6** 64 27N 39 58 E
Sudova Vyshnya, *Ukraine* **55 J10** 49 46N 23 22 E
Sudr, *Egypt* **106 B3** 29 40N 32 42 E
Sudzha, *Russia* **59 G8** 51 14N 35 17 E
Sue →, *Sudan* **107 F2** 7 41N 28 3 E
Sueca, *Spain* **41 F4** 39 12N 0 21W
Sŭedinenie, *Bulgaria* **51 D8** 42 16N 24 33 E
Suemez I., *U.S.A.* **142 B2** 55 15N 133 20W
Suez = El Suweis, *Egypt* **106 J8** 29 58N 32 31 E
Suez, G. of = Suweis, Khalîg el, *Egypt* **106 J8** 28 40N 33 0 E
Suez Canal = Suweis, Qanâ es, *Egypt* **106 H8** 31 0N 32 20 E
Suffield, *Canada* **142 C6** 50 12N 111 10W
Suffolk, *U.S.A.* **148 G7** 36 44N 76 35W
Suffolk □, *U.K.* **21 E9** 52 16N 1 0 E
Suga-no-Sen, *Japan* **72 B6** 35 25N 134 25 E
Şugag, *Romania* **53 E8** 45 47N 23 37 E
Sugar →, *U.S.A.* **156 B7** 42 26N 89 12W
Sugar Cr. →, *Ill., U.S.A.* **156 D7** 40 9N 89 38W
Sugar Cr. →, *Ind., U.S.A.* **157 E9** 39 50N 87 23W
Sugar Hill, *U.S.A.* **152 A5** 34 6N 84 2W
Sugar Loaf Pt., *St. Helena* **9 h** 15 54 S 5 42W
Sugargrove, *U.S.A.* **150 E5** 41 59N 79 21W
Sugarive →, *India* **93 F12** 26 16N 86 24 E
Sugbai Passage, *Phil.* **81 J3** 5 22N 120 33 E
Suğla Gölü, *Turkey* **100 D5** 37 20N 32 0 E
Sugluk = Salluit, *Canada* **139 B12** 62 14N 75 38W
Sugun, *China* **65 D8** 39 53N 76 47 E
Suhaia, Lacul, *Romania* **53 G10** 43 45N 25 15 E
Şuḩār, *Oman* **97 E8** 24 20N 56 40 E
Sühbaatar □, *Mongolia* **74 B8** 45 30N 114 0 E
Suheli Par, *India* **95 J1** 10 5N 72 17 E
Suhl, *Germany* **30 E6** 50 36N 10 42 E
Suhr, *Switz.* **32 B6** 47 22N 8 5 E
Şuhut, *Turkey* **49 C12** 38 31N 30 32 E
Sui, *Pakistan* **92 E3** 28 37N 69 19 E
Sui Xian, *China* **74 G8** 34 25N 115 2 E
Suiá Missu →, *Brazil* **173 C7** 11 13 S 53 15W
Šuica, *Bos.-H.* **52 G2** 43 52N 17 11 E
Suichang, *China* **77 C12** 28 29N 119 15 E
Suichuan, *China* **77 D10** 26 20N 114 32 E
Suide, *China* **74 F6** 37 30N 110 12 E
Suifenhe, *China* **75 B16** 44 25N 131 10 E
Suihua, *China* **69 B7** 46 32N 126 55 E
Suijiang, *China* **76 C4** 28 40N 103 59 E
Suining, *Hunan, China* **77 D8** 26 35N 110 10 E
Suining, *Jiangsu, China* **75 H9** 33 56N 117 58 E
Suining, *Sichuan, China* **76 B5** 30 26N 105 35 E
Suiping, *China* **74 H7** 33 10N 113 59 E
Suippes, *France* **27 C11** 49 8N 4 30 E
Suir →, *Ireland* **23 D4** 52 16N 7 9W
Suisse = Switzerland ■, *Europe* **32 D6** 46 30N 8 0 E
Suisun City, *U.S.A.* **160 G4** 38 15N 122 2W
Suita, *Japan* **73 C7** 34 45N 135 32 E
Suixi, *China* **77 G8** 21 19N 110 18 E
Suiyang, *Guizhou, China* **76 D6** 27 58N 107 18 E
Suiyang, *Heilongjiang, China* **75 B16** 44 30N 130 56 E
Suizhong, *China* **75 D11** 40 21N 120 20 E
Suizhou, *China* **77 B9** 31 42N 113 24 E
Sujangarh, *India* **92 F6** 27 42N 74 31 E
Sukabumi, *Indonesia* **84 D3** 6 56 S 106 50 E
Sukadana, *Kalimantan, Indonesia* **85 C4** 1 10 S 110 0 E
Sukadana, *Sumatera, Indonesia* **84 D3** 5 5 S 105 33 E
Sukagawa, *Japan* **71 F10** 37 17N 140 23 E
Sukaraja, *Indonesia* **85 C4** 2 28 S 110 25 E
Sukarnapura = Jayapura, *Indonesia* **83 B6** 2 28 S 140 38 E
Sukarno, Puntjak = Jaya, Puncak, *Indonesia* **83 B5** 3 57 S 137 17 E
Sukawati, *Indonesia* **79 K18** 8 35 S 115 17 E
Sukch'ŏn, *N. Korea* **75 E13** 39 22N 125 35 E
Sukhindol, *Bulgaria* **51 C9** 43 11N 25 10 E
Sukhinichi, *Russia* **58 E8** 54 8N 35 10 E
Sukhona →, *Russia* **56 C6** 61 15N 46 39 E
Sukhothai, *Thailand* **86 D2** 17 1N 99 49 E
Sukhoy Log, *Russia* **64 C9** 56 55N 62 1 E
Sukhum = Sokhumi, *Georgia* **61 J5** 43 0N 41 0 E
Sukhumi = Sokhumi, *Georgia* **61 J5** 43 0N 41 0 E
Sukkertoppen = Maniitsoq, *Greenland* **10 D5** 65 26N 52 55W
Sukkur, *Pakistan* **91 D3** 27 42N 68 54 E
Sukkur Barrage, *Pakistan* **92 F3** 27 40N 68 50 E
Sukma, *India* **94 E5** 18 24N 81 45 E
Sukovo, *Serbia & M.* **50 C6** 43 4N 22 37 E
Sukri →, *India* **92 G4** 25 4N 71 43 E
Sukumo, *Japan* **72 E4** 32 56N 132 44 E
Sukunka →, *Canada* **142 B4** 55 45N 121 15W
Sul, Canal do, *Brazil* **170 B2** 0 10 S 48 30W
Sula, *Norway* **18 C1** 61 7N 4 54 E
Sula →, *Ukraine* **59 H7** 49 40N 32 41 E
Sula, Kepulauan, *Indonesia* **82 B3** 1 45 S 125 0 E
Sulaco →, *Honduras* **164 C2** 15 2N 87 44W
Sulaiman Range, *Pakistan* **92 D3** 30 30N 69 50 E
Sulak →, *Russia* **61 J8** 43 20N 47 34 E
Sūlār, *Iran* **97 D6** 31 53N 51 54 E
Sulawesi □, *Indonesia* **82 B2** 2 0 S 120 0 E
Sulawesi Sea = Celebes Sea, *Indonesia* **82 A2** 3 0N 123 0 E
Sulawesi Selatan □, *Indonesia* **82 B1** 2 30 S 120 0 E
Sulawesi Tengah □, *Indonesia* **82 B2** 1 30 S 121 0 E
Sulawesi Tenggara □, *Indonesia* **82 B2** 3 50 S 122 0 E
Sulawesi Utara □, *Indonesia* **82 A2** 1 0N 124 0 E
Suldalsosen, *Norway* **18 E3** 59 29N 6 29 E
Sulechów, *Poland* **55 F2** 52 5N 15 40 E
Sulęcin, *Poland* **55 F2** 52 26N 15 10 E
Sulei, *Solomon Is.* **133 M10** 8 3 S 159 34 E
Sulejów, *Poland* **55 G6** 51 26N 19 53 E
Sulejówek, *Poland* **55 F8** 52 13N 21 17 E
Süleymanlı, *Turkey* **49 C9** 38 58N 27 47 E
Sulgen, *Switz.* **33 A8** 47 33N 9 7 E
Sulima, *S. Leone* **112 D2** 6 58N 11 32W
Sulina, *Romania* **53 E14** 45 10N 29 40 E
Sulina, Braţul →, *Romania* **53 E14** 45 10N 29 40 E
Sulingen, *Germany* **30 C4** 52 41N 8 48 E
Sulița, *Romania* **53 C11** 47 39N 26 59 E
Sulitjelma, *Norway* **14 C17** 67 9N 16 3 E
Sułkowice, *Poland* **55 J6** 49 50N 19 49 E
Sullana, *Peru* **172 A1** 4 52 S 80 39W
Süller, *Turkey* **49 C11** 38 9N 29 29 E
Sullivan, *Ill., U.S.A.* **154 F10** 39 36N 88 37W
Sullivan, *Ind., U.S.A.* **157 E9** 39 6N 87 24W
Sullivan, *Mo., U.S.A.* **156 F5** 38 13N 91 10W
Sullivan Bay, *Canada* **142 C3** 50 55N 126 50W
Sullivan I. = Lanbi Kyun, *Burma* **87 G2** 10 50N 98 20 E
Sullom Voe, *U.K.* **22 A7** 60 27N 1 20W
Sully, *U.S.A.* **156 C4** 41 34N 92 50W
Sully-sur-Loire, *France* **27 E9** 47 45N 2 20 E
Sulmierzyce, *Poland* **55 G4** 51 37N 17 32 E
Sulmona, *Italy* **45 F10** 42 3N 13 55 E
Süloğlu, *Turkey* **51 E10** 41 44N 26 53 E
Sulphur, *La., U.S.A.* **155 K8** 30 14N 93 23W
Sulphur, *Okla., U.S.A.* **155 H6** 34 31N 96 58W
Sulphur Pt., *Canada* **142 A6** 60 56N 114 48W
Sulphur Springs, *U.S.A.* **155 J7** 33 8N 95 36W
Sulsul, *Ethiopia* **120 C2** 5 5N 44 50 E
Sultan, *Canada* **140 C3** 47 36N 82 47W
Sultan, *U.S.A.* **160 C5** 47 52N 121 49W
Sultan Dağları, *Turkey* **100 C4** 38 20N 31 20 E
Sultan Kudarat, *Phil.* **81 H5** 7 16N 124 18 E
Sultan Kudarat □, *Phil.* **81 H5** 6 30N 124 10 E
Sultan Naga Dimaporo, *Phil.* **81 H4** 7 55N 123 44 E
Sultan sa Barongis, *Phil.* **81 H5** 6 45N 124 35 E
Sultanabad = Arāk, *Iran* **97 C6** 34 0N 49 40 E
Sultanhisar, *Turkey* **49 D10** 37 53N 28 9 E
Sultaniça, *Turkey* **51 F10** 40 37N 26 8 E
Sultaniye, *Turkey* **51 F12** 40 11N 28 12 E
Sultanpur, *Mad. P., India* **92 H8** 23 9N 77 56 E
Sultanpur, *Punjab, India* **92 D6** 31 13N 75 11 E
Sultanpur, *Ut. P., India* **93 F10** 26 18N 82 4 E
Sulu □, *Phil.* **81 J3** 5 30N 120 30 E
Sulu Arch., *Phil.* **81 J3** 6 0N 121 0 E
Sulu Sea, *E. Indies* **81 G3** 8 0N 120 0 E
Sülüklü, *Turkey* **100 C5** 38 53N 32 20 E
Sülüktü, *Kyrgyzstan* **65 D4** 39 56N 69 34 E
Sululta, *Ethiopia* **107 F4** 9 10N 38 43 E
Suluova, *Turkey* **100 B6** 40 46N 35 32 E
Suluq, *Libya* **108 B4** 31 44N 20 14 E
Suluru, *India* **95 H5** 13 42N 80 1 E
Sulütöbe, *Kazakhstan* **65 A3** 44 37N 66 3 E
Sulyukta = Sülüktü, *Kyrgyzstan* **65 D4** 39 56N 69 34 E
Sulzbach, *Germany* **31 F3** 49 18N 7 3 E
Sulzbach-Rosenberg, *Germany* **31 F7** 49 30N 11 44 E
Sulzberg, *Germany* **33 A10** 47 39N 10 39 E
Sulzberger Ice Shelf, *Antarctica* **7 E13** 78 0 S 150 0W
Sumaco -Napo Galeras △, *Ecuador* **168 D2** 0 34 S 77 38W
Sumalata, *Indonesia* **82 A2** 1 0N 122 31 E
Sumale □, *Ethiopia* **120 C2** 7 0N 45 0 E
Sumampa, *Argentina* **174 B3** 29 25 S 63 29W
Sumapaz △, *Colombia* **168 C3** 3 49N 74 13W
Sumatera, *Indonesia* **84 B2** 0 40N 100 20 E
Sumatera Barat □, *Indonesia* **78 E2** 1 0 S 101 0 E
Sumatera Utara □, *Indonesia* **78 D1** 2 30N 98 0 E
Sumatra = Sumatera, *Indonesia* **84 B2** 0 40N 100 20 E
Sumatra, *U.S.A.* **152 E5** 30 1N 84 59W
Sumava △, *Czech Rep.* **34 C6** 49 0N 13 49 E
Sumba, *Angola* **115 D2** 6 15 S 12 38 E
Sumba, *Indonesia* **82 C1** 9 45 S 119 35 E
Sumba, Selat, *Indonesia* **82 C1** 9 0 S 118 40 E
Sumbawa, *Indonesia* **85 D5** 8 26 S 117 30 E
Sumbawa Besar, *Indonesia* **85 D5** 8 30 S 117 26 E
Sumbe, *Angola* **115 E2** 11 10 S 13 48 E
Sumbu △, *Zambia* **119 D3** 8 43 S 30 22 E
Sumburgh Hd., *U.K.* **22 B7** 59 52N 1 17W
Sumdeo, *India* **93 D8** 31 26N 78 44 E
Sumdo, *China* **93 B8** 35 6N 78 41 E
Sumé, *Brazil* **170 C4** 7 39 S 36 55W
Sumedang, *Indonesia* **85 D3** 6 52 S 107 55 E
Sümeg, *Hungary* **52 D2** 46 59N 17 20 E
Sumeih, *Sudan* **107 F2** 9 50N 27 39 E
Šumen = Shumen, *Bulgaria* **51 C10** 43 18N 26 55 E
Sumenep, *Indonesia* **85 D4** 7 1 S 113 52 E
Sumgait = Sumqayıt, *Azerbaijan* **61 K9** 40 34N 49 38 E
Sumisu-Jima, *Japan* **73 F12** 31 27N 140 3 E
Sumiswald, *Switz.* **32 B5** 47 2N 7 44 E
Summer L., *U.S.A.* **158 E3** 42 50N 120 45W
Summerland, *Canada* **142 D5** 49 32N 119 41W
Summerland Key, *U.S.A.* **153 L8** 24 40N 81 27W
Summerside, *Canada* **141 C7** 46 24N 63 47W
Summersville, *U.S.A.* **148 F5** 38 17N 80 51W
Summerton, *U.S.A.* **152 B9** 33 36N 80 20W
Summertown, *U.S.A.* **152 C7** 32 45N 82 16W
Summerville, *Ga., U.S.A.* **149 H3** 34 29N 85 21W
Summerville, *S.C., U.S.A.* **152 B9** 33 1N 80 11W
Summit, *U.S.A.* **144 E10** 63 20N 149 7W
Summit Lake, *Canada* **142 C4** 54 20N 122 40W
Summit Peak, *U.S.A.* **159 H10** 37 21N 106 42W
Sumner, *N.Z.* **131 D7** 43 35 S 172 48 E
Sumner, *Ill., U.S.A.* **157 F9** 38 42N 87 53W
Sumner, *Iowa, U.S.A.* **156 B4** 42 51N 92 6W
Sumner, *Wash., U.S.A.* **160 C4** 47 12N 122 14W
Sumner, L., *N.Z.* **131 C7** 42 42 S 172 15 E
Sumoto, *Japan* **72 C6** 34 21N 134 54 E
Sumpangbinangae, *Indonesia* **82 B1** 4 24 S 119 36 E
Šumperk, *Czech Rep.* **35 B9** 49 59N 16 59 E
Sumprabum, *Burma* **90 B6** 26 33N 97 36 E
Sumqayıt, *Azerbaijan* **61 K9** 40 34N 49 38 E
Sumsar, *Kyrgyzstan* **65 C5** 41 18N 71 19 E
Sumter, *U.S.A.* **152 B9** 33 55N 80 21W
Sumy, *Ukraine* **59 G8** 50 57N 34 50 E
Sun City, *S. Africa* **116 D4** 25 17 S 27 3 E
Sun City, *Ariz., U.S.A.* **159 K7** 33 36N 112 17W
Sun City, *Calif., U.S.A.* **161 M9** 33 42N 117 11W
Sun City Center, *U.S.A.* **153 H7** 27 43N 82 18W
Sun Lakes, *U.S.A.* **159 K8** 33 10N 111 52W
Sun Prairie, *U.S.A.* **156 A7** 43 11N 89 13W
Sun Valley, *U.S.A.* **158 E6** 43 42N 114 21W
Sunagawa, *Japan* **70 C10** 43 29N 141 55 E
Sunan, *N. Korea* **75 E13** 39 15N 125 40 E
Sunart, L., *U.K.* **22 E3** 56 42N 5 43W

Sunburst, *U.S.A.* **158 B8** 48 53N 111 55W
Sunbury, *Australia* **129 D6** 37 35 S 144 44 E
Sunbury, *U.S.A.* **151 F8** 40 52N 76 48W
Sunchales, *Argentina* **174 C3** 30 58 S 61 35W
Suncho Corral, *Argentina* **174 B3** 27 55 S 63 27W
Sunch'ŏn, *S. Korea* **75 G14** 34 52N 127 31 E
Suncook, *U.S.A.* **151 C13** 43 8N 71 27W
Sunda, Selat, *Indonesia* **84 D3** 6 20 S 105 30 E
Sunda Is., *Indonesia* **62 K14** 5 0 S 105 0 E
Sunda Str. = Sunda, Selat, *Indonesia* **84 D3** 6 20 S 105 30 E
Sundance, *Canada* **143 B10** 56 32N 94 4W
Sundance, *U.S.A.* **154 C2** 44 24N 104 23W
Sundar Nagar, *India* **92 D7** 31 32N 76 53 E
Sundarbans, *Asia* **90 E2** 22 0N 89 0 E
Sundarbans △, *India* **93 J13** 22 0N 88 45 E
Sundargarh, *India* **94 C7** 22 4N 84 5 E
Sundays = Sondags →, *S. Africa* **116 E4** 33 44 S 25 51 E
Sunderland, *Canada* **150 B5** 44 16N 79 4W
Sunderland, *U.K.* **20 C6** 54 55N 1 23W
Sundi Lutete, *Dem. Rep. of the Congo* **115 C2** 4 34 S 14 14 E
Sundown △, *Australia* **127 D5** 28 49 S 151 38 E
Sundre, *Canada* **142 C6** 51 49N 114 38W
Sunds, *Denmark* **17 H3** 56 13N 9 1 E
Sundsvall, *Sweden* **16 B11** 62 23N 17 17 E
Sundsvallsbukten, *Sweden* **16 B11** 62 21N 17 25 E
Sung Hei, *Vietnam* **87 G6** 10 20N 106 2 E
Sungai Acheh, *Malaysia* **87 c** 5 8N 100 30 E
Sungai Kolok, *Thailand* **87 J3** 6 2N 101 58 E
Sungai Lembing, *Malaysia* **87 L4** 3 55N 103 3 E
Sungai Petani, *Malaysia* **87 K3** 5 37N 100 30 E
Sungaigerong, *Indonesia* **84 C2** 2 59 S 104 52 E
Sungailiat, *Indonesia* **84 C3** 1 51 S 106 8 E
Sungaipenuh, *Indonesia* **84 C2** 2 1 S 101 20 E
Sungaitiram, *Indonesia* **85 C5** 0 45 S 117 8 E
Sungari = Songhua Jiang →, *China* **69 B8** 47 45N 132 30 E
Sungguminasa, *Indonesia* **82 C1** 5 17 S 119 30 E
Sunghua Chiang = Songhua Jiang →, *China* **69 B8** 47 45N 132 30 E
Sungikai, *Sudan* **107 E2** 12 20N 29 51 E
Sungu, *Dem. Rep. of the Congo* **114 C3** 1 5 S 17 21 E
Sungurlu, *Turkey* **100 B6** 40 12N 34 21 E
Sunja, *Croatia* **45 C13** 45 21N 16 35 E
Sunland Park, *U.S.A.* **159 L10** 31 50N 106 40W
Sunnansjö, *Sweden* **16 D8** 60 13N 14 58 E
Sunndalsøra, *Norway* **18 B5** 62 40N 8 33 E
Sunne, *Sweden* **16 E7** 59 52N 13 5 E
Sunnemo, *Sweden* **16 E7** 59 53N 13 44 E
Sunnfjord, *Norway* **18 C2** 61 35N 5 45 E
Sunnmøre, *Norway* **18 B3** 62 35N 6 30 E
Sunnyside, *U.S.A.* **158 C3** 46 20N 120 0W
Sunnyvale, *U.S.A.* **160 H4** 37 23N 122 2W
Sunrise Manor, *U.S.A.* **159 H6** 36 12N 115 3W
Sunset Beach, *U.S.A.* **145 J13** 21 40N 158 3W
Suntar, *Russia* **67 C12** 62 15N 117 30 E
Suntrana, *U.S.A.* **144 E10** 63 52N 148 51W
Sunyani, *Ghana* **112 D4** 7 21N 2 22W
Suō-Nada, *Japan* **72 D3** 33 50N 131 30 E
Suomenselkä, *Finland* **14 E21** 62 52N 24 0 E
Suomi = Finland ■, *Europe* **14 E22** 63 0N 27 0 E
Suomussalmi, *Finland* **14 D23** 64 54N 29 10 E
Suoyarvi, *Russia* **58 A7** 62 3N 32 20 E
Supai, *U.S.A.* **159 H7** 36 15N 112 41W
Supamo →, *Venezuela* **169 B5** 6 48N 61 50W
Supaul, *India* **93 F12** 26 10N 86 40 E
Supe, *Peru* **172 C2** 11 0 S 77 30W
Superagüi △, *Brazil* **171 G2** 25 6 S 48 18W
Superior, *Ariz., U.S.A.* **159 K8** 33 18N 111 6W
Superior, *Mont., U.S.A.* **158 C6** 47 12N 114 53W
Superior, *Nebr., U.S.A.* **154 E5** 40 1N 98 4W
Superior, *Wis., U.S.A.* **154 B8** 46 44N 92 6W
Superior, L., *N. Amer.* **140 C2** 47 0N 87 0W
Supetar, *Croatia* **45 E13** 43 25N 16 32 E
Suphan Buri, *Thailand* **86 E3** 14 14N 100 10 E
Suphan Dağı, *Turkey* **101 C10** 38 54N 42 48 E
Supiori, *Indonesia* **83 B5** 1 0 S 136 0 E
Supraśl, *Poland* **55 E10** 53 13N 23 19 E
Supraśl →, *Poland* **55 E9** 53 11N 22 57 E
Supung Shuiku, *China* **75 D13** 40 35N 124 50 E
Sūq' Abs, *Yemen* **98 D3** 16 0N 43 12 E
Sūq Suwayq, *Si. Arabia* **96 E3** 24 23N 38 27 E
Suqian, *China* **75 H10** 33 54N 118 8 E
Suquṭra = Socotra, *Yemen* **99 D6** 12 30N 54 0 E
Sūr, *Lebanon* **103 B4** 33 19N 35 16 E
Ṣūr, *Oman* **99 B7** 22 34N 59 32 E
Sur, C., *Chile* **172 b** 27 12 S 109 26W
Sur, Pt., *U.S.A.* **160 J5** 36 18N 121 54W
Sura →, *Russia* **60 C8** 56 6N 46 0 E
Surab, *Pakistan* **91 C2** 28 25N 66 15 E
Surabaja = Surabaya, *Indonesia* **85 D4** 7 17 S 112 45 E
Surabaya, *Indonesia* **85 D4** 7 17 S 112 45 E
Surahammar, *Sweden* **16 E10** 59 43N 16 13 E
Suraia, *Romania* **53 E12** 45 40N 27 25 E
Surakarta, *Indonesia* **85 D4** 7 35 S 110 48 E
Surakhany, *Azerbaijan* **61 K10** 40 25N 50 1 E
Šurany, *Slovak Rep.* **35 C11** 48 6N 18 10 E
Surat, *Australia* **127 D4** 27 10 S 149 6 E
Surat, *India* **94 D1** 21 12N 72 55 E
Surat Thani, *Thailand* **87 H2** 9 6N 99 20 E
Suratgarh, *India* **92 E5** 29 18N 73 55 E
Suraż, *Poland* **55 F9** 52 57N 22 57 E
Surazh, *Belarus* **58 E6** 55 25N 30 44 E
Surazh, *Russia* **59 F7** 53 5N 32 27 E
Surduc, *Romania* **53 C8** 47 15N 23 25 E
Surduc Pasul, *Romania* **53 E8** 45 21N 23 23 E
Surdulica, *Serbia & M.* **50 D6** 42 41N 22 11 E
Surendranagar, *India* **92 H4** 22 45N 71 40 E
Surf, *U.S.A.* **161 L6** 34 41N 120 36W
Surfers Paradise, *Australia* **127 D5** 28 0 S 153 25 E
Surfside, *U.S.A.* **153 K9** 25 53N 80 8W
Surgana, *India* **94 D1** 20 34N 73 37 E
Surgères, *France* **28 B3** 46 7N 0 47W
Surgut, *Russia* **66 C8** 61 14N 73 20 E
Sùria, *Spain* **40 D6** 41 50N 1 45 E
Suriapet, *India* **94 F4** 17 10N 79 40 E
Surigao, *Phil.* **81 G5** 9 47N 125 29 E
Surigao del Norte □, *Phil.* **81 G5** 10 0N 125 40 E
Surigao del Sur □, *Phil.* **81 G6** 8 45N 126 0 E
Surigao Strait, *Phil.* **81 F5** 10 15N 125 23 E
Surin, *Thailand* **86 E4** 14 50N 103 34 E
Surin Nua, Ko, *Thailand* **87 H1** 9 30N 97 55 E
Surinam = Suriname ■, *S. Amer.* **169 C6** 4 0N 56 0W
Suriname ■, *S. Amer.* **169 C6** 4 0N 56 0W
Suriname →, *Suriname* **169 B6** 5 50N 55 15W
Surjagarh, *India* **94 E5** 19 36N 80 25 E
Surkhandarya →, *Uzbekistan* **65 E3** 37 12N 67 20 E
Surma →, *Bangla.* **90 C3** 24 34N 91 14 E
Sūrmaq, *Iran* **97 D7** 31 3N 52 48 E
Sürmene, *Turkey* **101 B9** 41 0N 40 1 E
Surna →, *Norway* **18 B5** 62 59N 8 40 E
Surnadalsøra, *Norway* **18 B5** 62 58N 8 40 E
Surovikino, *Russia* **61 F6** 48 32N 42 55 E
Surrency, *U.S.A.* **152 D7** 31 44N 82 12W
Surrey, *Canada* **160 A4** 49 10N 122 54W
Surrey □, *U.K.* **21 F7** 51 15N 0 31W
Sursand, *India* **93 F11** 26 39N 85 43 E
Sursar →, *India* **93 F12** 26 14N 87 3 E
Sursee, *Switz.* **32 B6** 47 11N 8 6 E
Sursk, *Russia* **60 D7** 53 3N 45 40 E
Surskoye, *Russia* **60 C8** 54 30N 46 44 E
Surt, *Libya* **108 B3** 31 11N 16 39 E
Surt □, *Libya* **108 B3** 30 0N 17 30 E
Surt, Al Hammadah al, *Libya* **108 C3** 30 0N 17 50 E
Surt, Khalīj, *Libya* **108 B3** 31 40N 18 30 E
Surtanahu, *Pakistan* **92 F4** 26 22N 70 0 E
Surte, *Sweden* **17 G6** 57 50N 12 1 E
Surtsey, *Iceland* **11 D6** 63 20N 20 30W
Surubim, *Brazil* **170 C4** 7 50 S 35 45W
Sürüç, *Turkey* **101 D8** 36 58N 38 25 E
Surud Ad, *Somali Rep.* **120 B3** 10 42N 47 9 E
Suruga-Wan, *Japan* **73 C10** 34 45N 138 30 E
Surumu →, *Brazil* **169 C5** 3 22N 60 19W
Susa = Sousse, *Tunisia* **108 A2** 35 50N 10 38 E
Susa, *Italy* **44 C4** 45 8N 7 3 E
Suså →, *Denmark* **17 J5** 55 12N 11 42 E
Sušac, *Croatia* **45 F13** 42 46N 16 30 E
Susak, *Croatia* **45 D11** 44 30N 14 18 E
Susaki, *Japan* **72 D5** 33 22N 133 17 E
Susam-Adasi = Sámos, *Greece* **49 D8** 37 45N 26 50 E
Susamyrtau, Khrebet = Suusamyr Kyrka Tooloru, *Kyrgyzstan* **65 B6** 42 8N 73 15 E
Sūsangerd, *Iran* **97 D6** 31 35N 48 6 E
Susanville, *U.S.A.* **158 F3** 40 25N 120 39W
Susch, *Switz.* **33 C10** 46 46N 10 5 E
Suşehri, *Turkey* **101 B8** 40 10N 38 6 E
Sušice, *Czech Rep.* **34 B6** 49 17N 13 30 E
Susleni, *Moldova* **53 C13** 47 25N 28 59 E
Susner, *India* **92 H7** 23 57N 76 5 E
Susong, *China* **77 B11** 30 10N 116 5 E
Susquehanna, *U.S.A.* **151 E9** 41 57N 75 36W
Susquehanna →, *U.S.A.* **151 G8** 39 33N 76 5W
Susques, *Argentina* **174 A2** 23 35 S 66 25W
Sussex, *Canada* **141 C6** 45 45N 65 37W
Sussex, *U.S.A.* **151 E10** 41 13N 74 37W
Sussex, E. □, *U.K.* **21 G8** 51 0N 0 20 E
Sussex, W. □, *U.K.* **21 G7** 51 0N 0 30W
Sussex Inlet, *Australia* **129 C9** 35 10 S 150 36 E
Sustut →, *Canada* **142 B3** 56 20N 127 30W
Susuman, *Russia* **67 C15** 62 47N 148 10 E
Susunu, *Indonesia* **83 B4** 3 7 S 133 39 E
Susurluk, *Turkey* **49 B10** 39 54N 28 8 E
Susuz, *Turkey* **101 B10** 40 46N 43 8 E
Susz, *Poland* **54 E6** 53 44N 19 20 E
Sütçüler, *Turkey* **100 D4** 37 29N 30 57 E
Şuţeşti, *Romania* **53 E12** 45 13N 27 27 E
Sutherland, *Australia* **129 C9** 34 2 S 151 4 E
Sutherland, *S. Africa* **116 E3** 32 24 S 20 40 E
Sutherland, *U.K.* **22 C4** 58 12N 4 50W
Sutherland, *U.S.A.* **154 E4** 41 10N 101 8W
Sutherland Falls, *N.Z.* **131 E2** 44 48 S 167 46 E
Sutherlin, *U.S.A.* **158 E2** 43 23N 123 19W
Suthri, *India* **92 H3** 23 3N 68 55 E
Sutjeska △, *Bos.-H.* **52 G3** 43 50N 18 32 E
Sutlej →, *Pakistan* **91 C3** 29 23N 71 3 E
Sutter, *U.S.A.* **160 F5** 39 10N 121 45W
Sutter Creek, *U.S.A.* **160 G6** 38 24N 120 48W
Sutton, *Canada* **151 A12** 45 6N 72 37W
Sutton, *N.Z.* **131 F5** 45 34 S 170 8 E
Sutton, *Nebr., U.S.A.* **154 E6** 40 36N 97 52W
Sutton, *W. Va., U.S.A.* **148 F5** 38 40N 80 43W
Sutton →, *Canada* **140 A3** 55 15N 83 45W
Sutton Coldfield, *U.K.* **21 E6** 52 35N 1 49W
Sutton in Ashfield, *U.K.* **20 D6** 53 8N 1 16W
Sutton L., *Canada* **140 B3** 54 15N 84 42W
Suttor →, *Australia* **126 C4** 21 36 S 147 2 E
Suttsu, *Japan* **70 C10** 42 48N 140 14 E
Sutwik I., *U.S.A.* **144 H8** 56 34N 157 12W
Suusamyr, *Kyrgyzstan* **65 B6** 42 12N 73 58 E
Suusamyr Kyrka Tooloru, *Kyrgyzstan* **65 B6** 42 8N 73 15 E
Suva, *Fiji* **133 B2** 18 6 S 178 30 E
Suva Gora, *Macedonia* **50 E5** 41 45N 21 3 E
Suva Planina, *Serbia & M.* **50 C6** 43 10N 22 5 E
Suva Reka, *Serbia & M.* **50 D4** 42 21N 20 50 E
Suvorov, *Russia* **58 E9** 54 7N 36 30 E
Suvorov Is. = Suwarrow Is., *Cook Is.* **135 J11** 13 15 S 163 5W
Suvorove, *Ukraine* **53 E13** 45 35N 28 59 E
Suvorovo, *Bulgaria* **51 C11** 43 20N 27 35 E
Suwa, *Japan* **73 A10** 36 2N 138 8 E
Suwa-Ko, *Japan* **73 A10** 36 3N 138 5 E
Suwałki, *Poland* **54 D9** 54 8N 22 59 E
Suwana, *Indonesia* **79 K18** 8 44 S 115 36 E
Suwanee, *U.S.A.* **152 A5** 34 3N 84 4W
Suwannaphum, *Thailand* **86 E4** 15 33N 103 47 E
Suwannee, *U.S.A.* **153 F6** 29 20N 83 9W
Suwannee →, *U.S.A.* **153 F6** 29 17N 83 10W
Suwannee Sd., *U.S.A.* **153 F6** 29 20N 83 15W
Suwanose-Jima, *Japan* **71 K4** 29 38N 129 43 E
Suwarrow Is., *Cook Is.* **135 J11** 13 15 S 163 5W
Suwayq aş Şuqban, *Iraq* **96 D5** 31 32N 46 7 E
Suweis, Khalîg el, *Egypt* **106 J8** 28 40N 33 0 E
Suweis, Qanâ es, *Egypt* **106 H8** 31 0N 32 20 E
Suwŏn, *S. Korea* **75 F14** 37 17N 127 1 E
Suzak = Sosaq, *Kazakhstan* **65 A4** 44 9N 68 27 E
Suzaka, *Japan* **73 A10** 36 39N 138 19 E
Suzdal, *Russia* **58 D11** 56 29N 40 26 E
Suzhou, *Anhui, China* **74 H9** 33 41N 116 59 E
Suzhou, *Jiangsu, China* **77 B13** 31 19N 120 38 E
Suzu, *Japan* **71 F8** 37 25N 137 17 E
Suzu-Misaki, *Japan* **71 F8** 37 31N 137 21 E
Suzuka, *Japan* **73 C8** 34 55N 136 36 E
Suzuka-Sammyaku, *Japan* **73 B8** 35 5N 136 30 E
Suzzara, *Italy* **44 D7** 44 59N 10 45 E
Svalbard, *Arctic* **6 B8** 78 0N 17 0 E
Svalbard Radio = Longyearbyen, *Svalbard* **6 B8** 78 13N 15 40 E
Svalbarð, *Norður-þingeyjarsýsla, Iceland* **11 A11** 66 12N 15 43W
Svalbarð, *Suður-þingeyjarsýsla, Iceland* **11 B8** 65 45N 18 5W
Svalöv, *Sweden* **17 J7** 55 57N 13 8 E
Svalyava, *Ukraine* **52 B7** 48 33N 22 59 E
Svaneke, *Denmark* **17 J9** 55 8N 15 8 E
Svängsta, *Sweden* **17 H8** 56 16N 14 47 E
Svanskog, *Sweden* **16 E6** 59 11N 12 33 E
Svappavaara, *Sweden* **14 C19** 67 40N 21 3 E
Svärdsjö, *Sweden* **16 D9** 60 45N 15 54 E
Svarstad, *Norway* **18 E6** 59 27N 9 56 E
Svartå, *Sweden* **16 E8** 59 8N 14 32 E
Svartárkot, *Iceland* **11 B9** 65 20N 17 15W
Svartevatn, *Norway* **18 E3** 59 10N 6 56 E
Svartisen, *Norway* **14 C15** 66 40N 13 59 E
Svartvik, *Sweden* **16 B11** 62 19N 17 24 E
Svatove, *Ukraine* **59 H10** 49 22N 38 15 E
Svatovo = Svatove, *Ukraine* **59 H10** 49 22N 38 15 E
Svatsum, *Norway* **18 C6** 61 20N 9 50 E
Svay Chek, *Cambodia* **86 F4** 13 48N 102 58 E
Svay Rieng, *Cambodia* **87 G5** 11 9N 105 45 E
Svealand □, *Sweden* **16 D9** 60 20N 15 0 E
Svedala, *Sweden* **17 J7** 55 30N 13 15 E
Sveg, *Sweden* **16 B8** 62 2N 14 21 E
Sveindal, *Norway* **18 F4** 58 29N 7 30 E
Sveinseyri, *Iceland* **11 B3** 65 38N 23 51W
Sveio, *Norway* **18 E2** 59 33N 5 23 E
Svelgen, *Norway* **18 C2** 61 46N 5 17 E
Svelvik, *Norway* **18 E7** 59 37N 10 24 E
Svendborg, *Denmark* **17 J4** 55 4N 10 35 E
Svene, *Norway* **18 E6** 59 45N 9 31 E
Svenljunga, *Sweden* **17 G7** 57 29N 13 5 E
Svenstavik, *Sweden* **16 B8** 62 45N 14 26 E
Svenstrup, *Denmark* **17 H3** 56 58N 9 50 E
Sverdlovsk = Yekaterinburg, *Russia* **64 C8** 56 50N 60 30 E
Sverdlovsk, *Ukraine* **59 H10** 48 5N 39 47 E
Sverdrup Is., *Canada* **6 B3** 79 0N 97 0W
Sverige = Sweden ■, *Europe* **15 G16** 57 0N 15 0 E
Svetac, *Croatia* **45 E12** 43 3N 15 43 E
Sveti Ivan = Zelina, *Croatia* **45 C13** 45 57N 16 16 E
Sveti Nikola, Prokhad, *Europe* **50 C6** 43 27N 22 6 E
Sveti Nikole, *Macedonia* **50 E5** 41 51N 21 56 E
Sveti Rok, *Croatia* **45 D12** 44 22N 15 39 E
Sveti Vrach = Sandanski, *Bulgaria* **50 E7** 41 35N 23 16 E
Svetlaya, *Russia* **70 A9** 46 33N 138 18 E
Svetlogorsk = Svyetlahorsk, *Belarus* **59 F5** 52 38N 29 46 E
Svetlogorsk, *Russia* **54 D7** 54 56N 20 10 E
Svetlograd, *Russia* **61 H6** 45 25N 42 58 E
Svetlovodsk = Svitlovodsk, *Ukraine* **59 H7** 49 2N 33 13 E
Svetlyy, *Russia* **54 D7** 54 41N 20 8 E
Svetlyy, *Russia* **64 F8** 50 48N 60 51 E
Svidník, *Slovak Rep.* **35 B14** 49 20N 21 37 E
Svignaskarð, *Iceland* **11 C5** 64 40N 21 42W
Svilaja Planina, *Croatia* **45 E13** 43 49N 16 31 E
Svilajnac, *Serbia & M.* **50 B5** 44 15N 21 11 E
Svilengrad, *Bulgaria* **51 E10** 41 49N 26 12 E
Svinafell, *Iceland* **11 D10** 63 59N 16 51W
Svir →, *Russia* **58 B7** 60 30N 32 48 E
Sviritsa, *Russia* **58 B7** 60 29N 32 51 E
Svishtov, *Bulgaria* **51 C9** 43 36N 25 23 E
Svislach, *Belarus* **55 E11** 53 3N 24 2 E
Svitava →, *Czech Rep.* **35 B9** 49 11N 16 37 E
Svitavy, *Czech Rep.* **35 B9** 49 47N 16 28 E
Svitlovodsk, *Ukraine* **59 H7** 49 2N 33 13 E
Svizzer △, *Switz.* **33 C10** 46 40N 10 10 E
Svizzera = Switzerland ■, *Europe* **32 D6** 46 30N 8 0 E
Svobodnyy, *Russia* **67 D13** 51 20N 128 0 E
Svoge, *Bulgaria* **50 D7** 42 59N 23 23 E
Svolvær, *Norway* **14 B16** 68 15N 14 34 E
Svorkmo, *Norway* **18 A6** 63 10N 9 46 E
Svoronáta, *Greece* **39 C2** 38 7N 20 31 E
Svratka →, *Czech Rep.* **35 B9** 49 11N 16 38 E
Svrljig, *Serbia & M.* **50 C6** 43 25N 22 6 E
Svullrya, *Norway* **18 D9** 60 25N 12 23 E
Svyatogorovsky Rudnik = Dobropole, *Ukraine* **59 H9** 48 25N 37 2 E
Svyetlahorsk, *Belarus* **59 F5** 52 38N 29 46 E
Swa, *Burma* **90 F6** 19 15N 96 17 E
Swa Tende, *Dem. Rep. of the Congo* **115 D3** 7 9 S 17 7 E
Swabian Alps = Schwäbische Alb, *Germany* **31 G5** 48 20N 9 30 E
Swaffham, *U.K.* **21 E8** 52 39N 0 42 E
Swains I., *Amer. Samoa* **135 J11** 11 11 S 171 4W
Swainsboro, *U.S.A.* **152 C7** 32 36N 82 20W
Swakop →, *Namibia* **116 C2** 22 38 S 14 36 E
Swakopmund, *Namibia* **116 C1** 22 37 S 14 30 E
Swale →, *U.K.* **20 C6** 54 5N 1 20W
Swamihalli, *India* **95 G3** 14 52N 76 38 E
Swan →, *Australia* **125 F2** 32 3 S 115 45 E
Swan →, *Canada* **143 C8** 52 30N 100 45W
Swan Hill, *Australia* **128 C5** 35 20 S 143 33 E
Swan Hills, *Canada* **142 C5** 54 43N 115 24W
Swan Is. = Santanilla, Is., *Honduras* **164 C3** 17 22N 83 57W
Swan L., *Canada* **143 C8** 52 30N 100 40W
Swan Peak, *U.S.A.* **158 C7** 47 43N 113 38W
Swan Ra., *U.S.A.* **158 C7** 48 0N 113 45W
Swan Reach, *Australia* **128 C3** 34 35 S 139 37 E
Swan River, *Canada* **143 C8** 52 10N 101 16W
Swanage, *U.K.* **21 G6** 50 36N 1 58W
Swansea, *N.S.W., Australia* **129 B9** 33 3 S 151 35 E
Swansea, *Tas., Australia* **127 G4** 42 8 S 148 4 E
Swansea, *Canada* **150 C5** 43 38N 79 28W
Swansea, *U.K.* **21 F4** 51 37N 3 57W
Swansea, *U.S.A.* **152 B8** 33 44N 81 6W
Swansea □, *U.K.* **21 F3** 51 38N 4 3W
Swanton, *U.S.A.* **157 C13** 41 35N 83 53W
Swar →, *Pakistan* **93 B5** 34 40N 72 5 E
Swartberge, *S. Africa* **116 E3** 33 20 S 22 0 E
Swartmodder, *S. Africa* **116 D3** 28 1 S 20 32 E
Swartnossob →, *Namibia* **116 C2** 23 8 S 18 42 E
Swartruggens, *S. Africa* **116 D4** 25 39 S 26 42 E
Swarzędz, *Poland* **55 F4** 52 25N 17 4 E
Swastika, *Canada* **140 C3** 48 7N 80 6W
Swatow = Shantou, *China* **77 F11** 23 18N 116 40 E
Swaziland ■, *Africa* **117 D5** 26 30 S 31 30 E
Sweden ■, *Europe* **15 G16** 57 0N 15 0 E
Swedru, *Ghana* **113 D4** 5 32N 0 41W
Sweet Home, *U.S.A.* **158 D2** 44 24N 122 44W
Sweet Springs, *U.S.A.* **156 F3** 38 58N 93 25W
Sweetgrass, *U.S.A.* **158 B8** 48 59N 111 58W
Sweetwater, *Nev., U.S.A.* **160 G7** 38 27N 119 9W
Sweetwater, *Tenn., U.S.A.* **149 H3** 35 36N 84 28W
Sweetwater, *Tex., U.S.A.* **155 J4** 32 28N 100 25W
Sweetwater →, *U.S.A.* **158 E10** 42 31N 107 2W
Swellendam, *S. Africa* **116 E3** 34 1 S 20 26 E
Swider →, *Poland* **55 F8** 52 6N 21 14 E
Świdnica, *Poland* **55 H3** 50 50N 16 30 E
Świdnik, *Poland* **55 G9** 51 13N 22 39 E
Świdwin, *Poland* **54 E2** 53 47N 15 49 E
Świebodzice, *Poland* **55 H3** 50 51N 16 20 E
Świebodzin, *Poland* **55 F2** 52 15N 15 31 E
Świecie, *Poland* **54 E5** 53 25N 18 30 E
Swierzawa, *Poland* **55 G2** 51 1N 15 54 E
Świętokrzyski △, *Poland* **55 H7** 50 53N 20 59 E
Świętokrzyskie □, *Poland* **55 H7** 50 45N 20 45 E
Świętokrzyskie, Góry, *Poland* **55 H7** 51 0N 20 30 E
Swift Current, *Canada* **143 C7** 50 20N 107 45W
Swift Current →, *Canada* **143 C7** 50 38N 107 44W
Swifts Creek, *Australia* **129 D7** 37 17 S 147 44 E
Swilly, L., *Ireland* **23 A4** 55 12N 7 33W
Swindon, *U.K.* **21 F6** 51 34N 1 46W
Swindon □, *U.K.* **21 F6** 51 34N 1 46W
Swinemünde = Świnoujście, *Poland* **54 E1** 53 54N 14 16 E
Swinford, *Ireland* **23 C3** 53 57N 8 58W
Świnoujście, *Poland* **54 E1** 53 54N 14 16 E
Switzerland ■, *Europe* **32 D6** 46 30N 8 0 E
Swords, *Ireland* **23 C5** 53 28N 6 13W
Swoyerville, *U.S.A.* **151 E9** 41 18N 75 53W
Syasstroy, *Russia* **58 B7** 60 9N 32 33 E
Sycamore, *Ill., U.S.A.* **157 C8** 41 59N 88 41W
Sycamore, *Ohio, U.S.A.* **157 D13** 40 57N 83 10W
Sychevka, *Russia* **58 E8** 55 59N 34 16 E
Syców, *Poland* **55 G4** 51 19N 17 40 E
Sydenham →, *Canada* **150 D2** 42 33N 82 25W
Sydney, *Australia* **129 B9** 33 53 S 151 10 E
Sydney, *Canada* **141 C7** 46 7N 60 7W
Sydney L., *Canada* **143 C10** 50 41N 94 25W
Sydney Mines, *Canada* **141 C7** 46 18N 60 15W
Sydprøven = Alluitsup Paa, *Greenland* **10 E6** 60 30N 45 35W
Sydra, G. of = Surt, Khalīj, *Libya* **108 B3** 31 40N 18 30 E
Syeverodonetsk, *Ukraine* **59 H10** 48 58N 38 35 E
Syfteland, *Norway* **18 D2** 60 14N 5 27 E
Syke, *Germany* **30 C4** 52 55N 8 50 E
Sykesville, *U.S.A.* **150 E6** 41 3N 78 50W
Sykkylven, *Norway* **18 B3** 62 23N 6 35 E
Syktyvkar, *Russia* **56 B9** 61 45N 50 40 E
Sylacauga, *U.S.A.* **152 B3** 33 10N 86 15W
Sylarna, *Sweden* **18 A9** 63 2N 12 13 E
Sylhet, *Bangla.* **90 C3** 24 54N 91 52 E
Sylt, *Germany* **30 A4** 54 54N 8 22 E
Sylte, *Norway* **18 B4** 62 18N 7 17 E
Sylva →, *Russia* **64 B6** 58 0N 56 54 E
Sylvan Beach, *U.S.A.* **151 C9** 43 12N 75 44W
Sylvan Lake, *Canada* **142 C6** 52 20N 114 3W
Sylvania, *Ga., U.S.A.* **152 C8** 32 45N 81 38W
Sylvania, *Ohio, U.S.A.* **157 C13** 41 43N 83 42W
Sylvester, *U.S.A.* **152 D6** 31 32N 83 50W
Sym, *Russia* **66 C9** 60 20N 88 18 E
Symón, *Mexico* **162 C4** 24 42N 102 35W
Synelnykove, *Ukraine* **59 H8** 48 25N 35 30 E
Synevyr △, *Ukraine* **53 B8** 48 30N 23 40 E
Synevyrska Polyana, *Ukraine* **53 B8** 48 35N 23 41 E
Synnfjell, *Norway* **18 C6** 61 5N 9 46 E
Synnott Ra., *Australia* **124 C4** 16 30 S 125 20 E
Synyak, *Ukraine* **52 B7** 48 35N 22 51 E
Syowa, *Antarctica* **7 C5** 68 50 S 12 0 E
Syracuse = Siracusa, *Italy* **47 E8** 37 4N 15 17 E
Syracuse, *Ind., U.S.A.* **157 C11** 41 26N 85 45W
Syracuse, *Kans., U.S.A.* **155 G4** 37 59N 101 45W
Syracuse, *N.Y., U.S.A.* **151 C8** 43 3N 76 9W
Syracuse, *Nebr., U.S.A.* **154 E6** 40 39N 96 11W
Syrdarinsky = Syrdarya, *Uzbekistan* **65 C4** 40 50N 68 40 E
Syrdarya, *Uzbekistan* **65 C4** 40 50N 68 40 E
Syrdarya →, *Kazakhstan* **66 E7** 46 3N 61 0 E
Syria ■, *Asia* **101 E8** 35 0N 38 0 E
Syriam, *Burma* **90 G6** 16 44N 96 19 E
Syrian Desert = Shām, Bādiyat ash, *Asia* **96 C3** 32 0N 40 0 E
Syrnovorossiysk = Syrdarya, *Uzbekistan* **65 C4** 40 50N 68 40 E
Syros = Síros, *Greece* **48 D6** 37 28N 24 57 E
Sysert, *Russia* **64 C8** 56 29N 60 49 E
Sysslebäck, *Sweden* **16 D6** 60 44N 12 52 E
Syvde, *Norway* **18 B2** 62 5N 5 44 E
Syzran, *Russia* **60 D9** 53 12N 48 30 E
Szabolcs-Szatmár-Bereg □, *Hungary* **52 B6** 48 2N 21 45 E
Szadek, *Poland* **55 G5** 51 41N 18 59 E
Szamocin, *Poland* **55 E4** 53 2N 17 7 E
Szamos →, *Hungary* **52 B7** 48 7N 22 20 E
Szamotuły, *Poland* **55 F3** 52 37N 16 33 E
Száraz →, *Hungary* **52 D6** 46 10N 21 15 E
Szarvas, *Hungary* **52 D5** 46 50N 20 38 E
Százhalombatta, *Hungary* **52 C3** 47 20N 18 58 E
Szczawnica, *Poland* **55 J7** 49 26N 20 30 E
Szczebrzeszyn, *Poland* **55 H9** 50 42N 22 59 E
Szczecin, *Poland* **54 E1** 53 27N 14 27 E
Szczecinek, *Poland* **54 E3** 53 43N 16 41 E
Szczeciński, Zalew = Stettiner Haff, *Germany* **30 B10** 53 47N 14 15 E
Szczekociny, *Poland* **55 H6** 50 38N 19 48 E
Szczucin, *Poland* **55 H8** 50 18N 21 4 E
Szczuczyn, *Poland* **54 E9** 53 36N 22 19 E
Szczyrk, *Poland* **55 J6** 49 43N 19 2 E
Szczytna, *Poland* **55 H3** 50 25N 16 28 E
Szczytno, *Poland* **54 E7** 53 33N 21 0 E
Szechuan Basin = Sichuan Pendi, *China* **76 B5** 31 0N 105 0 E
Szechwan = Sichuan □, *China* **76 B5** 30 30N 103 0 E
Szécsény, *Hungary* **52 B4** 48 7N 19 30 E
Szeged, *Hungary* **52 D5** 46 16N 20 10 E
Szeghalom, *Hungary* **52 C6** 47 1N 21 10 E
Székesfehérvár, *Hungary* **52 C3** 47 15N 18 25 E
Szekszárd, *Hungary* **52 D3** 46 22N 18 42 E
Szendrő, *Hungary* **52 B5** 48 24N 20 41 E
Szentendre, *Hungary* **52 C4** 47 39N 19 4 E
Szentes, *Hungary* **52 D5** 46 39N 20 21 E
Szentgotthárd, *Hungary* **52 D1** 46 58N 16 19 E
Szentlőrinc, *Hungary* **52 D3** 46 3N 18 1 E
Szeping = Siping, *China* **75 C13** 43 8N 124 21 E
Szerencs, *Hungary* **52 B6** 48 10N 21 12 E
Szigetszentmiklós, *Hungary* **52 C4** 47 21N 19 3 E
Szigetvár, *Hungary* **52 D2** 46 3N 17 46 E
Szikszó, *Hungary* **52 B5** 48 12N 20 56 E
Szklarska Poreba, *Poland* **55 H2** 50 50N 15 33 E
Szkwa →, *Poland* **55 E8** 53 11N 21 43 E
Szlichtyngowa, *Poland* **55 G3** 51 42N 16 15 E
Szob, *Hungary* **52 C3** 47 48N 18 53 E
Szolnok, *Hungary* **52 C5** 47 10N 20 15 E
Szombathely, *Hungary* **52 C1** 47 14N 16 38 E
Szprotawa, *Poland* **55 G2** 51 33N 15 35 E
Sztálinváros = Dunaújváros, *Hungary* **52 D3** 46 58N 18 57 E
Sztum, *Poland* **54 E6** 53 55N 19 1 E
Sztutowo, *Poland* **54 D6** 54 20N 19 15 E
Szubin, *Poland* **55 E4** 53 1N 17 45 E
Szydłowiec, *Poland* **55 G7** 51 15N 20 51 E
Szypliszki, *Poland* **54 D10** 54 17N 23 2 E

T

Ta Khli Khok, *Thailand* **86 E3** 15 18N 100 20 E
Ta Lai, *Vietnam* **87 G6** 11 24N 107 23 E
Ta Pieh Shan = Dabie Shan, *China* **77 B10** 31 20N 115 20 E
Tab, *Hungary* **52 D3** 46 44N 18 2 E
Tabacal, *Argentina* **174 A3** 23 15 S 64 15W
Tabaco, *Phil.* **80 E4** 13 22N 123 44 E
Tabagné, *Ivory C.* **112 D4** 7 59N 3 4W
Ţābah, *Si. Arabia* **96 E4** 26 55N 42 38 E
Tabajara, *Brazil* **173 B5** 8 56 S 62 8W
Tabalo, *Papua N. G.* **132 A5** 1 24 S 149 40 E
Tabalos, *Peru* **172 B2** 6 26 S 76 37W
Tabanan, *Indonesia* **79 K18** 8 32 S 115 8 E
Tabankort, *Niger* **113 B5** 17 44N 0 20 E
Tabar I., *Papua N. G.* **132 B7** 2 56 S 152 0 E
Tabar Is., *Papua N. G.* **132 B7** 2 50 S 152 0 E
Tabarka, *Tunisia* **108 A1** 36 56N 8 46 E
Ţabas, *Khorāsān, Iran* **97 C9** 32 48N 60 12 E
Ţabas, *Khorāsān, Iran* **97 C8** 33 35N 56 55 E
Tabasará, Serranía de, *Panama* **164 E3** 8 35N 81 40W
Tabasco □, *Mexico* **163 D6** 17 45N 93 30W
Tabāsīn, *Iran* **97 D8** 31 12N 57 54 E
Tabatinga, *Brazil* **172 A4** 4 16 S 69 56W
Tabatinga, Serra da, *Brazil* **170 D3** 10 30 S 44 0W
Tabayin, *Burma* **90 D5** 22 42N 95 20 E
Tabelbala, Kahal de, *Algeria* **111 C4** 28 47N 2 0W
Tabelembila, *Algeria* **111 D5** 24 43N 4 16 E
Taber, *Canada* **142 D6** 49 47N 112 8W
Taberg, *Sweden* **17 G8** 57 40N 14 6 E
Taberg, *U.S.A.* **151 C9** 43 18N 75 37W
Tabi, *Angola* **115 D2** 8 10 S 13 18 E
Tabira, *Brazil* **170 C4** 7 35 S 37 33W
Tabla, *Niger* **113 C5** 13 46N 3 1 E
Tablas de Daimiel △, *Spain* **43 F7** 39 9N 3 40W
Tablas I., *Phil.* **80 E4** 12 25N 122 2 E
Tablas Strait, *Phil.* **80 E3** 12 40N 121 48 E
Table, Pte. de la, *Réunion* **121 c** 21 14 S 55 48 E
Table B., *Canada* **141 B8** 53 40N 56 25W
Table B., *S. Africa* **116 E2** 33 35 S 18 25 E
Table C., *N.Z.* **130 F7** 39 6 S 178 0 E
Table Grove, *U.S.A.* **156 D6** 40 20N 90 27W
Table I., *Burma* **95 G11** 14 12N 93 22 E
Table Mt., *S. Africa* **116 E2** 34 0 S 18 22 E
Table Rock L., *U.S.A.* **155 G8** 36 36N 93 19W
Tabletop, Mt., *Australia* **126 C4** 23 24 S 147 11 E
Tabocal, *Brazil* **169 D6** 2 42 S 57 40W
Tábor, *Czech Rep.* **34 B7** 49 25N 14 39 E
Tabora, *Tanzania* **118 D3** 5 2 S 32 50 E
Tabora □, *Tanzania* **118 D3** 5 0 S 33 0 E
Taboshar, *Tajikistan* **65 C4** 40 34N 69 38 E
Tabou, *Ivory C.* **112 E3** 4 30N 7 20W
Tabrīz, *Iran* **101 C12** 38 7N 46 20 E
Tabuaeran, *Kiribati* **135 G12** 3 51N 159 22W
Tabubil, *Papua N. G.* **132 C1** 5 20 S 141 15 E
Tabuenca, *Spain* **40 D3** 41 42N 1 33W
Tabuk, *Phil.* **80 C3** 17 24N 121 25 E
Tabūk, *Si. Arabia* **96 D3** 28 23N 36 36 E
Taburno-Camposauro ⌓, *Italy* **47 A7** 41 8N 14 37 E
Tabwemasana, Mt., *Vanuatu* **133 E4** 15 20 S 166 44 E
Täby, *Sweden* **16 E12** 59 28N 18 4 E
Tacámbaro de Codallos, *Mexico* **162 D4** 19 14N 101 28W
Tacarigua, Laguna de, *Venezuela* **168 A4** 10 15N 65 50W
Tacheng, *China* **68 B3** 46 40N 82 58 E
Tach'i, *Taiwan* **77 E13** 24 46N 121 0 E
Tachia, *Taiwan* **77 E13** 24 25N 120 28 E
Tachibana-Wan, *Japan* **72 E2** 32 45N 130 7 E
Tachikawa, *Japan* **73 B11** 35 42N 139 25 E
Tach'ing Shan = Daqing Shan, *China* **74 D6** 40 40N 111 0 E
Táchira □, *Venezuela* **168 B3** 8 7N 72 15W
Tachov, *Czech Rep.* **34 B5** 49 47N 12 39 E
Tácina →, *Italy* **47 D9** 38 57N 16 55 E
Tacloban, *Phil.* **81 F5** 11 15N 124 58 E
Tacna, *Peru* **172 D3** 18 0 S 70 20W
Tacna □, *Peru* **172 D3** 17 40 S 70 20W
Tacoma, *U.S.A.* **160 C4** 47 14N 122 26W
Tacopaya = Zudáñez, *Bolivia* **173 D5** 19 6 S 64 44W
Tacuarembó, *Uruguay* **175 C4** 31 45 S 56 0W
Tacurong, *Phil.* **81 H5** 6 40N 124 41 E
Tacutu →, *Brazil* **169 C5** 3 1N 60 29W
Tada-u, *Burma* **90 E5** 21 49N 95 58 E
Tadahadi, *Solomon Is.* **133 N11** 10 18 S 161 35 E
Tademaït, Plateau du, *Algeria* **111 C5** 28 30N 2 30 E
Tadent, O. →, *Algeria* **111 D6** 22 25N 6 40 E
Tadéra, *Niger* **111 D6** 20 29N 8 18 E
Tadine, *N. Cal.* **133 U21** 21 33 S 167 52 E
Tadio, L., *Ivory C.* **112 D3** 5 10N 5 15W
Tadjerdjeri, O. →, *Algeria* **111 C6** 26 0N 8 0 E
Tadjerouna, *Algeria* **111 B5** 33 31N 2 3 E
Tadjettaret, O. →, *Algeria* **111 D6** 21 20N 7 22 E
Tadjmout, *Laghouat, Algeria* **111 B5** 33 52N 2 30 E
Tadjmout, *Saoura, Algeria* **111 C5** 25 37N 3 48 E
Tadjoura, *Djibouti* **107 E5** 11 50N 42 55 E
Tadjoura, Golfe de, *Djibouti* **107 E5** 11 50N 43 0 E
Tadmor, *N.Z.* **131 B7** 41 27 S 172 45 E
Tadoba △, *India* **94 D4** 20 30N 78 20 E
Tadotsu, *Japan* **72 C5** 34 16N 133 45 E
Tadoule L., *Canada* **143 B9** 58 36N 98 20W
Tadoussac, *Canada* **141 C6** 48 11N 69 42W
Tadpatri, *India* **95 G4** 14 55N 78 1 E
Tadrés ⌓, *Niger* **113 B6** 16 0N 7 10 E
Tadzhikistan = Tajikistan ■, *Asia* **65 D4** 38 30N 70 0 E
Taechŏn-ni, *S. Korea* **75 F14** 36 21N 126 36 E
Taegu, *S. Korea* **75 G15** 35 50N 128 37 E
Taegwan, *N. Korea* **75 D13** 40 13N 125 12 E
Taejŏn, *S. Korea* **75 F14** 36 20N 127 28 E
Taen, Ko, *Thailand* **87 b** 9 22N 99 57 E
Tafalla, *Spain* **40 C3** 42 30N 1 41W
Tafar, *Sudan* **107 F2** 6 52N 28 15 E
Tafassasset, O. →, *Algeria* **111 D6** 22 0N 9 57 E
Tafelbaai = Table B., *S. Africa* **116 E2** 33 35 S 18 25 E
Tafelney, C., *Morocco* **110 B3** 31 3N 9 51W
Tafermaar, *Indonesia* **83 C4** 6 47 S 134 10 E
Taffermit, *Morocco* **110 C3** 29 37N 9 15W
Tafí Viejo, *Argentina* **174 B2** 26 43 S 65 17W
Tafīhān, *Iran* **97 D7** 29 25N 52 39 E
Tafilalet, *Morocco* **110 B4** 31 20N 4 45W
Tafiré, *Ivory C.* **112 D3** 9 4N 5 4W
Tafjord, *Norway* **18 B4** 62 14N 7 24 E
Tafnidilt, *Morocco* **110 C2** 28 47N 10 58W

Tafo, *Ghana* **113 D4** 6 15N 0 20W
Tafraoute, *Morocco* . . **110 C3** 29 50N 8 58W
Tafresh, *Iran* . . . . **97 C6** 34 45N 49 57 E
Taft, *Iran* . . . . **97 D7** 31 45N 54 14 E
Taft, *Phil.* . . . . **81 F5** 11 57N 125 30 E
Taft, *U.S.A.* **161 K7** 35 8N 119 28W
Taftān, Kūh-e, *Iran* . . **97 D9** 28 40N 61 0 E
Tafwap, *India* . . . . **95 L11** 7 23N 93 43 E
Taga, *Samoa* . . . . **133 W23** 13 46 S 172 28W
Taga Dzong, *Bhutan* . . **90 B2** 27 5N 89 55 E
Tagana-an, *Phil.* . . . . . **81 G5** 9 42N 125 35 E
Taganrog, *Russia* . . . . . **59 J10** 47 12N 38 50 E
Taganrogskiy Zaliv,
Russia . . . . **59 J10** 47 0N 38 30 E
Tagânt, *Mauritania* . . . **112 B2** 18 20N 11 0W
Tagap Ga, *Burma* . . . . . **90 B6** 26 56N 96 13 E
Tagatay, *Phil.* . . . . **80 D3** 14 6N 120 56 E
Tagauayan I., *Phil.* . . . **81 F3** 10 58N 121 13 E
Tagaung, *Burma* . . . . . **90 D6** 23 30N 96 2 E
Tagawa, *Japan* . . . . . . **72 D2** 33 38N 130 51 E
Tagbilaran, *Phil.* . . . . . **81 G4** 9 39N 123 51 E
Tagdempt = Tiaret,
Algeria . . . . **111 A5** 35 20N 1 21 E
Tage, *Papua N. G.* . . . . **132 D2** 6 19 S 143 20 E
Tággia, *Italy* . . . . **44 E4** 43 52N 7 51 E
Taghzout, *Morocco* . . . **110 B4** 33 30N 4 49W
Tagish, *Canada* **142 A2** 60 19N 134 16W
Tagish L., *Canada* **142 A2** 60 10N 134 20W
Tagkawayan, *Phil.* . . . . **80 E4** 13 58N 122 32 E
Tagliacozzo, *Italy* . . . . **45 F10** 42 4N 13 14 E
Tagliamento →, *Italy* . **45 C10** 45 38N 13 6 E
Tàglio di Po, *Italy* . . . . **45 D9** 45 0N 12 12 E
Tagna, *Colombia* . . . . . **168 D3** 2 24 S 70 37W
Tago, *Phil.* . . . . **81 G6** 9 2N 126 13 E
Tago, Mt., *Phil.* . . . . . . **81 G5** 8 23N 125 5 E
Tagomago, *Spain* . . . . . **38 C2** 39 2N 1 39 E
Tagourãret, *Mauritania* **112 B3** 17 45N 7 45W
Taguatinga, *Brazil* . . . **171 D3** 12 16 S 42 26W
Tagudin, *Phil.* . . . . **80 C3** 16 56N 120 27 E
Taguenout Hagguerel,
Mali **111 D4** 21 14N 0 48W
Tagula, *Papua N. G.* . . **132 F7** 11 22 S 153 15 E
Tagula I., *Papua N. G.* **132 F7** 11 30 S 153 30 E
Tagum, *Phil.* . . . . **81 H5** 7 33N 125 53 E
Tagus = Tejo →,
Europe **43 F2** 38 40N 9 24W
Tahakopa, *N.Z.* . . . . . . **131 G4** 46 30 S 169 23 E
Tahala, *Morocco* **110 B4** 34 0N 4 28W
Tahan, Gunung,
Malaysia . . . . **87 K4** 4 34N 102 17 E
Tahānah-ye sūr Gol,
Afghan. . . . . **91 C2** 31 43N 67 53 E
Tahara, *Japan* . . . . **73 C9** 34 40N 137 16 E
Tahat, *Algeria* . . . . **111 D6** 23 18N 5 33 E
Tāherī, *Iran* . . . . **97 E7** 27 43N 52 20 E
Tahiti,
French Polynesia . . . **133 S16** 17 37 S 149 27W
Tahlab →, *Pakistan* . . **91 C1** 28 9N 62 45 E
Tahlequah, *U.S.A.* **155 H7** 35 55N 94 58W
Tahoe, L., *U.S.A.* **160 G6** 39 6N 120 2W
Tahoe City, *U.S.A.* . . . **160 F6** 39 10N 120 9W
Tahoka, *U.S.A.* **155 J4** 33 10N 101 48W
Taholah, *U.S.A.* **160 C2** 47 21N 124 17W
Tahora, *N.Z.* . . . . **130 F3** 39 2 S 174 49 E
Tahoua, *Niger* . . . . **113 C6** 14 57N 5 16 E
Tahrūd, *Iran* . . . . **97 D8** 29 26N 57 49 E
Tahsis, *Canada* **142 D3** 49 55N 126 40W
Tahta, *Egypt* . . . . **106 B3** 26 44N 31 32 E
Tahtaköprü, *Turkey* . . **51 G13** 39 57N 29 39 E
Tahtalı Dağları, *Turkey* **100 C7** 38 20N 36 0 E
Tahuamanu →, *Bolivia* **172 C4** 11 6 S 67 36W
Tahulandang, *Indonesia* **82 A3** 2 27N 125 23 E
Tahuna, *Indonesia* . . . **82 A3** 3 38N 125 30 E
Taï, *Ivory C.* **112 D3** 5 55N 7 30W
Taï △, *Ivory C.* **112 D3** 5 25N 7 5W
Tai Au Mun, *China* . . . **69 G11** 22 18N 114 17 E
Tai Hu, *China* . . . . **77 B12** 31 5N 120 10 E
Tai Mo Shan, *China* . . **69 G11** 22 25N 114 7 E
Tai O, *China* . . . . **69 G10** 22 15N 113 52 E
Tai Pang Wan, *China* . **69 F11** 22 33N 114 24 E
Tai Po, *China* . . . . **69 F11** 22 27N 114 10 E
Tai Rom Yen △,
Thailand . . . . **87 H2** 8 45N 99 30 E
Tai Shan, *China* . . . . . **75 F9** 36 25N 117 20 E
Tai Yue Shan = Lantau
I., *China* . . . . **69 G10** 22 15N 113 56 E
Tai'an, *China* . . . . **75 F9** 36 12N 117 8 E
Taiarapu, Presq. de,
Tahiti . . . . **133 S16** 17 47 S 149 14W
Taibei = T'aipei,
Taiwan . . . . **77 E13** 25 2N 121 30 E
Taibique, *Canary Is.* . . **9 e1** 27 42N 17 58W
Taibus Qi, *China* . . . . . **74 D8** 41 54N 115 22 E
Taicang, *China* . . . . . . **77 B13** 31 30N 121 5 E
Taichow = Taizhou,
China . . . . **77 A12** 32 28N 119 55 E
T'aichung, *Taiwan* . . . **77 E13** 24 9N 120 37 E
Taieri →, *N.Z.* . . . . . . **131 G5** 46 3 S 170 12 E
Taiga Madema, *Libya* . **108 D3** 23 46N 15 25 E
Taigu, *China* . . . . **74 F7** 37 28N 112 30 E
Taihang Shan, *China* . . **74 G7** 36 0N 113 30 E
Taihape, *N.Z.* . . . . **130 F4** 39 41 S 175 48 E
Taihe, *Anhui, China* . . **74 H8** 33 20N 115 42 E
Taihe, *Jiangxi, China* . **77 D10** 26 47N 114 52 E
Taihoku = T'aipei,
Taiwan . . . . **77 E13** 25 2N 121 30 E
Taihu, *China* . . . . **77 B11** 30 22N 116 20 E
Taijiang, *China* . . . . . . **76 D7** 26 39N 108 21 E
Taikang, *China* . . . . . . **74 G8** 34 5N 114 50 E
Taikkyi, *Burma* . . . . . . **90 G6** 17 20N 96 0 E
Tailem Bend, *Australia* **128 C3** 35 12 S 139 29 E
Tailfingen, *Germany* . . **31 G5** 48 15N 9 1 E
Tailuko, *Taiwan* . . . . . **77 E13** 24 9N 121 37 E
Taimyr Peninsula =
Taymyr, Poluostrov,
Russia . . . . **67 B11** 75 0N 100 0 E
Tain, *U.K.* **22 D4** 57 49N 4 4W
T'ainan, *Taiwan* . . . . . **77 F13** 23 0N 120 10 E
Taínaron, Ákra, *Greece* **48 E4** 36 22N 22 27 E
Tainggyo, *Burma* . . . . **90 G5** 17 49N 94 29 E
Taining, *China* . . . . . . **77 D11** 26 54N 117 9 E
Taiobeiras, *Brazil* . . . . **171 E3** 15 49 S 42 14W
Taipa, *China* . . . . **69 G10** 22 10N 113 35 E
T'aipei, *Taiwan* . . . . . **77 E13** 25 2N 121 30 E
Taiping, *China* . . . . . . **77 B12** 30 15N 118 6 E
Taiping, *Malaysia* . . . . **87 K3** 4 51N 100 44 E
Taipingzhen, *China* . . . **74 H6** 33 35N 111 42 E
Taipu, *Brazil* . . . . **170 C4** 5 37 S 35 36W
Tairbeart = Tarbert,
U.K. **22 D2** 57 54N 6 49W
Tairenpokpi, *India* . . . **90 C4** 24 39N 93 40 E
Tairua, *N.Z.* . . . . **130 D4** 37 0 S 175 51 E
Taisha, *Japan* . . . . **72 B4** 35 24N 132 40 E
Taishan, *China* . . . . . . **77 F9** 22 14N 112 41 E
Taishun, *China* . . . . . . **77 D12** 27 30N 119 42 E
Taita Hills, *Kenya* . . . . **118 C4** 3 25 S 38 15 E
Taitao, C., *Chile* . . . . . **176 C1** 45 53 S 75 5W
Taitao, Pen. de, *Chile* . **176 C2** 46 30 S 75 0W
T'aitung, *Taiwan* . . . . **77 F13** 22 43N 121 4 E
Taivalkoski, *Finland* . . **14 D23** 65 33N 28 12 E
Taiwan ■, *Asia* . . . . . **77 F13** 23 30N 121 0 E
Taiwan Strait, *Asia* . . . **77 E12** 24 40N 120 0 E
Taixing, *China* . . . . . . **77 A13** 32 11N 120 0 E
Taiyara, *Sudan* . . . . . . **107 E3** 13 12N 30 47 E
Taïyetos Óros, *Greece* . **48 D4** 37 0N 22 23 E
Taiyiba, *Israel* . . . . . . **103 C4** 32 36N 35 27 E
Taiyuan, *China* . . . . . . **74 F7** 37 52N 112 33 E
Taizhong = T'aichung,
Taiwan . . . . **77 E13** 24 9N 120 37 E
Taizhou, *China* . . . . . . **77 A12** 32 28N 119 55 E
Taizhou Liedao, *China* **77 C13** 28 30N 121 55 E
Ta'izz, *Yemen* . . . . **98 D4** 13 35N 44 2 E
Tājābād, *Iran* . . . . **97 D7** 30 2N 54 24 E
Tajapuru, Furo do,
Brazil . . . . **170 B1** 1 50 S 50 25W
Tajarḥī, *Libya* . . . . **108 D2** 24 21N 14 28 E
Tajikistan ■, *Asia* . . . . **65 D4** 38 30N 70 0 E
Tajima, *Japan* . . . . **71 F9** 37 12N 139 46 E
Tajimi, *Japan* . . . . **73 B9** 35 19N 137 8 E
Tajo = Tejo →, *Europe* **43 F2** 38 40N 9 24W
Tajrīsh, *Iran* . . . . **97 C6** 35 48N 51 25 E
Tājūrā, *Libya* . . . . **108 B2** 32 51N 13 21 E
Tak, *Thailand* . . . . **86 D2** 16 52N 99 8 E
Takāb, *Iran* . . . . **101 D12** 36 24N 47 7 E
Takachiho, *Japan* . . . . **72 E3** 32 42N 131 18 E
Takachu, *Botswana* . . . **116 C3** 22 37 S 21 58 E
Takada, *Japan* . . . . **71 F9** 37 7N 138 15 E
Takahagi, *Japan* . . . . . **71 F10** 36 43N 140 45 E
Takahashi, *Japan* . . . . . **72 C5** 34 51N 133 39 E
Takaka, *N.Z.* . . . . **131 A7** 40 51 S 172 50 E
Takaki = Yamato,
Japan . . . . **73 B11** 35 27N 139 25 E
Takamaka, *Seychelles* . **121 b** 4 50 S 55 30 E
Takamatsu, *Japan* . . . . **72 C6** 34 20N 134 5 E
Takanabe, *Japan* . . . . . **72 E3** 32 8N 131 30 E
Takaoka, *Japan* . . . . . . **73 A9** 36 47N 137 0 E
Takapau, *N.Z.* . . . . **130 G5** 40 2 S 176 21 E
Takapuna, *N.Z.* . . . . . . **130 C3** 36 47 S 174 47 E
Takasago, *Japan* . . . . . **72 C6** 34 45N 134 48 E
Takasaki, *Japan* . . . . . . **73 A11** 36 20N 139 0 E
Takatsuki, *Japan* . . . . . **73 C7** 34 51N 135 37 E
Takaungu, *Kenya* . . . . . **118 C4** 3 38 S 39 52 E
Takayama, *Japan* . . . . . **73 A9** 36 18N 137 11 E
Takayama-Bonchi,
Japan . . . . **73 B9** 36 0N 137 18 E
Take-Shima, *Japan* . . . **71 J5** 30 49N 130 26 E
Takefu, *Japan* . . . . **73 B8** 35 50N 136 10 E
Takehara, *Japan* . . . . . **72 C4** 34 21N 132 55 E
Takeli, *Tajikistan* . . . . **65 C4** 40 29N 69 26 E
Takengon, *Indonesia* . . **84 B1** 4 45N 96 50 E
Takeo, *Japan* . . . . **72 D2** 33 12N 130 1 E
Tåkern, *Sweden* . . . . . . **17 F8** 58 22N 14 45 E
Takeshima = Tok-do,
Asia . . . . **71 F5** 37 15N 131 52 E
Tākestān, *Iran* . . . . **97 C6** 36 0N 49 40 E
Taketa, *Japan* . . . . **72 E3** 32 58N 131 24 E
Takev, *Cambodia* . . . . . **87 G5** 10 59N 104 47 E
Takh, *India* . . . . **93 C7** 33 6N 77 32 E
Takhār □, *Afghan.* . . . . **91 A3** 36 40N 70 0 E
Takht-Sulaiman,
Pakistan . . . . **92 D3** 31 40N 69 58 E
Taki, *Papua N. G.* . . . . **132 D8** 6 29 S 155 52 E
Takikawa, *Japan* . . . . . **70 C10** 43 33N 141 54 E
Takla L., *Canada* **142 B3** 55 15N 125 45W
Takla Landing, *Canada* **142 B3** 55 30N 125 50W
Takla Makan =
Taklamakan Shamo,
China . . . . **68 C3** 38 0N 83 0 E
Taklamakan Shamo,
China . . . . **68 C3** 38 0N 83 0 E
Takotna, *U.S.A.* **144 E8** 62 59N 156 4W
Taku, *Japan* . . . . **72 D2** 33 18N 130 3 E
Taku →, *Canada* **142 B2** 58 30N 133 50W
Takua Thung, *Thailand* **87 a** 8 24N 98 27 E
Takum, *India* . . . . **90 B4** 27 47N 93 37 E
Takum, *Nigeria* . . . . . . **113 D6** 7 18N 9 36 E
Takundi, *Dem. Rep. of*
the Congo . . . . **115 C3** 4 45 S 16 34 E
Takutu →, *Guyana* . . . **169 C5** 3 1N 60 29W
Tal Halāl, *Iran* . . . . **97 D7** 28 54N 55 1 E
Tala, *Uruguay* . . . . **175 C4** 34 21 S 55 46W
Talachyn, *Belarus* . . . . **58 E5** 54 25N 29 42 E
Talacogan, *Phil.* . . . . . . **81 G5** 8 32N 125 39 E
Talagang, *Pakistan* . . . **92 C5** 32 55N 72 25 E
Talagante, *Chile* . . . . . **174 C1** 33 40 S 70 50W
Talahouhait, *Algeria* . . **111 D5** 24 52N 1 5 E
Talaimannar, *Sri Lanka* **95 K4** 9 6N 79 43 E
Talaïnt, *Morocco* **110 C3** 29 41N 9 40W
Talak, *Niger* . . . . **113 B6** 18 0N 5 0 E
Talakag, *Phil.* . . . . **81 G5** 8 16N 124 37 E
Talamanca, Cordillera
de, *Cent. Amer.* **164 E3** 9 20N 83 20W
Talant, *France* . . . . **27 E11** 47 19N 4 58 E
Talara, *Peru* . . . . **172 A1** 4 38 S 81 18W
Talas, *Kyrgyzstan* . . . . **65 B6** 42 30N 72 13 E
Talas, *Turkey* . . . . **100 C6** 38 41N 35 33 E
Talas →, *Kazakhstan* . . **65 B5** 44 0N 70 20 E
Talas Ala Too,
Kyrgyzstan . . . . **65 B6** 42 15N 72 0 E
Talasea, *Papua N. G.* . **132 C6** 5 20 S 150 2 E
Talasskiy Alatau =
Talas Ala Too,
Kyrgyzstan . . . . **65 B6** 42 15N 72 0 E
Talâta, *Egypt* . . . . **103 E1** 30 36N 32 20 E
Talata Mafara, *Nigeria* **113 C6** 12 38N 6 4 E
Talaud, Kepulauan,
Indonesia . . . . **82 A3** 4 30N 126 50 E
Talaud Is. = Talaud,
Kepulauan, *Indonesia* **82 A3** 4 30N 126 50 E
Talavera de la Reina,
Spain **42 F6** 39 55N 4 46W
Talavera la Real, *Spain* **43 G4** 38 53N 6 46W
Talawgyi, *Burma* . . . . . **90 C6** 25 4N 97 19 E
Talayan, *Phil.* . . . . **81 H5** 6 52N 124 24 E
Talayuela, *Spain* **42 F5** 39 59N 5 36W
Talbandh, *India* . . . . . . **93 H12** 22 3N 86 20 E
Talbert, Sillon de,
France **26 D3** 48 53N 3 5W
Talbot, *Australia* . . . . **128 D5** 37 10 S 143 44 E
Talbot, C., *Australia* . . **124 B4** 13 48 S 126 43 E
Talbotton, *U.S.A.* **152 C5** 32 41N 84 32W
Talbragar →, *Australia* **129 B8** 32 12 S 148 37 E
Talca, *Chile* . . . . **174 D1** 35 28 S 71 40W
Talcahuano, *Chile* . . . . **174 D1** 36 40 S 73 10W
Talcher, *India* . . . . **94 D7** 21 0N 85 18 E
Talcho, *Niger* . . . . **113 C5** 14 44N 3 28 E
Taldy Kurgan =
Taldyqorghan,
Kazakhstan . . . . **66 E8** 45 10N 78 45 E
Taldy-Suu, *Kyrgyzstan* **65 B9** 42 48N 78 26 E
Taldyqorghan,
Kazakhstan . . . . **66 E8** 45 10N 78 45 E
Talent, *U.S.A.* **158 E2** 42 15N 122 47W
Tālesh, *Iran* . . . . **97 B6** 37 58N 48 58 E
Tālesh, Kūhhā-ye, *Iran* **97 B6** 37 42N 48 55 E
Talgar = Talghar,
Kazakhstan . . . . **65 B8** 43 19N 77 15 E
Talgar, Pik, *Kazakhstan* **65 B8** 43 5N 77 20 E
Talghar, *Kazakhstan* . . **65 B8** 43 19N 77 15 E
Talguharai, *Sudan* . . . . **106 D4** 18 19N 35 56 E
Talguppa, *India* . . . . . . **95 G2** 14 13N 74 56 E
Tali Post, *Sudan* . . . . . **107 F3** 5 55N 30 44 E
Taliabu, *Indonesia* . . . **82 B2** 1 50 S 125 0 E
Talibon, *Phil.* . . . . **81 F5** 10 9N 124 20 E
Talibong, Ko, *Thailand* **87 J2** 7 15N 99 23 E
Talihina, *U.S.A.* **155 H7** 34 45N 95 3W
Talikota, *India* . . . . **95 F3** 16 29N 76 17 E
Talimardzhan,
Uzbekistan . . . . **65 D2** 38 17N 65 33 E
Talipao, *Phil.* . . . . **81 J3** 5 59N 121 7 E
Talisay, *Phil.* . . . . **81 F4** 10 44N 122 58 E
Talisayan, *Phil.* . . . . . . **81 G5** 9 0N 124 55 E
Talitsa, *Russia* . . . . **64 C9** 57 0N 63 43 E
Talitsky Zavod =
Talitsa, *Russia* . . . . . **64 C9** 57 0N 63 43 E
Taliwang, *Indonesia* . . **85 D5** 8 50 S 116 55 E
Talkeetna, *U.S.A.* **144 E10** 62 20N 150 6W
Tall 'Afar, *Iraq* . . . . . . **101 D10** 36 22N 42 27 E
Tall Kalakh, *Syria* . . . . **103 A5** 34 41N 36 15 E
Talla, *Egypt* . . . . **106 B3** 28 5N 30 43 E
Talladega, *U.S.A.* **152 B3** 33 26N 86 6W
Tallahassee, *U.S.A.* . . . **152 E5** 30 27N 84 17W
Tallangatta, *Australia* . **129 D7** 36 15 S 147 19 E
Tallapoosa, *U.S.A.* . . . **152 B4** 33 45N 85 17W
Tallapoosa →, *U.S.A.* . **152 C3** 32 30N 86 16W
Tallard, *France* . . . . . . **29 D10** 44 28N 6 3 E
Tallarook, *Australia* . . **129 D6** 37 5 S 145 6 E
Tallassee, *U.S.A.* **152 C4** 32 32N 85 54W
Tällberg, *Sweden* . . . . . **16 D9** 60 51N 15 2 E
Tallering Pk., *Australia* **125 E2** 28 6 S 115 37 E
Talli, *Pakistan* . . . . **92 E3** 29 32N 68 8 E
Tallinn, *Estonia* . . . . . . **15 G21** 59 22N 24 48 E
Tallmadge, *U.S.A.* **150 E3** 41 6N 81 27W
Tallulah, *U.S.A.* **155 J9** 32 25N 91 11W
Tălmaciu, *Romania* . . . **53 E9** 45 38N 24 19 E
Talmest, *Morocco* **110 B3** 31 48N 9 21W
Talmont-St-Hilaire,
France **28 B2** 46 27N 1 37W
Talne, *Ukraine* . . . . **59 H6** 48 50N 30 44 E
Talnoye = Talne,
Ukraine . . . . **59 H6** 48 50N 30 44 E
Taloda, *India* . . . . **94 D2** 21 34N 74 11 E
Talodi, *Sudan* . . . . **107 E3** 10 35N 30 22 E
Tāloqān, *Afghan.* . . . . . **65 E4** 36 44N 69 33 E
Talovaya, *Russia* . . . . . **60 E5** 51 6N 40 45 E
Taloyoak, *Canada* **138 B10** 69 32N 93 32W
Talpa de Allende,
Mexico **162 C4** 20 23N 104 51W
Talparo, *Trin. & Tob.* . **169 F9** 10 30N 61 17W
Talquin, L., *U.S.A.* . . . **152 E5** 30 23N 84 39W
Talsi, *Latvia* . . . . **15 H20** 57 10N 22 30 E
Talsi □, *Latvia* . . . . **54 A9** 57 20N 22 40 E
Talsinnt, *Morocco* **111 B4** 32 33N 3 27W
Taltal, *Chile* . . . . **174 B1** 25 23 S 70 33W
Taltson →, *Canada* . . . **142 A6** 61 24N 112 46W
Talwood, *Australia* . . . **127 D4** 28 29 S 149 29 E
Talyawalka Cr. →,
Australia . . . . **128 B5** 32 28 S 142 22 E
Tam Ky, *Vietnam* . . . . . **86 E7** 15 34N 108 29 E
Tam Quan, *Vietnam* . . . **86 E7** 14 35N 109 3 E
Tama, *U.S.A.* **156 C4** 41 58N 92 35W
Tama △, *Ethiopia* . . . . **107 F4** 5 55N 36 5 E
Tamada, *Algeria* . . . . . **111 D5** 21 34N 3 20 E
Tamalameque,
Colombia **168 B3** 8 52N 73 49W
Tamale, *Ghana* **113 D4** 9 22N 0 50W
Taman, *Russia* . . . . **59 K9** 45 14N 36 41 E
Taman Negara △,
Malaysia . . . . **87 K4** 4 38N 102 26 E
Tamana, *Japan* . . . . **72 E2** 32 58N 130 32 E
Tamana, *Kiribati* . . . . **123 A13** 2 30 S 175 59 E
Tamanar, *Morocco* **110 B3** 31 1N 9 46W
Tamani, *Mali* **112 C3** 13 20N 6 50W
Tamano, *Japan* . . . . **72 C5** 34 29N 133 59 E
Tamanrasset, *Algeria* . . **111 D6** 22 50N 5 30 E
Tamanrasset, O. →,
Algeria . . . . **111 D5** 22 0N 2 0 E
Tamanthi, *Burma* . . . . . **90 C5** 25 19N 95 17 E
Tamaqua, *U.S.A.* **151 F9** 40 48N 75 58W
Tamar →, *U.K.* **21 G3** 50 27N 4 15W
Támara, *Colombia* **168 B3** 5 50N 72 10W
Tamarac, *U.S.A.* **153 J9** 26 12N 80 10W
Tamarin, *Mauritius* . . . **121 d** 20 19 S 57 20 E
Tamarinda, *Spain* . . . . . **38 B4** 39 55N 3 49 E
Tamarite de Litera,
Spain . . . . **40 D5** 41 52N 0 25 E
Tamaroa, *U.S.A.* **156 F7** 38 8N 89 14W
Tamashima, *Japan* . . . . **71 G6** 34 32N 133 40 E
Tamási, *Hungary* . . . . . **52 D3** 46 40N 18 18 E
Tamaské, *Niger* . . . . . . **113 C6** 14 49N 5 43 E
Tamaulipas □, *Mexico* **163 C5** 24 0N 99 0W
Tamaulipas, Sierra de,
Mexico **163 C5** 23 30N 98 20W
Tamazula, *Mexico* **162 C3** 24 55N 106 58W
Tamazunchale, *Mexico* **163 C5** 21 16N 98 47W
Tamba-Dabatou,
Guinea **112 C2** 11 50N 10 40W
Tambacounda, *Senegal* **112 C2** 13 45N 13 40W
Tambaram, *India* . . . . . **95 H5** 12 55N 80 7 E
Tambea, *Solomon Is.* . . **133 M10** 9 16 S 159 41 E
Tambelan, Kepulauan,
Indonesia . . . . **84 B3** 1 0N 107 30 E
Tambellup, *Australia* . **125 F2** 34 4 S 117 37 E
Tambo, *Australia* . . . . **126 C4** 24 54 S 146 14 E
Tambo, *Peru* . . . . **172 C3** 12 57 S 74 1W
Tambo →, *Peru* . . . . . **172 C3** 10 42 S 73 47W
Tambo de Mora, *Peru* **172 C2** 13 30 S 76 8W
Tambobamba, *Peru* . . **172 C3** 13 54 S 72 8W
Tambohorano, *Madag.* **117 B7** 17 30 S 43 58 E
Tambopata →, *Peru* . . **172 C4** 13 21 S 69 36W
Tambora, *Indonesia* . . . **85 D5** 8 12 S 118 5 E
Tamboritha, Mt.,
Australia . . . . **129 D7** 37 31 S 146 40 E
Tambov, *Russia* . . . . . . **60 D5** 52 45N 41 28 E
Tambre →, *Spain* **42 C2** 42 49N 8 53W
Tambuku, *Indonesia* . . **85 D4** 7 8 S 113 40 E
Tambul, *Papua N. G.* . . **132 C2** 5 54 S 143 54 E
Tambura, *Sudan* . . . . . . **107 F2** 5 40N 27 25 E
Tambuyukan, Gunong,
Malaysia . . . . **85 A5** 6 13N 116 39 E
Tâmchekket,
Mauritania **112 B2** 17 25N 10 40W
Tamdybulak,
Uzbekistan . . . . **65 C2** 41 46N 64 36 E
Tame, *Colombia* **168 B3** 6 28N 71 44W
Tâmega →, *Portugal* . . **42 D2** 41 5N 8 21W
Tamelelt, *Morocco* **110 B3** 31 50N 7 32W
Tamenglong, *India* . . . . **90 C4** 25 0N 93 35 E
Tamerza, *Tunisia* . . . . . **108 B1** 34 23N 7 58 E
Tamgué, Massif du,
Guinea **112 C2** 12 0N 12 18W
Tami Is., *Papua N. G.* . **132 D4** 6 46 S 147 55 E
Tamiahua, L. de,
Mexico **163 C5** 21 30N 97 30W
Tamiami Canal, *U.S.A.* **153 K8** 25 50N 81 0W
Tamil Nadu □, *India* . . **95 J3** 11 0N 77 0 E
Tamis →, *Serbia & M.* **52 F5** 44 51N 20 39 E
Tamluk, *India* . . . . **93 H12** 22 18N 87 58 E
Tammerfors =
Tampere, *Finland* . . . **15 F20** 61 30N 23 50 E
Tammisaari, *Finland* . . **15 F20** 60 0N 23 26 E
Tämnaren, *Sweden* . . . **16 D11** 60 10N 17 25 E
Tamo Abu, Banjaran,
Malaysia . . . . **85 B5** 3 10N 115 5 E
Tampa, *Angola* . . . . . . **115 F2** 15 30 S 13 27 E
Tampa, *U.S.A.* **153 H7** 27 57N 82 27W
Tampa, Tanjung,
Indonesia . . . . **79 K19** 8 55 S 116 12 E
Tampa B., *U.S.A.* **153 H7** 27 50N 82 30W
Tampa International ✕
(TPA), *U.S.A.* **153 H7** 27 59N 82 32W
Tamparan, *Phil.* . . . . . **81 H5** 7 53N 124 20 E
Tampere, *Finland* . . . . **15 F20** 61 30N 23 50 E
Tampico, *Mexico* **163 C5** 22 20N 97 50W
Tampico, *U.S.A.* **156 C7** 41 38N 89 47W
Tampin, *Malaysia* . . . . **87 L4** 2 28N 102 13 E
Tampoi, *Malaysia* . . . . **87 d** 1 30N 103 39 E
Tamrah, *Si. Arabia* . . . **98 B4** 20 24N 45 25 E
Tamrau, Peg.,
Indonesia . . . . **83 B4** 0 30 S 132 27 E
Tamri, *Morocco* **110 B3** 30 49N 9 50W
Tamrida = Qādib,
Yemen . . . . **99 D6** 12 37N 53 57 E
Tamsweg, *Austria* . . . . **34 D6** 47 7N 13 49 E
Tamu, *Burma* . . . . **90 C5** 24 13N 94 12 E
Tamuja →, *Spain* **43 F4** 39 38N 6 29W
Tamworth, *Australia* . . **129 A9** 31 7 S 150 58 E
Tamworth, *Canada* . . . **150 B8** 44 29N 77 0W
Tamworth, *U.K.* **21 E6** 52 39N 1 41W
Tamyang, *S. Korea* . . . **75 G14** 35 19N 126 59 E
Tan An, *Vietnam* . . . . . **87 G6** 10 32N 106 25 E
Tan Chau, *Vietnam* . . . **87 G5** 10 48N 105 12 E
Tan Iddah, *Algeria* . . . **111 C6** 26 33N 9 42 E
Tan-Tan, *Morocco* **110 C2** 28 29N 11 1W
Tana →, *Kenya* . . . . . . **118 C5** 2 32 S 40 31 E
Tana →, *Norway* . . . . **14 A23** 70 30N 28 14 E
Tana, L., *Ethiopia* . . . . **107 E4** 13 5N 37 30 E
Tana River Primate △,
Kenya . . . . **118 C5** 1 55 S 40 7 E
Tanabe, *Japan* . . . . **73 D7** 33 44N 135 22 E
Tanabi, *Brazil* . . . . **171 F2** 20 37 S 49 37W
Tanacross, *U.S.A.* **144 E12** 63 23N 143 21W
Tanafjorden, *Norway* . . **14 A23** 70 45N 28 25 E
Tanaga I., *U.S.A.* **144 L3** 51 48N 177 53W
Tanaga Volcano, *U.S.A.* **144 L3** 51 53N 178 8W
Tanah Merah, *Malaysia* **84 A2** 5 48N 102 9 E
Tanahbala, *Indonesia* . **84 C1** 0 30 S 98 30 E
Tanahgrogot, *Indonesia* **85 C5** 1 55 S 116 15 E
Tanahjampea,
Indonesia . . . . **82 C2** 7 10 S 120 35 E
Tanahmasa, *Indonesia* **84 C1** 0 12 S 98 39 E
Tanahmerah, *Indonesia* **83 C6** 6 5 S 140 16 E
Tanakpur, *India* . . . . . . **93 E9** 29 5N 80 7 E
Tanakura, *Japan* . . . . . **71 F10** 37 10N 140 20 E
Tanamalwila, *Sri Lanka* **95 L5** 6 26N 81 8 E
Tanami, *Australia* . . . . **124 C4** 19 59 S 129 43 E
Tanami Desert,
Australia . . . . **124 C5** 18 50 S 132 0 E
Tanana, *U.S.A.* **144 D9** 65 10N 152 4W
Tanana →, *U.S.A.* . . . **144 D10** 65 10N 151 58W
Tananarive =
Antananarivo,
Madag. . . . . **117 B8** 18 55 S 47 31 E
Tananger, *Norway* . . . . **18 F2** 58 57N 5 37 E
Tanannt, *Morocco* **110 B3** 31 54N 6 56W
Tánaro →, *Italy* . . . . . **44 D5** 44 55N 8 40 E
Tanauan, *Phil.* . . . . **80 D3** 14 5N 121 10 E
Tanay, *Phil.* . . . . **80 D3** 14 30N 121 17 E
Tanba-Sanchi, *Japan* . . **73 B7** 35 7N 135 48 E
Tancheng, *China* . . . . . **75 G10** 34 25N 118 20 E
Tanch'ŏn, *N. Korea* . . . **75 D15** 40 27N 128 54 E
Tanda, *Ut. P., India* . . **93 F10** 26 33N 82 35 E
Tanda, *Ut. P., India* . . **93 E8** 28 57N 78 56 E
Tanda, *Ivory C.* **112 D4** 7 48N 3 10W
Tandag, *Phil.* . . . . **81 G6** 9 4N 126 9 E
Tandaia, *Tanzania* . . . . **119 D3** 9 25 S 34 15 E
Tăndărei, *Romania* . . . **53 F12** 44 39N 27 40 E
Tandaué, *Angola* . . . . . **116 B2** 16 58 S 18 5 E
Tandil, *Argentina* . . . . **174 D4** 37 15 S 59 6W
Tandil, Sa. del,
Argentina . . . . **174 D4** 37 30 S 59 0W
Tandin, *Burma* . . . . **90 F4** 19 33N 93 58 E
Tandjilé →, *Chad* . . . . **109 G3** 9 45N 15 50 E
Tandlianwala, *Pakistan* **92 D5** 31 3N 73 9 E
Tando Adam, *Pakistan* **92 G3** 25 45N 68 40 E
Tando Allahyar,
Pakistan . . . . **92 G3** 25 28N 68 43 E
Tando Bago, *Pakistan* . **92 G3** 24 47N 68 58 E
Tando Mohommed
Khan, *Pakistan* . . . . . **92 G3** 25 8N 68 32 E
Tando-Zinze, *Angola* . . **115 D2** 5 22 S 12 30 E
Tandou-Bengou, *Congo* **114 C2** 3 50 S 11 44 E
Tandou L., *Australia* . . **128 B5** 32 40 S 142 5 E
Tandragee, *U.K.* **23 B5** 54 21N 6 24W
Tandsjöborg, *Sweden* . **16 C8** 61 42N 14 43 E
Tandubas, *Phil.* . . . . . . **81 J3** 5 8N 120 20 E
Tandula →, *India* . . . . **94 D5** 21 6N 81 14 E
Tandula Tank, *India* . . . **94 D5** 20 40N 81 12 E
Tandur,
Andhra Pradesh,
India . . . . **94 E4** 19 11N 79 30 E
Tandur,
Andhra Pradesh,
India . . . . **94 F3** 17 14N 77 35 E
Tane-ga-Shima, *Japan* . **71 J5** 30 30N 131 0 E
Taneatua, *N.Z.* . . . . **130 E6** 38 4 S 177 1 E
Tanen Tong Dan =
Dawna Ra., *Burma* . . **86 D2** 16 30N 98 30 E
Tanew →, *Poland* . . . . **55 H9** 50 29N 22 16 E
Tanezrouft, *Algeria* . . . **111 D5** 23 9N 0 11 E
Tanezzuft, W. →,
Libya . . . . **108 C2** 25 51N 10 19 E
Tang, Koh, *Cambodia* . **87 G4** 10 16N 103 7 E
Tang, Ra's-e, *Iran* . . . . **97 E8** 25 21N 59 52 E
Tang Krasang,
Cambodia . . . . **86 F5** 12 34N 105 3 E
Tanga, *Tanzania* . . . . . **118 D4** 5 5 S 39 2 E
Tanga □, *Tanzania* . . . **118 D4** 5 20 S 38 0 E
Tanga Is., *Papua N. G.* **132 B7** 3 20 S 153 15 E
Tangail, *Bangla.* . . . . . . **90 C2** 24 15N 89 55 E
Tangalla, *Sri Lanka* . . . **95 L5** 6 1N 80 48 E
Tanganyika =
Tanzania ■, *Africa* . . **118 D3** 6 0 S 34 0 E
Tanganyika, L., *Africa* **118 D3** 6 40 S 30 0 E
Tangarare, *Solomon Is.* **133 M10** 9 36 S 159 41 E
Tangariro, Mt., *N.Z.* . . **130 F4** 39 8 S 175 38 E
Tangasseri, *India* . . . . . **95 K3** 8 53N 76 35 E
Tangaza, *Nigeria* . . . . . **113 C5** 13 19N 4 55 E
Tangen, *Norway* . . . . . . **18 D8** 60 37N 11 15 E
Tanger, *Morocco* **110 A3** 35 50N 5 49W
Tangerang, *Indonesia* . **84 D3** 6 11 S 106 37 E
Tangerhütte, *Germany* . **30 C7** 52 26N 11 48 E
Tangermünde,
Germany . . . . **30 C7** 52 33N 11 58 E
Tanggu, *China* . . . . **75 E9** 39 2N 117 40 E
Tanggula Shan, *China* . **68 C4** 32 40N 92 10 E
Tanghe, *China* . . . . **74 H7** 32 47N 112 50 E
Tanghla Range =
Tanggula Shan,
China . . . . **68 C4** 32 40N 92 10 E
Tangi, *India* . . . . **94 E7** 19 56N 85 24 E
Tangier = Tanger,
Morocco **110 A3** 35 50N 5 49W
Tangjia, *China* . . . . **69 G10** 22 22N 113 35 E
Tangjia Wan, *China* . . . **69 G10** 22 21N 113 36 E
Tangkeboke,
Indonesia . . . . **82 B2** 3 10 S 121 30 E
Tangorin, *Australia* . . . **126 C3** 21 47 S 144 12 E
Tangorombohitr'i
Makay, *Madag.* . . . . . **117 C8** 21 0 S 45 15 E
Tangshan, *China* . . . . . **75 E10** 39 38N 118 10 E
Tangtou, *China* . . . . . . **75 G10** 35 28N 118 30 E
Tangub, *Phil.* . . . . **81 G4** 8 3N 123 44 E
Tanguiéta, *Benin* . . . . . **113 C5** 10 35N 1 21 E
Tangxi, *China* . . . . **77 C12** 29 3N 119 25 E
Tangyan He →, *China* **76 C7** 28 54N 108 19 E
Tanimbar, Kepulauan,
Indonesia . . . . **83 C4** 7 30 S 131 30 E
Tanimbar Is. =
Tanimbar,
Kepulauan, *Indonesia* **83 C4** 7 30 S 131 30 E
Taninthari =
Tenasserim, *Burma* . **87 F2** 12 6N 99 3 E
Tanjay, *Phil.* . . . . **81 G4** 9 30N 123 5 E
Tanjong Malim,
Malaysia . . . . **87 L3** 3 42N 101 31 E
Tanjong Pelepas,
Malaysia . . . . **87 d** 1 21N 103 33 E
Tanjore = Thanjavur,
India . . . . **95 J4** 10 48N 79 12 E
Tanjung, *Indonesia* . . . **79 J19** 8 21 S 116 9 E
Tanjung, *Phil.* . . . . **85 C5** 2 10 S 115 25 E
Tanjung Tokong,
Malaysia . . . . **87 c** 5 28N 100 18 E
Tanjungbalai, *Indonesia* **84 B1** 2 55N 99 44 E
Tanjungbatu, *Indonesia* **85 B5** 2 23N 118 3 E
Tanjungkarang
Telukbetung,
Indonesia . . . . **84 D3** 5 20 S 105 10 E
Tanjungpandan,
Indonesia . . . . **85 C3** 2 43 S 107 38 E
Tanjungpinang,
Indonesia . . . . **84 B2** 1 5N 104 30 E
Tanjungpriok,
Indonesia . . . . **84 D3** 6 8 S 106 55 E
Tanjungredeb,
Indonesia . . . . **85 B5** 2 9N 117 29 E
Tanjungselor, *Indonesia* **85 B5** 2 55N 117 25 E
Tank, *Pakistan* . . . . **91 B3** 32 14N 70 25 E
Tankhala, *India* . . . . . . **92 J5** 21 58N 73 47 E
Tankwa-Karoo △,
S. Africa . . . . **116 E2** 32 14 S 19 50 E
Tanna, *Vanuatu* . . . . . **133 J7** 19 30 S 169 20 E
Tännäs, *Sweden* . . . . . **16 B6** 62 26N 12 42 E
Tannersville, *U.S.A.* . . **151 E9** 41 3N 75 18W
Tannis Bugt, *Denmark* **17 G4** 57 40N 10 15 E
Tannu-Ola, *Russia* . . . **67 D10** 51 0N 94 0 E
Tannum Sands,
Australia . . . . **126 C5** 23 57 S 151 22 E
Tano →, *Ghana* **112 D4** 5 7N 2 56W
Tanombella, *Algeria* . . **111 C5** 26 30N 5 49 E
Tanon Str., *Phil.* . . . . . **81 F4** 10 20N 123 30 E
Tanout, *Niger* . . . . **113 C6** 14 50N 8 55 E
Tanquinho, *Brazil* . . . . **171 D4** 11 58 S 39 6W
Tanshui, *Taiwan* . . . . . **77 E13** 25 10N 121 28 E
Tansilla, *Burkina Faso* **112 C4** 12 25N 4 23W
Tanta, *Egypt* . . . . **106 H7** 30 45N 30 57 E
Tantabin, *Burma* . . . . . **90 G5** 17 1N 95 59 E
Tantoyuca, *Mexico* . . . **163 C5** 21 21N 98 10W
Tantung = Dandong,
China . . . . **75 D13** 40 10N 124 20 E
Tanuku, *India* . . . . **94 F5** 16 45N 81 44 E
Tanumshede, *Sweden* . **17 F5** 58 42N 11 20 E
Tanunda, *Australia* . . . **128 C3** 34 30 S 139 0 E
Tanur, *India* . . . . **95 J2** 11 1N 75 52 E
Tanus, *France* . . . . **28 D6** 44 8N 2 19 E
Tanzania ■, *Africa* . . . **118 D3** 6 0 S 34 0 E
Tanzawa-Sanchi, *Japan* **73 B11** 35 27N 139 0 E
Tanzhou, *China* . . . . . . **69 G9** 22 16N 113 28 E
Tanzilla →, *Canada* . . **142 B2** 58 8N 130 43W
Tao, Ko, *Thailand* . . . . **87 G2** 10 5N 99 52 E
Tao'an = Taonan,
China . . . . **75 B12** 45 22N 122 40 E
Tao'er He →, *China* . . **75 B13** 45 45N 124 5 E
Taohua Dao, *China* . . . **77 C14** 29 50N 122 20 E
Taolanaro, *Madag.* . . . . **117 D8** 25 2 S 47 0 E
Taole, *China* . . . . **74 E4** 38 48N 106 40 E
Taonan, *China* . . . . **75 B12** 45 22N 122 40 E
Taora, *Solomon Is.* . . . **133 L9** 7 21 S 157 30 E
Taormina, *Italy* . . . . . . **47 E8** 37 51N 15 17 E
Taos, *U.S.A.* **159 H11** 36 24N 105 35W
Taoudenni, *Mali* **110 D4** 22 40N 3 55W
Taoudrart, Adrar,
Algeria . . . . **111 D5** 24 25N 2 24 E
Taounate, *Morocco* . . . **110 B4** 34 25N 4 41W
Taourir, Dj., *Algeria* . . **111 D6** 35 52N 1 46 E
Taourirt, *Algeria* . . . . . **111 C5** 26 37N 0 20 E
Taourirt, *Morocco* **111 B4** 34 25N 2 53W
Taouz, *Morocco* **110 B4** 30 53N 4 0W
Taoyuan, *China* . . . . . . **77 C8** 28 55N 111 16 E
T'aoyüan, *Taiwan* . . . . **77 E13** 25 0N 121 4 E
Tapa, *Estonia* . . . . **15 G21** 59 15N 25 50 E
Tapa Shan = Daba
Shan, *China* . . . . **76 B7** 32 0N 109 0 E
Tapachula, *Mexico* . . . **163 E6** 14 54N 92 17W
Tapah, *Malaysia* . . . . . **87 K3** 4 12N 101 15 E
Tapajós →, *Brazil* . . . **169 D7** 2 24 S 54 41W
Tapaktuan, *Indonesia* . **84 B1** 3 15N 97 10 E
Tapanahoni →,
Suriname **169 C7** 4 20N 54 25W
Tapanui, *N.Z.* . . . . **131 F4** 45 56 S 169 18 E
Tapauá, *Brazil* . . . . . . **173 B5** 5 40 S 64 20W
Tapauá →, *Brazil* . . . . **173 B5** 5 40 S 64 21W
Tapaz, *Phil.* . . . . **81 F4** 11 16N 122 32 E
Tapes, *Brazil* . . . . **175 C5** 30 40 S 51 23W
Tapeta, *Liberia* **112 D3** 6 29N 8 52W
Taphan Hin, *Thailand* . **86 D3** 16 13N 100 26 E
Tapi →, *India* . . . . **94 D1** 21 8N 72 41 E
Tapia de Casariego,
Spain **42 B4** 43 34N 6 56W
Tapiantana Group,
Phil. . . . . **81 H4** 6 20N 122 0 E
Tapiau = Gvardeysk,
Russia . . . . **15 J19** 54 39N 21 5 E
Tapilon =
Daanbantayan, *Phil.* **81 F5** 11 17N 124 2 E
Tapini, *Papua N. G.* . . **132 E4** 8 19 S 147 0 E
Tapiraí, *Brazil* . . . . **171 E2** 19 52 S 46 1W
Tapirapé →, *Brazil* . . . **170 D1** 10 41 S 50 38W
Tapirapecó, Serra,
Venezuela **169 C5** 1 10N 65 0W
Tapirapuã, *Brazil* . . . . **173 C6** 14 51 S 57 45W
Taplan, *Australia* . . . . . **128 C4** 34 33 S 140 52 E
Tapo-Capara △,
Venezuela **165 E5** 7 55N 71 15W
Tapoeripa, *Suriname* . . **169 B6** 5 22N 56 34W
Tapolca, *Hungary* . . . . **52 D2** 46 53N 17 29 E
Tapuae-o-Uenuku,
N.Z. . . . . **131 B8** 42 0 S 173 39 E
Tapul, *Phil.* . . . . **81 J3** 5 42N 120 55 E
Tapul Group, *Phil.* . . . **81 J3** 5 35N 120 50 E
Tapul I., *Phil.* . . . . **81 J3** 5 35N 120 55 E
Tapun, *India* . . . . **90 B6** 27 35N 96 22 E
Tapurucuará, *Brazil* . . **169 D4** 0 24 S 65 2W
Taqṭaq, *Iraq* . . . . **101 E11** 35 53N 44 35 E
Taquara, *Brazil* . . . . . . **175 B5** 29 36 S 50 46W
Taquari →, *Brazil* . . . **173 D6** 19 15 S 57 17W
Taquaritinga, *Brazil* . . **171 F2** 21 24 S 48 30W
Tara, *Australia* . . . . . . **127 D5** 27 17 S 150 31 E
Tara, *Canada* **150 B3** 44 28N 81 9W
Tara, *Japan* . . . . **72 D2** 33 2N 130 11 E
Tara, *Russia* . . . . **66 D8** 56 55N 74 24 E
Tara, *Zambia* . . . . **119 F2** 16 58 S 26 45 E
Tara △, *Serbia & M.* . . **50 C3** 43 55N 19 30 E
Tara →, *Serbia & M.* . **50 C2** 43 21N 18 51 E
Tara-Dake, *Japan* . . . . **72 E2** 32 58N 130 6 E
Taraba □, *Nigeria* . . . . **113 D7** 8 0N 10 30 E
Taraba →, *Nigeria* . . . **113 D7** 8 30N 10 15 E
Tarabuco, *Bolivia* . . . . **173 D5** 19 10 S 64 57W

Tarābulus, Lebanon 103 A4 34 31N 35 50 E
Tarābulus, Libya 108 B2 32 49N 13 7 E
Taraclia, Taraclia, Moldova 53 E13 45 54N 28 40 E
Taraclia, Tighina, Moldova 53 D14 46 34N 29 7 E
Taradale, N.Z. 130 F5 39 33 S 176 53 E
Taradehi, India 93 H8 23 18N 79 21 E
Taragi, Japan 72 E2 32 16N 130 56 E
Tarahouahout, Algeria 111 D6 22 41N 5 59 E
Tarajalejo, Canary Is. 9 e2 28 12N 14 7W
Tarakan, Indonesia 85 B5 3 20N 117 35 E
Tarakit, Mt., Kenya 118 B4 2 2N 35 10 E
Taralga, Australia 129 C8 34 26 S 149 52 E
Tarama-Jima, Japan 71 M2 24 39N 124 42 E
Taramakau →, N.Z. 131 C6 42 34 S 171 8 E
Taran, Mys, Russia 15 J18 54 56N 19 59 E
Taranagar, India 92 E6 28 43N 74 50 E
Taranaki □, N.Z. 130 F3 39 25 S 174 30 E
Taranaki, Mt., N.Z. 130 F3 39 17 S 174 5 E
Tarancón, Spain 40 E1 40 1N 3 1W
Tarangire △, Tanzania 118 C4 4 21 S 36 7 E
Taransay, U.K. 22 D1 57 54N 7 0W
Táranto, Italy 47 B10 40 28N 17 14 E
Táranto, G. di, Italy 47 B10 40 8N 17 20 E
Tarapacá, Colombia 168 D4 2 56 S 69 46W
Tarapacá □, Chile 174 A2 20 45 S 69 30W
Tarapoto, Peru 172 B2 6 30 S 76 20W
Taraquá, Brazil 168 C4 0 6N 68 28W
Tarare, France 29 C8 45 54N 4 26 E
Tararua Ra., N.Z. 130 G4 40 45 S 175 25 E
Tarasag, Vanuatu 133 D5 14 12 S 167 36 E
Tarascon, France 29 E8 43 48N 4 39 E
Tarascon-sur-Ariège, France 28 F5 42 50N 1 36 E
Tarashcha, Ukraine 59 H6 49 30N 30 31 E
Tarata, Peru 172 D3 17 27 S 70 2W
Tarauacá, Brazil 172 B3 8 6 S 70 48W
Tarauacá →, Brazil 172 B4 6 42 S 69 48W
Taravo →, France 29 G12 41 42N 8 49 E
Tarawa, Kiribati 134 G9 1 30N 173 0 E
Tarawai I., Papua N. G. 132 B2 3 13 S 143 15 E
Tarawera, N.Z. 130 F5 39 2 S 176 36 E
Tarawera, L., N.Z. 130 E5 38 13 S 176 27 E
Tarawera, Mt., N.Z. 130 E5 38 14 S 176 32 E
Taraz, Kazakhstan 65 B5 42 54N 71 22 E
Tarazona, Spain 40 D3 41 55N 1 43W
Tarazona de la Mancha, Spain 41 F3 39 16N 1 55W
Tarbagatay, Khrebet, Kazakhstan 66 E9 48 0N 83 0 E
Tarbat Ness, U.K. 22 D5 57 52N 3 47W
Tarbela Dam, Pakistan 92 B5 34 8N 72 52 E
Tarbert, Arg. & Bute, U.K. 22 F3 55 52N 5 25W
Tarbert, W. Isles, U.K. 22 D2 57 54N 6 49W
Tarbes, France 28 E4 43 15N 0 3 E
Tarboro, U.S.A. 149 H7 35 54N 77 32W
Tarbū, Libya 108 C3 26 0N 15 5 E
Tărcău, Munţii, Romania 53 D11 46 39N 26 7 E
Tarcento, Italy 45 B10 46 13N 13 13 E
Tarcoola, Australia 127 E1 30 44 S 134 36 E
Tarcoon, Australia 127 E4 30 15 S 146 43 E
Tarcutta, Australia 129 C7 35 16 S 147 44 E
Tardets-Sorholus, France 28 E3 43 8N 0 52W
Tardoire →, France 28 C4 45 52N 0 14 E
Taredjedja, Algeria 111 C5 25 12N 2 32 E
Taree, Australia 129 A10 31 50 S 152 30 E
Tarella, Australia 128 A5 31 2 S 143 2 E
Tarf, Ras, Morocco 110 A3 35 40N 5 11W
Ţarfā, Ra's aţ, Si. Arabia 98 C3 17 2N 42 22 E
Tarfa, W. el →, Egypt 106 B3 28 25N 30 50 E
Tarfaya, Morocco 110 C2 27 55N 12 55W
Târgovişte, Romania 53 F10 44 55N 25 27 E
Târgu Bujor, Romania 53 E12 45 52N 27 54 E
Târgu Cărbuneşti, Romania 53 F8 44 57N 23 31 E
Târgu Frumos, Romania 53 C12 47 12N 27 2 E
Târgu-Jiu, Romania 53 E8 45 5N 23 19 E
Târgu Lăpuş, Romania 53 C8 47 27N 23 52 E
Târgu Mureş, Romania 53 D9 46 31N 24 38 E
Târgu Neamţ, Romania 53 C11 47 12N 26 25 E
Târgu Ocna, Romania 53 D11 46 16N 26 39 E
Târgu Secuiesc, Romania 53 E11 46 0N 26 10 E
Targuist, Morocco 110 B4 34 59N 4 14W
Târguşor, Romania 53 F13 44 27N 28 25 E
Tărhăus, Vf., Romania 53 D11 46 40N 26 8 E
Tarhbalt, Morocco 110 B3 30 39N 5 20W
Tarhit, Algeria 111 B4 30 58N 2 0W
Tarhūnah, Libya 108 B2 32 27N 13 36 E
Tari, Papua N. G. 132 C2 5 54 S 142 59 E
Táriba, Venezuela 168 B3 7 49N 72 13W
Ţarif, U.A.E. 97 E7 24 3N 53 46 E
Tarifa, Spain 43 J5 36 1N 5 36W
Tarija, Bolivia 174 A3 21 30 S 64 40W
Tarija □, Bolivia 174 A3 21 30 S 63 30W
Tariku →, Indonesia 83 B5 2 55 S 138 26 E
Tarīm, Yemen 99 C5 16 3N 49 0 E
Tarim Basin = Tarim Pendi, China 68 B3 40 0N 84 0 E
Tarim He →, China 68 C3 39 30N 88 30 E
Tarim Pendi, China 68 B3 40 0N 84 0 E
Taritatu →, Indonesia 83 B5 2 54 S 138 27 E
Tarka →, S. Africa 116 E4 32 10 S 26 0 E
Tarkastad, S. Africa 116 E4 32 0 S 26 16 E
Tarkhankut, Mys, Ukraine 59 K7 45 25N 32 30 E
Tarko Sale, Russia 66 C8 64 55N 77 50 E
Tarkwa, Ghana 112 D4 5 20N 2 0W
Tarlac, Phil. 80 D3 15 29N 120 35 E
Tarlac □, Phil. 80 D3 15 30N 120 30 E
Tarm, Denmark 17 J2 55 56N 8 31 E
Tarma, Peru 172 C2 11 25 S 75 45W
Tarn □, France 28 E6 43 49N 2 8 E
Tarn →, France 28 D5 44 5N 1 6 E
Tarn-et-Garonne □, France 28 D5 44 8N 1 20 E
Tarna →, Hungary 52 C4 47 31N 19 59 E
Târnava Mare →, Romania 53 D8 46 10N 23 43 E
Târnava Mică →, Romania 53 D8 46 9N 23 55 E
Târnăveni, Romania 53 D9 46 19N 24 13 E
Tarnica, Poland 55 J9 49 4N 22 44 E
Tarnobrzeg, Poland 55 H8 50 35N 21 41 E
Tarnogród, Poland 55 H9 50 22N 22 45 E
Tarnopol = Ternopil, Ukraine 59 H3 49 30N 25 40 E
Tarnos, France 28 E2 43 32N 1 28W
Târnova, Moldova 53 B12 48 10N 27 40 E
Târnova, Romania 52 E6 45 23N 21 59 E
Tarnów, Poland 55 H8 50 3N 21 0 E
Tarnowitz = Tarnowskie Góry, Poland 55 H5 50 27N 18 54 E
Tarnowskie Góry, Poland 55 H5 50 27N 18 54 E
Tärnsjö, Sweden 16 D10 60 9N 16 56 E
Táro →, Italy 44 C7 45 2N 10 15 E
Ţārom, Iran 97 D7 28 11N 55 46 E
Taroom, Australia 127 D4 25 36 S 149 48 E
Taroudannt, Morocco 110 B3 30 30N 8 52W
Tarp, Germany 30 A5 54 39N 9 24 E
Tarpeena, Australia 128 D4 37 37 S 140 47 E
Tarpon Springs, U.S.A. 153 G7 28 9N 82 45W
Tarquínia, Italy 45 F8 42 15N 11 45 E
Tarrafal, C. Verde Is. 9 j 15 18N 23 39W
Tarragona, Spain 40 D6 41 5N 1 17 E
Tarragona □, Spain 40 D6 41 5N 1 0 E
Tarraleah, Australia 127 G4 42 17 S 146 26 E
Tarrasa = Terrassa, Spain 40 D7 41 34N 2 1 E
Tàrrega, Spain 40 D6 41 39N 1 9 E
Tarrytown, Ga., U.S.A. 152 C7 32 19N 82 34W
Tarrytown, N.Y., U.S.A. 151 E11 41 4N 73 52W
Târs, Denmark 17 G4 57 23N 10 7 E
Tarshiha = Me'ona, Israel 103 B4 33 1N 35 15 E
Tarsus, Turkey 100 D6 36 58N 34 55 E
Tartagal, Argentina 174 A3 22 30 S 63 50W
Tärtär, Azerbaijan 61 K8 40 20N 46 58 E
Tärtär →, Azerbaijan 61 K8 40 26N 47 20 E
Tartas, France 28 E3 43 50N 0 49W
Tartogay, Kazakhstan 65 A3 44 26N 66 15 E
Tartu, Estonia 15 G22 58 20N 26 44 E
Ţarţūs, Syria 100 E6 34 55N 35 55 E
Tarumirim, Brazil 171 E3 19 16 S 41 59W
Tarumizu, Japan 72 F2 31 29N 130 42 E
Tarussa, Russia 58 E9 54 44N 37 10 E
Tarutao = Ko Tarutao △, Thailand 87 J2 6 31N 99 26 E
Tarutao, Ko, Thailand 87 J2 6 33N 99 40 E
Tarutung, Indonesia 84 B1 2 0N 98 54 E
Tarutyne, Ukraine 53 D14 46 12N 29 9 E
Tarvísio, Italy 45 B10 46 30N 13 35 E
Tarxien, Malta 38 F8 35 52N 14 31 E
Tarz Ulli, Libya 108 C2 25 32N 10 8 E
Tasahku, Burma 90 B6 27 33N 97 52 E
Tasaret, O. →, Algeria 111 C5 26 25N 1 59 E
Tasāwah, Libya 108 C2 26 0N 13 30 E
Tasböget, Kazakhstan 65 A2 44 46N 65 33 E
Täsch, Switz. 32 D5 46 4N 7 46 E
Taseko →, Canada 142 C4 52 8N 123 45W
Tasgaon, India 94 F2 17 2N 74 39 E
Tash-Bashat, Kyrgyzstan 65 C8 41 23N 76 20 E
Tash-Kömür, Kyrgyzstan 65 C6 41 40N 72 10 E
Tash-Kumyr = Tash-Kömür, Kyrgyzstan 65 C6 41 40N 72 10 E
Tashauz = Dashhowuz, Turkmenistan 66 E6 41 49N 59 58 E
Tashi Chho Dzong = Thimphu, Bhutan 90 B2 27 31N 89 45 E
Tashino = Pervomaysk, Russia 60 C6 54 56N 43 58 E
Ţashk, Daryācheh-ye, Iran 97 D7 29 45N 53 35 E
Tashkent = Toshkent, Uzbekistan 65 C4 41 20N 69 10 E
Tashtagol, Russia 66 D9 52 47N 87 53 E
Tasiilaq, Greenland 10 D7 65 40N 37 20W
Tasikmalaya, Indonesia 85 D3 7 18 S 108 12 E
Tåsinge, Denmark 17 J4 55 0N 10 35 E
Tåsjön, Sweden 14 D16 64 15N 15 40 E
Task, Niger 109 F2 14 56N 10 46 E
Taskan, Russia 67 C16 62 59N 150 20 E
Tasker, Niger 113 C7 15 8N 10 40 E
Taşköprü, Turkey 100 B6 41 30N 34 15 E
Taskul, Papua N. G. 132 B6 2 32 S 150 27 E
Taşlâc, Moldova 53 C14 47 4N 29 24 E
Tasman □, N.Z. 131 B7 41 30 S 172 40 E
Tasman →, N.Z. 131 D5 43 48 S 170 8 E
Tasman, Mt., N.Z. 131 D5 43 34 S 170 12 E
Tasman B., N.Z. 131 A8 40 59 S 173 25 E
Tasman Basin, Pac. Oc. 134 M7 46 0 S 158 0 E
Tasman Mts., N.Z. 131 B7 41 3 S 172 25 E
Tasman Pen., Australia 127 G4 43 10 S 148 0 E
Tasman Plateau, S. Ocean 7 A10 48 0 S 146 0 E
Tasman Sea, Pac. Oc. 134 L8 36 0 S 160 0 E
Tasmania □, Australia 127 G4 42 0 S 146 30 E
Tăşnad, Romania 52 C7 47 30N 22 33 E
Tassili n'Ajjer, Algeria 111 C6 25 47N 8 1 E
Tassili-Oua-n-Ahaggar, Algeria 111 D6 20 41N 5 30 E
Tassili Tin-Rerhoh, Algeria 111 D5 20 5N 3 55 E
Tasty, Kazakhstan 65 A4 44 47N 69 7 E
Tata, Hungary 52 C3 47 37N 18 19 E
Tata, Morocco 110 C3 29 46N 7 56W
Tata Mai Lau, E. Timor 82 C3 8 58 S 125 30 E
Tatabánya, Hungary 52 C3 47 32N 18 25 E
Tatamá △, Colombia 168 B2 5 5N 76 9W
Tatamba, Solomon Is. 133 M10 8 21 S 159 51 E
Tataouine, Tunisia 108 B2 32 57N 10 29 E
Tatar-Pazardzhik = Pazardzhik, Bulgaria 51 D8 42 12N 24 20 E
Tatar Republic = Tatarstan □, Russia 60 C10 55 30N 51 30 E
Tatarbunary, Ukraine 53 E14 45 50N 29 39 E
Tatarsk, Russia 66 D8 55 14N 76 0 E
Tatarstan □, Russia 60 C10 55 30N 51 30 E
Tatatóváros = Tata, Hungary 52 C3 47 37N 18 19 E
Tatau, Malaysia 85 B4 2 53N 112 51 E
Tatau I., Papua N. G. 132 B6 2 48 S 151 57 E
Tatebayashi, Japan 73 A11 36 15N 139 32 E
Tateshina-Yama, Japan 73 A10 36 8N 138 11 E
Tateyama, Japan 73 C11 35 0N 139 50 E
Tathlina L., Canada 142 A5 60 33N 117 39W
Tathlīth, Si. Arabia 98 C3 19 32N 43 30 E
Tathlīth, W. →, Si. Arabia 98 B4 20 35N 44 20 E
Tathra, Australia 129 D8 36 44 S 149 59 E
Tatinnai L., Canada 143 A9 60 55N 97 40W
Tatitlek, U.S.A. 144 F11 60 52N 146 41W
Tatkon, Burma 90 E6 20 7N 96 13 E
Tatla L., Canada 142 C4 52 0N 124 20W
Tatlısu, Turkey 51 F11 40 24N 27 55 E
Tatnam, C., Canada 143 B10 57 16N 91 0W
Tatra = Tatry, Slovak Rep. 35 B13 49 20N 20 0 E
Tatranský △, Slovak Rep. 35 B13 49 10N 20 0 E
Tatry, Slovak Rep. 35 B13 49 20N 20 0 E
Tatshenshini →, Canada 142 B1 59 28N 137 45W
Tatsuno, Hyōgo, Japan 72 C6 34 52N 134 33 E
Tatsuno, Nagano, Japan 73 B10 35 58N 138 0 E
Tatta, Pakistan 91 D2 24 42N 67 55 E
Tätti, Kazakhstan 65 B6 43 13N 73 18 E
Tatuī, Brazil 175 A6 23 25 S 47 53W
Tatum, U.S.A. 155 J3 33 16N 103 19W
Tat'ung = Datong, China 74 D7 40 6N 113 18 E
Tatura, Australia 129 D6 36 29 S 145 16 E
Tatvan, Turkey 101 C10 38 31N 42 15 E
Ta'ū, Amer. Samoa 133 X25 14 15 S 169 30W
Tau, Norway 18 E2 59 3N 5 55 E
Tauá, Brazil 170 C3 6 1 S 40 26W
Taubaté, Brazil 175 A6 23 0 S 45 36W
Tauberbischofsheim, Germany 31 F5 49 37N 9 39 E
Taucha, Germany 30 D8 51 23N 12 29 E
Tauern, Austria 36 E7 47 15N 12 40 E
Tauern-tunnel, Austria 34 D6 47 0N 13 12 E
Taufikia, Sudan 107 F3 9 24N 31 37 E
Taulé, France 26 D3 48 37N 3 55W
Taumarunui, N.Z. 130 E4 38 53 S 175 15 E
Taumaturgo, Brazil 172 B3 8 54 S 72 51W
Taung, S. Africa 116 D3 27 33 S 24 47 E
Taungdwingyi, Burma 90 E5 20 1N 95 40 E
Taunggyi, Burma 90 E6 20 50N 97 0 E
Taungtha, Burma 90 E5 21 12N 95 25 E
Taungup, Burma 90 F5 18 51N 94 14 E
Taungup Pass, Burma 90 F5 18 40N 94 45 E
Taunsa, Pakistan 92 D4 30 42N 70 39 E
Taunsa Barrage, Pakistan 92 D4 30 42N 70 50 E
Taunton, U.K. 21 F4 51 1N 3 5W
Taunton, U.S.A. 151 E13 41 54N 71 6W
Taunus, Germany 31 E4 50 13N 8 34 E
Taupo, N.Z. 130 E5 38 41 S 176 7 E
Taupo, L., N.Z. 130 E4 38 46 S 175 55 E
Tauragė, Lithuania 15 J20 55 14N 22 16 E
Tauragė □, Lithuania 54 C9 55 15N 22 17 E
Tauranga, N.Z. 130 D5 37 42 S 176 11 E
Tauranga Harb., N.Z. 130 D5 37 30 S 176 5 E
Taureau, Rés., Canada 140 C5 46 46N 73 50W
Tauri →, Papua N. G. 132 E4 8 8 S 146 8 E
Taurianova, Italy 47 D9 38 21N 16 1 E
Taurus Mts. = Toros Dağları, Turkey 100 D5 37 0N 32 30 E
Taus = Domažlice, Czech Rep. 34 B5 49 28N 12 58 E
Tauste, Spain 40 D3 41 58N 1 18W
Tautira, Tahiti 133 S16 17 44 S 149 9W
Tauz = Tovuz, Azerbaijan 61 K7 41 0N 45 40 E
Tavaar, Somali Rep. 120 D3 3 6N 46 1 E
Tavannes, Switz. 32 B4 47 13N 7 12 E
Tavares, U.S.A. 153 G8 28 48N 81 44W
Tavas, Turkey 49 D11 37 34N 29 4 E
Tavastehus = Hämeenlinna, Finland 15 F21 61 0N 24 28 E
Tavda, Russia 66 D7 58 7N 65 8 E
Tavda →, Russia 66 D7 57 47N 67 18 E
Tavernes de la Valldigna, Spain 41 F4 39 5N 0 13W
Tavernier, U.S.A. 153 K9 25 1N 80 31W
Taveta, Tanzania 118 C4 3 23 S 37 37 E
Taveuni, Fiji 133 A3 16 51 S 179 58W
Taviano, Italy 47 C11 39 59N 18 5 E
Tavignano →, France 29 F13 42 7N 9 33 E
Tavildara, Tajikistan 65 D5 38 41N 70 29 E
Tavira, Portugal 43 H3 37 8N 7 40W
Tavistock, Canada 150 C4 43 19N 80 50W
Tavistock, U.K. 21 G3 50 33N 4 9W
Tavolara, Italy 46 B2 40 54N 9 42 E
Távora →, Portugal 42 D3 41 8N 7 35W
Tavoy, Burma 86 E2 14 2N 98 12 E
Tavşanlı, Turkey 49 B11 39 32N 29 30 E
Tavua, Fiji 133 A1 17 37 S 177 5 E
Tavuki, Fiji 133 B2 19 7 S 178 8 E
Taw →, U.K. 21 F3 51 4N 4 4W
Tawa →, India 92 H8 22 48N 77 48 E
Tawa Tawa Mal Reef, Papua N. G. 132 F7 11 3 S 152 55 E
Tawai, India 90 B6 27 48N 96 47 E
Tawas City, U.S.A. 148 C4 44 16N 83 31W
Tawau, Malaysia 85 B5 4 20N 117 55 E
Taweisha, Sudan 107 E2 12 19N 26 40 E
Tawi-Tawi □, Phil. 81 J3 5 0N 120 0 E
Tawitawi, Phil. 79 B6 5 10N 120 0 E
Tawitawi Group, Phil. 81 J3 5 10N 120 15 E
Tawngche, Burma 90 B5 26 34N 95 38 E
Tawu, Taiwan 77 F13 22 30N 120 50 E
Tāwurghā', Libya 108 B3 32 1N 15 2 E
Tāwurghā', Sabkhat, Libya 108 B3 31 51N 15 15 E
Taxco de Alarcón, Mexico 163 D5 18 33N 99 36W
Taxila, Pakistan 92 C5 33 42N 72 52 E
Taxkorgan He →, China 65 E8 37 45N 76 10 E
Taxkorgan Tajik Zizhixian, China 65 E7 37 49N 75 14 E
Tay ⌓, U.K. 22 E5 56 43N 3 59W
Tay →, U.K. 22 E5 56 37N 3 38W
Tay, Firth of, U.K. 22 E5 56 25N 3 8W
Tay, L., Australia 125 F3 32 55 S 120 48 E
Tay, L., U.K. 22 E4 56 32N 4 8W
Tay Ninh, Vietnam 87 G6 11 20N 106 5 E
Tayabamba, Peru 172 B2 8 15 S 77 16W
Tayabas = Quezon, Phil. 81 G1 9 15N 117 59 E
Tayabas, Phil. 80 D3 14 1N 121 35 E
Tayabas Bay, Phil. 80 E3 13 45N 121 45 E
Tayandu, Kepulauan, Indonesia 83 C4 5 30 S 132 15 E
Taylakova, Russia 66 D8 59 13N 74 0 E
Taylakovy = Taylakova, Russia 66 D8 59 13N 74 0 E
Taylor, Canada 142 B4 56 13N 120 40W
Taylor, Fla., U.S.A. 152 E7 30 26N 82 18W
Taylor, Mich., U.S.A. 157 B13 42 14N 83 16W
Taylor, Nebr., U.S.A. 154 E5 41 46N 99 23W
Taylor, Pa., U.S.A. 151 E9 41 23N 75 43W
Taylor, Tex., U.S.A. 155 K6 30 34N 97 25W
Taylor, Mt., N.Z. 131 D6 43 30 S 171 20 E
Taylor, Mt., U.S.A. 159 J10 35 14N 107 37W
Taylorsville, U.S.A. 157 F11 38 2N 85 21W
Taylorsville L., U.S.A. 157 G11 38 0N 85 15W
Taylorville, U.S.A. 156 E7 39 33N 89 18W
Taymā, Si. Arabia 96 E3 27 35N 38 45 E
Taymyr, Oz., Russia 67 B11 74 20N 102 0 E
Taymyr, Poluostrov, Russia 67 B11 75 0N 100 0 E
Tayport, U.K. 22 E6 56 27N 2 52W
Tayrona △, Colombia 165 D5 11 20N 74 2W
Tayshet, Russia 67 D10 55 58N 98 1 E
Taytay, Phil. 81 F2 10 45N 119 30 E
Taytay Bay, Phil. 81 F2 10 55N 119 35 E
Tayug, Phil. 80 C3 16 2N 120 45 E
Tāyyebād, Iran 97 C9 34 45N 60 45 E
Tayyebād □, Iran 97 C9 34 44N 60 44 E
Taz →, Russia 66 C8 67 32N 78 40 E
Taza, Morocco 110 B4 34 16N 4 6W
Tāza Khurmātū, Iraq 101 E11 35 18N 44 20 E
Tazawa-Ko, Japan 70 E10 39 43N 140 40 E
Taze, Burma 90 D5 22 57N 95 24 E
Tazenakht, Morocco 110 B3 30 35N 7 12W
Tazerbo, Libya 108 C4 25 45N 21 0 E
Tazin, Canada 143 B7 59 48N 109 55W
Tazin L., Canada 143 B7 59 44N 108 42W
Tazlina, U.S.A. 144 E11 62 4N 146 27W
Tazoult, Algeria 111 A6 35 29N 6 11 E
Tazovskiy, Russia 66 C8 67 30N 78 44 E
Tbilisi, Georgia 61 K7 41 43N 44 50 E
Tchad = Chad ■, Africa 109 F3 15 0N 17 15 E
Tchad, L., Chad 109 F2 13 30N 14 30 E
Tchaourou, Benin 113 D5 8 58N 2 40 E
Tch'eng-tou = Chengdu, China 76 B5 30 38N 104 2 E
Tchentlo L., Canada 142 B4 55 15N 125 0W
Tchetti, Benin 113 D5 7 50N 1 40 E
Tchibanga, Gabon 114 C2 2 45 S 11 0 E
Tchien, Liberia 112 D3 5 59N 8 15W
Tchin Tabaraden, Niger 113 B6 15 58N 5 56 E
Tchingou, Massif de, N. Cal. 133 T19 20 54 S 165 0 E
Tcholliré, Cameroon 114 A2 8 24N 14 10 E
Tch'ong-k'ing = Chongqing, China 76 C6 29 35N 106 25 E
Tczew, Poland 54 D5 54 8N 18 50 E
Te Anau, N.Z. 131 F2 45 25 S 167 43 E
Te Anau, L., N.Z. 131 F2 45 15 S 167 45 E
Te Araroa, N.Z. 130 D7 37 39 S 178 25 E
Te Aroha, N.Z. 130 D4 37 32 S 175 44 E
Te Awamutu, N.Z. 130 E4 38 1 S 175 20 E
Te Ika a Maui = North I., N.Z. 130 E4 38 0 S 175 0 E
Te Kaha, N.Z. 130 D6 37 44 S 177 52 E
Te Karaka, N.Z. 130 E6 38 26 S 177 53 E
Te Kauwhata, N.Z. 130 D4 37 25 S 175 9 E
Te Kopuru, N.Z. 130 C2 36 2 S 173 56 E
Te Kuiti, N.Z. 130 E4 38 20 S 175 11 E
Te-n-Dghâmcha, Sebkhet, Mauritania 112 B1 18 30N 15 55W
Te Puke, N.Z. 130 D5 37 46 S 176 22 E
Te Teko, N.Z. 130 E5 38 2 S 176 48 E
Te Waewae B., N.Z. 131 G2 46 13 S 167 33 E
Te Wai Pounamu = South I., N.Z. 131 E5 44 0 S 170 0 E
Tea →, Brazil 168 D4 0 30 S 65 9W
Teaca, Romania 53 D9 46 55N 24 30 E
Teague, U.S.A. 155 K6 31 38N 96 17W
Teano, Italy 47 A7 41 15N 14 4 E
Teapa, Mexico 163 D6 18 35N 92 56W
Teba, Spain 43 J6 36 59N 4 55W
Tebakang, Malaysia 78 D4 1 6N 110 30 E
Teberau, Malaysia 84 B2 1 32N 103 45 E
Teberda, Russia 61 J5 43 30N 41 46 E
Teberu, Malaysia 87 d 1 30N 103 42 E
Tébessa, Algeria 111 A6 35 22N 8 8 E
Tebicuary →, Paraguay 174 B4 26 36 S 58 16W
Tebingtinggi, Riau, Indonesia 84 B2 1 0N 102 45 E
Tebingtinggi, Sumatera Utara, Indonesia 84 B1 3 20N 99 9 E
Tébourba, Tunisia 108 A1 36 49N 9 51 E
Téboursouk, Tunisia 108 A1 36 29N 9 10 E
Tebulos, Georgia 61 J7 42 36N 45 17 E
Tecate, Mexico 161 N10 32 34N 116 38W
Tecer Dağları, Turkey 100 C7 39 27N 37 27 E
Tech →, France 28 F7 42 36N 3 3 E
Techa →, Russia 64 C9 56 13N 62 58 E
Techiman, Ghana 112 D4 7 35N 1 58W
Techirghiol, Romania 53 F13 44 4N 28 32 E
Techou = Dezhou, China 74 F9 37 26N 116 18 E
Tecka, Argentina 176 B2 43 29 S 70 48W
Tecomán, Mexico 162 D4 18 55N 103 53W
Tecopa, U.S.A. 161 K10 35 51N 116 13W
Tecoripa, Mexico 162 B3 28 37N 109 57W
Tecuala, Mexico 162 C3 22 23N 105 27W
Tecuci, Romania 53 E12 45 51N 27 27 E
Tecumseh, Canada 150 D2 42 19N 82 54W
Tecumseh, Mich., U.S.A. 157 B13 42 0N 83 57W
Tecumseh, Okla., U.S.A. 155 H6 35 15N 96 56W
Ted, Somali Rep. 120 D2 4 24N 43 55 E
Tedjert, Algeria 111 D6 21 23N 6 25 E
Tedzhen = Tejen, Turkmenistan 66 F7 37 23N 60 31 E
Tees →, U.K. 20 C6 54 37N 1 10W
Tees B., U.K. 20 C6 54 40N 1 9W
Teeswater, Canada 150 C3 43 59N 81 17W
Tefé, Brazil 169 D5 3 25 S 64 50W
Tefé →, Brazil 169 D5 3 35 S 64 47W
Tefenni, Turkey 49 D11 37 18N 29 45 E
Tegal, Indonesia 85 D3 6 52 S 109 8 E
Tegallalang, Indonesia 79 J18 8 27 S 115 17 E
Tegalsari, Indonesia 79 J17 8 25 S 114 8 E
Tegel, Berlin ✕ (TXL), Germany 30 C9 52 35N 13 14 E
Tegernsee, Germany 31 H7 47 43N 11 46 E
Teggiano, Italy 47 B8 40 23N 15 32 E
Tegid, L. = Bala, L., U.K. 20 E4 52 53N 3 37W
Tegina, Nigeria 113 C6 10 5N 6 11 E
Téglio, Italy 33 D10 46 10N 10 4 E
Tegua, Vanuatu 133 C4 13 15 S 166 37 E
Tegucigalpa, Honduras 164 D2 14 5N 87 14W
Teguidda i-n-Tessoum, Niger 113 B6 17 25N 6 37 E
Tehachapi, U.S.A. 161 K8 35 8N 118 27W
Tehachapi Mts., U.S.A. 161 L8 35 0N 118 30W
Tehamiyam, Sudan 106 D4 18 20N 36 32 E
Teheran = Tehrān, Iran 97 C6 35 44N 51 30 E
Tehilla, Sudan 106 D4 17 42N 36 6 E
Téhini, Ivory C. 112 D4 9 39N 3 40W
Tehoru, Indonesia 83 B3 3 23 S 129 30 E
Tehrān, Iran 97 C6 35 44N 51 30 E
Tehran □, Iran 97 C6 35 30N 51 30 E
Tehri, India 93 D8 30 23N 78 29 E
Tehuacán, Mexico 163 D5 18 30N 97 30W
Tehuantepec, Mexico 163 D5 16 21N 95 13W
Tehuantepec, G. de, Mexico 163 D5 15 50N 95 12W
Tehuantepec, Istmo de, Mexico 163 D6 17 0N 94 30W
Teide, Pico de, Canary Is. 9 e1 28 15N 16 38W
Teifi →, U.K. 21 E3 52 5N 4 41W
Teigebyen, Norway 18 D8 60 12N 11 0 E
Teign →, U.K. 21 G4 50 32N 3 32W
Teignmouth, U.K. 21 G4 50 33N 3 31W
Teiuş, Romania 53 D8 46 12N 23 40 E
Teixeira, Brazil 170 C4 7 13 S 37 15W
Teixeira Pinto, Guinea-Biss. 112 C1 12 3N 16 0W
Tejakula, Indonesia 79 J18 8 8 S 115 20 E
Tejam, India 93 E9 29 57N 80 11 E
Tejen, Turkmenistan 66 F7 37 23N 60 31 E
Tejen →, Turkmenistan 97 B9 37 24N 60 38 E
Tejo →, Europe 43 F2 38 40N 9 24W
Tejon Pass, U.S.A. 161 L8 34 49N 118 53W
Tekamah, U.S.A. 154 E6 41 47N 96 13W
Tekapo →, N.Z. 131 E5 44 13 S 170 21 E
Tekapo, L., N.Z. 131 D5 43 53 S 170 33 E
Tekax, Mexico 163 C7 20 11N 89 18W
Teke, Kazakhstan 65 B4 43 15N 68 10 E
Teke, Turkey 51 E13 41 4N 29 39 E
Tekeli, Kazakhstan 65 A9 44 50N 79 0 E
Tekeze →, Ethiopia 107 E4 14 20N 35 50 E
Tekija, Serbia & M. 50 B6 44 42N 22 26 E
Tekirdağ, Turkey 51 F11 40 58N 27 30 E
Tekirdağ □, Turkey 51 E11 41 0N 27 0 E
Tekirova, Turkey 49 E12 36 30N 30 32 E
Tekkali, India 94 E7 18 37N 84 15 E
Tekke, Turkey 100 B7 40 42N 36 12 E
Tekman, Turkey 101 C9 39 38N 41 29 E
Tekoa, U.S.A. 158 C5 47 14N 117 4W
Tekong Besar, Pulau, Singapore 87 d 1 25N 104 3 E
Tekouiât, O. →, Algeria 111 D5 22 25N 2 35 E
Tekro, Chad 109 E4 19 32N 20 56 E
Teku, Indonesia 82 B2 0 46 S 123 26 E
Tel →, India 94 D6 20 50N 83 54 E
Tel Aviv ✕ (TLV), Israel 103 C3 32 5N 34 49 E
Tel Aviv-Yafo, Israel 103 C3 32 4N 34 48 E
Tel Lakhish, Israel 103 D3 31 34N 34 51 E
Tel Megiddo, Israel 103 C4 32 35N 35 11 E
Tela, Honduras 164 C2 15 40N 87 28W
Télagh, Algeria 111 B4 34 51N 0 32W
Telanaipura = Jambi, Indonesia 84 C2 1 38 S 103 30 E
Telašćica ⌓, Croatia 45 E12 43 55N 15 10 E
Telavåg, Norway 18 D1 60 15N 4 58 E
Telavi, Georgia 61 J7 42 0N 45 30 E
Telč, Czech Rep. 34 B8 49 11N 15 28 E
Telciu, Romania 53 C9 47 25N 24 24 E
Telde, Canary Is. 9 e1 27 59N 15 25W
Tele →, Dem. Rep. of the Congo 114 B4 2 48N 23 54 E
Telefomin, Papua N. G. 132 C1 5 10 S 141 31 E
Telegraph Creek, Canada 142 B2 58 0N 131 10W
Telekhany = Tsyelyakhany, Belarus 59 F3 52 30N 25 46 E
Telemark, Norway 15 G12 59 15N 7 40 E
Telemark □, Norway 18 E5 59 25N 8 30 E
Telén, Argentina 174 D2 36 15 S 65 31W
Telen →, Indonesia 85 C5 0 10 S 117 20 E
Teleneşti, Moldova 53 C13 47 30N 28 22 E
Teleng, Iran 97 E9 25 47N 61 3 E
Teleño, Spain 42 C4 42 23N 6 22W
Teleorman □, Romania 53 G10 44 0N 25 0 E
Teleorman →, Romania 53 G10 43 52N 25 26 E
Teles Pires →, Brazil 173 B6 7 21 S 58 3W
Telescope Pk., U.S.A. 161 J9 36 10N 117 5W
Teletaye, Mali 113 B5 16 31N 1 30 E
Telfer Mine, Australia 124 C3 21 40 S 122 12 E
Telford, U.K. 21 E5 52 40N 2 27W
Telford and Wrekin □, U.K. 20 E5 52 45N 2 27W
Telfs, Austria 34 D4 47 19N 11 4 E
Telida, U.S.A. 144 E9 63 23N 153 16W
Télimélé, Guinea 112 C2 10 54N 13 2W
Teljo, J., Sudan 107 E2 14 42N 25 26 E
Telkwa, Canada 142 C3 54 41N 127 5W
Tell City, U.S.A. 157 G10 37 57N 86 46W
Teller, U.S.A. 144 D6 65 16N 166 22W
Tellicherry, India 95 J2 11 45N 75 30 E
Telluride, U.S.A. 159 H10 37 56N 107 49W
Telok Datok, Malaysia 84 B2 2 49N 101 31 E
Teloloapán, Mexico 163 D5 18 21N 99 51W
Telpos Iz, Russia 56 B10 63 16N 59 13 E
Telsen, Argentina 176 B3 42 30 S 66 50W
Telšiai, Lithuania 15 H20 55 59N 22 14 E
Telšiai □, Lithuania 54 C9 55 59N 22 15 E
Teltow, Germany 30 C9 52 24N 13 15 E
Teluk Anson = Teluk Intan, Malaysia 87 K3 4 3N 101 0 E
Teluk Bahang, Malaysia 87 c 5 28N 100 13 E
Teluk Betung = Tanjungkarang Telukbetung, Indonesia 84 D3 5 20 S 105 10 E
Teluk Cenderawasih, Indonesia 83 B5 2 30 S 135 20 E
Teluk Darvel, Malaysia 81 J2 4 45N 118 30 E
Teluk Intan, Malaysia 87 K3 4 3N 101 0 E
Teluk Kumbar, Malaysia 87 c 5 18N 100 14 E
Telukbutun, Indonesia 85 B3 4 13N 108 12 E
Telukdalem, Indonesia 84 B1 0 33N 97 50 E
Tema, Ghana 113 D5 5 41N 0 0W
Temanggung, Indonesia 85 D4 7 18 S 110 10 E
Temasint, Algeria 111 D6 23 18N 7 40 E
Temax, Mexico 163 C7 21 10N 88 50W
Temba, S. Africa 117 D4 25 20 S 28 17 E
Tembagapura, Indonesia 83 B5 4 20 S 137 0 E
Tembe, Dem. Rep. of the Congo 118 C2 0 16 S 28 14 E
Tembe ⌓, S. Africa 117 D5 26 51 S 32 24 E
Tembesi, Indonesia 84 C2 1 43 S 103 6 E
Tembilahan, Indonesia 84 C2 0 19 S 103 9 E
Temblador, Venezuela 169 B5 8 59N 62 44W
Tembleque, Spain 42 F7 39 41N 3 30W
Temblor Range, U.S.A. 161 K7 35 20N 119 50W
Teme →, U.K. 21 E5 52 11N 2 13W
Temecula, U.S.A. 161 M9 33 30N 117 9W
Temerloh, Malaysia 84 B2 3 27N 102 25 E
Teminabuan, Indonesia 83 B4 1 26 S 132 1 E
Temir, Kazakhstan 57 E10 49 1N 57 14 E
Temir, Kazakhstan 65 B4 42 49N 68 26 E
Temir-Khan-Shura = Buynaksk, Russia 61 J8 42 48N 47 7 E
Temirlan, Kazakhstan 65 B4 42 36N 69 17 E
Temirtau, Kazakhstan 66 D8 50 5N 72 56 E
Temirtau, Russia 66 D9 53 10N 87 30 E
Temiscamie →, Canada 141 B5 50 59N 73 5W
Témiscaming, Canada 140 C4 46 44N 79 5W
Témiscamingue, L., Canada 140 C4 47 10N 79 25W
Temnikov, Russia 60 C6 54 40N 43 11 E
Temo →, Italy 46 B1 40 17N 8 28 E
Temora, Australia 129 C7 34 30 S 147 30 E
Temosachic, Mexico 162 B3 28 58N 107 50W
Tempe, U.S.A. 159 K8 33 25N 111 56W
Tempelburg = Czaplinek, Poland 54 E3 53 34N 16 14 E
Témpio Pausánia, Italy 46 B2 40 54N 9 6 E
Tempiute, U.S.A. 160 H11 37 39N 115 38W
Templar Bank, S. China Sea 81 F1 9 0N 117 30 E
Temple, U.S.A. 155 K6 31 6N 97 21W
Temple B., Australia 126 A3 12 15 S 143 3 E
Temple Terrace, U.S.A. 153 G7 28 2N 82 23W
Templemore, Ireland 23 D4 52 47N 7 51W
Templeton, U.S.A. 160 K6 35 33N 120 42W
Templeton →, Australia 126 C2 21 0 S 138 40 E
Templin, Germany 30 B9 53 7N 13 28 E
Tempoal, Mexico 163 C5 21 31N 98 23W
Tempué, Angola 115 E3 13 27 S 18 49 E
Temryuk, Russia 59 K9 45 15N 37 24 E
Temska →, Serbia & M. 50 C6 43 17N 22 33 E
Temuco, Chile 176 A2 38 45 S 72 40W
Temuka, N.Z. 131 E6 44 14 S 171 17 E
Ten Degree Channel, India 95 K11 10 0N 92 30 E
Ten Thousand Is., U.S.A. 153 K8 25 55N 81 45W
Tena, Ecuador 168 D2 0 59 S 77 49W
Tenabo, Mexico 163 C6 20 2N 90 12W
Tenaha, U.S.A. 155 K7 31 57N 94 15W
Tenakee Springs, U.S.A. 142 B1 57 47N 135 13W
Tenali, India 95 F5 16 15N 80 35 E
Tenancingo, Mexico 163 D5 19 0N 99 33W

Tenango, *Mexico* **163 D5** 19 7N 99 33W
Tenaro, Ákra = Taínaron, Ákra, *Greece* **48 E4** 36 22N 22 27 E
Tenasserim, *Burma* **87 F2** 12 6N 99 3 E
Tenasserim □, *Burma* **86 F2** 14 0N 98 30 E
Tenby, *U.K.* **21 F3** 51 40N 4 42W
Tenda, Colle di, *France* **29 D11** 44 7N 7 36 E
Tendaho, *Ethiopia* **107 E5** 11 48N 40 54 E
Tende, *France* **29 D11** 44 5N 7 35 E
Tendelti, *Sudan* **107 E3** 13 1N 31 55 E
Tendjedi, Adrar, *Algeria* **111 D6** 23 41N 7 32 E
Tendrara, *Morocco* **111 B4** 33 3N 1 58W
Tendre, Mt., *Switz.* **32 C2** 46 35N 6 18 E
Tendrovskaya Kosa, *Ukraine* **59 J6** 46 16N 31 35 E
Tendukhera, *India* **93 H8** 23 24N 79 33 E
Tenebroûret, O. →, *Mauritania* **110 D1** 20 35N 16 0W
Teneguía, Volcanes de, *Canary Is.* **9 e1** 28 28N 17 51W
Teneida, *Egypt* **106 B2** 25 30N 29 19 E
Tenenkou, *Mali* **112 C4** 14 28N 4 55W
Tenente Marques →, *Brazil* **173 C6** 11 10 S 59 56W
Ténéré, *Niger* **113 B7** 19 0N 10 30 E
Ténéré, Erg du, *Niger* **109 E2** 17 35N 10 55 E
Tenerife, *Canary Is.* **9 e1** 28 15N 16 35W
Tenerife, Pico, *Canary Is.* **9 e1** 27 43N 18 1W
Tenerife Norte ✕ (TFN), *Canary Is.* **9 e1** 28 28N 16 17W
Tenerife Sur ✕ (TFS), *Canary Is.* **9 e1** 28 3N 16 33W
Ténès, *Algeria* **111 A5** 36 31N 1 14 E
Teng Xian, *Guangxi Zhuangzu, China* **77 F8** 23 21N 110 56 E
Teng Xian, *Shandong, China* **75 G9** 35 5N 117 10 E
Tengah, Kepulauan, *Indonesia* **85 D5** 7 5 S 118 15 E
Tengchong, *China* **76 E2** 25 0N 98 28 E
Tengchowfu = Penglai, *China* **75 F11** 37 48N 120 42 E
Tenggarong, *Indonesia* **85 C5** 0 24 S 116 58 E
Tenggol, Pulau, *Malaysia* **87 K4** 4 48N 103 41 E
Tengi-Kharam = Dekhkanabad, *Uzbekistan* **65 D3** 38 21N 66 30 E
Tengiz, Ozero, *Kazakhstan* **66 D7** 50 30N 69 0 E
Tenhult, *Sweden* **17 G8** 57 41N 14 20 E
Teniente Enciso △, *Paraguay* **174 A3** 21 5 S 61 8W
Teniente Rodolfo Marsh, *Antarctica* **7 C18** 62 30 S 58 0W
Tenigerbad, *Switz.* **33 C7** 46 42N 8 57 E
Tenille, *U.S.A.* **152 F6** 29 46N 83 19W
Tenino, *U.S.A.* **160 D4** 46 51N 122 51W
Tenkasi, *India* **95 K3** 8 55N 77 20 E
Tenke, *Katanga, Dem. Rep. of the Congo* **119 E2** 11 22 S 26 40 E
Tenke, *Katanga, Dem. Rep. of the Congo* **119 E2** 10 32 S 26 7 E
Tenkodogo, *Burkina Faso* **113 C4** 11 54N 0 19W
Tenna →, *Italy* **45 E10** 43 14N 13 47 E
Tennant Creek, *Australia* **126 B1** 19 30 S 134 15 E
Tennessee □, *U.S.A.* **149 H2** 36 0N 86 30W
Tennessee →, *U.S.A.* **148 G1** 37 4N 88 34W
Tennille, *U.S.A.* **152 C7** 32 56N 82 48W
Teno, Pta. de, *Canary Is.* **9 e1** 28 21N 16 55W
Tenom, *Malaysia* **85 A5** 5 4N 115 57 E
Tenosique, *Mexico* **163 D6** 17 30N 91 24W
Tenri, *Japan* **73 C7** 34 39N 135 49 E
Tenryū, *Japan* **73 C9** 34 52N 137 49 E
Tenryū-Gawa →, *Japan* **73 B9** 35 39N 137 48 E
Tensift, Oued →, *Morocco* **110 B3** 32 3N 9 28W
Tentelomatinan, *Indonesia* **82 A2** 0 56N 121 48 E
Tentena, *Indonesia* **82 B2** 1 47 S 120 39 E
Tenterden, *U.K.* **21 F8** 51 4N 0 42 E
Tenterfield, *Australia* **127 D5** 29 0 S 152 0 E
Tenuaiur, Uad →, *W. Sahara* **110 D1** 21 36N 16 0W
Teo, *Spain* **42 C2** 42 45N 8 30W
Teófilo Otoni, *Brazil* **171 E3** 17 50 S 41 30W
Tepa, *Indonesia* **83 C3** 7 52 S 129 31 E
Tepalcatepec →, *Mexico* **162 D4** 18 35N 101 59W
Tepecik, *Bursa, Turkey* **51 F12** 40 7N 28 25 E
Tepecik, *Kütahya, Turkey* **49 B11** 39 32N 29 28 E
Tepehuanes, *Mexico* **162 B3** 25 21N 105 44W
Tepelenë, *Albania* **50 F4** 40 17N 20 2 E
Tepequem, Serra, *Brazil* **169 C5** 3 45N 61 45W
Tepetongo, *Mexico* **162 C4** 22 28N 103 9W
Tepic = Nayarit □, *Mexico* **162 C4** 22 0N 105 0W
Tepic, *Mexico* **162 C4** 21 30N 104 54W
Teplá, *Czech Rep.* **34 B5** 49 59N 12 52 E
Teplice, *Czech Rep.* **34 A6** 50 40N 13 48 E
Teplitz = Teplice, *Czech Rep.* **34 A6** 50 40N 13 48 E
Teploklyuchenka, *Kyrgyzstan* **65 B9** 42 30N 78 30 E
Teplyk, *Ukraine* **53 B14** 48 40N 29 44 E
Tepoca, C., *Mexico* **162 A2** 30 20N 112 25W
Tequila, *Mexico* **162 C4** 20 54N 103 47W
Ter →, *Spain* **40 C8** 42 2N 3 12 E
Ter Apel, *Neths.* **24 B7** 52 53N 7 5 E
Téra, *Niger* **113 C5** 14 0N 0 45 E
Tera →, *Spain* **42 D5** 41 54N 5 44W
Teraina, *Kiribati* **135 G11** 4 43N 160 25W
Terakeka, *Sudan* **107 F3** 5 26N 31 45 E
Téramo, *Italy* **45 F10** 42 39N 13 42 E
Terang, *Australia* **128 E5** 38 15 S 142 55 E
Terang, Teluk, *Indonesia* **79 K19** 8 44 S 116 0 E
Terawhiti, C., *N.Z.* **130 H3** 41 16 S 174 38 E
Terazit, Massif de, *Niger* **111 D6** 20 2N 8 30 E
Tercan, *Turkey* **101 C9** 39 47N 40 23 E
Terceira, *Azores* **9 d1** 38 43N 27 13W
Tercero →, *Argentina* **174 C3** 32 58 S 61 47W
Terdal, *India* **94 F2** 16 33N 75 3 E
Terebovlya, *Ukraine* **59 H3** 49 18N 25 44 E
Teregova, *Romania* **52 E7** 45 10N 22 16 E
Tereida, *Sudan* **107 E3** 10 35N 31 17 E
Terek →, *Russia* **61 J8** 44 0N 47 30 E
Terek-Say, *Kyrgyzstan* **65 C5** 41 30N 71 11 E
Terengganu □, *Malaysia* **84 B2** 4 55N 103 0 E
Terengözek, *Kazakhstan* **65 A2** 45 3N 64 59 E
Terenos, *Brazil* **173 E7** 20 26 S 54 50W
Terepaima △, *Venezuela* **165 E6** 9 58N 69 17W
Tereshka →, *Russia* **60 E8** 51 48N 46 26 E
Teresina, *Brazil* **170 C3** 5 9 S 42 45W
Teresinha, *Brazil* **169 C7** 0 58N 52 2W
Terespol, *Poland* **55 F10** 52 5N 23 37 E
Teressa, *India* **95 K11** 8 15N 93 10 E
Teresva, *Ukraine* **53 B8** 48 0N 23 42 E
Terewah, L., *Australia* **127 D4** 29 52 S 147 35 E
Terges →, *Portugal* **43 H3** 37 49N 7 41W
Tergnier, *France* **27 C10** 49 40N 3 17 E
Terhazza, *Mali* **110 D3** 23 38N 5 22W
Teridgerie Cr. →, *Australia* **129 A8** 30 25 S 148 50 E
Teríjoki = Zelenogorsk, *Russia* **58 B5** 60 12N 29 43 E
Terlizzi, *Italy* **47 A9** 41 8N 16 32 E
Terme, *Turkey* **100 B7** 41 11N 37 0 E
Termez = Termiz, *Uzbekistan* **65 E3** 37 15N 67 15 E
Términi Imerese, *Italy* **46 E6** 37 59N 13 42 E
Términos, L. de, *Mexico* **163 D6** 18 35N 91 30W
Termiz, *Uzbekistan* **65 E3** 37 15N 67 15 E
Térmoli, *Italy* **45 F12** 42 0N 15 0 E
Ternate, *Indonesia* **82 A3** 0 45N 127 25 E
Terneuzen, *Neths.* **24 C3** 51 20N 3 50 E
Terney, *Russia* **67 E14** 45 3N 136 37 E
Terni, *Italy* **45 F9** 42 34N 12 37 E
Ternitz, *Austria* **34 D9** 47 43N 16 2 E
Ternivka, *Ukraine* **53 B14** 48 32N 29 58 E
Ternopil, *Ukraine* **59 H3** 49 30N 25 40 E
Ternopol = Ternopil, *Ukraine* **59 H3** 49 30N 25 40 E
Terowie, *Australia* **128 B3** 33 8 S 138 55 E
Terpní, *Greece* **50 F7** 40 55N 23 26 E
Terra Bella, *U.S.A.* **161 K7** 35 58N 119 3W
Terra Nova △, *Canada* **141 C9** 48 33N 53 55W
Terrace, *Canada* **142 C3** 54 30N 128 35W
Terrace Bay, *Canada* **140 C2** 48 47N 87 5W
Terracina, *Italy* **46 A6** 41 17N 13 15 E
Terralba, *Italy* **46 C1** 39 43N 8 39 E
Terranova di Sicilia = Gela, *Italy* **47 E7** 37 4N 14 15 E
Terranova Pausania = Ólbia, *Italy* **46 B2** 40 55N 9 31 E
Terrasini, *Italy* **46 D6** 38 10N 13 4 E
Terrassa, *Spain* **40 D7** 41 34N 2 1 E
Terrasson-la-Villedieu, *France* **28 C5** 45 8N 1 18 E
Terre Haute, *U.S.A.* **157 E9** 39 28N 87 25W
Terrebonne B., *U.S.A.* **155 L9** 29 5N 90 35W
Terrecht, *Mali* **111 D4** 20 10N 0 10W
Terrell, *U.S.A.* **155 J6** 32 44N 96 17W
Terrenceville, *Canada* **141 C9** 47 40N 54 44W
Terry, *U.S.A.* **154 B2** 46 47N 105 19W
Terryville, *U.S.A.* **151 E11** 41 41N 73 3W
Terschelling, *Neths.* **24 A5** 53 25N 5 20 E
Terskey Ala Too, *Kyrgyzstan* **65 C8** 41 50N 77 0 E
Terskey Alatau = Terskey Ala Too, *Kyrgyzstan* **65 C8** 41 50N 77 0 E
Tersko-Kumskiy Kanal, *Russia* **61 H7** 44 32N 44 38 E
Tertenía, *Italy* **46 C2** 39 42N 9 34 E
Terter = Tärtär →, *Azerbaijan* **61 K8** 40 26N 47 20 E
Teruel, *Spain* **40 E3** 40 22N 1 8W
Teruel □, *Spain* **40 E4** 40 48N 1 0W
Tervel, *Bulgaria* **51 C11** 43 45N 27 28 E
Tervola, *Finland* **14 C21** 66 6N 24 49 E
Teryaweyna L., *Australia* **128 B5** 32 18 S 143 22 E
Tešanj, *Bos.-H.* **52 F3** 44 38N 18 1 E
Teschen = Český Těšín, *Czech Rep.* **35 B11** 49 45N 18 39 E
Teschen = Cieszyn, *Poland* **55 J5** 49 45N 18 35 E
Teseney, *Eritrea* **107 D4** 15 5N 36 42 E
Tesha →, *Russia* **60 C6** 55 38N 42 9 E
Teshekpuk L., *U.S.A.* **144 A9** 70 35N 153 26W
Teshio, *Japan* **70 B10** 44 53N 141 44 E
Teshio-Gawa →, *Japan* **70 B10** 44 53N 141 45 E
Tešica, *Serbia & M.* **50 C5** 43 27N 21 45 E
Tesiyn Gol →, *Mongolia* **68 A4** 50 40N 93 20 E
Teslić, *Bos.-H.* **52 F2** 44 37N 17 54 E
Teslin, *Canada* **142 A2** 60 10N 132 43W
Teslin →, *Canada* **142 A2** 61 34N 134 35W
Teslin L., *Canada* **142 A2** 60 15N 132 57W
Tesouro, *Brazil* **173 D7** 16 4 S 53 34W
Tessalit, *Mali* **111 D5** 20 12N 1 0 E
Tessaoua, *Niger* **113 C6** 13 47N 7 56 E
Tessin, *Germany* **30 A8** 54 2N 12 26 E
Tessit, *Mali* **113 B5** 15 13N 0 18 E
Tessounfat, *Mali* **111 D5** 22 53N 0 32 E
Test →, *U.K.* **21 G6** 50 56N 1 29W
Testa del Gargano, *Italy* **45 G13** 41 50N 16 10 E
Testigos, Is. Las, *Venezuela* **165 D7** 11 23N 63 7W
Tét, *Hungary* **52 C2** 47 30N 17 33 E
Têt →, *France* **28 F7** 42 44N 3 2 E
Tetachuck L., *Canada* **142 C3** 53 18N 125 55W
Tetas, Pta., *Chile* **174 A1** 23 31 S 70 38W
Tete, *Mozam.* **119 F3** 16 13 S 33 33 E
Tete □, *Mozam.* **119 F3** 15 15 S 32 40 E
Tetenga, Caleta, *Chile* **172 b** 27 9 S 109 19W
Tetepare, *Solomon Is.* **133 M9** 8 45 S 157 35 E
Teterev →, *Ukraine* **59 G6** 51 1N 30 5 E
Teterow, *Germany* **30 B8** 53 46N 12 34 E
Teteven, *Bulgaria* **51 D8** 42 58N 24 17 E
Tethul →, *Canada* **142 A6** 60 35N 112 12W
Tetiyev, *Ukraine* **59 H5** 49 22N 29 38 E
Tetlin, *U.S.A.* **144 E12** 63 8N 142 31W
Tetlin Junction, *U.S.A.* **144 E12** 63 19N 142 36W
Teton →, *U.S.A.* **158 C8** 47 56N 110 31W
Tétouan, *Morocco* **110 A3** 35 35N 5 21W
Tetovo, *Macedonia* **50 D4** 42 1N 20 59 E
Tetschen = Děčín, *Czech Rep.* **34 A7** 50 47N 14 12 E
Tetyukhe = Dalnegorsk, *Russia* **67 E14** 44 32N 135 33 E
Tetyushi, *Russia* **60 C9** 54 55N 48 49 E
Teuco →, *Argentina* **174 B3** 25 35 S 60 11W
Teufen, *Switz.* **33 B8** 47 24N 9 23 E
Teulada, *Italy* **46 D1** 38 58N 8 46 E
Teulon, *Canada* **143 C9** 50 23N 97 16W
Teun, *Indonesia* **83 C3** 6 59 S 129 8 E
Teutoburger Wald, *Germany* **30 C4** 52 5N 8 22 E
Teutopolis, *U.S.A.* **157 E8** 39 8N 88 29W
Tevere ⌓, *Italy* **45 F9** 42 46N 12 14 E
Tevere →, *Italy* **45 G9** 41 44N 12 14 E
Teverya, *Israel* **103 C4** 32 47N 35 32 E
Teviot →, *U.K.* **22 F6** 55 29N 2 38W
Tewantin, *Australia* **127 D5** 26 27 S 153 3 E
Tewkesbury, *U.K.* **21 F5** 51 59N 2 9W
Texada I., *Canada* **142 D4** 49 40N 124 25W
Texarkana, *Ark., U.S.A.* **155 J8** 33 26N 94 2W
Texarkana, *Tex., U.S.A.* **155 J7** 33 26N 94 3W
Texas, *Australia* **127 D5** 28 49 S 151 9 E
Texas □, *U.S.A.* **155 K5** 31 40N 98 30W
Texas City, *U.S.A.* **155 L7** 29 24N 94 54W
Texel, *Neths.* **24 A4** 53 5N 4 50 E
Texline, *U.S.A.* **155 G3** 36 23N 103 2W
Texoma, L., *U.S.A.* **155 J6** 33 50N 96 34W
Teykovo, *Russia* **58 D11** 56 55N 40 30 E
Teyvareh, *Afghan.* **91 B2** 33 30N 64 24 E
Teza →, *Russia* **60 B5** 56 32N 41 53 E
Tezin, *Afghan.* **91 B3** 34 24N 69 30 E
Teziutlán, *Mexico* **163 D5** 19 50N 97 22W
Tezpur, *India* **90 B4** 26 40N 92 45 E
Tezzeron L., *Canada* **142 C4** 54 43N 124 30W
Tha-anne →, *Canada* **143 A10** 60 31N 94 37W
Tha Deua, *Laos* **86 D4** 17 57N 102 53 E
Tha Deua, *Laos* **86 C3** 19 26N 101 50 E
Tha Pla, *Thailand* **86 D3** 17 48N 100 32 E
Tha Rua, *Thailand* **86 E3** 14 34N 100 44 E
Tha Sala, *Thailand* **87 H2** 8 40N 99 56 E
Tha Song Yang, *Thailand* **86 D1** 17 34N 97 55 E
Thaba Putsoa, *Lesotho* **117 D4** 29 45 S 28 0 E
Thabana Ntlenyana, *Lesotho* **117 D4** 29 30 S 29 16 E
Thabaung, *Burma* **90 G5** 17 2N 94 48 E
Thabazimbi, *S. Africa* **117 C4** 24 40 S 27 21 E
Thabeikkyin, *Burma* **90 D5** 22 53N 95 59 E
Thādiq, *Si. Arabia* **96 E5** 25 18N 45 52 E
Thai Binh, *Vietnam* **76 G6** 20 35N 106 1 E
Thai Muang, *Thailand* **87 H2** 8 24N 98 16 E
Thai Nguyen, *Vietnam* **76 G5** 21 35N 105 55 E
Thailand ■, *Asia* **86 E4** 16 0N 102 0 E
Thailand, G. of, *Asia* **87 G3** 11 30N 101 0 E
Thakhek, *Laos* **86 D5** 17 25N 104 45 E
Thakurgaon, *Bangla.* **90 B2** 26 2N 88 34 E
Thal, *Pakistan* **91 B3** 33 28N 70 33 E
Thal Desert, *Pakistan* **92 D4** 31 10N 71 30 E
Thala, *Tunisia* **108 A1** 35 35N 8 40 E
Thalabarivat, *Cambodia* **86 F5** 13 33N 105 57 E
Thalkirch, *Switz.* **33 C8** 46 39N 9 17 E
Thallon, *Australia* **127 D4** 28 39 S 148 49 E
Thalu, Ko, *Thailand* **87 b** 9 26N 99 54 E
Thalwil, *Switz.* **33 B7** 47 17N 8 35 E
Thamarīt, *Oman* **99 C6** 17 39N 54 2 E
Thames, *N.Z.* **130 D4** 37 7 S 175 34 E
Thames →, *Canada* **140 D3** 42 20N 82 25W
Thames →, *U.K.* **21 F8** 51 29N 0 34 E
Thames →, *U.S.A.* **151 E12** 41 18N 72 5W
Thames, Firth of, *N.Z.* **130 D4** 37 0 S 175 25 E
Thames Estuary, *U.K.* **21 F8** 51 29N 0 52 E
Thamesford, *Canada* **150 C4** 43 4N 81 0W
Thamesville, *Canada* **150 D3** 42 33N 81 59W
Thāmit, W. →, *Libya* **108 B3** 31 11N 16 8 E
Thamūd, *Yemen* **99 C5** 17 18N 49 55 E
Than, *India* **92 H4** 22 34N 71 11 E
Than Uyen, *Vietnam* **86 B4** 22 0N 103 54 E
Thana Gazi, *India* **92 F7** 27 25N 76 19 E
Thanbyuzayat, *Burma* **90 G6** 15 58N 97 44 E
Thandaung, *Burma* **90 F6** 19 4N 96 41 E
Thandla, *India* **92 H6** 23 0N 74 34 E
Thane, *India* **94 E1** 19 12N 72 59 E
Thanesar, *India* **92 D7** 30 1N 76 52 E
Thanet, I. of, *U.K.* **21 F9** 51 21N 1 20 E
Thangool, *Australia* **126 C5** 24 38 S 150 42 E
Thanh Hoa, *Vietnam* **86 C5** 19 48N 105 46 E
Thanh Hung, *Vietnam* **87 H5** 9 55N 105 43 E
Thanh Pho Ho Chi Minh, *Vietnam* **87 G6** 10 58N 106 40 E
Thanh Thuy, *Vietnam* **86 A5** 22 55N 104 51 E
Thanjavur, *India* **95 J4** 10 48N 79 12 E
Thann, *France* **27 E14** 47 48N 7 5 E
Thano Bula Khan, *Pakistan* **92 G2** 25 22N 67 50 E
Thaolinta L., *Canada* **143 A9** 61 30N 96 25W
Thaon-les-Vosges, *France* **27 D13** 48 15N 6 24 E
Thap Lan △, *Thailand* **86 E4** 14 15N 102 16 E
Thap Sakae, *Thailand* **87 G2** 11 30N 99 37 E
Thap Than, *Thailand* **86 E2** 15 27N 99 54 E
Thar Desert, *India* **92 F5** 28 0N 72 0 E
Tharad, *India* **92 G4** 24 30N 71 44 E
Thargomindah, *Australia* **127 D3** 27 58 S 143 46 E
Tharrawaddy, *Burma* **90 G5** 17 38N 95 48 E
Tharrawaw, *Burma* **90 G5** 17 41N 95 28 E
Tharthār, Buḩayrat ath, *Iraq* **101 E10** 34 0N 43 15 E
Tharthar, L. = Tharthār, Buḩayrat ath, *Iraq* **101 E10** 34 0N 43 15 E
Tharthār, W. ath →, *Iraq* **101 E10** 33 59N 43 12 E
Thasopoúla, *Greece* **51 F8** 40 49N 24 45 E
Thásos, *Greece* **51 F8** 40 40N 24 40 E
That Khe, *Vietnam* **76 F6** 22 16N 106 28 E
Thatcher, *Ariz., U.S.A.* **159 K9** 32 51N 109 46W
Thatcher, *Colo., U.S.A.* **155 G2** 37 33N 104 7W
Thaton, *Burma* **90 G6** 16 55N 97 22 E
Thau, Bassin de, *France* **28 E7** 43 23N 3 36 E
Thaungdut, *Burma* **90 C5** 24 30N 94 40 E
Thawatti, *Burma* **90 F6** 19 32N 96 16 E
Thayer, *U.S.A.* **155 G9** 36 31N 91 33W
Thayetmyo, *Burma* **90 F5** 19 20N 95 10 E
Thayngen, *Switz.* **33 A7** 47 49N 8 43 E
Thazi, *Magwe, Burma* **90 F5** 19 59N 95 3 E
Thazi, *Mandalay, Burma* **90 E6** 21 0N 96 5 E
The Bight, *Bahamas* **165 B4** 24 19N 75 24W
The Briars, *St. Helena* **9 h** 15 56 S 5 43W
The Crane, *Barbados* **165 g** 13 6N 59 27W
The Dalles, *U.S.A.* **158 D3** 45 36N 121 10W
The Entrance, *Australia* **129 B9** 33 21 S 151 30 E
The Forks = Merritt, *Canada* **142 C4** 50 10N 120 45W
The Great Divide = Great Dividing Ra., *Australia* **126 C4** 23 0 S 146 0 E
The Hague = 's-Gravenhage, *Neths.* **24 B4** 52 7N 4 17 E
The Oaks, *Australia* **129 C9** 34 3 S 150 34 E
The Pas, *Canada* **143 C8** 53 45N 101 15W
The Range, *Zimbabwe* **119 F3** 19 2 S 31 2 E
The Rock, *Australia* **129 C7** 35 15 S 147 2 E
The Settlement, *Br. Virgin Is.* **165 e** 18 43N 64 22W
The Woodlands, *U.S.A.* **155 K7** 30 9N 95 27W
Thebes = Thívai, *Greece* **48 C5** 38 19N 23 19 E
Thebes, *Egypt* **106 B3** 25 40N 32 35 E
Thedaw, *Burma* **90 E6** 21 5N 96 4 E
Thedford, *U.S.A.* **154 E4** 41 59N 100 35W
Theebine, *Australia* **127 D5** 25 57 S 152 34 E
Thègon, *Burma* **90 F5** 18 39N 95 25 E
Thékli, Ayía, *Greece* **39 C1** 38 15N 20 23 E
Thekulthili L., *Canada* **143 A7** 61 3N 110 0W
Thelon →, *Canada* **143 A8** 64 16N 96 4W
Thénezay, *France* **26 F6** 46 44N 0 2W
Thenia, *Algeria* **111 A5** 36 44N 3 33 E
Thenon, *France* **28 C5** 45 9N 1 4 E
Theodore, *Australia* **126 C5** 24 55 S 150 3 E
Theodore, *Canada* **143 C8** 51 26N 102 55W
Theodore, *U.S.A.* **149 K1** 30 33N 88 10W
Theodore Roosevelt △, *U.S.A.* **154 B3** 47 0N 103 25W
Theodore Roosevelt L., *U.S.A.* **159 K8** 33 40N 111 10W
Thepha, *Thailand* **87 J3** 6 52N 100 58 E
Thérain →, *France* **27 C9** 49 15N 2 27 E
Theresa, *U.S.A.* **151 B9** 44 13N 75 48W
Theressa, *U.S.A.* **152 F7** 29 50N 82 4W
Therma = Eagle Nest, *U.S.A.* **159 H11** 36 33N 105 16W
Thermaïkós Kólpos, *Greece* **50 F6** 40 15N 22 45 E
Thermí, *Greece* **49 B8** 39 11N 26 29 E
Thermopolis, *U.S.A.* **158 E9** 43 39N 108 13W
Thermopylae P., *Greece* **48 C4** 38 48N 22 35 E
Thesprotía □, *Greece* **48 B2** 39 27N 20 22 E
Thessalía □, *Greece* **48 B4** 39 25N 22 0 E
Thessalon, *Canada* **140 C3** 46 20N 83 30W
Thessaloníki, *Greece* **50 F6** 40 38N 22 58 E
Thessaloníki □, *Greece* **50 F7** 40 45N 23 0 E
Thessaloníki ✕ (SKG), *Greece* **50 F7** 40 30N 23 0 E
Thessaloníki, Gulf of = Thermaïkós Kólpos, *Greece* **50 F6** 40 15N 22 45 E
Thessaly = Thessalía □, *Greece* **48 B4** 39 25N 22 0 E
Thetford, *U.K.* **21 E8** 52 25N 0 45 E
Thetford Mines, *Canada* **141 C5** 46 8N 71 18W
Theun →, *Laos* **86 C5** 18 19N 104 0 E
Theunissen, *S. Africa* **116 D4** 28 26 S 26 43 E
Thevenard, *Australia* **127 E1** 32 9 S 133 38 E
Thiámis →, *Greece* **48 B2** 39 15N 20 6 E
Thiberville, *France* **26 C7** 49 8N 0 27 E
Thibodaux, *U.S.A.* **155 L9** 29 48N 90 49W
Thicket Portage, *Canada* **143 B9** 55 19N 97 42W
Thief River Falls, *U.S.A.* **154 A6** 48 7N 96 10W
Thiel Mts., *Antarctica* **7 E16** 85 15 S 91 0W
Thiene, *Italy* **45 C8** 45 42N 11 29 E
Thiérache, *France* **27 C10** 49 51N 3 45 E
Thiers, *France* **28 C7** 45 52N 3 33 E
Thiès, *Senegal* **112 C1** 14 50N 16 51W
Thiesi, *Italy* **46 B1** 40 31N 8 43 E
Thiet, *Sudan* **107 F2** 7 37N 28 49 E
Thika, *Kenya* **118 C4** 1 1 S 37 5 E
Thille-Boubacar, *Senegal* **112 B1** 16 31N 15 5W
Thimphu, *Bhutan* **90 B2** 27 31N 89 45 E
Thingangyun, *Burma* **90 G6** 16 49N 96 12 E
Þingeyjarsýsla □, *Iceland* **11 B10** 65 40N 16 30W
Þingeyri, *Iceland* **11 B3** 65 52N 23 30W
Þingmúli, *Iceland* **11 B12** 65 2N 14 37W
Þingvallavatn, *Iceland* **11 C5** 64 11N 21 9W
Þingvellir, *Iceland* **11 C5** 64 15N 21 7W
Þingvellir △, *Iceland* **11 C5** 64 16N 21 5W
Thio, *N. Cal.* **133 U20** 21 37 S 166 14 E
Thionville, *France* **27 C13** 49 20N 6 10 E
Thíra, *Greece* **49 E7** 36 23N 25 27 E
Thirasía, *Greece* **49 E7** 36 26N 25 21 E
Third Cataract, *Sudan* **106 D3** 19 42N 30 20 E
Thirsk, *U.K.* **20 C6** 54 14N 1 19W
Thiruvananthapuram = Trivandrum, *India* **95 K3** 8 41N 77 0 E
Thiruvarur, *India* **95 J4** 10 46N 79 38 E
Thisted, *Denmark* **17 H2** 56 58N 8 40 E
Þistilfjörður, *Iceland* **11 A11** 66 18N 15 24W
Thistle I., *Australia* **128 C2** 35 0 S 136 8 E
Thitgy, *Burma* **90 F6** 18 15N 96 13 E
Thithia = Cicia, *Fiji* **133 A3** 17 45 S 179 18W
Thitpokpin, *Burma* **90 F5** 19 24N 95 58 E
Thiva = Thívai, *Greece* **48 C5** 38 19N 23 19 E
Thívai, *Greece* **48 C5** 38 19N 23 19 E
Thiviers, *France* **28 C4** 45 25N 0 54 E
Thizy, *France* **27 F11** 46 2N 4 18 E
Þjórsá →, *Iceland* **11 D6** 63 47N 20 48W
Thlewiaza →, *Canada* **143 A10** 60 29N 94 40W
Thmar Puok, *Cambodia* **86 F4** 13 57N 103 4 E
Tho Vinh, *Vietnam* **86 C5** 19 16N 105 42 E
Thoa →, *Canada* **143 A7** 60 31N 109 47W
Thoen, *Thailand* **86 D2** 17 43N 99 12 E
Thoeng, *Thailand* **86 C3** 19 41N 100 12 E
Tholdi, *Pakistan* **93 B7** 35 5N 76 6 E
Thomas, *U.S.A.* **155 H5** 35 45N 98 45W
Thomas, L., *Australia* **127 D2** 26 4 S 137 58 E
Thomas Hill Reservoir, *U.S.A.* **156 E4** 39 34N 92 39W
Thomaston, *U.S.A.* **152 C5** 32 53N 84 20W
Thomasville, *Ala., U.S.A.* **149 K2** 31 55N 87 44W
Thomasville, *Ga., U.S.A.* **152 E6** 30 50N 83 59W
Thomasville, *N.C., U.S.A.* **149 H5** 35 53N 80 5W
Thompson, *Canada* **143 B9** 55 45N 97 52W
Thompson, *U.S.A.* **151 E9** 41 52N 75 31W
Thompson →, *Canada* **142 C4** 50 15N 121 24W
Thompson →, *U.S.A.* **156 E3** 39 46N 93 37W
Thompson Falls, *U.S.A.* **158 C6** 47 36N 115 21W
Thompson Pk., *U.S.A.* **158 F2** 41 0N 123 0W
Thompson Sd., *N.Z.* **131 F1** 45 8 S 166 46 E
Thompson Springs, *U.S.A.* **159 G9** 38 58N 109 43W
Thompsontown, *U.S.A.* **150 F7** 40 33N 77 14W
Thomson, *Ga., U.S.A.* **152 B7** 33 28N 82 30W
Thomson, *Ill., U.S.A.* **156 C6** 41 58N 90 6W
Thomson →, *Australia* **126 C3** 25 11 S 142 53 E
Thomson's Falls = Nyahururu, *Kenya* **118 B4** 0 2N 36 27 E
Thônes, *France* **29 C10** 45 54N 6 18 E
Thong Yang, *Thailand* **87 b** 9 28N 99 56 E
Thongwa, *Burma* **90 G6** 16 45N 96 33 E
Thonon-les-Bains, *France* **27 F13** 46 22N 6 29 E
Thonze, *Burma* **90 G5** 17 38N 95 47 E
Thorez, *Ukraine* **59 H10** 48 4N 38 34 E
Þórisjökull, *Iceland* **11 C6** 64 32N 20 43W
Þórisvatn, *Iceland* **11 C8** 64 20N 18 55W
Þórkötlustaðir, *Iceland* **11 D4** 63 50N 22 24W
Þorlákshöfn, *Iceland* **11 D5** 63 51N 21 22W
Thorn = Toruń, *Poland* **55 E5** 53 2N 18 39 E
Thornaby on Tees, *U.K.* **20 C6** 54 33N 1 18W
Thornbury, *Canada* **150 B4** 44 34N 80 26W
Thornbury, *N.Z.* **131 G3** 46 17 S 168 9 E
Thorne, *U.K.* **20 D7** 53 37N 0 57W
Thornhill, *Canada* **142 C3** 54 31N 128 32W
Thornton, *Colo., U.S.A.* **154 F2** 39 52N 104 58W
Thornton, *Iowa, U.S.A.* **156 B3** 42 57N 93 23W
Thornton-Beresfield, *Australia* **129 B9** 32 50 S 151 40 E
Thorntown, *U.S.A.* **157 D10** 40 8N 86 36W
Thorold, *Canada* **150 C5** 43 7N 79 12W
Þórshöfn, *Iceland* **11 A11** 66 12N 15 20W
Thouarcé, *France* **26 E6** 47 17N 0 30W
Thouars, *France* **26 F6** 47 0N 0 15W
Thouet →, *France* **26 E6** 47 17N 0 6W
Thouin, C., *Australia* **124 D2** 20 20 S 118 10 E
Thousand Oaks, *U.S.A.* **161 L8** 34 10N 118 50W
Thrace, *Turkey* **51 F10** 41 0N 27 0 E
Thrakikón Pélagos, *Greece* **51 F8** 40 30N 25 0 E
Thredbo, *Australia* **129 D8** 36 30 S 148 21 E
Three Forks, *U.S.A.* **158 D8** 45 54N 111 33W
Three Gorges Dam, *China* **77 B8** 30 45N 111 15 E
Three Hills, *Canada* **142 C6** 51 43N 113 15W
Three Hummock I., *Australia* **127 G3** 40 25 S 144 55 E
Three Oaks, *U.S.A.* **157 C10** 41 48N 86 36W
Three Pagodas Pass, *Asia* **86 E2** 15 20N 98 30 E
Three Points, C., *Ghana* **112 E4** 4 42N 2 6W
Three Rivers, *Calif., U.S.A.* **160 J8** 36 26N 118 54W
Three Rivers, *Mich., U.S.A.* **157 C11** 41 57N 85 38W
Three Rivers, *Tex., U.S.A.* **155 L5** 28 28N 98 11W
Three Sisters, *U.S.A.* **158 D3** 44 4N 121 51W
Three Sisters Is., *Solomon Is.* **133 N11** 10 10 S 161 57 E
Three Springs, *Australia* **125 E2** 29 32 S 115 45 E
Throssell, L., *Australia* **125 E3** 27 33 S 124 10 E
Throssell Ra., *Australia* **124 D3** 22 3 S 121 43 E
Thrushton △, *Australia* **127 D4** 27 47 S 147 40 E
Thuamal Rampur, *India* **94 E6** 19 23N 82 56 E
Thuan Hoa, *Vietnam* **87 H5** 8 58N 105 30 E
Thubun Lakes, *Canada* **143 A6** 61 30N 112 0W
Thueyts, *France* **29 D8** 44 41N 4 9 E
Thuin, *Belgium* **24 D4** 50 20N 4 17 E
Thuir, *France* **28 F6** 42 38N 2 45 E
Thule = Qaanaaq, *Greenland* **10 B4** 77 40N 69 0W
Thule Air Base = Uummannaq, *Greenland* **6 B5** 70 58N 52 0W
Thun, *Switz.* **32 C5** 46 45N 7 38 E
Thunder B., *U.S.A.* **150 B1** 45 0N 83 20W
Thunder Bay, *Canada* **140 C2** 48 20N 89 15W
Thunderbolt, *U.S.A.* **152 C8** 32 3N 81 4W
Thunersee, *Switz.* **32 C5** 46 43N 7 39 E
Thung Salaeng Luang △, *Thailand* **86 D3** 16 43N 100 50 E
Thung Song, *Thailand* **87 H2** 8 10N 99 40 E
Thunkar, *Bhutan* **90 B3** 27 55N 91 0 E
Thuong Tra, *Vietnam* **86 D6** 16 2N 107 42 E
Thur →, *Switz.* **33 A8** 47 32N 9 10 E
Thurgau □, *Switz.* **33 A8** 47 34N 9 10 E
Thüringen □, *Germany* **30 D6** 51 0N 11 0 E
Thüringer Wald, *Germany* **30 E6** 50 35N 11 0 E
Thurles, *Ireland* **23 D4** 52 41N 7 49W
Thurn P., *Austria* **34 D5** 47 20N 12 25 E
Thurrock □, *U.K.* **21 F8** 51 31N 0 23 E
Thursday I., *Australia* **126 A3** 10 30 S 142 3 E
Thurso, *Canada* **140 C4** 45 36N 75 15W
Thurso, *U.K.* **22 C5** 58 36N 3 32W
Thurso →, *U.K.* **22 C5** 58 36N 3 32W
Thurston I., *Antarctica* **7 D16** 72 0 S 100 0W
Thury-Harcourt, *France* **26 D6** 48 59N 0 30W
Thusis, *Switz.* **33 C8** 46 42N 9 26 E
Thutade L., *Canada* **142 B3** 57 0N 126 55W
Thy, *Denmark* **17 H2** 56 52N 8 25 E
Thy ⌓, *N. Cal.* **133 V20** 22 10 S 166 31 E
Thyborøn, *Denmark* **17 H2** 56 42N 8 12 E
Þykkvabæjarklaustur, *Iceland* **11 D8** 63 30N 18 22W
Þykkvibær, *Iceland* **11 D6** 63 45N 20 37W
Thyolo, *Malawi* **119 F4** 16 7 S 35 5 E
Ti-n-Amzi →, *Niger* **113 B5** 18 20N 4 32 E
Ti-n-Barraouene, O. →, *Africa* **113 B5** 18 40N 4 5 E
Ti-n-Barraouene, O. →, *Algeria* **111 E5** 19 2N 4 45 E
Ti-n-Medjerdam, O. →, *Algeria* **111 C5** 25 45N 1 30 E
Ti-n-Rerhoh, *Algeria* **111 D5** 20 44N 4 2 E
Ti-n-Tanetfirt, *Algeria* **111 D5** 24 49N 3 48 E
Ti-n-Tarabine, O. →, *Algeria* **111 D6** 21 16N 7 25 E
Ti-n-Toumma, *Niger* **109 E2** 16 4N 12 40 E
Ti-n-Zaouatene, *Algeria* **111 E5** 19 55N 2 55 E
Ti Tree, *Australia* **126 C1** 22 5 S 133 22 E
Tiadiaye, *Senegal* **112 C1** 14 25N 16 40W
Tiahuanacu, *Bolivia* **172 D4** 16 33 S 68 42W
Tian Shan, *Asia* **65 C8** 40 30N 76 0 E
Tianchang, *China* **77 A12** 32 40N 119 0 E
Tiandeng, *China* **76 F6** 23 6N 107 7 E
Tiandong, *China* **76 F6** 23 36N 107 8 E
Tian'e, *China* **76 E6** 25 1N 107 9 E
Tianguá, *Brazil* **170 B3** 3 44 S 40 59W
Tianhe, *China* **76 E7** 24 48N 108 40 E
Tianjin, *China* **75 E9** 39 8N 117 10 E
Tiankoura, *Burkina Faso* **112 C4** 10 47N 3 17W
Tianlin, *China* **76 E6** 24 21N 106 12 E
Tianmen, *China* **77 B9** 30 39N 113 9 E
Tianquan, *China* **76 B4** 30 7N 102 43 E
Tianshui, *China* **74 G3** 34 32N 105 40 E
Tiantai, *China* **77 C13** 29 10N 121 2 E
Tianyang, *China* **76 F6** 23 42N 106 53 E
Tianyar, *Indonesia* **79 J18** 8 12 S 115 30 E
Tianzhen, *China* **74 D8** 40 24N 114 5 E
Tianzhu, *China* **76 D7** 26 54N 109 11 E
Tianzhuangtai, *China* **75 D12** 40 43N 122 5 E
Tiaret, *Algeria* **111 A5** 35 20N 1 21 E
Tiassalé, *Ivory C.* **112 D4** 5 58N 4 57W
Tibagi, *Brazil* **175 A5** 24 30 S 50 24W
Tibagi →, *Brazil* **175 A5** 22 47 S 51 1W
Tībastī, Sarīr, *Libya* **108 D3** 22 50N 18 30 E
Tibati, *Cameroon* **113 D7** 6 22N 12 30 E
Tibe, *Ethiopia* **107 F4** 9 2N 37 12 E
Tiber = Tevere →, *Italy* **45 G9** 41 44N 12 14 E
Tiberias = Teverya, *Israel* **103 C4** 32 47N 35 32 E
Tiberias, L. = Yam Kinneret, *Israel* **103 C4** 32 45N 35 35 E
Tibesti, *Chad* **109 D3** 21 0N 17 30 E
Tibet = Xizang Zizhiqu □, *China* **68 C3** 32 0N 88 0 E
Tibet, Plateau of, *Asia* **62 F12** 32 0N 86 0 E
Tibiao, *Phil.* **81 F4** 11 17N 122 2 E
Tibiri, *Niger* **113 C6** 13 34N 7 4 E
Ţibleş, Vf., *Romania* **53 C9** 47 32N 24 15 E
Ţibleşului, Munţii, *Romania* **53 C9** 47 38N 24 5 E
Tibnī, *Syria* **101 E8** 35 36N 39 50 E
Tibooburra, *Australia* **127 D3** 29 26 S 142 1 E
Tibro, *Sweden* **17 F8** 58 28N 14 10 E
Tibugá, G. de, *Colombia* **168 B2** 5 45N 77 20W
Tiburón, I., *Mexico* **162 B2** 29 0N 112 30W
Ticao I., *Phil.* **80 E4** 12 31N 123 42 E
Tice, *U.S.A.* **153 J8** 26 40N 81 49W
Tîchît, *Mauritania* **112 B3** 18 21N 9 29W
Tichla, *Mauritania* **110 D2** 21 36N 14 58W
Ticho, *Ethiopia* **107 F4** 7 50N 39 32 E
Ticino □, *Switz.* **33 D7** 46 20N 8 45 E
Ticino →, *Italy* **31 J4** 45 9N 9 14 E
Ticleni, *Romania* **53 F8** 44 53N 23 24 E
Ticonderoga, *U.S.A.* **151 C11** 43 51N 73 26W
Ticul, *Mexico* **163 C7** 20 20N 89 31W

Tidaholm, *Sweden* **17 F7** 58 12N 13 58 E
Tidan, *Sweden* **17 F8** 58 34N 14 1 E
Tiddim, *Burma* **90 D4** 23 28N 93 45 E
Tiden, *India* **95 L11** 7 15N 93 33 E
Tideridjaouine, Adrar, *Algeria* **111 D5** 23 0N 2 15 E
Tidikelt, *Algeria* **111 C5** 26 58N 1 30 E
Tidioute, *U.S.A.* **150 E5** 41 41N 79 24W
Tidjikja, *Mauritania* **112 B2** 18 29N 11 35W
Tidmore = Seminole, *U.S.A.* **155 H6** 35 14N 96 41W
Tidore, *Indonesia* **82 A3** 0 40N 127 25 E
Tiébissou, *Ivory C.* **112 D3** 7 9N 5 10W
Tiéboro, *Chad* **109 D3** 21 20N 17 7 E
Tiefencastel, *Switz.* **33 C9** 46 40N 9 33 E
Tiegang Shuiku, *China* **69 F10** 22 37N 113 53 E
Tiel, *Neths.* **24 C5** 51 53N 5 26 E
Tiel, *Senegal* **112 C1** 14 55N 15 5W
Tieling, *China* **75 C12** 42 20N 123 55 E
Tielt, *Belgium* **24 C3** 51 0N 3 20 E
Tien Shan = Tian Shan, *Asia* **65 C8** 40 30N 76 0 E
Tien-tsin = Tianjin, *China* **75 E9** 39 8N 117 10 E
Tien Yen, *Vietnam* **86 B6** 21 20N 107 24 E
T'ienching = Tianjin, *China* **75 E9** 39 8N 117 10 E
Tienen, *Belgium* **24 D4** 50 48N 4 57 E
Tiéngbé, *Ivory C.* **112 D3** 8 11N 5 43W
Tientsin = Tianjin, *China* **75 E9** 39 8N 117 10 E
Tieri, *Australia* **126 C4** 23 2 S 148 21 E
Tieroko, Tarso, *Chad* **109 D3** 20 45N 17 52 E
Tierp, *Sweden* **16 D11** 60 20N 17 30 E
Tierra Amarilla, *Chile* **174 B1** 27 28 S 70 18W
Tierra Amarilla, *U.S.A.* **159 H10** 36 42N 106 33W
Tierra Colorada, *Mexico* **163 D5** 17 10N 99 35W
Tierra de Barros, *Spain* **43 G4** 38 40N 6 30W
Tierra de Campos, *Spain* **42 C6** 42 10N 4 50W
Tierra del Fuego □, *Argentina* **176 D3** 54 0 S 67 45W
Tierra del Fuego △, *Argentina* **176 D3** 54 50 S 68 23W
Tierra del Fuego, I. Gr. de, *Argentina* **176 D3** 54 0 S 69 0W
Tierralta, *Colombia* **168 B2** 8 11N 76 4W
Tiétar →, *Spain* **42 F4** 39 50N 6 1W
Tieté →, *Brazil* **175 A5** 20 40 S 51 35W
Tifarati, *W. Sahara* **110 C2** 26 9N 10 33W
Tiffin, *U.S.A.* **157 C13** 41 7N 83 11W
Tiffin →, *U.S.A.* **157 C12** 41 20N 84 24W
Tiflèt, *Morocco* **110 B3** 33 54N 6 20W
Tiflis = Tbilisi, *Georgia* **61 K7** 41 43N 44 50 E
Tifton, *U.S.A.* **152 D6** 31 27N 83 31W
Tifu, *Indonesia* **82 B3** 3 39 S 126 24 E
Tiga, Î., *N. Cal.* **133 U21** 21 7 S 167 49 E
Tigalda I., *U.S.A.* **144 J6** 54 6N 165 5W
Tigaon, *Phil.* **80 E4** 13 38N 123 30 E
Tigbauan, *Phil.* **81 F4** 10 41N 122 27 E
Tighina, *Moldova* **53 D14** 46 50N 29 30 E
Tigil, *Russia* **67 D16** 57 49N 158 40 E
Tigiria, *India* **94 D7** 20 29N 85 31 E
Tignall, *U.S.A.* **152 B7** 33 52N 82 44W
Tignish, *Canada* **141 C7** 46 58N 64 2W
Tigray □, *Ethiopia* **107 E4** 13 35N 39 15 E
Tigre →, *Peru* **168 D3** 4 30 S 74 10W
Tigre →, *Venezuela* **169 B5** 9 20N 62 30W
Tigris = Dijlah, Nahr →, *Asia* **96 D5** 31 0N 47 25 E
Tiguentourine, *Algeria* **111 C6** 27 52N 9 8 E
Tigveni, *Romania* **53 E9** 45 10N 24 31 E
Tigyaing, *Burma* **90 D6** 23 45N 96 10 E
Tigzerte, O. →, *Morocco* **110 C3** 28 10N 9 37W
Tîh, Gebel el, *Egypt* **106 B3** 29 32N 33 26 E
Tihodaine, Erg de, *Algeria* **111 C6** 25 15N 7 15 E
Tihwa = Ürümqi, *China* **66 E9** 43 45N 87 45 E
Tijara, *India* **92 F7** 27 56N 76 31 E
Tîjî, *Libya* **108 B2** 32 0N 11 18 E
Tijuana, *Mexico* **161 N9** 32 30N 117 10W
Tijuca △, *Brazil* **171 F3** 22 56 S 43 12W
Tikal, *Guatemala* **164 C2** 17 13N 89 24W
Tikal △, *Guatemala* **164 C2** 17 23N 89 34W
Tikamgarh, *India* **93 G8** 24 44N 78 50 E
Tikaré, *Burkina Faso* **113 C4** 13 15N 1 43W
Tikchik Lakes, *U.S.A.* **144 G8** 60 0N 159 0W
Tikhonkaya = Birobidzhan, *Russia* **67 E14** 48 50N 132 50 E
Tikhoretsk, *Russia* **61 H5** 45 56N 40 5 E
Tikhvin, *Russia* **58 C7** 59 35N 33 30 E
Tikiraqjuaq = Whale Cove, *Canada* **143 A10** 62 10N 92 34W
Tikkadouine, Adrar, *Algeria* **111 D5** 24 28N 1 30 E
Tiko, *Cameroon* **113 E6** 4 4N 9 20 E
Tikrīt, *Iraq* **101 E10** 34 35N 43 37 E
Tiksi, *Russia* **67 B13** 71 40N 128 45 E
Tilamuta, *Indonesia* **82 A2** 0 32N 122 23 E
Tilburg, *Neths.* **24 C5** 51 31N 5 6 E
Tilbury, *Canada* **140 D3** 42 17N 82 23W
Tilbury, *U.K.* **21 F8** 51 27N 0 22 E
Tilcara, *Argentina* **174 A2** 23 36 S 65 23W
Tilden, *U.S.A.* **154 D6** 42 3N 97 50W
Tilemses, *Niger* **113 B5** 15 37N 4 44 E
Tilemsi, Vallée du, *Mali* **113 B5** 17 42N 0 15 E
Tilhar, *India* **93 F8** 28 0N 79 45 E
Tilia, O. →, *Algeria* **111 C5** 27 32N 0 55 E
Tilichiki, *Russia* **67 C17** 60 27N 166 5 E
Tililane, *Algeria* **111 C4** 27 49N 0 6W
Tilin, *Burma* **90 E5** 21 41N 94 6 E
Tílissos, *Greece* **39 E6** 35 20N 25 1 E
Till →, *U.K.* **20 B5** 55 41N 2 13W
Tillabéri, *Niger* **113 C5** 14 28N 1 28 E
Tillamook, *U.S.A.* **158 D2** 45 27N 123 51W
Tillanchong I., *India* **95 K11** 8 30N 93 37 E
Tillberga, *Sweden* **16 E10** 59 40N 16 39 E
Tillia, *Niger* **113 B5** 16 8N 4 47 E
Tillman, *U.S.A.* **152 C8** 32 28N 81 6W
Tillsonburg, *Canada* **140 D3** 42 53N 80 44W
Tillyeria, *Cyprus* **39 E8** 35 6N 32 40 E
Tilogne, *Senegal* **112 B2** 16 0N 13 40W
Tílos, *Greece* **49 E9** 36 27N 27 27 E
Tilpa, *Australia* **128 A6** 30 57 S 144 24 E
Tilrhemt, *Algeria* **111 B5** 33 9N 3 22 E
Tilsit = Sovetsk, *Russia* **15 J19** 55 6N 21 50 E
Tilt →, *U.K.* **22 E5** 56 46N 3 51W
Tilton, *U.S.A.* **151 C13** 43 27N 71 36W
Tiltonsville, *U.S.A.* **150 F4** 40 10N 80 41W
Tim, *Denmark* **17 H2** 56 12N 8 19 E
Timagami, L., *Canada* **140 C3** 47 0N 80 10W
Timanah, *Asia* **98 C3** 19 0N 41 0 E
Timanfaya △, *Canary Is.* **9 e2** 29 0N 13 46W
Timanskiy Kryazh, *Russia* **56 A9** 65 58N 50 5 E
Timaru, *N.Z.* **131 E6** 44 23 S 171 14 E
Timashevo, *Russia* **60 D10** 53 22N 51 9 E
Timashevsk, *Russia* **61 H4** 45 35N 39 0 E
Timau, *Kenya* **118 B4** 0 4N 37 15 E
Timbákion, *Greece* **39 E5** 35 4N 24 45 E
Timbaúba, *Brazil* **170 C4** 7 31 S 35 19W
Timbedgha, *Mauritania* **112 B3** 16 17N 8 16W
Timber Creek, *Australia* **124 C5** 15 40 S 130 29 E
Timber Lake, *U.S.A.* **154 C4** 45 26N 101 5W
Timber Mt., *U.S.A.* **160 H10** 37 6N 116 28W
Timbío, *Colombia* **168 C2** 2 20N 76 40W
Timbiquí, *Colombia* **168 C2** 2 46N 77 42W
Timbo, *Guinea* **112 C2** 10 35N 11 50W
Timbo, *Liberia* **112 D3** 5 35N 9 45W
Timboon, *Australia* **128 E5** 38 30 S 142 58 E
Timbuktu = Tombouctou, *Mali* **112 B4** 16 50N 3 0W
Timdjaouine, *Algeria* **111 D5** 21 37N 4 30 E
Timeiaouine, *Algeria* **111 D5** 20 27N 1 50 E
Timellouline, *Algeria* **111 C6** 29 22N 8 55 E
Timétrine, Mts., *Mali* **113 B4** 19 25N 1 0W
Timfi Óros, *Greece* **48 B2** 39 59N 20 45 E
Timfristós, Óros, *Greece* **48 C3** 38 57N 21 50 E
Timhadit, *Morocco* **110 B3** 33 15N 5 4W
Timi, *Cyprus* **39 F8** 34 44N 32 31 E
Tîmia, *Niger* **113 B6** 18 4N 8 40 E
Timika, *Indonesia* **83 B5** 4 47 S 136 32 E
Timimoun, *Algeria* **111 C5** 29 14N 0 16 E
Timimoun, Sebkha de, *Algeria* **111 C5** 28 50N 0 46 E
Timirist, Râs, *Mauritania* **112 B1** 19 21N 16 30W
Timiş = Tamis →, *Serbia & M.* **52 F5** 44 51N 20 39 E
Timiş □, *Romania* **52 E6** 45 40N 21 30 E
Timiskaming, L. = Témiscamingue, L., *Canada* **140 C4** 47 10N 79 25W
Timişoara, *Romania* **52 E6** 45 43N 21 15 E
Timmersdala, *Sweden* **17 F7** 58 32N 13 46 E
Timmins, *Canada* **140 C3** 48 28N 81 25W
Timmonsville, *U.S.A.* **152 A10** 34 8N 79 57W
Timok →, *Serbia & M.* **50 B6** 44 10N 22 40 E
Timon, *Brazil* **170 C3** 5 8 S 42 52W
Timor, *Asia* **82 C3** 9 0 S 125 0 E
Timor Leste = East Timor ■, *Asia* **82 C3** 8 50 S 126 0 E
Timor Sea, *Ind. Oc.* **124 B4** 12 0 S 127 0 E
Timrå, *Sweden* **16 B11** 62 29N 17 18 E
Timucuan ⌂, *U.S.A.* **152 E8** 30 28N 81 27W
Tin, Ra's at, *Libya* **108 B4** 32 37N 23 8 E
Tin Alkoum, *Algeria* **111 D7** 24 42N 10 17 E
Tin Amzi, O. →, *Algeria* **111 D6** 18 20N 4 32 E
Tin Atanai, *Algeria* **111 C5** 25 52N 1 37 E
Tin Can Bay, *Australia* **127 D5** 25 56 S 153 0 E
Tin Ethisane, *Mali* **113 B4** 19 3N 0 52W
Tin Gornai, *Mali* **113 B4** 16 38N 0 38W
Tin Mt., *U.S.A.* **160 J9** 36 50N 117 10W
Tina →, *S. Africa* **117 E4** 31 18 S 29 13 E
Tîna, Khalîg el, *Egypt* **106 A3** 31 20N 32 42 E
Tinaca Pt., *Phil.* **81 J5** 5 30N 125 25 E
Tinaco, *Venezuela* **168 B4** 9 42N 68 26W
Tinafak, O. →, *Algeria* **111 C6** 27 10N 7 0 E
Tinajo, *Canary Is.* **9 e2** 29 4N 13 42W
Tinca, *Romania* **52 D6** 46 46N 21 58 E
Tindal, *Australia* **124 B5** 14 31 S 132 22 E
Tindivanam, *India* **95 H4** 12 15N 79 41 E
Tindouf, *Algeria* **110 C3** 27 42N 8 10W
Tinée →, *France* **29 E11** 43 55N 7 11 E
Tineo, *Spain* **42 B4** 43 21N 6 27W
Tinerhir, *Morocco* **110 B3** 31 29N 5 31W
Tinfouchi, *Algeria* **110 C3** 28 52N 5 49W
Tinfunque △, *Paraguay* **174 A3** 23 55 S 60 17W
Ting Jiang →, *China* **77 E11** 24 45N 116 35 E
Tinggi, Pulau, *Malaysia* **87 L5** 2 18N 104 7 E
Tingkawk Sakan, *Burma* **90 B6** 26 4N 96 44 E
Tinglayan, *Phil.* **80 C3** 17 15N 121 9 E
Tinglev, *Denmark* **17 K3** 54 57N 9 13 E
Tingo Maria, *Peru* **172 B2** 9 10 S 75 54W
Tingrela, *Ivory C.* **112 C3** 10 27N 6 25W
Tingsryd, *Sweden* **17 H9** 56 31N 15 0 E
Tingstäde, *Sweden* **17 G12** 57 44N 18 37 E
Tingvoll, *Norway* **18 B5** 62 55N 8 12 E
Tingwon Group, *Papua N. G.* **132 B5** 2 37 S 149 42 E
Tinh Bien, *Vietnam* **87 G5** 10 36N 104 57 E
Tinharé, I. de, *Brazil* **171 D4** 13 30 S 38 58W
Tinian, *N. Marianas* **134 F6** 15 0N 145 38 E
Tinigua △, *Colombia* **168 C3** 2 30N 74 8W
Tiniguiban, *Phil.* **81 F2** 11 22N 119 30 E
Tinjar →, *Malaysia* **85 B4** 4 4N 114 18 E
Tinn = Atrå, *Norway* **18 E5** 59 59N 8 45 E
Tinnevelly = Tirunelveli, *India* **95 K3** 8 45N 77 45 E
Tinnoset, *Norway* **18 E6** 59 43N 9 3 E
Tinnsjø, *Norway* **18 E5** 59 55N 8 54 E
Tinogasta, *Argentina* **174 B2** 28 5 S 67 32W
Tínos, *Greece* **49 D7** 37 33N 25 8 E
Tiñoso, C., *Spain* **41 H3** 37 32N 1 6W
Tinpahar, *India* **93 G12** 24 59N 87 44 E
Tinputz, *Papua N. G.* **132 C8** 5 33 S 155 0 E
Tinsukia, *India* **90 B5** 27 29N 95 20 E
Tinta, *Peru* **172 C3** 14 3 S 71 20W
Tintina, *Argentina* **174 B3** 27 2 S 62 45W
Tintinara, *Australia* **128 C4** 35 48 S 140 2 E
Tintioulé, *Guinea* **112 C3** 10 13N 9 12W
Tinto →, *Spain* **43 H4** 37 12N 6 55W
Tinui, *N.Z.* **130 G5** 40 52 S 176 5 E
Tinwald, *N.Z.* **131 D6** 43 55 S 171 43 E
Tioga, *N. Dak., U.S.A.* **154 A3** 48 23N 102 56W
Tioga, *Pa., U.S.A.* **150 E7** 41 55N 77 8W
Tioman, Pulau, *Malaysia* **87 L5** 2 50N 104 10 E
Tione di Trento, *Italy* **44 B7** 46 2N 10 43 E
Tionesta, *U.S.A.* **150 E5** 41 30N 79 28W
Tior, *Sudan* **107 F3** 6 26N 31 11 E
Tioulilin, *Algeria* **111 C4** 27 1N 0 2W
Tipp City, *U.S.A.* **157 E12** 39 58N 84 11W
Tippecanoe →, *U.S.A.* **157 D10** 40 30N 86 45W
Tipperary, *Ireland* **23 D3** 52 28N 8 10W
Tipperary □, *Ireland* **23 D4** 52 37N 7 55W
Tipton, *Calif., U.S.A.* **160 J7** 36 4N 119 19W
Tipton, *Ind., U.S.A.* **157 D10** 40 17N 86 2W
Tipton, *Iowa, U.S.A.* **156 C5** 41 46N 91 8W
Tipton, *Mo., U.S.A.* **156 F4** 38 39N 92 47W
Tipton Mt., *U.S.A.* **161 K12** 35 32N 114 12W
Tiptonville, *U.S.A.* **155 G10** 36 23N 89 29W
Tiptur, *India* **95 H3** 13 15N 76 26 E
Tiquié →, *Brazil* **168 C4** 0 5N 68 25W
Tiracambu, Serra do, *Brazil* **170 B2** 3 15 S 46 30W
Tirahart, O. →, *Algeria* **111 D5** 23 45N 3 10 E
Tīrān, *Iran* **97 C6** 32 45N 51 8 E
Tīrān, *Si. Arabia* **106 B3** 27 57N 34 32 E
Tiranë, *Albania* **50 E3** 41 18N 19 49 E
Tiranë ✈ (TIA), *Albania* **50 E3** 41 57N 19 42 E
Tirano, *Italy* **44 B7** 46 13N 10 10 E
Tiraspol, *Moldova* **53 D14** 46 55N 29 35 E
Tiratimine, *Algeria* **111 C5** 25 56N 3 37 E
Tirau, *N.Z.* **130 D4** 37 58 S 175 46 E
Tirdout, *Mali* **113 B4** 16 7N 1 5W
Tire, *Turkey* **49 C9** 38 5N 27 45 E
Tirebolu, *Turkey* **101 B8** 40 58N 38 45 E
Tiree, *U.K.* **22 E2** 56 31N 6 55W
Tiree, Passage of, *U.K.* **22 E2** 56 30N 6 30W
Tîrgovişte = Târgovişte, *Romania* **53 F10** 44 55N 25 27 E
Tîrgu-Jiu = Târgu-Jiu, *Romania* **53 E8** 45 5N 23 19 E
Tîrgu Mureş = Târgu Mureş, *Romania* **53 D9** 46 31N 24 38 E
Tirgua △, *Venezuela* **168 A4** 10 5N 68 48W
Tirich Mir, *Pakistan* **91 A3** 36 15N 71 55 E
Tiriolo, *Italy* **47 D9** 38 57N 16 30 E
Tiririca, Serra da, *Brazil* **171 E2** 17 6 S 47 6W
Tiriro, *Guinea* **112 C3** 10 27N 8 40W
Tiris, *W. Sahara* **110 D2** 23 10N 13 20W
Tiritiri o te Moana = Southern Alps, *N.Z.* **131 D5** 43 41 S 170 11 E
Tirlyanskiy, *Russia* **64 D7** 54 14N 58 35 E
Tirna →, *India* **94 E3** 18 4N 76 57 E
Tírnavos, *Greece* **48 B4** 39 45N 22 18 E
Tirodi, *India* **94 D4** 21 40N 79 44 E
Tirol □, *Austria* **34 D3** 47 3N 10 43 E
Tiros, *Brazil* **171 E2** 19 0 S 45 58W
Tirrukkovil, *Sri Lanka* **95 L5** 7 7N 81 51 E
Tirschenreuth, *Germany* **31 F8** 49 53N 12 19 E
Tirschtiegel = Trzciel, *Poland* **55 F2** 52 23N 15 50 E
Tirso →, *Italy* **46 C1** 39 53N 8 32 E
Tirstrup, *Denmark* **17 H4** 56 18N 10 42 E
Tirthahalli, *India* **95 H2** 13 42N 75 14 E
Tirua Pt., *N.Z.* **130 E3** 38 25 S 174 40 E
Tiruchchendur, *India* **95 K4** 8 30N 78 11 E
Tiruchchirappalli, *India* **95 J4** 10 45N 78 45 E
Tirukkoyilur, *India* **95 J4** 11 57N 79 12 E
Tirumangalam, *India* **95 K3** 9 49N 77 58 E
Tirumayam, *India* **95 J4** 10 14N 78 45 E
Tirunelveli, *India* **95 K3** 8 45N 77 45 E
Tirupati, *India* **95 H4** 13 39N 79 25 E
Tiruppattur, *Tamil Nadu, India* **95 J4** 10 8N 78 37 E
Tiruppattur, *Tamil Nadu, India* **95 H4** 12 30N 78 30 E
Tiruppur, *India* **95 J3** 11 5N 77 22 E
Tirur, *India* **95 J2** 10 54N 75 55 E
Tiruttani, *India* **95 H4** 13 11N 79 58 E
Tirutturaippundi, *India* **95 J4** 10 32N 79 41 E
Tiruvadaimarudur, *India* **95 J4** 11 2N 79 27 E
Tiruvalla, *India* **95 K3** 9 23N 76 34 E
Tiruvallar, *India* **95 H4** 13 9N 79 57 E
Tiruvannamalai, *India* **95 H4** 12 15N 79 5 E
Tiruvettipuram, *India* **95 H4** 12 39N 79 33 E
Tiruvottiyur, *India* **95 H5** 13 10N 80 22 E
Tisa, *India* **92 C7** 32 50N 76 9 E
Tisa →, *Serbia & M.* **52 E5** 45 15N 20 17 E
Tisdale, *Canada* **143 C8** 52 50N 104 0W
Tishomingo, *U.S.A.* **155 H6** 34 14N 96 41W
Tisjön, *Sweden* **16 D7** 60 56N 13 0 E
Tisnaren, *Sweden* **17 F9** 58 58N 15 56 E
Tišnov, *Czech Rep.* **35 B9** 49 21N 16 25 E
Tisovec, *Slovak Rep.* **35 C12** 48 41N 19 56 E
Tissamaharama, *Sri Lanka* **95 L5** 6 17N 81 17 E
Tissemsilt, *Algeria* **111 A5** 35 35N 1 50 E
Tissint, *Morocco* **110 C3** 29 57N 7 16W
Tista →, *India* **90 C2** 25 23N 89 43 E
Tistedal, *Norway* **18 E8** 59 8N 11 27 E
Tisza = Tisa →, *Serbia & M.* **52 E5** 45 15N 20 17 E
Tiszaföldvár, *Hungary* **52 D5** 46 58N 20 14 E
Tiszafüred, *Hungary* **52 C5** 47 38N 20 50 E
Tiszalök, *Hungary* **52 B6** 48 1N 21 20 E
Tiszavasvári, *Hungary* **52 C6** 47 58N 21 18 E
Tit, *Ahaggar, Algeria* **111 D6** 23 0N 5 10 E
Tit, *Tademait, Algeria* **111 C5** 27 0N 1 29 E
Tit-Ary, *Russia* **67 B13** 71 55N 127 2 E
Titabar, *India* **90 B5** 26 36N 94 12 E
Titaguas, *Spain* **40 F3** 39 53N 1 6W
Titao, *Burkina Faso* **113 C4** 13 45N 2 5W
Titel, *Serbia & M.* **52 E5** 45 10N 20 18 E
Tithwal, *Pakistan* **93 B5** 34 21N 73 50 E
Titicaca, L., *S. Amer.* **172 D4** 15 30 S 69 30W
Titisee, *Germany* **31 H4** 47 54N 8 10 E
Titiwa, *Nigeria* **113 C7** 12 14N 12 53 E
Tititira Hd., *N.Z.* **131 D4** 43 36 S 169 25 E
Titlagarh, *India* **94 D6** 20 15N 83 11 E
Titlis, *Switz.* **33 C6** 46 46N 8 27 E
Tito, *Italy* **47 B8** 40 35N 15 40 E
Titograd = Podgorica, *Serbia & M.* **50 D3** 42 30N 19 19 E
Titova Korenica, *Croatia* **45 D12** 44 45N 15 41 E
Titu, *Romania* **53 F10** 44 39N 25 32 E
Titule, *Dem. Rep. of the Congo* **118 B2** 3 15N 25 31 E
Titusville, *Fla., U.S.A.* **153 G9** 28 37N 80 49W
Titusville, *Pa., U.S.A.* **150 E5** 41 38N 79 41W
Tivaouane, *Senegal* **112 C1** 14 56N 16 45W
Tivat, *Serbia & M.* **50 D2** 42 28N 18 43 E
Tivedens △, *Sweden* **17 F8** 58 45N 14 35 E
Tiverton, *U.K.* **21 G4** 50 54N 3 29W
Tivoli, *Italy* **45 G9** 41 58N 12 45 E
Tīwī, *Oman* **99 B7** 22 45N 59 12 E
Tiyo, *Eritrea* **107 E5** 14 41N 40 15 E
Tiyo, Peg., *Indonesia* **83 B5** 4 0 S 135 30 E
Tizga, *Morocco* **110 B3** 32 1N 5 9W
Ti'zi N'Isli, *Morocco* **110 B3** 32 28N 5 47W
Tizi-Ouzou, *Algeria* **111 A5** 36 42N 4 3 E
Tizimín, *Mexico* **163 C7** 21 0N 88 1W
Tiznados →, *Venezuela* **168 B4** 8 16N 67 47W
Tiznap He →, *China* **65 D8** 38 23N 77 24 E
Tiznit, *Morocco* **110 C3** 29 48N 9 45W
Tjæreborg, *Denmark* **17 J2** 55 28N 8 36 E
Tjällmo, *Sweden* **17 F9** 58 43N 15 21 E
Tjeggelvas, *Sweden* **14 C17** 66 37N 17 45 E
Tjieggelvas = Tjeggelvas, *Sweden* **14 C17** 66 37N 17 45 E
Tjirebon = Cirebon, *Indonesia* **85 D3** 6 45 S 108 32 E
Tjluring, *Indonesia* **79 J17** 8 25 S 114 13 E
Tjøme, *Norway* **18 E7** 59 8N 10 26 E
Tjörn, *Sweden* **17 F5** 58 0N 11 35 E
Tkibuli = Tqibuli, *Georgia* **61 J6** 42 26N 43 0 E
Tkvarcheli = Tqvarcheli, *Georgia* **61 J5** 42 47N 41 42 E
Tlacolulan, *Mexico* **163 D5** 18 37N 95 40W
Tlahualilo, *Mexico* **162 B4** 26 20N 103 30W
Tlaquepaque, *Mexico* **162 C4** 20 39N 103 19W
Tlaxcala, *Mexico* **163 D5** 19 20N 98 14W
Tlaxcala □, *Mexico* **163 D5** 19 30N 98 20W
Tlaxiaco, *Mexico* **163 D5** 17 18N 97 40W
Tlemcen, *Algeria* **111 B4** 34 52N 1 21W
Tleta Sidi Bouguedra, *Morocco* **110 B3** 32 16N 9 59W
Tlumach, *Ukraine* **53 B10** 48 51N 25 0 E
Tłuszcz, *Poland* **55 F8** 52 25N 21 25 E
Tlyarata, *Russia* **61 J8** 42 9N 46 26 E
Tmassah, *Libya* **108 C3** 26 19N 15 51 E
Tnine d'Anglou, *Morocco* **110 C3** 29 50N 9 50W
To Bong, *Vietnam* **86 F7** 12 45N 109 16 E
To-Shima, *Japan* **73 C11** 34 31N 139 17 E
Toa Payoh, *Singapore* **87 d** 1 20N 103 51 E
Toad →, *Canada* **142 B4** 59 25N 124 57W
Toad River, *Canada* **142 B3** 58 51N 125 14W
Toamasina, *Madag.* **117 B8** 18 10 S 49 25 E
Toamasina □, *Madag.* **117 B8** 18 0 S 49 0 E
Toay, *Argentina* **174 D3** 36 43 S 64 38W
Toba, *China* **76 B1** 31 19N 97 42 E
Toba, *Japan* **73 C8** 34 30N 136 51 E
Toba, Danau, *Indonesia* **84 B1** 2 30N 97 30 E
Toba Kakar, *Pakistan* **91 C3** 31 30N 69 0 E
Toba Tek Singh, *Pakistan* **92 D5** 30 55N 72 25 E
Tobago, *Trin. & Tob.* **169 E10** 11 10N 60 30W
Tobarra, *Spain* **41 G3** 38 37N 1 44W
Tobelo, *Indonesia* **82 A3** 1 45N 127 56 E
Tobermory, *Canada* **140 C3** 45 12N 81 40W
Tobermory, *U.K.* **22 E2** 56 38N 6 5W
Tobi, *Pac. Oc.* **83 A4** 2 40N 131 10 E
Tobias Fornier, *Phil.* **81 F3** 10 30N 121 57 E
Tobin, *U.S.A.* **160 F5** 39 55N 121 19W
Tobin, L., *Australia* **124 D4** 21 45 S 125 49 E
Tobin L., *Canada* **143 C8** 53 35N 103 30W
Toblach = Dobbiaco, *Italy* **45 B9** 46 44N 12 14 E
Toboali, *Indonesia* **84 C3** 3 0 S 106 25 E
Tobol, *Kazakhstan* **64 E9** 52 40N 62 39 E
Tobol →, *Russia* **66 D7** 58 10N 68 12 E
Toboli, *Indonesia* **82 B2** 0 38 S 120 5 E
Tobolsk, *Russia* **66 D7** 58 15N 68 10 E
Tobor, *Senegal* **112 C1** 12 40N 16 15W
Toboso, *Phil.* **81 F4** 10 43N 123 31 E
Tobruk = Tubruq, *Libya* **108 B4** 32 7N 23 55 E
Tobyhanna, *U.S.A.* **151 E9** 41 11N 75 25W
Tobyl = Tobol →, *Russia* **66 D7** 58 10N 68 12 E
Tocache Nuevo, *Peru* **172 B2** 8 9 S 76 26W
Tocantínia, *Brazil* **170 C2** 9 33 S 48 22W
Tocantinópolis, *Brazil* **170 C2** 6 20 S 47 25W
Tocantins □, *Brazil* **170 D2** 10 0 S 48 0W
Tocantins →, *Brazil* **170 B2** 1 45 S 49 10W
Toccoa, *U.S.A.* **149 H4** 34 35N 83 19W
Toce →, *Italy* **44 C5** 45 56N 8 29 E
Tochi →, *Pakistan* **92 C4** 32 49N 70 41 E
Tochigi, *Japan* **73 A11** 36 25N 139 45 E
Tochigi □, *Japan* **73 A11** 36 45N 139 45 E
Tocina, *Spain* **43 H5** 37 37N 5 44W
Töcksfors, *Sweden* **16 E5** 59 31N 11 52 E
Toco, *Chile* **172 E4** 22 5 S 69 35W
Toco, *Trin. & Tob.* **169 F10** 10 49N 60 57W
Toconao, *Chile* **174 A2** 23 11 S 68 1W
Tocopilla, *Chile* **174 A1** 22 5 S 70 10W
Tocqueville = Rass el Oued, *Algeria* **111 A6** 35 57N 5 2 E
Tocumwal, *Australia* **129 C6** 35 51 S 145 31 E
Tocuyo →, *Venezuela* **168 A4** 11 3N 68 23W
Tocuyo de la Costa, *Venezuela* **168 A4** 11 2N 68 23W
Todal, *Norway* **18 B5** 62 49N 8 44 E
Todd →, *Australia* **126 C2** 24 52 S 135 48 E
Todeli, *Indonesia* **82 B2** 1 40 S 124 29 E
Todenyang, *Kenya* **118 B4** 4 35N 35 56 E
Todgarh, *India* **92 G5** 25 42N 73 58 E
Todi, *Italy* **45 F9** 42 47N 12 24 E
Tödi, *Switz.* **33 C7** 46 48N 8 55 E
Todos os Santos, B. de, *Brazil* **171 D4** 12 48 S 38 38W
Todos Santos, *Mexico* **162 C2** 23 27N 110 13W
Todtnau, *Germany* **31 H3** 47 49N 7 56 E
Toe Hd., *U.K.* **22 D1** 57 50N 7 8W
Toecé, *Burkina Faso* **113 C4** 11 50N 1 16W
Toetoes B., *N.Z.* **131 G3** 46 42 S 168 41 E
Tofield, *Canada* **142 C6** 53 25N 112 40W
Tofino, *Canada* **142 D3** 49 11N 125 55W
Töfsingdalens △, *Sweden* **16 B6** 62 10N 12 28 E
Tofte, *Norway* **18 E7** 59 33N 10 34 E
Tofua, *Tonga* **133 P13** 19 45 S 175 5W
Toga, *Vanuatu* **133 C4** 13 26 S 166 42 E
Tōgane, *Japan* **73 B12** 35 33N 140 22 E
Togba, *Mauritania* **112 B2** 17 26N 10 12W
Togbo, *C.A.R.* **114 A3** 6 0N 17 27 E
Toggenburg, *Switz.* **33 B8** 47 16N 9 9 E
Togiak, *U.S.A.* **144 G7** 59 4N 160 24W
Togian, Kepulauan, *Indonesia* **82 B2** 0 20 S 121 50 E
Togliatti, *Russia* **60 D9** 53 32N 49 24 E
Togo ■, *W. Afr.* **113 D5** 8 30N 1 35 E
Togtoh, *China* **74 D6** 40 15N 111 10 E
Toguzak →, *Kazakhstan* **64 D9** 54 3N 62 44 E
Tohma →, *Turkey* **100 C7** 38 29N 38 23 E
Tōhoku □, *Japan* **70 E10** 39 50N 141 45 E
Töhöm, *Mongolia* **74 B5** 44 27N 108 2 E
Tohopekaliga, L., *U.S.A.* **153 G8** 28 12N 81 24W
Toi, *Japan* **73 C10** 34 54N 138 47 E
Toibalewe, *India* **95 J11** 10 32N 92 30 E
Toili, *Indonesia* **82 B2** 1 24 S 122 26 E
Toinya, *Sudan* **107 F2** 6 17N 29 46 E
Toiyabe Range, *U.S.A.* **158 G5** 39 30N 117 0W
Tojikiston = Tajikistan ■, *Asia* **65 D4** 38 30N 70 0 E
Tojo, *Indonesia* **82 B2** 1 20 S 121 15 E
Tōjō, *Japan* **72 C5** 34 53N 133 16 E
Tok, *U.S.A.* **144 E12** 63 20N 142 59W
Tok →, *Russia* **64 E4** 52 46N 52 22 E
Tok-do, *Asia* **71 F5** 37 15N 131 52 E
Toka, *Guyana* **169 C6** 3 58N 59 17W
Tokaanu, *N.Z.* **130 E4** 38 58 S 175 46 E
Tokachi-Dake, *Japan* **70 C11** 43 17N 142 5 E
Tokachi-Gawa →, *Japan* **70 C11** 42 44N 143 42 E
Tokai, *Japan* **73 B8** 35 2N 136 55 E
Tokaj, *Hungary* **52 B6** 48 8N 21 27 E
Tokala, *Indonesia* **82 B2** 1 30 S 121 40 E
Tōkamachi, *Japan* **71 F9** 37 8N 138 43 E
Tokanui, *N.Z.* **131 G3** 46 34 S 168 56 E
Tokar, *Sudan* **106 D4** 18 27N 37 56 E
Tokara-Rettō, *Japan* **71 K4** 29 37N 129 43 E
Tokarahi, *N.Z.* **131 E5** 44 56 S 170 39 E
Tokashiki-Shima, *Japan* **71 L3** 26 11N 127 21 E
Tokat, *Turkey* **100 B7** 40 22N 36 35 E
Tŏkch'ŏn, *N. Korea* **75 E14** 39 45N 126 18 E
Tokeland, *U.S.A.* **160 D3** 46 42N 123 59W
Tokelau Is., *Pac. Oc.* **134 H10** 9 0 S 171 45W
Toki, *Japan* **73 B9** 35 18N 137 8 E
Tokmak, *Kyrgyzstan* **65 B7** 42 49N 75 15 E
Tokmak, *Ukraine* **59 J8** 47 16N 35 42 E
Toko Ra., *Australia* **126 C2** 23 5 S 138 20 E
Tokomaru Bay, *N.Z.* **130 E7** 38 8 S 178 22 E
Tokoname, *Japan* **73 C8** 34 53N 136 51 E
Tokoro-Gawa →, *Japan* **70 B12** 44 7N 144 5 E
Tokoroa, *N.Z.* **130 E4** 38 13 S 175 50 E
Tokorozawa, *Japan* **73 B11** 35 47N 139 28 E
Toksook Bay, *U.S.A.* **144 F6** 60 32N 165 0W
Toktogul, *Kyrgyzstan* **65 C6** 41 50N 72 50 E
Toktogul Suu Saktagychy, *Kyrgyzstan* **65 C6** 41 48N 72 51 E
Toku, *Tonga* **133 P13** 18 10 S 174 11W
Tokuji, *Japan* **72 C3** 34 11N 131 42 E
Tokuno-Shima, *Japan* **71 L4** 27 56N 128 55 E
Tokushima, *Japan* **72 C6** 34 4N 134 34 E
Tokushima □, *Japan* **72 D6** 33 55N 134 0 E
Tokuyama, *Japan* **72 C3** 34 3N 131 50 E
Tōkyō, *Japan* **73 B11** 35 45N 139 45 E
Tōkyō □, *Japan* **73 B11** 35 40N 139 30 E
Tokyo Haneda ✈ (HND), *Japan* **73 B11** 35 33N 139 46 E
Tokyo Narita ✈ (NRT), *Japan* **73 B12** 35 45N 140 25 E
Tōkyō-Wan, *Japan* **73 B11** 35 25N 139 47 E
Tokzār, *Afghan.* **91 B2** 35 52N 66 26 E
Tolaga Bay, *N.Z.* **130 E7** 38 21 S 178 20 E
Tolageak, *U.S.A.* **144 A7** 70 3N 162 27W
Tolbukhin = Dobrich, *Bulgaria* **51 C11** 43 37N 27 49 E
Tolé, *C.A.R.* **114 A3** 6 3N 16 1 E
Töle Bī, *Kazakhstan* **65 B6** 43 42N 73 46 E
Toledo, *Brazil* **175 A5** 24 44 S 53 45W
Toledo, *Phil.* **81 F4** 10 23N 123 38 E
Toledo, *Spain* **42 F6** 39 50N 4 2W
Toledo, *Ill., U.S.A.* **157 E8** 39 16N 88 15W
Toledo, *Iowa, U.S.A.* **156 C4** 42 0N 92 35W
Toledo, *Ohio, U.S.A.* **157 C13** 41 39N 83 33W
Toledo, *Oreg., U.S.A.* **158 D2** 44 37N 123 56W
Toledo, *Wash., U.S.A.* **158 C2** 46 26N 122 51W
Toledo, Montes de, *Spain* **43 F6** 39 33N 4 20W
Toledo Bend Reservoir, *U.S.A.* **155 K8** 31 11N 93 34W
Tolentino, *Italy* **45 E10** 43 12N 13 17 E
Tolfa, *Italy* **45 F8** 42 9N 11 56 E
Tolga, *Algeria* **111 B6** 34 40N 5 22 E
Tolga, *Australia* **126 B4** 17 15 S 145 29 E
Tolga, *Norway* **18 B8** 62 26N 11 1 E
Tolhuaca △, *Chile* **176 A2** 38 15 S 71 50W
Toliara, *Madag.* **117 C7** 23 21 S 43 40 E
Toliara □, *Madag.* **117 C8** 21 0 S 45 0 E
Tolima, *Colombia* **168 C2** 4 40N 75 19W
Tolima □, *Colombia* **168 C2** 3 45N 75 15W
Tolitoli, *Indonesia* **82 A2** 1 5N 120 50 E
Tolkmicko, *Poland* **54 D6** 54 19N 19 31 E
Tollarp, *Sweden* **17 J7** 55 55N 13 58 E
Tollensesee, *Germany* **30 B9** 53 30N 13 13 E
Tollhouse, *U.S.A.* **160 H7** 37 1N 119 24W
Tolmachevo, *Russia* **58 C5** 58 56N 29 51 E
Tolmezzo, *Italy* **45 B10** 46 24N 13 1 E
Tolmin, *Slovenia* **45 B10** 46 11N 13 45 E
Tolna, *Hungary* **52 D3** 46 25N 18 48 E
Tolna □, *Hungary* **52 D3** 46 30N 18 30 E
Tolo, *Dem. Rep. of the Congo* **114 C3** 2 55 S 18 34 E
Tolo, Teluk, *Indonesia* **82 B2** 2 20 S 122 10 E
Tolo Harbour, *China* **69 G11** 22 27N 114 12 E
Tolochin = Talachyn, *Belarus* **58 E5** 54 25N 29 42 E
Tolokiwa I., *Papua N. G.* **132 C4** 5 19 S 147 37 E
Tolong Bay, *Phil.* **81 G4** 9 20N 122 49 E
Tolono, *U.S.A.* **157 E8** 39 59N 88 16W
Tolosa, *Spain* **40 B2** 43 8N 2 5W
Tolox, *Spain* **43 J6** 36 41N 4 54W
Toltén, *Chile* **176 A2** 39 13 S 74 14W
Toluca, *Mexico* **163 D5** 19 20N 99 40W
Toluca, *U.S.A.* **156 C7** 41 0N 89 9W
Tolybay, *Kazakhstan* **64 F9** 50 31N 62 19 E
Tom Burke, *S. Africa* **117 C4** 23 5 S 28 0 E
Tom Price, *Australia* **124 D2** 22 40 S 117 48 E
Toma, *Burkina Faso* **112 C4** 12 45N 2 53W
Tomah, *U.S.A.* **154 D9** 43 59N 90 30W
Tomahawk, *U.S.A.* **154 C10** 45 28N 89 44W
Tomai, *Moldova* **53 D13** 46 34N 28 19 E
Tomakomai, *Japan* **70 C10** 42 38N 141 36 E
Tomales, *U.S.A.* **160 G4** 38 15N 122 53W
Tomales B., *U.S.A.* **160 G3** 38 15N 123 58W
Tomanlivi, *Fiji* **133 A2** 17 37 S 178 1 E
Tomar, *Portugal* **43 F2** 39 36N 8 25W
Tómaros, Óros, *Greece* **48 B2** 39 29N 20 48 E
Tomarza, *Turkey* **100 C6** 38 27N 35 48 E
Tomás Barrón, *Bolivia* **172 D4** 17 35 S 67 31W
Tomashevka, *Belarus* **55 G10** 51 33N 23 36 E
Tomashpil, *Ukraine* **53 B13** 48 32N 28 31 E
Tomaszów Lubelski, *Poland* **55 H10** 50 27N 23 25 E
Tomaszów Mazowiecki, *Poland* **55 G7** 51 30N 20 2 E
Tomatlán, *Mexico* **162 D3** 19 56N 105 15W
Tombadonkéa, *Guinea* **112 C2** 11 0N 14 25W
Tombador, Serra do, *Brazil* **173 C6** 12 0 S 58 0W
Tombe, *Sudan* **107 F3** 5 53N 31 40 E
Tombel, *Cameroon* **114 B1** 4 45N 9 40 E
Tombigbee →, *U.S.A.* **149 K2** 31 8N 87 57W
Tombôco, *Angola* **115 D2** 6 48 S 13 18 E
Tombouctou, *Mali* **112 B4** 16 50N 3 0W
Tombstone, *U.S.A.* **159 L8** 31 43N 110 4W
Tombua, *Angola* **116 B1** 15 55 S 11 55 E
Tomé, *Chile* **174 D1** 36 36 S 72 57W
Tomé-Açu, *Brazil* **170 B2** 2 25 S 48 9W
Tomelilla, *Sweden* **17 J7** 55 33N 13 58 E
Tomelloso, *Spain* **43 F7** 39 10N 3 2W
Tömenaryk, *Kazakhstan* **65 A3** 44 2N 67 1 E
Tomingley, *Australia* **129 B8** 32 26 S 148 16 E
Tomini, *Indonesia* **82 A2** 0 30N 120 30 E
Tomini, Teluk, *Indonesia* **82 B2** 0 10 S 121 0 E
Tominian, *Mali* **112 C4** 13 17N 4 35W
Tomiño, *Spain* **42 D2** 41 59N 8 46W
Tomintoul, *U.K.* **22 D5** 57 15N 3 23W
Tomioka, *Japan* **73 A10** 36 15N 138 54 E
Tomislavgrad, *Bos.-H.* **52 G2** 43 42N 17 13 E
Tomkinson Ranges, *Australia* **125 E4** 26 11 S 129 5 E
Tommot, *Russia* **67 D13** 59 4N 126 20 E
Tomnop Ta Suos, *Cambodia* **87 G5** 11 20N 104 15 E
Tomo, *Colombia* **168 C4** 2 38N 67 32W
Tomo →, *Colombia* **168 B4** 5 20N 67 48W
Tomobe, *Japan* **73 A12** 36 20N 140 20 E
Tomra, *Norway* **18 B3** 62 34N 6 56 E
Toms Place, *U.S.A.* **160 H8** 37 34N 118 41W
Toms River, *U.S.A.* **151 G10** 39 58N 74 12W
Tomsk, *Russia* **66 D9** 56 30N 85 5 E
Tomtabacken, *Sweden* **17 G8** 57 30N 14 30 E
Tona, *Spain* **40 D7** 41 51N 2 14 E
Tonalá, *Mexico* **163 D6** 16 8N 93 41W
Tonale, Passo del, *Italy* **44 B7** 46 16N 10 35 E
Tonami, *Japan* **73 A8** 36 40N 136 58 E
Tonantins, *Brazil* **168 D4** 2 45 S 67 45W
Tonasket, *U.S.A.* **158 B4** 48 42N 119 26W
Tonate, *Fr. Guiana* **169 C7** 5 0N 52 28W
Tonawanda, *U.S.A.* **150 D6** 43 1N 78 53W
Tonb, *Iran* **97 E7** 26 15N 55 15 E
Tonbo, *Burma* **90 F5** 18 31N 95 25 E
Tonbridge, *U.K.* **21 F8** 51 11N 0 17 E
Tonda, *Papua N. G.* **132 E1** 8 55 S 141 34 E
Tondabayashi, *Japan* **73 C7** 34 30N 135 36 E
Tondano, *Indonesia* **82 A2** 1 35N 124 54 E
Tondela, *Portugal* **42 E2** 40 31N 8 5W
Tønder, *Denmark* **17 K2** 54 58N 8 50 E
Tondern = Tønder, *Denmark* **17 K2** 54 58N 8 50 E
Tondi, *India* **95 K4** 9 45N 79 4 E
Tondi Kiwindi, *Niger* **113 C5** 14 28N 2 2 E
Tondibi, *Mali* **113 B4** 16 39N 0 14W

Tondoro, *Namibia* **116 B2** 17 45 S 18 50 E
Tone →, *Australia* **125 F2** 34 25 S 116 25 E
Tone-Gawa →, *Japan* **73 B12** 35 44N 140 51 E
Tonekābon, *Iran* **97 B6** 36 45N 51 12 E
Tong I., *Papua N. G.* **132 B4** 2 2 S 147 47 E
Tong Xian, *China* **74 E9** 39 55N 116 35 E
Tôngâ, *Sudan* **107 F3** 9 28N 31 3 E
Tonga ■, *Pac. Oc.* **133 P13** 19 50 S 174 30W
Tonga Trench, *Pac. Oc.* **134 J10** 18 0 S 173 0W
Tongaat, *S. Africa* **117 D5** 29 33 S 31 9 E
Tongala, *Australia* **129 D6** 36 14 S 144 56 E
Tong'an, *China* **77 E12** 24 37N 118 8 E
Tongareva, *Cook Is.* **135 H12** 9 0 S 158 0W
Tongariro △, *N.Z.* **130 F4** 39 8 S 175 33 E
Tongatapu, *Tonga* **133 Q14** 21 10 S 174 0W
Tongatapu Group, *Tonga* **133 Q13** 21 0 S 175 0W
Tongbai, *China* **77 A9** 32 20N 113 23 E
Tongcheng, *Anhui, China* **77 B11** 31 4N 116 56 E
Tongcheng, *Hubei, China* **77 C9** 29 15N 113 50 E
Tongchŏn-ni, *N. Korea* **75 E14** 39 50N 127 25 E
Tongchuan, *China* **74 G5** 35 6N 109 3 E
Tongdao, *China* **76 D7** 26 10N 109 42 E
Tongeren, *Belgium* **24 D5** 50 47N 5 28 E
Tonggu, *China* **77 C10** 28 31N 114 20 E
Tonggu Jiao, *China* **69 G10** 22 22N 113 37 E
Tongguan, *China* **74 G6** 34 40N 110 25 E
Tonghae, *S. Korea* **75 F15** 37 29N 129 7 E
Tonghai, *China* **76 E4** 24 10N 102 53 E
Tonghua, *China* **75 D13** 41 42N 125 58 E
Tongjiang, *China* **76 B6** 31 58N 107 11 E
Tongjosŏn Man, *N. Korea* **75 E15** 39 30N 128 0 E
Tongkil, *Phil.* **81 H3** 6 4N 121 48 E
Tongking, G. of = Tonkin, G. of, *Asia* **68 E5** 20 0N 108 0 E
Tongliang, *China* **76 C6** 29 50N 106 3 E
Tongliao, *China* **75 C12** 43 38N 122 18 E
Tongling, *China* **77 B11** 30 55N 117 48 E
Tonglu, *China* **77 C12** 29 45N 119 37 E
Tongnae, *S. Korea* **75 G15** 35 12N 129 5 E
Tongnan = Anyue, *China* **76 B5** 30 9N 105 50 E
Tongoa, *Vanuatu* **133 F6** 16 54 S 168 34 E
Tongobory, *Madag.* **117 C7** 23 32 S 44 20 E
Tongoy, *Chile* **174 C1** 30 16 S 71 31W
Tongquil I., *Phil.* **81 H3** 6 2N 121 51 E
Tongren, *China* **76 D7** 27 43N 109 11 E
Tongres = Tongeren, *Belgium* **24 D5** 50 47N 5 28 E
Tongsa Dzong, *Bhutan* **90 B3** 27 31N 90 31 E
Tongshi, *China* **86 C7** 18 30N 109 20 E
Tongue, *U.K.* **22 C4** 58 29N 4 25W
Tongue →, *U.S.A.* **154 B2** 46 25N 105 52W
Tongwei, *China* **74 G3** 35 0N 105 5 E
Tongxiang, *China* **77 B13** 30 39N 120 34 E
Tongxin, *China* **74 F3** 36 59N 105 58 E
Tongyang, *N. Korea* **75 E14** 39 9N 126 53 E
Tongyu, *China* **75 B12** 44 45N 123 4 E
Tongzi, *China* **76 C6** 28 9N 106 49 E
Tonica, *U.S.A.* **156 C7** 41 13N 89 4W
Tonj, *Sudan* **107 F2** 7 20N 28 44 E
Tonj →, *Sudan* **107 F2** 7 31N 28 55 E
Tonk, *India* **92 F6** 26 6N 75 54 E
Tonkawa, *U.S.A.* **155 G6** 36 41N 97 18W
Tonkin = Bac Phan, *Vietnam* **86 B5** 22 0N 105 0 E
Tonkin, G. of, *Asia* **68 E5** 20 0N 108 0 E
Tonle Sap, *Cambodia* **86 F4** 13 0N 104 0 E
Tonnay-Charente, *France* **28 C3** 45 56N 0 55W
Tonneins, *France* **28 D4** 44 23N 0 19 E
Tonnerre, *France* **27 E10** 47 51N 3 59 E
Tönning, *Germany* **30 A4** 54 19N 8 56 E
Tono, *Japan* **70 E10** 39 19N 141 32 E
Tonopah, *U.S.A.* **159 G5** 38 4N 117 14W
Tonoshō, *Japan* **72 C6** 34 29N 134 11 E
Tonosí, *Panama* **164 E3** 7 20N 80 20W
Tons →, *Haryana, India* **92 D7** 30 30N 77 39 E
Tons →, *Ut. P., India* **93 F10** 26 1N 83 33 E
Tønsberg, *Norway* **18 E7** 59 19N 10 25 E
Tonsina, *U.S.A.* **144 F11** 61 39N 145 11W
Tonstad, *Norway* **18 F3** 58 40N 6 45 E
Tonto ⌂, *U.S.A.* **159 K8** 33 39N 111 7W
Tonumea, *Tonga* **133 Q13** 20 30 S 174 30W
Tonya, *Turkey* **101 B8** 40 53N 39 16 E
Tonzang, *Burma* **90 D4** 23 36N 93 42 E
Tonzi, *Burma* **90 C5** 24 39N 94 57 E
Toobanna, *Australia* **126 B4** 18 42 S 146 9 E
Toodyay, *Australia* **125 F2** 31 34 S 116 28 E
Tooele, *U.S.A.* **158 F7** 40 32N 112 18W
Toompine, *Australia* **127 D3** 27 15 S 144 19 E
Toomsboro, *U.S.A.* **152 C6** 32 50N 83 5W
Toora, *Australia* **129 E7** 38 39 S 146 23 E
Toora-Khem, *Russia* **67 D10** 52 28N 96 17 E
Toowoomba, *Australia* **127 D5** 27 32 S 151 56 E
Top-ozero, *Russia* **56 A5** 65 35N 32 0 E
Top Springs, *Australia* **124 C5** 16 37 S 131 51 E
Topalu, *Romania* **53 F13** 44 31N 28 3 E
Topaz, *U.S.A.* **160 G7** 38 41N 119 30W
Topeka, *U.S.A.* **154 F7** 39 3N 95 40W
Topl'a →, *Slovak Rep.* **35 C14** 48 45N 21 45 E
Topley, *Canada* **142 C3** 54 49N 126 18W
Toplica →, *Serbia & M.* **50 C5** 43 15N 21 49 E
Topliţa, *Romania* **53 D10** 46 55N 25 20 E
Topo, *Azores* **9 d1** 38 33N 27 45W
Topo, Pta. do, *Azores* **9 d1** 38 33N 27 46W
Topocalma, Pta., *Chile* **174 C1** 34 10 S 72 2W
Topock, *U.S.A.* **161 L12** 34 46N 114 29W
Topola, *Serbia & M.* **50 B4** 44 17N 20 41 E
Topolčani, *Macedonia* **50 E5** 41 14N 21 25 E
Topol'čany, *Slovak Rep.* **35 C11** 48 35N 18 12 E
Topolnitsa →, *Bulgaria* **51 D8** 42 11N 24 18 E
Topolobampo, *Mexico* **162 B3** 25 40N 109 4W
Topoloveni, *Romania* **53 F10** 44 49N 25 5 E
Topolovgrad, *Bulgaria* **51 D10** 42 5N 26 20 E
Topolvăţu Mare, *Romania* **52 E6** 45 46N 21 41 E
Topornino = Kushnarenkovo, *Russia* **64 D5** 55 6N 55 22 E
Toppenish, *U.S.A.* **158 C3** 46 23N 120 19W
Topraisar, *Romania* **53 F13** 44 1N 28 27 E
Topusko, *Croatia* **45 C12** 45 18N 15 59 E
Toquepala, *Peru* **172 D3** 17 24 S 70 25W
Torà, *Spain* **40 D6** 41 49N 1 25 E
Tora Kit, *Sudan* **107 E3** 11 2N 32 36 E
Toraka Vestale, *Madag.* **117 B7** 16 20 S 43 58 E
Torata, *Peru* **172 D3** 17 23 S 70 1W
Torbalı, *Turkey* **49 C9** 38 10N 27 21 E
Torbat-e Heydārīyeh, *Iran* **97 C8** 35 15N 59 12 E
Torbat-e Jām, *Iran* **97 C9** 35 16N 60 35 E
Torbay, *Canada* **141 C9** 47 40N 52 42W
Torbay □, *U.K.* **21 G4** 50 26N 3 31W
Tørberget, *Norway* **18 C9** 61 8N 12 7 E
Torbjörntorp, *Sweden* **17 F7** 58 12N 13 36 E
Tordesillas, *Spain* **42 D6** 41 30N 5 0W
Töreboda, *Sweden* **17 F8** 58 41N 14 7 E
Torekov, *Sweden* **17 H6** 56 26N 12 37 E
Torellò, *Spain* **40 C7** 42 3N 2 16 E
Toreno, *Spain* **42 C4** 42 42N 6 30W
Torfaen □, *U.K.* **21 F4** 51 43N 3 3W
Torfajökull, *Iceland* **11 D7** 63 54N 19 0W
Torgau, *Germany* **30 D8** 51 34N 13 0 E
Torgelow, *Germany* **30 B10** 53 37N 14 1 E
Torgovaya = Salsk, *Russia* **61 G5** 46 28N 41 30 E
Torhamn, *Sweden* **17 H9** 56 6N 15 50 E
Torhout, *Belgium* **24 C3** 51 5N 3 7 E
Torhovytsya, *Ukraine* **53 B10** 48 36N 25 26 E
Tori, *Ethiopia* **107 F3** 7 53N 33 35 E
Tori-Shima, *Japan* **71 J10** 30 29N 140 19 E
Torigni-sur-Vire, *France* **26 C6** 49 3N 0 58W
Torija, *Spain* **40 E1** 40 44N 3 2W
Torin, *Mexico* **162 B2** 27 33N 110 15W
Torino, *Italy* **44 C4** 45 3N 7 40 E
Torit, *Sudan* **107 G3** 4 27N 32 31 E
Torkamān, *Iran* **101 D12** 37 35N 47 23 E
Torkovichi, *Russia* **58 C6** 58 51N 30 21 E
Tormac, *Romania* **52 E6** 45 30N 21 30 E
Tormes →, *Spain* **42 D4** 41 18N 6 29W
Tornado Mt., *Canada* **142 D6** 49 55N 114 40W
Tornal'a, *Slovak Rep.* **35 C13** 48 25N 20 20 E
Torneå = Tornio, *Finland* **14 D21** 65 50N 24 12 E
Torneälven →, *Europe* **14 D21** 65 50N 24 12 E
Torneträsk, *Sweden* **14 B18** 68 24N 19 15 E
Tornio, *Finland* **14 D21** 65 50N 24 12 E
Tornionjoki = Torneälven →, *Europe* **14 D21** 65 50N 24 12 E
Tornquist, *Argentina* **174 D3** 38 8 S 62 15W
Toro, *Baleares, Spain* **38 B5** 39 59N 4 8 E
Toro, *Zamora, Spain* **42 D5** 41 35N 5 24W
Torö, *Sweden* **17 F11** 58 48N 17 50 E
Toro ⌂, *Uganda* **118 C3** 0 5 S 30 22 E
Toro, Cerro del, *Chile* **174 B2** 29 10 S 69 50W
Toro Pk., *U.S.A.* **161 M10** 33 34N 116 24W
Torokina, *Papua N. G.* **132 D8** 6 14 S 155 3 E
Törökszentmiklós, *Hungary* **52 C5** 47 11N 20 27 E
Toronίos Kólpos, *Greece* **50 F7** 40 5N 23 30 E
Toronto, *Australia* **129 B9** 33 0 S 151 30 E
Toronto, *Canada* **140 D4** 43 39N 79 20W
Toronto, *U.S.A.* **150 F4** 40 28N 80 36W
Toronto Lester B. Pearson International ✈ (YYZ), *Canada* **150 C5** 43 40N 79 34W
Toropets, *Russia* **58 D6** 56 30N 31 40 E
Tororo, *Uganda* **118 B3** 0 45N 34 12 E
Toros Dağları, *Turkey* **100 D5** 37 0N 32 30 E
Torotoro, *Bolivia* **173 D4** 18 7 S 65 46W
Torotoro △, *Bolivia* **173 D4** 18 8 S 65 46W
Torpa, *India* **93 H11** 22 57N 85 6 E
Torpo, *Norway* **18 D5** 60 40N 8 43 E
Torquay, *Australia* **128 E6** 38 20 S 144 19 E
Torquay, *U.K.* **21 G4** 50 27N 3 32W
Torquemada, *Spain* **42 C6** 42 2N 4 19W
Torrais, Pta., *Azores* **9 d2** 39 43N 31 7W
Torrance, *U.S.A.* **161 M8** 33 50N 118 19W
Torrão, *Portugal* **43 G2** 38 16N 8 11W
Torre Annunziata, *Italy* **47 B7** 40 45N 14 27 E
Torre de Moncorvo, *Portugal* **42 D3** 41 12N 7 8W
Torre del Campo, *Spain* **43 H7** 37 46N 3 53W
Torre del Greco, *Italy* **47 B7** 40 47N 14 22 E
Torre del Mar, *Spain* **43 J6** 36 44N 4 6W
Torre-Pacheco, *Spain* **41 H4** 37 44N 0 57W
Torre Péllice, *Italy* **44 D4** 44 49N 7 13 E
Torreblanca, *Spain* **40 E5** 40 14N 0 12 E
Torrecampo, *Spain* **43 G6** 38 29N 4 41W
Torrecilla en Cameros, *Spain* **40 C2** 42 15N 2 38W
Torredembarra, *Spain* **40 D6** 41 9N 1 24 E
Torredonjimeno, *Spain* **43 H7** 37 46N 3 57W
Torrejón de Ardoz, *Spain* **42 E7** 40 27N 3 29W
Torrejoncillo, *Spain* **42 F4** 39 54N 6 28W
Torrelaguna, *Spain* **42 E7** 40 50N 3 38W
Torrelavega, *Spain* **42 B6** 43 20N 4 5W
Torremaggiore, *Italy* **45 G12** 41 41N 15 17 E
Torremolinos, *Spain* **43 J6** 36 38N 4 30W
Torrens, L., *Australia* **128 A2** 31 0 S 137 50 E
Torrens Cr. →, *Australia* **126 C4** 22 23 S 145 9 E
Torrens Creek, *Australia* **126 C4** 20 48 S 145 3 E
Torrent, *Spain* **41 F4** 39 27N 0 28W
Torrenueva, *Spain* **43 G7** 38 38N 3 22W
Torreón, *Mexico* **162 B4** 25 33N 103 26W
Torreperogil, *Spain* **43 G7** 38 2N 3 17W
Torres, *Brazil* **175 B5** 29 21 S 49 44W
Torres, *Mexico* **162 B2** 28 46N 110 47W
Torres, Is., *Vanuatu* **133 C4** 13 15 S 166 37 E
Torres del Paine △, *Chile* **176 D2** 51 3 S 72 58W
Torres Novas, *Portugal* **43 F2** 39 27N 8 33W
Torres Strait, *Australia* **132 E2** 9 50 S 142 20 E
Torres Vedras, *Portugal* **43 F1** 39 5N 9 15W
Torrevieja, *Spain* **41 H4** 37 59N 0 42W
Torrey, *U.S.A.* **159 G8** 38 18N 111 25W
Torricelli Mts., *Papua N. G.* **132 B2** 3 23 S 142 15 E
Torridge →, *U.K.* **21 G3** 51 0N 4 13W
Torridon, L., *U.K.* **22 D3** 57 35N 5 50W
Torrijos, *Phil.* **80 E4** 13 19N 122 5 E
Torrijos, *Spain* **42 F6** 39 59N 4 18W
Tørring, *Denmark* **17 J3** 55 52N 9 29 E
Torrington, *Conn., U.S.A.* **151 E11** 41 48N 73 7W
Torrington, *Wyo., U.S.A.* **154 D2** 42 4N 104 11W
Torroella de Montgrì, *Spain* **40 C8** 42 2N 3 8 E
Torrox, *Spain* **43 J7** 36 46N 3 57W
Torsås, *Sweden* **17 H9** 56 24N 16 0 E
Torsby, *Sweden* **16 D6** 60 7N 13 0 E
Torshälla, *Sweden* **16 E10** 59 25N 16 28 E
Tórshavn, *Færoe Is.* **14 E9** 62 5N 6 56W
Torslanda, *Sweden* **17 G5** 57 44N 11 45 E
Torsö, *Sweden* **17 F7** 58 48N 13 45 E
Törtköl, *Kazakhstan* **65 B4** 42 55N 68 57 E
Tortola, *Br. Virgin Is.* **165 e** 18 19N 64 45W
Tórtoles de Esgueva, *Spain* **42 D6** 41 49N 4 2W
Tortolì, *Italy* **46 C2** 39 55N 9 39 E
Tortona, *Italy* **44 D5** 44 54N 8 52 E
Tortorici, *Italy* **47 D7** 38 2N 14 49 E
Tortosa, *Spain* **40 E5** 40 49N 0 31 E
Tortosa, C., *Spain* **40 E5** 40 41N 0 52 E
Tortosendo, *Portugal* **42 E3** 40 15N 7 31W
Tortue, I. de la, *Haiti* **165 B5** 20 5N 72 57W
Tortuguero △, *Costa Rica* **164 D3** 10 31N 83 29W
Tortum, *Turkey* **101 B9** 40 19N 41 35 E
Toru-Aygyr, *Kyrgyzstan* **65 B8** 42 30N 76 26 E
Ţorūd, *Iran* **97 C7** 35 25N 55 5 E
Torul, *Turkey* **101 B8** 40 34N 39 18 E
Toruń, *Poland* **55 E5** 53 2N 18 39 E
Torun, *Ukraine* **53 B8** 48 40N 23 34 E
Tory I., *Ireland* **23 A3** 55 16N 8 14W
Torysa →, *Slovak Rep.* **35 C14** 48 39N 21 21 E
Torzhok, *Russia* **58 D8** 57 5N 34 55 E
Torzym, *Poland* **55 F2** 52 19N 15 5 E
Tosa, *Japan* **72 D5** 33 24N 133 23 E
Tosa-Shimizu, *Japan* **72 E4** 32 52N 132 58 E
Tosa-Wan, *Japan* **72 D5** 33 15N 133 30 E
Tosa-Yamada, *Japan* **72 D5** 33 36N 133 38 E
Toscana □, *Italy* **44 E8** 43 25N 11 0 E
Toscanella = Tuscánia, *Italy* **45 F8** 42 25N 11 52 E
Toscano, Arcipelago, *Italy* **44 F7** 42 30N 10 30 E
Toshkent, *Uzbekistan* **65 C4** 41 20N 69 10 E
Tosno, *Russia* **58 C6** 59 38N 30 46 E
Tossa de Mar, *Spain* **40 D7** 41 43N 2 56 E
Tösse, *Sweden* **17 F6** 58 58N 12 39 E
Tostado, *Argentina* **174 B3** 29 15 S 61 50W
Tostedt, *Germany* **30 B5** 53 17N 9 42 E
Tostón, Pta. de, *Canary Is.* **9 e2** 28 42N 14 2W
Tosu, *Japan* **72 D2** 33 22N 130 31 E
Tosya, *Turkey* **100 B6** 41 1N 34 2 E
Toszek, *Poland* **55 H5** 50 27N 18 32 E
Totak, *Norway* **18 E5** 59 40N 8 0 E
Totana, *Spain* **41 H3** 37 45N 1 30W
Totebo, *Sweden* **17 G10** 57 38N 16 12 E
Toteng, *Botswana* **116 C3** 20 22 S 22 58 E
Tôtes, *France* **26 C8** 49 41N 1 2 E
Tótkomlós, *Hungary* **52 D5** 46 24N 20 45 E
Totland, *Norway* **18 C2** 61 56N 5 23 E
Totma, *Russia* **56 C7** 60 0N 42 40 E
Totnes, *U.K.* **21 G4** 50 26N 3 42W
Totness, *Suriname* **169 B6** 5 53N 56 19W
Toto, *Nigeria* **113 D6** 8 26N 7 5 E
Totonicapán, *Guatemala* **164 D1** 14 58N 91 12W
Totora, *Bolivia* **173 D4** 17 42 S 65 9W
Totoya, I., *Fiji* **133 B3** 18 57 S 179 50W
Totskoye, *Russia* **64 E4** 52 32N 52 45 E
Totten Glacier, *Antarctica* **7 C8** 66 45 S 116 10 E
Tottenham, *Australia* **129 B7** 32 14 S 147 21 E
Tottenham, *Canada* **150 B5** 44 1N 79 49W
Tottori, *Japan* **72 B6** 35 30N 134 15 E
Tottori □, *Japan* **72 B6** 35 30N 134 12 E
Touaret, *Niger* **111 D6** 20 17N 7 8 E
Touat, *Algeria* **111 C5** 27 27N 0 30 E
Touba, *Ivory C.* **112 D3** 8 22N 7 40W
Touba, *Senegal* **112 C1** 14 50N 15 55W
Toubkal △, *Morocco* **110 B3** 31 0N 8 2W
Toubkal, Djebel, *Morocco* **110 B3** 31 0N 8 0W
Toucy, *France* **27 E10** 47 44N 3 15 E
Tougan, *Burkina Faso* **112 C4** 13 11N 2 58W
Touggourt, *Algeria* **111 B6** 33 6N 6 4 E
Tougouri, *Burkina Faso* **113 C4** 13 20N 0 30W
Tougué, *Guinea* **112 C2** 11 25N 11 50W
Touho, *N. Cal.* **133 T19** 20 47 S 165 14 E
Toukmatine, *Algeria* **111 D6** 24 49N 7 11 E
Toukoto, *Mali* **112 C3** 13 27N 9 52W
Toul, *France* **27 D12** 48 40N 5 53 E
Toulepleu, *Ivory C.* **112 D3** 6 32N 8 24W
Toulon, *France* **29 E9** 43 10N 5 55 E
Toulon, *U.S.A.* **156 C7** 41 6N 89 52W
Toulouse, *France* **28 E5** 43 37N 1 27 E
Toulouse Blagnac ✈ (TLS), *France* **28 E5** 43 37N 1 22 E
Toummo, *Niger* **108 D2** 22 45N 14 8 E
Toummo Dhoba, *Niger* **108 D2** 22 30N 14 31 E
Toumodi, *Ivory C.* **112 D3** 6 32N 5 4W
Tounan, *Taiwan* **77 F13** 23 41N 120 28 E
Tounassine, Hamada, *Algeria* **110 C4** 28 48N 5 0W
Toungo, *Nigeria* **113 D7** 8 20N 12 3 E
Toungoo, *Burma* **90 F6** 19 0N 96 30 E
Touques →, *France* **26 C7** 49 22N 0 8 E
Touraine, *France* **26 E7** 47 20N 0 30 E
Tourane = Da Nang, *Vietnam* **86 D7** 16 4N 108 13 E
Tourcoing, *France* **27 B10** 50 42N 3 10 E
Touriñán, C., *Spain* **42 B1** 43 3N 9 17W
Tourine, *Mauritania* **110 D2** 22 23N 11 50W
Tournai, *Belgium* **24 D3** 50 35N 3 25 E
Tournan-en-Brie, *France* **27 D9** 48 44N 2 46 E
Tournay, *France* **28 E4** 43 13N 0 13 E
Tournon-St-Martin, *France* **26 F7** 46 45N 0 58 E
Tournon-sur-Rhône, *France* **29 C8** 45 4N 4 50 E
Tournus, *France* **27 F11** 46 35N 4 54 E
Touros, *Brazil* **170 C4** 5 12 S 35 28W
Tours, *France* **26 E7** 47 22N 0 40 E
Touside, Pic, *Chad* **109 D3** 21 1N 16 29 E
Touws →, *S. Africa* **116 E3** 33 45 S 21 11 E
Touwsrivier, *S. Africa* **116 E3** 33 20 S 20 2 E
Tovar, *Venezuela* **168 B3** 8 20N 71 46W
Tovarkovskiy, *Russia* **58 F10** 53 40N 38 14 E
Tovdal, *Norway* **18 F5** 58 47N 8 10 E
Tovdalselva →, *Norway* **18 F5** 58 11N 8 7 E
Tovste, *Ukraine* **53 B10** 48 50N 25 44 E
Tovuz, *Azerbaijan* **61 K7** 41 0N 45 40 E
Towada, *Japan* **70 D10** 40 37N 141 13 E
Towada-Hachimantai △, *Japan* **70 D10** 40 20N 140 55 E
Towada-Ko, *Japan* **70 D10** 40 28N 140 55 E
Towanda, *Ill., U.S.A.* **157 D8** 40 36N 88 53W
Towanda, *Pa., U.S.A.* **151 E8** 41 46N 76 27W
Tower, *U.S.A.* **154 B8** 47 48N 92 17W
Tower, I. = Genovesa, I., *Ecuador* **172 a** 0 20N 89 58W
Towerhill Cr. →, *Australia* **126 C3** 22 28 S 144 35 E
Towner, *U.S.A.* **154 A4** 48 21N 100 25W
Townsend, *Ga., U.S.A.* **152 D8** 31 33N 81 31W
Townsend, *Mont., U.S.A.* **158 C8** 46 19N 111 31W
Townshend I., *Australia* **126 C5** 22 10 S 150 31 E
Townsville, *Australia* **126 B4** 19 15 S 146 45 E
Towraghondi, *Afghan.* **91 B1** 35 13N 62 16 E
Towson, *U.S.A.* **148 F7** 39 24N 76 36W
Towuti, Danau, *Indonesia* **82 B2** 2 45 S 121 32 E
Toxkan He →, *China* **65 C9** 41 8N 80 11 E
Toya-Ko, *Japan* **70 C10** 42 35N 140 51 E
Toyama, *Japan* **73 A9** 36 40N 137 15 E
Toyama □, *Japan* **73 A9** 36 45N 137 30 E
Toyama-Wan, *Japan* **71 F8** 37 0N 137 30 E
Toyapakeh, *Indonesia* **79 K18** 8 41 S 115 29 E
Tōyo, *Ehime, Japan* **72 D5** 33 56N 133 5 E
Tōyō, *Kōchi, Japan* **72 D6** 33 26N 134 16 E
Toyohara = Yuzhno-Sakhalinsk, *Russia* **67 E15** 46 58N 142 45 E
Toyohashi, *Japan* **73 C9** 34 45N 137 25 E
Toyokawa, *Japan* **73 C9** 34 48N 137 27 E
Toyonaka, *Japan* **73 C7** 34 50N 135 28 E
Toyooka, *Japan* **72 B6** 35 35N 134 48 E
Toyota, *Japan* **73 B9** 35 3N 137 7 E
Toyoura, *Japan* **72 C2** 34 6N 130 57 E
Toytepa, *Uzbekistan* **65 C4** 41 3N 69 20 E
Tozeur, *Tunisia* **108 B1** 33 56N 8 8 E
Tozkhurmato, *Iraq* **101 E11** 34 56N 44 38 E
Tqibuli, *Georgia* **61 J6** 42 26N 43 0 E
Tqvarcheli, *Georgia* **61 J5** 42 47N 41 42 E
Trá Li = Tralee, *Ireland* **23 D2** 52 16N 9 42W
Tra On, *Vietnam* **87 H5** 9 58N 105 55 E
Trabancos →, *Spain* **42 D5** 41 36N 5 15W
Traben-Trarbach, *Germany* **31 F3** 49 57N 7 7 E
Trabzon, *Turkey* **101 B8** 41 0N 39 45 E
Tracadie-Sheila, *Canada* **141 C7** 47 30N 64 55W
Trachenburg = Żmigród, *Poland* **55 G3** 51 28N 16 53 E
Tracy, *Calif., U.S.A.* **160 H5** 37 44N 121 26W
Tracy, *Minn., U.S.A.* **154 C7** 44 14N 95 37W
Tradate, *Italy* **44 C5** 45 43N 8 54 E
Trade Town, *Liberia* **112 D3** 5 40N 9 50W
Traer, *U.S.A.* **156 B4** 42 12N 92 28W
Trafalgar, *Australia* **129 E7** 38 14 S 146 12 E
Trafalgar, C., *Spain* **43 J4** 36 10N 6 2W
Trāghān, *Libya* **108 C2** 26 0N 14 30 E
Traian, *Brăila, Romania* **53 E12** 45 11N 27 44 E
Traian, *Tulcea, Romania* **53 E13** 45 2N 28 15 E
Traiguén, *Chile* **176 A2** 38 15 S 72 41W
Trail, *Canada* **142 D5** 49 5N 117 40W
Traill Ø, *Greenland* **10 C8** 72 30N 23 0W
Trainor L., *Canada* **142 A4** 60 24N 120 17W
Traíra →, *Brazil* **168 D4** 1 4 S 69 26W
Trákhonas, *Cyprus* **39 E9** 35 12N 33 21 E
Tralee, *Ireland* **23 D2** 52 16N 9 42W
Tralee B., *Ireland* **23 D2** 52 17N 9 55W
Tramelan, *Switz.* **32 B4** 47 13N 7 7 E
Tramore, *Ireland* **23 D4** 52 10N 7 10W
Tramore B., *Ireland* **23 D4** 52 9N 7 10W
Tran Ninh, Cao Nguyen, *Laos* **86 C4** 19 30N 103 10 E
Tranås, *Sweden* **17 F8** 58 3N 14 59 E
Tranbjerg, *Denmark* **17 H4** 56 6N 10 9 E
Tranby, *Norway* **18 E7** 59 49N 10 15 E
Trancas, *Argentina* **174 B2** 26 11 S 65 20W
Trancoso, *Portugal* **42 E3** 40 49N 7 21W
Tranebjerg, *Denmark* **17 J4** 55 51N 10 36 E
Tranemo, *Sweden* **17 G7** 57 30N 13 20 E
Trang, *Thailand* **87 J2** 7 33N 99 38 E
Trangahy, *Madag.* **117 B7** 19 7 S 44 31 E
Trangan, *Indonesia* **83 C4** 6 40 S 134 20 E
Trangie, *Australia* **129 B8** 32 4 S 148 0 E
Trångsviken, *Sweden* **16 A7** 63 19N 13 59 E
Trani, *Italy* **47 A9** 41 17N 16 25 E
Tranoroa, *Madag.* **117 C8** 24 42 S 45 4 E
Tranqueras, *Uruguay* **175 C4** 31 13 S 55 45W
Transantarctic Mts., *Antarctica* **7 E12** 85 0 S 170 0W
Transilvania, *Romania* **53 D9** 46 30N 24 0 E
Transilvanian Alps = Carpaţii Meridionali, *Romania* **53 E9** 45 30N 25 0 E
Transjordan = Jordan ■, *Asia* **103 E5** 31 0N 36 0 E
Transnistria = Stînga Nistrului □, *Moldova* **53 C14** 47 20N 29 15 E
Transtrand, *Sweden* **16 C7** 61 6N 13 20 E
Transtrandsfjällen, *Sweden* **16 C6** 61 8N 13 0 E
Transylvania = Transilvania, *Romania* **53 D9** 46 30N 24 0 E
Trápani, *Italy* **46 D5** 38 1N 12 29 E
Trapper Pk., *U.S.A.* **158 D6** 45 54N 114 18W
Traralgon, *Australia* **129 E7** 38 12 S 146 34 E
Trarza, *Mauritania* **112 B2** 17 30N 15 0W
Trás-os-Montes = Cucumbi, *Angola* **115 E3** 10 17 S 19 5 E
Trasacco, *Italy* **45 G10** 41 57N 13 32 E
Trăscău, Munţii, *Romania* **53 D8** 46 14N 23 14 E
Trasimeno, L., *Italy* **45 E9** 43 8N 12 6 E
Träslövsläge, *Sweden* **17 G6** 57 4N 12 16 E
Trasvase Tajo-Segura, Canal de, *Spain* **40 E2** 40 15N 2 55W
Trat, *Thailand* **87 F4** 12 14N 102 33 E
Tratani →, *Pakistan* **92 E3** 29 19N 68 20 E
Traun, *Austria* **34 C7** 48 14N 14 15 E
Traunreut, *Germany* **31 H8** 47 57N 12 36 E
Traunsee, *Austria* **34 D6** 47 55N 13 50 E
Traunstein, *Germany* **31 H8** 47 52N 12 37 E
Traveller's L., *Australia* **128 B5** 33 20 S 142 0 E
Travemünde, *Germany* **30 B6** 53 57N 10 52 E
Travers, Mt., *N.Z.* **131 C7** 42 1 S 172 45 E
Traverse City, *U.S.A.* **148 C3** 44 46N 85 38W
Travis, L., *U.S.A.* **155 K5** 30 24N 97 55W
Travnik, *Bos.-H.* **52 F2** 44 17N 17 39 E
Trbovlje, *Slovenia* **45 B12** 46 12N 15 5 E
Treasure Island, *U.S.A.* **153 H7** 27 46N 82 46W
Treasury Is., *Solomon Is.* **133 L8** 7 22 S 155 37 E
Trébbia →, *Italy* **44 C6** 45 4N 9 41 E
Trebel →, *Germany* **30 B9** 53 54N 13 2 E
Trébeurden, *France* **26 D3** 48 46N 3 35W
Trebević △, *Bos.-H.* **52 G3** 43 20N 18 45 E
Třebíč, *Czech Rep.* **34 B8** 49 14N 15 55 E
Trebinje, *Bos.-H.* **50 D2** 42 44N 18 22 E
Trebisacce, *Italy* **47 C9** 39 52N 16 32 E
Trebišnjica →, *Bos.-H.* **50 D2** 42 47N 18 8 E
Trebišov, *Slovak Rep.* **35 C14** 48 38N 21 41 E
Trebitsch = Třebíč, *Czech Rep.* **34 B8** 49 14N 15 55 E
Trebižat →, *Bos.-H.* **45 E14** 43 15N 17 30 E
Trebnitz = Trzebnica, *Poland* **55 G4** 51 20N 17 1 E
Trebnje, *Slovenia* **45 C12** 45 54N 15 1 E
Třeboň, *Czech Rep.* **34 B7** 49 1N 14 48 E
Trebonne, *Australia* **126 B4** 18 37 S 146 5 E
Třeboňsko ⌂, *Czech Rep.* **34 B7** 49 1N 14 49 E
Trebujena, *Spain* **43 J4** 36 52N 6 11W
Trecate, *Italy* **44 C5** 45 26N 8 44 E
Tregaron, *U.K.* **21 E4** 52 14N 3 56W
Tregnago, *Italy* **45 C8** 45 31N 11 10 E
Tregrosse Is., *Australia* **126 B5** 17 41 S 150 43 E
Tréguier, *France* **26 D3** 48 47N 3 16W
Trégunc, *France* **26 E3** 47 51N 3 51W
Treherne, *Canada* **143 D9** 49 38N 98 42W
Tréia, *Italy* **45 E10** 43 19N 13 19 E
Treignac, *France* **28 C5** 45 32N 1 48 E
Treinta y Tres, *Uruguay* **175 C5** 33 16 S 54 17W
Treis-karden, *Germany* **31 E3** 50 10N 7 18 E
Treklyano, *Bulgaria* **50 D6** 42 33N 22 36 E
Trelawney, *Zimbabwe* **117 B5** 17 30 S 30 30 E
Trélazé, *France* **26 E6** 47 26N 0 30W
Trelew, *Argentina* **176 B3** 43 10 S 65 20W
Trélissac, *France* **28 C4** 45 11N 0 47 E
Trelleborg, *Sweden* **17 J7** 55 20N 13 10 E
Tremadog Bay, *U.K.* **20 E3** 52 51N 4 18W
Trembowla = Terebovlya, *Ukraine* **59 H3** 49 18N 25 44 E
Tremedal = Monte Azul, *Brazil* **171 E3** 15 9 S 42 53W
Tremezzo, *Italy* **33 E8** 45 59N 9 15 E
Trémiti, *Italy* **45 F12** 42 8N 15 30 E
Tremonton, *U.S.A.* **158 F7** 41 43N 112 10W
Tremp, *Spain* **40 C5** 42 10N 0 52 E
Trenche →, *Canada* **140 C5** 47 46N 72 53W
Trenčiansky □, *Slovak Rep.* **35 C11** 48 45N 18 20 E
Trenčín, *Slovak Rep.* **35 C11** 48 52N 18 4 E
Trengereid, *Norway* **18 D2** 60 26N 5 37 E
Trenggalek, *Indonesia* **85 D4** 8 3 S 111 43 E
Trenque Lauquen, *Argentina* **174 D3** 36 5 S 62 45W
Trent →, *Canada* **150 B7** 44 6N 77 34W
Trent →, *U.K.* **20 D7** 53 41N 0 42W
Trentino-Alto Adige □, *Italy* **45 B8** 46 30N 11 20 E
Trento, *Italy* **44 B8** 46 4N 11 8 E
Trento, *Phil.* **81 G6** 8 3N 126 2 E
Trenton = Quinte West, *Canada* **140 D4** 44 10N 77 34W
Trenton, *Fla., U.S.A.* **153 F7** 29 37N 82 49W
Trenton, *Mich., U.S.A.* **157 B13** 42 8N 83 11W
Trenton, *Mo., U.S.A.* **156 D3** 40 5N 93 37W
Trenton, *N.J., U.S.A.* **151 F10** 40 14N 74 46W
Trenton, *Nebr., U.S.A.* **154 E4** 40 11N 101 1W
Trenton, *Ohio, U.S.A.* **157 E12** 39 29N 84 28W
Trenton, *S.C., U.S.A.* **152 B8** 33 45N 81 51W
Trepassey, *Canada* **141 C9** 46 43N 53 25W
Treptow an der Rega = Trzebiatów, *Poland* **54 D2** 54 3N 15 18 E
Trepuzzi, *Italy* **47 B11** 40 24N 18 4 E
Tres Arroyos, *Argentina* **174 D3** 38 26 S 60 20W
Três Casas, *Brazil* **173 B5** 6 59 S 62 41W
Três Corações, *Brazil* **171 F2** 21 44 S 45 15W
Tres Equinas, *Colombia* **168 C2** 0 43N 75 16W
Três Lagoas, *Brazil* **171 F1** 20 50 S 51 43W
Tres Lagos, *Argentina* **176 C2** 49 35 S 71 25W
Tres Lomas, *Argentina* **174 D3** 36 27 S 62 51W
Tres Marías, Islas, *Mexico* **162 C3** 21 25N 106 28W
Três Marias, Reprêsa, *Brazil* **171 E2** 18 12 S 45 15W
Tres Montes, C., *Chile* **176 C1** 46 50 S 75 30W
Tres Pinos, *U.S.A.* **160 J5** 36 48N 121 19W
Três Pontas, *Brazil* **171 F2** 21 23 S 45 29W
Três Pontas, C. das, *Angola* **115 E2** 10 28 S 13 32 E
Tres Puentes, *Chile* **174 B1** 27 50 S 70 15W
Tres Puntas, C., *Argentina* **176 C3** 47 0 S 66 0W
Três Rios, *Brazil* **171 F3** 22 6 S 43 15W
Tres Valles, *Mexico* **163 D5** 18 15N 96 8W
Tresco, *U.K.* **21 H1** 49 57N 6 20W
Tresfjord, *Norway* **18 B4** 62 31N 7 7 E
Treska →, *Macedonia* **50 E5** 42 0N 21 20 E
Treskavica, *Bos.-H.* **52 G3** 43 40N 18 20 E
Trespaderne, *Spain* **42 C7** 42 47N 3 24W
Tresticklan △, *Sweden* **17 F5** 59 0N 11 42 E
Trets, *France* **29 E9** 43 27N 5 41 E
Treuburg = Olecko, *Poland* **54 D9** 54 2N 22 31 E
Treuchtlingen, *Germany* **31 G6** 48 58N 10 54 E
Treuenbrietzen, *Germany* **30 C8** 52 5N 12 52 E
Treungen, *Norway* **18 E5** 59 1N 8 31 E
Trèves = Trier, *Germany* **31 F2** 49 45N 6 38 E
Trevi, *Italy* **45 F9** 42 52N 12 45 E
Trevíglio, *Italy* **44 C6** 45 31N 9 35 E
Trevínca, Peña, *Spain* **42 C4** 42 15N 6 46W
Treviso, *Italy* **45 C9** 45 40N 12 15 E
Trévoux, *France* **29 C8** 45 57N 4 47 E
Trgovište, *Serbia & M.* **50 D6** 42 20N 22 10 E
Triabunna, *Australia* **127 G4** 42 30 S 147 55 E
Triánda, *Greece* **38 E12** 36 25N 28 10 E
Triangle, *Zimbabwe* **117 C5** 21 2 S 31 28 E
Triaucourt-en-Argonne, *France* **27 D12** 48 59N 5 2 E
Tribal Areas □, *Pakistan* **91 B3** 33 0N 70 0 E
Tribly, *U.S.A.* **153 G7** 28 28N 82 12W
Tribsees, *Germany* **30 A8** 54 5N 12 44 E
Tribulation, C., *Australia* **126 B4** 16 5 S 145 29 E
Tribune, *U.S.A.* **154 F4** 38 28N 101 45W
Tricárico, *Italy* **47 B9** 40 37N 16 9 E
Tricase, *Italy* **47 C11** 39 56N 18 22 E
Trichinopoly = Tiruchchirappalli, *India* **95 J4** 10 45N 78 45 E
Trichur, *India* **95 J3** 10 30N 76 18 E
Trida, *Australia* **129 B6** 33 1 S 145 1 E
Trier, *Germany* **31 F2** 49 45N 6 38 E
Trieste, *Italy* **45 C10** 45 40N 13 46 E
Trieste, G. di, *Italy* **45 C10** 45 40N 13 35 E
Trieux →, *France* **26 D3** 48 43N 3 9W
Triggiano, *Italy* **47 A9** 41 4N 16 55 E
Triglav, *Slovenia* **45 B10** 46 21N 13 50 E
Triglavski △, *Slovenia* **45 B10** 46 20N 13 50 E
Trigno →, *Italy* **45 F11** 42 4N 14 48 E
Trigo de Morais = Guijá, *Mozam.* **117 C5** 24 27 S 33 0 E
Trigueros, *Spain* **43 H4** 37 24N 6 50W
Tríkeri, *Greece* **48 B5** 39 6N 23 5 E
Trikhonis, Límni, *Greece* **48 C3** 38 34N 21 30 E
Tríkkala, *Greece* **48 B3** 39 34N 21 47 E
Tríkkala □, *Greece* **48 B3** 39 41N 21 30 E
Trikomo, *Cyprus* **39 E9** 35 17N 33 52 E
Trikora, Puncak, *Indonesia* **83 B5** 4 15 S 138 45 E
Trilj, *Croatia* **45 E13** 43 38N 16 42 E
Trillo, *Spain* **40 E2** 40 42N 2 35W
Trim, *Ireland* **23 C5** 53 33N 6 48W
Trimbak, *India* **94 E1** 19 56N 73 33 E
Trincomalee, *Sri Lanka* **95 K5** 8 38N 81 15 E
Trindade, *Brazil* **171 E2** 16 40 S 49 30W
Trindade, I., *Atl. Oc.* **8 J9** 20 20 S 29 50W
Třinec, *Czech Rep.* **35 B11** 49 41N 18 39 E
Trinidad = Jose Abad Santos, *Phil.* **81 J5** 5 55N 125 39 E
Trinidad, *Bolivia* **173 C5** 14 46 S 64 50W
Trinidad, *Colombia* **168 B3** 5 25N 71 40W
Trinidad, *Cuba* **164 B4** 21 48N 80 0W
Trinidad, *Trin. & Tob.* **169 F9** 10 30N 61 15W
Trinidad, *Uruguay* **174 C4** 33 30 S 56 50W
Trinidad, *U.S.A.* **155 G2** 37 10N 104 31W
Trinidad →, *Mexico* **163 D5** 17 49N 95 9W
Trinidad, G., *Chile* **176 C1** 49 55 S 75 25W
Trinidad, I., *Argentina* **176 A4** 39 10 S 62 0W
Trinidad & Tobago ■, *W. Indies* **165 D7** 10 30N 61 20W
Trinitápoli, *Italy* **47 A9** 41 21N 16 5 E
Trinity, *Canada* **141 C9** 48 59N 53 55W
Trinity, *U.S.A.* **155 K7** 30 57N 95 22W
Trinity →, *Calif., U.S.A.* **158 F2** 41 11N 123 42W
Trinity →, *Tex., U.S.A.* **155 L7** 29 45N 94 43W
Trinity B., *Canada* **141 C9** 48 20N 53 10W
Trinity Hills, *Trin. & Tob.* **169 F9** 10 7N 61 7W
Trinity Is., *U.S.A.* **144 H9** 56 33N 154 25W
Trinity Range, *U.S.A.* **158 F4** 40 15N 118 45W
Trinkat, *India* **95 K11** 8 5N 93 30 E
Trinkitat, *Sudan* **106 D4** 18 45N 37 51 E

Trino, Italy 44 C5 45 12N 8 18 E
Trinway, U.S.A. 150 F2 40 9N 82 1W
Triolet, Mauritius 121 d 20 4 S 57 32 E
Trionto, C., Italy 47 C9 39 37N 16 43 E
Triora, Italy 44 D4 44 1N 7 46 E
Tripoli = Tarābulus, Lebanon 103 A4 34 31N 35 50 E
Tripoli = Tarābulus, Libya 108 B2 32 49N 13 7 E
Tripoli = Trípolis, Greece 48 D4 37 31N 22 25 E
Tripoli, U.S.A. 156 B4 42 49N 92 16W
Trípolis, Greece 48 D4 37 31N 22 25 E
Tripolitania, N. Afr. 104 C5 31 0N 13 0 E
Tripura □, India 90 D3 24 0N 92 0 E
Tripylos, Cyprus 39 F8 34 59N 32 41 E
Trischen, Germany 30 A4 54 4N 8 40 E
Tristan da Cunha, Atl. Oc. 8 K10 37 6 S 12 20W
Trisul, India 93 D8 30 19N 79 47 E
Trivandrum, India 95 K3 8 41N 77 0 E
Trivento, Italy 45 G11 41 47N 14 33 E
Trnava, Slovak Rep. 35 C10 48 23N 17 35 E
Trnavský □, Slovak Rep. 35 C10 48 30N 17 45 E
Troarn, France 26 C6 49 11N 0 11W
Trobriand Is., Papua N. G. 132 E6 8 30 S 151 0 E
Trochu, Canada 142 C6 51 50N 113 13W
Trodely I., Canada 140 B4 52 15N 79 26W
Troezen, Greece 48 D5 37 25N 23 15 E
Trogen, Switz. 33 B8 47 24N 9 28 E
Trogir, Croatia 45 E13 43 32N 16 15 E
Troglav, Croatia 45 E13 43 56N 16 36 E
Tróia, Italy 47 A8 41 22N 15 18 E
Troilus, L., Canada 140 B5 50 50N 74 35W
Troina, Italy 47 E7 37 47N 14 36 E
Trois Fourches, Cap des, Morocco 111 A4 35 26N 2 58W
Trois-Pistoles, Canada 141 C6 48 5N 69 10W
Trois-Rivières, Canada 140 C5 46 25N 72 34W
Trois-Rivières, Guadeloupe 164 b 15 57N 61 40W
Troisdorf, Germany 30 E3 50 48N 7 11 E
Troitsk, Russia 64 D8 54 10N 61 35 E
Troitskiy, Russia 64 C9 57 5N 63 43 E
Troitsko Pechorsk, Russia 56 B10 62 40N 56 10 E
Troitskosavsk = Kyakhta, Russia 67 D11 50 30N 106 25 E
Troitskoye, Russia 61 G7 46 26N 44 15 E
Troitsky = Troitsk, Russia 64 D8 54 10N 61 35 E
Trölladyngja, Iceland 11 C9 64 54N 17 16W
Trollhättan, Sweden 17 F6 58 17N 12 20 E
Trollheimen, Norway 18 B6 62 46N 9 1 E
Trombetas →, Brazil 169 D6 1 55 S 55 35W
Tromelin I., Ind. Oc. 121 F4 15 52 S 54 25 E
Tromøy, Norway 18 F5 58 27N 8 51 E
Tromsø, Norway 14 B18 69 40N 18 56 E
Trona, U.S.A. 161 K9 35 46N 117 23W
Tronador, Mte., Argentina 176 B2 41 10 S 71 50W
Trøndelag, Norway 14 D14 64 17N 11 50 E
Trondheim, Norway 18 A7 63 36N 10 25 E
Trondheimsfjorden, Norway 14 E14 63 35N 10 30 E
Trondheimsleia, Norway 18 A5 63 25N 8 30 E
Trondhjem = Trondheim, Norway 18 A7 63 36N 10 25 E
Trönninge, Sweden 17 H6 56 37N 12 51 E
Tronto →, Italy 45 F10 42 54N 13 55 E
Troodos, Cyprus 39 F8 34 55N 32 52 E
Troon, U.K. 22 F4 55 33N 4 39W
Tropea, Italy 47 D8 38 41N 15 54 E
Tropic, U.S.A. 159 H7 37 37N 112 5W
Tropojë, Albania 50 D4 42 23N 20 10 E
Troppau = Opava, Czech Rep. 35 B10 49 57N 17 58 E
Trosa, Sweden 17 F11 58 54N 17 33 E
Trostan, U.K. 23 A5 55 3N 6 10W
Trostberg, Germany 31 G8 48 1N 12 33 E
Trostyanets, Ukraine 53 B14 48 31N 29 11 E
Trostyanets, Ukraine 59 G8 50 33N 34 59 E
Trotsk = Chapayevsk, Russia 60 D9 53 0N 49 40 E
Trotsk = Gatchina, Russia 58 C6 59 35N 30 9 E
Trou Gras Pt., St. Lucia 165 f 13 51N 60 53W
Trout →, Canada 142 A5 61 19N 119 51W
Trout L., N.W.T., Canada 142 A4 60 40N 121 14W
Trout L., Ont., Canada 143 C10 51 20N 93 15W
Trout Lake, Canada 142 B6 56 30N 114 32W
Trout Lake, U.S.A. 160 E5 46 0N 121 32W
Trout River, Canada 141 C8 49 29N 58 8W
Trout Run, U.S.A. 150 E7 41 23N 77 3W
Trouville-sur-Mer, France 26 C7 49 21N 0 5 E
Trowbridge, U.K. 21 F5 51 18N 2 12W
Troy, Turkey 49 B8 39 57N 26 12 E
Troy, Ala., U.S.A. 152 D4 31 48N 85 58W
Troy, Ill., U.S.A. 156 F7 38 44N 89 54W
Troy, Ind., U.S.A. 157 G10 37 59N 86 55W
Troy, Kans., U.S.A. 154 F7 39 47N 95 5W
Troy, Mich., U.S.A. 157 B13 42 37N 83 9W
Troy, Mo., U.S.A. 156 F6 38 59N 90 59W
Troy, Mont., U.S.A. 158 B6 48 28N 115 53W
Troy, N.Y., U.S.A. 151 D11 42 44N 73 41W
Troy, Ohio, U.S.A. 157 D12 40 2N 84 12W
Troy, Pa., U.S.A. 151 E8 41 47N 76 47W
Troyan, Bulgaria 51 D8 42 57N 24 43 E
Troyes, France 27 D11 48 19N 4 3 E
Trpanj, Croatia 45 E14 43 1N 17 15 E
Trstenik, Serbia & M. 50 C5 43 36N 21 0 E
Trubchevsk, Russia 59 F7 52 33N 33 47 E
Truchas Peak, U.S.A. 155 H2 35 58N 105 39W
Truchas Pk., U.S.A. 159 J11 36 0N 105 30W
Trucial States = United Arab Emirates ■, Asia 97 F7 23 50N 54 0 E
Truckee, U.S.A. 160 F6 39 20N 120 11W
Trudfront, Russia 61 H8 45 56N 47 40 E
Trudovoye, Russia 70 C6 43 17N 132 5 E
Trujillo, Colombia 168 C2 4 10N 76 19W
Trujillo, Honduras 164 C2 16 0N 86 0W
Trujillo, Peru 172 B2 8 6 S 79 0W
Trujillo, Spain 43 F5 39 28N 5 55W
Trujillo, U.S.A. 155 H2 35 32N 104 42W
Trujillo, Venezuela 168 B3 9 22N 70 38W
Trujillo □, Venezuela 168 B3 9 25N 70 30W
Trujillo Mtn. = Duarte, Pico, Dom. Rep. 165 D5 19 2N 70 59W
Truk, Micronesia 134 G7 7 25N 151 46 E
Trumann, U.S.A. 155 H9 35 41N 90 31W
Trumansburg, U.S.A. 151 D8 42 33N 76 40W
Trumbull, Mt., U.S.A. 159 H7 36 25N 113 8W
Trŭn, Bulgaria 50 D6 42 51N 22 38 E
Trun, France 26 D7 48 50N 0 2 E
Trun, Switz. 33 C7 46 45N 8 59 E
Trundle, Australia 129 B7 32 53 S 147 35 E
Trung-Phan = Annam, Vietnam 86 E7 16 0N 108 0 E
Truro, Australia 128 C3 34 24 S 139 9 E
Truro, Canada 141 C7 45 21N 63 14W
Truro, U.K. 21 G2 50 16N 5 4W
Truskavets, Ukraine 59 H2 49 17N 23 30 E
Trŭstenik, Bulgaria 51 C8 43 31N 24 28 E
Trustrup, Denmark 17 H4 56 20N 10 46 E
Trutch, Canada 142 B4 57 44N 122 57W
Truth or Consequences, U.S.A. 159 K10 33 8N 107 15W
Trutnov, Czech Rep. 34 A8 50 37N 15 54 E
Truxton, U.S.A. 151 D8 42 45N 76 2W
Truyère →, France 28 D6 44 38N 2 34 E
Tryavna, Bulgaria 51 D9 42 54N 25 25 E
Tryonville, U.S.A. 150 E5 41 42N 79 48W
Tryphena, N.Z. 130 C4 36 18 S 175 28 E
Trysilelva →, Norway 18 C9 61 2N 12 35 E
Trzcianka, Poland 55 E3 53 3N 16 25 E
Trzciel, Poland 55 F2 52 23N 15 50 E
Trzcińsko Zdrój, Poland 55 F1 52 58N 14 35 E
Trzebiatów, Poland 54 D2 54 3N 15 18 E
Trzebiez, Poland 54 E1 53 38N 14 31 E
Trzebnica, Poland 55 G4 51 20N 17 1 E
Trzemeszno, Poland 55 F4 52 33N 17 48 E
Tržič, Slovenia 45 B11 46 22N 14 18 E
Tsagan Aman, Russia 61 G8 47 34N 46 43 E
Tsakarisiánon, Greece 39 C2 38 10N 20 40 E
Tsala Apopka L., U.S.A. 153 G7 28 53N 82 19W
Tsamandás, Greece 48 B2 39 46N 20 21 E
Tsamkong = Zhanjiang, China 77 G8 21 15N 110 20 E
Tsandi, Namibia 116 B1 17 42 S 14 50 E
Tsangpo = Brahmaputra →, Asia 68 D3 23 40N 90 35 E
Tsaratanana, Madag. 117 B8 16 47 S 47 39 E
Tsaratanana △, Madag. 117 A8 13 57 S 48 52 E
Tsaratanana, Mt. de = Maromokotro, Madag. 117 A8 14 0 S 49 0 E
Tsarekonstantinovka = Kuybyshevo, Ukraine 59 J9 47 25N 36 40 E
Tsarevo = Michurin, Bulgaria 51 D11 42 9N 27 51 E
Tsarevo, Bulgaria 51 D9 42 28N 25 52 E
Tsaribrod = Dimitrovgrad, Serbia & M. 50 C6 43 2N 22 48 E
Tsaritsáni, Greece 48 B4 39 53N 22 14 E
Tsarskoye Selo = Pushkin, Russia 58 C6 59 45N 30 25 E
Tsaryovokokshaysk = Yoshkar Ola, Russia 60 B8 56 38N 47 55 E
Tsau, Botswana 116 C3 20 8 S 22 22 E
Tsavo East △, Kenya 118 C4 2 44 S 38 47 E
Tsavo West △, Kenya 118 C4 3 19 S 37 57 E
Tsebrykove, Ukraine 59 J6 47 9N 30 10 E
Tselinograd = Astana, Kazakhstan 66 D8 51 10N 71 30 E
Tsementny = Fokino, Russia 58 F8 53 30N 34 22 E
Tsentralnyy □, Russia 60 D4 52 0N 40 0 E
Tses, Namibia 116 D2 25 58 S 18 8 E
Tsetserleg, Mongolia 68 B5 47 36N 101 32 E
Tsévié, Togo 113 D5 6 25N 1 20 E
Tshabong, Botswana 116 D3 26 2 S 22 29 E
Tshabuta, Dem. Rep. of the Congo 115 D4 7 42 S 23 7 E
Tshane, Botswana 116 C3 24 5 S 21 54 E
Tshela, Dem. Rep. of the Congo 115 C2 4 57 S 13 4 E
Tshesebe, Botswana 117 C4 21 51 S 27 32 E
Tshibeke, Dem. Rep. of the Congo 118 C2 2 40 S 28 35 E
Tshibinda, Dem. Rep. of the Congo 118 C2 2 23 S 28 43 E
Tshikapa, Dem. Rep. of the Congo 115 D4 6 28 S 20 48 E
Tshilenge, Dem. Rep. of the Congo 118 D1 6 17 S 23 48 E
Tshindjambo, Dem. Rep. of the Congo 115 E4 10 52 S 22 43 E
Tshinota, Dem. Rep. of the Congo 115 D4 7 2 S 20 58 E
Tshinsenda, Dem. Rep. of the Congo 119 E2 12 20 S 28 0 E
Tshitadi, Dem. Rep. of the Congo 115 D4 6 46 S 21 43 E
Tshofa, Dem. Rep. of the Congo 118 D2 5 13 S 25 16 E
Tshuapa →, Dem. Rep. of the Congo 114 C4 0 14 S 20 42 E
Tshumbiri, Dem. Rep. of the Congo 114 C3 2 38 S 16 18 E
Tshwane, Botswana 116 C3 22 24 S 22 1 E
Tsiaotso = Jiaozuo, China 74 G7 35 16N 113 12 E
Tsigara, Botswana 116 C4 20 22 S 25 54 E
Tsihombe, Madag. 117 D8 25 10 S 45 41 E
Tsiigehtchic, Canada 138 B6 67 15N 134 0W
Tsimlyansk, Russia 61 G6 47 40N 42 6 E
Tsimlyansk Res. = Tsimlyanskoye Vdkhr., Russia 61 F6 48 0N 43 0 E
Tsimlyanskoye Vdkhr., Russia 61 F6 48 0N 43 0 E
Tsinan = Jinan, China 74 F9 36 38N 117 1 E
Tsineng, S. Africa 116 D3 27 5 S 23 5 E
Tsing Yi, China 69 G11 22 21N 114 6 E
Tsínga, Greece 51 E8 41 23N 24 44 E
Tsinghai = Qinghai □, China 68 C4 36 0N 98 0 E
Tsingshih = Jinshi, China 77 C8 29 40N 111 50 E
Tsingtao = Qingdao, China 75 F11 36 5N 120 20 E
Tsingy de Bemaraha △, Madag. 117 B8 18 35 S 45 25 E
Tsingy de Namoroka △, Madag. 117 B8 16 29 S 45 25 E
Tsining = Jining, China 74 G9 35 22N 116 34 E
Tsinjoarivo, Madag. 117 B8 19 37 S 47 40 E
Tsinjomitondraka, Madag. 117 B8 15 40 S 47 8 E
Tsinling Shan = Qinling Shandi, China 74 H5 33 50N 108 10 E
Tsiroanomandidy, Madag. 117 B8 18 46 S 46 2 E
Tsiteli-Tsqaro, Georgia 61 K8 41 33N 46 0 E
Tsitondroina, Madag. 117 C8 21 19 S 46 0 E
Tsitsihar = Qiqihar, China 67 E13 47 26N 124 0 E
Tsitsikamma △, S. Africa 116 E3 34 3 S 23 40 E
Tsivilsk, Russia 60 C8 55 50N 47 25 E
Tsivory, Madag. 117 C8 24 4 S 46 5 E
Tskhinvali, Georgia 61 J7 42 14N 44 1 E
Tsna →, Russia 60 C6 54 55N 41 58 E
Tsnori, Georgia 61 K7 41 40N 45 57 E
Tso Moriri, L., India 93 C8 32 50N 78 20 E
Tsobis, Namibia 116 B2 19 27 S 17 30 E
Tsodilo Hill, Botswana 116 B3 18 49 S 21 43 E
Tsogni, Gabon 114 C2 2 48 S 10 10 E
Tsogttsetsiy = Baruunsuu, Mongolia 74 C3 43 43N 105 35 E
Tsolo, S. Africa 117 E4 31 18 S 28 37 E
Tsomo, S. Africa 117 E4 32 0 S 27 42 E
Tsoukaládes, Greece 39 B2 38 41N 20 47 E
Tsu, Japan 73 C8 34 45N 136 25 E
Tsu L., Canada 142 A6 60 40N 111 52W
Tsubata, Japan 73 A8 36 40N 136 44 E
Tsuchiura, Japan 73 A12 36 5N 140 15 E
Tsuen Wan, China 77 F10 22 22N 114 6 E
Tsugaru-Kaikyō, Japan 70 D10 41 35N 141 0 E
Tsukuba, Japan 73 A12 36 2N 140 4 E
Tsukumi, Japan 72 D3 33 4N 131 52 E
Tsukushi-Sanchi, Japan 72 D2 33 25N 130 30 E
Tsumeb, Namibia 116 B2 19 9 S 17 44 E
Tsumis, Namibia 116 C2 23 39 S 17 29 E
Tsuna, Japan 72 C6 34 28N 134 56 E
Tsuno-Shima, Japan 72 C2 34 21N 130 52 E
Tsuru, Japan 73 B10 35 31N 138 57 E
Tsuruga, Japan 73 B8 35 45N 136 2 E
Tsuruga-Wan, Japan 73 B8 35 50N 136 3 E
Tsurugi, Japan 73 A8 36 29N 136 37 E
Tsurugi-San, Japan 72 D6 33 51N 134 6 E
Tsurumi-Saki, Japan 72 E4 32 56N 132 5 E
Tsuruoka, Japan 70 E9 38 44N 139 50 E
Tsurusaki, Japan 72 D3 33 14N 131 41 E
Tsushima, Ehime, Japan 72 D4 33 7N 132 32 E
Tsushima, Gifu, Japan 73 B8 35 10N 136 43 E
Tsushima, Nagasaki, Japan 72 C1 34 20N 129 20 E
Tsuyama, Japan 72 B6 35 3N 134 0 E
Tsvetkovo, Ukraine 59 H6 49 8N 31 33 E
Tsyelyakhany, Belarus 59 F3 52 30N 25 46 E
Tu →, Burma 90 E6 21 50N 96 15 E
Tua, Dem. Rep. of the Congo 114 C3 3 38 S 16 38 E
Tua →, Papua N. G. 132 D3 6 30 S 144 28 E
Tua →, Portugal 42 D3 41 13N 7 26W
Tuaheni Pt., N.Z. 130 E7 38 43 S 178 4 E
Tuai, N.Z. 130 E6 38 47 S 177 10 E
Tuakau, N.Z. 130 D3 37 16 S 174 59 E
Tual, Indonesia 83 C4 5 38 S 132 44 E
Tuam, Ireland 23 C3 53 31N 8 51W
Tuamarina, N.Z. 131 B8 41 25 S 173 59 E
Tuamotu Arch. = Tuamotu Is., French Polynesia 135 J13 17 0 S 144 0W
Tuamotu Is., French Polynesia 135 J13 17 0 S 144 0W
Tuamotu Ridge, Pac. Oc. 135 K14 20 0 S 138 0W
Tuanfeng, China 77 B10 30 38N 114 52 E
Tuanxi, China 76 D6 27 28N 107 8 E
Tuao, Phil. 80 C3 17 55N 121 22 E
Tuapse, Russia 61 H4 44 5N 39 10 E
Tuas, Singapore 87 d 1 19N 103 39 E
Tuatapere, N.Z. 131 G2 46 8 S 167 41 E
Tuba City, U.S.A. 159 H8 36 8N 111 14W
Tuban, Indonesia 85 D4 6 54 S 112 3 E
Tubani, Botswana 116 C3 24 46 S 24 18 E
Tubarão, Brazil 175 B6 28 30 S 49 0W
Tūbās, West Bank 103 C4 32 20N 35 22 E
Tubas →, Namibia 116 C2 22 54 S 14 35 E
Tubau, Malaysia 85 B4 3 10N 113 40 E
Tubbataha Reefs △, Phil. 81 G2 8 53N 119 53 E
Tubigon, Phil. 81 G4 9 57N 123 58 E
Tübingen, Germany 31 G5 48 31N 9 4 E
Tubod, Phil. 81 G4 8 3N 123 48 E
Tubou, Fiji 133 B3 18 13 S 178 48W
Tubruq, Libya 108 B4 32 7N 23 55 E
Tubruq □, Libya 108 B4 30 0N 24 0 E
Tubuai Is., French Polynesia 135 K13 25 0 S 150 0W
Tuburan, Basilan, Phil. 81 H4 6 39N 122 16 E
Tuburan, Cebu, Phil. 81 F4 10 44N 123 49 E
Tuc Trung, Vietnam 87 G6 11 1N 107 12 E
Tucacas, Venezuela 168 A4 10 48N 68 19W
Tucano, Brazil 170 D4 10 58 S 38 48W
T'uch'ang, Taiwan 77 E13 24 42N 121 25 E
Tuchodi →, Canada 142 B4 58 17N 123 42W
Tuchola, Poland 54 E4 53 33N 17 52 E
Tuchów, Poland 55 J8 49 54N 21 1 E
Tuckanarra, Australia 125 E2 27 7 S 118 5 E
Tucker, U.S.A. 152 B5 33 51N 84 13W
Tuckers Town, Bermuda 9 a 32 20N 64 42W
Tucson, U.S.A. 159 K8 32 13N 110 58W
Tucumán □, Argentina 174 B2 26 48 S 66 2W
Tucumcari, U.S.A. 155 H3 35 10N 103 44W
Tucunaré, Brazil 173 B6 5 18 S 55 51W
Tucupido, Venezuela 168 B4 9 17N 65 47W
Tucupita, Venezuela 169 B5 9 2N 62 3W
Tucuruí, Brazil 170 B2 3 42 S 49 44W
Tucuruí, Represa de, Brazil 170 B2 4 0 S 49 30W
Tuczno, Poland 55 E3 53 13N 16 10 E
Tuddal, Norway 18 E5 59 46N 8 49 E
Tudela, Spain 40 C3 42 4N 1 39W
Tudmur, Syria 101 E8 34 36N 38 15 E
Tudor, L., Canada 141 A6 55 50N 65 25W
Tudora, Romania 53 C11 47 31N 26 45 E
Tuella →, Portugal 42 D3 41 30N 7 12W
Tuen Mun, China 69 G10 22 24N 113 59 E
Tueré →, Brazil 170 B1 2 48 S 50 59W
Tuffer = Laško, Slovenia 45 B12 46 10N 15 16 E
Tufi, Papua N. G. 132 E5 9 8 S 149 19 E
Tufsingdalen, Norway 18 B8 62 18N 11 44 E
Tugalan = Kolkhozobod, Tajikistan 65 E4 37 35N 68 40 E
Tugela →, S. Africa 117 D5 29 14 S 31 30 E
Tugidak I., U.S.A. 144 H9 56 30N 154 40W
Tuguegarao, Phil. 80 C3 17 35N 121 42 E
Tugur, Russia 67 D14 53 44N 136 45 E
Tui, Spain 42 C2 42 3N 8 39W
Tuineje, Canary Is. 9 e2 28 19N 14 3W
Tukangbesi, Kepulauan, Indonesia 82 C2 6 0 S 124 0 E
Tukarak I., Canada 140 A4 56 15N 78 45W
Tukayyid, Iraq 96 D5 29 47N 45 36 E
Tûkh, Egypt 106 H7 30 21N 31 12 E
Tukhlya, Ukraine 53 B8 48 55N 23 28 E
Tukituki →, N.Z. 130 F5 39 36 S 176 56 E
Tukkae, Ao, Thailand 87 a 7 51N 98 25 E
Tukobo, Ghana 112 D4 5 1N 2 47W
Tūkrah, Libya 108 B4 32 30N 20 37 E
Tuktoyaktuk, Canada 138 B6 69 27N 133 2W
Tukums, Latvia 15 H20 56 58N 23 10 E
Tukums □, Latvia 54 B10 56 55N 23 0 E
Tukuran, Phil. 81 H4 7 51N 123 34 E
Tukuyu, Tanzania 119 D3 9 17 S 33 35 E
Tula, Hidalgo, Mexico 163 C5 20 5N 99 20W
Tula, Tamaulipas, Mexico 163 C5 23 0N 99 40W
Tula, Nigeria 113 D7 9 51N 11 27 E
Tula, Russia 58 E9 54 13N 37 38 E
Tulagi, Solomon Is. 133 M11 9 5 S 160 10 E
Tülak, Afghan. 91 B1 33 55N 63 40 E
Tulancingo, Mexico 163 C5 20 5N 99 22W
Tulangbawang →, Indonesia 84 C3 4 24 S 105 52 E
Tulare, Serbia & M. 50 D5 42 48N 21 28 E
Tulare, U.S.A. 160 J7 36 13N 119 21W
Tulare Lake Bed, U.S.A. 160 K7 36 0N 119 48W
Tularosa, U.S.A. 159 K10 33 5N 106 1W
Tulbagh, S. Africa 116 E2 33 16 S 19 6 E
Tulcán, Ecuador 168 C2 0 48N 77 43W
Tulcea, Romania 53 E13 45 13N 28 46 E
Tulcea □, Romania 53 E13 45 0N 28 30 E
Tulchyn, Ukraine 53 B13 48 41N 28 49 E
Tūleh, Iran 97 C7 34 35N 52 33 E
Tulemalu L., Canada 143 A9 62 58N 99 25W
Tulgheş, Romania 53 D10 46 58N 25 45 E
Tuli, Zimbabwe 119 G2 21 58 S 29 13 E
Tulia, U.S.A. 155 H4 34 32N 101 46W
Tuliszków, Poland 55 F5 52 5N 18 18 E
Tulita, Canada 138 B7 64 57N 125 30W
Ţulkarm, West Bank 103 C4 32 19N 35 2 E
Tülkibas, Kazakhstan 65 B5 42 29N 70 17 E
Tulla, Ireland 23 D3 52 53N 8 46W
Tullahoma, U.S.A. 149 H2 35 22N 86 13W
Tullamore, Australia 129 B7 32 39 S 147 36 E
Tullamore, Ireland 23 C4 53 16N 7 31W
Tulle, France 28 C5 45 16N 1 46 E
Tulln, Austria 34 C9 48 20N 16 4 E
Tullow, Ireland 23 D5 52 49N 6 45W
Tullus, Sudan 107 E1 11 7N 24 31 E
Tully, Australia 126 B4 17 56 S 145 55 E
Tully, U.S.A. 151 D8 42 48N 76 7W
Ţulmaythah, Libya 108 B4 32 40N 20 55 E
Tulnici, Romania 53 E11 45 51N 26 38 E
Tulovo, Bulgaria 51 D9 42 33N 25 32 E
Tulsa, U.S.A. 155 G7 36 10N 95 55W
Tulsequah, Canada 142 B2 58 39N 133 35W
Tulu Milki, Ethiopia 107 F4 9 55N 38 20 E
Tulu Welel, Ethiopia 107 F3 8 56N 34 47 E
Tulua, Colombia 168 C2 4 6N 76 11W
Tuluceşti, Romania 53 E13 45 34N 28 2 E
Tuluksak, U.S.A. 144 F7 61 6N 160 58W
Tulun, Russia 67 D11 54 32N 100 35 E
Tulungagung, Indonesia 85 D4 8 5 S 111 54 E
Tuma, Russia 58 E11 55 10N 40 30 E
Tuma →, Nic. 164 D3 13 6N 84 35W
Tumacacori △, U.S.A. 159 L8 31 34N 111 3W
Tumaco, Colombia 168 C2 1 50N 78 45W
Tumaco, Ensenada, Colombia 168 C2 1 55N 78 45W
Tumatumari, Guyana 169 B6 5 20N 58 55W
Tumauini, Phil. 80 C3 17 17N 121 49 E
Tumba, Dem. Rep. of the Congo 114 C4 3 10 S 23 36 E
Tumba, Sweden 16 E11 59 12N 17 48 E
Tumba, L., Dem. Rep. of the Congo 114 C3 0 50 S 18 0 E
Tumbarumba, Australia 129 C8 35 44 S 148 0 E
Tumbaya, Argentina 174 A2 23 50 S 65 26W
Tumbes, Peru 172 A1 3 37 S 80 27W
Tumbes □, Peru 172 A1 3 50 S 80 30W
Tumbur, Sudan 107 G3 4 20N 31 34 E
Tumbwe, Dem. Rep. of the Congo 119 E2 11 25 S 27 15 E
Tumby Bay, Australia 128 C2 34 21 S 136 8 E
Tumd Youqi, China 74 D6 40 30N 110 30 E
Tumen, China 75 C15 43 0N 129 50 E
Tumen Jiang →, China 75 C16 42 20N 130 35 E
Tumeremo, Venezuela 169 B5 7 18N 61 30W
Tumiritinga, Brazil 171 E3 18 58 S 41 38W
Tumkur, India 95 H3 13 18N 77 6 E
Tump, Pakistan 91 D1 26 7N 62 16 E
Tumpat, Malaysia 87 J4 6 11N 102 10 E
Tumsar, India 94 D4 21 26N 79 45 E
Tumu, Ghana 112 C4 10 56N 1 56W
Tumucumaque, Serra, Brazil 169 C7 2 0N 55 0W
Tumupasa, Bolivia 172 C4 14 9 S 67 55W
Tumut, Australia 129 C8 35 16 S 148 13 E
Tumwater, U.S.A. 160 C4 47 1N 122 54W
Tuna, India 92 H4 22 59N 70 5 E
Tunadal, Sweden 16 B11 62 26N 17 22 E
Tunapuna, Trin. & Tob. 169 F9 10 38N 61 24W
Tunas de Zaza, Cuba 164 B4 21 39N 79 34W
Tunbridge Wells = Royal Tunbridge Wells, U.K. 21 F8 51 7N 0 16 E
Tunçbilek, Turkey 49 B11 39 37N 29 29 E
Tunceli, Turkey 101 C8 39 6N 39 31 E
Tuncurry, Australia 129 B10 32 17 S 152 29 E
Tundla, India 92 F8 27 12N 78 17 E
Tundubai, Sudan 106 D2 18 36N 28 35 E
Tunduru, Tanzania 119 E4 11 8 S 37 25 E
Tundzha →, Bulgaria 51 E10 41 40N 26 35 E
Tung Chung, China 69 G10 22 17N 113 57 E
Tung Lung Chau, China 69 G11 22 15N 114 17 E
Tunga →, India 95 G2 15 0N 75 50 E
Tunga Pass, India 90 A5 29 0N 94 14 E
Tungabhadra →, India 95 G4 15 57N 78 15 E
Tungabhadra Dam, India 95 G2 15 0N 75 50 E
Tungaru, Sudan 107 E3 10 9N 30 52 E
Tungawan, Phil. 81 H4 7 30N 122 20 E
Tungch'uan = Dongchuan, China 76 D4 26 8N 103 1 E
Tunghwa = Tonghua, China 75 D13 41 42N 125 58 E
Tungi, Bangla. 90 D3 23 53N 90 24 E
Tungla, Nic. 164 D3 13 24N 84 21W
Tungnafellsjökull, Iceland 11 C9 64 45N 17 55W
Tungsha Tao = Dongsha Dao, China 77 G11 20 45N 116 43 E
Tungshih, Taiwan 77 E13 24 12N 120 43 E
Tungsten, Canada 142 A3 61 57N 128 16W
Tungufell, Iceland 11 C6 64 17N 20 10W
Tungurahua □, Ecuador 168 D2 1 15 S 78 35W
Tunguska, Nizhnyaya →, Russia 67 C9 65 48N 88 4 E
Tunguska, Podkamennaya →, Russia 67 C10 61 50N 90 13 E
Tuni, India 94 F6 17 22N 82 36 E
Tunia, Colombia 168 C2 2 41N 76 31W
Tunica, U.S.A. 155 H9 34 41N 90 23W
Tunis, Tunisia 108 A2 36 50N 10 11 E
Tunis ✈ (TUN), Tunisia 46 F3 36 52N 10 14 E
Tunis, Golfe de, Tunisia 108 A2 37 0N 10 30 E
Tunisia ■, Africa 108 B1 33 30N 9 10 E
Tunja, Colombia 168 B3 5 33N 73 25W
Tunkhannock, U.S.A. 151 E9 41 32N 75 57W
Tunliu, China 74 F7 36 13N 112 52 E
Tunnel Creek △, Australia 124 C4 17 41 S 125 18 E
Tunnsjøen, Norway 14 D15 64 45N 13 25 E
Tunø, Denmark 17 J4 55 57N 10 27 E
Tuntutuliak, U.S.A. 144 F7 60 22N 162 38W
Tununak, U.S.A. 144 F6 60 37N 165 15W
Tunungayualok I., Canada 141 A7 56 0N 61 0W
Tunuyán, Argentina 174 C2 33 35 S 69 0W
Tunuyán →, Argentina 174 C2 33 33 S 67 30W
Tuo Jiang →, China 76 C5 28 50N 105 35 E
Tuolumne, U.S.A. 160 H6 37 58N 120 15W
Tuolumne →, U.S.A. 160 H5 37 36N 121 13W
Tüp, Kyrgyzstan 65 B9 42 45N 78 20 E
Tūp Āghāj, Iran 101 D12 36 3N 47 50 E
Tupã, Brazil 175 A5 21 57 S 50 28W
Tupaciguara, Brazil 171 E2 18 35 S 48 42W
Tupelo, U.S.A. 149 H1 34 16N 88 43W
Tupik, Russia 58 E7 55 42N 33 22 E
Tupinambaranas, Brazil 169 D6 3 0 S 58 0W
Tupirama, Brazil 170 C2 8 58 S 48 12W
Tupiratins, Brazil 170 C2 8 23 S 48 8W
Tupiza, Bolivia 174 A2 21 30 S 65 40W
Tupižnica, Serbia & M. 50 C6 43 43N 22 10 E
Tupman, U.S.A. 161 K7 35 18N 119 21W
Tupper, Canada 142 B4 55 32N 120 1W
Tupper Lake, U.S.A. 151 B10 44 14N 74 28W
Tupungato, Cerro, S. Amer. 174 C2 33 15 S 69 50W
Tuquan, China 75 B11 45 18N 121 38 E
Túquerres, Colombia 168 C2 1 5N 77 37W
Tura, India 90 C3 25 30N 90 16 E
Tura, Russia 67 C11 64 20N 100 17 E
Turabah, Ḥā'il, Si. Arabia 96 D4 28 20N 43 15 E
Turabah, Makkah, Si. Arabia 98 B3 21 15N 41 34 E
Turagua, Serranía, Venezuela 169 B5 7 20N 64 35W
Turakina, N.Z. 130 G4 40 3 S 175 16 E
Turakina →, N.Z. 130 G4 40 5 S 175 8 E
Turakirae Hd., N.Z. 130 H3 41 26 S 174 56 E
Turakŭrghan, Uzbekistan 65 C5 41 0N 71 31 E
Turama →, Papua N. G. 132 D2 7 40 S 143 50 E
Turān, Iran 97 C8 35 39N 56 42 E
Turan, Russia 67 D10 51 55N 95 0 E
Turangi, N.Z. 130 E4 38 59 S 175 48 E
Turar Rysqulov, Kazakhstan 65 B5 42 32N 70 20 E
Ţurayf, Si. Arabia 96 D3 31 41N 38 39 E
Turbaco, Colombia 168 A2 10 21N 75 25W
Turbacz, Poland 55 J7 49 30N 20 8 E
Turbat, Pakistan 91 D1 25 59N 63 4 E
Turbe, Bos.-H. 52 F2 44 15N 17 35 E
Turbenthal, Switz. 33 B7 47 27N 8 51 E
Turbeville, U.S.A. 152 B9 33 54N 80 1W
Turbo, Colombia 168 B2 8 6N 76 43W
Turčianske Teplice, Slovak Rep. 35 C11 48 52N 18 52 E
Turco, Bolivia 172 D4 18 10 S 68 11W
Turcoaia, Romania 53 E13 45 7N 28 11 E
Turda, Romania 53 D8 46 34N 23 47 E
Turek, Poland 55 F5 52 3N 18 30 E
Turfan = Turpan, China 68 B3 43 58N 89 10 E
Turfan Basin = Turpan Pendi, China 62 E12 42 40N 89 25 E
Turfan Depression = Turpan Pendi, China 62 E12 42 40N 89 25 E
Turgayskaya Stolovaya Strana, Asia 64 F8 51 0N 63 0 E
Turgeon →, Canada 140 C4 50 0N 78 56W
Tŭrgovishte, Bulgaria 51 C10 43 17N 26 38 E
Turgut, Turkey 49 D10 37 22N 28 4 E
Turgutlu, Turkey 49 C9 38 30N 27 43 E
Turgwe →, Zimbabwe 117 C5 21 31 S 32 15 E
Turhal, Turkey 100 B7 40 24N 36 5 E
Turia →, Spain 41 F4 39 27N 0 19W
Turiaçu, Brazil 170 B2 1 40 S 45 19W
Turiaçu →, Brazil 170 B2 1 36 S 45 19W
Turiec →, Slovak Rep. 35 B11 49 7N 18 55 E
Turin = Torino, Italy 44 C4 45 3N 7 40 E
Turinsk, Russia 64 B9 58 3N 63 42 E
Turinskaya Kultbaza = Tura, Russia 67 C11 64 20N 100 17 E
Turka, Ukraine 55 J10 49 10N 23 2 E
Turkana, L., Africa 118 B4 3 30N 36 5 E
Türkeli, Turkey 51 F11 40 30N 27 30 E
Turkestan = Türkistan, Kazakhstan 65 B4 43 17N 68 16 E
Turkestan Range, Asia 65 D4 39 35N 69 0 E
Túrkeve, Hungary 52 C5 47 6N 20 44 E
Turkey ■, Eurasia 100 C7 39 0N 36 0 E
Turkey →, U.S.A. 156 B5 42 43N 91 2W
Turkey Creek, Australia 124 C4 17 2 S 128 12 E
Turki, Russia 60 D6 52 0N 43 15 E
Türkistan, Kazakhstan 65 B4 43 17N 68 16 E
Türkmenbashi, Turkmenistan 57 G9 40 5N 53 5 E
Turkmenistan ■, Asia 66 F6 39 0N 59 0 E
Türkmenli, Turkey 49 B8 39 45N 26 30 E
Türkoğlu, Turkey 100 D7 37 23N 36 50 E
Turks & Caicos Is. ☑, W. Indies 165 B5 21 20N 71 20W
Turks Island Passage, W. Indies 165 B5 21 30N 71 30W
Turku, Finland 15 F20 60 30N 22 19 E
Turkwel →, Kenya 118 B4 3 6N 36 6 E
Turlock, U.S.A. 160 H6 37 30N 120 51W
Turnagain →, Canada 142 B3 59 12N 127 35W
Turnagain, C., N.Z. 130 G5 40 28 S 176 38 E
Turneffe Is., Belize 163 D7 17 20N 87 50W
Turner, U.S.A. 158 B9 48 51N 108 24W
Turner Pt., Australia 126 A1 11 47 S 133 32 E
Turner Valley, Canada 142 C6 50 40N 114 17W
Turners Falls, U.S.A. 151 D12 42 36N 72 33W
Turnhout, Belgium 24 C4 51 19N 4 57 E
Türnitz, Austria 34 D8 47 55N 15 29 E
Turnor L., Canada 143 B7 56 35N 108 35W
Turnov, Czech Rep. 34 A8 50 34N 15 10 E
Tŭrnovo = Veliko Tŭrnovo, Bulgaria 51 C9 43 5N 25 41 E
Turnu Măgurele, Romania 53 G9 43 46N 24 56 E
Turnu Roşu, P., Romania 53 E9 45 33N 24 17 E
Turobin, Poland 55 H9 50 50N 22 44 E
Tuross Head, Australia 129 D9 36 3 S 150 8 E
Turpan, China 68 B3 43 58N 89 10 E
Turpan Pendi, China 62 E12 42 40N 89 25 E
Turrawan, Australia 129 A8 30 28 S 149 53 E
Turrës, Kala e, Albania 50 E3 41 10N 19 28 E
Turriff, U.K. 22 D6 57 32N 2 27W
Tursāq, Iraq 101 F11 33 27N 45 47 E
Tursi, Italy 47 B9 40 15N 16 28 E
Tursunzade, Tajikistan 65 D4 38 30N 68 14 E
Turtle Head I., Australia 126 A3 10 56 S 142 37 E
Turtle Is., Phil. 81 H2 6 7N 118 14 E
Turtle Is., S. Leone 112 D2 7 40N 13 0 E
Turtle L., Canada 143 C7 53 36N 108 38W
Turtle Lake, U.S.A. 154 B4 47 31N 100 53W
Turtleford, Canada 143 C7 53 23N 108 57W
Turtucaia = Tutrakan, Bulgaria 51 B10 44 2N 26 40 E
Turua, N.Z. 130 D4 37 14 S 175 35 E
Turuépano △, Venezuela 165 D7 10 34N 62 43W
Turugart Pass, Kyrgyzstan 65 C7 40 32N 75 24 E
Turukhansk, Russia 67 C9 65 21N 88 5 E

Turyinskiye Rudniki =
  Krasnoturinsk,
  Russia .... **64 B8** 59 46N 60 12 E
Turzovka, *Slovak Rep.* . **35 B11** 49 25N 18 35 E
Tuscaloosa, *U.S.A.* **149 J2** 33 12N 87 34W
Tuscánia, *Italy* .... **45 F8** 42 25N 11 52 E
Tuscany = Toscana □,
  Italy .... **44 E8** 43 25N 11 0 E
Tuscarawas ➔, *U.S.A.* . **150 F3** 40 24N 81 25W
Tuscarora Mt., *U.S.A.* . **150 F7** 40 55N 77 55W
Tuscola, *Ill., U.S.A.* ... **157 E8** 39 48N 88 17W
Tuscola, *Tex., U.S.A.* .. **155 J5** 32 12N 99 48W
Tuscumbia, Ala., U.S.A. **149 H2** 34 44N 87 42W
Tuscumbia, Mo., U.S.A. **156 F4** 38 14N 92 28W
Tuskegee, *U.S.A.* **152 C4** 32 25N 85 42W
Tusket Wedge =
  Wedgeport, *Canada* **141 D6** 43 44N 65 59W
Tustin, *U.S.A.* **161 M9** 33 44N 117 49W
Tustna, *Norway* ...... **18 A5** 63 10N 8 5 E
Tuszyn, *Poland* ...... **55 G6** 51 36N 19 33 E
Tutak, *Turkey* .... **101 C10** 39 32N 42 46 E
Tutayev, *Russia* ...... **58 D10** 57 53N 39 32 E
Tuticorin, *India* ...... **95 K4** 8 50N 78 12 E
Tutin, *Serbia & M.* .... **50 D4** 42 58N 20 20 E
Tutóia, *Brazil* .... **170 B3** 2 45 S 42 20W
Tutong, *Brunei* ...... **85 B4** 4 47N 114 40 E
Tutova ➔, *Romania* .. **53 D12** 46 7N 27 30 E
Tutrakan, *Bulgaria* ... **51 B10** 44 2N 26 40 E
Tuttle Creek L., *U.S.A.* **154 F6** 39 22N 96 40W
Tuttlingen, *Germany* . **31 H4** 47 58N 8 48 E
Tutuala, *E. Timor* ..... **83 C3** 8 25 S 127 15 E
Tutuala, *E. Timor* ..... **83 C3** 8 25 S 127 15 E
Tutubeia, Papua N. G. **132 E6** 9 34 S 150 40 E
Tutuila, *Amer. Samoa* **133 X24** 14 19 S 170 50W
Tutuko, Mt., N.Z. ..... **131 E3** 44 35 S 168 1 E
Tutun, *Egypt* .... **106 J7** 29 9N 30 46 E
Tututepec, *Mexico* ... **163 D5** 16 9N 97 38W
Tütz = Tuczno, Poland **55 E3** 53 13N 16 10 E
Tuva □, *Russia* ...... **67 D10** 51 30N 95 0 E
Tuvalu ■, *Pac. Oc.* ... **134 H9** 8 0 S 178 0 E
Tuvuca, Fiji .... **133 A3** 17 40 S 178 48W
Tūwal, *Si. Arabia* .... **98 B2** 22 17N 39 6 E
Tuxer Alpen, *Austria* . **34 D4** 47 10N 11 45 E
Tuxpan, *Mexico* **163 C5** 20 58N 97 23W
Tuxtla Gutiérrez,
  Mexico **163 D6** 16 50N 93 10W
Tuy = Tui, Spain **42 C2** 42 3N 8 39W
Tuy An, *Vietnam* ...... **86 F7** 13 17N 109 16 E
Tuy Duc, *Vietnam* ..... **87 F6** 12 15N 107 27 E
Tuy Hoa, *Vietnam* ..... **86 F7** 13 5N 109 10 E
Tuy Phong, *Vietnam* .. **87 G7** 11 14N 108 43 E
Tuya L., *Canada* **142 B2** 59 7N 130 35W
Tuyen Hoa, *Vietnam* .. **86 D6** 17 50N 106 10 E
Tuyen Quang, *Vietnam* **76 G5** 21 50N 105 10 E
Tuymazy, *Russia* ..... **64 D4** 54 36N 53 42 E
Tuyun = Duyun, China **76 D6** 26 18N 107 29 E
Tuz Gölü, *Turkey* .... **100 C5** 38 42N 33 18 E
Tūz Khurmātū =
  Tozkhurmato, *Iraq* . **101 E11** 34 56N 44 38 E
Tuzi, *Serbia & M.* ..... **50 D3** 42 22N 19 20 E
Tuzigoot △, *U.S.A.* ... **159 J7** 34 46N 112 2W
Tuzla, Bos.-H. .... **52 F3** 44 34N 18 41 E
Tuzlov ➔, *Russia* ..... **59 J10** 47 17N 39 57 E
Tuzluca, *Turkey* ...... **101 B10** 40 3N 43 39 E
Tuzly, *Ukraine* ...... **53 E15** 45 54N 30 6 E
Tvååker, *Sweden* ..... **17 G6** 57 4N 12 25 E
Tvärditsa, *Bulgaria* ... **51 D9** 42 42N 25 53 E
Tved, *Moldova* ...... **53 D13** 46 9N 28 58 E
Tvedestrand, *Norway* . **18 F5** 58 38N 8 58 E
Tver, *Russia* .... **58 D8** 56 55N 35 55 E
Tvrdošín, Slovak Rep. . **35 B12** 49 21N 19 35 E
Tvrdošovce,
  Slovak Rep. ...... **35 C11** 48 6N 18 4 E
Tvŭrditsa, *Bulgaria* ... **51 D9** 42 42N 25 53 E
Twain, *U.S.A.* **160 E5** 40 1N 121 3W
Twain Harte, *U.S.A.* .. **160 G6** 38 2N 120 14W
Twann, *Switz.* .... **32 B4** 47 6N 7 9 E
Twardogóra, *Poland* .. **55 G4** 51 23N 17 28 E
Tweed ➔, *Canada* **150 B7** 44 29N 77 19W
Tweed ➔, *U.K.* **22 F6** 55 45N 2 0W
Tweed Heads, Australia **127 D5** 28 10 S 153 31 E
Tweedsmuir ➔, Canada **142 C3** 54 0N 126 20W
Twentynine Palms,
  U.S.A. **161 L10** 34 8N 116 3W
Tweya, Dem. Rep. of
  the Congo .... **114 C3** 0 54 S 18 58 E
Twillingate, Canada ... **141 C9** 49 42N 54 45W
Twin Bridges, U.S.A. .. **158 D7** 45 33N 112 20W
Twin City, *U.S.A.* **152 C7** 32 35N 82 10W
Twin Falls, Canada **141 B7** 53 30N 64 32W
Twin Falls, U.S.A. **158 E6** 42 34N 114 28W
Twin Hills, *U.S.A.* **144 G8** 59 23N 159 58W
Twin Lakes, U.S.A. **152 E6** 30 43N 83 13W
Twin Valley, U.S.A. ... **154 B6** 47 16N 96 16W
Twinnge, Burma ...... **90 D6** 23 10N 96 2 E
Twinsburg, U.S.A. **150 E3** 41 18N 81 26W
Twistringen, Germany . **30 C4** 52 48N 8 37 E
Twitchell Reservoir,
  U.S.A. **161 L6** 34 59N 120 19W
Two Boats Village,
  Ascension I. ...... **9 g** 7 56 S 14 22W
Two Harbors, U.S.A. .. **154 B9** 47 2N 91 40W
Two Hills, Canada **142 C6** 53 43N 111 52W
Two Rivers, U.S.A. **148 C2** 44 9N 87 34W
Two Rocks, Australia .. **125 F2** 31 30 S 115 35 E
Two Thumbs Ra., N.Z. **131 D5** 43 45 S 170 44 E
Twofold B., Australia .. **129 D8** 37 8 S 149 59 E
Ty Ty, *U.S.A.* **152 D6** 31 28N 83 39W
Tyachiv, *Ukraine* .... **59 H2** 48 1N 23 35 E
Tybee Island, U.S.A. .. **152 C9** 32 1N 80 51W
Tychy, *Poland* ...... **55 H5** 50 9N 18 59 E
Tyczyn, *Poland* ...... **55 J9** 49 58N 22 2 E
Tydal, *Norway* ...... **18 A3** 63 4N 11 34 E
Tyin, *Norway* .... **18 C5** 61 18N 8 15 E
Tykocin, *Poland* ..... **55 E9** 53 13N 22 46 E
Tyler, Minn., U.S.A. .. **154 C6** 44 18N 96 8W
Tyler, Tex., U.S.A. **155 J7** 32 21N 95 18W
Tyligul ➔, *Ukraine* .. **59 J6** 47 4N 30 57 E
Tylldal, *Norway* ..... **18 B7** 62 4N 10 48 E
Tymanivka, *Ukraine* . **53 B14** 48 34N 28 50 E
Týn nad Vltavou,
  Czech Rep. ...... **34 B7** 49 13N 14 26 E
Tynda, *Russia* ...... **67 D13** 55 10N 124 43 E
Tyndall, *U.S.A.* **154 D6** 43 0N 97 50W
Tyndinsky = Tynda,
  Russia .... **67 D13** 55 10N 124 43 E
Tyne ➔, *U.K.* **20 C6** 54 59N 1 32W
Tyne & Wear □, U.K. . **20 B6** 55 6N 1 17W
Týnec nad Sázavou,
  Czech Rep. ...... **34 B7** 49 50N 14 36 E
Tynemouth, *U.K.* **20 B6** 55 1N 1 26W
Tynset, *Norway* ...... **18 B7** 62 17N 10 47 E
Tyonek, *U.S.A.* **144 F10** 61 4N 151 8W
Tyre = Sūr, Lebanon .. **103 B4** 33 19N 35 16 E
Tyresta, *Sweden* ..... **16 E12** 59 12N 18 14 E
Tyrifjorden, *Norway* .. **18 D7** 60 2N 10 8 E
Tyringe, *Sweden* ..... **17 H7** 56 9N 13 35 E
Tyristrand, *Norway* ... **18 D7** 60 4N 10 6 E
Tyrnavaz, *Russia* .... **59 J7** 43 21N 42 45 E
Tyrol = Tirol □, Austria **34 D3** 47 3N 10 43 E
Tyrone, U.S.A. **150 F6** 40 40N 78 14W
Tyrone □, *U.K.* **23 B4** 54 38N 7 11W
Tyrrell ➔, Australia ... **128 C5** 35 26 S 142 51 E
Tyrrell, L., Australia ... **128 C5** 35 20 S 142 50 E
Tyrrell L., Canada **143 A7** 63 7N 105 27W
Tyrrhenian Sea,
  Medit. S. .... **12 G8** 40 0N 12 30 E
Tysfjorden, *Norway* .. **14 B17** 68 7N 16 25 E
Tysmenytsya, *Ukraine* **53 B9** 48 54N 24 51 E
Tysnes, *Norway* ...... **18 D2** 60 1N 5 30 E
Tysnesøya, *Norway* ... **18 D2** 60 0N 5 35 E
Tysse, *Norway* ...... **18 D2** 60 23N 5 47 E
Tyssedal, *Norway* .... **18 D3** 60 7N 6 35 E
Tystberga, *Sweden* ... **17 F11** 58 51N 17 15 E
Tytuvėnai, *Lithuania* . **54 C10** 55 36N 23 12 E
Tyub Karagan, Mys,
  Kazakhstan ...... **61 H10** 44 40N 50 19 E
Tyuleni, Ostrova,
  Kazakhstan ...... **61 H10** 45 20N 50 16 E
Tyuleniy, *Russia* ..... **61 H8** 44 28N 47 30 E
Tyuleniy, Mys,
  Azerbaijan .... **61 K10** 40 12N 50 22 E
Tyulgan, *Russia* ..... **64 E6** 52 22N 56 12 E
Tyumen, *Russia* ..... **66 D7** 57 11N 65 29 E
Tyumen-Aryk =
  Tömenaryk,
  Kazakhstan ...... **65 A3** 44 2N 67 1 E
Tyup = Tüp,
  Kyrgyzstan .... **65 B9** 42 45N 78 20 E
Tywi ➔, *U.K.* **21 F3** 51 48N 4 21W
Tywyn, *U.K.* **21 E3** 52 35N 4 5W
Tzaneen, S. Africa .... **117 C5** 23 47 S 30 9 E
Tzermiádhes, *Greece* . **39 E6** 35 12N 25 29 E
Tzia = Kéa, Greece .... **48 D6** 37 35N 24 22 E
Tzoumérka, Óros,
  Greece .... **48 B3** 39 30N 21 26 E
Tzukong = Zigong,
  China .... **76 C5** 29 15N 104 48 E
Tzupo = Boshan, China **75 F9** 36 28N 117 49 E

U

U Taphao, *Thailand* .. **86 F3** 12 35N 101 0 E
U.S.A. = United States
  of America ■,
  N. Amer. **137 F10** 37 0N 96 0W
U.S.S. Arizona △,
  U.S.A. **145 K14** 21 22N 157 57W
U.S. Virgin Is. ☑,
  W. Indies .... **165 e** 18 20N 65 0W
Uacalla Iero,
  Somali Rep. ...... **120 D2** 1 48N 42 38 E
Uachadi, Sierra =
  Uasadi-jidi,
  Venezuela **169 C4** 4 54N 65 18W
Uad Atui ➔,
  W. Sahara **110 D2** 20 4N 15 59W
Uad el Jat ➔,
  W. Sahara **110 C2** 26 47N 13 3W
Uad Erni, O. ➔,
  W. Sahara **110 D2** 26 45N 10 47W
Uainambi, Colombia .. **168 C4** 1 43N 69 51W
Uamba, Angola ...... **115 D3** 7 21 S 16 10 E
Uanle Uen,
  Somali Rep. ...... **120 D2** 2 37N 44 54 E
Uarsciek, Somali Rep. . **120 D3** 2 28N 45 55 E
Uasadi-jidi, Venezuela **169 C4** 4 54N 65 18W
Uascen, Somali Rep. .. **120 D2** 4 11N 43 13 E
Uatumã ➔, Brazil .... **169 D6** 2 26 S 57 37W
Uauá, Brazil .... **170 C4** 9 50 S 39 28W
Uaupés, Brazil ...... **168 D4** 0 8 S 67 5W
Uaupés ➔, Brazil **168 C4** 0 2N 67 16W
Uaxactún, Guatemala . **164 C2** 17 25N 89 29W
Ub, Serbia & M. ...... **50 B4** 44 28N 20 6 E
Uba, Brazil .... **171 F3** 21 8 S 43 0W
Uba, Nigeria .... **113 C7** 10 29N 13 13 E
Ubai, Papua N. G. .... **132 C6** 5 39 S 150 38 E
Ubaitaba, Brazil ...... **171 D4** 14 18 S 39 20W
Ubajara △, Brazil .... **170 B3** 3 55 S 40 50W
Ubangi = Oubangi ➔,
  Dem. Rep. of
  the Congo .... **114 C3** 0 30 S 17 50 E
Ubaté, Colombia **168 B3** 5 19N 73 49W
Ubauro, Pakistan ..... **92 E3** 28 15N 69 45 E
Ubay, Phil. .... **81 F5** 10 3N 124 28 E
Ubaye ➔, France .... **29 D10** 44 28N 6 18 E
Ubayyiḍ, W. al ➔, Iraq **101 F10** 32 34N 43 48 E
Ube, Japan .... **72 D3** 33 56N 131 15 E
Úbeda, Spain **43 G7** 38 3N 3 23W
Uberaba, Brazil ...... **171 E2** 19 50 S 47 55W
Uberaba, L., Brazil ... **173 D6** 17 30 S 57 50W
Uberlândia,
  Minas Gerais, Brazil **171 E2** 19 0 S 48 20W
Uberlândia, Roraima,
  Brazil **169 C6** 0 48N 59 20W
Überlingen, Germany . **31 H5** 47 46N 9 10 E
Überlinger See,
  Germany .... **33 A8** 47 45N 9 9 E
Ubiaja, Nigeria ...... **113 D6** 6 41N 6 22 E
Ubin, Pulau, Singapore **87 d** 1 25N 103 56 E
Ubolratna Res.,
  Thailand .... **86 D4** 16 45N 102 30 E
Ubombo, S. Africa .... **117 D5** 27 31 S 32 4 E
Ubon Ratchathani,
  Thailand .... **86 E5** 15 15N 104 50 E
Ubondo, Dem. Rep. of
  the Congo .... **118 C2** 0 55 S 25 42 E
Ubort ➔, Belarus .... **59 F5** 52 6N 28 30 E
Ubrique, Spain **43 J5** 36 41N 5 27W
Ubud, Indonesia ..... **79 J18** 8 30 S 115 16 E
Ubuna, Solomon Is. .. **133 N11** 10 11 S 161 24 E
Ubundu, Dem. Rep. of
  the Congo .... **118 C2** 0 22 S 25 30 E
Ucayali ➔, Peru ...... **172 A3** 4 30 S 73 30W
Uchab, Namibia ...... **116 B2** 19 47 S 17 42 E
Uchaly, Russia ...... **64 D7** 54 19N 59 27 E
Uchiko, Japan ...... **72 D4** 33 33N 132 39 E
Uchiura-Wan, Japan .. **70 C10** 42 25N 140 40 E
Uchiza, Peru .... **172 B2** 8 25 S 76 20W
Uchquduq, Uzbekistan **66 E7** 41 50N 62 50 E
Uchqŭrghon,
  Uzbekistan .... **65 C6** 41 6N 72 4 E
Uchte, Germany ...... **30 C4** 52 30N 8 54 E
Uchur ➔, Russia ..... **67 D14** 58 48N 130 35 E
Uckermark, Germany . **30 B9** 53 15N 13 30 E
Uckkulach, Uzbekistan **65 C3** 40 33N 67 1 E
Ucluelet, Canada **142 D3** 48 57N 125 32W
Úcua, Angola .... **116 A2** 8 48 S 13 26 E
Uda ➔, Russia ...... **67 D14** 54 42N 135 14 E
Uda Walawe △,
  Sri Lanka .... **95 L5** 6 20N 81 0 E
Udagamandalam, India **95 J3** 11 30N 76 44 E
Udainagar, India ..... **92 H7** 22 33N 76 13 E
Udaipur, Raj., India .. **92 G5** 24 36N 73 44 E
Udaipur, Tripura, India **93 H18** 23 32N 91 30 E
Udaipur Garhi, Nepal **93 F12** 27 0N 86 35 E
Udala, India .... **93 J12** 21 35N 86 34 E
Udalguri, India ...... **90 B4** 26 46N 92 8 E
Udayagiri,
  Andhra Pradesh,
  India .... **95 M4** 14 52N 79 19 E
Udayagiri, Orissa, India **94 D7** 20 8N 84 23 E
Udbina, Croatia ...... **45 D12** 44 31N 15 47 E
Uddeholm, Sweden ... **16 D7** 60 1N 13 38 E
Uddevalla, Sweden ... **17 F5** 58 21N 11 55 E
Uddjaure, Sweden ... **14 D17** 65 56N 17 49 E
Uden, Neths. .... **24 C5** 51 40N 5 37 E
Udgir, India .... **94 E3** 18 25N 77 5 E
Udhampur, India .... **93 C6** 33 0N 75 5 E
Udi, Nigeria .... **113 D6** 6 17N 7 21 E
Údine, Italy .... **45 B10** 46 3N 13 14 E
Udmurtia □, Russia .. **64 C4** 57 30N 52 30 E
Udon Thani, Thailand **86 D4** 17 29N 102 46 E
Udu Pt., Fiji .... **133 A3** 16 9 S 179 57W
Udupi, India .... **95 H2** 13 25N 74 42 E
Udva, India .... **94 D1** 20 5N 73 0 E
Udvoy Balkan,
  Bulgaria .... **51 D10** 42 50N 26 50 E
Udzungwa △, Tanzania **118 D4** 7 52 S 36 35 E
Udzungwa Range,
  Tanzania .... **119 D4** 9 30 S 35 10 E
Ueckermünde,
  Germany .... **30 B10** 53 44N 14 1 E
Ueda, Japan .... **73 A10** 36 24N 138 16 E
Uedineniya, Os., Russia **6 B12** 78 0N 85 0 E
Uel Scimbirro,
  Somali Rep. ...... **120 D2** 2 23N 44 14 E
Uele ➔, Dem. Rep. of
  the Congo .... **114 B4** 3 45N 24 45 E
Uelen, Russia **67 C19** 66 10N 170 0W
Uelzen, Germany .... **30 C6** 52 57N 10 32 E
Ueno, Japan .... **73 C8** 34 45N 136 8 E
Uetendorf, Switz. ... **32 C5** 46 47N 7 34 E
Uetersen, Germany .. **30 B5** 53 40N 9 40 E
Uetze, Germany ..... **30 C6** 52 28N 10 11 E
Ufa, Russia .... **64 D6** 54 45N 55 55 E
Ufa ➔, Russia ...... **64 D6** 54 40N 56 0 E
Uffenheim, Germany . **31 F6** 49 33N 10 14 E
Ugab ➔, Namibia .... **116 C1** 20 55 S 13 30 E
Ugalla ➔, Tanzania .. **118 D3** 5 8 S 30 42 E
Ugalla River △,
  Tanzania .... **118 D3** 5 50 S 31 54 E
Ugam Tizmasi,
  Kazakhstan ...... **65 B5** 42 20N 70 30 E
Uganda ■, Africa .... **118 B3** 2 0N 32 0 E
Ugento, Italy .... **47 C11** 39 56N 18 10 E
Ugep, Nigeria ...... **113 D6** 5 53N 8 2 E
Ughelli, Nigeria ..... **113 D6** 5 33N 6 0 E
Ugie, S. Africa ...... **117 E4** 31 10 S 28 13 E
Ugíjar, Spain **43 J7** 36 58N 3 7W
Ugine, France ...... **29 C10** 45 45N 6 25 E
Uglegorsk, Russia ... **67 E15** 49 5N 142 2 E
Uglich, Russia ...... **58 D10** 57 33N 38 20 E
Ugljan, Croatia ...... **45 D12** 44 12N 15 10 E
Ugljane, Croatia ..... **45 E13** 43 35N 16 46 E
Ugolny = Beringovskiy,
  Russia .... **67 C18** 63 3N 179 19 E
Ugolny = Karpinsk,
  Russia .... **64 B8** 59 45N 60 1 E
Ugolnyye Kopi =
  Kopeysk, Russia ... **64 D8** 55 7N 61 37 E
Ugra ➔, Russia ...... **58 E9** 54 30N 36 7 E
Ugŭrchin, Bulgaria .. **51 C8** 43 6N 24 26 E
Uh ➔, Slovak Rep. ... **35 C15** 48 37N 22 0 E
Uherské Hradiště,
  Czech Rep. ...... **35 B10** 49 4N 17 30 E
Uherský Brod,
  Czech Rep. ...... **35 B10** 49 1N 17 40 E
Úhlava ➔, Czech Rep. **34 B6** 49 45N 13 24 E
Uhlenhorst, Namibia . **116 C2** 23 45 S 17 55 E
Uhniv, Ukraine ...... **55 H10** 50 22N 23 45 E
Uhrichsville, U.S.A. .. **150 F3** 40 24N 81 21W
Uibhist a Deas = South
  Uist, U.K. **22 D1** 57 20N 7 15W
Uibhist a Tuath =
  North Uist, U.K. ... **22 D1** 57 40N 7 15W
Uíche, Angola ...... **115 E4** 12 5 S 30 51 E
Uig, U.K. **22 D2** 57 35N 6 21W
Uíge, Angola .... **115 D2** 7 30 S 14 40 E
Uíge □, Angola ...... **115 D3** 7 0 S 16 0 E
Uiha, Tonga .... **133 P13** 19 54 S 174 25W
Uijŏngbu, S. Korea ... **75 F14** 37 48N 127 0 E
Uiju, N. Korea ...... **75 D13** 40 15N 124 35 E
Uinta Mts., U.S.A. ... **158 F8** 40 45N 110 30W
Uis, Namibia .... **116 C1** 21 8 S 14 49 E
Uitenhage, S. Africa .. **116 E4** 33 40 S 25 28 E
Uithuizen, Neths. .... **24 A6** 53 24N 6 41 E
Ujazd, Poland ...... **55 H5** 50 23N 18 21 E
Újfehértó, Hungary .. **52 C6** 47 49N 21 41 E
Uji ➔, India .... **92 C6** 32 10N 75 18 E
Ujhani, India .... **93 F8** 28 0N 79 6 E
Uji, Japan .... **73 C7** 34 53N 135 48 E
Uji-guntō, Japan ..... **71 J4** 31 15N 129 25 E
Ujiyamada = Ise, Japan **73 C8** 34 25N 136 45 E
Ujjain, India .... **92 H6** 23 9N 75 43 E
Ujście, Poland ...... **55 E3** 53 3N 16 45 E
Újszász, Hungary .... **52 C5** 47 19N 20 7 E
Ujung Pandang,
  Indonesia .... **82 C1** 5 10 S 119 20 E
Uka, Russia .... **67 D17** 57 50N 162 0 E
Ukara I., Tanzania ... **118 C3** 1 50 S 33 0 E
Uke-Shima, Japan ... **71 K4** 28 2N 129 14 E
Ukerewe I., Tanzania . **118 C3** 2 0 S 33 0 E
Ukholovo, Russia .... **60 D5** 53 47N 40 30 E
Ukhrul, India ...... **90 C5** 25 10N 94 25 E
Ukhta, Russia ...... **6 C9** 63 34N 53 41 E
Uki Ni Masi,
  Solomon Is. ...... **133 N11** 10 15 S 161 47 E
Ukiah, U.S.A. **160 F3** 39 9N 123 13W
Ukmergė, Lithuania .. **15 J21** 55 15N 24 45 E
Ukraine ■, Europe ... **59 H7** 49 0N 32 0 E
Uku, Angola .... **115 E2** 11 24 S 14 22 E
Ukwi, Botswana ..... **116 C3** 23 29 S 20 30 E
Ulaan-Uul, Mongolia . **74 B4** 44 13N 111 10 E
Ulaanbaatar, Mongolia **67 E11** 47 55N 106 53 E
Ulaangom, Mongolia . **68 A4** 50 5N 92 10 E
Ulaanjirem, Mongolia **74 B4** 45 5N 105 30 E
Ulak I., U.S.A. **144 L3** 51 22N 178 57W
Ulala = Gorno-Altaysk,
  Russia .... **66 D9** 51 50N 86 5 E
Ulamambri, Australia . **129 A8** 31 19 S 149 23 E
Ulamba, Dem. Rep. of
  the Congo .... **119 D1** 9 3 S 23 38 E
Ulamona, Papua N. G. **132 C6** 5 0 S 151 15 E
Ulan Bator =
  Ulaanbaatar,
  Mongolia .... **67 E11** 47 55N 106 53 E
Ulan Erge, Russia .... **61 G7** 46 19N 44 53 E
Ulan Khol, Russia ... **61 H8** 45 18N 46 37 E
Ulan Ude, Russia .... **67 D11** 51 45N 107 40 E
Ulanbel, Kazakhstan . **65 B5** 44 50N 71 9 E
Ulanów, Poland ..... **55 H9** 50 30N 22 16 E
Ulaş, Sivas, Turkey .. **100 C7** 39 27N 37 2 E
Ulaş, Tekirdağ, Turkey **51 E11** 41 14N 27 42 E
Ulaya, Morogoro,
  Tanzania .... **118 D4** 7 3 S 36 55 E
Ulaya, Tabora,
  Tanzania .... **118 C3** 4 25 S 33 30 E
Ulcinj, Serbia & M. .. **50 E3** 41 58N 19 10 E
Ulco, S. Africa ...... **116 D3** 28 21 S 24 15 E
Ule träsk = Oulujärvi,
  Finland .... **14 D21** 64 25N 27 15 E
Ule älv = Oulujoki ➔,
  Finland .... **14 D21** 65 1N 25 30 E
Uleåborg = Oulu,
  Finland .... **14 D21** 65 1N 25 29 E
Ulefoss, Norway .... **18 E6** 59 17N 9 16 E
Ulëz, Albania ...... **50 E3** 41 46N 19 54 E
Ulfborg, Denmark ... **17 H2** 56 16N 8 20 E
Ulhasnagar, India ... **94 E1** 19 15N 73 10 E
Uliastay, Mongolia .. **68 B4** 47 56N 97 28 E
Uljma, Serbia & M. .. **52 E6** 45 2N 21 10 E
Ulla ➔, Spain **42 C2** 42 39N 8 44W
Ulladulla, Australia .. **129 C9** 35 21 S 150 29 E
Ullapool, U.K. **22 D3** 57 54N 5 9W
Ullared, Sweden .... **17 G6** 57 8N 12 42 E
Ulldecona, Spain ... **40 E5** 40 36N 0 20 E
Ullswater, U.K. **20 C5** 54 34N 2 52W
Ullŭng-do, S. Korea . **71 F5** 37 30N 130 30 E
Ulm, Germany ...... **31 G5** 48 23N 9 58 E
Ulmarra, Australia ... **127 D5** 29 37 S 153 4 E
Ulmeni, Buzău,
  Romania .... **53 E11** 45 4N 26 40 E
Ulmeni, Maramureş,
  Romania .... **53 C8** 47 28N 23 18 E
Ulonguè, Mozam. .... **119 E3** 14 37 S 34 19 E
Ulricehamn, Sweden . **17 G7** 57 46N 13 26 E
Ulriksdal, Sweden ... **16 A4** 53 19N 13 21 E
Ulrika, Sweden ..... **17 F9** 58 5N 15 23 E
Ulsan, S. Korea ..... **75 G15** 35 20N 129 15 E
Ulsberg, Norway .... **18 B6** 62 45N 10 0 E
Ulsta, U.K. **22 A7** 60 30N 1 9W
Ulster □, U.K. **23 B5** 54 35N 6 30W
Ulstein, Bulgaria ... **50 A3** 42 23N 16 27 E
Ultima, Australia .... **128 C5** 35 30 S 143 18 E
Ulubat Gölü, Turkey **51 F12** 40 9N 28 35 E
Ulubey, Turkey ..... **49 C11** 38 25N 29 18 E
Uluborlu, Turkey .... **49 C12** 38 4N 30 28 E
Uludağ, Turkey ..... **51 F13** 40 4N 29 13 E
Uludağ △, Turkey ... **51 F13** 40 0N 29 12 E
Uludere, Turkey .... **101 D10** 37 28N 42 42 E
Ulugqat, China ...... **65 D7** 39 48N 74 15 E
Uluguru Mts., Tanzania **118 D4** 7 15 S 37 40 E
Ulukışla, Turkey .... **100 D6** 37 33N 34 28 E
Ulungur He ➔, China **68 B3** 47 1N 87 24 E
Ulupalakua, U.S.A. .. **145 C5** 20 39N 156 24W
Uluru = Ayers Rock,
  Australia .... **125 E5** 25 23 S 131 5 E
Uluru-Kata Tjuta △,
  Australia .... **125 E5** 25 19 S 131 1 E
Ulutau, Kazakhstan . **66 E7** 48 39N 67 1 E
Uluwatu, Indonesia .. **79 K18** 8 50 S 115 5 E
Ulva, U.K. **22 E2** 56 29N 6 13W
Ulverston, U.K. **20 C4** 54 13N 3 5W
Ulverstone, Australia . **129 G4** 41 11 S 146 11 E
Ulvik, Norway ...... **18 D3** 60 35N 6 54 E
Ulya ➔, Russia ...... **67 D15** 60 35N 142 0 E
Ulyanovsk = Simbirsk,
  Russia .... **60 C9** 54 20N 48 25 E
Ulyasutay = Uliastay,
  Mongolia .... **68 B4** 47 56N 97 28 E
Ulysses, U.S.A. **155 G4** 37 35N 101 22W
Umag, Croatia ...... **45 C10** 45 26N 13 31 E
Umala, Bolivia ...... **172 D4** 17 25 S 68 5W
'Umān = Oman ■, Asia **99 B7** 23 0N 58 0 E
Uman, Ukraine ...... **59 H6** 48 40N 30 12 E
Umarkhed, India .... **94 E3** 19 37N 77 46 E
Umarpada, India .... **92 J5** 21 73N 73 33 E
Umatac, Guam ...... **133 R15** 13 18N 144 39 E
Umatilla, U.S.A. **158 D4** 45 55N 119 21W
Umba, Russia ...... **56 A5** 66 42N 34 11 E
Umbagog L., U.S.A. .. **151 B13** 44 46N 71 3W
Umbakumba, Australia **126 A2** 13 47 S 136 50 E
Umbértide, Italy ..... **45 E9** 43 18N 12 20 E
Umboi I., Papua N. G. **132 C4** 5 40 S 148 0 E
Umbrella Mts., N.Z. .. **131 F4** 45 35 S 169 5 E
Umbria □, Italy ..... **45 F9** 42 53N 12 30 E
Umeå, Sweden ...... **14 E19** 63 45N 20 20 E
Umeälven ➔, Sweden **14 E19** 63 45N 20 20 E
Umera, Indonesia ... **83 E3** 0 12 S 129 37 E
Umfolozi △, S. Africa . **117 D5** 28 18 S 31 50 E
Umfuli ➔, Zimbabwe **119 F2** 17 30 S 29 23 E
Umfurudzi △,
  Zimbabwe .... **119 F3** 17 6 S 31 40 E
Umgusa, Zimbabwe . **119 F2** 19 29 S 27 52 E
Umiat, U.S.A. **144 B9** 69 22N 152 8W
Umim Urûmah,
  Si. Arabia .... **106 B4** 25 43N 36 35 E
Umka, Serbia & M. ... **50 B4** 44 40N 20 19 E
Umkomaas, S. Africa . **117 E5** 30 13 S 30 48 E
Umm ad Daraj, J.,
  Jordan .... **103 C4** 32 18N 35 48 E
Umm al Aranib, Libya **108 C2** 26 10N 14 43 E
Umm al Qaywayn,
  U.A.E. .... **97 E7** 25 30N 55 35 E
Umm al Qittayn,
  Jordan .... **103 C5** 32 18N 36 40 E
Umm al'Abid, Libya . **108 C3** 27 31N 15 2 E
Umm Arda, Sudan ... **107 D3** 15 17N 32 31 E
Umm Bāb, Qatar .... **97 E6** 25 12N 50 48 E
Umm Badr, Sudan ... **107 E2** 14 13N 27 58 E
Umm Baiyud, Sudan . **107 E3** 14 25N 28 1 E
Umm Bel, Sudan .... **107 E2** 13 35N 28 0 E
Umm Birkah,
  Si. Arabia .... **106 B4** 27 44N 36 31 E
Umm Boim, Sudan .. **107 E2** 11 43N 25 27 E
Umm Dam, Sudan .. **107 E3** 13 45N 30 59 E
Umm Debi, Sudan .. **107 E3** 14 37N 30 23 E
Umm Dubban, Sudan **107 D3** 15 23N 32 52 E
Umm Durman =
  Omdurmân, Sudan **107 D3** 15 40N 32 28 E
Umm el Fahm, Israel . **103 C4** 32 31N 35 9 E
Umm Gafala, Sudan . **107 E2** 13 27N 28 22 E
Umm Ginana, Sudan **107 E3** 11 27N 28 52 E
Umm Inderaba, Sudan **107 D3** 17 30N 33 13 E
Umm Keddada, Sudan **107 E2** 13 33N 26 35 E
Umm Koweika, Sudan **107 E3** 13 10N 27 48 E
Umm Lajj, Si. Arabia . **96 E3** 25 0N 37 23 E
Umm Merwa, Sudan . **106 D3** 18 4N 32 30 E
Umm Qantur, Sudan . **107 E2** 11 31N 26 53 E
Umm Qurein, Sudan . **107 E2** 11 58N 26 9 E
Umm Ruwaba, Sudan **107 E3** 12 50N 31 20 E
Umm Saiyala, Sudan . **107 E3** 14 26N 31 57 E
Umm Shanqa, Sudan **107 E2** 13 14N 27 14 E
Umm Shutur, Sudan . **107 E2** 11 30N 25 10 E
Umm Sidr, Sudan ... **107 E2** 12 25N 26 10 E
Umm Zehrtir, Egypt . **106 J8** 28 40N 33 23 E
Umnak I., U.S.A. **144 K5** 53 15N 168 20W
Umniati ➔, Zimbabwe **119 F2** 16 49 S 28 45 E
Umnugovĭ, Mongolia **74 C4** 44 35N 109 0 E
Umpang, Thailand ... **86 E2** 16 3N 98 54 E
Umpqua ➔, U.S.A. .. **158 E1** 43 40N 124 12W
Umpulo, Angola ..... **115 E3** 12 8 S 17 30 E
Umred, India .... **94 D3** 20 51N 79 18 E
Umreth, India ...... **92 H5** 22 41N 73 4 E
Umri, India .... **92 J2** 21 9N 77 39 E
Umtata, S. Africa .... **116 E4** 31 36 S 28 49 E
Umtentweni, S. Africa **117 E5** 30 48 S 30 44 E
Umuahia, Nigeria ... **113 D6** 5 31N 7 26 E
Umuarama, Brazil ... **175 A5** 23 45 S 53 20W
Umuda I., Papua N. G. **132 E2** 8 23 S 143 46 E
Umurbey, Turkey ... **51 F10** 40 17N 26 21 E
Umvukwe Ra.,
  Zimbabwe .... **119 F3** 16 45 S 30 45 E
Umzimvubu, S. Africa **117 E4** 31 38 S 29 33 E
Umzingwane ➔,
  Zimbabwe .... **119 G2** 22 12 S 29 56 E
Umzinto, S. Africa ... **117 E5** 30 15 S 30 45 E

Una, India .... **92 J4** 20 46N 71 8 E
Una ➔, Bos.-H. ..... **45 C13** 45 0N 16 20 E
Unac ➔, Bos.-H. .... **45 D13** 44 30N 16 9 E
Unaðsdalur, Iceland . **11 A4** 66 7N 22 36W
Unadilla, Ga., U.S.A. . **152 C5** 32 16N 83 44W
Unadilla, N.Y., U.S.A. **151 D9** 42 20N 75 19W
Unaí, Brazil ...... **171 E2** 16 23 S 46 53W
Unalakleet, U.S.A. .. **144 F7** 63 52N 160 47W
Unalaska, U.S.A. **144 K6** 53 53N 166 32W
Unalaska I., U.S.A. .. **144 K6** 53 35N 166 50W
'Unayzah, Si. Arabia . **96 E4** 26 6N 43 58 E
'Unayzah, J., Asia .... **101 F8** 32 12N 39 18 E
Uncastillo, Spain **40 C3** 42 21N 1 8W
Uncía, Bolivia ...... **172 D4** 18 25 S 66 40W
Uncompahgre Peak,
  U.S.A. **159 G10** 38 4N 107 28W
Uncompahgre Plateau,
  U.S.A. **159 G9** 38 20N 108 15W
Undara Volcanic △,
  Australia .... **126 B3** 18 14 S 144 41 E
Unden, Sweden ..... **17 F8** 58 45N 14 25 E
Underbool, Australia . **128 C4** 35 10 S 141 51 E
Undersaker, Norway . **16 A7** 63 19N 13 21 E
Undredal, Norway ... **18 D4** 60 57N 7 6 E
Unea I., Papua N. G. . **132 C5** 4 53 S 149 9 E
Unecha, Russia ..... **59 F7** 52 50N 32 37 E
Uneiuxi ➔, Brazil ... **168 D4** 0 37 S 65 34W
Unga I., U.S.A. **144 J7** 55 15N 160 40W
Ungarie, Australia ... **129 B7** 33 38 S 146 56 E
Ungarisch-Hradisch =
  Uherské Hradiště,
  Czech Rep. ...... **35 B10** 49 4N 17 30 E
Ungarisch-Ostra =
  Uherský Brod,
  Czech Rep. ...... **35 B10** 49 1N 17 40 E
Ungarra, Australia ... **128 C2** 34 12 S 136 2 E
Ungava, Pén. d',
  Canada **139 C12** 60 0N 74 0W
Ungava B., Canada ... **139 C13** 59 30N 67 30W
Ungeny = Ungheni,
  Moldova .... **53 C12** 47 11N 27 27 E
Unggi, N. Korea ..... **75 C16** 42 16N 130 28 E
Ungheni, Moldova .. **53 C12** 47 11N 27 51 E
Unguala ➔, Ethiopia **107 F5** 8 6N 41 9 E
Ungvár = Uzhhorod,
  Ukraine .... **52 B7** 48 36N 22 18 E
Ungwana B., Kenya .. **118 C5** 2 40 S 40 20 E
Ungwatiri, Sudan ... **107 D4** 16 52N 36 10 E
Uni, Russia .... **60 B10** 57 46N 51 31 E
União, Brazil ...... **170 B3** 4 35 S 42 52W
União da Vitória,
  Brazil .... **175 B5** 26 13 S 51 5W
União dos Palmares,
  Brazil .... **170 C4** 9 10 S 36 2W
Uničov, Czech Rep. . **35 B10** 49 46N 17 8 E
Uniejów, Poland .... **55 G5** 51 59N 18 46 E
Unije, Croatia ...... **45 D11** 44 40N 14 15 E
Unimak I., U.S.A. ... **144 J7** 54 45N 164 0W
Unimak Pass, U.S.A. . **144 J6** 54 15N 164 30W
Unini ➔, Brazil .... **169 D5** 1 61 S 61 31W
Union, Miss., U.S.A. . **155 J10** 32 34N 89 7W
Union, Mo., U.S.A. .. **156 F6** 38 27N 91 0W
Union, Ohio, U.S.A. . **157 E12** 39 55N 84 12W
Union, S.C., U.S.A. .. **149 H5** 34 43N 81 37W
Union City, Calif.,
  U.S.A. **160 H4** 37 36N 122 1W
Union City, Ga., U.S.A. **152 B5** 33 35N 84 33W
Union City, N.J., U.S.A. **151 F10** 40 45N 74 2W
Union City, Ohio,
  U.S.A. **157 D12** 40 12N 84 48W
Union City, Pa., U.S.A. **150 E5** 41 54N 79 51W
Union City, Tenn.,
  U.S.A. **155 G10** 36 26N 89 3W
Union Gap, U.S.A. ... **158 C3** 46 33N 120 28W
Union Grove, U.S.A. . **157 B8** 42 41N 88 3W
Union Park, U.S.A. .. **153 G8** 28 34N 81 17W
Union Point, U.S.A. . **152 B6** 33 37N 83 4W
Union Springs, U.S.A. **152 C4** 32 9N 85 43W
Union Star, U.S.A. .. **156 E2** 39 59N 94 36W
Uniondale, S. Africa . **116 E3** 33 39 S 23 7 E
Uniontown, Ky., U.S.A. **157 G9** 37 47N 87 56W
Uniontown, Pa., U.S.A. **148 F6** 39 54N 79 44W
Unionville, Ga., U.S.A. **152 D6** 31 26N 83 30W
Unionville, Mo., U.S.A. **156 D3** 40 29N 93 1W
Unirea, Romania .... **53 F12** 44 15N 27 35 E
United Arab
  Emirates ■, Asia .. **97 F7** 23 50N 54 0 E
United Arab
  Republic = Egypt ■,
  Africa .... **106 B3** 28 0N 31 0 E
United Kingdom ■,
  Europe **19 E6** 53 0N 2 0W
United Provinces =
  Uttar Pradesh □,
  India .... **93 F9** 27 0N 80 0 E
United States of
  America ■, N. Amer. **137 F10** 37 0N 96 0W
Unity, Canada **143 C7** 52 30N 109 5W
Universales, Mtes.,
  Spain **40 E3** 40 18N 1 33W
University City, U.S.A. **156 F6** 38 40N 90 20W
University Park, U.S.A. **159 K10** 32 17N 106 45W
Unjha, India .... **92 H5** 23 46N 72 24 E
Unmet, Vanuatu ..... **133 F5** 16 8 S 167 15 E
Unna, Germany ...... **30 D3** 51 32N 7 42 E
Unnao, India .... **93 F9** 26 35N 80 30 E
Uno, Ilha, Guinea-Biss. **112 C1** 11 15N 16 13W
Unnukki, Finland ... (not present)
Unpongkor, Vanuatu **133 H6** 18 50 S 168 59 E
Unruhstadt = Kargowa,
  Poland .... **55 F2** 52 5N 15 51 E
Unsengedsi ➔,
  Zimbabwe .... **119 F3** 15 43 S 31 14 E
Unst, U.K. **22 A8** 60 44N 0 53W
Unstrut ➔, Germany **30 D7** 51 10N 11 48 E
Unter-engadin, Switz. **33 C9** 46 48N 10 20 E
Unterägeri, Switz. ... **32 B7** 47 8N 8 36 E
Unterdrauburg =
  Dravograd, Slovenia **45 B12** 46 36N 15 5 E
Unterfranken □,
  Germany .... **31 F5** 50 0N 10 0 E
Unterkulm, Switz. ... **32 B6** 47 18N 8 7 E
Unterseen, Switz. ... **32 C5** 46 41N 7 50 E
Unterwalden ob dem
  Wald □, Switz. .... (not present)
Unterwaldner Alpen,
  Switz. .... **33 B8** 46 55N 8 15 E
Unterwasser, Switz. . **33 B8** 47 13N 9 19 E
Unuk ➔, U.S.A. **142 B2** 56 5N 131 3W
Ünye, Turkey ...... **100 B7** 41 5N 37 15 E
Unzen-Amakusa △,
  Japan .... **72 C2** 32 15N 130 10 E
Unzen-Dake, Japan . **72 C2** 32 45N 130 17 E
Unzha, Russia ...... **60 A7** 58 0N 44 0 E
Unzha ➔, Russia .... **60 B6** 57 30N 43 40 E
Uong Bi, Vietnam ... **86 B6** 21 2N 106 24 E
Uozu, Japan .... **73 A8** 36 48N 137 24 E
Upata, Venezuela ... **169 B5** 8 1N 62 24W
Upatoi Cr. ➔, U.S.A. **152 C5** 32 25N 84 58W
Upemba, L., Dem. Rep.
  of the Congo ..... **119 D2** 8 30 S 26 20 E
Upemba, Dem. Rep.
  of the Congo ..... **119 D2** 9 0 S 26 35 E

Upernavik, *Greenland* **10 C5** 72 49N 56 20W
Upington, *S. Africa* **116 D3** 28 25 S 21 15 E
Upleta, *India* **92 J4** 21 46N 70 16 E
'Upolu, *Samoa* **133 W24** 13 58 S 172 0W
Upolu Pt., *U.S.A.* **145 C6** 20 16N 155 52W
Upper □, *Ghana* **113 C4** 10 30N 1 30W
Upper Alkali L., *U.S.A.* **158 F3** 41 47N 120 8W
Upper Arlington, *U.S.A.* **157 E13** 40 0N 83 4W
Upper Arrow L., *Canada* **142 C5** 50 30N 117 50W
Upper Austria = Oberösterreich □, *Austria* **34 C7** 48 10N 14 0 E
Upper Darby, *U.S.A.* **148 F8** 39 58N 75 16W
Upper Foster L., *Canada* **143 B7** 56 47N 105 20W
Upper Hutt, *N.Z.* **130 H4** 41 8 S 175 5 E
Upper Juba, *Somali Rep.* **120 D2** 3 0N 43 0 E
Upper Klamath L., *U.S.A.* **158 E3** 42 25N 121 55W
Upper Lake, *U.S.A.* **160 F4** 39 10N 122 54W
Upper Manilla, *Australia* **129 A9** 30 38 S 150 40 E
Upper Manzanilla, *Trin. & Tob.* **169 F9** 10 31N 61 4W
Upper Missouri River Breaks ⌂, *U.S.A.* **158 C9** 47 50N 108 55W
Upper Musquodoboit, *Canada* **141 C7** 45 10N 62 58W
Upper Preoria L., *U.S.A.* **156 D7** 40 55N 89 27W
Upper Red L., *U.S.A.* **154 A7** 48 8N 94 45W
Upper Sandusky, *U.S.A.* **157 D13** 40 50N 83 17W
Upper Senegal & Niger = Mali ■, *Africa* **112 B4** 17 0N 3 0W
Upper Sheikh, *Somali Rep.* **120 C3** 9 56N 45 13 E
Upper Volta = Burkina Faso ■, *Africa* **112 C4** 12 0N 1 0W
Upphärad, *Sweden* **17 F6** 58 9N 12 19 E
Uppland, *Sweden* **16 D12** 59 59N 17 48 E
Upplands-Väsby, *Sweden* **16 E11** 59 31N 17 54 E
Uppsala, *Sweden* **16 E11** 59 53N 17 38 E
Uppsala län □, *Sweden* **16 D11** 60 0N 17 30 E
Upshi, *India* **93 C7** 33 48N 77 52 E
Upstart, C., *Australia* **126 B4** 19 41 S 147 45 E
Upton, *U.S.A.* **154 C2** 44 6N 104 38W
Uqsuqtuuq = Gjoa Haven, *Canada* **138 B10** 68 38N 95 53W
Ur, *Iraq* **96 D5** 30 55N 46 25 E
Ura-Tyube = Uroteppa, *Tajikistan* **65 D4** 39 55N 69 1 E
Urabá, G. de, *Colombia* **168 B2** 8 25N 76 53W
Urad Qianqi, *China* **74 D5** 40 40N 108 30 E
Uraga-Suidō, *Japan* **73 B11** 35 13N 139 45 E
Urakawa, *Japan* **70 C11** 42 9N 142 47 E
Ural = Uralskiy □, *Russia* **66 C7** 64 0N 70 0 E
Ural = Zhayyq →, *Kazakhstan* **57 E9** 47 0N 51 48 E
Ural, *Australia* **129 B7** 33 21 S 146 12 E
Ural Mts. = Uralskie Gory, *Eurasia* **64 C7** 60 0N 59 0 E
Uralla, *Australia* **129 A9** 30 37 S 151 29 E
Uralmedstroy = Krasnouralsk, *Russia* **64 B8** 58 21N 60 3 E
Uralsk = Oral, *Kazakhstan* **60 E10** 51 20N 51 20 E
Uralskie Gory, *Eurasia* **64 C7** 60 0N 59 0 E
Uralskiy □, *Russia* **66 C7** 64 0N 70 0 E
Urambo, *Tanzania* **118 D3** 5 4 S 32 0 E
Urana, *Australia* **129 C7** 35 15 S 146 21 E
Urana, L., *Australia* **129 C7** 35 16 S 146 10 E
Urandangi, *Australia* **126 C2** 21 32 S 138 14 E
Uranga, *Australia* **129 A10** 30 31 S 153 1 E
Uranium City, *Canada* **143 B7** 59 34N 108 37W
Uraricaá →, *Brazil* **169 C5** 3 20N 61 56W
Uraricoera, *Brazil* **169 C5** 3 27N 60 59W
Uraricoera →, *Brazil* **169 C5** 3 2N 60 30W
Uravakonda, *India* **95 G3** 14 57N 77 12 E
Urawa, *Japan* **73 B11** 35 50N 139 40 E
Uray, *Russia* **66 C7** 60 5N 65 15 E
'Uray'irah, *Si. Arabia* **97 E6** 25 57N 48 53 E
Urbakh = Pushkino, *Russia* **60 E8** 51 16N 47 0 E
Urbana, *Ill., U.S.A.* **157 D8** 40 7N 88 12W
Urbana, *Ohio, U.S.A.* **157 D13** 40 7N 83 45W
Urbandale, *U.S.A.* **156 C3** 41 38N 93 43W
Urbánia, *Italy* **45 E9** 43 40N 12 31 E
Urbano Santos, *Brazil* **170 B3** 3 12 S 43 23W
Urbel →, *Spain* **42 C7** 42 21N 3 40W
Urbino, *Italy* **45 E9** 43 43N 12 38 E
Urbión, Picos de, *Spain* **40 C2** 42 1N 2 52W
Urcos, *Peru* **172 C3** 13 40 S 71 38W
Urdaneta, *Phil.* **80 D3** 15 59N 120 34 E
Urdinarrain, *Argentina* **174 C4** 32 37 S 58 52W
Urdos, *France* **28 F3** 42 51N 0 35W
Urdzhar, *Kazakhstan* **66 E9** 47 5N 81 38 E
Ure →, *U.K.* **20 C6** 54 5N 1 20W
Uren, *Russia* **60 B7** 57 35N 45 55 E
Ureparapara, *Vanuatu* **133 C5** 13 32 S 167 20 E
Ures, *Mexico* **162 B2** 29 30N 110 30W
Ureshino, *Japan* **72 D1** 33 6N 129 59 E
Urewera △, *N.Z.* **130 E6** 38 29 S 177 7 E
Urfa = Sanliurfa, *Turkey* **101 D8** 37 12N 38 50 E
Urga = Ulaanbaatar, *Mongolia* **67 E11** 47 55N 106 53 E
Urganch, *Uzbekistan* **66 E7** 41 40N 60 41 E
Urgench = Urganch, *Uzbekistan* **66 E7** 41 40N 60 41 E
Ürgüp, *Turkey* **96 B2** 38 38N 34 56 E
Urgut, *Uzbekistan* **65 D3** 39 23N 67 15 E
Uri, *India* **93 B6** 34 8N 74 2 E
Uri □, *Switz.* **33 C7** 46 43N 8 35 E
Uribante →, *Venezuela* **168 B3** 7 25N 71 50W
Uribe, *Colombia* **168 C3** 3 13N 74 24W
Uribia, *Colombia* **168 A3** 11 43N 72 16W
Uricani, *Romania* **52 E8** 45 20N 23 9 E
Urimba, *Angola* **115 E3** 10 56 S 16 32 E
Uriondo, *Bolivia* **174 A3** 21 41 S 64 41W
Urique, *Mexico* **162 B3** 27 13N 107 55W
Urique →, *Mexico* **162 B3** 26 29N 107 58W
Urirotstock, *Switz.* **33 C7** 46 52N 8 32 E
Urk, *Neths.* **24 B5** 52 39N 5 36 E
Urkiola ⌂, *Spain* **40 B3** 43 6N 1 2W
Urla, *Turkey* **49 C8** 38 20N 26 47 E
Urlaţi, *Romania* **53 F11** 44 59N 26 15 E
Urmia = Orūmīyeh, *Iran* **101 D11** 37 40N 45 0 E
Urmia, L. = Orūmīyeh, Daryācheh-ye, *Iran* **101 D11** 37 50N 45 30 E
Urnäsch, *Switz.* **33 B8** 47 19N 9 17 E
Urner Alpen, *Switz.* **33 C7** 46 45N 8 45 E
Uroševac, *Serbia & M.* **50 D5** 42 23N 21 10 E
Uroteppa, *Tajikistan* **65 D4** 39 55N 69 1 E
Uroyan, Montanas de, *Puerto Rico* **165 d** 18 12N 67 0W
Urrao, *Colombia* **168 B2** 6 20N 76 11W
Ursatyevskaya = Khavast, *Uzbekistan* **65 C4** 40 10N 68 49 E
Urshult, *Sweden* **17 H8** 56 31N 14 50 E
Uruaçu, *Brazil* **171 D2** 14 30 S 49 10W
Uruana, *Brazil* **171 E2** 15 30 S 49 41W
Uruapan, *Mexico* **162 D4** 19 30N 102 0W
Uruará, *Brazil* **169 D7** 3 42 S 53 51W
Uruará →, *Brazil* **169 D7** 2 6 S 53 38W
Urubamba, *Peru* **172 C3** 13 20 S 72 10W
Urubamba →, *Peru* **172 C3** 10 43 S 73 48W
Urubaxi →, *Brazil* **169 D5** 0 31 S 64 50W
Urubu →, *Brazil* **169 D6** 2 55 S 58 25W
Uruçara, *Brazil* **169 D6** 2 32 S 57 45W
Uruçuí, *Brazil* **170 C3** 7 20 S 44 28W
Uruçuí, Serra do, *Brazil* **170 C3** 9 0 S 44 45W
Uruçuí Prêto →, *Brazil* **170 C3** 7 20 S 44 38W
Urucuia →, *Brazil* **171 E2** 16 8 S 45 5W
Urucurituba, *Brazil* **169 D6** 2 41 S 57 40W
Uruguai →, *Brazil* **175 B5** 26 0 S 53 30W
Uruguaiana, *Brazil* **174 B4** 29 50 S 57 0W
Uruguay ■, *S. Amer.* **174 C4** 32 30 S 56 30W
Uruguay →, *S. Amer.* **174 C4** 34 12 S 58 18W
Urumchi = Ürümqi, *China* **66 E9** 43 45N 87 45 E
Ürümqi, *China* **66 E9** 43 45N 87 45 E
Urundi = Burundi ■, *Africa* **118 C3** 3 15 S 30 0 E
Urup →, *Russia* **61 H5** 45 0N 41 10 E
Urup, Ostrov, *Russia* **67 E16** 46 0N 151 0 E
Urutaí, *Brazil* **171 E2** 17 28 S 48 12W
Uryupinsk, *Russia* **60 E5** 50 45N 41 58 E
Urzhum, *Russia* **60 B9** 57 10N 49 56 E
Urziceni, *Romania* **53 F11** 44 40N 26 42 E
Usa, *Japan* **72 D3** 33 31N 131 21 E
Usa →, *Russia* **56 A10** 66 16N 59 49 E
Uşak, *Turkey* **49 C11** 38 43N 29 28 E
Uşak □, *Turkey* **49 C11** 38 30N 29 0 E
Usakos, *Namibia* **116 C2** 21 54 S 15 31 E
Usborne, Mt., *Falk. Is.* **9 f** 51 40 S 59 55W
Ušće, *Serbia & M.* **50 C4** 43 30N 20 39 E
Usedom, *Germany* **30 B10** 53 55N 14 2 E
Usedom ⌂, *Germany* **30 B10** 53 55N 14 0 E
Useless Loop, *Australia* **125 E1** 26 8 S 113 23 E
'Usfān, *Si. Arabia* **98 B2** 21 58N 39 27 E
Ush-Tobe, *Kazakhstan* **66 E8** 45 16N 78 0 E
Ushakova, Ostrov, *Russia* **6 A12** 82 0N 80 0 E
Ushakovo, *Russia* **54 D7** 54 37N 20 16 E
Ushant = Ouessant, Î. d', *France* **26 D1** 48 28N 5 6W
Usharal, *Kazakhstan* **65 B5** 43 53N 70 31 E
Ushashi, *Tanzania* **118 C3** 1 59 S 33 57 E
Ushat, *Sudan* **107 F2** 7 59N 29 28 E
'Ushayrah, *Si. Arabia* **106 C5** 21 46N 40 42 E
Ushibuka, *Japan* **72 E2** 32 11N 130 1 E
Ushuaia, *Argentina* **176 D3** 54 50 S 68 23W
Ushumun, *Russia* **67 D13** 52 47N 126 32 E
Ushytsya →, *Ukraine* **53 B12** 48 35N 27 8 E
Usino, *Papua N. G.* **132 C3** 5 32 S 145 23 E
Usk, *Canada* **142 C3** 54 38N 128 26W
Usk →, *U.K.* **21 F5** 51 33N 2 58W
Uska, *India* **93 F10** 27 12N 83 7 E
Uskedal, *Norway* **18 E2** 59 56N 5 53 E
Üsküb = Skopje, *Macedonia* **50 D5** 42 1N 21 26 E
Üsküdar, *Turkey* **51 F13** 41 0N 29 5 E
Uslar, *Germany* **30 D5** 51 39N 9 38 E
Usman, *Russia* **59 F10** 52 5N 39 48 E
Usmat, *Uzbekistan* **65 D3** 39 45N 67 38 E
Usoke, *Tanzania* **118 D3** 5 8 S 32 24 E
Usolye, *Russia* **64 B6** 59 28N 56 31 E
Usolye Sibirskoye, *Russia* **67 D11** 52 48N 103 40 E
Usolye-Solikamskoye = Berezniki, *Russia* **64 B6** 59 24N 56 46 E
Usoro, *Nigeria* **113 D6** 5 33N 6 11 E
Uspallata, P. de, *Argentina* **174 C2** 32 37 S 69 22W
Uspenka = Kirovskiy, *Russia* **70 B6** 45 7N 133 30 E
Uspenskiy, *Kazakhstan* **66 E8** 48 41N 72 43 E
Ussel, *France* **28 C6** 45 32N 2 18 E
Usson-du-Poitou, *France* **28 B4** 46 16N 0 31 E
Ussuriysk, *Russia* **67 E14** 43 48N 131 59 E
Ussurka, *Russia* **70 B6** 45 12N 133 31 E
Ust-Aldan = Batamay, *Russia* **67 C13** 63 30N 129 15 E
Ust-Amginskoye = Khandyga, *Russia* **67 C14** 62 42N 135 35 E
Ust-Bolsheretsk, *Russia* **67 D16** 52 50N 156 15 E
Ust-Buzulukskaya, *Russia* **60 E6** 50 8N 42 11 E
Ust-Chaun, *Russia* **67 C18** 68 47N 170 30 E
Ust-Chorna, *Ukraine* **53 B8** 48 19N 23 56 E
Ust-Donetskiy, *Russia* **61 G5** 47 35N 40 55 E
Ust-Ilimpeya = Yukta, *Russia* **67 C11** 63 26N 105 42 E
Ust-Ilimsk, *Russia* **67 D11** 58 3N 102 39 E
Ust-Ishim, *Russia* **66 D8** 57 45N 71 10 E
Ust-Kamchatsk, *Russia* **67 D17** 56 10N 162 28 E
Ust-Kamenogorsk = Öskemen, *Kazakhstan* **66 E9** 50 0N 82 36 E
Ust-Khayryuzovo, *Russia* **67 D16** 57 15N 156 45 E
Ust-Kut, *Russia* **67 D11** 56 50N 105 42 E
Ust-Kuyga, *Russia* **67 B14** 70 1N 135 43 E
Ust-Labinsk, *Russia* **61 H4** 45 15N 39 41 E
Ust-Luga, *Russia* **58 C5** 59 35N 28 20 E
Ust-Maya, *Russia* **67 C14** 60 30N 134 28 E
Ust-Medveditskaya = Serafimovich, *Russia* **60 F6** 49 36N 42 43 E
Ust-Mil, *Russia* **67 D14** 59 40N 133 11 E
Ust-Nera, *Russia* **67 C15** 64 35N 143 15 E
Ust-Nyukzha, *Russia* **67 D13** 56 34N 121 37 E
Ust-Olenek, *Russia* **67 B12** 73 0N 120 5 E
Ust-Omchug, *Russia* **67 C15** 61 9N 149 38 E
Ust-Port, *Russia* **66 C9** 69 40N 84 26 E
Ust-Sysolsk = Syktyvkar, *Russia* **56 B9** 61 45N 50 40 E
Ust-Tsilma, *Russia* **56 A9** 65 28N 52 11 E
Ust Urt = Ustyurt Plateau, *Asia* **66 E6** 44 0N 55 0 E
Ust-Usa, *Russia* **56 A10** 66 2N 56 57 E
Ust-Vorkuta, *Russia* **56 A11** 67 24N 64 0 E
Ust-Zhuya = Chara, *Russia* **67 D12** 56 54N 118 20 E
Ustaoset, *Norway* **18 D5** 60 30N 8 2 E
Ustaritz, *France* **28 E2** 43 24N 1 27W
Ustecký □, *Czech Rep.* **34 A7** 50 30N 14 0 E
Uster, *Switz.* **33 B7** 47 22N 8 43 E
Ústí nad Labem, *Czech Rep.* **34 A7** 50 41N 14 3 E
Ústí nad Orlicí, *Czech Rep.* **35 B9** 49 58N 16 24 E
Ústica, *Italy* **46 D6** 38 42N 13 11 E
Ustinov = Izhevsk, *Russia* **64 C4** 56 51N 53 14 E
Ustka, *Poland* **54 D3** 54 35N 16 55 E
Ustroń, *Poland* **55 J5** 49 43N 18 48 E
Ustrzyki Dolne, *Poland* **55 J9** 49 27N 22 40 E
Ustupo, *Panama* **168 B2** 9 27N 78 34W
Ustyluh, *Ukraine* **55 H11** 50 51N 24 10 E
Ustyurt Plateau, *Asia* **66 E6** 44 0N 55 0 E
Ustyuzhna, *Russia* **58 C9** 58 50N 36 32 E
Usu, *China* **68 B3** 44 27N 84 40 E
Usuki, *Japan* **72 D3** 33 8N 131 49 E
Usulután, *El Salv.* **164 D2** 13 25N 88 28W
Usumacinta →, *Mexico* **163 D6** 17 0N 91 0W
Usumbura = Bujumbura, *Burundi* **118 C2** 3 16 S 29 18 E
Usure, *Tanzania* **118 C3** 4 40 S 34 22 E
Usutuo →, *Mozam.* **117 D5** 26 48 S 32 7 E
Usva, *Russia* **64 B6** 58 41N 57 37 E
Uta, *Indonesia* **83 B5** 4 33 S 136 0 E
Utah □, *U.S.A.* **158 G8** 39 20N 111 30W
Utah L., *U.S.A.* **158 F8** 40 10N 111 58W
Utansjö, *Sweden* **16 B11** 62 46N 17 55 E
Utara, Selat, *Malaysia* **87 c** 5 28N 100 20 E
Utarni, *India* **92 F4** 26 5N 71 58 E
Utatlan, *Guatemala* **164 C1** 15 2N 91 11W
Ute Creek →, *U.S.A.* **155 H3** 35 21N 103 50W
Utebo, *Spain* **40 D3** 41 43N 1 0W
Utemurat, *Uzbekistan* **65 B2** 42 6N 65 42 E
Utena, *Lithuania* **15 J21** 55 27N 25 40 E
Utete, *Tanzania* **118 D4** 8 0 S 38 45 E
Uthai Thani, *Thailand* **86 E3** 15 22N 100 3 E
Uthal, *Pakistan* **92 G2** 25 44N 66 40 E
Utiariti, *Brazil* **173 C6** 13 0 S 58 10W
Utica, *N.Y., U.S.A.* **151 C9** 43 6N 75 14W
Utica, *Ohio, U.S.A.* **150 F2** 40 14N 82 27W
Utiel, *Spain* **41 F3** 39 37N 1 11W
Utikuma L., *Canada* **142 B5** 55 50N 115 30W
Utinga, *Brazil* **171 D3** 12 6 S 41 5W
Utkela, *India* **94 D6** 20 6N 83 10 E
Utne, *Norway* **18 D3** 60 25N 6 37 E
Utnur, *India* **94 E4** 19 22N 78 46 E
Uto, *Japan* **72 E2** 32 41N 130 40 E
Utö, *Sweden* **16 F12** 58 56N 18 16 E
Utopia, *Australia* **126 C1** 22 14 S 134 33 E
Utraula, *India* **93 F10** 27 19N 82 25 E
Utrecht, *Neths.* **24 B5** 52 5N 5 8 E
Utrecht, *S. Africa* **117 D5** 27 38 S 30 20 E
Utrecht □, *Neths.* **24 B5** 52 6N 5 7 E
Utrera, *Spain* **43 H5** 37 12N 5 48W
Utría △, *Colombia* **168 B2** 5 57N 77 21W
Utsira, *Norway* **18 E1** 59 19N 4 53 E
Utsjoki →, *Finland* **14 B22** 69 51N 26 59 E
Utsunomiya, *Japan* **73 A11** 36 30N 139 50 E
Uttar Pradesh □, *India* **93 F9** 27 0N 80 0 E
Uttaradit, *Thailand* **86 D3** 17 36N 100 5 E
Uttaranchal □, *India* **93 D8** 30 0N 79 30 E
Uttoxeter, *U.K.* **20 E6** 52 54N 1 52W
Utuado, *Puerto Rico* **165 d** 18 16N 66 42W
Utva →, *Kazakhstan* **64 F4** 51 28N 52 40 E
Uummannaq, *Greenland* **10 B4** 77 0N 69 0W
Uummannaq, *Greenland* **6 B5** 70 58N 52 0W
Uummannarsuaq = Nunap Isua, *Greenland* **10 F6** 59 48N 43 55W
Uusikaarlepyy, *Finland* **14 E20** 63 32N 22 31 E
Uusikaupunki, *Finland* **15 F19** 60 47N 21 25 E
Uva, *Russia* **60 B11** 56 59N 52 13 E
Uvá →, *Colombia* **168 C3** 3 41N 70 3W
Uvac →, *Serbia & M.* **50 C3** 43 35N 19 30 E
Uvalda, *U.S.A.* **152 C7** 32 2N 82 31W
Uvalde, *U.S.A.* **155 L5** 29 13N 99 47W
Uvarovo, *Russia* **60 E6** 51 59N 42 14 E
Uvat, *Russia* **66 D7** 59 5N 68 50 E
Uvdal, *Norway* **18 D5** 60 17N 8 48 E
Uvelskiy, *Russia* **64 D8** 54 26N 61 22 E
Uvinza, *Tanzania* **118 D3** 5 5 S 30 24 E
Uvira, *Dem. Rep. of the Congo* **118 C2** 3 22 S 29 3 E
Uvs Nuur, *Mongolia* **68 A4** 50 20N 92 30 E
Uwa, *Japan* **72 D4** 33 22N 132 31 E
'Uwairidh, Ḩarrat al, *Si. Arabia* **96 E3** 26 50N 38 0 E
Uwajima, *Japan* **72 D4** 33 10N 132 35 E
Uwanda ⌂, *Tanzania* **118 D3** 7 46 S 32 0 E
Uweinat, Jebel, *Sudan* **106 C1** 21 54N 24 58 E
Uwekuli, *Indonesia* **82 B2** 1 25 S 121 6 E
Uxbridge, *Canada* **150 B5** 44 6N 79 7W
Uxin Qi, *China* **74 E5** 38 50N 109 5 E
Uxmal, *Mexico* **163 C7** 20 22N 89 46W
Uyak, *U.S.A.* **144 H9** 57 38N 154 0W
Üydzin, *Mongolia* **74 B4** 44 9N 107 0 E
Uyo, *Nigeria* **113 D6** 5 1N 7 53 E
Uyu →, *Burma* **90 C5** 24 51N 94 57 E
Uyuk = Oyyq, *Kazakhstan* **65 B5** 43 36N 71 16 E
Üyüklü Tepe, *Turkey* **49 D9** 37 5N 27 21 E
Uyûn Mûsa, *Egypt* **103 F1** 29 53N 32 40 E
Uyuni, *Bolivia* **172 E4** 20 28 S 66 47W
Uzbekistan ■, *Asia* **65 C2** 41 30N 65 0 E
Uzen, *Kazakhstan* **57 F9** 43 29N 52 54 E
Uzen, Bolshoi →, *Kazakhstan* **61 F9** 49 6N 49 56 E
Uzen, Mal →, *Kazakhstan* **61 F9** 49 4N 49 44 E
Uzerche, *France* **28 C5** 45 25N 1 34 E
Uzès, *France* **29 D8** 44 1N 4 26 E
Uzgen = Özgön, *Kyrgyzstan* **65 C6** 40 46N 73 18 E
Uzh →, *Ukraine* **59 G6** 51 15N 30 12 E
Uzhgorod = Uzhhorod, *Ukraine* **52 B7** 48 36N 22 18 E
Uzhhorod, *Ukraine* **52 B7** 48 36N 22 18 E
Uzhok, *Ukraine* **52 B7** 48 59N 22 52 E
Užice, *Serbia & M.* **50 C3** 43 55N 19 50 E
Uzlovaya, *Russia* **58 F10** 54 0N 38 5 E
Üzümlü, *Turkey* **49 E11** 36 44N 29 14 E
Uzunköprü, *Turkey* **51 E10** 41 16N 26 43 E
Uzunkuyu, *Turkey* **49 C8** 38 17N 26 33 E
Uzwil, *Switz.* **33 B8** 47 26N 9 9 E
Uzynaghash, *Kazakhstan* **65 B8** 43 35N 76 20 E
Uzynaghash, *Kazakhstan* **65 B8** 43 13N 76 19 E

V

Vaal →, *S. Africa* **116 D3** 29 4 S 23 38 E
Vaal Dam, *S. Africa* **117 D4** 27 0 S 28 14 E
Vaalbos △, *S. Africa* **116 D3** 28 22 S 24 20 E
Vaalwater, *S. Africa* **117 C4** 24 15 S 28 8 E
Vaasa, *Finland* **14 E19** 63 6N 21 38 E
Vabkent, *Uzbekistan* **65 C2** 40 1N 64 30 E
Vabre, *France* **28 E6** 43 42N 2 24 E
Vác, *Hungary* **52 C4** 47 49N 19 10 E
Vacaria, *Brazil* **175 B5** 28 31 S 50 52W
Vacata, *Fiji* **133 A3** 17 15 S 179 31W
Vacaville, *U.S.A.* **160 G5** 38 21N 121 59W
Vaccarès, Étang de, *France* **29 E8** 43 32N 4 34 E
Vach = Vakh →, *Russia* **66 C8** 60 45N 76 45 E
Vache, Î. à, *Haiti* **165 C5** 18 2N 73 35W
Väckelsång, *Sweden* **17 H8** 56 37N 14 58 E
Vacoas, *Mauritius* **121 d** 20 18 S 57 29 E
Vada, *India* **94 E1** 19 39N 73 8 E
Väddö, *Sweden* **16 D12** 60 0N 18 50 E
Väderstad, *Sweden* **17 F8** 58 19N 14 55 E
Vadheim, *Norway* **18 C2** 61 13N 5 49 E
Vadnagar, *India* **92 H5** 23 47N 72 40 E
Vado Lígure, *Italy* **44 D5** 44 17N 8 26 E
Vadodara, *India* **92 H5** 22 20N 73 10 E
Vadret, Piz, *Switz.* **33 C9** 46 51N 9 58 E
Vadsø, *Norway* **14 A23** 70 3N 29 50 E
Vadstena, *Sweden* **17 F8** 58 28N 14 54 E
Vaduj, *India* **94 F2** 17 36N 74 27 E
Vaduz, *Liech.* **33 B9** 47 8N 9 31 E
Værlandet, *Norway* **18 C1** 61 18N 4 44 E
Værøy, *Norway* **14 C15** 67 40N 12 40 E
Vagalat, *Albania* **38 B10** 39 44N 20 8 E
Vågåmo, *Norway* **18 C6** 61 52N 9 6 E
Vágar, *Færoe Is.* **14 E9** 62 5N 7 15W
Vagarshapat = Yejmiadzin, *Armenia* **61 K7** 40 12N 44 19 E
Vaggeryd, *Sweden* **17 G8** 57 30N 14 10 E
Vaghena, *Solomon Is.* **133 L9** 7 25 S 157 45 E
Vagney, *France* **27 D13** 48 1N 6 43 E
Vagnhärad, *Sweden* **17 F11** 58 57N 17 33 E
Vagos, *Portugal* **42 E2** 40 33N 8 42W
Vågsfjorden, *Norway* **14 B17** 68 50N 16 50 E
Váh →, *Slovak Rep.* **35 D11** 47 43N 18 7 E
Vahsel B., *Antarctica* **7 D1** 75 0 S 35 0W
Váhtjer = Gällivare, *Sweden* **14 C19** 67 9N 20 40 E
Vái, *Greece* **39 E7** 35 15N 26 18 E
Vaigach, *Russia* **66 B6** 70 10N 59 0 E
Vaigai →, *India* **95 K4** 9 15N 79 10 E
Vaiges, *France* **26 D6** 48 2N 0 30W
Vaihingen, *Germany* **31 G4** 48 54N 8 57 E
Vaijapur, *India* **94 E2** 19 58N 74 45 E
Vaikam, *India* **95 K3** 9 45N 76 25 E
Vail, *U.S.A.* **146 C5** 39 40N 106 20W
Vailala →, *Papua N. G.* **132 D3** 7 57 S 145 25 E
Vailly-sur-Aisne, *France* **27 C10** 49 24N 3 31 E
Vaippar →, *India* **95 K4** 9 0N 78 25 E
Vaisali →, *India* **93 F8** 26 28N 78 53 E
Vaison-la-Romaine, *France* **29 D9** 44 14N 5 4 E
Vaitogi, *Amer. Samoa* **133 X24** 14 24 S 170 44W
Vajpur, *India* **94 D1** 21 24N 73 17 E
Vakaga →, *C.A.R.* **114 A4** 9 48N 21 32 E
Vakarai, *Sri Lanka* **95 K5** 8 8N 81 26 E
Vakarel, *Bulgaria* **50 D7** 42 35N 23 40 E
Vakfikebir, *Turkey* **101 B8** 41 2N 39 17 E
Vakh →, *Russia* **66 C8** 60 45N 76 45 E
Vakhsh, *Tajikistan* **65 E4** 37 43N 68 50 E
Vakhsh →, *Tajikistan* **65 E4** 37 6N 68 18 E
Vakhshstroy = Vakhsh, *Tajikistan* **65 E4** 37 43N 68 50 E
Vakhtan, *Russia* **60 B8** 57 53N 46 47 E
Vaksdal, *Norway* **18 D2** 60 29N 5 45 E
Vakuta I., *Papua N. G.* **132 E6** 8 51 S 151 10 E
Vál, *Hungary* **52 C3** 47 22N 18 40 E
Val-de-Marne □, *France* **27 D9** 48 45N 2 28 E
Val-d'Isère, *France* **29 C10** 45 27N 6 59 E
Val-d'Oise □, *France* **27 C9** 49 5N 2 10 E
Val-d'Or, *Canada* **140 C4** 48 7N 77 47W
Val Grande △, *Italy* **44 B5** 46 3N 8 25 E
Val Marie, *Canada* **143 D7** 49 15N 107 45W
Val Thorens, *France* **29 C10** 45 20N 6 33 E
Valaam, *Russia* **58 B6** 61 22N 30 57 E
Valadares, *Portugal* **42 D2** 41 5N 8 38W
Valahia, *Romania* **53 F9** 44 35N 25 0 E
Valaichenai, *Sri Lanka* **95 L5** 7 54N 81 32 E
Valais □, *Switz.* **32 D5** 46 12N 7 45 E
Valais, Alpes du, *Switz.* **32 D5** 46 5N 7 35 E
Valandovo, *Macedonia* **50 E6** 41 19N 22 34 E
Valašské Meziříčí, *Czech Rep.* **35 B10** 49 29N 17 59 E
Valáxa, *Greece* **48 C6** 38 50N 24 29 E
Vålberg, *Sweden* **16 E7** 59 23N 13 11 E
Valbo, *Sweden* **16 D10** 60 40N 17 0 E
Valbondione, *Italy* **44 B7** 46 2N 10 1 E
Vălcani, *Romania* **52 D5** 46 0N 20 26 E
Vâlcea □, *Romania* **53 F9** 45 0N 24 10 E
Valcheta, *Argentina* **176 B3** 40 40 S 66 8W
Valdagno, *Italy* **45 C8** 45 39N 11 18 E
Valdahon, *France* **27 E13** 47 8N 6 21 E
Valdai Hills = Valdayskaya Vozvyshennost, *Russia* **58 D7** 57 0N 33 30 E
Valday, *Russia* **58 D7** 57 58N 33 9 E
Valdayskaya Vozvyshennost, *Russia* **58 D7** 57 0N 33 30 E
Valdeazogues →, *Spain* **43 G6** 38 45N 4 55W
Valdecañas, Embalse de, *Spain* **42 F5** 39 45N 5 25W
Valdemarsvik, *Sweden* **17 F10** 58 14N 16 40 E
Valdemoro, *Spain* **42 E7** 40 12N 3 40W
Valdepeñas, *Spain* **43 G7** 38 43N 3 25W
Valderaduey →, *Spain* **42 D5** 41 31N 5 42W
Valdérice, *Italy* **46 D5** 38 4N 12 37 E
Valderrobres, *Spain* **40 E5** 40 53N 0 9 E
Valdés, Pen., *Argentina* **176 B4** 42 30 S 63 45W
Valdez, *Ecuador* **168 C2** 1 15N 79 0W
Valdez, *U.S.A.* **144 F11** 61 7N 146 16W
Valdgeym = Dobropole, *Ukraine* **59 H9** 48 25N 37 2 E
Valdivia, *Chile* **176 A2** 39 50 S 73 14W
Valdivia, *Colombia* **168 B2** 7 11N 75 27W
Valdobbiádene, *Italy* **45 C8** 45 54N 12 0 E
Valdosta, *U.S.A.* **152 E6** 30 50N 83 17W
Valdoviño, *Spain* **42 B2** 43 36N 8 8W
Valdres, *Norway* **18 C6** 61 5N 9 5 E
Vale, *Georgia* **61 K6** 41 30N 42 58 E
Vale, *U.S.A.* **158 E5** 43 59N 117 15W
Vale of Glamorgan □, *U.K.* **21 F4** 51 28N 3 25W
Valea lui Mihai, *Romania* **52 C7** 47 32N 22 11 E
Valea Mărului, *Romania* **53 E12** 45 49N 27 42 E
Valemount, *Canada* **142 C5** 52 50N 119 15W
Valença = Valença do Piauí, *Brazil* **170 C3** 6 20 S 41 45W
Valença, *Brazil* **171 D4** 13 20 S 39 5W
Valença, *Portugal* **42 C2** 42 1N 8 34W
Valença do Piauí, *Brazil* **170 C3** 6 20 S 41 45W
Valençay, *France* **27 E8** 47 9N 1 34 E
Valence, *France* **29 D8** 44 57N 4 54 E
Valence d'Agen, *France* **28 D4** 44 6N 0 53 E
Valencia, *Phil.* **81 H5** 7 57N 125 3 E
Valencia, *Spain* **41 F4** 39 27N 0 23W
Valencia, *Trin. & Tob.* **169 F9** 10 39N 61 11W
Valencia, *U.S.A.* **159 J10** 34 48N 106 43W
Valencia, *Venezuela* **168 A4** 10 11N 68 0W
Valencia □, *Spain* **41 F4** 39 20N 0 40W
Valencia ✕ (VLC), *Spain* **41 F4** 39 20N 0 26W
Valencia, G. de, *Spain* **41 F5** 39 30N 0 20 E
Valencia de Alcántara, *Spain* **43 F3** 39 25N 7 14W
Valencia de Don Juan, *Spain* **42 C5** 42 17N 5 31W
Valencia I., *Ireland* **23 E1** 51 54N 10 22W
Valenciennes, *France* **27 B10** 50 20N 3 34 E
Văleni, *Romania* **53 F9** 44 15N 24 45 E
Vălenii de Munte, *Romania* **53 E11** 45 11N 26 2 E
Valensole, *France* **29 E9** 43 50N 5 59 E
Valentigney, *France* **27 E13** 47 27N 6 51 E
Valentim, Sa. do, *Brazil* **170 C3** 6 0 S 43 30W
Valentin, *Russia* **70 C7** 43 8N 134 17 E
Valentine, *Nebr., U.S.A.* **154 D4** 42 52N 100 33W
Valentine, *Tex., U.S.A.* **155 K2** 30 35N 104 30W
Valenza, *Italy* **44 C5** 45 1N 8 38 E
Våler, *Hedmark, Norway* **18 D8** 60 41N 11 50 E
Våler, *Østfold, Norway* **18 E7** 59 29N 10 51 E
Valera, *Venezuela* **168 B3** 9 19N 70 37W
Valesdir, *Vanuatu* **133 F6** 16 47 S 168 10 E
Valestrand, *Norway* **18 E2** 59 40N 5 26 E
Valga, *Estonia* **15 H22** 57 47N 26 2 E
Valguarnera Caropepe, *Italy* **47 E7** 37 30N 14 23 E
Valier, *U.S.A.* **158 B7** 48 18N 112 16W
Valinco, G. de, *France* **29 G12** 41 40N 8 52 E
Valjevo, *Serbia & M.* **50 B3** 44 18N 19 53 E
Valka, *Latvia* **15 H21** 57 46N 26 3 E
Valkeakoski, *Finland* **15 F20** 61 16N 24 2 E
Valkenswaard, *Neths.* **24 C5** 51 21N 5 29 E
Vall de Uxó = La Vall d'Uixó, *Spain* **40 F4** 39 49N 0 15W
Valla, *Sweden* **16 E10** 59 2N 16 20 E
Valladolid, *Mexico* **163 C7** 20 40N 88 11W
Valladolid, *Spain* **42 D6** 41 38N 4 43W
Valladolid □, *Spain* **42 D6** 41 38N 4 43W
Vallata, *Italy* **47 A8** 41 2N 15 15 E
Valldemossa, *Spain* **38 B3** 39 43N 2 37 E
Valle, *Norway* **18 E4** 59 13N 7 33 E
Valle d'Aosta □, *Italy* **44 C4** 45 45N 7 15 E
Valle de Arán, *Spain* **40 C5** 42 50N 0 55 E
Valle de la Pascua, *Venezuela* **168 B4** 9 13N 66 0W
Valle de las Palmas, *Mexico* **161 N10** 32 20N 116 43W
Valle de Santiago, *Mexico* **162 C4** 20 25N 101 15W
Valle de Suchil, *Mexico* **162 C4** 23 38N 103 55W
Valle de Zaragoza, *Mexico* **162 B3** 27 28N 105 49W
Valle del Cauca □, *Colombia* **168 C2** 3 45N 76 30W
Valle del Ticino ⌂, *Italy* **44 C6** 45 22N 9 0 E
Valle Fértil, Sierra del, *Argentina* **174 C2** 30 20 S 68 0W
Valle Gran Rey, *Canary Is.* **9 e1** 28 5N 17 20W
Valle Hermoso, *Mexico* **163 B5** 25 35N 97 40W
Valledupar, *Colombia* **168 A3** 10 29N 73 15W
Vallehermoso, *Canary Is.* **9 e1** 28 10N 17 15W
Vallejo, *U.S.A.* **160 G4** 38 7N 122 14W
Vallenar, *Chile* **174 B1** 28 30 S 70 50W
Vallentuna, *Sweden* **16 E12** 59 32N 18 5 E
Valleraugue, *France* **28 D7** 44 6N 3 39 E
Vallet, *France* **26 E5** 47 10N 1 15W
Valletta, *Malta* **38 F8** 35 54N 14 31 E
Valley Center, *U.S.A.* **161 M9** 33 13N 117 2W
Valley City, *U.S.A.* **154 B6** 46 55N 98 0W
Valley Falls, *Oreg., U.S.A.* **158 E3** 42 29N 120 17W
Valley Falls, *R.I., U.S.A.* **151 E13** 41 54N 71 24W
Valley Junction = West Des Moines, *U.S.A.* **156 C3** 41 35N 93 43W
Valley of Flowers △, *India* **93 D8** 30 50N 79 40 E
Valley of the Kings, *Egypt* **106 B3** 25 41N 32 34 E
Valley Springs, *U.S.A.* **160 G6** 38 12N 120 50W
Valley Station, *U.S.A.* **157 F11** 38 6N 85 52W
Valley View, *U.S.A.* **151 F8** 40 39N 76 33W
Valley Wells, *U.S.A.* **161 K11** 35 27N 115 46W
Valleyview, *Canada* **142 B5** 55 5N 117 17W
Valli di Comácchio, *Italy* **45 D9** 44 40N 12 15 E
Vallimanca, Arroyo, *Argentina* **174 D4** 35 40 S 59 10W
Vallo della Lucánia, *Italy* **47 B8** 40 14N 15 16 E
Vallon-Pont-d'Arc, *France* **29 D8** 44 24N 4 24 E
Vallorbe, *Switz.* **32 C2** 46 42N 6 20 E
Valls, *Spain* **40 D6** 41 18N 1 15 E
Valmaseda = Balmaseda, *Spain* **40 B1** 43 11N 3 12W
Valmeyer, *U.S.A.* **156 F6** 38 18N 90 19W
Valmiera, *Latvia* **15 H21** 57 37N 25 29 E
Valnera, *Spain* **42 B7** 43 9N 3 40W
Valognes, *France* **26 C5** 49 30N 1 28W
Valona = Vlorë, *Albania* **50 F3** 40 32N 19 28 E
Valongo, *Portugal* **42 D2** 41 8N 8 30W
Valozhyn, *Belarus* **58 E4** 54 3N 26 30 E
Valpaços, *Portugal* **42 D3** 41 36N 7 17W
Valparai, *India* **95 J3** 10 22N 76 58 E
Valparaíso, *Chile* **174 C1** 33 2 S 71 40W
Valparaíso, *Mexico* **162 C4** 22 50N 103 32W
Valparaiso, *Fla., U.S.A.* **153 E3** 30 29N 86 30W
Valparaiso, *Ind., U.S.A.* **157 C9** 41 28N 87 4W
Valparaíso □, *Chile* **174 C1** 33 2 S 71 40W
Valpovo, *Croatia* **52 E3** 45 39N 18 25 E
Valpoy, *India* **95 G2** 15 32N 74 8 E
Valréas, *France* **29 D9** 44 24N 5 0 E
Vals, *Switz.* **33 C8** 46 39N 9 11 E
Vals →, *S. Africa* **116 D4** 27 23 S 26 30 E
Vals, Tanjung, *Indonesia* **83 C5** 8 26 S 137 25 E
Vals-les-Bains, *France* **29 D8** 44 42N 4 24 E
Valsad, *India* **94 D1** 20 40N 72 58 E
Valsamáta, *Greece* **39 C2** 38 10N 20 36 E
Valtellina, *Italy* **44 B6** 46 11N 9 55 E
Valþjofsstaður, *Iceland* **11 B12** 65 1N 14 59W
Valtí, *Greece* **39 C3** 38 27N 21 7 E
Valuyki, *Russia* **59 G10** 50 10N 38 5 E
Valverde, *Canary Is.* **9 e1** 27 48N 17 55W
Valverde del Camino, *Spain* **43 H4** 37 35N 6 47W
Valverde del Fresno, *Spain* **42 E4** 40 15N 6 51W
Vama, *Romania* **53 C10** 47 34N 25 42 E
Vambori, *India* **94 E2** 19 17N 74 44 E
Vamdrup, *Denmark* **17 J3** 55 25N 9 17 E
Våmhus, *Sweden* **16 C8** 61 7N 14 29 E
Vammala, *Finland* **15 F20** 61 20N 22 54 E
Vámos, *Greece* **39 E5** 35 24N 24 13 E
Vamsadhara →, *India* **94 E7** 18 21N 84 8 E
Van, *Turkey* **101 C10** 38 30N 43 20 E
Van, L. = Van Gölü, *Turkey* **101 C10** 38 30N 43 0 E
Van Alstyne, *U.S.A.* **155 J6** 33 25N 96 35W
Van Blommestein Meer, *Suriname* **169 C6** 4 45N 55 5W
Van Buren = Kettering, *U.S.A.* **157 E12** 39 41N 84 10W
Van Buren, *Canada* **141 C6** 47 10N 67 55W

Van Buren, *Ark., U.S.A.* **155 H7** 35 26N 94 21W
Van Buren, *Maine, U.S.A.* **149 B11** 47 10N 67 58W
Van Buren, *Mo., U.S.A.* **155 G9** 37 0N 91 1W
Van Canh, *Vietnam* **86 F7** 13 37N 109 0 E
Van Diemen, C., *N. Terr., Australia* **124 B5** 11 9 S 130 24 E
Van Diemen, C., *Queens., Australia* **126 B2** 16 30 S 139 46 E
Van Diemen G., *Australia* **124 B5** 11 45 S 132 0 E
Van Gölü, *Turkey* **101 C10** 38 30N 43 0 E
Van Horn, *U.S.A.* **155 K2** 31 3N 104 50W
Van Horne, *U.S.A.* **156 B4** 42 1N 92 4W
Van Meter, *U.S.A.* **156 C3** 41 32N 93 57W
Van Ninh, *Vietnam* **86 F7** 12 42N 109 14 E
Van Rees, Pegunungan, *Indonesia* **83 B5** 2 35 S 138 15 E
Van Tivu, *India* **95 K4** 8 51N 78 15 E
Van Wert, *U.S.A.* **157 D12** 40 52N 84 35W
Van Yen, *Vietnam* **76 G5** 21 4N 104 42 E
Vanadzor, *Armenia* **61 K7** 40 48N 44 30 E
Vanavara, *Russia* **67 C11** 60 22N 102 16 E
Vanceburg, *U.S.A.* **157 F13** 38 36N 83 19W
Vancouver, *Canada* **142 D4** 49 15N 123 10W
Vancouver, *U.S.A.* **160 E4** 45 38N 122 40W
Vancouver, C., *Australia* **125 G2** 35 2 S 118 11 E
Vancouver, Mt., *U.S.A.* **144 F13** 60 20N 139 41W
Vancouver I., *Canada* **142 D3** 49 50N 126 0W
Vancouver International ✈ (YVR), *U.S.A.* **160 A3** 49 10N 123 10W
Vanda = Vantaa, *Finland* **15 F21** 60 18N 24 58 E
Vandalia, *Ill., U.S.A.* **156 F7** 38 58N 89 6W
Vandalia, *Mo., U.S.A.* **156 E5** 39 19N 91 29W
Vandalia, *Ohio, U.S.A.* **157 E12** 39 54N 84 12W
Vandavasi, *India* **95 H4** 12 30N 79 30 E
Vandeloos B., *Sri Lanka* **95 L5** 8 0N 81 45 E
Vandenburg, *U.S.A.* **161 L6** 34 35N 120 33W
Vanderbijlpark, *S. Africa* **117 D4** 26 42 S 27 54 E
Vandergrift, *U.S.A.* **150 F5** 40 36N 79 34W
Vanderhoof, *Canada* **142 C4** 54 0N 124 0W
Vanderkloof Dam, *S. Africa* **116 E3** 30 4 S 24 40 E
Vanderlin I., *Australia* **126 B2** 15 44 S 137 2 E
Vänern, *Sweden* **17 F7** 58 47N 13 30 E
Vänersborg, *Sweden* **17 F6** 58 26N 12 19 E
Vang, *Norway* **18 C5** 61 7N 8 34 E
Vang Vieng, *Laos* **86 C4** 18 58N 102 32 E
Vanga, *Kenya* **118 C4** 4 35 S 39 12 E
Vangaindrano, *Madag.* **117 C8** 23 21 S 47 36 E
Vangsnes, *Norway* **18 C3** 61 9N 6 39 E
Vanguard, *Canada* **143 D7** 49 55N 107 20W
Vangunu, *Solomon Is.* **133 M10** 8 40 S 158 5 E
Vanimo, *Papua N. G.* **83 B6** 2 42 S 141 21 E
Vanino, *Russia* **67 E15** 48 50N 140 5 E
Vanivilasa Sagara, *India* **95 H3** 13 45N 76 30 E
Vaniyambadi, *India* **95 H4** 12 46N 78 44 E
Vanj, *Tajikistan* **65 D5** 38 22N 71 27 E
Vânju Mare, *Romania* **52 F7** 44 25N 22 52 E
Vanna, *Norway* **14 A18** 70 6N 19 50 E
Vännäs, *Sweden* **14 E18** 63 58N 19 48 E
Vannes, *France* **26 E4** 47 40N 2 47W
Vannovsky = Khamza, *Uzbekistan* **65 C5** 40 25N 71 29 E
Vanoise, Massif de la, *France* **29 C10** 45 25N 6 40 E
Vanrhynsdorp, *S. Africa* **116 E2** 31 36 S 18 44 E
Vansada, *India* **94 D1** 20 47N 73 25 E
Vansbro, *Sweden* **16 D8** 60 32N 14 15 E
Vanse, *Norway* **18 F3** 58 6N 6 41 E
Vansittart B., *Australia* **124 B4** 14 3 S 126 17 E
Vantaa, *Finland* **15 F21** 60 18N 24 58 E
Vanua Balavu, *Fiji* **133 A3** 17 12 S 178 55W
Vanua Lava, *Vanuatu* **133 C5** 13 50 S 167 30 E
Vanua Levu, *Fiji* **133 A2** 16 33 S 179 15 E
Vanua Vatu, *Fiji* **133 B3** 18 22 S 179 15W
Vanuatu ■, *Pac. Oc.* **133 E6** 15 0 S 168 0 E
Vanwyksvlei, *S. Africa* **116 E3** 30 18 S 21 49 E
Vanzylsrus, *S. Africa* **116 D3** 26 52 S 22 4 E
Vapnyarka, *Ukraine* **53 B13** 48 32N 28 45 E
Var □, *France* **29 E10** 43 27N 6 18 E
Var →, *France* **29 E11** 43 39N 7 12 E
Vara, *Sweden* **17 F6** 58 16N 12 55 E
Vara, Pico da, *Azores* **9 d3** 37 48N 25 13W
Varada →, *India* **95 G2** 15 0N 75 40 E
Varades, *France* **26 E5** 47 25N 1 1W
Varáita →, *Italy* **44 D4** 44 9N 7 53 E
Varaldsøy, *Norway* **18 D2** 60 6N 5 59 E
Varallo, *Italy* **44 C5** 45 49N 8 15 E
Varāmīn, *Iran* **97 C6** 35 20N 51 39 E
Varāmīn □, *Iran* **97 B6** 35 18N 51 35 E
Varanasi, *India* **93 G10** 25 22N 83 0 E
Varangerfjorden, *Norway* **14 A23** 70 3N 29 25 E
Varangerhalvøya, *Norway* **14 A23** 70 25N 29 30 E
Varano, Lago di, *Italy* **45 G12** 41 53N 15 45 E
Varaždin, *Croatia* **45 B13** 46 20N 16 20 E
Varazze, *Italy* **44 D5** 44 22N 8 34 E
Varberg, *Sweden* **17 G6** 57 6N 12 20 E
Varcar Vakuf = Mrkonjić Grad, *Bos.-H.* **52 F2** 44 26N 17 4 E
Vardak □, *Afghan.* **91 B3** 34 0N 68 0 E
Vardar = Axiós →, *Greece* **50 F6** 40 57N 22 35 E
Varde, *Denmark* **17 J2** 55 38N 8 29 E
Varde Å →, *Denmark* **17 J2** 55 35N 8 19 E
Vardø, *Norway* **14 A24** 70 23N 31 5 E
Varel, *Germany* **30 B4** 53 23N 8 8 E
Varella, Mui, *Vietnam* **86 F7** 12 54N 109 26 E
Varėna, *Lithuania* **15 J21** 54 12N 24 30 E
Varennes-sur-Allier, *France* **27 F10** 46 19N 3 24 E
Varennes-Vauzelles, *France* **27 E10** 47 3N 3 9 E
Vareš, *Bos.-H.* **52 F3** 44 12N 18 23 E
Varese, *Italy* **44 C5** 45 48N 8 50 E
Vârfurile, *Romania* **52 D7** 46 19N 22 31 E
Vårgårda, *Sweden* **17 F6** 58 2N 12 49 E
Vargem Bonita, *Brazil* **171 F2** 20 20 S 46 22W
Vargem Grande, *Brazil* **170 B3** 3 33 S 43 56W
Varginha, *Brazil* **175 A6** 21 33 S 45 25W
Vargön, *Sweden* **17 F6** 58 22N 12 20 E
Varhaug, *Norway* **18 F2** 58 37N 5 41 E
Varillas, *Chile* **174 A1** 24 0 S 70 10W
Varkaus, *Finland* **15 E22** 62 19N 27 50 E
Värmdölandet, *Sweden* **16 E12** 59 20N 18 33 E
Värmeln, *Sweden* **16 E6** 59 35N 12 54 E
Värmlands län □, *Sweden* **16 E6** 60 0N 13 20 E
Värmlandsbro, *Sweden* **16 E7** 59 11N 13 0 E
Varna, *Bulgaria* **51 C11** 43 13N 27 56 E
Varna, *Russia* **64 E8** 53 24N 60 58 E
Varna □, *Bulgaria* **51 C11** 43 20N 27 30 E
Varna →, *India* **94 F2** 16 48N 74 32 E
Värnamo, *Sweden* **17 G8** 57 10N 14 3 E
Varnsdorf, *Czech Rep.* **34 A7** 50 55N 14 35 E
Varnville, *U.S.A.* **152 C8** 32 51N 81 5W
Várpalota, *Hungary* **52 C3** 47 12N 18 8 E
Vars, *Canada* **151 A9** 45 21N 75 21W
Vars, *France* **29 D10** 44 37N 6 42 E
Vartdal, *Norway* **18 B3** 62 20N 6 8 E
Varto, *Turkey* **101 C9** 39 10N 41 27 E
Varvarin, *Serbia & M.* **50 C5** 43 43N 21 20 E
Varysburg, *U.S.A.* **150 D6** 42 46N 78 19W
Varzaneh, *Iran* **97 C7** 32 25N 52 40 E
Várzea Alegre, *Brazil* **170 C4** 6 47 S 39 17W
Várzea da Palma, *Brazil* **171 E3** 17 36 S 44 44W
Várzea Grande, *Brazil* **173 D6** 15 39 S 56 8W
Varzi, *Italy* **44 D6** 44 49N 9 12 E
Varzo, *Italy* **44 B5** 46 12N 8 15 E
Varzob, *Tajikistan* **65 D4** 38 46N 68 49 E
Varzy, *France* **27 E10** 47 22N 3 20 E
Vas □, *Hungary* **52 C1** 47 10N 16 55 E
Vasa = Vaasa, *Finland* **14 E19** 63 6N 21 38 E
Vasa Barris →, *Brazil* **170 D4** 11 10 S 37 10W
Vásárosnamény, *Hungary* **52 B7** 48 9N 22 19 E
Vascâo →, *Portugal* **43 H3** 37 31N 7 31W
Vaşcău, *Romania* **52 D7** 46 28N 22 30 E
Vascongadas = País Vasco □, *Spain* **40 C2** 42 50N 2 45W
Vāshīr, *Afghan.* **91 B1** 32 16N 63 51 E
Vashkivtsi, *Ukraine* **53 B10** 48 23N 25 31 E
Vasht = Khāsh, *Iran* **91 C1** 28 15N 61 15 E
Vasilevichi, *Belarus* **59 F5** 52 15N 29 50 E
Vasilikí, *Greece* **39 B2** 38 37N 20 36 E
Vasiliko = Michurin, *Bulgaria* **51 D11** 42 9N 27 51 E
Vasilikón, *Greece* **48 C5** 38 25N 23 40 E
Vasilikós, *Greece* **39 D2** 37 43N 20 59 E
Vasilkov = Vasylkiv, *Ukraine* **59 G6** 50 7N 30 15 E
Vasilyova Sloboda = Chkolovsk, *Russia* **60 B6** 56 50N 43 10 E
Vasilyovo = Chkolovsk, *Russia* **60 B6** 56 50N 43 10 E
Vaslui, *Romania* **53 D12** 46 38N 27 42 E
Vaslui □, *Romania* **53 D12** 46 30N 27 45 E
Väsman, *Sweden* **16 D9** 60 9N 15 5 E
Vassar, *Canada* **143 D9** 49 10N 95 55W
Vassar, *U.S.A.* **148 D4** 43 22N 83 35W
Vassfaret, *Norway* **18 D6** 60 38N 9 28 E
Västerås, *Sweden* **16 E10** 59 37N 16 38 E
Västerbotten, *Sweden* **14 D18** 64 36N 20 4 E
Västerdalälven →, *Sweden* **16 D8** 60 30N 14 7 E
Västergötland, *Sweden* **17 F7** 58 0N 13 10 E
Västerhaninge, *Sweden* **16 E12** 59 7N 18 6 E
Västervik, *Sweden* **17 G10** 57 43N 16 33 E
Västmanland, *Sweden* **15 G16** 59 45N 16 20 E
Västmanlands län □, *Sweden* **16 E10** 59 45N 16 20 E
Vasto, *Italy* **45 F11** 42 8N 14 40 E
Västra Götalands Län □, *Sweden* **17 F6** 58 0N 13 0 E
Vasvár, *Hungary* **52 C1** 47 3N 16 47 E
Vasylivka, *Ukraine* **53 E13** 45 38N 28 50 E
Vasylkiv, *Ukraine* **59 G6** 50 7N 30 15 E
Vatan, *France* **27 E8** 47 4N 1 50 E
Vaté = Efate, I., *Vanuatu* **133 G6** 17 40 S 168 25 E
Vatersay, *U.K.* **22 E1** 56 55N 7 32W
Vathí, *Greece* **39 B2** 38 41N 20 47 E
Váthia, *Greece* **48 E4** 36 29N 22 29 E
Vatican City ■, *Europe* **45 G9** 41 54N 12 27 E
Vaticano, C., *Italy* **47 D8** 38 37N 15 50 E
Vatili, *Cyprus* **39 E9** 35 6N 33 40 E
Vatin, *Serbia & M.* **52 E6** 45 12N 21 20 E
Vatiu = Atiu, *Cook Is.* **135 J12** 20 0 S 158 10W
Vatnajökull, *Iceland* **11 C10** 64 30N 16 48W
Vatnås, *Norway* **18 E6** 59 58N 9 37 E
Vatneyri, *Iceland* **11 B2** 65 35N 24 0W
Vatnsfjörður, *Iceland* **11 B4** 65 56N 22 30W
Vatólakkos, *Greece* **39 E4** 35 27N 23 53 E
Vatoloha, *Madag.* **117 B8** 17 52 S 47 48 E
Vatomandry, *Madag.* **117 B8** 19 20 S 48 59 E
Vatra-Dornei, *Romania* **53 C10** 47 22N 25 22 E
Vatrak →, *India* **92 H5** 23 9N 73 2 E
Vättern, *Sweden* **17 F8** 58 25N 14 30 E
Vättis, *Switz.* **33 C8** 46 55N 9 27 E
Vatu Vara, *Fiji* **133 A3** 17 26 S 179 31W
Vatulele, *Fiji* **133 B1** 18 33 S 177 37 E
Vaucluse □, *France* **29 E9** 43 50N 5 20 E
Vaucouleurs, *France* **27 D12** 48 37N 5 40 E
Vaud □, *Switz.* **32 C3** 46 35N 6 30 E
Vaudreuil-Dorion, *Canada* **151 A10** 45 23N 74 3W
Vaughn, *Mont., U.S.A.* **158 C8** 47 33N 111 33W
Vaughn, *N. Mex., U.S.A.* **159 J11** 34 36N 105 13W
Vaujours L., *Canada* **140 A5** 55 27N 74 15W
Vaulruz, *Switz.* **32 C3** 46 38N 6 58 E
Vaupés = Uaupés →, *Brazil* **168 C4** 0 2N 67 16W
Vaupes □, *Colombia* **168 C3** 1 0N 71 0W
Vauvert, *France* **29 E8** 43 42N 4 17 E
Vauxhall, *Canada* **142 C6** 50 5N 112 9W
Vav, *India* **92 G4** 24 22N 71 31 E
Vavatenina, *Madag.* **117 B8** 17 28 S 49 12 E
Vava'u, *Tonga* **133 P14** 18 36 S 174 0W
Vava'u Group, *Tonga* **133 P14** 18 40 S 174 0W
Vavoua, *Ivory C.* **112 D3** 7 23N 6 29W
Vavuniya, *Sri Lanka* **95 K5** 8 45N 80 30 E
Vawkavysk, *Belarus* **59 F3** 53 9N 24 30 E
Vaxholm, *Sweden* **16 E12** 59 25N 18 20 E
Växjö, *Sweden* **17 H8** 56 52N 14 50 E
Våxtorp, *Sweden* **17 H7** 56 25N 13 8 E
Vayalpad, *India* **95 H4** 13 39N 78 38 E
Vayenga = Severomorsk, *Russia* **56 A5** 69 5N 33 27 E
Vaygach, Ostrov, *Russia* **66 C6** 70 0N 60 0 E
Váyia, *Greece* **48 C5** 38 19N 23 11 E
Váyia, Ákra, *Greece* **38 E12** 36 15N 28 11 E
Veadeiros, *Brazil* **171 D2** 14 7 S 47 31W
Veaikevárri = Svappavaara, *Sweden* **14 C19** 67 40N 21 3 E
Vechelde, *Germany* **30 C6** 52 16N 10 22 E
Vechta, *Germany* **30 C4** 52 44N 8 17 E
Vechte →, *Neths.* **24 B6** 52 34N 6 6 E
Vecsés, *Hungary* **52 C4** 47 26N 19 19 E
Vedaranniyam, *India* **95 J4** 10 25N 79 50 E
Vedavågen, *Norway* **18 E2** 59 17N 5 12 E
Veddige, *Sweden* **17 G6** 57 17N 12 20 E
Vedea →, *Romania* **53 G10** 43 42N 25 41 E
Vedia, *Argentina* **174 C3** 34 30 S 61 31W
Vedrette di Ries-Aurina ⌓, *Italy* **45 B9** 46 54N 12 5 E
Vedum, *Sweden* **17 F7** 58 11N 13 0 E
Veedersburg, *U.S.A.* **157 D9** 40 7N 87 16W
Veendam, *Neths.* **24 A6** 53 5N 6 52 E
Veenendaal, *Neths.* **24 B5** 52 2N 5 34 E
Vefsna →, *Norway* **14 D15** 65 48N 13 10 E
Vega, *Norway* **14 D14** 65 40N 11 55 E
Vega, *U.S.A.* **155 H3** 35 15N 102 26W
Vega Baja, *Puerto Rico* **165 d** 18 27N 66 23W
Vega de Ribadeo = Vegadeo, *Spain* **42 B3** 43 27N 7 4W
Vegadeo, *Spain* **42 B3** 43 27N 7 4W
Vegårshei, *Norway* **18 F5** 58 44N 8 51 E
Vegas Verde = North Las Vegas, *U.S.A.* **161 J11** 36 12N 115 7W
Veggli, *Norway* **18 D6** 60 3N 9 9 E
Veglia = Krk, *Croatia* **45 C11** 45 8N 14 40 E
Vegorrítis, Límni, *Greece* **50 F5** 40 45N 21 45 E
Vegreville, *Canada* **142 C6** 53 30N 112 5W
Veidholmen, *Norway* **18 A4** 63 31N 7 58 E
Veinge, *Sweden* **17 H7** 56 33N 13 4 E
Veisiejai, *Lithuania* **54 D10** 54 6N 23 42 E
Vejbystrand, *Sweden* **17 H6** 56 19N 12 45 E
Vejen, *Denmark* **17 J3** 55 30N 9 9 E
Vejer de la Frontera, *Spain* **43 J5** 36 15N 5 59W
Vejle, *Denmark* **17 J3** 55 43N 9 30 E
Vejle Amtskommune □, *Denmark* **17 J3** 55 45N 9 20 E
Vejle Fjord, *Denmark* **17 J3** 55 40N 9 50 E
Vela Luka, *Croatia* **45 F13** 42 59N 16 44 E
Velachha, *India* **94 D1** 21 26N 73 1 E
Velanai I., *Sri Lanka* **95 K4** 9 45N 79 45 E
Velas, *Azores* **9 d1** 38 41N 28 13W
Velas, C., *Costa Rica* **164 D2** 10 21N 85 52W
Velasco, Sierra de, *Argentina* **174 B2** 29 20 S 67 10W
Velay, Mts. du, *France* **28 D7** 45 0N 3 40 E
Velbert, *Germany* **30 D3** 51 20N 7 3 E
Velddrif, *S. Africa* **116 E2** 32 42 S 18 11 E
Velebit ⌓, *Croatia* **45 D12** 44 30N 15 15 E
Velebit Planina, *Croatia* **45 D12** 44 50N 15 20 E
Velebitski Kanal, *Croatia* **45 D11** 44 45N 14 55 E
Veleka →, *Bulgaria* **51 D11** 42 4N 27 58 E
Velencei-tó, *Hungary* **52 C3** 47 13N 18 36 E
Velenje, *Slovenia* **45 B12** 46 23N 15 8 E
Veles, *Macedonia* **50 E5** 41 46N 21 47 E
Velestínon, *Greece* **48 B4** 39 23N 22 43 E
Vélez, *Colombia* **168 B3** 6 1N 73 41W
Vélez-Málaga, *Spain* **43 J6** 36 48N 4 5W
Vélez Rubio, *Spain* **41 H2** 37 41N 2 5W
Velhas →, *Brazil* **171 E3** 17 13 S 44 49W
Velika, *Croatia* **52 E2** 45 27N 17 40 E
Velika Gorica, *Croatia* **45 C13** 45 44N 16 5 E
Velika Kapela, *Croatia* **45 C12** 45 10N 15 5 E
Velika Kikinda = Kikinda, *Serbia & M.* **52 E5** 45 50N 20 30 E
Velika Kladuša, *Bos.-H.* **45 C12** 45 11N 15 48 E
Velika Kruša, *Serbia & M.* **50 D4** 42 19N 20 39 E
Velika Morava →, *Serbia & M.* **50 B5** 44 43N 21 3 E
Velika Plana, *Serbia & M.* **50 B5** 44 20N 21 4 E
Velikaya →, *Russia* **58 D5** 57 48N 28 10 E
Velikaya Kema, *Russia* **70 B8** 45 30N 137 12 E
Velikaya Lepetikha, *Ukraine* **59 J7** 47 2N 33 58 E
Veliké Kapušany, *Slovak Rep.* **35 C15** 48 34N 22 5 E
Velike Lašče, *Slovenia* **45 C11** 45 49N 14 45 E
Veliki Jastrebac, *Serbia & M.* **50 C5** 43 25N 21 30 E
Veliki Kanal, *Serbia & M.* **52 E4** 45 45N 19 15 E
Veliki Popović, *Serbia & M.* **50 B5** 44 8N 21 18 E
Veliki Ustyug, *Russia* **56 B8** 60 47N 46 20 E
Velikiye Luki, *Russia* **58 D6** 56 25N 30 32 E
Veliko Gradište, *Serbia & M.* **50 B5** 44 46N 21 29 E
Veliko Tŭrnovo, *Bulgaria* **51 C9** 43 5N 25 41 E
Velikonda Range, *India* **95 G4** 14 45N 79 10 E
Vélingara, *Kolda, Senegal* **112 C2** 13 12N 14 5W
Vélingara, *Louga, Senegal* **112 B2** 15 0N 14 40W
Velingrad, *Bulgaria* **50 D7** 42 4N 23 58 E
Velino, Mte., *Italy* **45 F10** 42 9N 13 23 E
Velizh, *Russia* **58 E6** 55 36N 31 11 E
Velké Karlovice, *Czech Rep.* **35 B11** 49 20N 18 17 E
Velké Meziříčí, *Czech Rep.* **34 B9** 49 21N 16 1 E
Vel'ký Javorník, *Slovak Rep.* **35 B11** 49 19N 18 22 E
Vel'ký Krtíš, *Slovak Rep.* **35 C12** 48 12N 19 21 E
Vel'ký Meder, *Slovak Rep.* **35 D10** 47 52N 17 46 E
Vel'ký Tribeč, *Slovak Rep.* **35 C11** 48 28N 18 15 E
Vella G., *Solomon Is.* **133 M9** 8 0 S 156 50 E
Vella Lavella, *Solomon Is.* **133 L9** 7 45 S 156 40 E
Vellar →, *India* **95 J4** 11 30N 79 36 E
Velletri, *Italy* **46 A5** 41 41N 12 47 E
Vellinge, *Sweden* **17 J6** 55 29N 13 0 E
Vellmar, *Germany* **30 D5** 51 22N 9 28 E
Vellore, *India* **95 H4** 12 57N 79 10 E
Velsk, *Russia* **58 B11** 61 10N 42 5 E
Velten, *Germany* **30 C9** 52 42N 13 10 E
Veluwezoom △, *Neths.* **24 B6** 52 5N 6 0 E
Velva, *U.S.A.* **154 A4** 48 4N 100 56W
Velvendós, *Greece* **50 F6** 40 15N 22 6 E
Velyka Mykhaylivka, *Ukraine* **53 C14** 47 4N 29 52 E
Velyki Luchky, *Ukraine* **52 B7** 48 25N 22 34 E
Velykyy Bereznyy, *Ukraine* **52 B7** 48 54N 22 28 E
Velykyy Bychkiv, *Ukraine* **53 C9** 47 58N 24 1 E
Vemb, *Denmark* **17 H2** 56 21N 8 21 E
Vembanad L., *India* **95 K3** 9 36N 76 15 E
Vemdalen, *Sweden* **16 B7** 62 27N 13 51 E
Ven, *Sweden* **17 J6** 55 55N 12 45 E
Venaco, *France* **29 F13** 42 14N 9 11 E
Venado Tuerto, *Argentina* **174 C3** 33 50 S 62 0W
Venafro, *Italy* **47 A7** 41 29N 14 2 E
Venarey-les-Laumes, *France* **27 E11** 47 32N 4 26 E
Venaría, *Italy* **44 C4** 45 8N 7 38 E
Venčane, *Serbia & M.* **50 B4** 44 24N 20 28 E
Vence, *France* **29 E11** 43 43N 7 6 E
Vendas Novas, *Portugal* **43 G2** 38 39N 8 27W
Vendée □, *France* **26 F5** 46 50N 1 35W
Vendée →, *France* **26 F5** 46 20N 1 10W
Vendéen, Bocage, *France* **28 B2** 46 40N 1 20W
Vendeuvre-sur-Barse, *France* **27 D11** 48 14N 4 28 E
Vendôme, *France* **26 E8** 47 47N 1 3 E
Vendrell = El Vendrell, *Spain* **40 D6** 41 10N 1 30 E
Vendsyssel, *Denmark* **17 G4** 57 22N 10 0 E
Vendychany, *Ukraine* **53 B12** 48 38N 27 48 E
Venelles, *France* **29 E9** 43 35N 5 28 E
Véneta, L., *Italy* **45 C9** 45 23N 12 25 E
Venetie, *U.S.A.* **144 C11** 67 1N 146 25W
Véneto □, *Italy* **45 C9** 45 30N 12 0 E
Venev, *Russia* **58 E10** 54 22N 38 17 E
Venézia, *Italy* **45 C9** 45 27N 12 21 E
Venézia, G. di, *Italy* **45 C10** 45 15N 13 0 E
Venezia Tridentina = Trentino-Alto Adige □, *Italy* **45 B8** 46 30N 11 20 E
Venezuela ■, *S. Amer.* **168 B4** 8 0N 66 0W
Venezuela, G. de, *Venezuela* **168 A3** 11 30N 71 0W
Vengurla, *India* **95 G1** 15 53N 73 45 E
Vengurla Rocks, *India* **95 G1** 15 55N 73 22 E
Venice = Venézia, *Italy* **45 C9** 45 27N 12 21 E
Venice, *U.S.A.* **153 H7** 27 6N 82 27W
Vénissieux, *France* **29 C8** 45 42N 4 53 E
Venjansjön, *Sweden* **16 D8** 60 54N 14 0 E
Venkatagiri, *India* **95 H4** 14 0N 79 35 E
Venkatapuram, *India* **94 E5** 18 20N 80 30 E
Venlo, *Neths.* **24 C6** 51 22N 6 11 E
Vennesla, *Norway* **18 F4** 58 15N 7 59 E
Venosa, *Italy* **47 B8** 40 58N 15 49 E
Venray, *Neths.* **24 C6** 51 31N 6 0 E
Vent, Îs. du, *French Polynesia* **133 S16** 17 30 S 149 30W
Venta, *Lithuania* **54 B9** 56 12N 22 42 E
Venta →, *Latvia* **54 A8** 57 24N 21 33 E
Venta de Baños, *Spain* **42 D6** 41 55N 4 30W
Venta de Cardeña = Cardeña, *Spain* **43 G6** 38 16N 4 20W
Ventana, Punta de la, *Mexico* **162 C3** 24 4N 109 48W
Ventana, Sa. de la, *Argentina* **174 D3** 38 0 S 62 30W
Ventersburg, *S. Africa* **116 D4** 28 7 S 27 9 E
Ventersburgweg = Hennenman, *S. Africa* **116 D4** 27 59 S 27 1 E
Venterstad, *S. Africa* **116 E4** 30 47 S 25 48 E
Ventimíglia, *Italy* **44 E4** 43 47N 7 36 E
Ventnor, *U.K.* **21 G6** 50 36N 1 12W
Ventoténe, *Italy* **46 B6** 40 47N 13 25 E
Ventoux, Mt., *France* **29 D9** 44 10N 5 17 E
Ventspils, *Latvia* **15 H19** 57 25N 21 32 E
Ventspils □, *Latvia* **54 A8** 57 20N 21 50 E
Ventuarí →, *Venezuela* **168 C4** 3 58N 67 2W
Ventucopa, *U.S.A.* **161 L7** 34 50N 119 29W
Ventura, *U.S.A.* **161 L7** 34 17N 119 18W
Venus, *U.S.A.* **153 H8** 27 4N 81 22W
Venus B., *Australia* **129 E6** 38 40 S 145 42 E
Vera, *Argentina* **174 B3** 29 30 S 60 20W
Vera, *Spain* **41 H3** 37 15N 1 51W
Veracruz, *Mexico* **163 D5** 19 10N 96 10W
Veracruz □, *Mexico* **163 D5** 19 0N 96 15W
Veraval, *India* **92 J4** 20 53N 70 27 E
Verbánia, *Italy* **44 C5** 45 56N 8 33 E
Verbicaro, *Italy* **47 C8** 39 45N 15 55 E
Verbier, *Switz.* **32 D4** 46 6N 7 13 E
Verceia, *Italy* **33 D8** 46 12N 9 27 E
Vercelli, *Italy* **44 C5** 45 19N 8 25 E
Verchovchevo, *Ukraine* **59 H8** 48 32N 34 10 E
Vercors ⌓, *France* **29 D9** 45 0N 5 25 E
Verdalsøra, *Norway* **14 E14** 63 48N 11 30 E
Verde →, *Argentina* **176 B3** 41 56 S 65 5W
Verde →, *Goiás, Brazil* **171 E1** 19 11 S 50 44W
Verde →, *Goiás, Brazil* **171 E1** 18 1 S 50 14W
Verde →, *Mato Grosso, Brazil* **173 C6** 11 54 S 55 48W
Verde →, *Mato Grosso do Sul, Brazil* **173 E7** 21 25 S 52 20W
Verde →, *Chihuahua, Mexico* **162 B3** 26 29N 107 58W
Verde →, *Oaxaca, Mexico* **163 D5** 15 59N 97 50W
Verde →, *Veracruz, Mexico* **162 C4** 21 10N 102 50W
Verde →, *Paraguay* **174 A4** 23 9 S 57 37W
Verde →, *U.S.A.* **146 D4** 33 33N 111 40W
Verde, Cay, *Bahamas* **164 B4** 23 0N 75 5W
Verde Grande →, *Brazil* **171 E3** 16 13 S 43 49W
Verde I., *Phil.* **80 E3** 13 33N 121 5 E
Verde Island Pass, *Phil.* **80 E3** 13 34N 120 51 E
Verde Pequeno →, *Brazil* **171 D3** 14 48 S 43 31W
Verden, *Germany* **30 C5** 52 55N 9 14 E
Verdhikoúsa, *Greece* **48 B3** 39 47N 21 59 E
Verdi, *U.S.A.* **160 F7** 39 31N 119 59W
Verdon ⌓, *France* **29 E10** 43 50N 6 5 E
Verdon →, *France* **29 E9** 43 43N 5 46 E
Verdun, *France* **27 C12** 49 9N 5 24 E
Verdun-sur-le-Doubs, *France* **27 F12** 46 54N 5 2 E
Vereeniging, *S. Africa* **117 D4** 26 38 S 27 57 E
Vereshchagino, *Russia* **64 B5** 58 5N 54 40 E
Verga, C., *Guinea* **112 C2** 10 30N 14 10W
Vergara, *Uruguay* **175 C5** 32 56 S 53 57W
Vergato, *Italy* **44 D8** 44 17N 11 7 E
Vergemont Cr. →, *Australia* **126 C3** 24 16 S 143 16 E
Vergennes, *U.S.A.* **151 B11** 44 10N 73 15W
Vergt, *France* **28 C4** 45 2N 0 43 E
Veria = Véroia, *Greece* **50 F6** 40 34N 22 12 E
Verín, *Spain* **42 D3** 41 57N 7 27W
Verkhne-Saldinsky Zavod = Verkhnyaya Salda, *Russia* **64 C8** 58 2N 60 33 E
Verkhnedvinsk = Vyerkhnyadzvinsk, *Belarus* **58 E4** 55 45N 27 58 E
Verkhneufaleysky Zavod = Verkhniy Ufaley, *Russia* **64 C8** 56 4N 60 14 E
Verkhneuralsk, *Russia* **64 E7** 53 53N 59 13 E
Verkhnevilyuysk, *Russia* **67 C13** 63 27N 120 18 E
Verkhniy Avzyan, *Russia* **64 E6** 53 32N 57 33 E
Verkhniy Baskunchak, *Russia* **61 F8** 48 14N 46 44 E
Verkhniy Tagil, *Russia* **64 C7** 57 22N 59 56 E
Verkhniy Ufaley, *Russia* **64 C8** 56 4N 60 14 E
Verkhniye Kigi, *Russia* **64 D7** 55 25N 58 37 E
Verkhnyaya Salda, *Russia* **64 C8** 58 2N 60 33 E
Verkhnyaya Tura, *Russia* **64 B7** 58 22N 59 50 E
Verkhoturye, *Russia* **64 B8** 58 52N 60 48 E
Verkhovye, *Russia* **59 F9** 52 55N 37 15 E
Verkhovyna, *Ukraine* **53 B9** 48 9N 24 47 E
Verkhoyansk, *Russia* **67 C14** 67 35N 133 25 E
Verkhoyansk Ra. = Verkhoyanskiy Khrebet, *Russia* **67 C13** 66 0N 129 0 E
Verkhoyanskiy Khrebet, *Russia* **67 C13** 66 0N 129 0 E
Verma, *Norway* **18 B5** 62 21N 8 3 E
Vermenton, *France* **27 E10** 47 40N 3 42 E
Vermilion, *Canada* **143 C6** 53 20N 110 50W
Vermilion, *U.S.A.* **150 E2** 41 25N 82 22W
Vermilion →, *Canada* **143 C6** 53 22N 110 51W
Vermilion →, *Ill., U.S.A.* **156 C7** 41 19N 89 4W
Vermilion →, *Ind., U.S.A.* **157 E9** 39 57N 87 27W
Vermilion B., *U.S.A.* **155 L9** 29 45N 91 55W
Vermilion Bay, *Canada* **143 D10** 49 51N 93 34W
Vermilion L., *U.S.A.* **154 B8** 47 53N 92 26W
Vermillion, *U.S.A.* **154 D6** 42 47N 96 56W
Vermillion →, *Canada* **140 C5** 47 38N 72 56W
Vermont, *U.S.A.* **156 D6** 40 18N 90 26W
Vermont □, *U.S.A.* **151 C12** 44 0N 73 0W
Vermosh, *Albania* **50 D3** 42 35N 19 42 E
Verna, *U.S.A.* **153 H7** 27 23N 82 16W
Vernadsky, *Antarctica* **7 C17** 65 0 S 64 0W
Vernal, *U.S.A.* **158 F9** 40 27N 109 32W
Vernalis, *U.S.A.* **160 H5** 37 36N 121 17W
Vernayaz, *Switz.* **32 D4** 46 8N 7 3 E
Vernazza, *Italy* **44 D6** 44 10N 9 45 E
Verner, *Canada* **140 C3** 46 25N 80 8W
Verneuil-sur-Avre, *France* **26 D7** 48 45N 0 55 E
Verneukpan, *S. Africa* **116 E3** 30 0 S 21 0 E
Vernier, *Switz.* **32 D2** 46 11N 6 12 E
Vérnio, *Italy* **44 D8** 44 3N 11 9 E
Vernon, *Canada* **142 C5** 50 20N 119 15W
Vernon, *France* **26 C8** 49 5N 1 30 E
Vernon, *Ill., U.S.A.* **156 F7** 38 48N 89 5W
Vernon, *Ind., U.S.A.* **157 F11** 38 59N 85 36W
Vernon, *Tex., U.S.A.* **155 H5** 34 9N 99 17W
Vernonia, *U.S.A.* **160 E3** 45 52N 123 11W
Verny = Almaty, *Kazakhstan* **65 B8** 43 15N 76 57 E
Vero Beach, *U.S.A.* **153 H9** 27 38N 80 24W
Véroia, *Greece* **50 F6** 40 34N 22 12 E
Véroli, *Italy* **45 G10** 41 41N 13 25 E
Verona, *Canada* **151 B8** 44 29N 76 42W
Verona, *Italy* **44 C7** 45 27N 10 59 E
Verona, *U.S.A.* **156 B7** 42 59N 89 32W
Verrès, *Italy* **44 C4** 45 40N 7 42 E
Verron Ra., *Papua N. G.* **132 C7** 4 21 S 152 46 E
Versailles, *France* **27 D9** 48 48N 2 8 E
Versailles, *Ill., U.S.A.* **156 E6** 39 53N 90 39W
Versailles, *Ind., U.S.A.* **157 E11** 39 4N 85 15W
Versailles, *Ky., U.S.A.* **157 F12** 38 3N 84 44W
Versailles, *Mo., U.S.A.* **156 F4** 38 26N 92 51W
Versailles, *Ohio, U.S.A.* **157 D12** 40 13N 84 29W
Versalles, *Bolivia* **173 C5** 12 44 S 63 18W
Versmold, *Germany* **30 C4** 52 2N 8 9 E
Versoix, *Switz.* **32 D2** 46 17N 6 10 E
Vert, C., *Senegal* **112 C1** 14 45N 17 30W
Vertou, *France* **26 E5** 47 10N 1 28W
Vertus, *France* **27 D11** 48 54N 4 2 E
Verulam, *S. Africa* **117 D5** 29 38 S 31 2 E
Verviers, *Belgium* **24 D5** 50 37N 5 52 E
Vervins, *France* **27 C10** 49 50N 3 53 E
Veržej, *Slovenia* **45 B13** 46 34N 16 13 E
Verzy, *France* **27 C11** 49 9N 4 10 E
Vescovato, *France* **29 F13** 42 30N 9 27 E
Veselí nad Lužnicí, *Czech Rep.* **34 B7** 49 12N 14 43 E
Veselie, *Bulgaria* **51 D11** 42 18N 27 38 E
Veselovskoye Vdkhr., *Russia* **61 G5** 46 58N 41 25 E
Veshenskaya, *Russia* **60 F5** 49 35N 41 44 E
Vesle →, *France* **27 C10** 49 23N 3 28 E
Veslyana →, *Russia* **64 A4** 60 20N 54 0 E
Vesoul, *France* **27 E13** 47 40N 6 11 E
Vessigebro, *Sweden* **17 H6** 56 58N 12 40 E
Vest-Agder □, *Norway* **18 F4** 58 30N 7 15 E
Vestbygd, *Norway* **18 F3** 58 6N 6 34 E
Vesterålen, *Norway* **14 B16** 68 45N 15 0 E
Vestfjorden, *Norway* **14 C15** 67 55N 14 0 E
Vestfold □, *Norway* **18 E7** 59 15N 10 0 E
Vestfossen, *Norway* **18 E6** 59 44N 9 52 E
Vestgrønland = Kitaa □, *Greenland* **10 C6** 70 0N 47 0W
Vestmannaeyjar, *Iceland* **11 D6** 63 27N 20 15W
Vestnes, *Norway* **18 B4** 62 39N 7 5 E
Vestre Gausdal, *Norway* **18 C7** 61 12N 10 8 E
Vestre Slidre, *Norway* **18 C5** 61 5N 8 58 E
Vestsjællands Amtskommune □, *Denmark* **17 J5** 55 30N 11 20 E
Vestspitsbergen, *Svalbard* **6 B8** 78 40N 17 0 E
Vestur-skaftafellssýsla □, *Iceland* **11 D8** 63 50N 18 30W
Vestvågøy, *Norway* **14 B15** 68 18N 13 50 E
Vesul Spitze, *Austria* **33 C10** 47 0N 10 21 E
Vesuvio, *Italy* **47 B7** 40 49N 14 26 E
Vesuvius, Mt. = Vesuvio, *Italy* **47 B7** 40 49N 14 26 E
Vesyegonsk, *Russia* **58 C9** 58 40N 37 16 E
Veszprém, *Hungary* **52 C2** 47 8N 17 57 E
Veszprém □, *Hungary* **52 C2** 47 5N 17 55 E
Vésztő, *Hungary* **52 D6** 46 55N 21 16 E
Vetapalem, *India* **95 G5** 15 47N 80 18 E
Vetlanda, *Sweden* **17 G9** 57 24N 15 3 E
Vetluga, *Russia* **60 B7** 57 53N 45 45 E
Vetlugu →, *Russia* **60 B8** 56 36N 46 4 E
Vetluzhskiy, *Kostroma, Russia* **60 A7** 58 23N 45 26 E
Vetluzhskiy, *Nizhniy Novgorod, Russia* **60 B7** 57 17N 45 12 E
Vetovo, *Bulgaria* **51 C10** 43 42N 26 16 E
Vetralla, *Italy* **45 F9** 42 20N 12 2 E
Vetren, *Bulgaria* **51 D8** 42 15N 24 3 E
Vettore, Mte., *Italy* **45 F10** 42 49N 13 16 E
Veurne, *Belgium* **24 C2** 51 5N 2 40 E
Vevay, *U.S.A.* **157 F11** 38 45N 85 4W
Veveno →, *Sudan* **107 F3** 6 40N 32 58 E
Vevey, *Switz.* **32 D3** 46 28N 6 51 E
Vévi, *Greece* **50 F5** 40 47N 21 38 E
Vex, *Switz.* **32 D4** 46 12N 7 24 E
Veynes, *France* **29 D9** 44 32N 5 49 E
Veys, *Iran* **97 D6** 31 30N 49 0 E
Vézelay, *France* **27 E10** 47 27N 3 45 E
Vézelise, *France* **27 D13** 48 30N 6 5 E
Vézère →, *France* **28 D4** 44 53N 0 53 E
Vezhen, *Bulgaria* **51 D8** 42 50N 24 20 E
Vezirköprü, *Turkey* **100 B6** 41 8N 35 27 E
Vezzani, *France* **29 F13** 42 10N 9 15 E
Vi Thanh, *Vietnam* **87 H5** 9 42N 105 26 E
Viacha, *Bolivia* **172 D4** 16 39 S 68 18W
Viadana, *Italy* **44 D7** 44 56N 10 31 E
Vialar = Tissemsilt, *Algeria* **111 A5** 35 35N 1 50 E
Viamão, *Brazil* **175 C5** 30 5 S 51 0W
Viana, *Brazil* **170 B3** 3 13 S 44 55W
Viana, *Spain* **40 C2** 42 31N 2 22W
Viana do Alentejo, *Portugal* **43 G3** 38 17N 7 59W
Viana do Bolo, *Spain* **42 C3** 42 11N 7 6W
Viana do Castelo, *Portugal* **42 D2** 41 42N 8 50W
Viana do Castelo □, *Portugal* **42 D2** 41 50N 8 30W
Vianden, *Lux.* **24 E6** 49 56N 6 12 E

Viangchan = Vientiane, Laos 86 D4 17 58N 102 36 E
Vianópolis, Brazil 171 E2 16 40 S 48 35W
Viar →, Spain 43 H5 37 36N 5 50W
Viaréggio, Italy 44 E7 43 52N 10 14 E
Viaur →, France 28 D5 44 8N 1 58 E
Vibble, Sweden 17 G12 57 37N 18 16 E
Vibo Valéntia, Italy 47 D9 38 40N 16 6 E
Viborg, Denmark 17 H3 56 27N 9 23 E
Viborg Amtskommune □, Denmark 17 H3 56 30N 9 30 E
Vibraye, France 26 D7 48 3N 0 44 E
Vic, Spain 40 D7 41 58N 2 19 E
Vic, Étang de, France 28 E7 43 29N 3 50 E
Vic-en-Bigorre, France 28 E4 43 24N 0 3 E
Vic-Fezensac, France 28 E4 43 47N 0 19 E
Vic-le-Comte, France 27 G10 45 39N 3 14 E
Vic-sur-Cère, France 28 D6 44 59N 2 38 E
Vícar, Spain 41 J2 36 50N 2 38W
Vicente Pérez Rosales ∆, Chile 176 B2 41 11 S 72 12W
Vicenza, Italy 45 C8 45 33N 11 33 E
Vich = Vic, Spain 40 D7 41 58N 2 19 E
Vichada □, Colombia 168 C4 5 0N 69 30W
Vichada →, Colombia 168 C4 4 55N 67 50W
Vichuga, Russia 60 B5 57 12N 41 55 E
Vichy, France 27 F10 46 9N 3 26 E
Vicksburg, Ariz., U.S.A. 161 M13 33 45N 113 45W
Vicksburg, Mich., U.S.A. 157 B11 42 7N 85 32W
Vicksburg, Miss., U.S.A. 155 J9 32 21N 90 53W
Vico, France 29 F12 42 10N 8 49 E
Vico, L. di, Italy 45 F9 42 19N 12 10 E
Vico del Gargano, Italy 45 G12 41 54N 15 57 E
Viçosa, Brazil 170 C4 9 28 S 36 14W
Viçosa do Ceará, Brazil 170 B3 3 34 S 41 5W
Vicosoprano, Switz. 33 D9 46 22N 9 38 E
Vicovu de Sus, Romania 53 C10 47 56N 25 41 E
Victor, India 92 J4 21 0N 71 30 E
Victor, U.S.A. 150 D7 42 58N 77 24W
Victor Emanuel Ra., Papua N. G. 132 C2 5 20 S 142 15 E
Victor Harbor, Australia 128 C3 35 30 S 138 37 E
Victor Hugo = Hamadia, Algeria 111 A5 35 28N 1 57 E
Victoria = Labuan, Malaysia 85 A5 5 20N 115 14 E
Victoria, Argentina 174 C3 32 40 S 60 10W
Victoria, Canada 142 D4 48 30N 123 25W
Victoria, Chile 176 A2 38 13 S 72 20W
Victoria, China 69 G1 22 17N 114 9 E
Victoria, Guinea 112 C2 10 50N 14 32W
Victoria, Malta 38 E6 36 3N 14 14 E
Victoria, Mind. Or., Phil. 80 E3 13 12N 121 12 E
Victoria, Tarlac, Phil. 80 D3 15 35N 120 41 E
Victoria, Romania 53 E9 45 44N 24 41 E
Victoria, Seychelles 121 b 4 38 S 55 28 E
Victoria, Kans., U.S.A. 154 F5 38 52N 99 9W
Victoria, Tex., U.S.A. 155 L6 28 48N 97 0W
Victoria □, Australia 128 D6 37 0 S 144 0 E
Victoria →, Australia 124 C4 15 10 S 129 40 E
Victoria, Grand L., Canada 140 C4 47 31N 77 30W
Victoria, L., Africa 118 C3 1 0 S 33 0 E
Victoria, L., Australia 128 B4 33 57 S 141 15 E
Victoria, Mt. = Tomanlivi, Fiji 133 A2 17 37 S 178 1 E
Victoria, Mt., Burma 90 E4 21 14N 93 55 E
Victoria, Mt., Papua N. G. 132 E4 8 55 S 147 32 E
Victoria Beach, Canada 143 C9 50 40N 96 35W
Victoria de Durango = Durango, Mexico 162 C4 24 3N 104 39W
Victoria de las Tunas, Cuba 164 B4 20 58N 76 59W
Victoria Falls, Zimbabwe 119 F2 17 58 S 25 52 E
Victoria Harbour, Canada 150 B5 44 45N 79 45W
Victoria I., Canada 138 A8 71 0N 111 0W
Victoria L., Canada 141 C8 48 20N 57 27W
Victoria Ld., Antarctica 7 D11 75 0 S 160 0 E
Victoria Nile →, Uganda 118 B3 2 14N 31 26 E
Victoria Peaks, Phil. 81 G2 9 22N 118 20 E
Victoria Ra., N.Z. 131 C7 42 12 S 172 7 E
Victoria River, Australia 124 C5 16 25 S 131 0 E
Victoria Str., Canada 138 B9 69 31N 100 30W
Victoria West, S. Africa 116 E3 31 25 S 23 4 E
Victorias, Phil. 81 F4 10 54N 123 5 E
Victoriaville, Canada 141 C5 46 4N 71 56W
Victorica, Argentina 174 D2 36 20 S 65 30W
Victorville, U.S.A. 161 L9 34 32N 117 18W
Vicuña, Chile 174 C1 30 0 S 70 50W
Vicuña Mackenna, Argentina 174 C3 33 53 S 64 25W
Vidal, U.S.A. 161 L12 34 7N 114 31W
Vidal Junction, U.S.A. 161 L12 34 11N 114 34W
Vidalia, U.S.A. 152 C7 32 13N 82 25W
Vidamlya, Belarus 55 F10 52 19N 23 47 E
Vidauban, France 29 E10 43 25N 6 27 E
Videbæk, Denmark 17 H2 56 6N 8 38 E
Videle, Romania 53 F10 44 17N 25 31 E
Videseter, Norway 18 C4 61 57N 7 14 E
Vidette, U.S.A. 152 B7 33 2N 82 15W
Vídho, Greece 38 B9 39 38N 19 55 E
Vidigueira, Portugal 43 G3 38 12N 7 48W
Vidin, Bulgaria 50 C6 43 59N 22 50 E
Vidio, C., Spain 42 B4 43 35N 6 14W
Vidisha, India 92 H7 23 28N 77 53 E
Vidra, Romania 53 E11 45 56N 26 55 E
Viduša, Bos.-H. 50 D2 42 55N 18 21 E
Vidzy, Belarus 15 J22 55 23N 26 37 E
Viechtach, Germany 31 F8 49 4N 12 53 E
Viedma, Argentina 176 B4 40 50 S 63 0W
Viedma, L., Argentina 176 C2 49 30 S 72 30W
Vieira do Minho, Portugal 42 D2 41 38N 8 8W
Vielha, Spain 40 C5 42 43N 0 44 E
Viella = Vielha, Spain 40 C5 42 43N 0 44 E
Vielsalm, Belgium 24 D5 50 17N 5 54 E
Vienenburg, Germany 30 D6 51 57N 10 34 E
Vieng Pou Kha, Laos 76 G3 20 41N 101 4 E
Vienna = Wien, Austria 35 C9 48 12N 16 22 E
Vienna, Ga., U.S.A. 152 C6 32 6N 83 47W
Vienna, Ill., U.S.A. 155 G10 37 25N 88 54W
Vienna, Mo., U.S.A. 156 F5 38 11N 91 57W
Vienne, France 29 C8 45 31N 4 53 E
Vienne □, France 28 B4 46 30N 0 42 E
Vienne →, France 26 E7 47 13N 0 5 E
Vientiane, Laos 86 D4 17 58N 102 36 E
Vientos, Paso de los, Caribbean 165 C5 20 0N 74 0W
Vieques, Isla de, Puerto Rico 165 d 18 8N 65 25W
Vierge Pt., St. Lucia 165 f 13 49N 60 53W
Viernheim, Germany 31 F4 49 31N 8 35 E
Viersen, Germany 30 D2 51 15N 6 23 E
Vierwaldstättersee, Switz. 33 C7 47 0N 8 30 E
Vierzon, France 27 E9 47 13N 2 5 E
Vieste, Italy 45 G13 41 53N 16 10 E
Vietnam ■, Asia 86 C6 19 0N 106 0 E
Vietz = Witnica, Poland 55 F1 52 40N 14 54 E
Vieux-Boucau-les-Bains, France 28 E2 43 48N 1 23W
Vieux Fort, St. Lucia 165 f 13 46N 60 58W
Vif, France 29 C9 45 5N 5 41 E
Viga, Phil. 80 E5 13 52N 124 18 E
Vigan, Phil. 80 C3 17 35N 120 28 E
Vigévano, Italy 44 C5 45 19N 8 51 E
Vigia = Almenara, Brazil 171 E3 16 11 S 40 42W
Vigia, Brazil 170 B2 0 50 S 48 5W
Vigía Chico, Mexico 163 D7 19 46N 87 35W
Vigla, Greece 39 A2 39 7N 20 50 E
Víglas, Ákra, Greece 38 F11 35 54N 27 51 E
Vignemalle, France 28 F3 42 47N 0 10W
Vigneulles-lès-Hattonchâtel, France 27 D12 48 59N 5 43 E
Vignola, Italy 44 D8 44 29N 11 1 E
Vigo, Spain 42 C2 42 12N 8 41W
Vigo, Ría de, Spain 42 C2 42 15N 8 45W
Vigrestad, Norway 18 F2 58 34N 5 42 E
Vigsø Bugt, Denmark 17 G2 57 5N 8 47 E
Vihiers, France 26 E6 47 10N 0 30W
Vihowa, Pakistan 92 D4 31 8N 70 30 E
Vihowa →, Pakistan 92 D4 31 8N 70 41 E
Viipuri = Vyborg, Russia 58 B5 60 43N 28 47 E
Vijayadurg, India 94 F1 16 30N 73 25 E
Vijayawada, India 94 F5 16 31N 80 39 E
Vijosë →, Albania 50 F3 40 37N 19 24 E
Vík, Iceland 11 D7 63 25N 19 1W
Vik, Norway 18 C3 61 21N 6 6 E
Vika, Sweden 16 D8 60 57N 14 28 E
Vikarabad, India 94 E3 17 20N 77 54 E
Vikarbyn, Sweden 16 D9 60 55N 15 1 E
Vike, Norway 18 D2 60 23N 5 35 E
Vikedal, Norway 18 E2 59 30N 5 55 E
Vikeke = Viqueque, E. Timor 82 C3 8 52 S 126 23 E
Vikeland, Norway 18 F4 58 5N 7 18 E
Viken, Skåne, Sweden 17 H6 56 9N 12 34 E
Viken, Västra Götaland, Sweden 17 F8 58 39N 14 20 E
Vikersund, Norway 18 E6 59 58N 9 59 E
Vikeså, Norway 18 F3 58 38N 6 3 E
Vikevåg, Norway 18 E2 59 5N 5 41 E
Viking, Canada 142 C6 53 7N 111 50W
Vikmanshyttan, Sweden 16 D9 60 18N 15 50 E
Vikna, Norway 14 D14 64 55N 10 58 E
Vikos-Aoos ∆, Greece 48 B2 40 0N 20 45 E
Viksøyri, Norway 18 C3 61 4N 6 34 E
Vila Alferes Chamusca = Guijá, Mozam. 117 C5 24 27 S 33 0 E
Vila António Enes = Angoche, Mozam. 119 F4 16 8 S 39 55 E
Vila Bela da Santissima Trindade, Brazil 173 C6 15 0 S 59 57W
Vila Cabral = Lichinga, Mozam. 119 E4 13 13 S 35 11 E
Vila Cabral = Niassa □, Mozam. 119 E4 13 30 S 36 0 E
Vila da Maganja, Mozam. 119 F4 17 18 S 37 30 E
Vila da Ribeira Brava, C. Verde Is. 9 j 16 32N 24 25W
Vila de Rei, Portugal 42 F2 39 41N 8 9W
Vila do Bispo, Portugal 43 H2 37 5N 8 53W
Vila do Conde, Portugal 42 D2 41 21N 8 45W
Vila do Porto, Azores 9 d4 36 56N 25 9W
Vila Franca de Xira, Portugal 43 G2 38 57N 8 59W
Vila Franca do Campo, Azores 9 d3 37 43N 25 26W
Vila Gamito, Mozam. 119 E3 14 12 S 33 0 E
Vila Gomes da Costa, Mozam. 117 C5 24 20 S 33 37 E
Vila Machado, Mozam. 119 F3 19 15 S 34 14 E
Vila Mouzinho, Mozam. 119 E3 14 48 S 34 25 E
Vila Nova de Famalicão, Portugal 42 D2 41 25N 8 32W
Vila Nova de Fos Côa, Portugal 42 D3 41 5N 7 9W
Vila Nova de Gaia, Portugal 42 D2 41 4N 8 40W
Vila Nova de Gaza = Xai-Xai, Mozam. 117 D5 25 6 S 33 31 E
Vila Nova de Ourém, Portugal 42 F2 39 40N 8 35W
Vila Nova do Corvo, Azores 9 d2 39 40N 31 8W
Vila Pereira de Eça = Ondjiva, Angola 116 B2 16 48 S 15 50 E
Vila Pery = Manica, Mozam. 117 B5 18 58 S 32 59 E
Vila Pouca de Aguiar, Portugal 42 D3 41 30N 7 38W
Vila Real, Portugal 42 D3 41 17N 7 48W
Vila Real □, Portugal 42 D3 41 36N 7 35W
Vila-real de los Infantes, Spain 40 F4 39 55N 0 3W
Vila Real de Santo António, Portugal 43 H3 37 10N 7 28W
Vila Teixeira da Silva = Luau, Angola 115 E4 10 40 S 22 10 E
Vila Vasco da Gama, Mozam. 119 E3 14 54 S 32 14 E
Vila Velha, Amapá, Brazil 169 C7 3 13N 51 13W
Vila Velha, Espírito Santo, Brazil 171 F3 20 20 S 40 17W
Vila Viçosa, Portugal 43 G3 38 45N 7 27W
Vilafranca del Maestrat, Spain 40 E4 40 26N 0 16W
Vilafranca del Penedès, Spain 40 D6 41 21N 1 40 E
Vilagarcía de Arousa, Spain 42 C2 42 34N 8 46W
Vilaine →, France 26 E4 47 30N 2 27W
Vilakalaka, Vanuatu 133 E5 15 25 S 167 42 E
Vilanandro, Tanjona, Madag. 117 B7 16 11 S 44 27 E
Vilanculos, Mozam. 117 C6 22 1 S 35 17 E
Vilanova de Castelló, Spain 41 F4 39 5N 0 31W
Vilanova i la Geltrú, Spain 40 D6 41 13N 1 40 E
Vilar Formosa, Portugal 42 E4 40 38N 6 45W
Vilaseca, Spain 40 D6 41 7N 1 9 E
Vilaseca-Salou = Vilaseca, Spain 40 D6 41 7N 1 9 E
Vilbjerg, Denmark 17 H2 56 12N 8 46 E
Vilcabamba, Cordillera, Peru 172 C3 13 0 S 73 0W
Vilcanchos, Peru 172 C3 13 40 S 74 25W
Vilcheka, Zemlya, Russia 6 A11 80 30N 60 30 E
Vilches, Spain 43 G7 38 12N 3 30W
Vileyka, Belarus 58 E4 54 30N 26 53 E
Vilhelmina, Sweden 14 D17 64 35N 16 39 E
Vilhena, Brazil 173 C5 12 40 S 60 5W
Viliya = Neris →, Lithuania 15 J21 55 8N 24 16 E
Viljandi, Estonia 15 G21 58 28N 25 30 E
Viljoensdorp = Newcastle, S. Africa 117 D4 27 45 S 29 58 E
Vilkaviškis, Lithuania 54 D10 54 39N 23 2 E
Vilkija, Lithuania 54 C10 55 3N 23 35 E
Vilkitskogo, Proliv, Russia 67 B11 78 0N 103 0 E
Vilkomir = Ukmergė, Lithuania 15 J21 55 15N 24 45 E
Vilkovo = Vylkove, Ukraine 53 E14 45 28N 29 32 E
Villa Abecia, Bolivia 174 A2 21 0 S 68 18W
Villa Ahumada, Mexico 162 A3 30 38N 106 30W
Villa Ana, Argentina 174 B4 28 28 S 59 40W
Villa Ángela, Argentina 174 B3 27 34 S 60 45W
Villa Bella = Serra Talhada, Brazil 170 C4 7 59 S 38 18W
Villa Bella, Bolivia 173 C4 10 25 S 65 22W
Villa Bruzual, Venezuela 168 C4 9 20N 69 6W
Villa Cañás, Argentina 174 C3 34 0 S 61 35W
Villa Cecilia = Ciudad Madero, Mexico 163 C5 22 19N 97 50W
Villa Cisneros = Dakhla, W. Sahara 110 D1 23 50N 15 53W
Villa Colón, Argentina 174 C2 31 38 S 68 20W
Villa Constitución, Argentina 174 C3 33 15 S 60 20W
Villa de Cura, Venezuela 168 A4 10 2N 67 29W
Villa de María, Argentina 174 B3 29 55 S 63 43W
Villa del Nevoso = Ilirska-Bistrica, Slovenia 45 C11 45 34N 14 14 E
Villa del Río, Spain 43 H6 37 59N 4 17W
Villa del Rosario, Venezuela 168 A3 10 19N 72 19W
Villa Dolores, Argentina 174 C2 31 58 S 65 15W
Villa Frontera, Mexico 162 B4 26 56N 101 27W
Villa Grove, U.S.A. 157 E8 39 52N 88 10W
Villa Guillermina, Argentina 174 B4 28 15 S 59 29W
Villa Hayes, Paraguay 174 B4 25 5 S 57 20W
Villa Iris, Argentina 174 D3 38 12 S 63 12W
Villa Juárez, Mexico 162 B4 27 37N 100 44W
Villa María, Argentina 174 C3 32 20 S 63 10W
Villa Mazán, Argentina 174 B2 28 40 S 66 30W
Villa Minozzo, Italy 44 D7 44 22N 10 28 E
Villa Montes, Bolivia 174 A3 21 10 S 63 30W
Villa Ocampo, Argentina 174 B4 28 30 S 59 20W
Villa Ocampo, Mexico 162 B3 26 29N 105 30W
Villa Ojo de Agua, Argentina 174 B3 29 30 S 63 44W
Villa Rica, U.S.A. 152 B5 33 44N 84 55W
Villa San Giovanni, Italy 47 D8 38 13N 15 38 E
Villa San José, Argentina 174 C4 32 12 S 58 15W
Villa San Martín, Argentina 174 B3 28 15 S 64 9W
Villa Sanjurjo = Al Hoceïma, Morocco 110 A4 35 8N 3 58W
Villa Santina, Italy 45 B9 46 24N 12 55 E
Villa Unión, Mexico 162 C3 23 12N 106 14W
Villaba, Phil. 81 F5 11 13N 124 24 E
Villablino, Spain 42 C4 42 57N 6 19W
Villacarlos, Spain 38 B5 39 53N 4 17 E
Villacarriedo, Spain 42 B7 43 14N 3 48W
Villacarrillo, Spain 43 G7 38 7N 3 3W
Villacastín, Spain 42 E6 40 46N 4 25W
Villach, Austria 34 E6 46 37N 13 51 E
Villacidro, Italy 46 C1 39 27N 8 44 E
Villada, Spain 42 C6 42 15N 4 59W
Villadiego, Spain 42 C6 42 31N 4 1W
Villadóssola, Italy 44 B5 46 4N 8 16 E
Villafeliche, Spain 40 D3 41 10N 1 30W
Villafranca, Spain 40 C3 42 17N 1 46W
Villafranca de los Barros, Spain 43 G4 38 35N 6 18W
Villafranca de los Caballeros, Spain 43 F7 39 26N 3 21W
Villafranca del Cid = Vilafranca del Maestrat, Spain 40 E4 40 26N 0 16W
Villafranca del Panadés = Vilafranca del Penedès, Spain 40 D6 41 21N 1 40 E
Villafranca di Verona, Italy 44 C7 45 21N 10 50 E
Villafranca Tirrena, Italy 47 D8 38 20N 15 25 E
Villagio Mussolini = Arboréa, Italy 46 C1 39 46N 8 35 E
Villagrán, Mexico 163 C5 24 29N 99 29W
Villaguay, Argentina 174 C4 32 0 S 59 0W
Villaharta, Spain 43 G6 38 9N 4 54W
Villahermosa, Mexico 163 D6 17 59N 92 55W
Villahermosa, Spain 41 G2 38 46N 2 52W
Villaines-la-Juhel, France 26 D6 48 21N 0 20W
Villajoyosa, Spain 41 G4 38 30N 0 12W
Villalba, Spain 42 B3 43 26N 7 40W
Villalba de Guardo, Spain 42 C6 42 42N 4 49W
Villalón de Campos, Spain 42 C5 42 5N 5 4W
Villalpando, Spain 42 D5 41 51N 5 25W
Villaluenga, Spain 42 E7 40 2N 3 54W
Villamanán, Spain 42 C5 42 19N 5 35W
Villamartín, Spain 43 J5 36 52N 5 38W
Villamayor de Santiago, Spain 40 F2 39 50N 2 59W
Villamblard, France 28 C4 45 2N 0 32 E
Villanova Monteleone, Italy 46 B1 40 30N 8 28 E
Villanueva, Colombia 168 A3 10 37N 72 59W
Villanueva, U.S.A. 155 H2 35 16N 105 22W
Villanueva de Castellón = Vilanova de Castelló, Spain 41 F4 39 5N 0 31W
Villanueva de Córdoba, Spain 43 G6 38 20N 4 38W
Villanueva de la Fuente, Spain 41 G2 38 42N 2 42W
Villanueva de la Serena, Spain 43 G5 38 59N 5 50W
Villanueva de la Sierra, Spain 42 E4 40 12N 6 24W
Villanueva de los Castillejos, Spain 43 H3 37 30N 7 15W
Villanueva de los Infantes, Spain 43 G7 38 43N 3 1W
Villanueva del Arzobispo, Spain 41 G2 38 10N 3 0W
Villanueva del Fresno, Spain 43 G3 38 23N 7 10W
Villanueva y Geltrú = Vilanova i la Geltrú, Spain 40 D6 41 13N 1 40 E
Villaputzu, Italy 46 C2 39 26N 9 34 E
Villaquilambre, Spain 42 C5 42 39N 5 33W
Villar del Arzobispo, Spain 40 F4 39 44N 0 50W
Villar del Rey, Spain 43 F4 39 7N 6 50W
Villard-de-Lans, France 29 C9 45 3N 5 33 E
Villarramiel, Spain 42 C6 42 2N 4 55W
Villarreal = Vila-real de los Infantes, Spain 40 F4 39 55N 0 3W
Villarrica, Chile 176 A2 39 15 S 72 15W
Villarrica, Paraguay 174 B4 25 40 S 56 30W
Villarrica ∆, Chile 176 A2 39 24 S 71 46W
Villarrobledo, Spain 41 F2 39 18N 2 36W
Villarroya de la Sierra, Spain 40 D3 41 27N 1 46W
Villarrubia de los Ojos, Spain 43 F7 39 14N 3 36W
Villars-les-Dombes, France 27 F12 46 0N 5 3 E
Villasayas, Spain 40 D2 41 24N 2 39W
Villaseca de los Gamitos = Villaseco de los Gamitos, Spain 42 D4 41 2N 6 7W
Villaseco de los Gamitos, Spain 42 D4 41 2N 6 7W
Villasimíus, Italy 46 C2 39 8N 9 31 E
Villastar, Spain 40 E3 40 17N 1 9W
Villatobas, Spain 42 F7 39 54N 3 20W
Villavicencio, Argentina 174 C2 32 28 S 69 0W
Villavicencio, Colombia 168 C3 4 9N 73 37W
Villaviciosa, Spain 42 B5 43 32N 5 27W
Villazón, Bolivia 174 A2 22 0 S 65 35W
Ville-Marie, Canada 140 C4 47 20N 79 30W
Ville Platte, U.S.A. 155 K8 30 41N 92 17W
Villedieu-les-Poêles, France 26 D5 48 50N 1 13W
Villefort, France 28 D7 44 28N 3 56 E
Villefranche-de-Lauragais, France 28 E5 43 25N 1 44 E
Villefranche-de-Rouergue, France 28 D6 44 21N 2 2 E
Villefranche-du-Périgord, France 28 D5 44 38N 1 5 E
Villefranche-sur-Saône, France 29 C8 45 59N 4 43 E
Villegrande, Bolivia 173 D5 18 30 S 64 10W
Villel, Spain 40 E3 40 14N 1 12W
Villemur-sur-Tarn, France 28 E5 43 51N 1 31 E
Villena, Spain 41 G4 38 39N 0 52W
Villenauxe-la-Grande, France 27 D10 48 35N 3 33 E
Villenave-d'Ornon, France 28 D3 44 46N 0 33W
Villeneuve, Switz. 32 D3 46 24N 6 56 E
Villeneuve-d'Ascq, France 27 B10 50 38N 3 9 E
Villeneuve-l'Archevêque, France 27 D10 48 14N 3 32 E
Villeneuve-lès-Avignon, France 29 E8 43 58N 4 49 E
Villeneuve-sur-Allier, France 27 F10 46 40N 3 13 E
Villeneuve-sur-Lot, France 28 D4 44 24N 0 42 E
Villeneuve-sur-Yonne, France 27 D10 48 5N 3 18 E
Villeréal, France 28 D4 44 38N 0 45 E
Villers-Bocage, France 26 C6 49 3N 0 40W
Villers-Cotterêts, France 27 C10 49 15N 3 4 E
Villers-sur-Mer, France 26 C6 49 21N 0 2W
Villersexel, France 27 E13 47 33N 6 26 E
Villerupt, France 27 C12 49 28N 5 55 E
Villeurbanne, France 29 C8 45 46N 4 55 E
Villiers, S. Africa 117 D4 27 2 S 28 36 E
Villingen-Schwenningen, Germany 31 G4 48 3N 8 26 E
Villisca, U.S.A. 156 D2 40 56N 94 59W
Villmanstrand = Lappeenranta, Finland 15 F23 61 3N 28 12 E
Villupuram, India 95 J4 11 59N 79 31 E
Vilna = Vilnius, Lithuania 15 J21 54 38N 25 19 E
Vilna, Canada 142 C6 54 7N 111 55W
Vilnius, Lithuania 15 J21 54 38N 25 19 E
Vils, Austria 34 D3 47 33N 10 38 E
Vils →, Bayern, Germany 31 G9 48 37N 13 11 E
Vils →, Bayern, Germany 31 F7 49 10N 11 57 E
Vilsbiburg, Germany 31 G8 48 26N 12 22 E
Vilshofen, Germany 31 G9 48 37N 13 11 E
Vilusi, Serbia & M. 50 D2 42 44N 18 34 E
Vilvoorde, Belgium 24 D4 50 56N 4 26 E
Vilyuy →, Russia 67 C13 64 24N 126 26 E
Vilyuysk, Russia 67 C13 63 40N 121 35 E
Vimianzo, Spain 42 B1 43 7N 9 2W
Vimioso, Portugal 42 D4 41 35N 6 31W
Vimmerby, Sweden 17 G9 57 40N 15 55 E
Vimoutiers, France 26 D7 48 57N 0 10 E
Vimperk, Czech Rep. 34 B6 49 3N 13 46 E
Vina →, Cameroon 114 A3 7 45N 15 36 E
Viña del Mar, Chile 174 C1 33 0 S 71 30W
Vinarós, Spain 40 E5 40 30N 0 27 E
Vincennes, U.S.A. 157 F9 38 41N 87 32W
Vincent, U.S.A. 161 L8 34 33N 118 11W
Vinces, Ecuador 168 D2 1 32 S 79 45W
Vinchina, Argentina 174 B2 28 45 S 68 15W
Vindava = Ventspils, Latvia 15 H19 57 25N 21 32 E
Vindelälven →, Sweden 14 E18 63 55N 19 50 E
Vindeln, Sweden 14 D18 64 12N 19 43 E
Vinderup, Denmark 17 H2 56 29N 8 45 E
Vindhya Ra., India 92 H7 22 50N 77 0 E
Vine Grove, U.S.A. 157 G11 37 49N 85 59W
Vineland, U.S.A. 148 F8 39 29N 75 2W
Vineuil, France 26 47 35N 1 22 E
Vinga, Romania 52 D6 46 1N 21 14 E
Vingåker, Sweden 16 E9 59 2N 15 52 E
Vingelen, Norway 18 B7 62 25N 10 52 E
Vingnes, Norway 18 C7 61 7N 10 26 E
Vinh, Vietnam 86 C5 18 45N 105 38 E
Vinh Linh, Vietnam 86 D6 17 4N 107 2 E
Vinh Loi = Bac Lieu, Vietnam 87 H5 9 17N 105 43 E
Vinh Long, Vietnam 87 G5 10 16N 105 57 E
Vinh Yen, Vietnam 76 G5 21 21N 105 35 E
Vinhais, Portugal 42 D3 41 50N 7 5W
Vinica, Croatia 45 B13 46 20N 16 9 E
Vinica, Macedonia 50 E6 41 53N 22 30 E
Vinica, Slovenia 45 C12 45 28N 15 16 E
Vinita, U.S.A. 155 G7 36 39N 95 9W
Vinje, Hordaland, Norway 18 D3 60 48N 6 30 E
Vinje, Sør-Trøndelag, Norway 18 A5 63 12N 9 0 E
Vinje, Telemark, Norway 18 E4 59 37N 7 51 E
Vinkovci, Croatia 52 E3 45 19N 18 48 E
Vinnitsa = Vinnytsya, Ukraine 59 H5 49 15N 28 30 E
Vinnytsya, Ukraine 59 H5 49 15N 28 30 E
Vinodelnoye = Ipatovo, Russia 61 H6 45 45N 42 50 E
Vinslöv, Sweden 17 H7 56 7N 13 55 E
Vinson Massif, Antarctica 7 D16 78 35 S 85 25W
Vinstra, Norway 18 C6 61 37N 9 44 E
Vinstra →, Norway 18 C6 61 37N 9 44 E
Vintar, Phil. 80 B3 18 14N 120 39 E
Vintjärn, Sweden 16 D10 60 50N 16 4 E
Vinton, Calif., U.S.A. 160 F6 39 48N 120 10W
Vinton, Iowa, U.S.A. 156 B4 42 10N 92 1W
Vinton, La., U.S.A. 155 K8 30 11N 93 35W
Vinţu de Jos, Romania 53 D8 46 0N 23 30 E
Vinukonda, India 95 F4 16 4N 79 45 E
Viöl, Germany 30 A5 54 34N 9 11 E
Viola, U.S.A. 156 C6 41 12N 90 35W
Violet Town, Australia 129 D6 36 38 S 145 42 E
Vipacco = Vipava, Slovenia 45 C10 45 51N 13 58 E
Vipava, Slovenia 45 C10 45 51N 13 58 E
Vipiteno, Italy 45 B8 46 54N 11 26 E
Viqueque, E. Timor 82 C3 8 52 S 126 23 E
Vir, Croatia 45 D12 44 17N 15 3 E
Vira, Switz. 33 D7 46 8N 8 50 E
Virac, Phil. 80 E5 13 30N 124 20 E
Virachey, Cambodia 86 F6 13 59N 106 49 E
Virachey ∆, Cambodia 86 E6 14 14N 106 55 E
Virago Sd., Canada 142 C2 54 0N 132 30W
Virajpet = Virarajendrapet, India 95 H2 12 10N 75 50 E
Viramgam, India 92 H5 23 5N 72 0 E
Viranşehir, Turkey 101 D8 37 13N 39 45 E
Virarajendrapet, India 95 H2 12 10N 75 50 E
Virawah, Pakistan 92 G4 24 31N 70 46 E
Virbalis, Lithuania 54 D9 54 39N 22 49 E
Virden, Canada 143 D8 49 50N 100 56W
Virden, U.S.A. 156 E7 39 30N 89 46W
Vire, France 26 D6 48 50N 0 53W
Vire →, France 26 C5 49 20N 1 7W
Virei, Angola 115 F2 15 43 S 12 52 E
Virgem da Lapa, Brazil 171 E3 16 49 S 42 21W
Vírgenes, C., Argentina 176 D3 52 19 S 68 21W
Virgin →, U.S.A. 159 H6 36 28N 114 21W
Virgin Gorda, Br. Virgin Is. 165 e 18 30N 64 26W
Virgin Is. (British) ☒, W. Indies 165 e 18 30N 64 30W
Virgin Is. (U.S.) ☒, W. Indies 165 e 18 20N 65 0W
Virgin Islands ∆, U.S. Virgin Is. 165 C7 18 21N 64 43W
Virginia, S. Africa 116 D4 28 8 S 26 55 E
Virginia, Ill., U.S.A. 156 E6 39 57N 90 13W
Virginia, Minn., U.S.A. 154 B8 47 31N 92 32W
Virginia □, U.S.A. 148 G7 37 30N 78 45W
Virginia Beach, U.S.A. 148 G8 36 51N 75 59W
Virginia City, Mont., U.S.A. 158 D8 45 18N 111 56W
Virginia City, Nev., U.S.A. 160 F7 39 19N 119 39W
Virginia Falls, Canada 142 A3 61 38N 125 42W
Virginiatown, Canada 140 C4 48 9N 79 36W
Virje, Croatia 45 B13 46 4N 16 59 E
Viroqua, U.S.A. 154 D9 43 34N 90 53W
Virovitica, Croatia 52 E2 45 51N 17 21 E
Virpazar, Serbia & M. 50 D3 42 14N 19 6 E
Virpur, India 92 J4 21 51N 70 42 E
Virserum, Sweden 17 G9 57 20N 15 35 E
Virton, Belgium 24 E5 49 35N 5 32 E
Virú, Peru 172 B2 8 25 S 78 45W
Virudunagar, India 95 K3 9 30N 77 58 E
Virunga ∆, Dem. Rep. of the Congo 118 B2 0 5N 29 38 E
Vis, Croatia 45 E13 43 4N 16 10 E
Visalia, U.S.A. 160 J7 36 20N 119 18W
Visayan Sea, Phil. 81 F4 11 30N 123 30 E
Visby, Sweden 17 G12 57 37N 18 18 E
Viscount Melville Sd., Canada 6 B2 74 10N 108 0W
Visé, Belgium 24 D5 50 44N 5 41 E
Višegrad, Bos.-H. 52 G4 43 47N 19 17 E
Viseu, Brazil 170 B2 1 10 S 46 5W
Viseu, Portugal 42 E3 40 40N 7 55W
Viseu □, Portugal 42 E3 40 40N 7 55W
Vişeu de Sus, Romania 53 C9 47 45N 24 25 E
Vishakhapatnam, India 94 F6 17 45N 83 20 E
Vishera →, Russia 64 A6 59 55N 56 25 E
Vişina, Romania 53 G9 43 52N 24 27 E
Vişineşti, Moldova 53 D13 46 20N 28 27 E
Visingsö, Sweden 17 F8 58 2N 14 20 E
Viskafors, Sweden 17 G6 57 37N 12 50 E
Viskan →, Sweden 17 G6 57 14N 12 12 E
Viški Kanal, Croatia 45 E13 43 4N 16 5 E
Vislanda, Sweden 17 H8 56 46N 14 30 E
Visnagar, India 92 H5 23 45N 72 32 E
Višnja Gora, Slovenia 45 C11 45 58N 14 45 E
Viso, Mte., Italy 44 D4 44 38N 7 5 E
Viso del Marqués, Spain 43 G7 38 32N 3 34W
Visoko, Bos.-H. 52 G3 43 58N 18 10 E
Visokoi I., Antarctica 7 B1 56 43 S 27 15W
Visp, Switz. 32 D5 46 17N 7 52 E
Vispa →, Switz. 32 D5 46 9N 7 48 E
Vissefjärda, Sweden 17 H9 56 32N 15 35 E
Visselhövede, Germany 30 C5 52 59N 9 34 E
Vissenbjerg, Denmark 17 J4 55 23N 10 7 E
Vissoie, Switz. 32 D5 46 13N 7 36 E
Vista, U.S.A. 161 M9 33 12N 117 14W
Vistonikos, Ormos = Vistonís, Límni, Greece 51 E9 41 0N 25 7 E
Vistonís, Límni, Greece 51 E9 41 0N 25 7 E
Vistula = Wisła →, Poland 54 D5 54 22N 18 55 E
Vistula Lagoon = Zalew Wiślany, Poland 54 D6 54 20N 19 50 E
Vit →, Bulgaria 51 C8 43 30N 24 30 E
Vita, India 94 F2 17 17N 74 33 E
Vitanje, Slovenia 45 B12 46 25N 15 18 E
Vitebsk = Vitsyebsk, Belarus 58 E6 55 10N 30 15 E
Viterbo, Italy 45 F9 42 25N 12 6 E
Vitez, Bos.-H. 52 F2 44 10N 17 48 E
Viti Levu, Fiji 133 A1 17 30 S 177 30 E
Vitiaz Str., Papua N. G. 132 C4 5 40 S 147 10 E
Vitigudino, Spain 42 D4 41 1N 6 26W
Vitim, Russia 67 D12 59 28N 112 35 E
Vitim →, Russia 67 D12 59 26N 112 34 E
Vitina, Bos.-H. 45 E14 43 17N 17 29 E
Vitína, Greece 48 D4 37 40N 22 10 E
Vítkov, Czech Rep. 35 B10 49 46N 17 45 E
Vitória = Vitória de São Antão, Brazil 170 C4 8 10 S 35 20W
Vitória, Espírito Santo, Brazil 171 F3 20 20 S 40 22W

Vitória, *Pará, Brazil* **169 D7** 2 54 S 52 1W
Vitória da Conquista, *Brazil* **171 D3** 14 51 S 40 51W
Vitória de São Antão, *Brazil* **170 C4** 8 10 S 35 20W
Vitoria-Gasteiz, *Spain* **40 C2** 42 50N 2 41W
Vitória Seamount, *India* **8 J8** 20 0 S 44 0W
Vitorino Friere, *Brazil* **170 B2** 4 4 S 45 10W
Vitosha △, *Bulgaria* **50 D7** 42 36N 23 18 E
Vitré, *France* **26 D5** 48 8N 1 12W
Vitry-le-François, *France* **27 D11** 48 43N 4 33 E
Vitry-sur-Seine, *France* **27 D9** 48 47N 2 24 E
Vitsand, *Sweden* **16 D7** 60 20N 13 0 E
Vitsi, Óros, *Greece* **50 F5** 40 40N 21 25 E
Vitsyebsk, *Belarus* **58 E6** 55 10N 30 15 E
Vittaryd, *Sweden* **17 H7** 56 58N 13 57 E
Vitteaux, *France* **27 E11** 47 24N 4 30 E
Vittel, *France* **27 D12** 48 12N 5 57 E
Vittória, *Italy* **47 F7** 36 57N 14 32 E
Vittório = Vittório Véneto, *Italy* **45 C9** 45 59N 12 18 E
Vittório Véneto, *Italy* **45 C9** 45 59N 12 18 E
Vittoriosa, *Malta* **38 F8** 35 54N 14 31 E
Vittsjö, *Sweden* **17 H7** 56 20N 13 40 E
Vitznau, *Switz.* **33 B6** 47 1N 8 29 E
Viveiro, *Spain* **42 B3** 43 39N 7 38W
Vivian, *U.S.A.* **155 J8** 32 53N 93 59W
Viviers, *France* **29 D8** 44 30N 4 40 E
Vivonne, *Australia* **128 C2** 35 59 S 137 9 E
Vivonne, *France* **28 B4** 46 25N 0 15 E
Vivonne B., *Australia* **128 C2** 35 59 S 137 9 E
Viwa, *Fiji* **133 A1** 17 10 S 177 58 E
Vizagapatam = Vishakhapatnam, *India* **94 F6** 17 45N 83 20 E
Vizcaíno, Desierto de, *Mexico* **162 B2** 27 40N 113 50W
Vizcaíno, Sierra, *Mexico* **162 B2** 27 30N 114 0W
Vizcaya □, *Spain* **40 B2** 43 15N 2 45W
Vize, *Turkey* **51 E11** 41 34N 27 45 E
Vizianagaram, *India* **94 E6** 18 6N 83 30 E
Vizille, *France* **29 C9** 45 5N 5 46 E
Viziňada, *Croatia* **45 C10** 45 20N 13 46 E
Viziru, *Romania* **53 E12** 45 0N 27 43 E
Vizlinsky Zaliv = Zalew Wiślany, *Poland* **54 D6** 54 20N 19 50 E
Vizzini, *Italy* **47 E7** 37 10N 14 45 E
Vlaardingen, *Neths.* **24 C4** 51 55N 4 21 E
Vlădeasa, Vf., *Romania* **52 D7** 46 47N 22 50 E
Vladičin Han, *Serbia & M.* **50 D6** 42 42N 22 1 E
Vladikavkaz, *Russia* **61 J7** 43 0N 44 35 E
Vladimir, *Russia* **58 D11** 56 15N 40 30 E
Vladimir Volynskiy = Volodymyr-Volynskyy, *Ukraine* **59 G3** 50 50N 24 18 E
Vladimirci, *Serbia & M.* **50 B3** 44 36N 19 50 E
Vladimirovac, *Serbia & M.* **52 E5** 45 1N 20 53 E
Vladimirovka = Yuzhno-Sakhalinsk, *Russia* **67 E15** 46 58N 142 45 E
Vladimirovka, *Russia* **61 F8** 48 27N 46 10 E
Vladimirovo, *Bulgaria* **50 C7** 43 32N 23 22 E
Vladimorvka, *Kazakhstan* **60 E10** 50 51N 51 8 E
Vladislavovka, *Ukraine* **59 K8** 45 12N 35 29 E
Vladivostok, *Russia* **67 E14** 43 10N 131 53 E
Vlăhiţa, *Romania* **53 D10** 46 21N 25 31 E
Vlakhiótis, *Greece* **48 E4** 36 52N 22 42 E
Vlasenica, *Bos.-H.* **52 F3** 44 11N 18 59 E
Vlašić, *Bos.-H.* **52 F2** 44 19N 17 37 E
Vlašim, *Czech Rep.* **34 B7** 49 40N 14 53 E
Vlasinsko Jezero, *Serbia & M.* **50 D6** 42 44N 22 22 E
Vlasotince, *Serbia & M.* **50 D6** 42 59N 22 7 E
Vlieland, *Neths.* **24 A4** 53 16N 4 55 E
Vlissingen, *Neths.* **24 C3** 51 26N 3 34 E
Vlorë, *Albania* **50 F3** 40 32N 19 28 E
Vlorës, Gjiri i, *Albania* **50 F3** 40 29N 19 27 E
Vltava →, *Czech Rep.* **34 A7** 50 21N 14 30 E
Vo Dat, *Vietnam* **87 G6** 11 9N 107 31 E
Vobarno, *Italy* **33 E11** 45 39N 10 30 E
Voćin, *Croatia* **52 E2** 45 37N 17 33 E
Vöcklabruck, *Austria* **34 C6** 48 1N 13 39 E
Vodice, *Croatia* **45 E12** 43 47N 15 47 E
Vodňany, *Czech Rep.* **34 B7** 49 9N 14 11 E
Vodnjan, *Croatia* **45 D10** 44 59N 13 52 E
Vodopyanovo = Donskoy, *Russia* **58 F10** 53 55N 38 15 E
Voe, *U.K.* **22 A7** 60 21N 1 16W
Vogar, *Iceland* **11 D4** 63 58N 22 22W
Vogel Pk., *Nigeria* **113 D7** 8 24N 11 47 E
Vogelkop = Doberai, Jazirah, *Indonesia* **83 B4** 1 25 S 133 0 E
Vogelsberg, *Germany* **30 E5** 50 31N 9 12 E
Voghera, *Italy* **44 D6** 44 59N 9 1 E
Vogorno, *Switz.* **33 D7** 46 13N 8 52 E
Voh, *N. Cal.* **133 T18** 20 58 S 164 42 E
Vohibinany, *Madag.* **117 B8** 18 49 S 49 4 E
Vohilava, *Madag.* **117 C8** 21 4 S 48 0 E
Vohimarina = Iharana, *Madag.* **117 A9** 13 25 S 50 0 E
Vohimena, Tanjon' i, *Madag.* **117 D8** 25 36 S 45 8 E
Vohipeno, *Madag.* **117 C8** 22 22 S 47 51 E
Voi, *Kenya* **118 C4** 3 25 S 38 32 E
Void-Vacon, *France* **27 D12** 48 40N 5 36 E
Voineşti, *Iaşi, Romania* **53 C12** 47 5N 27 27 E
Voineşti, *Prahova, Romania* **53 E10** 45 5N 25 14 E
Voíotía □, *Greece* **48 C5** 38 20N 23 0 E
Voiron, *France* **29 C9** 45 22N 5 35 E
Voisey B., *Canada* **141 A7** 56 15N 61 50W
Voitsberg, *Austria* **34 D8** 47 3N 15 9 E
Vojens, *Denmark* **17 J3** 55 16N 9 18 E
Vojmsjön, *Sweden* **14 D17** 65 0N 16 24 E
Vojnić, *Croatia* **45 C12** 45 19N 15 43 E
Vojnik, *Italy* **45 B12** 46 18N 15 19 E
Vojvodina □, *Serbia & M.* **52 E5** 45 20N 20 0 E
Vokeo I., *Papua N. G.* **132 B3** 3 14 S 144 2 E
Vokhtoga, *Russia* **58 C11** 58 46N 41 8 E
Volary, *Czech Rep.* **34 C6** 48 54N 13 52 E
Volborg, *U.S.A.* **154 C2** 45 51N 105 41W
Volcán de Colima △, *Mexico* **162 D4** 19 30N 103 40W
Volcano, *U.S.A.* **145 D6** 19 26N 155 14W
Volcano Is. = Kazan-Rettō, *Pac. Oc.* **134 E6** 25 0N 141 0 E
Volcans △, *Rwanda* **118 C2** 1 30 S 29 26 E
Volcans d'Auvergne ⌓, *France* **28 C6** 45 20N 2 40 E
Volchansk = Vovchansk, *Ukraine* **59 G9** 50 17N 36 58 E
Volchansk, *Russia* **64 B8** 59 56N 60 4 E
Volchya →, *Ukraine* **59 H8** 48 32N 36 0 E
Volda, *Norway* **18 B3** 62 9N 6 5 E
Volga = Privolzhskiy □, *Russia* **60 B10** 56 0N 50 0 E
Volga, *Russia* **58 C10** 57 58N 38 16 E
Volga →, *Russia* **61 G9** 46 0N 48 30 E
Volga Hts. = Privolzhskaya Vozvyshennost, *Russia* **60 E7** 51 0N 46 0 E
Volgo-Baltiyskiy Kanal, *Russia* **58 B9** 60 0N 38 0 E
Volgo-Donskoy Kanal, *Russia* **61 F7** 48 40N 43 37 E
Volgodonsk, *Russia* **61 G6** 47 33N 42 5 E
Volgograd, *Russia* **61 F7** 48 40N 44 25 E
Volgogradskoye Vdkhr., *Russia* **60 E8** 50 0N 45 20 E
Volgorechensk, *Russia* **60 B5** 57 28N 41 14 E
Volímai, *Greece* **39 D2** 37 52N 20 39 E
Volintiri, *Moldova* **53 D14** 46 26N 29 37 E
Volissós, *Greece* **49 C7** 38 29N 25 54 E
Volkach, *Germany* **31 F6** 49 52N 10 14 E
Völkermarkt, *Austria* **34 E7** 46 39N 14 39 E
Volkhov, *Russia* **58 C7** 59 55N 32 15 E
Volkhov →, *Russia* **58 B7** 60 8N 32 20 E
Volkhovstroy = Volkhov, *Russia* **58 C7** 59 55N 32 15 E
Völklingen, *Germany* **31 F2** 49 15N 6 50 E
Volkovysk = Vawkavysk, *Belarus* **59 F3** 53 9N 24 30 E
Volksrust, *S. Africa* **117 D4** 27 24 S 29 53 E
Voll, *Norway* **18 B4** 62 31N 7 27 E
Volnansk, *Ukraine* **59 H8** 48 2N 35 29 E
Volnovakha, *Ukraine* **59 J9** 47 35N 37 30 E
Volochanka, *Russia* **67 B10** 71 0N 94 28 E
Volodarsk, *Russia* **60 B6** 56 12N 43 15 E
Volodymyr-Volynskyy, *Ukraine* **59 G3** 50 50N 24 18 E
Vologda, *Russia* **58 C10** 59 10N 39 45 E
Volokolamsk, *Russia* **58 D8** 56 5N 35 57 E
Volokonovka, *Russia* **59 G9** 50 33N 37 52 E
Vólos, *Greece* **48 B4** 39 24N 22 59 E
Vološinovo = Novi Bečej, *Serbia & M.* **52 E5** 45 36N 20 10 E
Volosovo, *Russia* **58 C5** 59 27N 29 32 E
Volovets, *Ukraine* **53 B8** 48 43N 23 11 E
Volovo, *Russia* **58 F10** 53 35N 38 1 E
Volozhin = Valozhyn, *Belarus* **58 E4** 54 3N 26 30 E
Volsk, *Russia* **60 D8** 52 5N 47 22 E
Volta □, *Ghana* **113 D5** 7 0N 0 30 E
Volta →, *Ghana* **113 D5** 5 46N 0 41 E
Volta, L., *Ghana* **113 D5** 7 30N 0 0W
Volta Blanche = White Volta →, *Ghana* **113 D4** 9 10N 1 15W
Volta Redonda, *Brazil* **171 F3** 22 31 S 44 5W
Voltaire, C., *Australia* **124 B4** 14 16 S 125 35 E
Volterra, *Italy* **44 E7** 43 24N 10 51 E
Voltri, *Italy* **44 D5** 44 26N 8 45 E
Volturno →, *Italy* **46 A6** 41 1N 13 55 E
Volubilis, *Morocco* **110 B3** 34 2N 5 33W
Vólvi, L., *Greece* **50 F7** 40 40N 23 34 E
Volyně, *Czech Rep.* **34 B6** 49 10N 13 53 E
Volzhsk, *Russia* **60 C9** 55 57N 48 23 E
Volzhskiy, *Russia* **61 F7** 48 56N 44 46 E
Vomo, *Fiji* **133 A1** 17 30 S 177 15 E
Vonavona, *Solomon Is.* **133 M9** 8 15 S 157 5 E
Vondrozo, *Madag.* **117 C8** 22 49 S 47 20 E
Vónitsa, *Greece* **39 B2** 38 55N 20 53 E
Vopnafjörður, *Iceland* **11 B12** 65 45N 14 50W
Vorarlberg □, *Austria* **34 D2** 47 20N 10 0 E
Vóras Óros, *Greece* **50 F5** 40 57N 21 45 E
Voray-sur-l'Ognon, *France* **32 B2** 47 20N 6 1 E
Vorbasse, *Denmark* **17 J3** 55 39N 9 6 E
Vorchdorf, *Austria* **34 C6** 48 0N 13 55 E
Vorderrhein →, *Switz.* **33 C8** 46 49N 9 25 E
Vordingborg, *Denmark* **17 J5** 55 0N 11 54 E
Vorë, *Albania* **50 E3** 41 23N 19 40 E
Voreio Aigaio = Vórios Aiyaíon □, *Greece* **49 C7** 38 50N 25 30 E
Voreppe, *France* **29 C9** 45 18N 5 39 E
Vóriai Sporádhes, *Greece* **48 B5** 39 15N 23 30 E
Vórios Aiyaíon □, *Greece* **49 C7** 38 50N 25 30 E
Vórios Evvoïkos Kólpos, *Greece* **48 C5** 38 45N 23 15 E
Vorkuta, *Russia* **56 A11** 67 48N 64 20 E
Vorma →, *Norway* **18 D8** 60 9N 11 29 E
Vormsi, *Estonia* **15 G20** 59 1N 23 13 E
Vóroi, *Greece* **39 E5** 35 4N 24 49 E
Vorona →, *Russia* **60 E6** 51 22N 42 3 E
Voronezh, *Russia* **59 G10** 51 40N 39 10 E
Voronezh, *Ukraine* **59 G7** 51 47N 33 28 E
Voronezh →, *Russia* **59 G10** 51 32N 39 10 E
Vorontsovo-Aleksandrovskoye = Zelenokumsk, *Russia* **61 H6** 44 24N 44 0 E
Voroshilov = Ussuriysk, *Russia* **67 E14** 43 48N 131 59 E
Voroshilovgrad = Luhansk, *Ukraine* **59 H10** 48 38N 39 15 E
Voroshilovsk = Alchevsk, *Ukraine* **59 H10** 48 30N 38 45 E
Voroshilovsk = Stavropol, *Russia* **61 H6** 45 5N 42 0 E
Vorpommersche Boddenlandschaft △, *Germany* **30 A8** 54 25N 12 32 E
Vorskla →, *Ukraine* **59 H8** 48 50N 34 10 E
Võrts Järv, *Estonia* **15 G22** 58 16N 26 3 E
Võru, *Estonia* **15 H22** 57 48N 26 54 E
Vosges, *France* **27 D14** 48 20N 7 10 E
Vosges □, *France* **27 D13** 48 12N 6 20 E
Vosges du Nord ⌓, *France* **27 D14** 49 0N 7 30 E
Voskopojë, *Albania* **50 F4** 40 35N 20 33 E
Voskresensk, *Russia* **58 E10** 55 19N 38 43 E
Voskresenskoye, *Russia* **60 B7** 56 51N 45 30 E
Voss, *Norway* **18 D3** 60 38N 6 26 E
Vostok = Neftegorsk, *Russia* **61 H4** 44 25N 39 45 E
Vostok, *Antarctica* **7 D8** 78 30 S 106 50 E
Vostok I., *Kiribati* **135 J12** 10 5 S 152 23W
Votice, *Czech Rep.* **34 B7** 49 38N 14 39 E
Votkinsk, *Russia* **64 C4** 57 0N 53 55 E
Votkinskoye Vdkhr., *Russia* **64 C5** 57 22N 55 12 E
Votsuri-Shima, *Japan* **71 M1** 25 45N 123 29 E
Votuporanga, *Brazil* **171 F2** 20 24 S 49 59W
Vouga →, *Portugal* **42 E2** 40 41N 8 40W
Vouillé, *France* **26 F7** 46 38N 0 10 E
Voulou, *C.A.R.* **114 A4** 8 33N 22 36 E
Vouma →, *Cameroon* **114 B2** 3 19N 14 9 E
Vouvry, *Switz.* **32 D3** 46 21N 6 51 E
Voúxa, Ákra, *Greece* **39 E4** 35 37N 23 32 E
Vouzela, *Portugal* **42 E2** 40 43N 8 7W
Vouziers, *France* **27 C11** 49 22N 4 40 E
Vovchansk, *Ukraine* **59 G9** 50 17N 36 58 E
Vovodo →, *C.A.R.* **114 A4** 5 40N 24 21 E
Vowchyn, *Belarus* **55 F10** 52 18N 23 18 E
Voyageurs △, *U.S.A.* **154 A8** 48 32N 93 0W
Vozhe, Ozero, *Russia* **58 B10** 60 45N 39 0 E
Vozhega, *Russia* **58 B11** 60 29N 40 12 E
Voznesensk, *Ukraine* **59 J6** 47 35N 31 21 E
Voznesenye, *Russia* **58 B8** 61 0N 35 28 E
Vrå, *Denmark* **17 G3** 57 21N 9 56 E
Vráble, *Slovak Rep.* **35 C11** 48 15N 18 16 E
Vraćevšnica, *Serbia & M.* **50 B4** 44 2N 20 34 E
Vrådal, *Norway* **18 E5** 59 20N 8 25 E
Vrakhnéïka, *Greece* **48 C3** 38 10N 21 40 E
Vrancea □, *Romania* **53 E11** 45 50N 26 45 E
Vrancei, Munţii, *Romania* **53 E11** 46 0N 26 30 E
Vrang, *Tajikistan* **65 E6** 37 0N 72 22 E
Vrangelya, Ostrov, *Russia* **67 B19** 71 0N 180 0 E
Vranica, *Bos.-H.* **52 G2** 43 55N 17 50 E
Vranje, *Serbia & M.* **50 D5** 42 34N 21 54 E
Vranjska Banja, *Serbia & M.* **50 D6** 42 34N 22 1 E
Vranov nad Topl'ou, *Slovak Rep.* **35 C14** 48 53N 21 40 E
Vransko, *Slovenia* **45 B11** 46 17N 14 58 E
Vransko Jezero, *Croatia* **45 E12** 43 53N 15 34 E
Vrapčište, *Macedonia* **50 E4** 41 50N 20 53 E
Vratsa, *Bulgaria* **50 C7** 43 15N 23 30 E
Vråvatn, *Norway* **18 E5** 59 20N 8 8 E
Vrbas, *Serbia & M.* **52 E4** 45 40N 19 40 E
Vrbas →, *Bos.-H.* **52 E2** 45 8N 17 29 E
Vrbnik, *Croatia* **45 C11** 45 4N 14 40 E
Vrbovec, *Croatia* **45 C13** 45 53N 16 28 E
Vrbovsko, *Croatia* **45 C12** 45 24N 15 5 E
Vrchlabí, *Czech Rep.* **34 A8** 50 38N 15 37 E
Vrede, *S. Africa* **117 D4** 27 24 S 29 6 E
Vredefort, *S. Africa* **116 D4** 27 0 S 27 22 E
Vreden, *Germany* **30 C2** 52 2N 6 50 E
Vredenburg, *S. Africa* **116 E2** 32 56 S 18 0 E
Vredendal, *S. Africa* **116 E2** 31 41 S 18 35 E
Vretstorp, *Sweden* **16 E8** 59 1N 14 53 E
Vrgorac, *Croatia* **45 E14** 43 12N 17 20 E
Vrhnika, *Slovenia* **45 C11** 45 58N 14 15 E
Vriddhachalam, *India* **95 J4** 11 30N 79 20 E
Vrïdi, *Ivory C.* **112 D4** 5 15N 4 3W
Vrigstad, *Sweden* **17 G8** 57 22N 14 28 E
Vrin, *Switz.* **33 C8** 46 39N 9 6 E
Vrindavan, *India* **92 F7** 27 37N 77 40 E
Vríses, *Greece* **39 E5** 35 23N 24 13 E
Vrnograč, *Bos.-H.* **45 C12** 45 10N 15 57 E
Vrondádhes, *Greece* **49 C8** 38 25N 26 7 E
Vrpolje, *Croatia* **52 E3** 45 13N 18 24 E
Vršac, *Serbia & M.* **52 E6** 45 8N 21 20 E
Vrsacki Kanal, *Serbia & M.* **52 E5** 45 15N 21 0 E
Vrútky, *Slovak Rep.* **35 B11** 49 7N 18 55 E
Vryburg, *S. Africa* **116 D3** 26 55 S 24 45 E
Vryheid, *S. Africa* **117 D5** 27 45 S 30 47 E
Vsetín, *Czech Rep.* **35 B11** 49 20N 18 0 E
Vu Liet, *Vietnam* **86 C5** 18 43N 105 23 E
Vŭcha →, *Bulgaria* **51 D8** 42 10N 24 26 E
Vučitrn, *Serbia & M.* **50 D4** 42 49N 20 59 E
Vukovar, *Croatia* **52 E3** 45 21N 18 59 E
Vulcan, *Canada* **142 C6** 50 25N 113 15W
Vulcan, *Romania* **53 E8** 45 23N 23 17 E
Vulcaneşti, *Moldova* **53 E13** 45 41N 28 18 E
Vulcano, *Italy* **47 D7** 38 24N 14 58 E
Vŭlchedruma, *Bulgaria* **50 C7** 43 42N 23 27 E
Vulkaneshty = Vulcaneşti, *Moldova* **53 E13** 45 41N 28 18 E
Vunduzi →, *Mozam.* **119 F3** 18 56 S 34 1 E
Vung Tau, *Vietnam* **87 G6** 10 21N 107 4 E
Vunidawa, *Fiji* **133 A2** 17 50 S 178 21 E
Vunisea, *Fiji* **133 B2** 19 3 S 178 10 E
Vuntut △, *Canada* **144 B13** 68 25N 139 41W
Vuranggo, *Solomon Is.* **133 L9** 6 39 S 156 38 E
Vŭrbitsa, *Bulgaria* **51 D10** 42 59N 26 40 E
Vurshets, *Bulgaria* **50 C7** 43 13N 23 23 E
Vutcani, *Romania* **53 D12** 46 26N 27 59 E
Vuya, *Sudan* **107 F2** 5 21N 29 40 E
Vuzlove, *Ukraine* **52 B7** 48 22N 22 24 E
Vwaza ⌓, *Malawi* **119 E3** 10 58 S 33 25 E
Vyara, *India* **94 D1** 21 8N 73 28 E
Vyartsilya, *Russia* **58 A6** 62 8N 30 45 E
Vyatka = Kirov, *Russia* **64 B2** 58 35N 49 40 E
Vyatka →, *Russia* **60 C10** 55 37N 51 28 E
Vyatskiye Polyany, *Russia* **60 B10** 56 14N 51 5 E
Vyazemskiy, *Russia* **67 E14** 47 32N 134 45 E
Vyazma, *Russia* **58 E8** 55 10N 34 15 E
Vyazniki, *Russia* **60 B6** 56 10N 42 10 E
Vyborg, *Russia* **58 B5** 60 43N 28 47 E
Vychegda →, *Russia* **56 B8** 61 18N 46 36 E
Vychodné Beskydy, *Europe* **35 B15** 49 20N 22 0 E
Vyerkhnyadzvinsk, *Belarus* **58 E4** 55 45N 27 58 E
Vyg-ozero, *Russia* **56 B5** 63 47N 34 29 E
Vyhoda, *Ukraine* **53 B8** 48 56N 23 55 E
Vyksa, *Russia* **60 C6** 55 19N 42 11 E
Vylkove, *Ukraine* **53 E14** 45 28N 29 32 E
Vylok, *Ukraine* **52 B7** 48 6N 22 50 E
Vynohradiv, *Ukraine* **52 B8** 48 9N 23 2 E
Vypin, *India* **95 J3** 10 10N 76 15 E
Vyrnwy, L., *U.K.* **20 E4** 52 48N 3 31W
Vyshkiv, *Ukraine* **53 B8** 48 44N 23 39 E
Vyshkove, *Ukraine* **53 B8** 48 3N 23 25 E
Vyshniy Volochek, *Russia* **58 D8** 57 30N 34 30 E
Vyshzha = imeni 26 Bakinskikh Komissarov, *Turkmenistan* **97 B7** 39 22N 54 10 E
Vyškov, *Czech Rep.* **35 B9** 49 17N 17 0 E
Vysokaye, *Belarus* **55 F10** 52 22N 23 22 E
Vysoké Mýto, *Czech Rep.* **35 B9** 49 58N 16 10 E
Vysokovsk, *Russia* **58 D9** 56 22N 36 30 E
Vyšší Brod, *Czech Rep.* **34 C7** 48 37N 14 19 E
Vytegra, *Russia* **58 B9** 61 0N 36 27 E
Vyzhnytsya, *Ukraine* **53 B10** 48 15N 25 11 E
Vyzhnytsya ⌓, *Ukraine* **53 B10** 48 7N 25 15 E

W

W du Benin △, *Benin* **113 C5** 11 57N 2 43 E
W du Burkina Faso △, *Burkina Faso* **113 C4** 11 52N 2 50W
W du Niger △, *Niger* **113 C5** 13 31N 2 28 E
W.A.C. Bennett Dam, *Canada* **142 B4** 56 2N 122 6W
Wa, *Ghana* **112 C4** 10 7N 2 25W
Waal →, *Neths.* **24 C5** 51 37N 5 0 E
Waalwijk, *Neths.* **24 C5** 51 42N 5 4 E
Waar, *Indonesia* **83 B4** 2 5 S 134 23 E
Waat, *Sudan* **107 F3** 8 10N 32 7 E
Wabag, *Papua N. G.* **132 C2** 5 32 S 143 40 E
Wabakimi △, *Canada* **140 B2** 50 43N 89 29W
Wabana, *Canada* **141 C9** 47 40N 53 0W
Wabao, *N. Cal.* **133 U21** 21 36 S 167 57 E
Wabao, C., *N. Cal.* **133 U21** 21 35 S 167 53 E
Wabasca →, *Canada* **142 B5** 58 22N 115 20W
Wabasca-Desmarais, *Canada* **142 B6** 55 57N 113 56W
Wabash, *U.S.A.* **157 D11** 40 48N 85 49W
Wabash →, *U.S.A.* **157 G8** 37 48N 88 2W
Wabasso, *U.S.A.* **153 H9** 27 45N 80 26W
Wabawng, *Burma* **90 B6** 26 20N 97 25 E
Wabi →, *Ethiopia* **107 F5** 7 45N 40 50 E
Wabigoon L., *Canada* **143 D10** 49 44N 92 44W
Wabowden, *Canada* **143 C9** 54 55N 98 38W
Wąbrzeźno, *Poland* **55 E5** 53 16N 18 57 E
Wabu Hu, *China* **77 A11** 32 20N 116 50 E
Wabuda I., *Papua N. G.* **132 E2** 8 23 S 143 37 E
Wabuk Pt., *Canada* **140 A2** 55 20N 85 5W
Wabush, *Canada* **141 B6** 52 55N 66 52W
Waccasassa B., *U.S.A.* **153 F7** 29 10N 82 50W
Wąchock, *Poland* **55 G8** 51 4N 21 1 E
Wächtersbach, *Germany* **31 E5** 50 14N 9 17 E
Wacissa, *U.S.A.* **152 E6** 30 22N 83 59W
Waco, *U.S.A.* **155 K6** 31 33N 97 9W
Waconichi, L., *Canada* **140 B5** 50 8N 74 0W
Wad Ban Naqa, *Sudan* **107 D3** 16 32N 33 9 E
Wad Banda, *Sudan* **107 E2** 13 10N 27 56 E
Wad el Haddad, *Sudan* **107 E3** 13 50N 33 30 E
Wad en Nau, *Sudan* **107 E3** 14 10N 33 34 E
Wad Hamid, *Sudan* **107 D3** 16 30N 32 45 E
Wad Medanî, *Sudan* **107 E3** 14 28N 33 30 E
Wad Thana, *Pakistan* **91 D2** 27 22N 66 23 E
Wadai, *Africa* **104 E5** 12 0N 19 0 E
Wadayama, *Japan* **72 B6** 35 19N 134 52 E
Wadbilliga △, *Australia* **129 D8** 36 25 S 149 35 E
Waddān, *Libya* **108 C3** 29 9N 16 10 E
Waddeneilanden, *Neths.* **24 A5** 53 25N 5 10 E
Waddenzee, *Neths.* **24 A5** 53 6N 5 10 E
Waddi, Chappal, *Nigeria* **113 D7** 7 2N 11 43W
Waddington, *U.S.A.* **151 B9** 44 52N 75 12W
Waddington, Mt., *Canada* **142 C3** 51 23N 125 15W
Waddy Pt., *Australia* **127 C5** 24 58 S 153 21 E
Wadebridge, *U.K.* **21 G3** 50 31N 4 51W
Wadena, *Canada* **143 C8** 51 57N 103 47W
Wadena, *U.S.A.* **154 B7** 46 26N 95 8W
Wädenswil, *Switz.* **33 B7** 47 14N 8 40 E
Wadern, *Germany* **31 F2** 49 32N 6 53 E
Wadeye, *Australia* **124 B4** 14 28 S 129 52 E
Wadgaon, *India* **94 E1** 18 44N 73 39 E
Wadhams, *Canada* **142 C3** 51 30N 127 30W
Wadhwan = Surendranagar, *India* **92 H4** 22 45N 71 40 E
Wadi, *India* **94 F3** 17 4N 76 59 E
Wādī as Sīr, *Jordan* **103 D4** 31 56N 35 49 E
Wādī Banī Walīd, *Libya* **108 B2** 31 49N 14 0 E
Wadi Gemâl, *Egypt* **106 C4** 24 35N 35 10 E
Wadi Halfa, *Sudan* **106 C3** 21 53N 31 19 E
Wadi Rum △, *Jordan* **103 F4** 29 30N 35 20 E
Wadian, *China* **77 A9** 32 42N 112 29 E
Wadlew, *Poland* **55 G6** 51 31N 19 23 E
Wadley, *Ala., U.S.A.* **152 B4** 33 7N 85 34W
Wadley, *Ga., U.S.A.* **152 C7** 32 52N 82 24W
Wadowice, *Poland* **55 J6** 49 52N 19 30 E
Wadsworth, *Nev., U.S.A.* **158 G4** 39 38N 119 17W
Wadsworth, *Ohio, U.S.A.* **150 E3** 41 2N 81 44W
Waegwan, *S. Korea* **75 G15** 35 59N 128 23 E
Waeplau, *Indonesia* **82 B3** 3 8 S 126 55 E
Wafangdian, *China* **75 E11** 39 38N 121 58 E
Wafania, *Dem. Rep. of the Congo* **114 C4** 1 23 S 20 22 E
Wafrah, *Si. Arabia* **96 D5** 28 33N 47 56 E
Wagadugu = Ouagadougou, *Burkina Faso* **113 C4** 12 25N 1 30W
Wagener, *U.S.A.* **152 B8** 33 39N 81 22W
Wageningen, *Neths.* **24 C5** 51 58N 5 40 E
Wageningen, *Suriname* **169 B6** 5 50N 56 50W
Wager B., *Canada* **139 B11** 65 26N 88 40W
Wagga Wagga, *Australia* **129 C7** 35 7 S 147 24 E
Waghai, *India* **94 D1** 20 46N 73 29 E
Waghete, *Indonesia* **83 B5** 4 10 S 135 50 E
Wagin, *Australia* **125 F2** 33 17 S 117 25 E
Wagner, *U.S.A.* **154 D5** 43 5N 98 18W
Wagon Mound, *U.S.A.* **155 G2** 36 1N 104 42W
Wagoner, *U.S.A.* **155 H7** 35 58N 95 22W
Wagrowiec, *Poland* **55 F4** 52 48N 17 11 E
Wah, *Pakistan* **91 B4** 33 45N 72 40 E
Wahai, *Indonesia* **83 B3** 2 48 S 129 35 E
Waharoa, *N.Z.* **130 D4** 37 46 S 175 45 E
Wahiawa, *U.S.A.* **145 K13** 21 30N 158 2W
Wahiawa Reservoir, *U.S.A.* **145 K13** 21 30N 158 3W
Wâḥid, *Egypt* **103 E1** 30 48N 32 21 E
Wahnai, *Afghan.* **92 C1** 32 40N 65 50 E
Wahni, *Ethiopia* **107 E4** 12 40N 36 39 E
Wahoo, *U.S.A.* **154 E6** 41 13N 96 37W
Wahpeton, *U.S.A.* **154 B6** 46 16N 96 36W
Wahx, Ras il-, *Malta* **38 F7** 35 56N 14 20 E
Wai, *India* **94 F1** 17 56N 73 57 E
Waiai →, *N.Z.* **131 G2** 46 12 S 167 38 E
Waialee, *U.S.A.* **145 J13** 21 41N 158 1W
Waialua, *U.S.A.* **145 J13** 21 34N 158 8W
Waialua B., *U.S.A.* **145 J13** 21 35N 158 5W
Waianae, *U.S.A.* **145 K13** 21 27N 158 11W
Waianae Mts., *U.S.A.* **145 K13** 21 30N 158 10W
Waiapu →, *N.Z.* **130 D7** 37 47 S 178 29 E
Waiau, *N.Z.* **131 C8** 42 39 S 173 5 E
Waiau →, *N.Z.* **131 C8** 42 47 S 173 22 E
Waiawa →, *U.S.A.* **145 K14** 21 23N 157 59W
Waiawe Ganga →, *Sri Lanka* **95 L5** 6 15N 81 0 E
Waibeem, *Indonesia* **83 B4** 0 30 S 132 59 E
Waiblingen, *Germany* **31 G5** 48 49N 9 18 E
Waidhofen an der Thaya, *Austria* **34 C8** 48 49N 15 17 E
Waidhofen an der Ybbs, *Austria* **34 D7** 47 57N 14 46 E
Waigeo, *Indonesia* **83 B4** 0 20 S 130 40 E
Waihao →, *N.Z.* **131 E6** 44 52 S 171 11 E
Waihao Downs, *N.Z.* **131 E5** 44 48 S 170 55 E
Waiheke I., *N.Z.* **130 C4** 36 48 S 175 6 E
Waihi, *N.Z.* **130 D4** 37 23 S 175 52 E
Waihi Beach, *N.Z.* **130 D7** 37 25 S 175 57 E
Waihola, *N.Z.* **131 G5** 46 1 S 170 8 E
Waihola L., *N.Z.* **131 F5** 45 59 S 170 8 E
Waihou →, *N.Z.* **130 D4** 37 15 S 175 40 E
Waika, *Dem. Rep. of the Congo* **118 C2** 2 22 S 25 42 E
Waikabubak, *Indonesia* **82 C1** 9 45 S 119 25 E
Waikaia, *N.Z.* **131 F3** 45 44 S 168 51 E
Waikaka, *N.Z.* **131 F4** 45 55 S 169 1 E
Waikare, L., *N.Z.* **130 D4** 37 26 S 175 13 E
Waikareiti, L., *N.Z.* **130 E6** 38 43 S 177 10 E
Waikaremoana, *N.Z.* **130 E6** 38 42 S 177 12 E
Waikaremoana, L., *N.Z.* **130 E6** 38 49 S 177 9 E
Waikari, *N.Z.* **131 C7** 42 58 S 172 41 E
Waikato →, *N.Z.* **130 D3** 37 23 S 174 43 E
Waikelo, *Indonesia* **82 C1** 9 24 S 119 19 E
Waikerie, *Australia* **128 C4** 34 9 S 140 0 E
Waikiekie, *N.Z.* **130 B3** 35 57 S 174 16 E
Waikiki, *U.S.A.* **145 K14** 21 17N 157 50W
Waikokopu, *N.Z.* **130 F6** 39 3 S 177 52 E
Waikouaiti, *N.Z.* **131 F5** 45 36 S 170 41 E
Waikouaiti Downs, *N.Z.* **131 F5** 45 30 S 170 30 E
Wailingding Dao, *China* **69 G11** 22 6N 114 2 E
Wailua, *Hawaii, U.S.A.* **145 A2** 22 3N 159 20W
Wailua, *Hawaii, U.S.A.* **145 C5** 20 51N 156 8W
Wailuku, *U.S.A.* **145 C5** 20 53N 156 30W
Waimakariri →, *N.Z.* **131 D7** 43 24 S 172 42 E
Waimanalo, *U.S.A.* **145 K14** 21 21N 157 43W
Waimanalo B., *U.S.A.* **145 K14** 21 20N 157 40W
Waimanalo Beach, *U.S.A.* **145 K14** 21 21N 157 42W
Waimangaroa, *N.Z.* **131 B6** 41 43 S 171 46 E
Waimano →, *U.S.A.* **145 K14** 21 25N 157 58W
Waimarie, *N.Z.* **131 B6** 41 35 S 171 58 E
Waimate, *N.Z.* **131 E6** 44 45 S 171 3 E
Waimea, *Hawaii, U.S.A.* **145 B2** 21 58N 159 40W
Waimea, *Hawaii, U.S.A.* **145 J13** 21 39N 158 3W
Waimea B., *U.S.A.* **145 J13** 21 40N 158 5W
Waimea Plain, *N.Z.* **131 F3** 45 55 S 168 35 E
Wainganga →, *India* **94 E4** 18 50N 79 55 E
Waingapu, *Indonesia* **82 C2** 9 35 S 120 11 E
Waingmaw, *Burma* **90 C6** 25 21N 97 26 E
Waini →, *Guyana* **169 B6** 8 20N 59 50W
Wainuiomata, *N.Z.* **130 H3** 41 17 S 174 56 E
Wainwright, *Canada* **143 C6** 52 50N 110 50W
Wainwright, *U.S.A.* **144 A7** 70 38N 160 2W
Waiotapu, *N.Z.* **130 E5** 38 21 S 176 25 E
Waiouru, *N.Z.* **130 F4** 39 28 S 175 41 E
Waipa →, *N.Z.* **130 E4** 38 16 S 175 21 E
Waipahi, *N.Z.* **131 G4** 46 6 S 169 15 E
Waipahu, *U.S.A.* **145 K13** 21 23N 158 1W
Waipapa Pt., *N.Z.* **131 G3** 46 40 S 168 51 E
Waipara, *N.Z.* **131 D7** 43 3 S 172 46 E
Waipawa, *N.Z.* **130 F5** 39 56 S 176 38 E
Waipio Acres, *U.S.A.* **145 K13** 21 28N 158 1W
Waipio Peninsula, *U.S.A.* **145 K14** 21 20N 158 0W
Waipiro, *N.Z.* **130 E7** 38 2 S 178 22 E
Waipiro Bay, *N.Z.* **130 E7** 38 1 S 178 21 E
Waipoua Forest, *N.Z.* **130 B2** 35 39 S 173 33 E
Waipu, *N.Z.* **130 B3** 35 59 S 174 29 E
Waipukurau, *N.Z.* **130 G5** 40 1 S 176 33 E
Wairakei, *N.Z.* **130 E5** 38 37 S 176 6 E
Wairarapa, L., *N.Z.* **130 H4** 41 14 S 175 15 E
Wairau →, *N.Z.* **131 B9** 41 32 S 174 7 E
Wairio, *N.Z.* **131 F3** 45 59 S 168 3 E
Wairoa, *N.Z.* **130 F6** 39 3 S 177 25 E
Wairoa →, *Hawke's Bay, N.Z.* **130 F6** 39 4 S 177 25 E
Wairoa →, *Northland, N.Z.* **130 C2** 36 5 S 173 59 E
Waïsisi, *Vanuatu* **133 J7** 19 32 S 169 22 E
Waita Reservoir, *U.S.A.* **145 B2** 21 55N 159 28W
Waitaki →, *N.Z.* **131 E6** 44 56 S 171 7 E
Waitaki Plains, *N.Z.* **131 E5** 44 22 S 170 0 E
Waitangi, *N.Z.* **130 B3** 35 16 S 174 5 E
Waitara, *N.Z.* **130 E3** 38 59 S 174 15 E
Waitara →, *N.Z.* **130 E3** 38 59 S 174 14 E
Waitoa, *N.Z.* **130 D4** 37 37 S 175 35 E
Waitomo Caves, *N.Z.* **130 E4** 38 16 S 175 7 E
Waitotara, *N.Z.* **130 F3** 39 49 S 174 44 E
Waitotara →, *N.Z.* **130 F3** 39 51 S 174 41 E
Waitsburg, *U.S.A.* **158 C5** 46 16N 118 9W
Waitzen = Vác, *Hungary* **52 C4** 47 49N 19 10 E
Waiuku, *N.Z.* **130 D3** 37 15 S 174 45 E
Wajima, *Japan* **71 F8** 37 30N 137 0 E
Wajir, *Kenya* **118 B5** 1 42N 40 5 E
Waka, *Dem. Rep. of the Congo* **114 B4** 1 1N 20 13 E
Waka, *Ethiopia* **107 F4** 7 2N 37 20 E
Wakai, *Suriname* **169 B6** 5 18N 57 14W
Wakarusa, *U.S.A.* **157 C10** 41 32N 86 1W
Wakasa, *Japan* **72 B6** 35 20N 134 24 E
Wakasa-Wan, *Japan* **73 B7** 35 40N 135 30 E
Wakatipu, L., *N.Z.* **131 F3** 45 5 S 168 33 E
Wakaw, *Canada* **143 C7** 52 39N 105 44W
Wakaya, *Fiji* **133 A2** 17 37 S 179 0 E
Wakayama, *Japan* **73 C7** 34 15N 135 15 E
Wakayama □, *Japan* **73 D7** 33 50N 135 30 E
Wake, *Japan* **72 C6** 34 48N 134 8 E
Wake Forest, *U.S.A.* **149 H6** 35 59N 78 30W
Wake I., *Pac. Oc.* **134 F8** 19 18N 166 36 E
WaKeeney, *U.S.A.* **154 F5** 39 1N 99 53W
Wakefield, *Jamaica* **164 a** 18 26N 77 42W
Wakefield, *N.Z.* **131 B8** 41 24 S 173 5 E
Wakefield, *U.K.* **20 D6** 53 41N 1 29W
Wakefield, *Mass., U.S.A.* **151 D13** 42 30N 71 4W
Wakefield, *Mich., U.S.A.* **154 B10** 46 29N 89 56W
Wakema, *Burma* **90 G5** 16 30N 95 11 E
Waki, *Japan* **72 C6** 34 4N 134 9 E
Wakkanai, *Japan* **70 B10** 45 28N 141 35 E
Wakkerstroom, *S. Africa* **117 D5** 27 24 S 30 10 E
Wakool, *Australia* **128 C6** 35 28 S 144 23 E
Wakool →, *Australia* **128 C5** 35 5 S 143 33 E
Wakre, *Indonesia* **83 B4** 0 19 S 131 5 E
Waku, *Papua N. G.* **132 D5** 6 5 S 149 9 E
Wakuach, L., *Canada* **141 A6** 55 34N 67 32W
Wakulla, *U.S.A.* **152 E5** 30 14N 84 14W
Wakunai, *Papua N. G.* **132 C8** 5 52 S 155 13 E
Walamba, *Zambia* **119 E2** 13 30 S 28 42 E
Wałbrzych, *Poland* **55 H3** 50 45N 16 18 E
Walbury Hill, *U.K.* **21 F6** 51 21N 1 28W
Walcha, *Australia* **129 A9** 30 55 S 151 31 E
Walcheren, *Neths.* **24 C3** 51 30N 3 35 E
Walckenaer, Teluk, *Indonesia* **83 B5** 2 20 S 139 50 E
Walcott, *U.S.A.* **158 F10** 41 46N 106 51W
Wałcz, *Poland* **55 E3** 53 17N 16 27 E
Wald, *Switz.* **33 B7** 47 17N 8 56 E
Waldbröl, *Germany* **30 E3** 50 52N 7 37 E
Waldburg Ra., *Australia* **125 D2** 24 40 S 117 35 E
Waldeck, *Germany* **30 D5** 51 12N 9 4 E
Walden, *Colo., U.S.A.* **158 F10** 40 44N 106 17W
Walden, *N.Y., U.S.A.* **151 E10** 41 34N 74 11W
Waldenberg = Wałbrzych, *Poland* **55 H3** 50 45N 16 18 E
Waldenburg, *Switz.* **32 B5** 47 23N 7 45 E
Waldkirch, *Germany* **31 G3** 48 5N 7 58 E
Waldkirchen, *Germany* **31 G9** 48 43N 13 36 E
Waldkraiburg, *Germany* **31 G8** 48 11N 12 24 E
Waldo, *U.S.A.* **152 F7** 29 48N 82 10W
Waldport, *U.S.A.* **158 D1** 44 26N 124 4W
Waldron, *U.S.A.* **155 H7** 34 54N 94 5W
Waldviertel, *Austria* **34 C8** 48 30N 15 30 E
Walebing, *Australia* **125 F2** 30 41 S 116 13 E
Walembele, *Ghana* **112 C4** 10 30N 1 58W
Walensee, *Switz.* **33 B8** 47 7N 9 13 E
Walenstadt, *Switz.* **33 B8** 47 8N 9 19 E
Wales, *U.S.A.* **144 D5** 65 37N 168 5W
Wales □, *U.K.* **21 E3** 52 19N 4 43W
Walewale, *Ghana* **113 C4** 10 21N 0 50W
Walgett, *Australia* **127 E4** 30 0 S 148 5 E
Walgreen Coast, *Antarctica* **7 D15** 75 15 S 105 0W
Walhalla, *Australia* **129 D7** 37 56 S 146 29 E

Walis I., *Papua N. G.* **132 B2** 3 14 S 143 18 E
Walker, *Mich., U.S.A.* **157 B11** 42 58N 85 46W
Walker, *Minn., U.S.A.* **154 B7** 47 6N 94 35W
Walker, L., *Canada* **141 B6** 50 20N 67 11W
Walker L., *Canada* **143 C9** 54 42N 95 57W
Walker L., *U.S.A.* **158 G4** 38 42N 118 43W
Walkerston, *Australia* **126 K7** 21 11 S 149 8 E
Walkerton, *Canada* **140 D3** 44 10N 81 10W
Walkerton, *U.S.A.* **157 C10** 41 28N 86 29W
Wall, *U.S.A.* **154 D3** 44 0N 102 8W
Walla Walla, *Australia* **129 C7** 35 45 S 146 54 E
Walla Walla, *U.S.A.* **158 C4** 46 4N 118 20W
Wallace, *Idaho, U.S.A.* **158 C6** 47 28N 115 56W
Wallace, *N.C., U.S.A.* **149 H7** 34 44N 77 59W
Wallaceburg, *Canada* **140 D3** 42 34N 82 23W
Wallacetown, *N.Z.* **131 G3** 46 21 S 168 19 E
Wallachia = Valahia, *Romania* **53 F9** 44 35N 25 0 E
Wallal, *Australia* **127 D4** 26 32 S 146 7 E
Wallam Cr. →, *Australia* **127 D4** 28 40 S 147 20 E
Wallambin, L., *Australia* **125 F2** 30 57 S 117 35 E
Wallan, *Australia* **129 D6** 37 26 S 144 59 E
Wallangarra, *Australia* **127 D5** 28 56 S 151 58 E
Wallaroo, *Australia* **128 B2** 33 56 S 137 39 E
Walldürn, *Germany* **31 F5** 49 34N 9 22 E
Wallenhorst, *Germany* **30 C4** 52 21N 8 1 E
Wallenpaupack, L., *U.S.A.* **151 E9** 41 25N 75 15W
Wallerawang, *Australia* **129 B9** 33 25 S 150 4 E
Wallingford, *U.S.A.* **151 E12** 41 27N 72 50W
Wallis & Futuna, Is., *Pac. Oc.* **134 J10** 13 18 S 176 10W
Wallisellen, *Switz.* **33 B7** 47 25N 8 36 E
Wallowa, *U.S.A.* **158 D5** 45 34N 117 32W
Wallowa Mts., *U.S.A.* **158 D5** 45 20N 117 30W
Walls, *U.K.* **22 A7** 60 14N 1 33W
Walls of Jerusalem △, *Australia* **127 G4** 41 56 S 146 15 E
Wallsend, *Australia* **129 B9** 32 55 S 151 40 E
Wallula, *U.S.A.* **158 C4** 46 5N 118 54W
Wallumbilla, *Australia* **127 D4** 26 33 S 149 9 E
Walmsley, L., *Canada* **143 A7** 63 25N 108 36W
Walney, I. of, *U.K.* **20 C4** 54 6N 3 15W
Walnut, *U.S.A.* **156 C7** 41 33N 89 36W
Walnut Canyon ⌓, *U.S.A.* **159 J8** 35 15N 111 20W
Walnut Creek, *U.S.A.* **160 H4** 37 54N 122 4W
Walnut Grove, *U.S.A.* **152 A3** 34 4N 86 18W
Walnut Hill, *U.S.A.* **153 E2** 30 53N 87 30W
Walnut Ridge, *U.S.A.* **155 G9** 36 4N 90 57W
Walpeup, *Australia* **128 C5** 35 7 S 142 2 E
Walpole, *Australia* **125 F2** 34 58 S 116 44 E
Walpole, *U.S.A.* **151 D13** 42 9N 71 15W
Wals, *Austria* **34 D5** 47 47N 12 58 E
Walsall, *U.K.* **21 E6** 52 35N 1 58W
Walsenburg, *U.S.A.* **155 G2** 37 38N 104 47W
Walsh, *U.S.A.* **155 G3** 37 23N 102 17W
Walsh →, *Australia* **126 B3** 16 31 S 143 42 E
Walsrode, *Germany* **30 C5** 52 51N 9 35 E
Walt Disney World, *U.S.A.* **153 G8** 28 25N 81 35W
Waltair, *India* **94 F6** 17 44N 83 23 E
Walter F. George Reservoir, *U.S.A.* **152 D4** 31 38N 85 4W
Walterboro, *U.S.A.* **152 C9** 32 55N 80 40W
Walters, *U.S.A.* **155 H5** 34 22N 98 19W
Waltershausen, *Germany* **30 E6** 50 54N 10 33 E
Waltham, *U.S.A.* **151 D13** 42 23N 71 14W
Waltman, *U.S.A.* **158 E10** 43 4N 107 12W
Walton, *Ky., U.S.A.* **157 F12** 38 52N 84 37W
Walton, *N.Y., U.S.A.* **151 D9** 42 10N 75 8W
Walton-on-the-Naze, *U.K.* **21 F9** 51 51N 1 17 E
Waltonville, *U.S.A.* **156 F7** 38 13N 89 2W
Walu, *Burma* **90 B7** 26 28N 98 2 E
Walvis Bay, *Namibia* **116 C1** 23 0 S 14 28 E
Walvis Ridge, *Atl. Oc.* **8 J12** 26 0 S 5 0 E
Walvisbaai = Walvis Bay, *Namibia* **116 C1** 23 0 S 14 28 E
Walwa, *Australia* **129 C7** 35 59 S 147 44 E
Wamba, *Équateur, Dem. Rep. of the Congo* **114 C4** 1 37 S 22 30 E
Wamba, *Orientale, Dem. Rep. of the Congo* **118 B2** 2 10N 27 57 E
Wamba, *Kenya* **118 B4** 0 58N 37 19 E
Wamba, *Nigeria* **113 D6** 8 57N 8 42 E
Wamba →, *Dem. Rep. of the Congo* **115 C3** 3 56 S 17 12 E
Wamego, *U.S.A.* **154 F6** 39 12N 96 18W
Wamena, *Indonesia* **83 B5** 4 4 S 138 57 E
Wamsutter, *U.S.A.* **158 F9** 41 40N 107 58W
Wamulan, *Indonesia* **82 B3** 3 27 S 126 7 E
Wan Hat, *Burma* **90 E6** 20 14N 97 53 E
Wan Kinghao, *Burma* **90 E7** 21 34N 98 17 E
Wan Lai-kam, *Burma* **90 E7** 21 21N 98 22 E
Wan Tup, *Burma* **90 E7** 21 13N 98 42 E
Wan Xian, *China* **74 E8** 38 47N 115 7 E
Wana, *Pakistan* **91 B3** 32 20N 69 32 E
Wanaaring, *Australia* **127 D3** 29 38 S 144 9 E
Wanaka, *N.Z.* **131 E4** 44 42 S 169 9 E
Wanaka, L., *N.Z.* **131 E4** 44 33 S 169 7 E
Wan'an, *China* **77 D10** 26 26N 114 49 E
Wanapiri, *Indonesia* **83 B5** 4 30 S 135 59 E
Wanapitei L., *Canada* **140 C3** 46 45N 80 40W
Wanbi, *Australia* **128 C4** 34 46 S 140 17 E
Wandaik, *Guyana* **169 C6** 4 27N 59 35W
Wandel Sea = McKinley Sea, *Arctic* **10 A11** 82 0N 0 0W
Wandérama, *Ivory C.* **112 D4** 8 37N 4 25W
Wanderer, *Zimbabwe* **119 F3** 19 36 S 30 1 E
Wandhari, *Pakistan* **92 F2** 27 42N 66 48 E
Wanding, *China* **76 E2** 24 5N 98 4 E
Wandoan, *Australia* **127 D4** 26 5 S 149 55 E
Wandur Marine △, *India* **95 J11** 11 30N 92 30 E
Wanfu, *China* **75 D12** 40 8N 122 38 E
Wang →, *Thailand* **86 D2** 17 8N 99 2 E
Wang Kai, *Sudan* **107 F2** 9 3N 29 23 E
Wang Noi, *Thailand* **86 E3** 14 13N 100 44 E
Wang Saphung, *Thailand* **86 D3** 17 18N 101 46 E
Wang Thong, *Thailand* **86 D3** 16 50N 100 26 E
Wanga, *Dem. Rep. of the Congo* **118 B2** 2 58N 29 12 E
Wangal, *Indonesia* **83 C4** 6 8 S 134 9 E
Wanganella, *Australia* **129 C6** 35 6 S 144 49 E
Wanganui, *N.Z.* **130 F4** 39 56 S 175 3 E
Wanganui →, *W. Coast, N.Z.* **131 D5** 43 3 S 170 26 E
Wanganui →, *Wanganui-Manawatu, N.Z.* **130 F4** 39 55 S 175 4 E
Wangaratta, *Australia* **129 D7** 36 21 S 146 19 E
Wangary, *Australia* **127 E2** 34 35 S 135 29 E
Wangcang, *China* **76 A6** 32 18N 106 20 E
Wangcheng, *China* **77 C9** 28 22N 112 49 E
Wangdu, *China* **74 E8** 38 40N 115 7 E
Wangdu Phodrang, *Bhutan* **90 B2** 27 28N 89 54 E
Wangen, *Germany* **31 H5** 47 41N 9 50 E
Wangerin = Węgorzyno, *Poland* **54 E2** 53 32N 15 33 E
Wangerooge, *Germany* **30 B3** 53 47N 7 54 E
Wängi, *Switz.* **33 B7** 47 30N 8 57 E
Wangiwangi, *Indonesia* **82 C2** 5 22 S 123 37 E
Wangjiang, *China* **77 B11** 30 10N 116 42 E
Wangmo, *China* **76 E6** 25 11N 106 5 E
Wangolodougou, *Ivory C.* **112 D3** 9 55N 5 10W
Wangqing, *China* **75 C15** 43 12N 129 42 E
Wani, *India* **94 D4** 20 5N 78 55 E
Wanigela, *Papua N. G.* **132 E5** 9 21 S 149 9 E
Wankaner, *India* **92 H4** 22 35N 71 0 E
Wanlaweyne = Uanle Uen, *Somali Rep.* **120 D2** 2 37N 44 54 E
Wanless, *Canada* **143 C8** 54 11N 101 21W
Wanneroo, *Australia* **125 F2** 31 42 S 115 46 E
Wannian, *China* **77 C11** 28 42N 117 4 E
Wanning, *China* **86 C8** 18 48N 110 22 E
Wanon Niwat, *Thailand* **86 D4** 17 38N 103 46 E
Wanqinsha, *China* **69 F10** 22 43N 113 33 E
Wanquan, *China* **74 D8** 40 50N 114 40 E
Wanrong, *China* **74 G6** 35 25N 110 50 E
Wansen = Wiązów, *Poland* **55 H4** 50 50N 17 10 E
Wanshan, *China* **76 D7** 27 30N 109 12 E
Wanshan Qundao, *China* **69 G10** 21 57N 113 45 E
Wanshengchang, *China* **76 C6** 28 57N 106 53 E
Wanstead, *N.Z.* **130 G5** 40 8 S 176 30 E
Wantage, *U.K.* **21 F6** 51 35N 1 25W
Wanxian, *China* **76 B7** 30 42N 108 20 E
Wanyin, *Burma* **90 E6** 20 23N 97 15 E
Wanyuan, *China* **76 A7** 32 4N 108 3 E
Wanzai, *Guangdong, China* **69 G10** 22 12N 113 31 E
Wanzai, *Jiangxi, China* **77 C10** 28 7N 114 30 E
Wapakoneta, *U.S.A.* **157 D12** 40 34N 84 12W
Wapato, *U.S.A.* **158 C3** 46 27N 120 25W
Wapawekka L., *Canada* **143 C8** 54 55N 104 40W
Wapello, *U.S.A.* **156 C5** 41 11N 91 11W
Wapikopa L., *Canada* **140 B2** 52 56N 87 53W
Wapinda, *Dem. Rep. of the Congo* **114 B4** 3 41N 22 48 E
Wapiti →, *Canada* **142 B5** 55 5N 118 18W
Wappingers Falls, *U.S.A.* **151 E11** 41 36N 73 55W
Wapsipinicon →, *U.S.A.* **156 C6** 41 44N 90 19W
Wapusk △, *Canada* **143 B10** 57 46N 93 22W
Warab □, *Sudan* **107 F2** 7 30N 28 30 E
Warabi, *Japan* **73 B11** 35 49N 139 41 E
Warangal, *India* **94 F4** 17 58N 79 35 E
Waraseoni, *India* **93 J9** 21 45N 80 2 E
Waratah, *Australia* **127 G4** 41 30 S 145 30 E
Waratah B., *Australia* **129 E7** 38 54 S 146 5 E
Warburg, *Germany* **30 D5** 51 28N 9 11 E
Warburton, *Vic., Australia* **129 D6** 37 47 S 145 42 E
Warburton, *W. Austral., Australia* **125 E4** 26 8 S 126 35 E
Warburton, The →, *Australia* **127 D2** 28 4 S 137 28 E
Warburton Ra., *Australia* **125 E4** 25 55 S 126 28 E
Ward, *N.Z.* **131 B9** 41 49 S 174 11 E
Ward →, *Australia* **127 D4** 26 28 S 146 6 E
Ward Hunt, C., *Papua N. G.* **132 E5** 8 2 S 148 10 E
Ward Hunt Str., *Papua N. G.* **132 E6** 9 30 S 150 0 E
Ward Mt., *U.S.A.* **160 H8** 37 12N 118 54W
Wardang I., *Australia* **128 C2** 34 30 S 137 20 E
Warden, *S. Africa* **117 D4** 27 50 S 29 0 E
Wardha, *India* **94 D4** 20 45N 78 39 E
Wardija Point, *Malta* **38 E6** 36 2N 14 11 E
Wardo, *Indonesia* **83 B5** 1 2 S 135 50 E
Ware, *Canada* **142 B3** 57 26N 125 41W
Ware, *U.K.* **21 F8** 51 49N 0 0W
Ware, *U.S.A.* **151 D12** 42 16N 72 14W
Waregem, *Belgium* **24 D3** 50 53N 3 27 E
Wareham, *U.S.A.* **151 E14** 41 46N 70 43W
Waremme, *Belgium* **24 D5** 50 43N 5 15 E
Waren, *Germany* **30 B8** 53 31N 12 40 E
Waren, *Indonesia* **83 B5** 2 16 S 136 20 E
Warendorf, *Germany* **30 D4** 51 57N 8 1 E
Waresboro, *U.S.A.* **152 D7** 31 15N 82 29W
Waria →, *Papua N. G.* **132 D4** 7 49 S 147 41 E
Warialda, *Australia* **127 D5** 29 29 S 150 33 E
Wariap, *Indonesia* **83 B4** 1 30 S 134 5 E
Warin Chamrap, *Thailand* **86 E5** 15 12N 104 53 E
Warka, *Poland* **55 G8** 51 47N 21 12 E
Warkopi, *Indonesia* **83 B4** 1 12 S 134 9 E
Warkworth, *N.Z.* **130 C3** 36 24 S 174 41 E
Warm Baths = Bela Bela, *S. Africa* **117 C4** 24 51 S 28 19 E
Warm Springs, *Ga., U.S.A.* **152 C5** 32 53N 84 41W
Warm Springs, *Nev., U.S.A.* **159 G5** 38 10N 116 20W
Warman, *Canada* **143 C7** 52 19N 106 30W
Warmandi, *Indonesia* **83 B4** 0 22 S 132 39 E
Warmbad = Bela Bela, *S. Africa* **117 C4** 24 51 S 28 19 E
Warmbad, *Namibia* **116 D2** 28 25 S 18 42 E
Warmińsko-Mazurskie □, *Poland* **54 D8** 54 0N 21 0 E
Warminster, *U.K.* **21 F5** 51 12N 2 10W
Warminster, *U.S.A.* **151 F9** 40 12N 75 6W
Warnemünde, *Germany* **30 A8** 54 10N 12 4 E
Warner Mts., *U.S.A.* **158 F3** 41 40N 120 15W
Warner Robins, *U.S.A.* **152 C6** 32 37N 83 36W
Warnes, *Bolivia* **173 D5** 17 30 S 63 10W
Warnow →, *Germany* **30 A8** 54 6N 12 9 E
Waroona, *Australia* **125 F2** 32 50 S 115 58 E
Warora, *India* **94 D4** 20 14N 79 1 E
Warracknabeal, *Australia* **128 D5** 36 9 S 142 26 E
Warragul, *Australia* **129 E6** 38 10 S 145 58 E
Warrego →, *Australia* **127 E4** 30 24 S 145 21 E
Warrego Ra., *Australia* **126 C4** 24 58 S 146 0 E
Warren, *Australia* **129 A7** 31 42 S 147 51 E
Warren, *Ark., U.S.A.* **155 J8** 33 37N 92 4W
Warren, *Ill., U.S.A.* **156 B7** 42 29N 90 0W
Warren, *Ind., U.S.A.* **157 D11** 40 41N 85 26W
Warren, *Mich., U.S.A.* **157 B13** 42 30N 83 0W
Warren, *Minn., U.S.A.* **154 A6** 48 12N 96 46W
Warren, *Ohio, U.S.A.* **150 E4** 41 14N 80 49W
Warren, *Pa., U.S.A.* **150 E5** 41 51N 79 9W
Warrenpoint, *U.K.* **23 B5** 54 6N 6 15W
Warrensburg, *Ill., U.S.A.* **156 E7** 39 56N 89 4W
Warrensburg, *Mo., U.S.A.* **156 F3** 38 46N 93 44W
Warrensburg, *N.Y., U.S.A.* **151 C11** 43 29N 73 46W
Warrenton, *S. Africa* **116 D3** 28 9 S 24 47 E
Warrenton, *Ga., U.S.A.* **152 B7** 33 24N 82 40W
Warrenton, *Mo., U.S.A.* **156 F5** 38 49N 91 9W
Warrenton, *Oreg., U.S.A.* **160 D3** 46 10N 123 56W
Warrenville = Gloverville, *U.S.A.* **152 B8** 33 32N 81 48W
Warri, *Nigeria* **113 D6** 5 30N 5 41 E
Warrina, *Australia* **127 D2** 28 12 S 135 50 E
Warrington, *N.Z.* **131 F5** 45 43 S 170 35 E
Warrington, *U.K.* **20 D5** 53 24N 2 35W
Warrington, *U.S.A.* **153 E2** 30 23N 87 17W
Warrington □, *U.K.* **20 D5** 53 24N 2 35W
Warrnambool, *Australia* **128 E5** 38 25 S 142 30 E
Warroad, *U.S.A.* **154 A7** 48 54N 95 19W
Warrumbungle △, *Australia* **129 A8** 31 18 S 149 1 E
Warruwi, *Australia* **126 A1** 11 36 S 133 20 E
Warsa, *Indonesia* **83 B5** 0 47 S 135 55 E
Warsak Dam, *Pakistan* **92 B4** 34 11N 71 19 E
Warsaw = Warszawa, *Poland* **55 F8** 52 13N 21 0 E
Warsaw, *Ill., U.S.A.* **156 D5** 40 22N 91 26W
Warsaw, *Ind., U.S.A.* **157 C11** 41 14N 85 51W
Warsaw, *Ky., U.S.A.* **157 F12** 38 47N 84 54W
Warsaw, *Mo., U.S.A.* **156 F3** 38 15N 93 23W
Warsaw, *N.Y., U.S.A.* **150 D6** 42 45N 78 8W
Warsaw, *Ohio, U.S.A.* **150 F3** 40 20N 82 0W
Warstein, *Germany* **30 D4** 51 26N 8 22 E
Warszawa, *Poland* **55 F8** 52 13N 21 0 E
Warszawa ✈ (WAW), *Poland* **55 F7** 52 9N 20 59 E
Warta, *Poland* **55 G5** 51 43N 18 38 E
Warta →, *Poland* **55 F1** 52 35N 14 39 E
Wartenburg = Barczewo, *Poland* **54 E7** 53 50N 20 42 E
Warth, *Austria* **33 B10** 47 15N 10 11 E
Warthbrücken = Koło, *Poland* **55 F5** 52 14N 18 40 E
Warthe = Warta →, *Poland* **55 F1** 52 35N 14 39 E
Warthen, *U.S.A.* **152 B7** 33 6N 82 48W
Warthenau = Zawiercie, *Poland* **55 H6** 50 30N 19 24 E
Waru, *Indonesia* **83 B4** 3 30 S 130 36 E
Warud, *India* **94 D4** 21 30N 78 16 E
Warwick, *Australia* **127 D5** 28 10 S 152 1 E
Warwick, *U.K.* **21 E6** 52 18N 1 35W
Warwick, *Ga., U.S.A.* **152 D6** 31 50N 83 57W
Warwick, *N.Y., U.S.A.* **151 E10** 41 16N 74 22W
Warwick, *R.I., U.S.A.* **151 E13** 41 42N 71 28W
Warwickshire □, *U.K.* **21 E6** 52 14N 1 38W
Wasaga Beach, *Canada* **150 B4** 44 31N 80 1W
Wasagaming, *Canada* **143 C9** 50 39N 99 58W
Wasatch Ra., *U.S.A.* **158 F8** 40 30N 111 15W
Wasbank, *S. Africa* **117 D5** 28 15 S 30 9 E
Wasco, *Calif., U.S.A.* **161 K7** 35 36N 119 20W
Wasco, *Oreg., U.S.A.* **158 D3** 45 36N 120 42W
Wase, *Nigeria* **113 D6** 9 4N 9 54 E
Waseca, *U.S.A.* **154 C8** 44 5N 93 30W
Wasekamio L., *Canada* **143 B7** 56 45N 108 45W
Wasgomura △, *Sri Lanka* **95 L5** 7 45N 81 0 E
Wash, The, *U.K.* **20 E8** 52 58N 0 20 E
Washago, *Canada* **150 B5** 44 45N 79 20W
Washburn, *Ill., U.S.A.* **156 D7** 40 55N 89 17W
Washburn, *N. Dak., U.S.A.* **154 B4** 47 17N 101 2W
Washburn, *Wis., U.S.A.* **154 B9** 46 40N 90 54W
Washim, *India* **94 D3** 20 3N 77 0 E
Washington, *U.K.* **20 C6** 54 55N 1 30W
Washington, *D.C., U.S.A.* **148 F7** 38 54N 77 2W
Washington, *Ga., U.S.A.* **152 B7** 33 44N 82 44W
Washington, *Ill., U.S.A.* **156 D7** 40 42N 89 24W
Washington, *Ind., U.S.A.* **157 F9** 38 40N 87 10W
Washington, *Iowa, U.S.A.* **156 C5** 41 18N 91 42W
Washington, *Mo., U.S.A.* **156 F5** 38 33N 91 1W
Washington, *N.C., U.S.A.* **149 H7** 35 33N 77 3W
Washington, *N.J., U.S.A.* **151 F10** 40 46N 74 59W
Washington, *Pa., U.S.A.* **150 F4** 40 10N 80 15W
Washington, *Utah, U.S.A.* **159 H7** 37 8N 113 31W
Washington □, *U.S.A.* **158 C3** 47 30N 120 30W
Washington, Mt., *U.S.A.* **151 B13** 44 16N 71 18W
Washington Court House, *U.S.A.* **157 E13** 39 32N 83 26W
Washington I., *U.S.A.* **148 C2** 45 23N 86 54W
Washington Land, *Greenland* **10 A4** 80 30N 66 0W
Washougal, *U.S.A.* **160 E4** 45 35N 122 21W
Washpool △, *Australia* **127 D5** 29 22 S 152 20 E
Washuk, *Pakistan* **91 D2** 27 42N 64 45 E
Wasian, *Indonesia* **83 B4** 1 47 S 133 19 E
Wasilków, *Poland* **55 E10** 53 12N 23 13 E
Wasilla, *U.S.A.* **144 F10** 61 35N 149 26W
Wasior, *Indonesia* **83 B4** 2 43 S 134 30 E
Wāsiţ □, *Iraq* **96 C5** 32 30N 46 0 E
Waskaganish, *Canada* **140 B4** 51 30N 78 40W
Waskaiowaka, L., *Canada* **143 B9** 56 33N 96 23W
Waskesiu Lake, *Canada* **143 C7** 53 55N 106 5W
Wassaw I., *U.S.A.* **152 D9** 31 53N 80 58W
Wassaw Sd., *U.S.A.* **152 D9** 31 55N 80 55W
Wassen, *Switz.* **33 C7** 46 42N 8 36 E
Wasserauen, *Switz.* **33 B8** 47 17N 9 26 E
Wasserburg, *Germany* **31 G8** 48 3N 12 14 E
Wasserkuppe, *Germany* **30 E5** 50 29N 9 55 E
Wassy, *France* **27 D11** 48 30N 4 58 E
Wasu, *Papua N. G.* **132 C4** 5 58 S 147 12 E
Wasua, *Papua N. G.* **132 E2** 8 18 S 142 52 E
Waswanipi, *Canada* **140 C4** 49 40N 76 29W
Waswanipi, L., *Canada* **140 C4** 49 35N 76 40W
Watam, *Papua N. G.* **132 B3** 3 55 S 144 33 E
Watampone, *Indonesia* **82 B2** 4 29 S 120 25 E
Watamu, *Kenya* **118 C5** 3 23 S 40 0 E
Watansoppeng, *Indonesia* **82 B1** 4 10 S 119 56 E
Watarrka △, *Australia* **124 D5** 24 20 S 131 30 E
Watee, *Solomon Is.* **133 N12** 10 30 S 162 2 E
Watenstadt-Salzgitter = Salzgitter, *Germany* **30 C6** 52 9N 10 19 E
Water Park Pt., *Australia* **126 C5** 22 56 S 150 47 E
Water Valley, *U.S.A.* **155 H10** 34 10N 89 38W
Waterberg Plateau ⌓, *Namibia* **116 C2** 20 25 S 17 18 E
Waterberge, *S. Africa* **117 C4** 24 10 S 28 0 E
Waterbury, *Conn., U.S.A.* **151 E11** 41 33N 73 3W
Waterbury, *Vt., U.S.A.* **151 B12** 44 20N 72 46W
Waterbury L., *Canada* **143 B8** 58 10N 104 22W
Waterdown, *Canada* **150 C5** 43 20N 79 53W
Wateree →, *U.S.A.* **152 B9** 33 45N 80 37W
Waterford, *Canada* **150 D4** 42 56N 80 17W
Waterford, *Ireland* **23 D4** 52 15N 7 8W
Waterford, *Calif., U.S.A.* **160 H6** 37 38N 120 46W
Waterford, *Mich., U.S.A.* **157 B13** 42 45N 83 32W
Waterford, *Pa., U.S.A.* **150 E5** 41 57N 79 59W
Waterford, *Wis., U.S.A.* **157 B8** 42 46N 88 13W
Waterford □, *Ireland* **23 D4** 52 10N 7 40W
Waterford Harbour, *Ireland* **23 D5** 52 8N 6 58W
Waterhen L., *Canada* **143 C9** 52 10N 99 40W
Waterloo, *Belgium* **24 D4** 50 43N 4 25 E
Waterloo, *Ont., Canada* **140 D3** 43 30N 80 32W
Waterloo, *Qué., Canada* **151 A12** 45 22N 72 32W
Waterloo, *S. Leone* **112 D2** 8 26N 13 8W
Waterloo, *Ill., U.S.A.* **156 F6** 38 20N 90 9W
Waterloo, *Ind., U.S.A.* **157 C11** 41 26N 85 1W
Waterloo, *Iowa, U.S.A.* **156 B4** 42 30N 92 21W
Waterloo, *N.Y., U.S.A.* **150 D8** 42 54N 76 52W
Waterloo, *Wis., U.S.A.* **156 A8** 43 11N 88 59W
Waterman, *U.S.A.* **157 C8** 41 46N 88 47W
Watersmeet, *U.S.A.* **154 B10** 46 16N 89 11W
Waterton Lakes △, *Canada* **142 D6** 48 45N 115 0W
Watertown, *Conn., U.S.A.* **151 E11** 41 36N 73 7W
Watertown, *Fla., U.S.A.* **152 E7** 30 11N 82 36W
Watertown, *N.Y., U.S.A.* **151 C9** 43 59N 75 55W
Watertown, *S. Dak., U.S.A.* **154 C6** 44 54N 97 7W
Watertown, *Wis., U.S.A.* **154 D10** 43 12N 88 43W
Waterval-Boven, *S. Africa* **117 D5** 25 40 S 30 18 E
Waterville, *Canada* **151 A13** 45 16N 71 54W
Waterville, *Maine, U.S.A.* **149 C11** 44 33N 69 38W
Waterville, *N.Y., U.S.A.* **151 D9** 42 56N 75 23W
Waterville, *Pa., U.S.A.* **150 E7** 41 19N 77 21W
Waterville, *Wash., U.S.A.* **158 C3** 47 39N 120 4W
Watervliet, *Mich., U.S.A.* **157 B10** 42 11N 86 18W
Watervliet, *N.Y., U.S.A.* **151 D11** 42 44N 73 42W
Wates, *Indonesia* **85 D4** 7 51 S 110 10 E
Watford, *Canada* **150 D3** 42 57N 81 53W
Watford, *U.K.* **21 F7** 51 40N 0 24W
Watford City, *U.S.A.* **154 B3** 47 48N 103 17W
Wathaman →, *Canada* **143 B8** 57 16N 102 59W
Wathaman L., *Canada* **143 B8** 56 58N 103 44W
Watheroo, *Australia* **125 F2** 30 15 S 116 0 E
Watheroo △, *Australia* **125 F2** 30 19 S 115 48 E
Wating, *China* **74 G4** 35 40N 106 38 E
Watkins Glen, *U.S.A.* **150 D8** 42 23N 76 52W
Watkinsville, *U.S.A.* **152 B6** 33 52N 83 25W
Watling I. = San Salvador I., *Bahamas* **165 B5** 24 0N 74 40W
Watmuri, *Indonesia* **83 C4** 7 25 S 131 42 E
Watom I., *Papua N. G.* **132 C7** 4 7 S 152 4 E
Watonga, *U.S.A.* **155 H5** 35 51N 98 25W
Watrous, *Canada* **143 C7** 51 40N 105 25W
Watrous, *U.S.A.* **155 H2** 35 48N 104 59W
Watsa, *Dem. Rep. of the Congo* **118 B2** 3 4N 29 30 E
Watseka, *U.S.A.* **157 D9** 40 47N 87 44W
Watsi Kenga, *Dem. Rep. of the Congo* **114 C4** 0 49 S 20 34 E
Watson, *Australia* **125 F5** 30 29 S 131 31 E
Watson, *Canada* **143 C8** 52 10N 104 30W
Watson Lake, *Canada* **142 A3** 60 6N 128 49W
Watsontown, *U.S.A.* **150 E8** 41 5N 76 52W
Watsonville, *U.S.A.* **160 J5** 36 55N 121 45W
Wattenwil, *Switz.* **32 C5** 46 46N 7 31 E
Wattiwarriganna Cr. →, *Australia* **127 D2** 28 57 S 136 10 E
Wattwil, *Switz.* **33 B8** 47 18N 9 6 E
Watu, *Dem. Rep. of the Congo* **114 C4** 3 18 S 20 3 E
Watuata = Batuata, *Indonesia* **82 C2** 6 12 S 122 42 E
Watubela, Kepulauan, *Indonesia* **83 B4** 4 28 S 131 35 E
Watubela Is. = Watubela, Kepulauan, *Indonesia* **83 B4** 4 28 S 131 35 E
Wau = Wâw, *Sudan* **107 F2** 7 45N 28 1 E
Wau, *Papua N. G.* **132 D4** 7 21 S 146 47 E
Waubamik, *Canada* **150 A4** 45 27N 80 1W
Waubay, *U.S.A.* **154 C6** 45 20N 97 18W
Waubra, *Australia* **128 D5** 37 21 S 143 39 E
Wauchope, *N.S.W., Australia* **129 A10** 31 28 S 152 45 E
Wauchope, *N. Terr., Australia* **126 C1** 20 36 S 134 15 E
Wauchula, *U.S.A.* **153 H8** 27 33N 81 49W
Waukarlycarly, L., *Australia* **124 D3** 21 18 S 121 56 E
Waukeenah, *U.S.A.* **152 E6** 30 25N 83 57W
Waukegan, *U.S.A.* **157 B9** 42 22N 87 50W
Waukesha, *U.S.A.* **154 D10** 43 1N 88 14W
Waukon, *U.S.A.* **154 D9** 43 16N 91 29W
Waupaca, *U.S.A.* **154 C10** 44 21N 89 5W
Waupun, *U.S.A.* **154 D10** 43 38N 88 44W
Waurika, *U.S.A.* **155 H6** 34 10N 98 0W
Wausau, *Fla., U.S.A.* **152 E4** 30 38N 85 35W
Wausau, *Wis., U.S.A.* **154 C10** 44 58N 89 38W
Wauseon, *U.S.A.* **157 C12** 41 33N 84 8W
Wautoma, *U.S.A.* **154 C10** 44 4N 89 18W
Wauwatosa, *U.S.A.* **157 A9** 43 3N 88 0W
Waveland, *U.S.A.* **157 E9** 39 53N 87 3W
Waveney →, *U.K.* **21 E9** 52 35N 1 39 E
Waverley, *N.Z.* **130 F3** 39 46 S 174 37 E
Waverley Hall, *U.S.A.* **152 C5** 32 41N 84 44W
Waverly, *Ala., U.S.A.* **152 C4** 32 44N 85 35W
Waverly, *Fla., U.S.A.* **153 H8** 27 59N 81 37W
Waverly, *Ga., U.S.A.* **152 D8** 31 6N 81 43W
Waverly, *Ill., U.S.A.* **156 E7** 39 36N 89 57W
Waverly, *Iowa, U.S.A.* **156 B4** 42 44N 92 29W
Waverly, *Mo., U.S.A.* **156 E3** 39 13N 93 31W
Waverly, *N.Y., U.S.A.* **151 E8** 42 1N 76 32W
Wavre, *Belgium* **24 D4** 50 43N 4 38 E
Waw, *Burma* **90 G6** 17 28N 96 41 E
Wâw, *Sudan* **107 F2** 7 45N 28 1 E
Wāw al Kabīr, *Libya* **108 C3** 25 20N 16 43 E
Wāw an Nāmūs, *Libya* **108 D3** 24 55N 17 46 E
Wawa, *Canada* **140 C3** 47 59N 84 47W
Wawa, *Nigeria* **113 D5** 9 54N 4 27 E
Wawa, *Sudan* **106 C3** 20 30N 30 22 E
Wawanesa, *Canada* **143 D9** 49 36N 99 40W
Wawasee, L., *U.S.A.* **157 C11** 41 24N 85 42W
Wawoi →, *Papua N. G.* **132 D2** 7 48 S 143 16 E
Wawona, *U.S.A.* **160 H7** 37 32N 119 39W
Waxahachie, *U.S.A.* **155 J6** 32 24N 96 51W
Way, L., *Australia* **125 E3** 26 45 S 120 16 E
Waya, *Fiji* **133 A1** 17 19 S 177 10 E
Wayabula, *Indonesia* **82 A3** 2 29N 128 17 E
Waycross, *U.S.A.* **152 D7** 31 13N 82 21W
Wayi, *Sudan* **107 F3** 5 8N 30 10 E
Wayland, *Mich., U.S.A.* **157 B11** 42 40N 85 39W
Wayland, *N.Y., U.S.A.* **150 D7** 42 34N 77 35W
Wayne, *Nebr., U.S.A.* **154 D6** 42 14N 97 1W
Wayne, *W. Va., U.S.A.* **148 F4** 38 13N 82 27W
Wayne City, *U.S.A.* **157 F8** 38 21N 88 35W
Wayne County, Detroit ✈ (DTW), *U.S.A.* **157 B13** 42 13N 83 21W
Wayne Lakes, *U.S.A.* **157 D12** 40 1N 84 40W
Waynesboro, *Ga., U.S.A.* **152 B7** 33 6N 82 1W
Waynesboro, *Miss., U.S.A.* **149 K1** 31 40N 88 39W
Waynesboro, *Pa., U.S.A.* **148 F7** 39 45N 77 35W
Waynesboro, *Va., U.S.A.* **148 F6** 38 4N 78 53W
Waynesburg, *U.S.A.* **148 F5** 39 54N 80 11W
Waynesville, *Mo., U.S.A.* **156 G4** 37 50N 92 12W
Waynesville, *N.C., U.S.A.* **149 H4** 35 28N 82 58W
Waynesville, *Ohio, U.S.A.* **157 E12** 39 32N 84 5W
Waynoka, *U.S.A.* **155 G5** 36 35N 98 53W
Wayside, *U.S.A.* **152 B6** 33 4N 83 37W
Waza, *Afghan.* **91 B3** 33 22N 69 26 E
Waza △, *Cameroon* **109 F2** 11 15N 14 38 E
Wazikhwah, *Afghan.* **91 B3** 32 11N 68 21 E
Wāzin, *Libya* **108 B2** 31 58N 10 40 E
Wazirabad, *Pakistan* **92 C6** 32 30N 74 8 E
Wda →, *Poland* **54 E5** 53 25N 18 29 E
We, *Indonesia* **84 A1** 5 51N 95 18 E
Wé, *N. Cal.* **133 K5** 20 55 S 167 16 E
Weald, The, *U.K.* **21 F8** 51 4N 0 20 E
Weam, *Papua N. G.* **132 E1** 8 37 S 141 8 E
Wear →, *U.K.* **20 C6** 54 55N 1 23W
Weatherford, *Okla., U.S.A.* **155 H5** 35 32N 98 43W
Weatherford, *Tex., U.S.A.* **155 J6** 32 46N 97 48W
Weaubleau, *U.S.A.* **156 G3** 37 54N 93 32W
Weaverville, *U.S.A.* **158 F2** 40 44N 122 56W
Webb City, *U.S.A.* **155 G7** 37 9N 94 28W
Webequie, *Canada* **140 B2** 52 59N 87 21W
Weber, *N.Z.* **130 G5** 40 24 S 176 20 E
Webo = Nyaake, *Liberia* **112 E3** 4 52N 7 37W
Webster, *Mass., U.S.A.* **151 D13** 42 3N 71 53W
Webster, *N.Y., U.S.A.* **150 C7** 43 13N 77 26W
Webster, *S. Dak., U.S.A.* **154 C6** 45 20N 97 31W
Webster City, *U.S.A.* **156 B3** 42 28N 93 49W
Webster Springs, *U.S.A.* **148 F5** 38 29N 80 25W
Weda, *Indonesia* **79 D7** 0 21N 127 50 E
Weda, Teluk, *Indonesia* **82 A3** 0 20N 128 0 E
Weddell I., *Falk. Is.* **9 f** 51 50 S 61 0W
Weddell Sea, *Antarctica* **7 D1** 72 30 S 40 0W
Wedderburn, *Australia* **128 D5** 36 26 S 143 33 E
Weddin Mts. △, *Australia* **129 C8** 33 59 S 148 0 E
Wedel, *Germany* **30 B5** 53 34N 9 42 E
Wedemark, *Germany* **30 C5** 52 32N 9 43 E
Wedgeport, *Canada* **141 D6** 43 44N 65 59W
Wednesday I., *Australia* **132 F2** 10 31 S 142 16 E
Wedowee, *U.S.A.* **152 B4** 33 19N 85 29W
Wedza, *Zimbabwe* **119 F3** 18 40 S 31 33 E
Wee Waa, *Australia* **127 E4** 30 11 S 149 26 E
Weed, *U.S.A.* **158 F2** 41 25N 122 23W
Weed Heights, *U.S.A.* **160 G7** 38 59N 119 13W
Weedsport, *U.S.A.* **151 C8** 43 3N 76 35W
Weedville, *U.S.A.* **150 E6** 41 17N 78 30W
Weeki Wachee, *U.S.A.* **153 G7** 28 32N 82 35W
Weenen, *S. Africa* **117 D5** 28 48 S 30 7 E
Weener, *Germany* **30 B3** 53 9N 7 20 E
Weert, *Neths.* **24 C5** 51 15N 5 43 E
Weggis, *Switz.* **33 B6** 47 2N 8 26 E
Węgierska-Górka, *Poland* **55 J6** 49 36N 19 7 E
Węgliniec, *Poland* **55 G2** 51 18N 15 10 E
Węgorzewo, *Poland* **54 D8** 54 13N 21 43 E
Węgorzyno, *Poland* **54 E2** 53 32N 15 33 E
Węgrów, *Poland* **55 F9** 52 24N 22 0 E
Wehda □, *Sudan* **107 F3** 8 30N 30 0 E
Wei He →, *Hebei, China* **74 F8** 36 10N 115 45 E
Wei He →, *Shaanxi, China* **74 G6** 34 38N 110 15 E
Weichang, *China* **75 D9** 41 58N 117 49 E
Weichuan, *China* **74 G7** 34 20N 113 59 E
Weida, *Germany* **30 E8** 50 46N 12 2 E
Weiden, *Germany* **31 F8** 49 41N 12 10 E
Weifang, *China* **75 F10** 36 44N 119 7 E
Weihai, *China* **75 F12** 37 30N 122 6 E
Weil, *Germany* **31 H3** 47 35N 7 37 E
Weilburg, *Germany* **30 E4** 50 28N 8 17 E
Weilheim, *Germany* **31 H7** 47 50N 11 9 E
Weimar, *Germany* **30 E7** 50 58N 11 19 E
Weinan, *China* **74 G5** 34 31N 109 29 E
Weinfelden, *Switz.* **33 A8** 47 34N 9 6 E
Weingarten, *Germany* **31 F4** 49 3N 8 31 E
Weinheim, *Germany* **31 F4** 49 32N 8 39 E
Weining, *China* **76 D5** 26 50N 104 17 E
Weipa, *Australia* **126 A3** 12 40 S 141 50 E
Weir →, *Australia* **127 D4** 28 20 S 149 50 E
Weir →, *Canada* **143 B10** 56 54N 93 21W
Weir, L., *U.S.A.* **153 F8** 29 0N 81 57W
Weir River, *Canada* **143 B10** 56 49N 94 6W
Weirsdale, *U.S.A.* **153 G8** 28 59N 81 55W
Weirton, *U.S.A.* **150 F4** 40 24N 80 35W
Weiser, *U.S.A.* **158 D5** 44 10N 117 0W
Weishan, *Shandong, China* **75 G9** 34 47N 117 5 E
Weishan, *Yunnan, China* **76 E3** 25 12N 100 20 E
Weissenbach, *Austria* **33 B11** 47 26N 10 39 E
Weissenburg, *Germany* **31 F6** 49 2N 10 58 E
Weissenfels, *Germany* **30 D7** 51 11N 12 0 E
Weisshorn, *Switz.* **32 D5** 46 7N 7 43 E
Weisskirchen = Hranice, *Czech Rep.* **35 B10** 49 34N 17 45 E
Weisskugel, *Austria* **33 C11** 46 48N 10 44 E
Weissmies, *Switz.* **32 D6** 46 8N 8 1 E
Weisstannen, *Switz.* **33 C8** 46 59N 9 22 E
Weisswasser, *Germany* **30 D10** 51 30N 14 36 E
Weistritz = Bystrzyca →, *Dolnośląskie, Poland* **55 G3** 51 12N 16 55 E
Weistritz = Bystrzyca →, *Lubelskie, Poland* **55 G9** 51 21N 22 46 E
Wéitra, *Austria* **34 C7** 48 41N 14 54 E
Weixi, *China* **76 D2** 27 10N 99 10 E
Weixin, *China* **76 D5** 27 48N 105 3 E
Weiyuan, *China* **74 G3** 35 7N 104 10 E
Weiz, *Austria* **34 D8** 47 13N 15 39 E
Weizhou Dao, *China* **76 G7** 21 0N 109 5 E
Wejherowo, *Poland* **54 D5** 54 35N 18 12 E
Wekusko L., *Canada* **143 C9** 54 40N 99 50W
Welch, *U.S.A.* **148 G5** 37 26N 81 35W
Weldya, *Ethiopia* **107 E4** 11 50N 39 34 E
Welega, *Ethiopia* **107 F3** 9 25N 34 20 E
Welford △, *Australia* **126 D3** 25 5 S 143 16 E
Weligama, *Sri Lanka* **95 M5** 5 58N 80 25 E
Welkite, *Ethiopia* **107 F4** 8 15N 37 42 E
Welkom, *S. Africa* **116 D4** 28 0 S 26 46 E
Welland, *Canada* **140 D4** 43 0N 79 15W
Welland →, *U.K.* **21 E7** 52 51N 0 5W
Wellawaya, *Sri Lanka* **95 L5** 6 44N 81 6 E
Wellesley Is., *Australia* **126 B2** 16 42 S 139 30 E
Wellingborough, *U.K.* **21 E7** 52 19N 0 41W
Wellington, *Australia* **129 B8** 32 35 S 148 59 E
Wellington, *Canada* **150 C7** 43 57N 77 20W

Wellington, N.Z. **130 H3** 41 19 S 174 46 E
Wellington, S. Africa **116 E2** 33 38 S 19 1 E
Wellington, Somst., U.K. **21 G4** 50 58N 3 13W
Wellington, Telford & Wrekin, U.K. **21 E5** 52 42N 2 30W
Wellington, Colo., U.S.A. **154 E2** 40 42N 105 0W
Wellington, Kans., U.S.A. **155 G6** 37 16N 97 24W
Wellington, Mo., U.S.A. **156 E3** 39 8N 93 59W
Wellington, Nev., U.S.A. **160 G7** 38 45N 119 23W
Wellington, Ohio, U.S.A. **150 E2** 41 10N 82 13W
Wellington, Tex., U.S.A. **155 H4** 34 51N 100 13W
Wellington □, N.Z. **130 G4** 41 0 S 175 30 E
Wellington, I., Chile **176 C2** 49 30 S 75 0W
Wellington, L., Australia **129 E7** 38 6 S 147 20 E
Wellman, U.S.A. **156 C5** 41 28N 91 50W
Wells, U.K. **21 F5** 51 13N 2 39W
Wells, Maine, U.S.A. **151 C14** 43 20N 70 35W
Wells, N.Y., U.S.A. **151 C10** 43 24N 74 17W
Wells, Nev., U.S.A. **158 F6** 41 7N 114 58W
Wells, L., Australia **125 E3** 26 44 S 123 15 E
Wells, Mt., Australia **124 C4** 17 25 S 127 8 E
Wells Gray ⌂, Canada **142 C4** 52 30N 120 15W
Wells-next-the-Sea, U.K. **20 E8** 52 57N 0 51 E
Wells River, U.S.A. **151 B12** 44 9N 72 4W
Wellsboro, U.S.A. **150 E7** 41 45N 77 18W
Wellsburg, U.S.A. **150 F4** 40 16N 80 37W
Wellsford, N.Z. **130 C3** 36 16 S 174 32 E
Wellston = Warner Robins, U.S.A. **152 C6** 32 37N 83 36W
Wellsville, Mo., U.S.A. **156 E5** 39 4N 91 34W
Wellsville, N.Y., U.S.A. **150 D7** 42 7N 77 57W
Wellsville, Ohio, U.S.A. **150 F4** 40 36N 80 39W
Wellsville, Utah, U.S.A. **158 F8** 41 38N 111 56W
Wellton, U.S.A. **159 K6** 32 40N 114 8W
Welmel, Wabi →, Ethiopia **107 F5** 5 38N 40 47 E
Welo, Ethiopia **107 E4** 11 50N 39 48 E
Welo, Somali Rep. **120 C3** 9 25N 48 55 E
Wels, Austria **34 C7** 48 9N 14 1 E
Welshpool, Australia **129 E7** 38 42 S 146 26 E
Welshpool, U.K. **21 E4** 52 39N 3 8W
Welungen = Wieluń, Poland **55 G5** 51 15N 18 34 E
Welwitschia = Khorixas, Namibia **116 C1** 20 16 S 14 59 E
Welwyn Garden City, U.K. **21 F7** 51 48N 0 12W
Wem, U.K. **20 E5** 52 52N 2 44W
Wembere →, Tanzania **118 C3** 4 10 S 34 15 E
Wemindji, Canada **140 B4** 53 0N 78 49W
Wen Xian, China **74 G7** 34 55N 113 5 E
Wenatchee, U.S.A. **158 C3** 47 25N 120 19W
Wenchang, China **86 C8** 19 38N 110 42 E
Wencheng, China **77 D13** 27 46N 120 4 E
Wenchi, Ghana **112 D4** 7 46N 2 8W
Wenchow = Wenzhou, China **77 D13** 28 0N 120 38 E
Wenchuan, China **76 B4** 31 22N 103 35 E
Wenden, U.S.A. **161 M13** 33 49N 113 33W
Wendeng, China **75 F12** 37 15N 122 5 E
Wendesi, Indonesia **83 B4** 2 30 S 134 17 E
Wendo, Ethiopia **107 F4** 6 40N 38 27 E
Wendover, U.S.A. **158 F6** 40 44N 114 2W
Weng'an, China **76 D6** 27 5N 107 25 E
Wengcheng, China **77 E9** 24 22N 113 50 E
Wengen, Switz. **32 C5** 46 37N 7 55 E
Wengyuan, China **77 E10** 24 20N 114 9 E
Wenjiang, China **76 B4** 30 44N 103 55 E
Wenling, China **77 C13** 28 21N 121 20 E
Wenlock →, Australia **126 A3** 12 2 S 141 55 E
Wenona, U.S.A. **156 C7** 41 3N 89 3W
Wenshan, China **76 F5** 23 20N 104 18 E
Wenshang, China **74 G9** 35 45N 116 30 E
Wenshui, China **74 F7** 37 26N 112 1 E
Wensleydale, U.K. **20 C6** 54 17N 2 0W
Wensu, China **68 B3** 41 15N 80 10 E
Wensum →, U.K. **20 E8** 52 40N 1 15 E
Wentworth, Australia **128 C4** 34 2 S 141 54 E
Wentzel L., Canada **142 B6** 59 2N 114 28W
Wentzville, U.S.A. **156 F6** 38 49N 90 51W
Wenut, Indonesia **83 B4** 3 11 S 133 19 E
Wenxi, China **74 G6** 35 20N 111 10 E
Wenxian, China **74 H3** 32 43N 104 36 E
Wenzhou, China **77 D13** 28 0N 120 38 E
Weott, U.S.A. **158 F2** 40 20N 123 55W
Wepener, S. Africa **116 D4** 29 42 S 27 3 E
Werda, Botswana **116 D3** 25 24 S 23 15 E
Werdau, Germany **30 E8** 50 44N 12 22 E
Werder, Ethiopia **120 C3** 6 58N 45 1 E
Werder, Germany **30 C8** 52 23N 12 55 E
Werdohl, Germany **30 D3** 51 15N 7 46 E
Wereilu, Ethiopia **107 E4** 10 40N 39 28 E
Weri, Indonesia **83 B4** 3 10 S 132 38 E
Werneck, Germany **31 F6** 49 58N 10 5 E
Wernigerode, Germany **30 D6** 51 50N 10 47 E
Werra →, Germany **30 D5** 51 24N 9 39 E
Werribee, Australia **128 D6** 37 54 S 144 40 E
Werrikimbee △, Australia **129 A10** 31 11 S 152 15 E
Werrimull, Australia **128 C4** 34 25 S 141 38 E
Werris Creek, Australia **129 A9** 31 18 S 150 38 E
Werschetz = Vršac, Serbia & M. **52 E6** 45 8N 21 20 E
Wertach →, Germany **31 G6** 48 22N 10 54 E
Wertheim, Germany **31 F5** 49 45N 9 32 E
Wertingen, Germany **31 G6** 48 33N 10 41 E
Wesel, Germany **30 D2** 51 39N 6 37 E
Weser →, Germany **30 B4** 53 36N 8 28 E
Weser-Ems □, Germany **30 C3** 53 0N 7 30 E
Weserbergland, Germany **30 C5** 52 12N 9 7 E
Weserbergland Schaumburg Hameln ⌂, Germany **30 C5** 52 8N 9 20 E
Wesermünde = Bremerhaven, Germany **30 B4** 53 33N 8 36 E
Wesiri, Indonesia **82 C3** 7 30 S 126 30 E
Weslaco, U.S.A. **155 M6** 26 10N 97 58W
Weslemkoon L., Canada **150 A7** 45 2N 77 25W
Wesleyville, U.S.A. **150 D4** 42 9N 80 0W
Wessel, C., Australia **126 A2** 10 59 S 136 46 E
Wessel Is., Australia **126 A2** 11 10 S 136 45 E
Wesselburen, Germany **30 A4** 54 13N 8 54 E
Wessington Springs, U.S.A. **154 C5** 44 5N 98 34W
West, U.S.A. **155 K6** 31 48N 97 6W
West →, U.S.A. **151 D12** 42 52N 72 33W
West Allis, U.S.A. **157 B8** 43 1N 88 0W
West Antarctica, Antarctica **7 D15** 80 0 S 90 0W
West Baines →, Australia **124 C4** 15 38 S 129 59 E
West Bank ☒, Asia **103 C4** 32 6N 35 13 E
West Bend, U.S.A. **148 D1** 43 25N 88 11W
West Bengal □, India **93 H13** 23 0N 88 0 E
West Berkshire □, U.K. **21 F6** 51 25N 1 17W
West Beskids = Západné Beskydy, Europe **35 B12** 49 30N 19 0 E
West Branch, U.S.A. **148 C3** 44 17N 84 14W
West Branch Susquehanna →, U.S.A. **151 F8** 40 53N 76 48W
West Bromwich, U.K. **21 E6** 52 32N 1 59W
West Burra, U.K. **22 A7** 60 5N 1 21W
West Canada Cr. →, U.S.A. **151 C10** 43 1N 74 58W
West Cape Howe, Australia **125 G2** 35 8 S 117 36 E
West Carrollton, U.S.A. **157 E12** 39 40N 84 17W
West Chazy, U.S.A. **151 B11** 44 49N 73 28W
West Chester, U.S.A. **151 G9** 39 58N 75 36W
West Chicago, U.S.A. **157 C8** 41 53N 88 12W
West Coast ⌂, Namibia **116 C1** 21 53 S 14 14 E
West Coast □, N.Z. **131 D5** 43 15 S 170 30 E
West Coast △, S. Africa **116 E2** 33 13 S 18 0 E
West Columbia, S.C., U.S.A. **152 B8** 33 59N 81 4W
West Columbia, Tex., U.S.A. **155 L7** 29 9N 95 39W
West Covina, U.S.A. **161 L9** 34 4N 117 54W
West Des Moines, U.S.A. **156 C3** 41 35N 93 43W
West Dunbartonshire □, U.K. **22 F4** 55 59N 4 30W
West End, Bahamas **164 A4** 26 41N 78 58W
West Falkland, Falk. Is. **9 f** 51 40 S 60 0W
West Fargo, U.S.A. **154 B6** 46 52N 96 54W
West Farmington, U.S.A. **150 E4** 41 23N 80 58W
West Fjord = Vestfjorden, Norway **14 C15** 67 55N 14 0 E
West Fork Trinity →, U.S.A. **155 J6** 32 48N 96 54W
West Frankfort, U.S.A. **156 G8** 37 54N 88 55W
West Grand L., U.S.A. **149 C12** 45 14N 67 51W
West Green, U.S.A. **152 D7** 31 37N 82 44W
West Hartford, U.S.A. **151 E12** 41 45N 72 44W
West Haven, U.S.A. **151 E12** 41 17N 72 57W
West Hazleton, U.S.A. **151 F9** 40 58N 76 0W
West Helena, U.S.A. **155 H9** 34 33N 90 38W
West Hurley, U.S.A. **151 E10** 41 59N 74 7W
West I., India **95 H11** 13 35N 92 54 E
West Ice Shelf, Antarctica **7 C7** 67 0 S 85 0 E
West Indies, Cent. Amer. **165 D7** 15 0N 65 0W
West Jefferson, U.S.A. **157 E12** 39 57N 83 17W
West Jordan, U.S.A. **158 F8** 40 36N 111 56W
West Lafayette, U.S.A. **157 D10** 40 27N 86 55W
West Lamma Channel, China **69 G11** 22 13N 114 4 E
West Liberty, Iowa, U.S.A. **156 C5** 41 34N 91 16W
West Liberty, Ky., U.S.A. **157 G13** 37 55N 83 16W
West Liberty, Ohio, U.S.A. **157 D13** 40 15N 83 45W
West Lorne, Canada **150 D3** 42 36N 81 36W
West Lothian □, U.K. **22 F5** 55 54N 3 36W
West Lunga △, Zambia **115 E4** 12 49 S 24 47 E
West Lunga →, Zambia **119 E1** 13 6 S 24 39 E
West MacDonnell △, Australia **124 D5** 23 38 S 132 59 E
West Memphis, U.S.A. **155 H9** 35 9N 90 11W
West Midlands □, U.K. **21 E6** 52 26N 2 0W
West Mifflin, U.S.A. **150 F5** 40 22N 79 52W
West Milton, Ohio, U.S.A. **157 E12** 39 58N 84 20W
West Milton, Pa., U.S.A. **150 E8** 41 1N 76 50W
West Monroe, U.S.A. **155 J8** 32 31N 92 9W
West New Britain □, Papua N. G. **132 C5** 5 0 S 149 30 E
West Newton, U.S.A. **150 F5** 40 14N 79 46W
West Nicholson, Zimbabwe **119 G2** 21 2 S 29 20 E
West Odessa, U.S.A. **155 K3** 31 50N 102 31W
West Palm Beach, U.S.A. **153 J9** 26 43N 80 3W
West Palm Beach Canal, U.S.A. **153 J9** 26 40N 80 15W
West Pensacola, U.S.A. **153 E2** 30 25N 87 16W
West Plains, U.S.A. **155 G9** 36 44N 91 51W
West Point, Ga., U.S.A. **152 C4** 32 53N 85 11W
West Point, Iowa, U.S.A. **156 D5** 40 43N 91 27W
West Point, Ky., U.S.A. **157 G11** 37 59N 85 57W
West Point, Miss., U.S.A. **155 J10** 33 36N 88 39W
West Point, N.Y., U.S.A. **151 E11** 41 24N 73 58W
West Point, Nebr., U.S.A. **154 E6** 41 51N 96 43W
West Point, Va., U.S.A. **148 G7** 37 32N 76 48W
West Point L., U.S.A. **152 B4** 33 0N 85 5W
West Pt. = Ouest, Pte. de l', Canada **141 C7** 49 52N 64 40W
West Pt., Australia **128 C1** 35 1 S 135 56 E
West Ra., Papua N. G. **132 C1** 4 55 S 141 30 E
West Road →, Canada **142 C4** 53 18N 122 53W
West Rutland, U.S.A. **151 C11** 43 38N 73 5W
West Salem, U.S.A. **157 F8** 38 31N 88 1W
West Schelde = Westerschelde →, Neths. **24 C3** 51 25N 3 25 E
West Seneca, U.S.A. **150 D6** 42 51N 78 48W
West Sepik □, Papua N. G. **132 B2** 3 30 S 142 0 E
West Siberian Plain, Russia **62 C11** 62 0N 75 0 E
West Sussex □, U.K. **21 G7** 50 55N 0 30W
West Terre Haute, U.S.A. **157 E9** 39 28N 87 27W
West-Terschelling, Neths. **24 A5** 53 22N 5 13 E
West Union, Iowa, U.S.A. **156 B5** 42 57N 91 49W
West Union, Ohio, U.S.A. **157 F13** 38 48N 83 33W
West Unity, U.S.A. **157 C12** 41 35N 84 26W
West Valley City, U.S.A. **158 F8** 40 42N 111 57W
West Virginia □, U.S.A. **148 F5** 38 45N 80 30W
West-Vlaanderen □, Belgium **24 D2** 51 0N 3 0 E
West Walker →, U.S.A. **160 G7** 38 54N 119 9W
West Wyalong, Australia **129 B7** 33 56 S 147 10 E
West Yellowstone, U.S.A. **158 D8** 44 40N 111 6W
West Yorkshire □, U.K. **20 D6** 53 45N 1 40W
Westall, Pt., Australia **127 E1** 32 55 S 134 4 E
Westbay, U.S.A. **152 E4** 30 18N 85 52W
Westbrook, U.S.A. **149 D10** 43 41N 70 22W
Westbury, Australia **127 G4** 41 30 S 146 51 E
Westby, U.S.A. **154 A2** 48 52N 104 3W
Westend, U.S.A. **161 K9** 35 42N 117 24W
Westerland, Germany **15 J13** 54 54N 8 17 E
Westerly, U.S.A. **151 E13** 41 22N 71 50W
Western □, Ghana **112 D4** 5 30N 2 30W
Western □, Kenya **118 B3** 0 30N 34 30 E
Western □, Papua N. G. **132 D2** 7 30 S 142 0 E
Western □, S. Leone **112 D2** 8 30N 13 20W
Western □, Zambia **119 F1** 15 0 S 24 4 E
Western Australia □, Australia **125 E2** 25 0 S 118 0 E
Western Cape □, S. Africa **116 E3** 34 0 S 20 0 E
Western Dvina = Daugava →, Latvia **15 H21** 57 4N 24 3 E
Western Ghats, India **95 H2** 14 0N 75 0 E
Western Highlands □, Papua N. G. **132 C3** 5 45 S 144 30 E
Western Isles □, U.K. **22 D1** 57 30N 7 10W
Western Sahara ■, Africa **110 D2** 25 0N 13 0W
Western Samoa = Samoa ■, Pac. Oc. **133 X24** 14 0 S 172 0W
Westernport, U.S.A. **148 F6** 39 29N 79 3W
Westerschelde →, Neths. **24 C3** 51 25N 3 25 E
Westerstede, Germany **30 B3** 53 15N 7 55 E
Westerwald, Germany **30 E3** 50 38N 7 56 E
Westfield, Ill., U.S.A. **157 E8** 39 27N 88 0W
Westfield, Ind., U.S.A. **157 D10** 40 2N 86 8W
Westfield, Mass., U.S.A. **151 D12** 42 7N 72 45W
Westfield, N.Y., U.S.A. **150 D5** 42 20N 79 35W
Westfield, Pa., U.S.A. **150 E7** 41 55N 77 32W
Westhill, U.K. **22 D6** 57 9N 2 19W
Westhope, U.S.A. **154 A4** 48 55N 101 1W
Westland, U.S.A. **157 B13** 42 15N 83 20W
Westland △, N.Z. **131 D5** 43 16 S 170 16 E
Westland Bight, N.Z. **131 C5** 42 55 S 170 5 E
Westlock, Canada **142 C6** 54 9N 113 55W
Westmar, Australia **127 D4** 27 55 S 149 44 E
Westmeath □, Ireland **23 C4** 53 33N 7 34W
Westminster, Colo., U.S.A. **154 F2** 39 50N 105 2W
Westminster, Md., U.S.A. **148 F7** 39 34N 76 59W
Westmont, U.S.A. **150 F6** 40 19N 78 58W
Westmoreland, Barbados **165 g** 13 13N 59 37W
Westmorland, U.S.A. **161 M11** 33 2N 115 37W
Weston, Malaysia **85 A5** 5 10N 115 35 E
Weston, Ohio, U.S.A. **157 C13** 41 21N 83 47W
Weston, Oreg., U.S.A. **158 D4** 45 49N 118 26W
Weston, W. Va., U.S.A. **148 F5** 39 2N 80 28W
Weston I., Canada **140 B4** 52 33N 79 36W
Weston-super-Mare, U.K. **21 F5** 51 21N 2 58W
Westover, U.S.A. **150 F6** 40 45N 78 40W
Westphalia, U.S.A. **156 F5** 38 26N 92 0W
Westport, Canada **151 B8** 44 40N 76 25W
Westport, Ireland **23 C2** 53 48N 9 31W
Westport, N.Z. **131 B6** 41 46 S 171 37 E
Westport, Ind., U.S.A. **157 E11** 39 11N 85 34W
Westport, N.Y., U.S.A. **151 B11** 44 11N 73 26W
Westport, Oreg., U.S.A. **160 D3** 46 8N 123 23W
Westport, Wash., U.S.A. **160 D2** 46 53N 124 6W
Westray, Canada **143 C8** 53 36N 101 24W
Westray, U.K. **22 B5** 59 18N 3 0W
Westree, Canada **140 C3** 47 26N 81 34W
Westville, Calif., U.S.A. **160 F6** 39 8N 120 42W
Westville, Fla., U.S.A. **152 E4** 30 46N 85 51W
Westville, Ill., U.S.A. **157 D9** 40 2N 87 38W
Westville, Ind., U.S.A. **157 C10** 41 35N 86 55W
Westwood, U.S.A. **158 F3** 40 18N 121 0W
Wetar, Indonesia **82 C3** 7 48 S 126 30 E
Wetar, Selat, Indonesia **82 C3** 8 20 S 126 30 E
Wetaskiwin, Canada **142 C6** 52 55N 113 24W
Wetherby, U.K. **20 D6** 53 56N 1 23W
Wethersfield, U.S.A. **151 E12** 41 42N 72 40W
Wetlet, Burma **90 D5** 22 20N 95 53 E
Wetteren, Belgium **24 D3** 51 0N 3 53 E
Wettingen, Switz. **33 B6** 47 28N 8 20 E
Wetumpka, U.S.A. **152 C3** 32 32N 86 13W
Wetzikon, Switz. **33 B7** 47 19N 8 48 E
Wetzlar, Germany **30 E4** 50 32N 8 31 E
Wevok, U.S.A. **144 B6** 68 53N 166 13W
Wewahitchka, U.S.A. **152 E4** 30 7N 85 12W
Wewak, Papua N. G. **132 B2** 3 38 S 143 41 E
Wewoka, U.S.A. **155 H6** 35 9N 96 30W
Wexford, Ireland **23 D5** 52 20N 6 28W
Wexford □, Ireland **23 D5** 52 20N 6 25W
Wexford Harbour, Ireland **23 D5** 52 20N 6 25W
Weyburn, Canada **143 D8** 49 40N 103 50W
Weyer Markt, Austria **34 D7** 47 51N 14 40 E
Weyhe, Germany **30 C4** 52 58N 8 49 E
Weyib →, Ethiopia **107 F5** 7 15N 40 15 E
Weymouth, Canada **141 D6** 44 30N 66 1W
Weymouth, U.K. **21 G5** 50 37N 2 28W
Weymouth, U.S.A. **151 D14** 42 13N 70 58W
Weymouth, C., Australia **126 A3** 12 37 S 143 27 E
Wha Ti, Canada **138 B8** 63 8N 117 16W
Whakaari = White I., N.Z. **130 D6** 37 30 S 177 13 E
Whakamaru, N.Z. **130 E4** 38 23 S 175 50 E
Whakatane, N.Z. **130 D6** 37 57 S 177 1 E
Whakatane →, N.Z. **130 D6** 37 57 S 177 1 E
Whale →, Canada **141 A6** 58 15N 67 40W
Whale Cove, Canada **143 A10** 62 10N 92 34W
Whale Pt., Ascension I. **9 g** 7 57 S 14 18W
Whales, B. of, Antarctica **7 D12** 78 0 S 165 0W
Whalsay, U.K. **22 A8** 60 22N 0 59W
Whangaehu →, N.Z. **130 G4** 40 3 S 175 6 E
Whangamata, N.Z. **130 D4** 37 12 S 175 53 E
Whangamomona, N.Z. **130 F3** 39 8 S 174 44 E
Whanganui △, N.Z. **130 F3** 39 17 S 174 53 E
Whangaparaoa Pen., N.Z. **130 C4** 36 40 S 174 45 E
Whangarei, N.Z. **130 B3** 35 43 S 174 21 E
Whangarei Harb., N.Z. **130 B3** 35 45 S 174 28 E
Whangaroa Harb., N.Z. **130 B2** 35 4 S 173 46 E
Whangaruru Harb., N.Z. **130 B3** 35 24 S 174 23 E
Wharanui, N.Z. **131 B9** 41 55 S 174 6 E
Wharekauri = Chatham Is., Pac. Oc. **130 a** 44 0 S 176 40W
Wharfe →, U.K. **20 D6** 53 51N 1 9W
Wharfedale, U.K. **20 C5** 54 6N 2 1W
Wharton, N.J., U.S.A. **151 F10** 40 54N 74 35W
Wharton, Pa., U.S.A. **150 E6** 41 31N 78 1W
Wharton, Tex., U.S.A. **155 L6** 29 19N 96 6W
Wharton Basin, Ind. Oc. **134 J3** 22 0 S 92 0 E
Whataroa, N.Z. **131 D5** 43 18 S 170 24 E
Whataroa →, N.Z. **131 D5** 43 7 S 170 16 E
Whatcom = Bellingham, U.S.A. **160 B4** 48 46N 122 29W
Wheatfield, U.S.A. **157 C9** 41 13N 87 4W
Wheatland, Calif., U.S.A. **160 F5** 39 1N 121 25W
Wheatland, Ind., U.S.A. **157 F9** 38 40N 87 19W
Wheatland, Wyo., U.S.A. **154 D2** 42 3N 104 58W
Wheatley, Canada **150 D2** 42 6N 82 27W
Wheaton, Ill., U.S.A. **157 C8** 41 52N 88 6W
Wheaton, Md., U.S.A. **148 F7** 39 3N 77 3W
Wheaton, Minn., U.S.A. **154 C6** 45 48N 96 30W
Wheelbarrow Pk., U.S.A. **160 H10** 37 26N 116 5W
Wheeler, Oreg., U.S.A. **158 D2** 45 41N 123 53W
Wheeler, Tex., U.S.A. **155 H4** 35 27N 100 16W
Wheeler →, Canada **141 A6** 57 2N 67 13W
Wheeler L., U.S.A. **149 H2** 34 48N 87 23W
Wheeler Pk., N. Mex., U.S.A. **159 H11** 36 34N 105 25W
Wheeler Pk., Nev., U.S.A. **159 G6** 38 57N 114 15W
Wheeler Ridge, U.S.A. **161 L8** 35 0N 118 57W
Wheelersburg, U.S.A. **148 F4** 38 44N 82 51W
Wheeling, U.S.A. **150 F4** 40 4N 80 43W
Whernside, U.K. **20 C5** 54 14N 2 24W
Whirlwind Reef, Papua N. G. **132 C5** 4 42 S 148 16 E
Whiskey Jack L., Canada **143 B8** 58 23N 101 55W
Whiskeytown-Shasta-Trinity ⌂, U.S.A. **158 F2** 40 45N 122 15W
Whistleduck Cr. →, Australia **126 C2** 20 15 S 135 18 E
Whistler, Canada **142 C4** 50 7N 122 58W
Whitby, Canada **150 C6** 43 52N 78 56W
Whitby, U.K. **20 C7** 54 29N 0 37W
Whitcombe Pass, N.Z. **131 D5** 43 13 S 170 55 E
White →, Ark., U.S.A. **155 J9** 33 57N 91 5W
White →, Ind., U.S.A. **157 F9** 38 25N 87 45W
White →, S. Dak., U.S.A. **154 D5** 43 42N 99 27W
White →, Tex., U.S.A. **155 J4** 33 14N 100 56W
White →, Utah, U.S.A. **158 F9** 40 4N 109 41W
White →, Vt., U.S.A. **151 C12** 43 37N 72 20W
White →, Wash., U.S.A. **160 C4** 47 12N 122 15W
White, East Fork →, U.S.A. **157 F9** 38 33N 87 14W
White, L., Australia **124 D4** 21 9 S 128 56 E
White B., Canada **141 C8** 50 0N 56 35W
White Bird, U.S.A. **158 D5** 45 46N 116 18W
White Butte, U.S.A. **154 B3** 46 23N 103 18W
White City, Fla., U.S.A. **152 F4** 29 53N 85 13W
White City, Oreg., U.S.A. **158 E2** 42 26N 122 51W
White Cliffs, Australia **128 A5** 30 50 S 143 10 E
White Hall, U.S.A. **156 E6** 39 26N 90 24W
White Haven, U.S.A. **151 E9** 41 4N 75 47W
White Horse, Vale of, U.K. **21 F6** 51 37N 1 30W
White I., N.Z. **130 D6** 37 30 S 177 13 E
White L., Canada **151 A8** 45 18N 76 31W
White L., U.S.A. **155 L8** 29 44N 92 30W
White Mountain, U.S.A. **144 D7** 64 41N 163 24W
White Mountain Peak, U.S.A. **159 G4** 37 38N 118 15W
White Mts., Alaska, U.S.A. **144 D11** 65 30N 146 30W
White Mts., Calif., U.S.A. **160 H8** 37 30N 118 15W
White Mts., N.H., U.S.A. **151 B13** 44 15N 71 15W
White Mts. △, Australia **126 C4** 20 43 S 145 12 E
White Nile = Nîl el Abyad →, Sudan **107 D3** 15 38N 32 31 E
White Nile Dam = Khazzān Jabal al Awliyā, Sudan **107 D3** 15 24N 32 20 E
White Oak, U.S.A. **152 D8** 31 2N 81 43W
White Otter L., Canada **140 C1** 49 5N 91 55W
White Pass, U.S.A. **160 D5** 46 38N 121 24W
White Pigeon, U.S.A. **157 C11** 41 48N 85 39W
White Plains, Ga., U.S.A. **152 B6** 33 28N 83 1W
White Plains, N.Y., U.S.A. **151 E11** 41 2N 73 46W
White River, Canada **140 C2** 48 35N 85 20W
White River, S. Africa **117 D5** 25 20 S 31 0 E
White River, U.S.A. **154 D4** 43 34N 100 45W
White Rock, Canada **160 A4** 49 2N 122 48W
White Rock, U.S.A. **159 J10** 35 50N 106 12W
White Russia = Belarus ■, Europe **58 F4** 53 30N 27 0 E
White Sands ⌂, U.S.A. **159 K10** 32 46N 106 20W
White Sea = Beloye More, Russia **56 A6** 66 30N 38 0 E
White Springs, U.S.A. **152 E7** 30 20N 82 45W
White Sulphur Springs, Mont., U.S.A. **158 C8** 46 33N 110 54W
White Sulphur Springs, W. Va., U.S.A. **148 G5** 37 48N 80 18W
White Swan, U.S.A. **160 D6** 46 23N 120 44W
White Volta →, Ghana **113 D4** 9 10N 1 15W
Whitecliffs, N.Z. **131 D6** 43 26 S 171 55 E
Whitecourt, Canada **142 C5** 54 10N 115 45W
Whiteface Mt., U.S.A. **151 B11** 44 22N 73 54W
Whitefield, U.S.A. **151 B13** 44 23N 71 37W
Whitefish, U.S.A. **158 B6** 48 25N 114 20W
Whitefish Bay, U.S.A. **157 A9** 43 23N 87 54W
Whitefish L., Canada **143 A7** 62 41N 106 48W
Whitefish Point, U.S.A. **148 B3** 46 45N 84 59W
Whitegull, L. = Goélands, L. aux, Canada **141 A7** 55 27N 64 17W
Whitehall, Mich., U.S.A. **148 D2** 43 24N 86 21W
Whitehall, Mont., U.S.A. **158 D7** 45 52N 112 6W
Whitehall, N.Y., U.S.A. **151 C11** 43 33N 73 24W
Whitehall, Wis., U.S.A. **154 C9** 44 22N 91 19W
Whitehaven, U.K. **20 C4** 54 33N 3 35W
Whitehorse, Canada **142 A1** 60 43N 135 3W
Whiteman Ra., Papua N. G. **132 C5** 5 55 S 150 0 E
Whitemark, Australia **127 G4** 40 7 S 148 3 E
Whiteplains, Liberia **112 D2** 6 28N 10 40W
Whiteriver, U.S.A. **159 K9** 33 50N 109 58W
Whitesand →, Canada **142 A5** 60 9N 115 45W
Whitesands, S. Africa **116 E3** 34 23 S 20 50 E
Whitesboro, N.Y., U.S.A. **151 C9** 43 7N 75 18W
Whitesboro, Tex., U.S.A. **155 J6** 33 39N 96 54W
Whiteshell ⌂, Canada **143 D9** 50 0N 95 40W
Whiteside, Canal, Chile **176 D2** 53 55 S 70 15W
Whitesville, U.S.A. **150 D7** 42 2N 77 46W
Whiteville, U.S.A. **149 H6** 34 20N 78 42W
Whitewater, U.S.A. **157 B8** 42 50N 88 44W
Whitewater B., U.S.A. **153 K9** 25 15N 81 0W
Whitewater Baldy, U.S.A. **159 K9** 33 20N 108 39W
Whitewater L., Canada **140 B2** 50 50N 89 10W
Whitewood, Australia **126 C3** 21 28 S 143 30 E
Whitewood, Canada **143 C8** 50 20N 102 20W
Whitfield, Australia **129 D7** 36 42 S 146 24 E
Whithorn, U.K. **22 G4** 54 44N 4 26W
Whitianga, N.Z. **130 C4** 36 47 S 175 41 E
Whiting, U.S.A. **157 C9** 41 41N 87 29W
Whitman, U.S.A. **151 D14** 42 5N 70 56W
Whitmore Village, U.S.A. **145 J13** 21 31N 158 1W
Whitney, Canada **140 C4** 45 31N 78 14W
Whitney, Mt., U.S.A. **160 J8** 36 35N 118 18W
Whitney Point, U.S.A. **151 D9** 42 20N 75 58W
Whitstable, U.K. **21 F9** 51 21N 1 3 E
Whitsunday I., Australia **126 J7** 20 15 S 149 4 E
Whitsunday Islands △, Australia **126 J7** 20 15 S 149 0 E
Whitsunday Passage, Australia **126 J6** 20 16 S 148 51 E
Whittemore, U.S.A. **156 A2** 43 4N 94 26W
Whittier, Alaska, U.S.A. **144 F10** 60 47N 148 41W
Whittier, Calif., U.S.A. **161 M8** 33 58N 118 3W
Whittlesea, Australia **129 D6** 37 27 S 145 9 E
Wholdaia L., Canada **143 A8** 60 43N 104 20W
Whyalla, Australia **128 B2** 33 2 S 137 30 E
Wiang Kosai △, Thailand **86 D2** 17 54N 99 29 E
Wiarton, Canada **140 D3** 44 40N 81 10W
Wiawso, Ghana **112 D4** 6 10N 2 25W
Wiay, U.K. **22 D1** 57 24N 7 13W
Wiązów, Poland **55 H4** 50 50N 17 10 E
Wibaux, U.S.A. **154 B2** 46 59N 104 11W
Wichabai, Guyana **169 C6** 2 57N 59 35W
Wichian Buri, Thailand **86 E3** 15 39N 101 7 E
Wichita, U.S.A. **155 G6** 37 42N 97 20W
Wichita Falls, U.S.A. **155 J5** 33 54N 98 30W
Wick, U.K. **22 C5** 58 26N 3 5W
Wicked Pt., Canada **150 C7** 43 52N 77 15W
Wickenburg, U.S.A. **159 K7** 33 58N 112 44W
Wickepin, Australia **125 F2** 32 50 S 117 30 E
Wickham, Australia **124 D2** 20 42 S 117 11 E
Wickham, C., Australia **127 F3** 39 35 S 143 57 E
Wickliffe, U.S.A. **150 E3** 41 36N 81 28W
Wicklow, Ireland **23 D5** 52 59N 6 3W
Wicklow □, Ireland **23 D5** 52 57N 6 25W
Wicklow Hd., Ireland **23 D6** 52 58N 6 0W
Wicklow Mts., Ireland **23 C5** 52 58N 6 26W
Wicklow Mts. △, Ireland **23 C5** 53 6N 6 21W
Widawa, Poland **55 G5** 51 27N 18 51 E
Widawka →, Poland **55 G5** 51 27N 18 52 E
Wide B., Papua N. G. **132 C7** 5 5 S 152 5 E
Widgeegoara Cr. →, Australia **127 D4** 28 51 S 146 34 E
Widgiemooltha, Australia **125 F3** 31 30 S 121 34 E
Widi, Kepulauan, Indonesia **82 B3** 0 33 S 128 24 E
Widnau, Switz. **33 B9** 47 24N 9 38 E
Widnes, U.K. **20 D5** 53 23N 2 45W
Więcbork, Poland **55 E4** 53 21N 17 30 E
Wiehengebirge = Nördlicher Teutoburger Wald-Wiehengebirge ⌂, Germany **30 C4** 52 18N 8 10 E
Wiehl, Germany **30 E3** 50 56N 7 34 E
Wiek, Germany **30 A9** 54 37N 13 17 E
Wielbark, Poland **54 E7** 53 24N 20 55 E
Wieleń, Poland **55 F3** 52 53N 16 9 E
Wielichowo, Poland **55 F3** 52 7N 16 22 E
Wieliczka, Poland **55 J7** 50 0N 20 5 E
Wielkopolski △, Poland **55 F3** 52 18N 16 45 E
Wielkopolskie □, Poland **55 F4** 52 10N 17 30 E
Wieluń, Poland **55 G5** 51 15N 18 34 E
Wien, Austria **35 C9** 48 12N 16 22 E
Wien ✕ (VIA), Austria **35 C9** 48 7N 16 35 E
Wiener Neustadt, Austria **35 D9** 47 49N 16 16 E
Wieprz →, Poland **55 G8** 51 34N 21 49 E
Wieprza →, Poland **54 D3** 54 26N 16 25 E
Wieruszów, Poland **55 G5** 51 19N 18 9 E
Wiesbaden, Germany **31 E4** 50 4N 8 14 E
Wiesen, Switz. **33 C9** 46 42N 9 43 E
Wiesental, Germany **31 F4** 49 13N 8 31 E
Wiesloch, Germany **31 F4** 49 18N 8 41 E
Wiesmoor, Germany **30 B3** 53 24N 7 47 E
Wieżyca, Poland **54 D5** 54 14N 18 8 E
Wigan, U.K. **20 D5** 53 33N 2 38W
Wiggins, Colo., U.S.A. **154 E2** 40 14N 104 4W
Wiggins, Miss., U.S.A. **155 K10** 30 51N 89 8W
Wight, I. of □, U.K. **21 G6** 50 40N 1 20W
Wigierski △, Poland **54 D10** 54 23N 23 5 E
Wigry, Jezioro, Poland **54 D10** 54 2N 23 8 E
Wigston, U.K. **21 E6** 52 35N 1 6W
Wigton, U.K. **20 C4** 54 50N 3 10W
Wigtown, U.K. **22 G4** 54 53N 4 27W
Wigtown B., U.K. **22 G4** 54 46N 4 15W
Wil, Switz. **33 B8** 47 28N 9 3 E
Wilamowice, Poland **55 J6** 49 55N 19 9 E
Wilber, U.S.A. **154 E6** 40 29N 96 58W
Wilberforce, Canada **150 A6** 45 2N 78 13W
Wilberforce, C., Australia **126 A2** 11 54 S 136 35 E
Wilburton, U.S.A. **155 H7** 34 55N 95 19W
Wilcannia, Australia **128 A5** 31 30 S 143 26 E
Wilcox, U.S.A. **150 E6** 41 35N 78 41W
Wildbad, Germany **31 G4** 48 45N 8 32 E
Wildcat →, U.S.A. **157 D10** 40 28N 86 52W
Wildenschwert = Ústí nad Orlicí, Czech Rep. **35 B9** 49 58N 16 24 E
Wildeshausen, Germany **30 C4** 52 54N 8 27 E
Wildeshauser Geest ⌂, Germany **30 C4** 52 54N 8 30 E
Wildhorn, Switz. **32 D4** 46 22N 7 21 E
Wildon, Austria **34 E8** 46 52N 15 31 E
Wildrose, U.S.A. **161 J9** 36 14N 117 11W
Wildspitze, Austria **34 E3** 46 53N 10 53 E
Wildstrubel, Switz. **32 D5** 46 24N 7 32 E
Wildwood, U.S.A. **153 G7** 28 52N 82 2W
Wilga →, Poland **55 G8** 51 52N 21 18 E
Wilge →, S. Africa **117 D4** 27 3 S 28 20 E
Wilhelm, Mt., Papua N. G. **132 C3** 5 50 S 145 1 E
Wilhelm II Coast, Antarctica **7 C7** 68 0 S 90 0 E
Wilhelmina Geb., Suriname **169 C6** 3 50N 56 30W
Wilhelmina Top = Trikora, Puncak, Indonesia **83 B5** 4 15 S 138 45 E
Wilhelmsburg, Austria **34 C8** 48 6N 15 36 E
Wilhelmshaven, Germany **30 B4** 53 31N 8 7 E
Wilhelmstal, Namibia **116 C2** 21 58 S 16 21 E
Wilkes-Barre, U.S.A. **151 E9** 41 15N 75 53W
Wilkes Land, Antarctica **7 D9** 69 0 S 120 0 E
Wilkie, Canada **143 C7** 52 27N 108 42W
Wilkinsburg, U.S.A. **150 F5** 40 26N 79 53W
Wilkinson Lakes, Australia **125 E5** 29 40 S 132 39 E
Willacoochee, U.S.A. **152 D6** 31 20N 83 3W
Willandra △, Australia **129 B6** 33 12 S 145 0 E
Willandra Creek →, Australia **128 B6** 33 22 S 145 52 E
Willapa B., U.S.A. **158 C2** 46 40N 124 0W
Willapa Hills, U.S.A. **160 D3** 46 35N 123 25W
Willard, N.Y., U.S.A. **150 D8** 42 40N 76 50W

Willard, *Ohio, U.S.A.* . **150 E2** 41 3N 82 44W
Willaumez Pen.,
  Papua N. G. . . . . **132 C6** 5 15 S 150 2 E
Wilbriggie, *Australia* . . **129 C7** 34 28 S 146 2 E
Wilcox, *U.S.A.* **159 K9** 32 15N 109 50W
Willemstad, *Neth. Ant.* . **165 D6** 12 5N 69 0W
Willenberg = Wielbark,
  Poland . . . . **54 E7** 53 24N 20 55 E
Willet, *U.S.A.* **151 D9** 42 28N 75 55W
William →, *Canada* . . . **143 B7** 59 8N 109 19W
William, Mt., *Australia* . **128 D5** 37 17 S 142 35 E
William B. Hartsfield
  International,
  Atlanta ✈ (ATL),
  U.S.A. **152 B5** 33 38N 84 26W
William 'Bill' Dannelly
  Res., *U.S.A.* **149 J2** 32 10N 87 10W
William Creek,
  Australia . . . . **127 D2** 28 58 S 136 22 E
Williams, *Australia* . . . **125 F2** 33 2 S 116 52 E
Williams, *Ariz., U.S.A.* . **159 J7** 35 15N 112 11W
Williams, *Calif., U.S.A.* **160 F4** 39 9N 122 9W
Williams Harbour,
  Canada **141 B8** 52 33N 55 47W
Williams Lake, *Canada* . **142 C4** 52 10N 122 10W
Williamsburg, *Iowa,*
  U.S.A. **156 C4** 41 40N 92 1W
Williamsburg, *Ky.,*
  U.S.A. **149 G3** 36 44N 84 10W
Williamsburg, *Pa.,*
  U.S.A. **150 F6** 40 28N 78 12W
Williamsburg, *Va.,*
  U.S.A. **148 G7** 37 17N 76 44W
Williamsfield, *U.S.A.* . . **156 D6** 40 55N 90 1W
Williamson, *N.Y.,*
  U.S.A. **150 C7** 43 14N 77 11W
Williamson, *W. Va.,*
  U.S.A. **148 G4** 37 41N 82 17W
Williamsport, *Ind.,*
  U.S.A. **157 D9** 40 17N 87 17W
Williamsport, *Pa.,*
  U.S.A. **150 E7** 41 15N 77 0W
Williamston, *Mich.,*
  U.S.A. **157 B12** 42 41N 84 17W
Williamston, *N.C.,*
  U.S.A. **149 H7** 35 51N 77 4W
Williamstown, *Australia* **127 F3** 37 51 S 144 52 E
Williamstown, *Ky.,*
  U.S.A. **157 F12** 38 38N 84 34W
Williamstown, *Mass.,*
  U.S.A. **151 D11** 42 41N 73 12W
Williamstown, *N.Y.,*
  U.S.A. **151 C9** 43 26N 75 53W
Williamsville, *U.S.A.* . . **156 E7** 39 57N 89 33W
Willimantic, *U.S.A.* . . . **151 E12** 41 43N 72 13W
Willingboro, *U.S.A.* . . . **148 E8** 40 3N 74 54W
Willis Group, *Australia* **124 B4** 16 18 S 150 0 E
Willisau, *Switz.* . . . . . . **32 B6** 47 7N 8 0 E
Willisburg, *U.S.A.* **157 G11** 37 49N 85 8W
Williston, *S. Africa* . . . **116 E3** 31 20 S 20 53 E
Williston, *N. Dak.,*
  U.S.A. **154 A3** 48 9N 103 37W
Williston, *S.C., U.S.A.* . **152 B8** 33 24N 81 25W
Williston L., *Canada* . . **142 B4** 56 0N 124 0W
Willits, *U.S.A.* **158 G2** 39 25N 123 21W
Willmar, *U.S.A.* **154 C7** 45 7N 95 3W
Willmore
  Wilderness △,
  Canada **142 C5** 53 45N 119 30W
Willoughby, *U.S.A.* . . . **150 E3** 41 39N 81 24W
Willow, *U.S.A.* **146 C5** 61 45N 150 3W
Willow Bunch, *Canada* . **143 D7** 49 20N 105 35W
Willow L., *Canada* **142 A5** 62 10N 119 8W
Willow Tree, *Australia* . **129 A9** 31 40 S 150 45 E
Willow Wall, The,
  China . . . . **75 C12** 42 10N 122 0 E
Willowick, *U.S.A.* **150 E3** 41 38N 81 28W
Willowlake →, *Canada* . **142 A4** 62 42N 123 8W
Willowmore, *S. Africa* . **117 E4** 33 15 S 23 30 E
Willows, *U.S.A.* **160 F4** 39 31N 122 12W
Willowvale = Gatyana,
  S. Africa . . . . **117 E4** 32 16 S 28 31 E
Wills, L., *Australia* . . . **124 D4** 21 25 S 128 51 E
Wills Cr. →, *Australia* . **126 C3** 22 43 S 140 2 E
Willsboro, *U.S.A.* **151 B11** 44 21N 73 24W
Willunga, *Australia* . . . **128 C3** 35 15 S 138 30 E
Wilma, *U.S.A.* **152 E5** 30 9N 84 58W
Wilmette, *U.S.A.* **157 B9** 42 5N 87 42W
Wilmington, *Australia* . **128 B3** 32 39 S 138 7 E
Wilmington, *Del.,*
  U.S.A. **148 F8** 39 45N 75 33W
Wilmington, *Ill., U.S.A.* **157 C8** 41 18N 88 9W
Wilmington, *N.C.,*
  U.S.A. **149 H7** 34 14N 77 55W
Wilmington, *Ohio,*
  U.S.A. **157 E13** 39 27N 83 50W
Wilmington, *Vt., U.S.A.* **151 D12** 42 52N 72 52W
Wilmslow, *U.K.* **20 D5** 53 19N 2 13W
Wilna = Vilnius,
  Lithuania . . . . **15 J21** 54 38N 25 19 E
Wilpattu △, *Sri Lanka* . **95 K4** 8 20N 79 50 E
Wilpena, *Australia* . . . . **128 A3** 31 5 S 138 1 E
Wilpena Cr. →,
  Australia . . . . **128 A3** 31 25 S 139 29 E
Wilsall, *U.S.A.* **158 D8** 45 59N 110 38W
Wilson, *N.C., U.S.A.* . . **149 H7** 35 44N 77 55W
Wilson, *N.Y., U.S.A.* . . **150 C6** 43 19N 78 50W
Wilson, *Pa., U.S.A.* . . . **151 F9** 40 41N 75 15W
Wilson →, *Australia* . . **124 C4** 16 48 S 128 16 E
Wilson Bluff, *Australia* . **125 F4** 31 41 S 129 0 E
Wilson Inlet, *Australia* . **125 G2** 35 0 S 117 22 E
Wilson Str., *Solomon Is.* **133 M9** 8 0 S 156 39 E
Wilsons Promontory,
  Australia . . . . **129 E7** 38 55 S 146 25 E
Wilsons Promontory △,
  Australia . . . . **129 D7** 37 59 S 146 23 E
Wilster, *Germany* . . . . . **30 B5** 53 55N 9 23 E
Wilton, *Iowa, U.S.A.* . . **156 C5** 41 34N 91 4W
Wilton, *N. Dak., U.S.A.* **154 B4** 47 10N 100 47W
Wilton →, *Australia* . . **126 A1** 14 45 S 134 33 E
Wiltshire □, *U.K.* **21 F6** 51 18N 1 53W
Wiltz, *Lux.* . . . . **24 E5** 49 57N 5 55 E
Wiluna, *Australia* . . . . . **125 E3** 26 36 S 120 14 E
Wimborne Minster,
  U.K. **21 G6** 50 48N 1 59W
Wimereux, *France* . . . . **27 B8** 50 45N 1 37 E
Wimmera →, *Australia* **128 D4** 36 8 S 141 56 E
Winam G., *Kenya* . . . . . **118 C3** 0 20 S 34 15 E
Winamac, *U.S.A.* **157 C10** 41 3N 86 36W
Winburg, *S. Africa* . . . . **116 D4** 28 30 S 27 2 E
Winchelsea, *Australia* . . **128 E6** 38 10 S 144 1 E
Winchendon, *U.S.A.* . . . **151 D12** 42 41N 72 3W
Winchester, *N.Z.* . . . . . **131 E6** 44 11 S 171 17 E
Winchester, *U.K.* **21 F6** 51 4N 1 18W
Winchester, *Conn.,*
  U.S.A. **151 E11** 41 53N 73 9W
Winchester, *Idaho,*
  U.S.A. **158 C5** 46 14N 116 38W
Winchester, *Ill., U.S.A.* **156 E6** 39 38N 90 27W
Winchester, *Ind.,*
  U.S.A. **157 D12** 40 10N 84 59W
Winchester, *Ky., U.S.A.* **157 G12** 38 0N 84 11W
Winchester, *N.H.,*
  U.S.A. **151 D12** 42 46N 72 23W

Winchester, *Nev.,*
  U.S.A. **161 J11** 36 6N 115 10W
Winchester, *Ohio,*
  U.S.A. **157 F13** 38 57N 83 40W
Winchester, *Tenn.,*
  U.S.A. **149 H2** 35 11N 86 7W
Winchester, *Va., U.S.A.* **148 F6** 39 11N 78 10W
Wind →, *U.S.A.* **158 E9** 43 12N 108 12W
Wind Cave △, *U.S.A.* . . **154 D3** 43 32N 103 17W
Wind Point, *U.S.A.* **157 B9** 42 47N 87 46W
Wind River Range,
  U.S.A. **158 E9** 43 0N 109 30W
Windamere, L.,
  Australia . . . . **129 B8** 32 42 S 149 44 E
Windau = Ventspils,
  Latvia . . . . **15 H19** 57 25N 21 32 E
Windber, *U.S.A.* **150 F6** 40 14N 78 50W
Winder, *U.S.A.* **152 A6** 34 0N 83 45W
Windermere, *U.K.* **20 C5** 54 23N 2 55W
Windermere, *U.S.A.* . . . **153 G8** 28 29N 81 32W
Windfall, *U.S.A.* **157 D11** 40 22N 85 57W
Windhoek, *Namibia* . . . **116 C2** 22 35 S 17 4 E
Windischbad, *Switz.* . . . **32 B6** 47 28N 8 14 E
Windisch-Feistritz =
  Slovenska Bistrica,
  Slovenia . . . . **45 B12** 46 24N 15 35 E
Windischgarsten,
  Austria . . . . **34 D7** 47 42N 14 21 E
Windischgratz =
  Slovenj Gradec,
  Slovenia . . . . **45 B12** 46 31N 15 5 E
Windom, *U.S.A.* **154 D7** 43 52N 95 7W
Windorah, *Australia* . . . **126 D3** 25 24 S 142 36 E
Window Rock, *U.S.A.* . . **159 J9** 35 41N 109 3W
Windrush →, *U.K.* **21 F6** 51 43N 1 24W
Windsor, *Australia* . . . . **129 B9** 33 37 S 150 50 E
Windsor, *N.S., Canada* . **141 D7** 44 59N 64 5W
Windsor, *Ont., Canada* . **140 D3** 42 18N 83 0W
Windsor, *N.Z.* . . . . **131 E5** 44 59 S 170 49 E
Windsor, *U.K.* **21 F7** 51 29N 0 36W
Windsor, *Calif., U.S.A.* . **158 G2** 38 33N 122 49W
Windsor, *Colo., U.S.A.* . **154 E2** 40 29N 104 54W
Windsor, *Conn., U.S.A.* **151 E12** 41 50N 72 39W
Windsor, *Ill., U.S.A.* . . . **156 F9** 39 26N 88 36W
Windsor, *Mo., U.S.A.* . . **156 F3** 38 32N 93 31W
Windsor, *N.Y., U.S.A.* . **151 D9** 42 5N 75 37W
Windsor, *Vt., U.S.A.* . . . **151 C12** 43 29N 72 24W
Windsor &
  Maidenhead □, *U.K.* . **21 F7** 51 29N 0 40W
Windsorton, *S. Africa* . . **116 D3** 28 16 S 24 44 E
Windward Is., *W. Indies* **165 D7** 13 0N 61 0W
Windward Passage =
  Vientos, Paso de los,
  Caribbean **165 C5** 20 0N 74 0W
Winefred L., *Canada* . . **143 B6** 55 30N 110 30W
Winejok, *Sudan* . . . . . . **107 F2** 9 1N 27 30 E
Winfield, *Iowa, U.S.A.* . **156 C5** 41 7N 91 26W
Winfield, *Kans., U.S.A.* . **155 G6** 37 15N 96 59W
Winfield, *Mo., U.S.A.* . . **156 F6** 39 0N 90 44W
Wingate Mts., *Australia* **124 B5** 14 25 S 130 40 E
Wingham, *Australia* . . . **129 A10** 31 48 S 152 22 E
Wingham, *Canada* **140 D3** 43 55N 81 20W
Winisk →, *Canada* **140 A2** 55 20N 85 15W
Winisk L., *Canada* **140 A2** 55 17N 85 5W
Winisk L., *Canada* **140 B2** 52 55N 87 22W
Wink, *U.S.A.* **155 K3** 31 45N 103 9W
Winkler, *Canada* **143 D9** 49 10N 97 56W
Winklern, *Austria* . . . . . **34 E5** 46 52N 12 52 E
Winlock, *U.S.A.* **160 D4** 46 30N 122 56W
Winneba, *Ghana* **113 D4** 5 25N 0 36W
Winnebago, L., *U.S.A.* . **156 D1** 44 0N 88 26W
Winnecke Cr. →,
  Australia . . . . **124 C5** 18 35 S 131 34 E
Winnemucca, *U.S.A.* . . . **158 F5** 40 58N 117 44W
Winnemucca L., *U.S.A.* **158 F4** 40 7N 119 21W
Winner, *U.S.A.* **154 D5** 43 22N 99 52W
Winnett, *U.S.A.* **158 C9** 47 0N 108 21W
Winnfield, *U.S.A.* **155 K8** 31 56N 92 38W
Winnibigoshish, L.,
  U.S.A. **154 B7** 47 27N 94 13W
Winnipeg, *Canada* **143 D9** 49 54N 97 9W
Winnipeg →, *Canada* . . **143 C9** 50 38N 96 19W
Winnipeg, L., *Canada* . . **143 C9** 52 0N 97 0W
Winnipeg Beach,
  Canada **143 C9** 50 30N 96 58W
Winnipegosis, *Canada* . **143 C9** 51 39N 99 55W
Winnipegosis L.,
  Canada **143 C9** 52 30N 100 0W
Winnipesaukee, L.,
  U.S.A. **151 C13** 43 38N 71 21W
Winnisquam L., *U.S.A.* **151 C13** 43 33N 71 31W
Winnsboro, *La., U.S.A.* . **155 J9** 32 10N 91 43W
Winnsboro, *S.C., U.S.A.* **149 H5** 34 23N 81 5W
Winnsboro, *Tex.,*
  U.S.A. **155 J7** 32 58N 95 17W
Winokapau, L., *Canada* **141 B7** 53 15N 62 50W
Winona, *Minn., U.S.A.* . **154 C9** 44 3N 91 39W
Winona, *Miss., U.S.A.* . **155 J10** 33 29N 89 44W
Winooski, *U.S.A.* **151 B11** 44 29N 73 11W
Winooski →, *U.S.A.* . . . **151 B11** 44 32N 73 17W
Winschoten, *Neths.* . . . . **24 A7** 53 9N 7 3 E
Winsen, *Germany* . . . . . **30 B6** 53 22N 10 13 E
Winsford, *U.K.* **20 D5** 53 12N 2 31W
Winslow, *Ariz., U.S.A.* . **159 J8** 35 2N 110 42W
Winslow, *Ind., U.S.A.* . . **157 F9** 38 23N 87 13W
Winslow, *Wash., U.S.A.* **160 C4** 47 38N 122 31W
Winsted, *U.S.A.* **151 E11** 41 55N 73 4W
Winston-Salem, *U.S.A.* . **149 G5** 36 6N 80 15W
Winter Garden, *U.S.A.* . **153 G8** 28 34N 81 35W
Winter Haven, *U.S.A.* . . **153 G8** 28 1N 81 44W
Winter Park, *U.S.A.* . . . **153 G8** 28 36N 81 20W
Winterberg, *Germany* . . **30 D4** 51 11N 8 33 E
Winterhaven, *U.S.A.* . . . **161 N12** 32 47N 114 39W
Winters, *U.S.A.* **160 G5** 38 32N 121 58W
Winterset, *U.S.A.* **156 C3** 41 20N 94 1W
Wintersville, *U.S.A.* . . . **150 F4** 40 23N 80 42W
Winterswijk, *Neths.* . . . **24 C6** 51 58N 6 43 E
Winterthur, *Switz.* . . . . **33 B7** 47 30N 8 44 E
Winthrop, *U.S.A.* **158 B3** 48 28N 120 10W
Winton, *Australia* . . . . . **126 C3** 22 24 S 143 3 E
Winton, *N.Z.* . . . . **131 G3** 46 8 S 168 20 E
Wintua, *Vanuatu* . . . . . **133 F5** 16 30 S 167 26 E
Wipper →, *Germany* . . . **30 D7** 51 16N 11 12 E
Wirraminna, *Australia* . **128 A2** 31 12 S 136 13 E
Wirrulla, *Australia* . . . . **127 E1** 32 24 S 134 31 E
Wisbech, *U.K.* . . . . **21 E8** 52 41N 0 9 E
Wisconsin □, *U.S.A.* . . **154 C10** 44 45N 89 30W
Wisconsin →, *U.S.A.* . . **156 A5** 43 0N 91 15W
Wisconsin Rapids,
  U.S.A. **154 C10** 44 23N 89 49W
Wisdom, *U.S.A.* **158 D7** 45 37N 113 27W
Wiseman, *U.S.A.* **146 B4** 67 25N 150 6W
Wishaw, *U.K.* **22 F5** 55 46N 3 54W
Wishek, *U.S.A.* **154 B5** 46 16N 99 33W
Wisła, *Poland* . . . . **55 J5** 49 38N 18 53 E
Wisła →, *Poland* . . . . . **54 E5** 54 22N 18 55 E
Wisłok →, *Poland* . . . . **55 H9** 50 13N 22 32 E
Wisłoka →, *Poland* . . . **55 H8** 50 27N 21 23 E
Wismar, *Germany* . . . . **30 B7** 53 54N 11 29 E
Wismar, *Guyana* **169 B6** 5 59N 58 18W
Wisner, *U.S.A.* **154 E6** 41 59N 96 55W
Wissant, *France* . . . . . . **27 B8** 50 52N 1 40 E
Wissembourg, *France* . . **27 C14** 49 2N 7 57 E
Wisznice, *Poland* . . . . . **55 G10** 51 48N 23 13 E

Witbank, *S. Africa* . . . . **117 D4** 25 51 S 29 14 E
Witdraai, *S. Africa* . . . . **116 D3** 26 58 S 20 48 E
Witham →, *U.K.* . . . . . . **21 F8** 51 48N 0 40 E
Witham, *U.K.* **20 E7** 51 59N 0 2W
Withernsea, *U.K.* . . . . . **20 D8** 53 44N 0 1 E
Withlacoochee →, *Fla.,*
  U.S.A. **152 E6** 30 24N 83 10W
Withlacoochee →, *Fla.,*
  U.S.A. **153 G7** 29 0N 82 45W
Witjira △, *Australia* . . . **127 D2** 26 22 S 135 37 E
Witkowo, *Poland* . . . . . **55 F4** 52 26N 17 45 E
Witney, *U.K.* **21 F6** 51 48N 1 28W
Witnossob →, *Namibia* **116 D3** 23 55 S 18 45 E
Witten, *Germany* . . . . . **30 D3** 51 26N 7 20 E
Wittenberge, *Germany* . **30 B7** 53 0N 11 45 E
Wittenburg, *Germany* . . **30 B7** 53 31N 11 4 E
Wittenheim, *France* . . . **27 E14** 47 44N 7 20 E
Wittenoom, *Australia* . . **124 D2** 22 15 S 118 20 E
Witti, Banjaran,
  Malaysia . . . . **85 A5** 5 11N 116 29 E
Wittingau = Třeboň,
  Czech Rep. . . . . **34 B7** 49 1N 14 48 E
Wittingen, *Germany* . . . **30 C6** 52 44N 10 44 E
Wittlich, *Germany* . . . . **31 F2** 49 59N 6 53 E
Wittmund, *Germany* . . . **30 B3** 53 34N 7 46 E
Wittow, *Germany* . . . . . **30 A9** 54 38N 13 21 E
Wittstock, *Germany* . . . **30 B8** 53 10N 12 28 E
Witu Is., *Papua N. G.* . . **132 C5** 4 50 S 149 25 E
Witvlei, *Namibia* . . . . . **116 C2** 22 23 S 18 32 E
Witzenhausen,
  Germany . . . . **30 D5** 51 20N 9 51 E
Wixom, *U.S.A.* **157 B13** 42 32N 83 32W
Wkra →, *Poland* . . . . . **55 F7** 52 27N 20 44 E
Władysławowo, *Poland* **54 D5** 54 48N 18 25 E
Wleń, *Poland* . . . . **55 G2** 51 2N 15 39 E
Wlingi, *Indonesia* . . . . . **85 D4** 8 5 S 112 25 E
Włocławek, *Poland* . . . . **55 F6** 52 40N 19 3 E
Włodawa, *Poland* . . . . . **55 G8** 51 33N 23 31 E
Włoszczowa, *Poland* . . . **55 H6** 50 50N 19 55 E
Woburn, *U.S.A.* **151 D13** 42 29N 71 9W
Wodian, *China* . . . . **74 H7** 32 50N 112 35 E
Wodonga = Albury-
  Wodonga, *Australia* . . **129 D7** 36 3 S 146 56 E
Wodonga, *Australia* . . . **129 D7** 36 5 S 146 50 E
Wodzisław Śląski,
  Poland . . . . **55 H5** 50 1N 18 26 E
Wœrth, *France* . . . . **27 D14** 48 57N 7 45 E
Wohlau =
  Wołów, *Poland* . . . . . **55 G3** 51 20N 16 38 E
Wohlen, *Switz.* . . . . **32 B6** 47 21N 8 17 E
Woinbogoin, *China* . . . . **76 A2** 32 51N 98 39 E
Woinui, Selat,
  Indonesia . . . . **83 B4** 1 10 S 134 36 E
Woippy, *France* . . . . **27 C13** 49 10N 6 8 E
Woitape, *Papua N. G.* . . **132 E4** 8 33 S 147 15 E
Wojcieszów, *Poland* . . . **55 H2** 50 58N 15 55 E
Wokam, *Indonesia* . . . . **83 C4** 5 45 S 134 28 E
Wokha, *India* . . . . **90 B5** 26 6N 94 16 E
Woking, *U.K.* **21 F7** 51 19N 0 34W
Wokingham, *U.K.* **21 F7** 51 24N 0 49W
Wokingham □, *U.K.* . . . **21 F7** 51 25N 0 51W
Woko △, *Australia* . . . . **129 A9** 31 46 S 151 49 E
Wolbrom, *Poland* . . . . . **55 H6** 50 24N 19 45 E
Wolcottville, *U.S.A.* . . . **157 C11** 41 32N 85 22W
Wołczyn, *Poland* . . . . . . **55 G5** 51 1N 18 3 E
Woldegk, *Germany* . . . . **30 B9** 53 27N 13 34 E
Woldenberg =
  Dobiegniew, *Poland* . . **55 F2** 52 59N 15 45 E
Wolf →, *Canada* **142 A2** 60 17N 132 33W
Wolf Creek, *U.S.A.* **158 C7** 47 0N 112 4W
Wolf L., *Canada* **142 A2** 60 24N 131 40W
Wolf Point, *U.S.A.* **154 A2** 48 5N 105 39W
Wolfe I., *Canada* **140 D4** 44 7N 76 20W
Wolfeboro, *U.S.A.* **151 C13** 43 35N 71 13W
Wolfen, *Germany* . . . . . **30 D8** 51 39N 12 15 E
Wolfenbüttel, *Germany* . **30 C6** 52 10N 10 33 E
Wolfratshausen,
  Germany . . . . **31 H7** 47 54N 11 24 E
Wolfsberg, *Austria* . . . . **34 E7** 46 50N 14 52 E
Wolfsburg, *Germany* . . . **30 C6** 52 25N 10 48 E
Wolfurt, *Austria* . . . . . . **33 B9** 47 28N 9 45 E
Wolgast, *Germany* . . . . **30 A9** 54 3N 13 44 E
Wolhusen, *Switz.* . . . . . **32 B6** 47 4N 8 4 E
Wolin, *Poland* . . . . **54 B1** 53 50N 14 37 E
Woliński △, *Poland* . . . . **54 B1** 53 57N 14 28 E
Wollaston, Is., *Chile* . . . **176 E3** 55 40 S 67 30W
Wollaston Forland,
  Greenland **10 C9** 74 25N 19 40W
Wollaston L., *Canada* . . **143 B8** 58 7N 103 10W
Wollaston Lake,
  Canada **143 B8** 58 3N 103 33W
Wollaston Pen., *Canada* **138 B8** 69 30N 115 0W
Wollemi △, *Australia* . . **129 B9** 33 0 S 150 36 E
Wollongong, *Australia* . **129 C9** 34 25 S 150 54 E
Wolmar = Valmiera,
  Latvia . . . . **15 H21** 57 37N 25 29 E
Wolmaransstad,
  S. Africa . . . . **116 D4** 27 12 S 25 59 E
Wolmirstedt, *Germany* . **30 C7** 52 14N 11 37 E
Wolomin, *Poland* . . . . . **55 F8** 52 19N 21 15 E
Wołów, *Poland* . . . . **55 G3** 51 20N 16 38 E
Wolseley, *Australia* . . . **128 D4** 36 23 S 140 54 E
Wolseley, *S. Africa* . . . . **116 E2** 33 26 S 19 7 E
Wolsey, *U.S.A.* **154 C5** 44 24N 98 28W
Wolstenholme, C.,
  Canada **136 C12** 62 35N 77 30W
Wolsztyn, *Poland* . . . . . **55 F3** 52 8N 16 5 E
Wolvega, *Neths.* . . . . . . **24 B6** 52 52N 6 0 E
Wolverhampton, *U.K.* . **21 E5** 52 35N 2 7W
Wondai, *Australia* . . . . . **126 D5** 26 20 S 151 49 E
Wonenara, *Papua N. G.* **132 D3** 6 48 S 145 53 E
Wonga Wongué △,
  Gabon . . . . **114 C1** 0 29 S 9 25 E
Wongalarroo L.,
  Australia . . . . **128 A6** 31 32 S 144 0 E
Wongan Hills, *Australia* **125 F2** 30 51 S 116 37 E
Wŏnju, *S. Korea* . . . . . . **75 F14** 37 22N 127 58 E
Wonosari, *Indonesia* . . . **85 D4** 7 58 S 110 36 E
Wonosobo, *Indonesia* . . **85 D3** 7 22 S 109 54 E
Wonowon, *Canada* **142 B4** 56 44N 121 48W
Wŏnsan, *N. Korea* . . . . **75 E14** 39 11N 127 27 E
Wonthaggi, *Australia* . . **129 E6** 38 37 S 145 37 E
Wood Buffalo △,
  Canada **142 B6** 59 0N 113 41W
Wood Is., *Australia* . . . . **124 C3** 16 24 S 123 19 E
Wood L., *Canada* **143 B8** 55 17N 103 17W
Wood River, *U.S.A.* . . . **156 F6** 38 52N 90 5W
Woodah, I., *Australia* . . **126 A2** 13 27 S 136 10 E
Woodbine, *U.S.A.* **153 F5** 30 58N 81 44W
Woodbourne, *U.S.A.* . . . **151 E10** 41 46N 74 36W
Woodbridge, *Canada* . . **150 C5** 43 47N 79 36W
Woodbridge, *U.K.* . . . . . **21 E9** 52 6N 1 20 E
Woodburn, *U.S.A.* **160 D2** 45 9N 122 51W
Woodbury, *U.S.A.* **152 C5** 32 59N 84 35W
Woodenbong, *Australia* . **127 D5** 28 24 S 152 39 E
Woodford, *Australia* . . . **127 D5** 26 58 S 152 47 E
Woodfords, *U.S.A.* **160 G7** 38 47N 119 50W
Woodlake, *U.S.A.* **160 J7** 36 25N 119 6W
Woodland, *Calif.,*
  U.S.A. **160 G5** 38 41N 121 46W

Woodland, *Maine,*
  U.S.A. **149 C12** 45 9N 67 25W
Woodland, *Pa., U.S.A.* . **150 F6** 40 59N 78 21W
Woodland, *Wash.,*
  U.S.A. **160 E4** 45 54N 122 45W
Woodland Caribou △,
  Canada **143 C10** 51 0N 94 45W
Woodlands, *Singapore* . **87 d** 1 27N 103 47 E
Woodlark I.,
  Papua N. G. . . . . **132 E7** 9 10 S 152 50 E
Woodridge, *Canada* . . . **143 D9** 49 20N 96 9W
Woodroffe, Mt.,
  Australia . . . . **125 E5** 26 20 S 131 45 E
Woods, L., *Australia* . . . **126 B1** 17 50 S 133 30 E
Woods, L. of the,
  Canada **143 D10** 49 15N 94 45W
Woodside, *S. Austral.,*
  Australia . . . . **128 C3** 34 58 S 138 52 E
Woodside, *Vic.,*
  Australia . . . . **129 E7** 38 31 S 146 52 E
Woodson, *U.S.A.* **156 E6** 39 37N 90 14W
Woodstock, *N.S.W.,*
  Australia . . . . **129 B8** 33 45 S 148 53 E
Woodstock, *Queens.,*
  Australia . . . . **126 B4** 19 35 S 146 50 E
Woodstock, *N.B.,*
  Canada **141 C6** 46 11N 67 37W
Woodstock, *Ont.,*
  Canada **140 D3** 43 10N 80 45W
Woodstock, *U.K.* **21 F6** 51 51N 1 20W
Woodstock, *Ga., U.S.A.* **152 B4** 34 6N 84 31W
Woodstock, *Ill., U.S.A.* **154 D10** 42 19N 88 27W
Woodstock, *Vt., U.S.A.* **151 C12** 43 37N 72 31W
Woodsville, *U.S.A.* **151 B13** 44 9N 72 2W
Woodville, *N.Z.* . . . . . . **130 G4** 40 20 S 175 53 E
Woodville, *Fla., U.S.A.* . **152 E5** 30 19N 84 15W
Woodville, *Ga., U.S.A.* . **152 B3** 33 40N 83 7W
Woodville, *Miss.,*
  U.S.A. **155 K9** 31 6N 91 18W
Woodville, *Ohio,*
  U.S.A. **157 C13** 41 27N 83 22W
Woodville, *Tex., U.S.A.* **155 K7** 30 47N 94 25W
Woodward, *U.S.A.* **155 G5** 36 26N 99 24W
Woody, *U.S.A.* **161 K8** 35 42N 118 50W
Woody →, *Canada* **143 C8** 52 31N 100 51W
Woolamai, C., *Australia* **129 E6** 38 30 S 145 23 E
Woolbrook, *Australia* . . **129 A9** 30 56 S 151 25 E
Woomera, *Australia* . . . **128 A2** 31 5 S 136 50 E
Woonsocket, *R.I.,*
  U.S.A. **151 E13** 42 0N 71 31W
Woonsocket, *S. Dak.,*
  U.S.A. **154 C5** 44 3N 98 17W
Wooramel →, *Australia* **125 E1** 25 47 S 114 10 E
Wooramel Roadhouse,
  Australia . . . . **125 E1** 25 45 S 114 17 E
Wooster, *U.S.A.* **150 F3** 40 48N 81 56W
Worb, *Switz.* . . . . **32 C5** 46 56N 7 33 E
Worcester, *S. Africa* . . . **116 E2** 33 39 S 19 27 E
Worcester, *U.K.* **21 E5** 52 11N 2 12W
Worcester, *Mass.,*
  U.S.A. **151 D13** 42 16N 71 48W
Worcester, *N.Y., U.S.A.* **151 D10** 42 36N 74 45W
Worcestershire □, *U.K.* **21 E5** 52 13N 2 10W
Wörgl, *Austria* . . . . **34 D5** 47 29N 12 3 E
Workai, *Indonesia* . . . . . **83 C4** 6 40 S 134 40 E
Workington, *U.K.* **20 C4** 54 39N 3 33W
Worksop, *U.K.* **20 D6** 53 18N 1 7W
Workum, *Neths.* . . . . . . **24 B5** 52 59N 5 26 E
Worland, *U.S.A.* **158 D10** 44 1N 107 57W
Wormhout, *France* . . . . **27 B9** 50 52N 2 28 E
Worms, *Germany* . . . . . **31 F4** 49 37N 8 21 E
Worsley, *Australia* **142 B5** 56 31N 119 8W
Wörth, *Germany* . . . . . . **31 F8** 49 1N 12 24 E
Wortham, *U.S.A.* **155 K6** 31 47N 96 28W
Wörther See, *Austria* . . **34 E7** 46 37N 14 10 E
Worthing, *Barbados* . . . **165 g** 13 5N 59 35W
Worthing, *U.K.* **21 G7** 50 49N 0 21W
Worthington, *Ind.,*
  U.S.A. **157 E10** 39 7N 86 59W
Worthington, *Minn.,*
  U.S.A. **154 D7** 43 37N 95 36W
Worthington, *Ohio,*
  U.S.A. **157 D13** 40 5N 83 1W
Worthington, *Pa.,*
  U.S.A. **150 F5** 40 50N 79 38W
Wosi, *Indonesia* . . . . . . **82 B3** 0 15 S 128 0 E
Wosimi, *Indonesia* . . . . **83 B4** 2 54 S 134 31 E
Wotu, *Indonesia* . . . . . . **82 B2** 2 35 S 120 48 E
Wou-han = Wuhan,
  China . . . . **77 B10** 30 31N 114 18 E
Wour, *Chad* . . . . **109 D3** 21 14N 16 0 E
Wousi = Wuxi, *China* . . **77 B13** 31 33N 120 18 E
Wowoni, *Indonesia* . . . . **82 B2** 4 5 S 123 5 E
Woy Woy, *Australia* . . . **129 B9** 33 30 S 151 19 E
Wrangel I. = Vrangelya,
  Ostrov, *Russia* . . . . . **67 B19** 71 0N 180 0 E
Wrangell, *U.S.A.* **142 B2** 56 28N 132 23W
Wrangell Mts., *U.S.A.* . **144 F12** 61 30N 142 0W
Wrangell-St. Elias △,
  U.S.A. **144 D12** 61 0N 142 0W
Wrath, C., *U.K.* **22 C3** 58 38N 5 1W
Wray, *U.S.A.* **154 E3** 40 5N 102 13W
Wrekin, The, *U.K.* **21 E5** 52 41N 2 32W
Wrens, *U.S.A.* **152 B7** 33 12N 82 23W
Wrexham, *U.K.* **20 D4** 53 3N 3 0W
Wrexham □, *U.K.* **20 D5** 53 1N 2 58W
Wright, *Fla., U.S.A.* . . . **149 K2** 30 27N 86 38W
Wright, *Wyo., U.S.A.* . . **154 D2** 43 47N 105 30W
Wright Pt., *Canada* . . . **150 C3** 43 48N 81 44W
Wrightmyo, *India* . . . . . **95 J11** 11 47N 92 43 E
Wrightsville, *U.S.A.* . . . **152 C7** 32 44N 82 43W
Wrightwood, *U.S.A.* . . . **161 L9** 34 21N 117 38W
Wrigley, *Canada* **138 B7** 63 16N 123 37W
Wrocław, *Poland* . . . . . **55 G4** 51 5N 17 5 E
Wronki, *Poland* . . . . **55 F3** 52 41N 16 10 E
Września, *Poland* . . . . . **55 F4** 52 21N 17 36 E
Wschowa, *Poland* . . . . . **55 G3** 51 48N 16 20 E
Wu Jiang →, *China* . . . . **76 C6** 29 40N 107 20 E
Wu Kau Tang, *China* . . **69 F11** 22 30N 114 14 E
Wu'an, *China* . . . . **74 F8** 36 40N 114 15 E
Wubin, *Australia* . . . . . **125 F2** 30 6 S 116 37 E
Wubu, *China* . . . . **74 F6** 37 28N 110 42 E
Wuchang, *China* . . . . . . **75 B14** 44 55N 127 5 E
Wuchow = Wuzhou,
  China . . . . **77 F8** 23 30N 111 18 E
Wuchuan, *Guangdong,*
  China . . . . **77 G8** 21 33N 110 43 E
Wuchuan, *Guizhou,*
  China . . . . **76 C7** 28 25N 108 3 E
Wuchuan,
  Nei Monggol Zizhiqu,
  China . . . . **74 D6** 41 5N 111 28 E
Wudi, *China* . . . . **75 F9** 37 40N 117 35 E
Wuding, *China* . . . . **76 E4** 25 24N 102 21 E
Wuding He →, *China* . . **74 F6** 37 2N 110 23 E

Wudu, *China* . . . . **74 H3** 33 22N 104 54 E
Wufeng, *China* . . . . **77 B8** 30 12N 110 42 E
Wugang, *China* . . . . **77 D8** 26 44N 110 35 E
Wugong Shan, *China* . . **77 D9** 27 30N 114 0 E
Wuguishan, *China* . . . . **69 G9** 22 25N 113 25 E
Wuhan, *China* . . . . **77 B10** 30 31N 114 18 E
Wuhe, *China* . . . . **75 H9** 33 10N 117 50 E
Wuhsi = Wuxi, *China* . . **77 B13** 31 33N 120 18 E
Wuhu, *China* . . . . **77 B12** 31 22N 118 21 E
Wujiang, *China* . . . . . . **77 B13** 31 10N 120 38 E
Wukari, *Nigeria* . . . . . . **113 D6** 7 51N 9 42 E
Wulajie, *China* . . . . **75 B14** 44 6N 126 33 E
Wulanbulang, *China* . . **74 D6** 41 5N 110 55 E
Wular L., *India* . . . . **93 B6** 34 20N 74 30 E
Wulehe, *Ghana* . . . . **113 D5** 8 39N 0 0 E
Wulff Land, *Greenland* . **10 A6** 82 0N 52 0W
Wulian, *China* . . . . **75 G10** 35 40N 119 12 E
Wuliang Shan, *China* . . **76 E3** 24 30N 100 40 E
Wuliaru, *Indonesia* . . . . **83 C4** 7 27 S 131 0 E
Wuling Shan, *China* . . . **76 C7** 30 0N 110 0 E
Wulong, *China* . . . . **76 C6** 29 25N 107 43 E
Wuluk'omushih Ling,
  China . . . . **68 C3** 36 25N 87 25 E
Wulumuchi = Ürümqi,
  China . . . . **66 E9** 43 45N 87 45 E
Wuming, *China* . . . . **76 F7** 23 12N 108 18 E
Wuning, *China* . . . . **77 C10** 29 17N 115 5 E
Wunna →, *India* . . . . . . **94 D2** 20 18N 78 48 E
Wunnummin L.,
  Canada **140 B2** 52 55N 89 10W
Wunsiedel, *Germany* . . **31 E8** 50 2N 12 0 E
Wunstorf, *Germany* . . . **30 C5** 52 25N 9 26 E
Wuntho, *Burma* . . . . . . **90 D5** 23 55N 95 45 E
Wupatki △, *U.S.A.* **159 J8** 35 35N 111 20W
Wuping, *China* . . . . **77 E11** 25 5N 116 5 E
Wuppertal, *Germany* . . **30 D3** 51 16N 7 12 E
Wuppertal, *S. Africa* . . **116 E2** 32 13 S 19 12 E
Wuqia, *China* . . . . **65 D7** 39 40N 75 7 E
Wuqing, *China* . . . . **75 E9** 39 23N 117 4 E
Würenlingen, *Switz.* . . . **33 A6** 47 32N 8 16 E
Wurtsboro, *U.S.A.* **151 E10** 41 35N 74 29W
Würzburg, *Germany* . . . **31 F5** 49 46N 9 55 E
Wurzen, *Germany* . . . . . **30 D8** 51 22N 12 44 E
Wushan, *China* . . . . **74 G3** 34 43N 104 53 E
Wushishi, *Nigeria* . . . . . **113 D6** 9 46N 6 7 E
Wusi, *Vanuatu* . . . . **133 E4** 15 21 S 166 40 E
Wusih = Wuxi, *China* . . **77 B13** 31 33N 120 18 E
Wutach →, *Germany* . . **31 H4** 47 37N 8 15 E
Wutai, *China* . . . . **74 E7** 38 40N 113 12 E
Wuting = Huimin,
  China . . . . **75 F9** 37 27N 117 28 E
Wutongqiao, *China* . . . . **58** 25 24N 110 4 E
Wutongqiao, *China* . . . . **75 C11** 42 50N 120 5 E
Wutung, *Papua N. G.* . . **132 B1** 2 37 S 141 1 E
Wuwei, *Anhui, China* . . **77 B11** 31 18N 117 54 E
Wuwei, *Gansu, China* . . **68 C5** 37 57N 102 34 E
Wuxi, *Jiangsu, China* . . **77 B13** 31 33N 120 18 E
Wuxi, *Sichuan, China* . . **76 B7** 31 23N 109 35 E
Wuxiang, *China* . . . . . . **74 F7** 36 49N 112 50 E
Wuxuan, *China* . . . . **76 F7** 23 34N 109 39 E
Wuyang, *China* . . . . **74 H7** 33 25N 113 35 E
Wuyi, *Hebei, China* . . . **74 F8** 37 46N 115 56 E
Wuyi, *Zhejiang, China* . **77 C12** 28 52N 119 50 E
Wuyi Shan, *China* . . . . **77 D11** 27 0N 117 0 E
Wuyishan, *China* . . . . . **77 D12** 27 45N 118 0 E
Wuyo, *Nigeria* . . . . **113 C7** 10 23N 11 50 E
Wuyuan, *China* . . . . **77 C11** 29 15N 117 50 E
Wuyuan,
  Nei Mongol Zizhiqu,
  China . . . . **74 D5** 41 2N 108 20 E
Wuzhai, *China* . . . . **74 E6** 38 54N 111 48 E
Wuzhi Shan, *China* . . . . **86 C7** 18 45N 109 45 E
Wuzhong, *China* . . . . . . **74 E4** 38 2N 106 12 E
Wuzhou, *China* . . . . **77 F8** 23 30N 111 18 E
Wyaaba Cr. →,
  Australia . . . . **126 B3** 16 27 S 141 35 E
Wyalkatchem, *Australia* **125 F2** 31 8 S 117 22 E
Wyalusing, *U.S.A.* **151 E8** 41 40N 76 16W
Wyandotte, *U.S.A.* **157 B13** 42 12N 83 9W
Wyandra, *Australia* . . . . **127 D4** 27 12 S 145 56 E
Wyangala, L., *Australia* **129 B8** 33 54 S 149 0 E
Wyara, L., *Australia* . . . **127 D3** 28 42 S 144 14 E
Wycheproof, *Australia* . **129 D6** 36 5 S 143 17 E
Wye →, *U.K.* **21 F5** 51 38N 2 40W
Wyemandoo, *Australia* . **125 E2** 28 28 S 118 29 E
Wyk, *Germany* . . . . **30 A4** 54 41N 8 33 E
Wymondham, *U.K.* . . . . **21 E9** 52 35N 1 7 E
Wymore, *U.S.A.* **154 E6** 40 7N 96 40W
Wyndham, *Australia* . . . **124 C4** 15 33 S 128 3 E
Wyndham, *N.Z.* . . . . . . **131 G3** 46 20 S 168 51 E
Wynne, *U.S.A.* **155 H9** 35 14N 90 47W
Wynyard, *Australia* . . . **127 G4** 41 5 S 145 44 E
Wynyard, *Canada* **143 C8** 51 45N 104 10W
Wyola L., *Australia* . . . . **125 E5** 29 8 S 130 17 E
Wyoming = Plympton-
  Wyoming, *Canada* . . . **150 D2** 42 57N 82 7W
Wyoming, *Ill., U.S.A.* . . **156 C7** 41 4N 89 47W
Wyoming, *Iowa, U.S.A.* **156 B6** 42 4N 91 0W
Wyoming, *Mich.,*
  U.S.A. **157 B11** 42 54N 85 42W
Wyoming □, *U.S.A.* . . . **158 E10** 43 0N 107 30W
Wyomissing, *U.S.A.* . . . **151 F9** 40 20N 75 59W
Wyong, *Australia* . . . . . **129 B9** 33 14 S 151 24 E
Wyperfeld △, *Australia* . **128 C4** 35 35 S 141 42 E
Wyrzysk, *Poland* . . . . . **55 E4** 53 10N 17 17 E
Wyśmierzyce, *Poland* . . **55 G7** 51 37N 20 50 E
Wysokie, *Poland* . . . . . . **55 H9** 50 55N 22 40 E
Wysokie Mazowieckie,
  Poland . . . . **55 F9** 52 55N 22 25 E
Wyszków, *Poland* . . . . . **55 F8** 52 36N 21 25 E
Wyszogród, *Poland* . . . **55 F7** 52 23N 20 9 E
Wytheville, *U.S.A.* **148 G5** 36 57N 81 5W

X

Xa-Cassau, *Angola* . . . . **115 D4** 9 5 S 20 15 E
Xa-Muteba, *Angola* . . . . **115 D3** 9 34 S 17 50 E
Xaafuun, *Somali Rep.* . . **120 B4** 10 25N 51 16 E
Xaçmaz, *Azerbaijan* . . . **61 K9** 41 31N 48 42 E
Xadded, *Somali Rep.* . . . **120 C3** 9 46N 48 2 E
Xaghra, *Malta* . . . . **38 E7** 36 3N 14 16 E
Xai-Xai, *Mozam.* . . . . . . **117 D5** 25 6 S 33 31 E
Xaidulla, *China* . . . . **65 E8** 36 28N 77 59 E
Xainza, *China* . . . . **68 C3** 30 58N 88 35 E
Xalapa, *Mexico* . . . . **170 C2** 6 25 S 48 40W
Xambioá, *Brazil* . . . . . . **170 C2** 6 25 S 48 40W
Xangongo, *Angola* . . . . **116 B2** 16 45 S 15 5 E
Xankändi, *Azerbaijan* . . **101 C12** 39 52N 46 49 E
Xanlar, *Azerbaijan* . . . . **61 K8** 40 34N 46 12 E
Xanten, *Germany* . . . . . **30 D2** 51 39N 6 26 E
Xánthi, *Greece* . . . . **51 E8** 41 10N 24 58 E
Xánthi □, *Greece* . . . . . **51 E8** 41 10N 24 58 E
Xanthos, *Turkey* . . . . . . **49 E11** 36 19N 29 18 E
Xanxerê, *Brazil* . . . . . . **175 B5** 26 53 S 52 23W

Xapuri, *Brazil* .... **172 C4** 10 35 S 68 35W
Xar Moron He →,
  China .... **75 C11** 43 25N 120 35 E
Xarrë, *Albania* ...... **38 B10** 39 44N 20 3 E
Xàtiva, *Spain* **41 G4** 38 59N 0 32W
Xau, L., *Botswana* ... **116 C3** 21 15 S 24 44 E
Xavantina, *Brazil* .... **175 A5** 21 15 S 52 48W
Xenia, *U.S.A.* **157 E13** 39 41N 83 56W
Xeropotamos →,
  Cyprus .... **39 F8** 34 42N 32 33 E
Xertigny, *France* ..... **27 D13** 48 3N 6 24 E
Xewkija, *Malta* ...... **38 E7** 36 2N 14 15 E
Xhora, *S. Africa* ..... **117 E4** 31 55 S 28 38 E
Xhumo, *Botswana* .... **116 C3** 21 7 S 24 35 E
Xi Jiang →, *China* .... **77 F9** 22 5N 113 20 E
Xi Xian, *Henan, China* **77 A10** 32 20N 114 43 E
Xi Xian, *Shanxi, China* **74 F6** 36 41N 110 58 E
Xia Xian, *China* ...... **74 G6** 35 8N 111 12 E
Xiachengzi, *China* .... **75 B16** 44 40N 130 18 E
Xiachuan Dao, *China* . **77 G9** 21 40N 112 40 E
Xiaguan, *China* ...... **68 D5** 25 32N 100 16 E
Xiajiang, *China* ...... **77 D10** 27 30N 115 10 E
Xiajin, *China* .... **74 F9** 36 56N 116 0 E
Xiamen, *China* .... **77 E12** 24 25N 118 4 E
Xi'an, *China* .... **74 G5** 34 15N 109 0 E
Xianfeng, *China* ...... **76 C7** 29 40N 109 8 E
Xiang Jiang →, *China* . **77 C9** 28 55N 112 50 E
Xiangcheng, *Henan,*
  China .... **74 H8** 33 29N 114 52 E
Xiangcheng, *Henan,*
  China .... **74 H7** 33 50N 113 27 E
Xiangcheng, *Sichuan,*
  China .... **76 C2** 28 53N 99 47 E
Xiangdu, *China* ...... **76 F6** 23 13N 106 58 E
Xiangfan, *China* ...... **77 A9** 32 2N 112 8 E
Xianggang = Hong
  Kong □, *China* .... **77 F10** 22 11N 114 14 E
Xianghuang Qi, *China* **74 C7** 42 2N 113 50 E
Xiangning, *China* ..... **74 G6** 35 58N 110 50 E
Xiangquan, *China* .... **74 F7** 36 30N 113 1 E
Xiangquan He =
  Sutlej →, *Pakistan* .. **91 C3** 29 23N 71 3 E
Xiangshan, *China* ..... **77 C13** 29 29N 121 51 E
Xiangshui, *China* ..... **75 G10** 34 12N 119 33 E
Xiangtan, *China* ...... **77 D9** 27 51N 112 54 E
Xiangxiang, *China* .... **77 D9** 27 43N 112 28 E
Xiangyin, *China* ...... **77 C9** 28 38N 112 54 E
Xiangzhou, *China* .... **76 F7** 23 58N 109 40 E
Xianju, *China* .... **77 C13** 28 51N 120 44 E
Xianshui He →, *China* **76 B3** 30 10N 100 59 E
Xiantao, *China* .... **77 B9** 30 25N 113 25 E
Xianyang, *China* ...... **74 G5** 34 20N 108 40 E
Xianyou, *China* .... **77 E12** 25 22N 118 38 E
Xiao Hinggan Ling,
  China .... **69 B7** 49 0N 127 0 E
Xiao Xian, *China* ..... **74 G9** 34 15N 116 55 E
Xiaofeng, *China* ...... **77 B12** 30 35N 119 45 E
Xiaogan, *China* ...... **77 B9** 30 52N 113 55 E
Xiaojin, *China* .... **76 B4** 30 59N 102 21 E
Xiaolan, *China* .... **77 F9** 22 38N 113 13 E
Xiaoshan, *China* ..... **77 B13** 30 12N 120 18 E
Xiaoyi, *China* .... **74 F6** 37 8N 111 48 E
Xiapu, *China* .... **77 D12** 26 54N 119 59 E
Xiawa, *China* .... **75 C11** 42 35N 120 38 E
Xiayi, *China* .... **74 G9** 34 15N 116 10 E
Xichang, *China* ...... **76 D4** 27 51N 102 19 E
Xichong, *China* ...... **76 B5** 30 57N 105 54 E
Xichou, *China* .... **76 E5** 23 25N 104 42 E
Xichuan, *China* ...... **74 H6** 33 0N 111 30 E
Xide, *China* .... **76 C4** 28 18N 102 43 E
Xiemahe, *China* ...... **77 B8** 31 38N 111 12 E
Xieng Khouang, *Laos* . **86 C4** 19 17N 103 25 E
Xifei He →, *China* .... **77 H9** 32 45N 116 40 E
Xifeng, *Gansu, China* . **74 G4** 35 40N 107 40 E
Xifeng, *Guizhou, China* **76 D6** 27 7N 106 42 E
Xifeng, *Liaoning, China* **75 C13** 42 42N 124 45 E
Xifengzhen = Xifeng,
  China .... **74 G4** 35 40N 107 40 E
Xigazê, *China* .... **68 D3** 29 5N 88 45 E
Xihe, *China* .... **74 G4** 34 2N 105 20 E
Xihua, *China* .... **74 H8** 33 45N 114 30 E
Xilaganí, *Greece* ..... **51 F9** 40 58N 25 28 E
Xiliao He →, *China* ... **75 C12** 22 36N 123 57 E
Xilin, *China* .... **76 E5** 24 30N 105 6 E
Xilókastron, *Greece* .. **48 C4** 38 5N 22 38 E
Ximana, *Mozam.* ..... **119 F3** 19 24 S 33 58 E
Xime, *Guinea-Biss.* ... **112 C2** 11 59N 14 57W
Ximeng, *China* .... **76 F2** 22 50N 99 27 E
Xin Jiang →, *China* ... **77 C11** 28 45N 116 35 E
Xin Xian = Xinzhou,
  China .... **74 E7** 38 22N 112 46 E
Xinavane, *Mozam.* .... **117 D5** 25 2 S 32 47 E
Xinbin, *China* .... **75 D13** 41 40N 125 2 E
Xincai, *China* .... **77 A10** 33 15N 114 51 E
Xinchang, *China* ..... **77 C13** 29 28N 120 52 E
Xincheng,
  Guangxi Zhuangzu,
  China .... **76 E7** 24 5N 108 39 E
Xincheng, *Jiangxi,*
  China .... **77 D10** 26 48N 114 6 E
Xindu, *China* .... **76 B5** 30 50N 104 10 E
Xinfeng, *Guangdong,*
  China .... **77 E10** 24 5N 114 16 E
Xinfeng, *Jiangxi, China* **77 D11** 27 7N 116 11 E
Xinfeng, *Jiangxi, China* **77 E10** 25 27N 114 58 E
Xinfengjiang Skuiku,
  China .... **77 F10** 23 52N 114 30 E
Xing Xian, *China* ..... **74 E6** 38 27N 111 7 E
Xing'an,
  Guangxi Zhuangzu,
  China .... **77 E8** 25 38N 110 40 E
Xingan, *Jiangxi, China* **77 D10** 27 46N 115 20 E
Xingcheng, *China* .... **75 D11** 40 40N 120 45 E
Xingguo, *China* ...... **77 D10** 26 21N 115 21 E
Xinghe, *China* .... **74 D7** 40 55N 113 55 E
Xinghua, *China* ...... **75 H10** 32 58N 119 48 E
Xinghua Wan, *China* . **77 E12** 25 15N 119 20 E
Xinglong, *China* ..... **75 D9** 40 25N 117 30 E
Xingping, *China* ...... **74 G5** 34 20N 108 28 E
Xingren, *China* .... **76 E5** 25 24N 105 11 E
Xingshan, *China* ..... **77 B8** 31 15N 110 45 E
Xingtai, *China* .... **74 F8** 37 3N 114 32 E
Xingu →, *Brazil* ..... **169 D7** 1 30 S 51 53W
Xingwen, *China* ...... **76 C5** 28 22N 104 50 E
Xingyang, *China* ..... **74 G7** 34 45N 112 52 E
Xinhe, *China* .... **74 F8** 37 30N 115 15 E
Xinhua, *China* .... **77 D8** 27 42N 111 13 E
Xinhuang, *China* ..... **76 D7** 27 20N 109 12 E
Xinhui, *China* .... **77 F9** 22 25N 113 0 E
Xining, *China* .... **68 C5** 36 34N 101 40 E
Xinjiang, *China* ...... **74 G6** 35 34N 111 11 E
Xinjiang Uygur
  Zizhiqu □, *China* .. **68 C3** 42 0N 86 0 E
Xinjie, *China* .... **68 D5** 26 48N 101 15 E
Xinjin = Pulandian,
  China .... **75 E11** 39 25N 121 58 E
Xinjin, *China* .... **76 B4** 30 24N 103 47 E
Xinkai He →, *China* ... **75 C12** 43 32N 123 35 E
Xinken, *China* .... **69 F10** 22 39N 113 36 E

Xinle, *China* .... **74 E8** 38 25N 114 40 E
Xinlitun, *China* ...... **75 D12** 42 0N 122 8 E
Xinlong, *China* .... **76 B3** 30 57N 100 12 E
Xinmin, *China* .... **75 D12** 41 59N 122 50 E
Xinning, *China* ...... **77 D8** 26 28N 110 50 E
Xinshao, *China* ...... **76 E3** 24 5N 101 59 E
Xinshao, *China* ...... **77 D8** 27 21N 111 26 E
Xintai, *China* .... **75 G9** 35 55N 117 45 E
Xintian, *China* .... **77 E9** 25 55N 112 13 E
Xinwan, *China* .... **69 F10** 22 47N 113 40 E
Xinxian, *China* .... **77 D10** 31 36N 113 51 E
Xinxiang, *China* ..... **74 G7** 35 18N 113 50 E
Xinxing, *China* .... **77 F9** 22 35N 112 35 E
Xinyang, *China* ...... **77 A10** 32 6N 114 3 E
Xinye, *China* .... **77 A9** 32 25N 112 45 E
Xinyi, *China* .... **77 F8** 22 25N 111 0 E
Xinyu, *China* .... **77 D10** 27 49N 114 58 E
Xinzhan, *China* ...... **75 C14** 43 50N 127 18 E
Xinzheng, *China* ..... **74 G7** 34 20N 113 45 E
Xinzhou, *Hubei, China* **77 B10** 30 50N 114 48 E
Xinzhou, *Shanxi, China* **74 E7** 38 22N 112 46 E
Xinzo de Limia, *Spain* **42 C3** 42 3N 7 47W
Xiongyuecheng, *China* **75 D12** 40 12N 122 5 E
Xiping, *Henan, China* . **74 H8** 33 22N 114 5 E
Xiping, *Henan, China* . **74 H6** 33 25N 111 8 E
Xiping, *Zhejiang, China* **77 C12** 28 16N 119 29 E
Xique-Xique, *Brazil* .. **170 D3** 10 50 S 42 40W
Xiruá →, *Brazil* ..... **172 B4** 6 3 S 67 50W
Xisha Qundao =
  Paracel Is.,
  S. China Sea ...... **78 A4** 15 50N 112 0 E
Xishui, *Guizhou, China* **76 C6** 28 19N 106 9 E
Xishui, *Hubei, China* . **77 B10** 30 30N 115 15 E
Xitole, *Guinea-Biss.* .. **112 C2** 11 43N 14 50W
Xiu Shui →, *China* ... **77 C10** 29 13N 116 0 E
Xiuning, *China* ...... **77 C12** 29 45N 118 10 E
Xiuren, *China* .... **77 E8** 24 27N 110 12 E
Xiushan, *China* ...... **76 C7** 28 25N 108 57 E
Xiushui, *China* ...... **77 C10** 29 2N 114 33 E
Xiuwen, *China* .... **76 D6** 26 49N 106 32 E
Xiuyan, *China* .... **75 D12** 40 18N 123 11 E
Xixia, *China* .... **74 H6** 33 25N 111 29 E
Xixiang, *China* ...... **74 H4** 33 0N 107 44 E
Xixing, *China* .... **77 E13** 37 38N 113 38 E
Xizang Zizhiqu □,
  China .... **68 C3** 32 0N 88 0 E
Xlendi, *Malta* .... **38 E6** 36 2N 14 13 E
Xochob, *Mexico* **163 D7** 19 28N 89 45W
Xu Jiang →, *China* ... **77 D10** 28 0N 116 25 E
Xuan Loc, *Vietnam* ... **87 G6** 10 56N 107 14 E
Xuan'en, *China* ...... **76 C7** 30 0N 109 30 E
Xuanhan, *China* ...... **76 B6** 31 18N 107 38 E
Xuanhua, *China* ...... **74 D8** 40 40N 115 2 E
Xuanwei, *China* ...... **76 C5** 26 15N 103 59 E
Xuanzhou, *China* .... **77 B12** 30 56N 118 43 E
Xuchang, *China* ...... **74 G7** 34 2N 113 48 E
Xudat, *Azerbaijan* .... **61 K9** 41 38N 48 41 E
Xuddur = Oddur,
  Somali Rep. ...... **120 D2** 4 11N 43 52 E
Xuefeng Shan, *China* . **77 D8** 27 5N 110 35 E
Xuejiaping, *China* .... **77 B8** 31 39N 110 16 E
Xun Jiang →, *China* .. **77 F8** 23 35N 111 30 E
Xun Xian, *China* ..... **74 G8** 35 42N 114 33 E
Xundian, *China* ...... **76 E4** 25 36N 103 15 E
Xunwu, *China* .... **77 E10** 24 54N 115 37 E
Xunyang, *China* ...... **74 H5** 32 48N 109 22 E
Xunyi, *China* .... **74 G5** 35 8N 108 20 E
Xupu, *China* .... **77 D8** 27 53N 110 32 E
Xúquer →, *Spain* **41 F4** 39 5N 0 10W
Xushui, *China* .... **74 E8** 39 2N 115 40 E
Xuwen, *China* .... **77 G8** 20 20N 110 10 E
Xuyen Moc, *Vietnam* . **87 G6** 10 34N 107 25 E
Xuyong, *China* ...... **76 C5** 28 10N 105 22 E
Xuzhou, *China* ...... **75 G9** 34 18N 117 10 E
Xylophagou, *Cyprus* .. **39 F9** 34 54N 33 51 E

Y

Ya Xian = Sanya, *China* **86 C7** 18 14N 109 29 E
Yaamba, *Australia* ... **126 C5** 23 8 S 150 22 E
Ya'an, *China* .... **76 C4** 29 58N 103 5 E
Yaapeet, *Australia* .... **128 C5** 35 45 S 142 3 E
Yabassi, *Cameroon* ... **113 E6** 4 30N 9 57 E
Yabelo, *Ethiopia* ..... **107 G4** 4 50N 38 8 E
Yabelo □, *Ethiopia* ... **107 F4** 6 0N 37 50 E
Yablanitsa, *Bulgaria* .. **51 C8** 43 2N 24 5 E
Yablonovy Ra. =
  Yablonovyy Khrebet,
  Russia .... **67 D12** 53 0N 114 0 E
Yablonovyy Khrebet,
  Russia .... **67 D12** 53 0N 114 0 E
Yabluniv, *Ukraine* .... **53 B9** 48 24N 24 57 E
Yablunytsya, *Ukraine* . **53 B9** 48 19N 24 29 E
Yabrai Shan, *China* ... **74 E4** 39 40N 103 0 E
Yabrūd, *Syria* .... **103 B5** 33 58N 36 39 E
Yabucoa, *Puerto Rico* . **165 d** 18 3N 65 53W
Yacambú △, *Venezuela* **168 E6** 9 42N 69 27W
Yacheng, *China* ...... **76 C7** 18 22N 109 6 E
Yackandandah,
  Australia .... **129 D7** 36 18 S 146 52 E
Yacuiba, *Bolivia* ..... **174 A3** 22 0 S 63 43W
Yacuma →, *Bolivia* ... **174 C3** 13 38 S 65 23W
Yadgir, *India* .... **94 F3** 16 45N 77 5 E
Yadkin →, *U.S.A.* **149 H5** 35 29N 80 9W
Yadua, *Fiji* .... **133 A2** 16 49 S 178 18 E
Yaeyama-Rettō, *Japan* **71 M1** 24 30N 123 40 E
Yafran, *Libya* .... **108 B2** 32 4N 12 31 E
Yafran □, *Libya* ..... **108 B2** 32 0N 12 0 E
Yagaba, *Ghana* **113 C4** 10 14N 1 20W
Yagasa Cluster, *Fiji* ... **133 B3** 18 57 S 178 28W
Yağcılar, *Turkey* ..... **49 B10** 39 58N 28 23 E
Yagodnoye, *Russia* ... **67 C15** 62 33N 149 40 E
Yagoua, *Cameroon* ... **109 F3** 10 20N 15 13 E
Yaguas →, *Peru* ...... **168 D3** 2 45 S 70 10W
Yahila, *Orientale,*
  Dem. Rep. of
  the Congo .... **114 B4** 1 48N 23 37 E
Yahila, *Orientale,*
  Dem. Rep. of
  the Congo .... **118 B1** 0 13N 24 28 E
Yahk, *Canada* **142 D5** 49 6N 116 10W
Yahotyn, *Ukraine* .... **59 G6** 50 17N 31 46 E
Yahuma, *Dem. Rep. of*
  the Congo .... **114 B4** 1 0N 23 10 E
Yahyalı, *Turkey* ...... **100 C6** 38 5N 35 2 E
Yaita, *Japan* .... **71 F9** 36 48N 139 56 E
Yaiza, *Canary Is.* **9 e2** 28 57N 13 46W
Yaizu, *Japan* .... **73 C10** 34 52N 138 20 E
Yajiang, *China* ...... **76 B3** 30 2N 100 57 E
Yajua, *Nigeria* ...... **113 C7** 11 27N 12 49 E
Yakage, *Japan* ...... **72 C6** 34 37N 133 35 E
Yakamba, *Dem. Rep. of*
  the Congo .... **114 B3** 2 42N 19 38 E
Yakima, *U.S.A.* **158 C3** 46 36N 120 31W
Yakima →, *U.S.A.* ... **158 C3** 47 0N 120 30W
Yakkabag, *Uzbekistan* **65 D3** 38 55N 66 51 E
Yako, *Burkina Faso* ... **112 C4** 12 59N 2 15W
Yakobi I., *U.S.A.* **142 B1** 58 0N 136 30W
Yakoma, *Dem. Rep. of*
  the Congo .... **114 B4** 4 5N 22 27 E

Yakoruda, *Bulgaria* .. **50 D7** 42 1N 23 39 E
Yakossi, *C.A.R.* ..... **114 A4** 5 37N 23 19 E
Yakovlevka, *Russia* ... **70 B6** 44 26N 133 28 E
Yakovlevskoye =
  Privolzhsk, *Russia* .. **60 B5** 57 23N 41 16 E
Yakshur Bodya, *Russia* **64 C4** 57 11N 53 7 E
Yaku-Shima, *Japan* ... **71 J5** 30 20N 130 30 E
Yakumo, *Japan* ...... **70 C10** 42 15N 140 16 E
Yakutat, *U.S.A.* **144 G13** 59 33N 139 44W
Yakutat B., *U.S.A.* ... **144 G12** 59 45N 140 45W
Yakutia = Sakha □,
  Russia .... **67 C13** 66 0N 130 0 E
Yakutsk, *Russia* ...... **67 C13** 62 5N 129 50 E
Yala, *Thailand* .... **87 J3** 6 33N 101 18 E
Yala △, *Sri Lanka* .... **95 L5** 6 33N 81 30 E
Yalboroo, *Australia* ... **126 J6** 20 50 S 148 40 E
Yale, *U.S.A.* **150 C2** 43 8N 82 48W
Yalgoo, *Australia* .... **125 E2** 28 16 S 116 39 E
Yalgorup △, *Australia* **125 D2** 24 34 S 115 2 E
Yali, *Dem. Rep. of*
  the Congo .... **114 B4** 0 4N 21 3 E
Yaligimba, *Dem. Rep.*
  of the Congo ..... **114 B4** 2 13N 22 56 E
Yalikanda, *Dem. Rep.*
  of the Congo ..... **114 B4** 0 23N 24 47 E
Yalinga, *C.A.R.* ..... **114 A4** 6 33N 23 10 E
Yalkubul, Punta,
  Mexico **163 C7** 21 32N 88 37W
Yalleroi, *Australia* .... **126 C4** 24 3 S 145 42 E
Yalobusha →, *U.S.A.* . **155 J9** 33 33N 90 10W
Yaloké, *C.A.R.* ...... **114 A3** 5 19N 17 5 E
Yalong Jiang →, *China* **76 D3** 26 40N 101 55 E
Yalova, *Turkey* ...... **51 F13** 40 41N 29 15 E
Yalpuh, Ozero, *Ukraine* **53 E13** 45 30N 28 41 E
Yalta, *Ukraine* ...... **59 K8** 44 30N 34 10 E
Yalu Jiang →, *China* .. **75 E13** 40 0N 124 22 E
Yalvaç, *Turkey* ...... **100 C4** 38 17N 31 10 E
Yam Ha Melah = Dead
  Sea, *Asia* .... **103 D4** 31 30N 35 30 E
Yam Kinneret, *Israel* . **103 C4** 32 45N 35 35 E
Yamada, *Japan* ...... **72 D2** 33 33N 130 49 E
Yamaga, *Japan* ...... **72 D2** 33 1N 130 41 E
Yamagata, *Japan* .... **70 E10** 38 15N 140 15 E
Yamagata □, *Japan* .. **70 E10** 38 30N 140 0 E
Yamagawa, *Japan* .... **72 F2** 31 12N 130 39 E
Yamaguchi, *Japan* ... **72 C3** 34 10N 131 32 E
Yamaguchi □, *Japan* . **72 C3** 34 20N 131 40 E
Yamal, Poluostrov,
  Russia .... **66 B8** 71 0N 70 0 E
Yamal Pen. = Yamal,
  Poluostrov, *Russia* .. **66 B8** 71 0N 70 0 E
Yamanaka, *Japan* .... **73 A8** 36 15N 136 22 E
Yamanashi, *Japan* ... **73 B10** 35 40N 138 40 E
Yamanashi □, *Japan* . **73 B10** 35 40N 138 40 E
Yamanie Falls △,
  Australia .... **126 B4** 18 29 S 146 9 E
Yamantau, Gora,
  Russia .... **64 D7** 54 15N 58 6 E
Yamasaki, *Japan* .... **72 C6** 35 0N 134 32 E
Yamato, *Japan* ...... **73 B11** 35 27N 139 25 E
Yamatotakada, *Japan* **73 C7** 34 31N 135 45 E
Yamba, *Australia* .... **127 D5** 29 26 S 153 23 E
Yambarran Ra.,
  Australia .... **124 C5** 15 10 S 130 25 E
Yambata, *Dem. Rep. of*
  the Congo .... **114 B4** 2 26N 21 58 E
Yambéring, *Guinea* ... **112 C2** 11 50N 12 18 E
Yâmbiô, *Sudan* ...... **107 G2** 4 35N 28 16 E
Yambol, *Bulgaria* .... **51 D10** 42 30N 26 30 E
Yamboyo, *Dem. Rep. of*
  the Congo .... **114 B4** 0 40N 22 18 E
Yambuya, *Dem. Rep. of*
  the Congo .... **114 B4** 1 17N 24 34 E
Yamdena, *Indonesia* .. **83 C4** 7 45 S 131 20 E
Yame, *Japan* .... **72 D2** 33 13N 130 35 E
Yamethin, *Burma* .... **90 E6** 20 29N 96 18 E
Yamma-Yamma, L.,
  Australia .... **127 D3** 26 16 S 141 20 E
Yamoussoukro,
  Ivory C. **112 D3** 6 49N 5 17W
Yampa →, *U.S.A.* **158 F9** 40 32N 108 59W
Yampi Sd., *Australia* .. **124 C3** 16 8 S 123 38 E
Yampil, *Moldova* ..... **59 H5** 48 15N 28 15 E
Yampol = Yampil,
  Moldova .... **59 H5** 48 15N 28 15 E
Yamrat, *Nigeria* ..... **113 C6** 10 11N 9 55 E
Yamrukchal = Botev,
  Bulgaria .... **51 D8** 42 44N 24 52 E
Yamuna →, *India* .... **93 G9** 25 30N 81 53 E
Yamunanagar, *India* .. **92 D7** 30 7N 77 17 E
Yamzho Yumco, *China* **68 D4** 28 48N 90 35 E
Yan →, *Sri Lanka* .... **95 K5** 9 0N 81 10 E
Yan Oya →, *Sri Lanka* **95 K5** 9 0N 81 10 E
Yana →, *Russia* ...... **67 B14** 71 30N 136 0 E
Yanagawa, *Japan* .... **72 D2** 33 10N 130 24 E
Yanahara, *Japan* ..... **72 C6** 34 58N 134 2 E
Yanai, *Japan* .... **72 D4** 33 58N 132 7 E
Yan'an, *China* .... **74 F5** 36 35N 109 26 E
Yanaul, *Russia* ...... **64 C5** 56 25N 55 0 E
Yanbian, *China* ...... **76 D3** 26 47N 101 31 E
Yanbu 'al Baḥr,
  Si. Arabia .... **96 F3** 24 0N 38 5 E
Yanchang, *China* ..... **74 F6** 36 43N 110 1 E
Yancheng, *Henan,*
  China .... **74 H8** 33 35N 114 0 E
Yancheng, *Jiangsu,*
  China .... **75 H11** 33 23N 120 8 E
Yanchep Beach,
  Australia .... **125 F2** 31 33 S 115 37 E
Yanchi, *China* .... **74 F4** 37 48N 107 20 E
Yanchuan, *China* ..... **74 F6** 36 51N 110 10 E
Yanco, *Australia* ..... **129 C7** 34 58 S 146 27 E
Yanco Cr. →, *Australia* **129 C6** 35 14 S 145 35 E
Yandé, Î., *N. Cal.* .... **133 T17** 20 3 S 163 49 E
Yandicoogina, *Australia* **124 D2** 22 49 S 119 12 E
Yandina, *Solomon Is.* . **133 M10** 9 7 S 159 13 E
Yandja, *Dem. Rep. of*
  the Congo .... **114 C3** 1 41 S 17 43 E
Yandoon, *Burma* ..... **90 G5** 17 0N 95 40 E
Yanfeng, *China* ...... **76 E3** 25 52N 101 8 E
Yanfolila, *Mali* **112 C3** 11 11N 8 9W
Yang Xian, *China* .... **74 H4** 33 15N 107 30 E
Yang-Yang, *Senegal* .. **112 B1** 15 0N 15 20W
Yangambi, *Dem. Rep.*
  of the Congo ..... **118 B1** 0 47N 24 24 E
Yangbi, *China* .... **76 E3** 25 38N 99 59 E
Yangcheng, *China* .... **74 G7** 35 28N 112 22 E
Yangchow = Yangzhou,
  China .... **77 A12** 32 21N 119 26 E
Yangchuan =
  Yangquan, *China* .. **74 F7** 37 58N 113 31 E
Yangchun, *China* ..... **77 F8** 22 11N 111 48 E
Yanggao, *China* ...... **74 D7** 40 21N 113 55 E
Yanggu, *China* .... **74 F8** 36 8N 115 43 E
Yangi-Nishan,
  Uzbekistan .... **65 D2** 38 49N 65 47 E
Yangiabad, *Uzbekistan* **65 C5** 41 7N 70 6 E
Yangibazar =
  Kofarnikhon,
  Tajikistan .... **65 D4** 38 34N 69 1 E

Yangikishlak,
  Uzbekistan .... **65 C3** 40 25N 67 10 E
Yangirabad, *Uzbekistan* **65 C2** 40 2N 65 58 E
Yangiyer, *Uzbekistan* . **65 C4** 40 16N 68 48 E
Yangiyul, *Uzbekistan* . **65 C4** 41 0N 69 3 E
Yangjiang, *China* ..... **77 G8** 21 50N 111 59 E
Yangliuqing, *China* ... **75 E9** 39 2N 117 5 E
Yangon = Rangoon,
  Burma .... **90 G6** 16 45N 96 20 E
Yangonde, *Dem. Rep.*
  of the Congo ..... **114 B4** 0 22 N 22 43 E
Yangping, *China* ..... **77 B8** 31 12N 111 25 E
Yangpingguan, *China* . **74 H4** 32 58N 106 5 E
Yangquan, *China* ..... **74 F7** 37 58N 113 31 E
Yangshan, *China* ..... **77 E9** 24 30N 112 40 E
Yangshuo, *China* ..... **77 E8** 24 48N 110 29 E
Yangtse = Chang
  Jiang →, *China* .... **77 B13** 31 48N 121 10 E
Yangtze Kiang = Chang
  Jiang →, *China* .... **77 B13** 31 48N 121 10 E
Yangudi Rassa △,
  Ethiopia .... **107 E5** 10 50N 40 42 E
Yangxin, *China* ...... **77 C10** 29 50N 115 12 E
Yangyang, *S. Korea* ... **75 E15** 38 4N 128 38 E
Yangyuan, *China* ..... **74 D8** 40 1N 114 10 E
Yangzhong, *China* .... **77 A12** 32 21N 119 59 E
Yangzhou, *China* ..... **77 A12** 32 21N 119 26 E
Yanhe, *China* .... **76 C7** 28 48N 108 18 E
Yanji, *China* .... **75 C15** 42 59N 129 30 E
Yanjin, *China* .... **76 C5** 28 5N 104 18 E
Yanjing, *China* .... **76 C2** 29 7N 98 33 E
Yankari △, *Nigeria* ... **113 D7** 9 50N 10 28 E
Yankton, *U.S.A.* **154 D6** 42 53N 97 23W
Yanonge, *Dem. Rep. of*
  the Congo .... **118 B1** 0 35N 24 38 E
Yanov = Ivanava,
  Belarus .... **59 F3** 52 7N 25 29 E
Yanqi, *China* .... **68 B3** 42 5N 86 35 E
Yanqing, *China* ...... **74 D8** 40 30N 115 58 E
Yanshan, *Hebei, China* **75 E9** 38 4N 117 22 E
Yanshan, *Jiangxi, China* **77 C11** 28 15N 117 41 E
Yanshan, *Yunnan,*
  China .... **76 F5** 23 35N 104 20 E
Yanshou, *China* ...... **75 B15** 45 28N 128 22 E
Yantabulla, *Australia* . **127 D4** 29 21 S 145 0 E
Yantai, *China* .... **75 F11** 37 34N 121 22 E
Yantarnyy, *Russia* .... **54 D6** 54 52N 19 57 E
Yantian, *China* .... **69 F11** 22 35N 114 16 E
Yanting, *China* .... **76 B5** 31 11N 105 24 E
Yantra →, *Bulgaria* ... **51 C9** 43 40N 25 37 E
Yanuca, *Fiji* .... **133 B1** 18 24 S 178 0 E
Yanwa, *China* .... **76 D2** 27 35N 98 55 E
Yanykurgan =
  Zhangaqŭrghan,
  Kazakhstan .... **65 A3** 43 50N 68 48 E
Yanyuan, *China* ...... **76 D3** 27 25N 101 30 E
Yanzhou, *China* ...... **74 G9** 35 35N 116 49 E
Yao, *Chad* .... **109 F3** 12 56N 17 33 E
Yao, *Japan* .... **73 C7** 34 32N 135 36 E
Yao Noi, Ko, *Thailand* **87 a** 8 7N 98 37 E
Yao Xian, *China* ..... **74 G5** 34 55N 108 59 E
Yao Yai, Ko, *Thailand* **87 a** 8 0N 98 35 E
Yao'an, *China* .... **76 E3** 25 31N 101 18 E
Yaodu, *China* .... **76 A5** 32 45N 105 22 E
Yaoundé, *Cameroon* .. **113 E7** 3 50N 11 35 E
Yaowan, *China* ...... **75 G10** 34 15N 118 3 E
Yap, *Pac. Oc.* .... **134 G5** 9 30N 138 10 E
Yapacana △, *Venezuela* **168 C4** 3 49N 66 44W
Yapehe, *Dem. Rep. of*
  the Congo .... **114 C4** 0 13 S 24 28 E
Yapen, *Indonesia* ..... **83 B5** 1 50 S 136 0 E
Yapen, Selat, *Indonesia* **83 B5** 1 20 S 136 10 E
Yapero, *Indonesia* .... **83 B5** 4 59 S 137 11 E
Yappar →, *Australia* .. **126 B3** 18 22 S 141 16 E
Yaqaga, *Fiji* .... **133 A2** 16 35 S 178 36 E
Yaqui →, *Mexico* **162 B2** 27 37N 110 39W
Yar, *Russia* .... **64 B4** 58 14N 52 5 E
Yar-Sale, *Russia* ..... **66 C8** 66 50N 70 50 E
Yaracuy □, *Venezuela* . **168 A4** 10 20N 68 45W
Yaracuy →, *Venezuela* . **168 A4** 10 38N 68 15W
Yaraka, *Australia* .... **126 C3** 24 53 S 144 3 E
Yaransk, *Russia* ...... **60 B8** 57 22N 47 49 E
Yarbasan, *Turkey* .... **49 C10** 38 59N 28 49 E
Yardımcı Burnu,
  Turkey .... **49 E12** 36 13N 30 25 E
Yare →, *U.K.* .... **21 E9** 52 35N 1 38 E
Yaremcha, *Ukraine* ... **53 B9** 48 27N 24 33 E
Yarensk, *Russia* ...... **56 B8** 62 11N 49 15 E
Yarfa, *Si. Arabia* ..... **106 C4** 24 37N 38 35 E
Yarí →, *Colombia* .... **168 D3** 0 20 S 72 20W
Yarım, *Yemen* .... **98 E4** 14 20N 44 22 E
Yaritagua, *Venezuela* . **168 A4** 10 5N 69 8W
Yarkand = Shache,
  China .... **65 D8** 38 20N 77 10 E
Yarker, *Canada* **151 B8** 44 23N 76 46W
Yarkhun →, *Pakistan* . **93 A5** 36 17N 72 30 E
Yarlung Ziangbo
  Jiang =
  Brahmaputra →,
  Asia .... **68 D3** 23 40N 90 35 E
Yarmouth, *Canada* ... **141 D6** 43 50N 66 7W
Yarmūk →, *Syria* ..... **103 C4** 32 42N 35 40 E
Yarqa, W. →, *Egypt* .. **103 F2** 30 0N 33 49 E
Yarra Ranges △,
  Australia .... **129 D7** 37 40 S 146 3 E
Yarra Yarra Lakes,
  Australia .... **125 E2** 29 40 S 115 45 E
Yarram, *Australia* .... **129 E7** 38 29 S 146 39 E
Yarraman, *Australia* .. **127 D5** 26 50 S 152 0 E
Yarras, *Australia* ..... **129 A10** 31 25 S 152 20 E
Yarrawonga, *Australia* **129 D7** 36 1 S 146 0 E
Yartsevo, *Sib., Russia* . **67 C10** 60 20N 90 0 E
Yartsevo, *Smolensk,*
  Russia .... **58 E7** 55 6N 32 43 E
Yarumal, *Colombia* ... **168 B2** 6 58N 75 24W
Yasawa, *Fiji* .... **133 A1** 16 47 S 177 31 E
Yasawa Group, *Fiji* ... **133 A1** 17 0 S 177 23 E
Yaselda, *Belarus* ..... **59 F4** 52 7N 26 28 E
Yasen, *Ukraine* ...... **53 B9** 48 45N 24 10 E
Yashbum, *Yemen* .... **98 D4** 14 19N 46 56 E
Yashi, *Nigeria* .... **113 C6** 12 23N 7 54 E
Yashikera, *Nigeria* ... **113 D5** 9 44N 3 15 E
Yashiro-Jima, *Japan* .. **72 D4** 33 55N 132 15 E
Yashkul, *Russia* ...... **61 G7** 46 11N 45 21 E
Yasin, *Pakistan* ...... **93 A5** 36 24N 73 23 E
Yasinovataya, *Russia* . **59 H9** 48 7N 37 57 E
Yasinski, L., *Canada* .. **140 B4** 53 16N 77 35W
Yasinya, *Ukraine* ..... **53 B9** 48 16N 24 21 E
Yasnyy, *Russia* ...... **64 F7** 51 1N 59 58 E
Yasothon, *Thailand* ... **86 C4** 15 50N 104 10 E
Yass, *Australia* ...... **129 C8** 34 49 S 148 54 E
Yasugi, *Japan* .... **72 B5** 35 26N 133 15 E
Yāsūj, *Iran* .... **101 D6** 30 31N 51 31 E
Yasuní △, *Ecuador* ... **168 D2** 1 19 S 76 3W
Yat, *Niger* .... **109 D2** 20 28N 13 27 E
Yata →, *Bolivia* ...... **173 C4** 10 29 S 65 26W
Yata, *C.A.R.* .... **114 A4** 10 29N 23 25 E
Yata-Ngaya △, *C.A.R.* **114 A4** 9 15N 23 15 E
Yataǧan, *Turkey* ..... **49 D10** 37 20N 28 10 E
Yatakala, *Niger* ...... **113 C5** 14 50N 0 22 E
Yaté, *N. Cal.* .... **133 V20** 22 9 S 166 57 E
Yates Center, *U.S.A.* . **155 G7** 37 53N 95 44W

Yates Pt., *N.Z.* ...... **131 E2** 44 29 S 167 49 E
Yathkyed L., *Canada* . **143 A9** 62 40N 98 0W
Yathong, *Australia* ... **129 B6** 32 37 S 145 33 E
Yatolemu, *Dem. Rep.*
  of the Congo ..... **114 B4** 0 25N 24 35 E
Yatsuo, *Japan* .... **73 A9** 36 34N 137 8 E
Yatsushiro, *Japan* .... **72 E2** 32 30N 130 40 E
Yatta Plateau, *Kenya* . **118 C4** 2 0 S 38 0 E
Yatua →, *Venezuela* .. **168 C4** 1 30N 66 30W
Yauca, *Peru* .... **172 D3** 15 39 S 74 35W
Yauco, *Puerto Rico* ... **165 d** 18 2N 66 51W
Yauri, *Peru* .... **172 C3** 14 47 S 71 25W
Yauyos, *Peru* .... **172 B2** 8 59 S 77 17W
Yaval, *India* .... **94 D2** 21 10N 75 42 E
Yavan, *Tajikistan* ..... **65 D4** 38 19N 69 2 E
Yavari →, *Peru* ...... **172 A3** 4 21 S 70 2W
Yávaros, *Mexico* **162 B3** 26 42N 109 31W
Yavatmal, *India* ...... **94 D4** 20 20N 78 15 E
Yavero →, *Peru* ...... **172 C3** 12 6 S 72 57W
Yavne, *Israel* .... **103 D3** 31 52N 34 45 E
Yavoriv, *Ukraine* ..... **55 J10** 49 55N 23 20 E
Yavorov = Yavoriv,
  Ukraine .... **55 J10** 49 55N 23 20 E
Yavuzeli, *Turkey* ..... **100 D7** 37 18N 37 24 E
Yawatahama, *Japan* .. **72 D3** 33 27N 132 24 E
Yawnghwe, *Burma* ... **90 E6** 20 39N 96 56 E
Yawri B., *S. Leone* ... **112 D2** 8 22N 13 0W
Yaxi, *China* .... **76 D6** 27 33N 106 41 E
Yaxian = Sanya, *China* **86 C7** 18 14N 109 29 E
Yazagyo, *Burma* ..... **90 D5** 23 30N 94 6 E
Yazd, *Iran* .... **97 D7** 31 55N 54 27 E
Yazd □, *Iran* .... **97 D7** 32 0N 55 0 E
Yazd-e Khvāst, *Iran* .. **97 D7** 31 31N 52 7 E
Yazdān, *Iran* .... **91 B1** 33 30N 60 50 E
Yazıköy, *Turkey* ..... **49 E9** 36 40N 27 20 E
Yazman, *Pakistan* .... **92 E4** 29 8N 71 45 E
Yazoo →, *U.S.A.* **155 J9** 32 22N 90 54W
Yazoo City, *U.S.A.* ... **155 J9** 32 51N 90 25W
Ybbs, *Austria* .... **34 C8** 48 12N 15 4 E
Ybycuí, *Paraguay* .... **174 B4** 26 5 S 56 46W
Ybytyruzú △, *Paraguay* **175 B4** 25 51 S 56 11W
Yding Skovhøj,
  Denmark .... **17 J3** 55 59N 9 46 E
Ye, *Burma* .... **86 E1** 15 15N 97 15 E
Ye-ngan, *Burma* ..... **90 E6** 21 9N 96 27 E
Ye-u, *Burma* .... **90 D5** 22 46N 95 26 E
Ye Xian = Laizhou,
  China .... **75 F10** 37 8N 119 57 E
Ye Xian, *China* ...... **74 H7** 33 35N 113 25 E
Yea, *Australia* ...... **129 D6** 37 14 S 145 26 E
Yebawmi, *Burma* .... **90 C5** 25 15N 95 45 E
Yebbi-Souma, *Chad* .. **109 D3** 21 7N 17 54 E
Yebyu, *Burma* .... **86 E2** 14 15N 98 13 E
Yecheng, *China* ...... **65 E8** 37 54N 77 26 E
Yechon, *S. Korea* .... **75 F15** 36 39N 128 27 E
Yecla, *Spain* **41 G3** 38 35N 1 5W
Yécora, *Mexico* **162 B3** 28 20N 108 58W
Yedashe, *Burma* ..... **90 F6** 19 10N 96 20 E
Yedebub Biheroch
  Bihereseboch na
  Hizboch □, *Ethiopia* **107 F4** 12 0N 36 0 E
Yedintsy = Edineț,
  Moldova .... **53 B12** 48 9N 27 18 E
Yedri, *Chad* .... **109 D3** 22 25N 17 30 E
Yedseram →, *Nigeria* . **113 C7** 12 30N 14 5 E
Yefremov, *Russia* .... **58 F10** 53 8N 38 3 E
Yeghegnadzor,
  Armenia .... **101 C11** 39 44N 45 19 E
Yegorlyk →, *Russia* ... **61 G5** 46 35N 41 57 E
Yegorlykskaya, *Russia* **61 G5** 46 33N 40 35 E
Yegoryevsk, *Russia* ... **58 E10** 55 27N 38 55 E
Yegri-Dere = Ardino,
  Bulgaria .... **51 F9** 41 34N 25 9 E
Yegros, *Paraguay* .... **174 B4** 26 20 S 56 25W
Yehbuah, *Indonesia* .. **84 a** 8 23 S 114 45 E
Yehuda, Midbar, *Israel* **103 D4** 31 35N 35 15 E
Yei, *Sudan* .... **107 G3** 4 9N 30 40 E
Yei, Nahr →, *Sudan* .. **107 F3** 6 15N 30 13 E
Yejmiadzin, *Armenia* . **61 K7** 40 12N 44 19 E
Yekaterinburg, *Russia* **64 C8** 56 50N 60 30 E
Yekaterinoslav =
  Dnipro, *Ukraine* ... **59 H8** 48 30N 35 0 E
Yekaterinstadt =
  Marks, *Russia* ..... **60 E8** 51 45N 46 50 E
Yekaterinodar =
  Krasnodar, *Russia* .. **61 H4** 45 5N 39 0 E
Yekumbe, *Dem. Rep. of*
  the Congo .... **114 C4** 1 2 S 23 27 E
Yelabuga, *Russia* ..... **60 C11** 55 45N 52 0 E
Yelan, *Russia* .... **60 E6** 50 55N 43 43 E
Yelandur, *India* ...... **95 H3** 12 6N 77 0 E
Yelarbon, *Australia* ... **127 D5** 28 33 S 150 38 E
Yelatma, *Russia* ...... **60 C5** 55 0N 41 45 E
Yelcho, L., *Chile* ..... **176 B2** 43 18 S 72 18W
Yelenovskiye
  Karyery =
  Dokuchayevsk,
  Ukraine .... **59 J9** 47 44N 37 40 E
Yelets, *Russia* .... **59 F10** 52 40N 38 30 E
Yélimané, *Mali* **112 B2** 15 9N 10 34W
Yelizavetgrad =
  Kirovohrad, *Ukraine* **59 H7** 48 35N 32 20 E
Yelizavetgrad =
  Kirovohrad, *Ukraine* **59 H7** 48 35N 32 20 E
Yelizavetinka, *Russia* . **64 F7** 51 46N 59 45 E
Yell, *U.K.* **23 A7** 60 35N 1 5W
Yell Sd., *U.K.* **22 A7** 60 33N 1 15W
Yellamanchili =
  Elamanchili, *India* . **94 F6** 17 33N 82 50 E
Yellandu, *India* ...... **94 F5** 17 39N 80 23 E
Yellapur, *India* ...... **95 G2** 14 58N 74 43 E
Yellareddi, *India* ..... **94 E4** 18 12N 78 2 E
Yellow = Huang He →,
  China .... **75 F10** 37 55N 118 50 E
Yellow Sea, *China* .... **75 G12** 35 0N 123 0 E
Yellowhead Pass,
  Canada **142 C5** 52 53N 118 25W
Yellowknife, *Canada* . **142 A6** 62 27N 114 29W
Yellowknife →,
  Canada **142 A6** 62 31N 114 19W
Yellowstone △, *U.S.A.* **158 D9** 44 40N 110 30W
Yellowstone →, *U.S.A.* **154 B2** 47 59N 103 59W
Yellowstone L., *U.S.A.* **158 D8** 44 27N 110 22W
Yelnya, *Russia* ...... **58 E7** 54 35N 33 15 E
Yelsk, *Belarus* .... **59 G5** 51 50N 29 10 E
Yelwa, *Nigeria* ...... **113 C5** 10 49N 4 41 E
Yemanzhelinsk, *Russia* **64 D8** 54 58N 61 18 E
Yemassee, *U.S.A.* **152 C9** 32 41N 80 51W
Yembongo, *Dem. Rep.*
  of the Congo ..... **114 B3** 3 12N 19 2 E
Yemen ■, *Asia* ...... **98 D4** 15 0N 44 0 E
Yemmiganur, *India* .. **95 G3** 15 44N 77 29 E
Yen Bai, *Vietnam* .... **76 G5** 21 42N 104 52 E
Yenagoa, *Nigeria* .... **113 E6** 4 58N 6 16 E
Yenakiyeve, *Ukraine* . **59 H10** 48 15N 38 15 E
Yenakiyevo =
  Yenakiyeve, *Ukraine* **59 H10** 48 15N 38 15 E
Yenangyat, *Burma* ... **90 E5** 21 6N 94 48 E
Yenangyaung, *Burma* **90 E5** 20 30N 94 59 E
Yenanma, *Burma* .... **90 F5** 19 46N 94 49 E
Yenbo = Yanbu 'al
  Baḥr, *Si. Arabia* ... **96 F3** 24 0N 38 5 E

Yenda, *Australia* **129 C7** 34 13 S 146 14 E
Yende Millimou,
Guinea **112 D2** 8 55N 10 10W
Yendéré, *Burkina Faso* **112 C4** 10 12N 4 59W
Yendi, *Ghana* **113 D4** 9 29N 0 1W
Yengisar, *China* **65 D8** 38 56N 76 9 E
Yengo, *Congo* **114 B3** 0 22N 15 29 E
Yengo △, *Australia* **129 B9** 33 0 S 150 55 E
Yéni, *Niger* **113 C5** 13 30N 3 1 E
Yeni-Pazar = Novi
Pazar, *Serbia & M.* **50 C4** 43 12N 20 28 E
Yenice, *Ankara, Turkey* **100 C5** 39 14N 32 42 E
Yenice, *Aydın, Turkey* **49 D10** 37 49N 28 35 E
Yenice, *Çanakkale,*
Turkey **49 B9** 39 55N 27 17 E
Yenice, *Edirne, Turkey* **51 F10** 40 42N 26 9 E
Yenice →, *Turkey* **100 D6** 37 37N 35 33 E
Yenifoça, *Turkey* **49 C8** 38 44N 26 51 E
Yenihisar, *Turkey* **49 D9** 37 22N 27 16 E
Yeniköy, *Bursa, Turkey* **51 F13** 40 31N 29 22 E
Yeniköy, *Çanakkale,*
Turkey **49 B8** 39 55N 26 10 E
Yeniköy, *Kütahya,*
Turkey **49 C11** 38 52N 29 17 E
Yenipazar, *Turkey* **49 D10** 37 49N 28 11 E
Yenisaía, *Greece* **51 E8** 41 1N 24 57 E
Yenişehir, *Turkey* **51 F13** 40 16N 29 38 E
Yenisey →, *Russia* **66 B9** 71 50N 82 40 E
Yeniseysk, *Russia* **67 D10** 58 27N 92 13 E
Yeniseyskiy Zaliv,
Russia **66 B9** 72 20N 81 0 E
Yenki = Yanji, *China* **75 C15** 42 59N 129 30 E
Yennádhi, *Greece* **38 E11** 36 2N 27 56 E
Yenne, *France* **29 C9** 45 43N 5 44 E
Yenotayevka, *Russia* **61 G8** 47 15N 47 0 E
Yenyuka, *Russia* **67 D13** 57 57N 121 15 E
Yeo →, *U.K.* **21 G5** 51 2N 2 49W
Yeo, L., *Australia* **125 E3** 28 0 S 124 30 E
Yeo I., *Canada* **150 A3** 45 24N 81 48W
Yeola, *India* **94 D2** 20 2N 74 30 E
Yeoryioúpolis, *Greece* **39 E5** 35 20N 24 15 E
Yeovil, *U.K.* **21 G5** 50 57N 2 38W
Yepes, *Spain* **42 F7** 39 55N 3 39W
Yeppoon, *Australia* **126 C5** 23 5 S 150 47 E
Yérakas, *Ákra, Greece* **39 D2** 37 42N 20 59 E
Yeráki, *Greece* **48 D4** 37 0N 22 42 E
Yerbent, *Turkmenistan* **66 F6** 39 30N 58 50 E
Yerbogachen, *Russia* **67 C11** 61 16N 108 0 E
Yerevan, *Armenia* **61 K7** 40 10N 44 31 E
Yerington, *U.S.A.* **158 G4** 38 59N 119 10W
Yerkesik, *Turkey* **49 D10** 37 7N 28 19 E
Yerköy, *Turkey* **100 C6** 39 38N 34 28 E
Yerla →, *India* **94 F2** 16 50N 74 30 E
Yermak, *Kazakhstan* **66 D8** 52 2N 76 55 E
Yermo, *U.S.A.* **161 L10** 34 54N 116 50W
Yerólakkos, *Cyprus* **39 E9** 35 11N 33 15 E
Yeropol, *Russia* **67 C17** 65 15N 168 40 E
Yeropótamos →,
Greece **39 E5** 35 3N 24 50 E
Yeroskipos, *Cyprus* **39 F8** 34 46N 32 28 E
Yershov, *Russia* **60 E9** 51 23N 48 27 E
Yerupaja, Cerro, *Peru* **172 C2** 10 16 S 76 55W
Yerushalayim =
Jerusalem, *Israel* **103 D4** 31 47N 35 10 E
Yerville, *France* **26 C7** 49 40N 0 53 E
Yerzhar = Gagarin,
Uzbekistan **65 C4** 40 39N 68 10 E
Yes Tor, *U.K.* **21 G4** 50 41N 4 0W
Yesagyo, *Burma* **90 E5** 21 38N 95 14 E
Yesan, *S. Korea* **75 F14** 36 41N 126 51 E
Yeshin, *Burma* **90 D5** 23 43N 95 6 E
Yeşilhisar, *Turkey* **100 C6** 38 20N 35 5 E
Yeşilırmak →, *Turkey* **100 B7** 41 22N 36 37 E
Yeşilkent, *Turkey* **100 D7** 36 57N 36 12 E
Yeşilköy, *Turkey* **51 F12** 40 57N 28 49 E
Yeşilova, *Turkey* **49 D11** 37 31N 29 46 E
Yeşilyurt, *Manisa,*
Turkey **49 C10** 38 22N 28 40 E
Yeşilyurt, *Muğla,*
Turkey **49 D10** 37 10N 28 20 E
Yeski Dzhumaya =
Târgovişte, *Romania* **53 F10** 44 55N 25 27 E
Yesnogorsk, *Russia* **58 E9** 54 32N 37 38 E
Yeso, *U.S.A.* **155 H2** 34 26N 104 37W
Yessentuki, *Russia* **61 H6** 44 5N 42 53 E
Yessey, *Russia* **67 C11** 68 29N 102 10 E
Yeste, *Spain* **41 G2** 38 22N 2 19W
Yetman, *Australia* **127 D5** 28 56 S 150 48 E
Yetti, *Mauritania* **110 C3** 26 10N 7 50W
Yeu, Î. d', *France* **26 F4** 46 42N 2 20W
Yevdokimovskoye =
Krasnogvardeyskoye,
Russia **61 H5** 45 52N 41 33 E
Yevlakh = Yevlax,
Azerbaijan **61 K8** 40 39N 47 7 E
Yevlax, *Azerbaijan* **61 K8** 40 39N 47 7 E
Yevpatoriya, *Ukraine* **59 K7** 45 15N 33 20 E
Yeya →, *Russia* **59 J10** 46 40N 38 40 E
Yeysk, *Russia* **59 J10** 46 40N 38 12 E
Yezd = Yazd, *Iran* **97 D7** 31 55N 54 27 E
Yezerishche, *Belarus* **58 E5** 55 50N 29 59 E
Yhati, *Paraguay* **174 B4** 25 45 S 56 35W
Yhú, *Paraguay* **175 B4** 25 0 S 56 0W
Yi →, *Uruguay* **174 C4** 33 7 S 57 8W
Yi 'Allaq, G., *Egypt* **103 E2** 30 22N 33 32 E
Yi He →, *China* **75 G10** 34 10N 118 8 E
Yi Xian, *Anhui, China* **77 C11** 29 55N 117 57 E
Yi Xian, *Hebei, China* **74 E8** 39 20N 115 30 E
Yi Xian, *Liaoning,*
China **75 D11** 41 30N 121 22 E
Yialí, *Greece* **49 E9** 36 41N 27 11 E
Yialiás →, *Cyprus* **39 E9** 35 9N 33 44 E
Yi'allaq, G., *Egypt* **106 A3** 30 21N 33 31 E
Yialousa, *Cyprus* **39 E10** 35 32N 34 10 E
Yiáltra, *Greece* **48 C4** 38 51N 22 59 E
Yianisádhes, *Greece* **39 E7** 35 20N 26 10 E
Yiannitsa, *Greece* **50 F6** 40 46N 22 24 E
Yibin, *China* **76 C5** 28 45N 104 32 E
Yichang, *China* **77 B8** 30 40N 111 20 E
Yicheng, *Henan, China* **77 B9** 31 41N 112 12 E
Yicheng, *Shanxi, China* **74 G6** 35 42N 111 40 E
Yichuan, *China* **74 F6** 36 2N 110 10 E
Yichun, *Heilongjiang,*
China **69 B7** 47 44N 128 52 E
Yichun, *Jiangxi, China* **77 D10** 27 48N 114 22 E
Yidu, *China* **75 F10** 36 43N 118 28 E
Yidun, *China* **76 B2** 30 22N 99 21 E
Yifag, *Ethiopia* **107 E4** 12 4N 37 46 E
Yifeng, *China* **77 C10** 28 22N 114 45 E
Yihuang, *China* **77 D11** 27 30N 116 12 E
Yijun, *China* **74 G5** 35 28N 109 8 E
Yıldız Dağları, *Turkey* **51 E11** 41 48N 27 36 E
Yıldızeli, *Turkey* **100 C7** 39 51N 36 36 E
Yilehuli Shan, *China* **69 A7** 51 20N 124 20 E
Yiliang, *Yunnan, China* **76 D5** 27 38N 104 2 E
Yiliang, *Yunnan, China* **76 E4** 24 56N 103 11 E
Yilong, *China* **76 B6** 31 34N 106 23 E
Yimen, *China* **76 E4** 24 40N 102 10 E
Yimianpo, *China* **75 B15** 45 7N 128 2 E
Yinchuan, *China* **74 E4** 38 30N 106 15 E
Yindaik, *Burma* **90 G6** 23 35N 95 22 E
Yindargooda, L.,
Australia **125 F3** 30 40 S 121 52 E
Ying He →, *China* **74 H9** 32 30N 116 30 E
Ying Xian, *China* **74 E7** 39 32N 113 10 E
Yingcheng, *China* **77 B9** 30 56N 113 35 E
Yingde, *China* **77 E9** 24 10N 113 25 E
Yingjiang, *China* **76 E1** 24 41N 97 55 E
Yingjing, *China* **76 C4** 29 41N 102 52 E
Yingkou, *China* **75 D12** 40 37N 122 18 E
Yingkow = Yingkou,
China **75 D12** 40 37N 122 18 E
Yingshan, *Henan,*
China **77 B9** 31 35N 113 50 E
Yingshan, *Hubei, China* **77 B10** 30 41N 115 32 E
Yingshan, *Sichuan,*
China **76 B6** 31 4N 106 35 E
Yingshang, *China* **77 A11** 32 38N 116 12 E
Yingtan, *China* **77 C11** 28 12N 117 0 E
Yining, *China* **66 E9** 43 58N 81 10 E
Yinjiang, *China* **76 C7** 28 1N 108 21 E
Yinmabin, *Burma* **90 D5** 22 10N 94 55 E
Yiofiros →, *Greece* **39 E6** 35 20N 25 6 E
Yioúra, *Nótios Aiyaíon,*
Greece **48 D6** 37 32N 24 40 E
Yioúra, *Thessalía,*
Greece **48 B6** 39 23N 24 10 E
Yipinglang, *China* **76 E3** 25 10N 101 52 E
Yirápetra, *Ákra,*
Greece **39 B2** 38 51N 20 41 E
Yirba Muda, *Ethiopia* **107 F4** 6 12N 38 42 E
Yirga Alem, *Ethiopia* **107 F4** 6 48N 38 22 E
Yirol, *Sudan* **107 F3** 6 33N 30 30 E
Yirrkala, *Australia* **126 A2** 12 14 S 136 56 E
Yishan, *China* **76 E7** 24 28N 108 38 E
Yishui, *China* **75 G10** 35 47N 118 30 E
Yishun, *Singapore* **87 d** 1 26N 103 50 E
Yíthion, *Greece* **48 E4** 36 46N 22 34 E
Yitong, *China* **75 C13** 43 13N 125 20 E
Yiwu, *China* **77 C13** 29 20N 120 3 E
Yixing, *China* **77 B12** 31 21N 119 48 E
Yiyang, *Henan, China* **74 G7** 34 27N 112 10 E
Yiyang, *Hunan, China* **77 C9** 28 35N 112 18 E
Yiyang, *Jiangxi, China* **77 C11** 28 22N 117 20 E
Yizhang, *China* **77 E9** 25 27N 112 57 E
Yizheng, *China* **77 A12** 32 18N 119 10 E
Yli-Kitka, *Finland* **14 C23** 66 8N 28 30 E
Ylitornio, *Finland* **14 C20** 66 19N 23 39 E
Ylivieska, *Finland* **14 D21** 64 4N 24 28 E
Yngaren, *Sweden* **17 F10** 58 50N 16 35 E
Yoakum, *U.S.A.* **155 L6** 29 17N 97 9W
Yob △, *Eritrea* **107 D4** 17 15N 37 50 E
Yobe □, *Nigeria* **113 C7** 12 0N 11 30 E
Yobuko, *Japan* **72 D1** 33 32N 129 54 E
Yog Pt., *Phil.* **80 D5** 14 6N 124 12 E
Yogan, *Togo* **113 D5** 6 23N 1 30 E
Yoğuntaş, *Turkey* **51 E11** 41 50N 27 4 E
Yogyakarta, *Indonesia* **85 D4** 7 49 S 110 22 E
Yogyakarta □,
Indonesia **85 D4** 7 48 S 110 22 E
Yoho △, *Canada* **142 C5** 51 25N 116 30W
Yojoa, L. de, *Honduras* **164 D2** 14 53N 88 0W
Yŏju, *S. Korea* **75 F14** 37 20N 127 35 E
Yok Don △, *Vietnam* **86 F6** 12 50N 107 40 E
Yokadouma, *Cameroon* **114 B2** 3 26N 14 55 E
Yokkaichi, *Japan* **73 B8** 35 6N 136 12 E
Yŏkaichiba, *Japan* **73 B12** 35 42N 140 33 E
Yokkaichi, *Japan* **73 C8** 34 55N 136 38 E
Yoko, *Cameroon* **113 D7** 5 32N 12 20 E
Yokohama, *Japan* **73 B11** 35 27N 139 28 E
Yokosuka, *Japan* **73 B11** 35 20N 139 40 E
Yokote, *Japan* **70 E10** 39 20N 140 30 E
Yola, *Nigeria* **113 D7** 9 10N 12 29 E
Yolaina, Cordillera de,
Nic. **164 D3** 11 30N 84 0W
Yolombo, *Dem. Rep. of*
the Congo **114 C4** 1 36 S 23 12 E
Yoloten, *Turkmenistan* **97 B9** 37 18N 62 21 E
Yom →, *Thailand* **78 A2** 15 35N 100 1 E
Yombi, *Gabon* **114 C2** 1 26 S 10 37 E
Yonago, *Japan* **72 B5** 35 25N 133 19 E
Yonaguni-Jima, *Japan* **71 M1** 24 27N 123 0 E
Yŏnan, *N. Korea* **75 F14** 37 55N 126 11 E
Yonezawa, *Japan* **70 F10** 37 57N 140 4 E
Yong Peng, *Malaysia* **87 L4** 2 0N 103 3 E
Yong Sata, *Thailand* **87 J2** 7 8N 99 41 E
Yongama, *Dem. Rep. of*
the Congo **114 B4** 0 2N 24 35 E
Yongamp'o, *N. Korea* **75 E13** 39 56N 124 23 E
Yong'an, *China* **77 E11** 25 59N 117 25 E
Yongcheng, *China* **74 H9** 33 55N 116 20 E
Yŏngch'ŏn, *S. Korea* **75 G15** 35 58N 128 56 E
Yongchuan, *China* **76 C5** 29 17N 105 55 E
Yongchun, *China* **77 E12** 25 16N 118 20 E
Yongde, *China* **76 E2** 24 5N 99 25 E
Yongdeng, *China* **74 F2** 36 38N 103 25 E
Yongding, *China* **77 E11** 24 43N 116 45 E
Yŏngdŏk, *S. Korea* **75 F15** 36 24N 129 22 E
Yŏngdŭngpo, *S. Korea* **75 F14** 37 31N 126 54 E
Yongfeng, *China* **77 D10** 27 20N 115 22 E
Yongfu, *China* **76 E7** 24 59N 109 59 E
Yonggyap Pass, *India* **90 A5** 29 17N 95 37 E
Yonghe, *China* **74 F6** 36 46N 110 38 E
Yonghong, *India* **90 B5** 26 28N 94 58 E
Yŏnghŭng, *N. Korea* **75 E14** 39 31N 127 18 E
Yongji, *China* **74 G6** 34 52N 110 28 E
Yongjia, *China* **77 C13** 28 10N 120 45 E
Yŏngju, *S. Korea* **75 F15** 36 50N 128 40 E
Yongkang, *Yunnan,*
China **76 E2** 24 9N 99 20 E
Yongkang, *Zhejiang,*
China **77 C13** 28 55N 120 2 E
Yongnian, *China* **74 F8** 36 47N 114 29 E
Yongning,
Guangxi Zhuangzu,
China **76 F7** 22 44N 108 28 E
Yongning,
Ningxia Huizu, China **74 E4** 38 15N 106 14 E
Yongping, *China* **76 E2** 25 27N 99 38 E
Yongqing, *China* **74 E9** 39 25N 116 28 E
Yongren, *China* **76 D3** 26 4N 101 40 E
Yongshan, *China* **76 C4** 28 11N 103 35 E
Yongsheng, *China* **76 D3** 26 38N 100 46 E
Yongshun, *China* **76 C7** 29 2N 109 51 E
Yongtai, *China* **77 E12** 25 49N 118 58 E
Yŏngwŏl, *S. Korea* **75 F15** 37 11N 128 28 E
Yongxin =
Jinggangshan, *China* **77 D10** 26 58N 114 15 E
Yongxing, *China* **77 D9** 26 9N 113 8 E
Yongxiu, *China* **77 C10** 29 2N 115 42 E
Yongzhou, *China* **77 D8** 26 17N 111 37 E
Yonibana, *S. Leone* **112 D2** 8 30N 12 19W
Yonkers, *U.S.A.* **151 F11** 40 56N 73 54W
Yonne □, *France* **27 E10** 47 50N 3 40 E
Yonne →, *France* **27 D9** 48 23N 2 58 E
Yopal, *Colombia* **168 B3** 5 21N 72 23W
Yopurga, *China* **65 D8** 39 15N 76 45 E
York, *Australia* **125 F2** 31 52 S 116 47 E
York, *U.K.* **20 D6** 53 58N 1 6W
York, *Ala., U.S.A.* **155 J10** 32 29N 88 18W
York, *Nebr., U.S.A.* **154 E6** 40 52N 97 36W
York, *Pa., U.S.A.* **148 F7** 39 58N 76 44W
York, C., *Australia* **126 A3** 10 42 S 142 31 E
York, City of □, *U.K.* **20 D6** 53 58N 1 6W
York, Kap, *Greenland* **10 B4** 75 55N 66 25W
York, Vale of, *U.K.* **20 C6** 54 15N 1 25W
York Haven, *U.S.A.* **150 F8** 40 7N 76 46W
York Sd., *Australia* **124 C4** 15 0 S 125 5 E
Yorke Pen., *Australia* **128 C2** 34 50 S 137 40 E
Yorketown, *Australia* **128 C2** 35 0 S 137 33 E
Yorkshire Dales △,
U.K. **20 C5** 54 12N 2 10W
Yorkshire Wolds, *U.K.* **20 C7** 54 8N 0 31W
Yorkton, *Canada* **143 C8** 51 11N 102 28W
Yorkville, *Calif., U.S.A.* **160 G3** 38 52N 123 13W
Yorkville, *Ga., U.S.A.* **152 B5** 33 55N 84 58W
Yorkville, *Ill., U.S.A.* **157 C8** 41 38N 88 27W
Yoro, *Honduras* **164 C2** 15 9N 87 7W
Yoron-Jima, *Japan* **71 L4** 27 2N 128 26 E
Yorosso, *Mali* **112 C4** 12 17N 4 55W
Yos Sudarso, Pulau =
Dolak, Pulau,
Indonesia **83 C5** 8 0 S 138 30 E
Yos Sudarso, Teluk,
Indonesia **83 B6** 2 35 S 140 45 E
Yosemite △, *U.S.A.* **160 H7** 37 45N 119 40W
Yosemite Village,
U.S.A. **160 H7** 37 45N 119 35W
Yoshida, *Japan* **72 C4** 34 40N 132 42 E
Yoshimatsu, *Japan* **72 F2** 32 0N 130 47 E
Yoshino-Kumano △,
Japan **73 C7** 34 12N 135 55 E
Yoshkar Ola, *Russia* **60 B8** 56 38N 47 55 E
Yŏsu, *S. Korea* **75 G14** 34 47N 127 45 E
Yotala, *Bolivia* **173 D4** 19 10 S 65 17W
Yotvata, *Israel* **103 F4** 29 55N 35 2 E
You Jiang →, *China* **76 F6** 22 50N 108 6 E
You Xian, *China* **77 D9** 27 1N 113 17 E
Youbou, *Canada* **160 B2** 48 53N 124 13W
Youghal, *Ireland* **23 E4** 51 56N 7 52W
Youghal B., *Ireland* **23 E4** 51 55N 7 49W
Youkounkoun, *Guinea* **112 C2** 12 35N 13 11W
Young, *Australia* **129 C8** 34 19 S 148 18 E
Young, *Canada* **143 C7** 51 47N 105 45W
Young, *Uruguay* **174 C4** 32 44 S 57 36W
Young Ra., *N.Z.* **131 E4** 44 10 S 169 30 E
Younghusband, L.,
Australia **128 A2** 30 50 S 136 5 E
Younghusband Pen.,
Australia **128 D3** 36 0 S 139 25 E
Youngstown, *Canada* **143 C6** 51 35N 111 10W
Youngstown, *Fla.,*
U.S.A. **152 E4** 30 22N 85 26W
Youngstown, *N.Y.,*
U.S.A. **150 C5** 43 15N 79 3W
Youngstown, *Ohio,*
U.S.A. **150 E4** 41 6N 80 39W
Youngsville, *U.S.A.* **150 E5** 41 51N 79 19W
Youngwood, *U.S.A.* **150 F5** 40 14N 79 34W
Youssoufia, *Morocco* **110 B3** 32 16N 8 31W
Youxi, *China* **77 D12** 26 10N 118 13 E
Youyang, *China* **76 C7** 28 47N 108 42 E
Youyu, *China* **74 D7** 40 10N 112 20 E
Yozgat, *Turkey* **100 C6** 39 51N 34 47 E
Ypacaraí △, *Paraguay* **174 B4** 25 18 S 57 19W
Ypané →, *Paraguay* **174 A4** 23 29 S 57 19W
Yport, *France* **26 C7** 49 45N 0 15 E
Ypres = Ieper, *Belgium* **24 D2** 50 51N 2 53 E
Ypsilanti, *U.S.A.* **157 B13** 42 14N 83 37W
Yreka, *U.S.A.* **158 F2** 41 44N 122 38W
Ysabel Chan.,
Papua N. G. **132 B5** 2 0 S 150 0 E
Yssingeaux, *France* **29 C8** 45 9N 4 8 E
Ystabø, *Norway* **18 E2** 59 3N 5 23 E
Ystad, *Sweden* **17 J7** 55 26N 13 50 E
Ysyk-Köl = Balykchy,
Kyrgyzstan **65 B8** 42 26N 76 12 E
Ysyk-Köl, *Kyrgyzstan* **65 B8** 42 25N 77 15 E
Ythan →, *U.K.* **22 D7** 57 19N 1 59W
Ytre Arna, *Norway* **18 D2** 60 27N 5 25 E
Ytre Enebakk, *Norway* **18 E5** 59 44N 11 0 E
Ytre Rendal, *Norway* **18 C8** 61 46N 11 8 E
Ytterhogdal, *Sweden* **16 B8** 62 12N 14 56 E
Ytyk-Kyuyel, *Russia* **67 C14** 62 30N 133 45 E
Yu Jiang →, *China* **76 F7** 23 22N 110 3 E
Yu Shan, *Taiwan* **77 F13** 23 30N 120 58 E
Yu Xian = Yuzhou,
China **74 G7** 34 10N 113 28 E
Yu Xian, *Hebei, China* **74 E8** 39 50N 114 35 E
Yu Xian, *Shanxi, China* **74 E7** 38 5N 113 20 E
Yuan Jiang →, *Hunan,*
China **77 C8** 28 55N 111 50 E
Yuan Jiang →,
Yunnan, China **76 F4** 22 20N 103 59 E
Yuan'an, *China* **77 B8** 31 3N 111 34 E
Yuanjiang, *Hunan,*
China **77 C9** 28 47N 112 21 E
Yuanjiang, *Yunnan,*
China **76 F4** 23 32N 102 0 E
Yüanli, *Taiwan* **77 E13** 24 27N 120 39 E
Yüanlin, *Taiwan* **77 F13** 23 58N 120 30 E
Yuanling, *China* **77 C8** 28 29N 110 22 E
Yuanmou, *China* **76 E3** 25 42N 101 53 E
Yuanqu, *China* **74 G6** 35 18N 111 40 E
Yuanyang, *Henan,*
China **74 G7** 35 3N 113 58 E
Yuanyang, *Yunnan,*
China **76 F4** 23 10N 102 43 E
Yuat →, *Papua N. G.* **132 C2** 4 10 S 143 52 E
Yuba →, *U.S.A.* **160 F5** 39 8N 121 36W
Yuba City, *U.S.A.* **160 F5** 39 8N 121 37W
Yūbari, *Japan* **70 C10** 43 4N 141 59 E
Yubdo, *Ethiopia* **107 F4** 8 58N 35 24 E
Yūbetsu, *Japan* **70 B11** 44 13N 143 50 E
Yubo, *Sudan* **107 F2** 5 23N 27 25 E
Yucatán □, *Mexico* **163 C7** 21 30N 86 30W
Yucatán, Canal de,
Caribbean **164 B2** 22 0N 86 30W
Yucatán, Península de,
Mexico **136 H11** 19 30N 89 0W
Yucatan Basin,
Cent. Amer. **136 H11** 19 0N 86 0W
Yucatan Channel =
Yucatán, Canal de,
Caribbean **164 B2** 22 0N 86 30W
Yucca, *U.S.A.* **161 L12** 34 52N 114 9W
Yucca Valley, *U.S.A.* **161 L10** 34 8N 116 27W
Yucheng, *China* **74 F9** 36 55N 116 32 E
Yuci, *China* **74 F7** 37 42N 112 46 E
Yudu, *China* **77 E10** 25 59N 115 30 E
Yuechi, *China* **76 B6** 30 34N 106 25 E
Yuen Long, *China* **69 G11** 22 26N 114 2 E
Yuendumu, *Australia* **124 D5** 22 16 S 131 49 E
Yueqing, *China* **77 C13** 28 9N 120 59 E
Yueqing Wan, *China* **77 D13** 28 5N 121 20 E
Yuexi, *Anhui, China* **77 B11** 30 50N 116 20 E
Yuexi, *Sichuan, China* **76 C4** 28 37N 102 26 E
Yueyang, *China* **77 C9** 29 21N 113 5 E
Yufu-Dake, *Japan* **72 D3** 33 17N 131 33 E
Yugan, *China* **77 C11** 28 43N 116 37 E
Yugoslavia = Serbia &
Montenegro ■,
Europe **50 C4** 43 20N 20 0 E
Yuhuan, *China* **77 C13** 28 9N 121 12 E
Yuhuan Dao, *China* **77 C13** 28 5N 121 15 E
Yujiang, *China* **77 C11** 28 10N 116 43 E
Yukhnov, *Russia* **58 E8** 54 44N 35 15 E
Yūki, *Japan* **73 A11** 36 18N 139 53 E
Yukon, *U.S.A.* **155 H6** 35 31N 97 45W
Yukon →, *U.S.A.* **144 E7** 62 32N 163 54W
Yukon-Charley
Rivers △, *U.S.A.* **144 C12** 65 15N 144 0W
Yukon Territory □,
Canada **138 B6** 63 0N 135 0W
Yüksekova, *Turkey* **101 D11** 37 34N 44 16 E
Yukta, *Russia* **67 C11** 63 26N 105 42 E
Yukuhashi, *Japan* **72 D2** 33 44N 130 59 E
Yulara, *Australia* **125 E5** 25 10 S 130 55 E
Yule →, *Australia* **124 D2** 20 41 S 118 17 E
Yuleba, *Australia* **127 D4** 26 37 S 149 24 E
Yulee, *U.S.A.* **152 E8** 30 38N 81 36W
Yuli, *Nigeria* **113 D7** 9 44N 10 12 E
Yuli, *Taiwan* **77 F13** 23 20N 121 18 E
Yulin,
Guangxi Zhuangzu,
China **77 F8** 22 40N 110 8 E
Yulin, *Hainan, China* **86 C7** 18 10N 109 31 E
Yulin, *Shaanxi, China* **74 E5** 38 20N 109 30 E
Yuma, *Ariz., U.S.A.* **161 N12** 32 43N 114 37W
Yuma, *Colo., U.S.A.* **154 E3** 40 8N 102 43W
Yuma, B. de,
Dom. Rep. **165 C6** 18 20N 68 35W
Yumali, *Australia* **128 C3** 35 32 S 139 45 E
Yumbe, *Uganda* **118 B3** 3 28N 31 15 E
Yumbi, *Équateur,*
Dem. Rep. of
the Congo **114 C3** 1 53 S 16 34 E
Yumbi, *Maniema,*
Dem. Rep. of
the Congo **118 C2** 1 12 S 26 15 E
Yumbo, *Colombia* **168 C2** 3 35N 76 28W
Yumen, *China* **68 C4** 39 50N 97 30 E
Yumurtalık, *Turkey* **100 D6** 36 45N 35 43 E
Yun Gui Gaoyuan,
China **76 E3** 26 0N 104 0 E
Yun Ho →, *China* **75 E9** 39 10N 117 10 E
Yun Ling, *China* **76 D2** 27 0N 99 20 E
Yun Xian, *Hubei,*
China **77 A8** 32 50N 110 46 E
Yun Xian, *Yunnan,*
China **76 E3** 24 27N 100 8 E
Yuna, *Australia* **125 E2** 28 20 S 115 0 E
Yunak, *Turkey* **100 C4** 38 49N 31 43 E
Yunan, *China* **77 F8** 23 12N 111 30 E
Yunaska I., *U.S.A.* **144 K5** 52 38N 170 40W
Yuncheng, *Henan,*
China **74 G8** 35 36N 115 57 E
Yuncheng, *Shanxi,*
China **74 G6** 35 2N 111 0 E
Yunfu, *China* **77 F9** 22 50N 112 5 E
Yungas, *Bolivia* **173 D4** 17 0 S 66 0W
Yungay, *Chile* **174 D1** 37 10 S 72 5W
Yungay, *Peru* **172 B2** 9 2 S 77 45W
Yungki = Jilin, *China* **75 C14** 43 44N 126 30 E
Yungning = Nanning,
China **76 F7** 22 48N 108 20 E
Yunhe, *China* **77 C12** 28 8N 119 33 E
Yunkai Dashan, *China* **77 F8** 22 30N 111 0 E
Yunlin, *Taiwan* **77 F13** 23 42N 120 30 E
Yunlong, *China* **76 E2** 25 57N 99 13 E
Yunmeng, *China* **77 B9** 31 2N 113 43 E
Yunnan □, *China* **76 E4** 25 0N 102 0 E
Yunotsu, *Japan* **72 B4** 35 5N 132 21 E
Yunquera de Henares,
Spain **40 E1** 40 47N 3 11W
Yunt Dağı, *Turkey* **49 C9** 38 56N 27 13 E
Yunta, *Australia* **127 E2** 32 34 S 139 36 E
Yunxi, *China* **74 H6** 33 0N 110 22 E
Yunxiao, *China* **77 F11** 23 59N 117 18 E
Yuping, *China* **76 D7** 27 13N 108 56 E
Yupukarri, *Guyana* **169 C6** 3 45N 59 20W
Yupyongdong,
N. Korea **75 D15** 41 49N 128 53 E
Yuqing, *China* **76 D6** 27 13N 107 53 E
Yuraygir △, *Australia* **127 D5** 29 45 S 153 15 E
Yurga, *Russia* **66 D9** 55 42N 84 51 E
Yurimaguas, *Peru* **172 B2** 5 55 S 76 7W
Yurkiyka, *Ukraine* **53 B13** 48 42N 28 35 E
Yurla, *Russia* **64 B5** 59 22N 54 21 E
Yurubí △, *Venezuela* **165 D6** 10 26N 68 42W
Yurya, *Russia* **64 B2** 59 1N 49 13 E
Yuryev = Tartu,
Estonia **15 G22** 58 20N 26 44 E
Yuryev-Polskiy, *Russia* **58 D10** 56 30N 39 40 E
Yuryevets, *Russia* **60 B6** 57 25N 43 2 E
Yuryuzan, *Russia* **64 D7** 54 57N 58 28 E
Yuscarán, *Honduras* **164 D2** 13 58N 86 45W
Yūsef, Bahr →, *Egypt* **106 B3** 28 25N 30 35 E
Yushan, *China* **77 C12** 28 42N 118 10 E
Yushanzhen, *China* **76 C7** 29 28N 108 22 E
Yushe, *China* **74 F7** 37 4N 112 58 E
Yushu, *Jilin, China* **75 B14** 44 43N 126 38 E
Yushu, *Qinghai, China* **68 C4** 33 5N 96 55 E
Yusufeli, *Turkey* **101 B9** 40 50N 41 33 E
Yutai, *China* **74 G9** 35 0N 116 45 E
Yutian, *China* **75 E9** 39 53N 117 45 E
Yütze = Yuci, *China* **74 F7** 37 42N 112 46 E
Yuxarı Qarabağ =
Nagorno-
Karabakh □,
Azerbaijan **101 C12** 39 55N 46 45 E
Yuxi, *China* **76 E4** 24 30N 102 35 E
Yuyao, *China* **77 B13** 30 3N 121 10 E
Yuzawa, *Japan* **70 E10** 39 10N 140 30 E
Yuzha, *Russia* **60 B6** 56 34N 42 1 E
Yuzhno-Sakhalinsk,
Russia **67 E15** 46 58N 142 45 E
Yuzhnouralsk, *Russia* **64 D8** 54 26N 61 15 E
Yuzhnyy □, *Russia* **61 H5** 44 0N 40 0 E
Yuzhou, *China* **74 G7** 34 10N 113 28 E
Yuzovka = Donetsk,
Ukraine **59 J9** 48 0N 37 45 E
Yvelines □, *France* **27 D8** 48 40N 1 45 E
Yverdon-les-Bains,
Switz. **32 C3** 46 47N 6 39 E
Yvetot, *France* **26 C7** 49 37N 0 44 E
Yvonand, *Switz.* **32 C3** 46 48N 6 44 E
Yzeure, *France* **27 F10** 46 33N 3 22 E

Z

Zaalayskiy Khrebet,
Tajikistan **65 D6** 39 20N 73 0 E
Zaanstad, *Neths.* **24 B4** 52 27N 4 50 E
Zab, Monts du, *Algeria* **111 B6** 34 55N 5 0 E
Zāb al Kabīr →, *Iraq* **101 D10** 36 1N 43 24 E
Zāb aş Şaghīr →, *Iraq* **101 E10** 35 17N 43 29 E
Žabalj, *Serbia & M.* **52 E5** 45 21N 20 5 E
Žabari, *Serbia & M.* **50 B5** 44 22N 21 15 E
Zabarjad, *Egypt* **106 C4** 23 40N 36 12 E
Zabaykalsk, *Russia* **67 E12** 49 40N 117 25 E
Zabbar, *Malta* **38 F8** 35 53N 14 32 E
Zabīd, *Yemen* **98 D3** 14 0N 43 10 E
Zabīd, W. →, *Yemen* **98 D3** 14 7N 43 6 E
Zabki, *Poland* **55 F8** 52 17N 21 6 E
Ząbkowice Śląskie,
Poland **55 H3** 50 35N 16 50 E
Žabljak, *Serbia & M.* **50 C3** 43 18N 19 5 E
Zabłudów, *Poland* **55 F9** 53 0N 23 19 E
Žabno, *Poland* **55 H7** 50 9N 20 53 E
Zābol, *Iran* **97 D9** 31 0N 61 32 E
Zābol □, *Afghan.* **91 B2** 32 0N 67 0 E
Zābolī, *Iran* **97 E9** 27 10N 61 35 E
Zabolotiv, *Ukraine* **53 B10** 48 28N 25 18 E
Zabolottya, *Ukraine* **55 G11** 51 38N 24 16 E
Zabré, *Burkina Faso* **113 C4** 11 12N 0 36W
Zábřeh, *Czech Rep.* **35 B9** 49 53N 16 52 E
Zabrze, *Poland* **55 H5** 50 18N 18 50 E
Zabuzhzhya, *Ukraine* **55 G10** 51 21N 23 42 E
Zabzuga, *Ghana* **113 D5** 9 20N 0 30 E
Zacapa, *Guatemala* **164 D2** 14 59N 89 31W
Zacapu, *Mexico* **162 D4** 19 50N 101 43W
Zacatecas, *Mexico* **162 C4** 22 49N 102 34W
Zacatecas □, *Mexico* **162 C4** 23 30N 103 0W
Zacatecoluca, *El Salv.* **164 D2** 13 29N 88 51W
Zachary, *U.S.A.* **155 K9** 30 39N 91 9W
Zachodnio-
Pomorskie □, *Poland* **54 E2** 53 40N 15 50 E
Zacoalco, *Mexico* **162 C4** 20 14N 103 33W
Zacualtipán, *Mexico* **163 C5** 20 39N 98 36W
Zadar, *Croatia* **45 D12** 44 8N 15 14 E
Zadawa, *Nigeria* **113 C7** 11 33N 10 19 E
Zadetkyi Kyun, *Burma* **87 G2** 10 0N 98 25 E
Zadonsk, *Russia* **59 F10** 52 25N 38 56 E
Zafarqand, *Iran* **97 C7** 33 11N 52 29 E
Zafora, *Greece* **49 E8** 36 5N 26 24 E
Zafra, *Spain* **43 G4** 38 26N 6 30W
Żagań, *Poland* **55 G2** 51 39N 15 22 E
Zagaoua, *Chad* **109 E4** 16 0N 21 10 E
Žagarė, *Lithuania* **54 B10** 56 21N 23 15 E
Zagazig, *Egypt* **106 H7** 30 40N 31 30 E
Zāgheh, *Iran* **97 C6** 33 30N 48 42 E
Zaghouan, *Tunisia* **108 A2** 36 23N 10 10 E
Zaglivérion, *Greece* **50 F7** 40 36N 23 15 E
Zaglou, *Algeria* **111 C4** 27 17N 0 3W
Zagnanado, *Benin* **113 D5** 7 18N 2 28 E
Zagorá, *Greece* **48 B5** 39 27N 23 6 E
Zagora, *Morocco* **110 B3** 30 22N 5 51W
Zagorje, *Slovenia* **45 B11** 46 8N 15 0 E
Zagórów, *Poland* **55 F4** 52 10N 17 54 E
Zagorsk = Sergiyev
Posad, *Russia* **58 D10** 56 20N 38 10 E
Zagorsky =
Krasnozavodsk,
Russia **58 D10** 56 27N 38 25 E
Zagórz, *Poland* **55 J9** 49 30N 22 14 E
Zagreb, *Croatia* **45 C12** 45 50N 15 58 E
Zagreb ✕ (ZAG),
Croatia **45 C13** 45 45N 16 4 E
Zāgros, Kūhhā-ye, *Iran* **97 C6** 33 45N 48 5 E
Zagros Mts. = Zāgros,
Kūhhā-ye, *Iran* **97 C6** 33 45N 48 5 E
Žagubica, *Serbia & M.* **50 B5** 44 15N 21 47 E
Zaguinaso, *Ivory C.* **112 C3** 10 1N 6 14W
Zagyva →, *Hungary* **52 C5** 47 5N 20 4 E
Zahamena △, *Madag.* **117 B8** 17 37 S 48 49 E
Zāhedān, *Fārs, Iran* **97 D7** 28 46N 53 52 E
Zāhedān,
Sīstān va Balūchestān,
Iran **97 D9** 29 30N 60 50 E
Zahirabad, *India* **94 F3** 17 43N 77 37 E
Zahlah, *Lebanon* **103 B4** 33 52N 35 50 E
Zahna, *Germany* **30 D8** 51 55N 12 49 E
Záhony, *Hungary* **52 B7** 48 25N 22 11 E
Zahrān, *Si. Arabia* **98 C3** 17 40N 43 30 E
Zainsk, *Russia* **60 C11** 55 18N 52 4 E
Zaïre = Congo →,
Africa **115 D2** 6 4 S 12 24 E
Zaïre = Congo, Dem.
Rep. of the ■, *Africa* **115 C4** 3 0 S 23 0 E
Zaire □, *Angola* **115 D2** 7 0 S 14 0 E
Zaječar, *Serbia & M.* **50 C6** 43 53N 22 18 E
Zaka, *Zimbabwe* **117 C5** 20 20 S 31 29 E
Zakamensk, *Russia* **67 D11** 50 23N 103 17 E
Zakani, *Dem. Rep. of*
the Congo **114 B4** 2 33N 23 16 E
Zakarpatska □,
Ukraine **53 B8** 48 20N 23 20 E
Zakataly = Zaqatala,
Azerbaijan **61 K8** 41 38N 46 35 E
Zakbayemé, *Cameroon* **114 B2** 4 2N 10 34 E
Zakháro, *Greece* **48 D3** 37 30N 21 39 E
Zakhmatabad = Ayni,
Tajikistan **65 D4** 39 23N 68 32 E
Zakhodnaya Dzvina =
Daugava →, *Latvia* **15 H21** 57 4N 24 3 E
Zākhū, *Iraq* **101 D10** 37 10N 42 50 E
Zákinthos, *Greece* **39 D2** 37 47N 20 54 E
Zákinthos □, *Greece* **48 D2** 37 47N 20 57 E
Zákinthos ✕ (ZTH),
Greece **39 D2** 37 45N 20 50 E
Zakopane, *Poland* **55 J6** 49 18N 19 57 E
Zakouma, *Chad* **109 F3** 10 54N 19 49 E
Zakouma △, *Chad* **109 F3** 10 52N 19 45 E
Zakroczym, *Poland* **55 F7** 52 26N 20 38 E
Zákros, *Greece* **39 E7** 35 6N 26 10 E
Zakynthos = Zákinthos,
Greece **39 D2** 37 47N 20 54 E
Zala, *Angola* **115 D2** 7 52 S 13 42 E
Zala, *Ethiopia* **107 F4** 6 28N 37 13 E
Zala □, *Hungary* **52 D1** 46 42N 16 50 E
Zala →, *Hungary* **52 D2** 46 43N 17 16 E
Zalaegerszeg, *Hungary* **52 D1** 46 53N 16 47 E
Zalakomár, *Hungary* **52 D2** 46 33N 17 10 E
Zalalövő, *Hungary* **52 D1** 46 51N 16 35 E
Zalamea de la Serena,
Spain **43 G5** 38 40N 5 38W
Zalamea la Real, *Spain* **43 H4** 37 41N 6 38W
Zalău, *Romania* **52 C8** 47 12N 23 3 E
Zalazna, *Russia* **64 B4** 58 39N 52 31 E
Žalec, *Slovenia* **45 B12** 46 16N 15 10 E
Zaleshchiki =
Zalishchyky, *Ukraine* **53 B10** 48 45N 25 45 E
Zalesye, *Russia* **54 D8** 54 50N 21 31 E
Zalew Wiślany, *Poland* **54 D6** 54 20N 19 50 E
Zalewo, *Poland* **54 E6** 53 50N 19 41 E
Zalīm, *Si. Arabia* **98 B3** 22 43N 42 10 E
Zalingei, *Sudan* **109 F4** 12 51N 23 29 E
Zalishchyky, *Ukraine* **53 B10** 48 45N 25 45 E
Zaltan, *Ajdābiyā, Libya* **108 C3** 28 51N 19 52 E
Zaltan, *Zuwārah, Libya* **108 B2** 32 57N 11 52 E
Zaltan, Jabal, *Libya* **108 C3** 28 46N 19 45 E
Zalun, *Burma* **90 G5** 17 29N 95 34 E
Zama L., *Canada* **142 B5** 58 45N 119 5W
Zambales □, *Phil.* **80 D3** 15 20N 120 10 E
Zambales Mts., *Phil.* **80 D3** 15 45N 120 5 E
Zambeke, *Dem. Rep. of*
the Congo **118 B2** 2 8N 25 17 E
Zambeze →, *Africa* **119 F4** 18 35 S 36 20 E
Zambezi =
Zambeze →, *Africa* **119 F4** 18 35 S 36 20 E
Zambezi, *Zambia* **115 E4** 13 30 S 23 15 E
Zambezi △, *Zimbabwe* **119 F2** 17 54 S 25 41 E
Zambezia □, *Mozam.* **119 F4** 16 15 S 37 30 E
Zambia ■, *Africa* **119 F2** 15 0 S 28 0 E
Zamboanga, *Phil.* **81 H4** 6 59N 122 3 E
Zamboanga del
Norte □, *Phil.* **81 H4** 8 0N 123 0 E
Zamboanga del Sur □,
Phil. **81 H4** 7 40N 123 0 E
Zambrano, *Colombia* **168 B3** 9 45N 74 49W
Zambrów, *Poland* **55 F9** 52 59N 22 14 E
Zametchino, *Russia* **60 D6** 53 30N 42 30 E
Zamfara □, *Nigeria* **113 C6** 12 10N 6 0 E
Zamfara →, *Nigeria* **113 C5** 12 5N 4 2 E
Zamora, *Ecuador* **168 D2** 4 4 S 78 58W
Zamora, *Mexico* **162 D4** 20 0N 102 21W
Zamora, *Spain* **42 D5** 41 30N 5 45W
Zamora □, *Spain* **42 D5** 41 30N 5 46W
Zamora →, *Ecuador* **168 D2** 2 59N 78 13W
Zamora-Chinchipe □,
Ecuador **168 D2** 4 15 S 78 50W

Zamość, Poland .... 55 H10 50 43N 23 15 E
Zams, Austria .... 33 B11 47 9N 10 35 E
Zamtang, China .... 76 A3 32 26N 101 6 E
Zamuro, Sierra del, Venezuela 169 C5 4 0N 62 30W
Zamzam, W. →, Libya .... 108 B2 30 58N 14 48 E
Zan, Ghana 113 D4 9 26N 0 17W
Zanaga, Congo .... 114 C2 2 48 S 13 48 E
Záncara →, Spain 41 F1 39 18N 3 18W
Zanderij, Suriname 169 B6 5 20N 55 16W
Zandu, Dem. Rep. of the Congo .... 115 D3 5 11 S 18 16 E
Zandvoort, Neths. .... 24 B4 52 22N 4 32 E
Zanesville, U.S.A. 150 G2 39 56N 82 1W
Zangābād, Iran .... 96 B5 38 26N 46 44 E
Zangue →, Mozam. .... 119 F4 17 50 S 35 21 E
Zanjān, Iran .... 97 B6 36 40N 48 35 E
Zanjān □, Iran .... 97 B6 37 20N 49 30 E
Zanjān →, Iran .... 97 B6 37 8N 47 47 E
Zannone, Italy .... 46 B6 40 58N 13 3 E
Zanow = Sianów, Poland .... 54 D3 54 13N 16 18 E
Zante = Zákinthos, Greece .... 39 D2 37 47N 20 54 E
Zanthus, Australia .... 125 F3 31 2 S 123 34 E
Zanzibar, Tanzania .... 118 D4 6 12 S 39 12 E
Zanzūr, Libya .... 108 B2 32 55N 13 1 E
Zaouatallaz, Algeria .... 111 D6 24 52N 8 30 E
Zaouiet El-Kala = Bordj Omar Driss, Algeria .... 111 C6 28 10N 6 40 E
Zaouiet Reggâne, Algeria .... 111 C5 26 32N 0 3 E
Zaoyang, China .... 77 A9 32 10N 112 45 E
Zaozhuang, China .... 75 G9 34 50N 117 35 E
Zap Suyu = Zâb al Kabîr →, Iraq .... 101 D10 36 1N 43 24 E
Zapadna Morava →, Serbia & M. .... 50 C5 43 38N 21 30 E
Zapadnaya Dvina → Daugava →, Latvia .... 15 H21 57 4N 24 3 E
Zapadnaya Dvina, Russia .... 58 D7 56 15N 32 3 E
Západné Beskydy, Europe .... 35 B12 49 30N 19 0 E
Zapadni Rodopi, Bulgaria .... 50 E7 41 50N 24 0 E
Západočeský □, Czech Rep. .... 34 B6 49 35N 13 0 E
Zapala, Argentina .... 176 A2 39 0 S 70 5W
Zapaleri, Cerro, Bolivia .... 174 A2 22 49 S 67 11W
Zapata, U.S.A. 155 M5 26 55N 99 16W
Zapatón →, Spain 43 F4 39 0N 6 49W
Zapiga, Chile .... 172 D4 19 40 S 69 55W
Zapolyarnyy, Russia .... 56 A5 69 26N 30 51 E
Zaporizhzhya, Ukraine .... 59 J8 47 50N 35 10 E
Zaporozhye = Zaporizhzhya, Ukraine .... 59 J8 47 50N 35 10 E
Zaqatala, Azerbaijan .... 61 K8 41 38N 46 35 E
Zara, Turkey .... 100 C7 39 58N 37 43 E
Zarafshan, Uzbekistan .... 65 C2 41 34N 64 12 E
Zaragoza, Colombia 168 B3 7 30N 74 52W
Zaragoza, Coahuila, Mexico 162 B4 28 30N 101 0W
Zaragoza, Nuevo León, Mexico 163 C5 24 0N 99 46W
Zaragoza, Spain 40 D3 41 39N 0 53W
Zaragoza □, Spain 40 D3 41 35N 1 0W
Zarand, Kermān, Iran .... 97 D8 30 46N 56 34 E
Zarand, Markazī, Iran .... 97 C6 35 18N 50 25 E
Zărandului, Munții, Romania .... 52 D7 46 14N 22 7 E
Zaranj, Afghan. .... 91 C1 30 55N 61 55 E
Zarasai, Lithuania .... 15 J22 55 40N 26 20 E
Zárate, Argentina .... 174 C4 34 7 S 59 0W
Zaratsiz, Spain 40 B2 43 17N 2 10W
Zaraysk, Russia .... 58 E10 54 48N 38 53 E
Zaraza, Venezuela 169 B4 9 21N 65 19W
Zarbdar, Uzbekistan .... 65 C4 40 3N 68 10 E
Zard, Kūh-e, Iran .... 97 C6 32 22N 50 4 E
Zāreh, Iran .... 97 C6 35 7N 49 9 E
Zari, Nigeria .... 113 C7 13 4N 12 45 E
Zaria, Nigeria .... 113 C6 11 0N 7 40 E
Zarki, Poland .... 55 H6 50 38N 19 23 E
Zárkon, Greece .... 48 B4 39 38N 22 6 E
Zarneh, Iran .... 96 C5 33 55N 46 10 E
Zărneşti, Romania .... 53 E10 45 33N 25 18 E
Zarós, Greece .... 39 E5 35 8N 24 54 E
Zarów, Poland .... 53 H4 50 56N 16 29 E
Zarqā', Nahr az →, Jordan .... 103 C4 32 10N 35 37 E
Zarrīn, Iran .... 97 C7 32 46N 54 37 E
Zaruma, Ecuador .... 168 D2 3 40 S 79 38W
Żary, Poland .... 55 G2 51 37N 15 10 E
Zarza de Granadilla, Spain 42 E4 40 14N 6 3W
Zarzaïtine, Algeria .... 111 C6 28 15N 9 34 E
Zarzal, Colombia 168 C2 4 24N 76 4W
Zarzis, Tunisia .... 108 B2 33 31N 11 2 E
Zas, Spain 42 B2 43 4N 8 53W
Zaskar →, India .... 93 B7 34 13N 77 20 E
Zaskar Mts., India .... 93 C7 33 15N 77 30 E
Zastavna, Ukraine .... 53 B10 48 31N 25 51 E
Zastron, S. Africa .... 116 E4 30 18 S 27 7 E
Zátec, Czech Rep. .... 34 A6 50 20N 13 32 E
Zaterechnyy, Russia .... 61 H7 44 48N 45 11 E
Zatishye = Elektrostal, Russia .... 58 E10 55 41N 38 32 E
Zator, Poland .... 55 J6 49 59N 19 28 E
Zatyshshya, Ukraine .... 53 C14 47 20N 29 51 E
Zavala, Bos.-H. .... 50 D1 42 50N 17 59 E
Zavāreh, Iran .... 97 C7 33 29N 52 28 E
Zave, Zimbabwe .... 117 B5 17 6 S 30 1 E
Zavérdhas, Kólpos, Greece .... 39 B2 38 47N 20 51 E
Zavetnoye, Russia .... 61 G6 47 13N 43 50 E
Zavidovići, Bos.-H. .... 52 F3 44 27N 18 10 E
Zavitaya = Zavitinsk, Russia .... 67 D13 50 10N 129 20 E
Zavitinsk, Russia .... 67 D13 50 10N 129 20 E
Zavodovski, I., Antarctica .... 7 B1 56 0 S 27 45W
Zavodskoy = Komsomolskiy, Russia .... 60 C7 54 27N 45 33 E
Zavolzhsk, Russia .... 60 B6 57 30N 42 0 E
Zavolzhye = Zavolzhsk, Russia .... 60 B6 57 30N 42 0 E
Zavolzhye, Russia .... 60 B6 57 30N 42 0 E
Zawadzkie, Poland .... 55 H5 50 37N 18 28 E
Zawichost, Poland .... 55 H8 50 48N 21 51 E
Zawidów, Poland .... 55 G2 51 1N 15 1 E
Zawiercie, Poland .... 55 H6 50 30N 19 24 E
Zāwiyat al Baydā = Al Baydā, Libya .... 108 B4 32 50N 21 44 E
Zāwiyat Masūs, Libya .... 108 B4 31 35N 21 1 E
Zawyet Shammas, Egypt .... 106 A2 31 30N 26 37 E
Zawyet Um el Rakham, Egypt .... 106 A2 31 18N 27 1 E
Zawyet Ungeîla, Egypt .... 106 A2 31 23N 26 42 E
Zāyā, Iraq .... 96 C5 33 33N 44 13 E
Zāyandeh →, Iran .... 97 C7 32 35N 52 0 E

Zaymah, Si. Arabia .... 98 B3 21 37N 40 6 E
Zaysan, Kazakhstan .... 66 E9 47 28N 84 52 E
Zaysan, Oz., Kazakhstan .... 66 E9 48 0N 83 0 E
Zayü, China .... 76 C1 28 48N 97 27 E
Zazafotsy, Madag. .... 117 C8 21 11 S 46 21 E
Zāzamt, W. →, Libya .... 108 B2 30 29N 14 30 E
Zazir, O. →, Algeria .... 111 D6 22 0N 5 40 E
Zázrivá, Slovak Rep. .... 35 B12 49 16N 19 7 E
Zbarazh, Ukraine .... 59 H3 49 43N 25 44 E
Zbąszyń, Poland .... 55 F2 52 14N 15 56 E
Zbąszynek, Poland .... 55 F2 52 16N 15 51 E
Zblewo, Poland .... 54 E5 53 56N 18 19 E
Zbruch →, Ukraine .... 53 B11 48 32N 26 27 E
Žďár nad Sázavou, Czech Rep. .... 34 B8 49 34N 15 57 E
Zdolbuniv, Ukraine .... 59 G4 50 30N 26 15 E
Żdrelo, Serbia & M. .... 50 B5 44 16N 21 28 E
Zduńska Wola, Poland .... 55 G5 51 37N 18 59 E
Zduny, Poland .... 55 G4 51 39N 17 21 E
Zearing, U.S.A. 156 B3 42 10N 93 18W
Zeballos, Canada 142 D3 49 59N 126 50W
Zēbāk, Afghan. .... 65 E5 36 31N 71 20 E
Zebediela, S. Africa .... 117 C4 24 20 S 29 17 E
Zebila, Ghana 113 C4 10 55N 0 30W
Zebulon, U.S.A. 152 B5 33 36N 84 21W
Zeebrugge, Belgium .... 24 C3 51 19N 3 12 E
Zeehan, Australia .... 127 G4 41 52 S 145 25 E
Zeeland, U.S.A. 157 B10 42 49N 86 1W
Zeeland □, Neths. .... 24 C3 51 30N 3 50 E
Zeerust, S. Africa .... 116 D4 25 31 S 26 4 E
Zefat, Israel .... 103 C4 32 58N 35 29 E
Zegdou, Algeria 110 C4 29 51N 4 45W
Zege, Ethiopia .... 107 E4 11 43N 37 18 E
Zeggerene, Iracher, Mali .... 113 B5 16 49N 2 16 E
Zégoua, Mali 112 C3 10 32N 5 35W
Zehden = Cedynia, Poland .... 55 F1 52 53N 14 12 E
Zehdenick, Germany .... 30 C9 52 58N 13 20 E
Zeigler, U.S.A. 156 G7 37 54N 89 3W
Zeil, Mt., Australia .... 124 D5 23 30 S 132 23 E
Zeila = Saylac, Somali Rep. .... 120 B2 11 21N 43 30 E
Zeist, Neths. .... 24 B5 52 5N 5 15 E
Zeitz, Germany .... 30 D8 51 2N 12 7 E
Zejtun, Malta .... 38 F8 35 51N 14 32 E
Zelechów, Poland .... 55 G8 51 49N 21 54 E
Zelena, Ukraine .... 53 B9 48 3N 24 45 E
Zelengora, Bos.-H. .... 50 C2 43 22N 18 30 E
Zelenodolsk, Russia .... 60 C9 55 55N 48 30 E
Zelenogorsk, Russia .... 58 B5 60 12N 29 43 E
Zelenograd, Russia .... 58 D9 56 1N 37 12 E
Zelenogradsk, Russia .... 15 J19 54 53N 20 29 E
Zelenokumsk, Russia .... 61 H6 44 24N 44 0 E
Železná Ruda, Czech Rep. .... 34 B6 49 8N 13 15 E
Železnik, Serbia & M. .... 50 B4 44 43N 20 23 E
Zelfana, Algeria .... 111 B5 32 27N 4 15 E
Zelienople, U.S.A. 150 F4 40 48N 80 8W
Želiezovce, Slovak Rep. .... 35 C11 48 3N 18 40 E
Zelina, Croatia .... 45 C13 45 57N 16 16 E
Zell, Baden-W., Germany .... 31 H3 47 42N 7 52 E
Zell, Rhld-Pfz., Germany .... 31 E3 50 1N 7 10 E
Zell am See, Austria .... 34 D5 47 19N 12 47 E
Zella-Mehlis, Germany .... 30 E6 50 39N 10 40 E
Zellersee, Germany .... 33 A8 47 45N 9 2 E
Zelmen = Rovnoye, Russia .... 60 E8 50 52N 46 3 E
Zelów, Poland .... 55 G6 51 28N 19 14 E
Zeltweg, Austria .... 34 D7 47 11N 14 45 E
Zelyony Dol = Zelenodolsk, Russia .... 60 C9 55 55N 48 30 E
Zemaitijos △, Lithuania .... 54 B8 56 21 55 E
Zembra, I., Tunisia .... 108 A2 37 5N 10 56 E
Zemgale = Jelgava, Latvia .... 15 H20 56 41N 23 49 E
Zémio, C.A.R. .... 118 A2 5 2N 25 5 E
Zemlya Imperatora Nikolaya II = Severnaya Zemlya, Russia .... 67 B10 79 0N 100 0 E
Zemmora, Algeria .... 111 A5 35 44N 0 51 E
Zemmur, W. Sahara 110 C2 25 5N 12 0W
Zemongo △, C.A.R. .... 114 A5 6 45N 25 5 E
Zemoul, O. →, Algeria 110 C3 29 15N 7 0W
Zempelburg = Sępólno Krajeńskie, Poland .... 54 E4 53 26N 17 30 E
Zempléni-hegység, Hungary .... 52 B6 48 25N 21 25 E
Zemplínska šírava, Slovak Rep. .... 35 C15 48 48N 22 0 E
Zempoala, Mexico 163 D5 19 27N 96 24W
Zemun, Serbia & M. .... 50 B4 44 51N 20 25 E
Zendeh Jān, Afghan. .... 91 B1 34 21N 61 45 E
Zengbé, Cameroon .... 113 D7 5 46N 13 4 E
Zengcheng, China .... 77 F9 23 13N 113 52 E
Zenica, Bos.-H. .... 52 F2 44 10N 17 57 E
Zennisūji, Japan .... 72 C5 34 14N 133 47 E
Zenza →, Angola .... 115 D2 9 16 S 14 13 E
Zepče, Bos.-H. .... 52 F3 44 28N 18 2 E
Zephyrhills, U.S.A. 153 G7 28 14N 82 11W
Zepu, China .... 65 D8 38 12N 77 18 E
Zeraf, Bahr ez →, Sudan .... 107 F3 9 42N 30 32 E
Zeravshan, Tajikistan .... 65 D3 39 20N 68 39 E
Zeravshan →, Asia .... 65 D1 39 22N 63 45 E
Zeravshanskiy Khrebet, Tajikistan .... 65 D4 39 20N 69 0 E
Zerbst, Germany .... 30 D8 51 58N 12 5 E
Zerków, Poland .... 55 F4 52 4N 17 32 E
Zermatt, Switz. .... 32 D5 46 2N 7 46 E
Zernez, Switz. .... 33 C10 46 42N 10 7 E
Zernograd, Russia .... 61 G5 46 52N 40 19 E
Zernovoy = Zernograd, Russia .... 61 G5 46 52N 40 19 E
Zerqan, Albania .... 50 E4 41 27N 20 20 E
Zestaponi, Georgia .... 61 J6 42 6N 43 0 E
Zetel, Germany .... 30 B3 53 25N 7 58 E
Zetland = Shetland □, U.K. 22 A7 60 30N 1 30W
Zeulenroda, Germany .... 30 E7 50 39N 11 59 E
Zeven, Germany .... 30 B5 53 17N 9 16 E
Zevenaar, Neths. .... 24 C6 51 56N 6 5 E
Zévio, Italy .... 44 C8 45 22N 11 8 E
Zeya, Russia .... 67 D13 53 48N 127 14 E
Zeya →, Russia .... 67 D13 51 42N 128 53 E
Zeytinbaği, Turkey .... 51 F12 40 24N 28 47 E
Zeytindağ, Turkey .... 49 C9 38 58N 27 4 E
Zghartā, Lebanon .... 103 A4 34 21N 35 53 E
Zgierz, Poland .... 55 G6 51 50N 19 27 E
Zgorzelec, Poland .... 55 G2 51 10N 15 0 E
Zgurita, Moldova .... 53 B13 48 8N 28 1 E
Zhabasak, Kazakhstan .... 64 F6 50 52N 64 41 E
Zhabinka, Belarus .... 55 F11 52 13N 24 2 E
Zhabokrych, Ukraine .... 53 B14 48 23N 28 59 E
Zhailma, Kazakhstan .... 64 F6 51 37N 61 33 E
Zhalanash, Kazakhstan .... 65 B9 43 9N 78 38 E
Zhambyl = Taraz, Kazakhstan .... 65 B5 42 54N 71 22 E

Zhanatas, Kazakhstan .... 65 B4 43 35N 69 35 E
Zhangaly, Kazakhstan .... 61 G10 47 1N 50 37 E
Zhangaqazaly, Kazakhstan .... 66 E7 45 48N 62 6 E
Zhangaqūrghan, Kazakhstan .... 65 A4 43 50N 68 48 E
Zhangatas = Zhanatas, Kazakhstan .... 65 B4 43 35N 69 35 E
Zhangbei, China .... 74 D8 41 10N 114 45 E
Zhangguangcai Ling, China .... 75 B15 45 0N 129 0 E
Zhangjiaban, China .... 69 F9 22 33N 113 28 E
Zhangjiagang, China .... 75 B13 31 55N 120 30 E
Zhangjiakou, China .... 74 D8 40 48N 114 55 E
Zhangping, China .... 77 E11 25 17N 117 23 E
Zhangpu, China .... 77 E11 24 30N 117 35 E
Zhangshu, China .... 77 C10 28 4N 115 29 E
Zhangwu, China .... 75 C12 42 43N 123 52 E
Zhangye, China .... 68 C5 38 50N 100 23 E
Zhangzhou, China .... 77 E11 24 30N 117 35 E
Zhanhua, China .... 75 F10 37 40N 118 8 E
Zhanjiang, China .... 77 G8 21 15N 110 20 E
Zhannetty, Ostrov, Russia .... 67 B16 76 43N 158 0 E
Zhanyi, China .... 76 E4 25 38N 103 48 E
Zhanyu, China .... 75 B12 44 30N 122 30 E
Zhao Xian, China .... 74 F8 37 43N 114 45 E
Zhao'an, China .... 77 F11 23 41N 117 10 E
Zhaocheng, China .... 74 F6 36 22N 111 38 E
Zhaojue, China .... 76 C4 28 1N 102 49 E
Zhaoping, China .... 77 E8 24 11N 110 48 E
Zhaoqing, China .... 77 F9 23 0N 112 20 E
Zhaotong, China .... 76 D4 27 20N 103 44 E
Zhaoyuan, Heilongjiang, China .... 75 B13 45 27N 125 0 E
Zhaoyuan, Shandong, China .... 75 F11 37 20N 120 23 E
Zharkovskiy, Russia .... 58 E7 55 56N 32 19 E
Zhashkiv, Ukraine .... 59 H6 49 15N 30 5 E
Zhashui, China .... 74 H5 33 40N 109 8 E
Zhayyq →, Kazakhstan .... 57 E9 47 0N 51 48 E
Zhdanov = Mariupol, Ukraine .... 59 J9 47 5N 37 31 E
Zhdanovo, Kazakhstan .... 65 B5 43 40N 71 6 E
Zhecheng, China .... 74 G8 34 7N 115 20 E
Zhegao, China .... 77 B11 31 46N 117 45 E
Zhejiang □, China .... 77 C13 29 0N 120 0 E
Zheleznodorozhny = Qŭnghirot, Uzbekistan .... 66 E6 43 6N 58 54 E
Zheleznodorozhny, Russia .... 54 D8 54 22N 21 19 E
Zheleznodorozhnyy, Russia .... 56 B9 62 35N 50 55 E
Zheleznogorsk, Russia .... 59 F8 52 22N 35 23 E
Zheleznogorsk-Ilimskiy, Russia .... 67 D11 56 34N 104 8 E
Zheltyye Vody = Zhovti Vody, Ukraine .... 59 H7 48 21N 33 31 E
Zhen'an, China .... 74 H5 33 27N 109 9 E
Zhenba, China .... 74 H5 32 34N 107 58 E
Zhenfeng, China .... 76 E5 25 22N 105 40 E
Zheng'an, China .... 76 C6 28 32N 107 27 E
Zhengding, China .... 74 E8 38 8N 114 32 E
Zhenghe, China .... 77 D12 27 20N 118 50 E
Zhengyang, China .... 77 C9 32 37N 114 1 E
Zhengyangguan, China .... 74 G7 34 45N 113 34 E
Zhengzhou, China .... 77 C13 29 59N 121 42 E
Zhenhai, China .... 77 A12 32 11N 119 26 E
Zhenjiang, China .... 77 A12 32 11N 119 26 E
Zhenkang, China .... 76 F2 23 58N 99 0 E
Zhenlai, China .... 75 B12 45 50N 123 5 E
Zhenning, China .... 76 D5 26 4N 105 45 E
Zhenping, Henan, China .... 74 H7 33 10N 112 16 E
Zhenping, Shaanxi, China .... 76 B7 31 59N 109 31 E
Zhenxiong, China .... 76 D5 27 27N 104 50 E
Zhenyuan, Gansu, China .... 74 G4 35 35N 107 30 E
Zhenyuan, Guizhou, China .... 76 D7 27 4N 108 21 E
Zherdevka, Russia .... 60 E5 51 56N 41 29 E
Zherebkove, Ukraine .... 53 C14 47 50N 29 52 E
Zhetigen, Kazakhstan .... 65 B8 43 40N 77 6 E
Zhetiqara, Kazakhstan .... 64 F6 52 11N 61 12 E
Zhezqazghan, Kazakhstan .... 66 E7 47 44N 67 40 E
Zhicheng, China .... 77 B8 30 25N 111 27 E
Zhidan, China .... 74 F5 36 48N 108 48 E
Zhigansk, Russia .... 67 C13 66 48N 123 27 E
Zhigulevsk, Russia .... 60 D9 53 28N 49 30 E
Zhijiang, Hubei, China .... 77 B8 30 28N 111 45 E
Zhijiang, Hunan, China .... 76 D7 27 27N 109 42 E
Zhijin, China .... 76 D5 26 37N 105 45 E
Zhilinda, Russia .... 67 C12 70 0N 114 20 E
Zhilino, Russia .... 54 D8 54 54N 21 54 E
Zhirnovsk, Russia .... 60 E7 50 57N 44 49 E
Zhirnovsky = Zhirnovsk, Russia .... 60 E7 50 57N 44 49 E
Zhirnovsky = Zhirnovsk, Russia .... 60 E7 50 57N 44 49 E
Zhitomir = Zhytomyr, Ukraine .... 59 G5 50 20N 28 40 E
Zhizdra, Russia .... 58 E9 53 45N 34 40 E
Zhlobin, Belarus .... 59 F6 52 55N 30 0 E
Zhmerinka = Zhmerynka, Ukraine .... 59 H5 49 2N 28 2 E
Zhmerynka, Ukraine .... 59 H5 49 2N 28 2 E
Zhob, Pakistan .... 91 C3 31 20N 69 31 E
Zhob →, Pakistan .... 92 C3 32 4N 69 50 E
Zhodino = Zhodzina, Belarus .... 59 E5 54 5N 28 17 E
Zhodzina, Belarus .... 58 E5 54 5N 28 17 E
Zhokhova, Ostrov, Russia .... 67 B16 76 4N 152 40 E
Zholkva = Nesterov, Ukraine .... 59 G2 50 4N 23 58 E
Zholkva = Nesterov, Ukraine .... 59 G2 50 4N 23 58 E
Zhongdian, China .... 76 D2 27 48N 99 42 E
Zhongdong, China .... 76 E7 24 48N 107 47 E
Zhongdu, China .... 76 E7 24 40N 109 44 E
Zhongning, China .... 74 F3 37 29N 105 40 E
Zhongshan, Antarctica .... 7 C6 69 0 S 39 50 E
Zhongshan, Guangdong, China .... 77 F9 22 26N 113 20 E
Zhongshan, Guangxi Zhuang, China .... 77 E8 24 29N 111 18 E
Zhongshankong, China .... 69 F9 22 35N 113 28 E
Zhongtiao Shan, China .... 74 G6 35 0N 111 10 E
Zhongwei, China .... 74 F3 37 30N 105 12 E
Zhongxiang, China .... 77 B9 31 12N 112 34 E
Zhongyang, China .... 74 F6 37 20N 111 11 E
Zhoran, Ukraine .... 55 G10 51 9N 23 57 E
Zhoucun, China .... 75 F9 36 47N 117 48 E
Zhouning, China .... 77 D12 27 7N 119 23 E
Zhoushan, China .... 77 B14 30 1N 122 6 E
Zhoushan Dao, China .... 77 C14 29 56N 122 22 E
Zhouzhi, China .... 74 G5 34 10N 108 12 E
Zhovti Vody, Ukraine .... 59 H7 48 21N 33 31 E

Zhovtneve, Ukraine .... 55 H11 50 42N 24 12 E
Zhovtnevoye = Zhovtneve, Ukraine .... 59 J7 46 54N 32 3 E
Zhu Jiang →, China .... 77 F9 22 45N 113 37 E
Zhuanghe, China .... 75 E12 39 40N 123 0 E
Zhūcheng, China .... 75 G10 36 0N 119 27 E
Zhugqu, China .... 74 H3 33 40N 104 30 E
Zhuhai, China .... 77 F9 22 17N 113 34 E
Zhuji, China .... 77 C13 29 40N 120 10 E
Zhujiang Kou, China .... 77 G10 22 20N 113 45 E
Zhukovka, Russia .... 58 F7 53 35N 33 50 E
Zhumadian, China .... 74 H8 32 59N 114 2 E
Zhuo Xian = Zhuozhou, China .... 74 E8 39 28N 115 58 E
Zhuolu, China .... 74 D8 40 20N 115 12 E
Zhuozhou, China .... 74 E8 39 28N 115 58 E
Zhuozi, China .... 74 D7 41 0N 112 25 E
Zhushan, China .... 77 A8 32 15N 110 13 E
Zhuxi, China .... 76 A7 32 25N 109 40 E
Zhuzhou, China .... 77 D9 27 49N 113 12 E
Zhvanets, Ukraine .... 53 B11 48 33N 26 30 E
Zhytomyr, Ukraine .... 59 G5 50 20N 28 40 E
Zi Shui →, China .... 77 D9 28 40N 112 30 E
Žiar nad Hronom, Slovak Rep. .... 35 C11 48 35N 18 53 E
Zīārān, Iran .... 97 B6 36 7N 50 32 E
Ziarat, Pakistan .... 92 D2 30 25N 67 49 E
Zibo, China .... 75 F10 36 47N 118 3 E
Zichang, China .... 74 F5 37 18N 109 40 E
Zidani Most, Slovenia .... 45 B12 46 6N 15 6 E
Zidarovo, Bulgaria .... 51 D11 42 20N 27 24 E
Zībel = Wandhari, Pakistan .... 92 F2 27 42N 66 48 E
Ziębice, Poland .... 55 H4 50 37N 17 2 E
Ziebingen = Cybinka, Poland .... 55 F1 52 12N 14 46 E
Ziegenhals = Głuchołazy, Poland .... 55 H4 50 19N 17 24 E
Zielenzig = Sulęcin, Poland .... 55 F2 52 26N 15 10 E
Zielona Góra, Poland .... 55 G2 51 57N 15 31 E
Zierikzee, Neths. .... 24 C3 51 40N 3 55 E
Ziesar, Germany .... 30 C8 52 16N 12 17 E
Zifta, Egypt .... 106 H7 30 43N 31 14 E
Zigey, Chad .... 109 F3 14 43N 15 50 E
Zigon, Burma .... 90 F5 18 20N 95 37 E
Zigong, China .... 76 C5 29 15N 104 48 E
Ziguinchor, Senegal 112 C1 12 35N 16 20W
Zihuatanejo, Mexico 162 D4 17 38N 101 33W
Zijin, China .... 77 F10 23 30N 115 8 E
Zile, Turkey .... 100 B6 40 15N 35 52 E
Žilina, Slovak Rep. .... 35 B11 49 12N 18 42 E
Žilinský □, Slovak Rep. .... 35 B11 49 10N 19 0 E
Zillah, Libya .... 108 C3 28 30N 17 33 E
Zillertaler Alpen, Austria .... 34 A4 47 6N 11 45 E
Zima, Russia .... 67 D11 54 0N 102 5 E
Zimane, Adrar in, Algeria .... 111 D5 22 10N 4 30 E
Zimapán, Mexico 163 C5 20 54N 99 20W
Zimba, Zambia .... 119 F2 17 20 S 26 11 E
Zimbabwe, Zimbabwe .... 119 G3 20 16 S 30 54 E
Zimbabwe ■, Africa .... 119 F3 19 0 S 30 0 E
Zimi, S. Leone 112 D2 7 20N 11 20W
Zimnicea, Romania .... 53 G10 43 40N 25 22 E
Zimovniki, Russia .... 61 G6 47 10N 42 25 E
Zina, Cameroon .... 109 F2 11 19N 14 54 E
Zinal, Switz. .... 32 D5 46 8N 7 38 E
Zinave △, Mozam. .... 117 C5 21 35 S 33 40 E
Zinder, Niger .... 113 C6 13 48N 9 0 E
Zinga, Tanzania .... 119 D4 9 16 S 38 49 E
Zingaro △, Italy .... 46 D5 38 6N 12 53 E
Zingst, Germany .... 30 A8 54 26N 12 39 E
Ziniaré, Burkina Faso 113 C4 12 35N 1 18W
Zinnowitz, Germany .... 30 A9 54 4N 13 54 E
Zinovyevsk = Kirovohrad, Ukraine .... 59 H7 48 35N 32 20 E
Zion, U.S.A. 157 B9 42 27N 87 50W
Zion △, U.S.A. 159 H7 37 15N 113 5W
Zionsville, U.S.A. 157 E10 39 57N 86 16W
Zipaquirá, Colombia 168 C3 5 0N 74 0W
Zirbitzkogel, Austria .... 34 D7 47 4N 14 22 E
Zirc, Hungary .... 52 C2 47 17N 17 52 E
Žiri, Slovenia .... 45 B11 46 3N 14 4 E
Žirje, Croatia .... 45 E12 43 39N 15 42 E
Zirke = Sieraków, Poland .... 55 F3 52 39N 16 2 E
Zirl, Austria .... 34 D4 47 17N 11 14 E
Zirndorf, Germany .... 31 F6 49 27N 10 57 E
Ziros, Greece .... 39 E7 35 5N 26 8 E
Zirreh, Gowd-e, Afghan. .... 91 C1 29 45N 62 0 E
Zisterdorf, Austria .... 35 C9 48 33N 16 45 E
Zitácuaro, Mexico 162 D4 19 28N 100 21W
Žitava →, Slovak Rep. .... 35 C11 48 14N 18 21 E
Žitište, Serbia & M. .... 50 E5 45 30N 20 32 E
Zitong, China .... 76 B5 31 37N 105 10 E
Zitsa, Greece .... 48 B2 39 47N 20 40 E
Zittau, Germany .... 30 E10 50 57N 14 48 E
Zitundo, Mozam. .... 117 D5 26 48 S 32 47 E
Živinice, Bos.-H. .... 52 F3 44 27N 18 36 E
Ziwa Magharibi = Kagera □, Tanzania .... 118 C3 2 0 S 31 30 E
Ziway, L., Ethiopia .... 107 F4 8 0N 38 50 E
Zixi, China .... 77 D11 27 45N 117 4 E
Zixing, China .... 77 E9 25 59N 113 21 E
Ziyang, Shaanxi, China .... 74 H5 32 32N 108 31 E
Ziyang, Sichuan, China .... 76 B6 30 6N 104 40 E
Ziyuan, China .... 77 D8 26 30N 110 26 E
Ziyun, China .... 76 E6 25 45N 106 5 E
Ziz, Oued →, Morocco 110 B4 31 4N 4 15W
Zizhong, China .... 76 C5 29 48N 104 47 E
Zlarin, Croatia .... 45 E12 43 42N 15 49 E
Zlatar, Croatia .... 45 B13 46 5N 16 2 E
Zlatar, Serbia & M. .... 50 C3 43 25N 19 47 E
Zlataritsa, Bulgaria .... 51 C9 43 2N 25 55 E
Zlaté Moravce, Slovak Rep. .... 35 C11 48 23N 18 37 E
Zlatibor, Serbia & M. .... 50 C3 43 45N 19 43 E
Zlatitsa, Bulgaria .... 51 D8 42 41N 24 7 E
Zlatna, Romania .... 53 D8 46 8N 23 11 E
Zlatna Panega, Bulgaria .... 51 C8 43 5N 24 9 E
Zlatni Pyasŭtsi, Bulgaria .... 51 C12 43 17N 28 3 E
Zlatograd, Bulgaria .... 51 F8 41 22N 25 7 E
Zlatoust, Russia .... 64 D7 55 10N 59 40 E
Zletovo, Macedonia .... 50 E6 41 59N 22 14 E
Zlín, Czech Rep. .... 35 B10 49 14N 17 40 E
Zlínský □, Czech Rep. .... 35 B10 49 20N 17 40 E
Zlītan, Libya .... 108 B2 32 32N 14 1 E
Złocieniec, Poland .... 55 E3 53 30N 16 1 E
Złoczew, Poland .... 55 G5 51 25N 18 37 E
Zlot, Serbia & M. .... 50 B5 44 1N 21 59 E
Złotoryja, Poland .... 55 G3 51 8N 15 55 E
Złotów, Poland .... 55 E4 53 22N 17 2 E
Złoty Potok, Poland .... 55 H6 50 42N 19 27 E

Znamensk, Russia .... 54 D8 54 36N 21 16 E
Znamyanka, Ukraine .... 59 H7 48 45N 32 30 E
Znin, Poland .... 55 F4 52 51N 17 44 E
Znojmo, Czech Rep. .... 34 B8 48 50N 16 2 E
Zobeyrī, Iran .... 96 C5 34 10N 46 40 E
Zobia, Dem. Rep. of the Congo .... 118 B2 3 0N 25 59 E
Zobten = Sobótka, Poland .... 55 H3 50 54N 16 44 E
Zoetermeer, Neths. .... 24 B4 52 3N 4 30 E
Zofingen, Switz. .... 32 B5 47 17N 7 56 E
Zogang, China .... 76 C1 29 55N 97 42 E
Zogno, Italy .... 44 C6 45 48N 9 40 E
Zogqên, China .... 76 A2 32 19N 98 47 E
Zolfo Springs, U.S.A. 153 H8 27 30N 81 48W
Zolikofen, Switz. .... 32 C4 47 11N 7 28 E
Zollikon, Switz. .... 33 B7 47 21N 8 34 E
Zolochev = Zolochiv, Ukraine .... 59 H3 49 45N 24 51 E
Zolochiv, Ukraine .... 59 H3 49 45N 24 51 E
Zolotonosha, Ukraine .... 59 H7 49 39N 32 5 E
Zolotyy Potik, Ukraine .... 53 B10 48 54N 25 20 E
Zomba, Malawi .... 119 F4 15 22 S 35 19 E
Zongo, Dem. Rep. of the Congo .... 114 B3 4 20N 18 35 E
Zonguldak, Turkey .... 100 B4 41 28N 31 50 E
Zongyang, China .... 77 B11 30 42N 117 12 E
Zonqor Pt., Malta .... 38 F8 35 52N 14 34 E
Zonza, France .... 29 G13 41 45N 9 11 E
Zorgo, Burkina Faso 113 C4 12 15N 0 35W
Zorita, Spain 43 F5 39 17N 5 39W
Zörbig, Germany .... 30 D8 51 38N 12 7 E
Zorleni, Romania .... 53 D12 46 14N 27 44 E
Zornitsa, Bulgaria .... 51 D10 42 23N 26 58 E
Zorritos, Peru .... 172 A1 3 43 S 80 40W
Zory, Poland .... 55 H5 50 3N 18 44 E
Zorzor, Liberia 112 D3 7 46N 9 28W
Zossen, Germany .... 30 C9 52 13N 13 27 E
Zou Xiang, China .... 74 G9 35 30N 116 58 E
Zouan-Hounien, Ivory Coast 112 D3 6 55N 8 15W
Zouar, Chad .... 109 D3 20 30N 16 32 E
Zouérate = Zouîrât, Mauritania 110 D2 22 44N 12 21W
Zouîrât, Mauritania 110 D2 22 44N 12 21W
Zouri, Gabon .... 114 C1 1 1 S 8 53 E
Zourika, Niger .... 113 B6 19 16N 7 52 E
Zourma, Burkina Faso 113 C5 12 3N 0 50W
Zousfana, O. →, Algeria .... 111 B4 31 28N 2 04 E
Zoutkamp, Neths. .... 24 A6 53 20N 6 18 E
Zrenjanin, Serbia & M. .... 52 E5 45 22N 20 23 E
Zuba, Nigeria .... 113 D6 9 11N 7 12 E
Zubayr, Yemen .... 98 D3 15 3N 42 10 E
Zubtsov, Russia .... 58 D8 56 10N 34 34 E
Zudáñez, Bolivia .... 173 D5 19 6 S 64 44W
Zuenoula, Ivory C. 112 D3 7 34N 6 3W
Zuera, Spain 40 D4 41 51N 0 49W
Zuetina = Az Zuwaytīnah, Libya .... 108 B4 30 58N 20 7 E
Zufār, Oman .... 99 C6 17 40N 54 0 E
Zug, Switz. .... 33 B7 47 10N 8 31 E
Zug, W. Sahara 110 D2 21 36N 14 9W
Zug □, Switz. .... 33 B7 47 9N 8 30 E
Zugdidi, Georgia .... 61 J5 42 30N 41 55 E
Zugersee, Switz. .... 33 B7 47 7N 8 35 E
Zugspitze, Germany .... 31 H6 47 25N 10 59 E
Zuid-Holland □, Neths. .... 24 C4 52 0N 4 35 E
Zuidbeveland, Neths. .... 24 C3 51 30N 3 50 E
Zuidhorn, Neths. .... 24 A6 53 15N 6 23 E
Zújar, Spain 43 H8 37 34N 2 50W
Zújar →, Spain 43 G5 39 1N 5 47W
Zukowo, Poland .... 54 D5 54 21N 18 27 E
Żukowo, Poland .... 54 D5 54 21N 18 27 E
Zula, Eritrea .... 107 D4 15 17N 39 40 E
Zulia □, Venezuela 168 B3 10 0N 72 10W
Züllichau = Sulechów, Poland .... 55 F2 52 5N 15 40 E
Zülpich, Germany .... 30 E2 50 41N 6 39 E
Zülz = Biała, Poland .... 55 H4 50 24N 17 40 E
Zumaia, Spain 40 B2 43 19N 2 15W
Zumárraga, Spain 40 B2 43 19N 2 19W
Zumbo, Mozam. .... 119 F3 15 35 S 30 26 E
Zummo, Nigeria .... 113 D7 9 51N 12 59 E
Zumpango, Mexico 163 D5 19 48N 99 6W
Zunhua, China .... 75 D9 40 18N 117 58 E
Zuni, U.S.A. 159 J9 35 4N 108 51W
Zunyi, China .... 76 D6 27 42N 106 53 E
Zuo Jiang →, China .... 76 F6 22 50N 108 6 E
Zuozhou, China .... 76 E6 22 42N 107 27 E
Zupanja, Croatia .... 52 E3 45 4N 18 43 E
Zur, Serbia & M. .... 50 D4 42 13N 20 34 E
Zura, Russia .... 64 C7 57 36N 53 24 E
Zurbātīyah, Iraq .... 101 F12 33 9N 46 3 E
Zürich, Switz. .... 33 B7 47 22N 8 32 E
Zürich □, Switz. .... 33 B7 47 26N 8 40 E
Zürich ✈ (ZRH), Switz. .... 33 B7 47 27N 8 33 E
Zürichsee, Switz. .... 33 B7 47 18N 8 40 E
Zuromin, Poland .... 55 E6 53 4N 19 51 E
Zurrieq, Malta .... 38 F8 35 50N 14 28 E
Zurzach, Switz. .... 33 A7 47 35N 8 18 E
Zut, Croatia .... 45 E12 43 52N 15 17 E
Zutphen, Neths. .... 24 B6 52 9N 6 12 E
Zūzan, Iran .... 91 C9 34 22N 59 53 E
Zvenigorodka = Zvenyhorodka, Ukraine .... 59 H6 49 4N 30 56 E
Zvenyhorodka, Ukraine .... 59 H6 49 4N 30 56 E
Zverinogolovskoye, Russia .... 66 D7 54 26N 64 50 E
Zvezdets, Bulgaria .... 51 D11 42 6N 27 26 E
Zvishavane, Zimbabwe .... 119 G3 20 17 S 30 2 E
Zvolen, Slovak Rep. .... 35 C12 48 33N 19 10 E
Zvonce, Serbia & M. .... 50 C6 42 57N 22 34 E
Zvornik, Bos.-H. .... 52 F4 44 26N 19 10 E
Zwedru = Tchien, Liberia 112 D3 5 59N 8 15W
Zweibrücken, Germany .... 31 F3 49 15N 7 21 E
Zweisimmen, Switz. .... 32 C4 46 33N 7 22 E
Zwenkau, Germany .... 30 D8 51 13N 12 20 E
Zwettl, Austria .... 34 C8 48 35N 15 9 E
Zwickau, Germany .... 31 E8 50 44N 12 30 E
Zwierzyniec, Poland .... 55 H9 50 36N 22 58 E
Zwiesel, Germany .... 31 F9 49 1N 13 13 E
Zwittau = Svitavy, Czech Rep. .... 35 B9 49 47N 16 28 E
Zwoleń, Poland .... 55 G8 51 21N 21 36 E
Zwolle, U.S.A. 155 K8 31 38N 93 39W
Zwolle, Neths. .... 24 B6 52 31N 6 6 E
Zyrardów, Poland .... 55 F7 52 3N 20 28 E
Zyryan, Kazakhstan .... 66 E9 49 43N 84 20 E
Zyryanka, Russia .... 67 C16 65 45N 150 51 E
Zyryanovsk = Zyryan, Kazakhstan .... 66 E9 49 43N 84 20 E
Żywiec, Poland .... 55 J6 49 42N 19 10 E

WORLD: REGIONS IN THE NEWS

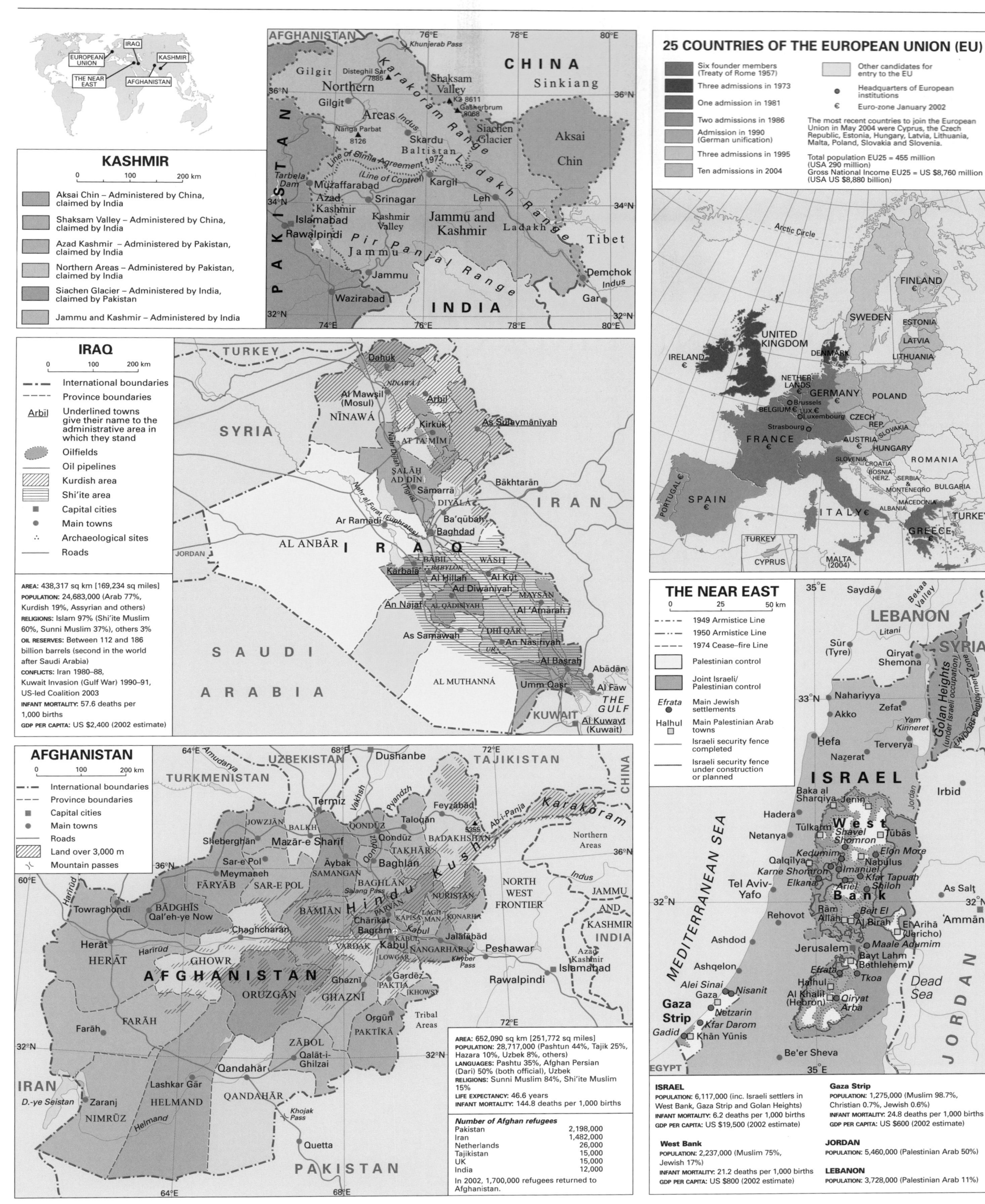

 **Large scale maps**
(>1:3 900 000)

 Medium scale maps
(1:4 000 000 – 1:9 900 000)

 Small scale maps
(<1:10 000 000)

Arctic Circle

11

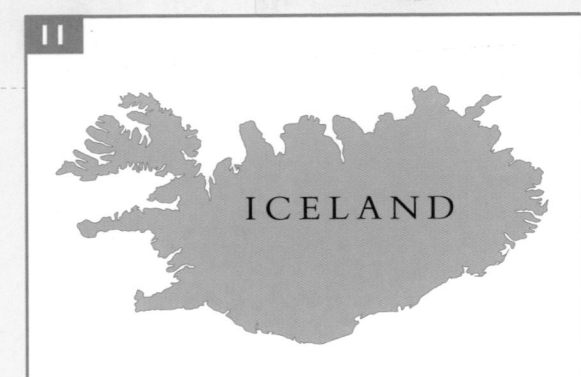

ICELAND

14

19

22

22

20

23

UNITED KINGDOM

IRELAND

24

26

28

FRA...

ANDORRA

42

40

PORTUGAL

SPAIN

38

MOROCCO

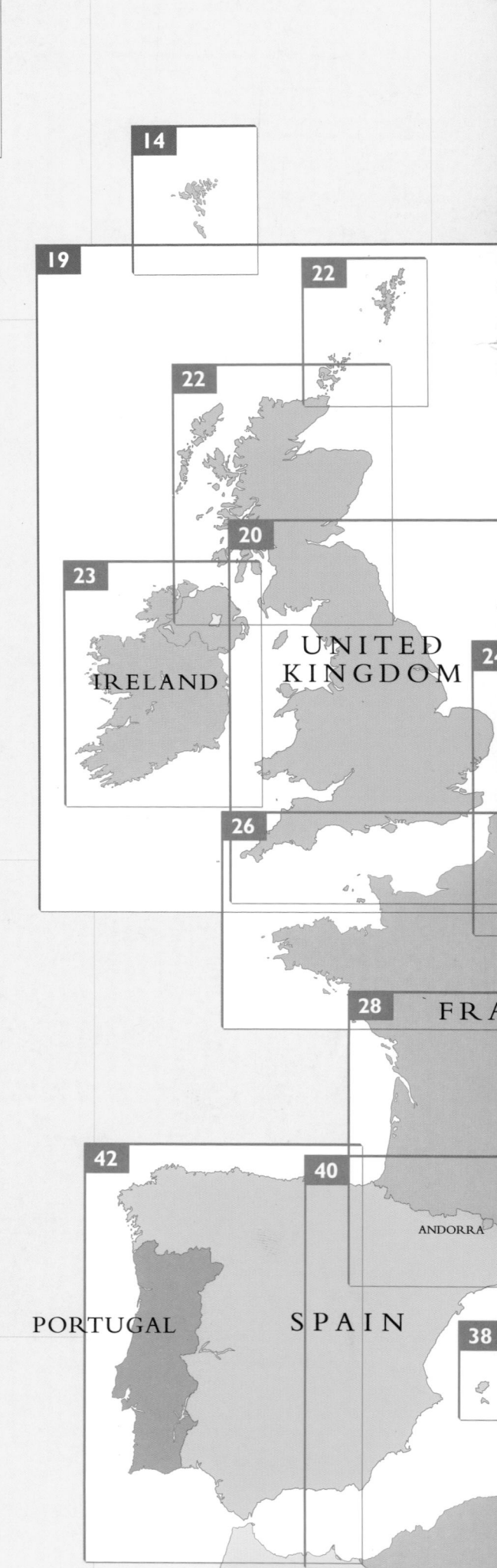

WORLD COUNTRY INDEX

Afghanistan 91
Albania 50
Algeria 110–111
Angola 115
Argentina 174, 176
Armenia 101
Australia 124–129
Austria 34–35
Azerbaijan 101
Azores 9

Bahamas 164–165
Bahrain 99
Bangladesh 90
Barbados 165
Belarus 58–59
Belgium 24
Belize 164
Benin 113
Bhutan 90
Bolivia 172–173
Bosnia-Herzegovina 45, 50
Botswana 116
Brazil 168–175
Brunei 85
Bulgaria 50–51
Burkina Faso 112–113
Burma (Myanmar) 86–87, 90
Burundi 118

Cambodia 86–87
Canary Is. 9
Cameroon 109, 114
Canada 138–143
Cape Verde Is. 9
Central African Republic 114
Chad 109
Chile 172, 174, 176
China 68–69, 74–77
Colombia 168
Comoros 121
Congo 114–115
Congo, Dem. Rep. of the 114–115, 118–119
Costa Rica 164
Croatia 45, 52
Cuba 164–165
Cyprus 39
Czech Republic 34–35

Denmark 17
Djibouti 120
Dominican Republic 165

Ecuador 168
Egypt 106
El Salvador 164
England 20–21
Equatorial Guinea 114
Eritrea 106–107
Estonia 58
Ethiopia 107, 120

Fiji 133
Finland 14–15
France 26–29
French Guiana 169

Gabon 114
Gambia 112
Georgia 101

Germany 30–31
Ghana 112–113
Greece 48–51
Greenland 10
Guadeloupe 164
Guatemala 164
Guinea 112
Guinea-Bissau 112
Guyana 169

Haiti 165
Honduras 164
Hungary 52

Iceland 11
India 90, 92–95
Indonesia 82–85
Iran 96–97
Iraq 96–97
Irish Republic 23
Israel 103
Italy 44–47
Ivory Coast 112

Jamaica 164
Japan 70–73
Jordan 103

Kazakhstan 65, 66
Kenya 118
Korea, North 75
Korea, South 75
Kuwait 96–97
Kyrgyzstan 65

Laos 86
Latvia 58
Lebanon 103
Lesotho 117
Liberia 112
Libya 108
Lithuania 58
Luxembourg 24

Macedonia 50
Madagascar 117
Malawi 119
Malaysia 84–85
Mali 110–111, 112–113
Malta 38
Martinique 164
Mauritania 110, 112
Mauritius 121
Mexico 162–163
Moldova 53
Mongolia 68–69
Morocco 110–111
Mozambique 117, 119

Namibia 116
Nepal 93
Netherlands 24
New Zealand 130–131
Nicaragua 164
Niger 109, 113
Nigeria 113
Northern Ireland 23
Norway 14–15, 18

Oman 99

Pakistan 91
Panama 164
Papua New Guinea 132
Paraguay 174–175
Peru 168, 172
Philippines 80–81
Poland 54–55
Portugal 42–43
Puerto Rico 165

Qatar 99

Réunion 121
Romania 52–53
Russia 56–61, 64, 66–67
Rwanda 118

St. Lucia 165
Samoa 133
Saudi Arabia 96–99
Scotland 22
Senegal 112
Serbia and Montenegro 50, 52
Seychelles 121
Sierra Leone 112
Singapore 87
Slovak Republic 35
Slovenia 45
Solomon Is. 133
Somali Republic 120
South Africa 116–117
Spain 40–43
Sri Lanka 95
Sudan 106–107
Suriname 169
Swaziland 117
Sweden 14–17
Switzerland 32–33
Syria 100–101, 103

Taiwan 77
Tajikistan 65
Tanzania 118–119
Thailand 86–87
Togo 113
Tonga 133
Trinidad and Tobago 169
Tunisia 111
Turkey 100–101
Turkmenistan 65, 66

Uganda 118
Ukraine 59
United Arab Emirates 99
United Kingdom 20–23
USA 144–161
Uruguay 174–175
Uzbekistan 65, 66

Vanuatu 133
Venezuela 168–169
Vietnam 86–87

Wales 20–21

Yemen 98–99

Zambia 115, 119
Zimbabwe 119